MEDICAL ONCOLOGY

Basic Principles and
Clinical Management of Cancer

EDITORS

PAUL CALABRESI
M.D.

Professor and Chairman, Department of
Medicine, Brown University; Physician-in-Chief,
Roger Williams General Hospital, Providence,
Rhode Island

PHILIP S. SCHEIN
M.D.

Adjunct Professor of Medicine and
Pharmacology, University of Pennsylvania,
Philadelphia, Pennsylvania; Adjunct Professor of
Medicine, Brown University, Providence, Rhode
Island; Professor of Medicine and Pharmacology,
Georgetown University, Washington, D.C.;
Vice-President, Clinical Research and
Development, Smith Kline and French
Laboratories, Philadelphia, Pennsylvania

SAUL A. ROSENBERG
M.D.

Professor of Medicine and Radiology; American
Cancer Society Professor of Clinical Oncology;
Chief, Division of Medical Oncology, Stanford
University, Stanford, California

MEDICAL ONCOLOGY

Basic Principles and
Clinical Management of Cancer

Macmillan Publishing Company
NEW YORK

Collier Macmillan Canada, Inc.
TORONTO

Collier Macmillan Publishers
LONDON

Macmillan Publishing Company
866 Third Avenue, New York, New York 10022

Collier Macmillan Canada, Inc.
Collier Macmillan Publishers · London

Library of Congress Cataloging in Publication Data

Main entry under title:

Medical oncology.

  Bibliography: p.
  Includes index.
  1. Cancer. I. Calabresi, Paul. II. Schein, P. S.
III. Rosenberg, Saul A. [DNLM: 1. Neoplasms. 2. Neoplasms—
therapy. QZ 266 M4888]
RC261.M469 1984   616.99'4   84–20189
ISBN 0–02–318040–4

Printing: 1 2 3 4 5 6 7 8   Year: 5 6 7 8 9 0 1 2 3

THIS VOLUME IS DEDICATED

To our parents and teachers,
who showed us the way;

To our wives and colleagues,
who have traveled it with us;

To our children and students,
who will lead us into the future.

Paul Calabresi
Philip S. Schein
Saul A. Rosenberg

Preface

Medical oncology became an established specialty during the 1970s, although its roots were firmly planted a decade or so before. The American Board of Internal Medicine recognized this important field of endeavor by offering, in 1973, subspecialty certification to qualified candidates who completed formal training in the discipline and passed a written examination. For several years, the three editors worked together on the test committees of the Board, carefully defining the appropriate body of knowledge required of the diplomates, and each served successively as chairman of the new Subspecialty Board of Medical Oncology. During this time, the need for a textbook that embraced comprehensively the fundamental and practical aspects of this specialty became increasingly apparent.

By the end of the decade, the American College of Physicians also recognized a growing need for all broadly trained internists to be appropriately knowledgeable and clinically competent in the area of neoplastic disorders by dedicating a separate section of its Medical Knowledge Self-Assessment Program (MKSAP-V) to medical oncology. After participating in the writing of the Syllabus for MKSAP-V, the editors began to outline in detail the contents of the present book.

Although *Medical Oncology: Basic Principles and Clinical Management of Cancer* is written primarily for the medical oncologist, its style and organization make this extensive volume of information easily accessible to a much broader audience. It is anticipated that the book will be used by surgeons, radiation oncologists, oncology nurses, general internists, family physicians, pathologists, pediatricians, psychiatrists, radiologists, other specialists and subspecialists, residents, and medical students involved in the management of the patient with cancer. In addition, it should be of value to selected allied medical personnel, particularly nurses, dietitians, pharmacists, and other health-care workers in psychosocial and rehabilitation medicine. Finally, basic scientists interested in cancer research will find important information about the biology and clinical manifestations of cancer that may have relevant and far-reaching implications for their studies.

In selecting the eighty-six contributors, the editors sought broad representation of opinion by choosing authors from many institutions with wide geographic distribution who are recognized nationally and internationally as experts in their fields. Special attention has been devoted to the details of organization, integration, illustrations, and writing style. The book is divided into three sections, which contain comprehensive but lucid discussions of the subject matter, accompanied by abundant current references.

Section One, "Basic Principles," consists of 14 chapters and explores our current understanding of the underlying molecular, cellular, and biologic phenomena that are responsible for the etiology, pathogenesis, and clinical aspects of the disease. This section also emphasizes the fundamental principles of integrated management for the patient with cancer and the specific contributions and limitation of the various diagnostic and therapeutic modalities. While stressing the cardinal importance of the multidisciplinary approach to the patient with cancer, the book is directed at medical oncologists and describes the principles, but not the technical details, of surgical and radiotherapeutic interventions. A thorough description of current tumor immunology and clinical pharmacology of chemotherapeutic agents is provided, however, since these are essential for understanding the acute and late effects of antineoplastic therapy on the delicate interactions of tumor and host, which affect the medical care of the patient.

Section Two, "Specific Neoplasms," presents authoritative descriptions of various neoplastic diseases that encompass the field of medical oncology. This portion contains 25 chapters arranged systemically by regions in a convenient sequence, which begins with neoplasms of the hematopoietic system, followed by those of the integument, oro- and nasopharynx, respiratory system, alimentary tract, endocrine glands, genitourinary systems, and ultimately tumors of the nervous system, supporting structures, and childhood. In order to orient the reader and to facilitate quick reference to specific information, each individual disorder is presented according to the following organizational format: incidence and epidemiology, etiology and pathogenesis, pathology and natural history, diagnosis, staging, specific and supportive management, and future prospects.

Section Three, "Supportive Care," includes 12 chapters and is concerned with the vital medical, nursing, and psychosocial supportive measures required for optimal care of the patient with cancer and the family. The medical management of life-threatening oncologic emergencies, special complications, infections, and hematologic problems are discussed in detail. The control of pain and nutritional factors are major responsibilities for all clinical oncologists. The unique problems of the rapidly growing elderly population make the chapter on the geriatric patient with cancer a particularly important topic. In recognition of the essential role of oncologic nurses, a special chapter is dedicated to this crucial area. Finally, one of two eventual outcomes faces the patient with cancer and the family: survival or death. The last portion of this section addresses the extremely difficult and challenging considerations involved. The complex problems and often agonizing decisions that derive from the terminal care of these patients and their families are approached in a sensitive and professional manner. In recent years, however, medical oncology has led the way in achieving cures for several types of previously fatal human cancers. A decrease in cancer deaths is particularly evident in the younger age groups and, with improved availability of existing technology or anticipated advances, even greater improvements in survival are predicted for other populations. It is because of these optimistic expectations that the editors elected to end the book with chapters on coping and rehabilitation, as an expression of their concern for the survivors and their families, as well as admiration for their courage, tenacity, and hope!

Paul Calabresi, M.D.
Philip S. Schein, M.D.
Saul A. Rosenberg, M.D.

Contributors

Abeloff, Martin D., M.D. Chief, Medical Oncology, Johns Hopkins Oncology Center, Johns Hopkins Hospital, Baltimore, Maryland

Ahlgren, James D., M. D. Assistant Professor of Medicine, Vincent T. Lombardi Cancer Research Center, Georgetown University School of Medicine, Washington, D.C.; Executive Director, Mid-Atlantic Oncology Program, Potomac, Maryland

Alford, Bobby R., M.D. Professor and Chairman, Department of Otorhinolaryngology and Communicative Sciences, Baylor College of Medicine, Houston, Texas

Bertram, Juergen H., M.D., Ph.D. Assistant Professor of Medicine, University of Southern California, Los Angeles, California

Blackburn, George L., M.D., Ph.D. Associate Professor of Surgery, Harvard Medical School; Director, Nutrition Support Service, New England Deaconess Hospital; Chief, Nutrition/Metabolism Laboratory, Cancer Research Institute, New England Deaconess Hospital, Boston, Massachusetts

Bloomfield, Clara D., M.D. Professor of Medicine, Section of Medical Oncology, University of Minnesota Health Sciences Center, Minneapolis, Minnesota

Bonadonna, Gianni, M.D. Director, Division of Medical Oncology, Instituto Nazionale per lo Studio e la Cura dei Tumori, Milan, Italy

Bothe, Albert, Jr., M.D. Assistant Professor of Surgery, Department of Surgery, Harvard Medical School, Boston, Massachusetts

Busch, Harris, M.D., Ph.D. Distinguished Professor and Chairman, Department of Pharmacology, Baylor College of Medicine, Houston, Texas

Calabresi, Paul, M.D. Professor and Chairman, Department of Medicine, Brown University; Physician-in-Chief, Roger Williams General Hospital, Providence, Rhode Island

Callen, Jeffrey P., M.D. Associate Professor of Medicine, Department of Dermatology, University of Louisville School of Medicine, Louisville, Kentucky

Carbone, Paul P., M.D. Professor and Chairman, Department of Human Oncology; Director, Wisconsin Clinical Cancer Center, University of Wisconsin Medical School, Madison, Wisconsin

Carter, Stephen K., M.D. Vice President, Anticancer Research, Pharmaceutical Research and Development Division, Bristol-Myers Company, New York, New York

Coffey, Robert J., Jr., M.D. Fellow in Gastroenterology, Mayo Clinic, Rochester, Minnesota

Cummings, Frank J., M.D. Associate Professor of Medicine and Director of Medical Oncology, Brown University and Roger Williams General Hospital, Providence, Rhode Island

Daly, John M., M.D., F.A.C.S. Associate Professor of Surgery, Cornell University Medical College; Associate Attending Surgeon, Memorial Sloan-Kettering Cancer Center, New York, New York

DeCosse, Jerome J., M.D. Chairman, Department of Surgery, Memorial Sloan-Kettering Cancer Center; Professor of Surgery, Cornell University Medical College, New York, New York

Dexter, Daniel, L. Ph.D. Research Associate, E. I. du Pont de Nemours and Co., Inc., Wilmington, Delaware; Adjunct Associate Professor of Medicine, Brown University, Providence, Rhode Island

Dietz, J. Herbert, Jr., M.D. Late Consultant in Rehabilitation, Memorial Hospital, Memorial Sloan-Kettering Cancer Center; Honorary Physician, The New York Hospital-Cornell Medical Center, New York, New York

Donovan, Donald T., M.D. Assistant Professor of Otorhinolaryngology and Communicative Sciences, Baylor College of Medicine, Houston, Texas

Durant, John R., M.D. President and Medical Director, Fox Chase Cancer Center, Philadelphia, Pennsylvania

Einhorn, Lawrence H., M.D. Professor of Medicine, Indiana University Medical Center, Indianapolis, Indiana

Fefer, Alexander, M.D. Professor of Medicine, University of Washington School of Medicine; Member, Fred Hutchinson Cancer Research Center, Seattle, Washington

Foley, Kathleen M., M.D. Associate Professor of Neurology and Pharmacology, Cornell University Medical College, New York, New York

Frenkel, Eugene P., M.D. Professor of Internal Medicine and Radiology; Director, Division of Hematology-Oncology, University of Texas Health Science Center at Dallas, Dallas, Texas

Gelber, Richard D., Ph.D. Associate Professor of Biostatistics, Harvard School of Public Health and Dana-Farber Cancer Institute, Boston, Massachusetts

Glick, John H., M.D. Professor of Medicine, Department of Medicine, University of Pennsylvania School of Medicine; Associate Director for Clinical Research, University of Pennsylvania Cancer Center, Philadelphia, Pennsylvania

Glicksman, Arvin S., M.D. Professor of Medical Science, Chairman, Department of Radiation Medicine, Brown University; Chairman, Department of Radiation Oncology, Rhode Island Hospital, Providence, Rhode Island

Glover, Donna J., M.D. Assistant Professor of Medicine, University of Pennsylvania School of Medicine, Philadelphia, Pennsylvania

Goldberg, Richard J., M.D. Assistant Professor, Section of Psychiatry and Human Behavior, Brown University, Providence, Rhode Island

Goodman, Robert L., M.D. Professor and Chairman, Department of Radiation Therapy, University of Pennsylvania School of Medicine, Philadelphia, Pennsylvania; Fox Chase Cancer Center, Philadelphia, Pennsylvania

Gunderson, Leonard L., M.D. Associate Professor of Oncology, Mayo Medical School; Consultant in Radiation Therapy, Mayo Clinic, Rochester, Minnesota

Hajdu, Steven I., M.D. Attending Pathologist and Chief of Cytology Service, Memorial Sloan-Kettering Cancer Center, New York, New York

Herr, Harry W., M.D. Associate Attending Surgeon, Memorial Sloan-Kettering Cancer Center; Associate Professor of Surgery, Cornell University Medical College, New York, New York

Hilderley, Laura J., R.N., M.S. Clinical Specialist and Nursing Coordinator, Department of Radiation Oncology, Rhode Island Hospital, Providence, Rhode Island

Holyoke, E. Douglas, M.D. Chief, Department of Surgical Oncology, Roswell Park Memorial Institute, State University of New York at Buffalo, Buffalo, New York

Howarth, Cathryn B., M.B., Ch.B., M.R.C.P. Associate Professor, Department of Pediatrics, Temple University, Philadelphia, Pennsylvania

Hurd, David D., M.D. Assistant Professor of Medicine, Section of Medical Oncology, University of Minnesota, Minneapolis, Minnesota

Isom, Harriet C., Ph.D. Associate Professor, Department of Microbiology, The Pennsylvania State University College of Medicine, Hershey, Pennsylvania

Kennedy, B. J., M.D. Professor of Medicine and Masonic Professor of Oncology; Head, Division of Medical Oncology, University of Minnesota Medical School, Minneapolis, Minnesota

Klastersky, Jean, M.D. Professor and Chief of Medicine, Department of Medicine, Institut Jules Bordet, Brussels, Belgium

Kornblith, Paul L., M.D. Chief, Surgical Neurology Branch, National Institute of Neurological and Communicative Disorders and Stroke, National Institutes of Health, Bethesda, Maryland

Lane, Montague, M.D. Professor of Pharmacology and Medicine; Head, Division of Clinical Oncology, Department of Pharmacology; Head, Section of Oncology, Department of Medicine, Baylor College of Medicine, Houston, Texas

Levin, Bernard, M.D. Professor of Medicine, University of Texas Medical School at Houston; Chief, Section of Digestive Diseases and Gastrointestinal Oncology, M.D. Anderson Hospital and Tumor Institute, Houston, Texas

Lipsett, Mortimer B., M.D. Director, National Institute of Arthritis, Diabetes, Digestive and Kidney Diseases, National Institutes of Health, Bethesda, Maryland

McDonald, Charles J., M.D. Professor and Head, Division of Dermatology, Department of Medicine, Brown University and Roger Williams General Hospital, Providence, Rhode Island

McIntyre, O. Ross, M.D. James J. Carroll Professor of Oncology and Director, Norris Cotton Cancer Center, Dartmouth-Hitchcock Medical Center, Hanover, New Hampshire

McKechnie, John C., M.D. Clinical Professor, Department of Medicine, Baylor College of Medicine, Houston, Texas

Miller, Marijean M., A.B. Clinical Coordi-

nator, Nutrition/Metabolism Laboratory, Cancer Research Institute, New England Deaconess Hospital, Boston, Massachusetts

Miller, Robert W., M.D., Dr.P.H. Chief, Clinical Epidemiology Branch, National Cancer Institute, Bethesda, Maryland

Mitchell, Malcolm S., M.D. Professor of Medicine and Microbiology; Chief, Division of Medical Oncology, University of Southern California School of Medicine, and U.S.C. Comprehensive Cancer Center, Los Angeles, California

Odell, William D., M.D., Ph.D. Professor of Medicine and Physiology, Chairman, Department of Medicine, University of Utah School of Medicine, Salt Lake City, Utah

Oldfield, Edward H., M.D. Deputy Chief for Clinical Neurosurgery, Surgical Neurology Branch, National Institute of Neurological and Communicative Disorders and Stroke, National Institutes of Health, Bethesda, Maryland

Omura, George A., M.D. Professor of Medicine, University of Alabama in Birmingham, Birmingham, Alabama

Owens, Albert H., Jr., M.D. Professor of Oncology and Professor of Medicine, Johns Hopkins University School of Medicine; Director, The Johns Hopkins Oncology Center, Baltimore, Maryland

Passero, Michael A., M.D. Assistant Professor of Medicine, Department of Medicine, Brown University; Director of Allergy and Occupational Medicine, Roger Williams General Hospital, Providence, Rhode Island

Peterson, Bruce A., M.D. Associate Professor of Medicine, Division of Medical Oncology, Department of Medicine, University of Minnesota Health Sciences Center, Minneapolis, Minnesota

Pinkel, Donald, M.D. Professor and Chairman, Department of Pediatrics, St. Christopher's Hospital for Children, Temple University School of Medicine, Philadelphia, Pennsylvania

Posner, Jerome B., M.D. Chairman, Department of Neurology, Memorial Sloan-Kettering Cancer Center; Professor of Neurology, Columbia University College of Physicians and Surgeons, New York, New York

Rapp, Fred, Ph.D Professor and Chairman, Department of Microbiology, The Pennsylvania State University College of Medicine, Hershey, Pennsylvania

Richter, Melvyn P., M.D. Assistant Professor of Radiation Therapy, University of Pennsylvania School of Medicine; Clinical Director, Department of Radiation Therapy, Fox Chase Cancer Center, Philadelphia, Pennsylvania

Rosen, Gerald, M.D. Medical Director, Comprehensive Cancer Centers, Inc., Beverly Hills, California; Attending Physician, Cedar Sinai Medical Center, Los Angeles, California; Associate Clinical Professor of Pediatrics and Hematology/Oncology, UCLA, Los Angeles, California

Rosenberg, Saul A., M.D. Professor of Medicine and Radiology; American Cancer Society Professor of Clinical Oncology; Chief, Division of Medical Oncology, Stanford University, Stanford, California

Rubin, Philip, M.D. Professor and Chairman, Division of Radiation Oncology, University of Rochester Cancer Center, Rochester, New York

Schein, Philip S., M.D. Adjunct Professor of Medicine and Pharmacology, University of Pennsylvania, Philadelphia, Pennsylvania; Adjunct Professor of Medicine, Brown University, Providence, Rhode Island; Professor of Medicine and Pharmacology, Georgetown University, Washington, D.C.; Vice-President, Clinical Research and Development, Smith Kline and French, Philadelphia, Pennsylvania

Schiffer, Charles A., M.D. Professor of Medicine and Oncology; Head, Division of Hematologic Malignancies, University of Maryland Cancer Center; Head, Division of Hematology, Department of Medicine, University of Maryland School of Medicine, Baltimore, Maryland

Schreiner, George E., M.D. Professor of Medicine, Director, Division of Nephrology, Georgetown University School of Medicine, Washington, D.C.

Shackney, Stanley E., M.D. Associate Physician, Division of Medical Oncology, Alleghany General Hospital, Pittsburgh, Pennsylvania

Share, Frederick S., M.D. Assistant Professor of Radiation Therapy, University of Pennsylvania School of Medicine, Philadelphia, Pennsylvania; Medical Director, Community Cancer Center, North Shore Medical Center, Miami, Florida

Slaby, Andrew E., M.D., Ph.D., M.P.H. Professor of Psychiatry and Human Behavior in the Department of Psychiatry and Human Behavior, Brown University; Psychiatrist-in-Chief, Rhode Island Hospital, Roger Williams General Hospital, and Women and Infants Hospital, Providence, Rhode Island

Smith, Barry H., M.D., Ph.D Senior Staff Fellow, Neurosurgery, Memorial Sloan-Kettering Cancer Center, New York, New York

Smith, Frederick P., M.D. Clinical Associate Professor of Medicine, Division of Medical Oncology, Department of Medicine, Georgetown University, Washington, D.C.

Spremulli, Ellen N., M.D. Medical Oncologist, Anniston Medical Clinic, Anniston, Alabama

Tartaglia, Charles R., M.D. Assistant Professor of Psychiatry; Director, Psychiatric Consultation-Liaison Service, Georgetown University Medical Center, Washington, D.C.

Tecala, Mila, M.S.W., A.C.S.W. Center for Loss and Grief, Washington, D.C.

Tew, Kenneth D., Ph.D. Head, Molecular Pharmacology, Lombardi Cancer Center, Georgetown University, Washington, D.C.

Upton, Arthur C., M.D. Professor and Chairman, Department of Environmental Medicine, New York University Medical Center, New York, New York

Weinstein, I. Bernard, M.D. Professor of Medicine and Public Health; Director, Division of Environmental Sciences, School of Public Health; and Deputy Director, Cancer Center/Institute of Research, Columbia University College of Physicians and Surgeons, New York, New York

Wiemann, Michael C., M.D. Assistant Professor of Medicine, Department of Medicine, Brown University and Division of Oncology-Hematology, Roger Williams General Hospital, Providence, Rhode Island

Wiernik, Peter H., M.D. Gutman Professor of Medicine, Albert Einstein College of Medicine; Chairman, Department of Oncology, Montefiore Medical Center; Associate Director, Cancer Center, Albert Einstein College of Medicine, New York, New York

Williams, Stephen D., M.D. Associate Professor, Department of Medicine, Indiana University, Indianapolis, Indiana

Woolley, Paul V., M.D. Professor of Medicine and Pharmacology, Georgetown University School of Medicine, Lombardi Cancer Research Center, Washington, D.C.

Yagoda, Alan, M.D. Attending, Department of Medicine, Memorial Sloan-Kettering Cancer Center, Associate Professor of Clinical Medicine, Cornell University Medical College, New York, New York

Zelen, Marvin, Ph.D. Professor and Chairman, Department of Biostatistics, Harvard School of Public Health and Division of Biostatistics and Epidemiology, Dana-Farber Cancer Institute, Boston, Massachusetts

Zimmerman, Jack M., M.D. Associate Professor of Surgery, Johns Hopkins University School of Medicine; Chief of Surgery, Church Hospital, Baltimore, Maryland

Zinner, Stephen H., M.D. Professor of Medicine and Head, Division of Infectious Diseases, Brown University and Roger Williams General Hospital, Providence, Rhode Island

Acknowledgments

The editors want to express their thanks to the contributors of the 51 chapters in this volume, and to acknowledge the advice and enthusiasm received from several other individuals, particularly: Drs. Michael H. Kroll, M. Peter Lance, W. P. L. Meyers, Robert M. White, and Michael C. Wiemann, who reviewed specific chapters; editorial assistants Katherine B. Terrell, Susan J. Berman, and Claudia F. Dennis, who helped with manuscript preparation, proofreading, and many other tasks; and Joan C. Zulch, Publisher and Editor-in-Chief, Medical/Nursing/Health Sciences Department, Macmillan Publishing Company, whose interest and support have been evident from the beginning of this endeavor.

Contents

Section Three *SUPPORTIVE CARE*

Section One
Basic Principles

1

Molecular and Cell Biology of Cancer

HARRIS BUSCH, KENNETH D. TEW, and PHILIP S. SCHEIN

INTRODUCTION

The motivating premise behind most research in the area of cancer cell biology has been to discover differences between tumor and normal cells that could be exploited to achieve a selective therapeutic advantage. Although a number of obvious changes occur in transformed cells, the fundamental biochemical mechanisms by which a tumor cell survives are largely the same as those of a normal cell. The answer to the question of what causes a normal, differentiated euploid cell to assume the cancerous characteristics of uncontrolled growth, tissue invasiveness, and metastasis remains enigmatic. The phenotypic expression of cancer is an inheritable Mendelian trait, therefore it is not surprising that much emphasis has been placed on the study of the genetic storehouse of a cell, the nucleus. An alteration in the chromatin of a cancer cell is probably responsible for the neoplastic phenotype.

Concomitant with the changed growth characteristics of a transformed cell are a number of other differences. One of the earliest differences, discovered by Warburg (1926), was an abnormally high rate of glycolysis in some tumor cells. Other recognized differences that have been described for certain cancers include the following: An increased glucose transport potential, altered adenosinetriphosphatases (ATPases), changes in cytoskeletal structure, anchorage independence of growth, loss of contact inhibition, lack of intercellular connections through gap junction deficiencies, development of tumor-specific membrane antigens, loss of fibronectin, lowered requirements for calcium and for other serum factors, cyclic nucleotide variabilities, intra-cellular pH, sodium flux, polyamine differences, and a number of nuclear alterations that can manifest themselves through the presence of specific marker chromosomes. In cancer, there exists an extraordinary degree of cellular heterogeneity. No consistent pattern of an altered state of metabolism has been identified that completely distinguishes cancer cells from

Table 1–1. Nuclear Products

DNA

    Complete DNA replication during cell division
    Gene amplification or repetition

RNA
  mRNA
    mRNA sequences
    poly(A) 3'-termini
    The 5'-cap (? nucleus)

  rRNA
    28S rRNA
    18S rRNA
    5.8S rRNA
    5S rRNA

  tRNA
    tRNA nucleotide sequence
    Many modified tRNA nucleotides

  LMWN RNA
    Uridine-rich nuclear RNA U1, U2, U3, U4, U5, U6
    Other species including 4.5S RNA_{I-III}, 7S RNA, 8S RNA, Alu RNA

  Precursor-processing reactions for each RNA species

RNP particles (see Table 1–4)
  mRNP particles
    Informosomes
    Polysomes

  rRNA particles
    Granular nucleolar elements
    Completed ribosomes

normal cells, and, as a consequence, the goal of curing cancer through exploitation of the imbalanced glycolytic pathways has been impossible to achieve. This finding has not diminished the hopes of many biologists who seek to identify an exploitable and definitive difference in the biochemistry and cell biology of tumor cells that could lead to less empirical approaches to the treatment of cancer.

Both the progressive nature of neoplasia and the ultimately fatal outcome of the disease result from the growth, invasiveness, and metastasis of cancer cells, as well as their ability to alter adversely the metabolism of the host. Regardless of the site of origin of the disease, enlargement of the neoplastic masses alone produces compression effects that, in either sensitive or enclosed sites, produce serious restrictions of normal organ function. Even benign tumors or neoplasms of relatively low orders in the heart and brain result in marked

functional alterations. Other tumors exhibit serious pathophysiologic effects only after multiple metastases to the lung, liver, or other organs compromise the reserve functional capacity of these organs.

It is the aim of this chapter to cover some of the basic aspects of cell biology that control cell survival and to highlight differences in the way a tumor cell exists when compared to its normal, or preneoplastic, progenitor.

THE NUCLEUS

The cell nucleus is part of an integrated system by which cells of all organs respond to extracellular and intracellular stimuli. The stimuli interact with the nuclear informational system to produce specific products (see Table 1–1) that permit response by the cytoplasm and cell membrane to the environment and its

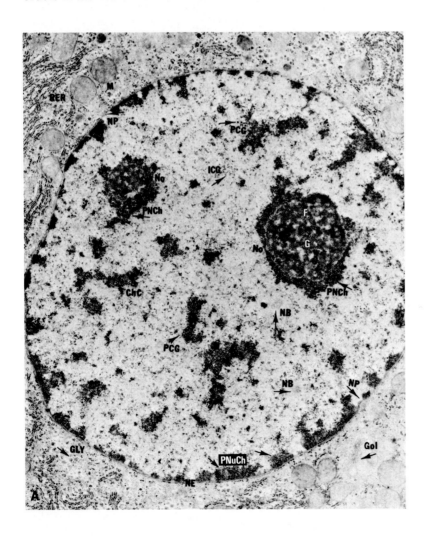

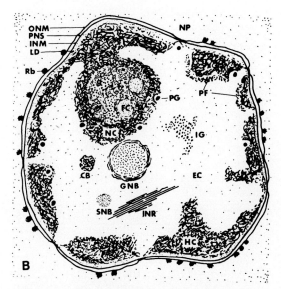

Figure 1–1B. Ideal section of a nucleus, showing the main components. The nucleus is surrounded by the outer nuclear membrane (ONM) and inner nuclear membrane (INM) that enclose the perinuclear space (PNS), which is a part of the rough endoplasmic reticulum and has ribosomes (Rb) attached. Between the chromatin and the inner membrane lies the lamina densa (LD), which is thinner in front of the nuclear pores (NP). The chromatin is found as heterochromatin (HC), nucleolus-associated chromatin (NC), and euchromatin (EC). The nucleolus shows the granular (g) components and fibrillar centers (FC). In the borderline of the chromatin, many perichromatin granules (PG) and a layer of perichromatin fibrils (PF)—of which only a portion has been drawn—are found. Finally, in the interchromatin space, a cluster of interchromatin granules (IG), a granular nuclear body (GNB), a simple nuclear body (SNB), a coiled body (CB), and an intranuclear rodlet (INR) have been drawn. From Bouteille, M.; Laval, M.; and Dupuy-Coin, A. M.: Localization of nuclear functions as revealed by ultrastructural autoradiography and cytochemistry. In Busch, H. (ed.): *The Cell Nucleus,* Vol. 1. Academic Press, New York, 1974.

functional demands. A remarkable feature of normal nuclear function is the variety, from tissue to tissue and from organ to organ, of nuclear products that profoundly alter cellular metabolism.

The nucleus is the major repository of chromatin, which is composed of DNA and its associated proteins. Very small amounts of DNA are also present in mitochondria. If there is any DNA in the cell membrane or endoplasmic reticulum, the levels are so low that uniform reports of its presence have not been possible. The genetic information of the cell nucleus becomes operational in the form of polysomes that contain messenger RNA (template RNA), ribosomes, and associated biosynthetic elements (see Table 1–1).

Figures 1–1A and 1–1B show an electron micrograph and an illustration of a eukaryotic cell nucleus. The elements labeled compose the nuclear morphology of both normal and cancerous cells; however, their proportions and arrangements may be markedly changed in some tumor cells. In an interphase nucleus chromatin is present in two major forms, euchromatin and heterochromatin. The latter is a darkly staining, electron-dense material that is located at the periphery of the nucleus, contiguous with the inner nuclear membrane. Euchromatin is more electron lucent and is spread throughout the remainder of the nucleus. The staining properties of these fractions are governed by the degree of "compactness" of the chromatin fibers. During mitosis, after chromosomes have formed, the chromatin arrangement alters drastically, after chromatin has combined with residual inner nuclear membrane proteins and nuclear matrix proteins to form metaphase chromosomes (see Figure 1–2). The scanning electron micrograph shows clearly how chromatin becomes supercoiled and compacted during cell division. Table 1–2 indicates how the arrangement of chromatin can influence its higher order structure and size.

The precise mechanisms that control chromosome formation and chromatin segregation are not presently understood. The obvious degree of fidelity, however, that accompanies the normal division of genetic material at mitosis predetermines that whatever

Figure 1–1A. Electron micrograph of a rat liver cell nucleus (×18,000). Within the nucleus, nucleoli (No) are surrounded by perinucleolar chromatin (PNCh). The nucleoli consist of granular (G) and fibrillar (F) elements. Chromocenters (ChC) are distributed randomly within the nucleoplasm. Perichromatin granules (PCG) are frequently associated with these chromocenters. Nuclear bodies (NB) and interchromatin granules (ICG) are occasionally seen; these are apparently cross-sections of the nuclear ribonucleoprotein network. The inner layer of the nuclear envelope (NE) surrounds a conspicuous layer of dense chromatin (PNuCh). The clear areas within this heterochromatin layer usually mark the location of the nuclear pores (NP). In the cytoplasm glycogen elements (GLY) are present. Mitochondria (M) and rough endoplasmic reticulum (RER) are distributed throughout the cytoplasm. Golgi complexes (Gol) are occasionally seen around the nuclear periphery. Lead citrate-uranyl acetate staining. From Busch, H.: The eukaryotic nucleus. In O'Malley, B. W., and Birnbaumer, L. (eds.): *Receptors and Hormone Action,* Vol. 1. Academic Press, Inc., New York, 1977.

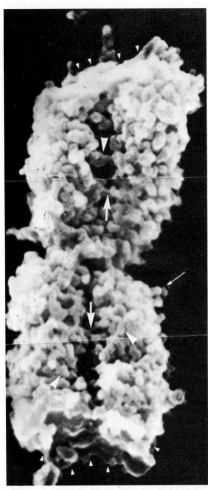

Figure 1-2. Scanning electron micrograph of whole-mount isolated CHO metaphase chromosome 2 (×65,000). Membranous platelike structures (small arrowheads) connect both chromatids only at their distal ends. Multiple interchromatidal connections (large arrows) are seen in the interchromatidal furrow. Highly coiled topical microconvules (large arrowheads) and axial coilings (small arrows) are present. From Daskal, Y.; Mace, M. L., Jr.; Wray, W.; and Busch, H.: Use of direct current sputtering from improved visualization of chromosome topology by scanning electron microscopy. *Exp. Cell Res.,* **100**:204–212, 1976.

the mechanism, a high degree of molecular stability and control exist. Recently, evidence has been presented to demonstrate a role for the structural protein elements of the nucleus, the nuclear matrix, in the organization of chromatin during replication and cell division.

The Structure of Chromatin and Domains

Electron microscopy reveals that the most basic chromatin structure resembles "beads on a string" (see Figure 1–3). If this structure is

dissected biochemically, each bead, or nucleosome, is seen to be composed of a double tetramer of histones H2A, H2B, H3, and H4 with DNA wrapped around these core histones (see Figure 1–4). The areas between nucleosomes are relatively protein free, and are referred to as "linker regions." Histone H1 and a number of nonhistone proteins are located on this internucleosomal linker DNA and serve to maintain an ordered structural domain through charge interactions between basic amino acid substituents and the highly negative phosphate groups of the DNA. The amino acids involved and their location within the tailed-globular structure of these histone proteins are the subject of a great deal of research in the molecular biology of chromatin structure.

The relevance of the structure of nucleosomes to their function is not yet clear. There is a phase distribution of nucleosomes in both transcriptional and nontranscriptional chromatin. Virtually all DNA sequences transcribed into mRNA are present as nucleosome-associated DNA. Apparently, these structures are potentially random with respect to DNA sequence, and, at the very least, do not interfere with the transcription process. It is possible that topoisomerases or other nuclease enzymes release the protein-DNA restraints of the nucleosome region before, or during, transcription, thereby permitting access of the RNA polymerase system to the DNA. If this does occur, there must be an immediate reformation of the nucleosome structure following transcription, since transcribed chromatin retains the beads-on-a-string appearance.

Nucleosomes certainly have a role in higher-ordered chromatin structures, such as solenoids and superbeads. These structures can determine the biological activity of chromatin regions, since tightly packed, supercoiled chromatin does not permit easy access to the DNA for the enzymes responsible for nuclear function. Evidence that specific protein species may be associated with activated chromatin (*i.e.,* that which is undergoing transcription) has been reported, although it is not yet known how these proteins control the transcriptional process. These proteins include ubiquinated histones H2A and H2B (Busch and Goldknopf, 1981) and high mobility group (HMG) proteins.

The structural domains of chromatin are continually modified and maintain a state of biologic fluidity throughout the cell cycle, presumably in response to physiologic control. The relationship of structure to function is not

Table 1–2. Higher-Order Structure of DNA

STRUCTURE (unit)	NUMBER OF BASE PAIRS	DIMENSIONS	NUMBER OF NUCLEOSOMES	NUMBER OF LOOPS*	NUMBER OF BANDS (high resolution)
Double helix (turn)	10.4	3.2 nm pitch 2.0 nm diam.	—	—	—
Nucleosomes −HI	146	$11 \times 11 \times 5.5$ nm	1	—	—
+HI	166				
Fibril (core + linker)	200	10 nm diam	1	—	—
Fiber (turn)	−1,200	10 nm pitch 30 nm diam.	−6	—	—
Gene (intron, exon)	−1,000–10,000	?	−50	—	—
Loop −histones	30,000–100,000	$10–30\mu$ contour length	0	1	—
+histones		$0.2–1.0\mu$ contour length	−150–500		
Metaphase band (average)	$2–4 \times 10^6$	100–150 nm axial length	$−1–2 \times 10^4$	30–100	1
Metaphase chromatid	$0.5–2.4 \times 10^8$	$1–10\mu$ length $0.5\ \mu$ diam.	$0.25–1 \times 10^6$	500–2000	15–75
Interphase nucleus	7×10^9	10μ diam.	3.5×10^7	20,000–50,000	—

* Loops detected by electron microscopy where two DNA anchor points occur on the matrix, after chromatin spreading.
Adapted from Feinberg, A. P., and Coffey, D. S.: The topology of DNA loops: A possible link between the nuclear matrix structure and nucleic and function. In Maul, G. C. (ed.): *The Nuclear Envelope and The Nuclear Matrix.* Alan R. Liss, Inc., New York, 1982.

well understood, but it is possible that differences exist between normal and tumor cell chromatins and that these differences may be exploited.

The Nuclear Membrane and Nuclear Matrix

The periphery of the nucleus is separated from the cytoplasm by a highly permeable, double-layered envelope that encloses the semihomogeneous internal milieu of the nucleoplasm (see Figure 1–5). Macromolecular transfer between the nucleus and the cytoplasm is facilitated by the nuclear pore complexes, which vary in size dependent upon cell type but are nanometers in diameter. A typical nucleus has three to four thousand nuclear pores, and transfer of even large macromole-

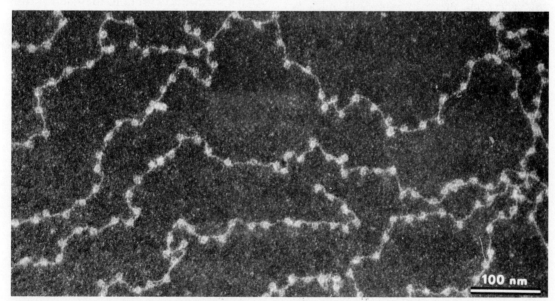

Figure 1–3. Nucleosomes. Chromatin fibers streaming out of a rat thymocyte nucleus. The spheroid chromatin units (nucleosomes) exhibit local variations in arrangement and separation, possibly due to differential stretching of the fibers. Negative stain 0.5% ammonium molybdate; pH 7.4 (×260,800). From Olins, A. L.; Breillant, J. T.; Carlson, R. D.; Senior, M. B.; Wright, E. B.; and Olins, D. E.: On nu models for chromatin structure. In Ts'o, P. (ed.): *The Molecular Biology of the Mammalian Genetic Apparatus,* Vol. 1. Elsevier/North-Holland Biomedical Press, Amsterdam, 1977.

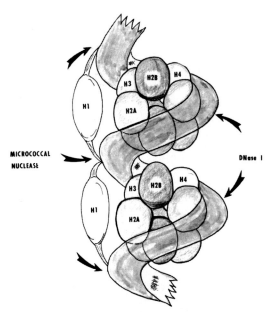

Figure 1–4. Diagrammatic representation of nucleosomal structure. The core histones (H2A, H2B, H3, and H4) are surrounded by approximately 140 base pairs (bp) of DNA. Between nucleosomes, histone H1 is associated with the linker DNA region that is up to 60 bp in length. Histone H1 together with other nonhistone protein species are thought to stabilize the chromatin structure through specific interactions with DNA. The specificities of the two enzymes, micrococcal nuclease (preferential digestion of internucleosomal DNA) and DNase I (relative lack of preferential digestion site), are indicated.

cules between the cytoplasm and nucleus should not be limited by adequate supply channels. The nuclear envelope breaks down during mitosis and is partially conserved in the nucleoprotein scaffold of chromosomes. The membrane, in addition, possesses a high degree of flexibility that permits the nucleus to swell or contract, to invaginate, and even to breakdown and reform, under physiologic control.

The connections between the peripheral heterochromatin and the inner nuclear membrane may be critical to the organization of genetic material within the nucleus. The binding of chromatin to membrane is reversible and therefore probably electrostatic in nature, involving the nucleic acid components of the chromatin and the protein components of the inner nuclear membrane. The overall charge on the membrane may be altered by radiation. During the autolytic stages of cell death, the chromatin becomes detached from the membrane.

Although the nuclear envelope controls the

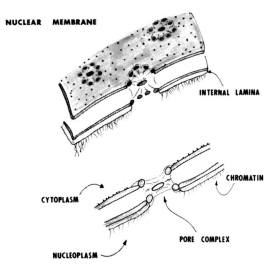

Figure 1–5. Diagrammatic representation of the nuclear membrane showing bilayer structure and nuclear pores.

outer constraints of the nucleus, increasing evidence suggests that the overall nuclear architecture is controlled, at least in part, by a nucleoprotein scaffold: The nuclear matrix. This structure (see Figure 1–6) remains after isolated nuclei are stripped of chromatin through high salt buffer and nuclease treatments (Berezney and Coffey, 1973). The structural framework is composed of the residual nuclear envelope (pore complex and lamina), and interchromatinic network that includes the re-

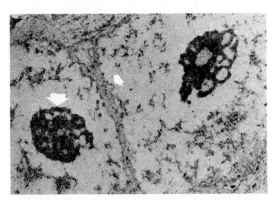

Figure 1–6. Electron micrograph of two isolated HeLa cell nuclear matrices ($\times$15,000). The spongelike protein matrix resulted from removing virtually all chromatin components. Remnants of the nucleolus (large arrow) are surrounded by the residual nonhistone protein fibrillar matrix. Residual inner nuclear membrane (small arrow) is also present. From Tew, K. D.: Chromatin associated nuclear components as potential drug targets. In Serrou, B.; Schein, P.S.; and Imbach, J.-L. (eds.): *Nitrosoureas in Cancer Treatment.* Elsevier/North-Holland Biomedical Press, New York, 1981.

sidual nucleolus and a small amount of residual chromatin. The matrix represents approximately 5% of the total nuclear protein, together with small quantities of phospholipids, carbohydrates, RNA, and DNA (Berezney and Coffey, 1976). Its flexible structural properties permit chromatin organization, condensation, and segregation. Evidence suggests that the matrix mediates, or at least participates in, many of the processes that constitute nuclear function, including DNA replication (DNA polymerase alpha is known to be associated with the matrix), RNA processing and transport (through nucleolar associations), and nuclear hormone receptors (which play a role in hormone activity). The potential biologic importance of the nuclear matrix is yet to be defined (for a review of the nuclear matrix, see Maul, 1982). As part of the nonhistone protein complement of the nucleus, the possibility that differences in the matrix protein composition may exist between tumor and normal cells and between various tumor cells has been suggested (Tew et al., 1982b).

The Nonhistone Proteins of the Nucleus

Early progress in the identification of nonhistone nuclear proteins was hindered by their comparatively low solubility properties (Busch, 1965). By using 6 to 8 mol urea and two-dimensional gel electrophoresis, identification of over nine hundred subunits and species of nuclear polypeptides has been possible (Takami et al., 1979).

Researchers (Paul and Gilmour, 1966a, b, 1968) have provided evidence to suggest that the nonhistone proteins were the gene-control elements in the nucleus. Reasoning that the three elements involved in gene transcription (producing messenger DNA [mRNA]) included (1) DNA, (2) histones, and (3) nonhistone proteins, they added histones and/or nonhistone proteins from liver, kidney, spleen, and brain to DNA from liver, spleen, and brain. The DNA or histones did not affect the gene transcription, but the nonhistone proteins did. When nonhistone proteins of spleen were added, for example, spleen RNA was produced regardless of the origin of the DNA or histones.

A key experiment would be to add a single, highly purified nonhistone protein to chromatin and demonstrate that it produces a specific and definitive gene transcription. Several groups have found that with radiolabeled hormones, protein-receptor hormone complexes form in the cytoplasm and undergo modifications in transit to the nucleus. Subsequently, labeled hormone-receptor complexes are found in the chromatin (O'Malley and Means, 1974). Addition of hormone-receptor complexes to chromatin has been reported to activate specific genes, but the key experiment noted above has yet to be performed (Thrall et al., 1978).

Histones are the most abundant nuclear proteins; each major histone species is present in amounts of approximately 2 pg (10^{-12} gram)/nucleus (Busch, 1965). Proteins C23 to C25, which are among the most abundant of the more than two hundred species of nucleolar nonhistone proteins, are present in amounts of approximately 10 to 100 fg (10^{-15} gram) or 1000 to 10,000 molecules per nucleus. Such proteins are now readily visualized by staining on two-dimensional gels, particularly after fractionation and purification. When ^{32}P and immunological methods are used, the levels of detection are 10- to 100-fold greater, approaching 50 attagrams (10^{-18} gram)/nucleus. Such amounts approximate the levels that are probably important in gene control. For molecules of approximately 50,000 molecular weight, amounts of 100 attagrams would equal 200 to 1000 molecules per nucleus. The increasing information on nuclear enzymes and immunologically active nuclear elements suggests that many nuclear proteins are present in very small amounts; the task of their purification and functional analysis is clearly a difficult one.

It has been possible to compare the nonhistone protein components of normal and tumor cells by using a combination of two-dimensional isoelectric focusing and sodium dodecyl sulfate gel electrophoresis. Extraction of nuclei with increasing salt concentrations provides a much improved approach to the analysis of the number and types of nuclear proteins. In Novikoff tumor nuclei, 483 different polypeptides were identified by dye staining; 427 polypeptides were found in normal liver nuclei. The sensitivity of the method was such that spots containing 0.1 μg of protein were readily identified on these gels; such proteins are present in approximately 500 copies per nucleus (Hirsch et al., 1978).

Other studies compared the nuclear proteins of regenerating adult and fetal liver, and slow- and fast-growing tumors. The protein patterns of the regenerating liver and a slow-growing tumor were similar to that of a normal liver. Many similarities were found between the fetal liver and the fast-growing tumors. Only four proteins common to the rat tumors were absent from the nontumor tissues, and it is possible that they have special nuclear functions (Takami *et al.,* 1979).

When nuclear proteins from four human tumor cell lines (HeLa, Namalwa, acute myelogenous leukemia, and lymphoma) and four normal cells (IMR 90, WI 38, liver, and lymphocytes) were compared, two protein spots, 140/7.7 and 54/6.6, were found in the four tumors but not in the normal cells. Interestingly, two protein spots, 56/6.7 and 56/6.9, were found in all four normal cells but not in any of the tumors. These proteins differed from those of the rat tissues. These techniques are time consuming, but may eventually define different polypeptides from tumors that have a role in their uncontrolled growth.

The Nucleolus

Special Features of the Nucleolus of the Cancer Cell. The role of the nucleolus is in the synthesis of ribosomes, which are essential for growth and new cell formation (see Figure 1–7). Pleomorphism and enlargement of the nucleoli of cancer cells are cytologic markers of cancer (Busch and Smetana, 1970). One researcher (MacCarty and Haumeder, 1934; MacCarty, 1936) reported that enlargement and variation in size and morphology of nucleoli in cancer cells were pathognomonic of this disease. Another study (Caspersson and Santession, 1942) indicated that aberrations in size and shape of nucleoli in cells were pathognomonic of cancer.

Studies have been designed to analyze the mechanisms of alteration in nucleolar size and shape in neoplasia (Busch *et al.,* 1963; Busch and Smetana, 1970). This approach required analysis of the nucleolar RNA products, par-

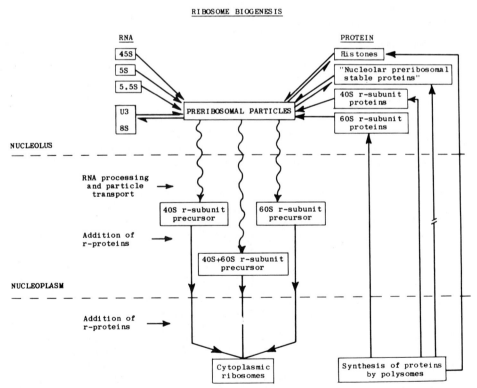

Figure 1–7. Diagram of the role of the nucleolus in the biogenesis of ribosomes. Reprinted with permission from Prestayko, A. W.; Klomp, G. R.; Schmoll, D. J.; and Busch, H.: Comparison of proteins of ribosomal subunits and nucleolar preribosomal particles from Novikoff hepatoma ascites cells by two-dimensional polyacrylamide gel electrophoresis. *Biochemistry,* **13:**1945–1951, 1974. Copyright 1982 American Chemical Society.

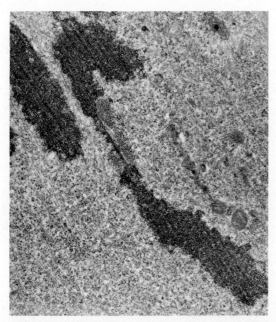

Figure 1–8. The X-chromosome of the kangaroo rat *(Potorous tridactylus)* showing the nucleolus organizer region (secondary constriction) (×25,700). The continuity of the dense deoxyribonucleoprotein structure in the region of the secondary constriction is apparent. There is another element of lighter density around the constriction. The preparation was fixed in glutaraldehyde, postfixed in osmium, and embedded in EPON. From Busch, H., and Smetana, K.: *The Nucleolus.* Academic Press, New York, 1970.

Table 1–3. Specific Nucleolar Components

I. rDNA
II. U3 low molecular weight RNP
III. Specific elements
    A. Fibrillar elements
    B. Granular elements
    C. Interelement spacers
IV. Phosphoproteins
    A. C23
    B. B23
V. Specific nucleolar antigens

ticularly the 12,000 nucleotide 45S precursor of ribosomal RNA, and the small 5.8S, and U3-RNA, and 7S nucleolar RNAs, the nucleolar histones and the changes in their conjugates during activation of function, the preribosomal proteins of the nucleolus, the special nucleolar RNA polymerase (A or I) and the "silver-staining" nucleolar, nucleolus organizer region (NOR) (see Figure 1–8) phosphoproteins B23 and C23 (the "silver-staining" proteins).

The nucleolus synthesizes about 85% of all the cellular RNA. The NORs of chromatin (see Figure 1–8) on which the nucleolus originates contain the repetitive nucleolar DNA (rDNA) and the specific structural organization for interlocking nucleolar protein and RNA products.

The nucleolus is the sole cellular location of some highly specific cellular and nuclear components (see Table 1–3). One of the most remarkable facets of nucleolar function is the production of the enormous numbers of nucleotide chains (12,000) of 45S nRNA that are

synthesized by RNA polymerase I with great rapidity on rDNA (see Figure 1–9); they are methylated, cleaved, and modified as the ribosomal RNA (rRNA) molecules are formed. The nucleolus, in addition, is a site of protein binding to the newly synthesized RNA to form the nucleolar granular elements (see Figure 1–1A). The fibrillar elements of the nucleolus are the matrix composed of the rDNA, the RNA polymerase I, and juxtaposed enzymes that provide the beginnings of synthesis of preribosomal RNP particles. The granular elements are the mature ribonucleoprotein particles of the nucleolus that contain preribosomal RNA chains, proteins that migrate to the cytoplasm in the nascent ribosomes and others that are involved in maturation processes. Some drugs, such as actinomycin D, produce a remarkable "segregation" of these granular and fibrillar structures, although the precise relevance of this phenomenon to cell viability is unclear.

Further maturation of nucleolar products occurs in the nuclear ribonucleoprotein network (Busch and Smetana, 1970), the locus for joining other ribosomal proteins and polysomal elements to these preribosomal elements to complete the fully matured polysomes.

The "secondary constrictions" or NOR in chromosomes contain the rDNA and its flanking regions (see Figure 1–8). Nucleolar DNA (rDNA) is "geographically" segregated as perinucleolar chromatin and intranucleolar chromatin. Much of the rDNA has been sequenced and studies on its transcription controls are in progress.

Improved hybridization techniques have established that the concentration of rDNA in the nucleolus of Novikoff hepatoma ascites cells is ten to 12 times that of the rDNA throughout the remainder of the nucleus. Accordingly, it appears that the nucleoli contain 90% or more of the total rDNA.

The initial RNA product of the nucleolus is 45S pre-RNA and oligomers with sedimenta-

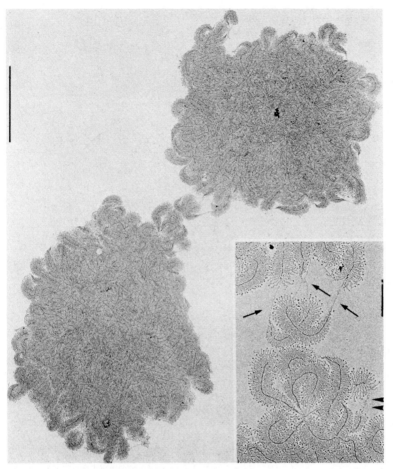

Figure 1–9. Electron micrograph spread preparations, from *Rana pipiens,* of readouts of nucleolar fibrillar regions showing condensed masses of dense rDNA filaments and the packed RNA polymerases along their surfaces. The branches are preribosomal RNA filaments. *Inset:* High magnification of spread preparation showing Christmas-tree-like patterns with miniparticles at the termini of the newly forming rRNA threads. From Trendelenburg, M. F., and McKinnell, O. O.: Transcriptionally active and inactive regions of nucleolar chromatin in amplified nucleoli of fully grown oocytes of hibernating frogs, *Rana pipiens* (Amphibia, Anura). A quantitative electron microscopic study. *Differentiation,* **15:**73– 95, 1979.

tion coefficients of up to 85S. Through a series of unique and specific endonucleolytic cleavages, these giant nucleolar RNAs are cleaved to three major ribosome species, 28S, 18S, and 5.8S rRNA (Busch and Smetana, 1970).

Nucleolar Proteins and Control of Nucleolar Function. Nucleolar proteins can be divided as follows:

1. Structural elements including histones, special proteins of the preribosomal particles and ribosomal proteins;
2. Enzymes of RNA synthesis (RNA polymerase I) and RNA processing (exonucleases and endonucleases); and
3. Gene control proteins.

Gene control of nucleolar function may re-side in specific elements that are either phosphoproteins or other specific types of nonhistone proteins. The participation of the nucleolus in important regulatory and phase-specific events indicates that its controls are highly responsive to cellular activity.

Improved methods for determining their numbers and types have shown that the nucleolus contains approximately 400 species of proteins. Another group of proteins is acid-insoluble, but is extractable under conditions that require solvents that dissociate hydrogen bonds and destroy hydrophobic molecular interactions. RNA polymerase I that is uniquely localized in the nucleolus alone accounts for ten to 12 polypeptides that are presumably enzyme subunits. Many nonhistone nucleolar proteins are elements of the nucleolar ribonucleoproteins of the fibrillar granular elements, the ribosomes, and the nucleolar matrix.

Two nuclear phosphoproteins referred to as protein C23 and B23 are nucleolus-specific phosphoproteins, and represent the major silver-staining proteins of the nucleolus (Busch *et al.,* 1979; Lischwe *et al.,* 1979, 1981). One researcher (Kleinsmith, 1978) has reviewed the roles of phosphoproteins in nuclear function. Phosphoproteins are present in every nuclear subfraction and, accordingly, may serve roles as enzymes or enzyme subunits, elements of RNP particles, gene control proteins, chromatin structural proteins, or matrix proteins. The nuclear kinases are also phosphorylated. A large number of systems involved in growth and development, hormonal stimulation, neoplastic and transformed cells, and cells stimulated by chemical agents are all associated with increased nonhistone protein phosphorylation or overall kinase activity (Kleinsmith, 1978). In addition, others (Langan, 1969; Gurley *et al.,* 1973) showed histone phosphorylation occurs with cell cycle specificity and in some systems that have been stimulated with hormones. These findings suggested a relationship of chromatin activation to either phosphorylation of histones or nonhistone proteins.

Replication and Transcription

The property of uncontrolled growth elicited by cancer cells implies that the process of DNA replication and transcription will be different in cancer cells when compared with their normal counterparts. Such differences are most likely related to alterations in the rate and frequency of nucleic acid synthesis, rather than changes in the enzymatic mechanisms that underlie the processes.

Most of the early work on replication and transcription was carried out in prokaryotes. Because eukaryotic cells have DNA organized into nucleosomes and other higher-ordered chromatin superstructures, the initial steps of nucleic acid syntheses will be complicated by the requirement of a destabilization of DNA-protein interactions within the chromatin. The basic enzymes involved in the processes, however, are similar in both eukaryotes and prokaryotes.

DNA is replicated with a high degree of fidelity by the process of semiconservative replication, whereby each of the two parent duplex DNA molecules acts as a template for the synthesis of complementary daughter strands. The end-point of the synthesis is the production of two complete daughter duplex DNA molecules containing one parental strand and one daughter strand. The regions of DNA where replication begins are referred to as *origins.* In prokaryotes, replication forks can move away from the origin in a bidirectional manner, synthesizing DNA in two directions. Because eukaryotic cells contain considerably more DNA, replication must occur simultaneously at a number of different origin sites, otherwise, replication of each chromosome would take months. Recent theories (Feinberg and Coffey, 1982) have suggested that DNA replication occurs at fixed sites located on the nuclear matrix (structural proteins of the nucleus). It has been proposed that loops of chromatin are replicated simultaneously (as many as 10,000 at a time) and that the enzymes involved are localized and stationary on the matrix. Synthesis is believed to occur by movement of the DNA, producing replication forks and daughter strands in a manner similar to that described for prokaryotes. Replication in this manner permits the duplication of the entire eukaryotic cell genome in a matter of hours.

Eukaryotic cell nuclei contain DNA polymerases, DNA ligases, a variety of topoisomerase enzymes (such enzymes are capable of unwinding DNA), and other undefined protein factors. This enzyme complement is responsible for the net synthesis of DNA, although the precise mechanisms by which they function are not clearly understood. It has been estimated that 20 or more enzymes and protein factors are involved in the replication of prokaryotic DNA (Kornberg. 1980). It is likely that at least the same number are involved in eukaryotic replication. Sequentially, replication involves: Origin recognition; separation of DNA from nucleosome conformation; parent duplex unwinding and template separation; daughter strand synthesis initiation; strand elongation; rewinding of the double helix; and termination of the replication process. A replication unit, consisting of the DNA template and associated enzymes, is termed a *replisome.* For replication to begin, one strand of parent DNA is required as a primer with DNA polymerase adding nucleotides sequentially to the 3′ end of the primer strand. Synthesis of the new strand thus proceeds in a $5' \rightarrow 3'$ direction.

During replication, it is possible to detect short pieces of DNA (in prokaryotes about 1000 to 2000 bases long; in eukaryotes less than 200 bases). The replication intermediates are termed *Okazaki fragments* and represent DNA that is replicated in a discontinuous manner and then spliced together. One DNA strand is replicated continuously in a $5' \rightarrow 3'$ direction. This is called the *leading strand.* The other strand is called the *lagging strand* and is made discontinuously in short pieces, also by adding nucleotides to the 3′ end, but in the direction opposite to that of the replication fork. These small pieces are eventually spliced together enzymatically to form the daughter strand. DNA ligase can form a phosphodiester bond between the 3′-hydroxyl group at the end of the DNA undergoing elongation and the 5′-phosphate group of the Okazaki fragment, thereby producing a continuous DNA strand.

The process of transcription is the first processing step whereby DNA is used as a template for the enzymatic synthesis of RNA. Transcription of the entire genome does not occur. Instead, transcriptionally active chromatin regions are transcribed by DNA-directed RNA polymerase. It is common to have as little as 10 to 20% of the DNA transcribed by a cell. This transcriptionally active chromatin differs from the remaining 80 to 90% in its nonhistone protein complement and its struc-

tural configuration. There are also differences in the susceptibility of active chromatin to cleavage by nuclease enzymes. DNase I, for example, is known to cleave preferentially those regions of DNA that code for actively transcribed gene sequences. It should be apparent, therefore, that transcription of DNA is a selective process, controlled, at least in part, by specific DNA regulatory sequences.

The majority of the DNA is transcribed into mRNA with smaller quantities of other RNA species. These RNA species and their processing are discussed in more detail in the following sections.

Nuclear RNA

Messenger RNA. Synthesis of mRNA is a specific function of the cell nucleus. Through interaction of specific control factors with the genome, a defined number of mRNA species are produced, transported to the cytoplasm (see Figure 1–10) and translated by polysomes into special cellular products. The polysomes that ultimately translate mRNA into proteins are associated with a host of initiation and elongation factors (Busch, 1976).

Synthesis of mRNA. The elongation processes involved in messenger RNA synthesis are apparently very similar to those in ribosomal RNA (rRNA) synthesis, but the initiation

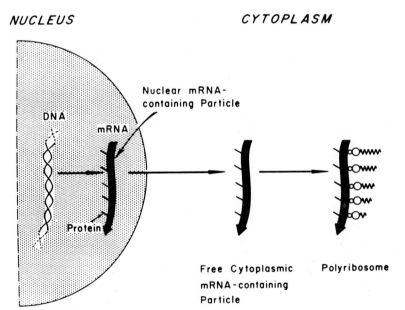

Figure 1–10.   Scheme of synthesis and transport of mRNA from the nucleus to the cytoplasm where it functions as part of the polyribosome complex. From Busch, H.: Messenger RNA and other high molecular weight RNA. In Busch (ed.): *The Molecular Biology of Cancer.* Academic Press, New York, 1974.

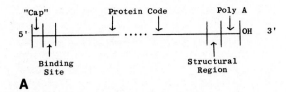

A

Figure 1-11A.   General arrangement of the structure of mRNA. Reprinted by permission of the University of Chicago Press from Busch, H.: The function of the 5′ cap of mRNA and nuclear RNA species. *Perspect. Biol. Med.,* **19**:549-567, 1976. © 1976 by the University of Chicago.

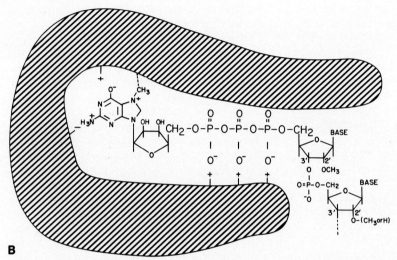

B

Figure 1-11B.   5′ cap of mRNA. Originally discovered on the small nucleolar RNAs, the 5′ cap is the only constant structural feature of messenger RNA. The cap protein is shaded. Reprinted by permission of the University of Chicago Press from Busch, H.: The function of the 5′ cap of mRNA and nuclear RNA species. *Perspect. Biol. Med.* **19**:549-567, 1976. © 1976 by the University of Chicago.

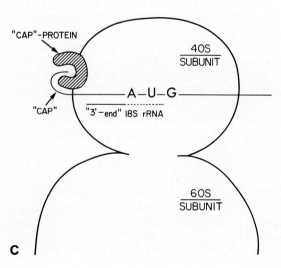

C

Figure 1-11C. Relationship of the cap structure (shaded) and mRNA to the ribosome. From Busch, H.; Hirsch, F.; Gupta, K. K.; Rao, M.; Spohn, W.; and Wu, B. C.: Structural and functional studies on the "5-cap": a survey method for m-RNA. *Prog. Nucleic Acid Res.,* **19**:39-61, 1976.

processes are not well defined for eukaryotes. The enzyme RNA polymerase II catalyzes the elongation of heterogenous nuclear RNA (hnRNA), which may contain several long introns in addition to the exons or coding regions. Closely associated in these transcriptional events are methylases, pyrophosphorylases for formation of the 5′ cap (see Figure 1–11A) and poly(A) polymerases that are responsible for the synthesis of the 3′ poly A terminus (see Figure 1–11B). These events all occur on heterogenous ribonucleoprotein (hnRNP) particles that are complexes of hnRNA and proteins. RNA polymerase II and its associated factors link nucleoside triphosphates covalently into 3′,5′-phosphodiester bonds of mRNA. Termination of the mRNA occurs when appropriate triplet codons such as UAA, UAG, or UGA are encountered by RNA polymerase II, but recognition proteins are apparently important to the termination process.

The 5′ cap is added by a series of reactions involving guanylyl transferases and methylating enzymes that form the $m_7(5')ppp(5')Y_mpZ_mp$ cap. The formation of this cap occurs mainly in the nucleus; it is modified in the cytoplasm. The 5′ cap serves as a binding site for protein complexes involved in the initiation of protein synthesis or for mRNA binding directly to special ribosomal proteins (see Figure 1–11C). Recent reviews on mRNA (Abelson, 1979; Breathnach and Chambon, 1981) emphasize that an mRNA is usually made up of a 5′-cap leader sequence, a coding sequence, and a poly A 3′ end. Only the 5′-cap (Banerjee, 1980) and the coding sequence are invariant elements of mRNA (Darnell, 1978).

Splicing of Pre-mRNA. During the analysis of these genes, the process of splicing of intervening sequences (IVS) or introns was discovered (Berget et al., 1977; Sharp, 1981). Many questions have arisen about IVS (Breathnach and Chambon, 1981). For example, is there any consistency or logic to IVS? They are random, and with the exception of the splice sites, heterogeneous in lengths, sequences, or time of cleavage, even for any given gene readout. In some genes, the IVS are far longer than the exon or coding regions. In others, like collagen genes, there are many IVS. In some cases, either one or no IVS may be present. Mutational potential, either ancient or ongoing, may exist in these regions (Darnell, 1978; Gilbert, 1978), but some argue that the IVS are filler for the genes (Chow et al., 1977).

Surprisingly simple mechanisms may exist for removing the IVS from the coding products. These may involve the U-snRNA species (Hodnett and Busch, 1968; Lerner et al., 1980; Busch et al., 1982). The finding by one research team (Breathnach and Chambon, 1981) of consensus IVS terminal sequences, and their possible recognition role in the IVS led another team (Lerner et al., 1980) to suggest that the binding of U-1 snRNA to these regions provided a guide for subsequent attack by cleavage and splicing enzymes.

Other important elements of the genes, particularly Alu sequences (Jelinek et al., 1980; Weiner, 1980) are widely distributed and may be related to processes for gene amplification or rearrangement by transposons. As noted earlier, some genes involved in the cancer process may be related to segments of the retroviruses such as lymphoid leukosis, which is induced by ALV (avian leukemia virus) (Hayward et al., 1981) (see Chapter 3D). If the inserted segment is a promoter, it might activate cellular genes. One published study (Hayward et al., 1981) reported the cellular "onc" gene myc was activated by an ALV promoter.

Cancer cell gene transcription may not be abnormal but, because the active genes are not controllable by normal cell feedback mechanisms, may simply be excessive. Such mechanisms may relate to activation of previously suppressed fetal genes or random activation of a variety of genes in rapidly growing tumors. The finding by researchers (Illmensee and Mintz, 1976) that passage of a neoplasm through blastocysts eliminated the neoplastic state requires an explanation other than viral gene insertion; an epigenetic mechanism may exist for cancer.

In most tumors, only the phenotypically active genes of the tissue of origin are expressed, rather than a broad range of genes. Accordingly, gene activation is specific rather than general and many genes are repressed rather than activated. Many hepatomas, for example, synthesize little or no albumin (Nakhasi et al., 1981).

Gene control has been extremely resistant to direct experimental attack in eukaryotic systems, mainly because of the large number of genes and the difficulties in reliable reconstitution of chromatin (Darnell, 1978). In some systems, such as the adenovirus synthetic system, mutational analysis has permitted evaluation of a control system in which a 72,000 DNA-binding protein affects translation rather than transcription of the adenovirus mRNA (Jay *et al.*, 1981). This effect is presumably indirect via interaction with a cellular component.

Small Nuclear RNA. A series of investigations has linked the small nuclear RNAs (snRNA) and small ribonucleoprotein particles (snRNP) to splicing of premessenger RNA (pre-mRNA) transcripts (Lerner and Steitz, 1979; Reddy and Busch, 1981; Busch *et al.*, 1982) and to autoimmune diseases that produce antibodies defined by specialists in arthritis and rheumatology (Tan, 1979). The important hypothesis emerged that the U-snRNP class of small nuclear RNP particles guides the elimination of IVS, or introns, of pre-mRNA, by binding to splice sites of the IVS in hnRNP particles (see Figure 1–12). The mechanisms of excision of the IVS and ligation of the useful portions of the mRNA are not yet known. Further studies have suggested that the snRNPs are involved in transport of mRNA to the cytoplasm and incorporation into polysomes (Lerner *et al.*, 1980).

The evidence for the involvement of U1-RNP in splicing of hnRNA is: (1) The complementarity between conserved consensus sequences and U1-RNA is unlikely to be a coincidence; (2) U1-RNPs lacking the 5′-terminal sequence were not associated with hnRNPs; (3) in studies on effects of anti-snRNP antibodies on splicing reactions (Yang *et al.*, 1981), splicing of adenovirus hnRNA in HeLa cell nuclei was inhibited when they were preincubated with anti-Sm or anti-RNP antibodies. When the nuclei were incubated with anti-Ro or anti-La antibodies, splicing was not inhibited. Because other cellular functions (*e.g.*, polyadenylation) were not inhibited, and since anti-RNA or anti-Sm antibodies react with and presumably inactivate the U-snRNPs, it was suggested that U-snRNPs are required for splicing.

Nuclear Particles

The cell nucleus polymerizes RNA structures and arranges specific genetic information in sequences with remarkable fidelity. This information is packaged in ribonucleoprotein (RNP) particles (see Table 1–4), which are now a topic of intense interest (Busch *et al.*, 1982).

The nuclear RNP particles are divisible into: Nucleolar rRNP precursors of ribosomes; hnRNP nuclear precursors of polysomal mRNP; snRNP particles that include U-snRNP particles of the nucleoplasm and U3 RNP particles of the nucleolus; a variety of particles associated with small 7-8S and 4.5S nuclear RNAs, some of which may be associated with processing of ribosomal RNA. Each of these elements is involved in production of systems for production of cellular proteins.

The 5′-cap of the U-snRNAs differs from that of the mRNAs in its two extra methyl groups on the 2′ N of the guanine base. This methylation may offer special binding properties to the hnRNP structure. The binding of snRNP to the hnRNP particles is not random, despite the fact that homologies were found for other regions of the U1-RNA, particularly since most of the U1-RNA is largely shielded from interaction with macromolecules by proteins. The mechanism for the binding reactions is under study.

Electron microscopic studies employing antibodies from systemic lupus erythematosus (SLE) patients have also provided supportive evidence for such binding. Inasmuch as only one (or two) U-snRNP particle is visualized on

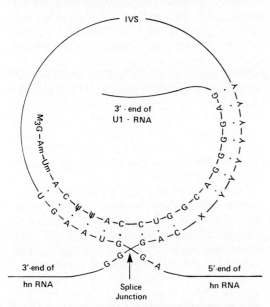

Figure 1–12. A proposed model for splicing of hnRNA involving U1-snRNA. The consensus sequences for the splice junctions and the sequence of U1-snRNA exhibit remarkable complementarity. Adapted, with permission, from Busch, H.; Reddy, R.; Rothblum, L.; and Choi, Y. C.: SnRNAs, SnRNPs and RNA processing. *Annu. Rev. Biochem.*, **51**:617–654, 1982. © 1982 by Annual Reviews Inc.

Table 1–4. Nuclear Particles

I. Large

  hnRNP particles: contain pre-mRNA in varying sizes from the original long (exons + introns) readout to the processed molecule with 5′ cap ± poly A termini

  rRNP particles: contain pre-rRNA in varying sizes from the origin 45S readout to processed preribosome containing 18S and 28S large and 5S and 5.8S small rRNAs

II. Small

  U-snRNP particles: containing U1-, U2-, U4-, U5-, and U6-RNA; bound to Sm and other proteins; found associated with hnRNP particles or "free" in the nucleoplasm

  U3-snRNP particles: found in nucleoli; associated temporally with pre-rRNP particles during processing of pre-rRNA

  perichromatin granules: definitive dense core structures containing U6-snRNA; associated with early transcripts from chromosomes

  snRNP containing other RNA species: Alu type 4.5S and 7S RNA: 8S RNA; "To" RNA of nucleolus

  "miniparticles": particles with doughnut shapes, composed of 8 subunits; multiple protein components with MW 15,000–30,000.

each hnRNP particle at any one time, presumably only one intron is cleaved out of these structures at a time. The turnover rate of hnRNA is rapid and that of U-snRNA is very slow, and, accordingly, the U-snRNP particles have catalytic rather than substrate functions. The enzymes associated with the hnRNP intron cleavage reactions have not been identified; whether these enzymes act after the binding of U-snRNP to hnRNP is not known.

Perichromatin Granules. These granules (see Figure 1–13) that have a special electron microscopic appearance were described by Watson (1962). They accumulate in cells treated with some anticancer agents such as doxorubicin (Daskal, 1981). Their presence in the juxtachromatin and intrachromatin elements of the nucleus suggests that they play an early role in either the transport or processing of newly synthesized hnRNP particles. When these particles were isolated (Daskal *et al.,* 1980), they were found to contain U6-RNA, a small and interesting species of the U-snRNA series.

Gene Regulation

It has become increasingly apparent over the last five years that control of transcription in eukaryotic cells differs greatly from that in prokaryotes. Although DNA sequences play an integral role in the regulation process, the structural properties of the chromatin fiber is a predeterminant for the initiation of transcription. It is known that actively transcribed regions of chromatin are more sensitive to the cleaving activity of DNase I, a nuclease enzyme. Studies have shown that when some genes are active, a region of DNase I hypersen-

sitivity is found "upstream" from the gene. These regions have been found in yeast, *Drosophila,* rat, and chicken cells, and are known to be in a configuration that is more open or exposed than bulk chromatin. It is likely that the DNA in these regions is more relaxed and less covered with proteins than the remaining chromatin. Specific DNA sequences are associated with these nuclease-sensitive sites, although these need not be proximate in location to the actual cleavage site. The first of the two sequences, TATA (thymine, adenine repeat), has been found in front of nearly 60 different genes that are essential for transcription *in vitro.* The TATA sequence (also known as the TATA box or Hogness box) is well conserved, which is suggestive of an important control function. It is located between the hypersensitive region and the gene.

The second sequence, CCAAT, is within the hypersensitive region, upstream from the gene. This sequence is also evolutionarily conserved; together with its location, this finding suggests it has a regulatory role.

Transcription is a complex multistep process in eukaryotic cells. Because control is not mediated by a DNA sequence specificity at the 5′ end of a gene, it is tempting to deduce that to initiate transcription, the configuration of the chromatin at the DNase I hypersensitive site is a prerequisite for the binding of the RNA polymerase system. The TATA box probably assists in ensuring that the polymerase starts at the correct place towards the 5′ end of the gene. Transcription of many genes begins with a leader sequence that codes for amino acids that are not found in the final protein product. The gene itself is composed of alternating exons and introns. After transcription, the intron se-

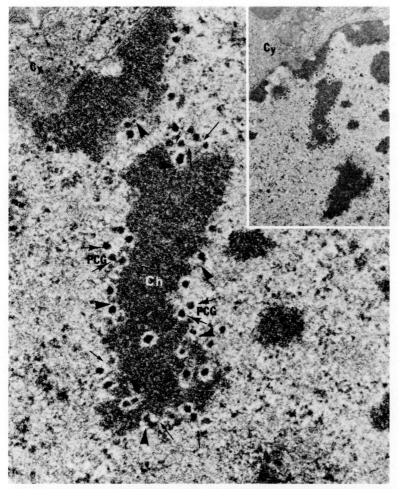

Figure 1 – 13. High magnification (×69,000; inset ×17,500) perichromatin granule (PCG) complexes in a rat hepatocyte nucleus treated with 200 mg/kg cycloheximide. Perichromatin fibrils (arrow heads) connect the PCG to the chromocenter (Ch). Finer filaments (arrows) interconnect the PCGs proper. From Daskal, Y: Perichromatin granules. In Busch, H. (ed.): *The Cell Nucleus,* Vol. 8. Academic Press, New York, 1981.

quences are spliced out, leaving a messenger RNA made up of exons that are expressed in the mature message.

The fact that cancer is a syndrome of inappropriate and/or uncontrolled gene expression suggests that a knowledge of the mechanisms underlying transcription is valuable to our understanding of the disease state.

Cancer-Related DNA Repair Defects

There are many ways that DNA can be damaged by carcinogens (see Chapter 3B). Essentially, all of these lesions, which can include strand breakage (single or double), base alkylation or hydroxylation, chemical adduct for-

mation, DNA-DNA or DNA-protein cross-linking, and pyrimidine dimerization, are deleterious and often fatal to the host cell unless efficiently repaired. In eukaryotic cells, the repair process involves a number of nuclear enzymes. The repair of a pyrimidine dimer formed through cellular exposure to short wave ultraviolet light, for example, requires a process known as excision repair. Initially, endonuclease activity breaks the DNA backbone at a site contiguous to the base damage. Excision of the damaged strand is achieved by a $5' \rightarrow 3'$ exonuclease activity and is followed by a synthesis of a strand complementary in sequence to the undamaged strand of the helix by a $5' \rightarrow 3'$ polymerase activity. Finally, a polynucleotide ligase seals the two ends of a new strand. If damaged DNA reaches a replication fork before its repair, postreplicational repair mechanisms can initiate a correction of the damaged DNA. Evidence for an error-prone repair in bacteria involves a special DNA polymerase that is more tolerant of mutations in template DNA and is able to replicate the altered DNA by observing the base pairing rules less strictly than the normal polymerase. Recent evidence for an inducible repair system that involves special methyl-acceptor proteins has been reported. During a period of low carcinogen exposure level, proteins that have sterically, favorably located cysteine residues are induced. These are able to remove electrophilic alkyl groups from DNA by the interaction of the sulfhydryl groups with the alkyl residue, thereby repairing the damaged DNA. Other enzymes, such as glycosylases, are also able to aid in the repair of specific DNA damage (for a review of DNA repair, see Howard-Flanders, 1981).

A number of human disorders are linked to defects in the repair potential of cells. In patients with xeroderma pigmentosum, there is an excessive susceptibility to skin cancer through exposure to UV light. The disorder is due to a homozygous recessive mutation in one or several genetic loci, and results in a 50 to 90% deficiency in excision repair. The particular defect is in the incision step of the repair process that leads to a defective removal of thymine dimers when an individual is exposed to sunlight. Other diseases that are linked to hereditary repair defects are ataxia-telangiectasia, in which fibroblasts from affected individuals are three to four times more susceptible to x-rays and other carcinogens. Fanconi's anemia is a rare disorder leading to bone marrow deficiencies and skeletal, heart, and kidney abnormalities. The recognized predisposition towards leukemia may result from a defect in the cell's ability to repair cross-linked DNA. In Bloom's syndrome, in which repair deficiencies lead to a high frequency of chromosome aberrations, DNA synthesis proceeds more slowly than in normal cells. Individuals affected with this disorder have an increased sensitivity to skin cancer, leukemias, and gastrointestinal tumors. Finally, progeria is a syndrome characterized by a reduced rate of DNA single-strand damage repair, which results in a greatly accelerated aging process. Interestingly, there is no apparent increase in the susceptibility of these individuals to cancer.

Nuclear Structure and Chemotherapy

The Concept of Nuclear Target Specificity. Although there is much evidence that the cytotoxic properties of nuclear-reactant drugs such as nitrogen mustards, nitrosoureas, anthracycline antibiotics, vinca alkaloids, steroid hormones, and even radiation are mediated through interactions with DNA, less consideration has been given to the relative importance of nuclear macromolecules as potential drug targets. The complexity of chromatin organization and the presence of regions of functional redundancy provide the basis for the theory that the site of drug interaction within the nucleus is as important, or more important, than the type of lesion. The potential for cell survival may be determined by the type, number, or diversity of drug lesions, their location within the chromatin, and the speed and efficiency of their repair. These factors may be closely interrelated, and it is important to understand which regions of the nucleus are susceptible to drug attack, in order that specific macromolecules may be considered as potential sites for drug-mediated cytotoxicity. In addition to the variety of nuclear macromolecules, a high degree of heterogeneity of structural chromatin domains exists.

The binding of nuclear-reactant drugs with macromolecules involves the interaction of an electrophilic drug species with a nucleophilic site within the cell. Chemical nucleophiles that are present in biologic molecules include amino, carboxyl, sulfhydryl, imidazole, and phosphate groups. Such groups are predominantly localized in amino acids and nucleosides, which comprise the protein and nucleic acid components of the nucleus.

Although histone and nonhistone proteins and nuclear RNA are alkylated by several anticancer drugs, the extent of duplication and rate of turnover of many protein and RNA species may decrease their role in the drug's cytotoxic properties. Of course, for certain proteins present in very low amounts, such modifications could be of great importance.

With nuclease enzyme digestion studies, it has been possible to demonstrate that certain drugs show a specificity for chromatin regions at the subnucleosomal level (Green *et al.,* 1982). Four nitrosoureas were incubated with either murine bone marrow cells or the cells of the murine leukemia, L1210. Two, chlorozotocin and GANU, have limited bone marrow toxicity in the mouse, but retain antitumor activity. Both CCNU and ACNU have marked bone marrow toxicity combined with antitumor activity. Figure 1–14 shows that all four drugs bind preferentially to DNA in the nucleosomal regions of L1210 chromatin, but only CCNU and ACNU were found on the core particle of bone marrow chromatin. In contrast, the two drugs with low myelotoxicity preferentially alkylated the linker chromatin in bone marrow. The alkylation of linker chromatin may be of less cytotoxic consequence because it is more readily repaired. The qualitative differences in drug binding found for these drugs may be of relevance for the differences observed in their tissue-specific cytotoxic properties.

Of relevance to drug therapy is the observation that some members of this class of drug preferentially alkylate transcriptionally active chromatin (Tew *et al.,* 1980). By increasing the transcriptional activity of tumor cells with corticosteroids, it is possible to increase subsequent cell kill with alkylating agents (Wilkinson *et al.,* 1979) or nitrosoureas (Tew *et al.,* 1982a). These observations may help to explain the relative success of empirically designed hormone-chemotherapy combinations in the treatment of human neoplasms.

The implication that the nuclear membrane or matrix may be a critical drug target is supported by the fact that it is preferentially attacked by nitrosoureas (Tew, 1982), which results in disproportionate amounts of alkylation and carbamoylation of the structural macromolecules. The membrane and matrix, in addition, have the following properties that are of potential relevance to drug interactions: (1) Both present structural barriers through which drug species must pass to reach chromatin; (2) they contain large numbers of nucleophilic macromolecular species; (3) their structure is dynamic rather than fixed; (4) the ultimate target, chromatin, is contiguous with both structures; (5) there is flexibility in the ratio of phospholipids to proteins; (6) there is a possibility for morphologic differences between different cell types; (7) the manifestations of cell death are accompanied by a breakdown of nuclear membrane integrity accompanied by disruption of inner nuclear membrane-chromatin attachments.

Gene Amplification. Because of their abnormally high growth rate, tumor cell populations provide an opportunity to observe evolutionary processes, which for normal eukaryotic cells could take many years and many generations. Exposure to chemotherapeutic agents can provide an external selective pressure that can stress the already unstable genetic apparatus of tumor cells. The high degree of genetic heterogeneity combined with the inherent genetic instability of tumor cells allows for the selection of clones of cells that can resist the cytotoxic effects of a drug. Following chemotherapy, the repopulation of a tumor by resistant cell clones can (and usually does) exacerbate the problem of successful eradication of a patient's cancer. Some biochemical mechanisms by which cells can develop resistance are listed in Table 1–5. By repeated exposure of cultured Chinese hamster ovary (CHO) cells to incrementally increased concentrations of methotrexate, researchers were able to select cell lines that were hundreds of times more resistant to the drug (Schimke *et al.,* 1978). Methotrexate is an analog of folic acid and kills cells by binding tightly to the enzyme dihydrofolate reductase; this effectively inhibits the

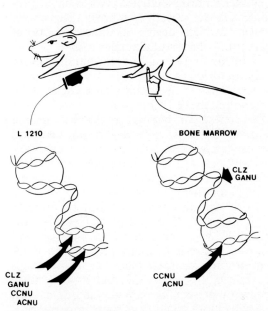

Figure 1–14. Qualitative site specificity of chloroethylnitrosourea alkylation in murine bone marrow and L1210 cells. 2-(3-[2-chloroethyl]-3-nitrosoureido)-D-glucopyranose (CLZ) and 1-(2-chloroethyl)-3-(β-D-glucopyranosyl)-1-nitrosourea (GANU) are relatively nonmyelotoxic compared to 1-(2-chloroethyl)-3-cyclohexyl-1-nitrosourea (CCNU) and 3-(4-amino-2-methylpyrimidin-5-yl)methyl-3-(2-chloroethyl)-3-nitrosourea (ACNU), whereas all four drugs possess great antitumor activity in L1210 leukemia.

Table 1–5. Mechanisms of Drug Resistance

1. Altered plasma membrane properties: impaired uptake of drug
2. Intracellular enzyme changes: nonactivation of drug
3. Intracellular enzyme changes: increased catabolism of drug
4. Increase in intracellular protective thiols
5. Increased DNA repair potential
6. Increased production of antimetabolite target enzymes through gene amplification

conversion of dihydrofolate to tetrahydrofolate in the cell, thereby interfering with DNA and protein synthesis.

The resistant CHO cells have been found to have up to 400 times the quantity of dihydrofolate reductase found in the parent cell line. Because the normal intracellular levels of methotrexate are insufficient to saturate the enzyme's active sites, the extra, unblocked enzyme (which can account for up to 5% of the total cellular protein) results in the phenotypic expression of drug resistance. The overproduction of the target enzyme has been attributed to the amplification of those genes coding for dihydrofolate reductase. Up to 400 extra copies of the enzyme gene have been found, located on the terminal arm of the no. 2 chromosome. Some of the resistant cell lines have an unstable resistance, which is progressively lost over several generations. Amplification of the dihydrofolate reductase was found to be localized in extrachromosomal, double-minute chromatin fragments, which do not have centromeres and cannot obey the rules of Mendelian inheritance. In daughter cells, therefore, the extrachromosomal material may not be inherited equally following mitosis. Over a number of generations this would lead to a progressive decrease in the resistance properties of the cell line.

The presence of double-minute chromosomes and homogenous staining regions, together with the genetic instability in Walker 256 carcinoma cells, may provide an interesting correlate to the methotrexate-resistant CHO cells, since the targets for alkylating agents are less specific than the dihydrofolate system. Clearly, gene amplification in eukaryotes may have important consequences to the evolution of drug-resistant cells.

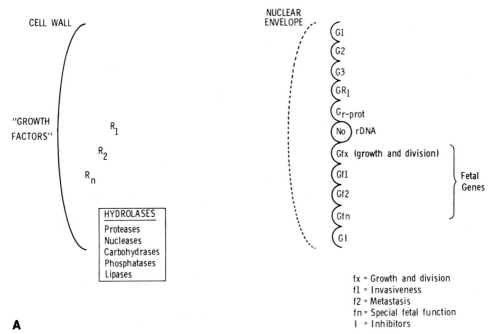

A

Figure 1–15A. Elements of the cellular response to external stimuli in the resting or ground state. It is envisaged that growth factors and other stimuli are almost continuously present in the cell periphery in equilibrium with intracellular elements. The symbols are: R_1–R_n, cytoplasmic receptor proteins; G1–GR_1, structural genes including genes for receptor proteins (GR_1); Gfx–Gfn, fetal genes with functions indicated; GI represents inhibitor genes; No, rDNA genes; and $G_{r\text{-prot}}$, genes for ribosomal proteins. From Busch, H.: A general concept for molecular biology of cancer. *Cancer Res.,* 36:4291–4294, 1976.

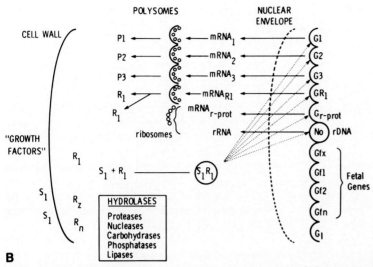

Figure 1–15B.   Response of cells to stimulus (S_1) with formation of stimulus-receptor complex (S_1R_1) that impinges on a group of genes—G1–GR_1, G_{r-prot}, and No(rDNA)—to produce a series of mRNAs, ribosomes, and polysomes; these in turn synthesize specific products including R_1. The "battery" of fetal genes is not involved in these normal responses. P1–P3 are protein readouts. See Figure 1–15A for other symbols. From Busch, H.: A general concept for molecular biology of cancer. *Cancer Res.,* **36:**4291–4294, 1976.

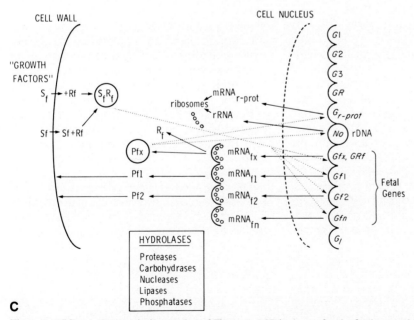

Figure 1–15C.   A pattern similar to that of Figure 1–15B is shown for the fetal state where a variety of fetal genes are activated by stimulus S_f (fetal stimulus factors) and receptor Rf to form S_fR_f, which acts in the same way as the factors controlling structural genes in the adults. See Figure 1–15A for other symbols. From Busch, H.: A general concept for molecular biology of cancer. *Cancer Res.,* **36:**4291–4294, 1976.

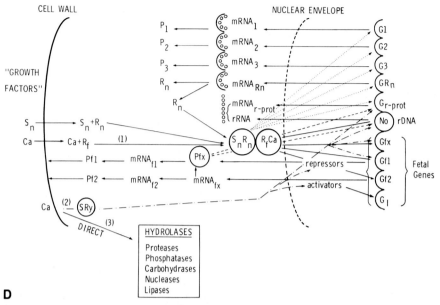

D

Figure 1-15D. Effects of carcinogenic agents on cellular responses. It is envisaged that carcinogens permit structural genes to function in the production of normal products but that, through several mechanisms, fetal genes are activated to produce a variety of fetal products, including Pf1 and Pf2, which are important for invasiveness and metastasis. The carcinogen may act with a fetal receptor to interact directly with the genome, or it may cause a new stimulus within the cell to interact with a receptor that will interact with the genome. Alternatively, the carcinogen may interfere with degradative reactions that are involved in normal growth controls. Ca represents a carcinogen; see Figure 1-15A for other symbols. From Busch, H.: A general concept for molecular biology of cancer. *Cancer Res.*, **36**:4291-4294, 1976.

REGULATION OF CELLULAR DIFFERENTIATION: FETAL GENE PRODUCTS

One of the major advances of the last decade has been the progression and development of evidence for the presence of "oncofetal," "oncoembryonic," or "oncodevelopmental" proteins in cancer cells (see Chapter 6A). Along with the work of Abelev and his associates (1979) on "oncoembryonic antigens," and the studies of Weinhouse (1972) and Sugimura (Sato and Sugimura, 1974) of fetal isoenzymes in cancer cells, there has been a profusion of studies on specific enzymes and other proteins that represent fetal gene readouts and that clearly were not designed to be produced in the normal adult.

As recently pointed out in studies from many laboratories (Fishman and Sells, 1976; Fishman and Busch, 1979), the tumor antigens of human cells and nonviral animal tumors frequently represent fetal gene readouts (see Figures 1-15A and 1-15B) ranging from late fetal stages to early elements of sperm and ovum. Along with neoplastic transformation, there may be fetal gene activation that is

apparently random with respect to tissue development and maturation. It is not clear whether such fetal gene derepression has meaningful effects on neoplastic processes, because activation of genes for production of the many isozymes appears to be quite random (Weinhouse, 1972; Sato and Sugimura, 1974). As Figure 1-15C indicates, fetal cells operate with special sets of signals coupled with a high degree of fidelity to produce the array of events that involve growth, specialization, and migration of cells as well as specification of organogenesis.

Special events occur at precise times in ontogenesis that do not recur during normal life. The processes involved in limb bud formation, including initiation, elongation, and termination of growth, for example, can be interfered with by thalidomide resulting in the arrested states characteristic of phocomelia. Even if the drug was removed, there would be no repetition of the phenomenon; that is, the limb buds would not continue to grow. Thus, there is only a defined "time window" during which limb bud growth and development are destined to occur.

These special time points in the biologic

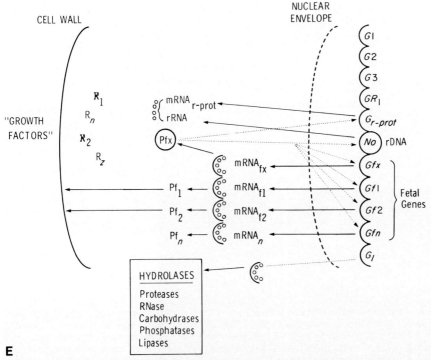

Figure 1–15E. This diagram indicates the expression of cancer as a continuous production of gene products involved in growth, invasiveness and metastasis. Such cells no longer produce R_1, R_2 (R_1 and R_2 are blocked out), or other products that may have phenotypic specificity. It is envisaged that these gene products and their derepressors are produced or maintained in high concentration through mitosis and that they keep these genes' new cell formation. In addition, the lack of fetal extracellular regulatory mechanisms does not permit these genes to be inactivated as they would be during normal fetal growth and development. See Figure 1–15A for other symbols. From Busch, H.: A general concept for molecular biology of cancer. *Cancer Res.*, **36:**4291–4294, 1976.

clock must be under the control of special start and stop signals that are probably active only during specific phases of ontogenesis. There is a rigid timing of these events in embryogenesis; either a series of feedback loops, specific activators, or inhibitors exist that control specific fetal functions.

Among the types of "shutoff mechanisms" that could exist are (1) loss of a fetal stimulus (Sf); or (2) inhibition of Sf by fetal factors. When special fetal genes are activated in cancer cells (see Figure 1 – 15C), suppression of their function may not occur in the adult because the corresponding control factors have long been inoperative. It is conceivable that a variety of functions of neoplastic cells could be controlled if specific fetal control elements were available as therapeutic agents. This concept was supported by Illmensee and Mintz (1976), who injected tumor cells from neoplastic rat testicular teratoma into rat blastocytes; the teratoma cells then grew like normal cells.

Figure 1 – 15D indicates that, at the time of exposure to carcinogens, several major effects

may occur in which a carcinogen interacts (1) with receptors, (2) with activators, (3) with cellular or chromatin enzymes or other proteins, or (4) directly or indirectly with the genome. The primordial cell that becomes a cancer cell is thrown into genomic disarray, leading to the phenotypic dysplasia (Sugimura, 1976). Carcinogens may well destroy most of the affected cells. Others undergo a wide variety of phenotypic alterations ranging from total loss to excessive production of specialized products. At some time, the genome becomes "set" for its altered functional activity in which both fetal and specialized genes are expressed. Recent studies have suggested that in daughter cancer cells the genome "set" may occur even before telophase has been completed (Busch *et al.*, 1979).

The cancer cells that emerge from the oncogenic events have fixed gene functions that include the operation of fetal genes. In these cells, many normal receptors are deleted (see Figure 1 – 15E). Other receptors (Rn or Rz) may be produced. The key genes, however, Pfx, Pf1, and Pf2, that are derepressed probably represent fetal gene elements that are vital to the biology of cancer, including the phenotypes of cell growth and division, invasiveness, and metastasis.

ANTIGENS OF CANCER CELLS

Oncoembryonic Antigens

The discovery (Gold and Freedman, 1965; Abelev *et al.,* 1979) that specific embryonic

markers could be detected in colon cancer and hepatoma rekindled interest in the possibility that derepressed fetal or developmental antigens in cancer cells could serve as immunodiagnostic aids for both detection and evaluation of the progress of the disease (see Chapter 6A). No cancer-specific antigen has yet been identified. This search has been ongoing for more than 30 years, and the chances for finding cancer-specific antigens seem to be diminishing. The increasingly accurate ultramicro-

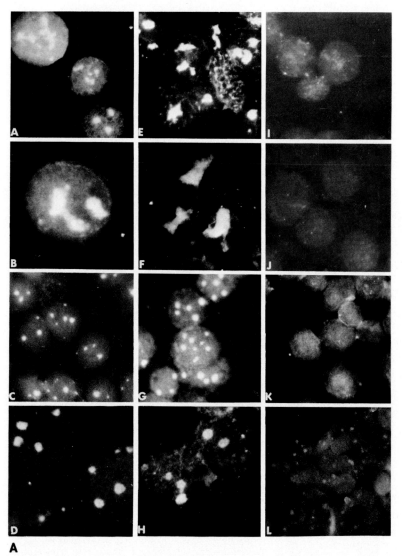

A

Figure 1–16A. Photomicrographs of nuclei analyzed with antisera or normal sera by the indirect immunofluorescent technique. Tumor antinucleolar antisera were incubated with Novikoff hepatoma nuclei (A × 1800; B × 4500) and liver nuclei (C × 1800; D × 4500). Liver antinucleolar antisera were incubated with Novikoff hepatoma nuclei (E × 1800; F × 4500) and liver nuclei (G × 1800; H × 4500). Normal rabbit sera were incubated with Novikoff hepatoma nuclei (I × 1800) and liver nuclei (J × 1800). Tumor antinucleolar antiserum absorbed with Novikoff tumor nucleoli was incubated with Novikoff nuclei (K × 1800), and liver antinucleolar antiserum absorbed with liver nucleoli was incubated with liver nuclei (L × 1800). From Busch, R.; Daskal, I.; Spoh, W. H.; Kellermayer, M.; and Busch, H.: Rabbit antibodies to nucleoli of Novikoff hepatoma and normal liver of the rat. *Cancer Res.,* **34:**2362–2367, 1974.

technology related to this question, however, precludes either optimism or pessimism. Specific antigens may be found intracellularly in the nucleus, nucleolus, or cytoplasm at any time. As one researcher (Old, 1981) pointed out, intensive and precise work is required to evaluate each proposed cancer-specific candidate. In the dysplastic state of cancer cells, common fetal or adult enzyme and other proteins and antigens are selected for survival, growth, invasiveness, and metastasis. Some may differ from their normal counterparts. Others may be markers from the tissue of origin or from the random activation of fetal or other tissue genes.

Nucleolar Antigens

It has been possible to produce nucleolus-specific antibodies in rabbits immunized with whole nucleoli as part of the studies on the proteins of the nucleolus (see Figure 1–16A). Some antigens (such as NoAg-1) were found in the nucleolar chromatin of Novikoff hepa-toma ascites cells, but not in those of normal liver cells (Busch and Busch, 1977). Other nucleolar antigens were present in normal liver cells but not in tumor cells (see Figure 1–16B).

In studies designed to purify nucleolar antigens by differential solubilization of nucleolar proteins, antigens were isolated from normal liver and Novikoff hepatoma nucleoli and compared by Ouchterlony double immunodiffusion and immunoelectrophoresis (Busch and Busch, 1977; Davis et al., 1978). The various extracts differed both in the number of antigenic species precipitated and in the density of immunoprecipitin bands.

Studies were carried out to determine whether antigens were present mainly in either normal liver (L) or Novikoff hepatoma (T) nucleoli, or in extracts of fetal liver nuclei (F). As shown in Figure 1–17, one antigen was present in the tumor only, and two were present in the tumor and fetal liver and may be referred to as oncofetal antigens (Davis et al., 1978).

In extended studies on human nucleolar antigens, rabbit antibodies to nucleoli isolated from HeLa cells produced bright nucleolar immunofluorescence in human cancer cells. After absorption with fetal bovine serum, placental, and liver nuclear extracts, the IgG still produced bright nucleolar fluorescence in

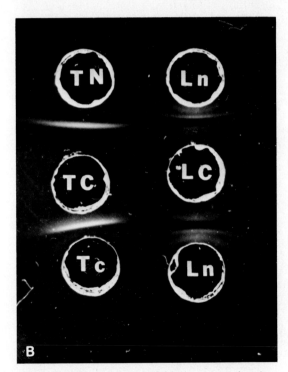

Figure 1–16B. Immunoprecipitin bands showing that antibodies to tumor chromatin (TC) and liver chromatin (LC) formed specific immunoprecipitates with liver (Ln) and tumor (TN) nucleolar extracts. Only one dense band was found in the tumor where three (or four) were found for the liver. There was no cross immunoreactivity in these preparations. From Busch, R. K., and Busch, H.: Antigenic proteins of nucleolar chromatin of Novikoff hepatoma ascites cells. *Tumori,* **63**:347–357, 1977.

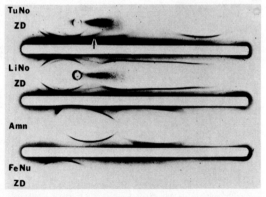

Figure 1–17. Immunoelectrophoretic profile of liver, tumor, and fetal Zubay-Doty extracts and amniotic fluid. Zubay-Doty extract (20 μg) from tumor nucleoli (TuNoZD), liver nucleoli (LiNoZD), fetal nuclei (FeNuZD), and amniotic fluid (Amn) were analyzed by electrophoresis at 75 V for 35 min on 1% agarose. Antitumor nucleolar immunoglobulin (50 μL), at 80 mg protein per ml, were placed in the antiserum troughs and precipitin arcs that developed in 24 hours were stained with Coomassie brilliant blue. The arrow shows a precipitin arc in the extract from Novikoff nucleoli that was not detected in the other fractions. From Davis, R. M.; Busch, R. K.; Yeoman, L. C.; and Busch, H.: Differences in nucleolar antigens of rat liver and Novikoff hepatoma ascites cells. *Cancer Res.,* **38**:1906–1915, 1978.

human tumor cells. Bright nucleolar fluorescence was not observed in most non-neoplastic human cells. With these antisera to HeLa cell nucleoli, positive nucleolar fluorescence was obtained in 94% of the neoplastic tumors studied. Very similar results have been obtained in several laboratories. Together, these data show the nucleolar antigen may be the most widespread human neoplastic tumor antigen found thus far.

In early studies, positive nucleolar fluorescence was noted in sections of a gastric ulcer and chronic ulcerative colitis; these conditions have tendencies to undergo neoplastic change, and the areas studied may have been undergoing such changes, but the positive effects may also reflect common nucleolar antigens in proliferating epithelial cells such as PCNA, the proliferating cell nucleolar antigen that is distributed throughout the nucleus in interphase and most of G1 phase; it migrates into the nucleolus during late G1 and early S phase (Deng *et al.,* 1981; Takasaki *et al.,* 1982).

The localization of the antigens suggests that they are involved either in the early reactions of the transcription of the rDNA genes and the production of rRNA or that they are involved in transport of the newly synthesized pre-rRNP particles. They may represent fetal elements involved in activation or acceleration of ribosome synthesis.

THE PLASMA MEMBRANE AND CELL SURFACE

The cell biology of the plasma membrane is complex, not only in regard to the molecules that form the membrane itself, but also in terms of its functional significance in transport, cell communication, cell adherence, and immune recognition. The inner plasma membrane, in addition, has important enzymatic associations (both synthetic and degradative), as well as cytoskeletal attachments, which serve to control cell shape and communication between cellular organelles. Many differences are known to exist between the outer plasma membrane of tumor cells as compared to normal cells. Table 1–6 illustrates some of these differences.

General Membrane Structure

The plasma membrane is a supramolecular structure composed of lipid, protein, and car-

Table 1–6. Differences in Cell Surface Properties of Normal and Tumor Cells

1. Modified surface charge densities
2. Lost exoskeletal fibronectin
3. Depletion or loss of glycoproteins and glycolipids
4. Modified permeability and transport of some molecules
5. Depletion or absence of cell gap junctions, with concomitant impairment of cell-cell communication
6. Increased lectin agglutinability
7. Differences in surface enzyme characteristics
8. Altered endocytotic and phagocytotic functions
9. Reduced thickness of hyaluronate-containing coat on cell surface
10. Modified mobility of membrane macromolecules
11. Altered adhesion and contact inhibition properties
12. Increased secretion of proteases and other lytic enzymes
13. Novel production of tumor-associated antigens
14. Periodic release of cell surface antigens

bohydrate. Sixty to eighty-five percent of the membrane mass is protein that is highly diversified, both structurally and functionally. The ratio of protein to lipid remains fairly constant for a given membrane, but can vary with differentiation, physiologic state, aging, and disease state. Structurally, membrane lipids are arranged in a bilayer with proteins distributed throughout the bilayer asymmetrically. These proteins may be classified as intrinsic, those located within the membrane bilayer and stabilized by hydrophobic interaction, and extrinsic, those located on the membrane surface and stabilized primarily by polar bonds. Less than 1% of the total membrane lipids are glycolipids. Among these, gangliosides are composed of neutral sugars and sialic acids and function as receptors or binding sites for toxins, polypeptide hormones, lymphokines, and interferon. Gangliosides, too, contribute to the antigenic properties of the cell surface. Cholesterol is a major sterol present in both normal and tumor cell membranes. The molar ratio of cholesterol to polar lipid approximates to unity. The presence of cholesterol serves to alter the permeability of membranes and interferes with the activity of a number of membrane-bound enzymes. Abnormal levels of cellular cholesterol are prominent in many disease states, which include atherosclerosis and erythrocyte disorders, as well as neoplasia (Wallach, 1975).

Many intrinsic proteins are covalently attached to chains of oligosaccharide carbohydrates via specific amino acid linkages. These oligosaccharide groups participate in a number of biologic recognition processes, including antigen-antibody, hormone-receptor, and cell contact inhibition.

The organization of these molecules to give an overall membrane architecture has been the subject of much research over the past decade. At present, two basic models have been proposed for membrane structure: The fluid mosaic model (Singer and Nicolson, 1972), which predicated fluidity of structural components with the bilayers constrained primarily by their mutual interactions and by their associations with peripheral proteins and cytoskeletal elements; and the lattice model (Changeux and Thiery, 1968), which proposed that repeated arrays of lipoproteins exist in two interconvertible states, which can be triggered by external stimuli. Effects are transmitted through the membrane by molecular cooperativity.

Each of these models helps to explain some membrane properties, but, obviously, much work remains before an accurate structure-function model can be determined.

Membrane Changes in Transformed Cells

The large number of phenotypic differences that have been identified in the membranes of tumor cells (see Table 1–6) suggests that some of these will be of relevance to the expression of the neoplastic process. Although it has been suggested that cancer is a disease of cellular membranes (Wallach, 1975), this suggestion has not been validated. The finding of a number of antigenic membrane surface alterations in tumor cells has given encouragement for the effort to couple antitumor agents with tumor-specific antibodies in an attempt to deliver cytotoxic drugs directly to tumor cells with minimal normal tissue toxicity. Such technology is dependent upon tumor-specific cell surface antigens and may prove to be limited to specific tumor types, or even to individual tumor cells.

Any of the changes in membrane structure that are listed in Table 1–6 either alone or in combination may be responsible for the expression of tumor cell characteristics. Because of the paucity of good experimental models, it has not been possible to attribute unequivocally any of the observed changes with, for example, loss of contact inhibition, tissue invasiveness, metastatic potential, or immune recognition. Additional complexity results from the heterogeneous properties and behavior of many tumor cells that are derived from a

single type of cancer, since these may exhibit different membrane properties.

Whether the large number of membrane changes that have been observed in transformed cells are the cause or effect of the neoplastic process is unclear. Obviously, these alterations are under genomic control, and thus, should be a function of prior modifications of DNA. The importance of the membrane to cellular integrity and the fact that tumor cells can be killed by drugs that interact solely with the membrane (Tritton and Yee, 1982) are indicative of the value of continued research into plasma membrane structure and function.

METABOLIC IMBALANCE: GLYCOLYSIS

One of the most studied discoveries of the last fifty years is the discovery that neoplasms exhibit a high rate of aerobic glycolysis (Warburg, 1926; Burk et al., 1967). A number of studies have attempted to relate this increased glycolysis with the transformation process, suggesting that the pleiotropic manifestations of the biochemical anomalies expressed in tumor cells may result from a gene mutation of enzymes involved in the control of glycolysis (Racker, 1976). Changes in intracellular pH are known to influence the rate of glycolysis (see the section on Other Properties of Tumor Cells later in this chapter), although the precise site of action of pH is unknown. Interestingly, many of the enzymes involved in glycolysis are attached to the plasma membrane interior through specific receptor sites. For example, glyceraldehyde-3-phosphate dehydrogenase (G-3-PDH), glucose-6-phosphate dehydrogenase (G-6-PDH), phosphoglycerate kinase (PK), phosphofructokinase (PFK), aldolase, and at least some of the purported protein kinases (Racker, 1981; Racker and Spector, 1981) are known to undergo tight, reversible, physiologic pH-dependent binding with integral membrane proteins. Because of the high degree of heterogeneity between the plasma membranes of tumor cells and their normal counterparts, it would be worthwhile to study further the interrelationships between membrane enzymes and the aberrant glycolytic rates of tumor cells. By analyzing the fermentation of glucose to lactic acid in a number of cancerous tumors, a high rate of adenosine triphosphate hydrolysis (ATP hydrolysis yielding adenosine diphosphate [ADP] and inorganic phosphate) was found to be a common denominator for all tumors. ADP and inorganic phosphate (Pi) are rate limiting for glycolysis and in Ehrlich ascites tumor cells. An inefficient Na^+, K^+ pump results in excesses of both ADP and Pi, which can be linked with the increased glycolytic rate. The precise mechanism by which the Na^+, K^+ pump is rendered inefficient is the subject of extensive research and controversy (Racker, 1981). It was thought that phosphorylation of tyrosine residues in the beta-subunit of sodium-potassium dependent adenosine triphosphatase (Na^+, K^+ ATPase) is catalyzed by a protein kinase, which is present in the plasma membrane of tumor cells. It may be possible to design drugs that make use of the manifest aberrant kinase in order to achieve a great chemotherapeutic advantage.

GROWTH FACTORS

An understanding of the mechanism of action of growth factors may assist in explaining the altered growth control of tumor cells. In tissue culture, malignant cells usually have a lowered growth requirement for serum than do their normal counterparts, and in some instances, tumor cells produce their own growth factors. In most cases, growth factors are polypeptides that are essential to cellular proliferation and may even influence the differentiation of specific target cells. By definition, these factors are distinct from nutrient chemicals that are required as substrates for growth. Their absolute requirement by tissue culture cells accounts for the inclusion of animal sera (which usually have high levels of growth factors) in the growth media for normal and transformed cells. Table 1–7 gives examples of some growth factors and their target cells.

The degree of mitogenic activity (potential to stimulate cell growth) of these growth factors is variable. Insulin alone, for example, is a comparatively inefficient growth stimulator, but can potentiate the activity of other factors, presumably because it is required for optimal uptake and utilization of other nutrient substrates.

The mechanism (or mechanisms) by which

Table 1–7. Some Characteristics of Various Growth Factors

FACTOR	SOURCE	TARGET CELL	MOLECULAR WEIGHT
Insulin	Beta cell of pancreas	General	6000
IGF-1	Human plasma	General	7650
IGF-2	Human plasma	General	7470
NSILA-P	Human plasma	General	100,000
Somatomedin A	Human plasma	Cartilage	7000
	Bovine plasma	Fibroblasts	
Somatomedin B	Human plasma	Glial cells	—
	Bovine plasma	Lung fibroblasts	
Somatomedin C	Human plasma	Cartilage	7000
	Bovine plasma	Fibroblasts	
MSA	Calf serum, liver, cell culture medium	Fibroblasts	10,000
FGF	Bovine pituitary	Fibroblasts, myoblasts, smooth muscle, chondrocytes, glial cells, vascular endothelium	13,400
NGF	Mouse submaxillary gland, snake venoms, cultured cells	Sympathetic ganglia cells and sensory neurons	26,500
EGF	Mouse submaxillary gland, human urine	Epidermal cells, mammary epithelial cells, vascular endothelial cells, chondrocytes, fibroblasts, glial cells	6045
PDGF	Human platelets	Fibroblasts, glial cells, arterial smooth muscle cells	13,000–16,000
TAF	Tumor tissues	Capillary endothelium	Unknown
SGF	Murine sarcoma, virus-transformed fibroblasts	Normal and transformed fibroblasts	9000

Abbreviations: IGF = insulinlike growth factor; NSILA-P = nonsuppressible insulinlike activity (ethanol-precipitable); MSA = multiplication-stimulating activity; FGF = fibroblast growth factor; NGF = nerve growth factor; EGF = epidermal growth factor; PDGF = platelet-derived growth factor; TAF = tumor angiogenesis factor; SGF = sarcoma growth factor.
Adapted from Ruddon, R. W.: *Cancer Biology.* Oxford University Press, New York, 1981.

growth factors control cellular proliferation is not well understood. Epidermal growth factor (EGF) is one of the more studied mitogens. Isolated by Cohen, EGF was demonstrated to be capable of promoting the proliferation and differentiation of epidermal tissue in newborn mice (Cohen, 1962; Cohen and Carpenter, 1975). When EGF binds to cell surface receptors, the receptor-EGF complexes are then internalized by an endocytotic mechanism. Degradation of EGF by lysosomal activity may follow this uptake phenomenon and may control the intracellular growth factor concentration.

Studies on a human epidermoid carcinoma cell line (Carpenter *et al.,* 1979) have shown that receptor-mediated uptake of EGF stimulates the phosphorylation of endogenous plasma membrane proteins via activation of an adenosine 3′, 5′-cyclic monophosphate (cAMP)-independent protein phosphorylating activity, more specifically, tryrosine-specific protein kinase. The importance of protein phosphorylation as a regulatory mechanism is discussed in this chapter in relationship to the oncogene theory. The fact that certain oncogenic virus genomes carry a gene coding for a cAMP-independent protein kinase, referred to as the src product, emphasizes further the possible implication of phosphorylation as a metabolic growth regulator (see Chapters 3A and 3D).

Tumor growth factors (TGFs) are under intensive study because of their ability to stimulate the division of cancer cells. Some of these factors bind to EGF receptors, others act on different surface factors. The future characterization of TGF peptides may offer opportunities for the development of new methods for controlling neoplastic cell proliferation.

OTHER PROPERTIES OF TUMOR CELLS

A number of less well-studied biochemical features of neoplastic cells have been found to be different from the same properties in their normal counterparts. The relevance of these differences to the causation or maintenance of the transformed state is unclear. Uncertainties of the cause-and-effect relationship stem partly from the relative lack of in-depth studies in these areas and partly because of a plethora of ambiguous data that are interesting and suggestive but indefinite. The following sections will offer a brief summary of some areas of interest that have contributed to our knowledge of the neoplastic process, without as yet explaining the phenomenon.

Cyclic Nucleotides

Although many *in vivo* and *in vitro* models are available to study the role of cyclic nucleotides as biochemical regulatory molecules, major problems in assessing their relevance in transformation are encountered through problems of tumor cell heterogeneity. The possible roles of the two main nucleotides, cAMP and guanosine 3′,5′-cyclic monophosphate (cGMP) can vary within the individual cellular populations that constitute a single solid tumor. No single unifying theory of the role of these molecules in neoplastic cells, or the maintenance of the transformed state, has yet been formulated.

A number of tumor cells have low levels of intracellular cAMP compared to normal cells. These include a chemically transformed embryonic fibroblast cell line, Morris hepatoma, and an asbestos-induced rat peritoneal mesothelioma. Conversely, the following tumors have demonstrated elevated cAMP levels relative to normal cells: A dimethyl benzanthracene (DMBA)-induced rat mammary carcinoma, rat neoplastic hepatic nodules, and a human adrenocortical carcinoma. In some of these cases, rapid degradation of free cyclic nucleotide by cyclic nucleotide phosphodiesterase may be responsible for intracellular differences. In a Walker 256 rat mammary carcinoma, acquired resistance to bifunctional alkylating agents has been associated with lowered phosphodiesterase activity and modified structural properties of cAMP binding proteins in the resistant cell population (Tisdale and Philips, 1976). Once again, it is not clear whether these differences are the *sine qua non* for resistance or a consequence of the selective genetic process.

Some problems relating to the role of cyclic nucleotides on transformation, growth, and differentiation have been raised elsewhere (Prasad, 1981), and are worthy of consideration: (1) The role of cAMP in maintaining a normal phenotype in some cells and not in others; (2) the possible modulating activity of cGMP on the cAMP system; (3) the effect of cAMP and cGMP on macromolecular transport; (4) the role of cAMP binding proteins during differentiation and transformation; and (5) the importance of specific protein cAMP-mediated phosphorylation in controlling these same processes.

Polyamine Metabolism

A further class of molecules affects both normal and neoplastic cellular metabolisms through a functional role in the synthesis of macromolecules. The polyamines, putrescine, spermidine, and spermine are ubiquitous in living cells. These polycations are of interest with respect to their potential role in cell growth and proliferation. Not only are elevated polyamine levels found in many tumor cells of diverse origin (Sunkara and Rao, 1981), but, clinically, urinary excretion of polyamines was reported to be higher in cancer patients than in normal individuals (Russell, 1971). Although the requirement for polyamines for DNA replication is well appreciated, no precise molecular mechanism by which control is mediated has been established. Limited data suggest that two enzymes, putrescine oxidase and polyamine oxidase, regulate the catabolism of polyamines throughout the cell cycle. Whether an imbalance in these enzymes occurs in tumor cells or not has yet to be established.

Intracellular pH

Variations in the intracellular pH (pH_i) of cells has been linked with cell growth. Glycolysis, in addition, has been shown to be sensitive to changes in pH_i *in situ.* This may be linked with the imbalanced glycolysis found in many tumor cells. It has been suggested that the proton is sufficiently pleiotropic and cellularly ubiquitous enough to be a candidate for the altered cell growth factor found in tumor cells (Gillies, 1981). Although the internal milieu of a cell is subject to control of pH within a physiologic range, localized alterations of pH_i are known to occur, and these may create specialized microenvironments affecting cellular metabolism. This may be especially important at the inner plasma membrane where local pH_i changes may influence cellular transport or membrane-associated enzyme activity.

Intracellular Sodium

Through studies on cellular transmembrane potential (Em) of normal and tumor cells, it has been found that the Em level of actively proliferating, neoplastic cells is greatly reduced in comparison with normal cells (Cone, 1969). Substantial changes in the cellular Na^+ level have been shown, with tumor cells possessing markedly elevated levels of Na^+. Concentrations of Cl^-, in addition, are significantly higher in dividing populations when compared to mitotically quiescent ones. Mitotic activity in nontumor cells is accompanied by elevated potassium and magnesium levels (Cameron *et al.,* 1980). These requirements are lost in transformed cells. Furthermore, treatment of both normal and transformed cells with the drug amiloride inhibits Na^+ flux and suppresses tumor cell division *in vivo.* A concomitant decrease in intracellular sodium accompanies this drug treatment, and it is of interest that this alteration in ion flux may be relevant to the control of cell division. Conclusive evidence is not yet available regarding the importance of this control mechanism to the maintenance of either the transformed or normal states.

Nuclear Magnetic Resonance (NMR) Difference in Normal and Neoplastic Cells

In 1916, reports presented evidence that the percentage of water in tumors was higher than in the host tissues of origin (Cramer, 1916). Furthermore, it was possible to correlate faster growth rates in tumors with increased water content; these faster growth rates were the result of increased uptake of water by transformed cells (McEwen and Haven, 1941). These observations led to a number of studies that, through NMR techniques, demonstrated that differences in the extent and type of water-macromolecular interactions occur in tumor cells when they are compared to their normal counterparts.

In mouse mammary epithelial cells, more than twenty biologic properties were found to be similar between normal, preneoplastic, and neoplastic cells (Beall *et al.,* 1981). Measurement of spin-lattice and spin-spin NMR values, however, showed that significant differences were apparent among all three cellular development stages. In common with the other biologic variables discussed in this section, the importance of these NMR differences to the process of transformation or the maintenance of the transformed phenotype remains poorly understood.

TUMOR CELL HETEROGENEITY

The heterogeneous nature of cancer cells has been stressed throughout most of this chapter. This property arises from the inherent genetic instability of tumor cells, which in most cases are derived from a single cell. By using glucose-6-phosphate dehydrogenase (G-6-PDH) as a biochemical marker, the clonality (or single cell origin) of human cancer has been studied in at least 25 different benign and neoplastic tumors (Fialkow, 1974). In a study of over 300 neoplasms, fewer than 10% were found to be of multicellular origin, supporting the concept that transformation of a single cell is sufficient to lead to the formation of a multicellular neoplasm.

Most advanced tumors share the property of increased DNA synthetic rates and continuous proliferation. As tumor progression occurs, the macro- and microenvironment to which individual tumor cells are exposed becomes variable. This results in "speeding up" selective pressures and, in effect, creates a microcosm of natural selection. The rate of emergence of sublines of tumor cells is dependent upon the host environment and the particular selective pressures that yield metabolic advantage for a tumor cell variant. Over a period of time, those cells that are not eliminated by host immunity, or by metabolic disadvantage, usually proliferate and become dominant. Subsequently, further genetic instability results in sequential selection of cells that are abnormal with respect to karyotype, differentiation, invasiveness, metastatic potential (see Chapter 4), and a plethora of biochemical and pharmacologic properties. These changes are of considerable importance to the successful eradication of tumors by chemotherapeutic and immunotherapeutic approaches, since the unique biochemical properties of particular sublines within an individual tumor may preclude the successful use of one treatment modality (see Chapter 10). Intrinsic and acquired resistance to chemotherapeutic agents in patients who are undergoing treatment is one of the major problems in the successful eradication of tumors.

Karyotype Heterogeneity

The discovery of the Philadelphia chromosome, in which a portion of chromosome 22 has been attached to chromosome 9 in chronic myelogenous leukemia cells, led to the hope that specific chromosome changes might characterize neoplastic disease. Recently, a number of acquired chromosome abnormalities have been discovered in solid tumors as well as leukemias and lymphomas (see Chapter 18). In addition to the Philadelphia chromosome, a translocation of the long arm of 17 to chromosome 15 has been found in acute promyelocytic leukemia and the long arm of 21 to chromosome 8 in acute myeloblastic leukemia. Three related translocations have been seen in Burkitt's lymphoma and B-cell acute lymphocytic leukemia; in each, one chromosome 8 is involved with chromosome 2, 14, or 22. These are essentially constant rearrangements (Rowley, 1982). In human small cell lung cancer cultures, a specific acquired deletion has been found in at least one chromosome 3 in 100% of 12 separate cell lines (Whang-Peng *et al.,* 1982). This deletion was not found in other types of cultured human tumor cells, including non-small-cell lung cancers. In addition to these specific examples, however, a wide spectrum of chromosome variants has been discovered, and they lack specificity for particular types of cancer or for cancer cells as a whole. It is clear that the first cancer cell is a euploid normal cell that has been subjected to DNA damage or other stimuli. Whether the subsequent clones of neoplastic cells that derive from the original cell have deranged chromosome patterns or not probably depends upon enzymes such as DNases and other DNA-related enzymes such as topoisomerases, transposonases, or repair systems that influence the integrity of the DNA and the chromosomes. Repetitive arrangements develop so that portions of the genome can become amplified.

Karyotypic changes may also relate to alterations in the neoplastic behavior of a tumor. Meningiomas (tumors of the brain lining) are usually localized tumors, which in rare cases may evolve into highly invasive and lethal sarcomas. This change can be correlated with karyotypic alterations. Some ordinary meningiomas are characterized by the loss of chromosome 22, but the mutated sarcoma has many other chromosome abnormalities, which are not apparent in the parent meningioma. In other cases, increased lethality of prostate cancer in rats can be correlated with a doubling of chromosome number. Tumor progression from benign to neoplastic is accompanied by a higher rate of spontaneous mutation, suggesting concomitant genetic instability.

At present, there is no definitive evidence that karyotypic alterations are the cause of normal cell transformation, rather than the result of tumor progression. The relevance of observed chromosome heterogeneity to the cancer phenotype, therefore, may not be clear. It is interesting to note, however, that by genetic mapping studies in human cells, 13 chromosomes are known to contain genes that regulate nucleic acid synthesis. Eleven of these (chromosomes 1, 5, 9, 13, 14, 15, 16, 17, 20, 21, and 22) are frequently involved in abnormal rearrangements in cancer cells. Other genes on these chromosomes are known to regulate intermediary metabolism; therefore, it is possible that mutation of these genes, with concomitant alteration of the chromosome, may provide selective advantage for the growth of tumor cells. Abnormalities of chromosome 1 are more readily detected than most because it is the largest human chromosome and has a distinctive chromosome banding pattern. Chromosome 1 has more chromatin than other chromosomes and thus would be more likely to be affected by a carcinogenic insult. The conformation of chromatin is known to influence the interaction of both drugs and carcinogens.

Chromosome banding has limits of application for detecting genetic alteration. An average stained band on a chromosome contains 5×10^6 nucleotide pairs, and deletions or duplications of approximately half this size are at the limit of detection (Rowley, 1977). Since an average polypeptide (MW = 50,000 daltons) is encoded by approximately 1200 nucleotide pairs, deletions or duplications of up to 1000 genes could occur without detection (Ruddon, 1981). If cellular transformation is a function of large alterations in genetic information, then these would show up as aberrations of the chromosome. The chromosomal alterations would be too subtle to distinguish a cancerous state if point mutations or base-patch mutations are critical.

A unique form of selective pressure is applied to tumor cell populations during exposure to chemotherapeutic agents. In a rat mammary carcinoma (Walker 256), acquired resistance to the alkylating agent chlorambucil is accompanied by alteration in both karyotype and nuclear structure (Tew and Wang, 1982; see Table 1–8). Although some studies of brain tumors have indicated that a statisti-

Table 1–8. Karyotype Analysis of Walker 256 Carcinoma Cells Sensitive (WS) and Resistant (WR) to Alkylating Agents

ANALYSIS	TYPE OF CELL	
	WR	WS
Polyploid percentage	10	10
Modal chromosome number	54	62
DNA (pg/cell)	1.19	1.49
RNA (pg/cell)	13.7	19.1
Marker Chromosomes		
Double minutes	+	−
Large metacentric	++	++
Large acrocentric	−	+
Acrocentric H2 with terminal arm, homogeneously staining region (HSR)	+*	+†
Submetacentric H1	−	+
Submetacentric H3	+	−
Submetacentric variable banding	++	++
Chromosome breaks	−	++
Interarm exchanges	−	+
Intraarm exchanges	−	+

* Short HSR
† Long HSR

cal correlation between drug sensitivity and tumor karyotype does not exist (Shapiro *et al.,* 1981), it is too early to predict that nuclear structural differences do not influence chemosensitivity, especially since gene amplification can be identified through homogeneously staining regions (HSR) and double minutes.

The Walker 256 rat mammary carcinoma, for example, has a degree of chromosome number heterogeneity that is illustrated in Table 1–8. The modal chromosome number per cell was statistically different for the resistant cell line (WR) that was derived from the parent line (WS) by selective exposure to chlorambucil. For both WR and WS, the chromosome numbers were aneuploid (polysomic) with respect to the normal diploid rat cell where 2n = 42. In addition to the numerical differences, the extra chromosomes are reflected in the DNA and RNA content of each cell (see Table 1–8). A number of marker chromosomes were present in each cell line. Double minutes (see Figure 1–18) were found only in WR, a situation consistent with the karyotypes of methotrexate-resistant tumor cell lines in which variable numbers of minutes are present (Schimke, 1980). These minutes are pieces of chromatin that are not true chromosomes, as they lack centromeres and are not passed to daughter cells by normal Mende-

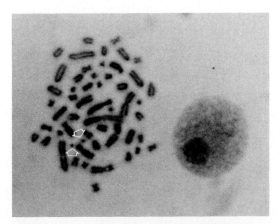

Figure 1–18. Chromosome spread of Walker 256 rat mammary carcinoma that expresses acquired resistance to bifunctional alkylating agents. The presence of nonchromosomal double minutes (arrows) distinguishes the resistant cell line from the parent-sensitive cell line.

lian genetics. Thus, the mechanism of inheritance determine that nuclear heterogeneity will be increased, because the random segregation of the chromatin will cause an uneven distribution of genetic information.

A further analysis of the chromosomes of the parent WS cell line revealed genetic instability that was not found in WR cells. Figure 1–19 shows a number of chromosome aberrations that were found in WS cells. By monitoring chromosome breaks and inter- and intra-arm exchanges, 42% of WS cells were found to contain chromosomal aberrations. Intra-arm exchanges are rare in most tumor cells; this further emphasizes the high degree of genetic instability for this tumor cell line. The selective pressures supplied by exposure to the alkylating agent chlorambucil have produced a cell line with a more stable chromosome complement, as none of the chromosomal aberrations found in the WS cells were present in the WR cell line. These findings serve to emphasize the problem of tumor cell heterogeneity, because in an *in vivo* situation, the resistant subpopulation of cells would thrive and reestablish the tumor following chemotherapy.

Other Forms of Cancer Cell Heterogeneity

Within a cancer, there may be subsets of cells that are neoplastic but nevertheless retain some of the differentiated properties of the tissue of origin. Such cells may have varying physiologic activities; for example, production of calcitonin in medullary carcinoma of the thyroid, insulin or gastrin from islet cell carci-

nomas, and melanin in melanomas. In other tumors, functions not expressed in the cell of origin are derepressed with the production of ectopic products that include many hormones and hormone-like materials (antidiuretic hormone [ADH], parathyroid hormone [PTH], adrenocorticotropic hormone [ACTH], and erythropoietin). If the neoplasm is efficient in this autonomous secretion of hormones, clinical syndromes will be produced that may provide the initial evidence for the presence of the disease or may cause devastating consequences.

Tumors also differ in their relative sensitivities to growth factors such as insulin, estrogen, epithelial growth factor (EGF), and tumor growth factor (TGF). This heterogeneity accounts for differences in requirements for growth *in vitro* and probably *in vivo* as well. The variation with respect to these factors is in part related to the quantity and the qualitative form of the receptors for hormones such as estrogen, progesterone, androgens, glucocorticoids, and others. In each of these cases, there may be a heterogeneity range from complete absence of receptors to quantitative excesses. An important example is human breast cancer wherein the content of estrogen receptors may vary greatly among the primary tumor and metastases and within relapsing sites. The receptor status of an individual patient may affect the chemotherapeutic regimen employed in the treatment of the disease.

There have been many pathologic analyses of variations in the desmoplastic responses in cancers, particularly in breast cancer, which may provide the consistency of forms of the neoplasms that is used clinically in the diagnosis of a possible tumor. Tumors may have large amounts of surrounding fibrous tissue or very little. They may also demonstrate relative degrees of lymphocytosis (melanoma) or vascularization. Correlations between rates of growth and degrees of vascular and desmoplastic reaction have been made, but no precise relationship has been proven.

The growth rates of various forms of cancer can differ considerably. Some tumors such as embryonic germ cell neoplasms and non-Hodgkin's lymphoma of diffuse histology are generally characterized by rapid growth rates, and others such as epidermal carcinomas and basal cell carcinomas have low growth rates. Some breast carcinomas may kill in six months and others may not result in death for 20 years despite the fact that their comparative

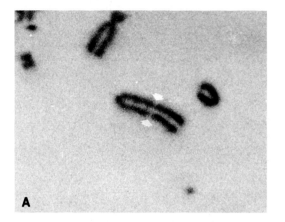

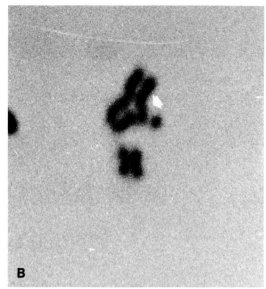

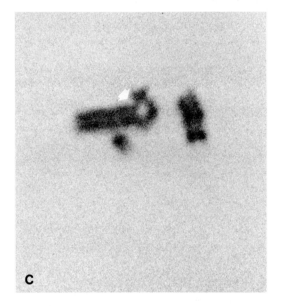

Figure 1–19. Examples of spontaneous chromosome aberrations in the Walker 256 alkylating-agent-sensitive cell line. The genetic instability of tumor cells is exemplified by three types of aberration: *(A)* Chromosome strand breakage; *(B)* intra-arm exchange; and *(C)* inter-arm exchange.

histologies appear identical. In part, this variation may result from differences in cell cycle time of individual tumor cells, growth fractions, rate of cell death, or variations in sensitivity to growth factors. This variation may also reflect cell-cell interactions within the tumor mass or cellular and humoral reactions to the tumor cells.

The sites in which the metastases localize are also variable. Some gastrointestinal neoplasms metastasize primarily to the liver and others may exhibit hematogenous spread to a variety of distal sites, with examples of solitary metastases localizing in the lung, brain, or bone suprascapular fossa. In terms of the total cellular mass of the malignant neoplasms, the number of cells that metastasize is usually small. Frequently, the metastases may be far larger than the primary tumor mass and, in rare cases, the primary may be difficult to find, as in the cases of a carcinoid tumor of the ileum or the generic category of carcinomas of unknown origin.

In experimental melanomas, there is a remarkable specificity of the sites of metastasis. Specific clones have been obtained that metastasize primarily to the lung or to the brain. Apparently, elements of the tissue substrate are critical to the deposition and growth of the cells in these loci. Although some evidence has suggested that metastasis is related to the presence of platelets either at the site of cell localization or at the surface of the tumor cells, it is not clear that there is a definitive relationship between the platelets and the metastases.

Although one hope of immunochemistry has been that common surface markers might exist for tumors in general or for specific tissues, the heterogeneity exhibited is bewildering. Variants are notable for leukemic cells for which B, T, lymphocyte, fetal, and other markers may be useful in defining the origins of the neoplastic cells, but these do not distinguish between the benign and malignant state. Many new markers are being investigated to identify the cells, particularly "Calla" and variations in lectin binding. No common surface marker for neoplasia has yet been defined.

In a specific tumor there are variations from clone to clone with respect to oxidative metabolism, macromolecular synthesis, production of endocrine factors, metastasis, and overall growth. In tumors that exhibit the presence of, or production of, CEA, the total amount of production of CEA is the average of synthetic efficiency of the cell populations within the mass. Colonic tumors that have a well-differentiated histology, for example, will produce more CEA when compared to their anaplastic counterparts. As different cell clones dominate within a metastatic mass, changes in rates of growth and product formation will reflect the changing cellular composition of the tumor. The altered population of cells producing prostatic acid phosphatase in secondary populations of prostatic carcinomas is an example of this change. Some metastases or tumor clones may produce none, others some, and still others more than the original tumors. As with CEA, this may depend upon the differentiation of the tumor.

High levels of the enzyme acid phosphatase were produced by tumors with well-differentiated cells whereas little if any enzyme was detected in undifferentiated cell masses. Depending upon the types of cells that metastasize out of the original tumor mass, a varying amount of acid phosphatase is produced and the levels in the blood vary accordingly. This emphasizes the deficiencies encountered in the use of these tumor products as indicators either of the presence of cancer or of relative changes in tumor mass.

Production of endocrine products has been related to the efficiency of clones of secretory cells and the relative mass of such cells within the tumor mass. If the majority of cells in a given tumor maintain a high rate of hormonal production and secretion, the amount of hormones produced per gram of tumor will be high. If the clone does not actively secrete hormones or produces hormones at a slow rate, changes in the plasma hormone level may not be detectable. In the case of an insulinoma, a 1-cm neoplasm may cause life-threatening hy-

Table 1–9.   Viral oncogenes.

RETROVIRAL ONCOGENES (V-ONC GENES)		TRANSFORMATION IN CELL CULTURE		
	Abbreviation viral gene	Acute leukemia	373 fibroblasts	Sarcoma/ carcinoma
Acute viruses				
1. Rous sarcoma (chicken)	v-src	−	+	+/−
2. Fujinami sarcoma* (chicken, rat)	v-fps	−	+	+/−
3. Yamaguchi sarcoma* (chicken)	v-yes	−	+	+/−
4. Rochester-2 sarcoma* (chicken)	v-ros	−	+	+/−
5. Myelocytomatosis MC29* (chicken)	v-myc	+	+	+/+
6. Carcinoma MH2*	v-mht/myc	+	+	+/+
7. Avian erythroblastosis* (chicken)	verb^A/verb^B	+	+	+/+
8. Myeloblastosis and erythroblastosis-E26* (chicken)	v-myb (v-amv or v-ets)	+	−	−/−
9. Reticuloendotheliosis (turkey)	v-rel	+	−	−/?
Mammalian viruses				
10. Moloney murine sarcoma	v-mos	−	+	+/v
11. Harvey and Kirsten rat sarcoma (also mouse)	v-ras$^{HA \text{ or } Ki}$	+	+	+/−
12. Abelson murine leukemia* (also cat)	v-abl	+	+	−/−
13. FBJ murine osteosarcoma	v-fos	−	+	+/−
14. ST and GA feline sarcoma*	v-fes	−	+	+/+
15. SM feline sarcoma*	v-fms	−	+	+/−
16. Simian sarcoma* (also cat)	v-sis	−	+	+/−

*Δgag
†Δenv
From Busch, H.: Molecular lesions in cancer. *Mol. Cell. Biochem.*, **61**:111–130, 1984.

poglycemia, whereas an adrenal corticocarcinoma may become massive and heavily involve the liver but still not produce viralization or Cushing's syndrome.

For further discussion of the biology and patterns of metastases, see Chapter 4.

The recent spectacular developments in the field of oncogenes (see Table 1–9) have markedly changed the perspectives of experimental oncologists. The demonstration that a variety of retroviral genes exists in cancer cells, frequently in activated states, has led to the conclusion that part of the heterogeneity of cancer resides in the many mechanisms for activation of these genes and varying levels of their specific products in many kinds of experimental and human cancers. Their precise roles in oncogenesis and neoplasia are being intensively studied.

REFERENCES

Abelev, G. I.; Engelhardt, N. V.; and Elgort, D. A.: Immunochemical and immunohistochemical micromethods in the study of tumor-associated embryonic antigens (α-fetoprotein). In Fishman, W. H., and Busch, H. (eds.): *Methods in Cancer Research,* Vol. XVIII. Academic Press, New York, 1979.

Abelson, J.: RNA processing and the intervening sequence problem. *Annu. Rev. Biochem.,* **48:**1035–1069, 1979.

Banerjee, A. K.: 5′-terminal cap structure in eucaryotic messenger ribonucleic acids. *Microbiol. Rev.,* **44(2):**175–205, 1980.

Beall, P. T.; Asch, B. B.; Medina, D.; and Hazelwood, C.: Distinction of normal, preneoplastic and neoplastic mouse mammary cells and tissues by nuclear magnetic resonance techniques. In Cameron, I. L., and Pool, T. B. (eds.): *The Transformed Cell.* Academic Press, New York, 1981.

Berezney, R., and Coffey, D. S.: Isolation of a nuclear structural complex from mammalian nuclei. *J. Cell Biol.,* **59 (Part 2):**22a, 1973.

Berezney, R., and Coffey, D. S.: The nuclear protein matrix: isolation, structure and functions. *Adv. Enzyme Regul.,* **14:**63–100, 1976.

Berget, S. M.; Berk, A. J.; Harrison, T.; and Sharp, P.: Spliced segments at the 5′ termini of adenovirus-2 late mRNA: A role for heterogeneous nuclear RNA in mammalian cells. *Cold Spring Harbor Symp. Quant. Biol.,* **42:**523–529, 1977.

Bouteille, M.; Kalifat, S. R.; and Delarne, J. J.: Ultrastructural variations of nuclear bodies in human diseases. *J. Ultrastruct. Res.,* **19:**474–486, 1967.

Breathnach, R., and Chambon, P.: Organization and expression of eucaryotic split genes coding for proteins. *Annu. Rev. Biochem.,* **50:**349–383, 1981.

Burk, D.; Woods, M.; and Hunter, J.: On the significance of glucolysis for cancer, with special reference to Morris rat hepatomas. *J.N.C.I.,* **38:**839–863, 1967.

Busch, H.: *Histones and Other Nuclear Proteins.* Academic Press, New York, 1965.

Busch, H.: Messenger RNA and other high molecular

weight RNA. In Busch, H. (ed.): *The Molecular Biology of Cancer.* Academic Press, New York, 1974.

Busch, H.: The function of the 5′ "cap" of mRNA and nuclear RNA species. *Perspect. Biol. Med.,* **19:**549–567, 1976.

Busch, H.: The eukaryotic nucleus. In O'Malley, B. W., and Birnbaumer, L. (eds.): *Receptors and Hormone Action,* Vol. 1. Academic Press, New York, 1977.

Busch, H.; Byvoet, P.; and Smetana, K.: The nucleolus of the cancer cell: A review. *Cancer Res.,* **23:**323–339, 1963.

Busch, H.; Daskal, Y.; Gyorkey, F.; and Smetana, K.: Silver staining of nucleolar granules in tumor cells. *Cancer Res.,* **39:**857–863, 1979.

Busch, H., and Goldknopf, I. L.: Ubiquitin-protein conjugates. *Mol. Cell. Biochem.,* **40:**173–187, 1981.

Busch, H.; Hirsch, F.; Gupta, K. K.; Rao, M.; Spohn, W.; and Wu, B. C.: Structural and functional studies on the "5-cap": a survey method for m-RNA. *Prog. Nucleic Acid Res.,* **19:**39–61, 1976.

Busch, H.; Reddy, R.; Rothblum, L.; and Choi, Y. C.: SnRNA's, SnRNP's and RNA processing. *Annu. Rev. Biochem.,* **51:**617–654, 1982.

Busch, H., and Smetana, K.: *The Nucleolus.* Academic Press, New York, 1970.

Busch, R. K., and Busch, H.: Antigenic proteins of nucleolar chromatin of Novikoff hepatoma ascites cells. *Tumori,* **63:**347–357, 1977.

Cameron, I. L.; Pool, T. B.; and Smith, N. K.: Intracellular concentration of potassium and other elements in vaginal epithelial cells stimulated by estradiol administration. *J. Cell. Physiol.,* **104(1):**121–125, 1980.

Carpenter, G.; King, L.; and Cohen, S.: Rapid enhancement of protein phosphorylation in A-431 cell membrane preparations by epidermal growth factor. *J. Biol. Chem.,* **254:**4884–4891, 1979.

Caspersson, T., and Santession, L.: Studies on protein metabolism in the cells of epithelial tumors. *Acta Radiol. [Suppl.],* **46:**5–105, 1942.

Changeux, J. P., and Thiery, J.: On the excitability and cooperativity of biological membranes. In Jarnefelt, J. (ed.): *Regulatory Functions of Biological Membranes,* Vol. 2. Elsevier, Amsterdam, 1968.

Chow, L. T.; Gelinas, R. E.; Broker, T. R.; and Roberts, R. J.: An amazing sequence arrangement at the 5′ ends of adenovirus 2 messenger RNA. *Cell,* **12:**1–8, 1977.

Cohen, S.: Isolation of a mouse submaxillary gland protein accelerating incisor eruption and eyelid opening in the newborn animal. *J. Biol. Chem.,* **237:**1555–1562, 1962.

Cohen, S., and Carpenter, G.: Human epidermal growth factor: Isolation and chemical biological properties. *Proc. Natl. Acad. Sci. USA,* **72:**1317–1321, 1975.

Cone, C. D.: Electroosmotic interactions accompanying mitosis initiations in sarcoma cells *in vitro. Trans. N.Y. Acad. Sci.,* **31:**404–427, 1969.

Cramer, W.: On the biochemical mechanism of growth. *J. Physiol.,* **50:**322–334, 1916.

Darnell, J.: Implications of RNA-RNA splicing in evolution of eukaryotic cells. *Science,* **202:**1257–1260, 1978.

Daskal, Y.: Perichromatin granules. In Busch, H. (ed.): *The Cell Nucleus,* Vol. 8. Academic Press, New York, 1981.

Daskal, Y.; Komaromy, L.; and Busch, H.: Isolation and partial characterization of perichromatin granules: A unique class of nuclear RNP particles. *Exptl. Cell Res.,* **126:**39–46, 1980.

Daskal, Y.; Mace, M. L., Jr.; Wray, W.; and Busch, H.: Use

of direct current sputtering from improved visualization of chromosome topology by scanning electron microscopy. *Exp. Cell Res.,* **100:**204–212, 1976.

Davis, R. M.; Busch, R. K.; Yeoman, L. C.; and Busch, H.: Differences in nucleolar antigens of rat liver and Novikoff hepatoma ascites cells. *Cancer Res.,* **38:**1906–1915, 1978.

Deng, J. S.; Takasaki, T.; and Tan, E. M.: Nonhistone nuclear antigens reactive with autoantibodies. Immunofluorescent studies of distribution in synchronized cells. *J. Cell Biol.,* **91:**654–660, 1981.

Feinberg, A. P., and Coffey, D. S.: The topology of DNA loops: A possible link between the nuclear matrix structure and nucleic acid function. In Maul, G. C. (ed.): *The Nuclear Envelope and the Nuclear Matrix.* Alan R. Liss, Inc., New York, 1982.

Fialkow, P. J.: The origin and development of human tumors studied with cell markers. *N. Engl. J. Med.,* **291:**26–35, 1974.

Fishman, W. H., and Busch, H. (eds.): *Methods in Cancer Research,* Vol. XVIII. Academic Press, New York, 1979.

Fishman, W. H., and Sells, S.: In *Oncodevelopmental Gene Expression.* Academic Press, New York, 1976.

Gilbert, W.: Why genes in pieces? *Nature,* **271:**501, 1978.

Gillies, R. J.: Intracellular pH and growth control in eukaryotic cells. In Cameron, I. L., and Pool, T. B. (eds.): *The Transformed Cell.* Academic Press, New York, 1981.

Gold, P., and Freedman, S. O.: Specific carcinoembryonic antigens of the human digestive system. *J. Exp. Med.,* **122:**467–481, 1965.

Green, D.; Tew, K. D.; Hisamatsu, T.; and Schein, P. S.: Correlation of nitrosourea murine bone marrow toxicity with DNA alkylation and chromatin binding sites. *Biochem. Pharmacol.,* **31:**1671–1679, 1982.

Gurley, L. R.; Enger, M. D.; and Walters, R. A.: The nature of histone f1 isolated from polysomes. *Biochemistry,* **12:**237–245, 1973.

Hayward, W. S.; Neel, B. G.; and Astrin, S. M.: Activation of a cellular oncogene by promoter insertion in ALU-induced lymphoid leukosis. *Nature,* **290:**475–479, 1981.

Hirsch, F. W.; Nall, K. N.; Busch, F. N.; Morris, H. P.; and Busch, N.: Comparison of abundant cytosol proteins in rat liver, Novikoff hepatoma, and Morris hepatoma by two-dimensional gel electrophoresis. *Cancer Res.,* **38:**1514–1522, 1978.

Hodnett, J. L., and Busch, H.: Isolation and characterization of the uridylic acid-rich RNA of rat liver nuclei. *J. Biol. Chem.,* **243:**6334–6342, 1968.

Howard-Flanders, P.: Inducible repair of DNA. *Sci. Am.,* **245:**72–80, 1981.

Illmensee, K., and Mintz, B.: Totipotency and normal differentiation of single teratocarcinoma cells cloned by injection into blastocysts. *Proc. Natl. Acad. Sci. USA,* **73:**549–553, 1976.

Jay, F. T.; Laughlin, C. A.; and Carter, B. J.: Eukaryotic translational control: Adeno-associated virus protein synthesis is affected by a mutation in the adenovirus DNA-binding protein. *Proc. Natl. Acad. Sci. USA,* **78:**2927–2931, 1981.

Jelinek, W. R.; Toomey, T. P.; Leinwand, L.; Duncan, C. H.; Bird, P. A.; Choudary, P. V.; Weissman, S. M.; Rubin, C. M.; Housck, C. M.; Deininger, P. L.; and Schmid, C. W.: Ubiquitous, interspersed repeated sequences in mammalian genomes. *Proc. Natl. Acad. Sci. USA,* **77:**1398–1402, 1980.

Kleinsmith, L. J.: Phosphorylation of nonhistone proteins. In Busch, H. (ed.): *The Cell Nucleus, Chromatin, Part C,* Vol. 6. Academic Press, New York, 1978.

Kornberg, A.: *DNA Replication.* Freeman, San Francisco, 1980.

Langan, T. A.: Phosphorylation of liver histone following the administration of glucagon and insulin. *Proc. Natl. Acad. Sci. USA,* **64:**1276–1283, 1969.

Lerner, M. R.; Boyle, J. A.; Mount, S. M.; Wolin, S. L.; and Steitz, J. A.: Are snRNPs involved in splicing? *Nature,* **283:**220–224, 1980.

Lerner, M. R., and Steitz, J. A.: Antibodies to small nuclear RNAs complexed with proteins are produced by patients with systemic lupus erythematosus. *Proc. Natl. Acad. Sci. USA,* **76:**5495–5499, 1979.

Lischwe, M. A.; Richards, R. L.; Busch, R. K.; and Busch, H.: Localization of phosphoprotein C23 to nucleolar structures and to the nucleolus organizer regions. *Exp. Cell Res.,* **136:**101–109, 1981.

Lischwe, M. A.; Smetana, K.; Olson, M. O. J.; and Busch, H.: Proteins C23 and B23 are the major nucleolar silver staining proteins. *Life Sci.,* **25:**701–708, 1979.

MacCarty, W. C.: The value of the macronucleolus in the cancer problem. *Am. J. Cancer,* **26:**529–532, 1936.

MacCarty, W. C., and Haumeder, E.: Has the cancer cell any differential characteristics? *Am. J. Cancer,* **20:**403–407, 1934.

McEwen, H. D., and Haven, F. L.: The effect of carcinosarcoma 256 on the water content of liver. *Cancer Res.,* **1:**148–150, 1941.

Maul, G. G. (ed.): *The Nuclear Envelope and the Nuclear Matrix.* Alan R. Liss, Inc., New York, 1982.

Nakhasi, H. L.; Lynch, K. R.; Dolan, K. P.; Unterman, R. D.; and Feigelson, P.: Covalent modification and repressed transcription of a gene in hepatoma cells. *Proc. Natl. Acad. Sci. USA,* **78:**834–837, 1981.

Old, L. J.: Cancer immunology: The search for specificity: G.H.A. Clowes Memorial Lecture. *Cancer Res.,* **41:**361–375, 1981.

Olins, A. L.; Breillant, J. T.; Carlson, R. D.; Senior, M. B.; Wright, E. B.; and Olins, D. E.: On nu models for chromatin structure. In Ts'o, P. (ed.): *The Molecular Biology of the Mammalian Genetic Apparatus,* Vol. 1. Elsevier/North-Holland Biomedical Press, Amsterdam, 1977.

O'Malley, B. W., and Means, A. R.: Effects of female steroid hormones on target cell nuclei. In Busch, H. (ed.): *The Cell Nucleus,* Vol. 3. Academic Press, New York, 1974.

Paul, J., and Gilmour, R. S.: Template activity of DNA is restricted in chromatin. *J. Mol. Biol.,* **16:**242–244, 1966a.

Paul, J., and Gilmour, R. S.: Restriction of deoxyribonucleic acid template activity in chromatin is organ specific. *Nature,* **210:**992–993, 1966b.

Paul, J., and Gilmour, R. S.: Organ-specific restriction of transcription in mammalian chromatin. *J. Mol. Biol.,* **34:**305–316, 1968.

Prasad, K. N.: Involvement of cyclic nucleotides in transformation. In Cameron, I. L., and Pool, T. B. (eds.): *The Transformed Cell.* Academic Press, New York, 1981.

Prestayko, A. W.; Klomp, G. R.; Schmoll, D. J.; and Busch, H.: Comparison of proteins of ribosomal subunits and nucleolar preribosomal particles from Novikoff hepatoma ascites cells by two-dimensional polyacrylamide gel electrophoresis. *Biochemistry,* **13:**1945–1951, 1974.

Racker, E.: *A New Look at Mechanisms in Bioenergetics.* Academic Press, New York, 1976.

Racker, E.: Warburg effect revisited: Letter. *Science,* **213:**1313, 1981.

Racker, E., and Spector, M.: Warburg effect revisited: merger of biochemistry and molecular biology. *Science,* **213:**303–307, 1981.

Reddy, R., and Busch, H.: U snRNA's of nuclear snRNP's. In Busch, H. (ed.): *The Cell Nucleus,* Vol. VIII. Academic Press, New York, 1981.

Rowley, J. D.: Mapping of human chromosomal regions related to neoplasia: evidence from chromosomes 1 and 17. *Proc. Natl. Acad. Sci. USA,* **74:**5729–5733, 1977.

Rowley, J. D.: Identification of the constant chromosome regions involved in human hematologic malignant disease. *Science,* **216:**749–751, 1982.

Ruddon, R. W.: *Cancer Biology.* Oxford University Press, New York, 1981.

Russell, D. H.: Increased polyamine concentrations in the urine of human cancer patients. *Nature; New Biol.,* **233:**144–145, 1971.

Sato, S., and Sugimura, T.: Isozymes of carbohydrate enzymes. In Busch, H. (ed.): *Methods in Cancer Research,* Vol. 12. Academic Press, New York, 1974.

Schimke, R. T.: Gene amplification and drug resistance. *Sci. Am.,* **243:**60–69, 1980.

Schimke, R. T.; Kaufman, R. J.; Alt, F. W.; and Kellems, R. F.: Gene amplification and drug resistance in cultured murine cells. *Science,* **202:**1051–1055, 1978.

Shapiro, J. R.; Yung, W. A.; and Shapiro, W. R.: Isolation, karyotype and clonal growth of heterogeneous subpopulations of human malignant gliomas. *Cancer Res.,* **41:**2349–2359, 1981.

Sharp, P. A.: Speculations on RNA splicing. *Cell,* **23:**643–646, 1981.

Singer, S. J., and Nicolson, G. L.: The fluid mosaic model of the structure of cell membranes. *Science,* **175:**720–731, 1972.

Sunkara, P. S., and Rao, P. N.: Role of polyamines in the regulation of the cell cycle in normal and transformed mammalian cells. In Cameron, I. L., and Pool, T. B. (eds.): *The Transformed Cell.* Academic Press, New York, 1981.

Takami, H.; Busch, F. N.; Morris, H. P.; and Busch, H.: Comparison of salt-extractable nuclear proteins of regenerating liver, fetal liver, and Morris hepatomas 9618A and 3924A. *Cancer Res.,* **39:**2096–2105, 1979.

Takasaki, Y.; Deng, J. S.; and Tan, E. M.: A nuclear antigen associated with cell proliferation and blast-transformation. *J. Exp. Med.,* **154(6):**1899–1909, 1982.

Tan, E. M.: Autoimmunity to nuclear antigens. In Busch, H. (ed.): *The Cell Nucleus,* Vol. 7. Academic Press, New York, 1979.

Tew, K. D.: Chromatin associated nuclear components as potential drug targets. In Serrou, B.; Schein, P. S.; and Imbach, J.-L. (eds.): *Nitrosoureas in Cancer Treatment.* Elsevier/North Holland Biomedical Press, New York, 1981.

Tew, K. D.: The interaction of nuclear reactant drugs with the nuclear membrane and nuclear matrix. In Maul, G. C. (ed.): *The Nuclear Envelope and the Nuclear Matrix.* Alan R. Liss, Inc., New York, 1982.

Tew, K. D.; Schein, P. S.; Lindner, D. J.; Wang, A. L.; and Smulson, M. E.: Influence of hydrocortisone on the binding of nitrosoureas to nuclear chromatin subfractions. *Cancer Res.,* **40:**3697–3703, 1980.

Tew, K. D., and Wang, A. L.: Selective cytotoxicity of haloethylnitrosoureas in a carcinoma cell line resistant to bifunctional nitrogen mustards. *Mol. Pharmacol.,* **21:**729–738, 1982.

Tew, K. D.; Wang, A. L.; Lindner, D. J.; and Schein, P. S.: Enhancement of nitrosourea cytotoxicity in vitro using hydrocortisone. *Biochem. Pharmacol.,* **31:**1179–1180, 1982a.

Tew, K. D.; Wang, A. L.; Macdonald, J. S.; and Moy, B. C.: Differences in the nuclear morphologies of a carcinoma cell line with or without acquired resistance to bifunctional alkylating agents. *Proc. Am. Assoc. Cancer Res.,* **23:**167, 1982b.

Thrall, C. L.; Webster, R. A.; and Spelsberg, T. C.: Steroid receptor interaction with chromatin. In Busch, H. (ed.): *The Cell Nucleus, Chromatin,* Part C, Vol. VI. Academic Press, New York, 1978.

Tisdale, M. J., and Philips, B. J.: Alterations in adenosine 3′,5′ monophosphate-binding protein in Walker carcinoma cells sensitive or resistant to alkylating agents. *Biochem. Pharmacol.,* **25:**1831–1836, 1976.

Trendelenburg, M. F., and McKinnell, R. G.: Transcriptionally active and inactive regions of nucleolar chromatin in amplified nucleoli of fully grown oocytes of hibernating frogs, *Rana pipiens* (Amphibia, Anura). A quantitative electron microscopic study. *Differentiation,* **15:**73–95, 1979.

Tritton, T. R., and Yee, G. L.: The anticancer agent adriamycin can be actively cytotoxic without entering cells. *Science,* **217:**248–250, 1982.

Wallach, D. F. H.: *Membrane Molecular Biology of Neoplastic Cells.* Elsevier, Amsterdam, 1975.

Warburg, O.: *Über den Stoffwechsel der Tumoren.* Springer, Berlin, 1926.

Watson, M. L.: Observations on a granule associated with chromatin in the nuclei of cells of rat and mouse. *J. Cell Biol.,* **13:**162–167, 1962.

Weiner, A.: An abundant cytoplasmic 7S RNA is complementary to the dominant interspersed middle repetitive DNA sequence family in the human genome. *Cell,* **22:**209–218, 1980.

Weinhouse, S.: Glycolysis, respiration and anomalous gene expression in experimental hepatomas: G.H.A. Clowes Memorial Lecture. *Cancer Res.,* **32:**2007–2016, 1972.

Whang-Peng, J.; Kao-Shan, C. S.; Lee, E. C.; Bunn, P. A.; Carney, D. N.; Gazdar, A. P.; and Minna, J. D.: Specific chromosome defect associated with human small-cell lung cancer: deletion 3p (14–23). *Science,* **215:**181–182, 1982.

Wilkinson, R.; Birbeck, M.; and Harrap, K. R.: Enhancement of nuclear reactivity of alkylating agents by prednisolone. *Cancer Res.,* **39:**4256–4261, 1979.

Yang, V. W.; Lerner, M.; Steitz, J. A.; and Flint, S. J.: A small nuclear ribonucleoprotein is required for splicing of adenoviral early RNA sequences. *Proc. Natl. Acad. Sci. USA,* **78:**1371–1375, 1981.

2

Cell Kinetics and Cancer Chemotherapy

STANLEY E. SHACKNEY

INTRODUCTION

The field of cell kinetics deals with quantitative aspects of the growth behavior of normal and abnormal cell populations and their responses to cytotoxic agents. Clinical experience has shown that rapidly proliferating human tumors are often more responsive to systemic treatment than are slowly proliferating tumors (Shackney et al., 1978). The increased susceptibility of rapidly proliferating cells to cytotoxic drugs has also been demonstrated in numerous experimental tumor cell systems. Thus, it might be expected that the proper application of principles of cell kinetics would result in more effective forms of cancer treatment. Indeed, there has been considerable interest in recent years in clinical protocols that are designed with principles of cell kinetics in mind. Therapeutic regimens employing late treatment intensification (Norton et al., 1982; Cabanillas et al., 1983) and newer therapeutic approaches to the problem of emergence of genetic drug resistance (Fisher et al., 1983) have relied on basic kinetic concepts of tumor growth and drug response. Such concepts are likely to assume increasing importance as the emphasis of clinical investigative therapeutics shifts more and more from empirical trials to the development and testing of rational clinical treatment strategies.

In this chapter, the basic principles and methods of cell kinetics will be presented, with emphasis on principles that bear on clinical treatment.

TUMOR GROWTH

The Clonal Nature of Human Cancers

It is likely that most, if not all, human tumors arise from a single genetically abnormal cell that multiplies and eventually kills the host, usually when the body burden of tumor approaches or exceeds 1×10^{12} cells (one trillion cells; approximately 1 kg of tumor). Evidence for the clonal nature of human cancers comes from a variety of sources:

1. Karyotype studies reveal abnormal marker chromosomes and abnormal modal chromosome numbers in approximately 70% to 80% of human solid tumors, and 20% to 40% of human leukemias;

2. Characteristic translocations are commonly observed in the non-Hodgkin's lymphomas and leukemias, and in some solid tumors as well;

3. Intrachromosomal gene rearrangements and viral oncogene insertions have been demonstrated in human tumors using molecular genetic methods; and

4. Human tumors, and particularly lymphoid cancers, exhibit monoclonal patterns of expression of enzyme markers and monoclonal immunologic determinants on the cell surface.

One might expect that these genetically abnormal populations overgrow all others because they have a proliferative advantage; indeed, recent flow cytometry studies have demonstrated a higher rate of proliferation in the aneuploid component of diploid-aneuploid human tumor cell mixtures (Braylan *et al.*, 1982; Shackney *et al.*, 1983, 1984).

The clonal overgrowth of human neoplasms has major therapeutic implications. It is clear, for example, that the goal of curative therapy must be to eradicate the last genetically abnormal neoplastic cell.

Clonal Evolution

Many human tumors are cytogenetically unstable. Such tumors often produce a sequence of progressively more malignant clonal overgrowths, which indicate their presence clinically in relation to both their natural histories and their patterns of therapeutic responses. For example, the clinical development of blastic transformation in chronic myelogenous leukemia is accompanied and often preceded by new chromosomal abnormalities. Low-grade neoplasms often evolve into high-grade neoplasms (*e.g.*, the non-Hodgkin's lymphomas, bladder carcinoma); the high-grade neoplasms often exhibit more extensive genetic abnormalities than their low-grade counterparts (Reeves, 1973; Tribukait *et al.*, 1979; Shackney *et al.*, 1983, 1984). The transition from carcinoma *in situ* to invasive and metastatic solid tumors is also marked by the appearance of new cytogenetic abnormalities (Kirkland *et al.*, 1967; Sandberg and Wake, 1981). The rapid development of clinical drug resistance following initial responsiveness may also be due to clonal evolution, with the overgrowth of drug-resistant clones under the selection pressure of continuous therapy.

Before dealing with the complexities of multiclonal populations, we might begin with simpler models.

Simple Exponential Growth

The simplest model for mammalian cell population growth is one in which a cell divides to produce two daughter cells, each of which subsequently divides, producing four cells, eight cells, and so on. Thus, cell number would increase in powers of 2. That is,

$$N = 2^{n(t)}, \tag{1}$$

where N is the total number of cells, and $n(t)$ is the number of cell divisions that have occurred by time t. For simplicity, we are assuming in Equation 1 that the time elapsed from one cell

division to the next is the same for all cells in the population. This is called the cell cycle time (T_c) or the cell generation time.

Such a population can also be said to grow exponentially:

$$N = N_o e^{kt}, \tag{2}$$

where N_o is the starting number of cells (one cell, in our case), and k is the *fraction* of the population dividing per unit time (hours, commonly). The latter is also known as the growth rate constant.

Most investigators refer to *fractional* changes and rates of change in population size for the same reason that investors prefer to assess the rate of return on investment by considering *percent* yield, or annual *percentage* rate. This is apparent not only in the use of fractional growth rates but also in the use of surviving cell *fractions* in radiation dose response curves and clonogenic assays, and in the log kill concept (first proposed by Skipper *et al.*, 1964).

Some investigators refer to changes in tumor *mass* or cell *number* per unit time rather than changes in the *fraction* of the population per unit time to assess population growth (Laird, 1969; Norton and Simon, 1977). By analogy, they assess the rate of return on investment by considering actual *dollars* per year rather than annual *percentage* rate. This distinction will be important later on, when we consider the conceptual basis for late treatment intensification.

If all cells in the population are proliferating, if they all have the same cell cycle time, and if there is no cell loss, then the cell cycle time is equivalent to the time required for the entire population to double in size. This is called the population doubling time, or T_D, and is given by

$$T_D = T_C = \frac{0.693}{k}. \tag{3}$$

Of course, many of the simple assumptions that have been used up to this point are not really valid for biological populations, and more realistic ones must now be considered.

Cell Loss

Cell loss occurs in all biological cell populations, and can take one of several forms. In normal cell populations, cells may undergo end-stage differentiation and removal or they may die without differentiating. In tumors, dead cells often lyse and their products accu-

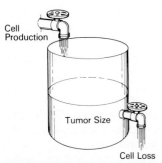

Cell Production

Tumor Size

Cell Loss

Figure 2–1. Analogous representation of the relationships among the rate of cell production (water inflow), the rate of cell loss (water outflow), and observable tumor size (water level in the tank). If water flows rapidly into the tank (high rate of cell production) and water flows out just as rapidly (high rate of cell loss), the water level in the tank will not change (stable cell population size) although the overall rate of flow of water is high (high rate of cell turnover). If a trickling inflow is balanced by a trickling outflow, again the water level will not change; in this case the turnover rate is low. If the rate of inflow exceeds the rate of outflow then the water level will rise progressively (tumor growth).

mulate in regions of cell necrosis. It is important to recognize that cell production and cell loss go on all the time, and that the observed size of a tumor represents the balance between these two processes. This is shown schematically in Figure 2–1, where tumor size is represented by the amount of water in a tank that has an inflow and an outflow tap. If the rate of inflow (cell production) exceeds the rate of outflow (cell loss), then the water level in the tank rises (*i.e.*, the tumor grows).

Thus, when one performs serial measurements of tumor size and calculates a fractional growth rate, one actually obtains an estimate of *net* fractional growth rate. That is,

$$k_{net} = k_{cell\ production} - k_{cell\ loss}. \tag{4}$$

In the presence of cell loss, the *net* fractional growth rate would be less than the fractional rate of cell production. It follows from this that the observed population doubling time would be longer than the cell cycle time. This can be readily appreciated from an investment analogy. If the annual percentage rate of return on investment (the fractional rate of money production) is 10%, one can expect that principal will double in seven years. This is easily verified using Equation 3. However, if half of the interest is withheld for tax purposes (for an overall rate of money loss of 5%), the *net* annual percentage rate of return is only 5%, and the actual doubling time of principal will lengthen to 14 years.

If the rate of cell production and the rate of cell loss were truly constant and the former were greater than the latter, then normal and tumor cell populations would still satisfy the equation for simple exponential growth. In reality, the rate of cell production decreases and the rate of cell loss usually increases as population size increases and net growth rate decreases.

Normal cell populations at steady-state equilibrium can be thought of as being in plateau phase growth, where the rate of new cell production is just balanced by the rate of differentiation and/or cell loss, and the net growth rate is zero. If the rate of cell production is high, as in the gut and bone marrow, the rate of cell differentiation and/or cell loss is also high; when the rate of cell production is low, the balancing rate of cell differentiation and/or cell loss is also low. For cell populations at their equilibrium size in plateau phase, the rate of cell production is called the cell turnover rate. Normal host tissues with high cell turnover rates are highly susceptible to the effects of cytotoxic drugs, and the acute toxic effects of drugs in these tissues often limit the dosage and frequency of administration of these agents.

Tumors also undergo growth retardation as they enlarge, and in this respect they *do* obey "laws" of growth. Whether they achieve a true plateau phase is a moot point. Certainly, the body burden of indolent human tumors may not appear to change appreciably over the course of several years. Yet, it has recently been shown in the Sézary syndrome that the magnitude of the daily turnover rate of malignant *T* cells is comparable to that of the normal bone marrow (Shackney and Schuette, 1983). More generally, human tumors in clinically advanced stages of disease have cell loss rates that approach their respective rates of cell production (Malaise *et al.*, 1973). Thus, in tumors with high rates of cell production, the rates of cell loss are also high; in slowly proliferating tumors, the rates of cell loss are also low.

One often finds that the rate of cell loss in experimental tumors is expressed as a fraction of the rate of cell production (Steel, 1968); this is known as the cell loss *factor*. The cell loss factor may not be useful, especially in reference to advanced human tumors at or near plateau phase, where the cell loss factor can be expected to approach 1 as a matter of course. Under these circumstances, the cell turnover rate may provide more useful information.

The Graphic Representation of Tumor Growth; Simple Exponential Growth and the Gompertzian Function

Figure 2–2A shows a plot of the number of tumor cells, N, as a function of time in a population that obeys the simple exponential growth equation (Equation 2). The curve bows upward, with an ever-increasing slope. In this case, the slope represents the change in cell *number* per unit time.

If one takes the natural logarithm of both sides of Equation 2, one obtains

$$\log_e N = kt + \log_e N_o, \qquad (5)$$

which, as every high school algebra student knows, is the slope-intercept form of the equation for a straight line. Figure 2–2B shows a plot of $\log_e N$ as a function of time. This is a straight line whose slope is k, the *fractional* growth rate constant. This is what makes semilog plots of tumor growth curves so useful. A semilog plot of the simple exponential growth curve can serve as a useful reference, even when tumor growth behavior is more complex.

It was noted in the previous section that real tumor cell populations exhibit a reduction in net fractional growth rate with increasing population size. The Gompertz function is a mathematical equation for tumor growth that exhibits this property. It is given as:

$$N = N_o e^{\frac{\beta}{a}(1 - e^{-\alpha t})} \qquad (6)$$

The mathematical details of this equation need not be of concern here. It is sufficient to note that the simple growth rate constant of Equation 2 has been replaced by a more complicated expression, resulting in growth curves of the form shown in Figure 2–3A; the simple exponential curve (dashed line) is also shown for comparison. Initially, the behavior of the Gompertz growth curve bows upward, much as the simple exponential curve does. However, at longer times, the increase in the number of cells per unit time becomes smaller and smaller, and the Gompertz curve levels off, approaching a plateau asymptotically.

A semilog plot of the Gompertz function is shown in Figure 2–3B; a semilog plot of a simple exponential growth curve is also shown for comparison (dashed line). It is readily apparent that the Gompertz curve exhibits a steady and progressive decrease in the *fractional* growth rate, as the curve bows toward its plateau. Indeed, the distinctive feature of the Gompertz function is that the fractional growth rate decreases exponentially with time; thus, a semilog plot of the fractional growth rate over time describes a straight line with a negative slope (see Figure 2–3C). By comparison, a semilog plot of the fractional growth rate over time for simple exponential growth (dashed line in Figure 2–3C) describes a horizontal straight line.

The Gompertz function is not the only equation that can be used to describe growth retardation. Indeed, the simple exponential decrease in fractional growth rate with time that characterizes the Gompertz equation (see Figure 2–3C) may be an unrealistic constraint for human tumors.

Human Tumor Growth Curves

Idealized human tumor growth curves are shown in Figure 2–4 (see curve C). A representation of the tumor growth curve of mouse L 1210 leukemia also is shown for comparison (curve A).

The minimum detectable body burden of tumor in man is commonly taken to be 1×10^9 cells (1 gm). The range, however, is relatively broad. Small cutaneous nodules in solid tumors may contain as few as 2 to 3×10^8 cells at the time of detection. The minimum detectable body tumor burden in acute leukemia is in the range of 5 to 7.5×10^{10} cells (assuming a bone marrow cell mass of 1 to 1.5 kg and the requirement that the percentage of blast cells in the marrow must exceed 5% for diagnosis); tumors in the mediastinum or retroperitoneum might achieve a weight of several hundred grams before becoming detectable.

The lethal body burden of tumor in man is

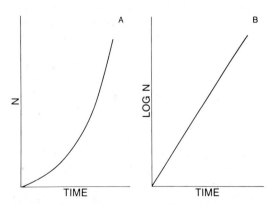

Figure 2–2. *(A)* A linear plot of simple exponential growth where N (cell number) is on the ordinate and time is on the abscissa. *(B)* A semilog plot of simple exponential growth, where $\log_e$ N is on the ordinate and time is on the abscissa.

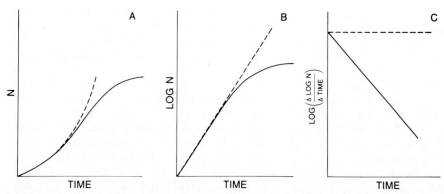

Figure 2–3. *(A)* A linear plot of the Gompertz function (solid line). A linear plot of simple exponential growth (dashed line) is shown for comparison. *(B)* A semilog plot of the Gompertz function (solid line). A semilog plot of simple exponential growth (dashed line) is shown for comparison. *(C)* A semilog plot of the slope of the Gompertz function (solid line) over time. A semilog plot of the slope of the simple exponential function (dashed line) over time is shown for comparison.

taken to be approximately 1×10^{12} cells (1 kg of tumor). Again, considerable variability exists, depending on the type and location of a given tumor and its metastases.

Human tumor doubling times within the clinically observable range of tumor growth can be calculated directly from measurements of tumor size over a period of time. Representative clinical doubling times for a variety of solid tumors are given in Table 2–1. Subclinical tumor doubling times can be calculated when the time of onset of the tumor can be estimated, as in gestational choriocarcinoma (Shackney *et al.*, 1978). The time from earliest possible onset to diagnosis is assumed to span at least 30 tumor doublings (producing approximately 1×10^{9} cells). Thus, in choriocarcinoma, with an average span of 11 months (330 days) from onset of gestation to diagnosis, the average subclinical tumor doubling time

can be calculated as 11 days per tumor doubling (330 days/30 tumor doublings). In breast cancer, the time elapsed from mastectomy to the appearance of a tumor nodule in the surgical scar (750 days on the average) can also be used to estimate the subclinical tumor doubling time (750 days/30 doublings, or 25 days). In making this calculation, one assumes that a single tumor cell was deposited in the incision at the time of surgery. If, for example, as many as a million (1×10^{6}) cells were left behind, the subclinical doubling time would be 75 days (the reader can verify this using the fact that every thousandfold increase in cell number represents 10 cell divisions). By comparison, the average doubling time in advanced breast cancer is 130 days (see Table 2–1). This confirms the principle that all growing cell populations, including human tumors, undergo growth retardation in late stages of growth.

Given that all tumors undergo growth retardation sooner or later, how can one distinguish between slowly growing human tumors and

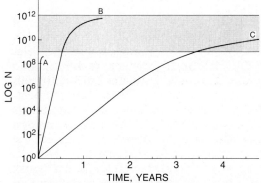

Figure 2–4. Schematic representation of the growth curve of a rapidly growing human tumor (B), and a slowly growing human tumor (C). The growth curve of mouse L 1210 leukemia (A) is shown for comparison.

Table 2–1.   Mean Clinical Doubling Times of Human Tumors

TUMOR TYPE	DOUBLING TIME
Burkitt's lymphoma	2–5 days
Testicular cancer	21 days
Ewing's sarcoma	22 days
Non-Hodgkin's lymphoma (predominantly large cell)	25 days
Osteogenic sarcoma	34 days
Hodgkin's disease	38 days
Small cell carcinoma, lung	81 days
Squamous cell carcinoma, lung	87 days
Adenocarcinoma, colon	96 days
Adenocarcinoma, breast	129 days
Adenocarcinoma, lung	134 days

rapidly growing ones? In operational terms, slowly growing tumors undergo much of their growth retardation when they are still below the level of clinical detection. Thus, when one measures clinical tumor doubling times, they are usually relatively long (> 70 days). Rapidly growing tumors are defined operationally by the fact that their short subclinical doubling times are maintained well into the clinically detectable range of tumor sizes (see curve B, Figure 2–4). Burkitt's lymphoma, for example, has a subclinical doubling time that is less than six days, and an early clinical doubling time that is also in the range of two to five days (Shackney *et al.,* 1978).

It is important to recognize that when one assigns 30 tumor doublings to a population of 1×10^9 cells, one assumes a minimum of 30 cell doublings. Because of cell loss, there must be many more cell divisions than actual population doublings. Thus, although clinical tumor doubling time measurements are relatively easy to perform, and although in practice they do tend to reflect the rates of tumor cell production in a general way, they provide only very crude estimates of rates of tumor cell production. More direct techniques for assessing rates of tumor cell prodution are described in the next section.

The Cell Cycle

The cell cycle can be subdivided into phases in relation to DNA synthesis. DNA synthesis occurs predominantly during S phase (see Figure 2–5). This phase was originally defined by radiotracer methods and autoradiography (Howard and Pelc, 1953). The G_1 phase of the cell cycle precedes S, and the G_2 phase follows S (see Figure 2–5); these two phases of the cell cycle were originally defined, using radiotracer labeling techniques (Howard and Pelc, 1953), by the absence of demonstrable DNA synthesis early and late in the cell cycle. M, or the mitotic phase of the cell cycle (see Figure 2–5), is defined morphologically. The durations of the G_1, S, G_2, and M phases of the cell cycle are commonly denoted by T_{G_1}, T_S, T_{G_2}, and T_M, respectively.

The fraction of cells in S phase can be obtained by one of two methods: Tritiated thymidine ([³H]dTh) labeling or autoradiography. Cells that are actively synthesizing DNA and are exposed briefly to tritiated thymidine will incorporate this radiotracer exclusively into DNA. Representative samples of cells from the population under study are fixed, placed on glass slides, coated with a photosensitive emulsion, and stored in the dark for periods ranging from several days to several months. Tritiated thymidine emits weak β particles that travel only 1 to 2 μm. These β particles activate the emulsion overlying the cell nucleus from which they originated. Thus, when the slide is developed and fixed like a photographic negative, cells in S phase are identified by the presence of silver grains overlying their nuclei (see Figure 2–6). The fraction of labeled cells is known as the pulse labeling index (LI). That is,

$$LI = \frac{\text{number of labeled cells}}{\text{total number of cells}}. \qquad (7)$$

Flow Cytometry. The fraction of cells in S can also be determined from measurements of cell DNA content. Cell DNA content can be determined rapidly and accurately for large numbers of cells by means of flow cytometry (see Figure 2–7). To use this technique, one must disperse cells into a single cell suspension, stain them with a fluorescent dye that binds stoichiometrically to DNA, and pass

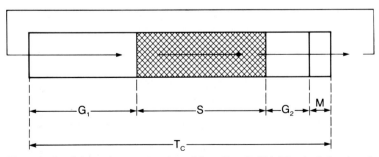

Figure 2–5. Schematic representation of the cell cycle (T_c). The shaded region, S, represents the period of active DNA synthesis. G_1 and G_2 represent postmitotic and premitotic phases of the cell cycle, respectively, during which there is no detectable DNA synthesis. M represents mitosis.

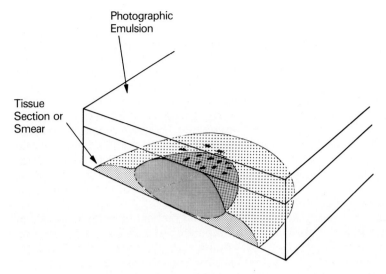

Figure 2-6. Diagrammatic representation of an autoradiograph.

them one cell at a time through a strong monochromatic light source (commonly a laser beam). The amount of fluorescence emitted by each cell is proportional to its DNA content.

A typical DNA content frequency distribution, or DNA histogram, is shown in Figure 2-8A. G_1 cells have a 2N DNA content, and G_2 cells have a 4N DNA content. Cells with intermediate DNA contents are those that were in the process of DNA synthesis at the time the sample was obtained. The fraction of cells in S phase can be estimated from the DNA histogram (middle zone, Figure 2-8A). This value is comparable with, but not necessarily identical to, the tritiated thymidine labeling index. Cells that would show up in the S region of the DNA histogram may have been synthesizing DNA at rates that would be too

low to allow the cells to incorporate a sufficient amount of tritiated thymidine to be detected by autoradiography. Some cells might stop synthesizing DNA altogether while they are still in S; such cells would not incorporate tritiated thymidine but would also come to rest in the S region of the DNA histogram. In general, then, the S fraction by flow cytometry is likely to be equal to or greater than the tritiated thymidine pulse labeling index, but not less.

Generally speaking, the fraction of cells in S (or the tritiated thymidine labeling index) reflects the relative rate of cell production in a population. The higher the S fraction, the higher the rate of cell production. That is, under ideal conditions, the S fraction would be approximately equal to T_S/T_C, and this ratio would be high when T_C is short. From the S fraction alone, however, one cannot obtain a quantitative estimate of the actual duration of

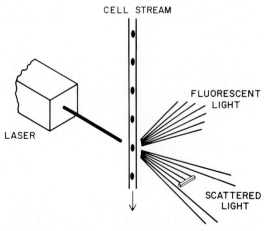

Figure 2-7. Diagrammatic representation of a flow cytometer.

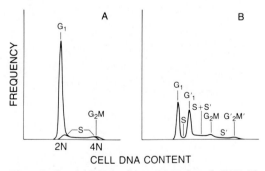

Figure 2-8. *(A)* Schematic representation of a DNA histogram obtained by flow cytometry. Cell DNA content ranges from 2N to 4N. *(B)* A DNA histogram with two overlapping populations, one diploid and the other hyperdiploid.

the cell cycle, T_C, or the durations of the phases of the cell cycle. Under ideal conditions, this can be determined from the percent labeled mitosis (PLM) curve.

DNA measurements by flow cytometry are also useful in detecting and characterizing cytogenetically abnormal tumor cell populations. Clinical samples with tumor cell populations that have abnormal chromosome numbers often produce composite DNA histograms, with a shifted histogram of the aneuploid line overlapping the diploid histogram (see Figure 2–8B).

The PLM Curve. When a population is pulse labeled with tritiated thymidine, only the cells in S are labeled. Under ideal circumstances, as this cohort of labeled cells progresses through mitosis and on to the next cell cycle, a wave of labeled mitoses appears and then subsides (see Figure 2–9A). When the still-labeled daughter cells go through mitosis in turn, a second wave of labeled mitoses is inscribed (Quastler and Sherman, 1959). The durations of S, G_2, and T_C can be estimated from such a curve (Wimber, 1963) (see Figure 2–9A). The duration of G_1 can be obtained from the relation,

$$T_{G_1} + T_S + T_{G_2} + T_M = T_C. \qquad (8)$$

This analysis is highly idealized in that it assumes that the cell cycle and its phases are of uniform duration. In reality, human tumors have a broad range of cell cycle times, and real PLM curves deviate significantly from the ideal curves (see Figure 2–9B). Comprehensive analyses of human adult leukemia and melanoma have indicated that in a given patient the T_Cs of the neoplastic cells can range

from 12 hours to many hundreds of hours (Shackney, 1977). Phase durations are also highly variable, and in slowly proliferating cells with low rates of DNA synthesis the phase durations are difficult to determine. Because slowly proliferating cells contribute relatively few cells to the mitotic cell pool, the PLM curve features are generally determined by the most rapidly proliferating component of a kinetically heterogeneous population. Published estimates of average cell cycle times of the rapidly proliferating components of human tumors are in the range of two to three days (Tannock, 1978).

The Growth Fraction. The rapidly proliferating component of human tumors is commonly known as the growth fraction (GF) (Mendelsohn, 1962). One can assign a numerical value to the growth fraction from the relation,

$$GF = \frac{\text{observed fraction of cells in } S}{\text{expected fraction of cells in } S}, \qquad (9)$$

where the expected fraction of cells in S is determined from PLM-curve-based estimates of T_S and T_C. Given the difficulties in estimating T_S and T_C in the slowly proliferating component of human tumors using the PLM curve method, however, the GF should not be thought of as a discrete population compartment with intrinsically well-defined properties; rather, it represents a region of the cell cycle time distribution whose boundary is arbitrarily determined by the method of calculation (see Figure 2–10). Thus, the retardation of tumor growth in advanced disease can be understood either in terms of a decrease in the growth fraction or in terms of a shift in the cell cycle time distribution to longer values. Cell loss, of course, is superimposed on this phenomenon.

The G_0 State. Cells that are excluded from the growth fraction have been assigned to what has come to be known as the G_0 state (Quastler, 1963). Of course, truly nondividing cells would be very difficult to distinguish from very slowly proliferating cells with very long cell cycle times by any experimental method, since both types might exhibit comparable morphologic or biochemical differences from rapidly dividing cells. Thus, the G_0 state might best be taken to represent the slowly proliferating region of the cell cycle time distribution (see Figure 2–10A), rather than a well-defined nonproliferative state. Thus, the transition of cells into G_0 (growth retardation) or out of G_0 into

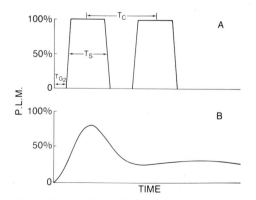

Figure 2–9. *(A)* An idealized percent-labeled mitosis (PLM) curve. *(B)* Schematic representation of a PLM curve that is typical of human tumors.

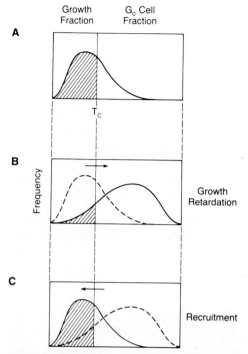

Figure 2-10. *(A)* The relationship among the growth fraction, the nonproliferating pool, and the cell cycle time distribution. *(B)* The conceptual equivalence of entry into G_0 and a shift of the cell cycle time distribution to longer values. *(C)* The conceptual equivalence of recruitment from G_0 into rapid cycle and a shift of the cell cycle time distribution to shorter values.

the proliferating cell pool (recruitment) can be understood in terms of shifts in the cell cycle time distribution (see Figures 2-10B and 2-10C).

Cell Clonogenicity

The malignant nature of neoplastic cell populations depends on the capacity of their cells to proliferate indefinitely. The capacity to undergo cyclical growth and perpetual cell division defines the tumor stem cell. Assays for human tumor stem cells have been developed and are commonly known as clonogenic assays, since they rely on the ability of individual stem cells to produce separate cloned proliferations in soft agar (Hamburger and Salmon, 1977a,b). The yields of human tumor stem cells (colonies observed per total cells plated) are commonly very low, usually in the range of 0.1%–1%. Since assay efficiency (colonies observed per *stem* cells plated) is unknown, it is difficult to know the true stem cell content of human tumors. For therapeutic

purposes, one should assume that all cells are potential stem cells until proven otherwise; thus, the kinetic behavior of the tumor cell population as a whole should serve as the basis for treatment planning. This is supported by experimental studies in normal tissues that have suggested that the kinetic heterogeneity of the measurable clonogenic cell fraction in the bone marrow parallels the kinetic heterogeneity of the entire marrow cell population (Shackney, 1978).

Composite Growth Curves; Clonal Evolution

Up to this point, various aspects of kinetic heterogeneity in populations that are genetically homogeneous have been considered. As noted earlier, however, human tumor cells are cytogenetically unstable. In a given tumor, genetic variants are produced over the course of time, one of which may turn out to have a proliferative advantage over the parent line; this new, aggressive variant eventually becomes the dominant cell population. This process can repeat itself, resulting in a succession of clonal overgrowths.

At first, it might seem natural to think of proliferative advantage only in terms of increased relative rates of tumor cell production. It should be kept in mind, however, that all cell populations undergo growth retardation sooner or later. Thus, it is the *net* growth rates (the rate of cell production minus the rate of cell loss) for each cell population that must be considered in relation to total population size, along with the degree of competition among subpopulations that must be taken into account.

Several simple examples might be considered. In the first case, two subpopulations with identical Gompertzian growth rate characteristics compete directly with one another for the same host resources. If both subpopulations are established at the same time, each subpopulation will approach a plateau population size that is half that that would be achieved by either one alone. If one population is established before the other, it will achieve a higher plateau level (see Figure 2-11, upper panel). If one population is established long before the other, the first population will effectively suppress the growth of the second population (see Figure 2-11, middle panel), even though the intrinsic growth properties of both populations are identical.

If the first subpopulation has an intrinsically

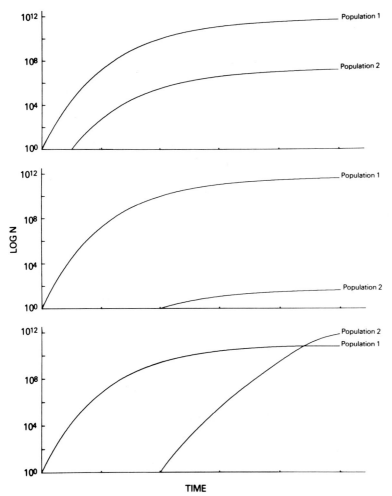

Figure 2–11. Composite growth curves. *(Upper panel)* Two subpopulations with identical Gompertzian growth characteristics competing for the same host resources. Population 2 originates during log phase growth of population 1. *(Middle panel)* Same as in upper panel, but population 2 originates at a time when population 1 is approaching plateau phase growth. *(Lower panel)* Population 2 originates during plateau phase of population 1, but population 2 has a higher plateau level.

lower plateau level than the second subpopulation, then the second subpopulation will overgrow the first, regardless of when the second subpopulation was established (see Figure 2–11, lower panel). If the first subpopulation is near its plateau level when the second population overtakes it, one would expect that the second population might exhibit a higher rate of cell production than the first. Indeed, in mixed diploid-aneuploid clinical tumor samples, the aneuploid component usually does have a higher S fraction than the diploid component (Braylan *et al.,* 1982; Shackney *et al.,* 1983, 1984). This finding suggests that the aneuploid subpopulations have higher plateau levels than the diploid ones.

With regard to possible mechanisms for cy-

togenetic instability in human tumors, it is a common observation that the *degree* of aneuploidy in human tumors (either the quantity of abnormal cell DNA revealed by flow cytometry or the abnormal modal chromosome number per cell shown in karyotype studies) often ranges between diploid and tetraploid. Many tumors are slightly hyperdiploid, while others are tetraploid or near tetraploid (Barlogie *et al.,* 1978; Atkin and Kay, 1979; Tribukait *et al.,* 1979; Vindelov *et al.,* 1980). This would suggest that the abrupt step-up to tetraploidization is a relatively common event in human tumors, presumably by cell endoreduplication or cell fusion. Evidence also suggests that tetraploid human tumors may be cytogenetically unstable, and that they lose chromosomes during the course of tumor progression (Kirk-land *et al.,* 1967). This series of events is now well documented in experimental tumor systems (Isaacs *et al.,* 1982). The cytogenetic instability of tetraploid cells might well fuel clonal evolution in human neoplasms, and could account for the rapid clinical development of tumor resistance to multiple drugs under the selection pressure of continuing drug treatment. Other possible mechanisms include gene amplification (Schimke, 1984) and point mutation. The latter are considered below.

THE EFFECTS OF CYTOTOXIC DRUGS

The Concept of Log Kill

The log kill concept was developed (Skipper *et al.,* 1964) to account for the observations in mouse L1210 leukemia that multiple courses of treatment with cytotoxic drugs could be curative although individual courses of treatment were not.

The log kill concept expresses the notion that, quite apart from any other forms of drug resistance that might be present, cells can survive a course of treatment purely by chance, even though they are essentially no different in their susceptibility from the cells that are killed. The same surviving cells might be killed by a dose of the same drug in a subsequent course of treatment. A simplified example taken from the field of radiation biology is described below.

Let us assume that a given dose of radiation produces a given average number of randomly distributed "active events" per unit area within the radiation field and that the number of "active events" greatly exceeds the initial number of cells in the field. Let us assume further in this example that any cell within the field has a 50% chance of being "hit" by an "active event" and killed. When there are 20 cells within the field, ten cells are killed by a given radiation dose (see Figure 2–12A). The ten cells that survive are intrinsically no different in their susceptibility to radiation from the cells that were killed. A second dose of radiation will be just as effective as the first and is likely to kill another 50 percent of the population (see Figure 2–12B).

It is clear from this example that a treatment regimen that reduces a population of 20 cells by 75% overall is hardly curative, because even

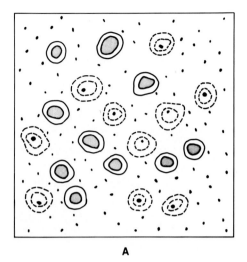

A

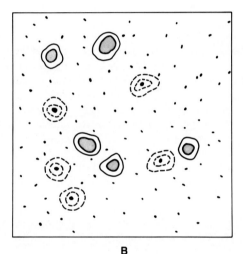

B

Figure 2–12. Schematic illustration of log kill. Small dots represent "active" radiation "events" randomly distributed throughout the radiation field. Cells shown with broken lines represent lethally damaged cells. Each treatment is assumed to kill half of the viable cells that are present at the time of exposure. If 20 viable cells are present initially, 10 viable cells will be killed by the first treatment *(A)*. A second treatment will also kill half of the remaining cells *(B)*, but the absolute number of cells killed (five) by the second treatment is smaller than the number killed by the first treatment.

one surviving viable cell can regenerate the entire population. If the cell fraction killed per treatment were higher, say 90% (or 0.9), then approximately two cells, on the average, would survive the first dose, and the probability of at least one viable cell surviving a second dose would be low. When the cell population is large (*e.g.,* 1×10^9 cells), a much greater fractional cell kill, or many more courses of ther-

Table 2–2. The Relationship of Fractional Cell Kill to Log Kill

CELL FRACTION KILLED	SURVIVING CELL FRACTION	LOG SURVIVING CELL FRACTION	LOG KILL
.9	.1	−1	1
.99	.01	−2	2
.999	.001	−3	3
.999999999	.000000001	−9	9

apy, would be needed to achieve cure. Large overall fractional cell kills (*e.g.,* 0.99999) can be cumbersome to deal with in decimal notation. Hence, the log kill notation where

$$\text{log kill} = -\log (\text{surviving cell fraction}). \qquad (10)$$

Sample calculations are shown in Table 2–2. Thus, for example, to eradicate a tumor containing 1×10^9 cells, one must achieve a log kill that exceeds 9.

The example shown in Figure 2–12 implies that a given dose of drug will kill a constant fraction of the population *regardless* of population size. Originally, the developers of the log kill concept did, in fact, make this assumption in interpreting their drug response data for cytosine arabinoside treatment. For simplicity, they also assumed the ideal case of simple exponential growth for L 1210 leukemia, as shown schematically in Figure 2–13A. Detailed computer modeling studies of the L 1210 leukemia data, however, have demonstrated the importance of growth retardation even in this rapidly proliferating cell system,

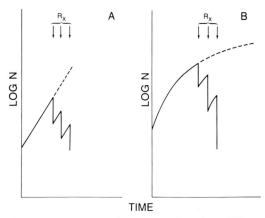

TIME

Figure 2–13. Schematic representation of log kill in relation to tumor growth. *(A)* Simple exponential growth and constant log kill are assumed. *(B)* Gompertzian growth and a log kill that varies with tumor growth rate are assumed.

and have indicated that log kill varies with population growth rate (see Figure 2–13B) (Shackney, 1970). In late stages of growth a progressive decrease in log kill takes place that accompanies a progressive decrease in fractional growth rate. These modeling studies suggest that inability to cure large inocula of L 1210 cells ($> 1 \times 10^6$ cells) with cytosine arabinoside is due at least in part to the decreased responsiveness of slowly proliferating cells to the lethal effects of the drug.

The Proliferation Rate Dependence of Drug Cytotoxicity

Extensive studies in experimental tumor cell systems have shown that most cytotoxic drugs in common clinical use are more effective against rapidly proliferating cells than against slowly proliferating cells. This statement is valid, however, only when one compares the effects of the same drug given at the same dose and on the same schedule in rapidly and slowly proliferating cells. Representative one-hour dose-survival curves showing the effects of cytosine arabinoside and doxorubicin on sarcoma 180 cells in log phase and plateau phase are shown in Figure 2–14. The lethal effects of cytosine arabinoside (see Figures 2–14A and 2–14B) are dose-dependent and drug-exposure-duration-dependent, but above a concentration of 1 μmol, drug-exposure-duration-dependence is the predominant factor. For any given drug concentration and drug exposure duration, log phase cells are always more sensitive to the lethal effects of the drug than plateau phase cells. The lethal effect of doxorubicin is also dependent on drug concentration and drug exposure duration. No plateau in dose response is evident over the range of doses studied. Again, for any given drug concentration and drug exposure duration, log phase cells are more sensitive than plateau phase cells.

It should be apparent from these data that drug resistance is not simply an all-or-none phenomenon; rather, it is defined by the criteria that are used for drug response in relation to dose, schedule, and the proliferative state of the cells. Thus, for example, if one were to choose a surviving fraction of 0.1 (a one-log cell kill) to distinguish drug sensitivity from resistance, then cytosine arabinoside would be considered effective against sarcoma 180 cells only in log phase, and then only after prolonged drug exposure. Doxorubicin might not

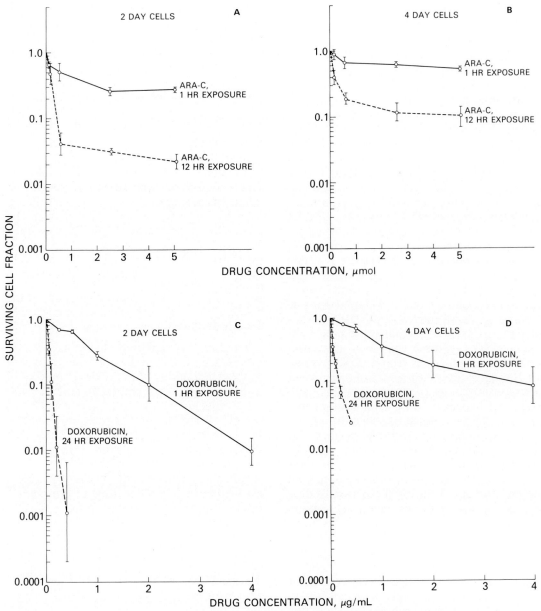

Figure 2–14. (A) Surviving cell fractions in log phase (two-day) sarcoma 180 cells after exposure to cytosine arabinoside. (B) Surviving cell fractions in plateau phase (four-day) cells after exposure to cytosine arabinoside. (C) Cell survival in log phase cells after exposure to doxorubicin. (D) Cell survival in plateau phase cells after exposure to doxorubicin.

be considered effective after brief exposure to plateau phase cells except at drug concentrations that are much higher than those that can be achieved in plasma with current clinical drug regimens. On the other hand, the drug *would* be considered effective against plateau phase cells after prolonged exposure to low drug concentrations.

The clinical implications of such studies are clear. A slowly proliferating tumor that appears to be resistant to a drug at a given dose or on a given drug schedule might be responsive at a higher dose or on a different schedule. Thus, for example, high-dose *cis*-platinum has been shown to produce a longer median duration of response in non-small-cell carcinoma of the lung than conventional doses (Gralla *et al.*, 1981).

Phase Specificity of Drug Lethality

Given the long-standing interest of cell kineticists in such processes as mitosis and DNA synthesis, it was only natural, in early studies, to ascribe the greater drug sensitivity of rapidly proliferating cells to cell cycle phase-specific effects (Bruce et al., 1966, 1969). It is now known, however, that the effects of tubulin binding agents like the vinca alkaloids are not restricted to mitosis (Madoc-Jones and Mauro, 1968; Camplejohn et al., 1980; Lengsfeld et al., 1981; Mujagic et al., 1983a,b), and an exclusive causal relation between drug-induced inhibition of DNA synthesis and drug lethality has not been clearly established for most chemotherapeutic agents in current clinical use. Two drugs for which there is strong evidence for DNA synthesis-rate-dependent lethality are hydroxyurea (Mauro and Madoc-Jones, 1970; Bhuyan et al., 1973) and cytosine arabinoside (Bhuyan et al., 1972, 1973). Antimetabolites such as methotrexate and 5-FU inhibit DNA synthesis, but they also affect other cellular processes such as RNA synthesis. It is not entirely clear which of these effects is responsible for drug lethality, or whether different mechanisms of drug lethality come into play in relation to dose and schedule.

In general, claims of S-phase specificity for drug lethality should be evaluated critically. Such claims are often made on the basis of the decreased cell survival in synchronized cells passing through S during the period of drug exposure. Many other biochemical processes are going on concurrently with DNA synthesis, any one of which could be responsible for drug lethality in S. Furthermore, all cells that are killed by cytotoxic drugs will stop synthesizing DNA sooner or later, regardless of the mechanism of drug lethality; thus, it is important to establish whether drug-induced inhibition of DNA synthesis is a cause of cell death or is one of its effects.

Flow cytometry studies have demonstrated that antitumor antibiotics such as doxorubicin and daunomycin (Linden et al., 1974; Barlogie et al., 1976b; Krishan and Frei, 1976; Tobey et al., 1976; Ritch et al., 1982) and bleomycin (Barlogie et al., 1976a), as well as alkylating agents (Barlogie and Drewinko, 1977), the nitrosoureas (Ritch et al., 1982), and other anticancer drugs cause cells to accumulate in the premitotic region of the DNA histogram. Whatever the intracellular lethal mechanisms

are for these drugs, they do not prevent cells from synthesizing their full complement of DNA; thus, it seems unlikely that the lethality of these drugs is dependent on the inhibition of active DNA synthesis. Nonetheless, when cells accumulate in G_2, the flow of daughter cells through subsequent cell cycles is interrupted, resulting in a delayed secondary "inhibition" of DNA synthesis (Ritch et al., 1982; Mujagic et al., 1983a,b).

In addition, early expectations of cell kineticists that human tumor cells could be synchronized in S phase have not been borne out, because of the high degree of kinetic heterogeneity in human tumors. Thus, given the relatively low fractions of cells in S in most human tumors (see Table 2–3), clinical treatment strategies that are based on S-phase specificity of drug lethality would not appear to hold great promise.

Cell Recruitment

The fact that rapidly proliferating cells are more susceptible than slowly proliferating cells to the lethal effects of many drugs may be of some importance in clinical treatment planning, quite apart from DNA synthesis. When tumor cell population size is reduced rapidly, slowly proliferating cells are often mobilized into rapid cell cycle. This shift in the cell cycle time distribution from longer to shorter values is called cell recruitment. Thus, if an initial cytoreductive treatment leads to a mobilization of slowly proliferating cells, a second treatment might be most effective if it is timed to coincide with the period of maximum cell recruitment after the priming dose. In human cell populations, the period of maximum recruitment occurs approximately 8 to 18 days after a priming dose of drugs (Burke et al.,

Table 2–3. The Pulse Labeling Index (LI) in Human Tumors

TUMOR TYPE	LI
Burkitt's lymphoma	0.29
Lymphoma, pooled data	0.09
Small cell carcinoma of the lung	0.11–0.24
Squamous cell carcinoma, head and neck	0.05–0.11
Squamous cell carcinoma, lung	0.08
Sarcomas, pooled data	0.05
Adenocarcinoma of lung	0.05
Adenocarcinoma of colon	0.03
Adenocarcinoma of breast	0.02
Multiple myeloma	0.02

1973, 1977; Shackney *et al.,* 1980). The improvement in recent treatment results of the non-Hodgkin's lymphomas with such regimens as M-BACOD (Skarin *et al.,* 1983), and ProMACE-MOPP (Fisher *et al.,* 1983) may be due at least in part to the nonmyelosuppressive drug treatment on day 14, a feature common to both of these regimens.

Kinetic Drug Resistance; Late Treatment Intensification

The decreased susceptibility of slowly proliferating cells to chemotherapy can be considered to be a form of kinetic drug resistance. One pair of researchers has used the concept of kinetic drug resistance as a justification for late cancer treatment intensification (Norton and Simon, 1977). It was assumed that growth was Gompertzian and that susceptibility to drugs (a decrease in cell *number* per treatment) varied directly with tumor growth rate (number of cells per unit time, *not* fractional growth rate). They concluded that smaller tumors actually were more *resistant* to therapy and, therefore, that patients who achieve good clinical therapeutic responses should then receive more intensive treatment to eradicate the more resistant residual tumor.

In order to better appreciate this rationale, consider the following analogy. An interest-free loan of $1000 is repaid in annual installments, as shown in Table 2–4. Is the loan being repaid more efficiently in later years, or less efficiently? One could say that the loan is being repaid more efficiently, since each successive payment represents a larger *fraction* of the outstanding balance. On the other hand, one could also take the aforementioned researchers' position and claim that the loan is being repaid *less* efficiently, because the *dollar amount* of each payment decreases progressively.

Ultimately, the validity of judgments of this type can be determined only by carefully controlled prospective clinical studies that are designed to assess the clinical value of late treatment intensification. Now, kinetic drug resistance *per se* might be overcome by treatment intensification regardless of when it is given. Thus, in order to validate the kinetic drug resistance concept specifically, one would have to show prospectively that *late* treatment intensification is more effective than *early* intensification or intensification throughout the course of treatment.

Genetic Drug Resistance

A great deal of evidence in experimental systems suggests that mammalian cell populations can undergo genetic changes that result in resistance to one or more cytotoxic drugs (Bech-Hansen *et al.,* 1976; Flintoff *et al.,* 1976; Alt *et al.,* 1978; Lewis and Wright, 1978; Ling and Baker, 1978; Cabral *et al.,* 1980; Elliot and Ling, 1981; Tyler-Smith and Anderson, 1981). Recent modeling studies (Goldie and Coldman, 1979; Goldie *et al.,* 1982) have emphasized the importance of genetic drug resistance in the design of cancer treatment regimens in man. These authors based their model on a number of simple assumptions that include the following:

1. All cells in the population are proliferating;
2. Genetic drug resistance is an all-or-none phenomenon;
3. For each cell there is some probability per cell generation that a mutation at some genetic locus will produce resistance to a given drug. This mutation rate, α, might range between 1×10^{-3} and 1×10^{-6}, and is estimated to be close to 1×10^{-6}, based on a study in L 1210 mouse leukemia (Skipper *et al.,* 1974); and
4. Although one group of researchers (Gol-

Table 2–4.   Two Measures of Rate of Change Compared
Initial loan (interest-free): $1000

END OF YEAR	PRINCIPAL	PAYOFF RATE, DOLLARS/YEAR	PAYOFF RATE, PERCENT/YEAR
1	$500	$500	50%
2	$200	$300	60%
3	$50	$150	75%
4	$5	$45	90%
5	$0.10	$4.90	98%
6	0	$0.10	100%

die *et al.,* 1982) claimed that their model is independent of the form of the growth curve, they have relied primarily on the simple exponential growth model.

This research team (Goldie and Coldman, 1979) drew a number of simple but powerful conclusions from their model. First, the likelihood that a tumor cell population will contain at least one cell that is genetically drug resistant increases with the total number of cell divisions in the population. In the absence of cell loss, this is virtually the same as the number of cells in the population. For example, if α is 1×10^{-6}, then as the size of the population approaches and exceeds 1×10^6 cells, the probability of encountering at least one cell that is resistant to drug approaches 1.

These researchers showed that the transition from low probability of encountering a resistant cell ($P < .05$) to a high probability of encountering a resistant cell ($P > .95$) occurs over a relatively small range of tumor growth (1.77 logs). This, the authors claim, calls for the earliest possible institution of cytoreduction therapy (Goldie and Coldman, 1979). Although the principle of early treatment is clearly a sound one when effective therapy is available, it should be kept in mind that 1.77 logs represent almost six tumor doublings, and that human tumor doubling times in the clinically observable range vary from 2 to 4 months among the commonly encountered tumors (see Table 2–1).

These researchers (Goldie *et al.,* 1982) have also considered resistance to more than one drug. If α is on the order of 1×10^{-6}, then clinically detectable human tumors will almost certainly contain cells that are resistant to single drugs, and may contain cells that are resistant to two agents. Based on their modeling studies, the authors recommend the use of alternating cycles of non-cross-resistant regimens to minimize the development of resistance to multiple agents (Goldie *et al.,* 1982).

Clinical applications of this model are limited by the fact that α, the mutation rate per cell generation, is difficult to define and measure in practice. Because of extensive cell loss, there are many more cell generations than there are tumor doublings (see the section on Cell Loss above); this would undermine any relationship between the mutation rate per cell generation and actual tumor cell number. A nominal value for α of 1×10^{-6} might seem reasonable for many experimental cell sys-

tems, but it would be too high to account for the curability of some human tumors by single agents (*e.g.*, choriocarcinoma) and too low to account for the rapid development of clinical resistance to up to six agents simultaneously in other tumors, such as small cell carcinoma of the lung or breast cancer. Values for α in the range of 1×10^{-6} might be consistent with clinical observations if a single mutation could produce resistance to multiple drugs. Although there is evidence for this phenomenon in experimental cell systems (Alt *et al.,* 1978) this phenomenon is not well studied in human tumors. Alternative mechanisms for the development of multidrug resistance for which there *is* evidence in human tumors include gene amplification (Curt *et al.,* 1983; Carman *et al.,* 1984; Horns *et al.,* 1984; Trent *et al.,* 1984) and the development of tetraploidy with associated cytogenetic instability.

The Clinical Distinction Between Kinetic and Genetic Drug Resistance

Clinical drug resistance might be due to kinetic factors, genetic factors, or both. Indeed, the two may be difficult to distinguish clinically. Genetic resistance may not be an all-or-none phenomenon; rather, it may involve a change in the slope of the dose-response curve such that a higher dose of drug might achieve the same fractional cell kill in a resistant tumor that a lower dose would achieve in a sensitive one. That is, treatment intensification might produce a clinical response in a tumor that might otherwise have been considered resistant either on a kinetic basis or on a genetic basis.

The favorable responses to chemotherapy that are observed in experimental systems when tumor body burden is small might be attributed to the greater fractional cell kills in smaller, more rapidly growing tumors. But then, the principle that genetically resistant cells are less likely to be found in smaller tumors than in larger ones might also be applicable, regardless of the presumed mechanism underlying the development of drug resistance. Indeed, it seems likely that the curability of small tumors by chemotherapy may be due to both kinetic and genetic factors operating simultaneously.

Because kinetic drug resistance might be amenable to drug-schedule optimization (optimization of the sequences and intervals between drugs), whereas absolute genetic drug resistance presumably would not, the distinction between the two would be worthwhile. Clonogenic assays might be helpful in this regard, but low clonogenic cell yields may limit the usefulness of such assays.

CLINICAL APPLICATIONS

The role of cell kinetics in the development of improved cancer chemotherapeutic regimens might be considered on two levels. Principles of cell kinetics can be used to develop strategies to deal with such broad problems as treatment intensification (see the section on Kinetic Drug Resistance; Late Treatment Intensification above), the role of low-dose maintenance therapy, and early versus late initiation of treatment of indolent disease. Principles of cell kinetics might also be useful on the tactical level to aid in choosing the types of drugs and determining the best sequences and intervals for these drugs in individual courses of therapy.

Strategic Considerations

The Intensity and Duration of Successful Therapy. One recurrent problem in cancer treatment design is knowing when to stop chemotherapy in patients who have achieved what appear to be durable complete responses. One might continue treatment, often at reduced therapeutic intensity for an indefinite time or for an arbitrarily set long time period (*e.g.*, one to two years). One has good reason to question the cell-killing effectiveness of prolonged low-intensity treatment, and, moreover, reason to be concerned also that such treatment might actually provide a selection pressure for the overgrowth of drug-resistant cells.

In dealing with the question of protracted, low-intensity therapy, it might be helpful to keep in mind the distinction between palliative therapy and treatment with curative intent. For palliative purposes, one might choose to devise a long-term regimen of low to moderate therapeutic intensity that is intended primarily to delay tumor recurrence or to slow the progression of disease. In designing regimens with curative intent, however, one would not want to treat longer than is necessary to eradicate the last tumor cell in most patients. Thus, for example, 12 cycles of CMF adjuvant therapy in breast cancer have not been shown to be better

than 6 cycles of therapy (Tancini *et al.*, 1983). Well-crafted regimens of cytosine arabinoside and daunorubicin can produce prolonged disease-free survival in adult acute leukemia even after only one or two courses of therapy (Vaughan *et al.*, 1982).

One useful early clinical guide to the effectiveness of therapy that can be used to tailor therapy for individual patients is the rate of tumor regression. Patients who achieve complete responses within the first two or three cycles are likely to do better than patients whose tumors regress more slowly (see Figure 2 – 15). The latter group might benefit from an early shift to more intensive and/or more prolonged therapy, or from a complete change in treatment regimen.

The duration of complete response is a major retrospective indicator of treatment effectiveness. Patients who achieve complete responses but who relapse within months after the cessation of therapy undoubtedly had tumors that already contained relatively large numbers of resistant cells at the start of therapy (see Figure 2 – 15, curve D). Patients with rapidly growing tumors who achieve complete responses and relapse more than one to two years after the cessation of therapy are likely to have experienced considerable treatment-induced reductions in body tumor burden (see Figure 2 – 15, curve C). In such patients, more intensive and/or more prolonged initial ther-

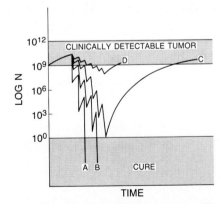

Figure 2 – 15. Schematic representation of heterogeneity of drug response in a "responsive" human cancer. Some patients will be cured with three courses of therapy (A); others will be cured with five courses (B); in some patients who achieve clinical complete responses one or more viable tumor cells will survive even after six courses of therapy, and late recurrences will be observed (C); log kills are small in relatively unresponsive tumors, and even if clinical complete responses are observed they will be of short duration (D).

apy might have been curative in retrospect. Such patients often respond well a second time when given the same regimen they were treated with originally (Fisher *et al.,* 1979; Batist *et al.,* 1983). Since complete response durations tend to be shorter with second complete remissions (Fisher *et al.,* 1979; Vaughan *et al.,* 1982), the development of genetic drug resistance may also be a late factor.

From a kinetic standpoint, one can expect a considerable degree of intertumor variability in the fractional cell kills produced by a given drug regimen in a particular disease. A regimen that is curative for most patients is likely to overtreat some individuals and undertreat others (see Figure 2–15). Thus, an optimum regimen must always represent a compromise. For a given level of treatment intensity and for a given number of treatment courses, there will always be *some* proportion of the responding patient population in whom early and late relapses will be observed. The proportion of patients with late relapses might be decreased by increasing the number of courses and/or the intensity of treatment (see Figure 2–15).

The Management of Indolent Disease. Such neoplasms as the favorable-histology non-Hodgkin's lymphomas often follow an indolent clinical course. Chemotherapy is effective, but not curative. Should treatment be instituted early or should it be withheld until the patient's clinical course requires therapeutic intervention? The results of empirical studies indicate that the latter strategy is a reasonable option (Portlock and Rosenberg, 1979).

Again, it is important to define therapeutic objectives. If the goal is to develop new curative regimens in an investigative setting, then the earlier that treatment is started, the better. If, however, the goal is optimal management using currently available treatment regimens that are known to be effective but noncurative, then a good case can be made for watchful waiting for as long as the patient's clinical course remains indolent. This course of treatment might be justified on the grounds that prolonged treatment with noncurative therapy might provide a selective pressure favoring the development and overgrowth of genetically resistant cells. That is, an indolent tumor with a low cell turnover rate at or near its plateau level might have a lower incidence of mutations and a decreased likelihood of developing genetic resistance *de novo* in comparison with a partially treated tumor that is in a state of active regrowth. Furthermore, the presence of an es-

tablished, indolent, drug-responsive tumor might actually suppress the growth of small numbers of genetically drug-resistant cells that might already be present (see Figures 2–11A and 2–11B).

Tactical Considerations

The area of drug schedule optimization has not been adequately explored and offers what may be the most exciting opportunities for the clinical application of principles of cell kinetics. Kinetically optimized schedules of cytosine arabinoside and daunorubicin in adult acute leukemia have been mentioned earlier (Vaughan *et al.,* 1982). The possible advantages of nonmyelosuppressive treatment on day 14 in the non-Hodgkin's lymphomas were also mentioned earlier in relation to cell recruitment (Fisher *et al.,* 1983; Skarin *et al.,* 1983).

Progress in this area will depend in large measure on the systematic exploration of cellular processes other than DNA synthesis in relation to cell proliferation, and on the availability of more extensive data on the magnitude and time course of drug-induced changes in these processes in man.

REFERENCES

Alt, F. W.; Kellems, R. E.; Bertino, J. R.; and Schimke, R. T.: Selective multiplication of dihydrofolate reductase genes in methotrexate-resistant variants of cultured murine cells. *J. Biol. Chem.,* **253:**1357–1370, 1978.

Atkin, N. B., and Kay, R.: Prognostic significance of modal DNA value and other factors in malignant tumors, based on 1465 cases. *Br. J. Cancer,* **40:**210–221, 1979.

Barlogie, B., and Drewinko, B.: Cell cycle-related induction of cell progression delay. In Drewinko, B., and Humphrey, R. M. (eds.): *Growth Kinetics and Biochemical Regulation of Normal and Malignant Cells.* The Williams & Wilkins Company, Baltimore, 1977.

Barlogie, B.; Drewinko, B.; Johnston, D. A.; and Freireich, E. J.: The effect of adriamycin on the cell cycle traverse of a human lymphoid cell line. *Cancer Res.,* **36:**1975–1979, 1976b.

Barlogie, B.; Drewinko, B.; Schumann, J.; and Freireich, E. J.: Pulse cytophotometric analysis of cell cycle perturbation with bleomycin in vitro. *Cancer Res.,* **36:**1182–1187, 1976a.

Barlogie, B.; Gohde, W.; Johnston, D. A.; Smallwood, L.; Schumann, J.; Drewinko, B.; and Freireich, E. J.: Determination of ploidy and proliferative characteristics of human solid tumors by pulse cytophotometry. *Cancer Res.,* **38:**3333–3339, 1978.

Batist, G.; Ihde, D. C.; Zabell, A.; Lichter, A. S.; Veach, S. R.; Cohen, M. H.; Carney, D. N.; and Bunn, P. A.: Small cell carcinoma of the lung: Reinduction therapy after late relapse. *Ann. Intern. Med.,* **98:**472–474, 1983.

Bech-Hansen, N. T.; Till, J. E.; and Ling, V.: Pleiotropic phenotype of colchicine-resistant CHO cells: Cross-resistance and collateral sensitivity. *J. Cell Physiol.,* **88:**23–31, 1976.

Bhuyan, B. K.; Fraser, T. J.; Gray, L. G.; Kuentzel, S. L.; and Neil, G. L.: Cell-kill kinetics of several S-phase-specific drugs. *Cancer Res.,* **33:**888–894, 1973.

Bhuyan, B. K.; Scheidt, L. G.; and Fraser, T. J.: Cell cycle phase specificity of antitumor agents. *Cancer Res.,* **32:**398–407, 1972.

Braylan, R. C.; Benson, N. A.; and Nourse, V. A.: Flow cytometry: A new approach toward characterizing lymphomas. In Vitetta, E. S., and Fox, C. F. (eds.): *B and T Cell Tumors.* Academic Press, New York, 1982.

Bruce, W. R.; Meeker, B. E.; Powers, W. E.: Comparison of the dose- and time-survival curves for normal hematopoietic and lymphoma colony-forming cells exposed to vinblastine, vincristine, arabinosylcytosine, and amethopterin. *J.N.C.I.,* **42:**1015–1025, 1969.

Bruce, W. R.; Meeker, B. E.; and Valeriote, F. A.: Comparison of the sensitivity of normal hematopoietic and transplanted lymphoma colony-forming cells to chemotherapeutic agents administered in vivo. *J.N.C.I.,* **37:**233–245, 1966.

Burke, P. J.; Diggs, C. H.; and Owens A. H., Jr.: Factors in human serum affecting the proliferation of normal and leukemic cells. *Cancer Res.,* **33:**800–806, 1973.

Burke, P. J.; Karp, J. E.; Braine, H. G.: Timed sequential therapy of human leukemia based upon the response of leukemic cells to humoral growth factors. *Cancer Res.,* **37:**2138–2146, 1977.

Cabanillas, F.; Burgess, M. A.; Bodey, G. P.; and Freireich, E. J.: Sequential chemotherapy and late intensification for malignant lymphomas of aggressive histologic type. *Am. J. Med.,* **74:**382–388, 1983.

Cabral, F.; Sobel, M. E.; and Gottesman, M. M.: CHO mutants resistant to colchicine, colcemid, or griseoofulvin have an altered beta-tubulin. *Cell,* **20:**29–36, 1980.

Camplejohn, R. S.; Schultze, B.; and Maurer, W.: An in vivo double-labeling study with the JF-1 mouse ascites tumour of the subsequent fate of cells arrested in metaphase by vincristine. *Cell Tissue Kinet.,* **13:**239–250, 1980.

Carman, M. D.; Schornagel, J. H.; Rivest, R. S.; Srimatkandada, S.; Portlock, C. S.; Duffy, T.; and Bertino, J. R.: Resistance to methotrexate due to gene amplification in a patient with acute leukemia. *J. Clin. Oncol.,* **2:**16–20, 1984.

Curt, G. A.; Carney, D. M.; Cowan, K. H.; Jolivet, J.; Bailey, B. D.; Drake, J. C.; Kad-Shan, C. W.; Minna, J. D.; and Chabner, B. A.: Unstable methotrexate resistance in human small-cell carcinoma associated with double minute chromosomes. *New Engl. J. Med.,* **308:**199–202, 1983.

Elliot, E. M., and Ling, V.: Selection and characterization of Chinese hamster ovary mutants resistant to melphalan. *Cancer Res.,* **41:**393, 1981.

Fisher, R. I.; DeVita, V. T.; and Hubbard, S. P.: Prolonged disease-free survival in Hodgkin's disease with MOPP reinduction after first relapse. *Ann. Intern. Med.,* **90:**761–763, 1979.

Fisher, R. I.; DeVita, V. T.; Hubbard, S. M.; Longo, D. L.; Wesley, R.; Chabner, B. A.; and Young, R. C.: Diffuse aggressive lymphomas: Increased survival after alternating flexible sequences of ProMACE and MOPP chemotherapy. *Ann. Intern. Med.,* **98:**304–309, 1983.

Flintoff, W. F.; Davidson, S. V.; and Siminovitch, L.: Isolation and partial characterization of three methotrex-ate-resistant phenotypes from Chinese hamster ovary cells. *Somatic Cell Genet.,* **2:**245–261, 1976.

Goldie, J. H., and Coldman, A. J.: A mathematical model for relating the drug sensitivity of tumors to their spontaneous mutation rate. *Cancer Treat. Rep.,* **63:**1727–1733, 1979.

Goldie, J. H.; Coldman, A. J.; and Gudauskas, G. A.: Rationale for the use of alternating non-cross-resistant chemotherapy. *Cancer Treat. Rep.,* **66:**439–449, 1982.

Gralla, R.; Casper, E. S.; Kelsen, D. P.; Braun, D. W., Jr.; Dukeman, M. E.; Martin, N.; Young, C. W.; and Golby, R. B.: Cisplatin and vindesine combination chemotherapy for advanced carcinoma of the lung: A randomized trial investigating two dosage schedules. *Ann. Intern. Med.,* **95:**414–420, 1981.

Hamburger, A. W., and Salmon, S. E.: Primary bioassay of human tumor stem cells. *Science,* **197:**461–463, 1977a.

Hamburger, A. W., and Salmon, S. E.: Primary bioassay of human myeloma stem cells. *J. Clin. Invest.,* **60:**846–854, 1977b.

Horns, R. C., Jr.; Dower, W. J.; and Schimke, R. T.: Gene amplification in a leukemic patient treated with methotrexate. *J. Clin. Oncol.,* **2:**2–7, 1984.

Howard, A., and Pelc, S. R.: Synthesis of desoxyribonucleic acid in normal and irradiated cells and its relation to chromosome breakage. *Heredity* (Suppl.), **6:**261–273, 1953.

Isaacs, J. T.; Wake, N.; Coffey, D. S.; and Sandberg, A. A.: Genetic instability coupled to clonal selection as a mechanism for tumor progression in the Dunning R-3327 rat prostatic adenocarcinoma system. *Cancer Res.,* **42:**2353–2361, 1982.

Kirkland, J. A.; Stanley, M. A.; and Cellier, K. M.: Comparative study of histologic and chromosomal abnormalities in cervical neoplasia. *Cancer,* **20:**1934–1952, 1967.

Krishan, A., and Frei E., III: Effect of adriamycin on the cell cycle traverse and kinetics of cultured human lymphoblasts. *Cancer Res.,* **36:**143–150, 1976.

Laird, A. K.: Dynamics of growth in tumors and in normal organisms. In Perry, S. (ed.): National Cancer Institute Monograph 30. U.S. Government Printing Office, Washington, D.C., 1969.

Lengsfeld, A. M.; Schultze, B.; and Maurer, W.: Time-lapse studies on the effect of vincristine on HeLa cells. *Eur. J. Cancer,* **17:**307–319, 1981.

Lewis, W. H., and Wright, J. W.: Genetic characterization of hydroxyurea resistance in Chinese hamster ovary cell. *J. Cell Physiol.,* **97:**87–97, 1978.

Linden, W. A.; Baisch, H.; and Canstein, L. V.: Impulse cytophotometric studies on the effects of daunomycin on synchronized L-cells. *Eur. J. Cancer,* **10:**647–651, 1974.

Ling, V., and Baker, R. M.: Dominance of colchicine resistance in hybrid CHO cells. *Somatic Cell Genet.,* **4:**193–200, 1978.

Madoc-Jones, H., and Mauro, F.: Interphase action of vinblastine and vincristine: Differences in their lethal action through the mitotic cycle of cultured mammalian cells. *J. Cell Physiol.,* **72:**185–196, 1968.

Malaise, E. P.; Chavaudra, N.; and Tubiana, M.: The relationship between growth rate, labeling index and histologic type of human solid tumors. *Eur. J. Cancer,* **9:**305–312, 1973.

Mauro, F., and Madoc-Jones, H.: Age responses of cultured mammalian cells to cytotoxic drugs. *Cancer Res.,* **30:**1397–1408, 1970.

Mendelsohn, M. L.: Autoradiographic analysis of cell proliferation in spontaneous breast cancer of C3H mouse. III. The growth fraction. *J.N.C.I.,* **28**:1015–1029, 1962.

Mujagic, H.; Chen, S. S.; Geist, R.; Occhipinti, S. J.; Conger, B. M.; Smith, C. A.; Schuette, W. H.; and Shackney, S. E.: The effects of vincristine on cell survival, cell cycle progression and mitotic accumulation in asynchronously growing sarcoma 180 cells. *Cancer Res.,* **43**:3591–3597, 1983.

Mujagic, H.; Conger, B; Smith, C. A.; Occhipinti, S. J.; Schuette, W. H.; and Shackney, S. E.: The schedule dependence of vincristine lethality in sarcoma 180 cells following partial synchronization with hydroxyurea. *Cancer Res.,* **43**:3598–3603, 1983.

Norton, L.; Green, M.; Pajak, T. F.; Gottlieb, A.; Bloomfield, C.; Cooper, R. M.; Cuttner, J.; and Holland, J. F.: Feasibility of late-intensification chemotherapy of advanced Hodgkin's disease in complete remission. *Blood,* 60, Suppl. **1**:162a, 1982 (abstract).

Norton, L., and Simon, R.: Tumor size, sensitivity to therapy, and design of treatment schedules. *Cancer Treat. Rep.,* **61**:1307–1317, 1977.

Portlock, C. S., and Rosenberg, S. A.: No initial therapy for stage III and IV non-Hodgkin's lymphomas of favorable histologic types. *Ann. Intern. Med.,* **90**:10–13, 1979.

Quastler, H.: The analysis of cell population kinetics. In Lamerton, L. F., and Fry, R. J. M. (eds.): *Cell Proliferation.* Blackwell Scientific Publications, Oxford, 1963.

Quastler, H., and Sherman, F. G.: Cell population kinetics in the intestinal epithelium of the mouse. *Exp. Cell Res.,* **17**:420–438, 1959.

Reeves, B. R.: Cytogenetics of malignant lymphomas. *Hum. Genet.,* **20**:231–250, 1973.

Ritch, P. S.; Occhipinti, S. J.; Skramstad, K.; and Shackney, S. E.: Increased relative effectiveness of adriamycin with prolonged drug exposure in sarcoma 180 in vitro. *Cancer Treat. Rep.,* **66**:1159–1168, 1982.

Sandberg, A. A., and Wake, N.: Chromosomal changes in primary and metastatic tumors and in lymphoma: Their non-randomness and significance. In Arrighi, F. E., and Rao, P. N. (eds.): *Genes, Chromosomes and Neoplasia.* Raven Press, New York, 1981.

Schimke, R. T.: Gene amplification, drug resistance, and cancer. *Cancer Res.,* **44**:1735–1742, 1984.

Shackney, S. E.: A computer model for tumor growth and chemotherapy, and its application to L1210 leukemia treated with cytosine arabinoside. *Cancer Chemother. Rep.,* **54**:399–429, 1970.

Shackney, S. E.: A cytokinetic model for heterogeneous mammalian cell populations. III. Tritiated thymidine studies. Correlations among multiple kinetic parameters in human tumours. *J. Theor. Biol.,* **65**:421–464, 1977.

Shackney, S. E.: The orderliness of cell proliferation and cell differentiation in relation to kinetic heterogeneity in mouse bone marrow. In Clarkson, B.; Marks, P. A.; and Till, J. E. (eds.): *Differentiation of Normal and Neoplastic Hematopoietic Cells.* Cold Spring Harbor Laboratory, Cold Spring Harbor, N. Y., 1978.

Shackney, S. E.; Bunn, P. A.; Ford, S. S.: A study of drug-induced kinetic perturbations in the marrow of a patient with neuroblastoma. *Cancer,* **45**:882–892, 1980.

Shackney, S. E.; Levine, A. M.; Fisher, R.; Smith, C. A.; Nichols, P.; Jaffe, E.; Simon, R.; Parker, J.; Cossman, J.; Schuette, W. H.; Young, R. C.; Occhipinti, S. J.; and Lukes, R. J.: The biology of tumor growth in the non-Hodgkin's lymphomas: A dual parameter flow cytometry study of 220 cases. *J. Clin. Invest.,* **73**:1201–1214, 1984.

Shackney, S. E.; Levine, A.; Simon, R.; Nichols, P.; Fisher, R.; Jaffe, E.; Parker, J.; Schuette, W.; Smith, C.; Young, R.; Occhipinti, S.; and Lukes, R.: Dual parameter flow cytometry studies in 220 cases of non-Hodgkin's lymphoma. *Proc. Am. Soc. Clin. Oncol.,* **2**:8, 1983 (abstract).

Shackney, S. E.; McCormack, G. W.; and Cuchural, G. J.: Growth rates of solid tumors and their relation to responsiveness to therapy. An analytical review. *Ann. Intern. Med.,* **89**:107–121, 1978.

Shackney, S. E., and Schuette, W. H.: Multicompartment analysis of cell proliferation and cell migration in the Sezary syndrome. *Hematol. Oncol.,* **1**:31–48, 1983.

Skarin, A. T.; Canellos, G. P.; Rosenthal, D. S.; Case, D. C., Jr.; MacIntire, J. M.; Pinkus, G. S.; Moloney, W. C.; and Frei, E., III: Improved prognosis of diffuse histiocytic and undifferentiated lymphoma by use of high-dose methotrexate alternating with standard agents (M-BACOD). *J. Clin. Oncol.,* **1**:91–98, 1983.

Skipper, H. E.; Schabel, F. M., Jr.; and Wilcox, W. S.: Experimental evaluation of potential anticancer agents. XIII. On the criteria and kinetics associated with "curability" of experimental leukemia. *Cancer Chemother. Rep.,* **35**:1–111, 1964.

Steel, G. G.: Cell loss from experimental tumors. *Cell Tissue Kinet.,* **1**:193–207, 1968.

Tancini, G.; Bonadonna, G.; Valagussa, P.; Marchini, S.; and Veronesi, U.: Adjuvant CMF in breast cancer: Comparative 5-year results of 12 versus 6 cycles. *J. Clin. Oncol.,* **1**:2–10, 1983.

Tannock, I.: Cell kinetics and cancer chemotherapy: A critical review. *Cancer Treat. Rep.,* **62**:1117–1133, 1978.

Tobey, R. A., and Crissman, H. A.: Comparative effects of three nitrosourea derivatives on mammalian cell cycle progression. *Cancer Res.,* **35**:460–470, 1975.

Tobey, R. A.; Crissman, H. A.; and Oka, M. S. Arrested and cycling CHO cells as a kinetic model: Studies with adriamycin. *Cancer Treat. Rep.,* **60**:1829–1837, 1976.

Trent, J. M.; Buick, R. N.; Olson, S.; Horns, R. C., Jr.; and Schimke, R. T.: Cytologic evidence for gene amplification in methotrexate-resistant cells obtained from a patient with ovarian adenocarcinoma. *J. Clin. Oncol.,* **2**:8–15, 1984.

Tribukait, B.; Gustafson, H.; and Esposti, P.: Ploidy and proliferation in human bladder tumors as measured by flow cytofluorometric DNA-analysis and its relations to histopathology and cytology. *Cancer,* **43**:1742–1751, 1979.

Tyler-Smith, C., and Anderson, T.: Gene amplification in methotrexate-resistant mouse cells. I. DNA rearrangement accompanies dihydrofolate reductase gene amplification in a T-cell lymphoma. *J. Mol. Biol.,* **153**:203–218, 1981.

Vaughan, W. P.; Karp, J. E.; and Burke, P. J.: Two-cycle timed-sequential chemotherapy for adult acute myelocytic leukemia. *Blood,* **60**:158a, 1982.

Vindelov, L. L.; Hansen, H. H.; Christensen, J. J.; Spang-Thomsen, M.; Hirsch, F. R.; Hansen, M.; and Nissen, N. I.: Clonal heterogeneity of small cell anaplastic carcinoma of the lung demonstrated by flow cytometric DNA analysis. *Cancer Res.,* **40**:4295–4300, 1980.

Wimber, D. E.: Methods for studying cell proliferation with emphasis on DNA labels. In Lamerton, L. F., and Fry, R. J. M. (eds.): *Cell Proliferation.* Blackwell Scientific Publications, Oxford, 1963.

3

Etiology of Cancer

A. INTRODUCTION

Philip S. Schein

Progress in the elucidation of the complex mechanisms of carcinogenesis is being made at a rate that defies the capacity of the medical oncologist to remain informed of major new advances as they are rapidly developed and refined. A full understanding of this field in its entirety requires a basic appreciation of such diverse disciplines as molecular biology and epidemiology. The initiating agent may be chemical, viral, or radiation related, and the event takes place in a complex milieu of factors, including the genetic composition and the immunologic status of the host, that may either promote or retard the process of transformation.

Epidemiology has made substantial contributions through the empirical identification of risk factors in our environment that have been implicated as causative factors (Doll, 1977). The magnitude of the task is placed into perspective by our recognition that "cancer" is a generic term that serves to describe no less than 100 different disease-states, each with its intrinsic natural history, methods of diagnosis and treatment, as well as etiologies. The latter are described in the relevant sections of each disease-specific chapter of this book. Several basic concepts must, nevertheless, be appreciated. Most important is the estimate that 60% to 90% of cancers are environmental in origin. To cite several important examples, the role of cigarette smoking (lung cancer), asbestos (lung cancer and mesothelioma), vinyl chloride (hepatic angiosarcoma), and benzidine (leukemia) have been demonstrated. In specific cases, the identification of these im-portant carcinogens has resulted in responsible action on the part of Congress and industry, with a resultant reduction in incidence of specific tumors. It is regrettable, however, that society as a whole has not always responded appropriately to information provided from cancer research, most notably in our continued production and use of tobacco.

Continued interdisciplinary investigation will undoubtedly identify the exogenous factors that account for the dramatic decreased incidence of gastric carcinoma in the United States, and the equally important simultaneous increase in other tumors, such as cancer of the pancreas. Dietary nitrates, for example, have been implicated in the formation of nitrosamines, as well as other N-nitroso chemicals, which may have a role in the etiology of gastrointestinal neoplasms (see Chapters 26 and 27). The chapters dealing with molecular and cellular biochemistry and chemical carcinogenesis provide detailed information about the mechanisms of carcinogen binding to specific DNA bases and the process of repair for cellular transformation. An association with specific forms of trauma, such as burns (carcinoma of the skin), lye injury (esophageal carcinoma), and pulmonary infection ("scar carcinomas"), has also been established (see Chapters 20, 23, and 25).

The field of viral oncology has attracted increasing interest during the past three years as a result of new information implicating an infectious etiology for certain human cancers. It has long been recognized that viruses could cause leukemia in inbred mice, and that they could result in horizontal spread of cancer in many animal species. Although many investigators remain unconvinced that a specific viral etiology for human cancer has been demonstrated conclusively, the correlations of hepatitis B with hepatoma, herpes simplex II with cervical cancer, the Epstein-Barr virus with Burkitt's lymphoma, and more recently the identification of a retrovirus association with specific T-cell lymphomas make an increasingly convincing case for infectious causation. Further credence is given to an infectious etiology by the diagnosis of Kaposi's sarcoma and certain lymphomas in patients with the acquired immunodeficiency syndrome (AIDS), a disorder that can be transmitted through transfusion of blood products (see Chapter 11).

One of the most important by-products of the recent research efforts in viral carcinogenesis has been the evolution of the oncogene theory. It is widely accepted that cellular transformation must result from an alteration in the genetic information that controls the processes of cellular maturation and proliferation, modulated by exogenous influences such as hormones, growth factors, and the immunologic milieu. It has been clearly demonstrated that viruses, like specific classes of chemicals and radiation, can alter the genetic code of a cell by the integration and replication of viral DNA. In the case of retroviruses, this requires the initial transcription of the viral genome into DNA by reverse transcriptase. Some viruses, notably the Rous sarcoma virus, contain a single gene that codes for a specific protein that may mediate the transformation process. In this case the product is a protein kinase that can phosphorylate tyrosine, a now-recognized common characteristic of oncogene-coded enzymes. Further research, using the tools of molecular hybridization, have shown that apparently normal human cells contain genes that are closely related to the viral oncogene, in essence cellular oncogenes that may have a function similar to their viral counterpart.

This finding supports the hypothesis that all cells contain "cancer genes" that produce regulatory proteins that control cellular proliferation. The integration of viral oncogenes may

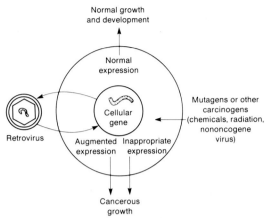

Figure 3–1. Cancer-gene concept, supported by oncogene data and other preliminary evidence, suggests a unifying explanation for various forms of carcinogenesis. The common central element is a group of cellular genes required for normal growth and development. Transplanted into a retrovirus genome (left), such a gene becomes an oncogene. Cancer can also result if the cellular gene is affected by any of a wide variety of mutagens or other carcinogens (right). From Bishop, J. M.: Oncogenes. *Sci. Am.*, **246**:80–92, 1982. Copyright © 1982 by Scientific American, Inc. All rights reserved.

result in an augmented expression of this transforming factor, which under basal conditions is otherwise limited and controlled in production. It is possible that this concept will ultimately provide one part of a unified hypothesis for cancer induction whereby chemicals, viruses, and radiation, as well as specific cancer-related genetic disorders, may be shown to promote or augment the activity of preexisting cancer genes in normal cells (see Figure 3–1) (Bishop, 1982). This represents a challenge worthy of the current level of investigation, which, if successful, may ultimately result in the birth of a new field of preventive and therapeutic molecular intervention.

REFERENCES

Bishop, J. M.: Oncogenes. *Sci. Am.*, **246**:80–92, 1982.
Doll, R.: Introduction. In Hiatt, H. H.; Watson, J. D.; and Winsten, J. A. (eds.): *Origins of Human Cancer.* Cold Spring Harbor Laboratory, Cold Spring Harbor, New York, 1977.

B. CHEMICAL CARCINOGENESIS
I. Bernard Weinstein

INTRODUCTION: MAGNITUDE AND EPIDEMIOLOGY OF CANCER

Cancer is the second leading cause of death in the United States (see Table 3-1), accounting for approximately 440,000 deaths per year (for detailed figures on cancer incidence and mortality see: Mason *et al.*, 1975; National Cancer Institute, 1982; *Ca*, 1983). Approximately 20% of all deaths in the United States are due to cancer. About 855,000 new cases of cancer are diagnosed each year in the United States, exclusive of nonmelanoma skin cancers and *in situ* cervical cancer. Nearly 200,000 of these cases have, or will, develop disseminated disease. Although major progress is being made in cancer therapy, it is apparent that efforts leading to the primary prevention of only a fraction of these cases could have a major impact on human health.

Cancer is many different diseases, and efforts at cancer prevention must be addressed to specific types of tumors. In the adult American man, the most common form is lung cancer; in the woman, breast cancer; and in both sexes considered together, colon and rectal cancer. Nonmelanoma skin cancers (squamous and basal cell carcinomas), and carcinoma *in situ* of the uterine cervix are the most common

tumors in terms of incidence, but these types rarely produce major clinical problems. In the adult, more than 80% of cancers are carcinomas arising from epithelial tissues, whereas leukemias and sarcomas are relatively rare. This may reflect the greater exposure of epithelial tissues to environmental agents that readily contact the lining surfaces of the body, both internal and external, and/or the accumulation of these agents in glandular tissues.

The incidence of cancer in children is low when compared with that of adults. Cancer deaths during the ages from one to 14 account for only 1% of the cancers observed in all age groups in the United States. Within that age group, cancer is the second leading cause of death and is exceeded only by accidents. Leukemias, tumors of the central nervous system, and soft tissue tumors account for the majority of cancers in children.

Time Trends

It is instructive to examine the changing pattern of cancer mortality rates in the United States during the past 40 years. Figures 3-2 and 3-3 indicate the astonishing increase in lung cancer death rate in males and females. These increases parallel the increase in cigarette

Table 3-1. Mortality for Leading Causes of Death: United States, 1978

RANK	CAUSE OF DEATH	NUMBER OF DEATHS	DEATH RATE PER 100,000 POPULATION	PERCENT OF TOTAL DEATHS
1.	Heart diseases	729,510	300.4	37.8
2.	Cancer	396,992	169.9	20.6
3.	Cerebrovascular diseases	175,629	70.8	9.1
4.	Accidents	105,561	45.8	5.5
5.	Pneumonia & influenza	58,319	23.6	3.0
6.	Chronic obstructive lung disease	50,488	21.2	2.6
7.	Diabetes mellitus	33,841	14.2	1.8
8.	Cirrhosis of liver	30,066	13.4	1.6
9.	Arteriosclerosis	28,940	11.1	1.5
10.	Suicide	27,294	11.6	1.4
11.	Diseases of infancy	22,033	12.1	1.1
12.	Homicide	20,432	8.7	1.1
13.	Aortic aneurysm	14,028	5.8	0.8
14.	Congenital anomalies	12,968	6.8	0.7
15.	Pulmonary infarction	10,941	4.6	0.6
	Other & ill-defined	210,606	89.9	10.8
All causes		1,927,788	809.9	100.0

From *Ca—A Cancer Journal for Clinicians*, **33**, 1983.

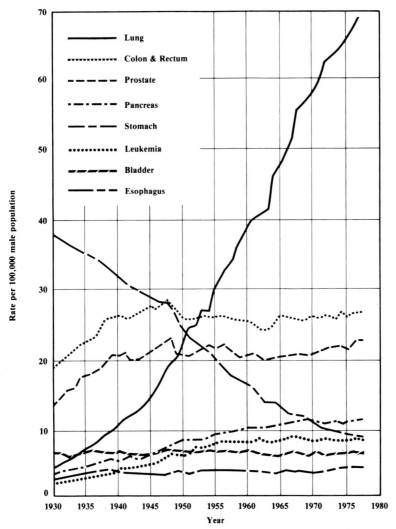

Figure 3-2. Male cancer death rates by site, United States, 1930–1977. (Rate for male population standardized for age on the 1940 U.S. population. Sources of Data: National Vital Statistics Division and Bureau of the Census, United States). Reprinted from *CA: A Cancer Journal for Clinicians,* 30, 1980.

smoking and reflect a lag of about 20 years between the increase in smoking and lung cancer occurrence. Death rates from cancer of the pancreas and ovary have gradually increased during this time, but there has been a striking decrease in stomach and uterine cancer. The mortality rates and the incidence rates of breast, colon, and rectal cancer have remained essentially unchanged.

Stomach cancer has become a relatively rare disease in the United States. This presumably reflects a decrease in human exposure to an exogenous agent(s). The causative agent has not been identified with certainty, but the decrease has been attributed by some investiga-

tors to a general decrease in dietary nitrite, and an increase in dietary vitamins. This illustrates the potential for decreasing the incidence of specific cancers by appropriate modification of the human environment. Generally, the occurrence of specific cancers is not inborn. Studies on migrant populations also support this conclusion.

In the past 25 years, the overall age-specific total cancer death rates in the United States have remained fairly stable in the older adult population. The incidence of and mortality from lung cancer, however, continue to increase, particularly in women, for whom mortality is increasing at a rate of about 6% per

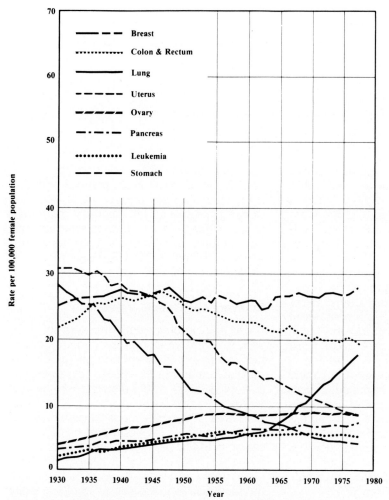

Figure 3–3. Female cancer death rates by site, United States 1930–1977. (Rate for female population standardized for age on the 1940 U.S. population. Sources of Data: National Vital Statistics Division and Bureau of the Census, United States). Reprinted from *CA: A Cancer Journal for Clinicians,* 30, 1980.

year. If this trend continues, within 10 years lung cancer will be more prevalent in American women than breast cancer. This is a shocking figure given the fact that currently about one in twelve American women develop breast cancer. The impact of lung cancer is so great that if lung cancer deaths are subtracted from total cancer mortality, the data suggest that there has actually been a decline in deaths from cancer in the past few years. Because most of the cases of lung cancer in both men and women can be attributed to cigarette smoking, these facts present an important challenge to the medical profession and the general public in terms of primary cancer prevention.

Geographic Differences

There are remarkable differences in the incidence of and mortality from specific types of cancer in different countries (see Table 3-2). In the United States and Western Europe, a high mortality from lung, colon, and breast cancer, and a low mortality from stomach cancer is evident. In Japan, stomach cancer predominates, but colon and breast cancer are relatively rare. Liver cancer occurs more frequently in Africa and in Japan than it does in the United States. Epidemiologic studies have demonstrated that as Japanese migrate from Japan to Hawaii or to the mainland United States, within one or two generations the high

Table 3-2. Cancer Around the World: Age-Adjusted Death Rates Per 100,000 Population

COUNTRIES	ALL SITES		COLON & RECTUM		LUNG		STOMACH		BREAST	PROSTATE
	M	F	M	F	M	F	M	F	F	M
United States	214	136	26	20	68	17	9	4	27	22
England	252	156	30	23	97	19	25	12	34	18
Japan	187	109	15	11	28	8	70	35	6	4

M = Males; F = Females.
Data from *Ca—A Cancer Journal for Clinicians*, **33**, 1983.

incidence of stomach cancer characteristic of Japan abates, and the high incidence of colon cancer characteristic of the United States is acquired. A similar trend among urban Japanese in Japan who have adopted a more Western diet and lifestyle is evident. These trends remain constant, even though Japanese continue to marry Japanese, indicating that genetic factors are not primarily involved. These, and other migrant population studies, reinforce the argument for the predominant role of environmental factors (in contrast to genetic or inborn factors) in the etiology of most human cancers.

The development of a U.S. atlas of cancer mortality by county has highlighted geographic differences in the mortality from specific cancers within the United States and has provided important clues to human cancer etiology (Mason *et al.,* 1975). A similar atlas has been prepared for the Peoples Republic of China, which also shows striking geographic variations in mortality from cancer.

Socioeconomic and Lifestyle Factors

Considerable variation is evident in the incidence of specific cancers in different subsets of the American population. The black population in the United States has a higher incidence of cancer of the prostate, uterine cervix, lung, esophagus, and oropharynx and a lower incidence of breast cancer and cancer of the corpus uteri than does the white population. The pattern of some of the cancers seen in the black population is, however, gradually shifting towards that of the white population, suggesting that changes in diet and environment related to changing socioeconomic factors play an important role. Variations in the incidence of some cancers in the white population are also related to geographic and socioeconomic factors.

Cigarette smoking, diet, and reproductive behavior markedly influence cancer risks, em-

phasizing the role of lifestyle in cancer causation. Although certain occupations and synthetic chemicals are important risk factors, it would appear that the majority of human cancer is due to more common aspects of our diet, culture, and personal behavior (Armstrong and Doll, 1975; Higginson and Muir, 1976; Hiatt *et al.,* 1977).

Relevance to Cancer Prevention

The epidemiologic data discussed above, as well as extensive laboratory studies, seem to indicate that a great proportion (as high as 80%) of human cancer is due to environmental (*i.e.,* exogenous), rather than endogenous (hereditary), factors (Hiatt *et al.,* 1977). This suggests that if the exogenous causative factors were identified, a major proportion of human cancer could be prevented, either by reducing human exposure or by protecting the host. Great progress has already been made through the identification of cigarette smoking as the major cause of lung cancer. At least seven industrial processes or occupational exposures and 23 chemicals or groups of chemicals have been implicated in various forms of human cancer (IARC, 1982) (see Table 3-3). The specific causes of other major cancers (*i.e.,* cancers of the large bowel and breast), however, have not been identified with certainty. A number of important questions remain unanswered. The current controversies concerning the extent to which human cancers are due to naturally occurring versus man-made chemicals, the relative contribution of initiators and promoters, the roles of chemical versus viral agents, the role of general nutritional factors (*i.e.,* fat, fiber, and vitamins), and the role of multifactor interactions are being studied (Weinstein, 1981a, 1981b). It is likely that specific answers to these questions will come mainly from two sources: (1) Fundamental research on mechanisms of chemical carcinogenesis at the cellular and molecular levels,

Table 3-3. Chemicals and Industrial Processes That Are Carcinogenic for Humans

GROUP 1

Chemicals and Processes for Which Convincing
Epidemiological Evidence of Carcinogenicity in Humans Appears

Industrial processes and occupational
    exposures
    Auramine manufacture
    Boot and shoe manufacture and re-
      pair (certain occupations)
    Furniture manufacture
    Isopropyl alcohol manufacture
      (strong-acid process)
    Nickel refining
    Rubber industry (certain occupa-
      tions)
    Underground hematite mining (with
      exposure to radon)

Chemicals and groups of chemicals
    4-Aminobiphenyl
    Analgesic mixtures containing phena-
      cetin*
    Arsenic and arsenic compounds*
    Asbestos
    Azathioprine
    Benzene
    Benzidine

N,N-*bis*(2-chloroethyl)-2-naphthyla-
    mine (Chlomaphazine)
Bis(chloromethyl)ether and techni-
    cal-grade chloromethyl methyl
    ether
1,4-Butanediol dimethanesulphonate
    (MYLERAN)
Certain combined chemotherapy for
    lymphomas* (including MOPP†)
Chlorambucil
Chromium and certain chromium
    compounds*
Conjugated estrogens*
Cyclophosphamide
Diethylstilbestrol (DES)
Melphalan
Methoxsalen with ultraviolet A ther-
    apy (PUVA)
Mustard gas
2-Naphthylamine
Soots, tars, and oils*‡
Treosulphan
Vinyl chloride

GROUP 2

Chemicals and Compounds That Are Probably Carcinogenetic in Humans.
The Evidence for the Compounds in Group A Is Stronger Than That for
the Compounds in Group B
Group A

Acrylonitrile
Aflatoxins
Benzo[*a*]pyrene
Beryllium and beryllium compounds*
Combined oral contraceptives*
Diethyl sulphate
Dimethyl sulphate

Manufacture of magenta*
Nickel and certain nickel compounds
Nitrogen mustard
Oxymetholone
Phenacetin
Procarbazine
ortho-Toluidine

Group B

Actinomycin D
Amitrole
Auramine (technical grade)
Benzotrichloride
Bischloroethylnitrosourea (BCNU)
Cadmium and cadmium compounds
Carbon tetrachloride
Chloramphenicol
1-(2-Chloroethyl)-3-cyclohexyl-1-nitro-
    sourea (CCNU)
Chloroform
Chlorophenols (occupational exposure
    to)*
Cisplatin
Dacarbazine
DDT
3,3'-Dichlorobenzidine
Dienestrol
3,3'-Dimethoxybenzidine (*ortho*-diani-
    sidine)
Dimethylcarbamoyl chloride
Epichlorohydrin

Estradiol 17β
Estrone
Ethinylestradiol
Ethylene dibromide
Ethylene oxide
Ethylene thiourea
Formaldehyde (gas)
Hydrazine
Mestranol
Metronidazole
Norethisterone
Phenazopyridine
Phenytoin
Phenoxyacetic acid herbicides (occupa-
    tional exposure to)*
Polychlorinated biphenyls (PCBs)
Progesterone
Propylthiouracil
Sequential oral contraceptives*
Tetrachlorodibenzo-para-dioxin
    (TCDD)

continued

Table 3-3. *(continued)*

GROUP 2

*Chemicals and Compounds That Are Probably Carcinogenetic in Humans.
The Evidence for the Compounds in Group A Is Stronger Than That for
the Compounds in Group B*
Group B

1,4-Dioxane	2,4,6-Trichlorophenol
Direct black 38 (technical grade)	Tris(aziridinyl)-para-benzoquinone
Direct blue 6 (technical grade)	(Triaziquone)
Direct brown 95 (technical grade)	Tris(1-aziridinyl)phosphine sulphide
Doxorubicin hydrochloride (ADRIAMY-	(Thiotepa)
CIN)	Uracil mustard

*The compound(s) responsible for the carcinogenic effect in humans cannot be specified.
†Procarbazine, nitrogen mustard, vincristine, and prednisone
‡Mineral oils may vary in composition, particularly in relation to their content of carcinogenic
polycyclic aromatic hydrocarbons.
Note: This list does not include known human carcinogens such as tobacco smoke, betel, and
alcoholic beverages. Ionizing and ultraviolet radiation are also recognized carcinogens in humans.
Modified from IARC: *IARC Monographs on the Evaluation of the Carcinogenic Risk of Chemicals to
Humans: Chemicals and Industrial Processes Associated with Cancer in Humans, Supplement 4.*
IARC, Lyon, France, 1982.

and (2) clinical and epidemiologic studies that utilize newly emerging laboratory methods for identifying potential carcinogens in environmental samples and human tissues, assessing various host factors and interindividual variations.

Along with organized research efforts, physicians and health professionals as well as patients can play a major role in providing clues to causes of human cancer. Indeed, one of the first associations between an occupational exposure and cancer was made by the English Surgeon Sir Percival Pott in his classic description, over 200 years ago, of cancer of the scrotum in chimney sweeps (Pott, 1775). Since then, astute clinical observations provided the first clues to a number of human carcinogens, including the association between cigarette smoking and lung cancer, asbestos exposure and mesothelioma, and transplacental exposure to diethylstilbestrol (DES) and vaginal carcinoma. It is important that physicians who treat patients with cancer continue to provide new clues to etiologic factors by asking the question: Was this patient exposed to anything that might have caused this cancer?

DIVERSITY OF STRUCTURE AND SOURCES OF CHEMICAL CARCINOGENS

When the list (see Table 3-3) of known human (and animal) carcinogens is examined, the broad diversity of the compounds, both in terms of their chemical structures and sources, is obvious. They include polycyclic aromatics, aromatic amines, nitrosamines and nitro-

soureas, alkylating agents, alkyl and aryl halides, steroid hormones, mycotoxins, metals, asbestos fibers, and others. A discussion is presented in relevant chapters dealing with tumors for which these agents have been implicated as etiologic factors. Some carcinogens are synthetic, and others (*e.g.,* aflatoxin) occur naturally.

Several carcinogens enountered in the work-place are listed in Table 3-4 (National Cancer Institute, 1980). A detailed occupational history is essential for all patients with cancer. Physicians must be aware that radiation and certain drugs administered for therapeutic purposes are also potentially carcinogenic. A detailed history of radiation and drug exposure is important in evaluation of patients with cancer. The fetus is extremely sensitive to carcinogens. Carcinogenesis can occur transplacentally, and the tumor may not manifest itself in the offspring until adolescence or adulthood. Diethylstilbestrol-induced vaginal carcinoma is an example. Ideally, it would be useful to know which medications the patient's mother received during pregnancy; whether she was exposed to radiation; whether she was a cigarette smoker; and her occupation. Table 3-5 lists a number of therapeutic agents known to be carcinogenic in experimental animals (see also Weinstein, 1980). Some, but not all of these agents are also known to be carcinogenic in humans. When prescribing medication, physicians must carefully weigh benefits versus risks, and must maintain constant surveillance to determine whether the drugs being used pose a significant carcinogenic risk to humans. With the increas-

Table 3–4.   Common Occupational Carcinogens

AGENT	ORGAN(S) AFFECTED	OCCUPATION
Wood	Nasal cavity and sinuses	Woodworkers
Leather	Nasal cavity and sinuses, urinary bladder	Leather and shoe workers
Iron oxide	Lung, larynx	Iron ore miners, metal grinders and polishers, silver finishers, iron foundry workers
Nickel	Nasal sinuses, lung	Nickel smelters, mixers, and roasters, electrolysis workers
Arsenic	Skin, lung, liver	Miners, smelters, insecticide makers and sprayers, tanners, chemical workers, oil refiners, vintners
Chromium	Nasal cavity and sinuses, lung, larynx	Chromium producers, processers, and users, acetylene and aniline workers, bleachers, glass, pottery, and linoleum workers, battery makers
Asbestos	Lung (pleural and peritoneal mesothelioma)	Miners, millers, textile, insulation, and shipyard workers
Petroleum, petroleum coke, wax, creosote, anthracene, paraffin, shale, and mineral oils	Nasal cavity, larynx, lung, skin, scrotum	Those who came into contact with lubricating, cooling, paraffin, or wax fuel oils or coke, rubber fillers, retort workers, textile weavers, diesel jet testers
Mustard gas	Larynx, lung, trachea, bronchi	Mustard gas workers
Vinyl chloride	Liver, brain	Plastic workers
Bis-chloromethyl ether, chloromethyl, methyl ether	Lung	Chemical workers
Isopropyl oil	Nasal cavity	Isopropyl oil producers
Coal soot, coal tar, and other products of coal combustion	Lung, larynx, skin, scrotum, urinary bladder	Gashouse workers, stokers, and producers, asphalt, coal tar, and pitch workers, coke oven workers, miners, still cleaners
Benzene	Bone marrow	Explosives, benzene, or rubber cement workers, distillers, dye users, painters, shoemakers
Auramine, benzidine, alpha-Naphthyl-amine magenta, 4-Amino-diphenyl, 4-Nitro-diphenyl	Urinary bladder	Dyestuffs manufacturers and users, rubber workers (pressmen, filtermen, laborers), textile dyers, paint manufacturers

Source: National Cancer Institute

Table 3–5.   Examples of Diagnostic and Therapeutic Agents with Known or Suspected Carcinogenic Activity in Animals or Humans

Adriamycin
Alkylating agents: Chlornaphazin, cyclophosphamide
Androgens
Arsenicals (inorganic)
Dapsone
Diethylstilbestrol (DES)
Diphenylhydantoin (DILANTIN)
Drugs as precursors of nitrosamines
Estrogens and oral contraceptives
Griseofulvin
Hycanthone
Hydrazines
Isonicotinic acid hydrazide
Metronidazole (FLAGYL), and other nitro-heterocycles
Nitrofurans: FANFT (N-[4-(5-nitro-2-furyl)-2-thiazolyl]formamide)
Phenacetin
Phenylbutazone
Radiation: x ray and UV
Reserpine
Tars
Thorotrast

ing use of long-term therapy in the treatment of chronic diseases (for example, hypertension), this aspect takes on increasing importance.

Aflatoxin B_1, the product of a mold that frequently contaminates peanuts, cereals, and grains is an important example of a naturally occurring carcinogen. It is thought to contribute (probably in combination with hepatitis B virus infection) to the high incidence of liver cancer in certain parts of Africa (see Chapter 28). Aflatoxin is the most potent carcinogen known in any experimental animal system. Certain plant and fungal products and certain cooking and food preservation practices may generate carcinogenic substances. Highly potent mutagens have recently been identified in pyrolysis products of certain amino acids. These compounds can be generated during the broiling of fish or meat (Sugimura, 1982). Whether the latter substances are carcinogenic in humans or not is not yet known.

BASIC BIOLOGIC AND BIOCHEMICAL PRINCIPLES OF CARCINOGENESIS

Certain biologic and biochemical principles pertaining to chemical (and radiation) carcinogenesis are listed in Table 3-6 (see also

Weinstein, 1980). In terms of human exposure, an apparent lack of a threshold along with an increasing incidence with increasing dose, and a long lag between exposure and the appearance of tumors should be emphasized. These principles are reinforced in the case of cigarette smoking and lung cancer; the lag in the occurrence of leukemias (and an even longer lag for carcinomas) in Hiroshima and Nagasaki survivors; the occurrence of cancers in patients following radiation for therapeutic or diagnostic purposes; and various occupationally related cancers. The explanation for the lag appears to be mainly the multistep nature of the process. The diversity in phenotypes between individual tumors, even those produced by the same carcinogen in the same tissue, has thwarted efforts to identify a single biochemical or immunologic characteristic that might provide a universal marker for the detection of cancers or one that might be used as a general target or strategy in cancer therapy.

Metabolic Activation

A basic principle in the biochemistry of carcinogenesis is that several environmental carcinogens are not active in their native form. They undergo metabolic activation by the host and are converted to highly reactive electro-

Table 3-6. Chemical Carcinogens—Basic Biologic and Biochemical Facts

1. Carcinogenesis is *dose dependent*—the larger the dose the greater the incidence of tumors and the shorter the lag. There is no evidence of a *threshold dose* below which a carcinogen is safe.
2. There is a long *lag* between exposure and the appearance of tumors. In humans this is about five to 30 years. In various species, the lag is generally proportional to the lifespan of the species. Carcinogens can act transplacentally, with tumors appearing only later in the adult progeny.
3. Conversion of a normal tissue to a malignant neoplasm is a *multistep process.*
4. The action of certain types of carcinogens, so-called initiating agents, is markedly enhanced by *promoting agents, hormonal agents,* and various *cofactors.*
5. Cellular *proliferation enhances* carcinogenesis.
6. Neoplasms induced by the same chemical carcinogen often display *antigenic diversity,* as well as a general *diversity of phenotypes* in terms of growth rate, degree of differentiation, cell surface properties, enzyme profiles, etc.
7. Carcinogens are subject to both *metabolic activation* and *detoxification in vivo.*
8. The metabolically activated forms of carcinogens are highly reactive *electrophiles* that bind covalently to nucleophilic residues in cellular proteins and nucleic acids.

Modified from Weinstein, I. B.: Molecular and cellular mechanisms of chemical carcinogenesis. In Crooke, S., and Prestayko, A. (eds.): *Cancer and Chemotherapy, Vol. 1: Introduction to Neoplasia and Anti-Neoplastic Chemotherapy.* Academic Press, New York, 1980.

philic species. These can then react with nucleophilic residues in cellular proteins and nucleic acids to form covalent adducts (Heidelberger, 1975; Miller, 1978; Weinstein, 1981a). The polycyclic aromatic hydrocarbon benzo(a)pyrene, for example, is not highly reactive chemically. The endoplasmic reticulum, however, present in a variety of tissues and species, including humans, contains a group of enzymes, the so-called cytochrome P-450 system or microsomal monooxygenase system, that convert benzo(a)pyrene and related polycyclic aromatic hydrocarbons to a variety of derivatives, including phenols and dihydrodiols. The intermediates in this oxidative process are epoxides, which can be subsequently hydrated or can form complexes with various substrates. The normal role of this system is to convert lipid-soluble foreign substances to more water-soluble substances that can be excreted (for a review of the metabolism of benzo(a)pyrene and several other types of carcinogens by the microsomal monooxygenase system, see Gelboin and Ts'o, 1978; Nebert and Negishi, 1982).

In a sense, carcinogenesis can be interpreted as an error in drug detoxification. In the process of detoxification, the highly reactive intermediates can accumulate, and, unless further metabolized, will react with cellular DNA and other macromolecules to form covalent adducts, thereby disrupting macromolecular synthesis and function. In the case of benzo(a)pyrene, the reactive intermediate is a specific diol epoxide. Its reaction with DNA is shown schematically in Figure 3–4. This pathway can be influenced by a variety of other biochemical pathways and indirectly with several aspects of intermediary metabolism. Various dietary and host factors will determine whether the diol epoxide derivative of benzo(a)pyrene will be detoxified by conjugation with glutathione or glucuronic acid, converted to a tetrol, or react with cellular DNA. The enzymes in these pathways are also induced by their substrates and by a variety of drugs. Genetic variations as well as tissue-specific factors influence the inducibility and absolute levels of these drug metabolizing enzymes. The host's genetic background, previous exposure history and nutritional status, a parallel exposure to other agents, and some tissue-specific factors will influence the likelihood that benzo(a)pyrene will flow through this pathway and attack cellular macromolecules or will be detoxified and excreted so that it is not carcinogenic. These principles can be generalized for a number of other carcinogens that are activated by the microsomal monooxygenase system (Miller, 1978; Gelboin and Ts'o, 1978; Weinstein, 1981a; Nebert and Negishi, 1982).

The complete chemical structures of the adducts formed between benzo(a)pyrene diol epoxide and nucleic acids have been documented in rodent and human cell systems (Jeffrey et al., 1980; Weinstein, 1981a). The major derivative (see Figure 3–5) consists of a guanine residue, linked via its 2-amino group to the 10 position of benzo(a)pyrene. The same adduct is formed in the DNAs of both rodent and human cells after exposure to the parent compound benzo(a)pyrene.

Structures of Carcinogen-DNA Adducts

The chemistry, metabolism, and nucleic acid interactions of several other types of carcinogens have been elucidated in considerable detail (Miller, 1978; Grover, 1979; Grunberger and Weinstein, 1979). The simple alkylating agents can methylate or ethylate any of the nitrogen or oxygens in all four bases in DNA, as well as the sugar residues and phosphates of the DNA backbone (Singer and Kroger, 1979). Although the N-7 position of guanine is generally the most extensive site of modification, current evidence indicates that the O-6 position of guanine is the most important site of attack with respect to mutagenesis and carcinogenesis. Because the O-6 position is involved in Watson-Crick base pairing, alkylation of O-6 interferes with hydrogen bonding, and thus produces base-pairing errors during nucleic acid replication.

The interaction of the larger polycyclic carcinogens is more complex, as illustrated by the aromatic amine carcinogen N-2-acetylaminofluorene (AAF), which, like benzo(a)pyrene, undergoes metabolic activation. Activation of AAF occurs on the amino group, and the major nucleic acid adduct results from linkage to the C-8 position of guanine residues (see Figure 3–5). This presents steric (or space-filling) problems in terms of accommodating the bulky AAF residue within the nucleic acid helix. AAF modification of DNA results in a distortion in the conformation of the DNA helix known as base displacement (Grunberger and Weinstein, 1979). The activated derivative of aflatoxin, which is also an epoxide, attacks the N-7 position of guanine

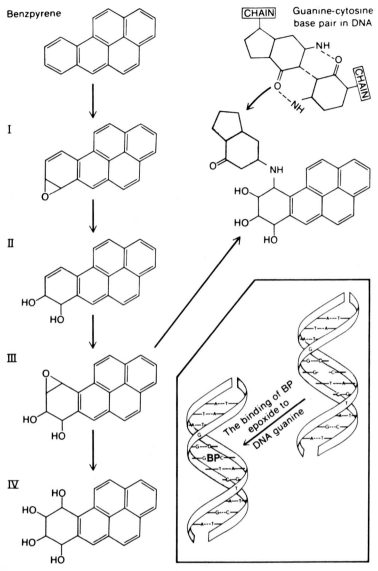

Figure 3–4. The detoxification and metabolic activation of benzo(a)pyrene. The detoxification of the carcinogen benzo(a)pyrene (BP) goes through several steps as it is made more water-soluble prior to excretion. One of the intermediate steps in this process (III) is capable of reacting with guanine in DNA (as shown in the diagram). This leads to a distortion in the structure and function of the DNA molecule. From Cairns, J.: *Cancer, Science and Society*. Freeman Press, San Francisco, 1978.

(see Figure 3–5). The conformational effects of this modification have not been documented in detail.

Different carcinogens can attack different sites on the DNA, and even a single carcinogen can form multiple types of adducts (see Figure 3–5). This complicates attempts to formulate a unified or simple theory relating specific types of DNA damage to the mechanism of carcinogenesis. The major carcinogen-DNA adducts are generally the same in diverse spe-

cies and tissues. This evidence provides some unity to the comparative chemistry of carcinogen-DNA adducts (Weinstein, 1981a). Studies with benzo(a)pyrene have emphasized the stereoselective aspects of carcinogen metabolism and DNA binding (Jeffrey *et al.*, 1980), and this principle is likely to apply to other polycyclic carcinogens.

In addition to carcinogens that form covalent adducts with DNA, it appears that certain carcinogenic agents (ionizing radiation, free

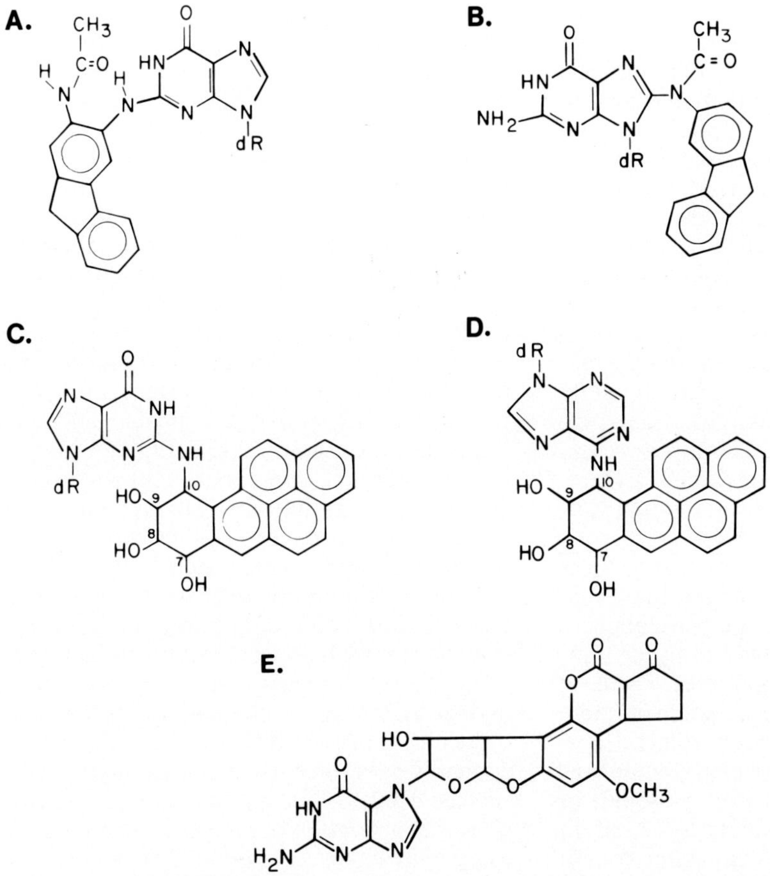

Figure 3–5.   The structures of several carcinogen-nucleoside adducts. *(A)* 2-Acetamido-3-(2′-deoxy-N²-guanosyl)-fluorene. *(B)* 3-[N-(2′-Deoxy-8-guanosyl)acetaamido]fluorene. *(C)* 2′-Deoxy-N²-(7,8,9,10-tetrahydro-7,β,8α,9α-trihydroxy-benzo[a]pyren-10-yl)guanosine. *(D)* 2′-Deoxy-N⁶(7,8,9,10-tetrahydro-7β,8α,9α,-tridroxybenzo[a]pyren-10-yl)adenosine. *(E)* 7-Guanyl-dihydro-hydroxyaflatoxin B₁. From Grunberger, D., and Weinstein, I. B.: Biochemical effects of the modification of nucleic acids by certain polycyclic aromatic carcinogens. In Cohn, W. E. (ed.): *Progress in Nucleic Acid Research and Molecular Biology.* Academic Press, New York, 1979.

radicals, activated oxygen, and others) produce their effects by a "hit-and-run" attack on the DNA. The resulting DNA damage can include single and double strand breaks and oxidation of the base residues. The detection and quantification of these effects is much more difficult than in the case of covalently bound chemical carcinogens.

Although most of the studies on carcinogen-DNA interactions have focused on nuclear DNA, it has been found that carcinogens also cause extensive modification of mitochondrial DNA (Backer and Weinstein, 1982). The functional importance of carcinogen attack on mitochondrial DNA is not known. This could cause disturbance in energy metabolism and/or perturbations in intracellular ion homeostasis, contributing to alterations in growth control in carcinogen-exposed cells. The modification of specific regions of chromatin by carcinogens is also an area of current research interest.

DNA Repair

The types of nucleic acid damage induced by environmental chemicals and radiation are not a *fait accompli,* because bacterial and mammalian cells are capable of repairing damaged DNA (for a detailed review of DNA repair, see Hanawalt *et al.,* 1982). Biochemical studies have revealed a multiplicity of DNA excision repair mechanisms, including N-glycosylases, phosphodiesterases, and even a transferase enzyme that simply removes an alkyl adduct from the O-6 position of guanine, thus restoring the normal nucleic acid structure. Little is known, however, about the enzymatic mechanisms by which polycyclic carcinogens like AAF, benzo(a)pyrene, or aflatoxin are removed. *In vivo* studies indicate that excision does occur in rodent and human cells (Cerutti, 1982). The multiplicity of excision mechanisms and enzymes that nature has evolved to protect our DNA from the onslaught of environmental chemicals is somewhat reassuring, but obviously our environment should not become so polluted that it overtaxes this defense mechanism. Patients with the autosomal recessive disease xeroderma pigmentosum are deficient in enzymes that excise thymine dimers, and are therefore highly susceptible to skin carcinogenesis induced by solar radiation (Hanawalt *et al.*, 1982). Other types of deficiencies in DNA repair may, in part, explain interindividual variations in carcinogen susceptibility.

Much less is known about the consequences of persistent lesions — for example, those that elude excision repair — and the consequences these have on DNA replication and gene transcription, particularly in eukaryotes. The level and duration of persistence of some of these adducts is appreciable (Cerutti, 1982). Complex host responses to such lesions, analogous to those controlled by the Rec A system in bacteria (Witkin, 1976), likely do exist in higher organisms and may play a key role in carcinogenesis (Ivanovic and Weinstein, 1980; Weinstein, 1981a). More detailed information regarding mechanisms of DNA repair can be found in Chapter 1.

Carcinogen-DNA Modification and the Mechanism of Initiation

Considerable evidence that the modification of DNA, RNA, and synthetic nucleic acids by carcinogens impairs their template activities during *in vitro* replication, transcription, and translation has been reported (Grunberger and Weinstein, 1980). These and other findings suggest several possible mechanisms by which covalent modification of DNA by carcinogens might initiate the carcinogenic process (see Table 3–7). The most frequently cited theory is random mutation, but there are several reasons to believe the mechanism is more complex (Weinstein, 1981a). These include: (1) the complex effects on template function; (2) the *in vitro* transformation of rodent cells by chemical carcinogens and radiation can occur with much greater efficiency than random mutation; (3) although human and rodent cell cultures are equally susceptible to mutagenesis, human cells appear to be much more resistant to cell transformation; (4) the notable lag between carcinogen exposure and tumor formation; and (5) the striking parallels between differentiation and multistage carcinogenesis. It appears that the induction of gene rearrangements, gene amplification, and/or alterations in the state of methylation of specific genes are likely to play a key, though probably not an exclusive, role in carcinogenesis (see Table 3–7). Increasing evidence suggests that activation of gene expression is often associated with a decrease in 5-methylcytidine content of the expressed gene, although other mechanisms also appear to be involved in the control of gene expression (Razin and Riggs, 1980).

Because of the diversity in types of chemical carcinogens, and the multistep nature of the carcinogenic process, it is possible that the types of responses to DNA damage by chemical carcinogens described earlier may not be mutually exclusive.

Table 3–7. Possible Molecular Mechanisms of Intiation of the Carcinogenesis Process

---

With permanant changes in DNA sequence
  Random point mutations
    Direct: Base substitution, frame shift, deletion in structural or regulatory gene
    Indirect: Induction of "SOS-type" error-prone DNA synthesis
  Ordered gene rearrangements: Transposition, amplification, deletion, integration of exogenous sequences, etc.

Without permanent changes in DNA sequence
  Altered chromatin structure, altered feedback loops, altered DNA methylation, etc.

Note: These mechanisms need not be mutually exclusive.
Note: For a detailed discussion, see Weinstein, I. B.: Current concepts and controversies in chemical carcinogenesis. *J. Supramol. Struct. Cell Biochem.,* **17**:99–120, 1981a.

TUMOR PROMOTION AND MULTIFACTOR INTERACTIONS

Two-Stage Skin Carcinogenesis

In the intact animal, carcinogenesis is a multistage process that can proceed over a considerable fraction of the lifespan of the individual, and the evolution of a fully malignant tumor is subject to a variety of promoting, as well as inhibitory, factors (Foulds, 1969; Slaga *et al.*, 1978; Weinstein, 1980, 1981a). The most powerful paradigm for understanding these complex phenomena has been the model of two-stage carcinogenesis on mouse skin (see Figure 3-6). In this model, at least two stages, initiation and promotion, have been defined clearly (Berenblum, 1975; Slaga *et al.*, 1978). Each of these stages is elicited or inhibited by different types of agents. The two-stages, in addition, have quite different biologic properties (see Table 3-8): The major difference is that initiation appears to involve DNA damage, which is not the case in promotion. The two-stage mouse skin carcinogenesis system has also served as a paradigm for studies on the multistage aspects of carcinogenesis in several other tissues and species. Evidence is available to show that hepatocellular cancer, bladder cancer, colon cancer, and breast cancer proceed via processes analogous to initiation and promotion (Slaga *et al.*, 1978; Greenebaum and Weinstein, 1981). The concept of promotion appears to be particularly relevant to the development of human breast cancer (Weinstein, 1981c). The striking synergistic interaction between cigarette smoking and asbestos exposure in the causation of human lung cancer (as reported by Selikoff

and Hammond, 1979) may also reflect interactions between initiating and promoting factors, although other explanations have not been excluded.

Very few specific cellular or biochemical markers for the action of tumor promoters were available until recently. Important advances have been made in studies on the biochemical effects of the phorbol ester tumor promoters in cell culture systems, and on mouse skin. A number of biologic effects of these compounds have been documented that can be classified into three categories: (1) Mimicry of transformation, (2) modulation of differentiation, and (3) membrane effects (for a review see Slaga *et al.*, 1978; Weinstein *et al.*, 1980).

Mimicry of Transformation and Modulation of Differentiation

Perhaps the most intriguing capacities of the potent tumor promoter 12-0-tetradecanoyl-phorbol-13-acetate (TPA) and related phorbol esters are their abilities to induce in normal cells the expression of several phenotypic traits characteristic of tumor cells and to enhance the further expression of some of these traits in cells that are already transformed (Weinstein *et al.*, 1980). These findings reinforce a recurring theme in cancer biology: That the individual phenotypic properties of tumor cells preexist but may be dormant in the normal tissue of origin. The phorbol esters provide potent pharmacologic agents for studying the cellular mechanisms that control the expression of these genes.

Since it is likely that carcinogenesis involves major disturbances in differentiation, it is of interest that TPA is a highly potent inhibitor or

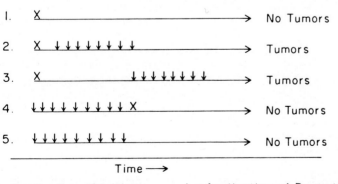

X = Application of Initiator   ↓ = Application of Promoter

Figure 3-6. Schematic diagram of experiments demonstrating the characteristic properties of two-stage carcinogenesis on mouse skin. See also Table 3-8. From Pitot, H. C.; Barsness, L.; and Kitigawa, T.: Stages in the process of hepatocarcinogenesis in rat liver. In Slaga, T. J.; Sivak, A.; and Boutwell, R. K. (eds.): *Carcinogenesis, Volume 2: Mechanisms of Tumor Promotion and Cocarcinogenesis.* Raven Press, New York, 1978.

Table 3–8. Biologic Properties of Initiating and Promoting Agents

INITIATING AGENTS	PROMOTING AGENTS
1. Carcinogenic by themselves — "solitary carcinogens"	1. Not carcinogenic alone
2. Must be given before the promoting agent	2. Must be given after the initiating agent
3. Single exposure sufficient	3. Require prolonged exposure
4. Action "irreversible" and additive	4. Action reversible (at early stage) and not additive
5. No apparent threshold	5. Possible threshold
6. Yield electrophiles — bind covalently to cell macromolecules	6. No evidence of covalent binding
7. Mutagenic	7. Not mutagenic

Adapted from Weinstein, I. B.; Mufson, R. A.; Lee, L.-S.; Fisher, P. B.; Laskin, J.; Horowitz, A. D.; and Ivanovic, V.: Membrane and other biochemical effects of the phorbol esters and their relevance to tumor promotion. In Pullman, B.; Ts'o, P. O. P.; and Gelboin, H. (eds.): *Carcinogenesis: Fundamental Mechanisms and Environmental Effects.* D. Reidel, Boston, 1980.

inducer of differentiation in a variety of cell systems (Weinstein *et al.,* 1980). The basal cells in the adult epidermis are continually dividing, yet the tissue is in a state of balanced growth because of asymmetric division of stem cells. One daughter cell remains a stem cell, and the other is committed to keratinize and terminally differentiate, irreversibly losing its growth potential. If an "initiated" stem cell were restrained to this mode of division, it could not increase its proportion in the stem cell pool. If this mode of tissue renewal were interrupted by a tumor promoter, however, the initiated cell could undergo exponential division, yielding a clone of similar cells. Because TPA can also induce phenotypic changes in cells that mimic those of transformed cells, the microenvironment of a clone of such cells might itself enhance their further outgrowth and development into a tumor. Clonal expansion of the population of initiated cells would provide, in addition, a larger population from which variants that have progressed to later stages of neoplasia might emerge.

Phorboid Receptors and Membrane Effects

Studies of the cell culture effects of the phorbol ester tumor promoters suggest that they act by binding to and usurping the function of membrane-associated receptors normally utilized by an endogenous growth factor. Specific high-affinity phorbol ester receptors have been demonstrated in a variety of both normal and transformed cell cultures and in a variety of normal tissues (Driedger and Blumberg, 1980; Shoyab and Todaro, 1980; Horowitz *et al.,* 1981). Recent studies indicate that these re-

ceptors are actually a complex between membrane lipid and a calcium- and phospholipid-dependent enzyme designated protein kinase C (Castagna *et al.,* 1982; Nishizuka, 1984). Indeed, TPA and related compounds are potent activators of protein kinase C (Castagna *et al.,* 1982; Nishizuka, 1984). In general, the abilities of a series of TPA analogs and two recently discovered tumor promoters — teleocidin and aplysia toxin (Sugimura, 1982) — to bind to these receptors and to activate protein kinase C correlates with their known potencies in cell culture and with their activities as tumor promoters on mouse skin (Weinstein, 1981a; Horowitz *et al.,* 1981; Nishizuka, 1984). These results provide evidence that these receptors mediate the biologic action of the phorbol esters. It is possible that the phorboid receptor-protein kinase C system might play a role during normal development by enhancing the outgrowth of new stem cell populations. In the adult, this same system might enhance expansion of stem cell populations during hyperplasia, wound healing, and regeneration. During tumor promotion, aberrant stem cells (generated during initiation) might undergo preferential clonal expansion as a result of excessive stimulation of the phorboid receptor system. This model has obvious implications in terms of the normal control of proliferation of stem cell populations, and the possible role of hormones, growth factors, and protein kinases in the carcinogenic process.

The earliest responses of cells to the phorbol ester tumor promoters involve alterations in membrane function. These include altered ion flux and nutrient uptake, increased phospholipid turnover, and altered function of certain membrane-associated receptors (Weinstein *et al.,* 1980). Some of these membrane effects occur within minutes and are not blocked by inhibitors of protein or RNA synthesis. They are mediated directly at the level of the cell membrane, presumably through the activation of protein kinase C and possibly other membrane-associated proteins. A variety of mitogens and polypeptide growth factors induce somewhat similar membrane effects, perhaps by direct or indirect activation of protein kinases; the resultant phosphorylation of specific membrane and cytoplasmic proteins presumably alters gene expression, growth, and differentiation.

Little is known about the mechanism of action of other classes of tumor promoters and the specific biochemical events associated with tumor promotion in tissues other than skin (Greenebaum and Weinstein, 1981). The results obtained with the phorbol esters suggest several hypotheses. It is possible, for example, that the important role of dietary lipid as a cofactor in carcinogenesis (as reviewed by Carroll and Khor, 1975) may be mediated via changes in membrane lipid metabolism and activation of cellular protein kinase activity, analogous to the effects induced by the phorbol ester tumor promoters (Weinstein, 1981a, 1981c). Table 3-9 lists various hypotheses to explain the effects of dietary lipid on incidence of breast and colon cancer. There is considerable interest in the possibility that a reduction in total dietary lipid might decrease the incidence of these two diseases.

Chemical-Viral Interactions

Several examples in which initiating carcinogens, tumor promoters, or other chemical and physical agents interact synergistically with viruses in the carcinogenic process, both

Table 3-9. Possible Roles of Dietary Fat in Carcinogenesis

Breast cancer
1. Fat depots convert androstenedione to estrone
2. High dietary fat → ↑ pituitary prolactin secretion
3. Direct effect on membrane lipids in target tissue

Colon cancer
1. ↑ Fecal cholesterol metabolites and bile salts and altered microflora → initiating carcinogens
2. ↑ Bile salts act as tumor promoters
3. Altered formation of fecal mutagens
4. Direct effect on membrane lipids in target tissue

Adapted from Weinstein, I. B.: Studies on the mechanism of action of tumor promoters and their relevance to mammary carcinogenesis. In McGrath, C. M.; Brennan, M. J.; and Rich, M. A. (eds.): *Cell Biology of Breast Cancer.* Academic Press, New York, 1981.

in vivo and in cell culture, have been reported (Fisher and Weinstein, 1980; Greenebaum and Weinstein, 1981). It seems likely that certain human cancers may be due to interactions between chemical agents and types of viruses that have little or no oncogenic potential independently. This may be the case for liver cancer in Africa, nasopharyngeal cancer in Asia, and Burkitt's lymphoma. Hepatitis B virus infection, perhaps in combination with exposure to aflatoxin, appears to be an important factor in the former case; and Epstein-Barr virus in combination with unknown environmental factors have been implicated in the latter two cases (see Chapter 3D). The primary effects of the phorbol ester tumor promoters seem to be a result of alterations in cell surface membrane structure and function. Current evidence suggests that the proteins coded for by several tumor viruses responsible for neoplastic transformation act at or near the cell surface membrane. These findings suggest that alterations in membrane function play a central role not only in chemical carcinogenesis, but also during maintenance of the tumor cell phenotype in cells transformed by oncogenic viruses. Greater progress might be made in further studies on human cancer causation and prevention if it is assumed that certain human cancers result from complex interactions between viruses and chemicals and that the final pathways by which both classes of agents produce cell transformation may be quite similar.

A UNIFIED THEORY OF MULTISTAGE CARCINOGENESIS

A unified theory of multistage carcinogenesis explains carcinogenesis within the framework of normal development and differentiation and links to current theories about the origins and mechanisms of action of certain tumor viruses.

It has been postulated (Herskowitz *et al.,* 1980; Finnegan, 1981) that the establishment of normal populations of stem cells involves gene rearrangements and that DNA damage by initiating carcinogens might induce aberrant gene rearrangement and aberrant stem cells (Weinstein, 1981a). The subsequent role of tumor promoters, hormones, and certain growth factors could be to enhance the outgrowth of these aberrant stem cells, as well as to "switch on" their abnormal programs of differentiation, just as normal growth factors appear to induce normal stem cells to proliferate and express their specialized functions. The phorbol ester tumor promoters presumably accomplish this by binding to and activating protein kinase C, an enzyme system that might play a role in the normal control of stem cell replication and differentiation. Following repeated exposure of initiated cells to a tumor promoter, a neoplastic population might eventually emerge that grows autonomously in the absence of the promoter, possibly due to further changes in genome structure.

The mechanism by which the transformed phenotype is eventually "locked in" with respect to constitutive expression is not known.

Tumor progression and the further evolution of tumors into a more heterogeneous cell population may involve additional steps occurring by mechanisms similar to those described above as well as by the acquisition of chromosomal anomalies. The list of specific chromosomal abnormalities associated with specific types of human cancer is rapidly growing (Klein, 1981; Rowley and Testa, 1982). Gross chromosomal changes may play an important role in multistep carcinogenesis although it seems likely that they are primarily associated with the latter stages of the carcinogenic process, particularly tumor progression (Wolman, 1983). Recent evidence suggests that oncogene amplification may also play a role in tumor progression (Robertson, 1984).

A major challenge to future research in carcinogenesis is to identify the specific host genes involved in the transformation of cells by chemical and physical agents and to utilize recombinant DNA techniques in analyzing the state of integration and/or expression of these genes in normal and carcinogen-transformed cells. Recent studies (Cooper, 1982; Weinberg, 1983) indicate that the technique of DNA transfection may prove to be extremely useful for this research. Studies of the RNA sarcoma viruses have led to the theory that they originated from the recombination of retroviruses with specific oncogenes (also called protooncogenes) endogenous to normal vertebrate species (Bishop, 1983). Infection of cells by these viruses leads to the integration of these oncogenes into aberrant sites in the host genome, where they are expressed at high levels, leading to the transformed state. It is possible that the homologous cellular protooncogenes are involved in the transformation of cells by chemical carcinogens. In this case, however, DNA damage might trigger various types of changes in cellular oncogenes including point mutations, sequence deletions or insertions, chromosome translocation, amplification, and/or constitutive expression. If this hypothesis is correct, then, by utilizing the technique of DNA transfection and nucleic acid probes derived from cloned oncogenes, it might be possible to rapidly identify the host genes that play a role in the causation of a variety of human cancers. Recent studies utilizing these techniques have implicated specific protooncogenes in the causation of several types of human cancer (Der *et al.*, 1982; Goldfarb *et al.*, 1982; Parada *et al.*, 1982; Weinberg, 1983). More extensive studies utilizing a variety of approaches will be required, however, to fully understand the roles of cellular oncogenes in specific stages of the carcinogenic process. It seems likely that the widespread disturbances in gene expression seen in cancer cells may also reflect abnormalities in DNA methylation and in the function of DNA promoter and enhancer sequences (Weinstein *et al.*, 1984).

MOLECULAR EPIDEMIOLOGY AND CANCER PREVENTION

Limitations of Current Approaches

Although major progress has been made, there are still great gaps in our understanding of the fundamental mechanisms involved in the carcinogenic process. Several concepts and methods have already emerged that provide new approaches to identifying potential human carcinogens and improve the science of risk assessment and extrapolation in the field of environmental carcinogenesis. Although conventional approaches in cancer epidemiology have provided a wealth of information, they have serious limitations for identifying specific causal factors, particularly in human cancers that result from multifactor interactions. Such studies are largely retrospective rather than predictive, and unless very large numbers of individuals are studied, they are not highly sensitive. Although animal bioassays and the newly developed short-term tests (as described by Ames, 1979; Hollstein *et al.*, 1979; Fisher and Weinstein, 1981) are extremely sensitive and useful for detecting potential human carcinogens, a paucity of information on how such data can be applied to humans still exists (Weinstein, 1981b; Perera and Weinstein, 1982).

Molecular Cancer Epidemiology

This problem will not be resolved by continued research utilizing the same types of studies. A different type of methodology should be developed in which studies on human cancer causation combine epidemiologic methods with laboratory techniques; a methodology whereby specific biochemical and molecular quantities are measured in human tissues and in various biologic fluids. This approach is known as "molecular cancer epidemiology" (Perera and Weinstein, 1982). A variety of highly sensitive and specific laboratory procedures are now available that can be used in humans as markers or indicators of specific factors relating to (1) genetic and acquired host susceptibility; (2) metabolism and tissue levels of carcinogens; (3) levels of covalent adducts formed between carcinogens and cellular macromolecules; and (4) markers of early cellular responses to carcinogen exposure; for example, sister chromatid exchange, DNA repair, altered gene expression, and mutation.

A promising tool for studies on molecular cancer epidemiology has been provided by the recent development of highly sensitive immunoassays for carcinogen-DNA adducts (Poirier et al., 1980; Muller and Rajewsky, 1981; Poirier, 1981; Perera and Weinstein, 1982). This approach might provide a tissue dosimeter for carcinogen exposure that would be more valid than assays of ambient levels and total dosage and that would take into account complex pharmacodynamic variables including metabolic activation of the substance in question. Surgical specimens, autopsy material, skin biopsies, peripheral white blood cells, and placental tissue are all possible sources of material for study. Detection and quantification of certain carcinogen-DNA adducts in the urine, as a result of their excision from DNA, should also be possible, greatly facilitating epidemiologic studies. Within the next few years these methods should become available in clinical and epidemiologic studies.

These laboratory methods, along with clinical and epidemiologic studies, as well as further advances in our understanding of basic methods of carcinogenesis, will bring us closer to the goal of primary cancer prevention.

REFERENCES

Ames, B.: Identifying environmental chemicals causing mutations and cancer. Science, **204:**587–593, 1979.

Armstrong, B., and Doll, R.: Environmental factors and cancer incidence and mortality in different countries with special references to dietary practices. Int. J. Cancer, **15:**617–631, 1975.

Backer, J., and Weinstein, I. B.: Interaction of benzo(a)pyrene and its dihydrodiol epoxide derivative with nuclear and mitochondrial DNA in C3H 10T1/2 cell cultures. Cancer Res., **42:**2764–2769, 1982.

Berenblum, I.: Sequential aspects of chemical carcinogenesis: Skin. In Becker, F. F. (ed): Cancer: A Comprehensive Treatise, Vol. 1. Plenum Press, New York, 1975.

Bishop, J. M.: Cellular oncogenes and retroviruses. Ann. Rev. Biochem., **52:**301–354, 1983.

Ca: A Cancer Journal for Clinicians, **33:**10, 1983.

Cairns, J.: Cancer, Science and Society. W. H. Freeman & Company, Publishers, San Francisco, 1978.

Carroll, K. K., and Khor, H. T.: Dietary fat in relation to tumorigenesis. Prog. Biochem. Pharmacol., **10:**308–353, 1975.

Castagna, M.; Takai, U.; Kaibuchi, K.; Sano, K.; Kikkawa, U.; and Nishizuka, Y.: Direct activation of calcium-activated, phospholipid-dependent protein kinase by tumor promoting phorbol esters. J. Biol. Chem, **257:**7847–7851, 1982.

Cerutti, P. A.: Persistence of carcinogen-DNA adducts in cultured mammalian cells. In Harris, C. C., and Cerutti, P. A. (eds): Mechanisms of Chemical Carcinogenesis. Alan R. Liss, Inc., New York, 1982.

Cooper, G. M.: Cellular transforming genes. Science, **218:**801–806, 1982.

Der, C. J.; Krontiris, T. G.; and Cooper, G. M.: Transforming of human bladder and lung carcinoma cell lines are homologous to the ras gene of Harvey and Kirsten sarcoma viruses. Proc. Natl. Acad. Sci. USA, **79:**3637–3640, 1982.

Driedger, P. E., and Blumberg, P. M.: Specific binding of phorbol ester tumor promoters. Proc. Natl. Acad. Sci. USA, **77:**567–571, 1980.

Finnegan, J.: Transposable elements and proviruses. Nature, **292:**800–801, 1981.

Fisher, P. B., and Weinstein, I. B.: Chemical viral interactions and multistep aspects of cell transformation. In Montesano, R.; Bartsch, H.; and Tomatis, L. (eds.): Molecular and Cellular Aspects of Carcinogen Screening Tests. IARC Scientific Publications, Lyon, France, 1980.

Fisher, P. B., and Weinstein, I. B.: In Vitro screening tests for potential carcinogens. In Sontag, J. M. (ed.): Carcinogens in Industry and the Environment. Marcel Dekker, Inc., New York, 1981.

Foulds, L.: Neoplastic Development, Vol. 1. Academic Press, New York and London, 1969.

Gelboin, H. V., and Ts'o, P.O.P. (eds.): Polycyclic Hydrocarbons and Cancer, Vols. 1 and 2. Academic Press, New York, 1978.

Goldfarb, M.; Shimizu, K.; Perucho, M.; and Wigler, M.: Isolation and preliminary characterization of a human transforming gene from T24 bladder carcinoma cells. Nature, **296:**404–409, 1982.

Greenebaum, E., and Weinstein, I. B.: Relevance of the concept of tumor promotion to the causation of human cancer. In Fenoglio, C. M., and Wolff, M. (eds.): Progress in Surgical Pathology. Masson Publishing USA, Inc., New York, 1981.

Grover, P. L. (ed): Chemical Carcinogens and DNA. CRC Press, Boca Raton, Florida, 1979.

Grunberger, D., and Weinstein, I. B.: Conformational changes in nucleic acids modified by chemical carcinogens. In Grover, P. L. (ed.): *Chemical Carcinogens and DNA.* CRC Press, Boca Raton, Florida, 1979.

Grunberger, D., and Weinstein, I. B.: Biochemical effects of the modification of nucleic acids by certain polycyclic aromatic carcinogens. In Cohn, W. E. (ed.): *Progress in Nucleic Acid Research and Molecular Biology.* Academic Press, New York, 1979.

Hanawalt, P. C.; Cooper, P. K.; Ganesan, A. K.; Lloyd, R. S.; Smith, C. A.; and Zolan, M. E.: Repair responses to DNA damage: Enzymatic pathways in *E. coli* and human cells. In Harris, C. C., and Cerutti, P. A. (eds.): *Mechanisms of Chemical Carcinogenesis.* Alan R. Liss, Inc., New York, 1982.

Heidelberger, C.: Chemical carcinogenesis. *Annu. Rev. Biochem.,* **44:** 79–121, 1975.

Herskowitz, I.; Blair, L.; Forbes, D.; Hicks, J.; Kassir, Y.; Kushner, P.; Rine, J.; Sprague, G.; and Strathern, J.: Control of cell type in the yeast *Saccharomyces cerevisiae* and a hypothesis for development in higher eukaryotes. In Leighton, T., and Loomis, W. F. (eds.): *Molecular Genetics of Development.* Academic Press, New York, 1980.

Hiatt, H. H.; Watson, J. D.; and Winsten, J. A. (eds.): *Origins of Human Cancer.* Cold Spring Harbor Laboratory, Cold Spring Harbor, New York, 1977.

Higginson, J., and Muir, C. S.: The role of epidemiology in elucidating the importance of environmental factors in human cancer. *Cancer Detect. Prev.,* **1:**79–105, 1976.

Hollstein, M.; McCann, J.; Angelosanta, F. A.; and Nichols, W. W.: Short-term tests for carcinogens and mutagens. *Mutat. Res.,* **65:**133–226, 1979.

Horowitz, A. D.; Greenebaum, E.; and Weinstein, I. B.: Identification of receptors for phorbol ester tumor promoters in intact mammalian cells and of an inhibitor of receptor binding in biologic fluids. *Proc. Natl. Acad. Sci. USA,* **78:**2315–2319, 1981.

IARC: *IARC Monographs on the Evaluation of the Carcinogenic Risk of Chemicals to Humans: Chemicals and Industrial Processes Associated with Cancer in Humans, Supplement 4.* IARC, Lyon, France, 1982.

Ivanovic, V., and Weinstein, I. B.: Genetic factors in *Escherichia coli* that affect cell killing and mutagenesis induced by benzo(a)pyrene-7, 8-dihydrodiol 9, 10-oxide. *Cancer Res.,* **40:**3508–3510, 1980.

Jeffrey, A. M.; Kinoshita, T.; Santella, R. M.; Grunberger, D.; Katz, L.; and Weinstein, I. B.: The chemistry of polycyclic aromatic hydrocarbon-DNA adducts. In Pullman, B.; Ts'o P.O.P.; and Gelboin, H. (eds.): *Carcinogenesis: Fundamental Mechanisms and Environmental Effects.* R. Reidel Pub. Co., Amsterdam, 1980.

Klein, G.: The role of gene dosage and genetic transpositions in carcinogenesis. *Nature,* **294:**313–318, 1981.

Mason, T. J.; McKay, F. W.; Hoover, R.; Blot, W. J.; and Fraumeni, J. F.: *Atlas of Cancer Mortality for U. S. Counties 1950–1969,* DHEW Publication No. (NIH)75–780. U. S. Dept. Health, Education and Welfare, Washington, D. C., 1975.

Miller, E. C.: Some current perspectives on chemical carcinogenesis in humans and experimental animals: Presidential address. *Cancer Res.,* **38:**1479–1496, 1978.

Muller, R., and Rajewsky, M. F.: Antibodies specific for DNA components structurally modified by chemical carcinogens. *J. Cancer Res. Clin. Oncol.,* **102:**99–113, 1981.

National Cancer Institute: *Monograph 59 — Cancer Mortality in the United States 1950–1977,* NIH Publication No. 82-2435, U. S. Dept. of Health and Human Services, Washington, D. C., 1982.

National Cancer Institute, Common Occupational Cancers, personal communication, 1980.

Nebert, D. W., and Negishi, M.: Multiple forms of cytochrome P-450 and the importance of molecular biology and evolution. *Biochem. Pharmacol.,* **31:**2311–2317, 1982.

Nishizuka, Y.: The role of protein kinase C in cell surface signal transduction and tumor promotion. *Nature,* **308:**693–698, 1984.

Parada, L. F.; Tabin, C. J.; Shih, C.; and Weinberg, R. A.: Human EJ bladder carcinoma oncogene is homologue of Harvey Sarcoma virus *ras* gene. *Nature,* **297:**474–478, 1982.

Perera, F. P., and Weinstein, I. B.: Molecular epidemiology and carcinogen-DNA adduct detection: New approaches to studies of human cancer causation. *J. Chron. Dis.,* **35:**581–600, 1982.

Pitot, H. C.; Barsness, L.; and Kitigawa, T.: Stages in the process of hepatocarcinogenesis in rat liver. In Slaga, T. J.; Sivak, A.; and Boutwell, R. K. (eds.): *Carcinogenesis, Volume 2: Mechanisms of Tumor Promotion and Cocarcinogenesis.* Raven Press, New York, 1978.

Poirier, M. C.: Antibodies to carcinogen-DNA adducts. *J. N. C. I.,* **67:**515–519, 1981.

Poirier, M. C.; Santella, R. S.; Weinstein, I. B.; Grunberger, D.; and Yuspa, S. H.: Quantitation of benzo(a)pyrene-deoxyguanosine adducts by radioimmunoassay. *Cancer Res.,* **40:**412–416, 1980.

Pott, P.: Cancer scroti. *Chirurgical Observations.* Hawes, Clarke and Collins, London, 1775.

Razin, A., and Riggs, A.: DNA methylation and gene function. *Science,* **210:**604–610, 1980.

Robertson, M.: Progress in malignancy. *Nature,* **309,** 812–813, 1984.

Rowley, J., and Testa, J. R.: Chromosome abnormalities in malignant hematologic diseases. *Adv. Cancer Res.,* **36:**103–143, 1982.

Selikoff, I. J., and Hammond, E. C.: Asbestos and smoking (editorial). *J.A.M.A.,* **242:**458–459, 1979.

Shoyab, M., and Todaro, G.: Specific high affinity cell membrane receptors for biologically active phorbol and ingenol esters. *Nature,* **288:**451–455, 1980.

Singer, B., and Kroger, B.: Participation of modified nucleosides in translation and transcription. *Prog. Nucleic Acid Res. Mol. Biol.,* **23:**151–194, 1979.

Slaga, T. J.; Sivak, A.; and Boutwell, R. K. (eds.): *Carcinogenesis, Volume 2: Mechanisms of Tumor Promotion and Cocarcinogenesis.* Raven Press, New York, 1978.

Sugimura, T.: A view of a cancer researcher on environmental mutagens. In Sugimura, T.; Kondo, S.; and Takebe, H. (eds.): *Environmental Mutagens and Carcinogens.* University of Tokyo Press, Tokyo; Alan R. Liss, Inc., New York, 1982.

Weinberg, R. A.: A molecular basis of cancer. *Sci. Am.,* **249:**126–142, 1983.

Weinstein, I. B.: Molecular and cellular mechanisms of chemical carcinogenesis. In Crooke, S., and Prestayko, A. (eds.): *Cancer and Chemotherapy, Vol. 1: Introduction to Neoplasia and Anti-Neoplastic Chemotherapy.* Academic Press, New York, 1980.

Weinstein, I. B.: Current concepts and controversies in chemical carcinogenesis. *J. Supramol. Struct. Cell. Biochem.,* **17:**99–120, 1981a.

Weinstein, I. B.: The scientific basis for carcinogen detection and primary cancer prevention. *Cancer,* **47:**1133–1141, 1981b.

Weinstein, I. B.: Studies on the mechanism of action of tumor promoters and their relevance to mammary carcinogenesis. In McGrath, C. M.; Brennan, M. J.; and Rich, M. A. (eds.): *Cell Biology of Breast Cancer.* Academic Press, New York, 1981c.

Weinstein, I. B.; Gattoni-Celli, S.; Kirschmeier, P.; Hsiao, W.; Horowitz, A.; and Jeffrey, A.: Cellular targets and host genes in multistage carcinogenesis. *Fed. Proc.,* **43**:2287–2294, 1984.

Weinstein, I. B.; Mufson, R. A.; Lee, L. -S.; Fisher, P. B.; Laskin, J.; Horowitz, A. D.; and Ivanovic, V.: Membrane and other biochemical effects of the phorbol esters and their relevance to tumor promotion. In Pullman, B.; Ts'o, P.O.P.; and Gelboin, H. (eds.): *Carcinogenesis: Fundamental Mechanisms and Environmental Effects.* D. Reidel, Boston, 1980.

Witkin, E. M.: ultraviolet mutagenesis and inducible DNA repair in *E. coli. Bacteriol. Rev.,* **40**:869–907, 1976.

Wolman, S. R.: Karyotypic progression in human tumors. *Cancer Metastasis Reviews,* **2**:257–293, 1983.

C. RADIATION

Arthur C. Upton

INTRODUCTION

Carcinogenic effects of ionizing radiation, discovered at the turn of the century, have been investigated more thoroughly than those of any other environmental agent. The study of these effects received its initial impetus from the growing use of radiation in medicine, science, and industry. More recently, far-reaching developments in atomic energy, notably the production of nuclear weapons and the expanding utilization of atomic energy for electric power, have created a climate of concern about the potential carcinogenic risks of low-level irradiation.

Because of the wealth of our information about the carcinogenic effects of ionizing radiation, including extensive epidemiologic as well as experimental data, our knowledge of such effects is helpful in considering the carcinogenic effects of other cancer-causing agents.

HISTORIC BACKGROUND

The first cancer attributed to radiation was an epidermoid carcinoma involving the hand of a radiologist (Frieben, 1902). In ensuing decades, before adequate steps were taken to curtail exposure, scores of similar cases were reported (Furth and Lorenz, 1954; Upton, 1975). The cancers were predominantly squamous cell and basal cell carcinomas but also included fibrosarcomas. Their clinical appearance was characteristically preceded by a long

The author thanks Ms. Jean Smith for assistance in preparation of this manuscript.

history of radiation dermatitis (Furth and Lorenz, 1954).

Leukemia was another occupational disease noted in pioneer radiologists, in whom the first cluster of cases was reported as early as 1911 (von Jagie *et al.,* 1911). Although the incidence of the disease in U.S. radiologists who entered practice in the first decades of the century was several times higher than normal (Henshaw and Hawkins, 1944; Lorenz, 1944), the excess has virtually disappeared in recent cohorts owing to improved safety standards (Matanoski, 1981).

The increased frequency of osteosarcomas and cranial sinus carcinomas in radium-dial painters that was noted as early as 1929 (Martland, 1931) is also of historic interest. The induction of such growths in these workers resulted from their practice of pointing their fine-tipped camel's hair brushes between their lips, gradually ingesting sufficient quantities of radium and mesothorium to cause radiation osteitis in many victims (Martland, 1931).

Cancer of the lung in miners of radioactive ore is another historic example. Known for centuries as an occupational disability among pitchblende miners in Czechoslovakia, this disease was not attributed to their inhalation of radon until fairly recently (Furth and Lorenz, 1954). The incidence of lung cancer in uranium miners, fluorspar miners, and other underground miners who are exposed occupationally to high concentrations of radon is also increased in relation to the intensity and duration of exposure (NAS, 1980).

Cancers of many types and sites have been observed to be increased in frequency in atomic-bomb survivors of Hiroshima and Nagasaki (Beebe *et al.,* 1978). Leukemia was the first cancer to be noted: The increase in the disease became evident within five years after the bombs were dropped. Cancers of the breast, lung, thyroid gland, stomach, lymphoid tissues, and other organs have also increased in frequency, to a degree that has varied with the type of cancer in question, the dose of radiation received, age at the time of irradiation, and sex (NAS, 1980; Beebe, 1982).

The increased incidence of various cancers in atomic-bomb survivors is paralleled by similar increases in patients who have received varying doses of radiation to different organs in medical treatment or diagnosis. These patients include (1) Patients given x-ray therapy to the spine for ankylosing spondylitis, in whom an excess of leukemias and tumors in certain of the irradiated sites (*e.g.,* bone, lung, pharynx, stomach, and pancreas) has subsequently been observed (Smith and Doll, 1981); (2) patients given x-ray therapy to the breast for mastitis and other benign diseases, in whom an excess of carcinomas in the irradiated breast tissue has been observed (Shore *et al.,* 1977); (3) women treated for menorrhagia by ovarian irradiation, in whom an excess of leukemias and gastrointestinal tumors has been observed (Smith and Doll, 1976); (4) patients given x-ray therapy to the mediastinum in infancy for enlargement of the thymus or other non-neoplastic conditions, in whom an excess of thyroid tumors, leukemias, osteochondromas, salivary gland tumors, and other neoplasms in irradiated sites has been observed (Hempelmann *et al.,* 1975); (5) patients treated with x-rays for various non-neoplastic lesions, in whom solid tumors (chiefly sarcomas) have been observed to arise subsequently at the site of irradiation (Jones, 1953; Pinkston and Sekine, 1982); (6) patients treated with radium 226 for ankylosing spondylitis or tuberculous osteitis, in whom an excess of skeletal tumors has been observed (Mays *et al.,* 1978); (7) patients given x-ray therapy to the scalp in childhood for treatment of tinea capitis, in whom an excess of skin, thyroid, and brain tumors has been observed (Shore *et al.,* 1976); (8) patients treated with phosphorus 32 for polycythemia vera, in whom an excess of leukemias has been observed (Modan and Lilienfeld, 1965); (9) patients treated with iodine 131 for adenocarcinoma of the thyroid gland, in whom an excess of leukemias has been observed (Pochin, 1960); (10) patients injected intravascularly with colloidal thorium oxide (thorotrast) for

angiographic examination, in whom an excess of leukemias, hepatic hemangioendotheliomas, and other tumors has been observed (Faber, 1978; Mole, 1978); (11) women subjected to repeated fluoroscopic examination of the lungs in the treatment of pulmonary tuberculosis with artificial pneumothorax, in whom an excess of breast cancers has been observed (Boice *et al.,* 1979); and (12) children exposed prenatally during the radiographic examination of their mothers, in whom an excess of childhood leukemias and other cancers has been observed (UN, 1977; NAS, 1980).

In natives of the Marshall Islands who were exposed accidentally to nuclear fallout in 1954 an excess of thyroid tumors has been observed. In those who were heavily exposed at less than 10 years of age the incidence of thyroid nodules increased from zero to more than 80% between eight and 16 years after exposure. The development of tumors was associated with hypothyroidism in some of these islanders, in whom the dose to the thyroid was estimated at approximately 7 to 14 Sv from internally deposited radioiodine and 1.75 Sv from external gamma rays (Conard *et al.,* 1980).

Confirming early observations on the carcinogenic effects of radiation in human populations were parallel studies of radiation carcinogenesis in laboratory animals (see Table 3-10) (The early literature has been reviewed by Lacassagne, 1945a,b; Brues, 1951; Furth and Lorenz, 1954. More recent surveys have been published by Casarett, 1965; Upton, 1967; UN, 1972, 1977.)

NATURE, TYPES, AND LEVELS OF RADIATION

Ionizing radiations include: (1) Those radiations of the electromagnetic spectrum that are characterized by relatively short wavelength and high frequency; and (2) electrons, protons, neutrons, alpha particles, and other particulate radiations of varying masses and charges. When such radiations penetrate matter, they lose their energy through interactions with atoms in their path, resulting in the formation of ions and reactive radicals. These, in turn, damage molecules in their vicinity and thereby cause biochemical lesions.

In general, the density of ionizations along the path of an impinging radiation or their rate of linear energy transfer (LET) increase with

Table 3-10. Incidence of Leukemia in Japanese Atomic-Bomb Survivors in Life Span Study, Hiroshima and Nagasaki, 1950-1971 (Cases from Leukemia Registry)

T65 DOSE rads (kerma)	AVERAGE KERMA		NO. PERSON-YEARS	NO. CASES*			NO. CASES PER 100,000 PY†		
	Gamma	Neutron		AL	CGL	All	AL	CGL	All
Hiroshima									
400-600	381	144	9,535	10	2	12	104.9	21.0	125.9
200-399	211	70	19,614	8	7	15	40.8	35.7	76.5
100-199	109	30	32,384	9	3	12	27.8	9.3	37.1
50-99	57	13	51,456	3	4	7	5.8	7.8	13.6
1-49	9	2	469,060	11	14	25	2.3	3.0	5.3
<1	0	0	569,266	16	4	20	2.8	0.7	3.5
Total			1,151,315	57	34	91	5.0	3.0	7.9
Nagasaki									
400-600	514	11	6,981	6	1	7	85.9	14.3	100.3
200-399	264	4	20,151	7	1	8	34.7	5.0	39.7
100-199	143	1	27,355	4	0	4	14.6	0.0	14.6
50-99	71	0	25,643	0	0	0	0.0	0.0	0.0
1-49	10	0	200,417	6	3	9	3.0	1.5	4.5
<1	0	0	90,944	2	0	2	2.2	0.0	3.3c
Total			371,491	25	5	30	6.7	1.3	8.3c

* AL = acute leukemia; CGL = chronic granulocytic leukemia
† One case of chronic lymphocytic leukemia was included
From Ishimaru, T.; Otake, M.; and Ichimaru, M.P: Dose-response relationship of neutrons and gamma rays to leukemia incidence among atomic bomb survivors in Hiroshima and Nagasaki by type of leukemia, 1950-1971. *Radiat. Res.,* 77:377-394, 1979; and NAS, National Academy of Sciences Advisory Committee on the Biological Effects of Ionizing Radiation (BEIR): *The Effects on Populations of Exposure to Low Levels of Ionizing Radiation.* National Academy Press, Washington, D.C., 1980.

the mass and charge of the radiation. X-rays, for example, tend to deposit relatively little energy along their paths and to penetrate deeply; while alpha particles are densely ionizing and penetrate poorly.

Because the biologic effects of radiation result from the chemical changes caused by ionization of atoms and molecules in cells, the traversal of a cell by an alpha particle involves a higher probability of injury than traversal by an x-ray.

Levels and doses of radiation are measured in various units (ICRU, 1980). The roentgen (R) is a unit of exposure. The unit for expressing absorbed dose is the rad (1 rad = 100 ergs per gram of tissue) and the gray (1 Gy = 1 joule per kilogram of tissue = 100 rad). The dose imparted to tissue by exposure to one roentgen approximates one rad. Because one rad of particulate radiation generally produces greater injury than one rad of x-rays, the rem and the sievert (Sv) have been introduced to enable doses of different radiations to be normalized for biologic effects. One rem is that dose of any radiation that produces a biologic effect equivalent to one rad of x-rays or gamma rays. One

sievert is that amount of any radiation that produces a biologic effect equivalent to one gray of x-rays or gamma rays (1 Sv = 100 rem). The millirem (mrem) (1 millirem = 1/1000 rem) is also used. The units used for expressing the collective dose to a population are the person-rem and person-sievert, which denote the product of the number of people exposed times the average dose per person (*e.g.,* 1 rem to each 1000 people = 1000 person-rem = 10 person-sievert).

The general population is exposed to ionizing radiation from various sources, man-made as well as natural. Natural background radiation comes from (1) cosmic rays; (2) thorium, radium, and other radionuclides in the earth's crust; and (3) potassium 40, carbon 14, and other naturally occurring radioactive elements in the body (see Table 3-11). Collectively, the average dose received from these sources by a person living at sea level is about 0.80 mSv per year; however, doses at least twice as large are received by populations at higher elevations, where cosmic rays are more intense, or in areas where the content of radioactive material in the soil and subterranean rock is increased.

Table 3–11. Estimated Annual Whole-Body Radiation Doses to the U.S. Population

SOURCE OF RADIATION	AVERAGE DOSE RATES (mSv/year)
Natural	
Environmental	
Cosmic Radiation	0.28 (0.26 to 1.0)*
Terrestrial Radiation	0.26 (0.15 to 1.4)†
Internal Radioactive Isotopes	0.26
Subtotal	0.80
Man-Made	
Environmental	
Technologically Enhanced	0.04‡
Global Fallout	0.04
Nuclear Power	0.003
Medical	
Diagnostic	0.78
Radiopharmaceuticals	0.14
Occupational	0.01
Consumer Products and Miscellaneous	0.05
Subtotal	1.06
Total	1.86

* Values in parentheses indicate range over which average levels for different states vary with elevation.
† Range of variation (shown in parentheses) attributable largely to geographic differences in the content of potassium 40, radium, thorium, and uranium in the earth's crust.
‡ Average dose to the population from mine- and mill-tailings, crushed rock, phosphate fertilizers, and comparable sources of naturally-occurring radioactivity introduced into the human environment through various technological activities.
From Department of Health, Education and Welfare, Interagency Task Force on the Health Effects of Ionizing Radiation: *Report of the Work Group on Science.* U.S. Dept. of Health, Education, and Welfare, Washington, D.C., 1979; and NAS, National Academy of Sciences Advisory Committee on the Biological Effects of Ionizing Radiation (BEIR): *The Effects on Populations of Exposure to Low Levels of Ionizing Radiation.* National Academy Press, Washington, D.C., 1980.

Man-made sources are estimated to deliver an average of 106 mrem per year to each member of the population (see Table 3–11). The largest man-made contribution comes from medical diagnosis. Smaller contributions come from "technologically enhanced" sources, such as the use of phosphate fertilizers and building materials containing small amounts of radioactivity, global fallout from atmospheric testing of atomic weapons, nuclear power, high-altitude jet flight, occupational exposure, and consumer products (color TV sets, smoke detectors, luminescent clock and instrument dials, and so forth).

In comparison with the average dose to the general population from cosmic radiation, which approximates 0.28 mSv per year, the average dose to the thorax from a standard x-ray examination of the chest is of the order of 0.1 mSv. Other diagnostic procedures may involve substantially larger doses; *e.g.,* the average dose to the bone marrow from a barium enema examination of the colon is of the order of 50 to 80 mSv.

CARCINOGENIC EFFECTS ON SPECIFIC ORGANS AND TISSUES

Hemopoietic and Reticular Tissues

The incidence of all major forms of leukemia, except the chronic lymphocytic form, has been observed to be increased in human populations after irradiation of the whole body or a major part of the hemopoietic bone marrow. The increase, which becomes detectable within two to five years after irradiation, is dose-dependent and persists for 15 years or longer, depending on the hematologic type in question and age at irradiation (see Figure 3–7).

The combined incidence of all forms of leukemia other than the chronic lymphatic form,

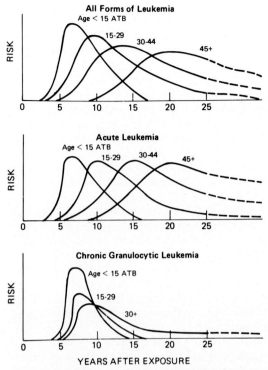

Figure 3–7. Relationship between age at time of bombing and calendar time on leukemogenic effect of radiation in heavily exposed atomic-bomb survivors. From NAS, National Academy of Sciences Advisory Committee on the Biological Effects of Ionizing Radiation (BEIR): *The Effects on Populations of Exposure to Low Levels of Ionizing Radiation.* National Academy Press, Washington, D. C., 1980.

averaged over the first 25 years after irradiation in atomic-bomb survivors, patients treated with spinal irradiation for ankylosing spondylitis, and women treated with pelvic irradiation for menorrhagia, approximates one case per 10,000 persons per year per Sv to the bone marrow (NAS, 1972, 1980). A somewhat higher rate, approximating three cases per 10,000 persons per year per Sv, has been observed in persons given x-ray therapy to the scalp in childhood for tinea capitis or x-ray therapy to the neck in infancy for thymic enlargement or other non-neoplastic conditions (NAS, 1972, 1980).

While it is clear that the overall incidence of leukemia increases with increasing dose (see Table 3–10), the data are not adequate to define unambiguously the shape of the dose-incidence curve. Until recently, there appeared to be differences between Hiroshima and Nagasaki in dose-incidence relationships, which

were attributed to differences in the relative contributions of neutrons to the dose in each city (see Table 3–10). Now, however, based on revised dose calculations, which have greatly lowered the estimated neutron doses in both cities, the dose incidence curves appear similar (see Figure 3–8). This interpretation must remain tentative, pending more thorough analysis of the dosimetry. Comparison of the curves for the two cities is also complicated by differences in the ratio between chronic and acute leukemia, chronic granulocytic leukemia being appreciably more common at Hiroshima than at Nagasaki (see Table 3–10).

Irradiation *in utero* is associated with an increased incidence of acute leukemia in British and U. S. children who were exposed prenatally during the radiographic examination of their mothers (NAS, 1980). No such excess of leukemia is evident in Japanese children who were exposed *in utero* to atomic-bomb radiation (NAS, 1980), and there is evidence that other risk factors, such as a maternal history of untoward pregnancy outcomes, may also be involved (Gibson *et al.,* 1968). Nevertheless, the interpretation that irradiation plays a causal role in the etiology of the disease is supported by evidence that the magnitude of the

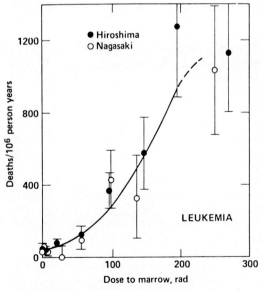

Figure 3–8. Leukemia in atomic-bomb survivors, in relation to dose. From Straume, T., and Dobson, R. L.: Implications of new Hiroshima and Nagasaki dose estimates: cancer risks and neutron RBE. *Health Phys.,* **41**:666–671, 1981. Reproduced from *Health Physics* by permission of the Health Physics Society.

excess increases with the radiation dose to the embryo or fetus, as measured by the number of radiographs of the mother's pelvis, and by the fact that the excess is as large in irradiated twins as in singleton births (Mole, 1974). The excess roughly corresponds to a 5% increase in the relative risk of childhood leukemia per mSv or to approximately 25 cases per 10,000 children at risk per Sv per year during the first 12 years of life (NAS, 1980).

It is evident from these observations that the magnitude of any radiation-induced increase in the relative risk of leukemia depends on age at irradiation. The increase appears to be larger with prenatal irradiation than with postnatal irradiation, and to be larger with irradiation in childhood than with irradiation during adolescence or adult life. In atomic-bomb survivors (see Figure 3–9) and spondylitics (Doll, 1970) irradiated during adolescence or adult life, the number of radiation-induced cases, or the absolute excess in incidence, has been observed to increase with age at irradiation.

The relative risk is increased in atomic-bomb survivors and other irradiated populations for other radiation-induced hematologic

cancers including lymphomas of the non-Hodgkin's type (as reported by NAS, 1980) and multiple myeloma (NAS, 1980; Cuzick, 1981). The average latency of these neoplasms appears to be longer than that of juvenile or chronic granulocytic leukemia (NAS, 1980). Too few cases of these diseases have been observed to indicate their dose-incidence relations, but both types of diseases were increased in frequency in U. S. radiologists dying between 1930 and 1949 (Matanoski, 1981), suggesting that these neoplasms may be induced by chronic, low-level irradiation as well as by more intensive exposure.

Confirming and amplifying the carcinogenic effects of radiation on human hemopoietic and reticular tissues are studies in several species of laboratory animals (UN, 1977; Upton, 1977). These have demonstrated that virtually all species are susceptible to some degree to the induction of leukemias and lymphomas by irradiation, but that the effects of radiation on the frequency of a given neoplasm vary with the growth in question, the conditions of irradiation (total dose and temporal and spatial distribution of the dose), host

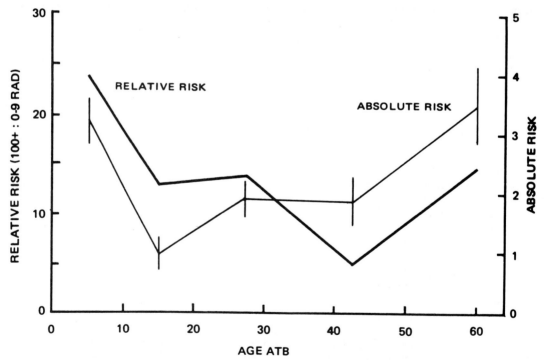

Figure 3–9. Age-specific relative-risk estimates and absolute-risk estimates for leukemia (excess deaths per 10^6 PYR) with 90% confidence intervals. From Beebe, G. W.; Kato, H.; and Land, C. E.: Studies of the mortality of A-bomb survivors. 6. Mortality and radiation dose, 1950–1974. *Radiat. Res.,* **75**:138–201, 1978; and NAS, National Academy of Sciences Advisory Committee on the Biological Effects of Ionizing Radiation (BEIR): *The Effects on Populations of Exposure to Low Levels of Ionizing Radiation.* National Academy Press, Washington, D. C., 1980.

factors (species, strain, sex, age at irradiation, and physiological condition), and other variables (microbial flora, viruses, and extraneous environmental agents). These variations cannot be adequately explained on the basis of present knowledge.

It may be concluded, nevertheless, from the available data that: (1) The neoplasms induced by irradiation include examples of virtually all hematologic forms; (2) not all of the hematologic neoplasms that occur naturally are increased in frequency by irradiation in a given population; (3) the dose-incidence curves for radiation-induced neoplasms generally rise less steeply with low-linear energy transfer (LET) irradiation than with high-LET irradiation in the low-to-intermediate dose region; (4) the dose-incidence curves also rise less steeply with low-LET irradiation at low dose rates than at high dose rates; (5) at high dose rates, the incidence usually passes through a maximum at some intermediate dose and decreases with further increase in the dose; (6) although considerable data are available on the dose-incidence relationships for various hematologic neoplasms at low-to-intermediate doses and dose rates, the relationships are not sufficiently well defined nor the mechanisms of carcinogenesis sufficiently well understood to enable accurate prediction of the effects of low doses; and (7) uncertainties about dose-incidence relationships and causative mechanisms (the role of viruses, hormones, and other growth factors) complicate extrapolation of the animal data to man (UN, 1977).

Breast

Since 1965, when MacKenzie first reported an increased incidence of breast cancer in Canadian women subjected to multiple fluoroscopic examinations of the chest, the female breast has come to be recognized as one of the organs most susceptible to radiation carcinogenesis (UN, 1977; NAS, 1980). This conclusion derives from epidemiologic studies on: (1) Women surviving atomic-bomb irradiation (McGregor et al., 1977; Tokunaga et al., 1979); (2) women given radiation therapy to the breast for acute post-partum mastitis or other benign diseases (Baral et al., 1977; Shore et al., 1977); and (3) women subjected to repeated fluoroscopic examinations of the chest during treatment for pulmonary tuberculosis with artificial pneumothorax (Myrden and Hiltz, 1969; Boice and Manson, 1977).

The incidence of carcinoma of the breast in each of the above groups became demonstrably elevated within five to 10 years after irradiation, depending on age at exposure, and remained elevated for the duration of follow-up. Averaged over all ages, the excess increases with dose similarly in each group (see Figure 3–10) in spite of marked differences among the three groups in the rapidity with which the radiation doses were accumulated. The absence of a diminished carcinogenic effect in the multiply fluoroscoped women, who accumulated their doses in numerous, small, widely separated increments, implies that the individual exposures in such women were fully additive in their cancer-causing effects. In view of the low dosage of the individual exposures, which are estimated to have averaged about 15 mSv each (Boice et al., 1978), the absence of intervening repair implies that there is no threshold for carcinogenic effects of radiation on the breast. The data argue in favor of the linear, nonthreshold hypothesis: the concept that the incidence is proportional to the radiation dose, down to zero dose. The data do not exclude other dose-incidence relationships, such as a linear-quadratic function with a negative exponential term to account for saturation at high doses (NAS, 1980; Land, 1981), as suggested in the curve for the mastitis series (see Figure 3–10).

Complicating interpretation of the curves illustrated (see Figure 3–10) is evidence that the increase in incidence induced by a given dose of radiation and the latent period preceding the appearance of the radiation-induced tumors may vary in relation to age at the time of irradiation. The excess in women irradiated in adolescence appears higher than that in women irradiated at older ages, despite the longer latency of tumors in the younger age group (Boice et al., 1979). While the excess became evident within five to nine years after irradiation in the older age group, it was not evident until 15 to 20 years after irradiation in the women irradiated during adolescence (Land, 1981). This difference, coupled with the fact that no excess has yet appeared in atomic-bomb survivors who were irradiated at younger than 10 years of age, implies that expression of the carcinogenic changes depends on the promoting effects of age-related endocrinological stimulation of breast tissue (Land, 1981).

The high susceptibility of the female breast to radiation carcinogenesis has also been

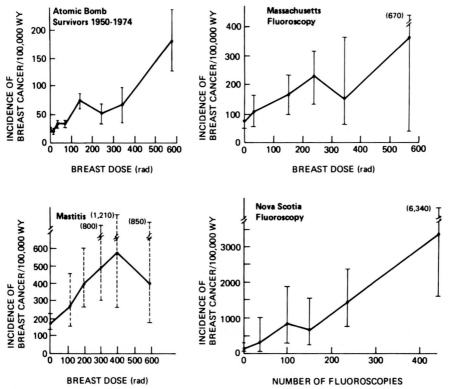

Figure 3-10. Incidence of breast cancer in relation to radiation dose. From Boice, J. D., Jr.; Land, C. E.; Shore, R. E.; Norman, J. E.; and Tokunaga, M.: Risk of breast cancer following low-dose exposure. *Radiology,* **131**:589-597, 1979.

found in experimental animals of certain genetic backgrounds (UN, 1977; Dethlefsen *et al.*, 1978). In female rats of the Sprague-Dawley strain, for example, which naturally develop a high incidence of mammary gland tumors during senescence, a small dose of radiation accelerates the development of these tumors and increases their incidence (Shellabarger, 1976). These effects are detectable after a dose as low as 250 mSv of gamma radiation or 2.5 mSv of fast neutrons (Vogel and Zaldivar, 1969; Shellabarger *et al.*, 1974). As in the human female, susceptibility is influenced by age at irradiation, endocrine stimuli, and other variables (Shellabarger *et al.*, 1976). Also affecting susceptibility is genetic background; responses vary widely among animals of different species and strains (Shellabargar *et al.*, 1976; UN, 1977; Dethlefsen *et al.*, 1978).

Thyroid and Other Endocrine Glands

Thyroid. Epidemiologic studies have revealed the thyroid gland to be highly susceptible to radiation carcinogenesis. The incidence of thyroid tumors is increased in atomic-bomb

survivors (Parker *et al.*, 1974; Beebe *et al.*, 1978); patients given radiation therapy to the neck region in infancy for thymic enlargement and other non-neoplastic conditions (Hempelmann, 1977; Webber, 1977; Shore *et al.*, 1980); patients given x-ray therapy to the scalp in childhood for treatment of tinea capitis (Shore *et al.*, 1976; Modan *et al.*, 1977); Marshall Islanders exposed to radioactive fallout from a weapons test in 1954 (Conard *et al.*, 1980); and other populations with a history of thyroid irradiation (DeGroot *et al.*, 1977; UN, 1977; NAS, 1980).

The cancers in question are chiefly of the papillary type and are characterized by a low rate of mortality. Adenomas are also included. The data imply that the probability of carcinoma is twice as high in the presence of radiation-induced nodular disease as in spontaneous nodular disease (Schneider *et al.*, 1978). Development of the tumors is generally preceded by a latent period of 15 to 25 years or longer. Susceptibility is two to four times higher in females than in males and possibly somewhat higher in children than in adults (UN, 1977; NAS, 1980). The data also suggest that susceptibility may be increased in people of Jewish extraction (NAS, 1980).

The excess of thyroid tumors has been observed over a wide range of doses, from 1.5 to 2.0 Sv down to 65 mSv (UN, 1977; NAS, 1980). Although the shape of the dose-incidence curve cannot be defined precisely from the available evidence, the data are consistent with a linear, nonthreshold relationship, corresponding to an excess of approximately four cancers per 10,000 persons per year per Sv and 12 adenomas per 10,000 persons per year per Sv (UN, 1977; NAS, 1980). No excess of tumors has been observed in populations treated with iodine 131 for hyperthyroidism. The data are inconclusive, however, and the doses in question are large enough (40 Sv) to have caused substantial cell death (Safa et al., 1975; UN, 1977; NAS, 1980).

In laboratory animals, tumors of the thyroid gland have been induced by internal as well as external irradiation (UN, 1977). With external irradiation, the dose-incidence curve appears to increase in slope with increasing dose in the region below 15 Sv, and then to pass through a maximum, and then to decrease with further increase in the dose, presumably due to excessive damage of the follicular epithelium (Lindsay and Chaikoff, 1964; Walinder, 1972). Protracted irradiation from internally deposited iodine 131 is several times less tumorigenic for a given dose than x-radiation administered in a single, brief exposure (Doniach, 1974). The carcinogenic effects of a given dose of radiation may be subsequently enhanced by hormonally stimulated hyperplasia of follicular epithelium (Doniach, 1974).

Other Endocrine Glands. Adenomas of the pituitary gland are increased in frequency by whole-body irradiation in mice of certain strains. The incidence is higher in females than in males, and the increase per Gy is larger with neutrons than with gamma rays. The tumors develop after a long latency, appearing predominantly in the longest-lived animals of a given dose group (Upton et al., 1960).

Other endocrine gland tumors observed with increased frequency in irradiated mice and rats include adenomas of the adrenal cortex, pancreatic islets, and parathyroid glands. Such growths have been observed too rarely, however, to enable quantitative inferences about their precise relationship to dose (Upton et al., 1960; Berdjis, 1972; UN, 1977).

In irradiated human populations, no increase in the incidence of endocrine tumors other than those of the thyroid gland has been reported.

Respiratory Tract

An increased incidence of lung cancer has been observed in atomic-bomb survivors (Beebe et al., 1978); patients treated with spinal irradiation for ankylosing spondylitis (Doll and Smith, 1977; Smith and Doll 1978, 1982); and hard-rock miners exposed to radon in the air of underground mines in Czechoslovakia (Sevc et al., 1976), Canada (Ham, 1976), the United States (Archer et al., 1974), and Sweden (Jorgensen, 1973). The tumors involved include epidermoid carcinomas and small cell anaplastic carcinomas, with only a smaller excess of adenocarcinomas and cancers of other types (Archer et al., 1974; Horacek et al., 1977).

Development of the tumors is preceded by a latent period of 10 years or more, depending on age at exposure. In atomic-bomb survivors, the excess of lung cancer did not become evident until after 10 years in those who were more than 50 years old at the time of irradiation, after 15 years in those who were 35 to 49 years at exposure, and after 25 years in those who were 20 to 34 years old at exposure (NAS, 1980). In cigarette smokers the latency is shorter than in nonsmokers (NAS, 1980).

The excess of lung cancer in atomic-bomb survivors and irradiated spondylitics, adjusted for age and duration of follow-up, corresponds to two to three cases per 10,000 persons per year per Sv (NAS, 1980). The excess in underground miners appears comparable, if adjusted similarly and based on appropriate normalization of the dose from radon (NAS, 1980). Although the data do not define precisely the shape of the dose-incidence curve, they are consistent with a nonthreshold response. The excess per Sv in miners appears larger at low-to-intermediate doses than at higher doses (NAS, 1980).

In cigarette smokers, the absolute excess of lung cancer is larger than in nonsmokers. Although the carcinogenic effects of smoking and irradiation are more than merely additive, they do not appear to be fully multiplicative if appropriate allowances are made for differences in the latency of the induced tumors (NAS, 1980).

Carcinogenic effects of radiation on the respiratory tract have been observed in experimental animals of many species and strains

(UN, 1977; Kennedy and Little, 1978). The tumors include benign and malignant growths of various types, and have been observed to occur at all levels of the respiratory tract, from the nasal mucosa to the peripheral bronchoalveolar parenchyma, depending on the animals irradiated and the conditions of irradiation (Kennedy *et al.*, 1978). The anatomic distribution of tumors tends to correspond to the distribution of the radiation dose within the respiratory system: The neoplasia occur preferentially in those sites most heavily irradiated. Susceptibility varies among the different types of cells in the respiratory tract, however, and no one dose-incidence relationship applies to all patterns of response. The data indicate that the probability of tumor formation may also be increased by proliferative stimuli applied after irradiation (Little *et al.*, 1978).

Skeletal System

An excess of bone tumors, both benign and cancerous, has been observed in radium-dial painters (Rowland and Stehney, 1978); patients treated for ankylosing spondylitis by intravenous injection of radium 224 (Mays *et al.*, 1978); patients injected intravenously with thorotrast for angiographic examination (Harrist *et al.*, 1979; Mays and Spiess, 1979), and patients exposed to therapeutic x-irradiation (UN, 1977; Yoshizawa *et al.*, 1977; Kim *et al.*, 1978; NAS, 1980).

In patients injected with radium 224 or treated with x-rays and receiving their radiation over a relatively brief period, the excess of osteosarcomas has been evident as early as four years after irradiation, has reached a maximum at six to eight years, and has declined thereafter, virtually disappearing after 20 to 25 years (NAS, 1980). This time distribution differs from that seen in radium dial painters, who continue to accumulate their dose from internally deposited radium 226 throughout their lives, and in whom osteosarcomas have appeared as late as 52 years after the start of exposure (Rowland and Stehney, 1978).

Susceptibility to the induction of osteosarcomas varies with age at irradiation, being higher in children than in adults (Spiess and Mays, 1970). It also varies from one part of the skeleton to another, being highest in sites where naturally occurring sarcomas occur most frequently (*e.g.*, near the knee) and lowest in the vertebrae (Thurman *et al.*, 1973).

The relation between the incidence of osteosarcomas and the cumulative dose to the endosteum is consistent with a linear, nonthreshold response in patients injected with radium 224, corresponding to an excess of about one case per 10,000 persons per year per Sv in the dose region below 10 Sv (Mays and Spiess, 1978; NAS, 1980). The data for radium 226 and for x-rays are more complicated, however, indicating that these radiations pose a far smaller risk per Sv in the low-dose region (NAS, 1980). It is not surprising, therefore, that no excess of bone tumors has been evident in atomic-bomb survivors (Beebe *et al.*, 1978).

The carcinogenic effects of radiation on bone have been studied extensively in experimental animals of several species, with results that confirm and amplify the observations in humans summarized above (Mays *et al.*, 1969). The animal studies have been useful in elucidating metabolic differences among bone-seeking radionuclides; relationships between the doses delivered by different radionuclides to the skeleton and their patterns of uptake, distribution, and retention in bone; and, ultimately, differences among radionuclides in their carcinogenic activities (Mays *et al.*, 1969).

Gastrointestinal System

Cancers of the pharynx, esophagus, stomach, colon, rectum, liver, pancreas, and salivary glands have been observed with increased frequency in irradiated human and animal populations, depending on the conditions of exposure.

Pharynx. An excess of carcinomas of the pharynx has been observed in patients treated with x-rays for ankylosing spondylitis (Court Brown and Doll, 1965; Smith and Doll, 1982) and other diseases (Yoshizawa and Takeuchi, 1974). The clinical appearance of the tumors has characteristically followed a long induction period, averaging more than 20 years. While the data are too sparse to enable a precise estimate of the dose-incidence relationship, they imply that the cumulative excess would not exceed 0.25 to 0.5 case per 10,000 persons per year per Sv (NAS, 1980).

Esophagus. Carcinoma of the esophagus has been reported as a cause of death at almost twice the expected frequency in patients treated with spinal irradiation for ankylosing spondylitis (Smith and Doll, 1982). In atomic-bomb survivors of Hiroshima who were 35 years of age or older at the time of irradiation, the incidence increases with increasing dose (Beebe *et al.,* 1978). A crude linear estimate of 0.39 excess cancers per 10,000 persons per year per Gy has been derived from the latter experience (NAS, 1980).

In laboratory rodents of several species, carcinomas of the esophagus and forestomach have been induced by irradiation (Cosgrove *et al.,* 1968; Gates and Warren, 1968; Warren and Gates, 1968). The excess of such tumors has been detectable generally only after relatively high doses (more than 5 Sv), and the yield of such tumors for a given dose has been larger with fast neutron irradiation than with x- or gamma-irradiation (Cosgrove *et al.,* 1968).

Stomach. The frequency of gastric carcinoma is increased by roughly 50% in patients treated with x-rays for ankylosing spondylitis (Smith and Doll, 1982) and in atomic-bomb survivors exposed to similarly large doses of radiation (Beebe *et al.,* 1978). The Tumor Registry data for Hiroshima, averaged over the period 1950 to 1974, are consistent with the interpretation that the incidence increases linearly with dose, at a rate corresponding to about 1.6 excess fatal cancers per 10,000 persons per year per Gy (NAS, 1980). The excess attributable to radiation in this population is small in comparison with the natural incidence; *i.e.,* 20 out of a total of 1,228 deaths from stomach cancer (NAS, 1980). The precise nature of the dose-incidence relationship, therefore, remains highly uncertain.

In laboratory rodents, carcinoma of the glandular stomach has also been induced by irradiation (Nowell *et al.,* 1958; Cosgrove *et al.,* 1968; Hirose, 1969; Upton *et al.,* 1969). The incidence of such tumors is usually low and is detectably increased only after relatively high doses, the increase for a given dose being appreciably larger with fast neutrons than with x-rays or gamma rays (Upton *et al.,* 1969).

Colon and Rectum. An excess of carcinomas of the colon and rectum has been observed in atomic-bomb survivors (NAS, 1980); patients treated with x-rays for ankylosing spondylitis (Smith and Doll, 1982); women treated with abdominal irradiation for benign pelvic disorders (Doll and Smith, 1968; Brinkley and Haybittle, 1969); and radium-dial painters (Polednak *et al.,* 1978). Although the data are not sufficient to define the dose-incidence relation, the incidence in these populations corresponds to a radiation-induced excess of about 0.6 cancer per 10,000 persons per year per Sv (NAS, 1980).

In laboratory rats, intensive, localized x-irradiation of the exteriorized bowel has been reported to induce intestinal carcinomas with predictable regularity (Coop *et al.,* 1974). Rats and dogs exposed to neutron beams or subjected to irradiation of the bowel by polonium 210 or cerium 144 administered in the diet have been observed to develop an excess of benign and cancerous polypoid tumors of the colon (Lebedeva, 1973). Under other conditions of irradiation, however, the frequency of such tumors in experimental animals has been too low to permit inferences about their dose-incidence relationships (Cosgrove *et al.,* 1968; Upton *et al.,* 1970).

Liver. The incidence of primary cancers of the liver is increased in patients injected intravascularly with thorotrast for angiographic examination (da Silva Horta *et al.,* 1978; Faber, 1978; van Kaick *et al.,* 1978; Mori *et al.,* 1979) and in atomic-bomb survivors (Beebe *et al.,* 1978). The increase is more pronounced in the thorotrast patients, who have a large excess of bile duct carcinomas and hepatocellular carcinomas as well as angiosarcomas. The latency for the induced tumors is typically long, averaging considerably more than 10 years.

Although the precise relation between dose and incidence cannot be inferred from the available data, the overall cumulative lifetime excess of liver cancers in the above populations is estimated to approximate 15 cases per 10,000 persons per Sv (NAS, 1980).

Radiation-induced liver tumors have also been observed in experimental animals injected intravascularly with colloidal radionuclides (Upton *et al.,* 1956; Taylor *et al.,* 1972; Benjamin *et al.,* 1975) or exposed to external radiation (UN, 1977). From these observations, it may be inferred that primary tumors of virtually all histologic types may be induced, depending on the species exposed and the conditions of irradiation, but that few such tumors are produced in the low-to-intermediate dose range.

Pancreas. Carcinoma of the pancreas has been recorded with increased frequency in atomic-bomb survivors (Beebe *et al.,* 1978; NAS, 1980) and in patients treated with x-rays for ankylosing spondylitis (Smith and Doll, 1978; Smith and Doll, 1982) or carcinoma of the cervix (Dickson, 1972). The shape of the dose-incidence curve is not evident from the available data, but the excess per unit dose approximates 0.6 cases per 10,000 persons per Sv per year in the irradiated spondylitics and 0.8 cases per 10,000 persons per Sv per year in the atomic-bomb survivors for whom tumor registry data are most complete (*i.e.,* those of Nagasaki) (NAS, 1980).

An excess of pancreatic cancer has also been reported in nuclear workers of the Hanford plant, and has been interpreted to imply that the risk per unit dose is larger than the above estimates (Mancuso *et al.,* 1977; Kneale *et al.,* 1978). Although the excess appears real, the interpretation that it is attributable to occupational irradiation has been questioned (NAS, 1980).

In experimental animals, tumors of the glandular pancreas have been observed too infrequently after irradiation to enable inferences about their dose-incidence relationships.

Salivary Glands. Tumors of the salivary glands have appeared with increased frequency in persons treated with x-rays to the head and neck in childhood for various benign conditions (Saenger *et al.,* 1960; Modan *et al.,* 1974; Hempelmann *et al.,* 1975; Shore *et al.,* 1976) and in atomic-bomb survivors (Belsky *et al.,* 1975).The tumors have included benign as well as cancerous types, and their clinical appearance has generally been preceded by a latency period of 15 to 25 years. The data are too sparse to define precisely the magnitude of the increase for a given dose, but they imply that the cumulative excess of such neoplasms would not exceed 0.5 case per 10,000 persons per year per Sv (NAS, 1980).

These tumors have been observed infrequently in irradiated animal populations (Glucksmann and Cherry, 1962; Takeichi, 1975), indicating a relatively low susceptibility of the salivary glands to radiation carcinogenesis in those species.

Genitourinary System

Ovary. The incidence of carcinoma of the ovary is increased in women who have received radiotherapy for benign diseases of the pelvic organs (Palmer and Spratt, 1956; Smith and Doll, 1976) and in atomic-bomb survivors (Beebe *et al.,* 1978). The data are too sparse to provide quantitative estimates of the dose-incidence relation, but they imply that the risk is probably less than 1 case per 100,000 persons per year per Sv (NAS, 1980).

In mice, tumors of the ovary are induced at high frequency by doses that sterilize both

ovaries. The neoplasms produced, which include tumors of granulosa cells, lutein cells, theca cells, and other stromal elements, are attributed to disturbance of hormonal regulation from radiation-induced cessation of ovulation (Upton, 1968).

Testis. Interstitial tumors of the testis have been observed to be increased in frequency in rats exposed to whole-body irradiation (Berdjis, 1972).

Uterus. An excess of cancers of the uterus and uterine cervix has been observed in women treated with radiation for benign pelvic diseases (Palmer and Spratt, 1956; Smith and Doll, 1976) and, to a lesser extent, in atomic-bomb survivors (Beebe *et al.,* 1978). While the data are too limited to indicate the dose-incidence relation, they imply a risk of less than one fatal uterine cancer per 10,000 persons per year per Sv (NAS, 1980).

Kidney. Cancers of the kidney and urinary bladder are increased in frequency in atomic-bomb survivors (Beebe *et al.,* 1978); patients treated with radiation for ankylosing spondylitis (Smith and Doll, 1982), uterine bleeding (Smith and Doll, 1976), or other pelvic diseases (McIntyre and Pointor, 1971); and patients examined by retrograde pyelography with thorotrast (da Silva Horta *et al.,* 1974). The tumors have characteristically been preceded by a long latency period (25 to 30 years), depending on the conditions of irradiation and age at exposure.The data are insufficient to define the dose-incidence relation, but they imply that the risk of death from such neoplasms may approximate 0.13 per 10,000 persons per year per Sv (NAS, 1980).

In laboratory mice and rats, tumors of the kidney are readily induced by irradiation (Berdjis, 1972; Hamilton, 1975). The tumors include benign as well as cancerous growths, and their incidence for a given dose varies, depending on the conditions of irradiation and on physiologic variables (Hamilton, 1975; NAS, 1980).

Central Nervous System

An excess of brain tumors has been reported in patients treated with scalp irradiation for tinea capitis in childhood (Modan *et al.,* 1974; Shore *et al.,* 1976); in patients treated with radiation to the head and neck in childhood for tonsillitis, adenoiditis, and other benign conditions (Colman *et al.,* 1978); and in children exposed to diagnostic irradiation *in utero*

(MacMahon, 1962; Diamond *et al.,* 1973; Bithell and Stewart, 1975). No deaths from brain tumors have been observed in atomic-bomb survivors who were irradiated *in utero,* but because the number of such survivors is small, their lack of brain tumors does not contradict the excess noted in the other populations (NAS, 1980). The data do not provide a firm indication of the dose-incidence relation, but they are consistent with a risk of about one case per 10,000 persons per year per Sv during the first 30 years following postnatal irradiation, and about six cases per 10,000 persons per year per Sv during the first 10 years after prenatal irradiation (NAS, 1980).

The experimental induction of brain tumors has been described in primates exposed to intensive thermal neutron or proton irradiation (Haymaker *et al.,* 1972).

Skin

As noted above, cancer of the skin has occurred as a late complication of long-standing radiation dermatitis in scores of pioneer radiation workers. Although chronic radiodermatitis used to be regarded as a prerequisite for the induction of the disease (Furth and Lorenz, 1954), it is now well established that basal cell carcinomas can be induced with little or no evidence of radiation damage (Albert *et al.,* 1968; UN, 1972). In addition to basal cell carcinomas, which predominate at lower doses, the neoplasms at higher doses include squamous cell carcinomas and smaller numbers of fibrosarcomas, melanomas, and sweat gland tumors (Traenkle, 1963; Shore *et al.,* 1976; NAS, 1980).

Most of the early literature on radiation-induced skin cancer consists of case reports, which do not permit quantitative inferences about the relation between incidence and dose. More recently, epidemiologic studies have shown an excess of skin cancer in patients treated with x-rays to the scalp for tinea capitis in childhood (Shore *et al.,* 1976); patients treated with x-rays to the chest in infancy for enlargement of the thymus (Hempelmann *et al.,* 1975); patients treated with x-rays to various parts of the body for other conditions (Takahashi, 1964); U. S. radiologists entering practice between 1920 and 1959 (Matanoski *et al.,* 1975); and Czechoslovakian uranium miners (Secova *et al.,* 1978). None of the studies provide the basis for confident estimates of the dose-incidence relationship, but analysis of the populations irradiated for tinea capitis and thymus enlargment implies that the excess may approximate 0.4 to 1.0 case per 10,000 persons per year per Sv (NAS, 1980). Although epidemiologic studies of the atomic-bomb survivors have failed to detect any such excess, the discrepancies are attributable to methodologic or other variables (NAS, 1980).

The induction of skin tumors has been studied extensively in experimental animals. In mice and rats, the incidence rises steeply with dose in the range of more than 20 Sv (Hulse *et al.,* 1968; Mole, 1975). At doses of less than 5 Sv, however, the incidence is too low to be readily investigated, indicating that the skin is not as susceptible to radiation carcinogenesis as many other tissues.

DOSE-INCIDENCE RELATIONSHIPS

Total Dose

A wide variety of relationships between tumor incidence and radiation dose has been observed in experimental animals for which data for different species and strains are available over a broad range of doses. While the cumulative incidence of neoplasms of most types is increased by irradiation, this is not true of all types (see Figure 3-11). In human populations, as noted above, the incidence of chronic lymphocytic leukemia, in contrast to leukemias of all other types, has not been detectably increased by irradiation.

For radiation-induced neoplasms, the dose-incidence curve usually passes through a maximum in the intermediate dose range and decreases with further increase in the dose (*e.g.,* see Figure 3-11, curves A, D, E, and F). The saturation of the curve at high doses is attributed to cell killing or other forms of damage that interfere with expression of the carcinogenic effects of radiation (Upton, 1961, 1977; UN, 1977; NAS, 1980).

The exact shape of the dose-incidence curve in the low-dose region is not known for any type of neoplasm. In theory, if a single radiation-induced mutation or chromosome aberration in a somatic cell was sufficient to initiate neoplasia, the curve for carcinogenesis would be expected on radiobiological grounds to conform to a linear quadratic function of the form:

$$I_D = (C + \alpha_1 D + \alpha_2 D^2)\, \exp^{-(\beta_1 D + \beta D^2)},$$

where I_D is the incidence at dose D, C is the

natural incidence, and α_1, α_2, β_1, and β_2 are constant coefficients (Upton, 1977). The ratios of the coefficients for DNA damage, chromosomal aberrations, and cell killing are such that the resulting dose-effect curve for low-LET radiation should be linear in the low-dose region; it should bend upward with increasing dose and dose rate in the intermediate-dose region; and it should pass through a maximum and decline with further increase in dose in the high-dose region (Upton, 1977).

Whereas some of the observed dose-incidence curves conform to the pattern described above (see Figure 3-11, curves A, D, E, and F), the multicausal, multistage nature of the cancer process is so complex that any simple model is unlikely to characterize the dose-incidence relationship adequately over a wide range of doses. At intermediate-to-high doses, radiation can be expected to exert promoting effects as well as initiating effects on tumor formation through alterations in cell population kinetics, hormonal relationships, immunologic reactivity, and other changes. Without better understanding of the mechanisms of carcinogenesis, any attempt to predict dose-incidence relationships for low-level irradiation must remain highly speculative.

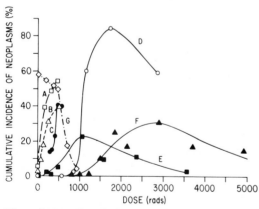

Figure 3–11. Dose-incidence curves for different neoplasms in animals exposed to external radiation. (A) Myeloid leukemia in x-irradiated mice; (B) mammary gland tumors at 12 months in gamma-irradiated rats; (C) thymic lymphoma in x-irradiated mice; (D) kidney tumors in x-irradiated rats; (E) skin tumors in alpha-irradiated rats (percentage incidence × 10); (F) skin tumors in electron-irradiated rats (percentage incidence × 10); (G) reticulum-cell sarcoma in x-irradiated mice. Modified from UN, United Nations: *Ionizing Radiation: Levels and Effects. A Report of the United Nations Scientific Committee on the Effects of Atomic Radiation.* General Assembly, Official Records: 27th Session, Suppl. Number 25 (A/8725), New York, 1972.

Dose Rate

In experimental animals, the dose-incidence curve for low-LET radiation generally decreases in slope with decreasing dose rate; that is, with increasing duration of exposure (NCRPM, 1980). The overall age-specific mortality from radiation-induced neoplasms and the associated reduction in life expectancy are therefore several times lower for a given dose of low-LET radiation if it is accumulated in small increments over a period of weeks than if it is accumulated in a single, brief exposure (see Figure 3-12).

With high-LET radiation, on the other hand, this type of dose rate dependency is not observed (see Figure 3-12). The dose-incidence curve may rise even more steeply with an increase in the duration of exposure (Thomson et al., 1981).

The influence of dose rate also varies in magnitude from one type of neoplasm to another. In the induction of breast tumors in Sprague-Dawley female rats, for example, the effectiveness of a given dose of x-rays or gamma rays changes relatively little with variation in the dose rate (Shellabarger, 1976).

Age-related changes in susceptibility to carcinogenesis may also complicate the situation if the period of irradiation is greatly protracted. In the induction of ovarian tumors in the mouse, both a protraction effect and an aging effect are observed.

With respect to the influence of dose rate on carcinogenesis in human populations, the data for low-LET radiation are insufficient to permit firm conclusions (UN, 1977; NAS, 1980; NCRPM, 1980). The data for carcinogenesis in the female breast (Figure 3-10) argue against the existence of a dose rate effect for the induction of this neoplasm, as noted above. For high-LET radiation, the data on osteosarcomas in patients injected with radium 224 for treatment of aklylosing spondylitis indicate a two- to threefold increase in carcinogenicity per Gy of alpha radiation when the duration of exposure to this bone-seeking radionuclide is prolonged.

Radiation Quality

As noted above, high-LET radiations (alpha particles, protons, neutrons) are generally more carcinogenic per unit dose than are low-LET radiations (x-rays, gamma rays), the differential increasing with increasing LET. The

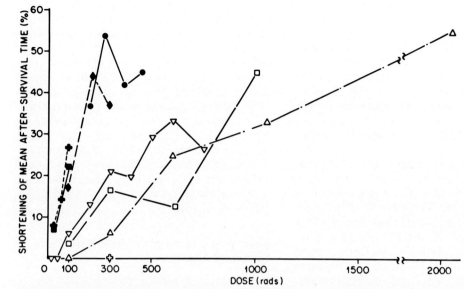

Figure 3–12. Shortening of mean after-survival time in RF female mice as influenced by dose and dose rate of neutron or gamma irradiation. The after-survival time is defined as the interval elapsing between the end of irradiation and the mean age at death; hence, groups irradiated until 50% or more of the animals had died are excluded. Hollow symbols represent results of gamma-rays; filled symbols are neutron results. ● = 85 rad/min; ▽ = 6.7 rad/min; △ = 0.01 to 0.02 rad/min (14 to 30 rad/day); □ = 0.0028 to 0.0038 rad/min (3.8 to 5.3 rad/day); ◆ = 0.00098 to 0.00199 rad/min (1.3 to 2.9 rad/day); + = 0.0004 to 0.0007 rad/min (0.5 to 1.1 rad/day). From Upton, A. C.; Randolph, M. L.; and Conklin, J. W.: Late effects of fast neutrons and gamma-rays in mice as influenced by the dose rate of irradiation. *Radiat. Res.,* **32:**493–509, 1967.

carcinogenic effectiveness of radiation per unit dose generally decreases with decreasing dose and dose rate in the case of low-LET radiation, although it remains relatively constant or may even increase with decreasing dose and dose rate in the case of high-LET radiation (Figure 3-12). The difference in relative biologic effectiveness (RBE) is maximal at low doses and low dose rates. There are few data on the magnitude of the RBE for high-LET radiation in the low-dose region (at doses as low as 10 mSv), but the available evidence implies that the magnitude of the RBE lies in the range of 20 to 200 mSv (UN, 1977; NAS, 1980; Shellabarger et al., 1980; Thomson et al., 1981).

Some of the previously reported differences between Hiroshima and Nagasaki in the rates of radiation-induced cancers in atomic-bomb survivors, which have been attributed to a larger relative neutron dose in Hiroshima (UN, 1977; NAS, 1980), are no longer evident since revision of the radiation dose estimates for the two cities (Straume and Dobson, 1981). Pending more complete analysis of the atomic-bomb dosimetry, the data cannot be used to derive valid inferences about the RBE of neutrons for carcinogenic effects in humans.

Internal Emitters

Although in principle the carcinogenic effects on a given tissue are the same, regardless of whether the radiation is received from a source outside the body or from within, certain aspects of the effects of internal emitters deserve special comment.

First, the anatomic distribution and temporal distribution of the radiation dose from an internal emitter are likely to be highly nonuniform (Smith et al., 1968; ICRP, 1979). The uptake, distribution, and retention of a radionuclide can vary profoundly, depending on the radionuclide in question, its physicochemical state, and its route of entry into the body. In the case of radioiodine, for example, the element rapidly concentrates and deposits the bulk of its emitted energy in the thyroid gland. The uptake of radioiodine by the thyroid gland is so predictable that it can be used as a test for thyroid function. In the case of radium, on the other hand, the element concentrates in the skeleton. The microscopic distribution of a radionuclide within its target organ is also often highly nonuniform, resulting in localized "hot spots." In the case of alpha emitters, the average dose in the hot spots can be orders of magnitude higher than that in neighboring areas, with the result that the "mean" tissue dose can be misleading.

Similarly, the distribution of the dose from an internally deposited radionuclide tends to be highly nonuniform in time, depending on the physical half-life and the biologic half-life of the element in question. Radionuclides that disintegrate slowly but are excreted rapidly are less hazardous than those having the opposite properties.

Because of the above nonuniformities in the spatial and temporal distribution of the dose, it is frequently difficult with internal emitters to determine precisely the dose to which a given carcinogenic effect should be attributed. In the case of long-lived, persistently retained internal emitters, the problem is further compounded by the fact that irradiation continues even after the cancer becomes clinically detectable, with the result that some fraction of the total cumulative dose is irrelevant to carcinogenesis and hence "wasted."

Host Factors Affecting Susceptibility

Susceptibility to the induction of a given type of neoplasm varies markedly among laboratory animals of different species and inbred strains (Upton, 1967; UN, 1977). It also varies with sex and with age at the time of irradiation (UN, 1977; NAS, 1980).

Patients treated in infancy with x-rays for familial retinoblastoma have shown a high incidence of second primary cancers in the radiation field, which has been interpreted as evidence for their heightened susceptibility (Knudson, 1977; Strong, 1977). A similarly heightened susceptibility to radiation-induced basal cell carcinoma has been reported in patients with the nevoid basal cell carcinoma syndrome (Strong, 1977).

The influence of age on susceptibility to radiation carcinogenesis shows a pattern that appears to vary slightly from one neoplasm to another (UN, 1977; NAS, 1980). The overall excess of cancers induced in adults by irradiation at a given age seems to resemble more closely a constant multiple of the natural incidence at that age than a constant number of additional cases irrespective of age (NAS, 1980). The radiation-induced increase in relative risk appears to be larger, however, in those irradiated during childhood or prenatal development than in those irradiated during adult life (NAS, 1980).

Analysis of the extent to which the carcinogenic effects of radiation on the human breast are influenced by other risk factors implies that there is no synergism between the effects of radiation and a family history of breast cancer, late parity, use of oral contraceptives, menopausal use of estrogens, or various ovarian-related factors; however, women given postpartum irradiation at their first childbirth appear to incur greater risk than those irradiated at a subsequent childbirth, even after allowance for the age differences. The data also indicate a particularly high risk in women with cystic disease of the breast and a history of irradiation (Shore *et al.*, 1980).

Modifying Effects of Other Physical and Chemical Agents

The carcinogenic effects of radiation may be enhanced or inhibited by a variety of other environmental agents. The promoting effects of hormonal stimulation on radiation carcinogenesis in endocrine glands and their target organs are well documented (Clifton and Sridharan, 1975; Furth, 1982). The excess of lung cancers in uranium miners who smoke cigarettes is higher, at least during early adult life, than would be predicted merely by adding the effects of smoking alone to those of uranium mining alone (NAS, 1980).

A variety of additional interactive effects between irradiation and other agents have been reported. These include a synergistic interaction with asbestos in the induction of mesotheliomas in rats (Warren *et al.*, 1981), and interactive effects with various chemical carcinogens in experimental animals (Elkind, 1980). Depending on the conditions of exposure to a given agent, additive, synergistic, or antagonistic interactions may be observed, for reasons that remain to be determined.

MECHANISMS

The carcinogenic effects of ionizing radiation result from molecular lesions caused by random interactions of impinging radiations with atoms and molecules in their path. Most of the molecular lesions induced in this way are of little consequence to the affected cell. It is well known, however, that damage to DNA is not repaired with 100% efficiency, and that the frequency of mutations and chromosomal aberrations increases with increasing radiation dose, presumably without any threshold (UN, 1977; NAS, 1980). These changes in genes and chromosomes have been postulated to account for the carcinogenic effects of radiation (UN, 1977; Upton, 1982a). The molecular mechanisms of radiation carcinogenesis, however, remain to be determined precisely.

Because the development of a neoplasm is a multicausal, multistage process (as described by Upton, 1982b), some observers have postulated that carcinogenesis involves sequential mutations, one or more of which may be inherited via the germ cells (Armitage and Doll, 1957; Knudson, 1977; Strong, 1977). To elucidate the mechanisms of radiation carcinogenesis at the molecular level and to explore the extent to which gene mutations, chromosomal aberrations, and other genetic alterations may be involved, research is now being focussed on the effects of radiation on cell transformation *in vitro* (Borek, 1980). The study of cell transformation in culture enables neoplastic changes, mutations, chromosomal aberrations, and other effects to be analyzed simultaneously in the same cell population. Although the results of such studies do not yet provide a definitive identification of the mechanism(s) of carcinogenesis, they point to the following important interim conclusions: (1) The frequency of transformed cells increases with increasing dose, reaching a plateau in the region of 1.5 to 4.0 Sv; (2) the transforming effectiveness per Sv of high-LET radiation is greater than that of low-LET radiation; (3) depending on the cell system used, transforming effects are detectable with doses as low as 1 mSv of fast neutrons or 10 mSv of x-rays; (4) the rate of transformation varies, depending on the cell system, radiation dose, and culture conditions used; (5) the rate of transformation may be modified after irradiation by agents that promote or inhibit carcinogenesis *in vivo* (Kennedy *et al.,* 1978; Borek *et al.,* 1979); (6) a dose of 0.5 to 3.0 Sv of x-rays divided into two fractions separated by an interval of five hours can cause a higher rate of transformation than the same dose delivered in a single exposure (Borek, 1979; Hall and Miller, 1981); and (7) essentially 100% of cells are potentially transformable under certain conditions of irradiation (Kennedy *et al.,* 1980).

The observations on transformation of cells *in vitro* are consistent with those on carcinogenesis *in vivo* and are helpful in amplifying some of the stages and relationships that are involved at the cellular and subcellular levels.

In vivo, however, additional homeostatic processes must also be taken into account in any consideration of the mechanisms of carcinogenesis. Effects of radiation on these processes (*e.g.,* cell population kinetics, hormonal regulation, and immunologic reactivity have been invoked as possible mechanisms of tumor promotion, at least with irradiation at high-dose levels (Cole and Nowell, 1965; UN, 1977; Upton, 1977).

ASSESSMENT OF OVERALL CANCER RISK

Estimates of the effects of whole-body irradiation on the cumulative overall risk of cancer must be highly tentative in our present state of knowledge. The majority of the atomic-bomb survivors are still alive, and the excess of cancers in this population continues to increase. Further analysis of the atomic-bomb dosimetry will be needed before the dose-incidence relationships can be assessed with confidence. Analysis of the data from patients irradiated for ankylosing spondylitis also involves uncertainties; *i.e.,* many of the patients are still alive; the irradiated fields did not include all tissues of the body; and the dose-distribution cannot be specified precisely in most instances.

In spite of the above sources of uncertainty, attempts have been made to derive crude estimates of the overall risk of radiation-induced cancer in populations exposed to low-level ionizing radiation, by extrapolation from observations at higher doses and dose rates, based on assumptions about the relevant dose-incidence relationships. The most widely used extrapolation model is based on the assumption that the cumulative incidence of cancer varies as a linear, nonthreshold function of the radiation dose (NAS, 1972), although other hypothetical dose-incidence models have also been used (UN, 1977; NAS, 1980).

Based on the use of these models, a range of risk estimates has been presented for cancers of various types and for the overall risk of cancers of all types combined (see Table 3-12). From these estimates, it is inferred that less than 2% of all cancers in the general population are attributable to natural background radiation (Jablon and Bailar, 1980), although as many as 20% of lung cancers in nonsmokers may be attributable to inhalation of naturally occurring radon in the atmosphere (Harley and Pasternack, 1980; Evans *et al.,* 1981).

Table 3–12.   Estimated Lifetime Cancer Risks from Low-Level
Radiation

	RISK PER 10,000 PERSONS/SV	
SITE	*Fatal Cancers*	*All Cancers*
Bone marrow (leukemia)	15–40	15–50
Thyroid	1–10	25–120
Breast (women only)	30–100	40–200
Lung	25–130	25–140
Stomach	3–50	5–60
Liver	3–50	5–60
Colon	3–50	5–60
Bone	2–15	5–30
Esophagus	2–15	5–30
Small intestine	2–15	5–30
Urinary bladder	2–15	5–30
Pancreas	2–15	5–30
Lymphatic tissue	2–15	5–30
Skin	—	1–2
Total (both sexes)	70–500	140–1000

From NAS, National Academy of Sciences, Advisory Committee on the Biological Effects of Ionizing Radiation (BEIR): *The Effects on Populations of Exposure to Low Levels of Ionizing Radiation.* National Academy Press, Washington, D.C., 1972, 1980; and UN, United Nations, Scientific Committee on the Effects of Atomic Radiation: *Sources and Effects of Ionizing Radiation.* Report to the General Assembly, with Annexes. United Nations, New York, 1977.

RADIOLOGIC PROTECTION

Until 20 years ago, genetic damage to future generations was thought to be the principal risk associated with low-level radiation. Epidemiologic studies of irradiated populations in recent years have implied that the risk of carcinogenic effects may be comparable in magnitude to the risk of genetic effects (UN, 1977; NAS, 1980). Any exposure to radiation is now assumed to cause some increase in the risk of cancer, therefore, strict limitation of exposure is clearly called for.

For purposes of radiologic protection (ICRP, 1977), a system of dose limitation has evolved, based on the principle that: (1) No practice involving radiation exposure should be undertaken unless it produces a net benefit; (2) all exposures should be kept as low as reasonably achievable, taking economic and social factors into account; and (3) the dose to any individual should not exceed the limits specified for the circumstances by the appropriate authority.

Since the average dose to the population from medical exposure now exceeds that from natural background, growing attention is being given to limitation of the doses involved in medical and dental practice (UN, 1977; NAS, 1980). Methods for reducing the dose to the patient from medical exposure include: (1)

Reduction of the number of radiographs per patient, with avoidance of unnecessary exposures; (2) reduction of the duration and intensity of exposure per radiograph; (3) use of radiography in preference to fluoroscopy whenever possible; (4) reduction of field size to a minimum; (5) shielding of tissues outside the field to be examined, especially the gonads; (6) proper training of staff engaged in radiologic examinations; and (7) proper calibration and operation of radiologic apparatus (ICRP, 1960). In the use of radiographic procedures for mass screening of asymptomatic populations, an appropriate balance between risk and benefit needs to be maintained, as illustrated in the guidelines for x-ray mammography in mass screening for early detection of breast cancer (Breslow *et al.,* 1977).

REFERENCES

Albert, R. E.; Omran, A. R.; Brauer, E. E.; Cohen, N. C.; Schmidt, H.; Dove, D. C.; Becker, M.; Baumring, R.; and Baer, R. L.: Follow-up study of patients treated by x-ray epilation for tinea capitis. II. Results of clinical and laboratory examinations. *Arch. Environ. Health,* **17:**919–934, 1968.

Archer, V. E.; Saccamanno, G.; and Jones, J. H.: Frequency of different histologic types of bronchogenic carcinoma as related to radiation exposure. *Cancer,* **34:**2056–2060, 1974.

Armitage, P., and Doll, R.: A two-stage theory of carcinogenesis in relation to the age distribution of human cancer. *Br. J. Cancer,* **11:**161–169, 1957.

Baral, E.; Larsson, L. E.; and Mattsson, B.: Breast cancer following irradiation of the breast. *Cancer,* **40:**2905–2910, 1977.

Beebe, G. W.: Ionizing radiation and health. *Am. Sci.,* **70:**35–44, 1982.

Beebe, G. W.; Kato, H.; and Land, C. E.: Studies of the mortality of A-bomb survivors. 6. Mortality and radiation dose, 1950–1974. *Radiat. Res.,* **75:**138–201, 1978.

Belsky, J. L.; Takeichi, N.; Yamamoto, T.; Cihak, R. W.; Hirose, F.; Ezaki, H.; Inoue, S.; and Blot, W. J.: Salivary gland neoplasms following atomic radiation. Additional cases and reanalysis of combined data in a fixed population, 1957–1970. *Cancer Res.,* **35:**555–559, 1975.

Benjamin, S. A.; Brooks, A. L.; and McClellan, R. O.: The biological effectiveness of Pu-239, Ce-144, and Sr-90 citrate in producing chromosome damage, bone-related tumors, liver tumors, and life shortening in the Chinese hamster. *Inhalation Toxicology Research Institute Annual Report LF-52.* Inhalation Toxicology Research Institute, Albuquerque, N.M., pp. 241–244, 1975.

Berdjis, C. C.: *Pathology of Irradiation.* The Williams & Wilkins Company, Baltimore, 1972.

Bithell, J. F., and Stewart, A. M.: Prenatal irradiation and childhood malignancy: A review of British data from the Oxford Survey. *Br. J. Cancer,* **31:**271–287, 1975.

Boice, J. D., Jr.; Land, C. E.; Shore, R. E.; Norman, J. E.; and Tokunaga, M.: Risk of breast cancer following low-dose exposure. *Radiology,* **131:**589–597, 1979.

Boice, J. D., Jr., and Monson, R. A.: Breast cancer in women after repeated fluoroscopic examinations of the chest. *J.N.C.I.,* **59:**823–832, 1977.

Boice, J. D., Jr.; Rosenstein, M.; and Trout, E. D.: Estimation of breast doses and breast cancer risk associated with repeated fluoroscopic chest examinations of women with tuberculosis. *Radiat. Res.,* **73:**373–390, 1978.

Borek, C.: Neoplastic transformation following split doses of x-rays. *Br. J. Radiol.,* **50:**845–846, 1979.

Borek, C.: X-ray induced in vitro neoplastic transformation of human diploid cells. *Nature,* **283:**776–778, 1980.

Borek, C.; Miller, R.; Pain, C.; and Troll, W.: Conditions for inhibiting and enhancing the protease inhibitor antipain on x-ray-induced neoplastic transformation in hamster and mouse cells. *Proc. Natl. Acad. Sci. USA,* **76:**1800–1803, 1979.

Breslow, L.; Henderson, B.; Massey, F., Jr.; Pike, M.; and Winkelstein, W., Jr.: Report of NCI ad hoc working group on the gross and net benefits of mammography in mass screening for the detection of breast cancer. *J.N.C.I.,* **59:**474–478, 1977.

Brinkley, D., and Haybittle, J. L.: The late effects of artificial menopause by x-radiation. *Br. J. Radiol.,* **42:**519–521, 1969.

Brues, A. M.: Carcinogenic effects of radiation. *Adv. Biol. Med. Phys.,* **2:**171–191, 1951.

Burns, F. J.; Albert, R. E.; and Heimbach, R. D.: RBE for skin tumors and hair follicle damage in the rat following radiation with alpha particles and electrons. *Radiat. Res.,* **36:**225, 1968.

Casarett, C. W.: Experimental radiation carcinogenesis. *Prog. Exp. Tumor Res.,* **7:**82, 1965.

Clifton, K. H., and Sridharan, B. N.: Endocrine factors and growth. In Becker, F. F. (ed.): *Cancer: A Compre-hensive Treatise,* Vol. 3. Plenum Press, New York, 1975.

Cole, L. J., and Nowell, P. C.: Radiation carcinogenesis: the sequence of events. *Science,* **150:**1782–1786, 1965.

Colman, M.; Kirsch, M.; and Creditor, M.: Tumours associated with medical x-ray therapy exposure in childhood. In *Late Biological Effects of Ionizing Radiation,* Vol. 1. International Atomic Energy Agency, Vienna, Austria, 1978.

Conard, R. A.; Paglia, D. E.; Larsen, P. R.; Sutow, W. W.; Dobyns, B. M.; Robbins, J.; Krotosky, W. A.; Field, J. B.; Rall, J. E.; and Wolff, J.: *Review of Medical Findings in a Marshallese Population Twenty-six Years After Exposure to Radioactive Fallout.* Brookhaven National Laboratory, Upton, New York, 1980.

Coop, K. L.; Sharp, J. G.; Osborne, J. W.; and Zimmerman, G. R.: An animal model for the study of small-bowel tumors. *Cancer Res.,* **34:**1487–1494, 1974.

Cosgrove, G. E.; Walburg, H. E.; and Upton, A. C.: Gastro-intestinal lesions in aged conventional and germfree mice exposed to radiation as young adults. *Monogr. Nucl. Med. Biol.,* **1:**302–312, 1968.

Court Brown, W. M., and Doll, R.: Mortality from cancer and other causes after radiotherapy for ankylosing spondylitis. *Br. Med. J.,* **2:**1327–1332, 1965.

Cuzick, J.: Leukemia occurrence compared with myeloma occurrence. *N. Engl. J. Med.,* **304:**204, 1981.

da Silva Horta, J. (organizer): International meeting on the toxicity of thorotrast and other alpha-emitting heavy elements. *Environ. Res.,* **18:**1–255, 1979.

da Silva Horta, J.; da Motta, L. C.; and Tavares, M. H.: Thorium dioxide effects in man. Epidemiological, clinical, and pathological studies (experience in Portugal). *Environ. Res.,* **8:**131–159, 1974.

da Silva Horta, J.; da Silva Horta, M. E.; da Motta, L. C.; and Tavares, M. H.: Malignancies in Portugese thorotrast patients. *Health Phys.,* **35:**137–151, 1978.

DeGroot, L. J.; Frohman, L. A.; Kaplan, E. L.; and Refetoff, S. R.: *Radiation-Associated Thyroid Carcinoma.* Grune & Stratton, Inc., New York, 1977.

Department of Health, Education and Welfare, Interagency Task Force on the Health Effects of Ionizing Radiation: *Report of the Work Group on Science.* U. S. Dept. of Health, Education and Welfare, Washington, D.C., 1979.

Dethlefsen, L. A.; Brown, J. M.; Carrano, A. V.; and Nandi, S.: Report of the BCTF *ad hoc* committee on x-ray mammography screening for human breast cancer. Can animal and *in vitro* studies give new, relevant answers? *J.N.C.I.,* **61:**1537–1545, 1978.

Diamond, E. L.; Schmerler, H.; and Lilienfeld, A. M.; The relationship of intrauterine radiation to subsequent mortality and development of leukemia in children. *Am. J. Epidemiol.,* **97:**283–313, 1973.

Dickson, R. J.: Late results of radium treatment of carcinoma of the cervix. *Clin. Radiol.,* **23:**528–535, 1972.

Doll, R.: Cancer following therapeutic external irradiation. Paper presented to the 10th International Cancer Congress, Houston, 1970.

Doll, R., and Smith, P. G.: The long term effects of x-irradiation in patients treated for metropathia haemorrhagica. *Br. J. Radiol.,* **41:**362–368, 1968.

Doll, R., and Smith, P. G.: Mortality from cancer and other causes after radiotherapy for ankylosing spondylitis. Further observations. In United Nations Scientific Committee on the Effects of Atomic Radiation: *Sources and Effects of Ionizing Radiation.* United Nations, New York, 1977.

Doniach, I.: Carcinogenesis effect of 100, 120 and 500 rad x-rays on the rat thyroid gland. *Br. J. Cancer,* **30:**487–495, 1974.

Elkind, M. M.: Combined effects, ionizing radiation plus other agents. In Interagency Radiation Research Committee: Proceedings of the Public Meeting to address a proposed Federal Radiation Research Agenda, Vol. 1, Issue Papers, 1980.

Evans, R. D.; Harley, J. H.; Jacobi, W.; McLean, A. S.; Mills, W. A.; and Stewart, C. G.: Estimate of risk from environmental exposure to radon-222 and its decay products. *Nature,* **290:**98–100, 1981.

Faber, M.: Malignancies in Danish thorotrast patients. *Health Phys.,* **35:**153–158, 1978.

Frieben, A.: Demonstration lines cancroids des rechten Handruckens, das sich nach langdauernder Einwirkung von Röntgenstrahlen entwickett hatte. *Fortschr. Geb. Rontgenstr. Nuklearmed. Erganzungsband,* **6:**106, 1902.

Furth, J.: Hormones as etiological agents in neoplasia. In Becker, F. F. (ed.): *Cancer: A Comprehensive Treatise, Vol. 1,* 2nd ed. Plenum Press, New York, 1982, pp. 89–134.

Furth, J., and Lorenz, E.: Carcinogenesis by ionizing radiations. In Hollaender, A. (ed.): *Radiation Biology, Vol. 1.* McGraw-Hill, Inc., New York, 1954.

Gates, O., and Warren, S.: Radiation-induced experimental cancer of the esophagus. *Am. J. Pathol.,* **53:**667–685, 1968.

Gibson, R. W.; Bross, D. J.; Graham, S.; Lilienfeld, A. M.; Schuman, L. M.; Levin, M. L.; and Dowd, J. E.: Leukemia in children exposed to multiple risk factors. *N. Engl. J. Med.,* **279:**906–909, 1968.

Glucksmann, A., and Cherry, C. P.: The induction of adenomas by the irradiation of salivary glands of rats. *Radiat. Res.,* **17:**186–202, 1962.

Hall, E. J., and Miller, R. C.: The how and why of *in vitro* oncogenic transformation. *Radiat. Res.,* **87:**208–223, 1981.

Ham, J. M.: *Report of the Royal Commission on the Health and Safety of Workers in Mines.* Ministry of the Attorney General, Province of Ontario, Toronto, Canada, 1976.

Hamilton, J. M.: Renal carcinogenesis. *Adv. Cancer Res.,* **22:**1–56, 1975.

Harley, N. H., and Pasternack, B. S.: A model for predicting lung cancer risks induced by environmental levels of radon daughters. *Health Phys.,* **40:**307–316, 1980.

Harrist, T. J.; Schiller, A. L.; Trelstad, R. L.; Mankin, H. J.; and Mays, C. W.: Thorotrast associated sarcoma of bone. *Cancer,* **44:**2049–2058, 1979.

Haymaker, W.; Rubinstein, L.; and Miquel, J.: Brain tumors in irradiated monkeys. *Acta Neuropathol.,* **20:**267–277, 1972.

Hempelmann, L. H.: Thyroid neoplasms following irradiation in infancy. In DeGroot, L. J.; Frohman, L. A.; Kaplan, E. L.; and Refetoff, S. R. (eds.): *Radiation-Associated Thryoid Carcinoma.* Grune & Stratton, New York, 1977.

Hempelmann, L. H.; Hall, W. J.; Phillips, M.; and Ames, W. R.: Neoplasms in persons treated with x-rays in infancy: Fourth survey in 20 years. *J.N.C.I.,* **55:**519–530, 1975.

Henshaw, P. S., and Hawkins, J. W.: Incidence of leukemia in physicians. *J.N.C.I.,* **4:**339–346, 1944.

Hirose, F.: Induction of gastric adenocarcinoma in mice by localized x-irradiation. *Gann,* **60:**253–260, 1969.

Horacek, J.; Placek, V.; and Sevc, J.: Histologic types of bronchogenic cancer in relation to different conditions of radiation exposure. *Cancer,* **40:**832–835, 1977.

Hulse, E.; Mole, R.; and Papworth, D.: Radiosensitivities of cells from which rad-induced skin tumors are derived. *Int. J. Radiat. Biol.,* **14:**437–444, 1968.

ICRP, International Commission on Radiological Protection: *Report of Committee III: Protection Against X-rays up to energies of 3 Mev and Beta- and Gamma-rays from Sealed Sources.* Pergamon Press, Inc., New York, 1960.

ICRP, International Commission on Radiological Protection: *Recommendations of the International Commission on Radiological Protection.* Pergamon Press, Oxford, 1977.

ICRP, International Commission on Radiological Protection: *Limits for Intakes of Radionuclides by Workers. A report of Committee 2 of the International Commission on Radiological Protection.* Pergamon Press, Inc., New York, 1979.

ICRU, International Commission on Radiation Units. *Radiation Quantities and Units.* International Commission on Radiation Units and Measurements, Washington, D.C., 1980.

Ishimaru, T.; Otake, M.; and Ichimaru, M.: Dose-response relationship of neutrons and gamma rays to leukemia incidence among atomic bomb survivors in Hiroshima and Nagasaki by type of leukemia, 1950–1971. *Radiat. Res.,* **77:**377–394, 1979.

Jablon, S., and Bailar, J. C., III: The contribution of ionizing radiation to cancer mortality in the United States. *Prev. Med.,* **9:**219–226, 1980.

Jones, A.: Irradiation sarcoma. *Br. J. Radiol.,* **26:**273–284, 1953.

Jorgensen, H. S.: A study of mortality from lung cancer among miners in Kiruna 1950–1970. *Work Environ. Health,* **10:**125–133, 1973.

Kaplan, H. S., and Brown, M. B.: A quantitative dose response study of lymphoid-tumor development in irradiated C57 black mice. *J.N.C.I.,* **13:**185–208, 1952.

Kennedy, A.; Fox, M.; Murphy, G.; and Little, J. B.: On the relationship between x-ray exposure and malignant transformation in C3H 10T 1/2 cells. *Proc. Natl. Acad. Sci. USA,* **77:**7262–7266, 1980.

Kennedy, A., and Little, J. B.: Radiation carcinogenesis in the respiratory tract. In Harris, C. C. (ed.): *Pathogenesis and Therapy of Lung Cancer.* Marcel Dekker, Inc., New York, 1978.

Kennedy, A.; Mondal, S.; Heidelberger, C.; and Little, J. B.: Enhancement of x-ray transformation by 12-O-tetradecanoyl-phorbol-13-acetate in a cloned line of C3H mouse embryo cells. *Cancer Res.,* **38:**439–443, 1978.

Kim, J. H.; Chu, F. C.; Woodard, H. Q.; Melamed, M. R.; Huvos, A.; and Cantin, J.: Radiation induced soft-tissue and bone sarcoma. *Radiology,* **129:**501–508, 1978.

Kneale, G. W.; Stewart, A. M.; and Mancuso, T. F.: Reanalysis of data relating to the Hanford study of the cancer risks of radiation workers. In *Late Biological Effects of Ionizing Radiation, Vol. 1.* International Atomic Energy Agency, Vienna, Austria, 1978.

Knudson, A. G.: Genetics and etiology of human cancer. *Adv. Hum. Genet.,* **1:**66, 1977.

Lacassagne, A.: Les cancers produits par les rayonnements corpusculaires; mécanisme présumable de la cancerisation par les rayons. *Actualities Scientifiques et Industrielles,* **981:**1–137, 1945a.

Lacassagne, A. Les cancers produits par les rayonnements électromagnetiques. *Actualities Scientifiques et Industrielles,* **975:**1–102, 1945b.

Land, C. E.: A-bomb survivor studies, immunity, and the epidemiology of radiation carcinogenesis. In Dubnois, J. B.; Serrou, B.; and Rosenfeld, C. (eds.): *Immunopharmacologic Effects of Radiation Therapy.* Raven Press, New York, 1981.

Lebedeva, G. A.: Intestinal polyps arising under the influence of various kinds of ionizing radiations. *Vopr. Onkol.,* **19:**47–51, 1973.

Lindsay, S., and Chaikoff, I. L.: The effects of irradiation on the thyroid gland with particular reference to the induction of thyroid neoplasms: A review. *Cancer Res.,* **24:**1099–1107, 1964.

Little, J. B.: Biological consequences of x-ray induced DNA damage and repair processes in relation to cell killing and carcinogenesis. In Hanawalt, P.; Friedbert, E. C.; and Fox, C. F. (eds.): *DNA Repair Mechanisms. ICN-UCLA Symposia on Molecular and Cellular Biology, Vol. 9.* Academic Press, Inc., New York, 1978.

Little, J. B.; McGrandy, R. B.; and Kennedy, A. R.: Interactions between polonium-210, α-radiation, benzo(a)pyrene, and 0.9% NaCl solution installations in the induction of experimental lung cancer. *Cancer Res.,* **38:**1929–1935, 1978.

Lorenz, E.: Radioactivity and lung cancer: a critical review of lung cancer in the miners of Schneeberg and Joachimsthal. *J.N.C.I.,* **5:**1–5, 1944.

McGregor, D. H.; Land, C. E.; Choi, K.; Tokuoka, S.; Liv, P. I.; Wakabayaski, T.; and Beebe, G. W.: Breast cancer incidence among bomb survivors, Hiroshima and Nagasaki, 1950–1969. *J.N.C.I.,* **59:**799–811, 1977.

McIntyre, D., and Pointor, R. C. S.: Vesical neoplasms occurring after radiation treatment for carcinoma of the uterine cervix. *J. R. Coll. Surg. Edinb.,* **16:**141–146, 1971.

MacKenzie, I.: Breast cancer following multiple fluoroscopies. *Br. J. Cancer,* **19:**1–8, 1965.

MacMahon, B.: Prenatal x-ray exposure and childhood cancer. *J.N.C.I.,* **28:**1173–1191, 1962.

Maldague, P.: Comparative study of experimentally induced cancer of the kidney in mice and rats with x-rays. In *Radiation-Induced Cancer.* International Atomic Energy Agency, Vienna, Austria, 1969.

Mancuso, T. F.; Stewart, A.; and Kneale, G.: Radiation exposure of Hanford workers dying from cancer and other causes. *Health Phys.,* **33:**369–385, 1977.

Martland, H. S. The occurrence of malignancy in radioactive persons. *Am. J. Cancer,* **15:**2435, 1931.

Matanoski, G. M.: Risk of cancer associated with occupational exposure in radiologists and other radiation workers. In Burchenal, J. H., and Oettgen, H. F. (eds.): *Cancer: Achievements, Challenges and Prospects for the 1980s.* Grune & Stratton, Inc., New York, 1981.

Matanoski, G. M.; Seltser, R.; Sartwell, P. E.; Diamond, E. L.; and Elliott, E. A.: The current mortality rates of radiologists and other physician specialists. Deaths from all causes and from cancer. *Am. J. Epidemiol.,* **101:**188–198, 1975.

Mays, C. W.; Jee, W. S. S.; Lloyd, R. D.; Stover, B. J.; Dougherty, J. H.; and Taylor, G. N. (eds.): *Delayed Effects of Bone-Seeking Radionuclides.* University of Utah Press, Salt Lake City, Utah, 1969.

Mays, C. W., and Spiess, H.: Bone sarcoma risks to man from ^{224}Ra, ^{226}Ra, and ^{239}Pu. In Muller, W. A., and Ebert, H. G. (eds.): *Biological Effects of ^{224}Ra: Benefit and Risk of Therapeutic Application.* Nijhoff Medical Division, The Hague, 1978.

Mays, C. W., and Spiess, H.: Bone tumors in Thorotrast patients. *Environ. Res.,* **18:**88–93, 1979.

Mays, C. W.; Spiess, H.; and Gerspach, A.: Skeletal effects following ^{224}Ra injections into humans. *Health Phys.,* **35:**83–90, 1978.

Metalli, P.; Covelli, V.; DiPaola, M.; and Silini, G.: Dose-incidence data for mouse reticulum cell sarcoma. *Radiat. Res.,* **59:**21, 1974.

Modan, B.; Baidatz, D.; Mart, H.; Steinitz, R.; and Levin, S. G.: Radiation-induced head and neck tumors. *Lancet,* **1:**277–279, 1974.

Modan, B., and Lilienfeld, A. M.: Polycythemia vera and leukaemia—the role of radiation treatment. *Medicine,* **44:**305–344, 1965.

Modan, B.; Ron, E.; and Werner, A.: Thyroid cancer following scalp irradiation. *Radiology,* **123:**741–744, 1977.

Mole, R. H.: Antenatal irradiation and childhood cancer. Causation or coincidence? *Br. J. Cancer,* **30:**199–208, 1974.

Mole, R. H.: Ionizing radiation as a carcinogen: practical questions and academic pursuits. *Br. J. Radiol.,* **48:**157–169, 1975.

Mole, R. H.: The radiobiological significance of the studies with ^{224}Ra and Thorotrast. *Health Phys.,* **35:**167–174, 1978.

Mori, T.; Kato, Y.; Shimamine, T.; and Watanabe, S.: Statistical analysis of Japanese Thorotrast-administered autopsy cases. In International Meeting on the Toxicity of Thorotrast and Other Alpha-Emitting Heavy Elements. Lisbon. *Environ. Res.,* **18:**231–244, 1979.

Myrden, J. A., and Hiltz, J. E.: Breast cancer following multiple fluoroscopies during artificial pneumothorax treatment of pulmonary tuberculosis. *Can. Med. Assoc. J.,* **100:**1032–1034, 1969.

NAS, National Academy of Sciences Advisory Committee on the Biological Effects of Ionizing Radiation (BEIR): *The Effects on Populations of Exposure to Low Levels of Ionizing Radiation.* National Academy Press, Washington D.C., 1972, 1980.

NCRPM, National Council on Radiation Protection and Measurements: *Influence of Dose and Its Distribution in Time on Dose-Response Relationships for Low-Let Radiations.* National Council on Radiation Protection and Measurements, Washington, 1980.

Nowell, P. C.; Cole, L. J.; and Ellis, E.: Neoplasms of the glandular stomach in mice irradiated with x-rays or fast neutrons. *Cancer Res.,* **18:**257–260, 1958.

Okada, S.; Hamilton, H. F.; Egami, N.; Okajima, S.; Russell, W. J.; and Takeshita, K. (eds.): A review of thirty years study of Hiroshima and Nagasaki atomic bomb survivors. *J. Radiat. Res. (Tokyo),* **16**(Suppl.):1–164, 1975.

Palmer, J. P., and Spratt, D. W.: Pelvic carcinoma following irradiation for benign gynaecological diseases. *Am. J. Obstet. Gynecol.,* **72:**497–505, 1956.

Parker, L. N.; Belsky, J. L.; Yamamoto, T.; Kawamoto, S.; and Keehn, R. J.: Thyroid carcinoma diagnosed between 13 and 26 years after exposure to atomic radiation. A study of the ABCC-HNIH Adult Health Study Population Hiroshima and Nagasaki 1958–71. Technical Report 5-73. *Ann. Intern. Med.,* **80:**600–604, 1974.

Pinkston, J. A., and Sekine, I.: Postirradiation sarcoma (malignant fibrous histiocytoma) following cervix cancer. *Cancer,* **49:**434–438, 1982.

Pochin, E. E.: Leukaemia following radioiodine treatment of thyrotoxicosis. *Br. Med. J.,* **5212:**1545–1550, 1960.

Polednak, A. P.; Stehney, A. F.; and Rowland, R. E.: Mortality among women first employed before 1930 in the U.S. radium dial painting industry. A group ascertained from employment lists. *Am. J. Epidemiol.,* **107:**179–195, 1978.

Rowland, R. E., and Stehney, A. F.: Radium-induced malignancies. In Argonne National Laboratory Report ANL-78-65, Part II, 259–264, 1978.

Saenger, E. L.; Silverman, F. N.; Sterling, T. D.; and Turner, M. E.: Neoplasia following therapeutic irradiation for benign conditions in childhood. *Radiology,* **74:**889–904, 1960.

Safa, A. M.; Schumacher, O. P.; and Rodriquez-Antunez, A.: Long-term follow-up results in children and adolescents treated with radioactive iodine (^{131}I) for hyperthyroidism. *N. Engl. J. Med.,* **292:**167–171, 1975.

Schneider, A. B.; Favus, M. J.; Stachuro, M. E.; Arnold, J.; Arnold, M. J.; and Frohman, L. A.: Incidence, prevalence and characteristics of radiation-induced thyroid tumors. *Am. J. Med.,* **64:**243–252, 1978.

Secova, M.; Sevc, J.; and Thomas, J.: Alpha irradiation of the skin and the possibility of late effects. *Health Phys.,* **35:**803–806, 1978.

Sevc, J.; Kunz, E.; and Placek, V.: Lung cancer in uranium miners and long-term exposure to radon daughter products. *Health Phys.,* **30:**433–437, 1976.

Shellabarger, C. J.: Radiation carcinogenesis. *Cancer,* **37:**1090–1096, 1976.

Shellabarger, C. J.; Bond, V. P.; Cronkite, E. P.; and Aponte, G. E.: Relationship of dose of total body ^{60}Co radiation to incidence of mammary neoplasia in female rats. In *Radiation-Induced Cancer.* International Atomic Energy Agency, Vienna, Austria, 1969.

Shellabarger, C. J.; Brown, R. D.; Rao, A. R.; Shanley, J. P.; Bond, V. P.; Kellerer, A. M.; Rossi, H. H.; Goodman, L. J.; and Mills, R. E.: Rat mammary carcinogenesis following neutron or x-radiation. In *Biological Effects of Neutron Irradiation.* International Atomic Energy Agency, Vienna, Austria, 1974.

Shellabarger, C. J.; Chmelevsky, D.; and Kellerer, A. M.: Induction of mammary neoplasms in the Sprague-Dawley rat by 430 keV neutrons and x-rays. *J.N.C.I.,* **64:**821–833, 1980.

Shellabarger, C. J.; Stone, J. P.; and Holtzman, S.: Synergism between neutron radiation and diethylstilbestrol in the production of mammary adenocarcinomas in the rat. *Cancer Res.,* **36:**1019–1022, 1976.

Shore, R. E.; Albert, R.E.; and Pasternack, B. S.: Follow-up study of patients treated by x-ray epilation for tinea capitis. Resurvey of post-treatment illness and mortality experience. *Arch. Environ. Health,* **31:**17–28, 1976.

Shore, R. E.; Hempelmann, L. H.; Kowaluk, E.; Mansur, P.; Pasternack, B.; Albert, R.; and Haughie, G.: Breast neoplasms in women treated with x-rays for acute post-partum mastitis. *J.N.C.I.,* **59:**813–822, 1977.

Shore, R. E.; Woodard, E. D.; Hempelmann, L. H.; and Pasternack, B. S.: Synergism between radiation and other risk factors for breast cancer. *Rev. Med.,* **9:**815–822, 1980.

Smith, E. M.; Brownell, G. L.; and Ellett, W. H.: Radiation dosimetry. In Wagner, H. N., Jr. (ed.): *Principles of Nuclear Medicine.* W. B. Saunders Company, Philadelphia, 1968.

Smith, P. G., and Doll, R.: Later effects of x-irradiation in patients treated for metropathia haemorrhagica. *Br. J. Radiol.,* **49:**224–232, 1976.

Smith, P. G., and Doll, R.: Age- and time-dependent changes in the rates of radiation-induced cancers in patients with ankylosing spondylitis following a single course of x-ray treatment. In *Late Biological Effects of Ionizing Radiation.* International Atomic Energy Agency, Vienna, Austria, 1978.

Smith, P. G., and Doll, R.: Mortality from cancer and all causes among British radiologists. *Br. J. Radiol.,* **54:**187–194, 1981.

Smith, P. G., and Doll, R.: Mortality among patients with ankylosing spondylitis after a single treatment course with x-rays. *Br. Med. J.,* **284:**449–460, 1982.

Spiess, H., and Mays, C. W.: Bone cancers induced by ^{224}Ra (ThX) in children and adults. *Health Phys.,* **19:**713–729, 1970.

Straume, T., and Dobson, R. L.: Implications of new Hiroshima and Nagasaki dose estimates: cancer risks and neutron RBE. *Health Phys.,* **41:**666–671, 1981.

Strong, L. C.: Theories of pathogenesis: mutation and cancer. In Mulvihill, J. H.; Millers, R. W.; and Fraumeni, J. F., Jr. (eds.): *Genetics of Human Cancer.* Raven Press, New York, 1977.

Takahashi, S.: A statistical study on human cancer induced by medical irradiation. *Acta. Radiol. (Nippon),* **23:**1510–1530, 1964.

Takeichi, N.: Induction of salivary gland tumours following x-ray examination. II. Development of salivary gland tumours in long-term experiments. *Med. J. Hiroshima Univ.,* **23:**391–411, 1975 (in Japanese).

Taylor, G. N.; Jee, W. S. S.; Williams, J. L.; and Shabestari, L.: Hepatic changes induced by ^{239}Pu. In Stover, B. J., and Jee, W. S. S. (eds.): *Radiology of Plutonium.* J. W. Press, University of Utah, Salt Lake City, 1972.

Thomson, J. F.; Williamson, F. S.; Grahn, D.; and Ainsworth, E. J.: Life shortening in mice exposed to fission neutrons and γ rays. *Radiat. Res.,* **86:**559–572, 1981.

Thurman, G. B.; Mays, C. W.; Taylor, G. N.; Keane, A. T.; and Sissons, H. A.: Skeletal location of radiation-induced and naturally occurring osteosarcomas in man and dog. *Cancer Res.,* **33:**1604–1607, 1973.

Tokunaga, M.; Norman, J. E., Jr.; Asano, M.; Tokuoka, S.; Ezaki, H.; Nishimori, I.; and Tsuji, Y.: Malignant breast tumors among atomic bomb survivors, Hiroshima and Nagasaki, 1950–1974. *J.N.C.I.,* **62:**1347–1359, 1979.

Traenkle, H. L.: X-ray induced skin cancer in man. In *Biology of Cutaneous Cancer. Natl. Cancer Inst. Monogr.,* **10:**423–432, 1963.

UN, United Nations: *Ionizing Radiation: Levels and Effects. A Report of the United Nations Scientific Committee on the Effects of Atomic Radiation.* General Assembly, Official Records: 27th Session, Suppl. Number 25 (A/8725), New York, 1972.

UN, United Nations, Scientific Committee on the Effects of Atomic Radiation: Sources and Effects of Ionizing Radiation. Report to the General Assembly, With Annexes. United Nations, New York, 1977.

Upton, A. C.: The dose-response relation in radiation induced cancer. *Cancer Res.,* **21:**717–729, 1961.

Upton, A. C.: Comparative observations on radiation carcinogenesis in man and animals. In *Carcinogenesis: A Broad Critique.* The Williams & Wilkins Company, Baltimore, 1967.

Upton, A. C.: Radiation carcinogenesis. In Busch, H. (ed.): *Methods in Cancer Research, Vol. IV.* Academic Press, New York, 1968.

Upton, A. C.: Physical carcinogenesis: Radiation—

history and sources. In Becker, F. F. (ed.): *Cancer, Vol. 1.* Plenum Publishing Corporation, New York, 1975.

Upton, A. C.: Radiobiological effects of low doses: implications for radiological protection. *Radiat. Res.,* **71**:51–74, 1977.

Upton, A. C.: Principles of tumor biology. Etiology and prevention. In DeVita, V. T.; Hellman, S.; and Rosenberg, S. A. (eds.): *Principles and Practices of Oncology.* J. B. Lippincott Company, Philadelphia, 1982a.

Upton, A. C.: Role of DNA damage in radiation and chemical carcinogenesis. In Sugimura, T.; Kondo, S.; and Takebe, H. (eds.): *Proceedings of the Third International Conference on Environmental Mutagens.* University of Tokyo Press, Tokyo, 1982b.

Upton, A. C.; Cosgrove, G. E.; and Lushbaugh, C. C.: Induction of carcinoma of the glandular stomach in mice by whole-body irradiation. *Gann Monogr.,* **8**:63–74, 1969.

Upton, A. C.; Furth, J.; and Burnett, W. T., Jr.: Liver damage and hepatomas in mice produced by radioactive colloidal gold. *Cancer Res.,* **16**:211–215, 1956.

Upton, A. C.; Kimball, A. W.; Furth, J.; Christenberry, K. W.; and Benedict, W. H.: Some delayed effects of atom bomb radiations in mice. *Cancer Res.,* **20**:1–62, 1960.

Upton, A. C.; Randolph, M. L.; and Conklin, J. W.: Late effects of fast neutrons and gamma-rays in mice as influenced by dose rate of irradiation. *Radiat. Res.,* **32**:493–509, 1967.

Upton, A. C.; Randolph, M. L.; and Conklin, J. W.: Late effects of fast neutrons and gamma-rays in mice as influenced by the dose rate of irradiation: induction of neoplasia. *Radiat. Res.,* **41**:467–491, 1970.

Upton, A. C.; Wolff, F. F.; Furth, J.; and Kimball, A. W.: A comparison of the induction of myeloid and lymphoid

leukemias in x-radiated RF mice. *Cancer Res.,* **18**:842–848, 1958.

van Kaick, G.; Lorentz, D.; Muth, H.; Kaul, A.: Malignancies in German thorotrast patients and estimated tissue dose. *Health Phys.,* **35**:127–136, 1978.

Vogel, H. H., and Zaldivar, R.: Experimental mammary neoplasms: A comparison of effectiveness between neutrons, x- and gamma-radiation. In *Proceedings of the Symposium on Neutrons in Radiobiology.* USAEC, Oak Ridge, Tenn., 1969.

von Jagie, N.; Schwarz, G.; and Von Siebenrock, L.: Blutbefunde bei Röntgenologon. *Berl. Klin. Wschr.,* **48**:1220–1222, 1911.

Walinder, G.: Late effects of irradiation on the thyroid gland of mice. I. Irradiation of adult mice. *Acta Radiol. Ther. Phys. Biol.* **11**:433–451, 1972.

Warren, S.; Brown, C. E.; Chute, R. N.; and Federman, M.: Mesothelioma relative to asbestos, radiation, and methylcholanthrene. *Arch. Pathol. Lab. Med.,* **105**:304–312, 1981.

Warren, S., and Gates, O.: Radiation-induced cancer on the esophagus as an experimental model. *Cancer Bull.,* **20**:57–59, 1968.

Webber, B. M.: Radiation therapy for pertussis. A possible etiologic factor in thyroid carcinoma. *Ann. Intern. Med.,* **86**:449–450, 1977.

Yoshizawa, Y.; Kusama, T.; and Morimoto, K.: Search for the lowest irradiation dose from literatures on radiation induced bone tumours. *Acta Radiol.* (Nippon), **37**:377–386, 1977.

Yoshizawa, Y., and Takeuchi, T.: Search for the lowest irradiation dose from literatures on radiation induced cancer in pharynx and larynx. *Acta Radiol.* (Nippon), **34**:903–909, 1974.

D.   VIRAL

Fred Rapp and Harriet C. Isom

INTRODUCTION

The role of viruses in the etiology of neoplasia has been studied for over 70 years, but it still cannot be stated unequivocally that viruses cause tumors in humans. A great deal of information concerning the relationship between viruses and cancer has been amassed, but many questions remain unanswered. Virologists have clearly demonstrated that inoculation of animals with certain viruses produces tumors. Indeed, certain cancers occurring naturally in animals, such as the Lucké renal adenocarcinoma of frogs, Marek's lymphomatous disease in chickens, and leukemia in cats and cattle, are transmitted horizontally from animal to animal by viruses. In humans, some papillomavirus infections produce warts that can become cancerous, and particles resembling viruses associated with the transmission of leukemia in animals have been found in human cancer patients. In addition, in Burkitt's lymphoma, nasopharyngeal carcinoma (NPC), human cervical cancer, and hepatocellular carcinoma a definite correlation between the disease, viral infection, and the presence and retention of specific virus nucleic acid sequences and virus proteins in the tumor cells has been found. This chapter examines the role of specific viruses in certain animal and human cancers. The reader is directed to medical virology textbooks for detailed information on structure, macromolecular synthesis, and replication of the various tumor viruses.

Historical Background of Viral Oncology

The conclusion that pathogenic microorganisms were the causative agents of anthrax, tuberculosis, diphtheria and other infectious diseases and the discovery of viruses as infectious agents led to speculation that cancer might be caused by viruses. Ellermann and Bang (1908) demonstrated in 1908 that cell-free extracts could be used to transmit leukemia in chickens. Shortly thereafter, Rous (1911) published observations revealing that a solid tumor (a sarcoma) of chickens could be similarly transmitted. Speculation that these findings were simply isolated events related to avian cancer was resolved when Shope (1932) discovered that a virus isolated from wild cottontail rabbits produced highly neoplastic carcinomas in domestic rabbits. The same virus, however, produced a wartlike growth in wild rabbits that remained benign or regressed. Interest in the viral etiology of cancer mounted as Bittner (1936) showed that milk consumed by suckling mice could contain a virus responsible for transmission of mammary tumors from mother to offspring. In retrospect, this observation was probably made possible by newly developed inbred lines of mice. Two years later, Lucké (1938) reported observations suggesting a virus as the cause of a naturally occurring renal adenocarcinoma in leopard frogs. Research in viral oncology, however, was hampered by technical difficulties involved in studying viruses in the laboratory. This obstacle was overcome in the early 1950s with the development of techniques for widespread cultivation of animal cells *in vitro*. The findings (by Gross, 1951) that leukemia in mice was of viral origin initiated the modern era of viral oncology.

DNA and RNA Tumor Viruses

DNA viruses associated with cancer are listed by family in Table 3–13 and are represented in all DNA virus groups except the parvovirus family. This distribution reveals that all DNA tumor viruses contain double-stranded DNA; the parvoviruses contain only single-stranded DNA. DNA tumor viruses range in size (see Figure 3–13) from the small human papovaviruses (38 to 40 nm) and hepatitis B virus (42 nm) to the herpesviruses (180 to 200 nm). The DNA of the human BK virus (BKV) has a molecular weight of 3.45×10^6 daltons, whereas the molecular weight of human cytomegalovirus (CMV) DNA is more than fortyfold (150×10^6 daltons) greater. All DNA tumor viruses are icosahedral and some are enveloped (the herpesviruses), whereas

others, such as the papovaviruses and adenoviruses, are not.

The RNA viruses are subdivided into nine families, but only one, the retroviruses, is associated with oncogenicity. Retroviruses differ from all other RNA viruses because they require a DNA intermediate to replicate. All retroviruses contain and specify reverse transcriptase, an enzyme that, in the presence of the four nucleoside triphosphates, can synthesize DNA complementary to the single-stranded RNA contained in the virion. About 30 molecules of reverse transcriptase are packaged in each virion. Early after infection, DNA synthesis can be detected in the cytoplasm as an RNA-DNA hybrid is synthesized. The virus RNA is then degraded and a double-stranded linear DNA molecule forms, which moves to the nucleus and is integrated into the cellular DNA as provirus. Transcription of the integrated provirus yields progeny RNA. The reverse transcriptase most likely performs three enzymatic functions: (1) Formation of the RNA-DNA hybrid; (2) degradation of the RNA in the RNA-DNA hybrid; and (3) formation of the DNA-DNA double strand. The retrovirus virions are spherical, enveloped particles 70 to 100 nm in diameter. The capsid is icosahedral and contains the single-stranded RNA genome, a 70S RNA that, like cellular mRNA, has a poly(A) tail at the 3' end and a cap at the 5' end. The surface envelope possesses antigenic glycoprotein spikes that function in adsorption of the virus to the host cell. Retroviruses associated with a viral etiology of cancer are listed in Table 3–14.

Comparison of Viruses with Chemicals as Carcinogens

Our current knowledge of how viruses act as carcinogens indicates that the mechanism of viral carcinogenesis may be quite different from that of chemical carcinogenesis. Many viruses act as carcinogens by adding specific virus genes to the cell genome. It has often been demonstrated that cells transformed by a variety of DNA or RNA tumor viruses contain viral DNA sequences integrated into the cellular DNA. In addition, in some cases, *i.e.,* lymphocytes transformed by the DNA-containing Epstein-Barr virus (EBV), the virus DNA can also be present and persist in daughter cells in the form of a nonintegrated plasmid. In papova- and adenovirus-transformed cells, a

Table 3–13. DNA Viruses Associated with Cancer

VIRUS GROUP (OR FAMILY)	VIRUS MEMBER	ABBREVIATION	NATURAL HOST	ASSOCIATION WITH ONCOGENICITY
Papovaviruses	Polyomavirus	Py	Mouse	Wide variety of tumors (particularly sarcomas) in hamsters, mice, and rats
	Simian virus 40	SV 40	Monkey	Lymphocytic leukemia, ependymomas, lymphosarcoma, reticulum cell sarcoma, and osteogenic sarcoma in hamsters; tumors in mice and rats
	BK virus	BKV	Human	Fibrosarcomas and ependymomas in hamsters
	JC virus	JCV	Human	Brain tumors in hamsters and owl monkeys
	Papillomaviruses Human	HPV 5	Human	Squamous cell carcinoma in humans
		HPV 6	Human	Squamous cell carcinoma in humans
		HPV ?	Human	Laryngeal papilloma in humans
	Shope		Rabbit	Squamous cell carcinoma in domestic rabbits
	Bovine	BPV	Cow	Esophageal papilloma in cow
	Mastomys		*Mastomys natalensis*	Invasive acanthomas in mastomys
Hepatitis B virus	Hepatitis B virus	HBV	Human	Primary hepatocellular carcinoma in humans
Adenoviruses	Human types 3, 7, 11, 12, 14, 16, 18, 21, 31		Human	Undifferentiated sarcomas and neoplastic lymphomas in hamster, mouse, rat, and mastomys
	Simian		Monkey	Sarcomas in hamster, rat, and mouse
	Bovine type 3		Cow	Sarcomas in hamster
	Avian	CELO	Chicken	Sarcomas in hamster
Herpesviruses	Herpes simplex virus (types 1 and 2)	HSV HSV 1, HSV 2	Human	Uterine cervical and vulvar carcinoma in humans; adenocarcinoma and fibrosarcoma in hamsters
	Cytomegalovirus	CMV	Human	Prostatic carcinoma, Kaposi's sarcoma, uterine cervical carcinoma in humans
	Epstein-Barr virus	EBV	Human	Burkitt's lymphoma, nasopharyngeal carcinoma, and Hodgkin's disease in humans
	Lucké herpesvirus	LHV	Frogs	Lucké adenocarcinoma in frogs
	Marek's disease virus	MDV	Chickens	Neurolymphomatosis in chickens
	Herpesvirus ateles	HVA	Spider monkeys	Lymphoma in marmosets, owl monkeys, and rabbits
	Herpesvirus saimiri	HVS	Squirrel monkeys	Lymphoma in marmosets, owl monkeys, and rabbits
	Herpesvirus sylvilagus		Rabbit	Lymphoma in rabbits
	Guinea pig herpesvirus	GPHV	Guinea pig	Lymphocytic leukemia in guinea pigs
Poxviruses	Yaba monkey tumor virus		Monkey	Benign skin tumors of monkeys and other primates
	Rabbit fibroma virus		Rabbit	Fibromas in cottontail and domestic rabbits
	Myxomavirus		Rabbit	Fibromas in South American forest rabbit and lethal disease in domestic European rabbits

DNA viruses

Poxvirus

Herpesvirus

Hepatitis B virus

Adenovirus

Papovavirus

RNA viruses

Retrovirus

|———————|
100 nm

Figure 3–13 Diagram illustrating the shapes and relative sizes of DNA and RNA tumor viruses.

large number of sites in the viral sequence can be joined to cellular DNA, indicating the absence of specificity in the choice of viral sequences that participate in integration. Of equal importance is the finding that a large number of cellular sequences function as satis-

factory targets for papova- and adenovirus integration. Specifically, in human cells transformed by the DNA-containing papovavirus simian virus 40 (SV 40), the virus sequences can integrate not only into different sites within the same chromosome but also into different chromosomes (Croce, 1981). Molecular biologists have concluded that the integration of DNA tumor virus genes into cell DNA is inefficient. Although integration of DNA tumor virus sequences is accomplished in the laboratory under manipulated conditions, the low efficiency of integration raises questions about how this process occurs in nature. Integration events are not controlled, are dependent upon illegitimate (nonhomologous) recombination events, and therefore, generate inactive configurations of viral sequences with great frequency.

In contrast to the low efficiency of integration of DNA viruses, integration of retrovirus sequences into the cell genome is often efficient. It is possible that this efficiency has evolved because integration of retrovirus sequences into the cell genome is mandatory for replication of RNA tumor viruses, whereas integration is not required in the life cycle of DNA viruses. In addition, retrovirus infection of cells harboring silent endogenous retrovirus sequences can result in exogenous retrovirus sequences integrating adjacent to silent endogenous sequences or recombining with them.

The presence of integrated virus sequences within cells cannot be equated with transformation. Support for this statement comes from at least two major findings. First, inte-

Table 3–14. RNA Viruses Associated with Cancer

VIRUS GROUP (OR FAMILY)	VIRUS MEMBER	ABBREVIATION	NATURAL HOST	ASSOCIATION WITH ONCOGENICITY
Avian retroviruses	Sarcoma (Rous)	RSV	Chicken	Sarcoma in chicken, quail, turkey, duck, hamster, monkey
	Leukemia	ALV	Chicken	Leukemia in chicken, turkey
Murine retroviruses	Sarcoma	MSV	Mouse	Sarcoma in mouse, rat, hamster, cat
	Leukemia	MuLV	Mouse	Leukemia, lymphoma in mouse, rat, hamster
	Murine mammary tumor (Bittner)	MMTV	Mouse	Adenocarcinoma in mouse
Feline retroviruses	Sarcoma	FeSV	Cat	Sarcoma in cat, dog, rabbit, monkey
	Leukemia	FeLV	Cat	Leukemia and lymphoma in cat
Primate retroviruses	Simian sarcoma	SiSV	Woolly monkey	Fibrosarcomas in marmoset monkey
	Gibbon ape leukemia	GALV	Gibbon ape	Lymphosarcoma in ape
	Mason-Pfizer	MPMV	Monkey	Mammary carcinoma in monkey
Human retroviruses	T-cell leukemia	$HTLV_{CR}$	Human	Cutaneous adult T-cell leukemia/lymphoma

grated parvovirus DNA has been found in cells that are persistently infected but are not transformed. Second, retrovirus genes are present in the DNA of normal cells of many different animals. Virus genes integrated into cell DNA may be regulated as though they were cell genes. Evidence for the existence of cellular controls on exogenously added and endogenous virus genomes stems from the finding that cells can contain viral genomes with complete genes for transformation and not be transformed. The cell may be able to protect itself from oncogenic transformation by possessing devices for selectively preventing the expression of integrated virus sequences. Identifying the virus protein(s) or enzyme(s) coded for by integrated sequences and establishing the link between the primary product(s) and the neoplastic phenotype are the subjects of current research.

Molecular Basis of Neoplastic Transformation

Effort has shifted dramatically in recent years to defining the molecular basis of neoplastic transformation, both viral and nonviral. The development of numerous new techniques in the last decade has enabled molecular biologists to address the question of which virus genes are capable of causing the transformation of a normal cell to a cancer cell (Helling et al., 1974; Maniatis et al., 1975; Swanstrom and Shenk, 1978). Molecular cloning made it possible to rapidly and relatively inexpensively obtain milligram quantities of virus DNA fragments. Coupled with the Southern and northern blot transfer procedures (see Figures 3–14A and 3–14B), the sensitivity of detecting virus DNA and RNA in transformed and tumor cells was greatly increased (Southern, 1975; Alwine et al., 1977). Techniques have been developed to allow the introduction of DNA into cells. The most commonly used method is calcium phosphate precipitation (Graham and van der Eb, 1973; Graham et al., 1980). When Ca^{2+} is added to a phosphate-containing DNA solution, DNA in association with calcium phosphate crystals is precipitated. When the crystals settle on the gel monolayer and appose the cell surface, uptake of DNA occurs. This process is referred to as transfection. Only a small proportion of the cells in a culture are competent to be transfected. Using this technique, the genomic regions necessary for transformation by several

other DNA tumor viruses have also been localized (see Table 3–15).

Transfection can be used to introduce whole cell DNA isolated from tumors or transformed cells into normal cells and to transform the normal cells (Copeland et al., 1979; Weinberg, 1981). Such a process can be sequentially repeated and the DNA of the newly derived transformants can be analyzed for new or altered genes. Cellular DNA isolated from mouse, rabbit, and human bladder carcinoma lines, a series of rat neuroblastomas, and the mouse Lewis lung carcinoma line have been used successfully to transform normal cells (Weinberg, 1981). Studies show that the transforming functions can be transferred across species and tissue barriers; that is, the DNA from both rabbit and human bladder carcinoma (a tumor of epithelial origin) transforms recipient normal mouse fibroblasts. In separate studies, DNA for transfection was obtained from 15 (independently derived) transformed mouse cell lines. The DNAs from five 3-methylcholanthrene (3-MC)-transformed mouse fibroblast cell lines were biologically active and induced foci in normal mouse cell monolayers. No foci were observed when DNA from normal mouse fibroblasts was used. Further studies with this system suggest that the transforming gene is carried in a BamHI fragment of approximately 20 kilobases.

Molecular cloning enables determination of an altered gene within the large cellular genome. The cellular genome can be fragmented with restriction endonuclease enzymes and resulting fragments can be introduced into bacteriophage (lambda) vectors. Selection of the appropriate restriction enzyme requires determining which restriction enzymes do not cleave within the critical fragment. For example, it was shown that the transforming ability of DNA from 3-MC-transformed donor cell lines remained intact when the DNA was cleaved with BamHI, XhoI, or SalI, but was destroyed when cleaved with EcoRI or HindIII. If the cellular genome is 3×10^6 kilobases and each fragment is 15 kilobases, then at least 2×10^5 independent bacteriophages are required to have a cell library of the entire genome. To initiate such an experiment, the library is divided first into 10 to 20 sublibraries to delineate which sublibraries contain the genome fragment able to transform a normal cell. By exponentially narrowing the search, identification of the bacteriophage carrying

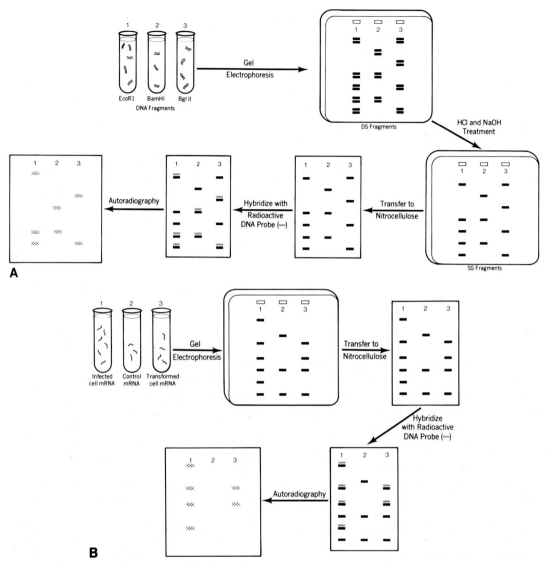

Figure 3–14. Techniques for identification and analysis of nucleic acids. *(A)* Identification of specific DNA sequences by electrophoresis, denaturation of double-stranded DNA to form single-stranded molecules, Southern blot transfer, nucleic acid hybridization, and autoradiography. This method allows detection of a DNA fragment of several hundred base pairs in the diploid cell genome. *(B)* Detection of virus-specific mRNA from infected and transformed cells using electrophoresis, "northern" blot transfer, nucleic acid hybridization, and autoradiography.

the genes of interest can be achieved in four or five cycles of transfection.

This technique can be used to determine the role of viruses in the etiology of cancer. The putative transforming genes (oncogenes) of many viruses have been identified; these include the *src* gene of many RNA tumor viruses and the A gene of SV 40. A transforming gene, however, has not been found for avian leukosis virus (ALV), even though the virus produces leukemia in chickens. Apparently, the ALV genome contains genetic information for repli-

cation functions but not for oncogenic transformation. Transfection of DNA from ALV-induced tumors induces foci in mouse embryo fibroblast (NIH 3T3) monolayer cultures. Serial passage of the DNA results in foci, but the DNA lacks ALV sequences present in the parental tumor cells (see Figure 3–15). These findings suggest that (1) the ALV genes and the transforming genes are probably not linked in the DNA of the parental tumor, otherwise cotransfection would have occurred, and (2) ALV leukemogenesis involves the creation of

Table 3–15. Localization of Genomic Region Necessary for Transformation by Several DNA Tumor Viruses

VIRUS	TOTAL DNA SIZE (Kb)*	PORTION OF GENOME ASSOCIATED WITH TRANSFORMATION		PROTEINS ASSOCIATED WITH REGION	FUNCTION
		Map Units (0 to 100)	Size (Kb)*		
BKV	5.2	9.9–72.3	3.2	97K 17K	Transformation of hamster kidney cells
SV 40	5.24	14.9–72 (except 54–59)	2.7	94K (large T)	Transformation of rat cells
Polyomavirus	5.29	65.4–100 58–100	1.8	55K (middle T) 22K (small T)	Transformation of rat cells Tumors in newborn hamsters
BPV	8.0	31–100	5.5	?	Transformation of mouse cells
Adenovirus types 2, 5, and 12	36	0–11	4.1	32K 30K (0–4.5) 26K 24K 55K 19K (4.5–11)	Transformation of rat and human cells
HSV 1	160	31–42	15.8	?	Transformation of hamster embryo fibroblast cells
HSV 2	160	58–62	7.1	?	Transformation of rat, hamster, and mouse cells

* Kb = kilobases

novel, nonviral-transforming genes. Similar transfection studies are being carried out with DNA from cells transformed by other viruses and with DNA from tumors induced directly by the virus or by virus-transformed cells. It will be interesting to use this method to isolate the transforming gene from a particular human cancer and ask the following questions: If the same experiment is reproduced with human tumors of a histologically similar type, will the same transforming gene be isolated and will the transforming gene(s) contain any sequence homology to the virus associated with that cancer or with any known virus (see Figure 3-16)? It has already been demonstrated that DNAs from five mouse tumors induced by mouse mammary tumor virus (MMTV), two mouse mammary tumors induced by a chemical carcinogen, and one human mammary tumor cell line all contain transforming genes that must have a similar structure because their activity can be inactivated by the same restriction enzymes.

DNA TUMOR VIRUSES

DNA viruses that can induce proliferative lesions either in their natural host or upon experimental inoculation into a foreign host have been identified in five families: Papovaviridae, Adenoviridae, Herpesviridae, Poxvi-

ridae, and hepatitis B virus (as yet unclassified and in a miscellaneous family). This chapter will be restricted to a discussion of those viruses associated with naturally occurring neoplasia in animals (Lucké herpesvirus and Marek's disease virus) and human viruses associated with human neoplasia (human polyoma- and papillomaviruses, hepatitis B virus, and human herpesviruses). In so doing, only viruses from the Papovaviridae, Herpesviridae, and hepatitis B virus groups will be discussed. Two poxviruses, fibroma virus and Yaba monkey tumor virus, cause benign tumors that soon regress. A third poxvirus, myxomavirus, produces localized gelatinous swellings similar to benign fibromas in some rabbit species, but produces a rapidly fatal disease (myxomatosis) in European rabbits. The poxviruses have been included in Table 3–13. The papovaviruses, polyomavirus, SV 40, adenoviruses, and the simian herpesviruses have been extensively used as models to study tumorigenicity and a vast amount of knowledge on growth control, induction of DNA synthesis, integration and recombination of virus and cellular genes, and regulation of gene expression has been obtained (Martin, 1981). Polyomavirus is found ubiquitously in wild and laboratory mouse populations, and when inoculated into newborn mice results in the formation of many tumors. A structurally similar virus, SV 40, does not produce any known

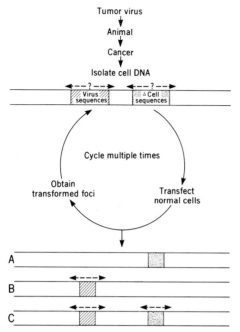

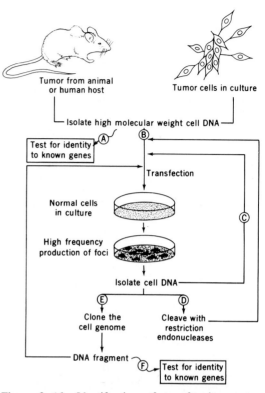

Figure 3–15. Use of sequential cell DNA transfer to study the mechanism of virus transformation. Viruses can transform by altering cell sequences (A), introducing virus sequences into the cell genome (B), or a combination of these two events (C). When virus sequences are introduced into the cell genome (B) they may have a direct effect or they may code for the production of a gene product that alters the normal cell. The method of transfection to carry out sequential cell DNA transfer has been used to study the mechanism of avian leukosis virus (ALV)-induced leukemogenesis. The cell DNA of parental tumor cells from ALV-infected chickens contains ALV sequences. These sequences are lost after sequential DNA transfer and altered cell genes are found in the resulting transformants. These altered cell sequences are also most likely in the DNA of the parental tumor cells. These studies suggest that ALV genes and transforming cell genes are not linked in the parental tumor cell DNA and that ALV leukemogenesis involves the creation of novel, nonviral transforming genes (the mechanism illustrated in A). The technology for ALV-leukemogenesis analysis can be used to establish whether other tumor viruses use the same (A) or other (B, C, etc.) mechanisms. Dashed arrows (◄ – – – ►) indicate that for different viruses the amount of virus or altered cell sequences and whether or not the sequences are linked may vary.

Figure 3–16. Identification of transforming genes. DNA isolated from tumor tissue or cells in culture can be analyzed directly for the presence of virus DNA sequences (A). The identity of specific genes within the tumor cell DNA can also be determined using a biologic approach in combination with molecular techniques. Calcium phosphate precipitation of DNA is used to introduce (transfect) intact cell DNA into normal cells (B). Focal colony formation is used to score for the transfer of transforming genes. Reisolation of transformed cell DNA and transfection of normal cells can be sequentially repeated to further limit and identify transforming sequences (C). Fragmenting the cellular genome with several different restriction endonuclease enzymes determines those enzymes that do not cleave within a sequence critical for transformation (D). The cell genome can then be cloned to form a cell library (E). The library is first divided into ten to 20 sublibraries to delineate sublibraries that contain the genome fragment that will transform a normal cell. By this method the search is narrowed exponentially, and in four or five cycles of transfection the cloned DNA sequences required for transformation can be established. The method of transfection is used to introduce intact high molecular weight cell DNA (B and C), restriction endonuclease-cleaved DNA (D), or cloned DNA fragments (E). Once the fragment is isolated it can be tested for identity to virus DNA sequences or to known cell DNA sequences associated with transformation (F).

disease in its natural host the cynomolgus monkey, but produces numerous different types of tumors when inoculated into newborn hamsters (see Table 3–16). Both polyomavirus and SV 40 can also transform mammalian cells in culture.

Human adenoviruses frequent the upper respiratory tract and can cause human respiratory disease and other infections, especially in crowded or institutional situations. Adeno-

virus types 12, 18, and 31 cause tumors rapidly and at high frequency when injected into newborn hamsters, whereas serotypes 3, 7, 14, 16, and 21 produce tumors at low frequency and only after a long latency period. Serotypes 2

Table 3-16. DNA Viruses Causing Tumors in Foreign Species But Not in the Host of Origin

VIRUS	NATURAL HOST	SUSCEPTIBLE HOST FOR TUMOR INDUCTION
SV 40	Monkey	Hamster, rat, mouse
BKV	Human	Hamster
JCV	Human	Hamster, owl monkey
Adenoviruses	Human	Hamster, mouse, rat, mastomys
	Monkey	Hamster
	Cow	Hamster
	Chicken	Hamster

and 5 are not oncogenic when inoculated into hamsters. Viruses from any of these serotypes (nononcogenic and highly oncogenic) transform rodent cells *in vitro*. Human cells are killed by adenovirus but can be transformed by subgenomic viral DNA fragments. Extensive studies using sensitive hybridization techniques to search for adenovirus sequences in numerous human tumors indicate that such sequences are not present. Although adenovirus is a ubiquitous human virus, it probably is not associated with human cancer. Animal model studies have continued to yield important information on the molecular aspects of transformation.

In animal models for tumorigenicity, the most extensively used simian lymphotropic herpesviruses have been Herpesvirus saimiri (HVS) and Herpesvirus ateles (HVA). HVS is indigenous in squirrel monkeys but induces T cell lymphomas in owl or marmoset monkeys. HVA is ubiquitous in spider monkeys and induces lymphomas in New World monkeys. In contrast to EBV, large amounts of either of these two viruses and their DNA or other structural components can be obtained easily from *in vitro* cultures in the laboratory. Interest in these viruses exists for several reasons. First, both HVS and HVA can transform lymphocytes *in vitro*. Second, virus-induced tumor models in nonhuman primates may be more applicable to cancer in man than other animal model systems. Third, the reproducibility and rapid course of tumor formation *in vivo* facilitates chemotherapeutic studies.

Naturally Occurring Animal Cancers

Lucké Herpesvirus. The Lucké tumor is a well-differentiated renal adenocarcinoma that develops spontaneously in the leopard frog, *Rana pipiens*. The natural occurrence of this tumor is geographically restricted to frogs in the northeastern and northcentral United States and adjacent areas of southern Canada.

The Lucké tumor invades and destroys the kidney and can metastasize to the liver and lung, although metastases are not common. The theory that this tumor was caused by a virus was first advanced by Lucké in 1938 (Lucké, 1938). Almost 20 years later, in 1956, herpesviruslike particles were detected in cells of the Lucké tumor by electron microscopy. The Lucké herpesvirus (LHV) was isolated from *R. pipiens* and tumor induction by the virus is observed in the same species.

Because the Lucké tumor is a naturally occurring animal cancer, it is possible to show a causal relationship by introducing the suspect etiological agent into a normal animal. The first experiments of this type were carried out by Tweedell in 1967. Cytoplasmic fractions from Lucké tumors containing inclusion bodies were inoculated into *R. pipiens* embryos. If the embryos were held at 20°C, renal adenocarcinomas developed as the animals underwent metamorphosis. Cytoplasmic fragments from virus-free or inclusion-free tumors failed to produce tumors. The experiment, however, was not conclusive because the cytoplasmic fractions contained many factors in addition to the Lucké herpesvirus. This problem was easily overcome in later investigations. The design of the experiment was critical and fortuitous because of the temperature chosen, and because embryos were used. The natural occurrence of the Lucké tumor in frogs three years of age or older varies from less than 1% to 9% in the temperatures the frog naturally experiences. If frogs are kept at a constant 25°C, the incidence increases to 25 to 50%. Transmission of the Lucké tumor in animals is difficult. The tumor is not transplantable to adult or immunosuppressed animals and is only transplantable when inoculated into embryos or at a privileged site such as the anterior eye chamber.

Although the original frog embryo inoculation experiments fulfilled, to some extent, the Koch-Henle postulates for LHV as the etiologic agent of the Lucké tumor, reisolation of the agent from the induced disease was not reported. With increasing time, the properties of LHV became known and it was possible to more clearly define an association between LHV and the Lucké tumor (Naegele *et al.,* 1974):

1. LHV cannot be grown in cells in culture, but the virus can be isolated and purified from tumor cells. The tumor-inducing activity of LHV in embryos is pronase-sensitive, is retained after sonication or storage at -70 °C for two years, and can be demonstrated with crude or purified virus preparations;

2. The Lucké tumor can exist either in a form containing inclusion bodies and virus or in a virus- and inclusion-body-free form. Whether the tumor cells contain virus or are virus-free is temperature dependent; when the tumor is in the natural site (the kidney) or transplanted to the anterior eye chamber, the tumor cells are virus-free above 11.5 °C. If the temperature is lowered to 7.5 to 9.5 °C, induction of virus occurs (with a three-month delay when the tumor is in the anterior eye chamber and a five- to seven-month delay for renal tumors). It should be noted that although tumor incidence increases when frogs are held at warmer temperatures (22 °C), the presence of virus only occurs at low temperature (7.5 °C);

3. The effect of temperaure on virus induction can be duplicated *in vitro* with tumor fragment explants.

This knowledge, particularly point 3, made it possible to design embryo inoculation experiments to fulfill the Koch-Henle postulates for LHV as the etiologic agent of the Lucké tumor (see Figure 3–17 and Table 3–17). The results of these experiments provide some of the strongest data demonstrating that a virus (LHV) causes cancer (Lucké tumor).

Biologic studies with LHV have been limited because LHV has not been cultivated successfully *in vitro* in homogeneous cell populations. LHV will not replicate at 7.5 °C or 25 °C in insect, fish, amphibian, or mammalian cell lines even with the aid of helper viruses. Failure to cultivate the virus has made it difficult to answer critical questions regarding virus-cell interactions associated with oncogenicity. It is not known, for example, whether the effect of temperature on LHV replication is due to a

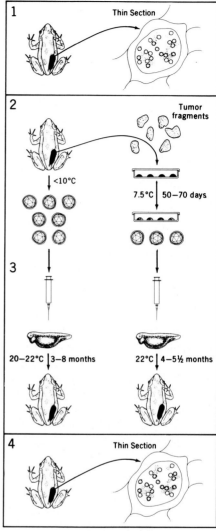

Figure 3–17. Diagrammatic representation of Table 3–17.

property of the virus or the cell in which the virus is replicating.

LHV DNA isolated from inclusion-containing tumors has a molecular weight of 66×10^6 daltons, with a base composition of 45 to 47% guanine plus cytosine. Hybridization studies show that virus-free tumors contain LHV RNA, suggesting that virus-free tumors contain LHV DNA sequences. Clearly, further work in this area will await development of systems in which LHV can be replicated; some of the obstacles will be overcome shortly by cloning LHV DNA and studying its properties.

Marek's Disease Virus (MDV): A Vaccine Against a Lymphoproliferative Disease. Marek's disease (MD) is a lymphoproliferative

Table 3–17. Koch's Postulates and the Role of the Lucké Herpesvirus in the Etiology of the Lucké Tumor

POSTULATE	CRITERIA	APPLICATION TO LUCKÉ TUMOR
1	Regular association of the microorganism with the disease	Virus particles are found in tumor cells of naturally occurring disease
2	Isolation of the organism and growth in pure culture	Virus can be isolated from the urine and ascitic fluid of tumor-bearing frogs, especially at the time of hibernation. Virus can be obtained from fragments of tumor explants maintained *in vitro* at 7.5 °C. The virus cannot be grown in pure culture
3	Reproduction of the disease in a susceptible animal after inoculation with a pure culture of the microorganism	Inoculation of frog embryos with virus excreted by tumor-bearing frog in hibernation or from fragment explants results in the formation of Lucké tumor as the animals metamorphose
4	Recovery of the organism from the lesion of the experimentally infected animal	Virus particles can be observed and virus isolated from experimentally induced tumors

See Figure 3–17 for diagrammatic representation of this table.

disease of chickens seen worldwide and was originally thought to be an inflammatory disease (Calnek, 1980). The disease has three phases. In the first phase, atrophic changes occur in the thymus, bursa of Fabricus, and bone marrow. During this phase and extending into the second phase, reticular- and lymphoid-cell proliferation is observed. These proliferative changes in lymphoid cells may progress to lymphomas that can be lethal to the chicken as early as three weeks after infection. Lymphomas are seen most commonly in the gonads, liver, spleen, kidneys, lungs, and heart. Lymphomas occur less frequently in the muscle, proventriculus, and feather follicles and can be present in any organ or tissue. Interestingly, the lymphomas regress in some birds. In the third phase of disease, proliferative lesions are replaced by chronic inflammatory lesions, particularly in the peripheral nerves. In the chronic disease, which is the classic and less acute form, nerve enlargement is followed by paresis and paralysis. Marek's disease occurs naturally, but the frequency of disease in commercial chicken flocks became markedly elevated after intensive systems of poultry farming were introduced. Without vaccination, 50 to 60% of chickens could be lost to MD.

Although MD was described initially in 1907 (Marek, 1907), not until the 1960s was it realized that the disease was infectious and that the transmissible agent was a herpesvirus. The first criterion of Koch's postulates was ful-

filled after a cell-associated herpesvirus was isolated from chickens with MD. Stronger support for MDV in the etiology of MD came from two findings. First, cell-free virus was prepared and when inoculated into genetically defined virus-free chickens, the animals developed MD. Second, chickens immunized with attenuated strains of MDV did not develop lymphomas characteristic of MD when exposed to nonattenuated virus.

Not all strains of MDV are tumorigenic. Isolates of MDV and herpesvirus of turkeys (HVT) are classified into three serotypes. The viruses in each serologic group demonstrate their own characteristic cytopathology and preference for fibroblastic or epithelial cells. All tumorigenic isolates belong to serotype 1; however, within this serotype, there are strains with low, medium, and high levels of oncogenicity. In addition, *in vitro* passage can decrease and eventually eliminate oncogenicity but does not eliminate immunogenicity. Indeed, an attenuated strain was developed that was no longer pathogenic and became the first effective MD vaccine (Churchill *et al.,* 1969).

In contrast to the Lucké tumor, it is not common to observe MDV particles in tumor tissue. Although research has shown evidence of virus gene expression in tumor cells, no association of virus replication with tumorigenicity has been observed. Virus infection and replication can, however, be detected in other cells of a bird destined to succumb to lymphoma. The feather follicle epithelium (FFE) is the only tissue of the bird in which cell-free, infectious enveloped virus is produced. Naked virions are visible in the nucleus and enveloped virions are evident in the cytoplasm of cells of the FFE. Release of infectious virus from the FFE occurs between 13 and 14 days after exposure to MDV and is a more passive than active process since it accompanies normal breakup of the keratinized cells. It is also possible that MDV can only replicate in keratinizing cells undergoing death.

In contrast to LHV, MDV can be grown in culture in a wide variety of chicken cells. Virus prepared from cultured cells is primarily cell-associated. It has not been possible, however, to demonstrate *in vitro* transformation of fibroblasts or epithelial cells with MDV. Virus-induced MD lymphomas can be transplanted *in vivo.* Although most attempts to derive continuous lymphoblastoid cell lines from lymphomas have failed, several lines have been derived. The success rate has been improved by using transplantable instead of primary lymphomas and by incubating the cultures at high temperature (40 to 41 °C).

Normal turkeys carry cell-associated HVT which is highly protective against MD in chickens. Six MDV proteins have been found in productively infected cells but only three are seen regularly and are termed A, B, and C. The A and B antigens are common to MDV and HVT, but the C antigen is MDV-specific. Biochemical and molecular comparisons of MDV with HVT are important because HVT is the most widely used MD vaccine. HVT is similar to MDV in terms of virus localization and infection after exposure of the chicken, but differs in that infected lymphocytes do not undergo cytolytic infection, and infection of FFE is very restricted. Immunization with HVT does not prevent superinfection of the bird with oncogenic MDV, but does prevent cytolytic infection in lymphoid organs, reduces virus shedding from the FFE, and eliminates formation of neoplastic lesions. Although MDV and HVT are antigenically similar, studies on the molecular biology of the two viruses reveal that their nucleic acids have very little (1 to 4%) or no homology. Characterization of MDV DNA and molecular studies of transformed tumor cells or lymphoblastoid cell lines have been limited by low yields of MDV (hence low yields of MDV DNA) in cell culture systems, as a result of its cell-associated nature. Molecular cloning of MDV DNA has

been reported recently and should enable rapid progress. Before cloning, investigators used classical techniques to draw the following conclusions: (1) The lymphoblastoid cell line derived from the strain JM-induced transplantable lymphoma most likely does not have a complete genome as no virus can be rescued; (2) other lymphoblastoid cell lines have the complete genome present in multiple copies; (3) in cell lines from which virus can be rescued, the virus genome can be detected in two forms: integrated into the cell genome or free as a nonintegrated circular plasmid; and (4) in cell lines from which virus cannot be rescued, the virus DNA is most likely present only in the integrated form. These findings can now be confirmed and extended with technical advances and recombinant DNA techniques.

Human Viruses and their Association with Human Neoplasms

The previous sections discussed the roles of LHV in the frog Lucké tumor and of MDV in Marek's disease. LHV and MDV are of particular interest because they are the only DNA viruses unequivocally shown to cause cancer in animals under natural conditions. At this time, there is no reason to believe that LHV or MDV is linked to the induction of any human tumors. The LHV and MDV systems are valuable because their existence strengthens the possibility of a viral etiology for certain human tumors. The experimental approaches used to demonstrate the viral etiology of the Lucké tumor and MD can serve as a guide for determining viral etiologies for other cancers. Certain approaches, however, cannot be used to study human cancers. It is not possible, for example, to fulfill the third criterion of Koch's postulates; that is, reproducing the disease by inoculating humans with the putative oncogenic human virus. For this reason, the ability of a human virus to produce tumors in animals or to transform mammalian (or human) cells, in particular, in culture is critical in evaluating its oncogenic potential. In this section, four groups of human viruses associated with human cancers will be discussed. Ordered by increasing size, they are the human polyomaviruses, papillomaviruses, hepatitis B virus (HBV), and the herpesviruses. These viruses have the following properties in common: (1) Each has been identified and studied as an agent of nononcogenic human disease; and (2) there is often a significant period of time be-

tween initial infection of the host and development of the tumor thought to be associated
with the virus. Of the four groups, the evidence
at this time showing a relationship between the
human papovaviruses and cancer is the weak-
est, but there is sufficient interest to warrant a
brief discussion in this section.

Human Polyomaviruses. The polyoma
subgroup of papovaviruses contains small viruses with supercoiled, circular, double-
stranded DNA with an approximate molecu-
lar weight of 3×10^6 daltons. In 1971, it was
realized that the polyoma subgroup also includes human viruses: BK and JC viruses (designated by the patients' initials) cultured from
human fluids and tissues. BKV was initially
isolated from the urine of an immunologically
suppressed renal transplant patient (Gardner
et al., 1971) and subsequently has been isolated from the urine of other renal transplant
patients and from patients treated for cancer.
JCV was originally isolated from the brain of a
man with progressive multifocal leukoencephalopathy (PML) and, as a result of subsequent
similar isolations, is thought to be the causal
agent of this neurologic disease.

Primary infection of humans with BKV and
JCV apparently occurs in childhood: 60 to
90% of all children have antibodies to BKV
and JCV by age ten. The clinical features of the
primary infection are unknown. Isolation of
BKV from immunocompromised patients
and JCV from PML patients is most likely indicative of virus reactivated from a latent state
and not of a primary infection. Current interest in BKV and JCV as human tumor viruses
stems from the following: (1) These viruses are
found ubiquitously in the human population;
(2) they are members of the polyoma subgroup
that contains animal viruses known to transform cells in culture and to produce tumors in
animal hosts; (3) inoculation of either BKV or
JCV into animals results in the formation of
tumors; (4) BKV proteins and nucleic acids
have been found in several human tumors;
and (5) transplant recipients have an increased
probability of reticulum cell sarcoma as well as
an increased likelihood of excreting BKV. One
report has been published describing the isolation of a strain of BKV from a brain tumor and
from the urine of a child with Wiskott-Aldrich
syndrome, an immunodeficiency disease. This
finding may suggest that the human polyomaviruses, like their animal counterparts, can
only induce tumors in the immunologically
suppressed host (Mäntyjärvi, 1979).

BKV DNA sequences have been found in
DNA of certain human tumors. This finding,
published in 1976 by Fiori and diMayorca,
was not supported by a similar study two years
later in a different laboratory (Wold et al.,
1978). Studies of this nature should be repeated using more sensitive technology to detect specific DNA sequences. Results of nucleic acid hybridization indicate some
sequence homology between BKV and SV 40,
particularly in the late region of the DNA coding for capsid proteins. Blot hybridization
DNA-DNA reassociation kinetic techniques
have also determined the presence and number of BKV genome equivalents in transformed and tumors cells (from 0.4 to 6.0
copies). BKV can be rescued from cell lines
(particularly BKV-transformed mouse cells)
with at least one copy of the genome present
per cell.

Human Papillomaviruses (HPV). The
papillomaviruses are small viruses containing
supercoiled, covalently closed, circular, double-stranded DNA with a molecular weight of
approximately 5×10^6 daltons. The genome is
slightly larger than that of the polyomaviruses.
Papillomaviruses are found in the epithelia of
man and in several animal species. In fact, the
original association between papillomavirus
and cancer was made in rabbits in 1932
(Shope, 1932). The papillomaviruses are host-
specific, with the exception of bovine papillomavirus, which can induce tumors in unrelated species. Bovine papillomavirus DNA has
also been identified in naturally occurring
equine tumors. Evidence for an association between some HPV strains and human tumors is
considerably greater than for the human polyomaviruses (zur Hausen, 1980). In animal or
HPV-induced cancers, however, the virus is
clearly not the only carcinogen involved. The
genetic makeup and immunologic competence of the host play a definite role, as do
numerous chemical and environmental
agents. The cocarcinogenic nature of human
papillomavirus-induced tumors is significant
because it complicates the question of viral etiology.

In human warts, the known critical synergistic factors that favor malignant conversion
are sunlight and x-irradiation (see Chapter
3C). The significance of environmental factors
as cocarcinogens for animal papillomaviruses
has also been noted (see Chapter 3B). Early
studies showed that simultaneous administration of chemical carcinogens either topically or

systemically in animals with Shope papillomavirus reduced the period of latency for conversion to malignancy and increased the percentage of invasive papillomas (zur Hausen, 1980). One type of bovine papillomavirus undergoes malignant conversion, producing esophageal papillomatous and urinary bladder tumors in cattle that consume bracken fern, a foliage that contains a potent carcinogen.

At least six distinct types of HPV have been identified, and they are conveniently named HPV 1 through HPV 6. Not all HPVs are carcinogenic; HPV 1, HPV 2 and HPV 4 are responsible for common warts that remain benign and do not convert into cancerous tumors. Even when x-irradiation is employed as a therapeutic regimen for common warts, the combined impact of virus and x-irradiation does not induce cancerous conversion. In contrast, HPV 5 is routinely associated with the rare disease epidermodysplasia verruciformis (EV) in which skin warts undergo neoplastic conversion to Bowen's carcinoma or squamous or basal cell carcinoma. Sensitivity to EV and subsequent neoplastic conversion is genetically determined and probably transmitted by an autosomal recessive gene. Patients with this predisposition also demonstrate abnormal cell-mediated immunity. In addition, conversion of warts induced by HPV 5 only occurs in lesions exposed to sunlight, suggesting the importance of ultraviolet irradiation as a cocarcinogenic environmental factor. HPV 3 has also been associated with flat, wartlike lesions in patients with EV; these warts generally do not undergo neoplastic conversion unless both HPV 3 and HPV 5 are present simultaneously. HPV 6 is responsible for condylomata acuminata, the typical genital wart. Papillomavirus particles recently have been found in superficial layers of mild dysplastic lesions of the uterine cervix. The dysplastic lesions, called condyloma planum, have a flat surface and a predilection for localizing in the uterine cervix and vagina, which distinguishes them from condylomata acuminata. In addition, electron micrographs of virion particles in dysplastic lesions show that the particles differ in appearance from those in condylomata acuminata. Although the virus associated with condylomata of the cervix is a papillomavirus, it most likely is either a variant of HPV 6 or a separate, distinct type. An HPV as yet unclassified is also most likely responsible for human laryngeal papillomas. In general, juvenile multifocal papillomas of the larynx are benign but can undergo neoplastic conversion. The risk of cancer is enhanced if the papilloma is x-irradiated. Generations ago, x-irradiation was the therapeutic treatment for laryngeal papillomas and, as a result of therapy as long as 40 years ago, cancers are sometimes seen today.

HPV type can be identified by immunofluorescence using antisera specific to each type or by molecular methods, that is, hybridization of the unknown sample virus DNA to complementary RNA probes transcribed from the known HPV DNAs. Restriction enzyme analysis of the virus DNA can also be used to ascertain HPV type. Hybridization studies of the viral DNA in condylomata of the uterine cervix and in laryngeal papilloma indicate that the viruses represent previously unclassified papillomaviruses.

In a recent study of cervical biopsy specimens, papillomavirus antigens were demonstrated by the peroxidase-antiperoxidase staining technique in 60% of patients with condylomata of the uterine cervix (Morin et al., 1981). Electron microscopic analysis of five antigen-positive sections revealed HPV particles in the nuclei. The papillomavirus antigen was not found in normal cervixes or in women with moderate dysplasia, carcinoma in situ, or invasive carcinoma. It is interesting to note that in Shope papillomavirus-induced warts in wild rabbits, the nuclei of the keratohyalin and keratinizing layers contain virus capsid, antigen, and virus particles. In contrast, the proliferating connective tissue and basal epidermis contain neither antigen nor virus but do contain virus DNA.

Hepatitis B Virus (HBV). The hepatitis B virus or the "Dane particle" is composed of two protein coats surrounding a nicked, double-stranded, circular DNA with a single-stranded region of variable length (Tiollais et al., 1981). HBV is the causative agent of serum (or B) hepatitis and is infectious to close contacts of carriers. The virus is strongly associated with chronic liver disease, including primary hepatocellular carcinoma (PHC) (Maupas and Melnick, 1981). In the United States and Western Europe, the incidence of HBV infection in the population is low (0.1 to 1%) and PHC is an uncommon cancer (1 to 3 cases per 100,000). In other parts of the world, including the Mediterranean basin, the Middle East, Southeast Asia, China, Japan, and some parts of Africa, the incidence of HBV infection is much higher (10 to 25%) and PHC is more prevalent (150 cases per 100,000). Not all PHC is associated with HBV infection; certain drugs and chemical pollutants are also associated with induction of this cancer. In opposition to the evidence supporting HBV as the causal agent of certain PHCs are observations that (1) PHC occurs in patients who are HBV negative, and (2) not all PHC cell lines contain HBV DNA or express it as RNA or proteins. The strengths for the association, however, far outweigh the weaknesses.

Studies on HBV have been limited for two reasons. First, all attempts to propagate the virus in cell culture have been unsuccessful. There is no infectivity assay for direct identification of infectious virus. Even hepatoma-derived cell lines that contain virus DNA and actively produce the virus protein HBsAg (hepatitis B surface antigen) (Blumberg *et al.,* 1965) do not synthesize virions. Second, until recently a good animal model system was unavailable for studying HBV. In 1978, HBV-like viruses were isolated from woodchucks, squirrels, and Pekin ducks. The woodchuck virus is indistinguishable from human HBV and shares nucleotide sequences and antigenic determinants with the human virus. Infection of woodchucks with woodchuck virus results in hepatic symptoms, and a substantial percentage of infected animals subsequently develop PHC (Summers *et al.,* 1978).

The unavailability of *in vitro* systems for propagation of HBV has been partially overcome by cloning of the HBV genome in *Escherichia coli* and by successful transfection of mammalian cells with cloned HBV DNA. When mouse cells are transfected with HBV DNA, the virus genome is integrated and the cells secrete HBsAg into the medium; no other antigens are detected. When HeLa cells are transfected with a cloned and recircularized HBV genome, the cells synthesize HBsAg, HBcAg (hepatitis B internal core antigen), and Dane-like particles are observed in cell-free supernatants. HBsAg obtained from transformed cells may be a possible source of antigen for vaccine production. Adaptation of nucleic acid extraction techniques has made it possible to obtain sufficient DNA for two or three hybridization analyses from percutaneous liver biopsy samples (10 to 20 mg of tissue). Studies with either autopsy or biopsy material indicated that in all hepatocellular carcinomas in which HBV DNA was present the DNA was integrated into the host genome (Shafritz *et al.,* 1981). In each tumor the integration pattern was unique. In one tumor, "extrachromosomal" DNA was also present. Analysis of these tumors, however, is complicated by partial degradation of DNA as a result of tissue necrosis and markedly abnormal liver functions in the host. In some specimens, hepatic parenchyma surrounding the tumor also contained integrated and extrachromosomal DNA, suggesting that integration of HBV DNA into hepatocytes may precede development of gross neoplasms.

In tissue from HBV carriers, virus DNA was not integrated into the host genome but instead was present in two molecular forms: (1) As the full genome of double-stranded HBV DNA (possibly a replication form of HBV DNA), and (2) as a double-stranded HBV DNA molecule in which one strand was complete but nicked (as in Dane particle DNA). Continued studies of this nature will make it possible to determine whether HBV integration naturally accompanies persistent virus infection or heralds the initiation of a tumor. Although hybridization techniques have been used primarily to determine whether HBV plays a role in the cause of PHC, they are sufficiently sensitive to also become important diagnostic tools for evaluating HBV in serum, blood products, body fluids, and biopsy specimens.

Human Herpesviruses. The herpesviruses are large, complex enveloped viruses approximately 150 Å in size that contain linear, double-stranded DNA with molecular weights varying from less than 80×10^6 to approximately 150×10^6 daltons. The strong evidence of the causal relationship of LHV in the etiology of the Lucké renal adenocarcinoma of the frog and MDV in lymphoma in chickens prompted interest in the relationship between other herpesviruses and cancers. Of the five known human herpesviruses, four are associated with human tumors: EBV, herpes simplex virus types 1 and 2 (HSV 1 and HSV 2), and cytomegalovirus CMV. The fifth, varicella-zoster virus (VZV), has not been shown to be related to any specific human cancer by epidemiologic, virologic, biochemical, or molecular techniques; however, recent reports indicate that VZV can transform normal mouse cells into tumor cells in culture. Perhaps it is only a matter of time before it too is associated with a human cancer. Human herpesviruses are suspect carcinogenic agents because they are found ubiquitously in the human population (see Table 3-18) and have been associated with a variety of human tumors by epidemiologic methods. In addition, because the viruses often enter the host early in life, the virus genes and gene products can interact with host cells over long periods of time before a tumor arises.

The cancers most closely linked to EBV infection are Burkitt's lymphoma (Henle *et al.,* 1969) and nasopharyngeal carcinoma (NPC). Burkitt's lymphoma is a B-cell lymphoma of the jaw found in children between the ages of 1 and 15 living in equatorial Africa and in New Guinea. Tumors can also arise in the ovaries, thyroid, testes, and abdominal viscera. Burkitt's lymphoma is endemic in geographic regions with warm, wet climates and in areas in which malaria is endemic. It is possible that malaria injures the reticuloendothelial system such that the host cannot restrict the proliferation of virus-stimulated lymphocytes. In contrast to the frog Lucké tumor, Burkitt's tumors do not contain virions. When the tumor cells are removed and placed in culture, however, 5 to 20% of the cells produce virus particles (Epstein *et al.,* 1964). This observation was first made by Epstein and Barr (1964), hence the name of the herpesvirus (Epstein-Barr virus; EBV). EBV shed by tumor cells is capable of transforming normal human lymphocytes into immortal or transformed lymphoblastoid lines. Inoculation of purified EBV into owl monkeys or cottontop marmosets induces multifocal lymphomas with many of the characteristics of Burkitt's lymphoma except that jaw tumors are not produced. EBV can be reisolated from tumors induced in test animals, thereby fulfilling Koch's postulates to the extent that it can be fulfilled for a human tumor virus.

EBV infection has also been implicated in undifferentiated NPC, a squamous cell carcinoma with lymphocytic infiltration and a high prevalence in the Southern Chinese and to a lesser extent in the populations of East Africa, Tunisia, and in Alaskan eskimos. Sporadic cases occur throughout the world. Familial aggregation of NPC suggests that a genetic predisposition and EBV infection act together to induce this human cancer. EBV particles are not present in NPC biopsies, but they do appear when cultured NPC cells are treated with halogenated pyrimidines or are injected into nude mice. The virus obtained from NPC cells can transform normal lymphocytes into lymphoblastoid cells. The virus rescued from these lymphoblastoid lines demonstrates no important biologic or biochemical difference from EBV isolated from patients with Burkitt's lymphoma or infectious mononucleosis. Attempts to fulfill Koch's postulates to demonstrate an EBV etiology for NPC are inhibited to date by the lack of a suitable primate animal model for induction of NPC-like tumors. No *in vitro* cell culture system has yet been found to propagate EBV to high titer. The EBV genome recently has been cloned, permitting generation of large quantities of DNA fragments and enabling investigators to carry out studies previously not feasible.

Although HSV 1 and HSV 2 are associated with a variety of human tumors (listed in Table 3-18), the greatest interest lies in the causal relationship of HSV 2 with uterine cervical carcinoma (Rapp, 1980). Antibodies against HSV 2 are found more frequently and at higher titers in women with uterine cervical carcinoma, dysplasia, and carcinoma *in situ*

Table 3–18. Diseases Associated With Human Herpesviruses

VIRUS	HUMAN ILLNESSES CAUSED BY HUMAN HERPESVIRUSES	TYPES OF CANCER ASSOCIATED WITH SPECIFIC HUMAN HERPESVIRUSES
Epstein-Barr virus	Infectious mononucleosis	Burkitt's lymphoma, nasopharyngeal carcinoma
Herpes simplex virus type 1	Gingivostomatitis, encephalitis, keratoconjunctivitis, neuralgia, labialis, traumatic herpes	Carcinoma of lip and oropharynx ?
Herpes simplex virus type 2	Genital herpes, disseminated neonatal herpes, encephalitis, neuralgia	Carcinoma of the uterine cervix, vulva, kidney, and nasopharynx
Cytomegalovirus	Cytomegalic inclusion disease, transfusion mononucleosis, interstitial pneumonia, congenital defects	Prostate cancer, Kaposi's sarcoma, carcinoma of bladder and uterine cervix
Varicella-zoster virus	Chickenpox, shingles, varicella pneumonia	?

than in healthy women or women with other cancers. HSV 2 is transmitted sexually so it is important to note that the same women who epidemiologically are at high risk for uterine cervical cancer because of early sexual exposure and poor genital hygiene are more likely to acquire HSV-2 infections. This information may provide support for the role of HSV 2 in the development of uterine cervical cancer; however, it raises the question of whether HSV 2 infection parallels tumor formation with no causal relationship.

HSV 2 inactivated photodynamically or with ultraviolet light can transform a variety of different rodent cells. The original studies (by Duff and Rapp, 1971) demonstrated that ultraviolet-irradiated HSV 2 transforms hamster cells and that these transformants produce tumors that metastasize to the lung and other organs when inoculated into newborn hamsters. Transformation has also been accomplished with temperature-sensitive mutant virus, virus at supraoptimal temperatures, sheared virus DNA, and defined virus DNA fragments. Live virus cannot be used for transformation because it is lytic. Because it is highly virulent in newborn rodents, live virus cannot be used to demonstrate oncogenic potential in animals.

Investigators have attempted to induce uterine cervical carcinoma in test animals by vaginal inoculation of HSV 2 (Wentz et al., 1981). Unless the animals are immunized or the virus is inactivated, the mortality rate is high. In one study, 10% of cebus monkeys inoculated repeatedly in the uterine cervix with HSV 2 developed cellular atypia 14 to 50 months after infection (Palmer et al., 1976). In another study, when the vaginas of mice were repeatedly exposed (three to five times a week) to sterile cotton pledgets saturated with inactivated virus or control fluid for periods of 20 to 90 weeks, precancerous or cancerous lesions of the uterine cervix similar to those in women were found in 78 to 91% of virus-exposed animals (Wentz et al., 1981). All controls were normal; no primary lesions were found in the vagina or ovaries. When the virus was formalin inactivated, invasive adenocarcinoma was detected in 30.2% of the mice. A more recent study indicates that if HSV 2 is inactivated by ultraviolet light instead of formalin, the frequency of invasive cancer is twice as great. Whether these results can be translated to the human population is unknown at this time.

The acute clinical manifestations of congenital CMV infections have been known and extensively studied for years, but the role of CMV in the cause of human cancer has received less attention. Human CMV has been detected in patients with many types of neoplasias, but it is possible that the virus is an adventitious passenger reactivated from a latent state as a result of the immunologic condition of the host. CMV has been isolated from the urine of leukemia, Hodgkin's disease, and lymphosarcoma patients, and from cell cultures derived from biopsies of cervical carcinoma. In addition, lymphoblastoid cell lines have been established from patients with CMV mononucleosis.

CMV has recently been implicated in human prostatic cancer and Kaposi's sarcoma, a rare multiple hemorrhagic sarcoma with an epidemiologic distribution in Africa reminiscent of that of African Burkitt's lymphoma (Giraldo et al., 1980). The concept that CMV plays a role in the etiology of prostate cancer requires further investigation but has received support from serologic surveys showing higher CMV antibody titers in prostatic cancer patients than age-matched controls. In addition, in one study, 82% of prostatic carcinoma patients possessed peripheral lymphocytes cytotoxic to CMV-transformed human cells, whereas only 35% of benign prostatic hyperplasia patients reacted to the cells (Sanford et al., 1978). CMV has also been isolated in cell cultures derived from tumor biopsies of patients with Kaposi's sarcoma (Giraldo et al., 1972). Kaposi's sarcoma can also be found in other parts of the world. Surprisingly, serologic studies indicate that patients with European Kaposi's sarcoma possess elevated CMV-neutralizing and complement-fixing antibody in their sera, whereas those with African Kaposi's sarcoma do not. Kaposi's sarcoma is rare in the United States, where the annual incidence is between 0.02 to 0.06 per 100,000 and where most cases are seen in elderly males. During a 30-month period ending in 1981, however, Kaposi's sarcoma was diagnosed in 26 men who are homosexual (20 in New York City, six in California) ranging in age from 26 to 51 years. The occurrence of this number of Kaposi's sarcoma cases during this period of time is highly unusual (see Chapter 20).

More evidence is now available to support the association of CMV with Kaposi's sarcoma. This is particularly disturbing considering the presence of CMV in patients suffering from acquired immune deficiency syndrome

(AIDS), as many of these patients also suffer from Kaposi's sarcoma. There are some important common features in individuals who have AIDS: (1) They are most often young homosexual men who live in large cities and use drugs; (2) the infectious agents are pathogens that cause opportunistic infections in immunocompromised hosts; and (3) the death rate is very high. The association of CMV with AIDS is strengthened by evidence of a current or previous CMV infection in almost all cases reported (Durak, 1981). In addition, CMV is known to immunosuppress mice and humans, and the virus will persist in semen for several months. Kaposi's sarcoma afflicts young Africans, elderly Americans, renal transplant recipients, and men who are homosexual. It is not known why this disease strikes members of these groups, but it is now known that CMV DNA and CMV RNA are present in tumor biopsies from patients with Kaposi's sarcoma.

Although human CMV can only be propagated in human cells, the virus can abortively infect cells derived from nonhuman sources, for example, hamster cells. Although human CMV has not shown oncogenicity after inoculation into test animals, the virus can malignantly transform cells in culture. Hamster embryo fibroblast cells can be transformed by ultraviolet-inactivated and by noninactivated CMV. Human CMV-transformed hamster cells after continued passage *in vitro* produce fibrosarcomas when inoculated into newborn hamsters. Infection of human embryo lung fibroblasts with CMV yields persistently infected cells and transformants that are tumorigenic in nude mice (Geder *et al.*, 1976). CMV has not been rescued from these cells by cocultivation with sensitive cells, exposure to ultraviolet radiation, or pretreatment with iododeoxyuridine.

The major evidence associating human herpesviruses with human cancer stems from biochemical and, more recently, from molecular approaches. The technology is currently available to determine which virus DNA sequences are required to trigger transformation, and studies with EBV, CMV, HSV 2, and HSV 1 are in progress. More than 95% of histologically typical Burkitt's lymphoma tumors derived from individuals in endemic areas of Africa contain detectable amounts of EBV DNA. Virus DNA is present in multiple copies (four to 113 virus genome equivalents), and although a small portion may be integrated, most of the virus DNA is recovered as free plasmids. Virus DNA is present in multiple copies in episomal form in lymphoblastoid cell lines derived from Burkitt's lymphoma, as well as in almost all tumor biopsies from patients with undifferentiated NPC. EBV DNA is found in the epithelial cells of NPC tumors and not in infiltrating lymphocytes.

New molecular methods to probe tumor tissue for HSV nucleic acids have yielded more satisfactory results than examination of tumor tissue or transformed cells for virus protein. The presence of HSV-2 DNA and RNA in invasive cervical carcinoma biopsies has only been reported for a single specimen (Frenkel *et al.*, 1972). Many of the original researchers, however, examined biopsy specimens by nucleic acid hybridization in solution, a method not sufficiently sensitive to detect small amounts of DNA. More recently, *in situ* hybridization has been used to measure HSV-2 RNA in tumor tissue. In one study, HSV-2 RNA was found in five of eight uterine cervical intraepithelial neoplasia samples. In a recent and more extensive study, HSV-2 RNA was found in 72% of cervical intraepithelial neoplasia, 60% of squamous uterine cervical carcinomas, 2% of nonneoplastic uterine cervices, and 9% of primary adenocarcinomas of the uterine cervix. Infectious HSV 2 was isolated from ectocervical swabs or cell-free tissue extracts in only 2% of the patients, suggesting that the HSV RNA detected was not due to overt infection (Eglin *et al.*, 1981).

One problem in detecting the HSV-2 genome and its gene products is that the genome is large and it is difficult to develop a sensitive nucleic acid probe of this size. For this reason studies have been carried out (1) to investigate HSV-transformed cells for the retention of specific gene sequences and expression of specific proteins (Reyes *et al.*, 1980); and (2) to use DNA fragments to accomplish *in vitro* transformation (see Table 3–15) (Jariwalla *et al.*, 1980; Galloway and McDougall, 1981). The results of these two types of studies may not be comparable since the genes maintained by transformants may not be identical to those required to initiate transformation. Cells transformed by HSV 2 express HSV information at least for a limited period of time, and preliminary results indicate that the genes expressed map to the left of 0.62 map units on the HSV genome. One limitation is that the most extensively studied HSV-transformed cells (derived with ultraviolet-irradiated virus) initially retain considerable amounts of genetic information but then lose variable quantities after extensive subculturing or cloning.

Although the information is not as extensive as that for EBV and HSV, some molecular evidence has been obtained for the role of CMV in neoplasia. DNA-DNA renaturation experiments demonstrated 0.4 genome equivalents of CMV per early passage CMV-transformed human cell. CMV gene expression has also been noted in several human neoplasms. CMV antigens have been observed in uterine cervical cancer cells, and CMV DNA has been detected in four of seven tumors of the colon. CMV antigens have been detected by anti-complement immunofluorescence in cell nuclei from seven of 31 Kaposi's sarcoma biopsies and four of 12 cell lines derived from the biopsies. Antigen was only found in 0.5 to 2% of the cell populations; however, this is not surprising because Kaposi's sarcoma cell lines contain a low percentage of tumor cells mixed with fibroblasts and cells of the mononuclear phagocytic system. In the same study, CMV DNA was detected at low levels in three of eight tumor biopsies from patients with Kaposi's sarcoma by DNA-DNA renaturation kinetics.

RNA TUMOR VIRUSES

Retroviruses associated with a viral etiology of cancer are primarily in the type-C group (Bishop, 1978). The only type-B retrovirus of interest is the mouse mammary tumor virus (MMTV). Isolates of MMTV either are exogenous and transmitted from one mouse to another or are endogenous and transmitted genetically. The most familiar MMTV is the milk factor of Bittner's virus. C3H and A-strain mice (high incidence strains for MMTV) carry large numbers of MMTV proviruses in their genomes. The virus is present in many cells of these animals, but particularly high numbers are present in lactating mammary tissues that are easily passed to progeny animals. Low-incidence strains of mice nursed by foster mothers of high-incidence strains develop tumors at a high frequency. MMTV produces adenocarcinomas, whereas the C-type viruses induce sarcomas and leukemias. In addition, not only is expression of the virus genetically controlled (low- and high-incidence mice), but transcription of MMTV provirus is also hormonally regulated. Mammary cancer normally occurs only in female mice,

but males of high-incidence strains develop the tumor if given estrogens. In addition, transcription of virus RNA and MMTV can be extensively induced by the addition of gluco-corticoids *in vitro* in cell culture and *in vivo*. Halogenated pyrimidines that induce the yield of many C-type retroviruses do not induce MMTV. Interest in MMTV stems from detection of particles containing 70S RNA (reverse transcriptase) and antigens related to the viral core antigen of MMTV in human breast cancer tissue.

The only type-D retroviruses associated with a viral etiology of cancer have been isolated from nonhuman primates (Nooter and Bentvelzen, 1980). Exogenous and endogenous type-C viruses have also been isolated from simian tumors. Several retroviruses of nonhuman primates are mentioned in Table 3–14; however, Table 3–19 shows a more detailed list of type-C and -D isolates.

Avian and Mammalian Retroviruses

Retroviruses have been implicated in tumors in several animal species for more than 70 years. The first breakthrough associating retroviruses with the etiology of cancer came in 1951, when Ludwik Gross demonstrated that C3H mice, which naturally have a low incidence of leukemia, developed the disease after being inoculated as newborns with cell-free extracts from AKR mice, which develop leukemia early in life and at a high frequency (Gross, 1951). Previous attempts to transmit leukemia in mice with filtered extracts had failed because the inoculated recipients had been adult mice. Similar studies with cell-free extracts have demonstrated that cat leukemia, bovine leukemia, and lymphosarcomas of Northern pike and gibbon apes are also transmissible; in each case C-type virus particles can be detected in tumor cells. The discovery that bovine leukemia had a viral origin was based on an unexpected observation. When blood from cattle was used to vaccinate sheep against fibroplasmosis, some sheep developed leukemia. Examination of the cattle blood revealed bovine leukemia virus. The successful transmission of lymphosarcoma in the Northern pike suggests that leukemias and cancerous lymphomas are caused by transmissible viruses not only in warm-blooded but also in poikilothermic animals.

Retroviruses implicated as the causes of cancer differ from DNA viruses in two major

Table 3–19. Retroviruses of Nonhuman Primates

VIRUS TYPE	ISOLATE DESIGNATION	NATURAL HOST	TISSUE SOURCE
Endogenous type C	M28	Live baboon	Testis
	Bab 455K		Kidney
	Bab 8-K		Kidney
	Bab 587-T		Testis
	M7	Yellow baboon	Placenta
	B1LN	Sacred baboon	Lymph node
	PP-1-Lu	Guinea baboon	Lung
	TG-1-K	Gelada baboon	Kidney
	MAC-1	Stumptail monkey	Spleen
	OMC-1	Owl monkey	Kidney
Exogenous type C	SiSV	Woolly monkey	Fibrosarcoma
	GALV-SF	White-handed gibbon ape	Lymphosarcoma
	GALV-SEATO		Myelogenous leukemia
	GALV-H		Lymphatic leukemia
Endogenous type D	PO-1-Lu	Langur	Lung
	SMRV	Squirrel monkey	Lung
Exogenous type D	MPMV	Rhesus monkey	Breast carcinoma

ways. First, retroviruses have considerably less genetic information in the virus genome. The largest genome, that of nondefective avian sarcoma viruses, is 10,000 nucleotides long and codes for at most 3×10^5 daltons of protein (see Figure 3–18). The small size of the genome has enabled investigators to learn a great deal about its structure and function (Duesberg, 1979). Second, retroviruses can replicate without causing cell injury or death. Thus, in contrast to DNA viruses that require restriction of virus replication for transformation to occur, some RNA viruses replicate and transform simultaneously. The retrovirus genome contains at most four different genes and a "common" (c) region (see Figure 3–19). The *gag* gene codes for a precursor, which is cleaved to yield four internal structural proteins of the virion (Pr65 *gag*:5′-p15-p12-p30-p10-3′). The *pol* gene codes for virion reverse transcriptase, the *env* gene for virion envelop glycoproteins, and the *onc* (or *src*) gene for the transformation-related protein. One current theory is that the *src* gene was added to the virus genome during evolution as a result of recombination with host cell information. Similar host cell sequences are designated *sarc*. The C region is found in most retroviruses but is not identified as a fifth gene because no mRNA or gene product for the C region has been detected. It is possible that the C region includes a promoter that regulates virus gene expression; during replication and integration, the C region is thought to be redundantly transcribed from viral RNA at both ends of the proviral DNA.

Avian and mammalian retroviruses associated with neoplasia in animals can be divided into three groups: (1) Sarcoma viruses,

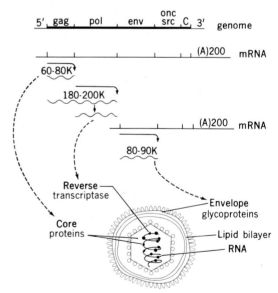

Figure 3–18. Expression of retrovirus genes. Retrovirus genes encoding replicative functions have been assigned three letter names: *gag* for the internal structural proteins; *pol* for the reverse transcriptase; and *env* for the envelope glycoproteins. The diagram illustrates the location of the gene products in the virion. The transforming-specific sequences are generally referred to as *onc* genes. There are at least 13 distinct *onc* genes identified in about 20 isolates of transforming retroviruses. The three-letter designation *src* has been given to the viral *onc* gene insert from Rous sarcoma virus. The *src* region codes for a 60,000-dalton phosphoprotein (pp60[src]), which is a protein kinase that transfers phosphate from the γ position of ATP to the hydroxyl position of tyrosine.

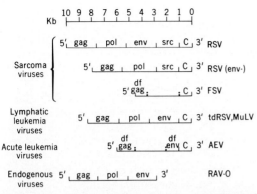

Figure 3-19. Relative genome sizes in various classes of retroviruses. Abbreviations: RSV = Rous sarcoma virus; env⁻ = envelope-negative; FSV = Fujinama avian sarcoma virus; td = transformation defective; MuLV = murine leukemia virus; AEV = avian erythroblastosis virus; RAV = Rous-associated virus; df = defective elements of specific genes; Kb = kilobases. See Table 3-13 for more information on each of these classes of viruses.

(2) lymphatic leukemia viruses, and (3) acute leukemia viruses (see Table 3-20). Sarcoma viruses can cause solid tumors, hemorrhagic disease, erythroblastosis, and lymphoblastomas in animals and can transform fibroblasts in cell culture in one to two weeks. The avian sarcoma viruses, Rous sarcoma virus (RSV), and B 77 virus are the only C-type viruses that possess and express all four genes. They are not defective for replication and can transform cultured fibroblasts and other cells. Through the use of mutants with defects in the transforming (src) gene, the product of the gene has been isolated and characterized. The src protein is a phosphorylated protein with a molecular weight of 60,000 and protein kinase activity. There are also defective avian sarcoma viruses. The Bryan RSV(−) and Schmidt-Ruppin RSV(−) N8 viruses have env deletions. The Fujinama sarcoma virus is defective in all three essential virion genes, gag, pol, and env, and has a unique onc gene unrelated to the RSV src gene. Defective avian sarcoma viruses produce sarcomas and transform fibroblasts in culture but cannot replicate without a helper virus. The leukemia viruses can provide the necessary gene products to function as helper viruses.

In contrast to the avian sarcoma viruses, all mammalian sarcoma viruses are defective for replication (Andersson, 1980). Included in this group are the Moloney, Kirsten, and Harvey murine sarcoma viruses (Mo-MSV, Ki-MSV, and Ha-MSV) and the feline sarcoma virus (FeSV). The mammalian sarcoma viruses rapidly cause a variety of sarcomas in vivo and can transform cells in vitro, even though they do not possess the src gene or any sequences related to the src gene. All known sarcoma viruses of feline origin were isolated from naturally occurring sarcomas in outbred cats. The genome of these defective viruses is about 5700 nucleotides and lacks the pol, env, and src genes. The 3' terminal half of the gag gene is also missing; hence, these viruses code for no more than two of the gag proteins. Like defective avian sarcoma viruses, defective mamma-

Table 3-20. Properties of Various Avian and Mammalian Leukemia and Sarcoma Viruses

VIRUS GROUP	VIRUS	ONCOGENICITY IN VIVO	TRANSFORMATION IN VITRO
Sarcoma viruses	RSV RSV(−) Mo-MSV Ki-MSV Ha-MSV FeSV	Produce sarcomas; all but RSV produce acute leukemia; lymphatic leukemia may be due to helper virus	Fibroblasts
Lymphatic leukemia viruses	ALV td RSV G-MuLV (FMR) MuLV FeLV	Produce lymphatic leukemia; sarcoma and carcinomas seen at low frequency after long latency periods	No transformation
Acute leukemia viruses	avian MC29 AEV Ab-MuLV	Produce acute leukemia; all but Ab-MuLV produce sarcoma and carcinoma; lymphatic leukemia may be due to helper virus	Fibroblasts and hematopoietic cells
	AMV SFFV-(F-MuLV)	Produce acute leukemia; sarcoma, carcinoma, and lymphatic leukemia may be due to helper virus	Hematopoietic cells

lian sarcoma viruses require helper viruses for replication. Helper viruses are generally present in excess and strains of all of these viruses consist of virus mixtures including helper virus and pseudotype particles containing components of the defective and the helper virus, for example, Moloney murine leukemia virus (Mo-MuLV) can act as a helper for Mo-MSV yielding Mo-MSV (Mo-MuLV).

Only a few murine sarcoma virus isolates have been obtained from naturally occurring tumors. These include the FJB murine osteosarcoma virus and the Gazdar murine spindle cell sarcoma virus (found to be similar to Mo-MSV). The murine sarcoma viruses have been developed in the laboratory and probably arose as a result of recombination between leukemia viruses and host genetic material. Ki-MSV and Ha-MSV were isolated from rats inoculated with Mo-MuLV, whereas Mo-MSV was isolated from a rhabdomyosarcoma induced in BALB/c mice infected with Mo-MuLV. One problem with this theory is that one must assume that nondefective leukemia virus RNA is deleted and that some of the deleted RNA is substituted by cellular genes to generate defective sarcoma virus transforming genes.

The lymphatic leukemia viruses possess the *gag, pol,* and *env* genes and the C region but lack the *src* gene and cannot transform fibroblasts or other cells *in vitro.* They are weakly oncogenic *in vivo* and produce leukemia in animals only after long latency periods. The avian lymphatic leukemia viruses (Rous-associated viruses) produce lymphocytic leukemia, osteopetrosis, nephroblastomas, and erythroblastomas late in the life of the bird or, if injected into uninfected birds, after a prolonged latency period. Tumor formation is not an inevitable consequence of infection with these viruses because viremias may be observed without pathologic effects. Included in this group is the transformation defective (td) RSV, a *src* deletion mutant.

The murine lymphatic leukemia viruses have been studied most extensively. The naturally occurring MuLV, Gross-AKR subgroup, typically gives rise to thymic lymphosarcomas and myeloid leukemia after a latent period of several months. A separate serologic subgroup, FMR (Friend, Moloney, Rauscher), composed of laboratory virus strains, causes erythroblastic leukemias after a latency of only a few weeks. Leukemia viruses have also been isolated from cats, hamsters, rats, and monkeys.

FeLV is contagious among cats and causes generalized lymphosarcoma, can cause leukemia in dogs, and replicates readily in human cells. Because lymphatic leukemia viruses lack a *src* gene, they may transform indirectly by affecting cellular gene expression as a consequence of provirus integration, or they may activate preexisting defective transforming genes in the animal (endogenous RNA virus sequences). The lymphatic leukemia viruses are nondefective for replication and hence can function as helper viruses for defective sarcoma and acute leukemia viruses.

All acute leukemia viruses are defective for replication and can be divided into two subgroups based on *in vitro* transforming properties. The first subgroup includes viruses that transform fibroblasts as well as hematopoietic cells in culture and contains the avian myelocytomatosis virus (NC 29), avian erythroblastosis virus, and Abelson murine leukemia virus (Ab-MuLV). The avian leukemia viruses rapidly cause erythroblastosis, myelocytomatosis, neurolymphomatosis, endotheliomas, sarcomas, and carcinomas; whereas the Abelson virus quickly induces reticulum cell sarcomas and thymus-independent lymphomas. Transformation after infection with these viruses is inevitable, occurs in culture within several days after exposure, and seems to be a direct consequence of the virus. Viruses in this acute leukemia virus group are defective in *gag, pol,* and *env* and require helper viruses (usually lymphatic leukemia viruses) for replication.

The second subgroup of acute leukemia viruses is distinguished from the first by the inability to transform fibroblasts in culture and includes avian myeloblastosis virus (AMV) and Friend murine leukemia virus. AMV causes erythroblastosis, myelocytomatosis, and neurolymphomatosis, and the Friend virus complex induces splenomegaly, granulocytic myelogenous leukemia, and erythroleukemia. Viruses in this subgroup cause acute leukemias *in vivo,* induce proliferation of hematopoietic cells in culture, and, like the mammalian sarcoma viruses and other acute leukemia viruses, are defective and require helper viruses for replication.

The oncogene hypothesis was first proposed by Huebner and Todaro (1969). They suggested that retrovirus oncogenes are part of the genetic makeup of all cells and that they were possibly acquired through viral infection early in evolution. These oncogenes were harmless as long as they existed in a dormant state. If stimulated by a carcinogenic agent, however, they could convert normal cells to cancer cells. In 1976, Bishop and colleagues (Stehelin *et al.,* 1976) used radioactive DNA copied solely from *src* (the oncogene of the Rous sarcoma virus) by reverse transcriptase as a probe for cellular DNA with a nucleotide sequence similar to that of *src.* The copy of *src* could hybridize with DNA from uninfected chickens and other birds. A later study (Spector *et al.,* 1978) continued these studies and found DNA related to *src* in mammals, including humans, and in fish. The conclusion was that all vertebrates probably contain a gene related to *src.* The gene proved, however, not to be a retrovirus gene at all but, rather, a cellular gene called *sarc.* This gene is not only present in normal cells, it is also active in them; the gene is transcribed into mRNA, and the RNA is translated into protein.

The product of the transforming gene (oncogene) of the avian sarcoma viruses (*src*) is a 60,000 dalton phosphoprotein (pp60^{src}), which is a protein kinase that transfers phosphate from the γ position of ATP to the hydroxyl position of tyrosine. The amount of phosphorylated tyrosine within cells increases tenfold as a result of transformation by *src;* pp60^{src} is unusual in that most protein kinases phosphorylate the amino acids serine and threonine. Since the function of pp60^{src} became known, it has been demonstrated that phosphorylation of tyrosine may have a role in the regulation of normal cell growth. The finding that pp60^{src} protein kinase activity is temperature sensitive when isolated from virions of a temperature-sensitive transformation mutant of RSV, suggests a role of the phosphotransferase activity in transformation by this virus. A single protein kinase could generate the cellular changes associated with transformation either by interacting directly with a single primary target that subsequently induces multiple changes or by acting on several different primary targets.

The importance of phosphotransferase activities became even more apparent with the finding that at least six other retroviruses possess proteins with this enzymatic activity. Included in this group are the *onc* gene product p15 of the mammalian sarcoma virus Mo-MSV, p21 of Ha-MSV and Ki-MSV, and the *gag* polyproteins of FeSV and Ab-MuLV. Not only are these proteins similar in enzymatic activity, but they also are similar in their compartmentalization within the cells, a factor that may be highly significant in ascertaining their function. The bulk of pp60^{src} in ASV transformation accumulates at the inner surface of the plasma membrane. Ha-MSV p21 is found almost exclusively at the inner surface of the plasma membrane, while the *gag* polyproteins of FeSV and Ab-MuLV can be detected at the cell surface. The Mo-MSV p15 protein can interact with cytoskeletal structures *in vitro.* Location at the cell surface would be important if the protein kinases interact with the cytoskeleton, with receptors for cell growth factors, or affect the ability of cells to adhere to surfaces. Any or all of these cellular elements have a role in the conversion of the normal cell to the cancer cell. A protein extremely similar in size and chemical structure has been found in much lower quantities in normal chicken, rodent, amphibian, fish, and human cells. This protein, denoted pp60^{sarc}, also catalyzes the phosphorylation of tyrosine. Finding pp60^{sarc} in normal cells further suggests that proteins of this nature are important in differentiation and growth control.

Almost all retrovirus oncogenes identified to date have close relatives in the normal genomes of vertebrate species. Most of these cellular homologs of viral oncogenes adhere to the principles first established for *sarc:* (1) They have the structural organization of cellular genes rather than viral genes; (2) they have apparently survived long periods of evolution; and (3) they are active in normal cells.

Most virologists agree that retrovirus oncogenes are copies of cellular genes. It is possible that the oncogenes were added to the already existing retrovirus genomes not too long ago. It is still not known how and why retroviruses have copied cellular genes. It is clear that cellular genes have transforming potential.

Two explanations have been proposed to account for the effects of retrovirus oncogenes on infected cells. One explanation, the mutational hypothesis, proposes that viral oncogenes differ from their cellular ancestors in subtle but important ways resulting from mutations that occurred when the cellular genes were copied into the retrovirus genome. The second hypothesis, the alternative dosage, proposes that retrovirus oncogenes act by overburdening cells with too many normal proteins conducting normal functions. With this hypothesis, the origin of cancer by retrovirus oncogenes is related to the amount of the viral proteins rather than to any unique property(ies) that they have. It would now appear that the first hypothesis is most probably correct. Very recently, observations at the molecular level have suggested that the transforming oncogenes derived from human tumor cells differ from the normal homologs by a single amino acid and that this change is reflected in the DNA of the gene. The change is reflected by the incorporation of valine instead of glycine (Reddy *et al.*, 1982; Tabin *et al.*, 1982).

Endogenous Retroviruses

Evidence for endogenous RNA tumor provirus within the cellular genome has been compiled for virtually every species, including rodents, birds, cats, monkeys, and primates. Proviruses are not normally expressed, but anywhere from one to 100 copies per cell may be present. A variety of methods has been used to detect endogenous viruses and endogenous virus sequences. When intact provirus is present, the endogenous virus can be reactivated by (1) treatment of cells with a variety of substances or radiation, or (2) by cocultivation with cell lines from heterologous species. The first reported endogenous type-C retrovirus from a rhesus monkey, for example, was obtained by cocultivation of a rhesus monkey esophageal carcinoma cell line with a canine osteosarcoma cell line. Similarly, baboon endogenous virus has been obtained by cocultivation of baboon tissues with human, monkey, dog, and bat cell lines. Induction and expression of endogenous retroviruses also depend upon the age of the animal and the state of differentiation of the cells tested. The most important endogenous RNA tumor virus of chickens is RAV-O. The genomes of RAV-O and RSV, an exogenous virus, are virtually identical in their *gag* and *pol* genes but have substantial sequence differences in the central portion but not the terminal regions of the *env* gene. Most of these differences are due to a single base change.

Normal cells may not only harbor multiple copies of a single provirus, but a single cell may harbor multiple proviruses, each of which may be reactivated by different conditions. Mice in particular have numerous proviruses in their genome; wild-type mice may harbor as many as ten different proviruses. How do such cells express a normal phenotype in the presence of virus-transforming genes such as *onc* or *src*? In addition, not only are the genes present, but transcription and translation of cellular *onc-*

related sequences have been detected. In certain chicken cells designated chf$^+$, a glycoprotein coded for by the *env* gene of RAV-O is expressed. This information was revealed by examination of certain chicken cells that permit replication of the Bryan strain (*env-*) of RSV. That is, chf$^+$ cells contain a functional, endogenous RAV-O *env* gene which produces the *env* protein complementary to the defect in the exogenous RSV mutant. It is possible that differences in regulation are sufficient to explain how endogenous virus-transforming sequences can be present and even expressed. For example, the size of *src* mRNA of RSV is 21S, whereas the endogenous cellular mRNA-carrying sequences related to *src* are 26 to 30S. Similarly a protein related to the 60K *src* gene of RSV is found in many vertebrate cells, yet several of these vertebrates distinguish between their own 60K *src* protein and the RSV protein because they produce antibodies to the RSV protein.

Retroviruses and Human Cancer

Two distinct approaches have been used to determine whether RNA tumor viruses play a role in the etiology of human cancer. The first looked for animal retrovirus information in tissues and fluids of human cancer patients; the second attempted to isolate a human cancer retrovirus. Until recently, attempts to isolate human C-type cancer viruses failed or yielded viruses later found to be reisolations of known animal retroviruses, in particular, nonhuman primate viruses. In 1980 the isolation of a putative human leukemia retrovirus generated renewed interest in the scientific community (Poiesz *et al.*, 1980; Hinuma *et al.*, 1981). Gallo, at the National Cancer Institute (U.S.A.), and Hinuma, at Kyoto University (Japan), identified a type-C retrovirus associated with adult T-cell leukemia/lymphoma (ATLL). This rare disease is accompanied by acute or chronic leukemia, lymphadenopathy, hepatosplenomegaly, hypercalcemia, and frequent skin lesions (erythroderma and nodule formation) but mediastinal tumor is absent. Pleomorphic leukemic cells with markedly deformed nuclei and T-cell surface markers appear in the blood of ATLL patients. The onset of ATLL occurs in adulthood, and the disease, which appears to be endemic to one region of southwestern Japan (the islands of Kyushu and Shikoku), is resistant to currently available antileukemic agents.

The human cutaneous T-cell lymphoma virus strain CR ($HTLV_{CR}$) was isolated in Gallo's laboratory from two T-cell lymphoblastoid cell lines from a patient with cutaneous T-cell lymphoma (mycoses fungoides). The recently devised method for *in vitro* culture of human T lymphoblasts, made possible by purification of T-cell growth factor, enabled establishment of normal T-cell lines and T-lymphoblastoid lines from cancer patients. Without such lines, $HTLV_{CR}$ would not have been found. The fact that the virus was also successfully isolated directly from fresh peripheral blood lymphocytes obtained from the same patient indicated that $HTLV_{CR}$ was not a cell culture contaminant. Characterization has shown that it is a C-type retrovirus that replicates poorly in the lymphoblastoid cell lines and contains a reverse transcriptase with a preference for Mg^{2+}, which is structurally similar but not identical to simian sarcoma virus-gibbon ape leukemia virus (SiSV-GALV) reverse transcriptase. Extensive studies have shown that $HTLV_{CR}$ is not a known avian, murine, rat, feline, or nonhuman primate type-C retrovirus. Since the original isolation, $HTLV_{CR}$ has been isolated from three other patients in the United States with cutaneous ATLL. In addition, an antibody to $HTLV_{CR}$ has been identified in the four patients and in two relatives of patients but not in healthy individuals. The virus is integrated into the genome of leukemic cells but has not been found in normal cells from the same patients.

Hinuma found that individuals with ATLL and more than 25% of healthy adults living in the region of Japan where the cancer is endemic have antibodies to a cytoplasmic antigen present in a T-cell lymphoblastoid line derived from an ATLL patient. Hinuma also reported that type-C virus particles are present in this cell line and that *in vitro* cocultivation of normal umbilical cord blood with cells infected with this type-C virus results in transformation of normal human blood cells. Obviously, these are potentially exciting findings and may represent the beginning of a new era relating retroviruses to human cancer.

ACKNOWLEDGMENT

The authors thank Frank Jenkins for assistance in illustrating the Southern and "northern" blot diagrams and Melissa Reese for editorial assistance.

REFERENCES

Alwine, J. C.; Kemp, D. J.; and Stark, G. R.: Method for detection of specific RNAs in agarose gels by transfer to diazobenzyloxymethyl-paper and hybridization with DNA probes. *Proc. Natl. Acad. Sci. USA,* **74**:5350–5354, 1977.

Andersson, P.: The oncogenic function of mammalian sarcoma viruses. *Adv. Cancer Res.,* **33**:109–171, 1980.

Bishop, J. M.: Retroviruses. *Annu. Rev. Biochem.,* **47**:35–88, 1978.

Bittner, J. J.: Some possible effects of nursing on the mammary gland tumor incidence in mice. *Science,* **84**:162, 1936.

Blumberg, B. S.; Alter, H. J.; and Visnich, S.: A "new" antigen in leukemia sera. *J.A.M.A.,* **191**:541–546, 1965.

Calnek, B.W.: Marek's disease virus and lymphoma. In Rapp, F. (ed.): *Oncogenic Herpesviruses.* CRC Press, Boca Raton, 1980.

Churchill, A. E.; Payne, L. N.; and Chubb, R. C.: Immunization against Marek's disease using a live attenuated vaccine. *Nature,* **211**:744–747, 1969.

Copeland, N. G.; Zelenetz, A. D.; and Cooper, G. M.: Transformation of NIH/3T3 mouse cells by DNA of Rous Sarcoma virus. *Cell,* **17**:993–1002, 1979.

Croce, C. M.: Integration of oncogenic viruses in mammalian cells. *Int. Rev. Cytol.,* **71**:1–17, 1981.

Duesberg, P. H.: Transforming genes of retroviruses. *Cold Spring Harbor Symp. Quant. Biol.,* **44**:13–29, 1979.

Duff, R., and Rapp, F.: Oncogenic transformation of hamster cells after exposure to herpes simplex virus type 2. *Nature New Biol.,* **233**:48–50, 1971.

Durak, D. T.: Opportunistic infections and Kaposi's sarcoma in homosexual men. *N. Engl. J. Med.,* **305**:1465–1467, 1981.

Ellermann, V., and Bang, O.: Experimentelle leukämie bei hühnern. *Zentralbl. Bakteriol. Mikrobiol. Hyg. [A],* **46**:595, 1908.

Eglin, R. P.; Sharp, F.; MacLean, A. B.; Macnab, J. C. M.; Clements, J. B.; and Wilkie, N. M.: Detection of RNA complementary to herpes simplex virus DNA in human cervical squamous cell neoplasms. *Cancer Res.,* **41**:3597–3603, 1981.

Epstein, M. A.; Achong, B. G.; and Barr, Y.: Virus particles in cultured lymphoblasts from Burkitt's lymphoma. *Lancet,* **1**:702–703, 1964.

Epstein, M. A., and Barr, Y. M.: Cultivation in vitro of human lymphoblasts from Burkitt's malignant lymphoma. *Lancet,* **1**:252–253, 1964.

Fiori, M., and diMayorca, G.: Occurrence of BK virus DNA in DNA obtained from certain human tumors. *Proc. Natl. Acad. Sci. USA,* **73**:4662–4666, 1976.

Frenkel, N.; Roizman, B.; Cassai, E.; and Nahmias, A.: DNA fragment of herpes simplex virus type 2 and its transcription in human cervical cancer tissue. *Proc. Natl. Acad. Sci. USA,* **69**:3784–3789, 1972.

Galloway, D. A., and McDougall, J. K.; Transformation of rodent cells by a cloned DNA fragment of herpes simplex virus type 2. *J. Virol.,* **38**:749–760, 1981.

Gardner, S. D.; Field, A. M.; Coleman, D. V.; and Hulme, B.: New human papovavirus (BK) isolated from urine after renal transplantation. *Lancet,* **1**:1253–1257, 1971.

Geder, L.; Lausch, R.; O'Neill, F.; and Rapp, F.: Oncogenic transformation of human embryo lung cells by human cytomegalovirus. *Science,* **492:**1134–1137, 1976.

Giraldo, G.: Beth, E.; Coeur, P.; Vogel, C. L.; and Dhru, D. S.: Kaposi's sarcoma: A new model in the search for viruses associated with human malignancies. *J. Natl. Cancer Inst.,* **49:**1495–1507, 1972.

Giraldo, G.; Beth, E.; and Huang, E. S.: Kaposi's sarcoma and its relationship to cytomegalovirus (CMV). III. CMV DNA and CMV early antigens in Kaposi's sarcoma. *Int. J. Cancer,* **26:**23–29, 1980.

Graham, F. L.; Bacchetti, S.; McKinnon, R.; Stanners, C.; Cordell, B.; and Goodman, H. M.: Transformation of mammalian cells with DNA using the calcium technique. In Baserga, R.; Croce, C.; and Rovera, G. (eds.): *Introduction of Macromolecules into Viable Mammalian Cells.* Alan R. Liss, Inc., New York, 1980.

Graham, F. L., and van der Eb, A. J.: A new technique for the assay of infectivity of human adenovirus 5 DNA. *Virology,* **52:**456–467, 1973.

Gross, L.: Spontaneous leukemia developing in C3H mice following inoculation in infancy with AK leukemic extracts or AK embryos. *Proc. Soc. Exp. Biol. Med.,* **76:**27–32, 1951.

Helling, R. B.; Goodman, H. M.; and Boyer, H. W.: Analysis of endonuclease R. Eco RI fragments of DNA from lamboid bacteriophages and other viruses by agarose gel electrophoresis. *J. Virol.,* **14:**1235–1244, 1974.

Henle, G.; Henle, W.; Clifford, P.; Diehl, V.; Kafuko, G. W.; Kirya, B. G.; Klein, G.; Morrow, R. H.; Munube, G. M. R.; Pike, P.; Tukei, P. M.; and Ziegler, J. L.: Antibodies to Epstein-Barr virus in Burkitt's lymphoma and control groups. *J.N.C.I.,* **43:**1147–1157, 1969.

Hinuma, Y.; Nagata, K.; Kanaoka, M.; Nakai, M.; Matsumoto, T.; Kinoshita, K.; Shirakawa, S.; and Miyoshi, I.: Adult T-cell leukemia: Antigen in an ATL cell line and detection of antibodies to the antigen in human sera. *Proc. Natl. Acad. Sci. USA,* **78:**6476–6480, 1981.

Huebner, R. J., and Todaro, G. J.: Oncogenes of RNA tumor viruses as determinants of cancer. *Proc. Natl. Acad. Sci. USA,* **64:**1087–1094, 1969.

Jariwalla, R. J.; Aurelian, L.; and Ts'o, P. O. P.: Tumorigenic transformation induced by a specific fragment of DNA from herpes simplex virus type 2. *Proc. Natl. Acad. Sci. USA,* **77:**2279–2283, 1980.

Lucké, B.: Carcinoma in the leopard frog: Its probable causation by a virus. *J. Exp. Med.,* **68:**457–468, 1938.

Maniatis, T.; Jeffrey, A.; and van deSande, H.: Chain length determination of small double- and single-stranded DNA molecules by polyacrylamide gel electrophoresis. *Biochemistry,* **14:**3787–3794, 1975.

Mäntyjärvi, R. A.: New oncogenic human papovaviruses. *Med. Biol.,* **57:**29–35, 1979.

Marek, J.: Multiple nervenentzundung (polyneuritis) bei hühnern. *DTW,* **15:**417–421, 1907.

Martin, R. G.: The transformation of cell growth and transmogrification of DNA synthesis by simian virus 40. *Adv. Cancer Res.,* **34:**1–68, 1981.

Maupas, P., and Melnick, J. L.: Hepatitis B infection and primary liver cancer. *Prog. Med. Virol.,* **27:**1–5, 1981.

Morin, C.; Braun, L.; Casas-Cordero, M.; Shah, K.; Roy, M.; Fortier, M.; and Meisels, A.: Confirmation of the papillomavirus etiology of condylomatous cervix lesions by the peroxidase-antiperoxidase technique. *J.N.C.I.,* **66:**831–835, 1981.

Naegele, R. F.; Granoff, A.; and Darlington, R. W.: The presence of the Lucké herpesvirus genome in induced tadpole tumors and its oncogenicity. Koch-Henle postulates fulfilled. *Proc. Natl. Acad. Sci. USA,* **71:**830–834, 1974.

Nooter, K., and Bentvelzen, P.: Primate type C oncoviruses. *Biochim. Biophys. Acta,* **605:**461–487, 1980.

Palmer, A. E.; London, W. T.; Nahmias, A. J.; Naib, Z. M.; Tunea, J.; Fuccillo, D. A.; Ellenburg, J. H.; and Sever, J. L.: A preliminary report on investigation of oncogenic potential of herpes simplex virus type 2 in cebus monkeys. *Cancer Res.,* **36:**807–809, 1976.

Poiesz, B. J.; Ruscetti, F. W.; Gazdar, A. F.; Bunn, P. A.; Minna, T. D.; and Gallo, R. C.: Detection and isolation of type C retrovirus particles from fresh and cultured lymphocytes of a patient with cutaneous T-cell lymphoma. *Proc. Natl. Acad. Sci. USA,* **77:**7415–7419, 1980.

Rapp, F.: Transformation by herpes simplex viruses. In Essex, M.; Todaro, G.; and zur Hausen, H. (eds.): *Viruses in Naturally Occurring Cancers.* Cold Spring Harbor Laboratory, Cold Spring Harbor, New York, 1980.

Reddy, E. P.; Reynolds, R. K.; Santos, E.; and Barbacid, M.: A point mutation is responsible for the acquisition of transforming properties by the T24 human bladder carcinoma oncogene. *Nature,* **300:**149–152, 1982.

Reyes, G. R.; LaFemina, R.; Hayward, S. D.; and Hayward, G. S.: Morphological transformation by DNA fragments of human herpesviruses: Evidence for two distinct transforming regions in herpes simplex virus types 1 and 2 and lack of correlation with biochemical transfer of the thymidine kinase gene. *Cold Spring Harbor Symp. Quant. Biol.,* **44:**629–641, 1980.

Rous, P.: A sarcoma of the fowl transmissible by an agent separable from the tumor cells. *J. Exp. Med.,* **13:**397–411, 1911.

Sanford, E. J.; Geder, L.; Dagen, J. E.; Laychock, A. E.; Rohner, T. J.; and Rapp, F.: Humoral and cellular immune response of prostatic cancer patients to cytomegalovirus-related antigens of cytomegalovirus-transformed human cells. *J. Surg. Res.,* **24:**404–408, 1978.

Shafritz, D. A.; Showval, D.; Sherman, H. I.; Hadziyannis, S. J.; and Kew, M. C.: Integration of hepatitis B virus DNA into the genome of liver cells in chronic liver disease and hepatocellular carcinoma. *N. Engl. J. Med.,* **305:**1067–1073, 1981.

Shope, R. E.: A filtrable virus causing a tumor-like condition in rabbits and its relationship to virus myxomatosum. *J. Exp. Med.,* **56:**803–822, 1932.

Southern, E. M.: Detection of specific sequences among DNA fragments separated by gel electrophoresis. *J. Mol. Biol.,* **98:**503–517, 1975.

Spector, D. H.; Varmus, H. E.; and Bishop, J. M.: Nucleotide sequences related to the transforming gene of avian sarcoma virus are present in DNA of uninfected vertebrates. *Proc. Natl. Acad. Sci. USA,* **75:**4102–4106, 1978.

Stehelin, D.; Varmus, H. E.; Bishop, J. M.; and Vogt, P. K.: DNA related to the transforming gene(s) of avian sarcoma viruses is present in normal avian DNA. *Nature,* **260:**170–173, 1976.

Summers, J. A.; Smolec, J. M.; and Snyder, R.: A virus similar to human hepatitis B virus associated with hepatitis and hepatoma in woodchucks. *Proc. Natl. Acad. Sci. USA,* **75:**4533–4537, 1978.

Swanstrom, R., and Shenk, P.: X-ray intensifying screens greatly enhance the detection by autoradiography of the radioactive isotopes ^{32}P and ^{125}I. *Anal. Biochem.,* **86:**184–192, 1978.

Tabin, C. J.; Bradley, S. M.; Bargmann, C. I.; Weinberg,

R. A.; Papageorge, A. G.; Scolnic, E. M.; Dhar, R.; Lowy, D. R.; and Chang, E. H.; Mechanism of activation of a human oncogene. *Nature,* **300:**143–149, 1982.

Tiollais, P.; Charnay, P.; and Vyas, G. N.: Biology of hepatitis B virus. *Science,* **213:**406–411, 1981.

Tweedell, K. S.: Induced oncogenesis in developing frog kidney cells. *Cancer Res.,* **27:**2042–2052, 1967.

Weinberg, R. A.: Use of transfection to analyze genetic information and malignant transformation. *Biochim. Biophys. Acta,* **651:**25–35, 1981.

Wentz, W. B.: Reagan, J. W.; Heggie, A. D.; Fu, Y.; and Anthony, D. D.: Induction of uterine cancer with inactivated herpes simplex virus types 1 and 2. *Cancer,* **48:**1783–1790, 1981.

Wold, W. S. M.; Mackey, J. K.; Brackmann, K. H.; Takemori, N.; Rigden, P.; and Green, M.: Analysis of human tumors and human malignant cell lines for BK virus-specific DNA sequences. *Proc. Natl. Acad. Sci. USA,* **75:**454–458, 1978.

zur Hausen, H.: The role of viruses in human tumors. *Adv. Cancer Res.,* **33:**77–107, 1980.

E.   GENETICS AND FAMILIAL PREDISPOSITION

Robert W. Miller

Each form of cancer has a heritable component. For some it is important (*e.g.,* colon cancer) and for others it is less meaningful (*e.g.,* esophageal cancer). As we learn about host susceptibility, we will be able to define mechanisms of human carcinogenesis for which no animal models presently exist. A variety of approaches may be used, from population studies to studying etiology at the bedside, paying particular attention to the family history.

ETHNIC DIFFERENCES

The conventional classification for coding death-certificate diagnoses of bone sarcoma did not separate Ewing's tumor from osteosarcoma. In 1968, this separation became possible for the first time, when all death-certificate diagnoses were recoded by histologic type for children who died of cancer from 1960 to 1966 (Miller, 1968). The results revealed a surprise: Ewing's tumors rarely occurred in nonwhites (Glass and Fraumeni, 1970). Nonwhites in Africa also seldom developed Ewing's tumor. The failure for rates to rise with migration of nonwhites to an area where the rates were higher (the United States) indicates a genetic resistance to this form of cancer.

Other population data (reviewed by Miller, 1977), show that teenage nonwhites have low rates for testicular cancers, all forms, and no childhood age-peak at four years for mortality from acute lymphocytic leukemia. Their genetically determined skin color protects them against melanoma and other skin neoplasms caused by ultraviolet light. Rates for multiple myeloma, by contrast, are higher in nonwhites than in whites, presumably for immunogenetic reasons.

Chinese and Japanese seldom develop chronic lymphocytic leukemia in their homelands or upon immigration to the United States. Again, the explanation appears to be genetic resistance to this form of cancer. The same is true of prostatic cancer. Among a substantial portion of the Japanese population, pineal tumors are about 12 times more common than they are elsewhere in the world. The excess seems to persist among Japanese who have migrated to Hawaii.

About 14% of North African children who die of neoplasia have skin cancer due to xeroderma pigmentosum. In this genetic disorder, inability to repair DNA damage from exposure to ultraviolet light apparently accounts for the tremendous increase in the frequency of skin cancer.

INBREEDING

Cousin marriage increases the chance for the pairing of autosomal recessive genes detrimental to health. Diseases associated with a high risk of cancer that are transmitted as autosomal recessive traits include ataxia-telangiectasia, xeroderma pigmentosum, Bloom's syndrome, and Fanconi's anemia. In theory, one might study the frequency of cousin marriage among the parents of persons affected with a specific neoplasm to determine the influence of autosomal recessive inheritance. In Japan, where about 5% of marriages involve first cousins, such studies could be made, looking for a frequency of consanguinity significantly greater than 5%.

TWINS

No excess for concordance of cancer in identical versus fraternal twins has yet been found in a study of about 15,000 pairs of twins who served in the military during World War II (Hrubec and Neel, 1982). The only data that suggest a carcinogenic effect due to monozygosity are from individual case reports.

A diminishing concordance with age at diagnosis of leukemia in young identical twins has been reported. If one member of the pair develops leukemia before one year of age, the other twin is virtually certain to develop the neoplasm. The frequency of leukemia in the second twin diminishes progressively thereafter and disappears at about six years of age. The explanation is not in the genetic identity of the twins, but in the circulation they share in utero. Through this circulation in common, leukemia cells are transplanted, as shown by chromosome markers present in both members of an identical pair with leukemia (Chaganti *et al.,* 1979).

SINGLE GENE DISORDERS

Retinoblastoma

In the 1950s, retinoblastoma was thought to be entirely due to the action of an autosomal dominant gene because patients with the disease, usually curable, lived to have their own children, some of whom were affected. In the late 1960s, case studies revealed that only about 40% of retinoblastoma was familial. In 1971, Knudson, by study of his own series and those in the literature, formulated a hypothesis based on the observation that hereditary retinoblastoma was usually multifocal (bilateral), and on the average occurred earlier in life than the sporadic form of the disease, which is unilateral. The differences in age at diagnosis when shown graphically and studied mathematically gave rise to the hypothesis that two steps were involved. In hereditary retinoblastoma, the first step is prezygotic and affects all cells in the body. The second step is postzygotic. The chance that a cell will sustain both steps is large — 100,000 times greater than in the nonhereditary form of the disease, in which both steps are thought to be postzygotic and would rarely affect the same cell by chance

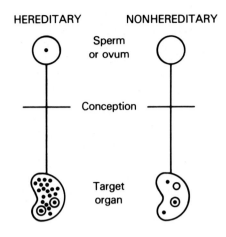

- • First mutation (pre- or post conception)
- ○ Second mutation (postconception only)

Figure 3–20. Knudson's hypothesis and Wilms' tumor. In the hereditary form (left) the first hit is a dominant germ-cell mutation. All derivative somatic (body) cells have this mutation. Those in the kidney undergo neoplastic transformation when a second, postconception hit occurs. In the nonhereditary form of Wilms' tumor (right) both hits occur after conception. These hits are rare and very unlikely to occur in the same cell. Modified from Li, F. P.: Cancers in children. In Schottenfeld, D., and Fraumeni, J. F., Jr. (eds.): *Cancer Epidemiology and Prevention.* W. B. Saunders Co., Philadelphia, 1982.

(Knudson, 1971). Figure 3-20 illustrates this hypothesis.

As cytogenetic techniques improved, a syndrome was delineated in which retinoblastoma, usually bilateral but not familial, occurred with mental retardation and other congenital disorders. The cytogenetic abnormality was a deleted part of the long arm of a D chromosome, later identified as chromosome 13. We now know that the site involved when retinoblastoma occurs is 13q14. A family in which the deletion was passed from generation to generation through 16 members, some of whom had balanced translocations without retinoblastoma, has been described (Strong *et al.,* 1981). The findings rule out the possibility that a chromosomal rearrangement or unmasking of retinoblastoma gene was responsible for development of retinoblastoma in this family. The deletion seems to function as though a dominant mutation had occurred.

In the course of heritable retinoblastoma, the gene action apparently affects retinocytes wherever they are: In the eye, the pineal body, or ectopically, in the cheek (Bader *et al.,* 1982). The pineal body is usually affected after bilateral retinoblastoma has occurred. Because the pineal in lower animals has been called "the third eye," involvement of both eyes and the pineal has been referred to as "trilateral retinoblastoma."

There may be multiple alleles for retinoblastoma, some of which are pleiotropic; that is, they induce more than one form of cancer, osteosarcoma in particular. Most of the osteosarcomas described to date have occurred in the lower femur of children with bilateral retinoblastoma. In several families, hereditary retinoblastoma has occurred in some children and osteosarcoma in another member of the family. The same tumors that occur as double primaries, therefore, may be dispersed as individual tumors among several members of the family (reviewed by Strong, 1977a).

The person with heritable retinoblastoma may be unusually susceptible to the carcinogenic effects of radiotherapy for the eye tumor: (periorbital) second primary tumors occur after a shorter latency period and more frequently than in persons given radiotherapy for nonhereditary cancers (Strong, 1977b). A defect in repair of radiogenic damage to DNA may be involved (Weichselbaum and Little, 1980).

This array of observations has implications for other cancers, and illustrates that from rarities in human oncology come generalizations concerning etiology and pathogenesis.

Nephroblastoma

The earlier age at diagnosis for familial or multifocal nephroblastoma versus sporadic nephroblastoma is consistent with Knudson's hypothesis (Knudson and Strong, 1972a). The tumor occurs excessively in children with congenital absence of the iris of the eye (aniridia) or hemihypertrophy or genitourinary anomalies (Miller *et al.,* 1964). Improvement in cytogenetic techniques led to the identification of a chromosomal deletion in 11p13 in the syndrome (Francke *et al.,* 1979). The deletion has been found in children with sporadic aniridia who did not develop nephroblastoma. Notable among them is a pair of identical twins, only one of whom developed nephroblastoma, despite their genetic identity, the same chromosomal deletion, and identical malformations (Riccardi *et al.,* 1980). Even in this most genetic of situations, some other influence was still necessary for tumor development.

The heritability of nephroblastoma is less well defined than that of retinoblastoma. Now that children with nephroblastoma are curable, the lineal transmissibility of the tumor is being evaluated. Second primaries have been observed, with hepatoblastoma for example, but not to the extent that has been reported for retinoblastoma. The hemihypertrophy-nephroblastoma syndrome, which is not due to deletion involving 11p13, has been seen distributed over members of a family: A woman with the malformation had three children who developed nephroblastoma and a fourth who had a double collecting system of the left kidney (Meadows *et al.,* 1974). Children with familial or multifocal nephroblastoma are not known to be unusually susceptible to the carcinogenic effects of radiotherapy.

Neuroblastoma

Knudson's hypothesis seems to apply also to neuroblastoma (Knudson and Strong, 1972b). An excessive occurrence with congenital malformations, however, has not been demonstrated (Miller *et al.,* 1968). No constitutional chromosomal anomaly has been linked to neuroblastoma. The frequency of second primaries is not remarkable, and radiosensitivity of the host has not been observed.

The peculiarities in neuroblastoma occurrence relate to its spontaneous disappearance, especially in type IV S (widely disseminated soon after birth, but not in the bone marrow), and the disappearance of *in situ* neuroblastoma by three months of age (Ikeda *et al.,* 1981). Regression or differentiation to normal tissue may explain the peculiar near absence of the neoplasm in Central Africa (Miller, 1977).

Cancer of the Colon

From 12 to 26% of colon cancer is familial, with or without adenomatous polyps. Persons with familial polyposis over 40 years of age have a very high risk, almost 100% of developing neoplastic transformation (Anderson, 1982). Polyposis occurs with other tumors, particularly in the syndromes of Gardner, Turcot, Peutz-Jeghers, and Cowden, but is especially prone to malignancy only in Gardner's syndrome. All these disorders are transmitted as autosomal dominant traits.

Tetraploidy occurs in fibroblasts in Gardner's syndrome (Danes, 1981), but other consistent chromosomal anomalies have not been reported. Presumably the inherent predisposition to colon cancer is brought out by environmental (dietary) exposures.

Breast Cancer

Cancer of the breast in women is now known to be genetically influenced in certain families. As shown in Table 3-21, the risk increases with the number of female relatives previously affected, the more so if they had bilateral disease early in life (Anderson, 1977). Genetic linkage studies of familial breast cancer have indicated a locus for a breast cancer gene linked to that for glutamate-pyruvate transaminase (King et al., 1980).

Leukemia

Leukemia seldom aggregates in families except in certain autosomal recessive chromosomal instability syndromes; for example, Fanconi's anemia (acute monomyelogenous leukemia) and ataxia-telangiectasia (acute lymphocytic leukemia). Leukemia also occurs excessively in Down's syndrome and Bloom's syndrome and in persons exposed to ionizing radiation or benzene, (see review by Miller, 1976), or therapeutically to alkylating agents. A feature in common is chromosomal abnormality, either inborn or acquired. These special circumstances anticipated the finding of chromosomal anomalies generally in leuke-

mia. With improvement in cytogenetic techniques (prophase banding), all cases in a series with acute myelogeneous leukemia were found to have chromosomal anomalies, (Yunis et al., 1981), and at times in acute lymphocytic leukemia (in which the chromosomes are less easily visualized) (Rowley, 1981). In leukemia at large, genetics plays a part in somatic rather than in germ cells.

Lymphoma

Lymphoma occurs excessively in persons with single gene disorders characterized by immunodeficiency, for example, ataxia-telangiectasia (autosomal recessive) and Wiskott-Aldrich syndrome (X-linked recessive). Of particular importance in this category is the X-linked lymphoproliferative syndrome with increased susceptibility to the effects of Epstein-Barr virus (EBV) on B-cell lymphocytes (Purtilo, 1981). In this disorder, host susceptibility and a virus interact in the induction of lymphoproliferative diseases—all of which are disorders of B-cell lymphocytes. Lymphoma also occurs excessively in patients who are heavily immunosuppressed for renal transplantation (Hoover, 1977), and in those patients for whom African lymphoma is induced by EBV (in conjunction with malaria). Translocations involving chromosomes 8 and/or 14 have been described in African lymphoma and other lymphomas (by Rowley, 1981), so immunosuppression, specific cytogenetic abnormalities, and a carcinogen play roles in the genesis of lymphoma.

Table 3-21. Risk of Breast Cancer in Women in Relation to Their Family History

RELATIVES WITH BREAST CANCER	BILATERAL?	POSTMENOPAUSAL AT DIAGNOSIS?	PROBABILITY OF BREAST CANCER	
			BEFORE 50 YEARS	LIFETIME
	One or both	Neither	0.11	0.51
		One	0.11	0.23
		Both	<0.001	0.28
	Neither	Neither	0.02	0.33
		One or both	<0.01	0.13
	One or both	Neither	0.04	0.50
		One or both	<0.001	0.11
	Neither	Neither	0.02	0.20
		One or both	<0.01	0.07
None*			<0.001	0.07

* None, but at least 2 other relatives with cancer not of the breast
Adapted from Petrakis, N. L.; Ernstner, V. L.; King, M.-C.: Breast. In Shottenfeld, D., and Fraumeni, J. F., Jr. (eds.) *Cancer Epidemiology and Prevention.* W. B. Saunders Company, Philadelphia, 1982.

Skin Cancer and DNA Repair

The dysplastic nevus syndrome (DNS) was first delineated by W. H. Clark, Jr. in 1976 and described in the literature by Reimer et al., (1978). The skin lesion is a clinically distinguishable precursor of familial or sporadic melanoma. DNS is transmitted as an autosomal dominant trait and has been found or its presence inferred in a series of heavily immunosuppressed renal-transplant patients who developed melanoma (Greene et al., 1981). Genetically determined light skin color predisposes people to skin cancer from sunlight, as previously noted.

The basal cell nevus syndrome, an autosomal dominant disorder of skin, bone, and brain, leads to basal cell carcinoma early in life. Medulloblastoma may occur before other evidence of the syndrome becomes apparent (Combined Clinical Staff Conference, 1966).

The marked sensitivity of the skin to cancer from ultraviolet light in xeroderma pigmentosum, an autosomal recessive disease, is due to defective repair of DNA (Kraemer, 1977). A DNA repair defect is also thought to exist for damage from gamma radiation in the autosomal recessive disorder, ataxia-telangiectasia (AT) (Bridges and Harnden, 1982). Lymphoma, the neoplasm most frequently observed in AT, is not induced by ionizing radiation and is probably related to the immunodeficiency characteristic of the syndrome (Kraemer, 1977). The relevance of DNA repair defects to cancer and aging remains to be determined.

Ovary

Genetic disorders in which ovarian tumors, usually benign, occur excessively include two polyposis syndromes (Gardner's and Peutz-Jeghers), the basal cell nevus syndrome, the Stein-Leventhal syndrome, and ataxia-telangiectasia (Schimke, 1978).

Teratomas

Apparently, autosomal dominant transmission of sacrococcygeal teratomas occurs in some families and is associated with pelvic anomalies (reviewed by Gilman, 1983). No other teratomas suggest heritable transmission. Benign teratomas of the ovary (dermoid cysts), however, are derived from a single germ cell after the first meiotic division, as revealed by studies of chromosome markers and enzyme variants (Linder et al., 1975b). Similar studies of extragonadal teratomas suggested that these tumors develop from a mitotic cell — either a somatic cell or a misplaced germ cell that failed to undergo meiosis and proceeded directly to mitosis (Linder et al., 1975a).

In experimental studies, teratocarcinomas have yielded spectacular findings. When transplanted subcutaneously in mice, they cause teratocarcinomas at the site of injection. Microinjection of teratocarcinoma cells into a blastocyst fertilizes it, and the mouse so conceived has characteristics of both parents. The teratocarcinoma is totipotent; therefore, its effect is the same as that of a sperm (reviewed by Mintz and Fleischmann, 1981). As previously noted by others, in effect, the father of the mouse was a cancer cell.

The Multiple Endocrine Neoplasias (MEN)

In the MEN type-I syndrome, tumors affect the pituitary, pancreas, and parathyroids, among other endocrine organs. In MEN type-II, pheochromocytoma occurs in patients with medullary carcinoma of the thyroid. Both syndromes are transmitted as autosomal dominant traits, as MEN type-III also seems to be. The findings are as in MEN type II, but with multiple small neuromas of the mucosa of the eye, gastrointestinal tract, and mouth, leading to the designation of "blubbery lip syndrome" (Schimke, 1976). These and other endocrine tumors derived from the neural crest fall into the APUD series, so named because they are a histochemical entity the characteristics of which include amine precursor uptake and decarboxylation (Tischler et al., 1977). Tumors of cells with this property are called APUDomas, a concept useful for probing the explanation for neoplasia in widely dispersed organs.

Neurofibromatosis (NF)

The clinical findings in NF derive from the neural crest, but not the APUD system. NF, an autosomal dominant trait, is characterized by multiple neurofibromas and café-au-lait spots of the skin. Tumors in this disease include neurofibrosarcomas, gliomas—especially optic, pheochromocytoma, and meningiomas (Hope and Mulvihill, 1981). The excessive occurrence of nonlymphocytic leukemia, rhabdomyosarcoma, and Wilms' tumor in children with NF was unexpected because the cells from which these tumors originate are not known to be derived from the neural crest. An estimated 1% of childhood cancer is associated with NF (Bader *et al.*, 1980).

Other Hamartomatous Syndromes

NF, the basal cell nevus syndrome, and the polyposis syndromes are hamartomatous disorders; that is, they have developmental benign tumors (single- or multiple-tissue elements usually in a normal anatomic location) (Schimke, 1978). The other two major disorders in this group are tuberous sclerosis and von Hippel-Lindau syndrome. Both are autosomal dominant disorders. In tuberous sclerosis, the tumors may develop in the skin, retina, kidneys, heart (rhabdomyoma), and the central nervous system and may undergo neoplastic degeneration. In von Hippel-Lindau disease, hemangioblastomas occur in the retina and central nervous system, especially in the cerebellum. These tumors, though cancerous, rarely metastasize (Vinken and Bruyn, 1972).

Genetic Repertory of Human Disease

It is impossible to cover in this narrative the 200 single-gene traits with benign or cancerous neoplasia as a feature, as culled from 1142 proven single-gene traits (Mulvihill, 1977). Individually and in combination they offer opportunities for new insights into the carcinogenic process.

FAMILY STUDIES

Cancer aggregates in a nonrandom fashion in certain families. The cancers may be of the same type or of dissimilar types and may be associated with diseases other than cancer. Population-based studies are a very slow and difficult method of evaluating family aggregation (Weiss *et al.*, 1980). Death certificates for all children in the United States from 1960 to 1967 revealed that when a child died of brain cancer the probability that a sibling would also die of brain cancer was 18 times the national rate (Miller, 1971). A similar increase was found for bone or soft tissue cancer in siblings of children who died of brain cancer. It re-

quired data from the entire nation to show these sibship aggregates.

The experienced oncologist can often judge whether or not family aggregation is likely to be due to chance. Two families in which six members had respiratory cancer, and in each a young member had a probable radiogenic cancer, are not likely to have had this aggregation by chance (Goffman *et al.*, 1982).

Cancers that cluster in families for reasons other than chance need not be of the same type, as exemplified by the Li-Fraumeni syndrome (Li and Fraumeni, 1969). Typically, more than one child in a family has soft-tissue sarcoma and relatives have a variety of cancers, especially of the breast in young women. In one family, sisters of the boys with sarcoma were thought to be at high risk. Examination revealed breast cancer in both (Li and Fraumeni, 1975). Recognition of family cancer syndromes thus permits early detection that may be life saving. Such observations also provide an opportunity to develop new understanding of carcinogenesis through laboratory research. The basis for the Li-Fraumeni syndrome is still unknown, but in other family cancer clusters, it has been revealed dramatically through laboratory research.

In Boston, for example, a medical student called attention to a family cluster of renal cell carcinomas. When the pedigree was complete, it showed seven members with the tumor. X-ray examination of the descendants of affected persons revealed three more with the tumor, not yet symptomatic. Cytogenetic study showed that members with the neoplasm had a constitutional translocation from chromosome 3 to 8. This abnormality also occurred in several members too young to have developed the tumor. Their probability of developing renal cell carcinoma is very high and they are being closely watched to allow early detection (Cohen *et al.*, 1979). The family members have no other abnormality linked to the translocation, so the high risk of renal cell carcinoma appears to be due to the equivalent of a point mutation.

CYTOGENETICS

From the foregoing, it is clear that chromosomal abnormalities are an important feature in a variety of cancers, some of which are associated with single-gene disorders. In other instances, inborn chromosomal anomalies (*i.e.,* not limited to a single gene) predispose to certain cancers (see Table 3-22). Such anomalies are features of certain syndromes that predispose to leukemia, nephroblastoma, and retinoblastoma, among other tumors. The chromosomal anomaly when transmitted from one generation to another can cause a cancer-malformation syndrome in one child and different malformations without cancer in a sibling. Prometaphase banding has identified such cases.

Retinoblastoma due to the 13q14 deletion (monosomy) was found in a boy, for example, whose sister had other malformations due to trisomy of the same portion of chromosome 13 that was deleted in her brother (Riccardi *et al.,* 1979). This finding illustrates the value of the family history with regard to cancer as well as to other diseases. Study of other diseases may open new avenues to our understanding of the biology of cancer.

Gonadoblastoma is peculiar in that it requires not only a dysgenetic ovary for its development, but at least a portion of a Y chromosome in the dysgenetic tissue (Schellhas, 1974).

CLONAL EVOLUTION

One laboratory procedure seems to indicate that most tumors studied to date are monoclonal in origin. The test is applied to specimens from persons with mosaicism (two or more genetically distinct cell types in each so-

Table 3-22. Chromosomal Anomalies Associated with Cancer

CHROMOSOME NUMBER	BLOOD/LYMPH DISEASES*†	OTHER CANCER†	OF SPECIAL INTEREST
1	+	+	
2			
3	+	+	3,8 translocation and renal cell carcinoma
4			
5	+		
6	+	+	
7	+		
8	+	+	See chromosome 3; 8,14 translocation and Burkitt's lymphoma
9	+		9,22 translocation and CLL
10			
11	+	+	11p- and Wilms' tumor-aniridia syndrome
12	+		
13		+	13q- and retinoblastoma-malformation syndrome
14	+	+	See chromosome 8; 14,14 translocation, and Burkitt's lymphoma
15			
16			
17	+		
18			
19			
20	+		
21	+		Trisomy 21 and Down's syndrome (high risk of leukemia)
22	+	+	See chromosome 9; monosomy and meningioma
X		+	XXY (Klinefelter's) syndrome and mediastinal teratoma
Y		+	Absent in gonadoblastoma associated with gonadal dysgenesis

* Adapted from Mitelman, F., and Levan, G.: Clustering of aberrations to specific chromosomes in human neoplasms. IV. A survey of 1871 cases. *Hereditas,* 95: 79–139, 1981.
† Adapted from Mulvihill, J. J., and Robinette, S. M.: Neoplasia of man (*Homo sapiens*). In O'Brien, S. J. (ed.): *Genetic Maps, Vol 2.* National Cancer Institute, Frederick, Maryland, 1982.

matic cell). The X-linked glucose-6-phosphate dehydrogenase (G-6-PD) locus is a useful marker in this respect. About one out of three black women in the United States is heterozygous for the usual G-6-PD gene (type A) and a variant allele (type B). They have two distinguishable populations of cells, whereas other people have only one. The two populations arise because of the natural inactivation of one X chromosome (the Lyon hypothesis) in each body cell of females. Some of the cells will be of type A and others of type B, when heterozygosity occurs. The enzymes, type A or type B, are readily measured by electrophoresis. Normal tissue from these women contains both enzymes. If a tumor is monoclonal in origin it will contain only one of the enzymes. The exceptions to unicellular origin are certain hereditary tumors: neuromas in neurofibromatosis and trichoepitheliomas. Burkitt's lymphoma is notable because it is monoclonal when first diagnosed and on early recurrence, but a clone from the other G-6-PD cell-type may give rise to late recurrences (Fialkow, 1977). Classifying tumors as to their unicellular or multicellular origin provides new insight into the carcinogenic process.

IN PERSPECTIVE

Genetic effects may involve germ cells or somatic cells. Study of germ cell mutations may provide new understanding of cancer biology that may extend from rarities to the population at large; for example, from leukemia in Down's syndrome to leukemia in the general population. Study of somatic cell mutations will probably clarify the pathogenesis of a substantial proportion of all cancers. An interaction of clinical, epidemiologic, and laboratory research will provide the most rapid progress in our knowledge and understanding. The results should lead to improved prevention, detection, and therapy.

REFERENCES

Anderson, D. E.: Breast cancer in families. *Cancer*, **40**:1855–1860, 1977.

Anderson, D. E.: Familial predisposition. In Schottenfeld, D., and Fraumeni, J. F., Jr. (eds.): *Cancer Epidemiology and Prevention.* W. B. Saunders Company, Philadelphia, 1982.

Bader, J. L.; Meadows, A. T.; Lemerle, J.; Voute, P. A.; Morris-Jones, P.; Newton, W. A.; Banfi, A.; and Baum, E. S.: Neurofibromatosis (NF) and other genetic defects associated with childhood cancer (abstr). *Proc. Am. Sci. Hum. Genet.*, **295**:97A, 1980.

Bader, J. L.; Meadows, A. T.; Zimmerman, L. E.; Rorke, L. B.; Voute, P. A.; Champion, L. A.; and Miller, R. W.: Bilateral retinoblastoma with ectopic intracranial retinoblastoma: trilateral retinoblastoma. *Cancer Genet. Cytogenet.*, **5**:203–213, 1982.

Bridges, B. A., and Harnden, D. G. (eds): *Ataxia-Telangiectasia—A Cellular and Molecular Link between Cancer, Neuropathology and Immune Deficiency.* John Wiley & Sons, Ltd., Sussex, England, 1982.

Chaganti, R. S. K.; Miller, D. R.; Meyers, P. A.; and German, J.: Cytogenetic evidence of the intrauterine origin of acute leukemia in monozygotic twins. *N. Engl. J. Med.*, **300**:1032–1034, 1979.

Cohen, A. J.; Li, F. P.; Berg, S.; Marchetto, D. J.; Tsai, S.; Jacobs, S. C.; and Brown, R. S.: Hereditary renal-cell carcinoma associated with a chromosomal translocation. *N. Engl. J. Med.*, **301**:592–595, 1979.

Combined Clinical Staff Conference, NIH: Basal cell nevus syndrome. *Ann. Intern. Med.*, **64**:403–421, 1966.

Danes, B. S.: Occurrence of in vitro tetraploidy in the heritable colon cancer syndrome. *Cancer,* **48**:1596–1601, 1981.

Fialkow, P. J.: Clonal origin and stem cell evolution of human tumors. In Mulvihill, J. J.; Miller, R. W.; and Fraumeni, J. F., Jr. (eds): *Genetics of Human Cancer.* Raven Press, New York, 1977.

Francke, U.; Holmes, L. B.; Atkins, L.; and Riccardi, V. M.: Aniridia-Wilms tumor association: Evidence for specific deletion of 11p13. *Cytogenet. Cell Genet.*, **24**:185–192, 1979.

Gilman, P. A.: Epidemiology of human teratomas. In Damjanov, I.; Knowles, B. B.; and Solter, D. (eds.): *The Biology of Human Teratomas.* Humana Press, Clifton, New Jersey, 1983.

Glass, A. G., and Fraumeni, J. F., Jr.: Epidemiology of bone cancer in children. *J.N.C.I.*, **44**:187–199, 1970.

Goffman, T. E.; Hassinger, D. D.; and Mulvihill, J. J.: Familial respiratory tract cancer. Opportunities for research and prevention. *J.A.M.A.*, **247**:1020–1023, 1982.

Greene, M. H.; Young, T. I.; and Clark, W. H. Jr.: Malignant melanoma in renal-transplant patients. *Lancet,* **1**:1196–1199, 1981.

Hoover, R.: Effects of drugs—immunosuppression. In Hiatt, H. H.; Watson, J. D.; and Winsten, J. A. (eds): *Origins of Human Cancer: Book A. Incidence of Cancer in Humans.* Cold Spring Harbor Conferences on Cell Proliferation, Vol 4. Cold Spring Harbor Laboratory, Cold Spring Harbor, New York, 1977.

Hope, D. G., and Mulvihill, J. J.: Malignancy in neurofibromatosis. In Riccardi, V. M., and Mulvihill, J. J. (eds.): *Neurofibromatosis (von Recklinghausen Disease): Genetics, Cell Biology, and Biochemistry,* Vol 29. Raven Press, New York, 1981.

Hrubec, Z., and Neel, J. V.: Contribution of familial factors to the occurrence of cancer (before old age) in twin veterans. *Am. J. Hum. Genet.*, **34**:658–671, 1982.

Ikeda, Y.; Lister, J.; Bouton, J. M.; and Buyukpamukcu, M.: Congenital neuroblastoma, neuroblastoma in situ, and the normal fetal development of the adrenal. *J. Pediatr. Surg.*, **16**(Suppl):636–644, 1981.

King, M.-C.; Go, R. C. P.; Elston, R. C.; Lynch, H. T.; and Petrakis, N. L.: Allele increasing susceptibility to human breast cancer may be linked to the glutamate-pyruvate transaminase locus. *Science,* **208**:406–408, 1980.

Knudson, A. G., Jr.: Mutation and cancer. Statistical study of retinoblastoma. *Proc. Natl. Acad. Sci. USA,* **68:**820–823, 1971.

Knudson, A. G., Jr., and Strong, L. C.: Mutation and cancer: A model for Wilms' tumor of the kidney. *J.N.C.I.,* **48:**313–324, 1972a.

Knudson, A. G., Jr., and Strong, L. C.: Mutation and cancer: Neuroblastoma and pheochromocytoma. *Am. J. Hum. Genet.,* **24:**514–532, 1972b.

Kraemer, K. H.: Progressive degenerative diseases associated with defective DNA repair: Xeroderma pigmentosum and ataxia telangiectasia. In Nichols, W. W., and Murphy, D. G. (eds.): *DNA Repair Processes: Cellular Senescence and Somatic Cell Genetics.* Symposia Specialists, Miami, Florida, 1977.

Li, F. P.: Cancers in children. In Schottenfeld, D., and Fraumeni, J. F., Jr. (eds.): *Cancer Epidemiology and Prevention.* W. B. Saunders Company, Philadelphia, 1982.

Li, F. P., and Fraumeni, J. F., Jr.: Soft-tissue sarcomas, breast cancer, and other neoplasms: A familial syndrome? *Ann. Intern. Med.,* **71:**747–752, 1969.

Li, F. P., Fraumeni, J. F., Jr.: Letter: Familial breast cancer, soft-tissue sarcomas, and other neoplasms. *Ann. Intern. Med.,* **83:**833–834, 1975.

Linder, D.; Hecht, F.; McCaw, B. K.; and Campbell, J. R.: Origin of extragonadal teratomas and endodermal sinus tumours. *Nature,* **254:**597–598, 1975a.

Linder, D.; McCaw, B. K.; and Hecht, F.: Parthenogenic origin of benign ovarian teratomas. *N. Engl. J. Med.,* **292:**63–66, 1975b.

Meadows, A. T.; Lichtenfeld, J. L.; and Koop, C. E.: Wilms's tumor in three children of a woman with congenital hemihypertrophy. *N. Engl. J. Med.,* **291:**23–24, 1974.

Miller, R. W.: Deaths from childhood cancer in sibs. *N. Engl. J. Med.,* **279:**122–126, 1968.

Miller, R. W.: Deaths from childhood leukemia and solid tumors among twins and other sibs in the United States, 1960–67. *J.N.C.I.,* **46:**203–209, 1971.

Miller, R. W.: The feature in common among persons at high risk of leukemia. In Yuhas, J. M.; Tennant, R. W., and Regan, J. D. (eds): *Biology of Radiation Carcinogenesis.* Raven Press, New York, 1976.

Miller, R. W.: Ethnic differences in cancer occurrence: Genetic and environmental influences with particular reference to neuroblastoma. In Mulvihill, J. J.; Miller, R. W.; and Fraumeni, J. F.; Jr (eds): *Genetics of Human Cancer.* Raven Press, New York, 1977.

Miller, R. W.; Fraumeni, J. F., Jr.; and Hill, J. A.: Neuroblastoma: Epidemiologic approach to its origin. *Am. J. Dis. Child.,* **115:**253–261, 1968.

Miller, R. W.; Fraumeni, J. F., Jr.; and Manning, M. D.: Association of Wilms's tumor with aniridia, hemihypertrophy and other congenital malformations. *N. Engl. J. Med.,* **270:**922–927, 1964.

Mintz, B., and Fleischmann, R. A.: Teratocarcinoma and other neoplasms as developmental defects in gene expression. *Adv. Cancer Res.,* **34:**211–278, 1981.

Mitelman, F., and Levan, G.: Clustering of aberrations to specific chromosomes in human neoplasms. IV. A survey of 1871 cases. *Hereditas,* **95:**79–139, 1981.

Mulvihill, J. J.: Genetic repertory of human neoplasia. In Mulvihill, J. J.; Miller, R. W.; and Fraumeni, J. F., Jr. (eds.): *Genetics of Human Cancer.* Raven Press, New York, 1977.

Mulvihill, J. J., and Robinette, S. M.: Neoplasia of man *(Homo sapiens).* In O'Brien, S. J. (ed.): *Genetic Maps, Vol. 2.* National Cancer Institute, Frederick, Maryland, 1982.

Petrakis, N. L.; Ernstner, V. L.; King, M.-C.: Breast. In Schottenfeld, D., and Fraumeni, J. F., Jr. (eds.): *Cancer Epidemiology and Prevention.* W. B. Saunders Company, Philadelphia, 1982.

Purtilo, D. T.: Immune deficiency predisposing to Epstein-Barr virus-induced lymphoproliferative diseases: The X-linked lymphoproliferative syndrome as a model. *Adv. Cancer Res.,* **34:**279–312, 1981.

Reimer, R. R.; Clark, W. H., Jr.; Green, M. H.; Ainsworth, A. M.; and Fraumeni, J. R., Jr.: Precursor lesions in familial melanoma, a new genetic preneoplastic syndrome. *J.A.M.A.,* **239:**744–746, 1978.

Riccardi, V. M.; Hittner, H. M.; Francke, U.; Pippin, S.; Holmquist, G. P.; Kretzer, F. L.; and Ferrell, R.: Partial triplication and deletion of 13q: Study of a family presenting with bilateral retinoblastoma. *Clin. Genet.,* **15:**332–345, 1979.

Riccardi, V. M.; Hittner, H. M.; Franke, U.; Yunis, J. J.; Ledbetter, D.; and Borges, W.: The aniridia-Wilms tumor association: The critical role of the chromosome band 11p13. *Cell Genet. Cytogenet.,* **2:**131–137, 1980.

Rowley, J. D.: Nonrandom chromosome changes in human leukemia. In Arrighi, F. E.; Rao, P. N.; and Stubblefield, E. (eds.): *Genes, Chromosomes, and Neoplasia.* Raven Press, New York, 1981.

Schellhas, H. F.: Malignant potential of the dysgenetic gonad. Part I. *Obstet. Gynecol.,* **44:**298–309, 1974.

Schimke, R. N.: Multiple endocrine adenomatosis syndromes. *Adv. Intern. Med.,* **21:**249–265, 1976.

Schimke, R. N.: *Genetics and Cancer in Man.* Churchill Livingstone, Edinburgh, 1978.

Strong L. C.: Genetic considerations in pediatric oncology. In Sutow, W. W.; Vietti, T. J.; and Fernbach, D. J. (eds.): *Clinical Pediatric Oncology,* 2nd ed. The C. V. Mosby Company, St. Louis, 1977a.

Strong, L. C.: Theories of pathogenesis: Mutation and cancer. In Mulvihill, J. J.; Miller, R. W.; and Fraumeni, J. F., Jr. (eds.): *Genetics of Human Cancer.* Raven Press, New York, 1977b.

Strong, L. C.; Riccardi, V. M.; Ferrell, R. E.; and Sparkes, R. S.: Familial retinoblastoma and chromosome 13 deletion transmitted via an insertional translocation. *Science,* **213:**1501–1503, 1981.

Tischler, A. S.; Dichter, M. A.; Biales, B.; and Greene, L. A.: Neuroendocrine neoplasms and their cells of origin. *N. Engl. J. Med.,* **296:**919–925, 1977.

Vinken, P. J., and Bruyn, G. W. (eds.): *The Phakomatoses. Handbook of Clinical Neurology,* Vol 14. American Elsevier, New York, 1972.

Weichselbaum, R. R., and Little, J. B.: Familial retinoblastoma and ataxia telangiectasia: Human models for the study of DNA damage and repair. *Cancer,* **45:**775–779, 1980.

Weiss, K. M.; Chakraborty, R.; Schull, W. J.; Rossman, D. L.; and Norton, S. L.: The Laredo epidemiology project. *Banbury Report,* **4:**267–282, 1980.

Yunis, J. J.; Bloomfield, C. D.; and Ensrud, K.: All patients with acute nonlymphocytic leukemia may have a chromosomal defect. *N. Engl. J. Med.,* **305:**135–139, 1981.

4

Biology and Patterns of Metastases

ELLEN N. SPREMULLI, DANIEL DEXTER, and PAUL CALABRESI

The development of metastases is a major obstacle to the successful treatment of the patient with cancer. Few patients die from their primary neoplasm; but the discovery of even a single secondary deposit generally signals a more guarded prognosis. Frequently, this finding means that multiple metastases exist and that death is inevitable. Their occurrence and the sites in which they develop vary greatly. The clinical oncologist must have detailed knowledge of the patterns of metastases in order to: (1) Discuss realistically the prognosis with the patient and the family; (2) assess the possible need for adjuvant therapy after resection of the primary tumor; and (3) plan appropriately for the continuing care of the patient.

Joseph Claude Recormier (Wilder, 1956) first used the term metastasis to describe growth of secondary tumors not contiguous with the primary. The appearance of these remote colonies is the result of several steps that include detachment of cells from the primary tumor, infiltration of lymphatic or vascular systems, regional or systemic circulation, invasion of distant organs, and, finally, the development of secondary proliferations. The etiology, biology, consequences, and potential prevention of metastases have received increasing attention both in laboratory and clinical investigations.

THE CLINICAL BACKGROUND

Clinically relevant aspects of metastases include variability in the likelihood that a primary tumor will metastasize and an understanding of where and when the secondary tumors will appear. These factors are important for determining both prognosis and treatment strategy.

Variability in the Expression of Metastatic Potential

Virtually all cancers possess metastatic potential. They express this potential, however, with considerable variability. The probability that metastases will develop depends on several factors, including the site of the primary tumor, its histologic characteristics, and its size. The importance of the type of tumor is illustrated by data indicating a greater than 50% probability of distant metastases developing in patients with breast cancer whose primary tumors are greater than 3 cm in size (Fisher *et al.*, 1969). By contrast, basal-cell carcinomas may become locally extensive without metastases developing (Klein *et al.*, 1973). In general, a large tumor that is poorly differentiated histologically has a high propensity to metastasize, whereas small, well-differentiated tumors do not tend to metastasize. Section II of this book discusses specific neoplasms and should be consulted for a better understanding of the relationship between site, size, histologic grade, and the incidence of metastases.

Different neoplasms exhibit considerable temporal variations in the occurrence of metastases (Sugarbaker, 1979). In patients with malignant melanoma, the risk of rapid development of local and regional metastases is high, with 95% of such lesions appearing by 24 months. Distant metastases from melanoma, however, may be latent, and recurrences more than ten years after removal of the primary lesion are not rare. After local treatment of squamous cell carcinoma of the oropharynx,

Table 4-1. Growth Potential of Occult Lymph Node Metastasis

NEOPLASM	SURGICAL SPECIMEN % POSITIVE	EVOLUTION OF NODES IN OBSERVED PATIENTS	GROWTH POTENTIAL
Thyroid carcinoma	61%	<10%	<10
Breast carcinoma	40%	15%	37.5
Malignant melanoma	19.7%	24.2%	~100
Squamous cell carcinoma of the tongue	23-46%	27-50%	~100

Adapted from Sugarbaker, E. V.: Cancer Metastasis: A product of tumor host interactions. *Curr. Probl. Cancer,* **3**:1-59, 1979.

more than 95% of relapses develop within three years. For patients with carcinoma of the breast, 40% of recurrences are detected within the first 18 months after mastectomy; in the remainder, metastases may be latent and recurrence, even after ten years, is not unusual.

Evidence suggests that, at least for lymph node metastases, the presence of microscopic foci of tumor may not always correlate with the development of macroscopic disease (Sugarbaker, 1979) (see Table 4-1). In patients with melanoma or squamous-cell carcinoma of the tongue, comparison of the frequency of microscopic lymph node metastases in surgical node dissection specimens with the evolution of grossly palpable nodes in observed patients indicates that these microscopic foci almost uniformly become macroscopic tumors. On the other hand, micrometastases from carcinoma of the breast become grossly palpable in the lymph nodes of less than 50% of patients, and less than 10% of nodes microscopically involved with papillary carcinoma of the thyroid become clinically palpable (Sugarbaker, 1979).

Location of Secondary Sites

Two basic hypotheses have been proposed to explain patterns of hematogenous metastases: The direct and the cascade. The direct hypothesis postulates that dissemination of neoplastic cells from a given primary site is a one-step process, in which distant metastases are the result of direct hematogenous seeding from the primary tumor. The cascade hypothesis, on the other hand, favors a multi-step process. A careful analysis of the pattern of metastases in 4728 autopsies suggests that: (1) A multi-step or cascade process is involved in metastases, and (2) the cascade involves one or more intermediate sites, usually the lung or the liver (see Figures 4-1A and 4-1B) (Bross *et al.,* 1975). Accordingly, hematogenous metas-

tases generally first develop in specific sites, which are dependent on the location of the primary tumor. These metastases may then act as a source of further metastases.

Although the sites of metastases vary widely, typical patterns of spread for various primary neoplasms have been documented (Sugarbaker, 1981). The predominant sites of metastases for some common neoplasms are summarized here.

Patients with lung cancer generally have metastases at the time of diagnosis, which may involve nearly every organ system of the body. At *post mortem* examination, the frequency of extrathoracic metastases is 25 to 54% for epidermoid carcinoma, 50 to 82% for adenocarcinoma, 48 to 86% for large-cell carcinoma, and 74 to 96% for small-cell carcinoma. For epidermoid carcinoma and adenocarcinoma, the most common sites of metastases are the hilar and mediastinal lymph nodes, pleura, chest wall, opposite lung, pericardium, and liver. For small cell carcinoma, the most frequently involved organs are the hilar and mediastinal lymph nodes, pleura, opposite lung, adrenals, bone, kidney, and central nervous system (Esrael and Chahanion, 1976).

The presence of positive axillary lymph nodes in patients with breast cancer serves as a "marker" for hematogenous spread. Approximately 67% of patients who have one to three positive lymph nodes at mastectomy will exhibit distant metastases within 10 years, whereas this risk increases to 87% for patients who have four or more nodes involved (Hellman *et al.,* 1982). Common distant sites of metastases for patients with cancer of the breast are lung, liver, bone, adrenal glands, skin, and ovary (Brennan, 1973).

Gastric cancer spreads via the lymphatics to involve surrounding structures. When vascular invasion occurs, the resultant metastases commonly involve the liver, with later development of pulmonary and osseous metastases

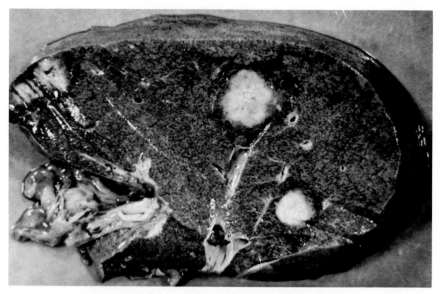

Figure 4–1A. Metastases to the liver from carcinoma of the breast.

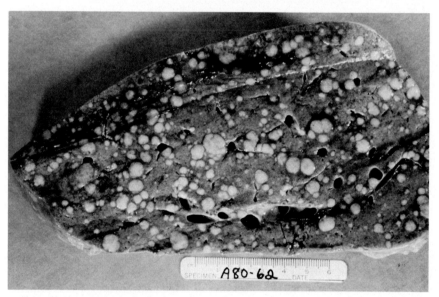

Figure 4–1B. Liver with multiple metastases from carcinoma of the colon.

(Glassman, 1970). One third of patients with carcinoma of the large bowel have clinical evidence of hematogenous spread at the time of diagnosis. Patients whose tumors recur after resection of the primary usually have regional, hepatic, or pulmonary disease (Warren, 1933; Warwick, 1928).

Ovarian cancer most commonly disseminates intraperitoneally; hematogenous metastases occur later in the disease (Feldman and Knapp, 1974). Uterine cervical cancer usually spreads locally; liver, lung, bone, and supraclavicular node involvement may occur later (Badib et al., 1968; Carlson et al., 1967).

Metastatic involvement of bones occurs in approximately 80% of patients with prostatic carcinoma. Osteoblastic, rather than osteolytic, lesions predominate (Prout, 1973). Because many of the neoplastic cells circulate via the paravertebral venous plexus, bones of the pelvis and lumbosacral spine are most frequently affected (Batson, 1957).

Unusual patterns of metastases may provide diagnostic or biologic clues to the site of the primary neoplasm. In a review of 19,675 cases, 222 patients demonstrated relatively rare sites of involvement (Brady *et al.,* 1977). In 30 patients, metastases occurred to the eye from primary sites that included breast, lung, esophagus, uterine cervix, and bladder. In addition, melanoma, cylindroma, osteosarcoma, and fibrosarcoma also metastasized to the eye. Seventeen patients whose primary tumors originated in the lung, breast, esophagus, tonsil, prostate, ovary, or uterus developed metastatic lesions of the kidneys. Of eight patients who had metastases to the heart, six had a primary tumor of the lung (see Figure 4–2), one of the kidney, and one had a leiomyosarcoma. Nineteen women developed metastases to the lower genitourinary tract; the common primaries were in the breast, ovary, lung, and uterus. Nine men whose carcinomas originated in the urinary bladder, prostate, kidney, rectum, or lung had metastases to the lower urinary tract with the penis the most common structure involved. Kaposi's sarcoma and melanoma were also responsible for metastases to this site. Sixteen patients exhibited metastases to the upper gastrointestinal tract; their primary carcinomas originated in the lung, breast, ovary, and uterine cervix. Melanoma may also metastasize to the small bowel, often with a characteristic "bullseye" pattern (Luce *et al.,* 1973).

TUMOR CELL HETEROGENEITY AND METASTASES

Etiology of Intraneoplastic Diversity

The cells found within a single tumor display considerable variability. This heterogeneity can result in notable differences between a primary tumor and its metastases. The phenomenon of intraneoplastic diversity has important clinical implications, especially with respect to disseminated cancer.

Cancer cells are usually of monoclonal origin, although polyclonal tumors may occur (Fialkow, 1976). The concept of tumor-cell progression, initially defined by Foulds (1954) and later examined mechanistically by Nowell (1976), provides an explanation for how a cell population that was monoclonal in origin becomes heterogenous. Progression is defined as the tumor's stepwise evolution of increasingly autonomous and neoplastic characteristics. Developed originally from morphological examination of heterogeneous murine mammary carcinomas, Fould's description of the progression of these tumors formed the bases of subsequent theories on the etiology of intraneoplastic diversity (Foulds, 1954, 1956a,b,c,d).

Cancer may evolve as a sequential series of heritable changes (Nowell, 1976). Evidence to support this concept comes from the observation that human neoplasms sometimes appear to change their behavior during their clinical courses. A tumor that originally appears relatively benign may progress to a much more aggressive neoplasm during a period of months or years. This does not necessarily involve either an increase in the size or extent of the tumor, nor an alteration in the patient's immune system, but rather represents a change in the intrinsic biologic properties of the neoplastic cells (Prehn, 1976). Nowell (1976), in an attempt to explain this progression on a molecular level, developed the theory that, although cancers are indeed unicellular in origin, intraneoplastic diversity occurs because the neoplastic cell is genetically unstable.

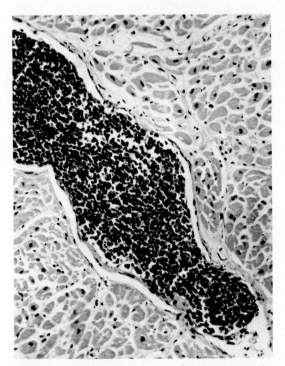

Figure 4–2.   Small cell carcinoma of the lung metastatic to the myocardium. The tumor lies lodged in a distended vessel.

Thus, the inherent genetic instability of the neoplastic cell allows mutant cell populations to arise that differ in many characteristics, including their antigenicity, growth rates, sensitivity to various treatment modalities, and metastatic potential. Numerous factors, including the growth rate and antigenicity of the various subpopulations, then determine their proportions in the evolving tumor. Thus, tumor cell heterogeneity is a dynamic process that may change during the lifetime of the tumor.

If the general concept of genetic instability is correct, then artificially increasing the mutation rate should result in the appearance of more "progressed" cells, that is, those with a higher metastatic potential. The mutation rate of UV2237 sarcoma cells was increased by exposing them to ultraviolet radiation (Fisher and Cifone, 1981). Animals bearing tumors produced by the inoculation of ultraviolet-treated sarcoma cells demonstrated more metastases than animals inoculated with untreated sarcoma cells. In addition, when Cifone and Fidler (1981) compared the spontaneous mutation frequencies of cells obtained from neoplastic tumors with high metastatic potential to cells derived from tumors with low metastatic potential, they found that mutations at the genetic loci for 6-thioguanine and oubain resistance occurred more often in the cells from tumors with high metastatic potential. Their data support Nowell's (1976) hypothesis that neoplastic cells that behave aggressively are more genetically unstable than are the more "benign" cells in the tumor.

Phenotypic Expression of Intratumor Heterogeneity

Clinical problems may arise because tumors have intraneoplastic variations in several phenotypic characteristics (Abeloff et al., 1979; Dunn, 1959; Sugarbaker, 1979). Therapy may selectively reduce one subpopulation of cells, allowing more resistant subpopulations to emerge. This perturbation of intratumor heterogeneity may account for the development of refractoriness to further treatment. Intraneoplastic diversity also provides an explanation for the differences in biologic characteristics between a primary tumor and its metastases, as well as for heterogeneity among metastases originating from the same primary neoplasm.

Heterogeneity Within the Primary Tumor. From the clinical standpoint, two of the most important phenotypic expressions of heterogeneity are the differential therapeutic sensitivity of the subpopulations, and variations in their metastatic potential. Intraneoplastic diversity has been demonstrated with respect to drug sensitivity and radiation (Calabresi, 1980; Calabresi et al., 1979; Dexter, 1981; Dexter et al., 1981; Dexter and Calabresi, 1982; Hakansson, 1974a, 1974b; Heppner et al., 1978; Leith et al., 1982; Trope et al., 1975, 1979).

Subpopulations of cells with differing metastatic propensity were isolated from a single B16 melanoma in a classic experiment performed by Fidler and Kripke (1977). These investigators demonstrated that clones of cells derived from a single tumor differed in abilities to form experimental lung metastases,* thus indicating that metastatic potential of the parent tumor was heterogenous. One group of researchers (Kripke et al., 1978) has reported similar results using an ultraviolet-light-induced murine fibrosarcoma. Heterogeneity in metastatic ability among cell subpopulations has also been demonstrated in a murine KHT sarcoma. Cloned lines were obtained from this tumor and injected into syngeneic mice; varying numbers of metastases developed from the clones (Chambers et al., 1981).

The studies cited above document heterogeneity within primary tumors; there is much less evidence for heterogeneity within single metastatic lesions. Many metastases are clonal in origin. Talmadge and associates (1982) irradiated neoplastic cells to induce the formation of marker chromosomes, inoculated mice with these cells, and demonstrated that experimental and most spontaneous metastases were monoclonal in origin. Fialkow (1976) analyzed the glucose-6-phosphate dehydrogenase isoenzyme type found in several liver metastases from patients with metastatic colon carcinoma and reported only a single isoenzyme type present in most of the metastases.

By contrast, flow cytometric DNA analysis

---

* The difference between spontaneous and experimental metastases should be noted. Spontaneous metastases develop from a primary tumor and must complete all the steps in the metastatic process. Experimental metastases arise from tumor cells that are injected intravenously, thus avoiding several of the steps in the metastatic process. Stackpole (1981) has shown that metastases detected after intravenous injection of cells do not necessarily have an increased ability to metastasize spontaneously.

of cells obtained by needle biopsy from metastases in patients with small cell carcinoma showed the existence of more than one subpopulation. This heterogeneity could reflect either a polyclonal origin of the metastasis or, more likely, the genetic instability of the neoplastic cells with the resultant emergence of variant subpopulations (Vindeløv *et al.*, 1980, 1982).

Heterogeneity Among the Primary Tumor and Its Metastases and Among Metastases Originating from the Same Primary Tumor. Heterogeneity between a primary tumor and its metastases has been demonstrated with methyl-cholanthrene-induced sarcoma in mice (Sugarbaker and Cohen, 1972). Greatly different growth characteristics and patterns of antigenicity were noted among the metastases. Tumors derived from several clones grew at the same rate in mice immunized to the primary tumor as in naive mice, indicating that immunologic resistance to the primary tumor does not protect from challenge by metastatic sublines.

Interlesional heterogeneity has also been found within patients (see Figure 4 – 3). Significant differences for several characteristics including growth kinetics and mucin production were found to exist between cell lines developed from two separate noncontiguous metastases obtained at exploratory laparatomy on a patient with a primary carcinoma of the colon (Spremulli *et al.*, 1982, 1983).

A metastasis may consist of cells with quantities of DNA differing from that present in the stemline of the primary tumor (Stitch and Steele, 1962). Using flow cytometric DNA analysis of biopsies of human small-cell carcinoma of the lung, differences among discrete metastasic foci found within the same patient have been documented (Vindeløv *et al.*, 1980). Differences among primary tumors and their metastases have been documented in markers, such as histaminase and L-dopa decarboxylase (Abeloff *et al.*, 1979; Baylin *et al.*, 1978). Clinically important differences in estrogen receptor (ER) protein concentration may exist between primary breast cancers and their metastases as well as among different metastases originating from the same tumor (Brennan *et al.*, 1979). These findings could account both for the lack of responsiveness of some of the metastases from ER positive primary tumors and for variable responses to endocrine therapy not infrequently observed among metastatic foci. In addition, primary and metastatic tumors differ in their responses to cytotoxic agents. Cells from ovarian cancers have exhibited differences in sensitivity to cytotoxic agents (Siracky, 1979).

Neoplastic cell heterogeneity provides a plausible explanation for clinical variation in therapeutic responsiveness between a primary tumor and its metastases.

Treatment-Induced Changes in Heterogeneity. Antineoplastic therapy may selectively reduce one or more subpopulations of cells within a tumor, thereby altering its intrinsic heterogeneity. Serial transplantation of the Dunning R-3327-H prostatic adenocarcinoma in castrated rats results in selective deletion of the androgen-dependent cells (Isaacs *et al.*, 1982). Treatment of nude mice hosting a heterogeneous human colon carcinoma with graded doses of x-irradiation selectively decreased the percentage of one of the clones (Calabresi and Dexter, 1982). Two clinical studies provide further information on this topic. Siracky (1979) successively sampled human ovarian cancer while patients were receiving cytostatic treatment and reported changes in the ploidy distribution, indicating, in some cases, selective reduction of one subpopulation of cells. Chemotherapy can also induce a shift in the ploidy distribution of cells from metastatic small-cell carcinoma (Vindelov *et al.*, 1980).

These perturbations are important in facilitating the emergence of treatment-resistant tumors; they also have the potential to influ-

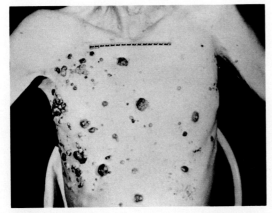

Figure 4 – 3.   Malignant melanoma with multiple superficial metastases. Note marked heterogeneity in size and pigmentation of lesions, ranging from deeply pigmented to amelanotic. Courtesy of Dr. James F. Holland.

ence subsequent metastases. Cytotoxic therapy may selectively destroy cell subpopulations with high or low metastatic potential or, by reducing specific cell lines, could lead to the loss of stabilizing clonal interactions resulting in the emergence of variant clones, some of which may have increased metastatic potential (Poste *et al.,* 1982).

STEPS IN METASTASIS

In order to produce a metastasis, a neoplastic cell must undergo a complex series of events that includes initial detachment from the main tumor mass, invasion of surrounding tissue, access to blood or lymphatic vessels, circulation in the blood stream or lymphatic channels, arrest at a target site, attachment at that site, egression, implantation in the organ, proliferation, and establishment of a new blood supply (see Figure 4–4). During each step, host defense mechanisms or mechanical factors may irreparably damage the neoplastic cell and render it incapable of successfully developing a secondary deposit. Accordingly, metastasis is a rare event in the biologic life of a malignant tumor. Neoplasms that contain billions of cells seldom produce more than a few dozen metastases. Within a neoplasm con-

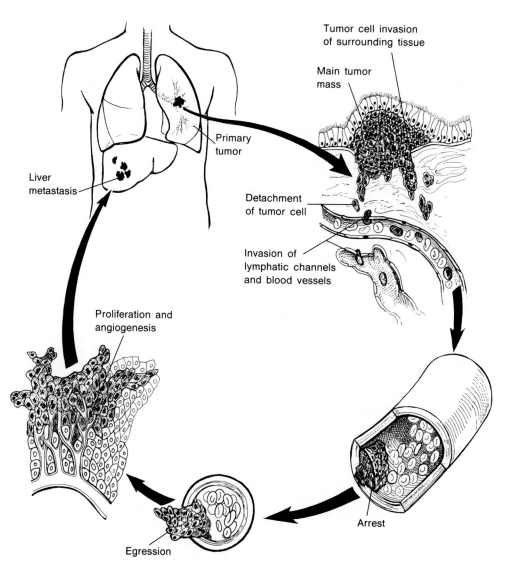

Figure 4–4. Steps in the development of a metastasis.

taining a heterogeneous population of cancer cells, only those cells functionally suited and fortuitously destined for dissemination will successfully complete the metastatic process. For reviews on this subject, see Fidler (1979), Roos and Dingemans (1979), and Sugarbaker (1979).

Detachment of Cells

The first step in metastasis, detachment of the cell from the main tumor mass, may be accomplished by active locomotion or by the enzymatic degradation of surrounding tissue. Neoplastic cells may migrate by means of ameboid motility. A major factor enabling neoplastic cells to become motile is decreased adhesiveness (Coman, 1953). Tumor interstitial fluid contains hydrolases that originate in the central necrotic areas present in large tumors (Sylven, 1973). These hydrolases allow neoplastic cells to detach more easily from the necrotic portion of a tumor than from its healthy, well-vascularized portion (Weiss, 1977). Because the number of circulating neoplastic cells, however, is generally proportional to the size of the primary tumor (Roos and Dingemans, 1979), the precise role of lysosomal hydrolases in producing a large increase in hematogenous dissemination is not clear.

Tumor Cell Invasion of Surrounding Tissue

Neoplastic cells may spread by direct invasion of host tissue. The factors involved in this process can be classified as mechanical or chemical. (For a review of tumor invasiveness, see Mareel, 1980.)

Mechanical factors resulting from cell proliferation have been implicated in the process of invasion (Willis, 1960; Hart, 1981). The increased hydrostatic pressure found within tumors may physically force neoplastic cells into surrounding structures. Rapid proliferation of neoplastic tissue in experimental systems can elevate the tumor's interstitial hydrostatic pressure to approximately 30 cm H_2O. Pressure in normal surrounding subcutaneous tissue is less than 5 cm H_2O (Butler and Gullino, 1975b).

Chemical factors are also involved in tumor cell invasion. Cancerous neoplasms possess higher levels of degradative enzymes than do benign tumors of corresponding normal tissues (Dresden et al., 1972; Strauch, 1972; Syl-

ven, 1973; Yamanishi et al., 1973). During the process of tissue invasion, neoplastic cells must traverse barriers of collagen and elastic structures in the interstitial tissues and basement membrane. The production of enzymes capable of degrading extracellular matrix may be important in this process (Dabbous et al., 1977; Fidler et al., 1977). Because neoplastic cell invasion is probably hindered most effectively by type IV (basement membrane) collagen, the presence of enzymes that degrade this substance may enhance invasion. Collagenolytic activity has been reported in human neoplasms (Dresden et al., 1972), and production of collagenase has been demonstrated in cell lines obtained from patients with melanoma and carcinoma of the breast (Paranjpe et al., 1980; Yamanishi et al., 1973). The amount of type IV collagenase present in several neoplastic cell lines established from tumors that develop spontaneous metastases has been determined, and a positive correlation has been found between the incidence of metastases and the level of enzyme production in cell culture medium (Garbison et al., 1980; Liotta et al., 1977, 1980).

Invasive cells do not necessarily have the potential to form a metastasis. Evidence suggests that a direct correlation between metastatic potential and invasiveness for several variant B16 melanoma lines does not necessarily exist (Hart, 1979), emphasizing the fact that invasiveness is only one of a number of variables in the metastatic process.

Invasion of Lymphatic Channels and Blood Vessels

Neoplasms frequently spread via the lymphatic system. Invasion of lymphatics is thought to correlate with the same factors responsible for tissue invasion: Cell motility, lack of adhesiveness, release of lytic enzymes, increase in primary tumor size, and changes in tissue hydrostatic pressure (Gullino, 1966; Van de Velde and Carr, 1977).

Considerable controversy exists concerning the fate of neoplastic cells encountering lymph nodes. Three possibilities are summarized below.

Destruction in the Node. Animal studies have demonstrated significant neoplastic cell destruction in the lymph nodes, and have led to the filter barrier concept of lymphatic metastases (Fisher and Fisher, 1967b). Ludwig and Titus (1967) injected labeled Walker 256 tumor cells into rat foot pads and found that the majority of the cells that reached the sub-capsular sinuses were destroyed. In support of the filter barrier function, Zeidman and Buss (1954) showed that some neoplastic cells are destroyed in lymphatics.

Free Passage Through the Node. Some neoplastic cells, however, can pass relatively freely through lymph nodes and between lym-phatic and blood vessels (Hewitt and Blake, 1975). Madden (1968) obtained direct evi-dence for the free passage of neoplastic cells through lymph nodes by injecting tumor cells into the mesenteric lymphatic system and used a bioassay technique to determine cell num-bers at the jugulosubclavian junction. When 5×10^5 cells were injected, the great majority traversed the lymph nodes in two to three hours. These data suggest that not all neoplas-tic cells are detained in lymph nodes but in-stead that many may traverse lymphatics and enter the vascular system.

Ineffective Destruction by the Node. Within 24 hours after inoculation of Rd/2 car-cinoma cells into the foot pads of rats, invasion of local lymphatics and access to both the sub-capsular and medullary sinuses of the regional nodes was observed (Carr and McGinty, 1974). The sinus macrophages in these nodes showed a proliferative response. In spite of this reaction, however, the lymph nodes were re-placed by neoplastic cells. Five days later, me-tastases were also observed in the paraaortic nodes, which were contiguous with the af-fected nodes.

Though each of these three possibilities de-serves consideration, the clinical relevance of the data used to support them is open to ques-tion. Fidler *et al.* (1977) pointed out that these experiments used normal animals injected with transplantable tumors. In this artificial situation, the lymph node may be suddenly confronted with a large number of neoplastic cells; when spontaneous tumors arise, only a few tumor cells probably metastasize to the lymph node initially. Accordingly, whether re-sults obtained from experiments using trans-planted tumors are applicable to clinical situa-tions is questionable (Fidler *et al.*, 1977). Unfortunately, animal models in which spon-taneous tumors arise with a high enough fre-quency to stimulate human neoplastic disease can rarely be identified. Perhaps lymph nodes provide a mechanical barrier to some neoplas-

tic cells, whereas others may pass through the nodes freely, and still other neoplastic cells are capable of resisting destruction by the nodes.

Poor development of the vascular endothe-lium in tumors may facilitate hematogenous dissemination of neoplastic cells (Burrage, 1970). Tumor-bearing animals treated with ICRF-159, a drug that promotes development of vascular endothelium, in concentrations too low to inhibit neoplastic growth developed fewer metastases than did control animals. Histologic examination of tumors from treated animals revealed better-developed vas-cular endothelium than in control animals.

Invasion of blood vessels, however, does not necessarily correlate with the successful devel-opment of metastases. Although a 1 g mam-mary tumor transplanted to the ovary releases as many as $3.2 (\pm 1.4) \times 10^6$ cells in 24 hours, relatively few metastatic lesions are observed (Gullino, 1977).

Circulation, Arrest, Redistribution, Tropism, and Egression

Once a neoplastic cell has invaded the host's circulatory system, it must survive in this hos-tile environment. When cells are separated from solid tissues and placed into suspension cultures, they usually die as a result of the envi-ronmental change (Weiss, 1977). Circulating tumor cells are also subject to considerable mechanical damage and limited survival.

Studies with radiolabeled cells show that cells usually arrest in the first capillary bed en-countered. Whether the cells remain there de-pends on several factors including the cell's ability to adhere to the vascular endothelium and to the cells of the organ in which they are trapped. Nicolson and Winkelhake (1975) ex-amined and compared the adhesive properties of two variant lines of B16 melanoma, which differed in the capacity to form experimental lung metastases: B16F10, which forms many lung colonies and B16F1 which forms only a few lung colonies. When mixed with dispersed lung cells, B16F10 cells form aggregates more readily than do B16F1 cells. In addition, the B16F10 cells adhered more strongly to mono-layers of 3T3 cells, which are considered endo-thelial cells. Nicolson (1979) also examined cell-surface properties important in the lung colonizing ability of B16 melanoma, and re-ported that B16F10 cells in culture shed bits of cell membrane in the form of small, closed vesicles. These vesicles were harvested, purified by centrifugation, and added to a culture of B16F1 cells along with polyethylene glycol, which causes the fusion of the B16F10 vesicles with the membrane of the B16F1 cells. When the B16F1 cells, enriched with these vesicles, were injected intravenously, their metastatic frequency approached that of the B16F10 cell line. These experiments suggest that the greater ability of B16F10 cells to produce pulmonary colonies is related to cell-membrane properties that allow them to adhere both to lung cells and to vascular endothelium. Neoplastic cells, as mentioned above, do not necessarily form metastases at the site of their initial arrest. Frequently, these cells are redistributed to other organs. Using Chromium-tagged Walker 256 tumor cells and similarly-tagged Brown Pierce and V-2 carcinoma cells to study distribution after jugular vein or intraportal injection, Fisher and Fisher (1967a) found that the majority of cells were not in the lung or liver 24 hours later, but had recirculated. Intravenous injection of cells from the M5076 ovarian tumor results in rapid initial arrest in the lungs, followed by slow release and subsequent localization in the liver three to four days later (Hart *et al.,* 1981).

Tropism is the preferential colonization in specific organs by neoplastic cells (Hart and Fidler, 1980; Kinsey, 1960; Sugarbaker, 1981). Kinsey (1960) and Sugarbaker *et al.* (1971) implanted various organs subcutaneously, injected lung-colonizing neoplastic cells, and later autopsied the host mice. Metastatic foci developed in the lungs and in grafted lung tissue, but not in other organs grafted as controls. Hart and Fidler (1980) labeled B16 cells with [125]IUdR and studied their initial arrest and redistribution. They found that the B16 cells, which formed metastatic foci in the ectopic lungs, did not originally arrest at that site but gained access after recirculation.

Egression of Walker 256 tumor cells from the circulation has been studied after intravenous inoculation into Sprague-Dawley rats (Jones *et al.,* 1971). The neoplastic cells were arrested singly, or in small groups, in capillaries or arterioles and were surrounded by a meshwork of platelets and fibrin. The tumor cells remained localized in the intravascular channels for about eight hours; subsequently the cells progressively breached the endothelial lining, and after 24 to 48 hours the cells were clearly perivascular and lying in direct apposition to connective tissue.

Tumor Angiogenesis

Once neoplastic cells egress from the circulation, they must develop a blood supply in order to undergo significant growth. Solid tumors may increase in size as much as 16,000-fold in two weeks and must continually recruit new blood vessels (Ausprunk, 1979). The new vasculature is derived from the host and not from the tumor (Folkman, 1975). The mechanism responsible for tumor angiogenesis is believed to be chemically mediated and does not require cell-to-cell contact (Folkman *et al.,* 1971). A soluble, diffusible extract, capable of inducing neovascularization from solid animal tumors and from neoplastic cells in culture has been reported (Folkman *et al.,* 1971). A protein extract has been partially purified and designated tumor angiogenesis factor (TAF).

TUMOR AND HOST FACTORS THAT MODULATE THE DEVELOPMENT OF METASTASES

Tumor Factors

A number of important tumor factors are recognized in the development of metastases. Among these are the site of the primary tumor, its size, its presence or absence, and tumor-associated antigens.

Site of Primary Tumor. The location of the primary tumor is important in determining not only whether metastases will occur, but also in which organ they will occur. Clinical variability in the expression of metastatic potential and in the location of secondary sites was discussed previously in this chapter (see "The Clinical Background" above). Animal experiments have explored the relationship between the location of the primary neoplasm and the development of metastases. Subcutaneous injection of murine reticulum sarcoma cells results in direct invasion of the peritoneum. When the same neoplastic cells, however, are inoculated into the external ear or foot pad, fewer metastases occur and these are primarily hepatic. Lewis lung carcinoma cells are widely metastatic when inoculated subcutaneously but do not metastasize when injected intraperitoneally (Sugarbaker, 1979). The direct clinical relevance of these interesting experiments is uncertain, both because of the necessarily artificial nature of the neoplastic cell injections and because the variability in number and site of metastases found among patients afflicted with different types of primary tumors may largely depend upon the intrinsic cellular properties of the subpopulations composing these neoplasms.

Size of Primary Tumor. A common belief is that patients whose cancers are relatively "small" when first detected have a better prognosis than those whose tumors are larger at diagnosis. The assumption is that smaller tumors are more curable than larger tumors since they have not yet metastasized. The reader is referred to the chapters that discuss each tumor type for statistics relating the size of the primary tumor to prognosis.

The probability of metastasis, however, does not necessarily correlate with the size of the primary tumor. Some neoplasms frequently exhibit metastases when the primary is still microscopic in size, while others rarely metastasize, regardless of the extent of the primary tumor. For example, Lewis lung carcinomas may become metastatic when the primary tumor is less than 0.5 cm in size, whereas several MCA-induced sarcomas do not metastasize and cause death by local extension. For other MCA-induced murine sarcomas, primary tumor size correlates with the likelihood of metastases (Sugarbaker, 1979).

Apparently, size is not an important factor in modulating the development of metastases in tumors of very high or very low metastatic potential. For tumors of moderate potential, however, increasing size is correlated with an increase in metastases. Two explanations for this are that increasing size is usually associated with increasing numbers of released cells and probably with more heterogeneity (Butler and Gullino, 1975a; Kleinerman and Liotta, 1977).

Presence of the Primary Tumor. Considerable evidence suggests that the presence of the primary tumor influences the growth rate of its metastases. Synchronous slowing of the growth rate of a primary tumor, the Lewis lung carcinoma, and its metastases has been demonstrated (DeWys, 1972). Early after transplantation, the implanted primary and its metastases grew exponentially at a similar rate. Later, as the growth rate of the primary tumor

decreased, that of the metastases also diminished, even though these metastatic foci were microscopic in size and continued rapid growth would have been expected. The Cloudman S91 melanoma, after it reaches a certain size, can inhibit the growth of its distant metastases (Schatten, 1958). When mice were inoculated with S91 cells, and the tumor-bearing extremity was subsequently amputated, the metastases grew more rapidly. The operative procedure itself was evidently not responsible for the observed results, since amputating the contralateral leg did not affect the frequency, number, or size of pulmonary metastases. Excision of a primary Lewis lung tumor performed on day seven or later results in an increase in the thymidine-labeling index and growth rate of the pulmonary metastases (Simpson-Herren, *et al.*, 1976).

The relationship between the presence or absence of the primary tumor and the number and size of the metastatic foci has been examined in five tumor systems (Ketcham *et al.*, 1961). Amputation of the limb bearing the primary tumor can result in a reduced number, but increased size, of pulmonary colonies. The reduced number of lung metastases probably results from cessation of shedding of neoplastic cells after removal of the primary. The larger metastatic tumors observed in animals after removal of the primary could reflect either a direct effect of the primary tumor on its metastases or could be the result of such indirect factors as better health of the animals after limb amputation or of reduced competition for nutrients among the fewer lung metastases.

In a clinical study involving eight patients with testicular cancer, cytoreductive surgery was followed by an acceleration in the growth rate of some metastatic foci (Lange *et al.*, 1980), suggesting that reduction of tumor burden may alter the growth kinetics of the remaining neoplastic cells.

The reason for the suppressive influence of the primary tumor upon its metastases is not known, although interaction of tissue chalones and polyamines has been suggested (Bichel *et al.*, 1975; Sugarbaker *et al.*, 1977). More work is needed to establish the overall clinical importance of the interrelationships between a primary tumor and its metastases, as well as the mechanisms involved.

Tumor-Associated Antigens. Tumor-associated antigens have been described for a wide variety of human and animal neoplasms.

Many of these antigens are capable of evoking either a humoral or cell-mediated immune response. Chapter 11 describes a review of this subject.

Host Factors

Host factors, immunologic, trauma-related, and hormonal, are important influences on the development of metastases.

Immunologic. Considerable evidence supports the view that the biologic behavior of tumors and, in particular, their capacity to metastasize, is in part determined by immunologic factors requiring the participation of T lymphocytes, macrophages, B lymphocytes, and natural killer (NK) cells (Alexander, 1976a, 1976b). (For a review of this topic see Nicolson and Poste, 1982, 1983). NK cells and macrophages appear to inhibit metastases, whereas blocking antibodies produced by lymphocytes may increase the likelihood of metastases. No simple correlation between the development of experimental metastases and the immune status of the host has been found; immune responses may either suppress or enhance disseminated disease (Fidler and Hart, 1982).

Transplanted syngeneic tumors that do not metastasize in normal animals do so in animals that have been exposed to whole-body x-irradiation or antilymphocyte serum (Barnes et al., 1957; Fisher et al., 1969). Enhancement of metastases by such treatment appears to be related to a T-cell deficit and not to bone marrow damage, as depletion of T cells by thymectomy or by drainage of thoracic duct lymphocytes markedly increases the frequency of metastases (Alexander, 1976b).

Immunologic factors also influence the circulation, initial arrest, organ distribution, and survival of tumor cells. Syngeneic animals sensitized to the murine B16 melanoma exhibit patterns of tumor cell arrest and survival that differ from those of normal syngeneic hosts (Fidler, 1977). The presence of a sensitizing tumor does not appear to affect the distribution pattern of intravenously injected cells from a second immunologically unrelated tumor. Therefore, immunologic factors appear to influence the shifts in arrest pattern observed in tumor-bearing mice after injection of cells of the same type as the sensitizing tumor (Weiss and Glaves, 1976). Accordingly,

normal animals, in contrast to immunized animals, may not be the best model system to use for studying the pathogenesis of metastases (Fidler, 1977).

Macrophages are important in the host's ability to prevent the development of metastases. They may be involved either as nonspecific antitumor agents or as agents that cooperate with lymphocytes in a cell-mediated immune response. Wood and Gillespie (1975) depleted a murine solid tumor of macrophages and injected the macrophage-free tumor-cell suspension subcutaneously into normal syngeneic mice, resulting in primary tumors that produced an increased number of metastases. The survival times of mice injected with macrophage-depleted tumor-cell suspensions were significantly shorter than those of mice inoculated with tumor-cell suspensions not depleted of macrophages. Additional studies documenting the ability of macrophages to affect neoplastic cells have been performed (Eccles and Alexander, 1974; Fidler, 1978; Fidler et al., 1982). Further evidence of the importance of macrophages in preventing the development of metastases was obtained in a study of the function of the reticuloendothelial system in mice bearing Lewis lung carcinomas (Otu et al., 1977). These studies confirm the existence of a substantial number of macrophages within syngeneic murine solid tumors and strongly suggest a regulatory function for macrophages in preventing metastases.

NK cells appear to play a major role in host defense against neoplastic disease. They do not require prior exposure to a particular tumor antigen, as do cytotoxic T lymphocytes. NK cells are not specific for individual tumors and can destroy spontaneously both tumor cells and cells infected with viruses (Marx, 1980). In addition, nude mice, which have increased numbers of NK cells, show a lower incidence of metastatic tumors than do normal mice. Human tumor xenografts growing in nude mice rarely metastasize and this failure is thought to be related to the high levels of natural killer cells in these animal hosts (Marx, 1980).

Trauma-Related. Radiation therapy or surgery may produce tissue damage. Tumor-bearing animals subjected to whole-body irradiation develop an increased number of metastases. This enhancement of metastases may be related to vascular endothelial damage resulting from treatment (Peters, 1975). The influence of trauma on development of metastases was also investigated using rabbits. Injury to the splenic and perisplenic tissue was accomplished by perfusion of the isolated spleen with a solution of nitrogen mustard or by controlled ischemia. The abdominal wall musculature was then injured by surgical incision. During the postoperative period, the thoracic aortas were inoculated with suspensions of VX-2 carcinoma cells. The number of metastases to the damaged tissues increased strikingly. About 60% of the test animals developed metastases to the spleen and perisplenic tissue compared with 8% of the controls. Metastases to the operative wound increased an average of 20 times their expected numbers when the intra-aortic inoculations were made one week after injury. Ischemic injury also results in an increase in hematogenous metastases to the injured part (Alexander and Altemeier, 1964). Other studies indicate that celiotomy increases the number of lung metastases in mice bearing the T241 sarcoma (Romsdahl, 1964) and that partial hepatectomy increases metastases in rats inoculated intraportally with Walker 256 carcinoma cells (Fisher and Fisher, 1959).

Accordingly, injured tissue appears to provide a better "soil" for metastases, regardless of how the local tissue is damaged.

Hormonal. Hormonal factors also influence the development of metastases (Zeidman, 1957). In some tumor-host systems, cortisone treatment increases metastases; this is probably explained by its ability to alter immune responsiveness. Transplanted mammary carcinomas in cortisone-treated mice produce widespread metastases, while no metastases appear in untreated mice. Krebs-2 cells injected intravenously produce only pulmonary metastases unless the animal is pretreated with cortisone, in which case large numbers of metastases are also found in the abdominal viscera (Agosin et al., 1952; Pomeroy, 1954). Treatment with pituitary growth hormone increases the number of lung metastases in mice after intravenous injection of a suspension of neoplastic cells, but does not affect the number of spontaneous metastases (Wood, 1955).

Clinical studies underscore the importance of the hormonal environment on the control of cancer. The use of exogenous thyroxine to suppress pituitary TSH frequently reduces the growth of metastatic, well-differentiated carcinoma of the thyroid (Sugarbaker, 1979). Prostatic neoplasms are often androgen-dependent

and changes in the hormonal milieu, such as castration or estrogen administration, will sometimes cause temporary regression of metastatic disease (Blackard et al., 1973; Emmett et al., 1960; Huggins et al., 1941). Furthermore, in both experimental and clinical breast cancers that contain the estrogen or progesterone receptor proteins, metastatic disease may be at least temporarily controlled by ovarian or adrenal ablation, by hypophysectomy, or by the administration of a variety of hormones (Heel et al., 1978; Kiang and Kennedy, 1977; Legha et al., 1978; Luft et al., 1958; Moore et al., 1974; Schweitzer, 1980; Silverstein et al., 1975; Smith et al., 1978; Sugarbaker, 1979).

EXPERIMENTAL APPROACHES TO THE PREVENTION OF METASTASES

Potentiation of Host Immunity

In order to increase the host's defense against metastases, many investigators have tried nonspecific stimulating agents such as bacillus Calmette-Guérin (BCG) and *Corynebacterium parvum* (*C. parvum*). In addition, Fidler (1978) recently reported the results of studies designed to evaluate the efficacy of activated macrophages in controlling metastases. The results from many laboratories can be summarized as follows. Treatment with BCG, *C. parvum*, or activated macrophages in animal systems has frequently been efficacious. Unfortunately, BCG, *C. parvum*, and other immunostimulating agents have not, in general, demonstrated great antineoplastic activity when used clinically (Borden et al., 1981; Budzar et al., 1981; Cohen et al., 1979; Heyn et al., 1975; Klefstrom et al., 1981; Leukemia Committee and the Working Party on Leukemia in Childhood, 1971; Mathe et al., 1969; Woodruff, 1975). Patient trials with macrophage activating agents are anticipated with great interest.

Interference with Blood Coagulation

Thrombocytopenia. Results with murine tumors indicate that thrombocytopenia may be associated with a decreased number of metastases. Thrombocytopenia, produced in mice by injecting mouse antiplatelet serum, reduced the number of metastases produced by a wide variety of murine tumors. Thrombocytopenia was most effective against metastases produced by tumors with the capacity to aggregate platelets *in vitro* but was also effective against metastases produced by tumors lacking such capacity (Gasic *et al.,* 1973; Mehta, 1984).

Heparin. Data regarding the effect of heparin on the formation of metastases are conflicting. Heparin can either increase or decrease lung metastases depending on the system studied. Daily subcutaneous injections of depoheparin in mice bearing T241 sarcomas or DBA-49 sarcomas does not inhibit growth of these primary sarcomas. Development of metastases from the T241 sarcoma was identical in treated and control mice. In treated mice hosting the DBA-49 sarcoma, however, fewer metastases were found, suggesting an antimetastatic effect for heparin only for the latter tumor. Thus, the effect of heparin may depend on the neoplastic cell line studied (Retik *et al.,* 1962). Heparin therapy has also been reported to decrease the number of pulmonary metastases from the Walker 256 carcinoma (Agostino and Cliffton, 1962).

The effect of heparin treatment was studied in four other experimental tumor systems (Maat, 1978). When neoplastic cells were inoculated by tail-vein injection, the heparin-treated animals had a reduced number of lung colonies. In three of the four tumors used, however, the number of extrapulmonary colonies was increased. These data suggest that heparin treatment may reduce the capacity of lung capillaries to trap tumor cells, thus facilitating tumor-cell circulation. Hagmar and Boeryd (1969) studied the effect of heparin on spontaneous metastasis formation using a syngeneic methylcholanthrene-induced rhabdomyosarcoma in CBA mice. The tumor was transplanted to the tail and heparin was administered for six days after metastatic spread began. Heparin treatment increased the average number of metastases to the lung. This effect was ascribed to promotion of neoplastic cell release (Hagmar, 1969). The inconsistencies in work with heparin from different laboratories suggest that additional investigations are warranted.

Coumadin. Coumadin affects the development of metastases in certain experimental systems. Coumadin treatment resulted in a significant decrease in metastases and an increase in the length of survival of rats bearing the Walker 256 carcinoma (Agostino *et al.,* 1966). Three separate experimental tumor-host systems in mice were used to study the growth rate of an implanted tumor; in each case, the size of the primary was significantly reduced with Coumadin-induced anticoagulation. In these tumor systems, animals with a prothrombin time prolongation of two to three times normal had an increase in their long-term survival and decrease in the number of metastases (Ketcham *et al.,* 1971).

Aspirin. On the basis of previous work indicating a relationship between platelet aggregation and the development of metastases, Gasic and colleagues (Gasic *et al.,* 1972) reasoned that drugs, such as aspirin, that inhibit platelet aggregation should inhibit tumor spread. These investigators inoculated T241 tumors intramuscularly; seven days later, the inoculated leg was amputated and subsequently the animals were necropsied. Aspirin-treated animals had a significant reduction in the number of pulmonary metastases. Initial data of this type suggest a need for further studies in this area.

Adjuvant Therapy

Background. Numerous preclinical experiments established that radiation therapy and antineoplastic agents are often more effective against small foci of tumors than against larger ones (Skipper, 1978; Martin, 1981). The response of micrometastases to therapy depends upon several factors, including size, anatomic location, growth kinetics, vascularization, and interaction with host defense mechanisms. These considerations led to the development of animal tumor models that could be used to study the efficacy of adjuvant therapy.

Steel and associates (1976) treated mice that had been inoculated intramuscularly or intravenously with Lewis cell carcinoma cells with a single injection of BCNU. Survival of cells from primary tumors hosted by treated animals was measured by colony formation in soft agar or by an *in vivo* assay, in which lung metastases were counted. BCNU was found to be ineffective against palpable intramuscular tumors but considerably effective against experimental lung metastases.

Shaeffer and associates (1973) administered a dose of 2100 rads to the lungs of mice 24 hours after intravenous injection of C3HBA adenocarci noma cells. All control mice had visible lung colonies at autopsy 28 days later, while 83% of treated mice appeared tumor free. In a separate experiment, primary C3HBA tumors were treated with graded doses of irradiation when they were between 300 and

500 mm³ in size (much larger than the microscopic pulmonary metastases treated in the previous experiment). A tumor dose of 6000 rads was required to control the disease in 75% of the animals. These experiments support the concept that micrometastatic disease is much easier to eradicate with radiation than macroscopic disease.

In an investigation of the effectiveness of adjuvant chemotherapy in murine lung, breast, and colon cancers after surgical removal of the primary (Schabel, 1977), survival rate improved with adjuvant chemotherapy compared to that expected with either surgery or chemotherapy alone. In dose-response studies using 6-mercaptopurine (6MP), alone or in combination with surgery, for treating murine carcinoma 755 tumors 10 to 29 mm in size, the combination yielded better survival rates than simply adding the effects expected from chemotherapy alone and those from surgery alone (Chirigos et al., 1962). Cyclophosphamide only slightly inhibited the growth of a spontaneous mouse mammary tumor when administered alone. The drug, however, doubled the surgical cure rate when used as an adjuvant after removal of the primary tumor (Martin, 1961). Enhanced rates of cure of spontaneous murine mammary carcinomas with surgery and a five-drug chemotherapy regimen have been reported (Fugmann et al., 1970). Studies such as these provide the rationale and impetus for the many clinical trials now in progress that employ chemotherapy as an adjuvant. For a detailed discussion of adjuvant chemotherapy in specific human neoplasms, refer to chapters describing the individual neoplasms.

REFERENCES

Abeloff, M. D.; Eggleston, J. C.; Mendelsohn, G.; Ettinger, D. S.; and Baylin, S. B.: Changes in morphologic and biochemical characteristics of small cell carcinoma of the lung. *Am. J. Med.,* **66**:757–764, 1979.

Agosin, M.; *et al.:* Cortisone-induced metastases of adenocarcinoma in mice. *Proc. Soc. Exp. Biol. Med.,* **80**:128–131, 1952.

Agostino, D., and Cliffton, E. E.: Decrease of metastases of carcinoma Walker 256 with irradiation and heparin or fibrinolytic agents. *Radiology,* **79**:848–855, 1962.

Agostino, D.; Cliffton, E. E.; and Girolami, A.: Effect of prolonged Coumadin treatment on the production of pulmonary metastases in the rat. *Cancer,* **19**:284–288, 1966.

Alexander, J. W., and Altemeier, W. A.: Susceptibility of injured tissues to hematogenous metastases: An experimental study. *Ann. Surg.,* **159**:933–944, 1964.

Alexander, P.: Dormant metastases which manifest on immunosuppression and the role of macrophages in tumours. In Weiss, L. (ed.): *Fundamental Aspects of Metastasis.* North-Holland Publishing Company, Amsterdam, 1976a.

Alexander, P.: Metastatic spread and "escape" from the immune defenses of the host. *Natl. Cancer Inst. Monograph,* **44**:125–129, 1976b.

Ausprunk, D. H.: Tumor angiogenesis. In Houck, J. C. (ed.): *Chemical Messengers of the Inflammatory Process.* Elsevier North-Holland, Inc. New York, 1979.

Badib, A. O.; Kurohara, S. S.; Webster, J. H.; and Pickren, J. W.: Metastases to organs in carcinoma of the uterine cervix; influence of treatment on incidence and distribution. *Cancer,* **21**:434–439, 1968.

Barnes, D. W. H.; Ford, C. E.; Ilbery, P. T. L.; Koller, P. C.; and Loutit, J. F.: Tissue transplantation of the radiation chimera. *J. Cell Comp. Physiol,* Number 50 supplement, 123–138, 1957.

Batson, O. V.: The vertebral vein system. Caldwell lecture, 1956. *Am. J. Roentgenol. Radium Ther. Nucl. Med.,* **78**:195–212, 1957.

Baylin, S. B.; Weisburger, W. R.; Eggleston, J. C.; Mendelsohn, G.; Beaven, M. A.; Abeloff, M. D.; and Ettinger, D. S.: Variable content of histaminase, L-dopa decarboxylase and calcitonin in small cell carcinoma of the lung: biologic and clinical implications. *N. Engl. J. Med.,* **229**:105–110, 1978.

Bichel, P.; Barford, N. M.; and Jakobsen, A.: Employment of synchronized cells and flow microfluorometry in investigations on the JB-I tumor cell chalones. *Virchows Arch. Cell Pathol.,* **19**:127–133, 1975.

Blackard, C. E.; Byar, D. P.; and Jordan, W. P.: Orchiectomy for advanced prostatic carcinoma. *Urology,* **1**:553–560, 1973.

Borden, E. C.; Davis, T. E.; Crowley, J. J.; Wolberg, W. H.; McKnight, B.; and Chirigos, M. A.: Interim analysis of a trial of levamisole and 5-fluorouracil in metastatic colorectal carcinoma. In Terry, W. D., and Rosenberg, S. A. (eds.): *Immunotherapy of Human Cancer.* Elsevier North-Holland, Inc., New York, 1981.

Brady, L. W.; O'Neill, E. A.; and Farber, S. H.: Unusual sites of metastases. *Semin. Oncol.,***4**:59–64, 1977.

Brennan, M. J.: Breast cancer. In Holland, J. F., and Frei, E., III (eds.): *Cancer Medicine.* Lea & Febiger, Philadelphia, 1973.

Brennan, M. J.; Donegan, W. L.; and Appleby, D. E.: The variability of estrogen receptors in metastatic breast cancer. *Am. J. Surg.,* **137**:260–262, 1979.

Bross, I. D.; Viadana, E.; and Pickren, J.: Do generalized metastases occur directly from the primary? *J. Chronic Dis.,* **28**:149–159, 1975.

Burrage, K.; Hellmann, K.; and Salsbury, A. J.: Drug-induced inhibition of tumour cell dissemination. *Br. J. Pharmacol.,* **39**:205–206, 1970.

Butler, T. P., and Gullino, P. M.: Quantitation of cell shedding into efferent blood of mammary adenocarcinoma. *Cancer Res.,* **35**:512–516, 1975a.

Butler, T. P., and Gullino, P. M.: Bulk transfer of fluid in the interstitial compartment of mammary tumors. *Cancer Res.,* **35**:3084–3088, 1975b.

Buzdar, A. V.; Blumenstein, G. R.; Hortibagyi, G. N.; Legha, S. S.; Hap, H-Y; Campos, L. T.; and Hersh, E. M.: Adjuvant chemotherapy with 5-fluorouracil, adriamycin, and cyclophosphamide with or without BCG immunotherapy in Stage II or III breast cancer. In Terry, W. D., and Rosenberg, S. A. (eds.): *Immunother-*

apy of Human Cancer. Elsevier North-Holland, Inc., New York, 1981.

Calabresi, P.: Crab or chimera? The clinical implications of cancer cell heterogeneity. *Trans. Am. Clin. Climatol. Assoc.,* **92:**49–65, 1980.

Calabresi, P., and Dexter, D. L.: Clinical implications of cancer cell heterogeneity. In Owens, A. H.; Coffey, D. S.; Baylin, S. B. (eds.): *Tumor Cell Heterogeneity: Origins and Implications.* Academic Press, New York, 1982.

Calabresi, P.; Dexter, D. L.; and Heppner, G. H.: Clinical and pharmacological implications of cancer cell differentiation and heterogeneity. *Biochem. Pharmacol.,* **28:**1933–1941, 1979.

Carlson, V.; Delclos, L.; and Fletcher, G. H.: Distant metastases in squamous-cell carcinoma of the uterine cervix. *Radiology,* **88:**961–966, 1967.

Carr, I., and McGinty, F.: Lymphatic metastasis and its inhibition: An experimental model. *J. Pathol,* **113:**85–95, 1974.

Chambers, A. F.; Hill, R. P.; and Ling, V.: Tumor heterogeneity and stability of the metastatic phenotype of mouse KHT sarcoma cells. *Cancer Res.,* **41:**1368–1372, 1981.

Chirigos, M. A.; Colsky, J.; Humphreys, S. R.; Glynn, J. P.; and Goldin, A.: Evaluation of surgery and chemotherapy in the treatment of mouse mammary adenocarcinoma 755. *Cancer Chemother. Rep.,* **22:**49–53, 1962.

Cifone, M. A., and Fidler, I. J.: Increasing metastatic potential is associated with increasing genetic instability of clones isolated from murine neoplasms. *Proc. Natl. Acad. Sci. USA,* **78:**6949–6952, 1981.

Cohen, M. H.; Chretien, P. B.; Ihde, D. C.; Fossieck, B. E.; Makuch, R.; Bunn, P. A.; Johnston, A. V.; Shackney, S. E.; Matthews, M. J.; Lipson, S. D.; Kenady, D. E.; and Minna, J. D.: Thymosin fraction V and intensive combination chemotherapy. *J.A.M.A.,* **241:**1813–1815, 1979.

Coman, D. R.: Mechanisms responsible for the origin and distribution of blood-borne tumor metastases: A review. *Cancer Res.,* **13:**397–404, 1953.

Dabbous, M. K.; Roberts, A. N.; and Brinkley, B.: Collagenase and neutral protease activities in cultures of rabbit VX-2 carcinoma. *Cancer Res.,* **37:**3537–3544, 1977.

DeWys, W. D.: Studies correlating the growth rate of a tumor and its metastases and providing evidence for tumor-related systemic growth-retarding factors. *Cancer Res.,* **32:**374–379, 1972.

Dexter, D. L.: Neoplastic subpopulations in carcinomas. *Ann. Clin. Lab. Sci.,* **11:**98–108, 1981.

Dexter, D. L. and Calabresi, P.: Cancer cell differentiation. In Humphrey, G. B.; Grindey, B. G.; Dehner, L. P.; Acton, R. T.; and Pysher, T. J. (eds.): *Pancreatic Tumors in Children.* Martinus Nijhoff, Boston, 1982.

Dexter, D. L.; Spremulli, E. N.; Fligiel, Z.; Barbosa, J. A.; Vogel, R.; Van Voorhees, A.; and Calabresi, P.: Heterogeneity of cancer cells from a single human colon carcinoma. *Am. J. Med.,* **71:**949–956, 1981.

Dresden, M. H.; Heilman, S. A.; and Schmidt, J.: Collagenolytic enzymes in human neoplasms. *Cancer Res.,* **32:**993–996, 1972.

Dunn, T.: Morphology of mammary tumors in mice. In Homburger, F., and Fishman, N. H. (eds.): *Physiopathology of Cancer,* 2nd ed. Paul B. Hoeber, Inc., New York, 1959.

Eccles, S. A., and Alexander, P.: Macrophage content of

tumours in relation to metastatic spread and host immune reaction. *Nature,* **250:**667–669, 1974.

Emmett, J. L.; Green, L. F.; and Papantonious, A.: Endocrine therapy in carcinoma of the prostate gland; 10-year survival studies. *J. Urol.,* **83:**471–484, 1960.

Esrael, L.; and Chahanion, P. (eds.): *Lung Cancer, Natural History and Prognosis.* Academic Press, New York, 1976.

Feldman, G. B., and Knapp, R. C.: Lymphatic drainage of the peritoneal cavity and its significance in ovarian cancer. *Am J. Obstet. Gynecol.,* **119:**991–994, 1974.

Fialkow, P. J.: Clonal origin of human tumors. *Biochim. Biophys. Acta.,* **458:**283–321, 1976.

Fidler, I. J.: 125 IUdR sensitized cells differential kinetics of tumor arrest and survival. *Cancer,* **40:**46–55, 1977.

Fidler, I. J.: Recognition and destruction of target cells by tumoricidal macrophages. *Isr. J. Med. Sci.,* **14:**177–191, 1978.

Fidler, I. J.; Barnes, Z.; Fogler, W. E.; Kirsh, R.; Bugelski, P.; and Poste, G.: Involvement of macrophages in the eradication of established metastases following intravenous injection of liposome containing macrophage activators. *Cancer Res.,* **42:**496–501, 1982.

Fidler, I. J.; Gersten, D. M.; and Hart, I. R.: The biology of cancer invasion and metastasis. *Adv. Cancer Res.,* **28:**149–250, 1977.

Fidler, I. J., and Hart, I. R.: Principles of cancer biology: Biology of cancer metastasis. In DeVita, V. T., Jr.; Hellman, S.; and Rosenberg, S. A. (eds.): *Cancer Principles and Practice of Oncology.* J. B. Lippincott Company, Philadelphia, 1982.

Fidler, I. J., and Kripke, M. L.: Metastasis results from preexisting variant cells within a malignant tumor. *Science,* **197:**893–895, 1977.

Fisher, B., and Fisher, E. R.: Experimental studies of factors influencing hepatic metastases. II. Effect of partial hepatectomy. *Cancer,* **12:**929–932, 1959.

Fisher, B., and Fisher, E. R.: Barrier function of lymph node to tumor cells and erythrocytes. *Cancer,* **20:**1907–1912, 1967a.

Fisher, B., and Fisher, E. R.: The organ distribution of disseminated 51CR-labeled tumor cells. *Cancer Res.,* **27:**412–420, 1967b.

Fisher, B.; Slack, N. H.; Bross, I. D.; and Cooperating Investigators: Cancer of the breast: Size of neoplasm and prognosis. *Cancer* **24:**1071–1080, 1969.

Fisher, B.; Soliman, O.; and Fisher, E. R.: Effect of anti-lymphocyte serum on parameters of tumor growth in a syngeneic tumor-host system. *Proc. Soc. Exp. Biol. Med.,* **131:**16–18, 1969.

Fisher, M. S., and Cifone, M. A.: Enhanced metastatic potential of murine fibrosarcomas treated in vitro with ultraviolet radiation. *Cancer Res.,* **41:**3018–3023, 1981.

Folkman, J.: Tumor angiogenesis. In Becker, F. F. (ed.): *Cancer,* Vol. 3. Plenum Publishing Corporation, New York, 1975.

Folkman, J.; Merler, E.; Abernathy, C.; and Williams, G.: Isolation of a tumor factor responsible for angiogenesis. *J. Exp. Med.,* **133:**275, 1971.

Foulds, L.: The experimental study of tumor progression: A review. *Cancer Res.,* **14:**327–339, 1954.

Foulds, L.: The histologic analysis of mammary tumors of mice. I. Scope of investigations and general principles of analysis. *J.N.C.I.,* **17:**701–712, 1956a.

Foulds, L.: The histological analysis of mammary tumors of mice. II. The histology of responsiveness and progression. The origins of tumors. *J.N.C.I.,* **17:**713–754, 1956b.

Foulds, L.: The histologic analysis of mammary tumors of mice. III. Organoid tumors. *J.N.C.I.,* **17:**755–782, 1956c.

Foulds, L.: The histological analyses of mammary tumors of mice. IV. Secretion. *J.N.C.I.,* **17:**783–802, 1956d.

Fugmann, R. A.; Martin, D. S.; Hayworth, P. E.; and Stolfi, R. L.: Enhanced cures of spontaneous mammary carcinomas with surgery and five compound combination chemotherapy, and their immunotherapeutic interrelationship. *Cancer Res.,* **30:**1931–1936, 1970.

Garbison, S.; Kniska, K.; Tryggvason, K.; Foltz, C.; and Liotta, L. A.: Quantitation of basement membrane collagen degradation by living tumor cells *in vitro. Cancer Lett.,* **9:**359–366, 1980.

Gasic, G. J.; Gasic, T. B.; Galanti, N.; Johnson, T.; and Murphy, S.: Platelet-tumor-cell interactions in mice. The role of platelets in the spread of malignant disease. *Int. J. Cancer,* **11:**704–718, 1973.

Gasic, G. J.; Gasic, T. B.; and Murphy, S.: Antimetastatic effect of aspirin. *Lancet,* **2:**932–933, 1972.

Glassman, J. A.: *Stomach Surgery.* C C Thomas, Springfield, Illinois, 1970.

Gullino, P. M.: In vivo release of neoplastic cells by mammary tumors. *Gann Monograph on Cancer Res.,* **20:**49–55, 1977.

Gullino, P. M.: The internal milieu of tumors. *Prog. Exp. Tumor Res.,* **8:**1–25, 1966.

Hagmar, B.: Effect of heparin, coumarin, and ε-aminocaproic acid (EACA) on spontaneous metastasis formation, possible cytotoxic effect of heparin and coumarin. *Pathol. Eur.,* **4:**283–292, 1969.

Hagmar, B., and Boeryd, B.: Distribution of intravenously induced metastases in heparin- and coumarin-treated mice. *Pathol. Eur.* **4:**103–111, 1969.

Hakansson, L., and Trope, C.: Cell clones with different sensitivity to cytostatic drugs in methylcholanthrene-induced mouse sarcomas. *Acta Pathol. Microbiol. Scand.* **82:**41–47, 1974a.

Hakansson, L., and Trope, C.: On the presence within tumors of clones that differ in sensitivity to cytostatic drugs. *Acta Pathol. Microbiol. Scand.,* **82:**35–40, 1974b.

Hart, I. R.: Selection and characterization of an invasive variant of the B16 melanoma. *Am. J. Pathol.,* **97:**587–600, 1979.

Hart, I. R.: Mechanisms of tumor cell invasion. *Cancer Biol. Rev.,* **2:**29–58, 1981.

Hart, I. R., and Fidler, I. J.: The role of organ selectivity in the determination of metastatic patterns of B16 melanoma. *Cancer Res.,* **40:**2281–2287, 1980.

Hart, I. R.; Talmadge, J. E.; and Fidler, I. J.: Metastatic behavior of a murine reticulum cell sarcoma exhibiting organ-specific growth. *Cancer Res.,* **41:**1281–1287, 1981.

Heel, R. C.; Brogden, R. N.; Speight, T. M.; and Avery G. S.: Tamoxifen: A review of its pharmacologic properties and therapeutic use in the treatment of breast cancer. *Drugs,* **16:**1–24, 1978.

Hellman, S.; Harris, J. R.; Canellos, G. P.; and Fisher, B.: Cancer of the breast. In DeVita, V. T., Jr.; Hellman, S.; and Rosenberg, S. A. (eds.): *Cancer Principles and Practice of Oncology.* J. B. Lippincott Company, Philadelphia, 1982.

Heppner, G. H.; Dexter, D. L.; DeNucci, T.; Miller, F. R.; and Calabresi, P.: Heterogeneity in drug sensitivity among tumor cell subpopulations of a single mammary tumor. *Cancer Res.,* **38:**3758–3763, 1978.

Hewitt, H. B., and Blake, E.: Quantitative studies of trans-lymphnodal passage of tumour cells naturally disseminated from a non-immunogenic murine squamous carcinoma. *Br. J. Cancer,* **31:**25–35, 1975.

Heyn, R. M.; Joo, P.; Karon, M.; Nesbit, M.; Shore, N.; Breslow, N.; Weiner, J.; Reed, A.; and Hammond, D.: BCG in the treatment of acute lymphatic leukemia. *Blood,* **46:**431–442, 1975.

Huggins, C.; Stevens, R. E.; and Hodges, C. V.: Studies on prostatic cancer. II. The effects of castration on advanced carcinoma of the prostate gland. *Arch. Surg.,* **43:**209, 1941.

Isaacs, J. T.; Wake, N.; Cofey, D. S.; and Sandberg, A. A.: Genetic instability coupled to clonal selection as a mechanism for progression in the Dunning R-3327 rat prostatic adenocarcinoma system. *Cancer Res.* **42:**2353–2371. 1982.

Jones, D. S.; Wallace, A. C.; and Fraser, E. E.: Sequence of events in experimental metastases of Walker 256 tumor: Light, immunofluorescent, and electron microscopic observations. *J.N.C.I.,* **46:**493–504, 1971.

Ketcham, A. S.; Kinsey, D. L.; Wexler, H.; and Mantel, N.: The development of spontaneous metastases after the removal of a "primary" tumor. II Standardization protocol of 5 animal tumors. *Cancer* **14:**875–882, 1961.

Ketcham, A. S.; Sugarbaker, E. V.; Ryan, J. J.; and Orme, S. K.: Clotting factors and metastasis formation. *Am. J. Roent.,* **111:**42–47, 1971.

Kiang, D. T., and Kennedy, B. J.: Tamoxifen (antiestrogen) therapy in advanced breast cancer. *Ann. Intern. Med.,* **87:**687–690, 1977.

Kinsey, D. L. An experimental study of preferential metastasis. *Cancer,* **13:**674–676, 1960.

Klefstrom, P.; Holsti, P.; Grohn, P.; and Heinonen, E.: Combination of levamisole immunotherapy with conventional treatment in breast cancer. In Terry, W. P., and Rosenberg, S. A. (eds.): *Immunotherapy of Human Cancer.* Elsevier North-Holland, Inc., New York, 1981.

Klein, E.; Burgess, G. H.; and Helm, F.: Neoplasms of the skin. In Holland, J. F., and Frei, E. (eds.): *Cancer Medicine.* Lea & Febiger, Philadelphia, 1973.

Kleinerman, J., and Liotta, L.: Release of tumor cells. In Day, S. (ed.): *Progress in Cancer Research and Therapy.* Raven Press, New York, 1977.

Kripke, M. L.; Gruys, E.; and Fidler, I. J.: Metastatic heterogeneity of cells from an ultraviolet light-induced murine fibrosarcoma of recent origin. *Cancer Res.,* **38:**2962–2967, 1978.

Lange, P. H.; Hekmat, K.; Bosl, G.; Kennedy, B. J.; and Fraley, E. E.: Accelerated growth of testicular cancer after cytoreductive surgery. *Cancer,* **45:**1498–1506, 1980.

Legha, S. S.; Davis, H. L.; and Muggia, F. M.: Hormonal therapy of breast cancer: New approaches and concepts. *Ann. Intern. Med.,* **88:**69–77, 1978.

Leith, J. T.; Dexter, D. L.; DeWyngaert, J. K.; Zeman, E. M.; Chu, M. Y.; Calabresi, P.; and Glicksman, A. S.: Differential responses to x-irradiation of subpopulations of two heterogeneous human carcinomas *in vitro. Cancer Res.,* **42:**2556–2561, 1982.

Leukemia Committee and the Working Party on Leukemia in Childhood: Treatment of acute lymphoblastic leukemia. *Br. Med. J.,* **48:**189–194, 1971.

Liotta, L. A.; Kleinerman, J.; Catanzaro, P.; and Rynbrandt, D.: Degradation of basement membrane by murine tumor cells. *J.N.C.I.,* **58**:1427–1431, 1977.

Liotta, L. A.; Tryggvason, K.; Garbison, S.; Hart, I.; Foltz, C. M.; and Slafie, A.: Metastatic potential correlates with enzymatic degradation of basement membrane collagen. *Nature,* **284**:67–68, 1980.

Luce, K. J.; McBride, C. M.; and Frei, E., III: Melanoma. In Holland, J. F., and Frei, E., III (eds.): *Cancer Medicine.* Lea & Febiger, Philadelphia, 1973.

Ludwig, J., and Titus, J. L.: Experimental tumor cell emboli in lymph nodes. *Arch. Pathol.,* **84**:304–311, 1967.

Luft, R.; Olivacrona, H.; Ikkos, D.; Milsson, L. B.; and Mossberg, H.: Hypophysectomy in the management of metastatic disease of the breast. In Carrie, A. (ed.): *Endocrine Aspects of Breast Cancer.* Livingstone, Edinburgh, Scotland, 1958.

Maat, B.: Extrapulmonary colony formation after intravenous injection of tumor cells into heparin treated animals. *Br. J. Cancer,* **37**:369–376, 1978.

Madden, R. E., and Gyure, L.: Translymphnodal passage of tumor cells. *Oncology,* 22, 281–289, 1968.

Mareel, M.: Recent aspects of tumor invasiveness. *Int. Rev. Exp. Pathol.,* **22**:65–125, 1980.

Martin, D. S.: Experimental design for chemotherapeutic cure of spontaneous mammary mouse cancer. *Proc. Am. Assoc. Cancer Res.,* **3**:248, 1961.

Martin, D. S.: The scientific basis for adjuvant chemotherapy. *Cancer Treat. Rev.,* **8**:169–189, 1981.

Marx, J. L.: Natural killer cells help defend the body. *Science,* 210, 624–626, 1980.

Mathe, G.; Amiel, J. L.; Schwarzenberg, L.; Schneider, M.; Cattan, A.; Schlumberger, J. R.; Hayat, M.; and de Vassal, F.: Active immunotherapy for acute lymphoblastic leukemia. *Lancet,* **1**:697–699, 1969.

Mehta, P.: Potential role of platelets in the pathogenesis of tumor metastasis. *Blood,* **63**:55–63, 1984.

Moore, F. D.; VanDevanter, S. B.; Boyden, C. M.; Lokich, J.; and Wilson, R. E.: Adrenalectomy with chemotherapy in the treatment of advanced breast cancer: objective and subjective response rates: Duration and quality of life. *Surgery,* **76**:376–390, 1974.

Nicolson, G. L.: Cancer metastasis. *Sci. Am.,* **240**:66–76, 1979.

Nicolson, G. L., and Poste, G.: Tumor cell diversity and host responses in cancer metastasis. Part I: Properties of metastatic cells. *Curr. Probl. Cancer,* **7**:1–83, 1982.

Nicolson, G. L., and Poste, G.: Tumor cell diversity and host responses in cancer metastasis. Part II: Host immune responses and therapy on metastases. *Curr. Probl. Cancer,* **7**:1–42, 1983.

Nicolson, G. L., and Winkelhake, J. L.: Organ specificity of blood-borne tumour metastasis determined by cell adhesion? *Nature,* **255**:2300–2332, 1975.

Nowell, P. C.: The clonal evolution of tumor cell populations. *Science,* **194**:23–28, 1976.

Otu, A. A.; Russell, R. J.; Wilkinson, P. C.; and White, R. G.: Alterations of mononuclear phagocyte function induced by Lewis lung carcinoma in C57BL mice. *Br. J. Cancer,* **36**:330–340, 1977.

Paranjpe, M.; Engel, L.; Young, N.; and Liotta, L. A.: Activation of human breast carcinoma collagenase through plasminogen activator. *Life Sci.,* **26**:1223–1231, 1980.

Peters, L. J.: Enhancement of syngeneic murine tumour transplantability by whole body irradiation—A nonimmunological phenomenon. *Br. J. Cancer,* **31**:293–300, 1975.

Pomeroy, T. C.: Studies on mechanisms of cortisone-induced metastases of transplantable mouse tumors. *Cancer Res.,* **14**:201–204, 1954.

Poste, G.; Doll, J.; Brown, A. E.; Tzing, J.; and Zeidman, I.: Comparison of the metastatic properties of B16 melanoma clones, subcutaneous tumors, and individual lung metastases. *Cancer Res.,* **42**:2770–2778, 1982.

Prehn, R. T.: Tumor progression and homeostasis. *Adv. Cancer Res.,* **23**:203–236, 1976.

Prout, G. R., Jr.: Prostate gland. In Holland, J. F., and Frei, E., III (eds.): *Cancer Medicine.* Lea & Febiger, Philadelphia, 1973.

Retik, A. B.; Arons, M. S.; Ketcham, A. S.; and Mantel, N.: The effect of heparin on primary tumors and metastases. *J. Surg. Res.,* **2**:49–53, 1962.

Romsdahl, M. M.: Influence of surgical procedures on development of spontaneous lung metastases. *J. Surg. Res.,* **4**:363–370, 1964.

Roos, K., and Dingemans, K. P.: Mechanisms of metastasis. *Biochim. Biophys. Acta,* **560**:135–166, 1979.

Schabel, F. M., Jr.: Rationale for adjuvant chemotherapy. *Cancer,* **39**:2875–2882, 1977.

Schatten, W. E.: An experimental study of postoperative tumor metastases. I. Growth of pulmonary metastases following total removal of primary leg tumor. *Cancer,* **2**:455–459, 1958.

Schweitzer, R. J.: Oophorectomy/adrenalectomy. *Cancer,* **46**:1061–1065, 1980.

Shaeffer, J.; El-Mahdi, A. M.; and Constable, W. C.: Radiation control of microscopic pulmonary metastases in C3H mice. *Cancer,* **32**:346–351, 1973.

Silverstein, M. J.; Byron, R. L., Jr.; Yonemoto, R. H.; Riihimaki, D. V.; and Schuster, G.: Bilateral adrenalectomy for advanced breast cancer: A 21-year experience. *Surgery,* **77**:825–831, 1975.

Simpson-Herren, L.; Sanford, A. H.; and Holmquist, J. P.: Effects of surgery on the cell kinetics of residual tumor. *Cancer Treat. Rep.,* **60**:1749–1760, 1976.

Siracky, J.: An approach to the problem of heterogeneity of human tumor cell populations. *Br. J. Cancer,* **39**:570–577, 1979.

Skipper, H. E.: Adjuvant chemotherapy. *Cancer,* **41**:936–940, 1978.

Smith, I. E.; Fitzharris, B. M.; McKinna, J. A.; Fahmy, D. R.; Nash, A. G.; Neville, A. M.; Gazet, J.-C.; Ford, H. T.; and Powles, T. J.: Aminoglutethimide in treatment of metastatic breast carcinoma. *Lancet,* **2**:646–649, 1978.

Spremulli, E. N.; Dexter, D. L.; Scott, C.; Libby, N. P.; Shochat, D.; Gold, D. V.; and Calabresi, P.: Characterization of two metastatic subpopulations from a human colon carcinoma. *Am. Fed. Clin. Res.,* 424A, 1982.

Spremulli, E. N.; Scott, C.; Campbell, D. E.; Libby, N. P.; Shochat, D.; Gold, D. V.; and Dexter, D. L.: Characterization of two metastatic subpopulations originating from a single human colon carcinoma. *Cancer Res.,* **43**:3828–3835, 1983.

Stackpole, C. W.: Distinct lung-colonizing and lung-metastasizing cell populations in B16 mouse melanoma. *Nature,* **289**:798–800, 1981.

Steel, G. G.; Adams, J.; and Stanely, J.: Size dependence of the response of Lewis lung tumors to BCNU. *Cancer Treat. Rep.,* **60**:1743–1748, 1976.

Stitch, H. F., and Steele, H. D.: DNA content of tumor cells. III. Mosaic composition of sarcomas and carcinomas in man. *J.N.C.I.,* **28**:1207–1218, 1962.

Strauch, L.: The role of collagenases in tumour invasion.

In Tarin, D. (ed.): *Tissue Interactions in Carcinogenesis.* Academic Press, London, 1972.

Sugarbaker, E. V.: Cancer metastasis: A product of tumor host interactions. *Curr. Probl. Cancer,* **3**:1–59, 1979.

Sugarbaker, E. V. Patterns of metastasis in human malignancies. *Cancer Biol. Rev.,* **2**:235–278, 1981.

Sugarbaker, E. V., and Cohen A. M.: Altered antigenicity in spontaneous pulmonary metastases from an antigenic murine sarcoma. *Surgery,* **72**:155–161, 1972.

Sugarbaker, E. V.; Cohen, A. M.; and Ketcham, A. S.: Do metastases metastasize? *Ann. Surg.* **174**:161–166, 1971.

Sugarbaker, E. V.; Thornthwaite, J.; and Ketcham, A. S.: Inhibitory effect of a primary tumor on metastasis. In Day, S. B.; Myers, W. P. L.; Stanely, P.; Garattini, S; and Lewis, M. G. (eds.): *Biologic Mechanisms and Therapy.* Raven Press, New York, 1977.

Sylven, B.: Biochemical and enzymatic factors involved in cellular detachment. In Garattini, S.; and Franchi, G. (eds.): *Chemotherapy of Cancer Dissemination and Metastasis.* Raven Press, New York, 1973.

Talmadge, J. E.; Wolman, S. R.; and Fidler, I. J.: Evidence for the clonal origin of spontaneous metastases. *Science,* **217**:361–362, 1982.

Trope, C.; Aspergen, K.; Kullander, S.; and Astredt, B.: Heterogeneous response of disseminated human ovarian cancers to cytostatics *in vitro. Acta Obstet. Gynecol. Scand.,* **58**:543–546, 1979.

Trope, C.; Hakansson, L.; and Dencker, H.: Heterogeneity of human adenocarcinomas of the colon and the stomach as regards sensitivity to cytostatic drugs. *Neoplasma,* **22**:423–430, 1975.

van de Velde, C., and Carr, I.: Lymphatic invasion and metastasis. *Experientia,* **33**:837–978, 1977.

Vindeløv, L. L.; Hansen, H. H.; Christensen, I. J.; Spang-Thompson, M.; Hirsch, F. R.; Hanson, M.; and Nissen, N. I.: Clonal heterogeneity of small cell anaplastic carcinoma of the lung demonstrated by flow-cytometric DNA analysis. *Cancer Res.,* **40**:4295–4300, 1980.

Vindeløv, L. L.; Hansen, H. H.; Gersel, A.; Hirsch, F. R.; and Nissen, N. I.: Treatment of small-cell carcinoma of the lung monitored by sequential flow cytometric DNA analyses. *Cancer Res.,* **42**:2499–2505, 1982.

Warren, S.: Studies on tumor metastasis. IV. Metastases of cancer of the stomach. *N. Engl. J. Med.,* **209**:825, 1933.

Warwick, M.: Analysis of one hundred and seventy-six cases of carcinoma of the stomach submitted to autopsy *Ann. Surg.,* **88**:216, 1928.

Weiss, L.: A pathobiologic overview of metastasis. *Semin. Oncol.,* **4**:5–17, 1977.

Weiss, L., and Glaves, D.: The immunospecificity of altered initial arrest patterns of circulating cancer cells in tumor-bearing mice. *Int. J. Cancer,* **18**:744–777, 1976.

Wilder, R. J.: The historical development of the concept of metastasis. *J. Mt. Sinai Hosp.,* **23**:728–734, 1956.

Willis, R. A.: *The Pathology of Tumors.* Butterworth, London, 1960.

Wood, G. W.: Pit. growth hormone. *Bull. Johns Hopkins Hosp.,* **96**:95, 1955.

Wood, G. W., and Gillespie, G. Y.: Studies on the role of macrophages in regulation of growth and metastasis in murine chemically induced fibrosarcomas. *Int. J. Cancer,* **16**:1022–1029, 1975.

Woodruff, M. F. A.: Tumor inhibitory properties of anaerobic Corynebacteria. *Transplant Proc.,* **7**:229–232, 1975.

Yamanishi, Y.; Maeyens, E.; Kabbous, M. K.; Ohyama, H.; and Hashimoto, K: Collagenolytic activity in malignant melanoma: Physicochemical studies. *Cancer Res.,* **33**:2507–2512, 1973.

Zeidman, I.: Metastasis: A review of recent advances. *Cancer Res.,* **17**:157–162, 1957.

Zeidman, I., and Buss, J. M.: Experimental studies on the spread of cancer in the lymphatic system. I: Effectiveness of the lymph node as a barrier to the passage of embolic tumor cells. *Cancer Res.,* **14**:403–410, 1954.

5

Concepts of Cancer Staging

PHILIP RUBIN

INTRODUCTION

The decision-making process in the multimodal approach to cancer treatment requires a precise description of the cancer in its various extensions. The initial decision is most often the one that determines whether the treatment is a success or failure. The ability to stage the cancer is central to this decision-making process. Each discipline has different capabilities and acts according to the stage of the cancer in attempting to achieve individualization of treatment.

It is important to distinguish the classification from the staging of a cancer. Classification is an all-encompassing system of viewing cancer spread in a multi-dimensional and multi-temporal fashion. Staging refers to a specific time, usually the time of initial diagnosis, when an attempt is made to define the tumor in its various compartments. The stage is a step in the evolution of the cancer spread, particularly if untreated.

Accurate and precise staging is the essential first act for all oncologic disciplines before undertaking treatment. For the surgeon, opportunities exist at each anatomic site for using exploratory and biopsy procedures and for setting the stage for a multidisciplinary design. Often, operative specimens or multiple biopsies are required to be certain of the degree of involvement. For the radiation oncologist, the ability to plan treatment demands that the cancer be confined to the primary site and regional nodal disease. The presence of metastases or the high risk of dissemination is the signal for the medical oncologist to employ chemotherapy.

The term stages of cancer does not imply a progression from stage I to stage IV; rather, these stages are arbitrary divisions, often related to treatment and prognosis. Diagnostic studies must be similarly applied in all cases before placement into a category. Occasionally, host factors preclude the use of more aggressive diagnostic studies. On the other hand, radical surgical treatment could preclude certain diagnostic procedures and circumvent good clinical staging. A balance needs to be maintained in using clinical-diagnostic studies prior to surgical pathologic procedures.

The main purpose of this chapter is to familiarize the clinical oncologist with the current staging systems of the American Joint Committee (AJC) and other schema from international societies that are widely used. The adoption of common systems allows for precise communication among disciplines, assists the multimodal approach to cancer treatment, and allows for accurate reporting of end results. The design of protocols requires a well-defined target group of patients with stratifications to accommodate variations. The key component to treatment decision and selection is most often the stage of the cancer.

HISTORY OF STAGING AND CLASSIFICATION

The terms early and late, operable and inoperable had endless, individualized definitions and meanings. The need for a universally acceptable scheme to classify cancers based on anatomic, histologic, and temporal variables became evident as soon as end results began to

157

be reported. The literature reflected these differences in language and made cross-comparisons of different patient series impossible.

In the 1920s, under the auspices of the League of Nations, gynecologists developed a system of classification and staging of cervical cancer (Dorland's, 1965). This scheme was used to characterize survival data from major cancer institutes worldwide. The concept of developing a consistent classification/staging system for all cancers, however, remained largely dormant until after World War II. The Commission on Stage Grouping and Presentation of Results (ICPR) of the International Congress of Radiology (1953) and the International Union Against Cancer (UICC) consequently did pioneering work in this field. The TNM (tumor, node, metastases) system was an outgrowth of these activities. Denoix (NRCCP, 1950) introduced the TNM language in an attempt to make the classification of cancer more consistent and accurate.

The American Joint Committee for Cancer Staging and End-Results Reporting (AJCCS) was formally organized in 1959. The sponsoring organizations of the committee included The American Cancer Society, The American College of Pathologists, The American College of Physicians, The American College of Radiology, The American College of Surgeons, and the National Cancer Institute. The American College of Surgeons has served as the administrative sponsor of this committee since its inception. The charge of the committee was to develop a system of clinical staging of cancer by body site, acceptable to the practicing community in the United States. Each of the sponsoring organizations nominated members to

serve on this committee. Development of the individual classification and staging systems was the product of various task forces, appointed by the committee to consider cancers of various anatomic sites. The scope of the American Joint Committee for Cancer Staging and End-Results Reporting gradually expanded to include the development of other staging systems (*e.g.*, surgical evaluative staging, postsurgical treatment, pathologic staging), and the creation of checklists to allow more uniform characterization of each cancer site and course, thus promoting the widespread use and appropriate application of classification-staging systems. In the interest of this expanded role, its name was changed in 1980 to the American Joint Committee on Cancer (AJC).

The older UICC, through its TNM Committee, adopted the TNM language for its classification system and began publication of its manual (UICC, 1978). With the formation of the American Joint Committee for Cancer Staging and End-Results Reporting in 1959, a decision was made to adopt the TNM language in the development of its classification system. This was a landmark agreement in the history of staging and classification of cancers. For the first time, the foundation for an international language was laid and the potential for developing a unified staging classification system existed. Hours of effort on the parts of the UICC and the AJC have continued to refine this system and gain its widespread acceptance. Both organizations have published pamphlets summarizing their systems of classification and staging. The first AJC manual for staging cancer (AJC, 1978) was published

Table 5–1. Staging in Cancer of the Larynx

STAGE	UICC*	AJC†	NEILSON	LEDERMAN	TASKINEN AND HOLSTI	GARLAND	BRYCE et al.
I	$T_1N_0M_0$	$T_1N_0M_0$	$T_1N_0M_0$	$T_1N_0M_0$	$T_1N_0M_0$	$T_1N_0M_0$	$T_1N_0M_0$
II	$T_2N_0M_0$ $T_1N_1M_0$	$T_{2-4}N_0M_0$	$T_2N_0M_0$‡	$T_2T_3N_0M_0$§	$T_2N_0M_0$ $T_1N_1M_0$	$T_{2-3}N_0M_0$	$T_2N_0M_0$ $T_1N_1M_0$
III	$T_{3-4}N_0M_0$ $T_{2-4}N_1M_0$ $T_{1-4}N_2M_0$	$T_{1-3}N_1M_0$	$T_2T_3N_0M_0$	$T_{2-4}N_0M_0$‖ $T_1T_4N_1M_0$	$T_3N_0M_0$ $T_{2-3}N_1M_0$ $T_{1-3}N_2M_0$	$T_{1-3}N_1M_0$	$T_3N_0M_0$ $T_{2-3}N_1M_0$ $T_{1-3}N_2M_0$
IV	$T_{1-4}N_3M_0$ $T_{1-4}N_{0-3}M_1$	$T_1N_1M_0$ $T_{1-4}N_2M_0$ $T_{1-4}N_{1-2}M_1$	$T_4N_0M_0$ $T_{1-4}N_{1-3}M_0$ $T_{1-4}N_{0-3}M_1$	$T_{1-4}N_{2-3}M_0$ $T_{1-4}N_{0-3}M_1$	$T_4N_{0-2}M_0$ $T_{1-4}N_3M_0$ $T_{1-4}N_{0-3}M_1$	$T_{1-4}N_2M_0$ $T_{1-4}N_{0-3}M_1$	$T_4N_0M_0$ $T_{1-4}N_3M_0$ $T_{1-4}N_{0-3}M_1$

* Unio Internationalis Contra Cancru.
† American Joint Committee on Cancer Staging and End-Results Reporting.
‡ Excluding cases with a fixed cord from stage II even though the tumor may still be confined to the cords. Such cases are placed in stage III.
§ Mobility of larynx impaired but not lost, or tumor extends beyond its tissue of origin.
‖ Tumor with fixation of larynx or unilateral mobile cervical lymph node metastases or extralaryngeal infiltration.

From Vermund, H.: Role of radiotherapy in cancer of the larynx as related to the TNM system of staging. *Cancer,* 25:485–504, 1970.

in 1978 and republished in 1982. Copies of this manual, as well as booklets characterizing each anatomic site may be obtained free of charge through the offices of the American College of Surgeons (AJC, 1978; UICC, 1978).

The AJC and UICC have worked cooperatively to develop compatible classification systems. Differences remain, but with continued efforts toward unification, these are disappearing (see Table 5–1). These differences are in the interests of recognition of other staging schemes already in widespread use and accepted by the surgical and medical specialists. As one reads the past literature, it is important to be aware that the *same* symbolism of TNM and Roman numeral designation of stages is applied to *different* extents of tumors as shown in Table 5–1. For certain sites staging recommendations have not yet been developed (adrenal, small intestine, urethra, and penis). Incomplete recommendations are present for other areas (pancreas, brain, and bone) for a number of reasons.

The incorporation of widely used systems of international societies representing certain oncologic specialities reduced confusion and conflict. Thus, the FIGO (International Federation of Gynecologic Oncology) classification of all gynecologic cancers was adopted by both the AJC and the UICC and translated into the TNM language (Ulfeder, 1981).

OBJECTIVES OF CLASSIFICATION-STAGING SYSTEMS

The complexities of cancer classification and staging are enormous and it is a tribute to the efforts of the UICC and AJC that they have developed a system that can be easily understood and applied in an unambiguous manner. It is only in this way that the information can be readily communicated to others, both to assist in institutional comparisons and to aid in the subsequent management of patients. As Feinstein has indicated, the purpose of any classification is to affect the treatment decision and prognosis (Feinstein, 1974).

The objectives for a staging system can be briefly summarized as: (1) Aiding the clinician in planning treatment; (2) giving some indication of prognosis; (3) assisting in the evaluation of end results; (4) facilitating the exchange of information between treatment centers; and (5) assisting in the continuing investigation of cancer (Rouvier, 1932; UICC, 1978).

DEFINITION OF TERMINOLOGY AND APPLICATION OF THE TNM SYSTEM

For the purposes of this book, the AJC classification system will be utilized, with notes commenting on other systems in broad use when appropriate. A proposed technique of description and classification applicable to all sites of cancer involves five basic steps:

1. Identification of the extent of disease by the use of the following symbols: T = extent of the primary tumor; N = condition of regional nodes; M = distant metastases: either present or not evident;
2. Assignment of a series of subscripts to each of these three components, indicating ascending degrees of involvement (*e.g.,* T_1, T_2, etc., and N_1, N_2, etc.);
3. Indication of the presence of metastatic disease by M_+, and absence by M_0. For certain sites, a number of specific M categories (M_1, M_2) may be desirable;
4. Grouping of the TNM assignments into a smaller number of clinical stages — usually four. This system makes it possible to regroup multiple categories (approximately 50) into similar staging systems; and
5. Addition of supplementary information based upon the results of histologic examination by attaching the symbol $_+$ or symbols designating specific radiologic studies, such as lymphangiography (*e.g.,* N_{L+}).

Histopathology is a vital attribute of any classification-staging system. The pattern of spread of a particular cancer often is the reflection of the specific cell type, its stage of differentiation, and degree of anaplasia. The language for describing histopathology is now being standardized from two major sources: the multiple columns constituting the *Atlases of Tumor Pathology* published by the Armed Forces Institute of Pathology and the World Health Organization's efforts entitled *International Classification of Tumors* (NRCCP, 1950; WHO, 1976).

Temporal values are defined in the TNM classification scheme to allow an update to occur after certain data have been obtained as follows:

1. *$_c$TNM clinical-diagnostic staging:* This allows for the pretreatment characteriza-

tion by clinical examination and specific diagnostic studies to define the tumor and allow its comparison following treatment;

2. *sTNM surgical-evaluative staging:* This terminology is applied following a major surgical exploration or biopsy;

3. *tTNM postsurgical treatment-pathologic staging:* This term characterizes the extent of the cancer following thorough examination of the resected surgical specimen;

4. *rTNM retreatment staging:* In instances in which the initial therapy has failed and additional treatment decisions are being considered, the disease is restaged under this terminology; and

5. *aTNM autopsy staging:* Final staging, after the post mortem, is the terminology reserved for this designation.

ONCOTAXONOMY — A UNIFIED CLASSIFICATION

Oncotaxonomy is the concept of one standard set of TNM definitions based on uniform criteria for all sites. The criteria are identified in Table 5 – 1 and are based upon an analysis of the numerous TNM systems in which specific words defining extent of disease are associated with certain categories (Rubin, 1973). The order of tumor progression is reflected in T_1, T_2, T_3, T_4, N_0, N_1, etc. A consistent cancer language allows for a uniform approach to tumor imaging and eventually to the cancer staging and management decisions. Modifications will be required at individual sites, but the basic features will remain similar, if not identical.

Tumor (T) Categories

The criterion for categorizing a primary tumor (T) is the apparent anatomic extent of the disease (see Table 5 – 2), based on clinical, diagnostic-imaging, surgical, or pathologic data. The extent commonly is dependent upon three features: depth of invasion, surface spread, and size. With the application of computed tomography (CT), ultrasound, and digital imaging techniques and, in the near future, nuclear magnetic resonance (NMR) imaging, these features should be more easily quantifiable.

Depth of invasion is a difficult yet critical criterion to be evaluated in defining any tumor. This is the main criterion utilized and primarily consists of the degree of invasion into adjacent or surrounding structures such as muscle, capsule, bone, cartilage, and the viscera. The loss of mobility or the fixation of the tumor to another structure is utilized in many schema. Figure 5 – 1 illustrates, in a unified fashion, the variety of tissues often involved at different primary sites. The fibrous capsule in solid organs, in contrast to the intrinsic muscle wall of hollow organs, is often the first tissue invaded by the cancer.

Surface spread is even more difficult to categorize, but may be related to the size of the tumor as well as to the organ of origin. Whether the organ is solid or hollow also determines its description. In solid organs, the largest dimension of the measured tumor is the one most often used. In hollow organs, the size of the primary tumor is given in terms of the tumor's circumferential or longitudinal spread. In some organs, arbitrary divisions into regions where a percentage of surface area

Table 5 – 2.   Specific Criteria Related to T Categories

CRITERIA	T_1	T_2	T_3	T_4
Depth of invasion				
Solid organs	Confined	Capsule muscle	Bone cartilage	Viscera
Hollow organs	Submucosa	Muscularis	Serosa	
Mobility	Mobile	Partial mobility	Fixed	Fixed and destructive
Neighboring structures	Not invaded	Adjacent (attached)	Surrounding (detached)	Viscera
Surface spread				
Regions (R)	½ or R_1	R_1	$R_1 + R_2$	$R_1 + R_2 + R_3$
Circumference	< ⅓	⅓ to ½	> ½ to ⅔	> ⅔
Size				
Diameter	< 2 cm	2 to 4 or 5 cm	> 4 to 5 cm	> 10 cm

From Rubin, P.: A unified classification of cancers: An oncotaxonomy with symbols. *Cancer,* **31:**963–982, 1973.

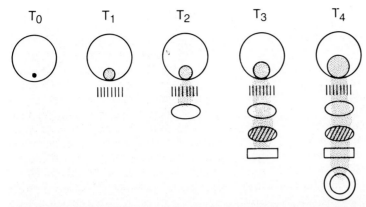

Figure 5–1. Classification of solid viscera. This series of symbols portrays the organ as a large circle and the dotted, smaller circles as the cancer. The vertical lines are adjacent muscle; the clear oval is an adjacent attached structure; the lined oval is a surrounding, often detached structure. The rectangle stands for bone or cartilage, and the double circle for another viscera. The gravity of cancer spread or progress is identified in the sequential spread shown symbolically in most sites and is the basis of most classifications of T_1, T_2, T_3, and T_4. For a solid structure or site: T_1 = Confined to the organ of origin, usually 2.0 cm in its largest diameter, localized, and mobile; T_2 = Deeply involving, usually 2.0 cm up to 4.0 cm in its largest diameter, localized, and mobile or partially mobile; T_3 = Regionally confined, usually greater than 4.0 or 5.0 cm but less than 10 cm, and fixed; and T_4 = A massive lesion, greater than 10 cm in diameter, destructive, and not confined to organ. From Rubin, P.: A unified classification of cancers: An oncotaxonomy with symbols. *Cancer,* **31**:963–982, 1973.

involved can be used in an attempt to quantify extent of tumor spread (see Table 5–1).

The size of a tumor is related to the number of cells present. This is more true earlier in the life of the tumor rather than later, when features of hemorrhage, necrosis, and other factors have intervened. Rate of tumor growth, cell removal or loss, and host resistance are obvious factors that will affect spread patterns. Even under the most controlled conditions in the laboratory, measurement of tumor volume used as an estimate of growth is fraught with error. As soon as the tumor becomes grossly palpable, changes in growth fraction, cell cycle, and cell loss occur. Nonetheless, these estimates are often provided as guidelines of tumor behavior and determine the stage.

Factors not used in categorizing primary tumors are location of the tumor within an organ, rate of tumor growth, multiplicity, and appearance of the tumor as either exophytic or endophytic. The reasons for these omissions are due to the difficulties in the relative weighing of each of these characteristics as well as in their evaluation subsequent to treatment and in prognosis.

To understand the applications of this tumor classification, a model system is presented as an illustration. Two basic differences in application exist, depending upon whether the organ system in question is solid (see Figure 5–1) or hollow (see Figure 5–2) anatomically. The common example is as follows:

T_X: Tumor cannot be assessed;

T_0: No evidence of primary tumor, grossly or microscopically;

T_{is}: Carcinoma *in situ;*

T_1: A lesion confined to the organ of origin. The tumor is mobile, does not invade adjacent or surrounding structures or tissue, and is often superficial;

T_2: A localized lesion characterized by deep extension into adjacent structures or tissues. The invasion is into the surrounding capsules, ligaments, intrinsic muscles, and adjacent, attached structures or similar tissues. There is some loss of tumor mobility but it is not complete, therefore true fixation is not present;

T_3: An advanced tumor that is confined to the region rather than the organ of origin, whether that organ is solid or hollow. The critical determinant is the presence of fixation, which indicates invasion into the adjacent, surrounding structures. These structures most often are bone or cartilage, but invasion of the extrinsic muscle walls, serosa, and skin should also be included. Invasion of surrounding detached structures of a different anatomy or function are in this category; and

T_4: A massive lesion extending into another hollow organ causing a fistula, or into another solid organ, causing a sinus. Invasion into major nerves, arteries, and veins is also placed in this category. In addition

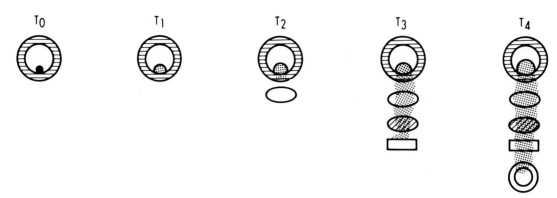

Figure 5–2. Classification of hollow organs. The model for classification of cancers of hollow viscera is illustrated by a linear arrangement of symbols for neighboring structures similar to the model for solid viscera (see Figure 5–1). The major exception is the placement of muscle in the wall of the viscera as compared to its juxtaposed relationship in numerous solid organs. The order of progression is: T_1 = Superficially invading, limited to mucosa or submucosa, less than one-third of circumference, localized, and occupying not more than one region; T_2 = Deeply invading into muscularis, more than one-third but less than one-half of the lumen circumference, and occupying more than one-half of the region, mobile; T_3 = Invading all layers of the visceral wall, through serosa, into surrounding structures, fixed but not necessarily to bone, covering more than one-half of circumference, and occupying more than one visceral site; and T_4 = A massive, destructive lesion, causing a fistula or sinus, covering more than two-thirds of circumference, resulting in complete luminal obstruction, and occupying more than two visceral regions. From Rubin, P.: A unified classification of cancers: An oncotaxonomy with symbols. *Cancer,* **31**:963–982, 1973.

to fixation, the destruction of bone is another advanced sign, placing the tumor in this category.

Nodal (N) Categories

The establishment of lymph node categories is as critical in design as the T classification; however, the criteria currently used are more varied, vague in definition, and, occasionally, arbitrarily assigned. A unified code needs to be agreed upon, and more consistency needs to be achieved.

The criteria of node evaluation consist of size; firmness; capsular invasion; depth of in-

vasion; mobility versus fixation; single versus multiple nodes; ipsilateral, contralateral, and bilateral distribution; as well as distant nodal metastases (see Table 5–3).

The *first station* is the cluster of lymph nodes receiving direct drainage of a specific site or organ; the regional nodes are considered the first station. The *second station* refers to those nodes that commonly receive lymph drainage from another lymph node rather than directly from the site or organ and are termed juxtaregional. This concept is a distinction with a meaningful clinical difference. Whether the drainage is unilateral or bilateral is important, as the designation for contralateral nodes de-

Table 5–3. Specific Criteria Related to N Categories

STATION	N_1 FIRST	N_2 FIRST	N_3 FIRST	N_4 SECOND
Drainage				
Unilateral	Ipsilateral	Ipsilateral	Ipsilateral	Contralateral
Bilateral	Ipsilateral	Contralateral or bilateral	Ipsilateral or contralateral	Distant
Number	Solitary	Multiple		
Size	<2 to 3 cm	>3 cm	>5 cm	>10 cm
Mobility	Mobile	Partial matted muscle invasion	Fixed to vessels, bone, skin	Fixed and destructive

To distinguish N_a from N_1 the specific criteria include: Size, between 1 and 2 cm; Firmness, soft to hard; Roundness, ½ cm to 1 cm.

From Rubin, P.: A unified classification of cancers: An oncotaxonomy with symbols. *Cancer,* **31**:963–982, 1973.

pends upon whether such contralateral nodes drain a site directly or indirectly, that is, whether they are N_2 or N_4. There are many variations in nodal drainage, and in some sites there are multiple first stations.

Size is one of the most important criteria, because a node must be palpable or detectable. When does a node reach a size to be considered noteworthy, disregarding its firmness? Most often this size threshold is considered somewhat greater than 1.0 cm but less than 3.0 cm. The use of size to categorize a progression of nodal categorization is not unlike the use of size in categorizing the primary tumor.

Firmness is another important criterion in differentiating the N_0 situation from N_1.

Roundness refers to the measurement of nodal thickness and implies a hard, pea-sized node. A discoid or flat node is usually a shoddy node. The rounder a node and the firmer the node, the more likely it is to be involved by tumor.

The *number* of involved nodes is another variable in categorization. Solitary nodal involvement, as distinct from multiple nodal involvement, is commonly considered. The presence of multiple nodes is often associated with invasion of the capsule of the node, resulting in matting or clustering and eventually in a loss of mobility.

Mobility versus fixation is an important criterion in considering progression. The term fixation is used but rarely defined in classification schema. The loss of mobility of a lymph node is due to invasion of the nodal capsule. Matted nodes or invasion into the fascia of muscle reduces lateral and vertical mobility; the oncologist can no longer roll the node in all directions. Invasion into muscle can be determined by loss of mobility upon contraction of the muscle. Complete fixation refers to the direct invasion of bone, major vessels, or skin.

As in the primary (T) category above, a model classification for illustrating the application of a unified system to lymph node (N) involvement is presented. Figure 5–3 summarizes this model classification.

N_x: Regional nodes cannot be assessed clinically;

N_0: Regional lymph nodes are not demonstrably abnormal. This category quite surprisingly represents a significant point of conflict between the classifications used by the UICC and the AJC. The issue is the absence of palpable nodes versus the finding of palpable but not clinically important adenopathy. In the latter situation, shoddy, soft nodes usually less than 1 cm in size are the clinical finding in question. These palpable, flat nodes of little importance are listed as N_0 in the AJC classification, but N_{1a} in the UICC system. In the interest of reaching a common agreement, the AJC has adopted the UICC designation;

N_1: Palpable, freely movable lymph nodes limited to the first station of involvement. A distinction must again be made between an uninvolved node and an involved node. Metastases are suggested but are based on lymph node firmness and roundness of the node, rather than its size alone. The presence of multiple lymph nodes does not change this category provided the nodes are confined to the regional primary station center and are not matter together;

N_2: Firm to hard lymph nodes, palpable yet partially movable, ranging in size from 3 cm to 5 cm. Such nodes may show microscopic evidence of capsular invasion and clinically they may be matted together, demonstrating partial fixation to adjacent muscle. These nodes may be contralateral or bilateral if the primary tumor drains to both sides because of its anatomy, but involvement is confined to the first station. Multiple lymph nodes tend to be in this category. Mobility is reduced and the nodes cannot be moved in all directions;

N_3: Fixation is now complete; with node invasion beyond the capsule with complete fixation to adjacent bone, to large blood vessels, to skin (dermal lymphatic invasion), or to the nerves (perineural invasion); and

N_4: This category is reserved for lymph node involvement beyond the first station, in second or more distant stations. Extensive nodal necrosis, leading to destruction of bone and skin (fistula formation), or massive size (10 cm or greater) should also be placed in this category.

Metastases (M) Categories

Some debate exists as to whether or not the metastatic category should be expanded to reflect solitary metastases as well as the number of metastatic lesions or anatomic sites in-

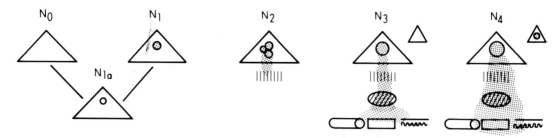

Figure 5–3. Classification of lymph nodes. The triangle stands for a node-bearing region. The large triangle represents the first station node or regional node, and the small triangle is the second station or juxtaregional node. The small, dotted circles are the cancer. The vertical lines are muscle, the lined oval is a surrounding, separate structure, the rectangle is bone or cartilage, the cylinder represents blood vessels, and the horizontal lines skin. The order of progression of the cancer extends as shown with increasing involvement of surrounding structures in N_1, N_2, N_3, and N_4. From Rubin, P.: A unified classification of cancers: An oncotaxonomy with symbols. *Cancer*, **31**:963–982, 1973.

volved. At the present time, the M category is dealt with simply as follows:

M_x = The presence of metastatic disease is not assessed;

M_0 = No evidence of metastatic disease; and

M_1 = Distant metastases are present. The specific sites for metastatic disease should be individually noted.

The lack of a consistent and thorough categorization of the anatomic extent of metastases is conspicuous in the current schema (see Table 5–4). The important feature is the presence or absence of metastases, that is, M_0 versus M_1. The reason for this reflects the poor prognosis if metastases are present. Nevertheless, cure, though rare, is possible for some solitary metastases. As chemotherapy becomes more effective and results are assessed, there will be a need to categorize and subclassify this group of patients.

One proposed classification of metastases (Rubin, 1973; Rubin and Keys, 1982) is based upon the criteria of number of metastases, the

number of organ systems involved, and the degree of functional impairment present. The designation of M_x for no metastatic work-up should be used, rather than M_0, only when the likelihood of metastatic disease is considered low.

The following classification schema for metastases to selected sites is offered (see also Figure 5–4):

M_0: No evidence of metastases;

M_1: Solitary, isolated metastasis confined to one organ or anatomic site;

M_2: Multiple metastatic foci confined to one organ system or one anatomic site; for example, lungs, skeleton, liver; no functional impairment to minimal functional impairment;

M_3: Multiple organs involved anatomically, no functional impairment or minimal to moderate functional impairment of involved organs;

M_4: Multiple organs involved anatomically, moderate to severe functional impairment of involved organs;

Table 5–4. Specific Criteria Related to M Categories

	M_1	M_2	M_3	M_4
Number of metastases	1	>1	Multiple	Multiple
Number of organs	1	1	Multiple	Multiple
Impairments	0	Minimal	Minimal to moderate	Moderate to severe

M: Modified to show viscera involved by lettered subscript as: pulmonary (M_p), hepatic (M_h), osseous (M_0), skin (M_s), brain (M_b), etc.
M_+: Microscopic evidence of suspected metastases, confirmed by pathologic examination.

From Rubin, P.: A unified classification of cancers: An oncotaxonomy with symbols. *Cancer*, **31**:963–982, 1973.

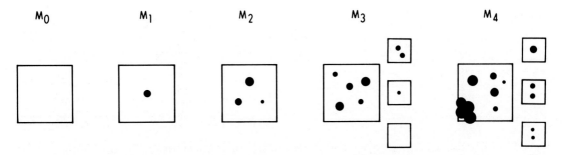

Figure 5–4. Metastatic taxonomy. Each box stands for a visceral organ or organs, and the black dots stand for the number of metastatic lesions. The stages are explained in the text, and the order of progression is M_1, M_2, M_3, and M_4. The number of organs and number of metastases increases. From Rubin, P.: A unified classification of cancers: An oncotaxonomy with symbols. *Cancer,* **31**:963–982, 1973.

M_x: No metastatic work-up;

M: Modified to show viscera involved by letter subscript: pulmonary metastases (M_p); hepatic (M_h); osseous (M_o); skin (M_s); brain (M_b).

M_+: Microscopic evidence of suspected metastases, confirmed by pathologic examination.

In considering this system of classification, note that visceral involvement by direct extension is not considered a metastases.

Stage Grouping

The problem of having four categories for the primary tumor (T), and four categories for regional nodes (N), plus two categories for metastases (M) means that each patient can be placed in 32 different categories.

The number of stages is unmanageable for the clinician, therefore the reduction to four stage groupings has become the clinical custom. Thus, the challenge in developing a unified stage grouping system is in determining which T and N categories to combine. The major clinical consideration is to determine which T and N categories have similar prognostic significance. Furthermore, the sum total of both components may be greater than either of its parts, or the nodal category may outweigh considerations at the primary site. Because of these varying circumstances, four possibilities with regard to the stage of the T lesion and its N_1 equivalent are shown in the grid analysis (see Figure 5–5), and those have been employed as shown in four different cancers:

$N_1 = T_1$ as in lung cancer (Feinstein, 1974; AJC, 1978);

$N_1 = T_2$ as in breast cancer (Feinstein, 1974; AJC, 1978);

$N_1 = T_3$ as in cervical cancer of the uterus (Feinstein, 1974; UICC, 1978); and

$N_1 = T_4$ as in laryngeal cancer (NRCCP, 1950; Feinstein, 1974).

Is there a common characteristic or feature? Prognostic outcome is the most obvious consideration. An alternate consideration relates to the resectability of the primary and its node stations.

THE PROCESSES OF CLASSIFICATION AND STAGING

There is a need to define both the minimum and optimum diagnostic work-ups that establish the extent or stage of the cancer. Differences exist here with respect to the UICC and AJC classification system. The UICC system declares all diagnostic radiologic procedures and endoscopy used in the evaluation of the cancer acceptable but does not include the operative findings. Operative findings are allowed in some specific sites that are otherwise inaccessible, as in ovarian tumor categories. The AJC allows inclusion of all types of examinations ordinarily available to the average specialist. Surgical and pathologic findings are not used in assigning a clinical stage, except in certain sites where specific procedures are necessary for the determination of the stage. One of the major sources of confusion is this use of different studies and criteria to arrive at the definition of extent of the cancer. Unless the criteria and examinations for definition are standardized, different groups of patients may be mistakenly placed in similar categories.

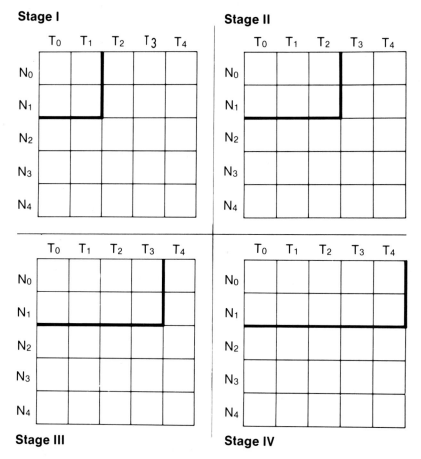

Figure 5–5. In this grid the stage grouping of N_1 with a T lesion varies with different sites so that stage I disease in lung is T_1N_1, stage II in breast is T_2N_1, stage III in uterine cervix is T_3N_1, and stage IV in larynx is T_4N_1. From Rubin, P.: A unified classification of cancers: An oncotaxonomy with symbols. *Cancer,* **31:**963–982, 1973.

In brief, there are four steps in the definition of the extent of any given tumor:

1. *Clinical staging:* The evaluation of the apparent extent of the tumor, based on physical examination, routine laboratory studies, and radiographic and endoscopic procedures;
2. *Radiographic staging:* The use of sophisticated radiographic procedures, such as selective arteriography, computed tomography, digital radiography, lymphangiography, and others, in tumor evaluation;
3. *Surgical staging:* Inclusion of the results of the exploratory procedure employed in the identification of the extent of a cancer, such as laparotomy in Hodgkin's disease or ovarian cancer. The use of a biopsy procedure and histologic evaluation to determine the depth of invasion,

histopathology, and presence or absence of nodal disease is also of importance here; and
4. *Pathologic staging:* Refers to a complete pathologic evaluation that implies total removal of the cancer and its site and organ of origin.

It is important to avoid interchanging clinical, surgical, or pathologic staging in reporting results unless doing so is specified and generally accepted. Categories for reporting these individual results are specified and summarized by the AJC system.

The inclusion of specific categories to modulate the classification system at different times using surgical, pathologic, and retreatment staging data is critical to the staging process. Often, there is a tendency to supplant these diseases.

For most *extensive diseases,* at that time

when the primary is locally invasive and is destructively eroding bone, fixing to blood vessels and viscera (T_3, T_4), and/or nodal disease is found (N_1, N_2, or N_3), there is a need to utilize procedures that provide the best oncologic images of these local and regional extensions. CT and ultrasound are utilized at most sites, particularly those that are inaccessible to direct physical examination or indirect endoscopic study. Most often, if the risk is high for metastatic disease, a thorough search for occult deposits is justified. In addition to those routine studies noted in the previous section, one should add CT scans or nuclear scans of the skeleton, liver, and brain.

When *metastatic disease* is found on presentation, it is quite often part of an advanced cancer with a large primary and/or nodal collection. There are times when the primary is smaller than the metastasis or even hidden, and a thorough search may be required. Most often, other remote sites such as liver, bone, lung, brain, and bone marrow are evaluated with appropriate studies.

The clinical oncologist must be aware of the history of the different neoplasms, their potential for spread, their distribution patterns, and their incidence of metastases. The search for occult metastases is often time consuming and costly; discrimination in ordering studies is both sensible and cost effective. The spread of tumors usually obeys the known anatomic paths of dissemination. Capitalizing on this knowledge, the oncologist should direct testing during his initial diagnosis and subsequent follow-up of cancer patients. The histopathology of each cancer and its site of origin determine in large part its pattern of spread and behavior. The subjective and objective findings are elicited by a thorough research of *history,* a *physical examination,* and direct subsequent clinical staging by surgical staging. This has been one of the missed opportunities in guiding clinical judgments because of the manner in which the data are recorded in the literature. If the clinical and radiologic assessments were made first, and then the restaging allocations into new categories based on surgical and pathologic findings were made, there would be improved accuracy of both clinical and radiologic evaluation. In fact, surgical exploration for staging rather than for resection is a redirection of surgical oncologic effort and is essential for multidisciplinary decision making. The criteria for each step in the staging sequence should be clearly indicated, and the oncologist

should not confuse these procedural steps and assignments. The transition from a clinical-diagnostic radiologic to a post-surgical pathologic staging, for example, marks the transition from a unidisciplinary to a multidisciplinary cancer management strategy.

THE DECISION-MAKING PROCESS IN CANCER MANAGEMENT

The order or sequence of working-up patients depends on the stage of advancement.

For early, small, localized lesions, particularly those that have no overt evidence of extension to surrounding structures (T_1, T_2), the regional nodal compartment needs to be evaluated next. If the nodal compartment is negative (N_0), there may be no indication to extensively work-up the patient for metastatic disease, that is, chest films, liver chemistries, and routine hemograms are adequate. For some neoplasms such as oat cell cancer and non-Hodgkin's lymphomas, bone marrow studies are indicated, since dissemination occurs early in laboratory and tumor-imaging examinations. A brief description of commonly used staging procedures for uncovering metastatic disease follows, because these are of greatest interest to the medical oncologist and determine the use of chemotherapy.

Staging Procedures for Pulmonary Metastases

Radiography. The lung is the most common site of metastasis and, fortunately, is one of the most readily imaged organs. One should not minimize the usefulness of plain chest radiography. The multiple projection technique, as well as tomographic evaluation, frequently defines initial hematogenous dissemination from distant sites.

Tomography. Whole lung plain film tomography, as well as computed tomography of the thorax, is a useful adjunct to the initial staging procedures in a patient whose tumor is known to spread rapidly and early. Such tumors include malignant melanoma, hypernephroma, soft tissue sarcomas, and testicular tumors (Polga and Watnick, 1976; Muhm *et al.,* 1977; Sindelar *et al.,* 1978; Chang *et al.,* 1979). Although lesions slightly smaller than 1 cm can be distinguished on plain radiography, lesions half that size (5 mm) can be identified with careful film tomography or computed tomography. Each of these modalities can be useful in excluding an isolated pulmonary mass from concern by demonstrating central calcification, which usually denotes benign granulomatous disease (Neifeld *et al.,* 1977; Rubin, 1983). Because of a 50% false-positive rate, the CT scan should be used cautiously by itself, particularly if resection of isolated pulmonary nodules is being contemplated (Sindelar *et al.,* 1978).

Exfoliative Cytology. Exfoliative cytology of sputa and bronchial brushings has been useful in the diagnosis of primary lung cancer, which can be detected in 75% of such cases, whereas secondary foci can be detected in 50% of cases where the lesion exceeds 2.5 cm in diameter (Kern and Schweizer, 1976).

Staging Procedures for Bone Metastases

Technetium 99m Polyphosphate Isotopes. Technetium 99m polyphosphate isotopes demonstrate the reactive response to destructive processes within bone. Most metastases, whether they are osteoblastic or osteolytic, evoke a response that can be imaged using these radioisotopes (Peck, 1972; Mall *et al.,* 1976; McNeil, 1978). The sensitivity of the examination is extremely high, and findings predate destructive or osteoblastic disease as defined by plain radiography, frequently by as much as six months (Roberts *et al.,* 1976; Joo *et al.,* 1979). While the sensitivity of such studies is high, the specificity is rather low. Metabolic diseases, trauma, and infection can all result in similar appearance by bone scan. Solitary abnormalities in bone scans in asymptomatic patients can represent benign entities in 33% of patients (Corcoran *et al.,* 1976). This high false-positive rate makes bone scans unsuitable as a primary screen in early stage breast cancer.

Skeletal Radiography. Skeletal radiography can be targeted, following the lead of bone scans. Plain films of the skeleton, including tomograms, require 30% to 50% of bone deossification to be identified as abnormal (O'Mara, 1976). Once they are identified as abnormal, however, the specificity of the abnormality is greater than with isotope scanning. Some small-cell tumors such as Ewing's sarcoma, non-Hodgkin's lymphoma, and multiple myeloma fail to evoke a response in bone and frequently appear negative on bone scans, whereas x-ray identification may prove positive.

Bone Biopsy. Lesions identified because of an increased uptake of bone scanning agents and subsequently defined by radiography can be biopsied either percutaneously or through an open approach. Benign and confusing lesions of bone can occur in the patient with cancer and one cannot assume that all osseous abnormalities are manifestations of disseminated tumors. Biopsy can be employed to resolve the confusion faced in these cases but should be done with caution to avoid future fracture through the biopsy site.

Staging Procedures for Liver Metastases

Increase of Enzymes. Metastases to the liver, if large enough and numerous enough, manifest their presence by an increase of liver enzymes, particularly lactic dehydrogenase (LDH). Alkaline phosphatase and serum glutamic oxaloacetic transaminase (SGOT) lack the sensitivity of LDH elevation, but the LDH is falsely positive with greater frequency. In a patient with known normal liver enzymes, however, a subsequent elevation of any combination of these three may herald the presence of metastatic disease (Kim *et al.,* 1977).

Imaging Techniques. Common techniques currently employed for imaging the liver to substantiate metastatic disease include technetium 99m sulphur colloid (which is approximately 80% accurate), as well as the direct imaging techniques of computed tomography and ultrasound (Lunia *et al.,* 1975; Kagan and Gilbert, 1976; McArdle, 1976; Biello *et al.,* 1978). The size threshold with isotope remains in the 2 to 2½ cm range, although slightly smaller lesions can be detected with either computed tomography or ultrasound.

The high incidence of false-positive scans (up to 40%) can be explained by other entities such as the fatty replacement of the liver seen in alcoholics. Because other entities produce filling defects, the differential diagnosis includes adenomas, abscesses, and vascular abnormalities (Hooper *et al.,* 1978). CT and ultrasound share equal sensitivity and specificity attributes. Angiography can be useful for positive imaging of metastases when equivocal findings are encountered with CT and ultrasound (Bragg, 1976).

Staging Procedures for Brain Metastases

Computed Tomography. During the past three to four years, computed tomography has replaced angiography, pneumoencephalography, and technetium 99m sodium pertechnetate studies in the evaluation of metastatic disease (Aronson *et al.,* 1964; Deck *et al.,* 1976). Although computed tomography does detect metastases with greater reliability than do nuclear scans, it nevertheless fails to detect 40% of brain metastases seen at autopsy. Multiple foci rather than a solitary finding in a symptomatic patient increases its reliability (Weiss *et al.,* 1980).

Angiography. Multiple focal lesions seen on computed tomography pose no diagnostic dilemmas. The solitary intracranial metastasis, however, can be confused with other non-neoplastic processes, such as abscess and resolving infarction, thereby requiring angiography as an adjunctive tool for differentiation.

Staging Procedures for Lymph Node Metastases

Lymphangiography. Evaluation of pelvic lymph nodes is best studied with the use of lymphangiography, particularly when staging tumors of cervical, rectal, prostatic, and bladder origins.

Computed Tomography and Ultrasound. Lymph nodes in the superior abdominal chain such as the periaortic or celiac, are best visualized with the techniques of computed tomography and ultrasound. The obese patient may best be studied by computed tomography, whereas the thin patient, lacking adequate fat surrounding normal viscera, may best be studied by ultrasound (Lee *et al.,* 1978).

Laparotomy. None of these modalities, if negative, should preclude further evaluation if clinically indicated, particularly with specific tumors such as lymphomas. Under such circumstances, exploratory laparotomy with lymphadenectomy may be necessary for definitive staging.

Staging Procedures in Metastases of Unknown Origin

Approximately 3 to 5% of patients with neoplastic disease present with metastases although the primary is undetermined (Hobbs and Rodriquez, 1980; Holmes and Fouts, 1970; Kagan and Gilbert, 1976; Krementz *et al.,* 1977; Nystrom *et al.,* 1977; Nystrom *et al.,* 1979).

Adenopathy of the High- and Midneck. Cervical adenopathy (high- and midneck) of a squamous histology is usually found to be secondary to head and neck carcinomas. Lower neck and supraclavicular nodes with squa-

mous cell cancer always demand a search for a lung cancer primary. Supraclavicular lymph nodes of the adenocarcinoma variety frequently have spread from the thyroid, stomach, colon, or pancreas, although the lung must be considered as well.

Metastases of the Lung, Liver, and Skeleton. The preponderance, however, of metastases of adenocarcinomatous histology, manifesting themselves by metastases within the lungs, liver, or skeleton, pose a great diagnostic mystery. In fewer than 15% of such cases will the primary tumor ever be found, even at *post mortem* (Krementz *et al.,* 1977). In approximately 8% of such cases, the primary tumor will be diagnosed before the patient's death.

Random Searches for Primaries. With such dismal statistics, a random, assiduous search for the primary site is not indicated. With the possible exceptions of carcinomas of the breast, prostate, and thyroid, the remaining primary sites, by virtue of the known dissemination, become moot to explore, because no effective therapy exists. Therefore, under the circumstances of adenocarcinomatous metastases from sites unknown, breast, prostate, and thyroid examinations are indicated, but thorough total body evaluation of all other systems is not cost/benefit/risk effective.

Staging Procedures for Cancerous Effusions

Diagnosing Effusions. Effusions of the pericardial, pleural, or peritoneal space can develop in cancer patients and result from either neoplasms or other conditions, such as congestive heart failure. In patients presenting with an effusion, tumors also must be included in the differential diagnosis. In both of these situations, examination of the fluid is very important in reaching a diagnosis.

Characteristics of Exudates. Cytologic examination has a high degree of specificity, but false negative results occur quite frequently. Neoplasms usually manifest an exudative effusion; those characteristics of an exudate that are most reliable are (Light *et al.,* 1972):

1. A ratio of fluid protein/serum protein of 0.5;
2. A fluid LDH level of 200 IU; and
3. An LDH fluid/serum ratio of 0.6.

Closed-Needle Biopsy. One then must differentiate on other grounds between neoplastic and inflammatory causes of an exudative effusion. For pleural or peritoneal effusions, a closed-needle biopsy with Cope's needle may clarify the diagnosis. In certain situations, a recurrent tumor may cause a transudate with a low protein content because of obstruction of the venous system (Witte *et al.,* 1972). Disease in these patients may be delineated angiographically.

Staging Procedures in Spinal Cord Compression

This is still a commonly missed diagnosis even with the patient under the direct observation of a physician. Metastatic tumors usually do not involve the spinal cord directly, but compress the cord from the epidural space.

Radicular Pain. Pain of a radicular nature is the usual presenting symptom and is almost always present to some degree. Radicular pain in the spine of a patient who is known to have a lymphoma or a cancer should be considered as evidence of cord compression until proven otherwise. Weakness of an extremity, easy fatigability, bladder or bowel dysfunction, and sensory changes, especially saddle anesthesia, all represent relatively late findings.

Physical Examination. Physical examination may reveal only minimal abnormalities, especially if pain is the only complaint. Differential weakness between lower and upper extremities is an important lead sign.

Myelography and CT Scans. Myelography and CT are the only definitive diagnostic procedures. Myelography should include cerebrospinal fluid (CSF) analysis for protein elevation and cytology. If a complete block is present, it is difficult to evaluate the entire longitudinal extent of involvement, particularly if skip areas exist. Contrast media from a cephalad approach may be required. An alternate procedure is CT, which can often clearly elucidate the soft tissue component and a myelogram may not be required.

Staging Procedures in Miscellaneous Metastatic Involvement

The search for occult metastases is the most important single factor in treatment decision-making for all cancer patients. The detection of metastatic spread for most cancers significantly alters the prognosis and makes cure unlikely.

Although not common at other sites, metastatic presentations should be suspected, particularly when they are the first and solitary events (Willis, 1952).

Skin Metastases. Skin metastases usually occur on the trunk or scalp or, less often, on the distal extremities. Usual primary tumors are breast, lung, colon, melanoma, and the lymphomas. Cutaneous seeding may occur at surgical incision or injection sites.

Eye Metastases. Eye metastases may be heralded by the development of a blind spot or loss of vision. Breast and lung are the common sites of origin.

Metastases to Breast, Uterus, Vagina, and Ovaries. Breast, uterus, and vagina can be involved by lymphomas and melanomas that can simulate a primary tumor. Ovaries are involved most frequently by colorectal, breast and genital neoplasms (Webb *et al.,* 1975).

Metastases to Kidney, Testis, and Bladder. Kidney and testis may be involved by lymphomas and leukemias. Retroperitoneal involvement from breast, lung, and other cancers may cause ureteral compression. Bladder involvement is rare, but occurs most often with melanoma or breast primaries. Retroperitoneal disease may offer particularly difficult problems in diagnosis until ureteral obstruction has occurred. Ultrasound B scans are useful in diagnosis and follow-up of intra-abdominal and retroperitoneal masses (Tolbert *et al.,* 1974).

SPECIFIC CANCERS

The application of these concepts for some cancer sites will be concisely covered and will be further amplified in each disease site chapter. In this section, however, a brief version of each classification schema will be presented in tabular form and analyzed as to its emphasis on certain criteria for categories that reflect the order of tumor progression. This will illustrate the principles outlined in the oncotaxonomy section; unifying aspects at each site will be stressed. Although the AJC systems (AJC, 1978) are recommended, agreement and differences between the UICC (UICC, 1978) and other schemas are noted where appropriate. Reference to these atlases (Feinstein, 1974; NRCCP, 1950; UICC, 1978) is advised.

Breast Cancer

The currently recognized anatomic staging system is discussed below (see Table 5–5 and Figure 5–6). Although it appears complex, the system is intended to be both accurately descriptive and all inclusive. It contains defi-

Table 5-5. Tumor (T) and Node (N) Classifications for Breast Cancer

CLASSIFICATION	CRITERIA
T_1	≤ 2 cm
T_2	> 2 to 5 cm a = Without fixation to fascia or muscle
T_3	> 5 cm b = With fixation to fascia or muscle
T_4	Extension to chest wall or skin:
	a = Chest Wall
	b = Skin edema/infiltration or ulceration
	c = Both
N_1	Mobile axillary
	a = Not considered metastatic
	b = Considered metastatic
N_2	Fixed axillary
N_3	Supraclavicular/edema of arm

Modified from UICC, International Union Against Cancer: *TNM Classification of Malignant Tumors,* 2nd ed. UICC, Geneva, Switzerland, 1978.

nitions for clinical, surgical, and pathologic staging.

Primary Tumor. Tumor (T) staging depends on tumor size and absence of fixation to skin, pectoral fascia, and underlying ribs. Primary tumors should be described as precisely as possible in terms of measured size in centimeters, shape, consistency, location, and involvement of adjacent structures. Palpable lymph nodes should also be carefully described by size, number, location, mobility, and consistency.

Regional Lymph Nodes. Axillary nodal metastases are present in 25% of T_1 breast cancers, in over 50% of T_3 tumors, and are unrelated to the location of the primary within the breast. Of those patients with axillary disease, 20% will have supraclavicular nodal metastases, whereas such metastases are almost unheard of with histologically negative axillae (Handley, 1975). Internal mammary node involvement varies in frequency with the location of the primary breast cancer; it is more common with central and internal quadrant cancers and with the presence of axillary nodal disease.

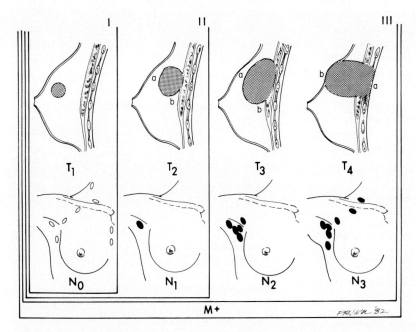

Figure 5-6.   Anatomic staging of cancer of the breast. From Rubin, P. (ed.): *Clinical Oncology for Medical Students and Physicians: A Multidisciplinary Approach,* 6th ed. American Cancer Society, New York, 1983. Copyright © 1983 by the American Cancer Society, Inc.

Lung Cancer

The definitions of tumor and node (T and N) categories for carcinoma of the lung, according to the AJC, follow (see Table 5–6 and Figure 5–7). Stage III cases, however, need to be divided into two categories: The stage at which the disease is still limited to the thorax, and the stage for which metastatic spread into mediastinal structures and outside the thorax has been proven (Carr and Mountain, 1977; AJC, 1978; Bitran *et al.*, 1978).

Tumor (T) Categories. Size and confinement to lung are the major considerations in the progression of non-oat-cell cancers, squamous cell cancer, and adenocarcinoma. A tumor's classification as T_1 versus T_2 depends on its mass being less or more than 3 cm. The depth of invasion is reflected by extension through the pleura, which is akin to an organ capsule (T_3). Further advancement into mediastinum or chest wall has been designated by the Radiation Therapy Oncology Group (RTOG) as T_4, although this is not part of the AJC or UICC criteria.

Node (N) Categories. Location of nodes within the lung hilum (N_1) or mediastinum (N_2) indicates the common progression. Supraclavicular nodes are considered metastatic, although an N_3 notation would be reasonable.

Stage Grouping. Stage grouping emphasizes the early resectable stages confined to a lobe or lung (T_1 and T_2) with or without hilar disease (N_1) as stages I and II respectively. Advanced disease (T_3), pleural invasion, and mediastinal nodes are stage III, with metastases reflecting stage IV. Special T_x and N_3 categories are not officially used by the AJC and UICC. Tumor (T) and node (N) equivalents are: $T_2 = N_1$; $T_3 = N_2$; and $T_4 = N_3$.

Table 5–6. Tumor (T) and Node (N) Classifications for Lung Cancer

CLASSIFICATION	CRITERIA
T_x	Positive cytology
T_1	≤ 3 cm or no invasion
T_2	> 3 cm or extension to hilar region
T_3	Gross extension or effusion or atalectasis
*T_4	Massive disease, unresectable
N_1	Hilar nodes
N_2	Mediastinal nodes
*N_3	Supraclavicular nodes

*From the Radiation Therapy Oncology Group classification of cancer.

Modified from UICC, International Union Against Cancer: *TNM Classification of Malignant Tumors,* 2nd ed. UICC, Geneva, Switzerland, 1978.

AJC Versus UICC Classifications. T_4 and N_3 are *not* official designations. Oat-cell carcinomas are usually metastatic or premetastatic and are categorized as intrathoracic or extrathoracic.

Rectal Cancer

Tumor (T) Categories. The depth of penetration is the most important criterion (see Figure 5–8). The order of progression is for hollow viscera, a stage for each layer: mucosa, muscle, serosa (T_1 to T_2 to T_3). Extension to extramural structures also characterizes T_3; fistula, T_4; and adjacent organs, T_5.

Node (N) Categories. The regional nodes are either negative or positive and are confined to the course of the inferior mesenteric artery and vein.

Stage Grouping. This is awkward but essential. It groups favorable T lesions (T_1 and T_2) as stage I because of ease of resection. Unfavorable T_3 to T_5 lesions are grouped as stage II. Positive nodes are stage III, and metastases, which include nodes beyond the inferior mesenteric, are stage IV.

AJC Versus UICC Classification. The UICC has approximately four categories (see Table 5–7) but differs from the standard categories of visceral organs by lumping muscle and serosal invasion into T_2, which in the AJC would be T_2 and T_3. The UICC T_3 category also corresponds to the AJC T_4. The UICC T_4 is equivalent to the AJC T_4 and T_5. There is an additional UICC N_4 category for juxtaregional nodes, whereas N_2 and N_3 are not applicable.

Carcinoma of the Prostate

Tumor (T) Categories. The extension of the cancer beyond the capsule (not size) and to surrounding structures determines the T category (see Table 5–8 and Figure 5–9). Nodules confined to the prostate depend upon distortion of proterine contour to determine T_1 or T_2 status. Tumor spread beyond the capsule laterally or superiorly into seminal vesicles is T_3 and fixation to the side wall is T_4.

Node (N) Categories. The regional nodes are pelvic nodes and advancement is measured from single homolateral (N_1) to multiple homolateral (N_2) to fixed nodules (N_3) and juxtaregional or paraortic (N_4).

Stage Grouping. This staging follows the T categories and is incorporated into the American Urologic System of stage A_1, B_1, C_1, D_1,

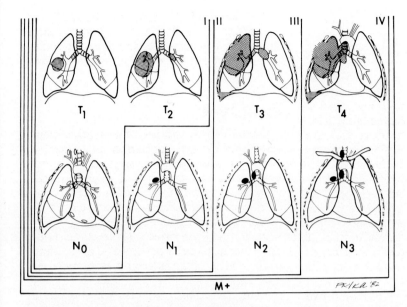

Figure 5–7. Anatomic staging of cancer of the lung. From Rubin, P. (ed.): *Clinical Oncology for Medical Students and Physicians: A Multidisciplinary Approach,* 6th ed. American Cancer Society, New York, 1983. Copyright © 1983 by the American Cancer Society, Inc.

and D_2. The AJC and UICC do not stage primary and group nodes. Regional pelvic nodes are N_1 to N_3, and juxtaregional nodes are considered N_4.

AJC Versus UICC Classification. The two systems are identical for classifying cancer of the prostate. The American Urologic (Jewett) system utilizes A, B, C, D designations that are translated to correspond to TNM categories.

Lymphomas

Hodgkin's Disease

Anatomic Staging. A generally accepted classification of anatomic staging of Hodgkin's disease is important to facilitate meaningful

Table 5–7. Tumor (T) and Node (N) Classifications for Rectal Cancer

CLASSIFICATION	CRITERIA
T_1/pT_1	Mucosa or submucosa only
T_2/pT_2	Muscle or serosa
T_{3a}/pT_{3a}	Extension to contiguous structures; no fistula
T_{3b}/pT_{3b}	Extension to contiguous structures; with fistula
T_4/pT_4	Extension beyond contiguous structures
N_0	No regional nodal involvement
N_1	Regional nodal involvement
N_4	Juxtaregional nodal involvement

Modified from UICC, International Union Against Cancer: *TNM Classification of Malignant Tumors,* 2nd. ed. UICC, Geneva, Switzerland, 1978.

communication and to aid in planning therapy (Symposium, 1966) (see Table 5–9 and Figure 5–10). The 1971 Ann Arbor Symposium on Staging in Hodgkin's Disease (Carbone *et al.,* 1971) recommended the following system utilizing clinical staging (CS) and pathologic staging (PS); the latter is based on surgical sampling of tissues, generally during laparotomy. Literature published before that symposium should be carefully interpreted because of varying definitions of stages.

1. *Stage I:* Involvement of a single lymph node region (I) or of a single extralymphatic organ or site (I_E);
2. *Stage II:* Involvement of two or more lymph nodes on the same side of the diaphragm (II) or localized involvement of extralymphatic organ or site and of one or more lymph node regions on the same side of the diaphragm (II_E). An optional recommendation is that the numbers of node regions involved be indicated by a subscript (*e.g.,* II_3);
3. *Stage III:* Involvement of lymph node regions on both sides of the diaphragm (III), which may also be accompanied by localized involvement of extralymphatic organ or site (III_E) or by involvement of the spleen (III_S) or both (III_{ES});
4. *Stage IV:* Diffuse or disseminated involvement of one or more extralymphatic organs or tissue with or without asso-

Table 5–8.　Tumor (T) and Node (N) Classifications for Cancer of the Prostate

AJC*	CRITERIA	AUS†
T_0	Incident carcinoma	0
T_1	Intracapsular; normal gland	A
T_2	Intracapsular; deformed gland	B
T_3	Extension beyond capsule	C
T_4	Extension fixed to neighboring organs	
N_1	Single homolateral regional	
N_2	Contra- or bilateral multiple regional	D_1
N_3	Fixed regional	
N_4	Juxtaregional	D_2

* AJC = American Joint Committee on Cancer Staging and End-Results Reporting.
† AUS = American Urologic System.
Modified from UICC, International Union Against Cancer: *TNM Classification of Malignant Tumors,* 2nd ed. UICC, Geneva, Switzerland, 1978.

ciated lymph node enlargement. The involved extralymphatic site should be identified by symbols used for pathologic staging: H^+ for liver (hepatic); L^+ for lung; M^+ for marrow; P^+ for pleura; O^+ for bone (osseous); and D^+ for skin (dermal);

5. *Symptoms A or B:* Each stage is subdivided into A and B categories: B for those with certain general symptoms and A for those without. B symptoms include: unexplained weight loss of more than 10% of body weight in the six months prior to admission; unexplained fever with temperatures above 38° C; and night sweats. (Note that pruritus alone will no longer qualify for a B classification.)

Non-Hodgkin's Lymphomas.　The staging system used for non-Hodgkin's lymphomas is the same as for Hodgkin's disease.

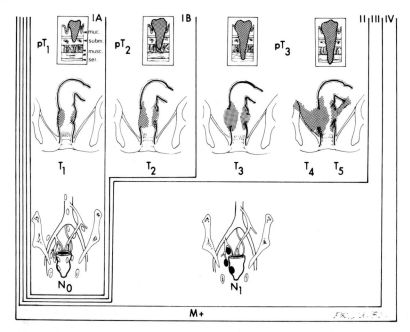

Figure 5–8.　Anatomic staging of cancer of the rectum. From Rubin, P. (ed.): *Clinical Oncology for Medical Students and Physicians: A Multidisciplinary Approach,* 6th ed. American Cancer Society, New York, 1983. Copyright © 1983 by the American Cancer Society, Inc.

Table 5-9. Stage and Substage Classifications for Hodgkin's Disease

STAGE	CRITERIA	SUBSTAGE
I	Single node region	I
	Single extralymphatic organ or site	I_E
II	Two or more node regions on the same side of the diaphragm	II
	Single node region + localized single extralymphatic organ or site	II_E
III	Node regions on both sides of the diaphragm	III
	Node regions on both sides of the diaphragm ± localized single extralymphatic organ or site	III_E
	Node regions on both sides of the diaphragm + involvement in spleen	III_S
	Both III_E and III_S	III_{ES}
IV	Diffuse involvement in extralymphatic organ or site ± node regions	IV
All stages	Without weight loss, fever, and sweats	A
All stages	With weight loss, fever, and sweats	B

Modified from Carbone, P. P.: Kaplan, H. S.: Musshoff, K.: Smithers, D. W.; and Tubiana, M.: Report of the committee on Hodgkin's disease, staging classification. *Cancer Res.,* 31:1860–1861, 1971.

CONCLUSION: NEW DIAGNOSTIC PROCEDURES

Oncologic imaging is undergoing rapid changes due to the new diagnostic procedures that have become available. The conventional radiographs of the head and neck, chest, abdomen, and pelvis have been supplemented and supplanted by computerized tomography and ultrasound (for pediatric tumors) for staging procedures. Sophisticated procedures such as lymphangiography and arteriography are utilized in special circumstances. The potential for three-dimensional reconstruction of tumor extensions and contours is having an important impact on decision making. Confirmation by thin-needle biopsies directed by imaging studies is both more accurate and is more

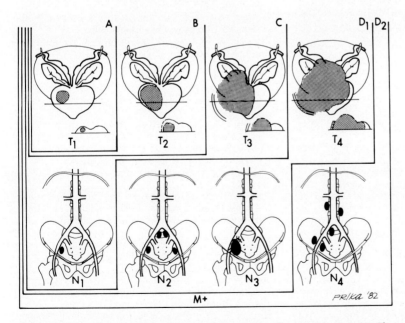

Figure 5-9. Anatomic staging of cancer of the prostate. From Rubin, P. (ed.): *Clinical Oncology for Medical Students and Physicians: A Multidisciplinary Approach,* 6th ed. American Cancer Society, New York, 1983. Copyright © 1983 by the American Cancer Society, Inc.

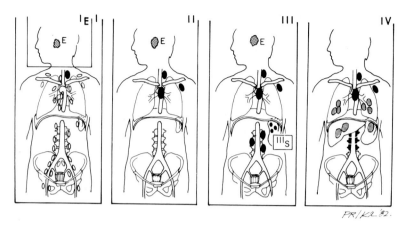

Figure 5-10. Anatomic staging of lymphomas. From Rubin, P. (ed.): *Clinical Oncology for Medical Students and Physicians: A Multidisciplinary Approach,* 6th ed. American Cancer Society, New York, 1983. Copyright © 1983 by the American Cancer Society, Inc.

widely made than thoracotomy and laparotomy; it is replacing invasive surgical procedures. In the immediate future, nuclear magnetic resonance and short-lived radioisotopes with positron emission tomography hold promise for detecting tumor extensions because of biochemical and metabolic features.

The use of decision trees and appropriate sequencing, of diagnostic studies individualized to meet each patient's presentation is essential. Blending of the knowledge of each cancer, its site of origin, and knowledge of its spreading patterns to direct staging procedures is vital to optimize the classification and staging of the patient with cancer (Bragg *et al.,* 1984).

REFERENCES

AJC, American Joint Committee on Cancer Staging and End-Results Reporting: *Manual for Staging Cancer.* AJC, Chicago, 1978.

Aronson, S. M.; Garcia, J. H.; and Aronson, B. E.: Metastatic neoplasms of the brain: Their frequency in relation to breast cancer. *Cancer,* 17:558–563, 1964.

Biello, D. R.; Levitt, R. G.; Siegel, B. A.; Sagel, S. S.; and Stanley, R. J.: Computed tomography and radionuclide imaging of the liver: A comparative evaluation. *Radiology,* 127:159–163, 1978.

Bragg, D. G.: Angiography of hepatic neoplasm: A review. *Int. J. Radiat. Oncol. Biol. Phys.,* 1:965–971, 1976.

Bragg, D. G.; Rubin, P.; and Youker, J. (eds.): *Oncologic Imaging.* Pergamon Press, Inc., New York, 1984.

Bitran, J. D.; Desser, R. K.; DeMesster, T.; and Golomb, H. M.: Metastatic non-oat cell bronchogenic carcinoma: Therapy with cyclophosphamide, doxorubicin, methotrexate and procarbazine (CAMP). *JAMA,* 240:2743–2746, 1978.

Carbone, P. P.; Kaplan, H. S.; Musshoff, K.; Smithers, D. W.; and Tubiana, M.: Report of the committee on Hodgkin's disease, staging classification. *Cancer Res.,* 31:1860–1861, 1971.

Carr, D. T., and Mountain, C.: Staging lung cancer. In Strauss, M. (ed.): *Lung Cancer: Clinical Diagnosis and Treatment.* Grune & Stratton, Inc., New York, 1977.

Chang, A. E.; Schaner, E. G.; Conkle, D. M.; Flye, M. W.; Doppman, J. L.; and Rosenberg, S. A.: Evaluation of computed tomography in the detection of pulmonary metastases: A prospective study. *Cancer,* 43:913–916, 1979.

Corcoran, R. J.; Thrall, J. H.; Kyle, R. W.; Kaminski, R. J.; and Johnson, M. C.: Solitary abnormalities in bone scans. *Radiology,* 121:663–667, 1976.

Deck, M. D.; Messina, A. V. A.; and Sackett, J. F.: Computed tomography in metastatic disease of the brain. *Radiology,* 119:115–120, 1976.

Dorland's Illustrated Medical Dictionary, 24th ed. W. B. Saunders Company, Philadelphia, 1965.

Feinstein, A. R.: *Clinical Judgement.* R. E. Kreiger Publishing Co., Inc., Huntington, New York, 1974.

Handley, R. S.: Carcinoma of the breast. *Ann. R. Coll. Surg. Engl.,* 57:59–66, 1975.

Hobbs, J., and Rodriquez, A. R.: Metastatic cancer of unknown primary site. *Am. Fam. Physician,* 22:164–168, 1980.

Holmes, F. F., and Fouts, T. L.: Metastatic cancer of unknown primary site. *Cancer,* 26:816–820, 1970.

Hooper, R. G.; Beechler, C. R.; and Johnson, M. D.: Radioisotope scanning in the initial staging of bronchogenic cancer. *Am. Rev. Respir. Dis.,* 118:279–286, 1978.

Joo, K. G.; Parthasaranthy, K. L.; Bakshi, S. P.; and Rosner, D.: Bone scintigrams: Their clinical usefulness in patients with breast carcinoma. *Oncology,* 36:94–98, 1979.

Kagan, A. R., and Gilbert, H. A.: The detection of occult metastases with imaging studies. *Int. J. Radiat. Oncol. Biol. Phys.,* 1:529–533, 1976.

Kern, W. H., and Schweizer, C. W.: Sputum cytology of metastatic carcinoma of the lung. *Acta Cytol. (Baltimore),* 20:514–520, 1976.

Kim, N. K.; Yasmineh, W. G.; Freier, E. F.; Goldman, A. I.; and Theologides, A.: Value of alkaline phosphatase, 5'-nucleotidase, gamma-glutamyltransference and glutamate dehydrogenase activity measurements (single and combined) in serum in diagnosis of metastases to the liver. *Clin. Chem.,* **23**:2034–2038, 1977.

Krementz, E. T.; Cerise, E. J.; Ciaravella, J. L., Jr.; and Morgan, L. R.: Metastases of undetermined source. *CA,* **27**:289–300, 1977.

Lee, J. K.; Stanley, R. J.; Sagel, S. S.; and McClennan, B. L.: Accuracy of CT in detecting intra-abdominal and pelvic lymph node metastases from pelvic cancers. *AJR,* **131**:675–679, 1978.

Light, R. W.; MacGregor, M. I.; Luchsinger, P. C.; and Ball, W. C.: Pleural effusions: The diagnostic separations of transudates and exudates. *Ann. Intern. Med.,* **77**:507–513, 1972.

Lunia, S.; Parthasarathykl, B.; and Blender, M. A.: An evaluation of ^{99}M technetium-sulfur colloid liver scintiscans and their usefulness in metastatic workup: A review of 1424 studies. *J. Nucl. Med.,* **16**:62–65, 1975.

Mall, J. C.; Bekerman, C.; Hoffer, P. B.; and Goffschalk, A.: A unified radiologic approach to the detection of skeletal metastases. *Radiology,* **118**:323–328, 1976.

McArdle, C. R.: Ultrasonic diagnosis of liver metastases. *J. Clin. Ultrasound,* **4**:265–268, 1976.

McNeil, B. J.: Rationale for the use of bone scans in skeletal metastatic and primary bone tumors. *Semin. Nucl. Med.,* **8**:336–345, 1978.

Muhm, J. R.; Brown, L. R.; and Croe, J. K.: Detection of pulmonary nodules by computed tomography. *AJR,* **128**:267–270, 1977.

Neifeld, J. P.; Michaelis, L. L.; and Doppman, J. L.: Suspected pulmonary metastases: Correlation to chest x ray, whole lung tomograms and operative findings. *Cancer,* **39**:383–387, 1977.

NRCCP, National Research Council Committee on Pathology: *Atlas of Tumor Pathology.* Armed Forces Institute of Pathology, Washington, D.C., 1950.

Nystrom, J. S.; Weiner, J. M.; and Heffelinger-Juttner, J.: Metastatic and histologic presentations in unknown primary cancer. *Semin. Oncol.,* **4**:53–58, 1977.

Nystrom, J. S.; Weiner, J. M.; Wolf, R. M.; Baleman, J. R.; and Viola, M. V.: Identifying the primary site in metastatic cancer of unknown origin: Inadequacy of roentgenographic procedures. *J.A.M.A.,* **241**:381–383, 1979.

O'Mara, R. E.: Skeletal scanning in neoplastic disease. *CA,* **37 (Suppl. 1)**:480–486, 1976.

Peck, A.: Emotional reactions to having cancer. *A. J. R. Radium Ther. Nucl. Med.,* **114**:591–599, 1972.

Polga, J. P., and Watnick, M.: Whole lung tomography in metastatic disease. *Clin. Radiol.,* **27**:53–56, 1976.

Roberts, J. G.; Gravalle, I. H.; and Baum, M.: Evaluation of radiography and isotopic scinitigraphy for detecting skeletal metastases in breast cancer. *Lancet,* **1**:237–239, 1976.

Rouvier, H.: *Anatomie des Lymphatiques des L'Homme.* Masson Press, Paris, 1932.

Rubin, P.: A unified classification of cancers: An oncotaxonomy with symbols. *Cancer,* **31**:963–982, 1973.

Rubin, P.: *TNM—An Illustrated Atlas,* to be published.

Rubin, P. (ed.): *Clinical Oncology for Medical Students and Physicians: A Multidisciplinary Approach,* 6th ed. American Cancer Society, New York, 1983.

Rubin, P., and Keys, H.: The staging and classification of cancer: A unified approach. In Carter, S. K.; Glatstein, E.; and Livingston, R. B. (eds.): *Principles of Cancer Treatment.* McGraw-Hill, Inc., New York, 1982.

Sindelar, W. F.; Bagley, B. H.; Felix, E. L.; Dopp, J. L.; and Ketcham, A. S.: Lung tomography in cancer patients: Full lung tomograms in screening for pulmonary metastases. *J.A.M.A.,* **240**:2060–2063, 1978.

Symposium: Obstacles to the control of Hodgkin's disease. *Cancer Res.,* **26**:1047–1311, 1966.

Tolbert, D. D.; Zagzebski, J. A.; Banjavic, R. A.; and Wiley, A. L., Jr.: Quantitation of tumor volumes and response to therapy with ultrasound b-scans. *Radiology,* **113**:705–708, 1974.

UICC, International Union Against Cancer: *TNM Classification of Malignant Tumors,* 2nd ed. UICC, Geneva, Switzerland, 1978.

Ulfeder, H.: Classification systems. *Int. J. Radiat. Oncol. Biol. Phys.,* **7**:1083–1086, 1981.

Vermund, H.: Role of radiotherapy in cancer of the larynx as related to the TNM system of staging. *Cancer,* **25**:485–504, 1970.

Webb, M. J.; Decker, D. G.; and Mussey, E.: Cancer metastatic to the ovary: Factors influencing survival. *Obstet. Gynecol.,* **45**:391–396, 1975.

Weiss, L.; Gilbert, H. A.; and Posner, J. (eds.): *Metastases: A Monograph Series, Vol. 2: Brain Metastases.* G. K. Hall and Company, Boston, 1980.

WHO, World Health Organization: *International Classification of Diseases for Oncology.* WHO, Geneva, Switzerland, 1976.

Willis, R. A.: *The Spread of Tumors in the Human Body.* Butterworth and Company, Ltd., London, 1952.

Witte, M. H.; Witte, C. L.; Davis, W. M.; Cole, W. R.; and Dumont, A. E.: Peritoneal transudate: A diagnostic clue to portal system obstruction in patients with intra-abdominal neoplasms or peritonitis. *J.A.M.A.,* **221**:1380–1383, 1972.

6

Paraneoplastic Phenomena

A. TUMOR MARKERS

E. Douglas Holyoke and Philip S. Schein

INTRODUCTION

When a cancer reaches the size of only 1 cm³ it has already completed approximately 30 doublings or two-thirds of its usual growth. It is estimated to contain one billion tumor cells, and it has reached a size where blood vessel or lymphatic invasion is likely and the number of viable cells shed into circulation may become great. Between the point in time when a neoplasm reaches this size, which is a realistic goal for early detection, and the time when most tumors are diagnosed due to symptoms or physical findings, the chance for containment decreases as microscopic metastases develop. In addition to our need to move the time of detection forward, we also require better means of identifying the presence of microscopic metastases that may be present even with the earliest possible diagnosis and treatment of primary tumor, using current methodology. Even in patients with advanced stages of disease, particularly with intra-abdominal cancer, it is often difficult to assess the extent of disease and its response or failure to treatment. Research has, therefore, been directed toward the identification of tumor-specific products in body tissues and fluids that might have three potential implications in clinical practice: (1) Early diagnosis of tumors, (2) the preoperative and postoperative assessment of prognosis of tumor staging, and (3) an assay of changing tumor cell burden.

An ideal tumor marker should not only signal the presence of tumor, but also should define the site of tumor and the morphological type of neoplasm. Unfortunately, most markers available now have not obtained a high enough degree of sensitivity and specificity to be useful for these functions, although sensitivity in the identification of small amounts of materials has been greatly improved through the use of radioimmunoassays that can measure nanogram quantities of antigen. The problem of specificity has been more difficult. The use of normally occurring hormones, enzymes, or proteins, or the use of oncofetal antigens, requires that the blood concentration of these materials be present in excess of an established normal range. This means that materials are being used as tumor markers that can only be quantitatively but not qualitatively separated from normal, thus requiring some determination as to when an individual value exceeds the range of normal. Increasingly, efforts are being directed towards the development and identification of specific monoclonal antibodies that can locate more precisely unique antigenic markers of cancer. The reader is referred to the appropriate chapters in this text that define the use of tumor markers in relationship to specific diseases.

ONCOFETAL ANTIGENS

Oncofetal antigens are gene products expressed during specific stages of the differentiation of fetal tissue and are thereafter largely repressed in the adult. With the state of dedifferentiation associated with cancer, dormant genomes may become derepressed and, consequently, embryonic antigens may appear again as an index of neoplastic transformation.

At the present time, three such oncofetal antigens have reached the stage of important clinical application, the carcinoembryonic antigen (CEA), the alpha fetoprotein (AFP), and the pancreatic oncofetal antigen (POA). These serve as important models for future developmental efforts in this field of investigation, but the current clinical results clearly demonstrate the considerable obstacles that are faced in an attempt to achieve specificity: the relatively high percentage of false positive and negative results serve as critical impediments to their use as diagnostic aids.

Carcinoembryonic Antigen (CEA)

The CEA, a glycoprotein with a molecular weight of 200,000 daltons, was described by Gold and Freedman (1965) as a specific product of colon carcinoma cells, which could be found in the plasma of almost all patients with this cancer. Since this initial report, concepts regarding the chemistry and biologic properties of CEA have been greatly refined. It is now recognized that the molecular structure of CEA is not uniform, but that there can be great variance in its carbohydrate content (Banjo et al., 1974; Gold et al., 1965; Coligan et al., 1973). Of great importance has been the demonstration that CEA is found in many tissues, both benign and neoplastic, and that the hoped-for specificity is not an attainable goal. This glycoprotein is present in glycocalyx of normal gastrointestinal cells, from which it is shed. CEA has been detected by radioimmunoassay in feces (Elias et al., 1974), in high concentration in intestinal secretions, particularly in the colorectal region, as well as in the normal secretion of the pancreatobiliary system (Go et al., 1975). It is of interest that mucosal production of this material increases as one moves distally in the intestinal tract. This glycocalyceal material can diffuse into the intestinal lymphatics and capillaries to enter the plasma, where it is readily measured in normal individuals using current radioimmunoassay methodology. Plasma CEA levels of 2.5 μg/mL or less, as measured by the Hoffman-La Roche assay, are generally regarded as normal values in a healthy nonsmoking population.

Plasma levels of CEA are elevated in cigarette smokers (Stevens and MacKay, 1973; Alexander et al., 1976). It is also well established that increased CEA concentrations are found in association with several additional nonmalignant conditions including alcohol-related hepatic cirrhosis and pancreatitis (Delwiche et al., 1973), inflammatory bowel disease (Moore et al., 1972b; Gardner et al., 1978), rectal polyps, and pulmonary infections. As a result, an abnormal plasma CEA level is not specific for cancer, although high concentrations in excess of 20 ng/ml are highly suggestive.

Continued emphasis is being placed on the use of plasma CEA concentration as a measure of monitoring the extent and progress of colorectal cancer (see Chapter 30). The frequency of abnormal values is dependent upon several well-recognized factors: Stage of disease, histologic differentiation, and extent and site of metastases. As the local tumor invades the bowel wall, with resultant destruction of basement membrane as well as cellular disintegration, neoplastic glycocalyx derivatives are absorbed into the local vascular and lymphatic channels. Patients with Duke's A and B tumors will have an abnormal plasma concentration in 25 to 40% of the cases, which emphasizes that insensitivity of CEA testing for early diagnosis (Patterson and Alpert, 1983). In contrast, 65 to 95% of patients with advanced metastatic colorectal cancer will demonstrate an abnormal plasma concentration. The efficiency of CEA production by a tumor may also demonstrate considerable variation, which has in some instances been correlated with histologic differentiation; colon carcinoma with poorly differentiated histology may produce little or no elevation of plasma CEA level, despite the presence of widespread tumor. This serves as a potential source of false-negative results and again emphasizes the obstacles faced when attempting to use CEA as an aid to cancer detection. The liver has a role in both the metabolism and excretion of CEA (Kupchik and Zamcheck, 1972; Moore et al., 1972a). With the onset of hepatic metastases there is often a striking and rapid increase in plasma CEA concentrations. In the setting of local-regional recurrence, in contrast, the general pattern of rise in CEA level is more gradual.

The principal role of CEA testing in colorectal cancer is its use as a monitor of tumor burden in patients with resected or advanced disease. Following a complete surgical resection, an elevated preoperative CEA concentration should decrease to a normal level within four to six weeks. If the plasma CEA remains elevated, assuming no intervening complications such as hepatitis, the presence of a residual

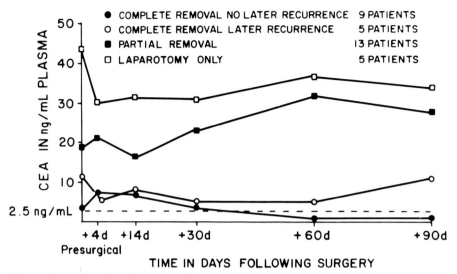

Figure 6-1. CEA following surgery for colorectal cancer. There is a change in plasma CEA following surgery. If preoperative values are low, there may be a rise as is seen for those with an initial normal value and complete tumor excision in this figure. It is also apparent that if preresection values are elevated, baseline may not be reached for 30 to 45 days after definitive surgery. It is also apparent that in this series of patients declared technically free of disease at surgery, a group with progressive disease was already demonstrating a rise in the plasma CEA.

tumor must be suspected (see Figure 6–1). A Consensus Development Panel convened by the National Institutes of Health (Goldenberg *et al.*, 1981) concluded that the regular and sequential assay of plasma CEA serves as the best available noninvasive test for postoperative surveillance of patients to detect disseminated recurrence of colorectal cancer. In ap-

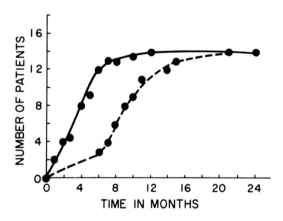

Figure 6-2. CEA and recurrence of colorectal cancer. In the aggregate of those patients (about one-third) demonstrating an elevation in plasma CEA prior to clinical detection by other means, the average lead time was four to five months, with some elevations occurring much earlier.

proximately one-third of patients, CEA values become greatly elevated months before metastatic tumor can be detected by conventional clinical or other diagnostic techniques (see Figure 6–2).

The presence of recurrent cancer is typically indicated by a consistently rising CEA value. In some centers, the CEA is being used as an indicator for the so-called second look surgery to identify an early relapse that may be resectable (Martin *et al.*, 1977; Wanebo, 1981). In an analysis of 117 patients, Patterson and Alpert (1983) found that a local resectable recurrence was found in only 30% of patients. The impact of such salvage procedures on the ultimate survival of this selected patient population remains to be determined (Rittgers *et al.*, 1978). It must also be recognized that an elevated CEA level may result from causes unrelated to tumor recurrence, such as smoking and intercurrent infection, and many patients may be subjected to unnecessary surgery.

For patients with a metastatic tumor, the plasma CEA level serves to complement standard clinical measurement of tumor response and provide an index of the effectiveness of chemotherapy or radiation therapy (Sugarbaker *et al.*, 1976; Mayer *et al.*, 1978). Instances of discordance between the measured changes in tumor size and the corresponding CEA levels do exist. As a consequence, the CEA assay has not as yet been fully accepted as objective measurement of tumor response and therefore cannot be substituted for the standard criteria of assessment.

The preoperative CEA concentration has been reported to have independent prognostic significance in patients with Duke's B and C colorectal cancer. Wanebo and others (1978) have found that patients with levels in excess of 5 μg/mL prior to resection had a significantly higher recurrence rate, and that the mean time to relapse demonstrated an inverse linear correlation with plasma concentration.

Abnormal plasma CEA levels are not specific to colorectal cancer but are found in association with a wide range of cancers particularly entodermally derived tumors of the gastrointestinal tract and lung. Elevation has been reported in 75 to 90% of patients with advanced pancreatic cancer, 60% with gastric cancer, 75% with lung cancer, especially small cell carcinoma, and in 50% with advanced breast cancer (Sugarbaker et al., 1977). The role of CEA testing in the postoperative and therapeutic monitoring of such cases has been less convincing than for colorectal cancer (Goldenberg et al., 1981). Changes in plasma levels have been used to monitor patients' metastatic breast disease to determine tumor burden and response to treatment (Haagensen et al., 1978; Tormey and Waalkes, 1978) and for staging in lung cancer as a predictor of survival (Dent et al., 1978), but these uses are more restricted than for colorectal cancer. Efforts have been made to utilize ^{131}I-antibody to CEA for immunodetection and radiolocalization of colon cancer (Goldenberg et al., 1978; Goldenberg et al., 1983). Primary colorectal cancers were demonstrated in 83% of patients evaluated preoperatively and between 87% and 92% of patients with known metastatic tumors. The false-negative rate was 9 to 14% and a false-positive rate of less than 4% was found. In 11 of 51 patients evaluated, tumor sites were detected that were not found by other clinical methods of cancer detection.

Alpha Fetoprotein

Alpha fetoprotein (AFP) is an alpha-globulin with a molecular weight of 70,000 daltons. It is normally synthesized by the endodermal cells of the liver and the yoke sac of the human fetus. Peak plasma AFP concentration occurs *in utero* during the 12th to 15th week of gestation. It declines to the normal adult level of less than 40 ng/mL between the sixth to twelfth

month following birth (Waldmann and McIntire, 1974). In general, a reciprocal relationship exists between the plasma concentrations of AFP and albumin, a protein with which AFP shares several physicochemical properties in pre- and postnatal development (Ruoslahti and Terry, 1975).

In 1963, Abelev and coworkers reported the production of AFP by a transplantable mouse hepatoma (Abelev et al., 1963). Abelev and others (1967) found increased concentrations of the same protein in the plasma of patients with hepatocellular carcinoma. AFP is an effective tumor marker for hepatoma as well as for germ cell neoplasms. As with CEA, AFP is measurable in the plasma of normal adults and in increased concentration in association with several benign conditions.

Cohen and colleagues (1973) reported that serum AFP levels in excess of 250 ng/mL may be found in pregnant women and are closely correlated with either fetal morbidity or death. The measurement of amniotic-fluid AFP is used for the diagnosis of fetal neural tube defects such as anencephaly and spina bifida (Brock, 1977). Elevated levels are also found in infants and children with ataxia telangiectasia (Simons and Hosking, 1974), hereditary tyrosinosis, and Indian childhood cirrhosis. Benign hepatic disorders are the principal noncancer sources of elevated AFP levels in adults; transient increases are observed in 20 to 30% of patients with acute viral and chronic active hepatitis (Alpert, 1976), which some have ascribed to AFP synthesis during the recovery phase of hepatocyte regeneration. In general, the elevations of serum AFP in association with benign disease are modest, whereas serum concentrations in excess of 500 ng/mL, in the absence of an obvious primary cancer of the gastrointestinal tract, strongly suggests the presence of either hepatocellular carcinoma or germ cell neoplasm. Nevertheless, the overall lack of specificity and sensitivity does not allow this tumor marker to serve as a diagnostic test for cancer.

With sensitive radioimmunoassay techniques, 70 to 95% of all patients with hepatocellular carcinoma are found to have serum AFP levels greater than 50 ng/mL. The principal application of AFP is in the use of serial measurements to determine the efficacy of chemotherapy or surgical resection (see Figure 6–3). The results of screening programs for groups with identified high risk for developing hepatoma have been quite variable. A survey of Bantu miners who were expected to have an incidence of 36/100,000/year failed to demonstrate a single case of hepatoma in over 5000 individual studies (Purves *et al.,* 1973). A similar mass screening survey carried out in China, however, resulted in the diagnosis of 300 cases of hepatoma with a resectability rate of 23% (Shangai Coordinating Group, 1979). A serious impediment is the inability of the test to distinguish between chronic benign disease and small hepatomas, particularly with serum AFP concentrations below 200 ng/mL. An abnormal level that demonstrates little fluctuation, however, must raise the suspicion of a minute hepatoma; an expontential rise usually occurs when the tumor has reached 3 to 5 cm. In the United States, serial AFP testing in patients with alcoholic cirrhosis or HB_sAG positive chronic liver disease is not regarded as cost-effective. The finding of a significant elevation in such cases does, however, warrant a complete evaluation, including CT scan, hepatic arteriography, and biopsy for the diagnosis of hepatoma (see Chapter 28).

The use of serum AFP levels, in conjunction with human chorionic gonadotropin (HCG), in the management of germ-cell neoplasms is described in the chapter dealing with testicular neoplasms (see Chapter 36). The majority of nonseminatous germ cell cancers secrete a tumor marker, either AFP, the beta-subunit of HCG, or both. The presence of yolk-sac elements within the tumor invariably results in serum AFP elevations. It is important to recognize that a germ cell cancer may contain several histologies within the primary tumor, as well as in sites of metastases, each with a distinct secretory nature. As a consequence, treatment of the neoplasm may result in discordant behavior of the AFP and beta-HCG; persistent elevation of one marker typically results from secretion of one histologic element within a treated mass or evidence of residual tumor in other sites (Waldmann and McIntire, 1974). After surgical removal of a teratocarcinoma producing AFP, the serum half-life of this marker is approximately five days. A two-week period should lapse before retesting for purposes of assessing the possible presence of residual cancer. Beta-HCG, in contrast, has a shorter half-life of 15 to 20 hours and should be undetectable within a few days in a nonpregnant female or in a male. These markers have proven to be an essential adjunct to the monitoring of the progress of disease and the effectiveness of treatment. The presence of a low titer of HCG in a male may result from a technical difficulty in completely distinguishing HCG and human luteinizing hormone (HLH). The initiation of suppressive doses of

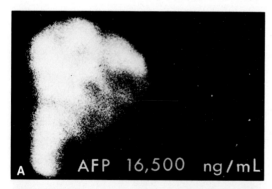

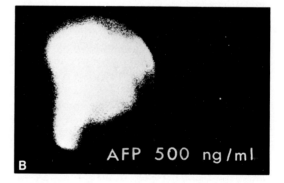

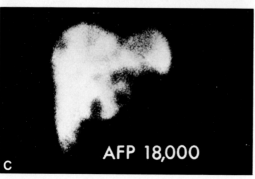

Figure 6–3. Alpha fetoprotein (AFP) as a marker. (*A*) There is obvious involvement of the liver in this scan. Note that the serum AFP value is 16,500 ng/mL. (*B*) There is evidence by scan as well as clinical evidence of a response of this patient's tumor and there has been a concomitant fall in serum AFP to 500 ng/mL. (*C*) The disease is out of remission, and the increased amount of tumor visible on scan is clear. It is accompanied by an increase in serum alpha fetoprotein to 18,000 ng/mL.

Table 6–1. Serum Alpha-Fetoprotein Levels in Patients with Cancer

DIAGNOSIS	NUMBER OF SAMPLES ASSAYED	PERCENT OF VALUES OVER 40 NG/ML
Hepatocellular carcinoma	130	72%
Testicular teratocarcinoma	101	75%
Pancreatic carcinoma	44	25%
Gastric carcinoma	91	18%
Colonic carcinoma	195	5%
Bronchogenic carcinoma	150	7%
Breast carcinoma	55	0%
Nonhepatic benign lesions	500	0.3%
Normal controls over one year of age	210	0%

From Waldmann, T. A., and McIntire, K. R.: The use of radioimmunoassay for alpha-fetoprotein in the diagnosis of malignancy. *Cancer,* **34**:1510–1515, 1974.

testosterone will not lower an autonomously secreted beta-HCG, in contrast to the reduction of contaminating HLH.

Waldmann and McIntire (1974), using a sensitive double antibody radioimmunoassay procedure, have reported the presence of elevated serum AFP levels in association with cancers of the gastrointestinal tract (see Table 6–1). Although in their initial report 23% of patients with pancreatic cancer and 18% of cases with gastric cancer presented with serum AFP levels in excess of 40 ng/mL, this marker has not received widespread acceptance as a monitor of these disease-sites.

Pancreatic Oncofetal Antigen

Because the need for improvement in the diagnosis of cancer of the pancreas is apparent, a considerable effort has been made to identify pancreatic cancer-specific antigens. Banwo and colleagues (1974) first reported a new putative pancreatic oncofetal antigen (POA) present in extracts of fetal pancreata, pancreatic tumor nodules, and sera from patients with pancreatic carcinoma. In contrast, the antigen was not detected in the sera of patients with cancer of the colon and other diseases. This report was followed by an extensive evaluation of this new tumor marker by Gelder and colleagues (1978). POA was characterized as a glycoprotein with a molecular weight of approximately 800,000 daltons, and migration in the alpha 2 beta region on electrophoresis. A monospecific antibody was developed that failed to react with CEA and other known tumor markers. POA was found in measurable levels in the sera of most normal individuals but in highest absolute measures and highest frequency in patients with pancreatic carcinoma (see Table 6–2). A lack of specificity for

this cancer was demonstrated; elevated serum concentration was also found in association with carcinoma of the stomach, biliary tract, colon, and lung. Lastly, increased values were measured in pregnant women and in patients with specific benign diseases, such as pancreatitis. While POA serves to complement other markers such as CEA, its overall lack of specificity and sensitivity serves to restrict its use to monitoring of a known disease during periods of treatment.

HUMAN CHORIONIC GONADOTROPIN

Human chorionic gonadotropin (HCG) is a glycoprotein that is normally secreted by the trophoblastic epithelium of the placenta (Rosen *et al.,* 1975). Its biologic properties are discussed in detail in Chapter 6F and referred to in the AFP section of this chapter. HCG is composed of alpha and beta subunits, which are dissimilar. The alpha subunit is identical in primary structure with the comparable alpha subunit of HLH, whereas their respective beta subunits have differences in chemical structure. Sensitive radioimmunoassays have been developed that utilize antisera produced against each beta subunit that allow for discrimination between HCG and HLH (Vaitukaitis *et al.,* 1972). HCG can be measured in both fetal and maternal serum during pregnancy and the immediate postpartum period. In the male or nonpregnant female, however, the presence of HCG has been regarded as indicative of underlying cancer. Historically, the principal application of HCG had been for diagnosis and management of trophoblastic tumors. It enabled the oncologist to assay chemically for the presence of retained trophoblastic neoplastic cells, and it also fur-

Table 6–2. Quantitative Serum Pancreatic Oncofetal Antigen (POA) Levels in Individuals with Various Conditions

DIAGNOSIS	NO. OF INDIVIDUALS STUDIED	NO. OF INDIVIDUALS WITH POA VALUES		
		0 to 14	*15 to 20*	*20*
Normal	102	99	3	0
Pancreatic disease				
Carcinoma of the pancreas	80	42	21	17
Pancreatitis	24	21	1	2
Islet cell or carcinoid tumor	6	6	0	0
Biliary disease				
Biliary tract carcinoma	14	9	4	1
Hepatoma	4	4	0	0
Benign biliary stone disease or cirrhosis	11	8	2	1
Bronchopulmonary disease				
Bronchogenic carcinoma	53	40	5	8
Small-cell carcinoma of lung	11	10	1	0
Adenocarcinoma of lung	26	22	3	1
Benign lung disease	12	11	1	0
Smokers	37	36	1	0
Gastrointestinal disease				
Carcinoma of colon or rectum	42	36	5	1
Inflammatory bowel disease	11	10	1	0
Carcinoma of stomach	16	12	3	1
Gastric ulcer	10	7	3	0
Duodenal ulcer	30	29	0	1
Other				
Breast cancer	23	20	1	2
Benign breast disease	27	25	2	0
Sarcoma	29	28	1	0
Malignant melanoma	20	20	0	0
Miscellaneous benign abdominal diseases	50	49	1	0
Pregnancy	87	76	6	5

From Gelder, F. B.; Reese, C. J.; Moossa, A. R.; Hall, T.; and Hunter, R.: Purification, partial characterization, and clinical evaluation of a pancreatic oncofetal antigen. *Cancer Res.,* **38**:313–324, 1978.

nished a sensitive guide for the follow-up of treated patients. HCG is secreted by germ-cell neoplasms of the testes or ovary as well as by extragonadal sites such as mediastinum or retroperitoneum. It is present in measurable levels in the plasma of 50 to 60% of patients with embryonal and teratocarcinoma of the testes, 40% of patients with seminoma, and virtually all patients with testicular choriocarcinoma (Braunstein *et al.,* 1973) (see Chapter 36). Detectable HCG has also been reported in 42% of patients with carcinoma of the ovary, in 33% of patients with pancreatic cancer, in 22% of patients with gastric cancer, and in 17% of patients with hepatoma (Braunstein *et al.,* 1973).

Human placenta lactogen (HPL) is a second placental hormone normally found in the serum of pregnant women. It is present in the serum of the majority of patients with trophoblastic neoplasms and is also found in a small percentage of patients with hepatoma, leukemia, lymphomas, endocrine tumors, and lung cancer (Rosen *et al.,* 1975). Placenta alkaline phosphatase (PAP), Regan isoenzyme, is also synthesized in the trophoblast, where it is located on the macrovilli membrane of the plasma membrane. It is readily distinguished from other isoenzymes of alkaline phosphatase by its heat stability, electrophoretic mobility, and immunochemical specificity. Its ectopic secretion was originally described in a patient with lung cancer. It is present in the serum of 5 to 15% of patients with cancer of the ovary (Fishman *et al.,* 1968; Rosen *et al.,* 1975). Unfortunately, the low incidence and sensitivity severely limits its use.

ECTOPIC POLYPEPTIDES

Many tumors that produce augmented quantities of hormones or proteins that are normally secreted by the cell of origin are known. Examples include the hypersecretion of insulin and gastrin by islet cell tumors, and the M spike of multiple myeloma. The abnormal plasma concentration of these markers must be distinguished from the phenomenon of augmented and autonomous secretion or ectopic secretion. The theory of ectopic secretion rests upon the concept that all somatic cells contain a complete genetic complement; with neoplastic transformation there may be a selective derepression of a previously dormant genome which is responsible for production of a specific polypeptide. The hormone can then be used as a tumor marker. As an example, small cell carcinoma of the lung may produce adrenocorticotropic hormone (ACTH), antidiuretic hormone, or calcitonin. This is covered in greater detail in Chapter 6F.

ENZYMES

Attention has been directed towards a number of enzymes identified with glycoprotein metabolism found in serum. Because sialic acid is an important component in cancer cells, sialyltransferase has been evaluated and has been found to be elevated in patients with metastatic breast cancer, ovarian cancer, and malignant melanoma. At present, however, the enzyme does not appear to be useful as a marker. Galactosyltransferase has been the subject of investigation, particularly its isoenzymes. A distinct isoenzyme designated GI II has been found in the serum of 75% of patients with gastrointestinal cancer. In patients with breast cancer, as well as in those with prostatic cancer and various lymphoproliferative disorders, it has been reported present (Podolsky et al., 1981). Interestingly, patients with Duke's B colonic carcinoma are reported to have detectable levels (see Figure 6–4). False-positive tests are uncommon, but do occur in association with celiac disease and severe alcoholic hepatitis.

The prostatic epithelium elaborates a specific tartrate-inhibitable acid phosphatase that has been used as a serum marker for metastatic cancer of the prostate. The standard enzymatic assays have not had sufficient specificity or sensitivity to diagnose patients with localized tumors. A solid phase radioimmunoassay for acid phosphatase has been developed. Approximately one-third of the patients with occult neoplasms and 75% of those with palpable tumors confined within or locally extending beyond the prostatic capsule (stages II and III) can now be detected. A small number of pa-

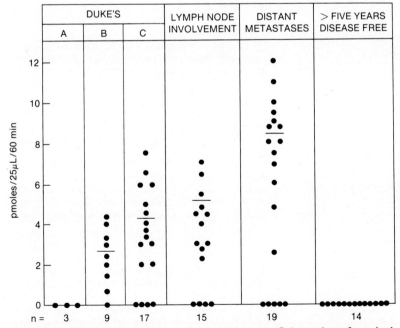

Figure 6–4.　Galactosyltransferase and colorectal cancer. Galactosyltransferase is elevated even in some patients with Duke's B cancer and is related to the presence of or absence of disease, and the amount of disease present. From Podolsky, D. K.; Weiser, M. M.; Isselbacher, K. J.; and Cohen, A. M.: *N. Engl. J. Med.,* **299**:703–705, 1978. Reprinted by permission of the *New England Journal of Medicine.*

tients with benign prostatic hypertrophy have also been demonstrated to have an elevated serum concentration. This assay for prostatic acid phosphatase does represent an improvement over prior methods and is of increased use in diagnosis and monitoring.

PROTEIN DEGRADATION PRODUCTS

A number of studies have indicated that increased protease activity is found in human cancerous tissues (Holyoke *et al.,* 1981). Plasminogen-dependent fibrinolytic activity has been found in melanomas, cervices, breasts, lungs, prostates, and ovaries. Research at present is directed towards attempting to isolate and purify human tumor plasminogen activator and to develop antibodies for radioimmunoassay of this material in body fluids as well as measurements of inter-alpha degradation products resulting from plasminogen activation. These include trypsin-inhibitor-derived peptides, alpha$_1$-microglycoprotein, alpha$_1$-microglobulin, complement component C3-derived peptide, fibronectin or cold-insoluble-globulin-derived peptides, and plasminogen-derived peptides.

EDC1, a polypeptide, has been identified in the urine of patients with desseminated disease using an RAI assay that indicates a correlation between EDC1 levels in the urine and response to chemotherapy for carcinomas of the breast, ovary, colon, and lung (Rudman *et al.,* 1977). Two cancers associated with DNA-binding proteins have been identified. One is derived from complement component C3 (C3DP), which is present in a variety of neoplastic diseases. The other is called malignancy-associated DNA binding protein (MAD-2). It has been found in serum of patients with carcinoma of the breast, colon, lung, and ovary. This polypeptide is known to be derived from fibronectin. At present, these materials remain objects of interest, but problems of stability and the technique of the assay continue to prevent them from being developed for use as clinical markers.

MISCELLANEOUS

A small class of hydrocarbon polycationic amine substances known as polyamines has been identified: putrescine, spermidine and spermine. They are found in highest concentration in rapidly proliferating tissues, and they have been linked to control of RNA metabolism and cell regulation. Elevated urinary secretion of polyamines has been demonstrated in approximately two-thirds of patients with metastatic cancer of the large intestine, breast, and lung (Russell *et al.,* 1971). These polyamines are not specific markers for neoplasia, as increased urinary excretion has also been documented in association with benign prostatic hypertrophy, bronchial adenomas, pernicious anemia, and acromegaly.

Methylated nucleosides and pseudouridine are found in transfer RNA (tRNA) and in ribosomal RNA. Increased tRNA methylase activity is a common characteristic of cancer. An elevated concentration of methylated bases has been demonstrated in the tRNA of human and animal tumors. Metabolism of these macromolecules results in the excretion of these nucleosides in the urine as free bases that can be measured as an index of tRNA methylation and turnover. Methylated nucleosides and pseudouridine have been found in abnormal amounts in patients with many forms of hematologic and solid cancer, including 60% of patients with advanced breast carcinoma.

REFERENCES

Abelev, G. I.; Assecritova, I. V.; Kraevsky, N. A.; Perova, S. D.; and Perevodchikova, N. I.: Embryonal serum alpha-globulin in cancer patients: Diagnostic value. *Int. J. Cancer,* **2**:551, 1967.

Abelev, G. I.; Perova, S. D.; Khramkova, N. I.; Postnikova, Z. A.; and Irlin, I. S.: Production of embryonal alpha-globulin by the transplantable mouse hepatoma. *Transplant. Bull.,* **1**:174, 1963.

Alexander, J. C.; Silverman, N. A.; and Chretien, P. B.: Effects of age and cigarette smoking on carcinoembryonic antigen levels. *J.A.M.A.,* **235**:1975–1979, 1976.

Alpert, E.: Alpha-1-fetoprotein. *Clin. Gastroenterol.,* **5**:639–644, 1976.

Banjo, C.; Shuster, J.; and Gold, P.: Intermolecular heterogeneity of the carcinoembryonic antigen. *Cancer Res.,* **34**:2114–2121, 1974.

Banwo, O.; Versey, J.; and Hobbs, J. R.: New oncofetal antigen for human pancreas. *Lancet,* **1**:643–645, 1974.

Braunstein, G. D.; Vaitukaitis, J. L.; Carbone, P. P.; and Ross, G. T.: Ectopic production of human chorionic gonadotrophin by neoplasms. *Ann. Intern. Med.,* **78**:39–45, 1973.

Brock, D. J.: Review: Prenatal diagnosis of neural tube defects. *Eur. J. Clin. Invest.,* **7**:465–472, 1977.

Cohen, H.; Graham, H.; and Lau, H. L.: Alpha-1-fetoprotein in pregnancy. *Am. J. Obstet. Gynecol.,* **7**:881–883, 1973.

Coligan, J. E.; Henkart, P. A.; Todd, C. W.; and Terry, W.

D.: Heterogeneity of the carcinoembryonic antigen. *Immunochemistry,* **10:**591–599, 1973.

Delwiche, R.; Zamcheck, N.; and Marcon, N.: Carcinoembryonic antigen in pancreatitis. *Cancer,* **31:**328–330, 1973.

Dent, P. B.; McColloch, P. B.; Wesley-James, O.; MacLaren, R.; Muirhead, W.; and Dunnett, C. W.: Measurement of carcinoembryonic antigen in patients with bronchogenic carcinoma. *Cancer,* **42:**1484–1491, 1978.

Elias, E. G.; Holyoke, E. D.; and Chu, T. M.: Carcinoembryonic antigen in feces and plasma of normal subjects and patients with colorectal cancer. *Dis. Colon Rectum,* **1:**38–41, 1974.

Fishman, W. H.; Inglis, N. I.; Stolbach, L. L.; and Krant, M. J.: A serum alkaline phosphatase isoenzyme of human neoplastic cell origin. *Cancer Res.,* **28:**150–154, 1968.

Gardner, R. C.; Feinerman, A. E.; Kantrowitz, P. A.; Guttblatt, S.; Lowenstein, M. S.; and Zamcheck, N.: Serial carcinoembryonic antigen (CEA) blood levels in patients with ulcerative colitis. *Am. J. Dig. Dis.,* **23:**129–133, 1978.

Gelder, F. B.; Reese, C. J.; Moossa, A. R.; Hall, T.; and Hunter, R.: Purification, partial characterization, and clinical evaluation of a pancreatic oncofetal antigen. *Cancer Res.,* **38:**313–324, 1978.

Go, V. L. W.; Ammon, H. V.; Holtermuller, K. H.; Krag, E.; and Phillips, S. F.: Quantification of carcinoembryonic antigen-like activities in normal human gastrointestinal secretions. *Cancer,* **36:**2346–2350, 1975.

Gold, P., and Freedman, S. O.: Demonstration of tumorspecific antigens in human colonic carcinomata by immunologic tolerance and absorption techniques. *J. Exp. Med.,* **122:**467–481, 1965.

Gold, P.; Shuster, J.; and Freedman, S. O.: Carcinoembryonic antigen (CEA) in clinical medicine. *Cancer,* **42:**1399–1405, 1982.

Goldenberg, D. M.; DeLand, F.; Kim, E.; Bennett, S.; Primus, F. J.; van Nagell, J. R., Jr.; Estes, N.; DeSimone, P.; and Rayburn, P.: Use of radiolabeled antibodies to carcinoembryonic antigen for the detection and localization of diverse cancers by external photoscanning. *N. Engl. J. Med.,* **298:**1384–1388, 1978.

Goldenberg, D. M.; Kim, E. E.; Bennett, S. J.; Nelson, M. O.; and Deland, F. A.: Carcinoembryonic antigen radioimmunodetection in the evaluation of colorectal cancer and in the detection of occult neoplasms. *Gastroenterology,* **84:**524–532, 1983.

Goldenberg, D. M.; Neville, A. M.; Carter, A. C.; Go, V. L. W.; Holyoke, E. D.; Isselbacher, K. J.; Schein, P.; and Schwartz, M.: Carcinoembryonic antigen: Its role as a marker in the management of cancer. *J. Cancer Res. Clin. Oncol.,* **101:**239–242, 1981.

Haagensen, D. E.; Kister, S. J.; Vandervoorde, J. P.; Grates, J. B.; Smart, E. K.; Hansen, H. J.; and Wells, S. A., Jr.: Evaluation of carcinoembryonic antigen as a plasma monitor for human breast carcinoma. *Cancer,* **42:**1512–1519, 1978.

Holyoke, E. D.; Block, G. E.; Jensen, E.; Sizemore, G. W.; Heath, H.; Chu, T. M.; Murphy, G. P.; Mittelman, A.; Rudden, R. W.; and Arnott, M. S.: Biological markers in cancer diagnosis and treatment. *Curr. Probl. Cancer,* **6(2):**1–68, 1981.

Kupchik, J. Z., and Zamcheck, N.: Carcinoembryonic antigen(s) in liver disease. II. Isolation from human cirrhotic liver and serum and from normal liver. *Gastroenterology,* **63:**95–101, 1972.

Martin, E. W.; James, K. K.; Hurtubise, P.; Catalano, P.; and Minton, J. P.: The use of CEA as an early indicator for gastrointestinal tumor recurrence and second-look procedures. *Cancer,* **39:**440–446, 1977.

Mayer, R. J.; Garnick, M. B.; Steele, G. D., Jr.; and Zamcheck, N.: Carcinoembryonic antigen (CEA) as a monitor of chemotherapy in disseminated colorectal cancer. *Cancer,* **42:**1428–1433, 1978.

Moore, T.; Dhar, P.; Zamcheck, N.; Keeley, A.; Gottlieb, L.; and Kupchik, H. Z.: Carcinoembryonic antigen(s) in liver disease. *Gastroenterology,* **63:**88–94, 1972a.

Moore, T. L.; Kantrowitz, P. A.; and Zamcheck, N.: Carcinoembryonic antigen (CEA) in inflammatory bowel disease. *J.A.M.A.,* **222:**944–947, 1972b.

Patterson, D. J., and Alpert, E.: Tumor markers of the gastrointestinal tract. In Hodgson, H. J. F., and Bloom, S. R. (eds.): *Gastrointestinal and Hepatobiliary Cancer.* Chapman and Hall, London, 1983.

Podolsky, D. K.; McPhee, M. S.; Alpert, E.; Warshaw, A. L.; and Isselbacher, K. J.: Galactosyl-transferase isoenzyme II in the detection of pancreatic cancer. *N. Engl. J. Med.,* **304:**1313, 1981.

Purves, L. R.; Manso, C.; and Torres, F. O.: Serum alphafetoprotein levels in people susceptible to primary liver cancer in Southern Africa. *GANN Monogr. Cancer Res.,* **14:**51–66, 1973.

Rittgers, R. A.; Steele, G.; Zamcheck, N.; Loewenstein, M. S.; Sugarbaker, P. H.; Mayer, R. J.; Lokich, J. J.; Maltz, J.; and Wilso, R. E.: Transient carcinoembryonic antigen (CEA) elevations following resection for colorectal cancer: A limitation in the use of serial CEA levels as an indicator for second look surgery. *J.N.C.I.,* **61:**315–318, 1978.

Rosen, S. W.; Weintraub, B. D.; Vaitukaitis, J. S.; Sussman, H. H.; Hershman, J. M.; and Muggia, F. M.: Placental proteins and their subunits as tumor markers. *Ann. Intern. Med.,* **82:**71–83, 1975.

Rudman, D.; Chawla, R. K.; Heymsfield, S. B.; Bethel, R. E.; Shoji, M.; Vogler, R.; and Nixon, D. W.: Urinary excretion of the cancer-related glycoprotein EDCI: Effect of chemotherapy. *Ann. Intern. Med.,* **86:**174, 1977.

Ruoslahti, E., and Terry, W. D.: Alpha-fetoprotein and serum albumin show sequence homology. *Nature,* **260:**804, 1975.

Russell, D. H.; Levy, C. C.; Schimpff, S. C.; and Hawk, I. A.: Urinary polyamines in cancer patients. *Cancer Res.,* **31:**1555, 1971.

Shanghai Coordinating Group for Research on Liver Cancer: Diagnosis and treatment of primary hepatocellular carcinoma in early stage: Report of 134 cases. *Chin. Med. J. [Engl.],* **92:**801, 1979.

Simons, M. J., and Hosking, C. S.: AFP and ataxia-telangiectasia. *Lancet,* **1:**1234, 1974.

Stevens, D. P., and MacKay, I. R.: Increased carcinoembryonic antigen in heavy cigarette smokers. *Lancet,* **1:**1238–1239, 1973.

Sugarbaker, P. H.; Beard, J. O.; and Drum, D. E.: Detection of hepatic metastases from cancer of the breast. *Am. J. Surg.,* **133:**531–535, 1977.

Sugarbaker, P. H.; Bloomer, W. D.; Corbett, E. D.; and Chaffey, J. T.: Carcinoembryonic antigen (CEA) monitoring of radiation therapy for colorectal cancer. *Am. J. Roentgenol.,* **127:**641–644, 1976.

Tormey, D. C., and Waalkes, T. P.: Clinical correlation between CEA and breast cancer. *Cancer,* **42:**1507–1511, 1978.

Vaitukaitis, J. L., Braunstein, G. D., and Ross, G. T.: A radioimmunoassay which specifically measures human

chorionic gonadotropin in the presence of human luteinizing hormone. *Am. J. Obstet. Gynecol.,* **113:**751–
758, 1972.
Waldmann, T. A., and McIntire, K. R.: The use of radioimmunoassay for alpha-fetoprotein in the diagnosis of
malignancy. *Cancer,* **34:**1510–1515, 1974.
Wanebo, H. J.: Are carcinoembryonic antigen levels of

value in the curative management of colorectal cancer?
Surgery, **89:**290, 1981.
Wanebo, H. J.; Rao, B.; Pinsky, C. M.; Hoffman, R. G.;
Stearns, M.; Schwartz, M. K.; and Oettgen, H. F.: Preoperative carcinoembryonic antigen level as a prognostic indicator in colorectal cancer. *N. Engl. J. Med.,*
299:448–457, 1978.

B. HEMATOLOGIC COMPLICATIONS OF CANCER

Paul V. Woolley

INTRODUCTION

The hematologic disorders that accompany neoplastic disease are complex and fascinating. Primary myeloproliferative diseases produce both quantitative and qualitative abnormalities in the formed elements of the marrow and peripheral blood, whereas solid tumors are associated with a spectrum of mechanical, metabolic, and paraneoplastic syndromes that can affect virtually any element of the blood-forming tissue and the vascular tree. These include, for example, effects on erythropoiesis, red cell survival, coagulation, and leukocyte function. Although this subject is separate from the hematologic effects of cancer treatment, the two topics on occasion overlap. In the following discussion the material is arranged in terms of the disorders that occur in each of the several hematologic cell lines.

DISORDERS OF ERYTHROPOIESIS

Several distinct ways exist in which solid tumors can alter the production of red cells and produce either anemia or polycythemia.

Anemia of Chronic Disease

A mild anemia may occur in the course of inflammatory, infectious, or cancerous diseases that persist for more than a few weeks (Cartwright, 1966). Once established, this anemia is nonprogressive, although its severity is related to the activity or extent of the underlying disorder. It is initially normochromic and normocytic, but hypochromia develops in 25 to 50% of cases. Microcytosis also occurs, but less frequently than hypochromia. It is not as marked as in iron deficiency anemia and usually the mean corpuscular volume (MCV) is greater than 72 μ^3. The bone marrow iron

stores are characteristically normal or increased, but sideroblasts are reduced in number. Serum iron is diminished to levels that may approach those of iron deficiency. Transferrin levels are also reduced, in contrast to the elevated levels found in iron deficiency. Because of the concurrent reduction in iron and transferrin levels, the saturation of transferrin binding sites is higher in anemia of chronic disease than in iron deficiency. In agreement with the normal or increased stores of marrow iron, serum ferritin levels are normal or increased. This has been demonstrated in various neoplasms, including breast cancer (Jacobs *et al.,* 1976a), leukemia (Jones *et al.,* 1973), and Hodgkin's disease (Jones *et al.,* 1973; Jacobs *et al.,* 1976b). An additional feature of the abnormalities in the peripheral blood is that free erythrocyte protoporphyrin levels rise (Krammer *et al.,* 1954; Jeffrey and Watson, 1954). Erythropoietin excretion is variably altered and does not correlate with the hematocrit (Douglas and Adamson, 1975).

Ferrokinetic studies in this disorder have shown that iron injected as a soluble salt disappears rapidly from plasma and is incorporated into erythrocytes in a normal fashion (Freireich *et al.,* 1957a, 1957b). Hence, the utilization of transferrin-bound iron is normal. By contrast, the reutilization of iron injected into humans as hemoglobin or senescent red cells is abnormally low, suggesting a block in its mobilization from the reticuloendothelial system (Freireich *et al.,* 1957a). This finding has not always been confirmed in animal studies, and some controversial aspects of the problem have been summarized (Zarrabi *et al.,* 1977). Finally, erythrocyte destruction is slightly accelerated.

The pathogenesis of this anemia is not completely defined. Its salient features are shortened erythrocyte survival, impaired iron release from reticuloendothelial stores, and an inadequate erythropoietic response to the shortened red cell lifetime (Cartwright, 1966; Wintrobe, 1981). Although the exact basis for any of these is not known, the accelerated erythrocyte destruction may be mediated by an extracorpuscular factor (Freireich et al., 1957b). The defect in iron metabolism may be related to the action of a soluble mediator such as leukocyte lactoferrin at the macrophage level (Van Snick et al., 1977; Wintrobe, et al., 1981). Finally, evidence that the bone marrow response to exogenous erythropoietin is subnormal in neoplasia but normal in inflammatory states has been established (Zucker, et al., 1974), suggesting different mechanisms of the anemia in the two classes of disease. In support of this hypothesis, Walker 256 carcinoma cells inhibit both erythropoietin-mediated erythroid colony formation in culture, and erythropoietin-mediated stimulation of bone marrow heme synthesis (Zucker et al., 1980). Cell-to-cell contact is not necessary for this effect, but a specific soluble mediator has not been identified. These several observations indicate that one or more soluble factors are involved in the development of anemia in chronic disease. In addition, the impaired marrow response may be in part due to the limited supply of serum iron (Douglas and Adamson, 1975).

This anemia usually does not require treatment. Replacement of iron, vitamin B_{12}, or folic acid is not necessary unless a specific deficiency is documented. Transfusions are given as needed, but usually the hematocrit is not so low that this is required.

Iron Deficiency Anemia

Carcinoma of the gastrointestinal tract can produce persistent blood loss that leads to iron deficiency anemia. To place this in perspective, gastrointestinal blood loss causes or contributes to 30 to 40% of all cases of hypochromic anemia related to iron deficiency (Beveridge et al., 1965; Fry, 1961). Furthermore, about 10 to 15% of the cases of gastrointestinal bleeding that result in iron deficiency anemia are caused by neoplastic disease (Beveridge et al., 1965; Fry, 1961). For example, in a series of 100 patients with gastrointestinal bleeding that was unexplained by procedures less radical than laparotomy (Retzlaff, et al., 1961), abdominal exploration established a definite diagnosis in 30, of which two were cecal carcinomas and six were small-bowel

neoplasms. While gastrointestinal carcinoma is responsible for only a fraction of the cases, it should be carefully excluded in any instance of iron deficiency anemia. Carcinoma of the right colon is a notorious source of gastrointestinal bleeding that produces blood in the stool in up to 70% of cases and anemia in 20 to 25% (Woolley, 1976). The older male with iron deficiency may be the most suspect for this source, but younger patients and females are also candidates.

Myelophthisis and Leukoerythroblastosis

Myelophthisis (from the Greek words meaning "wasting of the marrow") refers to the morphologic and functional consequences of bone marrow replacement by granuloma, fibrosis, metastatic tumor, or other abnormal tissue. In its simplest form this results in hypoplasia of one or more formed marrow elements, although sometimes accelerated, ineffective cell turnover occurs. The morphologic expression of myelophthisis in the peripheral blood is leukoerythroblastosis, meaning that immature granulocytic and erythrocytic cells are present in the general circulation.

Rohr and Hegglin (1936) were the first to recognize tumor cells in aspirates of sternal marrow. As this observation was confirmed (Jonsson and Rundles, 1951), the propensity of particular carcinomas, such as those of prostate, lung, and breast to involve marrow was recognized, as was the association of marrow invasion with characteristic morphologic abnormalities in the peripheral blood. A recent study (Anner and Drewinko, 1977) examined tumor infiltration of the marrow in 2877 cancer patients. Marrow metastases were found in 263 (9.1%) of these cases. Specific diseases that frequently spread to marrow were neuroblastoma (48% of cases studied) and Ewing's sarcoma (35%), breast carcinoma (20%), prostate carcinoma (20%), and undifferentiated carcinoma (19%). Bronchogenic carcinoma requires special consideration because the histologic subtypes invade bone marrow with different frequencies. Early studies (Rohr and Hegglin, 1936) remarked that the metastatic cells from lung tumors were smaller than those from prostate or stomach. The importance of this observation was realized with the description (Hansen and Muggia, 1971) of a high rate of bone marrow involvement by small-cell (oat cell) bronchogenic carcinoma. In a total of ten series (Hansen et al.,

1978), the frequency of bone marrow involvement by small-cell carcinoma was 23% (143 of 617 cases) with a range from 17 to 50% in the individual series. Comparable figures for squamous cell and adenocarcinoma of the lung are 15% and 5% (Anner and Drewinko, 1977). Furthermore, bone marrow involvement in small-cell carcinoma tends to be an early manifestation of the disease (Hirsch *et al.,* 1977) and a late occurrence in the other cell types.

Other tumors that may invade marrow include melanoma and gastric cancer (Jonsson and Rundles, 1951; Anner and Drewinko, 1977), whereas pancreatic carcinoma, colonic carcinoma, and soft tissue sarcomas are infrequent causes of myelophthisis. Bone marrow involvement has been reported in 5 to 28% of patients with Hodgkin's disease at the time at presentation (Webb *et al.,* 1970; Rosenberg, 1971; Moran and Ultmann, 1974), although the frequency is much higher if the disease progresses (Higgins, 1968). The same is true of diffuse histiocytic lymphoma (Chabner *et al.,* 1980). Some non-Hodgkin's lymphomas, particularly the nodular, poorly differentiated lymphocytic type, frequently involve bone marrow (50 to 80%) at presentation (Chabner *et al.,* 1976; see Chapter 16), but this involvement may be of minor clinical impact.

Leukoerythroblastic anemia is an anemia in which immature red cells and white cells circulate in the peripheral blood (Vaughn, 1936). An association with marrow infiltration is often made. Present use of the term leukoerythroblastosis refers only to the circulating cells and not to the anemia. Several studies have shown that one-third to one-half of all cases of leukoerythroblastosis are not caused by infiltration of the marrow (Retief, 1964; Weick, *et al.,* 1974). Nonetheless, nucleated red cells and metamyelocytes in the peripheral blood of a cancer patient strongly suggest bone marrow involvement, and an important segment of the differential diagnosis of unexplained leukoerythroblastosis is metastatic tumor, myeloma, or primary myeloproliferative disorder. Conversely, leukoerythroblastosis is not necessarily present in all patients with bone marrow metastases. In one series (Jonsson and Rundles, 1951), the incidence was 10 to 60% for various tumors with proven involvement.

Some diseases such as metastatic breast and prostatic carcinoma also produce myelofi-brosis, reflected morphologically by teardrop deformity and fragmentation of erythrocytes. Carcinoma metastatic to marrow, especially breast carcinoma, may simulate agnogenic myeloid metaplasia and myelofibrosis (Kiely and Silverstein, 1969). In these cases, anemia, thrombocytopenia, circulating normoblasts, reticulocytes, and splenomegaly are present. By contrast, oat cell carcinoma may present only slight thrombocytopenia as a manifestation of marrow involvement (Hirsch *et al.,* 1977).

Tumor metastases to bone marrow may also lead to multifocal bone marrow necrosis associated with bone pain, roentgenologic abnormalities, marrow fat emboli, and hypercalcemia (Kiraly and Wheby, 1976). The frequency of leukoerythroblastosis, anemia, and thrombocytopenia in these cases is very high.

The mechanistic relation between bone marrow infiltration and leukoerythroblastosis is partially understood. Although general terms such as crowding out and irritation of normal marrow have been used, a recent study (Lichtman, 1970) showed that white cells acquire deformability and fluidity during differentiation. Myeloblasts and promyelocytes are rather rigid and normally do not traverse pores in marrow sinuses smaller than their own diameter, but myelocytes and especially polymorphonuclear leukocytes are quite deformable and readily pass through these small openings to reach the peripheral circulation. Presumably, disruption of the selective system of marrow sinus pores by infiltrative processes allows the less deformable cells access to the peripheral blood.

Clinically, the recognition of tumor metastases in bone marrow establishes the stage of disease and is a guide to therapy. Patients with extensive marrow compromise need reduced doses of chemotherapy initially, but improvement in peripheral counts can be expected if the tumor regresses, allowing more drug to be given on subsequent courses. This will mean starting chemotherapy in the presence of low platelet or leukocyte counts in some cases, with the expectation that values will rise with therapy. The decision to include bone marrow aspirate and biopsy as part of the initial workup still depends upon the clinical situation. For leukemia, myeloma, lymphoma, and oat cell carcinoma it is routine, whereas for other diseases such as adenocarcinoma from various locations the need is assessed from clinical considerations including findings on bone scan, the morphology of the peripheral blood, and the statistical likelihood of tumor involvement.

Pure Red Cell Aplasia

Selective and profound erythroid hypoplasia can be a congenital lesion (Blackfan and Diamond anemia) or can occur after exposure to various chemicals or as an aplastic crisis in the course of hemolysis. It also occurs in association with neoplastic disease, the best known relation being with thymoma.

Pure red cell aplasia produces normochromic, normocytic anemia, complete depression of reticulocytes, and absent erythroid precursors in the marrow with maintenance of other cell lines (Hamilton and Conley, 1969). It is an unusual disease that occurs principally in middle-aged adults and is associated with a thymoma in about 50% of cases (Jacobs et al., 1959; Bernatz et al., 1961; Andersen and Ladefoged, 1963; Schmid et al., 1963; Schmid et al., 1965; Hirst and Robertson, 1967). The converse, the proportion of patients with thymoma who have pure red cell aplasia, is no more than 7% (Tsai and Levin, 1957; Jacobs et al., 1959; Havard and Scott, 1960; Andersen and Ladefoged, 1963; Schmid et al., 1965; Erslev, 1977). Sometimes, thymectomy produces remission of the aplasia (Andersen and Ladefoged, 1963; Al-Mondhiry et al., 1971). Pure red cell aplasia is a rare complication of carcinomas of the stomach, lung, and breast (Mitchell et al., 1971), of myeloma (Gilbert et al., 1968), and of chronic lymphocytic leukemia (Stohlman et al., 1971; Abeloff and Waterbury, 1974; Katz, et al., 1981; Nagasawa et al., 1981).

The association of thymoma with autoimmune disease including hypogammaglobulinemia, myasthenia gravis, thyroiditis, and rheumatoid arthritis is well known and suggests that pure red cell aplasia is also part of this spectrum of disorders (Erslev, 1977). The occasional disease remissions that accompany thymectomy, steroids, or cytotoxic drug therapy support this concept. Pure red cell aplasia without thymoma is also found in systemic lupus erythematosus and autoimmune hemolytic anemia, again making the association with an autoimmune etiology. Finally, clear evidence that IgG antibodies to erythroblast nuclei and inhibitors of heme synthesis are present in some patients with pure red cell aplasia has been reported (Krantz and Kao, 1967, 1969; Field et al., 1968; Krantz, 1973; Krantz et al., 1973; Jepson and Vas, 1974; Messner et al., 1981). In one patient (Krantz et al., 1973), removal of marrow cells from the host markedly increased their rate of heme synthesis, while the IgG fraction of his plasma inhibited heme synthesis by either his own marrow cells or those of a normal donor. Treatment of this patient with cyclophosphamide produced a progressive disappearance of the erythroblast cytoxicity activity in his serum IgG and led to increased marrow heme synthesis, reticulocytosis, and disease remission. More recently, a patient has been described (Messner et al., 1981) in whom antibodies were present that inhibited erythroid burst formation of normal and autologous bone marrow cells. Extensive plasmapheresis produced a prolonged disease remission after immunosuppressive therapy had failed.

The erythropoietin levels in these patients fall into two categories. Generally, the patients with cytotoxic IgG antibodies to erythroblasts have high erythropoietin levels and no inhibitor to erythropoietin itself (Krantz and Kao, 1967, 1969; Krantz et al., 1973; Krantz, 1976). A smaller number of patients, however, have been described in whom inhibitor activity against erythropoietin is present (Jepson and Lowenstein, 1968; Peschle et al., 1975), and the levels of erythropoietin are very low. This further illustrates the heterogeneity of this entity.

The approach to the treatment of pure red cell aplasia is to identify any underlying conditions and manage them effectively. If a thymoma is present it should be identified and removed. This results in about a 30% disease remission rate (Jacobs et al., 1959) and may potentiate the effect of steroids (Krantz, 1976). Thymic radiation is occasionally of benefit, especially if a thymoma is not resectable. Steroids and cytotoxic drugs also have a role (see Krantz, 1976 for review). Most recently, plasmapheresis of serum antibody has produced a disease remission (Messner, 1981).

Erythrocytosis

An absolute increase in circulating red cell mass, erythrocytosis, is the primary manifestation of polycythemia vera. The elevation in red cell count may be striking and is usually accompanied by increases in leukocytes and platelets, reflecting the underlying myeloproliferative disorder in which the marrow hyperplasia is independent of stimulation by erythropoietin.

Erythrocytosis is a secondary complication of various neoplasms, the most common site of origin being the kidney, followed in frequency by the liver, central nervous system, and uterus (see Table 6–3) (Golde *et al.*, 1981). An important mechanism of the increased red-cell production is the production by the tumor of erythropoietin or another factor that stimulates the marrow (Waldmann *et al.*, 1968; Hammond and Winnick, 1974; Balcerzak and Bromberg, 1975). This is supported both by direct measurements of erythropoietin in serum and tumor tissue of these patients and by the high frequency with which erythrocytosis disappears after tumor resection (Table 6–4) (Hammond and Winnick, 1974). Other mechanisms that involve disturbance of renal erythropoietin production by direct effects of the tumor on the kidney or the respiratory centers of the brainstem are also possible, however.

The renal tumors usually associated with erythrocytosis are hypernephromas (renal cell adenocarcinoma), but a few cases of other histologies such as Wilms' tumor, hemangioma, adenoma, and sarcoma have been reported (Thorling, 1972; Hammond and Winnick, 1974). Erythrocytosis occurs in 1 to 2% of cases of renal adenocarcinoma (Thorling, 1972) and is a less common complication of this tumor than is anemia. Thorling (1972) has summarized 118 reported cases of erythrocytosis and hypernephroma, using as a definition of erythrocytosis a hemoglobin of 18 g, a red count greater than $6.3 \times 10^6/mm^3$ and a hematocrit

Table 6–3. Tumor Sites Associated with Erythrocytosis

Kidney	179
(This group included 120 hypernephroma, 35 cystic kidney, 14 hydronephrosis, 3 Wilms' tumor, 3 hemangioma, 2 adenoma, 2 sarcoma.)	
Liver	64
Central nervous system	50
Uterus	25
Adrenal	11
Ovary	7
Lung	3
Pheochromocytoma	2
Thymus	1

From Hammond, D., and Winnick, S.: Paraneoplastic erythrocytosis and ectopic erythropoietins. *Ann. N.Y. Acad. Sci.*, **230**:219–227, 1974.

Table 6–4. Disappearance of Erythrocytosis after Tumor Resection

Hypernephroma	31/33 cases
Cerebellar hemangioblastoma	26/26 cases
Uterine fibromyoma	24/25 cases
Hydronephrosis	9/9 cases
Cystic kidney	5/5 cases
Pheochromocytoma	2/2 cases
Wilms'	2/2 cases

From Hammond, D., and Winnick, S.: Paraneoplastic erythrocytosis and ectopic erythropoietins. *Ann. N.Y. Acad. Sci.*, **230**:219–227, 1974.

over 55%. Men were three times as frequent as women in this series. The red count was usually between 6.3×10^6 and $8.5 \times 10^6/mm^3$ and the hematocrit 60 to 70%. No associated abnormalities of leukocytes and platelets were reported. Those bone marrow aspirates that were done showed erythroid hyperplasia. Erythropoietin levels, when reported, were elevated, and probably over 90% of these patients had increased erythropoietin in serum and in tumor tissue extracts (Hammond and Winnick, 1974). Removal of the tumor usually resulted in regression of the erythrocytosis. The increased red cell mass was a paraneoplastic expression of ectopic erythropoietin production by the tumor.

There have been several reports of erythrocytosis and hepatocellular carcinoma. The incidence was about 10% in cases of primary hepatoma (McFadzean, 1958; Brownstein and Ballard, 1966). Stimulus by erythropoietin was a likely mechanism for this erythrocytosis, but the reported measurements of erythropoietin have been equivocal (Thorling, 1972; Hammond and Winnick, 1974). A decreased erythropoietin clearance by the diseased liver could also play a role (Gordon *et al.*, 1970).

Erythrocytosis occurs with cerebellar hemangiomas, uterine myomas, and adrenal and ovarian tumors. At least 50 cases of erythrocytosis and cerebellar hemangiomas (Thorling, 1972) and material identical with renal erythropoietin have been identified in cyst fluid from some of these tumors. Respiratory depression, however, by pressure on the brainstem conceivably can also lead to hypoxia that will stimulate red cell production (Hammond and Winnick, 1974). Some tumors may produce mediators of erythropoiesis that are not erythropoietin. These include androgenic steroids from virilizing tumors of the adrenal cortex or the ovary (Waldmann *et al.*, 1968) or possibly prostaglandins (Hammond and Winnick, 1974). A few cases of erythrocytosis have occurred with pheochromocytoma (Waldmann and Bradley, 1961; Hammond and Winnick, 1974).

In summary, the erythrocytosis associated with solid tumors is most readily explained as a paraneoplastic syndrome in which a product secreted by the tumor stimulates red cell production. The product may be renal erythropoietin or an erythropoietinlike substance. It may also be a nonerythropoietin stimulator of erythropoiesis such as a steroid or conceivably a mediator of erythropoietin action such as a prostaglandin. Considerably more work will be required to fully understand this phenomenon.

HEMOLYTIC STATES

Hemolysis of various etiologies occurs in cancer patients and, in this setting, red cell destruction is a secondary or even tertiary manifestation of the underlying disease process. The most important immediate causes of erythrocyte destruction are red cell fragmentation, immune hemolysis, drug effects, sepsis, and hypersplenism.

Microangiopathic Hemolysis

This term refers to red cell destruction that occurs when erythrocytes are sheared and fragmented during passage through diseased, partially occluded small blood vessels. It occurs in various disease states that have the common feature of vascular endothelial damage or fibrin deposition. In oncology it is most commonly associated with mucin-secreting adenocarcinoma, particularly gastric carcinoma. Clinically, this process leads to the appearance of fragmented erythrocytes (schistocytes, "burr cells," "helmet cells") in the peripheral smear. These bits of red cell are morphologically drawn to two or three sharp points and are more irregular than the teardrop cells seen in myelofibrosis. Graphic microscopic descriptions of red cell shearing on fibrin strands have been published (Bull et al., 1968, 1970). Microspherocytes, produced from contraction of the schistocytes (Lohrmann et al., 1973), nucleated red cells, and reticulocytes are also present, frequently in large numbers. Microangiopathic hemolysis may produce mild changes consisting princi-

pally of the schistocytes in the peripheral blood or may abruptly lead to a clinically severe hemolytic anemia (MAHA) with high transfusion requirements (Cohan et al., 1972; Lohrmann et al., 1973, Ballas and Rubin, 1976; Antman et al., 1979). Thrombocytopenia is not invariably present but can be marked if the underlying disseminated intravascular coagulation or thrombotic thrombocytopenic purpura is severe.

M. C. Brain described microangiopathic hemolytic anemia in its present context (Brain et al., 1962) and postulated the vascular basis of red cell fragmentation. Before that time, the literature described the association of metastatic adenocarcinoma with severe hemolytic anemia in some cases (Antman et al., 1979). Of particular interest was a discussion by Jarcho (1936) of the coexistence of diffuse pulmonary infiltration by gastric carcinoma with anemia, thrombocytopenia, and purpura. The group described by Brain and colleagues (1962) included five cases of metastatic mucin-secreting adenocarcinomas. Subsequently, these five were analyzed together with seven additional cases (Brain et al., 1970). Seven of these 12 patients had gastric adenocarcinoma and the other five had either breast, lung, or pancreas adenocarcinoma. Many had evidence of active disseminated intravascular coagulation. They concluded that thromboplastins derived from mucin initiated intravascular coagulation, resulting in the microangiopathic hemolysis.

Many other reports have confirmed the close association of red cell fragmentation with adenocarcinoma of the stomach (Lynch et al., 1967; Seligsohn et al., 1968; Lohrmann et al., 1973; Antman et al., 1979), breast (Stratford and Tanaka, 1965; Propp, 1966; Ballas and Rubin, 1976), lung (Rodriguez and Stevenson, 1969), biliary tract (Joseph et al., 1967), and other sites (Antman et al., 1979). The typical patient has disseminated mucin-producing adenocarcinoma and develops severe hemolysis and a microangiopathic picture in the peripheral blood. Coombs' tests are negative. There is frequently simultaneous evidence of active disseminated intravascular coagulation with thrombocytopenia and hypofibrinogenemia. However, even when the plasma fibrinogen is normal, accelerated catabolism and turnover of ^{131}I-labeled fibrinogen are demonstrable (Baker et al., 1968; Brain et al., 1970). Antman and others (1979) collected 55 cases reported after 1962 and found evidence of disseminated intravascular coagulation in 28 of them. This raises the question of the fundamental processes of the red cell fragmentation. Apparently, three important mechanisms exist by which the vascular occlusion occurs in cancer patients, namely: (1) Fibrin deposition secondary to intravascular coagulation; (2) plugging of small vessels in pulmonary beds and elsewhere by tumor cell emboli; and (3) hyaline thrombus formation as part of thrombotic thrombocytopenic purpura. The first two of these may be interrelated. The clinical contribution of disseminated intravascular coagulation to many of these cases is well established. In some cases, however, widespread embolization of tumor cells to the microvasculature in the lungs and elsewhere takes place (Stratford and Tanaka, 1965; Lynch *et al.,* 1967; Antman *et al.,* 1979) without severe intravascular coagulation, suggesting that the red cell shearing occurred in small vessels occluded by tumor cells rather than by fibrin. A further possibility is that tumor cells in the microvasculature are the nidus for fibrin strand formation, perhaps by elaborating a procoagulant (Joseph *et al.,* 1967; Baker *et al.,* 1968; Cohan *et al.,* 1972; Ballas and Rubin, 1976), and that the combined vascular occlusion by tumor cells and fibrin strands provides the focus for erythrocyte shearing. This possibility is supported by the observation of tumor-cell emboli surrounded by a fibrinlike material in pulmonary arterioles and venules, as well as by the fact that tumor cell emboli *per se* are much more common than microangiopathic hemolysis (Cohan *et al.,* 1972). It is also in agreement with animal studies of microangiopathic hemolytic anemia. Hilgard and Gordon-Smith (1974) showed that the injection of Walker 256 carcinoma cells into rats produced a MAHA state accompanied by sequestration of fibrinogen and platelets in the lungs. Fibrin and platelets were deposited about tumor cell emboli and it was postulated that hemolysis resulted from contact of the red cell with the fibrin-tumor cell complex.

The balance between fibrin formation and fibrinolysis is also a determinant of the severity of red cell fragmentation. In animal models in which defibrination and MAHA are produced by injection of procoagulant (Rubenberg *et al.,* 1968; Hilgard and Gordon-Smith, 1974), the severity of the red cell fragmentation is increased by blocking fibrinolysis with epsilon-amino caproic acid. In humans, patients with microangiopathic hemolysis often do not show evidence of enhanced fibrinolysis (Baker *et al.,* 1968; Brain *et al.,* 1970; Ballas and Rubin, 1976). Presumably, complete lysis of the network of fibrin strands would reduce the sites available for erythrocyte shearing.

The other major association of microangiopathic hemolytic anemia in the cancer patient is with thrombotic thrombocytopenic purpura (TTP) or hemolytic-uremic syndrome (HUS). The fully developed TTP syndrome consists of hemolytic anemia, thrombocytopenia, renal disease, fluctuating neurologic signs, and fever (Amorosi and Ultmann, 1966). Hyaline thrombi are present in small blood vessels. The less severe hemolytic-uremic syndrome occurs principally in younger children (Gasser *et al.,* 1955; Kaplan, 1976) and is defined by the triad of acute nephropathy, microangiopathic hemolytic anemia, and thrombocytopenia. The distinction between these patients and those with disseminated intravascular coagulation is that they may have normal prothrombin time, partial thromboplastin time, thrombin time, and plasma fibrinogen in the presence of red cell fragmentation, markedly reduced platelets, and renal failure. The pathogenesis of TTP is not fully understood, but it is associated with an underlying neoplasm in some cases (Lohrmann *et al.,* 1973). It has also been described in association with infection (Mettler, 1969), vaccination (Brown, 1973), and lupus erythematosus (Levine and Shearn, 1964), which suggests an immune basis of the disease. The primary lesion may be focal damage to vascular endothelium that leads to accelerated platelet aggregation, small vessel occlusion, and red cell damage (Wintrobe *et al.,* 1981b).

Recently, a new cancer-related variant of thrombotic thrombocytopenic purpura has been noted. It has also been referred to as thrombotic microangiopathy, hemolytic-uremic syndrome (Harden *et al.,* 1982), chemotherapy-induced nephrotoxicity (Hanna *et al.,* 1981), and chronic glomerular microangiopathy (Laffay *et al.,* 1979). Typically, it consists of microangiopathic hemolytic anemia, thrombocytopenia, and renal failure. Less consistent features are neurologic defects such as seizures, pulmonary insufficiency, and adverse responses to blood transfusion (Jones *et al.,* 1980). Fever is unusual but may occur (Cantrell *et al.,* 1982). At present, at least 30 cases of this entity have been reported. Most have been patients with adenocarcinoma, frequently of gastric origin. Two cases, however, in patients with epidermoid cancer (Gulati *et al.,* 1980) and two in germ cell tumors (Jackson *et al.,* 1982) are known. In several instances the patients have been in complete remission following chemotherapy or have had only minimal residual disease demonstrated at autopsy. Results of coagulation tests in this disease have been variable. Some patients have prolonged thrombin times and elevated levels of fibrin split products, but in others these values are completely normal as are the prothrombin time and partial thromboplastin time. Coombs' tests are negative. The exact cause of the syndrome is unknown, although numerous etiologies have been proposed, including effects of chemotherapy, particularly mitomycin C, release of thromboplastin from tumor tissue, and immunologic aberrations. Of these, treatment with cytotoxic drugs, most notably mitomycin C, seems the most consistent initiator of the process (Krauss *et al.,* 1979; Karlin and Stroehlein, 1980; Kressel *et al.,* 1981; Pavy *et al.,* 1982; Rabani, 1982). Many of these patients have high levels of circulating immune complexes, but reduction of the levels of these complexes by plasmapheresis usually does not alter the clinical course (Cantrell *et al.,* 1982, 1983). In one case, however, a patient with high levels of circulating immune complexes that cross-reacted with gastric carcinoma tissue showed clinical improvement with plasmapheresis (Zimmerman *et al.,* 1982). Most patients affected with this syndrome are quite ill and the mortality rate exceeds 75% within six months of its onset. Therapeutic intervention has been of limited value. Occasional remissions have been attributed to treatment with heparin, corticosteroids, azathioprine, or plasmapheresis. No single modality, however, is clearly superior to others nor reliable in a large proportion of cases.

Treatment of microangiopathic hemolytic anemia in the patient with cancer is aimed at managing the immediate complications and reversing the underlying cause. Transfusion requirements may be substantial, even in the presence of brisk reticulocytosis. Management of disseminated intravascular coagulation involves the use of heparin and coagulation factor replacement, as the situation requires. As with consumptive coagulopathy of any cause, removal of the underlying disease is critical and chemotherapy may be beneficial in MAHA associated with cancer (Antman *et al.,* 1979). The proper treatment of TTP is controversial (Amorosi and Karpatkin, 1977). Splenectomy (Amorosi and Ultmann, 1966; Ber-

nard *et al.,* 1969; Goldenfarb and Finch, 1973), heparin (Allanby *et al.,* 1966; Carmichael and Medley, 1966), dextran infusions (Lerner *et al.,* 1967; Neame *et al.,* 1976), antiplatelet drugs (Amorosi and Karpatkin, 1977; Birgens *et al.,* 1979), steroids (Amorosi and Ultmann, 1966; Neame *et al.,* 1976), plasma infusion (Byrne and Khurana, 1977), plasmapheresis (Bukowski *et al.,* 1977; Ansell *et al.,* 1978), and prostacyclin infusion (Hensby *et al.,* 1979) all have their advocates, but no single regimen has been shown to be uniformly effective. At present, no absolute recommendation can be made, but judicious use of antiplatelet drugs such as acetylsalicylic acid and dipyridamole is appropriate, and if circulating immune complexes are present, plasmapheresis can be tried as well.

Immune Hemolysis

Antibody-mediated immune hemolysis is a relatively frequent complication of lymphoid neoplasia but is uncommon in patients with carcinoma. Autoimmune hemolytic anemia is present in up to 20% of patients with chronic lymphocytic leukemia and may be due either to a warm-reacting IgG antibody or, less commonly, a cold-reacting IgM antibody. Conversely, over half of patients with autoimmune hemolysis due to warm-reacting antibodies have an underlying lymphoreticular neoplasm, such as chronic lymphocytic leukemia, non-Hodgkin's lymphoma, multiple myeloma, or thymoma (Pirofsky, 1976). The antibodies in these cases are most frequently of the IgG_1 class and may be present either alone or with another subclass. They usually sensitize the red cell to phagocytosis by macrophages rather than producing overt, complement-mediated intravascular hemolysis. Cold IgM agglutinins with either anti-I or anti-i activity complicate many lymphoproliferative disorders, including Waldenström's macroglobulinemia, multiple myeloma, various non-Hodgkin's lymphomas, Hodgkin's disease, and chronic lymphocytic leukemia (Pruzanski and Shumak, 1977). They are frequently monoclonal and, in contrast to the IgG antibodies, fix complement. For this reason, if hemolysis occurs it is likely to be intravascular (Wintrobe, 1981c). Cold agglutinins can also be polyclonal as has been reported in angioimmunoblastic lymphadenopathy (Pruzanski and Shumak, 1977).

The association of autoimmune hemolytic

anemia with solid tumors is rare. Jones and Tillman (1945) described a case of hemolytic anemia that was resolved with removal of an ovarian cyst. It was suggested that a hemolysin from the tumor caused the anemia, but an antibody was not demonstrated. Several cases from the literature were cited of the association of dermoid cysts with hemolytic anemia. Subsequently, a small number of cases has been reported of autoimmune hemolysis with solid tumors. Spira and Lynch (1979) reviewed 16 cases of autoimmune hemolytic disease and carcinoma. Primaries were lung (five), ovary (three), kidney (two), large bowel (two), breast (one), stomach (one), cervix of the uterus (one), and testis (one). The antibody when specified was IgG without particular RBC antigenic specificity. One patient with ovarian cancer had an associated autoimmune thrombocytopenia. Resolution of hemolysis was seen in some cases by removal of the primary tumor. Steroids were less effective therapy in this situation than in idiopathic autoimmune hemolysis.

Acute Hemolysis Secondary to Drugs

Cytotoxic drugs commonly produce anemia due to myelosuppression; less frequently, they cause acute hemolysis. In some cases, particular drugs can be shown to damage the red cell *in vitro* or to cause hemolysis in animals, but these drugs have not been directly associated with clinical hemolysis. A summary of currently available data is presented in Table 6–5.

Nitrogen mustard has been studied when given in combination with other drugs and reported to depress levels of red cell superoxide dismutase. In some cases this is associated with hemolysis (Auclair, *et al.,* 1980). The nitrosoureas streptozotocin (Slonim *et al.,* 1976) and 1,3-*bis*(2-chloroethyl)-1-nitrosourea (BCNU) (Frischer and Ahmad, 1977) both lower the levels of erythrocyte reduced glutathione and allow hemolysis to occur due to oxidant stress.

The anthracyclines doxorubicin and daunorubicin do not cause oxidative hemolysis of normal human erythrocytes at therapeutic concentrations. At high concentrations *in vitro,* however, they increase the osmotic fragility of erythrocytes from several animal species (Schioppocassi and Schwartz, 1977) and hemolyze human erythrocytes (Shinohara and Tanaka, 1980). They produce peroxidation of thiols in red cell proteins and lipids, including

hemoglobin and membrane components, cause the generation of intracellular hydrogen peroxide, and produce instability of reduced glutathione (Henderson *et al.,* 1978; Shinohara and Tanaka, 1980). The hexose monophosphate shunt is stimulated in a process that utilizes oxyhemoglobin and reduced glutathione. It has been suggested that these phenomena could lead to *in vivo* hemolysis in G-6-PD deficient persons or if the anthracyclines are used in combination with agents such as BCNU that impair glutathione generation.

The plant alkaloid ellipticine has antitumor activity and has been used in clinical trials. It produces intravascular hemolysis in humans (Rouesse *et al.,* 1981) and in animals (Herman *et al.,* 1974; Lee, 1976). It also produces immediate hemolysis of erythrocytes *in vitro,* especially above a level of about 8 mg/mL (Herman *et al.,* 1974; Lee, 1976). These effects appear to be membrane-mediated and are blocked by agents such as citrate and EDTA that participate in Ca^{2+}-mediated uptake of the drug by the red cell. The complete mechanism remains to be established.

Cisplatin commonly produces a severe normochromic normocytic anemia without hemolysis (Rossof *et al.,* 1972; Rozencweig *et al.,* 1977; Kuzur and Greco, 1980; Najarian *et al.,* 1981). In addition, five cases of acute hemolysis due to cisplatin have been reported (Getaz *et al.,* 1980; Levi *et al.,* 1981; Nguyen *et al.,* 1981). In four of these, the direct Coombs' tests were positive, either with anti-IgG or anti-C3 sera. In one case, (Nguyen *et al.,* 1981) the Coombs' test became negative between cisplatin treatments and positive upon rechallenge. It is postulated that these cases represent antibody-mediated hemolysis with the antigen being a complex of cisplatin with the red cell membrane. Full characterization of the antibody or the precise mechanism of hemolysis has not been performed in any case.

At least two other cytotoxic drugs have been shown in isolated instances to produce antibody-mediated hemolysis. One case of acute hemolysis due to teniposide (VM26) was associated with a strongly positive Coombs' test and two IgG antibodies, one of which was IgG1 (Habibi *et al.,* 1981a, 1981b). The drug was required for the antibody reaction with RBC, but did not adhere to the red cell in the absence of antibody. Methotrexate has been associated with immune hemolysis in two cases. One patient developed antibody-mediated intravascular hemolysis secondary to

Table 6–5.   Cytotoxic Drugs Associated with Erythrocyte Destruction

DRUG	IN VITRO HEMOLYSIS	IN VIVO HEMOLYSIS	MECHANISMS	REFERENCE
Nitrogen mustard		Possible clinically	Depression of red cell superoxide dismutase	Auclair, *et al.*, 1980
Nitrosoureas Streptozotocin	In rat and human RBC	In rats	Lowering of erythrocyte-reduced glutathione; hemolysis due to oxidant stress protected by glucose, epinephrine, and nicotinamide	Slonim, *et al.*, 1976
1,3-bis(2-chloroethyl)-1-nitrosourea (BCNU)		Possible clinically	Lowering of erythrocyte-reduced glutathione by inhibition of glutathione reductase	Frischer and Ahmad, 1977
Procarbazine	In normal and G-6-PD deficient human cells	No	Oxidative changes similar to other hydrazines with decreased reduced glutathione, increased methemoglobin, and generation of intracellular hydrogen peroxide. Effects potentiated in G-6-PD deficient cells	Sponzo, *et al.*, 1974
Ellipticine	Yes	In humans and rodents		Herman, *et al.*, 1974; Lee, 1976
2-'Deoxycoformycin	In mice	In patients treated for leukemia	Inhibition of adenosine deaminase; fall in cellular ATP and rise in dATP. Exact mechanism of hemolysis not defined	Siaw, *et al.*, 1980; Spremulli, *et al.*, 1982; Prentice, *et al.*, 1981; Smith, *et al.*, 1980
Doxorubicin	In normal and G-6-PD-deficient human red cells and in several animal species (dog, monkey, rat)	No	Generation of oxygen radicals within cell; peroxidation of red cell proteins and lipids; decreased stability of reduced glutathione. Risk to patients at therapeutic concentrations in presence of G-6-PD deficiency or with concurrent inhibitor or glutathione such as BCNU	Schioppocossi, *et al.*, 1977; Henderson, *et al.*, 1978; Shinohara, and Tanaka, 1980
Cisplatin		Five clinical cases	Antibody directed against cisplatin-RBC membrane complex	Getaz, *et al.*, 1980; Levi, *et al.*, 1981; Nguyen, *et al.*, 1981
Teniposide (VM-26)		One clinical case	IgG antibody that requires the drug for binding to red cell membrane	Habibi, *et al.*, 1981a,b
Methotrexate		Two clinical cases	Antibody that requires the drug for binding to red cell membrane	Sacher, *et al.*, 1981; Woolley, *et al.*, 1983

triamterene with cross reactivity to methotrexate (Takahashi and Tsukada, 1979). A second had two episodes of hemolysis following methotrexate administration and was shown to have an IgG3 antibody that reacted with methotrexate but not folic acid or folinic acid. It did not fix complement, but sensitized macrophages to phagocytose erythrocytes, suggesting that the hemolysis was extravascular (Sacher *et al.,* 1981; Woolley *et al.,* 1983).

Sepsis

Septicemia involving various microorganisms can lead to disseminated intravascular coagulation and hemolysis. *Clostridium perfringens (C. welchii)* septicemia is associated with a particularly fulminant and catastrophic acute hemolysis that can result in virtually complete destruction of the circulating erythrocytes and severe depletion of coagulation factors within a few hours. Clostridial septicemia is well known as a complication of septic abortion (Mahn and Dantuono, 1955; Wallerstein and Aggeler, 1964) but also complicates disease of the biliary tract (Bennett and Healey, 1963) and leukemia (Boggs *et al.,* 1958). The clinical presentation includes high fever, mental irritability or delirium, dyspnea, marked tachycardia, intravascular hemolysis with burgundy-red serum and brown urine, and profound pallor as the hematocrit drops abruptly (Boggs *et al.,* 1958; Wallerstein and Aggeler, 1964). Microspherocytes are prominent on the peripheral blood film (Bennett and Healy, 1963). In leukemia patients who develop this problem, the source of the organisms is the gastrointestinal tract and other microbes such as enteric gram negative bacilli, or anaerobic streptococci may also be present (Boggs *et al.,* 1958). Of importance to the patient with cancer is the recent description of several cases of clostridial sepsis during or following drug infusion into the hepatic artery (Tully *et al.,* 1979). Although none of the cases cited was of *C. perfringens* hemolysis, it remains a potential complication of this procedure and of other invasive manipulations of the hepatobiliary tree such as percutaneous biliary drainage.

Some cases of clostridial sepsis occur without hemolysis, whereas in the others the hemolysis is of varying severity. The events leading to severe hemolysis are not completely clarified. A central role of bacterial alpha toxin, which is a lecithinase, has frequently been postulated, and in support of this are the demonstrable hemolytic properties of this toxin *in vitro* as well as in experimental animals. In one woman with *C. perfringens* sepsis, however, the changes in her red cell membranes did not correspond to those seen in lecithinase-treated cells inasmuch as there was less distortion of lipid content than of protein content (Simpkins *et al.,* 1971). These organisms produce several toxins, and it is possible that theta toxin, a hemolysin that does not hydrolyze erythrocyte membrane lipid, also has a role. Other toxins such as the delta toxin are hemolysins, and to ascribe the entire mechanism of the hemolysis (Alouf and Jolivet-Reynaud, 1981) to the alpha lecithinase may be simplifying the picture. Finally, synergy between *C. perfringens* and other organisms in *in vitro* hemolysis is recognized and also may be of clinical importance (Gubash, 1978, 1980; Choudhury, 1978).

The approach to these patients requires early clinical recognition and rapid intervention, including removal of instrumentation within the biliary tract, blood replacement, and antibiotics. Penicillin G is highly effective against clostridia. If a patient is allergic to penicillin, cefoxitin may be an appropriate alternative.

Erythrophagocytosis

Phagocytosis of erythrocytes is a normal function of the spleen. In the rare neoplasm, histiocytic medullary reticulosis (HMR) or malignant histiocytosis, this process is pathologically increased and contributes to the hematologic abnormalities of the disease. In HMR, hepatosplenomegaly, lymphoadenopathy, and pancytopenia are present (Scott and Robb-Smith, 1939; Warnke *et al.,* 1975), and a hemolytic anemia is present (Asher, 1946; Willcox, 1952; Marshall, 1956; Lynch and Alfrey, 1965; Natelson *et al.,* 1968). Abnormal histiocytes with active phagocytic properties proliferate widely in lymph nodes, spleen, liver, and bone marrow, and these ingest not only erythrocytes, but also white cells and platelets. The marrow is cellular and erythropoiesis is active but ineffective. The lifetime of ^{51}Cr-labeled red cells is markedly shortened; the isotope from these studies sequesters in the body and is not excreted (Lynch and Alfrey, 1965). Large quantities of stainable iron derived from red cells are present in the histiocytes. Ferrokinetic studies have shown that this iron does not reach the histiocytes via transferrin (Lynch and Alfrey, 1965; Natelson *et al.,* 1968). The conclusion is that the abnormal phagocytosis contributes significantly to the hemolytic anemia and to the accumulation of iron in the proliferating histiocytes (Lynch and Alfrey, 1965; Natelson *et al.,* 1968). Occasionally, a similar process is seen in other disorders, and a clinical picture closely resembling HMR has been reported in a patient with widespread gastric cancer (James *et al.,* 1979). This pathologic erythrophagocytosis is to be distinguished from erythrophagocytosis present in the spleen and liver during autoimmune hemolysis. In the first case, the proliferating histiocytes are cytologically abnormal, and the phagocytic process is the primary cause of the hemolysis. In other hemolytic states, the phagocytic cells are cytologically normal, and the phagocytosis is a secondary response to the hemolysis.

Hypersplenism

Hypersplenism is a clinical state in which the phagocytosis or sequestration of peripheral blood cells by the spleen occurs in excess of the ability of the marrow to compensate for their loss. A depression of one or more of the formed elements of the peripheral blood that responds to removal of the spleen is the result. Although historically there was a controversy as to whether or not a splenic hormone suppressed marrow function (Crosby, 1962a), it is now agreed that the phagocytic and filtering functions of the spleen are responsible for the decreases in peripheral cell counts. The diagnostic criteria for this disorder (set forth by Dameshek, 1955) are: (1) A decrease in the levels of one or more formed elements of the peripheral blood; (2) a reactive hyperplasia in the marrow corresponding to the deficient element(s); (3) splenomegaly; and (4) correction of the condition with splenectomy. Nonetheless, the definition of hypersplenism has long been controversial because of the problem of deciding where normal splenic function stops and hyperfunction begins. This has led Crosby (1962b) to state, "When a person is hematologically better off without his spleen, he had hypersplenism."

Historically, the subject of hypersplenism and the approach to the enlarged spleen in the patient with cancer has gone through several conceptual stages. Prior to 1940, splenectomy in patients with cancer, particularly those with

hematologic cancers, was regarded as a futile procedure because it had no impact upon the natural history of the disease (Fisher *et al.,* 1952). Subsequently, the question arose as to whether splenectomy was a useful procedure for therapy of Hodgkin's disease or for prevention of conversion of chronic myelogenous leukemia to an accelerated phase. Although not effective in these situations (Sykes *et al.,* 1954), opinion clearly favors the concept that hypersplenism is a correctable manifestation of some neoplasms, and that splenectomy is an appropriate procedure in some cases for the palliation of splenomegaly, hemolytic anemia, and hypersplenic thrombocytopenia (Fisher *et al.,* 1952; Duckett, 1963; Morris *et al.,* 1975). Splenectomy may also be diagnostic in some cases of lymphoma (Brown and Meynell, 1949; Rudders *et al.,* 1972; Ahmann *et al.,* 1966; Davey *et al.,* 1973) or histiocytic medullary reticulosis (Warnke *et al.,* 1975), and is a useful staging procedure in selected patients with Hodgkin's disease. Confining the discussion to the subject of hypersplenism and splenectomy, many studies show that properly selected patients with cancer can achieve a temporary or prolonged benefit from splenectomy. The question of proper selection raises some problems. Many of these patients have hematologic neoplasms that extensively involve the marrow, and the diagnostic criteria set forth by Dameshek may not be completely applicable because a limited marrow reserve precludes a full reactive response. The diagnosis of hypersplenism in these patients is then based upon the deficiency of cellular elements of the peripheral blood, splenomegaly, and response to splenectomy. Some attention has been given to basing the decision for splenectomy upon studies of splenic sequestration of ^{51}Cr-labeled red cells or platelets. Although a positive sequestration study almost always predicts a favorable outcome to splenectomy, a negative one does not preclude a good response (Adler *et al.,* 1975). In general, patients with larger spleens and more severe deficiencies respond best to splenectomy (Adler *et al.,* 1975). Bone marrow invasion by tumor does not preclude a favorable response. Hence, many recent authors have adopted a judiciously interventional approach to the patient with cancer with depressed peripheral counts (Adler *et al.,* 1975; Editorial, 1979; Gill *et al.,* 1981). Radiation of the spleen is an alternative in poor-risk patients who have splenomegaly and depressed peripheral counts, but the results are inferior to those of surgery (Adler *et al.,* 1975). Selective embolization of the splenic artery has also been used in poor operative risks. It may improve blood counts but produce severe symptoms from splenic infarction (Papadimitriou *et al.,* 1976).

Most patients with cancer with hypersplenism have a hematologic neoplasm such as chronic leukemia, lymphoma, or Hodgkin's disease. Some patients with breast cancer (Dunn and Goldwein, 1975; Woolley *et al.,* 1983) or other solid tumors may also be seen. It should be noted that splenectomy will raise peripheral counts and improve the tolerance of patients to radiation or chemotherapy, for example in Hodgkin's disease. It has not been shown, however, to be critical to achieving full doses of treatment or to improving survival in unselected patients, and therefore is not routine on that basis alone (Royster *et al.,* 1974; Editorial, 1979; Gill *et al.,* 1981). Because asplenic patients are at risk for systemic infections from organisms such as *Streptococcus pneumoniae* and *Haemophilus influenzae,* they should be carefully monitored for bacterial infection. The effective pneumococcal vaccine that is now available is only partially protective in this situation.

DISORDERS OF COAGULATION

The coagulation disorders that complicate neoplastic disease include both bleeding and thrombotic problems, both sometimes occurring in the same patient (Goodnight, 1974). While a small and rather infrequent set of abnormalities is associated with specific factor deficiencies or factor inhibitors, the most important group is related to disseminated intravascular coagulation (DIC). The subject is somewhat simplified by stating some general principles. First, disseminated intravascular coagulation occurs in two forms: acute, in which bleeding problems are common, and chronic, in which thrombotic complications predominate (Owen and Bowie, 1974; Colman *et al.,* 1979). In either case, the underlying mechanism is the introduction of procoagulant material into the circulation, resulting directly or indirectly in the generation of thrombin. Second, acute DIC is particularly associated with two neoplastic conditions, namely acute promyelocytic leukemia and prostatic carcinoma. In addition, both acute and chronic DIC can occur in conjunction with mucin-secreting adenocarcinoma. Finally, there exists a group of problems that have over the years been reported, often as separate entities, that includes disseminated intravascular coagulation, deep venous thrombosis, nonbacterial thrombotic endocarditis, and arterial emboli. Although these have sometimes been regarded as separate manifestations of cancer, particularly of mucin-secreting adenocarcinoma, current thinking places chronic DIC as the central problem and the other disorders as part of the presentation of chronic DIC (Sack *et al.,* 1977). An important remaining question is whether there exists a definable "hypercoagulable state" in patients with cancer that predisposes them to these problems.

With this as introduction, several specific topics need to be addressed, namely, (1) the overall state of the coagulation system in the patient with cancer; (2) the bleeding diathesis associated with acute promyelocytic leukemia, which is principally acute DIC; (3) the bleeding complications of prostatic carcinoma, which are related to acute or chronic DIC with an important additional component of fibrinolysis; and (4) the spectrum of disorders that are reported with adenocarcinoma, especially the mucin-secreting variety.

Many studies now show that the coagulation systems are not normal in patients with advanced cancer. The abnormalities include elevation of plasma levels of fibrinogen and other clotting factors, shortening of bleeding time and *in vitro* clotting time, prolonged prothrombin time, elevated levels of fibrin split products, and sometimes further evidence of fibrinolysis. A consistent finding is that plasma fibrinogen levels are elevated in 50 to 80% of patients (Miller *et al.,* 1967; Soong and Miller, 1970; Brugarolas *et al.,* 1973; Sun *et al.,* 1974; Hagedorn *et al.,* 1974). Often, these levels are in the range of 400 to 500 mg/100 mL, but they may be higher. The source of the fibrinogen is increased hepatic synthesis. Not only is plasma fibrinogen increased, but its turnover and destruction are accelerated as well (Slichter and Harker, 1974). Hence, a normal fibrinogen level in a patient with cancer may represent a balance between increased production and increased destruction, whereas if hypofibrinogenemia occurs, it represents accelerated consumption much more often than it represents impaired production.

Levels of other coagulation proteins can also

be abnormal, including marked elevations in factor VIII (Amundsen *et al.,* 1963; Miller *et al.,* 1967; Sun *et al.,* 1974). Prothrombin and factors V, IX, and X are variably increased (Waterbury and Hampton, 1967; Miller *et al.,* 1967). Factor XIII when examined has been normal or somewhat decreased (Miller *et al.,* 1967; Soong and Miller, 1970). Frequently, these altered levels of coagulation factors are associated with an abnormally short bleeding time (Miller *et al.,* 1967) or *in vitro* silicon tube clotting times (Miller *et al.,* 1967; Waterbury and Hampton, 1967; Soong and Miller, 1970). These findings have been interpreted as consistent with a hypercoagulable state that could predispose the patient to abnormal clotting. The prothrombin time in these cases is either normal or somewhat prolonged (Miller *et al.,* 1967; Hagedorn *et al.,* 1974; Sun *et al.,* 1974), and less frequently short (Soong and Miller, 1970). Likewise, the partial thromboplastin time and thrombin time are normal or slightly prolonged. Antithrombin III levels have been reported as normal (Miller *et al.,* 1967). Increases in fibrinolytic split products are also seen (Brugarolas *et al.,* 1973; Carlsson, 1973; Hagedorn *et al.,* 1974; Sun *et al.,* 1974) and are not necessarily accompanied by low fibrinogen levels or platelet counts. The increased FSP levels have been seen in between 38 and 82% of the cancer patients in these studies and in some cases the frequency of high levels is greater in patients with metastatic disease (Carlsson, 1973). Increased fibrinolytic activity is variably present. In those instances in which it is encountered, it is taken as evidence of intravascular coagulation (Owen and Bowie, 1974).

Overall, these observations show that patients with cancer exhibit a complex and far-ranging disturbance in the coagulation system. The percentage of patients in these studies with some abnormality is very high. Sun and colleagues (1974) found 3 of 61 patients with no abnormality, and others have confirmed this distribution (Soong and Miller, 1970; Miller *et al.,* 1967; Hagedorn *et al.,* 1974). They provide the background for the serious clinical problems of defibrination and thrombosis.

The clear description of acute promyelocytic leukemia as a clinical entity with a bleeding diathesis and a rapidly fatal course was made by Hillestad (1957) and acute disseminated intravascular coagulation leading to hypofibrinogenemia and bleeding in this disease is now well recognized. The coagulation dis-

order was first described as primary fibrinolysis, but as information accrued it became evident that the principal defect was disseminated intravascular coagulation. For example, Didisheim and colleagues (1964) reported two patients with acute promyelocytic leukemia. Both had decreased platelets, prolonged prothrombin and thrombin time, and low fibrinogen and factor V. Fibrinogen turnover was accelerated in one, but fibrinolysis was not abnormal. Baker and colleagues (1964) described a patient with acute leukemia and depressed levels of fibrinogen, factor V, and factor VIII. A clinical trial of epsilon aminocaproic acid failed, although heparin gave at least transient clinical improvement. Subsequently, Gralnick and colleagues (1972) established that patients with acute promyelocytic leukemia had coagulation abnormalities characteristic of disseminated intravascular coagulation with secondary fibrinolysis and that treatment with heparin could improve coagulation values and control the bleeding. The recommendation was made to treat these patients with heparin early in their course because cytoreductive chemotherapy would worsen the situation by releasing procoagulant material from cells. The dose of heparin was kept relatively low, for example, 100 to 200 μ/mg/day in divided doses or as an infusion, to avoid worsening the hemorrhage by excessive anticoagulation (Gralnick *et al.,* 1972; Gralnick and Sultan, 1975; Daly, *et al.,* 1980). The use of ϵ-aminocaproic acid was reserved for those situations where fibrinolysis was felt to play an important role and was used only in conjunction with heparin. Later work established that leukemic promyelocytes possess a procoagulant in the granular fraction that requires factors V, VII, and X for its activity and hence resembles tissue thromboplastin as an activator of the extrinsic pathway (Gralnick and Abrell, 1973). The protein moiety of this factor cross-reacts immunologically with human brain tissue thromboplastin (Gouault-Heilmann, *et al.,* 1975).

A bleeding diathesis has also been described in patients with prostatic carcinoma. The typical presentation is a person with metastatic prostatic carcinoma who develops bleeding, hypofibrinogenemia, and fibrinolytic activity in the plasma either spontaneously or after prostatic surgery. Initially, the fibrinolysis that occurs in these patients was emphasized, it now appears that many if not all of these cases have disseminated intravascular coagulation with secondary fibrinolysis. The earliest reports (Jurgens and Trautwein, 1930; Marder, et al., 1949) described the association of hypofibrinogenemia, bleeding, and prostate cancer. Later, both fibrinolysis and intravascular coagulation were mentioned as possible causes (Seale, et al., 1951), as was marked reduction in factor V (Cosgrieff and Leifer, 1952). Tagnon then described several cases emphasizing the fibrinolytic activity in the plasma (Tagnon et al., 1952, 1953a,b). The fibrinolytic activity and the bleeding resolved with estrogen therapy in some cases (Tagnon, et al., 1952, 1953a) and in one instance recurred when testosterone was administered (Tagnon et al., 1953b). It was also possible to demonstrate fibrinolytic activity in tissue extracts from primary tumors and metastases. When this was taken with the earlier demonstration that the chief proteolytic enzyme of human prostatic fluid is a fibrinolysin (Huggins and Neal, 1942; Huggins and Vail, 1942), the evidence seemed compelling that the release of fibrinolysins from prostatic tissue led to primary fibrinolysis. As more cases were described, however, it became clear that many, if not all, of these patients also had disseminated intravascular coagulation and that the fibrinolysis could be a secondary response (Rapoport and Chapman, 1959; Naeye, 1962). Furthermore, some cases that were described in terms of their fibrinolysis probably would be regarded today as disseminated intravascular coagulation (Bergen and Schilling, 1958; Brown et al., 1962). Nonetheless, the magnitude of the fibrinolytic response in prostatic carcinoma is out of proportion to that described in other neoplastic diseases that are accompanied by disseminated intravascular coagulation. One interpretation of the data suggests that acute disseminated intravascular coagulation can occur in patients with prostatic carcinoma, but that it may be accompanied by an exaggerated element of fibrinolysis, perhaps because of release of intrinsic fibrinolysins from prostatic tissue.

These considerations have implications regarding clinical management. Treatment of acute disseminated intravascular coagulation is directed at potentiation of antithrombin III activity with heparin and judicious coagulation factor replacement. Inhibition of fibrinolysis in these patients by ϵ-aminocaproic acid may be detrimental and may produce widespread thrombosis. This complication has been described as leading to renal failure in a patient with prostatic carcinoma (Naeye, 1962). A reasonable therapeutic approach would be to consider the severity of disseminated intravascular coagulation in a given case and to treat it accordingly with heparin. If fibrinolysis is excessive, if the patient does not have thrombotic complications, or if he is bleeding and hypofibrinogenemic, then ϵ-aminocaproic acid can be given with heparin. It seems unnecessary to risk provoking widespread thromboses with the use of ϵ-aminocaproic acid alone. Estrogen has been given during the acute disease process in these patients and is possibly of benefit (Tagnon et al., 1952, 1953a; Brown et al., 1962; Pellman et al., 1966). Theoretically, cell lysis by large doses of estrogen could worsen the basic process. The above syndromes are those that are associated with hemorrhagic acute disseminated intravascular coagulation. The long-term introduction of smaller amounts of procoagulant into the circulation results in a more chronic form of this disorder that is characterized by thrombotic manifestations.

Deep-vein thrombosis is by definition intravascular coagulation. The relation between cancer and venous thrombosis was made over a century ago by Armand Trousseau (Sack et al., 1977). More recent interest began with the description (Sproul, 1938) of venous thrombosis in 14 out of 47 (30%) autopsied cases of pancreatic carcinoma and 32 out of 147 (20%) cases of gastric cancer, as well as with carcinoma of lung, kidney, prostate, and ovary. Also described were fibrin vegetations on cardiac valves of several of these patients. Subsequently, the association of mucin-secreting cancers and venous thrombosis has been repeatedly confirmed (Jennings and Russell, 1948; Gore, 1953; Henderson, 1955; Perlow and Daniels, 1956; Lieberman et al., 1961; Rohner et al., 1966; Sack et al., 1977; Donati and Poggi, 1980). The pancreas is a common site of origin of these tumors, and so are the stomach, lung, and other organs.

The deep-vein thrombosis in these patients has some specific characteristics. It may precede the diagnosis of cancer by months to years (Lieberman et al., 1961). Most frequently, this time interval is two months or less, but cases in the range of two to four years have been reported. It is often migratory and recurrent and involves veins in unusual sites such as the upper extremity and the neck. It may be resistant to heparin treatment and carries a risk of pulmonary emboli. Finally, however, it should be noted that although the incidence of thrombophlebitis may be high in patients with certain types of cancer, the converse is not true.

Thus, the incidence of cancer in unselected patients with thrombophlebitis was 3% in one series (Byrne, 1960) and less than 1% in two others (Pineo *et al.*, 1974; Lieberman *et al.*, 1961).

Nonbacterial thrombotic endocarditis is a clinical and pathologic entity in which bland fibrinous vegetations, sometimes large, are present on cardiac values. Other names for this condition are marantic endocarditis and cachectic endocarditis. The initial complete description of the disease (Gross and Friedberg, 1936) pointed out its association with numerous underlying conditions, and, subsequently, there was some debate as to whether the vegetations were clinically important. It is currently clear, however, that nonbacterial thrombotic endocarditis is clinically noteworthy in the patient with cancer (Scotti, 1971). Its occurrence in patients with mucin-secreting adenocarcinoma is higher than would be expected in patients with non-neoplastic disease (Sproul, 1938; Rohner *et al.*, 1966; Barry and Scarpelli, 1962; Rosen and Armstrong, 1973a). In these patients, the vegetations may be particularly large. Located primarily on the mitral and aortic values, they are a source of arterial emboli to brain, kidney, coronary arteries, extremities, and other sites (Barry and Scarpelli, 1962; Rohner *et al.*, 1966; Rosen and Armstrong, 1973a). These large vegetations can also coexist with venous thrombosis in patients with mucin-secreting adenocarcinoma. For this reason, it is suggested that the release of procoagulant by the tumor and a state of chronic disseminated intravascular coagulation not only predispose to the valvular vegetations but are part of their pathogenesis. Consequently, nonbacterial thrombotic endocarditis and the associated arterial emboli are currently considered as part of the clinical spectrum of chronic disseminated intravascular coagulation (Sack *et al.*, 1977). In this regard, the nonbacterial lesion differs from infective endocarditis, which is probably not more common in patients with adenocarcinoma than in those with any other type of cancer (Rosen and Armstrong, 1973b; Sack *et al.*, 1977).

It may be possible to identify specific substances that contribute to intravascular coagulation in these patients. The procoagulant found in the granular fraction of promyelocytic leukemia cells is a thromboplastin that activates the extrinsic pathway and cross-reacts immunologically with brain thromboplastin. O'Meara and colleagues (O'Meara and

Thornes, 1961; Boggust *et al.*, 1963) have studied water soluble, thermolabile factors, extracted from human cancer tissue, that induce coagulation in recalcified plasma and that have electrophoretic mobility in the prealbumin region. These materials do not directly convert fibrinogen to fibrin. Svanberg (1975) found thromboplastic activity in human ovarian tumors that was significantly higher than in normal ovaries, and Sakuragawa and colleagues (1977) identified a thromboplastinlike substance from gastric cancer tissue that activated factor X but not prothrombin. Pineo and colleagues (1973) demonstrated procoagulant activity in extracts of human mucus. It had low phospholipid content and its action was mediated through activation of factor X. It differed from tissue thromboplastin because it did not require factor VII nor activate the intrinsic system. Gordon and colleagues (1975) have characterized a procoagulant from several neoplastic human tissues that was a serine protease rather than a thromboplastin. It activated factor X directly, did not require factors VII or VIII, did not activate prothrombin, and was inhibited by diisopropyl fluorophosphate. Although none of these substances has been fully characterized, many of them activate factor X (Curatolo *et al.*, 1979). None seems to have a direct action on either prothrombin or fibrinogen. These or other tissue constituents may be important in the initiation of clotting in patients with neoplastic disease. The treatment of the thrombotic disorders involves the decision as to anticoagulation. The use of fibrinolytic therapy with streptokinase or urokinase in acute deep vein thrombosis may be of value.

In summary, the introduction of procoagulant material from tumors into the circulation results in both acute and chronic DIC, and these manifest themselves differently. The situation with prostatic cancer is unique because the component of fibrinolysis seems greater than is seen in other tumors. Further identification of the tumor products responsible for the coagulation abnormalities will be of interest.

Bleeding Disorders in Dysproteinemia

Coagulation abnormalities and clinical bleeding frequently occur in macroglobulinemia, multiple myeloma, and other disorders that produce paraproteins (Fiddes *et al.*, 1971; Lackner, 1973). They result from many types of defects in the coagulation system, including vascular fragility, thrombocytopenia, qualitative changes in platelets or their interaction with vascular endothelium, impaired conversion of fibrinogen to fibrin, and inhibition or deficiency of specific coagulation factors. Presumably, these abnormalities are mediated by the physical interaction of the paraprotein with components of the coagulation system. Frequently, however, the specific mechanisms are poorly defined, so that only broad generalities can be made about the wide spectrum of disorders that have been reported (Perkins et al., 1970).

Epistaxis occurs in about 25% of patients with macroglobulinemia (McCallister et al., 1967) and purpura and ecchymoses are also common. Clinical bleeding is as frequent in patients with IgA myeloma as it is in macroglobulinemia, but is less common in IgG myeloma (Perkins et al., 1970). It is possible to draw some correlations between these hemorrhagic tendencies and general tests of hemostasis. Bleeding is most frequent in patients with high paraprotein levels and is best correlated with prolonged bleeding time and with abnormalities of platelet adhesiveness and platelet plug formation (Perkins et al., 1970; Penny et al., 1971). Although the platelet count, the prothrombin time, and the partial thromboplastin time are frequently abnormal in the presence of paraproteinemia, they are not directly related to the presence or absence of bleeding. Likewise, levels of coagulation factors may be low in the patients who bleed, but are not usually low enough to account for the hemorrhage (Perkins et al., 1970).

The abnormalities of platelet function in dysproteinemic patients fall into at least two categories. In the first, platelet aggregation is impaired and platelet factor III release is defective due to coating of the platelets by the abnormal protein (Pachter et al., 1959a,b). These defects may be reversible by washing the platelets free of the protein or by treating them with an antibody to it. In a second category are cases in which the aggregation of platelets is normal but their adhesion to vascular endothelium is inhibited by the interaction of the paraprotein with connective tissue collagen (Vigliano and Horowitz, 1967). Both types of defects can provide a basis for poor platelet plug formation.

Some patients with multiple myeloma have hemorrhagic problems, prolonged thrombin times, and poor clot retraction (Sanchez-Avalos et al., 1969). Frick (1955) reported that ten out of 45 cases of multiple myleloma had bleeding problems and 12 of the 45 had prolonged thrombin times. Six of the twelve with long thrombin times had hemorrhage. In one case that was studied in detail, an inhibitor of fibrinogen conversion to fibrin that precipated with the β-γ-globulin fraction was present. This confirmed earlier reports of such a phenomenon (Luscher and Labhard, 1949; Uehlinger, 1949; Craddock et al., 1953). Other studies have confirmed the direct prolongation of the thrombin time by myeloma proteins (Penny et al., 1971). It has further been shown (Coleman et al., 1972) that the Fab fragments of some myeloma proteins can inhibit fibrin monomer polymerization, as distinct from the conversion of fibrinogen to fibrin. This process presumably involved direct protein-protein interactions. A further mechanism by which the thrombin-catalyzed conversion of fibrinogen to fibrin can be impaired is the excessive binding of Ca^{2+} by the paraprotein (Glueck et al., 1962). In that instance, the addition of Ca^{2+} to in vitro assays and the in vivo infusion of ionized Ca^{2+} may improve the thrombin time.

Occasionally, inhibitors of specific coagulation factors arise in conjunction with dysproteinemias. The one that has been most studied is that of an antibody to factor VIII (Penny et al., 1971). Reductions in the levels of coagulation factors may also occur but are not clearly associated with the effects of the abnormal protein (Perkins et al., 1970; Lackner, 1973). Some of these changes may merge with the coagulation factor abnormalities described in the preceding section. Factor X deficiency is described in primary amyloidosis (Lackner, 1973). Overall, the bleeding disorders in dysproteinemias are multifactorial and it is entirely possible that further specific abnormalities will yet be described.

LEUKOCYTE ABNORMALITIES

A leukemoid reaction is a marked peripheral granulocytosis, sometimes accompanied by sufficient cellular immaturity to simulate leukemia. These reactions may be acute or chronic and are attributable to a variety of infectious and inflammatory causes. Leukemoid reactions with granulocyte counts in the range of 20 to 100 $\times$ 10^3 cells/mm^3 and not explainable by concurrent infection have been reported as part of the clinical course of various solid tumors (Meyer and Rotter, 1942; Fahey, 1951; Chen and Walz, 1958; Tveter, 1973; Robinson, 1974). The sites of primary tumors have included lungs, pancreas, stomach, kidney, adrenal gland, bladder, and colon. A few cases of melanoma (Robinson, 1974) and sarcoma (Chen and Walz, 1958) have also been reported.

The clinical features of these cases, apart from the primary tumor, have been rather nonspecific. Although some have had bone or bone marrow involvement, the majority in the recent literature have not. In the presence of marrow metastases, the designation of leukemoid reaction would merge with that of leukoerythroblastosis. Otherwise, another mechanism must be postulated for the increased peripheral white count. It is possible, for example, that the tumor could elaborate a product that either stimulated myelopoiesis in the marrow or released granulocytes from marginated peripheral pools. Evidence to favor the first mechanism in some cases has been made. The bone marrow may show myeloid hyperplasia with a particular increase in myelocytes (Chen and Walz, 1958). Robinson (1974) has reported a virtually linear relationship between peripheral white count and urinary-myeloid-colony-stimulating activity in 12 solid-tumor patients with leukemoid reactions. No evidence, however, that the colony-stimulating activity arose from the tumor was reported. It could have originated in the lung, which would agree with the large number of cases of bronchogenic primary tumor or pulmonary metastases included in these series.

Eosinophilia is also a complication of some neoplasms. It occurs with regularity in myeloproliferative disorders such as chronic myelogenous leukemia and polycythemia vera. Primary eosinophilic leukemia is an uncommon but particularly virulent disease. In chronic myelogenous leukemia there may be an absolute eosinophilia, even if the proportion of eosinophils in the total cell population is normal. Eosinophilia may occur in Hodgkin's disease (Major and Leger, 1939) and occasionally with solid tumors, such as adenocarcinoma from various sites (Isaacson and Rapoport, 1946; Banerjee and Narang, 1967). The mechanism of the eosinophilia is not clear but it may be a consequence of tumor necrosis or widespread metastases (Isaacson and Rapoport, 1946).

Basophilia occurs principally as a manifestation of various myeloproliferative diseases, especially chronic myelogenous leukemia.

PLATELET ABNORMALITIES

Abnormal platelet function occurs in myeloproliferative disorders and in paraproteinemia. Myeloproliferative disorders are associated with both hemorrhage and thrombosis in the presence of normal or increased platelet counts. Studies of platelet function in these diseases have detected defects that correlate with those tendencies. A consistent finding in polycythemia vera, chronic myelogeneous leukemia, essential thrombocytosis, and myelofibrosis is impaired platelet aggregation after stimulation by epinephrine, collagen, or adenosine diphosphate (ADP) (Nishimura et al., 1979; Phadke et al., 1981; Waddell et al., 1981). Of these, abnormal aggregation by epinephrine and collagen are most frequent, but all may occur together and all may occur in any of the myeloproliferative disorders. The frequency with which at least one of these abnormalities occurs in the platelets in a myeloproliferative disorder is 100% in some series (Phadke et al., 1981). The platelets that exhibit impaired aggregation may also have reduced levels of the adenine nucleotides adenosine triphosphate (ATP) and ADP, which creates a storage pool defect (Nishimura et al., 1979). Prostaglandin synthesis, however, can be normal (Phadke et al., 1981). Hence, the platelets in myeloproliferative disorders are biochemically and functionally abnormal, and this may contribute to the poor hemostasis in these diseases.

Two types of impaired platelet function are seen in paraproteinemia: (1) Abnormal aggregation and platelet factor III release due to coating by the protein, and (2) abnormal adhesion to endothelium due to the protein interaction with collagen (Pachter et al., 1959a,b; Vigliano and Horowitz, 1967). These are discussed above with bleeding disorders in dysproteinemias.

Thrombocytosis

Elevation of the platelet count above the normal upper limit of 400,000/mm^3 occurs in various myeloproliferative disorders as well as in other neoplastic disease (Gilbert, 1973).

Marked thrombocytosis is a cardinal feature of essential thrombocythemia, in which counts frequently exceed 10^6/mm^3 (Silverstein, 1968). The disease is associated with a high incidence of platelet functional abnormalities, hemorrhagic manifestations, and splenic infarction. In chronic myelogenous leukemia, elevated platelet counts are typical of early disease (Davis and Mendez Ross, 1973). As the disease progresses, the platelet counts tend to normalize and then become depressed. This reflects a combination of splenic destruction, disease evolution toward a marrow of less mature elements, and treatment. In polycythemia, vera megakaryocytic hyperplasia and expansion of the body platelet mass in virtually all patients is present (Gilbert, 1975). The circulating platelet levels may not completely reflect the total body mass because of shortened survival due to splenomegaly and, possibly, other factors. The platelets frequently show functional abnormality, usually decreased aggregation to one or more stimuli but sometimes hyperaggregability (Gilbert, 1975). Although thrombotic and hemorrhagic complications are common in polycythemia vera, the precise role of the platelet in their pathogenesis is unclear.

Thrombocytosis is often associated with disseminated solid tumors. In one study of 100 patients with thrombocytosis, (Davis and Mendez Ross, 1973), 36 had tumors, including carcinomas of ovary, pancreas, lung, colon, breast, and of undetermined origin. Seven also had either Hodgkin's disease or non-Hodgkin's lymphomas. In another study (Levin and Conley, 1964), 82 patients with thrombocytosis were identified in a population of 14,000. Of these 82, 31 had neoplasms, with stomach, colon, lung, breast, and ovary being the most common type. These authors then examined 268 patients with inoperable neoplasms and found that 40% of those with neoplasms of all types exclusive of carcinoma of the lung and 38% of those with carcinoma of the lung had thrombocytosis. In another series of 190 patients with carcinoma of the lung (Silvis, et al., 1970), 60% had thrombocytosis, usually in the range of 400,000 to 600,000/mm³. The incidence did not vary substantially among the histologic subgroups of squamous-cell carcinoma, adenocarcinoma, undifferentiated carcinoma, and small cell carcinoma. In a recent review of diffuse mesothelioma, 90% of the patients studied had elevated platelet counts during the disease and 10% had counts over 10^6/mm³ (Chahinian et al., 1982). The mechanism of thrombocytosis in these patients is not defined, although humoral releasing factors are postulated. Platelet function studies have not usually been evaluated in solid-tumor pa-

tients, but abnormalities are said to be most characteristic of myeloproliferative disorders. The elevated acid phosphatase and pseudohyperkalemia may occur from platelet elevation of any cause.

PROTEIN ABNORMALITIES

Hyperviscosity Syndrome

The hyperviscosity syndrome is a collection of clinical signs and symptoms that occur when the viscosity of the blood rises to sufficiently high levels. Because blood viscosity is determined both by its cell content and by the level of plasma protein, hyperviscosity appears in polycythemia vera, in leukemias with high peripheral white counts, and in myeloma and related B-cell neoplasms that produce large amounts of paraprotein.

The clinical presentation of the hyperviscosity syndrome is the same in all these cases (see Table 6–6), and consists of general signs and symptoms such as fatigue, decreased appetite, and weight loss, as well as vascular, ocular, and neurologic manifestations (Bloch and Maki, 1973; Hild and Myers, 1980; Verstraete, 1981). The etiology of the flushing and mucous membrane bleeding that occur is multifactorial and includes defects in platelet function produced by paraprotein coating and alterations in coagulation factors from complexing with these proteins. The ocular manifestations include retinopathy characterized by sausage-shaped retinal veins and vascular extravasation with flame-shaped hemorrhages. Other symptoms include alterations in vision and hearing, dizziness, gait disturbances, fainting, and mental dullness. Priapism may occur with either leukostasis or paraproteinemia. Raynaud's phenomenon and other cutaneous manifestations are not part of the hyperviscosity syndrome unless the paraprotein is a cryoglobulin (Jones, 1980). One case of ischemic digital necrosis associated with a white cell count of 256,000 mm³ has been reported (Hild and Myers, 1980).

The normal whole blood viscosity is about 3.5 centipoise when measured at a defined shear rate of 230 s⁻¹. The viscosity of serum is 1.4 to 1.8 times that of water (Tuddenham et al., 1974). Whole blood viscosity is determined by: (1) The properties of the red cell, including its membrane, the viscosity of its intracellular contents, and its concentration in

Table 6-6. Clinical Manifestations of Hyperviscosity

General:	Fatigue, decreased appetite, weight loss, nausea
Vascular:	Epistaxis, plethora, purplish palmar erythema, bruising, mucous membrane bleeding (*e.g.,* gums or rectum), priapism
Ocular:	Blurring or loss of vision, thickened, sausage-shaped retinal veins with extravasations or flame-shaped hemorrhages
CNS:	Tinnitus and decreased hearing, headache, dizziness, altered consciousness, gait disturbances

From Hild, D. H., and Myers, T. J.: Hyperviscosity in chronic granulocytic leukemia. *Cancer,* 46:1418–1421, 1980; and Verstraete, M.: The clinical relevance of hyperviscosity. *Acta Clin. Belg.,* **36**:269–273, 1981.

plasma; (2) the plasma protein concentration; and (3) the interplay between these two (Verstraete, 1981). In general, the packed cell volume is the most important of these determinants (Preston *et al.,* 1978), and significant elevations in packed cell volume (cytocrit), whether due to red cells or white cells, can produce clinical symptomatology. If a protein interacts with red cells to produce clumping or rouleau formations, this may accentuate the effects on viscosity.

Patients with high peripheral counts of either leukocytes or granulocytes usually develop symptoms of hyperviscosity in association with total cell counts in excess of 150,000/mm^3. Serum viscosities in these patients are normal. Some controversy has been noted in the literature as to the correlation between white cell count and whole blood viscosity, because various investigators either have (Stephens, 1936; Preston *et al.,* 1978; Hild and Myers, 1980) or have not (Steinberg and Charm, 1971) demonstrated a linear relation between whole blood viscosity and increasing white count. In general, however, these studies have shown the most marked effects of white cell count upon whole blood viscosity to be in chronic granulocytic leukemia. In these patients a disproportionate increase in whole blood viscosity occurs when the total packed cell volume is over 30% (Hild and Myers, 1980), especially if the leukocyte packed volume is over 6%. Anemia may be a protective factor (Steinberg and Charm, 1971; Lichtman, 1973) that obscures the relation between white count and viscosity. *In vitro* studies of leukocyte suspensions have shown that both lymphocytes and myelocytes have a higher viscosity than an equivalent volume of red cells (Steinberg and Charm, 1971). Under these conditions, equivalent concentrations of myelocytes and lymphocytes produce equivalent increments in whole blood viscosity (Licht-

man, 1973). This conflicts somewhat with those clinical studies that show greater increases in whole blood viscosity in myelocytic leukemia than in lymphocytic leukemia (Preston, 1978; Hild and Myers, 1980). The differences may be either methodologic (Lichtman, 1973) or due to other factors such as adhesiveness of granulocytes within vascular structures.

Patients with B-cell lymphoproliferative disorders that secrete paraproteins become symptomatic as the serum viscosity exceeds four times that of water (Verstraete, 1981). This may occur in patients with IgM secretion due to Waldenström's macroglobulinemia or with IgA or IgG myeloma. Of these three molecules, however, the increase in plasma viscosity with respect to a unit increase in protein is greatest for IgM, followed by IgA and then IgG (Tuddenham *et al.,* 1974). This is because IgM is a large pentameric structure composed of five subunits linked into a closed configuration by disulphide bonds; it has a high intrinsic viscosity and a high molecular weight. It also has a small volume of distribution and tends to remain 80 to 90% confined to the intravascular space. Partly for this reason, patients with IgM macroglobulinemia have an expanded plasma volume that correlates with the increase in relative serum viscosity (MacKenzie *et al.,* 1970). Although monomeric IgA has a lower intrinsic viscosity than IgM, over 80% of patients with IgA myeloma have an elevated relative plasma viscosity (Chandy *et al.,* 1981). Symptomatic hyperviscosity is infrequent in these patients and its occurrence relates to aggregation of IgA into dimers and higher polymeric forms (Cohen, 1968; Tuddenham *et al.,* 1974; Virella *et al.,* 1975; Roberts-Thompson *et al.,* 1976; Chandy *et al.,* 1981). A general but not perfect correlation does exist between the polymeric IgA in the plasma and the hyperviscosity symptoms (Virella *et al.,* 1975; Chandy *et al.,*

1981). Because some patients with large amounts of polymeric IgA are asymptomatic, other conformational features of the IgA polymers or their subunits may also determine viscosity (Virella *et al.*, 1975). One factor of possible importance is the ability of IgA to undergo association with other molecules such as albumin, β-lipoprotein, and alpha-1-antitrypsin. These complexes, however, do not always explain the asymptomatic patients with high polymerization and low viscosity (Chandy *et al.*, 1981).

Hyperviscosity is least frequent in patients with IgG myeloma. The relatively low molecular weight IgG monomer is distributed widely outside of the vascular system and its effects on blood viscosity are the least of those of the three immunoglobulin types. Hyperviscosity symptoms may occur when IgG polymerizes *in vivo* (Smith *et al.*, 1965). The IgG3 subtype is particularly prone to form large protein aggregates or polymers (Capra and Kunkel, 1970; Tuddenham *et al.*, 1974) and although only about 4% of patients with IgG myeloma develop hyperviscosity, more than 50% of those who do have an IgG3 paraprotein.

Two approaches to treatment of hyperviscosity syndrome are known. In paraproteinemic hyperviscosity the mainstay of treatment is plasmapheresis (Beck *et al.*, 1982). Treatment of the underlying disease with cytotoxic drugs will bring a slower resolution of the problem if the tumor responds. In leukostasis and hyperviscosity, the usual approach is to reduce the peripheral white count with drugs such as hydroxyurea or cytosine arabinoside. Leukapheresis is also effective, although inconvenient and expensive, but can be utilized for management of very acute cases (Vallejos *et al.*, 1973; Hadlock *et al.*, 1975; Ballas and Kiesel, 1979).

Cryoproteins

The paraproteins that are produced in multiple myeloma, macroglobulinemia, and other neoplasms sometimes have temperature-dependent solubility properties. Usually they are cryoproteins that gel or precipitate in the cold, but heat-insoluble pyroproteins also occur (Zinneman, 1980). The most clinically significant of these are cold-insoluble immunoglobulins, for example, cryoglobulins. They are of two general types: (1) homogeneous monoclonal proteins that lack a component with anti-γ-globulin properties, and (2) complexes

of two or more proteins in which one component has antibody activity to IgG, that is, rheumatoid factor activity (Grey and Kohler, 1973). Cryoglobulins of the first type are usually IgM or IgG and much less commonly are IgA or Bence Jones proteins. The monoclonal proteins present in multiple myeloma are cryoproteins in as many as 5% of cases and are most often IgG. The temperatures at which such proteins are insoluble vary from one specimen to another over the range from 5 to 37°C. The physical properties that render them cold-insoluble are not fully defined, but the process involves weak noncovalent forces and is highly dependent upon pH and ionic strength of the solvent. The monoclonal IgM of macroglobulinemia is cold-precipitable more frequently than is the IgG of multiple myeloma. Many of these macroglobulins have anti-IgG activity and circulate as complexes, that is, they are rheumatoid factors.

Clinically, patients are occasionally seen who have "essential" or unexplained cryoglobulinemia. Such persons are at risk for the development of plasma cell dyscrasias, perhaps after an interval of several years (Gordon-Smith *et al.*, 1968; Grey *et al.*, 1968). These proteins are responsible for a number of clinical manifestations, including Raynaud's phenomenon, cutaneous vasculitis, purpura, and both bleeding and thrombotic problems (Grey and Kohler, 1973; Zinneman, 1980). Treatment with plasmapheresis or longer-term chemotherapy may be effective management.

Pyroglobulins, that is immunoglobulins that are heat insoluble, are also reported but are rarely of clinical significance (Zinneman, 1980). Other cold-precipitable proteins include the cryofibrinogens. Unlike the cryoglobulins, they occur in association with solid tumors such as prostatic or lung carcinoma (Korst and Kratochvil, 1955; Kalbfleisch and Bird, 1960; Stathekis *et al.*, 1981). They may (Stathekis *et al.*, 1981) or may not (Korst and Kratochvil, 1955) be complexes of fibrinogen and a cold-insoluble globulin. Such proteins have been associated with clinical problems of phlebitis and rouleau formation in the peripheral blood (Korst and Kratochvil, 1955).

CONCLUSIONS

The diverse problems described here reflect the intimate association of the blood with the rest of the body and its pathologic states. In many cases, the phenomena are only descriptive and much remains to be learned of basic mechanisms.

REFERENCES

Abeloff, M. D., and Waterbury, L.: Pure red cell aplasia and chronic lymphocytic leukemia. *Arch. Intern. Med.,* **134:**721–724, 1974

Adler, S.; Stutzman, L.; Sokal, J. E.; and Mittelman, A.: Splenectomy for hematologic depression in lymphocytic lymphoma and leukemia. *Cancer,* **35:**521–528, 1975.

Ahmann, D. L.; Kiely, J. M.; Harrison, E. G.; and Payne, W. S.: Malignant lymphoma of the spleen: A review of 49 cases in which the diagnosis was made at splenectomy. *Cancer,* **19:**461–469, 1966.

Allanby, K. D.; Huntsman, R. G.; and Sacker, L. S.: Thrombotic microangiopathy: Recovery of a case after heparin and magnesium therapy. *Lancet,* **1:**237–239, 1966.

Al-Mondhiry, H.; Zonjani, E. D.; Spivack, M.; Zalusky, R.; and Gordon, A. S.: Pure red cell aplasia and thymoma: Loss of serum inhibitor of erythropoiesis following thymectomy. *Blood,* **38:**576–582, 1971.

Alouf, J. E., and Jolivet-Reynaud, C.: Purification and characterization of *clostridium perfringens* delta-toxin. *Infect. Immun.,* **31:**536–546, 1981.

Amorosi, E. L., and Ultmann, J. E.: Thrombotic thrombocytopenic purpura: Report of 16 cases and review of the literature. *Medicine* (Baltimore), **45:**139–159, 1966.

Amorosi, E. L., and Karpatkin, S.: Antiplatelet treatment of thrombotic thrombocytopenic purpura. *Ann. Intern. Med.,* **86:**102–106, 1977.

Amundsen, M. D.; Spittell, J. A.; Thompson, J. H.; and Owen, C. A.: Hypercoagulability associated with malignant disease and with the postoperative state: Evidence for elevated levels of antihemophiliac globulin. *Ann. Intern. Med.,* **58:**608–616, 1963.

Andersen, S. B., and Ladefoged, J.: Pure red cell anaemia and thymoma. *Acta Haematol. (Basel),* **30:**319–325, 1963.

Anner, R. M., and Drewinko, B.: Frequency and significance of bone marrow involvement by metastatic solid tumors. *Cancer,* **39:**1337–1344, 1977.

Ansell, J.; Beaser, R. S.; and Pechet, L.: Thrombotic thrombocytopenic purpura fails to respond to fresh frozen plasma infusion. *Ann. Intern. Med.,* **89:**647–648, 1978.

Antman, K. H.; Skarin, A. T.; Mayer, R. J.; Hargreaves, H. K.; and Canellos, G. P.: Microangiopatic hemolytic anemia and cancer: A review. *Medicine* **58:**377–384, 1979.

Asher, R.: Histiocytic medullary reticulosis—A case without lymphadenopathy. *Lancet,* **1:**650–651, 1946.

Auclair, C.; Dhermy, D.; and Boivin, P.: Superoxide dismutase deficiency in patients with nitrogen mustard therapy-induced intravascular hemolysis. *Cancer Chemother. Pharmacol.,* **4:**281–282, 1980.

Baker, L. R. I.; Rubenberg, M. L.; Dacie, J. V.; and Brain, M. C.: Fibrinogen catabolism in microangiopathic haemolytic anemia. *Br. J. Haematol.* **15:**617–625, 1968.

Baker, W.; Bang, N. U.; Nachman, R. L.; Raafat, F.; and Horowitz, H. I.: Hypofibrinogenemic hemorrhage in acute myelogenous leukemia treated with heparin. *Ann. Intern. Med.* **61:**116–123, 1964.

Balcerzak, S. P., and Bromberg, P. A.: Secondary polycythemia. *Semin. Hematol.,* **12:**353–382, 1975.

Ballas, S. K., and Kiesel, J. K.: Leukapheresis for hyperviscosity. *Transfusion,* **19:**787, 1979.

Ballas, S. K., and Rubin, R. N.: Microangiopathic hemolytic anemia and thrombocytopenia with disseminated cancer. *Postgrad. Med.,* **60:**180–181, 1976.

Banerjee, R. N., and Narang, R. M.: Haematological changes in malignancy. *Br. J. Haematol.,* **13:**829–843, 1967.

Barry, W. E., and Scarpelli, D.: Nonbacterial thrombotic endocarditis: A clinicopathologic study. *Arch. Intern. Med.,* **109:**151–156, 1962.

Beck, J. R.; Quinn, B. M.; Meier, F. A.; and Rawnsby, H. M.: Hyperviscosity syndrome in paraproteinemia, managed by plasma exchange, monitored by serum tests. *Transfusion,* **22:**51–53, 1982.

Bennett, J. M., and Healey, P. J. M.: Spherocytic hemolytic anemia and acute cholecystitis caused by *clostridium welchii.* *N. Engl. J. Med.,* **268:**1070–1072, 1963.

Bergen, S., and Schilling, F. J.: Circulating fibrinolysin in a case of prostatic carcinoma with bony metastases. *Ann. Intern. Med.,* **48:**389–398, 1958.

Bernard, R. P.; Bauman, A. W.; and Schwartz, S. I.: Splenectomy for thrombotic thrombocytopenic purpura. *Ann. Surg.,* **169:**616–624, 1969.

Bernatz, P. E.; Harrison, E. G.; and Clagett, O. T.: Thymoma: A clinicopathologic entity. *J. Thorac. Cardiovasc. Surg.,* **42:**424–444, 1961.

Beveridge, B. R.; Bannerman, R. M.; Evanson, J. M.; and Witts, L. J.: Hypochromic anaemia: A retrospective study and follow-up in 378 in-patients. *Q. J. Med.,* **34:**145–161, 1965.

Birgens, H.; Ernst, P.; and Hansen, M. S.: Thrombotic thrombocytopenic purpura: Treatment with a combination of antiplatelet drugs. *Acta Med. Scand.,* **205:**437–439, 1979.

Bloch, K., and Maki, D. G.: Hyperviscosity syndromes associated with immunoglobulin abnormalities. *Sem. Hematol.,* **10:**113–124, 1973.

Boggs, D. R.; Frei, E.; and Thomas, L. B.: Clostridial gas gangrene and septicemia in four patients with leukemia. *N. Engl. J. Med.,* **259:**1255–1258, 1958.

Boggust, W. A.; O'Brien, D. J.; O'Meara, R. A. Q.; and Thornes, R. D.: The coagulative factors of normal human and human cancer tissue. *Ir. J. Med. Sci.,* **6:**131–144, 1963.

Brain, M. C.; Azzopardi, J. G.; Baker, L. R. I.; Pineo, G. F.; Roberts, D. D.; and Dacie, J. V.: Microangiopathic haemolytic anaemia and mucin-forming adenocarcinoma. *Br. J. Haematol.,* **18:**183–193, 1970.

Brain, M. C.; Dacie, J. V.; and Hourihane, D. O'B.: Microangiopathic haemolytic anaemia: The possible role of vascular lesions in pathogenesis. *Br. J. Haematol.,* **8:**350–374, 1962.

Brown, R. C.: TTP after influenza vaccination. *Br. Med. J.,* **2:**3034, 1973.

Brown, R. C.; Campbell, D. C.; and Thompson, J. H.: Increased fibrinolysin with malignant disease. *Arch. Intern. Med.,* **109:**201–204, 1962.

Brown, R. J. K., and Meynell, M. J.: Hemolytic anemia associated with Hodgkin's disease. *Lancet,* **2:**835–836, 1949.

Brownstein, M. H., and Ballard, H.: Hepatoma associated with erythrocytosis: Report of eleven new cases. *Am. J. Med.,* **40:**204–210, 1966.

Brugarolas, A.; Elias, E. G.; Takita, H.; Mink, I. B.; Mittelman, A., and Ambrus, J. L.: Blood coagulation and fibrinolysis in patients with carcinoma of the lung. *J. Med.* (Basel), **4**:96–105, 1973.

Bukowski, R. M.; King, J. W.; and Hewlett, J. S.: Plasmapheresis in the treatment of thrombotic thrombocytopenic purpura. *Blood*, **50**:413–417, 1977.

Bull, B. S., and Kuhn, I. N.: The production of schistocytes by fibrin strands (A scanning electron microscope study). *Blood*, **35**:104–111, 1970.

Bull, B. S.; Rubenberg, M. L.; Dacie, J. V.; and Brain, M. C.: Microangiopathic haemolytic anaemia: Mechanisms of red-cell fragmentation: *In vitro* studies. *Br. J. Haematol.* **14**:643–652, 1968.

Byrnes, J. J.: Phlebitis—Study of 979 cases at Boston City Hospital: *JAMA,* **174**:113–118, 1960.

Byrnes, J. J., and Khurana, M.: Treatment of thrombotic thrombocytopenic purpura with plasma. *N. Engl. J. Med.,* **297**:1386–1389, 1977.

Cantrell, J. E.; Philips, T. M.; Smith, F. P.; and Schein, P. S.: Immune complex analysis and plasmapheresis in cancer related thrombotic thrombocytopenic purpura (TTP)/hemolytic uremic syndrome (HUS) syndrome. *Blood*, **60**:185a, 1982.

Cantrell, J. E.; Philips, T. M.; Winokur, S.; and Schein, P. S.: A cancer-related thrombotic microangiopathy: Natural history and therapy. *Proc. Am. Soc. Clin. Onc.,* **2**:12, 1983.

Capra, J. D., and Kunkel, H. G.: Aggregation of alphagammaG3 proteins: Relevance to the hyperviscosity syndrome. *J. Clin. Invest.,* **49**:610–621, 1970.

Carlsson, S.: Fibrinogen degradation products in serum from patients with cancer. *Acta Chir. Scand.,* **139**:499–502, 1973.

Carmichael, D. S., and Medley, D. R. K.: Heparin in thrombotic microangiopathy. *Lancet,* **1**:1421, 1966.

Cartwright, G. E.: The anemia of chronic disorders. *Semin. Hematol.,* **3**:351–375, 1966.

Chabner, B. A.; Fisher, R. I.; Young, R. C.; and DeVita, V. T.: Staging of non-hodgkin's lymphomas. *Semin. Oncol.,* **7**:285–291, 1980.

Chabner, B. A.; Johnson, R. E.; Young, R. C.; Canellos, G. P.; Hubbard, S. P.; Johnson, S. K.; and DeVita, V. T.: Sequential non-surgical and surgical staging of non-Hodgkin's lymphoma. *Ann. Intern. Med.,* **85**:149–154, 1976.

Chahinian, A. P.; Pajak, T. F.; Holland, J. F.; Norton, L.; Ambinder, R. M.; and Mandel, E. M.: Diffuse malignant mesothelioma: Prospective evaluation of 69 patients. *Ann. Intern. Med.,* **96**:746–755, 1982.

Chandy, K. G.; Stockley, R. A.; Leonard, R. C. F.; Crockson, R. A.; Burnett, D.; and Maclennan, I. C. M.: Relationship between serum viscosity and intravascular IgA polymer concentration in IgA myeloma. *Clin. Exp. Immunol.,* **46**:653–661, 1981.

Chen, H. P., and Walz, D. V.: Leukemoid reaction in the bone marrow, associated with malignant neoplasms. *Am. J. Clin. Pathol.* **29**:345–349, 1958.

Choudhury, T. K.: Synergistic lysis of erythrocytes by propionibacterium acnes. *J. Clin. Microbiol.,* **8**:238–241, 1978.

Cohan, M.; Pittman, G.; and Hoffman, G. C.: Hemolytic anemia, tumor cell emboli and intravascular coagulation. *Arch. Pathol.,* **93**:305–307, 1972.

Cohen, S.: The nature of myeloma proteins. *Br. J. Haematol.,* **15**:211–215, 1968.

Coleman, M.; Vigliano, E. M.; Weksler, M. E.; and Nachman, R. L.: Inhibition of fibrin monomer polymerization by lambda myeloma proteins. *Blood,* **39**:210–223, 1972.

Colman, R. W.; Robboy, S. J.; and Minna, J. D.: Disseminated intravascular coagulation: A reappraisal. *Ann. Rev. Med.,* **30**:359–374, 1979.

Cosgrieff, S. W., and Leifer, E.: Factor 5 deficiency in hemorrhagic diathesis (parahemophilia). *J.A.M.A.,* **148**:462–463, 1952.

Craddock, C. G.; Adams, W. S.; and Figueroa, W. G.: Interference with fibrin formation in multiple myeloma by an unusual protein found in blood and urine. *J. Lab. Clin. Med.,* **42**:847–859, 1953.

Crosby, W. H.: Is hypersplenism a dead issue? *Blood,* **20**:94–99, 1962a.

Crosby, W. H.: Hyperplenism. *Ann. Rev. Med.,* **13**:127–146, 1962b.

Curatolo, L.; Colucci, M.; Cambini, A. L.; Poggi, A.; Moraser, L.; Donati, M. B.; and Semeraro, N.: Evidence that cells from experimental tumors can activate coagulation factor X. *Br. J. Cancer,* **40**:228–233, 1979.

Daly, P. A.; Schiffer, C. A.; and Wiernik, P. H.: Acute promyelocytic leukemia—clinical management of 15 patients. *Am. J. Hematol.,* **8**:347–359, 1980.

Dameshek, W.: Hypersplenism. *Bull. N.Y. Acad. Sci.,* **31**:113–136, 1955.

Davey, F. R.; Skarin, A. T.; and Moloney, W. C.: Pathology of splenic lymphoma. *Am. J. Clin. Pathol.,* **59**:95–103, 1973.

Davis, W. M., and Mendez Ross, A. O.: Thrombocytosis and thrombocythemia: The laboratory and clinical significance of an elevated platelet count. *Am. J. Clin. Pathol.,* **59**:243–247, 1973.

Didisheim, P.; Trombold, J. S.; Vandervoort, R. L. E.; and Mibashan, R.: Acute promyelocytic leukemia with fibrinogen and factor V deficiencies. *Blood,* **23**:717–728, 1964.

Donati, M. B., and Poggi, A.: Malignancy and hemostasis. *Br. J. Haematol.,* **44**:173–182, 1980.

Douglas, S. W., and Adamson, J. W.: The anemia of chronic disorders: Studies of marrow regulation and iron metabolism. *Blood,* **45**:55–65, 1975.

Duckett, J. W.: Splenectomy in treatment of secondary hypersplenism. *Ann. Surg.,* **157**:737–746, 1963.

Dunn, M. A., and Goldwein, M. I.: Hypersplenism in advanced breast cancer: Report of a patient treated with splenectomy. *Cancer,* **35**:1449–1452, 1975.

Editorial: Splenectomy for massive splenomegaly. *Br. Med. J.* **2**:293–294, 1979.

Erslev, A.: Pure red cell aplasia. In Williams, W. J.; Beutler, E.; Erslev, A. J.; and Rundles, R. W. (eds.): *Hematology.* McGraw-Hill, Inc., New York, 1977.

Fahey, R. J.: Unusual leukocyte response in primary carcinoma of the lung. *Cancer,* **4**:930–935, 1951.

Fiddes, P.; Penny, R.; and Castaldi, P.: Protein-induced bleeding. *Med. J. Aust.,* **2**:667–671, 1971.

Field, E. O.; Caughi, M. N.; Blackett, N. M.; and Smithers, D. W.: Marrow-suppressing factors in the blood in pure red cell aplasia, thymoma and Hodgkin's disease. *Br. J. Haematol.,* **15**:101–110, 1968.

Fisher, J. H.; Welch, C. S.; and Dameshek, W.: Splenectomy in leukemia and lymphoma. *N. Engl. J. Med.,* **246**:477–484, 1952.

Freireich, E. F.; Miller, A.; Emerson, C. P.; and Ross, J. F.: The effect of inflammation on the utilization of erythrocyte and transferrin-bound radioiron for red cell production. *Blood,* **12**:972–983, 1957a.

Freireich, E. J., Raso, J. F.; Bayles, T. B.; Emerson, C. P.; and Finch, S. C.: Radioactive iron metabolism and erythrocyte survival studies of the mechanisms of the anemia associated with rheumatoid arthritis. *J. Clin. Invest.,* **36:**1043–1058, 1957b.

Frick, P. G.: Inhibition of conversion of fibrinogen to fibrin by abnormal proteins in multple myeloma. *Am. J. Clin. Pathol.,* **25:**1263–1273, 1955.

Frischer, H., and Ahmad, T.: Severe generalized glutathione reductase deficiency after antitumor chemotherapy with BCNU (1,3-bis(2-chloro-ethyl)-1-nitroso-urea). *J. Lab. Clin. Med.,* **89:**1080–1091, 1977.

Fry, J.: Clinical patterns and course of anemias in general practice. *Br. Med. J.,* **2:**1732–1736, 1961.

Gasser, C.; Gautier, E.; Steck, A.; Siebenmann, R. E.; and Oechslin, R.: Hamolytisch-uraemische Syndrome: Bilaterale Nierenrindennekrosen bei akuten Erworbenen hamolytischen Anamien. *Schweiz Med. Wochenschr.,* **85:**905–909, 1955.

Getaz, E. P.; Beckley, S.; Fitzpatrick, J.; and Dozier, A.: Cisplatin-induced hemolysis. *N. Engl. J. Med.;* **302:**334–335, 1980.

Gilbert, E. F.; Harky, J. B.; Anido. V.; Mengali, H. F.; and Hughes, J. T.: Thymoma, plasma cell myeloma, red cell aplasia and malabsorption syndrome. *Am. J. Med,* **44:**820–829, 1968.

Gilbert, H.: The spectrum of myeloproliferative disorders. *Med. Clin. North Am.,* **57:**355–393, 1973.

Gilbert, H.: Definition, clinical features and diagnosis of polycythemia vera. *Clin. Haematol.,* **4:**263–290, 1975.

Gill, P. G.; Sauter, R. G.; and Morris, P. J.: Splenectomy for hypersplenism in malignant lymphomas. *Br. J. Surg.,* **68:**29–33, 1981.

Glueck, H. I.; Wayne, L.; and Goldsmith, R.: Abnormal calcium binding associated with hyperglobulinemia, clotting defects and osteoporosis: A study of this relationship. *J. Lab. Clin. Med.,* **59:**40–64, 1962.

Golde, D. W.; Hocking, W. G.; Koeffler, H. P.; and Adamson, J. W.: Polycythemia: Mechanisms and management. *Ann. Int. Med.,* **95:**71–87, 1981.

Goldenfarb, P. B., and Finch, S. C.: Thrombotic thrombocytopenic purpura: A ten year survey. *J.A.M.A.,* **226:**644–647, 1973.

Goodnight, S. H.: Bleeding and intravascular clotting in malignancy: A review. *Ann. N.Y. Acad. Sci.,* **230:**271–288, 1974.

Gordon, A. S.; Zanjani, E. D.; and Zalusky, R.: A possible mechanism for the erythrocytosis associated with hepatocellular carcinoma in man. *Blood,* **35:**151, 1970.

Gordon, S. G.; Franks, J. J.; and Lewis, B.: Cancer procoagulant A: A factor X activating procoagulant from malignant tissue. *Thromb. Res.,* **6:**127–137, 1975.

Gordon-Smith, E. C.; Harrison, R. J.; and Hobbs, J. R.: Multiple myeloma presenting as cryoglobulinemia. *Proc. R. Soc. Med.,* **61:**1112–1115, 1968.

Gore, I.: Thrombosis and pancreatic carcinoma. *Am. J. Pathol.,* **29:**1093–1101, 1953.

Gouault-Heilmann, M.; Chardon, E.; Sultan, C.; and Jasso, F.: The procoagulant factor of leukemia promyelocytes: Demonstration of immunologic cross reactivity with human brain tissue factor. *Br. J. Haematol.,* **30:**151–158, 1975.

Gralnick, H. R., and Abrell, E.: Studies of the procoagulant and fibrinolytic activity of promyelocytes in acute promyelocytic leukemia. *Br. J. Haematol.,* **24:**89–99, 1973.

Gralnick, H. R.; Bagley, J.; and Abrell, E.: Heparin treat-

ment for the hemorrhagic diathesis of acute promyelocytic leukemia. *Am. J. Med.,* **52:**167–174, 1972.

Gralnick, H. R., and Sultan, C.: Acute promyelocytic leukemia: Haemorrhagic manifestation and morphologic criteria. *Br. J. Haematol.,* **29:**373–376, 1975.

Grey, H. M., and Kohler, P.: Cryoimmunoglobulins. *Semin. Hematol.,* **10:**87–112, 1973.

Grey, H. M.; Kohler, P. F.; Terry, W. D.; and Franklin, E. C.: Human monoclonal gammaG-cyroglobulins with anti-gamma-globulin activity. *J. Clin. Invest.,* **47:**1875–1884, 1968.

Gross, L., and Friedberg, C. K.: Nonbacterial thrombotic endocarditis. Classification and general description. *Arch. Intern. Med.,* **58:**620–240, 1936.

Gubash, S. M: Synergistic hemolysis phenomenon shown by an alpha-toxin-producing *clostridium perfringens* and streptococcal CAMP factor in presumptive streptococcal grouping. *J. Clin. Microbiol.,* **8:**480–488, 1978.

Gubash, S. M: Synergistic hemolysis test for presumptive indentification and differentiation of *Clostridium perfringens, C. bifermentans, C. sordelli* and *C. paraperfringens. J. Clin. Pathol.,* **33:**395–399, 1980.

Gulati, S. C.; Sordillo, P.; Kempin, S.; Reich, L.; Magill, G. B.; Scheiner, E.; and Clarkson, B.: Microangiopathic hemolytic anemia observed after treatment of epidermoid carcinoma with mitomycin-C and 5-fluorouracil. *Cancer,* **45:**2252–2256, 1980.

Habibi, B.; Baumelou, A.; and Serdaru, M.; Acute intravascular haemolysis and renal failure due to teniposide-related antibody. *Lancet.,* **1:**1434–1435, 1981a.

Habibi, B.; Lopez, M.; Serdaru, M.; Baumelou, A.; Vonlanthen, M.; Marteau, R.; and Salmon, C.: Immune hemolytic anemia and renal failure due to teniposide. *N. Engl. J. Med.,* **306:**1091–1093, 1981b.

Hadlock, D. C.; Fortuny, I. E.; McCullaugh, J. J.; and Kennedy, B. J.: Continuous flow centrifuge leukapheresis in the management of chronic myelogenous leukemia. *Br. J. Haematol.,* **29:**443–453, 1975.

Hagedorn, A. B.; Bowie, E. J. W.; Elveback, L. R.; and Owen, C. A.: Coagulation abnormalities in patients with inoperable lung cancer. *Mayo Clin. Proc.,* **49:**647–653, 1974.

Hamilton, C. R., and Conley, C. L.: Pure red cell aplasia and thymoma. *Johns Hopk. Med. J.,* **125:**262–269, 1969.

Hammond, D., and Winnick, S.: Paraneoplastic erythrocytosis and ectopic erythropoietins. *Ann. N.Y. Acad. Sci.,* **230:**219–227, 1974.

Hanna, W. T.; Krauss, S.; Resester, R. F., and Murphy, W. M.: Renal disease after mitomycin-C therapy. *Cancer,* **48:**2583–2588, 1981.

Hansen, H. H.; Dombernowsky, D.; and Hirsch, F. R.: Staging procedures and prognostic features in small cell anaplastic bronchogenic carcinoma. *Semin. Oncol.,* **5:**280–287, 1978.

Hansen, H. H., and Muggia, F. M.: Early detection of bone marrow invasion in oat cell carcinoma of the lung. *N. Engl. J. Med.,* **284:**962–963, 1971.

Harden, E.; Lucas, V. S.; Proia, A.; and Silberman, H. R.: Hemolytic uremic syndrome during therapy with mitomycin-C plus 5-fluorouracil. *Proc. Am. Assoc. Cancer Res.,* **1:**93, 1982.

Havard, C. W. H., and Scott, R. B.: Thymic tumor and erythroblastic aplasia: report of three cases and a review of the syndrome. *Br. J. Haematol.,* **6:**178–190, 1960.

Henderson, C. A.; Metz, E. N.; Balcerzak, S. P.; and Sagone, A. L.: Adriamycin and daunomycin generate reactive oxygen compounds in erythrocytes. *Blood,* **52:**878–885, 1978.

Henderson, P. H.: Multiple migratory thrombophlebitis associated with ovarian carcinoma. *Am. J. Obstet. Gynecol.,* **70:**452–453, 1955.

Hensby, C. N.; Lewis, P. J.; Hilgard, P.; Mufti, G. J.; Horos, J.; and Webster, J.: Prostacycline deficiency in thrombotic thrombocytopenic purpura. *Lancet,* **2:**748, 1979.

Herman, E. H.; Lee, I. P.; Mhatre, R. M; and Chadwick, D. P.: Prevention of hemolysis induced by ellipticine (NSC-71795) in rhesus monkeys. *Cancer Chemother. Repts. (Part 1),* **58:**171–179, 1974.

Higgins, G. K.: Pathologic anatomy. In Molander, D. W., and Pack, G. T., (eds.): *Hodgkin's Disease.* Charles C Thomas, Publisher, Springfield, Illinois, 1968.

Hild, D. H., and Myers, T. J.: Hyperviscosity in chronic granulocytic leukemia. *Cancer,* **46:**1418–1421, 1980.

Hilgard, P., and Gordon-Smith, E. C.: Microangiopathic hemolytic anemia and experimental tumor cell emboli. *Br. J. Haematol.,* **26:**651–659, 1974.

Hillestad, L. K.: Acute promyelocytic leukemia. *Acta Med. Scand. [Suppl].,* **159:**189–194, 1957.

Hirsch, F.; Hansen, H. H.; Dombernowsky, P.; and Hainau, B.; Bone marrow examination in the staging of small cell anaplastic carcinoma of the lung with special reference to subtyping. *Cancer,* **39:**2563–2567, 1977.

Hirst, E., and Robertson, T. I.: The syndrome of thymoma and erythroblastopenic anemia. *Medicine* (Baltimore), **46:**225–264, 1967.

Huggins, C., and Neal, W.; Coagulation and liquefaction of semen: Proteolytic enzymes and citrate in prostatic fluid. *J. Exp. Med.,* **76:**527–541, 1942.

Huggins C., and Vail, V. C.: Plasma coagulation and fibrinolysis by prostatic fluid and trypsin. *Am. J. Physiol.,* **139:**129–134, 1942.

Isaacson, N. H., and Rapoport, P.: Eosinophilia in malignant tumors: Its significance. *Ann. Intern. Med.,* **25:**893–902, 1946.

Jackson, A. M.; Graff, L. G.; Rose, B. D.; Jacobs, J. B.; Schwartz, J. H.; Strauss, G. M.; Yang, J. P. S.; Rudnick, M. R.; Bastl, C. P.; Narins, R. G.; and Elfenbein, I. B.: Thrombotic microangiopathy and renal failure associated with antineoplastic chemotherapy. *Clin. Res.,* **30:**419A, 1982.

Jacobs, A.; Jones, B.; Ricketts, C.; Bulbrook, R. D.; and Wang, D. Y.: Serum ferritin concentration in early breast cancer. *Br. J. Cancer,* **34:**286–290, 1976a.

Jacobs, A.; Slater, A.; Whittaker, J. A.; Canellos, G.; and Wiernik, P. H.: Serum ferritin concentration in untreated Hodgkin's disease. *Br. J. Cancer,* **34:**162–166, 1976b.

Jacobs, E. M.; Hutter, R. V. P.; Pool, J. L.; and Ley, A. B.: Benign thymoma and selective erythroid aplasia of the bone marrow. *Cancer,* **12:**47–57, 1959.

James, L. P.; Stass, S. A.; Peterson, V.; and Schumacher, H. R.: Abnormalities of bone marrow simulating histiocytic medullary reticulosis in a patient with gastric carcinoma. *Am. J. Clin. Pathol.,* **71:**600–602, 1979.

Jarcho, S.: Diffusely infiltrative carcinoma: A hitherto undescribed correlation of several varieties of metastasis. *Arch. Pathol.,* **22:**674–696, 1936.

Jeffrey, M. R. and Watson, D.: Free erythrocyte porphyrin and plasma copper in rheumatoid disease. *Acta Haematol* (Basel)., **12:**169–176, 1954.

Jennings, W. K., and Russell, W. O.: Phlebothrombosis associated with mucin-producing carcinomas of the tail

and body of the pancreas. *Arch. Surg.,* **56:**186–198, 1948.

Jepson, J. H., and Lowenstein, L.: Panhypoplasia of the bone marrow: I. Demonstration of a plasma factor with anti-erythropoietin-like activity. *Can. Med. Assoc. J.,* **99:**99–101, 1968.

Jepson, J. H., and Vas, M.: Decreased *in vivo* and *in vitro* erythropoiesis induced by plasma of ten patients with thymoma, lymphosarcoma or idiopathic erythroblastopenia. *Cancer Res.,* **34:**1325–1334, 1974.

Jones, B. G.; Fielding, T. W.; Newman, C. E.; Howell, A.; and Brookes, V. S.: Intravascular hemolysis and renal impairment after blood transfusion in two patients on long term 5-fluorouracil and mitomycin-C. *Lancet,* **1:**1275–1277, 1980.

Jones, E., and Tillman, C.: A case of hemolytic anemia relieved by removal of an ovarian tumor. *J.A.M.A.,* **128:**1225–1227, 1945.

Jones, P. A. E.; Miller, F.; Worwood, M.; and Jacobs, A.: Ferritinaemia in leukemia and Hodgkin's disease. *Br. J. Cancer,* **27:**212–217, 1973.

Jones, R. R.: The cutaneous manifestations of paraproteinemia. *Br. J. Dermatol.,* **103:**335–345, 1980.

Jonsson, U., and Rundles, R. W.: Tumor metastases in bone marrow. *Blood,* **6:**16–25, 1951.

Joseph, R. R.; Day, H. J.; Sherwin, R. M.; and Schwartz, H. G.: Microangiopathic haemolytic anaemia associated with consumption coagulopathy in a patient with disseminated carcinoma. *Scand. J. Haematol.,* **4:**271–282, 1967.

Jurgens, R., and Trautwein, H.: Uber Fibrinopenie (Fibrinogenopenie) beim Erwachsener, nebst Bemerkungen uber die Herkunft des Fibrinogens. *Dtsch. Arch. Klin. Med.,* **169:**28–43, 1930.

Kalbfleisch, J. M., and Bird, R. M.: Cryofibrinogenemia. *N. Engl. J. Med.,* **263:**881–886, 1960.

Kaplan, B. S.: The hemolytic uremic syndrome. *Pediatr. Clin. North Am.,* **23:**761–777, 1976.

Karlin, D. A., and Stroehlein, T. R.: Rash, nephritis, hypertension and hemolysis in patient on 5-fluorouracil, doxorubicin and mitomycin-C. *Lancet,* **2:**534–535, 1980.

Katz, L. J.; Hoffman, R.; Ritchey, A. K.; and Dainiak, N.: The proliferative capacity of pure red cell aplasia bone marrow cells. *Yale J. Biol. Med.,* **54:**89–94, 1981.

Kiely, J. M., and Silverstein, M. N.: Metastatic carcinoma simulating agnogenic myeloid metaplasia and myelofibrosis. *Cancer,* **24:**1041–1044, 1969.

Kiraly, J. F., and Wheby, M. S.: Bone marrow necrosis, *Am. J. Med.,* **60:**361–368, 1976.

Korst, D. R., and Kratochvil, C. H.: Cryofibrinogen in a case of lung neoplasm associated with thrombophlebitis migrans. *Blood,* **10:**945–953, 1955.

Krammer, A.; Cartwright, G. E.; and Wintrobe, M. M.: The anemia of infection XIX: Studies on free erythrocyte coproporphyrin and protoporphyrin. *Blood,* **9:**183–188, 1954.

Krantz, K. B., and Kao, V.: Studies on red cell aplasia: I. Demonstration of a plasma inhibitor to heme synthesis and an antibody to erythroblast nuclei. *Proc. Natl. Acad. Sci USA,* **68:**493–500, 1967.

Krantz, K. B., and Kao, V.: Studies on red cell aplasia: II. Report of a second patient with an antibody to erythroblast nuclei and a remission after immunosuppressive therapy. *Blood,* **34:**1–12, 1969.

Krantz, S. B.: Annotation: Pure red cell aplasia. *Br. J. Haematol.,* **25:**1–6, 1973.

Krantz, S. B.: Diagnosis and treatment of pure red cell aplasia. *Med. Clin. North Am.,* **60:**945–958, 1976.

Krantz, S. B.; Moore, W. H.; and Zaentz, S. D.: Studies on pure red cell aplasia: I. Presence of erythroblast cytotoxicity in G-globulin fraction of plasma. *J. Clin. Invest.,* **52:**324–336, 1973.

Krauss, S.; Sonoda, T.; and Solomon, A.: Treatment of advanced gastrointestinal cancer with 5-fluorouracil and mitomcyin-C. *Cancer,* **43:**1598–1603, 1979.

Kressel, B.; Ryan, K. P.; Duong, A. T.; Berenberg, J.: and Schein, P. S.: Microangiopathic hemolyic anemia, thrombocytopenia, and renal failure in patients treated for adenocarcinoma. *Cancer,* **48:**1738–1745, 1981.

Kuzur, M. E., and Greco, F. A.: Cisplatin-induced anemia. *N. Engl. J. Med.,* **303:**110–111, 1980.

Lackner, H.: Hemostatic abnormalities associated with dysproteinemia. *Semin. Hematol.* **10:**125–133, 1973.

Laffay, D. L.; Tubbs, R. R.; Valenzuela, R.; Hall, P. M.; and McCormack, L. J.: Chronic glomerular microangiopathy and metastatic carcinoma. *Hum. Pathol.,* **10:**433–438, 1979.

Lee, I. P.: A possible mechanism of ellipticine-induced hemolysis. *J. Pharmacol. Exp. Ther.,* **196:**525–535, 1976.

Lempert, K. D.: Hemolysis and renal impairment syndrome in patients on 5-fluorouracil and mitomycin-C. *Lancet,* **2:**369–370, 1980.

Lerner, R. G.; Rapoport, S. I.; and Meltzer, J.: Thrombotic thrombocytopenic purpura: Serial clotting studies, relation to the generalized Schwartzman reaction and remission after adrenal steroid and dextran therapy. *Ann. Intern. Med.,* **66:**1180–1190, 1967.

Levi, J. A.; Aroney, R. S.; and Dalley, D. N.: Haemolytic anemia after cisplatin treatment. *Br. Med. J.,* **282:**2003–2004, 1981.

Levin, J., and Conley, C. L.: Thrombocytosis associated with malignant disease. *Arch. Intern. Med.,* **114:**497–500, 1964.

Levine, S., and Shearn, M. A.: Thrombotic thrombocytopenic purpura and lupus erythematosus. *Arch. Intern. Med.,* **113:**826–836, 1964.

Lichtman, M. A.: Cellular deformability during maturation of the myeloblast: Possible role in marrow egress. *N. Engl. J. Med.,* **283:**943–948, 1970.

Lichtman, M. A.: Rheology of leukocytes, leukocyte suspensions and blood in leukemia: Possible relationship to clinical manifestations. *J. Clin. Invest.,* **52:**350–357, 1973.

Lieberman, J. L.; Borrero, J.; Urdoneta, E.; and Wright, I. S.: Thrombophlebitis and cancer. *J.A.M.A.,* **177:**542–545, 1961.

Lohrmann, H. P.; Adam, W.; Heymer, B.; and Kubanek, B.: Microangiopathic hemolytic anemia in metastatic carcinoma: Report of eight cases. *Ann. Intern. Med.,* **79:**368–375, 1973.

Luscher, E., and Labhard, A.: Bluterinnungsstorung durch beta-gamma Globuline: Zur Kenntnis der Gerinnungsstorungen durch korpereigene Antikoagulantien. *Schweiz Med. Wochenschr.,* **79:**598–604, 1949.

Lynch, E. C., and Alfrey, C. P.: Histiocytic medullary reticulosis: hemolytic anemia due to erythrophagocytosis by histiocytes. *Ann. Intern. Med.,* **63:**666–671, 1965.

Lynch, E. C.; Bakken, C. L.; Casey, T. H.; and Alfrey, C. P.: Microangiopathic hemolytic anemia in carcinoma of the stomach. *Gastroenterology,* **52:**88–93, 1967.

McCallister, B. D.; Bayrd, E. D.; Harrison, E. G.; and McGuckin, W. F.: Primary macroglobulinemia. *Am. J. Med.,* **43:**394–434, 1967.

McFadzean, A. J. S.; Todd, D.; and Tsang, K. C.: Polycythemia in primary carcinoma of the liver. *Blood,* **13:**427–435, 1958.

MacKenzie, M. R.; Brown, E.; Fudenberg, H. H. J.; and Goodenday, L.: Waldenstrom's macroglobulinemia: Correlation between expanded plasma: Volume and increased serum viscosity. *Blood,* **35:**394–408, 1970.

Mahn, E., and Dantuono, L. M.: Postabortal septicotoxemia due to *Clostridium welchii.* Seventy-five cases from the maternity hospital, Santiago, Chile, 1948–1952. *Am. J. Obstet. Gynecol.,* **70:**604–610, 1955.

Major, R. H., and Leger, L. H.: Marked eosinophilia in Hodgkin's disease. *J.A.M.A.,* **112:**2601–2602, 1939.

Marder, M.; Weiner, M.; Schulman, P.; and Shapiro, S.: Afibrinogenemia occurring in a case of malignancy of the prostate with bone metastases. *N.Y. State J. Med.,* **49:**1197–1198, 1949.

Marshall, A. H. E.: Histiocytic medullary reticulosis. *J. Pathol. Bact.,* **71:**61–71, 1956.

Messner, H. A.; Fauser, A. A.; Curtis, J. E.; and Dotten, D.: Control of antibody-mediated pure red cell aplasia by plasmapheresis. *N. Engl. J. Med.,* 1334–1338, 1981.

Mettler, N. E.: Isolation of a Microtatobiote from patients with hemolytic uremic syndrome and thrombotic thrombocytopenic purpura and from mites in the United States. *N. Engl. J. Med.,* **281:**1023–1027, 1969.

Meyer, L. M., and Rotter, S. D.: Leukemoid reaction (hyperleucocytosis) in malignancy. *Am. J. Clin. Pathol.,* **12:**218–222, 1942.

Miller, S. P.; Sanchez-Avolos, J.; Stefanski, T.; and Zuckerman, L.: Coagulation disorders in cancer. *Cancer,* **20:**1452–1465, 1967.

Mitchell, A. B. S.; Pinn, M. G.; and Pegrum, G. D.: Pure red cell aplasia and carcinoma. *Blood,* **37:**594–597, 1971.

Moran, E. M., and Ultmann, F. E.: Clinical features and course of Hodgkin's disease. *Semin. Haematol.,* **3:**91–129, 1974.

Morris, P. J.; Cooper, I. A.; and Madigan, J. P.: Splenectomy for haematological cytopenias in patients with malignant lymphoma. *Lancet,* **2:**250–253, 1975.

Naeye, R. L.: Thrombotic state after a hemorrhagic diathesis, a possible complication of therapy with epsilon-aminocaproic acid. *Blood,* **19:**694–701, 1962.

Nagasawa, T.; Abe, T.; and Nakegawa, T.: Pure red cell aplasia and hypogammaglobulinemia associated with Tr-cell chronic lymphocytic leukemia. *Blood,* **57:**1025–1031, 1981.

Najarian, T.; Miller, A.; Zimelman, A. P.; and Hong, W. K.: Hematologic effect of cis-platinum-bleomycin therapy. *Oncology,* **38:**195–197, 1981.

Natelson, E. A.; Lynch E. C.; Hettig, R. A.; and Alfrey, C. P.: Histiocytic medullary reticulosis: The role of phagocytosis in pancytopenia. *Arch. Intern. Med.,* **122:**223–229, 1968.

Neame, P. B.; Hirsh, J.; Browman, G.; Denburg, J.; D'Sauza, T. J.; Galbes, A.; and Brain, M. C.: Thrombotic thrombocytopenic purpura: A syndrome of intravascular platelet consumption. *Can. Med. Assoc. J.,* **114:**1108–1112, 1976.

Nguyen, B. V.; Jaffe, N.; and Lichtiger, B.: Cisplatin-induced anemia. *Cancer Treat. Rep.,* **65:**1121, 1981.

Nishimura, J.; Okamoto, S.; and Ibagashi, H.: Abnormalities of platelet adenine nucleotides in patients with myeloproliferative disorders. *Thromb. Haemost.,* **41**:787–795, 1979.

O'Meara, R. A. Q., and Thornes, R. D.: Some properties of the cancer coagulative factor. *Ir. J. Med. Sci.,* **423**:106–112, 1961.

Owen, C. A., and Bowie, E. J. W.: Chronic intravascular coagulation syndromes: A summary. *Mayo Clin. Proc.,* **49**:673–679, 1974.

Pachter, M. R.; Johnson, S. A.; and Basinski, D. H.: The effect of macroglobulins and their dissocation units on release of platelet factor 3. *Thromb. Diath. Hemorr.,* **3**:501–509, 1959a.

Pachter, M. R.; Johnson, S. A.; Neblett, T. R.; and Truant, J. P.: Bleeding platelets and macroglobulinemia. *Am. J. Clin. Pathol.,* **31**:467–482, 1959b.

Papadimitriou, J.; Tritakis, C.; Karatzas, G.; and Papaioannou, A.: Treatment of hypersplenism by embolus placement in the splenic artery. *Lancet,* **2**:1268–1270, 1976.

Pavy, M. D.; Wiley, E. L.; and Abeloff, M. D.: Hemolytic-uremic syndrome associated with mitomycin therapy. *Cancer Treat. Rep.,* **66**:457–466, 1982.

Pellman, C. M; Ridlon, H. C.; and Philips, L. L.: Manifestation and management of hypofibrinogenemia and fibrinolysis in patients with carcinoma of the prostate. *J. Urol.,* **96**:375–379, 1966.

Penny, R.; Castaldi, P. A.; and Whitsed, H. M.: Inflammation and haemostasis in paraproteinaemias. *Br. J. Haematol.,* **20**:35–44, 1971.

Perkins, H. A.; MacKenzie, M. A.; and Fudenberg, H. H.: Hemostatic defects in dysproteinemias. *Blood,* **35**:695–707, 1970.

Perlow, S.; and Daniels, J. L.: Venous thrombosis and obscure visceral carcinoma—Report of 10 cases. *Arch. Intern. Med.,* **97**:184–188, 1956.

Peschle, C.; Marmont, A. M.; Marone, G.; Genovese, A.; Sesso, G. F.; and Condorelli, M.: Pure red cell aplasia: Studies on an IgG serum inhibitor neutralizing erythropoietin. *Br. J. Haematol.,* **30**:411–417, 1975.

Phadke, K.; Dean, S.; and Pitney, W. R.: Platelet dysfunction in myeloproliferative syndromes. *Am. J. Hematol.,* **10**:57–64, 1981.

Pineo, G. F.; Brain, M. C.; Gallus, A. S.; Hirsh, J.; Hatton, M. W. C.; and Regoeczi, E.: Tumors, mucus production and hypercoagulability. *Ann. N.Y. Acad. Sci.,* **230**:289–296, 1974.

Pineo, G. F.; Regoeczi, E.; Hatton, M. W. C.; and Brain, M. C.: The activation of coagulation by extracts of mucus: A possible pathway of intravascular coagulation accompanying adenocarcinoma. *J. Lab. Clin. Med.,* **82**:255–266, 1973.

Pirofsky, B.: Clinical aspects of autoimmune hemolytic anemia. *Semin. Hematol.,* **13**:251–265, 1976.

Prentice, H. G.; Russell, N. H.; Lee, N.; Ganeshagaru, K.; Blacklock, H.; Piga, A.; Smyth, J. F.; and Hoffbrand, A. V.: Therapeutic selectivity of and prediction of response to 2′-deoxycoformycin in acute leukemia. *Lancet,* **2**:1250–1259, 1981.

Preston, F. E.; Sokol, R. J.; Lillyman, J. S.; Winfield, D. A.; and Blackburn, E. K.: Cellular hyperviscosity as a cause of neurological symptoms in leukemia. *Br. Med. J.,* **1**:476–478, 1978.

Propp, R.: Microangiopathic anemia and thrombocytopenia in disseminated breast cancer. Erythrocyte and platelet kinetics before and after steroid-associated remission. *Clin. Res.,* **14**:324, 1966.

Pruzanski, W., and Shumak, K. H.: Biologic activity of cold-reacting autoantibodies. *N. Engl. J. Med.,* **297**:538–542, 583–589, 1977.

Rabani, S. T.: Mitomycin-induced hemolytic uremic syndrome: Case presentation and review of literature. *Cancer Treat. Rep.,* **66**:1244–1248, 1982.

Rapoport, S. I., and Chapman, C. G.: Co-existent hypercoagulability and acute hypofibrinogenemia in a patient with prostatic carcinoma. *Am. J. Med.,* **27**:144–153, 1959.

Retief, F. P.: Leuco-erythroblastosis in the adult. *Lancet,* **1**:639–642, 1964.

Retzlaff, J. A.; Hagedorn, A. B.; and Bartholomew, L. G.: Abdominal exploration for gastrointestinal bleeding of obscure origin. *J.A.M.A.,* **177**:104–107, 1961.

Roberts-Thompson, P. J.; Mason, D. Y.; and MacLerman, I. C. M.: Relationship between paraprotein polymerization and clinical features in IgA myeloma. *Br. J. Haematol.,* **33**:117–130, 1976.

Robinson, W. A.: Granulocytosis in neoplasia. *Ann. N.Y. Acad. Sci.,* **230**:212–218, 1974.

Rodriguez, J., and Stevenson, T.: Chronic intravascular coagulation and microangiopathic hemolytic anemia in a patient with carcinoma of the lung. *Ohio State Med. J.,* **65**:1010–1016, 1969.

Rohner, R. F.; Prior, J. T.; and Sipple, J. H.: Mucinous malignancies, venous thrombosis and terminal endocarditis with emboli. A syndrome. *Cancer,* **19**:1805–1812, 1966.

Rohr, K. and Hegglin, R.: Tumorzellen in Stornalpunktat. *Dtsch. Arch. Klin. Med.,* **179**:61–79, 1936.

Rosen, P., and Armstrong, D.: Nonbacterial thrombotic endocarditis in patients with malignant neoplastic diseases. *Am. J. Med.,* **54**:23–29, 1973a.

Rosen, P., and Armstrong, D.: Infective endocarditis in patients treated for malignant neoplastic diseases. *Am. J. Clin. Pathol.,* **59**:241–250, 1973b.

Rosenberg, S. A.: Hodgkin's disease of the bone marrow. *Cancer Res.,* **31**:1733–1736, 1971.

Rossof, A. H.; Slayton, R. E.; and Perlia, C. P.: Preliminary clinical experience with cis-diamminedichloroplatinum (II). *Cancer,* **30**:1451–1456, 1972.

Rouesse, J.; Huertas, D.; Sancho-Garnier, H.; Chevalier, T.; Amiel, J. L.; Brule, G.; Tursz, T.; and Mondesir, J. M.: 2-N-methyl-9-hydroxy-ellipticine in treatment of metastatic breast cancer. *Bull. Cancer (Paris),* **68**:437–441, 1981.

Royster, R. L.; Wassim, J. A.; and King, E. R.: An evaluation of the effects of splenectomy in patients with Hodgkin's disease undergoing extended field or total lymph node irradiation. *Am. J. Roentgenol.,* **120**:521–530, 1974.

Rozencweig, M.; VonHoff, D. D.; Slavik, M.; and Muggia, F.: Cis-diamminedichloroplatinum (II): A new anticancer drug. *Ann. Intern. Med.,* **86**:803–812, 1977.

Rubenberg, M. L.; Regoeczi, E.; Bull, B. S.; Dacie, J. V.; and Brain, M. C.: Microangiopathic hemolytic anaemia: The experimental production of haemolysis and red-cell fragmentation by defibrination *in vivo. Br. J. Haematol.,* **14**:627–642, 1968.

Rudders, R. A.; Aisenberg, A.; and Schiller, A. L.: Hodgkin's disease presenting as "idiopathic" thrombocytopenic purpura. *Cancer,* **30**:220–230, 1972.

Rumpf, K. W.; Rieger, J.; Lankisch, P. G.; von Heyden, H. W.; Nagel, G. A.; and Scheler, F.: Mitomycin-induced haemolysis and renal failure. *Lancet,* **2**:1037–1038, 1980.

Sacher, R. A.; Woolley, P. V.; Priego, V. M.; Schanfield, M.; and Bonnem, E.: Methotrexate-induced. Hemolytic anemia. *Proc. Am. Assoc. Blood Bank,* 42, 1981.

Sack, G. H.; Levin, J.; and Bell, W. R.: Trousseau's syndrome and other manifestations of chronic disseminated coagulopathy in patients with neoplasms: Clinical, pathophysiologic and therapeutic features. *Medicine* (Baltimore), **56**:1–37, 1977.

Sakuragawa, N.; Takahashi, K.; Hashigama, M.; Jimbo, C.; Ashizawa, K.; Matsuaka, M.; and Ohnishi, Y.: The extract from the tissue of gastric cancer as procoagulant in disseminated intravascular coagulation syndrome. *Thromb. Res.,* **10**:457–463, 1977.

Sanchez-Avalos, J.; Soong, B. C. F.; and Miller, S. P.: Coagulation disorders in cancer: II. Multiple myeloma. *Cancer,* **29**:1388–1398, 1969.

Schioppocassi, G., and Schwartz, H. S.: Membrane actions of daunorubicin in mammalian erythrocytes. *Res. Commun. Chem. Pathol., Pharmacol.,* **18**:519–531, 1977.

Schmid, J. R.; Kiely, J. M.; Harrison, E. G.; Bayrd, E. D.; and Pease, G. L.: Thymoma associated with pure red cell aplasia. *Cancer,* **18**:216–230, 1965.

Schmid, J. R.; Kiely, J. M.; Pease, G. L.; and Hargraves, M. M.: Acquired pure red cell aplasia. Report of 16 cases and review of the literature. *Acta Haematol.* (Basel), **30**:255–270, 1963.

Scott, R. B., and Robb-Smith, A. H. T.: Histiocytic medullary reticulosis. *Lancet,* **2**:194–198, 1939.

Scotti, T. M.: In Anderson, W. A. D.: *Pathology.* The C. V. Mosby Company, St. Louis, 1971.

Seale, R. A.; Jampolis, R. W.; and Bargen, J. A.: Clotting defect in the presence of metastatic carcinoma of prostate: A case report. *S. Clin. North Am.,* **31**:1111–1119, 1951.

Seligsohn, U.; Weber, H.; Yoran, C.; Horowitz, A.; and Ramot, B.: Microangiopathic hemolytic anemia and defibrination syndrome in metastatic carcinoma of the stomach. *Isr. J. Med. Sci.,* **4**:69–75, 1968.

Shinohara, K., and Tanaka, K. R.: The effects of adriamycin (doxorubicin HCl) on human red blood cells. *Hemoglobin,* **4**:735–745, 1980.

Siaw, M. F. E.; Mitchell, B. S.; Keller, C. A.; Coleman, M. S.; and Hutton, J. J.: ATP depletion as a consequence of adenosine deaminase inhibition in man. *Proc. Natl. Acad. Sci. USA,* **77**:6157–6161, 1980.

Silverstein, M.: Primary or hemorrhagic thrombocythemia. *Arch. Intern. Med.,* **122**:18–22, 1968.

Silvis, S. E.; Turkbas, N.; and Doscherholmen, A.: Thrombocytosis in patients with lung cancer. *J.A.M.A.,* **211**:1852–1853, 1970.

Simpkins, H.; Kahlenberg, A.; Rosenberg, A.; Tay, S.; and Panko, E.: Structural and compositional changes in the red cell membrane during *Clostridium welchii* infection. *Br. J. Haematol.,* **21**:173–182, 1971.

Slichter, S. J., and Harker, L. A.: Hemostasis in malignancy. *Ann. N.Y. Acad. Sci.,* **230**:252–261, 1974.

Slonim, A. E.; Fletcher, T.; Burke, V.; and Burr, I. M.: Effect of streptozotocin on red blood cell reduced glutathione: Modification by glucose, nicotinamide and epinephrine. *Diabetes,* **25**:216–222, 1976.

Smith, C. M.; Belch, A.; and Henderson, J. F.: Hemolysis in mice treated with deoxycoformycin, an inhibitor of adenosine deaminase. *Biochem. Pharmacol.,* **29**:1209–1210, 1980.

Smith, E.; Kochwa, S.; and Wasserman, L. R.: Aggregation of IgG globulin *in vivo:* I. The hyperviscosity syndrome in multiple myeloma. *Am. J. Med.* **39**:35–48, 1965.

Soong, B. C. F., and Miller, S. P.: Coagulation disorders in cancer: III. Fibrinolysis and inhibitors. *Cancer,* **25**:867–874, 1970.

Spira, M. A., and Lynch, E. C.: Autoimmune hemolytic anemia and carcinoma: An unusual association. *Am. J. Med.,* **67**:753–758, 1979.

Sponzo, R. W.; Arseneau, J. C.; and Canellos, G. P.: Procarbazine induced oxidative haemolysis: Relationship to *in vivo* red cell survival. *Br. J. Haematol.,* **27**:587–595, 1974.

Spremulli, E.; Crabtree, G. W.; Dexter, D. L.; Diamond, I.; and Calabresi, P.: 2′-deoxycoformycin-induced hemolysis in the mouse. *J.N.C.I.,* **68**:1011–1014, 1982.

Sproul, E. E.: Carcinoma and venous thrombosis: The frequency of association of carcinoma in the body or tail of the pancreas with multiple venous thrombosis. *Am. J. Cancer,* **34**:566–585, 1938.

Stathekis, N. E.; Karamanolis, D.; Kaukoulis, G.; and Tsianos, E.: Characterization of cryofibrinogen isolated from patients' plasma. *Haemostasis,* **10**:195–202, 1981.

Steinberg, M. H., and Charm, S. E.: Effect of high concentrations of leukocytes on whole blood viscosity. *Blood,* **38**:299–301, 1971.

Stephens, D. J.: Relation of viscosity of blood to leucocyte count, with particular reference to chronic myelogenous leukemia. *Proc. Soc. Exp. Biol. Med.,* **35**:251–256, 1936.

Stohlman, F.; Quesenberry, P. J.; Howard, D.; Miller, M. E.; and Schur, P.: Erythroid hyperplasia as a complication of chronic lymphocytic leukemia? *Clin. Res.,* **19**:566, 1971.

Stratford, E. C., and Tanaka, K. R.: Microangiopathic hemolytic anemia in metastatic carcinoma. *Br. Intern. Med.,* **116**:346–350, 1965.

Sun, N. C. J.; Bowie, E. J. W.; Kazmier, F. J.; Elveback, L. R.; and Owen, C. A.: Blood coagulation studies in patients with cancer. *Mayo Clin. Proc.,* **49**:636–641, 1974.

Svanberg, L.: Thromboplastic activity of human ovarian tumors. *Thromb. Res.,* **6**:307–313, 1975.

Sykes, M. P.; Karnofsky, D. A.; McNeer, G. P.; and Craver, L. F.: Splenectomy in far-advanced Hodgkin's disease. Report of five cases. *Blood,* **9**:824–836, 1954.

Tagnon, H. J.; Schulman, P.; Whitmore, W. F.; and Leone, L. A.: Prostatic fibrinolysis. Study of a case illustrating role in hemorrhagic diathesis of cancer of the prostate. *Am. J. Med.,* **15**:875–884, 1953a.

Tagnon, H. J.; Whitmore, W. F.; Schulman, P.; and Kravitz, S. C.: The significance of fibrinolysis occurring in patients with metastatic cancer of the prostate. *Cancer,* **6**:63–67, 1953b.

Tagnon, H. J.; Whitmore, W. F.; and Shulman, N. R.: Fibrinolysis in metastatic cancer of the prostate. *Cancer,* **5**:9–12, 1952.

Takahashi, H., and Tsukada, T.: Triamterene-induced hemolytic anemia with acute intravascular hemolysis and acute renal failure. *Scand. J. Haematol.,* **23**:169–176, 1979.

Thorling, E. B.: Paraneoplastic erythrocytosis and inappropriate erythropoietin production. *Scand. J. Haematol. [Suppl.]* **17**:1–166, 1972.

Tsai, S. Y., and Levin, W. C.: Chronic erythrocytic hypoplasia: Review of literature and report of a case. *Am. J. Med.,* **22**:322–330, 1957.

Tuddenham, E. G. D.; Whittaker, J. A.; Lilleyman, J. S.; and James, D. R.: Hyperviscosity syndrome in IgA multiple myeloma. *Br. J. Haematol.*, 27:65–76, 1974.

Tully, J. L.; Lew, M. A.; Common, M.; and D'Orsi, C. J.: Clostridial sepsis following hepatic arterial infusion chemotherapy. *Am. J. Med.*, 67:707–710, 1979.

Tveter, K. J.: Unusual manifestations of renal carcinoma: A review of the literature. *Acta Chir. Scand.*, 139:401–412, 1973.

Uehlinger, E.: Uber eine Bluterinnungsstorung bei Dysproteinamie. Beitrag zur Kenntnis der Korperseigene Antikoagulantia. *Helv. Med. Acta,* 16:508–528, 1949.

Vallejos, C. S.; McCredie, K. B.; Brihin, G. M.; and Freireich, E. J.: Biological effects of leukapheresis of patients with chronic myelogenous leukemia. *Blood,* 42:925–933, 1973.

Van Snick, J. L.; Marcowetz, B.; and Masson, P. L.: The ingestion and digestion of human lactoferrin by mouse peritoneal macrophages and the transfer of its iron into ferritin. *J. Exp. Med.,* 146:817–827, 1977.

Vaughn, J. M.: Leuco-erythroblastic anemia. *J. Pathol. Bacteriol.,* 42:541–564, 1936.

Verstraete, M.: The clinical relevance of hyperviscosity. *Acta Clin. Belg.,* 36:269–273, 1981.

Vigliano, E. M., and Horowitz, H. I.: Bleeding syndrome in a patient with IgA myeloma: Interaction of protein and connective tissue. *Blood,* 29:823–836, 1967.

Virella, G.; Valadas,; Preto, R.; and Graca, F.: Polymerized monoclonal IgA in two patients with myelomatosis and hyperviscosity syndrome. *Br. J. Haematol.,* 30:479–487, 1975.

Waddell, C. C.; Brown, J. A.; and Repincz, Y. A.: Abnormal platelet function in myeloproliferative disorders. *Arch. Pathol. Lab. Med.,* 105:432–435, 1981.

Waldmann, T. A., and Bradley, J. E.: Polycythemia secondary to a pheochromocytoma with production of an erythropoiesis stimulating factor by the tumor. *Am. J. Med.,* 31:318–324, 1961.

Waldmann, T. A.; Rosse, W. F.; and Swarm, R. L.: The erythropoiesis-stimulating factors produced by tumors. *Ann. N.Y. Acad. Sci.,* 149:509–515, 1968.

Wallerstein, R. O., and Aggeler, P. M.: Acute hemolytic anemia. *Am. J. Med.,* 37:92–104, 1964.

Warnke, R. A.; Kim, H.; and Dorfman, R. F.: Malignant histiocytosis (histiocytic medullary reticulosis): I. Clinicopathologic study of 29 cases. *Cancer,* 35:215–230, 1975.

Waterbury, L. S., and Hampton, J. W.: Hypercoagulability with malignancy. *Angiology,* 18:197–203, 1967.

Webb, D. I.; Ubogy, G.; and Silver, R. T.: Importance of bone marrow biopsy in the clinical staging of Hodgkin's disease. *Cancer,* 26:313–317, 1970.

Weick, J. K.; Hagedorn, A. B.; and Linman, J. W.: Leukoerythroblastosis. Diagnostic and prognostic significance. *Mayo Clin. Proc.,* 49:110–113, 1974.

Willcox, D. R. C.: Hemolytic anemia and reticulosis. *Br. Med. J.,* 1:1322–1325, 1952.

Wintrobe, M. M.: *Clinical hematology.* Lea & Febiger, Philadelphia, 1981.

Wintrobe, M. M.; Lee, G. R.; Boggs, D. R.; Bithell, T. C.; Foerster, J.; Athens, J. W.; and Lukens, J. N.: *Clinical Hematology.* Lea & Febiger, Philadelphia, 1981, Chapter 24, pp 646–653; Chapter 40, pp 965–969; Chapter 38, pp 926–948.

Woolley, P. V.: Clinical manifestations of cancer of the colon and rectum. *Semin. Oncol.,* 3:373–376, 1976.

Woolley, P. V.; Sacher, R. A.; Priego, V. M.; Schanfield, M. S.; and Bonnem, E. M.: Methotrexate-induced haemolytic anaemia. *Br. J. Haematol.,* 54:543–552, 1983.

Zarrabi, M. H.; Lysik, R.; DiStefano, J.; and Zucker, S.: The anaemia of chronic disorders: Studies of iron reutilization in the anaemia of experimental malignancy and chronic inflammation. *Br. J. Haematol.,* 35:647–658, 1977.

Zimmerman, S. E.; Smith, F. P.; Phillips, T. M.; Coffey, R. J.; and Schein, P. S.: Gastric carcinoma and thrombotic thrombocytopenic purpura: Association with plasma immune complex concentrations. *Br. Med. J.,* 284:1432–1434, 1982.

Zinneman, H. H.: Cryoglobulins and pyroglobulins. *Pathobiol. Annu.* 10:83–104, 1980.

Zucker, S.; Friedman, S., and Lysik, R. M.: Bone marrow erythropoiesis in the anemia of infection, inflammation and malignancy. *J. Clin. Invest.,* 53:1132–1138, 1974.

Zucker, S.; Lysik, R.; and DiStefano, J. F.: Cancer cell inhibition of erythropoiesis. *J. Lab. Clin. Med.,* 96:770–782, 1980.

C.   RENAL COMPLICATIONS OF CANCER

Frederick P. Smith and George E. Schreiner

Renal complications are being encountered with increasing frequency in the management of patients with cancer. In an autopsy survey of 300 patients with malignant neoplasms, over 50% were found to have significant impairment of one or both kidneys (Pascal, 1980). Potential causes of such renal injury from neoplasia include the direct and remote effects of the tumor, as well as complications related to treating the neoplastic disease. A general listing of these complications is provided in Table 6–7. Some of the remote effects of neoplasia of the kidney have only recently been described and suggest an important immunologic pathogenesis to the resultant renal damage (Lee *et al.,* 1966; Lewis *et al.,* 1971; Costanza *et al.,* 1973; Gagliano *et al.,* 1976; Eagen and Lewis, 1977). The list of renal injuries related to treatment continues to rise with the continued search for new antineoplastic agents and with more prolonged use and experience with existing chemotherapeutic drugs. Potential interactions between antineoplastic agents and antibiotics, particularly the aminoglycosides, are

Table 6-7.   Causes of Renal Complications in Cancer

I.   Direct Effect of the Neoplasm:
   A.   Obstruction:
      Prostate, bladder, cervix, lymphoma
   B.   Metastatic nephropathy
      Leukemic, lymphomatous
   C.   Myeloma nephropathy
II.   Metabolic Nephropathy:
   A.   Uric acid precipitation
   B.   Hypercalcemia
   C.   "Tumor lysis" syndrome
III.   Remote Effect of the Neoplasm:
   A.   Nephrotic syndrome
      Carcinoma
      Hodgkin's disease
      Non-Hodgkin's lymphoma
   B.   Amyloid deposition
IV.   Treatment-Related:
   A.   Antineoplastic nephropathy
   B.   Radiation nephropathy
   C.   Immunotherapy nephropathy

Table 6-8.   Treatment-Related Renal Complications

Drug-Induced
   A.   Nitrosoureas
     1.   Streptozotocin
     2.   Methyl-CCNU, BCNU
     3.   Chlorozotocin
   B.   Methotrexate
   C.   *Cis*-diamminedichloroplatinum
Radiation Induced
Immunotherapy Induced
   C.   Parvum

only now being recorded (Gonzales-Vitale *et al.*, 1978). Table 6-8 outlines some of these iatrogenic complications that are detailed in the chapter on pharmacology (see Chapter 10). Whereas the end result of all these nephrotoxic factors may be varying degrees of azotemia, medical oncologists must recognize the potential contributing causes in their patients. Many are preventable, and the treatment of specific entities may be unique; for example, the use of plasmapheresis to reverse the hemolytic-uremic syndrome in a patient with gastric carcinoma (Zimmerman *et al.*, 1982a).

Elsewhere in this text, the renal consequences of metabolic disorders encountered with neoplasia and its therapy are described (see Chapters 6F and 40). Wiemann and Calabresi (see Chapter 10), have discussed nephrotoxicity due to antineoplastic chemotherapy. Consequently, in this section, we will only briefly review the direct effects of neo-plasia and metabolic disorders resulting in renal impairment, and will concentrate primarily on the paraneoplastic manifestations.

DIRECT EFFECTS OF THE NEOPLASM

Obstruction

Obstruction of the genitourinary tract may lead to azotemia, especially in patients with genitourinary or gynecologic neoplasms and lymphoma (Fallon *et al.*, 1980). Obstructive uropathy has been reported to account for 60 to 80% of deaths due to cervical cancer (Beach, 1952; Fallon *et al.*, 1980). With frequent cytologic examination and earlier detection, however, the frequency of ureteral obstruction from cervical cancer appears to be declining. Prostatic carcinoma accounts for less than 6% of obstructive uropathy related to prostatic disease; benign prostatic hypertrophy in contrast, accounts for 70% and inflammatory disease and other non-neoplastic entities make up the remainder (Randall, 1931; Fallon *et al.*, 1980). When carcinoma of the bladder involves the trigone, unilateral or bilateral ureteral obstruction may be produced. Less common causes of obstructive uropathy include lymphoma (Abeloff and Lenhard, 1974), seminoma (Johnson *et al.*, 1981), and retroperitoneal fibrosis secondary to neoplasm (Thomas *et al.*, 1973). This last entity can produce systemic symptoms such as diabetes insipidus and hypertension that can easily be mistaken for metastases (Knowlan *et al.*, 1960).

The treatment of obstructive uropathy in the patient with neoplasia as discussed earlier must entail consideration of the natural history of the underlying tumor as well as whether the obstruction is unilateral or bilateral and the acuteness of renal compromise. Surgery, radiotherapy, and chemotherapy may all represent appropriate treatment modalities. It is often a difficult ethical decision to decide whether or not to attempt a surgical bypass of an obstruction in a patient with an advanced, treatment-refractory tumor. For selected cases with a reasonable survival expectation and a good quality of life prognosis, percutaneous nephrostomies (Sing *et al.*, 1979; Fallon *et al.*, 1980; Ho *et al.*, 1980) and ureteral stents (Hepperlen *et al.*, 1979; Ho *et al.*, 1980) represent reasonable options for palliation, and substantial improvement in azotemia has been achieved with acceptably low morbidity.

Metastatic Nephropathy

Metastases to the kidneys by solid tumors are uncommon and are reported in less than 10% of patients autopsied (Willis, 1973; Wagle et al., 1975). Such direct involvement rarely results in functional impairment in spite of frequent bilateral and multifocal involvement. Melanoma, carcinomas of the breast, lung, kidney, and colon are the most frequently observed histologies producing renal metastases.

Lymphomas and leukemias are more likely to involve the kidneys but rarely result in renal failure (Lightwood et al., 1960; Richmond et al., 1962; Kiely et al., 1969; Nies et al., 1972). Renal involvement in lymphoma is more common with histiocytic lymphoma and other histologic types of non-Hodgkin's lymphoma than with Hodgkin's disease. Kidney involvement has been described in over 40% of autopsied patients with histiocytic lymphoma, in 28% of those with mycosis fungoides, and in 15% of Hodgkin's disease patients autopsied. Nevertheless, Richmond and colleagues report that uremia was the cause of death in only 0.7% of 690 autopsied patients with known lymphomatous involvement of the kidneys (Richmond et al., 1962).

Myelomatous Nephropathy

Renal insufficiency is an important unfavorable prognostic manifestation of multiple myeloma and is the second most frequent cause of death in these patients (see Chapter 17). Pathologic changes in the kidney have been identified in more than 50% of patients who die from multiple myeloma and make up a variety of abnormalities that have been termed "myeloma kidney" (Martinez-Maldonado et al., 1971). The most prominent features include tubular atrophy, dense eosinophilic casts within the tubules, and syncytial formation of epithelial cells surrounding proteinaceous material and nonspecific glomerular changes (Schubert et al., 1972).

Tubular dysfunction in myeloma patients is well recognized (Schubert et al., 1972; DeFronzo et al., 1978). Renal tubular acidosis and concentration defects are encountered frequently, particularly in the presence of urinary light chains or Bence Jones proteinuria. Bence Jones proteinuria has been implicated as a likely pathogenic factor in the development of "myeloma kidney" (Martinez-Maldonado et al., 1971; Maldonado et al., 1975).

Light chains, metabolized by mesangial cells and possibly renal tubular epithelium, may directly damage the tubular cells (Clyne et al., 1979).

These light chains can be one of two types: Kappa or lambda. The former is more frequently associated with the Fanconi syndrome with excessive urinary loss of amino acids, phosphate, bicarbonate, uric acid, and tubular proteins and a resultant proximal renal tubular acidosis (Maldonado et al., 1975). The Fanconi syndrome may presage the diagnosis of multiple myeloma by several years (Maldonado et al., 1975). Lambda chains, by contrast, are more frequently associated with acute renal failure (Maldonado et al., 1975). Patients with chronic renal failure due to myeloma may have a lower anion gap as a result of the cationic hyperglobulinemia (Murray et al., 1975). The importance of a low anion gap in diagnosing multiple myeloma has recently been disputed, ascribing it to laboratory error (Goldstein et al., 1980).

Amyloid deposition in the glomeruli may contribute to renal dysfunction in 10% of patients with long-standing myeloma (Walker et al., 1971). Additional contributions to acute renal insufficiency encountered in this disease include hypercalcemia and hyperuricemia. Acute tubular necrosis and myeloma have been reported with dehydration and also with an increased susceptibility to radiograph contrast material.

Dialysis in selected patients has been reported to ameliorate treatment results and should be carefully considered in these patients (Leech et al., 1972; Richards and Hines, 1973). The multi-factoral causes of renal failure in this disease make the contribution of potentially reversible complications difficult to separate. A trial of peritoneal dialysis or hemodialysis may allow the appropriate elucidation for pursuing further aggressive therapy.

METABOLIC NEPHROPATHY

Uric Acid Precipitation

In cancers with rapid turnover of cells and nucleic acid, hyperuricemia is likely to be encountered. For the most part, leukemias and lymphomas make up the most frequently encountered neoplasms associated with high serum uric acid levels (Richards and Hines, 1973). With effective treatment and rapid tumor lysis and release of purines into the blood, marked elevation of serum uric acid may be observed. Hyperuricemic nephropathy results from uric acid crystal deposits within the tubules. Very rarely, nephrolithiasis may be observed. Tophaceous gouty nephropathy is only encountered with prolonged and severe hyperuricemia. Hydration, maintaining an adequate alkaline urine higher than the dissociation constant for uric acid (pka = 5.4), and the use of allopurinol are well-established prophylactic measures for preventing urate nephropathy (Wienman, 1976; Crittenden and Ackerman, 1977).

Hypercalcemia

Hypercalcemia is a well-recognized complication of neoplasia and may arise by several different mechanisms. These include bone resorption by direct tumor involvement, production of parathormone-like substances, prostaglandins, osteoclast-stimulating factors, and, potentially, hormonal therapy of breast cancer (Stewart et al., 1980). The early clinical symptoms of hypercalcemia are polyuria and polydipsia with resultant hyposthenuria, anorexia, nausea, and constipation. In some cases, mental obtundation with a metabolic encephalopathy may prevail. Nephrocalcinosis with or without scarring and vascular changes may be seen depending upon the duration and severity of the elevated calcium; nephrolithiasis is uncommon. Management of the blood calcium depends in part on the severity of symptoms but should include hydration, diuresis, and, when necessary, mithramycin (Parsons et al., 1967) and calcitonin (Deftos and First, 1981).

"Tumor Lysis" Syndrome

Certain poorly differentiated lymphoproliferative cancers with their high growth fraction may respond to cytotoxic therapy with a rapid dissolution of tumor. This "tumor lysis" syndrome has been shown to result in rapid metabolic shifts from cellular destruction; hyperkalemia, hyperphosphatemia resulting in hypocalcemia, hyperuremia and lactic acidosis have been observed following treatment of Burkitt's lymphomas and acute lymphoblastic leukemia (Frei et al., 1963; Ettinger et al., 1978; Brereton et al., 1979; Cohen et al., 1980). Renal insufficiency frequently results from uric acid nephropathy or phosphate deposition in the renal tubules (Kaufer et al., 1979). Patients at greatest risk for developing the "tumor lysis" syndrome are those with large tumor burdens. Surgical resection of Burkitt's tumor masses reduces the likelihood of these metabolic complications (Tsokos et al., 1981). In individuals with large abdominal masses, abnormal renal function, and a relative contraindication for peritoneal dialysis, preparation for hemodialysis should be considered prior to the initiation of chemotherapy (Brereton et al., 1979).

REMOTE EFFECTS OF CANCER

In 1966, Lee and colleagues first reported the significant association of cancer with the nephrotic syndrome (Lee et al., 1966). They observed an 11% incidence of cancer in 100 adults with the nephrotic syndrome followed over a 10-year period. This paraneoplastic phenomenon antedated the diagnosis of cancer in 7 of the 11 patients. Lee and colleagues postulated that glomerular deposition of tumor antigen-antibody complex led to the proteinuria. Several other studies have since confirmed this association and confirm the links between immune complexes and the glomerular lesion associated with carcinoma (Eagen and Lewis, 1977). Lewis and associates (1971) have described a lung-tumor-specific antigen eluated from the glomeruli of a patient with epidermoid carcinoma of the lung. Costanza and colleagues have reported carcinoembryonic antigen antibody complexes in a patient with colon cancer and the nephrotic syndrome (Costanza et al., 1973). Other studies of tumor-specific or tumor-related immune complex glomerulopathy have been described for melanoma, hypernephroma, and gastric carcinoma (Ozawa et al., 1975; Olson et al., 1979; Wakashin et al., 1980).

With carcinomas, membranous glomerulopathy prevails as the principal paraneoplastic renal disorder. Carcinomas of the lung (Lee et al., 1966; Higgins et al., 1974; Row et al., 1975; Eagen and Lewis, 1977; Pascal, 1980) and colon (Costanaza et al., 1973; Couser et al., 1974; Row et al., 1975) represent the cancers most frequently associated with the nephrotic syndrome.

Associations have also been described with cancer of the stomach (Cantrell, 1969, Catane and Cantrell, 1969; Whitworth et al., 1976; Wakashin et al., 1980), kidney (Lee et al.,

1966; Hopper *et al.,* 1976; Grossman and Croker, 1978), pancreas (Denis *et al.,* 1978; Grossman and Croker, 1978; Pascal 1980), ovary (Lee *et al.,* 1966), melanoma (Eagen and Lewis, 1977), and prostate (Pascal, 1980). Glomerulonephritis has most recently been described in a homosexual man with Kaposi's sarcoma who had evidence of hepatitis-antigen-related immune-complex deposits in the glomerular basement membrane (Scully *et al.,* 1982).

Carcinoma-related nephrotic syndrome is more prevalent in older patients, in a range from 20 to 80 years of age; very few individuals under age 40 have been described with this syndrome. This age-related incidence may simply be a reflection of the increased incidence of carcinomas in older age. The clinical manifestation is heavy proteinuria, although renal failure has been reported with crescentic glomerulonephritis. Eagen and Lewis have suggested that the development of nephrotic syndrome in carcinoma is associated with a poor prognosis (Eagen and Lewis, 1977) with an average three-month survival. This may reflect the prognosis of the underlying disease more than the paraneoplastic phenomenon. In fact, reversal of the nephrotic syndrome with successful surgical or chemotherapeutic therapy of the tumor has been described (Cantrell, 1969; Barton *et al.,* 1980).

Hodgkin's disease represents the neoplasm most commonly associated with the nephrotic syndrome (Ghosh and Muehrcke, 1970; Sherman *et al.,* 1972; Lokich *et al.,* 1973; Gagliano *et al.,* 1976; Kaplan *et al.,* 1976; Eagen and Lewis, 1977; Ma *et al.,* 1978). The principal glomerular pathology encountered is minimal change or lipoid nephrosis. Zimmerman and associates reviewed 46 cases of histopathologically documented nephrotic syndrome associated with Hodgkin's disease (Zimmerman, S. W., *et al.,* 1982). Minimal change disease accounted for 33 (72%) of cases reported. Membranous glomerulopathy is reported in about 10% of nephrotic patients with Hodgkin's disease, in contrast to 80 to 90% of nephrotic patients with carcinoma. Antiglomerular basement disease has been reported in a case of Hodgkin's disease (Ma *et al.,* 1978), and focal glomerulosclerosis has been described in at least one patient (Scully *et al.,* 1982).

The nephrotic syndrome in Hodgkin's disease is rare with an incidence of 0.4% in a combined series of 1700 cases (Plager and Shutz-

man, 1971; Ma *et al.,* 1978, Scully, *et al.,* 1983). The age ranges from 6 to 60 years; all stages of the disease with and without systemic "B" symptoms have been described.

Massive proteinuria with normal renal function is the most frequent manifestation and is described as a selective albuminuria (Hansen *et al.,* 1972). Reversal of the nephrotic syndrome has been observed in almost all instances where direct treatment has resulted in a complete remission of the underlying Hodgkin's disease (Ghosh and Muehrcke, 1970; Sherman *et al.,* 1972; Eagen and Lewis, 1977; S. W. Zimmerman *et al.,* 1982). Recurrences of tumor have been associated with relapses of the nephrotic syndrome (Hyman *et al.,* 1973). Consequently, patients who redevolop clinically important proteinuria should be examined for relapse of their Hodgkin's diseases.

In contrast to the evidence for immune complexes in the pathogenesis of the nephrotic syndrome in carcinomas, the mechanism by which Hodgkin's disease may result in glomerulopathy is less well defined. It has been proposed that the T-cell disorder may result in the release of lymphokines, which results in increased glomerular permeability leading to the nephrotic syndrome with minimal change (Salhoub, 1974; Lagrue *et al.,* 1975). Experimental evidence for this pathogenic mechanism has been controversial (Couser *et al.,* 1974; Lagrue *et al.,* 1975). Experimental models of glomerular disease assumed to be mediated by immune complexes without demonstrable deposit on histologic analysis of the kidneys have been observed (Germuth *et al.,* 1975).

The nephrotic syndrome appears to occur less frequently in the non-Hodgkin's lymphomas, with one-tenth of the incidence in Hodgkin's disease (Ma *et al.,* 1978), and the histopathology is more frequently membranous or membranoproliferative glomerulopathies (Ghosh and Muehrcke, 1970; Gluck *et al.,* 1973; Petzel *et al.,* 1979; Zimmerman, S. W., *et al.,* 1982). In S. W. Zimmerman's review of ten patients with non-Hodgkin's lymphomas and adequate histopathologic proof of nephrotic syndrome, two had minimal change glomerulopathy, the remainder presented with membranous or membranoproliferatiave histology (Zimmerman, S. W. *et al.,* 1982). Remission of the nephrotic syndrome has been observed with successful treatment of patients with Burkitt's lymphoma (Hyman *et al.,* 1973), "lymphosar-coma" (Ghosh and Muehrcke, 1970), and his-tiocytic lymphoma (Muggia and Ultmann, 1971). Resistance of proteinuria and renal fail-ure to treatment, however, have been de-scribed more often in non-Hodgkin's lym-phoma than with than with Hodgkin's disease.

In summary, the nephrotic paraneoplastic syndrome is described with the highest fre-quency in Hodgkin's disease and less fre-quently with non-Hodgkin's lymphoma and carcinomas. The glomerular lesion is minimal change or lipoid nephropathy in over two-thirds of the cases of Hodgkin's disease; mem-branous glomerulopathy is the pathology more commonly seen (in about two-thirds of the cases) with carcinomas and non-Hodgkin's lymphoma. In keeping with the paraneoplastic nature of the association, the nephrotic syn-drome can antedate the diagnosis of neoplasia and reversal of the syndrome has been de-scribed with successful therapy of the underly-ing cancer. Finally, an immune mechanism has been strongly implicated for the develop-ment of this disorder.

Amyloidosis

Amyloidosis involving the kidneys is a rec-ognized feature of myeloma and, as previously noted, may be seen in 10% of such cases (Goldstein, 1980). Nonmyelomatous amyloi-dosis has also been described in 3 to 5% of hypernephroma patients (Berger and Sinkoff, 1957) as well as in 3 to 8% of patients with Hodgkin's disease (Kiely *et al.,* 1969). The overall incidence of amyloidosis in neoplastic disease is rare, however, and is found in less than .5% of over 4,000 autopsied cancer pa-tients (Kindall, 1961).

"TTP-like" Syndrome

Disseminated intravascular coagulation is an established complication of cancer and in a series by Siegal and colleagues was associated with renal failure in 25% of 118 such cases (Siegal *et al.,* 1978). Recently, a hemolytic ure-mic and "TTP-like" syndrome has been de-scribed in patients with adenocarcinoma of a variety of primary sites including stomach, colon, lung, and primaries of unknown origin (see Chapter 6B). An immune-complex patho-genesis has been suggested for this entity, and reversal of the syndrome with plasmaphoresis and immunosuppressive therapy was achieved

in a patient who was in apparent complete clinical remission from a linitis plastica cancer of the stomach (Zimmerman, S. E., *et al.,* 1982).

REFERENCES

Abeloff, M. D., and Lenhard, R. E.: Clinical management of ureteral obstruction secondary to malignant lym-phoma. *Johns Hopk. Med. J.,* **134**:34–42, 1974.

Barton, C. H.; Vaziri, N. D.; and Spear, G. S.: Nephrotic syndrome associated with adenocarcinoma of the breast. *Am. J. Med.,* **68**:308, 1980.

Beach, E. W.: Urologic complications of cancer of the uterine cervix. *J. Urol.,* **63**:178, 1952.

Berger, L., and Sinkoff, M. W.: Systemic manifestation of hypernephroma. A review of 273 cases. *Am. J. Med.,* **22**:791, 1957.

Brereton, H. D.; Anderson, T.; Johnson, R. E.; and Schein, P. S.: Hyperphosphatemia and hypocalcemia in Burkitt's lymphoma. *Arch. Intern. Med.,* **283**:354, 1979.

Cantrell, E. G.: Nephrotic syndrome cured by removal of gastric carcinoma. *Br. Med. J.,* **1**:739–740, 1969.

Clyne, D. H.; Perce, A. J.; and Thompson, R. E.: Nephro-toxicity of Bence Jones proteins in the rat: Importance of protein isoelectric point. *Kidney Int.,* **16**:345, 1979.

Cohen, L. F.; Balow, J. E.; Magralt, I.; Poplack, D.; and Ziegler, J.: Acute tumor lysis syndrome: A review of 37 patients with Burkitt's Lymphoma. *Am. J. Med.,* **68**:486, 1980.

Costanza, M. E.; Pinn, V.; Schwartz, R. S.; and Nathan-son, L.: Carcino-embryonic antigen-antibody com-plexes in a patient with colonic carcinoma and ne-phrotic syndrome. *N. Engl. J. Med.,* **289**:520–522, 1973.

Couser, W. G.; Wagonfeld, J. B.; Spargo, B. H.; and Lewis, E. J.: Glomerular deposition of tumor antigen in mem-branous nephropathy associated with colonic carci-noma. *Am. J. Med.,* **57**:962, 1974.

Crittenden, D. R., and Ackerman, G. L.: Hyperuricemic acute renal failure in disseminated carcinoma. *Arch. Intern. Med.,* **137**:97, 1977.

DeFronzo, R. A.; Cooke, R. C.; Wright, J. R.; and Humphrey, R. L.: Renal function in patients with mul-tiple myeloma. *Medicine* (Baltimore), **57**:151, 1978.

Deftos, L. J., and First, B. P.: Calcitonin as a drug. *Ann. Intern. Med.,* **95**:192–197, 1981.

Denis, J.; Mignon, F.; Ramee, M. P.; Morel-Margoert, L. J.; and Richet, G.: Glomerulites extra-membran-euses associees aux tumeurs malignes. *Nouv. Presse Med.,* **7**:991, 1978.

Eagen, J. W., and Lewis, E. J.: Glomerulopathies of neo-plasia. *Kidney Int.,* **11**:297–306, 1977.

Ettinger, D. S.; Harken, W. G.; Gerry, H. W.; Sanders, R. C.; and Sarod, R.: Hyperphosphatemia, hypocalce-mia, and transient renal failure. Results of cytotoxic treatment of acute lymphoblastic leukemia. *J.A.M.A.,* **239**:2472–2479, 1978.

Fallon, B.; Olney, L.; and Culp, D. A.: Nephorostomy in cancer patients: To do or not to do. *Br. J. Urol.,* **52**:237–242, 1980.

Frei, E.; Bentzel, C. J.; Rieselbach, R.; and Block, J. B.: Renal complications of neoplastic disease. *J. Chronic Dis.,* **16**:757, 1963.

Gagliano, R. G.; Costanzi, J. J.; Beathard, G. A.; Serles,

H. E.; and Bell, J. D.: The nephrotic syndrome associated with neoplasia: An unusual paraneoplastic syndrome. *Am. J. Med.,* **60:**1026, 1976.

Germuth, F. G., Jr.; Valdes, A. J.; Taylor, J. J.; Wise, O.; and Rodriguez, E.: Fatal immune complex glomerulonephritis without deposits. *Johns Hopk. Med. J.,* **136:**189–192, 1975.

Ghosh, L., and Muehrcke, R. C.: The nephrotic syndrome. A prodrome to lymphoma. *Ann. Intern. Med.,* **72:**379–382, 1970.

Gluck, M. C.; Gallo, G.; Lowenstein, J.; and Baldwin, D. S.: Membranous glomerulonephritis: Evaluation of clinical and pathologic features. *Ann. Intern. Med.,* **78:**1, 1973.

Goldstein, R. J.; Lichtenstein, N. S.; and Souder, D.: The myth of the low anion gap. *J.A.M.A.,* **243:**1737, 1980.

Gonzales-Vitale, J. C.; Hayes, D. M.; Cvitkovic, E.; and Sternberg, S. S.: Acute renal failure after cis-diamminedichloroplatinum (II) and gentamycin cephalothic therapies. *Cancer Treat. Rep.,* **62:**693, 1978.

Grossman, S., and Croker, B.: Additional studies of membranous glomerulonephritis, malignant tumors and carcinoembryonic antigen (Abstract). *Kidney Int.,* **14:**711, 1978.

Hansen, H. E.; Skov, P. E.; Askjaer, S. A.; and Albertsen, K.: Hodgkin's disease associated with nephrotic syndrome. *Acta Med. Scand.,* **91:**307, 1972.

Hepperlen, T. W.; Mardis, H. K.; and Kammandel, H.: The pigtail ureteral stent in the cancer patient. *J. Urol.,* **121:**17, 1979.

Higgins, M. R.; Randall, R. E.; and Still, W. J. S.: Nephrotic syndrome with oat cell carcinoma. *Br. Med. J.,* **3:**450, 1974.

Ho, P. C.; Talner, L. B.; Parson, C. L.; and Schmidt, J. D.: Percutaneous nephrostomy: experience in 107 kidneys. *Urology,* **16:**532–535, 1980.

Hopper, J.; Biava, C. B.; and Naughton, J. L.: Glomerular extracapillary proliferation (crescentic glomerulonephritis) associated with non-renal malignancies (Abstract). *Kidney Int.,* **10:**544, 1976.

Hyman, L. R.; Burkholder, P. M.; Joo, P. A.; and Seger, W. E.: Malignant lymphoma and nephrotic syndrome. *J. Pediatr.,* **82:**207, 1973.

Johnson, R. D.; Johnson, J. R.; and Bansayan, G. A.: Seminoma metastatic to ureter. *Urology,* **17:**281–283, 1981.

Kaplan, B. S.; Klassan, J.; and Gault, M. H.: Glomerular injury in patients with neoplasia. *Annu. Rev. Med.,* **27:**117, 1976.

Kaufer, A.; Richet, G.; Roland, J.; and Chatelet, F.: Extreme hyperphosphatemia causing acute anuric nephrocalcinosis in lymphosarcoma. *Br. Med. J.,* **1:**1320, 1979.

Kiely, J. M.; Wagoner, R. D.; and Holley, K. E.: Renal complications of lymphoma. *Ann. Intern. Med.,* **71:**1159, 1969.

Kindall, K. H.: Amyloidosis in association with neoplastic disease. *Ann. Intern. Med.,* **55:**958, 1961.

Knowlan, D.; Corrado, M.; Schreiner, G. E.; and Baker, R.: Perirenal fibroís, with a diabetes insipidus like syndrome occurring with progressive partial obstruction of the ureter unilaterally. *Am. J. Med.,* **28:**22, 1960.

Lagrue, G.; Xheneumont, S.; Branellec, A.; Hirbec, G.; and Weil, B.: A vascular permeability factor elaborated from lymphocytes. I. Demonstration in patients with nephrotic syndrome. *Biomedicine,* **23:**37–40, 1975.

Lee, J. C.; Yamauchi, H.; and Hopper, J., Jr.: The association of cancer and the nephrotic syndrome. *Ann. Intern. Med.,* **64:**41–51, 1966.

Leech, S. H.; Polesky, H. F.; and Shapiro, F. L.: Chronic hemodialysis in myelomatosis. *Ann. Intern. Med.,* **77:**239, 1972.

Lewis, M. G.; Loughridge, L. W.; and Philips, T. M.: Immunological studies in nephrotic syndrome associated with extra-renal malignant disease. *Lancet,* **2:**134–135, 1971.

Lightwood, R.; Barrie, H.; and Butler, N.: Observations on 100 cases of leukemia in childhood. *Br. Med. J.,* **1:**747, 1960.

Lokich, J. J.; Galvanek, E. G.; and Moloney, W. C.: Nephrosis of Hodgkin's disease. *Arch. Intern. Med.,* **132:**597–600, 1973.

Ma, K. W.; Golbus, S. M.; Kaufman, R.; Staley, N.; Londer, H.; and Brown, P. C.: Glomerulonephritis with Hodgkin's disease and herpes zoster. *Arch. Pathol. Lab. Med.,* **102:**527, 1978.

Maldonado, J. E.; Velosa, J. A.; Kyle, R. A.; Wagoner, R. D.; Holley, K. E.; and Salassa, R. M.: Fanconi syndrome in adults: A manifestation of a latent form of myeloma. *Am. J. Med.,* **58:**354, 1975.

Martinez-Maldonado, M.; Yium, J.; Suki, W. N.; and Eknoyan, G.: Renal complications in multiple myeloma: Pathophysiology and some clinical management. *J. Chronic Dis.,* **24:**221, 1971.

Muggia, F. M., and Ultmann, J. E.: Glomerulonephritis in malignant lymphoma, reticulum cell type. *Lancet,* **1:**805, 1971.

Murray, T.; Long, W.; and Navins, R. G.: Multiple myeloma and the anion gap. *N. Engl. J. Med.,* **292:**547, 1975.

Nies, B. A.; Bodey, G. P.; Thomas, L. B.; Brecher, G.; and Freireich, E. J.: The persistence of extramedullary leukemic infiltrates during bone marrow remissions of acute leukemia. *Blood,* **26:**133, 1972.

Olson, J. F.; Philips, T. M.; Lewis, M. G.; and Solez, K.: Malignant melanoma with renal deposits containing tumor antigens. *Clin. Nephrol.,* **12:**74–82, 1979.

Ozawa, T.; Pluss, R.; Lacher, J.; Boedecker, E.; Guggenhein, S.; Hammon, D. W.; and McIntosh, R.: Endogenous immune complex nephropathy associated with malignancy. *Q. J. Med.,* **44:**523–541, 1975.

Parsons, V.; Baum, M.; and Self, M.: Effect of mithramycin on calcium and hydroxiproline metabolism in patients with malignant disease. *Br. J. Med.,* **1:**474, 1967.

Pascal, R. R.: Renal manifestations of extra-renal neoplasms. *Hum. Pathol.,* **11:**7–17, 1980.

Petzel, R. A.; Brown, D. C.; Staley, N. A.; McMillen, J. J.; Stibley, R. K.; and Kjellstrand, C. M.: Crescentin glomerulonephritis and renal failure associated with malignant lymphoma. *Am. J. Clin. Pathol.,* **71:**728, 1979.

Plager, J., and Shutzman, L.: Acute nephrotic syndrome as a manifestation of active Hodgkin's disease: Report of four cases and review of the literature. *Am. J. Med.,* **50:**56–66, 1971.

Randall, A.: *Surgical Pathology of Prostatic Obstruction.* The Williams & Wilkins Company, Baltimore, 1931.

Richards, A. L., and Hines, J. D.: Recovery from acute renal failure in plasma cell leukemia. *Am. J. Med. Sci.,* **266:**293, 1973.

Richmond, J.; Sherman, R. S.; Diamond, H. D.; and Craver, L. F.: Renal lesions associated with malignant lymphomas. *Am. J. Med.,* **32:**184–207, 1962.

Row, P. G.; Cameron, J. S.; Turner, D. R.; Evans, D. J.;

White, R. H. R.; Ogg, C. S.; Chantler, C.; and Brown, C. B.: Membranous nephropathy. Long-term follow-up association with neoplasia. *Q. J. Med.,* **44:**207, 1975.

Schubert, G. E.; Veifel, J.; and Lennert, K.: Structure and function of the kidney in multiple myeloma. *Virchows Arch. [Pathol. Anat.],* **355:**135, 1972.

Scully, R. E.; Mark, E. J.; and McNeely, B. U. (eds.): Case records of the Massachusetts General Hospital (Case 11-1982). *N. Engl. J. Med.,* **306:**657–668, 1983.

Shaloub, R. J.: Pathogenesis of lipoid nephrosis: A disorder of T-cell function. *Lancet,* 2:556–560, 1974.

Sherman, R. L.; Swain, M.; Weksler, M. E.; and Baker, E. L.: Lipoid nephrosis in Hodgkin's disease. *Am. J. Med.,* 52:699–706, 1972.

Siegal, T.; Selig, J. V.; Aghai, E.; and Modan, M.: Clinical and laboratory aspects of disseminated intravascular coagulation (DIC) a study of 118 cases. *Thromb. Haemost.,* 39:122, 1978.

Sing, B.; Kim, H.; and Wax, S. H.: Stent versus nephrostomy: Is there a choice? *J. Urol.,* 121:268, 1979.

Stewart, A. F.; Horst, R.; Deftos, L. F.; Cadman, E. C.; Lang, R.; and Broadus, A. E.: Biochemical evaluation of patients with cancer associated hypercalcemia. *N. Engl. J. Med.,* **303:**1377–1383, 1980.

Thomas, M. H., and Chisholm, G. C.: Retroperitoneal fibrosis associated with malignant disease. *Br. J. Cancer,* 8:453, 1973.

Tsokos, G. C.; Balow, J. E.; Spiegel, R. J.; and Magrath, I. T.: Renal and metabolic complication of undifferentiated and lymphoblastic lymphomas. *Medicine,* 60:218–229, 1981.

Wagle, D. G.; Moore, R. H.; and Murphy, G. P.: Secondary carcinomas of the kidney. *J. Urol.,* **114:**30, 1975.

Walker, W. G.; Harvey, A. M.; Yardley, J. H.: Renal involvement in myeloma, amyloidosis, SLE and other connective tissue disorders. In Sharos, M. D., and Welt, L. G. (eds.): *Diseases of the Kidney.* Little, Brown & Company, Boston, 1971.

Wakashin, M.; Wakashin, Y.; Lesato, K.; Ueda, S.; Mori, Y.; Tsuchida, H.; Shigematsu, H.; and Okuda, K.: Association of gastric cancer and nephrotic syndrome. An immunologic study in three patients. *Gastroenterology,* 78:749–756, 1980.

Whitworth, J. A.; Morel-Maroger, L.; Mignon, F.; and Richet, G.: The significance of extra-capillary proliferation. *Nephron,* 16:1, 1976.

Wienman, E. J.: Uric acid and the kidney. In Suki, W. N., and Eknoyan, G. (eds.): *The Kidney in Systemic Disease.* John Wiley & Sons, Inc., New York, 1976.

Willis, R. A.: Secondary tumors of the kidneys. In Willis, R. A. (ed.): *The Spread of Tumors in the Human Body.* Butterworth, London, 1973.

Zimmerman, S. E.; Smith, F. P.; Philips, T. M.; Coffey, R.; and Schein, P. S.: Gastric carcinoma and thrombotic thrombocytopenic purpura: Association with plasma immune complex concentrations. *Br. Med. J.,* **284:**1432, 1982.

Zimmerman, S. W.; Moorthy, A. V.; Burkholder, P. M.; and Jenmkins, P. G.: Glomerulopathies associated with neoplastic disease. In Rieselbach, R. E., and Garnick, M. B. (eds.): *Cancer and the Kidney.* Lea & Febiger, Philadelphia, 1982.

D. CUTANEOUS COMPLICATIONS OF CANCER

Jeffrey P. Callen

The skin is a window through which the careful examiner may recognize an internal neoplasm. Unexplained rashes, growths, or other symptoms often raise the patient's concern about internal causes, in particular cancer (Curth, 1978; Callen, 1981). Although not always precise, unique, or fixed, certain dermatologic conditions or findings are suggestive of internal cancer (Shelley, 1974). Some are very specific (for example, metastases), whereas others are highly controversial (for example, Bowen's disease). In addition, several cutaneous disorders have accompanied the advent of newer and more aggressive therapies. This section will deal with cutaneous metastases, dermatoses associated with internal cancer, heritable cancer family syndromes with prominent skin disease, and the cutaneous complications of cancer chemotherapy. This chapter will highlight the more important associations, point out where important controversies remain, and list in tabular form those conditions not otherwise covered.

CUTANEOUS METASTASES

Metastatic disease to the skin represents a specific manifestation of cancer (Rosen, 1980). Metastases are a final stage of tumor spread that require a complex set of phenomena to take place. The tumor must spread via implantation or through the lymphatics or blood to a secondary site. Even when cells implant at a distant site, however, interactions with the host are necessary before these micrometastases grow into macroscopic lesions.

Invasion of tumors that allows subsequent spread is made possible by mechanical displacement of tumor cells, the capacity of the tumor cells to produce proteolytic enzymes, or their capacity to be mobile. In addition, the membranes of cancer cells seem to be less adherent to other cells, and this factor also promotes spread.

The localization of metastases on the cutaneous surface is an interesting but poorly understood phenomenon. Aside from direct im-

Table 6–9. Common Sites of Primary Tumor Based on Location of Metastases

LOCATION OF METASTASIS	LOCATION OF PRIMARY TUMOR
Scalp	Breast, renal cell
Chest wall	Breast, lung
Umbilicus	Stomach, colon
Lower abdomen	Genitourinary tract

plantation in a site of proximity, mechanisms that explain the metastatic site are rarely recognized. Table 6–9 shows by site of metastatic skin tumor the most likely site of internal neoplasm (Brownstein and Helwig, 1972). One can readily observe that there is no specificity of site on the body and probable primary lesions. Metastases do tend to occur in or on cutaneous surfaces near the site of the primary tumor. Lung and breast carcinomas, for example, frequently spread to the chest wall, whereas colonic, gastric, or ovarian lesions spread to the abdominal wall.

The cutaneous metastatic lesion may be represented by multiple clinical appearances. Frequently, the lesion or lesions arise as firm, nontender, subcutaneous nodules, which may be solitary or multiple (Reingold, 1966) (see Figures 6–5 and 6–6). They may vary in size from several millimeters to many centimeters, but most will range from 1 to 3 cm. The lesion may be skin colored, but shades of red, blue, purple, brown, or black may occur (Rosen, 1980; Toboada and Fred, 1960). The cutaneous configuration, shape or multiplicity seems to have little correlation to tumor type or site of primary lesion.

Several clinical variants are worthy of spe-

cial mention. Carcinoma erysipelatoides, or inflammatory metastatic carcinoma, is a rather poorly defined area of warm, erythematous, edematous, slightly tender skin (Rasch, 1931). This change simulates cellulitis or erysipelas, from which the name is derived. The clinical manifestation usually occurs in close proximity to the initial tumor and is most often reported with breast cancers on the anterior chest wall (Taylor and Meltzger, 1938). It has also been reported on the abdominal wall in conjunction with primary tumors of the vulva, ovary, uterus, stomach, pancreas, or rectum (Rosen, 1980). Pathogenetically, these may be local direct extensions rather than true metastases (Hazelrigg and Rudolph, 1977). Correct diagnosis is often delayed, due to the clinical features suggestive of an infective process. Another unusual variation is the zosteriform inflammatory metastatic carcinoma. Clinically, this lesion takes on a distribution resembling herpes zoster (Hodge *et al.,* 1979). The scalp is a frequently mentioned site of distant metastases. In the large series reported by Brownstein and Helwig (1972), however, it represented only 4% of cutaneous lesions. Breast, lung, and renal carcinomas are primary tumors that result in scalp metastases. The Sis-

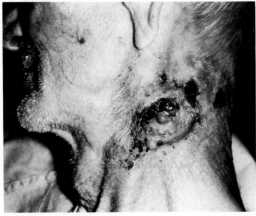

Figure 6–5. Metastatic squamous cell carcinoma from the larynx. Note that this lesion is in close proximity to the primary.

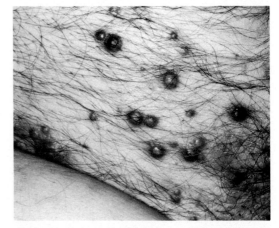

Figure 6–6. Lower abdomen—multiple nodules of metastatic squamous cell carcinoma of the vulva.

ter Joseph's nodule is the occurrence of a metastatic nodule in the umbilical area (Steck and Helwig, 1965). This lesion has most often been associated with gastric neoplasm but may occur in a variety of other abdominal and pelvic tumors. Iatrogenic cutaneous metastases occur from implantation during diagnostic, operative, or therapeutic manipulations. Thus, they have been reported in association with many types of procedures, including thoracentesis, mediastinoscopy, paracentesis, and percutaneous biopsy. In all cases, diagnosis of metastases is made by biopsy. In some instances, the primary tumor can be identified because the metastatic lesion has retained characteristic structural appearances.

In 15 to 20% of cases, the cutaneous metastatic lesion may be the initial sign of internal neoplasm or may occur in a patient with known previous neoplasm. Despite the type of

Table 6–10. Acquired Disorders Associated with Internal Neoplasia

DERMATOSIS	COMMENT
Acanthosis nigricans	Usually adenocarcinoma, in stomach or colon
Acquired ichthyosis	Occurs following diagnosis of tumor, usually lymphoma
Bowen's disease	Varied sites, controversial association
Bullous pemphigoid	Probably only related due to age
Carcinoid syndrome	Carcinoid tumor
Clubbing	Lung
Dermatitis herpetiformis	Lymphoma of the intestine
Myositis	
Dermatomyositis	Varied, only 25% of adults have neoplasm
Polymyositis	Probably coincidental occurrence
Diffuse plane xanthoma	Myeloma
Erythema annulare centrifugum	Rarely associated with tumors
Erythema gyratum repens	Varied types and sites. "Always" associated with a tumor
Exfoliative erythroderm	Lymphomas represent < 1% cases
Glucagonoma (necrolytic migratory erythema)	Glucagon-secreting tumor of pancreas
Herpes zoster	Probably not related other than coincidentally
Hypertrichosis lanuginosa	Varied sites, tumor almost always present
Leser-Trélat sign	Varied sites, unknown if truly a marker
Nodular fat necrosis	Pancreatic carcinoma
Paget's	
Mammary	Breast-ductal adenocarcinoma
Extramammary Paget's	Underlying tissue adenomatous, eccrine, or apocrine carcinomas
Palmar fasciitis	With arthritis, reported with ovarian cancer
Pemphigus group	Thymoma, often myasthenia gravis
Pinch purpura (amyloidosis)	Myeloma
Porphyria cutanea tarda	Hepatocellular carcinoma
Pruritus	Hodgkin's-lymphoma or polycythemia
Raynaud's phenomenon	Rarely associated with cryoglobulinemia as a manifestation of lymphoma or myeloma
Trousseau's sign (recurrent thrombophlebitis)	Pancreatic carcinoma
Vasculitis	Rare lymphomas, leukemias — in particular hairy cell leukemia

occurrence, skin metastases portend a poor prognosis, with most reviews suggesting average survival of three to seven months.

ACQUIRED DERMATOSES ASSOCIATED WITH INTERNAL NEOPLASM

Multiple dermatoses or cutaneous symptoms have been linked with internal neoplasm (see Table 6–10). Many past associations reported in the literature, however, are now being questioned. Not only is the frequency of neoplasm being reexamined but so too is the exact nature of the relationship. Curth (1978) made an important contribution by suggesting the following correlations that can be used to analyze the relationship of a dermatoses to internal neoplasm: a concurrent onset; a parallel course; a statistically important association; and a distinctive tumor associated with the dermatosis. Each of the following discussions will review the knowledge regarding the association of a dermatosis and internal neoplasm and its importance.

Acanthosis nigricans (AN) exists in multiple forms, including one variant associated with internal tumor. Clinically, the patient with neoplastic AN is usually easily recognized. AN is characterized by a hyperpigmented velvety thickening seen in the folds of the skin (in particular, at the nape of the neck and axilla) (see Figure 6–7). Occasionally, the AN can become generalized. It rarely, if ever, causes symptoms other than its appearance.

The appearance of AN in an adult who is not obese should raise the clinician's concern in regard to the presence of an underlying cancer. Neoplastic AN is thought to be related to a tumor secretion, a theory that is supported by the parallel course AN takes in relation to tumor growth. Curth and colleagues found that 61% of the cases of AN and neoplasm occurred concomitantly, whereas in 17% the AN antedated the cancer by up to 16 years, and in 22% AN followed the diagnosis of malignancy by up to 4½ years (Curth *et al.,* 1962). The histologic form of cancer associated with AN is almost always an adenocarcinoma, and 91% are located in the abdomen or pelvis. The occurrence of AN with internal malignancy is an ominous sign (Brown and Winkelmann, 1968). The tumors are usually very aggressive, with death occurring frequently within one to two years after diagnosis.

Bowen's disease is a form of squamous cell carcinoma (SCC) of the skin characterized by marked dysplasia. It usually presents as an *in situ* change, but it can become invasive. Not only has Bowen's type of SCC been linked with internal neoplasia, but other SCC and even basal cell epitheliomas are believed by some authorities to have an increased association (Carpenter *et al.,* 1963). Erythroplasia of Queyrat (EQ) has an histologic appearance identical to Bowen's disease but occurs on the male genitalia. The relation of EQ to internal cancer is not known.

The Bowen's lesion usually presents as a flat, erythematous, slightly scaly lesion (see Figure 6–8), which may be easily confused with, and treated as, localized eczema for months prior

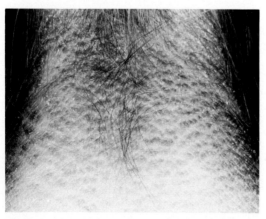

Figure 6–7. Posterior neck—confluent, reticulated lesions with velvety surface and hyperpigmentation, representative of acanthosis nigricans.

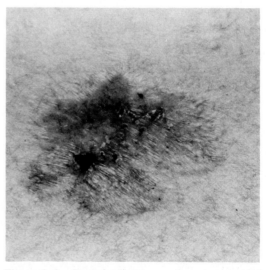

Figure 6–8. Bowen's disease—erythematous crusted lesion with undulating borders.

to diagnosis. The border of Bowen's lesions is irregular, undulating, and often crusted, and the lesions can become hyperkeratotic, nodular, or verrucous on rare occasions. Two-thirds of the time, the lesions are found on maximally exposed surfaces.

The relationship of Bowen's disease to internal neoplasms has been surrounded by controversy. Graham and Helwig (1959) first called attention to this association in a report of 35 patients with Bowen's disease, of whom 28 had visceral cancers; the rate most often reported is between 15 to 20%. Peterka and colleagues subsequently reported that the occurrence of the Bowen's lesion on nonexposed surfaces was associated with an increased incidence of cancer (Peterka *et al.,* 1961). In the Callen and Headington (1980) study, however, Bowen's disease was also associated with cancer, but not in any greater frequency than other varieties of SCC of the skin; and furthermore, the site of the lesion was found to be unimportant as to the risk of cancer. In contrast, Andersen and colleagues found no increased incidence of internal neoplasm in Bowen's disease or SCC (Andersen *et al.,* 1973). The types of neoplasms associated with Bowen's disease are varied, as are the onset and course. Although patients with Bowen's disease and SCC may have a disposition to internal neoplasia, the cancer may not be manifest for many years.

Several of the bullous dermatoses have been linked with internal cancer. Bullous pemphigoid (BP), a subepidermal blistering disease, is seen in the elderly, and is characterized by tense bullae on an erythematous base. Its relationship with cancer is probably related to the age of the patients alone, as shown by Stone and Schroeter (1975). Some authorities, however, believe that if the mucous membranes are involved or if the patient has negative immunofluorescence, there is an increased risk of cancer (Greer *et al.,* 1980; Hodge *et al.,* 1981). These views remain controversial, and thus current recommendations are to question closely and to perform a careful physical examination on all patients with BP.

Pemphigus, a group of disorders with intraepidermal blister formation, has been associated with thymomas (Callen, 1980). The relationship to other types of cancer seems to be coincidental.

Dermatitis herpetiformis (DH) (also called Duhring's disease) is an intensely pruritic subepidermal bullous disease in which small, grouped vesicles erupt symmetrically on the body (usually extensor surfaces). DH is linked with gluten-sensitive enteropathy and, possibly through this link, to intestinal lymphoma (Fowler and Thomas, 1976). The importance and incidence of this relationship is not established, as only a small number of cases have been reported.

Porphyria cutanea tarda (PCT) is a subepidermal blistering disease, resulting from abnormal porphyrin metabolism by the liver. It is characterized by tense vesicles and bullae on exposed surfaces (usually the hands), scarring with milia, hyperpigmentation, cutaneous sclerosis, and hypertrichosis. It is associated with hepatic disease, frequently cirrhosis secondary to excessive alcohol consumption. PCT has also been reported in association with primary hepatocellular carcinoma, thus, each patient with PCT should have a careful hepatic evaluation (Solis *et al.,* 1982).

Dermatomyositis (DM) is a skin and muscle disease that in adults has been linked to internal neoplasm (Callen *et al.,* 1980; Barnes, 1976). The muscle disease is characterized by a proximal symmetrical weakness that progresses over weeks or months. Electromyography and muscle biopsy may reveal a characteristic appearance and help to rule out other causes of a myopathy. The patients also have elevated muscle enzymes (that is, CPK, aldolase). The muscle disease is identical to polymyositis (PM). The skin lesions, which allow one to differentiate DM from PM, are the heliotrope rash, Gottron's papules, (see Figure 6–9) poikiloderma, periungual telangiectasias, and a photosensitive rash. The heliotrope is a violaceous edematous change surrounding the eyes. Gottron's papules are erythematous

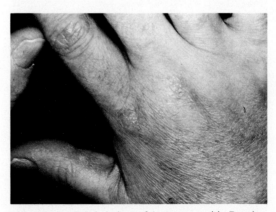

Figure 6–9. Subtle lesions of dermatomyositis. Papular violaceous changes were present over the bony prominences.

to violaceous lesions that occur over the bony prominences; often they contain telangiectasias. Both these lesions are felt to be pathognomonic for DM.

DM has been linked to cancer in adults, but only 25% of those with DM will have cancer (Callen, 1982). The cancer can be in any organ, and can precede, follow, or occur simultaneously with the DM. Careful evaluation of the DM patient for neoplasm is mandatory, but extensive search that is not directed by symptoms or signs is not recommended (Callen, 1982). Polymyositis, in itself, is rarely associated with neoplasm and may be a coincidental occurrence.

Several of the figurate erythemas may be linked to internal neoplasm (Willis, 1978). Erythema gyratum repens (EGR) is a bizarre eruption characterized by persistent erythematous bands that form a serpiginous or gyrate pattern. The bands migrate across the skin to give the appearance of "grains of wood" (Figure 6–10). A fine scale may also be present. The skin biopsy of EGR is not specific. Various types of internal cancers have been reported in almost all patients with EGR (Leavell *et al.,* 1967; Gammel, 1952). Although the onsets of EGR and internal cancers may not be concurrent, many patients demonstrate a parallel course. This eruption should trigger an extensive evaluation of the patient.

Erythema annulare centrifugum (EAC) is characterized by annular rings (with active borders) of erythema that migrate peripherally, with a trailing slight scale. They may coalesce to form polygyrate lesions (see Figure 6–11). EAC can occur in many other circumstances, and neoplasia is rarely present (Sum-

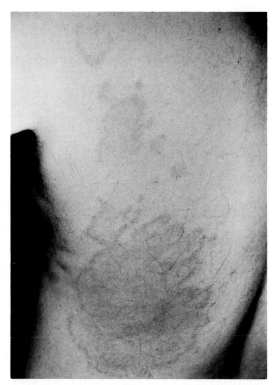

Figure 6–11. Erythema annulare centrifugum in a patient after irradiation of a malignant thymoma.

merly, 1964). The patient with EAC does not require an extensive neoplasm evaluation.

Necrolytic migratory erythema or the glucagonoma syndrome is a bizarre eruption usually associated with a glucagon-secreting neoplasm tumor of the pancreas (Mallinson *et al.,* 1974). The initial skin lesions are usually erythematous, angular, or irregular patches, often with an active border. Annular, circinate, or polycyclic lesions often develop, and flaccid vesicles and crusts may appear at a later stage (Lewis, 1979). The lesions tend to occur in the central area of the body with the pelvis and buttocks as the most common sites. Angular cheilitis or perianal dermatitis may be present. The cutaneous lesions are often misdiagnosed initially as seborrheic dermatitis or candidiasis. The other features that aid in diagnosis are painful glossitis, weight loss, anorexia, anemia, and mild to moderate glucose intolerance. The tumors are usually in the tail of the pancreas, and are frequently metastatic at the time of diagnosis. Surgical resection or effective chemotherapy of the tumor will cause resolution of the dermatitis (Marynick *et al.,* 1980).

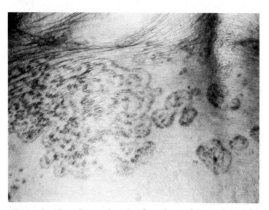

Figure 6–10. Gyrate bands of erythema in a patient with a presumed breast cancer. Biopsy and evaluation were refused by the patient.

Herpes zoster is a common, acute, painful cutaneous eruption due to a recrudescence of a dormant varicella-zoster-virus infection. The eruption consists of grouped vesicles arranged in a band that follows the dermatome. The previously healthy patient who develops herpes zoster does not seem to have an increased propensity for neoplasm (Ragozzino *et al.,* 1982). Controversy regarding those patients with disseminated zoster still remains. If associated with cancer, lymphomas or leukemia predominate.

Hypertrichosis lanuginosa acquista (HLA), also known as malignant down, is a rare but distinctive entity characterized by the excessive growth of fine lanugo hair (see Figure 6–12) (Fretzin, 1967). After considering endocrinopathies and porphyria cutanea tarda, the adult with HLA must have an extensive evaluation for cancer. The malignant down antedates the appearance of the tumor in most cases and is often accompanied by glossitis (Wadskov, 1976). The forms of underlying tumors are not uniform.

Acquired ichthyosis is a scaly dermatoses that appears similar to the inherited ichthyosis vulgaris. Rhomboidal scales with free edges on a noninflammatory base are usually found on the extremities. This must be differentiated from xerosis or hypothyroidism. When ichthyosis is acquired late in life, it may be associated with lymphomas, in particular Hodgkin's disease (Flint *et al.,* 1975). The ichthyosis, however, usually postdates the diagnosis of neoplasia, and, although interesting, rarely has been reported to be of practical significance.

Paget's disease and extramammary Paget's disease are almost always associated with an underlying cancer. It may be that Paget's dis-

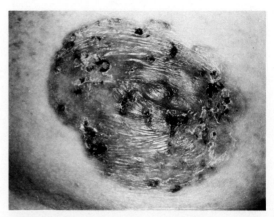

Figure 6–13. Erythematous, crusted, sharply marginated lesion of Paget's disease on the nipple.

ease represents epidermal involvement with adenocarcinomatous cells. Penneys and colleagues have shown evidence for this theory using the immunoperoxidase stain (Penneys *et al.,* 1982). Mammary Paget's disease is represented by an eczematous plaque on the nipple and surrounding skin (see Figure 6–13). Sharp margination of the border is usual. Extramammary Paget's disease is similar, but occurs in the pelvic or perianal areas.

Mammary Paget's disease is indicative of an underlying ductal adenocarcinoma of the breast (Paone and Baker, 1981). Metastatic disease to the axillary lymph nodes occurs in two-thirds of the patients with a palpable breast nodule, but also in one-third of those without a palpable tumor. Extramammary Paget's disease is associated with cancers of eccrine, apocrine, or adenomatous structures below or adjacent to the lesion (Helwig and Graham, 1963). Thus, if present in a perianal location, adenocarcinoma of the sigmoid colon or rectum must be considered. Metastases are common at the time of diagnosis, as is the case for mammary Paget's disease. A diagnosis of Paget's disease should be followed by a thorough search for a local neoplasm but portends a very poor prognosis.

The relationship of punctate palmar keratoses and arsenical keratoses (see Figure 6–14) to internal neoplasms remains steeped in controversy. Dobson and colleagues had reported that punctate palmar keratoses were more common in patients with cancer (Dobson *et al.,* 1965), but subsequent studies failed to confirm this relationship (Bean *et al.,* 1965). Little question exists that arsenical keratoses occur with multiple cutaneous cancers includ-

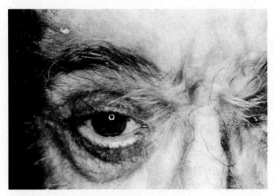

Figure 6–12. Hypertrichosis lanuginosa.

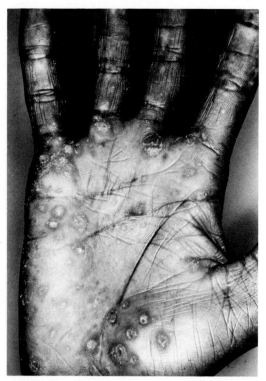

Figure 6–14. Arsenical keratoses—extensive palmar lesions are seen. To date this patient has not had an internal neoplasm.

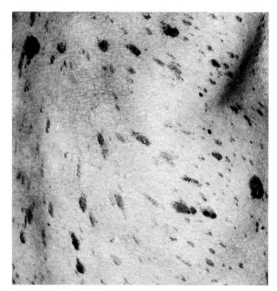

Figure 6–15. Multiple seborrheic keratoses.

ing Bowen's disease. Most studies, however, have failed to demonstrate an increased risk for internal carcinoma (Reymann *et al.*, 1978; Yeh *et al.*, 1968).

Pyoderma gangrenosum (PG) is characterized by necrotic ulcers with overhanging borders (Callen and Taylor, 1978). Its pathogenesis is not known. The lesions usually develop rapidly, beginning as an erythematous papule or pustule that spreads concentrically with necrosis and ulceration. Typical PG has been associated with paraproteinemias and occasionally with multiple myeloma. An atypical form that involves a more superficial lesion with bullous necrotic margin has been reported in conjunction with myelofibrosis and leukemia (Callen *et al.*, 1976; Perry and Winkelmann, 1972; Lewis *et al.*, 1978). Usually the leukemia is of the granulocytic series. The low incidence of PG and its rare association with cancer make this finding very unusual.

The Leser-Trélat sign refers to the sudden appearance and/or growth of multiple seborrheic keratoses (see Figure 6–15) in association with an underlying visceral cancer (Safai

et al., 1978). Schwartz (1981) has suggested that this may be similar mechanistically to acanthosis nigricans. No consistent tumor type has been found with this sign, and controversy still exists, because both cancer and seborrheic keratoses are commonly seen in an older population. Although the presence of multiple seborrheic keratoses alone is not sufficient to warrant investigation, a rapid increase in number and/or pruritis should raise the suspicion of an internal cancer.

Sweet's syndrome or acute febrile neutrophilic dermatosis is an acute or recurrent inflammatory disease characterized by painful erythematous plaques and/or nodules, fever, and leukocytosis. Females are usually affected, and arthritis is a commonly associated phenomenon. The lesions usually are present on the arms, face, or neck. Histologically, this entity is characterized by a massive infiltrate with polymorphonuclear leukocytes without evidence of vasculitis. Greer and Cooper (1982) have observed that 14 of the 88 cases reported have had an associated myeloproliferative disorder, either acute myelocytic or acute myelomonocytic leukemia. Additionally, three cases of other types of cancer have been reported. The onset and course of the Sweet's syndrome and the leukemia seem to be generally parallel (Soderstrom, 1981). A relationship of Sweet's syndrome and pyoderma gangrenosum has also been postulated.

INHERITED DERMATOSES ASSOCIATED WITH INTERNAL NEOPLASM

Cowden's syndrome or multiple hamartoma syndrome (MHS) has been associated with cancer, in particular, cancer of the breast (Weary *et al.*, 1972; Brownstein *et al.*, 1978) (see Table 6–11). This disorder is an autosomal, dominantly inherited condition characterized by multiple, warty, keratotic papules on the central face, neck, ears, and/or hands (see Figure 6–16). Similar lesions occur on the oral mucosa and may coalesce to form a cobblestone appearance. Multiple tumors are frequently found, including both benign and cancerous growths. Fibrocystic breast disease and bilateral adenocarcinoma of the breast have been reported. An association with thyroid adenomas, carcinomas, colonic polyps and adenocarcinoma, and lung cancers has also been described, but with a lesser frequency. Careful evaluation and early surgical intervention is necessary for the patient and affected family members with this disorder.

Gardner's syndrome is the combination of precancerous colonic polyposis with a variety of cutaneous lesions and bony abnormalities (Gardner & Richards, 1950), inherited as an autosomal dominant. The skin lesions usually precede the discovery of the colonic polyps and are characterized by multiple cutaneous epidermal cysts. In addition, fibromas, desmoid tumors, and lipomas may occur, as well

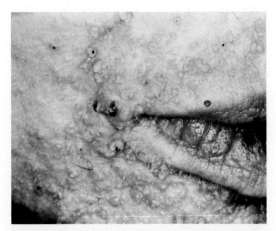

Figure 6–16. Cowden's disease—multiple warty lesions. This patient has had bilateral breast cancer and a thyroid adenoma.

as osteomas, which may be present. The polyps are adenomatous and will eventuate in adenocarcinoma if left untreated. Once the syndrome is recognized, consideration should be given to surgical resection of the entire colon and rectum (Weary *et al.*, 1964).

Peutz-Jeghers syndrome is characterized by the combination of multiple hamartomatous gastrointestinal polyps and melanotic macules of the lips, oral mucosa, and acral skin (see Figure 6–17). This disorder is an autosomal dominant. Although polyps are usually benign, 3 to 5% of these patients have developed duodenal, gastric, colonic, or proximal jejunal adenocarcinomas (Utsunomyia *et al.*, 1975;

Table 6–11. Inherited Disorders Associated with Prominent Cutaneous Features and Internal Cancer

INHERITED DISORDER	RELATED CANCER
Autosomal dominant	
Tylosis (hyperkeratosis of palms and soles)	Esophageal
Gardner's syndrome	Colonic
Cowden's syndrome (multiple hamartoma syndrome)	Breast, thyroid, and colon
Peutz-Jeghers syndrome	Intestinal, stomach breast (?), ovary (?)
Torre's syndrome	Colonic
Mucousal neuroma syndrome III	Medullary carcinoma of thyroid
Neurofibromatosis	Leukemia, neurofibrosarcoma
Blue rubber bleb nevus syndrome	Medulloblastoma
Autosomal recessive	
Ataxia-telangiectasia	Lymphoma
Wiscott-Aldrich syndrome	Lymphoma
Bloom's syndrome	Leukemia
Fanconi's anemia & dyskeratosis congenita	Leukemia
Chédiak-Higashi syndrome	Lymphoma

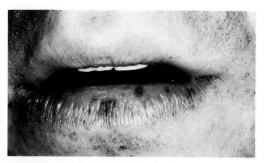

Figure 6–17. Peutz-Jeghers syndrome. Multiple melanotic macules. Photo courtesy of J. Chanda of Melbourne, Florida.

Hsu *et al.,* 1979). In addition, cases of breast carcinoma have been reported (Trau *et al.,* 1982). These patients should be followed closely, but preventive intervention is not indicated or practical.

Torre's syndrome is an autosomal dominant disorder characterized by sebaceous gland tumors of the skin and visceral neoplasms (Householder and Zeligman, 1980). In addition to sebaceous adenomas and carcinomas, multiple keratoacanthomas may be part of this syndrome (Lynch *et al.,* 1981). The internal tumors found are multiple and often the patient follows a more benign course than the histologic evaluation would predict. Colonic adenocarcinomas are by far the most frequent, but other organs may be involved. Recognition of this syndrome is important for other family members, because multiple internal cancers have usually occurred before recognition of this entity.

CUTANEOUS COMPLICATIONS OF CANCER CHEMOTHERAPY

Rapid advances have been made within the field of cancer chemotherapy in the last decade. The use of single and combinations of chemotherapeutic agents is aimed at decreasing the growth of tumors that are unresectable or not amenable to other local therapy. Unfortunately, normal tissues with rapidly dividing cells can also be affected by the chemotherapy. Thus, mucocutaneous reactions are often seen in chemotherapy patients (Adrian *et al.,* 1980).

Alopecia can be caused by many chemotherapeutic agents, such as doxorubicin and vincristine (see Chapter 10). All bodily hair may be affected, but the loss of scalp hair becomes cosmetically important to many patients. The damage that causes hair loss occurs to those hairs in an actively growing phase (anagen hairs); this causes weakened hairs that are easily fractured to grow. Most scalp hairs are in an anagen phase, so the hair loss may be quite extensive. The alopecia may be prevented or minimized by the use of a scalp tourniquet or by local hypothermia during the administration of the chemotherapeutic agents with a rapid, effective plasma disappearance (Soukop *et al.,* 1978; Edelstyn *et al.,* 1979).

The phenomenon of radiation recall (Phillips *et al.,* 1977; Adrian *et al.,* 1980) is characterized by acute dermatitis with vesiculation and erythema. Postinflammatory hyperpigmentation usually is seen following healing. The reaction takes place over the radiation portals and occurs mainly with actinomycin D, doxorubicin, bleomycin, 5-fluorouracil, and methotrexate (Adrian *et al.,* 1980).

Hyperpigmentation may occur with several chemotherapeutic agents including busulfan, cyclophosphamide, nitrogen mustard, doxorubicin, and bleomycin. In addition, localized hyperpigmentation of the nails may be seen with 5-fluorouracil.

MISCELLANEOUS

Although any of the agents can have cutaneous hypersensitive reactions, several agents have unique cutaneous side effects. Methotrexate-treated patients have been reported to develop severe sunburn reactions. This phenomenon may be pathogenetically similar to radiation recall (Møller, 1969). In addition, reactivation of a previous sunburn reaction may occur. Actinomycin D may cause an acneform eruption on the trunk. Bleomycin may cause sclerodermatous changes, Raynaud's phenomenon, and/or onycholysis (Bennett and Reich, 1979). A recent report of a "peculiar" acral erythema from bleomycin has been published (Burgdorf *et al.,* 1982). Linear hyperpigmentation over the veins has been reported with bleomycin and 5-fluorouracil.

In summary, the skin provides clues to the existence of cancer, to prognosis, and may exhibit changes related to the treatment of cancer. Careful and thoughtful analysis of the skin is necessary to fully appreciate the subtleties of these changes.

REFERENCES

Adrian, R. M.; Hood, A. F.; and Skarin, A. T.: Mucocutaneous reactions to antineoplastic agents. *CA,* **30:**143–157, 1980.

Andersen, S. L. C.; Nielsen, A.; and Reymann, F.: Relationship between Bowen's disease and internal malignant tumors. *Arch. Dermatol.,* **108:**367–370, 1973.

Barnes, B. E.: Dermatomyositis and malignancy. *Ann. Intern. Med.,* **84:**68–76, 1976.

Bean, S. F.; Foxley, F. G.; and Fusaro, R. M.: Palmar keratoses and internal malignancy. A negative study. *Arch. Dermatol.,* **97:**528–532, 1965.

Bennett, J. M. and Reich S. D.: Bleomycin. *Ann. Intern. Med.,* **90:**945–948, 1979.

Brown, J., and Winkelmann, R. K.: Acanthosis nigricans: A study of 90 cases. *Medicine,* **47:**33–51, 1968.

Brownstein, M. H., and Helwig, E. B.: Patterns of cutaneous metastasis. *Arch. Dermatol.,* **103:**862–868, 1972.

Brownstein, M. H.; Wolf, M.; and Bikowski, J. B.: Cowden's disease: A cutaneous marker of breast cancer. *Cancer,* **41:**2393–2398, 1978.

Burgdorf, W. H. C.; Gilmore, W. A.; and Ganinck, R. G.: Peculiar acral erythema secondary to high dose chemotherapy of acute myelogenous leukemia. *Ann. Intern. Med.,* **97:**61–62, 1982.

Callen, J. P.: The value of malignancy evaluation in patients with dermatomyositis. *J. Am. Acad. Dermatol.,* **6:**253–259, 1982.

Callen, J. P.: Skin signs of internal malignancy. In Callen, J. P. (ed): *Cutaneous Aspects of Internal Disease.* Year Book Medical Publishers, Inc., Chicago, 1981.

Callen, J. P.: Internal disorders associated with bullous diseases. *J. Am. Acad. Dermatol.,* **3:**107–119, 1980.

Callen, J. P.; Dubin, H. V.; and Gherke, C. F.: Pyoderma gangrenosum and agnogenic myeloid metaplasia. *Arch. Dermatol.,* **113:**1585–1586, 1976.

Callen, J. P., and Headington, J. T.: Bowen's and non-Bowen's squamous intraepidermal neoplasia of the skin: Relationship to internal malignancy. *Arch. Dermatol.,* **116:**422–427, 1980.

Callen, J. P.; Hyla, J. F.; Boles, G. G.; and Kay, D. R.: The relationship of dermatomyositis and polymyositis to internal malignancy. *Arch. Dermatol.,* **116:**295–298, 1980.

Callen, J. P., and Taylor, W. B.: Pyoderma gangrenosum. *Cutis,* **21:**61, 1978.

Carpenter, C. L.; Derbes, V. J.; and Jolly, H. W.: Carcinoma of the skin: A guidepost to internal malignancy. *J.A.M.A.,* **186:**621–623, 1963.

Curth, H. O.: Skin lesions and internal carcinoma. In Curth, H. O.; Andrade, R.; Gumport, S. L.; Popkin, G. L.; and Rees, T. D. (eds.): *Cancer of the Skin.* W. B. Saunders Company, Philadelphia, 1978.

Curth, H. O.; Hilberg, A. W.; and Machacek, G. F.: The site and histology of the cancer associated with malignant acanthosis nigricans. *Cancer,* **15:**364–382, 1962.

Dobson, R. L.; Young, M. R.; and Pinto, J. S.: Palmar keratoses and cancer. *Arch. Dermatol.,* **92:**553–556, 1965.

Edelstyn, G. A.; MacRae, K. D.; and MacDonald, F. M.: Improvement of life quality in cancer patients undergoing chemotherapy. *Clin. Oncol.,* **5:**43–49, 1979.

Flint, G. L.; Flam, M.; and Soter, N. A.: Acquired ichthyosis. *Arch. Dermatol.,* **111:**1446–1447, 1975.

Fowler, J. M., and Thomas, D. J. B.: Lymphoma in dermatitis herpetiformis. *Br. Med. J.,* **2:**757, 1976.

Fretzin, D. F.: Malignant down. *Arch. Dermatol.,* **95:**295–298, 1967.

Gammel, J. A.: Erythema gyratum repens. *Arch. Dermatol. Syphilol.,* **66:**494–499, 1952.

Gardner, E. J., and Richards, R. C.: Multiple cutaneous and subcutaneous lesions occurring with hereditary polyposis and osteomatosis. *Am. J. Hum. Genet.,* **5:**139–147, 1953.

Graham, J. H., and Helwig, F. B.: Bowen's disease and its relationship to systemic cancer. *Arch. Dermatol.,* **80:**133–159, 1959.

Greer, K. E.; Beacham, B. E.; and Askew, P. C.: Benign mucous membrane pemphigoid in association with internal malignancy. *Cutis,* **25:**183–185, 1980.

Greer, K. E., and Cooper, P. H.: Sweet's syndrome (acute febrile neutrophilic dermatosis). *Clin. Rheum. Dis.,* **8:**427–441, 1982.

Hazelrigg, D. E., and Rudolph, A. H.: Inflammatory metastatic carcinoma: carcinoma erysipelatoides. *Arch. Dermatol.,* **113:**69–70, 1977.

Helwig, E. B., and Graham, J. H.: Anogenital (extramammary) Paget's disease. A clinicopathologic study. *Cancer,* **16:**387, 1963.

Hodge, L.; Marsden, R. A.; Black, M. M.; Bhogal, B.; and Carbett, M. F.: Bullous pemphigoid: The frequency of mucosal involvement and concurrent malignancy related to indirect immunofluorescence findings. *Br. J. Dermatol.,* **105:**65–69, 1981.

Hodge, S. J.; Mackel, S.; and Owen, L. G.: Zosteriform inflammatory metastatic carcinoma. *Int. J. Dermatol.,* **19:**142–145, 1979.

Householder, M. S., and Zeligman, I.: Sebaceous neoplasms associated with visceral carcinomas. *Arch. Dermatol.,* **116:**61–64, 1980.

Hsu, S. D.; Zaharopoulos, P.; May, J. T.; and Costanzi, J. J.: Peutz-Jeghers syndrome with intestinal carcinoma. *Cancer,* **44:**1527–1532, 1979.

Kierland, R. R.: Cutaneous signs of internal malignancy. *South. Med. J.,* **65:**563–568, 1972.

Leavell, U. W.; Winternitz, W. W.; and Black, J. H.: Erythema gyratum repens and undifferentiated carcinoma. *Arch. Dermatol.,* **95:**69, 1967.

Lewis, A. E.: The glucagonoma syndrome. *Int. J. Dermatol.,* **18:**17, 1979.

Lewis, S. J.; Poh-Fitzpatrick, M. B.; and Walther, R. R.: Atypical pyoderma gangrenosum with leukemia. *J.A.M.A.,* **239:**935–938, 1978.

Lynch, H. T.; Lynch, P. M.; Pester, J.; and Fusaro, R. M.: The cancer family syndrome. *Arch. Intern. Med.,* **141:**607–611, 1981.

Mallinson, C. N.; Bloom, S. R.; Warin, A. P.; Salmon, P. R.; and Cox, B.: A glucagonoma syndrome. *Lancet,* **2:**1–5, 1974.

Marynick, S. P.; Fagadan, W. R.; and Duncan, L. A.: Malignant glucagonoma syndrome: Response to chemotherapy. *Ann. Intern. Med.,* **93:**453–454, 1980.

Møller, H.: Reactivation of acute inflammation by methotrexate. *J. Invest. Dermatol.,* **52:**437–441, 1969.

Paone, J. F., and Baker, R. R.: Pathogenesis and treatment of Paget's disease of the breast. *Cancer,* **48:**825–829, 1981.

Penneys, N. S.; Nadji, M.; Ziegels-Weissman, J.; Ketabchi, M.; and Morales, A.R.: Carcinoembryonic antigen in sweat-gland carcinomas. *Cancer,* **60:**1608, 1982.

Perry, H. O., and Winkelmann, R. K.: Bullous pyoderma

gangrenosum and leukemia. *Arch. Dermatol.,* **106**:901–905, 1972.

Peterka, E. S.; Lynch, F. W.; and Goltz, R. W.: An association between Bowen's disease and internal cancer. *Arch. Dermatol.,* **84**:139–145, 1961.

Phillips, T. L., and Fu, K. K.: Acute and late effects of multi-modal therapy on normal tissues. *Cancer,* **40**:489–494, 1977.

Ragozzino, M. W.; Melton, I.; Kurland, L. T.; Chu C. P.; and Perry, H. O.: Risk of cancer after herpes zoster. *N. Engl. J. Med.,* **307**:393–397, 1982.

Rasch, C.: Carcinoma erysipelatoides. *Br. J. Dermatol. Syphilol.,* **43**:351–354, 1931.

Reingold, I. M.: Cutaneous metastases from internal carcinoma. *Cancer,* **19**:162–168, 1966.

Reymann, F.; Møller, R.; and Nielsen, A.: Relationship between arsenic intake and internal malignant neoplasms. *Arch. Dermatol.,* **114**:378–381, 1978.

Rosen, T.: Cutaneous metastases. *Med. Clin. North Am.,* **64**:885–900, 1980.

Safai, B.; Grant, J. M.; and Good, R. A.: Cutaneous manifestation of internal malignancies II: The sign of Leser-Trélat. *Int. J. Dermatol.,* **17**:492–496, 1978.

Schwartz, R. A.: Acanthosis nigricans, florid cutaneous papillomatosis and the sign of Leser-Trélat. *Cutis,* **28**:319–334, 1981.

Shelley, W. B.: Cutaneous signs of internal malignancy. *Minn. Med.,* **57**:773–779, 1974.

Soderstrom, R. M.: Sweet's syndrome and acute myelogenous leukemia. *Cutis,* **28**:255–260, 1981.

Solis, J. A.: Betancor, P.; Campos, R.; deSalamanca, R.E.; Rojo, P.; Marin I.; and Schüller, A.: Association of porphyria cutanea tarda and primary liver cancer. *J. Dermatol.,* **9**:131–137, 1982.

Soukop, M.; Campbell, A.; Gray, M. M.; and Calman, K.

C.: Adriamycin, alopecia, and the scalp tourniquet. *Cancer Treat. Rep.,* **62**:489–490, 1978.

Steck, W. D., and Helwig, E. B.: Tumors of the umbilicus. *Cancer,* **18**:902–915, 1965.

Stone, S. P., and Schroeter, A. L.: Bullous pemphigoid and associated malignant neoplasms. *Arch. Dermatol.,* **111**:991, 1975.

Summerly, R.: Figurate erythemas and neoplasia. *Br. J. Dermatol.,* **76**:370, 1964.

Taboada, C. F., and Fred, H. L.: Cutaneous metastases. *Arch. Intern. Med.,* **117**:516–519, 1960.

Taylor, G. W., and Meltzer, A.: Inflammatory carcinoma of the breast. *Am. J. Cancer,* **33**:33–49, 1938.

Trau, H.; Schewach-Millet, M.; Fisher, B. K.; and Tsur, H.: Peutz-Jeghers syndrome and bilateral breast carcinoma. *Cancer,* **50**:788–792, 1982.

Utsunomyia, J.; Gocho, H.; Miyanaga, T.; Hamaguchi, E.; Kashimure, A.; Aoki, N.; and Kamatsu, I.: Peutz-Jeghers syndrome: Its natural course and management. *Johns Hopk. Med. J.,* **136**:71–82, 1975.

Wadskov, S.; Bro-Jorgensen, A.; and Sondergaard, J.: Acquired hypertrichosis lanuginosa. *Arch. Dermatol.,* **112**:1442–1444, 1976.

Weary, P. E.; Gorlin, R. J.; Gentry, W. C.; Comer, J. E.; and Greer, K. E.: Multiple hamartoma syndrome (Cowden's disease). *Arch. Dermatol.,* **106**:682–690, 1972.

Weary, P. E.; Linthicum, A.; Cawley, E. P.; Coleman, C. C. Jr.; and Graham, G. F.: Gardner's syndrome: A family group study and review. *Arch. Dermatol.,* **90**:20, 1964.

Willis, W. F.: The gyrate erythemas. *Int. J. Dermatol.,* **17**:698–702, 1978.

Yeh, S.; How, S. W.; and Lin, C. S.: Arsenical cancer of skin. *Cancer,* **21**:312–339, 1968.

E. NEUROLOGIC COMPLICATIONS OF CANCER

Frederick P. Smith and Jerome Posner

Direct involvement by metastasis is the most frequent cause of neurologic dysfunction in patients with cancer (Posner, 1971). Metastatic carcinoma to the brain and/or epidural space may be encountered at autopsy in up to 50% of patients with lung cancer (Chasen *et al.,* 1963) and 90% in one series of patients with melanoma (Aronson *et al.,* 1964). Diffuse leptomeningeal metastases, sometimes called "carcinomatous meningitis," is less frequent but occurred in 8% of 2375 patients examined pathologically at Memorial Sloan-Kettering Cancer Center (Posner and Chernik, 1978). Carcinomas of the breast and lung and malignant melanoma are the most common solid tumors associated with leptomeningeal metastases (Wasserstrom *et al.,* 1982). Meningeal metastases occur with greater frequency with specific hematologic cancers. The incidence is estimated to be approximately 50% in acute lymphoblastic leukemia of childhood (Aur *et al.,* 1972), 20 to 30% in aggressive histologies of non-Hodgkin's lymphoma (Sweet *et al.,* 1980), and 10 to 20% for acute nonlymphoblastic leukemia (Meyer *et al.,* 1980). As a consequence of this predilection, prophylactic central nervous system (CNS) therapy is standard for patients with acute lymphocytic leukemia (ALL), and is being studied in other hematologic cancers as well (Aur *et al.,* 1975; Sweet *et al.,* 1980; Meyer *et al.,* 1980) (see Chapter 37).

Less common, but equally devastating, are the nonmetastatic disorders of the central nervous system that affect patients with systemic cancer, the primary subject of this chapter. These abnormalities include infections, often by organisms that do not commonly affect the general medical population, with general medical vascular disorders (including brain infarction and hemorrhage), metabolic abnormalities (arising from failure of vital organs such as liver, lungs, kidney), toxicities of radiation therapy and chemotherapy, and remote effects of cancer on the nervous system.

For purposes of this chapter the term remote effects defines a group of neurologic disorders that occur either exclusively or with increased frequency in patients with cancer and are of unknown cause. The term paraneoplastic syndrome is sometimes used synonymously with remote effects but is encompassing and includes all indirect effects of cancer on the brain or any other organ.

Remote effects of cancer on the nervous system are rare. If one eliminates from consideration those disorders designated "neuromyopathy" as characterized by mild proximal muscle weakness and/or absent ankle jerks, and probably caused by weight loss and cachexia (Croft and Wilkinson, 1965), the incidence of remote effects is far less than their reported 16% (Croft and Wilkinson, 1965; Shapiro, 1976). Despite their rarity, however, remote effects are of interest because of their association with the underlying neoplasm, their potential for expression months to years prior to the diagnosis of cancer, and the possibility of reversal of these syndromes with the appropriate treatment of the neoplastic condition. Table 6–12 classifies these remote effects.

PROGRESSIVE MULTIFOCAL LEUKOENCEPHALOPATHY (PML)

Strictly speaking, progressive multifocal leukoencephalopathy (PML) is an infection of the nervous system by an opportunistic virus of the papova group. It is discussed here, however, because it is an important neurologic complication of certain cancers, particularly lymphomas. PML was first described in 1958 by Astrom and colleagues in patients with hematologic cancers (Astrom et al., 1958). Based on pathology findings, a virus was the likely cause and this theory has proved to be correct (ZuRhein and Chou, 1965, Weiner et al., 1972, Narayan et al., 1973). PML is strongly associated with lymphoreticular cancers and is limited to adults (ZuRhein and Chou, 1965). PML has also been reported in patients with severe systemic lupus, in the acquired immune deficiencies syndrome (AIDS) affecting homosexual men (Snider et al., 1983), and in an individual case report in which there is no known underlying immunosuppressive disease (Fermaglich et al., 1970). Approximately 100 cases have been described in the world's literature (ZuRhein and Chou, 1965), but most large cancer centers encounter one to two such patients a year.

Pathologic findings are distinctive, consisting of multiple foci of demyelination that ap-

Table 6–12. Remote Effects of Systemic Cancer on the Nervous System

Brain and cranial nerves
   Progressive multifocal leukoencephalopathy
   Dementia (limbic encephalitis)
   Bulbar encephalitis
   Subacute cerebellar degeneration — opsoclonus*
   Optic neuritis — retinal degeneration
Spinal cord
   Gray matter myelopathy
     Subacute motor neuropathy
     "Autonomic insufficiency"
     Amyotrophic lateral sclerosis (?)
Peripheral nerves and roots
   Subacute sensory neuropathy (dorsal root ganglionitis)*
   Sensorimotor peripheral neuropathy
   Acute polyneuropathy, Guillain-Barré type
   Autonomic neuropathy
Polymyositis and dermatomyositis (dermatomyositis in older men)*
   "Myathenic" syndrome (Lambert-Eaton)
   Myasthenia gravis (thymoma)
   Neuromyotonia

* Neurologic disorders that may precede diagnosis of cancer and strongly suggest its presence.

pear to the naked eye as granular and finely fenestrated tissue (see Figure 6–18). On microscopic examination, there is enlargement of oligodendroglial nuclei with loss of nuclear structure and ill-defined eosinophilic intranuclear inclusions. There is surrounding astroglial proliferation with bizarre transformation of their nuclei, assuming the appearance of neoplastic cells. This combination of microscopic findings makes the diagnosis of PML unequivocal. ZuRhein and Chou first demonstrated papova-like viral particles in the oligodendroglial cells on electron microscopy (ZuRhein and Chou, 1965). Since that time, the virus has been characterized and transmitted to animals (Walker, 1972; Weiner *et al.,*

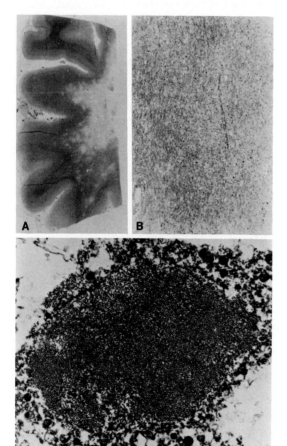

Figure 6–18. Progressive multifocal leukoencephalopathy in a patient with diffuse histiocytic lymphoma. (*A*) Multiple confluent foci of demyelination characteristic of PHL; (*B*) Demyelination and proliferation of macrophages; (*C*) An oligodendroglial nucleus packed with viruses of the papovirus group. From Manz, H. J.: Neuropathology of systemic malignant neoplasia. *Pathobiol. Annu.,* **12**:233–365, 1982.

1972; Padgett, 1976). The virus, termed the JC virus, is related to the SV 40 virus. Exposure to SV 40 may result from use of polio virus vaccines, which are prepared in rhesus monkey kidney cultures. In one population study in Wisconsin, antibodies to JC virus have been found in 17% of children before age 4, with increase to 60% by age 14 and 84% in the ninth decade. The development of PML could be the result of severe immunocompromise in the JC-virus-bearing patient.

The clinical presentation of PML is consistent with its name. The disease is an acutely to subacutely progressive disorder affecting multiple areas of the CNS, most consistently the cerebrum, with alterations of mental status, behavior, thinking, speech, movement, sensation, and special senses. Pyramidal tract signs occur in 76% of patients, intellectual impairment in 74%, visual deficits in 37%, aphasias and dysarthrias in 24%, brainstem signs in 20%, sensory deficits in 16%, and seizures in 11%.

The neurologic course is one of relentless progression, with coma and death usually occurring within three to four months. Occasional remissions, however, and long survivals have been reported (Price *et al.,* 1983). The cerebrospinal fluid (CSF) is normal in most cases, with mild mononuclear pleocytosis and mildly elevated CSF protein in a few patients. CT scans usually reveal multiple areas of white-matter lucency in the cerebral hemispheres. The abnormal areas usually do not contrast enhance with contrast material (Carroll *et al.,* 1977). The electroencephalogram (EEG) may be abnormal with diffuse slow waves and occasional focal abnormalities.

Limbic Encephalitis

This poorly defined syndrome has been reported in a small number of patients with bronchogenic carcinoma (Brierly *et al.,* 1960; Glasner and Pincus, 1969; Corsellis *et al.,* 1968). The syndrome presents with dementia characterized by prominent loss of recent memory. In addition, affected patients are often agitated, with dysarthria, occasional hallucinations, and seizures. The CSF is usually normal. The EEG may demonstrate slow waves localized to the temporal regions. Pathologic findings consist of extensive neuronal loss and astroglial proliferation, particularly evident in the temporal medial lobes.

The clinical picture may resemble herpes

encephalitis, but limbic encephalitis has a more subacute onset. The gross pathologic changes are not as marked, and in no case of limbic encephalitis have intranuclear inclusion bodies been found.

Bulbar Encephalitis

Bulbar or brainstem encephalitis was first established as an entity by Henson and colleagues (Henson *et al.,* 1954). In most instances, lung cancer has represented the underlying cancer; patients may present with dystonia, central hypoventilation, ophthalmoplegia, or seizures depending on the predominant site of the neurologic lesions (Reddy and Vakili, 1981; Deitl *et al.,* 1982). The most severe lesions have been seen in the medulla oblongata and the floor of the fourth ventricle, and also in motor nuclei of the cranial nerves (Henson and Urich, 1982).

Subacute Cerebellar Degeneration

Subacute cerebellar degeneration (SCD) is an unusual but well-established neurologic complication associated with neoplasia. Three percent of 96 patients with carcinomatous neuromyopathy in the series described by Brain and Wilkinson (1965) had these symptoms of SCD. Carcinoma of the lung, ovary, breast, fallopian tube, and stomach, as well as Hodgkin's disease, are the principal cancers that have been associated with SCD (Croft and Wilkinson, 1965; Bella, 1968). The average age of onset of cerebellar dysfunction is 50 years (Brain and Wilkinson, 1965, 1976).

Pathologically, there is panhemispheric loss of the Purkinje cell layer. This is in contrast to alcoholic cerebellar degeneration, in which there is a predilection for degeneration of the anterior and superior aspects of the vermis (see Figure 6–19). In paraneoplastic cerebellar degeneration, the disorder affects the molecular and granular layer of the cerebellum, the spinocerebellar tracts, and the pyramidal and dorsal columns (Brain and Wilkinson, 1965). A similarity in pathology between SCD and the "slow-virus" diseases of scrapie in sheep and kuru in the cannibal tribes of New Guinea has been recognized (Brain and Wilkinson, 1965).

The clinical manifestations of SCD include the subacute development of ataxia of the upper and lower extremities. An associated dementia has been noted in one half of reported cases; dysarthria and dysphagia may be

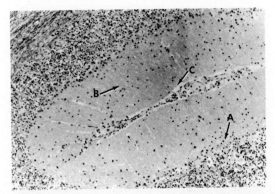

Figure 6–19. Subacute cerebellar degeneration (SCD), with a striking loss of Purkinje's cells (A), microglial and astroglial proliferation (B), and inflammatory cells in meninges characteristic of SCD (C). From Manz, H. J.: Neuropathology of systemic malignant neoplasia. *Pathobiol. Annu.,* **12:**233–365, 1982.

prominent findings. Motor weakness and reflex changes have been observed and are associated with involvement of the corticobulbar and corticospinal tracts. In half of the described cases, the tumor was discovered from two months to two years following the onset of SCD. Cerebrospinal fluid analysis may demonstrate mild pleocytosis and hyperproteinemia. This syndrome tends to be progressive, with a mean survival of three to four months.

Whereas remission of cerebellar dysfunction following resection of bronchogenic carcinomas has been recorded (McEntee, 1980), the case may represent a toxic syndrome as opposed to true cerebellar degeneration.

Optic Neuritis

Optic neuritis is a rare remote effect of cancer. It is characterized by decreased vision, central scotomas, and sometimes papilledema (Sawyer, 1976). It is important to differentiate true paraneoplastic optic neuritis from metastatic tumors to the optic nerves (Kattah *et al.,* 1980)

Spinal Cord Syndromes

A small percentage of remote neurological complications affect the spinal cord. In one series, amyotrophic lateral sclerosis (ALS) accounted for 9% of such cases (Croft and Wilkinson, 1965). Conversely, Norris and Engel have reported that 13 cases of ALS had an associated cancer, representing a 10% incidence (Norris and Engel, 1965). In most series of ALS, the incidence of cancer, however, is low and the specificity of the relationship is less clear (Henson, 1970).

The cardinal manifestations of ALS relate to the loss of lower motor neurons in the anterior horn region of the spinal cord. Fasciculations with muscle atrophy and weakness secondary to denervation and hyperreflexia are prominent features.

Subacute necrotic myelopathy, characterized by aggressive, fulminant ascending motor and sensory deficit is most often found in association with lung cancer (Mancall and Rosales, 1964). Degenerative changes in both white and gray matter are noted.

Subacute motor neuropathy characterized by a slowly progressive motor weakness has been described in patients with lymphoma (Walton et al., 1968).

Peripheral Nerve Syndromes

Disorders of the peripheral nerves are probably the most common neurological syndromes associated with cancer. Croft and associates defined two major groups of sensory motor neuropathies (Croft and Wilkinson, 1965). The first is a mild, symmetrical, peripheral sensory loss that occurs late in the course of neoplastic illness. The second is that of a subacute, severe sensory motor neuropathy that may antedate the diagnosis of cancer. These latter groups have a fluctuating course of neurologic impairment, which can progress to paralysis; steroid therapy has been reported to be beneficial. The CSF may demonstrate mild pleocytosis with an elevated protein. The pathology of the syndrome consists of a loss of both myelin and axis cylinder. These sensory lesions have been predominantly reported with lung cancer, but are also present with a variety of other primary sites of cancer (Tyler, 1974).

A pure sensory neuropathy has a strong association with neoplasms within the chest cavity (Horwich et al., 1977). Lung cancer, thymoma, lymphomas, esophageal and laryngeal cancers have been associated with this "dorsal root ganglionitis" (Tyler, 1974, Horwich et al., 1977, Henson et al., 1965). The neurologic symptoms of ataxia — severe sensory loss and normal muscle strength – usually precede the diagnosis of cancer and warrant a search for an underlying neoplasia. The CSF protein is often elevated and organ-specific antibrain antibodies have been reported in sera and CSF. The

syndrome is irreversible. Pathologically, there is loss of dorsal root ganglion cells with secondary changes in the peripheral nerves and dorsal root columns.

The Guillain-Barré syndrome, characterized by ascending acute polyneuropathy, has been reported in association with lymphomas and in particular with Hodgkin's disease (Lisak, 1977). The syndrome associated with cancer is indistinguishable from that encountered in the isolated neurologic illness, hence its relationship to neoplasia may be coincidental.

Polymyositis and Dermatomyositis

Whereas the association of polymyositis with cancer has been an oft debated subject (Kula, 1979; Bohan and Peter, 1975), patients with dermatomyositis may have a five- to sevenfold increased incidence of neoplasms (Barnes, 1976). Carcinomas of the lung, stomach, and ovary have predominated. It is generally considered imperative to evaluate a patient over 40 years in age who develops dermatomyositis for the presence of an underlying neoplasm. In contrast, an association of dermatomyositis with neoplastic disease in children is rare.

The pathologic features of dermatomyositis and polymyositis are identical to those encountered with the syndrome when it arises independent of cancer, and they consist of necrosis and phagocytosis of muscle fibers, with inflammatory cellular infiltration of perivascular tissue (Walton and Hudgson, 1979). Treatment with steroids has resulted in control of the syndrome in some cases (Kula, 1979).

Lambert-Eaton Syndrome

Lambert-Eaton syndrome is characterized by profound muscle weakness and fatigue, particularly in the pelvic limb girdle and lower extremities. Other symptoms include diplopia, dysarthria, ptosis, and paresthesias. This syndrome differs from myasthenia gravis in the lack of response to Tensilon and the potentiation of the muscle action potential on repetitive stimulation (Lambert et al., 1956; Lambert and Rooke, 1965). The syndrome is strongly associated with an underlying cancer, particularly small cell carcinoma of the lung, but it has also been encountered without an associated neoplasm and/or the subsequent development of a tumor (Elmquist and Lambert, 1968). In Lambert's series, 6% of patients with small cell cancer developed this myasthenic syndrome (Lambert *et al.,* 1956). The syndrome has also been observed in association with other histologic types of lung cancer, 1% of Lambert's lung cancer population, and in rare cases with cancers in other organ sites, including breast, prostate, rectum, and stomach. Recovery from the syndrome has been reported after a tumor response to therapy (Jenkyn *et al.,* 1980). A postulated mechanism for the Lambert-Eaton syndrome is the reduction in the quantity of acetylcholine secreted at the motor end-plate. Consequently, guanidine and calcium have been employed to improve the weakness (Cherrington, 1976).

Little evidence is available to link true myasthenia with neoplasia other than the one important exception of thymoma (Tyler, 1974). Pure neuromyotonia is an extremely rare manifestation described in patients with lung cancer (Humphrey *et al.,* 1976).

Remote effects of cancer on the nervous system are uncommon but important manifestations of systemic disease. Some of these neurologic syndromes, such as dorsal root ganglionitis and the Lambert-Eaton syndrome, are strongly associated with an underlying neoplasm and may presage the development of cancer. Successful treatment of the neoplasm may result in remission of the remote neurologic phenomenon, and consequently, a search for an underlying cancer is warranted in selected cases.

REFERENCES

Aronson, S. M.; Garcia, J. H.; and Aronson, B. E.: Metastatic neoplasms of the brain, colon: Their frequency and their relation to age. *Cancer,* **17**:558, 1964.

Astrom, K. K.; Mancall, E. L.; and Richardson, E. P.: Progressive multifocal leukoencephalopathy; hither to unrecognized complication of chronic lymphatic leukemia and Hodgkin's disease. *Brain,* **81**:93, 1958.

Aur, R. J. A.; Simone, J. V.; and Hustin, H. L.: A comparative study of central nervous irradiation and intensive chemotherapy early in remission of childhood acute lymphotic leukemia. *Cancer,* **29**:381–391, 1972.

Balla, J. I.: Cerebellar degeneration associated with carcinoma of the stomach. *Br. Med. J.,* **1**:34, 1968.

Barnes, B. E.: Dermatomyositis and malignancy. A review of the literature. *Ann. Intern. Med.,* **84**:68–76, 1976.

Bohan, A., and Peter, J. P.: Polymyositis and dermatomyositis. *New Engl. J. Med.,* **293**:344–347, 1975.

Brain, W. R., and Wilkinson, M.: Subacute cerebellar degeneration. In Brain, L., and Norris, F. (eds.): *Remote Effects of Cancer on the Nervous System.* Grune & Stratton, Inc., New York, 1965.

Brain, W. R., and Wilkinson, M.: Sub-acute cerebellar

degeneration as a remote of cancer. *Am. J. Ophthalmol.,* **81**:606–613, 1976.

Brierly, J. B.; Corsellis, J. M.; Hierons, R.; and Nevin, S.: Sub-acute encephalitis of late adult life mainly effecting the limbic areas. *Brain,* **83**:357, 1960.

Carroll, N. A.; Lane, B.; Norman, D.; and Enzmann, D.: Diagnosis of progressive multifocal leukoencephalopathy by computed tomography. *Radiology,* **122**:137–141, 1977.

Chasen, J. L.; Walker, F. B.; and Lander, J. W.: Metastatic carcinoma in the central nervous system and dorsal root ganglia. Prospective autopsy studies. *Cancer,* **16**:781, 1963.

Cherrington, M.: Guanidine and germine in Eaton-Lambert syndrome. *Neurology* (N.Y.), **26**:944–946, 1976.

Corsellis, J. N.; Goldberg, G. J.; and Norton, A. R.: Limbic encephalitis and its association with carcinoma. *Brain,* **91**:481, 1968.

Croft, P. B., and Wilkinson, M.: The incidence of carcinomatous neuromyopathy in patients with various types of carcinomas. *Brain,* **88**:427, 1965.

Dietl, H. W.; Pult, St.-M.; Enngelhardt, P.; and Mehrain, P.: Paraneoplastic brainstem encephalitis with acute dystonia and central hypoventilation. *J. Neurol.,* **227**:229–238, 1982.

Elmquist, D., and Lambert, E. H.: Detailed analysis of neuromuscular transmission in a patient with the myasthenic syndrome sometimes associated with bronchogenic carcinoma. *Mayo Clin. Proc.,* **43**:689–713, 1968.

Fermaglich, J.; Hardman, J. M.; and Earle, K. M.: Spontaneous progressive multifocal leukoencephalopathy. *Neurology* (N.Y.), **20**:479–484, 1970.

Glasner, G. J., and Pincus, J. H.: Limbic encephalitis. *J. Nerv. Ment. Dis.,* **149**:59, 1969.

Henson, R. A.: Non-metastatic neurological manifestations of malignant disease. In Williams, D. (ed.): *Modern Trends in Neurology.* Butterworth, London, 1970.

Henson, R. A.; Hoffman, H. L. K.; and Urich, H.: Encephalomyelitis with carcinoma. *Brain,* **88**:449–464, 1965.

Henson, R. A.; Russell, D. S.; and Wilkinson, M. I. P.: Carcinomatous neuropathy and myopathy. *Brain,* **77**:82, 1954.

Henson, R. A., and Urich, H.: *Cancer and the Nervous System.* Blackwell Scientific Publications, London, 1982.

Horwich, M. S.; Cho, L.; Porro, R. S.; and Posner, J. B.: Subacute sensory neuropathy: a remote effect of carcinoma. *Ann. Neurol.,* **1**:7–19, 1977.

Humphrey, J. G.; Hill, M. E.; Gordon, A. S.; and Kalow, W.: Myotonia associated with small cell carcinoma of the lung. *Arch. Neurol.,* **33**:575–576, 1976.

Jenkyn, L. R.; Brooks, P. L.; Forcier, R. J.; Maurer, L. H.; Ochoa, J.: Remission of the Lambert-Eaton syndrome and small cell anaplastic carcinoma of the lung induced by chemotherapy and radiotherapy. *Cancer,* **46**:1123–1127, 1980.

Kattah, J. G.; Suski, E. T.; Killen, J.; Smith, F. P.; and Limaye, S. R.: Optic neuritis and systemic lymphoma. *Am. J. Ophthalmol.,* **89**:431–436, 1980.

Kula, R. W.: Neuromuscular disorders associated with systemic disease. In Vincken, P. J., and Bruyn, G. W. (eds.): *Handbook of Clinical Neurology.* North-Holland Publishing Co., Amsterdam, 1979.

Lambert, E. H.; Eaton, L. M.; and Rooke, E. D.: Defect of neuromuscular conduction associated with malignant neoplasms. *Am. J. Physiol.,* **187**:612, 1956.

Lambert, E. H., and Rooke, E. D.: Myasthenic state and lung cancer. In Brain, W. R., and Norris, F. H., Jr. (eds.): *The Remote Effects of Cancer on the Nervous System*. Grune & Stratton, Inc., New York, 1965.

Lisak, R. P.: Guillain-Barré syndrome and Hodgkin's disease. Three cases with immunological studies. *Ann. Neurol.,* 1:72–78, 1977.

McEntee, W. J.: Remission of cerebellar dysfunction after pneumonectomy for bronchogenic carcinoma. *N. Engl. J. Med.,* **302:**1309, 1980.

Mancall, E. L., and Rosales, R. K.: Necrotizing myelopathy associated with visceral carcinoma. *Brain,* **876:**636–639, 1964.

Manz, H. J.: Neuropathology of systemic malignant neoplasia. *Pathobiol. Annu.,* **12:**233–365, 1982.

Meyer, R. F.; Ferreria, P. P.; Cuttner, J.; Greenberg, M. L.; Goldberg, J.; and Holland, J. F.: Central nervous system involvement at presentation in acute granulocytic leukemia. A prospective cytocentrifuge study. *Am. J. Med.,* **68:**69, 1980.

Narayan, O.; Penney, J. B.; Johnson, R. T.; Herndon, R. M.; and Weiner, L. P.: Etiology of progressive multifocal leukoencephalopathy. Identification of papova virus. *N. Engl. J. Med.,* **289:**1278, 1973.

Norris, F. H., and Engel, W. K.: Carcinomatous amyotrophic lateral sclerosis. In Brain, W. R., and Norris, F. H., Jr. (eds.): *The Remote Effects of Cancer on the Nervous System.* Grune & Stratton, Inc., New York, 1965.

Padgett, B. L.: JC papovirus in progressive multifocal leukoencephalopathy. *J. Infect. Dis.,* **113:**686–690, 1976.

Posner, J. B.: Neurologic complications of systemic cancer. *Med. Clin. North Am.,* **55:**625, 1971.

Posner, J. B., and Chernik, N. L.: Intracranial metastases. In Schoenberg, B. R. (ed.): *Advances in Neurology,* Vol. 19. Raven Press, New York, 1978.

Price, R. W.; Nielsen, S.; Horten, B.; Rubino, M.; Padgett, B.; and Walker, M.: Progressive multifocal leukoencephalopathy: a burnt-out case. *Ann. Neurol.,* **13:**485–490, 1983.

Reddy, R. V., and Vakili, S. T.: Midbrain encephalitis as a remote effect of a malignant neoplasm. *Arch. Neurol.,* **38:**781–789, 1981.

Sawyer, R.: Blindness caused by photoreceptor degeneration as a remote effect of cancer. *Am. J. Ophthalmol.,* **81:**606–690, 1976.

Shapiro, W. R.: Remote effects of neoplasm in the central nervous system: Encephalopathy. *Adv. Neurol.,* **15:**101, 1976.

Snider, W. D.; Simpson, D. M.; Nielsen, S.; Gold, J. W. M.; Metroka, C. E.; and Posner, J. B.: Neurological complications of acquired immune deficiency syndrome, analysis of fifty patients. *Ann. Neurol.,* 14, 1983.

Sweet, D. L.; Golomb, H. M.; Ultmann, J. E.; Miller, J. B.; Stein, R. S.; Lester, E. P.; Mintz, U.; Bitran, J. D.; Streuli, R. A.; Daly, K.; and Roth, N. O.: Cyclophosphamide, vincristine, methotrexate with leucovorin rescue, and cytarabine (COMLA) combination sequential chemotherapy for advanced diffuse histiocytic lymphoma. *Ann. Intern. Med.,* **92:**785–790, 1980.

Tyler, H. R.: Paraneoplastic syndromes of nerve, muscle and neuromuscular junction. *Ann. N.Y. Acad. Sci.,* **230:**348–357, 1974.

Walker, D. L.: Progressive multifocal leukoencephalopathy and opportunistic virus infection of the central nervous system. In Vincken, P. J., and Bruyn, G. W. (eds.): *Handbook of Clinical Neurology.* North Holland Publishing Co., Amsterdam, 1972.

Walton, J. N., and Hudgson, P.: Polymyositis and other inflammatory myopathies. In Vinken, P. J., and Bruyn, G. W. (eds.): *Handbook of Clinical Neurology.* North Holland Publishing Company, Amsterdam, 1979.

Walton, J. N.; Tomlinson, B. E.; and Pearce, G. W.: Subacute poliomyelitis and Hodgkin's disease. *J. Neurol. Sci.,* **6:**435–445, 1968.

Wasserstrom, W. R.; Glass, J. P.; and Posner, J. B.: Diagnosis and treatment of leptomeningeal metastases from solid tumours: Experience with 90 patients. *Cancer,* **49:**759–772, 1982.

Weiner, L. P.; Herndon, R. M.; Narayan, O.; Johnson, R. T.; Shah, K.; Rubenstein, L. J.; Preziosi, T. J.; and Conley, F. K.: Isolation of virus related to SV40 from patients with progressive multifocal leucoencephalopathy. *N. Engl. J. Med.,* **286:**385–390, 1972.

ZuRhein, G. M., and Chou, S. M.: Particles resembling papova viruses in human cerebral demyelinating disease. *Science* **148:**1477–1479, 1965.

F. ENDOCRINE COMPLICATIONS OF CANCER
William D. Odell

HUMORAL SYNDROMES CAUSED BY CANCER—ECTOPIC HORMONE PRODUCTION

Introduction

Cancers produce a wide variety of humoral substances, many of which are not biologically active or are weakly bioactive. When biologically active substances are produced, the clinical findings or symptoms are often striking.

The best understood of the clinical syndromes caused by cancer are the endocrine disorders—so-called ectopic endocrine syndromes. Table 6–13 lists the hormone or hormone-precursors reportedly secreted by cancers. Although this list is long, the biochemical natures of all but one (the prostaglandins) are similar; all are proteins or peptides. Wherever the cause is known, with the possible exception of prostaglandins, the humoral materials secreted by cancers are proteins or peptides (including glycoproteins). Prostaglandin secretion by cancers is discussed under the heading "Hypercalcemia and Cancer".

In this review will be discussed some of these syndromes and an attempt will be made to

Table 6–13.   Hormones and Related Substances Reported to be Secreted by Cancers

ACTH and related proteins	Calcitonin
Chorionic gonadotropin (CG),	Growth hormone
alpha and beta chains of CG	Prolactin
Vasopressin and related peptides	Gastrin
Somatomedins and related proteins	Secretin
Hypoglycemic-producing factors	Glucagon
Parathyroid hormone	Corticotropin-releasing hormone
Osteoclast-activating factor	Growth hormone-releasing hormone
Prostaglandins	Somatostatin
Erythropoietin	Chorionic somatotropin
Hypophosphatemia-producing factor	Neurophysins

offer a broad perspective of ectopic hormone syndromes, based on the available data.

Ectopic ACTH Syndromes

Cushing's syndrome caused by cancer production of biologically active ACTH was probably the first ectopic hormone syndrome to be described. In 1928, Brown reported the case of a patient with oat cell carcinoma of the bronchus and Cushing's syndrome (Brown, 1928). Liddle and colleagues in the 1960s published extensive studies concerning this syndrome; they demonstrated that extracts of the tumor and its metastases contained large amounts of biologically active ACTH (Liddle *et al.,* 1969). Several hundred cases of this syndrome subsequently have been described. Clinically, such patients often do not exhibit full Cushing's syndrome. Findings suggesting this syndrome include hypokalemia, abnormal glucose tolerance, psychosis, and weakness. Plasma cortisol concentrations are often very high.

These cases show a striking correlation with a few histologic types of neoplasms. Approximately 80% are associated with six histologic types of cancer: Small cell or oat cell carci-

noma of the lung, carcinoma of the pancreas, thymus carcinoma, neural crest tumors, medullary carcinoma of the thyroid, and bronchial adenoma or carcinoma (Odell, 1980). Although patients with Cushing's syndrome caused by these tumors usually show little or no suppression of plasma cortisol with high-dose dexamethasone treatment, those patients with bronchial adenoma often do (50%) show such suppression. This suggests that some of the bronchial adenomas secrete corticotropin-releasing hormone (CRH) rather than ACTH. Such production was first reported by Upton and Amatruda (1971). The action of CRH is at a pituitary level, and such action is inhibited by excess glucocorticoids. Table 6–14 lists the frequency of association with each type of neoplasm.

Although most patients with clinical evidence of ectopic ACTH production have one of these five carcinomas, only a small percentage of patients with these five neoplasms have Cushing's syndrome. For example, using the oat cell carcinoma as a model, Kato and associates (1969) demonstrated that 2.8% of patients with oat cell carcinoma of the lung have elevated plasma cortisol that fails to suppress

Table 6–14.   Neoplasms Associated with Bioactive Ectopic ACTH Production

TUMOR TYPE	APPROXIMATE PERCENTAGE OF CASES
Carcinoma of lung	50
Thymic carcinoma	10
Pancreatic carcinoma (including islet cell and carcinoid)	10
Neoplasms from neural crest tissue (pheochromocytoma, neuroblastoma, paraganglioma, ganglioma)	5
Bronchial adenoma (including carcinoid)	2
Medullary carcinoma of the thyroid	5
Miscellaneous*	each <2

* Carcinoma of ovary, prostate, breast, thyroid, kidney, salivary glands, testes, stomach, colon, gall bladder, esophagus, appendix, etc.
From Odell, W. D.: Humoral manifestations of cancer. In Williams, R. H. (ed.): *Textbook of Endocrinology,* 6th ed. W. B. Saunders Company, Philadelphia, 1980.

with dexamethasone. It thus appears that some factor other than the mere presence of a specific histologic type of neoplasm determines whether biologically active ACTH is produced in abnormal quantities.

During the past few years, a large number of studies have led to hypotheses that "most or all carcinomas produce large amounts of biologically inert (precursor) ACTH; selected carcinomas, depending on the histological type, metabolize such precursor ACTH to bioactive ACTH." (Odell, *et al.,* 1977). To understand these data, it is necessary to review the biochemistry of ACTH biosynthesis as it normally occurs in the pituitary gland. This biochemistry has been elucidated in Eipper and Mains (1976, 1980) and Mains and Eipper (1976), who used mouse pituitary tumor as well as primary pituitary cell cultures. The first messenger RNA product possessing ACTH immunoactivity is a 31,000 – molecular weight (mol wt) glycoprotein, which serves as a precursor to several secreted peptides. Figure 6–20 schematically shows the sequences of subsequent metabolism. The anterior lobe adrenotrophic cells preferentially form ProACTH, which is cleaved to bioactive ACTH (4500 mol wt) during secretion. Beta lipotropin (which contains the sequence of μg melanocyte-stimulating hormone) and the 16 K fragment may be metabolized within the adrenotrophic cell or secreted. They have no known biologic importance or functions. In other cells, lipotropin is metabolized to the endorphins, which are peptides that bind to opiate receptors and modulate pain responses. It is believed that cells in the central nervous system preferentially metabolize to these substances. Presumably, in such cell types, ProACTH and the 16 K fragments are degraded intracellularly or, if secreted, have poorly understood functions.

Studies (by Ratcliffe *et al.,* 1972; Bloomfield

Table 6–15. Immunoactive ACTH Content (pg/g wet weight)

| Carcinomas | 22,359 ± 163 | (N = 68) |
| Normal tissues | < 1000 | (N = 100) |

et al., 1977; Gewirtz and Yalow, 1974; Odell *et al.,* 1977; and Wolfsen and Odell, 1979) have shown that extracts from all carcinomas, whether or not associated with ectopic ACTH syndrome and regardless of histologic type, contain an immunoactive ACTH-like hormone (see Table 6–15). This immunoactive ACTH from carcinomas not causing ectopic ACTH syndrome has a higher molecular weight than standard ACTH: approximately 27,000. Wolfsen and Odell (1979) and Odell and colleagues (1977) have demonstrated that the amounts of immunoactive ACTH extractable from carcinomas are great, exceeding detectable amounts in normal tissues. This material is not reactive in a radioreceptor assay for ACTH (Wolfsen and Odell, 1979) or in *in vitro* dispersed adrenal cell bioassays (Gewirtz and Yalow, 1974), and thus has little or no bioactivity.

Wolfsen and Odell (1979) and Odell and colleagues (1977) performed a blind prospective clinical study of 100 consecutive patients admitted to the hospital with abnormal chest x-rays. Patients who were thought to have ectopic Cushing's syndrome (that is, those with hypokalemia, diabetes, or physical findings suggesting Cushing's syndrome) were excluded from the study. Twenty-four of the patients were found to have a benign disease; all had normal immunoactive ACTH. Seventy-four of the patients subsequently were found to have lung cancer, which included oat, squamous, alveolar, and undifferentiated cell types. Fifty-three of these patients (74%) had elevated immunoactive ACTH. Figure 6–21 shows the concentration of immunoactive

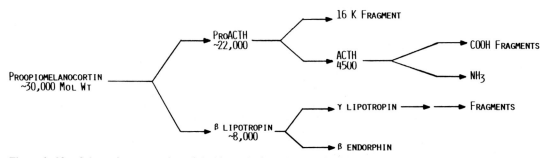

Figure 6–20. Schematic presentation of the biosynthetic pathways of ACTH and related peptides.

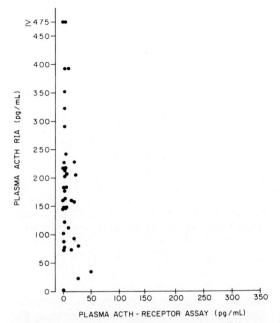

Figure 6-21. Plasma ACTH measured by radioimmunoassay and radioreceptor assay in patients with cancer but no clinically discernible ectopic ACTH syndrome. 100 pg/mL is the upper limit of normal in both assays. From Odell, W.; Wolfsen, A.; Yoshimoto, Y.; Weitzman, R.; Fisher, D.; and Hirose, F.: Ectopic peptide synthesis. A universal concomitant of neoplasia. *Trans. Assoc. Am. Physicians*, **90**:204–227, 1977.

ACTH plotted against receptor-active ACTH. This immunoactive receptor-inactive ACTH also has a molecular weight much greater than standard ACTH. These studies showed that a high–molecular weight ACTH-like material was present in abnormal amounts as measured by immunoassay in 74% of patients with lung cancer. This ACTH-like material was not

bioactive, as the patients did not have Cushing's syndrome even in subtle form, and the material did not react in the radioreceptor assay for ACTH. Thus, it is assumed that the high–molecular weight ACTH extractable from carcinomas is secreted into the blood. For these studies (Odell *et al.*, 1977; Wolfsen and Odell, 1979), the sensitivity of the ACTH immunoassay used was limited but permitted the statement that extracts of normal tissues contained less than 1000 pg/g.

Ectopic Production of Chorionic Gonadotropin (CG)

Chorionic gonadotropin (CG), until recently, has been considered to be produced only by the trophoblastic cells of the placenta, teratomas containing trophoblastic cells, hepatoblastomas, and an occasional carcinoma not related to the above. CG is a glycoprotein hormone composed of two peptide chains, an alpha and a beta, and is biochemically closely related to thyrotropin, luteinizing, and follicle-stimulating hormones. Figure 6–22 illustrates schematically the structure of CG. The alpha and beta chains of these glycoprotein hormones are not bound covalently, but associate based on charge-charge interaction. The beta chain of CG has a unique 47 amino acid carboxyl (COOH) tail not present on luteinizing, thyrotropic, or follicle-stimulating hormones, the so-called tail region of CG.

In 1964, Paul and Odell reported the first radioimmunoassay for CG using antisera produced against the whole molecule (Paul and Odell, 1969). In 1967, Odell and colleagues demonstrated the use of such an assay in

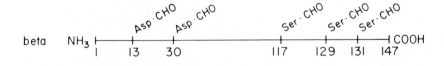

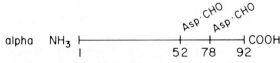

Figure 6-22. Chorionic gonadotropin (CG) structure shown schematically. The beta chain of placental CG possesses 147 amino acids. Complex carbohydrate moieties are linked via asparagines at positions 13 and 30 and via serines at positions 117, 131, and 147. The beta chain of CG is identical to that for human LH with the exception that the last 30 amino acids are not present on human LH. The alpha chain of CG contains 92 amino acids and two asparagine-linked complex carbohydrate moieties. The CG alpha differs from human LH alpha by a 2-amino acid inversion and a 3-residue deletion at the amino terminus. The carbohydrate moieties are made of a six different monosaccharides: D-mannose, *N*-acetylglucosamine, *N*-acetylgalactosamine, sialic acid, L-fucose, and D-galactose.

quantifying trophoblastic tumor production of CG. This assay, however, could not distinguish CG from luteinizing hormone. Thus in 1972, Vaitukaitis and colleagues used the purified beta HCG peptide to prepare antisera and develop the more specific beta CG assay. This assay is not entirely specific for CG and shows cross-reaction with luteinizing hormone at high concentrations. Nevertheless, the increased specificity permitted Braunstein and colleagues (1973) to screen a large number of sera collected from patients with various histologic types of cancer. Surprisingly, 6 to 15% of the samples had detectable CG in serum.

Because testicular teratocarcinomas also uniformly produce CG, Braunstein and colleagues in 1975 prepared extracts of normal human testes. Such extracts were partially purified by concanavalin A chromatography (Con A). Con A is a metalloprotein containing one carbohydrate binding site per molecule, directed towards hydroxyl groups at positions c-3, c-4, and c-6 of D-mannopyranose or D-glycopyranose rings. It thus binds glycoproteins such as CG by means of their carbohydrate structure. Braunstein and colleagues (1975) reported that all normal testes contained a CG-like material. Unfortunately, tissues other than testes were reported to contain no detectable CG.*

Yoshimoto and colleagues (1977) and Odell and colleagues (1977) reported that extracts of all normal tissues and carcinomas contained a CG-like material. This material was shown to be similar to placental CG using both the beta CG immunoassay and the CG radioreceptor assay. In contrast to ProACTH, for which concentrations were much greater in carcinomas, the concentrations of CG were similar in extracts of carcinomas and normal tissues in about two-thirds of the samples. About one-third of extracts from carcinomas contained CG in concentrations exceeding those in normal tissues. Con A binding of the CG-like material extracted from normal tissues, however, was extremely low, averaging about 5%. In contrast, Con A binding of the CG-like material extractable from carcinomas was variable, ranging from as low as 5% to as high as that for placental CG, over 90%. Figure 6–23 and Table 6–16 illustrate these data.

In order to explain the low Con A binding, Yoshimoto and associates (1979a) and Odell

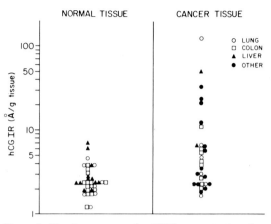

Figure 6–23. Immunoreactive HCG concentrations in normal and carcinoma tissues. From Yoshimoto, Y.; Wolfsen, A. R.; and Odell, W. D.: Glycosylation, a variable in the production of HCG by cancers. *Am. J. Med.,* 67:414–420, 1979.

and colleagues (1977) postulated that the CG-like material from normal tissues had a markedly altered carbohydrate structure. In further support of that, Odell and Evans (1980) reported that the molecular weight of the CG-like material extracted from normal human liver was about 27,000, which would be slightly smaller than carbohydrate-free placental CG.

The interpretation of Con A binding properties of normal tissue CG-like material, however, is controversial. Cole and Hussa (1981) evaluated the human CG (HCG) beta chain produced by cervical carcinoma cultures *in vitro.* They also reported poor Con A binding of the purified ectopic beta CG, but in addition found that Con A binding increased to 96% after digestion with N-acetylhexosaminidase. They suggested that the decreased Con A binding of the native ectopic beta CG was caused by the presence of an extra β-N-acetylglucosamine linked to a β-mannose, which blocked Con A binding.

Cole and colleagues (1982) reported the same ectopic beta chain CG to be composed of two molecular sizes, one similar to placental beta CG and a second, larger form that was more abundant. This larger form was shown not to possess the carboxyl amino acid sequence 116–145 (called carboxyl terminal peptide) that is unique to CG and not present on luteinizing hormone. These findings are in contrast to those of Odell and Evans, who reported that liver CG-like material did react in the COOH tail assay (thus possessing the amino acid sequence 116–145) and had a mo-

---

* Con A binding was used to prepare the tissue CG-like material. Normal tissue CG does not bind to Con A.

Table 6-16. HCG Binding to Concanavalin A

	% BOUND ± SEM	RANGE
Normal tissue (10)	6.1 ± 1.6	(0.0-14.6)
Cancer tissue (9)	31.2 ± 9.1	(4.0-86.0)
Placenta (4)	92.5 ± 0.9	(90.1-94.0)
Pregnant serum (3)	100.0	
Cancer serum (8)	54.7 ± 11.9	(3.1-92.5)

From Yoshimoto, Y.; Wolfson, A. R.; and Odell, W. D.: Glycosylation, a variable in the production of HCG by cancers. *Am. J. Med.,* **67**:414–420, 1979.

lecular weight small enough to suggest it was carbohydrate free (Odell and Evans, 1980). The cervical carcinoma cell line ectopic CG appears to differ from hepatic tissue CG. Further studies are required to resolve these issues. Tsuruhara and associates (1972) have shown that carbohydrate-free placental CG possesses very little *in vivo* bioactivity. It is cleared from the circulation due to a short half-life and is not able to achieve high blood concentrations.

Interestingly, a CG-like material has also been reported in nonmammalian and a few mammalian nonhuman tissues. Livingston and Livingston (1974) and Cohen and Strampp (1976) reported that a CG-like material was produced by some strains of bacteria. Maruo and colleagues in 1979 showed that a similar substance was produced by *Progenitor cryptocides.* Acevedo and colleagues, (1978a,b) and Slifkin and associates (1978) confirmed the findings of Livingston and Livingston and of Cohen and Strampp using immunohistologic identification and hypothesized that this CG-like material may be implicated in neoplastic development.

The relationship of protein hormone-like materials, which are produced by microorganisms, to endocrinology in general and more specifically to ectopic hormone production is of great current interest. In 1980, Yoshimoto and colleagues reported that a CG-like material was extractable from codfish, chickens, rats, rabbits, dogs, and cows (Yoshimoto *et al.,* 1980). In 1980, Rosenzweig and associates reported that insulin was extractable from all tissues of humans and rats. LeRoith and colleagues (1981a,b) showed an insulin-like material to be present in nonvertebrates such as insects, annelids, and bacteria. All these data indicating (1) widespread presence of protein hormone-like materials in non-endocrine tissues of vertebrates and (2) presence in and production of protein hormone-like materials by nonvertebrates, led to the suggestion that such materials are very early evolu-

tionary signals, probably autocrine, paracrine and later endocrine substances (Odell *et al.,* 1977; Odell and Wolfsen 1980; Odell and Saito 1982; Kolata *et al.,* 1982; Le Roith *et al.,* 1981a,b). Based on these findings for insulin, Roth (Kolata, 1982) and LeRoith and colleagues (1981a,b) independently came to the same hypothesis as Odell and associates (1977).

In summary:

1. A CG-like material appears to be widespread in nature. Relevant to ectopic production, such a material is extractable from all normal human tissues;
2. This normal tissue CG shows little binding to Con A, indicating that this material possesses little or no carbohydrate (as appears true for hepatic CG-like material) or has altered carbohydrate content (as appears true for cervical carcinoma CG-like material);
3. Such a CG-like material is also extractable from all carcinomas. Con A binding of carcinoma CG is variable, ranging from as low as normal tissue CG to as high as placental CG;
4. Carcinomas associated with increased blood CG either produce larger quantities of this CG-like material or have the additional property of glycosylating this material; and
5. "Ectopic" production of CG is not ectopic.

Hypercalcemia and Cancer

Hypercalcemia is commonly seen in patients with cancer. Warwick and associates (1961) reported that 9.1% of 438 patients admitted with cancer to Toronto General Hospital were hypercalcemic; Bender and Hansen (1974) reported that 12.5% of 200 patients with bronchogenic carcinoma were hypercalcemic. In contrast to most of the other humoral syndromes, hypercalcemia has several possible causes: (1) the production of a parathormonelike material; (2) production of prostaglandins that mobilize bone calcium; (3) production of osteoclast activating factor (OAF); and (4) the relatively common coincident occurrence of primary hyperparathyroidism in patients with cancer.

Since the coincident occurrence of hyperparathyroidism and cancer will not be discussed further, the reader is referred to Drezner and Lebovitz (1978), who studied 15 patients with hypercalcemia and cancer. Six patients had elevated renal excretion of cyclic adenosine monophosphate (cAMP) and were shown to have surgically proven hyperparathyroidism; nine had cAMP excretion that was not increased and presumably had cancer-caused hypercalcemia.

Albright (1941) first suggested cancers might produce a parathormonelike material. Subsequently, Tashjian and colleagues (1964), Berson and Yalow (1966), and Sherwood and associates (1967) found immunoactive parathormone (PTH) in extracts of a wide variety of carcinomas. The best evidence suggesting that cancer PTH production caused hypercalcemia was the patient with renal carcinoma studied by Buckle and colleagues (1970). This patient was found to have an arterial-venous difference for PTH across the kidney; the hypercalcemia disappeared following tumor resection.

Because PTH has been quantified using immunoassays, consideration of the assay is essential. Habener and colleagues (1972, 1975) have elucidated this sequence of biochemical events. During parathyroid gland synthesis, storage, secretion, and degradation, PTH undergoes metabolic changes similar to ACTH, as previously described. Figure 6–24 shows schematically the peptide cascade for PTH. PreProPTH possesses the 35 AA leader sequence that assists in directing this protein into the endoplasmic reticular space. The ProPTH is cleared to biologically active 84 AA PTH. This hormone then undergoes cleavage, either during secretion (dotted lines) or after secretion (solid lines), into COOH fragments that are not bioactive and amino (NH_3) fragments that may possess bioactivity. The metabolic clearance rate of the COOH fragments is considerably less than either the PTH or its NH_3 fragments, resulting in blood concentrations for the COOH fragment that are much greater than the PTH or the NH_3 fragment. It is for this practical reason that most immunoassays are directed towards measuring the COOH fragment.

Furthermore, Benson et al. (1974a) reported that the carboxyl terminal fragment of PTH is normally formed intracellularly by parathyroid tissue. Therefore, this fragment is usually highly elevated above normal in primary hyperparathyroidism. Arnaud (1981) has postulated that cancer-produced PTH is not directly produced by cancer tissue, but rather by peripheral metabolism. Because of this, Arnaud postulated carboxyl fragment PTH assays usually show highly elevated values in primary hyperparathyroidism and "normal" values in cancer-caused hypercalcemia.

The best discrimination between cancer-caused hypercalcemia and primary hyperparathyroidism is offered by carboxyl terminal PTH assays. Using such assays, approximately 80% of patients with primary hyperparathyroidism have "elevated" PTH, whereas most patients with cancer-caused hypercalcemia have low or "normal" values. Figure 6–25 illustrates such data.

Raisz and associates (1979) have directly compared several commercially available PTH assays used on 15 patients with hyperparathyroidism and 14 with hypercalcemia and cancer, further illustrating this point. Benson and colleagues (1974b) concluded that about 95% of patients with hypercalcemia of cancer had elevated PTH levels relative to their serum calcium levels, and that production of PTH by the cancer was the cause.

The hypothesis, however, that cancer production of PTH causes hypercalcemia has been challenged. Powell and associates (1973) carefully evaluated 11 patients with hypercalcemia, hypophosphatemia, and cancer with-

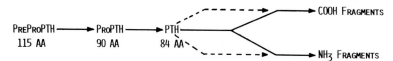

Figure 6–24. Schematic presentation of the biochemical sequences of parathormone synthesis, secretion, and degradation.

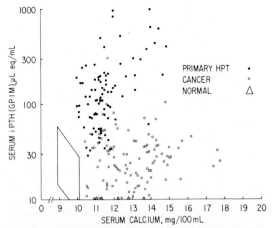

Figure 6–25. Relationship between serum iPTH (assayed using GP 1M) and serum calcium in primary hyperparathyroid (●) and in hypercalcemic patients with cancer (○). Serum iPTH is given in terms of equivalents of a standard hyperparathyroid plasma. For a given serum calcium value, serum iPTH was lower in patients with ectopic hyperparathyroidism and was undetectable (△) in five of the 108 patients with cancer. The parallelogram indicates area in which normal values would fall. From Benson, R. C., Jr.; Riggs, B. L.; Pickard, B. M.; and Arnaud, C. D.: Radioimmunoassay of parathyroid hormone in hypercalcemic patients with malignant disease. *Am. J. Med.,* **56:**821, 1974.

out bony metastases. In nine patients, treatment of the tumor by either surgical ablation or chemotherapy restored calcium to normal. PTH was quantified using several radioimmunoassays selected to react with intact PTH, as well as with the carboxyl and amino fragments. No PTH was detected in either blood or tumor extracts in these patients. The researchers postulated that a substance other than PTH was produced by these tumors to cause the hypercalcemia. Metz and colleagues (1981) confirmed that patients with hypercalcemia caused by cancer rarely have elevated PTH by amino terminal immunoassays, whereas carboxyl terminal assays usually show elevated values. The source of the carboxyl terminal biologically inert fragments remains uncertain. Using a cytochemical assay (based on the reaction of kidney cortex segments to parathormone), Goltzman and colleagues (1981) reported that plasma bioactivity was increased in 10 of 16 patients who had cancer and hypercalcemia associated with increased nephrogenous cAMP excretion. Mean levels were tenfold higher than in cancer patients who were normocalcemic or had hypercalcemia without increased cAMP excretion. Pros-

taglandins E_1 and E_2 showed no reaction in this bioassay. The active material had a molecular weight greater than 1-84 parathormone.

Skrabanek and colleagues (1980) reviewed 307 patients with hypercalcemia and cancer and analyzed the data for and against the hypothesis that PTH is produced by cancers. They report that 61 of 74 patients in whom the tumor was resected showed remission of hypercalcemia, demonstrating that the cancer caused the hypercalcemia. They summarize, however, that the evidence that ectopic PTH is produced is not solid and is in part based on conflicting radioimmunoassay results. They concluded, based on their data, that multiple causes of tumor hypercalcemia are likely.

The approximate percentage of histologic types of neoplasms associated with hypercalcemia from reports in the literature are listed in Table 6–17. This table is constructed without regard for the presence or absence of bone metastases. In earlier reviews by Odell (1980), histologic distribution was calculated for neoplasms without bone metastases.

A second postulated cause of hypercalcemia is cancer production of prostaglandins. This, too, is a disputed mechanism for human cancers. In 1972, Tashjian and colleagues studied an animal model, a fibrosarcoma producing hypercalcemia in mice. The tumor was shown to produce prostaglandins—probably PGE_2, a potent stimulant for bone resorption

Table 6–17. Approximate Percentage Distribution of Cancers Causing Hypercalcemia

TYPE OF CANCER	PERCENT
Kidney	14
Lung*	13
Leukemia	13
Breast	12
Lymphoma†	12
Urogenital‡	7
Gynecologic§	7
Liver	6
Esophagus	4
Pancreas	2
Pheochromocytoma‖	2
Head and neck	2
Miscellaneous#	6

* Predominantly squamous carcinoma
† Hodgkin's and non-Hodgkin's
‡ Renal pelvis, bladder, prostate, vulva, penis
§ Cervix, ovarian, uterine
‖ Pheochromocytoma is often associated with hyperparathyroidism as part of multiple endocrine neoplasias, but probably also less often directly causes hypercalcemia.
Skin, neoplastic melanoma, gall bladder, sarcoma, adrenal, parotid, seminoma

in vitro. The hypercalcemia was correctable by indomethacin treatment (an inhibitor of prostaglandin synthesis). Voelkel and associates (1975) also showed that prostaglandin secretion by a carcinoma in rabbits was a cause for hypercalcemia. Furthermore, Franklin and Tashjian (1975) demonstrated that intravenous infusion of PGE_2 raised serum calcium in rats; another prostaglandin, $PGF_{2\alpha}$, was inactive. The data for human cancers are suggestive, but less convincing than the animal models.

In 1975, Robertson and colleagues reported a patient with renal carcinoma and hypercalcemia who had elevated blood prostaglandin levels. Prostaglandin elevations in plasma coincided in time with increased serum. Ito and associates (1975) described a patient with renal carcinoma who responded to indomethacin treatment. In a larger study of 29 patients with solid tumors, 14 were hypercalcemic and 15 had normal blood calcium (Seyberth *et al.,* 1975). Twelve of the hypercalcemic patients had marked increases in urine prostaglandin metabolite excretion; seven of the eucalcemic patients had increased urine prostaglandin metabolite excretion, but this was slight to moderate. Six of the hypercalcemic patients were treated with aspirin or indomethacin, producing a fall in urinary prostaglandin metabolite excretion and a variable decrease (but not to normal in any) in blood calcium. Robertson and colleagues (1976) reported six patients treated with aspirin or indomethacin; all six had a decrease in prostagladin levels, but only two had a fall in serum calcium levels. These two patients also were the only ones with elevated blood prostaglandin and hypercalcemia. Combining the patients of Robertson and colleagues and Seyberth and associates, eight patients with elevated prostaglandin levels and hypercalcemia were studied. All eight patients had a lowering of blood calcium in response to indomethacin or aspirin. Since these reports, however, many clinicians have treated hypercalcemic patients with cancer with indomethacin and in general the results are disappointing: Few respond with a return of calcium to normal. Tashjian (1975), in an editorial, comments also that few patients with hypercalcemia and cancer respond to indomethacin.

Metz and colleagues (1981) have thoroughly reviewed the data concerning prostaglandins and hypercalcemia and have come to the conclusion that, considering the data for the animal models of cancer and hypercalcemia, the hypothesis stating prostaglandins produce hypercalcemia is sound. They are uncertain that prostaglandin production is a common cause of hypercalcemia in humans with cancer. Although a few selected patient reports are suggestive or even convincing, the majority of patients do not respond to indomethacin or aspirin. Furthermore, correlation of elevated or normal calcium with elevated or normal prostaglandin levels is poor. Caro and associates (1979) suggest prostaglandin in patients with breast cancer and hypercalcemia may be just a tumor marker, rather than a common cause for hypercalcemia.

A third cause for hypercalcemia of cancer is the production of osteoclast activating factor (OAF). Normally produced by white blood cells (Luben *et al.,* 1974), OAF is a protein of about 20,000 mol wt. Mundy and colleagues (1974) extracted multiple myeloma cells and found large quantities of OAF, using an *in vitro* bioassay based on the release of ^{45}Ca from prelabeled bone. PTH was also found by immunoassay in these extracts, but in amounts too small to produce bone resorption. Prostaglandins could not be detected. Thus, it is inferred that the hypercalcemia of multiple myeloma is caused by increased production of OAF by the neoplastic cells.

Mundy and colleagues (1978) also reported OAF by a lymphosarcoma that caused hypercalcemia. As indicated in Table 6–17, hypercalcemia caused by leukemias and lymphomas is relatively common. It appears likely that production of OAF is common in hematologic cancers.

In summary, three substances produced by cancers have been implicated as causes of hypercalcemia; the data for two of these (PTH and prostaglandin production) are not solid. The third, OAF, appears to be a cause in some hematological cancers producing hypercalcemia. This reviewer favors the hypothesis that most of the cancers causing hypercalcemia produce a substance with biologic properties similar to parathormone but which reacts poorly in immunoassays for parathormone. The latter fact suggests that this material is not structurally identical to parathormone. This hypothesis is based strongly on: (1) Bone biopsy data in patients with hypercalcemia and cancer, which indicate increased osteoclastic activity; (2) the cytochemical data of

Table 6–18. Types of Neoplasms Causing Hypoglycemia

TUMOR TYPES	APPROXIMATE PERCENTAGE OF CASES
Mesenchymal*	62
Hepatic	21
Adrenal carcinomas	6
Miscellaneous (anaplastic carcinomas, adenocarcinomas, pseudomyxomas, cholangiomas)	9

* Included in this category are fibrosarcomas, mesotheliomas, neurofibromas, neurofibrosarcomas, spindle cell sarcomas, rhabdomyosarcomas, and leiomyosarcomas.
From Odell, W. D.: Humoral manifestations of cancer. In Williams, R. H. (ed.): *Textbook of Endocrinology,* 6th ed. W. B. Saunders Company, Philadelphia, 1980.

Goltzman and associates (1981); and (3) the multiple publications of parathormone immunoassay data.

Hypoglycemia

Some neoplasms produce hypoglycemia, often extremely severe, in the host patients. The histologic types of neoplasms differ from the previously discussed syndromes. The approximate distribution of reported cases is listed in Table 6–18. Approximately two-thirds of these reported cases have what is loosely termed a mesothelioma, a designation that includes such entities as fibrosarcomas, neurofibromas, neurofibrosarcomas, rhabdomyosarcomas, leiomyosarcomas, and mesenchymomas. About one-fifth are hepatic carcinomas. The mesothelial tumors are unusually large, ranging from 800 to 10,000 g at the time that symptoms are produced.

The etiology of hypoglycemia, as was true for hypercalcemia, is not fully understood. In summary of many publications, extracts of 25 neoplasms causing hypoglycemia have been studied (Odell, 1974). Using *in vitro* bioassays (rat diaphragm and epididymal fat), insulinlike activity was demonstrated in ten of the 25 extracts. Using the insulin radioimmunoassay, six of the extracts were studied; insulin was not detected in any of these. In three instances, the assays were performed on the same extracts (Field *et al.,* 1963) and insulinlike activity was present by bioassay, but not by immunoassay. These data indicate that the material had biologic properties similar to insulin but was structurally different from insulin.

A family of peptide hormones fitting this description is the somatomedins, also called insulinlike growth factors (IGF) and nonsuppressible insulinlike factors (NSILF). These substances normally are produced by the liver and are intermediators of growth hormone stimulation of body growth. Two insulin-like growth factors are well-known: IGF-I and IGF-II.

Megyesi and associates (1974) studied plasmas from seven of these patients using a radioreceptor assay, developed from liver plasma membranes, that reacted with both IGFs. They reported that five of the seven samples had elevated IGF-like activity; these patients suffered from fibrosarcoma, adrenal cortical carcinoma, hepatoma, and malignant pheochromocytoma (two patients). Gorden and colleagues (1981) studied serum from 52 patients using a radioreceptor assay; 19 (37%) had elevated IGF-like material. Daughaday and associates (1981), using a placental cell membrane radioreceptor assay specific for IGF-II, found elevated IGF-II in ten of 14 serum samples from patients with tumor-related hypoglycemia. Froesch and colleagues (1982) developed separate radioimmunoassays for IGF-I and IGF-II. They reported IGF-II was not elevated in any of 22 patients with cancer-caused hypoglycemia. Furthermore, levels of IGF-I were generally below normal. These same workers, using a radioreceptor assay with receptor prepared from rat liver and iodinating the same NSILA-S preparation used by Gorden and colleagues, failed to show elevated IGF in any patients. Twelve of the same samples studied by Gorden's team were studied.

Thus, for now, the substance produced by these neoplasms causing hypoglycemia remains uncertain. Several substances could be involved. Such substances resemble the IGF in that they possess insulinlike bioactivity, but do not react in insulin radioimmunoassays. Also, according to Froesch and associates, they do not appear to react in IGF radioimmunoassays and are therefore *structurally* different from insulin, IGF-I, and IGF-II.

Hyponatremia Caused by Cancer: Sustained Inappropriate Antidiuretic Hormone (SIADH)

The Schwartz-Bartter syndrome was first described by Schwartz and colleagues (1957) as a tumor-caused humoral syndrome, consisting of hyponatremia, renal sodium loss, hypervolemia, and inappropriately high urine osmolality. Initially, lung cancer production of vasopressin (antidiuretic hormone) was described to cause this syndrome. Lung cancers are the most common type of neoplasm causing this syndrome, but the syndrome may be caused by a variety of neoplasms. SIADH can also be caused by factors other than cancer (*e.g.,* head trauma).

Amatruda and colleagues (1963) and Bower and Mason (1964) extracted tumors from two patients with this syndrome and demonstrated the presence of vasopressin (AVP) activity by means of a bioassay. Vorherr and colleagues (1968) demonstrated that the material extracted from tumors causing this syndrome also reacted in immunoassays for vasopressin. Hirata *et al.* (1976) characterized this vasopressinlike material, further demonstrating that using bioassays, immunoassays, and elution from Sephadex columns, the material was indistinguishable from native AVP. George *et al.* (1972) demonstrated synthesis of AVP by a lung cancer, based on *in vitro* incorporation of amino acids into a peptide that coeluted with AVP on gel chromatography.

The production of vasopressinlike materials by carcinoma of the lung is probably common. Gilby *et al.* (1975) reported that 40% of patients with oat cell carcinoma had SIADH secretion. Studies by Odell *et al.* (1977) showed that when controlled for body position and water intake, 41% of patients with carcinoma of the lung, regardless of histologic type, had elevated plasma ADH measured by radioimmunoassay. Most of the patients studied by Odell *et al.* did not present with the clinical syndrome of hyponatremia, renal sodium loss, hypervolemia, nor inappropriately high urine osmolality. This suggests that water intake and thirst are adjusted by normal control mechanisms in many patients with cancer ADH production.

Sustained ADH secretion in the absence of (excessive) water intake does not produce hyponatremia. Reasoning further, it is possible that patients who present with the clinical syndrome have an additional abnormality in thirst control, which then produces the clinical syndrome. Although lung cancer is the most common neoplasm causing the SIADH syndrome, other neoplasms such as prostate carcinoma, adrenal cortical carcinoma, and Hodgkin's disease also may be associated with the clinical syndrome.

It is important to emphasize that hypovolemia is a common cause of sustained *appropriate* ADH secretion, which at times is difficult to distinguish from SIADH. Although overt clinical signs of hypovolemia may make this diagnosis apparent for some patients, frequently this is not true. Volume control of vasopressin secretion is mediated through baroreceptors in two anatomic areas (*e.q.,* right atrium and carotids). In volume depletion not complicated by diuretic use or salt-losing nephritis, urine sodium concentration would be expected to be low at < 10 mEq/L. A plasma renin concentration is occasionally useful in distinguishing hypovolemia-stimulated sustained ADH secretion from SIADH syndromes. Treatment of the two diseases differs: Fluid restriction for SIADH and volume (saline) expansion for the former.

Growth Hormone (GH) and Growth Hormone Releasing Hormone (GHRH)

GH has been extracted from lung carcinomas (Steiner *et al.,* 1968; Cameron *et al.,* 1971; Beck and Burger, 1972; and Kaganowicz *et al.,* 1979), and gastric carcinoma (Beck and Burger, 1972). With the exception of rare examples of bronchial adenomas and carcinoids, however, neoplasms have not been reported to produce clinical syndromes of GH excess. Kaganowicz *et al.* (1979) studied extracts of numerous tumor and normal tissues. None of the 33 miscellaneous tissues (excluding ovary) contained immunoactive GH. Eight of 118 surgically-removed ovaries contained GH; seven of 29 ovaries with various types of benign tumors and neoplasias had GH at > 10 ng/g. Large amounts of GH (511,000, 350,000, 5000, and 4900 ng/g) were present in extracts from four tumors: An ovary in a patient with endometriosis, an ovary containing a serous cystadenoma, an ovarian metastases from breast cancer, and skin metastases from breast cancer. From these data, it seems reasonable to believe that GH is synthesized by some neoplasms in large quantities. Control data showed that this was not artifact due to ^{125}I-GH degradation by the extracts.

Studies by Kyle *et al.* (1981) showed that 30% ETOH–70% Tris buffer extracts of virtually every tissue obtained from normal human subjects dying traumatically contained small amounts of GH-like material. This GH was identical to highly purified pituitary GH as assessed by radioimmunoassay, radioreceptor assay using hepatic cell receptors, and by Sephadex chromatography. The amounts of GH-like material in human tissues averaged 5 to 10 ng/g tissue — much less than the tumor extracts discussed previously. The fact that normal tissues did not contain detectable GH in the studies of Kaganowicz *et al.* (1979), whereas all tissues did in the studies of Kyle and colleagues (1981), is probably explained by differences in extraction techniques and assay sensitivity.

Careful studies of GH plasma concentrations and control dynamics have not been performed in cancer patients. Thus, whether or not cancers secrete this GH-like material is uncertain. As indicated before, clinical signs and symptoms of excess GH secretion are not present in cancer patients.

In contrast to the previous discussion, a small number of patients have been described with acromegaly in association with bronchial carcinoids or gut carcinoids (Weiss and Ingram, 1961; Dabek, 1974; Sonksen *et al.,* 1976; Leveston *et al.,* 1978, 1981; Saeed uz Zafar *et al.,* 1979). In at least five patients, normal GH secretion was restored and/or the clinical syndrome of acromegaly subsided following removal of the carcinoid. In most of these patients, no therapy was directed against the pituitary gland itself, suggesting that the carcinoid tumor caused the pituitary adenoma and acromegaly.

Saeed uz Zafar and associates (1979) extracted a carcinoid from one patient with this syndrome and demonstrated potent GH-releasing factor (GHRF) activity. Frohman and colleagues (1980) partially purified this GHRF from carcinoid and pancreatic islet tumors from three patients with this syndrome, showing that it was a peptide with molecular weight of about 6000. The findings of Frohman and

associates (1980) are of major interest to endocrinologists because they demonstrate that constant excess of GHRF can lead to formation of a pituitary adenoma.

Corticotropin-Releasing Hormone

Cushing's syndrome has also been reported to be caused by bronchial carcinoids (Cohen *et al.,* 1960; Riggs and Sprague, 1961; Steel *et al.,* 1967; Strott *et al.,* 1968; Jones *et al.,* 1969; Mason *et al.,* 1972). Approximately half of the patients with this tumor and syndrome, and a few with carcinoma-caused Cushing's syndrome, show suppression of serum cortisol with high dose dexamethasone treatment or response to metyrapone (Cohen *et al.,* 1960; Riggs and Sprague, 1961, Steel *et al.,* 1967; Strott *et al.,* 1968; Jones *et al.,* 1969; Upton and Amatruda, 1971; Mason *et al.,* 1972). Neither the dexamethasone suppression nor response to metyrapone is expected in ectopic ACTH syndrome. Extracts of some bronchial carcinoids have contained large amounts of ACTH (Steel *et al.,* 1967; Strott *et al.,* 1968; Jones *et al.,* 1960). ACTH production, however, does not seem the likely cause in patients with bronchial carcinoids and Cushing's syndrome who show suppression of cortisol production with dexamethasone treatment or response to metyrapone. Carcinoid production of the hypothalamic peptide corticotropin-releasing hormone (CRH) would be compatible with these findings. As normally secreted by the hypothalamus, CRH is a 41 amino acid peptide that controls pituitary secretion of ACTH (Vale *et al.,* 1981). The action of CRH on the pituitary gland is inhibited at a pituitary level by either excess cortisol or dexamethasone. Upton and Amatruda (1971) extracted two tumors (a pancreatic and a small cell lung carcinoma) from patients responding to metyrapone and demonstrated the presence of CRH. Bronchial adenoma production of CRH has apparently not been proven directly. Thus far, a bronchial carcinoid-producing CRH, which in turn produces an ACTH-secreting pituitary adenoma, has not been described. Based on the acromegaly cases just reviewed, however, such cases may exist.

Calcitonin

This peptide hormone is normally secreted by the parafollicular cells of the thyroid and also by medullary carcinomas that develop from those cells. Medullary carcinoma occurs sporadically or as part of the multiple endocrine neoplasia syndromes, types IIA and IIB (hyperparathyroidism, medullary carcinoma, and pheochromocytoma). Calcitonin stimulates calcium incorporation into bone and, together with parathormone and the D vitamins, modulates serum calcium concentration. Hypersecretion of calcitonin in adults does not appear to produce symptoms or hypocalcemia, probably because parathormone and D vitamins can compensate to maintain calcium at normal values.

Calcitonin is also produced ectopically by a variety of neoplasms. The first series of patients with cancer in whom plasma calcitonin was studied was published by Coombes et al. (1974) and Hillyard et al. (1976). These workers reported that extracts of breast carcinoma contained immunoreactive calcitonin and that about 60% of patients with both carcinoma of the lung and breast had elevated plasma calcitonin. Schwartz et al. (1979) prospectively studied 240 patients admitted to the hospital for problems suggesting or possibly suggesting cancer. Of 123 patients subsequently shown to have a carcinoma, 40 had highly elevated calcitonin. Eight percent (19/49) of patients with carcinoma of the lung (regardless of histologic type), 24% with colon carcinoma (7/29), 38% with breast carcinoma (8/21), and 42% of patients with pancreatic carcinoma (6/14) had elevated values. No patient was hypocalcemic or hypercalcemic.

It is not certain that this calcitonin is being produced by the neoplasm in all cases. Silva et al. (1975) demonstrated, by selective thyroidal vein catheterization in a patient with cancer and hypercalcitonemia, that the normal thyroid was the source in this patient. Perhaps in some patients the cancer produces a substance that stimulates parafollicular cell secretion of calcitonin, whereas direct tumor production occurs in others. Further studies are required to resolve this issue.

Hypophosphatemia

A rare but clinically striking syndrome produced by tumor is hypophosphatemia. Symptoms usually consist of profound muscle spasm and osteopenia with bone fractures. The hypophosphatemia is caused by tumor production of a substance that produces profound phosphate loss in the urine. Parathormone and calcium concentrations are normal. It is likely that many patients with this syndrome have been erroneously reported in the literature to have adult onset vitamin D–resistant rickets. The types of neoplasms causing this syndrome are frequently unusual— pleomorphic sarcomas, mesenchymal (e.g., sclerosing hemangiomas) neoplasms, giant cell tumors of bone, and, rarely, leukemias or disseminated carcinomas. In the two latter cases, the mechanisms may or may not be the same. Drezner and Feinglos (1977) first suggested that the tumor produced a substance that inhibited one hydroxylation of vitamin D. Their patient was a 42-year-old woman with this syndrome caused by a giant cell tumor of bone. Plasma PTH, measured by both carboxyl and amino terminal immunoassays, was normal; serum 25 hydroxy vitamin D was normal, but concentrations of 1,25 dihydroxy vitamin D were consistently low in plasma. Treatment with high doses of 1,25 D (3 μg) abolished symptoms and returned phosphorus to normal. After relapse, when 1,25 D was discontinued, resection of the tumor again abolished hypophosphatemia and symptoms.

A second case caused by multicentric sclerosing hemangiomas of bone was studied by Daniels and Weisenfeld (1979). This patient was treated with phosphosoda and 100,000 units of vitamin D (probably vitamin D_2), with remission of hypophosphatemia. Fukumoto et al. (1979) had a patient with the same syndrome caused by a benign osteoblastoma. In addition to phosphaturia, however, this patient also had aminoaciduria and glycosuria, indicating more diffuse proximal renal tubular resorptive abnormalities. As in the patient tested by Drezner and Feinglos, serum 25 hydroxy vitamin D was normal, whereas 1,25 D was low. Treatment with 300,000 IU of ergocalciferol failed to improve phosphorus loss, whereas 1,25 vitamin D partially corrected the hypophosphatemia. When the tumor was resected, however, serum phosphorus returned to normal. The nature of the substance causing the phosphorus (and in some patients amino acid and glucose) wasting is unknown. Based on the data reviewed for other ectopic endocrine syndromes, it is presumably a protein or peptide affecting proximal renal tubular function.

The APUD Concept and Ectopic Endocrine Syndromes

An attractive hypothesis was derived from the work of Pearse in 1976 to explain the ectopic endocrine syndromes. This hypothesis, termed the APUD concept, stated that normal peptide hormone-secreting cells are derived from the neural crest and have some chemical and morphologic characteristics in common. They are capable of *amine precursor uptake and decarboxylation* (APUD). Because APUD cells are widely spread throughout tissues, it was suggested that when they become neoplastic they secrete peptide hormones ectopically. Not all APUD cells are derived from the neural crest; some, for example, are found in the gut and are of endodermal origin. Nevertheless, the hypothesis continues that such "endocrine" cells are present in many tissues that could be involved in ectopic hormone production.

Odell *et al.* (1977), Odell (1980), Odell and Wolfsen (1980) and Odell and Saito (1982) offer another hypothesis. The data leading to this hypothesis have been reviewed in part in this chapter. Protein hormonelike materials or protein hormone precursors have been extracted from virtually all normal human (and in some cases animal) tissues. The hormones now include hormones resembling or identical to HCG, ProACTH, GH, and calcitonin. Whereas a subgroup of cells (APUD) within these normal tissues could be responsible for the presence of these "normal tissue" hormones, we believe they are produced by these various tissues themselves. Furthermore, as was reviewed previously, insulin also has been recovered from virtually all tissues and was shown to be produced by white cells *in vitro* (Fukumoto *et al.,* 1979; LeRoith *et al.,* 1981a,b). Still again, HCG and insulin have been shown to be produced by several nonvertebrates, including bacteria, annelids, and protozoa (Rosenzweig *et al.,* 1980; LeRoith *et al.,* 1981a,b).

These data, taken together, suggest that protein hormones are widespread in nature and in normal tissues. Either they are old phylogenetically or a genetic exchange has occurred from mammals to these nonvertebrates at a later phylogenetic stage. Acevedo and colleagues (1978a,b) have suggested that the latter is true to explain HCG presence in bacteria, and, furthermore, they postulate that the bacterial HCG-like material promotes tumorogenesis. If one of these hypotheses is true, the APUD concept becomes less attractive.

HYPOTHESIS

Based on the data reviewed in this chapter, we hypothesize:

1. All normal tissues synthesize small amounts of protein hormonelike materials. Most are biologically inert or weakly biologically active;
2. Most neoplasms produce larger quantities of these same peptides or proteins;
3. Selected neoplasms metabolize these peptides to biologically active hormones. This metabolism property consists of increased specific enzyme activity (for example, to convert ProACTH to ACTH or to gycosylate HCG) and correlates with the histologic type of neoplasm; and
4. "Ectopic" hormone production is not ectopic.

REFERENCES

Acevedo, H. F.; Slifkin, M.; Pouchet, G. R.; and Pardo, M.: Immunohistochemical localization of a choriogonadotropin-like protein in bacteria isolated from cancer patients. *Cancer,* **41:**1217–1229, 1978a.

Acevedo, H. F.; Slifkin, M.; Pouchet, G. R.; and Rakhshan, M.: Human chorionic gonadotropin in cancer cells. I. Identification in in vitro and in vivo cancer cell systems. In Nieburgs, H. R. (ed.): *Detection and Prevention of Cancer.* Part 2, Vol. I. Marcel Dekker, Inc., New York, 1978b.

Albright, F. (discussant): Case records of the Massachusetts General Hospital. Case 27461. *N. Engl. J. Med.,* **225:**789–791, 1941.

Amatruda, T. T., Jr.; Mulrow, P. J.; Gallagher, J. C.; and Sawyer, W. H.: Carcinoma of the lung with inappropriate antidiuresis. *N. Engl. J. Med.,* **269:**544–549, 1963.

Arnaud, C. D.: Hypercalcemia. *Postgraduate Assembly of the Endocrine Society, Thirty-Third Annual Program, San Diego, California, November 9–13, 1981,* Endocrine Society, Bethesda, MD, 1981, p 430.

Beck, C., and Burger, H. G.: Evidence for the presence of immunoreactive growth hormone in cancers of the lung and stomach. *Cancer,* **30:**75–79, 1972.

Bender, R. A., and Hansen, H.: Hypercalcemia in bronchogenic carcinoma. A study of 200 patients. *Ann. Intern. Med.,* **80:**205–208, 1974.

Benson, R. C., Jr.; Riggs, B. L.; Pickard, B. M.; and Arnaud, C. D.: Immunoreactive forms of circulating parathyroid hormone in primary and ectopic hyperparathyroidism. *J. Clin. Invest.,* **54:**175–181, 1974a.

Benson, R. C., Jr.; Riggs, B. L.; Pickard, B. M.; and Arnaud, C. D.: Radioimmunoassay of parathyroid hormone in hypercalcemic patients with malignant disease. *Am. J. Med.,* **56:**821–826, 1974b.

Berson, S. A., and Yalow, R. S.: Parathyroid hormone in plasma in adenomatous hyperparathyroidism, uremia, and bronchogenic carcinoma. *Science,* **154:**907–909, 1966.

Bloomfield, G. A.; Holdaway, I. M.; Corrin, B.; Ratcliffe, J. G.; Rees, G. M.; Ellison, M.; and Rees, L. H.: Lung tumors and ACTH production. *Clin. Endocrinol.,* **6:**95–104, 1977.

Bower, B. F., and Mason, D. M.: Measurement of antidiuretic activity (ADA) in plasma and tumor in carcinoma of the lung with inappropriate antidiuresis. *Clin. Res.,* **12:**121(A), 1964.

Braunstein, G. D.; Rasor, J.; and Wade, M. E.: Presence in normal human testes of chorionic-gonadotropin-like substance distinct from human luteinizing hormone. *N. Engl. J. Med.,* **293**:1339–1343, 1975.

Braunstein, G. D.; Vaitukaitis, J. L.; Carbone, P. P.; and Ross, G. T.: Ectopic production of human chorionic gonadotrophin by neoplasms. *Ann. Intern. Med.,* **78**:39–45, 1973.

Brown, W. H.: A case of pluriglandular syndrome: Diabetes of bearded women. *Lancet,* **215**:1022–1023, 1928.

Buckle, R. M.; McMillan, M.; and Mallinson, C.: Ectopic secretion of parathyroid hormone by a renal adenocarcinoma in a patient with hypercalcaemia. *Br. Med. J.,* **4**:724–726, 1970.

Cameron, D. P.; Burger, H. G.; DeKretzer, D. M.; Catt, K. J.; and Best, J. B.: On the presence of immunoreactive growth hormone in a bronchogenic carcinoma. *Aust. Ann. Med.,* **18**:143–146, 1971.

Caro, J. F.; Besarab, A.; and Flynn, J. T.: Prostaglandin E and hypercalcemia in breast carcinoma: Only a tumor marker? *Am. J. Med.,* **66**:337–341, 1979.

Cohen, H., and Strampp, A.: Bacterial synthesis of substance similar to human chorionic gonadotropin. *Proc. Soc. Exp. Biol. Med.,* **152**:408–410, 1976.

Cohen, R. B.; Toll, G. D.; and Castleman, B.: Bronchial adenomas in Cushing's syndrome: Their relation to thymomas and oat cell carcinomas associated with hyperadrenocorticism. *Cancer,* **13**:812–817, 1960.

Cole, L. A.; Birken, S.; Sutphen, S.; Hussa, R. O.; and Patillo, R. A.: Absence of the COOH-terminal peptide on ectopic human chorionic gonadotropin β-subunit (hCGβ). *Endocrinology,* **110**:2198–2200, 1982.

Cole, L. A., and Hussa, R. O.: Use of glycosidase digested human chorionic gonadotropin beta-subunit to explain the partial binding of ectopic glycoprotein hormones to Con A. *Endocrinology,* **109**:2276–2278, 1981.

Coombes, R. C.; Hillyard, C.; Greenberg, P. B.; and MacIntyre, I.: Plasma-immunoreactive-calcitonin in patients with non-thyroid tumours. *Lancet,* **1**:1080–1083, 1974.

Dabek, J. T.: Bronchial carcinoid tumour with acromegaly in two patients. *J. Clin. Endocrinol. Metab.,* **38**:329–333, 1974.

Daniels, R. A., and Weisenfeld, I.: Tumorous phosphaturic osteomalacia. Report of a case associated with multiple hemangiomas of bone. *Am. J. Med.,* **67**:155–159, 1979.

Daughaday, W. H.; Trivedi, B.; and Kapadia, M.: Measurement of insulin-like growth factor II by a specific radioreceptor assay in serum of normal individuals, patients with abnormal growth hormone secretion, and patients with tumor-associated hypoglycemia. *J. Clin. Endocrinol. Metab.,* **53**:289–294, 1981.

Drezner, M. K., and Feinglos, M. N.: Osteomalacia due to 1α,25-dihydroxy-cholecalciferol deficiency. Association with a giant cell tumor of bone. *J. Clin. Invest.,* **60**:1046–1053, 1977.

Drezner, M. K., and Lebovitz, H. E.: Primary hyperparathyroidism in paraneoplastic hypercalcaemia. *Lancet,* **1**:1004–1006, 1978.

Eipper, B. A., and Mains, R. E.: Structure and biosynthesis of proadrenocorticotropin/endorphin and related peptides. *Endocr. Rev.,* **1**:1–27, 1980.

Eipper, B. A.; Mains, R. E.; and Guenzi, D.: High molecular weight forms of adrenocorticotropic hormone are glycoproteins. *J. Biol. Chem.,* **251**:4121–4126, 1976.

Field, J. B.; Keen, H.; Johnson, P.; and Herring, B.: Insulinlike activity of nonpancreatic tumors associated with hypoglycemia. *J. Clin. Endocrinol. Metab.,* **23**:1229–1236, 1963.

Franklin, R. B., and Tashjian, A. H., Jr.: Intravenous infusion of prostaglandin E_2 raises plasma calcium concentration in the rat. *Endocrinology,* **97**:240–243, 1975.

Froesch, E. R.; Zapf, J.; and Widmer, U.: Hypoglycemia associated with non-islet-cell tumor and insulin-like growth factors. *N. Engl. J. Med.,* **306**:1178, 1982.

Frohman, L. A.; Szabo, M.; and Berelowitz, M.: Partial purification and characterization of a peptide with growth hormone-releasing activity from extrapituitary tumors in patients with acromegaly. *J. Clin. Invest.,* **65**:43–54, 1980.

Fukumoto, Y.; Tarui, S.; Tsukiyama, K.; Ichihara, K.; Moriwaki, K.; Nonaka, K.; Mizushima, T.; Kobayashi, Y.; Dokoh, S.; Fukunaga, M.; and Morita, R.: Tumor-induced vitamin D-resistant hypophosphatemic osteomalacia associated with proximal renal tubular dysfunction and 1,25-dihydroxyvitamin D deficiency. *J. Clin. Endocrinol. Metab.,* **49**:873–878, 1979.

George, J. M.; Capen, C. C.; and Phillips, A. S.: Biosynthesis of vasopressin *in vitro* and ultrastructure of a bronchogenic carcinoma. Patient with the syndrome of inappropriate secretion of antidiuretic hormone. *J. Clin. Invest.,* **51**:141–148, 1972.

Gewirtz, G., and Yalow, R. S.: Ectopic ACTH production in carcinoma of the lung. *J. Clin. Invest.,* **53**:1022–1032, 1974.

Gilby, E. D.; Rees, L. H.; and Bondy, P. K.: Proceedings of the 6th International Symposium on Biology and Characterization of Human Tumours. In Davis, W.; Maltoni, C. (eds.): *Advances in Tumour Prevention, Detection and Characterization,* Vol. 3. Elsevier North-Holland, Inc., New York, 1975.

Goltzman, D.; Stewart, A. F.; and Broadus, A. E.: Malignancy-associated hypercalcemia: Evaluation with a cytochemical bioassay for parathyroid hormone. *J. Clin. Endocrinol. Metab.,* **53**:899–904, 1981.

Gorden, P.; Hendricks, C. M.; Kahn, C. R.; Megyesi, K.; and Roth, J.: Hypoglycemia associated with non-islet-cell tumor and insulin-like growth factors. *N. Engl. J. Med.,* **305**:1452–1455, 1981.

Habener, J. F.; Kemper, B.; Potts, J. T., Jr.; and Rich, A.: Proparathyroid hormone: Biosynthesis by human parathyroid adenomas. *Science,* **178**:630–633, 1972.

Habener, J. F.; Kemper, B.; Potts, J. T., Jr.; and Rich, A.: Pre-proparathyroid hormone identified by cell-free translation of messenger RNA from hyperplastic human parathyroid tissue. *J. Clin. Invest.,* **56**:1328–1333, 1975.

Hillyard, C. J.; Coombes, R. C.; Greenberg, P. B.; Galante, L. S.; and MacIntyre, I.: Calcitonin in breast and lung cancer. *Clin. Endocrinol.,* **5**:1–8, 1976.

Hirata, Y.; Matsukura, S.; Imura, H.; Yakura, T.; Ihjima, S.; Nagase, C.; and Itoh, M.: Two cases of multiple hormone-producing small cell carcinoma of the lung. *Cancer,* **38**:2575–2582, 1976.

Ito, H.; Sanada, T.; Katayama, T.; and Shimazaki, J.: Indomethacin-responsive hypercalcemia. *N. Engl. J. Med.,* **293**:558–559, 1975.

Jones, J. E.; Shane, S. R.; Gilbert, E.; and Flink, E. B.: Cushing's syndrome induced by the ectopic production of ACTH by a bronchial carcinoid. *J. Clin. Endocrinol. Metab.,* **29**:1–5, 1969.

Kaganowicz, A.; Farkouh, N. H.; Frantz, A. G.; and Blaustein, A. U.: Ectopic human growth hormone in ovaries and breast cancer. *J. Clin. Endocrinol. Metab.,* **48**:5–8, 1979.

Kato, Y.; Ferguson, T. B.; Bennett, D. E.; and Burford,

T. H.: Oat cell carcinoma of the lung. A review of 138 cases. *Cancer,* **23:**517–524, 1969.

Kolata, G.: New theory of hormones proposed. *Science,* **215:**1383, 1982.

Kyle, C. V.; Evans, M. C.; and Odell, W. D.: Growth hormone-like material in normal human tissues. *J. Clin. Endocrinol. Metab.,* **53:**1138–1144, 1981.

LeRoith, D.; Lesniak, M. A.; and Roth, J.: Insulin in insects and annelids. *Diabetes,* **30:**70–76, 1981.

LeRoith, D.; Shiloack, J.; Roth, J.; and Lesniak, M. A.: Insulin or a closely related molecule is native to *Escherichia coli. J. Biol. Chem.,* **256:**6533–6536, 1981b.

Leveston, S. A.; Lee, Y. C.; Jaffee, B. M.; and Daughaday, W. H.: Massive GH and ACTH hypersecretion associated with metastatic carcinoid tumor. *Program of the 60th Annual Endocrine Society Meeting,* 1978. Abstract #593. Endocrine Society, Bethesda, MD, 1978.

Leveston, S. A.; McKeel, D. W., Jr.; Buckley, P. J.; Deschryver, K.; Greider, M. H.; Jaffe, B. M.; and Daughaday, W. H.: Acromegaly and Cushing's syndrome associated with a foregut carcinoid tumor. *J. Clin. Endocrinol. Metab.,* **53:**682–689, 1981.

Liddle, G. W.; Nicholson, W. E.; Island, D. P.; Orth, D. N.; Abe, K.; and Lowder, S. C.: Clinical and laboratory studies of ectopic humoral syndromes. *Recent Prog. Horm. Res.,* **25:**283–314, 1969.

Livingston, V. W. C., and Livingston, A. M.: Some cultural, immunological, and biochemical properties of *Progenitor cryptocides. Trans. N.Y. Acad. Sci.,* **36:**569–582, 1974.

Luben, R. A.; Mundy, G. R.; Trummel, C. L.; and Raisz, L. G.: Partial purification of osteoclast-activating factor from phytohemagglutinin-stimulated human leukocytes. *J. Clin. Invest.,* **53:**1473–1480, 1974.

Mains, R. E., and Eipper, B. A.: Biosynthesis of adrenocorticotropic hormone in mouse pituitary tumor cells. *J. Biol. Chem.,* **251:**4115–4120, 1976.

Maruo, T.; Cohen, H.; Segal, S. J.; and Koide, S. S.: Production of choriogonadotropin-like factor by a microorganism. *Proc. Natl. Acad. Sci. USA,* **76:**6622–6626, 1979.

Mason, A. M. S.; Ratcliffe, J. G.; Buckle, R. M.; and Mason, A. S.: ACTH secretion by bronchial carcinoid tumours. *Clin. Endocrinol. (Oxf.),* **1:**3–25, 1972.

Megyesi, K.; Kahn, C. R.; Roth, J.; and Gorden, P.: Hypoglycemia in association with extrapancreatic tumors: Demonstration of elevated plasma NSILA-s by a new radioreceptor assay. *J. Clin. Endocrinol. Metab.,* **38:**931–934, 1974.

Metz, S. A.; McRae, J. R.; and Robertson, R. P.: Prostaglandins as mediators of paraneoplastic syndromes: Review and update. *Metabolism,* **30:**299, 1981.

Mundy, G. R.; Raisz, L. G.; Cooper, R. A.; Schechter, G. P.; and Salmon, S. E.: Evidence for the secretion of an osteoclast stimulating factor in myeloma. *N. Engl. J. Med.,* **291:**1041–1046, 1974.

Mundy, G. R.; Rick, M. E.; Turcotte, R.; and Kowalski, M. A.: Pathogenesis of hypercalcemia in lymphosarcoma cell leukemia. Role of an osteoclast activating factor-like substance and a mechanism of action for glucocorticoid therapy. *Am. J. Med.,* **65:**600–606, 1978.

Odell, W. D.: Humoral manifestations of non-endocrine neoplasms. In Williams, R. H. (ed.): *Textbook of Endocrinology,* 5th ed. W. B. Saunders Company, Philadelphia, 1974.

Odell, W. D.: Humoral manifestations of cancer. In Williams, R. H. (ed.): *Textbook of Endocrinology.* 6th ed. W. B. Saunders Company, Philadelphia, 1980.

Odell, W. D., and Evans, M. C.: Characterization of hepatic chorionic gonadotropin-like material. *Fertil. Steril.,* **34:**300, 1980 (abstract).

Odell, W. D.; Hertz, R.; Lipsett, M. B.; Ross, G. T.; and Hammond, C. B.: Endocrine aspects of trophoblastic neoplasms. *Clin. Obstet. Gynecol.,* **10:**290–302, 1967.

Odell, W. D., and Saito, E.: Protein hormone-like materials from normal and cancer cells—"Ectopic" hormone production. 13th International Cancer Congress, Part E. *Cancer Management,* Alan R. Liss, New York, 1983, p. 247.

Odell, W. D., and Wolfsen, A. R.: Hormones from tumors: Are they ubiquitous? (Editorial). *Am. J. Med.,* **68:**317–318, 1980.

Odell, W.; Wolfsen, A.; Yoshimoto, Y.; Weitzman, R.; Fisher, D.; and Hirose, F.: Ectopic peptide synthesis. A universal concomitant of neoplasia. *Trans. Assoc. Am. Physicians,* **90:**204–227, 1977.

Paul, W. E., and Odell, W. D.: Radiation inactivation of the immunological and biological activities of human chorionic gonadotropin. *Nature,* **203:**979–980, 1964.

Pearse, A. G. E., and Takor Takor, T.: Neuroendocrine embryology and the APUD concept. *Clin. Endocrinol.,* **5(suppl):**229–244, 1976.

Powell, D.; Singer, F. R.; Murray, T. M.; Minkin, C.; and Potts, J. T., Jr.: Nonparathyroid humoral hypercalcemia in patients with neoplastic diseases. *N. Engl. J. Med.,* **289:**176–181, 1973.

Raisz, L. G.; Yajnik, C. H.; Bockman, R. S.; and Bower, B. F.: Comparison of commercially available parathyroid hormone immunoassays in the differential diagnosis of hypercalcemia due to primary hyperparathyroidism or malignancy. *Ann. Intern. Med.,* **91:**739–740, 1979.

Ratcliffe, J. G.; Knight, R. A.; Besser, G. M.; Landon, J.; and Stansfeld, A. G.: Tumour and plasma ACTH concentrations in patients with and without the ectopic ACTH syndrome. *Clin. Endocrinol. (Oxf.),* **1:**27–44, 1972.

Riggs, B. L., Jr., and Sprague, R. G.: Association of Cushing's syndrome and neoplastic disease. *Arch. Intern. Med.,* **108:**841–849, 1961.

Robertson, R. P.; Baylink, D. J.; Marini, J. J.; and Adkison, H. W.: Elevated prostaglandins and suppressed parathyroid hormone associated with hypercalcemia and renal cell carcinoma. *J. Clin. Endocrinol. Metab.,* **41:**164–167, 1975.

Robertson, R. P.; Baylink, D. J.; Metz, S. A.; and Cummings, K. B.: Plasma prostaglandin E in patients with cancer with and without hypercalcemia. *J. Clin. Endocrinol. Metab.,* **43:**1330–1335, 1976.

Rosenzweig, J. L.; Havrankova, J.; Lesniak, M. A.; Brownstein, M.; and Roth, J.: Insulin is ubiquitous in extrapancreatic tissues of rats and humans. *Proc. Natl. Acad. Sci. USA,* **77:**572–576, 1980.

Saeed uz Zafar, M.; Mellinger, R. C.; Fine, G.; Szabo, M.; and Frohman, L. A.: Acromegaly associated with a bronchial carcinoid tumor: Evidence for ectopic production of growth hormone-releasing activity. *J. Clin. Endocrinol. Metab.,* **48:**66–71, 1979.

Saito, E., and Odell, W. D.: Widespread presence of large molecular weight adrenocorticotropin-like substances in normal rat extrapituitary tissues. *Endocrinology,* **113:**1010, 1983.

Saito, E., and Odell, W. D.: Corticotropin/lipotropin common precursor-like material in normal rat extrapituitary tissues. *Proc. Natl. Acad. Sci. USA,* **80:**3792, 1983.

Schwartz, K. E.; Wolfsen, A. R.; Forster, B.; and Odell,

W. D.: Calcitonin in nonthyroidal cancer. *J. Clin. Endocrinol. Metab.,* **49:**438–444, 1979.

Schwartz, W. B.; Bennett, W.; Curelop, S.; and Bartter, F. C.: A syndrome of renal sodium loss and hyponatremia probably resulting from inappropriate secretion of antidiuretic hormone. *Am. J. Med.,* **23:**529–542, 1957.

Seyberth, H. W.; Segre, G. V.; Morgan, J. L.; Sweetman, B. J.; Potts, J. T., Jr.; and Oates, J. A.: Prostaglandins as mediators of hypercalcemia associated with certain types of cancer. *N. Engl. J. Med.,* **293:**1278–1283, 1975.

Sherwood, L. M.; O'Riordan, J. L. H.; Aurbach, G. D.; and Potts, J. T., Jr.: Production of parathyroid hormone by nonparathyroid tumors. *J. Clin. Endocrinol. Metab.,* **27:**140–146, 1967.

Silva, O. L.; Becker, K. L.; Primack, A.; Doppman, J. L.; and Snider, R. H.: Hypercalcitonemia in bronchogenic cancer. Evidence for thyroid origin of the hormone. *J.A.M.A.,* **234:**183–185, 1975.

Skrabanek, P.; McPartlin, J.; and Powell, D.: Tumor hypercalcemia and "ectopic hyperparathyroidism." *Medicine (Baltimore),* **59:**262–282, 1980.

Slifkin, M.; Acevedo, H. F.; Pardo, M.; Pouchet, G. R.; and Rakhshan, M.: Human chorionic gonadotropin in cancer cells. II. Ultrastructural localization. In Nieburgs, H. R. (ed.): *Detection and Prevention of Cancer.* Part 2, Vol. I. Marcel Dekker, Inc., New York, 1978.

Sonksen, P. H.; Ayres, A. B.; Braimbridge, M.; Corrin, B.; Davies, D. R.; Jeremiah, G. M.; Oaten, S. W.; Lowy, C.; and West, T. E. T.: Acromegaly caused by pulmonary carcinoid tumours. *Clin. Endocrinol. (Oxf.),* **5:**503–513, 1976.

Sparagana, M.; Phillips, G.; Hoffman, C.; and Kucera, L.: Ectopic growth hormone syndrome associated with lung cancer. *Metabolism,* **20:**730–736, 1971.

Steel, K.; Baerg, R. D.; and Adams, D. O.: Cushing's syndrome in association with a carcinoid tumor of the lung. *J. Clin. Endocrinol. Metab.,* **27:**1285–1289, 1967.

Steiner, H.; Dahlback, O.; and Waldenstrom, J.: Ectopic growth-hormone production and osteoarthropathy in carcinoma of the bronchus. *Lancet,* **1:**783–785, 1968.

Strott, C. A.; Nugent, C. A.; and Tyler, F. H.: Cushing's syndrome caused by bronchial adenomas. *Am. J. Med.,* **44:**97–104, 1968.

Tashjian, A. H., Jr.: Prostaglandins, hypercalcemia and cancer (editorial). *N. Engl. J. Med.,* **293:**1317–1318, 1975.

Tashjian, A. H., Jr.; Levine, L.; and Munson, P. L.: Immunochemical identification of parathyroid hormone in non-parathyroid neoplasms associated with hypercalcemia. *J. Exp. Med.,* **119:**467–484, 1964.

Tashjian, A. H., Jr.; Voelkel, E. F.; Levine, L.; and Goldhaber, P.: Evidence that the bone resorption-stimulating factor produced by mouse fibrosarcoma cells is prostaglandin E_2. A new model for the hypercalcemia of cancer. *J. Exp. Med.,* **136:**1329–1343, 1972.

Tsuruhara, T.; Dufau, M. L.; Hickman, J.; and Catt, K. J.: Biological properties of hCG after removal of terminal sialic acid and galactose residues. *Endocrinology,* **91:**296–301, 1972.

Upton, G. V., and Amatruda, T. T., Jr.: Evidence for the presence of tumor peptides with corticotropin-releasing-factor-like activity in the ectopic ACTH syndrome. *N. Engl. J. Med.,* **285:**419–424, 1971.

Vaitukaitis, J. L.; Braunstein, G. D.; and Ross, G. T.: A radioimmunoassay which specifically measures human chorionic gonadotropin in the presence of human luteinizing hormone. *Am. J. Obstet. Gynecol.,* **113:**751–758, 1972.

Vale, W.; Spiess, J.; Rivier, C.; and Rivier, J.: Characterization of a 41-residue ovine hypothalamic peptide that stimulates secretion of corticotropin and β-endorphin. *Science,* **213:**1394–1397, 1981.

Voelkel, E. F.; Tashjian, A. H., Jr.; Franklin, R.; Wasserman, E.; and Levine, L.: Hypercalcemia and tumor-prostaglandins: The VX2 carcinoma model in the rabbit. *Metabolism,* **24:**973–986, 1975.

Vorherr, H.; Massry, S. G.; Utiger, R. D.; and Kleeman, C. R.: Antidiuretic principle in malignant tumor extracts from patients with inappropriate ADH syndrome. *J. Clin. Endocrinol. Metab.,* **28:**162–168, 1968.

Warwick, O. H.; Yendt, E. R.; and Olin, J. S.: The clinical features of hypercalcemia associated with malignant disease. *Can. Med. Assoc. J.,* **85:**719–723, 1961.

Weiss, L., and Ingram, M.: Adenomatoid bronchial tumors. A consideration of the carcinoid tumors and the salivary tumors of the bronchial tree. *Cancer,* **14:**161–178, 1961.

Wolfsen, A. R., and Odell, W. D.: ProACTH: Use for early detection of lung cancer. *Am. J. Med.,* **66:**765–772, 1979.

Yoshimoto, Y.; Odell, W. D.; and Fugita, T.: Human chorionic gonadotropin-like substance in non-mammalian vertebrates and mammalians other than humans. Program of the 6th International Congress of Endocrinology (Abstract), 1980.

Yoshimoto, Y.; Wolfsen, A.; Hirose, F.; and Odell, W. D.: Human chorionic gonadotropin-like material: Presence in normal human tissue. *Am. J. Obstet. Gynecol.,* **134:**729–733, 1979a.

Yoshimoto, Y.; Wolfsen, A. R.; and Odell, W. D.: Human chorionic gonadotropin-like substance in nonendocrine tissues of normal subjects. *Science,* **197:**575–577, 1977.

Yoshimoto, Y.; Wolfsen, A. R.; and Odell, W. D.: Glycosylation, a variable in the production of hCG by cancers. *Am. J. Med.,* **67:**414–420, 1979b.

7

Principles of Management

SAUL A. ROSENBERG, PHILIP S. SCHEIN, and PAUL CALABRESI

The oncologist should adhere to certain general principles of management to provide patients with the best possible care. These principles can be divided into the following considerations:

1. Establishment of the diagnosis
2. Determination of the extent of disease
3. Curative versus palliative therapy
4. Establishment of recurrence after potentially curative therapy
5. Supportive care
6. Record keeping and communications

These subjects are discussed, in more or less detail, in chapters that deal with specific disease sites, treatment modalities, and areas of supportive care. This is a general overview expressing the editors' principles of management.

The essential starting point in any case is the establishment of the diagnosis of cancer by a competent pathologist. The majority of patients are referred to the medical oncologist after a diagnosis of cancer has been made or is strongly suspected. The diagnosis of cancer, and the determination of the type of cancer, cannot be established without an appropriate biopsy and study by an experienced pathologist. There may be clinical presentations that make the diagnosis of cancer virtually certain, as well as the specific site of origin or histologic type, but despite these probabilities it is mandatory that an adequate biopsy be obtained. Increasingly disease-specific therapies are being developed that will have optimum application for only one tumor type, although representing ineffective and toxic treatment for others. It is also highly inappropriate to

employ the therapeutic modalities for cancer in patients who have benign disease but who, for lack of adequate biopsy material, are presumed to be harboring a neoplasm.

Rarely, a therapeutic program must be initiated without a tissue diagnosis of neoplasia. Life-threatening situations may precipitate such a choice, one in which an invasive procedure required for biopsy is thought to be more dangerous than the treatment itself, in a setting where the clinical evidence is virtually diagnostic of a particular neoplasm. As an example, this situation may occasionally arise in the presence of an intrathoracic tumor with superior vena caval obstruction, airway obstruction, or pericardial tamponade; with intracerebral tumors; tumors of the spinal cord; and perhaps others. Even in these settings, however, in the great majority of instances, an adequate biopsy can be obtained.

The oncologists should be confident that the best possible pathologic diagnosis has been obtained. Whenever possible, a formal signed pathologic report should be reviewed before proceeding with a management program. It is often very desirable to have a second pathologic opinion for difficult cases and for diagnoses that are in acknowledged areas of controversy. Most pathologists are willing and accustomed to exchanging slides and tissue blocks among their colleagues.

One of the most difficult clinical problems encountered by the medical oncologist is the newly diagnosed patient with a neoplasm of unknown origin. In some patients the primary site of disease will not be identified, despite the initiation of an exhaustive and costly diagnostic evaluation. Many studies have shown that this group of patients has, in general, a very poor prognosis following treatment with empirically derived drug combinations (Moertel *et al.,* 1972; Woods *et al.,* 1980; McKeen *et al.,* 1980). The principal responsibility of the oncologist is to diagnose correctly those tumors that have specific therapies that may result in cure or more effective palliation. In this regard, the opinion of a highly competent pathologist is invaluable for providing a focus on the probable diagnostic possibilities presented by the histologic appearance of the tumor.

As examples, the finding of an "undifferentiated carcinoma" in the mediastinum or retroperitoneum should immediately raise the possibilities of a curable germ cell neoplasm or a pleomorphic non-Hodgkin's lymphoma. In men, the diagnosis of prostate cancer should be considered because effective control of the disease is possible with endocrine therapy, in contrast to the nontherapeutic effects of less-specific forms of cytotoxic chemotherapy for other occult primary cancers. In women, breast cancer and ovarian cancer represent tumors where useful forms of treatment are available, especially hormonal therapies for the treatment of breast tumors. The pathologic findings of "Indian-file" appearance of adenocarcinoma may be an indication for mammography, or the presence of papillary features and psammoma bodies may direct the diagnostic evaluation to an occult ovarian primary. In many cases, unfortunately, the pathologist can provide no specific guidance. In this setting the oncologist must rely on judgment derived from experience, a detailed knowledge of the natural history of disease, as well as the cost-effectiveness of a planned evaluation in determining how aggressively to pursue a diagnosis and what forms of therapy to initiate.

If a neoplasm is limited in extent, usually involving lymph nodes or even a bone site, and after appropriate diagnostic studies cannot be identified as to its primary origin, then appropriate surgery and/or radiotherapy is recommended. In some instances, such as the involvement of high neck lymph nodes with an undifferentiated neoplasm, an occult nasopharyngeal or Waldeyer's ring primary may be suspected. In these patients, radiation therapy should be directed not only to the neck but also to Waldeyer's ring radiation fields. If lymph node involvement is found in the low neck, in particular in the supraclavicular fossae, it is more likely that an occult primary exists below the clavicles, very often in the abdomen. Even in these instances, however, if appropriate diagnostic studies are negative in identifying a primary tumor, the lymph node metastases should be irradiated to full tumoricidal doses. This is also recommended for neoplasms, in particular for carcinomas involving the axillary or inguinal lymph nodes without known primaries. In some instances these will represent amelanotic melanomas in which the primary tumor has spontaneously regressed. Such patients have a potential for being cured after appropriate surgical resection and radiation therapy. Depending on the location of the apparent metastatic disease, cure is possible after eradicative surgery and/or radiation in as many as 30% of patients of this type (Fu *et al.,* 1973).

The appropriate determination of the extent of the neoplasm, or staging of the disease, is the next requirement of the oncologist before the design and initiation of a treatment program. Knowledge of the usual sites of metastases of neoplasms, their recognition and documentation by the best available diagnostic methods and the efficient use of radiology, nuclear medicine, and surgical consultants are among the important skills of the clinical oncologist.

The presence of metastases in critical sites, which change the therapeutic philosophy, should be determined with accuracy. In many situations, biopsy confirmation of metastatic disease is required, even if major surgical procedures such as laparotomy and thoracotomy are necessary because of the impact such information has on the prognosis and therapeutic approach.

Staging procedures should be completed promptly, through efficient selection of tests and scheduling. This usually can be accomplished within one or two weeks after the diagnostic biopsy. During this period, appropriate review of the pathology, consultation with colleagues, review of the literature, and adjustment of the patient and family to the impact of the diagnosis can lead to formulation and presentation of a more informed and acceptable plan of therapy.

The critical initial decision that must be made by the clinical oncologist, with all the information available, is whether or not the neoplasm can be potentially cured. In this setting, therapy should be initiated promptly, whether or not the patient is symptomatic and justifies the use of potentially toxic treatment programs. If cure is not a reasonable goal, the therapeutic program should be designed to offer effective palliation. For the clinical oncologist, this is a major responsibility and challenge, emphasizing the importance of a comprehensive training experience that stresses a continued proficiency in internal medicine. The provision of effective forms of palliative therapy requires a complete knowledge of the natural history of the neoplasm, the tempo or pace of the disease in the particular patient, the risks of serious complications arising from tumor in particular sites, the differential diagnosis of various symptoms, signs of radiologic and laboratory abnormalities, the range of relative effectiveness of modalities for control of symptoms, and the psychologic needs of the patient.

Every patient with cancer can be offered effective palliative care with relief of symptoms of cancer and at times accompanied by a worthwhile prolongation of life. In the majority of other instances, even if an increased survival time is not possible, an improved functional status and quality of life is effected. Patients and families must recognize that it is the proper role of the oncologist to provide effective palliation and that they have the experience and methods to accomplish this important aspect of comprehensive care.

One of the most critical and important events in the management of a patient with cancer is the recurrence of a neoplasm despite the initiation or completion of a potentially curative treatment program.

As a general rule, the apparent recurrence of a neoplasm mandates that the clinical diagnosis be confirmed by biopsy. Biopsy confirmation is of special importance if the interval between treatment completion and apparent recurrence is long, if the site of recurrence is atypical, if the clinical findings are equivocal, and if the morbidity of the biopsy procedure is acceptable. As in the case of the original diagnosis, tumor relapse has a profound prognostic importance and usually necessitates a radical change in therapeutic strategy. For these reasons it is essential that the diagnosis be definitive, so as to exclude a complication of therapy that mimics tumor recurrence, such as intestinal obstruction after abdominal surgery, radiation pneumonitis or pleuritis, or chemotherapy-induced neurologic dysfunction. Similarly, typical or atypical infections can simulate tumor recurrence, especially granulomatous infections such as the mycoses.

Patients with cancer are at least at equivalent risk for developing a new cancer as other individuals. A second, unrelated, and poten-

tially curable neoplasm should always be considered when a patient presents with an apparent recurrence of cancer.

For some cancers, removal of a metastasis may result in cure of the neoplasm. Though these situations are uncommon, many primary tumor types are known in which this is a possibility, including cancer of the colon with an isolated hepatic metastasis, renal cancer, testicular cancer, melanoma, sarcomas, and others. Even if cure is not achieved, nor possible, surgical resection of metastases may provide effective palliation or delay serious complications.

Medical oncologists should establish a good working relationship with their colleagues in surgery and in radiation oncology. In many instances, consultation and discussion among individuals from different disciplines before embarking on the primary treatment program will be of great benefit to the patient. If cure has not been achieved, the appropriate and skillful use of palliative irradiation should be considered for all patients regardless of the type or extent of the neoplasm.

The appropriate use of supportive measures in the management of patients with cancer is discussed in detail in other chapters of the textbook. It is emphasized here that the skillful use of supportive care will allow curative treatment programs to be completed successfully and will contribute, immeasurably, to effective palliation.

The experienced clinical oncologist must recognize when specific anticancer treatment efforts will not be successful or useful. The study of experimental therapies, as emphasized in the chapter dealing with the design of clinical trials, requires a high degree of judgment and ethics to insure that patients are not needlessly subjected to harsh toxicities (see Chapter 12). The decision to withhold chemotherapy, irradiation, or surgery during the course of the neoplasm, and in some cases at the onset, is a very important and essential responsibility of the oncologist. For these patients, nonspecific supportive measures are always required and can be used with great benefit to the patient and family.

It is an essential principle of good medical oncology that accurate and detailed records be kept of the patient's course and therapy. The critical operative, pathologic, and radiotherapeutic reports should be preserved in the patient record or chart. Time-oriented flow sheets that summarize the laboratory findings, drug dosages, and toxicities are an absolute requirement for the provision of good oncologic care. Therapy flow sheets of the kind used by the cooperative clinical groups or major cancer centers are available to all practicing oncologists. These treatment records are necessary to make sequential therapy decisions, to give maximal but safe therapy, to judge treatment responses and duration. These records are essential for communication among oncologists, for transfer of information, and to facilitate the analyses of treatment results.

It is often desirable for patients or oncologists to seek second consultative opinions in the management of neoplastic disease. Of greatest benefit at the onset of illness, second consultation opinions should be obtained before treatment is initiated. It may also be of value near the end of the treatment program, especially if the response to treatment has been atypical or unexpected. Adequate records should always be made available for such consultations. Flow sheets, original biopsy slides, radiologic studies, and a concise consultation letter should be made available to the consultant, preferably in advance of the patient evaluation. These important records should always be returned promptly to the referring physician along with specific recommendations and opinions by the consultant.

These principles of management, combined with the factual and experiential knowledge about the various cancers are the essence of clinical oncology. The practice of the subspecialty is demanding and ever changing; an understanding of the general principles of cancer management is the basic core of this rewarding and respected discipline.

REFERENCES

Fu, K. K.; Stewart, J. R.; and Bagshaw, M. A.: Cervical node metastases from occult primary sites. *Rocky Mountain Med. J.,* **70:**31–35, 1973.

McKeen, E.; Smith, F.; Haidak, D.; Butler, T.; Hoth, D.; Woolley, P.; and Schein, P. S.: Fluorouracil, adriamycin and mitomycin-C (FAM) for adenocarcinoma of unknown origin. *Proc. Am. Soc. Clin. Oncol.,* **21:**358, 1980.

Moertel, C. G.; Reitemeier, R. J.; Schutt, A.; and Hahn, R. G.: Treatment of the patient with adenocarcinoma of unknown origin. *Cancer,* **30:**1469–1472, 1972.

Woods, R. L.; Fox, R. M.; Tattersall, M. H. N.; Levi, J. A.; and Brodie, G. N.: Metastatic adenocarcinomas of unknown primary site: A randomized study of two combination-chemotherapy regimens. *N. Engl. J. Med.,* **303:**87–89, 1980.

8

Principles of Surgical Oncology

JOHN M. DALY and JEROME J. DECOSSE

INTRODUCTION

The surgical oncologist occupies a unique position in the management of the patient with cancer. Approximately 90% of these patients undergo operative therapy for diagnosis, primary treatment, or management of complications during the course of treatment for their neoplastic disease. For about 75% of patients with cancer, resection is the initial curative treatment, because cancer is assumed to be a localized disease for a time, allowing cure following adequate surgical removal. Improved survival statistics of patients with cancer treated surgically have documented this assumption, but the leveling off of survival suggests that other forms of treatment should be applied to further improve cure rates.

The surgical oncologist bears the responsibility for initial diagnosis and management of many types of cancer. His knowledge of tumor staging and the natural history of the disease should be integrated into a multimodal approach to treatment of the patient in concert with the medical oncologist and the radiotherapist. The guiding principles of the surgical oncologist should be the accurate diagnosis and staging of the cancer with adequate operative removal of localized disease (see Table 8–1).

The surgical oncologist's role varies with the type of cancer. For example, primary curative operation may be performed on patients with melanoma, lung, ovarian, and large-bowel cancer. In other forms of cancer, such as lymphoma, the surgeon's role may be diagnostic, with a possible contribution to staging; in patients with leukemia, the only surgical role may be provision of vascular access or man-

agement of complications. Surgical pathology is important because accurate diagnosis and knowledge of the extent of tumors are essential to proper treatment; pathologic staging lends insight into the natural course of the neoplasm, which is necessary to determine further treatment plans and evaluate their efficacy.

The surgical oncologist uses physical examination and roentgenographic techniques to determine if the neoplasm is potentially curable by surgical removal. Studies to preclude metastases are indicated when they are cost-effective and would substantially alter surgical treatment. For example, the asymptomatic patient with a 1 cm breast mass and clinically negative regional lymph nodes should have serum hepatic enzymes measured. If these enzymes are normal, the probability of this patient having a positive liver or bone scan is very slight. Thus, these latter two tests would be cost-ineffective in this situation.

Surgical resectability is also determined by the tumor's relation to and degree of invasion into and around vital structures. Invasive and noninvasive radiology are extremely helpful in determining the goals of operative management and defining the operative approach in specific patients. In most centers, for example, portal vein occlusion indicates nonresectabil-

Table 8–1. Surgical Principles in Oncology

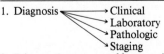

1. Diagnosis → Clinical
   → Laboratory
   → Pathologic
   → Staging
2. Primary therapy — *en bloc* resection
3. Adjunctive therapy — related to radiation therapy, chemotherapy
4. Therapy of complications due to disease/treatment

ity in patients with carcinoma of the pancreas, although surgical bypass may be necessary for biliary or gastric outlet obstruction. The extent of an operation may relate to the presence of additional precancerous lesions or to a strong family history of site-specific cancers, for example, in a patient with cancer of the colon and numerous colonic adenomas. Finally, operability and treatment decisions must take into account the medical status of the patient and the ability of the patient to tolerate the proposed operation. Assessment of cardiopulmonary status, hepatic and renal function, and nutritional status is vital to proper determination of operative risk.

SURGICAL ONCOLOGIST AS DIAGNOSTICIAN

Clinical Diagnosis

The surgeon, internist, or family practitioner is usually the first to examine the patient with cancer. A complete history and physical examination is indispensible before further judgments can be made regarding laboratory testing and treatment (see Table 8–2). Common symptoms range from anorexia, nausea, vomiting, hematemesis, abdominal pain, melana, and hematochezia in patients with gastrointestinal cancer to anorexia, productive cough, and hemoptysis in lung cancer to an enlarging mass in breast and soft-part tumors. Symptoms generally correspond to the sites involved, but nonspecific symptoms such as night sweats and weight loss may be the initial manifestations of an underlying neoplastic tumor. The duration of symptoms is important as it indicates the aggressiveness of the

Table 8–2. Surgical Principles in Oncology: Initial Management

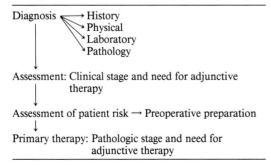

cancer. Finally, degree of impairment should be noted, as this will influence treatment decisions regarding palliation.

The patient's past medical history often lends clues to the diagnosis. Estrogen hormone use by the patient's mother during pregnancy, thymic irradiation for asthma or skin irradiation for acne in childhood, and a history of chronic inflammatory bowel disease are known to be associated with the later development of cancer. The medical history also reveals environmental factors such as smoking, alcohol ingestion, or exposure to asbestos or aniline dyes, which can be related to organ-specific sites of tumor development. Finally, a thorough medical history provides an important index of operative risk for the patient.

Inquiry into family history may reveal findings that support an initial diagnosis, suggest additional associated lesions, or influence the extent of surgical treatment. A patient with a thyroid nodule may have relatives with episodic hypertension, renal stones, or an "adrenal tumor" suggesting a multiple endocrine neoplasia syndrome. A patient with relatives who developed large-bowel cancer before the age of 40 should be screened for polyposis syndromes. Without a thorough history, these and other genetically influenced diseases will be missed.

Physical examination of the patient should begin with an overall assessment, should proceed through a systemic examination, then focus on the specific sites suggested by the medical history. Simple screening examinations, such as uterine cervical pap smear and fecal occult blood testing, should be performed routinely. Often, the surgeon is asked to evaluate a patient with a mass in a regional lymph node area such as the neck, axilla, or groin. Usually this mass represents one or more lymph nodes enlarged secondary to an inflammatory process originating in the area drained by the regional nodes. These nodes are often multiple and tender, and the primary area of inflammation is usually obvious. If the mass represents a solitary lymph node or several distinct painless nodes with no obvious cause, the question of biopsy to diagnose cancer is raised. Biopsy should be deferred until a thorough search for the source of a primary tumor has been made.

Excisional biopsy of lymph nodes containing metastatic cancer can release viable cancer cells into the biopsy wound because efferent and afferent lymphatics containing such cells are divided in the process of excising the lymph node. The incision of a node or group of nodes containing metastatic tumor may increase the risk of seeding the wound with cancer cells and violates the surgical principle of *en bloc* resection of the primary cancer, regional lymphatic channels, and regional lymph nodes. Once neoplastic disease is growing free in connective tissue and is no longer contained within the lymphatics or lymph nodes, operative eradication of tumor becomes difficult because the anatomic limits of the area containing cancerous tissue are broadened. With adenopathy in the head and neck region, the oral cavity, larynx, and pharynx should be thoroughly investigated. If the mass is in the axilla or groin, the breast and the skin of the corresponding extremity and portion of the trunk should be examined, and the patient should be queried as to previous removal of skin lesions, particularly moles. If a primary tumor is discovered, *en bloc* resection may be accomplished and the risk of regional recurrence minimized.

Laboratory Studies

In addition to the routine laboratory tests such as complete blood count, coagulation profile, multichannel serum biochemistry profile, and chest roentgenography, other studies are useful in determining primary site and extent of disease.

Evaluation of the patient with a suspicious breast lesion should include bilateral mammography. Roentgenographic characteristics may support the clinical diagnosis as well as reveal occult lesions in the contralateral breast. Clinically occult lesions may then undergo mammographically directed needle localization for biopsy. The patient with breast cancer who has abnormal liver function tests or palpable hepatomegaly should undergo a liver scan; those with skeletal symptoms should receive an isotopic bone scan. Metastatic lesions 3 cm in diameter can be detected on liver scintiscan, ultrasound, and CT scan with similar sensitivity, specificity, and accuracy (Smith *et al.,* 1982). The percentage of correct diagnoses reported for localized liver disease ranges from 72 to 94 (Sugarbaker, 1981).

Patients with symptoms or signs attributable to the gastrointestinal tract should receive an air contrast upper or lower barium study. Air contrast barium studies show greater mucosal detail than barium studies without air contrast and, although more demanding technically, they are also more sensitive to small lesions. Tomography is useful in evaluating suspicious lesions noted on chest roentgenography as well as skeletal and soft tissue lesions. Ultrasonic scanning is particularly useful in detection of abdominal cancer. Invasion of vascular structures and dilated extrahepatic and intrahepatic ducts secondary to biliary obstruction by a neoplasm can be demonstrated. Coexisting ascites also may be noted. Computed axial tomography has become valuable in determining the location and extent of a tumor and its relationship to adjacent structures; by quantitating x-ray absorption, the physical characteristics of tumors often can be determined.

Serum markers such as carcinoembryonic antigen (CEA), β-human chorionic gonadotropin (β-HCG), and α-fetoprotein are useful in the management of patients with specific tumors (see Chapter 6A). CEA is a tumor-associated glycoprotein found in the tissue of several different solid tumors: Breast, lung, gynecologic, and gastrointestinal cancers and sarcomas. Plasma CEA levels are neither sensitive nor specific enough to be of great value in diagnosis, particularly of early lesions. Sugarbaker noted that elevated plasma levels correlated with increasing tumor size, stage, and number of positive lymph node metastases in patients with large-bowel cancer (Sugarbaker, 1981). Herrera and associates (1976) and Wanebo and colleagues (1978) correlated the preoperative elevation of CEA with the later development of recurrent disease in patients with colorectal cancer. When surgical removal of the tumor was complete, circulating CEA returned to normal levels between 30 and 45 days after operative therapy (Sugarbaker, 1981). CEA monitoring is most useful in the follow-up of patients. Zamcheck has shown that there may be a rise in CEA before detection of recurrent cancer by other means (Zamcheck, 1975). Attiyeh and Stearns (1981) found a positive incidence of 89% when they explored, via laparotomy, patients with colorectal cancer solely because of a rising CEA.

SURGICAL PATHOLOGY

The importance of accurate pathologic diagnosis in the proper surgical treatment of cancer patients cannot be overstated. The determinations of cancer, histologic grade, primary site, and surgical resection margins provide critical information.

In 1934, Martin and Ellis reported needle aspiration with an 18-gauge needle to assess the histology of palpable tumors. Local anesthesia and skin incision were necessary. Schour and Chu (1974) reported that diagnosis using fine-needle (22-gauge) aspiration techniques concurred with surgical pathologic diagnosis in 97% of tested lymph nodes and 77% of breast tumors examined. This technique is rapid, minimally traumatic, and highly accurate for diagnosis of a clearly palpable mass or a radiographically visible lesion. False-positive results are rare; false negative results may occur due to small sample size and site of the lesion. With the use of fine-needle aspiration techniques in combination with roentgenography and ultrasound, deep, nonpalpable lesions have become amenable to diagnosis with minimal morbidity; examples include transthoracic aspiration of lung nodules using fluoroscopy and ultrasound, and computed tomography – directed aspiration of pancreatic masses. Tumor cell implantation of the aspiration site is rare; Frable (1982) noted only seven documented cases in the literature.

Aspiration cytology cannot be depended upon for grading of solid tumors, for subdividing types of lymphoma, or for accurate diagnosis following radiation treatment, but a positive diagnosis greatly facilitates diagnostic and treatment planning.

When an accurate diagnosis of tumor type and grade is necessary, an incisional or excisional biopsy is required. Care should be taken in the planning of a surgical biopsy so as not to jeopardize later surgical extirpation or the use of skin flaps. In general, large soft-tissue lesions (5 to 7 cm) that are deeper than the superficial fascia are best sampled by incisional biopsy. Small (<2 cm) superficial lesions can be managed by excisional biopsy with a view towards further treatment depending on tumor type, grade, and depth of invasion. Frozen section diagnosis should not be relied on to provide histologic grade and information about depth. Surgical margins of resection can and should be questioned on frozen section examination. In some instances (skin tumors and rectal polyps) local excisional therapy is all that is required if permanent histopathology determines superficial invasion, adequate resection margins, low-grade dedifferentiation, and absence of vascular or lymphatic invasion.

PREOPERATIVE PREPARATION

Appropriate preoperative preparation includes knowledge of the natural history of the patient's disease, evaluation of operative risk, decisions relevant to the need for and timing of operative intervention, estimate of the physiologic stress potentially imposed by the operation, and quantitative assessment of the patient's physiologic status (Polk, 1977). Comprehensive preparation of a patient for operative therapy requires both physiologic and psychologic support. During the preoperative period, the trust essential to an optimal physician-patient relationship is established. In the preoperative preparation of the surgical patient, the physician should consider potential abnormalities such as acid-base disorders, malnutrition, infection, respiratory insufficiency, hepatic and renal dysfunction, anemia, and clotting abnormalities.

The two aims of all treatment during the preoperative period should be preparing the patient to withstand the stresses of operative therapy and minimizing the risks of the surgical procedure. The appropriate duration of the preoperative period depends on the urgency of the operative procedure. The length of time feasible for correction of preexisting deficits may be *short* (hours), as in the case of massive gastrointestinal hemorrhage or free perforation of an obstructed colon; *intermediate,* as in complete but nonstrangulated bowel obstruction; or *prolonged* (days), as in jaundice due to pancreatic carcinoma. Determination of the urgency of a particular operative procedure requires knowledge of the operative risk and the natural history of the disease without immediate operative intervention. Included in this evaluation are factors such as age of the patient (chronologic and physiologic), degree of physiologic derangements and nutritional deficits, presence of organ system failure or insufficiency, and stage of the primary disease. Although the urgency of operative intervention may limit both the length of preoperative preparation and the methods available to the physician for correcting preexisting abnormalities, partial repair of deficiencies should be initiated promptly with plans made for more complete correction during and after operative therapy.

Months of chronic undernutrition cannot be corrected in a matter of hours, but anemia, dehydration, and electrolyte abnormalities can be ameliorated by early initiation of intensive intravenous support guided by appropriate laboratory monitoring (Duke and Miller, 1980).

Blood Disorders

Anemia is common among patients with cancer and should be corrected with packed red cell transfusions to a hematocrit equal to or greater than 35 before major operative intervention. The presence of continued bleeding and/or the existence of cardiopulmonary abnormalities greatly influence the rapidity of blood transfusions.

Clotting abnormalities can usually be determined by an adequate patient history, physical examination for evidence of hemostatic problems, and routine laboratory investigation (prothrombin time, partial thromboplastin time, and platelet count). Ascertainment of drug ingestion (especially aspirin, phenylbutazone, or indomethacin) is important because some medications result in qualitative platelet deficiencies leading to serious clotting abnormalities. Aspirin ingestion should be avoided for at least one week before elective hospital admission. In addition to drug ingestion, some conditions such as uremia, leukemia, and hepatic failure are associated with platelet dysfunction. The Mielke template bleeding time is a useful screening test for patients with suspected platelet dysfunction. It is generally agreed that 50,000 functionally active platelets per mm^3 are sufficient for operative procedures.

Cardiopulmonary Dysfunction

Evaluation of operative risk due to cardiopulmonary dysfunction begins with the patient's history; attention should focus on past respiratory infections, presence of morning sputum, smoking history, current level of physical activity, and history of chest pain, palpitations, or dyspnea upon exertion. The physical examination should concentrate on the dynamics of breathing to evaluate restrictive or obstructive disorders and on the cardiovascular system to evaluate function and congenital or acquired lesions. Pulmonary

function tests assess gas exchange and ventilatory function. Patients with a residual volume greater than 150% of predicted normal or a forced expiratory volume in one second (FEV_1) below one liter have marked degrees of pulmonary impairment and require extra attention perioperatively. The functional response of ventilation to bronchodilators can be useful in predicting the efficacy of perioperative pulmonary therapy.

Malnutrition

Protein-calorie malnutrition is a common associated problem in hospitalized patients with cancer (see Chapter 45). Several studies have shown that up to 30 to 50% of hospitalized patients suffer from moderate to severe degrees of malnutrition as a result of their primary tumor and/or the diagnostic and therapeutic regimens employed in the management of their primary disease (Bistrian et al., 1976; Willard et al., 1980). Protein-calorie malnutrition is generally a result of: (1) Decreased oral intake; (2) increased enteral losses secondary to malabsorption or intestinal fistula; and/or (3) increased nutritional requirements secondary to hypermetabolism or host inefficiency due to the presence of a tumor (see Table 8–3). Commonly, the patient's primary tumor leads to malnutrition resulting in impaired wound healing, reduced immunocompetence, anemia, decreased resistance to infection, generalized sepsis, and further malnutrition (Copeland and Dudrick, 1976). The end result may be multiple organ system failures and death.

Mullen et al. (1979) developed a "prognostic nutritional index" defined as follows:

$$(PNI = 158 - (16.6 \times \text{serum albumin [g\%]})$$
$$- (0.78 \times \text{triceps skinfold thickness [mm]})$$
$$- (0.20 \times \text{serum transferrin [mg\%]})$$
$$- (5.8 \times \text{delayed cutaneous hypersensitivity}).$$

In their series of surgical patients, $PNI \leq 30$ (low risk) was associated with an 11.7% complication rate and a 2% mortality rate, whereas $PNI \geq 60$ (high risk) was associated with an 81% complication rate and a 59% mortality rate. This study helped establish the relative importance of these nutritional indices as predictive factors for postoperative morbidity and mortality. Depressed skin test reactivity to a battery of recall skin test antigens in cancer patients also was shown to be associated with increased body weight loss, depressed serum

Table 8-3. Candidates for Perioperative Nutritional Support

PATIENTS UNABLE TO EAT	PATIENTS UNWILLING TO EAT	PATIENTS UNABLE TO EAT ENOUGH
1. Difficulties in swallowing 　a. Cancer of mouth, pharynx, larynx, or esophagus 　b. Trauma to mouth or throat 　c. Oropharyngeal or esophageal stricture 2. Upper gastrointestinal tract fistulas or obstruction	1. Anorexia secondary to malignancy, depression, chronic illness 2. Xerostomia 3. Radiation effects: Stomatitis, enteritis, intestinal stricture 4. Chemotherapy effects: Stomatitis, mucositis, enteritis	1. Increased nutritional requirements: severe catabolism 2° to sepsis 2. Impaired utilization of nutrients with host-tumor competition

albumin levels, and increased postoperative morbidity and mortality (Daly *et al.,* 1979).

After the need for preoperative nutritional support has been established, the most appropriate feeding regimen and duration of nutritional support are determined. The optimal duration of preoperative nutritional support varies with each patient and is ill-defined.

Holter and Fisher (1977) treated patients with carcinoma of the stomach by intravenous hyperalimentation (IVH) for two to three days preoperatively and five to seven days postoperatively and then compared these results with a group of patients who received "standard" intravenous therapy. No difference in postoperative morbidity or mortality was noted between these two groups during or following this short interval of nutritional support. Williams *et al.* (1977) randomly divided 74 patients with esophageal or stomach cancer into an enterally fed group who received 15 g nitrogen and 3000 calories per day and an IVH group who received 2 to 3 L of hypertonic dextrose and amino acids in addition to an oral diet. Postoperatively, the IVH group continued to receive parenteral nutrition, whereas the oral group was switched to parenteral nutrition if adequate oral intake was not possible within 48 hours. The incidence of wound infection was

significantly greater in the oral group compared to the IVH group, but postoperative mortality rates were similar. In a randomized comparative clinical trial, Muller *et al.* (1982) noted a signiicant reduction in postoperative morbidity and mortality in cancer patients given TPN for ten days preoperatively compared with a control group (see Table 8-4). Thus, to correct preexisting nutritional deficits, patients with moderate to severe malnutrition should receive a minimum of seven to ten days of preoperative nutritional therapy before an elective major operation and should continue to receive postoperative intravenous nutritional support until oral intake is adequate. The urgency of the operation dictates the time available to correct existing nutritional deficiencies.

The feeding regimen selected depends on the patient's nutritional status, the integrity of gastrointestinal function, and the type and magnitude of proposed treatment (Haffejee and Angorn, 1979). If the patient is unable to meet his or her daily nutritional requirements by voluntary oral ingestion of foodstuffs, the first step in nutritional support should be oral nutrient supplementation and intensive dietary counseling. Alert, well-motivated patients can often be encouraged to increase their

Table 8-4. Preoperative Total Parenteral Nutrition in Patients with Gastrointestinal Cancer: A Randomized Comparative Clinical Trial

	CONTROLS	TPN *(10 days preop)*
Number of patients	59	66
Change in mean body weight (kg) (between admission and surgery)	−1	+2
Number of patients with major postoperative complications	19(32%)	11(16%)*
Postoperative mortality	11(19%)	3(4%)*

* Difference between TPN group and controls is significant ($P < 0.05$).
Adapted from Muller, J. M.; Dienst, C.; Brenner, V.; and Pichlmaier, H.: Preoperative parenteral feeding in patients with gastrointestinal carcinoma. *Lancet,* **1**:68-71, 1982.

daily calorie and protein intakes through the ingestion of hospital or commercially prepared supplements or both. The patient who exhibits a moderate to severe degree of protein-calorie malnutrition, by definition, has failed to maintain himself or herself with spontaneous oral nutrient intake, and must be supplemented by an additional route and regimen of nutrition. A functional gastrointestinal tract is the best means to insure normal digestion and assimilation of foodstuffs; but the enteral route may be contraindicated by malabsorption, intestinal obstruction, upper gastrointestinal bleeding, or intractable vomiting or diarrhea. If the gastrointestinal tract is not available for use or if rapid nutritional repletion appears imperative, intravenous hyperalimentation should be initiated.

Prevention of Surgical Infection

After major elective operations, wound infection rates have varied from 0.5 to 40% depending on whether the procedure was "clean" or "contaminated" (see Table 8–5). Besides the added morbidity and potential mortality, surgical infection increased the average duration of hospitalization by at least ten days, resulting in a large increase in hospital costs. Resistance to infection (immune function) and dose and virulence of the invading bacteria are major factors determining the probability of wound infection (Cruse, 1977). Local wound resistance is aided by good surgi-cal technique: Gentle tissue handling, adequate hemostasis, debridement of dead tissue, good blood supply, avoidance of hematoma, and closure of the wound without tension (Keighley and Burdon, 1979).

Antibiotic prophylaxis has been used to reduce the incidence of postoperative wound infection in contaminated operations (Washington et al., 1974). The Veterans Administration ad hoc Interdisciplinary Advisory Committee on Antimicrobial Drug Usage (1977) suggested that antibiotics be used prophylactically both when prosthetic devices (valves, vascular grafts, joints, or cerebrospinal fluid shunts) are to be used and during genitourinary operations in which the urine is colonized or infected (more than 10^5 bacteria per milliliter). The committee also recommended chemoprophylaxis in other circumstances that might involve cancer patients including:

1. Head and neck surgery: Anticipation of cutting across a contaminated area or entering the dura mater
2. Chest surgery: Perforation or transection of the esophagus during mediastinal surgery; transection of a bronchus
3. Abdominal surgery: Anticipation of colotomy; enterotomy in the presence of blind loop syndrome or obstruction; operative procedure on the gallbladder in the high-risk patient (over 70 years of age or with common duct stones or obstructive jaundice); abdominal vascular catas-

Table 8–5. Operative Sites: Incidence of Postoperative Infections at the Operative Areas

OPERATION	INCIDENCE(%)	TYPE OF INFECTION	MAJOR PATHOGENS
Intradural craniotomy	4–8	wound	*Staphylococcus aureus*
	0.5–1	meningitis/abcess	gram negative
Head and neck	15–40	wound	*Staph. aureus*
			gram negative
			anaerobes
Pulmonary	0.5–6	wound	*Staph. aureus*
	1–2	empyema	gram negative
Laparotomy	2–4	wound	anaerobes
			gram negative
Gastric resection	5–10	wound	*Streptococcus*
			anaerobes
Biliary tract	3–10	wound	gram negative
			enterococci
			clostridia
Colon resection	8–40	wound	anaerobes
	2–10	abdominal abcess	gram negative
Mastectomy	1–3	wound	*Staph. aureus*
			gram negative

Adapted from Bartlett, J. G.: Choosing and using antibiotics. In Condon, R. E., and DeCosse, J. (eds): *Surgical Care.* Lea & Febiger, Philadelphia, 1980.

trophies; patients with cancer of the stomach, achlorhydria, or previous gastrectomy

4. Pelvic surgery: Hysterectomy
5. Cardiac and vascular surgery: Cardiopulmonary bypass; vascular graft

Use of antibiotics in these situations should be: (1) timed to allow adequate wound antibiotic levels before contamination; (2) only for a short time during the perioperative period; (3) specific for the most likely infecting organism(s); and (4) safe; that is, it should present minimal additional hazard to the patient (see Table 8–5).

DECISION FOR OPERATION

A decision for curative operation presupposes that the tumor is localized or confined regionally, that the area of the tumor can be encompassed by regional excision, that distant metastases cannot be documented, and that the tumor is appropriately treated by operation.

Given a decision for a curative operation, the extent of the surgical procedure must then be defined. In principle, an *en bloc* resection should be performed, encompassing the primary tumor, regional lymph nodes, and intervening lymphatic channels. Perhaps this principle is best illustrated by operations for large-bowel cancer, in which the regional lymphatics of the colon (but not the rectum) course in one direction with the major arteries and veins. This principle is less applicable in the rectum, where lateral spread and the limiting confines of the lateral pelvic wall preclude a wide margin. Similarly, the principle is less applicable for breast cancer, for which multiple pathways of lymphatic spread are well recognized.

As a result of these concepts, and partly due to emergence of earlier stage disease, the extents of various operations for cancer are undergoing change. This "remodeling" is perhaps best illustrated in breast cancer, for which the trend is toward a modified radical mastectomy or local excision with adjuvant radiation therapy and adjuvant chemotherapy (see Table 8–6). The therapeutic value of regional node dissection has been questioned by some, but performed properly it may establish the data base for precise staging for other adjuvant treatments.

Operation may be performed solely for staging purposes. An example is staging laparotomy in Hodgkin's disease, in which multiple lymph node biopsies, liver and bone marrow biopsies, and splenectomy are performed.

In a variety of settings, operative intervention is used for palliative treatment. Bypasses are performed around obstructed viscera, for example, gastrojejunostomy for obstructing carcinoma of the stomach, choledoduodenostomy or choledochojejunostomy for a carcinoma of the pancreas obstructing the common bile duct, or nephrostomy for an obstructed ureter. Plastic Celestine tubes may be inserted through an obstructing esophageal carcinoma; colon diversion may be performed for obstructing large-bowel cancer.

The use of cytoreductive surgery is controversial. This concept may be most relevant in ovarian cancer for which deliberate removal of as much ovarian tumor as possible may enhance the patient's response to subsequent

Table 8–6. Breast Carcinoma Less Than 2 cm: A Randomized Trial of Radical Mastectomy vs Quadrantectomy, Axillary Dissection, and Radiotherapy

	MASTECTOMY	QUADRANTECTOMY, AXILLARY DISSECTION, AND RADIOTHERAPY
Number of patients	349	352
Primary diameter ≤ 1 cm	44.4%	46.0%
Mean age (yr)	50.9	50.1
Local recurrences	3	1
Secondary primary tumors		
Ipsilateral breast	0	4
Contralateral breast	5	9
Distant metastases	30	22

Median follow-up = 3 years
Adapted from Veronesi, U.; Saccozzi, R.; Del Vecchio, M.; Banfi, A.; Clemente, C.; DeLena, M.; Grallus, G.; Greco, M.; Luini, A.; Marubini, E.; Muscolino, G.; Ruke, F.; Saboardori, B.; Zecchini, A.; and Zucali, R.: Comparing radical mastectomy with quadrantectomy, axillary dissection and radiotherapy in patients with small cancers of the breast. *N. Engl. J. Med.*, **305**:6–11, 1981.

chemotherapy or radiation therapy. Cytoreductive operations also may be valid in the treatment of some childhood tumors, such as neuroblastoma.

The extent of an operation should be dictated by precise staging. In many instances, a regional node dissection is carried out to remove all nodes in anticipation of metastases in some. With precise staging, and with the presence of effective chemotherapy, operative intervention may be more limited. For example, the traditional management of nonseminoma germ cell tumor of the testis has been radical orchiectomy and radical retroperitoneal lymph node dissection extending to the renal vasculature. The predictability of a normal beta subunit of human chorionic gonadotropin (βHCG) and alpha fetoprotein (αFP) with normal CT scans and ultrasound, backed by effective chemotherapy should dissemination occur, now may permit only radical orchiectomy without node dissection in those patients who are normal by these determinants. More precise pretreatment planning of tumors traditionally treated by operation is a main objective of current research. Research in areas such as lymphoscintigraphy is being exploited to achieve greater precision of staging.

SURGICAL ONCOLOGIST AS PRIMARY THERAPIST

The following sections describe the perspective of the surgical oncologist in regard to the management of specific tumors. They serve to complement, and in some cases differ with, the views of other authors who in their chapters have presented the same topics from the orientation of the medical oncologist. Presentation of these areas of difference is essential to a comprehensive discussion of the current concepts of patient management for these selected diseases.

Breast

If no evidence of distant metastases is found, the treatment plan for the patient with breast cancer is decided upon, often in consultation with a radiation therapist and a medical oncologist, based on the anatomic location of the lesion, its physical characteristics, and evidence of regional metastases (Wiseman *et al.*, 1982) (see Chapter 33). As a rule, excision or needle biopsy of the suspicious lesion and frozen section examination is done under general anesthesia, immediately before mastectomy. Excisional biopsy under local anesthesia, particularly as an office or outpatient procedure, can be difficult because the lesion may be deeper in the breast than initially anticipated. Needle biopsy or needle aspiration for cytology is much easier to perform under local anesthesia, but the lesion should be 1.5 cm or larger to obtain an adequate biopsy specimen.

Baker (1977) reported on 153 consecutive biopsies performed under local anesthesia. Patients found to have breast cancer were admitted to the hospital within one to three days for definitive treatment. An increase in local recurrence was not noted compared with patients having an open breast biopsy immediately before mastectomy.

The responsibility of the surgeon and radiation therapist is to provide the patient with the best chance for cure, for local chest wall control of tumor, and for minimal morbidity. Complete surgical dissection of the axilla should not be combined with radiation therapy to the axilla because the incidence of lymphedema of the arm is greatly increased. Major lymphatic channels should be removed surgically and remaining collateral channels may be destroyed by radiation therapy. If axillary metastases are multiple, large, or matted, a mastectomy is done in conjunction with a dissection of the lateral axilla, the medial limits of the dissection being the lateral border of the pectoralis minor muscle, an "extended simple mastectomy," and radiation therapy is applied to the apex of the axilla, chest wall, and peripheral lymphatics. In this way, the primary cancer and large lymph nodes ($>$ 1 cm in size), which are unlikely to be sterilized by radiation therapy, are removed surgically, and metastatic cancers in smaller, centrally located axillary lymph nodes, often intertwined around axillary structures and not adequately removed by operation, are sterilized by radiation therapy.

Circumscribed carcinoma less than 5 cm in diameter, limited to the lateral aspect of the breast, and without skin or pectoral fascia fixation can usually be treated by surgery alone, provided lymph node metastasis or lymphatic invasion is not found in the specimen. If lymph node metastasis is present or if the carcinoma is medially or centrally located, a combination of surgery and postoperative radiation therapy is often applied to insure local chest wall control of the tumor. The choice among options for both the surgical procedure and the radiation therapy depend upon the location and size of the primary tumor (Baker et al., 1979). In patients with stage I or II tumor, modified radical mastectomy is the treatment of choice. Laterally located cancer with axillary lymph node metastases may be associated with internal mammary or supra-clavicular lymph node metastases in as many as 25 to 30% of cases; consequently, radiation therapy is often used to treat these areas (this is called peripheral lymphatic radiation ther-apy). Medially located cancer is associated with internal mammary node metastases in 30% of patients; if axillary metastases are also present, the incidence may increase to 50%. At some centers, internal mammary nodes are biopsied before selecting radiation therapy as an adjuvant treatment.

Other approaches have been used to treat patients with small (<2 cm) cancers of the breast. Veronesi et al. (1981) compared radical mastectomy with quadrantectomy, axillary dissection, and radiotherapy in 701 patients with breast cancers measuring less than 2 cm in diameter (see Table 8–6). Local chest wall or ipsilateral breast recurrences and patient ac-tuarial survival were similar in both groups. The longest patient follow-up was seven and one-half years with a mean follow-up of three years.

In the National Surgical Adjuvant Project for Breast and Bowel Cancer (NASBP) trials, Fisher and colleagues (1980) have reported no difference in treatment failures between the group treated with total mastectomy plus local-regional radiation and the radical mas-tectomy group. Calle and associates (1978), however, reported on 120 patients with breast tumors less than 3 cm in diameter and without adenopathy who underwent "lumpectomy" and radiotherapy. The local-regional recur-rence rate was 13% at five years and 20% at ten years, with 14 of 16 cases requiring secondary surgery. This latter study emphasizes the im-portance of adequate duration of follow-up to determine breast cancer local recurrence.

A carcinoma larger than 5 cm in diameter but associated with minimal clinical axillary disease may be treated by operative therapy alone or by preoperative radiation therapy and either a radical, modified radical, or extended simple mastectomy, depending upon the loca-tion of the lesion and the amount of radiation therapy delivered to the apical axilla.

Minimal breast cancer, specifically, invasive cancer less than 5 mm in diameter or in situ intraductal or lobular breast cancer, is seldom associated with lymph node metastases (Fra-zier et al., 1977). A simple mastectomy with axillary sampling is performed for in situ breast cancer regardless of the location of the tumor in the breast; however, if cancer invades below the basement membrane, treatment is usually with a modified radical mastectomy, depending on location of the primary tumor.

Mirror image biopsy of the opposite breast should be done for lobular carcinoma, either in situ or invasive, but not for intraductal carci-noma unless the patient is under 40 years of age and has a strong family history.

All biopsy incisions should be encompassed with the specimen; therefore, the position of a biopsy incision should be planned. Ideally, a mastectomy should be done by a transverse incision. This incision is more cosmetically satisfying to the patient and breast reconstruc-tion is easier.

Sixty percent of recurrent breast cancer occurs within two years after mastectomy. If the initial local treatment for breast cancer is proper, local chest wall recurrence rates should be less than 5% in stage I disease and less than 10% in stage II disease. Breast reconstruction should probably not be performed simulta-neously with mastectomy in women with in-vasive breast cancer and should be discouraged for at least two years postoperatively in women who have had axillary lymph node metastases. The major criticism of breast reconstruction is the potential for delay in diagnosing local chest wall recurrence. The best defined role for im-mediate breast reconstruction may be in the treatment of in situ breast cancer. The cancer surgeon should plan his ablative operative procedure with reconstruction in mind, but he should not compromise the chance for local control of disease in order to preserve cosmetic appearance.

Esophagus and Stomach

Operative therapy for carcinomas of the esophagus has been associated with death rates as high as 30% (Rosenberg et al., 1981). The high mortality can be attributed to patient fac-tors such as preexisting cardiopulmonary dis-orders and malnutrition, and to anatomic fac-tors such as the lack of an esophageal serosal covering, tumor location, and extent of spread. Ellis and Gibb (1979) reported 82 esophageal cancer patients who underwent surgical resection with a mortality of 3% and a complication rate of 15%. They emphasized esophagogastric reconstruction and perioperative hyperalimentation to reduce complications in debilitated patients. Daly and associates (1982) reviewed the results of surgical therapy for esophageal cancer at M.D. Anderson Hospital from 1960 to 1980 and noted a great decrease in perioperative complications after 1973. This reduction in surgical morbidity was especially apparent in those patients who were supported preoperatively and postoperatively with total parenteral nutrition (TPN). Muller et al. (1982) recently demonstrated in a prospective randomized trial that perioperative TPN reduced postoperative mortality in patients with carcinoma of the esophagus and stomach (see Table 8–4).

In addition to intensive preoperative support to reduce postoperative complications, adjunctive radiotherapy and/or chemotherapy have been applied in an attempt to reduce local recurrence and increase patient survival. Marks and colleagues (1976) reported that preoperative radiation treatment to 4500 R produced tumor sterilization in 3% and reduction to in situ carcinomas in 10% of 101 patients. Kelson and associates (1981) treated 53 patients with preoperative combination chemotherapy consisting of cis-platinum (3 mg/kg), bleomycin (10 units/m² IV loading dose and 10 units/m² 24 hours × 4 day infusion), and vindesine (3 mg/m²) for one to two chemotherapy cycles and noted a partial response in 29 patients (55%). In addition, the surgical resectability rate was increased to 82% compared with 54% in historic control patients given preoperative radiation treatment.

In the event that resection for cure is impossible, resection of the tumor for palliation should be performed. If a patient can ingest adequate nutrients by mouth, the quality of remaining life is improved and the opportunity for further palliation from chemotherapy and radiation therapy is increased. In patients with large tumors, surgical palliation may include bypass by colon interposition. The risk of producing a major postoperative complication by doing a palliative resection must be weighed against the potential benefits of such a resection. The operating surgeon must consider life expectancy and quality of remaining life as he decides between palliative resection or bypass and nonoperative treatment.

Survival following gastric carcinoma and its treatment has not changed substantially in the past 50 years (Adashek et al., 1979). The surgical treatment of gastric cancer is based mainly on operative and pathologic observations (see Chapter 26). Carcinoma of the distal portion of the stomach (restricted to pylorus and antrum) should be treated by subtotal gastrectomy, omentectomy, and dissection of subpyloric, hepatic, and preaortic lymph nodes (Paulino and Roselli, 1973). Tumors located in the body of the stomach have been treated by either subtotal or total gastrectomy. Shiu et al. (1980) have reported significant improvement in five-year survival of patients with stage I or stage II tumors when they underwent radical total gastrectomy, splenectomy, and distal pancreatectomy, as compared with treatment by subtotal resection. Adenocarcinoma of the cardia has a worse prognosis than most gastric cancers (Buchholtz et al., 1978; Papachristou and Fortner, 1980). Proper management of clinical stage I or II resectable cancers of the cardia should include an extended total gastrectomy. Decisions regarding operative approaches are based on tumor size and proximal and distal extent of the cancer. Proximal submucosal spread of distal esophageal or proximal cardia adenocarcinoma mandates a minimum of 5 cm pathologic margin proximal to any resection.

Pancreas

If evidence of distant or regional metastases from carcinoma of the pancreas or periampullary region cannot be identified, the patient is a candidate for pancreaticoduodenectomy (see Chapter 27). Our practice has been to prepare the malnourished patient nutritionally with preoperative intravenous hyperalimentation, unless deteriorating liver function secondary to biliary obstruction necessitates immediate biliary decompression. Biliary decompression followed at a later date by a pancreaticoduodenectomy has not been recommended because adhesions secondary to the decompressive procedure make the excisional procedure more difficult. We have not found that elevated bilirubin and alkaline phosphatase in a well-nourished patient with normal hepatocellular function is associated with increased morbidity or mortality following pancreaticoduodenectomy. A histologic diagnosis of pancreatic carcinoma is desirable before undertaking a pancreaticoduodenectomy. Tissue can usually be obtained by transduodenal or direct needle biopsy of the pancreas. Preoperative

ERCP provides a useful alternative to achieve this objective. Pancreatic fistulas have not occurred when the biopsy needle avoided the major pancreatic ducts.

A surgeon should not operate upon a jaundiced patient unless he is prepared to treat definitively whatever pathologic process is discovered. Nevertheless, a resectable carcinoma of the pancreas is sometimes found by an operating surgeon and he may not wish to do the definitive procedure or a surgeon able to do it may not be immediately available. In that event, the operating surgeon should do a simple biliary bypass, refrain from mobilizing the duodenum and pancreas, and not biopsy the pancreas unless the lesion is easily accessible. Forrest and Longmire (1979) reported a median survival time of 20 months in patients who underwent pancreaticoduodenectomies for cure. The median survival after palliative resection was seven months; after bypass it was six months.

Liver

Advances in anesthesia, blood replacement, and surgical technique have made major hepatic resection feasible. Patients with primary hepatoma and certain solitary metastatic cancers — for example, from carcinoma of the colon — should be evaluated for possible curative resection (see Chapter 28). Adson and Van Heerden (1980) reported a 20 to 30% survival after resection of even large hepatic metastases. If liver function tests indicate any degree of hepatocellular malfunction in the normal liver, the patient is a borderline candidate for a major resection. Other contraindications such as advanced aged or other organ system disease militate against resection.

Isotopic hepatic scanning combined with serum alkaline phosphatase and CEA are the most effective tests for screening patients for liver disease, but their sensitivity is limited (Tartter et al., 1981). Arteriography may define deposits of metastatic cancer and also outlines the arterial blood supply to the liver. The variations in origin in the right and left hepatic artery must be known preoperatively, particularly if hepatic artery ligation or infusion chemotherapy is contemplated as an alternate procedure to resection. The venous phase of the arteriogram will identify the portal system. Cancer in the portal vein is a contraindication to major resection. Inferior vena cavography with identification of the hepatic veins aids in

evaluation of malignant tumor invading these structures, another contraindication to resection. Computerized axial tomography and ultrasonography also are sensitive tests that identify small metastatic deposits and are much better in detecting tumor in the lateral segment of the left hepatic lobe than is arteriography.

At exploration, metastases limited to one hepatic lobe should be considered for resection either by wedge excision or lobectomy. If the cancer is unresectable, hepatic arterial devascularization and/or chemotherapy infusion may be performed. The infusion catheter is placed through the gastroduodenal artery into the common hepatic artery. Once in place, fluoroscein dye is injected into the catheter to insure that both hepatic lobes are being perfused and that other structures supplied by branches of the celiac axis will receive negligible drug.

An implantable pump has been developed for chronic infusion chemotherapy. Chemotherapeutic infusion, usually with FUDR, is begun when the patient has recovered from the surgical procedure. To insure that the catheter has not been dislodged from the common hepatic artery during the postoperative period, a liver scan is obtained by injecting macroaggregates of technetium-labeled serum albumin directly into the catheter. In nonrandomized trials, a slight improvement in length of survival measured in months has been reported in patients undergoing chemotherapy by direct hepatic infusion when compared to systemic intravenous treatment. In one prospective randomized multiinstitutional trial, no difference in tumor response or patient survival was reported when intraarterial chemotherapy with 5-fluorouracil was compared with systemic intravenous 5-FU (Grage et al., 1979). Unfortunately, intraarterial treatment was given for only three weeks and patients were then switched to intravenous administration. Further studies are necessary to account for variations in mode of delivery, duration of treatment, proper staging, and drug pharmacology.

Large Bowel

Preoperative preparation of the patient with colorectal carcinoma requires thorough assessment by physical examination, radiographic methods, and/or endoscopic techniques to determine the size, mobility and histology of the primary tumor (see Chapters

30 and 31). Synchronous cancers of the large bowel have been noted in approximately 4% of patients (Copeland *et al.,* 1968). In the absence of obstruction, all patients should undergo a thorough mechanical bowel preparation with laxatives and enemas preoperatively. Currently, there is little debate regarding the need for antibiotic prophylaxis of some type, but controversy remains as to the length of time for perioperative administration and whether antibiotics should be given orally and/or intravenously. One center administers oral neomycin and erythromycin base at 1 PM, 2 PM, and 11 PM on the day prior to operation (Nichols *et al.,* 1973).

In colonic resection, the mesentery of the cancer-bearing bowel should be removed as completely as possible (Evans *et al.,* 1978). Turnbull and associates (1967) emphasized the "no-touch" technique with early high ligation of the vascular blood supply. Stearns and Schottenfeld (1971) encouraged wide mesenteric resection and suggested methods to minimize cancer cell contamination of the tumor bed, anastomosis, adjacent viscera, and abdominal wall. Polk (1975) noted that adjacent organ invasion did not always connote a hopeless prognosis; if an *en bloc* resection is performed in selected cases with acceptable operative risk, patient salvage is increased.

Good surgical judgment is necessary when operating on any part of the colon, but is required most when dealing with carcinoma of the rectum and rectosigmoid. The surgical oncologist should provide the best opportunity for cure and local control of disease combined with the least chance of postoperative morbidity, mortality, and loss of function. Sphincter-saving procedures should not be performed if the chance for local control is jeopardized. Cancerous lesions within 5 to 6 cm of the anal verge that invade through the muscularis propria usually should be removed by abdominoperineal resection. In women, a cancer cephalad from this level often can be managed with a low anterior resection or pull-through procedure. Use of automated suturing devices has been suggested to allow lower safer anastomosis to be performed. It should be emphasized, however, that attempts to perform a low anterior anastomotic repair should not compromise a wide pelvic dissection. Large rectal cancer in the 8 to 10 cm range that has invaded the pericolic fat and/or has clinically positive lymph node metastases may also require abdominoperineal resection.

Morson and colleagues (1977) have demonstrated the applicability of *local* excision for *early* cancer of the rectum in lesions that undergo complete excision with low grade histology and with tumor confined to the submucosal plane of the bowel wall without lymphatic or vascular invasion. This approach is preferable to electrosurgical diathermy, which destroys histologic markings and makes staging impossible. Electrocoagulation has been found useful only as palliation for selected patients. Adjunctive radiation treatment may be indicated because surgical therapy alone yielded the highest recurrence rates in Duke's C lesions with high-grade histology, size greater than 4 cm, and distance within 5 cm of the dentate line compared with other rectal tumors.

The Veterans Administration Surgical Oncology Group has entered 5,100 patients over 23 years into a series of trials in an effort to improve survival and decrease recurrence (Higgins *et al.,* 1981). Preoperative radiation therapy (2000 to 2500 R) reduced the percentage of patients having positive lymph nodes from 44 to 26% in those low-lying lesions requiring abdominoperineal resection. No significant increase in survival for patients who had undergone a resection with curative intent was observed.

A second trial applying 3150 R is currently underway. The Gastrointestinal Tumor Study Group has shown a significantly longer disease-free interval in rectal cancer patients given radiation therapy (4200 to 4800 R) postoperatively, although median followup is only three years (Enker *et al.,* 1981). Preoperative radiotherapy has been suggested to increase resectability, prevent seeding, and destroy cancer cells outside the operative field. On the other hand, postoperative radiotherapy "spares" those patients with more favorable pathologic lesions and can be given to a surgically "defined" area, but complications, particularly small-bowel radiation enteritis may be more frequent.

Approximately two-thirds of colorectal cancer recurrences are detected within 18 months of surgical resection (Rao *et al.,* 1981). Therefore, follow-up examination is extremely important if one is to identify recurrent tumor when it can be treated and possibly cured (MacKay *et al.,* 1974). Minton and Martin (1978) studied prospectively 18 patients who underwent second-look procedures based on elevated plasma CEA levels. Thirteen patients had localized disease, four patients had distant metastases, and in one patient no tumor was discovered. Attiyeh and Stearns (1981) performed second-look laparotomy in 32 asymptomatic patients with significant CEA elevations: Recurrent tumor was documented in 89%; liver metastases were evident in 18 patients, of whom seven had curative resections; and local abdominal disease was found in 15 patients with curative resection attempted in nine. Use of repeated physical examination, endoscopic and radiographic examinations, and serum biochemistries and markers such as CEA has improved the surgeon's ability to have an effect on recurrent disease when found at a localized stage (Holyoke et al., 1978).

Melanoma

Treatment of cancerous melanoma is based on depth of skin invasion, location on the body, and areas of metastatic spread (Davis, 1976) (see Chapter 21). Clark and colleagues (1969) has reported an 8.3% mortality with level II melanomas, 35% with level III, 46% with level IV, and 55% with level V. Breslow (1975) measured tumor thickness and found that lesions less than 0.76 mm in thickness rarely metastasized.

Punch biopsy may be satisfactory for histologic diagnosis, but excisional biopsy including a small amount of subcutaneous fat is preferable in order for the pathologist to define depth of invasion. Pathologic staging should be done on permanent sections, because interpretation of frozen section preparations can be misleading. Epstein and associates (1969) demonstrated that use of incisional biopsy rather than excisional biopsy does not alter the neoplastic potential of melanoma. Electrocauterization should be condemned because it destroys the lesion, leaving no tissue for microscopic examination.

Thin, cancerous melanoma that has not penetrated through the papillary dermis (Clark's levels I and II) or is less than 0.76 mm thick seldom metastasizes or recurs locally, and there is a 95% chance for initial cure by adequate local excision (Breslow, 1975; Lee, 1980). Usually, adequate local excision can be achieved by wide excision of the biopsy scar with margins sufficient to allow primary closure of the wound. Breslow and Macht (1977) evaluated the results of surgical excision of 62 "thin" melanomas and found that the width of

resection varied from 0.1 to 5.5 cm but none of the patients developed local recurrences or metastases. Some lesions, particularly the superficial spreading type, may be too large for excision and primary closure, and flap rotation or skin grafting may be necessary. Similarly, skin grafts may be needed in areas of the body where skin is not easily mobilized, for example, the sole of the foot.

Thick lesions that have penetrated to the reticular dermis (level III), into the reticular dermis (level IV), or through it and into the subcutaneous fat (level V) have a much higher cancerous potential that is directly proportional to the depth of invasion (especially when greater than 1.5 mm in thickness) and to the location on the body (the risk in head and neck tumors is greater than that in trunk tumors, which is greater than the risk in tumors of the extremities). All regional node-bearing areas and the area between the primary melanoma and the regional lymph nodes should be carefully evaluated in order to detect clinical regional lymph node metastases or in-transit metastases coursing to the regional lymph nodes through the intradermal or subdermal lymphatics (Copeland and McBride, 1973). In-transit metastases seldom are found unless stasis occurs in the regional lymphatics secondary to multiple lymph node metastases or previous resection of the regional lymph nodes.

Surgical treatment of all thick (1.5 to 2 mm) melanomas must be directed at eradication of the primary tumor, areas of potential in-transit metastases, and the regional lymph node-bearing areas. Treatment of regional lymph nodes also must be practical. A thick melanoma in the middle of the trunk may potentially metastasize to the axillary, inguinal, or supraclavicular lymph node areas on either side; prophylactic lymph node dissection of each of these locations would be impractical. Sugarbaker and McBride (1976a) found that Sappey's lines of lymphatic drainage predicted the site of regional lymph nodal metastases when metastasis occurred. Holmes et al. (1977) suggested colloidal gold scanning in situations where truncal lymphatic drainage was unclear. They found in 57 patients that lymph node metastasis did not occur at sites other than those taking up the colloidal gold.

Prophylactic lymph node dissection as treatment for stage I, thick melanomas is controversial (Ames et al., 1976). The incidence of subclinical lymph node metastases is between

20 and 40% in patients with thick melanomas. Some investigators believe that the prognosis for patients with resected subclinical lymph node metastases is the same as for patients with stage I disease and pathologically negative lymph nodes. Other investigators believe that subclinical lymph node metastases represent stage II disease and that disease in these patients will follow the course of stage II lesions.

Balch *et al.* (1979) retrospectively reviewed the incidence of subsequent regional lymph node metastases in patients treated initially by wide local excision. They found that the risk of lymphatic spread was 0% for primary tumors ≤0.76 mm in depth; 25% for 0.76 to 1.5 mm lesions; 51% for 1.5 to 3.99 mm lesions; and 62% for lesions ≥4.0 mm thick (Balch *et al.,* 1979). At five years, survival was 37% in patients with lesions 1.5 to 3.99 mm thick who underwent wide local excision alone, compared with 83% survival when regional lymph node dissection was performed simultaneously with wide excision. Regional lymph node dissection was not beneficial in thin (≤0.76 mm) or thicker (≥4.00 mm) lesions (see Table 8–7).

Similar trends have been reported by Breslow (1975) and Wanebo *et al.* (1975). In contrast, a prospective study by Veronesi *et al.* (1977), in which patients were randomized to excision of primary melanoma with prophylactic node dissection or wide excision with later therapeutic node dissection, found no difference in survival rates.

Thick melanomas on the extremity, not adjacent to the axilla or groin, present a special problem because it is not practical for the tissue between the primary lesion and the regional nodes to be excised in continuity with the primary lesion. The incidence of "trapped" in-transit metastases can be as high as 20% if the primary melanoma and regional lymph nodes are excised simultaneously. Isolated limb perfusion with phenylalanine mustard in conjunction with a limited excision of

the primary lesion has lowered the incidence of "trapped" in-transit metastascs to 2% compared to between 18 and 22% in historic control patients (Sugarbaker and McBride, 1976b).

Isolated limb perfusion with phenylalanine mustard, actinomycin D, and nitrogen mustard has been beneficial in increasing survival rates and providing adequate local control for patients with in-transit metastases. It is the treatment of choice for patients in these categories. Prophylactic perfusion for patients with stage I disease appears to improve ten-year survival rates and to lower regional recurrence when compared to historic controls. Unfortunately, randomized controlled studies have not been done and comparison with historic controls is difficult to interpret.

Malignant melanoma responds poorly to radiation therapy. Therefore, initial surgical procedures should be designed to totally eradicate local disease by *en bloc* dissection where possible. Lymph node biopsy should be avoided. If lymph nodes are palpably enlarged in the area of regional node drainage, dissection without biopsy is justified unless there is another reason for lymphadenopathy, such as BCG scarification in the immediate area. In this latter instance, lymphadenopathy will regress as the scarification wounds heal.

Adult Soft Tissue Sarcoma

Soft tissue sarcomas in adults may grow to a large size without detectable metastases (see Chapter 38). Prognosis has been shown to correlate with tumor size, site, histologic type, and degree of differentiation (Hajdu, 1981). Tumors that are small (less than 5 cm), superficial (not extending beyond the superficial fascia), and low grade are grouped together as tumors with a favorable prognosis. Tumors that are large (more than 5 cm), deep (extending beyond the superficial fascia), and high grade give a poor prognosis.

Table 8–7. Melanoma: Distant Metastases Following Wide Local Excision (WLE) + Regional Lymph Node Dissection (RND)

MELANOMA THICKNESS *(mm)*	WLE *(% metastases)*	WLE + RND *(% metastases)*
0.76	0	0
0.77–1.49	25	8
1.50–3.99	78*	15
4.0	80	70

* Difference between WLE and WLE + RND groups is significant. ($P < 0.001$)
Adapted from Balch, C. M.; Murad, T. M.; Soong, S.; Ingalls, A. L.; Richards, P. C.; and Maddox, W. A.: Tumor thickness as a guide to surgical management of clinical stage I melanoma patients. *Cancer,* **43:**883, 1979.

Traditionally, soft tissue sarcomas have been treated surgically. Experience has shown that "simple excision" results in a local recurrence rate of 90% due to the "pseudocapsule," an outer sheath of viable tumor cells that is stripped away and left behind after simple excision. Local recurrence rates approximate 39% after wide excision, 25% after muscle group soft part resection and 7 to 18% after radical amputation (Lindberg et al., 1981). In contrast, the local recurrence rate after radical radiation treatment alone was shown to be 66%.

In a series of 82 patients with extremity liposarcomas seen from 1949 to 1967, muscle group en bloc resection was applied in some patients and radical amputation in others; the overall rate of local recurrence was 27% (Shiu et al., 1975). Ten patients received wide soft part resection and adjunctive radiation therapy; the local recurrence rate was 10%. Lindberg et al. (1981) also emphasized use of postoperative radiation therapy in "unfavorable" lesions in an attempt to preserve a functional limb. The overall local recurrence rate was 22% with a functional limb preserved in 84% of patients. In a prospective randomized trial comparing amputation with wide local excision plus radiotherapy, local recurrences occurred in none of 16 patients treated with amputation and four of 26 undergoing combined treatment (Rosenberg et al., 1978). All local recurrences occurred in the thigh and generally in those with positive surgical margins. Finally, Eilber et al. (1980) reported a 3% local recurrence rate for extremity sarcomas treated with intraarterial doxorubicin, 3500 rads of external beam radiotherapy, followed by radical en bloc resection of primary tumor with limb salvage.

Thus, conservative surgery plus adjunctive radiation therapy with or without chemotherapy decreases local recurrence when complete operative removal with adequate surgical margins has been accomplished. Ideally, the surgeon and radiation therapist should plan their approach together. All areas of the operative site should be irradiated in order to minimize local recurrence. Brachytherapy has special appeal, because very high doses of radiation can be delivered to a precise field within a short time. Brachytherapy combined with wide regional resection has resulted in only one local recurrence in 23 patients (Hilaris, 1984).

The surgical approach to the management of soft tissue sarcomas must take into account the previously described prognostic criteria (Kearney et al., 1980). Adequate tumor material, usually by open surgical biopsy, should be obtained for histologic diagnosis by permanent section. Care must be taken in planning the biopsy approach so as not to compromise later surgical extirpative therapy. Ultrasound and extremity CT scans are useful in defining the gross limits of the tumor and proximity to vital structures. Angiography may be necessary to define both vascular supply and involvement of major blood vessels by sarcoma.

THE OPERATIVE TREATMENT OF COMPLICATIONS OF RADIATION THERAPY AND CHEMOTHERAPY

The surgeon is often called upon to perform surgery on a patient who has been treated with radiation therapy or chemotherapy. Relatively small amounts of radiation therapy have no impact on the nature or extent of an operation. More extensive amounts, such as 4000 to 5000 rads over five weeks in the preoperative treatment of sarcomas, breast, or rectal cancer, may require a delay of five to six weeks to allow resolution of erythema and edema. At the same time, operative risk is greater. The risk of an anastomotic disruption may be sufficiently high in the setting of extensive preoperative radiation therapy to require a temporary proximal colostomy. It may also be necessary to apply reinforcement to a wound closure. The concurrent application of radiomimetic drugs such as adriamycin or actinomycin D will augment the adverse side effects of radiation therapy to normal tissue.

The complications of radiation therapy, which occur infrequently, may include skin breakdown, fistulas, intestinal obstruction, and perforation. Radiation therapy as an adjunct in the management of gynecologic and urologic cancer may result in bladder and rectal injuries weeks to years after treatment. Anseline and associates (1981) reported 104 patients with radiation injury of the rectum; 50 patients required surgery for proctitis unresponsive to conservative measures (n = 14), rectal stricture or fistula (n = 32), or rectosigmoid perforation (n = 4). Diversion was considered the safest form of treatment for rectovaginal fistulas, rectal strictures, and proctitis; intestinal resection resulted in increased morbidity and mortality. Intestinal bypass or diversion is the safest approach to bowel obstruction or intestinal fistulae secondary to the late effects of pelvic irradiation. Diabetes mellitus, hypertension, and previous abdominal surgery predispose the bowel to radiation injury.

The surgeon may have to deal with the complications of chemotherapy. Patients with isolated areas of lymphomas in the gut may experience perforation during radiation therapy or chemotherapy; hence the principle of excision of these isolated areas before systemic treatment. Patients with leukemia may experience perforation in the gut or other areas of focal sepsis at the time of nadir white counts. In the presence of perforation in a hematopoietically depressed patient, exclusion of the perforated intestine may provide a better chance for survival than resection and anastomosis.

Chemotherapy may inhibit wound healing, resulting in increased complications. Devereux and colleagues (1979) found significant impairment in wound healing in rats when doxorubicin was given in the perioperative period (day seven before operation to day three after surgery). Corticosteroids, vincristine, methotrexate, actinomycin D, bleomycin, BCNU, and cyclophosphamide have also been shown to be deleterious in animal studies on wound healing (Cohen *et al.,* 1975).

INTRAOPERATIVE INTERACTIONS WITH CHEMOTHERAPY AND RADIATION THERAPY

The surgeon and the medical oncologist collaborate in regional chemotherapy in at least two particular areas. Cannulation of the gastroduodenal artery is necessary for infusion of the hepatic artery with chemotherapeutic drugs for patients with hepatic metastases, particularly from large-bowel cancer. The second area of interaction is that of limb perfusion in patients with melanoma or soft tissue sarcoma.

Surgical interaction with radiation therapists may include the application of interstitial therapy (brachytherapy) by implantation of radioactive isotopes or afterloading catheters in patients with lung cancer or after dissections for soft tissue sarcoma. Another area of growing interest is the application of intraoperative radiation therapy through the exposed viscera, hence permitting direct contact of radiation at the desired sites without need for penetration of intervening skin or soft tissue.

SUMMARY

The surgical oncologist bears the responsibility for initial diagnosis and management of patients with a variety of neoplasms. Accurate diagnosis and complete staging are coupled with adequate *en bloc* operative removal of localized disease. The surgical oncologist's role varies (curative, palliative, staging) with the type of cancer and should be integrated into a multimodal approach to the treatment of the patient with cancer.

REFERENCES

Adashek, K.; Sanger, J.; and Longmire, W. P.: Cancer of the stomach. *Ann. Surg.,* **189:**6, 1979.

Adson, M. A., and Van Heerden, J. A.: Major hepatic resections for metastatic colorectal cancer. *Ann. Surg.,* **191:**576, 1980.

Ames, F. C.; Sugarbaker, E. V.; and Ballantyne, A. J.: Analysis of survival and disease control in stage 1 melanoma of the head and neck. *Am. J. Surg.,* **132:**484–491, 1976.

Anseline, P. F.; Lavery, I. C.; Fazio, V. W.; Jagelman, D. G.; and Weakley, F. L.: Radiation injury of the rectum. *Ann. Surg.,* **194:**716, 1981.

Attiyeh, F. F., and Stearns, M. W.: Second-look laparotomy based on CEA elevations in colorectal cancer. *Cancer,* **47:**2119, 1981.

Baker, R. R.: Outpatient breast biopsies. *Ann. Surg.,* **185:**543, 1977.

Baker, R. R.; Montague, A.; and Childs, J. M.: A comparison of modified radical mastectomy to radical mastectomy in the treatment of operable breast cancer. *Ann. Surg.,* **189:**553, 1979.

Balch, C. M.; Murad, T.; Soong, S.; Ingalls, A. L.; Halpern, N. B.; and Maddox, W. A.: A multifactorial analysis of melanoma. *Ann. Surg.,* **188:**732, 1978.

Balch, C. M.; Murad, T. M.; Soong, S.; Ingalls, A. L.; Richards, P. C.; and Maddox, W. A.: Tumor thickness as a guide to surgical management of clinical stage I melanoma patients. *Cancer,* **43:**883, 1979.

Bartlett, J. G.: Choosing and using antibiotics. In Condon, R. E., and DeCosse, J. (eds.): *Surgical Care.* Lea & Febiger, Philadelphia, 1980.

Bartlett, J. G.; Condon, R. E.; Gorbach, S. L.; Clarke, J. S.; Nichols, R. L.; and Ochi, S.: VA cooperative study on bowel preparation for elective colorectal operations. *Ann. Surg.,* **188:**249, 1978.

Bistrian, B. R.; Blackburn, G. L.; Vitale, J.; Codran, D.; and Naylor, J.: Prevalence of malnutrition in general medical patients. *J.A.M.A.,* **235:**1567–1570, 1976.

Breslow, A.: Tumor thickness, level of invasion and node dissection in stage I cutaneous melanoma. *Ann. Surg.,* **182:**572, 1975.

Breslow, A., and Macht, S. D.: Optimal size of resection margin for thin cutaneous melanoma. *Surg. Gynecol. Obstet.,* **145:**691, 1977.

Buchholtz, T. W.; Welch, C. E.; and Malt, R. A.: Clinical correlates of resectability and survival in gastric carcinoma. *Ann. Surg.,* **188:**711, 1978.

Calle, R.; Pilleron, J. P.; Schlienger, P.; and Vilcoq, J. R.: Conservative management of operable breast cancer. *Cancer,* **42**:2045, 1978.

Cameron, J. L.; Gayler, B. W.; and Zuidema, G. D.: The use of silastic transhepatic stents in benign and malignant biliary strictures. *Ann. Surg.,* **188**:552, 1978.

Clark, W. H.; From, L.; Bernadino, E. A.; and Michm, M. C.: The histogenesis and biological behavior of primary human malignant melanomas of the skin. *Cancer Res.,* **29**:705, 1969.

Cohen, S. C.; Gabelnick, H. L.; Johnson, R. K.; and Goldin, A.: Effects of antineoplastic agents on wound healing in mice. *Surgery,* **78**:238, 1975.

Copeland, E. M., and Dudrick, S. J.: Nutritional aspects of cancer. *Curr. Probl. Cancer,* **1**, 1976.

Copeland, E. M., and McBride, C. M.: Axillary metastasis from an unknown primary site. *Ann. Surg.,* **178**:25–27, 1973.

Copeland, E. M.; Miller, L. D.; and Jones, R. S.: Prognostic factors in carcinoma of the colon and rectum. *Am. J. Surg.,* **116**:875–881, 1968.

Cruse, P.: Infection surveillance: Identifying the problems and the high-risk patient. *South. Med. J.,* **70**:4–10, 1977.

Daly, J. M.; Dudrick, S. J.; and Copeland, E. M.: Evaluation of nutritional indices as prognostic indicators in the cancer patient. *Cancer,* **43**:925–931, 1979.

Daly, J. M.; Massar, E.; Giacco, G.; Frazier, O. H.; Mountain, C. F.; Dudrick, S. J.; and Copeland, E. M.: Parenteral nutrition in esophageal cancer patients. *Ann. Surg.,* **193**:196–203, 1982.

Davis, N. C.: Cutaneous melanoma: The Queensland experience. *Curr. Probl. Surg.,* **13**:5, 1976.

Devereux, D. F.; Thilbault, L.; Bonetas, J.; and Brennan, M. F.: The quantitative and qualitative impairment of wound healing by adriamycin. *Cancer,* **43**:932, 1979.

Duke, J. H., and Miller, T. A.: Salt and water: Fluid and electrolyte problems. In Condon, R., and DeCosse, J. (eds.): *Surgical Care.* Lea & Febiger, Philadelphia, 1980.

Eilber, F. R.; Mirra, J. J.; Grant, T. T.; Weisenburger, T.; and Morton, D. L.: Is amputation necessary for sarcomas? *Ann. Surg.,* **192**:431, 1980.

Ellis, F. H., and Gibb, S.: Esophagogastrectomy for carcinoma. *Ann. Surg.,* **190**:699, 1979.

Enker, W. E.; Kemeny, N.; Shank, B.; and Rotstein, L.: Defining the needs for adjuvant therapy of rectal and colonic cancer. *Surg. Clin. North Am.,* **61**:1295, 1981.

Epstein, E.; Bragg, K.; and Linden, G.: Biopsy and prognosis of malignant melanoma. *J.A.M.A.,* **69**, 1969.

Evans, J. T.; Vana, J.; Aronoff, B. L.; Baker, H. W.; and Murphy, G. P.: Management and survival of carcinoma of the colon: Results of a national survey by the American College of Surgeons. *Ann. Surg.,* **188**:716, 1978.

Fisher, B.; Redmond, C.; Fisher, E.; and participating NASBP investigators: The contribution of recent NASBP clinical trials of primary breast cancer therapy to an understanding of tumor biology. *Cancer,* **46**:1009, 1980.

Fletcher, W.: The prognostic significance of estrogen receptors in human breast cancer. *Am. J. Surg.,* **135**:372, 1978.

Forrest, J. F., and Longmire, W. P.: Carcinoma of the pancreas and periampullary region. *Ann. Surg.,* **189**:129, 1979.

Frable, W. J.: Fine needle aspiration biopsy: Clinical applications. *Surg. Rounds,* **5**:40, 1982.

Frazier, T. G.; Copeland, E. M.; Gallager, H. S.; Paulus,

D. P.; and White, E. C.: Prognosis and treatment in minimal breast cancer. *Am. J. Surg.,* **133**:697, 1977.

Grage, T.; Vassilopoulos, P.; Shingleton, W.; Jubert, A. V.; Elias, E. G.; Aust, J. B.; and Moss, S. E.: Results of a prospective randomized study of hepatic artery infusion with 5-FU versus IV 5-FU in patients with hepatic metastases from colorectal cancer. *Surgery,* **86**:550, 1979.

Haffejee, A. A., and Angorn, I. B.: Nutritional status and the nonspecific cellular and humeral immune response in esophageal carcinoma. *Ann. Surg.,* **189**:475–480, 1979.

Hajdu, S. I.: Soft tissue sarcomas: Classification and natural history. *Cancer,* **31**:271, 1981.

Herrera, M.; Chu, T. M.; and Holyoke, E. D.: Carcinoembryonic antigens (CEA) as a prognostic and monitoring test in clinically complete resection of colorectal carcinoma. *Ann. Surg.,* **183**:5, 1976.

Higgins, G. A.; Donaldson, R. C.; Humphrey, E. W.; Rogers, L. S.; and Shields, T. W.: Adjuvant therapy for large-bowel cancer. *Surg. Clin. North Am.,* **61**:1311, 1981.

Hilaris, B.: Personal communication. 1984.

Holmes, E. C.; Moseley, H. S.; Morton, D. L.; Clark, W.; Robinson, D.; and Vrist, M.: A rational approach to the surgical management of melanoma. *Ann. Surg.,* **186**:481, 1977.

Holter, A. R., and Fischer, J. E.: The effects of perioperative hyperalimentation on complications in patients with carcinoma and weight loss. *J. Surg. Res.,* **23**:31–34, 1977.

Holyoke, E. D.; Evans, J. T.; and Chu, T. M.: CEA in the diagnosis and treatment of colon and rectal cancer. In Enker, W. E. (ed.): *Carcinoma of the Colon and Rectum.* Year Book Medical Publishers, Inc., Chicago, 1978.

Kearney, M. M.; Soule, E. H.; and Bivins, J. C.: Malignant fibrous histiocytoma. *Cancer,* **45**:167, 1980.

Keighley, M. R., and Burdon, D. W.: *Antimicrobial Prophylaxis in Surgery.* Pitman Medical, London, England, 1979.

Kelson, D. P.; Bains, M.; Hilaris, B.; Chapman, R.; McCormack, P.; Alexander, J.; Hopfan, S.; and Martini, N.: Combination chemotherapy of esophageal carcinoma using cisplatin, vindesine and bleomycin. *Cancer,* **49**:1174, 1981.

Launois, B.; Campion, J.; Brissot, P.; and Gosselin, M.: Carcinoma of the hepatic hilus. *Ann. Surg.,* **189**:151, 1979.

Lee, Y. N.: Diagnosis, treatment and prognosis of early melanoma. *Ann. Surg.,* **191**:87, 1980.

Lindberg, R. D.; Martin, R. G.; Romsdahl, M. M.; and Barkley, H. T.: Conservative surgery and postoperative radiotherapy in 300 adults with soft tissue sarcomas. *Cancer,* **47**:2391, 1981.

MacKay, A. M.; Patel, S.; Carter, S.; Stevens, O.; Lawrence, D. J.; Cooper, E. H.; and Neville, A. M.: Role of serial plasma CEA assays in detection of recurrent and metastatic colorectal carcinoma. *Br. Med. J.,* **4**:382, 1974.

Marks, R. D.; Scruggs, H. J.; and Wallace, K. M.: Preoperative radiation therapy for carcinoma of the esophagus. *Cancer,* **38**:84, 1976.

Martin, H., and Ellis, E.: Aspiration biopsy. *Surg. Gynecol. Obstet.,* **59**:578, 1934.

Minton, J. P., and Martin, E. W.: The use of serial CEA determinations to predict recurrence of colon cancer and when to do a second-look operation. *Cancer,* **42**:1422, 1978.

Morson, B. C.; Bussey, H. J. R.; and Samoorian, S.: Policy

of local excision for early cancer of the colorectum. *Gut,* **18:**1045, 1977.

Mullen, J. L.; Buzby, G. P.; Waldman, M. T.; Gertner, M. H.; Hobbs, C. L.; and Rosato, E. F.: Prediction of operative morbidity and mortality by preoperative nutritional assessment. *Surg. Forum,* **30:**80–81, 1979.

Muller, J. M.; Dienst, C.; Brenner, V.; and Pichlmaier, H.: Preoperative parenteral feeding in patients with gastrointestinal carcinoma. *Lancet,* **1:**68–71, 1982.

Nichols, R. L.; Broido, P.; Condon, R. E.; Gorbach, S. L.; and Nyhus, L. M.: Effect of preoperative neomycin-erythromycin intestinal preparation on the incidence of infectious complications following colon surgery. *Ann. Surg.,* **178:**453, 1973.

Papachristou, D. N., and Fortner, J. G.: Adenocarcinoma of the gastric cardia. *Ann. Surg.,* **192:**58, 1980.

Paulino, F., and Roselli, A.: Carcinoma of the stomach. *Curr. Probl. Surg.,* December, 1973.

Polk, H. C.: Extended resection for selected adenocarcinomas of the large bowel. *Ann. Surg.,* **175:**892, 1975.

Polk, H. C.: Principles of preoperative preparation of the surgical patient. In Sabiston, D. (ed.): Davis-Christopher's *Textbook of Surgery.* W.B. Saunders Company, Philadelphia, 1977.

Rao, A. R.; Kagan, A. R.; Chan, P. M.; Gilbert, H. A.; Nussbaum, H.; and Hintz, B. L.: Patterns of recurrence following curative resection alone for adenocarcinoma of the rectum and sigmoid colon. *Cancer,* **48:**1492, 1981.

Rosenberg, J. C.; Franklin, R.; and Steiger, Z.: Squamous cell carcinoma of the thoracic esophagus: an interdisciplinary approach. *Curr. Probl. Surg.,* **18:**5, 1981.

Rosenberg, S. A.; Kent, H.; Costa, J.; Webber, B. L.; Young, R.; Chabner, B.; Baker, A.; Brennan, M.; Cretian, P.; Cohen, M.; deMoss, E.; Sears, H.; Seipp, C.; and Simon, R.: Prospective randomized evaluation of the role of limb-sparing surgery, radiation therapy and adjuvant chemo-immunotherapy in the treatment of adult soft tissue sarcomas. *Surgery,* **84:**62, 1978.

Schour, L., and Chu, E.: Fine needle aspiration in the management of patients with neoplastic disease. *Acta Cytol.,* **18:**472, 1974.

Shiu, M. H.; Chu, F.; Castro, E. B.; Hajdu, S. I.; and Fortner, J. G.: Results of surgical and radiation therapy in the treatments of liposarcoma arising in an extremity. *Cancer,* **123:**577, 1975.

Shiu, M. H.; Papachristou, D.; Kosloff, C.; and Eliopoulos, G.: Selection of operative procedure for adenocarcinoma of the midstomach. *Ann. Surg.,* **192:**730, 1980.

Smith, T. J.; Kemeny, M. M.; Sugarbaker, P. H.; Jones, A. E.; Vermiss, M.; Shawker, T. H.; and Edwards, B.: A prospective study of hepatic imaging in the detection of metastatic disease. *Ann. Surg.,* **195:**486, 1982.

Stearns, M. W., and Schottenfeld, D.: Techniques for the surgical management of colon cancer. *Cancer,* **28:**165, 1971.

Sugarbaker, E. V., and McBride, C. M.: Melanoma of the trunk: The results of surgical excision and anatomic guidelines for predicting nodal metastases. *Surgery,* **80:**22, 1976a.

Sugarbaker, E. V., and McBride, C. M.: Survival and regional disease control after isolation-perfusion for invasive stage I melanoma of the extremities. *Cancer,* **37:**188, 1976b.

Sugarbaker, P. H.: Carcinoma of the colon: Prognosis and operative choice. *Curr. Probl. Surg.,* **18:**755–801, 1981.

Turnbull, R. B.; Kryle, K.; Watson, F. R.; and Spratt, J.: Cancer of the colon: The influence of the "no-touch" isolation technic on survival rates. *Ann. Surg.,* **166:**420, 1967.

Tartter, P.; Slater, G.; Gelernt, I.; and Aufses, A. H.: Screening for liver metastases from colorectal cancer with CEA and alkaline phosphatase. *Ann. Surg.,* **193:**357, 1981.

Veronesi, U.; Adamus, J.; Bandiera, D. C.; Brennhovd, I. O.; Caceres, E.; Cascinelli, N.; Claudio, F.; Ikonopison, R. L.; Javorskj, V. V.; Kirov, S.; Kulakowski, A.; Lacour, J.; Lejeune, F.; Mechl, A.; Morabito, A.; Rhode, I.; Sergeev, S.; van Slooten, E.; Szczygiel, K.; Trapenznikov, N. N.; and Wagner, R. I.: Inefficacy of immediate node dissection in stage 1 melanoma of the limbs. *N. Engl. J. Med.,* **297:**627–630, 1977.

Veronesi, U.; Saccozzi, R.; Del Vecchio, M.; Banfi, A.; Clemente, C.; DeLena, M.; Grallus, G.; Greco, M.; Luini, A.; Marubini, E.; Muscolino, G.; Ruke, F.; Saboardori, B.; Zecchini, A.; and Zucali, R.: Comparing radical mastectomy with quadrantectomy, axillary dissection and radiotherapy in patients with small cancers of the breast. *N. Engl. J. Med.,* **305:**6–11, 1981.

Veterans Administration ad hoc Interdisciplinary Advisory Committee on Antimicrobial Drug Usage. Prophylaxis in Surgery. *J.A.M.A.,* **237:**1003–1010, 1977.

Wanebo, H. J.; Woodruff, J.; and Fortner, J. G.: Malignant melanoma of the extremities: A clinicopathologic study using levels of invasion. *Cancer,* **35:**666, 1975.

Wanebo, H. J.; Rao, B.; Pinsky, C.; Hoffman, R.; Stearns, M.; Schwartz, M.; and Oettgen, H.: Preoperative carcinoembryonic antigen level as a prognostic indicator in colorectal cancer. *N. Engl. J. Med.,* **299:**448, 1978.

Washington, J. A.; Dearing, W. H.; Judd, E. S.; and Elveback, L. R.: Effect of preoperative antibiotic regimen on development of infection after intestinal surgery. *Ann. Surg.,* **180:**567, 1974.

Willard, M. D.; Gilsdorf, R. B.; and Price, R. A.: Protein-calorie malnutrition in a community hospital. *J.A.M.A.,* **243:**1720–1724, 1980.

Williams, R. H. P.; Heatley, R. V.; Lewis, M. H.; and Hughes, L. E.: Preoperative parenteral nutrition in patients with stomach cancer. In Baxter, D. H., and Jackson, G. M. (eds.): *Clinical Parenteral Nutrition.* Geistlich Education, Chester, England, 1977.

Wiseman, C.; Jessup, J. M.; Smith, T. L.; Hersh, E.; Biven, J.; and Blumenschein, G.: Inflammatory breast cancer treated with surgery, chemotherapy and allogenic tumor cell/BCG immunotherapy. *Cancer,* **49:**1266, 1982.

Zamcheck, N.: The present status of CEA in diagnosis, prognosis and evaluation of therapy. *Cancer,* **30:**2460, 1975.

9

Principles of Radiation Therapy

MELVYN P. RICHTER, FREDERICK S. SHARE, and
ROBERT L. GOODMAN

INTRODUCTION

Radiation oncology now represents the integration of knowledge obtained over an 80-year period from the physics and biology laboratories and the medical clinic. Such integration is recent; until the supervoltage era following World War II, the chief developments in these three areas for the most part were realized independently. The physics and engineering laboratories have now developed a dependable family of sources of ionizing radiations that can be precisely directed at tumor volumes at various depths within the body. The biology laboratory has provided the basic scientific support underlying the extensive clinical experience and currently is suggesting ways of using ionizing radiations more effectively, such as modified fractionation schedules relating to cell cycle kinetics and the use of drugs and chemicals as modifiers of radiation response and normal tissue reaction. The radiation therapy clinic has provided the patient stratum on which the acute and chronic effects of irradiation have been assessed, and the patterns of treatment success and failure identified. The radiation therapist has shared with the surgeon and medical oncologist the responsibility for clarifying the natural history of a large number of human neoplasms, and through such clarifications, has developed more effective treatment strategies. Several examples of this include the improved results in the treatment of Hodgkin's disease (Kaplan, 1980), squamous cell carcinoma of the cervix (Fletcher, 1980), seminoma (Maier and Sulak, 1973), and epithelial neoplasms of the upper aerodigestive tract (Fletcher, 1980).

HISTORY

Professor Wilhelm Roentgen of the University of Wurzburg discovered x-rays using a Hittorf-Crookes vacuum tube in 1895 (Roentgen, 1895). In 1898, Marie and Pierre Curie isolated radium and introduced the property of "radioactivity." In the same year, Villard demonstrated that gamma rays and x-rays were identical. Clinical applications with primitive equipment were begun almost immediately, consisting mainly of large single treatments of x-rays applied empirically against a broad spectrum of benign and neoplastic disease. One of the first inductive uses of therapeutic x-rays, the successful treatment of a benign hairy nevus, occurred in Vienna following the observation of local epilation produced by radiation exposure.

From a technical point of view, what was needed was the development of reliable x-ray sources of sufficient energy to treat tumors situated deep within the body. The development of the Coolidge hot filament tube in the United States in 1913 served as the model for the 220,000 volt orthovoltage x-ray generators developed in the 1920s. In the 1930s, the Cyclotron and Van de Graaff high-voltage generator were developed, and in the 1940s and thereafter, in the wake of nuclear weapons research, radioactive cobalt and the linear accelerator became available for medical use (Schulz, 1975).

As important to radiation therapy as the availability of higher energy equipment was the development of precise measurement of radiation dose. Initially, chemical dosimetry by colorimetry was used to estimate radiation exposure. This method was difficult to standardize and required correlation with empirically developed biologic end points, such as "skin erythema dose," a variable reddening of the skin occurring after one to two weeks following the irradiation event. By the 1920s, compact ionization chambers were available for the measurement of roentgen rays and radiations from radioactive sources. In 1928, the Roentgen (R), a measurement of ionizations in air, became the accepted unit of radiation exposure. The unit of radiation dose, equivalent to 100 ergs of absorbed energy per gram of tissue, the rad, was not introduced until 1954. Recently, a new unit of absorbed dose, the Gray (Gy), has been adopted; it is equal to 100 rads. See Chapter 3C for the definitions of other radiation units utilized in studies of carcinogenesis.

Paralleling advances in the technical delivery of ionizing radiations and their measurement was the clinical appreciation of the normal tissue benefits of dose fractionation. Claudius Regaud, Professor of Histology at Lyon and later Director of the Curie Foundation in Paris, demonstrated that although multiple low-dose fractions of irradiation on the ram's testis produced both cessation of spermatogenesis and preservation of the integrity of the overlying skin, single large doses produced not only the same physiologic result but also unacceptable damage to adjacent tissues (Regaud, 1977). Regaud appreciated the similarity between this response and that of tumor eradication and proposed that fractionated radiation therapy would be of clinical benefit (Regaud et al., 1922). His colleague, Henri Coutard, applied this principle of fractionated daily radiotherapy in the treatment of a variety of head and neck cancers (Coutard, 1932, 1934). Coutard's "protracted-fractional" method has essentially been adopted as a fundamental principle of clinical radiation therapy up to the present, and conventionally fractionated irradiation, 180–200 rads daily target dose, continues as the standard against which other dose schedules are measured (Peschel and Fischer, 1981).

Puck and Marcus (1956), using their technique of the clonal cultivation of mammalian cells in vitro, demonstrated the relationship of radiation dose to cell survival. Elkind and Sutton (1960) were able to show that mammalian cells were capable of repairing sublethal radiation damage. These findings, along with the appreciation of the clinical relevance of oxy-gen, a key radiation sensitizer, by L. H. Gray and his coworkers, enabled the discipline of radiation biology to become firmly linked to radiation oncology (Gray et al., 1953; Thomlinson and Gray, 1955).

PHYSICS

Ionizing radiations are composed of both electromagnetic waves such as x-rays and gamma rays and subatomic particles such as electrons, neutrons, protons, stripped nuclei, and pi-mesons (for general references, see Hendee, 1981; Johns and Cunningham, 1974; Meredith and Massey, 1977) (see Figure 9–1). Gamma rays are emitted spontaneously by the decay of unstable radioactive nuclei such as radium 226 or cobalt 60, and x-rays are produced by electronic devices such as diagnostic x-ray units and linear accelerators by the bombardment of a high-atomic-number target with an accelerated stream of electrons. High-energy electrons are produced by linear accelerators and betatrons, and some radioisotopes emit high-energy electrons called beta particles. Neutrons can be produced by fusing two isotopes of hydrogen, deuterium and tritium, or by accelerating protons or deuterons to high energy in a cyclotron. Research physics linear accelerators such as those at Vancouver and Berkeley are capable of producing high-energy heavy ions such as carbon, argon, and silicon that are being explored for treatment of neoplasms. Finally, exotic particles such as pi-mesons are being explored as a treatment modality at Los Alamos and elsewhere (Fowler, 1981).

Standard radiation therapy utilizes high energy x-rays and gamma rays and electrons. Einstein in 1905 demonstrated the direct proportional relationship between the energy of an x or gamma photon and its wave frequency by the formula $E = h\gamma$, where the constant of proportionality h is Planck's constant. All waves represent a transfer of energy from one

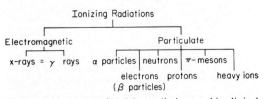

Figure 9–1. Types of ionizing radiation used in clinical radiation therapy.

locus to another. For electromagnetic radiation, this energy transfer occurs in a discontinuous fashion in *quanta,* which are finite "packets" of energy. The energy unit for electromagnetic radiations is the electron volt (eV), which is the amount of kinetic energy an electron would acquire if it were accelerated across a potential difference of one volt. By convention, x-rays of peak energy less than 1000 keV (1 MeV) are known as orthovoltage, and those greater than 1 MeV as supervoltage or megavoltage (see Figure 9–2).

The nature of the interaction of photons with matter is dependent on their energy: Low energy x-rays, generally below 30 keV, give up their energy to tissue by the photoelectric effect, in which the photon imparts all of its energy to an inner-shell electron. The photoelectric effect is most probable in high-atomic-number materials, increasing as the third power of the atomic number. For this reason, enhanced absorption is seen in bone versus soft tissue or air in a diagnostic radiograph. Above 30 keV, Compton scattering is the principal interaction of ionizing radiations with tissue, and it is essentially the only relevant interaction in the range of energies used in radiation therapy. Here the photon may impart only a portion of its energy to an orbital electron, resulting in a high-speed recoil elec-

tron and a scattered photon of lower energy. The greater the energy of the incoming photon, the higher the likelihood that the scatter will be in a forward direction and the higher the proportion of kinetic energy imparted to the recoil electron. Compton scattering interactions do not vary with atomic number as does the photoelectric effect. It depends on the number of electrons per gram, which is roughly equivalent for all elements except hydrogen. A third interaction, pair production, is seen with photon energies greater than 1.02 MeV. Such photons in the vicinity of the electric and magnetic forces of a nucleus may form an electron-positron pair. Though of great interest in physics, such pair production has limited clinical significance in radiation therapy.

The build-up of absorbed dose to a maximum value at a depth within tissue is related to the maximum range of the secondary electrons produced by the interaction of ionizing radiations with matter. For orthovoltage beams, the maximum dose is deposited at the surface of the absorbing medium as there is less forward scatter, and the range of the electrons produced is short. For supervoltage, the maximum absorbed dose occurs at some distance below the surface. The higher the energy of the ionizing radiation, the greater the skin sparing and the greater the degree of deep-tissue pene-

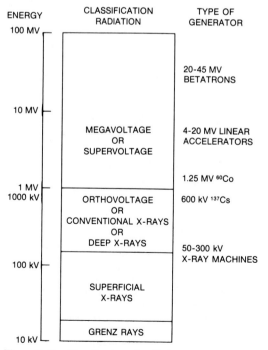

Figure 9–2. Classification of radiation beams.

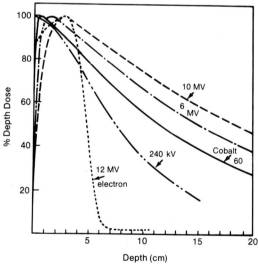

Figure 9–3. Typical depth dose curves for standard x-ray beams ranging from 240 kV to 10 MV contrasted with a 12 MV electron beam. Note the 240 kV has maximum dose at the skin surface, whereas the higher energy beams demonstrate the skin-sparing effect discussed in the text. The electron beam demonstrates slight skin-sparing properties.

Table 9–1. Skin-Sparing and Percentage Depth Doses for Commonly Used XRT Beams

	MAXIMUM BEAM ENERGY	DOSE MAXIMUM	50% DEPTH DOSE (10 × 10 CM FIELD)
Linacs	250 kV	Surface	7 cm
	1.25 MV (^{60}Co)	0.5 cm	11 cm
	4 MV	1.0 cm	14 cm
	6 MV	1.5 cm	16 cm
	10 MV	2.0 cm	18 cm
	15 MV	3.0 cm	20 cm
Betatrons	25 MV	4.0 cm	23 cm
	35 MV	5.0 cm	26 cm

tration (see Figure 9–3; Table 9–1). Without the property of skin sparing, radiation doses required to sterilize both microscopic and gross tumor could not be delivered to deep-seated disease without creating unacceptable skin and subcutaneous tissue changes, leading to ulceration and necrosis. This potential damage is one of the key factors that limits the efficacy of orthovoltage irradiation except in the treatment of tumors of the skin and superficial soft tissues and the occasional palliation of metastatic tumors involving the chest wall and ribs.

X-rays have an effect on matter through ionizations produced by secondary electrons. Electron beams generated by linear accelerators and betatrons have the same final effect as x-rays, but the depth dose characteristics of primary electron beams are quite different. Because electrons are charged particles, they cause ionizing interactions immediately upon entering tissue. The dose delivered by electrons has the dramatic characteristic of being relatively constant until a critical depth is reached and then the dose declines rapidly. The depth at which the dose is nearly zero depends on the initial energy of the beam. This property makes electron beams ideally suited for the treatment of superficially placed tumor volumes, such as cervical lymph nodes and the soft tissues of the chest wall, without giving a high dose to underlying normal tissue (Chu and Laughlin, 1981).

Once the maximum absorbed dose at depth is known, then other measured doses in tissue can be calculated as a percentage of that peak dose. These depth dose curves are developed from a knowledge of the central axis and off-axis dose measurements. For most deep-seated

tumors, it is not possible to deliver a reasonably homogeneous dose using a single field, as the relative dose decreases with depth. By combining fields, it is possible for the radiation therapist to optimize the dose distribution within the target volume while minimizing the dose delivered to adjacent normal tissues (see Figure 9–4). The radiation therapist, in conjunction with a radiation physicist and dosimetrist, can develop optimal plans of treatment, limited only by precise anatomic knowledge of the extent of the gross and microscopic tumor and the radiation tolerance of adjacent normal tissues.

In addition to external beam therapy, or teletherapy, certain tumor problems lend themselves to the direct application of radioactive materials either within a body cavity (intracavitary) or into tissues (interstitial) (Fletcher, 1980; Vaeth, 1978). Both intracavitary and interstitial therapy are collectively

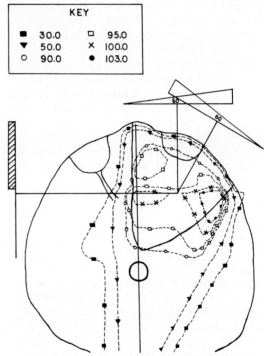

KEY			
■	30.0	□	95.0
▼	50.0	×	100.0
○	90.0	●	103.0

Figure 9–4. Cross-sectional radiation therapy treatment plan through the level of the mid orbits in a 75-year-old man with adenocarcinoma of the lacrimal gland and involvement of the posterior orbit. The patient was treated on a 6-MV linear accelerator utilizing a three-field plan consisting of an anterior oblique wedge pair supplemented by a contralateral open field posterior to eye. Target volumes were obtained by integrating clinical and CT anatomy. All doses were measured in rads (see key) and normalized to 100%.

known as brachytherapy. Such encapsulated radioactive materials act as point sources whose dose distribution behaves according to the inverse square law, decreasing inversely with the square of the distance from the radioactive source(s). This property allows for very high doses to be absorbed in close proximity to the radioactive device with markedly less dose delivered to structures more distant.

Certain organs such as the uterus and vagina are natural receptacles for the placement of intracavitary sources. The oral cavity, neck, breast, perineum, anus, and distal rectum lend themselves to interstitial placement. Both intracavitary and interstitial devices can be placed under fluoroscopic guidance to attain optimal anatomic position and radiation geometry. By the technique of afterloading, the device can be loaded with the radioactive material after the patient has been returned to an isolated environment. In such fashion, hardly any radiation exposure is received by supporting personnel and only minimal exposure is received by the radiation therapist, physicist, and nurses. Mechanisms and devices for intracavitary and interstitial placement of radioactive material parallel the historic development of radiation therapy and are associated with the major radiation therapy centers of Stockholm, Paris, and Manchester. Currently, cesium 137 has replaced radium 226 as the principal radioactive material for intracavitary encapsulated sources, and iridium 192 has replaced radium 226 as the principal material in interstitial work. The decline in the use of radium is related to problems of radiation protection, particularly the potential for encapsulated radium salts to leak radon gas, a daughter product. Permanent internal radiation placements are also available with gold 198, radon 222, and iodine 125. The latter has two special properties: A long half-life (60 days), permitting delivery of low-dose-rate gamma irradiation for an extended period of time. In addition, the gamma emitted by ^{125}I is of low energy, being almost exclusively absorbed within the implanted tumor, thereby allowing the patient to leave the hospital shortly after the implant procedure.

RADIATION BIOLOGY

The cellular response to irradiation is not due to heating. Exposing a 70 kg man to 1000 rads total body dose deposits less than 15.4 calories. Crowther (1924) and others developed a theory of cellular radiation damage based on injury to an unknown but specific target within the cell. As early as the 1930s, microirradiation studies indicated that the site of this damage resided in the nucleus. The site is now felt to be nuclear DNA (Kaplan, 1974). Radiation indirectly ionizes water molecules, resulting in the formation of superactive free radicals such as $\cdot OH$ (hydroxyl) that attack nuclear DNA, potentially interfering with cellular replication. When a radiation cell survival curve was developed, it was deduced that cell death was based on the radiation inactivation of at least two targets within the DNA molecule. Whereas cells have the capacity to accumulate and repair damage to a single target, a strand of DNA, inactivation of a second target, both DNA strands, leads to mitotic or, less often, to interphase cell death (for general references see Duncan and Nias, 1977; Hall, 1978; Ritter, 1981).

The technique of mammalian cell culture developed by Puck and Marcus (1956) has allowed for the development of a fundamental description of cellular radiation sensitivity, the dose-cell survival curve. This quantification of radiation sensitivity is a laboratory observation, not a direct statement of the *in vivo* radiation responsiveness of specific tissues and tumors to irradiation. A semilogarithmic graph of the percent of cell survival versus the radiation dose yields a plot with an initial sloping curve at low dose evolving into a straight line with higher dose (see Figure 9–5). The slope of the straight line portion is a measure of the radiation dose required to kill 63% of an initial number of cells beginning at some point on the linear part of the curve. This dose is expressed as the D_o or radiosensitivity of the cell type. An extrapolation of the linear portion of the curve to a point on the abscissa yields a theoretic target number referred to as *n*. The ordinate distance to the 100% survival point on this extrapolated line is an index of the radiation dose accumulated prior to the expression of lethal damage. This dose is expressed as the D_q or quasi-threshold dose. Both *n* and D_o provide a uniform means of comparing the sensitivity of cell types; the D_q provides the means of comparing accumulation and repair of sublethal damage. Surprisingly, along a broad spectrum, both normal and tumor cells demonstrate D_o's of approximately 100 to 200 rads, suggesting similar radiation sensitivity on an *in vitro* basis for both tumor and normal

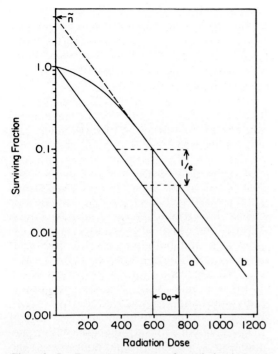

Figure 9–5. Dose-response curves for radiation-induced loss of reproductive capacity in cells. Curve a represents an exponential or single-event response, which appears as a straight line when displayed on a semilogarithmic plot. Curve b demonstrates a multiple-event survival response, typical of the response shown by most mammalian cells. Both curves are characterized by D_0, the dose necessary to reduce survival to $1/e$ or 37% on the straight portion of the curves. Curve b is further characterized by the extrapolation number, ñ, which is a measure of the initial shoulder. Reproduced by permission from Ritter, M.: Cellular radiobiology. *Semin. Oncol.,* **8:**3–17, 1981.

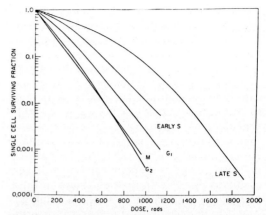

Figure 9–6. Survival curves for Chinese hamster cells at various stages of the cell cycle. From Sinclair, W. K., and Morton, R. A.: X-ray sensitivity during the cell generation cycle of cultured Chinese hamster cells. *Radiat. Res.,* **29:**450–474, 1966.

time of delivery of the total dose protracted, n decreases, D_0 increases, and the cells appear overall to be less sensitive per unit dose. This overall decrease in cellular sensitivity results from the allotment of sufficient time for intracellular repair of sublethal damage.

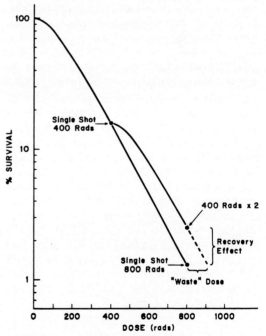

Figure 9–7. Theoretical split-dose experiment comparing cell survival for a single dose of 800 rads to two doses of 400 rads separated by several hours. Reproduced by permission from Peschel, R. E., and Fischer, J. J.: Optimization of the time-dose relationship. *Semin. Oncol.,* **8:**38–48, 1981.

cells. Lymphoid and bone marrow cells are exceptions, with D_0's averaging 95 rads. D_q's are known to vary widely from 10 rad for lymphocytes to 200 rads for melanocytes. Sensitivity to radiation is cell cycle-dependent (see Figure 9–6). Cells in late DNA synthesis (S) and at rest (G_o) are resistant, whereas cells in the premitotic phase (G_2) and in the mitotic phase (M) are most sensitive. A radiation exposure partially synchronizes a population of cells within the cycle by selectively destroying G_2 and M cells. Reassortment over time allows for the desynchronization of the surviving cells.

When a radiation dose is divided and delivered as two equal smaller fractions separated by a time delay, the cell kill of the combined dose of radiation is diminished (see Figure 9–7). Conceptually, the cells surviving the first radiation event respond as though no previous irradiation were experienced. As the total dose of radiation is further fractionated and the

Protraction of radiation by fractionation promotes cellular redistribution through the cell cycle, allowing uniform logarithmic cell kill with each fraction of radiation. This reassortment assures a more uniform distribution of cells throughout the phases of the cell cycle.

Following accumulated radiation damage to both tumor and adjacent tissues, repopulation of the normal tissues occurs more readily than with tumor tissues. Part of this differential repopulation is related to the recruitment or "turning on" of the stem cell compartment of rapidly proliferating tissues, such as the mucosa of the upper aerodigestive tract and gut. Acute radiation injury induces this recruitment, allowing for potential tumor sterilization while preserving the integrity of the normal tissues.

The most potent chemical modifier of radiation sensitivity is oxygen. Mammalian cells exposed to atmospheric oxygen during irradiation demonstrate a three-fold enhancement of cell kill as compared to cells irradiated under anoxic conditions. Tumor masses are known to contain hypoxic regions that may allow hypoxic cell fractions to preferentially survive radiation exposure. It is presumed that lysis and absorption of the more oxic radiation-killed cells allow remaining cells to become better oxygenated. Protraction of the radiation program through extended fractionation may thus gradually reduce the anoxic and hypoxic cell compartments as regression in tumor mass occurs. Reoxygenation would thereby reduce the more radiation-resistant hypoxic cell com-

ponent such that during a full course of therapy, 40 to 60 days, all tumor cells would have cycled through the oxic state. More densely ionizing radiations such as neutrons demonstrate smaller D_q's and reduce the oxygen dependence on cell kill.

PATHOPHYSIOLOGY OF LATE RADIATION EFFECTS

It is customarily assumed that acute radiation effects are secondary to the destruction of parenchymal cells and that the late chronic effects are secondary to vascular injury. Withers and others question this assumption, proposing "that both types of effect may result from radiation-induced parenchymal or stromal cell depletion or both" (Withers et al., 1980). The rate at which acute and chronic radiation changes in tissue develop would then be related to the individual turnover rates of the parenchymal and stromal cells within specific tissues. Rapidly proliferating tissues such as the crypt cells of the gastrointestinal mucosa or the stem cells of the bone marrow would manifest radiation damage almost immediately, whereas the vascular endothelium or connective tissue compartments, which are more slowly proliferating tissues, would manifest radiation damage at a later stage. It is the late effects that principally limit the total doses of irradiation that may be safely administered in attempting to obtain tumor sterilization of large volumes of gross disease (for general ref-

Table 9–2. Normal Tissue Tolerance (Estimated Doses for 5% and 50% Incidences of Injury Secondary to X-Irradiation* Without Chemotherapy)

ORGANS	COMPLICATION	$TD_{5/5}$† *(rad)*	$TD_{50/5}$‡ *(rad)*	WHOLE OR PARTIAL ORGAN (FIELD-SIZE OR LENGTH)
Bone marrow	aplasia, pancytopenia	250	450	whole
		3000	4000	segmental
Liver	acute and chronic hepatitis	2500	4000	whole
Stomach	ulcer, perforation, hemorrhage	4500	5500	100 cm²
Intestine	ulcer, perforation, hemorrhage	4500	5500	400 cm²
		5000	6500	100 cm²
Brain	infarction, necrosis	6000	7000	whole
Spinal cord	infarction, necrosis	4500	5500	10 cm
Heart	pericarditis and pancarditis	4500	5500	60%
		7000	8000	25%
Lung	acute and chronic pneumonitis	3000	3500	100 cm²
		1500	2500	whole
Kidney	acute and chronic nephrosclerosis	2000	2500	whole

* Dose given assuming 200 rads/fraction, 5 fractions/week.
† Dose for 5% injury in 5 years.
‡ Dose for 50% injury in 5 years.
Modified from Kramer, S., and the Committee for Radiation Oncology Studies: Research plan for radiation oncology, normal tissue tolerance, and damage. *Cancer (Suppl.)* **37**:2046–2055, 1976.

erences see Rubin and Casarett, 1968; Vaeth, 1972; White, 1975; Meyn and Withers, 1980). Tissue tolerances, pathogenic responses, and physiologic function are not only related to the total dose administered, but also to the volume of an individual organ that is encompassed by the primary high-dose radiation beam. Large single fractions can also produce physiologically impairing late effects without significant acute effects, a process known as dissociation (see Table 9–2).

THE CLINICAL BASIS OF RADIOTHERAPY

Both radiation and surgery are local as well as regional therapies. Though whole-body irradiation may be used effectively in the treatment of selected lymphomas and hemibody irradiation may be used for accelerated palliation of widespread osseous metastatic disease, the basic objective of radiation therapy is to obtain local and regional control. Accompanying radical or definitive treatment is the risk of normal tissue damage and physiologic alteration. A narrow therapeutic ratio exists that attempts to limit acute and chronic side effects while maximizing the potential for local-regional control (for general references see Fletcher, 1980; Gilbert and Kagan, 1978; Moss *et al.*, 1979).

Palliative programs are aimed at symptomatic relief generally delivered by a short treatment course (Richter, 1982). Planned doses of radiation in such instances should always remain well within the bounds of established normal tissue tolerances. In palliation, no attempt is made to sterilize the tumor. Palliation may also be directed prophylactically in an attempt to forestall potential complications of the tumor, including pain, pathologic fracture, obstruction, neurologic dysfunction, or disfigurement anticipated by the tumor's natural growth. Examples of such prophylactic palliation in an asymptomatic patient include treatment of atelectasis secondary to bronchial obstruction, extensive osseous involvement in a long bone or a vertebral body, and subclinical brain metastases. Reduction of tumor mass except when the mass produces disfigurement or organ dysfunction is not sought unless doing so contributes measurably to a patient's well being or longevity.

Curative radiotherapy in all instances requires tumor doses sufficient to sterilize all gross and microscopic disease. Differential doses are therefore required. Except for early lesions with little risk of lymphatic spread, such as T_1 lesions of the larynx and oral cavity, definitive irradiation requires a shrinking field technique with differentially prescribed doses to both the gross disease and its microscopic regional extensions. Fletcher (1980) and others have demonstrated that 4500 rads by conventional fractionation of 180 to 200 rads daily yields a greater than 90% likelihood of control of subclinical disease. Even for soft tissue sarcomas of distal extremities, 5000 to 5500 rads in conventional fractionation following wide-field surgical removal of gross disease produces a greater than 90% likelihood of local control. The corollary of this observation is that the greater the bulk, the higher the total dose needed for control. The effectiveness of increasingly graded doses in achieving local control has been well demonstrated in advanced tumors of the oropharynx and supraglottic larynx (Fletcher, 1980).

Another option for maximizing locoregional control is to combine surgery with regional irradiation. The timing of the irradiation, either preoperative or postoperative, depends on the clinical problem (Vaeth, 1970; Perez *et al.*, 1977). For tumors of the head and neck, without fixation of neck nodes to the underlying soft tissues, preoperative or postoperative irradiation may be equivalent relative to tumor control and complication (Snow *et al.*, 1981). For tumors of the pelvis, however, there may be an advantage to using preoperative irradiation in order to decrease the likelihood of small-bowel complications stemming from the surgical induction of small-bowel adhesions with bowel fixation within the pelvis. The rationale behind preoperative radiotherapy is to sterilize unrecognized microextensions of the tumor beyond the limits of the surgical resection, to cause partial or complete tumor regression, to decrease the ability of residual tumor cells to implant locally, and to eliminate subclinical disease in lymph nodes, thereby obviating the need for a regional lymphadenectomy. The only consistent disadvantage of preoperative irradiation is, perhaps, the increased incidence of delay in wound healing. A delay in the accomplishment of surgery may not always be necessary when using low doses of irradiation. For example, the placement of intracavitary radiation sources in the uterine cavity and upper vagina in partial treatment of adenocarcinoma of the endometrium may be followed within 24 hours to one week by a total abdominal hysterectomy and bilateral salpingo-oophorectomy. For carcinoma of the bladder, 2000 rads delivered in 400 rad daily fractions over one week to a limited pelvic portal may be followed immediately by definitive surgery. On the other hand, doses greater than 3000 rads produce extensive hyperemia, inflammation, and edema that necessitate a planned delay in surgery of four to six weeks. An additional benefit of this delay results from the concomitant tumor shrinkage that facilitates the definitive surgery. Such benefit may be seen following the preoperative irradiation of marginally resectable adenocarcinomas of the rectum (Pilepich et al., 1978). In all instances, however, the definitive surgery must not be compromised in its planned extent, regardless of the degree of tumor regression. Unless doses higher than 5000 rads are utilized, simple gross excision of residual disease is fraught with the hazard of tumor persistence or recurrence.

A chief advantage of postoperative irradiation is that full surgical staging provides precise pathologic information and clarification of the anatomic extent of gross and microscopic disease. This facilitates optimal placement of radiation portals and rational specification of differential doses.

Immediately following radiation therapy, the presence of tumor cells upon microscopic examination does not necessarily imply clonogenic viability, just as complete gross clearance of disease does not guarantee field sterilization (Suit and Gallagher, 1964; Suit et al., 1965). A long time interval for the clearance of necrotic debris may be inappropriately interpreted by the clinician as a poor radiation tumor response. Gradual and progressive reduction of tumor mass may continue immediately following the completion of a protracted course of treatment. Persistence of gross disease in head and neck cancer beyond day 90 from the inception of a definitive course of irradiation has been demonstrated by Rubin to be consistent with a high incidence of local radiation failure (Sobel et al., 1976). Hardt and coworkers (1982) have recently confirmed the observation of Marcial and Bosch (1970) by showing a direct relationship between radiation response and incidence of tumor nonrecurrence in all stages of carcinoma of the uterine cervix treated with definitive irradiation. Stage for stage, those with no visible or palpable tumor one month after the completion of definitive therapy were at much lower risk of

local recurrence than those who continued to have evidence of residual disease at that time. Such prognostic information might suggest the selective use of salvage surgery earlier in the course of follow-up.

THE TECHNICAL ART

The identification of the tumor-bearing areas to be treated precedes any therapeutic intervention with irradiation (for general references see Fletcher, 1980; Mould, 1981). Such tumor localization is based both on clinical and radiologic information, and has been greatly enhanced by the advent of computer assisted tomography. A precise knowledge of the natural history of the specific tumor will also allow radiation treatment to be directed to areas of potential micrometastatic spread. Treatment planning requires the immobilization of the patient in the proposed treatment position. For complex, large fields, such as the mantle for Hodgkin's disease or the intact breast with regional lymphatics, individually tailored casts are utilized in order to facilitate a reproducible set-up and to limit any motion during the radiation therapy event. CT scans may be taken as part of the simulation process, allowing the physician to determine more precisely the volume that will be homogenously irradiated. Computer dosimetric calculations of the spacial distribution of the dose to be delivered allow the physician, physicist, and dosimetrist an opportunity to develop an optimal plan. Combinations of selected radiation beams directed toward the target volume are tested by simulation using fluoroscopy and diagnostic quality x-ray films. For each ensuing radiation treatment a duplicate of the initial set-up must be obtained. It has been demonstrated that even a 5% decrease in planned total dose secondary to lack of immobilization and precise targeting can be associated with tumor persistence (Harwood et al., 1979).

The physician formulates a therapeutic plan based on the volume to be irradiated, the normal tissue tolerances within the target volume, and the total dose, fraction size, and interval of protraction necessary to accomplish the intended aim. Dose distributions are optimally specified to encompass a target volume consisting not only of the known gross and microscopic tumor volume, but also a margin of safety to compensate for the divergence of the external radiation beams and for uncontrolled patient movement such as that caused by respiration. The dose distribution within the portal fields is calculated using a variety of computer algorithms. Presentation of the dose distribution is by isodose curves, that is, lines connecting points of equal dose. One attempts to obtain a uniform dose distribution throughout the target volume by appropriate beam entry angles or beam modifiers, such as wedges. Even in the best of treatment plans, it is not always possible to obtain a uniform dose to the target volume. It is good practice in such cases to prescribe to a minimum tumor dose.

In the radiation treatment room, duplication of the simulation is accomplished through the assistance of laser beam markings and light fields that are coincident with the radiation beam. Gantry mounting of the radiation source allows radiation entry into the patient through any point in spherical space. With the patient in one position, the tube head of the treatment machine may rotate around a fixed point, the rotational axis of the machine, called an isocenter. Such isocentric technique insures greater precision by avoiding movement of the patient during multiportal therapy. "Port" or "check" films are obtained to confirm the treatment fields and patient positioning of the initially simulated set-up. Successful radiation therapy depends on precise reproduction of the initial planning set-up and a full knowledge of the doses delivered to both the target volume and the tissues treated. Such therapy can only be performed by an integrated team of physicians, physicists, dosimetrists, technologists, nurses, and machinists.

Treatment fields are often reduced during a course of therapy. By *"shrinking field technique"* or reduction of the volumes to be carried to high dose, one attempts to decrease potential radiation morbidity, both acute and chronic. Tumor control as well as normal tissue complications are both dose and volume related. For example, 5000 rads in five weeks may be administered to the whole pelvis after which a reduced target volume encompassing the known gross disease would be carried to tumoricidal doses of 6500 to 7000 rads.

FUTURE PROSPECTS

The future prospects in radiation therapy (for a general reference see Goodman and Krisch, 1981) are intimately connected with the future prospects in basic biologic research and in the development of more effective systemic agents for the treatment of micrometastatic disease. Both radiation and surgery alone and in combination are regional therapies and will continue to remain inadequate relative to disease-free survival as long as the major pattern of failure is metastatic. No longer should an adversarial relationship exist, however, between radiation and surgery. It is being clearly demonstrated that the combination of the two modalities can improve local and regional control in such settings as advanced head and neck cancer and carcinoma of the rectum, preserve function in soft tissue sarcomas of the extremities, and enhance cosmesis in the definitive management of clinical stages I and II carcinoma of the breast. Although the chief problem with irradiation is control of gross tumor larger than four to five centimeters, it is unquestionably effective in control of microscopic nodal disease and in sterilization of wide regional fields at high risk for microscopic extension.

For those tumor systems in which gross resection is neither possible nor desirable considering the associated severe cosmetic mutilation, interest is now being focused on the use of neutrons, heavy ions such as carbon, argon, and silicon, that produce in tissue a greater ionization density than x-rays that overcomes the oxygen dependency seen with conventional supervoltage x-ray beams (Catterall and Bewley, 1979; Castro, 1981; Munzenrider *et al.,* 1981). These so-called densely ionizing radiations are synonymous with the term high-LET (Linear Energy Transfer) radiations. Another potential advantage of particle irradiation is the lesser ability of irradiated cells to repair sublethal damage. Extensive tumors of the head and neck and salivary glands are currently being treated with neutrons in prospective randomized clinical trials under the supervision of the Radiation Therapy Oncology Group and the National Cancer Institute.

Another means of overcoming tissue hypoxia has been with the use of hypoxic cell sensitizers such as misonidazole (Brady, 1980). Such agents are capable of mimicking the effects of oxygen when used together with irradiation. Up to now, however, studies conducted by the Radiation Therapy Oncology Group with malignant astrocytomas and advanced cervical carcinoma have demonstrated no additional benefit with misonidazole.

Normal tissue protectors such as WR-2721

are completing phase I trials at this time. These compounds contain sulfhydryl groups capable of reductively reversing radiation-induced damage and are preferentially absorbed by normal but not tumor cells. Such compounds may allow for the delivery of higher radiation doses and, presumably, higher doses of certain chemotherapeutic agents as well (Brady, 1980; Phillips, 1981; Yuhas, 1980).

Intraoperative radiation therapy is undergoing clinical trials at multiple centers, including the National Cancer Institute, in the treatment of surgically unresectable carcinomas of the stomach and pancreas and extensive retroperitoneal soft tissue sarcomas. Large single doses of 1500 to 2000 rads are being delivered by electron beams in order to control limited disease while decreasing complications that would otherwise arise from high-dose radiotherapy administered by external beams to comparable volumes (Goldson, 1981).

Another interesting method of delivering a therapeutic dose of radiation is by using tissue-associated antibodies labeled with radioactive isotope. The Johns Hopkins group has developed experience in using antibodies labeled with radioactive iodine (^{131}I) in the treatment of hepatomas (Leibel et al., 1981).

Hyperthermia as a modifier of the radiation response has been well documented in the laboratory and is now undergoing clinical testing at many centers (Dritschillo and Piro, 1981). An additive effect with radiation has been demonstrated. Hyperfractionation, which allows for reduced normal tissue injury, is being studied in advanced tumors of the head and neck and pelvis.

Finally, more precise simulation combined with axial tomography and three-dimensional computer planning is being developed, which would make the delivery of radiation even more precise.

A renewed interest is being demonstrated in the use of interstitial radiotherapy in the definitive management of early carcinoma of the breast, adenocarcinoma of the prostate, and advanced cancers of the uterine cervix, rectum, and anus.

Last, but most important, earlier detection of tumors may be possible using positron and/or nuclear magnetic resonance (NMR) scanning (Doyle et al., 1981). These new diagnostic procedures could substantially increase the number of patients presenting with early-stage tumors. It is a corollary to our discipline that early-stage tumors can be well controlled with radiation therapy, whereas all oncologic modalities struggle with patients who have advanced disease.

REFERENCES

Bergonie, J., and Tribondeau, L.: Action des rayons X sur le testicle. *Archives d'electricite medicale.* **14**:779–791 *et sig.* 911–927, 1906.

Brady, L. W.: *Radiation Sensitizers: Their Use in the Clinical Management of Cancer.* Masson Publishing USA, Inc., New York, 1980.

Brown, J. M.: Exploitation of kinetic differences between normal and malignant cells. *Radiology,* **114**:189–197, 1975.

Castro, J. R.: Particle radiation therapy: The first forty years. *Semin. Oncol.,* **8**:103–109, 1981.

Catterall, M., and Bewley, D.: *Fast Neutrons in the Treatment of Cancer.* Grune & Stratton, Inc., New York, 1979.

Chu, F. C. H., and Laughlin, J. S.: *Proceedings of the Symposium on Electron Beam Therapy Conducted September 25–27, 1979,* Memorial Sloan-Kettering Cancer Center, New York, 1981.

Coutard, H.: Roentgenotherapy of epitheliomas of the tonsillar regions, hypopharynx and larynx. *A. J. R.,* **28**:313–331, 1932.

Coutard, H.: Principles of x-ray therapy of malignant disease. *Lancet,* **2**:1–8, 1934.

Crowther, J. A.: Some considerations relative to the action of x-rays on tissue cells. *Proc. R. Soc. Lond. [Biol.],* Series B, **96**:207–211, 1924.

Doyle, F. H.; Gore, J. C.; Pennock, J. M.; Bydder, G. M.; Orr, J. S.; Steiner, R. E.; Young, I. R.; Burl, M.; Clow, H.; Gildervale, D. J.; Bailes, D. R.; and Walters, P. E.: Imaging the brain by nuclear magnetic resonance. *Lancet,* **2**:53–57, 1981.

Dritschilo, A., and Piro, A. J.: Therapeutic implications of heat as related to radiation therapy. *Semin. Oncol.,* **8**:83–91, 1981.

Duncan, W., and Nias, A. H. W.: *Clinical Radiobiology.* Churchill Livingstone, Edinburgh, 1977.

Elkind, M. M., and Sutton, H.: Radiation response of mammalian cells grown in culture, I. Repair of x-ray damage in surviving Chinese hamster cells. *Radiat. Res.,* **13**:556–593, 1960.

Elkind, M. M., and Whitmore, G. F.: *The Radiobiology of Cultured Mammalian Cells.* Gordon and Breach, Science Publishers, Inc., New York, 1967.

Fletcher, G. H.: *Textbook of Radiotherapy,* 3rd ed. Lea & Febiger, Philadelphia, 1980.

Fowler, J. F.: *Nuclear Particles in Cancer Treatment: Medical Physics Handbook 8.* Adam Hilger Ltd., Bristol, England, 1981.

Galvin, J. M.: The physics of radiation therapy equipment. *Semin. Oncol.,* **8**:18–37, 1981.

Gilbert, H. A., and Kagan, A. R.: *Modern Radiation Oncology: Classic Literature and Current Management.* Harper & Row Publishers, Inc., New York, 1978.

Goldson, A. L.: Past, present, and prospects of intraoperative radiotherapy. *Semin. Oncol.,* **8**:59–64, 1981.

Goodman, R. L., and Krisch, R. E. (eds.): Future prospects in radiation therapy. *Semin. Oncol.,* **8**:1–2, 1981.

Gray, L. H.; Conger, A. H.; Ebert, M.; Hornsey, S.; and

Scott, O. C. A.: The concentrations of oxygen in dissolved tissues at the time of irradiation as a factor in radiotherapy. *Br. J. Radiol.,* **26**:638–648, 1953.

Hall, E. J.: *Radiobiology for the Radiologist,* 2nd ed. Harper & Row, Publishers, Inc., New York, 1978.

Hardt, N.; van Nagell, J. R.; Hanson, M.; Donaldson, E.; Yoneda, J.; and Maruyama, Y.: Radiation-induced tumor regression as a prognostic factor in patients with invasive cervical cancer. *Cancer,* **49**:35–39, 1982.

Harwood, A. R.; Hawkins, N. V.; Rider, W. D.; and Bryce, D. P.: Radiotherapy of early glottic cancer—I. *Int. J. Radiat. Oncol. Biol. Phys.,* **5**:473–476, 1979.

Hendee, W. R.: *Radiation Therapy Physics.* Year Book Medical Publishers, Inc., Chicago, 1981.

Howard, A., and Pelc, S. R.: Synthesis of deoxyribonucleic acid in normal and irradiated cells and its relationship to chromosome breakage. *Heredity,* Supp. No. **6**:261–273, 1953.

Johns, H. E., and Cunningham, J. R.: *The Physics of Radiology,* 3rd ed. Charles C. Thomas, Publisher, Springfield, Illinois, 1974.

Kaplan, H. S.: Repair of x-ray damage to bacterial DNA and its inhibition of chemicals. In Panel on Modification of Radiosensitivity in Biological Systems with Particular Emphasis on Chemical Radiation Sensitization and Its Use in Radiotherapy: *Advances in Chemical Radiosensitization.* International Atomic Energy Agency, Vienna, Austria, 1974.

Kaplan, H. S.: Basic principles in radiation oncology. *Cancer,* 39 (February Supp.): 689–693, 1977.

Kaplan, H. S.: Historic milestones in radiobiology and radiation therapy. *Semin. Oncol.,* **6**:479–489, 1979.

Kaplan, H. S.: *Hodgkin's Disease,* 2nd ed. Harvard University Press, Cambridge, Massachusetts, 1980.

Leibel, S. A.; Klein, J. L.; Sgagias, M.; Leichner, P.; and Order, S. E.: The integration of tumor associated antigens in cancer management. *Semin. Oncol.,* **8**:92–102, 1981.

Maier, J. G., and Sulak, M. H.: Radiation therapy in malignant testis tumors. Part 1: Seminoma. *Cancer,* **32**:1212–1216, 1973.

Marcial, V. A., and Bosch A.: Radiation-induced tumor regression in carcinoma of the uterine cervix: Prognostic significance. *A. J. R.,* **108**:113–123, 1970.

Meredith, W. J., and Massey, J. B.: *Fundamental Physics of Radiology,* 3rd ed. Year Book Medical Publishers, Inc., Chicago, 1977.

Meyn, R. E., and Withers, H. R.: *Radiation Biology in Cancer Research.* Raven Press, New York, 1980.

Moss, W. T.; Brand, W. N.; and Battifora, H.: *Radiation Oncology. Rationale, Technique, Results,* 5th ed. The C. V. Mosby Company, St. Louis, 1979.

Mould, R. F.: *Radiotherapy Treatment Planning: Medical Physics Handbook 7.* Adam Hilger Ltd., Bristol, England, 1981.

Munzenrider, J. E.; Shipley, W. V.; and Verhey, L. J.: Future prospects of radiation therapy with protons. *Semin. Oncol.,* **8**:110–124, 1981.

Perez, C. A.; Marks, J.; and Powers, W. E.: Preoperative irradiation in head and neck cancer. *Semin. Oncol.,* **4**:387–397, 1977.

Peschel, R. E., and Fischer, J. J.: Optimization of the time-dose relationship. *Semin. Oncol.,* **8**:38–48, 1981.

Phillips, T. L.: Sensitizers and protectors in clinical oncolgy, *Semin. Oncol.,* **8**:65–82, 1981.

Pilepich, M. V.; Munzenrider, J. E.; Tak, W. K.; and Miller, H. H.: Preoperative irradiation of primary unresectable colorectal carcinoma. *Cancer,* **42**:1077–1081, 1978.

Puck, T. T.; and Marcus, P. I.: Action of x-rays on mammalian cells. *J. Exp. Med.,* **103**:653–666, 1956.

Regaud, C.: The influence of the duration of irradiation on the changes produced in the testicles by radium. *Compt. Rend. Soc. Biol.,* **86**:787–790, 1922. Translated by Archambeau, J. O., and Del Regato, J. A., *Int. J. Radiat. Oncol. Biol. Phys.,* **2**:565–570, 1977.

Regaud, C.; Coutard, H.; and Hautant, A.: Contribution en traitement des cancers endo larynges par les rayons. Xth International Congress. *d/Otology,* 19–22, 1922.

Richter, M. P.: Palliative radiotherapy. In Cassileth, P., and Cassileth, B. (eds.): *Clinical Care of the Terminal Cancer Patient.* pp. 65–75. Lea & Febiger, Philadelphia, 1982.

Ritter, M. A.: The radiobiology of mammalian cells. *Semin. Oncol.,* **8**:13–17, 1981.

Roentgen, W. C.: Uber eine neue Art von Strahlen. Erste Mitteilung. Sitzungsberichte der Physikalische-Medizinischen Gesellschaft in Wurzburg, Physikalisches Institut der Universität, 132–141, 1895.

Rubin, P., and Casarett, G. W.: *Clinical Radiation Pathology.* W. B. Saunders Company, Philadelphia, 1968.

Schulz, M.: The supervoltage story: Janeway lecture, 1974. *A. J. R.,* **124**:541–559, 1975.

Sinclair, W. K., and Morton, R. A.: X-ray sensitivity during the cell generation cycle of cultured Chinese hamster cells. *Radiat. Res.,* **29**:450–474, 1966.

Snow, J. B.; Gilber, R. D.; Kramer, S.; Davis, L. W.; Marcial, V. A.; and Lowry, L. D.: Comparison of preoperative and postoperative radiation therapy for patients with carcinoma of the head and neck, interim report. *Acta Otolaryngol.* (Stockh.), **91**:611–626, 1981.

Sobel, S.; Rubin, P.; Keller, B.; and Poulter, C.: Tumor persistence as a predictor of outcome after radiation therapy of head and neck cancer. *Int. J. Radiat. Oncol. Biol. Phys.,* **1**:873–880, 1976.

Streffer, C.: *Cancer Therapy by Hyperthermia and Radiation.* Urban & Schwarzenberg, Inc., Baltimore, 1978.

Suit, H. D., and Gallagher, H. S.: Intact tumor cells in irradiated tissue. *Arch. Path.,* **78**:648, 1964.

Suit, H. D.; Lindberg, R. D.; and Fletcher, G. H.: Prognostic significance of extent of tumor regression at completion of radiation therapy. *Radiology,* **84**:1100, 1965.

Thomlinson, R. H., and Gray, L. H.: The histological structure of some human lung cancers and the possible implications for radiotherapy. *Br. J. Cancer,* **9**:539–549, 1955.

Vaeth, J. M.: The interrelationship of surgery and radiation therapy in the treatment of cancer. *Front. Radiat. Ther. Oncol.,* **5**: 1970.

Vaeth, J. M.: Radiation effect and tolerance, normal tissue. *Front. Radiat. Ther. Oncol.,* **6**: 1972.

Vaeth, J. M.: Renaissance of interstitial brachytherapy. *Front. Radiat. Ther. Oncol.,* **12**: 1978.

White, D. C.: *An Atlas of Radiation Histopathology.* National Technical Information Service, Springfield, Virginia, 1975.

Withers, H. R.; Peters, L. J.; and Kogelnik, H. D.: The pathobiology of late effects of irradiation in radiation biology. In Meyn, R. E., and Withers, H. R. (eds.) *Cancer Research.* Raven Press, New York, 1980.

Yuhas, J. M.: On the potential application of radioprotective drugs in radiotherapy. In Sokol, G. H. (ed.): *Radiation-Drug Interactions in Cancer Management.* John Wiley & Sons, Inc., New York, 1980.

10

Pharmacology of Antineoplastic Agents

MICHAEL C. WIEMANN and PAUL CALABRESI

Effective chemotherapy is available for many types of cancer. Although the list of neoplastic diseases that are curable by chemotherapy is still short, many patients achieve meaningful palliation and prolonged survival through the judicious use of these drugs.

The three principal entities involved in the chemotherapy of cancer are: (1) The host, (2) the drug, and (3) the tumor (Figure 10–1). An understanding of clinical pharmacology is essential for the practice of medical oncology. The oncologist must be knowledgable about pharmacologic considerations such as routes of administration, absorption, plasma kinetics, distribution, sites of metabolism, routes of excretion, and drug interactions. The use of drugs that possess both a narrow therapeutic index and the potential for serious and fatal toxicities is a continual challenge for the medical oncologist.

The effective use of these drugs also requires an understanding of the biology of the target cell population. In order to understand the mechanisms of action of chemotherapeutic agents, a knowledge of basic biochemical cell processes, such as the synthesis of nucleic acids and proteins, is required (see Chapter 1 and Figure 10–2). Acquired drug resistance is one example of a clinical problem that is based on the adaptive biochemical mechanisms of the tumor cell. Impaired transport of the drug into the cell, decreased production of activating enzymes, increased synthesis of catabolic enzymes, and elevated levels of target or repair enzymes are all potential mechanisms of resistance. Many, and possibly all, of these adaptive processes may be caused by drug-induced gene modulation. Because many chemotherapeutic agents are active only in a specific phase

of the cell cycle, tumor cell kinetics have important and practical implications for the design of drug treatment regimens (see Chapter 2). Differential toxic effects on normal tissues and tumor cells are often the result of variability between the kinetics of their constituent cell populations.

A variety of host factors are critical to the outcome of therapy. Knowledge of the function of the organs responsible for the absorption, metabolism, and excretion of the drug is essential. Other host factors that are of equal

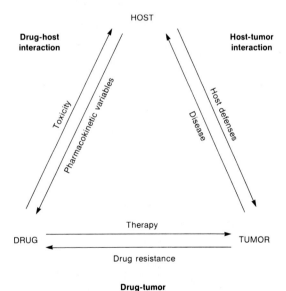

Figure 10–1. The chemotherapeutic triangle. Modified from Calabresi, P.: Principles of oncologic treatment: Irradiation, cytotoxic drugs, and immunostimulatory procedures. In Beeson, P. B.; McDermott, W.; and Wyngaarden, J. B. (eds.): *Textbook of Medicine.* W. B. Saunders, Philadelphia, 1979.

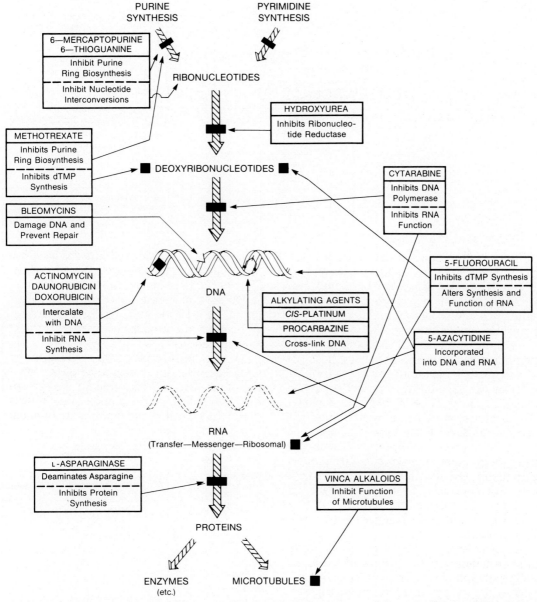

Figure 10-2. Summary of the mechanisms and sites of action of chemotherapeutic agents useful in neoplastic disease.*

importance include performance status, nutrition, and immune competence.

This chapter provides a discussion of the

* The artwork that appears in Figures 10-2, 10-3, 10-4, 10-5, 10-6, 10-7, 10-8, 10-9, 10-10, 10-19, 10-23, 10-24, 10-25, 10-26, 10-27, and 10-28 is reproduced from Calabresi, P., and Parks, R. E., Jr.: Antiproliferative agents and drugs used for immunosuppression. In Gilman, A. G.; Goodman, L. S.; and Gilman, A. (eds.): *Goodman and Gilman's The Pharmacological Basis of Therapeutics,* 6th ed. Macmillan Publishing Company, New York, 1980.

biochemical and clinical pharmacology of the most useful chemotherapeutic agents. Patterns of toxicity and strategies helpful in preventing or ameliorating these undesirable effects are presented. A synopsis of important clinical toxicities is provided in Table 10-1.

Most of the compounds discussed are clinically established and generally available. A few investigational agents of exceptional promise are included. The most common clinical indications for the use of each drug are listed in Table 10-2.

Table 10–1. Patterns of Toxicity of Chemotherapeutic Agents

		CARDIAC	CARCINOGENESIS	DERMATOLOGIC	GASTROINTESTINAL	HEMATOLOGIC	HEPATIC	HYPERSENSITIVITY	NEUROLOGIC	PULMONARY	RENAL	REPRODUCTIVE	OTHER
Alkylating Agents	Nitrogen mustard		★	x	★	★		x				★	
	Cyclophosphamide	x	★	x	★	★		x		x		★	Cystitis, hyponatremia, immunosuppression
	Melphalan		★		x	★				x		★	
	Chlorambucil		★	x	x	★				x		★	
	Busulfan		★	x	x	★				★		★	Weakness, weight loss
	Carmustine (BCNU)		★	x	★	★	x		x	x		★	
	Lomustine (CCNU)		★		★	★					x	★	
	Semustine (MeCCNU)		★		★	★					★	★	
	Streptozotocin				★	x					★		Glucose intolerance
	Dacarbazine	★		x	★	★	x	x	x			★	Flu-like syndrome
	Mitomycin	x	★	x	x	★	x	x		x	x	★	
Antimetabolites	Methotrexate			x	★	★	★	x	★	x	★	x	Immunosuppression
	5-Fluorouracil	x		x	★	★			x				
	Cytosine arabinoside				★	★	x	x	x	x			Immunosuppression
	5-Azacytidine			x	★	★			x				Fever
	6-Mercaptopurine			x	★	★	★			x			Immunosuppression
	6-Thioguanine				★	★	x						
	Hydroxyurea			x	x	★							
Natural Products	Vincristine			x					★				Inappropriate ADH secretion
	Vinblastine			x	x	★			x				
	Etoposide (VP-16-213)			x	★	★		x	x				Arterial hypotension
	Tenisopide (VM-26)			x	x	★		x	x				Arterial hypotension
	Doxorubicin	★			★	★		x					Radiation recall
	Daunorubicin	★			★	★		x					Radiation recall
	Bleomycin			★	x	x		★		★			Fever
	Actinomycin D			x	★	★							Radiation recall
	Mithramycin			x	★	★	★				★		Hemorrhagic diathesis
	Asparaginase			x	★		★	★	★				Hyperglycemia, pancreatitis, immunosuppression, coagulation defects
Miscellaneous Agents	Platinum			x	★	x		x	x		★	x	Ototoxicity, hypomagnesemia
	Procarbazine		★	x	★	★	x	x	★	x		★	Hypertension, adverse interaction with alcohol and drugs metabolized in the liver, immunosuppression
	Mitotane			x	★				★		x		Visual problems, hypertension, adrenal insufficiency

★ = major toxicity; x = uncommon toxicity

Table 10-2. Neoplastic Diseases Responsive to Chemotherapeutic Agents

CLASS	TYPE OF COMPOUND	AGENT	DISEASE*
Alkylating Agents	Nitrogen mustards	Nitrogen mustard	Hodgkin's disease
		Cyclophosphamide	Chronic lymphocytic leukemia, Hodgkin's disease, non-Hodgkin's lymphomas, multiple myeloma, breast, ovary, and lung
		Melphalan	Multiple myeloma, breast and ovary
		Chlorambucil	Chronic lymphocytic leukemia, Waldenström's macroglobulinemia, non-Hodgkin's lymphomas
	Alkyl sulfonates	Busulfan	Chronic granulocytic leukemia
	Nitrosoureas	Carmustine (BCNU)	Hodgkin's disease, non-Hodgkin's lymphoma, primary brain tumors, multiple myeloma
		Lomustine (CCNU)	Hodgkin's disease, non-Hodgkin's lymphoma, primary brain tumors, and small cell lung
		Semustine (MeCCNU)	Primary brain tumors, stomach and colon
		Streptozotocin	Islet cell tumors of the pancreas, carcinoid
	Triazenes	Dacarbazine	Hodgkin's disease, soft tissue sarcomas, melanoma
	Antibiotics	Mitomycin	Stomach, breast, cervix, lung, pancreas, head and neck
Antimetabolites	Folic acid analogs	Methotrexate	Acute lymphocytic leukemia, choriocarcinoma, mycosis fungoides, osteogenic sarcomas, breast, head and neck, lung, leukemic and carcinomatous meningitis
	Pyrimidine analogs	5-Fluorouracil	Colorectal, breast, ovary, stomach, bladder and pancreas
		Cytosine arabinoside	Acute myelogenous and acute lymphocytic leukemias, leukemic and carcinomatous meningitis
		5-Azacytidine	Acute myelogenous leukemia
	Purine analogs	6-Mercaptopurine	Acute lymphocytic leukemia
		6-Thioguanine	Acute myelogenous leukemia
	Substituted urea	Hydroxyurea	Chronic myelogenous leukemia, polycythemia vera, essential thrombocytosis, acute leukemia with high blast counts, head and neck, colon and cervix, and the hypereosinophilic syndrome

Adapted from Calabresi, P., and Parks, R. E., Jr.: Chemotherapy of neoplastic diseases: Introduction. In Gilman, A. G.; Goodman, L. S.; and Gilman, A. (eds.): *Goodman and Gilman's The Pharmacological Basis of Therapeutics,* 6th ed. Macmillan Publishing Company, New York, 1980.
* Neoplasms are carcinomas unless otherwise indicated.

Table 10–2. Neoplastic Diseases Responsive to Chemotherapeutic Agents (Continued)

CLASS	TYPE OF COMPOUND	AGENT	DISEASE*
Natural Products	Vinca alkaloids	Vincristine	Acute lymphocytic leukemia, Hodgkin's disease, non-Hodgkin's lymphomas, and breast
		Vinblastine	Testicular tumors, Hodgkin's disease, non-Hodgkin's lymphomas
		Vindesine	Chronic myelogenous leukemia, blastic phase; non-Hodgkin's lymphomas, systemic mastocytosis
	Epidophyllotoxins	Etoposide (VP-16-213)	Acute myelogenous leukemia, small cell lung, non-Hodgkin's lymphomas, testicular tumors
		Teniposide (VM-26)	Hodgkin's disease
	Antibiotics	Doxorubicin	Hodgkin's disease, non-Hodgkin's lymphomas, soft tissue sarcomas, acute lymphocytic leukemia, hepatoma, breast, lung, stomach, ovary, thyroid, pancreas, endometrium, and bladder
		Daunorubicin	Acute myelogenous leukemia
		Bleomycin	Testicular tumors, Hodgkin's disease, non-Hodgkin's lymphomas, head and neck, cervix, esophagus, skin, vulva, and lung
		Actinomycin D	Wilms' tumor, embryonal rhabdomyosarcoma, choriocarcinoma, Ewing's sarcoma, Kaposi's sarcoma, and testicular tumors
		Mithramycin	Hypercalcemia, testicular tumors
	Enzymes	Asparaginase	Acute lymphocytic leukemia
Miscellaneous Agents	Platinum coordination complexes	cis-platinum	Testicular tumors, head and neck, ovary, bladder, thyroid, uterine cervix, and lung
	Methyl hydrazine derivative	Procarbazine	Hodgkin's disease, lung cancer, primary brain tumors
	Adrenocortical suppressant	Mitotane	Adrenal cortex
Hormones and Antagonists	Adrenocorticosteroids	Prednisone; several other equivalent preparations	Acute and chronic lymphocytic leukemia, Hodgkin's disease, non-Hodgkin's lymphomas, breast
	Progestins	Hydroxyprogesterone caproate; medroxy-progesterone acetate; megestrol acetate	Breast and endometrium
	Estrogens	Diethylstilbestrol; ethinyl estradiol; other preparations	Breast and prostate

Table 10-2. Neoplastic Diseases Responsive to Chemotherapeutic Agents (Continued)

CLASS	TYPE OF COMPOUND	AGENT	DISEASE*
Hormones and Antagonists	Androgens	Testosterone propionate; fluoxymesterone; other preparations	Breast
	Antiestrogen	Tamoxifen	Breast

ALKYLATING AGENTS

The leukopenia and toxicity to lymphoid tissues observed following exposure to sulfur mustard in World War I prompted the laboratory studies that demonstrated the tumoricidal activity of nitrogen mustard to a murine lymphosarcoma. Activity against human cancers was initially shown in 1943 when a patient with Hodgkin's disease obtained a dramatic response after the administration of nitrogen mustard. Since that time, the diverse group of compounds with alkylating activity has proven useful in the treatment of a wide variety of neoplastic and non-neoplastic diseases (Gilman, 1963).

Many compounds with structural similarities to the nitrogen mustards have been synthesized, but only a few are clinically effective antitumor agents (see Figure 10-3). Five major classes of alkylating agents have been used in cancer therapy: (1) the nitrogen mustards, (2) the ethylenimines, (3) the alkyl sulfonates, (4) the nitrosoureas, and (5) the triazenes. The antibiotic mitomycin C also functions as an alkylating agent.

Biochemical Pharmacology

Chemically and functionally, the alkylating agents are characterized by the ability to form covalent bonds with nucleophilic, electron-rich, regions on biologically important macromolecules, such as nucleic acids and proteins (Ludlum, 1967; Rhaese and Freese, 1969; Bannon and Verly, 1972; Colvin, 1982). Phosphate, amino, sulfhydryl, and hydroxyl groups are frequent sites of attack. The most important target of the alkylating agents is the DNA molecule. Alterations of the structural integrity and function of DNA result in the cytotoxicity, mutagenicity, and carcinogenicity associated with these compounds.

The generation of an active alkylating species from the parent compound is most often mediated through the formation of a positively charged carbonium ion. For the chloroethyl alkylating groups, this is accomplished by an intramolecular cyclization and formation of an unstable ethylenimonium intermediate. Spontaneous opening of the ring then produces the active carbonium ion.

Any free oxygen and nitrogen in the purine and pyrimidine bases of DNA are targets for alkylation, the 7-nitrogen position of guanine, however, is particularly vulnerable (Brookes and Lawley, 1961; Lawley and Brookes, 1963). The 1-nitrogen and 3-nitrogen positions of adenine, the 6-oxygen position of guanine, and the 3-nitrogen position of cytosine are other

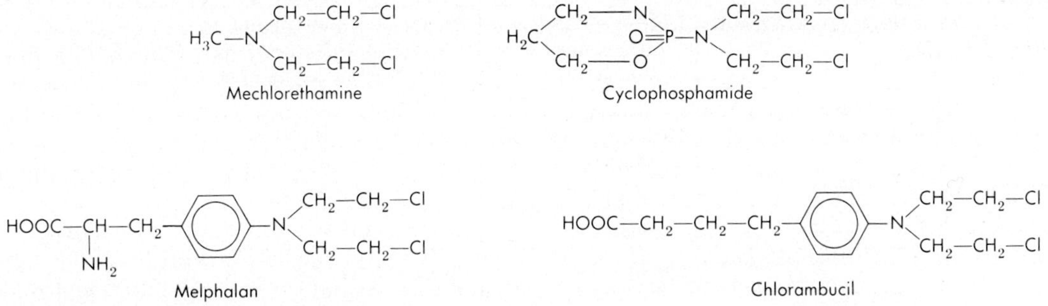

Figure 10-3. Nitrogen mustards used in clinical therapy.

frequently alkylated sites. The exact sites of alkylation that are responsible for cytotoxicity and mutagenicity are unclear. The differences in biologic effects among the alkylating agents probably result from individual patterns and frequencies of alkylation sites.

The ability of a compound to cross-link DNA correlates closely with cytotoxicity. Bifunctional alkylators, such as nitrogen mustard, can cross-link two nucleic acid chains as well as bind DNA to other macromolecules. Monofunctional alkylators, such as the chloroethylnitrosoureas, are also capable of cross-linking between DNA strands. Other physical and chemical factors that relate to clinical activity include lipophilicity, generation of the active moiety, and membrane transport kinetics.

The exact biologic damage produced by alkylation probably relates to the specific positions on the DNA bases that are affected. For example, when the 7-nitrogen of guanine is alkylated, inappropriate base pairing with thymidine may occur and ultimately lead to misreading of the DNA template. Alkylation may also lead to spontaneous depurination resulting from breakage of the sugar-base bond. Intracellular endonucleases, capable of recognizing damaged DNA, remove the alkylated base. Base removal may be followed by repair or by further enzymatically mediated damage to DNA (Papirmeister et al., 1970).

The alkylating agents are cytotoxic throughout the cell cycle; however, cells in late G_1 and early S phases are especially sensitive. Although nonproliferative G_0 cells are susceptible, toxicity is usually not expressed until the cell reenters the proliferative compartment and synthesizes DNA. Thus, neoplastic and normal host tissues that are rapidly proliferating will be most severely damaged. Tumors with relatively high growth fractions, such as lymphomas, are usually most responsive to therapy with alkylating agents. Similarly, leukopenia and thrombocytopenia, secondary to marrow suppression, frequently follow drug administration.

Resistance of tumors to alkylating agents probably results from an increased ability to repair damaged DNA. Other possible mechanisms of resistance include an increased production of nucleophilic substances that can compete with DNA for alkylation, diminished capacity for drug transport, and drug inactivation. The development of pleiotropic drug resistance is a common clinical problem (Shoemaker et al., 1983).

Although the mechanisms of action of the alkylating agents are similar, frequent examples of clinical non-cross-resistance, such as sensitivity to cyclophosphamide in melphalan-resistant multiple myeloma, suggest that important differences in alkylation patterns do exist. The following discussion will emphasize unique features of the clinical pharmacology and toxicity, as well as the clinical indications, for the individual drugs.

NITROGEN MUSTARD

Nitrogen mustard or mechlorethamine was the first alkylating agent introduced into clinical use. As described above, the activity of this bifunctional alkylator is mediated through the formation of a carbonium ion. The same carrier mechanism that transports choline into the cell is utilized by nitrogen mustard (Goldenberg et al., 1970; Goldenburg, 1975). Drug resistance may result from a loss of this transport mechanism but, more likely, is due to an increased ability to repair DNA (Lawlcy and Brookes, 1965).

Clinical Pharmacology

Mechlorethamine is unstable in solution and must be prepared immediately prior to administration. The compound rapidly undergoes spontaneous hydrolysis to produce 2-hydroxyethyl-2-chloroethylmethylamine and bis-2-hydroxyethylmethylamine. Within a few minutes after injection, active compounds cannot be detected in the plasma.

Clinical Toxicity

The drug is a powerful vesicant and should be administered carefully into a freely flowing intravenous line. Extravasation can produce necrosis and sloughing of the exposed tissues. If extravasation does occur, the area should be infiltrated with a sterile isotonic solution of sodium thiosulfate (⅙ M). Thiosulfate provides an ion that reacts avidly with nitrogen mustard and may ameliorate damage to tissues. Surgical debridement and skin grafting are frequently required to treat the resultant soft tissue ulceration.

Nausea and vomiting, frequently severe, invariably follow the administration of mechlorethamine within three to six hours and may persist for as long as 36 hours. Direct stimulation of the chemoreceptor trigger zone of the fourth ventricle and the vomiting center in the medullary reticular formation is the presumed mechanism. Leukopenia and thrombocytopenia are common. Gonadal dysfunction, including menstrual abnormalities, ovarian failure, testicular atrophy, azoospermia, and sterility have all been reported after the use of mechlorethamine alone and in multidrug combinations (Spitz, 1948; Sherins and DeVita, 1973). Uncommon toxicities include a type I hypersensitivity reaction (Weiss and Bruno, 1981) and a nonallergic maculopapular skin eruption. Significantly increased incidences of acute nonlymphocytic leukemia and non-Hodgkin's lymphomas have been reported after the use of the MOPP (mechlorethamine, vincristine [ONCOVIN], procarbazine, and prednisone) regimen for Hodgkin's disease (Toland et al., 1978).

Clinical Indications

Although active against non-Hodgkin's lymphomas and several solid tumors, the major indication for the use of nitrogen mustard today is in the treatment of Hodgkin's disease. Topical application of a dilute solution for mycosis fungoides and instillation into the pleural space for the palliation of malignant pleural effusions are other clinical uses. (For other clinical activity see Calabresi and Parks, 1985.)

CYCLOPHOSPHAMIDE

Cyclophosphamide, a bifunctional substituted nitrogen mustard, was synthesized in 1958 in an attempt to achieve greater selective toxicity for tumor tissue. The N-methyl moiety of nitrogen mustard is replaced with a cyclic phosphamide group, resulting in a stable, inactive compound. The bis-(2-chloroethyl) group cannot ionize until the cyclic phosphamide is opened at the phosphorus-nitrogen linkage. Because tumor tissues contain higher levels of the phosphatase and phosphamidase enzymes responsible for cleaving the P-N bond than do normal tissues, it was hoped that the toxic metabolites would be preferentially generated by tumor cells. It was subsequently realized that cyclophosphamide is activated primarily in the liver. Selective toxicity for tumor tissue has not been observed.

Clinical Pharmacology

Activation of cyclophosphamide is a multistep process (see Figure 10–4). The liver microsomal P-450 mixed-function oxidase system converts the parent drug to 4-hydroxycyclophosphamide. This metabolite is in a steady state with the acyclic tautomer, aldophosphamide. These compounds may be further oxidized by hepatic aldehyde oxidase to

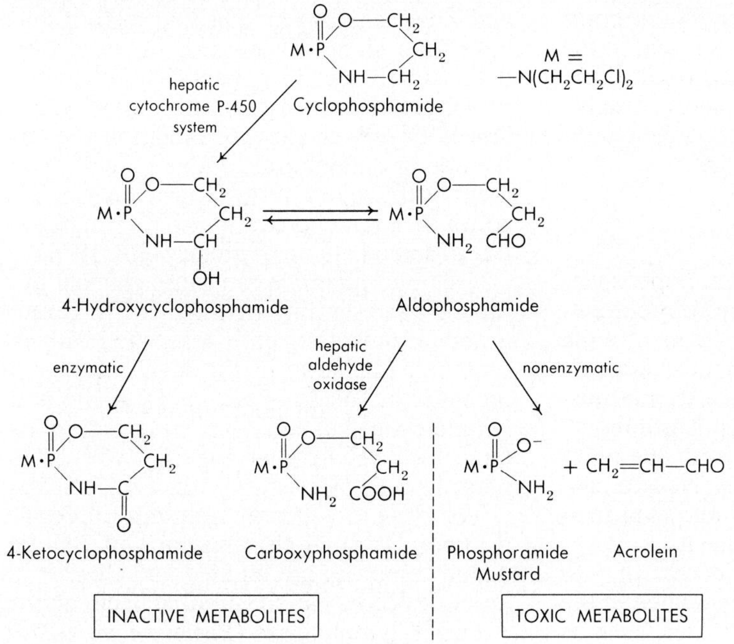

Figure 10–4. Metabolism of cyclophosphamide.

the inactive metabolites carboxyphosphamide and 4-ketocyclophosphamide. Nonenzymatic conversion to the cytotoxic compounds phosphoramide mustard and acrolein occurs in susceptible peripheral tissues.

The hepatic enzymes responsible for cyclophosphamide metabolism can be induced by barbiturates, corticosteroids, and other drugs. With repetitive daily administration, cyclophosphamide can stimulate its own metabolism. Neither increasing the rate of metabolism nor the plasma half-life affects the total amount of active alkylating metabolites generated. Because cytotoxicity relates best to the total amount of active metabolites produced rather than to their velocity of generation, the activity and therapeutic index are not significantly modified by these drugs (Sladek, 1972). High doses of barbiturates or corticosteroids, however, have been reported to increase acute toxicity (Field et al., 1972; Hayakawa et al., 1969).

Cyclophosphamide is well absorbed after oral administration. It is not a vesicant and intravenous administration does not produce local irritation. After an intravenous dose of 6 to 80 mg/kg, the plasma half-life ranges from 4 to 6.5 hours. (Mellett, 1971; Bagley et al., 1973). Fifty-six percent of the metabolites with alkylating activity are bound to plasma proteins. Less than 14% of the total dose is excreted unchanged in the urine and excretion of intact drug and metabolites in the stool is negligible. After oral administration, peak plasma levels are achieved in approximately one hour. A large amount of intact drug is found in the stool when the oral route is employed. If the glomerular filtration rate is markedly compromised, the dose should be reduced. (For additional references see Colvin, 1982.)

Clinical Toxicity

As with nitrogen mustard, cyclophosphamide is particularly toxic to rapidly proliferating cells. Myelosuppression is frequently the dose-limiting toxicity. The nadir of leukopenia occurs between 10 and 14 days after administration, with recovery by day 21. Thrombocytopenia is less common than with the other nitrogen mustard compounds. Nausea and vomiting also occur frequently and their incidence and severity are dose related.

Sterile hemorrhagic cystitis occurs in 5 to 10% of patients and is probably related to the concentration of active metabolites, such as acrolein, in the bladder. Adequate hydration and frequent voiding will usually prevent this complication. Irrigation of the bladder with an acetylcysteine solution reduces the incidence of hemorrhagic cystitis in dogs (Primack, 1971), but the effectiveness of this procedure in humans has not been demonstrated. Other sequelae of cyclophosphamide bladder toxicity may include bladder fibrosis with telangiectasia, abnormal cytology, and carcinoma of the bladder (Johnson and Meadows, 1971; Wall and Clausen, 1975).

Impaired water excretion, manifested by hyponatremia, decreased serum osmolarity, weight gain, and inappropriately concentrated urine may occur four to 12 hours after a parenteral dose of cyclophosphamide of greater than 50 mg/kg (DeFronzo et al., 1973). This self-limited impairment of renal diluting capacity is not caused by increased secretion of ADH and is probably secondary to a toxic effect on the distal renal tubules and collecting ducts. Because patients who receive large doses of cyclophosphamide are usually vigorously hydrated, they should be monitored for the development of water intoxication.

Although usual doses of cyclophosphamide are not associated with adverse cardiac effects, very high doses, 120 to 240 mg/kg, can produce a fatal pericardiomyopathy and cardiac necrosis (Gottdiener et al., 1981). Approximately 20 cases of interstitial pneumonitis have been reported after administration of cyclophosphamide. The time to onset is variable and no clear dose or schedule relationships have been identified. Because many of these patients were receiving other chemotherapeutic drugs with known pulmonary toxicity, prolonged oxygen therapy, or radiation therapy, the role of cyclophosphamide in the development of the injury to the lung is unclear. The administration of prednisone has been beneficial in some patients (Spector et al., 1979).

Cyclophosphamide can cause gonadal dysfunction and sterility (see Chapter 14). Teratogenesis is most frequently associated with exposure to the drug in the first trimester of pregnancy (Toledo et al., 1971). Acute nonlymphocytic leukemia has occurred in patients receiving long-term therapy with cyclophosphamide (Sieber and Adamson, 1975).

The drug is a potent immunosuppressive (Colvin, 1982). Both humoral and cell-mediated responses are blunted and there is an absolute decrease in the number of circulating B and T lymphocytes (Bagley et al., 1973).

Because of these immunosuppressive properties, it has been used in the treatment of non-neoplastic disorders associated with altered immunity, including rheumatoid arthritis, systemic lupus erythematosus, Wegener's granulomatosis, and the nephrotic syndrome in children. Cyclophosphamide has also been used as an immunosuppressive agent in organ transplantation. The increased incidence of second neoplasms after long-term administration may be, in part, a result of impaired immune surveillance (See Chapter 11).

Clinical Indications

A broad spectrum of clinical activity and the availability of oral and parenteral preparations have caused cyclophosphamide to become the most widely used alkylating agent. It is active in all of the lymphoproliferative diseases including Hodgkin's disease and chronic lymphocytic leukemia. Cyclophosphamide is a component of the regimens that have produced cures in patients with diffuse histiocytic lymphoma. Cures in patients with Burkitt's lymphoma have also been reported. Cyclophosphamide has also demonstrated significant activity against multiple myeloma, as well as ovarian and breast small-cell lung carcinoma. In combination with methotrexate and 5-fluorouracil (5-FU), it is useful in the adjuvant therapy of breast carcinoma. A cyclophosphamide analog, 4-hydroperoxycyclophosphamide, is being evaluated as part of an innovative approach to the treatment of acute leukemia (Kaizer et al., 1982). Bone marrow from patients in remission is harvested and incubated with the drug in an attempt to eliminate residual leukemic cells. After high-dose, marrow-ablative chemotherapy, hematopoiesis is restored by infusion of the autologous, treated marrow. The use of such drugs to selectively remove occult tumor cells from the bone marrow in vitro could greatly increase the usefulness of autologous bone marrow transplantation.

MELPHALAN

Melphalan, a nitrogen mustard derivative of the amino acid L-phenylalanine, was synthesized in 1953. Phenylalanine, a melanin precursor, was incorporated into the molecule with the expectation that the drug would be preferentially incorporated by malignant melanoma cells. Tumor amino acid utilization patterns, however, have not been shown to be responsible for the activity of this drug.

Clinical Pharmacology

The drug is usually administered in the oral form, although an intravenous preparation has been evaluated. Absorption after oral administration is variable. The plasma half-life is brief, 0.6 to 3 hours. The two major metabolites are products of hydrolysis. Between 20 to 50% of the drug is excreted in the feces (Tattersall et al., 1978), indicating poor absorption although biliary excretion may be partially responsible. Biliary excretion occurs in many animal species and a high concentration of drug is achieved in the bile. Only 10 to 15% of an oral dose is excreted unchanged in the urine (Alberts et al., 1978). Administration on an empty stomach and dissolving oral doses in an acidic solution have been advocated to improve absorption (Furner and Brown, 1980).

Melphalan may enter cells by the same active transport system that carries glutamine and leucine, because the addition of either of these amino acids reduces toxicity to cultured tumor cells (Temoshechkina and Budelina, 1976). Pretreatment with cysteine also has a protective effect in vitro (Ball and Connors, 1967). The clinical significance of these observations is still unclear.

Clinical Toxicity

Neutropenia and thrombocytopenia are common with melphalan but are not as profound as with other alkylating agents. Alopecia is unusual, but may occur with prolonged treatment. An autopsy study suggests that subclinical lung damage may occur in a substantial number of patients (Taetle et al., 1978), although less than five cases of clinical pulmonary toxicity have been reported. The relative risk for development of acute nonlymphocytic leukemia is increased after melphalan therapy.

Clinical Indications

Melphalan is used in combination with prednisone for multiple myeloma. Beneficial effects also occur in the therapy of patients with carcinomas of the ovary and breast. Activity against melanoma is marginal, but can be improved with high drug concentrations, such as can be achieved by isolated limb perfusion. Melphalan, in combination with 5-FU, is useful as adjuvant therapy after mastectomy in premenopausal breast cancer patients with axillary node involvement. High-dose (140 mg/m^2) intravenous melphalan, used in conjunction with autologous marrow reconstitution, has shown promising results against a variety of tumor types usually unresponsive to conventional doses.

CHLORAMBUCIL

Chlorambucil is a stable aromatic derivative of mechlorethamine.

Clinical Pharmacology

The drug is given orally and absorption is reliable. After a dose of 0.6 mg/kg, peak levels of 0.6 to 1.9 μg/ml of chlorambucil are achieved in the plasma within one hour of administration. Peak levels of the alkylating metabolite phenylacetic acid mustard range from 0.5 to 1.18 μg/ml and occur within two to four hours. The terminal phase plasma half-lives are 92 minutes and 145 minutes for chlorambucil and phenylacetic acid mustard, respectively. Approximately 50% of an administered dose is excreted in the urine within 24 hours as the monohydroxy and dihydroxy hydrolysis products of chlorambucil and phenylacetic acid mustard (Alberts et al., 1979a).

Clinical Toxicity

At usual doses, toxicity consists of moderate neutropenia and thrombocytopenia. Gastrointestinal and dermatologic toxicities occur infrequently. Chlorambucil-induced pulmonary toxicity is rare.

Clinical Indications

Chlorambucil is usually the primary treatment for chronic lymphocytic leukemia. It is also useful in the treatment of multiple myeloma, Waldenström's macroglobulinemia, and the more indolent nodular lymphomas. Although it has been effective in the therapy of polycythemia vera, its use is not advisable because of the marked increase in acute nonlymphocytic leukemia after prolonged administration.

BUSULFAN

Busulfan is an alkyl sulfonate structurally unrelated to nitrogen mustard (see Figure 10-5).

Clinical Pharmacology

After oral administration, the drug is well absorbed and rapidly metabolized to a bifunctional alkylator. Methanesulfonic acid and other metabolites are excreted in the urine.

Clinical Toxicity

Busulfan is a potent myelosuppressive agent. At lower doses, suppression of granulopoiesis is most prominent, but, with prolonged administration or with higher doses, the production of all hematopoietic elements is inhibited. Careful monitoring of the peripheral blood counts is required, particularly with daily therapy, because prolonged cytopenias and marrow aplasia can result. Acute leukemia and other neoplasms have been reported in patients previously treated with busulfan.

The occurrence of diffuse pulmonary fibrosis associated with busulfan therapy is well documented (Boyles, 1971). A relationship between dose or schedule of administration and the development of pulmonary toxicity has not been identified. Despite drug withdrawal and corticosteroid administration, progression to fatal pulmonary insufficiency usually occurs. A generalized increased pigmentation, sometimes accompanied by weakness, anorexia, and weight loss, may develop in patients receiving busulfan. Although suggestive of Addison's disease, adrenal function is normal (Kyle et al., 1961). Symptoms usually resolve with drug withdrawal. Other less common toxic manifestations include cataracts, cheilosis, glossitis, anhidrosis, and gynecomastia (Calabresi and Parks, 1985).

Clinical Indications

Busulfan is principally used in the treatment of chronic granulocytic leukemia. Initially, the

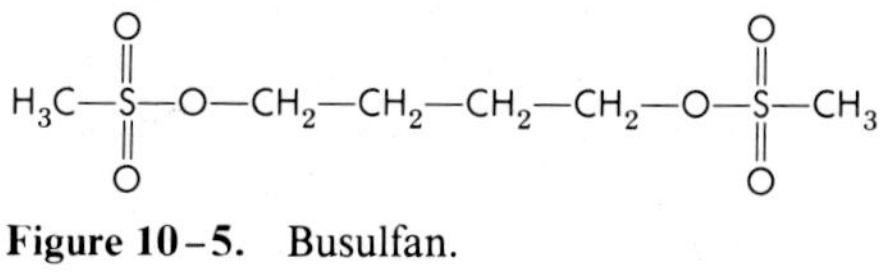

$$H_3C-\overset{\overset{\textstyle O}{\|}}{\underset{\underset{\textstyle O}{\|}}{S}}-O-CH_2-CH_2-CH_2-CH_2-O-\overset{\overset{\textstyle O}{\|}}{\underset{\underset{\textstyle O}{\|}}{S}}-CH_3$$

Figure 10-5. Busulfan.

drug is given daily until the white blood cell count decreases below 20,000/mm³. Thereafter, the drug is administered as needed to control the white cell count. Blood counts must be followed closely. The drug is not useful in the blastic crisis of the disease. Busulfan is also effective in myeloproliferative disorders such as myeloid metaplasia, essential thrombocytosis, and polycythemia vera.

NITROSOUREAS

The chloroethylnitrosoureas are a group of rationally designed antitumor compounds characterized by their lipophilic properties and chemical instability under physiologic conditions (see Figure 10–6). Their biologic effects include alkylation, carbamoylation, inhibition of repair of x-ray–induced DNA strand breaks, interference with the synthesis and processing of ribosomal and nucleoplasmic RNA, and inhibition of DNA polymerase II.

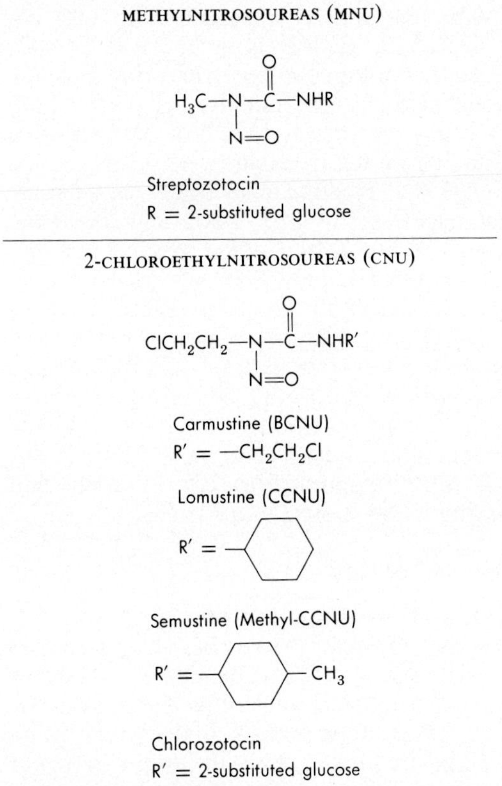

METHYLNITROSOUREAS (MNU)

Streptozotocin
R = 2-substituted glucose

2-CHLOROETHYLNITROSOUREAS (CNU)

Carmustine (BCNU)
R' = —CH₂CH₂Cl

Lomustine (CCNU)

R' =

Semustine (Methyl-CCNU)

R' =   CH₃

Chlorozotocin
R' = 2-substituted glucose

Figure 10–6. Classification and structures of some antineoplastic nitrosoureas.

Biochemical Pharmacology

These are highly reactive compounds with short plasma half-lives. Spontaneous decomposition occurs under physiologic conditions and generates a number of biologically active products capable of alkylation and carbamoylation (see Figure 10–7). The most important of these decomposition products are a chloroethyl diazohydroxide and an organic isocyanate (Montgomery et al., 1967; Brundrett and Colvin, 1977). The chloroethyl moiety further reacts to produce a chloroethyl carbonium ion that has the capability to alkylate DNA and produce interstrand cross-links and strand breaks. Isocyanates undergo carbamoylation reactions with intracellular proteins. In addition to spontaneous decomposition, nitrosoureas are metabolized to active hydroxylated products by the hepatic mixed-function oxidase system (Wang et al., 1981). Hydroxylated metabolites have higher in vitro alkylating activity than the decomposition products (Wheeler et al., 1977).

Alkylation is the primary mechanism responsible for the antitumor activity of the nitrosoureas (Colvin, 1982). Both the bifunctional, carmustine (BCNU), and the monofunctional, lomustine (CCNU) and semustine (MeCCNU), nitrosoureas alkylate DNA. For the monofunctional nitrosoureas, this multistep process first involves chloroethylation of a nucleophilic site on one strand of DNA. A chloride ion is then displaced on the opposite strand, a reactive carbonium ion is generated, and an ethyl bridge is formed between the two strands (Kohn, 1977). Cross-linking between DNA and nuclear proteins may also be produced.

The organic isocyanates produced by the decomposition of nitrosoureas are capable of undergoing carbamoylation reactions. The carbamoylating activity of the different nitrosoureas varies widely. BCNU and CCNU are potent carbamoylators, whereas chlorozotocin possesses only weak activity (Wheeler et al., 1974; Anderson et al., 1975). The repair of x-ray and ultraviolet irradiation damage to DNA is delayed by nitrosoureas that are strong carbamoylators. The repair of drug-induced alkylation of DNA is also inhibited by nitrosoureas with high carbamoylating activity. The contribution, however, of carbamoylation reactions to the cytotoxic and antitumor activity of the nitrosoureas is probably minor (DeVita et al., 1967; Panasci et al., 1979). Chloro-

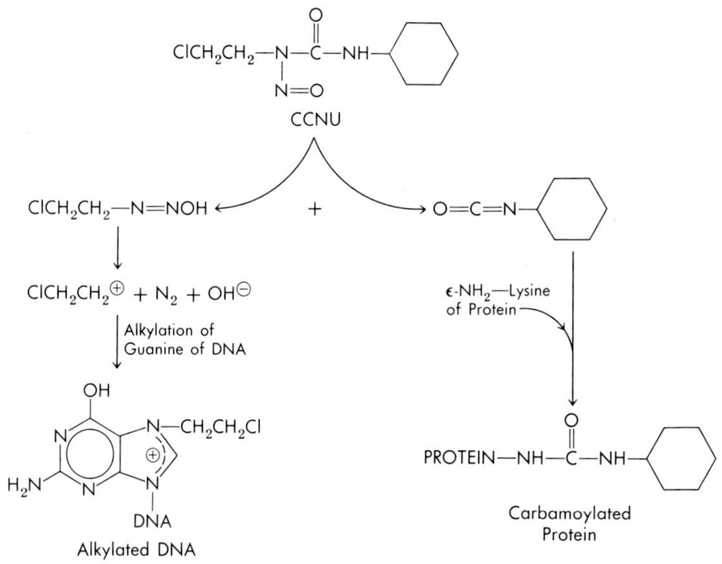

Figure 10-7. Degradation of lomustine (CCNU) with generation of alkylating and carbamoylating intermediates.

zotocin and streptozotocin are both weak carbamoylators but possess significant antitumor activity. Alkylating ability is the most important determinant of the antitumor activity of the individual nitrosoureas.

The sites of binding to specific regions of nuclear chromatin are determined by the structure of the nitrosourea molecule. For different nitrosoureas, there is preferential binding to either transcriptional regions of chromatin, nucleosomes, or to nontranscriptional linker regions (Wang *et al.,* 1981). The patterns of alkylation of chromatin for a particular nitrosourea may vary among different cell types and is an important determinant of cytotoxicity. For example, CCNU is a potent myelosuppressive drug, whereas chlorozotocin is relatively marrow sparing (Panasci *et al.,* 1979). Both agents are cytotoxic for L1210 cells and preferentially alkylate the nucleosome regions on L1210 chromatin. CCNU also preferentially alkylates the nucleosome regions of bone marrow cell chromatin, whereas the internucleosomal linker regions are alkylated by chlorozotocin (Green *et al.,* 1980). Thus, the reduced myelotoxicity of chlorozotocin, in comparison to CCNU, may result from tissue-specific differences in sites of alkylation. Streptozotocin, another glycosylated nitrosourea, is also minimally myelosuppressive. The presence of a glucose moiety appears to be an important structural determinant of myelosuppressive activity.

CARMUSTINE [BCNU; 1,3-*bis*(2-chloroethyl)-1-nitrosourea]

Clinical Pharmacology

Although rapidly absorbed after oral administration, BCNU is given intravenously because spontaneous decomposition and metabolism occur very quickly. The plasma half-life is five minutes and the biologic half-life is 15 to 30 minutes (Chirigos *et al.,* 1965; DeVita *et al.,* 1967). Hepatic microsomal enzymes are responsible for hydroxylation and denitrosation of BCNU to active and inactive metabolites. Approximately 80% of radioactive-labeled metabolic products are excreted in the urine within 24 hours. Biliary excretion and enterohepatic recirculation also occur. The high lipid solubility of BCNU is responsible for the entrance of active metabolites into the cerebrospinal fluid. Cerebrospinal fluid (CSF) concentrations are 15 to 30% of concurrent plasma levels (Levin *et al.,* 1978).

Clinical Toxicity

Delayed myelosuppression invariably follows the administration of BCNU. The nadirs of white blood cell and platelet counts occur between four to six weeks after therapy (Hoagland, 1982). Bone marrow toxicity is cumulative and frequently dose-limiting. Courses of therapy are usually given at six- to eight-week intervals.

Pulmonary fibrosis with interstitial pneumonitis has been reported after therapy with BCNU. Patients at greatest risk are those who receive large cumulative doses or high-dose BCNU in preparation for autologous bone marrow transplantation (Litam *et al.,* 1981; Ginsberg and Comis, 1982). After pulmonary toxicity develops, the mortality rate is high. Steroids have not been shown to be beneficial.

Self-limited nausea, vomiting, and diarrhea commonly occur within two hours of the administration of BCNU. Hepatotoxicity, usually manifested by transient elevations of alkaline phosphatase and serum transaminases, has been reported in as many as 26% of patients who receive BCNU (DeVita *et al.,* 1965). Acute hepatic necrosis has occurred with single doses of ≥ 1200 mg/m^2. Periorbital pain, conjunctival suffusion, lacrimation, confusion, disorientation, and seizures have occurred after infusion of BCNU into the carotid artery (Madajewicz *et al.,* 1981). High-dose BCNU may produce erythema of the skin and subsequent hyperpigmentation (DeVita *et al.,* 1965). BCNU is mutagenic and carcinogenic. Acute myelocytic leukemia has been reported after therapy with BCNU.

Clinical Indications

BCNU is useful in the therapy of Hodgkin's disease, non-Hodgkin's lymphomas, and multiple myeloma. Because of its lipophilic properties and ability to penetrate the blood-brain barrier, BCNU is used to treat primary and metastatic brain tumors. Intraarterial infusions, through either the carotid or vertebral arteries, have been utilized for this purpose. Marrow-ablative doses of BCNU have been used in association with autologous marrow transplantation. Using this approach, responses have been obtained in melanoma and in other solid tumors.

LOMUSTINE [CCNU; 1-(2-chloroethyl)-3-cyclohexyl-1-nitrosourea]

Clinical Pharmacology

CCNU is rapidly absorbed after oral administration. The plasma half-life of the intact drug is 15 minutes and ranges from 16 to 48 hours for its metabolites (Oliverio *et al.,* 1970). Approximately 50% of the administered dose is excreted in the urine within 24 hours and 75% within four days. Levels in the CSF range from 30 to 50% of concurrent plasma levels.

Clinical Toxicity

Nausea, vomiting, and delayed bone marrow suppression occur as with BCNU. Pulmonary toxicity has been reported in only one patient treated with CCNU (Macdonald *et al.,* 1981). Delayed nephrotoxicity occurs rarely. CCNU is mutagenic and acute myelocytic leukemia has been reported after long-term CCNU therapy.

Clinical Indications

Therapeutic indications include Hodgkin's disease, non-Hodgkin's lymphomas, brain tumors, and small cell lung carcinoma.

SEMUSTINE [MeCCNU; 1-(2-chloroethyl)-3-(4-methylcyclohexyl)-1-nitrosourea]

Clinical Pharmacology

MeCCNU is administered orally. Absorption and metabolism are rapid. Intact drug is not detectable in either plasma or urine. Metabolites and degradation products achieve peak plasma levels within one to six hours of administration and promptly enter the CSF (Sponzo *et al.,* 1973).

Clinical Toxicity

Delayed bone marrow suppression is the most common dose-limiting toxicity. Nausea and vomiting occur frequently. Progressive renal failure, occurring several years after completion of MeCCNU therapy, has been reported in children treated for brain tumors (Harmon *et al.,* 1979). In patients who receive more than 1500 mg/m^2 of MeCCNU, the incidence of chronic renal failure is high. A decrease in renal size may be the earliest manifestation of nephrotoxicity. Patients being treated with MeCCNU should have their renal size and function monitored. An increased incidence of acute leukemia occurred in patients who received MeCCNU as adjuvant therapy for gastrointestinal tract carcinomas (Boice *et al.,* 1983; Calabresi, 1983).

Clinical Indications

MeCCNU is currently used in the therapy of brain tumors and adenocarcinomas of the gastrointestinal tract.

STREPTOZOTOCIN

Streptozotocin, a naturally occurring glycosolated nitrosourea, is a product of the organism *Streptomyces achromogenes.*

Clinical Pharmacology

The cytotoxicity of streptozotocin is due to alkylation. In addition to its effects on DNA, streptozotocin depresses the intracellular concentrations of pyridine nucleotides. The diabetogenicity of streptozotocin is probably due to its inhibition of nicotinamide adenine dinucleotide in islet cells of the pancreas (Schein *et al.,* 1973; Anderson *et al.,* 1974).

After intravenous injection, the initial and terminal half-lives are 15 and 35 minutes, respectively (Bhuyan *et al.,* 1974; Adolphe *et al.,* 1975). Metabolites readily penetrate the CSF and, after two hours, CSF concentrations approach the levels in the plasma (Adolphe *et al.,* 1975). Excretion in the urine is almost complete by 24 hours. Only 10 to 20% of the drug is excreted intact.

Clinical Toxicity

Although diabetogenic in some species of animals, glucose intolerance is mild and occurs in only a small percentage of patients (Sadoff, 1972). Renal dysfunction is observed in 28 to 73% of patients and is the major dose-limiting toxicity (Weiss, 1982). Both glomerular and tubular damage may result. Hypophosphatemia, glycosuria, aminoaciduria, acetonuria, hyperchloremia, proteinuria, and renal tubular acidosis have been observed (Sadoff, 1970; Schein *et al.,* 1974). If therapy is discontinued, renal toxicity is reversible. Continuation of streptozotocin in the presence of renal dysfunction may result in irreversible renal failure. Vomiting, usually one to four hours after the administration of the drug, occurs in virtually every patient and is sometimes severe. Approximately 10% of patients experience leukopenia or thrombocytopenia (Schein *et al.,* 1974). The glucose moiety in the

structure of the compound is responsible for the low incidence of myelotoxicity.

Clinical Indications

Streptozotocin is the most effective agent for both functional and nonfunctional islet cell tumors of the pancreas. Beta and non-beta-cell tumors are responsive. The secretion of several hormones produced by tumors is decreased with streptozotocin therapy. Responses have been obtained in patients with carcinoid and other APUD tumors. Hodgkin's disease, colon, and pancreatic ductal carcinomas are other potentially responsive diseases.

CHLOROZOTOCIN

Chlorozotocin is a new glucose nitrosourea. It possesses high alkylating and low carbamoylating activity. Like streptozotocin, it has minimal bone marrow toxicity. Chlorozotocin is currently undergoing clinical trials.

TRIAZENES

DACARBAZINE

Dacarbazine [5-(3,3-dimethyl-1-triazeno)-imidazole-4-carboxamide; DTIC] was initially thought to be an antimetabolite. Its structural formula is similar to the metabolite 5-amino-imidazole-4-carboxamide (AIC), a precursor of inosinic acid in the purine biosynthetic pathway (see Figure 10–8). DTIC is now known to function as an alkylating agent.

Biochemical Pharmacology

DTIC is inactive and must be transformed in order to be cytotoxic. The hepatic microsomal cytochrome P-450 system activates DTIC. Conversion to the cytotoxic metabolite

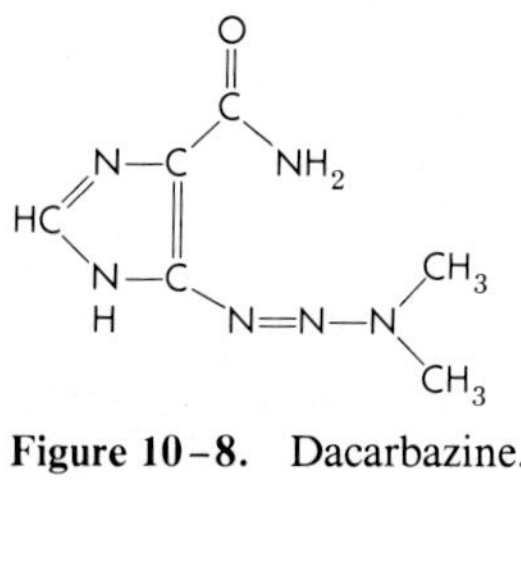

Figure 10–8.   Dacarbazine.

involves an enzymatic oxidative N-demethylation. The monomethyl derivative then spontaneously cleaves. This reaction yields AIC and an intermediate compound that decomposes to produce the methyl carbonium ion (Loo, 1974–1975). The methyl carbonium ion attacks nucleophilic groups on nucleic acids and other macromolecules. The 7-position of guanine on DNA is particularly susceptible to alkylation. The methylated residue of DNA, 7-methylguanine, has been detected in the urine of patients treated with DTIC.

The spontaneous photodegradation of DTIC is an alternate mechanism of activation. When exposed to the light, DTIC readily decomposes into 5-diazoimidazole-4-carboxamide and dimethylamine. 5-diazoimidazol-4-carboxamide is capable of attacking nucleophilic groups of DNA. This compound also undergoes structural rearrangement to form 2-azahypoxanthine. The products formed by the photodegradation of DTIC probably do not contribute greatly to its cytotoxicity *in vivo*. DTIC interferes with the synthesis of DNA, RNA, and proteins. The cytotoxicity of the drug is not specific for any phase of the cell cycle. DTIC is immunosuppressive in mice but not with the usual clinical schedules of administration (Chabner, 1982).

Clinical Pharmacology

DTIC is administered intravenously. After an intravenous injection, there is a biphasic pattern of clearance from the plasma. The initial and terminal half-lives are 20 minutes and 5 hours, respectively (Loo *et al.,* 1976). Clearance from the plasma is prolonged in patients with hepatic or renal disease. Excretion of the drug into the urine is by tubular secretion. Almost half of an intravenous dose is excreted as intact drug by this route within six hours. After the administration of DTIC, the urinary excretion of AIC is increased. The increased excretion of AIC is due to the catabolism of DTIC and not to inhibition of the metabolism of AIC. Concentrations of DTIC in the cerebrospinal fluid are 14% of the levels in plasma. The activity of DTIC may be adversely affected by prolonged exposure to light (Calabresi and Parks, 1985).

Clinical Toxicity

DTIC produces nausea and vomiting in virtually all patients. These symptoms usually develop within one to three hours after therapy. Patients treated on a daily schedule usually develop tolerance to the gastrointestinal side effects after two to three doses. The drug may be better tolerated if the amount of the initial dose is decreased. Leukopenia and thrombocytopenia are usually of only mild to moderate severity. During treatment, a flu-like syndrome characterized by fever, chills, malaise, and myalgias may occur. Less common toxicities include facial flushing, paresthesias, seizures, dementia, alopecia, dermatologic reactions, and hepatic dysfunction. DTIC is carcinogenic in rodents.

Clinical Indications

DTIC is useful in the treatment of melanoma and, combined with other drugs, in the therapy of soft tissue sarcomas and Hodgkin's disease.

ANTIBIOTICS

MITOMYCIN C

Mitomycin C is an antibiotic that is activated *in vivo* to an alkylating agent. Mitomycin has significant toxicities and important antitumor activity. Although in clinical trials in the United States for many years, only with the development of less toxic, high-dose intermittent schedules has it become widely used.

Mitomycin is isolated from *Streptomyces calspitosus* as blue-violet crystals (Wakaki *et al.,* 1958). Each molecule is composed of three active groups, a quinone, a urethane, and an aziridine (see Figure 10–9).

Biochemical Pharmacology

In vivo, an NADPH-dependent enzymatic reaction reduces the quinone, resulting in the loss of a methoxy group and the generation of a semiquinone and a hydroperoxy radical (Lown, 1979). After this activation reaction, mitomycin can act as a bifunctional or trifunc-

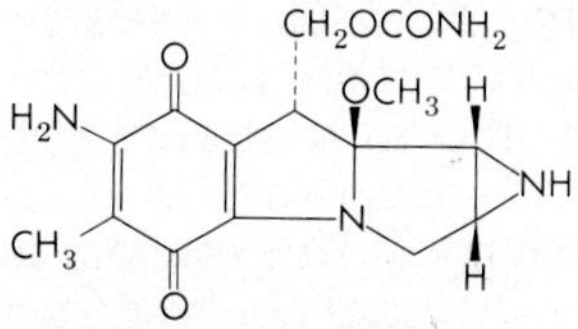

Figure 10–9.   Mitomycin.

tional alkylating agent. Mitomycin binds to DNA by covalent and noncovalent bonds. Inhibition of the synthesis of DNA, resulting from the production of interstrand and intrastrand DNA cross-links, is the primary mechanism of cytotoxicity. The extent of cross-linking is proportional to the guanine and cytosine content of DNA (Tomasz et al., 1974). Degradation of preformed DNA and inhibition of RNA synthesis are secondary and less important toxic effects. Chromosomal damage is prominent in cells treated with mitomycin. Although active throughout the cell cycle, inhibition of DNA synthesis and mitosis are maximal when cells are exposed to mitomycin during the late G_1 and early S phases.

Clinical Pharmacology

Because absorption from the gastrointestinal tract is erratic, mitomycin is administered intravenously. There is only minimal binding to plasma proteins. Clearance of an intravenous dose from the plasma is rapid and has a biphasic pattern. After a dose of 20 mg/m², the $t_{1/2} \alpha$ is approximately 10 minutes and $t_{1/2} \beta$ is 33 minutes (Reich, 1979). The peak plasma concentration after this dose is 1.5 μg/mL. Drug is not detectable in the serum six hours after administration. Mitomycin is widely distributed throughout the body but is not found in the brain.

Metabolism is the major mechanism for clearance of drug from the plasma. Many tissues are capable of metabolizing mitomycin, but the liver is thought to be the most important. Urinary excretion is low, accounting for less than 6% of a 20 mg intravenous dose, but may be an important mechanism for elimination of the drug when mitomycin is administered in high doses.

Clinical Toxicity

The most significant toxicity of mitomycin is myelosuppression. The hematologic toxicity is delayed, dose related, and cumulative. Nadir leukocyte and platelet counts generally occur four to six weeks after administration of the drug. With higher total cumulative doses, reductions in the dosage of mitomycin are frequently necessary in order to prevent dangerous cytopenias.

Interstitial pneumonitis and pulmonary fibrosis are uncommon toxicities resulting from mitomycin therapy. The incidence of pulmonary toxicity is apparently neither dose related nor correlated with the age of the patient. As with bleomycin, prior mitomycin therapy may predispose to the development of oxygen-induced lung damage (Ginsberg and Comis, 1982). The death rate from mitomycin lung toxicity is high. Fifty percent of patients eventually die of pulmonary insufficiency. Symptomatic and radiographic improvement have been reported with steroid therapy. Renal disease occurring after mitomycin therapy is uncommon but frequently fatal. Renal failure may be acute and accompanied by microangiopathic hemolytic anemia (Hanna et al., 1981; Pavy et al., 1982) (see Chapter 14). Pathologic examination of the kidneys reveals fibrin thrombi, cortical necrosis, focal glomerular sclerosis, and thickened glomerular basement membranes. This acute form of renal damage is apparently not dose related. Plasmapheresis and exchange-transfusions may be beneficial (Rabadi et al., 1982). A chronic form of progressive renal impairment, not associated with hemolysis, has also occurred after therapy with mitomycin. This type of chronic renal toxicity is delayed, occurring several months after initiation of therapy, and may be associated with high cumulative doses. Steroids have been proven to be helpful.

Extravasation of the drug can produce severe local ulceration and necrosis. Anorexia, nausea, vomiting, and diarrhea may accompany the administration of mitomycin. Hypersensitivity reactions, rashes, alopecia, and stomatitis occur infrequently. Cardiac and hepatic toxicities are rare (Ravry, 1979; Perry, 1982). When used in combination, mitomycin may potentiate the cardiotoxicity of doxorubicin (Sarna et al., 1982). Hepatic veno-occlusive disease has been reported in patients receiving high-dose mitomycin (Woods et al., 1980). Mitomycin is teratogenic and carcinogenic in rodents.

Clinical Indications

Mitomycin, in combination with 5-fluorouracil and doxorubicin (FAM), is useful for the palliative treatment of gastric adenocarcinoma (Macdonald et al., 1980). Activity has also been demonstrated in carcinomas of the breast, cervix, lung, pancreas, prostate, and head and neck. Instilled into the urinary bladder, mitomycin is effective in the therapy of superficial bladder tumors. Mitomycin has been administered in high doses, in conjunction with autologous bone marrow transplan-

tation, to treat a variety of solid tumors (Sarna *et al.,* 1982).

ANTIMETABOLITES

ANTIFOLATES

METHOTREXATE

Folic acid analogs have been used clinically for more than 30 years to treat neoplastic, as well as non-neoplastic diseases, such as psoriasis, and disorders with altered immunity. Methotrexate (2,4-diamino, N^{10}-methylpteroyl glutamic acid) is the most commonly used antifolate (Figure 10–10).

Biochemical Pharmacology

Methotrexate produces cytotoxicity by inhibition of the enzyme dihydrofolate reductase. This enzyme is required to maintain the intracellular pool of reduced folates. Reduced folates are essential cofactors required for the metabolic transfer of 1-carbon units in a number of synthetic reactions. The *de novo* syntheses of the purine precursor inosinic acid, the pyrimidine thymidylate and, ultimately, DNA and RNA are dependent upon a supply of reduced folates.

In the synthesis of thymidylate, catalyzed by the enzyme thymidylate synthetase, N^{5-10}-methylene tetrahydrofolate donates a methyl group to the uracil moiety of 2-deoxyuridylate. As a result of this reaction, tetrahydrofolate is metabolized to 5-6 dihydrofolic acid. To function again as a cofactor, dihydrofolate must be reduced to tetrahydrofolate by dihydrofolate reductase. As a tight-binding inhibitor of dihydrofolate reductase, methotrexate prevents the regeneration of the active tetrahydrofolate from the inactive dihydrofolate (Fig-

ure 10–11). Intracellular reduced folate pools are then rapidly depleted. This results in the cessation, first, of the synthesis of thymidylate and then of the *de novo* synthesis of purine nucleotides. Subsequently, the synthesis of DNA and, to a lesser extent, RNA are inhibited.

Methotrexate is cell-cycle dependent and is most toxic to cells during S phase. For methotrexate to produce cytotoxicity, the cell must be synthesizing thymidylate because this is the only reaction that oxidizes folates (Ayusawa *et al.,* 1981). Cells with low levels of thymidylate synthetase may be resistant to methotrexate (Washtien, 1982).

Methotrexate is transported into cells by an energy-dependent, carrier-mediated transport system. Circulating endogenous tetrahydrofolates and d1-5-formyl-tetrahydrofolate (leucovorin), a reduced folate used clinically to "rescue" cells from the toxic effects of methotrexate, share the same transport system. Leucovorin competes with extracellular methotrexate for transport by this common carrier and thereby slows the influx of methotrexate into the cell. This may contribute to the capability of leucovorin to reduce the toxicity of methotrexate. At low extracellular concentrations of methotrexate, influx is dependent solely upon this saturable mechanism. When the extracellular drug level is high, as is the case with high-dose methotrexate therapy, a second, low-affinity, transport mechanism is also employed (Hill *et al.,* 1979). Vincristine, the epipodophyllotoxins, and probenecid inhibit the efflux of methotrexate and produce increased intracellular concentrations (Yalowich *et al.,* 1982; Sirotnak *et al.,* 1981). The

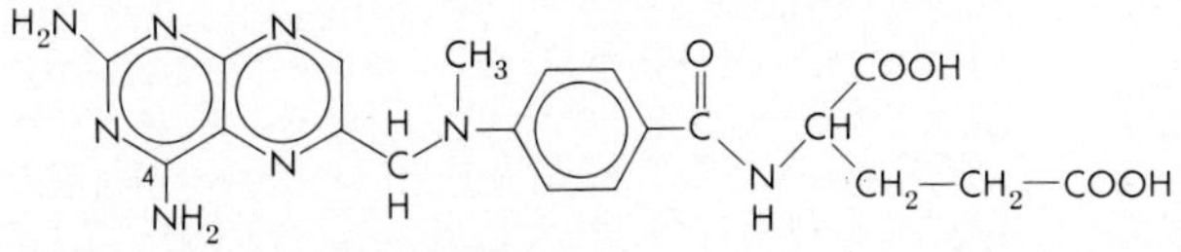

Figure 10–10. Methotrexate.

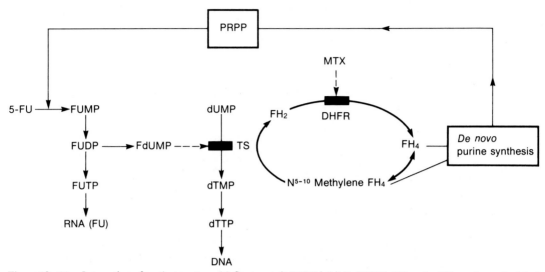

Figure 10–11. Interaction of methotrexate and 5-fluorouracil. MTX inhibits DHFR. When the FH_4 pools are depleted, the decrease in *de novo* purine synthesis results in increased concentrations of PRPP. Elevated PRPP levels increase the formation of FUMP. TS = thymidylate synthetase; DHFR = dihydrofolate reductase; PRPP = 5-phosphoribosyl-1-pyrophosphate; FH_2 = dihydrofolate; and FH_4 = tetrahydrofolate.

clinical importance of these drug interactions is uncertain.

Inhibition of nucleic acid and protein synthesis requires intracellular concentrations of methotrexate in excess of that needed to bind to all dihydrofolate reductase sites. Although methotrexate has a high affinity for dihydrofolate reductase and binds tightly to the enzyme, this binding is reversible. Methotrexate that is displaced from the enzyme can efflux out of the cell. As the extracellular concentration of methotrexate decreases, efflux of drug from the cell can become rapid (White, 1981). A high intracellular concentration of methotrexate is needed to overcome three other cellular mechanisms of protection: (1) The normal level of dihydrofolate reductase is in great excess of that required to maintain a sufficient pool of reduced folates. Even a small amount of uninhibited enzyme could protect the cell. (2) Inhibition of the enzyme results in an accumulation of dihydrofolates that compete with free methotrexate for binding sites on the enzyme. (3) Because the synthesis of new dihydrofolate reductase continues, successful inhibition of tetrahydrofolate-dependent processes requires the continued presence of unbound methotrexate. The attainment of high intracellular concentrations of methotrexate is dependent upon achieving even higher extracellular levels. This is a biochemical rationale for the use of high-dose methotrexate.

After entering the cell, both physiologic fo-late cofactors and methotrexate are conjugated with glutamic acid to form polyglutamyl derivatives (Fry *et al.*, 1982). Polyglutamates of methotrexate with as many as six extra glutamyl residues have been detected. The polyglutamates bind to dihydrofolate reductase with an affinity that is at least equal to the parent drug. The rate of efflux of the polyglutamates from the cell is slower than methotrexate and is related to the number of glutamyl residues. Considerable intracellular concentrations of polyglutamates with three and four extra glutamyl residues are maintained for prolonged periods even in the absence of methotrexate in the extracellular space. This preferential retention of the polyglutamates, with subsequent prolonged inhibition of dihydrofolate reductase, may lead to increased cytotoxicity. Cultured tumor cell lines that form long-chain glutamate residues are more susceptible to methotrexate than cells that do not form great amounts of polyglutamates (Jolivet *et al.*, 1982). The formation and retention of polyglutamates in the liver may be responsible for the hepatic toxicity observed in patients who receive long-term therapy with methotrexate (Jacobs *et al.*, 1977). Because the formation of polyglutamates is related to the dose and the duration of drug exposure, high-dose methotrexate infusion schedules may enhance their synthesis (Jolivet and Schilsky, 1981). In part, folic acid may reduce the toxicity of methotrexate by preventing the formation of long-chain polyglutamates (Galivan and Nimec, 1983).

Leucovorin is a fully reduced and metabolically functional coenzyme that can reverse the biologic effects of methotrexate. Leucovorin rescues cells by circumventing the inhibition of tetrahydrofolate synthesis. Because leucovorin uses the same specific carrier-mediated transport, it may also interfere with the entry of methotrexate into the cell.

By circumventing the inhibition of thymidylate synthesis, thymidine allows for the resumption of DNA synthesis and thereby provides a protective effect from methotrexate. The use of thymidine with methotrexate may provide a differential selectivity of rescue between tumor cells and normal tissue and produce increased tumor toxicity (Browman, 1982). Hypoxanthine, either alone or in combination with thymidine, may also protect against methotrexate toxicity (Howell and Wung, 1981).

Three distinct biochemical mechanisms of acquired resistance to methotrexate have been identified: (1) impaired transport of methotrexate into cells is associated with drug resistance in some cases; (2) tumor cells may become resistant by synthesizing dihydrofolate reductase that has a decreased binding affinity for methotrexate; and (3) alternatively, exposure to methotrexate may lead to a somatic cell mutation that results in the increased synthesis of dihydrofolate reductase. The chromosomes of these methotrexate-resistant cells may exhibit homogeneously staining regions (Biedler and Spengler, 1976). Homogeneously staining regions are the result of an increase in the number of genes that code for the mRNA responsible for the synthesis of dihydrofolate reductase (Melera et al., 1980; Alt et al., 1978). Amplification of the genes that code for the synthesis of dihydrofolate reductase is generally associated with the presence of either homogeneously staining regions or bits of extrachromosomal genetic material known as double minutes (Curt et al., 1983). The size of the homogeneously staining region and the number of double minutes correlate with the magnitude of increase in the synthesis of dihydrofolate reductase. These genetic changes are induced by exposure to methotrexate and may disappear in the absence of the drug. The importance of gene amplification in clinical drug resistance was suggested by the detection of increased levels of dihydrofolate reductase and numerous double minutes in the tumor cells of a patient with small cell carcinoma of the lung resistant to high-dose methotrexate (Curt et al., 1983).

Clinical Pharmacology

The two critical pharmacologic determinants of the biologic effects of methotrexate are the extracellular concentration of the drug and the duration of drug exposure. A variety of dose and administration schedules have been used in an attempt to maximize the clinical effects produced by manipulation of these pharmacokinetic factors. To inhibit thymidylate synthesis, an extracellular concentration of methotrexate of 10^{-8} mol is required (Chabner and Young, 1973). A concentration of 10^{-7} mol is needed to inhibit de novo purine synthesis (Zaharko et al., 1977). Toxicity is proportional to the dose of the drug and the duration of exposure. With prolonged exposure, increasing numbers of cells enter S phase and become susceptible to its toxic effects. Plasma concentrations of 10^{-6} mol maintained for more than 48 hours may produce fatal toxicities.

Methotrexate is readily absorbed from the gastrointestinal tract in doses up to 30 mg/m². As with physiologic folates, absorption occurs in the jejunum and is carrier-mediated (Strum, 1977). At higher doses, absorption after oral administration is erratic and varies among patients. The rate and completeness of absorption may be important determinants of remission duration in children with acute lymphocytic leukemia who receive oral methotrexate as maintenance therapy (Craft et al., 1981). Intramuscular, intravenous, intrathecal, and intracavitary routes of administration are also employed. There is a direct relationship between the dose of methotrexate and the plasma concentration.

Oral, low-dose methotrexate produces peak blood levels between one and five hours after administration. Absorption after an intramuscular injection is rapid and plasma levels are equivalent to that obtained by intravenous bolus administration. After intravenous administration, methotrexate disappears from the plasma in a triphasic pattern. The initial half-life of 45 minutes reflects the distribution of the drug. The second phase has a half-life of 2 to 3.5 hours and represents renal clearance. The terminal phase begins when the plasma concentration decreases to less than 1×10^{-7} mol and has a half-life of approximately ten hours. If the terminal phase is prolonged, and normal tissues are subjected to sustained plasma methotrexate concentrations of 10^{-8} mol or greater, severe toxicity may result.

Approximately 50% of circulating drug is bound to plasma proteins. Salicylates, sulfonamides and other drugs may displace methotrexate from albumin and produce increased levels of circulating free methotrexate (Calabresi and Parks, in preparation).

The influx of methotrexate into the cerebrospinal fluid and into third-space fluid collections, such as ascites and pleural effusions, is slow. Equilibrium of the concentration of the drug between plasma and third-space fluid collections occurs in approximately six hours (Chabner et al., 1981). When methotrexate is administered by intravenous infusion, only with high doses are cytocidal levels achieved in the cerebrospinal fluid (Jacobs et al., 1975). Clearance of methotrexate from the cerebrospinal fluid and from third-space fluid collections is also slow. Retention of methotrexate in third-space fluids may result in a prolonged terminal plasma half-life. Severe systemic toxicity may be caused by reentry of the drug into the circulation from such reservoirs. Patients with third-space fluids should have these removed prior to receiving methotrexate. Similarly, systemic toxicity may occur after intrathecal methotrexate administration.

The kidneys and the liver retain methotrexate longer than other organs. This may be due to specific transport mechanisms responsible for the uptake of drug and to high intracellular levels of dihydrofolate reductase in these tissues. In the liver, hepatic aldehyde oxidase metabolizes the parent drug to 7-hydroxy methotrexate and to polyglutamates (Jacobs et al., 1976). 7-hydroxy methotrexate is excreted in the urine. The polyglutamate forms may persist in tissues for long periods of time. Methotrexate that is retained in tumor tissues after the free drug disappears from the plasma is probably also in the form of polyglutamates. The metabolites of methotrexate do not possess great antifolate activity.

The majority of an administered dose of methotrexate is excreted unchanged in the urine within the first 12 hours. Methotrexate is filtered by the glomerulus and then undergoes tubular secretion and reabsorption. Two metabolites, 2,4-diamino N^{10}-methylpteroic acid, a product of bacterial metabolism in the gastrointestinal tract, and 7-hydroxy methotrexate, are excreted in the urine. Both of these metabolites are less soluble than the parent drug and may precipitate in the renal tubules during high-dose therapy. Weak organic acids, such as salicylates, may interfere with tubular excretion. Probenecid also interferes with the tubular secretion of methotrexate. There is a high potential for systemic toxicity in patients with diminished renal function. Such patients should be treated only with great caution and require careful monitoring of their methotrexate blood levels. Small amounts of methotrexate are secreted into the bile and then reabsorbed. Antibiotics that kill normal bowel flora may cause a decrease in this route of the metabolism of methotrexate and increase the enterohepatic recirculation. Small quantities of methotrexate are excreted in stools.

Clinical Toxicity

The plasma concentration of methotrexate and the duration of tissue exposure are important predictors of clinical toxicity. High plasma concentrations can be tolerated very well as long as the exposure is relatively brief. Conversely, modest plasma concentrations may be associated with severe toxicity if exposure is prolonged.

Because renal excretion is the primary route of elimination of methotrexate, pretreatment assessment of renal function is essential. When high-dose regimens are employed and in high-risk clinical settings, monitoring of plasma methotrexate concentrations may identify patients with delayed drug excretion. In these patients, toxicity may be ameliorated by the administration of high-dose leucovorin (100 mg/m^2 for levels of 10^{-6} mol methotrexate with proportional increases for higher methotrexate concentrations).

Rapidly proliferating tissues are the primary sites of methotrexate toxicity. The nadirs of leukopenia and thrombocytopenia occur seven to ten days after drug administration. Recovery is generally complete by 14 to 21 days. Mucositis is the most common gastrointestinal toxicity. If the clearance of drug is delayed, mucositis may be severe. The oral mucosae of patients who have received irradiation for carcinoma of the head and neck are particularly susceptible to this complication. Nausea, vomiting, and diarrhea occur less frequently. With delayed drug excretion, ulceration and bleeding of the gastrointestinal tract may occur.

With conventional doses of methotrexate, renal toxicity is infrequent. After high-dose therapy, renal damage may result from the precipitation of the parent drug or the metabolites 7-hydroxy methotrexate and 2,4-diamino N^{10}-methylpteroic acid in the renal tubules (Chabner, 1982). These metabolites are both several-fold less soluble than methotrexate. During high-dose infusions, the solubility of these compounds at the normal pH of urine may be exceeded. Increasing the rate of urine flow and raising the pH reduces the frequency of renal failure associated with high-dose methotrexate infusions. Vigorous intravenous hydration and alkalinization of the urine with intravenous sodium bicarbonate should precede the infusion of methotrexate by 12 hours. The pH of the urine should be 7 or higher. Urine output must be carefully monitored and urine flow should exceed 100 mL/hour. Hydration and alkalinization of the urine should continue for 36 hours. Methotrexate plasma levels should be monitored and high-dose leucovorin initiated if the clearance of the drug is delayed. Peritoneal dialysis and hemodialysis are not particularly effective in clearing methotrexate. The clearance rate of methotrexate by peritoneal dialysis is only 5 to 7 mL/min and clearance by hemodialysis is only 30 to 40 mL/min (Ahmad *et al.,* 1978; Harde *et al.,* 1977). Hemodialysis transiently lowers plasma methotrexate levels. When dialysis is stopped, however, there is a rapid influx of drug from tissue stores and a rebound of the plasma methotrexate concentration. Charcoal hemoperfusion columns are similarly ineffective. Extracorporeal circulation over immobilized carboxypeptidase G_1, a bacterial enzyme, cleaves and inactivates circulating methotrexate (Howell *et al.,* 1978). This enzyme is not readily available, however, and its use is still investigational. Acute renal failure induced by methotrexate usually resolves spontaneously within three weeks. The associated high mortality rate is secondary to toxicity to the bone marrow and gastrointestinal tract produced by prolonged exposure to high plasma concentrations of methotrexate. If renal toxicity occurs, methotrexate plasma levels should be monitored and leucovorin administered until the plasma level of methotrexate is less than 10^{-8} mol.

The chronic administration of methotrexate, such as is used in the treatment of psoriasis and acute lymphocytic leukemia of childhood, may produce hepatic toxicity (see Chapter 14).

The most common pathologic changes are those of portal fibrosis and cirrhosis. Hepatic damage occurs more frequently with daily administration schedules than with intermittent treatment regimens. The total cumulative dose of methotrexate may be another determinant of the development of hepatic toxicity. Liver function tests are not reliable indicators of hepatic injury. Patients with psoriasis who receive chronic methotrexate therapy require serial liver biopsies. The intracellular retention of methotrexate polyglutamates may be responsible for this clinical toxicity. High-dose methotrexate frequently produces transient elevations of the hepatic enzymes. Chronic hepatic toxicity associated with high-dose therapy, however, has not been observed.

The intrathecal administration of methotrexate can produce acute meningeal irritation. Associated symptoms usually begin within 48 hours and may include lethargy, stiff neck, headache, fever, nausea, and vomiting. A pleocytosis in the cerebrospinal fluid may occur either in the presence or absence of symptoms. Paraplegia, either transient or permanent, may occur after intrathecal methotrexate. This serious toxicity is probably related to persistently high levels of methotrexate in the cerebrospinal fluid and occurs most frequently after three to five intrathecal treatments (Bleyer, 1978). Other neurologic abnormalities associated with repetitive intrathecal administrations of methotrexate include sensory deficits, cranial nerve palsies, and seizures. Neurologic toxicities occur most frequently in patients receiving intrathecal methotrexate for meningeal leukemia. Patients receiving prophylactic intrathecal therapy are also susceptible to these complications. Patients who are treated with radiation therapy to the brain and then either intrathecal methotrexate or parenteral high-dose methotrexate are at risk for the development of necrotizing leukoencephalopathy. Clinical manifestations in these patients may include ataxia, spasticity, paresis, seizures, abnormalities on psychologic testing, and dementia. Neurologic impairment is usually progressive. Ventricular dilatation, enlargement of the subarachnoid space, and intracerebral calcifications may be seen on radiographic evaluation. Leukoencephalopathy may occur after only intravenous methotrexate, however, the frequency is highest in patients who receive both irradiation and drug. Cerebral atrophy has also been observed in patients who received the combination of brain irradiation and methotrexate. When both modalities are administered, patients who receive brain irradiation either prior to or simultaneously with the methotrexate have the highest incidence of leukoencephalopathy (Price and Jamieson, 1975). The administration of methotrexate prior to radiation therapy and the use of lower doses of cranial irradiation (1800 rads) may reduce the incidence of leukoencephalopathy and other manifestations of radiotherapy-chemotherapy toxicity. These approaches are still being evaluated.

An acute interstitial pneumonitis occurs rarely after the administration of methotrexate (Ginsberg and Comis, 1982) (see Chapter 14). This toxicity has been characterized as an allergic alveolitis and is typically associated with eosinophilia in the peripheral blood and in the parenchyma of the lungs. The incidence of pulmonary toxicity does not appear to be related to the dose of methotrexate or to the route of administration. Daily or weekly administration is more likely to result in toxicity than are less frequent treatment schedules. Spontaneous recovery after one to six weeks is usual, although progressive and lethal courses have been reported. High-dose corticosteroid therapy is frequently effective. Retreatment with methotrexate in recovered patients does not necessarily produce a recurrence of this uncommon toxicity.

A pruritic, erythematous, macular rash occurs in 10 to 15% of patients treated with methotrexate. Photosensitization and x-ray enhancement effects may also be seen. Acute hypersensitivity and anaphylactic reactions are rare.

Clinical Indications

Methotrexate has a broad range of clinical uses. The efficacy of methotrexate is well established in acute lymphocytic leukemia of childhood, choriocarcinoma, and cancers of the breast, bladder, and head and neck. Methotrexate is useful in the treatment of non-Hodgkin's lymphomas, including mycosis fungoides, Burkitt's lymphoma, and diffuse histiocytic lymphoma. High-dose methotrexate combined with leucovorin rescue has been evaluated against many types of tumors. This mode of administration effectively reduces the toxicity to normal tissues. The therapeutic superiority of high-dose therapy, however, has been convincingly demonstrated for only a few

neoplasms, particularly osteogenic sarcoma. Careful attention to hydration, urine flow and pH, and plasma methotrexate concentrations is essential when high-dose regimens are employed. The dose of leucovorin that is required to rescue normal tissues is dependent upon the plasma concentration of methotrexate. The leucovorin dose must be increased when methotrexate excretion is delayed. Other rescue methods include asparaginase, thymidine, and carboxypeptidase.

Methotrexate is injected intrathecally to treat meningeal leukemia, lymphoma, and other forms of carcinomatous meningitis. For children with acute lymphocytic leukemia, intrathecal methotrexate is administered prophylactically. The placement of an Ommaya reservoir allows direct instillation of drug into the ventricles and provides for better drug distribution. For patients with active meningeal disease, the use of an Ommaya reservoir is favored over injection into the lumbar region. The monitoring of methotrexate concentrations in the cerebrospinal fluid permits the appropriate modification of subsequent doses and may thereby reduce the incidence of neurotoxicity.

Methotrexate has been injected directly into the peritoneal cavity and into the pericardial and pleural spaces (Jones *et al.*, 1981). The usefulness of these approaches is still under evaluation.

PYRIMIDINE ANALOGS

5-FLUOROURACIL

In 1954, Rutman observed that rat hepatoma cells, in comparison to normal hepatocytes, utilized the base uracil more efficiently in the synthesis of nucleic acids (Rutman *et al.*, 1954). Heidelberger subsequently designed an analog of uracil with fluorine replacing hydrogen on position 5 of the pyrimidine ring (Heidelberger *et al.*, 1957). This fluorinated pyrimidine, 5-fluorouracil (5-FU), was one of the first rationally designed antitumor agents (Figure 10–12).

Biochemical Pharmacology

In order to be biologically active, 5-FU must first be converted enzymatically to the nucleo-

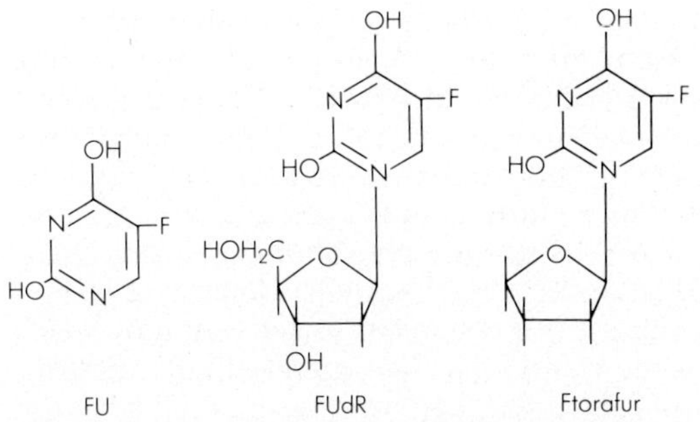

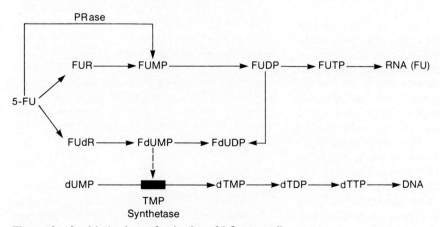

Figure 10–12. The clinically active fluoropyrimidines.

tide level. 5-FU produces cytotoxicity through two mechanisms: (1) the incorporation of the nucleotide fluorouridine triphosphate (FUTP) into RNA, and (2) inhibition of the enzyme thymidylate synthetase by fluorodeoxyuridine monophosphate (FdUMP) with subsequent inhibition of DNA synthesis. There are several mechanisms available for the activation of 5-FU to the nucleotide level (Figure 10–13). Fluorouridine monophosphate (FUMP) may be formed from the parent drug either in a single step by orotate phosphoribosyltransferase or by the sequential addition of, first, a ribose by uridine phosphorylase and then a phosphate by uridine kinase. FUMP may then be converted to the nucleotide triphosphate, FUTP. The incorporation of FUTP into RNA results in the alteration of the synthesis and function of RNA. All species of RNA are affected. In particular, FUTP inhibits the maturation of ribosomal RNA, interferes with the formation and function of ribosomes and causes miscoding during the translation of messenger RNA. Cytotoxicity may be produced by interference with protein synthesis and by the synthesis of abnormal proteins (Sawyer et al., 1981). Studies with cultured human tumor cells indicate that the incorporation of FUTP into RNA is an important mechanism of cytotoxicity (Kufe and Major, 1981).

Alternatively, FUMP may be converted to the diphosphate nucleotide and then reduced by ribonucleotide reductase to FdUMP. FdUMP is a potent inhibitor of thymidylate synthetase. Thymidylate synthetase catalyzes the methylation of dUMP to thymidylate. Thymidylate is essential for the synthesis of DNA. The most important determinant of the extent of inhibition of thymidylate synthetase by 5-FU is the amount of FdUMP formed in the target cell. FdUMP forms a stable, covalently bonded, ternary complex with thymidylate synthetase and N^{5-10} methylene tetrahydrofolate. Tetrahydrofolate is required for the tight binding of FdUMP to the enzyme. The depletion of intracellular reduced folates by methotrexate does not reduce the cytotoxicity of 5-FU because methotrexate is able to replace tetrahydrofolate in the ternary complex. Folic acid may enhance the toxicity of 5-FU by increasing the formation of the ternary complex. The inhibition of DNA synthesis that results from the inhibition of thymidylate synthetase is the principal mechanism of the toxicity of 5-FU in most cells. The sensitivity of tumor cells to 5-FU correlates best with a rapid and complete inhibition of thymidylate synthetase (Spears et al., 1982).

5-FU may also be converted directly to FdUMP by thymidine phosphorylase and thymidine kinase. This mechanism of activation results only in the inhibition of DNA synthesis. The route of 5-FU activation varies among

Figure 10–13. Mechanisms of activation of 5-fluorouracil.

different tissues. Residues of 5-FU have also been detected in the DNA of cultured human tumor cells exposed to the drug (Major *et al.,* 1982). The incorporation of 5-FU into DNA is enhanced by concurrent exposure to thymidine. The importance of this mechanism in producing cytotoxicity *in vivo* is unknown.

5-FU is catabolized to the inactive compound dihydrofluorouracil by the enzymes that breakdown physiologic pyrimidines, particularly dihydrouracil dehydrogenase. This catabolic process is rapid and occurs primarily in the liver. Degradative enzymes are also present in gastrointestinal tract mucosal cells. Tumor cells from colonic carcinomas may lack these catabolic enzymes. Thymidine is catabolized in the liver by the same enzymatic processes that degrade 5-FU. The infusion of high-doses of thymidine may protect 5-FU from enzymatic breakdown and produce higher levels of 5-FU in the plasma. Thymidine also stimulates the incorporation of 5-FU into RNA (Spiegelman *et al.,* 1980). By these two mechanisms, thymidine may enhance the antitumor activity of 5-FU.

Biochemical differences may be responsible for the innate and acquired variability among cells in sensitivity to 5-FU. The most important determinants of sensitivity to 5-FU are the amounts of FdUMP generated and the retention of the FdUMP pool. Resistance may result from decreases in the activities of enzymes that activate 5-FU, such as uridine phosphorylase, uridine kinase, and uracil phosphoribosyltransferase. dUMP competes favorably with FdUMP for newly synthesized thymidylate synthetase. Tissues, such as bone marrow, that are capable of generating high concentrations of dUMP after thymidylate synthetase is inhibited, may quickly recover from the inhibitory effects of the drug.

The administration of physiologic pyrimidine metabolites and other drugs in combination with 5-FU may increase antitumor activity and enhance the therapeutic ratio (Houghton and Houghton, 1980). Allopurinol and hypoxanthine may protect normal tissues from the toxic effects of 5-FU and permit the administration of higher doses of the drug. A metabolite of allopurinol, 1-oxypurinol-5'-monophosphate, inhibits orotidine 5'-monophosphate decarboxylase. Inhibition of this enzyme increases the intracellular concentration of orotic acid. Orotic acid competes with 5-FU for orotate phosphoribosyltransferase. As a result, the activation of 5-FU by this path-

way is decreased. This is the primary pathway of activation of 5-FU in most normal tissues. Allopurinol could thereby selectively protect normal tissues. Hypoxanthine depletes 5-phosphoribosyl-1-pyrophosphate (PRPP), the enzyme required for the conversion of 5-FU to FUMP by orotate phosphoribosyltransferase. Hypoxanthine selectively protects cells that utilize this mechanism of activation of 5-FU. Some tumor cell lines preferentially metabolize 5-FU to FUMP by the sequential activities of uridine phosphorylase and uridine kinase, utilizing ribose-1-phosphate. Cells that activate 5-FU by this mechanism would not be protected by either allopurinol or hypoxanthine. Despite this sound biochemical rationale, the increased effectiveness of either of these two combinations over 5-FU administered as a single agent remains to be demonstrated (Kroener *et al.,* 1982).

Physiologic pyrimidines, purines, and metabolites of these compounds, including uracil, uridine, deoxyuridine, thymine, thymidine, inosine, and deoxyinosine, may modulate the metabolism and toxicity of 5-FU (Rustum *et al.,* 1981). These substances can also reduce the rate of catabolism of 5-FU. Depending upon the compound employed, the activation of 5-FU may be selectively channeled into a particular pathway. At the present time, only thymidine is being clinically evaluated in combination with 5-FU.

The sequential combination of methotrexate administered prior to 5-FU has synergistic immunosuppressive and antitumor activity (Bareham *et al.,* 1974; Benz *et al.,* 1982). Pretreatment with methotrexate enhances the intracellular accumulation of 5-FU and, through its antipurine effect, increases the intracellular PRPP pools (see Figure 10–11). The increased levels of PRPP enhance the transfer of phosphoribosyl to 5-FU. The formation of FUMP and the subsequent incorporation of FUTP into RNA are increased. The administration of leucovorin may prevent this increase in intracellular 5-FU and PRPP levels. The synergistic cytotoxicity of this combination is strictly schedule dependent, methotrexate must precede 5-FU. Phase II clinical trials of this combination are now in progress.

Clinical Pharmacology

A variety of different routes and schedules of administration of 5-FU have been evaluated. After oral administration, 5-FU is erratically and incompletely absorbed. The bioavailability of the drug may be as low as 1 to 15%. Because the liver is the major site of metabolism of 5-FU, the availability of the drug to other organs may be compromised with oral administration. 5-FU is most frequently given as an intravenous bolus either once each week or daily for five days every four to six weeks. After an intravenous bolus injection, there is a monophasic pattern of disappearance of the drug from the plasma. The half-life is approximately ten minutes and reflects the rapid rate of metabolism (Fraile *et al.*, 1980). After an intravenous bolus dose of 15 mg/kg, peak plasma levels of 10^{-3} to 10^{-4} mol are achieved. Drug is undetectable in the plasma after two hours. When 5-FU is administered as a continuous intravenous infusion, a constant plasma concentration is achieved after 12 to 24 hours and is maintained for the duration of the infusion. Thereafter, 5-FU disappears from the plasma within one hour. The concentration of 5-FU in bone marrow cells and the incidence of myelosuppression are lower when the drug is given as a continuous infusion as compared to bolus administration. *In vitro* studies indicate that the administration of 5-FU at lower doses for longer time periods is more effective in producing cytotoxicity to human tumor cells than shorter periods of administration at higher doses (Calabro-Jones *et al.*, 1982). An enhanced therapeutic benefit for infusional schedules, however, has not been definitively demonstrated. 5-FU may be administered by infusion into the hepatic artery of patients with metastases in the liver. Because the liver is the primary site of catabolism of the drug, higher doses can be infused by this route without increasing systemic toxicity. The development of implantable infusion pumps may make this method of drug delivery more widely applicable.

5-FU readily enters effusions and ascites and, like methotrexate, persists in these third-spaces for prolonged periods. After intravenous administration, significant concentrations of 5-FU are achieved in the cerebrospinal fluid. An intravenous dose of 15 mg/kg produces concentrations in the cerebrospinal fluid of 6 to 8×10^{-6} mol within 30 minutes. The concentration of 5-FU then slowly declines during a period of nine hours (Bourke *et al.*, 1973).

Approximately 80% of an administered dose is catabolized in the liver. The pyrimidine ring is reduced by dihydrouracil dehydrogen-ase and then cleaved to yield α-fluoro-β-alanine, urea, ammonia, and carbon dioxide. Metabolism also occurs in the epithelium of the gastrointestinal tract. Small amounts of intact drug, 10 to 20%, are excreted in the urine. The dose of 5-FU does not need to be altered in patients with decreased hepatic or renal function.

In contrast to the rapid clearance of 5-FU from the plasma, the active metabolites, FdUMP and FUTP, may persist intracellularly for extended periods. The concentrations of these metabolites achieved by a particular schedule of administration of 5-FU may be a better predictor of clinical effectiveness than the plasma kinetics of the parent drug.

Clinical Toxicity

The route and schedule of administration of 5-FU are important determinants of the patterns of toxicity that are likely to occur. After intravenous bolus administration, myelosuppression is the predominant toxicity. The nadirs of the white blood cell and platelet counts occur between the ninth and fourteenth days after administration of the drug. A megaloblastic anemia may develop with prolonged therapy. With intravenous bolus administration, gastrointestinal tract toxicities are usually mild. Toxicity to the gastrointestinal tract is more common with bolus administration on five consecutive days than with once weekly schedules. Continuous intravenous infusions of 5-FU frequently produce stomatitis, nausea, vomiting, and diarrhea, whereas myelosuppression is less common. When 5-FU is given as an infusion into the hepatic artery, stomatitis and gastrointestinal tract toxicities predominate. Hepatotoxicity, characterized by elevations of serum transaminases, may be observed. If the tip of the catheter becomes displaced and the drug is inadvertently infused into vessels that supply the intestines, severe gastrointestinal tract toxicities, including pain, hemorrhage, ulceration, and perforation, may occur.

An acute and reversible cerebellar syndrome occurs in 3 to 7% of patients who receive 5-FU. Characteristic findings include somnolence, ataxia of the trunk or extremities, unsteady gait, slurred speech, and nystagmus. Patients who are treated with doses and schedules that produce high peak plasma levels of 5-FU are most susceptible. A metabolite of 5-FU, fluorocitrate, has been suspected to be the cause of this neurotoxicity. When fluorocitrate is injected into animals, neuropathologic lesions are produced that are nearly identical to those observed in patients. Other evidence, however, suggests that this may not be the mechanism. Because thymidine blocks the catabolism of 5-FU, its administration should result in the formation of less fluorocitrate. Combined therapy with 5-FU and thymidine, however, produces an increase rather than a decrease in the incidence of cerebellar toxicity (Cheng *et al.*, 1980).

Hyperpigmentation of the skin, particularly in areas exposed to sunlight, is frequently observed. Hyperpigmentation may be most prominent over the veins used for the administration of the drug. Photosensitivity may be manifested as an intense erythema that occurs after only brief periods of exposure to the sun. The toxic effects of irradiation to the skin may also be enhanced by 5-FU. Alopecia, acute and chronic conjunctivitis, and nail changes may be observed. Rarely, therapy with 5-FU has been associated with angina pectoris and myocardial infarction. The mechanism for this apparent drug-induced cardiotoxicity is unknown.

Clinical Indications

As a single agent, 5-FU is useful in the palliative therapy of advanced colorectal carcinoma. In combination with other drugs, 5-FU is used to treat breast cancer and carcinomas of the ovary, stomach, and pancreas. Activity against advanced head and neck cancer has been observed with the sequential combination of methotrexate and 5-FU. The utility of rational combinations of 5-FU with other agents, including physiologic nucleosides and bases, allopurinol, and N-phosphonoacetyl L-aspartate, is the subject of intense investigation.

FLUORODEOXYURIDINE

Fluorodeoxyuridine (FUdR) is a deoxyribonucleoside of 5-FU (see Figure 10–12). FUdR is a substrate for thymidine kinase and is converted to FdUMP in a single step. FUdR is also rapidly converted to 5-FU by both thymidine and deoxyuridine phosphorylases. FUdR is rapidly cleared from the plasma by the liver. FUdR has undergone extensive clinical evaluation. At the present time, the pri-

mary use for FUdR is in the treatment of patients with hepatic metastases by infusion into the hepatic artery.

FTORAFUR

Ftorafur is an analog of 5-FU that functions as a slow release depot form of the drug (see Figure 10–12). After intravenous administration, ftorafur undergoes a slow hydrolysis that results in low circulating levels of 5-FU that persist for several days. The half-life is approximately 16 hours. The toxicities produced by ftorafur are similar to the side effects of 5-FU administered by continuous infusion. Myelosuppression is mild and gastrointestinal tract toxicities may be significant. Ftorafur is more lipid soluble than 5-FU and penetrates into the cerebrospinal fluid more rapidly. Neurotoxicity, particularly with intravenous administration, may be dose limiting. Ftorafur does not appear to offer any clinical advantages over 5-FU.

CYTOSINE ARABINOSIDE

Cytosine arabinoside (1-β-D-arabinofuranosyl-cytosine; ara-C), a pyrimidine nucleoside, is an analog of 2′-deoxycytidine. Ara-C differs from deoxycytidine by the presence of a hy-

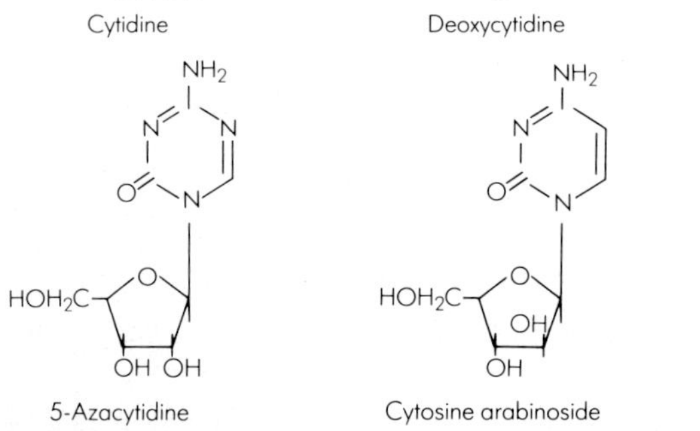

Figure 10–14. Structures of cytidine and related physiologic and analog nucleosides.

droxyl group, in the beta configuration, on the sugar moiety (see Figure 10–14).

Biochemical Pharmacology

As with most purine and pyrimidine antimetabolites, ara-C must first be enzymatically "activated" to a nucleotide in order to exert its biological effects. Ara-C rapidly enters cells by a carrier-mediated process. The enzyme deoxycytidine kinase then converts the parent drug to the 5'-monophosphate nucleotide, ara-CMP. This initial phosphorylation is the rate-limiting step in the activation of ara-C. Although this enzymatic conversion proceeds rapidly, deoxycytidine kinase has a higher affinity for its natural substrate, 2'-deoxycytidine. Sequential phosphorylations by deoxycytidylate kinase and nucleoside diphosphate kinase result in the formation of ara-CDP and ara-CTP, respectively (Figure 10–15).

Ara-CTP, the active nucleotide, is a competitive inhibitor of DNA polymerase and thus interferes with the synthesis of DNA (Momparler, 1972). The formation and retention of intracellular ara-CTP are the most important determinants of the cytotoxicity of ara-C. The concentration of ara-CTP is higher in the cells of sensitive tumors than in cells of unresponsive tumors and normal host tissue cells (Rustum, 1978). For patients with acute myeloid leukemia, the duration of the intracellular retention of ara-CTP correlates with the length of clinical remission (Rustum and Preisler, 1979). The amount of intracellular ara-CTP

generated is, in part, dependent upon the extracellular concentration of ara-C. With high-dose regimens, the concentration of intracellular ara-CTP is increased.

Nucleotides of ara-C are also incorporated into both RNA and DNA. The incorporation of ara-C into DNA results in the synthesis of abnormal DNA and may be the cause of the structural chromosome damage that is sometimes associated with the exposure of cells to the drug (Woodcock *et al.*, 1979). The importance of the incorporation of ara-C into DNA in producing cell death is unclear. Acute cellular toxicity, not reversible by deoxycytidine, is correlated with the number of nucleotides of ara-C incorporated into RNA (Chu, 1971). Since ara-C acts primarily by interfering with the synthesis and function of DNA, it is regarded as specific for the S phase of the cell cycle.

The degradative enzymes, cytidine deaminase and deoxycytidine monophosphate deaminase, deaminate ara-C and ara-CMP respectively. The products of these reactions, arabinosyl uracil (ara-U) and ara-UMP, are inactive. Cytidine deaminase has a high affinity for ara-C and is present in plasma, granulocytes, red blood cells, the mucosa of the gastrointestinal tract, the liver, spleen, and lungs. In human leukemia cells, cytidine deaminase is present in great excess to the activating enzyme deoxycytidine kinase (Coleman *et al.*, 1975). Deoxycytidine monophosphate deaminase is also present in higher concentrations in tumor tissues than is the competing

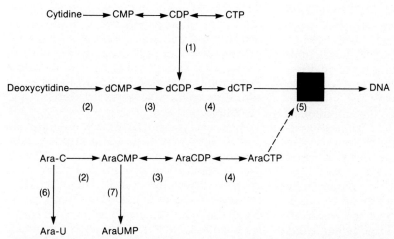

Figure 10–15. Activation and metabolism of cytidine, deoxycytidine, and cytosine arabinoside. (1) = Ribonucleoside diphosphate reductase; (2) = deoxycytidine kinase; (3) = deoxycytidylate kinase; (4) = nucleoside diphosphate kinase; (5) = DNA polymerase; (6) = cytidine deaminase; (7) = deoxycytidine monophosphate deaminase.

activating enzyme. The ratio of the concentrations of the activating to the deaminating enzymes is an important determinant of the susceptibility of tumor and normal tissues to ara-C. Tetrahydrouridine, a reduced pyrimidine, is a potent inhibitor of cytidine deaminase. When administered prior to ara-C, tetrahydrouridine prolongs the half-life of ara-C in the plasma. In human leukemia cells with high levels of cytidine deaminase, tetrahydrouridine also increases the net amount of ara-CTP generated (Ho *et al.*, 1980). The ability of tetrahydrouridine to improve the therapeutic index of ara-C has not yet been demonstrated.

Other mechanisms of resistance to ara-C include an increase in the production of the competitive substrate, dCTP; decreased activity or deletion of the activating enzyme, deoxycytidine kinase; increased concentrations of cytidine deaminase; and the synthesis of an altered DNA polymerase with a decreased affinity for ara-CTP.

Various methods of biochemical modulation are being devised to overcome these mechanisms of resistance. High intracellular levels of deoxycytidine triphosphate (dCTP) exert feed-back inhibition on the activity of deoxycytidine kinase. Reduced activity of deoxycytidine kinase leads to a decrease in the formation of ara-CTP. A decrease in the dCTP pool should, therefore, result in increased ara-CTP generation. The administration of high doses of thymidine elevates the intracellular concentration of deoxythymidine triphosphate (dTTP). High levels of dTTP decrease the activity of ribonucleotide reductase and, thereby, cause a decrease in the synthesis of dCDP from CDP. As a result, dCTP pools are reduced. The administration of high doses of thymidine, in combination with ara-C, should, therefore, decrease the feed-back inhibition on deoxycytidine kinase and increase the synthesis of ara-CTP. Because dCTP is also a competitive inhibitor of ara-CTP, high-dose thymidine may also increase the inhibition of DNA polymerase by ara-CTP. Studies in animals indicate that high-dose thymidine and other nucleosides do increase the intracellular pools of ara-CTP (Rustum *et al.*, 1981).

In contrast to the stimulation produced by very high intracellular levels of dTTP, compounds that lower dTTP pools also enhance the accumulation of ara-CTP (Cadman *et al.*, 1981). A reduction in dTTP increases the deamination of deoxycytidylate nucleotides to dUMP. As already discussed, methotrexate

and the fluoropyrimidines inhibit the formation of dTMP, the precursor of dTTP. Pretreatment with methotrexate, 5-FU, or FUdR prior to ara-C produces synergistic killing of tumor cells. The use of these and other compounds in combination with ara-C has the potential to favorably modulate the formation and retention of ara-CTP. The clinical effectiveness of these rational drug combinations remains to be established.

Clinical Pharmacology

Ara-C is poorly and unpredictably absorbed after oral administration. After intravenous administration, the drug is rapidly deaminated to the inactive compound ara-U, which is the predominant form of the drug in the plasma within minutes of administration. The clearance of ara-C from the plasma is biphasic. The half-life of the initial rapid phase ranges from 1.6 to 11.1 minutes (Harris *et al.*, 1979). The second phase of plasma decay has a half-life of 13.1 to 111 minutes. After a bolus injection of 30 to 300 mg/m^2, peak concentrations in the plasma of 2 to 50 μM are achieved. Within 24 hours, greater than 90% of an administered dose is excreted in the urine as ara-U. The remainder is excreted in the urine as intact drug.

With systemic administration, ara-C penetrates into the cerebrospinal fluid. A constant intravenous infusion of 400 mg/m^2/day produces an ara-C concentration of 1 μM in the cerebrospinal fluid (Ho and Frei, 1971). Ara-C may be administered intrathecally in the treatment of meningeal leukemia and carcinomatis meningitis. Because the level of cytidine deaminase activity is low in the cerebrospinal fluid, conversion of the parent drug to ara-U occurs slowly. An intrathecal injection of 50 mg/m^2 of ara-C produces peak concentrations of 1 to 2 mM. After 7 hours, only 10% of the total dose is metabolized to ara-U. The half-life of ara-C administered intrathecally is between two and 11 hours.

Because of the short plasma half-life and the S-phase specificity of ara-C, the drug is usually administered either as an intravenous bolus every 12 hours or as a continuous intravenous infusion. When the drug is administered by infusion, a steady-state concentration in the plasma is more rapidly achieved if an initial loading dose, equal to three times the hourly infusion dose, is given. Without a loading dose, steady-state levels of drug in the plasma are not achieved until 16 hours after the start of the infusion. Low-dose ara-C, administered by subcutaneous injection on a weekly schedule, is frequently included in maintenance regimens for patients with acute nonlymphocytic leukemia.

In order to overcome drug resistance and improve therapeutic results, high-dose ara-C regimens ($3 \ g/m^2$ given as a rapid intravenous infusion every 12 hours for a total of 12 doses) are being evaluated in patients with acute nonlymphocytic leukemia. Infusions of high-dose ara-C produce peak concentrations in the plasma ten to 100 times greater than are attained with conventional doses (Hande et al., 1982). The half-life of the drug in the plasma, however, is not prolonged. With high-dose therapy, the concentration of ara-C in the cerebrospinal fluid is ten times greater than that achieved with conventional doses. This is, however, still only 10% of the concentration produced by intrathecal administration. The role of high-dose ara-C in the therapy of patients with acute nonlymphocytic leukemia is the subject of intense investigation.

Clinical Toxicity

The primary toxicity of ara-C is to the rapidly proliferating cells of the bone marrow and gastrointestinal mucosa. The nadirs of granulocytopenia and thrombocytopenia usually occur between seven to 14 days. The bone marrow may recover within three weeks. This is dependent, however, upon the amount of previous exposure to cytotoxic drugs and the responsiveness of the disease infiltrating the marrow. In heavily pretreated patients with leukemia, the duration of myelosuppression may be prolonged. Megaloblastic anemia is another common hematologic abnormality.

Treatment with ara-C is frequently associated with nausea, vomiting, and diarrhea. Mild elevations of alkaline phosphatase and transaminases often occur. These enzyme changes are reversible. Hepatotoxicity induced by ara-C is rarely a significant clinical problem. Pulmonary edema after treatment with ara-C has been reported (Haupt et al., 1981). The occurrence of pulmonary edema does not appear to be dose related. Increased permeability of the alveolar capillaries, induced by ara-C, is thought to be responsible. Other infrequent toxicities include thrombophlebitis, stomatitis, and conjunctivitis. Ara-C suppresses both humoral- and cell-mediated immunity (Calabresi, 1967).

Intrathecal administration of ara-C may produce neurotoxic effects that are similar to those caused by methotrexate. Pathologic findings include arachnoiditis and necrotizing leukoencephalopathy. Clinical manifestations may include somnolence, altered mental status, seizures, and paraplegia.

Clinical Indications

Ara-C is used almost exclusively for the treatment of acute leukemia. When ara-C is used as a single agent, remission rates of 50% are achieved in patients with acute myeloid leukemia. Ara-C is most frequently used in combination with daunorubicin and 6-thioguanine. This combination produces remissions in 70 to 80% of previously untreated patients with acute myeloid leukemia. In high doses, ara-C may be effective in inducing remissions in patients who have relapsed and are refractory to conventional therapeutic approaches. High-dose ara-C may also be useful in the therapy of patients with secondary acute nonlymphocytic leukemia (Preisler et al., 1983). When ara-C is administered in low dosages, it has been reported to induce the morphologic maturation of leukemic cells to a more benign-appearing phenotype (Castaigne et al., 1983). Clinical trials are now in progress to evaluate the effectiveness of low-dose ara-C in patients with preleukemic disorders or refractory acute leukemia.

5-AZACYTIDINE

5-Azacytidine is an analog of cytidine that differs from that compound by the replacement of ring carbon 5 with nitrogen (see Figure 10–14).

Biochemical Pharmacology

Like ara-C, 5-azacytidine must be enzymatically activated. The initial phosphorylation of 5-azacytidine, a ribonucleoside, is catalyzed by uridine-cytidine kinase. The conversion to the active triphosphate, 5-aza CTP, is then accomplished by the same series of phosphorylating enzymes that act on ara-CMP. 5-azacytidine is also subject to rapid deamination.

5-Aza CTP is incorporated into RNA. Biochemical consequences of this incorporation include interference with the processing of ribosomal RNA and inhibition of the synthesis of protein (Čihák, 1979). 5-Aza CTP is also incorporated into DNA. This results in inhibition of the synthesis of DNA and RNA. Breakage of chromosomes may also occur. The incorporation of 5-aza CTP into DNA causes a reduction in the activity of DNA methyltransferase (Christman et al., 1983). As a result, hypomethylated sites appear on DNA. The demethylation of DNA by 5-azacytidine has been associated with altered gene expression and the morphologic differentiation of cultured tumor cells.

5-Azacytidine is specific for the S phase of the cell cycle. Resistance to the drug is usually due to the deletion of the initial activating enzyme.

Clinical Pharmacology

5-Azacytidine is administered by subcutaneous or intravenous injection. Intravenous administration produces high concentrations of the drug in plasma and tissues. Cytidine deaminase rapidly degrades the drug to 5-azauridine. Both the parent drug and this metabolite also undergo spontaneous decomposition. The terminal half-life of 5-azacytidine in the plasma is only 15 minutes. Ninety percent of an administered dose is excreted in the urine within 24 hours. 5-Azacytidine has a low lipid solubility and enters the cerebrospinal fluid by a nucleoside transport system. The drug is most frequently administered as a continuous intravenous infusion. 5-Azacytidine is markedly unstable in solutions with an alkaline or neutral pH and should be freshly prepared prior to administration. Ringer's solution, because of its slightly acidic pH, is frequently used as the vehicle of administration.

Clinical Toxicity

The most prominent toxicities of 5-azacytidine are myelosuppression and severe nausea, vomiting, and diarrhea. The gastrointestinal toxicities are reduced when the drug is given as a continuous intravenous infusion. Less frequent toxicities include abnormal liver function tests, myalgias, weakness, lethargy, confusion, fever, and rash.

Clinical Indications

5-Azacytidine is used primarily in the therapy of patients with refractory acute nonlymphocytic leukemia. Activity has also been re-

ported in patients with acute lymphocytic leukemia and lymphomas. Cross-resistance with ara-C has not been observed.

The use of 5-azacytidine to activate repressed genes is an exciting new approach to the treatment of patients with certain genetic disorders. After receiving 5-azacytidine, a patient with β thalassemia developed a significant increase in the synthesis of γ-globin (Ley et al., 1982). This was accompanied by a marked rise in the absolute reticulocyte count and in the concentration of hemoglobin. Hypomethylation of bone marrow DNA near the γ-globin and ϵ-globin genes was documented. These observations, however, are preliminary and require confirmation in large-scale trials. The use of 5-azacytidine for the favorable modulation of gene expression is, potentially, an important new approach to the treatment of patients with genetic disorders.

PURINE ANALOGS

In 1952, Hitchings developed the first purine analogs useful in the treatment of patients with neoplastic diseases. These two compounds, 6-mercaptopurine (6-MP) and 6-thioguanine (6-TG), continue to be used today to treat patients with acute leukemia (see Figure 10–16). During the past 30 years, many analogs of natural purine bases, nucleosides, and nucleotides have been synthesized and evaluated. These extensive investigations have produced several drugs that are important in the treatment of patients with cancer and other diseases. The hypoxanthine analog allopurinol, an inhibitor of xanthine oxidase, is used to prevent and treat hyperuricemic conditions. Azathioprine, a derivative of 6-MP, is a potent

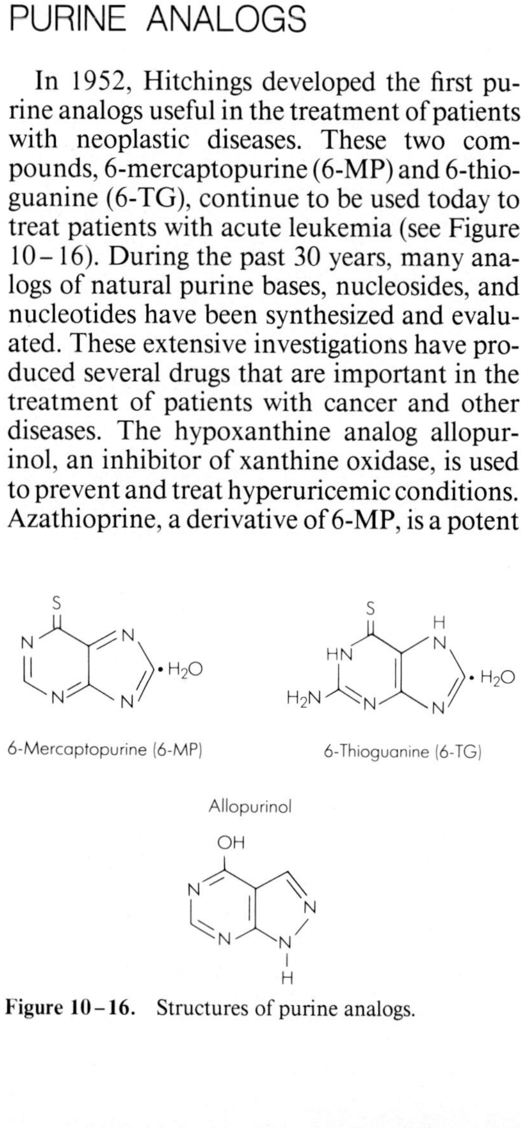

6-Mercaptopurine (6-MP)   6-Thioguanine (6-TG)

Allopurinol

Figure 10–16.   Structures of purine analogs.

immunosuppressive agent. Arabinosyladenine (ara-A) has antiviral and antitumor activity. Recently developed compounds with great potential are the inhibitors of adenosine deaminase, such as 2'-deoxycoformycin and erythrohydroxynonyladenine. When given in combination, inhibitors of adenosine deaminase potentiate the cytotoxic effects of analogs of adenosine, such as ara-A. As single agents, the inhibitors of adenosine deaminase show promise in the treatment of neoplastic disorders of T lymphocytes, such as mycosis fungoides. Some drugs of this class are also powerful immunosuppressive agents.

6-MERCAPTOPURINE

The antimetabolite 6-mercaptopurine (6-MP) is an analog of the natural purine hypoxanthine. The structure of 6-MP differs from hypoxanthine by the replacement of the keto group of carbon 6 of the purine ring with an atom of sulfur.

Biochemical Pharmacology

6-MP is inactive in its native state. In order to be cytotoxic, it must be enzymatically converted to the nucleotide level (see Figure 10–17). Hypoxanthine-guanine phosphoribosyltransferase (HGPRT) converts 6-MP to the ribonucleotide 6-thioinosine-5'-phosphate (T-IMP). Since T-IMP is a poor substrate for guanylate kinase, the analog diphosphate is not formed to any significant extent. As a result, T-IMP accumulates. High intracellular levels of T-IMP cause a "pseudofeedback" inhibition of the first committed step in the *de novo* pathway of purine biosynthesis. The inhibition of this reaction, the formation of ribosylamine-5-phosphate from glutamine and phosphoribosylpyrophosphate, leads to a major disruption in the biosynthesis of purine nucleotides. The accumulation of T-IMP also inhibits several other metabolic reactions that are essential to the conversion of inosinate to adenine and guanine nucleotides. 6-MP may also be converted to triphosphate nucleotides by enzymes of guanine metabolism. The slow incorporation of these analog nucleotides into DNA contributes to the cytotoxicity of 6-MP. An alternative pathway of metabolism of 6-MP involves the methylation of the sulfhydryl group. This methylated derivative is then oxidized to form 6-methylmercaptopurine (6-MMP). Nucleotides of 6-MMP, such as 6-MMP riboside-5'-triphosphate, may be slowly incorporated into DNA.

Xanthine oxidase, present in relatively large amounts in the liver, degrades 6-MP to the inactive compound 6-thiouric acid. Allopurinol, an inhibitor of xanthine oxidase, potentiates the biologic activity of 6-MP. When

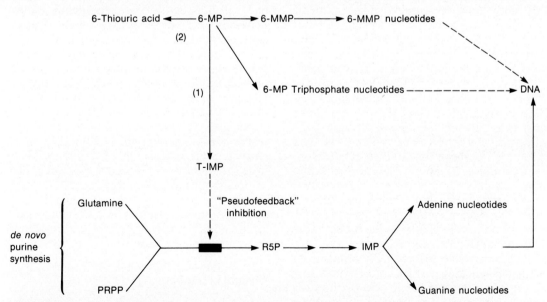

Figure 10–17. Activation and degradation of 6-mercaptopurine. (1) = hypoxanthine-guanine phosphoribosyltransferase; (2) = xanthine oxidase; R5P = ribosylamine-5-phosphate; PRPP = phosphoribosylpyrophosphate; 6-MMP = 6-methylmercaptopurine; T-IMP = 6-thioinosine-5'-phosphate.

these two drugs are administered concurrently, the catabolism of 6-MP is decreased and increased concentrations are available for conversion to the active nucleotide forms. 6-MP is also catabolized by desulfuration. The inorganic sulfates released by this process are excreted in the urine.

A common mechanism of biochemical resistance to 6-MP is a partial deficiency or total absence of the activating enzyme HGPRT. Resistance may also result from a decrease in the affinity of this enzyme for the drug. In human leukemia cells, an increase in the activity of a degradative enzyme, alkaline phosphatase, has been shown to confer resistance to 6-MP (Lee et al., 1978; Scholar and Calabresi, 1979). Other potential mechanisms of resistance include: (1) an increase in the rate of degradation of the ribonucleoside analog; (2) an alteration in the pseudofeedback inhibition of the synthesis of ribosylamine-5-phosphate; and (3) "exclusion" of 6-MP from contact with HGPRT (Brockman, 1974).

Clinical Pharmacology

The oral route is the usual mode of administration of 6-MP. Pharmacologic studies using radiolabeled 6-MP have previously suggested that, after oral administration, the drug is not completely absorbed. Using this analytical method, it was determined that approximately 50% of an administered dose of 6-MP reached the systemic circulation (Elion, 1967). A recent study, however, conducted with patients with acute lymphocytic leukemia, demonstrated that the absorption of 6-MP after oral administration is highly variable and that levels of the drug in the plasma are unexpectedly low (Zimm et al., 1983). Using a sensitive and specific HPLC assay, the mean bioavailability of an oral dose of 6-MP was found to be only 16%. After an oral dose of 75 mg/m^2, the mean peak plasma concentration of 6-MP was 0.89 μM. The mean time to peak plasma concentration was 2.2 hours. The mean elimination half-life was 1.5 hours. These values showed great variation among the patients evaluated. After a uniform oral dose of 6-MP, concentrations of the drug in the plasma were unpredictable. The low bioavailability of orally administered 6-MP probably results from metabolism in the intestinal epithelium during absorption and in the first pass of the drug through the liver. Additional studies of the pharmacokinetics of orally administered 6-MP are required.

Allopurinol is a potent inhibitor of xanthine oxidase. This enzyme is important for the catabolism of 6-MP. Patients concurrently treated with 6-MP and allopurinol may experience a significant increase in toxicity. Patients treated with both drugs should receive only 25% of the usual dose of 6-MP.

Clinical Toxicity

The rapidly dividing cells of the bone marrow and gastrointestinal tract mucosa are the most susceptible normal tissue cells. Nadir values for the peripheral blood cell counts usually occur between seven to ten days after treatment. Recovery from myelosuppression is generally complete by the fourteenth day. Nausea, vomiting, and mucositis, although common, are not severe. Diarrhea is a less frequent complication.

Hepatotoxicity may occur in as many as one-third of adult patients who receive 6-MP. In patients who receive continuous therapy with 6-MP, jaundice may appear within two weeks. Jaundice has developed as late as two years after the initiation of therapy with 6-MP administered on an intermittent schedule. There is not a clear relationship between the dose of 6-MP and the development of jaundice. Patients who receive greater than 2 mg/kg/day, however, are at the highest risk for hepatotoxicity. In addition to the direct bilirubin, serum transaminases and alkaline phosphatase may be elevated. The hepatotoxicity of 6-MP may be histologically manifested as hepatocellular or obstructive liver disease (Einhorn and Davidsohn, 1964). Features of either intrahepatic cholestasis or parenchymal cell necrosis may predominate. With cessation of the drug, the jaundice usually clears rapidly. Hepatotoxicity recurs with reinstitution of the drug. The hepatotoxicity of 6-MP is probably a direct toxic effect and not a hypersensitivity reaction. 6-MP should not be administered to patients with preexisting liver disease. The drug should be discontinued if the patient develops abnormal liver function tests during therapy.

Dermatologic toxicities have been reported. A rare complication of therapy with 6-MP is interstitial pneumonitis.

Clinical Indications

6-MP is used almost exclusively in the maintenance therapy of patients with acute lymphocytic leukemia of childhood. 6-MP, a potent inhibitor of cell-mediated immunity, has been successfully used in the therapy of Crohn's disease, ulcerative colitis, and auto-immune diseases (Present *et al.,* 1980).

6-THIOGUANINE

6-Thioguanine (6-TG) is an analog of guanine. In the structure of 6-TG, the keto group on carbon 6 of the purine ring of guanine is replaced by a sulfur atom.

Biochemical Pharmacology

6-TG is converted to the active nucleotide 5-thioguanosine-5'-phosphate (6-thio GMP) by HGPRT. 6-Thio GMP is slowly converted by guanylate kinase to 6-thio GDP and 6-thio GTP. 6-Thio GTP is then incorporated into RNA and DNA (Parks *et al.,* 1975). Incorporation of the analog nucleotide into DNA is the major mechanism for the cytotoxicity of 6-TG. Disturbances of other biochemical processes by the analog nucleotides also contribute to the toxic effects of the drug. Similar to T-IMP, 6-thio GMP produces pseudofeedback inhibition of the first step in the *de novo* pathway of purine biosynthesis. 6-Thio GMP also inhibits the interconversion of purine nucleotides. Through the inhibition of inosinate dehydrogenase, 6-thio GMP prevents the conversion of inosinate to adenine and guanine nucleotides.

The primary route of catabolism of 6-TG involves methylation of its sulfur atom. The product of this reaction is 2-amino-6-methylthiopurine. In another catabolic process, the enzyme guanase deaminates 6-TG to form 6-thioxanthine. Xanthine oxidase converts this compound to 6-thiouric acid. Because the substrate of xanthine oxidase, 6-thioxanthine, is not toxic, allopurinol does not increase the toxicity of 6-TG. When 6-TG and allopurinol are administered concurrently, the dosage of 6-TG does not have to be reduced. Metabolites of 6-TG excreted in the urine include 2-amino-6-methylthiopurine, 6-thiouric acid, and inorganic sulfate.

The mechanisms of natural and acquired resistance to 6-TG are the same as described for 6-MP.

Clinical Pharmacology

After oral administration, the adsorption of 6-TG is variable and incomplete. Peak con-centrations of 6-TG in the plasma are reached six to eight hours after an oral dose. Approximately 40% of the dose is excreted in the urine. After intravenous administration, the half-life in the plasma is 80 to 90 minutes. Seventy-five percent of an intravenous dose is excreted in the urine within the first 24 hours (LePage and Whitecar, 1971).

Clinical Toxicity

As with 6-MP, the major toxic effect of 6-TG is myelosuppression. Anorexia, nausea, vomiting, and mucositis may also occur. Hepatotoxicity is produced less frequently by 6-TG than by 6-MP.

Clinical Indications

In combination with other drugs, 6-TG is used in induction and maintenance therapies of patients with acute nonlymphocytic leukemia.

ADENOSINE ANALOGS

The adenosine analog arabinosyladenine (ara-A) is used to treat patients with certain viral diseases, particularly herpetic infections. In order to be toxic to mammalian cells, ara-A must be phosphorylated to ara-ATP. This analog nucleotide inhibits the synthesis of DNA by inhibiting DNA polymerase and ribonucleotide reductase. Ara-ATP may also be incorporated into DNA (White *et al.,* 1982). Ara-A is a substrate for adenosine deaminase. This enzyme rapidly deaminates ara-A to the inactive compound 9-β-D-arabinofuranosyl-hypoxanthine. This enzymatic degradation prevents the conversion of ara-A to the active nucleotide. Because of this rapid deamination and the limited solubility of the drug, the antitumor activity of ara-A is minimal.

A significant new development has been the discovery of inhibitors of adenosine deaminase (see Figure 10 – 18). 2'-Deoxycoformycin (DCF) is an analog of the natural nucleoside 2'-deoxyinosine. DCF is an extremely tight-binding inhibitor of adenosine deaminase. The affinity of DCF for the enzyme greatly exceeds that of the natural substrate. DCF blocks the deamination of natural nucleosides and analogs of adenosine. As a single agent, DCF is cytotoxic to cells that contain high concentrations of adenosine deaminase. Normal T-lymphocytes and their neoplastic coun-

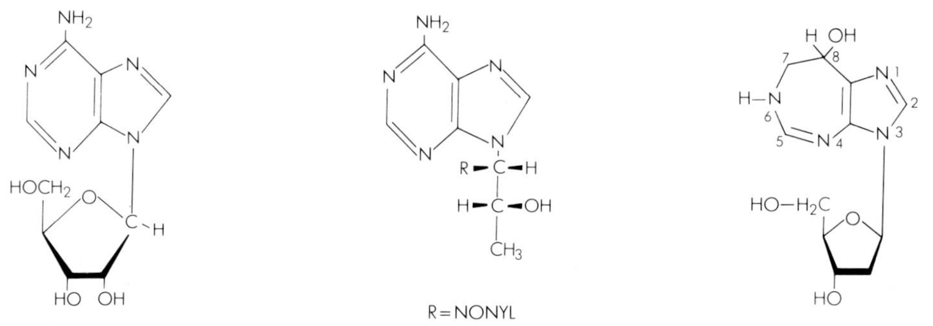

| Adenosine | Erythro-9-(2-hydroxy-3-nonyl) adenine (EHNA) | Deoxycoformycin |

Figure 10 – 18. Structures of adenosine and inhibitors of adenosine deaminase.

terparts contain particularly high concentrations of this enzyme. Responses to DCF have been observed in patients with T-cell acute lymphoblastic leukemia and mycosis fungoides. Leukemic cells from some patients with acute myelogenous leukemia also contain high levels of adenosine deaminase. These patients have been responsive to therapy with DCF.

The toxicity of DCF is due to the accumulation of deoxyadenosine and the resultant increase in the intracellular concentration of deoxyadenosine triphosphate (dATP) (Major *et al.,* 1981). dATP inhibits ribonucleotide reductase. Inhibition of this enzyme depletes the cell of the deoxyribonucleotides required for the synthesis of DNA. Deoxyadenosine also inactivates S-adenosyl homocysteine hydrolase. This results in the accumulation of S-adenosyl homocysteine, a compound toxic to lymphocytes.

In phase I trials of DCF, toxicity to the central nervous system was dose limiting. Other clinical toxicities included myalgias, arthralgias, and manifestations of nephrotoxicity. Serious infections, presumably precipitated by the immunosuppressive properties of the drug, have occurred after treatment with DCF.

The combination of DCF and ara-A is effective in animal tumor systems and will soon enter clinical trials. The antitumor activity of other adenosine analogs, such as 3′-deoxyadenosine and xylosyladenine, is also potentiated by DCF (Cass *et al.,* 1982).

The genetic deficiency of adenosine deaminase is associated with profound lymphopenia and a severe defect in both cellular and humoral immunity. Accumulation of the purine nucleoside substrates of adenosine deaminase is the cause of these toxic effects. DCF produces similar derangements of the immune

system. The clinical utility of DCF as an immunosuppressive agent is yet to be determined.

Erythro-9-(2-hydroxy-3-nonyl) adenine (EHNA) is another inhibitor of adenosine deaminase. There are several important differences between EHNA and DCF. The inhibitory effect of DCF on adenosine deaminase is more potent and prolonged as compared to EHNA. The half-life in the plasma of EHNA is less than DCF. The duration of biologic activity of EHNA is 50% of DCF. Because of its shorter duration of action, EHNA may be less toxic to normal tissues. In addition, EHNA is not as immunosuppressive as DCF.

2-Fluoro-ara-A, a derivative of ara-A, is an adenosine analog that is resistant to deamination. 2-Fluoro-ara-A inhibits the synthesis of DNA by the same mechanisms described for ara-A. This promising new compound has activity against cultured human leukemic cells that is comparable to the combination of DCF and ara-A. The monophosphate form of this compound, 2-fluoro-ara-AMP, is now in phase I trials.

SUBSTITUTED UREA

HYDROXYUREA

Hydroxyurea was first synthesized in 1869. Although the myelosuppressive properties of this drug were demonstrated in 1928, it is only within the past 20 years that hydroxyurea has been used to treat patients with cancer.

Biochemical Pharmacology

Hydroxyurea is a structurally simple compound (see Figure 10 – 19). Its mechanism of action is the inhibition of ribonucleotide reductase. The conversion of ribonucleotides to deoxyribonucleotides, catalyzed by this enzyme, is an essential and, probably, rate-limiting step in the biosynthesis of DNA. Cytotoxicity results from the inhibition of the synthesis of DNA. Hydroxyurea is specific for the S phase of the cell cycle.

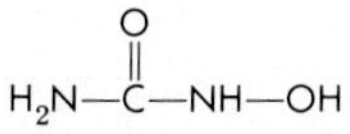

Clinical Pharmacology

Hydroxyurea is well absorbed after oral administration. Peak concentrations in the plasma are achieved in approximately one to two hours and the half-life is 100 minutes. Peak plasma levels are proportional to the administered dose and usually range from 30 to 150 μg/ml. The drug is undetectable in the plasma 24 hours after an oral dose. Eighty percent of an oral or intravenous dose is converted to urea by the liver and excreted in the urine within 12 hours.

Clinical Toxicity

Myelosuppression is the primary toxicity of hydroxyurea. Granulocytopenia and megaloblastic anemia are the most common manifestations. Thrombocytopenia only occasionally occurs. Patients who receive daily doses of hydroxyurea should have their blood counts monitored on a regular basis. The bone marrow usually recovers rapidly after the drug is discontinued. Other adverse effects include

$$H_2N-\overset{\overset{\displaystyle O}{\|}}{C}-NH-OH$$

Figure 10-19. Hydroxyurea.

gastrointestinal disturbances and mild dermatologic reactions. Alopecia, nail changes, stomatitis, and neurologic problems are rare occurrences.

Hydroxyurea enhances the toxic effect of irradiation. Enhancement of radiation injury to the skin, mucous membranes, esophagus, and other portions of the gastrointestinal tract have been reported (Landgren et al., 1974).

Clinical Indications

Hydroxyurea is useful in the management of certain myeloproliferative disorders, particularly chronic myelogenous leukemia, polycythemia vera, and essential thrombocytosis. It is also reported to be effective in the treatment of patients with the hypereosinophilic syndrome. It is frequently administered to patients with acute leukemia for the rapid reduction of high circulating blast counts. In combination with other drugs, hydroxyurea is used to treat patients with head and neck cancer and metastatic carcinoma of the colon. The use of hydroxyurea as a radiation sensitizer has demonstrated promising results in patients with cervical cancer (Hreshchyshyn et al., 1979).

NATURAL PRODUCTS

PLANT EXTRACTS

VINCA ALKALOIDS

The vinca alkaloids, vinblastine and vincristine, are extracts derived from the Madagascan periwinkle plant, Vinca rosea Linn. Desacetylvinblastine, vindesine, is a new derivative of vinblastine that is now in clinical trials.

The vinca alkaloids are asymmetrical dimeric indole derivatives composed of vindoline and catharanthine structures (see Figure 10-20). There are only minor structural differences among the clinically useful vinca alkaloids. Vinblastine differs from vincristine only by the presence of a methyl, rather than a

formyl side chain, on the indole nitrogen of the vindole moiety. Vinblastine and vindesine also only differ slightly in structure. At the C-23 position, vindesine has an amino group instead of the methoxy group in vinblastine and the C-4 position of vinblastine is deacetylated and bears an hydroxy group in the vindesine molecule. These minor structural variations result in important differences in antitumor activity and normal tissue toxicity. Structural requirements important for the retention of full antitumor activity include maintenance of the free hydroxyl functions. Partial reduction of the molecule or hydrogenation of the double bond may cause partial or complete loss of activity (Johnson et al., 1963).

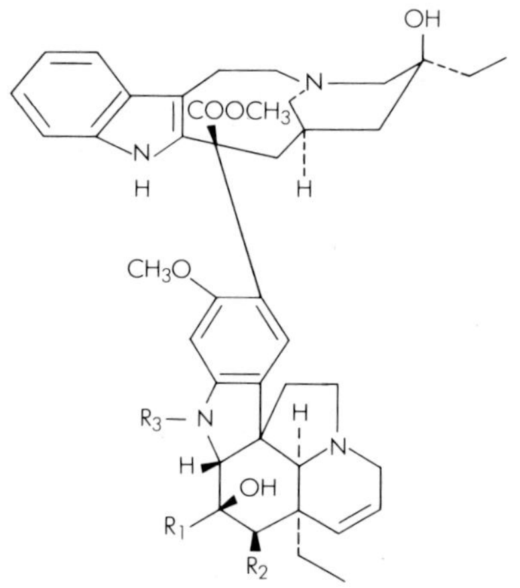

Figure 10–20. Vinca alkaloids.

Vindesine	Vinblastine	Vincristine
$R_1 = CONH_2$	$R_1 = COOCH_3$	$R_1 = COOCH_3$
$R_2 = OH$	$R_2 = OCOCH_3$	$R_2 = OCOCH_3$
$R_3 = CH_3$	$R_3 = CH_3$	$R_3 = CHO$

Biochemical Pharmacology

At the cellular level, the most conspicuous effect of the vinca alkaloids is the arrest of cell division in metaphase. Mitotic arrest results from dissolution of the mitotic spindle (Creasey, 1978). The mitotic spindle and other components of the cellular microtubule system are composed of tubulin. This dimeric protein exists in a soluble form that is in equilibrium with the formed microtubular structures. The vinca alkaloids act by binding to specific sites on the tubulin molecule. This interaction produces crystals that interfere with the formation of microtubules and cause the dissolution of the mitotic spindle. In the absence of an intact mitotic spindle, the chromosomes may disperse throughout the cytoplasm. The disruption of the synthesis and function of other cellular structures that are composed of microtubules is responsible for several of the other toxic effects produced by the vinca alkaloids. The disturbance of phagocytosis by polymorphonuclear leukocytes and certain neurologic toxicities result from interference with tubulin polymerization and the function of microtubules (Creasey, 1974–1975). Colchicine and podophyllotoxin bind to sites on the tubulin molecule that are distant from the sites specific for vinblastine. Although the vinca alkaloids arrest cell division in metaphase, S-phase cells are the most sensitive to the cytotoxic effects of these compounds (Madoc-Jones and Mauro, 1968).

The vinca alkaloids also interfere with the synthesis of nucleic acids, proteins, and lipids and impair the secretion of certain hormones (Cline, 1968). The significance of these actions in producing cytotoxicity is unknown.

The vinca alkaloids enter cells by a carrier-mediated transport system. The lack of cross-resistance among the vinca alkaloids and their different patterns of tumor sensitivity and normal tissue toxicity suggest that these compounds may differ in their ability to enter specific types of cells. Cross-resistance with several of the antitumor antibiotics suggests a shared transport mechanism for entry into cells (Dan, 1971). The mechanisms for resistance to the vinca alkaloids are not known.

Clinical Pharmacology

Because absorption after oral administration is unpredictable, both vincristine and vinblastine are administered intravenously.

After intravenous injection, vinblastine binds extensively to plasma proteins and to all of the cellular elements of the blood, particularly platelets. At usual clinical doses, the peak plasma concentration is 0.4 μM. Vinblastine has a triphasic pattern of clearance from the plasma. The α and β half-lives are 3.9 and 53 minutes, respectively. The γ half-life is 20 hours (Owellen et al., 1977). Metabolism of vinblastine to a biologically active product, desacetylvinblastine, occurs in the liver. Excretion in the bile results in approximately 10% of the administered dose appearing in the feces. Less than 20% of the drug is excreted intact in the urine.

Vincristine is also extensively bound to tissues. After intravenous bolus injection, there is a triphasic pattern of clearance from the plasma. The α half-life ranges from 0.85 to 2.9 minutes, β and γ half-lives range from 7.4 to 23.7 minutes and from 164 minutes to 18 hours, respectively. The peak plasma concentration is 0.4 μM. With a continuous intravenous infusion of vincristine, 0.5 mg/m^2/day for five days, the plasma half-life is 21.7 hours. Plasma concentrations of vincristine are maintained at consistently higher levels when the drug is administered by continuous infusion as compared to bolus administration (Jackson et al., 1981). The drug is metabolized in the liver and excreted in the bile. Biologically active metabolites have not been detected. Seventy percent of an administered dose of vincristine appears in the feces (Jackson et al., 1978).

Clinical Toxicity

Neurologic toxicities are frequently observed with vincristine and represent the most common dose-limiting factor for this drug. The neurotoxicity associated with the vinca alkaloids is probably secondary to interference with the function of the microtubules in axoplasmic transport and inhibition of neural secretory functions (Iqbal and Ochs, 1980). Peripheral neuropathies are the earliest and most common manifestations of the neurotoxicity of vincristine. Loss of the deep tendon reflexes, initially the Achilles tendon reflex, and paresthesias in the distal portions of the extremities are the earliest signs and symptoms. The neurotoxicity of vincristine is dose related and progressive abnormalities such as muscular pain, weakness, and sensory impairment may develop with continued administration of the drug. Manifestations of neurotoxicity are usually symmetrical. Severe jaw pain may occur with the initial dose of vincristine or vinblastine. Impairment of other cranial nerves occurs less frequently. Autonomic neuropathies, manifested by abdominal cramps, constipation, and, at higher doses, paralytic ileus, are common. Bladder atony and orthostatic hypotension have been reported (DiBella, 1980). The administration of vincristine may produce alterations in mental status, including confusion and coma. The more severe neurologic toxicities may be avoided by either suspending therapy or reducing the dosage upon occurrence of the earlier, milder abnormalities. Paresthesias and reflex abnormalities are usually reversible with discontinuation of the drug, but motor deficits may be permanent. Because neurotoxicity is dose related, vincristine is usually not administered in single doses greater than 2 mg. Adults are generally more susceptible to the neurologic toxicities of vincristine than are children. Patients with lymphomas may be particularly susceptible to the neurotoxicities of the vinca alkaloids although the reason for this finding is not clear. Patients who receive vincristine should be placed on a bowel care regimen that includes stool softeners and laxatives. Although vinblastine can produce neurologic toxicities identical to vincristine, this occurs infrequently, and only at high dosages. A significant incidence of neurotoxicities occurred in early clinical studies of vindesine (Valdivieso et al., 1981). The use of the vinca alkaloids in combination with other neurotoxic drugs, such as methotrexate, may produce additive or synergistic neurotoxicity (Taylor et al., 1978).

The most important toxicity of vinblastine is myelosuppression, particularly leukopenia. The nadir of the white blood cell count occurs four to seven days after administration of the drug. Recovery is usually complete by 14 days. Thrombocytopenia and anemia occur less frequently. Suppression of the bone marrow is uncommon with vincristine. This marrow-sparing property has led to the use of vincristine in many combination chemotherapy regimens. Myelosuppression is a common complication of therapy with vindesine. Vinblastine frequently produces stomatitis, nausea, vomiting, and diarrhea. These gastrointestinal disturbances are less common with vincristine.

Reversible alopecia occurs in about 20% of patients treated with vincristine and in a smaller number of patients who receive vinblastine. Extravasation of either drug will produce cellulitis and tissue necrosis. Therapy with vincristine may produce inappropriate secretion of antidiuretic hormone and dilutional hyponatremia. The dosage of the vinca alkaloids should be reduced in patients with hepatic failure or biliary obstruction.

Clinical Indications

Vincristine is employed in different combination chemotherapy regimens to treat a variety of neoplasms. Regimens that contain vincristine are effective in the treatment of acute lymphoblastic leukemia of childhood, Hodgkin's disease, and non-Hodgkin's lymphomas. Vincristine is able to promote the intracellular accumulation of methotrexate by inhibiting its efflux. Cytotoxic synergy in patients treated with the sequential combination of vincristine and methotrexate has not yet been demonstrated. In combination with other drugs, vinblastine is useful in the treatment of metastatic testicular tumors, Hodgkin's disease, and non-Hodgkin's lymphomas. The clinical spectrum of activity of vindesine is now being determined in clinical trials.

EPIPODOPHYLLOTOXINS

Podophyllotoxin is the crystalline extract of the plant *Podophyllum pelatum*, commonly known as the American mandrake. Etoposide

(VP-16-213) and teniposide (VM-26) are two synthetic derivatives of podophyllotoxin that have important antitumor activity.

The chemical structures of etoposide and teniposide differ only in the substitution on the 4,6-acetal carbon (Figure 10–21). Both drugs have limited stability in physiologic solutions.

Biochemical Pharmacology

Podophyllotoxin binds to microtubular proteins at the site of colchicine binding and arrests cells in metaphase (Wilson *et al.,* 1974). Etoposide and teniposide, however, do not interfere with the polymerization of tubulin and the assembly of microtubules. After an initial metaphase arrest, these derivatives cause a reduction of the mitotic index and an irreversible inhibition of cells entering into mitosis (Drewinko and Barlogie, 1976). The cytotoxic effects of epipodophyllotoxins *in vitro,* however, are greatest in S-phase-synchronized cultures. In cultured cells, etoposide and teniposide cause a reduction in nucleoside uptake and inhibit the incorporation of tritiated thymidine into DNA (Loike and Horwitz, 1976). Etoposide produces strand breaks in the DNA of cultured leukemic cells (Kalwinsky *et al.,* 1983). The production of DNA scission may be the key event that leads to cell death.

Clinical Pharmacology

Etoposide is administered either intravenously or orally as a hydrophilic soft gelatin capsule or as a drinking ampule. Gastrointestinal absorption is only 47 to 50% of an administered oral dose. When administered orally, the dosage must be appropriately adjusted to compensate for this incomplete absorption. After intravenous administration, a biphasic pattern of clearance of etoposide from the

plasma takes place. The mean half-life of the terminal phase is 11.5 hours (Allen and Creaven, 1975). After 72 hours, 44% of an administered dose is excreted in the urine, 29% as intact drug and 15% as metabolities. Cerebrospinal fluid levels range from 1 to 10% of the concurrent plasma levels.

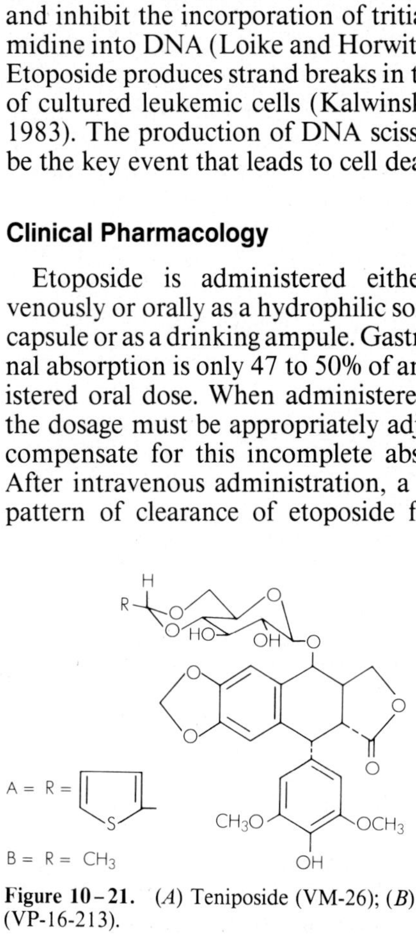

Teniposide is usually administered as a brief intravenous infusion. Teniposide exhibits a triphasic pattern of plasma decay. The half-life of the terminal phase ranges between 11 and 38 hours. After 72 hours, 44% of the drug can be recovered in the urine. Metabolism of teniposide is more extensive than etoposide. For teniposide, metabolites account for 78% of the drug detected in the urine. There is only minimal penetration of teniposide into the cerebrospinal fluid.

Clinical Toxicity

Leukopenia is the dose-limiting toxicity for both etoposide and teniposide. The time of the nadir of the white blood cell count is schedule dependent, but usually occurs in 10 to 14 days with recovery by days 16 to 21. Thrombocytopenia is less frequent and less severe. Cumulative marrow toxicity has not been observed. Gastrointestinal problems, such as nausea, vomiting, and diarrhea, occur in approximately 15% of patients treated with either drug by intravenous administration (Radice *et al.,* 1979). After oral administration of etoposide, gastrointestinal toxicity is more severe and may be dose-limiting. Reversible alopecia occurs commonly with both drugs. Mild peripheral neuropathy is observed in 10 to 20% of patients. Rapid intravenous infusion of either drug may produce acute arterial hypotension. This may be prevented by administering the drug as an infusion for at least 30 minutes. If either epipodophyllotoxin is given simultaneously with vincristine, severe, additive neurotoxicity may result. Anaphylactic reactions have been reported after administration of either etoposide or teniposide.

Clinical Indications

There appears not to be any difference in the spectrum of activity of these two compounds. Significant clinical activity has been demonstrated against Hodgkin's disease, testicular tumors, small cell carcinoma of the lung, acute nonlymphocytic leukemia, and non-Hodgkin's lymphomas. Optimal dosages and sched-

Figure 10–21. (*A*) Teniposide (VM-26); (*B*) Etoposide (VP-16-213).

ules are being determined in clinical trials (O'Dwyer *et al.*, 1985).

ANTITUMOR ANTIBIOTICS

ANTHRACYCLINES

The anthracycline antibiotics are among the most active compounds introduced into clinical use for the treatment of cancer in the past fifteen years. Although only doxorubicin (ADRIAMYCIN) and daunorubicin (daunomycin) are currently available for general use, a number of analogs are the subjects of intensive investigation.

The anthracyclines are products of the fungus *Streptomyces peucetius* var. caesius. Daunorubicin was isolated by DiMarco (Grein *et al.*, 1963) in 1963 and doxorubicin was identified by Arcamone in 1969 (Arcamone *et al.*, 1969).

The basic anthracycline structure consists of the amino sugar daunosamine linked through a glycosidic bond to a planar naphthacene-quinone nucleus at ring atom 7. Doxorubicin differs from daunorubicin only by a single hydroxyl group on carbon-14 (see Figure 10–22). By virtue of this structure, the anthracycline molecule possesses both lipophilic and hydrophilic characteristics. The presence of both the sugar moiety and the tetracycline ring are required to maintain antitumor activity. Cleavage of the molecule at the glycosidic bond produces an insoluble, inactive aglycone

(Driscoll *et al.*, 1974). Because the glycosidic bond is susceptible to enzymatic and acid-catalyzed cleavage, oral administration results in inactivation of the drug (Arena *et al.*, 1971).

Biochemical Pharmacology

The anthracyclines are capable of producing a number of biochemical effects. The killing of tumor cells is probably related to drug-induced alterations of nucleic acid synthesis, although the exact mechanisms of cytotoxicity are not yet clearly identified. The cause of toxicity may well vary among tumor cells and certain normal tissues.

Proposed mechanisms of action of the anthracyclines include: DNA intercalation, formation of free radicals and superoxide, chelation of divalent cations, the inhibition of sodium-potassium ATPase, and the binding of drug to certain constituents of cell membranes.

The anthracyclines rapidly enter cells (Egorin *et al.*, 1974). The largest intracellular concentration of drug is in the nucleus (DiMarco, 1975). After exposure to either doxorubicin or daunorubicin, a unique fluorescence can be detected in nuclear structures by fluorescent microscopy. In the nucleus, the anthracyclines bind to DNA with high affinity. The aglycone moiety intercalates in a parallel orientation between adjacent base pairs of DNA (Pigram *et al.*, 1972). The ionized amino group of the sugar moiety then binds to the sugar-phosphate backbone on DNA. The

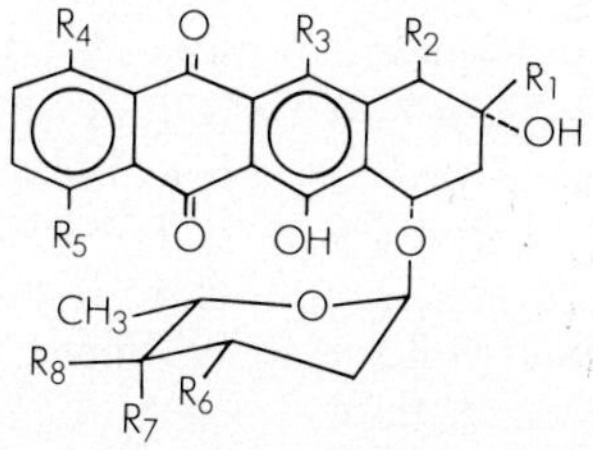

Compound	R_1	R_2	R_3	R_4	R_5	R_6	R_7	R_8
Daunorubicin	$COCH_3$	H_2	OH	H	OCH_3	NH_2	OH	H
Doxorubicin	$COCH_2OH$	H_2	OH	H	OCH_3	NH_2	OH	H
AD-32	$COCH_2OCO(CH_2)_3CH_3$	H_2	OH	H	OCH_3	$NHCOCF_3$	OH	H
Aclacinomycin A	CH_2CH_3	$COOCH_3$	H	H	OH	$N(CH_3)_2$	DF[a]-C[b]	H
Carminomycin	$COCH_3$	H_2	OH	H	OH	NH_2	OH	H
Idarubicin	$COCH_3$	H_2	OH	H	H	NH_2	OH	H
Epirubicin	$COCH_2OH$	H_2	OH	H	OCH_3	NH_2	H	OH

Figure 10–22. Structures of daunorubicin, doxorubicin, and some new anthracycline derivatives.

amino sugar moiety is thereby bound in the large groove of DNA. Through this process, a stable drug-DNA complex is formed. *In vitro,* the ability of anthracyclines to bind to DNA directly relates to their inhibitory effects on the synthesis of nucleic acids and cell proliferation.

Intercalation with DNA produces a number of important biochemical effects. DNA polymerase and DNA-dependent RNA polymerase are both inhibited, resulting in inhibition of the synthesis of DNA, RNA, and proteins (Painter, 1978). Depending upon their molecular structure, anthracyclines may affect mainly DNA or RNA synthesis (Crooke *et al.,* 1978). The synthesis of DNA is primarily inhibited by slowing the rate of chain elongation with only a small effect resulting from inhibition of replicon initiation. Ribosomal RNA appears to be the most sensitive of the various forms of RNA to the anthracyclines (Daskal *et al.,* 1978). Inhibition of the synthesis of ribosomal RNA is probably an important event in the production of cytotoxicity.

Anthracyclines not only inhibit DNA function by intercalation but also produce single-stranded breaks and subsequent fragmentation of DNA. The generation of reactive free radicals, such as superoxide, within the vicinity of the DNA molecule may be responsible for this form of damage. The mutagenicity, carcinogenicity, and teratogenicity of the anthracyclines may be secondary to this disruption of the structure of DNA. The relationship, however, between the production of single-stranded breaks in DNA and cytotoxicity is uncertain (Ross *et al.,* 1979).

By virtue of their quinone and hydroquinone groups, the anthracyclines have the potential to generate both peroxides and free radicals. As with other drugs that contain quinone groups, the microsomal enzyme P_{450} reductase catalyzes the reduction of the anthracycline molecule to a semiquinone free radical (Sato *et al.,* 1977). This semiquinone radical is then capable of donating an electron to molecular oxygen to form a superoxide radical and hydrogen peroxide. Other flavin-dependent oxireductases are also capable of catalyzing this reaction (Myers, 1980). The role of free-radical formation in the production of anthracycline toxicity is an area of active investigation.

The generation of free radicals is the probable mechanism responsible for anthracycline-induced cardiotoxicity. Myers showed that the antioxidant α-tocopherol could reduce lipid peroxidation in the heart and lessen cardiotoxicity without impairing tumor response (Myers *et al.,* 1976). Glutathione peroxidase, the enzyme that protects cells against such injury by catalyzing the reduction of hydrogen peroxide and lipid hydroperoxides, is lost from cardiac tissue after doxorubicin administration (Doroshow *et al.,* 1980). Doxorubicin also induces free-radical formation in platelets (Stuart *et al.,* 1978) and erythrocytes (Henderson *et al.,* 1978).

Inhibition of the synthesis of nucleic acids and disruption of the structure of DNA may not be the only mechanisms of cytotoxicity. In tissue culture, cells are killed at drug concentrations below those required to interfere with the activity of DNA. Inhibition of respiration in isolated mitochondria and alterations of cell membrane functions occur at low anthracycline concentrations (Gonsalves *et al.,* 1974). The protein spectrin and the phospholipid cardiolipin are binding sites for anthracyclines on the cell membrane (Mikkelsen *et al.,* 1977). Cardiolipin is an important constituent of the membranes of tumor cells and cardiac mitochondria. Tritton has suggested that binding of the anthracyclines to cardiolipin may produce toxicity to cardiac and tumor tissues (Tritton *et al.,* 1978). Anthracycline-induced alterations of the permeability of membranes to sodium and calcium are also associated with the development of cardiac toxicity.

Clinical Pharmacology

After intravenous administration, doxorubicin is cleared from the plasma in a triphasic pattern (Chan *et al.,* 1978). The initial half-life of ten to 30 minutes is due to the rapid distribution of the drug within the tissues. The intracellular concentration becomes significantly greater than the simultaneous plasma concentration (Bachur, 1975). The second half-life of ten hours is due to metabolism of the drug. Slow release from intracellular binding sites and excretion are responsible for the long terminal half-life of 24 to 48 hours.

The highest drug concentrations are attained in the lung, liver, spleen, kidney, heart, small intestine, and bone marrow. The blood-brain barrier is impermeable to the anthracyclines and they are not detected within the central nervous system. Tissue distribution patterns can be changed by altering the method of drug administration. When doxorubicin is given weekly at low doses or by continuous infusion, lower drug concentrations are achieved in cardiac muscle and cardiac toxicity is reduced (Garnick *et al.,* 1979; Chlebowski *et al.,* 1980).

The liver is an important site of metabolism and may clear as much as 40 to 50% of an administered dose (Chlebowski *et al.,* 1980). The bile is the primary route of elimination. Only a small proportion is eliminated by the kidneys. Renal excretion is greatest within the first six hours and produces a red discoloration of the urine. Dose modifications are necessary in patients with hepatic dysfunction, especially if the bilirubin is elevated. It is not necessary to reduce the dosage of drug in the presence of renal failure.

Doxorubicinol, the major metabolite of doxorubicin, is produced by the action of aldo-keto reductase on carbon atom 14. This compound retains approximately one-quarter of the therapeutic activity of the parent drug. Further metabolism occurs by cleavage of the glycosidic bond yielding 7 deoxy aglycones (Benjamin, 1981). These insoluble aglycones are conjugated with glucoronic or sulphonic acid and excreted in the bile. A small number of other metabolites of unknown significance have been identified in the urine (Takanashi and Bachur, 1976).

Clinical Toxicity

Suppression of the bone marrow, a frequent toxic manifestation of the anthracyclines, is dose related. Neutropenia is more pronounced than thrombocytopenia or anemia (Blum and Carter, 1974). The nadirs of the peripheral blood counts occur seven to ten days after treatment and recovery is usually complete by three weeks. Alopecia is virtually universal and complete. Vasoconstriction in the scalp, produced by local hypothermia, has been successfully employed to reduce hair loss (Dean *et al.,* 1979). Hypothermia or scalp tourniquets should not be used in patients with leukemia or other neoplasms in which tumor cells may be present in the scalp. Hair growth returns to normal after administration of the anthracycline is discontinued. Nausea and vomiting, lasting for 24 hours to 48 hours, occurs in 21 to 60% of patients. Mucositis develops in 4 to 70% of patients who receive anthracyclines.

Extravasation of anthracyclines is a serious problem that can lead to severe local necrosis and damage to underlying nerves, tendons, and muscles. Administrative techniques that can reduce the incidence and severity of this complication include the use of a freely flowing intravenous line and the avoidance of veins in the antecubital fossa and on the dorsum of the hand. If extravasation occurs, drug administration should be halted immediately. An attempt should be made to aspirate blood from the intravenous line in order to lower the concentration of drug in the local area. The application of ice and steroid cream and the local administration of sodium bicarbonate and hydrocortisone have all been reported to reduce the severity of the reaction (Barlock *et al.,* 1979). Unfortunately, surgical debridement, reconstructive surgery, and skin grafting are frequently necessary. A benign local allergic reaction, termed "ADRIAMYCIN flare," can sometimes be mistaken for extravasation. This reaction usually takes the form of erythematous streaking in the area of drug administration. "ADRIAMYCIN flare" may be associated with up to 3% of administered doses.

Radiation recall is a severe local toxicity that is produced in certain tissues by the interaction of doxorubicin and radiation. The skin, heart, lungs, esophagus, and intestinal mucosa are all susceptible to radiation-recall reactions (Aristizabal *et al.,* 1977; McInerney and Bullimore, 1977; Billingham *et al.,* 1979). Concurrent administration of radiation and drug or radiation given before or after drug administration can all produce this enhanced toxicity. Skin reactions can vary in intensity from erythema to ulceration and necrosis. Pulmonary fibrosis and sloughing of the esophageal mucosa have been reported (McInerney and Bullimore, 1977). Although not a contraindication to the use of these two agents in the same patient, close cooperation between the radiotherapist and the medical oncologist is required to minimize radiation-recall toxicity.

The potential for producing cardiotoxicity prevents the long-term administration of the anthracyclines. Anthracycline-induced cardiotoxicity can be manifested as an acute dysrhythmia, electrocardiographic abnormalities that are not dose dependent and as a cardiomyopathy that is related to the cumulative drug dose. Transient electrocardiographic abnormalities are the most common expression of acute anthracycline-induced cardiotoxicity. The incidence of electrocardiographic changes has been reported to be as high as 41%. A decrease in the voltage of the QRS complex, nonspecific ST-T wave changes, sinus tachycardia, premature atrial and ventricular contractions, and a variety of arrhythmias may occur during or shortly after the administration of either doxorubicin or daunorubicin (Von Hoff *et al.,* 1982). These changes are transient, unrelated to the cumulative anthracycline dose and, with the possible exception of reduced QRS voltage, not predictive of the later development of cardiomyopathy (Gilladoga *et al.,* 1975; Von Hoff *et al.,* 1979). Anthracycline administration can be safely continued in patients who develop such benign, transient electrocardiographic changes.

Another form of acute cardiotoxicity is the development of sudden and severe disturbances in impulse conduction and myocardial contractility (Bristow *et al.,* 1978). Pericardial effusions may develop as well as acute congestive heart failure. Such evidence of diffuse myocardial injury accompanied by pericardial effusion is referred to as the pericarditis-myocarditis syndrome. This acute syndrome may be fatal, but survival with and without permanent cardiac dysfunction has been reported (Greco *et al.,* 1976; Singer *et al.,* 1978).

The development of cardiomyopathy and congestive heart failure are the most serious manifestations of anthracycline-induced cardiotoxicity. The incidence of cardiomyopathy is related to the total cumulative dose of anthracycline administered. The frequency ranges from 0.3% at total doses of less than 500 mg/m^2 to 31% at total doses greater than 600 mg/m^2. The initial symptoms of congestive heart failure have been reported to develop from nine to 280 days after the last dose of anthracycline. Most frequently, symptoms first appear within a month of the last dose.

The pathologic changes that accompany anthracycline-induced cardiomyopathy are nonspecific but easily recognized (Ferrans, 1978). The most consistent findings on light microscopy include myofibrillar dropout and interstitial edema. Ultrastructural studies reveal swelling of the sarcoplasmic reticulum, vacuolar degeneration, and dilated mitochondria. These changes can proceed to overt cellular necrosis. Pathologic changes, noted on right ventricular endomyocardial biopsy, usually precede clinically detectable functional abnormalities. Biochemical abnormalities include an interference with myocyte-calcium exchange that results in an increased content of calcium in the myocardium (Olson *et al.,* 1974; Villani *et al.,* 1978). Decreased

contractility may result from these disturbances in calcium flux. Other biochemical mechanisms potentially responsible for anthracycline-induced cardiac damage have been discussed above.

A sensitive and specific method of monitoring patients receiving anthracyclines, in order to detect subtle changes in cardiac function before the symptoms of congestive heart failure became clinically apparent, would be of great benefit. The ability to confidently monitor patients would also be useful for the selection of individuals who could tolerate larger cumulative doses than those now considered to be safe. Clinical signs and symptoms of cardiac dysfunction occur too late to possess any useful predictive value. Patients who on electrocardiogram develop a decrease in the QRS voltage of greater than 30% of the pretreatment value have been reported to have an increased risk of developing congestive heart failure (Minow *et al.,* 1978). Unfortunately, this change may also occur too late to be helpful (Ali *et al.,* 1979). The determination of serial systolic time intervals, the ratio of the preejection period to the left ventricular ejection time, continues to be widely utilized for monitoring the early development of anthracycline-induced congestive heart failure. This technique is probably too sensitive and, if strictly relied upon, may often result in the premature termination of anthracycline therapy (Balcerzak *et al.,* 1978). Echocardiography also appears to be nonspecific and not predictive of subsequent congestive heart failure. Radionuclide cineangiography is the most promising noninvasive technique for the early prediction of anthracycline-induced congestive heart failure (Alexander *et al.,* 1979). Whether studies performed at rest or after exercise are most useful remains controversial. Percutaneous biopsy of the endomyocardium of the right ventricle is the most reliable method of assessing the cardiac damage produced by the anthracyclines. The frequency and severity of the pathologic changes detected on endomyocardial biopsy have been shown to relate directly to the total cumulative anthracycline dose. Pathologic changes occur earlier and are accurate predictors of subsequent physiologic abnormalities. Although the safety of this technique has been demonstrated in several centers, it is not generally available (Billingham *et al.,* 1978; Benjamin *et al.,* 1979).

In the absence of a reliable, noninvasive method to detect early anthracycline-induced cardiac damage, standard clinical practice is to discontinue therapy with doxorubicin after a cumulative dose of 450 to 550 mg/m². Although certain clinical situations may justify the high risk of cardiac toxicity that accompanies larger cumulative doses, it must be remembered that, in the majority of patients, drug-induced heart failure will be unresponsive to medical management (Von Hoff and Layard, 1981).

In addition to the cumulative dose of drug, other risk factors for the development of doxorubicin-induced cardiomyopathy have been identified. Patients of advanced age and young children are both more susceptible to drug-induced cardiomyopathy (Pratt et al., 1978; Von Hoff et al., 1979). Preexisting heart disease and uncontrolled hypertension have been reported to be potentiating factors (Minow et al., 1977). Previous radiotherapy to the mediastinum and concurrent administration of other antineoplastic drugs, particularly related anthracycline derivatives and cyclophosphamide, are other documented risk factors (Minow et al., 1977; Friedman et al., 1979).

The schedule of doxorubicin administration may be an important determinant of cardiotoxicity. When given in the usual every-three-week schedule, a cumulative doxorubicin dose greater than 600 mg/m² is associated with a 30% incidence of congestive heart failure. Weiss and colleagues (1976) administered doxorubicin in a weekly schedule and did not encounter a single instance of congestive heart failure even in 50 patients who received cumulative doses greater than 600 mg/m². This experience, and the results of other trials that employed weekly administration, suggest that doxorubicin-induced congestive heart failure may be schedule dependent (Chlebowski et al., 1980). This reduction in cardiotoxicity may be related to the lower doses employed when doxorubicin is administered on a weekly basis. The resulting lower peak levels of drug in the serum may be less toxic to the myocardium (Haskell and Sullivan, 1974). Continuous infusions of doxorubicin also result in lower peak serum levels and may produce less injury to the myocardium (Benjamin et al., 1981). The antitumor activity of doxorubicin appears not to be compromised with these newer methods of administration, but more experience is necessary.

A variety of pharmacologic methods designed to ameliorate anthracycline-induced cardiotoxicity are under evaluation. These include the administration of coenzyme Q10, a component of the mitochondrial electron-transport chain (Cortes et al., 1978); cardiac glycosides (Villani et al., 1978), calcium chelators, prednisone, carnitine, selenium, and α-tocopherol (Myers et al., 1976). The protective effects of any of these agents remain to be demonstrated.

The limitations imposed by cardiotoxicity have stimulated the development of new and potentially less toxic anthracycline analogs. Aclacinomycin A is a new anthracycline antibiotic isolated from cultures of *Streptomyces galilaeus* (Oki et al., 1975). Animal studies have suggested that cardiac toxicity may be less than that of doxorubicin. In a phase I study, clinically unimportant cardiac dysrhythmias occurred in a high proportion of patients (Van Echo, et al., 1982). Alopecia was minimal and tissue necrosis was not produced by extravasation. Activity against acute nonlymphocytic leukemia has been documented (Warrell et al., 1982). Zorubicin has also demonstrated activity against acute leukemia. Cardiotoxicity does occur with this drug and preliminary information suggests that cumulative doses should not exceed 3500 mg/m². N-trifluroacetyl adriamycin-14-valerate (AD32) is a new anthracycline of considerable interest (Israel et al., 1975). A broad spectrum of antitumor activity and much less cardiotoxicity than doxorubicin have been demonstrated in animal systems. Its insolubility in water renders this drug difficult to administer. Clinical trials with AD32 are now in progress. Carminomycin is an anthracycline antibiotic that appears to offer several advantages. Extravasation does not produce tissue necrosis. Alopecia is uncommon and drug-induced cardiomyopathy is yet to be encountered. Antitumor activity has been documented in early phase I and II trials (Gause et al., 1974; Perevodchikova et al., 1977). 4-Demethoxydaunorubicin (idarubicin) is an analog of daunorubicin that is active after intravenous or oral administration. Myelosuppression is the dose-limiting factor. Vomiting is a frequent problem with oral administration. Except for transient nonspecific electrocardiographic changes, cardiac toxicity has not been observed. Responses have been documented in patients with non-Hodgkin's lymphoma, breast cancer, melanoma, and carcinoma of the uterine cervix (Bonfante et al., 1983). 4'-Epi-doxorubicin (epirubicin) is another promising new anthracycline analog. In early clinical trials, epirubicin has been shown to be effective in the treatment of patients with non-Hodgkin's lymphomas, ovarian and pancreatic cancers, and sarcomas. Using equidosage regimens, the antitumor activity of epirubicin was comparable to doxorubicin. Epirubicin, however, was less myelosuppressive. As judged by clinical parameters and serial radionuclide cineangiography, epirubicin was also less cardiotoxic.

Another innovative approach is the development of anthracycline-DNA complexes. Theoretically, the linking of the drug to a digestible carrier would result in preferential uptake by cells capable of endocytosis. Cardiac myocytes would be spared exposure to the anthracycline and cardiac toxicity would be thereby reduced. In early phase I trials, the major toxic effects of doxorubicin-DNA complexes have been on the gastrointestinal tract and the bone marrow (Hall *et al.*, 1982). Tumor responses have been noted in phase I trials.

Clinical Indications

Doxorubicin has a broad spectrum of clinical activity. Hodgkin's disease, non-Hodgkin's lymphomas, sarcomas, acute leukemia, as well as breast, lung, and ovarian carcinomas are all responsive. Activity has also been observed in bladder tumors and carcinomas of the prostate, thyroid, endometrium, head and neck, and other solid tumors. Daunorubicin is primarily used in the treatment of acute nonlymphocytic leukemia. The clinical usefulness of the anthracyclines will increase as new strategies for the prevention of toxicity are developed and new, safer analogs are introduced.

BLEOMYCIN

Bleomycin, an antibiotic complex with an important spectrum of antitumor activity, was introduced into clinical trials in the United States in 1970. The commercial preparation is a mixture of small-molecular-weight, copper-chelating, glycopeptidic antibiotics isolated as fermentation products from a strain of *Streptomyces verticillus* (Umezawa *et al.*, 1966) (see Figure 10-23). Crude bleomycin can be purified by chromatography into several components, bleomycins A_{1-6} and B_{1-4}. The predominant species in the commercial preparation are bleomycins A_2 and B_2, making up greater than 50% and greater than 25%, respec-

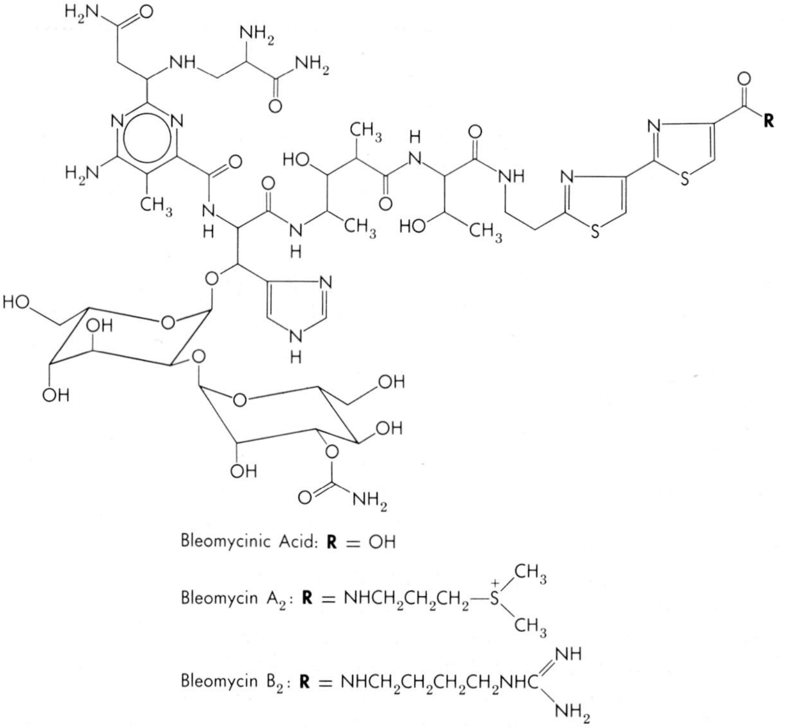

Bleomycinic Acid: **R** = OH

Bleomycin A_2: **R** = $NHCH_2CH_2CH_2-S^+(CH_3)_2$

Bleomycin B_2: **R** = $NHCH_2CH_2CH_2CH_2NHC(=NH)NH_2$

Figure 10-23. Structures of bleomycin A_2 and bleomycin B_2.

tively (Crooke and Bradner, 1976). The various species of bleomycin are structurally similar and many differ only in their terminal amine moiety. Structural and conformational changes within the bleomycin molecule significantly alter its capacity to interact with DNA (Asakura et al., 1975).

Biochemical Pharmacology

Bleomycin has antiviral, antibacterial, and antitumor activity. Cytotoxicity results from its interactions with DNA. Bleomycin binds with both double- and single-stranded DNA, producing site-specific and nonspecific double- and single-strand scissions (Huang et al., 1981; Mirabelli et al., 1979). DNA is cleaved preferentially at guanine-cytosine and guanine-thymine sequences (Mirabelli et al., 1982). DNA sequences in the open regions of chromatin are particularly susceptible to damage (Kuo, 1981). Double-strand breaks result from a number of single-strand breaks occurring in close proximity and are produced only at higher concentrations of bleomycin (Saunders et al., 1975).

Ferrous ions (Fe^{2+}) are chelated to nitrogen-containing groups, such as the pyrimidine ring, the imidazole of L-histidine and the carbamoyl group of mannose, on the bleomycin molecule. After bleomycin intercalates with DNA, the complexed Fe^{2+} is brought into close proximity to a deoxyribose moiety. The Fe^{2+} ion is then spontaneously oxidized to the Fe^{3+} state. This oxidation is associated with the release of a free purine or pyrimidine base from the DNA and is the critical reaction in the production of strand breakage. After dissociation from the DNA, the oxidized complex can be reduced to Fe^{2+}-bleomycin and then bind again to DNA. Free radicals, such as the superoxide or hydroxyl radical, are formed by a reduction of ambient O_2 as a result of this oxidative attack on DNA. These free radicals enhance DNA chain breakage by attacking the phosphodiester bonds of guanine-cytosine and guanine-thymine sequences (Povirk, 1979; Yamanaka et al., 1980). Other effects of bleomycin on DNA include the formation of noncovalent intermolecular cross-links, alteration of the activity of DNA-dependent DNA-polymerase, and inhibition of the reparative enzyme, DNA ligase (Müller et al., 1972; Ono et al., 1976; Lloyd et al., 1979). The enzyme ribonucleotide reductase may potentiate DNA

strand cleavage by bleomycin (Ayusawa et al., 1983). The activity or level of this enzyme may be a factor in determining the sensitivity of cells to bleomycin. Thus, bleomycin acts by degradation of preformed DNA, inhibition of the synthesis of DNA, and, to a lesser degree, by inhibition of the synthesis of RNA and proteins (Crooke, 1978). Cytotoxicity correlates best with the extent of breakage and degradation of DNA (Clarkson and Humphrey, 1976).

Morphologic changes seen in cells treated with bleomycin include a larger than normal size, multiple nuclei, and enlarged bizarre mitochondria and Golgi vesicles. Perichromatin granules may accumulate in association with the nucleolus. Chromosomes show prominent breaks and deletions.

Bleomycin demonstrates some cell-cycle specificity. Mitotic phase (M) and post-DNA synthesis phase (G_2) cells are most sensitive, whereas postmitotic phase cells (G_1) are the least sensitive. Progression through the cell cycle is blocked at the S-G_2 boundary causing an accumulation of cells in the G_2 phase (Barranco and Humphrey, 1976). This ability to produce partial synchronization has led to the development of sequential multiple drug regimens that contain bleomycin administered by continuous infusion.

Both ionizing radiation and local hyperthermia can enhance DNA strand breakage and the cytotoxicity of bleomycin (Meyn et al., 1979; Kimler, 1979). A decreased capacity to enzymatically repair damaged DNA may be an important factor in producing this synergism. In vitro, the addition of exogenous Fe^{2+} or ethanol increases the cytotoxicity of bleomycin by, respectively, accelerating the rate of breakage of DNA and inhibiting repair (Strong and Crooke, 1978; Mizuno, 1981). The metal chelator diethyldithiocarbamate enhances the ability of bleomycin to damage DNA by maintaining the Fe^{2+}-bleomycin complex in the reduced form that can generate free radicals (Lin et al., 1983). The effects of these substances on the activity of bleomycin in vivo is unknown.

In addition to enzymatic repair mechanisms, resistance to bleomycin may be mediated by an inactivating enzyme, bleomycin hydrolase. This enzyme hydrolyzes the amide group of the β-aminoalanine amide of the bleomycin molecule. Higher levels of bleomycin hydrolase are found in resistant tumor cells as compared to tumor cells sensitive to bleomycin (Umezawa, 1976). Low levels of this inactivating enzyme are found in normal lung and skin, tissues where bleomycin toxicity most frequently occurs (Fujita, 1971).

Clinical Pharmacology

Bleomycin is administered by subcutaneous, intramuscular, and intravenous injection as well as by intracavitary instillation. After parenteral administration, the highest tissue concentrations in animals are in the skin, spleen, kidney, lung, and heart (Fujita, 1971). Bleomycin does not penetrate the blood-brain barrier. Only a small amount of drug is bound to plasma proteins. There is a biphasic pattern of clearance from the plasma. After administration by intravenous bolus, the initial serum half-life is 24 minutes and the terminal half-life is four hours (Alberts et al., 1978). With continuous intravenous infusion, clearance from the plasma is prolonged, the $t_{1/2} \alpha$ increases to 80 minutes and $t_{1/2} \beta$ to nine hours. A steady-state concentration is achieved in the blood after 12 hours of continuous infusion (Kramer et al., 1978). A continuous infusion of 30 units of bleomycin daily for four to five days will produce an average steady-state concentration of approximately 150 mU/mL. When bleomycin is given as a continuous infusion, a loading dose, given by intravenous bolus, is frequently administered. The use of a loading dose more rapidly produces a steady-state concentration and may, thereby, reduce the development of resistance to the drug (Broughton et al., 1977). After an intramuscular injection, bleomycin has a half-life of two to three hours and the peak concentrations in the serum are dependent upon the dose. One hour after doses of 1 to 10 U/m² are injected, mean peak concentrations in the serum range from 0.133 to 0.587 mU/mL (Oken et al., 1981).

Several tissues, particularly the liver, are capable of degrading bleomycin. The degree of accumulation of bleomycin in normal and tumor tissue is inversely proportional to the activity of the degradative enzyme bleomycin hydrolase. Elimination of drug by enzymatic degradation is probably of importance only in patients with severely compromised renal function.

Bleomycin and its metabolites are primarily excreted in the urine. In patients with normal renal function, 70% of the dose was excreted after intravenous bolus or intramuscular injection and 63% after continuous infusion within the first 24 hours. The terminal half-life

of bleomycin is prolonged in the presence of severe renal failure. In patients with a creatinine clearance of less than 25 to 35 mL/min, the $t_{1/2} \beta$ was prolonged 375 to 1260 minutes (Crooke et al., 1977). In a patient with a creatinine clearance of 10 mL/min, however, bleomycin was undetectable in the serum 72 hours after intravenous injection (Crooke et al., 1977). Increased drug toxicity has been observed in patients with severe renal dysfunction after bleomycin administration (Perry et al., 1982). In the presence of severely compromised renal function, it is necessary to reduce the dose of bleomycin.

After intracavitary instillation, either intraperitoneal or intrapleural, of 60 U/m² of bleomycin, approximately 50% of the dose enters the systemic circulation. The terminal half-life then ranges from 3.5 to 5.5 hours and 17 to 23% of the administered dose is excreted in the urine within the first 24 hours (Alberts et al., 1979).

Clinical Toxicity

The organ systems most susceptible to the toxic effects of bleomycin are the lungs, skin, and mucous membranes. In contrast to most other antineoplastic agents, bleomycin has minimal myelosuppressive activity. Myelosuppression can occur when bleomycin is administered at high doses, and, when given as part of a combination drug regimen, bleomycin may enhance the marrow toxicity of other chemotherapeutic agents (Bennett and Reich, 1979).

Interstitial pneumonitis that may progress to pulmonary fibrosis is the primary dose-limiting toxicity of bleomycin. The initial damage may be related to injury to DNA and lipid peroxidation (Passero et al., 1983). The earliest pathologic changes in the lungs of mice after the administration of bleomycin are the development of blebs in the endothelium of alveolar capillaries. The formation of endothelial blebs is soon accompanied by interstitial edema, an infiltration of mononuclear cells, and the deposition of hyaline membranes (Adamson and Bowden, 1974). Concomitant with the development of these pathologic changes are increased activity of the enzyme collagen lysol oxidase, increased lung hydroxyproline, and an elevated rate of collagen synthesis (Kelley et al., 1980; Counts et al., 1981). In man, type I pneumocytes decrease and type II pneumocytes proliferate and migrate into the alveoli. Alveolar septae become thickened, collagen fibers are laid down, and there is a proliferation of dense fibrous tissue (Ginsberg and Comis, 1982). These anatomic abnormalities result in a decreased lung compliance and restrictive lung disease. Once pulmonary fibrosis develops, it is usually irreversible and sometimes fatal.

The overall incidence of clinically significant pulmonary toxicity due to bleomycin is 10% and the fatality rate is 1%. Symptoms and signs of lung damage may not occur until four to ten weeks after therapy is initated. Early symptoms of bleomycin pulmonary toxicity may include a nonproductive cough and exertional dyspnea. Fine rales may be present upon examination. Progressive pulmonary changes may be associated with dyspnea at rest, fever, and cyanosis. Coarse rales, rhonchii, and pleural friction rubs may develop. The chest film may be normal initially, but eventually will show bibasilar interstitial infiltrates that often progress to generalized lower lobe involvement and lobar consolidation. Arterial blood gases usually reveal hypoxemia and hypocapnia. Because the physical signs and radiographic findings may be nonspecific and not easily distinguished from other complications that commonly occur in patients with cancer, an open-lung biopsy is sometimes required to provide a diagnosis. Pulmonary function tests have been employed to detect the development of bleomycin-induced lung damage before symptoms and clinical signs appear. Decreases in the diffusing capacity (DLCO) and in the forced vital capacity (FVC) may be related to the total cumulative dose of bleomycin and may precede clinically detectable pulmonary toxicity (Comis *et al.*, 1979). Unfortunately, frequent false-positive and false-negative results can make interpretation of these studies difficult (Lewis and Izbicki, 1980). Despite these problems, it is generally recommended that pulmonary function studies be performed at regular intervals on all patients being treated with bleomycin. Therapy with this drug should be discontinued if either the DLCO falls below 40% or if the FVC falls below 25% of the pretreatment values, as well as if any of the physical signs, symptoms, or radiographic features of bleomycin toxicity develop.

The incidence of bleomycin pulmonary toxicity is dose-related. There is a 5% incidence with total cumulative doses of less than 300 mg (Brown *et al.*, 1980). This increases to 10%

with a total dose of 400 mg, and at cumulative doses of greater than 500 mg the incidence and mortality of pulmonary toxicity increase significantly (Brown *et al.*, 1980; Collis, 1980).

The method of administration may affect the incidence of bleomycin pulmonary toxicity. Continuous infusions may be less toxic than intermittent bolus injections (Cooper and Hong, 1981). Other risk factors include age of greater than 70 years, prior exposure to bleomycin, the use of bleomycin in certain combination chemotherapy regimens, and prior or concurrent radiation to the thorax (Schein *et al.*, 1976; Crooke *et al.*, 1978). Oxygen may potentiatate bleomycin lung toxicity (Toledo *et al.*, 1982). Patients who have received bleomycin are at risk for the development of postoperative adult respiratory distress syndrome when exposed to elevated but otherwise nontoxic concentrations of oxygen. Postoperatively, patients who have been exposed to bleomycin should receive reduced concentrations of oxygen and careful attention should be directed to the replacement of fluids (Allen *et al.*,1981).

No consistently effective therapy for bleomycin-induced lung toxicity is available. Steroids are reported to be beneficial in some patients (Brown *et al.*, 1980). Proline analogs and anti-inflammatory agents prevent collagen deposition and reduce the amount of lung fibrosis produced by bleomycin in experimental animals (Thrall *et al.*, 1979; Riley *et al.*, 1981). The efficacy of these drugs in humans has not been established.

Mucocutaneous reactions, including stomatitis, alopecia, erythema, hyperpigmentation, hyperkeratosis, edema, fibrosis, and vesiculation and ulceration of the skin, occur in approximately 50% of patients who receive bleomycin. The most common of these are stomatitis and alopecia; stomatitis may be dose limiting. The incidence of mucocutaneous toxicities is dose related and the severity may correlate with the total cumulative dose. Symptoms usually appear within three to four weeks or after a cumulative dose of 150 to 200 units of bleomycin. In patients with head and neck cancer, the incidence and severity of stomatitis is potentiated by concurrent radiation therapy and by the use of bleomycin in combination with other chemotherapeutic agents.

Pyrexia is a common occurrence after the administration of bleomycin and does not represent an allergic response (Spiegel, 1981). Another more serious toxic manifestation is an idiosyncratic reaction characterized by hyper-pyrexia, chills, nausea, vomiting, wheezing, hypotension, and cardiopulmonary collapse. Such reactions occur almost exclusively in patients with lymphoma. Patients who have fever as a symptom of their lymphoma may be particularly susceptible to this toxicity syndrome. The reaction is not antibody mediated and has occurred with the first exposure to bleomycin (Weiss and Bruno, 1981). A bleomycin-induced release of endogenous pyrogen from leukocytes is the probable mechanism of this reaction. Because the incidence of this toxicity syndrome is aproximately 1% in patients with lymphoma, the use of a one-unit test dose of bleomycin is recommended. Raynaud's phenomena and coronary artery disease have been reported in patients with testicular carcinoma treated with chemotherapeutic regimens that contain bleomycin (Vogelzang *et al.*, 1981; Ricci and Goldstein, 1982). The etiologic role of bleomycin in the development of these complications is uncertain. Hepatic and renal toxicities are rare.

Clinical Indications

Bleomycin is active against a broad range of squamous cell carcinomas, including head and neck cancer and tumors of the cervix, esophagus, skin, vulva, and lung (Ervin *et al.*, 1981; Kelsen *et al.*, 1981; Boice *et al.*, 1982; Rosenthal, 1982). Bleomycin has established activity in the therapy of germ cell testicular cancer, Hodgkin's disease, and non-Hodgkin's lymphoma (Vugrin *et al.*, 1981; Santoro *et al.*, 1982).

Because of its lack of toxicity to the bone marrow, bleomycin is frequently included in combination chemotherapy regimens. Bleomycin has been instilled in the pleural and peritoneal cavities to treat neoplastic effusions and into the urinary bladder in the treatment of superficial bladder tumors (Bracken *et al.*, 1977; Ostrowski and Halsall, 1982).

ACTINOMYCIN D

The actinomycins were the first crystalline antibiotics to be obtained from a species of *Streptomyces.* Actinomycin D is a chromopeptide that contains the phenoxazone ring chromophore *actinocin,* which is responsible for the drug's red color, and two cyclic polypeptides (see Figure 10–24).

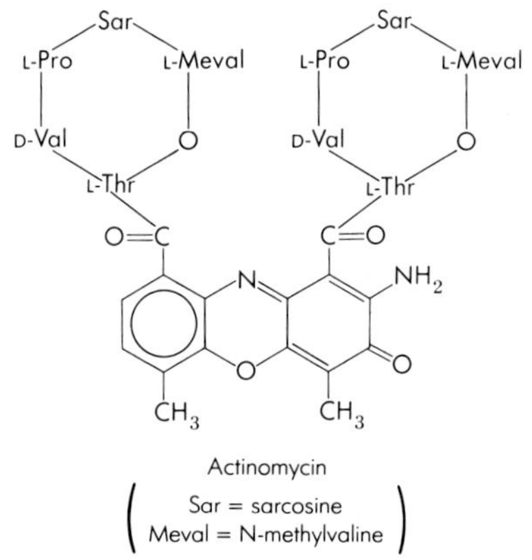

Figure 10–24.   Actinomycin.

Biochemical Pharmacology

The cytotoxic effects of actinomycin are primarily due to its ability to bind to DNA. The drug binds specifically to guanine bases of double-stranded DNA. The planar phenoxazone ring intercalates between adjacent guanine-cytosine sequences. Intercalation is dependent upon hydrogen bonding between the polypeptide portions of the actinomycin molecule and deoxyguanosines on the DNA chain (Sobell, 1973). The actinomycin-DNA complex does not permit the transcription of nucleic acids. DNA-dependent RNA polymerases are particularly sensitive to the effects of actinomycin and, even at low concentrations of the drug, the synthesis of RNA is inhibited. Inhibition of the synthesis of DNA requires higher concentrations of actinomycin (Reich *et al.*, 1962). The production of single-stranded breaks in DNA is another potential mechanism of cytotoxicity (Ross *et al.*, 1979). Although effective throughout the cell cycle, cells in early S phase may be particularly susceptible (Roots and Smith, 1976). Resistance to actinomycin may be related to membrane permeability, drug transport, and intracellular binding capacity (Goldstein *et al.*, 1966; Goldman *et al.*, 1981).

Clinical Pharmacology

Actinomycin D is administered intravenously. Clearance from the plasma is rapid. Little active drug is detectable in the plasma two minutes after administration. The drug is avidly bound by tissues. Subsequent release of bound drug produces a slow-phase half-life in the plasma of 36 hours (Tattersall *et al.*, 1975). Metabolic transformation does not occur. The drug is primarily excreted unchanged into the bile and urine. Actinomycin D does not appear to cross the blood-brain barrier.

Clinical Toxicity

Myelosuppression is the most frequent dose-limiting toxicity. Stomatitis is also common and sometimes severe. Other gastrointestinal toxicities include nausea, vomiting, and diarrhea. Dermatologic manifestations may include alopecia, erythema, and desquamation. Extravasation can produce local inflammation and tissue necrosis. Actinomycin can enhance radiation injury to the skin, mucous membranes, esophagus, liver, and gastrointestinal tract (Donaldson and Lenon, 1979; Mitchell and Schein, 1982). These radiation recall reactions can occur even if the drug is given weeks to months after irradiation, but are most severe when the two modalities are given together. Intercalation with DNA by actinomycin may inhibit the repair of irradiation-induced breaks in DNA and lead to this enhanced toxicity (Fox and Lajtha, 1973).

Clinical Indications

Actinomycin D has established activity against a defined group of tumors including Wilms' tumor, embryonal rhabdomyosarcoma, gestational choriocarcinomas, Ewing's sarcoma, testicular carcinomas, Kaposi's sarcoma, and lymphomas (Frei, 1974).

MITHRAMYCIN

Mithramycin is a cytotoxic antibiotic isolated from *Streptomyces plicatus* (see Figure 10–25). Although active against testicular carcinoma, it is most widely used in the treatment of hypercalcemia associated with cancer.

Biochemical Pharmacology

Mithramycin binds to DNA in a manner similar to actinomycin. Mg^{2+} is required for the formation of the mithramycin-DNA complex. The synthesis of DNA-dependent RNA is specifically inhibited (Yarbro *et al.,* 1966). The hypocalcemic effect is mediated through the inhibition of osteoclastic activity.

Clinical Pharmacology

Mithramycin is administered intravenously. Studies of its clinical pharmacology, metabolism, and excretion are incomplete.

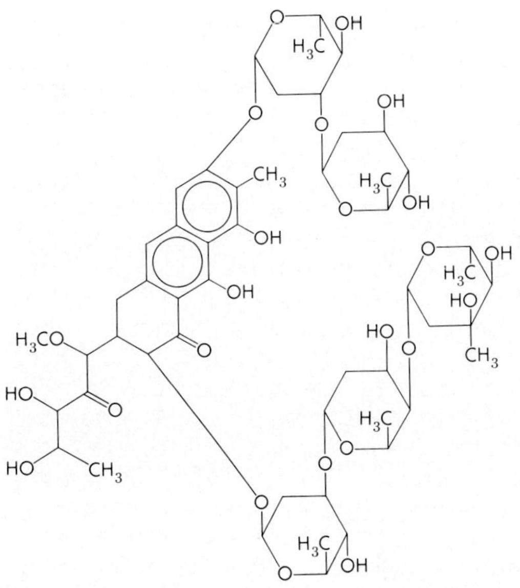

Figure 10–25.   Mithramycin.

Clinical Toxicity

The use of mithramycin to treat neoplastic diseases is limited by its severe toxicities. After a rapid infusion, almost all patients will acutely develop nausea and vomiting (Kennedy, 1970). Other gastrointestinal toxicities include diarrhea and stomatitis. Mithramycin may produce a serious hemorrhagic diathesis. Decreased synthesis of clotting factors II, V, VII, and X, abnormal platelet aggregation, and thrombocytopenia may lead to the development of severe bleeding (Ahr *et al.,*1978). The bleeding and prothrombin times are prolonged. Characteristically, bleeding is mucosal, such as epistaxis or gastrointesinal. Fatal hemorrhages have been associated with the administration of mithramycin in antitumor doses and on daily schedules. When mithramycin is administered in an alternate-day regimen, the incidence of hemorrhage is greatly reduced (Kennedy, 1972). The serum lactic dehydrogenase, blood urea nitrogen, prothrombin time, and platelet count must be checked prior to each dose in order to ensure the safety of this schedule of administration.

In addition to suppressing the synthesis of coagulation factors, hepatic damage by mithramycin may be manifested by marked elevations of serum transamines and lactic dehydrogenase levels. The histology reveals acute hepatic necrosis. Azotemia occurs in as many as 40% of patients treated with mithramycin on a daily schedule. Proteinuria and necrosis of both proximal and distal tubules may be present. Extravasation produces local inflammation and cellulitis.

The lower doses of mithramycin (25 μg/kg) used in the treatment of hypercalcemia are considerably safer than the usual antitumor doses. The serum calcium usually begins to decline within 12 hours after therapy and the peak effect occurs at 48 to 96 hours. Response from a single dose can extend from several days up to three weeks (Stewart, 1983). A rapid rebound in serum calcium levels, which may precipitate a hypercalcemic crisis, can occur after mithramycin therapy. Even at lower doses, the administration of mithramycin to patients with liver disease, renal disease, or thrombocytopenia is potentially dangerous.

ENZYMES

L-ASPARAGINASE

In 1953, Kidd observed that fresh guinea pig serum inhibited the growth of certain murine lymphoid tumors (Kidd, 1953). The enzyme L-asparaginase was subsequently shown to be the active antitumor component of guinea pig serum (Broome, 1963). Although L-asparaginase with antitumor activity can be isolated from many sources, the preparations in clinical usage are derived from *Escherichia coli* and *Erwinia carotovora.* The toxic effects of L-asparaginase were initially thought to be highly selective for tumor tissues. The current use of L-asparaginase, however, is limited by its significant clinical toxicities and narrow spectrum of antitumor activity.

Biochemical Pharmacology

The nonessential amino acid L-asparagine is present in abundance in the diet. In addition, the cells of most normal tissues can synthesize L-asparagine through the action of the enzyme L-asparagine synthetase. L-Asparaginase, a high-molecular-weight enzyme, catalyzes the hydrolysis of L-asparagine to L-aspartic acid and ammonia. Treatment with L-asparaginase results in the depletion of this amino acid. Cells with low levels of L-asparagine synthetase are dependent on exogenous sources of L-asparagine and are sensitive to the cytotoxic effects of L-asparaginase. L-Asparaginase derived from *E. coli* is capable of degrading 90,000 molecules of L-asparagine per minute.

L-Asparaginases derived from *E. coli* and *Erwinia carotovora,* although immunologically distinct, have similar antitumor activity. Of the two isoenzymes obtained from *E. coli,* only the fraction EC-2, with a high affinity for substrate, is active. Preparations of the enzyme derived from other strains of bacteria and from yeast have thus far proven to be inactive.

The toxicity of L-asparaginase is mediated through its depletion of L-asparagine. The lack of this amino acid results in an inhibition of the synthesis of protein. The synthesis of nucleic acids is also inhibited. Aspartic acid accumulates in cells that are sensitive to L-asparaginase. High concentrations of aspartic acid may inhibit basic cellular mechanisms of energy production and, thereby, contribute to the cytotoxicity produced by L-asparaginase (Broome, 1981). L-Asparaginase prepared from bacterial sources also possesses glutaminase activity. The depletion of glutamine may be responsible for the neurotoxic and immunosuppressive effects of L-asparaginase. Extracellular concentrations of glutamine far exceed asparagine. Enzymes that significantly deplete glutamine have relatively less asparaginase activity. A more specific asparaginase, without glutaminase activity, would probably be more specifically cytotoxic for sensitive tumor cells. Asparaginases without glutaminase activity are being evaluated.

Resistance to asparaginase can develop in a previously sensitive population of cells. Resistant cells are characterized by high levels of asparagine synthetase.

Clinical Pharmacology

The pharmacokinetics of L-asparaginases derived from *E. coli* and from *Erwinia carotovora* appear to be identical. L-Asparaginase may be administered by either intramuscular or intravenous injection. The frequency of hypersensitivity reactions is reduced when the intramuscular route is employed. After intramuscular administration, absorption is slow and the drug is not detectable in the plasma until one hour after injection. Peak levels in the plasma after intramuscular injection are only 25% of the concentrations achieved by intravenous administration (Ho *et al.,* 1981). The half-life in the plasma is dependent upon the specific preparation of enzyme used and generally ranges from 11 to 22 hours. Higher doses have more prolonged half-lives. Multiple doses may result in accumulation of the drug. Clearance from the plasma may be greatly accelerated in patients who experience a hypersensitivity reaction. Despite poor penetration across the blood-brain barrier, systemic administration of L-asparaginase does significantly decrease the concentration of L-asparagine in the cerebrospinal fluid.

Clinical Toxicity

Initially, L-asparaginase was thought to be essentially nontoxic to normal tissues. Unlike the majority of antitumor agents, L-asparaginase is not injurious to the stem cells of the bone marrow and does not damage oral or intestinal mucosa or hair follicles. Increased experience with the use of L-asparaginase has shown it to have important toxic effects.

The toxicities of L-asparaginase are due either to hypersensitivity reactions or to the consequences of the inhibition of the synthesis of protein. The dose and route of administration influence the frequency of hypersensitivity reactions. The intravenous route and widely spaced schedules of administration are most frequently associated with anaphylactic reactions.

Hypersensitivity reactions occur in approximately 10% of patients treated with L-asparaginase. The mortality rate from anaphylaxsis is estimated to be one percent. The immunoglobulin that mediates the reaction may be either an IgG or an IgE. Factors that increase the risk of hypersensitivity reactions include a history of atopy or allergy, prior exposure to L-asparaginase, widely spaced schedules of administration, high doses, and intravenous administration. Although hypersensitivity reactions usually occur after multiple doses, anaphylaxsis has been reported with the first injection of L-asparaginase. Hypersensitivity reactions may consist of only relatively mild symptoms, such as urticaria. Frequently, however, hypotension, laryngeal edema, bronchospasm, and other manifestations of anaphylactic shock occur. A physician experienced in the management of anaphylaxsis and cardiovascular collapse and appropriate emergency supplies should be readily available whenever L-asparaginase is administered. Since the L-asparaginases from the two commonly used bacterial sources are antigenically distinct, patients who demonstrate hypersensitivity to the enzyme derived from *E. coli* may be safely treated with the *Erwinia carotovora* preparation.

Hepatotoxicity, a frequent complication of therapy with L-asparaginase, is caused by inhibition of the synthesis of protein. Morphologically, the toxicity of L-asparaginase to the liver is manifested as a fatty metamorphosis. Biochemical changes include decreases in the concentrations of serum albumin, cholesterol, lipoproteins, transferrin, ceruloplasmin, haptoglobin, and β globulins, as well as, elevations of transaminases, alkaline phosphatase, and bilirubin. Decreased synthesis of the clotting factors II, VII, IX, X, and fibrinogen is another common manifestation of hepatotoxicity. Dysfunction of the liver quickly reverses when the drug is discontinued.

A decreased synthesis and defective release of insulin, induced by L-asparaginase, may result in hyperglycemia and hyperosmolarity. L-Asparaginase may also cause a decrease in the number of insulin receptors (Carpentieri and Balch, 1978). Pancreatitis occurs in 5% of patients treated with this drug. Fatal hemorrhagic pancreatitis has been reported. Other manifestations of pancreatic dysfunction may include malabsorption and elevations of serum amylase and lipase.

Neurotoxicity occurs in from 21 to 60% of patients that receive L-asparaginase and is more common in adults than in children. Encephalopathy that may be manifested by lethargy, depression, impaired sensorium, hallucinations, or coma is the most frequent form of dysfunction of the central nervous system. Seizures are uncommon. The electroencephalogram is frequently abnormal. Mild symptoms may develop after the first dose of L-asparaginase or the onset of cerebral dysfunction may be delayed. Neurologic toxicity is both more frequent and more severe with higher doses of the drug. Therapy may be continued in the presence of mild dysfunction of the central nervous system. The drug should be discontinued, however, if signs and symptoms are progressive. Neurologic abnormalities usually resolve when the drug is withheld. There are several possible causes for the neurotoxicity associated with L-asparaginase. Although the penetration of L-asparaginase into the cerebrospinal fluid is limited by its large molecular weight, it is sufficient to significantly decrease the concentration of L-asparagine. Depletion of L-asparagine and L-glutamine in the central nervous system decreases the synthesis of protein. The elevated levels of glutamic acid, L-aspartic acid, and ammonia that develop after therapy with L-asparaginase may be toxic to the brain. Symptoms that develop acutely are probably due to the accumulation of toxic metabolites, whereas delayed manifestations of neurotoxicity are most likely produced by the inhibition of the synthesis of protein in the brain.

Nausea, vomiting, fever, and chills frequently accompany the administration of L-asparaginase. These symptoms usually are not severe. L-Asparaginase is immunosuppressive and inhibits the functions of both T and B lymphocytes. The synthesis of antibodies, delayed hypersensitivity reactions, lymphocyte blastogenesis, and graft rejection are all affected.

Clinical Indications

Because the cytotoxicity of L-asparaginase is based upon a basic biochemical difference between sensitive and resistant cells, great optimism accompanied its introduction into clinical use. Unfortunately, only a limited number of neoplasms are susceptible to the toxic effects of this enzyme. At the present time, L-asparaginase is used almost exclusively in the treatment of patients with acute lymphoblastic leukemia. For the induction of remission in this disease, L-asparaginase is used in combination with vincristine and prednisone. L-Asparaginase may also be useful in the therapy of patients with other types of T-cell or null-cell leukemias and lymphomas. This drug has not proven to be effective in the treatment of patients with solid tumors.

When methotrexate is used in conventional doses to treat patients with acute lymphoblastic leukemia, the addition of L-asparaginase results in subadditive killing of cells. If the administration of methotrexate is followed in 24 hours by L-asparaginase, however, patients are able to tolerate larger doses of methotrexate and the therapeutic index of the drug is improved. When administered in this sequence, both drugs exert their antitumor effects. L-Asparaginase, by inhibiting the synthesis of protein and thereby preventing the progression of cells into S phase, attenuates the toxicity of the larger doses of methotrexate against bone marrow and intestinal mucosa cells (Capizzi, 1981). Patients with acute lymphoblastic leukemia refractory to both drugs may respond to the sequential combination of larger doses of methotrexate and L-asparaginase.

MISCELLANEOUS AGENTS

CIS-PLATINUM

Cis-dichlorodiammineplatinum (II) (*cis*-DDP) is the first member of a new class of compounds, the metal coordination complexes, to be used in cancer chemotherapy. Rosenberg *et al.,* (1965) observed that the growth of *E. coli* was inhibited in medium subjected to electrical currents delivered between platinum electrodes. The inhibition of bacterial replication was shown to be due to the formation of inorganic platinum-containing compounds (Rosenberg *et al.,* 1967). Of the several platinum compounds generated, *cis*-DDP was found to be the most effective in the treatment of a wide variety of animal tumors (Howle and Gale, 1970; Kociba *et al.,* 1970). In 1971, *cis*-DDP became the first metal coordination complex to be introduced into clinical trials.

Cis-DDP is an inorganic, water-soluble complex that contains a divalent, central atom of platinum bound to two chlorine and two ammonia ions in the *cis* position of the horizontal plane (see Figure 10–26). The biologic effects are dependent upon the geometry of the molecule. Only the *cis* configuration possesses antitumor activity. The corresponding *trans* isomer, although capable of producing interstrand crosslinks on DNA, is not cytotoxic (Zwelling and Kohn, 1979).

Biochemical Pharmacology

Cis-DDP enters cells by diffusion. Intracellularly, both chloride ions are displaced through hydrolysis. The resulting positively charged aquated complex has two active ligand sites. Thus, *cis*-DDP is transformed into a bifunctional compound with each molecule possessing two sites for reactions with nucleophiles. Aquated *cis*-DDP resembles the bifunctional alkylating agents such as nitrogen mustard. Activated *cis*-DDP is capable of

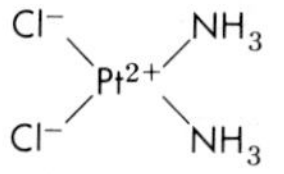

Figure 10–26.   *cis*-Platinum.

forming covalent crosslinks among or within DNA, RNA, and protein molecules. The formation of interstrand, intrastrand, and DNA-protein crosslinks have all been noted (Zwelling and Kohn, 1979). Intrastrand crosslinks may be particularly important in causing cell death because this is a lesion produced only by the active *cis* isomer. The amount of platinum bound to DNA is directly proportional to its guanine-cytosine content (Stone *et al.*, 1974). The N-7 position of guanine is usually the most nucleophilic site and is thus frequently attacked by the electrophilic aquated *cis*-DDP molecule. The N-3 position of cytosine is also particularly susceptible (Scovell and O'Connor, 1977).

Crosslinking with DNA continues to occur for several hours after exposure to the drug (Zwelling *et al.*, 1978). Thiourea has the potential to prevent or reverse interstrand crosslinking in preparations of isolated DNA (Filipski *et al.*, 1979). The high concentrations of thiourea required for this protective effect, however, have not been attainable in intact cells. DNA is the primary target of *cis*-DDP and cytotoxicity is caused by crosslinking DNA. Binding of *cis*-DDP to DNA results in a distortion of its macromolecular structure that leads to complete denaturation (Munchausen and Tahn, 1975; Cohen *et al.*, 1979). DNA can be repaired by the enzymatic excision of platinum adducts. Resistance to the cytotoxic effects of *cis*-DDP is related to the ability of the cell to excise platinum-induced lesions from its DNA (Roberts and Fraval, 1980).

Cis-DDP is not schedule dependent and has been generally considered to be cell-cycle-phase nonspecific. Different types of cultured cells, however, demonstrate enhanced sensitivity to the drug in specific stages of the cell cycle. For example, cultured human lymphoma cells demonstrate greater sensitivity to platinum in the G_1 phase compared to cells treated in mid-S phase (Drewinko and Barlogie, 1976).

Clinical Pharmacology

After intravenous administration, more than 90% of the platinum in the blood is bound to plasma proteins. This protein-bound component possesses little antitumor activity. Unbound or "free" platinum is probably the active species (Patton *et al.*, 1978). Radiopharmacokinetics of *cis*-DDP administered as a bolus show a biphasic pattern of excretion with a rapid initial plasma half-life ($t_{1/2}$ α 25 to 49 minutes) and a slower secondary half-life ($t_{1/2}$ β 59 to 73 hours) (DeConti *et al.*, 1973). Using whole body scanning, Lange determined the organ distribution of an injection of radioactive *cis*-DDP (Lange *et al.*, 1973). Three hours after injection, radioactivity was concentrated in the kidney and head, although not in the brain. After 40 hours, the kidney, liver, and intestine contained the highest concentrations of radioactivity. Animal studies have also shown little detectable platinum in brain tissue, suggesting poor penetrance of the blood-brain barrier (Lange *et al.*, 1972). A significant amount of platinum remains bound in the tissues for prolonged periods. Platinum has been detected in tissue samples at least four months after its administration (Piel *et al.*, 1974).

Urinary excretion is initially rapid but subsequent clearance is slow and incomplete. Fifteen to 27% of the drug is excreted in the first six hours. After 24 hours, only 18 to 39%, and after five days, only 27 to 45% of an administered dose is excreted (DeConti *et al.*, 1973). The extent of biliary excretion is unknown.

Recently developed flameless atomic absorption spectrophotometric (LeRoy *et al.*, 1977), high-pressure liquid chromatographic (Bannister *et al.*, 1979), and centrifugal ultrafiltration (Bannister *et al.*, 1977) techniques permit the separation and measurement of protein-bound and free drug as well as parent and aquated species. After a dose of 70 mg/m², the mean peak plasma level of free platinum is 30 μmol. The clearance of free platinum is biphasic with a $t_{1/2}$ α of 8 to 10 minutes and a $t_{1/2}$ β of 40 to 45 minutes (Gormley *et al.*, 1979).

The administration of platinum must be routinely accompanied by vigorous hydration and diuresis with mannitol or furosemide in order to minimize nephrotoxicity (Cvitkovic *et al.*, 1977; Hayes *et al.*, 1977). When platinum was administered as a six-hour infusion, pharmacokinetic factors including peak plasma concentration, terminal half-life, protein-bound fraction, and urinary excretion were similar in patients diuresed with either mannitol or furosemide (Ostrow *et al.*, 1981). Peak plasma levels of free platinum are lower, the elimination half-time shorter, and the amount of drug eliminated greater when platinum is given by infusion compared to bolus administration (Belt *et al.*, 1979). After a dose of 120 mg/m², administered by infusion with hydration and mannitol diuresis, the mean peak plasma level of free platinum was 18.7 μM and the mean $t_{1/2}\ \beta$ was 32 minutes (Ribaud *et al.,* 1981).

Clinical Toxicity

Nephrotoxicity is the most common dose-limiting toxic effect of *cis*-DDP. Pathologic changes associated with the nephrotoxicity of platinum include necrosis of both proximal and distal renal tubules (Gonzalez-Vitale *et al.,* 1977). The incidence and severity of nephrotoxicity are related to the dose. After a single dose of 50 mg/m^2, renal toxicity will develop in 25 to 30% of patients, but is mild and reversible. At higher doses or with multiple courses, toxicity may be more severe. Renal insufficiency may be cumulative and irreversible. Elevations in the BUN and serum creatinine usually occur within the first two weeks after therapy. Changes in the creatinine clearance may be a more sensitive indicator of early renal damage (Dentino *et al.,* 1978). The concurrent administration of nephrotoxic antibiotics with platinum may increase the risk of developing renal failure (Gonzalez-Vitale *et al.,* 1978). Hydration and diuresis with mannitol or furosemide reduce the incidence of platinum nephrotoxicity. A more rapid clearance of drug from the plasma, a decrease in urinary platinum concentration, and an accelerated passage of drug through the renal tubules are possible mechanisms of protection by hydration (Frick *et al.,* 1979). Saline hydration and furosemide or mannitol should be administered in order to maintain a urine output of 100 to 150 mL/hr.

Nausea and vomiting, frequently severe, are invariable consequences of therapy with *cis*-DDP. Symptoms usually begin one to two hours after therapy and resolve within 24 to 48 hours. Standard antiemetics are of little benefit. Droperidol (Grossman *et al.,* 1979) and metoclopramide (Gralla *et al.,* 1981) have been reported to be useful in controlling the nausea and vomiting induced by platinum.

Hypomagnesemia frequently occurs after the administration of platinum and results from a tubular defect in the magnesium reabsorption process with subsequent urinary loss (Schilsky and Anderson, 1979). Although usually asymptomatic, hypocalcemia and tetany, precipitated by hypomagnesemia, have occurred in children (Hayes *et al.,* 1979).

Serum magnesium levels should be routinely monitored.

Myelosuppression, manifested by transient leukopenia and thrombocytopenia, is usually mild. The nadir of peripheral blood counts is usually 14 days after therapy with recovery by day 21. Anemia has also been reported.

Ototoxicity, consisting of tinnitus and hearing loss in the high frequency range (4000 to 8000 Hz), occurs in from 11 to 70% of patients treated with *cis*-DDP (Lippman *et al.,* 1973; Reddel *et al.,* 1982). Elderly patients may be more susceptible. Audiometric abnormalities are dose related and cumulative (Piel *et al.,* 1974). Administration of *cis*-DDP by bolus injection or with furosemide may result in higher incidences of ototoxicity (Reddel *et al.,* 1982). Tinnitus is usually reversible but audiometric abnormalities may be permanent. Since audiometric changes, other than increased thresholds for tones above normal speech, are generally preceded by symptoms, the use of routine audiography may not be helpful. Vestibular symptoms rarely occur. Mixed sensory-motor peripheral neuropathies have been reported in a small percentage of patients. Paresthesias, dysesthesias, and disturbances of vibratory and position sense are the most common manifestations encountered (Becher *et al.,* 1980; Cowan *et al.,* 1980). Pathologic studies have suggested a segmental demyelination process (Von Hoff *et al.,* 1979).

Hypersensitivity reactions characterized by facial edema, bronchoconstriction, tachycardia, and hypotension have occurred immediately after *cis*-DDP administration in 1 to 20% of patients (Weiss and Bruno, 1981). These reactions are mediated through the release of IgE and other vasoactive substances (Khan *et al.,* 1975). Reactions are usually controlled by the intravenous administration of epinephrine, corticosteroids, or antihistamines. Premedication with corticosteroids and antihistamines and the administration of the drug as a very slow infusion may allow previously sensitive patients to tolerate further therapy with *cis*-DDP (Wiesenfeld *et al.,* 1979).

Clinical Indications

Cis-DDP is effective in the therapy of patients with testicular tumors, ovarian carcinoma, bladder tumors, and head and neck cancer. The use of *cis*-DDP as a radiation sensitizer is now being evaluated.

PROCARBAZINE

Procarbazine [N-isopropyl-a-(2-methylhydrazino)-p-toluamide hydrochloride], a derivative of methylhydrazine, was initially synthesized as an inhibitor of monoamine oxidase (see Figure 10–27). Antitumor activity was initially demonstrated in rodents. The usefulness of procarbazine has now been established in the therapy of several types of cancer in humans.

Biochemical Pharmacology

Procarbazine inhibits the synthesis of DNA, RNA, and proteins. Although procarbazine is thought to be cytotoxic due to its alkylating properties, the precise mechanisms of action have not yet been determined. Procarbazine requires conversion to its active metabolites in order to exert a cytotoxic effect. In aqueous solution, procarbazine undergoes a rapid nonenzymatic transformation to an azo derivative. *In vivo,* a similar enzymatically catalyzed activation occurs in erythrocytes and hepatic microsomes. Hydrogen peroxide is a byproduct of this oxidative process. Hydroxyl radicals, generated from the hydrogen peroxide, attack and degrade DNA. The action of the hydroxyl radicals on DNA is similar to the effects of ionizing radiation.

Azo-procarbazine is further metabolized by microsomal dependent N-hydroxylation or N-dimethylation to form unstable azoxy intermediates. Byproducts of these processes include formaldehyde, carbon dioxide, and methane. An active species, capable of alkylation, is generated from these intermediate compounds. An alternative mechanism of activation involves the formation of monomethyl hydrazine and the ultimate generation of an unstable methyldiazene free radical (Reed, 1974–1975). This metabolic pathway is quantitatively less important. The N-methyl group of procarbazine also selectively methylates the 7 position of guanine and the 1 position of adenine on nucleic acids.

When procarbazine is used as a single agent, resistance rapidly develops. The biochemical mechanisms of resistance are unknown. Procarbazine is not specific for any particular phase of the cell cycle.

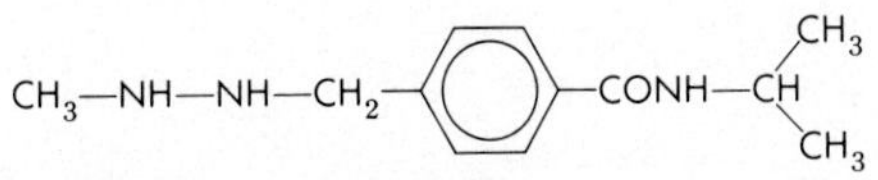

Clinical Pharmacology

Procarbazine may be administered orally or intravenously. The drug is absorbed almost completely from the gastrointestinal tract. Metabolism is rapid. After an intravenous injection, the half-life in plasma is seven minutes. Pretreatment with phenobarbital induces hepatic microsomal enzymes and increases the rate of conversion of procarbazine to the active azo form (Shiba *et al.,* 1979). Procarbazine readily crosses the blood-brain barrier and the concentration in the cerebrospinal fluid is rapidly in equilibrium with the plasma. Approximately 70% of an oral or parenteral dose is excreted in the urine during the first 24 hours after administration. The major excretory product is the inactive metabolite N-isopropylterephthalanic acid.

Clinical Toxicity

Nausea and vomiting occur in 75 to 95% of patients treated with procarbazine. With daily schedules of administration, anorexia is common. Leukopenia and thrombocytopenia are frequently observed.

As many as one-third of patients treated with the oral preparation will experience some manifestations of neurotoxicity. Mechanisms of neurotoxicity include the inhibition of monoamine oxidase and, possibly, decreased levels of pyridoxal phosphate. The administration of pyridoxine, however, does not reverse the neuropathy produced by procarbazine (Weiss *et al.,* 1974). Neurotoxic effects may include altered levels of consciousness, depression, agitation, psychosis, ataxia, and peripheral neuropathy. Even with continuation of therapy, mild symptoms may spontaneously resolve. Other toxic manifestations are reversible only upon discontinuation of the drug. The administration of intravenous procarbazine is associated with a high incidence of severe neurologic toxicities.

Since procarbazine is a weak inhibitor of monoamine oxidase, hypertension may occur if it is used concurrently with sympathomimetic agents, tricyclic antidepressants, or foods with a high content of tyramine. The

Figure 10–27. Procarbazine.

ingestion of alcohol by patients receiving procarbazine may produce symptoms, such as facial flushing, sweating, and headache, that resemble the acetaldehyde syndrome caused by disulfiram. Procarbazine inhibits the cytochrome P450 system. Drugs that are metabolized by hepatic microsomal enzymes have prolonged half-lives in patients who are receiving procarbazine. The sedative effects of phenothiazines, barbiturates, and narcotics are, therefore, potentiated. Patients being treated with procarbazine should be advised to avoid alcohol, foods with a high content of tyramine, such as bananas, cheese, and wine, and medications with the potential for adverse interactions.

A hypersensitivity pneumonitis, characterized by fever, cough, and bilateral interstitial infiltrates, has been associated with procarbazine. Symptoms usually resolve with discontinuation of the drug. Rash is another potential manifestation of hypersensitivity. The appearance of Heinz bodies in erythrocytes and hemolytic anemia have been reported.

Procarbazine is a potent immunosuppressive agent and is also highly teratogenic, mutagenic, and carcinogenic. An increased incidence of second neoplasms, including acute nonlymphocytic leukemia and non-Hodgkin's lymphomas, has been recorded in patients with Hodgkin's disease treated with the MOPP chemotherapy regimen and irradiation. Procarbazine in the MOPP combination is thought to be an important causative agent (see Chapter 19).

Clinical Indications

As a component of the MOPP regimen, procarbazine is useful in the treatment of advanced Hodgkin's disease. Procarbazine is also used to treat lung cancer and brain tumors. Procarbazine is not cross-resistant with the alkylating agents or with other classes of antitumor drugs.

MITOTANE

Toxicologic studies performed on dogs exposed to an insecticide similar to DDT revealed that the adrenal cortex was severely damaged. Mitotane (o, p'-DDD), a derivative of DDT, also causes necrosis and atrophy of the adrenal cortex and is useful in the therapy of neoplasms arising from this tissue (see Figure 10–28).

Biochemical Pharmacology

Mitotane is selectively toxic for normal and neoplastic cells of the adrenal cortex. Mitotane is bound to the mitochondria of adrenocortical cells. After the administration of this drug, the conversion of cholesterol to adrenal cortical steroids is inhibited and the metabolism of cortisol in peripheral tissues is stimulated.

Clinical Pharmacology

After oral administration, 40% of the dose is absorbed. Daily doses of 5 to 15 g produce concentrations in the plasma of 10 to 90 μg/mL of the parent compound and 30 to 50 μg/mL of a metabolite. The drug is concentrated in adipose tissue and detectable levels are present in the plasma six to nine weeks after therapy has been stopped. Approximately 25% of an oral or parenteral dose is excreted in the urine as a water-soluble metabolite. Spironolactone interferes with the adrenal suppression produced by mitotane and these two drugs should not be used together (Wortsman and Soler, 1977).

Clinical Toxicity

Gastrointestinal toxicities, including anorexia, nausea, and vomiting, occur in approximately 80% of patients treated with mitotane. Central nervous system effects, such as lethargy and somnolence, occur in 40%. Patients treated with mitotane should be warned about the possible impairment of their ability to perform tasks that require mental concentration and alertness. Dermatitis occurs in 15 to 20% of patients. These reactions are usually not severe and can be managed by lowering the dose of the drug. Other less common toxic reactions include orthostatic hypotension, proteinuria,

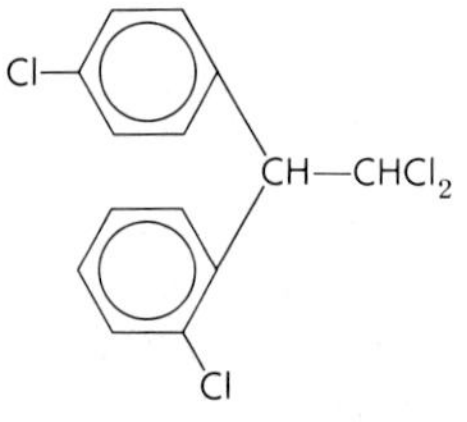

Figure 10–28. Mitotane.

hematuria, visual problems and hypertension. Because this drug damages the adrenal cortex, the administration of adrenocorticosteroids is frequently necessary. If the patient develops evidence of adrenal insufficiency, or in instances of severe trauma or shock, adrenocorticosteroids should be given.

Clinical Indications

Mitotane is useful in the treatment of patients with inoperable, residual, or metastatic adrenocortical carcinoma. The concentration of cortisol in the plasma should be monitored routinely in order to assess the antitumor response and to indicate the need for supplementation with exogenous adrenocorticosteroids. Because antitumor responses may occur only after prolonged therapy, treatment should be continued for a minimum of three months.

HORMONES AND ANTAGONISTS

The growth of certain cancers is influenced by hormones. Tumors that originate in the primary and secondary sex organs are particularly susceptible to hormonal control. Cytoplasmic receptors for several hormones have been identified in neoplastic cells. Receptors are proteins that bind avidly to specific hormones. The hormone-receptor complex undergoes a conformational change and is translocated into the nucleus. After binding to DNA, the complex induces gene transcription and directs the synthesis of specific RNA and protein molecules. The effect of the hormone-receptor complex may also be mediated by inducing fluctuations in the intracellular concentration of cyclic AMP. The measurement of hormone receptors in tumor tissues allows for a more selective and rational use of available endocrine therapies.

The remainder of this chapter will provide a brief summary of the hormones that have proven antitumor activity. For a more detailed discussion of the pharmacology of the hormones, the reader is referred to several comprehensive reviews (Calabresi and Parks, in preparation; Murad and Haynes, 1981). Details pertaining to the selection and use of endocrine therapies are provided in the chapters of this book that deal with specific diseases.

ADRENOCORTICOSTEROIDS

Adrenocorticosteroids have been used for many years in the therapy of advanced neoplasms and for the palliation of specific complications of cancer. The exact mechanisms responsible for the antitumor activity of the corticosteroids are uncertain and may vary among responding tumors. Certain palliative effects may be simply due to reduction of inflammation and tumor-associated edema. Corticosteroids are capable of inducing the synthesis of DNA, RNA, and proteins in tumor cells. The membranes of neoplastic cells may also be affected by corticosteroids. Due to their suppression of the function of the adrenal cortex, corticosteroids reduce the levels of circulating estrogens. In postmenopausal women, therapy with corticosteroids reduces the excretion of estrogen, androsterone, and etiocholanolone. The relationship between estrogen receptor levels and the response of women with breast cancer to therapy with corticosteroids is still unclear. Glucocorticoid receptors have been demonstrated on human breast cancer cells and on the surface of blast cells from patients with acute lymphocytic leukemia. The presence of receptors may help to identify patients who are likely to respond to therapy with glucocorticoids.

The side effects associated with glucocorticoid therapy have been well described and include glucose intolerance, fluid retention, proximal muscle weakness, immunosuppression, cushingoid appearance, increased appetite and weight gain. Lower doses and intermittent schedules of administration reduce the frequency and severity of these and other toxicities.

These drugs are useful in the symptomatic palliation of tumor-associated edema in critical areas such as the central nervous system. Hypercalcemia due to cancer may also respond to the administration of corticosteroids. Prednisone, in combination with cyclophosphamide, methotrexate, and 5-fluorouracil, is effective in the treatment of patients with advanced breast cancer. As a component of the MOPP regimen, prednisone is used to treat patients with Hodgkin's disease.

PROGESTINS

Progestins have been used for the treatment of cancer since the 1950s. Receptors for progesterone have been identified on tumor cells of patients with breast and endometrial cancers. In patients with breast carcinoma, there is a positive correlation between the response to hormonal therapy and the levels of both estrogen and progesterone receptors. In patients with endometrial carcinoma, progestins may act by decreasing the circulating levels of leutinizing hormone, the substance that stimulates endometrial proliferation. Progestational agents may also inhibit the synthesis of both DNA and RNA in tumor cells.

Parenteral and oral preparations are available. Side effects include weight gain, fluid retention, and a cushingoid appearance. Progestational agents are useful in the treatment of patients with advanced breast and endometrial cancers.

ESTROGENS

In 1944, Haddow and associates first reported the antitumor activity of estrogens in women with advanced breast cancer. Estrogens are now widely used in the therapy of postmenopausal women with breast cancer that is estrogen-receptor positive and in men with metastatic carcinoma of the prostate. In breast cancer, the effects of estrogen are dose dependent. At low doses, the growth of the tumor is stimulated. Tumor growth is inhibited, however, when higher, pharmacologic doses of estrogen are utilized.

The availability of the estrogen receptor assay has simplified the task of selecting the appropriate patients with breast cancer for endocrine therapies. The response rate to estrogen therapy in postmenopausal women with estrogen receptor positive tumors is 50 to 75%. Progesterone receptors are also present on a large number of tumors that contain estrogen receptors. The presence of both estrogen and progesterone receptors on breast tumor tissue identifies patients who are most likely to respond to treatment with estrogens. Estrogens inhibit the growth of prostate cancer by antagonizing the effect of endogenous androgens.

The adverse effects of estrogens are dose related. Toxicities may include nausea, vomiting, fluid retention, urinary stress incontinence, thrombophlebitis, thromboembolic disorders, hypertension, and, in men, impotence and gynecomastia. Gynecomastia may be prevented by low-dose irradiation to the breast tissue prior to initating hormone therapy. Women with breast cancer are also susceptible to hypercalcemia and a flare of the neoplastic process. A group of men treated with 5 mg of diethystilbestrol daily suffered a significant excess mortality from cardiac and cerebrovascular accidents (Bailar *et al.,* 1970). The frequency of these complications is significantly reduced at lower doses.

Compounds with estrogenic activity are numerous. Oral diethylstilbesterol and ethinyl estradiol are most commonly used. Estrogens have been conjugated to other chemotherapeutic agents in order to take advantage of the affinity of the estrogen receptor for the hormone. Conjugates such as estradiol mustard and estramustine are now in clinical use.

ANDROGENS

Androgens are useful in the therapy of postmenopausal women with hormone-responsive metastatic breast cancer. Their mechanism of antitumor activity is unclear. Androgens are known to affect the synthesis and function of endogenous estrogens.

Undesirable side effects include virilization, deepening of the voice, changes in libido, fluid retention, cholestatic jaundice, and other hepatic abnormalities such as peliosis hepatis. The degree of virilization is dependent upon the preparation used, the dose, and the duration of treatment. Women with breast cancer metastatic to bone may experience severe hypercalcemia.

Both oral and parenteral preparations are available. Halogenated derivatives of testosterone are absorbed from the gastrointestinal tract but may be hepatoxic. The most commonly used preparations are testosterone propionate, fluoxymesterone, and delta-1-testolactone.

ANTIESTROGENS

TAMOXIFEN

Antiestrogens were initially developed as antifertility drugs. One member of this class of compounds, tamoxifen, has been shown to be an effective and relatively nontoxic agent for the treatment of patients with breast cancer. Tamoxifen must bind to estrogen receptors on the tumor cell to be cytotoxic. The drug functions by competing for estrogen receptor sites and through the suppressive effect of the tamoxifen-receptor complex on the DNA of the tumor cell. Tamoxifen may also interfere with the synthesis of new receptors.

After oral administration, peak plasma concentrations of tamoxifen are present in four to seven hours. There is a biphasic pattern of clearance from the plasma. The initial half-life is seven to 14 hours and the terminal $t_{1/2}$ is longer than seven days. Tamoxifen undergoes extensive metabolic conversion. The monohydroxylated metabolite has more antiestrogenic activity than does the parent compound or the dihydroxylated metabolite. After enterohepatic circulation, glucuronides and other metabolites are excreted in the stool. Excretion in the urine is minimal.

Tamoxifen is almost completely free of side effects. Nausea, vomiting, and fluid retention are rare. Hypercalcemia, flare of the neoplastic process, and a mild, transient thrombocytopenia may occur. Menstrual irregularities, vaginal bleeding, and dermatitis have been reported.

Tamoxifen is useful in the palliative treatment of advanced carcinoma of the breast in postmenopausal women. Premenopausal women with estrogen receptor positive tumors may also respond.

Nafoxidine and clomiphene are other antiestrogens that have been evaluated in patients with metastatic breast cancer. Both of these drugs are more toxic than tamoxifen and appear not to offer any therapeutic advantage.

REFERENCES

Adamson, I. Y. R., and Bowden, D. H.: The pathogenesis of bleomycin-induced pulmonary fibrosis in mice. *Am. J. Pathol.,* **77**:185–198, 1974.

Adolphe, A. B.; Glasofer, E. D.; Troetel, W. M.; Ziegenfuss, J.; Stambaugh, J. E.; Weiss, A. J.; and Manthei,

R. W.: Fate of streptozotocin (NSC-85998) in patients with advanced cancer. *Cancer Chemother. Rep.,* **59**:547–556, 1975.

Ahmad, S.; Shen, F.; and Bleyer, W. A.: Methotrexate-induced renal failure and ineffectiveness of peritoneal dialysis. *Arch. Intern. Med.,* **138**:1146–1147, 1978.

Ahr, D. J.; Scialla, S. J.; and Kimball, D. B., Jr.: Acquired platelet dysfunction following mithramycin therapy. *Cancer,* **41**:448–454, 1978.

Alberts, D. S.; Chang, S. Y.; Chen, H.-S.; Gross, J. F.; Walson, P. D.; Moon, T. E.; and Salmon, S. E.: Variability of melphalan (M) absorption in man. *Proc. Am. Soc. Clin. Oncol.,* **19**:334, 1978.

Alberts, D. S.; Chang, S. Y.; Chen, H.-S.; Larcom, B. J.; and Jones, S. E.: Pharmacokinetics and metabolism of chlorambucil in man: A preliminary report. *Cancer Treat. Rev.,* 6, 9, 1979a.

Alberts, D. S.; Chen, H.-S. G.; Liu, R.; Himmelstein, K. J.; Mayersohn, M.; Perrier, D.; Gross, J.; Moon, T.; Broughton, A.; and Salmon, S. E.: Bleomycin pharmacokinetics in man. I. Intravenous administration. *Cancer Chemother. Pharmacol.,* **1**:177–181, 1978.

Alberts, D. S.; Chen, H.-S. G.; Mayersohn, M.; Perrier, D.; Moon, T. E.; and Gross, J. F.: Bleomycin pharmacokinetics in man. II. Intracavitary administration. *Cancer Chemother. Pharmacol.,* **2**:127–132, 1979b.

Alexander, J.; Dainiak, N.; Berger, H. J.; Goldman, L.; Johnstone, D.; Reduto, L.; Duffy, T.; Schwartz, P.; Gottschalk, A.; and Zaret, B. L.: Serial assessment of doxorubicin cardiotoxicity with quantitative radionuclide angiocardiography. *N. Engl. J. Med.,* **300**:278–283, 1979.

Ali, M. K.; Soto, A.; Maroongroge, D.; Bekheit-Saad, S.; Buzdar, A. U.; Blumenschein, G. R.; Hortobagyi, G. N.; Tashima, C. K.; Wiseman, C. L.; and Shullenberger, C. C.: Electrocardiographic changes after adriamycin chemotherapy. *Cancer,* **43**:465–471, 1979.

Allen, L. M., and Creaven, P. J.: Comparison of the human pharmacokinetics of VM-26 and VP-16, two antineoplastic epipodophyllotoxin glucopyranoside derivatives. *Eur. J. Cancer,* **11**:697–707, 1975.

Allen, S. C.; Riddell, G. S.; and Butchart, E. G.: Bleomycin therapy and anaesthesia: The possible hazards of oxygen administration to patients after treatment with bleomycin. *Anaesthesia,* **36**:60–63, 1981.

Alt, F. W.; Kellems, R. E.; Bertino, J. R.; and Schimke, R. T.: Selective multiplication of dihydrofolate reductase genes in methotrexate-resistant variants of cultured murine cells. *J. Biol. Chem.,* **253**:1357–1370, 1978.

Anderson, T.; Schein, P. S.; McMenamin, M.; Cooney, D. A.: Streptozotocin diabetes: Correlation with extent of depression and pancreatic islet nicotinamide adenine dinucleotide. *J. Clin. Invest.,* **54**:672–677, 1974.

Anderson, T.; McMenamin, M. G.; and Schein, P. S.: Chlorozotocin, 2-[3-(2-chloroethyl)-3-nitrosoureido]-D-glucopyranose, an antitumor agent with modified bone marrow toxicity. *Cancer Res.,* **35**:761–765, 1975.

Arcamone, F.; Cassinelli, G.; Franceschi, G.; Penco, S.; Pol, C.; Redaelli, S.; and Selva, A.: Structure and physicochemical properties of adriamycin (doxorubicin). In Carter, S. K.; Di Marco, A.; Ghione, M.; Krakoff, I. H.; and Mathé, G. (eds.): *International Symposium on Adriamycin.* Springer-Verlag New York, Inc., New York, 1972.

Arena, E.; d'Alessandro, N.; Dusonchet, L.; Gebbia, N.; Gerbasi, F.; Palazzoadriano, M.; Raineri, A.; Rausa, L.; and Tubaro, E.: Analysis of the pharmacokinetic characteristics, pharmacological and chemotherapeutic activity of 14-hydroxy-daunomycin (adriamycin), a new drug endowed with an antitumour activity. *Arzneimittelforsch.,* **21:**1258–1263, 1971.

Aristizabal, S. A.; Miller, R. C.; Schlichtemeier, A. L.; Jones, S. E.; and Boone, M. L. M.: Adriamycin-irradiation cutaneous complications. *Int. J. Radiat. Oncol. Biol. Phys.,* **2:**325–331, 1977.

Asakura, H.; Hori, M.; and Umezawa, H.: Characterization of bleomycin action on DNA. *J. Antibiot.* (Tokyo), **28:**537–542, 1975.

Ayusawa, D.; Iwata, K.; and Seno, T.: Unusual sensitivity to bleomycin and joint resistance to 9-*β*-D-arabionofuranosyladenine and 1-*β*-D-arabinofuranosylcytosine of mouse FM3A cell mutants with altered ribonucleotide reductase and thymidylate synthase. *Cancer Res.,* **43:**814–818, 1983.

Ayusawa, D.; Koyama, H.; and Seno, T.: Resistance to methotrexate in thymidylate synthetase-deficient mutants of cultured mouse mammary tumor FM3A cells. *Cancer Res.,* **41:**1497–1501, 1981.

Bachur, N. R.: Adriamycin (NSC-123127) pharmacology. *Cancer Chemother. Rep.,* **6:**153–158, 1975.

Bagley, C. M., Jr.; Bostick, F. W.; and DeVita, V. T., Jr.: Clinical pharmacology of cyclophosphamide. *Cancer Res.,* **33:**226–233, 1973.

Bailer, J. C.; Byar, D. P.; Veterans Administration Cooperative Urological Research Group: Estrogen treatment for cancer of the prostate: Early results with 3 doses of diethylstilbesterol and placebo. *Cancer,* **26:**257–261. 1970.

Balcerzak, S. P.; Christakis, J.; Lewis, R. P.; Olson, H. M.; and Malspeis, L.: Systolic time intervals in monitoring adriamycin-induced cardiotoxicity. *Cancer Treat. Rep.,* **62:**893–899, 1978.

Ball, C. R., and Connors, T. A.: Reduction of the toxicity of "radiomimetic" alkylating agents by thiol pretreatment—VI. The mechanism of protection by cysteine. *Biochem. Pharmacol.,* **16:**509–519, 1967.

Bannister, S. J.; Sternson, L. A.; and Repta, A. J.: Urine analysis of platinum species derived from *cis*-dichlorodiammineplatinum (II) by high-performance liquid chromatography following derivatization with sodium diethyldithiocarbamate. *J. Chromatogr.,* **173:**333–342, 1979.

Bannister, S. J.; Sternson, L. A.; Repta, A. J.; and James, G. W.: Measurement of free-circulating *cis*-dichlorodiammineplatinum (II) in plasma. *Clin. Chem.,* **12:**2258–2262, 1977.

Bannon, P., and Verly, W.: Alkylation of phosphates and stability of phosphate triesters in DNA. *Eur. J. Biochem.,* **31:**103–111, 1972.

Bareham, C. R.; Griswold, D. E.; and Calabresi, P.: Synergism of methotrexate with Imuran and with 5-fluorouracil and their effects on hemolysin plaque-forming cell production in the mouse. *Cancer Res.,* **34:**571–575, 1974.

Barlock, A. L.; Howser, D. M.; and Hubbard, S. M.: Nursing management of adriamycin extravasation. *Am. J. Nurs.,* **79:**94–96, 1979.

Barranco, S. C., and Humphrey, R. M.: The relevance of *in vitro* survival and cell cycle kinetics data to the clinical use of bleomycin. *Gann Monogr. Cancer Res.,* **19:**83–96, 1976.

Becher, R.; Schütt, P.; Osieka, R.; and Schmidt, C. G.: Peripheral neuropathy and ophthalmologic toxicity after treatment with *cis*-dichlorodiammineplatinum II. *J. Cancer Res. Clin. Oncol.,* **96:**219–221, 1980.

Belt, R. J.; Himmelstein, K. J.; Patton, T. F.; Bannister, S. J.; Sternson, L. A.; and Repta, A. J.: Pharmacoki-

netics of non-protein-bound platinum species following administration of *cis*-dichlorodiammineplatinum(II). *Cancer Treat. Rep.,* **63:**1515–1521, 1979.

Benjamin, R. S.: Clinical pharmacology of daunorubicin. *Cancer Treat. Rep.,* **65(Suppl. 4):**109–110, 1981.

Benjamin, R. S.; Ewer, M. S.; MacKay, B.; Ali, M. K.; Legha, S. S.; and Valdivieso, M.: An endomyocardial biopsy study of anthracycline-induced cardiomyopathy—detection, reversibility and potential amelioration. *Proc. Am. Soc. Clin. Oncol.,* **20:**372, 1979.

Benjamin, R.; Legha, S.; MacKay, B.; Ewer, M.; Wallace, S.; Valdivieso, M.; Rasmussen, S.; Blumenschein, G.; and Freireich, E.: Reduction of adriamycin cardiac toxicity using a prolonged intravenous infusion. *Proc. Am. Assoc. Cancer Res.,* **22:**179, 1981.

Bennett, J. M., and Reich, S. D.: Bleomycin. *Ann. Intern. Med.,* **90:**945–948, 1979.

Benz, C.; Tillis, T.; Tattelman, E.; and Cadman, E.: Optimal scheduling of methotrexate and 5-fluorouracil in human breast cancer. *Cancer Res.,* **42:**2081–2086, 1982.

Bhuyan, B. K.; Kuentzel, S. L.; Gray, L. G.; Fraser, T. J.; Wallach, D.; and Neil, G. L.: Tissue distribution of streptozotocin (NSC-85998). *Cancer Chemother. Rep.,* **58:**157–165, 1974.

Biedler, J. L., and Spengler, B. A.: Metaphase chromosome anomaly: Association with drug resistance and cell-specific products. *Science,* **191:**185–187, 1976.

Billingham, M. E.; Mason, J. W.; Bristow, M. R.; and Daniels, J. R.: Anthracycline cardiomyopathy monitored by morphologic changes. *Cancer Treat. Rep.,* **62:**865–872, 1978.

Bleyer, W. A.: The clinical pharmacology of methotrexate: New applications of an old drug. *Cancer,* **41:**36–51, 1978.

Blum, R. H., and Carter, S. K.: Adriamycin: A new anticancer drug with significant clinical activity. *Ann. Intern. Med.,* **80:**249–259, 1974.

Boice, C. R.; Freedman, R. S.; Herson, J.; Wharton, J. T.; and Rutledge, F. N.: Bleomycin and mitomycin-C (BLM-M) in recurrent squamous uterine cervical carcinoma. *Cancer,* **49:**2242–2245, 1982.

Boice, J. D.; Greene, M. H.; Killen, J. Y.; Ellenberg, S. S.; Keehn, R. J.; McFadden, E.; Chen, T. T.; and Fraumeni, J. F.: Leukemia and preleukemia after adjuvant treatment of gastrointestinal cancer with semustine (methyl-CCNU). *N. Engl. J. Med.,* **309:**1079–1084, 1983.

Bonfante, V.; Ferrari, L.; Villari, F.; and Bonadonna, G.: Phase I study of 4-demethoxydaunorubicin. *Invest. New Drugs,* **1:**161–168, 1983.

Bourke, R. S.; West, C. R.; Chheda, G.; and Tower, D. B.: Kinetics of entry and distribution of 5-fluorouracil in cerebrospinal fluid and brain following intravenous injection in a primate. *Cancer Res.,* **33:**1735–1746, 1973.

Boyles, P. W.: Interstitial pulmonary fibrosis after long term busulfan therapy. *Clin. Med.,* **76:**11–13, 1971.

Bracken, R. B.; Johnson, D. E.; Rodriquez, L; Samuels, M. L.; and Ayala, A.: Treatment of multiple superficial tumors of bladder with intravesical bleomycin. *Urology,* **9:**161–163, 1977.

Bristow, M. R.; Thompson, P. D.; Martin, R. P.; Mason, J. W.; Billingham, M. E.; and Harrison, D. C.: Early anthracycline cardiotoxicity. *Am. J. Med.,* **65:**823–832, 1978.

Brockman, R. W.: Resistance to purine analogs. Clinical Pharmacology Symposium. *Biochem. Pharmacol.* **23(Suppl. 2):**107–117, 1974.

Brookes, P., and Lawley, P. D.: The reaction of mono- and

di-functional alkylating agents with nucleic acids. *Biochem. J.,* **80:**496–503, 1961.

Broome, J. D.: Evidence that the L-asparaginase of guinea pig serum is responsible for its antilymphoma effects. I. Properties of the L-asparaginase of guinea pig serum in relation to those of the antilymphoma substance. *J. Exp. Med.,* **118:**99–120, 1963.

Broome, J. D.: L-Asparginase: Discovery and development as a tumor-inhibitory agent. *Cancer Treat. Rep.,* **65(Suppl. 4):**111–114, 1981.

Broughton, A.; Strong, J. E.; Holoye, P. Y.; and Bedrossian, C. W. M.: Clinical pharmacology of bleomycin following intravenous infusion as determined by radioimmunoassay. *Cancer,* **40:**2772–2778, 1977.

Browman, G. P.: Comparison of thymidine and folinic acid protection from methotrexate toxicity in human lymphoid cell lines. *Cancer Treat. Rep.,* **66:**2051–2059, 1982.

Brown, L. D.; Reimer, R. R.; Ahmad, M.; and Hewlett, J. S.: Successful treatment of bleomycin lung. *Cleve. Clin. Q.,* **47:**97–100, 1980.

Brundrett, R. B., and Colvin, M.: Chemistry of nitrosoureas. Decomposition of 1,3-bis(threo-3-chloro-2-butyl)-1-nitrosourea and 1,3-bis(erythro-3-chloro-2-butyl)-1-nitrosourea. *J. Org. Chem.,* **42:**3538–3541, 1977.

Bullen, B. R.; Giles, G. R.; Malhotra, A.; Bird, G. G.; Hall, R.; Bunch, G. A.; and Brown, G. J. A.: Randomized comparison of melphalan and 5-fluorouracil in the treatment of advanced gastrointestinal cancer. *Cancer Treat. Rep.,* **60:**1267–1271, 1976.

Cadman, E.; Grant, S.; Lehman, C.; and Rauscher, F., III: The modulation of cytosine arabinoside metabolism and cytotoxicity by altering deoxythymidine triphosphate levels. In Tattersall, M. H. N., and Fox, R. M. (eds.): *Nucleosides and Cancer Treatment: Rational Approaches to Antimetabolite Selectivity and Modulation.* Academic Press, Sydney, 1981.

Calabresi, P.: New techniques for measuring the effects of chemotherapeutic agents upon neoplastic and normal host cells. *Verlag Wien. Med. Akad.,* **7:**99–111, 1967.

Calabresi, P.: Principles of oncologic treatment: Irradiation, cytotoxic drugs, and immunostimulatory procedures. In Beeson, P. B.; McDermott, W.; Wyngaarden, J. B. (eds.): *Textbook of Medicine.* W. B. Saunders, Philadelphia, 1979.

Calabresi, P.: Leukemia after cytotoxic chemotherapy—A pyrrhic victory? *N. Engl. J. Med.,* **309:**1118–1119, 1983.

Calabresi, P., and Parks, R. E., Jr.: Antiproliferative agents and drugs used for immunosuppression. In Gilman, A. G.; Goodman, L. S.; and Gilman, A. (eds.): *The Pharmacological Basis of Therapeutics,* 6th ed. Macmillan Publishing Co., Inc., New York, 1980.

Calabresi, P., and Parks, R. E., Jr.: Antiproliferative agents and drugs used for immunosuppression. In Gilman, A. G.; Goodman, L. S.; Rall, T. W.; and Murad, F. (eds.): *Goodman and Gilman's The Pharmacological Basis of Therapeutics,* 7th ed. Macmillan Publishing Co., New York, 1985.

Calabro-Jones, P. M.; Byfield, J. E.; Ward, J. F.; and Sharp, T. R.: Time-dose relationships for 5-fluorouracil cytotoxicity against human epithelial cancer cells *in vitro. Cancer Res.,* **42:**4413–4420, 1982.

Capizzi, R. L.: Asparaginase-methotrexate in combination chemotherapy: Schedule-dependent differential effects on normal versus neoplastic cells. *Cancer Treat. Rep.,* **65(Suppl. 4):**115–121, 1981.

Carpentieri, V., and Balch, M. T.: Hyperglycemia asso-

ciated with the therapeutic use of L-asparaginase: Possible role of insulin receptors. *J. Pediatr.,* **93:**775–778, 1978.

Carter, S. K. (ed.): Proceedings of the seventh new drug seminar on the nitrosoureas (Washington, DC, December 15–16, 1975). *Cancer Treat. Rep.,* **60:**645–811, 1976.

Cass, C. E.; Selner, M.; Tan, T. H.; Muhs, W. H.; and Robins, M. J.: Comparison of the effects on cultured L1210 leukemia cells of the ribosyl, 2'-deoxyribosyl, and xylosyl homologs of tubercidin and adenosine alone or in combination with 2'-deoxycoformycin. *Cancer Treat. Rep.,* **66:**317–326, 1982.

Castaigne, S.; Daniel, M. T.; Tilly, H.; Herait, P.; and Degos, L.: Does treatment with ARA-C in low dosage cause differentiation of leukemic cells? *Blood,* **62:**85–86, 1983.

Chabner, B. A.: DTIC (dacarbazine), In Chabner, B. (ed.): *Pharmacologic Principles of Cancer Treatment.* W. B. Saunders, Philadelphia, 1982.

Chabner, B. A.; Donehower, R. C.; and Schilsky, R. L.: Clinical pharmacology of methotrexate. *Cancer Treat. Rep.,* **65(Suppl. 1):**51–54, 1981.

Chabner, B. A., and Young, R. C.: Threshold methotrexate concentration for *in vivo* inhibition of DNA synthesis in normal and tumorous target tissues. *J. Clin. Invest.,* **52:**1804–1811, 1973.

Chan, K. K.; Cohen, J. L.; Gross, J. F.; Himmelstein, K. J.; Bateman, J. R.; Tsu-Lee, Y.; and Marlis, A. S.: Prediction of adriamycin disposition in cancer patients using a physiologic, pharmacokinetic model. *Cancer Treat. Rep.,* **62:**1161–1171, 1978.

Cheng, E.; Woodcock, T.; Young, C.; and Golbey, R.: Enhanced neurotoxicity of 5 fluorouracil (FU) by thymidine (TdR). *Proc. Am. Assoc. Cancer Res.,* **21:**350, 1980.

Chirigos, M. A.; Humphreys, S. R.; and Goldin, A.: Duration of effective levels of three antitumor drugs in mice with leukemia L1210 implanted intracerebrally and subcutaneously. *Cancer Chemother. Rep.,* **49:**15–19, 1965.

Chlebowski, R. R.; Paroly, W. S.; Pugh, R. P.; Hueser, J.; Jacobs, E. M.; Pajak, T. F.; and Bateman, J. R.: Adriamycin given as a weekly schedule without a loading course: Clinically effective with reduced incidence of cardiotoxicity. *Cancer Treat. Rep.,* **64:**47–51, 1980.

Christman, J. K.; Mendelsohn, N.; Herzog, D.; and Schneiderman, N.: Effect of 5-azacytidine on differentiation and DNA methylation in human promyelocytic leukemia cells (HL-60). *Cancer Res.,* **43:**763–769, 1983.

Chu, M.-Y.: Incorporation of arabinosyl cytosine into 2-7S ribonucleic acid and cell death. *Biochem. Pharmacol.,* **20:**2057–2063, 1971.

Čihák, A.: Biological effects of 5-azacytidine in eukaryotes: A review. *Oncology,* **30:**405–422, 1979.

Clarkson, J. M., and Humphrey, R. M.: The significance of DNA damage in the cell cycle sensitivity of Chinese hamster ovary cells to bleomycin. *Cancer Res.,* **36:**2345–2349, 1976.

Cline, M. J.: Effect of vincristine on synthesis of ribonucleic acid and protein in leukaemic leucocytes. *Br. J. Haematol.,* **14:**21–30, 1968.

Cohen, G. L.; Bauer, W. R.; Barton, J. K.; and Lippard, S. J.: Binding of *cis-* and *trans-*dichlorodiammineplatinum (II) to DNA: Evidence for unwinding and shortening of the double helix. *Science,* **203:**1014–1016, 1979.

Coleman, C. N.; Johns, D. G.; and Chabner, B. A.: Studies

on mechanisms of resistance to cytosine arabinoside: Problems in the determination of related enzyme activities in leukemic cells. *Ann. N.Y. Acad. Sci.,* **255**:247–251, 1975.

Collis, C. H.: Lung damage from cytotoxic drugs. *Cancer Chemother. Pharmacol.,* **4**:17–27, 1980.

Colvin, M.: The alkylating agents. In Chabner, B. (ed.): *Pharmacologic Principles of Cancer Treatment.* W. B. Saunders, Philadelphia, 1982.

Comis, R. L.; Kuppinger, M. S.; Ginsberg, S. J.; Crooke, S. T.; Gilbert, R.; Auchincloss, J. H.; and Prestayko, A. W.: Role of single-breath carbon monoxide-diffusing capacity in monitoring the pulmonary effects of bleomycin in germ cell tumor patients. *Cancer Res.,* **39**:5076–5080, 1979.

Cooper, K. R., and Hong, W. K.: Prospective study of the pulmonary toxicity of continuously infused bleomycin. *Cancer Treat. Rep.,* **65**:419–425, 1981.

Cortes, E. P.; Gupta, M.; Chou, C.; Amin, V. C.; and Folkers, K.: Adriamycin cardiotoxicity: Early detection by systolic time interval and possible prevention by coenzyme Q10. *Cancer Treat. Rep.,* **62**:887–891, 1978.

Counts, D. F.; Evans, J. N.; DiPetrillo, T. A.; Sterling, K. M., Jr.; and Kelley, J.: Collagen lysyl oxidase activity in the lung increases during bleomycin-induced lung fibrosis. *J. Pharmacol. Exp. Ther.,* **219**:675–678, 1981.

Cowan, J. D.; Kies, M. S.; Roth, J. L.; and Joyce, R. P.: Nerve conduction studies in patients treated with *cis*-diamminedichloroplatinum (II): A preliminary report. *Cancer Treat. Rep.,* **64**:1119–1122, 1980.

Craft, A. W.; Rankin, A.; and Aherne, W.: Methotrexate absorption in children with acute lymphoblastic leukemia. *Cancer Treat. Rep.,* **65(Suppl. 1)**:77–81, 1981.

Creasey, W. A.: *Vinca* alkaloids and colchicine. In Sartorelli, A. C., and Johns, D. G. (eds.): *Antineoplastic and Immunosuppressive Agents, Pt. II* (Handbook of Experimental Pharmacology, New Series, Vol. 38/2). Springer-Verlag, Berlin, 1974–1975.

Creasey, W. A.: *Vinca* alkaloids. In Brodsky, I.; Kahn, S. B.; and Conroy, J. F. (eds.): *Cancer Chemotherapy III.* Grune & Stratton, Inc., New York, 1978.

Crooke, S. T.: Bleomycin: A brief review. In Carter, S. K.; Crooke, S. T.; and Umezawa, H. (eds.): *Bleomycin: Current Status and New Developments.* Academic Press, New York, 1978.

Crooke, S. T., and Bradner, W. T.: Bleomycin, a review. *J. Med.,* **7**:333–428, 1976.

Crooke, S. T.; Comis, R. L.; Einhorn, L. H.; Strong, J. E.; Broughton, A.; and Prestayko, A. W.: Effect of variations in renal function on the clinical pharmacology of bleomycin administered as an iv bolus. *Cancer Treat. Rep.,* **61**:1631–1636, 1977.

Crooke, S. T.; Duvernay, V. H.; Galvan, L.; and Prestayko, A. W.: Structure-activity relationships of anthracyclines relative to effects on macromolecular syntheses. *Mol. Pharmacol.,* **14**:290–298, 1978.

Crooke, S. T.; Einhorn, L. H.; Comis, R. L.; D'Aoust, J. C.; and Prestayko, A. W.: The effects of prior exposure to bleomycin on the incidence of pulmonary toxicities in a group of patients with disseminated testicular carcinomas. *Med. Pediatr. Oncol.,* **5**:93–98, 1978.

Crooke, S. T.; Luft, F.; Broughton, A.; Strong, J.; Casson, K.; and Einhorn, L.: Bleomycin serum pharmacokinetics as determined by a radioimmunoassay and a microbiologic assay in a patient with compromised renal function. *Cancer,* **39**:1430–1434, 1977.

Curt, G. A.; Carney, D. N.; Cowan, K. H.; Jolivet, J.; Bailey, B. D.; Drake, J. C.; Kao-Shan, C. S.; Minna,

J. D.; and Chabner, B. A.: Unstable methotrexate resistance in human small-cell carcinoma associated with double minute chromosomes. *N. Engl. J. Med.,* **308**:199–202, 1983.

Cvitkovic, E.; Spaulding, J.; Bethune, V.; Martin, J.; and Whitmore, W. F.: Improvement of *cis*-dichlorodiammineplatinum (NSC 119875): Therapeutic index in an animal model. *Cancer,* **39**:1357–1361, 1977.

Dan, K.: Development of resistance to daunomycin (NSC-82151) in Ehrlich ascites tumor. *Cancer Chemother. Rep.,* **55**:133–141, 1971.

Daskal, Y.; Woodard, C.; Crooke, S. T.; and Busch, H.: Comparative ultrastructural studies on nucleoli of tumor cells treated with adriamycin and the newer anthracyclines, carminomycin and marcellomycin. *Cancer Res.,* **38**:467–473, 1978.

Dean, J. C.; Salmon, S. E.; and Griffith, K. S.: Prevention of doxorubicin-induced hair loss with scalp hypothermia. *N. Engl. J. Med.,* **301**:1427–1429, 1979.

DeConti, R. C.; Toftness, B. R.; Lange, R. C.; and Creasey, W. A.: Clinical and pharmacological studies with *cis*-diamminedichloroplatinum (II). *Cancer Res.,* **33**:1310–1315, 1973.

DeFronzo, R. A.; Braine, H.; Colvin, O. M.; and Davis, P. J.: Water intoxication in man after cyclophosphamide therapy. *Ann. Intern. Med.,* **78**:861–869, 1973.

Dentino, M.; Luft, F. C.; Yum, M. N.; Williams, S. D.; and Einhorn, L. H.: Long term effect of *cis*-diamminedichloride platinum (CDDP) on renal function and structure in man. *Cancer,* **41**:1274–1281. 1978.

DeVita, V. T.; Carbone, P. P.; Owens, A. H., Jr.; Gold, G. L.; Krant, M. J.; and Edmonson, J.: Clinical trials with 1,3-bis(2-chloroethyl)-1-nitrosourea, NSC-409962. *Cancer Res.,* **25**:1876–1881, 1965.

DeVita, V. T.; Denham, C.; Davidson, J. D.; and Oliverio, V. T.: The physiological disposition of the carcinostatic 1,3-bis(2-chloroethyl)-1-nitrosourea (BCNU) in man and animals. *Clin. Pharmacol. Ther.,* **8**:566–577, 1967.

DiBella, N. J.: Vincristine-induced orthostatic hypotension: A prospective clinical study. *Cancer Treat. Rep.,* **64**:359–360, 1980.

DiMarco, A.: Adriamycin (NSC-123127): Mode and mechanism of action. *Cancer Chemother. Rep.,* **6**:91–106, 1975.

Donaldson, S. S., and Lenon, R. A.: Alterations of nutritional status: Impact of chemotherapy and radiation therapy. *Cancer,* **43**:2036–2052, 1979.

Doroshow, J. H.; Locker, G. Y.; and Myers, C. E.: Enzymatic defenses of the mouse heart against reactive oxygen metabolites: Alterations produced by doxorubicin. *J. Clin. Invest.,* **65**:128–135, 1980.

Drewinko, B., and Barlogie, B.: Survival and cycle-progression delay of human lymphoma cells *in vitro* exposed to VP-16-213. *Cancer Treat. Rep.,* **60**:1295–1306, 1976.

Drewinko, B.; Brown, B. W.; and Gottlieb, J. A.: The effect of *cis*-diamminedichloroplatinum(II) on cultured human lymphoma cells and its therapeutic implications. *Cancer Res.,* **33**:3091–3095, 1973.

Driscoll, J. S.; Hazard, G. F., Jr.; Wood, H. B., Jr.; and Goldin, A.: Structure-antitumor activity relationships among quinone derivatives. *Cancer Chemother. Rep.,* **4**:1–362, 1974.

Egorin, M. J.; Hildebrand, R. C.; Cimino, E. F.; and Bachur, N. R.: Cytofluorescence localization of adriamycin and daunorubicin. *Cancer Res.,* **34**:2243–2245, 1974.

Einhorn, M., and Davidsohn, I.: Hepatotoxicity of mercaptopurine. *J.A.M.A.*, **188**:802–806, 1964.

Elion, G. B.: Biochemistry and pharmacology of purine analogues. *Fed. Proc.*, **26**:898–904, 1967.

Ervin, T. J.; Weichselbaum, R.; Miller, D.; Meshad, M.; Posner, M.; and Fabian, R.: Treatment of advanced squamous cell carcinoma of the head and neck with cisplatin, bleomycin, and methotrexate (PBM). *Cancer Treat. Rep.*, **65**:787–791, 1981.

Ferrans, V. J.: Overview of cardiac pathology in relation to anthracycline cardiotoxicity. *Cancer Treat. Rep.*, **62**:955–961, 1978.

Field, R. B.; Gang, M.; Kline, I.; Venditti, J. M.; and Waravdekar, V. S.: The effect of phenobarbital or 2-diethylaminoethyl-2,2-diphenylvalerate on the activation of cyclophosphamide *in vivo*. *J. Pharmacol. Exp. Ther.*, **180**:475–483, 1972.

Filipski, J.; Kohn, K. W.; Prather, R; and Bonner, W. M.: Thiourea reverses cross-links and restores biological activity in DNA treated with dichlorodiammino-platinum(II). *Science*, **204**:181–183, 1979.

Fisher, B.; Carbone, P.; Economou, S. G.; Frelick, R.; Glass, A.; Lerner, H.; Redmond, C.; Zelen, M.; Band, P.; Katrych, D. L.; Wolmark, N.; Fisher, E. R.; and other cooperating investigators: L-Phenylalanine mustard (L-PAM) in the management of primary breast cancer: A report of early findings. *N. Engl. J. Med.*, **292**:117–122, 1975.

Fox, B. W., and Lajtha, L. G.: Radiation damage and repair phenomena. *Br. Med. Bull.*, **29**:16–22, 1973.

Fraile, R. J.; Baker, L. H.; Buroker, T. R.; Horwitz, J.; and Vaitkevicius, V. K.: Pharmacokinetics of 5-fluorouracil administered orally, by rapid intravenous and by slow infusion. *Cancer Res.*, **40**:2223–2228, 1980.

Frei, E., III: The clinical use of actinomycin. *Cancer Chemother. Rep.*, **58**:49–54, 1974.

Frick, G. A.; Ballentine, R.; Driever, C. W.; and Kramer, W. G.: Renal excretion kinetics of high dose *cis*-dichlorodiammineplatinum (II) administered with hydration and mannitol diuresis. *Cancer Treat. Rep.*, **63**:13–16, 1979.

Friedman, M. J.; Ewy, G. A.; Jones, S. E.; Cruze, D.; and Moon, T. E.: 1-Year followup of cardiac status after adriamycin therapy. *Cancer Treat. Rep.*, **63**:1809–1816, 1979.

Fry, D. W.; Yalowich, J. C.; and Goldman, I. D.: Rapid formation of poly-γ-glutamyl derivatives of methotrexate and their association with dihydrofolate reductase as assessed by high pressure liquid chromatography in the Ehrlich ascites tumor cell *in vitro*. *J. Biol. Chem.*, **257**:1890–1896, 1982.

Fujita, H.: Comparative studies on the blood level, tissue distribution, excretion and inactivation of anticancer drugs. *Jpn. J. Clin. Oncol.*, **12**:151–162, 1971.

Furner, R. L., and Brown, R. K.: L-Phenylalanine mustard (L-PAM): The first 25 years. *Cancer Treat. Rep.*, **64**:559–574, 1980.

Galivan, J., and Nimec, Z.: Effects of folinic acid on hepatoma cells containing methotrexate polyglutamates. *Cancer Res.*, **43**:551–555, 1983.

Garnick, M. B.; Ensminger, W. D.; and Israel, M.: A clinical-pharmacological evaluation of hepatic arterial infusion of adriamycin. *Cancer Res.*, **39**:4105–4110, 1979.

Gause, G. F.; Brazhnikova, M. G.; and Shorin, V. A.: A new antitumor antibiotic, carminomycin (NSC-180024). *Cancer Chemother. Rep.*, **58**:255–256, 1974.

Gilladoga, A. C.; Manuel, C.; Tan, C. C.; Wollner, N.; and

Murphy, M. L.: Cardiotoxicity of adriamycin (NSC-123127) in children. *Cancer Chemother. Rep.*, **6**:209–214, 1975.

Gilman, A.: The initial clinical trial of nitrogen mustard. *Am. J. Surg.*, **105**:574–578, 1963.

Ginsberg, S. J., and Comis, R. L.: The pulmonary toxicity of antineoplastic agents. *Semin. Oncol.*, **9**:34–51, 1982.

Goldenberg, G. J.: The role of drug transport in resistance to nitrogen mustard and other alkylating agents in L5178Y lymphoblasts. *Cancer Res.*, **35**:1687–1692, 1975.

Goldenberg, G. J.; Vanstone, C. L.; Israels, L. G.; Ilse, D.; and Bihler, I.: Evidence for a transport carrier of nitrogen mustard in nitrogen mustard-sensitive and -resistant L5178Y lymphoblasts. *Cancer Res.*, **30**:2285–2291, 1970.

Goldman, D.; Bowen, D.; and Gewirtz, D. A.: Some considerations in the experimental approach to distinguishing between membrane transport and intracellular disposition of antineoplastic agents, with specific reference to fluorodeoxyuridine, actinomycin D, and methotrexate. *Cancer Treat. Rep.*, **65(Suppl. 3)**:43–56, 1981.

Goldstein, M. N.; Hamm, K.; and Amrod, E.: Incorporation of tritiated actinomycin D into drug-sensitive and drug-resistant HeLa cells. *Science*, **151**:1555–1556, 1966.

Gonsalvez, M.; Blanco, M.; Hunter, J.; Miko, M.; and Chance, B.: Effects of anticancer agents on the respiration of isolated mitochondria and tumor cells. *Eur. J. Cancer*, **10**:567–574, 1974.

Gonzalez-Vitale, J. C.; Hayes, D. M.; Cvitkovic, E.; and Sternberg, S. S.: The renal pathology in clinical trials of *cis*-platinum (II) diamminedichloride. *Cancer*, **39**:1362–1371, 1977.

Gonzalez-Vitale, J. C.; Hayes, D. M.; Cvitkovic, E.; and Sternberg, S. S.: Acute renal failure after *cis*-dichlorodiammineplatinum (II) and gentamicin-cephalothin therapies. *Cancer Treat. Rep.*, **62**:693–698, 1978.

Gormley, P. E.; Bull, J. M.; LeRoy, A. F.; and Cysyk, R.: Kinetics of *cis*-dichlorodiammineplatinum. *Clin. Pharmacol. Ther.*, **25**:351–357, 1979.

Gottdiener, J. S.; Appelbaum, F. R.; Ferrans, V. J.; Deisseroth, A.; and Ziegler, J.: Cardiotoxicity associated with high-dose cyclophosphamide therapy. *Arch. Intern. Med.*, **141**:758–763, 1981.

Gralla, R. J.; Itri, L. M.; Pisko, S. E.; Squillante, A. E.; Kelsen, D. P.; Braun, D. W., Jr.; Bordin, L. A.; Braun, T. J.; and Young, C. W.: Antiemetic efficacy of high-dose metoclopramide: Randomized trials with placebo and prochlorperazine in patients with chemotherapy-induced nausea and vomiting. *N. Engl. J. Med.*, **305**:905–909, 1981.

Greco, F. A.; Brereton, H. D.; and Rodbard, D.: Noninvasive monitoring of adriamycin cardiotoxicity by "Sphygmo-Recording" of the pulse wave delay (QK$_d$ interval). *Cancer Treat. Rep.*, **60**:1239–1245, 1976.

Green, D.; Hisamatsu, T.; Tew, .; and Shein, P. S.: Correlation of nitrosourea bone marrow toxicity with DNA alkylation and chromatin binding sites. *Proc. Am. Assoc. Cancer Res.*, **21**:301, 1980.

Grein, A.; Spalla, C.; and DiMarco, A.: Descrizione e classificazione di un attinomicete (*Streptomyces peucetius* sp. nova) produttore di un sostanza ad attivita antitumorale: la Daunomicina. *G. Microbiol.*, **11**:109–115, 1963.

Grossman, B.; Lessin, L. S.; and Cohen, P.: Droperidol

prevents nausea and vomiting from *cis*-platinum. *N. Engl. J. Med.*, **301**:47, 1979.

Hall, S. W.; Benjamin, R. S.; Burgess, M. A.; Bodey, G. P.; Luna, M. A.; and Freireich, E. J.: Doxorubicin-DNA complex: A phase I clinical trial. *Cancer Treat. Rep.*, **66**:2033–2037, 1982.

Hande, K. R.; Balow, J. E.; Drake, J. C.; Rosenberg, S. A.; and Chabner, B. A.: Methotrexate and hemodialysis. *Ann. Intern. Med.*, **87**:495–496, 1977.

Hande, K. R.; Stein, R. S.; McDonough, D. A.; Greco, F. A.; and Wolff, S. N.: Effects of high-dose cytarabine. *Clin. Pharmacol. Ther.*, **31**:669–674, 1982.

Hanna, W. T.; Krauss, S.; Regester, R. F.; and Murphy, W. M.: Renal disease after mitomycin C therapy. *Cancer*, **48**:2583–2588, 1981.

Harmon, W. E.; Cohen, H. J.; Schneeberger, E. E.; and Grupe, W. E.: Chronic renal failure in children treated with methyl CCNU. *N. Engl. J. Med.*, **300**:1200–1203, 1979.

Harris, A. L.; Potter, C.; Bunch, C.; Boutagy, J.; Harvey, D. J.; and Grahame-Smith, D. G.: Pharmacokinetics of cytosine arabinoside in patients with acute myeloid leukaemia. *Br. J. Clin. Pharmacol.*, **8**:219–227, 1979.

Haskell, C. M., and Sullivan, A.: Comparative survival in tissue culture of normal and neoplastic human cells exposed to adriamycin. *Cancer Res.*, **34**:2291–2994, 1974.

Haupt, H. M.; Hutchins, G. M.; and Moore, G. M.: Ara-C lung: Noncardiogenic pulmonary edema complicating cytosine arabinoside therapy of leukemia. *Am. J. Med.*, **70**:256–261, 1981.

Hayakawa, T.; Kanai, N.; Yamada, R.; Kuroda, R.; Higashi, H.; Mogami, H.; and Jinnai, D.: Effect of steroid hormone on activation of endoxan (cyclophosphamide). *Biochem. Pharmacol.*, **18**:129–135, 1969.

Hayes, D. M.; Cvitkovic, E.; Goldberg, R. B.; Scheiner, E.; Helson, L.; and Krakoff, I. H.: High dose *cis*-platinum diammine dichloride: Amelioration of renal toxicity by mannitol diuresis. *Cancer*, **39**:1372–1381, 1977.

Hayes, F. A.; Green, A. A.; Senzer, N.; and Pratt, C. B.: Tetany: A complication of *cis*-dichlorodiammineplatinum (II) therapy. *Cancer Treat. Rep.*, **63**:547–548, 1979.

Heidelberger, C.; Chaudhuri, N. K.; Danneberg, P.; Mooren, D.; Griesbach, L.; Duschinsky, R.; Schnitzer, R. J.; Pleven, E.; and Scheiner, J.: Fluorinated pyrimidines, a new class of tumour-inhibitory compounds. *Nature*, **179**:663–666, 1957.

Henderson, C. A.; Metz, E. N.; Balcerzak, S. P.; and Sagone, A. L., Jr.: Adriamycin and daunomycin generate reactive oxygen compounds in erythrocytes. *Blood*, **52**:878–885, 1978.

Hill, B. T.; Bailey, B. D.; White, J. C.; and Goldman, I. D.: Characteristics of transport of 4-amino antifolates and folate compounds by two lines of L5178Y lymphoblasts, one with impaired transport of methotrexate. *Cancer Res.*, **39**:2440–2446, 1979.

Ho, D. H. W.; Carter, C. J.; Brown, N. S.; Hester, J.; McCredie, K.; Benjamin, R. S.; Freireich, E. J.; and Bodey, G. P.: Effect of tetrahydrouridine on the uptake and metabolism of 1-β-D-arabinofuranosylcytosine in human normal and leukemic cells. *Cancer Res.*, **40**:2441–2446, 1980.

Ho, D. H. W., and Frei, E., III: Clinical pharmacology of 1-β-D-arabinofuranosyl cytosine. *Clin. Pharmacol. Ther.*, **12**:944–954, 1971.

Ho, D. H. W.; Yap, H. Y.; and Brown, N.: Clinical pharmacology of intramuscularly administered L-asparaginase. *J. Clin. Pharmacol.*, **21**:72–78, 1981.

Hoagland, H. C.: Hematologic complications of cancer chemotherapy. *Semin. Oncol.*, **9**:95–102, 1982.

Houghton, J. A., and Houghton, P. J.: 5-Fluorouracil in combination with hypoxanthine and allopurinol: Toxicity and metabolism in xenografts of human colonic carcinomas in mice. *Biochem. Pharmacol.*, **29**:2077–2080, 1980.

Howell, S. B.; Blair, H. E.; Uren, J.; and Frei, E., III: Hemodialysis and enzymatic cleavage of methotrexate in man. *Eur. J. Cancer*, **14**:787–792, 1978.

Howell, S. B.; and Wung, W. E.: Effect of plasma hypoxanthine on the modulation of methotrexate toxicity by thymidine. In Tattersall, M. H. N., and Fox, R. M. (eds.): *Nucleosides and Cancer Treatment: Rational Approaches to Antimetabolite Selectivity and Modulation.* Academic Press, Sydney, 1981.

Howle, J. A., and Gale, G. R.: *Cis*-dichlorodiammineplatinum (II): Persistent and selective inhibition of deoxyribonucleic acid synthesis *in vivo. Biochem. Pharmacol.*, **19**:2757–2762, 1970.

Hreshchyshyn, M. M.; Aron, B. S.; Boronow, R. C.; Franklin, E. W., III; Shingleton, H. M.; and Blessing, J. A.: Hydroxyurea or placebo combined with radiation to treat stages IIIB and IV cervical cancer confined to the pelvis. *Int. J. Radiat. Oncol. Biol. Phys.*, **5**:317–322, 1979.

Huang, C.-H.; Mirabelli, C. K.; Jan, Y.; and Crooke, S. T.: Single-strand and double-strand deoxyribonucleic acid breaks produced by several bleomycin analogues. *Biochemistry*, **20**:233–238, 1981.

Iqbal, Z., and Ochs, S.: Uptake of *Vinca* alkaloids into mammalian nerve and its subcellular components. *J. Neurochem.*, **34**:59–68, 1980.

Israel, M.; Modest, E. J.; and Frei, E., III: N-trifluoroacetyladriamycin-14-valerate, an analog with greater experimental antitumor activity and less toxicity than adriamycin. *Cancer Res.*, **35**:1365–1368, 1975.

Jackson, D. V.; Castle, M. C.; and Bender, R. A.: Biliary excretion of vincristine. *Clin. Pharmacol. Ther.*, **24**:101–107, 1978.

Jackson, D. V., Jr.; Sethi, V. S.; Spurr, C. L.; White, D. R.; Richards, F., II; Stuart, J. J.; Muss, H. B.; Cooper, M. R.; and Castle, M. C.: Pharmacokinetics of vincristine infusion. *Cancer Treat. Rep.*, **65**:1043–1048, 1981.

Jacobs, S. A.; Bleyer, W. A.; Chabner, B. A.; and Johns, D. G.: Altered plasma pharmacokinetics of methotrexate administered intrathecally. *Lancet*, **1**:465–466, 1975.

Jacobs, S. A.; Derr, C. J.; and Johns, D. G.: Accumulation of methotrexate diglutamate in human liver during methotrexate therapy. *Biochem. Pharmacol.*, **26**:2310–2313, 1977.

Jacobs, S. A.; Stoller, R. G.; Chabner, B. A.; and Johns, D. G.: 7-Hydroxymethotrexate as a urinary metabolite in human subjects and rhesus monkeys receiving high dose methotrexate. *J. Clin. Invest.*, **57**:534–538, 1976.

Johnson, I. S.; Armstrong, J. G.; Gorman, M.; and Burnett, J. P., Jr.: The *Vinca* alkaloids: A new class of oncolytic agents. *Cancer Res.*, **23**:1390–1427, 1963.

Johnson, W. W., and Meadows, D. C.: Urinary-bladder fibrosis and telangiectasia associated with long-term cyclophosphamide therapy. *N. Engl. J. Med.*, **284**:290–294, 1971.

Jolivet, J., and Schilsky, R. L.: High-pressure liquid chromatography analysis of methotrexate polyglutamates in cultured human breast cancer cells. *Biochem. Pharmacol.*, **30**:1387–1390, 1981.

Jolivet, J.; Schilsky, R. L.; Bailey, B. D.; Drake, J. C.; and Chabner, B. A.: Synthesis, retention, and biological activity of methotrexate polyglutamates in cultured human breast cancer cells. *J. Clin. Invest.*, **70**:351–360, 1982.

Jones, R. B.; Collins, J. M.; Myers, C. E.; Brooks, A. E.; Hubbard, S. M.; Balow, J. E.; Brennan, M. F.; Dedrick, R. L.; and DeVita, V. T.: High-volume intraperitoneal chemotherapy with methotrexate in patients with cancer. *Cancer Res.*, **41**:55–59, 1981.

Kaizer, H.; Stuart, R. K.; Fuller, D. J.; Braine, H. G.; Saral, R.; Colvin, M.; Wharam, M. D.; and Santos, G. W.: Autologous bone marrow transplantation in acute leukemia: Progress report on a phase I study of 4-hydroperoxycyclo-phosphamide (4HC) incubation of marrow prior to cryopreservation. *Proc. Am. Soc. Clin. Oncol.*, **1**:131, 1982.

Kalwinsky, D. K.; Look, A. T.; Ducore, J.; and Fridland, A.: Effects of the epipodophyllotoxin VP-16-213 on cell cycle traverse, DNA synthesis, and DNA strand size in cultures of human leukemic lymphoblasts. *Cancer Res.*, **43**:1592–1597, 1983.

Kelley, J.; Newman, R. A.; and Evans, J. N.: Bleomycin-induced pulmonary fibrosis in the rat: Prevention with an inhibitor of collagen synthesis. *J. Lab. Clin. Med.*, **96**:954–964, 1980.

Kelsen, D. P.; Bains, M.; Chapman, R.; and Golbey, R.: Cisplatin, vindesine and bleomycin (DVB) combination chemotherapy for esophageal carcinoma. *Cancer Treat. Rep.*, **65**:781–785, 1981.

Kennedy, B. J.: Metabolic and toxic effects of mithramycin during tumor therapy. *Am. J. Med.*, **49**:494–503, 1970.

Kennedy, B. J.: Mithramycin therapy in testicular cancer. *J. Urol.*, **107**:429–432, 1972.

Khan, A.; Hill, J. M.; Grater, W.; Loeb, E.; MacLellan, A.; and Hill, N.: Atopic hypersensitivity to *cis*-dichlorodiammineplatinum (II) and other platinum complexes. *Cancer Res.*, **35**:2766–2770, 1975.

Kidd, J. G.: Regression of transplanted lymphomas induced *in vivo* by means of normal guinea pig serum. I. Course of transplanted cancers of various kinds in mice and rats given guinea pig serum, horse serum, or rabbit serum. *J. Exp. Med.*, **98**:565–581, 1953.

Kimler, B. F.: The effect of bleomycin and irradiation on G₂ progression. *Int. J. Radiat. Oncol. Biol. Phys.*, **5**:1523–1526, 1979.

Kociba, R. J.; Sleight, S. D.; and Rosenberg, B.: Inhibition of Dunning ascitic leukemia and Walker 256 carcinosarcoma with *cis*-diamminedichloroplatinum (NSC-119875). *Cancer Chemother. Rep.*, **54**:325–328, 1970.

Kohn, K. W.: Interstrand cross-linking of DNA by 1,3-bis(2-chlorethyl)-1-nitrosourea and other 1-(2-haloethyl)-1-nitrosoureas. *Cancer Res.*, **37**:1450–1454, 1977.

Kramer, W. G.; Feldman, S.; Broughton, A.; Strong, J. E.; Hall, S. W.; and Holoye, P. Y.: The pharmacokinetics of bleomycin in man. *J. Clin. Pharmacol.*, **18**:346–352, 1978.

Kroener, J. F.; Saleh, F.; and Howell, S. B.: 5-FU and allopurinol: Toxicity modulation and phase II results in colon cancer. *Cancer Treat. Rep.*, **66**:1133–1137, 1982.

Kufe, D. W., and Major, P. P.: 5-Fluorouracil incorporation into human breast carcinoma RNA correlates with cytotoxicity. *J. Biol. Chem.*, **256**:9802–9805, 1981.

Kuo, M. T.: Preferential damage of active chromatin by bleomycin. *Cancer Res.*, **41**:2439–2443, 1981.

Kyle, R. A.; Schwartz, R. S.; Oliner, H. L.; and Dameshek, W.: A syndrome resembling adrenal cortical insufficiency associated with long term busulfan (myleran) therapy. *Blood*, **18**:497–510, 1961.

Landgren, R. C.; Hussey, D. H.; Barkley, H. T., Jr.; and Samuels, M. L.: Split-course irradiation plus hydroxyurea in inoperable bronchogenic carcinoma—A randomized study of 53 patients. *Cancer*, **34**:1598–1601, 1974.

Lange, R. C.; Spencer, R. P.; and Harder, H. C.: Synthesis and distribution of a radiolabeled antitumor agent: *cis*-diamminedichloroplatinum (II). *J. Nucl. Med.*, **13**:328–330, 1972.

Lange, R. C.; Spencer, R. P.; and Harder, H. C.: The antitumor agent *cis*-Pt(NH₃)₂Cl₂: Distribution studies and dose calculations for ¹⁹³ᵐPt and ¹⁹⁵ᵐPt. *J. Nucl. Med.*, **14**:191–195, 1973.

Lawley, P. D., and Brookes, P.: Further studies on the alkylation of nucleic acids and their constituent nucleotides. *Biochem. J.*, **89**:127–138, 1963.

Lawley, P. D., and Brookes, P.: Molecular mechanism of the cytotoxic action of defunctional alkylating agents and of resistance to this action. *Nature*, **206**:480–483, 1965.

Lee, M. H.; Huang, Y.-M.; and Sartorelli, A. C.: Alkaline phosphatase activities of 6-thiopurine-sensitive and -resistant sublines of Sarcoma 180. *Cancer Res.*, **38**:2413–2418, 1978.

LePage, G. A., and Whitecar, J. P., Jr.: Pharmacology of 6-thioguanine in man. *Cancer Res.*, **31**:1627–1631, 1971.

LeRoy, A. F.; Wehling, M. L.; Sponseller, H. L.; Friauf, W. S.; Solomon, R. E.; and Dedrick, R. L.: Analysis of platinum in biological materials by flameless atomic absorption spectrophotometry. *Biochem. Med.*, **18**:184–191, 1977.

Levin, V. A.; Hoffman, W.; and Weinkam, R. J.: Pharmacokinetics of BCNU in man: A preliminary study of 20 patients. *Cancer Treat. Rep.*, **62**:1305–1312, 1978.

Lewis, B. M., and Izbicki, R.: Routine pulmonary function tests during bleomycin therapy: Tests may be ineffective and potentially misleading. *J.A.M.A.*, **243**:347–351, 1980.

Ley, T. J.; DeSimone, J.; Anagnou, N. P.; Keller, G. H.; Humphries, R. K.; Turner, P. H.; Young, N. S.; Heller, P.; and Nienhuis, A. W.: 5-Azacytidine selectively increases γ-globin synthesis in a patient with β+ thalassemia. *N. Engl. J. Med.*, **307**:1469–1475, 1982.

Lin, P.-S.; Kwock, L.; Hefter, K.; and Misslbeck, G.: Effects of iron, copper, cobalt, and their chelators on the cytotoxicity of bleomycin. *Cancer Res.*, **43**:1049–1053, 1983.

Lippman, A. J.; Helson, C.; Helson, L.; and Krakoff, I. H.: Clinical trials of *cis*-diamminedichloroplatinum (NSC-119875). *Cancer Chemother. Rep.*, **57**:191–200, 1973.

Litam, J. P.; Dail, D. H.; Spitzer, G.; Vellekoop, L.; Verma, D. S.; Zander, A. R.; and Dicke, K. A.: Early pulmonary toxicity after administration of high-dose BCNU. *Cancer Treat. Rep.*, **65**:39–44, 1981.

Lloyd, R. S.; Haidle, C. W.; and Robberson, D. L.: Noncovalent intermolecular crosslinks are produced by bleomycin reaction with duplex DNA. *Proc. Natl. Acad. Sci. USA*, **76**:2674–2678, 1979.

Loike, J. D., and Horwitz, S. B.: Effects of podophyllotoxin and VP-16-213 on microtubule assembly *in vitro* and nucleoside transport in HeLa cells. *Biochemistry*, **15**:5435–5443, 1976.

Loo, T. L.: Triazenoimidazole derivatives. In Sartorelli, A. C., and Johns, D. G. (eds.): *Antineoplastic and Immunosuppressive Agents, Pt. II* (Handbook of Experimental Pharmacology, New Series, Vol. 38/2). Springer-Verlag, Berlin, 1974–1975.

Loo, T. L.; Housholder, G. E.; Gerulath, A. H.; Saunders, P. H.; and Farquhar, D.: Mechanism of action and pharmacology studies with DTIC (NSC-45388). *Cancer Treat. Rep.,* **60:**149–152, 1976.

Lown, J. W.: The molecular mechanism of antitumor action of the mitomycins. In Carter, S. K., and Crooke, S. T. (eds.): *Mitomycin C: Current Status and New Developments.* Academic Press, New York, 1979.

Ludlum, D. B.: Reaction of nitrogen mustard with synthetic polynucleotides. *Biochim. Biophys. Acta,* **142:**282–284, 1967.

Macdonald, J. S.; Schein, P. S.; Woolley, P. U.; Smythe, T.; Ueno, W.; Hoth, D.; Smith, F.; Boiron, M.; Gisselbrecht, C.; Brunet, R.; and Lagarde, C.: 5-Fluorouracil, doxorubicin, and mitomycin (FAM) combination chemotherapy for advanced gastric cancer. *Ann. Intern. Med.,* **93:**533–536, 1980.

Macdonald, J. S.; Weiss, R. B.; Poster, D.; and Hammershaimb, L.: Subacute and chronic toxicities associated with nitrosourea therapy. In Prestayko, A. W.; Crooke, S. T.; Baker, L. H.; Carter, S. K.; and Schein, P. S. (eds.): *Nitrosoureas: Current Status and New Developments.* Academic Press, New York, 1981.

McInerney, D. P., and Bullimore, J.: Reactivation of radiation pneumonitis by adiamycin. *Br. J. Radiol.,* **50:**224–227, 1977.

Madajewicz, S.; West, C. R.; Park, H. C.; Ghoorah, J.; Avellanosa, A. M.; Takita, H.; Karakousis, C.; Vincent, R.; Caracandas, J.; and Jennings, E.: Phase II study—Intra-arterial BCNU therapy for metastatic brain tumors. *Cancer,* **47:**653–657, 1981.

Madoc-Jones, H., and Mauro, F.: Interphase action of vinblastine and vincristine: Differences in their lethal action through the mitotic cycle of cultured mammalian cells. *J. Cell. Physiol.,* **72:**185–196, 1968.

Major, P. P.; Agarwal, R. P.; and Kufe, D. W.: Clinical pharmacology of deoxycoformycin. *Blood,* **58:**91–96, 1981.

Major, P. P.; Egan, E.; Herrick, D.; and Kufe, D. W.: 5-Fluorouracil incorporation in DNA of human breast carcinoma cells. *Cancer Res.,* **42:**3005–3009, 1982.

Melera, P. W.; Lewis, J. A.; Biedler, J. L.; and Hession, C.: Antifolate-resistant Chinese hamster cells: Evidence for dihydrofolate reductase gene amplification among independently derived sublines overproducing different dihydrofolate reductases. *J. Biol. Chem.,* **255:**7024–7028, 1980.

Mellett, L. B.: Chemistry and metabolism of cyclophosphamide. In Varcil, M. (ed.): *Immunosuppressive Properties of Cyclophosphamide.* Meade Johnson, Evansville, Illinois, 1971.

Meyn, R. E.; Corry, P. M.; Fletcher, S. E.; and Demetriades, M.: Thermal enhancement of DNA strand breakage in mammalian cells treated with bleomycin. *Int. J. Radiat. Oncol. Biol. Phys.,* **5:**1487–1489, 1979.

Mikkelsen, R. B.; Lin, P.-S.; and Wallach, D. F. H.: Interaction of adriamycin with human red blood cells: A biochemical and morphological study. *J. Mol. Med.,* **2:**33–40, 1977.

Minow, R. A.; Benjamin, R. S.; Lee, E. T.; and Gottlieb, J. A.: Adriamycin cardiomyopathy-risk factors. *Cancer,* **39:**1397–1402, 1977.

Minow, R. A.; Benjamin, R. S.; Lee, E. T.; and Gottlieb, J. A.: QRS voltage change with adriamycin administration. *Cancer Treat. Rep.,* **62:**931–934, 1978.

Mirabelli, C. K.; Beattie, W. G.; Huang, C.-H.; Prestayko, A. W.; and Crooke, S. T.: Comparison of the sequences at specific sites on DNA cleaved by the antitumor anti-

biotics talisomycin and bleomycin. *Cancer Res.,* **42:**1399–1404, 1982.

Mirabelli, C. K.; Mong, S.; Huang, C.-H.; and Crooke, S. T.: Comparison of bleomycin A_2 and talisomycin A specific fragmentation of linear duplex DNA. *Biochem. Biophys. Res. Commun.,* **91:**871–877, 1979.

Mitchell, E. P., and Schein, P. S.: Gastrointestinal toxicity of chemotherapeutic agents. *Semin. Oncol.,* **9:**52–64, 1982.

Mizuno, S.: Ethanol-induced cell sensitization to bleomycin cytotoxicity and the inhibition of recovery from potentially lethal damage. *Cancer Res.,* **41:**4111–4114, 1981.

Momparler, R. L.: Kinetic and template studies with 1-β-D-arabinofuranosylcytosine 5'-triphosphate and mammalian deoxyribonucleic acid polymerase. *Mol. Pharmacol.,* **8:**362–370, 1972.

Montgomery, J. A.; James, R.; McCaleb, G. S.; and Johnston, T. P.: The modes of decomposition of 1,3-*bis*(2-chloroethyl)-1-nitrosourea and related compounds. *J. Med. Chem.,* **10:**668–674, 1967.

Müller, W. E. G.; Yamazaki, Z.; Breter, H.-J.; and Zahn, R. K.: Action of bleomycin on DNA and RNA. *Eur. J. Biochem.,* **31:**518–525, 1972.

Munchausen, L. L., and Kahn, R. O.: Biologic and chemical effects of *cis*-dichlorodiammineplatinum (II) (NSC-119875) on DNA. *Cancer Chemother. Rep.,* **59:**643–646, 1975.

Mundy, G. R.; Wilkinson, R.; and Heath, D. A.: Comparative study of available medical therapy for hypercalcemia of malignancy. *Am. J. Med.,* **74:**421–432, 1983.

Murad, F., and Haynes, R. C., Jr.: Estrogens and progestins. In Gilman, A. G.; Goodman, L. S.; and Gilman, A. (eds.): *The Pharmacological Basis of Therapeutics,* 6th ed. Macmillan Publishing Co., Inc., New York, 1980.

Myers, C. E.: Antitumor antibiotics I: Anthracyclines. In Pinedo, H. M. (ed.): *Cancer Chemotherapy 1980* (The EORTC Cancer Chemotherapy Annual 2). Excerpta Medica, Amsterdam, 1980.

Myers, C. E.; McGuire, W.; and Young, R.: Adriamycin: Amelioration of toxicity by α-tocopherol. *Cancer Treat. Rep.,* **60:**961–962, 1976.

O'Dwyer, P. J.; Leyland-Jones, B.; Alonso, M. T.; Marsoni, S.; and Wittes, R. E.: Etoposide (VP-16-213) Current status of an active anticancer drug. *N. Engl. J. Med.,* **312:**692–700, 1985.

Oken, M. M.; Crooke, S. T.; Elson, M. K.; Strong, J. E.; and Shafer, R. B.: Pharmacokinetics of bleomycin after im administration in man. *Cancer Treat. Rep.,* **65:**485–489, 1981.

Oki, T.; Matsuzawa, Y.; Yoshimoto, A.; Numata, K.; Kitamura, I.; Hori, S.; Takamatsu, A.; Umezawa, H.; Ishizuka, M.; Naganawa, H.; Suda, H.; Hamada, M.; and Takeuchi, T.: New antitumor antibiotics, aclacinomycins A and B. *J. Antibiot.* (Tokyo), **28:**830–834, 1975.

Oliverio, V. T.; Vietzke, W. M.; Williams, M. K.; and Adamson, R. H.: The absorption, distribution, excretion, and biotransformation of the carcinostatic 1-(2-chloroethyl)-3-cyclohexyl-1-nitrosourea in animals. *Cancer Res.,* **30:**1330–1337, 1970.

Olson, H. M.; Young, D. M.; Prieur, D. J.; LeRoy, A. F.; and Reagan, R. L.: Electrolyte and morphologic alterations of myocardium in adriamycin-treated rabbits. *Am. J. Pathol.,* **77:**439–454, 1974.

Ono, T.; Miyaki, M.; Taguchi, T.; and Ohashi, M.: Actions of bleomycin on DNA ligase and polymerases. *Prog. Biochem. Pharmacol.,* **11:**48–58, 1976.

Ostrow, S.; Egorin, M. J.; Hahn, D.; Markus, S.; Aisner, J.; Chang, P.; LeRoy, A.; Bachur, N. R.; and Wiernik,

P. H.: High-dose cisplatin therapy using mannitol versus furosemide diuresis: Comparative pharmacokinetics and toxicity. *Cancer Treat. Rep.,* **65:**73–78, 1981.

Ostrowski, M. J., and Halsall, G. M.: Intracavitary bleomycin in the management of malignant effusions: A multicenter study. *Cancer Treat. Rep.,* **66:**1903–1907, 1982.

Owellen, R. J.; Hartke, C. A.; and Hains, F. O.: Pharmacokinetics and metabolism of vinblastine in humans. *Cancer Res.,* **37:**2597–2602, 1977.

Painter, R. B.: Inhibition of DNA replicon initiation by 4-nitroquinoline 1-oxide, adriamycin, and ethyleneimine. *Cancer Res.,* **38:**4445–4449, 1978.

Panasci, L. C.; Green, D.; and Schein, P. S.: Chlorozotocin: Mechanism of reduced bone marrow toxicity in mice. *J. Clin. Invest.,* **64:**1103–1111, 1979.

Papirmeister, B.; Dorsey, J. K.; Davison, C. L.; and Gross, C. L.: Sensitization of DNA to endonuclease by adenine alkylation and its biological significance. *Fed. Proc.,* **29:**726, 1970.

Parks, R. E., Jr.; Crabtree, G. W.; Kong, C. M.; Agarwal, R. P.; Agarwal, K. C.; and Scholar, E. M.: Incorporation of analog purine nucleosides into the formed elements of human blood: Erythrocytes, platelets, and lymphocytes. *Ann. NY Acad. Sci.,* **255:**412–434, 1975.

Passero, M. A.; Held, J. K.; and Shearer, P. M.: Effects of bleomycin, O_2 concentration and H_2O_2 on peroxidation of arachidonic acid. *Am. Rev. Respir. Dis.,* **127:**287, 1983.

Patton, T. F.; Himmelstein, K. J.; Belt, R.; Bannister, S. J.; Sternson, L. A.; and Repta, A. J.: Plasma levels and urinary excretion of filterable platinum species following bolus injection and iv infusion of *cis*-dichlorodiammine-platinum(II) in man. *Cancer Treat. Rep.,* **62:**1359–1362, 1978.

Pavy, M. D.; Wiley, E. L.; and Abeloff, M. D.: Hemolytic-uremic syndrome associated with mitomycin therapy. *Cancer Treat. Rep.,* **66:**457–461, 1982.

Perevodchikova, N. I.; Lichinitser, M. R.; and Gorbunova, V. A.: Phase I clinical study of carminomycin: Its activity against soft tissue sarcomas. *Cancer Treat. Rep.,* **61:**1705–1707, 1977.

Perry, D. J.; Weiss, R. B.; and Taylor, H. G.: Enhanced bleomycin toxicity during acute renal failure. *Cancer Treat. Rep.,* **66:**592–593, 1982.

Perry, M. C.: Hepatotoxicity of chemotherapeutic agents. *Semin. Oncol.,* **9:**65–74, 1982.

Piel, I. J.; Meyer, D.; Perlia, C. P.; and Wolfe, V. I.: Effects of *cis*-diamminedichloroplatinum (NSC-119875) on hearing function in man. *Cancer Chemother. Rep.,* **58:**871–875, 1974.

Piel, I. J.; Rayadu, G. V. S.; Perlia, C. P.; Friedman, A. M.; and Fordham, E. W.: Use of neutron activation analysis to study excretion of *cis*-diamminedichloroplatinum (DDP) in cancer patients. *Proc. Am. Assoc. Cancer Res.,* **15:**111, 1974.

Pigram, W. J.; Fuller, W.; and Hamilton, L. D.: Stereochemistry of intercalation: Interaction of daunomycin with DNA. *Nature,* **235:**17–19, 1972.

Pinedo, H. M.; Zaharko, D. S.; Bull, J.; and Chabner, B. A.: The relative contribution of drug concentration and duration of exposure to mouse bone marrow toxicity during continuous methotrexate infusion. *Cancer Res.,* **37:**445–450, 1977.

Povirk, L. F.: Catalytic release of deoxyribonucleic acid bases by oxidation and reduction of an iron-bleomycin complex. *Biochemistry,* **18:**3989–3995, 1979.

Pratt, C. B.; Ransom, J. L.; and Evans, W. E.: Age-related adriamycin cardiotoxicity in children. *Cancer Treat. Rep.,* **62:**1381–1385, 1978.

Preisler, H. D.; Early, A. P.; Raza, A.; Vlahides, G.; Marinello, M. J.; Stein, A. M.; and Browman, G.: Therapy of secondary acute nonlymphocytic leukemia with cytarabine. *N. Engl. J. Med.,* **308:**21–23, 1983.

Present, D. H.; Korelitz, B. I.; Wisch, N.; Glass, J. L.; Sachar, D. B.; and Pasternack, B. S.: Treatment of Crohn's disease with 6-mercaptopurine: A long-term randomized, double-blind study. *N. Engl. J. Med.,* **302:**981–987, 1980.

Price, R. A., and Jamieson, P. A.: The central nervous system in childhood leukemia: II. Subacute leukoencephalopathy. *Cancer,* **35:**306–318, 1975.

Primack, A.: Amelioration of cyclophosphamide-induced cystitis. *J.N.C.I.,* **47:**223–227,1971.

Rabadi, S. J.; Khandekar, J. D.; and Miller, H. J.: Mitomycin-induced hemolytic uremic syndrome: Case presentation and review of literature. *Cancer Treat. Rep.,* **66:**1244–1247, 1982.

Radice, P. A.; Bunn, P. A., Jr.; and Ihde, D. C.: Therapeutic trials with VP-16-213 and VM-26: Active agents in small cell lung cancer, non-Hodgkin's lymphomas, and other malignancies. *Cancer Treat. Rep.,* **63:**1231–1239, 1979.

Ravry, M. J. R.: Cardiotoxicity of mitomycin C in man and animals. *Cancer Treat. Rep.,* **63:**555, 1979.

Reddel, R. R.; Kefford, R. F.; Grant, J. M.; Coates, A. S.; Fox, R. M.; and Tattersall, M. H. N.: Ototoxicity in patients receiving cisplatin: Importance of dose and method of drug administration. *Cancer Treat. Rep.,* **66:**19–23, 1982.

Reed, D. J.: Procarbazine. In Sartorelli, A. C., and Johns, D. G. (eds.): *Antineoplastic and Immunosuppressive Agents, Pt. II* (Handbook of Experimental Pharmacology, New Series, Vol. 38/2). Springer-Verlag, Berlin, 1974–1975.

Reich, E.; Franklin, R. M.; Shatkin, A. J.; and Tatum, E. L.: Action of actinomycin D on animal cells and viruses. *Proc. Natl. Acad. Sci. USA,* **48:**1238–1245, 1962.

Reich, S. D.: Clinical pharmacology of mitomycin C. In Carter, S. K., and Crooke, S. T. (eds.): *Mitomycin C: Current Status and New Developments.* Academic Press, New York, 1979.

Rhaese, H.-J., and Freese, E.: Chemical analysis of DNA alterations. IV. Reactions of oligodeoxynucleotides with monofunctional alkylating agents leading to backbone breakage. *Biochim. Biophys. Acta,* **190:**418–433, 1969.

Ribaud, P.; Gouveia, J.; Bonnay, M.; and Mathe, G.: Clinical pharmacology and pharmacokinetics of *cis*-platinum and analogs. *Cancer Treat. Rep.,* **65(Suppl. 3):**97–105, 1981.

Ricci, J. A., and Goldstein, L.: Coronary artery disease in the presence of bleomycin therapy. *Cancer Treat. Rep.,* **66:**410, 1982.

Riley, D. J.; Kerr, J. S.; Berg, R. A.; Ianni, B. D.; Pietra, G. G.; Edelman, N. H.; and Prockop, D. J.: Prevention of bleomycin-induced pulmonary fibrosis in the hamster by *cis*-4-hydroxy-L-proline. *Am. Rev. Respir. Dis.,* **123:**388–393, 1981.

Roberts, J. J., and Fraval, H. N. A.: Repair of *cis*-platinum (II) diammine dichloride-induced DNA damage and cell sensitivity. In Prestayko, A. W.; Crooke, S. T.; and Carter, S. K. (eds.): *Cisplatin: Current Status and New Developments.* Academic Press, New York, 1980.

Roots, R., and Smith, K. C.: Effects of actinomycin D on cell cycle kinetics and the DNA of Chinese hamster and mouse mammary tumor cells cultivated *in vitro. Cancer Res.,* **36:**3654–3658, 1976.

Rosenberg, B.; Van Camp, L.; Grimley, E. B.; and Thomson, A. J.: The inhibition of growth or cell division in *Escherichia coli* by different ionic species of platinum (IV) complexes. *J. Biol. Chem.,* **242:**1347–1352, 1967.

Rosenberg, B.; Van Camp, L.; and Krigas, T.: Inhibition of cell division in *Escherichia coli* by electrolysis products from a platinum electrode. *Nature,* **205:**698–699, 1965.

Rosenthal, C. J.; Ritter, S.; and Platica, O.: Bleomycin, cisplatin, vincristine, and methotrexate in advanced non-small cell bronchogenic carcinoma. *Cancer Treat. Rep.,* **66:**205–206, 1982.

Ross, W. E.; Glaubiger, D.; and Kohn, K. W.: Qualitative and quantitative aspects of intercalator-induced DNA strand breaks. *Biochim. Biophys. Acta,* **562:**41–50, 1979.

Ross, W. E.; Zwelling, L. A.; and Kohn, K. W.: Relationship between cytotoxicity and DNA strand breakage produced by adriamycin and other intercalating agents. *Int. J. Radiat. Oncol. Biol. Phys.,* **5:**1221–1224, 1979.

Rustum, Y. M.: Metabolism and intracellular retention of 1-β-D-arabinofuranosylcytosine as predictors of response of animal tumors. *Cancer Res.,* **38:**543–549, 1978.

Rustum, Y. M.; Danhauser, L.; Luccioni, C.; and Au, J. L.: Determinants of response to antimetabolites and their modulation by normal purine and pyrimidine metabolites. *Cancer Treat. Rep.,* **65(Suppl. 3):**73–82, 1981.

Rustum, Y. M., and Preisler, H.: Correlation between leukemic cell retention of 1-β-D-arabinofuranosylcytosine 5'-triphosphate and response to therapy. *Cancer Res.,* **39:**42–49, 1979.

Rutman, R. J.; Cantarow, A.; and Paschkis, K. E.: Studies in 2-acetylaminofluorene carcinogenesis. III. The utilization of uracil-2-C^{14} by preneoplastic rat liver and rat hepatoma. *Cancer Res.,* **14:**119–123, 1954.

Sadoff, L.: Nephrotoxicity of streptozotocin (NSC-85998). *Cancer Chemother. Rep.,* **54:**457–459, 1970.

Sadoff, L.: Patterns of intravenous glucose tolerance and insulin response before and after treatment with streptozotocin (NSC-85998) in patients with cancer. *Cancer Chemother. Rep.,* **56:**61–69, 1972.

Santoro, A.; Bonadonna, G.; Bonfante, V.; and Valagussa, P.: Alternating drug combinations in the treatment of advanced Hodgkin's disease. *N. Engl. J. Med.,* **306:**770–775, 1982.

Sarna, G. P.; Champlin, R.; Wells, J.; and Gale, R. P.: Phase I study of high-dose mitomycin with autologous bone marrow support. *Cancer Treat. Rep.,* **66:**277–282, 1982.

Sato, S.; Iwaizumi, M.; Handa, K.; and Tamura, Y.: Electron spin resonance study on the mode of generation of free radicals of daunomycin, adriamycin, and carboquone in NAD(P)H-microsome system. *Gann,* **68:**603–608, 1977.

Saunders, G. F.; Haidle, C. W.; Saunders, P. P.; and Kuo, M. T.: DNA-drug interactions. In *Pharmacological Basis of Cancer Chemotherapy.* The Williams & Wilkins Company, Baltimore, 1975.

Sawyer, R. C.; Stolfi, R. L.; Nayak, R.; and Martin, D. S.: Mechanism of cytotoxicity in 5-fluorouracil chemotherapy of two murine solid tumors. In Tattersall, M. H. N., and Fox, R. M. (eds.): *Nucleosides and Cancer Treatment: Rational Approaches to Antimetabolite Selectivity and Modulation.* Academic Press, Sydney, 1981.

Schein, P. S.; Cooney, D. A.; McMenamin, M., Anderson, T.: Streptozotocin diabetes: Further studies on the mechanism of depression of nicotinamide adenine dinucleotide concentrations in mouse pancreatic islets and liver. *Biochem. Pharmacol,* **22:**2625–2631, 1973.

Schein, P. S.; DeVita, V. T., Jr.: Hubbard, S.; Chabner, B. A.; Canellos, G. P.; Berard, C.; and Young, R. C.: Bleomycin, adriamycin, cyclophosphamide, vincristine, and prednisone (BACOP) combination chemotherapy in the treatment of advanced diffuse histiocytic lymphoma. *Ann. Intern. Med.,* **85:**417–422, 1976.

Schein, P. S.; O'Connell, M. J.; Blom, J.; Hubbard, S.; Magrath, I. T.; Bergevin, P.; Wiernik, P. H.; Ziegler, J. L.; and DeVita, V. T.: Clinical antitumor activity and toxicity of streptozotocin (NSC-85998). *Cancer,* **34:**993–1000, 1974.

Schilsky, R. L., and Anderson, T.: Hypomagnesemia and renal magnesium wasting in patients receiving cisplatin. *Ann. Intern. Med.,* **90:**929–931, 1979.

Scholar, E. M., and Calabresi, P.: Increased activity of alkaline phosphatase in leukemic cells from patients resistant to thiopurines. *Biochem. Pharmacol.,* **28:**445–446, 1979.

Scovell, W. M., and O'Connor, T.: Interaction of aquated cis-[$(NH_3)_2Pt^{II}$] with nucleic acid constituents. 1. Ribonucleosides. *J. Am. Chem. Soc.,* **99:**120–126, 1977.

Sherins, R. J., and DeVita, V. T., Jr.: Effect of drug treatment for lymphoma on male reproductive capacity: Studies of men in remission after therapy. *Ann. Intern. Med.,* **79:**216–220, 1973.

Shiba, D. A.; Weinkam, R. J.; and Levin, V. A.: Metabolic activation of procarbazine: Activity of the intermediates and the effects of pretreatment. *Proc. Am. Assoc. Cancer Res.,* **20:**139, 1979.

Shoemaker, R. H.; Curt G. A.; and Carney, D. N.; Evidence for multidrug-resistant cells in human tumor cells populations. *Cancer Treat. Rep.,* **67:**883–333, 1983.

Sieber, S. M., and Adamson, R. H.: Toxicity of antineoplastic agents in man: Chromosomal aberrations, antifertility effects, congenital malformations, and carcinogenic potential. In Klein, G.; Weinhouse, S.; and Haddow, A. (eds.): *Advances in Cancer Research.* Academic Press, New York, 1975.

Singer, J. W.; Narahara, K. A.; Ritchie, J. L.; Hamilton, G. W.; and Kennedy, J. W.: Time- and dose-dependent changes in ejection fraction determined by radionuclide angiography after anthracycline therapy. *Cancer Treat. Rep.,* **62:**945–948, 1978.

Sirotnak, F. M.; Moccio, D. M.; and Young, C. W.: Increased accumulation of methotrexate by murine tumor cells *in vitro* in the presence of probenecid which is mediated by a preferential inhibition of efflux. *Cancer Res.,* **41:**966–970, 1981.

Sladek, N. E.: Therapeutic efficacy of cyclophosphamide as a function of its metabolism. *Cancer Res.,* **32:**535–542, 1972.

Sobell, H. M.: The sterochemistry of actinomycin binding to DNA and its implications in molecular biology. *Prog. Nucleic Acid Res. Mol. Biol.,* **13:**153–190, 1973.

Spears, C. P.; Shahinian, A. H.; Moran, R. G.; Heidelberger, C.; and Corbett, T. H.: *In vivo* kinetics of thymidylate synthetase inhibition in 5-fluorouracil-sensitive and -resistant murine colon adenocarcinomas. *Cancer Res.,* **42:**450–456, 1982.

Spector, J. I.; Zimbler, H.; and Ross, J. S.: Early-onset cyclophosphamide-induced interstitial pneumonitis. *J.A.M.A.,* **242:**2852–2854, 1979.

Spiegel, R. J.: The acute toxicities of chemotherapy. *Cancer Treat. Rev.,* **8:**197–207, 1981.

Spiegelman, S.; Nayak, R.; Sawyer, R.; Stolfi, R.; and Martin, D.: Potentiation of the anti-tumor activity of 5FU by thymidine and its correlation with the formation of (5FU)RNA. *Cancer,* **45:**1129–1134, 1980.

Spitz, S.: The histological effects of nitrogen mustards on human tumors and tissues. *Cancer,* **1:**383–398, 1948.

Sponzo, R. W.; DeVita, V. T.; and Oliverio, V. T.: Physiologic disposition of 1-(2-chloroethyl)-3-cyclohexyl-1-nitrosourea (CCNU) and 1-(2-chloroethyl)-3-(4-methyl cyclohexyl)-1-nitrosourea (MeCCNU) in man. *Cancer,* **31:**1154–1159, 1973.

Stewart, A. F.: Therapy of malignancy-associated hypercalcemia: 1983. *Am. J. Med.,* **74:**475–480, 1983.

Stone, P. J.; Kelman, A. D.; and Sinex, F. M.: Specific binding of antitumor drug *cis*-Pt(NH$_3$)$_2$Cl$_2$ to DNA rich in guanine and cytosine. *Nature,* **251:**736–737, 1974.

Strong, J. E., and Crooke, S. T.: DNA breakage by tallysomycin. *Cancer Res.,* **38:**3322–3326, 1978.

Strum, W. B.: A pH-dependent, carrier-mediated transport system for the folate analog, amethopterin, in rat jejunum. *J. Pharmacol. Exp. Ther.,* **203:**640–645, 1977.

Stuart, M. J.; deAlacron, P. A.; and Barvinchak, M. K.: Inhibition of adriamycin-induced human platelet lipid peroxidation by vitamin E. *Am. J. Hematol.,* **5:**297–303, 1978.

Taetle, R.; Dickman, P. S.; and Feldman, P. S.: Pulmonary histopathologic changes associated with melphalan therapy. *Cancer,* **42:**1239–1245, 1978.

Takanashi, S., and Bachur, N. R.: Adriamycin metabolism in man: Evidence from urinary metabolites. *Drug Metab. Dispos.,* **4:**79–87, 1976.

Tattersall, M. H. N.; Jarman, M.; Newlands, E. S.; Holyhead, L.; Milstead, R. A. V.; and Weinberg, A.: Pharmaco-kinetics of melphalan following oral or intravenous administration in patients with malignant disease. *Eur. J. Cancer,* **14:**507–513, 1978.

Tattersall, M. H. N.; Sodergren, J. E.; Sengupta, S. K.; Trites, D. H.; Modest, E. J.; and Frei, E., III: Pharmaco-kinetics of actinomycin D in patients with malignant melanoma. *Clin. Pharmacol. Ther.,* **17:**701–708, 1975.

Taylor, S. G., IV; Desai, S. A.; and DeWys, W. D.: Phase II trial of a combination of cyclophosphamide, vincristine, and methotrexate in advanced colorectal carcinoma. *Cancer Treat. Rep.,* **62:**1203–1205, 1980.

Temoshechkina, M. E., and Budelina, G. I.: Amino acid conferred resistance to melphalan. I. Structure activity relationship in cultured murine L1210 leukemia cells. *Cancer Treat. Rep.,* **60:**1363–1367, 1976.

Thrall, R. S.; McCormick, J. R.; Jack, R. M.; McReynolds, R. A.; and Ward, P. A.: Bleomycin-induced pulmonary fibrosis in the rat: Inhibition by indomethacin. *Am. J. Pathol.,* **95:**117–127, 1979.

Toland, D. M.; Coltman, C. A., Jr.; and Moon, T. E.: Second malignancies complicating Hodgkin's disease: The Southwest Oncology Group experience. *Cancer Clin. Trials,* **1:**27–33, 1978.

Toledo, C. H.; Ross, W. E.; Hood, C. I.; and Block, E. R.: Potentiation of bleomycin toxicity by oxygen. *Cancer Treat. Rep.,* **66:**359–362, 1982.

Toledo, T. M.; Harper, R. C.; and Mosser R. H.: Fetal effects during cyclophosphamide and irradiation therapy. *Ann. Intern. Med.,* **74:**87–91, 1971.

Tomasz, M.; Mercado, C. M.; Olson, J.; and Chatterjie, N.: The mode of interaction of mitomycin C with deoxyribonucleic acid and other polynucleotides *in vitro. Biochemistry,* **13:**4878–4887, 1974.

Tritton, T. R.; Murphree, S. A.; and Sartorelli, A. C.:

Adriamycin: A proposal on the specificity of drug action. *Biochem. Biophys. Res. Commun.,* **84:**802–808, 1978.

Umezawa, H.: Structure and action of bleomycin. *Prog. Biochem. Pharmacol.,* **11:**18–27, 1976.

Umezawa, H.; Maeda, K.; Takeuchi, T.; and Okami, Y.: New antibiotics, bleomycin A and B. *J. Antibiot.* (Tokyo), **19:**200–209, 1966.

Valdivieso, M.; Richman, S.; Burgess, A. M.; Bodey, G. P.; and Freireich, E. J.: Initial clinical studies of vindesine. *Cancer Treat. Rep.,* **65:**873–875, 1981.

Van Echo, D. A.; Whitacre, M. Y.; Aisner, J.; Applefeld, M. M.; and Wiernik, P. H.: Phase I trial of aclacinomycin A. *Cancer Treat. Rep.,* **66:**1127–1132, 1982.

Villani, F.; Piccinini F.; Merelli, P.; and Favalli, L.: Influence of adriamycin on calcium exchangeability in cardiac muscle and its modification by ouabain. *Biochem. Pharmacol.,* **27:**985–987, 1978.

Vistica, D. T.; Toal, J. N.; and Rabinovitz, M.: Amino acid-conferred resistance to melphalan. I. Structure-activity relationship in cultured murine L1210 leukemia cells. *Cancer Treat. Rep.,* **60:**1363–1367, 1976.

Vogelzang, N. J.; Bosl, G. J.; Johnson, K.; and Kennedy, B. J.: Raynaud's phenomenon: A common toxicity after combination chemotherapy for testicular cancer. *Ann. Intern. Med.,* **95:**288–292, 1981.

Von Hoff, D. D., and Layard, M.: Risk factors for development of daunorubicin cardiotoxicity. *Cancer Treat. Rep.,* **65(Suppl. 4):**19–23, 1981.

Von Hoff, D. D.; Layard, M. W.; Basa, P.; Davis, H. L., Jr.; Von Hoff, A. L.; Rozencweig, M.; and Muggia, F. M.: Risk factors for doxorubicin-induced congestive heart failure. *Ann. Intern. Med.,* **91:**710–717, 1979.

Von Hoff, D. D.; Reichert, C. M.; Cuneo, R.; Reddick, R.; Gallagher, M.; and Rozencweig, M.: Demyelination of peripheral nerves associated with *cis*-diamminedichloroplatinum (II) (DDP) therapy. *Proc. Am. Assoc. Cancer Res.,* **20:**91, 1979.

Von Hoff, D. D.; Rozencweig, M.; and Piccart, M.: The cardiotoxicity of anticancer agents. *Semin. Oncol.,* **9:**23–33, 1982.

Vugrin, D.; Herr, H. W.; Whitmore, W. F., Jr.; Sogani, P. C.; and Golbey, R. B.: VAB-6 combination chemotherapy in disseminated cancer of the testis. *Ann. Intern. Med.,* **95:**59–61, 1981.

Wakaki, S.; Marumo, H.; Tomioka, K.; Shimizu, G.; Kato, E.; Kamada, H.; Kudo, S.; and Fujimoto, Y.: Isolation of new fractions of antitumor mitomycins. *Antibiot. Chemother.,* **8:**228–240, 1958.

Wall, R. L., and Clausen, K. P.: Carcinoma of the urinary bladder in patients receiving cyclophosphamide. *N. Engl. J. Med.,* **293:**271–273, 1975.

Wang, A. L.; Tew, K. D.; Byrne, P. J.; and Schein, P. S.: Biochemical and pharmacologic properties of nitrosoureas. *Cancer Treat. Rep.,* **65(Suppl. 3):**119–124, 1981.

Warrell, R. P., Jr.; Arlin, Z. A.; Kempin, S. J.; and Young, C. W.: Phase I–II evaluation of a new anthracycline antibiotic, aclacinomycin A, in adults with refractory leukemia. *Cancer Treat. Rep.,* **66:**1619–1623, 1982.

Washtien, W. L.: Thymidylate synthetase levels as a factor in 5-fluorodeoxyuridine and methotrexate cytotoxicity in gastrointestinal tumor cells. *Mol. Pharmacol.,* **21:**723–728, 1982.

Weiss, A. J.; Metter, G. E.; Fletcher, W. S.; Wilson, W. L.; Grage, T. B.; and Ramirez, G.: Studies of adriamycin using a weekly regimen demonstrating its clinical effectiveness and lack of cardiac toxicity. *Cancer Treat. Rep.,* **60:**813–822, 1976.

Weiss, H. D.; Walker, M. D.; and Wiernik, P. H.: Neurotoxicity of commonly used antineoplastic agents. *N. Engl. J. Med.,* **291:**75–81 (first of two parts), 127–133 (second of two parts), 1974.

Weiss, R. B.: Streptozocin: A review of its pharmacology, efficacy, and toxicity. *Cancer Treat. Rep.,* **66:**427–438, 1982.

Weiss, R. B., and Bruno, S.: Hypersensitivity reactions to cancer chemotherapeutic agents. *Ann. Intern. Med.,* **94:**66–72, 1981.

Wheeler, G. P.; Bowdon, B. J.; Grimsley, J. A.; and Lloyd, H. H.: Interrelationships of some chemical, physiochemical, and biological activities of several 1-(2-haloethyl)-1-nitrosoureas. *Cancer Res.,* **34:**194–200, 1974.

Wheeler, G. P.; Johnston, T. P.; Bowdon, B. J.; McCaleb, G. S.; Hill, D. L.; and Montgomery, J. A.: Comparison of the properties of metabolites of CCNU. *Biochem. Pharmacol.,* **26:**2331–2336, 1977.

White, E. L.; Shaddix, S. C.; Brockman, R. W.; and Bennett, L. L., Jr.: Comparison of the actions of 9-β-D-arabinofuranosyl-2-fluoroadenine and 9-β-D-arabinofuranosyl-adenine on target enzymes from mouse tumor cells. *Cancer Res.,* **42:**2260–2264, 1982.

White, J. C.: Recent concepts on the mechanism of action of methotrexate. *Cancer Treat. Rep.,* **65(Suppl. 1):**3–12, 1981.

Wiesenfeld, M.; Reinders, E.; Corder, M.; Yoo, T. J.; Dietz, B.; and Lovett, J.: Successful re-treatment with *cis*-dichlorodiammineplatinum (II) after apparent allergic reactions. *Cancer Treat. Rep.,* **63:**219–221, 1979.

Wilson, L.; Bamburg, J. R.; Mizel, S. B.; Grisham, L. M.; and Creswell, K. M.: Interaction of drugs with microtubule proteins. *Fed. Proc.,* **33:**158–166, 1974.

Woodcock, D. M.; Fox, R. M.; and Cooper, I. A.: Evidence for a new mechanism of cytotoxicity of 1-β-D-arabinofuranosylcytosine. *Cancer Res.,* **39:**1418–1424, 1979.

Woods, W. G.; Dehner, L. P.; Nesbit, M. E.; Krivit, W.; Coccia, P. F.; Ramsay, N. K.; Kim, T. H.; and Kersey, J. H.: Fatal veno-occlusive disease of the liver following high-dose chemotherapy, irradiation and bone marrow transplantation. *Am. J. Med.,* **68:**285–290, 1980.

Wortsman, J., and Soler, N. G.: Mitotane—Spironolactone antagonism in Cushing's syndrome. *J.A.M.A.,* **238:**2527–2529, 1977.

Yalowich, J. C.; Fry, D. W.; and Goldman, I. D.: Teniposide (VM-26)- and etopside (VP-16-213)-induced augmentation of methotrexate transport and polyglutamylation in Ehrlich ascites tumor cells *in vitro. Cancer Res.,* **42:**3648–3653, 1982.

Yamanaka, N.; Kato, T.; Nishida, K.; Shimizu, S.; Fukushima, M.; and Ota, K.: Increase of antitumor effect of bleomycin by reduced nicotinamide adenine dinucleotide phosphate and microsomes *in vitro* and *in vivo. Cancer Res.,* **40:**2051–2053, 1980.

Yarbro, J. W.; Kennedy, B. J.; and Barnum, C. P.: Mithramycin inhibition of ribonucleic acid synthesis. *Cancer Res.,* **26:**36–39, 1966.

Zaharko, D. S.; Fung, W.-P.; and Yang, K.-H.: Relative biochemical aspects of low and high doses of methotrexate in mice. *Cancer Res.,* **37:**1602–1607, 1977.

Zimm, S.; Collins, J. M.; Riccardi, R.; O'Neill, D.; Narang, P. K.; Chabner, B.; and Poplack, D. G.: Variable bioavailability of oral mercaptopurine. Is maintenance chemotherapy in acute lymphoblastic leukemia being optimally delivered? *N. Engl. J. Med.,* **308:**1005–1009, 1983.

Zwelling, L. A.; Anderson, T.; and Kohn, K. W.: DNA-protein and DNA interstrand cross-linking by *cis*- and *trans*-platinum (II) diamminedichloride in L1210 mouse leukemia cells and relation to cytotoxicity. *Cancer Res.,* **39:**365–369, 1979.

Zwelling, L. A., and Kohn, K. W.: Mechanism of action of *cis*-dichlorodiammineplatinum (II). *Cancer Treat. Rep.,* **63:**1439–1444, 1979.

Zwelling, L. A.; Kohn, K. W.; Ross, W. E.; Ewig, R. A. G.; and Anderson, T.: Kinetics of formation and disappearance of a DNA cross-linking effect in mouse leukemia L1210 cells treated with *cis*- and *trans*-diamminedichloroplatinum (II). *Cancer Res.,* **38:**1762–1768, 1978.

11

Immunology And Biomodulation of Cancer

MALCOLM S. MITCHELL and JUERGEN H. BERTRAM

INTRODUCTION

Tumor immunology is the study of the attempts by a tumor-bearing organism, the host, to reject its own tumor. Implicit in tumor immunology is the assumption that there are characteristics of the tumor that are so sufficiently different from those of corresponding normal tissues that the host can recognize the tumor as foreign and thus mount an immunologic reaction to it. The "foreignness" that is recognized by immunity is the definition of the *antigenicity* of a tumor cell. The *immunogenicity* of an antigen on the other hand means its ability to evoke an immune response in the host. Thus, a substance may have antigens that are only weakly immunogenic, making their identification and detection difficult. This appears to be the situation for tumor cells, which has created problems for immunologists attempting to prove conclusively the assumption of antigenicity upon which the entire field is built. More importantly, weak immunogenicity has made the problem of rejection of a tumor by the body extremely difficult.

Tumor cells are in fact antigenic, differing from the normal tissues from which they have arisen. Whether these antigens are unique in the individual or in nature is still a matter of some uncertainty. Nevertheless, since antigenicity exists, the scientific inquiry into the tumor-host relationship, including the means of using that relationship to advantage in overcoming (*i.e.*, curing) tumors, rests on a solid foundation. As with any body of knowledge, some concepts will undoubtedly have to be changed as further information accumulates, even those concepts that now appear unassailable. The struggle between the tumor and the host in all its aspects has engaged the attention of virologists, geneticists, chemists, biologists, and physicians. In this chapter the contributions of each of these types of worker to tumor immunology and the therapy based upon its principles, called "biomodulation," will be discussed.

IMMUNOLOGIC CONCEPTS

Tumor Antigens

Introduction. An intensive search for tumor specific antigens has spanned the last seven decades, since their presence was first postulated shortly after Landsteiner discovered the major blood group antigens in 1901 (Landsteiner, 1901). Tumor transplantation experiments were performed in which strong rejections of the transplanted tumors were observed. The similarity between a blood transfusion reaction and tumor rejection led to the hypothesis that tumor tissue is foreign and that the rejection is mediated by an immune response against "tumor-specific" antigens. The discovery of normal transplantation antigens (histocompatibility antigens), however, invalidated these early experiments. Because the tumors were transplanted across major histocompatibility barriers, the observed rejection reactions could not be ascribed to tumor-specific antigens.

Such antigens were finally demonstrated by

Foley in 1953 (Foley, 1953), and their presence later confirmed by Prehn (Prehn and Main, 1957). They injected inbred mice with methylcholanthrene, a polycyclic hydrocarbon. Soft tissue sarcomas developed, which eventually caused the death of the animals. If the tumors were removed before they had become too large, however, immunologic resistance to rechallenge with the same tumor developed. The availability of inbred mice genetically identical with one another insured that tumor rejection due to histoincompatibility would not occur to confuse the issue.

Today, a large number of chemically- and virally-induced tumor antigens have been demonstrated that lead to the rejection of tumors transplanted within inbred mice. These chemically and virally induced rejection antigens were once thought to be unique to the tumor, and were referred to as "tumor-specific transplantation antigens" (TSTA). More recent evidence, however, suggests a close relationship of all of these antigens with viral structural proteins. "Tumor-associated transplantation antigens" (TATA) is a more appropriate term. Tumor associated antigens (TAA), whether demonstrable by transplantation or other means, such as serology, are therefore not unique to the tumor but preferentially expressed on tumor tissue. Other examples of tumor-associated antigens are differentiation antigens and antigens also present on embryonic cells, so-called oncofetal antigens.

In human beings, no conclusive evidence has shown that tumor-specific antigens exist. Many claims of specific antigens have been reported in the literature, but careful research has found them to be tumor-associated at best.

Several reasons for the failure to demonstrate human tumor-specific antigens are possible. One could not demonstrate TSTA, even if they existed, because of ethical constraints. Their detection would necessitate transplantation of human tumors to other human beings. Tumor-specific antigens in man must be detected by other means, such as antisera. Because antisera are usually obtained by immunization of animals with tumor tissue, it may be that the animals do not possess the genetic repertoire to detect and to respond to the human neoantigens used as immunogens. In addition, the relatively weak antigens may be "hidden" on the cell membrane by their close proximity to strong antigens (*e.g.*, histocompatibility antigens) or may be present only in low concentrations.

Finally, if normal cell surface antigens form tumor-specific antigens simply by changing their physical state or configuration, they may not be detectable by routine methods of analysis, which depend upon chemical differences.

Monoclonal antibodies from hybridomas may be the means of resolving the issue of tumor-specific antigens (Mitchell and Oettgen, 1982). Their inherent specificity for a single antigenic determinant (epitope), makes them well suited for the detection of an unique antigenic molecule present among a myriad of others on the cell surface. The commonly used monoclonal antibodies against human cells generated by mouse-mouse hybridomas, however, may be encountering the same genetic restrictions as xenoantisera. Hence, *human* monoclonal antibodies should be far more likely to discern whether tumor-specific antigens exist on the surface of human neoplastic cells.

We should stress that even if such antigens do not exist, the current approach of using surface antigens for the diagnosis and therapy of neoplastic disease will not be invalidated. As long as the antigens in question are sufficiently restricted to neoplastic cells, as opposed to the normal tissues in which they are located, their usefulness as targets should be very similar to that of true tumor-specific antigens.

Virus-Induced and Chemically Induced Antigens. A variety of antigens are present on the surface of neoplastic cells, most of which are normal histocompatibility antigens, differentiation antigens, oncofetal antigens and viral structural antigens (see Figure 11-1). The leukemic T cells of the mouse are perhaps the most closely examined and may be used as an example (Old and Stockert, 1977). Histocompatibility antigens are governed by the $H-2^K$ and $H-2^D$ loci. Differentiation antigens belong to the Ly-series whose phenotypes

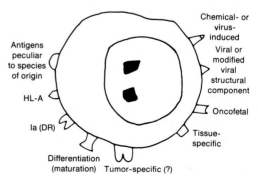

Figure 11-1. Schematic of possible range of antigens on a tumor cell membrane.

characterize these T cells as helper cells (Lyt-1) or suppressor cells (Lyt-2,3). Viral structural antigens are induced by C-type RNA viruses, which are a constant part of the mouse genome. Murine leukemia virus (MuLV) is the most important of these endemic RNA tumor viruses and expresses glycoproteins called GCSA and G_{IX} on the surface of both normal and transformed cells. GCSA is related to the pl5,30 virus core protein, whereas G_{IX} is identical to the p70 viral envelope protein. If DNA viruses such as polyoma or SV 40 are also present, a transformation (T) antigen is expressed on the nucleus and in the cytoplasm of the infected cell. This antigen is encoded by the early DNA region of these viruses and is virus-specific.

The virally or chemically induced TATA are expressed in addition to the antigens named above. Unfortunately, they usually cannot be defined by antisera. Hence, their ability to elicit rejection of the transplanted tumor is the only evidence for their existence. The inability to characterize these antigens by conventional means is a major limitation in their further biochemical characterization.

TATA can be induced by a large number of chemical carcinogens. Methylcholanthrene, other aromatic hydrocarbons, and aniline dyes are all potent inducers of soft tissue sarcomas or hepatomas. All of these chemically-induced TATA exhibit an extensive polymorphism. Thus, each tumor has its own unique transplantation antigens and even different primary tumors arising in a single animal may be antigenically dissimilar. A chemically induced tumor of this sort will elicit resistance only to itself (Klein, 1968).

In contrast, TATA induced by DNA or RNA viruses show extensive crossreactivity that even overrides species barriers. These virus-induced transplantation antigens are characteristic of all tumors induced by a particular virus regardless of the strain or species of the host. Therefore, they must contain at least one common antigen (Klein, 1968).

The central question is whether these TATA are true neoantigens or are related to viral structural protein. The latter possibility appears unlikely because immunity protecting against infection by the polyoma virus, for example, does not lead to rejection of a polyoma-induced transplanted tumor. Also RNA viral structural proteins are routinely expressed on mouse cells and their presence does not necessarily imply malignant conversion.

A definitive answer to the nature of viral (or chemical) TATA can be obtained only by biochemical analysis. The main difficulty is the unavailability of appropriate antisera. Tumor rejection experiments, therefore, must be performed at every purification step to document enrichment of the biological activity.

The TATA induced by SV 40 virus is the best characterized at the present time (Law *et al.,* 1980). At first it was thought that the TATA could not be identical with the T antigen of SV 40 because the latter is expressed mostly on the nucleus and in the cytoplasm, while TATA is a cell surface protein. TATA, however, has since been isolated in large quantities from nuclear material. Because its molecular weight is nearly identical with the T antigen, and one strain of SV 40 contains TATA activity within its T antigen, it is now almost certain that the T antigen and TATA of SV 40 are basically the same molecule. Antisera against the T antigen, however, are not crossreactive with TATA, implying some differences between the two. An additional processing step has been postulated to occur when the T antigen is inserted into the cell membrane. This would lead to loss of the T antigenicity and expression of TATA. Similar findings have now been obtained for the polyoma virus.

TATA induced by RNA viruses are also being examined on a molecular level. Available evidence suggests that these TATA are unique antigens unrelated to histocompatibility antigens or major viral structural proteins such as p15,30 and gp70. Their exact nature has not been clarified.

Chemically induced TATA have been regarded as the prototype of true tumor-specific neoantigens because of their seeming independence of virus. Their staggering polymorphism, however, has puzzled investigators for decades, suggesting that a relationship to ancient histocompatibility antigens was a likely possibility. Old and colleagues (Dubois *et al.,* 1981) found evidence against this assumption. They were able to produce syngeneic cytotoxic antisera against unrelated methylcholanthrene-induced tumors, called Meth A and CMSC 4. These antisera detect two molecules with molecular weights of 53,000 (p53) and 70,000 (p70). The molecule p53 was identified as a transformation protein that is present on all mouse cells transformed by chemicals, irradiation, or viruses. Its wide distribution and highly conserved nature excluded it from being the TATA, and leave p70 as a possible candidate. However, p70 is neither identical with histocompatibility antigens nor cross-reactive with antisera to MuLV.

A relationship of chemically-induced to virally-induced antigens is suggested by the work of Lennox *et al.* (1981), who used monoclonal antibodies for the characterization of TATA. They noted consistent reactivity with a 70,000 dalton protein. This protein was tentatively characterized as a variant of gp70, the retrovirus envelope protein. This important finding could imply that the chemically induced TATA are all virus related. By one schema, the chemical carcinogens may activate chromosomally integrated viral genes, which would provide the basic TATA molecule. This molecule may acquire its uniqueness from modification by the host cell.

Evidence exists that TATA induced both by viruses and chemical carcinogens may be basically viral structural proteins. Because the underlying cause of many cancers may be viruses, a unitary concept of tumor-specific antigens as essentially virally induced is appealing for its symmetry.

Human Melanoma Antigens. Neoplastic melanoma is the human tumor that has been examined most thoroughly for the presence of tumor-specific antigens. This tumor is of great immunologic interest because of occasional spontaneous regressions and its responsiveness to intradermal bacille Calmette Guérin (BCG) injections. Tumor specimens can often be propagated in tissue culture, thereby insuring a constant supply of tumor tissue for study.

A search for tumor-specific antigens on melanoma cells has been carried out at the Memorial Sloan-Kettering Cancer Center. Old and colleagues (Albino *et al.*, 1981; Old, 1981) have collected and characterized autologous sera to detect either unique ("private") antigens, present only on a patient's own tumor cells, or antigens shared by the group and characteristic of all melanomas. Private antigens are comparable with chemically induced TATA and are termed class 1 antigens.

Autologous typing avoids the complexities and false positives of allogeneic typing, and several class 1 antigens have been identified. Low antibody titers have prevented their biochemical analysis. The question still remains: Do these antigens belong to a common molecule that has many different epitopes, or do they represent totally unrelated molecules?

Allogeneic typing can more easily discover tumor-specific antigens shared by a class of tumor and/or a common tumor-associated

antigen not found on normal cells (class 2 antigens). A variety of class 2 tumor-associated melanoma antigens have been identified by this technique. MEL-1, AH, and B1-2 are well-known examples.

Monoclonal antibodies are now being used in the search for tumor-specific melanoma antibodies. They have detected a variety of differentiation antigens, with varying expression on different tissues (Old, 1981; Dippold *et al.*, 1982) (see Figure 11–2). R 24 appears to have one of the most restricted reactivities. It detects a glycolipid (GD_3) present in high concentrations on nearly all melanomas and is expressed only weakly on normal brain tissue, normal melanocytes, and astrocytoma cells. Still more specific may be an O-acetylated GD_3 apparently found only on melanoma (Cherish *et al.*, 1984). Gp 95 (also called p97 [Woodbury *et al.*, 1980]) and Gp 150 are more broadly represented but there is still a marked quantitative difference of expression between malignant melanoma cells and normal cells. Not indicated in the chart because it was discovered more recently (Reisfeld *et al.*, 1982), p250 appears highly specific for melanoma. It is more densely expressed on tumor cells than on normal tissue. These quantitative differences in expression of antigens are now being exploited for the diagnosis and therapy of patients with malignant melanoma.

Undoubtedly, new antigens will be discovered on melanoma cells, and human monoclonal antibodies to be developed may clarify whether tumor-specific antigens are present or not.

Other Human Tumor-Associated Antigens. A sarcoma-associated antigen has been described that was detected by autologous sera from patients. These sera cross-reacted with other sarcomas in different patients. An interesting finding was the reactivity of these antisera with genetically related normal family members. This finding suggests that the antigen detected was a normal differentiation antigen with restricted expression.

A variety of tumor-associated antigens have also been detected in patients with gastrointestinal cancers, testicular cancers, and hepatomas. Carcinoembryonic antigen (CEA) and alpha-fetoprotein are examples of such tumor-associated antigens. Normally expressed on embryonic cells during fetal life (oncofetal antigens), they are not present on mature adult tissue. These antigens may appear in high concentrations in the tumor tissue and are shed

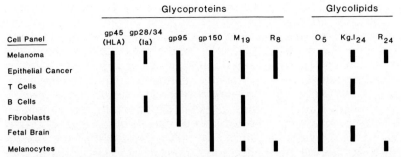

Figure 11–2. Cell surface antigens of melanoma defined by monoclonal antibodies. From Old, L. J.: Cancer immunology: The search for specificity—G. H. A. Clowes Memorial Lecture. *Cancer Res.,* **41:**361–375, 1981.

into the circulation, serving as useful markers for the presence of widespread disease.

Leukemias and lymphomas have also been scrutinized extensively for the presence of tumor antigens, leading to the identification of normal differentiation antigens. B lymphocytes carry the Ia-like (DR) antigen during their initial period of differentiation; the antigen disappears during the final maturation to the antibody-secreting plasma cell. Ia antigen is also present on the myeloid cell lineage and appears to be restricted to myeloid precursor cells and myeloblasts. Most of the so called AML-specific tumor antigens have now proved to be Ia antigens.

Human T cells carry a variety of differentiation antigens (Hansen and Martin, 1982), (see Figure 11–3). There are at least three distinct molecules present on all T cells and thymocytes (pan-T antigens). They are referred to as p50, p67, and p20–30 (the numbers represent the respective molecular weights $\times 10^{-3}$ daltons). The antigen identified by OK T1, Leu 1, T101, 10.2, and other commonly used pan-T reagents is p67. Several other T cell markers have been identified with the help of monoclonal antibodies. Helper T cells are characterized by reactivity with antibody OK-T4 and Leu-3a, whereas suppressor and cytotoxic T cells bind antibody OK-T8 and Leu2a. These antigens have not been defined biochemically. Often expressed in lymphocytic leukemias and lymphomas, they might aid in their differential diagnosis. The importance of these cells in the regulation of immunity will be discussed in the next section.

The Immune Response to Tumor Antigens

This section will deal with the host's immune response to antigens, especially tumor antigens. Many clinical anecdotes suggest that antitumor immunity exists and influences the course of neoplastic disease. The possible involvement of tumor immunity has been manifested in (1) spontaneous regressions of tumors, (2) prolonged survival or cure of patients after incomplete removal of neoplastic lesion, (3) sudden appearance of metastasis many years after successful therapy, and (4) regression of metastasis after local treatment of the primary lesion. Recently, much firmer evidence has documented an immune response to tumor antigens in patients with neoplastic disease. Measurements have been made of the cell-mediated and antibody reaction made by patients with cancer to the antigens on their own tumor or histologically similar tumors. Evidence for reactivity against autologous tumors would be most compelling to support tumor-associated immunity. In fact, the sera of cancer patients have been found to contain antibodies against the patient's own (autologous) tumors, most consistently in soft tissue

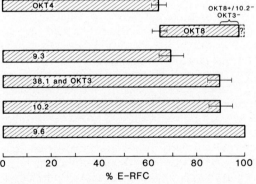

Figure 11–3. A graph of the human T-cell phenotypes, illustrating the subsets defined by several monoclonal antibodies. From Hansen, J. A., and Martin, P. J.: Human T-cell differentiation antigens. In Mitchell, M. S., and Oettgen, H. F. (eds.): *Hybridomas in Cancer Diagnosis and Treatment.* Raven Press, New York, 1982.

sarcoma, malignant melanoma, ovarian carcinoma, and lung cancer. Blood mononuclear cell-mediated cytotoxicity to autologous and second party (allogeneic) tumors has been demonstrated in a number of cancers (Hellstrom *et al.,* 1971) and leukocyte adherence inhibition testing has revealed reactivity to tumor extracts, particularly of breast cancer. The specificity of these cell-mediated reactions has been questioned, but, nevertheless, significant reactivity has frequently been observed. If sufficient attention is given to the details of the testing, such as the use of explanted tumor cells rather than cell lines, a considerable degree of discrimination between the antitumor reactivity of lymphocytes from normal patients versus those from patients with cancer is achievable (DeVries *et al.,* 1974; Mitchell *et al.,* 1980).

With the evidence of tumor transplantation immunity in animals and the demonstration of antitumor reactivity in man, the most important questions remaining are: How potent is antitumor immunity, and does it have any control over the initiation and development of cancer? These questions will be discussed after the components of the immune system have been described and their genetic control considered.

Overview. The two principal components of the immune response to tumor-associated antigens, and indeed to any antigen, are antibodies (humoral immunity) and leukocytes (cell-mediated immunity). Although their activities are separable, it should be emphasized that in the rejection of foreign cells, including cancers, the two components must act in concert. Often the two collaborate in a multifaceted process of killing, during which antibodies serve to prepare the tumor cell for destruction by the leukocytes.

The weight of evidence from animal experiments makes it seem very unlikely that antibodies act independently of leukocytes to kill tumor cells *in vivo.* Cytotoxic antibodies that bind *in vitro* complement and thus cause cytolysis of tumor cells have been demonstrated, particularly for mouse leukemias. *In vivo,* however, antibodies seem to serve principally to coat the tumor cells at their Fab combining sites, or "arm" leukocytes by attachment at their Fc end to receptors for this Fc on appropriate leukocytes. The white blood cells involved here are the macrophages and lymphoid cells, known as killer (K) cells, in a process termed antibody-dependent cell-mediated cytotoxicity (ADCC). Even antibodies that attach primarily to tumor cells must later be bound to macrophages at the Fc end. Thus, destruction of the tumor cells by the leukocytes occurs, after recognition is mediated by "cytophilic" antibodies, that is, those with the property of binding to leukocytes at their Fc end. The killing of tumor cells by macrophages occurs by a process of cytolysis or cytostasis rather than phagocytosis after the macrophages are brought into close proximity by the antibodies. The killing appears to be similar for both circulating macrophages and sessile macrophages in the reticuloendothelial system.

Cell-mediated cytotoxicity is the ultimate and major mechanism of destruction of tumor cells. In this process, macrophages appear to be the major effector cells, but other leukocytes such as thymus-derived (T) lymphocytes, natural killer cells, and even polymorphonuclear leukocytes play their roles, too. The interplay among various types of cells serves to modulate the immune response, often augmenting the response to immunogenic tumor cells, but sometimes leading to suppression. Macrophages are nonspecifically activated to kill tumor cells by soluble mediators from T lymphocytes, "lymphokines." Macrophages also make mediators, sometimes called "monokines," that can stimulate T lymphocytes. Although T cells have been shown to kill some tumor cells *in vitro* by direct cytotoxicity within four to 18 hours, it is likely that their major effect *in vivo* is to recruit and activate macrophages, judging from the preponderance of the latter at sites of rejection. Nonspecific killing is also a property of polymorphonuclear leukocytes, perhaps by mechanisms very similar to those employed by macrophages, and polymorphs may also be "armed" by cytophilic antibodies. Natural killer cells, which can lyse target cells within four to six hours *in vitro,* may also be active *in vivo,* perhaps as cells in surveillance against the emergence of tumor cells. Specific destruction of tumor antigens can be accomplished primarily through the stimulation of T cells, which leads either to specific antibody production and/or to cell-mediated reactions ultimately involving killer macrophages. The involvement of memory T cells insures that the long-lived immune recognition of the tumor will occur, with more than a nonspecific inflammatory exudate as effector cells (see Table 11-1).

Macrophages. Macrophages originate in

Table 11–1. Cells Involved in the Immune Response to Human Cancer

CELL	DERIVATION OR LINEAGE	CHARACTERISTIC SURFACE MARKER	KINETICS OF KILLING	SPECIFICITY
Macrophages	Bone marrow via blood monocyte	Receptors for Fc, DR, and complement (C3b)	Cytostasis; killing in 48 to 72 hrs	Nonspecific or determined by Fc receptor-bound antibody
T lymphocytes	Bone marrow differentiation induced by thymus	Receptors for sheep RBC. Have antigens reactive with monoclonal antibodies OK-T3 and Leu 1		Highly specific receptor for binding of antigen
Helper		OK-T4+, Leu 3a+. Some have receptors for Fc	Indirect by stimulation of cytotoxic T cells	
Cytotoxic		OK-T5/8+, Leu 2a+	Lysis in 4 to 18 hrs	
Suppressor		OK-T5/8+, Leu 2a+	—	
Natural killer (NK) cells	Lymphocyte, most likely; macrophage, possibly	Not yet completely defined. Receptors for Fc portion of antibody	Lysis in 4 hrs	Nonspecific, perhaps recognizes glycolipid in cell membrane
K cells	Lymphocyte, probably	Receptor for Fc portion of antibody	Lysis in 4 hrs	Determined by Fc receptor-bound antibody (ADCC)
B lymphocytes	Bone marrow, differentiation induced by "bursa" equivalent	Immunoglobulin on membrane; DR antigen; receptors for Fc and complement	Indirect through antibody secretion	Specificity of secreted antibody

369

the bone marrow from a myeloid stem cell. They circulate in the blood as monocytes and undergo final differentiation to mature tissue macrophages in lung, liver, and spleen, among other tissues. Macrophages are characterized by a variety of surface markers, most notably Fc and C3 receptors, and, in many locations such as the spleen, Ia (DR) antigen. Although Fc and C3 receptors are operative in the binding of antibody-coated antigens, the Ia antigen provides genetic control of the immune response. It is coded for by immune response (Ir) genes of the major histocompatibility complex, and restricts macrophage-T cell interactions to those carrying identical Ia molecules. Therefore, macrophages carrying the Ia molecule initiate a chain of cell-cell interactions, whereas macrophages lacking the Ia molecule perform roles such as killing and phagocytosis.

Effector (killer) macrophages destroy tumor cells by inhibiting their growth rather than by rapid cytolysis. Superoxide radicals, exoenzymes, and transfer of lysosomes have been some of the suggested mechanisms but none is conclusively proven. "Activated" effector macrophages are enlarged, and tightly adherent, and have ruffled membranes, making them easily distinguishable morphologically. Some macrophages, however, actively performing other functions, such as the production of mediators, may not have these features.

Afferent macrophages present antigens to helper T cells (Unanue, 1979). Antigenic material attached to the surface of a macrophage is handled in two different ways: It is either interiorized and then degraded by lysosomal enzymes or is presented to T cells. These dual functions are somewhat conflicting because destroyed antigen is unavailable for activation of T cells. Although only a small number of antigenic molecules remain on the surface for antigenic presentation, ingested molecules are only incompletely digested and later return to the surface by exocytosis. Antigens not bound to macrophages are usually poorly immunogenic and induce only a weak and transient immune response. Macrophages concentrate antigen on their surface, and thus present a large number of antigenic determinants to the T cell. The high concentration of antigenic molecules permits their steric interaction and aggregation, thus further enhancing their immunogenicity.

Macrophages initiate virtually every immune response by attaching antigenic material on their cell membrane and presenting it to helper T-lymphocytes. This antigenic presentation and the release of soluble mediators leads to the activation and clonal proliferation of T-cell subsets. Cytotoxic T cells are generated, B cells are turned into antibody-secreting cells by T cell-B cell interaction, and a comprehensive immune response is produced. This process is amplified by lymphokines from activated T cells, which in turn activate effector macrophages to participate in the specific immune response.

Macrophages produce soluble mediators such as interleukin 1 (lymphocyte-activating factor) and thereby nonspecifically stimulate proliferation. Extracts of primed macrophages can induce immunity even when the priming agent is itself immunogenic. Several soluble factors are released by macrophages, and some have been characterized chemically. All are potent T-cell mitogens, and some can also induce B-cell differentiation, with subsequent production of specific antibody.

The role of macrophages in regulating immunity is becoming increasingly evident (Oehler et al., 1978). A subset of macrophages that suppresses immunity has been identified. Ultimately, the existence of subsets fully analogous to those of T cells may be proved. Presently, macrophages are known to assist functions similar to T cells. Even unactivated bone marrow cells contain suppressor cells; some closely resemble macrophages.

T Cells. T-lymphocytes originate as stem cells in the bone marrow and migrate to the thymic cortex where they proliferate and differentiate into mature T cells under the influence of thymic hormones. They reside in all lymphatic organs of the body and are released into the circulation when stimulated by antigens. Their distribution in the lymphatic organs is quite distinctive. In the spleen, T cells are concentrated around the central arteriole, surrounded by a rim of B lymphocytes. In the cortex of lymph nodes, T cells fill the spaces between the postcapillary venules, while B cells populate the germinal centers. This normal distribution is severely disturbed in lymphomatous disease.

There are three major subsets of T-lymphocytes, designated cytotoxic, suppressor, and inducer helper T cells (Rich and Rich, 1977). Cytotoxic T cells, as their name states, exert a direct cytotoxic effect on tumor cells, lysing them within four to six hours in vitro. Suppressor T cells appear to be critically important in regulating the immune response to tumor antigens and might be excessively active in tumor-bearing hosts. Helper T cells can stimulate immunity by interacting with antigen on macrophages and then with B cells in the production of antibodies. They also interact with other T cells in cell-mediated responses. These inducer T cells are important in initiating suppressor reactions when stimulated by antigen-antibody complexes rather than antigens on macrophages (Rao *et al.,* 1980). Inducer T cells interact with naive T cells, called cooperator or acceptor cells. From this subset, two types of lymphocyte are recruited: Cytotoxic T cells and suppressor T cells. It is likely that suppressor cells are always activated by immunogens and their ratio to the effector cells, which are also induced through helper cells, determines the magnitude of the immune response.

Stimulation of T cells leads to their secretion of lymphokines. One of these, macrophage-activating factor (MAF) nonspecifically activates macrophages and recruits previously unstimulated monocytes. Some become cytotoxic effector cells, and others secrete monokines that augment the pool of activated lymphocytes. Migration inhibitory factor (MIF) is another lymphokine, chemically identical with MAF, which inhibits macrophage migration *in vitro* and probably *in vivo.*

Helper, suppressor, and cytotoxic T cells are distinct cells that can be differentiated by their surface markers. Mouse lymphocytes, for example, carry the "Lyt" differentiation (antigens Lyt 1, Lyt 2, and Lyt 3; Lyt 2 and Lyt 3 are always found together on cells). Helper cells exclusively carry the Lyt 1 antigen; suppressor cells and cytotoxic T cells are both positive for Lyt 2,3. These cells can be further differentiated with the help of the I-J marker, a product of the mouse immune response gene, which is found only on mouse suppressor T cells. Human lymphocytes also have characteristic phenotypes. Monoclonal antibodies of the Ortho-Kung (OK) or Leu series are now commonly used to subtype T cells. Reactivity with OK-T3 or Leu 1 defines T cells in general, whereas OK-T4 or Leu 3a reacts with helper T cells. OK T8 and Leu 2a define both cytotoxic T cells and suppressor cells.

Natural Killer Cells.   Natural killer (NK) cells (Herberman and Ortaldo, 1981), polymorphonuclear leukocytes, and non-Ia-bearing macrophages react against a wide variety of syngeneic, allogeneic, and xenogeneic cells. They therefore are not under genetic control and may provide the host with a "natural immunity," that is, immunoreactivity without prior immunization or sensitization. Nonadherent leukocytes of many normal persons, for example, can lyse selected tumor cells, especially from long-term tumor cell lines. NK cells have been separated on a per-coll gradient, where they appear to be large granular lymphocytes morphologically. Immunologically, however, they share characteristics of both T cells and macrophages. A large percentage of them carry the receptors for sheep RBC and a variety of antigenic structures defined by monoclonal anti-T-cell antibodies. Their reactivity with monoclonal antibody OKM1, defining monocytes and granulocytes, on the other hand, creates uncertainty as to their exact identity.

The importance of NK cells for controlling cancerous disease is unkown. Circumstantial evidence suggests they might perform a surveillance role. "Nude" mice, which are genetically deficient in T cells, nevertheless, are not unusually susceptible to spontaneous tumors. These mice have a high level of NK activity. "Beige" mice, which lack NK activity, are susceptible. *In vitro* NK cells have been greatly cytotoxic to certain human leukemias, a myeloma, and certain carcinomas, an activity that can be augmented by interferon. Transfer of NK cells leads to retardation of tumor growth in some animals, and NK cells have been found at the site of tumor growth. Their mechanism of cytotoxicity is unknown at present.

NK cells may be part of a nonspecific defense system, responding rapidly to foreign antigens before more potent and specific immunity is evoked.

Humoral Immunity.   Humoral immunity means the formation of antibodies to specific antigens by "bursa-dependent" lymphocytes. These cells originate from a progenitor pool in the bone marrow and develop to competent cells under the influence of a structure, called the bursa of Fabricius in birds, whose exact morphologic correlate in humans is not known. A possible role of lymphoid tissue of the gastrointestinal tract in this differentiation process is suspected.

B cell development occurs in several steps. First, isolated L (light) chains are expressed on the cell surface. This is followed by appearance of complete IgM molecules and finally IgD. Surface IgG is present only on approximately 10% of B cells, identifying them as the memory cells responsible for a secondary response to antigen. B cells differentiate to plasma cells under the influence of antigens and T-cell factors, then secrete antibodies. Antibodies produced by a given plasma cell are monoclonal and are identical with the surface-bound immunoglobulin except for the heavy chain that determines the subclass, such as IgM, IgG, etc.

Antigen alone will not induce B-cell proliferation and antibody production. Most antigens are known to be thymus-dependent; that is, T cells recognize the larger part of the molecule (carrier) and B cells, then produce antibodies against a few antigenic determinants (hapten) of this molecule. Elicitation of humoral immunity is now understood as a multistep event where antigen must be bound by macrophages and then presented to helper T cells. Proliferation of this T-cell subset occurs, helper cell factors are released, clonal expansion of the corresponding B-lymphocyte is induced, and, finally, antibody production occurs. It is unknown whether these helper cell factors also contain the stimulating antigen or whether B cells attach antigen-independently. Only a few thymus-independent molecules exist that can induce antibody production independently of the described cell-cell interaction. These are usually large molecules with identical repetitive determinants of which pneumococcal polysaccharide is an example. This immune response consists exclusively of IgM molecules and is brief in duration.

IgG antibodies are the principal cytophilic antibodies, which bind tightly to target cells and, at their opposite (Fc) end, to macrophages. The recognition of tumor antigens through "arming" of macrophages probably involves IgG antibodies, too. Armed effector cells, macrophages, and K cells kill by antibody-dependent cell-mediated cytotoxicity (ADCC). K cells, incidentally, appear to be lymphoid, and have receptors for Fc and complement, but not surface immunoglobulin. It is not known whether they are transient stages in B- or T-cell development or a distinct population of cells.

Antibodies can be detrimental to the cancer-bearing host by interacting with circulating tumor antigen, forming immune complexes, and then blocking antitumor immunity by eliciting suppressor T cells *in vivo*. This possibility will be discussed in a later section. Antibody *per se* is not detrimental to the host.

Genetic Control of Immunity

All specific immune responses, including those to cancer cells, are genetically controlled (Benacerraf and Germain, 1978). This was first appreciated in the early 1960s when laboratory animals were immunized with synthetic polypeptides. Some animal strains consistently responded to the antigenic challenge with high levels of specific antibodies; other strains were nonresponders. Crossbreeding experiments traced the genes controlling immune response to the histocompatibility region and are referred to as immune response (Ir) genes. These Ir genes exert their regulatory influence mostly on the T-cell level. Immunization with chemical (hapten)-protein (carrier) molecules, where the T cell recognizes the protein carrier and the B cell has made specific antibodies to the hapten, revealed a defect in T-cell recognition in nonresponders. Moreover, thymectomy converted animals that were genetically responders into nonresponders, again pinpointing the crucial importance of T-lymphocytes in antigenic recognition. Ir gene expression has also been documented on B cells, adding the regulation of cell-cell interaction to the duties of the Ir genes. The number of genes involved in controlling immunity has not been precisely defined, but crossbreeding experiments suggest at least two genes. Amino acid analysis of a human "DR" antigen, an Ia-like antigen coded for by the Ir gene, detected seven closely related DR molecules implying an extensive genetic polymorphism at the Ir gene locus.

Immune response genes were at first thought to influence only helper T cells, leading only to stimulation of immunity. Poor immunogenicity of an antigenic molecule was explained by poor stimulation of helper T cells. More recent evidence, however, shows that immunologic unresponsiveness is an active phenomenon due to genetically controlled stimulation of suppressor T cells. In several animal systems, antigenic stimulation lead to proliferation of suppressor cells alone and thus to complete suppression of immunity. It seems likely that within the immune response region, distinct antigen-specific immunosuppressive (Is) genes exist that serve as counterbalance to positive Ir genes.

A central question is: How is genetic control exerted? Mixing experiments with adequately primed T and B cells revealed that an immune response would occur only if these cells came from genetically identical animals. This genetic restriction is very important in the interaction of macrophages and helper T cells and in T-B cell interaction. The molecule responsible for genetic restriction is now believed to be the Ia antigen (mouse) that is termed Ia-like or

DR in humans. These molecules are both highly preserved in phylogeny, as shown by extensive interspecies crossreactivity.

Genetic control is, therefore, thought to occur by the recognition of the genetically appropriate Ia molecule by lymphocytes. It is believed that only Ia antigen-positive macrophages are capable of presenting antigen to T lymphocytes. T cells recognize two characteristics on the macrophage: Surface-bound antigen and the Ia molecule. Only T cells that carry the appropriate receptor to interact with this Ia molecule are able to proliferate and induce an immune response. This immune response is then carried forth by factors produced by helper and suppressor T cells. These factors contain Ia molecules that carry the genetic information to interactive cells. It appears likely that specific Ia molecules serve specific functions; that is, that certain Ia molecules activate T cells, whereas others primarily interact with suppressor T cells.

Cytotoxic T cells are not only subject to genetic restriction by the Ia molecule. In two animal models, T cell cytotoxicity was dependent on histocompatibility antigens other than Ia and the regulating genes were mapped to the $H-2^K$ and/or $H-2^D$ (class I) regions of the mouse histocompatibility complex. In these cases, the genetic restriction was the recognition of "self," *plus* viral antigens, which together were the target for the cytotoxic T cells. This mechanism may be important in anticancer immunity, where "self" *plus* TAA may be the stimulus to clonal expansion of cytotoxic T cell, as well as the target antigens.

Escape of Emerging Tumor Cells from Tumor Immunity

The role of immunity in controlling neoplastic disease is still poorly defined and is still a subject of controversy. Paul Ehrlich postulated the existence of antitumor immunity against established tumors in 1908. This concept was then modified by Thomas and later Burnet to a surveillance against the development of a tumor (Burnet, 1970). The immunosurveillance theory in its simplest form postulates that tumor cells arise frequently in every individual by somatic mutation but are recognized as foreign and destroyed by immunologic mechanisms before a frank tumor develops. This surveillance was believed by Burnet to be T cell-mediated and directed against tumor-specific surface antigens. Cellular immunity in animals, it was theorized, developed phylogenetically, mainly to prevent the emergence of cancer.

The distinction between the development of a tumor from a single cell and the continued growth and flourishing of established tumors is essential when considering the role of antitumor immunity. In both situations, a failure to eliminate tumor cells is evident. Patients with established tumors, however, unquestionably have antitumor immunity, which perhaps is inadequate but present nevertheless. This cannot be said with certainty for individuals with an early-developing tumor. Detection of the tumor at this early stage is literally impossible, therefore the degree of concomitant antitumor immunity at this time is unknown. Thus, "proof" of immunosurveillance consists mostly of examples where its predictions have been borne out clinically.

Patients with the various forms of immunodeficiency syndromes would be expected to develop cancer more frequently than normal individuals. Indeed, patients with ataxia telangiectasia, variable immunodeficiency, and Wiskott-Aldrich syndrome show an approximately 200-fold increase of cancer over age- and sex-matched controls. Patients receiving long-term immunosuppressive therapy after renal transplantation and cardiac transplantation have an approximately 300-fold increased incidence of neoplastic disease. Lymphomas predominate in both these groups, but renal transplant patients also have a very high incidence of epithelial neoplasms, lending credence to a generalized breakdown in surveillance rather than simply a derangement of lymphoid function. The most common forms of cancer might be expected to be the most frequent ones encountered in immunosuppressed patients. Breast, lung, and other common tumors, however, are clearly underrepresented. The same is true in children for whom an increased frequency of common childhood tumors has not been observed. These facts could be interpreted to mean either that immunosurveillance does not exist or that it has no role in controlling these types of neoplasms.

It does not mean that some form of surveillance has no role in oncogensis. Nude mice that lack effective T cells because of a genetic defect would be expected to have an increased incidence of spontaneous tumors. In fact, they do not, but it is known that NK cells and macrophages present in nude mice provide strong antitumor immunity that probably perform the surveillance function. "Beige" mice lacking NK cells indeed have increased susceptibility to cancer.

Kaposi's sarcoma in men who are homosexual may well be an example of a failure of classical T cell-mediated surveillance (see Chapter 20). In this disease, helper T cells are significantly reduced, and the functional activity of suppressor T cells is relatively increased. Severe viral and fungal infections occur in this setting of severe acquired cellular immunodeficiency. It is likely that a virus is involved in the etiology and that the immunodeficiency permits it to cause the tumor, which then develops unimpeded in this setting.

Surveillance against tumor cells by T cells, the Burnet version of the hypothesis, may require modification. Thus, non-T-cells may be more important in such nonspecific protection, and the target of the surveillance may be the etiologic agent rather than the transformed cell itself. Lymphomas, Kaposi's sarcoma in homosexuals, and carcinoma of the cervix uteri, all of which are increased in frequency in immunosuppressed patients, have been suspected to have a viral etiology. The virus may have been incorporated into the genome long before, but was dormant until immunodeficiency, either natural or iatrogenic, permitted it to be expressed.

Immunosurveillance remains an attractive theory with which to assess our observations of the occurrence of cancers. The constant testing of the validity of the hypothesis can lead to more precise understanding of the role of immunity in protecting against cancer, and justifies retaining the surveillance theory for now.

Escape of Established Tumors from Tumor Immunity

One of the most puzzling questions in tumor immunology is how neoplastic cells can grow in the face of an immune response. While few tumor-specific or tumor-associated antigens induce outright tumor rejection, many of them are somewhat immunogenic. Most experimental animals that develop cytotoxic lymphocytes or antibodies to their tumor nevertheless succumb to it. Yet when those lymphocytes are transferred to another syngeneic animal, a powerful antitumor immunity can often be demonstrated that protects the recipient when it is challenged with the specific tumor.

Such observations have led to the concept that tumors can escape antitumor immunity.

Ironically, mechanisms originally intended to regulate immunity or to control tumor growth are often subverted by the tumor to foster its growth. Many different mechanisms postulated or experimentally established partially explain why tumors escape immunologic destruction despite documented antitumor immunity. These mechanisms are not totally exclusive and undoubtedly combine to increase the tumor's chances of evading rejection.

Antigenic Modulation. Antigenic modulation was first noted in the thymus leukemia (TL) system. TL antigens are normal differentiation antigens on mouse thymocytes also present on their T cell-derived leukemias. Immunization against this surface antigen proved to be totally ineffective, resulting in unimpeded tumor growth in immunized animals. Analysis of tumor immunity revealed paradoxically strong cytotoxic antibodies after immunization. Rapid loss of the TL antigen could be demonstrated as soon as these tumor cells were incubated with an appropriate antibody, and TL antigens were resynthesized as soon as the antibody was removed. Antigenic modulation, therefore, is a transient or persistent loss of surface antigen after exposure of the antigen-bearing cell to specific antibody. Surface immunoglobulins on B cells can also be modulated. Antigenic modulation is the foremost theoretical concern in the treatment with monoclonal antibodies and has already been observed in a few patients with T-cell leukemias.

Blocking Factors. Tumor-bearing animals and patients are often substantially immunosuppressed. Removal of the bulk of the tumor often restores considerable immunity, and the suspicion arose that neoplastic disease can regulate immunity. This immunosuppression is most commonly a delayed-type hypersensitivity with skin test anergy. Enhancement of tumor growth has been noted in mice preimmunized with the same tumor. Such increased tumor growth was initially observed with allogeneic tumors in the early 1950s and can be transferred by serum from tumor-bearing mice to syngeneic recipients (Kaliss, 1958).

Enhancement of tumor growth and immunosuppression by serum factors were linked causally in one system when sera of syngeneic animals and human beings were demonstrated to abolish specifically antitumor activity of syngeneic lymphocytes *in vitro*. This phenomenon was attributed to the presence of "blocking factors" in the sera (Hellstrom and Hellstrom, 1974, 1978). Initially, tumor antibodies were implicated as the blocking principle; these antibodies were thought to coat the tumor cell surface, thus preventing sensitized lymphocytes from recognition of tumor antigen and its subsequent attack. Studies of tumor-bearing hosts, however, do not bear out this theory. During the time of rapid tumor growth, large amounts of tumor antigen are usually present in their circulation, whereas tumor-specific antibodies occur after tumor debulking. The presence of free tumor antibody, therefore, indicates restored immunity. It is now well established that soluble tumor antigens or specific immune complexes consisting of specific tumor antigens and tumor antibody are the blocking and tumor-enhancing principles in the serum.

The central question is how these specific antigen antibody complexes or free soluble tumor antigens suppress tumor immunity. Suppressor T cells induced by immune complexes are most likely the proximate mediators of this suppression of immunity. Thymectomy, for example, abolishes the suppressive effect of immune complexes in the mouse. Adoptive transfer of suppression by T cells further established the T cell dependence of this process (Mitchell and Rao, 1981). It is now established that helper/inducer T cells are initially evoked by immune complexes, which then induce the ultimate suppressor T cells. These suppressor cells then decrease cell-mediated responsiveness and perhaps even antibody synthesis.

Blocking factors are an excellent example of how a tumor can subvert antitumor immunity to perpetuate its own growth through the induction of a suppressed state. The shedding of tumor antigens exaggerates immunoregulation, leads to excessive activity of suppressor T cells, and thus to depression of antitumor immunity. Even though measurable cell-mediated and humoral immunities exist in tumor-bearing patients, they are, by this schema, lower than they should be because of this suppression.

Suppressor Cells. Suppressor cells, especially T cells, are probably the most important negative influence on antitumor immunity. In many animal models, suppressor lymphocytes can be demonstrated very shortly after tumor transplantation and usually persist during tumor growth. Immunization of mice with syngeneic methylcholanthrene-induced sarcoma predictably leads to strong tumor rejection. After tumor cells and suppressor T lymphocytes were given simultaneously to these

immunized animals, however, enhanced tumor growth was observed. Antibodies to T cells abolished this enhancement and caused regression of established tumors (Greene et al., 1977).

Available evidence suggests that these tumor-induced suppressor cells are generated and regulated exactly as are their "normal" immunoregulatory counterparts. A suppressor factor that causes clonal expansion of antigen-specific suppressor cells has recently been isolated. It also contains the I-J marker that is encoded by mouse Ir genes. Thus, the activation of tumor-induced suppressor lymphocytes is antigen-specific, whatever that tumor-associated antigen proves to be, and is under genetic control. Antibodies against the I-J marker in one mouse tumor model reacted strongly with the mouses's suppressor cells, inhibiting the suppressor cells and as a consequence causing tumor regression.

In addition to suppressor T lymphocytes, several other cells can suppress immunity, usually more nonspecifically. Macrophages, through their elaboration of prostaglandins, and lymphocytes without identifiable markers (null cells), have been shown to have suppressive activity. Macrophages seem to prevent the proliferation of T cells, inhibiting, for example, the development of cytotoxic T cells *in vitro*. Macrophages act nonspecifically to inhibit delayed hypersensitivity reactions by this means; their importance in regulating specific antitumor immunity is uncertain.

PRACTICAL APPLICATIONS

Hybridoma Technology and Monoclonal Antibodies

The development by Köhler and Milstein (1975) of techniques for creating stable clones from the fusion of immunized lymphocytes and myeloma cells, that is, "hybridomas," that produce monoclonal antibodies *in vitro* was a milestone in general immunology and certainly in tumor immunology. The ability afforded by this technique to obtain large amounts of pure antibodies to specific antigenic determinants (epitopes) will enable advances in all fields of biologic endeavor, as early results with the method have already amply demonstrated.

Figure 11–4 indicates schematically the formation and selection of hybridomas. It is extremely important to test for continued secretion of antibodies by the hybridomas at several

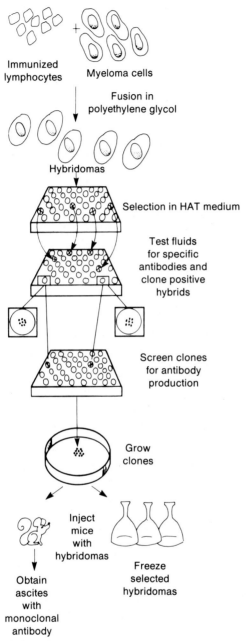

Figure 11–4. Production and selection of hybridomas.

points in the selection process in order to obtain antibody-producing clones that do not subsequently revert to wild type. Freezing ampules containing stocks of selected important hybridomas also insures against the loss of a critical fusion product. With these and related provisos, the hybridoma technology provides a large supply of stable, uniform, highly selective antibodies for a multitude of important different uses, many of which will be described in the

following section. A fuller consideration of these applications has recently appeared (Mitchell and Oettgen, 1982).

Immunologic Diagnosis of Cancer: Applications of Monoclonal Antibodies

The advent of monoclonal antibodies has increasingly made the diagnosis of cancer more secure, especially in situations where definitive diagnosis by conventional pathology has been impossible. With their intrinsic ability to discriminate between one antigenic specificity and another, monoclonal antibodies have the ability to detect a tumor-specific antigen characteristic of a class of tumor, if it exists. In melanoma and in colon carcinoma, reports of monoclonal antibodies that have recognized determinants not present on normal tissues or on neoplastic cells of other histologic types have been made (Hellstrom *et al.,* 1982; Reisfeld *et al.,* 1982; Steplewski and Koprowski, 1982). Diagnosis of a specific type of tumor, after attaching an immunoperoxidase label to the monoclonal antibody, is now possible, and should be helpful in distinguishing among such entities as the "round cell" tumors, the so-called LEMMON group (*L*ymphoma, *E*wing's sarcoma, *M*elanoma, *M*edulloblastoma, *O*at cell carcinoma, and *N*euroblastoma). Monoclonals against various subtypes of T- and B-lymphoma are available, as are antibodies with some degree of specificity for neuroblastoma and oat cell carcinoma. Thus, the entities that pathologists cannot easily separate with routine hematoxylin-eosin staining, or often even with histochemistry, frequently requiring electron microscopy, will soon be separable with ease by immunologic means. Breast cancer has been reported to be detectable in a setting of fibrocystic disease by monoclonal antibodies tagged with immunoperoxidase.

The antibodies need not be absolutely tumor specific; the antigens need only be present on the tumor but not on any other normal tissue in which the tumor is ordinarily found, nor on the tumors with which it may be commonly confused histologically (such as within the "round cell" tumor group). Panels of monoclonal antibodies may be necessary if there is no one characteristic antigen for the entire class. Only if it proves true that there are no class-specific antigens, only "private" antigens found on each tumor uniquely, would it be virtually impossible to use monoclonal antibodies diagnostically. Fortunately, this does not seem to be the case from many initial studies.

Serologic diagnosis of specific cancers would also be considerably aided by monoclonal antibodies, provided there were no circulating substances that were antigenically related to the tumor antigens. Antibodies to CEA and alpha-fetoprotein are already useful in detecting a variety of tumors that shed or secrete these substances. Better monoclonal antibodies might distinguish antigenic determinants that could separate the several tumors that shed CEA from one another. It is unlikely that even a panel of antibodies will be useful in screening for "cancer" in general, but a limited panel would be useful in screening patients at high risk for a specific type, for example, in the woman with a strong family history for breast cancer. Antigens or antibodies in the circulation can be detected by highly sensitive methods, such as radioimmunoassay or enzyme-linked immunosorption (ELISA). Immune complexes of tumor antigen and host antibodies have been detected more sensitively by improved methods, which permit dissociation of the complexes and analysis of each individual component.

Tagging of monoclonal antibodies with toxins or radioactive substances in order to kill tumor cells will be considered below. Tagged antibodies are potentially useful in the detection of deposits of tumor cells in the body. Technetium 99m pertechnetate and indium 111 have been used to label monoclonal antibodies, which in small amounts *in vivo* have localized in the tumor in twice the concentration of normal tissues (Hellstrom *et al.*, 1982). Because monoclonal antibodies "home" to tumor cells specifically, whereas radionuclides alone are taken up by inflammatory cells surrounding the tumor rather than the tumor itself, the selectivity and sensitivity of radionuclide scanning should be considerably improved in the future. There are already reports of improved detection of melanoma, colon cancer, and teratomas (Hellstrom *et al.*, 1982; Steplewski and Koprowski, 1982; Solter *et al.*, 1982) with labeled monoclonal antibodies to tumor-associated antigens injected *in vivo*. Polyclonal antibodies to substances that are associated with the tumor but are not tumor-specific, such as ferritin, have been tried as a conjugate with radionuclides, but monoclonal antibodies have not yet been used in this system.

BIOMODULATION (BIOLOGICAL RESPONSE MODIFICATION)

The area of cancer treatment that was formerly called "immunotherapy" might better be termed biologic response modification or "biomodulation," the latter being our abbreviated coinage. All approaches to cancer that attempt to modify the growth characteristics or antigenic structure of the tumor and thereby influence the host's response to the tumor can be included under this heading. Direct attempts to activate the cells involved in the immune response or improve the host's general ability to tolerate the treatment of the tumor are also included. Thus, the older field of immunotherapy is subsumed under the broader new heading of biomodulation. An agent is a biomodulator ("biomodulin," biological response modifier, BRM) if it does one or more of the following:

1. Augments the host's antitumor response directly, by stimulating an increase in the number or activity of effector ("killer") cells, or an increased production of soluble mediators, such as T-cell lymphokines or macrophage-made monokines. Examples include tumor antigens, nonspecific adjuvants such as BCG, thymic hormones, and interferons alpha and beta (leukocyte and fibroblast interferons respectively);

2. Decreases suppressor mechanisms and thus increases the host's immune reponse to the tumor indirectly. Examples: Low doses of cyclophosphamide, prostaglandin antagonists, and, perhaps, the immunosorbent *Staphylococcus* protein A column;

3. Increases the host's defenses by being itself a natural or synthetic effector or mediator. Examples: Bone marrow transplants; transfusions of leukocytes, especially lymphocytes; antibodies; interferon-gamma (T-cell interferon), and probably interferon-alpha and interferon-beta, too;

4. Increases the ability of the host to tolerate damage by cytotoxic modalities, such as by increasing bone marrow leukocyte precursors. Examples: Autologous bone marrow reinfusion and azimexone;

5. Changes the characteristics of the cell membrane of tumor cells sufficiently to

increase their immunogenicity, to alter their pattern of metastasis, or to make the tumor cells more susceptible to killing by immunologic mechanisms or cytotoxic drugs. Examples: Neuroaminidase (to augment immunogenicity); amphotericin B (to potentiate cytotoxic chemical agents);

6. Prevents or reverses transformation, or increases maturation of the "primitive" tumor cell. Examples: Retinoids, naturally occurring maturational factors.

It is most convenient to discuss biomodulation by beginning with "classical" immunotherapeutic agents, because many of the most common biomodulators are well-categorized into more narrowly restricted subgroups of immunotherapy than in the six broad areas of biomodulation just defined. Those agents that fall outside the immunotherapeutic categories will then be discussed.

Table 11–2 outlines the four broad classes of immunotherapy, derived principally from the categories of classic immunization: Active, adoptive, and passive, with the further addition of "restorative" immunotherapy, a more recent approach that has largely been developed as a form of antitumor treatment.

Active Immunotherapy

Active immunotherapy attempts to stimulate the host's intrinsic immune response to the tumor, either through a nonspecific approach with immunomodulators ("adjuvants"), or through the use of tumor-associated antigens on whole tumor cells or in extracts. Two broad subgroups will be considered separately, although there are compelling reasons for combining the two to provide maximally effective immunization.

Nonspecific. Nonspecific active immunotherapy is what many oncologists consider synonymous with "immunotherapy," because it has been the most exploited area thus far, but it is in fact only one subcategory. The nonspecific "adjuvants," better called "immunomodulators" because they can have both stimulatory and suppressive effects on immunity under various circumstances, include such common microbial agents as BCG and related mycobacteria, derivatives of BCG such as cell wall skeletons, "P3" (trehalose dimycolate), methanol extraction residue (MER), and muramyl dipeptide (MDP), the smallest structure with adjuvanticity in mycobacterial cell walls (Mitchell and Murahata, 1979). Other microbes include *Nocardia* and *Propionibacterium* acnes (formerly *Corynebacterium parvum*) and its fractions. Synthetic polyinosinic: cytidylic acid (Poly I:C) is also an adjuvant as are such diverse agents as the polyanion pyran copolymer (MVE, Diveema), the interferon-inducing fluorenones, such as tilorone, bacterial lipopolysaccharide (LPS, endotoxin), and interferon. These materials fundamentally act on macrophages, activating them so that they kill tumor cells and other foreign cells nonspecifically by cell-cell contact. Macrophages secondarily stimulate T lymphocytes to proliferate, through interleukin 1 (formerly lymphocyte-activating factor, LAF). The T cells can become cytotoxic after further stimulation by lymphokines. Activated T cells stimulate further interleukin 1 production from macrophages, and also make mediators that further activate macrophages, such as macrophage-activating factor (MAF). This bidirectional cycle of stimulatory events is set into motion by the nonspecific activating agents such as BCG (Mokyr and Mitchell, 1975). Introduction of either a "foreign" target cell or

Table 11–2. Types of Immunotherapy

1. Active: Stimulation of the host's intrinsic antitumor immunity
   a. Nonspecific: Use of microbial or chemical immunomodulators ("adjuvants"): Activates macrophages, NK cells, and other nonspecific effectors, T cells secondarily through macrophages
   b. Specific: Use of antigenic tumor cells or extracted tumor antigens, often altered by added chemical groups or treatment with enzymes: Activates specific effector cells such as T cells and "armed" macrophages.
2. Adoptive: Transfer of immunologic cells or informational molecules
3. Restorative: Repletion of deficient immunologic subpopulations (principally T cells) or inhibition of suppressor influences (T cells or macrophages)
4. Passive: Transfer of antibodies or short-lived antitumor "factors"

an antigen to be processed into this setting then leads to the well-known consequences of nonspecific stimulation noted earlier: Killing of foreign cells or adjuvanticity in antibody production. NK cells and the cells that mediate ADCC, which include macrophages and lymphocytes, K cells, are also stimulated by many of the nonspecific immunomodulators. Many or all of these cells, macrophages, T cells, NK, and K cells, probably play important roles in the reaction against the tumor.

Obviously there is nothing to preclude, and much to recommend, the *combined* use of specific immunization with nonspecific immunotherapy. In fact, the "adjuvants" have been used, as their name implies, as adjuncts to specific immunogens in animals, where their value in increasing the immune response was first demonstrated. Their use alone in man, by such schemes as vaccination by scarification into normal skin, has little or no precedent in preclinical experiments and has proved largely ineffective in prolonging the durations of remission in almost all clinical trials. Prolongation of survivals in nodular, poorly differentiated lymphocytic lymphoma and ovarian cancer by the addition of BCG to effective chemotherapy may be noteworthy exceptions (Biological Response Modifiers: Subcommittee Report, 1983).

The only consistently successful use of nonspecific immunotherapy in man has been the intratumoral injection of bacterial substances into intradermal lesions. BCG or any material to which a patient is able to make a delayed hypersensitivity reaction has seemed useful in causing the inflammatory rejection of "bystander" tumor cells, undoubtedly through the local activation of nonspecifically cytotoxic macrophages. These macrophages somehow recognize the foreignness of tumor cells and generally spare normal epithelial tissues with consequent good healing of the skin. Long-lived immunity to the tumor is usually not engendered, however, and the 50% of patients who reject tumorous skin lesions after intratumoral injection usually develop visceral metastases later. Disappointing long-term results despite an excellent initial local inflammatory response to intratumoral BCG have also been noted recently in lung cancer where BCG was given via fiberoptic bronchoscopy as an approach to generating an endogenous vaccine prior to definitive surgery for stage I non-oat-cell lung cancer (Matthay *et al.,* 1982). Granulomatous hepatitis and pulmonary granulomas are among the more serious complications of intratumoral immunotherapy with BCG, which is always accompanied by significant bacteremia and fever, making intralesional immunotherapy a procedure that requires very close attention and further limiting its application to cancer treatment.

Nonspecific active immunotherapy is a modulation of the immune response in all its aspects, not simply an augmentation. In fact, depression of the effective immune response can be produced if suppressor elements regulating immunity are activated. Suppressor macrophages, acting via prostaglandins, are particularly a problem because they can prevent the generation of cytolytic T cells (Bennett *et al.,* 1978; Klimpel and Henney, 1978). Whenever a nonspecific modulator is administered, its apparent effects represent the net effect of sometimes conflicting activities on various "positive" and "negative" arms of the immunoregulatory system.

Tables 11–3 and 11–4 illustrate the types of effects that nonspecific adjuvants might theoretically cause on macrophages and T cells. Most of these effects have now actually been

Table 11–3.   Potential Effects of Nonspecific Immunomodulators on T Cells

1. Helpful
    a. Activation of helper (inducer) T cells, causing increased cytotoxic and cytophilic antibody titers
    b. Activation of cytolytic T cells
    c. Elicitation of lymphokines, causing increased macrophage mediated cytotoxicity
2. Deleterious
    a. Activation of suppressor T cells, causing decreased antibody titers, decreased cytolytic T cells and decreased macrophage-mediated cytotoxicity
    b. Activation of the helper (inducer) T cells that induce suppressor T cells or those that increase the antibody component of "blocking factors"

Table 11-4. Potential Effects of Nonspecific Immunomodulators on Macrophages

1. Helpful
    a. Activation of effector macrophages, causing increased nonspecific cytotoxicity of unarmed macrophages and increased specific cytotoxicity of antibody-armed macrophages
    b. Activation of accessory macrophages, causing increased antibody titers and increased cytolytic T cells, via mediators (monokines) and direct cell interactions
2. Deleterious
    a. Activation of suppressor macrophages, causing decreased antibody synthesis, decreased generation of cytolytic T cells, and decreased delayed hypersensitivity reactions

noted with one or another of the agents (Berd, 1978; Mitchell and Murahata, 1979). Theoretically, suppressor macrophages or suppressor T cells, if stimulated out of proportion to other regulatory elements, could decrease immunity to a tumor, whereas the corresponding macrophage and T-cell effectors presumably aid in the rejection process. Although the theoretical problem of increasing the "blocking antibody" component of "blocking factors," thus enhancing tumor growth, has been included, this possibility is fairly small because shed tumor antigen is the predominant component of the blocking immune complex. Effects on antibody synthesis are far more likely to be beneficial to the host's rejection mechansim, particularly as "arming" substances for recognition of tumor cells by macrophages. Attention to dosage and scheduling is critical in dealing with any of the nonspecific activating agents. Unfortunately, however, these must often be determined by empiricism rather than by well-established rules. Attention to the source of adjuvant material, including the batch and lot, is also critical because diametrically opposite effects have been found with different lots of even the same bacterial modulator (Mokyr *et al.,* 1980). In fact, this extreme variation has caused whole microbial substances to be generally abandoned for therapeutic use, to be replaced by chemically defined derivatives or by synthetic chemicals such as pyran.

Specific. An area of treatment that is beginning to receive vigorous study is specific active immunotherapy. The use of killed autologous or allogeneic (second-party) tumor cells as immunogens has been attempted in the past as a way of increasing the reactivity of tumor-bearing subjects against their own tumor. Alteration of the tumor cells through the addition of haptenic groups or by treatment with neuraminidase to remove sialic acid and "unmask" antigens on the membrane has been proposed for increasing the immunogenicity of the tumor cells. Because the immunogenicity of "spontaneous" tumors is usually weak, such measures have been necessary to elicit a stronger rejection reaction. These approaches have met with varying degrees of success, as judged by the ability of the host to reject the tumor and survive without disease. Intralymphatic injections of killed (irradiated) vaccines have been used in human beings with melanoma and ovarian cancer with some success (Juillard *et al.,* 1978). Neuraminidase treatment has largely been abandoned, although some prolongation of lifespan (though not cure) with this interesting treatment method in animals with a chemically induced fibrosarcoma has been reported. The use of alkyl groups as haptens or the attachment of adjuvant substances directly to the tumor cells continues to be investigated (Prager *et al.,* 1976). One group of researchers (Hanna and Peters, 1981) has made whole tumor cell vaccines to treat the line 10 guinea pig hepatoma. These vaccines contain irradiated hepatoma cells and BCG and may work not only as immunogens provoking a direct antitumor response but also as means of disrupting the integrity of vascular barriers to the entry of antitumor drugs into the tumor. Preliminary (Phase I) trials in cancer patients suggest that autologous colon carcinoma vaccines can immunize patients who have recently undergone resection, and trials for prophylactic efficacy are imminent. More recently, with the advent of newer techniques for extracting antigenic materials from tumor cells, such as with 1-butanol (LeGrue *et al.,* 1980), and the ability to analyze the antigens contained in the extract through the use of monoclonal antibodies, it is now possible to pursue specific immunotherapy with renewed optimism. One research team has been able to cure mice with microscopic tumor cell deposits, and even those with gross skin lesions as large as 4 mm in diameter, by the injection of three weekly doses of a butanol extract of methylcholanthrene-induced sarcoma (Kahan *et al.,* 1982). With such large tumors, a dose of cyclophosphamide was required before the vaccination could be successful. The butanol extraction procedure can be applied to human beings, from whom several of the antigens associated with melanoma can be removed without loss of viability of the tumor, permitting reextraction if necessary. Application of this approach to the prophylaxis of patients with lymph node involvement, perhaps in a sequential combination of chemotherapy and concomitant with injection of the most appropriate nonspecific immunomodulator, may well form the basis for the approach to several cancers, including colon cancer, melanoma, and perhaps, breast cancer. Active specific immunotherapy, like active immunization for infectious disease, is likely to be the most durable form of immunologic treatment, because it elicits memory T cells that permit long-term recognition of the offending cells. Unlike the short-lived inflammatory response evoked by nonspecific immunotherapy, especially when given apart from the tumor site, the long-lived immunization afforded by specific immunization with tumor cells or extracts allows truly immunologic rejections to occur, which involve the combination of specific recognition, cell-cell interaction, and inflammatory cell migration.

A problem in immunizing patients with cancer may be the presence of tumor-specific suppressor elements (blocking factors and suppressor T cells). It may be necessary to remove suppressor influences by restorative immunotherapy before undertaking specific active approaches, particularly in patients who have a late-stage neoplasm and a heavy tumor burden. Another serious difficulty, perhaps more theoretical than actual, is the possibility of causing enhancement of tumor growth by attempts to immunize patients with tumor antigens. Induction of antibodies that form immune complexes (blocking factors) capable of eliciting suppressor T cells and that thereby depress immunity to the tumor is probably the mechanism of the "enhancement" phenomenon described in the 1950s (Hellstrom and Hellstrom, 1978; Kaliss, 1958; Mitchell and Rao, 1981). Whether or not tumor antigens will do this is uncertain, but the use of purified

extracts may well provide a means of selecting nonenhancing immunogens to circumvent the difficulty in any case.

The use of tumor antigen vaccines to prevent cancer in normal individuals is continually being proposed, but depends upon finding specific tumor antigens for each type of tumor and upon the identification of high-risk groups who should be given a particular vaccine. It seems very unlikely, however, that a universal preventive vaccine will be devised, at least one composed of tumor antigens, because no one single antigen or set of antigens that typifies all human cancers has been found. This is probably true for antiviral vaccines, as well, unless there proves to be a remarkably limited group of human tumorigenic viruses against which one would have to immunize (see Chapter 3-D).

Adoptive Immunotherapy

The transfer of immunologically competent cells, or their precursors, or immunologic information that can be incorporated into the host, constitutes adoptive immunotherapy. Transfusion of lymphocytes, particularly T lymphocytes, falls into this category and is likely to be exploited in the near future because of improved *in vitro* technology (Fefer and Goldstein, 1982). The ability to clone T cells and preserve their properties (such as cytotoxicity or helper function) while so doing has come about through the use of interleukin 2 (T-cell growth factor). It is now possible to select T cells that have a certain desirable characteristic, to clone them and expand the population sufficiently to have cells for adoptive transfer to an immunoincompetent host (Rosenberg *et al.,* 1982). Experiments in rodents have shown that the most effective T cells in adoptive transfer, whether of cytotoxicity or suppressor activity, are helper (inducer) T cells, of the Lyt 1+ phenotype in mice, the counterparts of OK T4+ in man (Mitchell and Rao, 1981; Greenberg *et al.,* 1982). In any event, it is essential to match donor and recipient carefully for histocompatibility antigens, because rejection of the transferred cells would otherwise occur.

A major ethical problem is circumvented by the use of autologous lymphocytes: The issue of whom to select as the donor of the lymphocytes for adoptive transfer. A few *in vitro* tests for immunologic reactivity against tumor cells are available, which may be of value in demonstrating who among potential donors of leukocytes might be most suitable. Cell-mediated cytotoxicity and leukocyte adherence inhibition or the production of mediators from T cells on restimulation with tumor antigens *in vitro* are possible *in vitro* tests, but none has proved completely correlative with *in vivo* reactivity. Arbitrary selection of parents or siblings of cancer patients as donors has been advocated in the past but often without evidence that the individual selected had any immunity to the patient's tumor. Certainly, one cannot immunize normal individuals or even patients with cancer in order to obtain immune cells, because of the danger that the supposedly "killed, antigenic" tumor might grow in the individual who was to be the immunized donor. Autologous lymphocytes from patients with cancer should be measured for their reactivity against the tumor *in vitro* with one or more available tests and can then be restimulated *in vitro* by incubation with killed tumor cells. This *in vitro* boost, followed by clonal selection and/or expansion, constitutes a useful strategy, the details of which are already well worked out and which should obviate the need for second-party donors (Cheever *et al.,* 1982).

Another very serious problem, circumvented only by autologous lymphocytes, is graft versus host disease, which occurs when the transferred cells recognize minor histocompatibility differences from the host and react against the host's tissues, especially the skin, gastrointestinal tract, and liver. Recruitment of host lymphocytes by transferred inducer cells compounds the problem. This graft versus host disease can be fatal if unsuccessfully treated with immunosuppressive agents for modifying the graft versus host reaction. Supportive care with antimicrobial drugs has vastly improved, bringing most patients through the infectious complications of the disease. Fortunately, too, new agents to treat graft versus host disease, such as cyclosporin A, have been added to the therapeutic armamentarium.

Bone marrow transplantation, although performed principally for the replacement of hematopoietic stem cells, should also be regarded as a type of adoptive immunotherapy, because human bone marrow contains immunocompetent T cells and their precursors. The critical requirement of careful tissue matching, through serologic and cell-mediated (mixed lymphocyte) reactivity, to prevent rejection, and the serious potential problem of graft versus host disease must be considered, just as with the transfer of pure lymphocyte populations. It has been suggested that one explanation for the documented failure of syngeneic (twin) bone marrow transplants to eradicate acute leukemia in contrast to the greater success with allogeneic transplants is that the identical twin's lymphocytes do not recognize the leukemic cells as sufficiently different from "self" to reject them (see Chapter 43). Allogeneic lymphocytes, on the other hand, it is further postulated, recognize minor alloantigens and leukemia antigens on the recipient's residual leukemic cells and can mediate a graft versus leukemia rejection reaction. The successful treatment of virally induced leukemias in rodents, by the transfer of T lymphocytes (Greenberg *et al.,* 1982) and by bone marrow transplantation, represents the only currently used adoptive immunotherapy involving the transfer of whole cells in man.

The transfer of subcellular immunologic information from one individual to another also constitutes adoptive immunotherapy. Although thymic hormones are immunologic informational molecules of a sort, they are categorized here as immunorestorative therapy because of that important property. During the 1970s, two substances were examined for their effect on cancer: "transfer factor" and "immune" RNA. "Transfer factor" is a 10,000-dalton protein extracted from leukocytes. "Immune" RNA is a phenal extract of cellular RNA from immune lymphocytes, not simply "messenger" RNA. Despite initial reports of efficacy for each of these materials, there was no convincing documentation of successful treatment of human tumors with either, and their use in cancer has largely been abandoned. *Bona fide* lymphokines, monokines (from macrophages), and well-characterized "factors" from lymphocytes are far more promising. Interleukins 1 (a monokine) and 2 (a lymphokine) are discrete biologic and chemical entities that can be isolated and administered. The clarification of which "activities" in supernatant fluids described by various investigators are merely different properties of the same mediator has been accomplished through physicochemical isolation of that mediator, aided by workshops (Goldstein and Chirigos, 1981). These strides afford the ability to transfer homogeneous, defined material to patients, in order to activate macrophages or lymphocytes *in vivo,* to cause leukocytes to proliferate or to migrate to a specific site. These activities have been evoked heretofore by a variety of nonspecific microbial substances that can stimulate lymphokines among their other properties. For example, BCG or its derivative MER, and other subcellular fractions of BCG prepared by removal of cellular lipids, are able to stimulate interleukin 1 production *in vitro* and *in vivo* (Mitchell and Murahata, 1979). It is preferable, however, to use the lymphokine or monokine itself rather than an elicitor to avoid the effects on the host of other mediators that a nonspecific active immunotherapeutic approach would also evoke. Interferon-gamma, a lymphokine, has been produced by recombinant DNA technology and should soon be available for activating lymphoid cells in patients with cancer far more precisely than the alpha and beta interferons, which are not lymphokines.

Restorative Immunotherapy

This subheading is one that comprises direct and indirect restoration of deficient immunologic function, through any means but direct adoptive transfer of cells. Repletion of competent effector cell populations is one form of restorative immunotherapy. Thymic hormones such as thymosin and thymopoietin, for example, can convert T-cell precursors, including some null cells in the blood, into functional T cells, a property that is shared by the antihelminthic agent levamisole and several of its congeners (Goldstein and Chirigos, 1981; Renoux, 1978). Thymosin, in particular, has been fractionated into fraction 5, and further into the alpha-1 component of fraction 5, and each fraction has been found to cause differentation of precursors into specific subsets of T cells in mice. It may soon be possible in man to augment helper T cells selectively as opposed to cytotoxic/suppressor cells, or vice versa. It is not yet possible to stimulate cytotoxic T cells independent of suppressor cells with thymosin or its subfractions alone, and indeed it is uncertain whether or not a distinct T-cell subpopulation with only one of the two properties exists. In those patients demonstrated to have deficient circulating T cells, perhaps as a consequence of the tumor — such as those patients with oat cell carcinoma of the lung or Kaposi's sarcoma — repletion of T cells with thymic hormones represents an interesting adjunctive approach. In oat cell carcinoma specifically, a randomized, though small-scale, study has

been done with thymosin fraction 5, which increased the median survival of patients with a complete response from chemotherapy (over 450 days versus 240). The subgroup of patients that benefited most was the one with the deficient T cell percentages, in whom the differences between thymosin-treated and placebo-treated patients was most pronounced (405-day median survival versus 180) (Chretien *et al.,* 1978). Further studies of the efficacy of thymosin in patients with head and neck cancer are in progress, although the deficient cell-mediated immunity in those patients is almost certainly due more to suppressor macrophage activity than to deficient T cells. One relevant activity of nonspecific immunomodulators might be mentioned here: The stimulation of macrophages or their precursors. Pretreatment with BCG has led both to the development of macrophagelike killer cells antagonizing immunosuppression by chemotherapy and to an expanded population of T cells (through interleukin 1), both representing varieties of restorative immunotherapy (Mitchell and Murahata, 1979).

In fact, antagonism of suppressor influences, both exogenous and particularly endogenous, is a major form of immunorestorative therapy. Cyclophosphamide in low doses, for example, 20 mg/kg in a mouse, where the LD_{10} is approximately 350 mg/kg, can specifically inhibit precursors or amplifiers of suppressor T cells, depressing suppressor T-cell activity and thereby augmenting cell-mediated immunity. It is likely that similar actions occur in human beings when low doses of cyclophosphamide are given rather than the conventionally large doses of $1g/m^2$ or greater. Antagonists of prostaglandin synthetase, such as indomethacin, inhibit the actions of suppressor macrophages that are mediated mainly through prostaglandin E. The anergy of Hodgkin's disease is due in part to the action of suppressor macrophages, as are the depressed skin reactivity in head and neck cancer and the decreased synthesis of normal immunoglobulins in myeloma. Prostaglandin antagonists, therefore, may play a role in several aspects of immunosuppression accompanying cancer.

A procedure recently introduced for removing suppressor influences in cancer patients is the immunosorbent *Staphylococcus* A protein column, developed principally by Terman and his colleagues (Terman *et al.,* 1981), although several investigators have reported on its use. In dogs and several women with breast cancer, a striking noninflammatory necrosis occurred after a series of sorptions of plasma. Not all the plasma had to be treated to produce the effect; sorption of a unit of plasma with reinfusion into the patient was sufficient. The presumption has been that immune complexes that block immunity are removed by the *Staphylococcus* A protein, which binds to the Fc end of IgG antibody. There may be something added to the plasma as well, although leaching of the *Staph* A protein itself has been ruled out. Infusion of plasma that has been treated by the column into a different individual from whom it was taken has also caused a necrotic response of the tumor in that person. Whether the delicate balance of immunoregulation is tipped in favor of the patient by the removal of only a portion of total blocking complexes from the plasma, or whether something that causes necrosis results from perfusion over the column, is uncertain. Nevertheless, the procedure does appear to be effective even in late-stage, heavily treated patients with cancer. One group of researchers reported a significant regression of disease in three of five patients with breast cancer treated by this means (Terman *et al.,* 1981). For now, it seems reasonable to consider the immunosorbent column a form of immunorestorative immunotherapy, although it may have to be put into another category of biomodulation after further studies on its effects are evaluated.

Passive Immunotherapy

This form of immunotherapy until recently seemed the least promising approach because it implied the transfer of antibodies in antisera from immunized individuals to tumorous recipients. Because antibodies are short-lived, and in most instances have seemed less important than cell-mediated immunity in tumor rejection, passive immunotherapy had very limited usefulness. The theoretical danger of enhancement of tumor growth through the formation of immune complexes with circulating tumor antigens was also recognized. The enhancement phenomenon was evoked in mice by the transfer of serum containing antibodies allogeneic to hosts bearing tumor grafts (Kaliss, 1958). The counterpart in the immunology of human autologous tumors may be "blocking" of cytotoxicity *in vitro* by serum-blocking factors (Hellstrom and Hellstrom, 1974). Whole serum contains tumor antibodies of different subclasses and binding properties, some of which might combine with tumor antigens and cause enhancement. Then, too, "blocking" immune complexes may already be present in the transferred serum.

Antibodies against immunologically foreign immunoglobulin allotypes, determinants that distinguish subtypes of the same class of antibody, and antibodies against idiotypes, the determinants on the antigen-combining portion, would lead to still more rapid clearance of the passively transferred antibodies. Technical problems exist in screening for the presence of antibodies in the serum of potential donors and there exist enormous ethical proscriptions against purposely immunizing an individual to raise high-titered antibody. These problems made passive immunotherapy one of the least desirable and most restricted approaches in this area of treatment, and it was used only as a stop-gap measure, analogous to the passive immunization for tetanus when time constraints preclude active immunization.

The situation has changed radically because of the development of hybridoma techniques for producing monoclonal antibodies. The potential utility of monoclonal antibodies in diagnosis and fuller coverage of monoclonals in cancer may be found in several recent sources (Kennett *et al.,* 1980; Mitchell and Oettgen, 1982). Monoclonal antibodies have not yet been fully explored in the treatment of patients with cancer, but it is possible to state some general principles of such therapy. The ability to make large amounts of pure antibody of a defined subclass against a specific antigenic determinant has made it unnecessary to administer large amounts of serum, which contain many different proteins and a number of irrelevant antibodies, that is, those not directed against the tumor. Immune complexes may still be formed after transfer of monoclonals, making enhancement a therapeutic problem, but at least they are not present in the material administered.

Monoclonal antibodies made against tumor-specific antigens, if they exist, against tumor-associated antigens, which clearly do exist, or against differentiation antigens shared also by certain normal cells are all of potential use against tumors. Monoclonal antibodies to melanoma and colon cancer are undergoing early trials in man, as are anti-T-cell antibodies in T-cell lymphomas and leukemia in man, supported by data on the efficacy of anti-T-cell antibodies in mouse leukemia.

It is likely that a dispersed tumor such as

leukemia and ascitic ovarian cancer will respond best to therapy with antibodies if experience in animals holds true. These dispersed tumors are accessible to antibodies that leave the circulation and to antibody-armed macrophages and K cells. As noted earlier, antibodies probably work through the arming of lymphoreticular effector cells rather than through a complement-mediated cytolysis. Thus, the IgG subclass (isotype) would predictably be the most useful because it is most cytophilic, as opposed to IgM, which is far less cytophilic although a better complement-fixing antibody. A combination of methods that activate macrophages nonspecifically, such as the local injection of *Propionibacterium* acnes intraperitoneally into ovarian ascites, together with the injection of monoclonal antibodies, holds considerable promise and is under current study in several centers.

Interferon

The categories of "classic" immunotherapy cannot adequately accommodate interferon or the retinoids, two of the newer agents in use for biomodulation. Interferon, or more properly interferons, because there are at least three types, were discovered by Isaacs and Lindermann in 1957, but only recently have been utilized in the treatment of cancer. The interferons are low-molecular-weight proteins of approximately 15,000 to 20,000 daltons. They are produced in response to a variety of stimuli, most familiarly a wide range of viruses. Double-stranded RNA, including synthetic RNA, can elicit interferon, but single-stranded RNA, double-stranded DNA, and even a few viruses cannot. A wide variety of interferon inducers are known, including poly I:C, poly A:U, pyran, and fluorenone derivatives such as tilorone. BCG can also induce interferon (Stewart, 1979). Interferon is the most potent biologic substance yet isolated, judged by its activity per milligram of protein, often with a potency of millions of units of antiviral activity per milligram. Alpha (leukocyte), beta (fibroblast), and gamma (T-cell-derived lymphokine) interferons have been distinguished from one another on the basis of their derivation and their reactivity with antibodies. Antibody to interferon gamma does not cross-react with either interferon alpha or beta (and vice versa). Antibody to alpha, however, does cross-react with beta. Stability at pH2 characterizes "classic" alpha and beta interferons, whereas gamma interferon is unstable at that pH (Stewart, 1979). Interferon is relatively species-specific but not at high doses. Many amino acid sequence homologies among the interferons of rodents and humans have been found.

Interferon stops the growth of viruses by interfering with the production of messenger RNA coded for by the virus. It has a cytostatic effect on tumor cells in tissue culture, halting their growth so that ultimately the cells will die. This cytostasis resembles the action of activated macrophages on tumor cells, perhaps not coincidentally. Some investigators believe interferon mediates the effects macrophages exert. The mechanisms underlying this effect are uncertain, but may be related to the antiviral effect. Interferons alpha and beta can also stimulate macrophages and T cells, and as such are active nonspecific immunomodulators. Interferon gamma, a true lymphokine from inducer T cells, influences other subsets of T cells, such as those destined to become cytotoxic (and suppressor), and it can activate macrophages. Because of its dual functions on the host and on the tumor, interferon appears particularly attractive for study against cancer *in vivo* apart from its continuing exploration as an antiviral substance.

The extraction of leukocytes or fibroblasts stimulated by a harmless virus was the original method of interferon production. Recombinant DNA technology has made it possible to obtain interferons in great quantities and in pure form from bacteria or yeasts to which the human gene for interferon is transferred. *E. coli* is the most common source and has permitted abundant supplies of pure interferon-alpha to be available for phase I and II testing. Interferon obtained by extraction is always mixed with a variety of other leukocyte- or fibroblast-derived materials, including lymphokines, and represents less than 1% of the mixture. In contrast, the recombinant-derived interferons are almost 100% pure and are nearly identical with the natural human material. Until the pure substance is tested thoroughly in cancer patients, one cannot be certain whether interferon *per se* has any effect on cancer cells or on the immunity of the tumor-bearing host, but at present some tentative conclusions can be drawn from trials with the extracted material.

Responses have been obtained, largely with extracted interferon-alpha, in breast cancer, multiple myeloma, nodular poorly differentiated lymphocytic lymphoma, and perhaps in osteosarcoma with micrometastatic residual tumor (Biological Response Modifiers: Subcommittee Report, 1983). Roughly one-third of the patients treated with each of the first three diseases have shown a response. Some of the responses have been complete, as in myeloma and lymphoma, but the one solid tumor consistently affected, breast cancer, has shown only partial responses. Because the patients treated had late-stage disease resistant to conventional chemotherapy, *any* response to a biomodulator such as interferon is impressive, and it is important to extend the studies to much earlier stages of cancer. Strander's studies in osteosarcoma at the Karolinska Hospital, which provided much of the impetus for exploration of interferon's role in cancer treatment, were nonrandom treatments of patients with interferon alpha after amputation for osteosarcoma. Control data were from contemporary patients at other Swedish hospitals treated only by amputation, as well as from historic controls treated only by surgery at Karolinska. At all times after surgery, the interferon-treated patients had a lesser incidence of metastases and a higher rate of survival. Interestingly, the contemporary controls had a better duration of survival and a lower incidence of metastases than the historic controls, indicating a change in the natural history of the untreated illness (Biological Response Modifiers: Subcommittee Report, 1983).

During phase I trials of recombinant interferon-alpha, clone A, there have been reports of responses in patients with small cell carcinoma of the lung, renal cell carcinoma, and the Kaposi's sarcoma occurring in homosexual men. Disease-directed phase II trials now in progress should clarify which tumors are in fact sensitive. Regardless of its ultimate role in cancer therapy, it should be noted that interferon will surely have a place in the treatment of viral diseases, including those that complicate cancer. Herpes simplex (of the lips and eyes but not the genitalia), varicella-zoster, hepatitis B, and cytomegalovirus infections have all responded to therapy with interferon. An unusual type of tumor, laryngeal papillomatosis, which may be more a viral disorder than a true tumor, has been remarkably well treated by interferon. This affliction of children, which otherwise would require repeated surgery, has been completely controlled in 14 patients by interferon given continuously for at least six weeks and then intermittently as maintenance.

Side effects of interferon include, in descending order of frequency, fever, malaise, lassitude, hypotension, leukopenia, thrombocytopenia, nausea, anorexia, alopecia, and interference with clotting *in vitro*. Fever, as high as 39 °C or more, occurs most typically with the first doses of a course and becomes progressively less pronounced with successive daily doses. Suppression of leukocyte and thrombocyte production is greatest in patients with preexistent bone marrow compromise, such as myeloma patients. The severity of each of the toxic effects varies with each patient and with the dose of interferon. In general, however, the toxicity of interferon is far lower than that of most conventional cytotoxic chemicals. Pure recombinant-generated interferon has had no less toxicity than the impure extracts, nor have fewer types of toxic effect been noted. Therefore, it appears that the side effects accompanying the use of interferon-containing mixtures were attributable to interferon itself.

As an agent that affects tumor cells both directly and through stimulation of the host's immunity, interferon is an excellent prototypical biomodulator. It is merely the first of a number of agents to be explored on a large scale, however, and its success or failure as an antitumor agent should not prejudice the acceptance of biomodulation as a valid concept.

Retinoids

The retinoids, derivatives of vitamin A, are effective against a gamut of afflictions ranging from acne to cancer. In adolescents and young adults 13-*cis*-retinoic acid (tretinoin) has been used successfully to treat pustular cystic acne by means of its ability to affect the maturation of squamous cells, thin the stratum corneum, and promote the proliferation of normal cells in the hair follicles assisting in expulsion of sebum. In addition, 13-*cis*-retinoic acid and the natural isomer beta-all-*trans*-retinoic (Figure 11–5) have been effective in promoting the maturation of cells that are dysplastic or metaplastic, thus preventing cancer from occurring (Biological Response Modifiers: Subcommittee Report, 1983). When administered with a carcinogenic chemical, retinoids can prevent and in some cases reverse progression of a precancerous lesion and can antagonize the promoters of carcinogens such as those in cigarette smoke. Some of the evidence on this point is epidemiologic, whereas other data are from direct experiments.

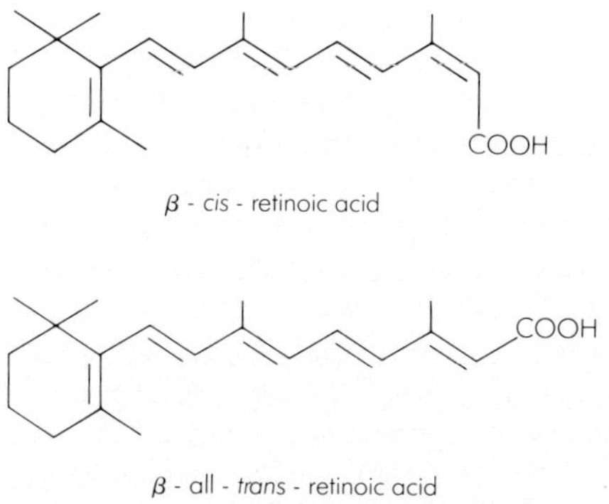

β - cis - retinoic acid

β - all - trans - retinoic acid

Figure 11–5.   Structure of two retinoids.

Vitamin A deficiency leads to an increased incidence of stomach cancer in rats. On the other hand, the incidence of lung cancer among light and heavy smokers was significantly influenced by their intake of vitamin A. Those with a high intake of vitamin A had a lower-than-expected incidence of both lung and bladder cancer, whereas those with a low intake had a twofold higher risk of lung cancer. Similarly, high vitamin A intake reduced the risk of bladder cancer in heavy coffee drinkers. Evidence for reversal of a carcinogenic stimulus in experimental animals comes from work with retinoids given to rats and mice who were also given nitrosomethylurea or butylhydroxybutyl nitrosamine. Retinoids given daily for a prolonged period of time after the carcinogen was administered delayed onset of the cancers. The cancers occurred, however, if retinoids were stopped. In rats, colon cancer can be induced in all with dimethylhydrazine, whereas 13-*cis*-retinoic acid reduced the incidence to 40%. As two other examples, retinoids have inhibited papilloma and carcinoma formation in the skin, and small doses have reduced the incidence of squamous cell carcinoma of the lung after intratracheal benzpyrene-ferric oxide from 10% to 1.9% (3/152). Tripling the dose completely eliminated the carcinomas. Metaplasia after methylcholanthrene in organ culture of prostate tissue or tracheal cultures was reversed by retinoids, and both metaplasia and hyperplasia after methylcholanthrene was prevented by retinoids (Biological Response Modifier: Subcommittee Report, 1983).

In human precancerous conditions, actinic keratoses were successfully treated by local retinoic acid application in 40% of 60 patients, and oral retinoic acid caused complete remissions in 22 of 33 bladder papillomas. Skin tumors have been treated with retinoids, particularly basal cell carcinoma, in which a 31% complete response rate was obtained in 16 patients. The treatment of frank carcinoma with retinoids, however, is not an established use nor is prevention of the recurrence of a tumor once it has been initially removed. Patients with transitional cell carcinoma of the bladder normally have a 70% relapse rate within six months after extirpative surgery. Patients treated with retinoic acid after surgery had an 88% recurrence rate, which was significantly higher, perhaps because cells that were already neoplastic or had progressed considerably through several stages of metaplasia were not susceptible to the action of the retinoids. Enhancement of tumor growth was uncertain, because the study was stopped after only 17 patients had been treated (Biological Response Modifiers: Subcommittee Report, 1983).

Retinoids can also augment the immune response, increasing both antibody production and cell-mediated cytotoxicity, acting as nonspecific, active agents through macrophages and T cells. Like interferon, retinoids have both direct and indirect effects on neoplastic cells. Retinoids uniquely have direct and indirect effects on preneoplastic cells.

A useful application of retinoids may be as a chemopreventive antineoplastic technique for dysplasia of the uterine cervix, and perhaps for fibrocystic disease and atypical ductal hyperplasia of the breast, in addition to the skin conditions mentioned above.

Agents that Alter the Cell Membrane and Behavioral Characteristics of Tumor Cells

Neuraminidase is an agent that changes the cell membrane of tumor cells. By reducing the sialic acid content of the membrane, the apparent immunogenicity of the cells is augmented, perhaps because the smaller "shrubs" are exposed after removal of the more abundant "trees." A more biophysical possibility is that sialic acid is highly negatively charged and repels the T cells that also have negative charges due to sialic acid. Removal of sialic acid may permit better recognition of antigenic structure by the lymphocytes according to this schema.

Since metastatic charge differences are involved in the migration of embryonic cells, the behavior of which is very like that of tumor cells, it is conceivable that the movement of tumor cells might also be affected by the electrostatic charges of their cell membrane. One research group found that the metastatic potential and precise location of specific sites of metastatic localization of tumor cells is clonally determined within a gross tumor (Fidler and Kripke, 1977). One researcher has clearly demonstrated that the surface structure of the membrane is an important determinant of metastatic spread, with differences among clones that migrate to different locations (Nicolson, 1981). An agent that could alter the cell membrane sufficiently to prevent or retard metastasis, perhaps by simply changing the membrane's electrostatic charge or destroying its complementarity with the site to which it homes, would be an important biomodulator whose activities fall well outside the realm of traditional immunotherapy.

Amphotericin B performs functions that lend themselves to this category. Although the immunogenicity of tumor cells is not altered by amphotericin, this substance, chemically a polyene, and its congeners bind to the cell membrane and enhance the transport of several chemotherapeutic agents across the membrane into the cell. Additive effects have been described with BCNU and vincristine in mice. Trials with patients have not yet been particularly successful, but the unusual activity of amphotericin is worth pursuing with other membrane-binding compounds.

Finally, although the agent has not yet been identified, an antagonist to the production of tumor angiogenesis factor (Folkman, 1975) responsible for vascularization and thus for continued growth of small tumors would be an extraordinary modifier of the behavior of tumor cells, too, one probably sufficient to lead to their rejection by conventional immunologic mechanisms. An antibody to the material has proved extraordinarily difficult to produce. Should that or any antagonist be developed, however, the impact on cancer therapy would be profound and far-reaching.

Agents that Improve the Ability of the Host to Tolerate Therapy

Many agents can increase the production of colony-stimulating factor (CSF), which has the effect of increasing the precursors of mature granulocytes and macrophages. Several of the classic nonspecific immunomodulators have been shown to have this property, which is not surprising, because CSF is one of a family of mediators released by resting or "activated" macrophages. *Propionibacterium*

acnes *(C. parvum)* have been studied fairly extensively, as has BCG, and both are effective stimulators of CSF (Wolmark and Fisher, 1974; Ladisch *et al.,* 1978). These agents have been used experimentally to protect animals against the deleterious effects of radiation therapy or chemotherapy with high doses of cyclophosphamide. BCG has also been shown to protect against the immunosuppressive effects of chemotherapy with cyclophosphamide or cytosine arabinoside (ara-C) (Mitchell and Murahata, 1979). Azimexone is a recently developed aziridine dye derivative that has been investigated more intensively than most newer agents for its ability to protect the bone marrow from cytoreductive therapy. Administration of azimexone for three days, beginning when a dose of cyclophosphamide was given, reduced the acute toxicity (mortality) of mice at all doses of the alkylating agent. Similarly, a single dose of azimexone given before or after 650 rads of total body irradiation decreased the mortality from 95% to 50 to 60%. These effects were achieved through stimulation of colony-forming cells, the proliferation of which enlarges the production of nucleated hematopoietic cells (Bicker, 1981). Azimexone is a moderate stimulator of macrophage activities other than CSF production and can activate suppressor T cells, putting it also in the general category of nonspecific immunomodulator. Lithium chloride and other lithium salts have been used for a similar purpose, also through the intermediary CSF.

Autologous bone marrow reinfusion clearly functions as a bone marrow protective maneuver. High-dose chemotherapy with drugs whose dose-limiting toxicity is bone marrow suppression is now possible with such a protective regimen. Although other types of bone marrow transplantation have the same effect, the problems associated with allogeneic transplantation, for example, make its selection for use solely as a protective regimen less likely.

Further attention to the host's tolerance of therapy will permit fully calculated doses of chemotherapy or radiation therapy to be administered, which will avoid the pitfall of calling an agent "ineffective" when it was really given at suboptimal doses.

COMMENTS ON BIOMODULATION

Although pertinent clinical results in trials of biomodulation have been mentioned under each section, it should be noted that the subject is discussed in considerable detail, particularly for the nonspecific immunomodulators, in the National Cancer Institute monograph, Biological Response Modifiers: Subcommittee Report, 1983). It is important to point out that many of the results to date were obtained before there was sufficient scientific knowledge concerning the properties of the agents used. Nevertheless, the promise of an approach that is far less toxic to the host than chemotherapy or radiation, yet still has experimental precedent in animal tumor models, is sufficient to merit continued exploration of biomodulation. The agents that affect both the tumor and host are of course the most promising, because they can conceivably be used to treat even later stages of a tumor's growth rather than solely micrometastatic disease. Even those biomodulators that affect the host alone, however, should be explored. This is particularly true where there is a well-defined lesion such as deficient T-cell subpopulations, as in some patients with oat cell carcinoma of the lung or Kaposi's sarcoma. Combined modality approaches involving surgery, chemotherapy, or radiation with biomodulation are worthy of thought. It is of great importance in planning treatment to consider the effects of any form of antitumor therapy on the ability of the patient to react against the tumor, because all standard types of treatment are at least to some degree immunosuppressive. Accordingly, an immunologic approach to cancer may be the most beneficial therapy, even if an immunotherapeutic agent is not involved.

REFERENCES

Albino, A. P., Lloyd, K. O., Houghton, A. N., Oettgen, H. F., and Old, L. J.: Heterogeneity in surface antigen and glycoprotein expression of cell lines derived from different melanoma metastases of the same patient. *J. Exp. Med.,* **154**:1764–1778, 1981.

Benacerraf, B., and Germain, R. N.: The immune response genes of the major histocompatibility complex. *Immunol. Rev.,* **28**:70–119, 1978.

Bennett, J. A., Rao, V. S., and Mitchell, M. S.: Systemic bacillus Calmette-Guérin (BCG) activates natural suppressor cells. *Proc. Natl. Acad. Sci. USA,* **75**:5142–5144, 1978.

Berd, D.: Effects of *Corynebacterium parvum* on immunity. *Pharmacol. Ther.,* **2**:373–396, 1978.

Bicker, U.: Aziridine dyes: Preclinical and clinical studies. In Hersh, E. M.; Chirigos, M. A.; and Mastrangelo, M. J. (eds.): *Augmenting Agents in Cancer Therapy.* Raven Press, New York, 1981.

Biological Response Modifiers: Subcommittee Report *Monogr. Natl. Cancer Inst.,* **63**, 1983.

Burnet, F. M.: The concept of immunological surveillance. *Prog. Exp. Tumor Res.,* **13**:1–23, 1970.

Cheever, M. A.; Greenberg, P. D.; Gillis, S.; and Fefer, A.: Specific adoptive transfer of murine leukemia with cells secondarily sensitized in vitro and expanded by culture with interleukin 2. In Fefer, A., and Goldstein, A. L. (eds.): *The Potential Role of T Cells in Cancer Therapy.* Raven Press, New York, 1982.

Cherish, D. A., Varki, A. P., Varki, N. M., Stallcup, W. B., Levine, J., and Reisfeld, R. A.: A monoclonal antibody recognizes an O-acylated sialic acid in a human melanoma-associated ganglioside. *J. Biol. Chem.,* **259**:7453–7459, 1984.

Chretien, P. B.; Lipson, S. D.; and Makuch, R.: Thymosin in cancer patients in vitro effects and correlations with clinical response to thymosin immunotherapy. *Cancer Treat. Rep.,* **62**:1787–1790, 1978.

DeVries, J. E.; Cornain, S.; and Rumke, P.: Cytotoxicity of non-T versus T-lymphocytes from melanoma patients and healthy donors on short- and long-term cultured melanoma cells. *Int. J. Cancer,* **14**:427–434, 1974.

Dippold, W. G.; Lloyd, N. O.; Houghton, A. N.; Li, L. T. C.; Ikeda, H.; Oettgen, H. F.; and Old, L. J.: Human melanoma antigens defined by monoclonal antibodies. In Mitchell, M. S., and Oettgen, H. F. (eds.): *Hybridomas in Cancer Diagnosis and Treatment.* Raven Press, New York, 1982.

DuBois, G. C.; Appella, E.; Lavin, L. S.; DeLeo, A. B.; and Old, L. J.: The soluble antigens of BALB/c sarcoma Meth A: A relationship between a serologically defined tumor specific surface antigen (TSSA) and the tumor associated transplantation anigen (TATA). *Transplant. Proc.,* **13**:1765–1773, 1981.

Fefer, A., and Goldstein, A. L. (eds.): *The Potential Role of T Cells in Cancer Therapy.* Raven Press, New York, 1982.

Fidler, I. J., and Kripke, M.: Metastasis results from pre-existing variant cells within a malignant tumor. *Science,* **197**:893–895, 1977.

Foley, E. J.: Antigenic properties of methylcholanthrene induced tumors in mice of strain of origin. *Cancer Res.,* **13**:835–838, 1953.

Folkman, J.: Tumor angiogenesis: A possible control point in tumor growth. *Ann. Intern. Med.,* **82**:96–100, 1975.

Goldstein, A. L., and Chirigos, M. A. (eds.): *Lymphokines and Thymic Hormones.* Raven Press, New York, 1981.

Greenberg, P. D.; Cheever, M. A.; and Fefer, A.: Prerequisite for successful adoptive immunotherapy: Nature of effector cells and role of H-2 restriction. In Fefer, A., and Goldstein, A. L. (eds.): *The Potential Role of T Cells in Cancer Therapy.* Raven Press, New York, 1982.

Greene, M. J.; Fujimoto, J.; and Sehon, H. N.: Regulation of the immune response to tumor antigens. III. Characterization of thymic suppressor factor(s) produced by tumor bearing hosts. *J. Immunol.* **119**:757–764, 1977.

Hanna, M. G., and Peters, L. C.: Morphologic and functional aspects of active specific immunotherapy of established pulmonary metastases in guinea pigs. *Cancer Res.,* **41**:4001–4009, 1981.

Hansen, J. A., and Martin, P. J.: Human T cell differentiation antigens. In Mitchell, M. S., and Oettgen, H. F. (eds.): *Hybridomas in Cancer Diagnosis and Treatment.* Raven Press, New York, 1982.

Hellstrom, J.; Hellstrom, K. E.; Sjogren, H. O.; and Warner, G. A.: Demonstration of cell-mediated immunity to human neoplasms of various histological types. *Int. J. Cancer,* **7**:1–16, 1971.

Hellstrom, K. E.; Brown, J. P.; and Hellstrom, I.: Four melanoma-associated antigens (3.1, p 97, P155, p 210) defined by monoclonal mouse antibodies. In Mitchell, M. S., and Oettgen, H. F. (eds.): *Hybridomas in Cancer Diagnosis and Treatment.* Raven Press, New York, 1982.

Hellstrom, K. E., and Hellstrom, I.: Lymphocyte-mediated cytotoxicity and blocking serum activity to tumor antigens. *Adv. Immunol.,* **18**:209–277, 1974.

Hellstrom, K. E., and Hellstrom, I.: Evidence that tumor antigens enhance tumor growth in vivo by interacting with a radiosensitive (suppressor?) cell population. *Proc. Natl. Acad. Sci. USA,* **75**:436–440, 1978.

Herberman, R. B., and Ortaldo, J. R.: Natural killer cells: Their role in defenses against disease. *Science,* **214**:24–29, 1981.

Juillard, G. J. F.; Boyer, P. J. J.; and Yamashiro, C. H.: A Phase I study of active specific intralymphatic immunotherapy (ASLI) *Cancer,* **41**:2215–2225, 1978.

Kahan, B. D.; Pellis, N. R.; LeGrue, S. J.; and Tanaka, T.: Immunotherapeutic effects of tumor-specific transplantation antigens released by 1-butanol. *Cancer,* **49**:1168–1173, 1982.

Kaliss, N.: Immunological enhancement of tumor homografts in mice. A review. *Cancer Res.,* **18**:992–1003, 1958.

Kennett, R. H.; McKearn, T. J.; and Bechtol, K. B. (eds.): *Monoclonal Antibodies. Hybridomas: A New Dimension in Biological Analysis.* Plenum Publishing Corporation, New York, 1980.

Klein, G.: Tumor specific transplantation antigens: G. H. A. Clowes Memorial Lecture. *Cancer Res.,* **28**:625–635, 1968.

Klimpel, G. R., and Henney, C. S.: BCG-induced suppressor cells. I. Demonstration of macrophage-like suppressor cell that inhibits cytotoxic T cell generation in vitro. *J. Immunol.,* **120**:563–569, 1978.

Kohler, G., and Milstein, C.: Continuous cultures of fused cells secreting antibody of predefined specificity. *Nature,* **256**:475–479, 1975.

Ladisch, S.; Poplack, D. G.; and Bull, J. M.: Acceleration of myeloid recovery from cyclophosphamide-induced leukopenia by pretreatment with Bacillus Calmette-Guérin. *Cancer Res.,* **38**:1049–1051, 1978.

Landsteiner, K.: Uber agglutinations erscheinungen des normalen menschlichen blutes. *Wien. Klin. Wochenschr.,* **14**:1132–1134, 1901.

Law, L. W.; Rogers, M. J.; and Appella, E.: Tumor antigens on neoplasms induced by chemical carcinogens and by DNA- and RNA-containing viruses: Properties of the solubilized antigens. *Adv. Cancer Res.,* **32**:201–235, 1980.

LeGrue, S. J.; Kahan, B. D.; and Pellis, N. R.: Extraction of a murine tumor-specific transplantation antigen with 1-butanol. I. Partial purification by isoelectric focusing. *J.N.C.I.,* **65**:191–196, 1980.

Lennox, E. S.; Lowe, A. D.; and Evan, G.: Specific antigens on methylcholanthrene-induced tumors of mice. *Transplant Proc.,* **13**:1759–1761, 1981.

Matthay, R. A.; Mahler, D. A.; Mitchell, M. S.; Carter, D. H.; Loke, J.; Beck, G. J.; Reynolds. H. Y.; and Baue, A. E.: Intratumoral BCG immunotherapy prior to surgery for carcinoma of the lung: Preliminary results. In Terry, W. D., and Rosenberg, S. A. (eds.): *Immunotherapy of Human Cancer.* Excerpta Medica, New York, 1982.

Mitchell, M. S., and Murahata, R. I.: Modulation of immunity by bacillus Calmette-Guérin (BCG). *Pharmacol. Ther.,* **4**:329–354, 1979.

Mitchell, M. S.; Nordlund, J. J.; and Lerner, A. B.: Comparison of cell-mediated immunity to melanoma cells in patients with vitiligo, halo nevi or melanoma. *J. Invest. Derm.,* **75**:144–147, 1980.

Mitchell, M. S., and Oettgen, H. F. (eds.): *Hybridomas in Cancer Diagnosis and Treatment.* Raven Press, New York, 1982.

Mitchell, M. S., and Rao, V. S.: The interrelationship of immune complexes and suppressor T cells in the suppression of macrophages. In Saunders, J. P.; Daniels, J. C.; Serrou, B.; Rosenfeld, C.; and Denney, C. B. (eds.): *Fundamental Mechanisms in Human Cancer Immunology.* Elsevier North-Holland, Inc., New York, 1981.

Mokyr, M. B.; Bennett, J. A.; Braun, D. P.; Hengst, J. C. D.; Mitchell, M. S.; and Dray, S.: Opposite effects of different strains or batch of same strain of BCG on in vitro generation of syngeneic and allogeneic antitumor cytotoxicity. *J.N.C.I.,* **64**:339–344, 1980.

Mokyr, M. B. and Mitchell, M. S.: Activation of lymphoid cells by BCG in vitro. *Cell Immunol.,* **15**:264–273, 1975.

Nicolson, G. L.: Tumor cell heterogeneity and bloodborne metastasis. In Saunders, J. P.; Daniels, J. C.; Serrou, B.; Rosenfeld, C.; and Denney, C. B. (eds.): *Fundamental Mechanisms in Human Cancer Immunology.* Elsevier North-Holland, Inc., New York, 1981.

Oehler, J. R.; Herberman, R. B.; and Holden, H. T.: Modulation of immunity by macrophages. *Pharmacol. Therap.,* **2**:551–594, 1978.

Old, L. J.: Cancer immunology: The search for specificity — G. H. A. Clowes Memorial Lecture. *Cancer Res.,* **41**:361–375, 1981.

Old, L. J., and Stockert, E.: Immunogenetics of cell surface antigens of mouse leukemia. *Annu. Rev. Genet.,* **17**:127–160, 1977.

Prager, M. D.; Gordon, W. C.; and Baechtel, F. S.: Immunogenicity of modified tumor cells in syngeneic hosts. *Ann. N.Y. Acad. Sci.,* **276**:61–74, 1976.

Prehn, R. T., and Main, J. M.: Immunity to methylcholanthrene-induced sarcomas. *J.N.C.I.,* **18**:769–778, 1957.

Rao, V. S.; Bennett, J. A.; Shen, F. W.; Gershon, R. K.; and Mitchell, M. S.: Antigen-antibody complexes generate Lyt 1 inducers of suppressor cells. *J. Immunol.,* **125**:63–67, 1980.

Reisfeld, R. A.; Morgan, A. C., Jr.; and Bumol, T. F.: Production and characterization of a monoclonal antibody to human melanoma associated antigens. In Mitchell, M. S., and Oettgen, H. F. (eds.): *Hybridomas in Cancer Diagnosis and Treatment.* Raven Press, New York, 1982.

Renoux, G.: Modulation of immunity by levamisole. *Pharmacol. Ther.,* **2**:397–424, 1978.

Rich, S. S., and Rich, R. R.: Modulation of immunity by thymus-derived lymphocytes. *Pharmacol. Ther.,* **2**:113-138, 1977.

Rosenberg, S. A.; Eberlin, T.; Grimm, E.; Mazumder, A.; and Rosenstein, M.: Adoptive transfer of lymphoid cells expanded in T-cell growth factor: Murine and human studies. In Fefer, A., and Goldstein, A. L. (eds.): *The Potential Role of T Cells in Cancer Therapy.* Raven Press, New York, 1982.

Solter, D.; Ballon, R.; Reilan, J.; Levine, G.; Hakala, T. R.; and Knowles, B. B.: Radioimmunodetection of tumors using monoclonal antibodies. In Mitchell, M. S., and Oettgen, H. F. (eds.): *Hybridomas in Cancer Diagnosis and Treatment.* Raven Press, New York, 1982.

Steplewski, Z., and Koprowski, H.: Anti-colorectal carcinoma monoclonal antibodies. In Mitchell, M. S., and

Oettgen, H. F. (eds.): *Hybridomas in Cancer Diagnosis and Treatment.* Raven Press, New York, 1982.

Stewart, W. E., II: *The Interferon System.* Springer-Verlag, New York, 1979.

Terman, D. S.; Young, J. B.; Shearer, W. T.; *et al.*: Preliminary observations of the effects on breast adenocarcinoma of plasma perfused over immobilized protein A. *New Engl. J. Med.,* **305:**1195-1200, 1981.

Unanue, E. R.: The macrophage as a regulator of lymphocyte function. *Hosp. Pract.,* 61–74, 1979.

Wolmark, N., and Fisher, B.: The effect of a single and repeated administration of *Corynebacterium parvum* on bone marrow macrophage colony production in syngeneic tumor-bearing mice. *Cancer Res.,* **34:**2869–2872, 1974.

Woodbury, R. G.; Brown, J. P.; Yeh, M.-Y.; Hellstrom, I.; and Hellstrom, K. E.: Identification of a cell surface protein, p 97, in human melanomas and certain other neoplasms. *Proc. Natl. Acad. Sci. USA,* **77:**2183–2187, 1980.

12

Clinical Evaluation of New Anticancer Agents

STEPHEN K. CARTER and PHILIP S. SCHEIN

INTRODUCTION

The clinical evaluation of new drugs takes place within a sequential framework of clinical trials of increasing complexity of design and analysis considerations. These trials are usually described with the designations of phases I, II, and III. Each of these studies has a desired endpoint that relates to decision making about whether the drug in question will be the subject of further evaluation. The concept of phase I, II, and III trials for neoplastic disease is complicated by the heterogeneity of disorders that are encompassed in the word "cancer." The new drug trial must be evaluated within the framework of the individualized data bases and clinical research strategies that exist for the many different types of cancer. In the phase I trial, the spectrum of diseases is numerous and the study design totally drug oriented, whereas in phase II and III trials, the evaluation must be disease oriented, and, therefore, individualized for colon cancer, lung cancer, breast cancer, and so forth.

New drugs can be divided into two generic categories: New chemical structures and analogs of existing known active compounds. Each requires a specific approach for the design of clinical trials and the analysis of results. The major difference is that the analog must be evaluated in comparative relationship to the efficacy and toxicity of the parent drug. Therapeutic activity *per se,* with an analog, is to be expected. What is hoped for is a superior level of therapeutic efficacy, at the cost of less clini-

cal toxicity. A new chemical structure is evaluated independently, and an opinion of the relative value of the drug for specific tumors must be arrived at with a perspective of what other forms of chemotherapy can accomplish in the given disease. This is ultimately accomplished in a phase III comparative trial.

It is the purpose of this chapter to review the basic principles of the design and analysis of phase I, II, and III trials for new anticancer drugs. Although the emphasis will be on the evaluation of new structures, the unique aspects of analogue trials will also be included.

PHASE I TRIALS

In the orderly process of drug development for cancer therapy, a drug that has shown antitumor activity in screening systems currently undergoes toxicologic studies in several species of animals, commonly rodents and dogs. The resulting data are used to predict the human toxicity of the new agent, to define its initial dose for clinical trials, and to anticipate the problems with its administration to humans. A phase I clinical trial represents the initial evaluation of the new drug in man. Its goal is to determine a safe dose for further studies of therapeutic activity, and to define the qualitative organ system toxicities associated with the compound. This includes an analysis of the intensity of adverse reactions and their rate of onset and reversibility. An important aspect of phase I testing is the investigation of clinical pharmacology, including drug uptake, metabolism, excretion, and organ distribution of the new drug. This permits evaluation of the effectiveness of different routes of administration and of the influence of liver and kidney function upon metabolism and excretion, as well as the anticipation of interactions with other drugs to be used in the design of later combinations.

Patient Selection

The toxicologic evaluation of an anticancer drug in human subjects is a clinical experiment that requires the highest standard of medical ethics. Care must be taken that patients do not relinquish their rights to established effective therapy, while at the same time insuring that the terminally ill are not subjected to needless toxicity. Several important criteria for the selection of patients for a phase I study must be considered. All patients should have histologically proven neoplastic disease that at the time of the study is no longer amenable to forms of treatment with established efficacy. This is a unique feature of the phase I testing of oncologic drugs, because the individuals who receive the new agent have the disease for which the drug may ultimately be indicated. By contrast, the phase I evaluation of most other classes of drugs is conducted in normal volunteers. To obtain meaningful results, the patient's clinical condition should be relatively stable in terms of disease progression and major organ function. Patients with acute lymphocytic leukemia are therefore inappropriate candidates for these trials, although they have been included in many studies in the past. An objective assessment of the bone marrow toxicity of a new agent is not possible in a patient with severely compromised hematologic function and a dynamic clinical state.

Most phase I protocols require that the patient have an estimated survival of at least one to two months, which is a minimum period of observation for drug-related effects. Physicians frequently overestimate survival, however, and many patients expire before drug effects can be fully evaluated. It may then be appropriate that the estimated survival of patients be increased to six months as a criterion for entry into a clinical trial. This emphasizes the need to separate the mortality associated with advanced disease from the possibly morbid effects of a new drug.

Other requirements exist for patient selection for phase I study. The toxicities of previous therapy must be sufficiently resolved so that the effects of the investigated agent are recognizable. In general, one month between therapies is required. Pregnant women are excluded from study because of teratogenic risks. Patients need not have objectively measurable disease, as is required in a phase II trial for which the primary goal is the determination of therapeutic effect.

The question remains, when should pediatric patients be subjects in these trials? In the past, there have been few well-designed phase I or phase II studies of cytotoxic drugs in children. This is the result of several factors, such as the special problems of patient consent, and the lack of both adequate patient populations and clinical investigators willing to carry out such studies. Nevertheless, new drugs with potential utility in children should be evaluated, especially in those cases where they have projected clinical use. Attention must be given to possible growth retardation if applicable. One approach to the overall problem would be to initiate pediatric clinical trials after the initial dose escalation studies in adults have been performed and tolerance has been established.

Informed Consent

There are relatively few issues related to the phase I testing of anticancer drugs that create as much controversy as that of informed consent. This may be traced to differing interpretations of the goals of the phase I trial. Traditionally for cytotoxic agents, and certainly for other classes of drugs, the phase I trial is a study of human toxicology. If this strict definition of a phase I trial is followed, then patients must clearly understand that they are volunteering for the sake of future cancer victims who may benefit from the results of the study. They must be informed of the experimental nature of the study and realize that in realistic terms they may be subjected to serious adverse reactions, without definite prospect for personal benefit.

The definitions of the phase I and phase II trials of anticancer drugs, however, tend to merge and cannot be readily separated. Because the study population has active cancer, it can be argued that all drug trials, phase I or otherwise, have therapeutic intent. The drug is routinely selected for evaluation because of some reasonable expectation of clinical activity, either from studies in predictive animal systems or because of structural analogy to an agent of known activity. The investigator is always searching for therapeutic as well as toxicologic effects. It has been stated that if no patients showed tumor regression during phase I study, then an agent would probably not be subjected to a vigorous phase II evaluation.

Nevertheless, the patients have in most instances been exposed to multiple courses of chemotherapy and possibly radiotherapy before becoming eligible for the phase I trial. Such cases are frequently resistant to all forms of treatment, as is substantiated by the negligible response rates reported for most phase I studies. Remissions, when observed, are of short duration and are usually not of sufficient quality to improve survival.

Because the major emphasis of the phase I trial is toxicologic, what should be the financial obligations of the patient as a result of his agreement to participate in the study? Optimally, all costs should be the responsibility of the sponsors of the new drug, be it the National Cancer Institute or a pharmaceutical company. Patients should also be fully informed of the financial liabilities that they assume by entering a trial.

Finally, the patients should not be coerced by inflated prospects of therapeutic benefit into entering a phase I study. They should have a complete understanding of therapeutic options if they choose not to take the new agent. They should be informed that they retain the right to revoke consent and to terminate their participation at any time, without prejudice or penalty. Conversely, their continuation in the study may be terminated by the investigators at any time.

Methodology

The patients selected for phase I study are those who present with clinical situations for which standard therapy has been either exhausted or is not known to exist. This means in many cases that they will have been extensively pretreated with some mixture of surgery, radiation, and more established chemotherapy. Despite this, the patients must be in a physical condition and performance status to undertake the trial, with a reasonable expectation that at least one course of treatment will be administered and evaluated. An example of the eligibility criteria is shown in Table 12–1, and is representative of what most institutions will utilize.

The following is an outline of some basic phase I study principles:

1. Initial dose is chosen from the maximum tolerated dose or a fraction of the LD10 dose in animal toxicology studies;
2. Doses are not escalated in the same patient;
3. Dose escalation is initially rapid with smaller increments of escalation as the toxic range is approached;
4. Three patients are treated at each nontoxic level and six at each level showing any toxicity; and
5. Antitumor response or lack thereof does not contribute directly to the decision to move the drug into phase II studies.

Drug doses are given in milligrams per square meter of body surface area, because this method achieves better correlation to certain metabolic and excretory functions than does

Table 12–1. General Patient Entry Criteria for a Phase I Study

1. Informed consent form must be signed and on file
2. Biopsy- or cytologically proven cancer
3. Tumor resect cannot be with curative intent and there must be no meaningful alternative forms of chemotherapy or radiotherapy available
4. Age $\leq$ 70 years
5. Karnofsky performance status $\geq$ 50
6. Life expectancy $\geq$ 6 weeks
7. Four-week lapse time since prior chemotherapy or irradiation, with complete reversal of myelosuppression from this therapy
8. Adequate hepatic, renal, and bone marrow function as defined by
   a. WBC $\geq$ 4,000/mm^3
   b. Platelet count $\geq$ 100,000/mm^3
   c. Creatinine $\leq$ 1.5 mg%
   d. BUN $\leq$ 25 mg%
   e. SGOT $<$ 3 times normal
   f. Bilirubin $<$ 2.0 mg%

body weight (Shirkey, 1965). Moreover, body surface area can be used as a common denominator for drug dosage in adults and children, as well as in different animal species (Freireich *et al.*, 1966; Shirkey, 1965; Zelen, 1974a; Zelen 1974b). The recommended starting dose for most initial clinical trials is one-third the minimal toxic dose in milligrams per square meter of body surface area to the most sensitive large animal species. It is important to keep in mind that calculations on a milligram per kilogram of body weight basis would not follow this one-third rule.

Three patients are entered at the starting dose level chosen, as described above. At least one week should pass between the entry of each of the three patients on treatment to decrease the risk of simultaneous toxicity. The patients are kept on the initial dose level for an arbitrary time period, such as six weeks, or less time if toxicity occurs.

Subsequent patients are entered at higher dose levels if no dose-limiting toxicity occurs at the preceding dose level. The dose escalations are initially rapid, with smaller increments the closer one gets to the toxic range (modified Fibonacci search scheme), an example of which is given (see Table 12–2). Other escalation schemes have been used but no single approach can be described as definitive. The modified Fibonacci scheme has been the most common one used in recent years, although it is not always necessary or possible to rigidly follow such a mathematical scheme. One research team showed that for 30 drugs analyzed, eight would have required more than six steps to reach maximum tolerated doses (MTD) in a phase I study if the initial dose had been chosen as one-third the lowest toxic dose (TDL) in dogs and a Fibonacci scheme had been employed (Goldsmith *et al.*, 1975). Three of these drugs would have required more than ten steps. Flexibility in dose escalation is necessary, and clinical judgment must be exercised in evaluating toxicity at one dose level and translating it into a subsequent higher dose. A useful estimate may be obtained from the slope of the animal toxicity curve, for example, for the increments in going from LD_{10} to LD_{50} to LD_{90} rodents. If this curve is steep, then small increments are necessary in human trials. If it is a more gradual slope, larger increments may be possible in these trials.

Some of the difficulties in this area may be circumvented by the consideration of pharmacokinetics. An important question, for example, is whether the blood levels that are achieved are within a toxic range based upon animal and *in vitro* studies of cytotoxicity. Pharmacokinetic studies can also help design intervals between successive drug doses in an individual patient, by defining the rate of clearance of the drug, and the relationship of the drug clearance to successive doses. Information may also be obtained from preexisting data on analogs of the drug under study.

From two to six weeks should pass before patients enter the next higher dose level to take advantage of the experience accrued at lower dose levels, especially when delayed and potentially dangerous types of toxicity are expected, as in the case of nitrosourea analogs.

The question of dose escalation within patients is controversial, although many investigators feel it is acceptable within a phase I study. The major argument in its favor is the rapidity with which information can be gained, as well as the fact that it maximizes the potential for therapeutic benefit to a given patient. The major argument against its usage is the danger of cumulative toxicity, particularly with a drug that produces delayed toxicity. In addition, dose escalation makes the prediction of a safe starting dose for phase II studies imprecise.

Three patients are placed on each nontoxic dose level and six at subtoxic levels. More patients can be treated at drug levels with acceptable, reversible toxicity, depending on individual variability of tolerance. Past experience dictates that the tolerated dose will be defined within five to eight dose steps. Hence, between ten and 30+ patients will be needed for exploration of the initial dose schedule.

It is usually desirable to explore more than one dose schedule of drug administration (*e.g.*, daily versus widely spaced doses). The starting

Table 12–2. Idealized Modified Fibonacci Search Scheme Approach to Dose Escalation in Phase I Study

DRUG DOSE	PERCENTAGE INCREASE ABOVE PRECEDING DOSE LEVEL
n*	—
2.0n	100
3.3n	67
5.0n	50
7.0n	40
9.0n	30 to 35
12.0n	30 to 35
16.0n	30 to 35

* Starting dose = n (mg/m²)

level for the drug dose on the second schedule is usually one to two dose steps below the level of expected toxicity, depending on the experience gained with the initial dose schedule (type of toxicity, reversibility of toxicity, variability of individual tolerance). Exploration of other dose schedules will probably require nine to 20 additional patients per schedule.

Toxicity should always be related to a given dose schedule, at a given dose level, for a given duration of time. Some toxicity definitions in phase I study are given (see Table 12–3).

As in any clincial study, the design of a phase I trial must encompass a number of critical variables, such as: (1) Selection of initial dose, (2) dose schedules, (3) pharmacology, and (4) dose escalation procedure.

Selection of Initial Dose

The initial dose for phase I studies may be chosen on the basis of rodent or large-animal data, clinical data obtained with an analog, or from foreign clinical trials.

Several investigators, particularly in Europe, the Soviet Union, and Japan, have used rodent data to predict an initial dose. For example, a protocol of the Pharmacology Committee of the Soviet Ministry of Health states that one-third of the maximum tolerated cumulative dose for rats, given over 15 days in milligrams per kilogram of body weight, is used for alkylating agents, whereas lower starting doses are recommended for drugs from other chemical classes.

Most European countries accept the approach of using three animal species, one of them nonrodent, in preclinical toxicity studies. Since the most sensitive species is used for prediction of the initial dose, a rodent species might become the predictive one.

In the United States, this problem has received major contributions (Pinkel, 1958; Freireich et al.,1966; Goldsmith et al.,1975). The critical observation was that of Pinkel, later refined by Freireich, showing that drug dosage could be more readily compared between species when doses were expressed on a milligrams per square meter of body surface basis rather than on a milligrams per kilogram basis. This concept of using body surface area as a basis for dose calculation has since become widely accepted in cancer chemotherapy. It is based upon the long-recognized fact that important physiologic variables, such as cardiac output and glomerular filtration rate, are more closely related to body surface area than to body weight. Pinkel was able to show that the toxic doses of five drugs (mechlorethamine, methotrexate, 6-mercaptopurine, actinomycin D, and triethylene thiophosphoramide) in animals and man were quite constant when calculated on a dose per square meter of surface area, but varied inversely with absolute body size when expressed on a dose per kilogram basis. Freireich and associates (1966) confirmed and extended this work by drawing upon the extensive toxicity data of the Cancer Chemotherapy National Service Center. Interspecies comparison was quantified by first converting drug dose to a uniform schedule of daily $\times$ 5, and then expressing these doses on a milligrams per square meter basis. When this was done, excellent comparisons could be made between LD_{10} doses in rodents, MTD in dogs and monkeys, and MTD in man. These values were close to constant for the various species when expressed as milligrams per

Table 12–3. Toxicity Definitions in Phase I Study

TERM	DEFINITION
Subtoxic dose	A dose that causes *consistent* changes of hematologic or biochemical variables and might thus herald toxicity at the next higher dose level or with prolonged drug administration (Example: Consistent, drug-related decrease of thrombocytes that do not drop below an arbitrarily defined "toxic" level of <100,000 per mm^3)
Minimal toxic dose	The smallest dose at which one or more of three patients show consistent, readily reversible drug toxicity
Recommended dose for therapeutic trial	The dose that causes moderate, reversible toxicity in most patients
Maximum tolerated dose	The highest safely tolerable dosage

square meter of body surface, but based on milligrams per kilogram they showed an inverse correlation with absolute body size. The authors' suggested that this correlation with body surface area was, in turn, related to the fact that the skin surface area was directly proportional to the true receptor target surface of the drug.

These and other authors (Goldsmith *et al.,*1975) have emphasized that direct translation of animal toxicity data into human MTD is not acceptable in practice. They believe that the human MTD must be derived from careful experimental trial. Nevertheless, the animal data provide an excellent basis upon which to estimate the initial dose for a phase I trial. Freireich *et al.,*(1966) underscored the importance of obtaining toxicity data from several species as a safety measure and then beginning human trials at about one-third the MTD of the most susceptible species, which is usually the dog or the monkey. The translation of this recommendation into practice at the National Cancer Institute (NCI) has usually been to use one-third of the TDL in the most susceptible animal species as the starting human dose.

Although one-third of the TDL in the most sensitive species, expressed in milligrams per square meter of body surface area, has been the approach for years, Goldsmith and associates (1975) and Guarino (1979) have analyzed the quantitative prediction of one-third the TDL from the most sensitive animal species as a safe starting dose. In both retrospective analyses of a large number of drugs tested by the National Cancer Institute Drug Development Program, this fraction was found to be generally safe, although not perfect. In Goldsmith's retrospective analysis of 30 drugs, it was found that if the phase I starting dose were taken as one-third the MTD in the most sensitive large-animal species, five of 30 drugs would have produced toxicity in the first patient (Goldsmith *et al.,*1975). As a result, many oncologists prefer to start at one-tenth the MTD in the most sensitive species, which would have a less than 1% chance of exceeding the human MTD.

The use of foreign clinical data entails different approaches for determining an initial dose. One may select the full dose or, particularly if there may be population differences in sensitivity to the drug, a fraction of the dose can be used. If the latter choice is made, then the proportion used must also be determined, and this often depends on the scientific quality of the original investigation.

Dose Schedules

The choice of an initial schedule for phase I study is aided by information from various sources, including schedule-dependency data in rodent tumor systems, data on cell-cycle sensitivity and mechanism of action, pharmacology investigations, and schedules used in studies of large-animal toxicology. Schedules usually followed in NCI-sponsored phase I studies are: (1) Single dose, (2) daily × 5 or 10, (3) twice weekly, (4) weekly, and (5) continuous infusion.

These schedules, which generally result from schedule-dependency studies in mice, raise the question of whether the extrapolation to man is relevant without correlation with metabolism and drug disposition. Are these really the optimal dose schedules? An important question remains as to whether to proceed in phase I study with only one schedule or with two, three, or all the schedules mentioned.

Pharmacology

The assessment of organ response to a toxic drug is best based upon measures of the functional state of the organ in question. In practice, the methodology may draw heavily upon chemical pathology and serum enzyme levels. Two important areas that require increased application in both preclinical and clinical toxicology are the measurement of blood levels of drug and correlation of plasma drug concentration as a function of time (C × t) with observed effects. This concept assumes that not only the concentration of drug to which an organ is exposed but also the duration of exposure are critical variables in determining toxicity. Therefore, the integral of serum drug concentration as a function of time is a quantity of importance for both animal and clinical toxicologic study. It has been generally recommended that: (1) Preclinical pharmacology should be defined before the drug is given for the first time in man, and (2) pharmacologic studies should be implemented in phase I trials.

A more complete discussion of the methodology of pharmacokinetics is presented in Chapter 10. Studies of pharmacokinetics in phase I trials may be initiated at the first dose level, at the level showing first toxicity, or at the MTD. The advantages of starting pharmacology at the initial dose level include early indications of unique pattern of drug distribution and excretion, early hints of improper choice of schedule, and early comparative pharmacology with other animal species. A disadvantage of starting at the initial dose level is the potential waste of resources in an investigation being performed at levels without biologic activity. In general, studies of pharmacologic disposition are optimally performed during the initial phase I studies, assuming that the analytical methods for determination of the parent drug and its metabolites are available.

Apart from the implications of pharmacokinetics to interspecies comparative toxicology, pharmacologic studies are of use in interpreting the results of early toxicity trials. The problem is basically that of explaining variations in observed toxicities among patients. There are a multitude of factors that may contribute to variability in plasma drug levels, as well as to clinically observed toxicity (see Table 12–4), and interpretation of toxicity requires an appreciation of these factors. The pertinent question in phase I trials is not whether all of the items in Table 12–4 can be defined, but whether there exists significant variation in plasma drug levels among different patients and whether these variations correlate with differences in toxicity. It is then a subject for later investigations to define the precise mechanisms by which such variations occur.

Dose Escalation Procedure

The basic approach of dose escalation until significant (life-threatening) and consistent toxicity has been observed has achieved an unchallengeable position in the thinking of many investigators. Inherent in this methodology is the risk that treatment-related deaths may result, despite the current advanced state of supportive care. This must be viewed in the context that a phase I study is primarily toxicologic in intent, and the patients selected often have little prospect of responding to any form of treatment.

It should be emphasized that the prerequisite of toxicology for therapeutic activity has rarely been subjected to a critical appraisal in tumors other than the adult form of acute myelogenous leukemia, for which the present goal of therapy is a virtual elimination of the bone marrow. A prospective trial of high- and low-dose alkylating agent treatment of ovarian cancer, and the retrospective analysis of 5-fluorouracil toxicity for therapeutic activity in colorectal cancer, however, fail to make a case for intensive, life-threatening therapy.

The severity of toxicity produced by an initial course of treatment has too infrequently been assessed in regard to its potential clinical application. Often the drug-related side effects are so harsh that repeated treatments at the

Table 12–4. Factors that may Alter Drug Pharmacokinetics and Contribute to Variability in Plasma Levels and Clinically Observed Toxicity among Patients

---

I. Alterations at the level of drug absorption
   a. Variability in absolute rate of gastrointestinal absorption
   b. Concurrent gastrointestinal disease—malabsorption, steatorrhea, neoplastic involvement, congestive heart failure
   c. Concurrent drugs that complex, precipitate, or otherwise interfere with absorption
   d. Failure to take the drug (noncompliance)
   e. Inappropriate pharmaceutical formulation
II. Acting at the level of drug distribution
   a. Altered level of protein binding due to increases or decreases in serum binding proteins
   b. Increased distribution due to displacement from protein binding sites by another drug
III. Factors that alter drug metabolism
   a. Genetic—produce alterations in levels of enzymatic systems, *e.g.,* acetylating systems that detoxify drugs
   b. Liver disease
   c. Concurrent drugs that induce drug-metabolizing enzymes, *e.g.,* phenobarbital
   d. Age-diminished drug conjugating ability
IV. Factors that alter drug excretion
   a. Liver disease
   b. Renal disease

From Woolley, P. V., and Schein, P. S.: Clinical pharmacology and phase I trial design. *Methods Cancer Res.,* **17**:177–198, 1979.

same dose level are not attempted, nor is this apparently considered an integral part of many phase I studies. Such an approach bears no relationship to how the same drug will ultimately be employed. In therapeutic trials, repeated courses are administered over an extended period of time. This is a situation where the cumulative toxicity in a sensitive organ may be as important as the acute effects. In addition, the majority of treatment programs for both solid tumors and hematologic neoplasms involve the use of drug combinations. In both instances, single-agent and combined therapy, the dose of the drug had to be lowered from that offered as the "traditional" MTD in the phase I trial.

How then shall the dose for a broad phase II study be chosen? One method is to extrapolate directly the MTD from the phase I studies. Two additional approaches, not mutually exclusive, can be considered. One involves pure clinical empiricism, whereas the other is based upon pharmacologic data. The first would depend upon the identification of a tumor sensitive to the action of a drug during the phase I studies. It is rare that an agent considered for phase II testing does not demonstrate antitumor activity during phase I testing. One could conduct a phase II trial in a sensitive tumor, randomizing a clinical dose of minimal toxicity against the more accepted MTD of moderate to severe toxicity from the phase I data. The question being asked is: How little drug is required for maximum therapeutic effect?

The second approach is pharmacologic and attempts to define the therapeutic dose range based upon knowledge of concentrations required for cytotoxicity, the metabolism, and pharmacokinetics of the specific agent. The blood levels achieved and the time the drug remains at cytotoxic levels can be determined for the dose range employed. Using this information, a therapeutic dose could be estimated and tested. Ultimately, as our understanding of the pharmacology of anticancer agents becomes increasingly more sophisticated, this approach should provide the most direct and rational method for dosage selection.

PHASE II TRIALS

Phase II of a New Drug

The phase II evaluation of a new anticancer drug is designed to determine whether or not the compound has objective antitumor activity in a well-defined patient population. The crucial decision at the end of the phase II study is whether more widespread (phase III) trials with the drug are indicated or not. Because it is rarely possible to perform a therapeutic study in every tumor type for which a new drug might have an indication, the phase II evaluation must be disease oriented. It is usual, therefore, to select a representative sample of tumor types for phase II study. Within the Drug Development Program of the National Cancer Institute's Division of Cancer Treatment, there has evolved the concept of "signal tumors," which constitute the minimum number of cancerous disorders for which the agent will be evaluated. If the drug has no therapeutic activity in these, it can be reasonably assumed that it would most likely be inactive in other tumor types. The current list of signal tumors includes breast cancer, colorectal cancer, lung cancer, melanoma, acute leukemia, and lymphoma.

Patient Selection

The patients must all have histologically confirmed neoplastic disease that is no longer amenable to conventional therapy or for which there is no established therapy. Because a phase II study is therapeutic in intent, the subjects *must have* objectively measurable neoplastic disease variables. Phase II studies should be carried out in patients who are expected to survive a required minimum period of observation, and whose physiologic function is compatible with the proposed therapeutic study. One must ensure that carry-over effects of antecedent therapies have been dissipated by the time the investigation begins and researchers must be reasonably certain that the effects of the investigated new drug can be separated from the effects of concurrently administered nonantineoplastic drugs as well as from effects of the disease itself.

The disease state should be carefully described in terms of the available prognostic factors that might affect the therapeutic outcome. For example, specification of the following factors may be necessary: Age, race, sex, histologic type of tumor, site of tumor, clinical extent of disease, rate of progression of the tumor, response to previous therapy, state of nutrition, and functional status of the subject.

Methodology

At the start of phase II study, the drug is used at the recommended dose level identified from the phase I study. In most cases, this is a close approximation to the MID with dosage regulation appropriate to the extent of prior therapy. It is common to choose a single schedule, although occasionally multiple schedules will be used when interest in the drug is extensive. Intermittent schedules are currently dominant in cancer chemotherapy, and the two most common schedules used for new drugs are either daily $\times 5$ or a single dose every three to four weeks, depending upon the expected recovery time from myelosuppression. It is highly unlikely that these intermittent schedules are optimal for every drug, but it hasn't been possible yet to rationally design an optimal schedule for a new drug from the pharmacokinetic data that may be obtained in phase I study.

The endpoints of a phase II study are response rate and toxicity. Limits of objective response must be selected, for example, a 50% reduction in the product of the lesion's maximum diameter and its maximum perpendicular, maintained for at least 30 days with no evidence of progressive disease elsewhere. Efficacy is determined by a denominator made up of the number of patients treated and/or evaluable and a numerator that is the number of responding patients utilizing the criteria of the study. The decision to be reached is whether the agent could be effective in a given percentage of patients (Gehan and Schneiderman, 1973). Because the number of patients in a phase II study is relatively small and the prognostic heterogeneity within tumors great, there is an expected probable error factor. A positive result in a phase II study will require further confirmation, and refinement, in subsequent trials. A negative phase II study is, however, rarely repeated. Therefore, we have some sense of the false-positive rate in phase II studies, but little, if any, about the false-negative rate. This is unfortunate, since a false-negative phase II study is a much more damaging error in drug development and clinical oncology than is a false positive evaluation.

One approach to the problem of determining the minimum size of sample for a phase II study has been provided (Gehan, 1961). Table 12–5 indicates the number of patients necessary for a decision as to whether an agent warrants further study or whether the sample size is not likely to give a true index of therapeutic effectiveness at given levels or within acceptable percentages of rejection error. Rejection error is the chance of inappropriately deciding that a drug should not be subjected to further study. Thus, if one is interested in an agent of 25% effectiveness and is willing to accept a 10% rejection error, a sample of nine patients is necessary. This number was derived by an assumption that the true effectiveness of the agent is 25% and calculating that the chance of nine consecutive failures is less than 10%. If all nine patients failed to respond, further study of the agent could be stopped, because with a true response rate of 25%, one or more responses would have been observed with a chance of over 90%.

This approach involves several simplifying assumptions. First, response is not an all-or-none phenomenon; there are varying degrees. Response must be defined so that when one or more responses have been observed, it is meaningful to say the agent is worth further study. The definition of response may not pose

Table 12–5. Number of Patients Required for Phase II Trials of an Agent for Given Levels of Therapeutic Effectiveness and Rejection Error

THERAPEUTIC EFFECTIVENESS (%)	NUMBER OF PATIENTS REQUIRED WITH A REJECTION ERROR OF	
	5%	10%
5	59	45
10	29	22
15	19	15
20	14	11
25	11	9
30	9	7
35	7	6
40	6	5
45	6	4
50	5	4

serious difficulties in diseases such as solid tumors, in which agents have been largely ineffective up to now. When transient regressions or partial benefits are regularly observed with currently available agents, it may be reasonable to define "response" as a marked objective improvement of some minimum duration in a patient's disease. Second, the number of patients given in Table 12 – 5 is based on the assumption that the probability of response is the same for each patient; however, patients' responses are not homogeneous, and they can often be subdivided into groups having different probabilities. Consequently, the numbers provided in Table 12 – 5 should be taken as approximate and as referring to an "average" level of therapeutic effectiveness of interest. Third, some prior knowledge may exist concerning the approximate level of effectiveness of the agent before the phase II study, and no allowance was made for this.

Agents with effectiveness of lower order than that of interest may have a substantial chance of being approved for further study based upon the results of a phase II trial. If one studies nine patients in search of an agent of 25% effectiveness (with 10% rejection error), for example, there is more than a 30% chance that one or more responses will be observed, even if the agent has only 5% true therapeutic effectiveness. Such a probability might be acceptable when no agent of any real effectiveness exists for a given disease, but it may not be satisfactory for diseases for which agents of a reasonably high order of effectiveness already exist.

The number of patients for a phase II study can be specified in many different ways. The *minimum* number of patients needed for an idealized phase II study (see Table 12 – 5) is one in which response rate is low and qualitative, patients' responses are homogeneous, and there is no correlation among response rates in various tumor categories. The plans are designed to reject ineffective agents quickly, and send on to further trial those that have some effectiveness.

When a regimen has passed a phase II trial or was sufficiently effective in a phase I trial, it will nearly always be desirable to study additional patients (in a follow-up trial) to obtain a more precise estimate of effectiveness. Usually, only a limited number of patients are needed in phase II (15 to 30), so more might be studied before starting a phase III trial. Gehan (1961) provided the number of additional patients to be studied to estimate the true therapeutic effectiveness with a specified (albeit approximate) precision.

Historically, two predominant designs for phase II studies have been used. A drug-oriented approach has been emphasized in the past, in which a large number of patients with a variety of diseases are treated with a particular drug. This has been the classic phase II investigation through which the active drugs such as 5-fluorouracil, cyclophosphamide, methotrexate, and, more recently, adriamycin (Schein et al., 1970), have been detected. Although the total patient numbers are sometimes quite large, there are often relatively few patients in each disease category. In addition, little information is obtained concerning the disease and patient characteristics that effect response.

Many limits of disease and patient population that influence the ability of a drug to induce objective response or to favorably alter survival have been reported. The performance status of the patient has a marked effect on survival in lung cancer (Woolley and Schein, 1979) and on response rate in colon cancer (Pinkel, 1958). Prior chemotherapy affects the objective response rate in solid tumors (O'Bryan et al., 1973), as well as in the hemotologic cancers (Frei et al., 1973). Various metastatic sites respond differently within the same disease category, such as soft tissue versus visceral disease in breast cancer (Broder and Tormey, 1974) and malignant melanoma (Carter and Freidman, 1972). The list of important variables is often unique for each major disease. It is not surprising, therefore, that patient selection factors could greatly alter the results of a small, uncontrolled drug-oriented trial.

These considerations have led to the second and current type of phase II trial: The disease-oriented study. The critical factor in this approach is that the prognostic variables that may affect response are accounted for in the study design. Currently, these studies are being performed in a nonrandomized sequential manner.

In the nonrandomized phase II study, consecutively entered patients are given a single treatment. The trial is directed to a specific disease category or subcategory; for example, pancreatic cancer versus all gastrointestinal cancer, or squamous cell carcinoma of the lung as opposed to lung cancer. Restrictions on patient entry may be imposed to limit the study to groups with specific prognostic variables, or, in large studies, specific prognostic groups may be analyzed separately after completion of the study. If possible, most studies should include patients with defined host and disease factors that may make them likely to respond to a reasonably active agent. The study design, priorities for drug testing, as well as the type of patients to be treated depend upon the therapy currently available for a given disease.

The disease-oriented decision about whether or not phase III comparative studies with a new drug are indicated depends upon the efficacy observed in phase II, against the background of what chemotherapy can accomplish in the particular tumor in question. In unresponsive tumors, such as large bowel cancer, non-oat-cell lung cancer, malignant melanoma, and pancreatic cancer, almost any level of activity can be considered as a positive phase II study. In responsive tumors, in contrast, this is not the case; not only must the response rate in general be higher, but toxicologic considerations are of greater importance. In responsive tumors, combination chemotherapy will be the general rule and a new drug should have toxicologic characteristics that would not preclude easy combination with other active drugs.

Phase II Testing of Analogs

Analogs pose specific problems in phase II study because their evaluation must be made in comparison with the therapeutic efficacy and toxicity of the parent structure and in relation to the rationale that was used in choosing the analogs for evaluation (Carter, 1978). An analog can be superior to its parent structure in three different ways: (1) It can have greater efficacy in responsive tumors, (2) it can have efficacy in unresponsive tumors (broader spectrum), or (3) it can have diminished acute or chronic toxicity. The endpoint for a positive phase II with an analog depends upon which of the potential measures of therapeutic superiority is being sought.

If the strategy assumes superior efficacy in a responsive tumor compared to the parent compound, the goal of the phase II trial will be to provide sufficient evidence to justify subsequent phase III trials. This approach can be complicated if the parent is a component of a primary combination with substantial therapeutic activity. The evaluation of a vincristine

analog in Hodgkin's disease is an example. There are two approaches to solving the problem: The analog may be evaluated after failure on a nonvincristine-containing combination; the second approach is to substitute the analog for vincristine in the MOPP combination. The major difficulty with this second approach is that it requires a phase III study to achieve the answer and in essence assumes a positive phase II.

The evaluation of an analog in a tumor intrinsically unresponsive to the parent drug is a great deal easier. In this situation, the evaluation becomes almost identical to that of a new drug structure, because any level of meaningful activity is indicative of the need for phase III study. The strategy for a demonstration of a lack of cross-resistance to the parent drug structure is also relatively simple. A positive phase II requires only noteworthy therapeutic activity in patients who have developed progressive disease while under treatment with the parent structure. This form of phase II evaluation, by definition, must occur as at least second-line drug treatment. This must be kept in mind in the analysis of a negative study that may have resulted from the inclusion of cases with far advanced disease beyond the hope of any response. Close attention must be given to the performance status of the patient population and other important response variables in the analysis.

The number of analogs developed in the hope of diminished toxicity have increased in importance in recent years. This has been particularly true with the analogs of: (1) Adriamycin (cardiac toxicity), (2) bleomycin (pulmonary toxicity), (3) cis-platinum (renal toxicity), and (4) nitrosoureas (marrow toxicity). If the desired endpoint for an analog is diminished toxicity, then the phase II study evaluation has two components: (1) In terms of efficacy, there should be presumptive evidence of at least comparable therapeutic activity to the parent structure, and (2) there should be presumptive evidence of diminished toxicity in this critical aspect.

PHASE III TRIALS

The principal objective of a phase III study is to compare definitively the new treatment with an established mode of therapy. For a new drug to be approved for a phase III evaluation, reasonable evidence must exist that the agent alone or in combination is either superior or at least comparable in effectiveness to that of an accepted standard of treatment for the specific tumor.

Patient Selection

The patient population consists of cases with histologically confirmed tumors of types that have been demonstrated to be responsive in prior phase II studies. Other disease categories may also be included based upon laboratory-derived rationale for the agent. Because of the large numbers of patients required for a phase III study, well controlled cooperative trials are required when a single investigator or institution cannot recruit a sufficient number of subjects over a reasonable period of time to complete the study (Zelen, 1974a, b). The disease state must be described in all cases, in terms of the available prognostic factors that might affect the therapeutic outcome. Specification of the following factors may be necessary: Age, race, sex, histologic type of tumor, site of tumor, clinical extent of the disease, response to previous therapy, state of nutrition, and functional status of the subject. The optimal patient population would include previously untreated cases, with excellent performance status.

Methodology

The determination of the dose and schedule for the phase III trial is based upon information derived from the phase II study. The preferred method of evaluation is the prospective randomized controlled trial, and there are two possibilities: (1) The new drug may be compared directly with an established agent or therapy or placebo; and (2) the new drug may be incorporated into an established regimen of treatment, usually a drug combination; a determination will then be made as to whether or not the new drug makes an added impact in terms of therapeutic effectiveness and tolerance.

An alternative method of comparison, the use of an historic control, is less desirable and its use should be justified. Historic control data must demonstrate close comparability with the clinical characteristics of the study population that are known to influence response and survival. A new drug that is not expected to exhibit independent therapeutic activity may be taken directly from phase I into phase III trial in a combination setting based upon rationale developed from biochemical, pharmacologic, or basic biologic studies. It must be anticipated, in this setting, that the experimental agent will enhance the therapeutic index of another drug or treatment.

The classic phase III study is one that directly compares a new drug with the standard drug with known efficacy for a given disease. The development of a new anticancer agent for colon cancer can be used as an example: This may take the form of a prospectively randomized comparison of the new drug against 5-fluorouracil, the standard treatment used by many oncologists for this disease. This classic phase III study, geared totally to answering a drug-related question, is becoming less common in clinical oncology. This is because the new drug, found active in a phase II study, is rapidly integrated into a disease-oriented clinical research strategy (see Figure 12–1), which puts the highest priority on combination chemotherapy and combined modality trials. New combination regimens have phase I, II, and III histories of their own against individual tumor types. These studies often lead to still newer combination regimens, therefore, the strategy for determining the independent therapeutic activity of the investigational drug becomes lost. This frustration can become particularly acute when multiple analogs are undergoing clinical evaluation at the same time. In recent years, examples of this occurrence include the nitrosoureas and anthracyclines. Currently, multiple analogs of *cis*-platinum diamminedichloride have entered clinical trial and the same difficulty will probably arise.

The clinical research superiority of a new drug, or regimen, must be established from a properly designed and executed study. This requires a comparative analysis—the *sine qua non* consists of direct assessment of the new treatment with the standard—in patient populations with identical prognostic features and appropriate stratifications (Zelen, 1974a, b).

A procedure termed stratification is employed before the patients are randomly allocated to two or more therapeutic regimens. Patients entering the study are categorized by sets of known important prognostic factors and the individuals falling within each set form a group or "stratum." Then the patients in each group are separately randomized to the treatment programs (Zelen, 1974b). This procedure attempts to ensure a balance of impor-

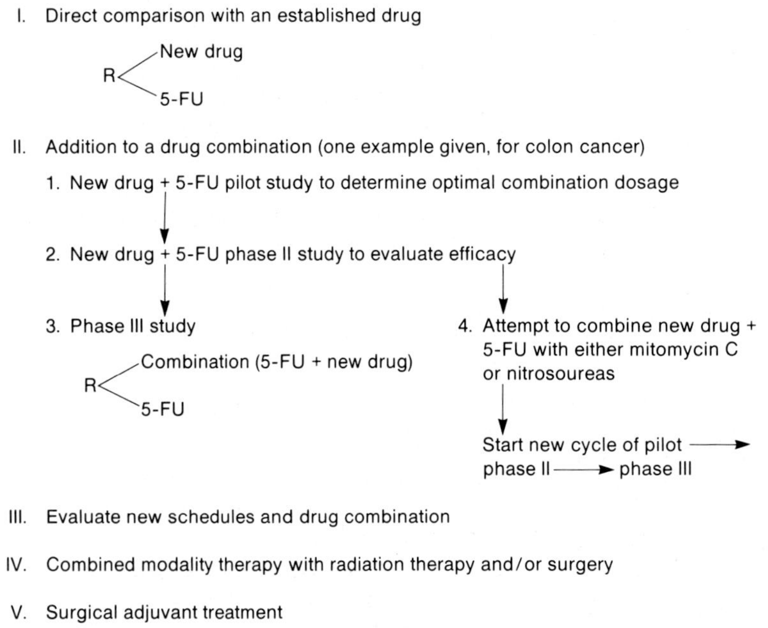

I. Direct comparison with an established drug

```
         New drug
    R
         5-FU
```

II. Addition to a drug combination (one example given, for colon cancer)

1. New drug + 5-FU pilot study to determine optimal combination dosage

2. New drug + 5-FU phase II study to evaluate efficacy

3. Phase III study

```
         Combination (5-FU + new drug)
    R
         5-FU
```

4. Attempt to combine new drug + 5-FU with either mitomycin C or nitrosoureas

Start new cycle of pilot ⟶
phase II ⟶ phase III

III. Evaluate new schedules and drug combination

IV. Combined modality therapy with radiation therapy and/or surgery

V. Surgical adjuvant treatment

Figure 12–1. Phase III trial study designs.

tant prognostic variables among the treatments being compared, so that no single treatment group is inordinately weighted with poor or favorable risk factors.

The biologic assumption that is made when a statistical significance test is performed is that all prognostic variables are exactly comparable in the two groups of patients, except for the therapies being compared. The methodology commonly used to achieve this comparability is prospective randomization. An alternative approach to the prospective randomized trial that has been proposed is the matched historic control. This approach has the attractiveness of increasing the efficiency of clinical research, as well as avoiding the difficulties of convincing patients to agree to be randomized. The increased efficiency comes from not having to place half the patients entered into a trial on a standard or older regimen. The difficulties in utilizing historic controls are, however, numerous. Historic controls assume that all important prognostic variables are known, and that the data that exist in the control group are identical to those recorded for the prospectively treated patient cohort. Neither of these two assumptions is likely valid. New prognostic variables are continuously being discovered, as a result of basic and clinical research. The estrogen receptor assay in breast cancer is a prime example. Historic controls in breast cancer, for which the

estrogen receptor data are not available, are open to question. Here the balance of ER+ and ER− patients in the prospectively treated group might be significantly different, thus making interpretation difficult.

In historic controls, an assumption is made that the baseline therapies have been comparably delivered. In a study of local control (surgery and/or radiation therapy) versus local control and adjuvant therapy, it is assumed that the measures for local control have been identically delivered in both groups. The assumption is impossible to verify and is probably not true. In a population drawn from an earlier point in time, the surgeons were different, as were their therapeutic concepts and measures for postoperative and supportive care.

Another problem with the use of historic controls relates to differential selection bias. In a prospectively treated group of patients on a protocol study, only a subset of eligible patients within an institution are actually placed on the study. Patients potentially eligible for a trial are excluded for a range of reasons, which have not been analyzed fully. Whatever the selection bias may be, prospective randomization offers the potential of this bias being equally distributed between two treatment options. In historically controlled studies, the selection bias in prospectively treated patients cannot be compared to problems that may have existed in the selection of the historic controls. These historic controls are either all patients treated in a set period of past time or a selected subset of the same. Even if selected prognostic variables are matched in historic controls, the potential imbalance in selection bias should make for extreme caution in interpretation.

The concept of selection bias in clinical trials also has its correlate in their translation into everyday practice. In a clinical trial, only a minority of potentially eligible patients within an institution are actually entered, and this population may be quite different from that treated in a community oncologic practice. The community oncologist, convinced by a clinical trial report, will treat all subsequent patients with the given disease and stage with the new regimen. The degree to which he can interpret and translate a clinical research finding will depend upon his ability to deliver the therapy at appropriate dose and schedule, combined with the comparability of prognostic variables of his specific patient population. It is probably a fair assumption that no regimen gives results in community practice equivalent to that reported from a specialized cancer center, but this assumption needs further analysis.

REFERENCES

Broder, L., and Tormey, D.: Combination chemotherapy of carcinoma of the breast. *Cancer. Treat. Rev.,* **1**: 183–205, 1974.

Carter, S. K.: The clinical evaluation of analogues I. The overall problem. *Cancer Chemother. Pharmacol.,* **1**: 69–72, 1978.

Carter, S. K., and Freidman, M. A.: 5–(3,3–dimethyl–1–triazeno)–imidazole–4–carboxamide (DTIC, DIC, NSC 45388)—a new antitumor agent with activity against malignant melanoma. *Eur. J. Cancer,* **8**: 85–92, 1972.

Carter, S. K.; Selawry, O.; and Slavik, M.: Phase I clinical trials: Methods of development of new anticancer drugs. *Natl. Cancer Inst. Monogr.,* **45**: 75–81, 1975.

Frei, E., III; Luce, J. K.; and Gamble, J. F.: Combination chemotherapy in advanced Hodgkin's disease: Induction and maintenance of remission. *Ann. Intern. Med.,* **79**: 376–382, 1973.

Freireich, E. J.; Gehan, E. A.; Rall, D. P.; Schmidt, L. H.; and Skipper, H. E.: Quantitative comparison of toxicity of anticancer agents in mouse, rat, hamster, dog, monkey and man. *Cancer Chemother. Rep.,* **50**: 219–244, 1966.

Gehan, E. A.: The determination of the number of patients required in a preliminary and a follow-up trial of a new chemotherapeutic agent. *J. Chronic. Dis.,* **13**: 346–353, 1961.

Gehan, E. A., and Schneiderman, M. A.: Experimental design of clinical trials. In Holland, J. F., and Frei, E., III (eds.): *Cancer Medicine.* Lea & Febiger, Philadelphia, 1973.

Goldsmith, M. A.; Slavik, M.; and Carter, S. K.: Quantitative prediction of drug toxicity in humans from toxicology in small and large animals. *Cancer Res.,* **35**: 1354–1364, 1975.

Guarino, A. M.: Pharmacologic and toxicologic studies of anticancer drugs: Of sharks, mice, and men (and dogs and monkeys). *Methods Cancer Res.,* **17(B)**: 92–168, 1979.

Kenis, Y.: Dose schedules and modes of administration of chemotherapeutic agents in man. *Recent Results Cancer Res.,* **21**: 54–61, 1969.

Knudtzon, S., and Nissen, N. I.: Clinical trial with mycophenolic acid (NSC–129185), a new antitumor agent. *Cancer Chemother. Rep.,* **56**: 221–227, 1972.

Mathe, G.: Clinical examination of drugs, a scientific and ethical challenge. *Biomedicine,* **18**: 169–172, 1973.

Moertel, C. G.; Schutt, A. J.; Hahn, R. G.; and Reitemeier, R. S.: Effects of patient selection on results on phase II chemotherapy trials in gastrointestinal cancer. *Cancer Chemother. Rep.,* **58**: 257–260, 1974.

O'Bryan, R. M.; Luce, J. K.; Talley, R. W.; Gottlieb, J. A.; Baker, L. H.; and Bonadonna, G.: Phase II evaluation of adriamycin in human neoplasia. *Cancer,* **32**: 1–8, 1973.

Pinkel, D.: The use of body surface area as a criterion of drug dosage in cancer chemotherapy. *Cancer Res.,* **18**: 853–856, 1958.

Schein, P. S.; Davis, R. D.; Carter, S. K.; Newman, J.; Schein, D. R.; and Rall, D. P.: The evaluation of anticancer drugs in dogs and monkeys for the prediction of qualitative toxicities in man. *Clin. Pharmacol. Ther.,* **11**: 3–49, 1970.

Shirkey, H. C.: Drug dosage for infants and children. *J.A.M.A.,* **193**: 443–446, 1965.

Woolley, P. V., and Schein, P. S.: Clinical pharmacology and phase I trial design. *Methods Cancer Res.,* **17**: 177–198, 1979.

Zelen, M.: Keynote address on biostatistics and data retrieval. *Cancer Chemother. Rep.,* **4**: 31–42, 1974a.

Zelen, M.: The randomization and stratification of patients to clinical trials. *J. Chron. Dis.,* **27**: 365–375, 1974b.

13

Planning and Reporting of Clinical Trials*

RICHARD D. GELBER and MARVIN ZELEN

INTRODUCTION

One of the most important modern advances in experimental therapeutics is the development and widespread adoption of the use of the clinical trial to evaluate the benefits of new therapies as well as to confirm the benefit of therapies that have long been used. We define a clinical trial as a scientific experiment that generates clinical data for the purpose of evaluating one or more therapies on a patient population. Implicit in the trial is the fact that the clinical investigator has control of the process by which a treatment is assigned to a patient. Clinical trials may be randomized, nonrandomized, multi-institutional, or only involve a single institution.

Among all of the chronic diseases, perhaps there is no greater activity in clinical investigations than in the field of cancer. One reason for this is that "cancer" refers to more than a hundred different disease sites, each with different etiologies and natural histories. Therapeutic decisions may not only differ for each disease site but are critically dependent upon whether the disease is local, regional, or metastatic. Decisions for secondary and tertiary treatment of disease are particularly difficult, owing to the conflicting opinion of "experts" and lack of unequivocal scientific evidence. The growing number of cancer clinical trials represents one direction for determining beneficial cancer treatments.

The beginning of the modern clinical trial owes much to the writings of the French physician P. C. A. Louis (1787–1872). In 1836, he published his studies on the effect of bloodletting to treat pneumonia, erysipelas, and other inflammations (Louis, 1836). Dr. Louis conducted a clinical trial in which he deliberately delayed the onset of bloodletting. Table 13–1 summarizes part of the results of his experiment. He concluded that there was no benefit from the bloodletting. This conclusion was contrary to the orthodox teaching of the time and could be considered a landmark in the development of the scientific basis of medicine. It is interesting that during the American Civil War bloodletting was still a popular therapy.

Dr. Louis called his approach to the scientific study of medicine the "numerical method." His views, as expressed in his *Essay on Clinical Instruction* (1834), are just as important today as when he wrote them. He wrote,

As to different methods of treatment, if it is possible for us to assure ourselves of the superiority of one or other among them in any disease whatsoever, having regard to the different circumstances of age, sex, and temperament, of strength and weakness, it is doubtless to be done by inquiring if under these circumstances a greater number of individuals have been cured by one means than another. Here again

Table 13–1. Pneumonia: Effects of Bloodletting (Deliberately delayed bloodletting)

DAY BLED AFTER ONSET	DIED	LIVED	PROPORTION SURVIVING
1 to 3	12	12	50%
4 to 6	12	22	65%
7 to 9	3	16	84%

From Louis, P. C. A.: Researches on the effects of bloodletting in some inflammatory diseases, and on the influence of tartarized antimony and vesication in pneumonitis. Translated by C. G. Putnam, with preface and appendix by James Jackson. Boston, 1836.

* Partial support from NIH grants CA-06516, CA-19589, and CA-23415.

it is necessary to count. And it is, in great part at least, because hitherto this method has been not at all, or rarely employed, that the science of therapeutics is still so uncertain, that when the application of the means placed in our hands is useful we do not know the bounds of this utility. . . . In order that the calculation may lead to useful or true results it is not sufficient to take account of the modifying powers of the individual; it is also necessary to know with precision at what period of the disease the treatment has commenced; and especially we ought to know the natural progress of the disease, in all its degrees, when it is abandoned to itself, and whether the subjects have or have not committed errors of regimen; with other particulars.

He further states,

The only reproach which can be made to the Numerical Method is that it offers real difficulties in its execution. For, on the one hand, it neither can, nor ought to be applied to any other than exact observations, and these are not common, and on the other hand, this method requires much more labor and time than the most distinguished members of our profession can dedicate to it. But what signifies this reproach, except that the research of truth requires much labor and is beset with difficulties.

The ideas of Dr. Louis on the numerical method and its applications are perhaps even more important today.

It is quite possible that Dr. Louis was influenced by the great French mathematician Pierre Simon Laplace, who in 1812 published his famous paper on probability entitled "Essai Philosophique sur la Probabilitié." This paper was written as a popular account of probability. In fact, Laplace wrote

. . . to recognize the best of the treatments in use for the cure of a malady, it suffices to prove each of them on the same number of such individuals, all other circumstances being made alike; the superiority of the most advantageous treatment will manifest itself more and more as the number to whom it is applied increases, and the calculus will make known the probability corresponding to its advantage and the ratio according to which it is superior to the others.

Thus, more than 150 years ago there was a clear recognition by both a distinguished physician and mathematician that scientific evidence for deciding on the superiority of treatment rested on quantitative methods.

The modern theory of clinical trials has evolved as a joint discipline involving medicine and statistical science. Many new statistical techniques have been developed to meet the special circumstances of clinical trials.

These have involved many new methods for planning and analyzing studies. The use of computers has allowed one to analyze highly complex data sets that even a decade ago could not be done properly.

In this chapter, the focus will be upon some aspects of the planning, analysis, and reporting of clinical trials. The chapter is not meant to be a substitute for a statistical text. The presentation stresses major ideas.

PLANNING OF CLINICAL TRIALS

A basic understanding of the objectives of statistical inference is important for an appreciation of the role of statistical science for medical research. Figure 13–1 illustrates the flow of statistical inference. A population is defined from which a sample is obtained. Ordinarily, a population consists of a very large number of patients, which for all practical purposes could be regarded as infinite. The observed data obtained from the sample of patients are then used to characterize the features of the population. Describing the characteristics of a population using the data from a sample always involves uncertainty and randomness. A different sample from the same population will always result in different numerical values. Hence, although the sample data can be used to estimate the population characteristics, they should never be interpreted to be the actual population values themselves. Statistical inference involves the study of randomness and variability in observations for the purpose of using the observed results to estimate the characteristics of the population.

The application of the ideas of statistical inference to clinical trials is illustrated in the lower portion of Figure 13–1. The example is a study of treatment for a specified population of patients with breast cancer. The sample is represented by the group of patients who are used in the analysis. The observed results are presented in terms of six-year relapse-free survival (RFS) estimates. It is important to distinguish these *observed* results (*e.g.*, 55.7% RFS with cyclophosphamide, methotrexate, 5-fluorouracil [CMF]) from the *population characteristic* being estimated (*e.g.*, six-year RFS of the population if treated with CMF). The observed results are estimates of the population RFS based on the sample. They are subject to fluctuations due to sampling. One role of statistical methods is to quantify the uncertainty of results due to sampling. Having a measurement of the uncertainty of reported results allows one to judge how closely different institutions should agree with one another when giving the same treatment as well as providing a standard for objectively deciding when two treatments differ. The recognition that observed results are simply *estimates* of population characteristics is fundamental to an appreciation of the objectives and rationale for statistical methods in clinical research.

The two main objectives for planning clinical trials are to eliminate systematic biases and to maximize the precision of the reported results. The concept of bias in clinical trials can be illustrated by the example in Figure 13–1. Recall that the observed clinical results (RFS) are being used to estimate the RFS for a defined population. It is implicit that any observed differences in RFS between the CMF and observation groups reflect differences in the effectiveness of the two regimens as well as sampling variation. Hypothetically, assume that the selection of evaluable patients for study was conducted so that patients with one to three positive axillary nodes received CMF, while those with four or more positive axillary nodes did not receive CMF. The long-run average of differences in RFS as estimated by

such experiments will tend to favor CMF by virtue of the biases introduced by the treatment selection criteria. Thus, the estimated treatment differences will be biased. This so-called prognostic factor bias is but one form of potential bias that can affect the results of a clinical trial.

In addition to bias, increasing the precision of the trial is the other main consideration for planning clinical trials. Even if the long-run averages of sample estimates approach the desired population quantity (*i.e.,* zero-bias situation), the result from any given experimental realization will exhibit a certain amount of variation around the desired population quantity. This variation or dispersion of the estimate consists of three major components:

1. Patient-to-patient variability, arising from the fact that patients do not represent homogeneous samples;
2. Random variability associated with the uncertainty of outcomes even from strictly homogeneous groups of patients;
3. Variability of the numerical estimate as a function of sample size and the manner in which observations are combined to calculate (estimate) population quantities.

THE GENERAL FLOW OF STATISTICAL INFERENCE

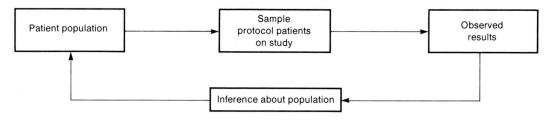

EXAMPLE OF STATISTICAL INFERENCES: BREAST CANCER (Bonadonna *et al.,* 1981)

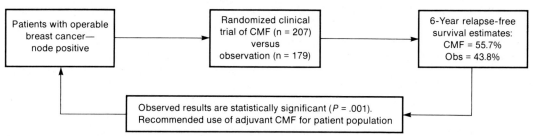

Figure 13–1. The flow of statistical inference.

The smaller the sampling variability of the estimate, the more likely it is to be close to the quantity being estimated. In this way, one can be more precise about making statements from the sample that apply to the *larger* population.

In an "idealized" experiment each experimental unit is alike, the treatments applied are exactly reproducible, and external environmental conditions are uniform. In this setting, which may exist in some areas of the physical sciences, the only variability encountered is usually due to the measuring instrument itself. Biases are eliminated by strict investigator control of experimental units and treatments. Observed differences between groups are easily ascribed to differences between the treatments, provided the magnitude of the differences is not "obscured" by measurement errors.

In clinical trials, however, the experimental units are patients who cannot be exactly alike. Furthermore, the treatments may not be exactly reproducible on every occasion, due to morbidity, toxicity, physical state of the patient, and so forth. Thus, the clinical trial must be carefully planned to eliminate biases and to control variability.

The Protocol Document

One of the most important items contributing to the quality of a clinical trial is a complete plan for the study as embodied in the protocol document. The main features of the protocol are listed in Table 13–2. A protocol document should be prepared for any clinical trial, whether it be phase I, II, or III. It is important to realize that whatever is not included in the protocol is left open to the vagaries of individual interpretation. Unless all of the essential elements of the study are clearly defined before the trial begins, the potential for biases in the results exists. A well-written protocol is an essential element for eliminating potential biases. In addition, the protocol document could provide much of the material required for a meaningful presentation of the results.

The Role of Randomization

The term randomization refers to the use of a chance mechanism as the means for allocating treatments (therapies) to experimental units (patients). By giving each patient the same opportunity of receiving any of the therapies under investigation, the characteristics of the different treatment groups will be "alike on the average" with respect to all factors that are likely to affect outcome. In this way, any observed differences in results between groups will tend to be due to the treatments. With the use of prospective randomization, neither the physician nor the patient knows in advance which therapy will be assigned. The principle advantages of randomization are:

1. It eliminates conscious bias; *e.g.*, physician selection of patients for trial or patient self-selection;
2. It eliminates unconscious bias; *e.g.*, un-

Table 13–2. Outline of Protocol Document

Schema: Pictorial summary of the essentials of the study design. Should be simple and logical and reflect the study objectives

Background: Prior results and rationale for the current study

Objectives: Few in number; relate to schema; feasible

Patient Population: Clearly defined, ideally homogeneous

Treatment Allocation: Randomization to avoid bias; stratification to achieve balance; placebo control; crossover plan; etc.

Treatment: Give all details to describe administration, schedule, potential toxicities, dose modification, and duration

Follow-Up Procedures: Schedules, clinical and laboratory data

Endpoints: Standardize and quantify criteria for evaluating treatment effect

Statistical Considerations: Study design and sample size

Forms Submission: Simple, efficient, and comparable schedules for all treatment arms

Informed Consent: Risks, benefits, alternative treatments, and right to withdraw

known factors affecting treatment groups, experimental environment related to diagnostic, supportive care, or treatment evaluation criteria;

3. It makes treatment groups "alike on the average" with respect to prognostic factors, nontreatment-related factors affecting the "drop-out" rate, and case evaluability; and

4. It establishes the validity of most of the statistical techniques used to analyze clinical data.

The use of randomization in clinical trials also has disadvantages. Randomization can interfere with the physician-patient relationship. The physician must tell the patient that he does not know which is the best treatment and that the therapy will be chosen by "computer" or the "toss of a coin." Another disadvantage is that some investigators regard having a control group as wasting resources because primary interest is in the group receiving the experimental therapy. Finally, since comparability of the groups is guaranteed only "on the average" by randomization, imbalances may be present in any single realization of the experiment.

Because of these disadvantages, the use of matched historic controls has been proposed as an alternative to prospective randomization. The numerous difficulties of using historic controls have been mentioned in Chapter 12. These include problems with both patient selection biases and experimental environment biases. The first category of biases arises because the treatment and control groups are selected via different mechanisms. Although some of the differences may be adjusted or controlled by matching of prognostic factors or by statistical modeling, many sources of bias cannot be controlled. The second category of biases is even more troublesome and generally arises because the treatment and control groups are treated and managed at different times under different sets of hospital conditions. Changes in supportive care, patient management, prior treatment, diagnostic and staging procedures, methods of evaluation, criteria for response, and quality of follow-up may differ among groups and will influence the treatment comparisons. This will certainly be true if the control group was treated at an earlier time. For example, by using routine CT scan to stage the primary disease, patients with occult metastases, who would have entered

adjuvant trials ten years ago, are being excluded from such trials today. It is impossible to adjust for these factors at the time of analysis, even if it were possible to quantify them. Nonrandomized studies have important roles in exploratory pilot studies and in protocols designed to stimulate new ideas. But if one requires credible data and unambiguous treatment comparisons, there is no substitute for a randomized clinical trial.

Additional Methods for Eliminating Bias

Additional study design strategies can be used in conjunction with randomization to eliminate bias in clinical trials. Prognostic factors that have a known significant influence on outcome may be balanced among treatment groups by using a stratified randomization study plan. Whereas simple randomization will provide groups that are "alike on the average," it is important to guarantee balance with respect to the most important factors. Patient subgroups defined by a set of these factors are referred to as strata. Stratified randomization refers to carrying out separate randomizations within each stratum. Overstratification of the population should be avoided as this may dilute resources (valid comparisons can only be made within strata) and may create unequal numbers of patients assigned to the treatments. Some authors have argued that stratified randomization should not be used for several reasons; for example, it adds to the complexity of the randomization process, prognostic factor imbalances can be adjusted in the analysis anyway, and imbalances among prognostic factors will be unlikely in trials with large numbers of patients. Nonetheless, the advantages of stratification far outweigh any claimed disadvantages.

The most reliable method of implementing randomization is to use a central randomization registrar. This can be carried out easily by adopting telephone randomization. To do this, the physician entering a patient on a study simply phones the registrar, gives some preliminary patient information, and receives a treatment assignment. Hence, any randomization complexity is unknown to the caller. Although imbalances in large trials when stratification is not used are unlikely, it is still possible for them to occur and compromise our ability to interpret the results. This would be particularly disastrous for a large trial. Furthermore, without stratification, imbalances are likely to occur at interim analyses or in small studies. In addition, the acceptance of results is more credible if the important factors are balanced between therapy groups. Thus, stratified randomization in clinical trials is strongly recommended.

Evaluation Criteria. Evaluation criteria must be comparable among all the treatment groups. The factors that are likely to influence the evaluation must be similar. Study designs that involve some aspects of "blinding" are often used to achieve this comparability. A single-blind study is one in which the patient is unaware of which treatment is being given. This controls for psychologic factors manifested by the patients that could influence evaluation. Blinding is especially important when the endpoint being measured requires the patient's subjective appraisal; for example, pain studies, attitudes, and the like. A double-blind study is one in which neither the physician nor the patient knows which treatment is being administered. Blinding the physician protects against unconscious biases that may influence the evaluation of response or the level of ancillary (nonprotocol) medication used. In addition to blinding, it is always necessary to have similar follow-up studies and comparable monitoring of patients.

When the control group involves no treatment, there is considerable risk that biases will be introduced by noncomparable follow-up and evaluation procedures. These biases can be reduced by using a placebo control and blinding. (The blinding of the placebo and treatment groups, however, may not always be feasible if the drug produces unique observable or measurable effects.) An example of the value of such a placebo control design is shown by the results of the Coronary Drug Project (see Table 13–3). The data apparently show that improved outcome is related to adherence to treatment (clofibrate), as measured by taking at least 80% of the protocol-specified number of capsules. Luckily, the trial was designed with a placebo control that showed an even larger favorable outcome associated with adherence to the placebo schedule. Apparently, adherence to treatment or placebo selected a more favorable patient subgroup rather than caused a more favorable outcome. Without the use of a placebo control, both treatment and no-treatment groups would have given the same overall results, but a benefit for the clofibrate might have been incorrectly claimed for those who adhere to the treatment schedule.

Crossover Designs. Crossover designs are also useful strategies for reducing biases that result from patient heterogeneity. A crossover design provides the opportunity for each patient to receive each of the treatments under study. These designs are generally of two types: (1) Crossover to the alternate treatment occurs at the time of failure on the initially assigned regimen; and (2) crossover to the alternate treatment occurs at a planned point in time (*e.g.*, on a cycle-by-cycle schedule). The first crossover design is generally adopted so that all patients who fail can expect to receive each treatment at some time during the course of their disease. This insures that there is some uniform program for the treating of failures. In this way, randomization does not deny potentially beneficial treatment to any patient. Crossover at failure provides data with which to assess response and time to failure of the initial treatment, evidence of the ability of a crossover therapy to induce benefit after an initial treatment failure, and, finally, an evaluation of the treatment program of A followed by B compared to B followed by A (in the case of two treatments).

In contrast, the second type of crossover design is potentially more useful. Although the order of the treatments is assigned at random, the time for the treatment crossover does not depend on the first outcome. Treatment comparisons can be made using each patient as his/her own control. If one assumes no carryover effect from cycle to cycle, all patient-to-patient biases are eliminated, each patient represents a separate stratum in the analysis, and treatments can be compared within homogeneous units. These designs are particularly useful when the criteria for evaluation are subjective, especially when the evaluation takes

Table 13–3. Value of a Placebo Control Group as Illustrated by the Coronary Drug Project Results

	ADHERENCE *(% of capsules taken)*	
TREATMENT	$\geq 80\%$	$< 80\%$
Clofibrate		
5-Year survival	85%	75%
Number of patients	708	357
Placebo		
5-Year survival	85%	72%
Number of patients	1813	882

From The Coronary Drug Project Research Group, Influence of adherence to treatment and response of cholesterol on mortality in the coronary drug project. *N. Engl. J. Med.*, **303**:1038–1041, 1980. Reprinted by permission of the *New England Journal of Medicine.*

the form of patient preferences for one or the other therapy. For example, this situation arises in studies of antiemetic agents that are designed to reduce chemotherapy side effects.

Randomized Consent and Preconsent Randomization Designs. Randomized consent and preconsent randomization designs have recently been suggested as methods for increasing the number of eligible patients who participate in clinical trials (Zelen, 1982). The preconsent or randomized consent designs involve randomizing the patients into two groups: A group where consent is to be obtained, and one in which consent is not necessarily sought. The patients assigned to this latter group receive best standard therapy (*i.e.,* the therapy that the patient would have received under normal circumstances). The patients assigned to the consent group are given the opportunity to receive the experimental therapy. If they give their consent, the patients receive the experimental therapy. Thus, the patients know about a departure from standard therapy in advance of consent.

A variant of the above occurs when all the therapies under study are considered experimental. The patients are prerandomized to each of these treatment groups and then consent must be obtained from the patients. Consent is necessary to receive the assigned treatment; if the patient declines, he or she receives best standard treatment or whatever the physician and patient agree is suitable. A high refusal to consent will, in itself, provide information about the treatment. The analysis compares the initial randomized groups, regardless of treatment actually received. This design has been used successfully when the natures of the available therapies involve different treatment modalities. A recent study by the National Surgical Adjuvant Breast Project (protocol B-06, Fisher *et al.,* 1985) uses preconsent randomization to assign total mastectomy, segmental mastectomy, or segmental mastectomy with local irradiation to patients with newly diagnosed resectable breast cancer. This protocol was initially planned as a classic randomized study. Due to low accrual, however, the preconsent randomization plan was introduced. A large increase in accrual followed.

Reducing Variability

One of the principal aims in designing clinical trials is to maximize the precision of the treatment comparisons that will result in a more sensitive trial. Increased precision may be attained by utilizing appropriate study designs that reduce the effects of the sources of variability on the treatment comparisons.

The effect of the variation arising from patient heterogeneity may be reduced by utilizing a stratified assignment of patients based on prognostic factors. Stratification will guarantee that prognostic factors are balanced among different treatment groups. In some instances, crossover designs can also be employed where each patient receives all treatments sequentially. Care must be taken, however, to design and analyze such studies to eliminate carryover effects. In both of these methods, treatment comparisons are made within relatively homogeneous subsets of the population (either a prognostic group or a comparison of different treatments using the same patient). The overall comparison of treatments is obtained by combining the results from the separate subsets using statistical methods appropriate for the purpose.

The variability of the measurements (random error) associated with patients depends on the endpoint being used. For example, in laboratory studies, the endpoint may be a measurement of serum drug concentration. These values may vary very little from patient to patient who receive the same drug dose. Contrast this to the situation in which the endpoint is treatment response. An individual patient either responds or does not respond. Hence, one compares the observed response rates among groups of patients receiving the same treatment. In this case, the individual measurements are either response or no response, making the patient-to-patient variability quite large. Thus, the variability associated with the endpoint selected for treatment evaluation will influence the precision of the comparison.

The final component of variability is that due to the estimation procedure itself. Both patient heterogeneity and the random error of the specific endpoint contribute to the variability of the observed result for individual patients. These individual results are then pooled (or combined) to obtain numerical estimates of the effects on patient populations. The precision of these treatment comparisons depends on both the variability of the individual measurements and on the actual number of patients. The greater the number of patients, the more precise the treatment comparison. Hence, the choice of sample size in a clinical trial is critical. Too few patients may result in an insensitive experiment; too many patients represent a waste of resources.

Sample Size Considerations. For clinical trials, considerations of sample size depend not only on statistical concepts but also on clinical considerations. Specific study objectives, acceptable error rates (false-positive and false-negative rates), and anticipated findings must be clinically important. It is not sufficient for a clinician to ask a statistician for the required number of patients without specifying the clinical objectives that the study is expected to meet. Therefore, it is important for clinical investigators to understand some of the basic principles that affect the determination of sample sizes for clinical trials.

Generally, in a comparative clinical trial, the larger the number of patients evaluated the greater the chance of finding differences (if they are real) between therapies. Although large treatment differences may be shown with relatively few patients, small or moderate differences require larger numbers of patients. The analysis is usually made using objective statistical tests. The results of a clinical trial may be inconclusive or misleading if an insufficient number of patients is entered. A lack of statistical significance may not necessarily mean that no treatment difference exists. It may simply mean that there was an insufficient number of patients in the trial to detect moderate or small treatment differences.

Four design criteria must be specified before objective estimates of sample size requirements can be determined. These are:

1. A clear statement of the *principal objective* of the study and which *principal endpoints* will be used to evaluate the effects of treatment. This establishes the statistical methods that will be used in the analysis and determines the rule that will be used to decide whether the study is positive (indicating an effect) or negative (failing to indicate an effect);
2. The *magnitude of treatment effects* (differences) that are considered to be of clinical or scientific relevance. This is given in terms of the principal endpoint and represents the minimum actual treatment effects for a positive study;
3. A value for the *false-positive rate* (significance level) of the statistical rule (test). This rate (usually denoted by α) is the probability that the test will show a treat-

ment effect when there is no real treatment difference. If the nonequivalence of treatment is possible only in one direction, then a one-sided error rate is used. Otherwise, a two-sided test is planned. (Generally, a two-sided test should be used unless significant results in one of the alternative directions would be ignored.) One-sided comparisons are made when a treatment is compared to a placebo where the treatment cannot result in any detrimental effects;
4. An acceptable level for the *false-negative rate*. This error rate (denoted by β) is the probability that the statistical test will fail to show a treatment effect even when the true treatment effects are different and clinically important (as defined by item 2 above). The *power* or *sensitivity* of the trial refers to the probability of finding a statistically significant result if indeed there is a real difference between the treatments. The power is the true-positive rate and is equal to $1 - \beta$.

All of the quantities mentioned above are related to one another. If the false-positive rate is kept constant (say at 5%), then an increase in the sample size will lower the false-negative rate (*i.e.,* increase the power) of the experiment. Alternatively, an increase in the false-positive rate (say from 5% to 10%) will raise the power of detecting smaller treatment differences.

It is a widely accepted practice to choose 5% as the false-positive rate or level of significance (α). To a lesser extent, the value of 1% is used. Sample sizes should be chosen so that there is *at least* an even chance ($\beta = 50\%$) of finding a treatment difference that is of clinical importance. The best experiments generally attempt to have values of β that are less than 20%.

The determination of clinically important treatment effects is illustrated by the following two examples. Consider a trial of single alkylating-agent therapy versus combination chemotherapy for the treatment of patients with advanced ovarian carcinoma in which the objective is to compare the regimens with respect to response rates. Because the combination is likely to represent an increased potential for severe toxicity, any increase in therapeutic efficacy would have to be "substantial" in order to be considered clinically important. If the current response rate were

Table 13–4. Number of Patients per Treatment for a Comparative Trial Based on Proportions (Assuming a two-sided false-positive rate of 5% and equal allocation of patients to each treatment)

MAGNITUDE OF CLINICALLY IMPORTANT DIFFERENCES BETWEEN PROPORTIONS			SENSITIVITY OR POWER				
r_1		r_2	.3	.5	.7	.8	.9
10%	vs	15%	182	337	538	680	910
10%	vs	20%	54	98	157	195	260
10%	vs	30%	17	31	49	59	79
10%	vs	40%	10	16	25	35	40
40%	vs	45%	406	752	1202	1530	2050
40%	vs	50%	103	190	304	390	520
40%	vs	60%	27	48	77	97	130
40%	vs	70%	12	22	34	44	56

For more extensive tables see Gehan, E. A., and Schneiderman, M. A.: Experimental design of clinical trials. In Holland, J. F., and Frei, E., III (eds.): *Cancer Medicine,* 2nd ed. Lea & Febiger, Philadelphia, 1982.

approximately 40%, then an improvement to at least 60% may be required by clinicians before the combination would be adopted. True differences less than 20% would be too small to be considered clinically important.

In contrast, consider a randomized trial designed to determine if the policy of changing IV tubing every 24 hours can be modified to allow changing IV tubing every 48 hours. The endpoint for comparison is the incidence of phlebitis. The experience with the 24-hour policy indicates a phlebitis incidence of about 10%. In order to justify the modified policy, it would be important to demonstrate that the two policies are "the same." On clinical grounds, "the same" might mean that the difference between phlebitis rates would be no greater than 5%. Thus, if the 48-hour policy meant an increase in the phlebitis rate to 15% and the 24-hour policy had a rate of 10%, we would want to be relatively certain that the statistical test of significance at the end of the trial would be positive (*i.e.,* would show a difference).

Table 13–4 summarizes the calculations for comparing response rate (or proportions) for a 5% two-sided significance level. For example, a comparison of two groups to detect rates of 40% vs 60% requires 130 patients in each treat-

ment group in order to have a power of 0.90; that is, a false-negative rate of 10%. In other words, if there were no real difference between the treatment effects, then 5% of the time one would falsely conclude that a difference existed. If the true difference, however, corresponded to 40% vs 60%, then the probability of concluding that the treatments are different is .90 when 130 patients are evaluated in each of two treatment groups.

Similar considerations apply when endpoints other than proportions are used for evaluations of treatment differences. Several references present sample sizes when time to some critical event (*i.e.,* survival time) is used to compare two treatments (George and Desu, 1974; Peto *et al.,* 1976; Lesser and Cento, 1981; Schoenfeld and Richter, 1982). When survival time is the endpoint, sample size calculations can be made on the basis of comparisons between medians (the median survival is that point in time that half of the patients reach). The planning of studies based on survival time (or any time-measured endpoint) must not only take into account numbers of patients but the follow-up time as well. The reason is that a complete observation requires the event (death or recurrence) to happen. The greater the number of events, the greater the informa-

Table 13–5. Sample Size Requirements per Treatment to Detect an 18-Month versus 12-Month Median Survival (Level of significance = .05; power = .80)

YEARS OF ACCRUAL	YEARS OF ADDITIONAL FOLLOW-UP		
	1	2	3
1	150	117	104
2	132	110	103
3	122	107	102

tion in the trial. In turn, the longer the follow-up, the more events are likely to take place.

Schoenfeld and Richter (1982) present nomograms that can be used to determine both total patient entry and follow-up time requirements for survival studies. Table 13–5 illustrates the influence of accrual rate and follow-up time on the number of patients required for a survival study. In this example, the calculations are based on comparing a 12-month median and an 18-month median survival. For comparisons involving longer median survival time, it would be necessary to have longer follow-up time.

ANALYSIS OF RESULTS

This section describes some of the basic ideas that are useful for the analysis of clinical trial data. This material is not intended to be a substitute for a statistics text but is designed to reduce some of the confusion that so often surrounds the application of statistical methods to clinical data. The concepts of point estimation, confidence intervals, and statistical tests of significance are discussed. Techniques for the analysis of proportions and the analysis of survival type data are presented.

The Analysis of Response Rates and Proportions

Measurements on patients in clinical trials often can take only one of two values, which we generally refer to as success or failure. Thus, the endpoint of a group of patients receiving the same treatment would be a success rate or the proportion of successes associated with a treatment. Success might be defined by objective tumor response, no severe toxicity, or disease-free survival for at least one year. For example, a recent trial conducted by the Eastern Cooperative Oncology Group (Rossoff and Creech, 1981) evaluated objective tumor response at 12 weeks following bilateral oophorectomy for premenopausal patients with advanced breast cancer. Twenty-one complete and partial responses were observed for 95 patients, giving an observed response rate of 22%.

It would not be surprising if another group of independent investigators reported a different observed proportion of success for the same procedure and the same patient population used in the example above. Both clinical trials would yield *estimates* of the same theoretical success rate. *Statistical inference* refers to the logic and reasoning of using estimates (based on data) and relating them to theoretical probabilities.

Confidence Limits. Placing confidence limits on an estimate is a statistical technique that enables one to infer how close the observed proportion is to the theoretical probability. In general, the greater the sample size, the closer the observed proportion will be to the theoretical probability. Often one can quote an uncertainty associated with an observed response rate that denotes limits within which the theoretical probability is likely to be.

In order to judge how far the observed or estimated proportion is from the theoretical success probability, one can calculate a confidence interval for the theoretical probability. Figure 13–2 can be used to calculate 95% confidence intervals as follows: The bowed lines correspond to sample size, the horizontal scales correspond to the observed proportion, and the vertical scales correspond to the theoretical probabilities representing the limits of the 95% confidence interval. For our example $21/95 = 22\%$, we first find .22 on the lower horizontal scale. Looking up the vertical .22 line, the lower confidence limit is found on the left vertical scale where the bowed line for 100 patients meets the .22 line, and the upper confidence limit is found where the upper 100 patient bow meets the .22 line. These limits are 14% and 31%, respectively. (The bowed lines corresponding to $n = 100$ are used as a convenient approximation to the real sample size of $n = 95$.)

The interpretation of the range of the interval 14% to 31% is that the observed rate may have been generated by any of the theoretical probabilities within this interval. That is, the observed oophorectomy success rate of 22% is consistent with theoretical rates that are as low as 14% and as high as 31%. The confidence interval is simply a declarative statement, giving the plausible values of the theoretical success probability that could have produced the observed result. In truth, the confidence interval either contains the true success probability or does not; that is, it is correct or false. The 95% figure associated with the confidence interval states the proportion of times these confidence statements are likely to be correct. It is as if we are talking to a person who does not tell the truth all of the time but only 95% of the time. We do not know whether any individual conversation is correct. Because, however, 95% of the statements are correct, we would

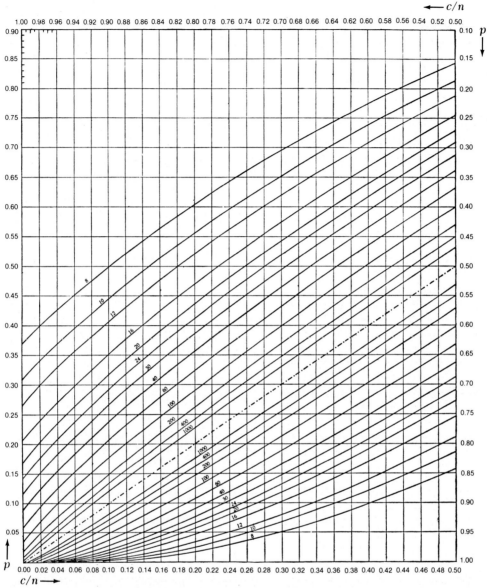

Figure 13–2. Chart providing confidence limits for P in binomial sampling, given a sample fraction c/n. Confidence coefficient: $1 - 2\alpha = 0.95$. The numbers printed along the curves indicate the sample size n. If for a given value of the abscissa c/n, P_A and P_B are the ordinates read from (or interpolated between) the appropriate lower and upper curves, then $\Pr\{P_A \leq P \leq P_B\} \geq 1 - 2\alpha$. From Biometrika: *Biometrika Tables for Statisticians* vol. 1, 3rd ed. Biometrika: London, 1976. Reprinted by permission of the Biometrika Trustees.

tend to believe everything the person says. The choice of a 95% confidence coefficient is arbitrary and one can choose different confidence coefficients. The value of 95% associated with confidence intervals, however, is widely used.

If the graph in Figure 13–2 is not readily available, approximate 95% confidence intervals can be calculated by taking the estimate $\pm 2 \times$ standard error of the mean (SEM). The SEM is a measure of the sampling variability

inherent in an observed response rate, and it is usually estimated by

$$\text{SEM} = \sqrt{r(1 - r)/n},$$

where r is the observed response rate and n is the number of patients observed. For values of the observed proportion between 20% and 80%, using $2 \times$ SEM provides reasonable approximations for the 95% confidence interval. For the example of the oophorectomy study, the approximate limits (14%, 30%) are almost the same as those obtained from Figure 13–2. A conservative way of calculating the 95% confidence limit is to use the value $1/n^{1/2}$ as the half-width of the interval. Hence, for our example, $n = 95$ and $1/95^{1/2} = 0.10$. Therefore, a conservative 95% confidence interval is $22\% \pm 10\%$. This gives 12% and 32% as the confidence limits.

Comparing Response Rates Using a Statistical Test of Significance. Using a statistical test of significance to compare response rates is also a common problem. For example, suppose that 13 patients are randomized and four of six respond on treatment A (67%) compared with one of seven on treatment B (14%). These results are often presented in a *2 × 2 contingency table* as shown in Table 13–6. The goal of the statistical analysis problem is to objectively decide whether the theoretical response probabilities are different for the two groups or whether the observed results could be due only to random variation when the treatments have the same theoretical response probabilities.

The logic for judging the evidence proceeds as follows. We assume that the theoretical success probabilities of both A and B are equal. Under this assumption, the probability of each possible outcome of the trial with fixed marginal totals (*i.e.,* five successes, eight failures, seven patients on treatment B, and six patients on treatment A) is computed. Trial outcomes can be enumerated explicitly by looking at "*a,*" the number of successes on treatment A, because, with fixed marginal totals, setting a value for "*a*" determines the remaining table entries. If the observed result ($a = 4$) is to be judged as evidence in favor of treatment A, then any stronger result (*i.e.,* $a = 5$) should also be judged as favoring A. Furthermore, the same reasoning would apply to treatment B, if the results had been reversed (*i.e.,* $a = 0$). Thus, by adding together the probabilities of all possible outcomes that are at least as extreme as the observed outcome, we obtain a probability that is called a *P* value or significance level. This probability assumes that the theoretical

success probabilities are the same for both treatments. The entire process is called significance testing. The operational interpretation of a test of significance is that if the *P* value is less than a small probability, either we have observed a result that would rarely occur or else the assumption of equality of treatments is incorrect. Because rare events occur infrequently (by definition), we would tend to place more credence in the second explanation and declare that the treatments are significantly different. It is commonly accepted that *P* values less than .05 are sufficiently small to "declare" that the treatments differ. *It is important to note that the P value is not the probability that the treatments are equal; rather, it is the chance of obtaining the observed result or one more extreme if we assume that the effects of the treatments are equal.*

The particular calculation described above (as applied to Table 13–6) is known as Fisher's exact test (see Fleiss, 1981). The *P* value for the example is 0.10. Although this method provides exact *P* values, a computer or specialized statistical tables are generally required to carry out the calculations. Because most scientists do not have easy access to these, the *P* value is often calculated using an approximation called the "chi-square test".

The chi-square statistic (corrected for continuity) is calculated by using the formula

$$\chi^2 = N(|ad - bc| - N/2)^2/(a + c)(b + d)(a + b)(c + d),$$

where *a, b, c,* and *d* refer to the entries in the 2 × 2 contingency table (Table 13–6), *N* is the total sample size, and the vertical bars in the numerator refer to absolute value. The approximate *P* value (two-sided) is the area under a chi-square distribution (1 degree of freedom) to the right of the value of χ^2. Values of χ^2 and corresponding two-sided *P* values are shown in Table 13–7. Values of χ^2 greater than 3.84 provide statistically significant evidence of a treatment difference (at the $P = .05$ level of significance). The approximate *P* value obtained for the example in Table 13–6 is 0.17.

Table 13–6. 2 × 2 Contingency Table

	SUCCESS	FAILURE	TOTAL	SUCCESS RATE
Treatment A	a = 4	b = 2	6	67%
Treatment B	c = 1	d = 6	7	14%
TOTAL	5	8	13	

Table 13–7. Table of Chi-Square (1 degree of freedom; P values are two-sided)

χ^2	P VALUE	χ^2	P VALUE	χ^2	P VALUE
.016	.90	.71	.40	3.17	.075
.06	.80	1.07	.30	3.84	.050
.15	.70	1.64	.20	5.02	.025
.27	.60	2.07	.15	6.63	.010
.46	.50	2.71	.10	7.88	.005
				10.83	.001

The Analysis of Survival Data

A common endpoint for the evaluation of treatment programs is the measurement of time to some critical event of interest. Although our presentation will refer to survival time, the principles discussed apply equally well to any time measurement endpoint including time to disease progression, duration of response, time to local failure, and so forth.

The survival characteristics of a patient population under study are usually described by what is called a survival curve. Time is displayed along the horizontal axis, and the height of the curve at each time represents the proportion of patients in the population who survive at least that length of time. The curve starts at height 1 at time 0 and cannot increase in height as time increases. The time at which the height of the survival curve equals ½ is the *median* survival time for the population. Half of the patients expire before the median and half survive beyond the median. Other summary measures used to characterize the population survival curve are the one-, two-, and five-year survival rates, which are simply the height of the survival curve intersecting the abscissa at 1, 2, and 5 years.

Occasionally, the shape of the survival curve may be described by a relatively simple mathematical equation. For example, if survival is determined by a constant *rate of mortality* (hazard function) over time, then survival is said to follow an exponential distribution. The survival curve for exponential survival is a straight line when displayed on a semilog plot; that is, when the survival probability on the vertical axis is presented on a logarithmic scale. The slope of the line corresponds to the constant mortality rate, with steeper lines indicating increased hazard function. If the semilog plot of the survival curve tends to be convex (leveling off), then a decreasing mortality rate (and potential cure) is indicated, whereas if the curve is concave (accelerates downward) an aging effect (increasing mortality rate) is

present. Hence, the shape of the survival curve on a logarithmic probability scale is valuable for assessing the qualitative behavior of mortality over time.

In practice, the survival curve for the entire patient population is not known exactly and must be estimated on the basis of the survival times observed in the clinical trial. If a specific functional form for the survival curve is postulated (*e.g.*, exponential survival), then the data are used to estimate the parameters of the distribution (*e.g.*, the constant exponential mortality rate). An example of such a parametric estimate is to use the total number of deaths (d) divided by the total follow-up time (T) as an estimate of the exponential mortality rate. For example, suppose that we had the five survival times 1, 5+, 7, 10, and 13, where 5+ refers to a patient still alive at 5 months. Then the total follow-up time (the sum of the observations) is $T = 36$ person-months and the number of failures is $d = 4$. The failure rate is $d/T = 4/36 = 0.11$ deaths per month. An approximation for the median survival is found by multiplying the reciprocal of the failure rate by 0.69. For our example, the median would be estimated as $.69/0.11 = 6.3$ months. This is based on the assumption that the survival law is described by an exponential probability distribution.

Distribution-free (or nonparametric) methods, which do not rely on assumptions about the shape of the survival curve, are also available. The *life-table* and *Kaplan-Meier* estimates are the most commonly used nonparametric estimates for a survival function. If all patients on a trial have died at the time of an analysis, then the estimated survival curve at any time t is simply the proportion of patients who survive beyond t. Because patients enter a clinical trial during an extended period of time, patients may still be alive at the time of analysis, may have been lost to follow-up, or may have withdrawn. The lengths of time these patients have been alive on study are known, but the eventual times to death are not known. The observations on these patients are *incomplete,* and the observed survival times for the patients are refered to as *censored observations.* Although we do not know the final survival time for the censored patients, we do know that these patients have survived at least as long as they have been followed. This incomplete information must be used in estimating the survival function. Discarding it will result in calculating biased survival curves. Both the life-table and Kaplan-Meier methods allow the censored observations to contribute appropriately to the survival curve estimate.

The Life-Table Method.   The life-table method is illustrated by the example shown in Table 13–8. In this method, fixed intervals of time (yearly in the example) are selected. For each interval, an estimate is obtained for the probability of surviving past the end of the interval conditional on survival to the start of the interval. The estimate is denoted by H_i for interval i and is shown in Table 13–8. The effective number at risk is shown in the column labeled F_i. The estimated survival probabilities at the end of each interval are denoted by I_i and are computed by taking the product of the probabilities of surviving all of the preceding intervals.

The Kaplan-Meier Product-Limit or Maximum Likelihood Estimator.   The Kaplan-Meier product-limit estimator is similar to the life-table procedure except that the lengths of the intervals are determined by the actual survival times. Probability calculations are made

at the time points where an event (say, death) has taken place. Consider the ten survival times (months) 3, 3, 3 +, 4, 6 +, 9, 10, 15 +, 20, and 21 +. The distinct time points at which a death has taken place correspond to 3, 4, 9, 10, and 20. The + to the right of a time point refers to an incomplete or censored observation, indicating that the individual was still alive at the follow-up time. The calculation of this estimate is simplified by calculating, at each time point where a death occurred, the number of patients who could have possibly died at that time. For example, all 10 patients were at risk to die at 3 months, whereas only 2 patients were at risk to die at 20 months. The outline of all the calculations is shown in Table 13–9, and the estimated survival curve is shown in Figure 13–3.

From the point of view of visualizing the estimated survival curves, it is important to realize that the precision of the curve at any given time point depends on the number of patients who survive until at least that time. Hence, the statistical variability in the curve will tend to increase with time and can be quite high for estimates in the tail of the curve. High survival probabilities at the end of the survival curve can drop appreciably with the registration of a few late occurring deaths. Another potential visual misrepresentation may appear when one observes a plateau in the tail of the estimated survival curve in an interim analysis. This "leveling-off" impression appears on survival curves plotted on a linear probability

Table 13–8.   Computation of the 5-Year Survival Rate by the Life-Table Method

INTERVAL NO. (i)	YEARS AFTER DIAGNOSIS (A_i)	ALIVE AT BEGINNING OF INTERVAL (B_i)	DIED DURING INTERVAL (C_i)	LOST TO FOLLOW-UP DURING INTERVAL (D_i)	CENSORED (E_i)
1	0 to 1	126	47	4	15
2	1 to 2	60	5	6	11
3	2 to 3	38	2	—	15
4	3 to 4	21	2	2	7
5	4 to 5	10	—	—	6

EFFECTIVE NUMBER EXPOSED TO THE RISK OF DYING $\left(F_i = B_i - \dfrac{1}{2}[D_i + E_i]\right)$	PROPORTION DYING $(G_i = C_i/F_i)$	PROPORTION SURVIVING $(H_i = 1 - G_i)$	CUMULATIVE PROPORTION SURVIVING FROM DIAGNOSIS THROUGH END OF INTERVAL $(I_i = H_i I_{i-1})$	STANDARD ERROR OF THE ESTIMATE $\left(J_i = I_i \sqrt{\sum_{j=1}^{i} \dfrac{G_j}{F_j - C_j}}\right)$
116.5	0.40	0.60	0.60	0.046
51.5	0.10	0.90	0.54	0.048
30.5	0.07	0.93	0.50	0.051
16.5	0.12	0.88	0.44	0.060
7.0	0.00	1.00	0.44	0.060

Adapted from Cutler, S. J., and Ederer, F.: Maximum utilization of the life table method in analyzing survival. *J. Chronic Dis.,* **8**:699–712, 1958, as presented in Miller, R. G.: *Survival Analysis.* John Wiley & Sons, Inc., New York, 1981.

Table 13–9. Calculation of the Product-Limit Estimate (Kaplan-Meier)

i	t_i (Survival Times)	A_i (No. of Deaths)	B_i (Censored Observations)	$C_i = A_i + B_i$	$D_i = C_i + D_{i+1}$* (No. at Risk)	$E_i = A_i/D_i$*	$F_i = 1 - E_i$*	$G_i = F_i G_{i-1}$* (Survival Curve)	$H_i = G_i \sqrt{\sum_{j=1}^{i} \dfrac{E_j}{D_j - A_j}}$*
1	3	2	0	2	10	2/10	8/10	.8	.127
2	3+	0	1	1	8	—	—	—	—
3	4	1	0	1	7	1/7	6/7	.69	.152
4	6+	0	1	1	6	—	—	—	—
5	9	1	0	1	5	1/5	4/5	.55	.173
6	10	1	0	1	4	1/4	3/4	.41	.175
7	15+	0	1	1	3	—	—	—	—
8	20	1	0	1	2	1/2	1/2	.21	.173
9	21+	0	1	1	1	—	—	—	—

Note: The number at risk (D_i) can be calculated by summing C_i from the bottom; *e.g.*, $D_9 = C_9$, $D_8 = C_8 + D_9$, $D_7 = C_7 + D_8$, etc. E_i = Probability of dying at time t_i; F_i = Probability of surviving past time t_i; and G_i = Estimate of survival curve for each failure point (usually denoted by S(t)); H_i is the estimated standard error for S(t).

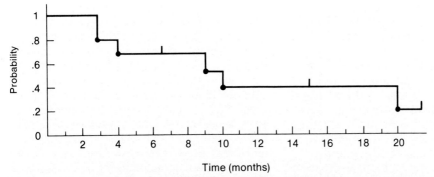

Figure 13–3.   Plot of product limit estimate S(t) based on calculation shown in Table 13–9. At time points at which a death occurred read lower value. Small vertical lines on plot refer to time points of censored observations.

and time scale even if there is a constant mortality rate. We can only be optimistic about the possibility of cure if the survival curve, plotted on a logarithmic probability scale, gives the impression of being convex when viewed from above. This impression must be predicated on having a reasonably large number of patients who have been followed for a long period of time. In all cases, caution should be exercised when interpreting the data based on the "tails" of the survival curve.

Greenwood's Formula. Greenwood's formula can be used to calculate the standard error (SE) of the life-table and Kaplan-Meier survival curve estimates. The interval given by the estimate at time t plus and minus twice the SE gives an approximate 95% confidence interval for the true survival probability at time t. The standard error should be calculated whenever an estimated survival probability is presented. For the life-table method, we first compute the ratio

$$w_j = \frac{\text{proportion dying}}{(\text{effective number} - \text{deaths})}$$

for each interval, j, in the life-table. The standard error for the survival estimate at the end of interval i is the survival estimate times the square root of the sum of the ratios w_j over all j from 1 to i. The standard errors for the example have been computed and are denoted by J_i in Table 13–8.

Greenwood's formula for the Kaplan-Meier estimates is similar, except that the ratios w_j are calculated at each death time and equal

$$w_j = \frac{(\text{no. of deaths at } t_j)/(\text{no. surviving to } t_j)}{(\text{no. surviving to } t_j) - (\text{no. of deaths at } t_j)}$$

The standard error for the estimate at time t is $S(t)$ times the square root of the sum of w_j for

all t_j less than or equal to t. The calculation for the Kaplan-Meier example is denoted by H_i in Table 13–9. Notice that although the ten-month estimated survival is .41, an approximate 95% confidence interval is [.06, .76].

Other factors, in addition to variability, influence the way in which calculated survival curves are interpreted. One important consideration is the origin or starting point for the time measurement. Possible starting points are the time of diagnosis, the time of randomization, the time of initial treatment, or the time of response to treatment. It is particularly important when survival curves are being compared that the same starting point be used.

Another important consideration is the mechanism by which patients' survival times have been censored. The assumption implicit in all the methods discussed above is that the censored patients are no different than the uncensored patients except for the follow-up time. Hence, if additional follow-up time were available on censored patients they would fail at the same rate as the patients who are not censored. If censoring is treatment related, however, the estimates may not be accurate for estimating the population survival curve. For example, suppose patients tend to be withdrawn from a treatment program just prior to failure. Then the patients' survival time is censored at that time point and the estimated survival curve will be biased towards the high side. Similar problems arise when deaths from causes other than cancer are considered as censored in the analysis. The cancer survival curves may look promising by virtue of the fact that patients are dying from other causes (and therefore being forever counted as successfully treated patients). This can be misleading, particularly if treatment cannot be absolutely ruled out as contributing to death. This is an example of the so-called *competing risk problem* in which patients who fail from causes other than the endpoint of interest are counted as censored in the life-table analysis. Consider the evaluation of CNS relapse in childhood acute lymphocytic leukemia. Ordinarily, patients with bone marrow relapse are considered censored. The interpretation of the time to CNS relapse curve, constructed in this way, is obscure because the estimated actuarial CNS relapse rates refer to a hypothetical situation where bone marrow relapses never occur. Although treatment comparisons on the basis of competing risk censoring are meaningful, the estimates obtained by such censoring should be interpreted with caution because the methodology requires other assumptions.

The Comparison of Survival Distributions Using Statistical Tests of Significance. The comparison of survival distributions using statistical tests of significance is based on similar principles as those described for the analysis of proportions. The comparison is based on consideration of the hazard function. Tests to obtain a P value based on the observed data under the assumption of equal hazard functions can be either parametric (F test, likelihood ratio test), or nonparametric (Wilcoxon-Gehan, logrank). Several references are available for a more in-depth discussion of these and other procedures (Lee, 1980; Miller, 1981). The idea behind the logrank test for comparing the survival times of two groups is to consider only times at which a failure has occurred and the number of people in each treatment group who were at risk for dying at those times. If there are no differences between the treatment groups, the *expected number* dying from each group is proportional to the number at risk in each group. For example, suppose there are eight patients from treatment A and 12 patients from treatment B who are alive and at risk for dying at 50 weeks. If the risk of death were the same for both treatments and one death is observed at 50 weeks, then the expected number of deaths for each treatment group is $8/20 = .40$ and $12/20 = .60$, respectively. The expectations are calculated for each time at which a failure occurs using a calculation similar to that just described.

Consider the following set of data that gives the survival time in months for two groups:

A: 1, 4, 5, 7+, 8, 10+, 12
B: 6, 8, 9, 10+, 12, 16

The + in the data refers to a censored observation. Table 13–10 outlines the calculation procedures. The steps are as follows.

1. *Column 1:* Combine the survival times for both groups (censored and uncensored) and write them in order from the smallest to the largest. It is only necessary to write the distinct times;
2. *Column 2:* In this column, record the number of individuals from group A who either died or were censored at each distinct time point. Note that the sum of column 2 is equal to the number of observations for group A;

Table 13–10. Computations for the Logrank Test

(1) TIMES	(2) A	(3) AT RISK	(4) B	(5) AT RISK	(6) NO. OF DEATHS	EXPECTATIONS (7) E_A	(8) E_B
1	1	7	0	6	1	7/13	6/13
4	1	6	0	6	1	6/12	6/12
5	1	5	0	6	1	5/11	6/11
6	0	4	1	6	1	4/10	6/10
7+	1	4	0	5	0	—	—
8	1	3	1	5	2	2(3/8)	2(5/8)
9	0	2	1	4	1	2/6	4/6
10+	1	2	1	3	0	—	—
12	1	1	1	2	2	2(1/3)	2(2/3)
16	0	0	1	1	*	—	—
TOTALS	7		6		9	$E_A = 3.64$	$E_B = 5.36$

$$\chi^2 = \frac{(O_A - E_A)^2}{E_A} + \frac{(O_B - E_B)^2}{E_B} = \frac{(5 - 3.64)^2}{3.64} + \frac{(4 - 5.76)^2}{5.36} = .85$$

$$P = .35$$

* Death not counted; see text.

3. *Column 3:* This column refers to the number at risk for A for each time point. It is easily calculated from column 2 by starting at the last line of column 2 and adding cumulatively from the bottom of this column. The last line in column 3 is the same as the last line in column 2. After that, one cumulatively adds upward;

4. *Column 4:* This is the same as column 2 but for group B;

5. *Column 5:* This column refers to the number at risk for B at each time point. It is calculated in the same way as described for column 3 for group A;

6. *Column 6:* Record the total number of deaths at each of the time points regardless of the group in which the death occurred;

7. *Column 7 and Column 8:* Calculate the expectation of death at each of the time points. This is calculated by defining for each time point: d = no. of deaths (column 6), a = no. of people at risk for A (column 3), and b = no. of people at risk for B (column 5). Then the expected number of deaths at each time point is calculated by

$$E_A = d[a/(a + b)], \; E_B = d[b/(a + b)]$$

For example, at 1 month we have $d = 1$, $a = 7$, $b = 6$, and $E_A = 7/13$, $E_B = 6/13$.

The expectations are only calculated at those time points for which there are people at risk in both treatment groups. For example, the death at 16 months has no one at risk from group A. Hence, no expectation is calculated. However, at 12 months, there are patients at risk from both groups and the expectation is thus calculated;

8. *Sums of Column 7 and Column 8:* These are the overall expectation of deaths for each group;

9. Record the number of deaths for each group, eliminating any deaths that occurred when only one group had individuals at risk for death. For example, A has five deaths and B also has five deaths. The 16-month death in group B, however, corresponds to the situation where only one individual is at risk for B and none for A. Hence, this death is eliminated from consideration. Label as O_A and O_B the number of deaths for each group, after eliminating deaths in

which only one group was at risk. In our example, we have $O_A = 5$ and $O_B = 4$.

10. Calculate the chi-square statistic, *e.g.*,

$$\chi^2 = \frac{(O_A - E_A)^2}{E_A} + \frac{(O_B - E_B)^2}{E_B}$$

11. Look up the *P* value in a chi-square table with one degree of freedom (cf. Table 13–7).

The logrank procedure is excellent for detecting survival differences when the failure rates (hazard functions) are proportional, but is insensitive to situations wherein the hazard ratio is not constant over time. These and other issues and procedures for comparing survival distributions are discussed in greater detail by others (Lee, 1980; Miller, 1981; Peto *et al.*, 1977).

REPORTING REQUIREMENTS

The field of cancer treatment appears to be moving too quickly for most oncologists to have a large personal experience with the "latest treatments." As a result, the practicing oncologist must rely heavily on the published literature to help make clinical therapeutic decisions. In this section, a discussion of the information that practicing oncologists should look for when relying on published papers to influence their practices is presented. Many of the issues previously discussed with respect to planning and analysis of clinical trials are reiterated here insofar as they bear on the interpretation of results.

Population Under Study

There should be clear statements describing the patient population under study. The conclusions of the study may not necessarily be valid for other patient populations having the same disease. Conclusions from single-institution studies may not necessarily transfer to other institutions as well as multi-institutional studies.

Therapy

The therapy actually received by patients should be discussed, as it may not necessarily correspond to the protocol therapy for all patients. This is especially true for chemotherapy studies where the full course of treatment as written in a protocol may not be given. The practicing oncologist should pay particular attention to the way drug doses are modified as a function of toxicity.

Study Design

Randomized studies are to be preferred to nonrandomized ones. There are many ways of carrying out a randomized trial, however, many of these are poor and often defeat the purposes of randomization. For example, the use of closed envelopes for executing the randomization procedure is not favored relative to having centralized randomization. Unfortunately, very few papers give sufficient details for the reader to determine whether the randomization procedures have been carried out satisfactorily.

Patient Accounting

The paper should have a detailed accounting of all patients registered for the study. This presupposes a registration system. If there is doubt about the registration system, the results of the paper should be seriously questioned. It is surprising to learn that, in some single-institution studies, registration may take place long after the first day of treatment. The paper should contain information on patients who are classified as cancelled or nonevaluable. A cancelled patient is a registered patient who withdrew from the study before the first day of treatment. An unevaluable patient may be one who has incomplete information. Some studies classify an unevaluable patient as one who has major deviations from the protocol treatment. If the reasons for patients being classified as cancelled or unevaluable are related to the treatment assignment, then it is mandatory that all patients be included in the analysis. Readers should become concerned when the number of patients evaluated on a complicated treatment regimen is smaller than the number evaluated in the control group. Selective exclusion of "noncompliant" patients may effect the conclusions of the study.

Follow-Up

If a major end-point is survival, disease-free survival, or a similar time metric, then it is mandatory that follow-up of patients be as complete as possible. If a relatively large number of patients is lost to follow-up (say 10%), then statements about long-term effects may be incorrect.

Data Quality

A discussion of the quality-control procedures used for the data should be provided. Were there any *second-party reviews?* A second-party review occurs when the patient data are reviewed by individuals other than the investigator generating the data in the clinic. Ordinarily, this could be carried out by panels, study chairmen, and/or data-management personnel. The discussion of patient-data quality control should be centered on answering three major questions for each patient: Was the patient eligible? Was the protocol followed? Was there objective documentation of major end-points?

End-Points and Censored Data

Trials in which the end-points are survival and/or disease-free survival may often have patients with incomplete data. Several situations arise where observations are incorrectly classified as censored observations that could seriously skew the results. When there are appreciable numbers of patients dying from competing causes of death, it could seriously alter the conclusions of a study if these patients were considered as censored observations. A second problem created in calling an observation censored is switching a patient off the study therapy onto another treatment. It is clear that if the change is made and the patient is taken off study just before the end-point is likely to be reached (say death), the poor therapy may be made to look good by classifying the time until the patient switches therapies as a censored observation.

Nonrandomized Studies

Nonrandomized studies require special discussion. The evaluation of the experimental therapy is usually made by comparing the results to an historical control group. In order for the analysis to be valid, the control group must be comparable to the experimental therapy group with regard to all major factors that affect the outcome. Publications on nonrandomized studies should include a *discussion* of the possible sources of bias that have the potential for altering the main conclusions of the study. Some potential biases requiring discussion include those relating to: (1) Physician selection; (2) patient selection (regarding consent); (3) diagnosis and staging; (4) supportive care and patient management; (5) endpoint evaluation and quality of follow-up; and (6) prognostic factor effects.

Patient Numbers

The outcome of a statistical analysis depends on both the existence of a true difference between the treatments and the number of patients on the study. If the number of patients is small, then the study will have poor sensitivity to detect differences of moderate magnitude between therapies. Hence, failure to demonstrate statistical significance may be due to small numbers of patients, rather than to the lack of a real difference.

Stopping of Accrual

One should keep in mind the reason(s) for terminating patient entry to the study. Was the trial terminated when the planned entry was completed or was it stopped because of an unusual outcome associated with a treatment? Some details of how the study was conducted and the rationale for terminating accrual and reporting results should be included in manuscripts on clinical trials.

All of the above factors should affect the reader's interpretation of the results of a clinical trial. Therefore, manuscripts should address each of the above points to enable the reader to adequately assess the evidence presented in a publication.

REFERENCES

Berkson, J., and Gage, R. P.: Survival curves for cancer patients following treatment. *J. Am. Stat. Assoc.,* **47**: 501–515, 1952.

Bonadonna, G.; Valagussa, P.; Rossi, A.; Tancini, G.; Brambilla, C.; Marchini, S.; and Veronesi, U.: Multimodal therapy with CMF in resectable breast cancer with positive axillary nodes: the Milan Institute experience. In Salmon, S. E., and Jones, S. E. (eds.): *Adjuvant Therapy for Cancer (III).* Grune & Stratton, Inc., New York, 1981.

Coronary Drug Project Research Group: Influence of adherence to treatment and response of cholesterol on mortality in the coronary drug project. *N. Engl. J. Med.,* **303**:1038–1041, 1980.

Cutler, S. J., and Ederer, F.: Maximum utilization of the life table method in analyzing survival. *J. Chronic Dis.,* **8**:699–712, 1958.

Dana-Farber Cancer Institute: *Lectures on Statistical Science for Oncologists.* Division of Biostatistics and Epidemiology, Dana-Farber Cancer Institute, Boston, 1979.

Fisher, B.; Bauer, M.; Margolese, R.; Poisson, R.; Pilch, Y.; Redmond, C.; Fisher, E.; Wolmark, N.; Deutsch, M.; Montague, E.; Saffer, E.; Wickerham, L.; Lerner, H.; Glass, A.; Shibata, H.; Deckers, P.; Ketcham, A.; Oishi, R.; and Russell, I.: Five-year results of a randomized clinical trial comparing total mastectomy and segmental mastectomy with or without radiation in the treatment of breast cancer. *N. Engl. J. Med.,* **312**:665–673, 1985.

Fleiss, J. L.: *Statistical Methods for Rates and Proportions,* 2nd ed. John Wiley & Sons, Inc., New York, 1981.

Gehan, E. A., and Schneiderman, M. A.: Experimental design of clinical trials. In Holland, J. F., and Frei, E., III (eds.): *Cancer Medicine,* 2nd ed. Lea & Febiger, Philadelphia, 1982.

George, S. L., and Desu, M. M.: Planning the size and duration of a clinical trial studying the time to some critical event. *J. Chronic Dis.,* **27**:15–24, 1974.

Kaplan, E. L., and Meier, P.: Nonparametric estimation from incomplete observations. *J. Am. Stat. Assoc.,* **53**: 457–481, 1958.

Lee, E. T.: *Statistical Methods for Survival Analysis.* Lifetime Learning Publications, Belmont, California, 1980.

Lesser, M. L.: Design and implementation of clinical trials. In Mike, V., and Stanley, K. E. (eds.): *Statistics in Medical Research: Methods and Issues, With Applications in Cancer Research.* John Wiley & Sons, Inc., New York, 1982.

Lesser, M. L., and Cento, S. J.: Tables of power for the F-test for comparing two exponential survival distributions. *J. Chronic Dis.,* **34**:533–544, 1981.

Louis, P. C. A.: *Essay on Clinical Instruction* (translated). P. Martin, London, 1834.

Louis, P. C. A.: Researches on the effects of bloodletting in some inflammatory diseases, and on the influence of tartarized antimony and vesication in pneumonitis. Translated by C. G. Putnam, with preface and appendix by James Jackson. Boston, 1836.

Miller, R. G.: *Survival Analysis.* John Wiley & Sons, Inc., New York, 1981.

Peto, R.; Pike, M. C.; Armitage, P.; Breslow, N. E.; Cox, D. R.; Howard, S. V.; Mantel, N.; McPherson, K.; Peto, J.; and Smith, P. G.: Design and analysis of clinical trials requiring prolonged observation of each patient. *Br. J. Cancer,* Part I, **34**:585–612, 1976; Part II, **35**:1–39, 1977.

Pocock, S. J.: *Clinical Trials: A Practical Approach,* John Wiley & Sons, Inc., Chichester, 1983.

Rossoff, A. H. and Creech, R. H.: Randomized evaluation of combination chemotherapy versus observation following oophorectomy for metastatic breast cancer. Abstract #C-349, American Society of Clinical Oncology Proceedings, Volume 22, 1980.

Schoenfeld, D.: Statistical considerations for pilot studies. *Int. J. Radiat. Oncol. Biol. Phys.,* **6**:371–374, 1980.

Schoenfeld, D. A., and Richter, J. R.: Nomograms for calculating the number of patients needed for a clinical trial with survival as an endpoint. *Biometrics,* **38**:163–170, 1982.

Zelen, M.: The randomization and stratification of patients to clinical trials. *J. Chronic Dis.,* **27**:365–375, 1974.

Zelen, M: Strategy and alternate randomized designs in cancer clinical trials. *Cancer Treat. Rep.,* **66**:1095–1100, 1982.

Zelen, M: Guidelines for publishing papers on cancer clinical trials: Responsibilities of editors and authors. *J. Clin. Oncol.,* **1**:164–169, 1983.

14

Acute and Late Effects of Cancer Therapy

ARVIN S. GLICKSMAN and PHILIP S. SCHEIN

As a direct result of recent advances in cancer treatment, an increased number of patients are achieving long term disease-free survival (DeVita *et al.,* 1981). This has been made possible largely through the use of intensive forms of combination chemotherapy and radiotherapy in patients with advanced disease, as in the case of Hodgkin's disease, non-Hodgkin's lymphoma, and testicular cancer. The same modalities, in addition, are being employed as surgical adjuvant therapies after curative surgery, a situation wherein a proportion of patients will have been rendered disease free by their primary treatment. Lastly, patients with benign disorders, such as collagen-vascular diseases and renal transplantation, are receiving antineoplastic agents and forms of immunosuppressive therapy (Skinner and Schwartz, 1972; Steinberg *et al.,* 1972; Hall, 1973; Kaplan and Calabresi, 1973; Schein and Winokur, 1975). As a consequence, a growing number of patients are being placed at risk for the development of both acute and chronic complications of treatment with radiotherapy and chemotherapy.

Anticancer agents and radiation therapy are distinguished by a relatively low therapeutic index, reflecting their inability to discriminate effectively between normal tissues and neoplasia. Because of their ability to inhibit the cell cycle, they function preferentially against rapidly proliferating cells, such as those of the bone marrow and gastrointestinal tract. Acutely, excessive treatment will cause nausea, vomiting, leukopenia, granulocytopenia, thrombocytopenia, and, with repeated insult, the bone marrow may eventually develop a state of chronic hypoplasia. Such toxicity is readily measured during the treatment period with simple clinical and laboratory techniques, thus allowing for dose reduction or cessation of therapy before the toxicity becomes severe. The consequences and management of these acute complications are of continued concern because none of the agents are casily removed once they have been introduced into the body, and antidotes, except in the case of methotrexate, are not available. Of equal importance are the long-term consequences of antineoplastic treatment that are now being increasingly appreciated, and, in particular, cumulative organ damage that is insidious in onset and manifested clinically after the effect has become severe and irreversible (Schein and Winokur, 1975).

PULMONARY TOXICITY

Radiation Therapy

The recognition of late pulmonary effects of cancer treatment has been sufficiently frequent to warrant judicious use of both radiation and chemotherapy. Asymptomatic pulmonary fibrosis limited to small segments of the lung is not infrequent after radiotherapy; however, when large segments of the lung are involved, incapacitating illness and death can result (Maier, 1972; Libshitz and Southard, 1974; Li *et al.,* 1979). Radiation fibrosis is associated with both small vessel and alveolar changes. Severely damaged lung tissue is characterized by endothelial thickening, loss of capillaries, as well as alveolar septal and basement membrane thickening with appreciable collagen deposition. This produces marked diminution in gas exchange (Travis *et al.,* 1980).

In the radiotherapy of Hodgkin's disease, using a standard mantle treatment of 3500 to 4000 rad, approximately 500 rads to the whole lung derived almost entirely from scatter and, to a lesser degree, from a small amount of radiation transmitted through the lung protective blocks. Less than 5% of the patients so treated developed symptomatic radiation pneumonitis (Wara et al., 1973). If careful respiratory function studies are performed, however, as many as 50% of the patients will show transient changes in total lung capacity, compliance, and gas diffusions. These changes are self-limited and usually disappear within two years. Only when a large amount of lung is included in the field will clinically noteworthy fibrosis occur and progress to chronic pulmonary insufficiency. Although steroids are frequently administered at this stage, their effectiveness has not been established (Host and Vale, 1973; Evans et al., 1974; Lassvik et al., 1977).

The progression of radiation pneumonitis to pulmonary fibrosis depends upon such factors as the volume of lung irradiated, the dose delivered, the overall time in which it is given, and the size of the individual fraction of radiation. Host factors are also important, including intercurrent infection and chronic obstructive lung disease. Furthermore, concurrent or sequential chemotherapy with any number of agents will potentiate the radiation effect (Jennings and Arden, 1962). Whole-lung radiotherapy in Wilms' tumor with doses of 1200 to 1300 rad in two to three weeks may be well tolerated. Concurrent doxorubicin hydrochloride (ADRIAMYCIN) or subsequent exposure to actinomycin D, however, can produce fatal pneumonitis (D'Angio et al., 1959) (see Figure 14–1). Cyclophosphamide and BCNU may also enhance the radiation effect, whereas bleomycin with its own pulmonary toxicity may have an additive effect (Phillips et al., 1975).

Chemotherapy

As cases of diffuse pulmonary disease associated with busulfan treatment were reported, the syndrome of "busulfan lung" was recognized as a distinct clinical entity (Leake et al., 1963; Kass et al., 1965; Feingold and Kass, 1969; Podall and Winbler, 1974). Clinically, an insidious onset of cough, dyspnea, and low-grade fever occurs. These symptoms may appear eight months to ten years after initiation of therapy, with an average of four years. Chest roentgenograms typically demonstrate diffuse interstitial and intra-alveolar infiltrates. Pulmonary function studies reveal diminished diffusing capacity, as well as changes of restrictive lung disease. The differential diagnosis of this clinical presentation requires that the syndrome be distinguished from opportunistic infections or leukemic infiltration of the lungs. Appropriate sputum cultures, viral serology, cytology, and biopsy are necessary to demonstrate the characteristic pathologic features of the syndrome and to exclude a potential infection.

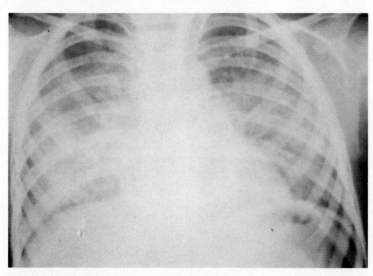

Figure 14–1. This three-year-old with Wilms' tumor received 1200 rads whole lung radiation and six months later actinomycin D. This resulted in a fatal pneumonitis.

Microscopically atypical alveolar and bronchiolar cells with large hyperchromatic nuclei are seen. Occasionally these dysplastic cells are identified in sputum by cytologic examination as being neoplastic (Kass et al., 1965). Of special interest in this regard are two case reports that describe patients with chronic granulocytic leukemia, treated with long-term busulfan, who developed diffuse interstitial pulmonary fibrosis, atypical alveolar cell hyperplasia, and bronchiolar cell carcinoma (Min and Gyorkey, 1968; Rosenaw, 1972).

The histologic findings associated with busulfan are similar to those seen with pulmonary irradiation, except for the absence of vascular-proliferative changes. Both conditions give rise to atypical alveolar lining cells and pulmonary fibrosis. The radiomimetic property of the alkylating agent may be responsible for damaging the alveolar lining cells and capillary epithelium. An increase in capillary permeability results in the development of interstitial and intra-alveolar fibrinous edema and hyaline membranes; the end result is progressive fibrosis (Heard and Cooke, 1968). The injury to the epithelium appears to result in proliferation and dysplasia of the large type II granular pneumocyte, as documented by electron microscopy (Littler et al., 1969).

Clinically, the course of busulfan lung is characterized by progressive deterioration in pulmonary function with arterial hypoxemia and decreased vital capacity, carbon monoxide diffusing capacity, and total lung capacity. Forced expiratory volume in one second (FEV1) frequently remains normal. The abnormalities of pulmonary function progress in spite of withdrawal of busulfan and administration of corticosteroids. In the majority of cases the patients have died within six months of the establishment of the diagnosis (Rosenaw, 1972).

Cyclophosphamide. Although of historic importance, the pulmonary abnormalities associated with busulfan are not unique for this compound, but are recognized as common to the alkylating agents as a group. A cyclophosphamide-induced pulmonary syndrome characterized by alveolar bronchiole lining hyperplasia is similar to that produced by busulfan (Rosenaw, 1972; Mark et al., 1978). Case reports have documented cyclophosphamide-associated pulmonary toxicity in a patient treated with high doses (40 mg/kg IV) and in a patient treated with prolonged low doses (50 to 150 mg/day orally for twenty-seven months) of cyclophosphamide (Robin et al., 1970; Topilow et al., 1973). Although it is clear that clinically significant cyclophosphamide pulmonary toxicity is uncommon, it is still important for the physician to be aware of the potential adverse effect of this frequently used antineoplastic agent.

Other Alkylating Agents. Since the initial reports of busulfan and cyclophosphamide pulmonary toxicity, it has become apparent that all members of this class of anticancer agents have a similar potential. Pulmonary fibrosis has been reported in association with treatment with melphalan (Codling and Chakera, 1972), chlorambucil (Cole et al., 1978) and mitomycin-C (Orwoll et al., 1978). The chloroethylnitrosoureas BCNU, methyl-CCNU, and chlorozotocin have been demonstrated to produce a similar interstitial pneumonitis and fibrosing alveolitis (Baily et al., 1978; Lee et al., 1978; Weiss et al., 1981), whereas the methylnitrosourea streptozotocin has not. A relationship between dose and treatment duration for the pulmonary toxicity of chloroethylnitrosoureas has not yet been demonstrated.

Bleomycin. Pulmonary toxicity is characteristically the most serious side-effect of bleomycin. The onset, which may be delayed for greater than one month after withdrawal of the drug, is frequently insidious and characterized by nonproductive cough, dyspnea, and tachypnea. Fine respiratory rales in both lungs may be an early finding (DeLena et al., 1972). Blood gases show arterial hypoxemia. Pulmonary function studies demonstrate a decreased diffusion capacity and restrictive pulmonary disease, perhaps the most sensitive indication of early toxicity. Roentgenography shows a pattern of diffuse interstitial disease with patchy basilar infiltrates, whereas pleural effusion and mediastinal or hilar adenopathy are unusual. Lung biopsies reveal atypical alveolar cells, fibrinous exudate, and hyaline membranes during the acute stages. These changes may progress to diffuse interstitial and intra-alveolar fibrosis, similar to the pattern observed with busulfan.

The pulmonary toxicity of bleomycin is difficult to characterize in its earliest stages because of the insensitivity of prevailing diagnostic tests. Furthermore, changes in pulmonary function are nonspecific. As a result, they are of little assistance in predicting or detecting the onset of pulmonary toxicity or in distinguishing it from either opportunistic infections or progression of disease (Yagoda et al., 1972).

The incidence of clinical toxicity is estimated to be 5 to 10% in patients receiving a total dose of less than 450 mg (Blum *et al.*, 1973). When a total dose of 550 mg is exceeded, current data indicate that fatal bleomycin pulmonary toxicity will occur in 10% of patients.

In patients older than 70 years, who appear to be at increased risk for bleomycin pulmonary toxicity, no correlation is evident between this complication and route of administration, nor with the type of tumor undergoing treatment.

Although a systematic study has not been conducted, it is the clinical impression of several investigators that bleomycin, like other specific antibiotic antitumor agents, has the capacity to enhance or exacerbate former irradiation damage in previously irradiated sites (Blum *et al.*, 1973). The treatment of bleomycin toxicity includes withdrawal of the drug and the administration of corticosteroids; the efficacy of the latter has not been adequately documented (Burgert *et al.*, 1969; Claryre *et al.*, 1969; Filip *et al.*, 1971; Goldman and Moschella, 1971; Sostman *et al.*, 1976).

Methotrexate. Several studies have reported diffuse pulmonary disease in association with intermittent therapy with methotrexate (Burgert *et al.*, 1969; Claryre *et al.*, 1969; Filip *et al.*, 1971; Goldman and Moschella, 1971; Sostman *et al.*, 1976). Clinically, one observes an abrupt onset of fever, a nonproductive cough, dyspnea, and hypoxemia. Chest roentgenograms show patchy intra-alveolar and interstitial infiltrates; hilar and mediastinal adenopathy has also been observed (Filip *et al.*, 1971). Peripheral eosinophilia has been a feature in some patients who were not receiving corticosteroids (Claryre *et al.*, 1969; Goldman and Moschella, 1971).

In childhood leukemia this syndrome invariably appears when the patient is in the maintenance stage of treatment and when one must rule out leukemia infiltration of the lung or an opportunistic pulmonary infection. The disorder usually occurs two weeks to three months after initiation of a course of therapy and does not appear to be related to total cumulative dose.

The histologic examination of the lung shows diffuse interstitial lymphocytic infiltrates, eosinophils, giant cells, and noncaseating granulomas, which serve to distinguish this form of toxicity from busulfan and bleomycin pulmonary toxicity (Schwartz and Kajani, 1969; Goldman and Moschella, 1971). Because of the peripheral eosinophilia, the pro-

cess has been thought to represent an allergic granulomatous pneumonitis. This process is usually reversible with the use of corticosteroids and withdrawal of methotrexate, further distinguishing it from the pulmonary toxicity associated with alkylating agents and bleomycin (Schwartz and Kajani, 1969; Goldman and Moschella, 1971).

CARDIOVASCULAR TOXICITY

Radiation Therapy

Radiation effects on the heart and great vessels following mediastinal irradiation are infrequent but extremely serious when they do occur (Grossman *et al.*, 1979). Between six months and one year after mantle therapy with doses in the range of 3500 to 4400 rad, 10% to 15% of the patients may develop a pericardial friction rub. When the dose is below 3000 rad, or if part of the heart is shielded by the introduction of a subcarinal block, the prospect of radiation pericarditis is essentially eradicated. Pericarditis may develop as late as four or five years after treatment (Haddain, 1947) (see Figure 14–2). The disease is usually self-limited, although for patients who develop persistent pericardial effusion or constrictive pericarditis, a pleuropericardial window or pericardial stripping may be required. In some cases, the process progresses to chronic pericardial disease (Masland *et al.*, 1968). The frequency of this has not been fully appreciated in the past. When careful cardiac studies were performed, 10 of 12 patients who had been treated ten to 16 years previously with radiotherapy using the mantle technique for Hodgkin's disease had abnormal echocardiographic studies, among others (Perrault *et al.*, 1980).

Anecdotal case reports of precocious myocardial infarction in patients who received radiation therapy to the chest have appeared regularly (Prentice, 1965; Boivin and Hutchinson, 1982). A number of these reports are of boys as young as 15 years of age with intervals of three to ten years after irradiation (Kopelson and Herwig, 1978). In a case-cohort of 957 patients treated for Hodgkin's disease, no increased risk of mortality from coronary heart disease was observed, although three males aged 18, 20, and 25 were reported as having coronary artery disease. This study was deficient in this respect because cardiovascular disease risk factors were not part of the original study design (Boivin and Hutchinson, 1982).

Diffuse interstitial myocardial fibrosis has

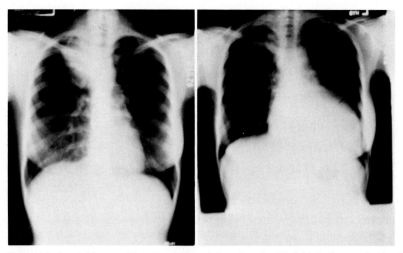

Figure 14 – 2. A 20-year-old woman with nodular sclerosing Hodgkin's disease who developed asymptomatic pericardial effusion nine months after mantle radiotherapy (3500 rads in four weeks — no subcarinal blocking).

been reported in patients who received doses of 4500 rad or greater to the heart. Vascular changes in these patients have been observed (Fajardo *et al.,* 1968). Intimal proliferation of small vessels is a response to irradiation. Whether or not these cells are more sensitive to even modest changes in cholesterol levels or other risk factors and, therefore, prone to atheromatous change is currently under investigation (Low, 1981).

Radiation can induce vascular changes in large vessels as well as in small arteries. Vascular changes of the aorta have been reported in patients who received total nodal irradiation. So called "pulseless disease," the aortic arch syndrome, and coronary artery disease have been reported after irradiation (Heidenberg *et al.,* 1966). Elevated serum cholesterol and hyperlipidemia as well as excessive cigarette smoking may contribute to the development of radiation-induced vascular changes. Successful surgical reconstructions have been possible, on occasion, if the problem was suspected clinically and investigated with arteriography. Vascular grafts may be more difficult because of the perivascular fibrosis, but have been successfully performed in many instances (Hayward, 1972).

Chemotherapy

The principal treatment-limiting effect of daunomycin and doxorubicin is cardiac toxicity. Isolated transient electrocardiographic changes without other evidence of cardiac abnormalities have been observed in 11% of pa-

tients receiving doxorubicin (Malpas and Scott, 1969; LeFrok *et al.,* 1973). These have included sinus tachycardia, ST segment depression, T-wave flattening, and occasional premature ventricular beats. These acute abnormalities are not related to the total dose of the drug administered and can occur during or immediately after intravenous administration. After withdrawal of the drug, the electrocardiogram usually returns to the pretreatment pattern. This is an acute reversible form of cardiac toxicity and has not been associated with any long-term sequelae.

Congestive heart failure is a second dose-related form of cardiac toxicity characterized by the onset of the classic symptoms and signs of biventricular failure. Histologic and ultrastructural studies of the hearts of patients who had received large doses have shown focuses of damaged and degenerating muscle cells, mitochondrial swelling and inclusion bodies, and alterations of nuclear chromatin (Rinehart *et al.,* 1974).

The relationship of dose and schedule of doxorubicin has been analyzed retrospectively, in a review of over 4000 patient records (Von Hoff *et al.,* 1979). The overall incidence of drug-related heart failure was 2.2%. The probability of incurring clinical cardiac toxicity was dose-related: 3% at 400 mg/m^2, 7% at 550 mg/m^2, and 18% at 700 mg/m^2. Cases of apparent doxorubicin-induced congestive heart failure were recorded at all dose levels, including less than 200 mg/m^2. Although the slope of the curve increased at a dose of 550 mg/m^2, there was a continuum of increased risk with increased dosage, and no absolutely safe cut-off dose could be identified. A weekly dose schedule of administration was associated with a significantly lower incidence of heart failure, compared to the more popular every-three-weeks schedule, with only a 2% probability at a total cumulative dose of 550 mg/m^2. An increased risk for clinical cardiac toxicity was also demonstrated in the elderly and, to a lesser extent, in children less than 15 years of age, as has been shown with daunorubicin (Halazun et al., 1974), and in patients with prior cardiac disease.

Radiotherapy to the heart, as in the case of mediastinal or left breast irradiation, potentiates the cardiotoxicity of the anthracyclines (Fajardo et al., 1976). The authors of this chapter recommend that a total cumulative dose of 350 mg/m^2 not be exceeded. The current administration of cyclophosphamide or mitomycin-C has been suggested as factors that can increase the risk of doxorubicin-induced congestive heart failure, but the data remain quite limited. An increased incidence of cardiac toxicity with the FAM regimen (5-fluorouracil, doxorubicin, and mitomycin-C) has not been observed.

A series of diagnostic tests have been used to monitor the changing cardiac function of patients receiving doxorubicin: A decrease in electrocardiographic voltage, a fall in ejection fraction measured from echocardiography, and first-pass radionucleotide angiography. All of these tests remain controversial regarding their prediction of developing cardiomyopathy, with literature suggesting that they are either too sensitive or insensitive in different series (Bonadonna and Monfardini, 1969; LeFrok et al., 1973; Rinehart et al., 1974; Von Hoff et al., 1982). The latter procedure has gained the widest acceptance as a noninvasive monitor, but it does not have the sensitivity of percutaneous endomyocardial biopsies.

One team of investigators has examined the role of endomyocardial biopsy as a measure for detecting doxorubicin cardiomyopathy and has compared this technique with phonocardiography (Bristow, 1978). Doxorubicin-associated myocyte degeneration was identified in almost all patients at doses equal to or greater than 240 mg/m^2. The preejection period to left ventricular ejection time ratio (PEP/LVET) did not begin to increase until a total dose of 400 mg/m^2 had been reached. It was concluded that myocardial degeneration antedates any functional abnormality and that

overt heart failure occurs only after a critical amount of damage has occurred.

The onset of congestive failure may occur within two weeks after therapy has been discontinued, but is commonly delayed one to six months (or perhaps years) following completion of treatment (LeFrok et al., 1973; Halazun et al., 1974). When congestive failure develops it is sometimes irreversible, but often responds to standard treatment with digitalis and diuretics. Early recognition and treatment have reduced morbidity and mortality.

A series of attempts to prevent anthracycline cardiac toxicity in laboratory models have been made using alpha tocopherol (Myers et al., 1977), or ICRF-159 (razoxane) (Herman et al., 1974), and liposomal delivery (Rahman et al., 1980), but none of these techniques have been clinically validated as of this writing. In addition to the weekly schedule, the use of a continuous intravenous infusion for 48 to 96 hours has been shown to decrease myocardial injury, perhaps by reducing the peak drug concentration delivered to the cardiac musculature (Legha et al., 1982).

Doxorubicin and daunomycin are important antitumor agents, however their dose-related cardiac toxicity limits their usefulness in maintaining remissions in patients who respond to these agents. A series of new anthracycline anticancer agents are now being developed in the hope of identifying a less toxic analog. At present, it is recommended that a total dose of 500 mg/m^2 of body surface not be exceeded in order to prevent serious or lethal cardiac toxicity. When there has been previous mediastinal or direct cardiac irradiation, the total dose should not exceed 350 mg/m^2.

NEUROLOGIC TOXICITY

Neurotoxicity of cancer treatment may be a major deterrent because the resultant morbidity may not be acceptable. Otherwise aggressive neurosurgeons will stop short of excising or even performing a biopsy of deep-seated tumors or tumors in vital areas of the brain. Radiation therapists understand the dose-limiting consequences of myelitis or brain necrosis, and chemotherapists are aware the dose reductions are required for drugs such as vincristine in the presence of neuropathy. Nevertheless, both acute and chronic late neurotoxicities have occurred. The late complications can be particularly serious. For radiation, the development of transverse myelitis is related to the dose and volume irradiated. Short lengths of the spinal cord, up to 5 cm long, appear to tolerate 5000 to 5500 rad. On the other hand, 15 cm of spinal cord will not tolerate doses in excess of 4500 rad (Maier, 1972). Even with careful attention to technical details, transverse myelitis can occur in .5% to 3% of patients (Kaplan and Stewart, 1973; Collaborative Study, 1976).

A growing concern has developed about the late effects of central nervous system (CNS) prophylaxis as a component of treatment of acute lymphocytic leukemia (ALL) in children. Standard treatment has included intrathecal methotrexate and cranial irradiation of 2400 rad. Some regimens include the use of cytosine arabinoside and hydrocortisone intrathecally in addition to the methotrexate and, more recently, increasingly high doses of methotrexate systemically to improve the cerebrospinal fluid level of methotrexate. Children who have successfully completed three to five years of maintenance chemotherapy have been found to manifest abnormalities in psychometric functions, neurologic status, and computerized tomography, as well as hypothalamic-pituitary dysfunction (Meadows and Evans, 1976; Brecher et al., 1981) (see Figure 14-3).

Based on age-appropriate IQ testing, achievement tests, and a neuropsychiatric battery of tests, it was found that patients' results were somewhat lower than normal both for verbal and performance IQs. This was particularly true for those children who received cranial irradiation and to a lesser extent for children whose CNS prophylaxis included only methotrexate. On the other hand, EEG changes in increasing numbers have been seen in the latter group of children. Significant CT scan abnormalities have been reported, including changes in ventricular size, hypodense areas, and calcifications. In a group of 106 children successfully treated for ALL in the Cancer and Acute Leukemia Group B (CALGB) study, mild and moderate abnormal CT scans were recorded in both irradiated and nonirradiated children. Abnormalities in growth hormones have been reported by Morris-Jones and coworkers in Manchester, England and have been confirmed by the CALGB. Growth hormone deficiency was twice as frequent in children who received cranial irradiation as in those whose prophylaxis did not include this treatment. Despite low

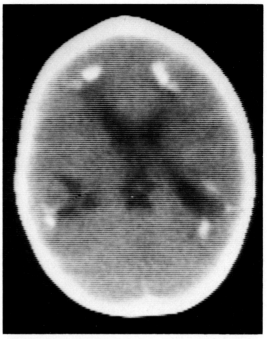

Figure 14-3. CT scan showing cortical calcifications and ventricular dilatation in a 14-year-old girl four years after CNS prophylaxis with 2400 rads and six cycles of intrathecal methotrexate for acute lymphocytic leukemia.

serum levels of growth hormone, linear growth has been undisturbed in these children. Because most of these children are currently prepubertal, a longer follow-up will be necessary to assess the significance of the serum growth hormone deficiency. Other hormone levels including T4, TSH, plasma cortisol, FSH, and LH have not been found to be altered by any form of CNS prophylaxis to date (Cohen et al., 1982; Rowland et al., 1982).

Comparable studies on children treated for medulloblastoma are in progress. Preliminary results indicate a similar pattern of verbal and performance IQ loss associated with a somewhat higher dose of cranial irradiation without either intrathecal or systemic chemotherapy. Somnolence syndrome characterized by lethargy, nausea, vomiting, mild diarrhea, low-grade fever, irritability, and weight loss has occurred in approximately half of the children six to eight weeks after completion of CNS irradiation and may be the prodrome of the late effects. Whether younger children are more likely to sustain permanent injury than older children is not established at this time, although some investigations have indicated a greater likelihood for the younger children to manifest a late effect of the radiation (Freeman *et al.,* 1973).

Chemotherapy

Neurotoxicity is most frequently associated with the vinca alkaloids (Weiss *et al.,* 1974; Weiss *et al.,* 1981; Whitehead *et al.,* 1982), procarbazine, L-asparaginase, and intrathecal administration of methotrexate (Weiss *et al.,* 1974). In addition, 5-fluorouracil (FU), *cis*-platinum, and the nitrosoureas may result in nervous system adverse effects, but with a much reduced frequency.

Vincristine

The earliest clinical findings of vincristine neurotoxicity are the diffuse loss of cutaneous sensation of the toes and fingertips without demonstrable abnormalities of tests of discrimination, position, or vibratory sense, and loss of Achilles reflex (Sandler *et al.,* 1969). Depression of other deep-tendon reflexes, progressing to complete areflexia, may occur. Maximal depression of reflexes usually occurs 17 days following administration, with return towards normal after one to three months.

Profound motor weakness is one of the most serious manifestations of vincristine neurotoxicity. Objective clinical findings characteristically reveal impairment of the extensors of the fingers, toes, and wrists (Sandler *et al.,* 1969; Rosenthal and Kaufman, 1975). Foot or wrist drop and a broad-based gait occurs. It may be severe in some cases, but in others completely reversible within several months. Cranial nerve dysfunction may result in ptosis and facial palsies. The earliest manifestation of autonomic nervous system disorder is usually abdominal colic and constipation , which may be accentuated in the elderly. Other neurologic abnormalities associated with vincristine administration include rare instances of seizures and, more frequently, myalgias of the jaw or throat. Inadvertent intrathecal injection of

vincristine results in rapid neurologic deterioration with peripheral neuropathies, cranial nerve palsies, paralytic ileus, bladder atony, hypertension or hypotension, seizures, and inappropriate ADH secretion progressing to death (Sandler *et al.,* 1969; Rosenthal and Kaufman, 1975).

All the above cited manifestations of vincristine neurotoxicity are usually more profound in the elderly and are dose related, being more severe with doses in excess of 1.5 mg/m^2. In general, total doses should be limited to 2 mg and less if there is evidence of hepatobiliary dysfunction that would limit excretion.

Methotrexate

Intrathecal administration of methotrexate may be accompanied by symptoms of meningeal irritation, transient or permanent paraparesis, and encephalopathy (Bleyer *et al.,* 1973). Sterile arachnoiditis with stiff neck, headache, vomiting, and cerebrospinal fluid pleocytosis has been reported in 10% to 40% of patients (Bleyer *et al.,* 1973; Geiser *et al.,* 1975). The symptoms usually begin two to four hours after the dose of intrathecal methotrexate and lasts 12 to 72 hours (Bleyer *et al.,* 1973; Geiser *et al.,* 1975; Rosenthal and Kaufman, 1975). Meningoencephalopathy can develop several months following therapy. Table 14 – 1 (from Weiss *et al.,* 1974) summarizes the symptoms and signs of methotrexate neurotoxicity.

L-Asparaginase

Cerebral dysfunction manifested as lethargy, somnolence, confusion, disorientation, hallucinations, and depression has been reported after the administration of L-asparaginase. These changes, described in 30% to 60% of patients (Haskell *et al.,* 1969), usually resolve following cessation of therapy. In addition to the acute toxicity, a delayed encephalopathy beginning approximately one week

Table 14 – 1. Symptoms and Signs of Methotrexate Neurotoxicity

COMMON *(5% to 50%)*	UNCOMMON *(1%)*

A. Subacute meningeal irradiation
  Stiff neck
  Nausea and vomiting
  Headache
  Fever
  Mild CSF pleocytosis
B. Decreased opening pressure
	A. Paraplegia
	  Transient
	  Permanent
	B. Seizures
	C. Encephalopathy

after therapy and lasting several weeks has been reported (Haskell *et al.,* 1969; Weiss *et al.,* 1974).

5-FU

Reversible cerebellar ataxia has been reported in less than 5% of patients receiving intravenous doses of 5-FU (Moertel *et al.,* 1964). Dizziness, gross dysmetria, coarse nystagmus, slurred speech, and truncal ataxia may occur. The syndrome appears unrelated to sex or age of patient or the total dose of 5-FU received. The incidence, however, does increase with higher single doses. The symptoms usually end one to six weeks after therapy is discontinued. These symptoms are more frequent with intravenous administration of ftorafur, a furanyl analog (Weiss *et al.,* 1974).

Other Agents

Irreversible ototoxicity and peripheral neuropathies may occur with *cis*-platinum. Tinnitus that occurs early may be followed by high-frequency hearing loss (Higby *et al.,* 1973). Central nervous system depression, which in rare cases may progress to profound stupor, has been described with oral procarbazine therapy and is greatly accentuated with intravenous therapy (Brunner and Young, 1965). Peripheral neuropathy, enhancement of barbiturates, narcotics, phenothiazines, and monamine oxidase inhibition have also been observed. Alcohol intolerance similar to that seen with disulfiram (ANTABUSE) has been reported and consequently patients should be warned of this complication (Brunner and Young, 1965; Weiss *et al.,* 1974).

GASTROINTESTINAL TOXICITY

The rapid proliferation of the cell population in the crypt epithelium makes the gastrointestinal tract extremely vulnerable to direct toxicity from chemotherapeutic agents. Other indirect effects such as anorexia, nausea, vomiting, and diarrhea are extremely common.

Nausea and Vomiting

Chemotherapy-induced nausea and vomiting are mediated by the vomiting center in the medullary reticular formation (Borison and Wang, 1953; Borison, 1974). The vomiting center lies structurally close to the chemoreceptor trigger zone (CTZ) in the area postrema of the fourth ventricle. Emesis results when the vomiting center is stimulated from the CTZ or afferent fibers located in the cerebral cortex, gastrointestinal tract (particularly the duodenum), heart, and vestibular apparatus (Scogna and Smalley, 1979). Vomiting induced by various chemicals, drugs, and toxic substances including apomorphine, cytotoxic agents, and radiation is mediated through the CTZ (Borison and Wang, 1953; Borison *et al.,* 1958; Wang *et al.,* 1958).

Nausea and vomiting are the most common early manifestations of toxicity of antineoplastic therapy and may result in dehydration, electrolyte imbalance, weakness, and weight loss, depending on the severity and duration. Great variability is evident in the emetogenic properties of anticancer drugs, although specific agents such as *cis*-platinum, DTIC, nitrogen mustard, and streptozotocin produce vomiting in virtually all patients.

Management of nausea and vomiting associated with chemotherapy requires judicious use of various classes of antiemetics by the most effective and convenient route. Compounds that exert an effect on the CTZ, such as the phenothiazines, have shown the greatest potential as antiemetics. Antihistamines, which may be beneficial in motion sickness, have shown limited effectiveness in emesis associated with cancer chemotherapy (Wang, 1965; Harris, 1978). The psychologic effect of treatment, however, is emphasized by the studies that have shown that placebo treatment may be effective. In a randomized double-blind study, one research team (Moertel *et al.,* 1963) compared the effectiveness of several antiemetic drugs to placebo therapy in patients receiving intravenous 5-FU. Ten milligrams of the phenothiazine derivatives thiopropazate and 5 mg of prochlorperzanine, given orally three times daily, demonstrated superior antiemetic effect compared to the placebo. Trimethobenzamide (TIGAN) showed only a slight advantage. In further investigations (Moertel and Reitemeier, 1969), researchers have reported superior therapeutic effectiveness of thiethylperazine—10 mg—and thiopropazate—10 mg—when tested against placebo. Metoclorpramide, which increases lower esophageal sphincter pressure and enhances the gastric emptying, showed no therapeutic advantage. The investigators concluded that thiopropazate, prochlorperazine, and thiethylperazine are effective antiemetics when administered orally in standard doses. These agents are, however, associated with extrapyramidal and sedative effects that do not correlate with their antiemetic activity. Other agents that have demonstrated efficacy in treating the nausea and vomiting associated with cancer chemotherapy are droperidol, (Grossman et al., 1979), haloperidol, (Plotkin et al., 1973) delta-9-tetrahydrocannabinol (THC) (Sallan et al., 1975).

In 1975, one research team followed reports from patients who described decreased nausea and vomiting from cancer chemotherapy while being "high" after smoking marijuana. This group (Sallan et al., 1975) subsequently reported the effectiveness of THC, a major constituent of marijuana, in relieving chemotherapy-associated nausea and vomiting. Orally administered THC (15 or 20 mg) demonstrated superior activity when compared to placebo. Complete or partial alleviation of symptoms was noted in 14 of 20 patients treated with THC, but in none of 22 treated with placebo. Another group (Chang et al., 1979) reported less nausea and vomiting in osteogenic sarcoma patients given high-dose methotrexate with THC (10 mg orally every three hours) when compared to placebo. Antiemetic activity correlated with increasing THC plasma concentrations. Plasma concentrations of 5.0, 5.0 to 10.0, and 10.0 ng/mL were associated with incidences of nausea and vomiting, or both, of 44%, 21%, and 6%, respectively. The incidence of nausea and vomiting after the use of placebo cigarettes was 96%, whereas the incidence of these symptoms was 83%, 38%, and 0% and corresponded to plasma concentrations of 5.0, 5.0 to 10.0, and 10.0 ng/mL respectively when marijuana cigarettes were used. Other patients receiving cyclophosphamide and doxorubicin, however, did not respond well to THC.

A third team (Lucas and Laszlo, 1980) reported on the effectiveness of THC for patients with nausea and vomiting refractory to standard antiemetics. Of 53 patients treated at doses of 5 to 15 mg/m^2 every four to six hours, 19% reported a complete alleviation of nausea and vomiting, 53% reported a 50% reduction of symptoms, and 28% experienced no relief. Patients receiving chemotherapy with cis-platinum, in general, did not respond well. A synthetic cannabinoid, nabilone, given orally has also demonstrated antiemetic effectiveness superior to prochlorperazine in patients receiving cancer chemotherapy (Herman et al., 1979).

McCabe and colleagues, (1981) have conducted a randomized study comparing THC to prochlorperazine in patients refractory to standard antiemetic therapy. Twenty-three of 36 (64%) patients reported THC superior to prochlorperazine, and nine (25%) experienced complete relief of symptoms with THC. Adverse reactions with THC include dizziness, somnolence, euphoria, and paranoid ideation. These occurred in patients receiving high doses (15 mg/m^2).

Frytak and associates (1979) reported THC equivalent to prochlorperazine but associated with a greater incidence of unpleasant side-effects. The age group of this latter study was older than in former trials, and it is now accepted that the elderly are at a greater risk for adverse reactions.

The mechanisms of the antiemetic effect of THC are unknown. It is clear that THC can be effectively used as an antiemetic in patients who experience nausea and vomiting from cancer chemotherapy. Because of problems with the extent of absorption of orally administering tablets, dosages and routes of administration deserve further study.

Mucositis

Gastrointestinal toxicity presenting as stomatitis, glossitis, esophagitis, and oral ulceration may severely decrease dietary intake. This form of toxicity is most commonly caused by methotrexate, the antibiotic antitumor agents, methylglyoxal, bisguanylhydrazone, 5-FU, and the vinca alkaloids. Single doses of methotrexate, 30 mg/m^2, rarely produce mucositis, whereas larger doses or repeated smaller doses may produce moderate to severe symptoms (Fajardo et al., 1968). Mucositis caused by high-dose, loading courses of 5-FU may be associated with bloody diarrhea and a high mortality (Hoston et al., 1970).

The toxicity of methotrexate to the gastrointestinal epithelium and other normal tissues depends on the duration of exposure to cytotoxic concentrations of the drug rather than peak levels achieved (Bleyer, 1978). The plasma concentration and time thresholds for gastrointestinal epithelium toxicity are approximately 2×10^{-8} mol and 42 hours, respectively (Chabner and Young, 1973; Young et al., 1973). Disappearance of methotrexate from plasma following an intravenous injection is triphasic (Young and Chabner, 1973; Huffman *et al.*, 1975; Stoller *et al.*, 1975). Studies have shown that the terminal half-life, which begins six to 24 hours following high-dose therapy, contributes the major portion of gastrointestinal and bone marrow toxicity (Stoller *et al.*, 1973).

Toxicity to the gastrointestinal tract can be diminished if citrovorum factor rescue is given within 42 hours of administration of methotrexate (Stoller *et al.*, 1977). Monitoring of methotrexate plasma concentrations may help identify those patients at risk for increased toxicity. Continuation of citrovorum rescue factor at standard doses six to 12 mg/m² every three to six hours for those patients with prolonged time thresholds, and augmentation of the dose to match the elevated plasma level of methotrexate may be necessary (Chabner *et al.*, 1972; Isacoff *et al.*, 1976; Bleyer, 1977). Intrathecal injection of methotrexate (Jacobs *et al.*, 1975) and distribution of this drug into third space compartments, such as ascitic fluid and pleural effusions, results in prolonged plasma levels because of slow drug removal from these reservoirs (Wan *et al.*, 1974).

Mucositis may preclude adequate oral nutrition. Treatment is usually conservative and symptomatic, including warm saline mouth rinses, topical anesthetics such as viscous xylocaine before fluid and food ingestion, and nystatin if moniliasis is evident. Fluid intake with a straw and intravenous nutritional support may be indicated.

Diarrhea and Constipation

Autonomic nerve dysfunction manifested as colicky abdominal pain, constipation, and adynamic ileus is frequently associated with vincristine treatment (Weiss *et al.*, 1974; Rosenthal and Kaufman, 1975). The elderly are particularly predisposed to these toxicities. The symptoms occur within three days of administration of the drug and may be unaccompanied by evidence of peripheral nerve dysfunction. One research team (Holland *et al.*, 1973) reported the presence of constipation in one-third of patients treated with vincristine. Symptoms were more frequent, more severe, and of earlier onset in the group receiving the highest dose (range 12.5 to 75 μ/kg). If treated conservatively, this condition usually resolves over a two-week period.

Profuse diarrhea may complicate treatment with 5-FU (Sherlock, 1979), and methyl GAG (Killen *et al.*, 1982).

HEPATIC TOXICITY

Radiation Effects

The liver, once considered relatively resistant to radiation, is now known to be intolerant of doses in excess of 3000 rads (Ingold *et al.*, 1965) Acute radiation hepatitis will appear two to six weeks following the completion of the radiotherapy. The liver enlarges and ascites generally occur. Abnormal liver chemistries are found, along with significant rises in alkaline phosphatase. Jaundice may also be present. The liver scan will show patchy uptake demarcating the irradiated volume (Tefft *et al.*, 1970). The characteristic histopathology is the finding of veno-occlusive disease. Atrophy of the liver cells is seen with progressive fibrosis, congestion, and hemorrhage (Reed and Cox, 1966). The fibrosis may resolve spontaneously, but can be fatal in about half of the patients. A chronic type of radiation effect may be seen as late as two to three years after the completion of treatment. In this situation, the patients will show the clinical syndrome and histologic picture of chronic liver insufficiency.

Chemotherapy

Liver damage is most frequently associated with the use of methotrexate and 6-mercaptopurine (6-MP). Azathioprine, which is metabolized *in vivo* to 6-MP (Elion, 1967), produces hepatic toxicity similar to that of 6-MP.

Methotrexate

Hepatic toxicity resulting from methotrexate was initially appreciated in patients being treated for acute lymphocytic leukemia and psoriasis. One of the earliest reports (Colsky *et al.*, 1955) described extensive hepatic fibrosis in five patients who had each received several hundred milligrams of methotrexate for leukemia therapy over periods of six to 14 months. The introduction of antifolates and steriods in the period 1948–1951 and the additional use of antipurines in 1952–1957 brought a marked increase in the incidence of hepatic fibrosis found at autopsy in leukemic children treated with these agents. It was concluded, therefore, that risk factors in the pathogenesis of hepatic fibrosis included both drug therapy and the duration of survival. Those children with fibrosis lived, on the average, twice as long as those with no fibrosis (Hutter *et al.*, 1960).

Hersh *et al.*, (1966) carried out a prospective study of 22 patients who received methotrexate for leukemia and other disorders. Reversible abnormalities of serum enzymes serum glutamic-oxaloacetic transaminase (SGOT), serum glutamic-pyruvic transaminase (SGPT), and lactic dehydrogenase (LDH) and prolongation of bromsulphthalein (BSP) retention were found in association with intensive methotrexate treatment. With an intermittent drug schedule, these abnormalities were less evident. Histologic abnormalities included portal inflammation and fatty changes. It has been observed that methotrexate can exacerbate pre-existing cirrhotic liver damage, with hepatic coma a potential consequence (Hansen *et al.*, 1971).

Following the initial use of methotrexate for psoriasis and with the use of the drug for long-term management of the disease, reports of liver damage began to appear (Muller *et al.*, 1969; Roenigk *et al.*, 1971; Dahl *et al.*, 1972). The primary association of cirrhosis and fibrosis was with prolonged small-dosage schedules, such as 2.5 mg/day for two to five days with a corresponding rest period. Significantly less cirrhosis was noted in those treated with intermittent large dosage, such as 10 to 25 mg every one to four weeks, even though the total monthly dose was the same as in the prolonged small-dose schedule. In addition, the speed of onset of liver damage appeared to be dose-dependent (Dahl *et al.*, 1972).

These findings have been confirmed and reported as the results of an international cooperative study (Weinstein *et al.*, 1973) consisting of 550 patients with severe psoriasis who underwent percutaneous liver biopsy while being treated with methotrexate. BSP, SGOT, and SGPT serum levels were frequently normal in biopsy-proven cases of drug-induced cirrhosis. Dosage schedule was important in determining liver damage. Daily oral methotrexate was associated with significantly greater nuclear variability, necrosis, and fibrosis when compared to more intermittent schedules, even at equivalent total cumulative dose. Total cumulative dose, however, was also important, and increasing the drug dose was correlated with significant worsening of the biopsy findings. In addition to schedule and total dose of drug, alcohol ingestion was significantly associated with periportal inflammation, fibrosis, and cirrhosis. Age, sex, and

severity of psoriasis, however, did not correlate with abnormal histologic changes.

Additional data on this subject have been reported (Warin *et al.*, 1975). A group of 25 psoriasis patients had liver biopsies before and after methotrexate therapies that in most instances were given on weekly schedules. None developed cirrhosis, and only one developed moderate fibrotic changes. A recent review of liver biopsy material in 328 patients treated with weekly or other intermittent schedules (Zachariae *et al.*, 1980) showed a strong correlation between the cumulative dose and the incidence of cirrhosis. The average total dose was 2200 mg with a range from 590 to 8150 mg. Impaired renal function and previous alcohol intake were also risk factors. Although daily oral methotrexate is particularly associated with cirrhosis, intermittent schedules that result in high cumulative doses are also implicated in this problem.

Methotrexate is frequently used in high dosage (100 to 400 mg/kg) followed by citrovorum factor rescue in certain chemotherapeutic applications (Bertino *et al.*, 1971). Liver damage may result from use of the drug in this manner, but this subject has not been systematically studied and conclusions remain anecdotal. Acute increases in SGOT and SGPT are commonly measured but resolve without apparent clinical significance. The duration of infusion may be an important variable, with less toxicity seen for a six-hour infusion than for a 24-hour infusion. The effect of citrovorum factor rescue upon long-term liver damage is not clear.

The mechanism of methotrexate damage remains a subject of continuing research. It is known that the liver can concentrate methotrexate to levels four to eight times that in plasma. This may be due partly to the presence of folate-binding proteins in the cytoplasm (Richter *et al.*, 1970), as well as conversion of methotrexate to polyglutamate forms with intracellular retention. The critical reaction(s) in the production of fatty liver is (are) suggested to be the limitation of methyl groups required for choline synthesis, and it has been demonstrated that exogenous choline has a protective effect on the liver in rats treated with methotrexate (Freeman-Narrod *et al.*, 1977).

Although liver function tests may be abnormal during a course of methotrexate treatment, there may not be a direct relationship of these abnormalities to the production of fibrosis. Furthermore, the incidence of false negatives makes routine liver function tests rather insensitive indicators of slowly progressive disease (Hersh *et al.*, 1966; Bertino *et al.*, 1971; Dahl *et al.*, 1971). When chronic therapy is used, the schedule should be intermittent and alcohol intake minimized. Although it is pertinent to follow serum enzyme levels as indicators of hepatic disease, percutaneous liver biopsy is the only reliable means for accurately assessing severity of hepatotoxicity.

6-Mercaptopurine

The onset of hepatotoxicity from 6-MP and azathioprine is more rapid than that seen with methotrexate, usually occurring one to two months after treatment. A range of one week to two or more years of treatment has been reported (McIlvanie and MacCarthy, 1959; Clarke *et al.*, 1960; Einhorn and Davidsohn, 1964; Krawitt *et al.*, 1967; Zarday *et al.*, 1972). Liver damage is manifested by elevated serum transaminase levels, at times with elevations also in alkaline phosphatase and bilirubin. In many cases, these abnormalities resolve upon cessation of therapy, but may reappear after rechallenge with the drug (Einhorn and Davidsohn, 1964). The histologic picture is hepatocellular necrosis and intrahepatic cholestasis and may resemble that of chlorpromazine damage (Krawitt *et al.*, 1967). Severe hepatic decompensation may occur with the use of 6-MP in the presence of preexisting liver disease (Krawitt *et al.*, 1967). It should be used cautiously, if at all, under these conditions.

The incidence of liver damage secondary to 6-MP is not known, but there have been estimates that 10% to 40% of patients treated for acute leukemia with 6-MP may develop icterus (McIlvanie and MacCarthy, 1959; Einhorn and Davidsohn, 1964). The appearance of jaundice in a child being treated for acute leukemia with both methotrexate and 6-MP may raise difficult questions as to its etiology, and the jaundice may be resolved only by empiric adjustments of drug dosage. In patients in whom azathioprine is used to control chronic active hepatitis, the complication rate is low, but toxicity may go undetected because it closely resembles the natural course of the disease.

Other Agents

Acute hepatoxicity from chemotherapeutic agents as evinced by mild transient elevations in enzymes may be seen with cytosine arabinoside (Bodey *et al.*, 1974), DTIC (Gottlieb and Serpick 1971), the nitrosoureas (Young *et al.*, 1973), streptozotocin (Schein *et al.*, 1974), and L-asparaginase (Haskell *et al.*, 1969).

The principal histopathologic change following asparaginase therapy is fatty metamorphosis, with some hepatocellular necrosis (Oettgen *et al.*, 1969). The distribution of fatty change may be peripheral rather than centrilobular and it tends to resolve over time after the drug is discontinued (Pratt and Johnson, 1971). In the dosage range between 10 IU/kg/day and 5000 IU/kg/day, no clear relationship between asparaginase dose and severe hepatic toxicity has been established. The lesion is not described as progressing to fibrotic change or cirrhosis.

The changes in serum chemistry include elevations of SGOT, SGPT, alkaline phosphastase, 5'-nucleotidase, and total bilirubin. In most cases the enzyme elevations are two to three times normal, but they may range higher. As with the fatty changes, there may be a better correlation with duration of treatment than with drug dose. L-Asparaginase produces several important biochemical alterations in the serum. Albumin levels fall significantly, as do other serum proteins such as transferrin, ceruloplasmin, and alpha-l-antitrypsin. Serum cholesterol and triglycerides fall, along with prebeta-, beta-, and alpha-lipoproteins. While the detailed mechanisms have not been studied, these effects are all consistent with a profound effect upon hepatic protein synthesis. Depression of other proteins leads to or contributes to coagulation abnormalities seen with L-asparaginase treatment. Hypofibrinogenemia occurs with prolongation of the thrombin time, and there may also be a prolongation of the prothrombin time and partial thromboplastin time.

Some of the highest elevations of LDH1, SGOT, and SGPT are seen with mithramycin. Approximately 50% of patients receiving 25 to 50 μg/kg per day for five days will show dramatic changes in liver function within one to four days (Kennedy, 1970). Microscopically, hepatic necrosis is visualized with fatty changes and vacuolization. In addition, synthesis of albumin and clotting factors II, V, VII, and X is depressed. Thus, transient prolongation of the prothrombin time is not uncommon, and this plus an associated thrombocytopenia may result in a serious bleeding diathesis.

URINARY TRACT TOXICITY

Radiation Effects on the Kidney

The effects of radiation on the kidney have been so well documented and are so catastrophic that it is rare that this complication of treatment now occurs (Clinical Pathological Conference, 1970). Renal tolerance of radiation is generally considered to be around 2000 rads to the entire renal mass. If one-third of the kidneys is shielded, however, clinical radiation nephritis will not occur. With radiation doses of 2500 to 3500 rad, approximately half the patients will develop acute radiation nephritis in six months to a year. This is characterized by the finding of proteinuria, both casts and red cells in the urine, and hypertension. Fatal uremia may occur or the clinical course may progress to chronic radiation nephritis characterized by progressive renal failure and severe hypertension. Some patients develop chronic radiation nephritis without a clinical acute phase. Histologically, late-stage radiation nephritis is characterized by gross, nonspecific, glomerular changes and tubular degeneration. Arteriolar narrowing is probably the most important lesion and is responsible for the renal injury. Unilateral radiation may result in a contracted kidney with malignant hypertension. This may be reversed by nephrectomy (Luxton and Kunkler, 1964).

Chemotherapy

Cyclophosphamide. In 1959 (Coggins *et al.,* 1959) the complication of hemorrhagic cystitis was first reported in patients who were treated with cyclophosphamide. This acute cystitis is more commonly observed in patients who are insufficiently hydrated when receiving large intermittent intravenous doses. The incidence of cystitis has been reported to range from 4% through 36% in patients. Dysuria frequency and urgency occur, and evidence of gross or microscopic hematuria and pyuria may be seen on urinalysis. The onset is extremely variable; it may occur early after the first dose (Coggins *et al.,* 1959; Host and Nissen-Mayer 1960), or it may be delayed until several weeks after the drug has been withdrawn (George, 1963). Cystoscopic examination shows a variety of changes, including mucosal hyperemia, telangiectatic blood vessels, focal or diffuse subepithelial bleeding sites,

and mucosal ulceration and necrosis (Anderson *et al.,* 1967; Riggenback *et al.,* 1968; Marsh *et al.,* 1971). Histologic examination of the urinary bladder by biopsy or at autopsy has shown numerous thin-walled vessels with capillary budding; the epithelium is edematous, and scattered areas of necrosis may be present. Urinary cytology commonly shows atypical epithelial cells, which may be misinterpreted as evidence of neoplasia (Wall and Clausen, 1975).

Acute cystitis usually resolves spontaneously with hydration and cessation of chemotherapy, but microscopic hematuria may persist for several months. Infrequently, the bleeding is massive and life threatening, and in such cases urologic intervention may be required. In reviewing the role of surgical management in patients with hemorrhagic cystitis, one research team has suggested that diverting urine from the bladder mucosa may be quite successful in controlling major bladder hemorrhage in patients who do not respond to conservative management (Berkson *et al.,* 1973). Urinary diversion bypasses the bladder epithelium and prevents further alkylation in patients still receiving the drug. A more common approach is the instillation of formalin. In patients who develop cystitis long after withdrawal of the drug, the continued flow of urine may prevent adequate healing and hemostasis in the damaged bladder epithelium.

Long-term treatment with cyclophosphamide has the potential for causing the development of chronic bladder fibrosis and vesicoureteral reflux (Johnson and Meadows, 1971; Marsh *et al.,* 1971; Bennett, 1974). Histologic examination of the bladder shows alterations similar to those seen after radiotherapy: capillary dilation, edema, inflammatory cells, and proliferating fibroblasts in the adjacent stroma. The telangiectatic vessels are predisposed to bleeding after minimal trauma. In the most systematic study of this problem, urinary bladder fibrosis was shown at autopsy in ten of 40 patients who had received long-term treatment with cyclophosphamide (Johnson and Meadows, 1971). Patients whose bladders were affected had received the largest doses, in excess of 6.0 g/m^2 body surface area, over the longest period of time. In approximately 50% of cases the process was entirely asymptomatic.

Patients receiving cyclophosphamide should be instructed to maintain a high urinary output during therapy. In addition, regular examination of the urine should be performed to detect evidence of microscopic hematuria. If cystitis develops it is recommended that cyclophosphamide therapy be discontinued and an alternative alkylating agent, such as chlorambucil or melphalan, which do not carry the risk of bladder toxicity, be utilized.

An unusual renal toxicity has been described in association with high-dose cyclophosphamide treatment and impaired water excretion after administration of intravenous doses in excess of 50 mg/kg body weight per day (DeFronzo et al., 1973). This syndrome is characterized by hyponatremia, decreased urine volume, and inappropriately concentrated urine, without associated glomerular or proximal tubular abnormalities. The damage is reversible after cessation of cyclophosphamide. This effect has been attributed to the alkylating metabolites of cyclophosphamide and their direct action on the distal renal tubule.

Cis-Platinum

The clinical usefulness of cis-diamminedichloroplatinum is limited by its dose-dependent nephrotoxicity (Korvach et al., 1973; Talley et al., 1973; Kuhn et al., 1980) (see Chapter 10). The renal insufficiency is characterized by a rise in serum creatinine that peaks at three to 14 days, may be irreversible, and is occasionally associated with transient proteinuria and hyperuricemia (Kuhn et al., 1980). Histologically, the findings are consistent with acute tubular necrosis. The incidence may vary from 25% at doses of 50 mg/m^2 to 100% at doses of 200 mg/m^2 (Korvach et al., 1973; Talley et al., 1973). The incidence decreases with preinfusion and postinfusion hydration and concomitant mannitol therapy and/or furosemide. Urinary β-glucuronidase activity may serve as a measure for monitoring the onset and progress of nephrotoxicity (Kuhn et al., 1980).

Streptozotocin

The principal treatment-limiting toxicity of streptozotocin is renal tubular damage (Schein et al., 1974). Great variability exists in the time until appearance of toxicity with respect to duration of treatment and total dose. The earliest manifestations are proteinuria, aminoaciduria, and hypophosphatemia, which are usually reversible in two to four weeks if therapy is discontinued. With continued treatment, or with the use of dose schedules in excess of 1.5 g/m^2 per week or 500 mg/m^2 per day for five days, a full Fanconi's syndrome, azotemia, or death from renal toxicity may result (Schein et al., 1974).

Ten to 20% of the total dose is excreted in the urine with an intact N-nitroso group within two hours after administration (Schein et al., 1974). The presence of active drug in the renal tubule under conditions that are known to lead to the release of an active alkylating agent may be responsible for the nephrotoxicity observed in these patients. Accordingly, it is recommended that adequate hydration and urine output be maintained during the administration of streptozotocin, and that patients with reduced creatinine clearance do not receive this drug.

Methotrexate

When used in small intravenous doses of 40 to 60 mg/m^2, methotrexate has not been associated with appreciable nephrotoxicity. Extensive trials of high dose treatment with citrovorum factor rescue at these larger doses, of 100 mg/kg and more, have been reported. Several investigators have reported severe kidney damage with oliguria, azotemia, and fatal renal failure (Bleyer, 1978).

This is a particularly ominous situation, because at least 90% of administered methotrexate is normally excreted as intact drug in the urine. The basis of the nephrotoxicity is thought to be precipitation of drug in the renal tubules. The solubility characteristics of methotrexate may compound the problem, because the drug is ten times less soluble at pH 5.5 than at pH 7.5 (Stoller et al., 1975; Bleyer, 1978). Methotrexate renal toxicity is far more likely to occur in older patients, and greater than 50% increases in serum creatinine has been reported in 19/33 (60%) of adults receiving high-dose methotrexate without intensive hydration and alkylinization regimens (Pitman et al., 1975). Ten percent or more of administered high-dose methotrexate is metabolized to 7-hydroxymethotrexate and excreted in the urine as this metabolite; 7-hydroxymethotrexate is three to five times less soluble than the parent compound (Jacobs et al., 1975).

REPRODUCTIVE INTEGRITY

Some of the most impressive gains in survival in the modern treatment era have been in young patients, particularly those with Wilms' tumor, acute lymphocytic leukemia, rhabdomyosarcoma in the pediatric group, Hodgkin's disease, and testicular tumors in young adults. Because many of these patients are of reproductive age, they may wish to have children. The effect of the cancer treatment on reproductive integrity may become a matter of concern to these young people once their survival has been assured.

In older patients, continuation of sexual activity may also become a concern. In this case, not only physiologic changes associated with the cancer treatment, but noteworthy psychologic aspects may be involved. This is particularly important for the patients with breast cancer, prostatic cancer, and colorectal cancer who require colostomy.

In the male, surgical treatment of some urologic cancers can affect both fertility and sexual function. Men with testicular cancer have been found to be subfertile before any type of treatment. Following orchiectomy and no other treatment, sperm counts in over half the men are in the subfertile range (Haubrich and Harmis, 1973). Interference with erection and ejaculation can be expected after pelvic and retroperitoneal surgical procedures that interrupt sympathetic or parasympathetic innervation. Abdominoperineal resection, cystectomy or total prostatectomy can result in loss of erection ability. Retroperitoneal lymphadenectomy with resection of the second lumbar sympathetic ganglia will result almost uniformly in loss of emission, and, therefore, dry ejaculation (Narayar and Lange, 1980). External radiation of the pelvis for carcinoma of the prostate may produce impotence in 25% to 50% of men. This complication is significantly reduced with interstitial radioactive implants (Fowler *et al.*, 1979).

Radiation Therapy

Patients treated with radiotherapy usually have some form of gonadal shielding. Internal scatter and a small percentage of transmission radiation, however, will effect the gonads. Radiation effects are sex-, age-, and dose-dependent. In men, fractionated doses of radiation appear to be more destructive than a single dose in terms of sperm production. In the treatment of Hodgkin's disease, periaortic irradiation will result in 20 to 50 rads to the testes from scatter and this may rise to as much as 100 rads depending upon the type of radiation equipment. When pelvic irradiation is added, the dose will increase to 300 to 500 rads unless special protective devices are used.

The usual treatment of seminoma delivers 3000 rads to the periaortic region in four weeks. This will result in 250 to 300 rads to the remaining testis. Low normal sperm counts will persist for four to five years after such treatment.

Fractionated radiation doses of 50 to 100 rads will produce temporary aspermia in 100% of the patients, but recovery usually begins within the first year. Some patients may have persistent oligospermia three to four years after this dose of radiation. With doses of 100 to 200 rads, aspermia will persist for two years or longer and in some cases as long as four years. After doses of 200 to 300 rads, azoospermia can be seen as early as two months after treatment and may persist for three to five years. Doses in excess of 300 rads are usually associated with permanent aspermia, although some recovery has been reported in a few cases four to five years after treatment (Lushbaugh and Casarett, 1976; Ash, 1980). Serum FSH levels will be elevated until damaged semniferous epithelium has been repaired and returns to normal function (Chapman *et al.*, 1979). In young men who may wish to have children some time in the future, the use of a sperm bank should be considered. Many of these young men with a diagnosis of cancer may be oligospermic before any treatment, greatly reducing the prospect of subsequent fatherhood.

In women, fractionated doses of radiation will result in temporary or permanent sterility depending upon the dose and age of the patient. Lower doses of radiation are frequently associated with permanent amenorrhea in older women. A fractionated dose of 150 rad over a four-year period appears to produce no permanent deleterious effects in younger women, but can produce sterilization in women over 35. Although doses of 250 to 500 rads are likely to permanently sterilize women over 35, only half of the women under 35 will have transient amenorrhea. Doses of 1000 to 3000 rads are likely to produce permanent sterility in all women (Lushbaugh and Casarett, 1976).

In Hodgkin's disease, preservation of ovarian function has been achieved by placing the ovaries in sites where only scatter radiation will effect them. Most widely used is the midline oophoropexy with shielding during irradiation. Approximately two-thirds of women maintain normal ovarian function and subsequent pregnancies are possible (Roy *et al.,* 1970). To date, the offspring appear to be normal (LeFloch *et al.,* 1976). Movement of the ovaries laterally to the iliac fossa has been used successfully for preservation of ovarian function and diminishes still further the dose that the ovaries will receive (Nahas *et al.,* 1971).

In young women with early-stage carcinoma of the cervix (stage IB), surgery may be considered preferable to radiotherapy treatment, because ovarian function can be preserved, even though the reproductive integrity of the patient will not. This prevents early menopausal symptoms and changes. Radiotherapy treatment of cervical cancer destroys ovarian function and will produce drying of the vaginal mucosa and stenosis of the vagina, unless specific measures to prevent this are undertaken soon after treatment.

Chemotherapy

Testicular Function. Azoospermia is well described in patients receiving alkylating agents and other classes of anticancer drugs (Richter *et al.,* 1970; Fairley *et al.,* 1972; Cheviakoff *et al.,* 1973). One research team (Richter *et al.,* 1970) studied the effect of chlorambucil on spermatogenesis in eight patients with malignant lymphomas. The observed dose-dependent oligospermia progressed to azoospermia when total doses of 400 mg were exceeded. Recovery from oligospermia occurred in one patient after the drug was withdrawn. Similar findings were reported in five patients who recovered spermatogenesis either partially or totally after withdrawal of chlorambucil (Cheviakoff *et al.,* 1973). Alterations in testicular function in 31 patients who received daily cyclophosphamide for more than six months were reported: 18 (60%) had azoospermia (Fairley *et al.,* 1972). Testicular biopsies showed tubular atrophy with markedly diminished or absent spermatogenesis. The problem is complex because of the potential influence of the specific disease state on testicular function.

Two researchers (Sherins and DeVita, 1973) analyzed the effect of intensive combination chemotherapy on reproductive function in 16 men with malignant lymphoma. Combination chemotherapy involving mechlorethamine or cyclophosphamide, vincristine, prednisone, and procarbazine had been completed six months to seven years previously and all patients were considered to be in complete remission. All had normal libido and potency. Only four of the men had normal spermatogenesis. The remainder showed partial or complete testicular failure as evidenced by biopsy-proven spermatogonial arrest associated with elevated levels of FSH. Within each treatment group, the men with normal spermatogenesis were those who had been experiencing remission, without chemotherapy, for the longest period of time. One patient observed at regular intervals over a period of three and one-half years had a rise in sperm count from almost zero to fifteen million/mL and was able to impregnate his wife. These findings, and those reported after chemotherapy with alkylating agents alone, indicate that return of normal spermatogenesis is possible in rare cases, but several years may be required after discontinuation of therapy (Richter *et al.,* 1970; Sherins and DeVita, 1973). In a follow-up study of 26 men with cyclophosphamide-related azoospermia, 12 patients experienced a return of spermatogenesis within 15 to 49 months (with median duration of 30 months); there was no significant association of recovery with age, duration of cyclophosphamide therapy, or total dose administered (Brickanan *et al.,* 1975).

In an English study of MVPP (nitrogen mustard, vinblastine, procarbazine, and prednisone) in adult men, a small number developed gynecomastia, and 93% of the men were found to have small testicles of soft consistency. Although most of the men had a temporary reduction in sexual interest during treatment, they usually recovered a few months after cessation of chemotherapy. In 15% of the men, however, this was incomplete; impotence and declining libido were reported. Only an occasional patient has been found to have an increase in libido after chemotherapy (Whitehead *et al.,* 1982).

It is of interest that the toxic effect of chemotherapy on the testes is specific for the tubular epithelium. The Sertoli and Leydig cells, in general, remain histologically and functionally normal, as evidenced by normal or near-normal levels of testosterone and luteinizing hormone (LH) (Van Thiel et al., 1972).

Of particular interest is the influence of chemotherapy on the quiescent or developing spermatogenic activity of prepubertal and pubescent boys. In prepubertal boys treated with cyclophosphamide, no abnormality of LH, FSH, or testosterone was found eight months to seven years after treatment (Sherins et al., 1979). Similarly, MOPP therapy in six prepubertal boys produced no change in serum gonadotropins, whereas nine of 13 pubescent boys had moderate to severe gynecomastia, germinal aplasia, elevation in FSH and LH, and reduced testosterone levels two years after combined chemotherapy (Kirkland et al., 1976).

Ovarian Function. Alterations in menstrual function have been associated with the administration of cytotoxic agents such as busulfan (Galton et al., 1958), chlorambucil (Nicholson, 1968), cyclophosphamide (Uldall et al., 1972) and vinblastine (Sobrinho et al., 1971). One group of investigators (Uldall et al., 1972) reported on a series of 34 women with glomerulonephritis treated with daily cyclophosphamide for an average of 18 months. Eighteen (53%) of the women developed amenorrhea an average of 17 months from the onset of therapy. Urinary estrogens were low and urinary gonadotropins were elevated, suggesting primary ovarian failure as the cause of the amenorrhea. Only 10% of patients observed for one year after withdrawal of cyclophosphamide experienced a return of menstrual periods. In a similar group of patients, ovarian biopsies were performed on several women with ovarian failure following long-term treatment with cyclophosphamide (Warne et al., 1973). Histologic findings included absence of ova with no evidence of follicular maturation. One study (Sobrinho et al., 1971) described nine women with Hodgkin's disease who developed oligomenorrhea or amenorrhea shortly after beginning chemotherapy with vinblastine. All nine had findings consistent with primary ovarian failure. It is probable that both total dose and duration of administration are important determinants of the reversibility of this complication.

Approximately half of the women receiving MOPP chemotherapy for Hodgkin's disease will develop persistent amenorrhea. This is more likely to occur in women over the age of 25. Some of the patients who developed irregular menses will have return of normal periods, and pregnancies can occur (Schilsky and Erlichman, 1982), whereas evidence of chemical sterilization may be evidenced by persistent elevations of serum FSH and LH levels (Sobrinho et al., 1971), and may be accompanied by "hot flashes" and other symptoms of menopause. The destruction of ovarian function by chemotherapy in the setting of adjuvant treatment of stage II breast cancer has raised the question, Does withdrawal of hormonal support of the neoplasm contribute to the positive results?

TERATOGENESIS

Chemotherapy

Widespread use of antineoplastic agents has caused increasing concern that these drugs will produce adverse effects on fetal development when administered to pregnant women during the first four months of gestation.

Folic Acid Antagonists. The antifolate agents are the chemotherapeutic drugs that have been consistently implicated as fetal toxins in women, to the extent that these agents have been used as abortifacients in some European centers. Successful termination of pregnancy has been reported in 10 of 12 cases in which aminopterin was used specifically for this purpose (Thiersch, 1952). Three of the fetuses in this series had malformations, including cleft palate, hydrocephalus, and meningoencephalocele.

Another researcher (Nicholson, 1968) reviewed the literature dealing with the effects of cytotoxic agents in pregnancy. Of 52 patients who were reported to have received aminopterin during the first trimester of pregnancy, in most cases as an abortifacient, 34 eventually aborted. The state of the fetus was described in 12 cases, and in 10 of these macroscopic malformation was detected with a predilection for the central nervous system. In three pregnancies during which women had received aminopterin after the first trimester, no fetal abnormalities were detected, although one fetus died from spontaneous abortion at the 26th week. In this latter case, the mother had been receiving concomitant treatment with 6-MP and desacetylmethylcolchicine. Five women had received methotrexate after the first trimester, and they delivered six normal babies.

6-Mercaptopurine and Azathioprine. Similar fetal abnormalities have been reported with other drugs. Of 20 women who received 6-MP during the first trimester of pregnancy, eight aborted (Skinner and Schwartz, 1972). There were one stillborn and one abortion in 28 pregnancies treated after the first trimester and no cases of macroscopic fetal abnormality.

Abortions are reported less frequently with azathioprine, a drug that is commonly used to prevent renal transplant rejection. In 1970, the Human Kidney Transplant Registry had on record 29 women who became pregnant while receiving azathioprine and corticosteroids, and 18 normal children were delivered (Golby, 1970). Seven women had spontaneous abortions, five of which occurred early in pregnancy. No evidence of fetal abnormality was noted. Another study (Penn et al., 1971) reported eight women with renal homografts who became pregnant ten times, of which eight pregnancies were allowed to come to term. One premature infant died from hyaline membrane disease. In the surviving infants, one had pulmonary valvular stenosis, two had transient adrenocortical insufficiency and lymphopenia, and one had respiratory distress syndrome.

Alkylating Agents. Aside from isolated case reports, this class of chemotherapeutic compounds does not appear to be a consistent cause of fetal abnormality, but does have the potential for terminating early pregnancy. In one review (Nicholson, 1968) of 60 pregnant women who had received alkylating agent chemotherapy, 34 during the first trimester, four cases of fetal malformation were reported. Fetal abnormalities have occurred after a combination of nitrogen mustard, vincristine, procarbazine, and prednisone (MVPP) was given in the first trimester to treat Hodgkin's disease (Garrett, 1974).

The overall problem of drug-induced congenital abnormalities is extremely complex. With the exception of methotrexate, the teratogenic potential of anticancer-immunosuppressive therapy in humans appears lower than one might have predicted from animal studies. Moreover, the overall risk of fetal malformation after cytotoxic therapy during the second and third trimesters does not appear to be greater than normal. Nevertheless, women should be encouraged to take measures to avoid becoming pregnant while receiving chemotherapy. A decision to allow an established pregnancy to continue or to interrupt therapy during the first trimester cannot be made using available criteria; it must ob-

viously take into account the wishes of the patient after she has been fully informed of the possible risks. In addition, the effect of cytotoxic drugs on subsequent fertility and possible teratogenecity needs clarification (Holmes and Holmes, 1978; Simon, 1980). In one study of 27 women with Hodgkin's disease successfully treated with MOPP, 13 children were born subsequent to chemotherapy. The children appeared to be entirely normal (Schilsky et al., 1981).

SKELETAL EFFECTS

Soon after the discovery of x-rays, the impairment that it can produce in growing bone was appreciated (Perthes, 1903). When children received even modest doses of radiation to epiphyseal plates, growth retardation occurred in long bones with significant limb shortening while the spine showed irregularity of growth pattern configurations, loss of overall height, and scoliosis and/or kyphosis (Newhauser et al., 1952). If doses of radiation commonly used with Hodgkin's disease are given to young children, subcutaneous fibrosis and muscle atrophy around the shoulders and neck will be seen. With somewhat high doses, severe growth disturbances will be seen (see Figure 14–4). Radiation osteitis resulting in fracture or bone necrosis has also been reported (Tefft, 1972).

Although growing bone appears to be more sensitive to radiation than mature bone, late effects including both sclerotic changes and

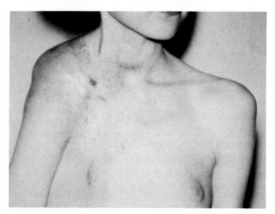

Figure 14–4. This 15-year-old girl during the first year of life received weekly radiation treatment for a benign cyst in the root of the neck. Agenesis of the hemithorax and breast is apparent as well as characteristic skin changes. She succumbed to an osteogenic sarcoma of the clavicle one year after this photograph was made.

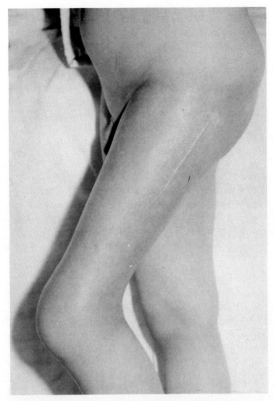

Figure 14–5. A seven-year-old boy with Ewing's sarcoma treated with intensive chemotherapy and radiotherapy showing marked soft tissue atrophy secondary to this combined treatment (Photo courtesy of Dr. Melvin Tefft, Rhode Island Hospital, Providence, RI.)

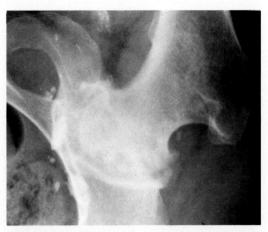

Figure 14–6. Roentgenogram of femoral head changes in an 18-year-old woman who received MOPP for advanced Hodgkin's disease.

bone reabsorption occur with higher doses of radiation. Radiation-induced soft tissue sarcomas with osteosarcomas have been reported regularly for more than half a century. The younger patients appear to be more likely to develop a malignancy than the older patients. Characteristically, a three-to-four-year delay occurs between treatment and the appearance of the sarcoma. The tumor will occur directly in the field of previous radiation and will be histologically distinct from the original tumor for which the treatment had been initially delivered (Cahan *et al.,* 1948).

The combined effects of many chemotherapeutic agents with radiation on muscle and bone will result in appreciably more intense late damage to those tissues than when either modality has been administered alone. This has been evident with intensive chemotherapy plus radiation for rhabdomyosarcoma or Ewing's sarcoma. Not infrequently, woody, hard pelvic induration and a malformed pelvis or extremity with crippling disabilities will be seen in the children who survive three to five

years or longer (Tefft *et al.,* 1976) (see Figure 14–5).

Another adverse effect on bone of combination chemotherapy used routinely in the management of lymphoma is avascular necrosis of the femoral head, which has been seen approximately one or two years or longer after both combination chemotherapy of MOPP and COPP (see Figure 14–6). It has been postulated that the steroid is the most likely agent responsible (Ihde and DeVita, 1975). Although only a small number of cases has been reported, a large number of unreported instances probably exists in the major centers using intermittent high-dose steroids to treat a large number of patients with lymphomas. Infrequent as it may be, correction by surgical intervention may be required because of the resultant incapacity.

PSYCHOSOCIAL PROBLEMS

In Chapter 50 of this book, Goldberg and Slaby discuss psychologic problems in cancer patients. One aspect of psychosocial support will be discussed here: The problems of adolescents and young adults. For them, a life-threatening illness is an implausible event. It is very difficult for them to accept their own mortality. An unusual form of denial is present and serves well as a coping mechanism. Rarely does it interfere with treatment. For the most part, these young people accept intensive treatment regimens faithfully. Almost apologetically they will admit to tiredness, loss of appetite, nausea, and vomiting. Frequently, they will resist changes in their lifestyle, supportive measures or even antinausea medications.

This cooperative attitude, along with trust and confidence in the treatment programs that cause transient disabilities but that are likely to be curative, may be shaken when the patient develops a recurrence of the disease. In many instances, salvage therapy has achieved excellent results, but for the young patient, the necessity of restarting treatment can be psychologically shattering. These patients may need special attention and extra psychosocial support measures.

The late psychologic impact in children up to the age of 15 has been studied ten years after treatment for cancer (Holmes and Holmes, 1975). It would appear that except for the physical disabilities associated with the cure of the neoplasm, most of the survivors made excellent adjustments and were living essentially normal lives. In another study of children treated for cancer, a high rate of adjustment problems was noted. In this study, there was a high degree of anxiety and depression (O'Malley et al., 1979). The early introduction of the adolescent and young adult patient to group sessions with psychosocial support staff may head off potential problems in later years.

SECOND NEOPLASMS

The appearance of a second neoplasm in a patient who has been successfully treated previously for a cancer can be one of the most difficult therapeutic problems for the oncologist. Multiple synchronous tumors in a single organ such as the oral passages, the colon, or bladder are frequent and may represent a combination of underlying host susceptibility and exposure to carcinogens. Whether simultaneous bilateral breast cancer is a sufficiently frequent occurrence to warrant bilateral treatment remains controversial. Less frequent is the appearance of multiple-organ, simultaneous primary cancers (Moertel, 1966).

Metachronous multiple primary neoplasms have been well documented. In general, patients with one primary neoplasm appear to have a high susceptibility to a second. Heredity, common exposure to carcinogens such as tobacco and alcohol, and endocrine stimulation may all play a role in the production of the second neoplasm (Schottenfeld, 1982). In studies of patients with Hodgkin's disease and

lymphoma treated before the era of intensive chemotherapy and/or radiation, there was a two- to threefold increase in second neoplasms, represented almost entirely by skin cancer (Berg, 1967). It is against this background that the influences of modern therapeutic intervention, radiation, and/or chemotherapy have to be assessed when examining the carcinogenicity of treatment.

Radiation-induced cancers have been known for over 75 years (Wolback, 1909). Postirradiation osteogenic sarcomas have been reported in patients treated for cancer of the breast, uterine cervix, and bladder and for seminoma and lymphomas, as well as in children with retinoblastoma, rhabdomyosarcoma, neuroblastoma, and Wilms' tumor, and, unfortunately, for a number of benign conditions (Glicksman and Toker, 1976). Chemotherapeutic agents were suspected of being carcinogenic by 1947 (Haddain, 1947). Mutagenic and carcinogenic effects have been documented in multiple laboratory tests, including the Ames test, sister chromatid exchanges, and in small-animal studies (Sieber and Adamson, 1975).

The oncogenic potentials of antineoplastic agents in man may arise through various mechanisms. Alkylating agents that bind DNA are perhaps the most important of the carcinogenic anticancer drugs. Chromosomal aberrations quite similar to those seen after irradiation have been produced by the alkylating agents. Similarly, a latent period of approximately four years can be expected between the onset of the use of these agents and the appearance of a new neoplasm. Secondly, long-term immunosuppression is another factor that leads to the appearance of a neoplasm both in patients treated for cancer and those treated for benign conditions. In addition, antineoplastic agents may be weak carcinogens in themselves, but in the presence of another chemical carcinogen, they may act as a cocarcinogen by activation of microsomal enzymes not clearly understood at this time. Agents such as actinomycin D in animal studies have been found to be both carcinogens and cocarcinogens, yet in a clinical study there was a decreased incidence of second neoplasms in children who received actinomycin D as part of their treatment for a wide variety of neoplasms (Chabner, 1982).

Recognition of the clinical implications became apparent only when chemotherapy for cancer became sufficiently successful that patients survived in appreciable numbers for relatively long periods of time. It is the consequences of this success that have led to the appreciation of the potential hazards of this cancer treatment.

In a study from Memorial Sloan-Kettering Cancer Center on second neoplasms in patients with Hodgkin's disease, three different time periods over the last 30 years were compared (Brody and Schottenfeld, 1980). A marked increase in second neoplasms in the more recent era was found, particularly leukemia. Arseneau and colleagues (1972) at the National Cancer Institute were the first to implicate the intensive radiotherapy and chemotherapy being used to cure patients with Hodgkin's disease in leukemogenesis.

Because increasing numbers of patients have been successfully treated for Hodgkin's disease, studies of the carcinogenic effects of antineoplastic treatment in patients are possible. For the most part, this treatment has included radiotherapy, combination chemotherapy, or both. Second neoplasms in the successfully treated patients are being seen much more frequently than in the preintensive-treatment era. The risk of acute myelogenous leukemia can be as high as 1000 times greater than in the normal population in patients who have had intensive chemotherapy, primarily including alkylating agents and intensive radiotherapy. The longer and more intensive the use of the alkylating agents, primarily chlorambucil and nitrogen mustard, the greater the risk of acute myelogenous leukemia. When nitrosoureas were used, leukemia was less frequent. Patients treated only with radiotherapy rarely develop leukemia. Cancers other than leukemia had a two- to threefold increase in these successfully treated patients. Contrary to the leukemogenesis observations, radiation *per se* was a significant hazard for other neoplasms and all the alkylating agents appeared to have a uniform risk. The median time to the development of leukemia was two and one-half to three years earlier than the appearance of the other second neoplasms (see Figure 14–7). It is possible that the full risk of second neoplasms has not been understood in these successfully treated patients. One early report on the use of ABVD, indicates that second neoplasms may not be as frequent in this group of patients (Glicksman *et al.,* 1982).

The development of a second neoplasm in patients successfully treated for Hodgkin's dis-

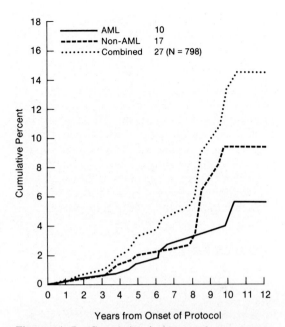

Figure 14-7. Cumulative incidence of second neoplasms in Hodgkin's disease patients while in continuous complete remission.

ease is now perceived as one of the major problems that must be addressed in the future. New strategies for treatment are being undertaken in the hope that the high rate of success in the eradication of the Hodgkin's disease can be achieved while the risk of a second neoplasm can be diminished.

It is important that adequate treatment be delivered so that the patient does not lose the prospect of cure. In a retrospective study of second neoplasms in patients successfully treated for Hodgkin's disease in the Cancer and Leukemia Group B, 1500 patients with stages III and IV Hodgkin's disease were entered on four protocols from 1966 to 1972. Of the 1332 patients evaluated, 798 achieved a complete remission. Of the complete responders, 27 developed a second neoplasm in the next decade. More serious, however, is the fact that 534 patients failed to respond to the combined treatments in these four studies. Although treatment regimens have improved over the last decade, 25% of the patients with either stages III or IV disease still fail to respond to treatment. The risk of dying of Hodgkin's disease far outweighs the risk of a second neoplasm.

Similarly, the risk of a late consequence of cancer treatment needs to be perceived in relationship to the risk of the cancer for which the treatment was initially delivered (D'Angio *et al.,* 1978). Untoward effects in perhaps 5% of the successfully treated patients must be weighed against an overall 50% failure to cure cancer with current available techniques. Attention to technical detail, improvement in understanding the toxicology of agents, and supportive care may reduce the untoward effects, and this is important. The risk of a late complication may have to be accepted to achieve a cure of the underlying neoplasm. It is hoped that new drugs, new radiotherapeutic techniques, new surgical techniques, and patient support systems may improve the risk/benefit equation in favor of the patient.

REFERENCES

Acute Leukemia Group B. Acute lymphocytic leukemia in children. *J.A.M.A.,* **207:**923–928, 1969.

Anderson, E. F.; Cobb, O. E.; and Glenn, J. F.: Cyclophosphamide hemorrhagic cystitis. *J. Urol.,* **97:**857, 1967.

Arseneau, J. C.; Sponzo, R. W.; Levin, D. L.; Schnipper, L. E.; Bonner, H.; Young, R. C.; Cancellos, G. P.; Johnson, R. E.; and DeVita, V. T.: Nonlymphomatous malignant tumors complicating Hodgkin's disease. *N. Engl. J. Med.,* **287:**1119–1122, 1972.

Ash, P.: The influence of radiation on fertility in man. *Br. J. Radiol.,* **53:**271–278, 1980.

Baily, C. C.; Marsden, H. B.; and Jones, P. H.: Fatal pulmonary fibrosis following BCNU therapy. *Cancer,* **42:**74–76, 1978.

Bennett, A. H.: Cyclophosphamide and hemorrhagic cystitis. *J. Urol.,* **111:**603, 1974.

Berg, J.: The incidence of multiple primary cancers in the development of further cancer in patients with lymphoma, leukemia and myeloma. *J.N.C.I.,* **38:**741–752, 1967.

Berkson, B. M.; Lome, L. G.; and Shapiro, I.: Severe cystitis induced by cyclophosphamide. *J.A.M.A.,* **225:**605, 1973.

Bertino, J. R.; Leavitt, M.; McCullough, J. L.; and Chabner, B. A.: New approaches to chemotherapy with folate antagonists: Use of leucovorin "rescue" and enzymatic folate depletion. *Ann. N.Y. Acad. Sci.,* **186:**486, 1971.

Bleyer, W. A.: Methotrexate: Clinical pharmacology, current status, and therapeutic guidelines. *Cancer Treat. Rev.,* **4:**87–101, 1977.

Bleyer, W. A.: The clinical pharmacology of methotrexate. *Cancer,* **41:**36–51, 1978.

Bleyer, W. A.; Drake, J. C.; and Chabner, B. A.: Neurotoxicity and elevated cerebrospinal fluid methotrexate concentration in meningeal leukemia. *N. Engl. J. Med.,* **289:**770, 1973.

Blum, R. H.; Carter, S. K.; and Agre, K.: A clinical review of bleomycin — new antineoplastic agent. *Cancer,* **31:**903, 1973.

Bodey, G. P.; Coltman, C. A.; Freireich, E. J.; Bonnet, J. J.; Gehan, E. A.; Haut, A. B.; Hewlett, J. S.; McCreditt, K. B.; Saiki, J. H.; and Wilson, H. E.: Chemotherapy of acute leukemia: Comparison of cytarabine alone and in combination with vincristine, prednisone, and cyclophosphamide. *Arch. Intern. Med.,* **133:**260, 1974.

Boivin, J. F., and Hutchinson, G. B.: Coronary heart disease mortality after irradiation for Hodgkin's disease. *Cancer,* **49:**2470–2475, 1982.

Bonadonna, G., and Monfardini, S.: Cardiotoxicity of daunomycin. *Lancet,* **1:**837, 1969.

Borison H. L.: Area postrema: chemoreceptor trigger zone for vomiting. Is that all? *Life Sci.,* **14:**1807–1817, 1974.

Borison, H. L.; Brand, E. D.; and Askind, R. K.: Emetic action of nitrogen mustard (mechloroethamine hydrochloride) in dogs and cats. *Am. J. Physiol.,* **192:**410–416, 1958.

Borison, H. L., and Wang, W. C.: Physiology and pharmacology of vomiting. *Pharmacol. Rev.,* **5:**193–230, 1953.

Brecher, M. L.; Freeman, A. L.; Glicksman, A. S.; Glidewell, O. J.; Rowland, J.; Duffner, P. K.; Cohen, M. E.; Voorhess, M.; Berger, P.; Harris, M.; Forman, E.; Jones, B.; Black, M.; Holland, J.; Sibley, R.; and Thomas, P. R. M.: Longterm toxicity of central nervous system prophylaxis in acute lymphocytic leukemia (for Cancer and Leukemia Group B). In Freeman, A., and Pochedly, C. (eds.): *Controversies in Pediatric and Adolescent Oncology.* Masson Publishing USA, Inc., New York, 1981.

Brickanan, J. D.; Fairley, K. F.; and Barrie, J. U.: Return of spermatogenesis after stopping cyclophosphamide therapy. *Lancet,* **2:**156, 1975

Bristow, M. R.; Mason, J. W.; Billingham, M. E.; and Daniels, J. R.: Doxorubicin cardiomyopathy: Evaluation by phonocardiography, endomyocardial biopsy and cardiac catheterization. *Ann. Intern. Med.,* **88:**168–175, 1978.

Brody, R. S., and Schottenfeld, D.: Multiple primary cancers in Hodgkin's disease. *Semin. Oncol.,* **7:**187–201, 1980.

Brunner, K. W., and Young, C. W.: A methyl-hydrazine derivative in Hodgkin's disease and other malignant neoplasms. *Ann. Intern. Med.,* **63:**69, 1965.

Burgert, E. O.; Glidewell, O.; Mills, S. D.; Nyhan, W. L.; Kung, F.; Lee, S. L.; Sawitsky, A.; Patterson, R. B.; Wolman, I. J.; Moon, J. H.; Jones, B.; Cortner, J.; Chevalier, L.; Selwary, O.; and Holland, J. O.: Acute leukemia group B, acute lymphocytic leukemia in children. Maintenance therapy with methotrexate administered intermittently. *J.A.M.A.,* **207:**923, 1966.

Cahan, W.; Woodward, H.Q.; Higgenbothan, N.L.; Stewart, F.W.; and Coley, B.I.: Sarcoma arising in irradiated bone. *Cancer,* **1:**3–29, 1948.

Chabner, B.: *Pharmacological Principles of Cancer Treatment.* W. B. Saunders Company, Philadelphia, 1982.

Chabner, B. A.; Johns, D. G.; and Bertino, J. R.: Enzymatic cleavage of methotrexate provides a method for prevention of drug toxicity. *Nature,* **239:**395–397, 1972.

Chabner, B. A.; Myers, C. E.; and Oliveria, V. T.: Clinical pharmacology of anticancer drugs. *Semin. Oncol.,* **2:**165–191, 1977.

Chabner, B. A., and Young, R. C.: Threshold methotrexate concentration for in vivo inhibition of DNA synthesis in normal and tumorous target tissues. *J. Clin. Invest.,* **52:**1104–1811, 1973.

Chang, A. E.; Shiling, D. J.; Stillman, R. C.; Nelson, H. G.; Seipp, C. A.; Barofsky, I.; Simon, R. M.; and Rosenberg, S. A.: Delta-9-tetrahydrocannabinol as an antiemetic in cancer patients receiving high-dose methotrexate. *Ann. Intern. Med.,* **91:**819–824, 1979.

Chapman, R. M.; Sutcliff, S. B.; Nees, L. H.; Edwards, C. R. W.; and Malpas, J. S.: Cyclic chemotherapy and gonadal function. *Lancet,* **1:**285–289, 1979.

Cheviakoff, S.; Calamera, J. C.; Morgenfeld, M.; and Mancini, R. E.: Recovery of spermatogenesis in patients with lymphoma after treatment with chlorambucil. *J. Reprod. Fertil.,* **33:**155, 1973.

Clarke, P. A.; Hsia, Y. E.; and Huntsman, R. G.: Toxic complications of treatment with 6-mercaptopurine: Two cases with hepatic necrosis and intestinal ulceration. *Br. Med. J.,* **1:**393, 1960.

Claryre, A. M.; Cathey, W. J.; Cartwright, G. E.; and Wintrobe, M. M.: Pulmonary disease complicating intermittent therapy with methotrexate. *J.A.M.A.,* **204:**1861, 1969.

Clinical Pathology Conference: Case 31-1970, Case Records of the Massachusetts General Hospital. *N. Engl. J. Med.,* **283:**191–201, 1970.

Codling, B. W., and Chakera, T. M.: Pulmonary fibrosis following therapy with melphalan for multiple myeloma. *J. Clin. Path.,* **25:**668–673, 1972.

Coggins, P. R.; Ravdin, R. G.; and Eisman, E. M.: Clinical pharmacology and preliminary evaluation of cytoxan. *Cancer Chemother. Rep.,* **3:**9, 1959.

Cohen, M. E.; Duffner, P. K.; Brecher, M. L.; Diamond, L. S.; Glicksman, A. S.; Forman, E.; Harris, M.; Jones, B.; Holland, J. F.; Glidewell, O.; and Freeman, A. (for Cancer and Leukemia Group B): EEGs in disease-free children with acute lymphocytic leukemia (ALL), *Proceedings, A.S.C.O.,* 1, Abstr. C-524, 135, 1982.

Cohn, K. E.; Steward, J. R.; Fajardo, L. F.; and Hancock, E. W.: Heart disease following radiation. *Medicine,* (Baltimore), **46:**281–297, 1967.

Cole, R. C.; Myers, T. J.; and Klatsky, A. V.: Pulmonary disease with chlorambucil therapy. *Cancer,* **41:**455–459, 1978.

Collaborative Study: Survival and complications of radiotherapy following involved and extended field therapy of Hodgkin's disease, stages I and II. *Cancer,* **38:**288–305, 1976.

Colsky, J.; Greenspan, E. M.; and Warren, T. N.: Hepatic fibrosis in children with acute leukemia after therapy with folic acid antagonists. *Arch. Pathol.,* **59:**198–206, 1955.

Dahl, M. G. C.; Gregory, M. M.; and Scheuer, P. J.: Liver damage due to methotrexate in patients with psoriasis. *Br. Med. J.,* **1:**625, 1971.

Dahl, M. G. C.; Gregory, M. M.; and Scheuer, P. J.: Methotrexate hepatotoxicity in psoriasis—comparison of different dose regimens. *Br. Med. J.,* **1:**654, 1972.

D'Angio, G. J.; Clatworthy, H. W.; Evans, A. E.; Newton, W. A.; and Tefft, M.: Is the risk of morbidity and rare mortality worth the cure? *Cancer,* **41:**377–380, 1978.

D'Angio, G. J.; Farber, S.; and Maddock, C. I.: Potentiation of x-ray effects by actinomycin D. *Radiology,* **73:**175, 1959.

DeFronzo, R. A.; Braine, H.; Colvin, O. M.; and Davis, P. J.: Water intoxication in man after cyclophosphamide therapy. *Ann. Intern. Med.,* **78:**861, 1973.

DeLena, M.; Guzzon, A.; Monfardini, S.; and Bonadonna, G.: Clinical, radiological, and histopathologic studies on pulmonary toxicity induced by treatment with bleomycin. *Cancer Chemother. Rep.,* **56:**343, 1972.

DeVita, V.; Henney, J.; and Hubbard, S. M.: Estimation of the numerical and economic impact of chemotherapy in the treatment of cancer. In Burchnell, J., and Oettgen, H. (eds.): *Cancer 1980 Symposium—Achievements, Challenges, Prospects.* Grune & Stratton, Inc., New York, 1981.

Einhorn, M., and Davidsohn, I.: Hepatotoxicity of mercaptopurine. *J.A.M.A.,* **188:**802, 1964.

Elion, G. B.: Biochemistry and pharmacology of purine analogues. *Fed. Proc.,* **26:**898, 1967.

Evans, R. F.; Sagerman, R. H.; Ringrose, J. H.; Auchincloss, J. H.; and Bowman, J.: Pulmonary function following mantle field irradiation for Hodgkin's disease. *Radiology,* **111:**729–731, 1974.

Fairley, K. F.; Barrie, T. U.; and Johnson, W.: Sterility and testicular atrophy related to cyclophosphamide therapy. *Lancet,* **1:**568, 1972.

Fajardo, L. F.; Eltringham, J. R.; and Stewart, J. R.: Combined cardiotoxicity of adriamycin and x-irradiation. *Lab. Invest.,* **34:**86–96, 1976.

Fajardo, L. F.; Stewart, J. R.; and Cohn, K. E.: Morphology of radiation induced heart disease. *Arch. Pathol.,* **86:**512–579, 1968.

Feingold, M. L., and Kass, L. G.: Effects of long term administration of busulfan. *Arch. Intern. Med.,* **124:**66, 1969.

Ferrans, V. J.: Overview of cardiac pathology in relation to anthracycline cardiotoxicity. *Cancer Treat. Rep.,* **62:**955–961, 1978.

Filip, D. J.; Logue, G. L.; Harle, T. S.; and Farrar, W. H.: Pulmonary and hepatic complications of methotrexate therapy of psoriasis. *J.A.M.A.* **215:**881, 1971.

Fowler, J. E.; Barzell, W.; Hilaris, B. S.; and Whitmore, W. F.: Complications of ^{125}iodine implantation and pelvic lymphadenopathy in the treatment of prostatic cancer. *J. Urol.,* **121:**447–451, 1979.

Freeman, J. E.; Johnston, P. G. B.; and Vore, J. M.: Somnolence after prophylactic cranial irradiation in children with acute lymphoblastic leukemia. *Br. Med. J.,* **4:**523–525, 1973.

Freeman-Narrod, M.; Narrod, S. A.; and Custer, R. P.: Chronic toxicity of methotrexate in rats: Partial to complete protection of the liver by choline. *J.N.C.I.,* **59:**1013–1017, 1977.

Frytak, S.; Moertel, C. G.; and O'Fallon, J. R.: Delta-9-tetrahydrocannabinol as an antiemetic for patients receiving chemotherapy. *Ann. Intern. Med.,* **91:**825–830, 1979.

Galton, D. A. G.; Till, M.; and Wiltshaw, E.: Busulfan: Summary of clinical results. *Ann. N.Y. Acad. Sci.,* **68:**967, 1958.

Garrett, M. J.: Teratogenic effect of combination chemotherapy. *Ann. Intern. Med.,* **80:**667, 1974.

Geiser, C. F.; Bishop, Y.; Jaffe, N.; Furman, L.; Traggis, D.; and Frei, E., III: Adverse effects of intrathecal methotrexate in children with acute leukemia in remission. *Blood,* **45:**189, 1975.

George, P: Hemorrhagic cystitic and cyclophosphamide. *Lancet,* **2:**942, 1963.

Glicksman, A. S., and Pajak, T. F.: Early and late effects of lymphoma treatment in the expectation of cure. In Rosenberg, S. A., and Kaplan, H. S. (eds.): *Malignant Lymphomas—Etiology, Immunology, Pathology, Treatment.* Academic Press, New York, 1982.

Glicksman, A. S.; Pajak, T. F.; Gottlieb, A.; Nissen, N.; Stutzman, L.; and Cooper, M. R.: Second malignant neoplasms in patients successfully treated for Hodgkin's disease—A CALGB study. *Cancer Treat. Rep.,* **66:**1035–1044, 1982.

Glicksman, A. S., and Toker, C.: Osteogenic sarcoma following radiotherapy for bursitis. *Mt. Sinai J. Med.* (N.Y.), **43:**163–167, 1976.

Golby, M.: Fertility after renal transplantation. *Transplantation,* **10:**201, 1970.

Goldman, G. C., and Moschella, S. L.: Severe pneumonitis occurring during methotrexate therapy. *Arch. Dermatol.,* **103**:194, 1971.

Gottlieb, J. A., and Serpick, A. A.: Clinical evaluation of 5-(3,3-dimethyl-l-triazone) imidazole-4-carboxamide in malignant melanoma and other neoplasms: Comparison of twice-weekly and daily administration schedules. *Oncology,* **25**:225, 1971.

Grossman, B.; Lessin, L. S.; and Cohen, P.: Droperidol prevents nausea and vomiting from cis-platinum. *N. Engl. J. Med.,* **301**:47, 1979.

Haddain, A.: Mode of action of chemical carcinogens. *Br. Med. Bull.,* **4**:331, 1947.

Halazun, J. F.; Wagner, H. R.; Gaeta, J. F.; and Sinks, L. F.: Daunorubicin cardiac toxicity in children with acute lymphocyte leukemia. *Cancer,* **33**:545, 1974.

Hall, T. C.: Uses of cancer chemotherapeutic agents in non-neoplastic diseases. *Cancer,* **31**:1256, 1973.

Hansen, H. H.; Selawry, O. S.; Holland, J. F.; and McCall, O. B.: The variability of individual tolerance to methotrexate in cancer patients. *Br. J. Cancer,* **25**:298, 1971.

Harris, J. G.: Nausea, vomiting and cancer treatment. *CA,* **28**:194–201, 1978.

Haskell, C. M.; Canellos, G. P.; and Levanthal, B. G.: L-Asparaginase toxicity. *Cancer Res.,* **29**:974, 1969.

Haskell, C. M.; Canellos, G. P.; Leventhal, B. G.; Carbone, P. P.; Block, J. B.; Serpick, A. A.; and Selawry, P. S.: *N. Engl. J. Med.,* **281**:1028, 1969.

Haubrich, R., and Harmis, I.: Unfruchtbarkeit bein eisertigen hadenkebs, malignoma testes orchiectomia, chemotherapy, radiotiosteriletos, post hoc aut propter hoc. *Strahlentherapie,* **146**:94, 1973.

Hayward, R. H.: Arteriosclerosis induced by radiation. *Surg. Clin. North. Am.,* **52**:359–366, 1972.

Heard, B. E., and Cooke, R. A.: Busulfan lung. *Thorax,* **23**:187, 1968.

Heidenberg, W. J.; Lupovitch, A.; and Tarr, N.: Pulseless disease complicating Hodgkin's disease. *J.A.M.A.,* **195**:488–491, 1966.

Henderson, I. C., and Frei, E.: Adriamycin and the heart. *N. Engl. J. Med.,* **300**:310–312, 1979.

Herman, E. H.; Mhatre, R. M.; and Chadwick, D. P.: Modification of some of the toxic effects of daunomycin (NSC-82151) by pretreatment with the antineoplastic agent ICRF 159 (NSC-129943). *Toxicol. Appl. Pharmacol.,* **27**:517–526, 1974.

Herman, T. S.; Einhorn, L.; Jones, S. E.: Superiority of nabilone over prochlorperazine as an antiemetic in patients receiving chemotherapy. *N. Engl. J. Med.,* **300**:1295–1297, 1979.

Hersh, E. M.; Wong, V. G.; Henderson, E. S.; and Freirich, E. J.: Hepatotoxic effects of methotrexate. *Cancer,* **19**:600, 1966.

Higby, D. J.; Wallace, H. J., Jr.; and Holland, J. F.: Diamminedichloroplatinum (NSC-119875): A phase I study. *Cancer Chemother. Rep.,* **57**:459–463, 1973.

Holland, J. F.; Scharlau, C.; Gailani, S.; Krant, M. J.; Olson, K. B.; Horton, J.; Shnider, B. I.; Lynch, J. J.; Owens, A.; Carbone, P. P.; Colsky, J.; Grob, D.; Miller, S. P.; and Hall, T. C.: Vincristine treatment of advanced cancer: A cooperative study of 392 cases. *Cancer Res.,* **33**:1258–1264, 1973.

Holmes, G. E., and Holmes, F. F.: Pregnancy outcome of patients treated for Hodgkin's disease. *Cancer,* **41**:1317–1322, 1978.

Holmes, H. A., and Holmes, F. F.: After ten years, what are the handicaps and lifestyles of children treated for cancer? *Clin. Pediatr.* (Phila.), **14**:819–823, 1975.

Host, H., and Nissen-Meyer, R.: A preliminary clinical study of cyclophosphamide. *Cancer Chemother. Rep.,* **9**:47, 1960.

Host, H., and Vale, J. R.: Lung function after mantle field irradiation in Hodgkin's disease. *Cancer,* **32**:329–332, 1973.

Hoston, J.; Olson, K. B.; Sullivan, J.; Reilly, C.; Shnider, B.; and The Eastern Cooperative Oncology Group: 5-fluorouracil in cancer: An improved regimen. *Ann. Intern. Med.,* **73**:897–900, 1970.

Huffman, D. H.; Wan, S. H.; Azarnoff, D. L.; and Hoogstraten, B.: Pharmacokinetics of methotrexate. *Cancer Chemother. Rep.,* **6**:19–24, 1973.

Hutter, R. V.; Shipkey, F. H.; Tan, C. T.; Murphy, M. L.; and Chowdhury, M.: Hepatic fibrosis in children with acute leukemia: A complication of therapy. *Cancer,* **13**:288–307, 1960.

Ihde, D. C., and DeVita, V. T.: Osteonecrosis of the femoral head in patients with lymphoma treated with intermittent combination chemotherapy. *Cancer,* **36**:1585–1588, 1975.

Ingold, J. A.; Reed, G. B.; Kaplan, H. S.; and Bagshaw, M. A.: Radiation hepatitis. *Am. J. Roentgen.,* **93**:200–208, 1965.

Isacoff, W. H.; Townsend, C. M.; Eilber, F. R.; Forster, T.; Morton, D. L.; and Block, J. B.: High-dose methotrexate therapy of solid tumors: Observations relating to clinical toxicity. *Med. Pediatr. Oncol.,* **2**:319–325, 1976.

Jacobs, S. A.; Bleyer, W. A.; Chabner, B. A.; and Johns, D. G.: Altered plasma pharmacokinetics of methotrexate administered intrathecally. *Lancet,* **1**:455–456, 1975.

Jennings, F. L., and Arden, A.: Development of radiation pneumonitis—Time and dose factors. *Arch. Pathol.,* **74**:351–360, 1962.

Johnson, W. W., and Meadows, D. C.: Urinary-bladder fibrosis and telangiectasia associated with long-term cyclophosphamide therapy. *N. Engl. J. Med.,* **284**:290, 1971.

Kaplan, H. S., and Stewart, J. R.: Complications of intensive megavoltage radiotherapy for Hodgkin's disease. *Natl. Cancer Inst. Monogr.,* **36**:439–444, 1973.

Kaplan, S. R., and Calabresi, P.: Drug therapy: Immunosuppressive agents. *N. Engl. J. Med.,* **289**:952, 1973.

Kass, L. G.; Melamed, M. R.; and Mayer, K.: The effect of busulfan on human epithelia. *Am. J. Clin. Pathol.,* **44**:385, 1965.

Kennedy, B. J.: Metabolic and toxic effects of mithramycin during tumor therapy. *Am. J. Med.,* **49**:494, 1970.

Killen, J.; Mitchell, E. P.; Woolley, P. V.; Phase II studies of methylglyoxal-bis-quanylhydrazone. *Cancer,* **50**:1258–1261, 1982.

Kirkland, R. T.; Bongiovanni, A. M.; Cornfeld, D.; McCormick, J. B.; Parks, J. S.; and Tenore, A.: Gonadotropin responses to luteinizing releasing factor in boys treated with cyclophosphamide for nephrotic syndrome. *J. Pediatr.,* **89**:941–944, 1976.

Kopelson, G., and Herwig, K. J.: Etiologies of coronary artery disease in cancer patients. *Int. J. Radiat. Oncol. Biol. Phys.,* **4**:895–906, 1978.

Kovach, J. S.; Moertel, C. G.; Schutt, A. J.; Reitemeier, R. G.; and Hahn, R. G.: Phase II study of cis-diamminedichloroplatinum (NSC-119875) in advanced carcinoma of the large bowel. *Cancer Chemother. Rep.,* **57**:357, 1973.

Krawitt, E. L.; Stein, J. H.; Kirkendall, W. M.; and Clifton, J. A.: Mercaptopurine hepatotoxicity in a patient with chronic active hepatitis. *Arch. Intern. Med.,* **120:**729, 1967.

Kuhn, J. A.; Argy, W. P.; Rakowski, T. A.; Moriarty, J. K., Jr.; Schreiner, G. E.; and Schein, P. S.: Nephrotoxicity of cis-diamminedichloroplatinum II as measured by urinary-glucoronidase. *Cancer Treat. Rep.,* **64:**1083–1086, 1980.

Lassvik, C.; Rosengren, B.; and Wranne, B.: Pulmonary gas exchange following irradiation of cervical, mediastinal, hilar and axillary nodes. *Acta Radiol. Ther. Phys. Biol.,* **16:**27–31, 1977.

Leake, E.; Smith, W. G.; and Woodliff, H. J.: Diffuse interstitial pulmonary fibrosis after busulfan therapy. *Lancet,* **2:**432, 1963.

LeFloch, O.; Donaldson, S. S.; and Kaplan, H. S.: Pregnancy following oophoropexy and total nodal irradiation in women with Hodgkin's disease. *Cancer,* **38:**2263–2268, 1976.

LeFrok, E. A.; Pitha, J.; and Rosenheim, S.: A clinicopathologic analysis of adriamycin cardiotoxicity. *Cancer,* **3:**302, 1973.

Legha, S. S.; Benjamin, R. S.; Eroy, M. S.; Mackay, B.; Ewer, M.; Wallace, S.; Valdiviesa, M.; Rasmussen, S. L.; Blumenschein, G. R.; and Freireich, E. J.: Reduction of doxorubicin cardiotoxicity by prolonged continuous intravenous infusion. *Ann. Intern. Med.,* **96:**133–139, 1982.

Lee, W.; Moore, R. P.; and Wampler, G. L.: Interstitial pulmonary fibrosis as a complication of prolonged methyl-CCNU therapy. *Cancer Treat. Rep.,* **62:**1355–1358, 1978.

Li, F. P.; Fine, W.; Jaffee, N.; Holmes, G. E.; and Holmes, F. F.: Offspring of patients treated for cancer in childhood. *J.N.C.I.,* **62:**1193–1197, 1979.

Libshitz, H. I., and Southard, M. E.: Complications of radiation therapy: The thorax. *Semin. Roentgenol.,* **9:**41–49, 1974.

Littler, W. A.; Kay, J. M.; and Hasleton, P. S.: Busulfan lung. *Thorax,* **24:**639, 1969.

Low, M. P.: Radiation-induced vascular injury and its relation to late effects in normal tissues. *Adv. Radiat. Biol.,* **9:**37–73, 1981.

Lucas, V. S., and Laszlo, J.: Delta-9-tetrahydrocannabinol for refractory vomiting induced by cancer chemotherapy. *J.A.M.A.,* **243:**1241–1243, 1980.

Lushbaugh, C. C., and Caserett, G. W.: The effects of gonadal irradiation in clinical radiation therapy: A review. *Cancer,* **37:**1111–1120, 1976.

Luxton, R. W., and Kunkler, P. B.: Radiation nephritis. *Acta Radiol. (Ther.),* (Stockh.), **2:**169–178, 1964.

McCabe, M.; Smith, F. P.; MacDonald, J. S.; Goldberg, D.; Woolley, P. V.; and Schein, P. S.: Comparative trial of oral delta-9-tetrahydrocannabinol (THC) and prochlorperazine (PCZ) for cancer chemotherapy-related nausea and vomiting. *Proc. Am. Soc. Clin. Oncol.,* **22:**4161, 1981.

McIlvanie, S. K., and MacCarthy, J. D.: Hepatitis in association with prolonged 6-mercaptopurine therapy. *Blood,* **14:**80, 1959.

Maier, J. G.: Radiation myelitis of the spinal cord. *Front. Radiat. Ther. Oncol.,* **6:**404–411, 1972.

Mark, G. J.; Lehinger-Zadeh, H.; and Ragsdale, B. D.: Cyclophosphamide pneumonitis. *Thorax,* **38:**89–93, 1978.

Marsh, F. P.; Vince, F. P.; Pollock, D. J.; Path, M. C.; Blandy, J. P.; and Chir, M.: Cyclophosphamide necrosis of bladder causing calcification, contracture and reflux; treated by colocystoplasty. *Br. J. Urol.,* **43:**324, 1971.

Masland, D. S.; Rotz, C. T.; and Harris, T. H.: Post radiation pericarditis with chronic pericardial effusion. *Ann. Intern. Med.,* **69:**97–102, 1968.

Meadows, A. T.; and Evans, A. E.: Effects of chemotherapy on the central nervous system. *Cancer,* **37:**1079–1085, 1976.

Min, K., and Gyorkey, F.: Interstitial fibrosis, atypical epithelial changes and brochiolar cell carcinoma following busulfan therapy. *Cancer,* **22:**1027, 1968.

Moertel, C. G.: *Multiple Primary Malignant Neoplasms: Their Incidence and Significance.* Springer-Verlag New York, Inc., New York, 1966.

Moertel, C. G., and Reitemeier, R. S.: Controlled clinical studies of orally administered antiemetic drugs. *Gastroenterology,* **57:**262–268, 1969.

Moertel, C. G.; Reitemeier, R. J.; and Gage, R. P.: A controlled clinical investigation of antiemetic drugs. *J.A.M.A.,* **186:**116–118, 1963.

Moertel, C. G.; Reitemeier, R. J.; and Hahn, R. G.: Fluorinated pyrimidine therapy of advanced gastrointestinal cancer. *Gastroenterology,* **46:**371, 1964.

Malpas, J., and Scott, M.: Daunomycin in acute myelocytic leukemia. *Lancet,* **1:**469, 1969.

Muller, S. A.; Farrow, G. M.; and Martalock, D. L.: Cirrhosis caused by methotrexate in the treatment of psoriasis. *Arch. Dermatol.,* **100:**523, 1969.

Myers, C. E.; McGuire, W. P.; Liss, R. H.; Grotzinger, K.; and Young, R. C.: Adriamycin: The role of lipid peroxidation in cardiac toxicity and tumor response. *Science,* **197:**165–167, 1977.

Nahas, W. A.; Nisce, L. Z.; D'Angio, G.; and Lewis, J. R.: Lateral ovarian transposition. *Obstet. Gynecol.,* **38:**785–788, 1971.

Narayar, P., and Lange, P. H.: Current controversies in the management of carcinoma of the prostate. *Semin. Oncol.,* **7:**460–467, 1980.

Newhauser, E. B. D.; Wittenberg, M. H.; Berman, C. Z.; and Cohen, J.: Irradiation effects of roentgen therapy on the growing spine. *Radiology,* **59:**637–650, 1952.

Nicholson, H. O.: Cytotoxic drugs in pregnancy. *J. Obstet. Gynaecol. Br. Commonw.,* **75:**307, 1968.

Oettgen, H. F.; Stephenson, P. A.; Schwartz, M. K.; Leeper, R. D.; Tallal, L.; and Burchenal, J. H.: Toxicity of E. coli L-asparaginase in man. *Cancer,* **25:**253–278, 1969.

O'Malley, J. E.; Koocher, G.; Foster, D.; and Slavin, L.: Psychiatric sequelae of surviving childhood cancer. *Am. J. Orthopsychiatry,* **49:**608–616, 1979.

Orwoll, E. S.; Kiessling, P. J.; and Paterson, J. R.: Interstitial pneumonia from mitomycin. *Ann. Intern. Med.,* **89:**352–355, 1978.

Penn, I.; Makowski, E.; Droegmueller, W.; Halgrimson, C. G.; and Starzl, T. E.: Parenthood in renal homograft recipients. *J.A.M.A.,* **216:**1755, 1971.

Perrault, D. J.; Gilbert, B. W.; Levy, M. D.; Herman, J.; and Adelman, A. G.: Longterm effects of upper mantle radiation on the heart in patients with lymphoma. *Proc. Am. Assoc. Cancer Res. Am. Soc. Clin. Oncol.,* ASCO 21, 349, Abstr. C-297, 1980.

Perthes, G.: Uber den eingluss der roentgenstrahlen auj epitheliale gewebe, inshesondere auj das carcinon. *Arch. Clin. Chir.,* **79:**955–1000, 1903.

Phillips, T.; Wharam, M. D.; and Margolis, L. W.: Modification of radiation injury to normal tissues by chemotherapeutic agents. *Cancer,* **35:**1678, 1684, 1975.

Pittman, S. W.; Parker, L. M.; Tattersall, M. H. N.; Jaffe, N.; and Frei, E.: Clinical trial of high-dose methotrexate (NSC-740) with citrovorum factor (NSC-3590). Toxicologic and therapeutic observations. *Cancer Chemother. Rep.,* **6**(Part 3):43, 1975.

Plotkin, D. A.; Plotkin, D.; and Okien, R.: Haloperidol in the treatment of nausea and vomiting due to cytotoxic drug administration. *Curr. Ther. Res.,* **15**:599–602, 1973.

Podall, L. N., and Winbler, S.: Busulfan lung. *A.J.R.,* **120**:151, 1974.

Pratt, C. B., and Johnson, W. W.: Duration and severity of fatty metamorphosis of the liver following L-asparaginase therapy. *Cancer,* **28**:361–364, 1971.

Prentice, R. T. W.: Myocardial infarction following radiation. *Lancet,* **2**:388–364, 1965.

Quershi, M. S. A.; Goldsmith, H.; Pennington, J.; Goldsmith, H. J.; and Cox, P. E.: Cyclophosphamide therapy and sterility. *Lancet,* **2**:1290, 1972.

Rahman, A.; Kessler, A.; More, N.; Sikic, B.; Rowden, G.; Woolley, P.; and Schein, P.: Liposomal protection of adriamycin-induced cardiac toxicity in mice. *Cancer Res.,* **41**:1532–1537, 1980.

Ray, G. R.; Trueblood, H. W.; Enright, L. P.; Kaplan, H. S.; and Nelson, T. S.: Oophoropexy: A means of preserving ovarian function following pelvic megavoltage radiotherapy for Hodgkin's disease. *Radiology,* **96**:175–180, 1970.

Reed, G. B.; and Cox, A. J.: The human liver after radiation injury. A form of veno-occlusive disease. *Am. J. Pathol,* **48**:597–611, 1966.

Richter, P.; Calamera, J. C.; Morgenfeld, M. C.; Kierszenbaum, A. L.; Lavieri, J. C.; and Mancini, R. E.: Effects of chlorambucil on spermatogenesis in the human with malignant lymphoma. *Cancer,* **25**:1026, 1970.

Riggenback, R.; Barrett, O.; and Shown, T.: Hemorrhagic cystitis due to cyclophosphamide. *South. Med. J.,* **61**:139, 1968.

Rinehart, J.; Lewis, R.; and Bolcerzak, S. P.: Adriamycin cardiotoxicity in man. *Ann. Intern. Med.,* **81**:475, 1974.

Robin, A. E.; Haggard, M. E.; and Travis, L. B.: Lung changes and chemotherapeutic agents in childhood: Report of a case associated with cyclophosphamide therapy. *Am. J. Dis. Child.,* **129**:337, 1970.

Roenigk, H. H., Jr.; Bergfield, W. F.; St. Jacques, R.; Owens, F. J.; and Hawk, W. A.: Hepatotoxicity of methotrexate in the treatment of psoriasis. *Arch. Dermatol.,* **103**:250, 1971.

Rosenaw, E. C., III: The spectrum of drug-induced pulmonary disease. *Ann. Intern. Med.,* **77**:977, 1972.

Rosenthal, S., and Kaufman, S.: Vincristine neurotoxicity. *Ann. Intern. Med.,* **80**:733–737, 1975.

Rowland, J.; Glidewell, O.; Sibley, J. R.; Holland, J. C.; Brecher, M.; Tull, R.; Berman, A.; Glicksman, A. S.; Forman, E.; Harris, M.; McSweeney, J.; Jones, B.; Black, M.; Cohen, M.; and Freeman, A. L.; for Cancer and Leukemia Group B (CALGB): Effect of cranial radiation (CRT) on neuropsychologic function in children with acute lymphocytic leukemia (ALL). *Proceedings, ASCO,* **1**:123, 1982.

Sallan, S.; Zinsberg, N.; and Frei, E. M.: Antiemetic effect of delta-9-tetrahydrocannabinol in patients receiving cancer chemotherapy. *N. Engl. J. Med.,* **293**:795–797, 1975.

Sandler, S. G.; Tobin, W.; and Henderson, E. S.: Vincristine induced neuropathy: A clinical study of fifty leukemia patients. *Neurology* (Minneapolis), **19**:367–374, 1969.

Schein, P. S.; O'Connell, M. J.; Blom, J.; Hubbard, S.; Magrath, I. T.; Bergevin, P.; Wiernik, P. H.; Ziegler, J. L.; and DeVita, V. T.: Clinical antitumor activity and toxicity of streptozotocin (NSC-85998). *Cancer,* **34**:993, 1974.

Schein, P. S., and Winokur, S. H.: Immunosuppressive and cytotoxic chemotherapy: Long term complications. *Ann. Intern. Med.,* **82**:84, 1975.

Schilsky, R. L., and Erlichman, C.: Late complications of chemotherapy: Infertility and carcinogens. In Chabner, B. (ed.): *Pharmacologic Principles of Cancer Treatment.* W. B. Saunders Company, Philadelphia, 1982.

Schilsky, R. L.; Sherins, R. J.; Hubbard, S. M.; Wesley, M. N.; Young, R. C.; and DeVita, V. T.: Longterm follow-up of ovarian function in women treated with MOPP chemotherapy for Hodgkin's disease. *Am. J. Med.,* **71**:552–556, 1981.

Schottenfeld, D.: Multiple primary cancers. In Schottenfeld, D., and Fraumeni, J. (eds.): *Cancer Epidemiology and Prevention.* W. B. Saunders Company, Philadelphia, 1982.

Schwartz, J. R., and Kajani, M. K.: Methotrexate therapy and pulmonary disease. *J.A.M.A.,* **210**:1924, 1969.

Scogna, D., and Smalley, R.: Chemotherapy induced nausea and vomiting. *Am. J. Nurs.,* **79**:1562–1564, 1979.

Sherins, R. J., and DeVita, V. T., Jr.: Effect of drug treatment for lymphoma on male reproduction capacity. Studies of men in remission after therapy. *Ann. Intern. Med.,* **79**:216, 1973.

Sherins, R. J.; Olweny, C. L.; and Siegler, J. L.: Gynecomastia and gonadal dysfunction in adolescent boys treated with combination chemotherapy for Hodgkin's disease. *N. Engl. J. Med.,* **229**:12–16, 1979.

Sherlock, P. (ed.): Effect of cancer treatment on nutrition and gastrointestinal function. *Clin. Bull.,* **9**:136–145, 1979.

Sieber, S. M., and Adamson, R. H.: Toxicity of antineoplastic agents in man: Chromosome aberrations, antifertility effects, congenital malformations and carcinogenic potential. *Adv. Cancer Res.,* **22**:57–155, 1975.

Simon, R.: Statistical methods for evaluating pregnancy outcomes in patients with Hodgkin's disease. *Cancer,* **45**:2890–2892, 1980.

Skinner, M. D., and Schwartz, R. S.: Immunosuppressive therapy. *N. Engl. J. Med.,* **287**:221–281, 1972.

Sobrinho, L. G.; Levine, R. A.; and DiConte, R. G.: Amenorrhea in patients with Hodgkin's disease treated with antineoplastic agents. *Am. J. Obstet. Gynecol.,* **109**:135–139, 1971.

Sostman, H. D.; Matthoy, R. A.; Putnam, C.; and Walker-Smith, G. J.: Methotrexate induced pneumonitis. *Medicine* (Baltimore), **55**:371–388, 1976.

Steinberg, A. D.; Plotz, P. H.; Wolff, S. M.; Wong, V. G.; Agus, S. G.; and Decker, J. L.: Cytotoxic drugs in treatment of non-malignant disease. *Ann. Intern. Med.,* **76**:619, 1972.

Stoller, R. G.; Hane, K. R.; and Jacobs, S. A.: Use of plasma pharmacokinetics to predict and prevent methotrexate toxicity. *N. Engl. J. Med.,* **297**:630–634, 1977.

Stoller, R. G.; Jacobs, S. A.; Drake, J. C.; Lutz, R. J.; and Chabner, B. A.: Pharmacokinetics of high-dose methotrexate (NSC-740). *Cancer Chemother. Rep.,* **6**:19–24, 1975.

Talley, P. N.; O'Bryan, R. M.; Gutterman, J. U.; Brownlee, R. W.; and McCredie, K. B.: Clinical evaluation of toxic effects of cis-diamminedichloroplatinum II (NSC-119875)—Phase I study. *Cancer Chemother. Rep.,* **57**:465, 1973.

Tefft, M.: Radiation effect on growing bone and cartilage. *Front. Radiat. Ther. Oncol.,* **6**:289–311, 1972.

Tefft, M.; Lattin, P. B.; Jereb, B.; Cham, W.; Ghavimi, F.;

Rosen, G.; Exclby, P.; Marcove, P.; Murphy, M. L.; and D'Angio, G. J.: Acute and late effects on normal tissues following combined chemotherapy and radiotherapy for childhood rhabdomyosarcoma and Ewing's sarcoma. *Cancer,* 37:1201–1213, 1976.

Tefft, M.; Mitus, A.; Das, L.; Vawter, G. F.; and Filler, R. M.: Irradiation of the liver in children: A review of experience in the acute and chronic phases, and in the intact normal and partically resected. *Am. J. Roentgenol.,* 108:365–385, 1970.

Thachiel, J. V.; Jewett, M. A. S.; and Rider, W. D.: The effects of cancer and cancer therapy on male fertility. *J. Urol.,* 126:141–145, 1981.

Thiersch, J. B.: Therapeutic abortions with a folic acid antagonist, 4-amino pteroylglutamic acid administered by the oral route. *Am. J. Obstet. Gynecol.,* 63:1298, 1952.

Topilow, A. A.; Rothenberg, S. P.; and Cottrell, T. S.: Interstitial pneumonia after prolonged treatment with cyclophosphamide. *Am. Rev. Respir. Dis.,* 108:114, 1973.

Travis, E. L.; Down, J. D.; Holmes, S. J.; and Hobson, B.: Radiation pneumonitis and fibrosis in mouse lung assayed by respiratory frequency and histology. *Radiat. Res.,* 84:133–143, 1980.

Uldall, P. R.; Kerr, D. N. S.; and Tacchi, D.: Sterility and cyclophosphamide. *Lancet,* 1:693, 1972.

Van Thiel, D. H.; Sherins, R. J.; Myers, G. H., Jr.: Evidence for a specific seminiferous tubular factor affecting follicle-stimulating hormone secretion in man. *J. Clin. Invest.,* 51:1009–1019, 1972.

Von Hoff, D. D.; Layard, M. W.; Basa, P.; Davis, H. L., Jr.; Von Hoff, A. L.; Rozencweig, M.; and Muggia, F. M.: Risk factors for doxorubicin-induced congestive heart failure. *Ann. Intern. Med.,* 91:710–717, 1979.

Von Hoff, D. D.; Rozencweig, M.; and Piccart, M.: The cardiac toxicity of anticancer agents. *Semin. Oncol.,* 9:23–33, 1982.

Wall, R. L., and Clausen, K. P.: Carcinoma of the urinary bladder in patients receiving cyclophosphamide. *N. Engl. J. Med.,* 293:271, 1975.

Wan, S. H.; Huffman, D. H.; Azarnoff, D. L.; Stephens, R.; and Hoogstreten, B.: Effect of route of administration and effusions on methotrexate pharmacokinetics. *Cancer Res.,* 34:3487–3491, 1974.

Wang, S. C.: Emetic and antiemetic drugs. In Root, W. C., and Hoffman, F. G. (eds.): *Physiological Pharmacology. The Nervous System. Part B.* Academic Press, New York, 1965.

Wang, S. C.; Rinz, A. A.; and Chinn, H. I.: Mechanism of emesis following irradiation. *Am. J. Physiol.,* 193:335–339, 1958.

Wara, W. M.; Phillips, T. L.; Margolis, L. W.; and Smith, V.: Radiation pneumonitis: A new approach to the derivation of time-dose factors. *Cancer,* 32:547–552, 1973.

Warin, A. P.; Landells, J. W.; Levene, G. M.; and Baker, H.: A prospective study of the effects of weekly oral methotrexate on liver biopsy. *Br. J. Dermatol.,* 93:321–327, 1975.

Warne, G. L.; Fairley, K. F.; Hobbs, J. B.; Martin, F. I. R.: Cyclophosphamide-induced ovarian failure. *N. Engl. J. Med.,* 289:1159, 1973.

Weinstein, G.; Roenigk, H.; Maibach, H.; Cosmides, J.; Almeyda, J.; Auerbach, R.; Bergfeld, W.; Clyde, D.; Dahl, M.; Frost, P.; Krueger, R.; Lee, J.; Lungquist, A.; Schaffner, F.; Scheuer, P.; and Zachariae, H.: Psoriasis-liver-methotrexate interactions. *Arch. Dermatol.,* 108:36, 1973.

Weiss, H.; Walker, M.; and Wiernik, P.: Neurotoxicity of commonly used antineoplastic agents. *N. Engl. J. Med.,* 291:75–81, 127–133, 1974.

Weiss, R. B.; Poster, D. S.; and Penta, J. S.: Nitrosoureas and pulmonary toxicity. *Cancer Treat. Rev.,* 8:111–125, 1981.

Whitehead, G.; Shalet, S. M.; Blackledge, G.; Todd, I.; Crowther, D.; and Beardwell, C. G.: The effects of Hodgkin's disease and combination chemotherapy. *Cancer,* 49:418–422, 1982.

Wolback, S. B.: Pathologic histology of chronic x-ray dermatitis and early x-ray carcinoma. *J. Med. Res.,* 21:415–450, 1909.

Yagoda, A.; Mukhirji, B.; Young, C.; Etcubanas, E.; Lamonte, C.; Smith, J. R.; Tan, T. C.; and Krakoff, I. H.: Bleomycin, an antitumor antibiotic: Clinical experiment in 274 patients. *Ann. Intern. Med.,* 77:861, 1972.

Young, R. C.; Walker, M. D.; Canellos, G.; and Schein, P. S.: Initial clinical trials with methyl-CCNU 1-(2-chloroethyl)-3-(4-methylcyclohexyl)-1-nitrosourea (McCCNU). *Cancer,* 31:1164, 1973.

Zachariae, H.; Kragballe, K.; and Sogaard, H.: Methotrexate induced liver cirrhosis. Studies including serial liver biopsies during continued treatment. *Br. J. Dermatol.,* 102:407–412, 1980.

Zarday, Z.; Veith, I. J.; Gliedman, M. L.; Soberman, R.: Irreversible liver damage after azathiaoprine. *J.A.M.A.,* 222:690, 1972.

Section Two
Specific Neoplasms

15

Hodgkin's Disease

SAUL A. ROSENBERG

Introduction

Hodgkin's disease is a primary neoplasm of lymphoid tissue. The characteristic pathologic findings of Hodgkin's disease distinguish it from the other primary lymphoid tumors, usually called the non-Hodgkin's lymphomas. The disease was first recognized by Thomas Hodgkin in 1832, when he described seven cases based on their peculiar clinical and gross pathologic findings. Subsequently, only three of Hodgkin's original cases were shown to contain the Reed-Sternberg giant cells now considered necessary to establish the diagnosis. The disease has been of great interest because of its infectious-disease-like symptoms and findings, its epidemiologic characteristics, its associated immunologic abnormalities, and its responsiveness to therapy. A uniformly fatal disorder when first recognized and if untreated, the majority of patients with Hodgkin's disease can now be cured of their neoplasms.

Incidence and Epidemiology

Approximately 7500 new patients with Hodgkin's disease are diagnosed in the United States annually. It is more common in males (sex ratio of ca. 1.4:1), especially before puberty (sex ratio 6 to 10:1). In the United States and other developed countries there is a bimodal age-specific incidence rate, with an early peak in young adulthood and another with advanced age (MacMahon, 1966). In Japan, the early peak is absent, presumably because of a reduced incidence of the nodular sclerosis pathologic subtype, which is discussed in the pathology section of this chapter.

A relatively high incidence of Hodgkin's disease among young men in undeveloped countries has been observed. These boys have the relatively aggressive histologic subtypes.

Important epidemiologic observations that correlate socioeconomic factors and the incidence of the disease have been reported. The disease is more common among individuals with few or no siblings, those with higher educational levels, and among urban rather than rural dwellers. Certain parallels with paralytic poliomyelitis have been emphasized in which there is an early common exposure to an infectious agent (Gutensohn and Cole, 1981).

Hodgkin's disease has a higher than expected incidence among siblings. It has been estimated that a sibling of a patient with Hodgkin's disease has a fivefold risk of developing the disease. If the sibling is of the same sex the risk is even greater, at ninefold. Preliminary studies suggest that there may be a region near the dR locus associated with familial Hodgkin's disease. All cases expressed this trait, and a higher incidence of the trait is present in nonfamilial Hodgkin's disease than in the general population (Tucker, *et al.*, 1980). These important observations need confirmation and analysis.

Other epidemiologic associations with the incidence of Hodgkin's disease, including tonsillectomy, appendectomy, infectious mononucleosis, and case clustering have been suggested. These associations or observations are not uniformly accepted or confirmed.

Etiology and Pathogenesis

Numerous attempts have been made to isolate a pathogenetic microorganism from patients with Hodgkin's disease. These efforts have been frustrated by the frequent infectious disease complications of patients with the disease. Among the leading candidates since the turn of the century have been mycobacterium tuberculosis, brucella, diphtheroids, and the herpes viruses. None of these potential causative agents have been confirmed, though initial reports by very qualified investigators were considered promising. The absence of an acceptable animal model for Hodgkin's disease has inhibited progress in our understanding of the etiology and pathogenesis of the disease. Similarities of the human disease to the graft versus host phenomenon in both animals and man have been observed by Kaplan and Smithers (1959).

Whether or not Hodgkin's disease is a "true" neoplasm corresponding to other human tumors has long been a matter of debate. It is noteworthy that the majority of the tumor mass, responsible for the major clinical findings, is composed of inflammatory, presumed non-neoplastic cells. Cells that meet the accepted criteria of being neoplastic are often very rare in Hodgkin's disease tissue. It may be that the mononuclear variant of the diagnostic Reed-Sternberg multinucleated giant cell is the major tumor cell in the disease. Current evidence favors that this cell is derived from the monocyte-macrophage system, rather than from a B or T lymphocyte precursor (Kaplan and Gartner 1977; Kadin et al., 1978).

The immunologic abnormalities of patients with Hodgkin's disease are unique and may have important implications relating to the etiology and pathogenesis of the disease. As newer immunologic methods and concepts have become available, greater insight and understanding of the abnormalities identified have resulted.

A defect in cell-mediated immunity has been recognized in patients with Hodgkin's disease since the detailed studies of Schier in the 1950s (Schier et al., 1954). A relative lymphocytopenia is characteristic of the disease, especially in patients with advanced and progressive disease. The immunologic abnormalities of patients with Hodgkin's disease are complicated by the acute and long-term effects of the therapy, especially of radiotherapy, used in the management of the disease. Previously untreated patients, however, can be shown to have a relative T-lymphocytopenia, T-lymphocyte dysfunction, and a serum factor that interferes with normal T-lymphocyte reactions (Hersh and Oppenheim, 1965; Fuks et al., 1976b; Hillinger and Herzig, 1978).

Despite the observations that an early and continuous abnormality of T-cell function exists in patients with Hodgkin's disease, B-cell function is relatively normal. Circulating immunoglobulin levels and antibody response are normal in Hodgkin's disease patients, at least until they enter the terminal phase of their illness.

Pathology

The minimum requirement for the pathologic diagnosis of Hodgkin's disease is the presence of characteristic giant cells of the Reed-Sternberg type in an appropriate histologic setting. The diversity of the morphologic findings, however, in the number and appearance of the giant cells, the variable presumptive inflammatory type of cellular proliferation, and degrees of necrosis and fibrosis are so great as to challenge the belief that Hodgkin's disease is in fact a single entity (Lukes et al., 1966a).

The most reliable characteristics of the Reed-Sternberg cell are the large inclusion-like nucleoli and the double or multiple nuclei of large size (see Figure 15-1). Mononuclear forms are also found in typical lesions of Hodgkin's disease, but cannot be considered as reliably diagnostic, because they may be confused with immunoblasts of viral and other antigenically stimulated reactions. A peculiar clear zone about the huge nucleolus is a distinctive feature of these cells. The nucleolus is typically large and spherical, with smooth margins and homogeneous eosinophilic or amphophilic staining characteristics. The Reed-Sternberg cells may vary considerably in

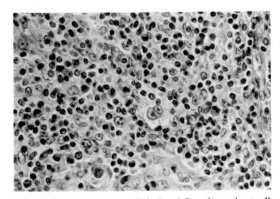

Figure 15-1. A characteristic Reed-Sternberg giant cell with a background of mixed cellularity Hodgkin's disease.

their morphologic appearance, depending on the histologic subtype.

When lymphocyte proliferation is prominent, the characteristic Reed-Sternberg cells are rare. When lymphocytes appear to be depleted, typical Reed-Sternberg cells with characteristic polyploid vesicular nuclei and huge inclusion-like nucleoli are numerous. The distinctive multinucleated giant cells associated with the nodular sclerosis variety are presumed to be variants of the Reed-Sternberg cell with abundant pale eosinophilic cytoplasm, well-defined cellular borders in lacuna-like spaces (in formalin-fixed tissue), with small- to medium-sized nucleoli, and an unusual degree of hyperlobation.

Cells indistinguishable from, or closely resembling, Reed-Sternberg cells may be found in conditions other than Hodgkin's disease, especially infectious mononucleosis (Lukes *et al.,* 1969). The appropriate cellular and architectural environment for these cells is required, therefore, to permit the diagnosis of Hodgkin's disease.

More than 30 years ago, Jackson and Parker put forward their classic histopathologic classification, which divided Hodgkin's disease into three categories: paragranuloma, granuloma, and sarcoma. This classification proved of little value in clinical practice, because nearly 90% of all cases were found to fall in the granuloma category. As a result of the work of Lukes and his colleagues, an important subgroup of the former granuloma category, designated nodular sclerosis, has been delineated (Lukes *et al.,* 1966a). This and other refinements have permitted the development of the Rye histopathologic classification (Lukes *et al.,* 1966b), the essential features of which are summarized in Table 15–1. The subtypes of the Rye classification have different prognoses and predict to a moderate degree certain clinical features of the disease. The lymphocyte predominance group has the best overall prognosis and the lymphocyte depletion group the worst. The nodular sclerosis group in general has a very good natural history and prognosis though some patients with this histopathologic type may be relatively resistant to therapy and have a very aggressive short course. The mixed cellularity picture identifies a relatively unfavorable group of patients. The prognostic variables of the histopathologic classification are not totally independent of other important variables such as the sites and extent of involvement, age, sex, and the presence or absence of systemic symptoms. The results of current, highly successful treatment programs are reducing the differences in survival formerly observed among the various histopathologic types of Hodgkin's disease (see Figures 15–2A and 15–2B).

The origin and neoplastic nature of the Reed-Sternberg cell has become increasingly defined. Cytogenetic studies show aneuploidy, often hypotetraploidy, together with structural changes in chromosomes, and perhaps marker chromosomes. These results and the suggestion of monoclonality are consistent with neoplasia. Cultures of Hodgkin's disease tissues have been difficult. Preliminary results yield Reed-Sternberg-like cells, which show aneuploidy and heterotransplantability consistent with a neoplastic origin. Cell marker studies, phagocytic activity, positive staining reactions for nonspecific esterase, and the capacity to excrete lysozymes suggest origin from the macrophage rather than from the lymphocyte (Kaplan and Gartner, 1977; Kadin *et al.,* 1978).

Table 15–1.   Rye Classification of Hodgkin's Disease

SUBGROUP	MAJOR HISTOLOGIC FEATURES	APPROXIMATE FREQUENCY
Lymphocyte predominance (LPHD)	Abundant normal-appearing lymphocytes with or without benign histiocytes; occasionally nodular; rare Reed-Sternberg (R-S) cells	2–10%
Nodular sclerosis (NSHD)	Nodules of lymphoid infiltrate of varying size, separated by bands of collagen and containing numerous "lacunar cell" variants of R-S cells	40–80%
Mixed cellularity (MCHD)	Pleomorphic infiltrate of eosinophils, plasma cells, histiocytes, and lymphocytes with numerous R-S cells	20–40%
Lymphocyte depletion (LDHD)	Paucity of lymphocytes with numerous R-S cells, often bizarre in appearance; may have diffuse fibrosis or reticulum fibers	2–15%

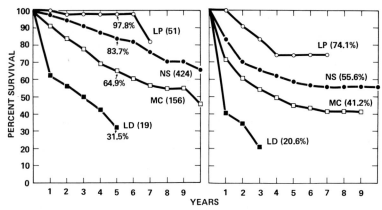

Figure 15–2A. Survival (left-hand graph) and freedom from progression (right-hand graph) actuarial curves of patients with Hodgkin's disease according to the Rye histopathologic type, treated prior to 1970.

Clinical Manifestations

The presenting and subsequent clinical manifestations of patients with Hodgkin's disease can be extremely varied and considerably influenced by the effects of therapy. A common typical presentation is the observation, usually by the patient, of a painless, enlarging mass, most commonly in the neck, but occa-

sionally in the axilla or inguinalfemoral region. Upon examination this is found to be a discrete, rubbery, painless lymphadenopathy, very often with enlarged lymph nodes in close proximity. In other patients, a chest roentgenogram, taken for an unrelated purpose, reveals a moderate or even massive mediastinal enlargement with associated lower cervical lymphadenopathy (see Figure 15–3), which was not apparent to the patient. Though these typical presentations may occur at any age for any histopathologic type, these patients are usually between 15 and 35 years of age and have the histologic subtype of nodular sclerosis.

As the typical asymptomatic patient is eval-

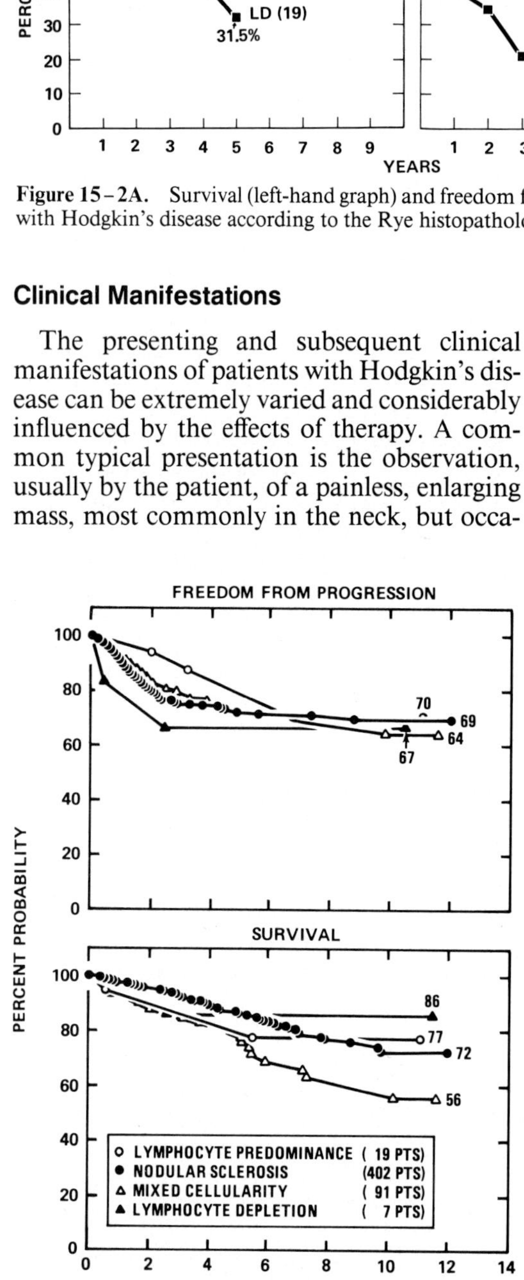

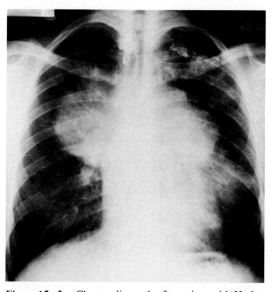

Figure 15–3. Chest radiograph of a patient with Hodgkin's disease, nodular sclerosis subtype.

Figure 15–2B. Survival (lower graph) and freedom from progression (upper graph) actuarial curves of patients with Hodgkin's according to the Rye histopathologic type, treated on protocol studies after 1968.

uated more thoroughly with indicated diagnostic methods, the anatomic extent of disease is usually more widespread than is apparent on physical examination. Frequently, mediastinal enlargement is found on routine or detailed radiologic examination, para-aortic lymphadenopathy is noted on lower extremity lymphography (see Figure 15–4), or splenic involvement is found at exploratory laparotomy in significant numbers of such patients.

The lymphadenopathy may become apparent to the patient or to the physician by producing local symptoms of pain, lymphatic, and/or venous obstruction of an extremity, vena caval obstruction, or airway narrowing. The duration of evident lymphadenopathy be-

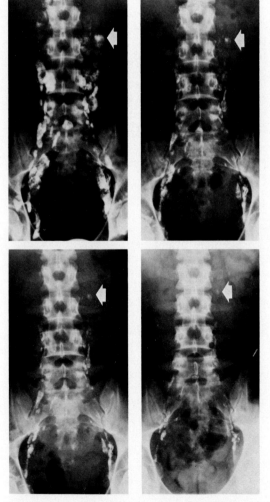

Figure 15–4. Bipedal lymphogram of a patient with stage II$_S$B Hodgkin's disease before (upper left) and during chemotherapy (upper right and lower left) and after para-aortic irradiation (lower right). Note the progressive reduction of lymphadenopathy.

fore diagnosis is extremely variable. Several weeks to several months often elapse between the time of the patient's first symptom and the diagnostic biopsy.

Some patients with Hodgkin's disease have unexplained and persistent fever and/or night sweats as their initial symptoms. Fatigue and weight loss may be associated complaints as these symptoms become more severe and prolonged. These patients tend to be in the older age group, more often male than female, and when evaluated are found to have obvious and more widespread disease than the other patients presenting without symptoms. In older patients, usually past the age of 40, one may see systemic symptoms that are severe, often with associated anemia, but the lymphadenopathy is minimal or occult. Extensive diagnostic efforts may be required to uncover the cause of the symptoms, including lymphography, bone marrow and liver biopsies, or even exploratory laparotomy. In rare cases, the diagnosis is not made before postmortem examination. These older patients, with a predominance of systemic symptoms at the onset of the disease, usually show the histologic varieties of mixed cellularity or lymphocyte depletion (Neiman *et al.*, 1973).

Some patients with Hodgkin's disease have intermittent evening fever lasting several days alternating with afebrile periods lasting days or weeks. The fever gradually becomes more severe and more continuous in most cases. The cyclic fever has been labeled as the Pel-Ebstein type and is rarely a presenting manifestation of the disease.

Pruritus, usually generalized and severe, is another characteristic systemic symptom of Hodgkin's disease. It may appear as a mild localized symptom, but, if due to Hodgkin's disease, it commonly progresses and becomes generalized. Initially, there are no associated skin lesions, but with chronic excoriations, secondary changes of thickening, infections, and pigmentation may be seen. The pruritus may be the only systemic symptom in the otherwise typical presentation of a young person, especially in women. It may also be seen, however, along with fever, sweats, and other systemic symptoms in any patient with Hodgkin's disease. Generalized severe pruritus may occur in patients with lymphoma other than Hodgkin's disease, and in other medical and dermatologic conditions, but the symptom should always suggest underlying Hodgkin's disease. Its cause is unknown.

A few patients complain of pain in the region of tissue involved with Hodgkin's disease within a few minutes after drinking alcoholic beverages. Although this is very suggestive of Hodgkin's disease, it is not diagnostic. Its mechanism is not known.

A wide variety of other symptoms may initially call the attention of the patient and the physician to the disease. These same problems occur more commonly as the course of the disease progresses. Involvement of bone may produce localized pain and tenderness. Epidural tumor masses producing spinal cord compression are rarely the first manifestation of the disease. Peripheral and cranial nerves may be compressed, producing unexplained neurologic deficits. Symptomatic involvement of the lung parenchyma, pleura, and liver, more common in the late stages of the disease, are occasionally responsible for the initial presentation of Hodgkin's disease. More uncommon is early involvement of the skin, gastrointestinal tract, genitourinary system, or central nervous system.

Clinical Course

The clinical course of patients with the disease can be extremely variable. Almost all patients, in addition, receive treatment that may profoundly affect the course of the disease, in many cases resulting in apparent cure, and in some instances resulting in complications that may be difficult to separate from the effects of the disease itself.

Commonly, in a young patient with uncontrolled Hodgkin's disease, the disease progresses at a variable rate, over a period of months or years, to involve lymph nodes adjacent to those initially involved. Extensions of the disease beyond the lymph nodes usually occur in time. Progressive intrathoracic problems may be seen with compression of the airway or great veins, involvement of the pleura and/or pericardium with resultant effusions, increasing pulmonary parenchymal involvement, or local osseous involvement of sternum, clavicle, ribs, pelvis, or vertebrae.

It has been observed that patients with early disease, apparently localized in the neck, may develop disease in the lymph nodes in the celiac, splenic hilar, upper para-aortic region, and/or spleen. Later in the course of the disease, even those patients with an initially favorable prognosis may develop widespread problems, indicating a loss of the host defense

mechanisms. At this stage of the disease, the bone marrow may become focally, then diffusely, involved, with resultant marrow failure. Multiple osseous lesions may occur, usually of an osteoblastic or mixed osteoblastic and osteolytic radiologic appearance. These may produce pain, but rarely pathologic, fractures. The liver may become progressively involved, with diffuse infiltration of the portal spaces resulting in serious and even fatal hepatic dysfunction and laboratory features of intrahepatic biliary obstruction. Liver involvement in Hodgkin's disease has been noted to be highly, if not uniformly, associated with involvement of the spleen (Kaplan, 1980). Peripheral neuropathies as a direct result of tumor growth and epidural cord compression are seen increasingly, as the disease progresses.

Almost all patients with Hodgkin's disease develop increasingly severe systemic symptoms as their disease progresses beyond control. High continuous fever, severe night sweats, malaise, fatigue, anorexia, and weight loss are all characteristics of the terminal picture of patients with Hodgkin's disease. Generalized pruritus is seen in a proportion of patients during their course.

Hematologic Abnormalities

It is difficult to distinguish the effects of therapy for Hodgkin's disease from the effects of the disease itself on hematologic bases. Both radiotherapy and chemotherapy used in the management of Hodgkin's disease may have profound acute effects on bone marrow function and chronic and late effects in some patients. In the untreated or minimally treated patient, however, hematologic abnormalities can be seen and become more obvious and severe as the disease progresses.

Anemia of a mild degree may be found in patients who present with widespread disease, often associated with systemic symptoms. This is usually anemia with normal indices, with a normal or low reticulocyte count, and with a negative Coombs' test. When the condition is analyzed in detail, there may be a shortened red blood cell survival, with inadequate marrow response, as seen in patients with advanced cancer or chronic infection.

Excluding the effects of therapy, which can greatly aggravate the situation, some patients develop severe anemia. This may be due to extensive bone marrow involvement with the disease, hypersplenism with splenomegaly, or, rarely, a Coombs' positive hemolytic picture. Combinations of these factors are responsible for the most profound anemias.

Bone marrow involvement by Hodgkin's disease cannot usually be demonstrated by the marrow aspirate technique and examination of marrow smears. The involvement is focal, often associated with fibrosis and can be discovered more readily by a marrow biopsy performed with a Jamshidi-type needle or open surgical technique. Bone marrow involvement is rarely, if ever, discovered in the favorable patient with limited nodal disease, unless systemic symptoms are present (Rosenberg, 1971; Brunning et al., 1975). It can be found with increasing frequency as the disease becomes more widespread with systemic symptoms and is often associated with an elevated serum alkaline phosphatase, radiologic evidence of bone lesions, and otherwise unexplained pancytopenia. Marrow involvement should always be suspected if the peripheral blood count depression is more extensive than expected after radiotherapy or chemotherapy.

Some patients with Hodgkin's disease develop typical findings of hypersplenism, including splenomegaly, peripheral blood cytopenia, and bone marrow hyperplasia. Even more uncommon is the patient who presents with a moderate or severe hemolytic anemia, elevated reticulocyte count, and positive Coombs' test. The typical findings of an idiopathic thrombocytopenia (ITP), with increased marrow megakaryocytes, may be found. Though sometimes difficult to recognize and manage, ITP may occur without evident disease activity and is not an ominous prognostic finding (Cohen, 1978; Waddell and Cimo, 1979).

The erythrocyte sedimentation is commonly elevated in patients with active disease and may be the only evidence that the disease has been inadequately treated or that clinical recurrence is imminent. It is a nonspecific abnormality, however, and is not always elevated, even when disease is evident. Numerous other laboratory abnormalities have been reported to be correlated with disease activity. These include elevations of serum alpha-2-globulin, fibrinogen, haptoglobin, copper, zinc, and ceruloplasmin; depression of serum iron and iron-binding capacity; elevation of leukocyte alkaline phosphatase; and increases in urinary hydroxyproline and lysozyme.

In the untreated patient, or in one for whom therapy has been minimal, a moderate to marked neutrophilic leukocytosis and thrombocytosis are characteristic of active, symptomatic Hodgkin's disease. The granulocytosis occasionally may be so marked as to suggest an associated complicating or unrelated chronic granulocytic leukemia.

Eosinophilia of a mild degree is not uncommon, but if moderate or marked, tends to occur in patients with severe and longstanding pruritus.

An absolute severe lymphopenia, even in untreated patients, is seen in a small percentage of cases and, when present, is a poor prognostic sign. An absolute lymphocytosis is rarely, if ever, seen in Hodgkin's disease and should always suggest an error in diagnosis, such as, lymphocytic lymphoma or infectious mononucleosis.

Reed-Sternberg cells have been found in the peripheral blood of patients by employing special techniques, but they are rarely seen with the usual hematologic tests.

Acute myelomonocytic leukemia is being reported more frequently in patients, usually with long-standing Hodgkin's disease, who have been treated with combination chemotherapy with or without irradiation (Coleman et al., 1982; Glicksman et al., 1982).

The severely neutropenic patient, no matter what the cause, will have serious problems with infection, which is often responsible for the death of the patient with Hodgkin's disease. With severe thrombocytopenia, whether due to the disease or therapy, hemorrhagic signs and symptoms characteristic of platelet lack are seen, but are only rarely fatal.

Pulmonary Infiltrates

The problem of the pulmonary infiltrate in the patient with Hodgkin's disease is a challenging one. The roentgenographic appearance of pulmonary Hodgkin's disease is variable. Diffuse irregular infiltrates extending from an obvious mediastinal or hilar nodal mass may be present. These may be difficult to distinguish from lymphatic obstruction, partial lung collapse, or infections related to airway obstruction. A typical radiologic appearance of Hodgkin's disease of the lung is multiple discrete pulmonary nodules. These are initially asymptomatic, and if untreated, progress to form large tumor masses. They rarely become excavated, presenting the appearance of a thick wall cavity.

The effects of radiotherapy on the lung and

pleura are important to recognize. Radiation pneumonitis, perihilar fibrosis, and pleural reactions may coexist with persistent or active Hodgkin's disease. The exuberant radiologic changes seen several months after irradiation, when the chest roentgenogram had previously returned to normal, frequently leads the inexperienced physician to conclude that Hodgkin's disease has recrudesced and has extended to the lungs or pleura.

Involvement of the lungs with Hodgkin's disease is common, however, in patients who progress with uncontrolled disease and must be distinguished not only from radiation effects but from a wide spectrum of pulmonary infections.

The most difficult pulmonary lesions to interpret are the linear or slightly nodular infiltrates. The tempo and progress of these infiltrates, the associated clinical status of the patients as regards fever, sputum production and character, and activity of other sites of Hodgkin's disease must be evaluated carefully before the nature of these infiltrates is determined. The therapeutic implications of these radiologic abnormalities are serious and in some instances a diagnostic thoracotomy is justified. The identification of *Pneumocystis carinii,* tuberculosis, the mycoses, or a drug-induced or nonspecific interstitial pneumonia can be of equal or greater therapeutic importance to the patient than the identification of Hodgkin's disease.

Infectious Complications

Almost all patients who have uncontrolled Hodgkin's disease and succumb to their disease will have episodes, usually serious, of infections. These infections occur most frequently during later stages of the disease and are well correlated with the more intensive use of therapy, especially of myelosuppressive drugs and corticosteroids.

At the turn of the century, tuberculosis was very common in patients with Hodgkin's disease and a causal relationship was proposed. Since tuberculosis has come under relative control in the United States and elsewhere, this infection is only rarely observed to coexist with Hodgkin's disease. Though bacterial infections are commonly identified and respond to the modern use of antibiotics, other infections complicate the late clinical course.

Fungal infections, especially of the lungs and meninges, with almost any species, but especially *Cryptococcus,* are encountered in most series of patients with hematologic neoplasms, especially when corticosteroids are administered. Pneumocystis carinii and toxoplasmosis are being recognized with increasing frequency and must be sought because effective therapy is now available. Viral infections, especially herpes zoster and cytomegaloviral infection, have frequently been described.

The occurrence of herpes zoster deserves special emphasis. The association of herpes zoster in patients with underlying illness is not limited to those with Hodgkins' disease. It also occurs with relatively high frequency in patients with other lymphomas, patients on immunosuppressive therapy, and to some extent in those with other neoplasms. The frequency, however, in patients with Hodgkin's disease, even in the young and relatively well individual, is striking. In carefully observed series, that frequency has approached 30%. It is probable that splenectomy and modern aggressive therapeutic approaches are responsible for an increased incidence of this infection. The frequency of disseminated varicella infection following a typical dermatome presentation may be much higher in patients with Hodgkin's disease than previously thought.

Speculation has been made that the pathogenesis and location of the dermatome involved in patients with herpes zoster may be related to involvement of the vertebra or other tissues by Hodgkin's disease in the same dermatome, or perhaps to radiotherapy used within the dermatome. The data are not sufficient to establish this causal relationship.

The prevention and treatment of infections in Hodgkin's disease are reviewed in the chapter on infectious complications (see Chapter 41). Splenectomized patients are at slightly increased risk of developing disseminated bacterial infections, particularly pneumococcal infections. Polyvalent pneumococcal vaccines have been administered, when possible, prior to splenectomy, but the protection resulting is uncertain (Siber *et al.,* 1978; Minor *et al.,* 1979). The prompt use of antibiotics for serious febrile episodes in previously splenectomized patients is indicated. Evidence that antiviral agents, such as interferon and arabinosyladenine, may limit the spread and hasten the resolution of localized herpes infections has been reported (Merigan *et al.,* 1978; Whitley *et al.,* 1982).

Diagnostic Evaluation

The progress being made in the treatment of Hodgkin's disease has paralleled the improvement of techniques for identifying the extent of the disease in the untreated patient. Given the current choices of therapy, it is essential that all patients with Hodgkin's disease be evaluated completely by physicians experienced with the disease before therapeutic decisions are made.

A careful history and physical examination to uncover the characteristic systemic symptoms of fever, night sweats, and pruritus, and to describe all of the lymph node areas of the body are essential. Special attention must be directed to the cervical, supraclavicular, infraclavicular, axillary, epitrochlear, iliac, inguinal, and femoral lymph node areas. Palpable lymph nodes are not all pathologic in the sense that they contain Hodgkin's disease. If, however, there are suspicious lymph nodes that, if involved, would change the therapeutic approach, biopsy should be done for confirmation. The lymphoid tissues in the oropharynx and nasopharynx are rarely involved by Hodgkin's disease, in contrast to other lymphomas. The size of the liver and spleen should be determined as carefully as possible. The bones should be examined for areas of tenderness.

Radiologic examinations should include routine chest films and whole lung tomography to identify mediastinal and hilar lymphadenopathy and pulmonary involvement. Lower extremity lymphography is recommended for all patients, unless pulmonary function is seriously limited. Bone scans complemented with skeletal x-rays are desirable to detect osteoblastic, or less commonly, osteolytic, lesions in symptomatic patients. Routine blood cell counts and determination of the sedimentation rate, serum alkaline phosphatase, urinalysis, and evaluation of renal function are the minimum laboratory studies required for evaluation. Bone marrow biopsy using a needle or an open technique should be performed in all patients with advanced lymph node involvement, systemic symptoms, or suggestive laboratory abnormalities.

The CT scan represents an important non-invasive approach for the evaluation of intrathoracic disease, mesenteric nodes, and other sites.

Exploratory laparotomy and splenectomy are widely used to identify and confirm the presence of Hodgkin's disease in the abdomen and pelvis. Studies have demonstrated that approximately half the patients with clinical or radiologic enlargement of the spleen do not have histologic involvement of that organ, and conversely, in approximately one case in four, spleens of normal size have demonstrable foci of Hodgkin's disease (Glatstein *et al.,* 1969).

The identification of involvement of the liver by Hodgkin's disease is especially difficult. When the organ is massively involved with significant nodular hepatomegaly, clinical jaundice, and an elevated alkaline phosphatase, a needle or open liver biopsy usually confirms nodular lesions or diffuse Hodgkin's disease involvement in the portal areas. In some cases, typical Reed-Sternberg cells may be difficult to identify in small biopsy specimens of the liver, despite the otherwise characteristic cellular infiltrates (Lukes *et al.,* 1971).

It is unusual for marked and obvious liver involvement to occur early in the course of the disease. Abnormalities of liver function tests, such as the serum alkaline phosphatase and other enzymes, modest hepatomegaly, and nonspecific hepatic scan abnormalities may all be misleading. These abnormalities may occur nonspecifically, especially in patients with systemic symptoms, and histologic verification of hepatic involvement should be sought. Conversely, liver involvement can be demonstrated, though rarely, at laparotomy, with no laboratory abnormalities thought to be characteristic of that condition.

Involvement of the spleen with Hodgkin's disease has more significance than involvement of just another lymph node area. An excellent correlation between the size of the spleen and the probability of liver involvement is evident, as documented at laparotomy. It is extremely rare to observe involvement of the liver or bone marrow with Hodgkin's disease without previous or concurrent splenic involvement (Kaplan, 1980).

The advances in our diagnostic ability and the results of detailed study of patients early in their courses provide strong evidence that Hodgkin's disease presents in relatively orderly patterns of involvement, suggesting a unifocal origin. Before the distribution of disease has been altered by treatment, the lymph node involvement is not random, but nodal disease occurs in contiguous regions (or those directly connected by lymphatic channels, such as the low neck and upper para-aortic lymph nodes) in 90% or more of the cases when a second node group is involved (Rosenberg and Kaplan, 1966).

Even after initial radiotherapeutic efforts have controlled the apparent disease, the next site of disease is not random. A high proportion of patients develop disease in untreated regions that are directly contiguous and connected via lymphatic channels to the initially treated regions (Rosenberg and Kaplan, 1966).

In advanced disease, orderliness of involvement and predictability of disease progression are lost, as if hematogenous spread has occurred. In a few cases this is noted earlier in the course of the disease.

Staging of Hodgkin's Disease

The definitive staging of Hodgkin's disease before initial treatment is critical because it is a major determinant of the selection of potentially curative treatment.

Peters (1950) was the first to introduce a rational clinical staging classification, which identified three prognostic groups depending on the extent of disease and recognized the poorer prognosis of patients with systemic symptoms. When lymphography made possible the earlier detection of retroperitoneal lymph node involvement, it became important to distinguish two subgroups within Peters' stage III: Those with widespread disease confined to lymphatic organs and those with spread of disease beyond the lymph nodes, thymus, spleen, and Waldeyer's ring to one or more extralymphatic organs or tissues. Recognition of this need led in 1965 to the adoption of the Rye or Paris four-stage clinical staging classification (Rosenberg, 1966).

As experience with the Rye classification increased, certain deficiencies became apparent. Of particular significance was the presentation of data indicating that localized involvement of extralymphatic organs or tissues, unlike disseminated involvement, did not carry the unfavorable prognosis that its allocation to stage IV in the Rye classification suggested. A new staging classification, therefore, was adopted at a conference held in Ann Arbor, Michigan in 1971 (Carbone *et al.*, 1971). This incorporated recommendations made by Musshoff and others (1968), recognizing that limited extranodal disease, the so-called E lesion, had a relatively favorable prognosis and must be distinguished from disseminated extranodal involvement. The systemic symptom of pruritus, in addition, though important and characteristic in patients with Hodgkin's disease, could not be shown to be associated with a poor prognosis, *per se*. The Ann Arbor staging system (see Table 15–2) still has deficiencies, especially in the definition of the E lesion and the lack of recognition of other prognostic factors. The Ann Arbor classification, however, is widely used and clinically valuable.

The prognosis in patients with Hodgkin's disease becomes less favorable with increasing stage (see Figure 15–5A and 15–5B) and with the presence of systemic symptoms (substage B). The histopathologic type of Hodgkin's disease correlates to some extent with the stage. The proportion of patients with early-stage disease is highest for lymphocyte-predominance and progressively decreases through nodular sclerosis, mixed cellularity, and lymphocyte-depletion.

Therapy

The treatment of patients with Hodgkin's disease has undergone radical changes since

Table 15-2. Ann Arbor Staging Classification of Hodgkin's Disease

Stage I	Involvement of a single lymph node region (I) or of a single extralymphatic organ or site (I_E).
II	Involvement of two or more lymph node regions on the same side of the diaphragm (II) or localized involvement of extralymphatic organ or site and of one or more lymph node regions on the same side of the diaphragm (II_E).
III	Involvement of lymph node regions on both sides of the diaphragm (III), which also may be accompanied by localized involvement of extralymphatic organ or site (III_E) or by involvement of the spleen (III_S) or both (III_{SE}).
IV	Diffuse or disseminated involvement of one or more extralymphatic organs or tissues with or without associated lymph node enlargement. The reason for classifying the patient as stage IV should be identified further by defining the site with symbols.
Symptoms A or B.	Each stage will be subdivided into A and B categories, B for those with defined general symptoms and A for those without. The B classification will be given to those patients with (1) unexplained weight loss of more than 10% of the body weight in the six months prior to admission; (2) unexplained fever with temperatures above 38°C; or (3) night sweats.

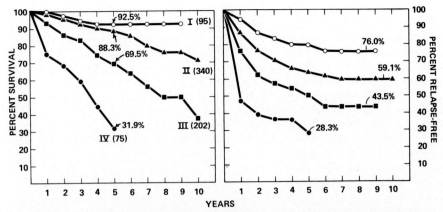

Figure 15–5A. Survival (left-hand graph) and freedom from progression (right-hand graph) actuarial curves of patients with Hodgkin's disease according to Ann Arbor stage, treated prior to 1970.

1940 and is continuing to evolve. These changes have resulted from advances in the availability and techniques of supervoltage radiotherapy, the effectiveness of combination chemotherapy programs, and the realization that patients can be cured of Hodgkin's disease (Easson and Russell, 1963).

The results of therapy now offer every new patient with Hodgkin's disease the probability of cure of the disease. Current successful therapeutic programs require the combined skills and cooperation of experienced pathologists, surgeons, radiotherapists, medical oncologists, surgeons, and oncology nurses. These programs are difficult and challenge the resources of the medical care team and the patient.

Radiotherapy

The major considerations in the radiotherapy of Hodgkin's disease are: The total radiation dose per field; the size, shape, and number of treatment fields; and the beam energy. Permanent eradication of any given site of involvement can be achieved in the great majority of patients with doses of 3500 to 4500 rad delivered at the rate of 1000 rad per week (Kaplan, 1966). Although enlarged lymph nodes may regress completely after substantially smaller doses, such responses are likely to be temporary and recurrences are common. Since reirradiation of recurrences is hazardous because of the poor tolerance of the normal tissues, it is important to use optimal dose levels for all involved sites in the first course of treatment.

When multiple chains of involved or potentially involved lymph nodes must be irradiated, the use of multiple small treatment fields is undesirable because of the risk of overlapping or of excessive gaps between fields. Current practice encompasses multiple lymph node chains within a few very large fields. Each such field must be carefully shaped to the contours of the lymph node chains, with lead shields placed to protect such vital structures

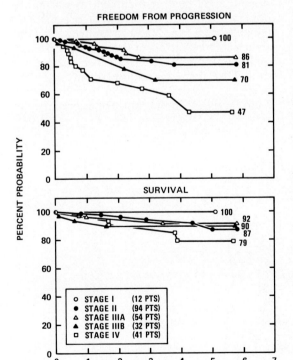

Figure 15–5B. Survival (lower graph) and freedom from progression (upper graph) actuarial curves of patients with Hodgkin's disease according to Ann Arbor stage, treated on protocol studies after 1974.

as the lungs, heart, liver, kidneys, and spinal cord. Encompassing all or most of the relevant lymph node chains within just two sets of matched anterior and posterior opposed fields is usually possible (see Figure 15–6): (1) The "mantle" field, covering the cervical, supraclavicular, infraclavicular, axillary, hilar, and mediastinal nodes down to the level of the diaphragm, and (2) the "inverted Y," covering the spleen or splenic pedicle, celiac, para-aortic, iliac, inguinal, and femoral nodes. At times it is necessary to divide the inverted Y field into two fields, the "spade" field, from the diaphragm to the level of aortic bifurcation, and the "pelvic" field. The mantle and inverted Y field together compose so-called total nodal irradiation (TNI) or total lymphoid irradiation (TLI). If the pelvis is not treated, the treatment fields are termed subtotal nodal irradiation (STNI) or lymphoid irradiation (STLI). It is essential to leave a gap between adjacent fields at the skin surface, its width calculated to permit perfect abutment of the two fields at the depth of the midplane to the body. In young female patients, surgical oophoropexy with fixation of the ovaries in the midline permits ovarian function to be preserved in up to 70% of women despite radiotherapy of the pelvic lymph nodes (Trueblood *et al.,* 1970; Le Floch *et al.,* 1976). When cervical lymphadenopathy extends into the upper neck, the possibility of spread to the preauricular nodes is of sufficient concern to justify adding small parallel opposed lateral fields covering this area.

Irradiating apparently uninvolved lymph node regions has long been advocated by experienced radiotherapists (Gilbert, 1939; Peters and Middlemiss, 1950; Kaplan, 1962). This approach is based on the knowledge of the clinical behavior of Hodgkin's disease, the inadequacies of our diagnostic techniques to discover minute or microscopic foci of the disease, and the advantage and efficiency of avoiding patchwork and overlapping fields of previously irradiated regions from unrecognized and untreated sites. Data are available that support this philosophy of therapy for stages I, II, and IIIA disease in providing prolonged relapse-free survival. Whether this is true for all histologic subtypes and to what degree intensive chemotherapy may be an alternative or supplemental therapeutic approach, is a subject of continued investigation.

Extended field, total lymphoid, or total nodal radiotherapy is technically demanding and potentially hazardous, and should not be attempted by inexperienced radiotherapists.

Mild to moderate dryness and soreness of the throat and dysphagia often occur during the treatment of the mantle field and occasionally may be severe enough to warrant a brief interruption of treatment or a decrease in the daily dose rate. Nausea, vomiting, and diarrhea are likely to occur during the treatment of the retroperitoneal and pelvic nodes and should be treated symptomatically. Leukopenia or thrombocytopenia usually reach nadir levels late in the course of treatment and

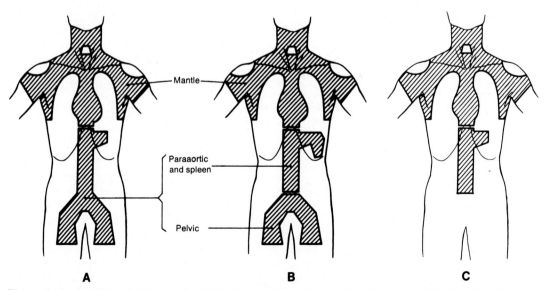

A **B** **C**

Figure 15–6. Total lymphoid irradiation (TLI) fields consisting of a mantle and an inverted Y (*A*) or three fields (*B*). Subtotal lymphoid irradiation (STLI) fields (*C*) after splenectomy consisting of a mantle and spade fields.

may necessitate temporary interruption of treatment. Hematologic tolerance has been reported to be better in those patients who have had a splenectomy (Salzman and Kaplan, 1971). Temporary alopecia may be expected in the occipital regions on either side of the mantle field.

Elevation of the thyroid-stimulating hormone (TSH) can be expected in about 50% of patients and hypothyroidism occurs in 10 to 20% of patients (Glatstein et al., 1971). Although some degree of radiographically recognizable radiation pneumonitis occurs in most patients after treatment to a mantle field, only about 10% of patients are symptomatic, and rarely is this serious. The usual clinical manifestations include a nonproductive cough, mild to moderate dyspnea on significant exertion, and fever. Chest films reveal accentuation of radiographic markings in the paramediastinal pulmonary zones corresponding to the treatment field contours. The clinical manifestations may persist for a few months and then gradually disappear, leaving little or no overt evidence of impaired ventilatory function, though careful physiologic measurements may continue to disclose evidence of restrictive phenomena and diffusion defects.

Radiation pericarditis, which occurs in about 6% of cases treated with 4400 rad or less to the mantle field, is usually asymptomatic and manifested primarily by the appearance of cardiomegaly on serial post-treatment roentgenograms of the chest. Diagnostic procedures usually confirm the presence of fluid in the pericardial sac, and a friction rub may be heard transiently. Although the usual course is benign, requiring little or no symptomatic therapy in the majority of cases, careful serial observation of these patients is essential to detect the occasional case in which the condition progresses to tamponade or chronic constrictive pericarditis, necessitating more aggressive therapy, including pericardiectomy. This complication can be reduced by appropriate shielding of the heart when there is no subcarinal lymph node disease and mediastinal disease is not marked (Carmel and Kaplan, 1976).

A common but minor complication is the Lhermitte syndrome, in which numbness, tingling, or "electric" sensations, without associated motor dysfunction, are experienced in the arms, legs, and lower back and are characteristically exacerbated by flexion of the neck. This symptom disappears gradually over a period of several months. Transverse myelitis is a much more serious, but fortunately quite rare, complication, that can usually be traced to technical errors such as an overlapping "hot spot" due to an inadequate and improperly planned gap at the junction of fields, or to ill-advised retreatment over the spinal cord.

Radiation pneumonitis or pericarditis may appear, sometimes years after radiotherapy, when the patient receives chemotherapy. The abrupt discontinuance of prednisone, as utilized in the MOPP regimen, may precipitate the symptoms and radiologic findings (Castellino et al., 1974). Radiation to the myocardium produces an increase in risk of doxorubicin cardiac toxicity, and, presumably, the use of bleomycin combinations in patients with prior lung irradiation would be harmful.

Total nodal irradiation and/or combination chemotherapy may produce amenorrhea, which, particularly in older patients, may be permanent (Horning et al., 1981). Aspermia following chemotherapy is common (Sherins and DeVita, 1973; Chapman, 1982) and occurs transiently in patients receiving pelvic radiotherapy. There is some evidence of an adverse effect on libido and sexual performance.

Chemotherapy

Numerous chemotherapeutic agents exist that individually have produced tumor regression in patients with Hodgkin's disease, and selected combinations of these agents have provided curative treatment for patients with the disease. Doses and toxicity of individual agents will not be presented in this chapter. Other than for patients with advanced refractory disease, combination chemotherapy has replaced single-agent chemotherapy. Although tumor regression may occur with single agent chemotherapy in as many as 50 to 60% of patients, complete remission is uncommon, and the duration of remission is in the range of two to five months; this is a major limitation of single-agent chemotherapy.

The most successful and widely employed combination was developed at the National Cancer Institute (NCI) and is referred to as the MOPP program (DeVita et al., 1970). This consists of mechlorethamine, vincristine, procarbazine, and prednisone. These agents are given in combination in a two-week course for a minimum of six cycles. A two-week rest period intervenes between courses or cycles of treatment (see Figure 15–7). A 15-year follow-up of the MOPP experience at NCI has been reported (DeVita *et al.,* 1980). The overall complete remission rate is 80% for patients with advanced (stages III and IV) disease. Sixty-eight percent of patients achieving complete remission remained disease-free for over ten years. Asymptomatic patients did significantly better than symptomatic patients in terms of disease-free survival. Prior treatment with some of the chemotherapeutic agents employed in the MOPP program adversely affected response. Previous treatment by radiotherapy, however, did not. The risk of relapse was relatively high in the first year and progressively decreased through the first four years after treatment, suggesting that patients who remain continuously disease-free for five years after treatment for Hodgkin's disease have a high probability of being cured.

Some of the principles involved in the application of the MOPP program are as follows. As much as possible, the dose rate prescribed in the MOPP program should be maintained. Reduction in dose or prolongation of the interval between courses of treatment may be required, particularly if myelosuppression is excessive, but should be minimized wherever possible (Carde *et al.,* 1983). Although six cycles of treatment is the standard prescribed, it is inadequate for some patients. Following four to six cycles of treatment, patients should be carefully restaged, including rebiopsy of sites of pretreatment organ involvement where possible. If microscopic disease persists, treatment should be continued. After patients enter a documented complete remission, treatment should be continued for a minimum of an additional two cycles. For certain patients who have poor prognostic findings, such as those

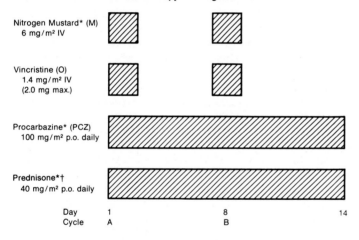

MOPP Chemotherapy for Hodgkin's Disease

Nitrogen Mustard* (M) 6 mg/m² IV

Vincristine (O) 1.4 mg/m² IV (2.0 mg max.)

Procarbazine* (PCZ) 100 mg/m² p.o. daily

Prednisone*† 40 mg/m² p.o. daily

Day 1 8 14
Cycle A B

MOPP Dosage Modification (Stanford)

		% calculated doses		
WBC	Platelets	M	O	PCZ
A cycle				
>3500	>120,000	100%	100%	100%
3000 to 3500	80,000 to 120,000	70	100	50
<3000	<80,000	No drugs, delay one or two weeks		
B cycle				
>3500	>120,000	100%	100%	100%
3000 to 3500	80,000 to 120,000	70	100	50
2500 to 3000	50,000 to 80,000	50	100	25
2000 to 2500		25	100	none
<2000	<50,000	No drugs, repeat cycle on day 29		

*It is sometimes preferable to begin the oral medications on day 2 through 15.
†Cycles 1 and 4 only; may be omitted if patient has received extensive prior mediastinal irradiation.

Figure 15–7. Schematic description of the MOPP chemotherapy regimen with the Stanford dose-reduction recommendations.

with bone marrow involvement, a longer course of treatment with MOPP or alternating MOPP with a non-cross-resistant regimen such as ABVD (which is discussed later in this section) should be considered (Santoro *et al.*, 1982a,b)

The acute toxicity of the MOPP program includes myelosuppression, which is usually dose-limiting, nausea, and vomiting, peripheral neuropathies associated with vincristine, and alopecia. The most serious long-term toxicity relates to the carcinogenic potential of the MOPP program. This has resulted in a significant increase in acute myelogenous leukemia as compared to that expected in age-matched control populations (Coleman *et al.*, 1982; Glicksman *et al.*, 1982).

Depressed cellular immunity may persist indefinitely following therapy for Hodgkin's disease (Levy and Kaplan, 1974; Fuks *et al.*, 1976a; Fisher *et al.*, 1980). This occurs following total nodal radiotherapy, as well as following chemotherapy, and it remains to be established to what degree this is due to the treatment or to the underlying original disease.

Aspermia, which is usually permanent, often occurs. This is not generally associated with other endocrinologic abnormalities, except perhaps in adolescent patients (Sherins *et al.*, 1978). Permanent amenorrhea is a risk that increases with the age of the woman at the time of treatment (Horning *et al.*, 1981).

Aseptic necrosis of the femoral heads, and rarely the humoral heads, is an unusual late complication, presumably related to the corticosteroid therapy.

Since the development of the MOPP program in 1964, additional active agents have been discovered for Hodgkin's disease, and other combinations have been developed (Coltman, 1980). Table 15–3 lists some of the regimens that have been reported. The most widely utilized of these is the ABVD program; a combination of doxorubicin, bleomycin, vinblastine, and dacarbazine (DTIC). This program, or variations of it, has produced complete remissions in 15% to 60% of MOPP failures with wide variations, depending on the study. In a comparative study of MOPP and ABVD as primary therapies conducted by the Milan group, the two programs were comparable in terms of high complete remission rates and durability of remissions (Bonadonna *et al.*, 1975). The usual use of ABVD, however, is for patients whose disease fails to be controlled by MOPP, so-called salvage therapy. The effectiveness of salvage therapies, including the reuse of MOPP, is directly related to the disease-free interval after the initial treatment with MOPP (Fisher *et al.*, 1979). If the initial complete remission was one year or more in duration, the response to salvage chemotherapy will be more satisfactory. The overall cure rate (five-year disease-free survival) for salvage therapies after MOPP relapse is no greater than 20%.

Various approaches to maintenance treatment following six to nine monthly courses of MOPP therapy have not improved the long-term disease-free survival rate or overall survival and are not recommended.

Numerous variations on these MOPP and ABVD programs have been studied without conclusive evidence that any are superior. One may vary the alkylating agent employed, the vinca alkaloid, and so forth. These substitutions or alterations in dose schedule may diminish the toxicity, at least in some studies. There is preliminary evidence that the ABVD program may be less carcinogenic than MOPP-like regimens, and result in a lower incidence of aspermia (Valagussa *et al.*, 1982).

Table 15–3. Primary MOPP-like Combination Chemotherapy Regimens used for Hodgkin's Disease

MOPP:	Mechlorethamine, vincristine, procarbazine, prednisone
MVPP:	Mechlorethamine, vinblastine, procarbazine, prednisone
C-MOPP:	Cyclophosphamide, vincristine, procarbazine, prednisone
BCVPP:	BCNU, cyclophosphamide, vinblastine, procarbazine, prednisone
MVVPP:	Mechlorethamine, vincristine, vinblastine, procarbazine, prednisone
ChlVPP:	Chlorambucil, vinblastine, procarbazine, prednisone
PAVe:	Melphalan, vinblastine, procarbazine
Alternatives*	
ABVD:	Doxorubicin, bleomycin, vinblastine, DTIC
B-DOPA:	Bleomycin, DTIC, vincristine, prednisone, doxorubicin
B-CAVe:	Bleomycin, CCNU, doxorubicin, vinblastine
SCAB:	Streptozotocin, CCNU, doxorubicin, bleomycin

* Alternative (salvage) combination chemotherapy regimens used for Hodgkin's disease.

The alternating MOPP-ABVD study of Bonadonna is especially promising in a preliminary report for patients with the poorest prognosis (Santoro *et al.,* 1982a).

Recommendations for Treatment by Stage

Patients with laparotomy-staged IA and IIA disease have a 90% probability of cure with subtotal lymphoid radiotherapy. For disease above the diaphragm, the fields include the mantle and spade fields. For patients with pretreatment bulk disease, particularly with large mediastinal disease greater than one-third the transverse diameter of the chest, a 60% risk of failure exists, and employment of combination chemotherapy in addition to radiotherapy is recommended (Mauch *et al.,* 1978).

For patients with IB and IIB disease, total nodal radiotherapy provides a five-year disease-free survival rate of 80%. Randomized trials have indicated that the addition of MOPP to such treatment does not improve the disease-free survival or the overall survival (Rosenberg *et al.,* 1982).

For patients with limited extranodal disease (E lesions), with or without systemic symptoms, radiotherapy alone is recommended if the entire extent of the extranodal involvement can be safely encompassed by full-dose irradiation (Torti *et al.,* 1981).

For patients with stage IIIB and IV disease, combination chemotherapy is the treatment of choice, producing a 25 to 60% five-year disease-free survival depending on the sites of disease. Patients with bone marrow involvement have the lowest probability of prolonged remissions following chemotherapy (Myers *et al.,* 1974; Carde *et al.,* 1983).

These generalizations are modified as follows: In children, irradiation to the bones would impair growth so that reduced radiotherapy fields and/or dose and supplementing the irradiation with combination chemotherapy is optimal (Donaldson and Kaplan, 1982; Jenkin *et al.,* 1982). Chemotherapy is recommended by some authors for patients with lung lesions or large mediastinal masses initially to substantially reduce the masses and thus the radiotherapy dose to substantial lung volumes (Levi and Wiernik, 1977).

For patients with IIIA disease, total nodal irradiation produces five-year disease-free survival of 40% to 80%. Patients with stage III_1A disease (splenic or upper abdominal involvement) in one study (Stein *et al.,* 1980; Stein *et al.,* 1982) had substantially better prognoses when irradiation was utilized than patients with stage III_2A disease (involvement of para-aortic, iliac, or mesenteric nodes, with or without upper abdominal involvement). This has not been confirmed, however, in the Stanford series (Hoppe *et al.,* 1980; Hoppe *et al.,* 1982), in which the extent of splenic involvement was the major prognostic variable in stage IIIA patients. Those with more than four splenic nodules had a relapse rate of greater than 60% following irradiation that included treatment to the liver (see Figure 15–8).

Combined modality therapy, utilizing combination chemotherapy such as MOPP or ABVD, and irradiation can be recommended for selected groups of patients, if administered by experienced treatment teams. As a generalization, if the primary treatment modality results in a prolonged (*i.e.,* for at least five years) disease-free survival of less than 50%, it is reasonable to use combined modality therapy.

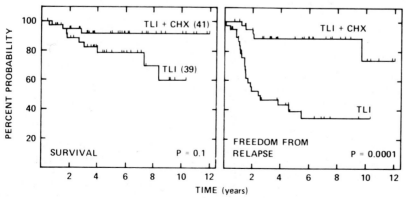

Figure 15–8. Survival (left-hand curve) and freedom from relapse (right-hand curve) actuarial curves of patients with pathologically stage III_SA Hodgkin's disease according to the extent of splenic involvement.

Table 15-4. Hodgkin's Disease: Stages and Clinical Situations Requiring Combined Modality Therapy

Stage III$_S$A with extensive involvement of the spleen (> 4 nodules)
Stage IIIB
Large mediastinal mass, > 1/3 transverse diameter of the chest, of any stage
Multiple E lesions, *i.e.,* lung, pleura, pericardium, and bone, of any stage
Children, usually age 15 and younger

The stages and clinical situations meeting this criteria are listed in Table 15-4. The details of management, including the sequence of treatments, the irradiation dose, the use of involved or wider radiation fields, and the choice of chemotherapeutic regimen and duration, will vary depending on the situation, the opinion of various experts, and whether or not the patient is being treated as part of a clinical trial. It must be emphasized that the bone marrow tolerance for chemotherapy is usually seriously reduced after full-dose total lymphoid irradiation, especially after treating the pelvic field.

Combined modality therapy results in a 4% to 10% incidence at 7 to 10 years after therapy of acute leukemia (Coleman *et al.,* 1982). This serious problem is primarily a result of chemotherapy of the MOPP type. It is not clear if irradiation adds to this risk, but there is reason for caution in utilizing chemotherapy in programs that have not resulted in improved survival.

Future Prospects

The treatment of patients with Hodgkin's disease can be very gratifying and successful. The disease and its management, however, are complex and treatment programs continue to evolve. A gradual improvement in cure rates for all stages of the disease and a reduction of acute and long-term toxicity and complications are possible. It is probable that chemotherapy regimens that do not utilize leukemogenic alkylating agents will replace the MOPP regimen for selected patient groups. Those with the poorest prognosis will need even more aggressive programs utilizing eight or more drugs, and in some centers, regimens with irradiation are being tested and show promise. Reductions in radiation dose, fields, and duration of chemotherapy are appropriate research questions, but are not yet standard practice for most patients.

The greatest advances in the control of Hodgkin's disease await an understanding of its etiology and pathogenesis. It seems very likely that before the turn of the next century, and perhaps within a decade, explanations of the unique epidemiologic, genetic, and immunologic characteristics of Hodgkin's disease will lead to its prevention or reversal.

REFERENCES

Bonadonna, G.; Zucali, R.; Monfardini, S.; DeLena, M.; and Uslenghi, C.: Combination chemotherapy of Hodgkin's disease with adriamycin, bleomycin, vinblastine and imidazole carboximide versus MOPP. *Cancer,* **36**:252-259, 1975.

Brunning, R. D.; Bloomfield, C. D.; McKenna, R. W.; and Peterson, L.: Bilateral trephine bone marrow biopsies in lymphoma and other neoplastic diseases. *Ann. Intern. Med.,* **82**:365-366, 1975.

Carbone, P. P.; Kaplan, H. S.; Musshoff, K.; Smithers, D. W.; and Tubiana, M.: Report of the committee on Hodgkin's disease staging. *Cancer Res.,* **31**:1860-1861, 1971.

Carde, P.; MacKintosh, F. R.; and Rosenberg, S. A.: A dose and time response analysis of the treatment of Hodgkin's disease with MOPP chemotherapy. *J. Clin. Oncol.,* **1**:146-153, 1983.

Carmel, R. J.; and Kaplan, H. S.: Mantle irradiation in Hodgkin's disease. An analysis of technique, tumor irradiation and complications. *Cancer,* **37**:2812-2825, 1976.

Castellino, R. A.; Glatstein, E.; Turbow, M. M.; Rosenberg, S. A.; and Kaplan, H. S.; Latent radiation injury of lungs or heart activated by steroid withdrawal. *Ann. Intern. Med.,* **80**:593-599, 1974.

Chapman, R. M.: Effect of cytotoxic therapy on sexuality and gonadal function. *Semin. Oncol.,* **9**:84-94, 1982.

Cohen, J. R.: Idiopathic thrombocytopenic purpura in Hodgkin's disease. *Cancer,* **41**:743-746, 1978.

Coleman, C. N.; Burke, J. S.; Varghese, A.; Rosenberg, S. A.; and Kaplan, H. S.: Secondary leukemia and non-Hodgkin's lymphoma in patients treated for Hodgkin's disease. In Rosenberg, S. A., and Kaplan, H. S. (eds.): *Malignant Lymphomas. Etiology, Immunology, Pathology, Treatment.* Bristol-Myers Cancer Symposia. Vol. 3, pp. 259-276. Academic Press, New York, 1982.

Coltman, C. A.: Chemotherapy of advanced Hodgkin's disease. *Semin. Oncol.,* **7**:155-173, 1980.

DeVita, V. T.; Serpick, A. A.; and Carbone, P. P.: Combination chemotherapy in the treatment of advanced Hodgkin's disease. *Ann. Intern. Med.,* **73**:891-895, 1970.

DeVita, V. T.; Simon, R. M.; Hubbard, S. M.; Young, R. C.; Berard, C. W.; Moxley, J. H., III; Frei, E., III;

Carbone, P. P.; and Canellos, G. P.: Curability of advanced Hodgkin's disease with chemotherapy: Long-term follow-up of MOPP treated patients at NCI. *Ann. Intern. Med.*, **92**:587–595, 1980.

Donaldson, S. S.; and Kaplan, H. S.: A survey of pediatric Hodgkin's disease at Stanford University: Results of therapy and quality of survival. In Rosenberg, S. A., and Kaplan, H. S. (eds.): *Malignant Lymphomas. Etiology, Immunology, Pathology, Treatment.* Bristol-Myers Cancer Symposia. Vol. 3, pp. 571–590, Academic Press, New York, 1982.

Easson, E. C., and Russell, M. H.: The cure of Hodgkin's disease. *Br. Med. J.,* **1**:1704, 1963.

Fisher, R. I.; DeVita, V. T., Bostick, F.; Van Haelen, C.; Howser, D. M.; Hubbard, S. M.; and Young, R. C.: Persistent immunologic abnormalities in long-term survivors of advanced Hodgkin's disease. *Ann. Intern. Med.,* **92**:595–599, 1980.

Fisher, R. I.; DeVita, V. T.; Hubbard, S. P.; Simon, R.; and Young, R. C.: Prolonged disease-free survival in Hodgkin's disease with MOPP reinduction after first relapse. *Ann. Intern. Med.,* **90**:761–763, 1979.

Fuks, Z.; Strober, S.; Bobrove, A. M.; Sasazuki, T.; McMichael, A.; and Kaplan, H. S.: Longterm effects of radiation on T and B lymphocytes in peripheral blood of patients with Hodgkin's disease. *J. Clin. Invest.,* **58**:803–814, 1976a.

Fuks, Z.; Strober, S.; and Kaplan, H. S.: Interaction between serum factors and T-lymphocytes in Hodgkin's disease. *N. Engl. J. Med.,* **295**:1273–1278, 1976b.

Gilbert, R.: Radiotherapy in Hodgkin's disease (Malignant granulomatosis): Anatomic and clinical foundations: Governing principles: results. *A.J.R.,* **41**:198–241, 1939.

Glatstein, E.; Guernsey, J. M.; Rosenberg, S. A.; and Kaplan, H. S.: The value of laparotomy and splenectomy in the staging of Hodgkin's disease. *Cancer,* **24**:709–718, 1969.

Glatstein, E.; McHardy-Young, S.; Brast, N.; Eltringham, J. R.; and Kriss, J. P.: Alterations in serum thyrotropin (TSH) and thyroid function following radiotherapy in patients with malignant lymphoma. *J. Clin. Endocrinol. Metab.,* **32**:833–841, 1971.

Glicksman, A. S.; Pajak, F.; Gottlieb, A.; Nissen, N.; Stutzman, L.; and Cooper, R.: Second malignant neoplasms in patients successfully treated for Hodgkin's disease: A Cancer and Leukemia Group B study. *Cancer Treat. Rep.,* **66**:1035–1044, 1982.

Gutensohn, N., and Cole, P.: Epidemiology of Hodgkin's disease. *N. Engl. J. Med.,* **304**:135–140, 1981.

Hersh, E. M., and Oppenheim, J. J.: Impaired lymphocyte transformation in Hodgkin's disease. *N. Engl. J. Med.,* **275**:1006–1012, 1965.

Hillinger, S. M., and Herzig, G. P.: Impaired cell-mediated immunity in Hodgkin's disease mediated by suppressor lymphocytes and monocytes. *J. Clin. Invest.,* **61**:1620–1621, 1978.

Hoppe, R. T.; Cox, R. S.; Rosenberg, S. A.; and Kaplan, H. S.: Prognostic factors in pathologic stage III Hodgkin's disease. *Cancer Treat. Rep.,* **66**:743–749, 1982.

Hoppe R. T.; Rosenberg, S. A.; Kaplan, H. S.; and Cox, R. S.: Prognostic factors in pathologic stage IIIA Hodgkin's disease. *Cancer,* **46**:1240–1246, 1980.

Horning, S. J.; Hoppe, R. T.; Kaplan, H. S.; and Rosenberg, S. A.: Female reproductive potential after treatment for Hodgkin's disease. *N. Engl. J. Med.,* **304**:1377–1382, 1981.

Jenkin, D.; Chan, H.; Freedman, M.; Greenberg, M.;

Gribbin, M.; McClure, P.; Saunders, F.; and Sonley, M.: Hodgkin's disease in children: Treatment results with MOPP and low-dose, extended-field irradition. *Cancer Treat. Rep.,* **66**:949–959, 1982.

Kadin, M. E.; Stites, D. P.; Levy, R.; and Warnke, R.: Exogenous immunoglobulin and the macrophage origin of Reed-Sternberg cells in Hodgkin's disease. *N. Engl. J. Med.,* **299**:1208–1214, 1978.

Kaplan, H. S.: The radical radiotherapy of regionally localized Hodgkin's disease. *Radiology,* **78**:553–561, 1962.

Kaplan, H. S.: Evidence for a tumorcidal dose level in the radiotherapy of Hodgkin's disease. *Cancer Res.,* **26**:1221–1224, 1966.

Kaplan, H. S.: *Hodgkin's Disease.* 2nd ed. Harvard University Press, Cambridge, Massachusetts, 1980.

Kaplan, H. S., and Gartner, S.: "Sternberg-Reed" giant cells of Hodgkin's disease: Cultivation in vitro, heterotransplantation, and characterization as neoplastic macrophages. *Int. J. Cancer,* **19**:511–525, 1977.

Kaplan, H. S., and Smithers, D. W.: Auto-immunity and homologous disease in mice in relation to the malignant lymphomas. *Lancet,* **2**:1–4, 1959.

LeFloch, O.; Donaldson, S. S.; and Kaplan, H. S.: Pregnancy following oophoropexy and total nodal irradiation in women with Hodgkin's disease. *Cancer,* **38**:2263–2268, 1976.

Levi, J. A., and Wiernik, P. H.: Limited extranodal Hodgkin's disease: unfavorable prognosis and therapeutic implications. *Am. J. Med.,* **63**:365–372, 1977.

Levy, R. A., and Kaplan, H. S.: Impaired lymphocyte function in untreated Hodgkin's disease. *N. Engl. J. Med.,* **290**:181–186, 1974.

Lukes, R. J.: Criteria for involvement of lymph node, bone marrow, spleen, and liver in Hodgkin's disease. *Cancer Res.,* **31**:1755–1767, 1971.

Lukes, R. J.; Butler, J. J.; and Hicks, E. D.: Natural history of Hodgkin's disease as related to its pathologic picture. *Cancer,* **19**:317–344, 1966(a).

Lukes, R. J.; Craver, L. F.; Hall, T. C.; Rappaport, H.; and Ruben, P.: Report of the nomenclature committee. *Cancer Res.,* **26(Part I)**:1311, 1966b.

Lukes R. J.; Tindle, B. H.; and Parker, J. W.: Reed-Sternberg-like cells in infectious mononucleosis. *Lancet,* **2**:1000–1004, 1969.

MacMahon, B.: Epidemiology of Hodgkin's disease. *Cancer Res.,* **26**:1189–1200, 1966.

Mauch, P.; Goodman, R.; and Hellman, S.: The significance of mediastinal involvement in early stage Hodgkin's disease. *Cancer,* **42**:1039–1045, 1978.

Merigan, T. C.; Rand, K. H.; Pollard, R. B.; Abdallah, P. S.; Jordan, G. W.; and Fried, R. P.: Human leukocyte interferon for the treatment of herpes zoster in patients with cancer. *N. Engl. J. Med.,* **298**:981–987, 1978.

Minor, D. R.; Schiffman, G.; and McIntosh, L. A.: Response of patients with Hodgkin's disease to pneumococcal vaccine. *Ann. Intern. Med.,* **90**:887–892, 1979.

Musshoff, K.; Renemann, H.; Boutis, L.; and Afknam, J.: Die extranodulare lymphogranulomatose. Diagnose, therapie und prognose bei zwei unterschiedlichen formen des organ befalls, Ein Beitrag zur Stadienein teilung des morbus Hodgkin *Forschr. Geb. Roentgenstr. Nuklearmed. Erganzunsbad,* **109**:776–786, 1968.

Myers, C. E.; Chabner, B. A.; DeVita, V. T.; and Gralick, H. R.: Bone marrow involvement in Hodgkin's disease: Pathology and response to MOPP chemotherapy. *Blood,* **44**:197–204, 1974.

Neiman, R. S.; Rosen, P. J.; and Lukes, R. J.: Lymphocyte-depletion in Hodgkin's disease: A clinicopathologic entity. *N. Engl. J. Med.,* **288:**751–755, 1973.

Peters, M. V., and Middlemiss, K. C. H.: A study of Hodgkin's disease treated by irradiation. *A.J.R.,* **63:**299–311, 1950.

Rosenberg, S. A.: Report of the committee on the staging of Hodgkin's disease. *Cancer Res.,* **26:**1310, 1966.

Rosenberg, S. A.: Hodgkin's disease of the bone marrow. *Cancer Res.,* **31:**1733–1736, 1971.

Rosenberg, S. A., and Kaplan, H. S.: Evidence for an orderly progression in the spread of Hodgkin's disease. *Cancer Res.,* **26:**1225–1231, 1966.

Rosenberg, S. A.; Kaplan, H. S.; Hoppe, R. T.; Kushlan, P.; and Horning, S. J.: The Stanford randomized trials of the treatment of Hodgkin's disease: 1967–1980. In Rosenberg, S. A., and Kaplan, H. S. (eds.): *Malignant Lymphomas. Etiology, Immunology, Pathology, Treatment.* Bristol-Myers Cancer Symposia. Vol 3. pp. 513–522, Academic Press, New York, 1982.

Salzman J., and Kaplan, H. S.: Effect of splenectomy on hematologic tolerance during total lymphoid radiotherapy of patients with Hodgkin's disease. *Cancer,* **27:**471–478, 1971.

Santoro, A.; Bonadonna, G.; Bonfante, V.; and Valagussa, P.: Alternating drug combinations in the treatment of advanced Hodgkin's disease. *N. Engl. J. Med.,* **306:**770–775, 1982a.

Santoro, A.; Bonfante, V.; and Bonadonna, G.: Salvage chemotherapy with ABVD in MOPP-resistant Hodgkin's disease. *Ann. Intern. Med.,* **96:**139–144, 1982b.

Schier, W. W.; Roth, A.; and Ostroff, J.: Hodgkin's disease and immunity. *Am. J. Med.,* **20:**94–99, 1954.

Sherins R. J., and DeVita, V. T.: Effects of drug treatment for lymphoma on male reproductive capacity. *Ann. Intern. Med.,* **79:**216–220, 1973.

Sherins, R. T.; Olweny, C. L. M.; and Ziegler, J. C.: Gynecomastia and gonadal dysfunction in adolescent boys treated with combination chemotherapy for Hodgkin's disease. *New Engl. J. Med.* **299:**12–16, 1978.

Siber, G. R.; Weitzman, S. A.; Aisenberg, A. C.; Weinstein, H. J.; and Schiffman, G.: Impaired antibody response to pneumococcal vaccine after treatment for Hodgkin's disease. *N. Engl. J. Med.,* **299:**442–448, 1978.

Stein, R. S.; Golomb, H. M.; Diggs, C. H.; Mauch, P.; Hellman, S.; Wiernik, P. H.; Ultmann, J. E.; and Rosenthal, D. S.: Anatomic substages of stage III-A Hodgkin's disease. *Ann. Intern. Med.,* **92:**159–165, 1980.

Stein, R. S.; Golomb, H. M.; Wiernik, P. H.; Mauch, P.; Hellman, S.; Ultmann, J. E.; Rosenthal., D. S.; and Flexner, J. M.: Anatomic substages of stage IIIA Hodgkin's disease: Follow-up of a collaborative study. *Cancer Treat. Rep.,* **66:**733–741, 1982.

Torti, F. M.; Portlock, C. S.; Rosenberg, S. A.; and Kaplan, H. S.: Extralymphatic Hodgkin's disease: Prognosis and response to therapy. *Am. J. Med.,* **70:**487–492, 1981.

Trueblood, H. W.; Enright, L. P.; Ray, G. R.; Kaplan, H. S.; and Nelsen, T. S.: Preservation of ovarian function in pelvic irradiation for Hodgkin's disease. *Arch. Surg.,* **100:**236–237, 1970.

Tucker, M. A.; Greene, M. H.; Mann, D.; Johnson, A. H.; and Fraumeni, J. F.: Histocompatability gene may play role in familial Hodgkin's disease. *Proc. Am. Soc. Clin. Onc.,* C–207, 1980.

Valagussa, P.; Santoro, A.; Fossati-Bellani, F.; Franchi, F.; Banfi, A.; and Bonadonna, G.: Absence of treatment-induced second neoplasms after ABVD in Hodgkin's disease. *Blood,* **59:**488–494, 1982.

Waddell, C. C., and Cimo, P. L.: Idiopathic thrombocytopenic purpura occurring in Hodgkin's disease after splenectomy. A report of two cases and review of the literature. *Am. J. Hematol.,* **7:**381–387, 1979.

Whitley, R. J.; Soong, S.-J.; Dolin, R.; Betts, R.; Linnemann, C.; and Alford, C. A.: NIAID Collaborative Antiviral Study Group: Early vidarabine therapy for control of herpes zoster. *N. Engl. J. Med.,* **307:**971–975, 1982.

16

Non-Hodgkin's Lymphomas

SAUL A. ROSENBERG

Introduction

The non-Hodgkin's lymphomas are a diverse group of neoplasms that have in common their origin from lymphoreticular cells. They usually arise or present in lymphoid tissues, such as the lymph nodes, spleen, bone marrow, or Waldeyer's ring, but may arise in almost any tissue of the body. They are distinguished from Hodgkin's disease by the absence of Reed-Sternberg giant cells and other pathologic features. They are distinguished from the lymphatic leukemias on the basis of relatively arbitrary clinical criteria. The spectrum of these lymphomas includes diseases that, at one extreme, are among the most rapidly progressive and fatal human neoplasms and at the other extreme are among the most indolent and well-tolerated human neoplasms, capable of prolonged stability and even spontaneous regression.

Study of the non-Hodgkin's lymphomas by laboratory and clinical investigators has been intense and productive because of:

1. Important epidemiologic characteristics, for example, Burkitt's lymphoma, Mediterranean (alpha heavy chain) lymphoma;
2. The strong evidence that viruses are associated with certain subtypes and may be etiologically important, for example, Epstein-Barr virus (EBV), human T-cell leukemia/lymphoma virus (HTLV);
3. They can be considered as neoplasms of the immune system and immunologic markers and methodologies can be applied to their study;

4. Many animal models exist that morphologically correspond to the human diseases; and
5. The neoplasms are highly responsive to therapy, often resulting in their cure.

Incidence and Epidemiology

A full discussion of the incidence and epidemiology of the non-Hodgkin's lymphomas is beyond the scope of this chapter. The data and observations vary considerably throughout the world and are complicated by variable morphologic criteria and terminology, to be discussed below.

In the United States, approximately 24,000 new patients per year develop one of these neoplasms and about half will die of their diseases. These lymphomas occur in all age groups. Among the ten major subtypes, however, the age ranges are more limited. Several are more common in children and young adults, but the majority are neoplasms of adults in the 40 to 70 year range. In general, men and women are affected equally, though there are striking male predominances for several subtypes. Table 16–1 lists the age range, median age, and sex ratio of the ten major subtypes of non-Hodgkin's lymphomas according to an international study of 1175 cases (NLPCP, 1982).

Several very important epidemiologic observations and differences among the various non-Hodgkin's lymphomas will be summarized. For a detailed review of this subject see Cantor and Fraumeni (1980).

An aggressive, high-grade lymphoma was

Table 16-1. Formulation of Non-Hodgkin's Lymphoma Selected Clinical Characteristics

SUBTYPE	AGE RANGE (years)	MEDIAN AGE (years)	SEX RATIO (M:F)
Small lymphocytic	26 to 79	60.5	1.2 to 1
Follicular, small cleaved cell	3 to 87	54.3	1.3 to 1
Follicular, mixed	26 to 99	56.1	0.8 to 1
Follicular, large cell	16 to 82	55.4	1.8 to 1
Diffuse, small cleaved cell	10 to 91	57.9	2.0 to 1
Diffuse, mixed	22 to 90	58.0	1.1 to 1
Diffuse, large cell	10 to 88	56.8	1.0 to 1
Immunoblastic	10 to 81	51.3	1.5 to 1
Lymphoblastic	11 to 90	16.9	1.9 to 1
Diffuse, small noncleaved	3 to 90	29.8	2.6 to 1

recognized by Denis Burkitt as the most common neoplasm of black African children (Burkitt, 1958). This tumor, also called a diffuse undifferentiated or small noncleaved cell lymphoma, was found to be almost epidemic in frequency, in certain parts of East Africa and in New Guinea. The association of this lymphoma with infection with an herpes virus, subsequently called the Epstein-Barr virus, has been a major discovery of biomedical research. The identical lymphoma is found sporadically throughout the world but its clinical characteristics and its association with the Epstein-Barr virus are different outside of the endemic areas (Klein, 1982).

Another high grade lymphoma, primarily localized in the abdomen with mesenteric and intestinal involvement, has been recognized among individuals of the Mediterranean region (Seligmann, 1975). Most common among North Africans and Sephardic Jews, the neoplasm is associated with the finding of the alpha heavy chain of immunoglobulin as a monoclonal secretory product of the neoplastic lymphoid cell. This neoplasm has a yet unexplained relationship to a non-neoplastic submucosal intestinal infiltration with relatively mature plasma cells. This same clinicopathologic and immunologic entity is rarely identified in individuals other than those of Mediterranean ethnic origin. Utilizing the terminology of the formulation of lymphoma pathology, the Mediterranean lymphoma is an immunoblastic lymphoma, with pyrinophilic features, a presumptive B-cell disease.

Non-Hodgkin's lymphomas that have the immunologic phenotypes corresponding to normal B cells are relatively uncommon in Japan and, presumably, in other Asian ethnic groups. In contrast, lymphomas with T-cell immunologic markers are more common in Japan. A spectrum of T-cell lymphoid neoplasms has been described in Japan varying from a T-cell type of chronic lymphatic leukemia to a very pleomorphic, aggressive neoplasm (Shimoyama and Watanabe, 1979). The discovery of an association of a new human C-type retrovirus with human T-cell leukemia and lymphoma in Japan and the United States is an important observation that, as with Epstein-Barr virus, has etiologic significance (Gallo and Wong-Staal, 1982).

One of the most common types of non-Hodgkin's lymphomas in the United States is the nodular or follicular lymphoma, as described by Rappaport (1956). This type of relatively low-grade neoplasm is less common in Europe and quite rare in Japan (NLPCP, 1982; Shimoyama and Watanabe, 1979).

In contrast to Hodgkin's disease, there is no good evidence that the non-Hodgkin's lymphomas are more frequent among family members. Familial disorders, however, such as immune deficiency syndromes may have as an associated complication the development of non-Hodgkin's lymphomas.

It may be that an intermediate-grade lymphoma, termed centrocytic by Lennert (Lennert *et al.*, 1975), and diffuse small cleaved cell type in the formulation (NLPCP, 1982), is found more commonly in Europe, predominantly among older men, with frequent involvement of the lymphoid tissues of Waldeyer's ring. This clinicopathologic entity has not been recognized in series from the United States.

It seems likely that as immunologic, genetic, and viral markers and probes become more refined and utilized, more unique epidemiologic observations of the non-Hodgkin's lymphomas will be made. These developments give great promise for a better understanding of the etiology and pathogenesis of these neoplasms and will be discussed in the following sections of this chapter.

Etiology and Pathogenesis

The cause of the human non-Hodgkin's lymphomas is not known. The information available, however, from animal model systems, epidemiologic, viral, and clinical associations is abundant and provocative.

The development of a non-Hodgkin's lymphoma, indistinguishable from a *de novo* neoplasm, is a recognized and sometimes frequent sequela of a variety of diseases and clinical settings. Patients who have a congenital or acquired immunodeficiency have a markedly increased risk of developing a non-Hodgkin's lymphoma (Talal *et al.,* 1967). An increased risk of these neoplasms is observed in a wide variety of collagen-vascular and autoimmune diseases, such as rheumatoid vasculitis, Sjögren's syndrome, systemic lupus erythematosis, chronic lymphocytic thyroiditis (Hashimoto's struma), angioimmunoblastic lymphadenopathy, and nontropical sprue (Banks *et al.,* 1979). The most common neoplasm to develop following renal or cardiac transplantation is a non-Hodgkin's lymphoma (Penn, 1975). It has also been described among the long-term survivors of Hodgkin's disease (Krikorian *et al.,* 1979).

Characteristic chromosome abnormalities are being described more frequently as more precise banding and other high-resolution techniques have been applied. In particular, chromosomes 8, 14, and 18 are often involved (Yunis *et al.,* 1982). The relationships of the observed chromosome abnormalities to gene function, neoplastic transformation, and etiology are not yet known.

No associated immunologic abnormalities, as known for Hodgkin's disease, have been recognized in any of the subtypes of non-Hodgkin's lymphomas. As these diseases become widespread and especially after extensive therapy, immunologic dysfunction, sometimes severe, can be demonstrated. No early or uniform defect, however, has presumed causal importance.

It is generally accepted that the non-Hodgkin's lymphomas are monoclonal neoplasms, presumably arising from a single neoplastic cell. Convincing data arguing for the single-cell origin of cancer has, in part, been derived from the study of lymphoid neoplasms. Yet, very often from clinical observations, many patients with non-Hodgkin's lymphomas have widespread, "systemic" disease from the onset of their clinical disease. In addition, even when the disease appears localized, and is treated as if it is a limited "primary" tumor, new involvement is found in widespread, often unpredictable sites. This behavior of the non-Hodgkin's lymphomas contrasts with Hodgkin's disease and many other human neoplasms. The prediction for spread of the non-Hodgkin's lymphomas and the likely sites correlate significantly with the particular subtype of lymphoma.

As described in the previous section, it seems very probable that viruses play an important etiologic role in human non-Hodgkin's lymphomas. Virtually every other mammal, including nonhuman primates, develop lymphomas that are virus induced. Problems of acquired viral infection in the immunocompromised patient and the inability to fulfill Koch's postulates have frustrated investigators in establishing the viral etiology of the human non-Hodgkin's lymphomas. The Epstein-Barr virus and the human T-cell leukemia/lymphoma virus (HTLV) are major and likely candidates for etiologic agents. The lymphomas they are associated with, however, are rare and may have other unique epidemiologic factors not shared by similar lymphomas.

Pathology and Classifications

It has been said that nowhere in the field of pathology has there been more confusion (and debate) than in the nomenclature and classification of the non-Hodgkin's lymphomas (Willis, 1953). The most widely used classification in the United States is the Rappaport system, which was modified in recent years (Rappaport *et al.,* 1956). Four or five other major classifications, however, are in use throughout the world (NLPCP, 1982).

A unique international study comparing six major pathologic classifications involving 1175 patients from the United States and Italy was reported in 1982 (NLPCP, 1982). This important study concluded that no classification was significantly superior to any other, including those that were based on more modern concepts of the immune system. The study identified ten major subtypes of non-Hodgkin's lymphomas, dividing them into low- , intermediate- , and high-grade neoplasms. By allowing additional subclassification of the ten major types, a formulation of terms was developed that could be used to translate among all the major proposed classifications. This so-called new formulation of non-Hodgkin's lymphomas was not proposed as still another classification but as a means of comparing different reports, studies, and trials utilizing different systems and terminology.

This international study confirmed the clinical importance of a nodular or follicular architectural pattern in lymph node material for identifying a relatively favorable group of patients. Those patients with a diffuse architectural pattern have a poorer prognosis within the same cytologic subtype. These conclusions were convincingly demonstrated in a multivariate analysis of prognostic factors.

The cytologic subtype is also very important, however, in prognosis and in predicting clinical characteristics and outcome. In general, those non-Hodgkin's lymphomas composed of small, mature-appearing lymphocytes or those with small cleaved cells have the most favorable prognoses. Those with a predominance of large cells have poorer prognoses. Patients with cells corresponding to lymphoblasts (Rappaport) or T cell convoluted (Lukes) or immunoblasts (Lukes, Lennert) or undifferentiated (Rappaport) or small noncleaved (Lukes) have the poorest prognoses (see Table 16–1).

A modification of the Rappaport classification, as listed in Table 16–2, can be recommended as clinically useful. Other major classification systems are shown in Table 16–3. The new formulation for clinical use is shown separately, in Table 16–4. It has the advantage

Table 16–3. Six Major Classification Systems of Non-Hodgkin's Lymphoma

British National Lymphoma Investigation (Henry, Bennett and Farrer-Brown)
Dorfman
Kiel (Lennert)
Lukes-Collins
Rappaport
WHO (Mathe)

of using terminology that is more currently acceptable than that of the Rappaport system proposed more than 20 years ago. The actuarial survival of patients treated in the late 1970s according to the ten subtypes of the formulation is shown in Figure 16–1.

Diagnostic Evaluation

In general, the same diagnostic procedures discussed in the evaluation of patients with Hodgkin's disease (see Chapter 15) are utilized in evaluating patients with the non-Hodgkin's lymphomas. Depending on the specific subtype, however, important clinical differences require evaluation by specific diagnostic methods. Involvement by the lymphoma of the following sites may be frequent and important: (1) bone marrow; (2) Waldeyer's ring; (3) mesenteric lymph nodes; (4) gastrointestinal tract; and (5) meninges.

Bone marrow involvement is frequent in certain subtypes, either at the onset or during the course of the disease (Rosenberg, 1975). Table 16–5 lists the frequency of bone marrow involvement at presentation in the ten sub-

Table 16–2. Modified Rappaport Classification of Non-Hodgkin's Lymphoma

Nodular subtypes
*Lymphocytic, poorly differentiated (NLPD)
*Mixed, lymphocytic and histiocytic (NM)
Histiocytic (NH)

Diffuse subtypes
*Lymphocytic, well differentiated (DLWD)
  with or without plasmacytic morphology
Lymphocytic, poorly differentiated (DLPD)
Mixed, lymphocytic and histiocytic (DM)
Lymphoblastic Lymphoma (LL)
Histiocytic (DH)
Undifferentiated (DU)
  Burkitt's or non-Burkitt's types

* Low-grade subtypes

Table 16–4. Formulation of Non-Hodgkin's Lymphoma

Low Grade
  A. Small lymphocytic*
  B. Follicular, predominantly small cleaved cell†
  C. Follicular, mixed small cleaved and large cells†

Intermediate Grade
  D. Follicular, predominantly large cell†
  E. Diffuse, small cleaved cell
  F. Diffuse, mixed small and large cells
  G. Diffuse, large cell
      cleaved or noncleaved cell

High Grade
  H. Large cell, immunoblastic*
  I. Lymphoblastic
      convoluted or nonconvoluted
  J. Small, noncleaved cell
      Burkitt's or non-Burkitt's

* May be plasmacytoid
† May have diffuse areas

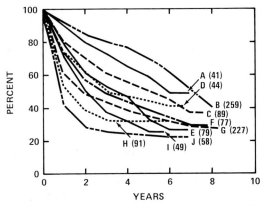

Figure 16–1. Actuarial survival curves for the ten subtypes of the formulation for non-Hodgkin's lymphoma classification. Subtypes A through J are identified in Table 16–4. Patient numbers in the international study are shown in parentheses.

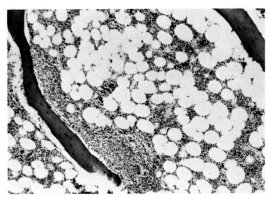

Figure 16–2. Bone marrow biopsy demonstrating focal, paratrabecular involvement by small cleaved lymphocytes.

types of the formulation. An adequate bone marrow biopsy, such as the type obtained with a Jamshidi needle, is required to demonstrate involvement by lymphoma. In contrast to the leukemias, bone marrow involvement lymphoma, especially early in the course of the disease, is focal. Pathologists recognize lymphomatous involvement by cellular atypia and the focal paratrabecular location of the infiltrate (see Figure 16–2). Several biopsies, or a larger open surgical biopsy, will improve the probability of identifying minimal involvement (Brunning *et al.,* 1975). In general, early and even moderate bone marrow involvement does not produce abnormalities in the peripheral blood or of the serum alkaline phosphatase level.

Involvement of the lymphoid tissues of Waldeyer's ring is relatively common in patients with the non-Hodgkin's lymphomas, especially in adult patients with intermediate and high-grade subtypes. The area should be examined by an experienced physician utiliz-

Table 16–5. Non-Hodgkin's
Lymphoma Bone Marrow Involvement

SUBTYPE	+ BM *(%)*
Small lymphocytic	71
Follicular, small cleaved cell	51
Follicular, mixed	30
Follicular, large cell	34
Diffuse, small cleaved cell	32
Diffuse mixed	14
Diffuse, large cell	10
Immunoblastic	12
Lymphoblastic	50
Diffuse, small noncleaved	14

ing direct and indirect techniques. The physician should remain alert to symptoms that may arise from lymphomatous involvement of the tonsil, base of tongue, and nasopharynx. If involvement of these tissues is suspected, computerized tomography and biopsy should be obtained to document the neoplasm and follow its response to therapy.

In contrast to Hodgkin's disease, the non-Hodgkin's lymphomas frequently involve the mesenteric lymph nodes and other abdominal lymph nodes outside of the para-aortic chain (Goffinet *et al.,* 1977). Enlargement of these lymph nodes may be responsible for the initial symptoms of the disease and lead to diagnostic laparotomy. It is recommended that all patients with non-Hodgkin's lymphoma be evaluated with abdominal computer tomography as well as bipedal lymphography. The two procedures are complementary (Castellino *et al.,* 1983). The lymphogram that evaluates the iliac and para-aortic lymph node chains to the level of the cysterna chyli is the most useful method to follow, with ordinary roentgenograms, during the course of the disease (see Figure 15–4 and 16–3).

Because retroperitoneal lymphadenopathy is common and may be bulky in low-grade lymphomas, there should be continued concern and evaluation of the renal collecting system. Abdominal ultrasonography is the most satisfactory, least invasive, method for studying this potential problem and should be done at intervals, depending on the clinical situation (Rochester *et al.,* 1977).

Neoplastic involvement of the gastrointestinal tract is a common problem in patients with the non-Hodgkin's lymphomas. Involvement

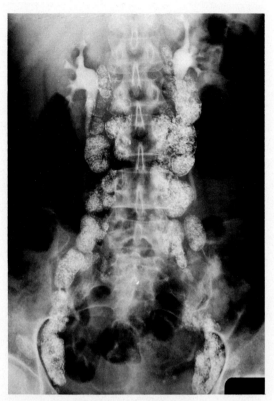

Figure 16–3. Lymphogram demonstrating characteristic diffuse involvement of retroperitoneal lymph nodes by follicular, small cleaved cell lymphoma. Note the relatively normal positions of the renal collecting system.

occurs much more frequently than is clinically appreciated, as demonstrated by autopsy series (Rosenberg *et al.*, 1961). The low-grade lymphomas, especially the small lymphocytic subtype, may involve the stomach and intestine extensively and be relatively asymptomatic and well tolerated. In contrast, the higher-grade subtypes may produce very serious symptoms of obstruction, ulceration, perforation, and hemorrhage. All patients who have gastrointestinal symptoms or mesenteric lymphadenopathy should have barium studies of the entire gastrointestinal tract. Endoscopy may be required to clarify the significance of prominent gastric rugae or ulcerations. The stomach and small intestine should be evaluated in all patients who have involvement of Waldeyer's ring (Hoppe *et al.*, 1978).

Meningeal lymphoma, much as meningeal leukemia, is being recognized as an increasingly serious problem for patients with certain subtypes of non-Hodgkin's lymphoma. As systemic chemotherapy regimens have become more successful, the meninges are emerging as an important site of the disease. All patients with the two highest-grade lymphomas, lymphoblastic and diffuse, small noncleaved (Burkitt's and non-Burkitt's), should have cerebrospinal fluid examination at the onset of the disease and during the course of the illness if symptoms or clinical findings are suggestive. Patients with a more common subtype, diffuse large-cell (diffuse histiocytic of Rappaport) lymphoma, have an increased probability of developing meningeal lymphoma during the course of the disease. As described below, patients with this subtype who present with or develop involvement of the sinuses, testes, bone marrow, or epidural space should have careful cerebrospinal fluid evaluation and monitoring (MacKintosh *et al.*, 1982).

Staging of Non-Hodgkin's Lymphomas

The Ann Arbor staging classification described in Chapter 15 is generally used for adult patients with the non-Hodgkin's lymphomas (Carbone *et al.*, 1971). Though no acceptable alternative to the Ann Arbor system is currently available, acknowledged deficiencies of this classification are evident when used for prognoses and therapeutic decisions.

For some of the subtypes, in particular the low-grade lymphomas, widespread stage III or IV disease is very common yet does not confer an ominous prognosis. In contrast, relatively localized disease of the higher-grade lymphomas is associated with fairly rapid, sometimes unpredictable, progression that limits the prognostic value of the staging designation. The size or bulk of the lymphoma mass, at presentation, especially for the higher-grade lymphomas is an important prognostic factor not considered in the Ann Arbor system (Gospodarowicz *et al.*, 1980). The site of involvement not acknowledged in the staging system, such as the mediastinum, bone marrow, or central nervous system, predicts important clinical and prognostic factors. The presence or absence of systemic symptoms, as defined for Hodgkin's disease in the Ann Arbor classification, has more limited value in the non-Hodgkin's lymphomas. These symptoms are less common at the onset for patients with these lymphomas, or when present may not be independent prognostic variables.

The limitations of the Ann Arbor system have led to different staging classifications for children with non-Hodgkin's lymphoma (see Table 16–6) and for patients with Burkitt's

Table 16-6. Murphy Staging System for Childhood Lymphoma

STAGE	CRITERIA FOR EXTENT OF DISEASE
I	A single tumor (extranodal) or single anatomic area (nodal), with the exclusion of mediastinum or abdomen.
II	A single tumor (extranodal) with regional node involvement. Two or more nodal areas on the same side of the diaphragm. Two single (extranodal) tumors with or without regional node involvement on the same side of the diaphragm. A primary gastrointestinal tract tumor, usually in the iliocecal area, with or without involvement of associated mesenteric nodes only.
III	Two single tumors (extranodal) on opposite sides of the diaphragm. Two or more nodal areas above and below the diaphragm. All the primary intrathoracic tumors (mediastinal, pleural, thymic). All extensive primary intra-abdominal disease. All paraspinal or epidural tumors, regardless of other tumor site(s).
IV	Any of the above with initial CNS and/or bone marrow involvement.

lymphoma (see Table 16-7) (Murphy, 1980; Ziegler and Magrath, 1974).

Clinical Symptomatology and Course

The symptoms and clinical courses of patients with the non-Hodgkin's lymphomas are so diverse that they cannot be completely reviewed in a chapter of this size. Therefore, general comments will be made about several of the most common or most unique subtypes and selected clinical problems will be reviewed. For convenience, the terminology of the modified Rappaport system will be used, but this can be easily translated into the subtypes of the formulation of other major classifications.

Diffuse Well-Differentiated Lymphocytic Lymphoma (DLWD). This lymphoma must be differentiated on relatively arbitrary clinical criteria from chronic lymphocytic leukemia. It includes the clinicopathologic variations with plasmacytoid histologic features often associated with serum immunogloulin abnormalities (Pangalis *et al.*, 1977).

Table 16-7. Burkitt's Lymphoma Staging System

STAGE	CRITERIA FOR EXTENT OF DISEASE
A	Single solitary extra-abdominal site
AR	Intra-abdominal tumor with >90% of tumor surgically resected
B	Multiple extra-abdominal sites
C	Intra-abdominal tumor
D	Intra-abdominal tumor with involvement of ≥ 1 extra-abdominal site

Of all the non-Hodgkin's lymphoma subtypes, this neoplasm affects the oldest age group, with a median age of 60 years, and is very rare in young adults and children. Men and women are affected equally. A biopsy diagnosis of DLWD in a child or young adult should always be questioned and may represent lymphocyte predominance Hodgkin's disease or a benign condition when examined more carefully.

A majority of patients with DLWD present with asymptomatic lymphadenopathy. When evaluated appropriately, the lymphadenopathy is often generalized and symmetric. The lymphogram may be diffusely abnormal with a characteristic foamy appearance. Mediastinal masses are uncommon, though hilar and paravertebral adenopathy may be found in the chest.

The bone marrow is involved in patients with DLWD in the majority of cases, usually at the onset or during the course of the disease. Despite involvement of the bone marrow, the typical patient does not show peripheral blood abnormalities. Patients may have a mild lymphocytosis, but if the absolute peripheral blood lymphocyte count exceeds 4000/ml^3 and the bone marrow is diffusely involved, a diagnosis of chronic lymphocytic leukemia (CLL) is usually made. Some patients will develop a serious peripheral blood lymphocytosis during the course of the disease and have a course typical of CLL. The majority do not, however, and despite considerable lymphadenopathy, splenomegaly, and serious disease progression have a relatively modest lymphocytosis, if any at all.

This subtype of lymphoma is the one that most frequently infiltrates many tissues, such as the skin, mucous membranes, and gastrointestinal tract. If biopsies are obtained of the liver, kidney, or other viscera, it is not unusual to demonstrate the lymphocytic infiltrate. It is rare, however, for DLWD to involve the meninges or central nervous system. Chylous pleural effusions or, more rarely, ascites, may result from paravertebral lymph nodes masses.

As with CLL, patients may develop increasing fatigue, low-grade evening fever, night sweats, and weight loss as the lymphadenopathy progresses. Occasionally, marked splenomegaly and hypersplenism produce serious clinical problems.

In general, the prognosis of DLWD is good, with median survivals in the range of six to ten years. Some patients have very stable lymphadenopathy, and a few undergo spontaneous regression.

A group of patients with DLWD, usually with plasmacytoid features, secrete immunoglobulins of the IgM class in the serum. When the macroglobulin level is high, and is detected early in the course, the entity of Waldenström's macroglobulinemia is usually diagnosed (Pangalis *et al.*, 1977). The major clinical differences between DLWD and Waldenström's macroglobulinemia are the presence of macroglobulin in the serum and the effects of hyperviscosity. These result in capillary and small-vessel stasis and thrombosis, platelet dysfunction with bleeding, hypervolemia, and often congestive heart failure. In addition to general approaches to management, plasmaphoresis is important for relieving serious symptoms and problems of the hyperviscosity state. The abnormalities of the retinal circulation due to hyperviscosity, producing "sausage or boxcar" venous enlargements, are characteristic of this condition.

Nodular, Lymphocytic, Poorly Differentiated Lymphoma (NLPD). The NLPD lymphoma (Rappaport) or follicular, small cleaved cell type of the formulation is the most common subtype of non-Hodgkin's lymphoma in the United States. The full array of clinical presentations and courses is quite varied, but a substantial number of patients have a characteristic course.

NLPD is a disease of adults with a median age of about 55 years. It is uncommon in individuals under 30 years of age and extremely rare in children. Men and women are affected equally. It is generally a low-grade neoplasm, often presenting with asymptomatic lymphadenopathy, which may wax and wane. More than any other subtype of lymphoma, patients with NLPD may have been aware of lymphadenopathy for years prior to diagnosis, or an enlarged lymph node may have been removed and thought to be a benign "hyperplasia;" on review years later, these are found to have been NLPD.

The initial lymphadenopathy, in contrast to Hodgkin's disease or high-grade non-Hodgkin's lymphomas, often is found in the femoral-inguinal, axillary, high cervical, epitrochlear, or mesenteric lymph nodes. Abnormalities in the chest x-ray are uncommon at onset, though some patients with very advanced disease will have hilar, paratracheal, or paravertebral enlargements, occasionally associated with chylous pleural effusions.

At the onset, the majority of patients are asymptomatic and a few remain so throughout the natural history of their disease. With time and progression, however, the majority of patients develop progressive lymphadenopathy, some developing systemic symptoms of fever, night sweats, fatigue, and weight loss. Local symptoms or problems develop resulting from the enlarged lymph nodes. Peripheral edema, neuropathies, abdominal pain, ureteral obstruction, ascites, and upper airway problems are all the type of symptoms that may occur as patients with NLPD are observed.

This type of lymphoma is the most common to undergo spontaneous regression (Horning and Rosenberg, 1984). These have been well documented in patients who have been observed without therapy. Occasionally, an infection, such as herpes zoster, precedes the spontaneous regression, but usually the regression occurs with no apparent cause. These patients will usually have a recurrence of their disease, but for others the regression may last for many years or indefinitely.

The bone marrow is frequently involved with NLPD. As many as 80% of patients with widespread lymphadenopathy have marrow infiltrates identifiable if adequate biopsies are obtained (Rosenberg, 1975). These patients usually have no peripheral blood abnormalities. Sometimes, characteristic cleaved or notched lymphocytes are found in the blood in small numbers. Special immunologic techniques and the use of the cell sorter may identify considerable numbers of neoplastic cells in these patients. Rarely, patients with NLPD develop a marked peripheral lymphocytosis, simulating chronic lymphocytic leukemia (CLL). Patients with CLL, however, do not have a nodular or follicular lymph node pattern when examined histologically.

The overall prognosis of patients with NLPD is good, with their median survival in the six-to-ten-year range. The patients (10% to 15% overall) who have relatively localized NLPD after detailed evaluation have an excellent prognosis, perhaps as a result of effective therapy (Paryani *et al.,* 1983).

Other than the characteristic slow progression of NLPD, the most serious clinical problem results from the frequent histologic transformation of the disease. It has been demonstrated that more than half of the patients with NLPD convert to a more aggressive type of lymphoma within five to seven years after diagnosis (Hubbard *et al.,* 1982; Acker *et al.,* 1983). The transformation is usually to a diffuse large-cell type — diffuse histiocytic (DH) of Rappaport. The clinical course and prognosis then changes for these patients, and the majority succumb to their disease within a few years. The few immunologic studies that have been done on tissues of patients who have converted from NLPD to DH indicate that they retain the same B-cell immunophenotype, the conversion representing a more rapidly proliferating state of the same neoplastic clone of cells (Woda and Knowles, 1979). This conversion seems to occur whether or not the patient has received therapy for the NLPD, and no matter what the type of therapy previously employed. The transition is similar to that in patients with CLL when they develop an aggressive large-cell lymphoma, the so-called Richter's syndrome.

Diffuse Large-Cell Lymphoma. The subtype designated as diffuse, large-cell type in the formulation corresponds most closely to the diffuse, histiocytic lymphoma (DH) of Rappaport. The formulation recognizes that the term histiocytic is scientifically inaccurate. In addition, another subtype, immunoblastic lymphoma, which has a slightly worse prognosis than the remainder of the group, is included in the Rappaport DH (NLPCP, 1982). The majority of the clinical data in the literature, however, corresponds most closely to the relatively heterogeneous subtype DH. For the purposes of this chapter, the two terms diffuse large-cell and DH will be used interchangeably.

DH is a relatively aggressive lymphoma with a wide spectrum of clinical presentations. It occurs in all age groups, with median age somewhat younger than that found in the low-grade subtypes. Males and females are affected equally. More than any other subtype, DH presents in extranodal sites. The neoplasm may be limited to the extranodal site (stage I_E) or include local draining lymph nodes (stage II_E). Overall, about half of patients have relatively localized stages I and II disease extent.

The most common sites of extranodal presentation of DH are the gastrointestinal tract, usually the stomach or small bowel, bone, and skin. Almost any tissue or organ, however, may be the site of a primary DH, including the thyroid, testes, lung, bone marrow, and even the brain.

DH lymphoma usually progresses rapidly and local tumor growth, often locally symptomatic, usually occurs without systemic symptoms of fever and night sweats. The presenting symptoms depend on the site of the tumor, but may result in pain, edema, bowel obstruction, or neurologic deficit. An abdominal presentation due to mesenteric adenopathy, with or without abdominal visceral involvement, is relatively common in DH, the diagnosis being made at exploratory laparotomy.

The prognosis of DH, more than the other subtypes of non-Hodgkin's lymphomas, is well correlated with the Ann Arbor stage. In addition, the size or bulk of the neoplasm is a prognostic variable (Gospodarowicz *et al.,* 1980). The larger the size, the worse the prognosis. Different series indicate that patients who have a mass greater than 5, 7, or 10 cm have a poorer survival. Tumor size is probably a continuous variable in this regard.

Computed tomography of the involved region, bipedal lymphography, and bone marrow biopsy are all important diagnostic procedures for patients with DH. Staging laparotomy is generally not recommended, because the yield is low and treatment decisions are usually not changed.

In contrast to low-grade lymphomas, in which cure by any therapy is unlikely, patients can be cured of DH lymphoma (Schein *et al.,* 1974). The overall median survival of patients with all stages of DH, before the advent of curative chemotherapy, was 12 to 18 months. As discussed below, the prognosis has considerably improved, depending on the stage and sites of disease.

All patients with lymphoma, especially uncontrolled DH, may develop epidural disease, with spinal cord or other neurologic compression. Patients with DH may develop meningeal lymphoma. Those patients at greatest risk for developing meningeal DH are those whose disease initially involves the bone marrow, testes, epidural space, sinuses, or the peripheral blood. Another major prognostic factor in the development of meningeal DH is recurrence or persistence of the disease after initial therapy (MacKintosh *et al.,* 1982).

DH lymphoma including the immunoblastic subtype (immunoblastic sarcoma of Lukes and Collins) is the type of lymphoma most often occurring in the setting of immune deficiency, collagen vascular disease, and post-transplantation (Talal *et al.,* 1967; Banks *et al.,* 1979; Penn, 1975).

Lymphoblastic Lymphoma. This clinico-pathologic entity, initally described by Barcos and Lukes, (1975) as convoluted T-cell lymphoma, is generally called lymphoblastic lymphoma (LL) (Nathwani *et al.,* 1981). This is a very aggressive neoplasm, more common in males than females, having a broad age range, and mainly affecting children and young adults. The median age was 16 years in the international study (see Table 16–1).

The cellular morphology of LL is indistinguishable from that seen in many patients with acute lymphocytic leukemia (ALL) particularly of the T-cell, or unfavorable, type. Patients with LL frequently present with, or subsequently develop, bone marrow involvement and meningeal disease. The clinical picture, therefore, overlaps with ALL.

The major clinical characteristic distinguishing LL from ALL is the extent of bone marrow involvement and the lymph node enlargement. Patients with LL do not usually present with a leukemic blood picture, and as many as half do not have bone marrow involvement at onset. In contrast, the majority have significant tumor masses, especially in the anterior mediastinum (see Figure 16–4). These intrathoracic tumors probably arise in the thymus. They may be massive and produce life-threatening problems such as superior vena caval obstruction, airway occlusion, pericardial and large pleural effusions.

When studied with immune markers, LL is usually a T-cell neoplasm (Lukes *et al.,* 1978). It is also terminal deoxytransferase (TDT) and focal acid phosphatase positive (Kung *et al.,* 1978). The lymphoma cells are kinetically very active, capable of rapid growth, a rapid response to therapy and may precipitate a tumor lysis syndrome.

Although LL is among the most aggressive and high-grade subtypes of non-Hodgkin's lymphomas, it is among the most curable with appropriate treatment programs (Weinstein *et al.,* 1979; Coleman *et al.,* 1981). Management, to be described below (and in Chapter 7), must take into account its early dissemination, especially to the bone marrow, its tendency to involve the meninges, and the need for intensive induction and consolidation therapy. Though the tumor is very radiosensitive, irradiation has only a limited role in the therapy program, even in the face of very large tumor masses.

Diffuse Small Noncleaved Cell Lymphoma. The most aggressive subtype of non-Hodgkin's lymphoma in the formulation are diffuse, small noncleaved cell types, both Burkitt's and non-Burkitt's. The Burkitt's type has a more uniform cytology, occurs in a younger age group and has important epidemiologic and viral associations. The non-Burkitt's type is more often seen in adults, is a more heterogeneous disease, but is also very high grade (Gro-

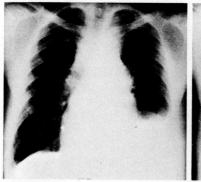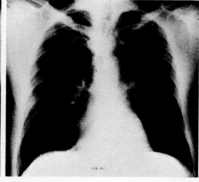

Figure 16–4. Chest roentgenogram demonstrating typical anterior mediastinal lymphoblastic lymphoma and a rapid response to chemotherapy.

gan *et al.*, 1982). More satisfactory clinical experience has been documented for the Burkitt's type than the non-Burkitt's type, but they will be described together.

Burkitt's lymphoma in its typical clinical form in African children affects boys more than girls and at a young age. Characteristically, the tumor involves the bones of the face, the mandibles, and maxillae, and may reach very large proportions. The lymphoma involves the gastrointestinal tract, ovaries, and breast, as well as lymph nodes. Bone marrow involvement is not an early or prominent feature, but meningeal spread occurs frequently.

A unique staging system has been described for patients with Burkitt's lymphoma (see Table 16–7), and is more useful than the Ann Arbor system. It recognizes that bulk of the tumor is an important prognostic variable and that surgical removal of the major tumor mass is beneficial (Ziegler and Magrath, 1974).

Tumor masses of patients with Burkitt's or non-Burkitt's subtypes are rapidly proliferating and respond dramatically to therapy. As a result, the tumor lysis syndrome must be anticipated in the therapeutic program. Patients with these high-grade lymphomas, if not responsive to therapy, have a median survival of less than a year, usually only a few months. Treatment, however, can be very successful and can result in cure for a significant proportion (see below) (Ziegler, 1981).

Other Clinicopathologic Subtypes. It is beyond the scope of this chapter to discuss, in detail, all the subtypes of non-Hodgkin's lymphomas or the wide variety of clinical problems that may occur. Brief comments, however, may be of value.

The low-grade lymphomas generally include the diffuse, well-differentiated (small lymphocytic) and the nodular or follicular subtypes with small cleaved or mixed small-cleaved and large-cell composition. A diffuse lymphoma, with intermediate differentiation (DLID), between a well-differentiated and small cleaved cell type has been described (Mann *et al.*, 1979). This DLID may not be recognized by other than the most experienced hematopathologists. DLID has been mistakenly called DLWD, accounting for those patients who have an unexpected, more aggressive, course. They may have also been included in series of patients with diffuse, lymphocytic, poorly differentiated subtypes of Rappaport, or the diffuse, small cleaved cell type of Lukes and Collins, accounting for a

more favorable course than expected. A follicular type composed of these intermediate cells has been described and called a mantle zone lymphoma (Weisenburger *et al.*, 1982). It identifies a relatively rare subtype that has a favorable natural history (low grade).

The nodular or follicular lymphomas include a morphologic and clinical spectrum from the most favorable or indolent type composed of small cleaved cells to a more aggressive type, though still follicular, composed of large follicular center cells. The most aggressive type corresponds to the nodular histiocytic (NH) subtype of Rappaport. This relatively uncommon lymphoma is called follicular large-cell lymphoma in the formulation and is of intermediate grade in its natural history. This group of patients differs from those at the indolent end of the spectrum, in that their disease is localized more often, with less frequent bone marrow involvement. They have poorer prognoses yet potential for prolonged remissions after appropriate therapy, resulting in probable cure of the neoplasms. In these regards, NH is similar to the diffuse histiocytic group of Rappaport (Osborne *et al.*, 1982). Yet NH usually presents in lymph nodes rather than extranodal sites, perhaps because the follicular architectural pattern is often lost in tissues other than the lymph nodes.

The nodular mixed (NM) subtype of Rappaport, follicular mixed, small cleaved, and large-cell subtype of the formulation, is intermediate in its behavior between NLPD and NH. The morphologic criteria separating NM from NLPD on the one hand and NH on the other, are not absolute and vary in interpretation by pathologists. In general, patients with NM behave more like patients with NLPD than with NH. In most series their prognosis is slightly worse and bone marrow involvement is less common. In one small series, prolonged disease-free survival was described in a proportion of patients treated for advanced disease (Longo *et al.*, 1981).

The diffuse mixed (DM) subtype of Rappaport is included in the formulation for morphologic reasons, without recognized clinical significance. In general, patients with DM behave like those who have the DH subtype and are included in these series. Lennert has described a group of patients with a component of benign epithelial histiocytes in the pathologic picture (Lennert and Mestdagh, 1968). Although the question of whether some of these patients have Hodgkin's disease remains, they generally are included in the DM category with an intermediate grade behavior.

Patients with immunoblastic lymphoma had been included in the DH subtype of Rappaport. As a group, these patients probably have a poorer prognosis and are considered high grade. Lukes and his colleagues have divided these patients into those with B-cell and T-cell types (Lukes and Collins, 1974). The B-cell type in its characteristic form is pyrinophilic and may correspond to an anaplastic or poorly differentiated plasma cell neoplasm. The T-cell type is composed of large clear cells but may be quite pleomorphic with smaller "wrinkled" lymphocytes admixed as described by Waldron (NLPCP, 1982). The clinical differences between these groups of patients with immunoblastic lymphoma are not established, and even their distinction from the larger group of patients with diffuse large cell lymphomas is not clear.

Management

The management of patients with non-Hodgkin's lymphomas is both challenging and satisfying. Generalizations are difficult because of the wide spectrum of histologic subtypes, the added variables of stage, site, and age, and especially because this is a field of very active clinical investigation and controversy. These patients, however, perhaps more so than any other group with neoplasms, are highly responsive to therapy, and a substantial proportion can be cured of their tumors. Even if cure is not achieved, almost all patients with non-Hodgkin's lymphomas can benefit from therapy with very good palliation and probable prolongation of life.

As a generalization, patients with the intermediate and high-grade lymphomas not only have relatively aggressive tumors, but they can be cured of their neoplasm. Therefore, therapy should be initiated promptly, after the appropriate diagnostic and staging procedures. Outside of the study or research setting, this is not the case for patients with the low-grade lymphomas. Despite their responsiveness to therapy, no satisfactory documentation has been made of cure of patients with advanced (stages III to IV) low-grade lymphomas. Because these patients tend to be older, with an average age of 55 to 60 years, a palliative program is usually indicated (Rosenberg, 1982).

Radiotherapy. The role of radiotherapy is relatively limited in the curative management of patients with the non-Hodgkin's lymphomas. In general, a dose of 3500 to 5000 rad is utilized to permanently irradicate the tumor. This is more often accomplished for the low-grade subtypes than for the higher-grade and for smaller rather than larger tumor masses.

The limitations of radiotherapy in managing patients with the non-Hodgkin's lymphomas, in contrast to Hodgkin's disease, is that these patients generally have unpredictable, often widespread, occult disease, which cannot be adequately encompassed with tolerable irradiation fields. The use of wide-field, high-dose irradiation in an attempt to cure patients with non-Hodgkin's lymphoma usually compromises the tolerance and timing of administration of chemotherapy, which has the potential of curing the disease.

The major indications for radiation therapy for patients with non-Hodgkin's lymphoma are:

1. Treatment of patients with low-grade lymphomas adequately staged, with disease of stage I or II extent, with curative intent (Paryani *et al.,* 1983);
2. Palliation of patients with low-grade lymphomas, of stage III or IV extent, individualized to the patient's problems and response to chemotherapy;
3. Whole brain irradiation, as part of meningeal and central nervous system prophylaxis, in the curative program for patients at high risk for this site of disease;
4. Combined modality programs for selected patients and disease settings, such as those with very bulky tumors, epidural cord compression, destructive bone lesions, and ureteral obstruction; and
5. Palliation of patients with all subtypes who have recurrences after initial potentially curative treatment programs.

When irradiation is considered as a potentially curative program for patients with relatively localized non-Hodgkin's lymphomas, different treatment fields must be considered than are usually utilized for patients with Hodgkin's disease. The lymphoid tissues of Waldeyer's ring must be considered as a potential site for occult disease, and the entire abdomen is at risk because of the involvement and mobility of mesenteric lymph nodes.

Chemotherapy. The mainstay of the treatment of patients with non-Hodgkin's lymphomas is chemotherapy. Many drugs and

Table 16-8. Palliative Single Agent Chemotherapy for Low Grade Non-Hodgkin's Lymphomas

Chlorambucil
    6 to 12 mg (po) daily
    30 mg/m² (po) twice monthly
    16 mg/m² (po) for 5 days, monthly

Cyclophosphamide
    75 to 150 mg (po) daily
    400 mg/m² (po) for 5 days, monthly

Note: Drug dosage must be adjusted to blood count tolerance and response. Prednisone, vincristine, or bleomycin may be added depending on blood count tolerance and response.

classes of agents are very active against this disease, and numerous combination chemotherapy regimens have been developed and are effective.

Single agent chemotherapy, usually with an oral alkylating agent, is an acceptable method of palliation for patients with low-grade non-Hodgkin's lymphomas (Hoppe *et al.*, 1981). This approach, however, has no potential for cure, which is the goal for patients with the higher-grade neoplasms. Table 16-8 lists several recommendations for the use of single agent palliative chemotherapy.

Numerous combination chemotherapy regimens have been developed for patients with the non-Hodgkin's lymphomas. Most include an alkylating agent, usually cyclophosphamide, vincristine, and prednisone. The initial experience with three drug regimens of this type, though producing high response rates, failed to result in adequate control of the more aggressive neoplasms. The addition of procarbazine, doxorubicin, bleomycin, methotrexate, the nitrosoureas, and podophylotoxins has provided a wide variety of combinations and schedule variations. These regimens have gradually resulted in improved complete re-

sponse rates and duration of responses. In some cases, particular regimens have been found to be more satisfactory for specific subtypes. The literature, however, is generally confusing and unsatisfactory in providing comparative treatment results that can be used to select the optimal chemotherapy regimen. The problem is further complicated by variable histologic criteria, groups and expertise in chemotherapy reports, and small series with short follow-up. Table 16-9 lists some of the major chemotherapy regimens used for the largest group of patients, those called DH according to Rappaport.

The CVP regimen or variations of it can be recommended for patients with low-grade histologic subtypes who require a relatively aggressive treatment program (Bagley *et al.*, 1972). This is indicated if a rapid response is required because of the severity of symptoms, rapid progression of disease, or serious local problems such as ureteral deviation or chylous effusion.

The CHOP regimen is probably the most widely used for intermediate-grade lymphomas, and, in particular, those with the more favorable settings of DH (McKelvey *et al.*, 1976). Generally, six cycles are given at three- to four-week intervals. At least two cycles should be administered after a complete remission has been documented. Patients who have slowly responsive disease or who, because of the site or bulk of the disease, have poorer prognoses, may require more prolonged chemotherapy to maximal doxorubicin tolerance.

Some patients with intermediate or high-grade subtypes have a rapidly growing tumor that must be treated more continuously than is achieved by the CHOP regimen. The BACOP

Table 16-9. Combination Chemotherapy Results for Previously Untreated Patients with Advanced Diffuse Histiocytic Lymphoma

REGIMEN	YEAR	COMPLETE RESPONSE FREQUENCY (%)	MEDIAN SURVIVAL (mo)	REFERENCE
CVP	1969	42	8	Nissen *et al.*, 1977
C-MOPP	1975	41	9	DeVita *et al.*, 1975
CHOP/HOP	1976	68/66	23	McKelvey *et al.*, 1976
BACOP	1976	48	>17	Schein *et al.*, 1976
BACOP	1977	56	9	Skarin *et al.*, 1977
COMLA	1980	55	>33	Sweet *et al.*, 1980
M-BACOD	1980	80	>21	Skarin *et al.*, 1980
ProMACE-MOPP	1980	63	>19	Fisher *et al.*, 1980
COP-BLAM	1981	73	>23	

Adapted from Laurence, J.; Coleman, M.; Allen, S. L.; Silver, R. T.; and Pasmantier, M.: Combination chemotherapy of advanced diffuse histiocytic lymphoma with the six-drug COP-BLAM regimen. *Ann. Intern. Med.*, **97:**190-195, 1982.

Table 16–10. Stanford Lymphoblastic Lymphoma (II) Regimen

WEEK	INDUCTION			CONSOLIDATION						REINFORCEMENT										MAINTENANCE				
	1	2	3	4	5	6	7	8	9	10	11	12	13	14	15	16	17	18	19	20	21	22	+	52
Cyclophosphamide—po 400 mg/m² × 3d	✓								✓			✓			✓			✓						
Doxorubicin—IV 50 mg/m²	✓	✓		✓	✓	✓			✓			✓			✓			✓						
Vincristine—IV 1.4 mg/m² (max. 2.0)	✓	✓	✓	✓	✓	✓			✓			✓			✓			✓						
Prednisone—po 40 mg/m²	daily → taper								5 days			5 days			5 days			5 days						
L-Asparaginase—IM 6000 U/m² (max. 10,000 U) 5 doses				WF ✓✓	MWF ✓✓✓	✓✓✓																		
Methotrexate—IT 12 mg/m² (max. 12 mg)	0		✓			MTh ✓	MTh ✓	M ✓																
Whole Brain—XRT							(5 doses) [2400/12fx]																	
6-Mercaptopurine—po 75 mg/m²																							Daily	
Methotrexate—po 30 mg/m²																							Weekly	

(Schein *et al.,* 1976) or M-BACOD (Skarin *et al.,* 1980) regimens provide more continuous therapy and use relatively non-marrow-suppressing drugs during the second half of the treatment cycle. An approach of increasing interest and popularity is the use of multiple drugs (six or eight) in alternating regimens. The ProMACE/MOPP and COP/BLAM regimens are such approaches with encouraging preliminary results (Fisher *et al.,* 1980; Laurence *et al.,* 1982).

Patients with the highest-grade lymphomas, lymphoblastic lymphoma, and the undifferentiated or small noncleaved cell type (Burkitt's and non-Burkitt's) require regimens that are more aggressive and continuous than those described above. These patients, often children or young adults, are managed most successfully with programs adapted from those employed for patients with relatively unfavorable acute lymphoblastic leukemia (Weinstein *et al.,* 1979; Coleman *et al.,* 1981). The Stanford regimen for patients with lymphoblastic lymphoma and the NCI program for patients with Burkitt's type lymphomas (MacGrath *et al.,* 1981) are shown in Tables 16–10 and 16–11. Chapter 39 should be consulted for a review of the experience of treating children with these high-grade lymphomas. Attention must be directed to the prevention of central nervous system (CNS) lymphomatous extension and growth in these patients. The CNS prophylaxis must be initiated early in the treatment program. Despite the very aggressive nature of these lymphomas and the difficulty of the treatment program, a majority of patients with these highest-grade lymphomas can be cured of their diseases.

No Initial Therapy. An area of continued controversy is the recommendation of therapy for patients with stages III and IV low-grade lymphomas. This is a common clinical problem in the United States.

The general experience is that despite high response rates to treatment programs, which have included combination chemotherapy, combined modality therapy (irradiation and chemotherapy), and whole body irradiation, relapse rate is continuous through ten years or more (Hoppe *et al.,* 1981). Because no plateau has been observed in the relapse-free or survival curves, cure cannot be claimed for patients with these relatively indolent neoplasms. Moreover, the several randomized trials that have been reported show no survival advantage of various treatment programs, including relatively conservative single agent treatment (Glick *et al.,* 1981).

Because of the relatively advanced age and asymptomatic state of these patients, a Stanford series of selected patients was reported in which therapy was withheld until required (Portlock and Rosenberg, 1979). This series has been updated at intervals and compared, when possible, to patients on various treatment protocols. The median survival of patients with low-grade lymphomas of stages III and IV extent managed initially without therapy, is approximately ten years (see Figure 16–5). Some of these patients undergo spontaneous regression and approximately 20% have never required therapy. As a group, these patients will require palliative treatment after a median period of observation of three to four years. Those with nodular mixed lymphomas, however, on the average require treatment within two years year of diagnosis.

No initial treatment is often difficult for the physician and patient to accept when a diagnosis of a neoplasm has been made. This is especially so when the evidence of disease can be markedly reduced in the majority of patients. Many patients, however, are best managed by delaying therapy until the tempo of the disease is assessed. Just as for patients with chronic lymphocytic leukemia, treatment

Table 16–11. Diffuse Small Noncleaved Cell (Burkitt's and non-Burkitt) Regimen (NCI)

Systemic therapy		
Cyclophosphamide (IV)	1200 mg/m^2	day 1*
Doxorubicin (IV)	40 mg/m^2	day 1
Vincristine (IV)	1.4 mg/m^2	day 1
Prednisone (po)	40 mg/m^2	days 1 through 5
Methotrexate (IV)†	2.7 g/m^2	day 10 (24-hr infusion)
Intrathecal therapy‡		
Methotrexate	12 mg/m^2	days 1 and 10 (12 mg max. dose)

* Six cycles are usually administered, at three-week intervals.
† With leucovorin rescue
‡ Cytosine arabinoside may be added.

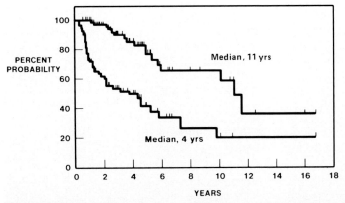

Figure 16–5. Actuarial survival curve of 83 patients with low-grade non-Hodgkin's lymphoma managed palliatively, delaying therapy until required (upper curve). Also shown is the actuarial probability of the time to requiring therapy (lower curve).

may be delayed for prolonged periods without compromising their comfort and survival.

Treatment Recommendations. It is difficult to provide precise treatment recommendations for the wide variety of clinical settings of patients with the non-Hodgkin's lymphomas. In some areas, controversy has not been settled by appropriate studies and in others, new, very promising treatment results are preliminary and unconfirmed. Nonetheless, it may be useful to have a general guide to management. Table 16–12 lists the major subtypes and management recommendations.

Related Clinical Entities

Several clinicopathologic entities are related to the non-Hodgkin's lymphomas but are not included in the usual description of these diseases. A limited discussion of these conditions follows, with more detailed reviews available in the literature referenced.

Angioimmunoblastic   Lymphadenopathy (AILD). This condition of adults, also called immunoblastic lymphadenopathy (Lukes and Tindle, 1975), lies on the borderline between a hypersensitivity disorder and a malignant lymphoma. The full syndrome includes symptoms of fever, skin rash, arthralgias or arthritis, polyclonal hypergammaglobulinemia, autoimmune hemolytic anemia, thrombocytopenia, pulmonary infiltrates, lymphadenopathy, and hepatosplenomegaly. The histologic picture is a marked immunoblastic reaction with eosinophilia, vascular proliferation, and a hyaline interstitial infiltrate (Frizzera *et al.,* 1975). Commonly, patients have only some of the symptoms and findings. Rarely, the disorder is self-limited. Most often it is progressive, the patient succumbing to episodes of infection and bone marrow failure. In a significant proportion of patients, the histologic and clinical picture transforms to a large-cell lymphoma of the histiocytic or immuno-

Table 16–12.   Management Recommendations* for Patients with Non-Hodgkin's Lymphomas

Low grade (DLWD, NLPD, NM)†	
Localized, stages I and II	Radiotherapy, modified involved fields
Generalized, stages III and IV	Palliative programs
Intermediate grade (NH, DLPD, DM, DH)	
Favorable localized, stages I, I_E, II	Radiotherapy (RT)
Unfavorable‡ localized, stages I, I_E, II	Combination chemotherapy *i.e.,* CHOP + RT
Generalized, stages III and IV	Combination chemotherapy, *i.e.,* CHOP
Generalized, unfavorable, stage IV	Combination chemotherapy, *i.e.,* M-BACOD
High grade (IBS, LL, DU)	
All stages	Combination chemotherapy with CNS prophylaxis (LL, DU)

* Patients staged with bone marrow biopsy, lymphogram, or abdominal CT scan
† Patients under age 40 or over age 70 should be individualized, younger patients might be treated more aggressively and older patients more conservatively.
‡ Bulky tumors (> 7 cm), multiple sites (> 2), systemic symptoms

blastic type. The overall prognosis of AILD is poor, with median survivals one to two years.

The usual treatment recommendation is to use corticosteroid therapy for symptomatic patients. This is generally of limited value, with eventually uncontrolled symptoms. Combination chemotherapy is then utilized including cyclophosphamide, vinca alkaloids, and doxorubicin, even in the absence of neoplastic transformation.

New therapeutic programs are required for these patients, perhaps utilizing approaches toward restoring the T-suppressor cell deficiency seen in AILD, or those regimens employed for autoimmune diseases or for organ transplantation.

Malignant Histiocytosis. Malignant histiocytosis is a neoplasm of the phagocytic histiocyte. It is a high-grade tumor often presenting with fever, lymphadenopathy, hepatosplenomegaly, and bone marrow infiltration. Erythrophagocytosis by the neoplastic cell in tissue sections of the bone marrow and spleen with involvement of the splenic red pulp helps distinguish this disease from the usual non-Hodgkin's lymphomas (Mann *et al.,* 1979).

The disease is usually rapidly progressive, may involve the skin, lung, and meninges, and results in death in less than a year in most patients.

Treatment can be successful for malignant histiocytosis with chemotherapy regimens like CHOP or M-BACOD. A series of patients, treated with CHOP and with high-dose methotrexate on days 10 to 14, achieved a high complete response rate in almost half of the patients, without relapse for two years or longer (Tseng *et al.,* 1983). The cure of this condition may be possible with aggressive treatment programs.

Mycosis Fungoides. A detailed description of this disorder is found in the discussion of cutaneous T-cell disorders in Chapters 6D and 21.

The classic clinical picture of mycosis fungoides overlaps with that of large-cell lymphoma. The cytologic and histologic findings in mycosis fungoides are characteristic, however, in the eyes of experienced hematopathologists (Mann *et al.,* 1979). A variant of mycosis fungoides in which the characteristic cerebriform, highly convoluted tumor cells are found in the blood is called the Sézary syndrome.

Rarely, the visceral manifestations of these cutaneous lymphomas predominate while skin problems are minimal. The prognoses of such patients is poor in contrast to those with disease confined to the skin. The treatment must be systemic chemotherapy of the type used for diffuse large-cell lymphoma. The results of therapy are in general unsatisfactory in these older patients, who are highly susceptible to infection and inanition.

Future Prospects

New developments in immunology, virology, bone marrow transplantation, and improved treatment programs predict considerable change in the near future in the understanding and control of the non-Hodgkin's lymphomas. Understanding and applying immunologic concepts, markers, probes, and therapies offers great promise. There has been a virtual explosion of knowledge and technology, from the realization that small lymphocytes were potential stem cells of either B- or T-cell lineage to the current use of monoclonal antibodies to dissect cell types, origins, and relationships. The initial efforts of Lukes and Collins (1974) to predict clinical behavior as a function of B- or T-cell phenotype was the beginning of what is now the very complex field of human lymphoid neoplasms. It seems likely that specific cell markers will improve the ability to predict clinical behavior of these diverse neoplasms and improve our abilities to identify minimal residual or occult disease and perhaps to direct therapies.

Monoclonal antibodies have already been used to treat patients with various lymphomas (Miller *et al.,* 1982). Their future application may be as adjuvants or as conjugates for directing cytotoxic therapy.

Interferon has been shown to have antitumor activity in the low-grade non-Hodgkin's lymphomas (Merigan *et al.,* 1978). The availability of relatively pure interferon of different types may provide a useful therapeutic approach and possibly a better understanding of normal lymphoproliferative control mechanisms.

As bone marrow transplantation, described in Chapter 43, becomes safer and more applicable, it is a logical approach to certain patients with non-Hodgkin's lymphomas (Applebaum *et al.,* 1981). Autologous bone marrow may be rendered free of lymphoma cells *in vitro* with monoclonal antibodies or other maneuvers and provide the margin of safety to provide curative chemotherapy and/or irradiation for these patients.

Finally, and of most importance and promise, is the likely identification of human viruses that are associated and are etiologically important in the human lymphomas. The Epstein-Barr virus and the type-C retrovirus, *e.g.,* human T-cell leukemia/lymphoma virus, are strong candidates for the study and the development of methods to prevent and possibly reverse the neoplastic process.

Nowhere in the field of oncology is there more ferment, excitement, and promise than in the understanding, control, and management of the non-Hodgkin's lymphomas.

REFERENCES

Acker, B.; Hoppe, R. T.; Colby, T. V.; Cox, R. S.; Kaplan, H. S.; and Rosenberg, S. A.: Histologic conversion in the non-Hodgkin's lymphomas. *J. Clin. Oncol.,* 1:11–16, 1983.

Applebaum, F. R.; Fefer, A.; Cheever, M. A.; Buckner, C. D.; Greenberg, P. D.; Kaplan, H.; Storb, R.; and Thomas, E. D.: Treatment of non-Hodgkin's lymphoma with marrow transplantation in identical twins. *Blood,* 58:509–513, 1981.

Bagley, C. M., Jr.; DeVita, V. T., Jr.; Berard, C. W.; and Canellos, G. P.: Advanced lymphosarcoma-intensive cyclical combination chemotherapy with cyclophosphamide, vincristine, and prednisone. *Ann. Intern. Med.,* 76:227–234, 1972.

Banks, P. M.; Witrak, G. A.; and Conn, D. L.: Lymphoid neoplasia following connective tissue disease. *Mayo Clin. Proc.,* 54:104–108, 1979.

Barcos, M. Q. P., and Lukes, R. J.: Malignant lymphoma of convoluted lymphocytes: A new entity of possible T-cell type. In Sinks, L., and Gooden, J. (eds.): *Conflicts in Childhood Cancer. An Evaluation of Current Management.* Alan R. Liss, Inc., New York, 1975.

Brunning, R. D.; Bloomfield, D. C.; McKenna, R. W.; and Peterson, L.: Bilateral trephine bone marrow biopsies in lymphoma and other neoplastic diseases. *Ann. Intern. Med.,* 82:365–366, 1975.

Burkitt, D.: A sarcoma involving the jaws in African children. *Br. J. Surg.,* 46:218–224, 1958.

Cantor, K. P., and Fraumeni, J. F.: Distribution of non-Hodgkin's lymphoma in the United States between 1950 & 1975. *Cancer Res.,* 40:2645–2652, 1980.

Carbone, P. P.; Kaplan, H. S.; Musshof, K.; Smithers, D. W.; and Tubiana, M: Report of the committee on Hodgkin's staging classification. *Cancer Res.,* 31:1860–1861, 1971.

Castellino, R. A.; Dunnick, N. R.; Goffinet, D. R.; Rosenberg, S. A.; and Kaplan, H. S.: Predictive value of lymphography for sites of subdiaphragmatic disease encountered at staging laparotomy in newly diagnosed Hodgkin's disease and non-Hodgkin's lymphoma. *J. Clin. Oncol.,* 1:532–536, 1983.

Coleman, C. N.; Cohen, J. C.; Burke, J. S.; and Rosenberg, S. A.: Lymphoblastic lymphoma in adults—results of a pilot protocol. *Blood,* 57:579–584, 1981.

Fisher, R. I.; DeVita, V. T.; Hubbard, S. M.; Brennan, M. F.; Chabner, B. A.; Simon, R.; and Young, R. C.: Pro-MACE-MOPP combination chemotherapy: Treatment of diffuse lymphomas. *Proc. Am. Soc. Clin. Oncol.,* 21:468, 1980.

Frizzera, G.; Moran, E. M.; and Rappaport, H.: Angioim-munoblastic lymphadenopathy. *Am. J. Med.,* 59:803–818, 1975.

Gallo, R. C., and Wong-Staal, F.: Retroviruses as etiologic agents of some animal and human leukemias and lymphomas and as tools for elucidating the molecular mechanisms of leukemogenesis. *Blood,* 60:545–557, 1982.

Glick, J. H.; Barnes, J. M.; Ezdinli, E. Z.; Berard, C. W.; Orlow, E. L. and Bennett, J. M.: Nodular mixed lymphoma: Results of a randomized trial failing to confirm prolonged disease-free survival with COPP chemotherapy. *Blood,* 58:920–925, 1981.

Goffinet, D. R.; Warnke, R.; Dunnick, N. R.; Castellino, R.; Glatstein, E.; Nelsen, T. S.; Dorfman, R. F.; Rosenberg, S. A.; and Kaplan, H. S.: Clinical and surgical (laparotomy) evaluation of patients with non-Hodgkin's lymphomas. *Cancer Treat. Rep.,* 61:981–992, 1977.

Gospodarowicz, M. K.; Bush, R. S.; Bergsagel, D. E.; and Brown, T. C.: Bulk of tumor as an important prognostic factor in non-Hodgkin's lymphomas. *Proc. Am. Soc. Clin. Oncol.,* 21:463, 1980.

Grogan, T. M.; Warnke, R. A.; and Kaplan, H. S.: A comparative study of Burkitt's and non-Burkitt's "undifferentiated" malignant lymphoma: Immunologic, cytochemical, ultrastructural, cytologic histopathologic, clinical and cell culture features. *Cancer,* 49:1817–1828, 1982.

Hoppe, R. T.; Burke, J. S.; Glatstein, E.; and Kaplan, H. S.: Non-Hodgkin's lymphoma: Involvement of Waldeyer's ring. *Cancer,* 42:1096–1104, 1978.

Hoppe, R. T.; Kushlan, P.; Kaplan, H. S.; Rosenberg, S. A.; and Brown, B. W.: The treatment of advanced stage favorable histology non-Hodgkin's lymphoma: A preliminary report of a randomized trial comparing single agent chemotherapy, combination chemotherapy and whole body irradiation. *Blood,* 58:592–598, 1981.

Horning, S. J., and Rosenberg, S. A.: Survival, spontaneous regression and histologic transformation in initially untreated non-Hodgkin's lymphomas of low grade. *New Eng. J. Med.,* 311:1471–1475, 1984.

Hubbard, S. M.; Chabner, B. A.; DeVita, V. T.; Simon, R.; Berard, C. W.; Jones, R. B.; Garvin, A. J.; Canellos, G. P.; Osborne, C. K.; and Young, R. C.: Histologic progression in non-Hodgkin's lymphomas. *Blood,* 59:258–264, 1982.

Klein, G.: The role of Epstein-Barr virus in the etiology of Burkitt's lymphoma and nasopharyngeal carcinoma. In Rosenberg, S. A., and Kaplan, H. S. (eds.): *Malignant Lymphomas. Etiology, Immunology, Pathology, Treatment.* Bristol-Myers Cancer Symposia. Vol. 3. Academic Press, New York, 1982.

Krikorian, J. G.; Portlock, C. S.; Cooney, D. P.; and Rosenberg, S. A.: Spontaneous regression of non-Hodgkin's lymphoma. A report of nine cases. *Cancer,* 46:2093–2099, 1980.

Kung, P. C.; Long, J. C.; McCaffrey, R. P.; Ratliff, R. L.; Harrison, T. A.; and Baltimore, D.: Terminal deoxynucleotidyl transferase in the diagnosis of leukemia and malignant lymphoma. *Am. J. Med.,* 64:788–794, 1978.

Laurence, J.; Coleman, M.; Allen, S. L.; Silver, R. T.; and Pasmantier, M.: Combination chemotherapy of advanced diffuse histiocytic lymphoma with the six-drug COP-BLAM regimen. *Ann. Intern. Med.,* 97:190–195, 1982.

Lennert, K., and Mestdagh, J.: Lymphogranulomatosen mit konstant hohem Epitheloidzellgehalt. *Virchows Arch. [Pathol. Anat.],* 344:1–20, 1968.

Lennert, K.; Mohri, N.; Stein, H.; and Kaiserling, E.: The

histopathology of malignant lymphoma. *Br. J. Haematol.,* **31(Suppl):**193–203, 1975.

Longo, D.; Hubbard, S.; Wesley, M.; Jaffe, E.; Chabner, B.; DeVita, V.; and Young, R.: Prolonged initial remission in patients with nodular mixed lymphoma (NML). *Proc. Am. Soc. Clin. Oncol.,* **22:**521, 1981 (abst).

Lukes, R. J., and Collins, R. D.: Immunological characterization of human malignant lymphomas. *Cancer,* **34:**1488–1503, 1974.

Lukes, R. J.; Parker, J. W.; Taylor, C. R.; Tindle, B. H.; Cramer, A. D.; and Lincoln, T. L: Immunologic approach to non-Hodgkin's lymphomas and related leukemias. Analysis of the results of multiparameter studies of 425 cases. *Semin. Hematol.,* **15:**322–351, 1978.

Lukes, R. J., and Tindle, B. H.: Immunoblastic lymphadenopathy: A hyperimmune entity resembling Hodgkin's disease. *N. Engl. J. Med.,* **292:**1–8, 1975.

MacGrath, I. T.; Spiegel, R. J.; Edwards, B. K.; and Janus, C.: Improved results of chemotherapy in young patients with Burkitt's (BL), undifferentiated (UL) and lymphoblastic lymphomas (LL). *Proc. Am. Soc. Clin. Oncol.,* **22:**520 abst C-736, 1981.

McKelvey, E. M.; Gottlieb, J. A.; Wilson, H. E.; Haut, A.; Talley, R. W.; Stephens, R.; Lane, M.; Gamble, J. F.; Jones, S. E.; Grozea, P. N.; Gutterman, J.; Coltman, C.; and Moon, T. E.: Hydroxyldaunomycin (adriamycin) combination chemotherapy in malignant lymphoma. *Cancer,* **38:**1484–1493, 1976.

MacKintosh, F. R.; Colby, T. V.; Podolsky, W. J.; Burke, J. S.; Hoppe, R. T.; Rosenfelt, F. P.; Rosenberg, S. A.; and Kaplan, H. S.: Central nervous system involvement in non-Hodgkin's lymphoma: An analysis of 105 cases. *Cancer,* **49:**586–595, 1982.

Mann, R. B.; Jaffe, E. S.; and Berard, C. W.: Malignant lymphomas: A conceptual understanding of morphologic diversity: A review. *Am. J. Pathol.,* **94:**105–192, 1979.

Merigan, T. C.; Sikora, K.; Breeden, J. H.; Levy, R.; and Rosenberg, S. A.: Preliminary observations on the effect of human leukocyte interferon in non-Hodgkin's lymphoma. *N. Engl. J. Med.,* **299:**1449–1453, 1978.

Miller, R. A.; Maloney, D. G.; Warnke, R.; and Levy, R.: Treatment of B-cell lymphoma with monoclonal antiidiotype antibody. *N. Engl. J. Med.,* **306:**517–522, 1982.

Murphy, S. B.: Classification, staging and end results of treatment of childhood non-Hodgkin's lymphomas: Dissimilarities from lymphomas in adults. *Semin. Oncol.,* **7:**332–339, 1980.

Nathwani, B. N.; Diamond, L. W.; Winberg, C. D.; Kim, H.; Bearman, R. M.; Glick, J.; Jones, S. E.; Gams, R. A.; Nissen, N. I.; and Rappaport, H.: Lymphoblastic lymphoma: A clinicopathologic study of 95 patients. *Cancer,* **48:**2347–2357, 1981.

(NLPCP), The Non-Hodgkin's Lymphoma Pathologic Classification Project National Cancer Institute sponsored study of classifications of non-Hodgkin's lymphomas. *Cancer,* **49:**2112–2135, 1982.

Osborne, C. K.; Norton, L.; Young, R. C.; Garvin, A. J.; Simon, R. M.; Berard, C. W.; Hubbard, S.; and DeVita, V. T.: Nodular histiocytic lymphoma: An aggressive nodular lymphoma with potential for prolonged disease-free survival. *Blood,* **56:**98–103, 1982.

Pangalis, G. A.; Nathwani, B. N.; and Rappaport, H.: Malignant lymphoma, well differentiated lymphocytic: Its relationship with chronic lymphocytic leukemia and macroglobulinemia of Waldenstrom. *Cancer,* **39:**999–1010, 1977.

Paryani, S. B.; Hoppe, R. T.; Cox, R. S.; Colby, T. V.; Rosenberg, S. A.; and Kaplan, H. S.: Analysis of non-Hodgkin's lymphomas with nodular and favorable histologies, Stage I and II *Cancer,* **52:**2300–2307, 1983.

Penn, I.: The incidence of malignancies in transplant recipients. *Transplant. Proc.,* **7:**323, 1975.

Portlock, C. S., and Rosenberg, S. A.: No initial therapy for stage III and IV non-Hodgkin's lymphomas of favorable histologic types. *Ann. Intern. Med.,* **90:**10–13, 1979.

Rappaport, H.; Winter, W. J.; and Hicks, E. B.: Follicular lymphoma—a reevaluation of its position in the scheme of malignant lymphoma, based on a survey of 253 cases. *Cancer,* **9:**792–821, 1956.

Rochester, D.; Bowie, J. D.; Kunzmann, A.; and Lester, E.: Ultrasound in the staging of lymphoma. *Radiology,* **124:**483–487, 1977.

Rosenberg, S. A.: Bone marrow involvement in the non-Hodgkin's lymphomata. *Br. J. Cancer,* **31:**261–264, 1975.

Rosenberg, S. A.: Is intensive treatment of favorable non-Hodgkin's lymphoma necessary? In Wiernik, P. H. (ed.): *Controversies in Oncology.* John Wiley & Sons, Inc., New York, 1982.

Rosenberg, S. A.; Diamond, H. D.; Jaslowitz, B.; and Craver, L. F.: Lymphosarcoma: A review of 1269 cases. *Medicine,* **40:**31, 1961.

Schein, P. S.; Chabner, B. A.; Canellos, G. P.; Young, R. C.; Berard, C. W.; and DeVita, V. T.: Potential for prolonged disease-free survival following combination chemotherapy of non-Hodgkin's lymphoma. *Blood,* **43:**181–189, 1974.

Schein, P. S.; DeVita, V. T.; Hubbard, S.; Chabner, B. A.; Canellos, G. P.; Berard, C. W.; and Young, R. C.: Bleomycin, adriamycin, cyclophosphamide, vincristine and prednisone (BACOP) combination chemotherapy in the treatment of advanced diffuse histiocytic lymphoma. *Ann. Intern. Med.,* **85:**417–422, 1976.

Seligmann, M.: Immunochemical, clinical and pathological features of α-chain disease. *Arch. Intern. Med.,* **135:**78–82, 1975.

Shimoyama, M., and Watanabe, S. (eds.): Symposium on T-cell malignancies. *Jap. J. Clin. Oncol.,* 9(Suppl I):1979.

Skarin, A.; Canellos, G.; Rosenthal, D.; Case, D.; Moloney, W.; and Frei, E., III: Therapy of diffuse histiocytic (DH) and undifferentiated (DU) lymphoma with M-BACOD. *Proc. Am. Soc. Clin. Oncol.,* **21:**463, abst C-568, 1980.

Talal, N.; Sokoloff, L.; and Barth, W.: Extra salivary lymphoid abnormalities in Sjögrens syndrome (reticulum cell sarcoma, "pseudolymphoma," macroglobulinemia). *Am. J. Med.,* **43:**50–65, 1967.

Tseng, A.; Coleman, C. N.; Cox, R. S.; Colby, T. V.; Turner, R. R.; Horning, S. J.; and Rosenberg, S. A.: Treatment of malignant histiocytosis. *Blood,* **64:**48–53, 1984.

Weisenburger, D. D.; Kim, H.; and Rappaport, H.: Mantle-zone lymphoma: A follicular variant of intermediate lymphocytic lymphoma. *Cancer,* **49:**1429–1438, 1982.

Weinstein, H. J.; Vance, L. B.; Jaffe, N.; Buell, D.; Cassady, J. R.; and Nathan, D. G.: Improved prognosis for patients with mediastinal lymphoblastic lymphoma. *Blood,* **53:**687–694, 1979.

Willis, R. A.: *Pathology of Tumours,* 2nd ed. The C. V. Mosby Company, St. Louis, 1953.

Woda, B. A., and Knowles, D. M.: Nodular lymphocytic

lymphoma eventuating into diffuse histiocytic lymphoma. Immunoperoxidase demonstration of monoclonality. *Cancer,* **43:**303–307, 1979.

Yunis, Y.; Oken, M. M.; Kaplan, M. E.; Ensrud, K. M.; Howe, R. R.; and Theologides, A.: Distinctive chromosomal abnormalities in histologic subtypes of non-

Hodgkin's lymphoma. *N. Engl. J. Med.,* 307, 1231–1236, 1982.

Ziegler, J. L.: Burkitt's lymphoma. *N. Engl. J. Med.,* **305:**735–745, 1981.

Ziegler, J. L., and Magrath, I. T.: Treatment of Burkitt's lymphoma. *Pathobiol. Annu.,* **4:**129–142, 1974.

17

Myeloma

O. ROSS McINTYRE

Introduction

Myeloma is a neoplastic B-cell disease initiated by the proliferation of a single clone of antibody-producing cells. The plasma cell morphology of this tumor and several additional characteristic features distinguish it from other B-cell cancers. Certain of its unusual variants, however, may occupy a place on an indistinct border with the B-cell lymphomas. In most patients, the disease is recognized as a diffuse or focal marrow plasmacytosis referred to as multiple myeloma or myelomatosis. In some patients, however, the disease occurs as a solitary plasmacytoma in bone or in an extramedullary site.

The plasma cell clone characteristically produces an excess of a single antibody molecule or portion of a molecule. The appearance of this tumor product, referred to as a monoclonal protein or M protein, in the serum or urine of patients is a clinically useful marker of the tumor. An M protein is found in 98% of patients with the disseminated form of the disease and in small amounts in about one quarter of patients with solitary or extra-medullary plasmacytomas. Apparently healthy individuals, however, may also produce an M protein. Three percent of the population over 70 years of age has been reported to have an M protein (Hallen, 1963; Axelsson *et al.*, 1966). Thus, the diagnosis of myeloma should be based upon all the clinical and laboratory evidence available. Table 17–1 shows diagnostic criteria often used in therapeutic studies.

Myeloma is remarkable for producing several clinical syndromes that pose difficulties in management. Osteolysis, hypercalcemia,

renal failure, and suppression of normal antibody production with infection are common findings. These abnormalities may be referred to as "secondary morbidity," because they derive from the action of tumor products upon the host or from the interaction of the disease with the regulation of the immune system. The extent of morbidity is related to the type and amount of tumor products synthesized and is characteristic for each individual tumor.

Once the disease becomes symptomatic it runs a rapid course, with median survival in untreated patients of less that one year (Feinleib and MacMahon, 1960; Holland *et al.*, 1966). Although vigorous treatment of multiple myeloma has not yet produced long-term unmaintained remissions or cures, current therapy is capable of achieving a three-year median survival. Appropriately treated soli-

Table 17–1. Criteria for the Diagnosis of Multiple Myeloma

Conditions I or II must be met
I. 1a *and* 1b
II. 1a or 1b *and* 2a or 2b or 2c or 2d
1. Tumor cells
a. Marrow plasma cells 10%
b. Biopsy-proven extramedullary plasmacytoma
2. Ancillary diagnostic criteria
a. Plasma myeloma protein
b. Urine myeloma protein
c. Osteolytic lesions (generalized osteoporosis will qualify if 1a is greater than 30%)
d. Plasma cells in peripheral blood smears

Note: Other diseases that are characterized by marrow plasmacytosis should be absent, *i.e.*, collagen-vascular disease, cirrhosis, metastatic carcinoma, and viral exanthemas. The presence of amyloid disease does not exclude the diagnosis of multiple myeloma.

Adapted from Chronic Leukemia-Myeloma Task Force: Proposed guidelines for protocol studies. II. Plasma cell myeloma. *Cancer Chemother. Rep.*, **4**:145–158, 1973.

tary and extramedullary myelomas, however, may often be cured, although late relapses with dissemination, in one instance more than 30 years after initial treatment, have been reported (Wanebo *et al.,* 1966).

Incidence and Epidemiology

Multiple myeloma ranks as the twentieth most frequently occurring cancer in whites, with an incidence approximately equal to Hodgkins disease (Cutler and Young, 1975). The age-adjusted incidence in males is 4.0 per 100,000 and 2.7 per 100,000 in females. Myeloma usually occurs in older individuals and only a few well-proven cases have been reported in individuals under 30 years of age (Hewell and Alexanian, 1976).

The incidence of myeloma in blacks is approximately twice as high as in whites. It is the eleventh most frequently occurring cancer, accounting for 7.2 percent of all cancers, and is the most common form of cancer of the lymphohemopoietic system in this group.

There is evidence that the incidence of the disease in blacks may be rising (Blattner *et al.,* 1981). The increase may be partly explained by improvements in health care and case ascertainment in this population group. For predominantly white Olmstead County, Minnesota, where case ascertainment is believed to be constant, there was no increase in average incidence for the period 1945 through 1964 compared to 1965 through 1977 (Linos *et al.,* 1981).

High-dose radiation received by atombomb survivors appears to increase the risk to 4.7 times the control for exposures over 100 rad (Ichimaru *et al.,* 1979). Chronic low-dose radiation exposure has been reported to increase the risk in nuclear industry workers (Mancuso *et al.,* 1977), but this study has been criticized on methodologic grounds (Hutchison *et al.,* 1979). When myeloma risk is examined in groups receiving various types of occupational, diagnostic, or therapeutic radiation, there appears to be an increased risk in most groups (Cuzick, 1981).

Although it has been suggested that the risk of myeloma is increased in petrochemical workers (Thomas *et al.,* 1980), other studies have not detected an association. An increased risk of myeloma has also been reported in farmers (Milham, 1971), smelter and lead workers (Axelson *et al.,* 1978), food workers, and those employed in woodworking. Myeloma may be increased in counties with plastics and related industries (Mason, 1975). These reports suggest associations that need further study.

It has been suggested that overstimulation of the immune system as a result of inflammation in patients with chronic cholecystitis and osteomyelitis is a causal factor (Wohlenberg; 1970; Isobe and Osserman, 1971; Schafer and Miller, 1979). These associations are not established because the incidence of myeloma in those with and without these chronic inflammatory states has not been ascertained. Individuals receiving multiple immunizations over several years because of exposure to germ-warfare agents are known to have increased levels of polyclonal immunoglobulin, but myeloma has not been described in this group (Peeler *et al.,* 1965).

Seventy-five cases of apparent familial myeloma have been reported (Blattner *et al.,* 1981). In two kindreds, three cases of myeloma and additional individuals with asymptomatic serum M protein have been reported (Meijers *et al.,* 1972; Maldonado and Kyle, 1974). Of 40 possible blood relationship pairs in familial cases, 28 sibling pairs have been reported. This predominance has suggests that familial susceptibility involves a recessive gene. On the other hand, myeloma in only one of monozygotic twins has been reported (Ogawa *et al.,* 1970). The unaffected twin has not developed myeloma over 12 years of observation. Although genetic predisposition may favor the emergence of the disease, it appears that environmental factors determine which of those in the population at risk will develop the disease.

Clusters of myeloma in small communities have been described on two occasions (Kyle *et al.,* 1972; Ende, 1979). Studies of these clusters have not detected a transmissible or environmental cause.

Etiology and Pathogenesis

Balb/c Mouse Model. The observation that myeloma could be induced in Balb/c mice by peritoneal implantation of plastic (Merwin and Algire, 1959) or by injection of mineral oil or Freund's adjuvant (Potter and Boyce, 1962) has provided insights into the etiology of myeloma. The mouse appears to require a sustained macrophage response, the presence of bacterial lipopolysaccharide in the gut, and a genetic susceptibility in order for the disease to be induced. Under these conditions, polyclonal expansion of the B-lymphocyte population occurs within the peritoneum, and peritoneal granulomas are induced. These changes apparently set the stage for the evolution of the neoplastic clone. Germ-free Balb/c mice that lack bacterial lipopolysaccharide in the gut mucosa do not develop peritoneal granulomas and myeloma doesn't occur with the same frequency despite implantation of plastic (McIntire and Princler, 1971). Although the relationship of these intraperitoneal changes to those in the human marrow are conjectural, a man has developed a solitary myeloma in the subcutaneous pocket that had previously held a silastic implanted pacemaker (Hamaker *et al.*, 1976). This suggests that the mouse model may indeed be relevant to the human disease. It will be important to observe the increasing number of individuals who have received implanted plastic devices for a possible increase in plasma cell neoplasia.

Regulation of B-Cell Clonal Proliferation. In patients with myeloma, IgM containing pre-B cells expressing the same idiotype as the myeloma plasma cells have been found. This finding indicates that the lesion responsible for the disease occurs at the earliest recognized stage of the B-cell lineage (Kubagawa *et al.*, 1979). Under normal circumstances, of course, the B-cell response to an antigen is polyclonal and also limited in degree. Therefore, one must postulate derangements in the regulation of one clone in a polyclonal response or an intrinsic cellular defect conferring unrestrained clonal plasma cell growth in order to explain the emergence of the disease. The mouse experiments are helpful in demonstating that the host's genetic background is of major importance in determining the frequency of the neoplastic event. Clinical evidence suggests that regulatory factors may be important as well.

Monoclonal Gammopathy of Undetermined Significance. As mentioned earlier, a number of otherwise healthy individuals, especially among the elderly, have serum M components that remain stable or increase slowly over long periods of follow-up. The name first given to this condition, "benign monoclonal gammopathy," has been revised recently to "monoclonal gammopathy of undetermined significance." This more accurate designation derives from the study done by Kyle (1978), who followed, for five or more years, 241 patients with serum monoclonal proteins who

lacked evidence of myeloma, macroglobulinemia, amyloidosis, or lymphoma. Fifty-seven percent of the patients showed no increase in monoclonal protein during this period. Two patients with monoclonal proteins were followed for 15 years without evidence of progressive disease. Nine percent showed a 50% increase in monoclonal protein during the observation period. Twenty-three percent died without serum studies at five years, and 11% developed myeloma, macroglobulinemia, or amyloidosis. The median interval between the detection of the monoclonal protein and the diagnosis of myeloma was 64 months. In two patients, one with sarcoidosis and another with degenerative arthritis, the monoclonal protein actually disappeared. Thus, once present, the expanded clone may persist without evidence of additional expansion, it may expand to give typical features of multiple myeloma, or, rarely, it may regress.

Two-Step Evolution and Kinetics. This has suggested to some that myeloma results from a two-step phenomenon: First, the emergence of the precancerous monoclonal B-cell proliferation that may be partially under the host's control, because clonal expansion is limited and may regress; and second, an event that converts a member of this clone to full neoplastic behavior (Salmon and Seligmann, 1974).

Some cases of myeloma progress slowly, taking from months to years to become symptomatic. These patients have been described as having smoldering myeloma (Kyle and Greipp, 1980), and are often diagnosed after a routine health examination has shown an elevated erythrocyte sedimentation rate or other evidence for disease. Most patients, however, present with acute symptoms.

Myeloma has been diagnosed in individuals who for other reasons had normal serum electrophoreses within several years prior to the diagnosis. This suggests that in most patients the preclinical phase of the disease is relatively brief. Studies of M-protein synthetic-rate measurements at various levels of tumor load tend to support this concept, because they indicate that tumor doubling time in myeloma is shorter at low tumor cell burdens than at high tumor cell levels (Salmon, 1973). This pattern of tumor growth, referred to as Gompertzian kinetics, has been discussed in detail in Chapter 2. Previous estimates of the length of myeloma's preclinical phase, which were based on the rate of tumor progression late in the disease, have been high (Hobbs, 1969).

The growth of human myeloma cells has been studied in patients receiving a continuous infusion of tritiated thymidine (Drewinko *et al.*, 1981). The percentage of cells with nuclear labeling at one hour (the labeling index) and the fraction of cells labeled after prolonged infusion (the growth fraction) were determined. These studies indicated that untreated patients and those in remission usually have a low labeling index (less than 1%) and a low growth fraction (usually less than 1%). A low growth fraction always correlated with a low labeling index, but a low labeling index was sometimes found in a patient with a high growth fraction. Patients in rapid relapse were likely to have a high labeling index, and all had a high growth fraction. Of interest was the observation that the growth fraction and labeling index did not appear to increase during remission as might be inferred from the Gompertzian model discussed above. This may be explained by the fact that remission is diagnosed when only about one log of tumor cells has been killed. The relatively low cell kill may not result in a tumor cell load representing the steep portion of the Gompertz curve, and therefore the model is not necessarily refuted. On the other hand, the high growth fraction seen in relapse, even in patients with high tumor loads, indicates a substantial change in the tumor cell kinetics, most likely arising from mutations in the original tumor clone. Thus, a model for the growth kinetics can be constructed that assumes that the tumor mass issues from a small proportion of proliferating cells and that relapsing patients have a marked expansion of the growth fraction. From these studies it is estimated that the plasma cell transit time through the proliferative compartment in untreated patients is 6.6 to 11.9 days with a calculated cell loss of 50 to 86% during the passage.

When marrow cells from myeloma patients are cultured in soft agar along with appropriate growth factors, colonies of plasma cells may be grown. This culture system, developed by Salmon, Hamburger, and their colleagues (Salmon *et al.*, 1978), is referred to as a "tumor stem cell assay" because linearity between the number of cells plated and the number of colonies generated has been established. The technique may be used for testing drug sensitivity of the cells. The plating efficiency in this assay is 0.001 to 0.1%, raising the possibility that not all cells shown to be in cycle in the *in vivo* studies described above are capable of forming recognizable colonies in this assay system.

Regulation by T-Cells. There is suggestive but unconfirmed work indicating that certain host factors might regulate the expansion of the neoplastic clone. Paglieroni and MacKenzie (1980) have described the occurrence of cytotoxic cells, in the peripheral blood of myeloma patients, that are capable of lysing autologous or allogeneic myeloma plasma cells. In these studies, peripheral blood mononuclear cells were isolated and cocultured with marrow enriched for plasma cells. Release of label from chromium-treated marrow plasma cells was taken as an indication of cytotoxicity. A proliferative response, indicated by a ^{125}IUDR uptake of 7 to 16 times that of control values, was found when peripheral blood lymphocytes were cultured with autologous marrow plasma cells. This was accompanied by chromium release values of 25 to 65% from autologous or allogeneic myeloma plasma cells but not from plasma cells isolated from patients with monoclonal gammopathy of undetermined significance. Cocultures of peripheral blood lymphocytes from patients with monoclonal gammopathy of undetermined significance, with allogeneic lymphocytes and myeloma cells, generated cells cytotoxic for neoplastic plasma cells. The proliferative response to allogeneic marrow plasma cells was generally somewhat less, as was the cytotoxicity.

In other experiments, these investigators demonstrated inhibition of proliferation in the one-way mixed tumor lymphocyte cultures when marrow T cells were added to the peripheral blood lymphocyte plasma cell cultures (Paglieroni and MacKenzie, 1979). If these experiments are confirmed, they suggest that a cytolytic host T-cell response is blocked by suppressor T cells in the region of the tumor. Interaction of the killer-suppressor functional populations may regulate proliferation of the malignant clone.

Regulation of Polyclonal Antibody Production. These experiments are also relevant to the mechanisms producing another distinctive pathophysiologic feature of myeloma: Patients with myeloma characteristically have significantly depressed levels of normal serum polyclonal immunoglobulins (Fahey *et al.*, 1963). The major cause of this decrease is impaired immunoglobulin synthesis (Waldmann and Strober, 1969). Broder and colleagues (1975) studied the *in vitro* production of polyclonal immunoglobulin by pokeweed-stimulated peripheral blood mononuclear cells from normal donors and from patients with myeloma. As anticipated, the peripheral blood mononuclear cells from most patients with myeloma showed a decreased number of normal B cells. Some patients, however, showed normal or only minimally reduced percentages of circulating B lymphocytes. In all patients studied, including those with normal numbers of B cells, polyclonal immunoglobulin production, as measured by specific competitive radioimmunoassays for IgM, IgA, and IgG, was markedly decreased. When lymphocytes from controls and from patients were cultured together, mononuclear cell populations from three of six patients studied effectively suppressed immunoglobulin production by cocultured normal lymphocytes. In two instances, this effect could be attributed to the phagocytic (monocyte) population in the cell preparations, because removal of these cells restored polyclonal immunoglobulin production in the coculture experiment. In three patients, it was not possible to demonstrate the presence of circulating inhibitory cells by the coculture technique, even though pokeweed-driven polyclonal immunoglobulin production by the patients' cells was impaired. Purified T cells from the patients were ineffective in suppressing polyclonal immunoglobulin production in the coculture experiments, in contrast to the results reported in studies of common variable hypogammaglobulinemia by the same group of investigators (Waldmann *et al.*, 1974). Studies by others (Hoover *et al.*, 1981),

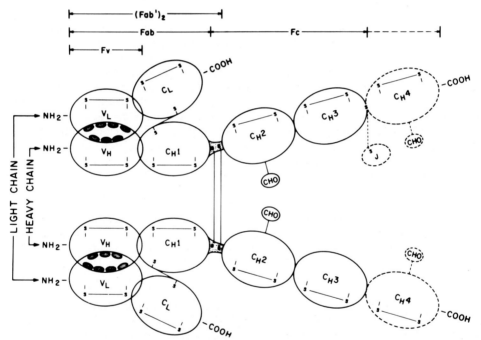

Figure 17–1. Schematic diagram of the basic domain structure of the light and heavy polypeptide chains of immunoglobulins. The domains in the amino-terminal (NH$_2$) portion of each chain, the variant regions, are designated V_L and V_H for the light chain and heavy chain, respectively; the hypervariable regions within the V_L and V_H are shown as discrete dark-stippled areas. The domains in the carboxyl-terminal (COOH) portion of each chain, the constant regions, are designated C_L and C_H for the light chain and heavy chain, respectively; the three C_H domains are designated C_H of immunoglobulins M and E and contain an additional domain designated C_H1, C_H2, and C_H3 (the C_H of immunoglobulins M and E contain an additional domain designated C_H4). An additional polypeptide chain, the J chain, is disulfide-linked to the C_H3 or C_H4 domains of polymeric immunoglobulins A and M, respectively. The carbohydrate moiety, usually exclusively on the heavy chain, is designated CHO. The polypeptide region between the C_H1 and C_H2 domains is termed the hinge region (indicated by the lightly stippled area); this region is particularly susceptible to proteolytic cleavage. Papain cleaves the heavy chain on the amino-terminal side of the interheavy chain disulfide bonds, resulting in the production of fragment Fc and the two monovalent antibody-combining fragments Fab; pepsin cleaves the heavy chain on the carboxyl-terminal side of the interheavy chain disulfide bonds, resulting in the production of the divalent antibody-combining fragment, (Fab')$_2$; and under special conditions of peptic cleavage the variant region (V_L and V_H) can be cleaved from the intact immunoglobulin molecule yielding the Fv fragment. (Reprinted, by permission of the *New England Journal of Medicine*, from Solomon, A.: Bence-Jones proteins and light chains of immunoglobulins. *N. Engl. J. Med.*, **294**:18, 1976.)

have shown an increased number of circulating T cells with Fc receptor specificity for the immunoglobulin heavy chain class of the M protein. These observations raise the possibility that such cells exert an immunoregulatory effect upon the myeloma cells.

Antibody Structure and Synthesis of M Protein. Patients with myeloma have provided immunologists with a source of homogeneous immunoglobulin for studies of antibody structure. In turn, fundamental studies of immunochemistry have provided considerable insight into the pathophysiology of the disease.

A general scheme for the structure of an immunoglobulin molecule is shown in Figure 17–1. Two heavy (H) and two light (L) chains are linked by disulfide bonds as shown. This molecule may be cleaved by papain into two fractions: One is referred to as the antigen binding fraction, or Fab; the other crystalizes upon standing and is referred to as the crystallizable fraction, or Fc. Twice as many Fab fragments are produced in this cleavage as are Fc fragments. Thus, the complete molecule, as predicted by earlier indirect studies, has two antigen-combining sites or is *divalent*. The Fc portion of the molecule is necessary for complement activation, cell binding, and placental transport.

Further studies, including amino acid sequence analysis, have shown that the molecule may be further divided into regions that are either constant or variable. The amino acid sequence of two unrelated κ myeloma light chains, for instance, gives a diverse amino acid composition in the amino terminal halves but nearly identical carboxy terminal halves (Hilschmann and Craig, 1965). On the basis of this information it has been deduced that anti-gen recognition and binding depends upon the conformation governed by the variable amino terminal portion.

The heavy chain of the immunoglobulin molecule can be divided into four units of about 110 amino acids each. Each unit is referred to as a "domain" (Edelman and Gall, 1969). Carbohydrate is bound to the second domain and varies from 3% (IgG) to 12% (IgM). It has been suggested that each domain fulfills a particular biologic function: For instance, the C_H2 region appears responsible for complement binding (Kehoe and Fougereau, 1969); and the C_H3 region for macrophage binding (Yasmeen *et al.*, 1973); and the variable regions of the light and heavy chains are responsible for the antigen binding function. The presence of both H- and L-chain variable regions is required for antibody activity because separation of the chains from each other greatly impairs antigen binding. Recombination of the chains restores antigen binding, but if either the H or L chain is substituted with a chain derived from antibody to an unrelated antigen, restoration does not occur.

Classes of Immunoglobulin. Five classes of immunoglobulin are recognized, namely, IgG, IgA, IgM, IgD, and IgE (see Table 17–2). These are distinguished from one another by the composition of the heavy chains γ, α, μ, δ, ϵ, respectively. Light chain structure is independent of immunoglobulin class. Certain properties of the immunoglobulin classes are summarized in Table 17–3.

Four subclasses of IgG are recognized. All occur as monomers comprised of two heavy and two light chains (H_2L_2). Although the subclasses are 95% homologous in amino acid sequence, they differ in important respects. IgG1

Table 17–2. Classification of Immunoglobulins of Normal Human Serum

IMMUNOGLOBULIN	IgG	IgA	IgM	IgD	IgE
Synonyms	γ, 7Sγ γ2, γG	βx, β2A, γ1A, γA	γ1, 19Sγ, β2M, γ1M, γM	γD	γE
Heavy chain classes	gamma (γ)	alpha (α)	mu (μ)	delta (δ)	epsilon (ϵ)
subclasses	IgG1, IgG2, IgG3, IgG4	IgA1, IgA2		Ja, La	
Light chain types	kappa (κ) lambda (λ)	κ λ	κ λ	κ λ	κ λ
Molecular formula	γ2κ2 γ2λ2	α2κ2* α2λ2	(μ2κ2)5 (μ2λ2)5	δ2κ2 δ2λ2	ϵ2κ2 ϵ2λ2
Designation	IgGκ IgGλ	IgAκ IgAλ	IgMκ IgMλ	IgDκ IgDλ	IgEκ IgEλ

* May form polymers
From Kyle, R. A.: Immunoglobulins and syndromes associated with monoclonal gammopathies. In Tice, F. (ed.): *Practice of Medicine.* Vol. 1. Harper & Row, Publishers, Inc., Hagerstown, Maryland, 1977.

Table 17-3. Properties of Immunoglobulins of Normal Human Serum

	IgG	IgA	IgM	IgD	IgE
Electrophoretic mobility	γ to $\alpha2$	γ to β	γ to $\gamma2$	γ to β	γ to β
Sedimentation coefficient	6.7S	7 to 15S*	19S	7S	8S
Molecular weight	150,000	170,000 to 500,000*	900,000	180,000	200,000
Carbohydrate (%)	2.6	5 to 10	9.8	10 to 12	11
Half-life (days)	23	5.8	5.1	2.8	2.3
Serum concentration, mean mg/ml	11.4	1.8	1.0	0.03	0.0003
Total serum immunoglobulin (%)	74	21	5	0.2	0.002
Total body pool in intravascular space (%)	45	42	76	75	51
Intravascular pool catabolized per day (% normal)	6.7	25	18	37	89
Normal synthetic rate (mg/kg/day)	33	24	6.7	0.4	0.02
Fixes complement	Yes	Alternate pathway	Yes	No	No
Crosses placenta	Yes	No	No	No	No

* Tends to form polymers of the monomer form
From Kyle, R. A.: Immunoglobulins and syndromes associated with monoclonal gammopathies. In Tice, F. (ed.): *Practice of Medicine.* Vol. 1. Harper & Row, Publishers, Inc., Hagerstown, Maryland, 1977.

and IgG3 interact more readily with complement than do IgG2 and IgG4. They also bind spontaneously to monocytes, neutrophils, and lymphocytes, whereas IgG2 and IgG4 require that the molecules be aggregated in order to bind (Andrews and Capra, 1980). IgG1, IgG2, and IgG4 bind to protein A derived from staphylococcal cell walls, whereas IgG3 fails to do so. IgG3 has an extended hinge region containing more than 100 amino acids, giving it a higher molecular weight than the other IgG sublcasses and inducing susceptibility to proteolytic degradation, the presumed cause of its shorter biologic half life *in vivo.*

IgA is the predominant immunoglobulin in secretions. It is thought to be synthesized locally in plasma cells near mucosal surfaces. Serum IgA in humans is predominantly in the form of a monomer (H_2L_2) (Tomasi, 1971). In secretions, the molecule is in the form of a dimer ($2 H_2L_2$) linked to two unique subunits attached by disulfide bonds. One of these two subunits is referred to as secretory component and the other the J ("joining") chain. Two subclasses of IgA are recognized. One of them, IgA1, predominates in serum; the other, IgA2, predominates in secretions. In contrast to IgA1, IgA2 is resistant to destruction by bacterial proteases because of a 13-amino-acid-residue deletion in the hinge region, the cleavage site for the protease (Plaut *et al.,* 1974).

IgM is usually a pentamer of five H_2L_2 structures linked by disulfide bonds in a radial fashion. Although rare cases of typical myeloma with IgM protein M components have been described, when monoclonal protein of the IgM class appears it is usually in association with a clinically different B-cell cancer, macroglobulinemia.

IgD is normally present in human serum in very small amounts and is distinguished by its localization on the membranes of B cells. The protein is highly susceptible to proteolysis. It is of interest that λ light chains are found on most monoclonal proteins of the IgD type.

IgE is present in extremely small amounts in human serum. The Fc portion of this immunoglobulin is bound to the membrane of basophils and tissue mast cells where it may be catabolized. When the antigen-combining site reacts with antigen, basophilic degranulation occurs, establishing this immunoglobulin's critical role in immediate hypersensitivity reactions (Ishizaka and Ishizaka, 1968). Because very few cells are normally at risk for malignant transformation, myeloma of the IgE type is encountered only very rarely.

Bence Jones Protein. Myeloma was first recognized as a distinct clinical entity when a patient was found to excrete a protein in the urine that had unique solubility properties on heating (Bence Jones, 1847; MacIntyre, 1850). This protein precipitates upon heating to 40 to 60 °C and redissolves near 100 °C. It is now recognized that Bence Jones protein consists of immunoglobulin light chains. Although, strictly speaking, the term refers to urinary protein with these solubility characteristics, solubility tests are often difficult to interpret and the term has come to be used for monoclonal light chain proteinuria as detected by immunologic methods. With these methods, light chain proteinuria is demonstrated in about 60% of patients with myeloma (Acute Leukemia Group B, 1975).

Overproduction of L chains with resultant Bence Jones proteinuria occurs because of derangements in the normal synthesis of immunoglobulin. The synthesis, assembly, and secretion of immunoglobulins has been studied in IgG-producing lymphoid cells and in cells obtained from a number of mouse myeloma lines. One characteristic of these lines, as well as of the neoplastic plasma cells of many patients with myeloma, is an unbalanced production of H versus L chains such that an excess of L chains is produced (Coffino and Scharff, 1971). The H and L chains are synthesized on two different classes of polyribosomes, and the assembly of H and L chains is presumed to occur in the cisternae of the rough endoplasmic reticulum following release from the polyribosomes. In mouse myelomas the pathway utilized for assembly depends on the subclass of the myeloma protein (Francus et al., 1978). For instance, pathways via $H + L \rightarrow HL + HL \rightarrow H_2L_2$ or via $H + H \rightarrow H_2 + L \rightarrow H_2L + L \rightarrow H_2L_2$ have been described. In addition, variants in which L chains, synthesized in excess, are secreted as free light chains, or light chain dimers, or are catabolized intracellularly have been described. Cell lines blocked with respect to assembly and secretion of H and L chains have been studied and evidence has been offered that if the L and H chains fail to combine, then H chains are not secreted (Cohn, 1967). Spontaneous mutants defective for H chain production as well as secretion are noted to arise in myeloma cell lines. This suggests that myelomas secreting L chain only may arise from a two-step mutation in which the cancerous cell first produces a complete M protein and then undergoes a second mutation leading to loss of H chain production or secretion (Morrison and Scharff, 1981).

A variety of structural abnormalities in the secreted tumor product have been described and have provided insight into the genetic and synthetic events taking place in normal as well as cancerous B cells. These include the secretion of H chain, or portions of H chain only, as well as other defective products. The most clinically important of these defects is that giving rise to imbalanced light chain secretion. Secreted κ excess chains are found primarily in the monomeric form, whereas λ proteins circulate as covalently linked dimers (Solomon, 1976).

Determination of Immunoglobulin Structure and Production of Immunoglobulin Genes. Antibody diversity depends on the amino acid sequence in the variable portions of the H and L chains. Once it was shown that the variable region was juxtaposed to a constant portion of the immunoglobulin molecule, speculation arose that a single protein was coded for by two separate genes. The controversy surrounding this possibility has been resolved by the application of gene-cloning techniques. These studies have demonstrated that immunoglobulin genes are created by a somatic recombination event that occurs during the maturation of antibody-producing cells. For the gene responsible for coding κ chain synthesis, this involves a single step in which one of a large number of germ-line variable-region genes is joined to one of four joining sequences (Seidman et al., 1979) (see Figure 17–2). The combination of the numerous variable-region genes with the four joining sequences imparts enormous diversity to the recombinant gene. Moreover, the joining is variable in its crossover point, creating additional diversity in a critical region of the light chain. Other studies have provided evidence that cloned heavy γ and μ chains have regions of conserved homology. These segments encompass regions in which μ/γ recombination occurs during the heavy chain class switch, and it is likely that the homology is relevant to this process.

Translational Regulation. Once messenger RNA has been synthesized, subsequent to the recombinant event, there are possibilities for further regulation of antibody production at the translational level. Messenger RNA for immunoglobulin synthesis has the unusual characteristics of a class of messengers responsible for the synthesis of certain specialized cell proteins, including hemoglobin (Nuss and Koch, 1976). These messengers display a high affinity for a component of the initiation complex, and, in contrast to messenger RNA for most protein, are translated in cells exposed to media of altered sodium chloride content or in the presence of lytic virus. It is of interest that translation mediated by messengers of this type is selectively inhibited by interferon (Garry et al., 1979; Garry and Waite, 1979).

Relationship of the M Protein to Disease Complications. The M protein, by its pres-

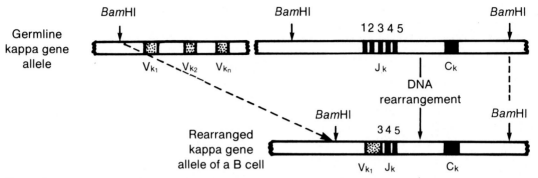

Figure 17-2. An example of immunoglobulin gene rearrangement. A germline kappa gene allele comprises separated DNA gene segments. These consist of multiple variable (V_κ), alternate joining (J_κ) sections, and a single constant (C_κ) region. Before transcription of κ chain messenger RNA, the gene undergoes a DNA rearrangement that recombines a single V_κ and J_κ region. This rearrangement introduces a new 5′ restriction endonuclease (*Bam*HI) site and allows discrimination between a rearranged and a germline allele by a C_κ-DNA probe. Redrawn, by permission of the *New England Journal of Medicine,* from Cossman, J.; Neckers, L. M.; Arnold, A.; and Korsmeyer, S. J.: Induction of differentiation in a case of common acute lymphoblastic leukemia. *N. Engl. J. Med.,* **307**:1251, 1982.

ence in the circulation, may produce various clinical syndromes related to the chemical or physical properties of the molecule. The severity of these syndromes is determined by the quantity of the abnormal tumor product and its structure. These syndromes can produce morbidity and mortality unrelated to the kinetics of tumor growth or total tumor cell burden.

Hyperviscosity. Hyperviscosity is the most common and often the most dramatic of the clinical syndromes related to the structure of the M protein. Common clinical features of this syndrome are hemorrhage, (especially into the mucous membranes), evidence of sludging of the blood seen on 40-power ophthalmoscopic examination of the small conjunctival vessels, progressive loss of cerebral function with coma, and a dramatic response to vigorous plasmapheresis (Pruzanski and Watt, 1972). The association of these findings with hyperviscosity was first appreciated in patients with macroglobulinemia. About 4% of patients with IgG myeloma have the syndrome. Although a higher incidence of hyperviscosity in myelomas of the IgG3 subtype was initially reported (Virella and Hobbs, 1971), a later report indicates that the syndrome may be more common in patients with IgG4 myeloma (Schur *et al.,* 1974). When the syndrome appears in patients with IgG or IgA myeloma, a relatively high concentration of the abnormal immunoglobulin and the formation of high-molecular-weight aggregates of the immunoglobulin molecules is implied (Smith *et al.,* 1965).

The relative viscosity of serum may be mea-

sured by using a simple apparatus, but unfortunately this does not correlate very well with the severity of clinical symptoms. This lack of correlation may result from the fact that the serum viscosity does not assess the impact of the abnormal protein on the viscosity of whole blood, where interactions between the abnormal protein and erythrocytes possibly occur. The determination of whole blood viscosity is technically more complex and there has been no report of a large series of myeloma patients studied with a whole blood viscosimeter at shear rates relevant to blood flow in small vessels. Measurement of serum viscosity, however, may provide some help in patient management, because the syndrome of hyperviscosity is rare in patients with relative viscosities of less than four, whereas many patients with relative viscosities higher than six will experience some symptoms. In addition, measurements of serum viscosity provide a useful guide when patients with hyperviscosity syndrome are treated with plasmapheresis, and they may be useful in predicting the need for additional plasmapheresis in chronic hyperviscosity states (Beck *et al.,* 1982).

Cryoglobulinemia. Certain of the abnormal IgG M components associated with hyperviscosity have also been shown to precipitate, or gel, in the cold. The clinical syndrome secondary to this phenomenon is far less common than hyperviscosity. Ischemia or infarction of the digits, leg ulcers, and perforation of the nasal septum due to cryoglobulinemia may occur in patients with myeloma, but these are more frequently seen in patients with lymphoma and cryoglobulinemia due to IgM pro-

teins. Although IgG M components often precipitate in the cold, the temperature at which
precipitation occurs is usually below that encountered in the areas of the body exposed to
cold. Patients with symptoms may be treated
with plasmapheresis to remove the abnormal
protein and by warming the patient's room to a
temperature above that at which the cryopre-
cipitate forms.

Coagulation Abnormalities. Although
thrombocytopenia is commonly observed in
patients with myeloma, some patients may
have problems of hemostasis unrelated to
thrombocytopenia. In some instances this has
been shown to result from inhibition of fibrin
aggregation (Cohen *et al.,* 1970) and platelet
function by large quantities of M protein.
Other coagulation abnormalities including deficient thromboplastin generation have also
been reported as secondary to the presence of
M protein.

Renal Failure. Renal failure is a prominent
feature of myeloma and is present in about
20% of patients at diagnosis. Although little
disagreement exists that M protein can initiate
the renal lesion, there is controversy about the
precise mechanisms involved. Renal failure is
encountered in patients without light chain
proteinuria, but most investigations of renal
failure in myeloma have centered on the role
played by urinary light chains. Defronzo and
colleagues (1975) reported that 19 of 27 patients with acute renal failure had Bence Jones
proteinuria. The group with Bence Jones proteinuria also had decreased creatinine clearance, PAH clearance, and concentrating ability compared with the group without urinary
light chains. Although renal failure develops
and progresses rapidly in some patients with
only modest amounts of urinary L chain, other
patients display impressive light chain proteinuria for years without deterioration of
renal function (Kyle and Greipp, 1982).

RENAL CATABOLISM OF LIGHT CHAINS.
Ordinarily, monomeric light chains (molecular weight about 22,000 daltons) are filtered at
the glomerulus and then cleared by the tubular
cells that catabolize the protein (Waldmann *et
al.,* 1972). Infusion of small amounts of radiolabeled light chains into normal individuals
demonstrates that under normal circumstances less than 1% of light chains reach the
distal nephron and are excreted. But when
large amounts of light chain are produced, as
in myeloma, the catabolic capacity of the tubular epithelial cell is exceeded, and high con-

centrations of light chains reach the distal
nephron.

Clyne and his colleagues (1979a) have proposed that in the distal tubule under aciduric
conditions, light chains interact with Tamm-
Horsfall mucoprotein, giving rise to tubular
casts. These casts, when found in the presence
of a giant cell response, are the hallmark of the
histopathology of myeloma kidney. Tubular
dilatation and interstitial fibrosis, presumably
secondary to plugging of the tubules by casts,
complete the picture. It is proposed that this
sequence is highly dependent upon the isoelectric point (pI) of the light chain; those with
$pI > 5.7$ react as cations in the acid conditions
of the distal nephron and precipitate with
Tamm-Horsfall protein in hydropenic conditions to form the casts. This sequence of events
has been verified in a model using aciduric
hydropenic rats where it was found that a direct relationship existed between the pI and
acute BUN elevations above a pI threshold of
5.7. These observations fit in well with clinical
experience. Acute renal failure in myeloma is
frequently precipitated by infection and dehydration, situations that are likely to result in
metabolic acidosis with renal changes resembling those of the rat model.

In Clyne's series renal failure was occasionally present in patients excreting light chains
with pIs less than 5.7. In addition, atrophy of
tubular cells, the most common pathologic
finding in myeloma patients with renal failure,
may be seen in the absence of tubular casts.
When mice were given large amounts of λ
Bence Jones protein it could be identified
shortly thereafter by immunofluorescence as
tubular casts. Tamm-Horsfall protein did not
appear in the casts until five days later (Koss *et
al.,* 1976).

Other mechanisms must therefore be invoked to explain renal failure in some patients.
Tubbs and colleagues (1981) have shown that
a small group of patients who develop renal
failure on the basis of light chain deposition
lack typical clinical features of myeloma and
do not excrete detectable myeloma light
chains. In these patients, light chains can be
identified by immunomicroscopy in deposits
found in the glomerular basement membrane,
mesangium, and tubular basement membrane
but not within the tubules. The distribution
pattern and the character of the deposits may
be influenced by light chain type. These findings suggest that renal failure may derive from
defects in the catabolism of the light chain or

from an affinity of the light chain for various renal structures.

The renal lesion appears to be highly selective, at times involving principally the proximal or the distal tubule, or, in other patients, producing the nephrotic syndrome.

Some of the renal failure seen in the 20% of patients who lack Bence Jones proteinuria is explained on the basis of pyelonephritis, nephrocalcinosis, and urate nephropathy, all of which arise as a consequence of the disease or its treatment.

URINARY LIGHT CHAIN AND PROGNOSIS. Controversy exists concerning the prognosis conferred by the type of urinary light chain excreted. Although some series have shown that light chain type has no effect on the patient's survival (Kyle and Elveback, 1976), other series have shown that patients excreting κ Bence Jones protein in the urine have responded to treatment better (Bergsagel et al., 1965) or survived longer than the patients excreting λ Bence Jones protein (Cornell et al., 1979). This survival advantage for those with κ Bence Jones protein excretion is demonstrated when the analysis is confined to those patients without substantial renal function abnormalities at the time of diagnosis.

Amyloidosis. Amyloidosis appears in some patients with multiple myeloma with a frequency that depends upon the diligence with which this complication has been sought (Hobbs, 1973). Although periorbital purpura and other evidence of skin fragility, macroglossia and hepatosplenomegaly are encountered in occasional patients, most — 98% in Kyle and Elveback's series (1976) — have proteinuria, and about one-fourth of these patients excrete mainly albumin. A history of previous treatment for carpal tunnel syndrome is a common finding, and in such cases amyloid is found in the surgically removed tissue. In patients with myeloma, amyloidosis is due to the formation of amyloid fibrils composed of a protein sequence probably identical to variable portions of the monoclonal light chain secreted by the tumor (Glenner et al., 1970, 1971, 1972; Isobe and Osserman, 1974). The reason fibrils are deposited in certain patients but not in others is not clear. A higher proportion of λ Bence Jones proteins is found in amyloidosis than would be expected on the basis of the observed frequency of κ vs λ monoclonal proteins. Selective tissue binding or precipitation of fibrils from protein with a particular variable chain structure may explain this finding.

Neurologic Syndromes. Uncharacterized tumor products or the antibody activity of the M protein itself are thought to cause a disabling sensorimotor neuropathy seen in 3 to 13% of patients with the disease (Davis and Drachman, 1972; Latov et al., 1980; Kelly et al., 1981). This neurologic condition may appear before myeloma is recognized. In about 25% of patients the syndrome is associated with a solitary myeloma. Definitive treatment of solitary lesions dramatically reverses the clinical syndrome in most instances. In one case, a solitary myeloma located in a vertebral body was associated with a cerebrospinal fluid (CSF) M protein that disappeared following radiation treatment at the time a neurologic response occurred (Acute Leukemia Group B, 1975). The relationship of the M protein to the syndrome, however, is conjectural. Progressive multifocal leukoencephalopathy has also been described in patients with myeloma, but is considerably less common than the neuropathy (DelDuca and Morningstar, 1967). Leptomeningeal infiltration as well as solitary intracranial plasmacytoma have been reported (Siegal et al., 1981).

Bone Disease. In addition to the syndromes caused by the interaction of the M protein with host tissues, there are features of myeloma that owe their existence to tumor products. Most prominent of these is the effect of the disease upon bone and calcium metabolism. About 70% of newly diagnosed patients have significant bone disease, and more than one-half of patients receiving their first treatment have painful bone lesions. (Kyle et al., 1975). About 15 to 30% of patients have elevated pretreatment serum calcium levels. The bone lesions in myeloma were for many years considered secondary to bone destruction by expanding tumor nodules. Examination of marrow biopsy specimens, however, frequently reveals increased osteoclastic activity and bone resorption without evidence of bone necrosis secondary to pressure of localized tumor.

Mundy and his colleagues (1974; Josse et al., 1981) have demonstrated a substance capable of stimulating osteoclastic activity in cultured bone in media from mitogen-stimulated normal B cells and in B-cell lines. This material, referred to as osteoclast-activating factor (OAF), is only partially characterized. OAF

production by cultured myeloma cells correlated with extent of bone disease in 33 patients
studied by Durie, Salmon, and Mundy
(1981b). The OAF studied by these investigators does not induce cyclic AMP formation, in
contrast to parathyroid hormone and its production or release from B cells is inhibited
by indomethacin. Other osteoclast-activating
factors may be present in B-cell neoplasia, at
least some of which appear to stimulate cyclic
AMP. A monoclonal antibody against one
such factor has been described (Luben *et al.,*
1979).

The lack of osteoblastic activity in areas
where bone destruction is taking place is a
curious feature of most patients with the disease. For this reason, bone scans are usually
negative. Even in patients showing objective
responses in other disease variables, bone
healing as detected by careful radiologic examination is observed in only 30% (Rodriguez *et
al.,* 1972). Most series report a considerably
lower fraction of patients showing some healing. Osteoblastic activity, however, is found in
a small fraction of myeloma patients often in
the subgroup of patients with peripheral neuropathy. In at least one instance an impressive
elevation of serum calcitonin presumably secondary to the tumor has been demonstrated
(Rousseau *et al.,* 1978).

Pathology and Natural History

Histopathology of Myeloma. Histologic
sections of solitary extramedullary myelomatous lesions show sheets of plasma cells. In
many instances the plasma cells are atypical,
and ballooning of the cytoplasm with intracellular protein (Russell bodies) is sometimes a
prominent finding. Bone marrow biopsies frequently show interruption of the normal architecture with focal collections of plasma cells
indistinguishable from those seen in solitary
extraosseous lesions. In other instances, the
marrow may be more diffusely involved, and
focal collections of cells, at least in those sites
susceptible to routine biopsy, may not be
found (see Figure 17–3).

At times, marrow aspirations and biopsies
from several sites or a surgical biopsy of an
osteolytic lesion are required to substantiate
the diagnosis. A detailed examination of cell
morphology on bone marrow smears may reveal a disassociation of nuclear and cytoplasmic maturation (Graham and Bernier, 1975;

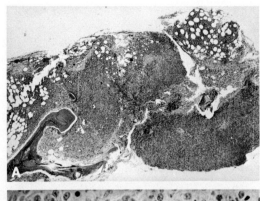
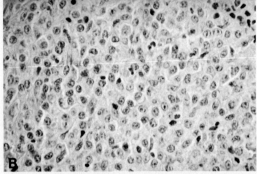
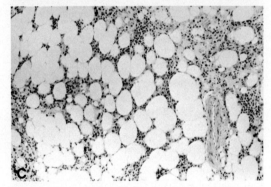

Figure 17–3. The bone marrow in multiple myeloma.
(*A*). Marrow biopsy of an untreated patient showing a
large mass of myeloma cells adjacent to areas of normocellular marrow (× 40). Large tumor masses such as this are
only rarely encountered in marrow biopsies. (*B*). Close-up
of mass shown in Figure 17–3A: Closely packed plasma
cells, many of which are atypical (× 1600). (*C*). Fixed
section of hypocellular marrow particle from untreated
patient with myeloma (× 160). Smears from this marrow
showed 38% plasma cells. This is a more typical distribution of myeloma cells in marrow.

Bernier and Graham, 1976) (see Figure 17–4).
In some series, marked nuclear immaturity
has been found to correlate with an adverse
prognosis, and, when taken with other evidence of plasma cell atypia, including the presence of multinucleated cells, is helpful in documenting the diagnosis. There is little problem

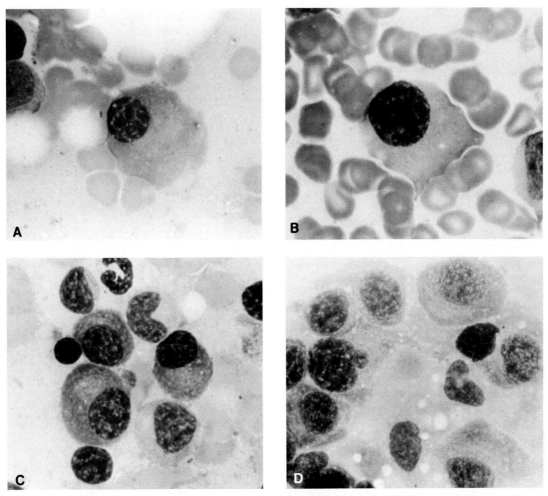

Figure 17–4. (*A*). Plasma cell from a normal bone marrow showing normal nuclear-cytoplasmic maturation. (*B*). Atypical plasma cell from patient with stable monoclonal gammopathy for two years and 9% plasma cells in marrow. (*C*). Three atypical plasma cells in patient with IgA myeloma. (*D*). Marked nuclear-cytoplasmic dissociation in clump of plasma cells from patient with IgG myeloma and 90% plasma cells in marrow.

with the diagnosis when more than 30% of the total cells examined are atypical plasma cells. Modest plasmacytosis, however, especially when a marked maturation defect is lacking, may present diagnostic difficulty. In these cases it is necessary to establish the diagnosis of myeloma by considering other important clinical and laboratory data as indicated in Table 17–1.

Benign plasmacytosis of the bone marrow may be seen in a variety of chronic inflammatory states such as collagen-vascular disease and neoplasms. In these diseases, biopsies may show the plasma cells to be concentrated in perivascular areas, in contrast to the diffuse pattern or focal collections more characteristic of myeloma.

Laboratory Diagnosis. The diagnosis of myeloma may be established on the basis of tests done to follow up on an abnormality found in routine health screening. A mild anemia, proteinuria, or elevation of the erythrocyte sedimentation rate commonly provoke investigations leading to the diagnosis of early stages of the illness.

Patients with more advanced disease may present with laboratory findings similar to those of patients with early disease but may also have extensive, painful osteolytic lesions or pathologic fractures. Azotemia, hypercalcemia, severe anemia, leukopenia, thrombocytopenia, and laboratory evidence for infection are common in this group of patients. Table 17–4 shows the results of pretreatment studies

Table 17–4. Laboratory Studies in 543 Patients with Myeloma before Specific Treatment

Leukocyte count/mm³	
Mean (×1000)	6.2
Percent <4,000	16
Platelet count/mm³	
Mean (×1000)	234
Percent <100,000	8
Hemoglobin g/dL	
Mean	10.4
Percent <8.5	16
Percent plasma cells in marrow, mean	47
Blood urea nitrogen mg/dL	27
percent >30	26
Serum calcium mg/dL*	9.8
percent >12.0	7

In some series up to one-third of patients are hypercalcemic at diagnosis (Kyle, 1975).
From Cornwell, G. G., III; Pajak, T. F.; Kochwa, S.; McIntyre, O. R.; Glowienka, L. P.; Brunner, K.; Rafla, S.; Coleman, M.; Cooper, M. R.; Henderson, E.; Kyle, R. A.; Haurani, F. I.; Cuttner, J.; Prager, D.; and Holland, J. F.: Vincristine and prednisone in the treatment of multiple myeloma: Prolonged survival in patients receiving melphalan. Cancer and Leukemia Group B Experience. In preparation, 1984; and Cornwell, G. G., III; Pajak, T. F.; Kochwa, S.; McIntyre, O. R.; Glowienka, L. P.; Brunner, K.; Rafla, S.; Silver, R. T.; Cooper, M. R.; Henderson, E.; Kyle, R. A.; Haurani, F. I.; and Cuttner, J.: Comparison of oral melphalan, CCNU, and BCNU with and without vincristine and prednisone in the treatment of multiple myeloma. Cancer, 50:1669–1675, 1982b.

performed on 543 patients with myeloma (Cornwell, 1982a,b).

The serum and urine electrophoresis, when coupled with the bone marrow or biopsy findings, is the most important diagnostic test for the disease. Only 1 or 2% of patients with myeloma fail to show evidence of a monoclonal protein in the serum or urine, and are said to have "nonsecreting" myeloma (Acute Leukemia Group B, 1975). Cellulose acetate serum or urine electrophoresis at pH 8.6 usually reveals a homogeneous band of protein with γ or β mobility. Immunoelectrophoresis provides additional evidence that the protein is homogeneous. In rare instances, about 0.2% (Cancer and Leukemia Group B, 1982) to 1% (Bihrer et al., 1974), biclonal gammopathies (for instance, IgG and IgA monoclonal proteins) are found. The amount of abnormal protein produced may be quantitated by immunodiffusion tests using known quantities of standard immunoglobulins (Mancini et al., 1965). Diffusion in these assays is influenced by the size of the M protein molecule and may not correlate exactly with measurements of the abnormal protein using other methods. For the purpose of following a patient's response to treatment, the area under the curve taken with a densitometer from the stained M protein on cellulose acetate electrophoresis is a useful and reproducible measure. The presence of M protein in the serum is responsible for another laboratory feature of the illness. The anion gap [serum sodium − (chloride + bicarbonate)] is normally equal to or over 12 mEq/L. In one series of patients with M proteins that had isoelectric points between 7.5 and 9.0, a significant reduction of the anion gap occurred, 28% having anion gaps below 6 mEq/L (Murray et al., 1975). At serum pH, these proteins act as cations, binding chloride and reducing the sodium-chloride difference. Although the existence of a decreased anion gap may suggest that a patient has occult myeloma, the finding is by no means specific for the disease.

Because dipsticks commonly used to screen urine for the presence of protein frequently fail to detect light chain proteinuria, methods based upon the acid precipitation of urinary protein should be applied (Watson, 1964; Gardner, 1971). In most laboratories, sulfosalicylic acid precipitation is used for this purpose. Methods capable of detecting 0.1 g of protein or more in a 24-hour urine sample should be employed and patients with proteinuria detectable under these conditions should have urine electrophoresis performed. Tests on a random urine sample may be done to establish the diagnosis, but 24-hour urine light chain–excretion values are required to assess tumor burden and response to treatment.

Serum alkaline phosphatase values, which are elevated in the small fraction of patients with osteoblastic lesions, may be helpful in following these patients. Serum uric acid determinations are important because renal damage can be accentuated if hyperuricemia occurs during therapy.

Urine calcium measurements may become more important as our knowledge concerning calcium metabolism in myeloma increases and as better means of coping with bone disease in these patients become available.

Radiologic Studies. X-rays of the axial skeleton and weight-bearing long bones are important in the assessment of a patient with suspected myeloma. "Punched-out" osteolytic lesions without evidence of osteoblastic activity are characteristic of the disease. These are seen most dramatically in lateral x-rays of the skull but they may occur in any bone. Identification of lesions in the weight-bearing bones is important if measures to prevent pathologic fracture are to be instituted. Extraosseous plasmacytomas may be visible on chest films as soft-tissue tumors projecting into the thorax from the ribs, especially in patients with high tumor loads (Edwards and Zawadzki, 1967).

Because about 60% of patients exhibit proteinuria, intravenous pyelograms are sometimes done before the diagnosis is established. This should be avoided, because the examination is not particularly helpful in the evaluation of proteinuria, and because dehydration is often involved in this procedure. The possible toxicity of the radiographic dye may also precipitate severe renal failure in a patient with myeloma. Even though the complication rate is low (Morgan and Hammack, 1966), it is an error to routinely order pyelography in the work-up of proteinuria without first considering myeloma.

Hazards of Diagnosis and Treatment

Patients with myeloma are often hospitalized for bed-rest and for the performance of diagnostic procedures. Because many patients with uncontrolled disease are already hypercalciuric (Siris *et al.,* 1980), increased mobilization of calcium as a result of inactivity can produce hypercalcemia and precipitate renal failure. Therefore, dehydration and immobilization are to be avoided in all patients admitted with a suspected diagnosis of myeloma.

It is usually not difficult to assign a diagnosis of myeloma on the basis of laboratory tests, histology, and other factors listed in Table 17–1. The diagnosis, however, may be very difficult to establish in some patients. For example, patients with a monoclonal protein, a modest bone marrow plasmacytosis, but with extensive symptomatic and progressive osteoporosis have been treated for myeloma, only to have retrospective judgments indicate that the patient had monoclonal gammopathy of undetermined significance as well as idiopathic osteoporosis. Errors of this sort are likely to be made from time to time in this difficult diagnostic area. Because treatment is associated with definite risks, considerable judgment is required when making the decision to treat indolent or slowly advancing disease.

Staging

Calculations of the tumor load in myeloma are possible because the M protein serves as a tumor marker. Because this protein can be easily quantitated, and because the fractional catabolic rate of homogeneous immunoglobulins at different serum concentrations is known (Waldmann and Strober, 1969), it is possible to calculate the number of tumor cells responsible for the observed serum level of M protein. In order to do this, the rate of protein production by each tumor cell must also be determined. Although studies by Salmon and Smith (1970) have shown that the rate of IgG synthesis per cell varies up to sevenfold, these investigators were, nevertheless, able to use this data to calculate tumor cell numbers, obtaining values consistent with tumor burdens estimated on the basis of clinical findings (Sullivan and Salmon, 1972).

In vitro determinations of myeloma globulin production and *in vivo* catabolism are not practical in large numbers of patients. For this reason, Durie and Salmon (1975) developed a myeloma staging system based on information from a small number of patients for whom *in vitro* data were available (see Table 17–5). Using the *in vitro* data, they related bone lesions, hemoglobin, serum calcium, and abnormal immunoglobulin levels in regression equations to tumor load. Later, general formulas were developed that estimate the body burden of myeloma cells for patients in whom the cellular rate of M-protein synthesis has not been measured (Salmon and Wampler, 1977). In addition, methods for calculating tumor load in the patients who excrete light chains

Table 17–5. Criteria for Estimating Myeloma Cell Mass

CELL MASS CATEGORY		HIGH	LOW	INTERMEDIATE
Number of myeloma cells		$>1.2 \times 10^{12}/m^2$	$<0.5 \times 10^{12}/m^2$	0.51 to $1.19 \times 10^{12}/m^2$
Requirements		One of A, B, or C	All of A, B, C, and D	Neither high nor low
Hemoglobin (gm/dl)	A	<8.5	>10.5	>8.5
Serum calcium (mg/dl)	B	>12	Normal	<12
M protein	C	IgG >7 g/dl	<5	<7
		IgA >5 g/dl	<3	<5
		BJ >12 g/day	<4	<12
Bone lesions	D	Scaled 3	0–1	2

Adapted from Durie, B. G. M., and Salmon, S. E.: A clinical staging system for multiple myeloma. *Cancer,* **36:**842–854, 1975.

only were also developed (Durie *et al.,* 1981a). It should not be surprising that attempts by other groups of investigators to determine pretreatment prognostic features have identified the factors on which these general formulas are based (Costa *et al.,* 1969; Medical Research Council, 1980b). When the staging system of Durie and Salmon (1975) was applied to 543 patients with myeloma, 8% were staged as low, 44% intermediate, and 48% as high tumor load (Cornwell, 1982a).

It should be emphasized that the response to treatment with reduction of tumor cell load and the reversibility of the initial abnormalities is a most important determinant of survival and is independent of the prognosis conferred by initial tumor cell load. Patients with high initial tumor cell loads who respond to treatment may survive longer than those with lower initial tumor cell loads who fail to respond.

Because tumor staging in myelomas is dependent upon the amount of abnormal protein produced, it is important to mention that an occasional patient will acquire subclones of tumor cells incapable of producing M protein as the disease advances. In such instances, it is not possible to relate changes in the M-protein level to burden of disease so other criteria for disease progression must be used (Sahasrabudhe and Parker, 1981).

Staging or assigning a prognosis for patients with myeloma will have major benefits only if this information is useful in guiding therapy. Evidence will be cited below that suggests that patients with large tumor cell burdens or a "poor risk" status respond better if treated with combination or intensive therapy.

Specific and Supportive Treatments

Chemotherapy. The oral alkylating agents, melphalan and cyclophosphamide, given either continuously or intermittently with prednisone, have been the standard treatment for myeloma since the mid-1960s (see review by Coleman and Silver, 1974). When cyclophosphamide and melphalan were compared in randomized studies, no significant differences were noted between the two in either response or patient survival (Rivers and Patno, 1969; Medical Research Council, 1971). A median survival for all patients treated with these agents is about 24 months (see Table 17–6). The response and survival results obtained in various series are dependent upon patient se-

lection and on the exclusion from analysis of patients who fail to respond or who die early. Recently, reported series suggest that objective response rates of approximately 60 to 70% and median survival of 30 to 36 months are possible (see Table 17–6).

The addition of prednisone to therapy with melphalan or cyclophosphamide increases the fraction of responders and improves survival (Alexanian *et al.,* 1969; Hoogstraten, 1973). This improvement has been noted with several different prednisone regimens. In one study, however, high-risk patients with large tumor burdens appeared to be adversely affected by prednisone at a dose of 1.2 mg/kg, probably because of increased mortality secondary to infection (Costa *et al.,* 1973; Cuttner *et al.,* 1975).

On the basis of experiments performed in mouse myeloma models in which non-cross-resistance to alkylating agents could be demonstrated (Ogawa *et al.,* 1973), various combinations of these drugs have been tested in myeloma patients. These include melphalan, cyclophosphamide, and nitrosoureas in various combinations and schedules (Alexanian *et al.,* 1977; Harley *et al.,* 1977; Bergsagel *et al.,* 1979). Although these efforts do not appear to have substantially improved the response or survival of all patients, one study using intravenously administered melphalan, cyclophosphamide, and lomustine found a significantly improved response and survival for patients with high tumor cell load (Harley *et al.,* 1979). In another study four drugs in combination also proved beneficial to patients with high tumor load (Salmon *et al.,* 1979). One study using a different schedule and route of administraion of the three alkylating agents, however, failed to show an advantage for high-risk or high tumor cell load patients (Bergsagel *et al.,* 1979; Medical Research Council, 1980a).

On the basis of theoretic considerations that suggest that the responding patient with myeloma may develop an increased number of myeloma cells in cycle (Salmon, 1975), several cycle-active agents have been tried in patients who have achieved partial remission. Azathioprine, cytosine arabinoside, and hydroxyurea are probably ineffective in this setting, but vincristine appears effective (Alberts *et al.,* 1977). Vincristine-containing multiple-drug regimens have been reported to be superior to other regimens (Alexanian *et al.,* 1977). It should be noted that responses equivalent to those achieved with multiple-agent regimens

Table 17–6. Response and Survival with Various Treatments in Selected Series

AUTHOR	TREATMENT	NUMBER OF PATIENTS	PROTEIN RESPONSE (%)[†]	MEDIAN SURVIVAL[*] (Months)
Feinleib & MacMahon, 1960	(Retrospective study only)	214	NA	10[‡]
Holland et al., 1966	Placebo	15	0	12
	Urethane (oral)	15	0	5
Bergsagel et al., 1962	Melphalan	165	24	25
Korst et al., 1964	Cyclophosphamide			
Hoogstraten et al., 1967	Melphalan "continuous"	64	45§	23
Hoogstraten et al., 1969	Melphalan "intermittent"	48	45§	26
Alexanian et al., 1969	Melphalan "daily"	31	31	18
	Melphalan "intermittent"	63	35‖	18
Costa et al., 1973	Melphalan "continuous"			
	"good risk"	35	20‖	30 }26
	"poor risk"	25	16‖	21
	Melphalan "continuous" plus prednisone			
	"good risk"	42	43‖	53 }35
	"poor risk"	29	31‖	9
	Melphalan "continuous" plus prednisone and testosterone			
	"good risk"	37	46‖	36 }24
	"poor risk"	21	33‖	4
Alexanian et al., 1977	MAP, MCP, CAP[#]		39 to 47**	22 to 26
	MPPV††		—	29
	VMCP + VACP‡‡		57 to 62**	30
Case et al., 1977	Melphalan prednisone cyslophosphamide BCNU vincristine	73	87	50[‡]
McIntyre et al., 1978	Melphalan "continuous" with prednisone	48	—	16
	Melphalan "IV" with prednisone	51	—	36
	Melphalan plus BCNU with prednisone	40	—	25
Bergsagel et al., 1979	Melphalan prednisone followed by cyclophosphamide BCNU on relapse	125	70	24
	Melphalan prednisone cyclophosphamide BCNU alternating	123	68	30
	Melphalan prednisone cyclophosphamide BCNU concurrent	116	72	30
Harley et al., 1977, 1979	Melphalan "continuous"			
	"good risk"	62	57	38
	"poor risk"	64	55	12
	IV Melphalan prednisone cyclophosphamide BCNU prednisone			
	"good risk"	71	70	30
	"poor risk"	53	64	24
Medical Research Council, 1980	Cyclophosphamide	124	—	20
	Melphalan "intermittent"	128	—	20
	Melphalan "intermittent" plus prednisone	120	20	
Salmon et al., 1979	VMCP, VABP plus Levamisole			36
Cooper et al., 1982	IV melphalan prednisone			36

* Survival from first treatment unless noted.
† Percent of patients achieving protein response as defined below.
‡Survival from first symptoms.
§ 2 g decrease.
‖ Myeloma task force criteria.
* MAP = melphalan, doxorubicin, prednisone; MCP = melphalan, cyclophosphamide, prednisone; CAP = cyclophosphamide, doxorubicin, prednisone.
** 75% reduction in M protein production, disappearance of urine M protein.
†† MPPV = melphalan, procarbazine, prednisone vincristine.
‡‡ VMCP = vincristine, melphalan, cyclosphosphamide, prednisone; VACP = vincristine, doxorubicin, cyclophosphamide, prednisone.

including vincristine have been achieved with melphalan given as a single agent intravenously with prednisone, as long as appropriate precautions are taken for azotemic patients entering the study (Cooper, 1982). Irregular absorption of oral melphalan provides the rationale for the use of the drug intravenously (Alberts et al., 1978). On the other hand, intravenous melphalan is associated with occasional instances of anaphylaxis (Cornwell *et al.*, 1979).

Measurement of Treatment Response. Response to treatment in myeloma is frequently expressed according to the Chronic Lymphocytic Leukemia-Myeloma Task Force (1973) recommendations. These recommendations define an objective response as a 50% reduction in M-protein or urinary Bence Jones protein. A decrease in the cross-sectional area of measured plasmacytomas of 50% or more and healing of bone lesions are also designated objective responses.

A more refined definition of response, namely, a 75% reduction in the rate of M-protein synthesis, has also been used (Alexanian *et al.*, 1972). Responses as defined by either of these two methods usually represent less than a one-log reduction in tumor cell burden. In occasional patients, the M-protein spike on serum electrophoresis is no longer demonstrable following treatment, but it is quite likely that if the patient's sera were tested by immunoelectrophoresis using antiserum to the M-protein idiotype, evidence of residual tumor would still be apparent. Long-term remissions are rare in myeloma, and eradication of the disease by the approaches used to date has not proved feasible. Thus, the search continues for treatments capable of further lowering the tumor cell burden in these patients.

Other Drugs with Possible Activity. New agents tested for activity in myeloma are usually tested in patients who have relapsed or who have failed to respond to initial therapy. The results of such trials are highly dependent upon the criteria used to define drug resistance or previous treatment failure. Doxorubicin and procarbazine, although having some activity in the disease, do not appear to contribute substantially to melphalan-prednisone regimens (Southwest Oncology Group, 1975; Alexanian *et al.*, 1977). The combination of doxorubicin and carmustine was reported as quite effective in relapsed patients in one series (Alberts and Salmon, 1975). When tested in patients where melphalan resistance was rigorously demonstrated, however, the doxorubicin-carmustine combination was no better than cyclophosphamide and carmustine in combination, and doxorubicin added nothing when included in combination with these agents (Kyle *et al.*, 1979, 1982). Some activity has been reported for galacitol, hexamethylmelamine, and *cis*-diamminedichloroplat-

inum, but it is not likely that these agents will come into common use. Some investigators are exploring the effect of the time of sequential drug administration in refractory patients who receive high-dose cyclo-phosphamide followed by doxorubicin (Karp *et al.*, 1981). The results from this study are encouraging but inconclusive.

Radiation Therapy. Radiation therapy is effective in the relief of localized pain caused by myelomatous lesions. For this purpose a small field can be applied to the painful lesion or pathologic fracture. Pain relief often begins with as little as 1000 rads, and doses of 2000 to 3000 rads are usually given; the larger doses are often directed at lesions of weight-bearing bones or at pathologic fractures. Because painful new lesions appear frequently in the patient with active disease, the physician may be tempted to treat disseminated disease by applying successive fields of radiation. Chemotherapy in such patients is preferable, often preventing the appearance of new lesions, whereas the application of radiation to successive fields will lead to hematosuppression, making chemotherapy more difficult.

Studies using systematic irradiation of all bone marrow-containing areas (Coleman *et al.*, 1982), as well as hemibody radiation are in progress (Salazar *et al.*, 1978). Although patients given this type of treatment have been observed to have significant reductions in M protein, the overall usefulness of this approach when combined with chemotherapy remains to be determined.

Biologic Response Modifiers. Previously untreated myeloma patients who received leukocyte interferon in the first clinical study of this agent responded with a frequency comparable to that seen with effective chemotherapy (Mellstedt *et al.*, 1979). The great excitement generated by this study abated as additional studies conducted with several interferon preparations produced much less satisfactory responses (Osserman and Sherman, 1980; Misset *et al.*, 1981). It should be mentioned that until interferon produced by recombinant techniques recently became available, all interferon trials had been conducted with impure material that probably contained a variety of biologically active materials. Whether the early results were due to interferon or the activity of contaminants in the interferon preparations remains uncertain. The possible specific effect of interferon upon the synthesis of immunoglobulin, mentioned earlier, has not been adequately excluded as a cause of M-protein reductions seen in the treated patients.

Levamisole has been used in a randomized study conducted by the Southwest Oncology Groups (Salmon and Dixon, 1981). The drug was given after an initial M-protein reduction had been achieved, and patients receiving the agent were observed to have an improved remission duration and survival. BCG was ineffective in prolonging remission in patients receiving combination therapy (Alexanian et al., 1981).

Treatment of Specialized Forms of Myeloma

Solitary Myeloma. Solitary myelomas of bone occur principally in the vertebrae but may occur in other bones, the ribs and pelvis being common. Such tumors are regarded as only the first manifestation of myeloma by some, because recurrence in a disseminated form is common following initial treatment. When restrictive criteria for the diagnosis of solitary myeloma are applied, response to treatment is satisfactory and long-term survival is good (Bataille and Sany, 1981). Criteria for this diagnosis include a biopsy showing localized disease, normal bone marrow examination, normal levels of polyclonal immunoglobulins, absence of anemia, hypercalcemia, renal involvement, and absence of monoclonal serum or urine protein (though small amounts may be detectable on immunoelectropheresis). Despite these criteria of localization, about 85% of patients will have evidence of dissemination at 10 years and more than 20% will have progression at two years. This is a favorable presentation, however, with nearly 70% of patients surviving 10 years following surgical resection of the lesion with or without postoperative radiation therapy.

Extramedullary Myeloma. Care must also be taken to distinguish solitary myeloma from multiple myeloma with extramedullary involvement. These single lesions are found most often in the upper airway where local symptoms lead to their diagnosis. Multiple myeloma develops despite treatment in about one-third of the patients, but the remainder may survive apparently cured following surgical excision or adequate radiation treatment (Webb et al., 1962).

Plasma Cell Leukemia. There are no features of this entity that distinguish it from multiple myeloma except that large numbers of plasma cells gain access to the circulation and that it may be more resistant to treatment (Pruzanski et al., 1969). At times, patients may respond well to initial therapy (Ogawa et al., 1969; Gailani et al., 1977), but responses, when seen, are usually brief. This has led to the use of drug regimens similar to those utilized for the treatment of acute leukemia, but this approach has been generally unrewarding.

Supportive Therapy. In addition to prompt initiation of chemotherapy for patients with advancing disease, it is important to begin specific therapy directed at various disease complications. These complications result in morbidity that severely limits the application of appropriate chemotherapy if not dealt with early and vigorously.

Hypercalcemia. Appropriate hydration with normal saline when given with a thiazide diuretic usually reverses symptomatic hypercalcemia. If the serum calcium is not reduced in several hours, prednisone, which has been shown to reduce calcium mobilization from the bone in myeloma (Bentzel et al., 1964), should be started at a dose of 0.6 to 1.2 mg/kg. These maneuvers alone are often successful in lowering the serum calcium. Specific treatment should also be started at this time because uncontrolled myeloma is the cause of the hypercalcemia. Rarely, treatment with mithramycin $25\mu g/kg$ IV for one to three doses is helpful, although marrow toxicity from this dose may further complicate chemotherapy. Treatment with oral inorganic phosphate solution has been advocated by some, although its use for this purpose has declined (Goldsmith, 1970). Dichloromethylene diphosphonate, which suppresses osteoclastic activity with little impairment of new bone formation in experimental animals, has been tested for its ability to lower serum calcium in myeloma (Siris et al., 1980). Seven of eight patients with hypercalciuria had sustained and highly significant decreases in urinary calcium.

It should be recognized that occasional M proteins have substantial calcium-binding activity. In these patients, the ionized calcium is much lower than predicted on the basis of the serum calcium, and these patients may exhibit impressive hypercalcemia with only minor clinical symptoms (Lindgarde and Zettervall, 1973).

Hypercalcemia may substantially aggravate preexisting or concurrent renal failure due to myeloma. Prompt reversal of hypercalcemia is usually beneficial in restoring some of the lost renal function.

Bone Disease. Symptomatic bone disease is the most common complaint of myeloma patients. Although roentgenograms reveal that osteolytic lesions heal in only about 15 to 30% of otherwise successfully treated patients, pain relief after initiation of appropriate chemotherapy is usually apparent within three to six weeks.

Pathologic fractures may prove to be highly disabling. Patients with osteolytic lesions in weight-bearing long bones should be considered for prophylactic orthopedic procedures aimed at reducing the possibility of such fractures. The morbidity following a pathologic fracture is often substantially greater than that attending prophylactic pinning or strengthening the bone otherwise. Radiation therapy following orthopedic stabilization and support is indicated.

Although collapse of vertebral bodies is common, cord compression is relatively less common. Early mobilization of the patient with a compression fracture of a vertebral body helps to diminish the risks of hypercalcemia and other myeloma complications. Fitting of a proper orthopedic appliance may assist in early ambulation.

Treatment of Renal Failure. As indicated earlier, renal failure is a major complication of the disease and frequently occurs in the setting of dehydration, sepsis, and shock. Prompt recognition of urinary tract sepsis or septicemia, treatment with appropriate antibiotics, and measures to improve renal blood flow may prevent an abrupt and profound loss of renal function. The appearance of chronic progressive renal failure in the absence of observed infection, dehydration, and shock poses a different and difficult problem. Slow reversal of the renal lesion is likely, and return of renal function toward normal may be expected if treatment substantially lowers the amount of the M protein (Martinez-Maldonado et al., 1971). Thus, in patients with azotemia, vigorous therapy directed at the tumor should be begun immediately. Whether plasmapheresis should be done to rapidly remove large quantities of a potentially toxic M component is controversial.

An even greater dilemma is posed by the untreated patient whose disease is accompanied by advanced renal failure. In such patients a trial of hemodialysis is sometimes justified if it seems likely that chemotherapy will control the disease (Johnson et al., 1980). A few patients with myeloma have received renal grafts and have survived sufficiently long to benefit from the procedure (Humphrey et al., 1975; DeLima et al., 1981).

Treatment of Infection. Urinary sepsis, frequently due to *Escherichia coli,* and pneumonia due to *Pneumococcus* or *Hemophilus* influenzae are the most common types of infections in previously untreated patients with myeloma. Standard laboratory screening often proves helpful in making a clinical decision about appropriate antibiotic therapy. Infection in the previously treated patient who may be leukopenic and on immunosuppressive drugs is likely to be secondary to a wider range of organisms that are often antibiotic resistant (Meyers et al., 1972).

Recurrent infection during treatment is a major cause of morbidity in some patients and is largely due to the decreased amounts of polyclonal immunoglobulin found in the disease (Lawson et al., 1955). Patients with repeated episodes of pneumococcal pneumonia, pneumococcal septicemia, and pneumococcal meningitis appear in most large series. Prophylactic administration of γ-globulin did not decrease the risk of infection in one randomized trial (Salmon et al., 1967). This trial was conducted before metabolic studies showed an increased catabolism of IgG in patients with increased amounts of IgG myeloma protein (Waldmann and Strober, 1969). Intravenous γ-globulin preparations may allow the administration of larger amounts of immunoglobulin and may prove beneficial in such patients.

Polyvalent pneumococcal vaccine has been administered to patients with myeloma (Lazarus et al., 1980; Schmid et al., 1981). As expected, the rise in antibody titer following the vaccine was substantially less than in normal individuals. Nevertheless, immunization with this vaccine may be of some help in management of the disease.

Infections with opportunistic organisms are less common in myeloma than in patients with lymphoma or leukemia. It has been suggested that despite the absence of normal polyclonal immunoglobulin in these patients, T-cell-mediated immunity to opportunistic organisms may be relatively intact.

Fluoride Treatment for Bone Lesions. In an effort to reduce bone pain and the progression of osteolytic lesions, various investigators have administered low-dose sodium fluoride either alone or with supplemental calcium (Cohen, 1966). Some patients have received androgen or vitamin D in addition. This approach is based on observations that mild skeletal fluorosis is associated with thickening of the trabeculae and increased bone density on x-ray examination. Conflicting results have been reported from these trials. A randomized placebo-controlled trial showed that sodium fluoride used alone did not prevent bone pain or fractures despite the induction of skeletal fluorosis in about 15% of patients receiving the high-dose regimen (Acute Leukemia Group B, 1972). Another randomized study, however, revealed that 50 mg of sodium fluoride twice daily plus 1.0 g calcium carbonate four times a day induced increases in bone density and decreased bone pain (Kyle *et al.*, 1975).

Neurologic Emergencies. In some instances, the spinal cord is injured by collapse of the vertebral neural arch or by protrusions of extradural myeloma tissue. A recent analysis of such patients has suggested that operative intervention to decompress the cord is not necessary, and it may in fact be associated with morbidity greater than the early institution of appropriate radiation therapy (Greipp and Kyle, 1980).

Leukemia. Although patients with multiple myeloma may rarely be diagnosed as having simultaneous acute myelogenous or acute monomyelogenous leukemia, it is clear that standard alkylating agent treatment of myeloma increases the risk of leukemia (Kyle *et al.*, 1970; Rosner and Grunwald, 1974). In one series, the actuarial risk of developing leukemia was 17% at 50 months of treatment (Bergsagel *et al.*, 1979). Other series suggest a somewhat lower but still substantial risk. It has been reported that bolus intravenous administration of alkylating agents in myeloma may decrease the risk of leukemic complications, at least during the early years of treatment, when compared to intermittent or continuous daily oral treatment with these agents (McIntyre *et al.*, 1981).

Other patients after variable periods of treatment develop a refractory pancytopenia, often with sideroblastic changes in the erythroid series. The relationship between this complication and leukemic transition is conjectural. The appearance of a refractory pancytopenia, however, greatly compromises the ability to successfully treat myeloma that can advance rapidly under these circumstances.

Maintenance Therapy. In an effort to diminish the toxic consequences of treatment, it has been suggested that after an initial response (for instance, a 75% reduction in protein synthetic rate) that therapy be discontinued and the patient be observed for signs of relapse (Southwest Oncology Group, 1975). Sixty percent of patients relapsing during an unmaintained maintenance phase have been found to respond to subsequent treatment (Alexanian *et al.*, 1978). It should be pointed out, however, that in this series some patients died or were lost to follow-up before treatment could be resumed. If patients are to be observed untreated following an initial response, it is imperative the follow-up be fastidious, and that prompt reinstitution of therapy occur once a relapse is documented.

Future Prospects

Eradication of the tumor by currently available treatments appears to be an elusive goal. New agents with greater selective effect on neoplastic B-cell clones, however, may yet be discovered and could have a substantial impact on this disease, and on the slowly growing low-grade B-cell lymphomas that pose a similar problem. This search may be assisted by the availability of soft agar culture systems in which tumor cell drug sensitivity may be tested (Hamburger and Salmon, 1977).

The fact that each myeloma cell produces a protein of the same unique idiotype presents an opportunity for immunotherapeutic approaches based on antiidiotypic mechanisms. These have been explored extensively in the mouse where idiotype-specific protection against tumor challenge has been conferred in mice immunized with myeloma protein (Lynch *et al.*, 1972). This protection was associated with the appearance of antiidiotype antibody in the protected mice. Protection could not be conferred by passive transfer of immune serum (Frikke *et al.*, 1977). An approach based upon passive administration of antiidiotype serum in humans may be limited by absorption of the antibody by the M protein before it reaches the neoplastic plasma cell and by the prospect of morbidity secondary to circulating antigen-antibody complexes, the result of reactions of the antiidiotype with the circulating M protein. Nevertheless, the encouraging initial results of treatment of a B-cell lymphoma with antiidiotype monoclonal antibody (Miller *et al.*, 1982) indicate that this approach deserves continued attention.

The factors that normally regulate expansion of B-cell clones are just coming under study (Lynch *et al.*, 1979). In the future, approaches to B-cell neoplasms may be based on methods that exploit regulatory molecules or their analogs. It is also possible that approaches based on enhancement of T-cell cytolytic activity for autologous myeloma cells, as described earlier, will become feasible. *In vivo* T-cell-mediated cytolysis may be inhibited by suppressor cells. Means of modifying this suppression may also be developed.

It is possible that improved supportive care will come from studies attempting to elucidate the precise mechanisms causing bone disease, renal failure, and polyclonal immunoglobulin suppression. If means are found to specifically reverse osteoclast activation, nephrotoxicity of the myeloma protein, and the suppression of normal polyclonal immunoglobulin production, substantial benefits will be achieved, even if complete eradication of the tumor burden is not feasible. The rapid progress of basic studies in these areas suggests that some of these goals will be reached in the near future.

REFERENCES

Acute Leukemia Group B: Ineffectiveness of flouride therapy in multiple myeloma. *N. Engl. J. Med.,* **286:**1283–1288, 1972.

Acute Leukemia Group B: Correlation of abnormal immunoglobulin with clinical features of myeloma. *Arch. Intern. Med.,* **135:**46–52, 1975.

Alberts, D. S.; Chang, S. Y.; Chen, H-S.; Gross, J. F.; Walson P. D.; Moon, T. E.; and Salmon, S. E.: Variability of melphalan (M) absorption in man. *ASCO Proc.,* **19:**C-112, 1978.

Alberts, D. S.; Durie, B. G. M.; and Salmon, S. E.: Treatment of multiple myeloma in remission with anticancer drugs having cell cycle specific characteristics. *Cancer Treat. Rep.,* **61:**381–388, 1977.

Alberts, D. S., and Salmon, S. E.: Adriamycin (NSC-123127) in the treatment of alkylator-resistant multiple myeloma: A pilot study. *Cancer Chemother. Rep.,* **59:**345–350, 1975.

Alexanian, R.; Bonnet, J.; Gehan, E.; Haut, A.; Hewlett, J.; Lane, M.; Monto, R.; and Wilson, H.: Combination chemotherapy for multiple myeloma. *Cancer,* **30:**382–389, 1972.

Alexanian, R.; Gehan, E.; Haut, A.; Saiki, J.; and Weick, J.: Unmaintained remissions in multiple myeloma. *Blood,* **51:**1005–1011, 1978.

Alexanian, R.; Haut, A.; Khan, A. U.; Lane, M.; McKelvey, E. M.; Migliore, P. J.; Stuckey, W. J., Jr.; and Wilson H. E.: Treatment for multiple myeloma. *J.A.M.A.,* **208:**1680–1685, 1969.

Alexanian, R.; Salmon, S.; Bonnet, J.; Gehan, E.; Haut, A.; and Weick, J.: Combination therapy for multiple myeloma. *Cancer,* **40:**2765–2771, 1977.

Alexanian, R.; Salmon, S.; Gutterman, J.; Dixon, D.; Bonnet, J.; and Haut, A.: Chemoimmunotherapy for multiple myeloma. *Cancer,* **47:**1923–1929, 1981.

Andrews, D. W., and Capra, J. D.: Structure and function of immunoglobulins. In Parker, C. W. (ed.): *Clinical Immunology.* W. B. Saunders company, Philadelphia, 1980.

Axelson, O.; Dahlgren, E.; Jansson, C.-D.; and Rehnlund, S. O.: Arsenic exposure and mortality: A case-referent study from a Swedish copper smelter. *Br. J. Ind. Med.,* **35:**8–15, 1978.

Axelsson, U.; Bachmann, R.; and Hallen, J.: Frequency of pathological proteins (M-components) in 6,995 sera from an adult population. *Acta Med. Scand.,* **179:**235–247, 1966.

Bataille, R.; and Sany, J.: Solitary myeloma: Clinical and prognostic features of a review of 114 cases. *Cancer,* **48:**845–851, 1981.

Beck, J. R.; Quinn, B. M.; Meier, F. A.; and Rawnsley, H. M.: Hyperviscosity syndrome in paraproteinemia. *Transfusion,* **22:**51–53, 1982.

Bence Jones, H.: Papers on chemical pathology. *Lancet,* **2:**254–257, 265–274, 360–369, 441–461, 1847.

Bentzel, C. J.; Carbone, P. P.; and Rosenberg, L.: The effect of prednisone on calcium metabolism and Ca^{47} kinetics in patients with multiple myeloma and hypercalcemia. *J. Clin. Invest.,* **43:**2132–2145, 1964.

Bergsagel, D. E.; Bailey, A. J.; Langley, G. R.; MacDonald, R. N.; White, D. F.; and Miller, A. B.: The chemotherapy of plasma-cell myeloma and the incidence of acute leukemia. *N. Engl. J. Med.,* **301:**743–748, 1979.

Bergsagel, D. E.; Migliore, P. J.; and Griffith, K. M.: Myeloma proteins and the clinical response to melphalan therapy. *Science,* **148:**376–377, 1965.

Bergsagel. D. E.; Sprague, C. C.; Austin, C,; and Griffith, K. M.: Evaluation of new chemotherapeutic agents in the treatment of multiple myeloma. IV. L-phenylalanine mustard (NC-8806). *Cancer Chemother. Rep.,* **21:**87–99, 1962.

Bernier, G. M., and Graham, R. C., Jr.: Plasma cell asynchrony in myeloma: Correlation of light and electron microscopy. *Semin. Hematol.,* **13:**239–245, 1976.

Bihrer R.; Flury, R.; and Morell, A.: Biklonale paraproteinamie. *Schweiz. Med. Wochenschr.,* **104:**39–45, 1974.

Blattner, W. A.; Blair, A.; and Mason, T. J.: Multiple myeloma in the United States, 1950–1975. *Cancer,* **48:**2547–2554, 1981.

Broder, S.; Humphrey, R.; Durm, M.; Blackman, M.; Meade, B.; Goldman, C.; Stober, W.; and Waldmann, T.: Impaired synthesis of polyclonal (nonparaprotein) immunoglobulins by circulating lymphocytes from patients with multiple myeloma. *N. Engl. J. Med.,* **293:**887–892, 1975.

Cancer and Leukemia Group B, 1982, unpublished.

Case, D. C.; Lee, B. J., III; and Clarkson, B. D.: Improved survival times in multiple myeloma treated with melphalan, prednisone, cyclophosphamide, vincristine and BCNU: M-2 protocol. *Am. J. Med.,* **63:**897–903, 1977.

Chronic Leukemia-Myeloma Task Force: Proposed guidelines for protocol studies. II. Plasma cell myeloma. *Cancer Chemother. Rep.,* **4:**145–158, 1973.

Clyne, D. H.; Kant, K. S.; Pesce, A. J.; and Pollak, V. E.: Nephrotoxicity of low molecular weight serum proteins: Physicochemical interactions between myoglobin, hemoglobin, Bence-Jones proteins and Tamm-Horsfall mucoprotein. In Dubach, V. C., and Schmidt, V. (eds.): *Diagnostic Significance of Enzymes and Proteins in Urine.* Hans Huber, Bern, 1979a.

Clyne, D. H.; Pesce, A. J.; and Thompson, R. E.: Nephrotoxicity of Bence Jones proteins in the rat: Importance of protein isoelectric point. *Kidney Int.,* **16**:345–352, 1979b.

Coffino, P., and Scharff, M. D.: Rate of somatic mutation in immunoglobulin production by mouse myeloma cells. *Proc. Natl. Acad. Sci. USA,* **68**:219–223, 1971.

Cohen, I.; Amir, J.; Ben-Shaul, Y.; Pick, A.; and De Vries, A.: Plasma cell myeloma associated with an unusual myeloma protein causing impairment of fibrin aggregation and platelet function in a patient with multiple malignancy. *Am. J. Med.,* **48**:766–776, 1970.

Cohen, P.: Fluoride and calcium therapy for myeloma bone lesions. *J.A.M.A.,* **198**:115–118, 1966.

Cohn, M.: Natural history of the myeloma. *Cold Spring Harbor Symp. Quant. Biol.,* **32**:211–221, 1967.

Coleman, M.; Saletan, S.; Wolf, D.; Nisce, L.; Wasser, J.; McIntyre, O. R.; and Tulloh, M.: Whole bone marrow irradiation for the treatment of multiple myeloma. *Cancer,* **49**:1328–1333, 1982.

Coleman, M., and Silver, R. T.: The chemotherapy of plasma cell myeloma and related disorders. In Schoenfeld, H.; Brockman, R. W.; and Hahn, F.E. (eds.): *Antibiotics and Chemotherapy.* S. Karger, Basel, 1974.

Cooper, M. R., personal communication, 1982.

Cornell, C. J., Jr.; McIntyre, O. R.; Kochwa, S.; Weksler, B. B.; and Pajak, T. F.: Response to therapy in IgG myeloma patients excreting lambda or kappa light chains: CALGB experience. *Blood,* **54**:23–29, 1979.

Cornwell, G. G.,III; Pajak, T. F.; Kochwa, S.; McIntyre, O. R.; Glowienka, L. P.; Brunner, K.; Rafla, S.; Coleman, M.; Cooper, M. R.; Henderson, E.; Kyle, R. A.; Haurani, F. I.; Cuttner, J.; Prager, D.; and Holland, J. F.: Vincristine and prednisone in the treatment of multiple myeloma: Prolonged survival in patients receiving melphalan. Cancer and Leukemia Group B Experience. In preparation, 1984.

Cornwell, G. G.,III; Pajak, T. F.; Kochwa, S.; McIntyre, O. R.; Glowienka, L. P.; Brunner, K.; Rafla, S.; Silver, R. T.; Cooper, M. R.; Henderson, E.; Kyle, R. A.; Haurani, F. I.; and Cuttner, J.: Comparison of oral melphalan, CCNU, and BCNU with and without vincristine and prednisone in the treatment of multiple myeloma. *Cancer,* **50**:1669–1675, 1982b.

Cornwell G. G.,III; Pajak, T. F.; and McIntyre, O. R.: Hypersensitivity reactions to IV melphalan during treatment of multiple myeloma: Cancer and Leukemia Group B experience. *Cancer Treat. Rep.,* **63**:399–403, 1979.

Cossman, J.; Neckers, L. M.; Arnold, A.; and Korsmeyer, S. J.: Induction of differentiation in a case of common acute lymphoblastic leukemia. *N. Engl. J. Med.,* **307**:1251–1254, 1982.

Costa, G.; Engle, R. L., Jr.; Schilling, A.; Carbone, P.; Kochwa, S.; Nachman, R. L.; and Glidewell, O.: Melphalan and prednisone: An effective combination for the treatment of multiple myeloma. *Am. J. Med.,* **54**:589–599, 1973.

Costa, G.; Engle, R. L., Jr.; and Taliente, P.: Criteria for defining risk groups and response to chemotherapy in multiple myeloma. *Proc. Am. Assoc. Cancer Res.,* **10**:15, 1969.

Cutler, S. J., and Young, J. L., Jr.: Third National Cancer Survey: Incidence data. *Natl. Cancer Inst. Monogr.,* **41**:1–454, 1975.

Cuttner, J.; Wasserman, L. R.; Martz, G.; Sonntag, R. W.; Kyle, R. A.; Silver, R. T.; Spurr, C.; Harley, J. B.; Wiernik, P. M.; Cornwell, G. G., III; Falkson, G.; Glidewell, O.; and Holland, J. F.: The use of low-dose prednisone

and melphalan in the treatment of poor-risk patients with multiple myeloma. *Med. Pediatr. Oncol.,* **1**:207–216, 1975.

Cuzick, J.: Radiation-induced myelomatosis. *N. Engl. J. Med.,* **304**:204–210, 1981.

Davis, L. E., and Drachman, D. B.: Myeloma neuropathy. *Arch. Neurol.,* **27**:507–511, 1972.

DeFronzo, R. A.; Humphrey, R. L.; Wright, J. R.; and Cooke, C. R.: Acute renal failure in multiple myeloma. *Medicine,* **54**:209–223, 1975.

DelDuca, V., Jr., and Morningstar, W. A.: Multiple myeloma associated with progressive multifocal leukoencephalopathy. *J.A.M.A.,* **199**:165–167, 1967.

De Lima, J. J. G.; Kourilsky, O.; Meyrier, A.; Morel-Maroger, L.; and Sraer, J.-D.: Kidney transplant in multiple myeloma. *Transplantation,* **31**:223–225, 1981.

Drewinko, B.; Alexanian, R.; Boyer, H.; Barlogie, B.; and Rubinow, S. I.: The growth fraction of human myeloma cells. *Blood,* **57**:333–338, 1981.

Durie, B. G. M.; Cole, P. W.; Chen, H.-S. G.; Himmelstein, K. J.; and Salmon, S. E.: Synthesis and metabolism of Bence Jones protein and calculation of tumor burden in patients with Bence Jones myeloma. *Br. J. Haematol.,* **47**:7–19, 1981a.

Durie, B. G. M., and Salmon, S. E.: A clinical staging system for multiple myeloma. *Cancer,* **36**:842–854, 1975.

Durie, B. G. M.; Salmon, S. E.; and Mundy, G. R.: Relation of osteoclast activating factor production to extent of bone disease in multiple myeloma. *Br. J. Haematol.,* **47**:21–30, 1981b.

Edelman, G. M., and Gall, W. E.: The antibody problem. *Annu. Rev. Biochem,* **38**:415–466, 1969.

Edwards, G. A., and Zawadzki, Z. A.: Extraosseous lesions in plasma cell myeloma. *Am. J. Med.,* **43**:194–205, 1967.

Ende, M.: Multiple myeloma: A cluster in Virginia? *Va. Med.,* **106**:115–116, 1979.

Fahey, J. L.; Scoggins, R.; Utz, J. P.; and Szwed, C. F.: Infection, antibody response and gamma globulin components in multiple myeloma and macroglobulinemia. *Am. J. Med.,* **35**:698–707, 1963.

Feinleib, M., and MacMahon, B.: Duration of survival in multiple myeloma. *J.N.C.I.,* **24**:1259–1269, 1960.

Francus, T.; Dharmgrongartama, B.; Campbell, R.; Scharff, M. D.; and Birshtein, B. K.: IgG$_{2a}$-producing variants of an IgG$_{2b}$-producing mouse myeloma cell line. *J. Exp. Med.,* **147**:1535–1550, 1978.

Frikke, M. J.; Bridges, S. H.; and Lynch, R. G.: Myeloma-specific antibodies: Studies of their properties and their relationship to tumor immunity. *J. Immunol.,* **118**:2206–2212, 1977.

Gailani, S.; Seon, B. K.; and Henderson, E. S.: Plasma cell leukemia: Response to conventional myeloma therapy. *J. Med.,* **8**:403–414, 1977.

Gardner, K. D., Jr.: Uromancy 1971: Tricks with sticks. *N. Engl. J. Med.,* **285**:1026–1027, 1971.

Garry, R. F.; Bishop, J. M.; Parker, S.; Westbrook, K.; Lewis, G.; and Waite, M. R. F.: Na$^+$ and K$^+$ concentrations and the regulation of protein synthesis in sindbis virus-infected chick cells. *Virology,* **96**:108–120, 1979.

Garry, R. F., and Waite, M. R. F.: Na$^+$ and K$^+$ concentrations and the regulation of the interferon system in chick cells. *Virology,* **96**:121–128, 1979.

Glenner, G. G.; Ein, D.; and Terry, W. D.: The immunoglobulin origin of amyloid. *Am. J. Med.,* **52**:141–147, 1972.

Glenner, G. G.; Harada, M.; Isersky, C.; Cuatrecasas, P.; Page, D.; and Keiser, H.: Human amyloid protein: Diversity and uniformity. *Biochem. Biophys. Res. Commun.,* **41:**1013–1019, 1970.

Glenner, G. G.; Terry, W.; Harada, M.; Isersky, C.; and Page, D.: Amyloid fibril proteins: Proof of homology with immunoglobulin light chains by sequence analyses. *Science,* **172:**1150–1151, 1971.

Goldsmith, R. S.: Multiple effects of phosphate therapy. *N. Engl. J. Med.,* **282:**927–928, 1970.

Graham, R. C., Jr., and Bernier, G. M.: The bone marrow in multiple myeloma: Correlation of plasma cell ultrastructure and clinical state. *Medicine* (Baltimore), **54:**225–243, 1975.

Greipp, P. R., and Kyle, R. A.: Spinal cord compression by extradural plasmacytoma—Mayo Clinic Experience. *Proc. Int. Soc. Hematol.,* 462, 1980.

Hallen, J.: Frequency of "abnormal" serum globulins (m-components) in the aged. *Acta Med. Scand.,* **173:**737–744, 1963.

Hamaker, W. R.; Lindell, M. E.; and Gomez, A. C.: Plasmacytoma arising in a pacemaker pocket. *Ann. Thorac. Surg.,* **21:**354–356, 1976.

Hamburger, A., and Salmon, S. E.: Primary bioassay of human myeloma stem cells. *J. Clin. Invest.,* **60:**846–854, 1977.

Harley, J.; McIntyre, O. R.; and Pajak, T. F.: Improved survival of poor risk myeloma patients receiving combination alkylating agent therapy. *Blood,* **50:**192, 1977.

Harley, J. B.; Pajak, T. F.; McIntyre, O. R.; Kochwa, S.; Cooper, M. R.; Coleman, M. R.; and Cuttner, J.: Improved survival of increased-risk myeloma patients on combined triple-alkylating-agent therapy: A study of the CALGB. *Blood,* **54:**13–22, 1979.

Hewell, G. M., and Alexanian, R.: Multiple myeloma in young persons. *Ann. Intern. Med.,* **84:**441–443, 1976.

Hilschmann, N., and Craig, L. C.: Amino acid sequence studies with Bence-Jones proteins. *Proc. Natl. Acad. Sci. USA,* **53:**1403–1409, 1965.

Hobbs, J. R.: Growth rates and responses to treatment in human myelomatosis. *Br. J. Haematol.,* **16:**607–617, 1969.

Hobbs, J. R.: An ABC of amyloid. *Proc. R. Soc. Med.,* **66:**705–710, 1973.

Holland, J. F.; Hosley, H.; Scharlau, C.; Carbone, P. P.; Frei, E.,III; Brindley, C. O.; Hall, T. C.; Shnider, B. I.; Gold, G. L.; Lasagna, L.; Owens A. H., Jr.; and Miller, S. P.: A controlled trial of urethane treatment in multiple myeloma. *Blood,* **27:**328–342, 1966.

Hoogstraten, B.: Steroid therapy of multiple myeloma and macroglobulinemia. *Med. Clin. North Am.,* **57:**1321–1330, 1973.

Hoogstraten, B., and Costa, J.: Intermittent melphalan therapy in multiple myeloma. *J.A.M.A.,* **209:**251–253, 1969.

Hoogstraten, B.; Sheehe, P. R.; Cuttner, J.; Cooper, T.; Kyle, R. A.; Oberfield, R. A.; Townsend, S. R.; Harley, J. B.; Hayes, D. M.; Costa, G.; and Holland, J. F.: Melphalan in multiple myeloma. *Blood,* **30:**74–83, 1967.

Hoover, R. G.; Hickman, S.; Gebel, H. M.; Reebe, N.; and Lynch, R. G.: Expansion of Fc receptor-bearing T lymphocytes in patients with immunoglobulin G and immunoglobulin A myeloma. *J. Clin. Invest.,* **67:**308–311, 1981.

Humphrey, R. L.; Wright, J. R.; Zachary, J. B.; Sterioff, S.; and DeFronzo, R. A.: Renal transplantation in multiple myeloma. *Ann. Intern. Med.,* **83:**651–653, 1975.

Hutchison G. B.; MacMahon, B.; Jablon, S.; and Land, C. E.: Review of report by Mancuso, Steward and Kneale of radiation exposure of Hanford workers. *Health Phys.,* **37:**207–220, 1979.

Ichimaru, M.; Ishimaru, T.; Mikami, M.; and Matsunaga, M.: *Multiple Myeloma Among Atomic Bomb Survivors and Controls in Hiroshima and Nagasaki, 1950–1976,* Hiroshima, Radiation Effects Research Foundation, 1979. (Radiation Effects Research Foundation technical report no. 9–79).

Ishizaka, K., and Ishizaka, T.: Reversed type allergic skin reactions by anti-E-globulin antibodies in humans and monkeys. *J. Immunol.,* **100:**554–562, 1968.

Isobe, T., and Osserman, E. F.: Pathologic conditions associated with plasma cell dyscrasias. A study of 806 cases. *Ann. N.Y. Acad. Sci.,* **90:**507–518, 1971.

Isobe, T., and Osserman, E. F.: Patterns of amyloidosis and their association with plasma-cell cyscrasia, monoclonal immunoglobulins and Bence-Jones proteins. *N. Engl. J. Med.,* **209:**473–477, 1974.

Johnson, W. J.; Kyle, R. A.; and Dahlberg, P. J.: Dialysis in the treatment of multiple myeloma. *Mayo Clin. Proc.,* **55:**65–72, 1980.

Josse, R. G.; Murray, T. M.; Mundy, G. R.; Jez, D.; and Heersche, J. N. M.: Observations on the mechanism of bone resorption induced by multiple myeloma marrow culture fluids and partially purified osteoclast-activating factor. *J. Clin. Invest.,* **67:**1472–1481, 1981.

Karp, J. E.; Humphrey, R. L.; and Burke, P. J.: Timed sequential chemotherapy of cytoxan-refractory multiple myeloma with cytoxan and adriamycin based on induced tumor proliferation. *Blood,* **57:**468–475, 1981.

Kehoe, J. M., and Fougereau, M.: Immunoglobulin peptide with complement fixing activity. *Nature,* **224:**1212–1213, 1969.

Kelly, J. J., Jr.; Kyle, R. A.; Miles, J. M.; O'Brien, P. C.; and Dyck, P. J.: The spectrum of peripheral neuropathy in myeloma. *Neurology,* **31:**24–31, 1981.

Korst, D. R.; Clifford, G. O.; Fowler, W. M.; Louis, J.; Will, J.; and Wilson, H. E.: Multiple myeloma. II. Analysis of cyclophosphamide therapy in 165 patients. *J.A.M.A.,* **189:**758–762, 1964.

Koss, M. N.; Pirani, C. L.; and Osserman, E. F.: Experimental Bence Jones case nephropathy. *Lab. Invest.,* **34:**579–591, 1976.

Kubagawa, H.; Vogler, L. B.; Capra, J. D.; Conrad, M. E.; Lawton, A. B.; and Cooper, M. D.: Studies on the clonal origin of multiple myeloma. *J. Exp. Med.,* **150:**792–807, 1979.

Kyle, R. A.: Multiple myeloma, review of 869 cases. *Mayo Clin. Proc.,* **50:**29–40, 1975.

Kyle, R. A.: Immunoglobulins and syndromes associated with monoclonal gammopathies. In Tice, F. (ed.): *Practice of Medicine.* Vol. 1. Harper & Row, Publishers, Inc., Hagerstown, Maryland, 1977.

Kyle, R. A.: Monoclonal gammopathy of undetermined significance. *Am. J. Med.,* **64:**814–826, 1978.

Kyle, R. A., and Elveback, L. R.: Management and prognosis of multiple myeloma. *Mayo Clin. Proc.,* **51:**751–760, 1976.

Kyle, R. A.; Finkelstein, S.; Elveback, L. R.; and Kurland, L. T.: Incidence of monoclonal proteins in a Minnesota community with a cluster of multiple myeloma. *Blood,* **40:**719–724, 1972.

Kyle, R. A.; Gailani, S.; Seligman, B. R.; Blom, J.; McIntyre, O. R.; Pajak, T. F.; and Holland, J. F.: Multiple myeloma resistant to melphalan: Treatment with cyclophosphamide, prednisone, and BCNU. *Cancer Treat. Rep.,* **63:**1265–1269, 1979.

Kyle, R. A., and Greipp, P. R.: Smoldering multiple myeloma. *N. Engl. J. Med.,* **301:**1347–1349, 1980.

Kyle, R. A., and Greipp, P. R.: "Idiopathic" Bence Jones proteinuria. *N. Engl. J. Med.,* **306:**564–567, 1982.

Kyle, R. A.; Jowsey, J.; Kelly, P. J.; and Taves, D. R.: Multiple-myeloma bone disease. *N. Engl. J. Med.,* **293:**1334–1338, 1975.

Kyle, R. A.; Pajak, T. F.; Henderson, E. S.; Nawabi, I. U.; Brunner, K.; Henry, P. H.; McIntyre, O. R.; and Holland, J. F.: Multiple myeloma resistant to melphalan: Treatment with doxorubicin, cyclophosphamide, carmustine (BCNU), and prednisone. *Cancer Treat. Rep.,* **66:**451–456, 1982.

Kyle, R. A.; Pierre, R. V.; and Bayrd, E. D.: Multiple myeloma and acute myelomonocytic leukemia. *N. Engl. J. Med.,* **283:**1121–1126, 1970.

Latov, N.; Sherman, W. H.; Nemni, R.; Galassi, G,; Shyong, J. S.; Penn, A. D.; Chess, L.; Olarte, M. R.; Rowland, L. P.; and Osserman, E. F.: Plasma-cell dyscrasia and peripheral neuropathy with a monoclonal antibody to peripheral-nerve myelin. *N. Engl. J. Med.,* **303:**618–621, 1980.

Lawson, H. A.; Stuart, C. A.; Paull, A. M.; Phillips, A. M.; and Phillips, R. W.: Observations on the antibody content of the blood in patients with multiple myeloma. *N. Engl. J. Med.,* **252:**13–18, 1955.

Lazarus, H. M.; Lederman, M.; Lubin, A.; Herzig, R. H.; Schiffman, G.; Jones, P.; Wine, A.; and Rodman, H. M.: Pneumococcal vaccination: The response of patients with multiple myeloma. *Am. J. Med.,* **69:**419–423, 1980.

Lindgarde, F., and Zettervall, O.: Hypercalcemia and normal ionized serum calcium in a case of myelomatosis. *Ann. Intern. Med.,* **78:**396–399, 1973.

Linos, A.; Kyle, R. A.; O'Fallon, W. M.; and Kurland, L. T.: Incidence and secular trend of multiple myeloma in Olmsted County, Minnesota: 1965–77. *J.N.C.I.,* **66:**17–20, 1981.

Luben, R. A.; Mohler, M. A.; and Nedwin, G. E.: Production of hybridomas secreting monoclonal antibodies against the lymphokine osteoclast activating factor. *J. Clin. Invest.,* **64:**337–341, 1979.

Lynch, R. G.; Graff, R. J.; Sirisinha, S.; Simms, E. S.; and Eisen, H. N.: Myeloma proteins as tumor-specific transplantation antigens. *Proc. Natl. Acad. Sci. USA,* **69:**1540–1544, 1972.

Lynch, R. G.; Rohrer, J. W.; Odermatt, B.; Gebel, H. M.; Autry, J. R.; and Hoover, R. G.: Immunoregulation of murine myeloma cell growth and differentiation: A monoclonal model of B cell differentiation. *Immunol. Rev.,* **48:**45–80, 1979.

McIntire, K. R., and Princler, G. L.: Plasma cell tumors (PCT) in germfree (GF) mice: Effect of subcellular extracts. *AACR Abstracts,* **12:**257, 1971.

McIntyre, O. R.; Leone, L.; and Pajak, T. F.: The use of intravenous melphalan (L-PAM) in the treatment of multiple myeloma. *Blood,* **52:**274, 1978.

McIntyre, O. R.; Pajak, T. F.; Wiernik, P.; Glowienka, L. P.; Cornwell, G. G.; Harley, J.; and Leone, L.: Delayed acute leukemia in myeloma patients receiving pulsed vs. continuous treatment. *Blood,* **58:**579, 1981.

MacIntyre, W.: Mollities and fragilitas ossium. *Medico Chir. Soc. Trans.,* **33:**211–232, 1850.

Maldonado, J. E., and Kyle, R. A.: Familial myeloma. *Am. J. Med.,* **57:**875–884, 1974.

Mancini, G.; Carbonara, A. O.; and Heremans, J. F.: Immunochemical quantitation of antigens by single radial immunodiffusion. *Immunochemistry,* **2:**235–254, 1965.

Mancuso, T. F.; Stewart A.; and Kneale, G.: Radiation exposures of Hanford workers dying from cancer and other causes. *Health Phys.,* **33:**369–385, 1977.

Martinez-Maldonado, M.; Yium, J.; Suki, W. N.; and Eknoyan, G.: Renal complications in multiple myeloma: Pathophysiology and some aspects of clinical management. *J. Chronic Dis.,* **24:**221–237, 1971.

Mason, T. J.: Cancer mortality in U.S. countries with plastics and related industries. *Environ. Health Perspect.,* **11:**79–84, 1975.

Medical Research Council's Working Party on Leukemia in Adults: Treatment comparison in the third MRC myelomatosis trial. *Br. J. Cancer,* **42:**823–830, 1980a.

Medical Research Council's Working Party on Leukaemia in Adults: Prognostic features in the third MRC myelomatosis trial. *Br. J. Cancer,* **42:**831–840, 1980b.

Medical Research Council's Working Party for Therapeutic Trials in Leukaemia: Myelomatosis: Comparison of melphalan and cyclophosphamide therapy. *Br. Med. J.,* **1:**640–641, 1971.

Meijers, K. A. E.; de Leeuw, B.; and Voormolen-Kalova, M.: The multiple occurrence of myeloma and asymptomatic paraproteinaemia within one family. *Clin. Exp. Immunol.,* **12:**185–193, 1972.

Mellstedt, H.; Bjorkholm, M.; Johansson, B.; Ahre, A.; Holm, G.; and Strander, H.: Interferon therapy in myelomatosis. *Lancet,* **1:**245–247, 1979.

Merwin, R. M., and Algire, G. H.: Induction of plasma-cell neoplasms and fibrosarcomas in BALB/c mice carrying diffusion chambers. *Proc. Soc. Exp. Biol. Med.,* **101:**437–439, 1959.

Meyers, B. R.; Hirschman, S. Z.; and Axelrod, J. A.: Current patterns of infection in multiple myeloma. *Am. J. Med.,* **52:**87–92, 1972.

Milham, S., Jr.: Leukemia and multiple myeloma in farmers. *Am. J. Epidemol.,* **94:**307–310, 1971.

Miller, R. A.; Maloney, D. G.; Warnke, R.; and Levy, R.: Treatment of B-cell lymphoma with monoclonal anti-idiotype antibody. *N. Engl. J. Med.,* **306:**517–522, 1982.

Misset, J. L.; Gastiaburu, J.; De Vassal, F.; and Mathe, G.: Phase II trial of interferon (IF) in malignant gammopathies meningeal leukemia on chronic lymphatic leukemia (CLL). *ASCO Abstracts,* **22:**C-621, 1981.

Morgan, C., Jr., and Hammack, W. J.: Intravenous urography in multiple myeloma. *N. Engl. J. Med.,* **275:**77–79, 1966.

Morrison, S. L., and Scharff, M. D.: Mutational events in mouse myeloma cells. *CRC Crit. Rev. Immunol.,* 1–22, September, 1981.

Mundy, G. R.; Raisz, L. R.; Cooper, R. A.; Schechter, G. P.; and Salmon, S. E.: Evidence for the secretion of an osteoclast stimulating factor in myeloma. *N. Engl. J. Med.,* **291:**1041–1046, 1974.

Murray, T.; Long, W.; and Narins, R. G.: Multiple myeloma and the anion gap. *N. Engl. J. Med.,* **292:**574–575, 1975.

Nuss, D. L., and Koch, G.: Variation in the relative synthesis of immunoglobulin G and non-immunoglobulin G proteins in cultured MPC-11 cells with changes in the overall rate of polypeptide chain initiation and elongation. *J. Mol. Biol.,* **102:**601–612, 1976.

Ogawa, M.; Bergsagel, D. E.; and McCulloch, E. A.:

Chemotherapy of mouse myeloma: Quantitative cell cultures predictive of response in vivo. *Blood,* **41**:7–15, 1973.

Ogawa, M.; Kochwa, S.; Smith, C.; Ishizaka, K.; and McIntyre, O. R.: Clinical aspects of IgE myeloma. *N. Engl. J. Med.,* **281**:1217–1220, 1969.

Ogawa, M.; Wurster, D. H.; and McIntyre, O. R.: Multiple myeloma in one of a pair of monozygotic twins. *Acta Haematol.* (Basel), **44**:295–304, 1970.

Osserman, E. F., and Sherman, W. H.: Preliminary results of the American Cancer Society (ACS)-sponsored trial of human leukocyte interferon (IF) in multiple myeloma (MM). *Proc. AACR,* **21**:643, 1980.

Paglieroni, T., and MacKenzie, M. R.: In vitro cytotoxic response to human myeloma plasma cells by peripheral blood leukocytes from patients with multiple myeloma and benign monoclonal gammopathy. *Blood,* **54**:226–237, 1979.

Paglieroni, T., and MacKenzie, M. R.: Multiple myeloma: An immunologic profile. III. Cytotoxic and suppressive effects of the EA rosette-forming cell. *J. Immunol.,* **124**:2563–2570, 1980.

Peeler, R. N.; Kadull, P. J.; and Cluff, L. E.: Intensive immunization of man. *Ann. Intern. Med.,* **63**:44–47, 1965.

Plaut, A. G.; Wistar, R., Jr.; and Capra, J. D.: Differential susceptibility of human IgA immunoglobulins to streptococcal IgA protease. *J. Clin. Invest.,* **54**:1295–1300, 1974.

Potter, M., and Boyce, C. R.: Induction of plasma-cell neoplasms in strain BALB/c mice with mineral oil and mineral oil adjuvants. *Nature,* **193**:1086–1087, 1962.

Pruzanski, W.; Platts, M. E.; and Ogryslo, M. A.: Leukemic form of immunocytic dyscrasia (plasma cell leukemia). *Am. J. Med.,* **47**:60–74, 1969.

Pruzanski, W., and Watt, J. G.: Serum viscosity and hyperviscosity syndrome in IgG multiple myeloma. *Ann. Intern. Med.,* **77**:853–860, 1972.

Rivers, S. L., and Patno, M. E.: Cyclophosphamide vs melphalan in treatment of plasma cell myeloma. *J.A.M.A.,* **207**:1328–1334, 1969.

Rodriguez, L. H.; Finkelstein, M. B.; Shullenberger, C. C.; and Alexanian, R.: Bone healing in multiple myeloma with melphalan chemotherapy. *Ann. Intern. Med.,* **76**:551–556, 1972.

Rosner, F., and Grunwald, H.: Multiple myeloma terminating in acute leukemia. *Am. J. Med.,* **57**:927–939, 1974.

Rousseau, J. J.; Granck, G.; Grisar, T.; Reznik, M.; Heynen, G.; and Salmon, J.: Osteosclerotic myeloma with polyneuropathy and ectopic secretion of calcitonin. *Eur. J. Cancer,* **14**:133–140, 1978.

Sahasrabudhe, D. M., and Parker, J. C.: Decreasing M spike with increasing tumor burden in multiple myeloma. *Arch. Intern. Med.,* **141**:1152–1158, 1981.

Salazar, O. M.; Rubin, P.; Keller, B.; and Scarantino, C.: Systemic (half-body) radiation therapy: Response and toxicity. *Int. J. Radiat. Oncol. Biol. Phys.,* **4**:937–950, 1978.

Salmon, S. E.: Immunoglobulin synthesis and tumor kinetics of multiple myeloma. *Semin. Hematol.,* **10**:135–147, 1973.

Salmon, S. E.: Expansion of the growth fraction in multiple myeloma with alkylating agents. *Blood,* **45**:119–129, 1975.

Salmon, S. E.; Alexanian, R.; and Dixon, D.: Non-cross resistant combination chemotherapy improves survival in multiple myeloma. *Blood,* **54**:207a (Suppl.), 1979.

Salmon, S. E., and Dixon, D.: Addition of levamisole to chemotherapy improves survival in multiple myeloma. *Blood,* **58**:583, 1981.

Salmon, S. E.; Hamburger, A. W.; Soehnlen, B.; Durie, B. G. M.; Alberts, D. S.; and Moon, T. E.: Quantitation of differential sensitivity of human-tumor stem cells to anticancer drugs. *N. Engl. J. Med.,* **298**:1321–1327, 1978.

Salmon, S. E.; Samal, B. A.; Hayes, D. M.; Hosley, H.; Miller, S. P.; and Schilling, A.: Role of gamma globulin for immunoprophylaxis in multiple myeloma. *N. Engl. J. Med.,* **227**:1336–1340, 1967.

Salmon, S. E., and Seligmann, M.: B-cell neoplasia in man. *Lancet,* **2**:1230–1233, 1974.

Salmon, S. E., and Smith, B. A.: Immunoglobulin synthesis and total body tumor cell number in IgG multiple myeloma. *J. Clin. Invest.,* **49**:1114–1121, 1970.

Salmon, S. E., and Wampler, S. B.: Multiple myeloma: Quantitative staging and assessment of response with a programmable pocket calculator. *Blood,* **49**:379–389, 1977.

Schafer, A. I., and Miller, J. B.: Association of IgA multiple myeloma with pre-existing disease. *Br. J. Haematol.,* **41**:19–24, 1979.

Schmid, G. P.; Smith, R. P.; Baltch, A. L.; Hall, C. A.; and Schiffman, G.: Antibody response to pneumococcal vaccine in patients with multiple myeloma. *J. Infect. Dis.,* **143**:590–597, 1981.

Schur, P. H.; Kyle, R. A.; Bloch, K. J.; Hammack, W. J.; Rivers, S. L.; Sargent, A.; Ritchie, R. F.; McIntyre, O. R.; Moloney, W. C.; and Wolfson, L.: IgG subclasses: Relationship to clinical aspects of multiple myeloma and frequency distribution among M-components. *Scand. J. Haematol.,* **12**:60–68, 1974.

Seidman, J. G.; Max, E. E.; and Leder, P.: A-immunoglobulin gene is formed by site-specific recombination without further somatic mutation. *Nature,* **280**:370–375, 1979.

Siegal, T.; Shorr, J.; Lubetzki-Korn, I.; Soffer, D.; Naparstek, E.; Tur-Kaspa, R.; and Abramsky, O.: Myeloma protein synthesis within the CNS by plasma cell tumors. *Ann. Neurol.,* **10**:271–273, 1981.

Siris, E. S.; Sherman, W. H.; Baquiran, D. C.; Schlatterer, J. P.; Osserman, E. F.; and Canfield, R. E.: Effects of dichloromethylene diphosphonate on skeletal mobilization of calcium in multiple myeloma. *N. Engl. J. Med.,* **302**:310–315, 1980.

Smith, E.; Kochwa, S.; and Wasserman, L. R.: Aggregation of IgG globulin in vivo. I. The hyperviscosity syndrome in multiple myeloma. *Am. J. Med.,* **39**:35–48, 1965.

Solomon, A.: Bence-Jones proteins and light chains of immunoglobulins. *N. Engl. J. Med.,* **294**:17–23, 1976.

Southwest Oncology Group Study: Remission maintenance therapy for multiple myeloma. *Arch. Intern. Med.,* **135**:147–152, 1975.

Sullivan, P. W., and Salmon, S. E.: Kinetics of tumor growth and regression in IgG multiple myeloma. *J. Clin. Invest.,* **51**:1697–1708, 1972.

Thomas, T. L.; Decoufle, P.; and Moure-Eraso, R.: Mortality among workers employed in petroleum refining and petrochemical plants. *J.O.M.,* **22**:97–103, 1980.

Tomasi, T. B., Jr.: Secretory immunoglobulins. *N. Engl. J. Med.,* **287**:500–506, 1971.

Tubbs, R. R.; Gephardt, G. N.; McMahon, J. T.; Hall,

P. M.; Valenzuela, R.; and Vidt, D. G.: Light chain nephropathy. *Am. J. Med.,* **71:**263–269, 1981.

Virella, G., and Hobbs, J. R.: Heavy chain typing in IgG monoclonal gammopathies with special reference to cases of serum hyperviscosity and cryoglobulinaemia. *Clin. Exp. Immunol.,* **9:**973–980, 1971.

Waldmann, T. A.; Broder, S.; Blaese, R. M.; Durm, M.; Blackman, M.; and Strober, W.: Role of suppressor T cells in pathogenesis of common variable hypogammaglobulinaemia. *Lancet,* **2:**609–613, 1974.

Waldmann, T. A., and Strober, W.: Metabolism of immunoglobulins. *Prog. Allergy,* **13:**1–110, 1969.

Waldmann, T. A.; Strober, W.; and Mogielnicki, R. P.: The renal handling of low molecular weight proteins. II. Disorders of serum protein catabolism in patients with tubular proteinuria, the nephrotic syndrome, or uremia. *J. Clin. Invest.,* **51:**2162–2174, 1972.

Wanebo, H.; Geller, W.; and Gerold, F.: Extramedullary plasmacytoma of upper respiratory tract. *N.Y. State J. Med.,* **66:**1110–1113, 1966.

Watson, D.: Limitations in clinical use of a screening test for protein. *Clin. Chem.,* **10:**559–562, 1964.

Webb, H. E.; Harrison, E. G.; Masson, J. K.; and ReMine, W. H.: Solitary extramedullary myeloma (plasmacytoma) of the upper part of the respiratory tract and oropharynx. *Cancer,* **15:**1142–1155, 1962.

Wohlenberg, H.: Osteomyelitis and plasmacytoma. *N. Engl. J. Med.,* **283:**822, 1970.

Yasmeen, D.; Ellerson, J. R.; Dorrington, K. J.; and Painter, R. H.: Evidence for the domain hypothesis: Location of the site of cytophilic activity toward guinea pig macrophages in the C_H3 homology region of human immunoglobulin G^1. *J. Immunol.,* **110:**1706–1709, 1973.

18

Leukemias

CLARA D. BLOOMFIELD, DAVID D. HURD,
and BRUCE A. PETERSON

The leukemias are a heterogeneous group of diseases characterized by infiltration of the peripheral blood, bone marrow, and other tissues by neoplastic cells of the hematopoietic system. Although all leukemias are disseminated at diagnosis, they comprise a spectrum of cancers that, untreated, range from among the rapidly fatal to among the most slowly growing and indolent. Based on the untreated course, the leukemias have traditionally been designated acute or chronic, and based on the morphologic appearance of the predominant cancer cell, myeloid (nonlymphocytic) or lymphoid. The incidence of the leukemias will be discussed as a group; however, it is convenient and traditional to consider the acute leukemias and chronic leukemias separately.

Incidence

Leukemia represents 2.8% of all new cases of cancer, and during 1982 an estimated 23,500 new cases were diagnosed in the United States (Silverberg, 1982). Acute and chronic leukemia make up roughly equal numbers. Three-fourths of the approximately 12,000 new cases of acute leukemia that occur annually are seen in adults. Eighty-five percent of these are nonlymphocytic. Among acute leukemias, the incidence of nonlymphocytic or myeloid leukemia (ANLL) is approximately twice that of lymphocytic leukemia (ALL) (Third National Cancer Survey, 1975). Almost all cases of chronic leukemia are found in adults. The incidence of chronic lymphocytic leukemic (CLL) is approximately twice that of chronic myelogenous leukemia (CML). In the past 20

years, the incidence of leukemia has remained relatively stable, with one major exception. The incidence of ANLL in men over 50 years of age has increased substantially (Linos *et al.,* 1978; Brandt *et al.,* 1979; Geary *et al.,* 1979). In the past 10 to 20 years the incidence of ANLL has almost doubled in this older male population while remaining stable in younger individuals.

Leukemia accounts for only 3.7% of all deaths related to cancer. Despite this low figure, it is the leading cause of cancer-related death in females through age 29 years and in males through age 34 years. Although with advancing age other cancers surpass leukemias in frequency, the incidence of leukemia increases steadily with age. By the age of 85 the incidence is 89 per 100,000 population (Third National Cancer Survey, 1975). A substantial increase in the incidence of leukemia is observed in the elderly and this finding is explained by the fact that the population is proportionately growing older, making leukemia in adults a major health problem.

A. ACUTE LEUKEMIA

Etiology

Heredity, environmental factors, and, most recently, viruses, have been implicated as causes of the development of human leukemia (Weiss, 1981; Heath, 1982b). For most patients, however, causally-related conditions or known exposures are not recognized. In the few patients in whom a cause or associated condition has been identified, the mechanisms by which these factors actually influence the development of the cancer process are not fully understood. Recent advances in our understanding of neoplastic transformation at the molecular level suggest a general mechanism for leukemogenesis, whether caused by viruses or environmental factors. It has been suggested that human cancers may result from structural changes in DNA adjacent to cellular oncogenes, which result in activation of these genes (Cairns, 1981; Klein, 1981a; Bishop, 1982).

Congenital Disorders and Heredity. Individuals, particularly children, with certain congenital or inherited syndromes develop acute leukemia at a frequency higher than expected (Mulvihill, 1977; Woods *et al.*, 1981; Heath, 1982b). Many of these syndromes are associated with somatic chromosome aneuploidy. This occurs most commonly in children with Down's syndrome, where trisomy number 21 is the result of nondisjunction of the chromosome. The occurrence of Down's syndrome is related to advancing maternal age that has also been recognized as a factor in the development of acute leukemia in children without Down's syndrome. The risk of individuals with Down's syndrome developing acute leukemia is nearly 20 times greater than would normally be expected and is higher for all ages, but particularly during the neonatal period. Younger patients with Down's syndrome and leukemia usually have ALL, whereas older patients usually have ANLL. Acute leukemia has also been described in other disorders associated with aneuploidy, including Klinefelter's syndrome (XXY and variants) and Patau's syndrome (trisomy D syndrome).

Inherited diseases in which chromatin from the patient's cells exhibits excessive fragility and rearrangement are also associated with a higher incidence of acute leukemia. Fanconi's syndrome, an autosomal recessive disorder that includes pancytopenia and characteristic physical abnormalities, often results in death from progressive marrow failure or leukemia, which may develop at any age. The leukemia is usually classified as acute myelomonocytic or acute monocytic leukemia (Bloomfield and Brunning, 1976). Other congenital syndromes in which spontaneous chromosomal breakage occurs are also associated with the development of acute leukemia or other neoplasms and include Bloom's syndrome, ataxia telangiectasia, and Kostman's syndrome (Louie

and Schwartz, 1978). The immunologic deficiencies that are present in Bloom's syndrome and ataxia telangiectasia may also contribute to the development of the leukemia.

Genetic factors other than those associated with inherited disorders or chromosomal breakage influence the occurrence of acute leukemia (Harris *et al.*, 1980; Knudson, 1981). Acute leukemia, primarily ALL, developing in one member of a pair of monozygotic twins raises the chance that the second twin will also develop leukemia: The concordance rate has been estimated at 20 to 25%. Reports of acute leukemia developing in dizygotic twins and in the siblings of patients with acute leukemia, however, make it difficult to totally distinguish genetic contributions from environmental factors.

Viruses. Viruses have a definite role in the development of leukemia in a variety of animal models. Recent virologic, serologic, and epidemiologic evidence strongly indicates that a newly observed retrovirus is the cause of certain types of adult T-cell leukemias (Gallo *et al.*, 1981; Klein, 1981b; Weiss, 1981; Deinhardt, 1982; Gallo *et al.*, 1982). Retroviruses account for most of the known leukemia viruses in animals. Some of these leukemias associated with viruses in animals are myeloid in appearance, but most are lymphoblastic. In some cases these viruses appear to have acquired cellular genes, which upon reinfection make them capable of inducing leukemia. An alternative molecular hypothesis suggests that these viruses may insert a very small part of their genome, which may act as a promoter for previously quiescent cellular oncogenic sequences.

Evidence for viruses acting as causal agents in the development of human acute leukemia has come from a variety of sources, and a resurgence of interest has developed following the isolation of a novel retrovirus called HTLV (human T-cell lymphoma-leukemia virus) from fresh and cultured T cells of two patients with T-cell lymphoproliferative disorders (Gallo *et al.*, 1981; Weiss, 1981; Gallo *et al.*, 1982). HTLV seems to be quite distinct from the numerous types of animal retroviruses previously described. The virus has been isolated from tumor cells of the patients, but not from non-neoplastic lymphocytes. Antibodies to the virus have been found in the sera of patients from whom the virus has been isolated and from the serum of a spouse. Serologic tests in hundreds of individuals and patients with other diseases have been negative for antibody, though many patients with T-cell leukemia also test negative. The virus appears to be associated with a particularly malignant, rapidly growing form of tumor. The causal role of HTLV is supported by epidemiologic studies from Japan, where antibodies to HTLV have been found in a cluster of Japanese patients with adult T-cell leukemia (Robert-Guroff *et al.,* 1982). HTLV appears to be a strong candidate for a true leukemogenic virus.

Radiation. Radiation is a definite causal agent in the development of acute leukemia, particularly ANLL (Upton, 1981; Heath, 1982a). Fewer cases of ALL secondary to radiation have been reported. Ionizing radiation damages nuclear chromatin, resulting in chromosome breakage. This damage is thought to precipitate the development of leukemia. The importance of radiation as a cause of leukemia is intensified because exposure can often be avoided or, at least, limited.

Survivors of the atom bomb explosions in Japan during World War II had a subsequent increased incidence of leukemia (Beebe, 1981). The risk of developing leukemia was related to age at exposure, with the greatest incidence for those under ten years and over 50 years of age, with the total body dose of radiation received also being important. The peak incidence occurred six to seven years following exposure, and the risk had essentially disappeared 30 years following the explosions. Survivors who received a calculated radiation dose of less than five rads did not have a detectable increase in the incidence of leukemia. Detecting a minor increase in incidence, especially in an uncommon disease, can be difficult. It should not be concluded that a threshold exists below which exposure to ionizing radiation will not result in an increased risk of leukemia.

Radiologists who are not adequately shielded in the course of their work and patients receiving radiotherapy are at increased risk of developing neoplasms, including acute leukemia (Matanoski, 1981; Upton, 1981; Coltman, 1982). Patients receiving high doses of localized irradiation for diseases such as Hodgkin's disease do not have the same increase in risk that is associated with lower doses of more generalized irradiation (Coltman and Dixon, 1982; Glicksman *et al.,* 1982). An elevated incidence of leukemia has been observed in patients treated for benign disorders such as ankylosing spondylitis as well

as for tumors (Beebe, 1981). Diagnostic roentgenography has not been generally associated with a detectable increase in the frequency of leukemia in either adults or children (Upton, 1981). If a threshold does not exist in the lower limit of radiation exposure that causes leukemia, then even low doses of radiation may occasionally cause leukemia.

Chemicals and Drugs. Bone marrow failure and transient aplasia resulting from exposure to drugs and chemicals have been reported to evolve into ANLL (Bloomfield and Brunning, 1976). Substances most commonly implicated include benzene, chloramphenicol, phenylbutazone, and, increasingly, antineoplastic drugs. Over 100 cases of acute leukemia have been attributed to chronic benzene exposure. Most of these patients have a period of bone marrow aplasia or symptoms compatible with anemia or pancytopenia preceding the development of leukemia, but the leukemia may intervene at any time, even ten years following the discontinuation of exposure. The acute leukemias following benzene exposure are nonlymphocytic, usually designated acute myelogenous leukemia or erythroleukemia. The development of leukemia may be related to the high incidence of chromosomal and chromatid abnormalities, similar to those induced by radiation, that occurs in individuals exposed to benzene. Although exposure to benzene has been reduced in the workplace since recognition of its causal role in the development of leukemia, acute leukemia in persons who have industrial exposure to other potential toxins is increasing. This may partially account for the rising incidence of leukemia in older men. Many of these patients have cytogenetic findings in their leukemic cells similar to those associated with leukemia following cytotoxic chemotherapy (Rowley, 1982). Rare cases of ANLL have also developed following marrow injury attributed to chloramphenicol. Chromosome abnormalities have been reported in some of these patients. An association between phenylbutazone-induced marrow injury and leukemia has also been described.

Currently, the major identifiable cause of acute leukemia is exposure to antineoplastic drugs (Coltman, 1982). Patients with treatment-associated acute leukemia constitute the largest group of patients in whom a cause can be identified. Alkylating agents, in particular, cause chromosomal damage and are clearly carcinogenic (Bloomfield and Brunning,

1976; Casciato and Scott, 1979). Phenylala-nine mustard and cyclophosphamide have both been associated with the development of acute leukemia following treatment in patients with multiple myeloma. These cases are often described as acute myelomonocytic leukemia and are accompanied by an elevated lysozyme. Acute nonlymphocytic leukemia is also being reported with increasing frequency in patients treated for Hodgkin's disease with drugs like mechlorethamine, cyclophosphamide, pro-carbazine, and nitrosoureas (Coltman, 1982; Coltman and Dixon, 1982; Glicksman et al., 1982). Leukemia has developed from eight months to 19 years after the diagnosis and treatment of Hodgkin's disease. Survival fol-lowing recognition of this type of leukemia is usually brief. The risk of developing leukemia increases with the intensity of chemotherapy, with or without radiotherapy (Coleman et al., 1977; Coltman, 1982). The risk continues to increase to 4 to 6% at seven years and, in pa-tients over 40 years of age, may reach 20%. ANLL also occurs in patients treated for a vari-ety of other cancers, including non-Hodgkin's lymphoma, ovarian carcinoma, and breast carcinoma (Coltman, 1982).

Although cytotoxic drugs should always be recognized as potentially leukemogenic, acute leukemia has also been diagnosed in patients whose original neoplasm was not treated with either chemotherapy or irradiation. Because slightly increased rates of leukemia are asso-ciated with a number of neoplasms, the pres-ence of the underlying tumor or the innate causes of its emergence may have a role in the development of an associated leukemia. Cyto-toxic drugs have also been used in the treat-ment of certain non-neoplastic diseases. Leu-kemia has developed following use in this situation as well. In all circumstances, but es-pecially in the treatment of non-neoplastic dis-eases, these drugs must be used with extreme caution.

The acute leukemia that develops following cytotoxic therapy is usually nonlymphocytic, and most frequently is subclassified as either erythroleukemia or acute myelomonocytic leukemia. The morphology of treatment-re-lated leukemia has been described in detail (Vardiman et al., 1978; Foucar et al., 1979). Generally, the abnormalities in the bone mar-row resemble a panmyelosis with involvement of all three hematopoietic cell lines. The pre-dominant neoplastic changes may be observed in the myeloid, erythroid, or megakaryocytic precursors. Clinically, pancytopenia or other evidence of incipient bone marrow failure is commonly the initial sign of this neoplasm and may arise suddenly or over a period of months.

Diagnosis and Classification

The categorization of acute leukemia into biologically distinct groups has been at-tempted since the time of Virchow. Tradition-ally, classification has been based on morphol-ogy, and most of the currently accepted morphologic forms were described more than 50 years ago using Romanovsky stains of blood specimens. In recent years, as therapeu-tic results have improved and the therapeutic options have increased, valid classification schemes have become increasingly important both for selecting therapy and for determining prognosis. The inclusion of histochemical, biochemical, cytogenetic, and immunologic techniques in addition to morphology has greatly improved precision in the classification of acute leukemia, and has increased our un-derstanding of the biology of the hematopoie-tic system.

Morphology. The recognition of charac-teristic morphologic features of leukemic blast cells has enabled hematopathologists to distin-guish two major categories of acute leukemia. Differences in epidemiology, clinical behav-ior, and response to specific therapy justify the separation of ALL from ANLL. It is difficult to differentiate between these two major groups solely on morphologic grounds. In general, lymphoblasts have a higher nuclear-cytoplas-mic ratio, the nuclear membrane is denser, and the chromatin pattern is coarser, with some areas of aggregated chromatin. Nucleoli are smaller and fewer in number (one to two per cell) in lymphoblasts than in myeloblasts. Myeloblasts have nuclear chromatin that is uniformly fine or lacelike in appearance and nucleoli that tend to be both larger and more numerous (two to five per cell). If specific cy-toplasmic granules, Auer rods, or the nuclear folding and clefting characteristic of monocy-toid cells are not present, the morphologic fea-tures observed under light microscopy may not be sufficient to clarify the diagnosis. Under these circumstances, ancillary studies are nec-essary to distinguish ALL from ANLL.

Further subclassification within each of these two major categories is also possible. Sev-eral classifications have been used in the past. Recently, a formal scheme for the characterization of the individual subtypes of acute leukemia, called the French-American-British (FAB) classification, was accepted (Bennett *et al.,* 1976; Bennett *et al.,* 1980; Bennett *et al.,* 1981). This scheme incorporates many of the criteria of previous classifications. The morphologic and histochemical criteria may be used in conjunction with other characteristics of leukemic blasts identified by enzyme determination, cytogenetics, and cell membrane surface markers to increase the specificity of diagnosis.

The FAB classification of acute leukemia is outlined in Tables 18–1 and 18–2. Lymphoblastic and myeloblastic leukemia are identified as the two major divisions of acute leukemia. ALL is divided into three subtypes. Subclassification is determined by cell size, the nuclear-cytoplasmic ratio, the presence and frequency of nucleoli, the regularity of nuclear membrane outline, and cell size. Although morphology alone cannot determine the cellular origin of most of the so-called lymphoblastic leukemias, immunologic, cytochemical, enzymatic, and cytogenetic determinations, as well as new molecular genetic techniques, confirm that they actually are lymphoid.

The three categories of ALL are designated L1, L2, and L3 (Table 18-1). L1 ALL is characterized by a rather homogeneous cell population of small cells that have a relatively coarse nuclear chromatin pattern and indistinct nucleoli. There is usually a sparse amount of cytoplasm. L2 ALL is characterized by larger cells with more abundant cytoplasm. The nuclear chromatin pattern is more delicate, and

nucleoli are fairly prominent. This is the type of ALL that is most frequently confused with ANLL. The final category of ALL is the L3 group. This is an uncommon morphologic variant in which the blasts resemble those found in Burkitt's lymphoma. These lymphoblasts have somewhat darker cytoplasm, frequently with numerous vacuoles that may stain positively for neutral lipids (oil red 0).

The majority of children have the L1 morphologic form. The Childrens Cancer Study Group evaluated 536 children with ALL and found the following frequencies of the FAB classes: L1, 85%; L2, 14%; L3, 1% (Miller et al., 1980). Several studies in adults suggest that FAB L2 is most common. Among 324 adult patients ($\geq$ 15 years of age), 29% were L1, 64% L2, and 7% L3 (Bloomfield, 1982). In its most recent study, the FAB group classified 39 adults (> 15 years) and found 44% L1, 49% L2, and 8% L3 (Bennett *et al.,* 1981).

The morphologic heterogeneity of the myeloid leukemias has been recognized for many years. The FAB classification differentiates six major types, M1 to M6 (see Table 18-2). The first three define morphologic types with predominantly granulocytic differentiation. Myeloblasts with evidence of granulocytic differentiation by virtue of the presence of peroxidase-positive cytoplasmic granules or Auer rods, but showing no maturation, are designated M1. These myeloblasts must be differentiated from the lymphoblasts of the L2 subtype, which are peroxidase negative. The M2 group shows both granulocytic differentiation and clear evidence of myeloid maturation.

Table 18–1. The French-American-British (FAB) Classification of Acute Leukemia

ACUTE LYMPHOBLASTIC LEUKEMIA (ALL)

L1: A relatively homogeneous cell population with 75% or more small cells with scanty cytoplasm, finely dispersed chromatin, and regular nuclear shape. Nucleoli are inconspicuous in more than 75% of the cells.*

L2: A heterogeneous cell population as regards size, chromatin pattern, and nuclear shape. The cells are usually large with the cytoplasm occupying 20% or more of the surface area of the cell. Nucleoli are frequently large in 25% or more of the cells.

L3: A large and relatively homogeneous cell population with regular nuclei and a fine chromatin pattern. Nucleoli are prominent. Cytoplasm is moderately abundant with vacuolization and deep basophilia. Lymphoblasts resemble those seen in Burkitt's lymphoma.

* A scoring system has recently been developed to assist in separating L1 from L2 (see Bennett, J. M.; Catovsky, D.; Daniel, M. T.; Flandrin, G.; Galton, D. A. G.; Gralnick, H. R.; and Sultan, C.: The morphological classification of acute lymphoblastic leukaemia: Concordance among observers and clinical correlations. *Br. J. Haematol.,* **47**:553–561, 1981).

Table 18-2. The French-American-British (FAB) Classification of Acute Leukemia

ACUTE NONLYMPHOCYTIC (MYELOID) LEUKEMIA (ANLL)

M1: Myeloblastic leukemia without maturation. Blasts show minimal evidence of myeloid differentiation with more than 3% of the blasts myeloperoxidase-positive and/or containing azurophilic granules, Auer rods, or both. No evidence of maturation is present.

M2: Myeloblastic leukemia with maturation. Some maturation of the granulocytic series is evident with more than 50% of the nucleated bone marrow cells consisting of myeloblasts and promyelocytes. In some cases, maturation may proceed beyond the promyelocyte stage, frequently with abnormal morphologic forms.

M3: Hypergranular promyelocytic leukemia. The predominant cells are abnormal promyelocytes packed with dense granulation and multiple Auer rods.
  M3 variant: "Microgranular" promyclocytic leukemia. An atypical form with minimal granulation in most cells. Nuclei of cells in blood are bilobed, multilobed, or reniform. Occasional typical cells are present.

M4: Myelomonocytic leukemia. Evidence of both granulocytic and monocytic differentiation is present in varying proportions. More than 20% of the nucleated cells in the blood and/or bone marrow are promonocytes and monocytes and at least 20% of the nucleated marrow cells are myeloblasts and promyelocytes.

M5: Monocytic leukemia*
  M5$_A$: Poorly differentiated (monoblastic) leukemia. Large monoblasts with abundant cytoplasm frequently exhibiting pseudopodia or budding. Promonocytes may be present but are uncommon.
  M5$_B$: Well-differentiated monocytic leukemia. Monoblasts, promonocytes, and monocytes are all found. The predominant cell in the bone marrow is the promonocyte.

M6: Erythroleukemia. Erythroblasts exceed 50% in the bone marrow, and bizarre morphologic variants are found. Many erythroid precursors are strongly periodic acid-Schiff positive. Auer rods may be seen in the myeloblasts.

* Diagnosis of monocytic leukemia must be confirmed by fluoride inhibition of the esterase reaction.

Maturation into promyelocytes, and even myelocytes, may be present, but myeloblasts and promyelocytes must constitute at least 50% of the cells in the marrow. Myeloblasts frequently contain azurophilic granules and Auer rods.

The M3 type is designated hypergranular promyelocytic leukemia. This was formerly called acute promyelocytic leukemia and is associated with markedly abnormal promyelocytes packed with dense azurophilic granules and multiple Auer rods. A number of morphologic variants of M3 have recently been described (Golomb et al., 1980; McKenna et al., 1982). One variant with minimal granulation and bilobed, multilobed, or reniform nuclei has been officially included in the FAB scheme as an M3 variant (Bennett et al., 1980). In the absence of careful examination of the blood and bone marrow, M3 variants may be mis-

diagnosed as atypical monocytic leukemias of M4 type. In contrast to typical M3, in which the leukocyte count usually varies from slightly above the normal range to subnormal levels, the M3 variant is commonly associated with very high leukocyte counts. The frequency of the M3 variant is unknown but in a recent study of M3 leukemias it constituted 23% of 30 consecutive cases (McKenna et al., 1982). M3 leukemias, regardless of morphology, are almost universally associated with a specific chromosome abnormality, t(15;17) (q24;q21) (Golomb, 1982; Hurd et al., 1982), and disseminated intravascular coagulation (DIC), either at diagnosis, or following the initiation of chemotherapy.

Two categories of ANLL, M4 and M5, contain cells that display evidence of monocytic differentiation. In acute myelomonocytic leukemia, M4, granulocytic and monocytic components coexist and independently may show varying degrees of maturation. Nuclei of the monocytoid cells are frequently folded or cleft. The monocytic component may be more apparent in the blood than in the bone marrow. The M5 category is acute monocytic leukemia. This category is further subdivided depending on the apparent maturity of the leukemic cells into M5$_A$, poorly differentiated (monoblastic), and M5$_B$, well-differentiated monocytic leukemia. Auer rods may occur in both the M4 and M5 subtypes, but are distinctly uncommon in M5$_A$. Clinically, the monocytic subtypes are associated with an increased frequency of tissue infiltration (especially the gingiva and skin) and central nervous system (CNS) involvement. DIC, though not to the degree seen with M3 leukemia, is also relatively common in M4 and M5 leukemias.

The final morphologic subtype is erythroleukemia, designated M6. This type was previously identified as DiGuglielmo's syndrome. Although dyserythropoiesis may be apparent in other types of ANLL, erythroleukemia is diagnosed when there is a marked degree of erythroid hyperplasia in the bone marrow with striking abnormalities of erythroid precursors. Nuclear changes consisting of karyorrhexis and karyolysis are accompanied by marked megaloblastoid changes. Erythroid cells may reach giant size and have multiple nuclei. Neoplastic changes in the granulocytic series are also present and Auer rods are often seen.

The distribution of adult ANLL according to the FAB classification has recently been reported in several large studies (Mertelsmann *et al.*, 1980; Bennett and Begg, Burn *et al.*, 1981; Sultan *et al.*, 1981). The frequencies in the various studies have been M1, 9 to 29%; M2, 28 to 32%; M3, 6 to 16%; M4, 8 to 37%; M5, 6 to 32%; and M6, 1 to 3%. The broad range in frequency of M3 probably reflects differences in referral patterns, but the broad range in M1, M4, and M5 appears to reflect problems in use of the classification by different investigators (Bennett and Begg, 1981; Dick *et al.*, 1982). Further studies are required to define the frequency of the M3 variant, and M5$_A$ and M5$_B$ leukemias.

Cytochemistry. The classification of the acute leukemias is facilitated by the identification of various cytoplasmic constituents with special cytochemical techniques (Catovsky *et al.*, 1981a; Bennett, 1982). The results of cytochemistry studies are considered when categorizing leukemias, especially ANLL, within the FAB classification. The more commonly used histochemical stains are listed in Table 18–3.

Peroxidases are cytoplasmic enzymes that catalyze the oxidation of various compounds by hydrogen peroxide. Myeloperoxidase activity is located in the azurophilic granules present in both granulocytes and monocytes but absent in lymphocytes. Myeloperoxidase is the single most useful stain for separating ALL from ANLL. In ANLL of the M1 variety a positive myeloperoxidase reaction may be the only distinguishing characteristic separating it from L2 ALL. The M2 and M3 subtypes are most strongly peroxidase positive. Myelomonocytic leukemia (M4) exhibits less intense activity and the peroxidase reaction occurs to a limited degree or not at all in monocytic leukemia (M5). Sudan black B activity closely parallels that of peroxidase.

A variety of different blasts, including lymphoblasts and myeloblasts with or without

Table 18–3. Cytochemical Profiles in Acute Nonlymphocytic Leukemia

CYTOCHEMICAL REACTION	MORPHOLOGIC SUBTYPES ACCORDING TO FAB CRITERIA					
	M1	*M2*	*M3*	*M4*	*M5*	*M6*
Peroxidase or Sudan black	+($\geq$3%)	+ to +++	+++	++ to +++	0 to ++	+ to +++
Naphthol ASD acetate esterase	+	++	++	+ to +++	+++	++
Napththol ASD acetate esterase-fluoride	+	++	++	+ to ++	0 to ±	++
Periodic acid-Schiff	0 to ±	0 to +	0 to +	0 to ++	0 to ++	± to +++*

Legend: 0 = negative; ± = equivocal; + = slight positivity; ++ = moderate positivity; +++ = strong positivity.
* Periodic acid-Schiff positivity may be found in the cancerous erythroid precursors.

monocytic components, contain nonspecific esterases. These esterases are detected by a number of tests and represent isoenzymes specific to the individual cell types. The usual reaction employed for the cytochemical detection of an esterase involves the splitting of naphthol from an ester. Naphthol then couples with a specific dye, resulting in the colored product that is detected under the microscope. Naphthol-ASD acetate is employed as the substrate for nonspecific esterase, and the reaction occurs most intensely in cells with monocytic differentiation. Also, in monocytes and monocytic precursors, sodium fluoride specifically inhibits the activity of this enzyme. Thus the inhibition of the cytochemical reaction for nonspecific esterase in monocytic leukemia (M5) may be helpful in establishing the diagnosis. Myelomonocytic leukemia (M4) shows a variable reduction in nonspecific esterase when incubated with sodium fluoride. The isoenzymes of nonspecific esterase present in myeloblasts (M1 to M3) or lymphoblasts are not inhibited by incubation with sodium fluoride.

The periodic acid-Schiff (PAS) reaction primarily identifies cytoplasmic carbohydrate and carbohydrate-containing proteins and lipids. Mature leukocytes contain substantial quantities of glycogen and the PAS reaction is usually strongly positive. Considerable quantities of PAS-positive material are found in the blast cells of ALL (L1 and L2), and, to a lesser extent, in the blasts of myeloid leukemias with a monocytic component (M4 and M5). Thus, the PAS reaction can help to distinguish lymphoblasts from myeloblasts (M1 and M2) that are usually PAS negative or have only small amounts of fine granular PAS-positive material. Although lymphoblasts often exhibit coarse cytoplasmic PAS activity, approximately 50% of cases will show complete nonreactivity. In erythroleukemia, the neoplastic erythroid precursors are frequently characterized by strikingly large aggregates of PAS positivity.

Additional cytochemical markers that are frequently used when studying lymphoid leukemias include acid phosphatase, β-glucuronidase, and methyl green pyronine (McKenna *et al.*, 1979; Bloomfield, 1982). T-cell leukemias often exhibit a strong acid-phosphatase reaction localized in the paranuclear region (Golgi zone) of the cytoplasm, whereas the majority of non-T ALL do not. Thus, a characteristic acid-phosphatase reaction suggests the possibility of T-ALL. β-Glucuronidase appears to have a distribution and utility similar to that of acid phosphatase. Cells of the L3 category frequently exhibit intense cytoplasmic staining with methyl green pyronine. The vacuoles prominently present in their cytoplasm characteristically stain with oil red 0, suggesting the presence of neutral lipid.

Biochemistry. Comparatively few enzymes are quantitatively assayed to aid in the classification of acute leukemias. Among those that should be routinely studied are serum lysozyme and terminal deoxynucleotidyl transferase. The enzyme lysozyme (muramidase) is present within monocytes and is released following cellular disruption. This results in elevated levels in the serum and/or urine detectable in some cases of ANLL. Significant elevations of the serum lysozyme level have been reported in the majority of cases of well-differentiated monocytic leukemia (M5$_B$) and, to a lesser extent, in acute myelomonocytic leukemia (M4). The serum lysozyme is not usually elevated in poorly differentiated monocytic leukemia (M5$_A$). Elevations are also detected in some cases of other subtypes of ANLL, but only rarely in ALL.

Terminal deoxynucleotidyl transferase (TdT) is a unique DNA polymerase that copies the deoxynucleotidyl sequences, but does not require nucleic acid template information. In normal tissues, TdT is found only in the cortex of the thymus and in rare small bone marrow cells of lymphoid appearance. It is not present in normal peripheral T or B lymphocytes. Elevated levels of TdT have been reported in most cases of non-T, non-B ALL and T ALL (Bloomfield, 1982). Elevated TdT levels have not been reported in any well-documented cases of B ALL and are detected in only 5 to 10% of leukemias of the granulocytic series (Catovsky *et al.*, 1981a; Mertelsmann *et al.*, 1982). TdT has been studied most extensively in leukemia with a biochemical assay. The recent development of a highly specific antibody to TdT has allowed the development of an indirect immunofluorescent (IF) assay that detects TdT in individual cells (Bollum, 1979). Preliminary studies suggest excellent correlation between the enzyme assay and immunocytochemical staining (IF assay) when there are more than 5% TdT positive cells as determined by IF (Bradstock *et al.*, 1981).

Adenosine-deaminase (ADA) activity has also been assayed in the leukemic blasts of patients with acute leukemia (Bloomfield, 1982).

ADA is a polymorphic enzyme that catalyzes the deamination of adenosine to inosine. ADA activity is high in normal mitogen-stimulated peripheral T lymphocytes and thymocytes and low in normal peripheral B lymphocytes. Most cases of both non-T, non-B ALL and T ALL have had elevated levels of ADA. ADA activity has been low in those cases of B ALL studied. Activity has been reported in cases of ANLL, but the enzyme has primarily been studied in ALL. Recently, a radioimmunoassay has been developed that appears to give results comparable to the enzymatic method.

The utility of hexosaminidase-isoenzyme profiles is currently being evaluated in ALL (Bloomfield, 1982). Hexosaminidase (N-acetyl-beta-glucosaminidase) is one of the lysozomal acid hydrolases. Three major isoenzymes (A, I, and B) have been identified and found to have characteristic profiles in normal granulocytes, lymphocytes, and thymocytes. The isoenzyme pattern, determined either by automated ion exchange chromatography or isoelectric focusing, has been reported to be useful in distinguishing immunologic types of ALL. In particular, the intermediate isoenzyme (hexosaminidase I) appears to be greatly increased, primarily in common ALL. Elevated levels have also been reported in some cases of "null" ALL, but not in T ALL or B ALL. Recently, other lysosomal enzymes (α-D-mannosidase, α-D-galactosidase, alphafucosidase, β-glucuronidase, acid phosphatase) have also been found to have unusual isoenzyme forms (or increased activity of forms present in normal cells at very low levels) in most cases of common ALL.

Cytogenetics. Considerable interest has recently been generated by newer techniques for the cytogenetic analysis of acute leukemia (Berger et al., 1981; Yunis et al., 1981; Bloomfield and Arthur, 1982b; Golomb, 1982). Older, less precise methods of analysis suggested that approximately 50% of patients with either ALL or ANLL had karyotype abnormalities in the leukemic cell populations. Previously, it was accepted that the chromosomal abnormalities detected were random rather than specific changes. The application of quinacrine fluorescence (Q) and Giemsa (G) banding techniques has permitted more detailed characterization of structural rearrangements within chromosomes. Gross morphologic alterations in the shape of the chromosome did not have to be present for abnormalities to be detected. Despite deletions and translocations it is now possible to precisely identify individual chromosomes. As a result of new techniques, nonrandom chromosome changes have been identified in the majority of patients with acute leukemia.

Cytogenetic analysis with banding techniques has identified clonal chromosome abnormalities in more than two-thirds of patients with ALL. In the largest series reported to date, abnormalities were found in 66% of 330 newly diagnosed patients (Third International Workshop on Chromosomes in Leukemia, 1981). Smaller studies have shown clonal abnormalities in over 80% of patients (Arthur et al., 1981). The chromosome abnormalities that have been observed in ALL generally differ from those seen in ANLL. The most common specific abnormalities identified in ALL have been the t(9;22), t(4;11), and the t(8;14) (Third International Workshop on Chromosomes in Leukemia, 1981). Other chromosome abnormalities have often been grouped by modal number (i.e., the predominant number of chromosomes in cells with a range of chromosome numbers). Some of these karyotypic subgroups appear to have distinctive clinical and hematologic features and response to treatment (see Table 18–4). The karyotype has also been demonstrated to be an independent variable for predicting duration of remission and survival in ALL.

Great differences in frequency of clonal chromosome abnormalities have been found among ALL immunologic classes (Bloomfield, 1982). All cases of B ALL have had abnormalities identified, compared with 68% of non-T, non-B ALL and only 45% of T ALL. The most common specific chromosomal abnormality in non-T, non-B ALL is a Philadelphia chromosome (Ph[1]), most commonly t(9;22)(q34;q11). Among adults with non-T, non-B ALL, as many as 30% have been found to have Ph[1] lymphoblasts. The presence in ALL of the Ph[1], which was previously thought to be specific for CML, suggests that a common stem cell may give rise to cancerous cells with lymphoid as well as myeloid characteristics. In non-T, non-B ALL, the second most common recurring chromosome abnormality is t(4;11)(q21;q23). The only other recurring translocation that has been noted in this group is t(11;14)(q23;q32). Among the nonspecific chromosome abnormalities, the only one usually restricted to non-T, non-B ALL is a modal number of more than 50. ALL with a modal number greater than 50 may occur in as many as 30% of childhood non-T, non-B ALL and appears to carry an unusually good prognosis (Third International Workshop on Chromosomes in Leukemia, 1981; Williams *et al.*, 1981). Recurring specific chromosome abnormalities have less frequently been reported in T ALL. Most cases of T ALL have had a modal number of 46. Rare cases with the Ph[1] or the t(4;11) have been reported. B ALL almost always demonstrated an 8q− or a 14q+. Results of studies of B ALL are similar to those reported in non-Hodgkin's lymphoma (Bloomfield *et al.*, 1982).

Using newer techniques, such as methotrexate synchronization, a clonal chromosome abnormality has been found in most cases of ANLL (Yunis *et al.*, 1981). In a number of recent series using more traditional culture techniques and studying metaphase chromosomes, 75 to 85% of cases were reported to have clonal chromosome abnormalities (Bloomfield and Arthur, 1982b). The most common nonrandom chromosome abnormalities reported in *de novo* ANLL are an additional chromosome number 8, deletions of part of the long arm, or absence of all of chromosomes 5 or 7, t(8;21)(q22;q22), t(15;17)(q24;q21), t(9;22)(q34;q11), and, recently, a partial deletion of the long arm of one chromosome 16 at band q22 (Bloomfield and

Arthur, 1982a,b). The majority of these chromosome abnormalities have been associated with specific clinical and other laboratory characteristics, as indicated in Table 18–4. In addition, it has been suggested that abnormalities of the long arm of chromosome 11 are associated with M5$_A$ leukemia (Berger *et al.*, 1980). Recently, a specific translocation, t(9;11)(p21;q23), has been reported (Hagemeijer *et al.*, 1982). Deletions of part of the long arm or absence of all of chromosomes 5 and 7 are present in an unusually high frequency in patients with secondary ANLL arising after exposure to radiation or cytotoxic agents used for treating other diseases (Golomb, 1982). It has been suggested that patients with *de novo* ANLL and these abnormalities may in fact have leukemia that results from unknown prior exposure to industrial toxins.

In addition to the obvious biologic importance of cytogenetic analyses in acute leukemia, the clinical associations summarized in Table 18–4 suggest that the results of these analyses will increasingly assist in the diagnosis and classification of acute leukemias. It also appears that they may improve our ability to predict the course of the leukemia and aid in the selection of therapy.

Cell Membrane Markers. The develop-

Table 18–4. Common Chromosome Abnormalities in *De Novo* Adult Acute Leukemia and Associated Clinical Findings

CHROMOSOME ABNORMALITY	USUAL FAB	APPROXIMATE FREQUENCY	CHARACTERISTIC PHYSICAL FINDINGS	CHARACTERISTIC LABORATORY FINDINGS	RESPONSE TO THERAPY AND SURVIVAL
Ph[1](22q−) t(9;22)	L2	20% adult ALL	Typical of ALL	Non-T, non-B, CALLA+ WBC > 50,000/μL in ⅓ of cases	CR rate low; moderately short remissions and survival
t(4;11)	L2	5% adult ALL	Splenomegaly; 20 to 30% CNS and mediastinal involvement	Non-T, non-B CALLA − WBC very high	CR rate low; short remissions and survival
t(8;14)	L3	<5% adult ALL	CNS involvement common	B-cell; WBC low	CR rate low; very short remissions and survival
t(8;21)	M2	5% adult ANLL	Young	Normal WBC	Relatively high CR rate and long survival with moderately intensive treatment
t(15;17)	M3	5% adult ANLL	Hemorrhage	DIC M3 typical: WBC low M3 variant: WBC high	M3: Long remissions and survival; M3 variant: Shorter survival
del(16)(q22)	M2 or M4	10% adult ANLL	Typical ANLL	Marrow eosinophilia	Long remissions and survival

Legend: CR: = complete remission.

ment of cell membrane surface markers to distinguish between B lymphocytes and T lymphocytes has further aided the classification of ALL (see reviews by Greaves, 1981; Bloomfield, 1982). As a result of changes that occur during neoplastic transformation, membrane markers on cancerous lymphoblasts may not exactly correspond to specific markers on normal lymphocytes. The characterization and classification of ALL on the basis of surface markers has greatly increased our understanding of their biologic nature. A large number of surface-marker techniques have been described, but relatively few have been applied clinically.

B lymphocytes are characterized by the presence of immunoglobulin on the surface of their cell membrane (SIg), which can be detected using fluorescein-conjugated anti-immunoglobulin antisera. Other markers characteristic of some B lymphocytes include receptors for complement and for the Fc portion of IgG. Monocytes and macrophages also have receptors for both complement and the Fc portion of IgG on their cell surface but do not have self-renewed SIg. Occasionally, when immunoglobulin is not detected on the cell membrane, a B-cell origin can still be determined by demonstrating immunoglobulin within the cytoplasm of the cell. ALL with only cytoplasmic immunoglobulin of IgM type (CIgM) has been designated as pre-B ALL. T

lymphocytes are traditionally identified by the spontaneous formation of rosettes upon incubation with nonsensitized sheep erythrocytes.

Recently, large numbers of monoclonal antibodies derived by cell hybridization have been developed for leukemic cell characterization (Greaves, 1981). These antibodies, which recognize the common-ALL antigen and other leukemia-associated antigens such as human B-lymphocyte antigens, an Ia-like antigen, and T-lymphocyte antigens, have been used to further define immunologic subsets of ALL. The use of these multiple immunologic markers has resulted in the classification of ALL into at least six groups (common ALL, pre-B ALL, B ALL, "null" ALL, pre-T ALL, T ALL).

When membrane surface markers are studied on the leukemic cells of adults, only a minority of cases demonstrate either T or B markers in ALL. Those that show spontaneous rosetting with nonsensitized sheep erythrocytes (T ALL) represent fewer than 20% of cases (see Table 18–5). Lymphoblasts, which have T-cell characteristics, often have strong acid-phosphatase activity located in the Golgi zone and low to intermediate levels of glucocorticoid receptors. TdT is elevated in these blast cells. T ALL is associated with either L1 or L2 morphology. Adults with T ALL tend to be younger and are usually male. Clinically the disease is similar to that found in children (see chapter 39). They frequently present with a

Table 18–5. Clinical and Laboratory Features of the Broad Immunologic Groups of Adult ALL

	NON-T, NON-B ALL	T-ALL	B-ALL
Approximate frequency (%)	75 to 80	15 to 20	5
FAB class (%) L1:L2:L3	35:64:1	41:59:0	0:44:56
Chromosome abnormalities (%)			
t(9;22)	25	Occasional	0
t(4;11)	5	Occasional	0
t(8;14)	0	0	60
Modal no. > 50	5	0	0
Glucocorticoid receptor levels	High	Intermediate	Low
Median age of patients (years)	30 to 35	20	40
Sex (% male)	55	75	80
Presenting signs (%)			
Lymphadenopathy	40	70	45
Splenomegaly	45	70	70
Hepatomegaly	30	30	55
Mediastinal mass	<5	50	15
CNS leukemia	10	25	50
Median WBC ($\times 10^9$/L)	5 to 15	40	5 to 15
Median % circulating blasts	25 to 60	70 to 75	5 to 20
Response to therapy			
Complete remission rate (%)	75	70	40
Median duration first CR	ca. 15 mos	5 to 10 mos	<5 mos
Median survival (mos)	15 to 26	9 to 17	1 to 9

high leukocyte count and/or a mediastinal mass. Patients with T ALL also tend to have lymphadenopathy, splenomegaly, and aggressive disease characterized by CNS and testicular relapses and, with conventional therapy, a relatively short survival time.

A small group of patients (approximately 5%) exhibit B-cell characteristics of their lymphoblasts. The lymphoblasts usually carry monoclonal SIg of the IgM class, with either kappa or lambda light chain specificity. Morphologically, these cases are often L3 leukemias, and the lymphoblasts resemble those seen in Burkitt's lymphoma. Patients with the L2 morphology may also have B-cell markers. Most of these may actually represent peripheralizing lymphomas. In either morphologic subtype, B cells are low in TdT and usually acid-phosphatase negative. B ALL of the L3 type has very low glucocorticoid receptor levels. Clinically, adults with B ALL tend to be older and predominantly male (Table 18–5). Hepatosplenomegaly and CNS leukemia at presentation are common. These patients tend to present with low leukocyte counts and few circulating lymphoblasts. Response to treatment is usually very poor, and few patients survive beyond six months.

Approximately 75% of adults with ALL do not have markers characteristic of either B or T lymphocytes on their lymphoblast membranes. These cases have been classified as non-T, non-B ALL. Non-T, non-B ALL has been further characterized with the common-ALL antisera. This antiserum (J5 or BA-3 monoclonal antibody) is positive in 50 to 75% of the cases of adult ALL where the usual B- and T-surface markers are not found. The common-ALL antigen is also present in B ALL and pre-B ALL, but rarely in T ALL and not in ANLL. Recent studies of the immunogobulin genes in lymphoblasts from patients with non-T, non-B ALL of common-ALL type demonstrate gene rearrangement and indicate that these cells are differentiating along the B-cell pathway (Korsmeyer et al., 1981).

Clinically, non-T, non-B ALL is quite heterogeneous (Table 18–5). Morphologically, these leukemias are most commonly L2, but more than one-third are L1. Cytogenetically, there are multiple subgroups, with the t(9;22) being the most common, occurring in about 25% of cases. Glucocorticoid receptor levels are often high, but a broad range has been reported (Bloomfield et al., 1981b). The age range is wide, and only a slight preponderance

of males is evident. Organomegaly is often not present and the presenting leukocyte count is frequently low. The response rate is similar to that for T ALL, and most patients achieve complete remissions with regimens that include vincristine, prednisone, and an anthracycline. Remissions are longer than for adults with T ALL or B ALL, but less than 50% of patients have prolonged survivals.

Antibodies specific for human T-lymphocyte antigens and B-lymphocyte antigens have provided additional methods for classifying ALL (Greaves, 1981; Nadler et al., 1982). Unlike the common-ALL antibody, these usually react with lymphoblasts that show the corresponding surface marker receptor. B-lymphocyte alloantigens have been recognized that are linked to the HLA-D locus. These antigens have been designated "Ia-like," and are present on most non-T ALL lymphoblasts. In addition, T-cell antibodies react with cells from some patients with non-T, non-B ALL. This suggests that some of these leukemias are derived from T cells but do not express the membrane receptors for nonsensitized sheep erythrocytes. Initial studies using monoclonal antibodies for phenotyping in adult ALL suggest that these leukemias are extremely heterogeneous (Sobol et al., 1982). The clinical utility of antibodies to these antigens for classification remains to be determined.

The development of surface marker characterization for ANLL has not occurred to an extent comparable to that in ALL. Although blasts with monocytic differentiation (M4 and M5) may express receptors for complement and the Fc portion of IgG, these receptors have not yielded additional information of clinical importance. Recently, a number of monoclonal antibodies to human myeloid leukemia cells have been developed (Civin et al., 1981; Griffin et al., 1981; Tatsumi et al., 1982). Their specificity and utility in the classification of ANLL is currently being studied.

Clinical Presentation

Symptoms. Most of the symptoms of patients with acute leukemia are nonspecific complaints that may begin gradually or abruptly but usually arise from the presence of anemia, leukocytosis, leukopenia or leukocyte dysfunction, and thrombocytopenia. One-half of the patients with ANLL have had symptoms for three months or more before the diagnosis of leukemia was made. This may be more common in older patients. A small proportion of patients with ALL have symptoms for longer periods, but they average a shorter symptomatic period prior to diagnosis than do patients with ANLL. It is rare that the initial symptoms of acute leukemia directly suggest the underlying disorder, because the common symptoms are observed in a variety of diseases.

The presenting features of adults with acute leukemia have been detailed in several large, older studies (Peterson and Bloomfield, 1982). Approximately one-half of the patients mention fatigue as their first symptoms, but almost all will complain of fatigue or weakness by the time of diagnosis. Other nonspecific complaints, such as anorexia and weight loss, also occur in one-half of patients. Fever, with or without an identifiable infection, is the first symptom in approximately 10% of patients. Fever, however, is present in the majority of patients at some time prior to diagnosis. Similarly, signs of abnormal hemostasis are noted first in 5% of all cases, but by the time of diagnosis, approximately one-half of the patients display ecchymoses, petechiae, or other overt signs of hemorrhage. Severe hemorrhage as the initial event is rare, except in those patients with M3 leukemia. Other symptoms, such as bone pain, lymphadenopathy, nonspecific cough, headaches, or diaphoresis, are rarely the first symptoms to direct a patient's attention to illness, but may be identified on closer examination.

Physical Findings.   Physical signs in patients with acute leukemia include fever, splenomegaly, hepatomegaly, lymphadenopathy, sternal tenderness, and evidence of infection and hemorrhagic tendencies. Most of these signs are also nonspecific, but some are more commonly associated with certain types of leukemias. Enlargement of lymph nodes, liver, and spleen is more frequent in ALL than in ANLL. The degree of lymphadenopathy or splenomegaly is also generally greater in ALL. Splenomegaly without accompanying hepatomegaly occurs in either type of leukemia, but hepatomegaly alone is usually limited to ANLL. No relationship has been established between the size of the spleen and the degree of leukocytosis. Enlargement of hilar or mediastinal lymph nodes is observed on chest x-ray in a small percentage of patients with ALL, most commonly in those with the T-cell type.

Skeletal findings on roentgenograms include osteoporosis, bands of radiolucency or of increased density in the metaphyseal region of long bones, discrete osteolytic lesions, and cortical destruction with or without periosteal elevation. These x-ray abnormalities are more commonly seen in children. Sternal tenderness is seen in patients with all types of acute leukemia, but localized bone or joint tenderness is more typical of patients with ALL.

Ecchymoses and/or petechiae are found in about one-half of patients at presentation, but signs of more serious hemorrhage are only occasionally present. Significant gastrointestinal blood loss, intrapulmonary hemorrhage, or the CNS findings of an acute intracranial hemorrhage occur most predictably and often with dire results in M3 leukemia. Bleeding is also associated with coagulopathies in other subtypes of acute leukemia, for example M5 leukemia, and with extreme degrees of leukocytosis or thrombocytopenia. Retinal hemorrhages are detected on ophthalmologic examination in 15% of patients.

Infiltration of gingivae, skin, soft tissues, or the meninges with leukemic blasts at diagnosis is especially characteristic of the monocytic subtypes of ANLL (M4 and M5). Approximately 10% of patients with ANLL will have gingival hypertrophy. This is almost totally accounted for by those with M4 and M5 leukemias, wherein as many as one-third of the patients will have gingival involvement. Similarly, skin infiltration resulting in reddish-purple, raised, firm nodules is found in 10% of patients with ANLL at diagnosis. Although symptomatic involvement of the CNS is uncommon at diagnosis in ANLL, the routine examination of cerebrospinal fluid prior to therapy reveals that nearly 40% of patients with M4 leukemia have leukemia cells present (Meyer *et al.,* 1980).

Hematologic Abnormalities.   Anemia is usually present at the time of diagnosis and can be severe. The degree varies considerably irrespective of other hematologic findings, splenomegaly, or the duration of symptoms. The anemia is usually normochromic and normocytic. Decreased erythropoiesis in ANLL often results in a reduced reticulocyte count and the survival of erythrocytes is decreased by accelerated destruction and active blood loss. In several large series, median leukocyte counts in patients with either ALL or ANLL were generally about 15,000/μL (Peterson and Bloomfield, 1982). The percentage of patients who have leukocyte counts less than 5000/μL ranges from 25 to 40%. Hyperleukocytosis, that is, leukocyte counts in excess of 100,000/

μL, is slightly more common in ANLL (20%) than in ALL (10 to 15%). Only 15% of patients have normal leukocyte counts, and fewer than 5% have no detectable leukemic cells in the blood. ANLL is often associated with granulocyte dysfunction. Neutrophil lobulation is frequently abnormal, and granulation is deficient. Phagocytosis and migration (chemotaxis) are impaired, which probably contributes to a greater susceptibility to infection.

Platelet counts less than 100,000/μL are found at diagnosis in three-fourths of patients with acute leukemia. Median platelet counts are approximately 50,000/μL in both ALL and ANLL, and about 25% of patients have less than 25,000/μL. Both morphologic and functional platelet abnormalities are observed in ANLL. Large and bizarre shapes, with abnormal granulation and inability of platelets to aggregate or adhere normally to one another, are characteristic findings. Severe active hemorrhage is not common at diagnosis, but when present is frequently associated with platelet counts less than 20,000/μL, infection, and/or extreme leukocytosis. Independent of the platelet counts, the leukocyte count alone can affect the tendency to bleed. The most serious and potentially disastrous hemorrhagic problems characteristically occur in patients with consumption coagulopathy. This occurs regularly in M3 leukemia, and, to a lesser extent, in M5 leukemia. It may occasionally be seen in patients with other morphologic types of leukemia, particularly when high leukocyte counts are present.

Pretreatment Evaluation. Once the diagnosis of acute leukemia is suspected, a rapid evaluation and initiation of appropriate therapy should follow (see Table 18–6). In addition to clarifying the subtype of leukemia, initial studies should evaluate the overall functional integrity of the major organ systems, including the cardiovascular, pulmonary, hepatic, and renal organs. Factors that have prognostic significance, either for achieving complete remission or predicting the duration of remission, should also be assessed before initiating therapy. Because many adults with acute leukemia are over 60 years of age, special attention should be directed towards detecting concomitant health problems. All patients should be evaluated for overt infection or an unapparent infection.

The majority of patients are anemic and thrombocytopenic at presentation. Immediately after obtaining the initial studies, prompt replacement of the appropriate blood components, if necessary, should begin. Because qualitative platelet dysfunction or the presence of an infection may increase the likelihood of bleeding, any evidence of hemorrhage justifies the immediate use of platelet transfusions, irrespective of the platelet count. The prophylactic administration of platelets is also

---

Table 18–6. Diagnostic Evaluation of Patients with Acute Leukemia

History and physical examination

Hemoglobin, leukocyte count (differential), platelet count

Bone marrow aspirate and biopsy
  Morphology
  Cytochemistry
  Cell membrane markers including monoclonal antibodies
  Terminal deoxynucleotidyl transferase
  Cytogenetics with banding

Blood chemistries
  Hepatic enzymes, creatinine, serum electrolytes, lactic dehydrogenase, uric acid, calcium, phosphorus, lysozyme

Coagulation profile
  Prothrombin time, partial thromboplastin time, thrombin time, factor V, fibrinogen, fibrin split products

Chest roentgenograph

EKG

Lumbar puncture for cytology (ALL)

Blood type and HL-A determination (evaluate family members as potential blood component and allogeneic bone marrow donors)

indicated in patients who have taken salicy-lates or who have thrombocytopenia below 50,000/μL.

A coagulation profile, including prothrom-bin time, partial thromboplastin time, throm-bin time, fibrinogen, factor V, and fibrin split products, should be obtained at the time of initial evaluation (Hasegawa and Bloomfield, 1981). Patients with M3 leukemia almost always display evidence of significant dissemi-nated intravascular coagulation. If the coagu-lopathy does not require intervention before the initiation of chemotherapy, it almost cer-tainly will during treatment (Collins et al., 1978). Studies of other morphologic subtypes of ANLL and ALL also indicate that con-sumptive coagulopathy may be present.

Blood chemistries should include an evalua-tion of liver and renal function. Approxi-mately 20% of patients will have some abnor-malities in their liver function tests prior to beginning therapy. Because some chemothera-peutic agents are detoxified and excreted by the liver, drug dosages in patients with hepatic dysfunction may require modification. Sev-eral drugs, such as purine analogs and anthra-cyclines, can also be hepatotoxic and aggravate underlying liver disease. Serum LDH has been found to have limited prognostic relevance. Approximately one-half of the patients have a mild to moderate elevation of serum uric acid at presentation. Only 10% have marked eleva-tions, but renal precipitation of uric acid and the nephropathy that may result are serious potential complications. The initiation of chemotherapy may further enhance the degree of hyperuricemia. In ALL, serum calcium and phosphorus should be measured. Occasion-ally, patients with acute leukemia may present with severe lactic acidosis, may be significantly hypokalemic, or have other electrolyte abnor-malities. In addition to being a possible marker for monocytic differentiation, lysozyme, when present in high concentrations, has been con-sidered a possible etiologic factor in causing renal tubular dysfunction, which could inten-sify other potential renal problems that often exist during the initial phases of therapy.

Acute Lymphoblastic Leukemia (ALL)

The survival of patients with ALL has im-proved dramatically in the past ten years. With appropriate treatment, more than 50% of chil-dren now appear to be cured (see Chapter 39).

Even among adults, 20 to 30% of patients re-main disease-free for longer than five years. Consequently, considerable emphasis is now placed on the identification at diagnosis of those patients likely to be long-term disease-free survivors with current therapeutic ap-proaches and those patients for whom present treatment is inadequate and new therapies must be developed.

Prognostic Factors. Prognostic factors for obtaining remission and for the duration of remission and survival have been evaluated. Clinical characteristics, morphology, and var-ious biologic markers such as lymphocyte surface markers and cytogenetic findings (Bloomfield, 1981) have been studied. Prog-nostic factors relating to children with leuke-mia have been more extensively evaluated than those of adults. Data are accumulating, however, to suggest that childhood prognostic factors have relevance for adults.

Many pretreatment clinical characteristics such as age, physical findings, and hematologic variables have been reported to be prognostic factors in ALL. The two features generally considered most important are age and initial leukocyte count (WBC). Prognostic factors de-rived from multivariate techniques have been developed for childhood ALL. In one of the largest recent studies, univariate analyses identified the following pretreatment features as significant predictors of the length of initial bone marrow remission and survival: WBC, age, hemoglobin, platelet count, sex, race, or-ganomegaly, CNS leukemia, and mediastinal mass (Robison et al., 1980). When multivar-iate techniques were used, the most important independent variables (listed in order of im-portance) were: Initial WBC, sex, age, lymph-adenopathy, hemoglobin, and platelet count. As a result of findings such as these, initial age and WBC are often used to select therapy for children with ALL.

Most of the large studies of adult ALL have determined age to be the most important prog-nostic factor affecting remission rate (Hender-son et al., 1979; Amadori et al., 1980; Omura et al., 1980; Garay et al., 1982; Mertelsmann et al., 1982). The response rate declines steadily with advancing age and is strikingly decreased in patients over 60 years of age. Age is not strongly predictive of remission duration in most studies. However, older patients are rarely long-term survivors.

The WBC observed at diagnosis is considered to be of major prognostic value among adults with ALL (Amadori et al., 1980; Bloomfield, 1982; Garay et al., 1982). In particular, adults with leukocyte counts over $50,000/\mu L$ have especially short remission durations and survival times. Variables that have not been established as prognostic factors include severe anemia and thrombocytopenia.

The sex of children with ALL has a bearing on survival time. Girls have a better prognosis than boys. Sex has not clearly been established as an important predictive factor in adults, although some have reported a higher response rate in women (Amadori et al., 1980; Mertelsmann et al., 1982).

A number of physical findings at presentation have been suggested as unfavorable prognostic factors, although the data in adults remain equivocal. Signs of an extensive leukemic cell burden, such as hepatomegaly and marked lymphadenopathy, have been associated with shorter remission time (Lister et al., 1978). The importance of a mediastinal mass as an independent predictive factor is being evaluated, because it is frequently accompanied by extreme leukocytosis and T-cell markers, both indicators of a poor prognosis. The presence of CNS involvement at diagnosis also appears to be an adverse prognostic finding.

The classification of ALL according to the FAB criteria appears to convey prognostic information. In most studies, patients with L2 cytology have been shown to survive a significantly shorter period than those with L1 cytology (Bloomfield, 1982). Patients with L3 leukemia have particularly dismal survivals, generally less than six months. Several studies evaluating the prognostic significance of the FAB system in a multivariate fashion suggest that FAB class is an independent prognostic factor, especially in childhood ALL (Coccia et al., 1979; Miller et al., 1980; Palmer et al., 1980; Third International Workshop on Chromosomes in Leukemia, 1981). The prognostic significance of the FAB classification in adult ALL requires further study.

The prognostic significance of immunologic phenotype has not yet been adequately evaluated by multivariate techniques. Many studies, however, have established important differences in duration of remission and survival according to immunologic class (Bloomfield, 1982). Important differences in rates of remission induction are not evident between patients with non-T, non-B ALL and those with

T-cell ALL in either children or adults. Similarly, among both children and adults with non-T, non-B ALL, no differences have been observed in response rate between patients with and without the common-ALL antigen on their lymphoblasts. Among the few children studied, the remission rate for pre-B ALL appears comparable to that for other common-ALL patients. However, comparisons of response rates among immunologic groups must be viewed with caution, because treatment is not always the same for all patients. Indeed, it appears quite likely that with some treatments the response rate will be comparable for non-T, non-B ALL and T ALL and that for others a given immunologic group will respond better. Remission rates of less than 50% have been reported in B ALL, both in children and in adults.

Remission duration is less dependent on immunologic phenotype (Bowman et al., 1981; Greaves, 1981; Bloomfield, 1982). In most early reports, remissions were significantly longer in children with non-T, non-B ALL than in those with T-ALL. By contrast, recent studies indicate that differences in prognosis attributed to this typing are not important (Greaves, 1981; Kersey et al., 1981). Whether these results represent recent changes in therapy or the effects of other prognostic factors awaits multivariate analysis of large numbers of patients.

Immunologic class has not been included in most published multivariate analysis of prognostic factors. In at least one study including both children and adults, which evaluated age, WBC, percent circulating blasts, FAB classification, the presence of a mediastinal mass, CNS leukemia, and immunologic class (non-T, non-B, T, and B), the independent prognostic factors were age, WBC, and immunologic class (Bloomfield, 1982). The results were similar for both survival and duration of first complete remission.

Several different features of cytogenetic analysis of the leukemic cell have been found to have prognostic significance in ALL, including: The presence of specific chromosome abnormalities; the chromosome number of the predominant abnormal clone; the presence of translocations; and the presence or absence of abnormal metaphases.

Certain specific chromosome abnormalities seem to be associated with a poor prognosis. ALL with the t(9;22) was first identified as having a poor prognosis in 1975, and multiple studies have now confirmed the short survival of such patients (Bloomfield *et al.*, 1977, Bloomfield *et al.*, 1980; Sandberg *et al.*, 1980; Third International Workshop on Chromosomes in Leukemia, 1981). More recently, both the t(4;11) and the t(8;14) have been found to predict poor response to treatment and short survival in ALL (Berger *et al.*, 1979; Bloomfield *et al.*, 1981a; Third International Workshop on Chromosomes in Leukemia, 1981; Arthur *et al.*, 1982).

The chromosome number of the predominant abnormal clone was first suggested to have prognostic significance in ALL by Secker-Walker and associates in 1978. They found that patients whose predominant abnormal clone was hyperdiploid (greater than 46 chromosomes) had the longest duration of remission. Patients whose predominant abnormal clone was pseudodiploid (46 chromosomes) had significantly shorter durations of first remission than other patients. Others have confirmed the short remission durations seen in patients with pseudodiploid leukemias (Bloomfield *et al.*, 1981a; Third International Workshop on Chromosomes in Leukemia, 1981; Williams *et al.*, 1981).

The fact that patients with a t(9;22), t(4;11), and t(8;14) responded poorly suggested that in ALL translocations were associated with a poor prognosis (Bloomfield *et al.*, 1981a). Data from the Third International Workshop on Chromosomes in Leukemia, however, suggest that it is only among children that patients with translocations survive a shorter period than patients with chromosome abnormalities other than translocations. Eventually, translocations that confer a favorable prognosis may be found in ALL, such as the t(8;21) in ANLL, but to date these have not been identified.

The Third International Workshop on Chromosomes in Leukemia identified a survival advantage, specifically in adults presenting with all normal metaphases. The presence or absence of abnormal metaphases was not found to be an independent prognostic variable when age, WBC, and FAB classification were considered.

The Third International Workshop on Chromsomes in Leukemia has demonstrated that subdividing the leukemic cell karyotype into ten groups based first on the presence or absence of specific chromosome abnormalities [*i.e.*, t(9;22), t(4;11), t(8;14), other 14q+, 6q−] and in the remaining cases considering clonal chromosome abnormalities on modal number

of the abnormal clone (less than 46, 46, 47 to 50, greater than 50) has independent prognostic importance, both with regards to duration of first remission and survival. Karyotypes grouped in this way seem to confer more prognostic information than modal number, the presence of translocations *per se,* or the presence or absence of abnormal metaphases. Indeed, among patients grouped according to the specific chromosome abnormalities noted above, survivals were similar for adults and children.

Therapy.   Currently, approximately 90% of children with ALL achieve complete remission, and 50 to 60% enjoy long-term relapse-free survival (see Chapter 39). Most of these latter children appear to be cured. Success in the therapy of adults has not paralleled that attained in children. Although 70 to 85% of adults achieve complete remission, the majority relapse within 24 months (see Table 18 – 7), and only 20 to 30% of patients enjoy long-term relapse-free survival (Esterhay and Wiernik, 1982; Garay *et al.,* 1982).

The clinical investigation of therapeutic approaches to ALL in adults is difficult because of the relative infrequency of the disease. An additional factor hindering progress is the marked heterogeneity of ALL in adults as determined by surface markers, enzymes, morphology, and cytogenetics (Bloomfield, 1982). This heterogeneity will certainly require the development of a variety of different therapies. Even when the cancerous lymphoblasts of adults are sensitive to the identical chemotherapeutic agents that are so effective in children, remission rates are lower and durations of response are relatively brief.

In childhood ALL, a variety of single agents regularly result in complete remissions in 20 to 50% of patients, including vincristine, prednisone, L-asparaginase, 6-mercaptopurine, and methotrexate. Combinations of these drugs have resulted in substantially higher complete remission rates. Although either vincristine or prednisone alone results in less than a 50% response rate, in combination they induce complete remissions in more than 85% of all children. Similar success with combinations of these drugs is not observed in adults. When vincristine and prednisone are used together, the response rate in adults is less than 50% (Willemze *et al.,* 1975; Lister *et al.,* 1978; Garay *et al.,* 1982). In adults, however, the addition of an anthracycline to vincristine and prednisone increases the complete remission

Table 18–7. Results of Selected Treatment Programs in Previously Untreated Adults with ALL

FIRST AUTHOR (ref)	AGE (yrs)	REMISSION INDUCTION REGIMEN	NO. PTS	% CR	PROPHYLACTIC CNS REGIMEN	CNS LEUKEMIA (%)	REMISSION CONTINUATION REGIMEN	MEDIAN DURATION CR (mos)	MEDIAN SURVIVAL (mos)
Omura, 1980	≥15	V + P + MTX	99 (≥21 yrs: 73%)	80	None vs IT-MTX + CI	32 11	Consolidation: ARA + TG, ASP + V + P; maintenance: MTX + MP + C; reinforcement: V + P	17	24
Henderson, 1979	≥20	V + P + ASP	149	58	IT-MTX + CI	8	Maintenance: MTX + MP Reinforcement: V + P	14	17
Sackmann-Muriel, 1981	>15	V + P + DNR	156	74	n.a.	n.a.	n.a.	n.a.	n.a.
Mertelsmann, 1982	≥20	V + P + DOX	72	85	IT-MTX* or OM-MTX	8	Consolidation: MTX + ARA + TG, ASP + C; maintenance: DOX, MTX + MP, DAC, BCNU, C; reinforcement: V + P	48+	46+
Gottlieb, 1979	≥20	V + P + DNR + ASP (CALGB 7612)	121	78	IT-MTX + CI	7	Maintenance: MTX + MP; reinforcement V + P	14	20
Lister, 1978	>15	V + P + DOX + ASP (OPAL)	51	71	IT-MTX + CI	7	Maintenance: MTX + MP + C	18.5	21

Legend: n.a. = data not available; * = nonrandomized study; CR = complete remission; ARA = cytarabine; ASP = asparaginase; BCNU = carmustine; CI = cranial irradiation; DAC = dactinomycin; DNR = daunorubicin; DOX = doxorubicin; IT-MTX = intrathecal methotrexate; MP = mercaptopurine; MTX = methotrexate; OM-MTX = methotrexate via Ommaya reservoir; P = prednisone; TG = thioguanine; V = vincristine.

rate to 70 to 85%. Results from the larger series (more than 50 patients) of representative chemotherapeutic regimens that have been utilized in adults with ALL are listed in Table 18–7.

Because of the results obtained with antileukemia therapy in adults, induction chemotherapy of greater intensity than is usually given to children is now routine for treating all adults with ALL. Many of the current programs used in adults resemble those used in ANLL. Frequently, they result in prolonged bone marrow hypoplasia, leukopenia, and anemia. Because of the hazards of induction therapy, these patients require access to experienced personnel and intensive supportive care. In both children and adults, even more intensive regimens, including marrow transplantation, are now being utilized at diagnosis in patients with adverse prognostic factors (Henze *et al.*, 1981; Dahl *et al.*, 1982; Kay, 1982; Weil *et al.*, 1982). The therapeutic approaches for children with T ALL and B ALL discussed by Pinkel and Howarth (see Chapter 39) are probably also applicable to adults with these leukemias. More intensive regimens may also be justified in adults with leukocyte counts at diagnosis of more than 50,000/μL. Whether these more intensive regimens should be used in patients who have age, cytogenetics, or morphology as their only adverse prognostic factor is currently unknown.

Early in the development of therapy for childhood ALL, it was recognized that complete remissions that were not maintained with additional chemotherapy were brief. As a result, maintenance chemotherapy is now routinely employed in adults as well as children, and most commonly consists of daily 6-mercaptopurine plus weekly methotrexate with or without the addition of periodic pulses of vincristine and prednisone. Even with maintenance chemotherapy, remission durations for adults have remained much shorter than those observed in children. Most series report median durations of complete remission ranging only from 1.5 to 2 years (see Table 18–7).

The optimal combination and intensity of maintenance chemotherapy for adult ALL remains unknown. More intensive programs, such as the L-10, L-10M protocol used at Memorial Sloan-Kettering Hospital in New York City (Mertelsmann *et al.*, 1982) or the program at the Sidney Farber Cancer Institute (Mayer *et al.*, 1982a), may produce longer remissions (median durations in excess of 24 months).

The question of whether or not to stop maintenance chemotherapy after two to five years, which is being systematically evaluated in children, is not yet pertinent to the majority of adults with ALL (George *et al.*, 1979; Nesbit *et al.*, 1982).

It was evident in children that although hematologic remissions could be easily achieved, a large proportion of remissions would be terminated prematurely by CNS relapses despite maintenance therapy. This appeared to be especially true in T ALL (Kersey *et al.*, 1981; Bloomfield, 1982). The CNS appears to serve as a sanctuary for leukemic cells where adequate concentrations of chemotherapeutic agents are not attained. In children, a steady increase of 4% per month in the incidence of CNS disease during the first year of complete marrow remission has been observed (Evans *et al.*, 1970). Although the rate decreases with time, 56% of children with ALL eventually develop CNS infiltration if they are not given prophylactic therapy. The routine presymptomatic use of adequate irradiation and/or intrathecal methotrexate has almost eliminated the CNS as a site of relapse.

In adults, the incidence of CNS leukemia appears to be similar to that in children. Wolk *et al.* (1974) found that clinically apparent CNS involvement occurred in 40% of adults with ALL. The median time from original diagnosis to the clinical evidence of meningeal disease was approximately 35 weeks. Seventy-four percent of the patients who responded to chemotherapy with a complete or partial remission developed evidence of CNS leukemia. At Memorial Sloan-Kettering Hospital, 22% of adults with ALL who had received an inadequate trial of intrathecal methotrexate as prophylaxis during hematologic remission relapsed with CNS involvement within 24 months (Gee *et al.*, 1976). These data suggest that all adults with ALL should receive CNS prophylaxis. Although craniospinal irradiation is effective, the more central distribution of active bone marrow in adults makes this approach excessively myelosuppressive. Cranial irradiation plus intrathecal methotrexate or intrathecal methotrexate alone has been shown to significantly reduce the incidence of CNS relapse in adults (see Table 18–7).

Unfortunately, all types of CNS prophylaxis may be associated with acute, subacute, or delayed neurotoxicity (Esterhay and Weirnik, 1982). Chemical arachnoiditis is the most common form of neurotoxicity. It presents as an acute syndrome, usually starting within hours after injection and resolving within one to five days. The symptoms and physical findings are due to meningeal irritation and increased intracranial pressure and include headache, backache, vomiting, fever, and leg pain. Both common intrathecal medications (cytarabine and methotrexate) can cause this syndrome, although it occurs more commonly with methotrexate. The subacute form of intrathecal methotrexate neurotoxicity occurs a few weeks after therapy is started. This form of neurotoxicity is rare and usually presents as brain or spinal cord motor dysfunction. It is more likely to occur in patients receiving more than two intrathecal injections per week and is apparently related to a continuously elevated concentration of methotrexate in the cerebrospinal fluid. This complication may be transient or permanent.

In childhood ALL, a delayed or chronic form of neurotoxicity, a demyelinating leukoencephalopathy, occurs months to years after the administration of intrathecal methotrexate. It presents insidiously and progresses to severe dementia, dysarthria, dysphagia, ataxia, spasticity, seizures, and coma. The risk of leukoencephalopathy depends not only on the combination of CNS therapeutic modalities used, but also on the dose of drug given. Children who develop leukoencephalopathy have usually received more than 2000 rads of cranial irradiation, more than 50 mg/m^2 of intrathecal methotrexate and/or more than 40 mg/m^2/week IV methotrexate. This CNS syndrome has also been observed in adults.

Although there are both acute and delayed side effects for both cranial irradiation and intrathecal methotrexate, the overall incidence is low compared to the high likelihood of CNS relapse without treatment. In the future, CNS irradiation and/or intrathecal chemotherapy may be replaced by systemic administration of antineoplastic agents that result in therapeutic cerebrospinal fluid levels. Intravenous highdose methotrexate appears promising in this regard (Esterhay et al., 1982).

The other major site of extramedullary relapse in children is the testes. It is not possible at this time to predict which, if any, adult men might benefit from prophylactic testicular irradiation. Because of this, testicular biopsies should be obtained prior to discontinuing maintenance therapy.

Despite the apparent normalization of bone marrow and blood counts that occur with the achievement of complete remission, adults with ALL remain at risk of developing opportunistic infections. Herpes zoster, cytomegalovirus, and fungi are the major pathogens. Of particular concern is Pneumocystis carinii, which can cause severe pneumonia. Pneumonias caused by Pneumocystis often have responded to therapy with trimethoprimsulfamethoxazole. This fixed combination antibiotic preparation has also been beneficial when used prophylactically in children. Many of the opportunistic infections can be life threatening, and all patients deserve close follow-up care to allow early diagnosis and proper therapy.

Few data are available on either the longterm survival or potential cure of adults with ALL (Esterhay and Wiernik, 1982). Approximately 20 to 30% of adult patients appear to survive five years disease free (Garay et al., 1982). Among favorable prognostic groups, more than 50% may survive at five years (Mertelsmann et al., 1982). It is clear from most studies, however, that the majority of adults will eventually suffer a relapse of their leukemia.

The reinduction of prolonged second complete remissions in adults with ALL is difficult (Esterhay and Wiernik, 1982). Approximately 60% of adults will achieve second remissions with drug programs that include vincristine, prednisone, and an anthracyline or asparaginase. This second remission, however, is usually short-lived. Intensive reinduction regimens may prolong remission duration in children (Rivera et al., 1982), but even in these cases bone marrow transplantation is usually recommended following achievement of a second remission, in order to achieve prolonged disease-free survival. Currently, allogeneic and autologous marrow transplantation for relapsed patients and those with poor prognostic factors at initial presentation are being investigated (Kay, 1982). Other promising experimental approaches involve the utilization of monoclonal antibodies for treatment (Ritz and Schlossman, 1982).

Acute Nonlymphocytic Leukemia (ANLL)

Although length of the median survival of adults with ANLL is still shorter than that of adults with ALL, dramatic changes have occurred in the past ten years. Major progress in achieving complete remissions in ANLL has resulted in median durations of initial remissions in many series that are comparable to those reported in adult ALL. Moreover, 10 to 20% of adults with ANLL now survive five years disease free and may be cured; this percentage is not substantially different from that seen in adult ALL. These improvements in survival in ANLL have resulted primarily from the development of more intensive and effective induction regimens and improved supportive care.

Prognostic Factors. Many clinical and laboratory findings at the time of diagnosis have been reported as prognostic factors in patients with ANLL (Ellison *et al.,* 1975; Gehan *et al.,* 1976; Keating, 1982; Mertelsmann *et al.,* 1982; Peterson, 1982). The single most important factor related to an improved survival is attaining a complete remission. As progress has been made in the treatment of leukemia and as the response rate has risen, many of the previously reported prognostic factors have become obsolete, whereas new ones may be emerging. Recently, factors specifically related to the length of remission and curability have been identified.

Age at diagnosis appears to remain the most important pretreatment clinical factor, with advanced age being associated with a poor prognosis primarily because of its influence on achieving a remission (Keating, 1982; Peterson, 1982). With current modes of therapy, however, less difference by age in the rates of complete remission is being seen than previously, and no noteworthy differences in remission duration have been reported. Originally, it appeared that leukemias in the elderly were more resistant to chemotherapy and that older patients could not survive the rigors of treatment. As supportive care has improved and the remission induction period has shortened as a result of more intensive chemotherapy, however, the frequency of complete remissions has increased in all age groups, with proportionately greater increases observed in the elderly.

Patient age provides only an estimation of the cumulative effects of both the aging process and intercurrent illness. Chronic and intercurrent diseases appear to impair tolerance to rigorous therapy. Acute medical problems at diagnosis also diminish survival rates. Performance status is probably more important than age and influences response to treatment and, ultimately, prognosis. Among those factors that affect performance status are the baseline physiologic function of a variety of organ systems and underlying or intercurrent illness. If the ability to perform normal activities is sufficiently impaired, the ability to withstand the added burdens of leukemia and to undergo treatment will be compromised.

The other pretreatment clinical features that with current induction regimens still seem associated with a lower remission rate and a shorter survival include a prolonged symptomatic interval preceding diagnosis, a history of treatment for a previous cancer, fever or a proven infection, and hepatomegaly. The duration of time that symptoms have been present before diagnosis and the presence of an antecedent hematologic disorder prior to the emergence of leukemia are related factors that have recently been linked to a compromised prognosis. The remission rate following treatment in patients who have anemia, leukopenia, and/or thrombocytopenia for more than one month before the diagnosis of acute leukemia has been lower when compared to those without such a history. In fact, responsiveness to chemotherapy appears to steadily decline as the duration of the antecedent disorder increases. Data would suggest that the leukemic cells in patients with a prolonged symptomatic interval preceding diagnosis, an antecedent hematologic disorder, or smouldering leukemia are relatively insensitive to current therapeutic programs (Cohen *et al.,* 1979; Keating *et al.,* 1981a, b).

The acute leukemias that occur in patients following treatment with cytotoxic drugs and/or irradiation for other cancers have proven difficult to treat successfully. Literature reviews suggest that approximately 10% of patients with treatment-associated leukemia will enter complete remission and that these remissions are often brief (Coltman, 1982). The Cancer and Leukemia Group B utilizing cytarabine-anthracycline induction chemotherapy, however, has found a complete remission rate of 24% in patients receiving only previous chemotherapy, 36% in patients receiving previous chemotherapy and radiotherapy, and 63% in patients receiving only previous radiotherapy. The median durations of remission were 12 months, five months, and 10.5 months, respectively (Rai *et al.,* 1981). Preliminary data suggest that patients with treatment-induced acute leukemia who have abnormalities of chromosomes 5 and 7 are those with the worst outcomes. Currently, when standard induction regimens are used, patients with treatment-induced ANLL who have previously received chemotherapy must be considered a poor risk group.

The results of certain laboratory tests also have prognostic significance (Berg et al., 1979; Keating, 1982). Hematologic factors, such as leukocyte count and hemoglobin, convey prognostic information and are easily determined at the time of diagnosis. The leukocyte count has been consistently linked both to response and survival. An inverse relationship between survival and total leukocyte or absolute myeloblast count has been reported. Before the advent of effective chemotherapy, extremely high leukocyte counts were associated with short survival. Patients with absolute blast counts in excess of $100,000/\mu L$ had the shortest survival. Early deaths were prevalent in this group. Although the overall prognostic importance of the initial leukocyte count in achieving complete remission has decreased with current therapy, it continues to be of value for predicting the duration of complete remission (Dutcher et al., 1981; Keating, 1982). Adults with hemoglobins higher than 12 gm/dl generally live longer than those who are severely anemic. Several other laboratory findings also appear to influence prognosis. The presence of Auer rods and/or an elevated lysozyme carries a favorable prognosis, whereas elevated TdT levels adversely influence response (Keating, 1982; Mertelsmann et al., 1982).

The relationship between FAB morphologic classes of ANLL and prognosis has not yet been completely delineated (Bennett and Begg, 1981; Sultan et al., 1981). In several studies, patients with M1, M2, M3, and M4 subtypes have had roughly equivalent response rates to induction chemotherapy. M3 leukemia, which was associated previously with a poor prognosis, now is associated with the longest survivals in some series (Keating, 1982). This has occurred after the development of successful programs for the management of the coagulopathy during initial therapy and the introduction of daunorubicin (Collins et al., 1978; Drapkin et al., 1978). Most studies find that patients with M5 leukemia, especially $M5_A$, have particularly short remissions and survivals, even if remission is achieved. M6 leukemia also appears to have a relatively poor prognosis.

Recently, a number of biologic characteristics of the leukemic cell have also been reported to have prognostic import, including chromosome abnormalities, in vitro growth characteristics, and in vitro chemotherapeutic sensitivity. In a number of studies, patients with ANLL and only normal karyotypes have had a more favorable prognosis when compared to those with all abnormal karyotypes or a mixture of both abnormal and normal karyotypes (Golomb, 1982). Because it has recently become apparent that abnormalities can be found in the chromosomes of most, if not all, cases of ANLL, the importance of the presence of all normal karyotypes using older techniques is unclear. Newer techniques for banded chromosomes have yielded specific chromosome abnormalities that appear to be associated with characteristic clinical features, response to therapy, and survival (see Table 18–4). Whether these nonrandom chromosomal changes will be independent prognostic variables remains to be determined.

In vitro laboratory tests have been employed to assess the proliferative activity or growth characteristics of leukemia by measuring the cancerous cells synthesizing DNA. Attempts have been made to correlate these data with prognosis. The labeling index of leukemic cells has been inconsistent in its ability to predict both the response to chemotherapy and the length of survival (Crowther et al., 1975; Hart et al., 1977). Similarly, differences related to prognosis have not been detected in the size of the S-phase compartment of myeloid leukemia cell populations when analyzed by DNA flow cytometry (Dosik et al., 1980). It is not clear whether the lack of findings in this instance reflects the absence of important biologic correlates or the preliminary status of investigation. Growth patterns of cells obtained at diagnosis from leukemic bone marrows as determined in short-term cultures can yield information of prognostic value. In vitro clonal cultures with a high ratio of small aggregates (< 40 cells) or "clusters" to larger "colonies" ($\geq$ 40 cells) are associated with a higher complete remission rate than other patterns (Mertelsmann et al., 1981). The efficiency with which cells from in vitro aggregates will grow and reproduce again when replated also correlates with the remission rate. Low efficiency or low capacity for such self-renewal is associated with a higher response rate (Buick et al., 1981).

Preliminary data are available concerning the in vitro interaction of chemotherapeutic agents with leukemic cells and subsequent response to chemotherapy (Park et al., 1980; Preisler, 1982). The uptake and retention of

1-β-D-arabinofuranosylcytosine triphosphate by leukemic cells appears to correlate positively with response to treatment regimens that include cytarabine (Preisler, 1982). Other drug effects *in vitro* on leukemic cells and the measurement of drug levels *in vivo* are also under evaluation. Investigations such as these will undoubtedly extend our understanding of the interaction of leukemic cells and cytotoxic drugs and may identify important pharmacologic determinants of response.

Most of the foregoing factors predict survival of patients with ANLL because they predict response to initial chemotherapy, the primary determinant of prognosis. However, they do not predict the length of remission or survival once a patient is in remission. Because most patients with ANLL now achieve complete remissions, several factors that correlate with the duration of remission have been identified (Ellison and Glidewell, 1979; Keating, 1982). Those pretreatment factors predicting a long remission include M3 leukemia, marrow eosinophilia $\geq 4\%$, lack of myeloid differentiation in the bone marrow, low serum calcium and fibrinogen levels. Among those pretreatment factors that predict a relatively short remission are a high initial blast count in the blood, and a high (> 400) pretreatment serum LDH. An elevated LDH probably reflects a large leukemic cell burden and rapid leukemic cell turnover.

Two additional treatment-related factors have been reported to correlate with remission duration. One is the rapidity with which the blast cells disappear from the blood after the institution of therapy. The more rapidly leukemic cells fall by 50%, the longer the remission. Several studies also suggest the importance for prolonged survival of cytarabine as part of the treatment.

Therapy. Advances in the management of ANLL have resulted in improved survival and the appearance of a small but definite percentage of cured patients. This is remarkable, because there were essentially no meaningful chemotherapeutic agents available for patients with ANLL prior to the 1960s, and even now there are relatively few. The initial goal in treatment of ANLL is to induce a quick, complete remission. Once a complete remission is obtained, further strategies must be applied to prolong survival and establish cure.

Induction Chemotherapy. The goal of induction chemotherapy is complete remission. A complete remission is reached following he-matologic recovery from induction chemotherapy when the bone marrow is normocellular and contains less than 5% myeloblasts, no residual morphologic evidence of leukemia exists in the marrow, and apparently normal precursors of erythrocytes, granulocytes, and platelets are present in normal percentages and quantities. Other hematologic factors, including the hemoglobin, leukocyte count, differential, and platelets must also be normal. When the post-treatment status does not meet these criteria, survival is not generally prolonged nor the quality of life improved.

The modern era in the treatment of ANLL began with agents such as vincristine, prednisone, 6-mercaptopurine, 6-thioguanine, and methotrexate (Henderson, 1968). These drugs were all relatively ineffective, producing complete remissions in less than 15% of patients. Utilization of these drugs alone usually did not alleviate symptoms or otherwise greatly alter the clinical course or survival time. Once these drugs were combined into multidrug regimens the effect on survival became apparent. Initial combinations produced complete remission in 20 to 25% of young adults, but responses were rarely observed in patients over 50 or 60 years of age.

Cytarabine (cytosine arabinoside) and the anthracycline antibiotic daunorubicin were the first chemotherapeutic agents that reliably yielded complete remissions in 25% or more of younger patients with ANLL when used as single agents, although response rates remained substantially lower in elderly patients (Foon and Gale, 1982; Peterson, 1982). These two drugs and, in the case of daunorubicin, other analogs, are now the standard agents for treatment of ANLL. The therapeutic progress that has come about in ANLL has arisen primarily from the optimization of the use of these two drugs. Initially, studies established the best schedules for these drugs individually and, subsequently, in combination. Newer dosage schedules such as high-dose cytarabine are being evaluated.

Schedule dependency for cytarabine has been clearly demonstrated. A variation in response dependent upon the schedule of administration was first seen in L1210 leukemia by Skipper and associates (1967). Frei and his colleagues (1969) demonstrated a similar schedule-dependent effect of cytarabine on normal marrow elements in humans when the drug was given as a continuous infusion. Marrow suppression was related to the length of the infusion or dose. In initial clinical studies of cytarabine alone in the treatment of ANLL, approximately 15% of patients achieved complete remissions. The Southwest Oncology Group subsequently demonstrated that the infusion of cytarabine continuously for 120 hours resulted in a higher response rate (36%) than treatment for only 48 hours (23%) (Bodey *et al.*, 1976). In studies of the combination of cytarabine plus daunorubicin, the superiority of the continuous infusion of cytarabine over an intermittent injection schedule, as well as the superiority of seven days of cytarabine over five days, was demonstrated (Rai *et al.*, 1981).

Daunorubicin has been shown to be the most effective single drug for the treatment of ANLL. As a single agent, it has produced complete remission rates as high as 50% (Peterson *et al.*, 1982b). When used as a single agent, the superiority of administering daunorubicin on successive days compared to administering it twice weekly or weekly, has been demonstrated. Using daunorubicin, remissions are obtained more readily in patients younger than 60 years of age (Peterson, 1982). Recent investigations have established the efficacy, although not the superiority, of other anthracy-clines, especially doxorubicin and zorubicin hydrochloride (Foon and Gale, 1982).

With the availability of these effective single agents, combinations of drugs could be devised in an attempt to achieve an additive therapeutic effect. Many different programs were attempted, and once the ability to deliver supportive care improved, substantial increments in response rates were documented (see Tables 18–8 and 18–9). One of the first successful combinations was that of cytarabine plus 6-thioguanine. This combination of drugs induced complete remissions in 45 to 55% of patients, as have other cytarabine-based treatment programs (Clarkson *et al.*, 1975; Coltman *et al.*, 1978). Most successful combinations currently in use and resulting in more than 50% complete remissions employ at least the two drugs cytarabine and an anthracycline. Representative regimens currently used in the treatment of ANLL are listed in Tables 18–8 and 18–9.

Initial attempts utilizing cytarabine and daunorubicin resulted in complete remission rates of 50% or less and were comparable to results obtained with daunorubicin alone. In these early combinations, doses of each drug

Table 18–8.   Cancer and Leukemia Group B (CALGB) Studies of Cytarabine and Anthracycline for ANLL

	AGE (yrs)	NO. PTS.	% CR
CALGB 7421 (Rai et al., 1981)			
Cytarabine 100 mg/m^2 every 12 hours IV on days 1 to 5	<60	39	36
Daunorubicin 45 mg/m^2/day days 1, 2	60–69	15	13
	≥70	12	8
Cytarabine 100 mg/m^2/day by continuous infusion days 1 to 5	<60	40	45
Daunorubicin 45 mg/m^2/day on days 1, 2	60–69	26	27
	≥70	9	0
Cytarabine 100 mg/m^2 every 12 hours IV days 1 to 7	<60	86	51
Daunorubicin 45 mg/m^2/day IV on days 1 to 3	60–69	11	27
	≥70	10	50
Cytarabine 100 mg/m^2/day by continuous infusion days 1 to 7	<60	82	59
Daunorubicin 45 mg/m^2 day IV days 1 to 3	60–69	12	50
	≥70	10	30
CALGB 7721 (Yates et al., 1980)			
Cytarabine 100 mg/m^2/day by continuous infusion days 1 to 7	<60	152	69
Daunorubicin 45 mg/m^2/day IV days 1 to 3	60–69	43	37
	≥70	23	17
Cytarabine 100 mg/m^2/day by continuous infusion days 1 to 7	<60	132	58
Daunorubicin 30 mg/m^2/day IV days 1 to 3	60–69	44	48
	≥70	26	42
Cytarabine 100 mg/m^2/day by continuous infusion on days 1 to 7	<60	124	56
Doxorubicin 30 mg/m^2/day IV days 1 to 3	60–69	63	41
	≥70	20	20

Table 18-9.   Results of Selected Induction Regimens in Previously Untreated Adults with ANLL

FIRST AUTHOR	REGIMEN	AGE (yrs)	NO. PTS	% CR
Vogler, 1982	ARA + DNR	—	314	63
Cassileth, 1982	ARA + DNR + TG	<60	153	67
		≥60	21	47
		Total	174	63
Gale, 1981	ARA + DNR + TG	<60	74	76
Foon, 1981		≥60	33	76
Rees, 1977; Rees, 1978	ARA + DNR + TG	—	40	85
Uzuka, 1976	ARA + DNR + MP + P	—	32	81
Glucksberg, 1975	ARA + DNR + TG + V + P	—	46	70
Peterson, 1980a	ARA + DOX + TG + V + P	—	22	82

Legend: ARA = cytarabine; DNR = daunorubicin; DOX = doxorubicin; MP = mercaptopurine; P = prednisone; TG = thioguanine; V = vincristine.

were reduced in an attempt to lessen the risks of bone marrow aplasia and sepsis. Subsequently, Yates *et al.,* (1973) increased the duration of infusion of cytarabine to seven days and administered daunorubicin on three successive days. They were thus able to increase the complete remission rate to 67% in a small number of patients. This response rate has since been confirmed in larger studies (see Tables 18-8, 18-9).

The Cancer and Leukemia Group B (CALGB) has undertaken a series of investigations of various combinations of cytarabine and either daunorubicin or doxorubicin (see Table 18-8). Its prospective evaluation of the combination of cytarabine and daunorubicin confirmed earlier observations regarding the requirement of an intensive induction regimen to achieve success (Rai *et al.,* 1981). Remission rates were found to be higher, irrespective of age, for patients treated for seven days with cytarabine and for three days with daunorubicin than for those treated for five days with cytarabine and for two days with daunorubicin. Fifty-two percent of all patients entered complete remission with the seven-and-three-day programs, compared to only 30% of those treated with the five-and-two-day programs. Even in patients over 60 years of age, 42% entered complete remission with the seven-and-three-day programs compared to only 16% of those treated with five-and-two-day programs. This study also demonstrated that cytarabine was more effective as a continuous infusion than when administered every 12 hours. The mean time to complete remission was 38 days on the seven-and-three-day schedules and 47 days with the five-and-two-day schedules. Only one course of the seven-and-three-day regimen was required to obtain

the remission in 71% of the responders. Only 36% of responders to the five-and-two-day regimen achieved remission after one course. The rapid and complete elimination of leukemic cells after a single course of more intensive therapy permitted earlier regeneration and recovery of normal marrow function than did repetitive shorter courses of treatment. The frequency of complications was similar. Mortality in the time period immediately following treatment, however, varied according to the treatment administered in patients over 60 years of age. Two-thirds of the patients over 60 years treated with the less intensive five-and-two-day regimens died during the remission induction attempt, compared to 35% treated with more intensive programs.

Another CALGB study in this series explored two dose levels of daunorubicin and a single dose level of doxorubicin in combination with seven days of cytarabine (see Table 18-8). When all of the patients were considered, daunorubicin administered at 45 mg/m²/day proved superior to either the lower dose of daunorubicin or doxorubicin in inducing complete remissions. The complete remission rates were 58%, 53%, and 48%, respectively. This result reflects primarily the higher rate of response with daunorubicin 45 mg/m²/day in patients who were less than 60 years of age. In patients older than 60 years, daunorubicin at the reduced dosage of 30 mg/m²/day together with cytarabine resulted in a higher complete remission rate, compared to either the standard dose of daunorubicin or doxorubicin. The greatest differences in response were seen in the patients older than 70 years of age. Another important finding in this study was the relatively high incidence of gastrointestinal toxicity that could be attributed to the doxorubicin. The results of the study suggest that daunorubicin, at the standard dose in patients younger than 60 years of age and at a slightly reduced dose in older patients, is more effective than doxorubicin in this combination.

Recently, in single-institution trials even higher complete response rates have been reported using more intensive chemotherapy (see Table 18–9). These regimens usually have added 6-thioguanine or 6-mercaptopurine to the combination of cytarabine and an anthracycline and have resulted in complete remissions in 70 to 85% of adults with leukemia. Despite the greater intensity of initial therapy, the period of leukopenia is shorter than that with less intensive programs that require repetitive courses of treatment to achieve remission. The great majority of patients enter remission following only one course of therapy. Elderly patients older than 60 or 70 years of age benefit from these newer regimens with response rates nearly comparable to those seen in younger patients (Foon et al., 1981; Peterson, 1982). Although these preliminary results are encouraging, further studies are necessary to prove that 6-thioguanine or 6-mercaptopurine add significantly to the use of cytarabine and daunorubicin for induction.

Induction treatment of the type just discussed is very hazardous. Serious complications are observed in almost every patient, and the mortality associated with therapy may range from 10 to 50%. The major complications of therapy are hemorrhage and infection. In one large series of patients, documented infection occurred in 44% of those under 60 years of age and 61% of those over 60 years (Rai et al., 1981). Clinically noteworthy hemorrhage occurred in 15% and 20%, respectively. Infection is clearly the major threat to patient survival during induction, because the availability of platelets for transfusion has essentially eliminated thrombocytopenia-induced hemorrhage as a cause of death (Chang et al., 1976). Although septicemia was at one time fatal to the majority of neutropenic patients within 48 to 72 hours, the early empiric use of broad-spectrum antibiotic combinations has permitted the salvage of over 70% of these patients (EORTC, 1978; Gurwith et al., 1978; Ketchel and Rodriguez, 1978). Other serious toxicities include hepatic, renal, and cardiac dysfunction. Hepatic dysfunction is seen in approximately 3% of patients. Clinically important renal dysfunction, which may often be antibiotic induced, is age related and occurs in 3 to 10% of patients (Rai et al., 1981). The anthracycline antibiotics are cardiotoxic and, although dosages are usually limited during the induction phase, 4% of patients over 60 years of age may show signs of cardiotoxicity.

In patients who present with extremely high leukocyte counts, cerebral leukostasis may result in a clouding of the sensorium, signs of increased intracranial pressure, or intracranial hemorrhage (McKee and Collins, 1974). Usually, leukostasis does not become a significant problem unless the leukocyte count is over $100,000/\mu L$. Clumps of leukemic blasts apparently embolize to the central nervous system and interfere with the vascular supply. Thus, a patient with ANLL and an elevated leukocyte count at diagnosis should be treated promptly to lower the leukocyte count. The desired result can be accomplished by the physical removal of cells by leukapheresis or by administering hydroxyurea. The leukapheresis results in a more prompt reduction of the leukocyte count (Berg et al., 1979; Cuttner et al., 1981; Kenyon et al., 1982). Once the leukocyte count has been initially reduced, standard induction chemotherapy should be initiated immediately. The rapid reduction in an elevated leukocyte count not only prevents problems associated with cerebral leukostasis, but also may lessen the coagulopathy associated with treatment of some patients with ANLL and very high leukocyte counts and help prevent metabolic abnormalities that may develop in this circumstance.

Patients with smouldering leukemia make up 6 to 10% of all adults with ANLL (Evensen and Stavem, 1978; Keating et al., 1981a,b). It is unclear whether waiting to initiate chemotherapy until there is obvious progression of the leukemia or until a complication such as hemorrhage or infection occurs is the correct approach in the management of these patients. This type of patient can only be recognized with confidence after several months of observation. Once the chronic nature of the leukemia has been established by close observation for several months, the median length of survival ranges from 16 to 29 months (Evensen and Stavem, 1978). The clinical status of these patients, however, is highly variable during their course. If an attempt is made to select patients at diagnosis for no immediate treatment, the median time to progression of the leukemia is six months, and survival is approximately nine months (Keating et al., 1978). Once disease progression has occurred and chemotherapy is instituted, the complete re-sponse rate to chemotherapy is only about 25%. The benefits of initiating therapy at diagnosis are not established.

Postremission Management. Because current treatment regimens enable the majority of patients with ANLL to achieve complete remission, efforts are being directed towards sustaining these remissions. When a patient enters a complete remission, it is estimated that there are 10^8 to 10^9 viable leukemic cells remaining. Most patients who enter complete remission will relapse within a few months if no efforts are made to prolong the remission. A number of different approaches to postremission management have been attempted, varying from no further therapy during the interval of remission to intensive treatment programs, including bone marrow transplantation. Although the data are preliminary, increasing evidence indicates that intensive postremission chemotherapy prolongs remission duration and survival.

Results of postremission therapy cannot be viewed in isolation from the induction chemotherapy. The initial induction treatment program appears to influence the duration of remission. In early trials with either cytarabine or daunorubicin alone, median durations of remission in unmaintained patients ranged from two to three months (Ellison *et al.,* 1968; Wiernik and Serpick, 1972). The use of more intensive induction schedules of cytarabine and daunorubicin has increased the median duration of unmaintained and nonconsolidated remissions to 9.5 months (Vaughan *et al.,* 1980). This suggests that more intensive therapy provides a greater reduction in the number of remaining leukemic cells, resulting in a longer period before the threshold of detectable leukemia is again passed. Even longer remissions have been obtained in unmaintained patients induced with daunorubicin, cytarabine, and 6-thioguanine, and in those given consolidation therapy (Büchner *et al.,* 1982; Sauter *et al.,* 1982; Zighelboim *et al.,* 1982).

Further evidence that the induction treatment program influences the duration of complete remission comes from a study of the Southwest Oncology Group, whose patients entered remission on different induction regimens and were randomized into identical maintenance chemotherapy (Coltman *et al.,* 1978). The complete response rates were similar, but the median duration of complete re-mission was twice as long in those patients who received the highest dose of cytarabine during induction.

Approaches to prolonging remission durations by postinduction manipulation have included maintenance, consolidation, or intensification chemotherapy, and bone marrow transplantation (Foon and Gale, 1982). The optimal form of therapy has not yet been determined. A number of interesting pilot studies and a few large prospective randomized trials that may help resolve these issues are currently underway (see Table 18–10).

Maintenance chemotherapy consists of relatively low doses of drug administered to patients in complete remission over a long period of time and often until relapse. It is designed to delay the reemergence of leukemia by suppressing the growth of residual leukemic cells. A variety of maintenance programs, including low-dose continuous or weekly chemotherapy and somewhat more intensive intermittent treatment regimens, have been used. Immunotherapy has also been used, but to date has not been of benefit (Vogler, 1980). In the past, maintenance chemotherapy generally yielded median remission durations ranging from ten to 18 months, but newer programs, in larger studies, sometimes accompanied by consolidation chemotherapy, have contributed to median durations of complete remission of 24 to 42 months in certain subgroups of patients (Rai *et al.,* 1981; Vogler *et al.,* 1982). The median durations of complete remission in patients who received no postremission therapy are less than ten months. The value of maintenance chemotherapy is established in patients who have not received consolidation, but alone it does not provide results comparable to early, intensive consolidation.

The benefit of adding consolidation or intensification chemotherapy, that is, repetitive cycles of intensive treatment during the immediate postremission period, may be substantial in patients treated early and intensively (see Table 18–10). Routine consolidation has provided only modest prolongation of remission in the past, but two-thirds of the patients treated by Weinstein and his colleagues were still in complete remission at one year, with a median duration of more than 2½ years (Mayer *et al.,* 1982b). These patients received multiple sequential courses of intensive chemotherapy after entering remission for a total of 14 months and then were followed without further treatment. Because most of the

Table 18–10. Postremission Chemotherapy in Previously Untreated Adults with ANLL

INDUCTION	% CR	CONSOLIDATION	MAINTENANCE	COMPLETE REMISSION no. in CR	COMPLETE REMISSION median mos.	COMPLETE REMISSION at 2 yrs.	FIRST AUTHOR
ARA, TG; ARA, DNR; or DNR, P	58	None	ARA, TG	26	17	42%	Peterson, 1981a
*V, ARA, P ± C or DNR	35 to 43	None	*{C, V, ARA, P	18	15	41%	Coltman, 1978
			V, ARA, P	21	19	43%	
*ARA, DNR (see Table 18–8)	26 to 56	None	*{TG, C, CCNU, DNR,	65	8	31%	Rai, 1981
			ARA (IV vs SQ)	60	18	37%	
ARA, DNR, TG	63	*{None	ARA, TG	42	8†	—	Cassileth, 1982
		ARA, DNR, TG	ARA, TG	38	11†	—	
ARA, DNR	63	{AZ, BTG	{ARA, DNR	16	42‡	—	Vogler, 1982
		*{AZ,	BCG	26	9	—	
		ARA, DNR, TG	*ARA, DNR, BCG	20	9	—	
ARA + DOX or DNR	82	§DOX, ARA, C	ARA, DOX, TG, C, MeG	22	37	—	‖Preisler, 1981
ARA, DNR, V	71	§ARA, DNR, V	*{ARA, TG, VP	67	16	—	Sauter, 1982
			None		16	—	
ARA, DNR, TG	71	§ARA, DNR, TG	None	66	13	—	Büchner, 1982
V, DOX, P, ARA	70	§DOX, ARA, AZ, MTX, MP, P, V	None	75	32†	55%	‖Weinstein, 1980; Mayer, 1982b

Legend: ARA = cytarabine; AZ = 5-azacytidine; BCG = bacillus Calmette-Guérin; BTG = betadeoxythioguanosine; C = cytoxan; CCNU = lomustine; DNR = daunorubicin; DOX = doxorubicin; HU = hydroxyurea; MeG = methyl-GAG; MP = 6-mercaptopurine; MTX = methotrexate; P = prednisone; TG = 6-thioguanine; V = vincristine.

* Point of randomization
† Actuarial projection
‡ Refers to maintenance arm ARA, DNR
§ Early intensive consolidation
‖ Predominantly young patients

patients in this series were young, the significance of this approach for patients with ANLL, irrespective of age, remains to be determined.

Allogeneic bone marrow transplantation is another form of postremission management, which, although promising, currently has limited applicability in ANLL (vida infra). Success in the employment of transplantation during first remission has generally been limited to patients under 30 years of age and especially to those under 20 years (Foon and Gale, 1982). In view of the comparable results in similarly aged patients treated with early, intensive consolidation chemotherapy, the role of transplantation needs to be better defined. Allogeneic transplantation now seems to be the appropriate treatment for young patients with ANLL in first remission who have an HLA-MLC compatible donor and whose leukemia has unfavorable clinical or biologic characteristics.

Central Nervous System Leukemia. Adults with ANLL are at risk for CNS relapse during bone marrow remission. The overall incidence of clinical CNS involvement is only 5 to 10% (Dawson *et al.,* 1973; Wolk *et al.,* 1974; Pippard *et al.,* 1979). Because of this relatively low rate it has not been possible to demonstrate that prophylactic CNS therapy is beneficial (Wiernik *et al.,* 1976; Gale *et al.,* 1981). Prophylactic CNS therapy has not prolonged the duration of complete hematologic remission.

The majority of adults with ANLL do not develop CNS leukemia, and identifying those at risk is highly desirable. CNS surveillance by regularly scheduled lumbar punctures during complete remission has been performed (Peterson and Bloomfield, 1977). No prophylactic CNS treatment was administered in these patients. Leukemic blasts were rarely detected in the cerebrospinal fluid immediately following the completion of induction chemotherapy, a finding possibly attributable to the use of systemic cytarabine in the induction treatment. Asymptomatic meningeal leukemia was subsequently documented in a small number of patients. The patients who developed CNS leukemia had an elevated serum lysozyme at diagnosis and either acute myelogenous or myelomonocytic leukemia. Treatment directed at the CNS successfully eliminated the blasts from the cerebrospinal fluid, and the patients continued in hematologic remission.

Patients known to be at increased risk (high initial leukocyte count, high lysozyme, and M4 or M5 morphology) should be considered for prophylactic therapy, but routine prophylactic CNS treatment cannot now be advocated. The only indication for CNS therapy is the detection of leukemic cells in the cerebrospinal fluid. When present, CNS leukemia is usually treated with intrathecal methotrexate or cytarabine and irradiation (Foon and Gale, 1982).

Relapsed or Refractory Leukemia. The median survival time for patients treated for ANLL is now approaching two years, compared to two or three months in untreated patients. These median survivals are occurring because more than 60% of patients enter complete remission. Median survival for those who do not enter complete remission remains only two to three months, similar to untreated patients. Several reasons for failing treatment exist for the 20 to 40% of patients who do not enter complete remission. The major reason is death during the induction period. Some patients may have leukemia that is resistant to the chemotherapy employed. These patients may either have persistent leukemia and never become aplastic following treatment or have regrowth of leukemic elements following marrow aplasia. It is this group of patients who present a special problem. In general, resistance to treatment cannot be predicted from the pretreatment evaluation, but the presence of resistance to standard agents augurs subsequent failure to most future chemotherapy.

Approximately 75% of patients who now enter complete remission eventually relapse and require reinduction chemotherapy. Therapy for these patients at relapse has been largely unsatisfactory. At one time, investigational single agents were frequently used, and subsequent complete remissions were rare. Nearly 60% of relapsed patients who undergo intensive reinduction chemotherapy with combinations of those drugs that are most effective in newly diagnosed patients may again enter complete remission. Unfortunately, second remissions are usually short, with median durations usually in the range of four to five months (Peterson and Bloomfield, 1981b).

Several new drugs, including m-AMSA (amsacrine) and VP-16-213 (etoposide), and the use of very high doses of cytarabine have begun to make an impact on both primary refractory and recurrent disease. One of these new drugs, m-AMSA [4'-(9-acridinylamino) methanesulfon-*m*-anisidide] is a synthetic acridine that binds preferentially to cellular

DNA (Legha *et al.*, 1980). Approximately 30% of patients with either refractory or recurrent leukemia treated with m-AMSA enter complete remission. Other investigational drugs, such as 5-azacitidine and zorubicin hydrochloride, are also active in acute leukemia, but rarely produce remissions in refractory patients (Peterson *et al.*, 1982a). VP-16-213, an epipodophylotoxin, like m-AMSA may be effective in refractory leukemia (Hurd *et al.*, 1981). Although VP-16-213 is not generally active in ANLL, it is effective in some patients whose leukemia has monocytic characteristics. The use of high doses of cytarabine has also proven effective in both refractory and relapsed acute leukemia (Rudnick *et al.*, 1979; Herzig *et al.*, 1981; Capizzi *et al.*, 1982; Early *et al.*, 1982). Usually, 3 g/m² are administered as a brief infusion every 12 hours until a maximum of 12 doses is reached. Toxicity, especially in older patients and those with liver dysfunction, can be substantial. Combinations of these drugs are also being evaluated. To date, none of these regimens in the relapsed or refractory patient commonly produces long-term remissions. Allogeneic bone marrow transplantation should be attempted in the young relapsed patient with an available donor.

Survival. A large number of patients with ANLL are now being cured of their disease. Reports from cooperative groups and single institutions alike have documented that 24 to 32% of patients achieving complete remission and 11 to 18% of all patients treated remain in continuous remission for five years or longer (see Table 18–11). Most of these patients are probably cured. A previous survey of long-term survivors showed that less than 1% of all patients survived for more than five years. All of the long-term survivors have been treated with some form of postremission chemotherapy. Whether the proportion of survivors will be further increased with the newer induction

treatment regimens and programs remains to be seen.

A full discussion of the management of patients with acute leukemia must include a review of the necessary supportive care required by these patients and the role of bone marrow transplantation. These subjects are covered in detail in Chapters 43 and 50.

B. CHRONIC LEUKEMIA

Chronic Myelogenous Leukemia (CML)

Definition, Incidence, and Etiology. Chronic myelogenous leukemia (CML) is a myeloproliferative disorder that is manifested clinically by a marked proliferation of the granulocyte series and cytogenetically by the presence of the Philadelphia chromosome (Ph¹). It is generally regarded as one of a group of proliferative disorders affecting the bone marrow that includes agnogenic myeloid metaplasia, polycythemia vera, and essential thrombocytosis. More is known about CML than the other myeloproliferative syndromes (for review see Koeffler and Golde, 1981).

CML is a relatively uncommon disorder, with a stable incidence of approximately one case per 100,000 people per year. It has a lower incidence than chronic lymphocytic leukemia and is about one-fourth as common as acute leukemia. CML is most frequently encountered between the ages of 20 and 60, with a median age of onset in the midforties. There appears to be no marked sex predominance, although some series report a slightly higher incidence in males.

Despite the wealth of knowledge on the behavior of CML, little is known about its cause. An increased incidence of CML has been noted in atomic-bomb survivors as well as in patients treated with radiation for ankylosing spondylitis (Beebe, 1981). Data on chemical carcinogenesis or viral oncogenesis for CML

Table 18–11. Five-Year Survival in Adult ANLL Treated with Chemotherapy

REFERENCE	TOTAL NO. PTS. TREATED	CR	SURVIVAL >5 YEARS	
			overall	*of CR*
Coltman *et al.*, 1979*	377	39%	11%	29%
Rai *et al.*, 1981	352	43%	12%	26%
Keating, 1982	224	52%	14%	24%
Peterson and Bloomfield, 1981a	45	58%	16%	27%
Mertelsmann *et al.*, 1982	67	57%	18%	32%

* Personal communication.

are lacking. The pathogenesis of CML is probably a multistep process (Fialkow *et al.,* 1981), and for the vast majority of patients no cause can be identified.

Chromosomal Abnormalities. Recent studies suggest that over 90% of patients who appear to have CML by usual clinical and hematologic criteria will demonstrate the Ph[1] chromosome on cytogenetic analysis of bone marrow and peripheral blood cells (First International Workshop on Chromosomes in Leukaemia, 1978; Fleischman *et al.,* 1981; Oshimura *et al.,* 1982). This abnormality most typically involves a translocation of chromosome material from the long arm (q) of a number 22 chromosome to the long arm of a number 9 chromosome. The Ph[1] is found in granulocytes, monocytes, eosinophils, basophils, platelets, and erythrocytes, suggesting derivation of all cell lines from a common hematopoietic stem cell. The standard translocation, abbreviated t(9;22)(q34;q11) in which the break points are indicated, is found in 95% of patients with Ph[1] positive CML. In the remaining cases of typical CML, the fragment of chromosome 22 is translocated to chromosomes other than number 9 or is involved in complex rearrangements. The clinical importance of variant translocations remains to be demonstrated.

Studies of chromosome abnormalities during the chronic phase of CML are somewhat difficult to interpret because most series include patients who have been evaluated at varying times since diagnosis. It appears that at diagnosis, however, the Ph[1] is usually present in almost all cells. In most series, less than 2% of patients will demonstrate normal metaphases, although Ph[1] negative metaphases may be seen in a higher percentage of cases when large numbers of metaphases are analyzed. At diagnosis, chromosome abnormalities in addition to the Ph[1] occur in less than 5% of cases. With the exception of loss of the Y chromosome in CML, which has been variably regarded as having no prognostic importance or as being a favorable prognostic sign, these additional chromosome changes are associated with a poorer prognosis.

Additional chromosome abnormalities occur in the majority of patients who undergo transformation. The most commonly recognized nonrandom changes are an extra Ph[1], trisomy 8, and structural rearrangements of chromosome 17, most frequently the formation of an isochromosome long arm (i17q)

(First International Workshop on Chromosomes in Leukaemia, 1978; Fleischman *et al.,* 1981; Alimena *et al.,* 1982). Successful treatment of the blastic transformation with reversion to the chronic phase is associated with the disappearance of the added abnormalities.

Approximately 10% of patients with the clinical picture of CML do not demonstrate the Ph[1]. In contrast to Ph[1] positive patients, patients without the Ph[1] chromosome are older, have a lower leukocyte and platelet count at presentation, have a poorer response to therapy, and a shorter survival (Canellos *et al.,* 1976b; Mintz *et al.,* 1979). No consistent karyotypic abnormality is present in Ph[1] negative CML, although trisomy 8 is seen in some patients (Kohno *et al.,* 1979; Mintz *et al.,* 1979). Although some patients will have features typical of Ph[1] CML such as low leukocyte alkaline phosphatase (LAP) scores and high serum B_{12} levels, Ph[1] negative CML appears to be a distinct entity among the myeloproliferative disorders that needs further definition.

Clonal Origin of CML. Evidence that CML is a clonal disorder arising at the level of the pluripotential bone marrow stem cell comes from cytogenetic, cell marker, and isoenzyme studies. *In vitro* studies of CML bone marrow cultures show that all metaphases from a single colony will be either Ph[1] positive or Ph[1] negative, rather than a mixed cell colony (Chervenick *et al.,* 1971). Studies on women who are heterozygous for glucose-6-phosphate dehydrogenase (G-6-PD) further support the clonal nature of CML (Fialkow *et al.,* 1977). This X-chromosome-linked enzyme will be either type A or type B depending on which X chromosome is active in a given cell. In heterozygous women with CML, type A and type B enzymes are found in equal quantities in skin and cultured skin fibroblasts, however, only single enzyme phenotypes (A or B) are found in the erythrocytes, granulocytes, macrophages, and platelets, suggesting a clonal derivation from a common progenitor cell. Granulocytes grown in culture from heterozygous women with CML likewise express only a single enzyme phenotype (Singer *et al.,* 1979). Recent studies of G-6-PD on peripheral blood lymphocytes in patients with CML suggest that at least some B lymphocytes may be involved in the cancerous process (Fialkow *et al.,* 1978). This is of particular interest in light of the demonstration of a pre-B phenotype of cells of some patients with CML who undergo a lymphoid transformation (Greaves *et al.,*

1979; LeBien *et al.,* 1979). This finding supports the concept of a common progenitor to both lymphoid and myeloid cell lines.

Clinical and Laboratory Features. The majority of patients with CML have an insidious onset to their disease (Koeffler and Golde, 1981). Symptoms may have been present for several months before the patient sought medical attention, or the disease may be discovered while the patient is undergoing evaluation for other reasons. A preclinical period probably exists for months to years before the patient becomes symptomatic. In fewer than 10% of cases patients will present in blast crisis with no antecedent history of CML (Peterson *et al.,* 1976; Gomez *et al.,* 1981).

Presenting symptoms are often nonspecific. Fatigue, malaise, night sweats, or weight loss are frequently the initial complaints. Fever, if present, is usually low grade. Abdominal discomfort, early satiety or nonspecific gastrointestinal symptoms may result from splenic enlargement. Less commonly bleeding or bruising due to abnormalities in either platelet function or numbers will be the presenting sign. Other uncommon presentations include symptoms secondary to hyperleukocytosis, with leukostasis and end organ dysfunction, or secondary gout related to hyperuricemia.

Physical findings at diagnosis usually include mild to moderate splenomegaly. Massive enlargement of the spleen is uncommon. Hepatomegaly is less common than splenomegaly and, if present, is generally only slight. Extramedullary leukemic tumor nodules are rare at diagnosis and herald a more aggressive disease with a poorer prognosis. Likewise, notable lymphadenopathy is unusual and often signifies accelerating disease (Stoll *et al.,* 1978).

The laboratory feature common to all patients with CML is granulocytic leukocytosis with the whole spectrum of myeloid maturation present in the blood. In a study of 50 newly diagnosed patients (Spiers *et al.,* 1977a), the leukocyte count ranged from 20,000 to 622,000/μL, with a mean of 225,000/μL. The mean percentage of mature neutrophils was 53%, metamyelocytes 8%, myelocytes 23%, promyelocytes 3%, and blasts 2%. Eosinophils, basophils, and lymphocytes each accounted for about 3% and monocytes for 2% of the cells. Absolute basophilia was present in all patients, with an absolute eosinophilia and monocytosis in 92% and 78% of the patients, respectively. A mild normochromic, normocytic anemia with a hemoglobin in the range of 9 to 10 g/dL is usually present in CML at diagnosis. Generally, an inverse relationship between the degree of leukocytosis and the hemoglobin level is observed.

Thrombocytosis is a frequent finding in CML at diagnosis, with over half the patients having a platelet count in excess of 450,000/μL. Platelet morphology is frequently abnormal, as is platelet function. Hemorrhagic problems, however, are uncommon. The most consistently observed abnormality in platelet function is diminished platelet aggregation in response to adenosine diphosphate, epinephrine, and collagen (Hasegawa and Bloomfield, 1981).

Cyclic oscillation of the leukocytes is a well-recognized feature of some patients with CML (Koeffler and Golde, 1981). The period of the cycle varies between 30 to 120 days and is relatively constant for any individual patient. Some patients, while undergoing therapy, will continue to display periodicity (Kennedy, 1970). An inverse relationship between the height of the leukocyte count and measured levels of colony-stimulating factor has been demonstrated in patients with cyclic oscillations, suggesting that normal regulatory feedback controls on the pleuripotential stem cell may be operational. Platelets may also show cyclic changes, although the cycle is usually different from that of the leukocytes.

Bone marrow evaluation shows hypercellularity with granulocytic and megakaryocytic hyperplasia and an elevated myeloid:erythroid (M:E) ratio. Basophilia and eosinophilia are invariably present. Noteworthy myelofibrosis at presentation is uncommon. A progressive accumulation of reticulum may occur, however, and appears to be part of the natural history of CML in many patients (Clough *et al.,* 1979). Cytogenetic analyses of the marrow fibroblasts fail to demonstrate the Ph[1] chromosome, suggesting that the stromal elements are not derived from the neoplastic clone, but represent a stromal reactive component in CML (Greenberg *et al.,* 1978). It has been hypothesized that platelet-derived growth factor may be playing an integral role in the genesis of the myelofibrosis (Groopman, 1980). Myelofibrosis in CML is associated with an elevation of the LAP and a poor prognosis. It is frequently identified in the terminal phase of the disease (Gralnick *et al.,* 1971).

Other laboratory features at diagnosis include an increased level of serum B$_{12}$, due to an increase in the serum B_{12} binding protein, transcobalamin I. This protein is derived from granulocytes and may represent an index of the total blood granulocyte pool, because levels of B_{12} and B_{12} binding protein parallel the degree of granulocytosis. The LAP is characteristically low in CML, and this feature has been cited to distinguish it from other myeloproliferative syndromes and leukemoid reactions. The decreased LAP activity appears to result from a low content of normally active enzyme, rather than from the presence of a structurally defective enzyme (Rosenblum and Petzold, 1975). The LAP will rise with treatment and control of the chronic phase or when the disease undergoes transformation. A rise in the LAP has also been noted when CML granulocytes were transfused into an infected neutropenic patient, suggesting that the LAP activity is inducible (Schiffer *et al.*, 1979). Observations on the functional activities of CML granulocytes in untreated patients have shown both normally functioning cells in some patients and abnormally functioning cells in others (Cramer *et al.*, 1977).

Low levels of factor V activity have been noted in some patients with CML as well as in others with myeloproliferative disorders (Hasegawa *et al.*, 1980). Hyperhistaminic syndromes have been associated with marked basophilia in CML (Youman *et al.*, 1973).

Clinical Course and Survival. The clinical course in CML is loosely divided into three stages: The chronic phase, the accelerated phase, and the terminal phase. The chronic phase generally lasts two to three years, during which time the disease can be fairly well controlled with chemotherapy. Eventually, the disease progresses through an accelerated phase, wherein hematologic variables become more difficult to manage, and, invariably, to the terminal phase. At least 80% of patients with CML die from their disease, almost always after undergoing transformation to the terminal phase (Spiers, 1979).

The terminal phase is characterized by either a progressive myeloproliferative pattern refractory to previously effective therapy or a blastic transformation that is indistinguishable from acute leukemia. The onset of the terminal phase can occur at any time during the course of the disease. Some patients will have terminal phase disease as their initial presentation, but most often terminal phase will evolve after a chronic phase of variable length. The term metamorphosis is preferred by some to encompass all transitions from the chronic phase with the precise variant specified by cytologic description (Spiers, 1979). The risk of metamorphosis occurring at any time increases with the time from diagnosis. What triggers an individual patient to transform from the chronic phase to the terminal phase at a specific time is entirely unknown. Although no precise definition determining the onset of metamorphosis is known, increasing basophilia, a rising LAP, the appearance of multiple Ph^1 chromosomes or the development of other chromosome abnormalities, myelofibrosis, lymphadenopathy, increasing splenomegaly, fever, extramedullary chloromas, and difficulties in controlling hematologic factors with increasing numbers of immature forms in the peripheral blood are all associated with transformation to the terminal phase (Theologides, 1972; Rosenthal *et al.*, 1977a).

Because CML arises from pluripotential stem cells, the morphologic appearance of the terminal phase can be quite variable. The majority of patients will have either a myeloblastic or lymphoblastic appearance to their cells. Erythroblastic (Rosenthal *et al.*, 1977b), megakaryoblastic (Bain *et al.*, 1977), basophilic (Rosenthal *et al.*, 1977d), and monoblastic (Ondreyco *et al.*, 1981) transformations have also been reported.

Prognostic features and survival data in CML have been evaluated (Theologides, 1972; Mason *et al.*, 1974; Sokal, 1976; Gomez *et al.*, 1981). A variety of factors reflecting the tumor load, including leukocyte count, serum B_{12} values, and the M : E ratio, do not predict outcome. Factors reflecting qualitative features of the disease, however, such as basophilia, marrow fibrosis, absence of the Ph^1 chromosome, chromosome changes in addition to the Ph^1 chromosome, thrombocytopenia or thrombocytosis, and an elevated percentage of circulating blasts adversely affect survival. Females survive much longer than males in some series, but not in others. Age at diagnosis does not appear to be an important prognostic factor. High serum LDH values appear to be one of the more reliable indicators of a poor prognosis, although moderate elevations have no prognostic value. Lymphadenopathy and the appearance of myeloblastomas carry a poor prognosis.

Therapy. The therapeutic approach to the patient with CML is dependent upon the phase of the disease. Treatments used during chronic phase are of little value once a patient enters the terminal phase. Recent studies employing allogeneic bone marrow transplantation suggest that some patients with CML may actually be cured by this approach.

Chronic Phase. Treatment during the chronic phase is directed at controlling the proliferation of the abnormal cell line and, hence, controlling symptoms and improving the quality of life (Canellos, 1977). Several effective agents are available for treating chronic phase disease, so that the choice of therapy is usually determined by factors other than the established superiority of one treatment over another. Median survival figures primarily reflect the initial patient population mix of both good and poor prognosis patients. It is only after the first two years that the annual mortality rate will reflect the influence of the antileukemic treatment (Sokal, 1976). Despite the number of effective agents introduced in the last 25 to 30 years since the introduction of busulfan therapy, no important changes in survival have been seen. The disease invariably progresses and most patients die of their disease.

Before the introduction of busulfan, radiation to the spleen was used as the primary mode of therapy for CML. Splenic irradiation, although somewhat effective in reducing splenomegaly and leukocytosis, did not prolong survival (Minot *et al.,* 1924). In studies comparing splenic irradiation to busulfan, busulfan consistently showed superior survival rates and better control of the disease (Medical Research Council, 1968). No difference in survival could be demonstrated between chemotherapy alone and chemotherapy plus splenic irradiation (Monfardini *et al.,* 1973). Currently, splenic irradiation should be reserved for patients with painful splenomegaly or with cytopenias secondary to hypersplenism in patients who are not candidates for splenectomy. Other forms of radiation therapy, such as ^{32}P or extracorporal irradiation of the blood, are not effective in the management of CML.

A variety of drugs are active in the therapy of chronic phase CML. Busulfan (dimethanesulfonyloxybutane) is classified as an alkylating agent, but its mechanism of action is not completely understood. It remains the most widely used drug and appears to be equally effective for achieving remission when administered on a continuous daily or an intermittent basis. Remission in chronic phase CML is loosely defined as control of the hematologic variables at near normal levels with regression of organomegaly. It has been suggested that the duration of the first unmaintained remission following intermittent busulfan therapy is directly related to the time interval between diagnosis and the onset of blast crisis (Bergsagel, 1967). An occasional patient has had an exceptionally long clinical remission following one or two courses of therapy with busulfan (Koeffler and Golde, 1981).

Typically, therapy with bulsulfan is begun at a dose of 0.1 mg/kg/day, or 4 mg/m^2/day and is continued until the leukocyte count has dropped to the 15,000 to 20,000/μL range, at which point therapy is discontinued. The leukocyte count will continue to fall after cessation of the drug. If therapy with busulfan is continued after the leukocyte count has fallen below 15,000/μL, the risk of irreversible marrow aplasia is significantly increased. Once in remission, no further therapy need be given until the leukocyte count is again elevated, generally above 50,000/μL, or until the patient becomes symptomatic. Subsequent remissions can usually be induced by following the same treatment schedule and stopping therapy when the leukocyte count again falls below 15,000 to 20,000/μL. Maintenance therapy can be employed while the disease is in remission, but it shows no clear advantage over intermittent therapy. The most important toxicities caused by busulfan are irreversible marrow suppression and pulmonary fibrosis.

Hydroxyurea, an inhibitor of DNA synthesis, is another effective agent for chronic phase CML (Kennedy, 1972; Schwartz and Canellos, 1975). Hydroxyurea administration usually results in a prompt fall in the leukocyte count, which will persist as long as the drug is administered. Once therapy is interrupted, the leukocyte count will begin to rise within several days. Unlike busulfan, hydroxyurea must be given on a continuous basis to maintain control. Although hydroxyurea has not been prospectively compared to busulfan therapy for effectiveness against CML, studies have suggested that it is equally efficacious. Hydroxyurea has been used successfully in patients who fail busulfan, and it may be particularly useful for patients who are entering the accelerated phase or who have experienced excessive myelosuppression from busulfan.

Therapy with hydroxyurea is initiated at 40 to 50 mg/kg/day until the leukocyte count is near normal. The dosage is then changed to 20 mg/kg/day on a continuous basis or 50 mg/kg/day given bi- or triweekly. The leukocyte count falls more rapidly after beginning therapy with hydroxyurea than with busulfan, and there appears to be less suppression of the platelet count with hydroxyurea. Continuous daily use has been associated with reversible atrophy of the skin (Kennedy *et al.,* 1975).

Dibromomannitol (Dibromomannitol Cooperative Study Group, 1973; Canellos *et al.,* 1975) and melphalan (Hauch *et al.,* 1978) are additional agents that are effective for chronic phase CML. Neither is widely used now.

The role of splenectomy in the management of CML is not clearly defined (Wolf *et al.,* 1978). It has been suggested that the spleen may be more important than the bone marrow in transformation of the disease and that splenectomy may improve survival by removing the abnormal clone of leukemic cells. Splenectomy early in chronic phase, however, has not improved survival nor delayed transformation. In addition, early splenectomy does not improve the response to blast phase chemotherapy. Splenectomy during chronic phase does allow better disease control of patients who are thrombocytopenic due to busulfan toxicity. Moreover, as a palliative procedure for acute splenic pain or symptomatic splenomegaly, splenectomy can be beneficial in either the chronic or terminal phase of disease. The morbidity and mortality of splenectomy during the terminal phase is higher than during the chronic phase, and in both instances the risks can be reduced when specialized support facilities are available and when the patients are managed by experienced personnel.

Leukapheresis may be of value in treating hyperleukocytosis at diagnosis and in special cases, such as in the pregnant patient, where chemotherapy should be avoided. For most patients, however, leukapheresis is a costly, time-consuming procedure that is of little value in the long-term management of CML (Vallejos *et al.,* 1973; Hadlock *et al.,* 1975; Lowenthal *et al.,* 1975).

Based on the observation that some patients with a mixed population of Ph[1] positive cells and cells that are karyotypically normal have had prolonged survival, several investigators have utilized intensive therapy during chronic phase CML in an attempt to reduce or eliminate the Ph[1] clone and improve survival. Only 20 to 50% of patients intensively treated, however, have experienced transient reductions in the proportion of Ph[1] positive cells. In the Memorial Sloan-Kettering experience it was concluded that although overall survival was not appreciably extended, patients showing a reduction in the Ph[1] positive cells may survive longer (Cunningham *et al.,* 1979). In another series, the mean survival of the entire group was improved over that of historic controls (Brodsky *et al.,* 1979). Others have concluded that the toxicity of the therapy did not justify the results obtained (Smalley *et al.,* 1977). Moreover, the favorable results of programs employing aggressive therapy may be biased by patient selection criteria. Further studies are needed to define the role of intensive chemotherapy during the chronic phase of CML.

Terminal Phase. Despite therapy for the chronic phase, nearly all patients will eventually enter a terminal phase of their disease. Multiple chemotherapeutic regimens have been used in the treatment of the blast crisis of CML (see Table 18–12). Because the majority of blast crises are morphologically myeloid, drugs that have been useful in inducing remissions in ANLL are generally employed. Response to therapy has been poor, however, and most patients die within two to three months. For those patients who do respond, median survival is much longer than for nonresponders, but the duration of response is still less than one year.

Patients who undergo a lymphoid transformation appear to respond better to chemotherapy than those who have myeloid transformations. Thirty percent of the acute transformations will be lymphoid on the basis of morphology, the presence of TdT, and detectable lymphoid membrane surface markers. It has been reported that about half of these patients will respond to treatment regimens that contain vincristine and prednisone (Rosenthal *et al.,* 1977c; Marks *et al.,* 1978; Janossy *et al.,* 1979). Patients whose blasts are hypodiploid appear to respond better than patients whose blasts have a pseudodiploid or hyperdiploid karyotype (Rosenthal *et al.,* 1977c).

Bone Marrow Transplantation. Although chemotherapy given during the chronic phase of CML may palliate symptoms, none of the current treatment programs are curative. The disease eventually progresses and patients die. Based on results of allogeneic bone marrow

Table 18–12. Representative Chemotherapy Regimens for CML in Blast Crisis

FIRST AUTHOR	NO. PTS	REGIMEN	RESPONSES		MEDIAN SURVIVAL *(days)*	
			Cr*	PR†	*responders*	*nonresponders*
Canellos, 1971	30	Vincristine, prednisone	6	3	315	75
Marks, 1978	22	Vincristine, prednisone	8		140	84
Canellos, 1976a	19	Vincristine, prednisone,	2	5	240	30 to 60
	13	Cytarabine, 6-thioguanine	1	3		
Schiffer, 1982	27	5-azacytidine, VP-16-213	1	15	231	73
Beard, 1976	24	Vincristine, prednisone, 6-thioguanine, cytarabine, L-asparaginase	5	12	240	30
Coleman, 1980	202	Hydroxyurea, 6-mercaptopurine, prednisone, vincristine, ±daunorubicin	38	41	210	49
Spiers, 1977b	19	6-Thioguanine, daunorubicin, cytarabine, methotrexate, prednisone, cyclophosphamide vincristine, L-asparaginase (TRAMPCOL)	8‡	—	203	—

* CR = return to chronic phase; <5% marrow blasts; normal peripheral blood counts; regression of organomegaly
† PR = marrow blasts <30%; normal peripheral blood counts
‡ Good responders = no circulating blasts; neutrophils > 1000/μL; platelets > 75,000/μL; regression of organomegaly; absence of symptoms

transplantation in acute leukemia, this approach has been attempted in CML and is discussed in Chapter 43.

Chronic Lymphocytic Leukemia (CLL)

Definition, Incidence, and Etiology. CLL is a neoplastic disease that has a persistent and usually progressive accumulation of immunologically defective lymphocytes. Typical CLL is a clonal disorder of the B lymphocyte, although T-cell CLL also occurs. CLL is the most common leukemia in the United States. The disease occurs more frequently in men than women (2 to 3 : 1) and has a median age of onset in the sixties. A marked increase in incidence occurs with advancing age. The reported age-adjusted incidence for men at ages 50 to 54 is 2.7/100,000. This increases to 53/100,000 at age 85 and older (Third National Cancer Survey, 1975). CLL is uncommon before the age of 30.

The cause of CLL is unknown. No increased incidence with radiation exposure has been reported, and environmental or infectious factors have not been clearly identified. Chronic antigenic stimulation has not been found to be a factor in the development of CLL. Chromosomal abnormalities have been difficult to demonstrate, although recently an extra number 12 chromosome has been found in as many as 50% of patients when the cells are stimulated by a polyclonal B-cell mitogen. Using such methods, other chromosome abnormalities are beginning to be identified. The relationship of chromosomal abnormalities to other features of CLL are currently unknown (Gahrton and Robert, 1982).

The genetic factors predisposing one to CLL have been recently reviewed (Conley *et al.,* 1980). CLL is more likely to be familial, occurring with greater frequency in relatives, most commonly siblings of patients, than other types of leukemia. In addition, a higher incidence of immunologic disorders and various autoimmune diseases in family members of patients with CLL has been reported. This suggests that genetic factors disturbing the regulation of the immune system may predispose one both to lymphoproliferative disorders and autoimmune diseases.

It has been suggested that abnormalities in T-cell function may be important in the etiology of B CLL. T cells normally participate in the orderly maturation of B lymphocytes. Because CLL represents an arrest in one stage of B-cell development, it has been hypothesized that abnormalities, which have been found in T-helper and T-suppressor function or their ratio, may play a role in the pathogenesis of CLL (Kay *et al.,* 1979; Catovsky *et al.,* 1981b; Semenzato *et al.,* 1981). Other researchers, however, have shown that T cells from patients with B CLL interact normally with B lymphocytes from normal individuals. This suggests that B CLL represents either an intrinsic defect in the B lymphocytes or their replacement by a neoplastic clone, rather than an abnormality of T-cell immunoregulatory function (Inoshita and Whiteside, 1981). It may be that CLL is heterogeneous with regard to abnormalities in T-cell function; studies of T-cell function may identify immunologically distinct subgroups of CLL patients that have clinical importance (Han *et al.,* 1981).

Laboratory and Clinical Features. The diagnosis of CLL is easily made. The finding of persistent lymphocytosis in a patient aged 40 or older should suggest the diagnosis. A bone marrow aspirate and biopsy will show an infiltration with the same cells as found in the blood. In the typical case, the diagnosis is confirmed by demonstrating the monoclonal B-cell nature of the lymphocytes. In the early stages of the disease, when slight lymphocytosis is present, the detection of a monoclonal proliferation of B cells is highly suggestive (Rudders and Howard, 1978).

The lymphocyte morphology is generally that of a small, uniform, and relatively mature-appearing cell with a high nuclear to cytoplasmic ratio. Larger, more reactive-appearing cells may also be present (Peterson *et al.,* 1975). Non-Hodgkin's lymphoma involving the peripheral blood (lymphosarcoma cell leukemia) can usually be distinguished from CLL by the presence of large cells with a nucleus that is clefted or folded and contains a distinct nucleolus. Circulating lymphoma cells can usually be distinguished from CLL cells by differences in distribution of surface membrane immunoglobulin (SIg). After incubation at 37 °C with fluoroscein-labeled anti-immunoglobulin, CLL cells most commonly show only faint uniform SIg, whereas lymphoma cells show intense SIg staining with cap formation (Cohen, 1978).

The characterization of membrane surface markers has been useful in demonstrating the monoclonal nature of CLL. The majority of cases are of B-cell lineage. They express a single light chain class (λ or κ) and, with the exception of δ, a single heavy chain class of immunoglobulin. Most commonly, both μ and δ heavy chains are found on the neoplastic cell. Mu is often seen, whereas δ only and γ are less frequent, and α is rare (Brouet and Seligmann, 1977; Said and Pinkus, 1981). Some patients with CLL will also demonstrate a monoclonal gammopathy, most commonly IgM. Cytoplasmic heavy and light chains have been demonstrated in CLL, both by immunofluorescence (Han *et al.,* 1982) and by immunoelectron microscopy (Gourdin *et al.,* 1982). The clinical importance of a specific SIg in CLL has been evaluated with conflicting results. In one series, SIg $\mu\kappa$ was associated with a less aggressive course than $\delta\mu$ (λ or κ) (Hamblin and Hough, 1977). This finding, however, could not be supported by other studies (Foa *et al.,* 1979).

CLL of T-cell origin (T CLL) has been described (Brouet *et al.,* 1975; Uchiyama *et al.,* 1977; Costello *et al.,* 1980b). It is a relatively uncommon disorder that appears to have a variable presentation and course. In Japan the clinical features include adult onset, a subacute or chronic leukemia with a rapidly progressive terminal course, frequent skin involvement, lymphadenopathy, hepatosplenomegaly, no mediastinal mass, and a clustering of the birthplaces. The cells have T-cell markers and can be killed by antithymocyte sera. Others have described a more indolent disease associated with T-cell lymphocytosis (McKenna *et al.,* 1977). Characterization by T-lymphocyte membrane markers suggest that some of the cases are disorders of mature T cells (Reinherz *et al.,* 1979; Boumsell *et al.,* 1981; Pandolfi *et al.,* 1982).

The clinical presentation of B CLL may be variable (Sweet *et al.,* 1977). In nearly 25% of the cases the disease is identified incidentally while the patient is undergoing routine evaluation. In other instances, systemic symptoms relating to the leukemia, local symptoms relating to the tumor bulk, immunologic manifestations of the disease, or a combination of these will cause the patient to seek medical attention. The demonstration of lymphadenopathy, hepatomegaly, splenomegaly, anemia, or thrombocytopenia helps determine the clinical stage of disease. Lymph node biopsies are generally not needed to establish the diagnosis. If, however, performed, the morphology is that of a well-differentiated lymphocytic lymphoma (Rappaport classification) or malignant lymphoma, small lymphocytic (Working Formulation for Clinical Usage). Some degree of immaturity of the cells in the lymph node is not uncommon and has no recognized clinical significance (Dick and Maca, 1978).

The direct antiglobulin test (Coombs' test) is positive in nearly one-third of patients, but a significant hemolytic anemia is less common. Hypogammaglobulinemia is found in the majority of patients, depending on the duration of disease. Neutropenia is a late manifestation, and the combination of neutropenia and hypogammaglobulinemia predisposes the patient to infection. Diffuse infiltration of CLL cells into any organ can lead to dysfunction, with specific symptoms relating to the degree of involvement.

An increased incidence of second neoplasms in patients with CLL has been reported: A frequency of from 4 to 34% has been reported in various series. The End Results Program of the National Cancer Institute found a greatly increased relative risk of developing melanoma, soft tissue sarcomas, and lung cancer in patients with CLL (Greene *et al.,* 1978). Nonmelanoma skin cancer was excluded from this study but has been reported by others to be increased. For all disease sites, the excess risk affected both men and women, treated and untreated patients, and patients throughout all stages of follow-up. In an Italian series, cancers of the head and neck and breast were the most frequently diagnosed second cancers (Santoro *et al.,* 1980). It is frequently postulated that an underlying impairment in immune surveillance in patients with CLL is the predisposing factor in the development of neoplasms.

Richter's syndrome is uncommon. It has been defined as a large cell lymphoreticular neoplasm supervening in the course of CLL.

The clinical findings at transformation include the abrupt onset of fever, asymmetric lymphadenopathy, hepatosplenomegaly, and a rapid clinical deterioration. Morphologic and immunologic studies suggest that this syndrome represents a dedifferentation or a clonal transformation of the CLL, rather than the occurrence of a second neoplasm (Foucar and Rydell, 1980; Trump *et al.,* 1980; Harosseau *et al.,* 1981).

Staging and Prognostic Factors. The prognosis in CLL varies considerably, with survival ranging from a few months to several years. Many factors have been suggested to influence survival. Based on some of these factors, a number of clinical staging systems have been developed, which appear to be quite useful for predicting the course of the disease (Rai *et al.,* 1975; Binet *et al.,* 1977; Rundles and Moore, 1978; Binet *et al.,* 1981). Currently, the most widely used system is the staging system devised by Rai and associates (see Table 18–13). It is based on the concept that CLL represents a progressive accumulation of lymphocytes. The usefulness of the Rai staging system has been confirmed by several groups (Phillips *et*

Table 18–13. Clinical Staging Systems for CLL

	MEDIAN SURVIVAL *(months)*
Rai *et al.,* 1975	
Blood: > 15,000/μL lymphocytes Bone marrow: > 40% lymphocytes	Stage 0: > 150
Blood and bone marrow lymphocytosis plus lymphadenopathy	Stage I: 101
Blood and bone marrow lymphocytosis plus liver and/or splenic enlargement with or without lymphadenopathy	Stage II: 71
Blood and bone marrow lymphocytosis plus anemia (hgb < 11 g/dL) regardless of type (hemolytic or otherwise), with or without hepatomegaly, splenomegaly, or lymphadenopathy	Stage III: 19
Blood and bone marrow lymphocytosis plus thrombocytopenia with or without anemia, hepatomegaly, splenomegaly, or lymphadenopathy	Stage IV: 19
Binet *et al.,* 1981	
No anemia or thrombocytopenia; less than 3 of the following 5 areas involved: *axillary, inguinal, cervical* lymphadenopathy (whether unilateral or bilateral), *liver, spleen*	Group A: same as age and sex matched population
No anemia or thrombocytopenia; 3 or more involved areas	Group B: 84
Anemia (hgb < 10 g/dL) and/or thrombocytopenia (platelet < 100,000/μL)	Group C: 24

al., 1977; Peterson *et al.,* 1980b). Other staging systems have been proposed, and each has been useful in separating patients into prognostic groups (Binet *et al.,* 1977; Rundles and Moore, 1978). Recently, a simplified staging system has been proposed by Binet and colleagues (1981), which separates patients into low-, intermediate-, and high-risk groups (see Table 18–13). The utility of this system has been confirmed (Rozman *et al.,* 1982).

All clinical staging systems agree on the adverse effects on prognosis of anemia and thrombocytopenia. It may be important, however, to differentiate between thrombocytopenia secondary to marrow replacement and that due to peripheral destruction of platelets. The latter patients, who may be treated by splenectomy, appear to survive better than other Rai stage IV patients (Rubinstein and Longo, 1981). Splenomegaly without lymphadenopathy appears to be a good prognostic sign and has been incorporated into some systems (Binet *et al.,* 1977; Baccarani *et al.,* 1982).

In addition to these clinical staging systems, a number of other laboratory features have been correlated with survival. Lymphocytosis of more than $40,000/\mu L$ or $50,000/\mu L$ may indicate a poor prognosis independent of stage of disease (Rozman *et al.,* 1980; Phillips *et al.,* 1977; Baccarani *et al.,* 1982). The degree and pattern of bone marrow involvement may also be important (Lipschutz *et al.,* 1980; Rozman *et al.,* 1981; Bartl *et al.,* 1982). An interstitial, nodular, or mixed interstitial/nodular pattern correlates with an earlier stage of disease and with a more favorable prognosis compared to a diffuse or mixed diffuse and nodular pattern, for which the course may be more rapidly progressive. Morphology of the circulating lymphocytes has been correlated with survival. Although survival differences were observed among the morphologic subgroups, they were less striking than those seen among the various clinical stages (Peterson *et al.,* 1980b).

Treatment. The optimal treatment program for CLL has not been identified. Due to the extreme survival variability it is generally accepted that not all patients with CLL require therapy at diagnosis. Treatment is usually initiated only when patients have active disease as defined by systemic symptoms, rapidly increasing or painful lymph node enlargement, autoimmune hemolytic anemia or thrombocytopenia, or progressive bone marrow failure secondary to infiltration and replacement by the CLL. Lymphocytosis without other symptoms is generally not an indication for therapy unless it is extreme (*i.e.,* a lymphocyte concentration $> 100,000$ to $200,000/\mu L$). Some researchers have proposed that treatment should be reserved for patients in Rai stages III and IV.

Alkylating agents (*e.g.,* chlorambucil and cyclophosphamide) with or without a corticosteroid have been effective in controlling disease in the majority of patients with CLL (Wiltshaw, 1977). Both continuous and intermittent treatment programs have been utilized. Response to therapy has correlated with prolonged survival in some series (Binet *et al.,* 1977; Burghouts *et al.,* 1980; Phillips *et al.,* 1977). In single-agent studies, intermittent chlorambucil administered every two weeks appears to be as effective as daily chlorambucil and has less hematotoxicity. Responses to an intermittent chlorambucil schedule are observed when the disease is refractory to daily therapy (Knospe *et al.,* 1974). The frequency of response and the number alive at two years have been higher when prednisone is combined with chlorambucil than when chlorambucil is used alone. No difference in median survival has been documented, however (Han *et al.,* 1973). Monthly chlorambucil with pulses of prednisone has shown improved patient response rates and survival when compared to prednisone alone (Sawitsky *et al.,* 1977). The addition of steroids to chlorambucil or cyclophosphamide or the use of steroids alone may be of particular benefit in the management of the immune cytopenias associated with CLL.

Other combination regimens have been studied for treatment of CLL. The regimen of cyclophosphamide, vincristine, and prednisone appears to be effective in many patients with advanced refractory disease (Oken and Kaplan, 1979) and may be beneficial as initial therapy for patients with advanced-stage disease (Liepman and Votaw, 1978). Vincristine, BCNU, cyclophosphamide, melphalan, and prednisone in combination have resulted in responses in previously treated patients. The morbidity and mortality of the treatment, however, have been substantial (Phillips *et al.,* 1977).

In some studies total body irradiation has shown results comparable to chemotherapy (Johnson, 1977). The specialized nature of this treatment, however, limits its usefulness for most patients. Splenic irradiation may be useful for palliation of painful spenomegaly, but its precise role in overall management compared to chemotherapy has not been evaluated (Byhardt et al., 1975). Mediastinal irradiation has shown beneficial effects (Richards et al., 1978), although a high incidence of toxicity has been reported (Sawitsky et al., 1976).

Splenectomy has been useful in the management of immune cytopenias or cytopenias due to hypersplenism and appears more effective than splenic irradiation for these conditions (Christensen et al., 1977). Plasma immunoabsorption to remove IgG may be of value for patients with hemolytic anemia unresponsive to other therapies (Besa et al., 1981). The role of chronic leukapheresis in CLL is limited (Curtis et al., 1972; Cooper et al., 1979; Goldfinger et al., 1980).

Other Chronic Leukemia

Prolymphocytic Leukemia. Prolymphocytic leukemia (PLL) is a rare, recently recognized disorder that is distinct from CLL (Galton et al., 1974). The disease predominantly affects males aged 60 or older. Fever, fatigue, weight loss, night sweats, and weakness are the common presenting symptoms. Massive splenomegaly, moderate hepatomegaly, and no significant lymphadenopathy are the major physical findings. The characteristic cell in PLL is a relatively large lymphoid cell with a prominent vesicular nucleus, well-condensed nuclear chromatin, and a moderate amount of cytoplasm. Leukocytosis (i.e., WBC > 100,000 μ/L) with 60 to 90% of the cells being prolymphocytes is present in nearly all cases (Bearman et al., 1978). Mild anemia and thrombocytopenia are usually observed.

The cells usually have surface markers of B cells, although T-cell cases have been described as well. Clinical and cytologic differences between the two immunologic subtypes have not been identified. Upon tissue section, the main characteristic of PLL is the almost complete absence of mitotic figures, despite an immature appearance of the nuclei (Bearman et al., 1978). Electron microscopy may be helpful in distinguishing PLL from CLL or follicular lymphoma (Costello et al., 1980a).

Prolymphocytic transformation of CLL has been described (Enno et al., 1979; Kjeldsberg and Marty, 1981). In these instances, patients with a history of typical CLL develop an increasing population of large lymphoid cells that often retain the same surface markers as the previous small lymphocytes. This progressive disease is usually refractory to conventional CLL therapy. This transformation may reflect the emergence of a new clone of more neoplastic cells or a change in the proliferative capacity of the CLL cells. Currently, the relationship of a prolymphocytoid transformation of CLL to PLL is unclear. They may represent different stages in the natural history of CLL or distinct clinical and pathologic entities.

The optimal therapy for PLL is not known. Patients may benefit from splenectomy and repeated leukapheresis as well as combination chemotherapy with anthracycline-based treatment regimens (Bearman et al., 1978; Catovsky, 1977; Enno et al., 1979; Kjeldsberg and Marty, 1981; Taylor et al., 1982). Splenic irradiation appears to be of little value in the overall management of PLL. Prognosis is generally poor, with a short survival in most cases.

Leukemic Reticuloendotheliosis (Hairy Cell Leukemia). Since first being described in 1958, leukemic reticuloendotheliosis [hairy cell leukemia (HCL)] has become an established clinical and pathologic entity (Catovsky, 1977; Golomb et al., 1978a; Bouroncle, 1979). Patients with HCL usually present with moderate to massive splenomegaly, minimal adenopathy, and pancytopenia. The characteristic cytologic feature is a mononuclear cell with cytoplasmic extensions ("hairy cell"), which cytochemically demonstrates tartrate-resistant acid phosphatase staining. HCL is uncommon, accounting for about 2% of all adult leukemias. The disease shows a marked male predominance, with most series reporting a ratio of males to females of 4 to 7 : 1. The median age of onset is in the fifties, with a diagnosis before the age of 30 being uncommon.

Cell of Origin and Pathogenesis. Etiologic factors in the development of HCL are unknown; no environmental exposures or consistent chromosomal changes have been identified. HCL has occasionally been described in members of the same family who share a common HLA haplotype (Ramseur et al., 1981; Wylin et al., 1982), but definite genetic linkage has not been proven.

The cell of origin has been variably claimed to be derived from a lymphocyte, monocyte/macrophage, lymphocyte-monocyte hybrid, or an as yet unidentified cell. The controversy surrounding the nature and origin of the hairy cell has been recently reviewed (Hooper et al., 1980). Evidence for a monocytic origin is based on the hairy cells' phagocytic and bactericidal properties, their ability to adhere, the presence of receptors for cytophilic antibody, and the finding of monocytopenia in patients with HCL. Arguments for the lymphocytic origin of the hairy cell are based on cell surface marker studies, the presence of surface immunoglobulin, and the ability of the cells to synthesize immunoglobulins both *in vivo* and *in vitro.* Although most of the data on a lymphocytic origin for HCL suggest a B-cell cancer, studies have demonstrated T-cell markers in some patients. Other studies have suggested that the hairy cell represents a particular B-lymphocyte subset that has phagocytic capability. Studies with monoclonal antibodies have demonstrated multiple phenotypes in HCL and have suggested that the disease represents a neoplastic proliferation of a lymphoid cell that is more mature than the cell in CLL (Jansen *et al.,* 1982a,b). It may be that the disease is derived from a pluripotential stem cell.

Clinical and Laboratory Features. The onset of HCL is insidious, with malaise, fatigue, and weakness being the commonest initial complaints. Abdominal symptoms relating to splenomegaly are frequent. Infection as the presenting problem is observed in 15% of patients, and bleeding manifestations at diagnosis have been reported in 9 to 34% of patients. HCL is discovered incidentally in about 10% of patients.

Moderate to massive splenomegaly is common, with some degree of splenic enlargement found in almost all patients. Hepatomegaly is seen in 25 to 50% of patients. Lymphadenopathy, if present, is usually minimal with nodes generally less than 2 cm in size.

Laboratory studies reveal a pancytopenia in most patients. In some instances only the leukocytes and platelets are depressed. Over half of the patients will have a leukocyte count of less than $3000/\mu L$ with the typical hairy cells being identifiable. At diagnosis, extreme leukocytosis (WBC $> 50,000/\mu L$) is unusual, as is absence of the characteristic cells on the peripheral blood smear. Granulocytopenia and an absolute depression of the monocytes are observed. Moderate thrombocytopenia is usually present (platelet count $< 100,000/\mu L$), however, a platelet count of less than $20,000/\mu L$ is uncommon. The hemoglobin concentration is generally between 5 and 12 g/dL, the anemia being normochromic and normocytic.

The results of liver function studies are generally normal, despite infiltration by hairy cells, but abnormalities may be found in 10 to 20% of patients. Abnormalities of renal function studies are seen in 10 to 25% of patients.

Serum and urine lysozyme concentrations are low or normal. Quantitative immunoglobulins are frequently normal, though increased and decreased levels of IgM, IgG, or IgA may be present. Rarely, patients show a monoclonal pattern by immunoelectrophoresis (Golde *et al.,* 1977).

The bone marrow is always involved by HCL, and in nearly half of the patients the aspirate will yield a "dry tap." On core biopsy, the pattern of distribution is generally diffuse, with patchy involvement in only 10% of cases. Some degree of fibrosis is usually present. In autopsy series, widespread involvement of the hematopoietic system, including spleen and lymph nodes, is characteristic. In addition, infiltration of the liver as well as of other organs is common. The pattern of infiltration tends to be diffuse and patchy rather than that of large tumor nodules. Unlike CLL, an absence of serious gastrointestinal tract involvement has been reported (Vardiman *et al.,* 1979).

Despite its distinctive clinicopathologic features, HCL is sometimes confused with CLL and non-Hodgkin's lymphoma (Neiman *et al.,* 1979). Difficulties arise in part because tartrate-resistant acid phosphatase staining can be positive in some cases of CLL and lymphoma (Hooper *et al.,* 1980) and in other instances because circulating "hairy cells" can be seen in perpheralized lymphomas (Palutke *et al.,* 1981). Occasionally the pathognomonic cell in HCL can only be demonstrated with supravital staining or with phase-contrast microscopy.

Prognosis and Treatment. HCL is a chronic disease with a reported median survival of nearly six years (Catovsky, 1977; Golomb *et al.,* 1978a; Bouroncle, 1979). An increase in the survival rate has been observed over the last ten to 15 years due to improvements in the management of the cytopenias and the infectious complications. Pnemonia and/or sepsis are still the most common causes of death; bleeding is the next most frequent. Gram-negative infections and infections with bizarre organisms are characteristic; the frequency of infections is directly related to the degree of granulocytopenia. No factors at diagnosis appear to reliably predict duration of survival. Patients who are older, however, have minimal splenomegaly, and have few circulating hairy cells, do better than those who require treatment.

Splenectomy remains the treatment of choice in HCL. The general treatment strategy for HCL has been to observe the rate of disease progression and the degree of cytopenia before doing a splenectomy. For patients who fail splenectomy or who are not surgical candidates, corticosteroids, alkylating agent chemotherapy, or interferon may be beneficial. For patients with refractory cases of HCL, more intensive chemotherapy may be indicated (Catovsky, 1977; Golomb *et al.*, 1978a; Stewart *et al.*, 1979).

In HCL, splenectomy is indicated when patients develop symptomatic hypersplenism with pancytopenia. Granulocytopenia ($<500/\mu$L) without other cytopenias may be an indication for early splenectomy to prevent infectious complications. Responses following splenectomy have been categorized as complete if the hemoglobin rises to more than 11/g/dL, the neutrophils to greater than 1000/μL, and the platelets to greater than 100,000/μL. A partial response is defined as improvement in only one or two of these cell lines, and if all three cell lines remain depressed then there is considered to be no response. Nearly all patients will achieve either a complete or partial response to splenectomy. All partial responders will eventually relapse, compared to a 50% relapse rate for the complete responders. Following splenectomy, patients have an improved survival compared to nonsplenectomized patients. Proper management in the perioperative period, however, is extremely important in reducing the morbidity and mortality associated with the procedure.

Chemotherapy in HCL has been reserved for patients who fail splenectomy or who are judged not to be surgical candidates. Responses to corticosteroids are occasionally seen. Other cytotoxic therapies, however, especially when administered before splenectomy, have yielded disappointing results and may be detrimental (Catovsky, 1977). Some patients who relapse after splenectomy will respond to alkylating agent chemotherapy (Golomb and Mintz, 1979). Leukapheresis may be useful for the rare patient with hyperleukocytosis (Fay *et al.*, 1979). Anecdotal reports have suggested that treatment with lithium may have a beneficial effect on the patient with pancytopenia in splenectomy failures (Blum, 1980; Paladine *et al.*, 1981).

Acknowledgement

The authors are indebted to Ms. Vivian Schultz for expert secretarial assistance in the preparation of this manuscript.

REFERENCES

Alavi, J. B.; Root, R. K.; Djerassi, I.; Evans, A. E.; Gluckman, S. J.; MacGregor, R. R.; Guerry, D.; Schreiber, A. D.; Shaw, J. M.; Koch, P.; and Cooper, R. A.: A randomized clinical trial of granulocyte transfusions for infection in acute leukemia. *N. Engl. J. Med.,* **296**:706–711, 1977.

Alimena, G.; Dallapiccola, B.; Gastaldi, R.; Mandelli, F.; Brandt, L.; Mitelman, F.; and Nilsson, P. G.: Chromosomal, morphological and clinical correlations in blastic crisis of chronic myeloid leukaemia; a study of 69 cases. *Scand. J. Haematol.,* **28**:103–117, 1982.

Amadori, S.; Montuoro, A.; Meloni, G.; Aloe Spiriti, M. A.; Pacilli, L.; and Mandelli, F.: Combination chemotherapy for acute lymphocytic leukemia in adults: Results of a retrospective study in 82 patients. *Am. J. Hematol.,* **8**:175–183, 1980.

Arthur, D. C.; Bloomfield, C. D.; Lindquist, L. L.; and Nesbit, M. E., Jr.: Translocation 4;11 in acute lymphoblastic leukemia: Clinical characteristics and prognostic significance. *Blood,* **59**:96–99, 1982.

Arthur, D. C.; Bloomfield, C. D.; Lindquist, L. L.; Peterson, B. A.; and Nesbit, M. E.: Chromosome abnormalities in acute lymphoblastic leukemia (ALL): Frequency and clinical implications. *Proc. Am. Soc. Clin. Oncol.,* **22**:345, 1981 (abstract).

Baccarani, M.; Cavo, M.; Gobbi, M.; Lauria, F.; and Tura, S.: Staging of chronic lymphocytic leukemia. *Blood,* **59**:1191–1196, 1982.

Bain, B.; Catovsky, D.; O'Brien, M.; Spiers, A. S. D.; and Richards, H. G.: Megakaryoblastic transformations in chronic granulocytic leukemia: An electron microscopy and cytochemical study. *J. Clin. Pathol.,* **30**:235–242, 1977.

Bartl, R.; Frisch, B.; Burkhardt, R.; Hoffmann-Fezer, G.; Demmler, K.; and Sund, M.: Assessment of marrow trephine in relation to staging in chronic lymphocytic leukaemia. *Br. J. Haematol.,* **51**:1–15, 1982.

Beard, M.; Gauci, C.; Sikora, E.; Kirk, B.; and Fairley, G. H.: Blast crisis of chronic myeloid leukaemia: The effect of intensive chemotherapy. *Scand. J. Haematol.,* **16**:258–262, 1976.

Bearman, R. M.; Pangalis, G. A.; and Rappaport, H.: Prolymphocytic leukemia. Clinical, histopathological, and cytochemical observations. *Cancer,* **42**:2360–2372, 1978.

Beebe, G. W.: Overall risks of cancer in A-bomb survivors and patients irradiated for ankylosing spondylitis. In Burchenal, J. H., and Oettgen, H. F. (eds.): *Cancer: Achievements, Challenges, and Prospects for the 1980s.* Grune & Stratton, Inc., New York, 1981.

Bennett, J. M.: The French-American-British classification of the acute adult myeloid leukemias: Its clinical relevance. In Bloomfield, C. D. (ed.): *Adult Leukemias 1.* Martinus Nijhoff Publishers, The Hague, 1982.

Bennett, J. M., and Begg, C. B.: Eastern Cooperative Oncology Group Study of the cytochemistry of adult acute myeloid leukemia by correlation of subtypes with response and survival. *Cancer Res.,* **41**:4833–4837, 1981.

Bennett, J. M.; Catovsky, D.; Daniel, M. T.; Flandrin, G.; Galton, D. A. G.; Gralnick, H. R.; and Sultan, C.: Proposals for the classification of the acute leukaemias. *Br. J. Haematol.,* **33**:451–458, 1976.

Bennett, J. M.; Catovsky, D.; Daniel M. T.; Flandrin, G.; Galton, D. A. G.; Gralnick, H. R.; Sultan, C.; (FAB 1980): A variant form of hypergranular promyelocytic leukemia (M3). *Ann. Intern. Med.,* **92:**261, 1980 (letter).

Bennett, J. M.; Catovsky, D.; Daniel, M. T.; Flandrin, G.; Galton, D. A. G.; Gralnick, H. R.; and Sultan, C.: The morphological classification of acute lymphoblastic leukaemia: Concordance among observers and clinical correlations. *Br. J. Haematol.,* **47:**553–561, 1981.

Berg, J.; Vincent, P. C.; and Gunz, F. W.: Extreme leucocytosis and prognosis of newly diagnosed patients with acute non-lymphocytic leukaemia. *Med. J. Aust.,* **1:**480–482, 1979.

Berger, R.; Bernheim, A.; Brouet, J. C.; Daniel, M. T.; and Flandrin, G.: t(8;14) translocation in a Burkitt's type of lymphoblastic leukaemia (L3). *Br. J. Haematol.,* **43:**87–90, 1979.

Berger, R.; Bernheim, A.; Daniel, M. T.; Valensi, F.; and Flandrin, G.: Karyotype and cell phenotypes in primary acute leukemias. *Blood Cells,* **7:**287–292, 1981.

Berger, R.; Bernheim, A.; Weh, H. J.; Daniel, M. T.; and Flandrin, G.: Cytogenetic studies on acute monocytic leukemia. *Leuk. Res.,* **4:**119–127, 1980.

Bergsagel, D.: The chronic leukemias. *Can. Med. Assoc. J.,* **96:**1616–1624, 1967.

Besa, E. C.; Ray, P. K.; Swami, V. K.; Idiculla, A.; Rhoads, J. E., Jr.; Bassett, J. G.; Joseph, R. R.; and Cooper, D. R.: Specific immunoadsorption of IgG antibody in a patient with chronic lymphocytic leukemia and autoimmune hemolytic anemia. A new form of therapy for the acute critical stage. *Am. J. Med.,* **71:**1035–1040, 1981.

Binet, J. L.; Auquier, A.; Dighiero, G.; Chastang, C.; Piguet, H.; Goasguen, J.; Vaugier, G.; Potron, G.; Colona, P.; Oberling, F.; Thomas, M.; Tchernia, G.; Jacquillat, C.; Boivin, P.; Lesty, C.; Duault, M. T.; Monconduit, M.; Belabbes, S.; and Gremy, F.: A new prognostic classification of chronic lymphocytic leukemia derived from a multivariate survival analysis. *Cancer,* **48:**198–206, 1981.

Binet, J. L.; Leporrier, M.; Dighiero, G.; Charron, D.; D'Athis, P. H.; Vaugier, G.; Beral, H. M.; Natali, J. C.; Raphael, M.; Nizet, B.; and Follezou, J. Y.: A clinical staging system for chronic lymphocytic leukemia. *Cancer,* **40:**855–864, 1977.

Bishop, J. M.: Oncogenes. *Sci. Am.,* **246:**80–92, 1982.

Bloomfield, C. D.: Classification and prognosis of acute lymphoblastic leukemia. *Prog. Clin. Biol. Res.,* **58:**167–183, 1981.

Bloomfield, C. D.: The clinical relevance of lymphocyte surface markers in adult acute lymphoblastic leukemia. In Bloomfield, C. D. (ed.): *Adult Leukemias 1.* Martinus Nijhoff Publishers, The Hague, 1982.

Bloomfield, C. D., and Arthur, D. C.: Del(16)(q21 or 22) and marrow eosinophilia in acute non-lymphoblastic leukemia (ANLL): A new cytogenetic-clinical association. *Proc. Am. Soc. Clin. Oncol.,* **1:**191, 1982a (abstract).

Bloomfield, C. D., and Arthur, D. C.: Evaluation of leukemic cell chromosomes as a guide to therapy. *Blood Cells,* **8:**501–518, 1982b.

Bloomfield, C. D.; Arthur, D. C.; Frizzera, G.; Peterson, B. A.; and Gajl-Peczalska, K.J.: Chromosomal abnormalities in non-Hodgkin's malignant lymphoma. In Vitetta, E., and Fox, C. F. (eds.): *B and T Cell Tumors: Biological and Clinical Aspects,* Volume XXIV. Academic Press, New York, 1982.

Bloomfield, C. D., and Brunning, R. D.: Acute leukemia as a terminal event in nonleukemia hematopoietic disorders. *Semin. Oncol.,* **3:**297–317, 1976.

Bloomfield, C. D.; Brunning R. D.; Smith, K. A.; and Nesbit, M. E.: Prognostic significance of the Philadel-

phia chromosome in acute lymphocytic leukemia. *Cancer Genet. Cytogenet.,* **1:**229–238, 1980.

Bloomfield, C. D.; Lindquist, L. L.; Arthur, D.; McKenna, R. W.; LeBien, T. W.; Peterson, B. A.; and Nesbit, M. E.: Chromosomal abnormalities in acute lymphoblastic leukemia. *Cancer Res.,* **41:**4838–4843, 1981a.

Bloomfield, C. D.; Peterson, L. C.; Yunis, J. J.; and Brunning, R. D.: The Philadelphia chromosome (Ph[1]) in adults presenting with acute leukaemia: A comparison of Ph[1]+ and Ph[1]− patients. *Br. J. Haematol.,* **36:**347–358, 1977.

Bloomfield, C. D.; Smith, K. A.; Peterson, B. A.; and Munck, A.: Glucocorticoid receptors in adult acute lymphoblastic leukemia. *Cancer Res.,* **41:**4857–4860, 1981b.

Blum, S. F.: Lithium in hairy-cell leukemia. *N. Engl. J. Med.,* **303:**464–465, 1980.

Blume, K. G.; Beutler, E.; Bross, K. J.; Chillar, R. K.; Ellington, O. B.; Fahey, J. L.; Farbstein, M. J.; Forman, S. J.; Schmidt, G. M.; Scott, E. P.; Spruce, W.E.; Turner, M. A.; and Wolf, J. L.: Bone marrow ablation and allogeneic marrow transplantation in acute leukemia. *N. Engl. J. Med.,* **302:**1041–1046, 1980.

Bodey, G. P.; Coltman, C. A.; Hewlett, J. S.; and Freireich, E. J.: Progress in the treatment of adults with acute leukemia. Review of regimens containing cytarabine studied by the Southwest Oncology Group. *Arch. Intern. Med.,* **136:**1383–1388, 1976.

Bollum, F. J.: Terminal deoxynucleotidyl transferase as a hematopoietic cell marker. *Blood,* **54:**1203–1215, 1979.

Boumsell, L.; Bernard, A.; Reinherz, E. L.; Nadler, L. M.; Ritz, J.; Coppin, H.; Richard, Y.; Dubertret, L.; Valensi, F.; Degos, L.; Lemerle, J.; Flandrin, G.; Dausset, J.; and Schlossman, S. F.: Surface antigens on malignant Sézary and T-CLL cells correspond to those of mature T cells. *Blood,* **57:**526–530, 1981.

Bouroncle, B. A.: Leukemic reticuloendotheliosis (hairy cell leukemia). *Blood,* **53:**412–436, 1979.

Bowman, W. P.; Melvin, S. L.; Aur, R. J. A.; and Mauer, A. M.: A clinical perspective on cell markers in acute lymphocytic leukemia. *Cancer Res.,* **41:**4794–4801, 1981.

Bradstock, K. F.; Janossy, G.; Hoffbrand, A. V.; Ganeshaguru, K.; Llewellin, P.; Prentice, H. G.; and Bollum, F. J.: Immunofluorescent and biochemical studies of terminal deoxynucleotidyl transferase in treated acute leukaemia. *Br. J. Haematol.,* **47:**121–131, 1981.

Brandt, L.; Nilsson, P. G.; and Mitelman, F.: Trends in incidence of acute leukemia. *Lancet,* **2:**1069, 1979.

Brodsky, I.; Fuscaldo, K. E.; Kahn, S. B.; and Conroy, J. F.: Myeloproliferative disorders: II CML: Clonal evolution and its role in management. *Leuk. Res.,* **3:**379–393, 1979.

Brouet, J.-C.; Flandrin, G.; Sasportes, M.; Preud'Homme, J.-L.; and Seligmann, M.: Chronic lymphocytic leukaemia of T-cell origin. Immunological and clinical evaluation in eleven patients. *Lancet,* **2:**890–893, 1975.

Brouet, J.-C., and Seligmann, M.: Chronic lymphocytic leukaemia as an immunoproliferative disorder. *Clin. Haematol.,* **6:**169–183, 1977.

Büchner, T.; Hiddemann, W.; Urbanitz, D.; Kamanabroo, D.; Schulte, H.; and van de Loo, J.: Intensified remission induction and consolidation without maintenance therapy for acute myeloid leukemia (AML). *Proc. Am. Soc. Clin. Oncol.,* **1:**135, 1982 (abstract).

Buckner, C. D.; Stewart, P.; Clift, R. A.; Fefer, A.; Neiman, P. E.; Singer, J.; Storb, N. R.; and Thomas, E. D.: Treatment of blastic transformation of chronic granulocytic leukemia by chemotherapy, total body irradiation and infusion of cryopreserved autologous marrow. *Exp. Hematol.,* **6:**96–109, 1978.

Buick, R. N.; Chang, L. J.-A.; Messner, H. A.; Curtis, J. E.; and McCulloch, E. A.: Self-renewal capacity of leukemic blast progenitor cells. *Cancer Res.,* **41:**4849–4852, 1981.

Burghouts, J.; Prüst, E.; and van Lier, J. J. H.: Response to therapy as prognostic factor in chronic lymphocytic leukemia: *Acta Haematol.* (Basel), **63:**217–221, 1980.

Burns, C. P.; Armitage, J. O.; Frey, A. L.; Dick, F. R.; Jordan, J. E.; and Woolson, R. F.: Analysis of the presenting features of adult acute leukemia: The French-American-British classification. *Cancer,* **47:**2460–2469, 1981.

Byhardt, R. W.; Brace, K. C.; and Wiernik, P. H.: The role of splenic irradiation in chronic lymphocytic leukemia. *Cancer,* **35:**1621–1625, 1975.

Cairns, J.: The origin of human cancers. *Nature,* **289:**353–357, 1981.

Canellos, G. P.: The treatment of chronic granulocytic leukaemia. *Clin. Haematol.,* **6:**113–128, 1977.

Canellos, G. P.; DeVita, V. T.; Whang-Peng, J.; and Carbone, P. P.: Hematologic and cytogenetic remission of blastic transformation in chronic granulocytic leukemia. *Blood,* **38:**671–679, 1971.

Canellos, G. P.; DeVita, V. T.; Whang-Peng, J.; Chabner, B. A.; Schein, P. S.; and Young, R. C.: Chemotherapy of the blastic phase of chronic granulocytic leukemia: Hypodiploidy and response to therapy. *Blood,* **47:**1003–1009, 1976a.

Canellos, G. P.; Whang-Peng, J.; and DeVita, V. T.: Chronic granulocytic leukemia without the Philadelphia chromosome. *Am. J. Clin. Pathol.,* **65:**467–470, 1976b.

Canellos, G. P.; Young, R. C.; Nieman, P. E.; and DeVita, V. T., Jr.: Dibromomannitol in the treatment of chronic granulocytic leukemia: A prospective randomized comparison with busulfan. *Blood,* **45:**197–203, 1975.

Capizzi, R. L.; Rudnick, S. A.; Gabriel, D. A.; Sakasrabudhe, D.; Tremont, S.; McClamrock, E.; Wells, R.; and Ross, D.: High-dose Ara-C (HiDAC) with sequential asparaginase (A'ase) (HiDAC → A'ase) for remission induction in acute leukemia. *Proc. Am. Soc. Clin. Oncol.,* **1:**130, 1982.

Casciato, D. A., and Scott, J. L.: Acute leukemia following prolonged cytotoxic agent therapy. *Medicine* (Baltimore), **58:**32–47, 1979.

Cassileth, P. A.; Begg, C. B.; Bennett, J. M.; Weiler, C.; and Glick, J. H.: A randomized study of the efficacy of consolidation therapy in adult acute nonlymphocytic leukemia (ANLL). *Proc. Am. Soc. Clin. Oncol.,* **1:**130, 1982 (abstract).

Catovsky, D.: Hairy-cell leukaemia and prolymphocytic leukaemia. *Clin. Haematol.,* **6:**245–267, 1977.

Catovsky, D.; de Salvo Cardullo, L.; O'Brien, M.; Morilla, R.; Costello, C.; Galton, D.; Ganeshaguru, K.; and Hoffbrand, V.: Cytochemical markers of differentiation in acute leukemia. *Cancer Res.,* **41:**4824–4832, 1981a.

Catovsky, D.; Lauria, F.; Matutes, E.; Foa, R.; Mantovani, V.; Tura, S.; and Galton, D. A. G.: Increase in Tγ lymphocytes in B-cell chronic lymphocytic leukaemia. *Br. J. Haematol.,* **47:**539–544, 1981b.

Champlin, R.; Arenson, E.; and Gale, R. P.: Allogeneic transplantation for patients with chronic myelogenous leukemia (CML) in chronic phase. *Blood,* **58**(suppl):171a, 1981 (abstract).

Chang, H. Y.; Rodriguez, V.; Narboni, G.; Bodey, G. P.;

Luna, M. A.; and Freireich, E. M.: Causes of death in adults with acute leukemia. *Medicine,* **55:**259–268, 1976.

Chervenick, P. A.; Ellis, L. D.; Pan, S. F.; and Lawson, A. L.: Human leukemic cells: *In vitro* growth of colonies containing the Philadelphia (Ph¹) chromosome. *Science,* **174:**1134–1136, 1971.

Christensen, B. E.; Hansen, M. M.; and Videbaek, A. A.: Splenectomy in chronic lymphocytic leukaemia. *Scand. J. Haematol.,* **18:**279–287, 1977.

Civin, C. I.; Mirro, J.; and Banquerigo, M. L.: My-1, a new myeloid-specific antigen identified by a mouse monoclonal antibody. *Blood,* **57:**842–845, 1981.

Clarkson, B. D.; Dowling, M. D.; Gee, T. S.; Cunningham, I. B.; and Burchenal, J. H.: Treatment of acute leukemia in adults. *Cancer,* **36:**775–795, 1975.

Clough, V.; Geary, C. G.; Hashmi, K.; Davson, J.; and Knowlson, T.: Myelofibrosis in chronic granulocytic leukaemia. *Br. J. Haematol.,* **42:**515–626, 1979.

Coccia, P. F.; Miller, D. R.; Kersey, J. H.; Bleyer, W. A.; Gross, S.; Siegel, S. E.; Sather, H. N.; and Hammond, G. D.: Relationship of blast cell surface markers and morphology (FAB classification) in childhood acute lymphocytic leukemia (ALL). *Blood,* **54:**182a, 1979 (abstract).

Cohen, H. J.: B-cell lymphosarcoma cell leukemia: Dynamics of surface-membrane immunoglobulin. Value for differentiation from chronic lymphocytic leukemia. *Ann. Intern. Med.,* **88:**317–322, 1978.

Cohen, H. J.; Creger, W. P.; Greenberg, P. L.; and Schrier, S. L.: Subacute myeloid leukemia: A clinical review. *Am. J. Med.,* **66:**959–966, 1979.

Coleman, C. N.; Williams, C. J.; Flint, A.; Glatstein, E. J.; Rosenberg, S. A.; and Kaplan, H. S.: Hematologic neoplasia in patients treated for Hodgkin's disease. *N. Engl. J. Med.,* **297:**1249–1252, 1977.

Coleman, M.; Silver, R. T.; Pajak, T. F.; Cavalli, F.; Rai, K. R.; Kostinas, J. E.; Glidewell, O.; and Holland, J. F.: Combination chemotherapy for terminal-phase chronic granulocytic leukemia: Cancer and Leukemia Group B Studies. *Blood,* **55:**29–36, 1980.

Collins, A. J.; Bloomfield, C. D.; Peterson, B. A.; McKenna, R. W.; and Edson, J. R.: Acute promyelocytic leukemia: Management of the coagulopathy during daunorubicin-prednisone remission induction. *Arch. Intern. Med.,* **138:**1677–1680, 1978.

Coltman, C. A., Jr.: Treatment related leukemia. In Bloomfield, C. D. (ed.): *Adult Leukemia 1.* Martinus Nijhoff Publishers, The Hague, 1982.

Coltman, C. A., Jr.; Bodey, G. P.; Hewlett, J. S.; Haut, A.; Bickers, J.; Balcerzak, S. P.; Costanzi, J. J.; Freireich, E. J.; McCredie, K. B.; Groppe, C.; Smith, T. L.; and Gehan, E. A.: Chemotherapy of acute leukemia: A comparison of vincristine, cytarabine, and prednisone alone and in combination with cyclophosphamide or daunorubicin. *Arch. Intern. Med.,* **138:**1342–1348, 1978.

Coltman, C. A., Jr., and Dixon, D. O.: Second malignancies complicating Hodgkin's disease: A Southwest Oncology Group 10-year followup. *Cancer Treat. Rep.,* **66:**1023–1033, 1982.

Coltman, C. A., Jr.; Freireich, E. J.; Savage, R. A.; and Gehan, E. A.: Long-term survival of adults with acute leukemia. *Proc. Am. Assoc. Cancer Res. and Am. Soc. Clin. Oncol.,* **20:**389, 1979 (abstract).

Conley, C. L.; Misiti, J.; and Laster, A. J.: Genetic factors predisposing to chronic lymphocytic leukemia and to autoimmune disease. *Medicine* (Baltimore), **59:**323–334, 1980.

Cooper, I. A.; Ding, J. C.; Adams, P. B.; Quinn, M. A.; and Brettell, M.: Intensive leukapheresis in the management of cytopenias in patients with chronic lymphocytic leukaemia (CLL) and lymphocytic lymphoma. *Am. J. Hematol.*, **6**:387–398, 1979.

Costello, C.; Catovsky, D.; O'Brien, M.; and Galton, D. A. G.: Prolymphocytic leukaemia: An ultrastructural study of 22 cases. *Br. J. Haematol.*, **44**:389–394, 1980a.

Costello, C.; Catovsky, D.; O'Brien, M.; Morilla, R.; and Varadi, S.: Chronic T-cell leukemias. I. Morphology, cytochemistry and ultrastructure. *Leuk. Res.*, **4**:463–476, 1980b.

Cramer, E.; Auclair, C.; Hakim, J.; Feliu, E.; Boucherot, J.; Troube, H.; Bernard, J. F.; Bergogne, E.; and Boivin, P.: Metabolic activity of phagocytosing granulocytes in chronic granulocytic leukemia: Ultrastructural observation of a degranulation defect. *Blood*, **50**:93–106, 1977.

Crowther, D.; Beard, M. D. J.; Bateman, C. J. T.; and Sewell, R. L.: Factors influencing prognosis in adults with acute myelogenous leukaemia. *Br. J. Cancer*, **32**:456–464, 1975.

Cunningham, I.; Gee, T.; Dowling, M.; Chaganti, R.; Bailey, R.; Hopfan, S.; Bowden, L.; Turnbull, A.; Knapper, W.; and Clarkson, B.: Results of treatment of Ph¹+ chronic myelogenous leukemia with an intensive treatment regimen (L-5 protocol). *Blood*, **53**:375–393, 1979.

Curtis, J. E.; Hersh, E. M.; and Freireich, E. J.: Leukapheresis therapy of chronic lymphocytic leukemia. *Blood*, **39**:163–175, 1972.

Cuttner, J.; Holland, J. F.; Norton, L.; Ambinder, E. M.; Button, G.; Greenberg, M. L.; and Meyer, R. J.: Therapeutic leukapheresis (TL), cytosine arabinoside (ara-C) and daunorubicin (DNR) in patients with acute myelogenous leukemia (AML) and hyperleukocytosis. Importance of 30% decrement in white blood count (WBC). *Blood*, **58**(Suppl.)**1**:138a, 1981 (abstract).

Dahl, G.; Kalwinsky, D.; McCallister, J.; Abromowitch, M.; and Rivera, G.: Initial therapy with VM-26 plus ARA-C for poor prognosis acute lymphocytic leukemia (ALL). *Proc. Am. Soc. Clin. Oncol.*, **1**:126, 1982 (abstract).

Dawson, D. M.; Rosenthal, D. S.; and Moloney, W. C.: Neurological complications of acute leukemia in adults: Changing rate. *Ann. Intern. Med.*, **79**:541–544, 1973.

Deinhardt, F.: Viral oncology in perspective. In Yohn, D. S., and Blakeslee, J.R. (eds.): *Advances in Comparative Leukemia Research.* Elsevier North-Holland, Inc., New York, 1982.

Dibromomannitol Cooperative Study Group: Survival of chronic myeloid leukaemia patients treated by dibromomannitol. *Eur. J. Cancer*, **9**:583–589, 1973.

Dick, F. R.; Armitage, J. O.; and Burns, C. P.: Diagnostic concurrence in the subclassification of adult acute leukemia using French-American-British criteria. *Cancer*, **49**:916–920, 1982.

Dick, F. R., and Maca, R. D.: The lymph node in chronic lymphocytic leukemia. *Cancer*, **41**:283–292, 1978.

Dicke, K. A.; Zander, A.; Spitzer, G.; Verma, D. S.; Peters, L.; Vellekoop, L.; McCredie, K. B.; and Hester, J.: Autologous bone-marrow transplantation in relapsed adult acute leukaemia. *Lancet*, **1**:514–517, 1979.

Doney, K.; Buckner, C. D.; Sale, G. E.; Ramberg, R.; Boyd, C.; and Thomas, E. D.: Treatment of chronic granulocytic leukemia by chemotherapy, total body irradiation and allogeneic transplantation. *Exp. Hematol.*, **6**:738–747, 1978.

Dosik, G. M.; Barlogie, B.; Smith, T. L.; Gehan, E. A.; Keating, M. J.; McCredie, K. B.; and Freireich, E. J.: Pretreatment flow cytometry of DNA content in adult acute leukemia. *Blood*, **55**:474–482, 1980.

Drapkin, R. L.; Gee, T. S.; Dowling, M. D.; Arlin, Z.; McKenzi, S.; Kempin, S.; and Clarkson, B.: Prophylactic heparin therapy in acute promyelocytic leukemia. *Cancer*, **41**:2484–2490, 1978.

Dutcher, J. P.; Schiffer, C. A.; Wesley, M.; and Wiernik, P. H.: Effect of hyperleukocytosis in acute leukemia on remission rate, duration and survival. *Proc. Am. Soc. Clin. Oncol.*, **1**:491, 1981 (abstract).

Early, A. P.; Preisler, H. D.; Slocum, H.; and Rustum, Y. M.: A pilot study of high-dose 1-β-D-arabinofuranosylcytosine for acute leukemia and refractory lymphoma: Clinical response and pharmacology. *Cancer Res.*, **42**:1587–1594, 1982.

Ellison, R. R., and Glidewell, O.: Improved survival in adults with acute myelocytic leukemia (AML). *Proc. Am. Assoc. Cancer Res. and Am. Soc. Clin. Oncol.*, **21**:161, 1979 (abstract).

Ellison, R. R.; Holland, J. F.; Weil, M.; Jacquillat, C.; Boiron, M.; Bernard, J.; Sawitsky, A.; Rosner, F.; Gussof, B.; Silver, R. T.; Karanas, A.; Cuttner, J.; Spurr, C. L.; Hayes, D. M.; Blom, J.; Leone, L. A.; Haurani, F.; Kyle, R.; Hutchinson, J. L.; Forcier, R. J.; and Moon, J. H.: Arabinosyl cytosine: A useful agent in the treatment of acute leukemia in adults. *Blood*, **32**:507–523, 1968.

Ellison, R. R.; Wallace, H. J.; Hoagland, H. C.; Woolford, D. C.; and Glidewell, O. J.: Prognostic parameters in acute myelocytic leukemia as seen in the Acute Leukemia Group B. In Fliedner, T. M., and Perry, S. (eds.): *Advances in the Biosciences 14, Workshop on Prognostic Factors in Human Acute Leukemia.* Pergamon Press, Inc., New York, 1975.

Enno, A.; Catovsky, D.; O'Brien, M.; Cherchi, M.; Kumaran, T. O.; and Galton, D. A. G.: "Prolymphocytoid" transformation of chronic lymphocytic leukaemia. *Br. J. Haematol.*, **41**:9–18, 1979.

EORTC International Antimicrobial Therapy Project Group: Three antibiotic regimens in the treatment of infection in febrile granulocytopenic patients with cancer. *J. Infect. Dis.*, **137**:14–29, 1978.

Esterhay, R. J., Jr., and Wiernik, P. H.: The therapy of adult acute lymphoblastic leukemia. In Bloomfield, C. D. (ed.): *Adult Leukemias 1.* Martinus Nijhoff Publishers, The Hague, 1982.

Esterhay, R. J., Jr.; Wiernik, P. H.; Grove, W. R.; Markus, S. D.; and Wesley, M. N.: Moderate dose methotrexate, vincristine, asparaginase and dexamethasone for treatment of adult acute leukemia. *Blood*, **59**:334–345, 1982.

Evans, A. E.; Gilbert, E. S.; and Zandstra, R.: The increasing incidence of central nervous system leukemia in children. *Cancer*, **26**:404–409, 1970.

Evensen, S. A., and Stavem, P.: Smouldering acute myelogenous leukemia. *Acta Med. Scand.*, **203**:305–407, 1978.

Fay, J. W.; Moore, J. O.; Logue, G. L.; and Huang, A. T.: Leukapheresis therapy of leukemic reticuloendotheliosis (hairy cell leukemia). *Blood*, **54**:747–749, 1979.

Fefer, A.; Cheever, M. A.; Greenberg, P. D.; Appelbaum, F. R.; Boyd, C. N.; Buckner, C. D.; Kaplan, H. G.; Ramberg, R.; Sanders, J. E.; Storb, R.; and Thomas, E. D.: Treatment of chronic granulocytic leukemia with chemoradiotherapy and transplantation of marrow from identical twins. *N. Eng. J. Med.*, **306**:63–68, 1982.

Fefer, A.; Cheever, M. A.; Thomas, E. D.; Appelbaum, F. R.; Buckner, C. D.; Clift, R. A.; Glucksberg, H.; Greenberg, P. D.; Johnson, F. L.; Kaplan, H. G.; Sanders, J. E.; Storb, R.; and Weiden, P. L.: Bone marrow transplants for refractory acute leukemia in 34 patients with identical twins. *Blood,* **57:**421–430, 1981.

Fialkow, P. J.; Denman, A. M.; Jacobson, R. J.; and Lowenthal, M. N.: Chronic myelocytic leukemia. Origin of some lymphocytes from leukemic stem cells. *J. Clin. Invest.,* **62:**815–823, 1978.

Fialkow, P. J.; Jacobson, R. J.; and Papayannopoulou, T.: Chronic myelocytic leukemia: Clonal origin in a stem cell common to the granulocyte, erythrocyte, platelet and monocyte/macrophage. *Am. J. Med.,* **63:**125–130, 1977.

Fialkow, P. J.; Martin, P. J.; Najfeld, V.; Penfold, G. K.; Jacobson, R. J.; and Hansen, J. A.: Evidence for a multistep pathogenesis of chronic myelogenous leukemia. *Blood,* **58:**158–163, 1981.

First International Workshop on Chromosomes in Leukaemia: Chromosomes in Ph^1-positive chronic granulocytic leukaemia. *Br. J. Haematol.,* **39:**305–309, 1978.

Fleischman, E. W.; Prigogina, E. L.; Volkova, M. A.; Frenkel, M. A.; Zakhartchenko, N. A.; Konstantinova, L. N.; Puchkova, G. P.; and Balakirev, S. A.: Correlations between the clinical course, characteristics of blast cells, and karyotype patterns in chronic myeloid leukemia. *Hum. Genet.,* **58:**285–293, 1981.

Foa, R.; Catovsky, D.; Brozovic, M.; Marsh, G.; Ooyirilangkumaran, T.; Cherchi, M.; and Galton, D. A. G.: Clinical staging and immunological findings in chronic lymphocytic leukemia. *Cancer,* **44:**483–487, 1979.

Foon, K. A., and Gale, R. P.: Controversies in the therapy of acute myelogenous leukemia. *Am. J. Med.,* **72:**963–979, 1982.

Foon, K. A.; Zighelboim, J.; Yale, C.; and Gale, R. P.: Intensive chemotherapy is the treatment of choice for elderly patients with acute myelogenous leukemia. *Blood,* **58:**467–470, 1981.

Foucar, K.; McKenna, R. W.; Bloomfield, C. D.; Bowers, T. K.; and Brunning, R. D.: Therapy-related leukemia: A panmyelosis. *Cancer,* **43:**1285–1296, 1979.

Foucar, K., and Rydell, R. E.: Richter's syndrome in chronic lymphocytic leukemia. *Cancer,* **46:**118–134, 1980.

Frei, E., III; Bicker, J. N.; Hewlett, J. S.; Lane, M.; Leary, W. V.; and Talley, R. W.: Dose schedule and antitumor studies of arabinosyl cytosine (NSC 63878). *Cancer Res.,* **29:**1325–1332, 1969.

Gahrton, G., and Robert, K. H.: Chromosomal aberrations in chronic B-cell lymphocytic leukemia. *Cancer Genet. Cytogenet.,* **6:**171–181, 1982.

Gale, R. P.; Foon, K. A.; Cline, M. J.; Zighelboim, J.; and the UCLA Acute Leukemia Study Group: Intensive chemotherapy for acute myelogenous leukemia. *Ann. Intern. Med.,* **94:**753–757, 1981.

Gallo, R. C.; Poiesz, B. J.; and Ruscetti, F. W.: Regulation of human T-cell proliferation: T-cell growth factor and isolation of a new class of type-C retroviruses from human T-cells. In Neth, R.; Gallo, R. C.; Graf, T.; Mannweiler, K.; and Winkler, K. (eds.): *Modern Trends in Human Leukemia IV.* Springer-Verlag New York, Inc., New York, 1981.

Gallo, R. C.; Wong-Staal, F.; and Ruscetti, F.: Viruses and adult leukemia-lymphoma of man and relevant animal models. In Bloomfield, C. D. (ed.): *Adult Leukemias 1.* Martinus Nijhoff Publishers, The Hague, 1982.

Galton, D. A. G.; Goldman, J. M.; Wiltshaw, E.; Catovsky, D.; Henry, K.; and Goldenberg, G. J.: Prolymphocytic Leukaemia. *Br. J. Haematol.,* **27:**7–23, 1974.

Garay, G.; Pavlovsky, S.; Eppinger-Helft, M.; Cavagnaro, F.; Saslavsky, J.; and Dupont, J.: Long-term survival in acute lymphoblastic leukemia. Evaluation of prognostic factors. *Proc. Am. Soc. Clin. Oncol.,* **1:**137, 1982 (abstract).

Geary, C. G.; Benn, R. T.; and Leck, I.: Incidence of myeloid leukaemia in Lancashire. *Lancet,* **2:**549–551, 1979.

Gee, T. S.; Haghbin, M.; Dowling, M. D., Jr.; Cunningham, I.; Middleman, M. P.; and Clarkson, B. D.: Acute lymphoblastic leukemia in adults and children: Differences in response with similar therapeutic regimens. *Cancer,* **37:**1256–1264, 1976.

Gehan, E. A.; Smith, T. L.; Freireich, E. J.; Bodey, G.; Rodriguez, V.; Speer, J.; and McCredie, K.: Prognostic factors in acute leukemia. *Semin. Oncol.,* **3:**271–282, 1976.

George, S. L.; Aur, R. J. A.; Mauer, A. M.; and Simone, J. V.: A reappraisal of the results of stopping therapy in childhood leukemia. *N. Engl. J. Med.,* **300:**269–273, 1979.

Glicksman, A. S.; Pajak, T. F.; Gottlieb, A.; Nissen, N.; Stutzman, L.; and Cooper, M. R.: Second malignant neoplasms in patients successfully treated for Hodgkin's disease: A Cancer and Leukemia Group B Study. *Cancer Treat. Rep.,* **66:**1035–1044, 1982.

Glucksberg, H.; Buckner, C. D.; Fefer, A.; DeMarsh, Q.; Coleman, D.; Dobrow, R. B.; Huff, J.; Kjobech, C.; Hill, A. S.; Dittman, W.; Neiman, P. E.; Cheever, M. A.; Einstein, A. B., Jr.; and Thomas, E. D.: Combination chemotherapy for acute nonlymphoblastic leukemia in adults. *Cancer Chemother. Rep.,* **59:**1131–1137, 1975.

Golde, D. W.; Saxon, A.; and Stevens, R. H.: Macroglobulinemia and hairy-cell leukemia. *N. Engl. J. Med.,* **296:**92–93, 1977.

Goldfinger, D.; Capostagno, V.; Lowe, C.; Sacks, H. J.; and Gatti, R. A.: Use of long-term leukapheresis in the treatment of chronic lymphocytic leukemia. *Transfusion,* **20:**450–454, 1980.

Goldman, J. M.; Catovsky, D.; Goolden, A. W. G.; Johnson, S. A.; and Galton, D. A. G.: Buffy coat autografts for patients with chronic granulocytic leukaemia in transformation. *Blut,* **42:**149–155, 1981.

Golomb, H. M.: Chromosome abnormalities in adult acute leukemias: Biologic and therapeutic significance. In Bloomfield, C. D. (ed.): *Adult Leukemias 1.* Martinus Nijhoff Publishers, The Hague, 1982.

Golomb, H. M.; Catovsky, D.; and Golde, D. W.: Hairy cell leukemia. A clinical review based on 71 cases. *Ann. Intern. Med.,* **89:**677–683, 1978a.

Golomb, H. M., and Mintz, U.: Treatment of hairy cell leukemia (leukemic reticuloendotheliosis) II. Chlorambucil therapy in postsplenectomy patients with progressive disease. *Blood,* **54:**305–309, 1979.

Golomb, H. M.; Rowley, J. D.; Vardiman, J. W.; Testa, J. R.; and Butler, A.: 'Microgranular' acute promyelocytic leukemia: A distinct clinical, ultrastructural, and cytogenetic entity. Blood, **55:**253–259, 1980.

Golomb, H. M.; Vardiman, J. W.; Rowley, J. D.; Testa, J. R.; and Mintz, U.: Correlation of clinical findings with quinacrine-banded chromosomes in 90 adults with acute nonlymphocytic leukemia: An eight-year study (1970–1977). *N. Engl. J. Med.,* **299:**613–619, 1978b .

Gomez, G. A.; Sokal, J. E.; and Walsh, D.: Prognostic

features at diagnosis of chronic myelocytic leukemia. *Cancer,* **47:**2470–2477, 1981.

Gottlieb, A. J., and Weinberg, V.: Efficacy of daunorubicin in induction therapy of adult acute lymphocytic leukemia (ALL): A controlled phase III study (CALGB #7612). *Blood,* **54:**188a, 1979.

Gourdin, M. F.; Farcet, J. P.; and Reyes, F.: The ultrastructural localization of immunoglobulins in human B cells of immunoproliferative diseases. *Blood,* **59:**1132–1140, 1982.

Gralnick, H. R.; Harbor, J.; and Vogel, C.: Myelofibrosis in chronic granulocytic leukemia. *Blood,* **37:**152–162, 1971.

Greaves, M. F.: Analysis of the clinical and biological significance of lymphoid phenotypes in acute leukemia. *Cancer Res.,* **41:**4752–4766, 1981.

Greaves, M. F.; Verbi, W.; Reeves, B. R.; Hoffbrand, A. V.; Drysdale, H. C.; Jones, L.; Sacker, L. S.; and Samaratunga, I.: "Pre-B" phenotypes in blast crisis of Ph[1] positive CML: Evidence for a pluripotential stem cell "target". *Leuk. Res.,* **3:**181–191, 1979.

Greenberg, B. R.; Wilson, F. D.; Woo, L.; and Jenks, H. M.: Cytogenetics of fibroblastic colonies in Ph[1] positive chronic myelogenous leukemia. *Blood,* **51:**1039–1044, 1978.

Greene, M. H.; Hoover, R. N.; and Fraumeni, J. F.: Subsequent cancer in patients with chronic lymphocytic leukemia—a possible immunologic mechanism. *J.N.C.I.,* **61:**337–340, 1978.

Griffin, J. D.; Ritz, J.; Nadler, L. M.; and Schlossman, S. F.: Expression of myeloid differentiation antigens or normal and malignant myeloid cells. *J. Clin. Invest.,* **68:**932–941, 1981.

Groopman, J. E.: The pathogenesis of myelofibrosis in myeloproliferative disorders (editorial). *Ann. Intern. Med.,* **92:**857–858, 1980.

Gurwith, M.; Brunton, J. L.; Lank, B. A.; Ronald, A. R.; Harding, G. K. M.; and McCullough, D. W.: Granulocytopenia in hospitalized patients. II. A prospective comparison of two antibiotic regimens in the empiric therapy of febrile patients. *Am. J. Med.,* **64:**127–132, 1978.

Hadlock, D. C.; Fortuny, I. E.; McCullough, J.; and Kennedy, B. J.: Continuous flow centrifuge leukapheresis in the management of chronic myelogenous leukaemia. *Br. J. Haematol.,* **29:**443–453, 1975.

Hagemeijer, A.; Hählen, K.; Sizoo, W.; and Abels, J.: Translocation (9;11)(p21;q23) in three cases of acute monoblastic leukemia. *Cancer Genet. Cytogenet.,* **5:**95–105, 1982.

Hamblin, T., and Hough, D.: Chronic lymphatic leukaemia: Correlation of immunofluorescent characteristics and clinical features. *Br. J. Haematol.,* **36:**359–365, 1977.

Han, T.; Ezdinli, E. Z.; Shimaoka, K.; and Desai, D. V.: Chlorambucil vs. combined chlorambucil-corticosteroid therapy in chronic lymphocytic leukemia. *Cancer,* **31:**502–508, 1973.

Han, T.; Ozer, H.; Bloom, M.; Sagawa. K.; and Minowada, J.: The presence of monoclonal cytoplasmic immunoglobulins in leukemic B cells from patients with chronic lymphocytic leukemia. *Blood,* **59:**435–438, 1982.

Han, T.; Ozer, H.; Henderson, E. S.; Dadey, B.; Nussbaum-Blumenson, A.; and Barcos, M.: Defective immunoregulatory T-cell function in chronic lymphocytic leukemia. *Blood,* **58:**1182–1189, 1981.

Hansen, J. A.; Clift, R. A.; Thomas, E. D.; Buckner, C. D.; Storb, R.; and Giblett, E. R.: Transplantation of marrow from an unrelated donor to a patient with acute leukemia. *N. Engl. J. Med.,* **303:**565–567, 1980.

Harousseau, J. L.; Flandrin, G.; Tricot, G.; Brouet, J. C.; Seligmann, M.; and Bernard, J.: Malignant lymphoma supervening in chronic lymphocytic leukemia and related disorders. Richter's syndrome: A study of 25 cases. *Cancer,* **48:**1302–1308, 1981.

Harris, C. C.; Mulvihill, J. J.; Thorgeirsson, S. S.; and Minna, J. D.: Individual differences in cancer susceptibility. *Ann. Intern. Med.,* **92:**809–825, 1980.

Hart, J. S.; George, S. L.; Frei, E., III.; Bodey, G. P.; Nickerson, R. C.; and Freireich, E. J.: Prognostic significance of pretreatment proliferative activity in adult acute leukemia. *Cancer,* **39:**1603–1617, 1977.

Hasegawa, D. K.; Bennett, A. J.; Coccia, P. F.; Ramsay, N. K. C.; Nesbit, M. E.; Krivit, W.; and Edson, J. R.: Factor V deficiency in Philadelphia-positive chronic myelogenous leukemia. *Blood,* **56:**585–595, 1980.

Hasegawa, D. K., and Bloomfield, C. D.: Thrombotic and hemorrhagic manifestations of malignancy. In Yarbro, J., and Bornstein, R. (eds.): *Oncologic Emergencies.* Grune & Stratton, Inc., New York, 1981.

Hauch, T.; Logue, G.; Laszlo, J.; Cox, E.; and Rundles, W.: Treatment of chronic granulocytic leukemia with melphalan. *Blood,* **51:**571–577, 1978.

Heath, C. W., Jr.: Leukemogenesis and low-dose exposure to radiation and chemical agents. In Yohn, D. S., and Blakeslee, J. R. (eds.): *Advances in Comparative Leukemia Research.* Elsevier North-Holland, Inc., New York, 1982a.

Heath, C. W., Jr.: The leukemias. In Schottenfeld, D., and Fraumeni, J. F., Jr., (eds.): *Cancer Epidemiology and Prevention.* W. B. Saunders Company, Philadelphia, 1982b.

Henderson, E. S.: Treatment of acute leukemia. *Ann. Intern. Med.,* **69:**628–632, 1968.

Henderson, E. S.; Scharlau, C.; Cooper, M. R.; Haurani, F. I.; Silver, R. T.; Brunner, K.; Carey, R. W.; Falkson, G.; Blom, J.; Nawab, I.; Levine, A. S.; Bank, A.; Cuttner, J.; Cornwell, G. G., III.; Henry, P.; Nissen, N. I.; Wiernik, P. H.; Leone, L.; Whol, H.; Rai, K.; James, G. W.; Weinberg, V.; Glidewell, O.; and Holland, J. F.: Combination chemotherapy and radiotherapy for acute lymphocytic leukemia in adults: Results of CALGB protocol 7113. *Leuk. Res.,* **3:**395–407, 1979.

Henze, G.; Langermann, H.-J.; Ritter, J.; Schellong, G.; and Riehm, H.: Treatment strategy for different risk groups in childhood acute lymphoblastic leukemia: A report from the BFM Study Group. In Neth, R.; Gallo, R. C.; Graf, T.; Mannweiler, K.; and Winkler, K. (eds.): *Modern Trends in Human Leukemia IV.* Springer-Verlag, Berlin, 1981.

Herzig, R. H.; Herzig, G. P.; Lazarus, H. M.; Wolff, S. N.; and Phillips, G. L.: Successful treatment of patients (pts) with refractory acute nonlymphocytic leukemia (ANLL) using high-dose cytosine arabinoside (HD AraC) with or without anthracycline. *Blood,* **58**(Suppl. 1):141, 1981.

Higby, D. J., and Burnett, D.: Granulocyte transfusions: Current status. *Blood,* **55:**2–8, 1980.

Hirsch, M. S., and Schwartz, M. S.: Antiviral agents. *N. Engl. J. Med.,* **302:**903–907, 949–953, 1980.

Hooper, W. C.; Buss, D. H.; and Parker, C. L.: Leukemic reticuloendotheliosis (hairy cell leukemia): A review of the evidence concerning the immunology and origin of the cell. *Leuk. Res.,* **4:**489–503, 1980.

Hurd, D. D.; Peterson, B. A.; McKenna, R. W.; and Bloomfield, C. D.: VP-16-213 and cyclophosphamide in the treatment of refractory acute nonlymphocytic leukemia with monocytic features. *Med. Pediatr. Oncol.,* **9:**251–255, 1981.

Hurd, D. D.; Vukelich, M.; Arthur, D. C.; Lindquist, L. L.; McKenna, R. W.; Peterson, B. A.; and Bloomfield, C. D.: 15;17 translocation in acute promyelocytic leukemia. *Cancer Genet. Cytogenet.,* **6:**331–337, 1982.

Inoshita, T., and Whiteside, T. L.: Imbalance of T-cell subpopulations does not result in defective helper function in chronic lymphocytic leukemia. *Cancer,* **48:**1754–1760, 1981.

Janossy, G.; Woodruff, R. K.; Pippard, M. J.; Prentice, G.; Hoffbrand, A. V.; Paxton, A.; Lister, T. A.; Bunch, C.; and Greaves, M. F.: Relation of "lymphoid" phenotype and response to chemotherapy incorporating vincristine-prednisolone in the acute phase of Ph^1 positive leukemia. *Cancer,* **43:**426–436, 1979.

Jansen, J.; LeBien, T. W.; and Kersey, J. H.: The phenotype of the neoplastic cells of hairy cell leukemia studied with monoclonal antibodies. *Blood,* **59:**609–614, 1982a.

Jansen, J.; Schuit, H. R. E.; Meijer, C. J. L. M.; van Nieuwkoop, J. A.; and Hijmans, W.: Cell markers in hairy cell leukemia studied in cells from 51 patients. *Blood,* **59:**52–60, 1982b.

Johnson, R. E.: Radiotherapy as primary treatment for chronic lymphocytic leukaemia. *Clin. Haematol.,* **6:**237–244, 1977.

Kaizer, H.; Stuart, R. K.; Colvin, M.; Korbling, M.; Wharam, M. D.; and Santos, G. W.: Autologous bone marrow transplantation in acute leukemia: A pilot study utilizing *in vitro* incubation of autologous marrow with 4-hydroperoxycyclophosphamide (4HC) prior to cryopreservation. *Exp. Hematol.,* **9**(Suppl.):190, 1981 (abstract).

Kay, H. E. M.: Bone marrow transplantation in adult acute leukaemia: Who should be transplanted, and when? In Bloomfield, C. D. (ed.): *Adult Leukemias 1.* Martinus Nijhoff Publishers, The Hague, 1982.

Kay, N. E.; Johnson, J. D.; Stanek, R.; and Douglas, S. D.: T-cell subpopulations in chronic lymphocytic leukemia: Abnormalities in distribution and in *in vitro* receptor maturation. *Blood,* **54:**540–544, 1979.

Keating, M. J.: Early identification of potentially cured patients with acute myelogenous leukemia—a recent challenge. In Bloomfield, C. D. (ed): *Adult Leukemias 1.* Martinus Nijhoff Publishers, The Hague, 1982.

Keating, M. J.; McCredie, K. B.; Benjamin, R. S.; Bodey, G. P.; Zander, A.; Smith, T. L.; and Freireich, E. J.: Treatment of patients over 50 years of age with acute leukemia. A combination of rubidazone and cytosine arabinoside, vincristine, and prednisone (ROAP). *Blood,* **53:**584–591, 1981a.

Keating, M. J.; McCredie, K.; and Freireich, E. J.: Prediction of progression and survival of untreated leukemia. *Proc. Am. Assoc. Cancer Res. and Am. Soc. Clin. Oncol.,* **19:**340, 1978.

Keating, M. J.; Smith, T. L.; McCredie, K. B.; Bodey, G. P.; Hersh, E. M.; Gutterman, J. U.; Gehan, E.; and Freireich, E. J.: A four-year experience with anthracycline, cytosine arabinoside, vincristine and prednisone combination chemotherapy in 325 adults with acute leukemia. *Cancer,* **47:**2779–2788, 1981b.

Kennedy, B. J.: Cyclic leukocyte oscillations in chronic myelogenous leukemia during hydroxyurea therapy. *Blood,* **35:**751–760, 1970.

Kennedy, B. J.: Hydroxyurea therapy in chronic myelogenous leukemia. *Cancer,* **29:**1052–1056, 1972.

Kennedy, B. J.; Smith, L. R.; and Goltz, R. W.: Skin changes secondary to hydroxyurea therapy. *Arch. Dermatol.,* **111:**183–187, 1975.

Kenyon, P. D.; Hurd, D. D.; Peterson, B. A.; McCullough, J.; and Bloomfield, C. D.: Therapeutic leukapheresis (TL) for hyperleukocytosis (HWBC) at diagnosis in acute non-lymphocytic leukemia (ANLL). *Proc. Am. Soc. Clin. Oncol.,* **1:**124, 1982 (abstract).

Kersey, J.; Coccia, P.; Siegel, S.; Bleyer, A.; Sather, H.; Lukens, J.; Gross, S.; and Hammond, D.: The presence of sheep erythrocyte receptors on leukemic lymphoblasts indicates extra medullary origin, lymphomatous presentation, and relapse in extra medullary sites. *Blood,* **58**(Suppl. 1):161a, 1981.

Ketchel, S. J., and Rodriguez, V.: Acute infections in cancer patients. *Semin. Oncol.,* **5:**167–179, 1978.

Kjeldsberg, C. R., and Marty, J.: Prolymphocytic transformation of chronic lymphocytic leukemia. *Cancer,* **48:**2447–2457, 1981.

Klein, G.: The role of gene dosage and genetic transpositions in carcinogenesis. *Nature,* **294:**313–318, 1981a.

Klein, G.: Viruses and cancer. In Burchenal, J. H., and Oettgen, H. F. (eds.): *Cancer: Achievements, Challenges, and Prospects for the 1980s.* Grune & Stratton, Inc., New York, 1981b.

Knospe, W. H.; Loeb, V., Jr.; and Huguley, C. M., Jr.: Bi-weekly chlorambucil treatment of chronic lymphocytic leukemia. *Cancer,* **33:**555–562, 1974.

Knudson, A. G., Jr.: Genetics and cancer. In Burchenal, J. H., and Oettgen, H. F. (eds.): *Cancer: Achievements, Challenges, and Prospects for the 1980s.* Grune & Stratton, Inc., New York, 1981.

Koeffler, H. P., and Golde, D. W.: Chronic myelogenous leukemia — new concepts. *N. Engl. J. Med.,* **304:**1201–1209, 1269–1274, 1981.

Kohno, S.; Abe, S.; and Sandberg, A. A.: The chromosomes and causation of human cancer and leukemia XXXVII. Cytogenetic experience in Ph^1 negative chronic myelogenous leukemia (CML). *Am. J. Hematol.,* **7:**281–291, 1979.

Körbling, M.; Burke, P.; Braine, H.; Elfenbein, G.; Santos, G.; and Kaizer, H.: Successful engraftment of blood derived normal hemopoietic stem cells in chronic myelogenous leukemia. *Exp. Hematol.,* **9:**684–690, 1981.

Korsmeyer, S. J.; Hieter, P. A.; Ravetch, J. V.; Poplack, D. G.; Waldmann, T. A; and Leder, P.: Developmental hierarchy of immunoglobulin gene rearrangements in human leukemic pre-B-cells. *Proc. Natl. Acad. Sci. USA,* **78:**7096–7100, 1981.

LeBien, T. W.; Hozier, J.; Minowada, J.; and Kersey, J. H.: Origin of chronic myelocytic leukemia in a precursor of pre-B lymphocytes. *N. Engl. J. Med.,* **301:**144–147, 1979.

Legha, S. S.; Keating, M. J.; Zander, A. R.; McCredie, K. B.; Bodey, G. P.; and Freireich, E. J.: 4'-(9-Acridinylamino) Methanesulfon-m-Anisidide (AMSA): A new drug effective in the treatment of adult acute leukemia. *Ann. Intern. Med.,* **93:**17–21, 1980.

Liepman, M., and Votaw, M. L.: The treatment of chronic lymphocytic leukemia with COP chemotherapy. *Cancer,* **41:**1664–1669, 1978.

Linos, A.; Kyle, R. A.; Elveback, L. R.; and Kurland, L. T.: Leukemia in Olmstead County, Minnesota, 1965–1974. *Mayo Clin. Proc.,* **53:**714–718, 1978.

Lipshutz, M. D.; Mir, R.; Rai, K. R.; and Sawitsky, A.: Bone marrow biopsy and clinical staging in chronic lymphocytic leukemia. *Cancer,* **46:**1422–1427, 1980.

Lister, T. A.; Whitehouse, J. M. A.; Beard, M. E. J.; Brearley, R. L.; Wrigley, P. F. M.; Oliver, R. T. D.; Freeman, J. E.; Woodruff, R. K.; Malpas, J. S.; Paxton, A. M.; and Crowther, D.: Combination chemotherapy for acute lymphoblastic leukemia in adults. *Br. Med. J.,* **1:**199–203, 1978 .

Louie, S., and Schwartz, R. S.: Immunodeficiency and the pathogenesis of lymphoma and leukemia. *Semin. Hematol.,* **15:**117–138, 1978.

Lowenthal, R. M.; Buskard, N. A.; Goldman, J. M.; Spiers, A. S. D.; Bergier, N.; Graubner, M.; and Galton, D. A. G.: Intensive leukapheresis as initial therapy for chronic granulocytic leukemia. *Blood,* **46:**835–844, 1975.

McGlave, P. B.; Hurd, D. D.; Ramsay, N. K. C.; Arthur, D. C.; Kim, T.; and Kersey, J.: Successful treatment of chronic myelogenous leukemia with allogeneic bone marrow transplantation. *Exp. Hematol.,* **10**(Suppl. 11):**18,** 1982.

McGlave, P. B.; Miller, W. J.; Hurd, D. D.; Arthur, D. C.; and Kim, T.: Cytogenetic conversion following allogeneic bone marrow transplantation for advanced chronic myelogenous leukemia. *Blood,* 1050–1055, 1981.

McKee, L. C., and Collins, R. D.: Intravascular leukocyte thrombi and aggregates as a cause of morbidity and mortality in leukemia. *Medicine,* **53:**463–478, 1974.

McKenna, R. W.; Brynes, R. K.; Nesbit, M. E.; Bloomfield, C. D.; Kersey, J. H.; Spanjers, E.; and Brunning R. D.: Cytochemical profiles in acute lymphoblastic leukemia. *Am. J. Pediatr. Hematol. Oncol.,* **1:**263–275, 1979.

McKenna, R. W.; Parkin, J.; Bloomfield, C. D.; Sundberg, R. D.; and Brunning, R. D.: Acute promyelocytic leukemia (APL): A study of 39 cases with identification of hyperbasophilic microgranular APL variant. *Br. J. Haematol.,* **50:**201–214, 1982.

McKenna, R. W.; Parkin, J.; Kersey, J. H.; Gajl-Peczalska, K. J.; Peterson, L.; and Brunning, R. D.: Chronic lymphoproliferative disorder with unusual clinical, morphologic, ultrastructural and membrane surface marker characteristics. *Am. J. Med.,* **62:**588–596, 1977.

Mahmood, T.; Robinson, W. H.; and Entringer, M.: Autologous bone marrow and peripheral blood buffy coat cell infusion in the treatment of chronic myeloid and acute leukemia. *Exp. Haematol.* 7(Suppl.):321–326, 1979.

Marks, S. M.; Baltimore, D.; and McCaffrey, R.: Terminal transferase as a predictor of initial responsiveness to vincristine and prednisone in blastic crisis chronic myelogeneous leukemia; a co-operative study. *N. Engl. J. Med.,* **298:**812–814, 1978.

Mason, J. E., Jr.; DeVita, V. T.; and Canellos, G. P.: Thrombocytosis in chronic granulocytic leukemia: Incidence and clinical significance. *Blood,* **44:**483–487, 1974.

Matanoski, G. M.: Risk of cancer associated with occupational exposure in radiologists and other radiation workers. In Burchenal, J. H., and Oettgen, H. F. (eds.): *Cancer: Achievements, Challenges, and Prospects for the 1980s.* Grune & Stratton, Inc., New York, 1981.

Mayer, R. J.; Coral, F. S.; Rosenthal, D. S.; Sallan, S. E.; and Frei, E., III: Treatment of non-T, non-B cell acute lymphocytic leukemia (ALL) in adults. *Proc. Am. Soc. Clin. Oncol.,* **1:**126, 1982a (abstract).

Mayer, R. J.; Weinstein, H. J.; Coral, F. S.; Rosenthal, D. S.; and Frei, E., III: The role of intensive post-induction chemotherapy in the management of patients with acute myelogenous leukemia. *Cancer Treat. Rep.,* **66:**1455–1462, 1982b.

Medical Research Council: Chronic granulocytic leukaemia: Comparison of radiotherapy and busulphan therapy. *Br. Med. J.,* **1:**201–208, 1968.

Mertelsmann, R.; Moore, M. A. S.; Broxmeyer, H. E.; Cirrincione, C.; and Clarkson, B.: Diagnostic and prognostic significance of the CFU-c assay in acute nonlymphoblastic leukemia. *Cancer Res.,* **41:**4844–4848, 1981.

Mertelsmann, R.; Moore, M. A. S.; and Clarkson, B.: Leukemia cell phenotype and prognosis: An analysis of 519 adults with acute leukemia. *Blood Cells,* **8:**561–583, 1982.

Mertelsmann, R.; Thaler, H. T.; To, L.; Gee, T. S.; McKenzie, S.; Schauer, P.; Friedman, A.; Arlin, Z.; Cirrincione, C.; and Clarkson, B.: Morphological classification, response to therapy, and survival in 263 adult patients with acute nonlymphoblastic leukemia. *Blood,* **56:**773–781, 1980.

Messner, H. A.; Curtis, J. E.; and Norman, C.: Allogeneic bone marrow transplantation in patients with CML prior to blastic crisis. *Blood,* **58**(Suppl.):175a, 1981 (abstract).

Meyer, R. J.; Ferreira, P. P. C.; Cuttner, J.; Greenberg, M. L.; and Holland, J. F.: Central nervous system involvement at presentation in acute granulocytic leukemia. *Am. J. Med.,* **68:**691–694, 1980.

Miller, D. R.; Leikin, S.; Albo, V.; Vitale, L.; Sather, H.; Coccia, P.; Nesbit, M.; Karon, M.; and Hammond, D.: Use of prognostic factors in improving the design and efficiency of clinical trials in childhood leukemia: Children's Cancer Study Group Report. *Cancer Treat. Rep.,* **64:**381–392, 1980.

Minot, G. R.; Buckman, T. E.; and Isaacs, R.: Chronic myelogenous leukemia: Age incidence, duration, and benefit derived from irradiation. *J.A.M.A.,* **82:**1489–1494, 1924.

Mintz, U. R. I.; Vardiman, J.; Golomb, H. M.; and Rowley, J. D.: Evolution of karyotypes in Philadelphia (Ph¹) chromosome-negative chronic myelogenous leukemia. *Cancer,* **43:**411–416, 1979.

Monfardini, S.; Gee, T.; Fried, J.; and Clarkson, B.: Survival in chronic myelogenous leukemia: Influence of treatment and extent of disease at diagnosis. *Cancer,* **31:**492–501, 1973.

Mulvihill, J. J.: Genetic repertory of human neoplasia. In Mulvihill, J. J.; Miller, R. W.; Fraumeni, J. F., Jr. (eds.): *Genetics of Human Cancer.* Raven Press, New York, 1977.

Nadler, L. M.; Ritz, J.; Griffin, J. D.; Todd, R. F.; Reinherz, E. L.; and Schlossman, S. F.: Diagnosis and treatment of human leukemias and lymphomas utilizing monoclonal antibodies. *Prog. Hematol.,* **12:**187–225, 1982.

Nauseef, W. M., and Maki, D. G.: A study of the value of simple protective isolation in patients with granulocytopenia. *N. Engl. J. Med.,* **304:**448–453, 1981.

Neiman, R. S.; Sullivan, A. L.; and Jaffe, R.: Malignant lymphoma simulating leukemic reticuloendotheliosis. A clinicopathologic study of ten cases. *Cancer,* **43:**329–342, 1979.

Nesbit, M.; Sather, H.; Robison, L.; Ortega, J.; Donaldson, M.; and Hammond, D.: The duration of chemotherapy for childhood acute lymphoblastic leukemia: A randomized study of 316 patients. *Proc. Am. Soc. Clin. Oncol.,* **1**:124, 1982 (abstract).

Netzel, B.; Haas, R. J.; Rodt, H.; Kolb, H. F.; and Thierfelder, S.: Immunological conditioning of bone marrow for autotransplantation in childhood acute lymphoblastic leukemia. *Lancet,* **l**:1330, 1980.

Newburger, P. E.; Latt, S. A.; Pesando, J. M.; Gustashaw, K.; Powers, M.; Chaganti, R. S. K.; and O'Reilly, R. J.: Leukemia relapse in donor cells after allogeneic bonemarrow transplantation. *N. Engl. J. Med.,* **304**:712–714, 1981.

Oken, M. M., and Kaplan M. E.: Combination chemotherapy with cyclophosphamide, vincristine, and prednisone in the treatment of refractory chronic lymphocytic leukemia. *Cancer Treat. Rep.,* **63**:441–447, 1979.

Omura, G. A.; Moffitt, S.; Vogler, W. R.; and Salter, M. M.: Combination chemotherapy of adult acute lymphoblastic leukemia with randomized central nervous system prophylaxis. *Blood,* **55**:199–204, 1980.

Ondreyco, S. M.; Kjeldsberg, C. R.; Fineman, R. M.; Vaninetti, S.; and Kushner, J. P.: Monoblastic transformation in chronic myelogenous leukemia. *Cancer,* **48**:957–963, 1981.

Oshimura, M.; Ohyashiki, K.; Terada, H.; Takaku, F.; and Tonomura, A.: Variant Ph[1] translocations in CML and their incidence, including two cases with sequential lymphoid and myeloid crises. *Cancer Genet. Cytogenet.,* **5**:187–201, 1982.

Paladine, W. J.; Price, L. M.; Williams, H. D.; and Jevtic, M. M.: Hairy-cell leukemia treated with lithium. *N. Engl. J. Med.,* **304**:1237–1238, 1981.

Palmer, M. K.; Hann, I. M.; Jones, P. M.; and Evans, D. I. K.: A score at diagnosis for predicting length of remission in childhood acute lymphoblastic leukemia. *Br. J. Cancer,* **42**:841–849, 1980.

Palutke, M.; Tabaczka, P.; Mirchandani, I.; and Goldfarb, S.; Lymphocytic lymphoma simulating hairy cell leukemia: A consideration of reliable and unreliable diagnostic features. *Cancer,* **48**:2047–2055, 1981.

Pandolfi, F.; De Rossi, G.; Semenzato, G.; Quinti, I.; Ranucci, A.; De Sanctis, G.; Lopez, M.; Gasparotto, G.; and Ajuti, F.: Immunologic evaluation of T chronic lymphocyte leukemia cells: Correlations among phenotype, functional activities, and morphology. *Blood,* **59**:688–695, 1982.

Park, C. H.; Amare, M.; Savin. M. A.; Goodwin, J. W.; Newcomb, M. M.; and Hoogstraten, B.: Prediction of chemotherapy response in human leukemia using an *in vitro* chemotherapy sensitivity test on the leukemic colony-forming cells. *Blood,* **55**:595–601, 1980.

Peterson, B. A.: Acute nonlymphocytic leukemia in the elderly: Biology and treatment. In Bloomfield, C. D. (ed.): *Adult Leukemia 1.* Martinus Nijhoff Publishers, The Hague, 1982.

Peterson, B. A., and Bloomfield, C. D.: Asymptomatic central nervous system (CNS) leukemia in adults with acute non-lymphocytic leukemia (ANLL). *Proc. Am. Assoc. Cancer Res. and ASCO,* **18**:341, 1977 (abstract).

Peterson, B. A., and Bloomfield, C. D.: Long-term disease-free survival in acute nonlymphocytic leukemia. *Blood,* **57**:1144–1147, 1981a.

Peterson, B. A., and Bloomfield, C. D.: Re-induction of complete remissions in adults with acute non-lymphocytic leukemia. *Leuk. Res.,* **5**:81–88, 1981b.

Peterson, B. A., and Bloomfield, C. D.: Acute leukemia in the adult. In Newcom, S. R., and Kadin, M. E. (eds.): *Hematologic Malignancies in the Adult.* Addison-Wesley Publishing Co., Inc., Reading, Massachusetts, 1982.

Peterson, B. A.; Bloomfield, C. D.; Bosl, G. J.; Gibbs, G.; and Malloy, M.: Intensive five-drug combination chemotherapy for adult acute nonlymphocytic leukemia. *Cancer,* **46**:663–668, 1980a.

Peterson, B. A.; Bloomfield, C. D.; Gottlieb, A. J.; Coleman, M.; and Greenberg, M. S.: 5-Azacitidine and zorubicin for patients with previously-treated acute nonlymphocytic leukemia: A Cancer and Leukemia Group B Pilot Study. *Cancer Treat. Rep.,* **66**:563–566, 1982a.

Peterson, B. A.; Bloomfield, C. D.; Theologides, A; and Kennedy, B. J.: Daunorubicin-prednisone in the treatment of acute non-lymphocytic leukemia. *Cancer Treat. Rep.,* **65**(Suppl. 4):29–33, 1981.

Peterson, L. C.; Bloomfield, C. D.; and Brunning, R. D.: Blast crisis as an initial or terminal manifestation of chronic myeloid leukemia: A study of 28 patients. *Am. J. Med.,* **60**:209–220, 1976.

Peterson, L. C.; Bloomfield, C. D.; and Brunning, R. D.: Relationship of clinical staging and lymphocyte morphology to survival in chronic lymphocytic leukaemia. *Br. J. Hematol.,* **45**:563–567, 1980b.

Peterson, L. C.; Bloomfield, C. D.; Sundberg, R. D.; Gajl-Peczalska, K. J.; and Brunning, R. D.: Morphology of chronic lymphocytic leukemia and its relationship to survival. *Am. J. Med.,* **59**:316–324, 1975.

Phillips, E. A.; Kempin, S.; Passe, S.; Mike, V.; and Clarkson, B.; Prognostic factors in chronic lymphocytic leukaemia and their implications for therapy. *Clin. Haematol.* **6**:203–222, 1977.

Pippard, M. J.; Callender, S. T.; and Sheldon, P. W. E.: Infiltration of central nervous system in adult acute myeloid leukemia. *Br. Med. J.,* **1**:227–229, 1979.

Pizzo, P. A.: The value of protective isolation in preventing nosocomial infections in high risk patients. *Am. J. Med.,* **70**:631–637, 1981.

Pizzo, P. A.; Robichaud, K. J.; Gill, F. A.; and Witebsky, F. G.: Empiric antibiotic and antifungal therapy for cancer patients with prolonged fever and granulocytopenia. *Am. J. Med.,* **72**:101–111, 1982.

Pizzo, P. A.; Robichaud, K. J.; Gill, F. A.; Witebsky, F. G.; Levine, A. S.; Deisseroth, A. B.; Glaubiger, D. L.; Maclowry, J. D.; Magrath, I. T.; Poplack, D. G.; and Simon, R. M.: Duration of empiric antibiotic therapy in granulocytopenic patients with cancer. *Am. J. Med.,* **67**:194–200, 1979.

Powles, R. L.; Clink, H. M.; Bandini, G.; Watson, J. G.; Spence, D.; Jameson, B.; Kay, H. E. M.; Morgenstern, G.; Hedley, D.; Lumley, H.; Lawson, D.; Barrett, A.; Lawler, S.; and McElwain, T. J.: The place of bone marrow transplantation in acute myelogenous leukemia. *Lancet,* **1**:1047–1050, 1980.

Preisler, H. D.; Brecher, M.; Browman, G.; Early, A. P.; Walker, I. R.; Raza, A.; and Freeman, A.: Treatment of AML in children and young adults. *Blood,* **58**:149a, 1981 (abstract).

Preisler, H.; Browman, G.; Henderson, E.; Hryniuk, W.; and Freeman, A.: Treatment of acute myelocytic leukemia: Effects of early intensive consolidation. *Proc. Am. Soc. Clin. Oncol.,* **21**:C493, 1980 (abstract).

Pullen, D. J.; Falletta, J. M.; Crist, W. M.; Vogler, L. B.; Dowell, B.; Humphrey, G. B.; Blackstock, R.; van Eys, J.; Cooper, M. D.; Metzger, R. S.; and Meydrech, E. F.: Southwest Oncology Group experience with immunological phenotyping in acute lymphocytic leukemia of childhood. *Cancer Res.,* **41**:4802–4809, 1981.

Rai, K. R.; Holland, J. F.; Glidewell, O. J.; Weinberg, V.; Brunner, K.; Obrecht, J. P.; Preisler, H. D.; Nawabi, I. W.; Prager, D.; Carey, R. W.; Cooper, M. R.; Haurani,

F.; Hutchinson, J. L.; Silver, R. T.; Falkson, G.; Wiernik, P.; Hoagland, H. C.; Bloomfield, C. D.; James, G. W.; Gottlieb, A.; Ramanan, S. V.; Blom, J.; Nissen, N. I.; Bank, A.; Ellison, R. R.; Kung, F.; Henry, P.; McIntyre, O. R.; and Kaan, S. K.: Treatment of acute myelocytic leukemia: A Study by Cancer and Leukemia Group B. *Blood*, **58**:1203–1212, 1981.

Rai, K. R.; Sawitsky, A.; Cronkite, E. P.; Chanana, A. D.; Levy, R. N.; and Pasternack, B. S.: Clinical staging of chronic lymphocytic leukemia. *Blood*, **46**:219–234, 1975.

Ramseur, W. L.; Golomb, H. M.; Vardiman, J. W.; Oleske, D.; and Collins, J. L.: Hairy cell leukemia in father and son. *Cancer*, **48**:1825–1829, 1981.

Rees, J. K. H., and Hayhoe, F. G. J.: D. A. T. (daunorubicin, cytarabine, 6-thioguanine) in acute myeloid leukaemia. *Lancet*, **1**:1360–1361, 1978.

Rees, J. K. H.; Sandler, R. M.; Challenger, J.; and Hayhoe, F. G. J.: Treatment of acute myeloid leukaemia with a triple cytotoxic regime: DAT. *Br. J. Cancer*, **36**:770–776, 1977.

Reinherz, E. L.; Nadler, L. M.; Rosenthal, D. S.; Moloney, W. C.; and Schlossman, S. F.: T-cell-subset characterization of human T-CLL. *Blood*, **53**:1066–1075, 1979.

Reisner, Y.; Kirkpatrick, D.; Dupont, B.; Kapoor, N.; Pollack, M. S.; Good, R. A.; and O'Reilly, R. J.: Transplantation for acute leukaemia with HLA-A and B nonidentical parenteral marrow cells fractionated with soy bean agglutinin and sheep red blood cells. *Lancet*, **2**:327–331, 1981.

Richards, F., II.; Spurr, C. L.; Ferree, C.; Blake, D. D.; and Raben, M.: The control of chronic lymphocytic leukemia with mediastinal irradiation. *Am. J. Med.*, **64**:947–1054, 1978.

Ritz, J.; Sallan, S. E.; Bast, R. E.; Lipton, J. M.; Nathan, D. G.; and Schlossman, S. F.: Autologous bone marrow transplantation in CALLA positive ALL following *in vitro* treatment with J5 monoclonal antibody and complement. *Blood*, **58**(Suppl.):175a, 1981 (abstract).

Ritz, J., and Schlossman, S. F.: Utilization of monoclonal antibodies in the treatment of leukemia and lymphoma. *Blood*, **59**:1–11, 1982.

Rivera, G.; Bowman, P.; Ochs, J.; Abromowitch, M.; and Pui, C. H.: Cyclic combination chemotherapy for recurrent childhood lymphocytic leukemia (ALL) after elective cessation of therapy. *Proc. Am. Soc. Clin. Oncol.*, **1**:126, 1982 (abstract).

Robert-Guroff, M.; Nakao, Y.; Notake, K.; Ito, Y.; Sliski, A.; and Gallo, R. C.: Natural antibodies to human retrovirus HTLV in a cluster of Japanese patients with adult T cell leukemia. *Science*, **215**:975–978, 1982.

Robison, L. L.; Nesbit, M. E.; Sather, H. N.; Hammond, G. D.; and Coccia, P. F.: Assessment of the interrelationship of prognostic factors in childhood acute lymphoblastic leukemia. A report from Childrens Cancer Study Group. *Am. J. Pediatr. Hematol. Oncol.*, **2**:5–13, 1980.

Rosenblum, D., and Petzold, S. J.: Neutrophil alkaline phosphatase: Comparison of enzymes from normal subjects and patients with polycythemia vera and chronic myelogenous leukemia. *Blood*, **45**:335–343, 1975.

Rosenthal, S.; Canellos, G. P.; DeVita, V. T., Jr.; and Gralnick, H. R.: Characteristics of blast crisis in chronic granulocytic leukemia. *Blood*, **49**:705–714, 1977a.

Rosenthal, S.; Canellos, G. P.; and Gralnick, H. R.: Erythroblastic transformation of chronic granulocytic leukemia. *Am. J. Med.*, **63**:116–124, 1977b.

Rosenthal, S.; Canellos, G. P.; Whang-Peng, J.; and Gralnick, H. R.: Blast crisis of chronic granulocytic leukemia; morphologic variants and therapeutic implications. *Am. J. Med.*, **63**:542–547, 1977c.

Rosenthal, S.; Schwartz, J. H.; and Canellos, G. P.: Basophilic chronic granulocytic leukemia with hyperhistaminaemia. *Br. J. Haematol.*, **36**:367–372, 1977d.

Rowley, J. D.: Chromosome abnormalities in human acute non-lymphocytic leukemia: Relationship to age, sex, and exposure to mutagens. *Natl. Cancer Inst. Monogr.*, **60**:17–23, 1982.

Rozman, C.; Hernandez-Nieto, L.; Montserrat, E.; and Brugues, R.: Prognostic significance of bone-marrow patterns in chronic lymphocytic leukaemia. *Br. J. Haematol.*, **47**:529–537, 1981.

Rozman, C.; Montserrat, E.; Feliu, E.; Grañena, A.; Marin, P.; Nomdedeu, B.; and Vives Corrons, J. L.: Prognosis of chronic lymphocytic leukemia: A multivariate survival analysis of 150 cases. *Blood*, **59**:1001–1005, 1982.

Rosman, C.; Montserrat, E.; Feliu, E.; and Woessner, S.: Lymphocyte size and survival of patients with chronic lymphocytic leukaemia (B-type). *Scand. J. Haematol.*, **24**:315–320, 1980.

Rubinstein, D. B., and Longo, D. L.: Peripheral destruction of platelets in chronic lymphocytic leukemia: Recognition, prognosis and therapeutic implications. *Am. J. Med.*, **71**:729–732, 1981.

Rudders, R. A., and Howard, J. P.: Clinical and cell surface marker characterization of the early phase of chronic lymphocytic leukemia. *Blood*, **52**:25–35, 1978.

Rudnick, S. A.; Cadman, E. C.; Capizzi, R. L.; Skeel, R. T.; Bertino, J. R.; and McIntosh, S.: High dose cytosine arabinoside (HDARAC) in refractory acute leukemia. *Cancer*, **44**:1189–1193, 1979.

Rundles, R. W., and Moore, J. O.: Chronic lymphocytic leukemia. *Cancer*, **42**:941–945, 1978.

Sackmann-Muriel, F.; Bustelo, P.; Pavlovsky, S.; Eppinger-Helft, M.; Svarch, E.; Braier, J. L.; Garay, G.; Vergara, B.; Birman, V.; Penalver, J.; Kvicala, R.; Divito, J.; Failace, R.; and Dibar, E.: Tratamiento de la leucemia linfoblastica aguda. Resultados en 1192 enfermos. *Medicina* (B. Aires), **41**:5–14, 1981.

Said, J. W., and Pinkus, G. S.: Immunologic characterization and ultrastructural correlations for 125 cases of B- and T-cell leukemias: Studies of chronic and acute lymphocytic, prolymphocytic, lymphosarcoma cell and hairy cell leukemia, Sézary's syndrome, and other lymphoid leukemias. *Cancer*, **48**:2630–2642, 1981.

Sallan, S. E.; Ritz, J.; Pesando, J.; Gelber, R.; O'Brien, C.; Hitchcock, S.; Coral, F.; and Schlossman, S. F.: Cell surface antigens: Prognostic implications in childhood acute lymphoblastic leukemia. *Blood*, **55**:395–402, 1980.

Sandberg, A. A.; Kohno, S.; Wake, N.; and Minowada, J.: Chromosomes and causation of human cancer and leukemia. XLII. Ph¹-positive ALL: An entity within myeloproliferative disorders. *Cancer Genet. Cytogenet.*, **2**:145–174, 1980.

Santoro, A.; Rilke, F.; Franchi, F.; and Monfardini, S.: Primary malignant neoplasms associated with chronic lymphocytic leukemia. *Tumori*, **66**:431–438, 1980.

Sauter, C.; Barrelet, L.; Berchtold, W.; Fopp, M.; Maurice, P.; Tschopp, L.; and Cavalli, F.: No advantage of maintenance treatment (MT) in acute myelogenous leukemia (AML) after intensive early consolidation (EC). *Proc. Am. Soc. Clin. Oncol.*, **1**:128, 1982 (abstract).

Sawitsky, A.; Rai, K. R.; Aral, I.; Silver, R. T.; Glicksman,

A. S.; Carey, R. W.; Scialla, S.; Cornell, C. J., Jr.; Seligan, B.; and Shapiro, L.: Mediastinal irradiation for chronic lymphocytic leukemia. *Am. J. Med.,* **61**:892–896, 1976.

Sawitsky, A.; Rai, K. R.; Glidewell, O.; Silver, R. T.; and CALGB: Comparison of daily versus intermittent chlorambucil and prednisone therapy in the treatment of patients with chronic lymphocytic leukemia. *Blood,* **50**:1049–1059, 1977.

Schiffer, C. A.; Aisner, J.; Daly, P. A.; and Wiernik, P. H.: Increased leukocyte alkaline phosphatase activity following transfusion of leukocytes from a patient with chronic myelogenous leukemia. *Am. J. Med.,* **66**:519–522, 1979.

Schiffer, C. A.; DeBellis, R.; Kasdorf, H.; and Wiernik, P. H.: Treatment of the blast crisis of chronic myelogenous leukemia with 5-azacitidine and VP-16-213. *Cancer Treat. Rep.,* **66**:267–271, 1982.

Schimpff, S. C.: Infection prevention during granulocytopenia. In Remington, J. S., and Swartz, M. N. (eds.): *Current Clinical Topics in Infectious Disease.* McGraw-Hill, Inc., New York, 1980.

Schubach, W. H.; Hackman, R.; Neiman, P. E.; Miller, G.; and Thomas, E. D.: A monoclonal immunoblastic sarcoma in donor cells bearing Epstein-Barr virus genomes following allogeneic marrow grafting for acute lymphoblastic leukemia. *Blood,* **60**:180–187, 1982.

Schwartz, J. H., and Canellos, G. P.: Hydroxyurea in the management of the hematologic complications of chronic granulocytic leukemia. *Blood,* **46**:11–16, 1975.

Secker-Walker, L. M.; Lawler, S. D.; and Hardisty, R. M.: Prognostic implications of chromosomal findings in acute lymphoblastic leukaemia at diagnosis. *Br. Med. J.,* **2**:1529–1530, 1978.

Semenzato, G.; Pezzutto, A.; Agostini, C.; Albertin, M.; and Gasparotto, G.: T-lymphocyte subpopulations in chronic lymphocytic leukemia: A quantitative and functional study. *Cancer,* **48**:2191–2197, 1981.

Silverberg, E.: Cancer statistics, 1982. *CA,* **32**:15–42, 1982.

Singer, J. W.; Fialkow, P. J.; Steinmann, L.; Najfeld, V.; Stein, S. J.; and Robinson, W. A.: Chronic myelocytic leukemia (CML): Failure to detect residual normal committed stem cells *in vitro. Blood,* **53**:264–268, 1979.

Skipper, H. E.; Schabel, F. M., Jr.; and Wilcox, W. S.: Experimental evaluation of potential anticancer agents. XXI. Scheduling of arabinosylcytosine to take advantage of its S-phase specificity against leukemic cells. *Cancer Chemother. Rep.,* **51**:125–165, 1967.

Smalley, R. V.; Vogel, J.; Huguley, C. M.; and Miller, D.: Chronic granulocytic leukemia: Cytogeneic conversion of the bone marrow with cycle specific chemotherapy. *Blood,* **50**:107–113, 1977.

Sobol, R. E.; Dillman, R. O.; Beauregard, J. C.; Yu, A. L.; Lea, J. W.; Collins, H.; Wormsley, S.; Green, M. R.; Ellison, R. R.; and Royston, I.: Clinical utility of monoclonal antibodies in the phenotyping of acute and chronic lymphocytic leukemia. In Peters, H. (ed.): *Protides of the Biologic Fluids: Proc. of 30th Colloquium.* Vol. 30, pp. 417–422. Pergamon Press, Oxford, 1983.

Sokal, J. E.: Evaluation of survival data for chronic myelocytic leukemia. *Am. J. Hematol.,* **1**:493–500, 1976.

Spiers, A. S. D.: Annotation: Metamorphosis of chronic granulocytic leukaemia: Diagnosis, classification and management. *Br. J. Haematol.,* **41**:1–7, 1979.

Spiers, A. S. D.; Bain, B. J.; and Turner, J. E.: The peripheral blood in chronic granulocytic leukaemia. Study of 50 untreated Philadelphia positive cases. *Scand. J. Haematol.,* **18**:25–38, 1977a.

Spiers, A. S. D.; Goldman, J. M.; Catovsky, D.; Costello, C.; Buskard, N. A.; and Galton, D. A. G.: Multiple drug chemotherapy for acute leukemia: The TRAMPCOL regimen: Results in 86 patients. *Cancer,* **40**:20–29, 1977b.

Stewart, D. J.; Benjamin, R. S.; McCredie, K. B.; Murphy, S.; and Keating, M.: The effectiveness of rubidazone in hairy cell leukemia (leukemic reticuloendotheliosis). *Blood,* **54**:298–304, 1979.

Stoll, C.; Oberling, F.; and Flori, E.: Chromosome analysis of spleen and/or lymph nodes of patients with chronic myeloid leukemia (CML). *Blood,* **52**:828–838, 1978.

Strauss, R. G.; Connett, J. E.; Gale, R. P.; Bloomfield, C. D.; Herzig, G. P.; McCullough, J.; Maguire, L. C.; Winston, D. J.; Ho, W.; Stump, D. C.; Miller, W. V.; and Koepke, J. A.: A controlled trial of prophylactic granulocyte transfusions during initial induction chemotherapy for acute myelogenous leukemia. *N. Engl. J. Med.,* **305**:597–603, 1981.

Sultan, C.; Deregnaucort, J.; Ko, Y. W.; Imbert, M.; D'Agay, M. F. R.; Gouault-Heilmann, M.; and Brun, B.: Distribution of 250 cases of acute myeloid leukaemia (AML) according to the FAB classification and response to therapy. *Br. J. Haematol.,* **47**:545–551, 1981.

Sweet, D. L., Jr.; Golomb, H. M.; and Ultmann, J. E.: The clinical features of chronic lymphocytic leukaemia. *Clin. Haematol.,* **6**:185–201, 1977.

Tatsumi, E.; Sugimoto, T.; Sagawa, K.; Minato, K.; Srivastava, B. I. S.; Han, T.; Ozer, H.; Preisler, H.; Freeman, A. I.; Henderson, E. S.; and Minowada, J.: Membrane phenotyping of human leukemias by murine monoclonal hybridoma antibodies: Comparative studies between 55 leukemia cell lines and 88 fresh leukemias. In Yohn, D. S., and Blakeslee, J. R. (eds.): *Advances in Comparative Leukemia Research 1981.* Elsevier North-Holland, Inc., New York, 1982.

Taylor, H. G.; Butler, W. M;, Rhoads, J.; Karcher, D. S.; and Detrick-Hooks, B.: Prolymphocytic leukemia: Treatment with combination chemotherapy to include doxorubicin. *Cancer,* **49**:1524–1529, 1982.

The Third International Workshop on Chromosomes in Leukemia. *Cancer Genet. Cytogenet.,* **4**:95–142, 1981.

Theologides, A.: Unfavorable signs in patients with chronic myelocytic leukemia. *Ann. Intern. Med.,* **76**:95–99, 1972.

Thiel, E.; Rodt, H.; Huhn, D.; Netzel, B.; Grosse-Wilde, H.; Ganeshaguru, K.; and Thierfelder, S.: Multimarker classification of acute lymphoblastic leukemia: Evidence for further T subgroups and evaluation of their clinical significance. *Blood,* **56**:759–772, 1980.

Third National Cancer Survey: Incidence data. In Cutler, S. J., and Young, J. L., Jr. (eds): *Natl. Cancer Inst. Monogr.,* **41**:1–454, 1975.

Thomas, E. D.; Buckner, C. D.; Banaji, M.; Clift, R. A.; Fefer, A.; Flournoy, N.; Goodell, B. W.; Hickman, R. O.; Lerner, K. G.; Neiman, P. E.; Sale, G. E.; Sanders, J. E.; Singer, J.; Stevens, M.; Storb, R.; and Weiden, P. L.: One hundred patients with acute leukemia treated by chemotherapy, TBI, and allogeneic marrow transplantation. *Blood,* **49**:511–533, 1977.

Thomas, E. D.; Buckner, C. D.; Clift, R. A.; Fefer, A.; Johnson, F. L.; Neiman, P. E.; Sale, G. E.; Sanders, J. E.; Singer, J. W.; Shulman, H.; Storb, R.; and Weiden, P. L.: Marrow transplantation for acute nonlymphoblastic leukemia in first remission. *N. Engl. J. Med.,* **301:**597–599, 1979a.

Thomas, E. D.; Sanders, J. E.; and Flournoy, N.: Marrow transplantation for patients with acute lymphoblastic leukemia in remission. *Blood,* **54:**468–476, 1979b.

Trump, D. L.; Mann, R. B.; Phelps, R.; Roberts, H.; and Conley, C. L.: Richter's syndrome: Diffuse histiocytic lymphoma in patients with chronic lymphocytic leukemia. A report of five cases and review of the literature. *Am. J. Med.,* **68:**539–548, 1980.

Uchiyama, T.; Yodoi, J.; Sagawa, K.; Takatsuki, K.; and Uchino, H.: Adult T-cell leukemia: Clinical and hematologic features of 16 cases. *Blood,* **50:**481–492, 1977.

UCLA Bone Marrow Transplantation Group: Bone marrow transplantation with intensive combination chemotherapy/radiation therapy (SCARI) in acute leukemia. *Ann. Inter Med.,* **86:**155–161, 1977.

Upton, A. C.: Radiation hazards. In Burchenal, J. H., and Oettgen, H. F. (eds.): *Cancer: Achievements, Challenges, and Prospects for the 1980s.* Grune & Stratton, Inc., New York, 1981.

Uzuka, Y.; Liong, S. K.; and Yamagata, S.: Treatment of adult acute nonlymphoblastic leukemia using intermittent combination chemotherapy with daunomycin, cytosine arabinoside, 6-mercaptopurine, and prednisolone-DCMP two step therapy. *Tohoku J. Exp. Med.,* **118:**217–225, 1976.

Vallejos, C. S.; McCredie, K. B., Button, G. M.; and Freireich, E. J.: Biologic effects of repeated leukapheresis of patients with chronic myelogenous leukemia. *Blood,* **42:**925–933, 1973.

Vardiman, J. W.; Golomb, H. M.; Rowley, J. D.; and Variakojis, D.: Acute non-lymphocytic leukemia in malignant lymphoma: A morphologic study. *Cancer,* **42:**229–242, 1978.

Vardiman, J. W.; Variakojis, D.; and Golomb, H. M.: Hairy cell leukemia. *Cancer,* **43:**1339–1349, 1979.

Vaughan, W. P.; Karp, J. E.; and Burke, P. J.: Long chemotherapy-free remissions after single-cycle timed-sequential chemotherapy for acute myelocytic leukemia. *Cancer,* **45:**859–865, 1980.

Vogler, W. R.: Results of randomized trials of immunotherapy for acute leukemia. *Cancer Immunol. Immunother.,* **9:**15–21, 1980.

Vogler, W. R.; Winton, E. F.; Gordon, D. S.; Lefante, J.; and Raney, M.: A randomized trial of post-remission therapy in acute myeloid leukemia. *Proc. Am. Soc. Clin. Oncol.,* **1:**138, 1982 (abstract).

Weil, M.; Jacquillat, C.; Auclerc, M. F.; Schaison, G.; Chastang, C.; and Bernard, J.: Poor-prognosis acute lymphoblastic leukemias. *Recent Results Cancer Res.,* **80:**36–41, 1982.

Weinstein, H. J.; Mayer, R. J.; Rosenthal, D. S.; Camitta, B. M.; Coral, F. S.; Nathan, D. G.; and Frei, E., III: Treatment of acute myelogenous leukemia in children and adults. *N. Engl. J. Med.,* **303:**473–478, 1980.

Weiss, R.: A virus associated with human adult T-cell leukaemia. *Nature,* **294:**212, 1981.

Wiernik, P. H., and Schimpff, S. C.: Therapy for infection in granulocytopenic patients. In Silver, R. T. (ed.): *Clinical Topics in Cancer Diagnosis and Management.* Le Jacq Publishing, Inc., New York, 1982.

Wiernik, P. H.; Schimpff, S. C.; Schiffer, C. A.; Lichtenfeld, J. L.; Aisner, J.; O'Connell, M. J.; and Fortner, C.: Randomized clinical comparison of daunorubicin (NSC-82151) alone with a combination of daunorubicin, cytosine arabinoside (NSC-63878), 6-thioguanine (NSC-752), and pyrimethamine (NSC-3061) for the treatment of acute nonlymphocytic leukemia. *Cancer Treat. Rep.,* **60:**41–53, 1976.

Wiernik, P. H., and Serpick, A. A.: A randomized clinical trial of daunorubicin and a combination of prednisone, vincristine, 6-mercaptopurine, and methotrexate in adult acute nonlymphocytic leukemia. *Cancer Res.,* **32:**2023–2026, 1972.

Willemze, R.; Hillen, H.; Hartgrink-Groeneveld, C. A.; and Haanen, C.: Treatment of acute lymphoblastic leukemia in adolescents and adults: A retrospective study of 41 patients (1970–1973). *Blood,* **46:**823–834, 1975.

Williams, D. L.; Tsiatis, A.; Brodeur, G. M.; Look, A. T.; Melvin, S. L.; Bowman, W. P.; Dahl, G. V.; Kalwinsky, D. K.; and Rivera, G.: Prognostic importance of pretreatment chromosome ploidy in 136 untreated children with acute lymphoblastic leukemia. *Blood,* **58:**156a, 1981 (abstract).

Wiltshaw, E.: Chemotherapy in chronic lymphocytic leukaemia. *Clin. Haematol.,* **6:**223–235, 1977.

Wolf, D. J.; Silver, R. T.; and Coleman, M.: Splenectomy in chronic myeloid leukemia. *Ann. Intern. Med.,* **89:**684–689, 1978.

Wolk, R. W.; Masse, S. R.; Conklin, R.; and Freireich, E. J.: The incidence of central nervous system leukemia in adults with acute leukemia. *Cancer,* **33:**863–869, 1974.

Woods, W. G.; Roloff, J. S.; Lukens, J. N.; and Krivit, W.: The occurrence of leukemia in patients with the Shwachman syndrome. *J. Pediatr.,* **99:**425–428, 1981.

Wright, D. G.; Robichaud, K. J.; Pizzo, P. A.; and Deisseroth, A. B.: Lethal pulmonary reactions associated with the combined use of amphotericin B and leukocyte transfusions. *N. Engl. J. Med.,* **304:**1185–1189, 1981.

Wylin, R. F.; Greene, M. H.; Palutke, M.; Khilanani, P.; Tabaczka, P.; and Swiderski, G.: Hairy cell leukemia in three siblings: An apparent HLA-linked disease. *Cancer,* **49:**538–542, 1982.

Yates, J. W.; Glidewell, O.; Wiernik, P.; and Holland, J. F.: A CALGB study of adriamycin vs daunorubicin induction and a four vs eight week maintenance in acute myelocytic leukemia. *Proc. Am. Assoc. Cancer. Res. and Am. Soc. Clin. Oncol.,* **21:**350, 1980 (abstract).

Yates, J. W.; Wallace, H. J., Jr.; Ellison, R. R.; and Holland, J. F.: Cytosine arabinoside (NSC-63878) and daunorubicin (NSC-83142) therapy in acute non-lymphocytic leukemia. *Cancer Chemother. Rep.,* **57:**485–488, 1973.

Youman, J. D.; Taddeini, L.; and Cooper, T.: Histamine excess symptoms in basophilic chronic granulocytic leukemia. *Arch. Intern. Med.,* **131:**560–562, 1973.

Yunis, J. J.; Bloomfield, C. D.; and Ensrud, K.: All patients with acute nonlymphocytic leukemia may have a chromosomal defect. *N. Engl. J. Med.,* **305:**135–166, 1981.

Zander, A. R.; Vellekoop, L.; Spitzer, G.; Verma, D. S.; Litam, J.; McCredie, K. B.; Keating, M.; Hester, J. P.; and Dicke, K. A.: Combination of high-dose cyclophosphamide, BCNU, and VP-16-213 followed by autologous marrow rescue in the treatment of relapsed leukemia. *Cancer Treat. Rep.,* **65:**377–381, 1981.

Zighelboim, J.; Foon, K.; Yale, C.; and Gale, R. P.: Treatment of acute myelogenous leukemia with intensive induction and consolidation chemotherapy. *Proc. Am. Soc. Clin. Oncol.,* **1:**128, 1982 (abstract).

Zwaan, F. E., and Hermans, J.: Bone marrow transplantation for leukaemia—European results in 264 cases. *Exp. Hematol.,* **10**(Suppl.):64–69, 1982.

19

Polycythemia Vera and Myelofibrosis

EUGENE P. FRENKEL

Introduction

The term myeloproliferative syndrome was popularized by Dameshek (1951) and has since been applied in a generic manner to explain similar clinical and laboratory findings and transitional relationships in polycythemia vera, primary thrombocythemia, and myelofibrosis. Conceptually, these interrelationships were posed by the observation that bone marrow cells in both benign and malignant circumstances of these lesions often proliferate *en masse* rather than as single elements. Thus, although an expansion of the erythron is considered a cardinal finding in polycythemia vera, even early in the clinical course increased proliferation of granulocytes and platelets is seen. Similar patterns of hyperplasia of cellular elements other than platelets occur in primary thrombocythemia, and patterns of hyperplasia of cellular elements other than fibroblasts occur in myelofibrosis. Pure proliferation of one cell type is less common than the nomenclature of the individual diseases suggests. Indeed, the structural changes found in the marrow in each of these entities can appropriately be described as "panmyelosis" to emphasize that hyperplastic changes involve multiple marrow elements. Two other circumstances have increased the use of this generic term. In some cases, particularly when first seen, it is difficult to define the specific subtype (*i.e.,* polycythemia vera, primary thrombocythemia, or myelofibrosis) because of the common clinical and laboratory features. In addition, transitions from one clinical form to another occur frequently enough to further blur specificity of diagnosis in some cases at first presentation. During these transitions it may be difficult to separate benign from their more neoplastic forms (Modan, 1975).

The term "myeloproliferative" has been controversial because each form is associated with clinical entities that are reactive or secondary to some underlying stimulus. Only a modest portion of the cases are associated with an autonomous or unrestricted drive to the cellular expansion that usually characterizes "proliferative" lesions. This semantic argument has even led to the use of the term "myelostimulatory" to circumvent the issue and yet acknowledge the commonality of clinical and laboratory features (Ward and Block, 1971). Because the etiology of none of these lesions is presently known and common aspects of these lesions exist, the use of the generic term "myeloproliferative disorder" appears reasonable and expedient (Laszlo, 1975). Where the clinical features permit an appropriate characterization of the specific diagnostic subtype, that specific term is preferable.

POLYCYTHEMIA VERA

Polycythemia or erythrocytosis is defined as an increased number of circulating red blood cells. Because a variety of altered physiologic states can result in increased red cell production, these "secondary forms" of polycythemia must first be excluded before one can denote polycythemia vera (or primary polycythemia), which indicates an autonomous proliferative abnormality that involves the multipotential stem cell unit and produces an expansion of the erythron.

Incidence and Epidemiology

Much of the data on incidence and demographic characteristics of polycythemia "vera" developed in the era preceding accurate quantification of the size of the red cell mass so that cases of relative polycythemia (*i.e.,* those that were found to have a normal red cell mass and a decreased plasma volume) were included. In addition, many forms of presently recognizable secondary types of polycythemia (*i.e.,* smokers' polycythemia, genetic abnormalities of the hemoglobin molecule, or disorders of erythropoietin production) were also included. Since more specific clinical and laboratory criteria of diagnosis have been applied, accurate information on incidence and the true demographic character is not available. One estimate has suggested an incidence of approximately five per million (Modan, 1965). Most of the described demographic features, such as predominance among Jews and a significantly greater occurrence in Caucasians than Blacks (Wintrobe *et al.,* 1974a), similarly antedate recent criteria of polycythemia vera (Lawrence, 1955). Virtually no data exist concerning the epidemiology of polycythemia vera.

Etiology and Pathogenesis

A better understanding of the pathogenesis of polycythemia vera has resulted from studies of *in vitro* cellular growth patterns (Golde *et al.,* 1981) and the recognition of cellular mosaicism of the expression of the enzyme glucose-6-phosphate dehydrogenase (Fialkow, 1982). The evidence suggests both normal and neoplastic pluripotential stem cells are present in the marrow early in the disease. Similar ratios of neoplastic and normal early progenitor cells and the cell cycle characteristics of the erythroid burst-forming cells (BFU-E) suggest that the events relating to *commitment* for both stem cell populations are the same (Golde *et al.,* 1981). An alteration in erythroid differentiation, however, is known to occur at some point between the erythroid burst-forming (BFU-E) cells and the colony-forming (CFU-E) cells of the normal clone, resulting in reduced production or release of normal erythrocytes to the circulation. Thus, the circulating red cells in patients with polycythemia vera arise largely from a neoplastic clone. The mechanism of inhibition of transition of BFU-E to CFU-E in the normal clone is unknown; nevertheless, it is clearly erythropoietin independent. The pattern of polycythemia is slowly progressive and during the course of the disease a parallel progressive suppression of the BFU-E to CFU-E transition occurs in the normal clone. Late in the course of polycythemia the transition is totally suppressed and all of the circulating cells are from the neoplastic erythroid clone. Because nonerythroid hematopoietic cells are also involved in polycythemia, studies of granulopoiesis in polycythemia vera have been performed and have shown a different mechanism than that found in the red cell clone. Only the neoplastic granulocyte/macrophage colony-forming cells were shown to be in active cell cycle. Thus, in polycythemia vera, all of the circulating granulocytes are from the neoplastic clone. The mechanisms whereby the suppression of the normal committed cell clone occurs are unknown but promise to provide important lessons regarding cellular differentiation.

Pathology and Natural History

Pathology. The primary structural changes in polycythemia vera involve the bone marrow. Nevertheless, no specific histologic changes establish the diagnosis; all of the findings are supportive or confirmatory in the appropriate clinical and laboratory setting. The most consistent findings include hypercellularity of the marrow (biopsy) (Ellis *et al.,* 1975) and an absence of stainable iron (Block and Bethard, 1952; Kurnick *et al.,* 1972). The hypercellularity of the marrow is associated with a great expansion of the erythron, as well as with increased granulocytes and eosinophils. These changes have resulted in the application of the term "panmyelosis" to describe the bone marrow. Megakaryocyte numbers and size are also increased and these changes correlate with the overall marrow cellularity (Ellis *et al.,* 1975). Less commonly seen (in approximately 15% of the cases) is increased reticulum in the marrow. When present, the myelofibrosis is generally not associated with disruption or replacement of the marrow, nor with peripheral blood evidence of extramedullary hematopoiesis (Ellis *et al.,* 1975). Further evidence of the "panmyelosis" is that active bone marrow can be found in areas of the axial skeleton that usually consist of fat spaces.

Late in the course of the disease extramedullary hematopoiesis may be seen. Although splenomegaly is commonly recognized early in the course of the disease (Gilbert, 1975), the histologic changes in the spleen are those of congestion until late in the disease when trilineage (extramedullary) hematopoiesis may be found. Similar changes of congestion and reticular endothelial hyperplasia may be found in the liver, particularly early in the clinical course; and, in time, extramedullary hematopoiesis may be recognized in the liver as it is in the spleen and even lymph nodes.

Natural History. Polycythemia vera is considered a chronic disorder, yet if untreated, approximately 50% of the patients will be dead at 18 months (Gilbert, 1975). Treatment intervention has prolonged that survival: 50% of the patients treated with only phlebotomy survive three to eight years. The application of myelosuppressive therapy has further improved survival to approximately 12 to 14 years (Lawrence, 1955).

Wasserman (1954, 1976) has clarified a pattern of "stages" or phases during the course of polycythemia vera. Although these stages are not crisply demarcated, they provide reference points for the consideration of those clinical problems that relate to the changing status of the disease. During the earliest stage of the disease, the "developmental stage," clearly evident erythrocytosis may not be identified and major complications do not occur unless thrombocythemia is present. Trivial symptoms, such as post-bathing pruritus, may be the only clinical features. The "erythrocytic stage" is thus clearly identifiable as one with increased red cell values and the clinical problems seen are the result of the increased red cell mass (*e.g.,* increased whole blood viscosity). Other changes that affect survival during this stage include thrombocytosis with thrombohemorrhagic phenomena. In time, the polycythemia gives way to a slowly progressive and symptomatic anemia and progressive splenomegaly is seen. This stage has been labeled the "spent phase" of polycythemia (Najean *et al.,* 1984) or, more appropriately, postpolycythemic myeloid metaplasia (Silverstein, 1976). This stage has many features of myelofibrosis, but with a somewhat more acute course. Finally, a leukemic stage (generally acute granulocytic leukemia) may occur. This final stage of polycythemia may result whether or not mitogenic therapeutic interventions have been used (Modan, 1975).

Special Problems Altering Natural History

Surgery. Patients with polycythemia vera subjected to operative procedures have greater morbidity and mortality than expected (Lawrence, 1955). Wasserman (1976) and Gilbert (1975) have described an 83% incidence of surgical complications in patients whose hemoglobin or packed red cell volume (or both) was greater than normal at the time of operation. These risks were considerably less (21%) when the peripheral red cell values were reduced to normal prior to the operation. The more effective and prolonged is control of the polycythemia, the more closely does the patient resemble a routine operative candidate. These observations urge caution in the approach to elective surgical procedures and emphasize the value of achieving good control of the polycythemia state prior to any invasive procedures (Wasserman, 1976; Gilbert, 1975). It is of particular importance that the increased risks of surgery correlate with the red cell values rather than any other feature or aspect.

Hyperuricemia. Increased uric acid production results from the expanded cell mass characteristic of polycythemia. Evidence of hyperuricemia and hyperuricosuria, as well as clinically symptomatic gout, may be seen even during the developmental stage of polycythemia vera. Gout and the potential for urate nephropathy represent special therapeutic problems during the course of the disease.

Symptoms and Signs

The clinical events in polycythemia vera are largely the result of an increased circulating red cell mass and expanded plasma volume. The symptoms at presentation usually have an insidious onset. The complaints reflect the cellular contribution to an increased whole blood viscosity and include headaches, visual disturbances, and dizziness or vertigo. Vascular sequelae range from plethora to clinical hypertension or virtually any form of arterial or venous occlusive lesion. Cerebrovascular thrombohemorrhagic events are more common than coronary artery occlusions (Gilbert, 1975).

Symptoms associated with bleeding are common. In general, the bleeding suggests a capillary lesion or a functional platelet defect resulting in epistaxis, superficial ecchymoses, or mucosal bleeding, primarily in the gastrointestinal tract.

Pruritus, particularly post-bathing pruritus, is commonly described by patients with polycythemia vera. The pruritus and an increased incidence of peptic ulcer disease have been related to increased histamine production and release associated with the expanded basophil cell mass seen in the panmyelosis of polycythemia vera (Brandt *et al.*, 1964).

Physical examination commonly reveals plethora of the skin, conjunctivae, and mucous membranes. Splenomegaly has been identified in approximately 75% of patients and hepatomegaly in about 50%. Both organs increase in size during the course of the disease.

Diagnosis

Absolute morphologic criteria do not exist to establish the diagnosis of polycythemia vera. The diagnosis is made on the grounds of a constellation of clinical and laboratory findings after identifiable causes for erythrocytosis are shown not to exist. The common basis for initial clinical evaluation of a patient with polycythemia vera is the recognition of increased peripheral red cell values (venous hematocrits in excess of 48 vol % in women and 52 vol % in men). Because the differential diagnosis of erythrocytosis includes the common circumstance of relative polycythemia, measurement of the red cell mass (Frenkel and McCall, 1978) should be done. This will identify those patients with a normal red cell mass and a constricted plasma volume (either acute or chronic) that results in an apparent increase in the peripheral venous hematocrit seen in relative polycythemia. True polycythemia can be defined by a measured red cell mass of greater than 36 mL/kg in men and 32 mL/kg in women (Berlin, 1975). A more appropriate way to express the range of normal for the measured red cell mass and/or plasma volume is to do so on the basis of surface area, because values expressed by weight apply only to those adults with a normal body habitus (Frenkel *et al.*, 1972).

In those individuals with an increase in red cell mass (true polycythemia), a variety of mechanisms capable of producing this change must be evaluated before a diagnosis of polycythemia vera can be considered (Erslev and Caro, 1984). Hypoxemia is the most common cause for erythrocytosis. Several mechanisms of "secondary" (hypoxic) polycythemia must be considered: (1) If the measured arterial oxygen saturation is less than 92%, the most common mechanism, those with arterial oxygen desaturation can be recognized; (2) an increased carboxyhemoglobin content (*i.e.*, one greater than 1%), particularly in absence of an expected compensatory increase in 2,3-diphosphoglycerate as is seen in hypoxia, identifies the common "smokers' polycythemia" (Sagonne and Balcerzak, 1975; Smith and Landaw, 1978); (3) circumstances of genetic abnormalities in the hemoglobin molecule exist that result in an increased affinity for oxygen. These congenital lesions are identified by reduced hemoglobin P_{50} (*i.e.*, the partial pressure of oxygen at which hemoglobin is half saturated) and a shift to the left of the oxygen dissociation curve (Stephens, 1977); (4) rarely, chronic cardiac failure can result in decreased tissue perfusion and secondary erythrocytosis.

Another mechanism capable of producing secondary polycythemia is inappropriately increased erythropoietin production. This may occur with renal lesions (cysts or renal cell carcinoma), liver lesions (cysts and hepatomas), and, less commonly, in patients with cerebellar hemangiosarcomas, pheochromocytomas and, rarely, large uterine leiomyomata. These are identified by erythropoietin measurement and the diagnostic selective radiographic examinations.

The National Polycythemia Vera Study Group in 1968 developed criteria (see Table 19-1) for the diagnosis of polycythemia vera in previously untreated patients. These criteria imply that the other causes described above have been eliminated. In addition, they help emphasize the lack of diagnostic specificity of the bone marrow and other related histologic materials. Finally, one rare form of polycythemia occurring in families must be considered in circumstances where the findings are consistent with polycythemia vera (Adamson, 1975).

Staging

As with other generalized lesions of the marrow, the usual concepts of staging utilized in nonhematopoietic tumors are not applicable, because these lesions are "disseminated" at the time of diagnosis.

Table 19-1. Criteria for Diagnosis of Polycythemia Vera

Category A	Category B
1. Measured increase in red cell mass: men $\geq$ 36 mL/kg women $\geq$ 32 mL/kg	1. Thrombocytosis: platelets $> 400,000/\mu$L
2. Normal arterial oxygen saturation: $\geq 92\%$	2. Leukocytosis: WBC $> 12,000/\mu$L (in absence of fever or infection)
3. Splenomegaly	3. Elevated leukocyte alkaline phosphatase score: > 100 (in absence of fever or infection)
	4. Elevated serum vitamin B_{12} content on unbound B_{12}-binding capacity: ($B_{12} > 900$ pg/mL; U B_{12}-binding capacity > 2200 pg/mL)

A diagnosis of polycythemia vera is acceptable if:
1. All three in category A are present, or
2. Only one or two in category A are present *plus* any two criteria in category B

Specific and Supportive Management

Specific Therapy. Therapy is designed to deal with the various phases in the sequential history of polycythemia vera, managing the specific complications of each of the phases (Wasserman, 1954, 1971, 1976). Because treatment has an important effect on the natural history of polycythemia vera and is a factor in some of the causes of death (Berk *et al.,* 1981; Wasserman *et al.,* 1981), the potential risks of any proposed therapeutic intervention must be seriously considered (Loeb, 1975).

Developmental Phase. The developmental phase is commonly recognized in retrospect because prominent symptoms or clinical findings are absent. Occasionally pruritus is recognized; cimetidine has provided symptomatic relief. Hyperuricemia or gouty symptoms should be managed with uricosuric therapy.

Erythremic or Erythrocytic Phase. Most patients with polycythemia vera are first identified during their early erythremic phase when the principal symptom complex results from the increased red cell mass, expanded plasma volume, and/or the increased numbers of platelets. The usual and appropriate management of this stage is a program of phlebotomies. Phlebotomies are capable of correcting the increased red cell mass and expanded plasma volume and those symptoms associated with these erythremic aspects. Phlebotomies of 1 unit of blood (500 mL) daily or every other day can promptly reduce the red cell mass to normal. A reduction of the peripheral venous hematocrit to below 48 vol % provides a convenient therapeutic standard and goal. In patients over the age of 50, particularly in those with cardiovascular abnormalities, the phlebotomies should be limited to smaller volumes (100 to 250 mL) and done only every other day, because cerebrovascular accidents have been precipitated by too vigorous a phlebotomy program. When the peripheral venous hematocrit has been reduced to the normal range, serial evaluation permits an evaluation of the tempo of the disease to determine the ability of a phlebotomy program to maintain a stable clinical state. In many patients, excellent control of the erythrocytic phase can be maintained with the removal of one unit of blood every four to eight weeks.

Simple removal of blood is not adequate to provide clinical stability in patients in whom increased platelets produce noteworthy clinical findings, or in those in whom the proliferative activities of the marrow establish a phlebotomy requirement in excess of 1 unit per month, or in patients with symptomatic hepatosplenomegaly. Myelosuppressive therapy has been utilized with success in these circumstances.

The best type of myelosuppressive therapy has been the subject of a multicenter study (Polycythemia Vera Study Group) over the past two decades (Wasserman, 1976). These studies considered the incidence of leukemia in patients with polycythemia vera treated with myelosuppressive agents, the effect of therapy on transitions to the spent stage, and other complications of therapy. In the initial studies, patients were randomized to one of three treatment regimens, that of phlebotomy, radiophosphorus, or chlorambucil. Kaplan-Meier actuarial survival curves in the three treatment groups demonstrated no significant difference when the cohort was followed for a minimum of seven years (with a maximum of 14 years). The median survival was 9.1 years in the chlorambucil-treated patients, 10.3 years in the radiophosphorus-treated group, and was not quite established for the phlebotomy group. Vascular thrombosis was the most frequent cause of death and accounted for a higher proportion of deaths in the phlebotomy-treated patients than in either of the other two groups (Wasserman *et al.,* 1981). The second most common cause of death was acute leukemia and the risk of leukemia in the chlorambucil group was 2.3 times that of the patients treated with radiophosphorus and 13 times that of the patients treated only with phlebotomy (Berk *et al.,* 1981). The increased incidence of leukemia with chlorambucil therapy was recognized early by the study group and its use discontinued in the treatment of polycythemia vera. Other neoplasms were also seen. Thus, of the initial 431 studied patients, 42 nonhematologic neoplasms were identified: 6 were in the phlebotomy-treated group and 18 each were in the radiophosphorus and chlorambucil-treated groups. Although not statistically significant, the incidences of the nonhematopoietic neoplasms seen with myelosuppressive therapy pose serious concern.

Thus, these careful studies have not yet provided a definitive myelosuppressive regimen that can be utilized without risk. Extensive experience with radiophosphorus (Lawrence, 1940; Osgood, 1968) supports its role as an effective myelosuppressive agent in the management of patients with polycythemia vera, and if its use is restricted to those over the age of 70 the concern over its carcinogenic potential is minimal. Although many dosage schedules have been utilized, the program of the Polycythemia Vera Study Group has wide use. After obtaining stable reduction of the peripheral venous hematocrit by phlebotomy, radiophosphorus (^{32}P) in a dose of 2.7 mCi/m^2 (not to exceed 5 mCi for a single dose) is given. Although intravenous administration has been advised to circumvent variable gastrointestinal absorption, extensive experience has shown adequate therapeutic effect when given orally. Radiophosphorus, which has a radioactive half-life of 14 days, provides total bone marrow radiation due to its uptake by the marrow. Following treatment, the effects are best evaluated after ten to 12 weeks. Second and even third doses of radiophosphorus may be required to provide a stable control of the disease. In general, these doses are in the range of 2 to 3 mCi.

A variety of other myelosuppressive agents have been utilized in the management of polycythemia vera. Busulfan has been used widely (Haanen and Mather, 1981; Brodsky, 1982); nevertheless, it does not appear to have important advantage over chlorambucil. A common therapy schedule for busulfan is 4 mg per day

orally. Blood counts should be monitored at approximately two-week intervals to identify patients with excessive reduction in circulating white cells or platelets. Therapy should be discontinued if the peripheral white cell counts fall below 5000/mL or the platelet counts fall below 100,000/mL. In general, treatment must be continued for three months to achieve a considerable myelosuppressive effect and a durable constraint of the polycythemic process. Other alkylating agents such as melphalan (using a dosage schedule and pattern similar to that of busulfan) or cyclophosphamide (usual dose of 2 mg/kg/day) have been used also. Because cyclophosphamide appears to be less suppressive of platelets than of white cells or red cells, it is a less desirable alkylating agent than the others in patients with serious thrombocytosis. Although only limited studies are available, hydroxyurea appears to be an effective myelosuppressive agent for patients under the age of 65. It appears not to be leukemogenic and is relatively safe and simple to use, so it currently provides promise for the therapy of the proliferative phase of polycythemia vera. In asymptomatic patients, 10 to 15 mg/kg of hydroxyurea per day orally and monitoring of blood counts have been done at two-week to three-week intervals. Unless serious granulocytopenia (less than 5000/mL) or thrombocytopenia (less than 100,000/mL) occur, therapy is continued for three to four months.

In spite of the studies to date, it is not known whether active myelosuppressive therapy will hasten the spent phase of polycythemia or whether the occurrence of hematopoietic and nonhematopoietic neoplasms is largely due to such therapy or part of the natural history of polycythemia vera.

Spent Phase (Postpolycythemia Myeloid Metaplasia). The symptomatic findings during this stage relate to the development of a slowly progressive anemia and to pressure symptoms due to the progressive splenomegaly and hepatomegaly. The management is at present entirely symptomatic. In some patients, particularly women, androgens have provided satisfactory stability of red cell values. In most, a progressive transfusion requirement develops. Symptoms related to the progressive splenomegaly have similarly been managed supportively. Splenic radiation and myelosuppressive agents have rarely been helpful and have frequently increased the severity of the anemia. Splenectomy has had serious morbidity and mortality, as discussed below.

Therapy of Selected Problems in Polycythemia Vera

Some events appear to be accentuated or caused by the therapeutic modalities utilized in the management of polycythemia vera.

Thrombotic Complications of Phlebotomy. Thrombotic complications are recognized as part of the natural history of the erythrocytic phase of polycythemia. The randomized therapeutic trials of the Polycythemia Vera Study Group, however, identified an excess incidence of thrombotic complications in those patients who were treated by phlebotomy alone. This excess was most marked during the first three years of the treatment program. Attempts to reduce the incidence of this treatment-associated complication with the use of inhibitors of platelet function (aspirin and dipyridamole) failed to prevent the thrombotic episodes in those polycythemia vera patients treated by phlebotomy alone (Tartaglia *et al.,* 1981).

Development of Iron-Deficient Erythropoiesis and Iron-Deficient Anemia. The development of a hypochromic microcytic anemia due to iron lack is commonly present in polycythemia vera. At presentation, it may be due to mucosal bleeding, especially from the gastrointestinal tract. At times the diagnosis of polycythemia may not be recognized because of the presence of anemia. The correct diagnosis is suggested by the presence of microcytic red cells in the absence of anemia; this implies an originally expanded erythron with limitation of iron stores. Other suggestive clues relate to the panmyelosis (*e.g.,* leukocytosis with increased eosinophils and basophils and increased platelets).

The development of iron-deficient erythropoiesis or an actual iron deficiency anemia is seen in virtually all polycythemia vera patients during the therapeutic program with phlebotomy. Because the iron lack helps reduce the proliferative activity of the erythron, it is a "complication" that can be used to therapeutic advantage. Rarely, nonhematologic symptoms of iron deprivation (*e.g.,* cheilosis, pica, and dysphagia) may occur and require iron therapy for replenishment of the tissue iron deficit.

PRIMARY (ESSENTIAL) THROMBOCYTHEMIA

Incidence and Epidemiology

Primary thrombocythemia is the least common of all the myeloproliferative lesions. Actual incidence data are lacking largely because the diagnostic criteria are least specific, and many categorize these patients as being in the developmental stage of polycythemia vera. No epidemiologic information exists.

Etiology and Pathogenesis

No etiologic factors are known. Pathogenetic data are largely descriptive and define an autonomous "drive" for platelet production that does not respond to expected regulatory mechanisms. Thus the net mass of megakaryocytes is increased and platelet production is increased manyfold. Autonomous endoproliferation of the megakaryocytes produces an increase in megakaryocyte volume, a finding that is the reverse of that classically seen in "reactive" thrombocytosis, wherein megakaryocyte volume decreases with increasing platelet numbers (Harker, 1971). It should be emphasized that our current knowledge of the regulatory mechanisms of thrombopoiesis is very limited (Harker and Finch, 1969).

Pathology and Natural History

Pathology. Panmyelosis of the marrow with hypercellularity and a prominent increase in megakaryocytes with increased megakaryocyte volume are seen. The megakaryocytes may actually occur in clusters and sheets, leading some to apply the term megakaryocytic leukemia (Gelin *et al.,* 1959). Hyperplasias of erythroid and granulocytic precursors provide further basis for the panmyelosis. All of the findings are consistent with the generic term myeloproliferative disorder; none of the findings can be used to imply morphologic specificity to the diagnosis of primary thrombocythemia. As in other myeloproliferative lesions, extramedullary hematopoiesis can be found in spleen, liver, and lymph nodes; these changes are usually late in the course of the disease. In spite of the potential for extramedullary hematopoiesis, the splenomegaly seen in patients with primary thrombocythemia is due to congestion and, commonly, to focal areas of infarction.

Natural History. Untreated patients with primary thrombocythemia have recurrent thrombotic and hemorrhagic (primarily mucosal) phenomena (Ozer *et al.*, 1960; Gunz, 1960). Inadequate information exists to define the true fate of untreated patients, but the risks of fatal thrombohemorrhagic lesions are commonly identified (Fanger *et al.*, 1954; Hardisty *et al.*, 1955; Silverstein, 1968). In addition to these risks, transitions to polycythemia vera, myelofibrosis, and even acute leukemia are recognized (Gunz, 1960), but temporal predictive patterns for these transitions are unknown (Frei-Lahr *et al.*, 1984).

Symptoms and Signs. Clinical symptoms are seen in less than 50% of patients with this diagnosis. In any given patient, it is difficult to predict risk from any given number of platelets. The symptoms commonly relate directly to the increased numbers of circulating platelets. Bleeding, particularly from the gastrointestinal tract or nose, is the most common symptom. Vascular thromboses and thromboembolic lesions are second only to bleeding; splenic vein thrombosis and pulmonary thromboembolic events are common. The symptoms resulting from these thrombohemorrhagic lesions depend on the sites of involvement and the extent (Schafer, 1984; Jabaily *et al.*, 1983).

Physical findings are usually limited to splenomegaly, seen in approximately 50% of patients, and the signs of easy bruising.

Diagnosis. Characteristic hematologic changes provide the major initial laboratory findings. Thrombocytosis, sometimes with the number of platelets in the millions per milliliter, with large and atypical platelet shapes, characterizes the disease. Platelet clumping may make actual enumeration difficult. An elevated total white blood cell count due to a polymorphonuclear leukocytosis is seen in most patients. Red blood cell values are normal or even sightly increased unless major bleeding has occurred. The common presence of bleeding is supported by the evidence of a microcytic hypochromic anemia of the iron deficient type in virtually all patients at least some time in the course of their disease.

Studies of the bleeding diathesis have not provided a consistent pathophysiologic mechanism. Clinical correlation of the total platelet number with bleeding appears to provide the best relationship in any given patient (Ozer *et al.*, 1960; Gunz, 1960). A clearly defined number (of platelets) that produces a defined risk of bleeding does not exist. The bleeding time is frequently prolonged and a variety of altered platelet functional properties have been seen (McClure *et al.*, 1966; Spaet *et al.*, 1969). These latter findings have not been consistent and are usually transient, disappearing when either the platelet numbers are diluted *in vitro* for testing or when the platelet numbers have been reduced by myelosuppresive therapy. Thus, physical factors relative to "crowding" and altered platelet plasma membrane interaction may have more importance in the platelet dysfunction and the bleeding diathesis. Studies of plasma coagulation factors have not helped elucidate the mechanism of bleeding.

Other laboratory abnormalities commonly include an elevated leukocyte alkaline phosphatase as seen in other myeloproliferative lesions. Similarly, an elevated serum uric acid is common and gout may occur. The serum potassium is usually increased and this is the result of the increased platelets and the liberation of potassium *in vitro*. This "pseudohyperkalemia" (Hartmann, 1971) must be identified as an *in vitro* event of cellular membrane injury to protect the patient from unnecessary therapeutic attempts to lower the *in vivo* potassium level.

The bone marrow findings described above stress that the diagnosis of primary thrombocythemia is a clinical-laboratory one. Specific morphologic findings do not exist (Case, 1984). The Polycythemia Vera Study Group has attempted to provide diagnostic criteria (see Table 19–2) to clarify the issues of specificity.

Specific and Supportive Management

Specific Therapy. The primary mechanism of the clinical findings in primary thrombocythemia is based on platelet numbers. Thus, therapy is directed toward reduction of the platelet excess.

Table 19–2. Criteria for Diagnosis of Primary Thrombocythemia

1. Platelet count $\geq 1,000,000/\mu L$ (on at least two separate occasions)
2. Absence of Philadelphia chromosome (from metaphase preparations of marrow aspirates)
3. Normal measured red cell mass (if hemoglobin is 13 g/dL or greater)
4. Present marrow iron stores
5. Absence of bone marrow fibrosis
6. Absence of a cause for the elevated platelet count

In circumstances of an acute or rapidly emerging crisis due to thrombotic or hemorrhagic events, thrombocytapheresis has proved of great value. Reduction in platelet numbers to near normal can be achieved in one or two days of platelet removal on a cell separator. This is of particular value with a developing abdominal crisis (*e.g.*, impending splenic vein thrombosis or possible splenic infarct) to separate possible intra-abdominal occlusive symptoms from those due to other intra-abdominal lesions. In addition, the rapid correction of hemostasis by platelet removal provides a safer milieu for any necessary surgical exploration.

Myelosuppression with radiophosphorus or alkylating agents has been used to control platelet numbers. Little comparative data between modalities exist. The Polycythemia Vera Study Group randomized patients with primary thrombocythemia to either melphalan or radiophosphorus (Murphy *et al.*, 1982). Although only a small number of cases was studied (31 patients), melphalan resulted in a higher complete remission rate than radiophosphorus early in the treatment course; but by 12 months of treatment the response rates were similar. Remission induction and maintenance were easily achieved with either agent. No data on sequelae of therapy are available.

Hydroxyurea has been effectively and safely used for both remission induction and maintenance (at platelet counts below 500,000/μL). In asymptomatic patients, 10 mg/kg of hydroxyurea per day have been used with evaluation weekly; when platelet values are normal, treatment can be stopped and then used intermittently, as needed. For symptomatic patients, 30 mg/kg/day has been used for remission induction and 5 to 10 mg/kg/day for maintenance.

Special Therapeutic Issues of Splenectomy. Splenectomy poses special risks in patients with primary thrombocythemia. There is a high operative mortality and morbidity, a remarkable postoperative increase in circulating platelets, and an exacerbation of thrombohemorrhagic phenomena (Hirsh and Dacie, 1966; Bensinger *et al.*, 1970; Ravich *et al.*, 1970).

Supportive Measures. Symptomatic hyperuricemia should be managed with allopurinol. The development of iron deficient anemia or iron deficient erythropoiesis is an indication for iron therapy.

The thromboembolic sequelae have been treated with anticoagulants; important evidence of therapeutic effectiveness has been uncertain (Conley *et al.*, 1948; Ravich *et al.*, 1970). Because bleeding may be a serious clinical feature, great caution should be exercised in the use of anticoagulants. In addition, anticoagulant therapy may be difficult to regulate because of the excessive amount of heparin required in the presence of high platelet numbers.

Recent enthusiasm for the use of antiplatelet agents (*e.g.*, aspirin and dipyridamole) is without supportive evidence of efficacy. If the lesson from polycythemia vera has a parallel in primary thrombocythemia, there exists little advantage in their use (Tartaglia *et al.*, 1981).

MYELOFIBROSIS

Myelofibrosis is a syndrome characterized by symptoms attributable to the sequelae of ineffective hematopoiesis with extramedullary sites of blood cell production. A plethora of names (*e.g.*, agnogenic myeloid metaplasia, primary myeloid metaplasia, myelosclerosis) help attest to our limited knowledge of the biology of this lesion. Although some have favored the term agnogenic myeloid metaplasia for the idiopathic form and myelofibrosis for the secondary forms of this lesion, there appears to be no rational basis for such an application.

Incidence and Epidemiology

No reliable incidence or epidemiologic data on myelofibrosis are available.

Etiology and Pathogenesis

A variety of mechanisms that produce marrow injury result in the clinical and laboratory findings characteristic of idiopathic myelofibrosis. This observation is the basis for the view that myeloproliferative disorders, particularly myelofibrosis, are non-neoplastic lesions (Ward and Block, 1971). The known causes of myelofibrosis include toxic injury such as those caused by benzene (Rawson *et al.*, 1941), infections (*e.g.*, typical and atypical forms of tuberculosis) (Andre *et al.*, 1961), neoplastic lesions (*e.g.*, metastatic carcinoma) (Kiely and Silverstein, 1969), radiation (Anderson *et al.*, 1964; Anderson and Yamamoto,

1970; Vaughan, 1970), and renal osteodystrophic changes associated with excess parathormone secretion (Weinberg *et al.,* 1977). Focal marrow injury (necrosis) appears to be the one important common aspect of all of these causes (Wyatt and Sommers, 1950; Peace, 1953).

Three major theories have been used to explain the pathogenesis of the clinical and laboratory findings in myelofibrosis. The first is that the extramedullary hematopoiesis is a compensatory response to some mechanism (known or unknown) of marrow injury (Donhauser, 1908). This compensatory concept is shaken by the presence of extramedullary hematopoiesis before evident marrow injury in some cases. In addition, panmyelosis with an expanded marrow mass may be present, yet foci of extramedullary hematopoiesis may already be identified. A second concept, that of a "myelostimulatory state," expresses the view that myelofibrosis represents a normal response of a normal stem cell to an unidentified stimulus (Ward and Block, 1971). The third concept, the original descriptive concept, is one that holds that myelofibrosis is a disorder associated with autonomous hematopoiesis (*i.e.,* the myeloproliferative concept) (Adamson, 1975); this theory appears to have an appropriate basis.

Recent studies of polycythemia vera with associated myelofibrosis and extramedullary hematopoiesis (Adamson and Fialkow, 1978) and of a case of idiopathic myelofibrosis (Jacobson *et al.,* 1978) have evaluated the clonal characteristics of the involved hematopoietic cells. Using glucose-6-phospate dehydrogenase isoenzyme types and chromosomal analyses, the hematopoietic cells at medullary and extramedullary sites appear to represent a lesion of a pluripotent stem cell with clonal characteristics. Thus, by inference, these hematopoietic changes in both the medullary and extramedullary sites are neoplastic. By contrast, the fibroblastic proliferation in the marrow, like that of the skin, had normal (two) isoenzymes and chromosomes, consistent with the view that the marrow fibrosis in myelofibrosis is not clonal but rather a secondary phenomenon (Jacobson *et al.,* 1978). It is now clear that the fibrosis (fibroblasts) in the marrow has mesenchymal rather than hematopoietic origin (Friedenstein *et al.,* 1978; Golde *et al.,* 1980).

Examination of the marrow in the panmyelosis seen in all myeloproliferative lesions has commonly demonstrated increased megakaryocytes, and where fibrosis is present the reticular fibers appear to envelop the megakaryocytes. The identification of the platelet-derived growth factor has now provided a conceptual basis for the fibrosis, because the platelet alpha granule is mitogenic for mesenchymal (fibroblasts) cells (Ross and Vogel, 1978; Scher *et al.,* 1979). Obviously, the presence of such a growth factor does not prove the relationship, because similar megakaryocyte numbers are seen in reactive thrombocytosis, but myelofibrosis does not occur. Nevertheless, increased or abnormal release of platelet-derived growth factor from megakaryocytes provides a now plausible pathogenetic basis for the fibroblastic aspects of myelofibrosis, whereas the clonal (neoplastic) nature of the interrelated hematopoietic elements appears certain (Hibbin *et al.,* 1984; Jacobs *et al.,* 1984).

Pathology and Natural History

Pathology. Bone marrow aspiration usually yields little or no material. Bone marrow biopsy material provides the evidence of fibrosis, although early in the course of the disease the fibrosis may not be recognizable in all specimens and multiple biopsies may be required. The typical histologic findings are those of a mesh of reticular fibers dividing the marrow into small compartments (Burkhardt *et al.,* 1982). The degree of marrow cellularity is quite variable within these "compartments." A prominent increase and clustering of megakaryocytes is seen with reticular fibrillar mesh appearing to "ensnare" the megakaryocytes. The increased reticulin is best identified with (methenamine) silver stains. Because aging is normally associated with an increase in fibrosis, the changes must be evaluated in the context of the age of the patient. Fat spaces are reduced. Late in the clinical course, myelosclerosis may be identified by the irregular spicules of woven bone with associated trabecular thickening (Burkhardt *et al.,* 1982).

Extramedullary hematopoiesis characterized by trilineal cellular infiltrates (precursors of red cells, white cells, and platelets) can be identified in spleen, liver, lymph nodes, and kidney. The foci of hematopoiesis in the spleen and liver are associated with congestive changes (*i.e.,* chronic passive congestion), and it is the combination of congestion and hematopoiesis that produces the organ enlargement. The hematopoietic foci in the liver are usually found in intrasinusoidal sites (Ligumski *et al.,* 1978).

During the course of myelofibrosis, ascites, portal hypertension, and portal vein thrombosis may occur. In some the clinical findings are associated with periportal fibrosis, whereas in many only extramedullary hematopoiesis is seen (Ligumski *et al.,* 1978). Recent recognition of nodular regenerative hyperplasia in myelofibrosis may help explain these findings (Shorey *et al.,* 1979).

Natural History. The clinical course of myelofibrosis is variable. Ward and Block (1971) described a median survival from the time of diagnosis of five years. They described a constant increase in spleen size (approximately 1 cm of splenic enlargement per year) with time. This suggested a very long presymptomatic period of the disease. Because therapeutic approaches in myelofibrosis are supportive, the "natural" history of the disease is that which is observed clinically.

The common complications that cause death are congestive heart failure (primarily right-sided failure) and thrombohemorrhagic phenomena, each in about one-third of cases. In addition, the development of acute granulocytic leukemia has been described in approximately 25% of patients with myelofibrosis (Silverstein and Linman, 1969; Takacsi-Nagy and Graf, 1975). This transition has been doubted because myeloblasts are commonly seen in myelofibrosis (Wintrobe *et al.,* 1974b). Therapy (employing either radiation or chemotherapeutic agents) has been implicated as the basis for some of the described cases (Stecher *et al.,* 1961). Chromosome changes during the evolution of peripheral blood changes, however, now provide important evidence that a true leukemic transition may occur (Jensen and Philip, 1970). Finally, intercurrent infection, often related to decreased immunologic competency or granulocyte dysfunction, had previously been the most common cause of death (Ward and Block, 1971); it now accounts for only about 10% of the deaths.

An uncommon complication affecting the course of myelofibrosis is hepatic vein thrombosis with resultant portal hypertension and esophageal varices (Shorey *et al.,* 1979). Painful splenic infarctions are not uncommon, but splenic rupture is very rare (Wintrobe *et al.,* 1974b).

Symptoms and Signs. The presymptomatic phase of myelofibrosis is identified by the presence of a large spleen on routine examination or abnormal peripheral blood findings in the absence of symptoms (Ward and Block, 1971; Takacsi-Nagy and Graf, 1975; Korst *et al.,* 1956; Linman and Bethell, 1957; Leonard *et al.,* 1957; Bouroncle and Doan, 1962; Pitcock *et al.,* 1962; Hickling, 1968; Rosenthal and Moloney, 1969; Silverstein, 1976).

The common clinical symptoms in myelofibrosis are shown in Table 19.3. Constitutional symptoms of malaise and weight loss are the most common complaints. Bleeding, either gastrointestinal or superficial cutaneous ecchymosis, is seen in one-third of patients. Ease of satiety or abdominal "fullness" can result from splenomegaly. Uncommonly, left upper quadrant pain results from splenic infarcts. Bone pain, particularly in the pelvis and long bones of the lower extremities, is a common symptom that is difficult to explain and often difficult to manage. Although gouty arthritis is

Table 19–3. Common Clinical Findings in Myelofibrosis

Case characteristics
Age: Average age 60 (range 35 to 80)
Sex: Equal ratio men : women

Symptoms	%	*(Range of values in %)*
Malaise	90	(65 to 100)
Weight loss	50	(30 to 70)
Bleeding	30	(20 to 50)
Splenic pain	30	(20 to 60)
Bone pain	10	(1 to 30)
Signs		
Splenomegaly	100	(90 to 100)
Hepatomegaly	80	(33 to 100)
Petechiae	20	(7 to 30)
Lymphadenopathy	15	(5 to 30)
Peripheral edema	15	(11 to 30)

Note: Values summarized from references below and unpublished data from The University of Texas Health Science Center at Dallas. The composite represents over 600 cases; the percentages and ranges represent estimates from these references because the stage of the disease was generally not recorded in the text.
Based on data from Takacsi-Nagy, L., and Graf, F.: Definition, clinical features and diagnosis of myelofibrosis. *Clin. Haematol.,* 4:291–308, 1975; Korst, D. R.; Clatanoff, D. V.; and Schilling, R. F.: On myelofibrosis. *Arch. Intern. Med.,* 97: 169–183, 1956; Linman, J. W., and Bethell, F. H.: Agnogenic myeloid metaplasia. Its natural history and present day management. *Am. J. Med.,* 22:107–122, 1957; Bouroncle, B. A., and Doan, C. A.: Myelofibrosis. Clinical, hematologic and pathologic study of 110 patients. *Am. J. Med. Sci.,* 243:697–715, 1962; Pitcock, J. A.; Reinhard, E. H.; Justus, B. W.; and Mendelsohn, R. S.: A clinical and pathological study of seventy cases of myelofibrosis. *Ann. Intern. Med.,* 57:73–84, 1962; Hickling, R. A.: The natural history of chronic non-leukaemic myelosis. *Q. J. Med.,* 37:267–279, 1968; Rosenthal, D. S., and Maloney, W. C.: Myeloid metaplasia. A study of 98 cases. *Postgrad. Med.,* 45:136–142, 1969; and Silverstein, M. N.: Primary or hemorrhagic thrombocythemia. *Arch. Intern. Med.,* 122:18–22, 1968.

seen in myelofibrosis, the bone pain described by these patients is usually easily separable from that of gout. In most, the skeletal pain increases late in the course of the disease, and it is particularly evident in those patients in transition to acute leukemia. Finally, an unexplained finding in as many as one-third of the patients is that of fever without identifiable cause; it often has an irregular but periodic pattern (Takacsi-Nagy and Graf, 1975).

The primary physical findings include splenomegaly (which may be massive) and hepatomegaly (see Table 19–3). The other findings are uncommon until late in the course of the disease.

Diagnosis

The diagnosis of myelofibrosis is established by the evidence of fibrosis in the bone marrow biopsy and the identification of extramedullary hematopoiesis involving the three classical committed stem cells, the erythroid, granulocytic, and megakaryocytic precursors. In practice, tissue examination of the extramedullary sites is not commonly performed.

The laboratory findings that further support and delineate the diagnosis are shown in Table 19–4. The anisocytosis and poikilocytosis (tear drop forms) of the red cells are often very remarkable. The evidence of leukoerythroblastosis in the peripheral blood strongly indicates an altered vascular sinusoidal structure in the marrow that allows egress of cells into the circulation prematurely. These findings are characteristic of marrow infiltrative lesions (*i.e.,* cancer, granulomatous disease, myelofibrosis, or lipid storage lesions), but are also seen in extramedullary hematopoiesis, because the absence of a (marrow) sinusoidal architecture similarly fails to control or affect cellular release from these abnormal sites of maturation.

An elevated leukocyte alkaline phosphatase helps differentiate myelofibrosis from chronic granulocytic leukemia, which may provide a difficult differential diagnosis. Although structural and numerical abnormalities of chromosomes have been described in myelofibrosis (Mitelman and Levan, 1981), the Philadelphia chromosomal translocation classically seen in chronic granulocytic leukemia is not present.

Laboratory evidence of ineffective hematopoiesis is seen in myelofibrosis. This includes ferrokinetic evidence of decreased radiolabeled iron utilization and extramedullary he-

Table 19–4.   Laboratory Findings in Myelofibrosis

Diagnostic features
 Bone marrow biopsy: Evidence of fibrosis; reticular mesh encompassing megakaryocytes
 Biopsy (aspiration) of spleen or liver: Evidence of trilineage extramedullary hematopoiesis (*i.e.,* erythrocytic, granulocytic, and megakaryocytic)
Supportive findings
 Peripheral blood: Leukoerythroblastic changes
  Red cells: Marked anisocytosis, poikilocytosis, and nucleated red cells
  White cells: Usually elevated with shift to left; increased eosinophils and basophils are common
  Platelets: Frequently (approximately 50%) increased in number with large atypical forms
Other laboratory findings
 RBC: 1. Ferrokinetic (radiolabeled [^{59}Fe] transferrin) demonstration of ineffective hematopoiesis (decreased iron utilization) and extramedullary (spleen or liver) hematopoietic sites
    2. "PNH-like defect": Evidence of a paroxysmal nocturnal hemoglobinuric-type defect with increased complement sensitive lysis (Kuo *et al.,* 1972)
 WBC: 1. Leukocyte alkaline phosphatase: Increased
 Platelets: 1. Platelet function: Abnormal bleeding time and clot retraction
 Other: 1. Serum uric acid: Elevated
    2. Serum lactic dehydrogenase: Elevated
    3. Chromosomes: Aneuploidy; structural and numerical abnormalities, but nonspecific and nonconsistent (Mitelman and Levan, 1981)
Radiologic findings
 1. Osteosclerosis of the axial and proximal long bones is found in approximately half of the patients
 2. Bone blood flow: Increased (^{133}Xe washout method) (Lahtinen *et al.,* 1982)

matopoiesis. In addition, serum lactic dehydrogenase, muramidase, uric acid, and vitamin B_{12} binding proteins are commonly elevated.

Radiographic changes are seen in 50% of the patients. The predominant changes involve the medullary region with preservation of the cortex of bone. Characteristically, there is a disorganization of the trabecular pattern with deposition of bone (osteosclerosis) throughout the marrow, which results in a "ground glass" appearance of the bone matrix and loss of the trabecular definition. The increase in bone density may be patchy or mottled, thereby simulating the mixed osteoblastic and osteolytic patterns of metastatic cancer.

Because the clinical and laboratory findings of myelofibrosis have been recognized as occurring with a variety of mechanisms of marrow injury, the diagnosis of idiopathic or primary myelofibrosis can be made only when identifiable causes of myelofibrosis have been eliminated.

Clinical Variants and Special Problems

Acute Myelofibrosis. An uncommon variant of classic myelofibrosis has been termed acute (or malignant) myelofibrosis (Fanger *et al.*, 1954; Lewis and Szur, 1963). The clinical pattern (see Table 19–5) in these cases separates them from those of classic myelofibrosis by the acute onset of symptoms, the presence of pancytopenia, and a rapid course with death secondary to complications of the pancytopenia (Fabich and Raich, 1977; Rojer *et al.*, 1978). The clinical presentation is often confused with that of acute leukemia. Indeed, the peripheral blood may be considered "consistent with leukemia" because of the presence of immature cells. The bone marrow examination provides the data for the correct diagnosis. Rappaport and coworkers (Bearman *et al.*, 1979) have provided evidence that this lesion can be separated from other myeloproliferative lesions as a distinct clinicopathologic entity; their diagnostic criteria are summarized in Table 19–5.

The fibrosis of the marrow has been shown to increase rapidly during the course of the disease. The brevity of the clinical course is emphasized by the similarity between the survival data expressed in terms of duration of symptoms and duration from diagnosis. Death has primarily been due to infections or bleeding. Although the clinical picture has features in common with acute leukemia, the therapeutic approaches effective in leukemia have been unsuccessful in acute myelofibrosis.

Table 19–5. Clinical and Laboratory Aspects of Acute (Malignant) Myelofibrosis

---

Clinical features
  1. Acute onset
  2. Symptoms secondary to circulating pancytopenia
  3. Minimal to absent splenomegaly
  4. Rapidly progressive clinical course
  5. Survival
     From onset of symptoms: Approximately six months
     From diagnosis: Approximately five months
Laboratory features
  1. Peripheral pancytopenia
  2. Minimal or absent red cell changes (*i.e., no* anisocytosis, poikilocytosis, or teardrop forms)
  3. Bone marrow hyperplasia with associated immaturity
  4. Bone marrow changes involve all three cell lines
  5. Pronounced increase in reticulin fiber content

Recent, but provisional, evidence that bone marrow transplantation may be an effective therapeutic modality in acute myelofibrosis makes the correct diagnosis important (Smith *et al.*, 1981; Wolf *et al.*, 1982).

Portal Hypertension and Nodular Regenerative Hyperplasia of the Liver. Portal venous hypertension has been noted during the course of myelofibrosis (Nakai *et al.*, 1962; Rosenbaum *et al.*, 1966; Shaldon and Sherlock, 1962; Shorey *et al.*, 1979). Both ascites and esophageal varices may develop as a result of the portal venous hypertension, and these complications require therapy. The pathophysiologic mechanism for the portal hypertension has been explained by the excessive blood flow through the large spleen. Abnormally high hepatic vascular resistance has been seen in myelofibrosis complicated by portal hypertension (Shaldon and Sherlock, 1962); and, despite this increased resistance, high rates of hepatic blood flow have been measured, suggesting that the increased transhepatic resistance may be the result of excessive splanchnic blood flow.

Another lesion, nodular regenerative hyperplasia of the liver, has been noted in myelofibrosis with associated portal venous hypertension (Shorey *et al.*, 1979). Nodular regenerative hyperplasia of the liver is an uncommon lesion in which the entire liver is coarsely nodular, the nodules being composed of hyperplastic hepatocytes. Evidence suggests that nodular regenerative hyperplasia of the liver may be a response to a high rate of portal venous blood flow resulting from increased blood flow through the enlarged spleen. Because portal venous hypertension is considered unusual on the basis of increased splanchnic blood flow alone (Shaldon and Sherlock, 1962), the development of nodular regenerative hyperplasia of the liver in myelofibrosis may help explain development of portal hypertension in myelofibrosis.

Familial Type. A nonprogressive form of myelofibrosis has been described in a familial pattern. The findings are relatively nonprogressive leukoerythroblastosis in the peripheral blood and extramedullary hematopoiesis in children and their parents (Randall *et al.*, 1965).

Specific and Supportive Management

Because the pathophysiologic mechanisms of myelofibrosis are not known, therapy is directed to the management of the clinical symptoms and complications. No specific therapy exists. Infection, bleeding, and congestive heart failure represent the common and life-threatening problems, and are managed in the classic clinical manner (*e.g.*, appropriate antibiotics, blood transfusions, or component therapy, and digitalis and diuretics as required).

Some of the specific symptoms have been successfully managed. Thus, episodes of gout can be controlled with allopurinol. Some improvement in the anemia has been achieved by the administration of androgens in an attempt to expand the erythron and to a lesser extent with adrenal corticosteroids (Silverstein, 1976).

Splenectomy has been considered a potential therapeutic intervention. Benbasset and colleagues (1979) reviewed the published data on splenectomy in myelofibrosis. Their survey of 321 cases failed to provide evidence that splenectomy (early or late in the course of disease) prolonged the survival or altered the rate of leukemic transformation of patients with myelofibrosis. Some palliation was achieved in about 65% of the patients, with improvement defined as reduced transfusion requirements, a lesser bleeding tendency, or disappearance of abdominal discomfort (Benbasset *et al.*, 1979). These palliative effects must be evaluated in terms of the high operative mortality of splenectomy in these patients, because 7% of the patients died within two days of splenectomy and 28% died within the first three months. The postoperative mortality was significantly higher in patients with platelet counts of less than 70,000 per microliter or when the weight of the spleen exceeded 2000 g; laboratory evidence of disseminated intravascular coagulation before surgery is also an unfavorable prognostic factor. Silverstein (1976) has formulated guidelines for splenectomy in myelofibrosis that include: (1) The presence of severe hemolysis that cannot be managed by available medical measures; (2) unacceptable abdominal pressure symptoms; (3) life-threatening thrombocytopenia; or (4) portal hypertension with life-threatening bleeding. These practical criteria appropriately recognize the risk and limited palliative value of splenectomy.

Splenic radiation to reduce the splenomegaly has been tried as an alternative to splenectomy, particularly in patients in whom the spleen is the major site of hematopoiesis (*i.e.*, associated with a hypoplastic marrow) or where the patient is a poor operative risk. Although pancytopenia is a common result of splenic radiation (Koeffler *et al.*, 1979), such therapy can provide modest palliation of pain and reduce the spleen size (Greenberger *et al.*, 1977). In general, the radiation is given at very low levels because of the risk of increasing the severity of the cytopenias.

REFERENCES

Adamson, J. W.: Familial polycythemia. *Semin. Hematol.,* **12:**383–396, 1975.

Adamson, J. W., and Fialkow, P. J.: The pathogenesis of myeloproliferative syndromes. *Br. J. Haematol.,* **38:**299–303, 1978.

Anderson, R. E.; Hoshino, T.; and Yamamoto, T.: Myelofibrosis with myeloid metaplasia in survivors of the atomic bomb in Hiroshima. *Ann. Intern. Med.,* **60:**1–18, 1964.

Anderson, R. E., and Yamamoto, T.: Myeloproliferative disorders in atomic bomb survivors. In Clarke, W. J.; Howard, E. B.; and Hackett, P. L. (eds.): *Myeloproliferative Disorders of Animals and Man.* U.S. AEC Sympos. Washington, D.C. Ser. 19, 1970.

Andre, J.; Schwartz, R.; and Dameshek, W.: Tuberculosis and myelosclerosis with myeloid metaplasia. *J.A.M.A.,* **178:**1169–1174, 1961.

Bearman, R. M.; Pangalis, G. A.; and Rappaport, H.: Acute ("malignant") myelosclerosis. *Cancer,* **43:**279–293, 1979.

Benbassat, J.; Penchas, S.; and Ligumski, M.: Splenectomy in patients with agnogenic myeloid metaplasia: An analysis of 321 published cases. *Br. J. Haematol.,* **42:**207–214, 1979.

Bensinger, T. A.; Logue, G. L.; and Rundles, R. W.: Hemorrhagic thrombocythemia: Control of postsplenectomy thrombocytosis with melphalan. *Blood,* **36:**61–69, 1970.

Berk, P. D.; Goldberg, J. D.; Silverstein, M. N.; Weinfeld, A.; Donovan, P. B.; Ellis, J. T.; Landaw, S. A.; Laszlo, J.; Najean, Y.; Pisciotta, A. V.; and Wasserman, L. R.: Increased incidence of acute leukemia in polycythemia vera associated with chlorambucil therapy. *N. Engl. J. Med.,* **304:**441–447, 1981.

Berlin, N. I.: Diagnosis and classification of the polycythemias. *Semin. Hematol.,* **12:**339–351, 1975.

Block, M., and Bethard, W.: Bone marrow studies in polycythemia. *J. Clin. Invest.,* **31:**618, 1952 (abstract).

Bouroncle, B. A., and Doan, C. A.: Myelofibrosis. Clinical, hematologic and pathologic study of 110 patients. *Am. J. Med. Sci.,* **243:**697–715, 1962.

Brandt, L.; Cederquist, E.; Rorsman, H.; and Tryding, N.: Blood histamine and basophil leukocytes in polycythemia. *Acta Med. Scand.,* **176:**745–750, 1964.

Brodsky, I.: Busulphan treatment of polycythaemia vera. *Br. J. Haematol.,* **52:**1–6, 1982.

Burkhardt, R.; Frisch, B.; and Bartl, R.: Bone biopsy in haematological disorders. *J. Clin. Pathol.,* **35:**257–284, 1982.

Case, D. C. Jr.: Absence of a specific chromosomal marker in essential thrombocythemia. *Canc. Genet. Cytogenet.,* **12:**163–165, 1984.

Conley, C. L.; Hartmann, R. C.; and Lalley, J. S.: The relationship of heparin activity to platelet concentration. *Proc. Soc. Exp. Biol. Med.,* **69:**284–287, 1948.

Dameshek, W.: Some speculations on the myeloproliferative syndromes. *Blood,* **6:**372–375, 1951.

Donhauser, J. L.: The human spleen as an haematoplastic organ, as exemplified in a case of splenomegaly with sclerosis of the bone marrow. *J. Exp. Med.,* **10:**559–574, 1908.

Ellis, J. T.; Silver, R. T.; Coleman, M.; and Geller, S. A.: The bone marrow in polycythemia vera. *Semin. Hematol.,* **12:**433–444, 1975.

Erslev, A. J., and Caro, J.: Pure erythrocytosis classified according to erythropoietin titers. *Am. J. Med.,* **76:**57–61, 1984.

Fabich, D. R., and Raich, P. C.: Acute myelofibrosis. A report of three cases. *Am. J. Clin. Pathol.,* **67:**334–338, 1977.

Fanger, H.; Cella, L. J., Jr.; and Litchman, H.: Thrombocythemia: Report of three cases and review of the literature. *N. Engl. J. Med.,* **250:**456–461, 1954.

Fialkow, P. J.: Cell lineages in hematopoietic neoplasia studied with glucose-6-phosphate dehydrogenase cell markers. *J. Cell. Physiol.,* **243:**(Suppl. 1):37–43, 1982.

Frenkel, E. P., and McCall, M. S.: Radioisotope techniques in hematology. In Race, G. J. (ed.): *Laboratory Medicine,* 5th ed. Harper & Row, Publishers, Inc., Hagerstown, Maryland, 1978.

Frenkel, E. P.; McCall, M. S.; Reisch, J. S.; and Minton, P. D.: An analysis of methods for the prediction of normal erythrocyte mass. *Am. J. Clin. Pathol.,* **58:**260–271, 1972.

Friedenstein, A. J.; Ivanov-Smolenski, A. A.; and Chajlakjan, R. K.: Origin of bone marrow stromal mechanocytes in radiochimeras and heterotopic transplants. *Exp. Hematol.,* **6:**440–444, 1978.

Frei-Lahr, D.; Barton, J. C.; Hoffman, R.; Burkett, L. L.; and Prchal, J. T.: Blastic transformation of essential thrombocythemia: Dual expression of myelomonoblastic/megakaryoblastic phenotypes. *Blood,* **63:**866–872, 1984.

Gelin, G., and Wasserman, L. R.: Remarques sur les megakaryocytoses malignes. *Sang,* **30:**829–847, 1959.

Gilbert, H.: Definition, clinical features and diagnosis of polycythemia vera. *Clin. Hematol.,* **4:**263–290, 1975.

Golde, D. W.; Hocking, W. G.; Quan, S. G.; Sparkes, R. S.; and Gale, R. P.: Origin of human bone marrow fibroblasts. *Br. J. Haematol.,* **44:**183–187, 1980.

Golde, D. W.; Hocking, W. G.; Koeffler, H. P.; and Adamson, J. W.: Polycythemia: Mechanisms and management. *Ann. Intern. Med.,* **95:**71–87, 1981.

Greenberger, J. S.; Chaffey, J. T.; Rosenthal, D. S.; and Moloney, W. C.: Irradiation for control of hypersplenism and painful splenomegaly in myeloid metaplasia. *Int. J. Radiat. Oncol. Biol. Phys.,* **2:**1083–1090, 1977.

Gunz, F. W.: Hemorrhagic thrombocythemia: A critical review. *Blood,* **15:**706–723 1960.

Haanen, C., and Mathe, G.: Treatment of polycythaemia vera by radiophosphorus or busulphan: A randomized trial. *Br. J. Cancer,* **44:**75–80, 1981.

Hardisty, R. M., and Wolff, H. H.: Haemorrhagic thrombocythaemia: A clinical and laboratory study. *Br. J. Haematol.,* **1:**390–405, 1955.

Harker, L. A.: Thrombokinetics. In Brinkhous, K. M.; Shermer, R. W.; and Mostofi, F. K. (eds.): *The Platelet.* The Williams & Wilkins Company, Baltimore, 1971.

Harker, L. A., and Finch, C. A.: Thrombokinetics in man. *J. Clin. Invest.,* **48:**963–974, 1969.

Hartmann, R. C.: Pseudohyperkaliemia. In Brinkhous,

K. M.; Shermer, R. W.; and Mostofi, F. K. (eds.): *The Platelet.* The Williams & Wilkins Company, Baltimore, 1971.

Hibbin, J. A.; Njoku, O. S.; Matutes, E.; Lewis, S. M.; and Goldman, J. M.: Myeloid progenitor cells in the circulation of patients with myelofibrosis and other myeloproliferative disorders. *Br. J. Haematol.,* **57:**495–503, 1984.

Hickling, R. A.: The natural history of chronic non-leukaemic myelosis. *Q. J. Med.,* **37:**267–279, 1968.

Hirsh, J., and Dacie, J. V.: Persistent post-splenectomy thrombocytosis and thrombo-embolism: A consequence of continuing anaemia. *Br. J. Haematol.,* **12:**44–53, 1966.

Jabaily, J.; Iland, H. J.; Laszlo, J.; Massey, E. W.; Faguet, G. B.; Briere, J.; Landaw, S. A.; and Pisciotta, A. V.: Neurologic manifestations of essential thrombocythemia. *Ann. Intern. Med.,* **99:**513–518, 1983.

Jacobs, P.; Le Roux, I.; and Jacobs, L.: Megakaryoblastic transformation in myeloproliferative disorders. *Cancer,* **54:**297–302, 1984.

Jacobson, R. J.; Salo, A.; and Fialkow, P. J.: Agnogenic myeloid metaplasia: A clonal proliferation of hematopoietic stem cells with secondary myelofibrosis. *Blood,* **51:**189–194, 1978.

Jensen, M. K., and Philip, P.: Cytogenetic studies in myeloproliferative disorders during transformation into leukaemia. *Scand. J. Haematol.,* **7:**330–335, 1970.

Kiely, J. M., and Silverstein, M. N.: Metastatic carcinoma simulating agnogenic myeloid metaplasia and myelofibrosis. *Cancer,* **24:**1041–1044, 1969.

Koeffler, H. P.; Cline, M. J.; and Golde, D. W.: Splenic irradiation in myelofibrosis: Effect on circulating myeloid progenitor cells. *Br. J. Haematol.,* **43:**69–77, 1979.

Korst, D. R.; Clatanoff, D. V.; and Schilling, R. F.: On myelofibrosis. *Arch. Intern. Med.,* **97:**169–183, 1956.

Kurnick, J. E.; Ward, H. P.; and Block, M. H.: Bone marrow sections in the differential diagnosis of polycythemia. *Arch. Pathol.,* **94:**489–499, 1972.

Kuo, C.; Van Voolen, G. A.; Morrison, A. N.: Primary and secondary myelofibrosis: Its relationship to "PNH-like" defect. *Blood,* **40:**875–880, 1972.

Lahtinen, R.; Lahtinen, T.; and Romppanen, T.: Bone and bone-marrow blood flow in chronic granulocytic leukemia and primary myelofibrosis. *J. Nucl. Med.,* **23:**218–224, 1982.

Laszlo, J.: Myeloproliferative disorders (MPD): Myelofibrosis, myelosclerosis, extramedullary hematopoiesis, undifferentiated MPD, and hemorrhagic thrombocythemia. *Semin. Hematol.,* **12:**409–432, 1975.

Lawrence, J. H.: Nuclear physics and therapy: Preliminary report on a new method for the treatment of leukemia and polycythemia. *Radiology,* **35:**51–60, 1940.

Lawrence, J. H.: Polycythemia: Physiology, diagnosis and treatment based on 303 cases. *Modern Medical Monographs,* Grune & Stratton, Inc., New York, 1955.

Leonard, B. J.; Israels, M. C. G.; and Wilkinson, J. F.: Myelosclerosis. A clinicopathological study. *Q. J. Med.,* **26:**131–147, 1957.

Lewis, S. M., and Szur, L.: Malignant myelosclerosis. *Br. Med. J.,* **2:**472–477, 1963.

Ligumski, M.; Polliack, A.; and Benbasset, J.: Nature and incidence of liver involvement in agnogenic myeloid metaplasia. *Scand. J. Haematol.,* **21:**81–93, 1978.

Linman, J. W., and Bethell, F. H.: Agnogenic myeloid metaplasia. Its natural history and present day management. *Am. J. Med.,* **22:**107–122, 1957.

Loeb, V., Jr.: Treatment of polycythaemia vera. *Clin. Haematol.,* **4:**441–456, 1975.

McClure, P. D.; Ingram, G. I. C.; Stacey, R. S.; Glass, U. H.; and Matchett, M. O.: Platelet function tests in thrombocythaemia and thrombocytosis. *Br. J. Haematol.,* **12:**478–498, 1966.

Mitelman, F., and Levan, G.: Clustering of aberrations to specific chromosomes in human neoplasms. IV. A survey of 1,871 cases. *Hereditas,* **95:**79–139, 1981.

Modan, B.: An epidemiological study of polycythemia vera. *Blood,* **26:**657–667, 1965.

Modan, B.: Inter-relationship between polycythaemia vera, leukaemia and myeloid metaplasia. *Clin. Haematol.,* **4:**427–439, 1975.

Murphy, S.; Rosenthal, D. S.; Weinfeld, A.; Briere, J.; Faguet, G. B.; Knospe, W. H.; Landaw, S. A.; Laszlo, J.; Pisciotta, A. V.; Tartaglia, A. P.; Goldberg, J. D.; Berk, P. D.; Donovan, P. B.; and Wasserman, L. R.: Essential thrombocythemia: Response during first year of therapy with melphalan and radioactive phosphorus: A polycythemia vera study group report. *Cancer Treat. Rep.,* **66:**1495–1500, 1982.

Najean, Y.; Arrago, J. P.; Rain, J. D.; and Dresch, C.: The "spent" phase of polycythaemia vera: hypersplenism in the absence of myelofibrosis. *Br. J. Haematol.,* **56:**163–170, 1984.

Nakai, G. S.; Craddock, C. G.; and Figueroa, W. G.: Agnogenic myeloid metaplasia. *Ann. Intern. Med.,* **57:**419–440, 1962.

Osgood, E. E.: The case for ^{32}P in treatment of polycythemia vera. *Blood,* **32:**492–499, 1968.

Ozer, F. L.; Truax, W. E.; Miesch, D. C.; and Levin, W. C.: Primary hemorrhagic thrombocythemia. *Am. J. Med.,* **28:**807–823, 1960.

Peace, R. J.: Myelonecrosis, extramedullary myelopoiesis, and leukoerythroblastosis. A mesenchymal reaction to injury. *Am. J. Pathol.,* **29:**1029–1057, 1953.

Pitcock, J. A.; Reinhard, E. H.; Justus, B. W.; and Mendelsohn, R. S.: A clinical and pathological study of seventy cases of myelofibrosis. *Ann. Intern. Med.,* **57:**73–84, 1962.

Randall, D. L.; Reiquam, C. W.; Githens, J. H.; and Robinson, A.: Familial myeloproliferative disease. *Am. J. Dis. Child.,* **110:**479–500, 1965.

Ravich, R. B. M.; Gunz, F. W.; Reed, C. S.; and Thompson, I. L.: The dangers of surgery in uncontrolled haemorrhagic thrombocythaemia. *Med. J. Aust.,* **1:**704–708, 1970.

Rawson, R.; Parker, F., Jr.; and Jackson, H., Jr.: Industrial solvents as possible etiologic agents in myeloid metaplasia. *Science,* **93:**541–542. 1941.

Rojer, R. A.; Mulder, N. H.; and Nieweg, H. O.: 'Classic' and 'acute' myelofibrosis. *Acta Haematol.* (Basel), **60:**108–116, 1978.

Rosenbaum, D. L.; Murphy, G. W.; and Swisher, S. N.: Hemodynamic studies of the portal circulation in myeloid metaplasia. *Am. J. Med.,* **41:**360–368, 1966.

Rosenthal, D. S., and Moloney, W. C.: Myeloid metaplasia. A study of 98 cases. *Postgrad. Med.,* **45:**136–142, 1969.

Ross, R., and Vogel, A.: The platelet-derived growth factor. *Cell,* **14:**203–210, 1978.

Sagonne, A. L., Jr., and Balcerzak, S. P.: Smoking as a cause of erythrocytosis. *Ann. Intern. Med.,* **82:**512–515, 1975.

Schafer, A. I.: Bleeding and thrombosis in the myeloproliferative disorders. *Blood,* **64:**1–12, 1984.

Scher, C. D.; Shepard, R. C.; Antoniades, H. N.; and Stiles, C. D.: Platelet-derived growth factor and the regulation of the mammalian fibroblast cell cycle. *Biochim. Biophys. Acta,* **560:**217–241, 1979.

Shaldon, S. and Sherlock, S.: Portal hypertension in the myeloproliferative syndrome and the reticuloses. *Am. J. Med.,* **32:**758–764, 1962.

Shorey, J.; Weinberg, M. N.; Frenkel, E. P.; and Fallis, B. D.: Nodular regenerative hyperplasia of the liver in a case of myelofibrosis with extramedullary hematopoiesis and secondary portal venous hypertension. *Am. J. Clin. Pathol.,* **72:**122–125, 1979.

Silverstein, M. N.: Primary or hemorrhagic thrombocythemia. *Arch. Intern. Med.,* **122:**18–22, 1968.

Silverstein, M. N.: The evolution into and the treatment of late stage polycythemia vera. *Semin. Hematol.,* **13:**79–84, 1976.

Silverstein, M. N., and Linman, J. W.: Causes of death in agnogenic myeloid metaplasia. *Mayo Clin. Proc.,* **44:**36–39, 1969.

Smith, J. R., and Landaw, S. A.: Smokers' polycythemia. *N. Engl. J. Med.,* **298:**6–10, 1978.

Smith, J. W.; Shulman, H. M.; Thomas, E. D.; Fefer, A.; Buckner, C. D.: Bone marrow transplantation for acute myelosclerosis. *Cancer,* **48:**2198–2203, 1981.

Spaet, T. H.; Lejnieks, I.; Gaynor, E.; and Goldstein, M. L.: Defective platelets in essential thrombocythemia. *Arch. Intern. Med.,* **124:**135–141, 1969.

Stecher, G.; Wolpers, H.; and Nettesheim, P.: Polycythemia vera-Leukose. *Deutsche Med. Woch.,* **86:**1861–1867, 1961.

Stephens, A. D.: Polycythaemia and high affinity haemoglobins. *Br. J. Haematol.,* **36:**153–159, 1977.

Takacsi-Nagy, L., and Graf, F.: Definition, clinical features and diagnosis of myelofibrosis. *Clin. Haematol.,* **4:**291–308, 1975.

Tartaglia, A. P.; Goldberg, J. D.; Silverstein, M. N.; Dresch, C.; Tatarsky, I.; Pisciotta, A. V.; Faguet, G.; Rosenthal, D.; Conjalka, M.; Donovan, P. B.; Berk, P. D.; and Wasserman, L. R.: Aspirin and persantine do not prevent thrombotic complications in patients with polycythemia vera treated with phlebotomy. *Blood,* **58:**240a, 1981.

Vaughan, J.: Radiation and myeloproliferative disorders in man. In Clarke, W. J.; Howard, E. B.; and Hackett, P. L. (eds.): *Myeloproliferative Disorders of Animals and Man.* U.S. AEC Sympos., Washington, D.C. **19:** 489–500, 1970.

Ward, H. P., and Block, M. H.: The natural history of agnogenic myeloid metaplasia (AMM) and a critical evaluation of its relationship with the myeloproliferative syndrome. *Medicine,* **50:**357–420, 1971.

Wasserman, L. R.: Polycythemia vera—Its course and treatment: Relation to myeloid metaplasia and leukemia. *Bull. N.Y. Acad. Med.,* **30:**343–375, 1954.

Wasserman, L. R.: The management of polycythemia vera. *Br. J. Haematol.,* **21:**371–376, 1971.

Wasserman, L. R.: The treatment of polycythemia vera. *Semin. Hematol.,* **13:**57–78, 1976.

Wasserman, L. R.; Balcerzak, S. P.; Berk, P. D.; Berlin, N. I.; Donovan, P. B.; Dresch, C.; Ellis, J. T.; Goldberg, J. D.; Landaw, S. A.; Laszlo, J.; McIntyre, O. R.; Najean, Y.; Pisciotta, A. V.; Silverstein, M. N.; Tartaglia, A. P.; Tatarsky, I.; and Weinfeld, A.: Influence of therapy on causes of death in polycythemia vera. *Trans. Assoc. Am. Physicians,* **94:**30–38, 1981.

Weinberg, S. G.; Lubin, A.; Wiener, S. N.; Deoras, M. P.; Ghose, M. K.; and Kopelman, R. C.: Myelofibrosis and renal osteodystrophy. *Am. J. Med.,* **63:**755–764, 1977.

Wintrobe, M. M.; Lee, G. R.; Boggs, D. R.; Bithell, T. C.; Athens, J. W.; and Foerster, J.: Polycythemia. In: Wintrobe, M. M. (ed.): *Clinical Hematology*. Lea & Febiger, Philadelphia, 1974a.

Wintrobe, M. M.; Lee, G. R.; Boggs, D. R.; Bithell, T. C.; Athens, J. W.; and Foerster, J.: Myelofibrosis. In Wintrobe, M. M. (ed.): *Clinical Hematology*. Lea & Febiger, Philadelphia, 1974b.

Wolf, J. L.; Spruce, W. E.; Bearman, R. M.; Forman, S. J.; Scott, E. P.; Fahey, J. L.; Farbstein, M. J.; Rappaport, H.: Blume, K. G.: Reversal of acute ("malignant") myelosclerosis by allogeneic bone marrow transplantation. *Blood,* **59:**191–193, 1982.

Wyatt, J. P., and Sommers, S. C.: Chronic marrow failure, myelosclerosis, and extramedullary hematopoiesis. *Blood,* **5:**329–347, 1950.

20

Dermatologic Neoplasms

CHARLES McDONALD and PAUL CALABRESI

Introduction

In all areas principally inhabited by members of the Caucasian races, malignant neoplasms of the skin occur at rates much higher than in any other site (Allen, 1954; Dorn and Cutler, 1958; Belisario, 1959; Pedersen and Magnus, 1959; Ringertz *et al.,* 1960; Eastcott, 1963; Haenszel, 1963). All of the component structures of skin, such as the epidermis, dermis, and adnexal structures, may give rise to malignant neoplasms (see Table 20–1). Except for cancer derived from epidermis, however, most are extremely rare. This chapter on cutaneous neoplasms will be limited to a discussion of: (1) the most commonly encountered neoplasms, basal cell and squamous cell carcinoma, and (2) two neoplasms that occur infrequently but offer clues to either the etiology, pathogenesis, diagnosis, and/or treatment of other human cancers (cutaneous T-cell lymphomas and Kaposi's sarcoma).

A large number of cutaneous lesions may be characterized as premalignant, meaning that given the proper conditions of lesion type, time, host, and location, an indeterminate number may progress or transform into malignant neoplasms (see Table 20–2). Some may develop characteristic malignant changes in morphology (changes such as disturbed cellular architecture, abnormal and frequent mitoses) from the onset, yet remain confined to the epidermis. These lesions are classified as carcinomas *in situ.* Rarely do they invade or

Table 20–1. Primary Tumors of the Skin

TUMOR TYPE	PRECURSOR LESION(S)	CELL OF ORIGIN	TISSUE OF ORIGIN
1. Basal cell carcinoma	—	Epidermis (germinative)	Epithelial
2. Squamous cell carcinoma	Actinic (solar) keratoses Tar and pitch keratoses Arsenical keratoses X-ray and radium keratoses Bowen's disease Erythroplasia of Queyrat	Epidermis (differentiating)	Epithelial
3. Keratoacanthoma	—	Epidermis (differentiating)	Epithelial
4. Paget's disease (extramammary)	—	Apocrine gland and goblet cells	Epithelial
5. Malignant melanoma	Lentigo maligna Congenital giant (garment type nevi) Junctional and compound nevi	Melanocyte	Neural
6. Kaposi's sarcoma	—	Endothelial	Vascular mesenchyme
7. T-cell lymphomas; mycosis fungoides lymphoma (Sézary syndrome)	Parapsoriasis and premycotic eczemas	Lymphocyte (thymus-derived)	Reticuloendothelial

Table 20-2. Precancerous Skin Lesions

Keratoses:
    Actinic (solar)
    X-ray and radium
    Arsenic
    Tar and pitch
Bowen's disease (precancerous dermatosis)
Erythroplasia of Queyrat
Paget's disease (extramammary)
Lentigo maligna

---

disrupt the basal lamina sufficiently to meet the ultimate criteria for being considered malignant. Each lesion, however, retains the ability to transform from a morphologic to a biologic cancer, principally squamous cell carcinoma, at any time during its history. Specific discussions of the important premalignant lesions are included in this Chapter.

Incidence and Epidemiology

Skin cancers are estimated to account for over 50% of all cancers in Australia (Belisario, 1959), 33% of all cancers in Texas (Phillips, 1941), but only 1.4% of all cancers in India (Mulay, 1963). The frequency of skin cancer in New Zealand and Australia is estimated to be three to ten times higher than in England and Wales, although the same ethnic groups (English, Welsh, Irish, Scottish) are affected (Eastcott, 1963; TenSeldam, 1963). In the United States, age adjusted incidence rates vary greatly depending upon the geographic region examined (Haenszel, 1963). According to Haenszel, the occurrence rate of skin cancer in northern white men is about 33.4/100,000, and in women it is 25.4/100,000, whereas in southern white men and women the rates are respectively 143.3/100,000 and 88/100,000 (Haenszel, 1963). Dorn and Cutler (1958) estimate the age adjusted morbidity incidence

Table 20-3. Some Etiologic Factors in Cutaneous Cancer

Endogenous
1. Heredity (skin color, genetic predisposition)
2. Race (skin color)
3. Age
4. Sex (occupational, recreational)

Exogenous
1. Physical agents (sunlight, x-ray, trauma)
2. Chemical agents (arsenic, polycyclic hydrocarbons)
3. Living agents (viruses, schistosomes)
4. Geographic and epidemiologic factors (occupational, recreational, ultraviolet light availability)

---

rates for whites versus nonwhites residing in the United States as follows: 56.1/100,000 for white men and 39.5/100,000 for white women; 4.5/100,000 for nonwhite men and 6.0/100,000 for nonwhite women.

Not only do these studies call to attention the influence of race, ethnic group, gender, and other individual factors, they also highlight the influence of environmental and physical factors on the development of skin cancer (see Table 20-3).

Etiology

External Factors. Ultraviolet light is the single most important external factor that influences development of cancer of the skin. The role of ultraviolet light in cancer induction has been recognized since the 1850s. Only since the middle and latter half of the twentieth century, however, have we begun to appreciate the exact role of ultraviolet light as an initiator and promoter in carcinogenesis (Grady *et al.*, 1941; Blum, 1959; Daniels, 1963; Cleaver, 1968; Painter and Cleaver, 1969; Kripke, 1982). Substantial evidence shows that sunburn and cancer are caused by ultraviolet radiation shorter than 3200 Å (320 nm), or the sunburn spectrum of ultraviolet (ultraviolet light B and C [UVB and UVC] within the ranges of 250 to 320 nm). Ultraviolet light A (UVA), a light spectrum from 320 to 440 nm, can also produce sunburn and augment the sunburn effects of UVB but is approximately 1000 times less effective than are UVB and UVC (Pathak, 1982). UVA may be considered protective rather than damaging to the skin because light within its spectrum is responsible for stimulating the production of melanin. Melanin pigment offers substantial protection to skin cells from the deleterious effects of sunburn radiation. Sunburn or carcinogenic wavelengths in sunlight that reach the earth occur principally in the UVB spectrum. Ultraviolet light of wavelengths less than 290 nm (UVC) is effectively blocked from reaching the earth's surface by a layer of ozone and molecular oxygen located at a stratospheric level between 15 to 35 kilometers. The ultimate destruction of this "protective" layer by physical means (high altitude supersonic aircraft) and chemical means (volatile hydrocarbons) would expose humans to sunburn and carcinogenic light of a much stronger magnitude than at present.

Tissue absorption of ultraviolet radiation in

the sunburn range appears to require the presence of chemicals with an aromatic ring structure found either in purines and pyrimidines of nucleic acids or tyrosine or tryptophan of proteins (Daniels, 1963). Absorption of ultraviolet light induces the formation of pyrimidine dimers that under normal circumstances are easily repaired (Painter and Cleaver, 1969; Trosko *et al.,* 1970). Under constant bombardment by ultraviolet light, as may occur with repeated sunburn, repair mechanisms are overwhelmed and become ineffective. Partial repair of defects eventually leads to cell death, mutation (carcinogenesis), or altered metabolism. Eventually (ten to 20 years later) cutaneous cancers occur in the sun-damaged skin of susceptible individuals. It has been postulated (Epstein, 1970) and there is some evidence to support the postulate (Hanawalt and Setlow, 1975) that skin cancer induction by UVB is initiated by early and initial repair of damaged DNA, and that cells survive but retain mechanisms favoring the subsequent development of errors in DNA replication and ultimately in neoplastic change. Basal cell replication occurring more frequently in the unaffected skin of patients with skin cancer than in normal controls has been noted by Gregg and Mansbridge (1982). The exact relationship of this observation to the development of skin cancer in a susceptible host is as yet undefined.

Kripke (1982) and many other investigators have identified an additional role of ultraviolet light in inducing skin cancer. UV irradiation seems to influence the immune system of the host (suppressor T-cell function) in a manner that favors the growth of tumors. The additive influence of increased temperature (Owens and Donald, 1977), wind and humidity (Owens and Donald, 1977), immunosuppression (Daynes *et al.,* 1979), UVA light (Sterns *et al.,* 1981), and chemical carcinogens (Epstein, 1970) have been shown.

The role of chemicals—topically and systemically administered—in inducing cutaneous cancer has been extensively studied since the concept of chemical carcinogenesis was introduced by Sir Percival Pott in 1775. Although the process of chemical carcinogenesis has been extensively studied, the true incidence of chemically related or induced cancers of the skin remains unknown. Most chemical carcinogens other than trivalent arsenic are complex substances, principally polycyclic and aromatic hydrocarbons. Tar, pitch, soot, tar oils, creosol, anthracine oil, coke, carbon blacks, asphalt, fuel oils, lubricating oils, greases, crude paraffin oils, and diesel oils are examples of chemical agents that may act as promoters and initiators of cancer. (For a comprehensive review of this subject the reader is referred to Brookes, 1980.) Other than arsenic-induced cancer, clear relationships between exposure to chemical carcinogens and the development of skin cancer are few, especially in comparison to the degree that ultraviolet exposure can be related to tumor development.

In the formation of skin cancer, a chemical carcinogen is activated within the cell by a variety of mechanisms and induces cellular responses similar to those after exposure to ultraviolet light and x-irradiation (Roberts, 1980; Sims, 1980). Activated chemical carcinogens are capable of interacting with cellular DNA and causing damage to DNA. Chemically damaged DNA is normally repaired by processes similar to those used by cells subsequent to damage by x-irradiation and UV light. Repair processes enable the cell to replicate its DNA past the induced lesions and to survive nucleic acid damage. Ultimately, and after repeated insult, the repair process becomes faulty and errors appear. Mutational (chromosomal) damage and carcinogenesis begin within the cell. Nitrogen mustards have been identified as human cutaneous carcinogens (Kravitz and McDonald, 1978; Lee *et al.,* 1982).

X-ray-induced cancers are encountered at a rate greatly reduced since the turn of the century. Most people in an environment associated with increased exposure to x-irradiation are well versed in the hazards of x-irradiation and in methods of self protection. New diagnostic and therapeutic instruments have considerably reduced the amount of radiation exposure during diagnostic procedures, as well as the amount of therapeutic x-irradiation delivered to sites other than the target tissue. Biologic x-irradiation, regardless of the delivery system, acts in a manner similar to that described for ultraviolet-induced carcinogenesis.

The role of viruses in the etiology of cutaneous cancer remains unclear. Human papilloma virus (HPV) has been associated with benign, self-regressing papillomas of the skin and mucous membrane (warts/condylomata acuminata). Papilloma viruses are also associated with a number of mammalian tumors, specifically the Shope virus in rabbits, the bovine virus in experimental animals, and at least two human syndromes. Epidermodysplasia verruciformis is a rare familial syndrome in which flat-to-dome-shaped warts are scattered over the face, neck, hands, and knees. (Approximately 25% of the patients with epidermodysplasia verruciformis develop cutaneous cancers in sun-exposed areas.) Very few HPV virus particles have been found in neoplastic tissue (Prunierais, 1976). In addition, the Buschke-Lowenstein tumor or verrucous carcinoma of the genital and perianal regions is associated with HPV positive benign and premalignant stages. Transition from a benign to a malignant state is a very unusual occurrence, and neoplastic lesions associated with the two diseases are probably malignant from the onset.

Host Factors. The single most important host factor in the development of skin cancer is skin color. Skin color depends on inherited (genetic) factors. Melanin pigment is the principal inherited sun protector. Inherited skin color relates directly to ethnicity. Celtic type skin usually has no melanin or contains reduced amounts of melanin pigment. Celtics are prone to develop severe sunburn after minimum sun exposure. They are also prone to develop malignant cutaneous neoplasms. Native black Africans have skin rich in melanin pigment. Only after long and intensive sun exposure will blacks develop sunburn. Cutaneous neoplasms are quite rare in black skin, particularly those that are attributed to sun exposure.

Hair color and eye color are similarly inherited and relate directly to skin color. A typical profile of a person prone to skin cancer is one whose skin color is very fair, eye color is pale blue, hair color is red, ethnic group is Celtic, and who reacts to sun by burning easily. Pathak (1982) and others have proposed a "sun-reactive skin typing system" as an aid for counseling people on the harmful effects of sunlight and for prevention of sunburn, solar skin changes, and skin cancer (see Table 20-4). Skin types are based on an individual's ability to sunburn and suntan, which are based principally upon intrinsic genetically endowed skin content of melanin, skin color, and facultative skin color (the genetically determined capacity of the skin to tan or produce protective melanin pigmentation). Skin types I and II describe persons of Northern European extraction, types III and IV, Southern Europeans, Northern Mongolians and Mediterraneans, and types V and VI describe African types, darker Mediterraneans, and Southern Mongolians.

Other inherited host factors yet to be defined are those related to the development of multiple basal cell carcinomas of the skin, such as in the basal cell nevus syndrome. In patients and families presenting with this syndrome, skin cancers occur at very early ages and at multiple sites. Most sites have not been exposed to excessive UV light (Gorlin et al., 1965). Individuals with xeroderma pigmentosum are born with the inability to repair effectively damaged DNA. As a result, even minimal exposure to sunlight results in the development of cutaneous cancers of all types, that is, basal cell and squamous cell cancers and malignant melanomas (Cleaver, 1968).

PRECANCEROUS LESIONS AND CARCINOMA IN SITU

Any discussion of cancers of the skin is incomplete without reference to certain precursor or precancerous lesions. The concept of precancer and precancerous lesions continues to be debated. Some believe an invasive squamous cell carcinoma of the skin begins as an

Table 20-4. Sun-Reactive Skin Types and Cutaneous Cancer

SKIN TYPE	HISTORY OF SUNBURN AND SUNTAN	UV SENSITIVITY	POTENTIAL FOR DEVELOPING SKIN CANCER
I	Always burns, never tans	Very sensitive	High
II	Always burns, tans minimally	Very sensitive	High
III	Sometimes burns, tans well	Sensitive	Moderate
IV	Burns minimally, always tans	Moderate sensitivity	Moderate
V	Rarely burns, tans darkly and well	Minimal sensitivity	Minimal
VI	Never burns, skin is black	Insensitive	Practically none

invasive squamous cell carcinoma; no intermediate stage exists between a clinically and histologically benign state and cancer. The number of proponents of this philosophy is rapidly shrinking. It is the rare dermatologist who has not observed the transformation of a benign solar or radiation keratosis into squamous cell cancer on a background of skin heavily damaged by sun or x-irradiation.

A classification of precancerous skin lesions could include all dermatoses having a potential to produce lesions of a neoplastic nature, including solar- and x-irradiation–damaged skin. Another classification could include only those specific lesions that have a very high degree of probability of undergoing malignant transformation: Actinic (solar) keratoses, radiation and arsenical keratoses, Bowen's tumor or Bowen's precancerous dermatitis, erythroplasia of Queyrat and kraurosis vulvae. On microscopic examination all of these show atypia or "malignant dyskeratosis" of epithelial cells while remaining confined to the epidermis. Some, such as Bowen's tumors, erythroplasia of Queyrat, and kraurosis vulvae, appear more malignant than others on histologic examination and are often referred to as "carcinoma *in situ*."

The frequency of neoplastic change is quite variable and principally depends on the specific type of precancerous lesion. For example, it has been estimated that less than 10% of all actinic (solar) keratoses will undergo malignant transformation (that is, will show dermal invasiveness), whereas it has been shown that upwards of 50% of untreated Bowen's tumors will eventually undergo malignant change (Graham and Helwig, 1961). The relative frequency of malignant degeneration in actinic keratoses, although low, still gives cause for concern because over the lifetime of a susceptible individual literally hundreds of actinic keratoses may occur. Montgomery and Dorffel (1932) estimate that 20 to 25% of patients with multiple actinic keratoses will develop one or more squamous cell carcinomas. The period of time required for malignant transformation of a typical precancerous lesion varies but appears to center around six to ten years after onset.

Specific Lesions

Keratoses. *Actinic Keratoses.* The true incidence of actinic keratoses is unknown, but they are extremely common. The average fair-skinned, red-haired, and freckled person rarely goes through life without developing one or more actinic keratoses. Most who experience several severe sunburns will develop numerous actinic keratoses. Actinic keratoses are rarely found in pigmented races. All of those etiologic factors that are outlined in the general discussion of cutaneous tumors, basal cell carcinoma, and malignant melanoma also apply to the development of actinic keratoses. Actinic keratoses are always found on sunlight-exposed areas of the skin and on a background of sun-damaged skin. The skin of patients with actinic keratoses is usually thin, wrinkled, and dry and is coursed by numerous telangiectatic blood vessels and large hyperpigmented frecklelike lesions (see Colorplate VII). The scalp, face, ears, lower lip, and dorsal surfaces of the arms and hands are the most frequently involved sites. The age of onset varies from 26 to 86 years (Graham and Helwig, 1963).

The clinical appearance of cutaneous lesions varies slightly with the age of the lesions. Early keratoses are flat, red macules with scaly surfaces. Their size varies from 2 to 5 mm and upward; the average lesion is about 1 cm in diameter. They are multiple but do not cover the entire cutaneous surface on the affected part. No explanation of why all sun-damaged areas of skin similarly exposed to sunlight do not develop sun-related keratoses has been reported. As each lesion ages, the surface becomes more keratotic. In old lesions, surface scaling may be so thick that the normal erythematous surface color is no longer apparent. Scaling may be so profuse that a "cutaneous horn" is produced (see Figure 20–1). Removal of scales reveals a red, bleeding surface. Older lesions also develop palpable induration at the bases. At this stage, clinical differentiation from frankly invasive squamous cell carcinoma is impossible. Although dermal invasiveness of squamous cell carcinomas derived from actinic keratoses does not differ from that of tumors derived from other precancerous lesions, the tendency to metastasize is considerably less (Lund, 1965).

Histologically, identifiable changes can be noted in the dermis and epidermis of each precancerous keratosis. Lever (1983) recognizes three primary histologic types, all of which may exist singly or in combination.

The Hypertrophic Type. This is the most commonly observed lesion (see Figure 20–2). Atrophic areas of the epidermis alternate with areas of hyperkeratosis, parakeratosis, and papillomatosis. Cells throughout the differentiating layers of the epidermis are irregularly ar-

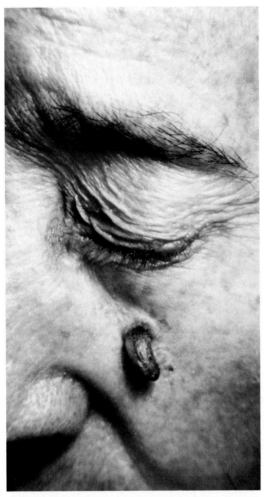

Figure 20–1. Cutaneous horn. A lesion characterized by an extreme degree of keratinization and retained epithelial cells. The histologic findings in this lesion may be typical of hypertrophic actinic keratosis or squamous cell carcinoma.

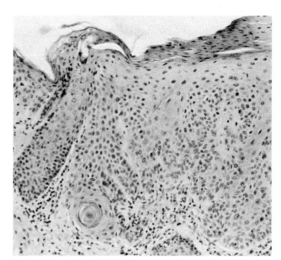

Figure 20–2. Hypertrophic actinic keratosis, showing a substantial amount of surface scale and atypia of the epithelial cells. There is a disturbance of normal maturation of epithelium, however the basement membrane remains intact. A sweat duct is contained within the lesion. Typical of this lesion, the epithelium of the sweat duct is not involved.

The Bowenoid Type. The histologic picture resembles one frequently seen in Bowen's tumor (see Figure 20–4).

Dermal changes in all three tumor types feature abnormalities (degeneration) in collagen and elastic tissue. Deposition of material that stains like elastin occurs in the upper portions of the dermis and proliferation of capillaries exists in the same region. A dense infiltrate containing large numbers of lymphocytes and plasma cells forms in the papillary dermis.

ranged and atypical, containing large, irregular, hyperchromatic nuclei. Individual cell keratinization, as well as downward proliferation of the epidermis, may also be present. In all cases, however, the basal laminae remain intact.

The Atrophic Type. Epidermal atrophy predominates, with, perhaps, minimal hyperkeratosis (see Figure 20–3). Cellular abnormalities are generally confined to the basal layer. Dyskeratosis of cells in this region may result in loss of intercellular connections and separation of basal layer from other layers of the epidermis, thereby forming lakes or "lacunae." Proliferation and downward growth of epithelium may also occur, but again the basement membrane remains intact.

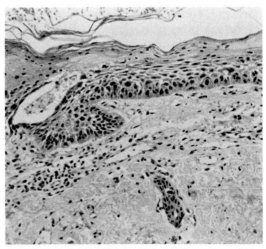

Figure 20–3. Atrophic actinic keratosis. Scaling is quite prominent. The epidermis is thin. Cellular abnormalities are confined to the basal layers of epidermis.

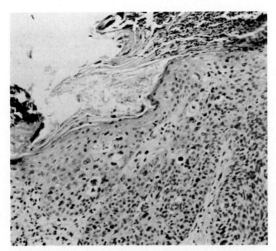

Figure 20–4. Bowenoid actinic keratosis. The epithelial abnormalities are characterized by the presence of numerous mitoses and ballooning of the epithelial cells, simulating to a degree those features found in Bowen's disease.

Treatment of Actinic Keratoses. Actinic keratoses may be treated effectively by a wide variety of methods. Solitary lesions can be treated with brief cryotherapy (application of liquid nitrogen using cotton-tipped applicators or cryospray; application of CO_2 slush). Curettage and electrodesiccation or excision are used principally on thick, scaling, and indurated lesions. Most patients with actinic keratoses have multiple superficial lesions. Two daily topical applications of various concentrations of 5-fluorouracil (5-FU, 1 to 5% ointments or lotions) to the entire affected integument has been found most useful and beneficial (Klein *et al.,* 1962; Dillaha *et al.,* 1965). In addition to eradicating all but the most hypertrophic lesions, topical application of 5-FU also uncovers and eradicates lesions that are not yet visible to the clinician's eyes. After one to four weeks, active lesions become inflammatory, firey red, pruritic (or burning), and exudative. If treatment is continued beyond 1½ to 2 weeks, sites without apparent involvement assume a similar appearance. Normal skin is not adversely affected. Treatment may be ended at any time after the appearance of eroded lesions. A sizable number of therapists, however, feel that treatment should extend up to six to eight weeks, at which time the entire face and/or other treated parts become firey red, eroded, and painful. Prolonged treatment purportedly reduces the incidence of new and recurrent lesions. Dermatologists have found that very few patients will tolerate treatment beyond three weeks.

The intensity of the reaction can be accelerated by exposure to sunlight (ultraviolet light) and by simultaneous applications of topical retinoic acid. Intensity can likewise be reduced by applying potent topical corticosteroids simultaneously with or after the development of reactive lesions. Contact dermatitis to 5-FU and/or its vehicles may complicate this form of treatment (Breza *et al.,* 1976). Lesions resistant to 5-FU may be treated by either of the techniques mentioned above except cryotherapy using cotton-tipped applicators.

The mechanism of action of 5-FU in the elimination of actinic keratoses is unknown, but a number of mechanisms have been hypothesized (Eaglstein *et al.,* 1970; Zelickson *et al.,* 1975). Medical oncologists have long been aware of the ability of systemically administered 5-FU to cause *reactive* changes in actinic keratoses of the skin of patients being treated for systemic cancers.

Radiation-Induced Keratoses. Cutaneous changes including premalignant keratoses may be induced by many forms of ionizing radiation (see Colorplates IX and X). Generally, premalignant lesions arise from improperly administered x-rays, especially in diagnostic procedures, or in the absence of proper shielding after inadvertently large doses administered for long periods of time. Very high doses when delivered therapeutically for short periods also result in precancerous lesions. Properly fractionated therapeutic x-rays that do not exceed a total dose of 4000 to 6000 rads administered for several weeks do not usually induce precancerous lesions.

A chronic radiation-induced dermatitis (Colorplate IX) always precedes the development of a precancerous lesion in the skin subsequent to ionizing radiation. The cutaneous changes associated with radiation dermatitis are identical to those seen after repeated overexposure to ultraviolet light. In fact, it is very difficult clinically to distinguish between sun-induced and radiation-induced dermatitides and keratoses.

Histologically, keratotic lesions produced by ionizing radiation appear similar to those occurring after sunlight and arsenic exposure. The dermis may differ slightly, showing more extensive replacement of collagen by elastic-type tissue, abnormal fibroblasts, and obliterative vascular changes. Treatment is essentially the same as for eradicating actinic keratoses.

Arsenical Keratoses. Arsenical keratosis is only one of several abnormal changes induced in the skin by chronic exposure to trivalent arsenic (see Colorplate VIII). These lesions are seen in all racial groups. Sources of inorganic arsenic include medications (Fowler's solution), insecticides, industry (foundaries, electroplating), contaminated water supplies, and foods (wines and fruits from vineyards treated with arsenic-containing insecticides). The total amount of arsenic required to induce keratoses and, subsequently, squamous cell carcinomas is unknown. There appears to be considerable individual variation in susceptibility, but a dose as small as 0.19 g has been shown to be carcinogenic (Neubauer, 1947). Exposure time varies but lesions usually become apparent one to ten years after exposure. Arsenical keratoses may occur at any age. Carcinomas secondary to arsenic have been reported in a young black child, and in Helwig and Grahams's series (1963) the average age of patients at the time of removal of cutaneous lesions was 49.

Although chronic arsenic poisoning is associated with hyperpigmentation and depigmentation, arsenic-induced keratoses most often develop on a background of normal skin. Arsenic-induced keratoses occur commonly on the extremities, particularly on the hands and feet. Areas subjected to friction and trauma, such as the palms and soles and ventral surfaces of the digits, are particularly vulnerable to the development of lesions. Multiple lesions are common. Arsenic-induced keratoses differ clinically from precancerous actinic and radiation keratoses not only in location but in appearance. Arsenic-induced keratoses generally do not exceed 5 mm in diameter and are often covered by a protuberant hard scale or crust. Some lesions are punctate in appearance. A rapidly appearing halo of erythema and thickening at the base of a keratosis often indicates transformation into an invasive lesion. Invasive squamous cell carcinoma arising in arsenic-induced keratoses is characterized by very rapid growth.

Histopathologically, *Bowenoid* changes in the cells are intermixed with areas of acanthosis, parakeratosis, and hyperkeratosis. Vacuolated cells with pyknotic nuclei are also observed. In the pathologic diagnosis of arsenic-induced keratoses, as well as in cancer related to arsenic, the finding of abnormally high concentrations of arsenic within involved tissues compared to normal surrounding skin is not unusual. The finding of nonspecific crystal formation in the skin after histochemical staining may be seen but may be misleading (Osborne test); direct chemical analysis is more reliable and will usually reveal arsenic values greater than the normal 0.00008 mg/g of tissue.

Treatment of arsenic-induced keratoses may prove difficult because the lesions are usually far too numerous for routine destructive techniques to be effective; nor do they respond to topical chemotherapeutic agents. Cryotherapy using the cryospray technique probably offers the best alternative. Patients should be examined frequently for malignant change in individual lesions and for the development of internal neoplasms. Pulmonary carcinomas are not commonly associated with arsenic ingestion.

Intraepidermal Squamous Cell Carcinoma. In addition to occurring as nonspecific cutaneous lesions, that is, actinic keratoses, arsenic-induced keratoses, and radiation-induced keratoses, some precancerous lesions— intraepidermal squamous cell carcinomas— may exist in clearly identifiable morphologic forms, such as Bowen's disease and erythroplasia of Queyrat. These two lesions, which differ histopathologically from other precancerous lesions because of their early involvement of the entire epidermis, can remain benign, confined within the epidermis for long periods of time. Eventually, and especially in certain locations such as Bowen's disease in and near the anal orifice, they become invasive and metastatic to regional lymph nodes and to distant sites.

Bowen's Disease. Most often, lesions of Bowen's disease (intraepidermal squamous cell carcinoma, or squamous cell carcinoma *in situ*) occur as solitary neoplasms on sun-exposed and covered areas of the body. It is often stated that if actinic keratoses with a Bowenoid histologic appearance are excluded, nearly all Bowen's tumors would be found on covered areas of the body. Bowen's tumors are most frequently found in fair-skinned Caucasians (Graham and Helwig, 1963). Because of a low index of suspicion, the generally asymptomatic nature of Bowen's disease, and the tendency to confuse Bowen's tumors with other dermatoses, they may be underreported in black patients (Mora *et al.,* 1984). Most lesions have a characteristic clinical appearance as sharply demarcated patches with little or no surface elevation. Color varies from intensely red to dull red to brown. The surface is usually covered with a very fine scale or crust. Most lesions are not indurated on palpation. Some that are probably on the borderline of transformation into invasive squamous cell carcinoma, however, may have an irregular surface and may be of variable thickness.

Lesions of the fingers are common and frequently do not present with the characteristic clinical appearance of Bowen's tumors. They often appear eczematous and are treated for long periods as nonresponsive eczematous eruptions. Lesions of moist intertriginous areas (glans penis, vulva, and oral mucosa) also differ in clinical appearance and at such sites are frequently called erthyroplasia of Queyrat. In these sites crusts do not form and the surface is red, friable, and oozing. Occasionally, lesions in these areas can be dry and deeply pigmented or papular and verrucous. Longstanding lesions may show ulceration of the surface epithelium; if so, the basement membrane has usually been invaded.

Several theories relative to the mode of development of Bowen's disease have been advanced. Very few lesions are thought to occur as a result of light exposure. Mounting epidemiologic evidence suggests that Bowen's tumors are a result of chronic ingestion of trivalent arsenic by one of several routes (Graham and Helwig, 1963; Miki *et al.,* 1982). These data are most convincing in patients with multiple lesions in non-sun-exposed sites. Additional evidence for a relationship to arsenic includes the high association of Bowen's disease and internal cancer. When internal cancers occur in association with Bowen's disease, they are in sites commonly involved after chronic arsenic ingestion (Graham and Helwig, 1961; Callen and Headington, 1980; Miki *et al.,* 1982).

Histopathologically, Bowen's disease has been referred to as squamous cell carcinoma *in situ* (Lever, 1983; Lever and Schaumberg-Lever, 1983) (see Figure 20-5). The lesion is confined to the epidermis. The upper epidermis shows hyperkeratosis and parakeratosis. Considerable acanthosis and enlargement of the rete ridges may obscure dermal papillae. The differentiating segment of the epidermis contains cells in complete disarray, which are atypical and contain large hyperchromatic nuclei. Many cells show marked vacuolization and individual cell keratinization. Multinucleated clusters of cells may be scattered throughout the epidermis. The dermis may show a moderate to heavy inflammatory cell infiltrate containing lymphocytes and plasma cells.

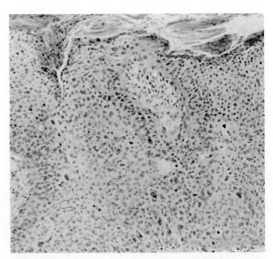

Figure 20-5. Bowen's disease or intraepidermal squamous cell carcinoma. The histology in this lesion should be compared to that seen in Figure 20-7. The epidermis is hyperkeratotic. There is considerable acanthosis. The atypical epithelial cells throughout are in complete disarray and contain large hyperchromatic nuclei. Many show vacuolization and individual cell keratinization.

Treatment of Bowen's tumors in the preinvasive stage is simple. Nearly all procedures prove satisfactory for eradicating the disease (see treatment of basal cell carcinoma). Care must be taken in treating sites that are prone to develop invasive carcinoma, such as the perianal region. Surgical excision of lesions in this area is often the preferred treatment so that all tissue may be submitted to pathology for examination of depth of tumor invasion and tumor margins.

Erythroplasia of Queyrat. Erythroplasia of Queyrat, a lesion that occurs principally on the glans penis, is often called Bowen's disease of the genitalia (or squamous cell carcinoma *in situ*). Graham and Helwig (1963), however, feel there is little evidence to support this concept. Although the histopathology of this lesion is the same as that described for Bowen's disease, Graham and Helwig believe the differing clinical behavior of each makes them different lesions. They cite a differing incidence of internal cancer among patients having the two diseases. The proneness of erythroplasia of Queyrat to invade underlying dermis (14%), as contrasted to Bowen's tumor (5.2%), may offer additional evidence for recognizing a difference between the two diseases. Erythroplasia of Queyrat, in spite of an increased tendency to become invasive, has a much more favorable outcome than does Bowen's tumor. Nearly all other observers are quite convinced that erythroplasia of Queyrat is Bowen's tumor situated on the glans penis (Lever, 1983).

Bowenoid Papulosis of the Genitalia. A discussion of precancerous lesions of the skin should include Bowenoid papulosis of the genitalia. Reported under a variety of names, such as multicentric Bowen's disease of the vulva, multicentric pigmented Bowen's disease, pigmented penile papules, and multiple Bowenoid papules of the penis, its true nature has been controversial for almost a decade. Is the primary lesion a wart, a precancerous variant of Bowen's disease, or does Bowenoid papulosis actually exist as a distinct entity?

Bowenoid papulosis does exist. It occurs principally in young adult men and women with a peak age of incidence in the third decade. The age range of reported cases is from one to 64 years (Kao and Graham, 1982). In Europe and the United States the disease occurs most frequently in men, whereas in Japan Bowenoid papulosis occurs with equal frequency in men and women. Typical lesions are multiple, 4 mm or less, reddish-brown to brown, flat to slightly dome-shaped papules found in clusters on the genitalia and perigenital skin (see Figure 20-6). They are usually asymptomatic, although an occasional patient may complain of burning and itching. Infrequently, lesions may coalesce to form plaques, some may become papillomatous or verrucous, but generally the surface is smooth in men, and smooth or velvety in women. Most males with this lesion have been circumcised in infancy. Nearly all patients report previous treatment for herpes progenitalis or condyloma acuminata or both. In some patients with

herpes progenitalis, light and dye therapy preceded the appearance of lesions. The tenuous relationship of light and dye treatment to the appearance of Bowenoid papules and unpublished reports of cancerous degeneration in some lesions in light- and dye-exposed skin have eliminated this method of treating herpetic lesions. Only two cases of Bowenoid papulosis progression to neoplastic lesions have been reported in the literature, one to invasive squamous cell carcinoma and the other to Bowen's intraepidermal squamous cell carcinoma (Kimura, 1982).

Based on recent clinical, histopathologic, ultrastructural, and immunofluorescent findings, Bowenoid papulosis of the genitalia may best be characterized as a disease caused by human papilloma viruses (Kimura, 1982). Histologically, lesions may show features similar to Bowen's disease and erythroplasia of Queyrat (see Figure 20-7). The most important microscopic feature that distinguishes Bowenoid papulosis from Bowen's disease and erythroplasia of Queyrat is the lack of full thickness involvement of the epithelium by atypical, pleomorphic keratinocytes; epithelial cells are more uniform in Bowenoid papulosis (Kao and Graham, 1982).

Bowenoid lesions can spontaneously regress, remain static, or enlarge progressively. Although treatment recommendations vary, Bowenoid papules are benign and should be treated conservatively by cryotherapy, curettage and electrodesiccation, and simple excision. Radical therapeutic procedures such as

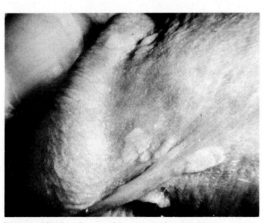

Figure 20-6. Bowenoid papulosis. Multiple, small, wartlike growths are clustered near the coronal sulcus.

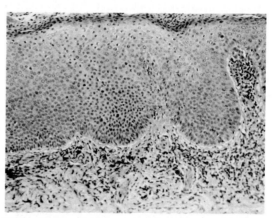

Figure 20-7. Histology of Bowenoid papulosis. This lesion shows hyperkeratosis and acanthosis of the epidermis. When contrasted with Figure 20-5 there is more uniformity of cells throughout the epidermis; there is less ballooning and vacuolization.

vulvectomy and amputation of the penis proposed by some are totally unwarranted.

SQUAMOUS CELL CANCER (EPIDERMOID CARCINOMA)

Incidence and Epidemiology

Squamous cell cancer is the second most common neoplasm among Caucasians (Eastcott, 1963; Haenszel, 1963; TenSeldam, 1963). In the United States the age adjusted incidence varies between men and women and between north and south (Haenszel, 1963). The age adjusted incidence in northern men and women is 8.9 and 5.3/100,000, respectively, whereas in southern men and women the incidence is 32.3 and 9.6/100,000, respectively. Squamous cell cancers are 15% of all skin cancers in New Zealand, 29% in London and 22% in Sydney (Eastcott, 1963). In nearly all other races, squamous cell cancer is the predominant skin cancer (Atkinson et al., 1963; Miyaji, 1963; Mulay, 1963; Oettle, 1963; Pringgoutomo and Pringgoutomo, 1963; Shanmugaratnam and LaBrooy, 1963; Yeh, 1963; Mora and Perniciaro, 1981).

In Caucasian men and women most squamous cell cancers are found on sun-exposed areas, principally the head and neck and extremities. Urbach (1966) has shown that squamous cell cancer of the skin in the head and neck occurs almost exclusively on those areas with maximum exposure to ultraviolet light. Squamous cell cancers often occur on the extremities in light-exposed areas whereas basal cell cancers are rarely found on the extremities. In pigmented races squamous cell cancers are much more frequent on the extremities than on other body areas. In the series by Mora and Perniciaro (1981), of 163 black patients treated at Charity Hospital in New Orleans the most common locations of squamous cell tumors were the face and lower extremities. Collectively, cutaneous tumors on non-sun-exposed areas were common. Although sunlight exposure may have been of etiologic significance in the 33.9% of tumors found on the faces of Moro and Perniciaro's black patients, the most common predisposing condition for all other sites appeared to be chronic scarring processes. The same observations have been recorded in reports from India (Mulay, 1963), Singapore (Shanmugaratnam and LaBrooy,

1963), New Guinea (Atkinson et al., 1963), Africa (Oettle, 1963), and Indonesia (Pringgoutomo and Pringgoutomo, 1963), among others.

Squamous cell cancers usually occur in middle-aged and elderly adults of all races, although squamous cell cancers as a result of exposure to topical and systemic chemical carcinogens tend to occur at an early age.

Etiology and Pathogenesis

Like basal cell carcinoma, squamous cell carcinoma often arises on skin that has suffered chronic overexposure to the sun. Based upon experimental and epidemiologic data, it is generally acknowledged that those factors relating to sunlight and skin color and the development of other cutaneous cancers also relate strongly to the development of squamous cell cancer (Hyde, 1906; Urbach et al., 1966). (See discussions in sections on Introduction to Cutaneous Cancers and Basal Cell Carcinoma.) Squamous cell cancer is a very common tumor in Celtics living in sunny climates such as Australia and New Zealand (Belisario, 1959; Eastcott, 1963; TenSeldam, 1963), as well as in sailors, fishermen, ranchers, farmers, and others who spend long hours engaged in outdoor occupations and avocations. The most common malignant tumor of the skin in pigmented races, squamous cell cancer, is quite rare in these groups. A relatively high incidence of squamous cell cancer is found on the skin of Negro albinos, yet the occurrence rate in blacks with vitiliginous (depigmented) skin is not increased (Oettle, 1963).

Other factors, such as exposure to noxious chemicals (internally and externally), external trauma (burns and chronic ulcers), and delayed effects of x-irradiation, play a minor role in the development of squamous cell cancer in white races, but appear of prime importance in pigmented races (Mulay, 1963; Oettle, 1963; Pringgoutomo and Pringgoutomo, 1963; Mora and Perniciaro, 1981). Considerable experimental, epidemiologic, and circumstantial evidence supports the role of all the etiologic factors cited above except repeated trauma. Evidence for the role of trauma is nearly all circumstantial (Treves and Pack, 1930; McAnally and Dockerty, 1949; Argyris and Sraga, 1981), but appears valid. The numerous reports of skin cancer occuring more frequently on body sites exposed to considerable trauma, particularly in pigmented races that are effectively protected from ultraviolet light damage, cannot be ignored. Pringgoutomo and Pringgoutomo (1963) have observed a marked reduction in squamous cell cancer of the foot in the Indonesian population. They attribute this reduced frequency to an improvement in social and hygienic conditions in general, and more specifically to "less people going barefooted." Several unusual skin cancers found principally in India are directly associated with trauma, both burns and local skin irritation. Kangri cancer is found in Kashmir, a region in the northernmost and coldest part of India (Mulay, 1963). To keep warm, natives of this region burn charcoal in earthenware pots that are then tied to the abdomen to produce warmth when in motion or placed between the thighs when sitting. In those body areas directly exposed to intense heat, dermatitis and burns of the skin are common. In this population cutaneous cancers, which are microscopically squamous cell cancers, tend to arise in old burn scars. Occasional lesions are seen in body areas that are not chronically exposed to heat. Kangri cancer has been reported to occur in the brick industry (Suindland, 1980). Dhoti cancers, also found in India, are associated with use of a loin cloth called a dhoti. Native populations wear this garment at all times asleep or awake, and it causes constant irritation to the skin, which, on inspection, appears hyperpigmented and lichenified. Some areas are devoid of pigment. Mulay (1963) described the histologic findings in the skin of these cases and he equates the changes as "being reminiscent of those described in the skin of mice after application of tar or methylcholanthrene." Oettle (1963) also describes squamous cell cancer occurring in chronic leg ulcers and after trauma, especially burns, in the South African black population.

Squamous cell carcinomas on the skin of immunosuppressed patients are an increasingly difficult problem (Hoxtell *et al.,* 1977). Immunosuppressed patients develop multiple squamous cell cancers over all areas of the body, particularly in sun-exposed areas. These tumors grow rapidly and appear to arise within solar keratoses and on skin that appears normal. Multiple verrucae may also occur over the entire integument of immunosuppressed patients.

Much has been written about the role of viruses in producing cutaneous cancers (Jablonska *et al.,* 1972; Yabe *et al,* 1978). To date,

no clear-cut evidence supports the direct role of viruses in producing human cutaneous squamous cell cancer.

Pathology and Natural History

Modes of Spread. In squamous cell cancer tumors arising in actinically damaged skin are very slow growing in both vertical and horizontal planes. Tumors arising on normal skin, or in precancerous lesions, are much more aggressive and malignant. They invade more frequently, and, once invasive, may grow very rapidly, involving the surrounding subcutaneous tissues and producing large, firm nodules. Local invasion and subsequent extension along peripheral nerves is quite common in lesions of the skin of the head and neck (Cottel, 1982).

The propensity to metastasize depends greatly on the site of origin and type of precursor lesions. Metastases rarely occur from lesions of actinically damaged skin, probably in less than 0.1% of cases in some studies (Helwig and Graham, 1963; Lund, 1965) or 2.6% in another (Katz, 1957). Squamous cell cancers arising in normal skin and on the lip and in other lesions such as Bowen's disease, erythroplasia of Queyrat, burn scars, chronic ulcers, sinus tracts, chemically injured skin, and late radiation dermatitis tend to metastasize frequently, 10 to 30% depending on site of origin. The frequency and aggressiveness of metastases also depend on the duration and histologic nature of the tumor.

Site of Metastases. Spread by lymphatic invasion is the principal mode of metastasis. As a result, regional lymph nodes become enlarged, firm, and, eventually, fixed to the surrounding tissues. Lesions that remain untreated for long periods may erode through contiguous tissues and into local vasculature. Spread to distant sites such as lungs, chest, and brain, although rare, may occur.

Symptoms and Signs. Symptoms and signs vary, depending principally on the site of origin and the type of precursor lesion. Tumors developing at the site of solar keratoses begin as flat, erythematous, scaling, and slightly elevated plaques. Most solar keratoses on palpation do not have "substance;" squamous cell carcinomas are slightly indurated early and become quite firm as they age and enlarge. Tumor borders that earlier are imperceptible become well defined as the tumor enlarges and occupies space above the surrounding skin.

The surface of the tumor may become smooth but most often is scaled. Further aging of the tumor is associated with ulceration of the surface and bleeding with minimal trauma. The skin surrounding squamous cell carcinoma is thin, dry, and keratotic. Telangiectasias are prominent and irregular hypo- and hyperpigmentation are noted (see Colorplate VII).

Tumors that arise in radiation-damaged skin (see Colorplate X) and subsequent to chronic exposure to chemical carcinogens (systemic and topical) often occur as multiple lesions. Those arising in chronic ulcers and in sinus tracts may be indistinguishable from other inflammatory tissue or may be hidden along the tract or beneath ulcer debris. In burn scars they usually occur at the border of the lesion in sites of extensive keratosis.

Tumors on the lip often appear innocuous. A small fissure of the lower lip within a white patch on a background of sun-damaged skin is all that may be observed. Ulceration is usually not prominent, and if present consists of a very small, friable or bleeding area on a patch of white skin. Palpable induration is found rarely and only in long-standing lesions, hence, this feature is not important in assessing the clinical nature of a lip lesion.

Diagnosis

Method and Yield. Biopsy of the skin is necessary to make a definitive diagnosis of squamous cell carcinoma. This is a very simple and rapid procedure. Punch biopsy should provide adequate tissue to make a diagnosis except in lesions within scars and ulcerations. In these lesions, large amounts of tissue are necessary to reveal patterns of tumor growth and cellular architecture sufficient to differentiate a tumor from a benign hyperplastic condition — pseudoepitheliomatous hyperplasia — which may occur at chronic ulcer margins (see Figure 20–8).

Histologically, squamous cell carcinoma shows downward proliferation of irregular masses of abnormal epithelial cells through the dermoepidermal junction and into the underlying dermis. In general, epithelial cells of varying shapes and sizes show hyperchromasia of the nuclei, atypical mitoses, individual cell keratinization and loss of intercellular bridges (see Figure 20–9). The degree of malignancy of the tumor is directly related to the degree of anaplasia demonstrated on histology. Tumors that show considerable differentiation (keratin

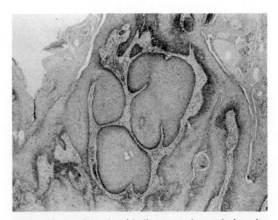

Figure 20–8. Pseudoepitheliomatous hyperplasia, a lesion that is often confused with well-differentiated squamous cell carcinoma. In this lesion, the squamous cells are well organized. Horn pearl formation, individual cell keratinization, and nuclear atypia occur infrequently. The basement membrane remains intact.

formation) are relatively benign or have low-grade malignancy. Tumors with low malignant potential show rather uniform-sized cells, infrequent mitoses, and infrequent nuclear irregularities. Intercellular bridges are often intact, and keratinization within the tumor mass is quite prominent (see Figure 20–10). Highly malignant tumors show many anaplastic cells, considerable nuclear hyperchromia, frequent and abnormal mitoses, loss of intercellular connections, and little or no keratinization (see Figure 20–11). Patterns of anaplasia and differentiation (keratinization) may vary throughout a single tumor, therefore, when as-

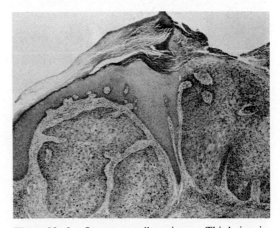

Figure 20–9. Squamous cell carcinoma. This lesion, in part, shows a moderately well-differentiated mixed cellular pattern. There is invasion into the dermis, particularly in the central part of the lesion. Poor horn cyst formation and individual cell keratinization, as well as nuclear atypia, are prominent.

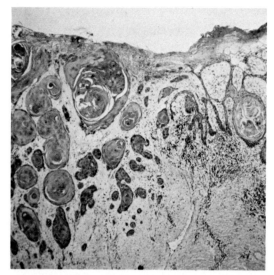

Figure 20–10. Squamous cell carcinoma—grade 1: A well-differentiated tumor. Individual cell keratinization, horn cyst formation, and nuclear atypia are prominent. Although well-differentiated histologically, this lesion is highly invasive.

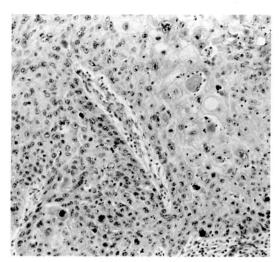

Figure 20–12. Squamous cell carcinoma—grade 2. The tumor is moderately well-differentiated. Epidermoid and spindle-type cells predominate. There is some evidence of individual cell keratinization without horn pear formation. Mitoses are moderate in number.

sessing the degree of malignancy displayed by an individual tumor, multiple tumor section must be examined before attempting to arrive at a firm diagnosis. In addition to tumor architecture, depth of tumor invasion also correlates well with degree of malignancy. Tumors that metastasize may show extensive invasion but may lack striking anaplasia. Tumors with a high potential for metastasis most often will

have invaded below the level of the sweat glands.

In 1932, Broders introduced a system of histologic grading of squamous cell carcinomas (Lever and Schaumberg-Lever, 1983). The degree of malignancy of a specific tumor was estimated according to the ratio of differentiated (keratinizing) cells to undifferentiated (anaplastic) cells. He established four grades in

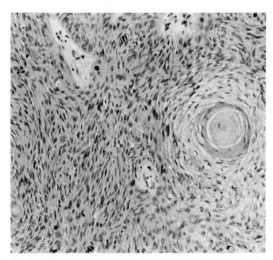

Figure 20–11. Squamous cell carcinoma—grade 4. Spindle cells predominate in this histologic section. There is a single foci of keratin pearl formation, and there is considerable mitotic activity throughout.

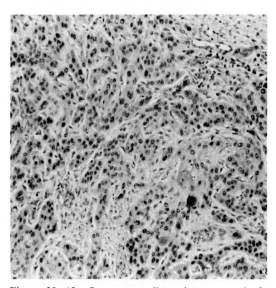

Figure 20–13. Squamous cell carcinoma—grade 3. This tumor contains a mixed cellular pattern. There is considerable dysplasia and individual cell keratinization. Mitoses are few. Cordlike extensions of epithelial cells are seen invading deeply into the dermis.

which the percentage of differentiated cells varied as follows: Grade 1, 75% differentiated (see Figure 20–10); grade 2, 50% differentiated (see Figure 20–12); grade 3, more than 25% differentiated (see Figure 20–13); and grade 4, less than 25% differentiated (all of the remaining cells within each tumor are classified as undifferentiated) (see Figure 20–11). In grade 1 tumors the cells are principally mature squamous cells that have not invaded the dermis below the level of sweat glands; in some areas the basal lamina may even remain intact. A marked inflammatory cell reaction in the dermis is present. In grade 4 carcinomas tumor cell atypia approaches 100%, keratinization is absent, and intercellular attachments are few. Elongated spindle-shaped cells often predominate, giving the tumor a histologic appearance much like that of malignant melanoma or fibrosarcoma. Inflammatory cell infiltrates are scanty. Grades 2 and 3 tumors show intermediate degrees of malignancy.

Staging

Clinical staging is not used in describing squamous cell cancer.

Specific and Supportive Management

Specific Therapy. Squamous cell carcinomas of the skin may be treated effectively by any of the methods described for basal cell carcinoma later in this chapter.

Surgical Excision. Surgical excision is probably the preferred method for treating most lesions, particularly in areas where surgical margins can be readily approximated along tissue cleavage lines, as in lesions of the face, scalp, eyelids, and ears, as well as in sites of radiation-damaged skin. Excisional surgery enables the physician to submit the entire lesion for histopathologic examination and estimation of the adequacy of the surgical margins. Electrosurgery (curettage and electrodesiccation), principally preferred by dermatologists, may be used to treat multiple small lesions that are not markedly invasive; carcinomas arising in actinic keratoses are prime examples. Large, invasive tumors, tumors within burn scars, ulcers, and regions of severe radiation dermatitis should not be treated by electrosurgery.

Cryosurgery may also be used for treating a variety of squamous cell carcinomas in various sites and of varying sizes. Few contraindications exist for the use of cryosurgery. Squamous cell carcinomas of the skin respond much more favorably to cryotherapy than do basal cell carcinomas. Cryosurgery is very effective for treating multiple superficial carcinomas. The procedure is rapid, and healing, although slow, is followed by very acceptable scar formation, far more so than in electrosurgery.

Radiation therapy, although effective in eradicating carcinomas of most sites, is not used very often and is reserved for special situations. It is contraindicated for treating patients under 50 years of age and for treating lesions arising in previously irradiated skin. Radiation therapy should be used with caution in severely sun-damaged skin and in areas devoid of substantial thickness in skin and subcutaneous tissues.

Moh's chemosurgery (fresh or fixed tissue) is quite effective in treating most lesions but is reserved for special situations. These are outlined in the section on treatment of basal cell carcinoma later in this chapter.

Future Prospects

The future prospects for squamous cell carcinoma are comparable to those for basal cell carcinoma. See this discussion in the following section.

BASAL CELL CARCINOMA

Basal cell carcinoma (basal cell epithelioma, rodent cancer, rodent ulcer) is the most commonly encountered cancer of the skin. Because of certain biologic properties, basal cell neoplasms are often referred to as benign epitheliomas or nonorganic (nonorganoid) hamartomas rather than true carcinomas (Lever and Schaumberg-Lever, 1983). Basal cell carcinomas tend to enlarge and remain confined to the epidermis, the tissue of origin, for very long periods. They grow slowly and are slow to invade surrounding tissues. If left untreated for long periods, however, basal cell carcinomas erode into and invade contiguous structures, including bone and cartilage. They may also metastasize (Safai and Good, 1977; Farmer and Helwig, 1980). It is because of their destructive and invasive properties that some dermatologists and pathologists prefer to classify the basal cell tumor as a true carcinoma (Allen, 1967; Pollack *et al.,* 1982).

Incidence and Epidemiology

Although basal cell cancer is clinically the most frequent human neoplasm in Caucasian populations, figures on the true incidence of basal cell cancer are difficult to obtain. Allen (1967) states that during his tenure in World War II at the Armed Forces Institute of Pathology, exclusive of neoplasms of the lower lip, one of every six lesions of the skin was basal cell cancer. Basal cell carcinomas were seen about five times as often as epidermoid carcinoma. Haenszel's data (1963) show that basal cell carcinomas occur in the United States about twice as often in both northern and southern men and women as do squamous cell carcinomas. The overall age adjusted basal cell cancer incidence per 100,000 people in eight United States cities (four northern, four southern) is: Northern men, 15.7; northern women, 12.4; southern men, 61.2; southern women, 40.6 (Haenszel, 1963). Basal cell carcinomas of the face, head, and neck are most frequent in both men and women. Unlike squamous cell carcinoma in Caucasian groups, however, a large number of basal cell carcinomas occur on skin that is not substantially exposed to sunlight (Haenszel, 1963; Urbach, 1966).

Basal cell carcinomas can occur in pigmented or non-Caucasian races, but the ratio of basal cell to squamous cell carcinomas is reversed (Oettle, 1963; Pringgoutomo and Pringgoutomo, 1963; Shanmugaratnam and LaBrooy, 1963). Basal cell carcinomas in pigmented races tend to localize on skin that has had substantial exposure to sunlight (Matsuoka *et al.,* 1981; Mora and Burris, 1981). A fair number of lesions, however, will present on the unexposed trunk and extremities.

As with most other cancers, basal cell carcinomas occur principally in older age groups. A significant incidence in basal cell cancer is first noted around age 40, with a sustained increase with advancing age.

Etiology and Pathogenesis

Considerable evidence supports the role of sunlight in the development of basal cell carcinoma: The overwhelming occurrence in sites subject to intense sunlight; the substantially reduced rate in pigmented races; and the apparent influence of geographic latitude on the rate of basal cell carcinoma in susceptible populations (Haenszel, 1963). Other studies have shown a tenfold increase of basal cell epithe-lioma in the Australian population over that found in similar ethnic groups in the British Isles (Belisario, 1959).

Factors other than sunlight, however, strongly influence the induction of basal cell carcinomas. Basal cell carcinomas are found at sites well removed from areas of maximum sunlight exposure, such as behind the ear and at the inner canthus of the eye. Often tumor density correlates poorly with ultraviolet light dose (Diffy *et al.,* 1979). Basal cell carcinomas tend to occur in families, particularly those of Irish, English, and Welsh origin. These three ethnic groups include large numbers of families with light blue eyes, very light hair, and skin that burns easily and freckles rather than tans. These factors are among the most common denominators in the development of basal cell carcinoma. Evidence is still insufficient to rule out other inherited factors. Genetic factors other than those that determine skin color act as strong etiologic influences. The basal cell nevus syndrome (Gorlin syndrome), is a genetically determined disorder (autosomal dominant) in which multiple basal cell carcinomas appear throughout life, beginning in the second decade or in adolescence. Other associated defects include palmar pits, dental cysts, bifid ribs, spinal cord defects, broad nasal root, hypertelorism, and a myriad of disorders of the central nervous system, gastrointestinal system, bone, and other organs and organ systems.

Exposure to carcinogens, externally applied and ingested, is associated with the development of basal cell carcinoma, but not to the same degree as with squamous cell carcinoma. A few studies, as well as practical experience, have linked the onset of basal cell carcinoma to the ingestion of trivalent arsenic and to skin damaged by ionizing radiation. Basal cell carcinomas also arise in areas of scarring induced by burns, vaccination, chicken pox, and chronic leg ulcers (Burns and Calnau, 1978; Hazelrigg, 1978; Hendricks, 1980; White, 1983).

Most basal cell carcinomas arise from surface epidermis. Other sites are the pilosebaceous ducts, the junction between epidermis and the pilosebaceous duct, epidermal and junctional nevi (Goldberg, 1980; Mehta, 1980), and other such organoid tumors as sebaceous nevus of Jadassohn (Domingo and Helwig, 1974). Tumors arising in sebaceous nevi tend to have a multifocal origin.

Histologically, the individual cells of a basal

cell neoplasm closely resemble those of the basal layer of normal epidermis and of the appendages. This similarity in morphologic appearance originally led to the belief that basal cell carcinomas originated predominately from basal cells of the epidermis. Pinkus (1953) postulated that basal cell carcinomas arise from immature pluripotential cells in the epidermis and that these cells can potentially form (or mature into) any of the characteristic appendages such as hair, sebaceous gland, and apocrine gland, or can become neoplastic. This differentiation probably occurs at about the time epithelial cells begin to proliferate. Aberrations in the relationship between proliferating primitive pluripotential cells and surrounding connective tissue (possibly induced by sunlight, other physical agents, chemicals, and injury) cause differentiation toward neoplasia. This postulate of Pinkus is now the most widely accepted. Retention of the basic ability to differentiate toward a variety of appendageal structures probably accounts for the wide range of histologic patterns seen in basal cell carcinoma.

Basal cell carcinomas are extremely stroma dependent. This concept was originally proposed by Pinkus (1953) and subsequently demonstrated in the laboratory by VanScott and Reinertson (1961) in human autotransplant experiments, by Flaxman (1972) and Kubilus and colleagues in tissue culture (1980), and in skin of other mammalian species by Pawlowski and Haberman (1979) and Gerstein (1963). Basal cell tumor cells transplanted without stroma either do not survive or convert back to normal keratinizing epithelium. Tumor-stromal dependence is thought to account for the very low incidence of metastasis experienced with basal cell carcinoma. Tumor cell-stromal interactions are probably responsible for the characteristic light microscopic appearance of basal cell carcinomas; tumor cells surrounded by well-organized stroma appear "palisading" at the periphery and disorganized and undifferentiated centrally. Tumor cell-stromal interactions may also account for basal cell cancer growth patterns, such as in scars (Mitrani, 1978) and along tissue fusion planes (*i.e.,* along medial canthus and nasolabial folds) where they tend to invade deeply and course along tissue planes rather than cross them.

There is considerable debate regarding the growth characteristics of basal cell carcinoma. Most basal cell carcinomas tend to grow slowly and mitotic figures are not very often observed in active tumors. When seen, mitotic figures are found throughout the tumor. According to Weinstein and Frost (1970), the typical cell within a basal cell carcinoma will replicate every nine days, compared to the 14 days required for replication of non-neoplastic basal cells of normal epidermis in persons at reduced risk of developing basal cell carcinomas. Basal cells of "normal" epidermis in individuals who are "cancer" prone or at risk appear to have a higher labeling index and tend to replicate more frequently than do basal cells in non-cancer-prone individuals (Gregg and Mansbridge, 1982). In spite of this obvious differential in normal-abnormal cell growth rate, basal cell carcinomas do not increase in size very rapidly. What accounts for this slow growth pattern? Possibilities are the prolongation of the DNA synthetic phase in tumor cells (Heenen *et al.,* 1973; Heenen and Galand, 1980), or that cells remain arrested in G_2 or G_0 for prolonged periods, or the fairly constant rate of cell death in each tumor (Iverson, 1967).

Cell death probably accounts for the presence of cylindromatous degeneration and pseudocyst and lacunae formation. Additionally, basal cell tumors usually begin as multiple independent clusters (buds) of cells emanating from the epidermis. These independent cell clusters grow and eventually merge into a single tumor mass and remain a single tumor mass for an indefinite period. In most tumors, some portions eventually separate from others forming individual tumor masses. In most cases these involute but once in a while grow into additional solitary tumors. This process may account in part for the visibly slow basal cell tumor growth. In areas of basal cell tumor degeneration connective tissue replication and replacement of tumor mass often occurs. This response plus an accompanying "fibroblastic" response to invading tumor cells occasionally give rise to the characteristic "morphea"-like basal cell carcinoma — a tumor type that has proven to be resistant to eradication by standard therapeutic techniques.

The surface of a basal cell carcinoma usually displays the characteristic identifying clinical feature of multiple telangiectatic vessels coursing over the surface. Like many solid tumors, basal cell carcinomas have been found to contain a number of chemical growth factors, including tumor angiogenesis factor (Wolf and Hubler, 1975). Tumor angiogenesis factor induces proliferation of blood vessels in and around tumor tissue, thereby providing a basis for an abundant supply of nutrients necessary for tumor growth. Perhaps surface telangiectatic vessels in basal cell carcinomas represent a local cutaneous response to tumor angiogenesis factor.

Pathology and Natural History

Modes of Spread. The aggressiveness of basal cell carcinoma is limited principally to the ability of an individual tumor to invade and destroy surrounding tissue, including cartilage and bone. Even local cutaneous metastases are rare (Kleinberg *et al.*, 1982). Local aggressiveness and spread can be attributed to a number of factors including: (1) The influence of tumor dependence on stroma; (2) contact inhibition (Flaxman, 1972); (3) host cell mediated immunity (Dellon, 1978; Weimar *et al.*, 1980; Burns *et al.*, 1980; Penn, 1980; Myskowski *et al.*, 1981); (4) host humoral immunity (Bustamante *et al.*, 1977); (5) the influence of tumor and sunlight on host immune response (Kripke, 1982); (6) locally induced biochemical reactions (Hashimoto *et al.*, 1972; Yamanishi *et al.*, 1972; Bauer *et al.*, 1977; Scalabrino *et al.*, 1980); (7) attachments between basal cell carcinoma and surrounding stroma (McNutt, 1976); and (8) the status of tumor cell locomotor activity (McNutt, 1976; Montandon *et al.*, 1982). Each of these factors will be discussed briefly below.

As pointed out above, basal cell carcinomas are very stromal dependent. Tumors in or around embryonal tissue planes, such as the nasolabial fold, medial canthus of the eye, the scalp, and the postauricular region tend to be very aggressive. They invade deeply and have a high rate of recurrence after apparently adequate therapy. Such aggressive behavior at these sites is attributed to the favorable stromal environment each site offers.

Numerous investigators (cited above) have noted a depression of cell-mediated immunity in persons prone to develop basal cell carcinomas. Diminished levels of peripheral blood T lymphocytes have been found in patients with basal cell carcinomas. The more aggressive a tumor proves to be, the more depressed are the T-cell levels in tissue and peripheral blood. The occurrence of large numbers of basal cell tumors in a single patient may be associated with decreased *in vitro* blastogenic responses to concanavalin A. To date no studies have found circulating antibodies to basal cell carcinomas. Large numbers of immunoglobulin-secreting cells, however, have been noted in the inflammatory infiltrates surrounding basal cell carcinomas. Basal cell carcinomas as well as squamous cell carcinomas may occur in abundance in patients who are immunosuppressed as a result of disease or pharmacologic manipulations. Tumors found in these circumstances are frequently very aggressive.

When present, the inflammatory infiltrate surrounding basal cell carcinomas contains large numbers of activated T cells in a ratio similar to that found in the classic delayed cutaneous hypersensitivity reaction (Eaglstein, *et al.*, 1982). Soluble extracts from basal cell carcinomas may stimulate *in vitro* lymphocyte transformation (Raffle *et al.*, 1980) as well as inhibit the *in vitro* lymphocyte response to mitogens (Sheretz *et al.*, 1982). Tumors that remain localized and are slow growing do not possess the ability to inhibit host immune response, whereas tumors that are aggressive in behavior or come from sites known to bear aggressive tumors abundantly produce inhibitors of the *in vitro* lymphocyte response to mitogens.

In recent years several studies have postulated the role of sunlight (ultraviolet A, B, and C) in inducing skin tumors. Up to 80% of all basal cell carcinomas occur in sun-exposed areas, and patients who are subjected to pharmacologic immunosuppression suffer an increased incidence of sunlight-associated skin cancers (Penn, 1975; Hoxtell *et al.*, 1977). In a recent series of experiments, Kripke (1982) and O'Dell and colleagues (1980) showed a decreased cutaneous reactivity to dinitrochlorobenzene and/or intradermally injected antigen in ultraviolet-damaged skin and that altered reactivity is due principally to the recruitment of suppressor T lymphocytes to the irradiated sites. Suppressor T cells whose transformation has been stimulated by ultraviolet radiation inhibit host immune response to tumor at the locally irradiated tissue site, making it more susceptible to tumor growth and invasion. Host immunologic mechanisms are probably intact early on in the course of tumor induction and growth because many tumors arising early in the course of irradiation may be destroyed and eliminated. Eventually the immune suppressor effect becomes dominant and tumors begin to appear. The long latency period for the appearance of cutaneous tumors after sunlight exposure may be accounted for by intact early immunologic surveillance and then elimination of this mechanism by constant exposure to damaging ultraviolet light.

Morphologic studies of basal cell carcinoma and surrounding stroma show disorganization and disruption of normal dermal architecture in the region of the advancing tumor border. The amount of collagenase found in extracts of basal cell carcinomas is nearly twice that found in normal tissue. The source of the collagenase is as yet unknown. It may come directly from tumor tissue or indirectly from tumor tissue through activated fibroblasts. In any case, disorganized, disrupted, and digested dermis (connective tissue) certainly offers fewer impediments to an advancing tumor than would an intact dermis.

Enzymes such as ornithine decarboxylase and s-adenosyl-L-methionine decarboxylase are required for polyamine synthesis and occur in very large quantities in basal cell tumor tissue. The presence of polyamines in tumor tissue has been linked directly to the tumor's ability to grow.

Morphologic studies have demonstrated the presence of actinlike microfilaments in cells that form at the periphery of basal cell tumors. These filaments have been linked to cell motility. The most abundant actinlike filaments have been detected in highly infiltrating tumors. These filaments are thought to enhance the ability of cytoplasmic extrusions to penetrate surrounding basement membrane and thus enhance tumor invasion. Externally, desmosomal and hemidesmosomal attachments between tumor cells and tumor basal cells and dermis are not as numerous as between basal cells and dermis in normal tissue. Additionally, basement membrane thickening and discontinuity are quite prominent around basal cell tumors. Anchoring filaments, fibrils, and elastic fibril attachments are also lost in abundance in the same region.

Sites of Metastases. The metastatic potential of basal cell carcinoma is practically nil. If left untreated, however, tumors may become deeply invasive in soft tissues, eroding bone, sinuses, and blood vessels. Thereafter, blood stream metastases may occur. Most highly erosive tumors occur on sun-exposed areas of the face or on the scalp, but a few may occur on the back and go untreated. From these areas tumors may spread to the regional lymph nodes, bones, lungs, liver, and other viscera. Metastases to the spinal cord have also been reported.

Symptoms and Signs. Fortunately, like most tumors of the skin, basal cell carcinomas are easily recognized by the trained observer. Most patients with basal cell carcinomas complain of bleeding and crusting of the lesion, but not of pain, pruritus, or other similar symptoms. Most will describe a recent onset, but, because of the slow growth rate of basal cell carcinomas, history in most instances can be disregarded. Most tumors, other than the smallest (2 to 3 mm), have probably been present for years. The patient may mistakenly assume them to be "moles" (dermal nevi), pustules, and chronic pimples. Bleeding, most often spontaneous, is frequently attributed to injury to the site subsequent to shaving, scratching, or other abrasions.

Clinically, early basal cell tumors appear as tiny translucent papules coursed by tiny telangiectatic blood vessels. In pigmented persons, principally Mediterranean races, the surface may be sprinkled with macular pigmentation or may be entirely covered by pigment, leading to confusion with superficial spreading malignant melanoma (see Colorplate V). As the lesion ages and grows peripherally, tumor borders become sharp and the surface flattened. Depressions may occur centrally in older lesions, as well as scaling, crusting, bleeding, and ulceration, all of which are generally associated with thinning and erosion of the overlying epidermis. Tumor color usually remains unchanged throughout the course and is often likened to the appearance of a pearl. Firm "pearly borders" are commonly seen in older basal cell carcinomas. Cystic tumors may have the appearance of pustules or epidermal cysts. Morphealike basal cell carcinomas may appear as localized patches of scleroderma. They are usually pale to white in color, devoid of telangiectasias, and only slightly elevated above the surrounding skin. The surface is usually smooth and "nonpearly" and the tumor may be depressed. Such lesions are quite firm.

Rodent ulcers are not special forms of basal cell carcinoma, but are usually long standing, and, therefore, their epithelial surfaces have thinned out and subsequently eroded (see Figure 20–14). Often tumor growth takes place vertically both externally and internally, giv-

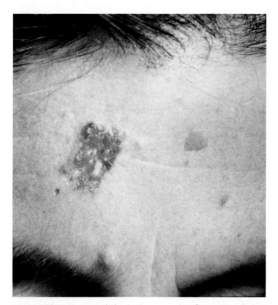

Figure 20–14. A clinical photograph of a rodent basal cell carcinoma.

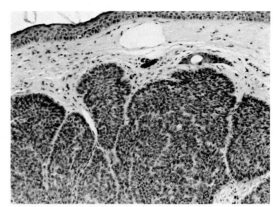

Figure 20–15. Basal cell carcinoma. Lying within the dermis is a well-differentiated tumor showing organized collections of cells having the characteristic features of epidermal basal cells. The thin atrophic epidermis and numerous blood vessels seen coursing throughout the dermis are features that are characteristic of actinically damaged skin.

ing such lesions the appearance of having thicker-than-normal tumor borders.

Infrequently, in some basal tumors very little vertical growth takes place and instead the tumor spreads horizontally. Borders are not well defined, the surface is scaly, and the color is erythematous. Telangiectasias are absent. These tumors are often confused with localized patches of eczema and Bowen's tumor.

Diagnosis

Methods and Yield. Most basal cell carcinomas are easily recognized clinically by the trained observer. Biopsy of the lesion is very simple and is used to confirm the clinical impression. Biopsy techniques vary from a simple excision to a shave technique to punch biopsy.

Histologic examination of appropriate tissue may show one of two histologic types, differentiated or undifferentiated (Lever, 1983). Differentiated tumors show transformation toward structures resembling cutaneous appendages such as hair or sebaceous glands. Most tumors contain both differentiated and undifferentiated areas (see Figure 20–15). Completely undifferentiated tumors are considered solid basal cell carcinomas. Differentiated tumors are called keratotic when resembling hair structures; cystic when appearing as sebaceous glands; adenoid when resembling apocrine or eccrine glands (see Figure 20–16);

and morphealike when containing large amounts of stroma (see Figure 20–17). It is generally believed that such diversity of histologic patterns has no relationship to tumor biology, clinical course, or state of differentiation.

Specific and Supportive Management

Albright (1982) offers a comprehensive review of the various techniques and modalities for treating basal cell carcinoma. Some of this material is summarized below.

Five primary techniques are used to treat basal cell carcinoma, the selection being based

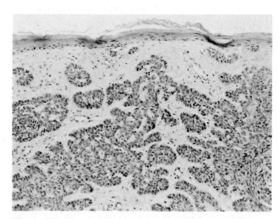

Figure 20–16. Adenoid basal cell carcinoma. In this lesion large sheets of basal-type cells are mixed with structures resembling apocrine- or eccrine-type glands. The epidermis is thin and hyperkeratotic. Many blood vessels are coursing through the lesion.

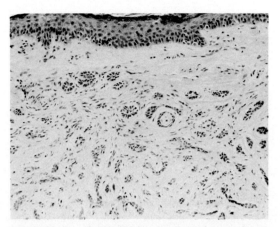

Figure 20-17. Sclerosing basal cell carcinoma. Small collections of basal-type cells are seen interspersed with dense bundles of collagen. The surface epithelium in this tumor appears quite normal and there is a paucity of blood vessels in the dermis. The clinical margins of this tumor may be difficult to perceive.

principally on the opinions and experience of the therapist. Excisional surgery, electrosurgery (curettage and fulguration), and cryosurgery are by far the most commonly used techniques. Radiation therapy is no longer looked upon with favor by most dermatologists (this applies to all lesions in all age groups and skin types) and Moh's fresh tissue and fixed-tissue chemosurgery are reserved principally for special cases. The experienced therapist can expect excellent cure rates no matter which technique is used. Therefore, important considerations in the selection of a particular therapeutic procedure include the age and general health of the patient, the cosmetic defect caused by a particular procedure, the anatomic location of the tumor, the size of the tumor, the clinical and histologic type of tumor, and the clinical status of the tumor (primary or recurrent). For example, both the patient and therapist are often less concerned about cosmetic appearance after treatment in an inactive or debilitated elderly patient than in a younger, more active patient. Tumor eradication is the sole objective of treatment. On the other hand, excellent cosmetic results are of considerable concern in a young patient. Therefore, for similar size and type lesions one may elect to use a single treatment of superficial filtered x-ray for the elderly patient (with curative but scarring results) and carefully perform cold-knife excisional surgery for the young patient (also curative but scarring is minimized). Additionally, one must be concerned about the late effects of radiation therapy in the young and in severely

sun-damaged skin. Treatment with x-ray is contraindicated in patients less than 50 years of age.

Some tumors, such as the sclerosing basal cell carcinoma, are not effectively treated using electrosurgery and/or radiation. Mohs-type surgery (fresh tissue and fixed chemosurgery), although potentially useful in all forms of basal cell cancer, requires special skills in both surgery and pathology. Therefore, it is best reserved for recurrent tumors, large sclerosing-type basal cell carcinomas, and tumors within embryonal tissue planes whose margins are indeterminate (Mohs, 1978).

Electrosurgery is the technique most commonly used by dermatologists. In this technique, requiring considerable skill and experience, a high-frequency monopolar electrical current is used to produce a spark that destroys tissue and aids in coagulation of blood. (Because the use of a high-frequency current is necessary, patients wearing pacemakers cannot be treated by this method.) The tumor is first curetted to a depth perceived adequate by the therapist. By touch with the curet the therapist can distinguish between the soft friable tissue of the tumor and the firm, rough tissue of normal dermis. Curetting is followed by fulguration. This combined procedure is repeated once or twice until the therapist is assured that all tumor is destroyed.

Cold-knife excisional surgery, used principally by general and plastic surgeons, is also becoming increasingly popular among dermatologists. Among the many advantages of this type of surgery are that the pathologist is provided with sufficient tissue to give a fairly reliable assessment of adequacy of tissue margins and the cosmetic appearance in a properly done procedure is extremely good, even when the size of the tumor makes it necessary to move adjacent tissues around.

Cryosurgery in dermatology is also becoming increasingly popular, probably due to its simplicity and ease of application in treating tumors of all types in nearly all locations. When using this technique, the therapist must be able to define with certainty both horizontal and vertical margins of the tumor. When removing thick, nodular tumors, many dermatologists will remove the protuberant portion of a tumor using a "shave" technique and then will apply cryotherapy to the remainder of the lesion. Cryosurgery is best performed with liquid nitrogen, because other cryogens such as freon, ethyl chloride, and solidified carbon dioxide cannot freeze tissue to the proper temperature to cause cell death. A large number of delivery systems are available, most using a container suitable for holding liquid nitrogen under pressure and an attached apparatus for delivering a stream of cold liquid nitrogen spray to the affected tissue. Cryoprobes, or solid brass attachments, once very popular, are used only in very inaccessible sites. Some apparatus for measuring temperature in the depths of the affected tissue should always be used in the treatment of basal cell tumors. A temperature in the range of -25 to -50 °C is sufficient to kill tumor tissue. At least two or more freeze-thaw cycles should be used on each lesion. The freeze time should be as rapid as possible and the tissue thaw time should exceed 120 seconds.

Although a very rapid, simple, and effective procedure when performed by an experienced therapist, cryosurgery has several major disadvantages. Healing time is very slow, varying from three to ten weeks depending on the size and depth of the lesion treated, and infection and bleeding may occur late in the course of healing. Healing may be accelerated by using one of the many semipermeable membranes for a dressing, as soon as the necrotic tumor tissue has sloughed.

X-irradiation to treat tumors of the skin has lost favor, but has a place in the management of certain lesions in patients more than 50 years of age. When used correctly, that is, when appropriate dose fractionation and adequate filtering are maintained, this technique can eradicate tumors with excellent cosmetic results. At present, radiation may be delivered by superficial x-ray apparatus, linear accelerators (electrons only) (Miller and Spittle, 1982), radon implants, and radon molds. X-ray therapy, in particular, has proven of value in treating lesions of the eyelids, inner canthus of the eye, ears, nose, lips, and in treating lesions in elderly, fragile, immobile patients.

Mohs' chemosurgery, a technique using microscopically controlled surgery (Mohs, 1978) for the eradication of tumors, was developed and introduced around 1936. In the original technique, tumor margins were estimated, a precise "map" of the lesion was made, the mapped lesion was divided into horizontal "quadrants," and a zinc chloride paste was applied for proper fixation of tissue. Fixed tissue quadrants were then excised, prepared, and examined microscopically to determine adequacy of excisional margins. Tumor tissue that

extended beyond the excised borders was then treated in a similar manner until all microscopic evidence of tumor was eliminated. About 20 years after introduction of the procedure, zinc chloride fixation of tissue was omitted and fresh, "mapped" tissue, after excision, was submitted to frozen tissue processing and examination (Mohs's chemosurgery, fresh tissue technique). Surgical defects may be allowed to heal with or without skin grafting.

As may be evident, Mohs' chemosurgery requires the skills of a properly trained surgeon or surgeons, pathologists, ancillary personnel, and considerable expenditures in time and equipment. Therefore, although useful for treating any type of cutaneous tumor, Mohs's technique is most often reserved for special circumstances, particularly for treating recurrent tumors, for which it is the technique of choice (Cottell and Proper, 1982).

A considerable body of literature has extolled the virtues of high concentrations (5 to 20%) of 5-fluorouracil applied to cutaneous tumors. Such practices, however, are to be condemned. An exceedingly large number of tumor recurrences accompany this technique. One of the most unfortunate after-effects is that the tumor tissue appears eradicated on the surface yet remains unobserved and deep to the surface epithelium to grow horizontally and vertically.

Follow-up care after treatment of basal cell tumors should take place at well-specified intervals, such as at three, six, and 18 months. This follow-up permits the therapist to perform additional examinations for tumor recurrence and to detect the development of new tumors and other precancerous lesions.

Future Prospects

Basal cell carcinomas are clearly visible as they occur, allowing early diagnosis and treatment, and are usually not malignant when treated early. Comparatively little interest in these tumors has been expressed except for examination of factors that relate to tumor occurrence and induction. This lack of interest is unfortunate because considerable information regarding the influence of physical and chemical agents such as sunlight, arsenic, and polycyclic hydrocarbons on the development of skin cancer needs to be identified. Much of this information may be applicable to cancers in other organ systems. We now know of the overwhelming effect of ultraviolet light on the development of basal cell carcinoma and the potential for preventing most of these tumors by educating the susceptible population at an early age to the proper use of sunscreens and avoidance of excessive exposure to the sun (Pathak, 1982).

Several new avenues of approach to the treatment and prevention of cutaneous cancers have been investigated in recent years. They include the use of systemic and topical retinoids to prevent the development of cancers in susceptible individuals (Meyskens, 1982); use of laser radiation to treat cutaneous tumors; use of localized injections of lymphokine fraction (Rhodes *et al.,* 1981); the use of human leukocyte interferon (Padovan *et al.,* 1981); and photoradiation (Dougherty, 1981).

KAPOSI'S SARCOMA

Kaposi's sarcoma (also called Kaposi's hemorrhagic sarcoma, multiple idiopathic hemorrhagic sarcoma [Kaposi], and idiopathic multiple pigmented sarcoma) is a rare neoplastic disorder that presents with very typical cutaneous lesions (see Colorplates XII and XIII). The cutaneous lesions are so typical that a definitive diagnosis may be made on the basis of clinical findings alone. Ninety percent of the people affected are Caucasians. The disease and its more typical manifestations were first described by the Hungarian dermatologist, Moricz Kaposi in 1872 (Kaposi, 1872). Until recent years Kaposi's sarcoma has been principally a medical oddity, largely unknown and of interest only to the dermatologist, the inquiring oncologist in equatorial Africa, and the occasional virologist with an interest in the viral etiology of cancer. Because these investigators were interested primarily in the study of Burkitt's lymphoma and the role of viruses in the etiology of lymphoma, observations of Kaposi's sarcoma were only secondary.

Within the past four years a "new disease" syndrome with a high mortality rate, characterized by the close association of neoplasms and opportunistic infections, has surfaced and with it an intensified interest in Kaposi's sarcoma. This serious new disease, named acquired immune deficiency syndrome (AIDS), has affected more than 8100 individuals with 3859 deaths, a 48% mortality rate. Ninety-five pediatric cases have been identified, with 62 deaths, a 65% mortality rate. One-third to one-half of patients with AIDS have developed a very malignant type of Kaposi's sarcoma. (CDC, 1981a,b,c, 1982a,b; Friedman-Kein, 1981; Gottlieb *et al.,* 1981; Hymes *et al.,* 1981; Report for the Center for Disease Control, 1985; CDC Briefings, 1983). The intensive investigations now taking place, particularly on the association and relationship among viruses, immunodeficiency, and the development of cancer, may uncover another substantial element in the puzzle of human neoplasia, its etiology, and pathogenesis.

Incidence and Epidemiology

Until the outbreak of Kaposi's sarcoma in young, promiscuous homosexual men with AIDS, Kaposi's sarcoma was seen predominately in two forms. In European populations, principally Central Europeans and Italians, Kaposi's sarcoma is a benign indolent disease of elderly men 50 to 60 years of age. In these people, 10 to 15 men develop Kaposi's sarcoma for every woman. Excluding disease associated with AIDS, in North America and Europe the reported incidence of Kaposi's sarcoma is 0.02 to 0.06 cases per 100,000 population (Oettle, 1962; Friedman-Kein, 1981). In North America, cases among Italian and Jewish men predominate, thus giving some credence to theories of racial and ethnic predispositions and the influence of genetics in the pathogenesis of this disease (Braverman [1981] offers a well-reasoned discussion of factors relative to racial and ethnic background in European cases of Kaposi's sarcoma). Kaposi's sarcoma in Africa occurs principally south of the Sahara in equatorial Africa. The highest incidence is found in the populations of Uganda, Tanzania, Zaire, Kenya and in the blacks of South Africa, where Kaposi's sarcoma accounts for 6 to 10% of all neoplasms in men (Rogoff, 1968; Slavin *et al.,* 1969; Taylor *et al.,* 1972; Templeton, 1981). In female populations of the same region Kaposi's sarcoma makes up less than 0.6% of all cancers. Thus, in African populations Kaposi's sarcoma also affects men most often, but here the similarities between African and North American disease end. In both African men and women the disease tends to occur at an earlier age than in Caucasians, principally at 30 to 40 years of age, and also appears to have a more aggressive and virulent nature, much like the disease now described in young men who are homosexual and in others with AIDS (Friedman-Kein, 1981; Templeton, 1981).

On numerous occasions it has been reported that black African children suffer a higher incidence of Kaposi's sarcoma than do children of other races; Templeton (1981) disagrees, stating that children account for approximately 4% of cases in both Caucasian (North American and European) and African groups. Dutz and Stout (1960) report that children under six years of age account for approximately 3.3% of all described cases and most of these have come from the African continent. In children the disease shows much less male over female frequency, occurring in a ratio of 1.3 : 1 males to females.

Even in regions of Africa where the prevalence of Kaposi's sarcoma is high in native blacks, the disease incidence is low or nonexistent in Caucasians. Considerable speculation exists on the disparity between incidence rates in black Americans, both North, Central, and Carribean, and in black Africans. In black populations in the Americas, Kaposi's sarcoma occurs at a rate equal to or somewhat lower than in the Caucasian population. Often, disparate incidence figures are used to refute genetic as well as racial factors that may be important in the pathogenesis of Kaposi's sarcoma. A closer look at these figures, however, keeping in mind earlier forced immigration patterns and the African region of origin of most blacks in the Americas, supports both genetic and racial factors in the development of Kaposi's sarcoma. With few exceptions blacks in the Americas are descendants of blacks from Western Africa. In the indigenous population of West Africa the incidence of Kaposi's sarcoma is about equal to that found in black Americans, and much lower than that found in black Equatorial Africa. In the Americas, recent reports of outbreaks of AIDS and Kaposi's sarcoma in Haitian immigrants (CDC, 1982a,b; Pitchenik et al., 1983) and Kaposi's sarcoma in the indigenous Haitian population are very thought provoking. Continuing migratory patterns and links between French Equatorial Africa and Haiti may shed light on the development of Kaposi's sarcoma and AIDS.

Etiology and Pathogenesis

The etiology of Kaposi's sarcoma remains obscure. The wealth of new observations on the role of infection, immunosuppression, and the immune deficiency state in recently described outbreaks of Kaposi's sarcoma, along with previously recorded observations, is beginning to provide important clues to the still obscure causes of Kaposi's sarcoma.

Because Kaposi's sarcoma lesions appear to have a predilection for acral parts, especially the lower extremities and below the knees, trauma and stasis associated with prolonged standing in outdoor occupations are often proposed as prime causal factors. There is, however, no good scientific evidence to support this.

In recent years excellent evidence has emerged to support the primary etiologic role of bacterial and viral infections, immunosuppression, or an immunodeficient state in genetically predisposed hosts (Masters et al., 1970; Haim et al., 1973; Taylor, 1973; Taylor and Ziegler, 1974; Giraldo et al., 1975, 1978, 1981; Boldogh et al., 1981; Ilie et al., 1981; Weiss and Serushan, 1982; Barré-Sinoussi et al., 1983; Essex et al., 1983; Gallo et al., 1983; Gelmann et al., 1983; Trainin et al., 1983).

In early 1981, the Centers for Disease Control Morbidity and Mortality Weekly Report (1981) called attention to a sudden outbreak of two rare diseases in homosexual males: *Pneumocystic carinii* pneumonia and Kaposi's sarcoma. Further observations and reports led to the development of a profile of a group of patients with the propensity to develop these diseases (Centers for Disease Control Briefings, 1981; Hymes et al., 1981; Report of the Centers for Disease Control, 1982). For the most part, susceptible individuals have been found to reside in large metropolitan coastal cities, principally New York City and in California. (Approximately 50% of all cases of Kaposi's sarcoma and AIDS have come from the metropolitan New York area.) Most are homosexual, have used drugs intravenously, have diffuse lymphadenopathy, have prolonged fevers of undetermined origin, and are susceptible to infections with low-grade pathogenic organisms — organisms known to cause opportunistic infections primarily in the immunocompromised host. In this population the incidence of sexually transmitted diseases and infections with intestinal parasites and viruses (herpes simplex, cytomegalovirus, hepatitis B) is very high, as is the number of homosexual partners, sexual encounters, and traumatic sexual acts. Recently a number of reports have described AIDS and Kaposi's sarcoma in women who use drugs intravenously, their offspring, heterosexual Haitian men, and hemophiliacs. Nearly all women with AIDS had either recent or remote intimate associations with bisexual males (Report of the Centers for Disease Control, 1982; Francis *et al.*, 1983). The probable role of each factor mentioned above in the development of Kaposi's sarcoma is discussed below.

Evidence for the association of an immunocompromised state in the pathogenesis of Kaposi's sarcoma is overwhelming, and epidemiologic data strongly suggest an infectious, probably viral, cause for AIDS. Infections of varying severity caused by at least a dozen different microorganisms have been detected in people with AIDS and Kaposi's sarcoma.

Kaposi's sarcoma occurs with an unusually high frequency in young homosexual men with *Pneumocystis pneumonia*. Previous studies have established that infection by *Pneumocystis carinii* is associated principally with the immunosuppressed state (Walzer *et al.*, 1974).

Among the viral infections, cytomegalovirus and herpes simplex predominate. Evidence for past or present cytomegalovirus infection was reported in more than 90% of a population of men who are homosexual (Drew *et al.*, 1981), over 7% of whom demonstrated cytomegaloviruria. In the same report only 54% of a control group of men who are heterosexual showed evidence of previous cytomegalovirus infection (positive serologic examination) and none demonstrated active shedding of virus in the urine. In the United Kingdom, where few cases of AIDS and Kaposi's sarcoma and only one case of Kaposi's sarcoma in a nonimmunosuppressed man who is homosexual have been reported, the incidence of cytomegalemia is 70% or less in men who are homosexual and 50% or less in men who are heterosexual. Cytomegaloviruria is rarely detected (Maurice *et al.*, 1982; Goldmeier *et al.*, 1983; Pinching *et al.*, 1983; Weber *et al.*, 1984). Cytomegalovirus also occurs in semen of men who are homosexual (Lang and Kummer, 1975). Cytomegalovirus infection can induce abnormalities of *in vitro* immune function in mice and human beings (Rinaldo *et al.*, 1980). Cytomegalovirus can induce transformation of lymphocytes, granulocytes, phagocytes, fibroblasts, and epithelial cells *in vitro* (Pagano, 1975). In an analysis of peripheral blood T-cell populations using a monoclonal antibody technique in patients with AIDS and cytomegalovirus infections as well as in homosexual men with Kaposi's sarcoma, the helper/inducer subset of T lymphocytes was virtually eliminated, the percentage of T lymphocytes

possessing suppressor/cytotoxic activity was increased, and the percentage of cells bearing thymocyte-associated antigen was increased (Gottlieb *et al.*, 1981).

Cytomegalovirus has been implicated as a primary etiologic agent in the pathogenesis of Kaposi's sarcoma based on findings in serologic studies (Giraldo *et al.*, 1975, 1978), on the finding of cytomegalogenome in Kaposi's sarcoma tissue (Boldogh *et al.*, 1981), and on the finding of virus particles in tissue culture of Kaposi's sarcoma material (Giraldo *et al.*, 1972). In a group of 13 male homosexual patients with AIDS, disseminated cytomegalovirus infection was found in 12 and Kaposi's sarcoma in 10. In two patients Kaposi's sarcoma was found in internal organs but not in skin (Guarda *et al.*, 1984). When seen in the tissues of human adults, cytomegalovirus inclusions have been found prominently in association with and within vascular endothelial cells (Wong and Warner, 1962), thus suggesting a cytomegalovirus tropism for endothelial cells. Strong evidence, discussed below, shows that Kaposi's sarcoma is a tumor of vascular endothelial cells. Although these findings strongly suggest that active cytomegalovirus may be the causal pathogen in Kaposi's sarcoma, its presence may represent an opportunistic infection in an immunocompromised host.

A human retrovirus infection may in some way participate actively in producing AIDS-associated Kaposi's sarcoma as recent data suggest (Barré-Sinoussi *et al.*, 1983; Essex *et al.*, 1983; Gallo *et al.*, 1983, 1984; Gelmann *et al.*, 1983; Sarngadharan *et al.*, 1984). Human T-cell leukemia-lymphoma virus (HTLV), a group of lymphotropic retroviruses that preferentially infect human T-helper lymphocytes and are associated with T-cell neoplasms (Poiesz *et al.*, 1980), was recently isolated from peripheral blood T cells in one person with AIDS (Gallo *et al.*, 1983). HTLV antigens were isolated from two patients with AIDS from France (Gallo *et al.*, 1983). A human C-type lymphotrophic retrovirus (LAV) distinctly different from those previously associated with human neoplasms was also isolated (Barré-Sinoussi *et al.*, 1983). Subsequently HTLV type III (HTLV-III) has been isolated from lymphocytes of patients with pre-AIDS (AIDS related complex [ARC] AIDS syndrome, and lymphadenopathy syndrome), normal mothers of children with AIDS, and adult and juvenile patients with

AIDS (Gallo *et al.*, 1984). HTLV-III has been isolated from peripheral blood, saliva, and semen of patients with AIDS and healthy homosexual men at risk for AIDS (Groopman *et al.*, 1984). Five of the six patients with AIDS had disseminated Kaposi's sarcoma. Proviral DNA of human T-cell lymphoma virus was found in two patients with AIDS (Gelmann *et al.*, 1983). In 19 of 75 patients with AIDS antibodies directed toward surface antigens of a reference T-cell lymphoid line, a line previously established from a patient with T-cell lymphoma, were identified (Essex *et al.*, 1983). Ten of 34 patients with Kaposi's sarcoma, and two of 11 patients with Kaposi's sarcoma and pneumocystis pneumonia were positive for HTLV-associated cell membrane antigen (HTLV-MA). Further studies of serum samples from 88% of patients with AIDS and 79% of homosexual men with pre-AIDS show antibodies reactive against antigens of HTLV-III (Sarngadharan *et al.*, 1984). Antibodies to LAV have been detected in African patients with AIDS. Seropositivity has been observed under these circumstances in a high proportion of heterosexual partners and children of AIDS patients, indicating familial transmission of AIDS in some African regions (Brun-Vézinet *et al.*, 1984).

These new data may represent an important link in the development of causal factors in Kaposi's sarcoma. Human Type C retroviruses may indeed play an important role in the etiology of Kaposi's sarcoma. Antibodies to HTLV are prevalent in the Haitian population, occurring in 4 to 5% of the general population (Blattner *et al.*, 1982; Schupbach, 1983). Antibodies to the same type virus, however, are found in up to 35% of the population in southern Japan. To date, AIDS has not been reported in Japan nor has an increased incidence of Kaposi's sarcoma. The method of spread supports the role of an infectious agent: Close intimate contact or transmission by blood products and fomites in contact with blood products are of utmost importance. The very fragile nature of the viral envelope surrounding human type-C retrovirus may make infection possible only by intimate cell-to-cell contact. Finally, HTLV infects only human helper T cells. Human helper T-cell defects are profound in patients with AIDS.

The linking of HTLV with AIDS and Kaposi's sarcoma does not prove that human C-type lymphotropic virus actually causes AIDS. Similar animal viruses, such as feline leukemia

virus, have been shown to impair T-cell function and diminish humoral antibody responses in the host (Trainin *et al.*, 1983). Cats naturally infected with feline leukemia virus are at increased risk of developing bacterial, viral, and parasitic diseases. The feline leukemia virus causes many more deaths by way of its immune suppression effects than by inducing leukemia. The immunosuppressed state caused by whatever means is crucial to the development of many cases of Kaposi's sarcoma. Hence, we may postulate that HTLV infection is associated with the development of Kaposi's sarcoma via its ability to cause the immunosuppressed state, rather than by its ability to cause neoplastic changes in infected tissue.

In the homosexual population in general, and the group affected with AIDS and Kaposi's sarcoma more specifically, a very high incidence of multiple infection with venereally acquired bacterial, viral, and parasitic diseases including syphilis, gonorrhea, hepatitis A and B, herpes simplex, condyloma, acuminata, amebiasis, *Campylobacter jejuni* and giardiasis is well documented. Other less frequent infections include pulmonary and intestinal candidiasis, *Klebsiella* pneumonia, tuberculosis, toxoplasmosis, cryptococcosis as well as infections by *Mycobacterium avium-intracellulare*. This vast array of infectious agents causing sequential or simultaneous disease, as well as the attendant chronic antigenic stimulation, severely taxes the immune system of a single host. Conceivably, continuous antigenic stimulation by these agents, including cytomegalovirus, "might result in the development of alloreactive suppressor T-cells and consequently in persistent and severe immunosuppression" (Koziner *et al.*, 1982).

Human seminal plasma may contain factors that are potent immunosuppressors *in vitro* and may have the potential for causing *in vivo* immunosuppression (Lord *et al.*, 1977). Rectal insemination of rabbit semen into normal male rabbits has produced a number of abnormal immune responses among which is a decreased ability to mount a humoral immune response to T-lymphocyte-dependent antigens (Richards *et al.*, 1984). Polyamines and prostaglandins along with mucosal injury have been identified as possible inciting factors. Those men who are homosexual who develop AIDS and Kaposi's sarcoma are estimated to have had, on the average, exposure to a large number of sexual partners (median of 50/year) and have a higher number of sexual encounters (in rare cases over 1000/year) than do nonaffected men who are homosexual (Jay and Young, 1979). A rational postulate is that the large number of sexual encounters, increased mucosal injury, and increased exposure to seminal fluid lead to substantial immunosuppressive effects and eventually to AIDS and Kaposi's sarcoma.

The role of drugs as etiologic agents in Kaposi's sarcoma and AIDS remains conjectural. Both groups of patients commonly use "street" drugs and "recreational" drugs of all types and via various routes. The intravenous use of heroin is often associated with acquiring active hepatitis B infection, which in turn may adversely affect host immunity. Psychoactive drugs such as the cannaboids produce the *in vivo* depression of cell mediated immunity (Morahan *et al.,* 1979). The effect of marijuana smoking on cellular immunity, however, is unclear (Nahas *et al.,* 1974; Rachelfski *et al.,* 1976). Amyl nitrite and butyl nitrite, vasoactive drugs frequently used by some men who are homosexual to enhance orgasm, appear to be associated with an increased risk of developing an altered immune state and of acquiring Kaposi's sarcoma (Marmor *et al.,* 1982; Goedert *et al.,* 1982). The actual role of these agents in inducing a state of altered immunity, however, remains under investigation.

The recent discovery of AIDS and Kaposi's sarcoma in native Haitians and Haitian immigrants largely supports the role of altered immunity, infection (including a high incidence of opportunistic infections), and drug use in the development of Kaposi's sarcoma (CDC, 1982a,b; Wormser *et al.,* 1983). To date, homosexual activity has not been found prevalent in this group. The observation that among residents of high incidence areas in equatorial Africa, Kaposi's sarcoma occurs almost exclusively in blacks, most of whom are in a very low socioeconomic class and who experience multiple infections from a wide variety of agents, also speaks for altered immunity and infection as prime causal agents in the development of the disease. The same reasoning may also apply to Kaposi's sarcoma in Haiti and in those affected Haitians who have recently immigrated to the United States. Haiti has one of the most underdeveloped economic and medical care systems and impoverished populations in the Americas.

There is a highly important association between the development of Kaposi's sarcoma and other neoplasms, principally those of the lymphoreticular system, such as lymphomas (particularly Hodgkin's disease), leukemias, and multiple myeloma (Reynolds *et al.,* 1965; Safai *et al.,* 1980; Ulbright and Santa Cruz, 1981). This association is particularly relevant in the (North American) Caucasian or non-African population in which second neoplasms are estimated to be the most common cause of death (Ulbright and Santa Cruz, 1981). Most of the neoplasms are derived from lymphoreticular tissues and Kaposi's sarcoma develops either simultaneously or subsequently in these patients. This mutual occurrence, therefore, may be associated with known immunodeficiencies in patients with lymphomas, leukemias, and myeloma.

Finally, a vast array of literature describes the initial onset of Kaposi's sarcoma in patients being treated actively with cytotoxic or immunosuppressive agents or both (Haim *et al.,* 1973; Ilie *et al.,* 1981; Weiss and Serushan, 1982). Many of these "acquired" tumors recede spontaneously upon tapering of or complete withdrawal from cytotoxic or immunosuppressive therapy.

Pathology and Natural History

Kaposi's sarcoma presents with a diversity of clinical features, the nature of presentation depending principally on the racial group affected and the age and gender of the patient (Table 20–5). In elderly men of European extraction the disease classically presents with solitary or multiple red, brown, blue, or purple macules, papules, nodules, and plaques (see Colorplate XII). Nodules and plaques vary in size and degree of firmness. Early lesions most often appear on acral parts, especially fingers and toes. Some are occasionally found on the face, scalp, or genitalia (see Colorplate XIII). Acute lesions most commonly occur, however, on the lower extremities, where they tend to be distributed bilaterally. As the lesions age, macules develop into plaques and papules into nodules. Large plaques frequently lose their characteristic color and become covered with a thick, pale hyperkeratotic (scaly) surface (see Colorplate XIV). Occasionally, plaquelike lesions resolve, disappearing spontaneously, leaving large atrophic telangiectatic and hyperpigmented patches. On the surface of some lesions the epidermis becomes atrophic and ulcerates, particularly on large nodular lesions or clusters of nodular lesions. Eventually, a

Table 20-5. Characteristics of Various Clinical Forms of Kaposi's Sarcoma

TYPE OF DISEASE	HISTOLOGIC PATTERN	AGE DISTRIBUTION	GENDER PREDOMINANCE	RACE PREDOMINANTLY AFFECTED	RESPONSE TO THERAPY*
1. Indolent					

A. Papules
    Plaques
    Nodules
	Mixed cellularity	>50 yrs.	Male	C	Good

B. Nodules	Mixed cellularity	>50 yrs.	Male	B	Good
2. Aggressive					
A. Florid (exophytic ulcerative)	Mixed cellularity; monocellular; anaplastic	>50 yrs.	Male	B	Excellent
B. Infiltrative	Monocellular	>50 yrs.	Male	B	Poor
C. Lymphadenopathic	Mixed cellularity	0-10 yrs.	Male, female	C,B	Excellent

D. Cutaneous;
    lymphadenopathic;
    systemic
	Mixed cellularity	20-40 yrs.	Male, female	B†	Poor

* Response to radiotherapy or chemotherapy.
† Now found to be the dominant disease type in patients with the acquired immune deficiency syndrome (AIDS), nearly all of whom are young Caucasian males.
Legend: C = Caucasian; B = blacks.

large fungating, necrotic tissue mass will become prominent at the site of ulceration. In spite of their diversity, the lesions are quite characteristic and are not difficult for the dermatologist to diagnose. These lesions are invariably misdiagnosed by other physicians. The differential diagnosis of Kaposi's cutaneous lesions include hemangioma, lymphangioma, granuloma pyogenicum, glomus tumor, and melanoma.

A brawny type of edema is often associated with upper and lower extremity lesions, particularly as the lesions enlarge. Edema may result from microscopic and macroscopic dermal lymphatic obstruction by the tumor.

In patients of European extraction visceral organ disease, though infrequent, may involve the gastrointestinal tract. This involvement may be so extensive that occult gastrointestinal bleeding may be the presenting complaint. In cases with gastrointestinal disease typical blue to purple blebs and nodules can be seen on the tongue, buccal mucosa, and throughout the gastrointestinal tract. Other organ involvement is rare and generally asymptomatic. Involvement of the central nervous system has not been reported.

In children, Kaposi's sarcoma rarely occurs on the skin, but most often involves the lymphoreticular system. Most children present with strikingly diffuse, discrete, nontender lymphadenopathy and hepatosplenomegaly. Occasionally the eyelids, lacrimal glands, and parotid glands are involved (Olweny *et al.,*

1974; Farrant, 1982). In young African and Haitian adults widespread cutaneous and systemic involvement is characteristic and is associated with a rapidly fatal course (Templeton, 1981). This pattern of disease is also seen in young men who are homosexual and in immunosuppressed patients (Friedman-Kein, 1981).

Although most patients with Kaposi's sarcoma present with clusters of lesions that develop at various times, the origin of distant disease is thought to be multicentric rather than metastatic. Regional lymph node metastases are rare, but aggressive lesions often diffusely infiltrate surrounding subcutaneous tissues and bone (Templeton, 1981).

Due to the variability of clinical expression in the African type of Kaposi's sarcoma, Taylor and colleagues (1971) developed a morphologic classification that identifies disease according to clinical presentation, histopathologic pattern, clinical course, and response to therapy (see Table 20-5). The four types identified include nodular, florid (exophytic or ulcerative), infiltrative, and lymphadenopathic. The *nodular* type is most commonly encountered and is indolent. Lesions occur most frequent on the extremities, occasionally internally, and may be solitary or multifocal. *Florid* disease occurs principally as rapidly growing exophytic ulcerating tumors. This type of tumor is often deeply invasive and frequently involves bone. *Infiltrative* disease, seen more often in European populations, re-

Table 20-6. Clinical Classification of Kaposi's Sarcoma

Indolent:	Cutaneous papules, plaques, nodules
Aggressive:	Florid (exophytic)
	Infiltrative
	Lymphadenopathic
	Cutaneous; lymphadenopathic; systemic

sults from widespread tumor infiltration of skin and subcutaneous tissues. It is usually confined to one or more extremities and is often associated with firm nonpitting edema in the affected part. Bone involvement may result from contiguous spread of disease. The *lymphadenopathic* type is seen most commonly in children. Tumor infiltrates are confined to lymphoreticular tissues. Cutaneous and other organ involvement are rare. To these four can be added an additional type best described as *cutaneous lymphadenopathic* Kaposi's sarcoma. This disease occurs almost exclusively in young adult men and women (Dutz and Stout, 1960; Taylor *et al.,* 1971; Haim *et al.,* 1973; Taylor, 1973). The prognosis is poor; the disease is very difficult to treat, and death occurs rapidly in a high percentage of cases.

In summary, based on clinical characteristics, that is, physical findings, distribution of lesions, clinical course, behavior, and response to treatment, a very simple uniform classification of nearly all forms of Kaposi's sarcoma, whether European, North American, or African type, has been developed (see Table 20-6).

Histopathologically, lesions of Kaposi's sarcoma show one of three basic cellular patterns: Mixed cellularity, monocellular or spindle cell, or anaplastic disease (Hutt, 1981; Lever and Schaumburg-Lever, 1983). The mixed cellular pattern is the most common and most typical pattern. Mixed tumors are composed of interlacing bundles of spindle-shaped cells, many having the appearance of endothelial cells, especially when lining well-defined vascular channels. Others will lie in aggregates.

Sometimes the tumor is composed predominantly of endothelial-lined vascular spaces (see Figures 20-18 and 20-19). Early lesions show an intense perivascular as well as diffuse cellular infiltrate composed of lymphocytes, plasma cells, and histiocytes. Clusters of extravasated red blood cells and hemosiderin may be scattered throughout the lesion (see Figures 20-20 and 20-21). As the tumor grows, spindle cells and vascular channels proliferate and the inflammatory component lessens (see Fig-

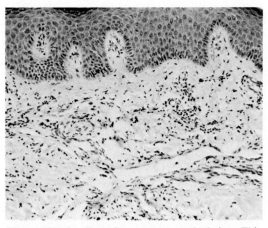

Figure 20-18. Kaposi's sarcoma—early lesion. This tumor is composed predominantly of endothelial-lined vascular spaces. A sparce inflammatory infiltrate may be seen scattered throughout.

ure 20-22). Lesions of mixed cellularity are seen in most patients with "nodular disease," in all patients with "lymphadenopathic disease," and in patients with "florid disease." Monocellular or spindle cell tumors are characterized by the predominance of spindle cells and a virtual absence of endothelial cell and vascular proliferation. In most of these lesions typical Kaposi's tissue may be seen at the periphery (Templeton, 1981). Histologically, this lesion is very difficult to distinguish from a number of other mesenchymal tumors. It may resemble a fibrosarcoma or leiomyosarcoma,

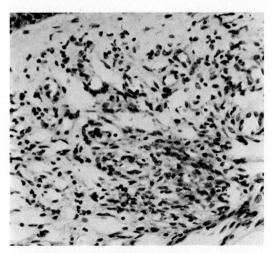

Figure 20-19. Kaposi's sarcoma—early lesion. Here vascular spaces lined by endothelial cells are quite prominent. There is a loose inflammatory infiltrate composed principally of lymphocytes, plasma cells, and histiocytes. Extravasated blood cells are found in abundance throughout the stroma of the lesion.

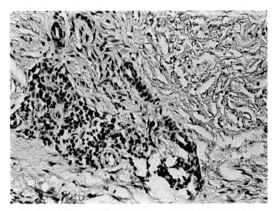

Figure 20–20. Kaposi's sarcoma. In this lesion there are normal blood vessels mixed with endothelial lined vascular spaces. There is a very heavy plasma cell infiltrate located in a perivascular position.

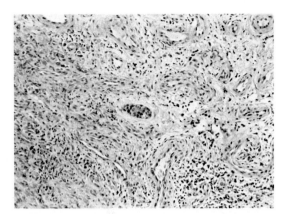

Figure 20–22. Late stage of Kaposi's sarcoma. In this tumor spindle cells predominate. Very small but well-defined vascular spaces are noted throughout the lesion. There is extravasation of red blood cells and also hemosiderin deposition.

as well as spindle cell variants of squamous cell carcinoma and spindle cell amelanotic melanoma (Hutt, 1981). The pleomorphic or anaplastic variant contains numerous anaplastic cells showing nuclear pleomorphism and multiple mitoses. Although the anaplastic pattern is associated almost exclusively with florid-type lesions, it is an unusual presentation in Kaposi's sarcoma tissue.

Origins of Tumor Cells. Since Kaposi's original description of the disease in which he proposed a vascular origin, numerous arguments have arisen over the exact origins of tumor cells. Both a lymphoreticular origin (Dorffel, 1932; Tedeschi, 1958; Dayan and Lewis, 1967) and tumor development from

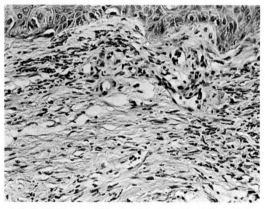

Figure 20–21. Kaposi's sarcoma. This lesion is dominated by the presence of endothelial lined vascular spaces, minimal inflammatory infiltrates, and some red cell extravasation. Other portions of the tumor are composed predominantly of dermal collections of inflammatory cells, many of which are plasma cells, and red blood cells. Very few vascular spaces are present.

Schwann cells have many proponents. (Mackee and Cipollaro, 1936; Becker, 1962). The more widely supported view now is that Kaposi's sarcoma originates from an angioformative or pluripotential endothelial cell (Hashimoto and Lever, 1964; Jaffee, 1977; Guarda et al., 1981; Nadji et al., 1981). A large body of evidence, including electron microscopic observations of tumor cell type, tends to support a vascular origin, at least in part. Two cell types have been identified in Kaposi's sarcoma tissue: (1) Cells with endothelial differentiation and (2) cells with fibroblastic differentiation. Factor VIII–related antigen was demonstrated in neoplastic cells in 52 cases of Kaposi's sarcoma (Guarda et al., 1981). Endothelial cells were shown to synthesize factor VIII (Jaffee, 1977). Finally, cytomegalovirus inclusions when found in the tissues of adults are nearly always prominent in vascular endothelial cells. Cytomegalovirus tropism for endothelial cells has been suggested (Wong and Warner, 1962), further adding to the evidence supporting the viral (cytomegalovirus) cause of Kaposi's sarcoma.

Diagnosis

The clinical diagnosis of Kaposi's sarcoma is not difficult in either the European or African variety. In 90% of cases the characteristic clinical features described above are present. In the other 10% of cases diagnosis can be made on the basis of characteristic histopathologic findings. In most cases the typical mixed cellular type of histologic pattern is seen, even in the clinically recognizable florid form of disease.

The pleomorphic or anaplastic type of Kaposi's sarcoma is rare and histologic diagnosis may be difficult.

In any diagnostic evaluation of patients with cutaneous lesions, the gastrointestinal and respiratory tracts must be examined, because extracutaneous involvement is most common in these systems. This is particularly true in the European or non-African variety. Endoscopy will show characteristic lesions throughout the gastrointestinal tract. In children all elements of the reticuloendothelial system may be involved; therefore, a thorough examination of the lymph nodes, liver, spleen, parotids, and so forth is in order. Rarely are other systems involved in this population. In young adults disseminated disease is most common; therefore, all organ systems must be examined.

Staging

The various types of Kaposi's sarcoma have been described above. The disease is multifocal in origin and is rarely metastatic.

Specific and Supportive Management

The indolent type of Kaposi's sarcoma, principally confined to limited areas of the skin, is radiosensitive to both gamma rays and electrons (Cohen et al., 1962; Nisce et al., 1981). X-irradiation is infrequently used in treating indolent nodular forms of this disease.

Patients with either form of indolent cutaneous disease who do not respond to radiation therapy may respond to one or more chemotherapeutic agents, as may patients with indolent disease involving other organ systems (Vogel et al., 1971, 1973; Olweny, 1981; Solan et al., 1981). Of the single agents reported to date, vinblastine appears to be the most widely used. Weekly intravenous vinblastine is effective in controlling both localized and generalized forms of the disease in elderly patients without inducing serious systemic toxicity. The major disadvantage of vinblastine therapy is the necessity for protracted use of the drug.

Various combinations of drugs have been used to control the more aggressive forms of disease as well as widespread indolent disease. The most impressive results have been reported by Olweny (1981). Of 32 patients receiving a three-drug combination of actinomycin D, vincristine, and DTIC, 30 achieved complete remission, one a partial remission, and one did not respond to therapy. Similar results were reported in children (Farrant, 1982). Two patients with very aggressive disease were treated with a three-drug combination consisting of vincristine, actinomycin D, and bleomycin. Both achieved complete disease remission (Olweny, 1981).

Patients with Kaposi's sarcoma and AIDS do not respond well to chemotherapy with over 50% succumbing to the disease within two years. The recently reported successful use of a purified human interferon in Kaposi's sarcoma with AIDS is encouraging (Brown et al., 1983) as is the recent report of AIDS-associated Kaposi's sarcoma responsive to dapsone (Poulsen et al., 1984). Withdrawal of immunosuppressive therapy in those patients who develop Kaposi's sarcoma appears to be accompanied by a diminution of tumor mass and in some cases complete resolution of disease. Drug combinations using prednisone appear to be ineffective in inducing remissions and are, thus, contraindicated.

Surgery is of limited use in localized disease.

Future Prospects

Recent observations and relevant data from intensive investigations of AIDS and Kaposi's sarcoma have led to the following: The association of acquired immune deficiency syndrome with Kaposi's sarcoma in young men who are homosexual and in Haitian immigrants; the association of altered immunity and the development of Kaposi's sarcoma; the identification of a common HLA phenotype in heterosexual or classic Kaposi's sarcoma, as well as in the homosexual type (Friedman-Kein, 1981); the high prevalence of cytomegalovirus and infections and human type-C retrovirus in affected populations; the findings of cytomegalovirus particles in tissues from affected patients; and the finding of human type-C retrovirus infections and cutaneous T-cell lymphomas in Haiti and their postulated role in causing other types of tumors. These and other rapidly unfolding clues should eventually provide us with solutions to the questions of etiology and pathogenesis of Kaposi's sarcoma and other human neoplasms.

CUTANEOUS T-CELL LYMPHOMAS

Cutaneous lymphomas are lymphoproliferative disorders that initially affect skin and structures derived from ectoderm primarily and internal organs secondarily. Cutaneous lymphomas demonstrate "epidermotropism" or "epitheliotropia" early in their clinical course (Altmeyer and Nodl, 1978; Edelson, 1980). Although B-cell lymphomas may occasionally demonstrate epidermotropism, most cutaneous lymphomas are of T-cell origin. Mycosis fungoides lymphoma and the Sézary's variant make up the bulk of lymphomas in the cutaneous T-cell lymphoma group. Although cutaneous T-cell lymphomas were once thought to be among the rarest of lymphomas, a recent review of clinical material, derived from the catchment area of the Cancer Center, Columbia University College of Physicians and Surgeons, shows that cutaneous T-cell lymphomas may occur more frequently than does Hodgkin's disease (Edelson, 1980).

Incidence and Epidemiology

Although mycosis fungoides was first described early in the eighteenth century (1806), until recently its existence as an entity had been challenged (Block et al., 1963; Clendenning et al., 1964). Mycosis fungoides is often very difficult to diagnose in its earliest stages; therefore, its true prevalence is probably not known.

The more easily recognized cutaneous lesions of mycosis fungoides lymphoma are frequently preceded by nonspecific chronic cutaneous eruptions clinically indistinguishable from a variety of benign eczematous and papulosquamous skin disorders. Some antecedent eruptions occur after chronic cutaneous stimulation, that is, the pruritic dermatitis of atopy, chronic allergic contact sensitivity, or chronic cutaneous photosensitivity (Buechner and Winkelmann, 1983). The early eczematous phase of the disease is called "premycotic" because there are no specific clinical or histopathologic features to identify it as a neoplasm. Each year in the United States approximately 200 people die from mycosis fungoides — about 1% of all deaths from lymphoma (Burbank, 1971). In the United States an estimated 1000 to 2000 new cases are reported each year (Oncology Overview, 1981). Mycosis fungoides has been reported from all areas of the world, with no overall regional, racial, or ethnic predilections. In the United States T-cell diseases as a group occur with equal frequency in Caucasians and blacks. An apparent male predominance gives some credence to theories of origin proposing a relationship between oc-

cupational exposure and etiology (Fischmann et al., 1979; Green et al., 1979; Cohen et al., 1980). "Subsets" of T-cell lymphomas and leukemias are extremely aggressive and carry a very poor prognosis for survival. These subsets are found most often in young adults, median age of 35, who are black, rural, West Indian, or Japanese living in southern Japan (Brigham et al., 1982; Catovsky et al., 1982; Robert-Guroff et al., 1982).

Etiology and Pathogenesis

To date, the specific etiologic agent or agents have not been identified in the development of mycosis fungoides. The most prominent theories point to (1) a nonneoplastic origin, and (2) viral etiology. In a report of seven cases of pre-Sézary erythroderma evolving to Sézary syndrome, Buechner and Winkelmann (1983) noted that the clinical course of the seven patients indicated "a consistent pattern of dermatitis-erythroderma, which implies that chronic antigen stimulation may lead to chronic T-cell disease." In two uncontrolled studies chronic cutaneous stimulation by commonly encountered environmental agents, such as petroleum products, rubber, metals, printing products, detergents, disinfectants, pesticides, solvents, air pollutants, as well as common drugs such as analgesics, thiazides, tobacco and tranquilizers, was linked to the development of mycosis fungoides (Fischmann et al., 1979; Green et al., 1979). Other studies attempted to show a correlation between disease, shortened survival, and trades peculiar to "heavy industry" (Cohen et al., 1980).

The finding of increased numbers of Langerhans cells in the skin of patients with mycosis fungoides provides evidence to support the mode of disease development from chronic benign dermatoses (Rowden and Lewis, 1976; Turbitt and Mackie, 1979; Chu et al., 1981; McMillan et al., 1981). Langerhans cells make up from 3 to 8% of all epidermal cell populations and are found localized principally in suprabasal and lower epidermal sites. Small numbers of Langerhans cells are also found in the dermis, other types of epithelia, lymph nodes, tonsils and thymus.

In most mammalian systems Langerhans cells apparently derive from bone marrow (Tamaki et al., 1980). They appear to share certain enzymatic reactions and immunologic features of other bone marrow-derived cells, specifically those of the monocytic/macrophage and granulocytic series (Berman and France, 1979; Berman and Gigli, 1980; Stingl et al., 1980). Langerhans cells are thought to play an important role in the development of certain types of cutaneous immunologic reactions (Silberberg-Sinakin et al., 1978). They have been observed aggregating in close apposition to mononuclear-lymphocyte cells within hours after the topical application of cutaneous contact allergens, regularly showing some evidence of cellular damage shortly thereafter. Silberberg (1971) has postulated, and to some degree has shown, that mononuclear cells apposed to Langerhans cells are specifically sensitized lymphocytes that are interacting with antigen on or near the surface of the Langerhans cell. Apposed lymphocytes release substances (lymphokines) that cause physical damage to the Langerhans cell; damaged Langerhans cells release substances that may in turn provoke additional inflammatory changes in skin, dermal lymphatics, and regional lymph nodes. These cell-to-cell interactions in skin reacting to contact allergens and the apparent local depletion of epidermal Langerhans cells through a process involving migration from skin to lymph node sites favor the concept that Langerhans cells play a prime role in the development of contact allergy. In contact allergy, Langerhans cells carry out a function (immune surveillance) analogous to conventional monocytic macrophages. Rowden and Lewis (1976) have reported frequently finding "mycosis cells" lying in close apposition to Langerhans cells in histopathologic material obtained from patients with stages II and III mycosis fungoides. Very prominent accumulations of Langerhans cells in Pautrier microabscesses, the *sine qua non* of pathologic findings in mycosis fungoides, and in the epidermis of patients with advancing disease have been described (Chu and McDonald, 1981). Others have found accumulations of Langerhans cells interspersed with cancerous T cells in dermal infiltrates of mycosis fungoides and suspected prelymphomatous lesions (Turbitt and Mackie, 1979; Chu et al., 1981; McMillan et al., 1981). Ultrastructural studies have uncovered physically damaged Langerhans cells in regions of close mycosis cell-Langerhans cell interaction.

The relationship of these findings to mycosis fungoides lymphoma suggests that the environmental antigens listed earlier may act as sources of chronic cutaneous antigenic stimulation. Chronic stimulation ultimately depletes cutaneous populations of Langerhans cells; diminished immune surveillance results as well as unrestricted proliferation of immunocytes and the eventual development of a cancerous clone of T-lymphocytes. In Buechner and Winkelmann's study (1983), prior to developing florid Sézary syndrome, four of the seven Sézary patients had histories of multiple contact allergies or drug reactions and one had severe atopic dermatitis.

In late 1980 and early 1981 Poiesz and coworkers, reporting from the Laboratory of Tumor Cell Biology, National Cancer Institute, called attention to the initial detection and isolation of type-C retrovirus particles from fresh peripheral blood lymphocytes and from two human T-lymphoblast cell lines. These materials had been obtained from a black male patient with the very aggressive variant of mycosis fungoides lymphoma (Poiesz et al., 1980, 1981). Other reported viral isolations were of dubious origin. Physical and biochemical characteristics showed them closely related to or indistinguishable from previously isolated primate type-C viruses. Further physical, biochemical, and immunologic studies of the type-C virus isolated by Poiesz showed that it differed in a number of qualitative and quantitative ways from primate type-C retroviruses. It had enough unique characteristics to identify it as a new virus associated intimately with certain types of human T-cell neoplasias (Kalyanaraman et al., 1982; Reitz et al., 1981). This virus was designated human T-cell lymphoma and leukemia virus (HTLV-I). In further reports by Catovsky and associates (1982), Robert-Guroff and colleagues (1982) and others, HTLV-I virus and antibody have been identified in patients with adult human T-cell lymphoma in nearly all parts of the world. Most patients harboring HTLV, however, reside in the southeastern United States, countries of the West Indies, and southwestern Japan. Other cases are sporadically identified in Africa, South America, Europe, and Alaska and other regions of the United States.

A characteristic profile of the typical patient with HTLV-associated lymphoma includes aggressive disease appearing in a young adult, usually black or Japanese, living in a rural environment. Cutaneous tumors are extensive, large numbers of malignant cells are found in the peripheral blood, lytic bone lesions are widespread, hypercalcemia is profound, and the patient is usually susceptible to opportunistic infections by *Pneumocystis carinii, Candida* species, and other deep fungi (Bunn *et al.,* 1983).

Of the 20 or so viral isolates so far described in patients from different parts of the world, many can transform T-lymphocytes. Infection of normal lymphocytes by HTLV-I *in vitro* results in the transformation of mature T cells and continuous proliferation of the T-cell line. HTLV is unique among transforming retroviruses in that there is no viral oncogene with a normal cellular homolog. Instead it appears that HTLV genomes contain a specific 3' region that is responsible for HTLV-induced cellular transformation. It has been shown that the 3' region of HTLV-I contains a gene-encoding protein that is responsible for cellular transformation (Lee *et al.,* 1984; Slamon *et al.,* 1984; Wachsman *et al.,* 1984). Transformed cells show a remarkable morphologic resemblance to malignant T cells obtained directly from active tumor tissue (Miyoshi *et al.,* 1981). Using a recombinant DNA cloning technique, it has been determined that HTLV-I infection may induce the expression of high levels of a normally repressed single copy gene (clone HT-3) (Manzari *et al.,* 1983). HT-3 may also be equated with a gene for T-cell growth factor or receptor or may be intimately involved in one of the steps leading to T-cell growth factor production. (T-cell growth factor is produced in abundance by a number of tumor cell lines and has been found to promote the growth of human T-lymphoblasts *in vitro* [Poiesz *et al.,* 1980]). HTLV-I may cause abnormal cell growth by inducing continuous expression of the gene HT-3 in infected cells, resulting in a cell producing both T-cell growth factor and receptor, which in turn produces autostimulation and increased cell proliferation.

Both these predominant but disparate postulates as to cause may have considerable merit. There are probably at least two variants and maybe more of cutaneous T-cell leukemia-lymphoma, and each variant may be provoked by differing stimuli: Contact irritants acting as the predominant etiologic agents in the chronic slowly progressive disease seen in most patients and type-C human retroviruses acting as the etiologic agents in the aggressive and rapidly fatal type seen in young adults. In some types both may act in concert or with other factors to produce cutaneous lymphoma. We generally acknowledge that human tumors are caused by multiple etiologic agents, physical, chemical, and viral.

Pathology and Natural History

With few exceptions, mycosis fungoides presents initially in the skin with slow but progressive involvement of lymph nodes and visceral organs secondarily. Visceral organ involvement was thought to occur only after a prolonged period of cutaneous disease; however, this concept has been recently challenged (Bunn *et al.,* 1980; Keller *et al.,* 1983). Intensive and extensive staging examinations have produced strong evidence to support the concept that systemic dissemination of cutaneous T-cell lymphoma is frequent, generally asymptomatic, and develops *early* by way of blood and lymphatics.

The various cutaneous lesions of mycosis fungoides may be observed singly, in combination, or may develop sequentially. Although several new methods of classification have been proposed, among which is the TNM (Bunn and Lamberg, 1979) (see Tables 20–7 and 20–8), the appearance of the characteristic cutaneous lesions is most often used by dermatologists to classify the disease into its various clinical stages (see Table 20–9). The disease progresses characteristically, moving from stage I through stage III. Stage I is the eczematous or premycotic stage. It is the least malignant of the four; treatment is often successful and prognosis for long-term survival is good. Stage I is characterized by a multiplicity of cutaneous eruptions most often of a nonspecific nature (see Colorplate XV). Scaling, macular, erythematous patches may predominate and may be localized or scattered over the entire integument. Some lesions in this stage may simulate an acute or chronic eczema, superficial fungus infection, seborrheic dermatitis, fixed drug eruption, poikiloderma, psoriasis, parapsoriasis en plaques, erythroderma, and

Table 20–7. Staging of Cutaneous T-Cell Lymphomas

	CUTANEOUS	NODES	VISCERA
Stage I			
A	T_1	N_0	M_0
B	T_2	N_0	M_0
Stage II			
A	T_{1-2}	N_1	M_0
B	T_3	N_{0-1}	M_0
Stage III	T_4	N_{0-1}	M_0
Stage IV			
A	T_{1-4}	N_{2-3}	M_0
B	T_{1-4}	N_{0-3}	M_1

Note: This table is based on the TNM description of extent of involvement in Table 20–8, according to criteria proposed by the National CTCL Workshop.

Table 20-8. TNM System to Describe Extent of Disease

Skin involvement (T)
- T_0 Clinically and/or histopathologically suspicious lesions
- T_1 Plaques, papules, or patches covering less than 10% of skin surface
- T_2 Plaques, papules, or patches covering more than 10% of skin surface
- T_3 Tumors
- T_4 Generalized erythroderma

Nodal involvement (N)
- N_0 Normal clinically and pathologically
- N_1 Abnormal clinically, normal pathologically
- N_2 Normal clinically, abnormal pathologically
- N_3 Clinically and pathologically abnormal

Peripheral blood (B)
- B_0 No evidence of atypical cells
- B_1 5% or more atypical cells

Visceral organs
- M_0 None
- M_1 Present

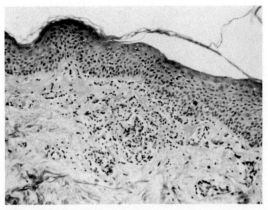

Figure 20-23. Mycosis fungoides—early stage I lesion. There is nothing to characterize this lesion or differentiate it from a nonspecific dermatitis. The epidermis is normal and scattered throughout the dermis are perivascular accumulations of round cells.

exfoliative dermatitis. Patients with total body redness of the skin (Indian skin, l'homme rouge) may also show loss of hair and thick hyperkeratotic palms and soles. It is often difficult to clinically separate this phase of stage I disease (erythroderma) from the early phase of Sézary's syndrome. The lesions of this stage can persist for months or years, even as long as several decades before progressing to more severe disease. In some cases spontaneous regression occurs. There is often a paucity of symptoms. The major symptom during this period is pruritus, usually very intense and unrelenting. Pruritus is so characteristic that mycosis fungoides should be suspected in any patient over 40 years of age with an acute or chronic dermatitis and therapeutically unresponsive pruritus.

In early stage I multiple skin biopsies from the same and multiple lesions are a necessity because histopathologic diagnosis is difficult. In the earliest lesions the epidermis is normal. In the dermis small perivascular accumulations of normal-appearing lymphocytes are seen (see Figure 20-23). Thus, "nonspecific" dermatitis is often diagnosed. In later lesions of

Table 20-9. Staging of Cutaneous T-Cell Lymphomas*

Stage I: Premycotic, eczematous lesions
- A. Without visceral or nodal involvement
- B. With visceral or nodal involvement

Stage II: Plaques, nodules, and eczematous lesions
- A. Without visceral or nodal involvement
- B. With visceral or nodal involvement

Stage III: Tumors and/or ulcerations

Stage IV: Sézary's or generalized erythroderma

* Based on cutaneous manifestations.

stage I the epidermis may be thickened and the rete ridges elongated, simulating psoriasis or a chronic lichenified dermatitis (see Figures 20-24 and 20-25). Focal spongiosis and microvesicles containing normal-appearing inflammatory cells may be noted in the epidermis. The stratum corneum is hyperkeratotic without parakeratosis. The dermal cellular infiltrate is nonspecific consisting of a loose polymorphous collection of lymphocytes, neutrophils, eosinophils, plasma cells, and histiocytes located perivascularly and throughout the dermis (see Figure 20-25). Occasionally in this stage, but more often in the infiltrated plaque and tumor stages, a specific cell appears in the dermal infiltrate that suggests the diagnosis of mycosis fungoides.

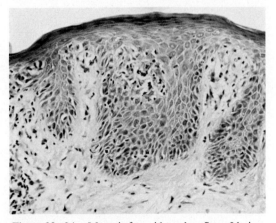

Figure 20-24. Mycosis fungoides—late Stage I lesion. The epidermis is somewhat acanthotic. There are collections of monocytic cells within the epidermis in the absence of obvious spongiosis.

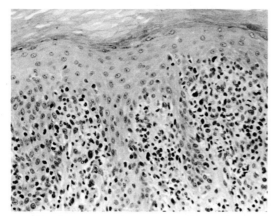

Figure 20–25. Mycosis fungoides. The epidermis shows considerable hyperkeratosis and elongation of some of the rete ridges. There is an intense bandlike infiltrate encroaching upon the epidermis. Scattered throughout the inflammatory infiltrate are cells with very large hyperchromatic nuclei; the so-called mycosis cells. The remainder of the infiltrate is quite pleomorphic in appearance.

This cell may be small but is often slightly larger than a monocyte. It contains a small amount of cytoplasm and a large hyperchromatic nucleus (see Figures 20–26, 20–27, and 20–28). Careful examination of this cell with routine light microscopy sometimes reveals multiple convolutions in the nucleus, giving it the characteristic "cerebriform" appearance. Single cells or collections of these abnormal cells may appear in the epidermis. Collections of closely packed, abnormal lymphoid cells within the epidermis make up the so-called

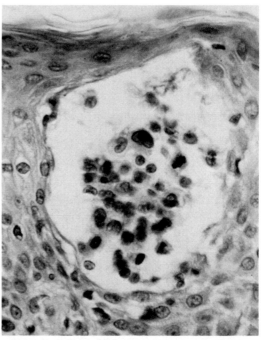

Figure 20–27. High-power view of a Pautrier microabscess. A collection of abnormal monocytic cells, some with very large folded nuclei, is seen.

Pautrier microabscess (see Figures 20–26 and 20–27). This micropathologic lesion is considered pathognomonic of mycosis fungoides.

In the "classic" progression of this disease stage II appears after a variable time period. Well-defined elevated plaques or nodules are seen alone or in an admixture of chronic eczematous-type lesions (see Colorplates XV and

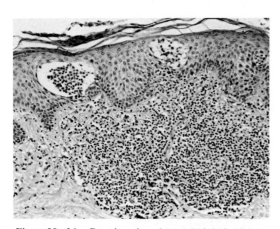

Figure 20–26. Pautrier microabscess. This lesion is considered pathognomonic of mycosis fungoides. The epidermis, though quite thin and hyperkeratotic, shows collections of round cells within spaces in a nonspongiotic epidermis. Within the dermis are a pleomorphic infiltrate and scattered cells containing large multilobulated nuclei.

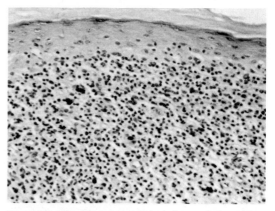

Figure 20–28. Plaque-type lesion of mycosis fungoides. The epidermis is thin and hyperkeratotic. The inflammatory infiltrate has invaded the epidermis and is obscuring the basal lamina as well as the basal layer of the epidermis. The intense inflammatory infiltrate is made up of pleomorphic cells, many of which have large hyperchromatic or large folded nuclei.

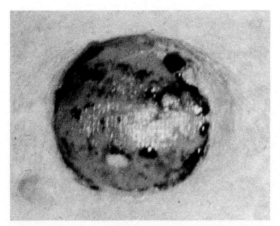

Figure 20-29. A clinical picture of tumor-stage mycosis fungoides.

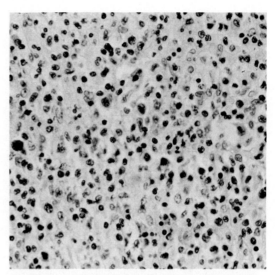

Figure 20-31. Tumor-stage mycosis fungoides. The inflammatory infiltrate in this tumor is pleomorphic, but the number of abnormal cells containing large hyperchromatic and folded nuclei is considerably greater than shown in previous photomicrographs.

XVI). They vary in color from bluish-red to brown and are indurated on palpation. In this stage, disease severity is intermediate between premycotic and tumor stages.

In stage II the histologic picture becomes more characteristic (see Figure 20-28). Lying in a compact zone in the subepidermal region is usually a cellular infiltrate somewhat similar to that seen in Hodgkin's disease. A multiplicity of cell types occurs: Neutrophils, lymphocytes, eosinophils, plasma cells, and a polymorphism of histiocytes. A so-called Grenz zone, or cell-free subepidermal region, may separate the infiltrate from the epidermis. The infiltrate, however, may be noted to be encroaching on and invading the epidermis. Greater numbers of abnormal mononuclear cells with large convoluted nuclei appear within the dermis. In the epidermis Pautrier microabscesses may appear in greater abundance. In some patients this pathognomonic microscopic lesion is never seen.

In stage III, the most ominous stage, tumors appear subsequent to the development of large plaques and nodules, except in the d'emblée type, in which the disease makes its initial appearance as tumors and nodules (see Figure 20-29). Tumors and nodules occur princi-

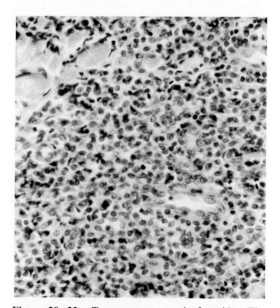

Figure 20-32. Tumor-stage mycosis fungoides. The predominant cellular infiltrate consists of T-lymphocytes, both large and small cell types. A small collection of giant cells may be seen in the upper left-hand corner of the photomicrograph.

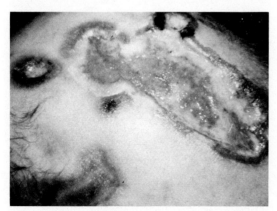

Figure 20-30. Mycosis fungoides—ulcerative lesion.

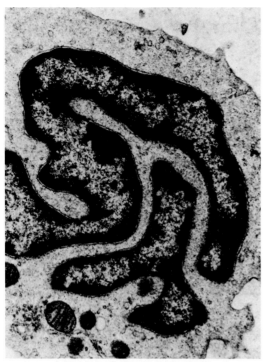

Figure 20–33. Electronmicrograph of a typical activated T cell found within the infiltrates of cutaneous T-cell lymphomas. The extensive infolding of the nucleus characterizes this type of cell.

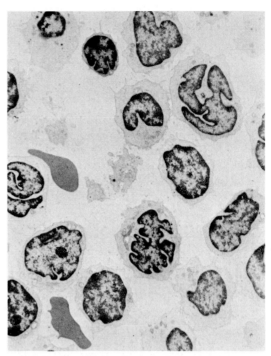

Figure 20–34. Electronmicrograph of activated T cells (Sézary's cells) in the peripheral blood.

pally in previously affected sites or occasionally in normal-appearing skin. They vary in size from 1 or 2 cm to several inches in diameter and are elevated above normal skin. In this stage the surface of these lesions, as well as the cutaneous surface of many plaque-type lesions, often spontaneously breaks down, forming deep ulcerations. Ulcerations can also appear on apparently normal skin (see Figure 20–30).

Histopathologically it is sometimes difficult to distinguish this clinical stage from the plaque stage except that cells containing large hyperchromatic and convoluted nuclei become more frequent (see Figure 20–31) and severe encroachment of the dermal infiltrate on the epidermis produces ulcerations. Often the cellular composition of the dermal infiltrate is almost exclusively T-lymphocytes (see Figure 20–32). Life expectancy is short after onset of the tumor stage. A few patients die of visceral organ involvement with lymphoma. Interestingly, many patients die simply of intercurrent infection and septicemia. Death from infection most certainly is associated with the numerous immunologic aberrations that occur in the late stages of disease. These will be addressed later in this discussion.

The Sézary syndrome, although previously classified as a distinctly different disease, is now widely acknowledged as a variety of cutaneous T-cell lymphoma whose neoplastic cells possess phenotypic characteristics of helper T cells (Broome *et al.,* 1973; Edelson *et al.,* 1974; Broder *et al.,* 1976; Zucker-Franklin, 1976; Davis and Simpkins, 1979; Edelson, 1980; Haynes *et al.,* 1981). Patients with classic Sézary's syndrome (Sézary and Bouvrain, 1938; Sézary, 1949) present with generalized erythroderma, often exfoliative in nature, generalized edema, increased pigmentation, alopecia,

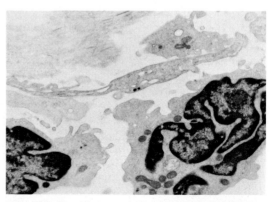

Figure 20–35. Electronmicrograph of activated T-lymphocytes in the skin of a patient with mycosis fungoides—Sézary's type.

dystrophic nails, keratoderma of the palms and soles, along with intense pruritus. Often, patients with stage I erythroderma are clinically confused with patients with Sézary's syndrome; in such cases, extensive cutaneous edema and peripheral blood leukocytosis are absent. Abnormal T-cell lymphocytes are found in abundance in the peripheral blood of patients with Sézary's syndrome (see Figure 20-34), but in patients with the erythroderma of mycosis fungoides, their absolute number is much lower. Because of increased white cell numbers in peripheral blood and large numbers of abnormal lymphocytes, the Sézary syndrome is often referred to as the leukemic variant of mycosis fungoides (Sézary and Bouvrain, 1938; Schein et al., 1976). Circulating Sézary cells may be found in up to 50% of patients in the various stages of mycosis fungoides. Their presence may be persistent or intermittent. In one study, circulating Sézary-type cells were present in 33% of patients with plaque stage disease, 36% of patients in the tumor stage, and 100% of patients with erythroderma (Moran et al., 1977).

Histologically, Sézary's syndrome does not differ from late stages of mycosis fungoides. In the skin the dermal infiltrate is composed of dense sheets of lymphocytes, eosinophils, and plasma cells. Pautrier microabscesses are commonly seen in the epidermis. Although the disease is best characterized as systemic- or leukemic-phase mycosis fungoides, patients with Sézary's syndrome may have no evidence of abnormal T-cell infiltration of sites other than skin and peripheral blood. Because of this phenomenon, skin rather than bone marrow is thought to be the source of the abnormal circulating cells in Sézary's syndrome. Disease that remains confined to skin and peripheral blood may account for the lack of aggressive behavior of Sézary's syndrome in a small number of patients.

Worringer-Kolepp's disease (epidermotropic reticulosis, pagetoid reticulosis), once considered a separate and distinct clinical entity, is probably an additional variant of cutaneous T-cell lymphoma. Patients with this disease present with rapidly enlarging, polycyclic, well-defined, erythematous scaling patches. Some lesions may resemble parapsoriasis variegata, others may become necrotic and show signs of central ulceration. Although slowly progressive disease in a few reported cases has been seen, the disease usually is rapidly fatal. Histologically the epidermis shows extensive invasion by a monomorphous cellular infiltrate. Electronmicroscopic examination and cytomorphologic studies of the cells invading epidermis have shown them to be similar in all respects to those seen in cutaneous T-cell lymphoma (Degreef et al., 1976; Haneke et al., 1977).

Despite numerous attempts to identify a specific cell type peculiar to mycosis fungoides that could be identified in early-stage disease all cell types observed to date populating the skin in mycosis fungoides have been found in abundance in other benign dermatoses (Flaxman et al., 1971; Orbaneja et al., 1976). Yet recent immunologic, cytochemical, and ultrastructural studies have clarified the controversy surrounding the nature of the predominant neoplastic cell types found in the peripheral blood, skin infiltrates, lymph nodes, and lung tissue of patients with cutaneous T-cell lymphoma (Lutzner et al., 1971; Broome et al., 1973; Broult et al., 1973; Lutzner et al., 1973; Edelson et al., 1974; Zucker-Franklin, 1976; Burg and Braun-Falco, 1978; Davis and Simpkins, 1979; Sterry et al., 1980; Haynes et al, 1981; Chu et al., 1983). Although occasionally debated (Thiers, 1982), considerable evidence supports the concept that the neoplastic cell found in the peripheral blood and tissue infiltrates of patients with Sézary's syndrome is in effect the same cell type found in patients with mycosis fungoides and T-cell leukemia. Two cell types or variants based on overall size have been described (Lutzner, 1973). The importance of size has yet to be determined because both cell sizes may be seen in the same patient. The most distinguishing feature of this cell is its highly convoluted (cerebriform) nucleus (Lutzner et al., 1971; Lutzner et al., 1973; Zucker-Franklin, 1976; Meyer et al., 1977), best seen on electronmicroscopic examination (see Figures 20–33, 20–34, 20–35, and 20–36). An additional distinguishing feature, large numbers of cytoplasmic filaments measuring approximately 100 nm in diameter, has been described. These neoplastic cells have membrane properties like those of normal thymus-derived lymphocytes. They readily form spontaneous rosettes with uncoated sheep erythrocytes. Their enzyme histochemical characteristics are those of thymus-derived lymphocytes (Burg and Braun-Falco, 1978; Davis and Simpkins, 1979). They produce many lymphokines, among which are macrophage migration inhibitory factor, leukocyte migration inhibitory factor, leukocyte migration enhancement factor, colony stimulating

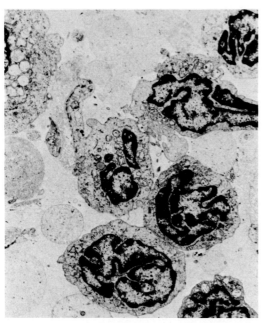

Figure 20–36. Electronmicrograph of activated T cells within the lymph node of a patient with cutaneous T-cell lymphoma.

factor, γ-interferon, and T-cell growth factor. (Yoshida *et al.,* 1975; Umbert *et al.,* 1976; Salahuddin *et al.,* 1984). They respond with blastogenic activity when stimulated by pokeweed mitogen and phytohemagglutinin (Burg *et al.,* 1978; Cooperrider and Roenigk, 1978), and they have been shown to possess membrane receptors for an antihuman T-lymphocyte globulin (Edelson *et al.,* 1974; Burg and Braun-Falco, 1978).

Although the neoplastic cells of cutaneous T-cell lymphomas have reportedly shown suppressor cell activity, or no activity when examined in coculture with B-lymphocytes, more recent studies, using panels of antihuman T-cell monoclonal antibodies capable of phenotyping lymphocytes *in situ* and in peripheral blood, clearly show that cutaneous T-cell lymphoma is a neoplasm of helper T cells (Edelson, 1980; Haynes *et al.,* 1981, Chu *et al.,* 1983, Kung *et al.,* 1983), confirming the earlier studies (Broder *et al.,* 1976; Waldman *et al.,* 1976). In very late-stage disease, and in some cases of rapidly progressive disease, characteristic T-cell markers may be lost (Kung *et al.,* 1981; Holden *et al.,* 1982). Loss of these markers is believed to relate to malignant dedifferentiation of tumor cells.

As mentioned earlier, cells with light and electron microscopic features similar to the neoplastic cell type found in cutaneous T-cell

lymphoma may appear in many benign cutaneous diseases, in the peripheral blood of normal healthy blood donors, and in human cord blood (Flaxman *et al.,* 1971; Orbaneja *et al.,* 1976; Meyer *et al.,* 1977; Chu *et al.,* 1983). Therefore, when randomly distributed in visceral organs or in peripheral blood, they are not diagnostic of T-cell lymphoma. When occurring in sheets and clusters in visceral organs and lymph nodes, or as 20% or more of the circulating peripheral blood cell population, however, they are diagnostic (Rappaport and Thomas, 1974; Rosas-Uribe *et al.,* 1974; Willemze *et al.,* 1983).

Cutaneous Lesions Associated With Mycosis Fungoides

Several cutaneous lesions, when observed in middle-aged or older persons, call for investigation. When data are insufficient to support a diagnosis of mycosis fungoides, these patients should be closely followed for its subsequent development.

Follicular Mucinosis. In 1954 Allen described mucinous changes in hair follicles in a case of mycosis fungoides. In 1957 Pinkus described a disease clinically characterized by erythematous, scaly, eczematous, coalescent papules and plaques scattered over several body areas including the scalp. He called this disease, also characterized by mucinous changes in hair follicles, alopecia mucinosa. Allen concluded that follicular mucinosis is a manifestation of mycosis fungoides or other malignant lymphomas. Pinkus and others believe that follicular mucinosis occurs as benign idiopathic alopecia mucinosa in patients with severe forms of atopic eczema and as a stage in the progression of mycosis fungoides and other malignant lymphomas.

Parapsoriasis En Plaques. The term parapsoriasis is applied to a variety of diseases (some of which have little clinical resemblance to the others and no resemblance to psoriasis) characterized by the development of red-to-brown scaling macules and patches of variable size. Some appear plaquelike and contain varying amounts of pigment. They are generally asymptomatic but persistent. Histologically the lesions do not show characteristic findings. Treatment to date is ineffective.

For an extensive review of the controversial subject of the progression of parapsoriasis, particularly the plaque types, to lymphoma refer to Lambert and Everett (1981). Mononuclear cells found in skin and peripheral blood of a single patient with parapsoriasis showed aneuploid DNA content (Keller *et al.,* 1983). Generally, patients with at least two varieties of parapsoriasis are at risk of developing malignant lymphoma, principally mycosis fungoides. Large plaque parapsoriasis develops into lymphoma in at least 10 to 20% of cases, and retiform parapsoriasis develops into lymphoma in nearly 100% of cases. Whether one believes that mycosis fungoides may develop from parapsoriasis or that cases of lymphoma that developed from parapsoriatic skin were cases of lymphomas originally misdiagnosed, one must attempt to differentiate active mycosis fungoides from parapsoriasis and to observe closely patients diagnosed as having parapsoriasis of the large plaque and/or retiform types.

Poikiloderma Vasculare Atrophicans. This cutaneous condition simulates, to a degree, radiation or solar damage. Skin shows areas of hyperpigmentation, depigmentation, atrophy and telangiectasia. It may appear as part of a number of dermatoses but is most commonly seen as a classic presentation in mycosis fungoides and dermatomyositis. In mycosis fungoides, poikiloderma occurs most commonly in a "bathing trunk" distribution, spreading gradually to involve large contiguous areas. In dermatomyositis the disease usually begins in areas of chronic sun exposure or over affected muscle groups. Histologically, epidermal atrophy is prominent and there is incontinence of melanin into the dermis, particularly after liquefactive degeneration of the basal layer. In the dermis there is a bandlike lymphohistiocytic infiltrate and dilatation of small blood vessels. In lymphomatous disease or in the transition stage from benign to lymphomatous disease, atypical lymphocytic cells are prominently distributed throughout the dermis.

Erythroderma. This is a nonspecific eruption that may occur in any lymphoma or leukemia but is principally seen in those of T-cell origin, particularly those displaying the phenomenon of epidermotropism. Erythroderma or red skin may be patchy or generalized. Generalized disease is usually associated with alopecia, hypertrophic nails, or loss of nails, hyperpigmentation, exfoliation, and keratoderma of the palms and soles. Pruritus is often the major symptomatic complaint. Erythroderma associated with lymphoma may occur without specific evidence of neoplastic change in the skin. The absence of lymphomatous change in the skin is considered an indicator of good "host resistance" (Cormia and Do-

monkos, 1965). When host resistance is overcome, infiltrates characteristic of the specific lymphoma appear and tumors begin to develop. Interestingly, pruritus often disappears with the onset of tumors.

Petechiae (Vasculitis). Eczematous, psoriasiform, bullous, erythrodermic, and other types of dermatoses have customarily preceded or accompanied the onset of mycosis fungoides. One researcher has described a number of patients with a dermatologic manifestation heretofore unrecognized in active mycosis fungoides (McDonald, 1969). These patients have petechiae as a major initial manifestation of active disease. Histologic changes include a small vessel vasculitis with endothelial destruction by malignant lymphophoma cells. One such case was followed for a number of years at another institution as vasculitis, thus preventing early initiation of adequate and appropriate therapy. Upon examination, a clinical and histopathologic diagnosis of mycosis fungoides was made. A review of the early biopsy material showed classic features of mycosis fungoides. The patient subsequently died of pulmonary, myocardial, and central nervous system disease.

Manifestations of Internal Organs

Internal organs are involved ultimately in all patients with mycosis fungoides. The degree of involvement varies and the time of onset has been debated. Many arguments for late involvement of sites other than skin were put forth prior to aggressive attempts at staging the disease. Recent prospective staging evaluations have highlighted early systemic dissemination of cutaneous T-cell lymphomas (Bunn *et al.,* 1980b; Keller, *et al.,* 1983). The organs of the reticuloendothelial system are the most commonly involved extracutaneous sites. Lymphadenopathy is the most common clinical manifestation of extracutaneous disease, occurring in up to 70% of all patients in one study. Two recent studies found the lung to be the most frequently involved visceral organ (Rappaport and Thomas, 1974; Marglin *et al.,* 1979) whereas other studies found the liver most frequently involved (Epstein *et al.,* 1972; Huberman *et al.,* 1980). Radiographic findings in patients with lung disease include pulmonary nodules, infiltrates, mediastinal and/or hilar adenopathy, and pleural effusion (Marglin *et al.,* 1979). Liver/spleen involvement often parallels lymph node involvement but to a lesser degree. Splenic enlargement occurs earlier and more frequently than does liver enlargement; liver/spleen scans often show early changes in the normal liver/spleen size ratio. Other viscera involved in decreasing order of frequency are kidney, thyroid, pancreas, bone marrow, and heart.

Despite early involvement, impairment of organ function is rare and generally occurs only in terminal disease. Internalization of disease including lymph nodes remains, however, a poor prognostic finding (Epstein *et al.*, 1972; Fuks *et al.*, 1973).

When dermal infiltrates become extensive or widespread visceral disease occurs, regional lymph nodes become enlarged and palpable. Such nodes, although often containing few recognizably abnormal T cells, show a characteristic histologic change that resembles that of active cutaneous disease (Rappaport and Thomas, 1974). There may be partial obliteration of the normal nodal architecture, scattered histocytic cells filled with melanin or fat, and isolated or abundant plasma cells and eosinophils. Occasionally, small patches or collections of abnormal T cells are seen. Dermatopathic lymphadenopathy describes these lymph node changes. Although characteristically seen in mycosis fungoides, dermatopathic lymphadenopathy may be noted in patients with other benign, longstanding, pruritic dermatoses. In benign disease the degree of paracortical involvement is more focal, the number of "reactive" follicles is smaller, and the number of small round lymphocytes is greater. Abnormal T cells are less abundant. Clinical lymph node enlargement is also much less evident in benign disease (Burke and Colby, 1981). Infrequently monomorphous infiltrates of abnormal T cells may be found in involved lymph nodes. Generally, dermatopathic lymph nodes drain sites in which nodules, plaques, and tumors predominate.

Histologic examination of other viscera is often less rewarding than examination of regional lymph nodes. Lesions found in visceral organs with other than terminal disease show typical features of cutaneous disease (Rappaport and Thomas, 1974). The presence of collections of cells with large convoluted, deeply indented, and cerebriform nuclei aids considerably in diagnosing visceral mycosis fungoides.

Symptoms and Signs

The characteristic clinical features of the different stages and variants of cutaneous T-cell lymphoma have already been described. Except in advanced disease the single most common complaint of patients with T-cell lymphoma is pruritus. It is constant, relentless, and in most instances not responsive to routine therapeutic measures. A popular belief is that pruritus and erythema, often the first clinical signs and symptoms of cutaneous T-cell lymphoma, are expressions of cutaneous immune defense mechanisms in action, attempting to divest the skin of highly antigenic neoplastic cells.

Diagnosis

Method and Yield. Despite the difficulty of diagnosing cutaneous T-cell lymphomas in the early stages, it is at this time that the most successful treatment can be initiated. Therefore, one must at all times suspect cutaneous T-cell lymphoma in any patient experiencing a chronic nonresponsive pruritic dermatosis. During frequent physical examinations the physician should look for changes in the clinical features of cutaneous lesions, hepatosplenomegaly, as well as peripheral lymph node enlargement. Multiple skin biopsies should be performed frequently at multiple lesion sites. Biopsy material should be submitted for routine light microscopic examination and for electron microscopy. In advanced disease, light microscopy of a single lesion may be sufficient for diagnosis.

Special Techniques Using Light Microscopy. Special studies using light microscopy extend our ability to diagnose cutaneous T-cell lymphomas more accurately. Special immunologic techniques using specific antihuman T-cell antiserum and indirect peroxidase staining can identify those tissue infiltrates composed predominantly of cells bearing specific T-cell antigen (Edelson *et al.*, 1974; Chu and MacDonald, 1981). Microscopic histochemical methods can ascertain and differentiate specific enzyme activity in tissue infiltrates of leukemias and lymphomas. Tissue infiltrates of cutaneous T-cell lymphomas generally show acid phosphatase, alpha-naphthyl butyrate esterase, alpha-naphthyl acetate esterase, adenisone deaminase, acid nonspecific esterase, and eccentric spotted, granular beta-glucoronidase activity (Harigaya, 1977; Buchner and Rufli, 1978; Burg and Braun-Falco, 1978; Davis and Simpkins, 1979; Sterry *et al.*, 1980). Several of these enzymes are characteristically found in normal active helper-type T-cells.

Cytogenic studies may be performed on tissues such as skin, lymph node, spleen, bone marrow, and peripheral blood (Erkman-Balis and Rappaport, 1974; Bunn et al., 1979a; Geraedts et al., 1980; Keller et al., 1983). Chromosome analysis may show abnormal karyotypes, as well as abnormal chromosome numbers. Aneuploidy may be extensive, and a wide range of heteroploidy may be observed. Often the degree of aneuploidy is proportional to the clinical stage of disease. Abnormal chromosomal patterns may range from hypodiploid to hypertetraploid. Generally, cytogenetic abnormalities are proportional to the degree of tissue infiltration with atypical convoluted lymphocytes and may be associated with the progression of disease, thus having possible prognostic, as well as diagnostic, importance (Keller et al., 1983). In each patient, specific chromosomal numerical and structural abnormalities appear similar, even when tissue samples are taken from multiple sites, supporting the concept that cutaneous T-cell lymphomas are indeed unifocal in origin (Nowell et al., 1982).

DNA cytophotometry, a method for quantitative analysis of the DNA content of normal and neoplastic cells, when combined with cytogenetic analysis, has added greatly to our ability to differentiate more accurately between abnormal T-cell infiltrates and those normal or inflammatory in origin (Lutzner et al., 1973; van Vloten et al., 1979; Willemze et al., 1983). Overall, abnormal T cells not only are larger, except in instances where small cells predominate (small cell variant of the Sézary cell), but are much more likely to have an abnormal DNA content than are normal cells or cells from benign dermatoses. Additionally, the number of cells in cutaneous infiltrates and peripheral blood containing abnormal amounts of DNA is usually higher in lymphomas than in benign dermatoses. The DNA content of cells in lymphomatous infiltrates may not at all times be abnormal, showing considerable variation from one biopsy specimen to another. Therefore, it is imperative that data obtained from cytometrics be combined with that from other investigative studies to arrive at conclusive diagnoses.

Other light microscopic techniques that may determine the malignant nature of cellular infiltrates include flow cytometry and multiparameter laser flow microfluorometry (Bunn et al., 1979; Vonderheid et al., 1981; Willemze et al., 1983). In fact, these techniques may also be of some use in determining

prognosis. Their usefulness in both regards has yet to be tested in large numbers of patients.

Special Techniques Using Electron Microscopy. Since Flaxman and associates (1971) identified abnormal "convoluted" nuclei in cells of a number of benign dermatoses, investigators have searched for electron microscopic methods to separate more effectively the cells of normal or inflammatory infiltrates from those of the cutaneous T-cell lymphomas. Extensive studies quantitating the nuclear contour index (NCI) of cells in benign and malignant infiltrates have shown that this technique may prove important in resolving this problem (Litovita and Lutzner, 1974; Meijer et al., 1980; McNutt and Crain, 1981; McNutt et al., 1981; Willemze et al., 1983). Electron microscopic quantification of the degree of nuclear indentation plus the number of cells with increased nuclear indentations appears to offer a much more sensitive estimate of malignancy than does DNA cytophotometry. Simply defined, the nuclear contour index is a measure of the perimeter of the nuclear profile in cross-section divided by the square root of the enclosed nuclear area, or NCI = perimeter measurement/area enclosed. A perfect circle would have a nuclear contour index equal to the number 3.54. The greater the degree of convolution or nuclear indentation the greater is the nuclear contour index. It has been concluded that patients with infiltrates containing cells having a mean nuclear contour index greater than 5.0 and having 6% or more of cells with nuclear contour indices greater than 9.0 are much more likely to have or develop T-cell lymphoma (Meijer et al., 1980; McNutt et al., 1981). When the nuclear contour index is combined with absolute measurements of nuclear profile area, it becomes even more useful as a diagnostic and predictive tool (McNutt et al., 1981). In early-stage disease McNutt and associates (1981) found values derived from a nomogram, which plots the proportion of cells having a nuclear contour index of 7 or more versus the proportion of cells with nuclear areas of 30 μm^2 or more, offers the best method of differentiating mycosis fungoides from nonmycosis fungoides infiltrates. In advanced disease, due to the presence of large numbers of large monomorphous cells containing large *nonconvoluted* nuclei, the nomogram may be found to be of little or no use. In such cases routine histologic examination is helpful.

Peripheral Blood Studies. In early-stage disease, patients with cutaneous T-cell lymphomas may not show peripheral blood abnormalities. Frequently, eosinophilia is the only abnormality. Intermittent examination of peripheral blood may prove helpful in identifying the percentage of cells capable of binding to sheep red blood cells, the number of cells having large convoluted or cerebriform nuclei, and the number of cells containing eccentrically spotted granular betaglucoronidase activity. These simple examinations, if positive, can aid in diagnosing early-stage disease. Leukopenia, leukocytosis, anemia, and thrombocytopenia are late signs of disease.

Antihuman T-cell monoclonal antibodies may also be used to characterize the predominant cell type in peripheral blood. T lymphocytes have distinctive cell-surface antigens that are not found on B cells or other peripheral blood cell types. A group of monoclonal antibodies has been developed that recognizes pan-T-cell markers. Monoclonal antibodies OKT1, OKT3, and OKT11 react with antigens of variable molecular weights that are present on all peripheral blood T lymphocytes. The predominant circulating and tissue T-cells in the cutaneous T-cell lymphomas are homogeneous in their antigen phenotype and are derived from a well-differentiated helper T-cell subset reactive with the monoclonal antibodies OKT1, OKT3, LEU-3a, BE1, and BE2 (BE1 and BE2 may be more useful in early-stage disease) (Haynes *et al.,* 1981; Kung *et al.,* 1981; Berger *et al.,* 1983). Varying numbers of OKT8, LEU-2a cells (T-cytotoxic, suppressor phenotype) have also been found in peripheral blood and tissue of mycosis fungoides patients, but not in those with Sézary's syndrome (Willemze *et al.,* 1983). The number of dendritic cells expressing HLA-DR and/or OKT6 antigens (Langerhans cells) are also increased in the tissue infiltrates and peripheral blood of patients with mycosis fungoides. Loss of reactivity of T-cell antisera appears to increase with disease severity (Willemze *et al.,* 1983). Because these reagents (monoclonal antibodies) are more reliable and much easier to work with, their use may well supplant the E-rosette technique in identifying T-cell populations in peripheral blood and tissue (Janossy *et al.,* 1980; Berger and Edelson, 1982).

Lymph Node Examination. Because lymph node involvement often precedes involvement of sites other than skin, every effort should be made to obtain adequate physical and histologic examinations of this tissue. The role of lymphangiography in diagnosis is often de-

bated. It has not produced sufficient or reliable information to warrant its use routinely, and some acute and long-term morbidity is associated with this procedure. Computerized tomography (CT) is a much less cumbersome procedure, offering better resolution and detail to assess internal organ involvement, and is not associated with acute or long-term morbidity.

Lymph node biopsy should be performed whenever possible. Palpable lymph nodes draining involved sites offer the best yield. Blind node biopsy of nonpalpable nodes, especially inguinal nodes, generally does not produce valuable diagnostic data except in advanced disease. Morbidity, however, following this procedure is minimal. In addition to routine histopathologic examination of lymph nodes, a multiplicity of diagnostic procedures are available: Enzyme histochemistry, cytogenetic, morphometric, light, and electronmicroscopic, cytophotometric, microfluorometric procedures, as well as fixed or fresh tissue monoclonal antibody techniques. Lymph node involvement of any degree generally portends a poor prognosis (Epstein *et al.,* 1972; Fuks *et al.,* 1973; Cohen *et al.,* 1980).

Liver and Spleen Examination. Liver and spleen are the viscera most frequently involved in cutaneous T-cell lymphoma. Therefore, examination of these organs should offer a reasonably high yield of positive results. Liver/spleen scan should be done routinely in all patients with suspected lymphoma. The procedure inflicts little discomfort on the patient and is associated with little or no acute or long-term morbidity. In patients with visceral cutaneous T-cell lymphoma, the most frequently noted abnormality on liver/spleen scan is a change in the liver/spleen size ratio. Splenic enlargement occurs long before visible evidence of disease is noted in the liver.

Liver biopsy is the only accurate method of detecting liver disease; however, liver biopsy by the percutaneous route cannot be recommended as a routine diagnostic procedure. Liver biopsy performed blindly does not yield positive results except in patients with far advanced disease (Huberman *et al.,* 1980).

Bone marrow examination, although often recommended as a routine diagnostic study in evaluating patients with T-cell lymphoma, offers a rather poor yield except in patients with far-advanced disease and in some cases of Sézary's syndrome (Woom *et al.,* 1978). Chest x-ray, also recommended in the routine examination of patients with lymphoma, similarly yields little useful information for assessing patients with early disease. Positive radiography, when seen, is found in patients with far-advanced disease. Nonspecific findings including pulmonary nodules, infiltrates mediastinal and/or hilar adenopathy, and pleural effusion must be differentiated from drug toxicity and/or parenchymal infection (Marglin *et al.,* 1979).

Staging

All of the above diagnostic procedures may help to determine the extent of disease and the proper form of treatment as well as prognosis. In recent years several staging methods have been proposed (Lamberg and Bunn, 1979; Vonderheid, 1980) (see Tables 20–7 and 20–8), yet the oldest and simplest classification retains its usefulness. In this system the cutaneous manifestations determine the stage of disease (see Table 20–9).

The old system of classification, although simple, is a very good prognostic indicator as well as a guide to the appropriate therapy. Disease at stages I or II without evidence of internal involvement offers a better prognosis for survival than with visceral involvement or stage III in any phase. Stage III disease offers a poor prognosis whether treated or untreated. Disease at stages I and II without evidence of visceral involvement may be treated with a number of topical agents and/or physical modalities. Patients with disease at stages I or II with internal involvement and all patients with stage III disease require more aggressive treatment, topical as well as systemic. Some controversy remains relative to treating unresponsive stages I and II disease without visceral involvement using systemic agents. At our institution, we treat those patients who have failed to respond to topical therapy with systemic agents.

Specific and Supportive Management

Stage I — Without Internal Disease. The topical application of potent fluorinated corticosteroids; shortwave or ultraviolet B (290 to 320 nm) exposure; topical and systemic psoralens combined with longwave or ultraviolet A (320 to 440 nm) exposure (PUVA); topical application of mechlorethamine; or x-rays and electrons all may effect cutaneous remissions.

Topical corticosteroids and ultraviolet B (UVB) are generally not used to induce remis-

sions but to relieve pruritus and to reduce tumor load in the skin, or for temporization, while a more definitive diagnostic and therapeutic plan is being formulated.

Topical Mechlorethamine. Since it was first introduced by VanScott and Kalmanson (1973), topical mechlorethamine for treating stage I disease has gained wide acceptance. In this method dilute solutions (20 mg/dL) of mechlorethamine are prepared and applied directly to the entire cutaneous surface for eight to 24 hours on a regular basis, starting daily and continuing until cutaneous remissions are induced. Applications may be repeated at longer intervals to maintain remissions.

Adverse reactions include hyperpigmentation, cutaneous carcinogenesis (Kravitz and McDonald, 1978; Lee *et al.,* 1982), and cutaneous "sensitization." Although attempts have been made to "desensitize" patients (VanScott and Kalmanson, 1973; Constantine *et a.,* 1975), patients who experience a mild to moderate cutaneous reaction after the initial application of topical mechlorethamine obtain the best therapeutic results. Price and colleagues (1982) have described reduced sensitization using an ointment-based mechlorethamine.

The ability of mechlorethamine to effect long-term remissions and cures in cutaneous T-cell lymphomas remains unclear.

PUVA. Topical or systemic psoralens and ultraviolet A light (PUVA) have effected remissions in up to 90% of patients (Gilchrest *et al.,* 1976; Molin *et al.,* 1981). Unfortunately, a number of these patients experienced rapidly fulminating visceral disease after cutaneous remissions. Although the temporal relationship between PUVA treatment and visceral dissemination appears real, in at least one of these studies the extent of disease (staging) was not determined before initiating PUVA. Therefore, at least some patients may have had visceral involvement prior to treatment. How long-wave ultraviolet light effects the cell remains in question, but probably its effects result from inhibition of nucleic acid synthesis in abnormal lymphocytes. PUVA has been shown to be directly cytotoxic to lymphocytes *in vitro* (Cripps *et al.,* 1978). Abnormal lymphocyte function has been described following long-term PUVA therapy for psoriasis (Morrison *et al.,* 1981).

Long-term use of PUVA may result in an increased incidence of cutaneous cancer (Stern *et al.,* 1981). PUVA effects on lymphocytes may be responsible for the development of cutaneous cancers in PUVA-treated patients (Morrison *et al.,* 1981). Elderly patients treated with standard PUVA apparatus can encounter cardiovascular stress (Ciafone *et al.,* 1980).

Radiation Therapy. Both superficial x-ray and high-energy electrons offer the best treatment to date for stage I disease. Localized lesions are effectively treated by a total dose of 1500 to 2000 rads when delivered by machines rated at 80 to 140 kV. X-ray treatment is, of course, limited by the amount of body surface area that can be effectively treated without producing severe local and systemic toxicity. Extensive disease, thus, cannot be treated by this method.

Since the introduction of total skin electron beam irradiation for mycosis fungoides in 1951 (Trump *et al.,* 1953), numerous reports of its efficacy, particularly in early-stage disease, have appeared (Fromer *et al.,* 1955; Fuks and Bagshaw, 1971; Fuks *et al.,* 1973; Meyler *et al.,* 1978; Lo *et al.,* 1979). The treatment programs reported vary in many aspects, such as total dosage of electrons, amount of radiation delivered per exposure, number of exposures per treatment course or per week, and the types of disease treated.

Total disease remissions may be expected in up to 80% of patients with stage I disease confined to the skin, and the rates are greatly reduced in diseases in stages II or III. Total electron dosages delivered to the integument at depths from 0.45 to 1.2 cm using linear accelerations with energy outputs between 2.5 and 6 million electron volts have averaged 2500 to 3600 rads per treatment course. Remissions have lasted for several months to many years. Response and recurrence rates appear to be related to the extent of skin involvement, the skin depth of involvement, and the presence or absence of an erythroderma.

Complications of electron beam therapy are acute or chronic. Acute toxicity includes radiation dermatitis (macular, erythematous, scaling patches of skin accompanied by swelling, burning, and itching), hyperpigmentation, blistering, as well as hair and nail loss. Long-term or chronic effects include thinning and wrinkling of the skin, telangiectasias, dry skin, increased and reduced skin pigmentation, permanent alopecia, and cutaneous cancers. Many of the late cutaneous radiation effects of electron beam therapy have been attributed to the small amount of x-irradiation inherently emitted along with electrons. Because electrons from currently used linear accelerators penetrate no further than a few millimeters into the skin, severe systemic toxicity rarely occurs.

With limited ability to penetrate skin, electrons cannot be used as the only treatment modality in patients with disease that has spread beyond the integument. Some investigators question its use as the sole agent even in disease apparently confined to the skin, because most patients with active disease actually have systemic involvement at a very early stage (Huberman *et al.,* 1979; Bunn *et al.,* 1980b). Therefore, if attempting to cure rather than palliate, any form of topical therapy, including radiation, should be accompanied or followed by some form of systemic therapy.

Systemic Agents. Systemic treatment of cutaneous T-cell lymphomas has consisted principally of administering one or more of the many cytotoxic agents that have yielded good to moderate success in treating other lymphomas (Wright, 1964; McDonald and Calabresi, 1971; Bernadou, 1972; Leavell and DeSimone, 1975; van Vloten and Polano, 1975; Levi *et al.,* 1977; Grozea *et al.,* 1978; McDonald and Bertino, 1978; Griem *et al.,* 1979; Kufe *et al.,* 1980). In recent years systemic treatment has used transfer factor (Zacharie *et al.,* 1979), antithymocyte and antilymphocyte globulin (Barrett *et al.,* 1976; Edelson *et al.,* 1979), leukapheresis (Tan *et al.,* 1975; Safai *et al.,* 1978), and monoclonal antibodies (Miller and Levy, 1981), but all have proved of limited usefulness.

Systemic cytotoxic agents used alone have received mixed degrees of enthusiasm. Of the single agents used, methotrexate, mechlorethamine, cyclophosphamide, bleomycin, and deoxycoformycin have been found most useful. In one study, a regimen of methotrexate plus leucovorin rescue has given the most consistent and complete remissions in patients with all stages of T-cell lymphomas. Response rates with this regimen have been as good or better than those of multiple-drug regimens reported. Remissions have been induced in higher percentages of patients with little systemic toxicity. Patients have been treated continuously using methotrexate and leucovorin for up to 2½ years without adverse effects. With this intensive treatment regimen, patients are treated until remissions are induced. Patients remain on an active, agressive treatment program for as long as evidence of continuing disease response is present (McDonald and Bertino, 1978; Alper *et al.,* 1985).

Limited toxicity to date has consisted of transient leukopenia and thrombocytopenia, cutaneous vasculitis, cutaneous recall phenomenon, ulcerations at sites of active disease, and a single death from sepsis in late-stage disease.

Deoxycoformycin, an inhibitor of adenosine deaminase, has tremendous potential for treating T-cell lymphomas but has not yet achieved a satisfactory level of safety (Kufe *et al.,* 1980; Cummings *et al.,* 1980). A number of unexpected and sudden deaths were experienced in patients treated with this agent. In earlier studies the drug may have been administered in quantities too large, too frequently. As a result, adenosine deaminase activity was completely inhibited in all body tissues and severe toxicity ensued. Infections were the most frequent cause of death. A better comprehension of the pharmacology of this agent has led to revised dosages and schedules of treatment.

More than a decade ago the use of combined radiation therapy and chemotherapy in a sequential manner was discussed (McDonald, 1969). In this regimen cutaneous remissions were induced using high-energy electron beam to the entire integument (total dose between 1000 to 1500 rads). Patients were given no further treatment until disease exacerbations occurred; remissions were again induced using high-energy electrons and were maintained with systemic cytotoxic agents. This combined approach effectively maintained a state of radiation-induced remission for a much longer period than did radiation therapy or chemotherapy alone. A more recent report has essentially confirmed these findings (Bunn *et al.,* 1980a).

Arguments against the use of systemic therapy in all but terminal disease include: (1) cytotoxic drugs interfere with or destroy the individual's basic immunologic mechanisms; (2) survival rates are not increased in patients treated, and (3) the severe toxicity experienced by most individuals is not warranted in the treatment of this chronic and benign disease. Those who have treated large numbers of patients recognize the many manifestations of the cutaneous T-cell lymphomas, acknowledge the limitation of the treatment regimens, and continue to strive to develop a therapeutic plan most appropriate for the individual patient.

In summary, a rational therapeutic approach to the patient with stage I cutaneous T-cell lymphoma confined to the skin is as follows: Topical nitrogen mustard is applied daily to the entire integument for periods up to 24 hours. If a remission is induced, the period of time between applications is lengthened. Many patients can maintain a good state of remission with applications once weekly. Patients who do not respond to this regimen are either given PUVA, or preferably a course of high-energy electrons. Patients who still do not respond to this regimen are then considered candidates for systemic cytotoxic therapy. A single-agent regimen, with methotrexate as the drug of choice, is preferred at some institutions. This may change with wider use of deoxycoformycin.

Stage I disease with evidence of systemic involvement — dermatopathic lymphadenopathy, splenic enlargement, abnormal cells in peripheral blood and/or lymph nodes — is considered appropriate for systemic cytotoxic therapy. In order to induce rapid and complete remissions, patients who are not on experimental drug protocols may also be treated simultaneously with topical nitrogen mustard, high energy electrons, or PUVA.

Stage II. Stage II disease confined to the skin, a relatively rare finding after an extensive and thorough examination, may be treated as recommended for stage I disease confined to the skin. Stage II disease with systemic involvement is also treated in a manner similar to systemic stage I disease.

Stage III. Stage III disease, as well as the Sézary form of cutaneous T-cell lymphoma, is treated with systemic therapy. Topical nitrogen mustard, local injections of dilute solutions of nitrogen mustard, total body electrons, and superficial x-ray may be added to a cytotoxic drug regimen. In patients with the Sézary's variant, leukapheresis may be added to reduce the number of abnormal T cells in the peripheral blood and skin, thereby reducing greatly the host tumor burden and increasing the potential for induction of a chemotherapeutic remission.

Future Prospects

Within the past five years, neoplastic diseases of T-cell origin have become the subject of intense interest among clinicians, researchers, and the public. Recent information demonstrating that retroviruses can infect human T cells and produce either a lympho-proliferative neoplasm or the acquired immune deficiency syndrome (AIDS) has brought this area of study to the forefront of medical research. The human T-cell leukemia virus HTLV-I was first isolated from two adult patients with aggressive forms of T-cell lymphoma by Gallo in 1981. HTLV-I has been identified as a causative agent in epidemiologic studies of patients with adult T-cell lymphoma in both Japan and the Caribbean. In 1983, Gallo's laboratory reported the association between HTLV-III and AIDS. The epidemiology of these diseases and the molecular biology of the responsible viruses are now being elucidated (Ratner *et al.*, 1985; Starcich *et al.*, 1985).

Within a brief period, a family of retroviruses tropic for human T cells has been identified. It is now clear that infection of T cells of patients with the same or closely related viruses may result in either a neoplastic proliferation (leukemia or lymphoma) or T-cell suppression and AIDS. These recent exciting findings regarding the etiology of certain T-cell neoplasms suggest that these diseases may serve as models for the elucidation of the causes of other cancers.

REFERENCES

Albright, S. D.: Treatment of skin cancer using multiple modalities. *J. Am. Acad. Dermatol.,* 7:143–171, 1982.

Allen, A. C.: *The Skin: A Clinicopathological Treatise.* The C. V. Mosby Company, St. Louis, 1954.

Allen, A. C.: *The Skin: A Clinicopathological Treatise,* 2nd ed. Grune & Stratton, Inc., New York, 1967.

Alper, J. C.; Kegel, M. F.; Wiemann, M. C.; Crabtree, G. W.; McDonald, C. J.; and Calabresi, P. C., A new form of combination chemotherapy for advanced mycosis fungoides. Meeting Abstract, *Am. Acad. Dermatol.,* 1985.

Altmeyer, P., and Nodl, F.: Specific epidermal characteristics of cutaneous lymphomas. *Arch. Dermatol. Res.,* 262:113–123, 1978.

Argyris, T. S., and Sraga, T. J.: Promotion of carcinoma by repeated abrasion in irritated skin of mice. *Cancer Res.,* 41:5193–5195, 1981.

Atkinson, L.; Farago, K.; Forbes, V. R. V.; and TenSeldam, R. E. J.: Skin cancer in New Guinea native peoples. *Natl. Cancer Inst. Monogr.,* 10:167–180, 1963.

Azcarian, S. A.: *Cryosurgical Advances in Dermatology and Tumors of the Head and Neck.* Charles C Thomas, Publisher, Springfield, Illinois, 1977.

Barré-Sinoussi, F.; Chermann, J. C.; Rey, F.; Nugeyre, M. T.; Chamaret, S.; Gruest, J.; Dauguet, C.; Axler-Blin, C.; Vezinet-Brun, F.; Rouzioux, C.; Rozenbaum, W.; and Montaginer, L.: Isolation of a T-lymphotropic retrovirus from a patient at risk for acquired immune deficiency syndrome (AIDS). *Science,* 220:868–871, 1983.

Barrett, A. J.; Brigden, D.; Roberts, J. T.; Staughton,

R. C. D.; Byrom, N.; and Hobbs, J. R.: Antilymphocyte globulin in the treatment of advanced Sézary syndrome. *Lancet,* 1:940–941, 1976.

Bauer, E. A.; Gordon, J. M.; Reddick, M. E.; and Eisen, A. Z.: Quantitation and immunocytochemical localization of human skin collagenase in basal cell carcinoma. *J. Invest. Dermatol.,* 69:363–369, 1977.

Becker, B. J. P.: The histogenesis of Kaposi's sarcoma. *Acta Un. Int. Cancer,* 18:477–486, 1962.

Belisario, J. C.: *Cancer of the Skin.* Butterworths, London, 1959.

Berger, C. L., and Edelson, R.: Monoclonal antibodies. Powerful new looks for the clinician. *Arch. Dermatol.,* 118:627–629, 1982.

Berger, C. L.; Edelson, R. L.; Spittle, M. F.; and Smith, N. P.: Cutaneous T cell lymphoma — Diagnosis using monoclonal antibodies against normal and malignant T cells. *J. Invest. Dermatol.,* 80:333a, 1983.

Berman, B., and France, D. S.: Histochemical analysis of Langerhans cells. *Am. J. Dermatopathol.,* 1:215–221, 1979.

Berman, B., and Gigli, I.: Complement receptors on guinea pig epidermal Langerhans cells. *J. Immunol.,* 124:685–690, 1980.

Bernadou, A.: Bleomycin in the reticuloses. *Br. Med. J.,* 1:285–286, 1972.

Blattner, W. A.; Kalyanaraman, V. S.; Robert-Guroff, M.; Lister, T. A.; Galton, D. A. G.; Sarin, P. S.; Crawford, M. H.; Catovsky, I.; Greaves, M.; and Gallo, R. C.: The human type-C retrovirus, HTLV, in blacks from the Caribbean region, and relation to adult T-cell leukemia lymphoma. *Int. J. Cancer,* 30:257–264, 1982.

Block, J. B.; Edgecomb, J.; Eisen, A.; and van Scott, E. J.: Mycosis fungoides. Natural history and aspects of its relationship to other malignant lymphomas. *Am. J. Med.,* 34:228–235, 1963.

Blum, H. F.: *Carcinogenesis by Ultraviolet Light.* Princeton University Press, Princeton, New Jersey, 1959.

Boldogh, I.; Beth, E.; Huang, E. S., Kyalwazi, S. K.; and Giraldo, G.: Kaposi's sarcoma IV. Detection of CMV DNA, CMV RNA and CMNA in tumor biopsies. *Int. J. Cancer,* 28:469–474, 1981.

Bosman, F. T., and van Vloten, W. A.: Sézary's syndrome: A cytogenetic, cytophotometric and autoradiographic study. *J. Pathol.,* 118:49–57, 1976.

Braverman, I. M.: Kaposi's hemorrhagic sarcoma. In Braverman, I. M. (ed.): *Skin Signs of Systemic Disease.* W.B. Saunders Company, Philadelphia, 1981.

Breza, T.; Taylor, R.; and Eaglstein, W. H.: Noninflammatory destruction of actinic keratoses by 5-fluorouracil. *Arch. Dermatol.,* 112:1256–1258, 1976.

Brigham, B. A.; Bunn, P. A.; Horton, J. E.; Schechter, G. P.; Wahl, L. M.; Bradley, E. C.; Dunnick, N. R.; and Mathews, M. J.: Skeletal manifestations in cutaneous T-cell lymphomas. *Arch. Dermatol.,* 118:461–467, 1982.

Broder, S.; Edelson, R. L.; Lutzner, M. A.; Nelson, D. L.; MacDermott, R. P.; Durm, M. E.; Goldman, C. K.; Meade, B. D.; and Waldman, T. A.: The Sézary syndrome: A malignant proliferation of helper T-cells. *J. Clin. Invest.,* 58:1297–1306, 1976.

Brookes, P. (ed.): Chemical carcinogenesis. *Br. Med. Bull.,* 36:1–100, 1980.

Broome, J. D.; Zucker-Franklin, D.; Weiner, M. S.; Bianco, C.; and Nussenzweig, V.: Leukemic cells with membrane properties of thymus-derived (T) lymphocytes in a case of Sézary's syndrome: Morphologic and immunologic studies. *Clin. Immunol. Immunopathol.,* 1:319–329, 1973.

Broult, J. C.; Flandrin, F.; and Seligmann, M.: Indications of the thymus-derived nature of the proliferating cells in six patients with Sézary's syndrome. *N. Engl. J. Med.,* **289:**341–344, 1973.

Brown, S. E.; Real, F. X.; Cunningham Rundles, S.; Myslowski, P. L.; Kozinger, B.; Fein, S. M.; Helman, A.; Oeitgen, H. F.; and Safa, B.: Preliminary observations on the effect of recombinant leucocyte A interferon in homosexual men with Kaposi's sarcoma. *N. Engl. J. Med.* **308:**1071–1076, 1983.

Brun-Vézinet, F.; Rouzioux, C.; Montagnier, L.; Chamaret, S.; Gruest, J.; Barrée-Sinoussi, F.; Geroldi, D.; Chermann, J. C.; McCormick, J.; Mitchell, S.; Piot, P., Taelman, H.; Mirlangu, K. B.; Wobin, D.; Mbendi, N.; Mazebo P.; Kalambayi, K.; Bridts, C.; Desmyter, J.; Feinsod, F. M.; and Quinn, T. C.: Prevalence of antibodies to lymphadenopathy-associated retrovirus in African patients. *Science,* **226:**453–456, 1984.

Buechner, S. A., and Winkelmann, R. K.: Pre-Sézary erythroderma evolving to Sézary syndrome. A report of seven cases. *Arch. Dermatol.,* **119:**285–291, 1983.

Bunn, P. A.; Fischmann, A.; Kumar, P.; Schechter, G.; Ihde, D.; Fossieck, B.; Cohen, M.; Matthews, M.; and Minna, J.: Combined electron beam irradiation (EBRT) and systemic chemotherapy for cutaneous T-cell lymphomas (CTCL). *Proc. Am. Assoc. Cancer Res.,* **21:**464, 1980a.

Bunn, P. A.; Huberman, M. S.; Whang-Peng, J.; Schechter, G. P.; Guccion, J. G.; Matthews, M. J.; Gazdar, A. F.; Dunnick, N. R.; Fischmann, A. B.; Ihde, D. C.; Cohen, M. H.; Fossieck, B.; and Minna, J. D.: Prospective staging evaluation of patients with cutaneous T-cell lymphomas. Demonstration of a high frequency of extracutaneous dissemination. *Ann. Intern. Med.,* **93:**223–230, 1980b.

Bunn, P. A.; Schechter, G. P.; Jaffe, E.; Blayney, D.; Young, R. C.; Mathews, M. J.; Blattner, W.; Broder, S.; Robert-Guroff, M.; and Gallo, R. C.: Clinical course of retrovirus-associated adult T-cell lymphoma in the United States. *N. Engl. J. Med.,* **309:**257–264, 1983.

Bunn, P. A., Jr., and Lamberg, S. I.: Report of the Committee on Staging and Classification of Cutaneous T-Cell Lymphomas. *Cancer Treat. Rep.,* **63:**725–728, 1979.

Bunn, P. A.; Whang-Peng, J.; Knutsen, T.; and Schlam, M.: Identification of aneuploidy in patients with cutaneous T-cell lymphoma (CTCL) with flow microfluorometry (FMF) and cytogenetics (CG). *Cell Tissue Kinet.,* **12:**673, 1979.

Burbank, F.: Patterns in cancer mortality in the United States: 1950–1967. *Natl. Cancer Inst. Monogr.,* **33:** 496–504, 1971.

Burg, G., and Braun-Falco, O.: Cutaneous non-Hodgkins lymphoma: Reevaluation of histology using enzyme cytochemical and immunologic studies. *Int. J. Dermatol.,* **17:**496–505, 1978.

Burg, G.; Rodt, H.; Grosne-Wild, H.; and Braun-Falco, O.: Surface markers and mitogen response of cells harvested from cutaneous infiltrates in mycosis fungoides and Sézary's syndrome. *J. Invest. Dermatol.,* **70:**257–259, 1978.

Burke, J. S., and Colby, T. V.: Dermatopathic lymphadenopathy: Comparison of cases associated and unassociated with mycosis fungoides. *Am. J. Surg. Pathol.,* **5:**343–352, 1981.

Burns, D. A., and Calnau, C. D.: Basal cell carcinoma in a chronic leg ulcer. *Clin. Exp. Dermatol.,* **3:**443–445, 1978.

Burns, J. E.; Eisenhauer, E. D., and Jabaley, M. D.: Cellu-

lar immune deficiency in black patients with basal cell carcinoma. *J. Surg. Oncol.,* **13:**129–134, 1980.

Bustamante, R.; Schmitt, D.; Pillet, C.; and Thivolet, J.: Immunoglobulin-producing cells in the inflammatory infiltrates of cutaneous tumors: Immunocytologic identification in situ. *J. Invest. Dermatol.,* **68:**346–349, 1977.

Callen, J. P., and Headington, J.: Bowen's and non-Bowen's squamous intraepidermal neoplasia of the skin. *Arch. Dermatol.,* **116:**422–426, 1980.

Catovsky, D.; Greaves, M. F.; Rose, M.; Galton, D. A. G.; Goolden, A. W. G.; McCluskey, D. R.; White, J. M.; Lampert, I.; Bousikas, G.; Ireland, R.; Brownell, A. F.; Bridges, J. A.; Blattner, W. A.; and Gallo, R. C.: Adult T-cell lymphoma-leukemia in blacks from the West Indies. *Lancet,* **1:**639–643, 1982.

Centers for Disease Control Briefings, AIDS Task Force, January 14, 1983. Centers for Disease Control *MMRW* RETS 9, 11, 13, 19, 25.

Centers for Disease Control Briefings: Opportunistic infections and Kaposi's sarcoma among Haitians in the United States. *MMWR,* **31:**353–361, 1982.

Centers for Disease Control Briefings: *Pneumocystis* pneumonia. Los Angeles. *MMWR,* **30:**250–251, 1981.

Centers for Disease Control Briefings: Follow up on Kaposi's sarcoma and *Pneumocystis* pneumonia. *MMWR,* **30:**409–410, 1981.

Centers for Disease Control Briefings: Kaposi's sarcoma and *Pneumocystis* pneumonia among homosexual men—New York City and California. *MMWR,* **30:**305–308, 1981.

Centers for Disease Control Briefings: A cluster of Kaposi's sarcoma and *Pneumocystis carinii* pneumonia among homosexual male residents of Los Angeles and Orange Counties, California. *MMWR,* **31:**305–307, 1982.

Chu, A. C.; Kung, P.; and Edelson, R.: Dermal Langerhans cells in cutaneous lymphoma: An in situ study using monoclonal antibodies. *J. Invest. Dermatol.,* **76:**324, 1981.

Chu, A. C., and MacDonald, D. M.: Identification in situ of T-lymphocytes in the dermal and epidermal infiltrates of mycosis fungoides. *Br. J. Dermatol.,* **76:**324, 1981.

Chu, A. C.; Robinson, D.; Smith, N. P.; Spittle, M. F.; Hawk, J. L. M.; and Catovsky, D.: The Sézary cell—A morphologically distinct but nonspecific cell type. *J. Invest. Dermatol.,* **80:**332a, 1983.

Ciafone, R. A.; Rhodes, A. R.; Audley, M.; Freedberg, I. M.; and Abelmann, W. H.: The cardiovascular stress of photochemotherapy (PUVA). *J. Am. Acad. Dermatol.,* **3:**499–505, 1980.

Cleaver, J. E.: Defective repair replication of DNA in xeroderma pigmentosum. *Nature,* **218:**652–656, 1968.

Clendenning, W. E.; Brecker, G.; and van Scott, E. J.: Mycosis fungoides. Relationship to malignant and cutaneous reticulosis and the Sézary syndrome. *Arch. Dermatol.,* **89:**785–792, 1964.

Cohen, L.; Palmer, P. E. S.; and Mickson, J. J.: Treatment of Kaposi's sarcoma by radiation. In Ackerman, L. V., and Murray, J. F. (eds.): *Symposium on Kaposi's Sarcoma.* New York, Karger, 1962.

Cohen, S. R.; Stenn, K. S.; and Braverman, I. M.: Mycosis fungoides: Clinicopathologic relationships, survival and therapy in 59 patients with observations on occupation as a new prognostic factor. *Cancer,* **46:**2645–2666, 1980.

Constantine, V. S.; Fuks, Z. Y.; and Farber, E. M.: Mechlorethamine desensitization in therapy for mycosis fungoides. Topical desensitization to mechlorethamine (nitrogen mustard) contact hypersensitivity. *Arch. Dermatol.,* **111:**484–488, 1975.

Cooperrider, P. A., and Roenigk, H. H., Jr.: Selective immunological evaluation of mycosis fungoides. *Arch. Dermatol.,* **114:**207–212, 1978.

Cormia, F. E., and Domonokos, A. N.: Cutaneous reactions to internal malignancy. *Med. Clin. North Am.,* **49:**655–680, 1965.

Cottel, W. I.: Perineural invasion by squamous cell carcinoma. *J. Dermatol. Surg. Oncol.,* **8:**589–600, 1982.

Cottell, W. I., and Proper, S.: Mohs surgery, fresh tissue technique. Our technique with a review. *J. Dermatol. Surg. Oncol.,* **8:**576–587, 1982.

Cripps, D. J.; Horowitz, S.; and Hong, R.: Spectrum of ultraviolet radiation of human B and T-lymphocyte viability. *Clin. Exp. Dermatol.,* **3:**43–50, 1978.

Cummings, F. J.; Crabtree, G. W.; Spremulli, E.; Rogler-Brown, T.; Parks, R. E., Jr.; and Calabresi, P., Studies with 2'-deoxycoformycin in man and subhuman primates. *Proc. Am. Soc. Clin. Oncol.,* **21,** 332, 1980.

Daniels, F., Jr.: Ultraviolet carcinogenesis in man. *Natl. Cancer Inst. Monogr.,* **10:**407–418, 1963.

Daniels, F., Jr.; Brophy, D.; and Lobitz, W. C., Jr.: Histochemical responses of human skin following ultraviolet irradiation. *J. Invest. Dermatol.,* **37:**351–356, 1961.

Davis, B. H., and Simpkins, H.: Mycosis fungoides and Sézary syndrome: Malignant cells with T-cell enzymatic properties. *Lab. Invest.,* **40:**251, 1979.

Dayan, A., and Lewis, P. D.: Origin of Kaposi's sarcoma from the reticuloendothelial system. *Nature,* **213:**889–890, 1967.

Daynes, R. A.; Harris, C. C.; Connor, R. J.; Eichwald, E. J.: Skin cancer development in mice exposed chronically to immunosuppressive agents. *J. Natl. Cancer Inst.,* **62:**1075–1081, 1979.

Degreef, H.; Holvoet, C.; VanVloten, W. A.; Desmet, V.; and DeWolf-Peeters, C.: Woringer-Kolopp disease: An epidermotropic variant of mycosis fungoides. *Cancer,* **38:**2154–2165, 1976.

Dellon, A. L.: Host tumor relationships in basal cell and squamous cancer of the skin. *Plast. Reconstr. Surg.,* **62:**37–48, 1978.

Deneau, D. G.; Wood, G. S.; Beckstead, J.; Hoppe, R. T.; Price, N.: Woringer-Kolopp disease (pagetoid reticulosis). Four cases with histopathologic, ultrastructural, and immunohistologic observations. *Arch. Dermatol.,* **120:**1045–1051, 1984.

Diffy, B. L.; Tate, T. J.; and Davis, A.: Solar dosimetry of the face: The relationship of natural ultraviolet radiation exposure to basal cell carcinoma localization. *Phys. Med. Biol.,* **24:**931–939, 1979.

Dillaha, C. J.; Jansen, G. T.; Honeycutt, M. W.; and Holt, G. A.: Further studies with topical 5-fluorouracil. *Arch. Dermatol.,* **92:**410–417, 1965.

Domingo, J., and Helwig, E. B.: Malignant neoplasia associated with nevus sebaceous of Jadassohn. *J. Am. Acad. Dermatol.,* **1:**545–556, 1974.

Dorffel, J.: Histogenesis of multiple idiopathic hemorrhagic sarcoma of Kaposi. *Arch. Dermatol. Syph.,* **26:**608–634, 1932.

Dorn, H. F., and Cutler, S. J.: *Morbidity from Cancer in the United States.* Washington, D.C., U.S. Gov't Print Office, 1958.

Dougherty, T. J.: Photoradiation therapy for cutaneous and subcutaneous malignancies. *J. Invest. Dermatol.,* **77:**122–124, 1981.

Drew, W. L.; Mintz, L.; Miner, R. C.; Sands, M.; and Ketterer, B.: Prevalence of cytomegalovirus infection in homosexual men. *J. Infect. Dis.,* **143:**188–192, 1981.

Dutz, W., and Stout, A. P.: Kaposi's sarcoma in infants and children. *Cancer,* **13:**684–694, 1960.

DuVivier, A.; Harper, R. A.; Vonderheid, E.; and Van-Scott, E. J.: Lymphocyte transformation in patients with staged mycosis fungoides and Sézary syndrome. *Cancer,* **42:**209–213, 1978.

Eaglstein, N. F.; Hernandez, A. D.; and Allen, J. E.: Lymphocytic response to basal cell carcinoma: In situ identification of functional subsets using monoclonal antibodies. *J. Dermatol. Surg. Onc.,* **8:**943–947, 1982.

Eaglstein, W. H.; Weinstein, G. D.; and Frost, P.: Fluorouracil: Mechanism of action in human skin and actinic keratoses. *Arch. Dermatol.,* **101:**132–139, 1970.

Eastcott, D. F.: Epidemiology of skin cancer in New Zealand. *Natl. Cancer Inst. Monogr.,* **10:**141–151, 1963.

Edelson, R. L.: Cutaneous T-cell lymphoma: Mycosis fungoides, Sézary syndrome and other variants. *J. Am. Acad. Dermatol.,* **2:**89–106, 1980.

Edelson, R. L.; Brown, J. A.; Grossman, M. E.; and Hardy, M. A.: Antithymocyte globulin in the management of cutaneous T-cell lymphoma. *Cancer Treat. Rep.,* **63:**675–680, 1979.

Edelson, R. L.; Kirkpatrick, C. H.; Shevach, E. M.; Schein, P. S.; Smith, R. W.; Green, I.; and Lutzner, M.: Preferential cutaneous infiltration by neoplastic thymus-derived lymphocytes. *Ann. Intern. Med.,* **80:**685–692, 1974.

Epstein, E. H., Jr.; Levin, D. L.; Croft, J. D.; and Lutzner, M. A.: Mycosis fungoides—Survival, prognostic features, response to therapy, and autopsy findings. *Medicine,* **51:**61–72, 1972.

Epstein, J. H.: Ultraviolet carcinogenesis. In Geise, A. C. (ed.): *Photophysiology,* Vol. 5. Academic Press, Inc., New York, 1970.

Erkman-Balis, B., and Rappaport, H.: Cytogenetic studies in mycosis fungoides. *Cancer,* **34:**626–633, 1974.

Essex, M.; McLane, M. F.; Lee, T. H.; Falk, L.; Howe, C. W. S.; Mullins, J. I.; Cubradilla, C.; and Francis, P. P.: Antibodies to cell membrane antigen associated with human T-cell leukemia virus in patients with AIDS. *Science,* **220:**859–862, 1983.

Farmer, E. R., and Helwig, E. B.: Metastatic basal cell carcinoma: A clinicopathologic study of seventeen cases. *Cancer,* **46:**748–757, 1980.

Fischmann, A. B.; Bunn, P. A., Jr.; Guccion, J. G.; Matthews, M. J.; and Minna, J. D.: Exposure to chemicals, physical agents, and biological agents in mycosis fungoides and the Sézary syndrome. *Cancer Treat. Rep.,* **63:**591–592, 1979.

Flaxman, B. A.: Growth in vitro and induction of differentiation in cells of basal cell cancer. *Cancer Res.* **32:**462–469, 1972.

Flaxman, B. A.; Zalazny, G.; and VanScott, E. J.: Nonspecificity of characteristic cells in mycosis fungoides. *Arch. Dermatol.,* **104:**141–147, 1971.

Flotte, T. J.; Hatcher, V. A.; and Friedman-Kein, A. E.: Factor VIII-related antigen in Kaposi's sarcoma in young homosexual men. *Arch. Dermatol.,* **120:**180–182, 1984.

Francis, D. P.; Curran, J. W.; and Essex, M.: Epidemic acquired immune deficiency syndrome. Epidemiologic evidence for a transmissible agent. *J.N.C.I.,* **71:**1–4, 1983.

Friedman-Kein, A. E.: Disseminated Kaposi's sarcoma syndrome in young homosexual men. *J. Am. Acad. Dermatol.,* **5:**468–471, 1981.

Fromer, J. L.; Smedal, M. I.; Trump, J. G.; and Wright,

K. A.: High energy electrons for generalized superficial dermatoses. *A.M.A. Arch. Dermatol.,* **71**:391–395, 1955.

Fuks, Z. Y., and Bagshaw, M. A.: Total-skin electron treatment of mycosis fungoides. *Radiology,* **100**:145–150, 1971.

Fuks, Z. Y.; Bagshaw, M. A.; and Farber, E. M.: Prognostic signs and the management of mycosis fungoides. *Cancer,* **32**:1385–1395, 1973.

Fukuhara, S.; Rowley, J. D.; and Variakojis, D.: Banding studies of chromosomes in a patient with mycosis fungoides. *Cancer,* **42**:2262–2268, 1978.

Gallo, R.; Sarin, P. S.; Gellmann, E. P.; Robert-Guroff, M.; Richardson, E.; Kalyanaramak, V. S.; Mann, D.; Sidhu, G. D.; Stahl, R. E.; Zolla-Panzer, S.; Leibowitch, J.; and Popovic, M.: Isolation of human T-cell leukemia virus in acquired immune deficiency syndrome (AIDS). *Science,* **220**:865–867, 1983.

Gallo, R. C.; Salahuddin, S. Z.; Popovic, M.; Shearer, G. M.; Kaplan, M.; Haynes, B. F.; Palker, T. J.; Redfield, R.; Oleske, J.; Safa, B.; White, G.; Foster, P.; and Markham, P. D.: Frequent detection and isolation of cytopathic retroviruses (HTLV-III) from patients with AIDS and at risk for AIDS. *Science* **224**:500–503, 1984.

Gelmann, E. P.; Popovic, M.; Blayney, D.; Masur, H.; Sidhu, G.; Stahl, R. E.; and Gallo, R.: Proviral DNA of a retrovirus human T-cell leukemia virus in two patients with AIDS. *Science,* **220**:862–865, 1983.

Geraedts, J. P.; Pet, E. A.; and van Vloten, W. A.: Chromosome abnormalities in mycosis fungoides. *Clin. Genet.,* **17**:67, 1980.

Gerstein W.: Transplantation of basal cell epitheliomas in the rabbit. *Arch. Dermatol.,* **88**:834–836, 1963.

Gilchrest, B. A.; Parrish, J. A.; Tannenbaum, L.; Haynes, H. A.; and Fitzpatrick, T. B.: Oral methoxsalen photochemotherapy of mycosis fungoides. *Cancer,* **38**:683–689, 1976.

Giraldo, G.; Beth, E.; and Haguenau, F.: Herpes-type virus particles in tissue culture of Kaposi's sarcoma from different geographic regions. *J. Natl. Cancer. Inst.,* **49**:1509–1526, 1972.

Giraldo, G.; Beth, E.; Herle, W.; Henle, G.; Mike, Y.; Safai, B.; Huraux, J. M.; McHardy, J.; and de The, G.: Antibody patterns to herpes virus in Kaposi's sarcoma II. Serological association of American Kaposi's sarcoma with cytomegalovirus. *Int. J. Cancer,* **22**:126–131, 1978.

Giraldo, G.; Beth, E.; Kourilsky, F. M.; Henle, G.; Mike, V.; Hurauy, J. M.; Andersen, H. K.; Gharbi, M. R.; Kyalwazi, S. K.; and Puissant, A.: Antibody patterns to herpes virus in Kaposi's sarcoma: Serological association of European Kaposi's sarcoma with cytomegalovirus. *Int. J. Cancer,* **15**:839–848, 1975.

Giraldo, G.; Beth, E.; and Kyalwazi, S. K.: Etiological implications of Kaposi's sarcoma. *Antibiot. Chemother.,* **29**:12–31, 1981.

Goedert, J. J.; Neuland, C. Y.; and Wallen, W. C.: Amyl nitrate may alter T lymphocytes in homosexual men. *Lancet,* **1**:412–415, 1982.

Goldberg, H. S.: Basal cell epitheliomas developing in a localized linear epidermal nevus. *Cutus,* **25**:295–299, 1980.

Goldmeier, D.; Linch, D.; and Mellars, B. J.: Immunocompromise syndrome in homosexual men: Prevalence of possible risk factors and screening for the prodrome using an accurate white cell count. *Br. J. Vener. Dis.,* **59**:127–130, 1983.

Gorlin, R.J.; Vickers, R. A.; Keller, E.; and Williamson,

J.J.: The multiple basal cell nevus syndrome. *Cancer,* **18**:89, 1965.

Gottlieb, M. S.; Schraff, R.; Schanker, H. M.; Weisman, J. D.; Fan, P. T.; Wolf, R. A.; and Saxon, A.: *Pneumocystis carinii* pneumonia and mucosal candidiasis in previously healthy homosexual men. Evidence of a new acquired cellular immunodeficiency. *N. Engl. J. Med.,* **305**:1425–1531, 1981.

Grady, H. G.; Blum, H. F.; and Kirby-Smtih, J. S.: Pathology of tumors of the external ear in mice induced by ultraviolet radiation. *J. Natl. Cancer Inst.,* **2**:269–275, 1941.

Graham, J. H., and Helwig, E. B.: Bowen's disease and its relationship to systemic cancer. *Arch. Dermatol.,* **83**:738–758, 1961.

Graham, J. H., and Helwig, E. B.: Cutaneous precancerous conditions in man. *Natl. Cancer Inst. Monogr.,* **10**:323–333, 1963.

Green, M. H.; Dalager, N. A.; Lamberg, S. I.; Argyropoulos, C. E.; and Fraumeni, J. F., Jr.: Mycosis fungoides: Epidemiologic observations. *Cancer Treat. Rep.,* **63**:596–601, 1979.

Gregg, K., and Mansbridge, J.: Epidermal characteristics related to skin cancer susceptibility. *J. Invest. Dermatol.,* **79**:178–182, 1982.

Griem, M. L.; Tokars, R. P.; Petras, V.; Variakojis, D.; Baron, J. M.; and Griem, S. F.: Combined therapy for patients with mycosis fungoides. *Cancer Treat. Rep.,* **63**:655–657, 1979.

Groopman, J. E.; Salahuddin, S.Z.; Sarngadharan, M. G.; Markham, P. D.; Gonda, M.; Sliski, A.; and Gallo, R.C.: HTLV-III in saliva of people with AIDS-related complex and healthy homosexual men at risk for AIDS. *Science,* **226**:447–449, 1984.

Grozea, P. N.; Jones, S. E.; and McKelvey, E. M.: Combination chemotherapy for the treatment of advanced stages of mycosis fungoides. *Proc. Am. Assoc. Cancer Res.,* **19**:66, 1978.

Guarda, L. G.; Silva, E. G.; Ordones, N. G.; and Smith, J. L.: Factor VIII in Kaposi's sarcoma. *Am. J. Clin. Pathol.,* **76**:197–200, 1981.

Guarda, L. G.; Luna, M. A.; Smith, J. L.; Mansell, P. W. A.; Gyorkoy, F.; and Nora, A. N.: Acquired immune deficiency syndrome; post mortem findings. *Am. J. Clin. Pathol.,* **81**:549–557, 1984.

Haenszel, W.: Variations in skin cancer incidence within the United States. *Natl. Cancer Inst. Monogr.,* **10**:225–243, 1963.

Haim, S.; Friedman-Birnbaum, R.; Better, O. S.; and Tuma, S.: Skin complications in immunosuppressed patients: Follow up of kidney recipients. *Br. J. Dermatol.,* **89**:169–173, 1973.

Hanawalt, P. C., and Setlow, R. B.: *Molecular Mechanisms for Repair of DNA.* Parts A and B. Plenum Publishing Company, New York, 1975.

Haneke, E.; Tulusan, A. H.; and Weidner, F.: Histological features of "pagetoid reticulosis" (Woringer-Kolopp) in premycosis fungoides. *Arch. Dermatol. Res.,* **258**:265–273, 1977.

Harigaya, K.: Enzyme histochemical characteristics on non-Hodgkins lymphomas. *Acta Pathol. Jpn.,* **27**:345–358, 1977.

Hashimoto, K., and Lever, W. F.: Kaposi's sarcoma: Histochemical and electron microscope studies. *J. Invest. Dermatol.,* **43**:539–549, 1964.

Hashimoto, K.; Yamanishi, K. Y.; and Dubbous, M. K.: Electron microscopic observations of collagenolytic activity of basal cell epithelioma of the skin in vivo and in vitro. *Cancer Res.,* **32**:2561–2567, 1972.

Haynes, B. F.; Metzgar, R. S.; Minna, J. D.; and Bunn, P. A.: Phenotypic characterization of cutaneous T-cell lymphoma. Use of monoclonal antibodies to compare to other malignant T-cells. *N. Engl. J. Med.,* **304**:1319–1323, 1981.

Hazelrigg, O. E.: Basal cell carcinoma arising in a vaccination scar. *Int. J. Dermatol.* **17**:723–725, 1978.

Helwig, E. B., and Graham, J. A.: Cutaneous precancerous conditions in man. *Natl. Cancer Inst. Monogr.,* **10**:323–334, 1963.

Heenen, M.; Achten, G.; and Galand, P.: Autoradiographic analysis of cell kinetics in human normal epidermis and basal cell carcinoma. *Cancer Res.* **33**:123–127, 1973.

Heenen, M., and Galand, P.: Decreased rate of DNA-chain growth in human basal cell carcinoma. *Nature,* **285**:265–267, 1980.

Hejna, W. F.: Squamous cell carcinoma developing in the chronic draining sinuses of osteomyelitis. *Cancer,* **18**:128–132, 1965.

Hendricks, W. M.: Basal cell carcinoma arising in a chicken pox scar. *Arch. Dermatol.,* **116**:1304–1305, 1980.

Ho, D. D.; Schooley, R. D.; Rota, T. R.; Kaplan, J. C.; Flynn, T.; Salahuddin, S. Z.; Gonda, M. A.; and Hirsch, M.: HTLV-III in the semen and blood of a healthy homosexual man. *Science,* **226**:451–453, 1984.

Holden, C. A.; Stoughton, R. C. D.; Campbell, M.; and MacDonald, D. M.: Differential loss of T-lymphocyte markers in advanced cutaneous T-cell lymphoma. *J. Am. Acad. Dermatol.,* **6**:507–513, 1982.

Hoxtell, E. O.; Mandel, J. S.; Murray, S. S.; Schuman, L. M.; and Goltz, R. W.: Incidence of skin carcinoma after renal transplant. *Arch. Dermatol.,* **113**:436–438, 1977.

Huberman, M. S.; Bunn, P. A.; Matthews, M. J.; Fischmann, A. B.; Guccion, J.; Dunnick, R.; Ihde, D.; Cohen, M.; and Minna, J.: Extracutaneous involvement in patients with cutaneous T-cell lymphomas (CTCL): Mycosis fungoides and Sézary syndrome. *Proc. Am. Assoc. Cancer Res.,* **20**:410, 1979.

Huberman, M. S.; Bunn, P. A., Jr.; Matthews, M. J.; Ihde, D. C.; Gasdar, A. F.; Cohen, M. H.; and Minna, J. D.: Hepatic involvement in the cutaneous T-cell lymphomas. Results of percutaneous biopsy and peritoneoscopy. *Cancer,* **45**:1683–1688, 1980.

Hueper, W. C.: The skin as an assay system for potential carcinogens. *Natl. Cancer Inst. Monogr.,* **10**:577–610, 1963.

Hutt, M. S. R.: Pathology of Kaposi's sarcoma. *Antibiot. Chemother.,* **29**:32–37, 1981.

Hyde, J. N.: On the influence of light in the production of cancer of the skin. *Am. J. Med. Sci.,* **131**:1–22, 1906.

Hymes, K. B.; Cheung, T.; Greene, J. B.; Prose, N. S.; Marcus, A.; Ballard, H.; William, D. C.; and Laubenstein, L. J.: Kaposi's sarcoma in homosexual men—a report of eight cases. *Lancet,* **2**:598–600, 1981.

Ilie, B.; Brenner, S.; Lipitz, R.; and Krakowski, A.: Kaposi's sarcoma after steroid therapy for pemphigus foliaceus. Case report and short review of literature. *Dermatologica,* **163**:455–459, 1981.

Iverson, O. H.: Kinetics of cellular proliferation and cell loss in human carcinoma. A discussion of methods available for in vivo studies. *Eur. J. Cancer,* **3**:389–394, 1967.

Jablonska, S.; Dabroski, J.; and Jakubowicz, K.: Epidermodysplasia verruciformis as a model in studies on the role of papovaviruses in oncogenesis. *Cancer Res.,* **32**:583–589, 1972.

Jaffee, E. A.: Endothelial cells and the biology of factor VIII. *N. Engl. J. Med.,* **296**:377–383, 1977.

Janossy, G.; Tidman, N.; Papageorgiou, E. S.; Kung, P. C.; and Goldstein, G.: Distribution of T-lymphocyte subsets in the human bone marrow and thymus: An analysis with monoclonal antibodies. *J. Immunol.,* **126**:1608–1613, 1980.

Jay, K., and Young, A.: *The Gay Report.* Summit Books, Inc., New York, 1979.

Kalyanaraman, V. S.; Sarngadharan, M. G.; Nakao, T.; Ito, Y.; Aoki, T.; and Gallo, R. C.: Natural antibodies to the structural core protein (p24) of the human T-cell leukemia (lymphoma) retrovirus found in sera of leukemia patients in Japan. *Proc. Natl. Acad. Sci. USA,* **79**:1653–1657, 1982.

Kaposi, M.: Idiopathisches multiples Pigmentsarkom der Haut. *Arch. Derm. Syph.,* **4**:265–273, 1872.

Katz, A. D.: The frequency and risk of metastases in squamous cell carcinoma of the skin. *Cancer,* **10**:1162–1166, 1957.

Keller, R. H.; Swartz, S.; Lyons, M.; Troy, J.; and Jordan, R. E.: Peripheral blood involvement in skin limited T-cell malignancy. *J. Invest. Dermatol.,* **80**:334a, 1983.

Kimura, S.: Bowenoid papulosis of the genitalia. *Int. J. Dermatol.,* **21**:432–436, 1982.

Klein, E.; Milgrom, H.; Helm, F.; Ambrus, J.; Traenkel, H. L.; and Stoll, H. S.: Tumors of the skin: Effect of local use of cytostatic agents. *Skin,* **1**:81–87, 1962.

Kleinberg, C.; Penetrante, R.; Milgrom, H.; Pickren, J. N.: Metastatic basal cell carcinoma of the skin. *J. Am. Acad. Dermatol.,* **7**:655–659, 1982.

Kord, J. P.; Cottel, W. I.; and Proper, S.: Metastatic basal cell carcinoma. *J. Dermatol. Surg. Oncol.,* **8**:604–608, 1982.

Koziner, B.; Denny, T.; Myskowski, P. L.; Kris, M.; and Safai, B.: Letter to the Editor. *New Engl. J. Med.,* **306**:933–934, 1982.

Kravitz, P., and McDonald, C. J.: Topical nitrogen mustard induced carcinogenesis. *Acta Derm. Venereol. (Stockh.),* **58**:421–425, 1978.

Kripke, M. L.: The role of UVR-induced immunosuppression in experimental photocarcinogenesis. In Epstein, Jr., E. (ed.): *Progress in Dermatology,* Vol. 16. Evanston, Illinois, Dermatology Foundation, 1982.

Kubilus, J.; Baden, H. P.; and McGilvray, N.: Filamentation protein of basal cell epithelioma: Characteristics in vivo and in vitro. *J.N.C.I.,* **65**:869–875, 1980.

Kufe, D.; Major, P.; Agarwal, R.; Reinherz, E.; and Frei, E., III.: Phase-I–Phase-II trial of deoxycoformycin (DCFP) in T-cell malignancies. *Proc. Am. Assoc. Cancer Res.,* **21**:328, 1980.

Kung, P. C.; Burger, C. L.; Estabrook, A.; and Edelson, R. L.: Monoclonal antibodies for clinical investigation on human T lymphocytes. *Int. J. Dermatol.,* **22**:67–74, 1983.

Kung, P. C.; Burger, C. L.; Goldstein, G.; LoGerfo, P.; and Edelson, R. L.: Cutaneous T-cell lymphoma: Characterization by monoclonal antibodies. *Blood,* **57**:261–266, 1981.

Lamberg, S. I., and Bunn, P. A.: Cutaneous T-cell lymphomas. Summary of the Mycosis Fungoides Cooperative Group—National Cancer Institute Workshop. *Arch. Dermatol.,* **115**:1103–1105, 1979.

Lambert, W. C., and Everett, M. A.: The nosology of parapsoriasis. *J. Am. Acad. Dermatol.,* **5**:373–395, 1981.

Lang, D. J., and Kummer, J.F.: Cytomegalovirus in semen: Observations in selected populations. *J. Infect. Dis.,* **132**:472–473, 1975.

Laubenstein, L. J.; Krigel, R. L.; Odajnyk, C. M.; Hymes,

K. B.; Friedman-Kien, A.; Wernz, J. C.; and Muggia, F. M.: Treatment of epidemic Kaposi's sarcoma with etoposide or a combination of doxorubicin, bleomycin, and vinblastine. *J. Clin. Oncol.,* **2:**1115–1120, 1984.

Leavell, U. W., and DeSimone, P.: Combination chemotherapy (COP) in treatment of mycosis fungoides: Report of four cases. *Arch. Dermatol.,* **111:**796, 1975.

Lee, L. A.; Fritz, K. A.; Golitz, L.; Fritz, T. J.; and Weston, W. L.: Second cutaneous malignancies in patients with mycosis fungoides treated with topical nitrogen mustard. *J. Am. Acad. Dermatol.,* **7:**590–598, 1982.

Lee, T. H.; Coligan, J. E.; Sodroski, J. G.; Haseltine, W. A.; Salahuddin, S. Z.; Wong-Staal, F.; Gallo, R. C.; and Essex, M.: Antigens encoded by the 3'-terminal region of human T-cell leukemia virus: Evidence for a functional gene. *Science,* **226:** 57–61, 1984.

Lever, W. F., and Schaumberg-Lever, G.: *Histopathology of the Skin,* 6th ed. J. B. Lippincott Company, Philadelphia, 1983.

Levi, J. A.; Diggs, C. H.; and Wiernik, P. H.: Adriamycin therapy in advanced mycosis fungoides. *Cancer,* **39:**1967–1970, 1977.

Litovita, T. L., and Lutzner, M. A.: Quantitative measurements of blood lymphocytes from patients with chronic lymphocytic leukemia and the Sézary syndrome. *J.N.C.I.,* **53:**75–77, 1974.

Lo, T. C.; Salzman, F. A.; Moschella, S. L.; Tolman, E. L.; and Wright, K. A.: Whole body surface electron irradiation in the treatment of mycosis fungoides. An evaluation of 200 patients. *Radiology,* **130:**453–457, 1979.

Lord, E. M.; Sensabaugh, G. F.; and Stites, D. P.: Immunosuppressive activity of human seminal plasma. I. Inhibition of in vitro lymphocyte activation. *J. Immunol.,* **118:**1704–1711, 1977.

Lowe, N. J.; Cripps, D. J.; Dufton, P. A.; and Vickers, C. F.: Photochemotherapy for mycosis fungoides. *Arch. Dermatol.,* **115:**50–53, 1979.

Lund, H. Z.: How often does squamous cell carcinoma of the skin metastasize? *Arch. Dermatol.,* **92:**635–637, 1965.

Lutzner, M. A.; Emerit, I.; Durepaire, R.; Flandrin, G.; Grupper, C. H.; and Prunieras, M.: Cytogenetic cytophotometric and ultrastructural study of large cerebriform cells of the Sézary syndrome and description of a small cell variant. *J.N.C.I.,* **50:**1145–1162, 1973.

Lutzner, M.; Hobbs, J.; and Horvath, P.: Ultrastructure of abnormal cells in Sézary syndrome, mycosis fungoides and parapsoriasis en plaque. *Arch. Dermatol.,* **103:**375–386, 1971.

McAnally, A. K., and Dockerty, M. S.: Carcinoma developing in chronic draining cutaneous sinuses and fistulas. *Surg. Gynecol. Obstet.,* **88:**87–96, 1949.

McDonald, C. J.: Mycosis fungoides: A malignant cutaneous lymphoma. *Conn. Med.,* **33:**37–41, 1969.

McDonald, C. J., and Bertino, J. R.: Treatment of mycosis fungoides lymphoma. Effectiveness of infusions of methotrexate followed by oral citrovorum factor. *Cancer Treat. Rep.,* **62:**1009–1014, 1978.

McDonald, C. J., and Calabresi, P.: Azaribine for mycosis fungoides. *Arch. Dermatol.,* **103:**158–167, 1971.

Mackee, G. M., and Cipollaro, A. C.: Idiopathic multiple hemorrhagic sarcoma (Kaposi). *Am. J. Cancer,* **26:**1, 1936.

McMillan, E.; Wasik, R.; and Everett, M. A.: In situ demonstration of OKT6-positive cells in cutaneous lymphoid infiltrates. *J. Am. Acad. Dermatol.,* **5:**274–279, 1981.

McNutt, N. S.: Ultrastructural comparison of the interface between epithelium and stroma in basal cell carcinoma

and control human skin. *Lab. Invest.,* **35:**132–142, 1976.

McNutt, N. S., and Crain, W. R.: Quantitative electron-microscopic comparison of lymphocyte nuclear contours in mycosis fungoides and in benign infiltrates in skin. *Cancer,* **47:**698–709, 1981.

McNutt, N. S.; Heilbron, D. C.; and Crain, W. R.: Mycosis fungoides: Diagnostic criteria based on quantitative electron microscopy. *Lab. Invest.,* **44:**466–474, 1981.

Manzari, V.; Wong-Staal, F.; Franchini, G.; Colombini, E. P.; Gelmann, S.; Oroszlaw, S.; Staal, R.; and Gallo, R. L.: Human T-cell leukemia/lymphoma virus (HTLV) cloning of an integrated defective provirus and flanking cellular sequences. *Proc. Natl. Acad. Sci. USA,* **80:**1574–1578, 1983.

Marglin, S. I.; Soulen, R. L.; Blank, N.; and Castellino, R. A.: Mycosis fungoides. Radiographic manifestations of extracutaneous intrathoracic involvement. *Radiology,* **130:**35–37, 1979.

Marmor, M.; Friedman-Kein, A. E.; Laubenstein, L.; Byrum, R. D.; William, D. C.; D'Onofrio, S.; and Dubin, N.: Risk factors for Kaposi's sarcoma in homosexual men. *Lancet,* **1:**1083–1087, 1982.

Masters, S. P.; Taylor, J. F.; Kyalwazi, S. K.; and Ziegler, J. L.: Immunological studies in Kaposi's sarcoma in Uganda. *Br. Med. J.,* **1:**600–602, 1970.

Matsuoka, L. Y.; Shaver, P. K.; and Sordillo, P. P.: Basal cell carcinoma in black patients. *J. Am. Acad. Dermatol.,* **4:**670–672, 1981.

Maurice, P. D.; Smith, N. P.; and Pincking, A. J.: Kaposi's sarcoma with a benign course in a homosexual. *Lancet,* **1:**571, 1982.

Mehta, V. R.: Basal cell epithelioma in a junctional nevus. A case report with ulceration and comedinous changes. *Indian J. Med. Sci.,* **34:**8–10, 1980.

Meijer, C. J.; van der Loo, E. M.; van Vloten, W. A.; van der Velde, E. A.; Scheffer, E.; and Cornelisse, C. J.: Early diagnosis of mycosis fungoides and Sézary's syndrome by morphometric analysis of lymphoid cells in the skin. *Cancer,* **45:**2864–2871, 1980.

Meyer, C. J.; vanLeeuwen, A. W.; van der Loo, E. M.; van de Putte, L. B.; and van Vloten, W. A.: Cerebriform (Sézary-like) mononuclear cells in healthy individuals: A morphologically distinct population of T-cells: Relationship with mycosis fungoides and Sézary's syndrome. *Virchows Arch. [Cell Pathol.],* **25:**95–104, 1977.

Meyler, T. S.; Blumberg, A. L.; and Purser, P.: Total skin electron beam therapy with hydridoma monoclonal antibody. *Cancer,* **42:**1171–1176, 1978.

Meyskens, F. L.: Studies of retinoids in the prevention and treatment of cancer. *J. Am. Acad. Dermatol.,* 6 (Part 2 Suppl.):824–827, 1982.

Miki, Y.; Kawatsu, T.; Matsuda, K.; Machino, H.; and Kubo, K.: Cutaneous and pulmonary cancers associated with Bowens disease. *J. Am. Acad. Dermatol.,* **6:**26–31, 1982.

Miller, R. A., and Levy, R.: Response of cutaneous T-cell lymphoma to therapy with hybridoma monoclonal antibody. *Lancet,* **2:**226–230, 1981.

Miller, R. A., and Spittle, M. F.: Electron beam therapy for difficult cutaneous basal and squamous cell carcinoma. *Br. J. Dermatol.,* **106:**429–435, 1982.

Mitrani, E.: Possible role of connective tissue in basal cell neoplasia. *Br. J. Dermatol.,* **99:**233–244, 1978.

Miyaji, T.: Skin cancer in Japan: A nationwide five year survey, 1956–1960. *Natl. Cancer Inst. Monogr.,* **10:**55–70, 1963.

Miyoshi, I.; Kubonishi, I.; Yoshimoto, S.; Akasi, T.; Ohtsuli, Y.; Shiraiski, Y.; Nagata, K.; and Hinuma, Y.:

Type C virus particles in a cord T-cell line derived by co-cultivating normal human cord leucocytes and human leukaemic T-cells. *Nature,* **294:**770–771, 1981.

Mohs, F. E.: *Chemosurgery: Microscopically Controlled Surgery for Skin Cancer.* Charles C Thomas, Publisher, Springfield, Illinois, 1978.

Molin, L.; Thomsen, K.; Volden, G.; and Groth, O.: Photochemotherapy (PUVA) in the tumor stage of mycosis fungoides: A report from the Scandinavian mycosis fungoides study group. *Acta Derm. Venereol.,* **61:**52–54, 1981.

Montandon, D.; Koche, O.; and Gabliani, G.: Cancer invasiveness: Immunofluorescent and ultrastructural methods of assessment. *Plast. Reconstr. Surg.,* **69:**365–371, 1982.

Montgomery, H., and Dorffel, J.: Verruca senilis and keratoma senile. *Arch. Dermatol.,* **116:**286–296, 1932.

Mora, R. G., and Burris, R.: Cancer of the skin in blacks: A review of 128 patients with basal cell carcinoma. *Cancer,* **47:**1436–1438, 1981.

Mora, R. G., and Perniciaro, C.: Cancer of the skin in Blacks: I. Review of 163 black patients with cutaneous squamous cell carcinoma. *J. Am. Acad. Dermatol.,* **5:**535–543, 1981.

Mora, R. G.; Perniciaro, C.; and Lee, B.: Cancer of the skin in blacks III. A review of 19 black patients with Bowen's disease. *J. Am. Acad. Dermatol.,* **11:**557–562, 1984.

Morahan, P. S.; Klykken, D. C.; Smith, S. A.; and Munson, A. E.: Effects of cannaboids on host resistance to listeria monocytogenes and herpes simplex virus. *Infect. Immun.,* **23:**674–678, 1979.

Moran, E. M.; Ealther, J. R.; Aronson, I. K.; and Variakojis, D.: Clinical significance of circulating Sézary cells in mycosis fungoides. Proc. Am. Soc. Clin. Oncol., **18:**276, 1977.

Morrison, W. L.; Parrish, J. A.; Moscicki, R.; and Block, K. J.: Abnormal lymphocyte function following long-term PUVA therapy for psoriasis. *Clin. Res.,* **29:**608a, 1981.

Morrtel, C. G., and Hagedorn, A. B.: Leukemia or lymphoma and coexisting primary malignant lesions. A review of the literature and a study of 120 cases. *Blood,* **12:**788, 1957.

Mottaz, J. H., and Zelickson, A. S.: Electron microscopic observations of Kaposi's sarcoma. *Acta Derm. Venereol* (Stockh.), **46:**195–200, 1966.

Mulay, D. M.: Skin cancer in India. *Natl. Cancer Inst. Monogr.,* **10:**215–223, 1963.

Myskowski, P. L.; Safai, B.; and Good, R. A.: Decreased lymphocyte blastogenic responses in patients with multiple basal cell carcinoma. *J. Am. Acad. Dermatol.,* **4:**711–714, 1981.

Nadji, M.; Morales, A. R.; Ziegles-Weissman, J.; and Pennys, N. S.: Kaposi's sarcoma: Immunohistologic evidence for an endothelial origin. *Arch. Pathol. Lab. Med.,* **105:**274–275, 1981.

Nahas, G. G.; Suciu-Foca, N.; Armand, J. P.; and Morishima, A.: Inhibition of cellular mediated immunity in marijuana smokers. *Science,* **183:**419–420, 1974.

Neubauer, O.: Arsenic cancer: A review. *Br. J. Cancer,* **1:**192–251, 1947.

Nisce, L. Z.; Safai, B.; and Kim, J. H.: Electron beam therapy for mycosis fungoides. *J. Dermatol. Surg.,* **4:**594–599, 1978.

Nisce, L. Z.; Safai, B.; and Poussin-Rosillo, H.: Once weekly total and subtotal skin electron beam therapy for Kaposi's sarcoma. *Cancer,* **47:**640–644, 1981.

Nowell, P. C.; Finan, J. B.; and Vonderheid, E. C.: Clonal

characteristics of cutaneous T-cell lymphomas: Cytogenetic evidence from blood, lymph nodes, and skin. *J. Invest. Dermatol.,* **78:**69–75, 1982.

O'Brien, P. H., and Brasfield, R. D.: Kaposi's sarcoma. *Cancer,* **19:**1497–1502, 1966.

O'Dell, B. L.; Jessen, R. T.; Becker, L. E.; Jackson, R. T.; and Smith, E. B.: Diminished immune response in sun-damaged skin. *Arch. Dermatol.,* **116:**559–561, 1980.

Oettle, A. G.: Geographical and racial differences in the frequency of Kaposi's sarcoma as evidence of environmental or genetic causes. *Acta Un. Int. Cancer,* **18:**330–363, 1962.

Oettle, A. G.: Skin cancer in Africa. *Natl. Cancer Inst. Monogr.,* **10:**197–214, 1963.

Olweny, C. L. M.: Management of Kaposi's sarcoma: Chemotherapy II. *Antibiot. Chemother.,* **29:**88–95, 1981.

Olweny, C. L. M.; Toya, T.; Katongole-Mbidde, E.; Lwanga, S. K.; Owor, R.; Kyalwazi, S.; and Vogel, C. B.: Treatment of Kaposi's sarcoma by combination of actinomycin-D, vincristine and imidazole carboxamide (NSC-45388): Results of a randomized clinical trial. *Int. J. Cancer,* **14:**649–656, 1974.

Oncology Overview: Selected abstracts on the diagnosis and treatment of mycosis fungoides. U.S. Department of Health and Human Services. July, 1981.

Orbaneja, J. G.; Diez, L. I.; Lozano, J. L. S.; and Salazar, L. C.: Lymphomatoid contact dermatitis. A syndrome produced by epicutaneous hypersensitivity with clinical features and a histopathologic picture similar to that of mycosis fungoides. *Contact Dermatitis,* **2:**139–143, 1976.

Owens, D., and Donald, W.: *The Influence of Heat, Wind, and Humidity on UV Injury. (Abstr.) International Conference on Ultraviolet Carcinogenesis.* National Cancer Institute, Bethesda, Maryland, 1977.

Padovan, I.; Brodarec, I.; Ikic, D.; Knezevic, M.; and Soos, E.: Effect of interferon in therapy of skin and head and neck tumors. *J. Cancer Res. Clin. Oncol.,* **100:**295–310, 1981.

Pagano, J. S.: Diseases and mechanisms of persistant DNA virus infection: Latency and cellular transformation. *J. Infect. Dis.,* **132:**209–223, 1975.

Painter, R. R., and Cleaver, J. E.: Repair replication, unscheduled DNA synthesis, and the repair of mammalian DNA. *Radiat. Res.,* **37:**451–466, 1969.

Pathak, M. A.: Sunscreens: Topical and systemic approaches for protection of human skin against harmful effects of solar radiation. *J. Am. Acad. Dermatol.* **7:**285–312, 1982.

Pawlowski, A., and Haberman, H. F.: Heterotransplantation of human basal cell carcinoma in "nude" mice. *J. Invest. Dermatol.,* **72:**310–313, 1979.

Pedersen, E., and Magnus, K.: *Cancer Registration in Norway. The Incidence of Cancer in Norway, 1953–1954.* The Norwegian Cancer Society, Oslo, 1959.

Penn, I.: The incidence of malignancies in transplant recipients. *Transplant Proc.,* **7:**323–326, 1975.

Penn, I.: Immunosuppression and skin cancer. *Clin. Plast. Surg.* **7:**361–368, 1980.

Phillips, C.: The relationship between skin cancer and occupation in Texas: A review of 1569 verified lesions occurring in 1190 patients. *Texas State J. Med.,* **36:**613–616, 1941.

Pinching, A. J.; McManus, T. J.; Jeffries, D. J.; Moshrael, D.; Donachy, M.; Parkin, J. M.; Munday, P. E.; and Harris, L. R. W.: Studies on cellular immunity in male homosexuals in London. *Lancet* **ii:**126–130, 1983.

Pinkus, H.: Alopecia mucinosa. *A.M.A. Arch. Dermatol.,* **76:**419–424, 1957.

Pinkus, H.: Premalignant fibroepithelial tumors of skin. *Arch Dermatol. Syph.,* **67:**598–615, 1953.

Pirchenik, A. E.; Fischl, M. A.; Dickinson, G. M.; Becker, D. M.; Fournier, A. M.; O'Connell, M. T.; Colton, R. M.; and Spira, J. J.: Opportunistic infections and Kaposi's sarcoma among Haitians: Evidence of a new acquired immunodeficiency state. *Ann. Intern. Med.,* **98:**277–284, 1983.

Poiesz, B. J.; Ruscetti, F. W.; Gazdur, A. F.; Bunn, P. A.; Minna, J. D.; and Gallo, R. C.: Detection and isolation of Type C retrovirus particles from fresh and cultured lymphocytes of a patient with cutaneous T-cell lymphoma. *Proc. Natl. Acad. Sci. USA,* **77:**7415–7419, 1980.

Poiesz, B. J.; Ruscetti, F. W.; Reitz, M. S.; Kalyanaraman, V. S.; and Gallo, R. C.: Isolation of a new type C retrovirus (HTLV) in primary uncultured cells of a patient with Sézary T-cell leukemia. *Nature,* **294:**268–271, 1981.

Pollack, S. V.; Goslen, J. B.; Sherertz, E. F.; and Jegasothy, B. V.: The biology of basal cell carcinoma: A review. *J. Am. Acad. Dermatol.,* **7:**569–577, 1982.

Pott, P.: Chirurgical observations relative to the cataract, the palypus of the nose, the cancer of the scrotum, the different kinds of rupture and the mortification of the toes and feet. London, Hawes, Clarke and Collins, 1775.

Poulsen, A.; Hultberg, B.; Thomsen, K.; and Wantzin, G. L.; Regression of Kaposi's sarcoma in AIDS after treatment with dapsone. Lancet, **i:**560, 1984.

Price, N. M.; Deneau, D. G.; and Hope, R. I.: The treatment of mycosis fungoides with ointment based mechlorethamine. *Arch. Dermatol.,* **118:**234–237, 1982.

Price, N. M.: Radiation dermatitis following electron beam therapy. *Arch. Dermatol.,* **114:**63–66, 1978.

Pringgoutomo, S., and Pringgoutomo S.: Skin cancer in Indonesia. *Natl. Cancer Inst. Monogr.,* **10:**191–195, 1963.

Prunierais, M.: Ultrastructure of the epidermis in epidermodysplasia verruciformis (EV). In Prunierais, M. (ed.): *Biomedical Aspects of Human Wart Virus Infection.* Merieux Foundation, Lyon, France, 1976.

Rachelefski, G. S.; Opelz, G.; Mickey, M. R.; Lessin, P.; Kiuchi, M.; Silverstein, M. J.; and Stieber, E. R.: Intact humoral and cell-mediated immunity in chronic marijuana smoking. *J. Allergy Clin. Immunol.,* **58:**483–490, 1976.

Raffle, E. J.; Macleod, T. M.; and Hutchinson, F.: Cell mediated immune response to basal cell carcinoma. *Acta Derm. Venerol.* (Stockh.), **61:**66–68, 1980.

Rappaport, H., and Thomas, L. B.: Mycosis fungoides: The pathology of extracutaneous involvement. *Cancer,* **34:**1198–1229, 1974.

Ratner, L.; Haseltine, W.; Patarca, R.; Livak, K. J.; Starcich, B.; Josephs, S. F.; Doran, E. R.; Rafalski, J. A.; Whitehorn, E. A.; Baumeister, K.; Ivanoff, L.; Petteway, S. R.; Pearson, M. L.; Lautenberger, J. A.; Papas, T. S.; Ghrayeb, J.; Chang, N. T.; Gallo, R. C.; and Staal, F. W.: Complete nucleotide sequence of the AIDS virus, HTLV-III. *Nature,* **313:**277–284, 1985.

Reitz, M. S.: Characterization and distribution of nucleic acid sequences of a novel retrovirus isolated from human neoplastic T lymphocytes. *Proc. Natl. Acad. Sci. USA,* **78:**1887–1891, 1981.

Report of the Center for Disease Control Task Force on Kaposi's sarcoma and Opportunistic Infections. Epidemiologic aspects of the current outbreak of Kaposi's sarcoma and opportunistic infections. *New Engl. J. Med.,* **306:**248–252, 1982.

Reynolds, W. A.; Winkelman, R. K.; and Soule, E. H.: Kaposi's sarcoma: A clinicopathologic study with particular reference to its relationship to the reticuloendothelial system. *Medicine,* **44:**419–443, 1965.

Rhodes, N. D.; McEntire, J. E.; Lopez, M.; Perez-Mesa C.; Gay, C.; Decker, M.; Kaltenbach, M. L.; and Papermaster, B. W.: Basal cell carcinomas: Treatment with intralesional injection of lymphokine fraction. *Missouri Med.,* **78:**737–739, 1981.

Richards, J. M.; Bedford, J. M.; and Witkin, S. S.: Rectal insemination modifies immune responses in rabbits. *Science,* **224:**390–392, 1984.

Rinaldo, C. R., Jr.; Carney, W. P.; Richter, B. S.; Black, P. H.; Hirsch, M. S.: Mechanisms of immunosuppression in cytomegaloviral mononucleosis. *J. Infect. Dis.,* **141:**488–495, 1980.

Ringertz, N.; Sjostrom, A.; Ericsson, J.; and Olinder, B.: *Cancer Incidence in Sweden 1958.* The Swedish Cancer Registry National Board of Health, Stockholm, 1960.

Robert-Guroff, M.; Nakas, Y.; Notake, K.; Ito, Y.; Sliski, A.; and Gallo, R. C.: Natural antibodies to human retrovirus HTLV in a cluster of Japanese patients with adult T-cell leukemia. *Science,* **215:**975–978, 1982.

Roberts, J. J.: Cellular responses to carcinogen-induced DNA damage and its repair. *Br. Med. Bull.,* **36:**25–31, 1980.

Roenigk, H. H., Jr.: Photochemotherapy for mycosis fungoides. *Arch. Dermatol.,* **113:**1047–1051, 1977.

Rogoff, M. G.: Kaposi's sarcoma: Age, sex, and tribal incidence in Kenya. In Clifford, P.; Linsell, C. A.; and Timms, G. L. (eds.): *Cancer in Africa. East African Medical Journal,* Nairobi, 1968.

Rosas-Uribe, A.; Variakojis, D.; Molnar, Z.; and Rappaport, H.: Mycosis fungoides: An ultrastructural study. *Cancer,* **34:**643–645, 1974.

Rowden, G., and Lewis, M. G.: Langerhans cells: Involvement in the pathogenesis of mycosis fungoides. *Br. J. Dermatol.,* **95:**665–672, 1976.

Safai, B., and Good, R. A.: Basal cell carcinoma with metastasis: Review of literature. *Arch. Pathol. Lab. Med.,* **101:**327–331, 1977.

Safai, B.; Mike, V.; Giraldo, G.; Betu, E.; and Good, R. A.: Association of Kaposi's sarcoma with secondary primary malignancies: Possible etiopathogenic implications. *Cancer,* **45:**1472–1479, 1980.

Safai, B.; Reich, L.; and Good, R. A.: Failure of lymphophoresis in the treatment of Sézary syndrome (SS) and mycosis fungoides (MF). *Clin. Res.,* **26:**57a, 1978.

Salahuddin, S. Z.; Markham, P. D.; Lindner, S. G.; Gootenberg, J.; Popovic, M.; Hemmi, H.; Sarin, P. S.; and Gallo, R. C.: Lymphokine production by cultured human T-cells transformed by human T-cell leukemialymphoma virus-I. *Science* **223:**703–707, 1984.

Sarngadharan, M. G.; Popovic, M.; Bruch, L.; Schüpbach, J.; and Gallo, R. C.: Antibodies reactive with human T-lymphotropic retroviruses (HTLV-III) in the serum of patients with AIDS. *Science,* **224:**506–508, 1984.

Scalabrino, G.; Pigatto, P.; Ferioli, M. E.; Modena, D.; Puerari, M.; and Carú, A.: Levels of activity of the polyamine biosynthetic decarboxylases as indicators of degree of malignancy of human cutaneous epitheliomas. *J. Invest. Dermatol.,* **74:**122–124, 1980.

Schein, P. S.; MacDonald, J. S.; and Edelson, R. L.: Cutaneous T-cell lymphoma. *Cancer,* **38:**1859–1861, 1976.

Schupbach, J.; Kalyanaraman, V. S.; Sarngadharan, M. G.; Blattner, W. A.; and Gallo, R. C.: Antibodies against three purified proteins of the human Type-C retrovirus, Human T-cell leukemia/lymphoma patients and healthy blacks from the Caribbean. *Cancer Res.,* **43:**886–891, 1983.

Sézary, A.: Une nouvelle reticulose cutanee. *Ann. Dermatol. Syph. VII,* **9:**5–22, 1949.

Sézary, A., and Bouvrain, Y.: Erythrodermie avec presence de cellules monstreuses dan terme et dans sang circulat. *Bull. Soc. Fr. Dermatol. Syphilig.,* **45:**254–260, 1938.

Shanmugaratnam, K., and LaBrooy, E. B.: Skin cancer in Singapore. *Natl. Cancer Inst. Monogr.,* **10:**127–140, 1963.

Sheretz, E. F.; Pollack, S. U.; and Jegasothy, V. B.: Correlation of basal cell aggressiveness with inhibition of host lymphocyte response. *Clin. Res.,* **30:**266A, 1982.

Silberberg, I.: Ultrastructural studies of Langerhans cells in contact sensitivity and primary irritant reactions to mercuric chloride. *Clin. Res.,* **19:**715, 1971.

Silberberg-Sinakin, I.; Baer, R. L.; and Thorbecke, G. J.: Langerhans cells. A review of their nature with emphasis on their immunologic functions. *Prog. Allergy,* **24:**268–294, 1978.

Sims, P.: Metabolic activation of chemical carcinogens. *Br. Med. Bull.,* **36:**11–18, 1980.

Slamon, D. J.; Shimotohno, K.; Cline, M. J.; Golde, D. W.; and Chen, I. S. Y.: Identification of the putative transforming protein of the human T-cell leukemia viruses HTLV-I and HTLV-II. *Science,* **226:**61–64, 1984.

Slavin, G.; Cameron, H. M.; and Singh, H.: Kaposi's sarcoma in mainland Tanzania: A report of 117 cases. *Br. J. Cancer,* **23:**349–357, 1969.

Solan, A. J.; Greenwald, E. S.; and Silvay, O.: Longterm complete remissions of Kaposi's sarcoma with vinblastine therapy. *Cancer,* **47:**637–639, 1981.

Starcich, B.; Ratner, L.; Josephs, S. F.; Okamoto, T.; Gallo, R. C.; and Staal, F. W.: Characterization of long terminal repeat sequences of HTLV-III. *Science,* **227:**538–540, 1985.

Sterns, R. S.; Parrish, J. A.; Bleich, H. L.; and Fitzpatrick, T. B.: PUVA (Psoralen and ultraviolet A) and squamous cell carcinoma in patients with psoriasis. *Clin. Res.,* **29:**615a, 1981.

Sterry, W.; Steigleder, G. K.; and Pullman, H.: In situ identification and enumeration of T-lymphocytes in cutaneous T-cell lymphomas by demonstration of granular activity of acid-nonspecific esterase. *Br. J. Dermatol.,* **103:**67–72, 1980.

Stingl, G.; Katz, S. I.; Green, I.; and Shevach, E. M.: The functional role of Langerhans cells. *J. Invest. Dermatol.,* **74:**315–318, 1980.

Suindland, H. B.: Kangri cancer in the brick industry. *Contact Dermatitis,* **6:**24–26, 1980.

Tamaki, K.; Stingl, G.; and Katz, S. I.: The origin of Langerhans cells. *J. Invest. Dermatol.,* **74:**309–311, 1980.

Tan, R. S.; Oon, C. J.; Barrett, A. J.; Hayes, J. P.; and Samman, P. D.: Sézary syndrome: Treatment of leukophoresis. *Proc. R. Soc. Med.,* **68:**648–649, 1975.

Taylor, J. F.: Lymphocyte transformation in Kaposi's sarcoma. *Lancet,* **1:**883–884, 1973.

Taylor, J. F.; Smith, P. G.; Bull, D.; and Pike, M. C.: Kaposi's sarcoma in Uganda: Geographic and ethnic distribution. *Br. J. Cancer,* **26:**483–497, 1972.

Taylor, J. F.; Templeton, A. C.; Vogel, C. L.; Zeigler, J. L.; and Kycelwazi, S. K.: Kaposi's sarcoma in Uganda: A clinicopathological study. *Int. J. Cancer,* **8:**122–135, 1971.

Taylor, J. F., and Zeigler, J. L.: Delayed cutaneous hypersensitivity reactions in patients with Kaposi's sarcoma. *Br. J. Cancer,* **30:**312–318, 1974.

Tedeschi, C. G.: Some considerations concerning the nature of the so-called sarcoma of Kaposi. *Arch. Pathol.,* **66:**656–684, 1958.

Templeton, A. C.: Kaposi's sarcoma. *Pathol. Annu.,* **16:**315–336, 1981.

TenSeldam, R. E. J.: Skin cancer in Australia. *Natl. Cancer Inst. Monogr.,* **10:**153–166, 1963.

Thiers, B. H.: Controversies in mycosis fungoides. *J. Am. Acad. Dermatol.,* **7:**1–16, 1982.

Trainin, Z.; Nernicke, D.; Ungar-Waron, H.; and Essex, M.: Suppression of the humoral antibody response in natural retrovirus infections. *Science,* **220:**858–859, 1983.

Treves, N., and Pack, G. T.: The development of cancer in burn scars. *Surg. Gynecol. Obstet.,* **51:**749–782, 1930.

Trosko, J. E.; Krause, D.; and Isoun, M.: Sunlight-induced pyrimidine dimers in human cells *in vitro. Nature,* **228:**358–359, 1970.

Trump, J. G.; Wright, K. A.; Evans, W. W.; and Anson, J. H.: High energy electrons for the treatment of extensive superficial malignant lesions. *Am. J. Roentgenol.,* **69:**623–629, 1953.

Turbitt, M., and Mackie, R.: Further evidence for the involvement of Langerhans cells in the pathogenesis of mycosis fungoides. *Br. J. Dermatol.,* **105**(Suppl 19):11–12, 1979.

Ulbright, T. M., and Santa Cruz, D. J.: Kaposi's sarcoma: Relationship with hematologic, lymphoid, and thymic neoplasia. *Cancer,* **47:**963–973, 1981.

Umbert, P.; Belcher, R. W.; and Winkelmann, R. K.: Macrophage inhibitor factor (MIF) in cutaneous lymphoproliferative diseases. *Br. J. Dermatol.,* **95:**475–480, 1976.

Urbach, F.; Davies, R. E.; and Forbes, P. D.: Ultraviolet radiation and skin cancer in man. In Montaglia, W., and Dobson, R. L. (eds.): Vol. III. Pergamon Press, Inc., New York, 1966.

VanScott, E. J., and Kalmanson, J. D.: Complete remission of mycosis fungoides lymphoma induced by topical nitrogen mustard (HN$_2$). Control of delayed hypersensitivity to HN$_2$ by desensitization and induction of specific immunologic intolerance. *Cancer,* **32:**18–30, 1973.

VanScott, E. J.; Reinertson, R. P.: The modulating influence of stromal environment on epithelial cells studied in human autotransplants. *J. Invest. Dermatol.,* **36:**109–117, 1961.

van Vloten, W. A., and Polano, M. K.: Bleomycin therapy in mycosis fungoides. *Dermatologica,* **150:**50–57, 1975.

van Vloten, W. A.; Scheffer, E.; and Meijer, C. J.: DNA cytophotometry of lymph node imprints from patients with mycosis fungoides. *J. Invest. Dermatol.,* **73:**275–277, 1979.

Vogel, C. L.; Primack, A.; and Dhru, D.: Treatment of Kaposi's sarcoma with actinomycin D and cyclophosphamide: Results of a randomized clinical trial. *Int. J. Cancer,* **8:**136–143, 1971.

Vogel, C. L.; Primack, A.; Owor, R.; and Kyalwazi, S. K.: Effective treatment of Kaposi's sarcoma with 5-(3,3-di methyl-l-triazeno)imidazole-4-carboxamide (NSC-45388). *Cancer Chemother. Rep., Part I,* **57:**65–71, 1973.

Vonderheid, E. C.: Evaluation and treatment of mycosis fungoides lymphoma. *Int. J. Dermatol.,* **19:**182–188, 1980.

Vonderheid, E. C.; Fang, S.; Helfrich, M. K.; Abraham, S. R.; and Nicolini, C. A.: Biophysical characterization of normal T-lymphocytes and Sézary cells. *J. Invest. Dermatol.,* **76**:28–37, 1981.

Wachsman, W.; Shimotohno, K.; Clark, S. C.; Golde, D. W.; and Chen, I. S. Y.: Expression of the 3' terminal region of human T-cell leukemia viruses. *Science,* **226**:177–179, 1984.

Waldman, T. A.; Broder, S.; Drum, M.; Meade, B.; Krakauer, R.; Blackman, M.; and Goldman, C.: T-cell suppression of pokeweed nitogen-induced immunoglobulin production. In Oppenheim, J. J., and Rosentreich, D. L.: (eds.): *Mitogens in Immunobiology.* Academic Press, Inc., New York, 1976.

Walzer, P. D.; Perl, D. P.; Krogstad, D. J.; Rawson, P. G.; and Schultz, M. G.: *Pneumocystis carinii* pneumonia in the United States. Epidemiologic, diagnostic and clinical features. *Ann. Intern. Med.,* **80**:83–93, 1974.

Weber, J. N.; Carmichael, D. J.; Sawyer, N.; Pinching, A. J.; and Harris, J. R. W.: Clinical aspects of the acquired immune deficiency syndrome in the United Kingdom. *Br. J. Vener. Dis.,* **60**:253–257, 1984.

Weimar, V. M.; Ceilley, R. I.; and Goeken, J. A.: Cell-mediated immunity in patients with basal and squamous cell skin cancer. *J. Am. Acad. Dermatol.,* **2**:143–147, 1980.

Weinstein, G. D., and Frost, P.; Cell proliferation in human body cell carcinoma. *Cancer Res.,* **30**:724–728, 1970.

Weiss, V. C., and Serushan, M.: Kaposi's sarcoma in a patient with dermatomyositis receiving immunosuppressive therapy. *Arch. Dermatol.,* **118**:183–185, 1982.

White, S. W.: Basal cell carcinoma arising in a burn scar: Case report. *J. Dermatol. Surg. Oncol.,* **9**:159–161, 1983.

Willemze, R.; deGraaff-Reitsma, J.; van Vloten, W. A.; and Meijer, C. J.: Characterization of T-cell subpopulations in skin and peripheral blood of patients with cutaneous T-cell lymphomas and benign inflammatory dermatoses. *J. Invest. Dermatol.,* **80**:60–66, 1983.

Wolf, J. E., Jr., and Hubler, W. R., Jr.: Tumor angiogenic factor and human skin tumors. *Arch. Dermatol.,* **111**:321–327, 1975.

Wong, T. W., and Warner, N. E.: Cytomegalic inclusion disease in adults: Report of 14 cases with review of literature. *Arch. Pathol.,* **74**:403–422, 1962.

Woom, A. M.; Hastrup, N.; Hou-Jensen, K.; and Thomsen, K.: Bone marrow involvement in mycosis fungoides demonstrated by needle biopsy. *J. Cutan. Pathol.,* **5**:31–32, 1978.

Wright, J. C.; Lyons, M. M.; Walker, D. G.; Golomb, F. M.; Gumport, S. L.; and Meorek, T. J.: Observations on the use of cancer chemotherapeutic agents in patients with mycosis fungoides. *Cancer,* **17**:1045–1062, 1964.

Yabe, Y.; Yasui, M.; Yoshino, H.; Fujiwana, T.; Ohukuma, N.; and Nohara, N.: Epidermodysplasia verruciformis: Viral particles in early malignant lesions. *J. Invest. Dermatol.,* **71**:225–228, 1978.

Yamanishi, Y.; Dubbous, M. K.; and Hashimoto, K.: Effect of collagenolytic activity in basal cell epithelioma of the skin on reconstituted collagen and physical properties and kinetics of the crude enzyme. *Cancer Res.,* **32**:2551–2560, 1972.

Yeh, S.: Relative incidence of skin cancer in Chinese in Taiwan: With special reference to arsenical cancer. *Natl. Cancer Inst. Monogr.,* **10**:81–105, 1963.

Yoshida, T.; Edelson, R. L.; Cohen, S.; and Green, I.: Migration inhibitory activity in serum and in cell supernatants of patients with Sézary syndrome. *J. Immunol.,* **114**:915–918, 1975.

Zacharie, H.; Grunnet, E.; Ellegaard, J.; and Thestrup-Pederson, K.: Transfer factor as an additional therapeutic agent in mycosis fungoides. In Kahn, A.; Kirkpatrick, C. H.; and Hill, N. O. (eds.): *Immune Regulators in Transfer Factor. Proceedings from the Third International Symposium on Transfer Factor.* Academic Press, Inc., New York, 1979.

Zagury, D.; Bernard, J.; Lebowitch, J.; Safai, B.; Groopman, J. E.; Feldman, M.; Sarngadharan, M. G.; and Gallo, R. C.: HTLV-III in cells cultured from semen of two patients with AIDS. *Science,* **226**:449–451, 1984.

Zelickson, A. S.; Motta, Z. J.; and Weissle, W.: Effects of topical fluorouracil on normal skin. *Arch. Dermatol.,* **111**:1301–1306, 1975.

Zucker-Franklin, D.: Thymus-dependent lymphocytes in lymphoproliferative disorders of the skin. *J. Invest. Dermatol.,* **67**:412–418, 1976.

21

Melanoma

FRANK J. CUMMINGS, CHARLES J. McDONALD, and PAUL CALABRESI

PRIMARY CUTANEOUS MALIGNANT MELANOMA

Primary cutaneous malignant melanoma, although detectable in more than 90% of patients at an early and curable stage, remains one of the most devastating of all cancers. Despite increased awareness and improved understanding of the biologic and clinical behavior of malignant melanoma, the incidence of the disease is rising and is associated with a high death rate (see Table 21–1) (Elwood and Lee, 1975; American Cancer Society, 1976, 1983; Lee et al., 1979; Silverberg, 1979; Holman et al., 1980).

Incidence and Epidemiology

Once considered rare, malignant melanoma is now estimated to represent 1 to 2% of all human cancers, excluding nonmelanoma skin cancer. Melanoma accounts for as many as 2% of all cancer deaths (Elwood et al., 1975; American Cancer Society, 1976; Silverberg, 1979). Age-adjusted death rates have increased from 1951 to 1975 by approximately 3% per year in the populations of Canada, England, and Wales and in the white population of the United States (Lee et al., 1979). Australian mortality rates have also risen steadily from 1931 to 1977 (see Table 21–2). Age-standardized mortality rates in Australia rose from 0.8/100,000 to 4.2/100,000 in men and in women from 0.6/100,000 to 2.5/100,000 (Holman et al., 1980).

Melanoma of the skin may occur at any age, but is extremely rare before puberty. In the prepubertal child it is almost always associated with a congenital melanocytic nevus (Trozak et al., 1974). The peak age of occurrence in women is 50 years. In men, disease incidence increases steadily with age. Melanoma occurs with equal frequency in men and women (Cutler and Young, 1975). Trunk melanomas are more prevalent in men, whereas melanomas of the extremities are more common in women.

Racial factors are of great importance in the occurrence rate of melanoma of the skin (Cutler and Young, 1975; Krementz et al., 1976a; Reddy et al., 1976). Factors that correlate with increased risk include skin pigmentation, eye color, hair color, and the tendency to sunburn rather than tan. The melanoma-prone patient may be characterized as being of Celtic or Northern European extraction, with

Table 21–1. Melanoma: Incidence and Mortality in the United States (1983 Estimate)

Number of new cases	
Men	8500
Women	8900
Total	17,400
Number of deaths	5200
Percent of all cancers	
Whites	1.5
Blacks	0.3
Annual age-adjusted incidence	
Rate/100,000	
Whites	4.5
Blacks	0.8
Relative 5-year survival	
Percent	
1960–1963	60
1970–1973	68

From *Cancer Patient Survival Report No. 5,* DHEW Publication No. (NIH) 77-992; Biometry Branch, National Cancer Institute; SEER Program, National Cancer Institute; American Cancer Society.

Table 21-2. Increases in Incidence and Mortality from Melanoma in Different Countries

	COUNTRY	GENDER	FIRST PERIOD OF OBSERVATION		SECOND PERIOD OF OBSERVATION		TOTAL % INCREASE	NO. OF YEARS	ANNUAL % INCREASE
			Time	RATE (per 1000)	Time	RATE (per 1000)			
Incidence	New York State	M	1941–1943	12.2	1967	33.7	176	25	7.0
		F	1941–1943	17.7	1967	29.3	65	25	2.6
Incidence	Norway	M	1955	17.9	1970	63.0	264	15	17.6
		F	1955	25.5	1970	68.4	195	15	13.0
Mortality	Norway	M	1956–1960	15.9	1966–1970	26.8	69	10	6.9
		F	1956–1960	13.3	1966–1970	18.1	36	10	3.6
Mortality	Canada	M	1951–1955	7.1	1966–1970	13.7	93	15	6.2
		F	1951–1955	5.9	1966–1970	12.2	107	15	7.1
Mortality	USA	Both	1950	9.3	1967	16.0	72	16	4.5
Mortality	UK	Both	1950	5.1	1967	10.2	100	16	6.3
Mortality	Australia	M	1931–1940	9.8	1961–1970	36.0	267	30	8.9
		F	1931–1940	7.6	1961–1970	24.9	227	30	7.8
Mortality	Denmark	M	1956–1960	15.9	1966–1969	23.7	49	10	4.9
		F	1956–1960	16.1	1966–1969	21.3	32	10	3.2
Mortality	Sweden	M	1956–1960	16.5	1966–1968	21.4	30	9	3.3
		F	1956–1960	10.6	1966–1968	14.8	40	9	4.4
Incidence	Connecticut	M	1935–1939	13.7	1965–1969	48.1	250	30	8.3
		F	1935–1939	10.5	1965–1969	47.7	354	30	11.8

Adapted from Elwood, J. M., and Lee, J. A. H.: Recent data on the epidemiology of malignant melanoma. *Semin. Oncol.*, 2:149–154, 1975.

651

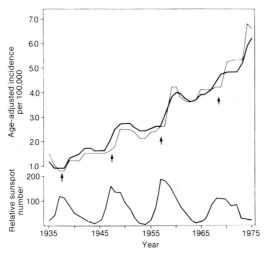

Figure 21–1. The age-adjusted incidence of melanoma related to sunspot activity per 100,000 persons in Connecticut between 1935 and 1975. From Houghton, A. N.; Munster, E. W.; and Viola, M. V.: Increased incidence of malignant melanoma after peaks of sunspot activity. *Lancet,* 1:759–760, 1978.

pale skin that sunburns easily and tans poorly, blue or gray eyes, and red or blonde hair and as being one who has had considerable sun exposure and frequent sun burns (Ancher *et al.,* 1966; Gellin *et al.,* 1969; Beitner *et al.,* 1981; Houghton and Viola, 1981). Collectively these factors relate to solar radiation exposure and

its effect on the skin. Whereas a few reports dispute earlier clinical impressions and observations linking the development of primary cutaneous melanoma to solar radiation (Kleep and Magnus, 1979; Sober *et al.,* 1979), more recent reports (Beitner *et al.,* 1981; Houghton and Viola, 1981) suggest that solar radiation acts as a cocarcinogen or promoter. As evidence for this relationship Houghton and colleagues (1978) cite a correlation between melanoma incidence and sunspot activity, with peak or excess melanoma cases observed every nine to twelve years after peak sunspot activity (see Figure 21–1). Beitner and coworkers (1981) have demonstrated lower minimal erythema dose (MED) responses in patients with melanoma than in normal controls. MED is the minimum amount of ultraviolet radiation necessary to produce minimally perceptible erythema in exposed skin. Other evidence includes higher occurrence rates of melanoma on anatomic sites receiving heavy doses of solar radiation and a correlation of higher incidence of melanoma and mortality with proximity of a susceptible population to the equator (see Figure 21–2).

Etiology and Pathogenesis

Melanomas are a result of biologic aberrations in normal melanocytes. Certain nevi that

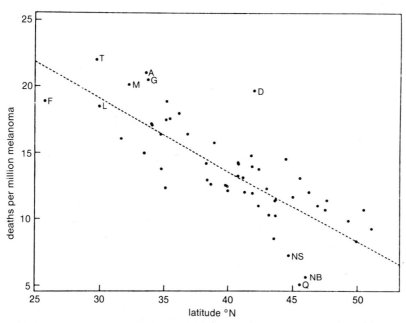

Figure 21–2. The relationship between death rate from melanoma and latitude-points for states of the United States and the Canadian provinces. Note the correlation of a higher melanoma mortality with proximity of a susceptible population to the equator. From Elwood, J. M., and Lee, J. A. H.: Recent data on the epidemiology of malignant melanoma. *Semin. Oncol.* 2:149–154, 1975.

are characterized histologically by atypical melanocytic dysplasia provide a possible link between the normal melanocytic nevus and melanoma. Except for the congenital melanocytic nevus, however, it is practically impossible to trace with assurance the development of a melanoma from benign melanocytic nevi. Good circumstantial evidence supports the role of genetic factors in the development of melanoma (Clark *et al.*, 1978; Lynch *et al.*, 1978; Reimer *et al.*, 1978). At least 6% of patients with melanoma report a family history of the disease (Sober *et al.*, 1980). Such families often possess a phenotypic marker consisting of atypical nevi characterized histologically by severe dysplasia of the melanocytes (the B-K mole or dysplastic nevus syndrome) (Sober *et al.*, 1979).

Actinic radiation, ultraviolet light (UV), may play an important role as a cocarcinogen or promoter in the etiology and pathogenesis of melanoma, but the mechanism of solar induction is a fairly complex and poorly understood process (Ancher *et al.*, 1966; Gellin *et al.*, 1969; Beitner *et al.*, 1981; Houghton and Viola, 1981). Higher rates of melanoma are found in fair-skinned persons living near the equator or in regions of prolonged intense solar radiation (McGovern and Mackie, 1959; Helwig, 1963; Crombie, 1981). Individuals with xeroderma pigmentosum, a disease characterized by defective excision repair of pyrimidine dimers induced by ultraviolet light in the DNA of skin cells, frequently develop melanomas and other cutaneous neoplasms (Robbins *et al.*, 1974). Melanomas, as well as severe solar damage, occur on sun-exposed body areas of men and women (Helwig, 1963; Sober *et al.*, 1980; Crombie, 1981). For example, melanomas tend to spare the legs and bathing trunk areas in men and the bathing suit areas in women. Primary cutaneous melanoma occurs less frequently in blacks, Orientals, and East Indians, whose skins are better protected from damaging ultraviolet light by melanin pigment. The usual sites of occurrence also differ between these races and Caucasians (White *et al.*, 1961; Cutler and Young, 1975; Krementz *et al.*, 1976a; Reddy *et al.*, 1976; Seiji *et al.*, 1979). In pigmented races, melanomas occur principally on non-sun-exposed sites such as palms, soles, nail beds, and mucous membranes. In these races neoplastic changes in nevi associated with the onset of melanoma are thought to be induced by repeated trauma.

The role of the environment, other than actinic radiation and occupation, in the pathogenesis of melanoma may also be important. Melanoma occurs with increased frequency in high-income groups and in certain occupations. Petrochemical and chemical workers, as well as those exposed to polychlorinated biphenyls or arsenic, appear to have a greater risk (Bahn *et al.*, 1976; Nathanson, 1983). The ingestion of birth control pills or levodopa has been implicated in the development of melanoma (Beral *et al.*, 1977; Skibba *et al.*, 1972). Unskilled workers appear to have a markedly poorer prognosis after the development of melanoma than more skilled employees. This may be due to more advanced disease at time of presentation for diagnosis and treatment (Shaw *et al.*, 1981).

Early detection and preventive measures offer the most substantial hope of improving the overall statistics for survival of melanoma. Education of the public and professionals to the clinical signs of preneoplastic and neoplastic lesions is an important goal for early diagnosis and effective treatment of localized disease. Susceptible persons should avoid excessive exposure to the sun and should apply sunscreens whenever undergoing prolonged sun exposure. Petrochemical workers, chemical workers, and persons exposed to polychlorinated biphenyls and arsenic may be at greater risk. Ways of avoiding exposure to potentially toxic compounds together with increased efforts in occupational safety education are needed (Bahn *et al.*, 1976; Nathanson, 1983). Physicians' awareness of hereditary factors associated with melanoma and their recognition of high-risk populations should be improved, including awareness of the clinical features of the dysplastic nevus syndrome, characterized by large, atypical melanocytic nevi with distinctive histologic changes (Elder *et al.*, 1980). The familial form of this, the B-K mole syndrome, underscores the need to examine relatives of individual melanoma patients for possible cancerous or precancerous lesions. Patients with xeroderma pigmentosum, congenital giant pigmented nevi and von Recklinghausen's disease are also more prone to develop primary cutaneous malignant melanoma. Equally important to preventive measures is regular, careful self-examination of the entire cutaneous surface, including the soles of the feet. This may allow an individual to detect early any suspicious moles that have changed in character. Thus, the medical profession and the public share the responsibility for preventive measures.

Pathology and Natural History

Primary cutaneous malignant melanoma is usually classified into four or five types based principally on clinical characteristics and biologic behavior: (1) lentigo maligna melanoma, (2) superficial spreading melanoma, (3) nodular melanoma, (4) polypoid, a variant of nodular melanoma, and (5) acral-lentiginous melanoma (palmar-plantar-subungual, mucosal melanoma) (see Table 21–3). Superficial spreading melanoma is most frequent, making up 50 to 70% of all cases; it is followed in frequency by nodular melanoma, 16 to 30%; lentigo maligna melanoma, 5 to 15%; acral-lentiginous melanoma, 5%; and polypoid melanoma, less than 1%. Polypoid melanomas, although rare, are the most aggressive of all melanomas (Manci *et al.,* 1981). Lentigo maligna melanoma is the least aggressive of the five types. Acral-lentiginous melanoma frequently simulates the clinical and histopathologic picture of lentigo maligna melanoma but is probably the second most aggressive form of melanoma. Overall, individuals with superficial spreading melanoma tend to have a more benign course than do those with nodular melanoma. When all lesions are of comparable thickness, however, differences in survival rates disappear even in lentigo maligna melanoma (Balch *et al.,* 1978; Balch *et al.,* 1979a,b; Koh *et al.,* 1984).

Lentigo Maligna Melanoma (Hutchinson's melanotic freckle, melanosis circumscripta preblastoma of Dubreuilh). Lentigo maligna melanoma almost always arises from a benign lesion, lentigo maligna, after a 10- to 20-year course (see Colorplate I). Lentigo maligna melanoma is often characterized as malignant melanoma *in situ.* A typical lesion arises on the sun-exposed skin of elderly individuals, especially on the face. The behavior of lentigo maligna melanoma is benign when contrasted to that of other melanocytic neoplasms. This concept, however, has been challenged recently (Koh *et al.,* 1984). Thick tumors grow

rather slowly from lentigo maligna and metastasize to regional lymph nodes late in the course of the disease. One-third of all lentigo malignas are estimated to develop a malignant (thick) component (Davis *et al.,* 1967). Only a small percentage metastasize (Peterson *et al.,* 1964). Lentigo maligna begins as a flat (macular) tan to darkly pigmented lesion with irregular borders, principally in sun-exposed areas. The depth of color may vary from one area to another within a single lesion (see Colorplates I and II). During a period ranging from months to many years, a single lesion progressively enlarges in the horizontal plane, often covering an area of 5 to 10 cm. As it enlarges papules and plaques gradually develop over the surface. Some of these areas become more darkly pigmented, others become amelanotic. The presence of papules and plaques implies that a transition to frankly malignant melanoma (lentigo maligna melanoma) has begun. In a few cases, lentigo maligna and lentigo maligna melanoma resolve spontaneously either in part or entirely. In most cases, however, if the lesion is untreated, continued progression with increased depth of tumor invasion is the rule.

The histologic picture of lentigo maligna melanoma varies, reflecting the portion of the tumor sampled, that is, an area of lentigo maligna or an area of early and late lentigo maligna melanoma (Clark and Mihn, 1969; Lever, 1975) (see Figures 21–3 and 21–4). An increased number of normal melanocytes or atypical melanocytes or an admixture of both may be observed in the lower epidermis of a representative area of lentigo maligna. Atypical melanocytes appear bizzare and often contain hyperchromatic, irregularly shaped single or multiple nuclei and heavily pigmented, vacuolated cytoplasm. Nests of normal intraepidermal melanocytes may be seen infrequently. Papillomatosis (thickening) of the epidermis may be noted, but frank disruption of the basement membrane with dermal invasion does not occur (see Figure 21–5).

In areas that have progressed to lentigo ma-

Table 21–3.   Primary Cutaneous Melanoma

	INCIDENCE *(approx. %)*	AGE *(Median)*	LATENCY *(Years)*	SURVIVAL *(% 5-year)*
Lentigo maligna	14	70	10–20	55–100
Superficial spreading	50	55	1–5	45–95
Nodular	30	48	.1–2	25–60
Polypoid	1	37		42
Acral-lentiginous	5	61	.1–2	5–10

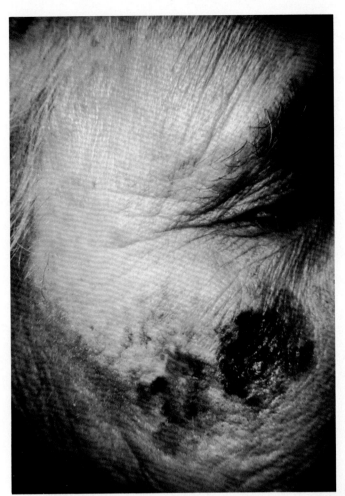

Colorplate I. Lentigo maligna. This lesion shows the typical features found in a lentigo maligna that has been present for a long time. The surface of the lesion is smooth and has not yet extended above the surrounding skin. The color of the lesion is varigated but does not show the "play" of colors typical of superficial spreading malignant melanoma. Treatment at this time would result in complete eradication of the lesion and its potential for malignant change.

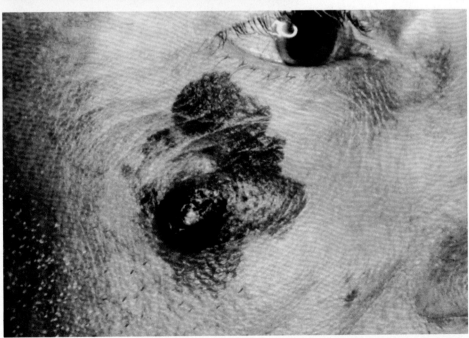

Colorplate II. Lentigo maligna melanoma. This photograph shows a lesion with the characteristic clinical features of lentigo maligna upon which a nodular melanoma is superimposed. Treatment in this case was not instituted at the appropriate time, and, as a result, the prognosis for cure is nil.

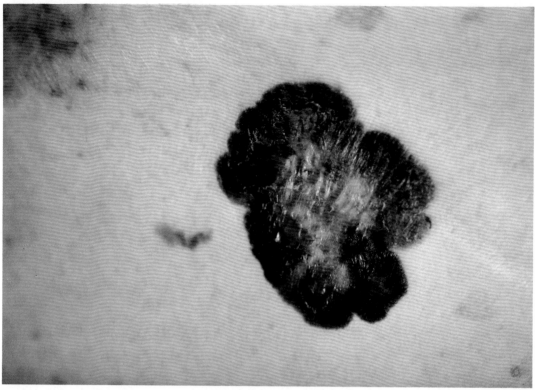

Colorplate III. Superficial spreading malignant melanoma. This photograph shows an almost classic appearance for this type of lesion. Within the lesion there is a "play" of colors—black, blue, slate gray, red, pink, and white—all of which lay on a background of skin that is virtually devoid of pigment (color). Growth in this lesion is principally on a horizontal plane. The prognosis for cure is good.

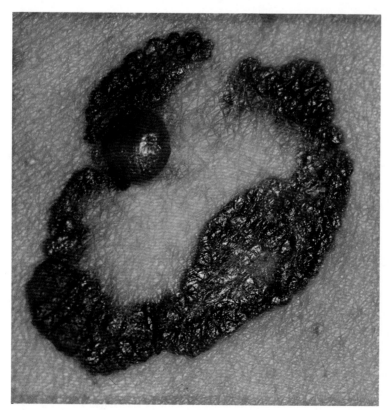

Colorplate IV. Superficial spreading malignant melanoma. This lesion shows virtually the same clinical features as are seen in Colorplate III. Although the borders of this lesion are fairly well defined, a closer look will reveal a substantial diffusion of pigment into skin that is not obviously involved with tumor. This is a clinical feature that may be used to differentiate benign from malignant lesions.

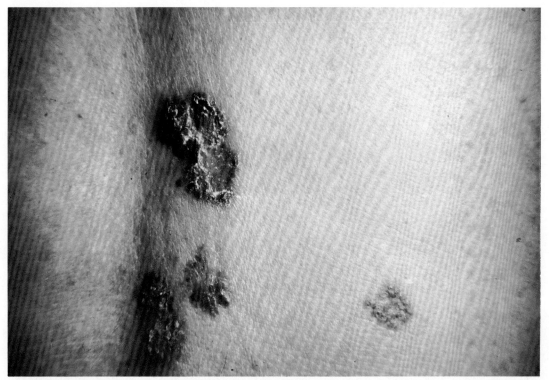

Colorplate V. Pigmented basal cell carcinoma. This is a lesion that is often confused with superficial spreading malignant melanoma. Close inspection of the lesion will reveal the characteristic features of basal cell carcinoma. These lesions are most commonly seen in heavily pigmented individuals. A simple 3-4-mm biopsy of this lesion is indicated so that an appropriate diagnosis can be made.

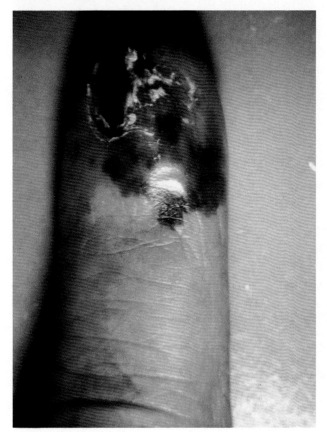

Colorplate VI. Acral lentiginous malignant melanoma. This lesion is generally found on the extremities. Clinically it is characterized by pigment diffusion throughout the involved skin. On palpation, there is little or no induration to be noted. Histologically this lesion may differ little from lentigo malignant melanoma, although it is considerably more difficult to cure. The malignant potential of this type of lesion closely approximates that of nodular melanoma.

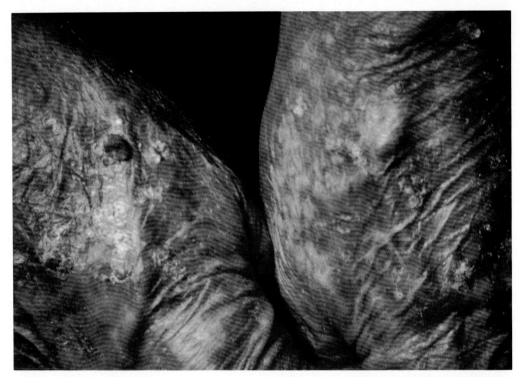

Colorplate VII. Actinic keratoses. Lesions of many ages and types are demonstrated in this photograph. Early lesions are red and slightly scaling. Old lesions are covered with a thick, hyperkeratotic crust. The hyperkeratotic lesions may have progressed to squamous cell cancer. All lesions exist on a background of sun-damaged skin.

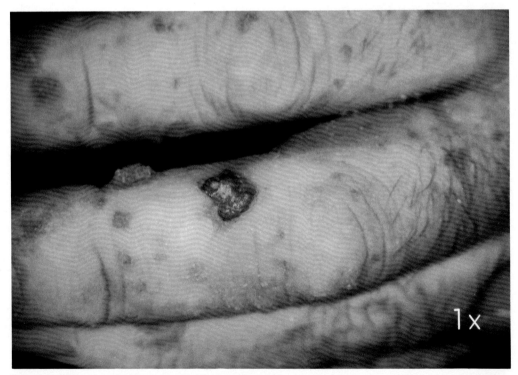

Colorplate VIII. Arsenical keratoses. In this photograph, the patient's skin shows none of the changes characteristic of sun-damaged skin. Arsenical keratoses usually are found on the extremities, especially the palms and soles. They most often occur as multiple protuberant lesions. The patient in this photograph died of generalized metastatic squamous cell carcinoma, site unknown.

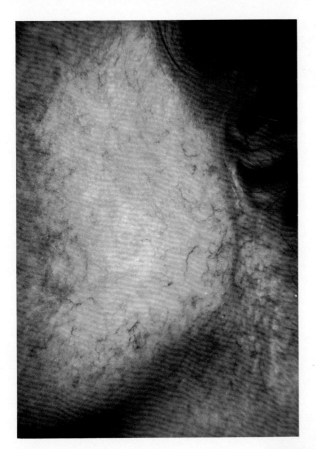

Colorplate IX. This photograph shows radiation-damaged skin containing several precancerous lesions. The most prominent of these may be seen near the left border, the upper left corner, and the center. Skin changes such as thinning of the epidermis, variegated color, and multiple telangiectasia may be seen following exposure to sun or ionizing radiation.

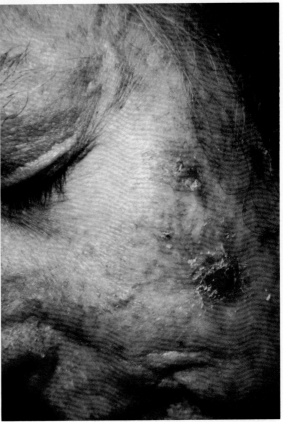

Colorplate X. This photograph shows squamous cell cancers arising in the precancerous lesions shown in Colorplate IX, approximately three years later.

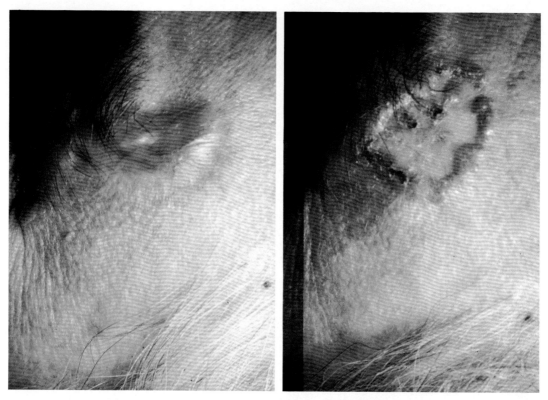

Colorplate XI. Basal cell cancer. Many typical clinical features of basal cell carcinoma may be seen in these photographs. In the photograph on the left an early lesion shows the pearllike border and extensive telangiectasia over the surface. On the right the lesion has remained to expand, and it now shows the clinical features of sclerosing basal cell carcinoma.

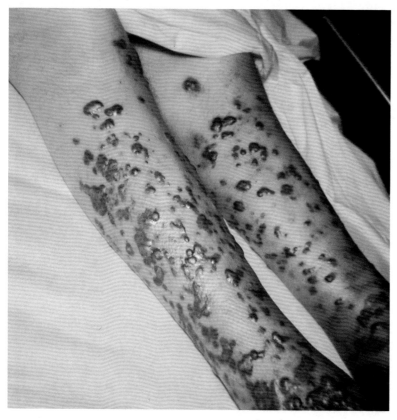

Colorplate XII. Kaposi's sarcoma. This photograph shows typical plaques and nodules that are characteristic of the European-type disease.

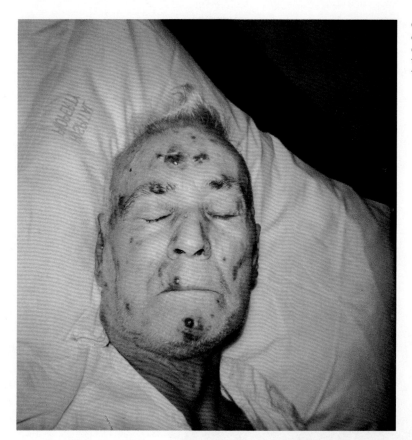

Colorplate XIII. Kaposi's sarcoma. These lesions are typical of those seen on body sites other than the lower extremities in the European-type disease.

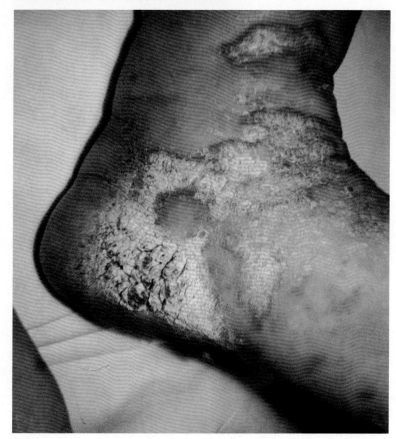

Colorplate XIV. Kaposi's sarcoma. A late stage in the disease in which nodules have enlarged and coalesced to form plaques is shown. The thick, hyperkeratotic surface appears to consist primarily of scale. Histopathologic examination, however, would show lesions typical of Kaposi's sarcoma. Note the extensive edema associated with this lesion.

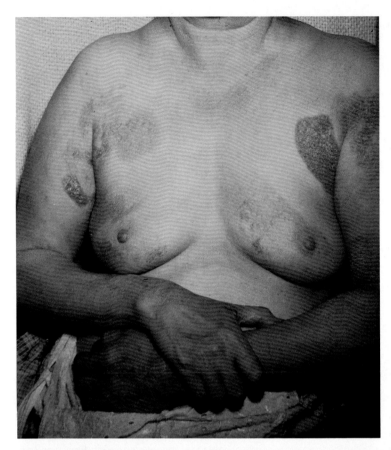

Colorplate XV. Cutaneous T-cell lymphoma. Eczematous lesions predominate on the skin of this patient. Variations in the color of each eczematous lesion are, although subtle, present. This is the so-called poikilodermatous appearance to the skin in this disease. Plaque-type lesions are found near the left axillary region and on the right upper arm. These lesions may be difficult to differentiate from large-plaque parapsoriasis en plaques.

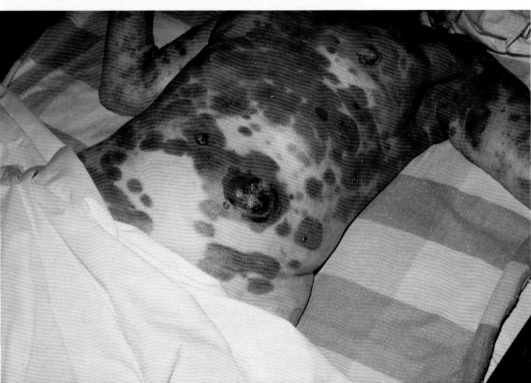

Colorplate XVI. Cutaneous T-cell lymphoma. The disease in this patient has progressed to the large-plaque, tumor, and ulcerative stages. The prognosis for this disease is poor.

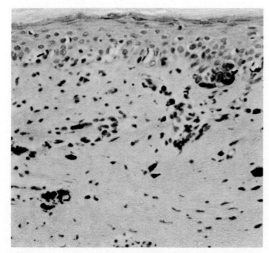

Figure 21-3. Preinvasive lentigo maligna. In this lesion, the epidermis appears thin and flattened. In the lower epidermis, melanocytic cells show evidence of anaplasia. Many show a vacuolated cytoplasm. Some of the nuclei are large and hyperchromatic. At the right-hand margin of this photomicrograph and within the epidermis is seen a collection of early melanized proliferating melanocytes. Scattered throughout the dermis are melanin-laden melanophores and inflammatory cells (×63).

ligna melanoma, sheets of malignant melanocytes have invaded the dermis. Nodular lesions often contain huge dermal nests of malignant melanocytes, with many of the spindle cell type. A dense mononuclear cell infiltrate may

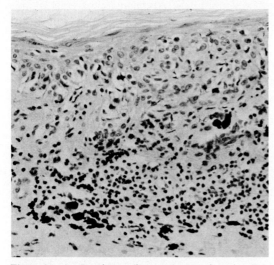

Figure 21-4. Lentigo maligna melanoma invasive. Beneath a totally disorganized and thin lower epidermis are seen many atypical nevus cells invading the upper dermis. Beneath and intermixed among these atypical cells is a dense collection of inflammatory cells. Melanophores are also intermixed with the inflammatory cells and atypical nevoid cells (×63).

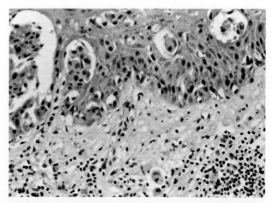

Figure 21-5. Intraepidermal malignant melanoma. In this view the tumor does not appear to have traversed the intact basal lamina. In the center of this photomicrograph, however, vascular invasion by tumor cells is seen. A dense collection of inflammatory cells lies beneath the tumor (×63).

be observed just beneath the sheets of neoplastic melanocytes; numerous pigment-ladened macrophages are frequently mixed with the mononuclear cell infiltrate within the dermis.

Superficial Spreading Melanoma. The most common of all melanomas is the superficial spreading type (see Figure 21-6). Early recognition and treatment of this neoplasm leads to a much more favorable prognosis than with nodular, acral-lentiginous, and polypoid melanomas. Favorable prognosis is directly related to the biologic characteristics of the tumor.

Superficial spreading melanoma proliferates through a lateral (horizontal) growth

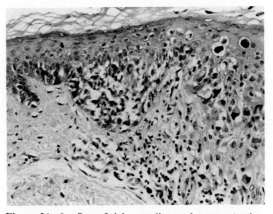

Figure 21-6. Superficial spreading melanoma. At the left-hand margin, considerable junctional activity is seen, whereas to the right, atypical nevus cells, both fusiform and cuboidal, are invading the dermis. Several tumor cells are in mitosis within the hyperplastic epidermis. The dermal inflammatory cell infiltrate appears sparse (×63).

phase during a considerable part of its evolution. During this period most of the characteristic clinical features of this tumor are evident. Nearly all superficial spreading melanomas have a variety of colors on the surface, which change as the lesion enlarges and evolves. Visible hues include pink, red, brown, blue, black, gray, slate gray, and white (see Colorplates III and IV). Each color represents a different stage of development for a specific portion of the tumor. Areas of intense inflammation are pink to red in appearance. Deep dermal deposits of pigment, containing active malignant melanocytes reflect a blue color. Intense superficial melanocytic activity produces black pigment, and areas of tumor regression or destruction appear white.

Most superficial spreading melanomas have irregular, often "notched" borders, which usually represent sites of tumor destruction or regression. Although the tumor is in its lateral growth phase, the surface appears flat. When it begins to penetrate internally, during its vertical growth phase, the external surface becomes irregular, and papular and nodular lesions appear. Tumors may grow to 2.5 cm in horizontal diameter and for several years before they begin a vertical growth phase. When this occurs, prognosis for prolonged survival of the person with cancer is markedly reduced. Superficial spreading melanoma may occur throughout the body and at all ages. Its distribution is that usually observed with melanoma, that is, the back and chest in both men and women, as well as the legs in women.

During the lateral growth phase, superficial spreading melanoma may closely resemble, histologically, an active junctional or compound nevus. The nuclei of melanoma cells, however, are larger, more hyperchromatic and contain prominent nucleoli, whereas the cytoplasm contains disproportionately large amounts of melanin. In such lesions, the atypical melanocytes are often confined to the lower epidermis and dermal-epidermal junction, either individually or in irregularly shaped nests. During the vertical growth phase, malignant melanocytes proliferate in both the upper epidermis and the dermis. Invasion of the upper epidermis often results in thinning and perforation. Ulceration is a late clinical sign. Early invasion of the dermis begins with migration of neoplastic cells into the papillary region and is accompanied by the appearance of large numbers of mononuclear inflammatory cells at the base of the tumor. As invasion progresses, sheets of neoplastic melanocytes migrate further into the dermis. At this stage, considerable variation in cellular morphology is evident, with cuboidal (epithelioid), fusiform (spindle-shaped), and nevuslike (small cell) cells present, but, as the tumor ages, a single cell type predominates. Tumor invasion of the dermis is often accompanied by downward proliferation of the rete ridges, whereas the inflammatory infiltrate becomes less intense and may disappear completely.

Nodular Melanoma. Nodular melanoma and its variant, polypoid melanoma, carry a poor prognosis for patient survival. A high death rate is probably related to the depth of invasion of the tumor at the time of diagnosis, the tendency for rapid tumor growth in a vertical plane, and the small size of the tumors during the initial vertical growth phase.

Most nodular melanomas occur as small, darkly pigmented, raised dome-shaped or polypoid lesions on any area of the body (see Figure 21-7). The color may vary from amelanotic to black with color changes being most prominent in the polypoid form. Nodular melanomas are frequently overlooked until the occurrence of such late clinical signs as bleeding and ulceration.

Histologically, nodular melanoma resembles the late stages of superficial spreading melanoma (see Figure 21-7), however, because no lateral growth phase occurs, the melanoma is well confined. Atypical nevus cells of the cuboidal and fusiform types are in abundance and appear in solid sheets streaming down-

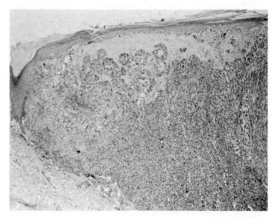

Figure 21-7. Nodular melanoma. Deeply invasive tumor with sparing of adjacent dermal papilla. There is very little evidence of horizontal growth in this type tumor. Vertical growth predominates and deep invasion of the dermis occurs very early (×10).

ward into the dermis and upward into the epidermis. The neoplastic cells appear to arise from the dermal-epidermal junction.

Polypoid Melanoma. Polypoid melanomas are generally thick, ulcerating lesions that may not invade deeply into the dermis (Manci *et al.*, 1981). Small numbers of mitotic figures are usually present. The presence and number of mitoses have been used with varying success to assess the neoplastic potential of melanomas (Balch *et al.*, 1978; Arrington *et al.*, 1977).

Acral-Lentiginous Melanoma. This type of melanoma occurs most often on the palms, soles, nailbeds, and mucous membranes and is considered to be an aggressive form of cutaneous melanoma (Arrington *et al.*, 1977) (see Colorplate VI). Acral-lentiginous melanomas are most frequently found in blacks and Orientals, but can occasionally be found in Caucasians (Seiji *et al.*, 1979; White *et al.*, 1961).

During the early phase of development, acral-lentiginous melanoma is difficult to distinguish from lentigo maligna. Lateral or horizontal spread of macular variegate pigmentation characterizes the lesion at this stage. During the initial vertical growth phase, papules, plaques, and nodules begin to appear but are not as prominent as in other types of melanoma.

Acral-lentiginous melanoma may resemble lentigo maligna melanoma histopathologically (see Figure 21–8). Macular areas show

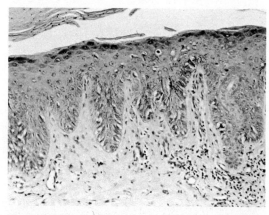

Figure 21–8. Acral lentiginous melanoma. In this lesion the epidermis appears acanthotic. There is considerable junctional activity extending high up into the epidermis. Several pigment cells are in mitosis. Throughout the lesion the basal lamina appears intact. In the dermis, a loose inflammatory infiltrate is scattered throughout. This lesion bears considerable resemblance to lentigo maligna melanoma but has a poor prognosis (×40).

proliferation of admixtures of normal and abnormal melanocytes at the dermal-epidermal junction. Other areas of macular pigmentation may demonstrate marked acanthosis and dermal invasion by atypical melanocytes. Papules and plaques manifest downward invasion by sheets of atypical spindle-shaped cells. A propensity for early dermal invasion and regional metastases is characteristic.

Microstaging of Primary Cutaneous Malignant Melanomas

Microstaging (Wanebo *et al.*, 1975) involves estimating the depth of invasion by primary cutaneous melanoma. It is of considerable value for predicting overall prognosis and for selecting appropriate clinical management in all types of lesions. A relationship between depth of neoplastic cell invasion and prognosis has been recognized for some time (Allen and Spitz, 1953). Mehnert and Heard (1965) proposed four prognostic stages of melanoma based on depth of cutaneous penetration. Subsequently, a number of additional systems of classification were suggested (Clark, 1967; Clark and Mihn, 1969; Breslow, 1970; McGovern, 1970). The classifications proposed by Clark and Breslow have gained wide acceptance.

Clark's system, initially proposed in 1967, includes five levels of invasion that reflect the depth of tumor penetration into the anatomic layers of the skin.

1. Level I lesions have not breached the integrity of the basement membrane and are, therefore, confined to the epidermis. The neoplastic nature of such lesions is nil, and they are often considered to be atypical melanocytic hyperplasia.
2. Level II lesions have violated the basement membrane but remain confined to the uppermost layer of the dermis, the papillary layer.
3. Level III lesions have penetrated the papillary dermis to the level of the interface of the papillary layer and the reticular dermis.
4. Level IV lesions have invaded beyond the interface between the papillary layer and the reticular dermis.
5. Level V lesions have invaded beyond the confines of the reticular dermis and into the subcutaneous fat.

Current overall five-year survival rates, after

adequate and appropriate treatment, in levels II to V are 95%, 75%, 60%, and 40% respectively.

In recent years numerous criticisms have been directed towards the Clark system of classification. Among these are: (1) differentiation between level III and IV lesions depends upon the correct identification of a junction between the papillary and reticular dermis. In many parts of the body the interface between the papillary and reticular dermis is obscure; (2) the exact definition of a level IV lesion is often impossible because isolated intrusions of tumor cells into the reticular dermis are not sufficient for classifying a lesion as level IV melanoma; (3) the level-of-invasion method of classification does not account for tumor growth above the epidermis; (4) Clark's method requires a precise interpretation of the exact level of tumor penetration of the dermis, but pathologists examining the same histopathologic material often differ in their opinions of the level of invasion (Suffin *et al.,* 1977).

These and other criticisms of Clark's level-of-invasion staging system, as well as impressions that the depth of tumor invasion is definitely related to prognosis, led to a more objective microstaging method (Breslow, 1970). With Breslow's method, the measurement of the maximum vertical tumor thickness is used to microstage the lesion. A measurement is made between upper (epidermal) and lower (dermal) reference points of tumor infiltration, using an ocular micrometer aligned at right angles to the adjacent normal skin. The granular cell layer of the epidermis in intact skin or the base of an ulcer crater in ulcerated skin is used as the upper reference point. The lower reference point may be the invading edge of a single tumor mass or an isolated cell or group of cells deep to the main tumor mass.

Most pathologists, dermatologists, and oncologists believe that Breslow's microstaging method has two major advantages over Clark's method: Ease of performance and reproducibility. With this method interpretations from different pathologists must be accepted with caution. Tumor thickness measurements of the same histopathologic material by different pathologists may vary significantly. When applied properly, Breslow's microstaging method shows good correlation between maximum tumor thickness and the rate of tumor metastases in patients with stage I melanoma

(Breslow, 1975; Hansen and McCarten, 1974). Patients with melanomas less than 0.76 mm in thickness have an estimated risk of 1 to 5% for developing metastatic disease. Patients with melanoma greater than 4 mm in thickness have an 80% or more chance of developing metastases beyond regional nodes. Patients with melanoma measuring between 0.76 and 3.99 mm in thickness are at increased risk of developing regional node metastases, 50 to 60%, but have a relatively lower risk of developing distant metastases, 10 to 20%. Measurements of thickness also reflect the risk of local recurrence at the primary excision site and help in determining the appropriate margins of primary surgical excision (Hansen and McCarten, 1974; Wanebo *et al.,* 1975; Breslow and Macht, 1977).

Many centers favor Breslow's microstaging techniques over Clark's. The data accumulated to date show that thickness measurements are more accurate and reproducible prognostic indicators than are Clark's levels of invasion (Wanebo *et al.,* 1975; Breslow and Macht, 1977; Balch *et al.,* 1978; Breslow *et al.,* 1978; Balch *et al.,* 1979b). Balch, in directly comparing the two microstaging methods, found a range of distribution of thickness measurements for each of the "Clark's levels" (see Figure 21–9) (Balch *et al.,* 1978). Statistically significant differences in survival rates within each of Clark's levels were noted when they were subgrouped by tumor thickness (Balch *et al.,* 1978). For example, level IV lesions, when compared for thickness, showed five-year sur-

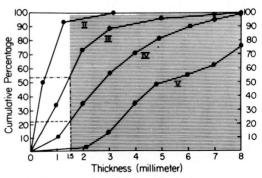

Figure 21–9. A comparison of the cumulative distribution of tumor thickness measurements with each of the Clark's levels of invasion. Note the range of distribution of thickness measurements for each level of invasion. As an example, 53% of level III and 22% of level IV melanomas had a thickness <1.5 mm (unshaded area). From Balch, C. M.; Murad, T. M.; Soong, S.-J.; Ingalls, A. L.; Halpern, N. B.; and Maddox, W. A.: A multifactorial analysis of melanoma. *Ann. Surg.,* **188:**732–742, 1978.

vival rates that ranged from 76% for thin lesions to 25% for thicker lesions. Similarly, survival rates for patients with melanomas of intermediate thickness demonstrated little difference regardless of the Clark's level of invasion.

Both methods continue to be used and reported by pathologists. Some centers prefer to combine Clark's level of invasion and Breslow's thickness measurements. Analysis of the histologic morphology of neoplastic melanocytes can complement these methods for determining prognosis and metastatic pattern (Day et al., 1982a).

Prognostic Indicators

The value of a number of prognostic variables, such as sex, location of tumor, age at diagnosis, diameter of the lesion, elevation of the lesion, history of bleeding, ulceration, pedunculation, number of mitoses, and the presence of a lymphocyte response at the base of the tumor, have been analyzed. Tumor thickness is the single most important prognostic factor with respect to the incidence of nodal occurrence, metastases, and death (Breslow, 1975; Cohen et al., 1976; Drzewiecki et al., 1980a,b; Day et al., 1981a,b,c; Kopf et al., 1981; LeDoussal et al., 1981; Levine et al., 1981; Palanzie et al., 1981; Pondes et al., 1981; Weidner, 1981).

Three categories of risk can be delineated on the basis of tumor thickness, as measured by Breslow's microstaging technique. These rates range from 100% five-year survival for those patients whose lesions measured less than 0.76 mm to 80% for those with lesions measuring between 0.76 to 4.0 mm to 20% for those with lesions larger than 4.0 mm (see Table 21 – 4). Age was considered the variable

that added the most information to the prognosis provided by thickness (Trozak et al., 1974). More recently, only sex and maximum thickness had an important effect on survival of patients in a multifactorial analysis by the WHO collaborating centers that followed 747 stage I patients for approximately nine years (Cascinelli et al., 1980). Furthermore, the effect of gender was not apparent in patients whose maximum tumor thickness did not exceed 2 mm, but women did significantly better when the maximum thickness of the primary was greater than 2 mm. Anatomic site may explain the sex difference noted in overall survival, because trunk lesions occur more frequently in men, and extremity melanomas, which have a better prognosis, are more prevalent in women (Day et al., 1981a; Weidner, 1981). Lesion ulceration and surgical treatment, as well as pathologic stage, location, and thickness were proposed to influence survival rates independently (Balch et al., 1978), but other investigators have not found any of these factors to be independent variables effecting survival (Day et al., 1980, 1982c,d,e; Sober et al., 1977). In stage I patients with a primary lesion thickness ≥ 3.65 mm, a combination of four variables best predicted bone or visceral metastases. These variables included nearly absent or minimal lymphocyte response at the base of the tumor, histologic type other than superficial spreading melanoma, trunk location and positive nodes, or no initial node dissection (Day et al., 1982c).

The clinical course of patients with disseminated melanoma is quite variable and unpredictable, ranging from early death to prolonged survival despite metastases. The variability in clinical presentations results, in part, from the tendency of melanoma to spread by both lymphatic and hematogenous

Table 21 – 4. Prognosis Based on Tumor Thickness

	Day et al., 1982a – e	Balch et al., 1979b, 1980	Cascinelli et al., 1980
Low risk (good prognosis)	<3.6 mm < 6 mitoses/mm² on lower trunk, **or** <3.6 mm on upper trunk < 6 mitoses/mm² + lymphocyte response	<0.76 mm maximum thickness; no ulceration	<2 mm
Intermediate risk (intermediate prognosis)	>3.6 mm thick on lower trunk > 6 mitoses/mm² <3.6 mm on upper trunk no lymphocyte response	0.76 to 3.99 mm maximum thickness	2.01 – 4.0 mm
High risk (poor prognosis)	>3.6 mm thick on upper trunk	>3.99 mm maximum thickness ulceration; >1 mitosis/HPF	>4.01 mm

routes. The marked heterogeneity in clinical manifestations of disseminated disease is depicted in several examples (see Figures 21–10A through 21–10D) that include patients with multiple cutaneous melanotic metastases (*A*), with both melanotic and amelanotic cutaneous lesions (*B*), with disabling leg edema secondary to extensive lymphatic obstruction (*C*), and with marked hepatomegaly and ascites from liver and peritoneal metastases (*D*).

Immunobiology

A number of host factors appear to influence melanoma growth, including the clinical phenomena of spontaneous regression, partial regression of primary melanoma, instances of prolonged *in situ* latency prior to metastases, prolonged intervals between tumor excision and recurrence, and depigmentation surrounding primary and metastatic lesions. Since a correlation was suggested between an-

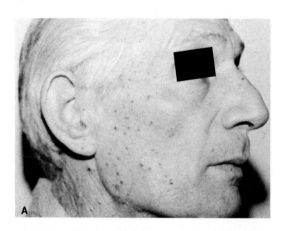

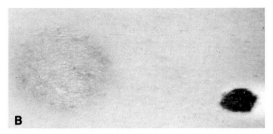

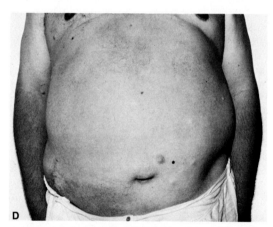

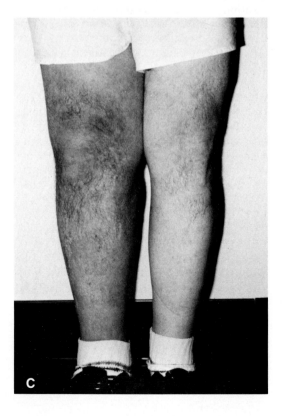

Figure 21–10. The clinical manifestations of disseminated melanoma. Note the marked heterogeneity in presentations, including an individual with multiple facial cutaneous melanotic lesions (*A*), coexistent melanotic and amelanotic cutaneous lesions (*B*), marked extremity lymphedema secondary to extensive lymphatic obstruction (*C*), and ascites with hepatomegaly from peritoneal and liver metastases (*D*).

tibody reactivity and prognosis in patients with melanoma in Uganda (Lewis, 1967), there has been considerable interest in the immunobiology of human melanoma. In this study two cohorts of patients were identified, one with rapid progression of disease until death and the other with prolonged survival. Cytotoxic antibody reactivity to cultured melanoma cells correlated with prolonged survival. Both cell-mediated reactivity and humoral responses, including the formation of antigen-antibody complexes that resulted in the abrogation of cell-mediated cytotoxicity, have been demonstrated (Sjogren *et al.,* 1971; Byrne *et al.,* 1973; Heppner *et al.,* 1973). The clinical importance of these observations is difficult to interpret, however, because of variability in patient and control reactivity when performing *in vitro* microcytotoxicity assays sequentially in the same individual (Heppner *et al.,* 1975). A variety of immunologic assays (see Table 21 – 5) have been performed with material from patients with melanoma in an effort to understand more fully host reactivity to localized, regional, and disseminated disease, as well as alterations induced by therapy.

Recently, more attention has been focused upon identifying and characterizing melanoma-cell associated antigens. These antigens may be identified by means of heterologous antisera or with the use of monoclonal antibodies generated by hybridoma technology (Herlyn *et al.,* 1980; Imai and Ferrone, 1980;

Imai *et al.,* 1981; Morgan *et al.,* 1980; Reisfeld and Ferrone, 1983). An intensive effort is underway to produce monoclonal antibodies with specificity and high affinity for melanoma tissue. One of the best characterized and most specific of these antigens is P97, a 97,000 molecular weight cell surface glycoprotein. Melanomas contain more than 100 times the amount of this glycoprotein compared to normal adult tissues. The P97 glycoprotein is also present in fetal tissue in large amounts, and is found, in lower concentrations, in normal serum and sebaceous glands (Brown *et al.,* 1981). Its amino acid sequence is homologous to serum transferrin. Whether the degree of specificity with this and related antigens can be exploited for potential diagnostic and therapeutic use remains to be determined. Preliminary studies have shown that ^{131}I-labeled Fab fragments of antibody to the P97 glycoprotein localize in metastatic sites of melanoma following intravenous injection. Thus, the monoclonal antibody generated may be sufficiently specific for melanoma tissues to allow selective identification of cancerous tissue. The role of melanoma cell-associated antigens is also of considerable interest in understanding the mechanism involved in regulation of tumor growth, particularly the complex relationships of helper and suppressor cells to antigenic modulation and antigen shedding (Bystryn, 1980).

Spontaneous Regression of Melanoma

A poorly understood phenomenon, which may influence survival in individual patients with melanoma, is spontaneous regression of tumor. Melanoma is the third most common neoplastic disease associated with spontaneous regression, exceeded only by hypernephroma and neuroblastoma and matched by choriocarcinoma. In 176 reported cases of spontaneous regression of neoplasms documented in the world literature between 1900 and 1966 were 19 cases of melanoma, 31 of hypernephroma, 29 of neuroblastoma, and 19 of choriocarcinoma (Everson and Cole, 1966). Spontaneous regression of melanoma has been more recently reviewed (Nathanson, 1976). Spontaneous regression may be more common in melanoma originating in the uveal tract, particularly chorodial melanoma. Halo nevi may somehow be related to the 5% of all melanomas that present with an unknown primary lesion.

Table 21 – 5. Immunologic Assays and Melanoma

Patient Reactivity
  Cytotoxicity
    Antibody-mediated
    Cell-mediated
    Antigen-antibody complexes
    Antibody-dependent (ADCC)
    Leukocyte-dependent
  Immunofluorescence
  Leukocyte adherence inhibition (LAI)
  Leukocyte migration inhibition (LMI)
  Mitogens
  Skin Testing
    Tumor-associated antigens
    DNCB and/or bacterial antigens
  Subpopulations
    T and non-T cells
    Macrophage/monocyte
    Suppressor cells
Detection of Antibody to Melanoma-Associated Antigens
  Antibody binding (and inhibition)
  Double antibody antigen binding
  Complement-dependent microcytotoxicity
  Double antibody radioimmunoassay
  Immune adherence (oncofetal antigen)

Criteria proposed to support the spontaneous regression of unknown primary lesions include: (1) clinical history of a pigmented lesion, compatible with primary melanoma in appearance, situated in an area drained by lymph nodes, involved with tumor; (2) absence of any other primary lesion identifiable on history or physical examination that could represent the original lesion; (3) presence of a typical pigmented or depigmented change in the skin at the site of the suspected primary lesion or histologic changes in the excised site of such a possible primary lesion that supports the clinical evidence of regression of a primary malignant melanoma; and (4) absence of a histologic configuration of primary neoplasm, with or without the presence of melanoma cells, in a typical distribution, in the dermis or subcutaneous tissue, at the site of the lesion (Smith and Stehlin, 1965).

The active phase of spontaneously regressing melanoma is characterized histologically by a dense infiltrate of lymphocytes that disappears when the regression process terminates, leaving vascular scar tissue with a variable number of pigment-containing phagocytes. Distinctive clinical patterns can be observed, including an inflammatory nodule with or without pigmentation, scarring in the tumor, multiple foci of melanoma simulating multi-centricity, a pigmented lesion with a depigmented halo, pigmented scarring with or without surviving melanoma cells, and metastatic melanomas with no demonstrable cutaneous primary (McGovern, 1975). Spontaneous regression of primary cutaneous melanoma has been observed in lesions associated with only radial growth phases, as defined by Clark. Evidence of spontaneous regression ranges from regression and depigmentation in clusters of cells of focal areas in primary cutaneous lesions to total regression of metastases. Thirty-three patients fit strict criteria for the regression of primary cutaneous lesions when reviewed by Nathanson (1976). Forty other patients demonstrated regression of metastatic lesions, but 13 of these 40 were considered doubtful. Regression of metastatic lesions is estimated to account for about 40% of all regressed melanomas.

The occurrence of spontaneous regression of melanoma has been attributed primarily to immunologic and hormonal factors. Six of the cases reported by Cole occurred after blood transfusions or after childbirth. Cytotoxic lymphocyte reactivity against two allogeneic melanoma target cell lines was reported during a clinically observed regression of metastatic melanoma, in the absence of major humoral cytotoxic or blocking activity (Bodurtha et al., 1976). In the immunologic profile of a patient with long-term spontaneous regression of malignant melanoma with visceral metastases (Bulkley et al., 1975), histologic sections of metastatic lesions revealed extensive necrosis of tumor and infiltration with lymphocytes and plasma cells. This patient had strongly positive delayed hypersensitivity responses to dinitrochlorobenzene (DNCB) and to a battery of standard bacterial and fungal antigens, as well as to several extracts prepared from melanoma tissues.

Paradoxically, melanomas with less than 0.76 mm thickness (low risk) may have an increased propensity to metastasize if areas of regression are noted in the specimen. In a series of 121 patients, 5 of 23 (21.7%) patients with evidence of regression had metastases, in contrast to only 2 of 98 (2%) who did not show focal regression (Gromet et al., 1978). Most of these spontaneously regressed lesions occurred in patients with cutaneous metastases, but this phenomenon has been reported in patients with cerebral, intestinal, and nodal involvement.

Modes of Spread

Primary malignant melanoma of the skin spreads by way of the lymphatics and blood stream in local, regional, and distant dissemination (McNeer and DasGupta, 1965). Local metastases generally occur within a 5 cm area around the primary site and may occasionally be amelanotic. Because amelanotic primary cutaneous melanomas are rare, occurring less than 5% of the time, they should be considered metastatic and stimulate a search for a remote primary. Locally recurrent disease, as well as additional primaries, may also mimic local metastatic disease. Spread to regional lymph nodes is most common, occurring in as many as 60% of patients with tumors thicker than 0.76 mm. Distant metastases, however, occur in less than 20% of such cases. Melanomas greater than 3.99 mm in thickness are almost always associated with regional lymph node metastases and a greater than 80% rate of distant metastatic disease. Lymphatic metastases often develop atypically, particularly when primary lesions occur on the trunk. The most frequent sites of visceral metastases include the lungs (70%), liver (68%), and gastrointestinal tract (58%). The heart, bones, and central nervous system (CNS) are also involved in approximately 40% of cases. One-third of patients with biopsy-proven melanoma develop central nervous system involvement, whereas pulmonary involvement and infections are the most common causes of death. The incidence of documented CNS metastases on *post mortem* examination was increased in a recent analysis performed at one institution (Budman *et al.,* 1978).

Local and regional recurrences of melanoma after definitive treatment represent distinct clinical entities. The natural history and pertinent clinical aspects of this subject were reviewed by Lee (1980). There are four types of recurrences: (1) local regrowth of melanoma near the original scar; (2) satellitosis or in-transit metastasis along the line of lymph drainage between the primary site and regional lymph nodes, including both cutaneous and subcutaneous lesions; (3) regional lymph node metastasis; and (4) distant cutaneous, subcutaneous, or visceral metastases. The incidence of local, in-transit, and distant recurrent melanoma ranges from 10 to 30%, whereas it is between 40 to 60% for involvement of the regional lymph nodes. Local and regional recurrences appear within two years in 80% of the stage I patients destined to fail, whereas in-transient and systemic metastases occur later. The likelihood of local and regional recurrences are greater when melanomas (1) occur in the head and neck region; (2) are located distal to the elbows and knees; (3) are in clinical stage II rather than I; and (4) present with pathologically proven metastases in regional nodes. The five-year disease-free percentage of survival after surgical retreatment is 40% for patients with local recurrence and 20 to 30% for those with nodal metastases, although it is more variable for those patients with recurrent satellitosis and is somewhat dependent upon the site of the primary.

Patients with melanoma of the head and neck have a poor prognosis when they develop in-transit regional recurrence, particularly if they present with clinically positive regional lymph nodes (Ames *et al.,* 1976).

Symptoms and Signs

Primary cutaneous melanoma offers few early diagnostic symptoms. Classic symptoms such as bleeding, ulceration, pruritus, and burning occur late in the course of the disease and are of little use for early detection. A number of signs, however, may aid in detecting the presence of malignant melanoma at an early stage in as many as 90% of patients (Mihn *et al.,* 1973). Most of these signs may be found during physical examination of patients with lentigo maligna melanoma, superficial spreading melanoma, and acral-lentiginous melanoma. Nodular melanoma offers few early signs and is generally discovered much too late to offer a good prognosis for cure. Early signs of melanoma include:

1. Irregular borders or "notching" in the peripheral border of a lesion ("notching" is believed to represent an area of tumor destruction or regression in an active melanoma);
2. Variation in color or a play of colors. Color differences represent a number of biophysical phenomena: Heavy deposits of melanin pigment in the dermis and epidermis (black, steel gray, and blue), regression of tumor (pink to white), inflammation (pink to red), and loss of pigment and reduced tumor activity in a previously active area (white). A clinical diagnosis of melanoma during pregnancy is difficult, however, because benign nevi often darken intensely at this time;
3. Change in surface characteristics, such as the development of an irregular surface in a formerly flat lesion; and
4. An increase in size of a previously static "mole."

The symptoms and signs of regional melanoma correlate primarily with the location and extent of nodal involvement. Symptoms may be minimal or absent in patients whose nodes are small or are only detected during a thorough physical examination. In other situations, extensive nodal involvement may cause disabling edema of an extremity, pain, weakness, muscular atrophy, deformity, ulceration, and bleeding as the involved lymph nodes become enlarged.

Symptoms and signs in patients with disseminated melanoma frequently include pain, organ dysfunction or failure, bleeding, swelling, or neurologic abnormalities. Many patients, however, are asymptomatic in spite of multiple, small, metastatic deposits.

Patients often present with symptoms referable to metastatic involvement. Frequently,

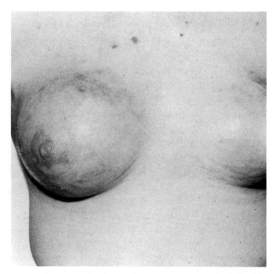

Figure 21-11. Malignant melanoma presenting with bilateral breast involvement.

although not always, a primary lesion can be found in these patients. If the primary lesion is not obvious, a thorough funduscopic examination and inspection of the nasal mucosa, subungual regions, perirectal and vaginal areas may be helpful. Rarely, melanoma presents in the breast (see Figure 21-11).

The symptoms and signs associated with metastatic melanoma may be as varied as the clinical presentation of the disease. With extensive hepatic metastases, anorexia, weight loss, and malaise are frequently noted; other patients with liver metastases, however, may be asymptomatic. In contrast to the relatively

frequent observation of multiple cutaneous deposits, an occasional patient may present with generalized hyperpigmentation, the "melanosis" syndrome usually associated with hepatic metastases (see Figure 21-12).

The etiology of the melanosis syndrome remains obscure. It has been attributed to several factors, including the oxidation of melanin precursors either in the circulation or in dermal histiocytes (Fitzpatrick *et al.,* 1954), the deposition in the skin of pigment granules originating from the primary tumor or from metastases (Silberberg *et al.,* 1968), or the cutaneous dissemination of individual melanoma cells capable of continued production of pigment (Konrad and Wolff, 1974; Schuler *et al.,* 1980). This syndrome is extremely rare, with about 20 well-documented cases. A nude mouse model, produced by heterotransplantation of a human primary malignant melanoma obtained from a patient with generalized melanosis, may help in our understanding of the etiology of this obscure syndrome (Spremulli *et al.,* 1983). The melanosis developed and became progressive as the tumor burden in the nude mice increased, similar to the clinical course of the patient from whom the melanoma was obtained. Light and electron micrographic examination of tissues from these animals showed disseminated tumor with pigment deposition in all organs with the ultrastructural features of melanoma cells, as described by Zelickson, 1962. Light and electron microscopic examination of melanotic skin obtained from both the donor patient and the mice hosting the tumor xenograft failed to re-

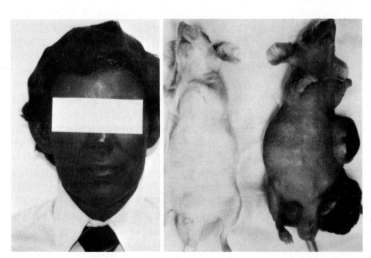

Figure 21-12. Human and murine examples of the generalized "melanosis" syndrome.

veal melanoma cells dispersed in the dermis but suggested that the hyperpigmentation was produced by melanosomes and melanin pigment within phagosomes of dermal macrophages, endothelial cells, pericytes, and, occasionally, fibroblasts.

Melanuria may also be seen in patients with widespread melanoma. Melanin is a pigment derived from tyrosine. A precursor of melanin, a conjugate of 5,6-dihydroxyindole, is excreted in the urine and polymerizes into a dark pigment on standing at room temperature. A ferric chloride test for melanin is positive if the urine precipitate turns black, and the nitroprusside test is positive if a red color in alkaline solution turns to green, blue, or black with acidification (Henry, 1979). Urine chromatography can also identify melanin or precursors (Blois and Banda, 1976).

Melanoma is the solid tumor with the greatest propensity to spread to the central nervous system, although this situation is more common in patients with metastatic lung or breast cancer, because these cancers occur with greater frequency (Aronson et al., 1964; Bullard et al., 1981; American Cancer Society, 1983). Changes in mental status are strongly suggestive of central nervous system metastases. Neurologic abnormalities found during physical examination often herald the onset of cerebral metastases. Cranial computerized transaxial tomography can usually confirm the presence of metastases. Metastases are frequently multiple. The longer the interval from the time of initial diagnosis to recurrence the greater the likelihood that a cerebral metastasis is solitary. In patients with lung metastases from melanoma, symptoms include cough, dyspnea, and hemoptysis. Pericardial or myocardial metastases should be suspected in patients who develop pericardial rubs or cardiac arrythmias. Gastrointestinal bleeding may indicate metastatic involvement of the bowel, particularly the small intestine. Characteristic lesions have been described on gastrointestinal roentgenograms. Resection of bowel may be necessary to control bleeding from this source. Bone pain may occur with osseous metastases, which can be disabling and refractory to treatment. Unexplained symptoms even many years later in patients with a history of primary melanoma should provoke a strong suspicion for recurrence because of the high risk of dissemination and the tendency for a long latency period.

Diagnosis

Although the incidence and mortality rates of melanoma are increasing, more early lesions are being detected. Increased curability is related to awareness of the four simple criteria for early detection and diagnosis listed above. Suspicious pigmented lesions should be removed, not observed for further development. Although a number of benign pigmented lesions will be removed, the outcome of advanced melanoma is so devastating that it is better to err on the side of caution. The entire lesion should be excised for histopathologic examination, because microstaging techniques are valid only for the entire lesion and are extremely valuable in determining the subsequent approach to treatment (Breslow and Macht, 1977; Balch et al., 1979a,b; Day et al., 1979; Day et al., 1981c). When a suspicious lesion is too large for total excisional biopsy, is cosmetically disfiguring, or is located in a hazardous area, an incisional biopsy for diagnostic purposes may be necessary. No evidence exists that a simple excisional biopsy or a resection close to the borders of a tumor mass decreases the rate of survival if followed within three weeks by a proper therapeutic surgical procedure (Jones et al., 1968; Epstein et al., 1969; Drzewiecki et al., 1980b). The depth of tumor invasion cannot be determined using material obtained by incisional biopsy.

The diagnosis of regional melanoma can only be confirmed by histologic examination of excised lymph nodes. It is often suspected clinically in the presence of one or more of the above symptoms and signs but may not be suspected if the lymph nodes are small and symptoms are absent. Regional tumor invasion should be suspected in all patients who present with a primary cutaneous melanoma. At times the diagnosis of stage II or regional melanoma is only established by histologic examination of nodal tissue removed in a prophylactic radical node dissection or after an abnormal lymphangiogram (LaMonica et al., 1976).

Confirmation of recurrence or metastasis in any suspicious area is obtained only by appropriate biopsy. This is not always feasible, however, and recurrence may be sufficiently documented by physical examination, routine chemical analysis of blood, and conventional roentgenograms, ultrasonography, computerized tomography, and radionuclide scans.

Once the diagnosis of primary cutaneous melanoma is established, further diagnostic studies may be indicated to determine the extent of extracutaneous involvement. Patients with lesions less than 0.76 mm thickness require no further investigation, because the incidence of extracutaneous or distant involvement is practically nonexistent. Patients with lesions thicker than 0.76 mm and patients with acral-lentiginous melanoma require more extensive staging procedures. Careful examination of the skin and regional lymph nodes is of great importance. Clinical involvement of the lymph nodes is associated with a high incidence of metastatic disease at distant sites.

Whether metastases are solely cutaneous and lymphatic or whether visceral organs, such as liver or lung, are involved is also important, because a much poorer prognosis is associated with the latter. Information concerning the location and extent of metastatic involvement is extremely helpful in determining the best overall approach to management of the patient.

Every new patient with melanoma (Clark's level III or greater or 0.76 mm or thicker by Breslow's criteria) should be evaluated for the presence of metastatic disease at diagnosis. Radionuclide scans of the liver, bones, and brain should be obtained routinely in addition to a chest x-ray film and a chemistry profile. Although metastases are not frequently detected (Felix *et al.,* 1975), and the percentage of false positive liver scans may be high (Hatfield, 1975), baseline studies are useful for later comparisons when the patient develops symptoms, particularly when symptoms are referable to bone or to the central nervous system. Abdominal and pelvic ultrasonography and computerized tomography may be the best methods to detect intra-abdominal and pelvic metastases (Meyer, 1978; Doiron and Bernardino, 1981).

Staging

Table 21–6 outlines the staging of melanoma. Disease limited to a single cutaneous site or associated with satellites within 3 cm of the primary lesion and without positive regional nodes or metastases is defined as stage I. Positive regional lymph nodes with histologic evidence of melanoma, in the absence of other evidence of spread, is considered stage II. Patients with disseminated melanoma are classified as stage III. Others prefer a four-stage system, in which stage II includes satellite lesions

Table 21–6. Clinical Stagings of Melanoma

Stage I: Localized melanoma
Stage II: Regional metastases
Stage III: Distant metastases

or

Stage I: Primary cutaneous melanoma
Stage II: Local satellitosis (≤ 5 cm from primary)
Stage III: Regional metastases (> 5 cm from primary)
  A: Intradermal, subcutaneous, in-transit (vascular and lymphatic)
  B: Lymph nodes
  AB: Both
Stage IV: Distant metastases

≤ 5 cm from the primary site and distant metastases represent stage IV. Patients with metastases more than 5 cm from the primary lesion are subdivided into: IIIA, representing intradermal, subcutaneous, and in-transit metastases; IIIB, which indicates regional lymph node involvement; and IIIAB, a designation for both types of metastases.

A staging system for malignant melanoma was proposed by the American Joint Committee for Cancer Staging and End-Results Reporting (see Table 21–7) (Ketcham and Christopherson, 1979). This classification, however, has yet to gain wide acceptance or usage. It is based upon an analysis of the noteworthy characteristics noted in 1700 cases, including levels of invasion, thickness of penetration, and the incidence of nodal involvement and distant metastases.

OTHER TYPES OF PRIMARY MELANOMA

Other forms of melanoma (see Table 21–8) are recognized by the American Joint Committee for Staging and the International Union Against Cancer (UICC) and are usually classified separately from the five cutaneous varieties described. Several generalizations regarding this group of diseases have been summarized (Clark *et al.,* 1975). Melanomas arising in small congenital nevi, blue nevi, or dermal nevi are rare, although melanoma arising in giant hairy nevi and in congenital nevi over 2 cm occur with greater frequency. Forty percent of childhood melanomas arise in congenital nevi, usually of the giant hairy type. Melanomas developing in many of these nevi are associated with rapid dissemination and a poor prognosis. Childhood melanomas are pathologically indistinguishable from adult melanomas and biologically behave like simi-

Table 21-7. Melanoma Staging System Proposed by the American Joint Committee for Cancer Staging End-Results

Primary tumor (T)
TX: No evidence of primary tumor (unknown primary, or primary tumor removed and not histologically examined)
T0: Atypical melanocytic hyperplasia (Clark's level I); not a malignant lesion
T1: Invasion of papillary dermis (level II) or 0.75 mm thick or less
T2: Invasion of the papillary-reticular-dermal interface (level III) or 0.76 to 1.5 mm thick
T3: Invasion of the reticular dermis (level IV) or 1.51 to 4.0 mm thick
T4: Invasion of subcutaneous tissue (level V) or 4.1 mm or greater thickness, or satellite(s) within 2 cm of any primary melanoma

Nodal involvement (N)
NX: Minimum requirements to assess the regional nodes cannot be met
N0: No regional lymph node involvement
N1: Involvement of only one regional lymph node station; node(s) movable and not over 5 cm in diameter, or negative regional lymph nodes and the presence of less than five in-transit metastases beyond 2 cm from the primary site
N2: Any one of the following: (1) Involvement of more than one regional lymph node station; (2) regional node(s) over 5 cm in diameter or fixed; (3) five or more in-transit metastases or any in-transit metastases beyond 2 cm from the primary site with regional lymph node involvement

Distant metastasis (M)
MX: Not assessed
M0: No known distant metastasis
M1: Involvement of skin or subcutaneous tissue beyond the site of primary lymph node drainage
Specify ————————————————
M2: Visceral metastasis (spread to any distant site other than skin or subcutaneous tissues)
Specify ————————————————

TNM STAGE GROUPS

Stage	TNM Group
Stage IA	T1, N0, M0
Stage IB	T2, N0, M0
Stage IIA	T3, N0, M0
Stage IIB	T4, N0, M0
Stage III	Any T, N1, M0
Stage IV	Any T, N2, M0
	Any T, N2, M0
	Any T, any N, M1 or M2

Table 21-8. Other Types of Melanoma

A. Extraocular
   1. Melanoma arising in a:
      (a) Giant-hairy nevus
      (b) Blue nevus
      (c) Visceral site
      (d) Dermal nevus
   2. Melanoma without demonstrable primary lesion
   3. Melanoma of childhood
B. Ocular

(Boutin, 1958). Most melanomas that present without a demonstrable primary usually originated from lesions that have spontaneously regressed, have been removed or destroyed previously without recollection, or are situated deep in the skin. The true incidence of spontaneously regressed melanoma is unknown, but the percent of occult primary lesions ranges from less than 4 to 15% in several collected series (DasGupta *et al.,* 1963; Smith and Stehlin, 1965; Brownstein and Helwig, 1972; Einhorn *et al.,* 1974; Baab and McBride, 1975).

Melanomas of the oral, nasal, vaginal, and anal cavities are of mucous membrane origin and are usually classified as acral-lentiginous melanoma. Ocular melanoma is also considered a separate entity. Each of these disorders has distinct clinical manifestations and unique principles of appropriate surgical management. A thorough discussion of these features is beyond the scope of this chapter. Additional references describe these conditions and their management in greater detail (Clark *et al.,* 1975, 1983; American Cancer Society, 1976; Graham and Duane, 1980; Ariel, 1981; Seigler, 1983).

Therapy

Surgical Considerations. *Localized Cutaneous Melanoma.* Historical surgical therapy for localized primary cutaneous melanoma is excisional biopsy, followed by wide resection with a margin of 4 to 5 cm surrounding the primary lesion. Skin grafting is often necessary to cover the resected area. Although this has been the accepted conventional surgical therapy for primary melanomas, recent publications suggest that a smaller, 1.5- to 3-cm, margin of resection might be acceptable for patients with superficial stage I lesions (Day *et al.,* 1982b). Several institutions are currently evaluating this approach.

More specialized sources discuss in detail surgical considerations for various localized noncutaneous melanomas, because therapeu-

lar lesions in adults. Melanomas in a visceral site are uncommon and may occur in unusual locations such as the tracheobronchial tree (Reid and Mehta, 1966), esophagus (Musher and Linder, 1974), gallbladder (Walsh, 1956), uterine cervix (Jones *et al.,* 1971), bladder (Ainsworth *et al.,* 1975), and leptomeninges

tic approaches may vary depending upon the site of the primary. It is important to understand that local wide excision affects local recurrence of tumor only and has no relationship to metastasis or distant spread of tumor.

Regional Melanoma. Clinically suspicious regional lymph nodes should be removed as a therapeutic procedure. Prophylactic lymph node resection in patients with small primaries of the extremity and clinically negative regional lymph nodes, however, is controversial. Prophylactic dissection has been advocated for prognostic information and because approximately 15% of clinically negative lymph nodes harbor microscopically positive metastases (Fortner *et al.*, 1977). The impact of these features upon results in patients with Clark's levels II and III has been examined, but little conclusive information is available regarding patients with deeper, level IV, primary lesions, that is, those at a greater risk for lymphatic and distant dissemination. Patients with level IV lesions may potentially benefit from prophylactic radical node dissection (Wanebo *et al.*,

1975; Holmes *et al.*, 1976; DasGupta, 1977; Fortner *et al.*, 1977; Goldsmith, 1979; Cascinelli, 1980). One randomized study does not support the concept of immediate prophylactic regional node dissection in clinical stage I melanoma (Veronesi *et al.*, 1977). In the largest prospective randomized trial designed to evaluate the efficacy of elective lymph node dissection in the treatment of small melanomas of the extremities, 553 cases underwent excision of primary melanoma and then either had an immediate regional lymph node dissection or a similar procedure when metastases in the nodes appeared. The overall results are shown in Figure 21–13. No statistical advantage was evident in terms of survival for the group undergoing an immediate lymph node dissection. These conclusions, however, apply only to those patients with melanomas of the extremities, without clinically palpable regional nodes, and only to those who can be followed closely to detect recurrence early. The conclusions based on this large trial have been challenged because of suggested inherent

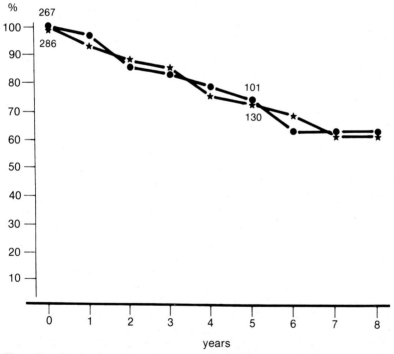

Figure 21–13. Survival of 553 melanoma patients with $T_{1.2.3}N_0M_0$ of the limb according to treatment with excision combined with immediate lymph node dissection (●) and excision (★) (node dissection at appearance of regional metastases). From Veronesi, U.; Adamus, J.; Bandeira, D. C.; Brennhovd, I. O.; Caceres, E.; Cascinelli, N.; Claudio, F.; Ikonopisov, R. L.; Javorski, V. V.; Kirov, S.; Kulakowski, A.; Lacour, J.; Lejeune, F.; Mechl, Z.; Morabito, A.; Rodi, I.; Serguv, S.; van Slooten, E.; Szczygiel, K.; Tropeznikov, N. N.; and Wagner, R. I.: Inefficacy of immediate node dissection in stage I melanoma of the limbs. *N. Engl. J. Med.,* **297**:627–630, 1977. Reprinted by permission of the *New England Journal of Medicine.*

weaknesses in the study. Criticisms include the high proportion of women in the study, the potential influences of geographic variations upon outcome, and the fact that only 60% of the cases had histologic review and analysis of the relative risk of recurrence based upon level of invasion, thickness of the tumor, and size of the primary lesion (Wanebo *et al.,* 1975; Krementz, 1977; Melanoma Cooperative Groups, 1978; Cascinelli, 1980). Several experienced surgeons have expressed reservations, particularly with respect to deeper, Clark's level IV, lesions, that the number of patients with deeper lesions included in the trial is too small to reach any definitive conclusions concerning the appropriate surgical approach in this situation. Because the risk of spread to regional lymph nodes is greatest in this group, these are the patients who potentially would benefit the most from an immediate lymph node dissection. Randomized studies to support these contentions, however, have yet to be performed.

Disseminated Melanoma. Radical surgical resection is usually not indicated in patients with disseminated melanoma. Surgical procedures, however, may be useful in conjunction with other therapeutic modalities (Bottino *et al.,* 1978). In specific situations, such as resection of a solitary pulmonary metastasis, 15 to 20% of patients can survive for at least five years (Cohan, 1973; Beattie, 1978).

Surgery also has a role in treating patients with disseminated cutaneous metastases restricted to a single extremity. These patients are candidates for isolated regional limb perfusion with chemotherapy alone or in conjunction with hyperthermia.

Systemic Therapies for Melanoma. *Immunotherapy.* Randomized trials with large numbers of patients have failed to demonstrate convincingly the benefits of adjuvant immunotherapy or immunochemotherapy for treating patients with local, regional or disseminated melanoma (Bajetta, 1982; Cunningham *et al.,* 1982; Quirt *et al.,* 1982; Terry *et al.,* 1982; Veronesi *et al.,* 1982). Veronesi and colleagues (1981), reporting for the World Health Organization, did not observe any differences in overall disease-free intervals (see Figure 21–14) and survivals for 761 patients randomly allocated to receive postoperative chemotherapy with dimethyl-triazeno-imidazole-carboxamide (DTIC), immunotherapy with BCG, combined BCG plus DTIC, or no postoperative treatment. This was disappoint-

ing in view of the initial report of Eilber *et al.* (1976) describing improved disease-free and overall survival rates in patients with a single positive axillary lymph node who received adjuvant BCG following excision and wide resection of their primary melanoma and an axillary lymph node dissection. Although a subsequent randomized study confirmed their results, the improved survival only followed recurrence (Morton *et al.,* 1982).

The current studies of specific immunotherapy, including the investigation of immune interferon for activity in melanoma, will extend the present approaches in this area. Modest antitumor activity observed in melanoma patients treated by various immunologic manipulations has raised the possibility that the early impure preparation, or more recent preparations of interferon obtained by recombinant DNA methodologies, may be useful for treating certain melanoma patients (Creagon *et al.,* 1984). The applicability and limitations of interferon in melanoma have yet to be fully described. More recent extensive clinical trials of purified interferon in other diseases have proven disappointing, although even these results are preliminary.

Intralesional injections of BCG, or the methanol extractable residue of BCG (MER), may result in tumor regression of small cutaneous lesions (Mastrangelo *et al.,* 1976; Krown *et al.,* 1978; Lokich *et al.,* 1979). For a thorough review of this subject see Rosenberg and Rapp (1976). Other reported studies used various immunotherapeutic compounds for intralesional injection, including dinitrochlorobenzene (DNCB) (Cohen *et al.,* 1978) and the cell wall skeleton of *Mycobacterium smegmatis* with trehalose dimycolate (Vosika *et al.,* 1979). Intralesional therapy is investigational and seems best suited for those patients with multiple small cutaneous lesions rather than those with nodal or visceral metastases or larger cutaneous or subcutaneous masses, although, on occasion, even injected pulmonary metastases will respond (Morton *et al.,* 1974). Interestingly, even uninjected lesions were noted to regress after intralesional injections of other cutaneous metastases.

Reports of adverse reactions after injection of BCG for immunotherapy include disseminated BCG infection associated with fever, liver function abnormalities, and hepatic and bone marrow granulomas, as well as impaired *in vitro* lymphocyte reactivity (Sparks *et al.,* 1976; Rosenberg *et al.,* 1978). After oral BCG,

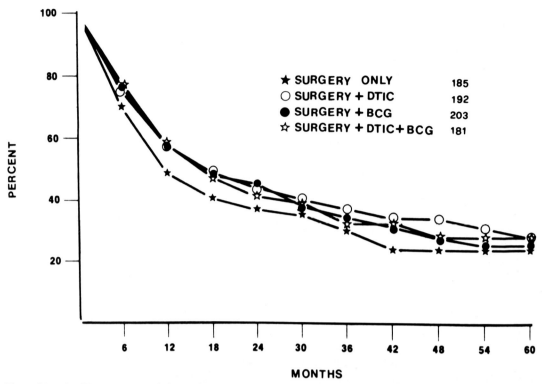

Figure 21–14. The percentage of disease-free patients of 761 evaluable cases, according to treatment with surgery only (☆), surgery plus DTIC (dacarbazine) (O), surgery plus BCG (●), or surgery plus combined DTIC and BCG (★). From Veronesi, U.; Adamus, J.; Aubert, C.; Bajetta, G.; Beretta, G.; Bonadonna, G.; Bufalino, R.; Cascinelli, N.; Cocconi, G.; Durand, J.; DeMarsillae, J.; Ikonopisov, R. L.; Kiss, B.; Lejeune, F.; MacKie, R.; Madej, G.; Mulder, H.; Mechl, Z.; Milton, G. W.; Morabito, A.; Peter, H.; Priario, J.; Paul, E.; Rumke, P.; Sertoli, R.; and Tomin, R.: A randomized trial of adjuvant chemotherapy and immunotherapy in cutaneous melanoma. *N. Engl. J. Med.,* **307**:913–916, 1982. Reprinted by permission of the *New England Journal of Medicine.*

pneumonitis and ascites were observed (Nutting and McPherson, 1976; Schapira and McPherson, 1977). Nephrotoxicity may result from intravenous administration of *Corynebacterium parvum* (Dosik *et al.,* 1978). The adverse effects of intralesional injections of BCG include severe thrombocytopenia (Norton *et al.,* 1978) and life-threatening allergic reactions (Robinson, 1977).

Chemotherapy. The overall results with systemic chemotherapy for managing disseminated melanoma are extremely disappointing, although occasional dramatic responses have been observed with individual patients. Chemotherapy is administered most frequently for palliation of stage III or IV disease, although it has also been used alone and in combination with immunotherapy as adjuvant postoperative therapy for patients with stage I or stage II disease. The most active single agents currently available are dimethyl-triazeno-imidazole carboxamide (DTIC),

and the nitrosoureas, (methylcyclohexyl-, bis-chloroethyl- and cyclohexyl-nitrosourea [MeCCNU, BCNU, and CCNU]). Response rates are in the range of 20% for each of these agents. The response rates reported with individual chemotherapeutic compounds, as well as various combinations, are listed in Table 21–9 and have been reviewed in the literature (Luce, 1975; Benjamin *et al.,* 1976; Lejeune and DeWasch, 1978; Nathanson, 1982).

Results with several chemotherapeutic agents with unique properties thought potentially useful in treating melanoma are generally disappointing. The diethyl derivative of imidazole carboxamide, TIC mustard, appeared more active than DTIC in preclinical studies but had an overall response rate of less than 10%. Melphalan, synthesized as an analog of phenylalanine, a precursor of melanin, also has a disappointingly low response rate of 10%. The same is true for bleomycin, which localizes in the skin. This agent, however, may

Table 21–9. Chemotherapy of Melanoma

SINGLE AGENTS	NUMBER OF RESPONSES/ NUMBER OF EVALUABLE PATIENTS	RESPONSE RATE (%)
Alkylating Agents		
Nitrogen mustard	2/40	5%
Cyclophosphamide	13/59	22
Melphalan	10/110	9
BCNU	22/122	18
CCNU	17/135	13
Methyl CCNU	15/87	17
DTIC	198/806	25
TIC mustard	7/87	8
Mitomycin C	11/68	16
Antimetabolites		
5-Fluorouracil	1/28	4%
Methotrexate	2/19	10
6-Mercaptopurine	4/59	7
Arabinosyl cytosine	3/27	11
Hydroxyurea	24/200	12
Vinca alkaloids		
Vincristine	6/30	20%
Vinblastine	28/137	20
Vindesine	15/96	16
Antibiotics		
Actinomycin D	14/80	18%
Podophyllotoxins		
VP-16	1/76	1%
VM-26	0/26	0
Miscellaneous		
Cisplatin	9/57	16%
Procarbazine	8/29	28
Tamoxifen	8/62	13
m-AMSA	2/62	3
Dibromodulcitol	5/25	20
Combinations		
BCNU + DTIC + vincristine (BVD)	82/305	27%
BCNU + DTIC + hydroxyurea (BHD)	24/89	27
BCNU + DTIC + actinomycin D (BAD)	12/36	33
BCNU + DTIC	12/61	20
Methyl CCNU + DTIC	6/26	23
DTIC + Cisplatin	16/75	21
Cisplatin + bleomycin + vinblastine	16/40	47

be useful in combination with other compounds. The acridine orange derivative, m-AMSA, binds to melanosomes, selectively concentrates in the liver, and has an overall response rate in melanoma of less than 5%. The antiestrogen tamoxifen may be a useful compound in selected patients with estrogen-receptor positive melanoma tissue, although the overall response rate is only 12%. Whether responses noted with tamoxifen are a direct antitumor effect of the drug or are related to alterations in gonadotrophic hormone levels is unclear. An oral synthetic nitrosourea, urea-chloroethyl - dioxo - piperidyl - nitrosourea (PCNU), showed some activity in early studies

of melanoma patients, but its activity and true response rate relative to other nitrosoureas will not be known until more patients are treated.

In an effort to improve upon the results with the most active single agents, a number of combination chemotherapy regimens have been devised. These include the combination of BCNU, vincristine, and DTIC (BVD); BCNU or methyl CCNU and DTIC; and BCNU or DTIC plus vincristine (Luce, 1975; Benjamin *et al.,* 1976; Cohen *et al.,* 1977). Unfortunately, the overall objective response rates with these combinations are not much higher than those observed with either DTIC,

BCNU, or methyl CCNU when taking into account important prognostic variables, such as sex, sites of disease, and performance status. Several three- and four-drug-combination chemotherapy regimens have suggested improved response rates with small numbers of patients, but the response rates drop dramatically to 20 to 25% when larger numbers of patients are evaluated.

Cis-platinum, one of the more active single agents available today, has a disappointingly low response rate of 16% when used alone. Recently, however, it was used in combination with DTIC and other compounds. Preliminary results in a small number of patients using *cis*-platinum in combination with vinblastine and bleomycin suggested an improved response rate (Nathanson *et al.*, 1981), but this has not been noted by others (Bajetta *et al.*, 1982).

Another chemotherapeutic approach used for a number of years by several institutions is regional perfusion. The chemotherapeutic agent common to all of these trials is phenylalanine mustard (melphalan). Some investigators have added hyperthermia to the regional perfusion technique (Stehlin *et al.*, 1977). Improved five-year and ten-year survival rates have been claimed with regional perfusion, with or without hyperthermia, for treating recurrent melanoma or metastases confined to a single extremity (Stehlin *et al.*, 1979) and for certain patients with stage I or regional melanoma (Krementz, 1976a). These provocative findings are extremely difficult to assess because none of the results were obtained in randomized controlled clinical trials that take into account more fully the important prognostic variables known to affect outcome. Regional perfusion following node dissection and wide excision and skin grafting can produce complications. Infectious or inflammatory in nature, they may include severe, persistent edema, thrombophlebitis, and leukopenia secondary to chemotherapy. Complications occurred in 28% of 726 perfusions reported by Krementz (1976a).

Hormone Therapy. Receptors for estrogen, progesterone, testosterone, and glucocorticoids have been found in human melanoma tissue (Neifeld and Lippman, 1980), and responses in melanoma patients treated with hormonal agents have been reported. Larger patient numbers are required, however, to determine the exact benefit of this approach when used alone or in combination with other drugs.

Radiation Therapy

Radiation therapy is not effective as a primary treatment for melanoma. It has been used occasionally with corticosteroids for the palliation of central nervous system metastases and for the relief of bone pain from osseous spread, but beneficial effects are minimal and may simply be related to anti-inflammatory reduction of edema and not to antineoplastic activity. Compared to other tumors, such as carcinoma of the breast or lymphomas, melanoma is a relatively radioresistant neoplasm. Although conventional dose fractionation schedules of radiation therapy have not been very effective in controlling melanoma, better control might be achieved with maximum individual treatment doses in the range of 600 to 1000 rads or higher (Habermalz and Fischer, 1976). Several clinical trials employing high-dose fractionation irradiation schedules are in progress.

Results of endolymphatic therapy using the radioactive isotope ^{32}P in a randomized trial of selected cases have suggested that this approach may reduce the number of regional node recurrences (Edwards, 1981).

Supportive Measures

In patients who develop central nervous system involvement, corticosteroids often reverse neurologic deficits by reducing cerebral swelling secondary to metastases.

Analgesics and narcotics are often needed to control the pain accompanying bone metastases. Usually oral medications in the form of narcotics, such as morphine, hydromorphone hydrochloride, Brompton's solution, or methadone are effective. Occasionally, parenteral medications are required to achieve sufficient analgesia. Recently, the instillation of morphine into the intraventricular or subarachnoid spaces, using either an Omaya reservoir or an implantable pump and catheter, has provided substantial pain relief. Other neurologic procedures, including chordotomy and rhizotomy, may be required for the management of pain.

Rehabilitation

Rehabilitation is an important aspect of management after resection of primary or regional disease. For individuals with ocular melanoma who require enucleation, a prosthesis often provides acceptable cosmetic results. Plastic surgery procedures can sometimes compensate for the defects incurred in achieving successful local control of a primary melanoma on the face, trunk, or an extremity. Physical therapy in patients who have had axillary node dissections often prevents the development of contractures and immobility of the shoulder girdle that sometimes results. Considerable psychosocial support is necessary for both hospitalized and ambulatory patients as well as for their families. A combination of professional and volunteer organizations, such as the American Cancer Society and the hospice movement, can often provide this support (see Chapters 48 and 49).

Follow Up. Appropriate follow-up for patients with primary melanomas requires regular, thorough cutaneous examinations as well as laboratory and radiologic evaluation to detect recurrences in the lung and liver early. Most recurrences after primary resections take place within the first two years. Patients should be examined four times a year for the first two years, then twice a year for several additional years, and eventually yearly. Quarterly chest roentgenograms and liver function tests, and yearly bone scans, are usually performed during the first two years. Occasionally, early detection of recurrence may allow successful resection of a solitary pulmonary metastasis or other accessible lesions.

Future Prospects

Melanoma continues to stimulate the interests of basic scientists and clinical investigators. Major efforts are being devoted to a variety of promising new approaches founded upon the development of modern technologies and a better understanding of the cellular mechanisms and immunobiology of this heterogeneous disease.

The reality of hybridoma technology has generated the hope that monoclonal antibodies specific for melanoma antigens can be developed and will prove useful in diagnosis and therapy. Additional immunotherapeutic and chemotherapeutic approaches are being explored in the experimental murine B-16 melanoma model that has proved useful to study the development of metastasis and the role of macrophages in the regression of metastases with liposome-encapsulated macrophage activating factor (MAF) (Fidler, 1980; Honn et al., 1981).

Recombinant DNA techniques for inserting a specific diphtheria gene sequence into the structural composition of melanin-stimulating hormone (MSH) could result in a product highly specific for melanoma cells, because MSH-specific receptors do exist exclusively on the surface of melanocytes (Bacha et al., 1983).

Modulation of melanoma growth and differentiation is being studied intensively, because a variety of hormonal and trophic factors including polypeptides, thymus-derived factors, and vitamins A and C exert effects upon melanoma cells (Meyskens, 1981). Cultured human melanoma cells can be stimulated into terminal differentiation by treatment with tumor-promoting agents, such as the phorbol esters and dimethyl sulfoxide (DMSO) (Huberman et al., 1979). Similar effects upon human colon carcinoma cells were noted using other maturational compounds (Dexter et al., 1979). Two derivatives of formamide, N-methyl (NMF) and di-methyl (DMF) also have antitumor activity in vitro and in vivo and influence response to radiation and to other chemotherapeutic compounds (Dexter et al., 1982; Leith et al., 1982). Clearly, further clinical and experimental studies of maturational agents are warranted to determine their potential usefulness in melanoma (Calabresi et al., 1979; Dexter and Calabresi, 1982). Planned studies will evaluate their effectiveness in terms of changing the melanoma cell characteristics and aggressiveness, including its potential for metastatic spread and susceptibility to pharmacologic and immunologic manipulations.

REFERENCES

Ainsworth, A. M.; Clark, W. H., Jr.; Mastrangelo, M. J; and Conger, K. B.: Primary malignant melanoma of the urinary bladder. *Cancer,* **37**:1928–1936, 1976.

Allen, A., and Spitz, S.: Malignant melanoma—A clinicopathologic analysis of the criteria for diagnosis and prognosis. *Cancer,* **6**:1–45, 1953.

Amer, M. H.; Al-Saffar, M.; Baker, L. H.; and Vaitkevicius, V. K.: Malignant melanoma and central nervous system metastases. *Cancer,* **42**:660–668, 1978.

American Cancer Society: *Cancer Facts and Figures.* American Cancer Society, New York, 1976.

Ames, F. C.; Sugarbaker, E. V.; and Ballantyne, A. J.: Analysis of survival and disease control in stage I melanoma of the head and neck. *Am. J. Surg.,* **132**:484–491, 1976.

Ancher, N.; Popov, I.; and Ikonopisov, R. L.: Epidemiology of malignant melanoma in Bulgaria in Della Porta. In Muehlbock, O. (ed.): *Structure and Control of the Melanocytes: Proceedings, International Pigment Cell Conference.* Springer-Verlag New York, Inc., New York, 1966.

Ariel, I. M.: *Malignant Melanoma.* Appleton-Century-Crofts, New York, 1981.

Aronson, S. M.; Garcia, J. H.; and Aronson, B. E.: Metastatic neoplasms of the brain: Their frequency in relation to age. *Cancer,* **17:**558–563, 1964.

Arrington, J. H., III; Reed, R. J.; Ichinose, H.; and Krementz, E. T.: Plantar lentiginous melanoma. A distinctive variant of human cutaneous malignant melanoma. *Am. J. Surg. Pathol.,* **1:**131–143, 1977.

Baab, G. H., and McBride, C. M.: Malignant melanoma: The patient with an unknown site of primary origin. *Arch. Surg.,* **110:**896, 1975.

Bacha, P.; Murphy, J. R.; and Reichlin, S.: Organ-specific binding of a thyrotropin-releasing hormone-diphtheria toxin complex after intravenous administration to rats. *Endocrinology,* **113:**1072–1076, 1983.

Bahn, A. K.; Rosenwaike, I.; Hermann, N.; Grover, P.; Stillman, J.; and O'Leary, K.: (letter) Melanoma after exposure to PCB's. *N. Engl. J. Med.,* **295:**450, 1976.

Bajetta, E.; Rovej, R.; Buzzoni, R.; Vaglini, M.; and Bonadonna, G.: Treatment of advanced malignant melanoma with vinblastine, bleomycin and cisplatin. *Cancer Treat. Rep.* **66:**1299–1302, 1982.

Balch, C. M.; Murad, T. M.; Soong, S.-J.; Ingalls, A. L.; Halpern, N. B.; and Maddox, W. A.: A multifactorial analysis of melanoma. *Ann. Surg.,* **188:**732–742, 1978.

Balch, C. M.; Murad, T. M.; Soong, S.-J.; Ingalls, A. L.; Richards, P. C.; and Maddox, W. A.: Tumor thickness as a guide to surgical management of clinical stage I melanoma patients. *Cancer,* **43:**883–888, 1979a.

Balch, C. M.; Soong, S.-J.; Murad, T. M.; Ingalls, A. L.; Richards, P. C.; and Maddox, W. A.: A multifactorial analysis of melanoma III. Prognostic features of clinical stage I disease. *Surgery,* **86:**343–351, 1979b.

Balch, C. M.; Soong, S.-J.; Murad, T. M.; Smith, J. W.; Maddox, W. A.; and Durant, J. R.: A multifactorial analysis of melanoma. IV. Prognostic factors in 200 melanoma patients with distant metastases (stage III). *J. Clin. Oncol.,* **1**(2):126–134, 1983.

Balch, C. M.; Wilkerson, J. A.; Murad, T. M.; Soong, S.-J.; Ingalls, A. L.; and Maddox, W. A.: The prognostic significance of ulceration of cutaneous melanoma. *Cancer,* **45:**3012–3017, 1980.

Beattie, E. J.: Thoracotomy and pulmonary metastases. *Ann. Thorac. Surg.,* **27:**294, 1979.

Beitner, H.; Ringborg, U.; Wennensten, G.; and Lagerlof, B.: Further evidence for increased light sensitivity in patients with malignant melanoma. *Br. J. Dermatol,* **104:**289–294, 1981.

Benjamin, R. S.; Gutterman, J. U.; McKelvey, E. M.; Einhorn, L. M.; Livingston, R. B.; and Gottlieb, J. A.: Systemic chemotherapy for melanoma. In *Neoplasms of the Skin and Malignant Melanoma.* Year Book Medical Publishers, Inc., Chicago, 1976.

Beral, V.; Ramcharan, S.; and Faris, R.: Malignant melanoma and oral contraceptives used among women in California. *Br. J. Cancer,* **36:**804–809, 1977.

Beretta, G., for WHO Collaborating Centres for Evaluation of Methods of Diagnosis and Treatment of Melanoma (Chairman: Umberto Veronesi): Progress report of a controlled study of prolonged chemotherapy, immunotherapy and chemotherapy plus immunotherapy as an adjuvant to surgery in malignant melanoma. In Terry, W. D., and Rosenberg, S. A. (eds.): *Immunotherapy of Human Cancer.* Elsevier North-Holland, Inc., New York, 1982.

Blois, M. S., and Banda, P. W.: Detection of occult metastatic melanoma by urine. *Cancer Res.,* **36:**3317–3323, 1976.

Bodurtha, A. J.; Berkelhammer, J.; Kim, Y. H.; Laucius,

J. F.; and Mastrangelo, M. J.: A clinical histologic and immunologic study of a case of metastatic malignant melanoma undergoing spontaneous remission. *Cancer,* **37:**735–742, 1976.

Bottino, J. C.; Rassen, R. D.; Hersh, E. M.; Rias, A.; Hester, J. P.; and McBride, C. M.: Response of malignant melanoma to plasma exchange, surgical debulking and corynebacterium parvum. *Int. J. of Artif. Organs* **1:**53–57, 1978.

Boutin, J.: Primary melanoma of the leptomeninges. *J. Clin. Pathol.,* **11:**122–127, 1958.

Breslow, A.: Thickness, cross-sectional areas and depth of invasion in the prognosis of cutaneous melanoma. *Ann. Surg.,* **172:**902–908, 1970.

Breslow, A.: Tumor thickness, level of invasion and node dissection in stage I cutaneous melanoma. *Ann. Surg.,* **182:**572–575, 1975.

Breslow, A.; Cascinelli, N.; VanderEsch, T. P.; and Morobito, A.: Stage I melanoma of the limbs: Assessment of prognosis by levels of invasion and maximum thickness. *Tumor,* **64:**273–284, 1978.

Breslow, A., and Macht, S. D.: Optimal size of resection margin for thin cutaneous melanoma. *Surg. Gynecol. Obstet.,* **145:**691–692, 1977.

Brown, J. P.; Woodbury, R. G.; Hart, C. E.; Hellstrom, I.; and Hellstrom, K. E.: Quantitative analysis of melanoma-associated antigen p97 in normal and neoplastic tissues. *Proc. Natl. Acad. Sci. USA,* **78:**539–543, 1981.

Brownstein, M. H., and Helwig, E. B.: Metastatic tumors of the skin. *Cancer,* **29:**1297–1307, 1972.

Budman, D. R.; Camacho, E.; and Wittes, R. E.: The current causes of death in patients with malignant melanoma. *Eur. J. Cancer,* **14:**327–330, 1978.

Bulkley, G. B.; Cohen, M. H.; Banks, P. M.; Char, D. H.; and Ketcham, A. S.: Long-term spontaneous regression of malignant melanoma with visceral metastases. *Cancer,* **36:**485–491, 1975.

Bullard, D. E.; Cox, E. B.; and Seigler, H. F.: Central nervous system metastases in malignant melanoma. *Neurosurgery,* **8:**26–30, 1981.

Byrne, M.; Heppner, G. H.; Stolbach, L.; Cummings, F.; McDonough, E.; and Calabresi, P.: Tumor immunity in melanoma patients as assessed by colony inhibition and microcytotoxicity methods: A preliminary report. *Natl. Cancer Inst. Monogr.,* **37:**3–8, 1973.

Bystryn, J.-C.: The immunobiology of human malignant melanoma. *Int. J. Dermatol.,* **19:**375–378, 1980.

Calabresi, P.; Dexter, D. L.; and Heppner, G. H.: Clinical and pharmacological implications of cancer cell differentiation and heterogeneity. *Biochem. Pharmacol.,* **28:**1933–1941, 1979.

Cascinelli, N.; Morabito, A.; Bufalino, E. P.; VanDerEsch, E. P.; Preda, F.; Vaglini, M.; Rovini, D.; and Orefice, S.: Prognosis of stage I melanoma of the skin. WHO Collaborating Centre for evaluation of methods of diagnosis and treatment of melanoma. *Int. J. Cancer,* **26:**733–739, 1980.

Clark, W. H., Jr.; Ainsworth, A. M.; Bernardino, E. A.; Yang, C.-H.; Mihm, M. C.; and Reed, R. J.: The developmental biology of primary human malignant melanomas. *Semin. Oncol.,* **2:**83–103, 1975.

Clark, W. H., Jr.; Reimer, R. R.; Greene, M.; Ainsworth, A. M.; and Mastroangelo, M. J.: Origin of familial malignant melanomas from heritable melanocytic lesions. *Arch. Dermatol,* **114:**732–738, 1978.

Clark, W. H., Jr.: A classification of malignant melanoma in man correlated with histogenesis and biologic behavior. In *Advances in Biology of the Skin: The Pigmentary*

System. Pergamon Press, Inc., Elmsford, New York, 1967.

Clark, W. H., Jr.; Mastrangelo, M.; and Goldman, L. I. (eds.): *Human Malignant Melanoma,* Grune & Stratton, Inc., New York, 1983.

Clark, W. H., Jr., and Mihn, M. D., Jr.: Lentigo maligna and lentigo maligna melanoma. *Am. J. Pathol.,* **55**:39–67, 1969.

Cohan, W.: Excision of melanoma metastases to lung. *Ann. Surg.,* **178**:703, 1973.

Cohen, M. H.; Jessup, J. M.; Felix, E. L.; Weese, J. L.; and Herberman, R. B.: Intralesional treatment of recurrent metastatic cutaneous malignant melanoma. *Cancer,* **41**:2456–2463, 1978.

Cohen, M. H.; Ketcham, A. S.; Felix, E. L.; Li, S. H.; Tomaszewski, M.-M.; Costa, J.; Robson, A. S.; Simon, R. M.; and Rosenberg, S. A.: Prognostic factors in patients undergoing lymphadenectomy for malignant melanoma. *Ann. Surg.,* **186**:635–642, 1976.

Cohen, S. M.; Greenspan, E. M.; Ratner, L. H.; and Weiner, M. J.: Combination chemotherapy of malignant melanoma with imidazole carboxamide, BCNU and vincristine. *Cancer,* **39**:41–44, 1977.

Creagan, E. T.; Ahmann, D. L.; Green, S. J.; Long, H. J.; Frytak, S.: O'Fallon, J. R.; and Itri, L. M.: Phase II study of low-dose recombinant leukocyte A interferon in disseminated malignant melanoma. *J. Clin. Oncol.,* **2**:1002–1005, 1984.

Crombie, I. K.: Distribution of malignant melanoma on the body surface. *Br. J. Cancer,* **43**:842–849, 1981.

Cunningham, T. J.; Schoenfeld, D.; Nathanson, L.; Wolter, J. M.; Patterson, W. B.; and Borden, E. C.: A controlled ECOG study of adjuvant therapy with BCG or BCG plus DTIC in patients with stage I and II malignant melanoma. In Terry, W. D., and Rosenberg, S. A. (eds.): *Immunotherapy of Human Cancer.* Elsevier North-Holland, Inc., New York, 1982.

Cutler, S. J., and Young, J. L. (eds): Third national cancer survey: Incidence data. *Natl. Cancer Inst. Monogr.,* **41**:1–454, 1975.

DasGupta, T. K.: Results of treatment of 260 patients with primary cutaneous melanoma: A five-year prospective study. *Ann. Surg.,* **186**:201–209, 1977.

DasGupta, T. K.; Bowden, L.; and Berg, J. W.: Malignant melanoma of unknown primary origin. *Surg. Gynecol. Obstet.,* **117**:341–346, 1963.

Davis, J.; Pack, G. T.; and Higgins, G. K.: Melanotic freckle of Hutchinson. *Am. J. Surg.,* **113**:457–463, 1967.

Day, C. L., Jr.; Sober, A. J.; Fitzpatrick, T. B.; and Mihm, M. C., Jr.: Prognosis in malignant melanoma. *J. Am. Acad. Dermatol.* **3**:525–526, 1980.

Day, C. L., Jr.; Sober, A. J.; Lopansri, S.; Mihm, M. C.; Kopf, A. W.; and Fitzpatrick, T. B.: Primary tumor thickness is the major determinant for recurrence in clinical stage I malignant melanoma patients with histologically positive nodes. *Clin. Res.,* **27**:383, 1979.

Day, C. L., Jr.; Harrist, T. J.; Lew, R. A.; and Mihm, Jr., M. C.: Classification of malignant melanomas according to the histologic morphology of melanoma nodules. *J. Dermatol. Surg. Oncol.,* **8**:874, 1982a.

Day, C. L., Jr.; Mihm, M. C.; Fitzpatrick, T. B.; and Malt, R. A.: Narrower margins for clinical stage I malignant melanomas. *N. Engl. J. Med.,* **306**:479–482, 1982b.

Day, C. L., Jr.; Lew, R. A.; Mihm, M. C., Jr.; Sober, A. J.; Harris, M. N.; Kopf, A. W.; Fitzpatrick, T. B.; Harrist, T. J.; Golomb, F. M.; Postel, A.; Hennessey, P.; Gumport, S. L.; Raker, J. W.; Malt, R. A.; Cosimi, A. B.;

Wood, W. C.; Roses, D. F.; Gorstein, F.; Rigel, D.; Friedman, R. J.; Mintzes, M. M.; and Grier, R. W.: A multivariate analysis of prognostic factors for melanoma patients with lesions ≧3.65 mm in thickness. *Ann. Surg.,* **195**:44–49, 1982c.

Day, C. L., Jr.; Mihm, M. C., Jr.; Lew, R. A.; Harris, M. N.; Kopf, A. W.; Fitzpatrick, T. B.; Harrist, T. J.; Golomb, F. M.; Postel, A.; Hennessey, P.; Gumport, S. J.; Raker, J. W.; Malt, R. A.; Cosimi, A. B.; Wood, W. C.; Roses, D. F.; Gorstein, F.; Rigel, D.; Friedman, R. J.; Mintzes, M. M.; and Sober, A. J.: Prognostic factors for patients with clinical stage I melanoma of intermediate thickness (1.51–3.99 mm). *Ann. Surg.,* **195**:35–43, 1982d.

Day, C. L., Jr.; Mihm, M. C., Jr.; Sober, A. J.; Harris, M. N.; Kopf, A. W.; Fitzpatrick, T. B.; Kew, R. A.; Harrist, T. J.; Bolomb, F. M.; Postel, A.; Hennessey, P.; Bumport, S. L.; Raker, J. W.; Malt, R. A.; Cosimi, A. B.; Wood, W. C.; Roses, D. F.; Gorstein, F.; Rigel, D.; Friedman, R. J.; and Mintzis, M. M.: Prognostic factors for melanoma patients with lesions 0.76–1.69 mm in thickness. *Ann. Surg.,* **195**:30–34, 1982e.

Day, C. L., Jr.; Sober, A. J.; Kopf, A. W.; Lew, R. A.; Mihm, M. C., Jr.; Golomb, F. M.; Hennessey, P.; Harris, M. N.; Gumport, S. L.; Raker, J. W.; Malt, R. A.; Cosimi, A. B.; Wood, W. C.; Roses, D. F.; Gorstein, F.; Fitzpatrick, T. B.; and Postel, A.: A prognostic model for clinical stage I melanoma of the lower extremity. *Surgery,* **89**:599–603, 1981a.

Day, C. L., Jr.; Sober, A. J.; Kopf, A. W.; Lew, R. A.; Mihm, M. C., Jr.; Golomb, F. M.; Postel, A.; Hennessey, P.; Harris, M. N.; Gumport, S. L.; Raker, J. W.; Malt, R. A.; Cosimi, A. B.; Wood, W. C.; Roses, D. F.; Gorstein, F.; and Fitzpatrick, T. B.: A prognostic model for clinical stage I melanoma of the trunk. *Am. J. Surg.* **142**:247–251, 1981b.

Day, C. L., Jr.; Sober, A. J.; and Lew, R. A.: Malignant melanoma patients with positive nodes and relatively good prognoses: Microstaging retains prognostic significance in clinical stage I melanoma patients with metastases to regional nodes. *Cancer,* **47**:955–962, 1981c.

DeVita, V. T., and Fisher, R. I.: Natural history of malignant melanoma as related to therapy. *Cancer Treat. Rep.,* **60**:153, 1976.

Dexter, D. L.; Barbosa, J. A.; and Calabresi, P.: N,N-Dimethylformamide-induced alteration of cell culture characteristics and loss of tumorigenicity in cultured human colon carcinoma cells. *Cancer Res.,* **39**:1020–1025, 1979.

Dexter, D. L., and Calabresi, P.: Cancer cell differentiation. In Humphrey, G. B. (ed.): *Pancreatic Tumors in Children.* Martinus Nijhoff Publishers, The Hague London, 1982.

Dexter, D. L.; Leith, J. T.; Crabtree, G. W.; Parks, R. E., Jr.; Glicksman, A. S.; and Calabresi, P.: N,N-Dimethylformamide-induced modulation of responses of tumor cells to conventional anticancer treatment modalities. In Moore, M. A. S. (ed): *Maturation Factors and Cancer.* Raven Press, New York, 1982.

Doiron, M. J., and Bernardino, M. E.: A comparison of non-invasive imaging modalities in the melanoma patient. *Cancer,* **47**:2581–2584, 1981.

Dosik, G. M.; Gutterman, J. U.; Hersh, E. M.; Akhtar, M.; Sonada, T.; and Horn, R. G.: Nephrotoxicity from cancer immunotherapy. *Ann. Intern. Med.,* **89**:41–46, 1978.

Drzewiecki, K. T.; Christensen, H. C.; Ladefoged, C.; and Poulsen, H.: Clinical course of cutaneous malignant melanoma related to histopathological criteria of primary tumor. *Scand. J. Plast. Reconstr. Surg.,* **14:**229–234, 1980a.

Drzewiecki, K. T.; Ladefoged, C.; and Christensen, H. C.: Biopsy and prognosis for cutaneous malignant melanomas in clinical stage I. *Scand. J. Plast. Reconstr. Surg.,* **14:**141–144, 1980b.

Edwards, J. M.: Treatment of malignant melanoma by endolymphatic therapy. In Ariel, I. M. (ed.): *Malignant Melanoma.* Appleton-Century-Crofts, New York, 1981.

Eilber, F. R.; Morton, D. L.; Holmes, E. C.; Sparks, F. C.; and Ramming, K. P.: Adjuvant immunotherapy with BCG in treatment of regional-lymph-node metastases from malignant melanoma. *N. Engl. J. Med.,* **295:**347–240, 1976.

Einhorn, L. H.; Burgess, M. A.; and Valleja, C. V.; Prognostic correlations and response of treatment in advanced metastatic malignant melanoma. *Cancer Res.,* **34:** 1995–2004, 1974.

Elder, D. E.; Goldman, L. I.; Goldman, S. C.; Greene, M. H.; and Clark, W. H. Jr.: Dysplastic nevus syndrome: A phenotypic association of sporadic cutaneous melanoma. *Cancer,* **46:**1787–1794, 1980.

Elwood, J. M., and Lee, J. A. H.: Recent data on the epidemiology of malignant melanoma. *Semin. Oncol.,* **2:**149–154, 1975.

Epstein, E.; Bragg, K.; and Linden, G.: Biopsy and prognosis of malignant melanoma. *J.A.M.A.,* **208:**1369–1371, 1969.

Everson, T. C., and Cole, W. H.: *Spontaneous Regression of Cancer.* W. B. Saunders Company; Philadelphia, 1966.

Felix, E. L.; Sindelar, W. F.; Bagley, D. H.; Johnston, G. S.; and Ketcham, A. S.: The use of bone and brain scans as screening procedures in patients with malignant lesions. *Surg. Gynecol. Obstet.,* **141:**867–869, 1975.

Fidler, I. J.: Therapy of spontaneous metastases by intravenous injection of liposomes containing lymphokines. *Science,* **208:**1469–1471, 1980.

Fitzpatrick, T. B.; Montgomery, H.; and Lerner, A. B.: Pathogenesis of generalized dermal pigmentation secondary to malignant melanoma and melanuria. *J. Invest. Dermatol.,* **22:**163–172, 1954.

Fortner, J. G.; Woodruff, J.; Schottenfeld, D.; and MacLean, B.: Biostatistical basis of elective node dissection for malignant melanoma. *Ann. Surg.,* **186:**100–103, 1977.

Gellin, G. A.; Kopf, A. W.; and Garfinkel, L.: Malignant melanoma—a controlled study of possible associated factors. *Arch. Dermatol.,* **99:**43–48, 1969.

Ghose, T.; Norvell, S. T.; Guclu, A.; Bodurtha, A.; Tai, J.; and MacDonald, A. S.: Immunochemotherapy of malignant melanoma with chlorambucil bound to anti-melanoma globulins: Preliminary results in patients with disseminated disease. *J.N.C.I.,* **58:**845–852, 1977.

Goldsmith, H. S.: Melanoma: An overview. *CA,* **29:**194–215, 1979.

Graham, B. J., and Duane, T. D.: Ocular Melanoma Task Force Report. *Am. J. Ophthalmol,* **90:**728–733, 1980.

Gromet, M. A.; Epstein, W. L.; and Blois, M. S.: The regressing thin malignant melanoma. *Cancer,* **42:**2282–2292, 1978.

Habermalz, H. J., and Fischer, J. J.: Radiation therapy of malignant melanoma. *Cancer,* **38:**2258–2262, 1976.

Hansen, M. G., and McCarten, A. B.: Tumor thickness and lymphocytic infiltration in malignant melanoma of the head and neck. *Am. J. Surg.,* **128:**557–561, 1974.

Hatfield, P. M.: Role of liver scanning in the diagnosis of hepatic metastases. *Med. Clin. North Am.,* **59:**247–276, 1975.

Hedley, D. W.; McElwain, T. J.; and Currie, G. A.: Specific active immunotherapy does not prolong survival in surgically treated patients with stage IIB malignant melanoma and may promote early recurrence. *Br. J. Cancer,* **37:**491–496, 1978.

Hellstrom, I.; Hellstrom, K. E.; Sjogren, H. O.; and Warner, G. A.: Demonstration of cell-mediated immunity to human neoplasms of various histological types. *Int. J. Cancer,* **7:**1–16, 1971.

Hellstrom, I.; Hellstrom, K. E.; Pierce, G. E.; and Yong, J. P. S.: Cellular and humoral immunity to different types of human neoplasms. *Nature,* **220:**1352–1354, 1968.

Helwig, E. B.: Malignant melanoma of the skin in man. *Natl. Cancer Inst. Mongr.* **10:**286–295, 1963.

Henry, J. B.: *Clinical Diagnosis and Management by Laboratory Methods.* W. B. Saunders Company, Philadelphia, 1979.

Heppner, G. H.; Henry, E.; Stolbach, L; Cummings, F. J.; McDonough, E.; and Calabresi, P.: Problems in the clinical use of microcytotoxicity assay for measuring cell-mediated immunity to tumor cells. *Cancer Res.,* **35:**1931, 1975.

Heppner, G. H.; Stolbach, L.; Byrne, M.; Cummings, F. J.; McDonough, E.; and Calabresi, P.: Cell mediated and serum blocking reactivity to tumor antigens in patients with malignant melanoma. *Int. J. Cancer,* **11:**245–260, 1973.

Herlyn, M.; Clark, W. H., Jr.; Mastrangelo, M. J.; Guerry, D. P., IV; Elder, D. E.; LaRossa, D.; Hamilton, R.; Bandi, E.; Tuthill, R.; Steplewski, Z.; and Kaprowski, H.: Specific immunoreactivity of hybridoma-secreted monoclonal anti-melanoma antibodies to cultured cells and freshly derived human cells. *Cancer Res.,* **40:**3602–3609, 1980.

Holman, C. D.; James, I. R.; Gattey, P. H.; and Armstrong, B. K.: An analysis of trends in mortality from malignant melanoma of the skin in Australia. *Int. J. Cancer,* **26:**703–709, 1980.

Holmes, E. C.; Clark, W.; Morton, D. I.; Eilber, F. R.; and Bachow, A. J.: Regional lymph node metastases and the level of invasion of primary melanoma. *Cancer,* **37:**199–201, 1976.

Honn, K. V.; Cicone, B.; and Skoff, A.: Prostacyclin: A potent antimetastatic agent. *Science,* **212:**1270–1272, 1981.

Houghton, A. N.; Munster, E. W.; and Viola, M. V.: Increased incidence of malignant melanoma after peaks of sunspot activity. *Lancet,* **i:**759–760, 1978.

Houghton, A. N., and Viola, M. V.: Solar radiation and malignant melanoma of the skin. *J. Am. Acad. Dermatol.,* **5:**477–483, 1981.

Huberman, E.; Heckman, C.; and Langenbach, R.: Stimulation of differentiated functions in human melanoma cells by tumor-promoting agents and dimethyl sulfoxide. *Cancer Res.,* **39:**2618–2624, 1979.

Imai, K., and Ferrone, S.: Indirect rosette microassay to characterize human melanoma-associated antigens recognized by operationally specific xenoantisera. *Cancer Res.,* **40:**628–631, 1980.

Imai, K.; Ng, A. K.; and Ferrone, S.: Characterization of monoclonal antibodies to human melanoma-associated antigens. *J.N.C.I.,* **66:**489–496, 1981.

Jones, H. W.; Druegemueller, W.; and Makowski, E. L.: A primary melanocarcinoma of the cervix. *Am. J. Obstet. Gynecol.,* **111:**959–963, 1971.

Jones, W. M.; Williams, W. J.; Roberts, M. M.; and Davies, K.: Malignant melanoma of the skin: Prognostic value of clinical features and the role of treatment in 111 cases. *Br. J. Cancer*, **22**:437–451, 1968.

Ketcham, A. S., and Christopherson, W. O.: A staging system for malignant melanoma. *World J. Surg.*, **3**:271–278, 1979.

Kleep, O., and Magnus, K.: Some environmental and bodily characteristics of melanoma patients. A case-control study. *Int. J. Cancer*, **23**:482–486, 1979.

Koh, H. K.; Michalik, E.; Sober, A. J.; Lew, R. A.; Day, C. L.; Clark, W.; Mihm, M. C.; Kopf, A. W.; Blois, M. S.; and Fitzpatrick, T. B.: Lentigo maligna melanoma has no better prognosis than other types of melanoma. *J. Clin. Oncology*, **2**:994–1000, 1984.

Konrad, K., and Wolff, K.: Pathogenesis of diffuse melanosis secondary to malignant melanoma. *Br. J. Dermatol.*, **91**:653–655, 1974.

Kopf, A. W.; Rigel, D.; and Bart, R. S.: Factors related to thickness of melanoma. Multifactorial analysis of variables correlated with thickness of superficial spreading malignant melanoma in man. *J. Dermatol. Surg. Oncol.*, **7**:645–650, 1981.

Krementz, E. T.: Node dissection for extremity melanoma. *N. Engl. J. Med.*, **297**:664–665, 1977.

Krementz, E. T.; Carter, R. D.; Sutherland, C. M.; and Ryan, R. F.: Malignant melanoma of the limbs: An evaluation of chemotherapy by regional perfusion. In *Neoplasms of the Skin and Malignant Melanoma*. Year Book Medical Publishers, Inc., Chicago, 1976a.

Krementz, E. T.; Sutherland, E. M.; Carter, R. D., Ryan, R. F.: Malignant melanoma in the American black. *Ann. Surg.*, **183**:533–542, 1976b.

Krown, S. E.; Hilal, E. Y.; Pinsky, C. M.; Hirshaut, Y.; Wanebo, H. J.; Hansen, J. A.; Huvos, A. G.; and Oettgen, H. F.: Intralesional injection of the methanol extraction residue of Bacillus Calmette-Guerin (MER) into cutaneous metastases of malignant melanoma. *Cancer*, **42**:2648–2660, 1978.

LaMonica, G.; Orefice, S.; and Paolucci, R.: Lymphographic evaluation of 250 patients with malignant melanoma. *Cancer* **38**:1563–1573, 1976.

LeDoussal, V.; Brunet, M.; Guérin, P.; Hacene, K.; Lasry, S.; Marcotorchino, F.; Michael, P.; and Herbert, H.: Prognostic histopathological features of malignant melanoma. New statistical approaches. *Nouv. Presse. Med.* **10**:2561–2563, 1981.

Lee, J. A.; Petersen, G. R.; Stevens, R. G.; and Vesanen, K.: The influence of age, year of birth, and date of mortality from malignant melanoma in the populations of England and Wales, Canada and the white population of the United States. *Am. J. Epidemiology*, **110**:734–739, 1979.

Lee, Y.-T. N.: Laco-regional recurrent melanoma: I. Natural history. *Cancer Treat. Rev.*, **7**:59–72, 1980.

Leith, J. T.; Gaskins, L. A.; Dexter, D. L.; Calabresi, P.; and Glicksman, A. S.: Alteration of the survival response of two human colon carcinoma subpopulations to x-irradiation by N,N-dimethylformamide. *Cancer Res.*, **42**:30–34, 1982.

Lejeune, F. J., and DeWasch, G.: Malignant melanoma. In Staquet, M. J. (ed.): *Randomized Trials in Cancer: A Critical Review by Sites*. Raven Press, New York, 1978.

Lever, W. F.: *Histopathology of the Skin*, 5th ed. J. B. Lippincott Company, Philadelphia, 1975.

Levine, J.; Kopf, A. Q.; Rigell, D. S.; Bart, R. S.; Hennessey, P.; Friedman, R. J.; and Mintzis, M. M.: Correlation of thickness of superficial malignant melanomas and ages of patients. *J. Dermatol. Surg. Oncol.*, **7**:311–316, 1981.

Lewis, M. G.: Possible immunological factors in human malignant melanoma in Uganda. *Lancet*, ii:921, 1967.

Lokich, J. J.; Garnick, M. B.; and Legg, M.: Intralesional immune therapy. *Oncology*, **36**:236–241, 1979.

Luce, J. K.: Chemotherapy of melanoma. *Semin. Oncol.*, **2**:179–185, 1975.

Lynch, H. T.; Frichot, B. C.; and Lynch, J. C.: Familial atypical multiple mole-melanoma syndrome. *J. Med. Genet.*, **15**:352–356, 1978.

McGovern, V. J.: The classification of melanoma and its relationship to prognosis. *Pathology*, **2**:85–98, 1970.

McGovern, V. J.: Spontaneous regression of melanoma. *Pathology*, **7**:91–99, 1975.

McGovern, V. J., and Mackie, B. S.: The relationship of solar radiation to melanoblastoma. *Aust. and New Zealand J. Surg.*, **28**:257–262, 1959.

McNeer, G., and DasGupta, T. D.: Routes of lymphatic spread of malignant melanoma. *CA*, **15**:168–174, 1965.

Manci, E. A.; Balch, C. M.; Murad, T. M.; and Soong, S.-J.: Polypoid melanoma. A virulent variant of the nodular growth pattern. *Am. J. Clin. Pathol.*, **75**:810–815, 1981.

Mastrangelo, M. J.; Sulit, H. L.; Prehn, L.; Bornstein, R. S.; Yarbro, J. W.; and Prehn, R. T.: Intralesional BCG in the treatment of metastatic malignant melanoma. *Cancer*, **37**:684–692, 1976.

Mehnert, J. H., and Heard, J. L.: Staging of malignant melanoma by depth of invasion. *Am. J. Surg.*, **110**:168–176, 1965.

Melanoma Cooperative Group, New York University School of Medicine: (letter) To do or not to do elective lymph-node dissections for certain malignant melanomas. *J. Dermatol. Surg. Oncol.*, **4**:493–497, 1978.

Meyer, J. E.: Radiographic evaluation of metastatic melanoma. *Cancer*, **42**:127–132, 1978.

Meyskens, F. L., Jr.: The endocrinology of malignant melanoma. *Rev. Endocr.-Rel. Cancer*, **9**:5–13, 1981.

Mihm, M. C.; Fitzpatrick, T. B.; Lane-Brown, M. M.; Raker, J. W.; Malt, R. A.; and Kaiser, J. S.: Early detection of primary cutaneous malignant melanoma: A color atlas. *N. Engl. J. Med.*, **289**:989–996, 1973.

Morgan, A. C., Jr.; Galloway, D. R.; Wilson, B. S.; and Reisfeld, R. A.: Human melanoma associated antigens: A solid-phase assay for detection of specific antibody. *J. Immunol. Methods*, **39**:233–246, 1980.

Morton, D. L.; Eilber, F. R.; Holmes, E. C.; Hunt, J. S.; Ketcham, A. S.; Silverstein, M. F.; and Sparks, F. C.: BCG immunotherapy of malignant melanoma: Summary of a seven year experience. *Ann. Surg.*, **180**:635–643, 1974.

Morton, D. L.; Holmes, E. C.; Eilber, F. R.; and Ramming, K. P.: Adjuvant immunotherapy of malignant melanoma: Results of a randomized trial in patients with node metastases. In Terry, W. D., Rosenberg, S. A. (eds.): *Immunotherapy of Human Cancer*. Elsevier North-Holland, Inc., New York, 1982.

Musher, D. R., and Linder, A. E.: Primary melanoma of the esophagus. *Dig. Dis.*, **19**:855–859, 1974.

Nathanson, L.: Spontaneous regression of malignant melanoma: A review of the literature on incidence, clinical features, and possible mechanisms. Conference on Spontaneous Regression of Cancer. *Natl. Cancer Inst. Monogr.*, **44**:67–77, 1976.

Nathanson, L.: Etiologic and epidemiologic considerations in human malignant melanoma. In Costanzi, J. (ed.): *Melanoma.* Martinus Nijhoff, The Hague, 1983.

Nathanson, L.; Kaufman, S. D.; and Carey, R. W.: Vinblastine infusion, bleomycin and *cis*-dichlorodiammine-platinum chemotherapy in metastatic melanoma. *Cancer,* **48:**1290–1294, 1981.

Neifeld, J. P., and Lippman, M. E.: Steroid hormone receptors and melanoma. *J. Invest. Dermatol.,* **74:**381–397, 1980.

Norton, J. A.; Shulman, N. R.; Carash, L.; Smith, R. L.; Au, F.; and Rosenberg, S. A.: Severe thrombocytopenia following intralesional BCG therapy. *Cancer,* **41:**820–826, 1978.

Nutting, M. G., and McPherson, T. A.: Ascites in malignant melanoma cells after oral BCG immunotherapy. *N. Engl. J. Med.,* **295:**395, 1976.

Palangie, A.; Lassau, R.; Moreau, T.; Noury-Duperrat, G.; and Cotterot, F.: Stage I malignant melanoma of the skin. Prognostic value of thickness and level. *Nouv. Presse Med.,* **10:**2337–2341, 1981.

Peterson, R. F.; Hazard, J. B.; Dykes, E. R.; Anderson, R.: Superficial malignant melanoma. *Surg. Gynecol. Obstet.,* **119:**37–41, 1964.

Pinsky, C. M.; Hirshaut, Y.; Wanebo, M. J.; Fortner, J. G.; Mike, V.; Schottenfeld, D.; and Oettgen, H. F.: Randomized trial of Bacillus Calmette-Guerin (percutaneous administration) as surgical adjuvant immunotherapy for patients with stage II melanoma. *Ann. N.Y. Acad. Sci.,* **277:**187–194, 1975.

Pondes, S.; Hunter, J. A.; White, H.; McIntyre, M. A.; and Prescott, R. J.: Cutaneous malignant melanoma in southeast Scotland. *Q. J. Med.,* **50:**103–121, 1981.

Quirt, I. C.; Kersey, P. A.; Baker, M. A.; Bodurtha, A. J.; King, M. H.; Norwell, S. T.; Osobo, P.; Dent, P. B.; McCulloch, P. B.; Ambus, U.; Blackstein, M. E.; Cowan, D. H.; Evans, W. K.; Talk, R. E.; Goldie, J. H.; Krieger, H.; Kutos, G. J.; and Tepperman, A. D.: Adjuvant chemoimmunotherapy with DTIC and BCG in patients with poor prognosis primary malignant melanoma and completely resected recurrent melanoma. In Terry, W. D., and Rosenberg, S. A. (eds.): *Immunotherapy of Human Cancer.* Elsevier North-Holland, Inc., New York, 1982.

Reddy, C. R.; Yellama, A.; Satyanarayana, B. V.; Sundareshwar, B.: Incidence and evolution of moles and the relationship to malignant melanoma in eastern India. *Int. Surg.,* **61:**469–471, 1976.

Reid, J. D.; and Mehta, V. T.: Melanoma of the lower respiratory tract. *Cancer,* **19:**627–631, 1966.

Reimer, R. R.; Clark, W. H., Jr.; Green, M. A.; Ainsworth, A. M.; and Fraumeni, J. F., Jr.: Precursor lesions in familial melanoma—a new genetic preneoplastic syndrome. *J. Am. Acad. Dermatol.,* **239:**744–746, 1978.

Reisfeld, R. A., and Ferrone, S. (eds.): *Melanoma Antigens and Antibodies.* Plenum Publishing Corporation, New York, 1983.

Robbins, J. H.; Kraemer, K. H.; Lutzner, M. A.; Festoff, B. W.; and Coon, H. G.: Xeroderma pigmentosum: An inherited disease with sun sensitivity, multiple cutaneous neoplasms and abnormal DNA repair. *Ann. Intern. Med.,* **80:**221–248, 1974.

Robinson, J. C.: Risks of BCG intralesional therapy: An experience with melanoma. *J. Surg. Oncol.,* **9:**587–593, 1977.

Rosenberg, S. A., and Rapp, H. J.: Intralesional immunotherapy of melanoma with BCG. *Med. Clin. North Am.,* **60:**419–430, 1976.

Rosenberg, S. A.; Seipp, C.; and Sears, H. F.: Clinical and immunologic studies of disseminated BCG infection. *Cancer,* **41:**1771–1780, 1978.

Schapira, D. V., and McPherson, T. A.: Pneumonitis with oral BCG. *N. Engl. J. Med.,* **296:**397, 1977.

Schuler, G.; Honigemann, H.; and Wolff, K.: Diffuse melanosis in metastatic melanoma. *J. Am. Acad. Dermatol.,* **3:**363–369, 1980.

Seigler, H. F. (ed.): *Clinical Management of Melanoma.* Martinus Nijhoff Medical Publishers, The Hague, 1983.

Seiji, M.; Mihm, M. C.; Sober, A. J.; Takahashi, M.; Kato, T.; and Fitzpatrick, T. B.: Malignant melanoma of the palmar-plantar-subungual-mucosal type: Clinical and histopathological features. *Pigment Cell,* **5:**95–104, 1979.

Shaw, H. M.; McGovern, V. J.; Milton, G. W.; and Farago, G. A.: Cutaneous malignant melanoma: Occupational and prognosis. *Med. J. Aust.,* **1:**37–38, 1981.

Silberberg, I.; Kopf, A. W.; and Gumport, S. L.: Diffuse melanosis in malignant melanoma. *Arch. Dermatol.,* **97:**671–677, 1968.

Silverberg, E.: Cancer statistics, 1979. *Cancer,* **29:**6–21, 1979.

Silverberg, E.: *Cancer Statistics, 1983. CA,* **33:**9–25, 1983.

Sjogren, H. O.; Hellstrom, I.; Bansal, S. C.; and Hellstrom, K. E.: Suggestive evidence that the "blocking antibodies" of tumor-bearing individuals may be antigen-antibody complexes. *Proc. Natl. Acad. Sci. USA,* **68:**1372–1375, 1971.

Skibba, J. L.; Pinckley, J.; Gilbert, E. F.; and Johnson, R. O.: Multiple primary melanoma following administration of levodopa. *Arch. Pathol.,* **93:**556–561, 1972.

Smith, J. L., and Stehlin, J. S.: Spontaneous regression of primary malignant melanoma with regional metastases. *Cancer,* **18:**1399, 1965.

Sober, A. J.; Blois, M. S.; Clark, W. H.; Fitzpatrick, T. B.; Kopf, A. W.; and Mihm, M. L.: Primary malignant melanoma of the skin—1130 cases from the melanoma clinical cooperative group. In González-Ochoa, A.; Dominquez-Soto, L.; and Ortiz, Y. (eds): *Proceedings of the XI International Congress of Dermatology,* Mexico City, October 16–22, 1977. Excerpta Medica, Amsterdam, *Excerpta Medical International Congress Series* 451, 1977.

Sober, A. J.; Fitzpatrick, T. B.; and Mihm, M. C.: Primary melanoma of the skin: Recognition and management. *J. Am. Acad. Dermatol.,* **2:**179–197, 1980.

Sober, A. J.; Lew, R. A.; Fitzpatrick, T. B.; and Marvell, R.: Solar exposure patterns in patients with cutaneous melanoma—a case control series. *Clin. Res.* **27:**383A, 1979.

Sparks, F. C.: Hazards and complications of BCG immunotherapy. *Med. Clin. North Am.,* **60:**499–509, 1976.

Spittler, L. E.; Sagebiel, R.; Allen, R.; Minor, D.; Dymott, C.; and Drake, T.: Levamisole in the treatment of melanoma. In Terry, W. D., and Rosenberg, S. A. (eds.): *Immunotherapy of Human Cancer.* Elsevier North-Holland, New York, 1982.

Spremulli, E. N.; Bogaars, H. A.; Dexter, D. L.; Matook, G. A.; Jolly, G. A.; Cummings, F. J.; Kuhn, R.; and Calabresi, P.: A nude mouse model of the melanosis syndrome. *J.N.C.I.,* **71:**933–939, 1983.

Stehlin, J. S.; Giovanella, B. C.; DeIpolyi, P. D.; and Anderson, R. F.: Results of eleven years experience with heated perfusion for melanoma of the extremities. *Cancer Res.,* **39:**2255–2257, 1979.

Stehlin, J. S., Jr.; Giovanella, B. C.; DeIpolyi, P. D.; Muenz, L. R.; Anderson, R. F.; and Gutierrez, A. A.:

Hyperthermic perfusion of extremities for melanoma and soft tissue sarcomas. *Recent Results Cancer Res.,* **59:**171–185, 1977.

Suffin, S. C.; Waisman, J.; Clark, W. H., Jr.; and Morton, D. L.: Comparison of the classification by microscopic level (stage) of malignant melanoma by three independent groups of pathologists. *Cancer,* **40:**3112–3114, 1977.

Terry, W. D.; Hodes, R. J.; Rosenberg, S. A.; Fisher, R. I.; Makuch, R.; Gordon, H. G.; and Fisher, S. G.: Treatment of stage I and II malignant melanoma with adjuvant immunotherapy or chemotherapy: Preliminary analysis of a prospective randomized trial. In Terry, W. D., and Rosenberg, S. A. (eds.): *Immunotherapy of Human Cancer.* Elsevier, North-Holland, Inc., 1982.

Trozak, D. J.; Roland, W. D.; and Hu, F.: Metastatic malignant melanoma in prepubertal children. *Pediatrics,* **55:**191–204, 1974.

Veronesi, U.; Adamus, J.; Aubert, C.; Bajetta, E.; Beretta, G.; Bonadonna, G.; Bufalino, R.; Cascinelli, N.; Cocconi, G.; Durand, J.; DeMarsillae, J.; Ikonopisov, R. L.; Kiss, B.; Lejeune, F.; MacKie, R.; Madej, G.; Mulder, H.; Mechl, Z.; Milton, G. W.; Morabito, A.; Peter, H.; Priario, J.; Paul, E.; Rumke, P.; Sertoli, R.; and Tomin, R.: A randomized trial of adjuvant chemotherapy and immunotherapy in cutaneous melanoma. *N. Engl. J. Med.,* **307:**913–916, 1982.

Veronesi, U.; Adamus, J.; Bandeira, D. C.; Brennhovd, I. O.; Caceres, E.; Cascinelli, N.; Claudio, F.; Ikonopisov, R. L.; Javorski, V. V.; Kirov, S.; Kulakowski, A.; Lacour, J.; Lejeune, F.; Mechl, Z.; Morabito, A.; Rodi, I.; Serguv, S.; van Slooten, E.; Szczygiel, K., Tropeznikov, N. N.; and Wagner, R. I.: Inefficacy of immediate node dissection in stage I melanoma of the limbs. *N. Engl. J. Med.,* **297:**627–630, 1977.

Vosika, G. J.; Schmidtke, J. R.; Goldman, A.; Ribi, E.; Parker, R.; and Gray, G. R.: Intralesional immunotherapy of malignant melanoma with mycobacterium smegmatis cell wall skeleton combined with trehalose dimycolate (P_3). *Cancer,* **44:**495–503, 1979.

Walsh, T. S.: Primary melanoma of the gall bladder with cervical metastasis and fourteen and a half year survival. *Cancer,* **9:**518–522, 1956.

Wanebo, H. J.; Woodruff, J.; and Fortner, J. G.: Malignant melanoma of the extremities: A clinicopathologic study using levels of invasion (microstage). *Cancer,* **35:**666–676, 1975.

Weider, F.: Eight year survival in malignant melanoma related to sex and tumour location. *Dermatologica,* **162:**51–60, 1981.

White, J. E.; Strudwick, W. J.; Ricketts, W. N.; Sampson, C.: Cancer in the skin of Negroes: A review of 31 cases. *J.A.M.A.,* **178:**845–847, 1961.

Zelickson, A. S.: The fine structure of human melanotic and amelanotic malignant melanoma. *J. Invest. Dermatol.,* **39:**605–613, 1962.

22

Neoplasms of the Head and Neck

MONTAGUE LANE, BOBBY R. ALFORD, and
DONALD T. DONOVAN

Introduction

The management of cancers of the head and neck has been conventionally the province of surgeons and radiotherapists. During the past 15 years medical oncologists have become increasingly interested in patients with these neoplasms. This reflects several factors, including recognition that some chemotherapeutic agents alone and in combination can produce partial and even complete clinical regression of these tumors, the high mortality of patients diagnosed in late stages of head and neck cancer, and the improved cure rates obtained in patients with other types of cancer treated with adjuvant chemotherapy. Multimodal management of head and neck cancer patients is now the *modus operandi* in most medical centers. Not only oncologists, but most physicians and dentists, should be familiar with these tumors in order to recognize symptoms and signs of early disease, thus improving the prospect of curative therapy.

This chapter considers tumors of the upper aerodigestive passages. They arise in closely adjacent sites: In the oral cavity, nasal cavity, paranasal sinuses, nasopharynx, oropharynx, hypopharynx and larynx, and the salivary glands. Cancers of the head and neck, with the exception of salivary gland tumors, often have similar etiologies, pathologies, and modes of dissemination because they usually originate in squamous epithelium and in relatively close proximity. The specific functions and anatomic relationships of the subdivisions of the upper aerodigestive tract, variations in the biologic activity of tumors in different sites, and host response factors, however, confer unique characteristics upon tumors arising in each site. This is reflected in distinctive symptoms, anatomic and physiologic derangements, physical findings, and clinical evolutions that influence tumor detectability and diagnosis, therapeutic approaches, and, ultimately, prognosis of these tumors at each primary location.

Incidence and Epidemiology

The National Cancer Institute's Surveillance Epidemiology and End-Results (SEER) Program estimates 27,100 new cases of buccal cavity and pharyngeal cancer and 11,000 cases of laryngeal cancer in the United States in 1983 (Silverberg, 1983). Cancers of the nasal cavity, paranasal sinuses, and nasopharynx are included in a group classified as "other and unspecified respiratory cancers," an estimated 3,100 cases. Cancers of the head and neck constitute approximately 6% of new cancer cases in men and 2% in women. At all sites except the salivary glands cases in men predominate, ranging from a male/female ratio of 2:1 for tongue to 5:1 for larynx and 9:1 for lip. Oral and pharyngeal cancer are more common in white men at every site, but the incidence of laryngeal cancer is somewhat higher in black men. Although the majority of head and neck cancers arise in the oral cavity region, the larynx is the most common specific anatomic site afflicted.

The geographic distribution pattern for head and neck cancer varies considerably and is site dependent. Cancers of the nasal cavity and paranasal sinuses are slightly more common in the South than in the rest of the United States (Cutler and Young, 1975), but the difference is not statistically significant. The average age adjusted incidence is 0.8/100,000 in men and 0.5/100,000 in women. These cancers are slightly more common (1/100,000) in England and in Scandinavian countries and three to four times more common in Japan and Africa than in this country (Muir and Nectoux, 1980). Nasopharyngeal cancer is a very common disease among the Chinese. The age-specific incidence rate in men from Kwangtung Province (Cantonese) is in excess of 30/100,000 (Waterhouse et al., 1976). This is two to three times the incidence in nearby Chinese provinces and is 40 times that of U.S. white men. Chinese men also have high incidence rates in the San Francisco Bay area, Singapore, Hong Kong, and Hawaii. Increased rates of nasopharyngeal cancer occur in Eskimos in Greenland, Alaska, and Canada and also in Malays (Shanmugaratnum, 1982). The rate in Alaskan Eskimos is 15 times higher than that in the United States' general population (Lanier et al., 1976).

Lip cancer is seven to ten times more common in white than in black men in the United States. It occurs with very high frequency in Newfoundland, Saskatchewan, and other Canadian provinces (Miller, 1974; Spitzer et al., 1975). Oral and pharyngeal cancers in the United States occur most frequently in urban areas. In women, however, oral cancer is highest in Southern rural areas (Blot and Fraumeni, 1977). Internationally the geographic incidence varies widely. Highest rates are seen in India, Southeast Asia, France, and Puerto Rico, intermediate rates in the United States, Canada, Australia, and England, and low rates in Japan, Israel, Mexico, and Egypt (Water-

house et al., 1976). Laryngeal cancer also has a varied international distribution. It is very common in men in São Paulo, Brazil (14.1/100,000), Bombay, France, Italy, Spain, and northern Thailand (Muir and Nectoux, 1982). The rate in the United States is somewhat lower (8.3/100,000) in white men but is higher (12.2/100,000) in black men (Young et al., 1978). The incidence rate is low in England.

Etiology and Pathogenesis

Epidemiologic studies of head and neck cancer have identified populations at higher risk for development of these diseases. Subsequent analysis of these populations compared to various control groups with respect to age, gender, race, genetics, diet, social habits, occupation, geography, customs, and other variables in conjunction with laboratory investigations of suspect potential carcinogen exposure identified risk factors for cancer at each site. One of the major difficulties in epidemiologic studies is to provide sufficient evidence that a particular association is causal. Suspected risk factors are often eventually proven to have no etiologic relationship to cancer. Documentation of a causally related risk factor, however, offers the potential for preventing some types of cancer through avoiding, eliminating, or modifying the factor.

The overwhelming majority of head and neck cancers have been related to prolonged exposure to environmental factors (Wynder et al., 1977). Although many associations between risk factors and various head and neck cancers are firm, others are questionable (see Table 22–1).

Table 22–1. Factors Associated with or Suspected of Causing Head and Neck Cancers

SITE	FACTOR
Lip	Sunlight; tobacco smoking; poor dentition; ionizing radiation
Oral cavity	Tobacco smoking, chewing; "reverse smoking;" betel (leaf, nut, ± lime, ± tobacco) chewing; alcohol consumption; iron deficiency (Plummer-Vinson syndrome); riboflavin deficiency; wool dust
Tongue	Tobacco smoking; alcohol consumption, poor dentition; poor oral hygiene; wool dust
Oropharynx	Tobacco smoking; alcohol consumption; wool dust
Nasal cavity and paranasal sinuses	Snuff; Thorotrast; nickel compounds; chromate compounds; wood dust; leather dust; radium; β,β-dichloroethyl sulfide; isopropyl oil, diisopropyl sulfate; hydrocarbons, nitrosamines; dioxane
Nasopharynx	Epstein-Barr virus; nitrosamines; genetic factors
Hypopharynx	Tobacco smoking; alcohol consumption; iron deficiency (Plummer-Vinson syndrome)
Larynx	Tobacco smoking; alcohol consumption; asbestos; nickel compounds; wood dust
Salivary glands	Ionizing radiation

Sunlight. Many studies have been documented that suggest that chronic and intense exposure to sunlight is a factor in the pathogenesis of lip cancer. The disease occurs primarily in fair- or ruddy-complected white men in the sixth and later decades of life. Generally, these men have had considerable solar exposure by virtue of outdoor occupations (Jørgensen et al., 1973; Molnár et al., 1974; Baker and Krause, 1981). Cancers arise on the lower lip 20 times more frequently than on the upper lip, which tends to be shaded from direct actinic exposure. The most common site involved on the lower lip is about halfway between the commissure and the midline on the vermilion surface that is below the line of contact with the upper lip (Batsakis, 1974). Lip cancer is nine to ten times more common in men than in women, probably reflecting occupational differences and perhaps also the protective effects of lipstick. The disease is rare in blacks, a fact that has been attributed to the protective effect of pigment. Finally, solar radiation damage has been found in the lips of most patients with lip cancer, regardless of their ages (Baker and Krause, 1981). As noted in a recent review (Decker and Goldstein, 1982), however, the Third National Cancer Survey did not demonstrate a correlation between lip and skin cancer (Szpak et al., 1977). There is a linear relationship between the incidence of skin cancer, but not lip cancer, and decreasing latitude. This raises some question regarding solar radiation in the pathogenesis of lip cancer and suggests a possible role for other contributory factors.

Jagged teeth, poorly fitting dentures, or chronically infected gingivae may cause lip irritation, and such findings are common in patients with lip cancer. Poor oral hygiene probably plays a contributory rather than a primary role in the etiology of lip cancer.

Tobacco. The two factors most consistently related to carcinoma of the oral cavity, oropharynx, hypopharynx, and larynx are chronic use of tobacco and alcohol (Wynder et al., 1957, 1977). Tobacco smoke contains many carcinogens, such as benzo[a]pyrene, 5-methylchrysene, and dibenz[a, h]anthracene, dimethyl, and other nitrosamines, cocarcinogens, and promoters (Hoffman et al., 1978). Tobacco tar also contains a variety of tumorigenic agents of which N′-nitrosonornicotine (NNN) is the most prevalent (Hoffman et al., 1978). This compound and other tobacco-specific N-nitrosamines are formed in the pro-

cesses of curing and fermenting tobacco and are present in snuff and chewing tobacco (Hecht et al., 1979). The risk of a tobacco user developing cancer at a specific site is a function of the degree of exposure and the inherent susceptibility of the site. The amount of exposure is related to years of use, type of use, smoking, chewing, snuffing, duration of contact, amount used daily, and specific composition of product. For smokers, the depth, mode, and frequency of inhalation are important (Wynder and Hoffman, 1982). This dose-response relationship accounts for the high incidence of these cancers in the sixth and later decades of life.

Many of the epidemiologic characteristics of cancer of the oral cavity, pharynx, and larynx can be explained in terms of cultural practices of tobacco use that influence the amount of exposure of various portions of the upper aerodigestive tract to the constituents of tobacco smoke, tar, and juice. The preponderance of these cancers in men in the United States probably reflects more widespread and generally more intensive cigarette smoking by men as well as their use of cigars and pipes. Snuff dipping is a common practice among women in some rural southern states, however, and is accompanied by a dramatic increase in the incidence of gingival and buccal mucosal cancer in these women (Winn et al., 1981). The higher incidence of laryngeal cancer in comparison to other sites in the oral cavity and oropharynx seems to be related to the depth of inhalation of cigarette smoke, as is the case for lung cancer as well.

Tobacco chewing is uncommon in the United States, but common in some parts of the world, such as Ceylon, Bombay, other parts of India and portions of Southeast Asia, which have some of the highest incidence rates of oral and pharyngeal cancer. Oral cavity cancer is the commonest form of cancer in Bombay. A mixture called pan (betel nut and leaf, lime, catechu, tobacco, and other additives) is very popular in India. It is chewed into a quid and buccal mucosa cancer usually develops at the site where the quid is kept. High incidences of buccal mucosa cancer have also been reported in tobacco-chewing populations of Soviet Central Asia and Afghanistan, where people chew a mixture similar to pan, called nass (Mahboubi and Sayed, 1982).

The smoking of a cigarette called "bidi," made of uncured tobacco, in Bombay and of a similar cigarette called "keego" in Northern

Thailand is associated with a high risk of cancer of the oropharynx (tonsil, base of tongue), hypopharynx, and esophagus (Mahboubi and Sayed, 1982).

Further evidence of the importance of type of exposure and site of cancer is the high incidence of cancer of the hard palate in populations that practice reverse smoking, keeping the burning end of the cigarette in the mouth during smoking, in parts of India, Sardinia, Venezuela, and Panama (Mahboubi and Sayed, 1982). Hard palate cancer is otherwise uncommon in most of the world.

Cancer of the lip has long been associated with pipe smoking, perhaps due to the high temperature of the pipe stem, to mechanical irritation, or to tobacco smoke (Broders, 1920; Ebenius, 1945; Jørgensen et al., 1973). Women pipe smokers have an increased incidence of lip cancer (Ebenius, 1945; Molnár et al., 1974). Even in pipe smokers, however, the upper lip is rarely involved despite thermal and mechanical contact with the pipe stem equal to the lower lip. Lesions rarely occur near the angle of the mouth, where pipes are generally held, and lip cancer is rare in black pipe smokers. These observations cast doubt on the importance of the hot pipe stem in the pathogenesis of lip cancer and suggests a more prominent role for tobacco smoke. Currently, cigarette smoke is much more frequently associated with lip cancer than is pipe smoking.

Alcohol. The relationship between chronic alcohol consumption and cancer of the oral cavity, oropharynx, hypopharynx, and larynx is long established (Wynder et al., 1957; Vogler et al., 1962; Martinez, 1969). Because the majority of patients with cancers at these sites are smokers and drinkers, assessing the relative importance of each factor was difficult. Now ample evidence shows that smoking and drinking are both risk factors and that their combined effects are synergistic. In the oral cavity and pharynx alcohol appears to be a more important factor than smoking. A recent study demonstrated that the relative risk of oral cancer for minimal drinkers who were heavy smokers is less than half of that for minimal smokers who were heavy drinkers (Mashberg, et al., 1981). Furthermore, the amount of alcohol consumed has a far greater effect on risk than does the number of cigarettes when both were used. This study also suggested that beer and wine consumption confer greater risks than do whiskey at equivalent levels of alcohol consumed. Alcohol consumption and cigarette smoking both demonstrate dose-response and multiplicative interactions in laryngeal cancer risks (Wynder and Stellman, 1977). Alcohol appears to increase the risks of supraglottic cancer to a greater extent than glottic cancer in smokers (Schottenfeld, 1979).

There is no evidence that ethanol itself is a carcinogen. The mechanism of its effects as a cocarcinogen may relate to other constituents in alcoholic beverages, nutritional deficiencies, tissue injury, or even interactions with trace constituents in alcoholic beverages. Various reports have suggested that one or another type of alcoholic beverage has a greater propensity for inducing oral cancer than others, that is, whiskey rather than beer, apple-based brandies and, as cited above, wine and beer rather than whiskey. Oral cancer has even been noted in chronic users of strong alcoholic mouthwashes. At this time alcohol itself and the amount of alcohol consumed appear to provide the principal risk.

Nutritional Deficiencies. Head and neck cancers often occur in patients with nutritional deficiencies. Many alcoholics suffer from malnutrition. Dietary deficiency of B vitamins, particularly riboflavin (Wynder and Chan, 1970), and in vitamin A and retinoids (Sporn, 1977) may play a role in the etiology of head and neck cancers, but this is not yet established definitively. Evidence suggests that dietary deficiencies are associated with esophageal cancer in some areas of the world, as also would reasonably be expected for squamous carcinomas of the aerodigestive tract proximal to the esophagus. Sideropenic dysphagia (Plummer-Vinson syndrome; Paterson-Brown-Kelly syndrome) occurs commonly in Scandinavia and England and has been related to a high frequency of carcinoma of the hypopharynx and esophagus, particularly in women (Wynder and Fryer, 1958). It appears to be a consequence of nutritional deficiencies of iron and B vitamins.

Occupational Factors. Various occupational exposures are associated with head and neck cancers (see Table 22–2). In some instances the suspect carcinogens are reasonably well defined (certain oxidation states of chromium and nickel, mustard gas, isopropyl alcohol, and/or diisopropylsulfate). In other instances, the epidemiologic association with these occupations is certain but the carcinogens remain undefined, for example, shoe manufacturing, woodworking, and textile manufacturing (Decouflé, 1982). In addition,

Table 22-2. Occupations Associated with an Increased Incidence of Head and Neck Cancer

SITE	OCCUPATION	SUSPECTED CARCINOGEN
Lip	Farming, ranching, fishing, other outdoor work	Ultraviolet light
Oral cavity	Textile manufacture	Wool dust
Tongue	Textile manufacture	Wool dust
Oropharynx	Textile manufacture	Wool dust
Larynx	Shipbuilding, insulating, asbestos mining or fabrication, other asbestos exposures	Asbestos
	Woodworking	Wood dust
	Nickel refining	Nickel compounds
	Mustard gas manufacture	β,β-dichloroethyl sulfide
Nasal cavity and paranasal sinuses	Woodworking	Wood dust
	Shoe manufacture	Leather or wood dust
	Nickel refining	Nickel compounds
	Chromate paint manufacture	Chromates
	Radium dial painting	Radium
	Mustard gas manufacture	β,β-dichloroethyl sulfide
	Isopropyl alcohol manufacture	Isopropyl oil, diisopropylsulphate
	Chemical and petroleum manufacture	Hydrocarbons, nitrosamines, dioxane

many of the occupation-associated cancers are primarily adenocarcinomas rather than epidermoid carcinomas, in contradistinction to tobacco- and alcohol-associated head and neck cancers.

Epstein-Barr Virus (EBV). Carcinoma of the nasopharynx occurs in younger patients than do other squamous carcinomas of the head and neck, with a peak incidence in the fifth decade. It is not associated with tobacco or alcohol use. The high frequency of serum antibodies to EBV in patients with nasopharyngeal carcinoma suggests a possible etiological role of this virus (de-Thé, 1981); this, however, has not yet been proven.

Genetic Factors. The high incidence of nasopharyngeal cancer (NPC) in Cantonese and the finding of a specific HLA antigen profile (A2-BW46) in Chinese NPC patients in Singapore, Malaysia, Hong Kong, and California suggest a genetic predisposition for the disease (Chan and Simons, 1977). Another haplotype, AW19-BW17, has been associated with poor survival in Chinese patients under 30 years of age with NPC (Simons et al., 1978). Interestingly, American-born Chinese have half the incidence of nasopharyngeal carcinoma of native-born Chinese. However, whether this is due to change in environment or marriage with Chinese from lower risk provinces is unclear (King and Haenzel, 1973). Although there seems to be considerable individual variation in susceptibility to head and neck cancer, no major genetic factors have yet been elucidated with the exception of the predisposition

of Chinese and other groups of Asian origin to NPC. Such factors continue to be sought.

Poor Oral Hygiene. The role of poor oral hygiene and bad teeth in oral cancer is uncertain. It is a common finding both in patients with oral cancer and in controls, although perhaps somewhat more common in those with cancer. Cancers of the tongue and buccal mucosa are frequently found at the site of irritation of a jagged tooth. Although poor hygiene and dentition may be independent or contributory risks, they certainly are of far less importance than tobacco and alcohol consumption.

Radiation. Exposure to radiation has been associated with an increased incidence of salivary gland tumors in survivors of the atomic-bomb explosion (Belsky et al., 1972).

In summary, the dose-response relationships of risk factors to the incidence of most head and neck cancers, the synergism observed between several of these factors, the tendency of head and neck cancers to occur more frequently with increasing age, the long latent periods for tumor development, and the high incidence of multiple head and neck primary cancers indicate that most of these risk factors behave either like carcinogens, cocarcinogens, or promoters. Furthermore, exposure to these factors is largely avoidable.

Pathology and Natural History

Squamous cell carcinomas are the most common malignant tumors of the head and neck. These tumors are derived from the epithelium that lines the upper airways and digestive tract. The gross pathologic appearance of squamous carcinomas of the head and neck is usually infiltrative (which is often ulcerative), exophytic (papillary), or verrucous. The latter has a pebbly surface and wartlike appearance and tends to spread superficially with little deep penetration.

The histopathologic characteristics of squamous carcinoma vary from well-differentiated keratinized lesions to those with nonkeratinizing, poorly differentiated features. The well- to moderately well-differentiated types predominate in the lip, nasal cavity, floor of the mouth, buccal mucosa, gingiva, hard palate, oropharynx, and glottic larynx. Tumors lacking cellular differentiation are characterized by increased mitotic activity, increased invasiveness, lack of a plasma lymphocytic response and, generally, a poorer prognosis than well-differentiated tumors (Lund *et al.,* 1977). These lesions have a greater tendency than well-differentiated tumors to metastasize to lymph nodes, which are often clinically involved at the time of diagnosis. They tend to have infiltrative rather than pushing margins. Less well- to poorly differentiated histologies predominate in cancers of the tongue, especially of the posterior third, the tonsil, the nasopharynx, the hypopharynx, and the supraglottic larynx. The squamous carcinomas of the maxillary sinus vary from well- to poorly differentiated. Only a small percentage of carcinomas of the nasopharynx are keratinized. The majority are nonkeratinizing and undifferentiated carcinomas. Those with incidental diffuse infiltration with normal lymphocytic elements have been called lymphoepitheliomas. These tumors are all variants of squamous cell carcinoma and may also be found in the base of the tongue, tonsil, and hypopharynx. They tend to be highly sensitive to radiation therapy.

Leukoplakia is often found on the mucous membranes of the oral cavity, tongue, oropharynx, and larynx, particularly in chronic users of alcohol and tobacco (see Figure 22–1). Such whitish patches may represent hyperkeratosis, hyperplasia, carcinoma *in situ,* or invasive carcinoma, that is, they may be benign, premalignant or malignant. Areas of leukoplakia are found in proximity to or at sites remote from obvious cancers. Early lesions may also present as erythroplasia—red,

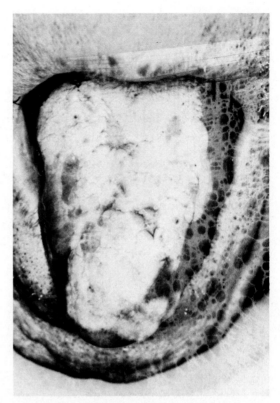

Figure 22–1. Extensive leukoplakia of the tongue. No malignancy detected in biopsies.

slightly elevated thickened areas of mucosa. Areas of leukoplakia and erythroplasia should be biopsied to establish whether they are benign or malignant.

Other tumors that may arise in the upper aerodigestive tract include lymphomas, melanomas, olfactory esthesioneuroblastomas, plasmacytomas, adenocarcinomas, adenoid cystic carcinomas, mucoepidermoid carcinomas, sarcomas, and various benign tumors. These include nasopharyngeal angiofibromas, which occur most commonly in adolescent and younger men, hamartomas, chemodectomas, some hemangiopericytomas, and glomus tumors. The head and neck region may contain metastatic carcinoma from the breast, lung, gastrointestinal tract, kidney, and other sites as well as metastases from myeloma, melanoma, and lymphoma.

Most salivary gland tumors arise from the parotid gland. Three-fourths of parotid tumors are benign. The commonest benign parotid tumor is the mixed tumor composed of multiple epithelial elements—glands, myxomatous areas, cartilaginous material, and stroma. The malignant parotid tumors include many cell types, that is, adenocarcinoma, adenoid cystic, mucoepidermoid, epidermoid, and undifferentiated. Mixed tumors occasionally undergo malignant transformation. Tumors of the submaxillary and sublingual glands are predominantly malignant, whereas minor salivary gland tumors, with the exception of those arising in the hard palate, are most commonly benign. Malignant tumors of these salivary glands have a histologic distribution similar to those of the malignant tumors of the parotid gland.

Modes of Spread. Epidermoid carcinomas of the head and neck tend to remain localized and to invade adjacent tissues progressively. Such invasion may extend submucosally as well as deeply into muscle and along tissue planes far beyond the limits of the apparent lesion. They may entrap and invade small blood vessels, lymphatic channels, and nerves. Intracranial spread may result from perineural extension of tumor along peripheral branches of cranial nerves. Direct invasion of the subcutaneous tissues and through the skin is not unusual. Lesions abutting cartilage and bone may spread along the perichondrium and periosteum and eventually may also invade and destroy cartilage and bone. Infiltrative and exophytic lesions tend to ulcerate, bleed, and become infected. Advanced lesions may invade large vessels such as the carotid artery and cause major and even fatal hemorrhage. Verrucous lesions may remain asymptomatic and achieve considerable size before they are noticed because of their bulk or as a consequence of symptoms related to tissue invasion and destruction.

The second most common mode of spread of epidermoid tumors is via extension into draining lymphatics to proximal and then to more remote lymph nodes. Thus, metastases from cancer of the mobile tongue often involve subdigastric nodes, cancer of the base of the tongue is associated with high jugular nodes, and hypopharyngeal cancer metastasizes primarily to midjugular nodes.

The head is supplied with extensive systems of superficial lymphatic vessels and nodes that drain into several major deep lymphatic systems in the neck. This superficial system of lymphatics terminates in occipital, postauricular, and preauricular nodes draining the scalp and ear region that connect with the upper deep jugular nodes. Lymph nodes that are superficial, within, and deep to the parotid gland collect afferent lymphatics from the gland, the eyelids, root of the nose, external ear, palate, and nasopharynx and drain into the upper deep jugular nodes. Facial lymph nodes draining the lids, nose, and cheek empty into the submaxillary nodes.

The major lymphatic groups in the neck include superficial, anterior and deep jugular, submental, submaxillary, spinal accessory, retropharyngeal, and supraclavicular groups.

Hematogenous metastases may occur via connection of the lymphatic trunks draining the head and neck with the venous system in the neck or by direct invasion of the vascular system.

Sites of Metastases. As previously noted, poorly differentiated and undifferentiated tumors are biologically more aggressive than well- to moderately well-differentiated tumors and involve lymph nodes more frequently and extensively. In addition, nodal involvement is more common in sites well supplied with lymphatics. Thus, node metastases are uncommon with well-differentiated carcinomas of the lip and hard palate, more common with well- to moderately well-differentiated lesions of the buccal mucosa and oropharynx, and very common with poorly differentiated tumors of the tonsil, base of the tongue, and hypopharynx. Additionally, if lesions attain a large size, they are likely to spread to draining lymph nodes.

As with lymphatic spread, hematogenous metastases are most common with the biologically aggressive tumors that arise in the tongue, tonsil, nasopharynx, hypopharynx and supraglottic larynx. The most prevalent metastatic sites are the lungs, bones, and liver, but other organs, such as the brain, may be involved. In apparent lung metastases, particularly if there is a solitary lesion, the possibility of a separate primary lung cancer must be considered. As patients survive longer due to more effective control of primary lesions and neck nodes and treatment of metastases with chemotherapy, the incidence of clinically evident hematogenous metastases increases. Malignant salivary gland tumors have a propensity for hematogenous metastases, particularly to lung and bone. Sarcomas, melanomas, and other non-squamous-cell carcinomas of the head and neck also have a high incidence of hematogenous spread.

Patients with recurrent or locally uncontrolled disease often suffer from anorexia, inability to chew or swallow, and other local problems that result in severe malnutrition. Cachexia, infection, hemorrhage, and aspiration pneumonia are common causes of death. In patients whose primary disease is controlled, death may result from metastases to other organs, such as the liver or lungs.

Symptoms and Signs

The symptoms and signs of head and neck cancers reflect the anatomic location of the primary tumor, the degree of advancement at the time of diagnosis, the growth characteristics of the tumor (infiltrative, exophytic, verrucous), and its biologic aggressiveness (see Figure 22-2). In some instances the presenting complaint or finding is sufficiently specific to clearly suggest the primary site, such as an

obvious lesion of the lip, a papillary tumor on the mobile tongue, or painful swelling of the anterior wall of the maxillary sinus. Some symptoms and signs are common to tumors of various sites because they share histopathologic features. Thus, infiltrative and exophytic lesions tend to ulcerate, become infected, and bleed. Patients with such cancers may note oral bleeding, malodorous breath, or odynophagia. Some signs or symptoms may be due to an early lesion of a particular site or an advanced tumor from another region that has invaded the site, that is, pain in the teeth from an early mucosal lesion of the superior alveolar ridge versus invasion of the alveolar bone by a carcinoma of the maxillary sinus. Symptoms in some areas may be the result of tumor invading that locus or may be referred by various

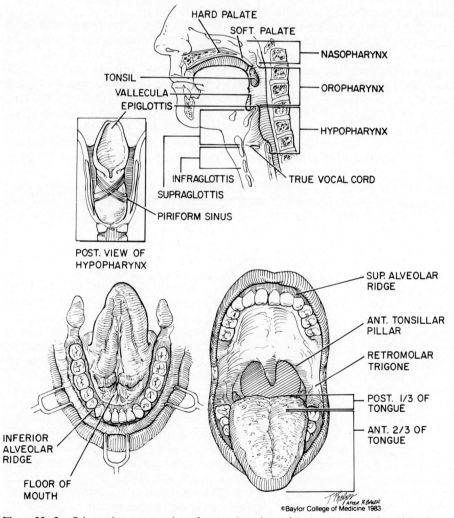

Figure 22-2. Schematic representation of anatomic regions of the head and neck in which primary cancers may arise.

mechanisms from tumors in more distant sites. Otalgia, for example, may be due to squamous carcinoma of the external auditory meatus, occlusion of the eustachian tube by carcinoma of the nasopharynx — producing a serous effusion in the middle ear, or may be a consequence of pain referred to the ear from other sites. Thus, tumors of the floor of the mouth and anterior tongue regions innervated by the lingual nerve may cause otalgia via connections with the auriculotemporal nerve. Pain from the inferior alveolar nerves may also be referred to the ear via the auriculotemporal nerve. Pain may be referred to the ear from distributions of the sensory division of the facial nerve (nervus intermedius), which also refers pain to the ear from lesions in the maxilla. The nervus intermedius communicates with branches of cranial nerves V, IX, and X and sends branches to the internal acoustic meatus. Pain from the posterior tongue, tonsil, and hypopharynx may be referred to the ear via auricular branches of the glossopharyngeal nerve. Auditory branches of the vagus nerve refer pain to the ear from the pharynx, supraglottic larynx, and larynx. Of course, otalgia may be due to benign processes such as otitis media.

Trismus is a late finding due to invasion of the muscles of mastication by tumors from several sites, including the buccal mucosa, base of tongue, maxillary sinus, and palatal arch.

Nasal stuffiness, unilateral nasal obstruction, postnasal drip, headache, and epistaxis are common symptoms of early tumors of the nasal cavity and more advanced tumors of the paranasal sinuses. These symptoms are also commonly associated with chronic sinusitis and should not be attributed to sinusitis without careful investigation for a neoplasm. Nasal speech may also be noted in these conditions and in nasopharyngeal carcinoma, whereas a "hot potato" speech occurs with large tumors of the posterior tongue.

Other symptoms commonly associated with head and neck cancer, as well as with other unrelated conditions, include poorly fitting dentures, loosening of teeth, dysphagia, hoarseness, stridor, and cranial nerve palsies. Cervical adenopathy may precede, appear simultaneously with, or follow the discovery of head and neck primary cancers.

Some of the more important symptoms of head and neck cancers and the tumors with which they are commonly associated are listed in Table 22–3. These symptoms, of course, can be due to many other disorders. Thus, bleeding from the nose may be due to trauma, vascular malformations, bleeding diatheses, leukemia, benign tumors, drugs, poor oral hygiene, or other etiologies. Hoarseness may be due to benign pathology of the vocal cords or to intrathoracic tumors involving the recurrent laryngeal nerve. A careful history, physical examination, and appropriate diagnostic studies are needed to lead to the correct diagnosis.

Systemic manifestations of head and neck cancers usually occur late in the course of disease and reflect protein-calorie malnutrition, infection and anemia, or are related to metastases to the lungs, liver, bones, or brain. Hypercalcemia may occur secondary to bone metastases or as a paraneoplastic syndrome in some patients with squamous cell carcinomas of the head and neck.

The usual signs and symptoms related to each primary site of head and neck cancer are catalogued below.

Oral Cavity. The anatomic structures that make up the oral cavity are the lips, the buccal mucosa, the upper and lower alveolar ridges, the floor of the mouth, the retromolar gingiva, the anterior two-thirds of the tongue, and the hard palate. The patient occasionally detects cancer in some of these sites, either visually or with the tongue. In other instances intraoral cancers may be asymptomatic until they achieve considerable local size or have advanced into structures beyond their sites of origin.

Lip. Approximately 95% of carcinomas of the lip occur on the lower lip (see Figure 22–3). They are usually located on the vermilion surface below the line of contact with the upper lip and about midway between the commissure and the midline. They may present as a sore that never heals completely, but repeatedly ulcerates, crusts over, and progressively enlarges. Ulcerated keratinizing tumors are often accompanied by an inflammatory reaction that may obscure their neoplastic nature, particularly if this reaction subsides temporarily after application of topical adrenocorticosteroid preparations. The underlying lesion will persist and must be biopsied. Some lip cancers may be exophytic or verrucous. These tumors tend to crack and bleed. They deform and swell the lip and are easily identifiable. Lymph node metastases are unusual except in advanced or recurrent cases of lip cancer. In these

Table 22-3.   Relationship of Common Symptoms and Signs of Head and Neck Cancer to Site of Primary Carcinoma

SYMPTOMS AND SIGNS	PRIMARY SITE OF CARCINOMA
Oral bleeding	Buccal mucosa, floor of mouth, mobile tongue, upper and lower alveolar ridges, hard palate
Persistent sore throat and/or odyno-phagia	Retromolar gingiva, tonsil, soft palate, base of tongue, periepiglottic region, lateral pharyngeal walls, hypopharynx, supraglottic larynx
Dysphagia	Hard palate, mobile tongue, soft palate, tonsil, base of tongue, periepiglottic region, lateral pharyngeal walls, hypopharynx
Malodorous breath	Buccal mucosa, floor of mouth, hard palate, mobile tongue, periepiglottic region, hypopharynx, other infected tumors
Pain in upper teeth or maxilla, loose teeth, or difficulty with dentures	Buccal mucosa, upper alveolar ridge, nasal cavity, maxillary sinus, hard palate
Pain in lower teeth or mandible, loose teeth, or difficulty with dentures	Buccal mucosa, floor of mouth, retromolar gingiva, inferior alveolar ridge
Facial pain	Upper and lower alveolar ridges, maxillary sinus, nasopharynx, soft palate, salivary gland
Facial swelling	Lip, buccal mucosa, upper and lower alveolar ridges, frontal sinus, axillary sinus, parotid gland
Trismus	Buccal mucosa, retromolar gingiva, maxillary sinus, soft palate, parotid gland
Hoarseness	Nasopharynx, periepiglottic region, hypopharynx, larynx
Otalgia	Upper and lower alveolar ridges, retromolar gingiva, mobile tongue, maxillary sinus, nasopharynx (chronic ache, unilateral hearing loss, and serous otitis), base of tongue, periepiglottic region, lateral pharyngeal walls, hypopharynx, subglottic larynx
Nasal swelling, bleeding, obstruction, discharge	Nasal cavity, paranasal sinuses, nasopharynx
Headache, chronic sinusitis	Nasal cavity, paranasal sinuses, nasopharynx
Excessive lacrimation	Nasal cavity, ethmoid sinus, maxillary sinus
Change in quality of speech	Floor of mouth, hard palate, mobile tongue, nasopharynx, base of tongue
Displacement of globe/diplopia	Nasal cavity, frontal ethmoid and maxillary sinuses, nasopharynx
Cranial nerve palsies	Paranasal sinuses, nasopharynx, parotid gland
Cervical adenopathy common at diagnosis	Buccal mucosa, floor of mouth, retromolar gingiva, mobile tongue, nasopharynx, soft palate, tonsil, base of tongue, periepiglottic region, lateral and posterior pharyngeal walls.

cases submental and submaxillary lymph node metastases from cancer of either lip may be observed or cancer of the upper lip may spread to preauricular and high anterior cervical nodes.

Buccal Mucosa.   The buccal mucosa lines the cheeks and lips and extends to the gingivae inferiorly and superiorly and terminates at the retromolar area posteriorly. Often these lesions are extensive before they become symptomatic (see Figure 22-4). They may first be detected subsequent to the appearance of submaxillary adenopathy. Verrucous carcinomas often appear benign, spread over a considerable area, and remain asymptomatic until they produce destruction of underlying tissues. Ulcerative lesions often extend submucosally anteriorly and posteriorly and invade the buccinator muscle. If the maxilla or the inferior alveolar ridge is invaded, the lesions may be associated with pain in these bones and with bleeding. They may cause difficulty with denture fit. Ulcerative and exophytic lesions often become infected. Foul breath, anorexia, and inanition are common consequences of in-

fected tumors. Large exophytic lesions can interfere with chewing. Buccal mucosa carcinomas may produce swelling of the cheek and even oral cutaneous fistulas. They can cause trismus by infiltration of the muscles of mastication. In most instances carcinomas of the buccal mucosa should be detected easily on an intraoral examination by a physician or dentist. These cancers may originate simultaneously in multiple primary sites and can be associated with leukoplakia and erythroplasia.

Floor of the Mouth.   Squamous cell carcinomas of the floor of the mouth are most often located close to the midline between the lower gum and the tongue (see Figure 22-5). They may be asymptomatic for some time. Occasionally the patient will detect the tumor with his tongue or notice it on self-examination. As these lesions enlarge and extend posteriorly, they may partially fix the tongue and interfere with speech or mastication. They may interfere with the fit of lower dentures. Ulcerative and exophytic lesions may bleed, become infected and painful, and be associated with foul breath and excessive salivation. These tumors

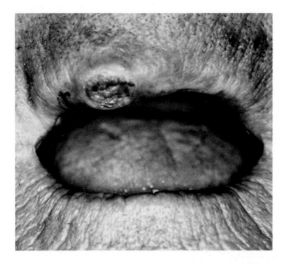

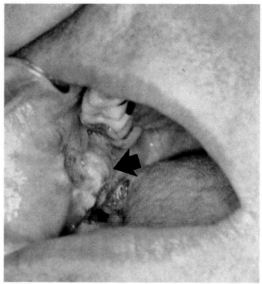

Figure 22-4. Papillary squamous cell carcinoma of the buccal mucosa (arrow).

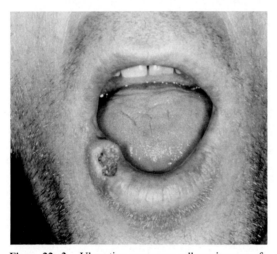

Figure 22-3. Ulcerative squamous cell carcinomas of the lips (upper and lower).

tend to spread along the periosteum of the mandible, but may invade the bone and produce severe pain. Metastatic spread to the submandibular nodes is often present at the time of diagnosis. The upper jugular nodes are usually involved later in the course of the disease.

Upper and Lower Alveolar Ridges. These squamous cell carcinomas arise in the gingiva, often in proximity to the premolar or molar teeth. They may be asymptomatic except for bleeding with tooth brushing or mastication. Difficulty in denture fit may cause the patient to seek dental consultation that can lead to recognition of a tumor as the basis of the problem. Cancers of the upper ridge spread to the hard palate, the gingivobuccal gutter, the soft

palate, and into the maxilla. They may perforate the maxillary sinus. Lesions of the lower ridge can extend to the gingivobuccal mucosa and floor of the mouth and may invade the mandible. Invasion of the maxillary bone or the mandible causes severe local pain and may produce unilateral otalgia.

Retromolar Gingiva (Retromolar Trigone). These tumors often remain unnoticed because of their location until they are advanced. The earliest symptom that usually leads to examination by a physician or dentist is persistent localized sore throat. Tumors of the retromolar gingiva (retromolar trigone) tend to be ul-

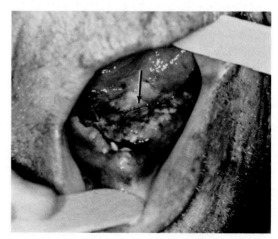

Figure 22-5. Squamous cell carcinoma of the floor of the mouth (arrow).

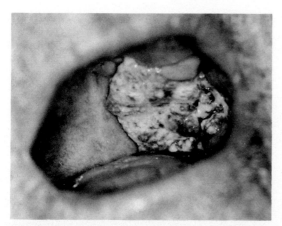

Figure 22–6. Squamous cell carcinoma of the left retromolar trigone extending to the soft palate.

cerative and invasive, with frequent spread to the anterior faucial pillar (see Figure 22–6). They invade the mandible, producing local pain, odynophagia, and unilateral otalgia. Trismus may result from invasion of the pterygoid muscle. Submandibular node metastases are often present at the time of initial diagnosis.

Hard Palate. Squamous cell carcinomas of the hard palate are infrequent. They tend to be ulcerative, to spread to the gingiva and soft palate, and to invade underlying bone. They may become infected and produce foul breath and local pain. Most of the tumors of the hard palate are benign salivary gland tumors that remain asymptomatic until large enough to interfere with speech, food passage, or the fit of dentures (see Figure 22–7). Upper jugular node metastases may occur. Malignant salivary gland tumors of the hard palate often have a similarly slow evolution and produce similar symptoms. They may also bleed and cause local pain. Hematogenous metastases to bone, lung, and liver may be present at initial diagnosis. Tumors of the hard palate are often detected by the patient.

Anterior Two-Thirds of the Tongue. The anterior two-thirds of the tongue is delineated from the base of the tongue by the circumvallate papillae. It is the most frequent site of oral cavity cancer. The squamous cell carcinomas of the mobile tongue are primarily ulcerative or papillary and frequently arise on the lateral tongue borders, where they may be adjacent to jagged and carious teeth (see Figure 22–8). Dorsal and ventral lesions also occur. Cancers of the mobile tongue are often asymptomatic until large. Speech and mastication may be impaired by bulky papillary lesions, which tend to bleed easily. Ulcerative tumors become infected easily and may cause local pain and malodorous breath. Involvement of the lingual nerve can produce ipsilateral otalgia via the auriculotemporal nerve. Laterally placed lesions may spread posteriorly toward the anterior pillar and cause dysphagia. Ventral lesions frequently invade deeply toward the floor of the mouth and may interfere with lingual mobility and speech; some may extend across the midline. Approximately one-half of patients have lymph node metastases to the upper jugular chain at the time of diagnosis. The subdigastric nodes are involved first and bilateral node metastases may be present. Metastases to lung, liver, and bone are noted commonly late in the course of this disease.

Nasal Cavity and Paranasal Sinuses. *Nasal Cavity.* The nasal cavities extend from the anterior to the posterior choanae and are separated medially by the nasal septum. The lateral

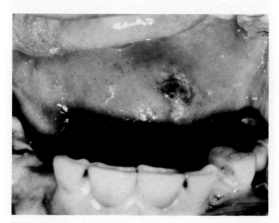

Figure 22–7. Benign ulcerating salivary gland tumor of the hard palate.

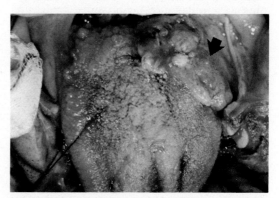

Figure 22–8. Squamous cell carcinoma of the left lateral tongue border (arrow).

wall of each cavity is formed by the turbinate bones. The nasolacrimal duct and the ostia of the paranasal sinuses open into the nasal cavity. The most frequent malignant tumor of this site is squamous cell carcinoma. The usual presenting symptoms of nasal cavity cancer are nasal obstruction, discharge, and bleeding. There may be unilateral swelling of the nose with tumors of the inferior and middle turbinates. If the ostia of the maxillary, ethmoid, or frontal sinuses are obstructed, these sinuses often become infected and patients will complain of unremitting headache in the region of the involved sinus and have other symptoms of sinusitis, such as fever and increased pain with movement of the head. Epiphora occurs if the lacrimal duct is obstructed. Tumors that arise near the anterior ethmoids may cause swelling close to the inner canthus, with displacement of the eye laterally, diplopia, and frontal headache. There may be severe pain from destruction of bone and invasion of the sinuses and cranial cavity. Perineural metastases can result in spread into the anterior fossa and severe frontal headache. Downward extension into the maxilla may produce pain in the upper teeth. With destruction of the nasal septum, the tumor may spread into the opposite nasal cavity. Fortunately, tumors of the nasal cavity are rare.

Paranasal Sinuses. FRONTAL SINUS CARCINOMA. Frontal sinus carcinoma is rare. Initial symptoms are similar to those of chronic frontal sinusitis, with a sensation of fullness or pressure between the eyes and above the brow, which may be referred to the temporal area. Often anterior or posterior nasal discharge of mucopurulent secretion offers some relief of discomfort. These symptoms are due to obstruction of the sinus by tumor and secondary infection. Anterior progression of the tumor produces unilateral bulging over the sinus. With destruction of the anterior wall of the sinus, the tumor enters the orbit and displaces the eye downward and laterally, producing diplopia. The lid is often swollen. A fistula may form between the sinus and the skin. With progression posteriorly, the tumor may enter the anterior fossa. Meningitis may occur.

ETHMOID SINUS CARCINOMA. Ethmoid sinus carcinoma often presents with persistent unilateral nasal discharge, epistaxis, nasal obstruction, and ache or pain near the inner canthus and just below the frontal sinus. Swelling of the nose and ulceration of the skin medial to the inner canthus may be present. Late in the disease, if the nasal septum is de-

stroyed, the bridge of the nose collapses. When the tumor invades the orbit, the eye is displaced laterally and the patient complains of diplopia (see Figure 22-9). Proptosis as well as obstruction of the lacrimal duct with excessive lacrimation may be noted. The tumor can spread directly through the cribriform plate and perineurally along olfactory nerve branches into the anterior fossa. Unilateral anosmia may occur.

SPHENOID SINUS CARCINOMAS. Sphenoid sinus carcinomas are rare, difficult to diagnose, and often far advanced when they become symptomatic. They may produce deep, poorly localized retro-orbital or occipital ache or pain. Other symptoms relate to invasion of the nasal cavity (unilateral obstruction, discharge), nasopharynx (discharge, fullness in the ear), sella turcica (visual field disturbances), or cavernous sinus and middle cranial fossa (cranial nerve III-VIII palsies.).

MAXILLARY SINUS CARCINOMAS. Maxillary sinus carcinomas are the most common neoplasms of the paranasal sinuses. These tumors are asymptomatic until they invade surrounding structures or obstruct the sinus ostia. Symptoms are related to the location of the primary tumor in the sinus and its direction of spread. Tumors of the lower half of the sinus (infrastructure) are far more common than those of the upper half (suprastructure). Lesions located inferiorly cause pain in the region of the upper posterior teeth. Destruction of the alveolar bone may result in loosening or even loss of teeth (see Figure 22-10). The gums and hard palate may become swollen

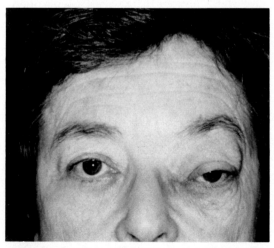

Figure 22-9. Squamous cell carcinoma of the left ethmoid sinus encroaching on the orbit and producing diplopia.

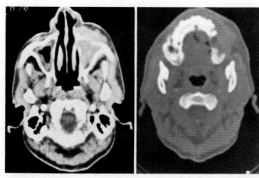

Figure 22–10. CT scans demonstrating squamous cell carcinoma of the maxillary sinus infrastructure with destruction of the maxilla and upper alveolar ridge; also note anterior facial swelling.

and impair the fit of dentures. There may be facial swelling, redness, and an anterolateral mass overlying the maxilla. Invasion of branches of the maxillary nerve may cause unilateral otalgia. Perineural extension along this division of the trigeminal nerve may result in invasion of the middle cranial fossa. When advanced cancers of the superior alveolar ridge rupture into the maxillary sinus, distinction between these lesions and maxillary sinus cancer may be difficult. Tumors of the infrastructure located posteriorly may extend into the pterygomaxillary fossa. They produce trismus with invasion of the pterygoid muscles and deep-seated diffuse pain and headache. They may also be associated with unilateral otalgia and hemianesthesia of the tongue, hard palate, and lower lip.

Lesions of the suprastructure may extend medially into the ethmoid sinuses and often present with epistaxis. These patients may have symptoms of chronic maxillary sinusitis with unilateral nasal obstruction, swelling, discharge, and aching pain over the maxillary sinus. If the lesion extends superiorly it invades the floor of the orbit and displaces the eye upward and laterally producing diplopia. Malar swelling occurs in the naso-orbital area. Infraorbital pain may be severe. Obstruction of the lacrimal duct results in excessive lacrimation. If the infraorbital nerve is invaded, sensory loss may occur in its distribution over the cheek and upper lip. These tumors may enter the middle fossa by extension through the openings in the base of the skull or by perineural metastases. Superiorly located antral tumors that extend laterally may invade the orbit and displace the eye medially and superiorly, with malar swelling that may extend to the temporal fossa. Diplopia, chemosis, and

proptosis may be present. Anteriorly located tumors usually produce malar swelling and pain.

Clinical involvement of lymph nodes and hematogenous metastases are uncommon with sinus carcinomas and occur late in the course of disease. Death is generally a result of local progression of tumor, secondary complication such as hemorrhage and infection, or intracranial metastases.

Nasopharynx. The nasopharynx begins anteriorly at the posterior choanae where it communicates with the nasal cavities. The floor of the nasopharynx is the upper surface of the soft palate. The roof extends along the occipital and sphenoid bones along the base of the skull and contains large amounts of lymphoid tissue. The lateral walls extend to form the posterior limit of Rosenmüller's fossa and include the openings of the eustachian tubes. The posterior wall extends from the roof to the posterior pharynx at the level of the second cervical vertebra.

Nasopharyngeal carcinomas most frequently present with unilateral cervical adenopathy. Characteristically, there is enlargement of a deep node under the upper posterior border of the sternocleidomastoid muscle. Often nodes enlarge rapidly and markedly in the spinal accessory chain and posterior triangle and involvement of the mid- and lower jugular and supraclavicular nodes can occur as well. Bilateral adenopathy is common. Anterior extension of the tumor causes nasal speech, nasal obstruction, and epistaxis. Rarely, eye displacement and diplopia are present. Occlusion of the eustachian orifice produces diminished hearing, a feeling of fullness in the ear, and chronic otalgia (see Figure 22–11). A serous otitis may be present. Invasion through the base of the skull results in

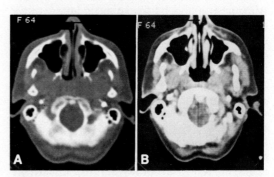

Figure 22–11. (*A*). CT scan demonstrating extensive carcinoma of the nasopharynx with obliteration of the eustachian orifices. (*B*). Complete regression of lesion after treatment with radiation.

cranial nerve involvement. Lateral rectus paralysis is characteristic. Blindness, complete ophthalmoplegia, ptosis, and severe pain in the distribution of the sensory divisions of the trigeminal nerve with invasion of the middle cranial fossa and cavernous sinus may occur. Extension of tumor into the retroparotid space can involve the cervical sympathetic nerve and cranial nerves IX to XII. This may produce Horner's syndrome, difficulty in swallowing, partial loss of taste, hemianesthesia of the soft palate, pharynx, and larynx, hoarseness, and unilateral paralysis of the trapezius and sternocleidomastoid muscles or of the tongue. Large lesions may be seen behind the soft palate on oral examination. More often the lesion requires mirror or nasopharyngoscopic examination for visualization. Hematogenous metastases to lungs, liver, and bones are occasionally present at diagnosis and are common if the primary lesion is controlled.

Oropharynx. The oropharynx consists of the soft palate, the tonsillar fossa and tonsil, the base of the tongue, the periepiglottic region, and the lateral pharyngeal walls. The posterior pharyngeal wall may be considered part of the oropharynx or the hypopharynx and is discussed with the hypopharynx.

Soft Palate. The soft palate extends from the posterior edge of the hard palate and forms the uvula in the midline. The anterior and posterior pillars originate from the base of the uvula and insert into the side of the base of the tongue and the lateral pharyngeal wall, respectively. The tonsillar fossa is formed between the base of the pillars and houses the palatine tonsil. Squamous cell carcinomas of the soft palate and pillars are usually ulcerative and invasive. They produce severe odynophagia as an early symptom. Dysphagia and severe local pain that may radiate to the face are common. Invasion of the pterygoid muscles produces trismus. Palpable high jugular nodes are often present at initial diagnosis.

Tonsil. Most tonsillar carcinomas are exophytic and tend to ulcerate. They may extend to the soft palate and anterior pillar (see Figure 22–12). Often they remain asymptomatic until large. Slight sore throat and a sticking sensation are common early symptoms. With disease progression, dysphagia and unilateral otalgia may occur. Palpable high jugular nodes are usually detected at initial diagnosis. Undifferentiated carcinomas tend to spread superficially without extensive ulceration or invasion. They produce little local symptomatology and present with cervical adenop-

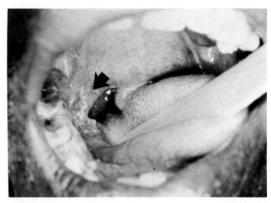

Figure 22–12. Squamous cell carcinoma of the tonsil (arrow).

athy. These tumors tend to metastasize hematogenously to lungs, liver, and bones.

Base of Tongue. Squamous cell carcinomas of the base of the tongue generally are poorly differentiated neoplasms that grow by infiltrating deep into the muscles of the tongue. Bilateral involvement by extension is common. These tumors characteristically produce diffuse and occasionally severe pain in the area. Odynophagia is common. Involvement of branches of the glossopharyngeal nerve leads to otalgia. The tongue may develop deep fissures. The patient may be unable to protrude the tongue, with resultant dysphagia and "hot potato" speech. Odynophagia and dysphagia lead to inanition. Palpable high jugular nodes, which may be bilateral, are often present at diagnosis. In contrast, undifferentiated carcinomas of the base of the tongue produce little infiltration or local symptomatology. They usually present with asymptomatic unilateral high jugular nodes. These tumors are difficult to diagnose and are characterized by a high propensity for hematogenous dissemination.

Periepiglottic Region. Perioepiglottic tumors often produce little in the way of early symptoms. Patients may note a mild sore throat that can progress to odynophagia. Extensive lesions can cause cough due to aspiration, dysphagia, and referred otalgia. Hoarseness from infiltration or swelling of the false cords may be noted with very extensive tumors. Tumors of the free epiglottis often are exophytic, ulcerated, and infected and cause foul breath. Tumors of the periepiglottic region produce mid- and upper jugular adenopathy early. These rapidly enlarging nodes usually lead to examination of the patient and discovery of the primary tumor.

Lateral Pharyngeal Walls. Tumors of the lateral pharyngeal walls tend to spread extensively before producing symptoms. Lateral wall lesions are invasive and usually infiltrate into the hypopharynx. They may also invade and destroy the thyroid cartilage or penetrate into the internal jugular artery. Chronic unilateral sore throat is often the first symptom. Other symptoms include odynophagia, dysphagia, and otalgia. Midjugular adenopathy is present in the majority of patients at initial presentation.

Hypopharynx. This region is bounded by the pyriform sinuses, the postcricoid area, and the posterior pharyngeal wall. Squamous cell carcinomas of the hypopharynx tend to be poorly differentiated. They may spread extensively prior to detection because this is a rather silent anatomic site. These tumors often are ulcerated and secondarily infected so that the breath has a foul odor. The pyriform sinus is the most commonly involved site (see Figure 22–13). Symptoms are similar to those of lateral pharyngeal wall lesions, that is, odynophagia, unilateral sore throat, dysphagia, and otalgia. Lateral wall extension of pyriform sinus carcinomas can destroy the thyroid cartilage and produce pain and neck swelling. Medial wall progression into the larynx may result

in hoarseness. Large lesions may cause frequent coughing because of aspiration of saliva and food.

Posterior Pharyngeal Wall. Tumors of the posterior pharyngeal wall cause progressive bulging of the posterior pharynx. They may develop longitudinal ulcerations and infection. Dysphagia and a sense of sticking in the back of the throat are common complaints. Most patients with hypopharyngeal cancer have midjugular adenopathy, which may be bilateral, at initial presentation. Death is usually due to complications of locally advanced disease, such as inanition, aspiration pneumonia, and hemorrhage. Distant hematogenous metastases occur in patients with controlled primary tumors.

Larynx. The anatomic subdivisions of the larynx are the supraglottic, glottic, and subglottic regions. Symptoms are related to the site of the primary lesion. The most common carcinomas of the larynx arise in the glottic region, that is, in the true vocal chords (see Figure 22–14.) These are well-differentiated squamous carcinomas that may have a papillary appearance. Hoarseness is the commonest presenting symptom and becomes constant and of increasing severity. This symptom often leads to early detection of these tumors. Advanced lesions may produce dyspnea and stri-

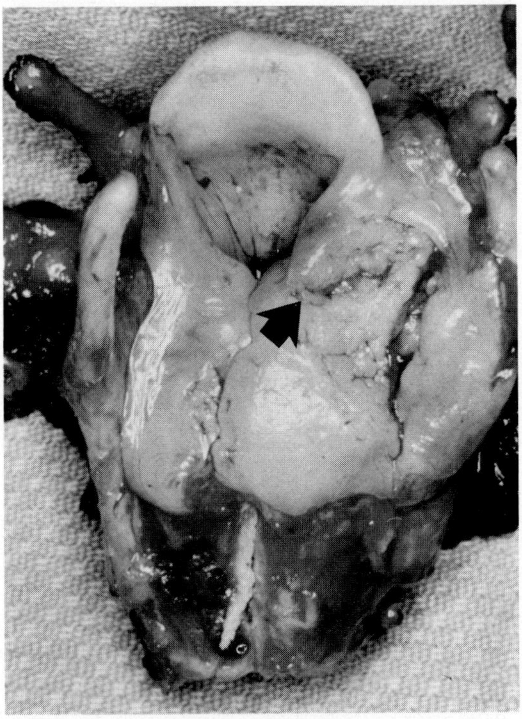

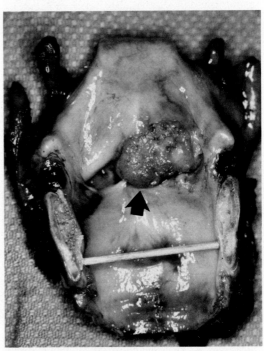

Figure 22–13. Extensive squamous cell carcinoma of the pyriform sinus (arrow).

Figure 22–14. Large squamous cell carcinoma of the true vocal cord (arrow).

dor and can also destroy the thyroid cartilage and produce lateral neck swelling and severe neck pain. Supraglottic lesions can cause intermittent hoarseness that may become persistent, as well as constant sore throat and odynophagia. Subglottic lesions often present with unilateral otalgia. They produce pain by invasion of the thyroid cartilage and can cause hoarseness by displacement of or extension to the true cord. Lymphatic and hematogenous metastases are uncommon.

Salivary Glands. The majority of salivary gland tumors are benign and are characterized by slow asymptomatic growth. Malignant tumors usually present as rapidly growing painful masses, most frequently located in the region of the parotid or submandibular glands. Adenoid cystic carcinomas may evolve more slowly and often are removed and recur locally repeatedly over several years. Adenoid cystic carcinomas, however, can follow an aggressive course as well. In the case of parotid tumors, local pain, trismus, or pain in the ear and neck may occur (see Figure 22-15). Peripheral paralysis of the facial nerve is common. The tumors are often fixed at the skin, which can appear tense and indurated and may ulcerate. Preparotid and upper cervical adenopathy is common. Extension into the retroparotid space may produce paralysis of cranial nerves IX to XII. Submaxillary gland carcinomas can produce severe mandibular pain and otalgia. Hematogenous metastases to lungs, bones, and liver are common and may occur early with salivary gland malignant.

Diagnosis

Definitive diagnosis of any cancer of the head and neck is ultimately established by a biopsy of the primary site to interpret the histopathologic characteristics of the tumor. When a patient is suspected of having a head and

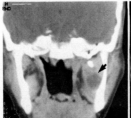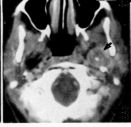

Figure 22-15. CT scans of deeply located (see arrows) adenoid cystic carcinoma of the left parotid gland with central calcification.

neck cancer, however, the diagnostic workup should be pursued logically and systematically, beginning with a careful history followed by thorough physical examination of the head and neck. Depending upon the information obtained, pertinent radiographic studies and appropriate laboratory studies can be ordered. When a head and neck cancer is strongly suspected, physicians skilled in the diagnosis and management of head and neck cancer should thoroughly examine the upper airways and digestive system, take appropriate biopsies, and determine the extent of the disease. A team approach from the outset should be used to conduct and interpret a complete diagnostic evaluation, plan effective primary therapy, and establish follow-up therapeutic and rehabilitative measures. This team should consist of the primary physician, a head and neck surgeon specializing in cancer, a radiotherapist, a medical oncologist, a pathologist, and a diagnostic radiologist. Other specialists may be required to plan treatment and rehabilitation. In most cases, these patients require considerable psychosocial support.

As in all facets of medicine, diagnosis begins with a careful history, paying careful attention to occupational risks and social habits, as well as to the patient's symptoms and signs. Most head and neck cancers are treatable and curable when discovered early, but many cancers of the head and neck are large and extensive when diagnosed. This late diagnosis appears to result from several factors. In some instances patient ignorance, denial, and procrastination may be responsible. On other occasions, rapidly growing tumors that pursue aggressive relentless growth patterns, such as anaplastic carcinoma of the nasopharynx or tumors in "silent" areas such as the parapharyngeal space, may assume considerable size before causing any symptoms or signs. Late diagnosis may sometimes be due to low index of suspicion or lack of sensitivity to early signs of head and neck cancer. The physicians or dentists consulted initially are more likely to render early diagnosis:

1. If they have a strong suspicion that these lesions are present in an abuser of alcohol and tobacco;
2. If they are familiar with the natural history and symptoms of these lesions. The most common symptoms of head and neck cancers are pain, bleeding, obstruction, or the presence of a mass. The mass

may be asymptomatic as in a neck node or a patient may develop a mass that contributes to malocclusion or ill-fitting dentures;

3. If they are familiar with the gross appearance of these lesions and pay careful attention on routine physical examination to the sites where they most commonly occur. With the exception of laryngeal carcinoma, which generally causes early symptomatology, the most common sites for head and neck cancers are the lip, tongue, and floor of mouth. These areas are all readily accessible on routine physical examination; and

4. If an adequate explanation of symptoms is sought in any patient with persistent symptomatology in the head and neck area. Approximately 85% of neck masses in the adult represent metastatic disease.

With these considerations in mind, the diagnostic workup will be reviewed briefly.

The evaluation of the patient begins with a good history, paying careful attention to symptoms, occupational characteristics, social habits, prior illnesses, general health, and use of medications. Subsequently, a thorough physical examination should be conducted, remembering several points. The head and neck are best examined with the patient seated, because this allows better visualization of the oral cavity and hypopharyngeal structures. Adequate light is mandatory to assess properly multiple contours of the mucosal folds of the upper aerodigestive tracts. A tongue blade should be used to manipulate the buccal mucosa, the tongue, and the palate to visualize hidden areas. A head light is of great help, because it frees both hands to manipulate instruments and tissues. Finally, the examiner should rely on both inspection and palpation in assessing head and neck lesions. This is especially true of suspected lesions of the oral cavity, base of the tongue, and palatal regions where palpation can give valuable information as to the submucosal extent of a lesion that may look small and inconsequential on inspection. Neck lesions should be evaluated from both in front of and behind the patient with the patient seated. They should also be examined with the patient supine and with the neck extended.

The otoscope, ophthalmoscope, and nasal speculum aid in examining the ears, eyes, and nasal cavity, respectively. With good light and manipulation of various structures with tongue blades, examination of the oral cavity for changes in color and shape, for ulcerations, or for mass effects can be carried out readily. Examination of the nasopharynx, hypopharynx, and larynx requires an indirect mirror or fiberoptic light systems, such as the Machida or Olympus flexible fiberoptic laryngoscope or nasopharyngoscope, which are introduced transnasally. An alternative to these scopes is the rigid Hopkins right angle telescope, which can be introduced transorally. These light systems allow excellent direct visualization of various cavities of the head and neck. They are very useful for examining the nasopharynx where any asymmetry, mucosal ulceration, or abnormally friable tissue is usually readily apparent. In examining the hypopharynx, one should look for alterations of cord mobility, mucosal lesions, or pooling of secretions in the pyriform sinus. The neck and major salivary glands are best examined by palpation and inspection. Careful evaluation of the function of the cranial nerves completes examination of the head and neck.

Examination of the head and neck should be followed by a thorough general physical examination. In addition to the nature and stage of the primary tumor, the presence of distant metastases, the patient's performance status, and coexisting medical problems must be evaluated. Also, an attempt should be made to assess the psychosocial status of the patient. The patient's motivation, will to live, and support systems are all critical in determining the best course of therapy.

Routine laboratory studies on all patients suspected of head and neck cancer should include a roentgenogram, complete blood and platelet counts, prothrombin time, partial thromboplastin time, SMA-15, urinalysis, and electrocardiogram. Specific radiographic and radioisotopic scanning studies should be based upon the suspected site of origin of the tumor and the probability of metastatic disease. Some general principles can be followed in this regard. Plain radiographs are best to determine any evidence of bone involvement of the mandible or paranasal sinus area. More definitive information regarding the bony architecture can be obtained by polytomography of the bone in question. This is most useful in evaluating paranasal sinuses and orbits. Soft tissues are best evaluated by more sophisticated computerized tomographic scanners. Radiographic contrast studies are most useful to determine functional compromise and the extent of lesions involving the oropharynx, hypopharynx, and cervical esophagus. Although angiographic studies are not generally indicated in the routine evaluation of head and neck tumors, they may be indicated in the evaluation of tumors of the nasopharynx, parapharyngeal space, or pulsatile neck masses to rule out juvenile nasopharyngeal angiofibromas, chemodectomas, or glomus tumors. In these lesions the angiogram can be diagnostic and may obviate the need for a biopsy. Angiographic studies for advanced head and neck lesions can also assess the involvement of the carotid artery or determine the accessibility of a large head and neck tumor mass to intra-arterial chemotherapeutic agents by delineating the feeding vessels.

Specific radiographic studies are determined by the patient's symptomatology and physical findings. In patients with facial swelling, proptosis, external or internal nasal lesions, or suspected lesions of the nasopharynx the most useful films are plain and stereo skull films, sinus series, polytomography, and computerized tomography of the head and paranasal sinuses. Computerized tomography (CT) adds an important dimension to the evaluation of head and neck cancers in that it provides excellent definition of soft tissue planes and may also demonstrate bone structure. Tumors of the oral cavity are best evaluated with panorex views of the mandible and CT scans to delineate soft tissue and bony interfaces. In tumors of the hypopharynx and larynx, the barium swallow is an excellent study to determine functional competence of deglutition and to approximate the extent of mucosal lesions in the hypopharynx and cervical esophagus. Submucosal extension of tumor, however, may be far beyond apparent radiographic limits.

In the past, lesions of the larynx were studied by tomograms or contrast laryngograms. Where computerized tomography is available, however, it has supplanted these older studies. Although a laryngogram can be a clinically useful study, it is technically difficult to perform, requires a considerable amount of experience on the part of the radiologist, and is uncomfortable for the patient. Evaluation of lesions of the major salivary glands is still probably best accomplished by physical examination. CT scan can be useful in delineating the gross limits of a lesion. No rigid criteria to differentiate benign from malignant lesions, however, have been elucidated and perineural extension of tumor may not be detected. Sialography does not add any additional information to the evaluation of a suspected parotid tumor.

The utility of radionuclide scanning depends upon the tumor location, size, and staging. Scanning can determine the presence of metastatic disease. Yet, in the patient with small (T_1 or T_2) lesions of most sites, especially with clinically negative nodes and moderately to well-differentiated tumors, extensive scanning of multiple organs for metastasis is not cost effective and is unwarranted. In general, metastatic work-up is indicated on any patient with advanced head and neck disease and should be carried out before instituting definitive therapy. An abnormal chest roentgenogram for a patient in this population may be due to metastases from a head and neck cancer, primary lung cancer, or benign diseases such as tuberculosis. Any patient with head and neck cancer who complains of persistant bone pain, has abnormal liver enzymes or hepatomegaly, or has had a change in mental status or abnormal findings on general neurologic examination should undergo bone scan, liver-spleen scan, and brain scan, respectively. The role of radioisotopic studies in salivary gland tumors is limited. They are not useful in delineating benign from malignant lesions with the exception that benign Warthin's tumor of the parotid gland has increased uptake of ^{99}Te and presents with a characteristic scanning pattern. Ultrasound is not of much value in head and neck tumors with the exception of suspected thyroid and orbital tumors.

After the initial evaluation is completed a biopsy should be performed for histologic diagnosis. Biopsy material may be obtained in a number of different ways. The exact method chosen often depends on the location and the accessibility of the lesion. Generally, four types of biopsies are used: Punch biopsy, needle biopsy, incisional biopsy, and excisional biopsy. The punch biopsy is the simplest technique, in which a small piece of tissue is obtained with punch or tissue biting forceps. This biopsy method is ideal for readily accessible lesions of the oral cavity, nasal cavity, or skin where tissue is ulcerated and the lesion is grossly evident. Adequate amounts of tissue must be taken for the pathologist and it is best to sample the tissue from several areas of the tumor, including deep areas.

There are two types of needle biopsy. Fine-needle biopsy consists of insertion of a small-gauge needle into the area of suspected tumor with aspiration of cellular contents. The aspirate is then placed on a glass slide, sprayed with CYTOFIX for fixation, and sent for pathologic examination. An alternative to fine-needle biopsy is a large-bore needle, such as the Silverman needle, in which a core of tissue is removed and placed in formalin. Needle biopsies are most useful in evaluating suspected cervical metastasis, parotid masses, or thyroid masses. Needle biopsies offer the advantage that tissue may be obtained under local anesthesia and that specimens may be provided quickly. They are useful when incisional or excisional biopsy is inadvisable. One disadvantage of the technique is the possible seeding of the surrounding tissue with tumor cells as the needle is withdrawn. Secondly, it may yield amounts of tissue inadequate for an accurate histopathologic diagnosis with resulting diagnostic errors. If a small-punch biopsy is not feasible or needle aspiration is unwarranted or fails to yield a diagnosis, an incisional biopsy can be performed. Incisional biopsies are indicated in supraclavicular masses when all diagnostic modalities have failed to establish a diagnosis and excisional biopsy of the supraclavicular mass is not technically feasible. Incisional biopsy is also used in large head and neck tumors when a diagnosis has not been obtained previously and a physician is ready to carry out a definitive procedure simultaneously. Incisional biopsies can also sample submucosal lesions of the oral cavity or pharynx. Although sometimes useful, incisional biopsy should be performed with a full understanding of the ramifications of violating the tumor capsule. The possibility of seeding the open wound with tumor cells is real and one must be prepared to deal with the consequences of this procedure.

Excisional biopsy consists of removal of a suspected tumor mass in its entirety without violating the tumor itself. Excisional biopsies that involve resection of the tumor and surrounding normal tissue, such as in tumors of the salivary gland and thyroid gland, often provide definitive therapy as well as diagnosis. Most squamous cell carcinomas of the upper aerodigestive tract, however, are not encapsulated and excisional biopsy is not indicated.

This procedure is inadequate for such lesions, because the biopsy leaves residual tumor and may make definitive therapy more difficult. These lesions are best diagnosed by simple punch biopsy.

The method of choice for obtaining histologic material ultimately depends upon the location and character of the lesion, the age and status of the patient, and the suspicions and experience of the physician treating the patient. Regardless of the method employed, histologic confirmation of the diagnosis is mandatory before proceeding with any definitive therapy, because all of the treatment modalities used in head and neck cancers can produce major and even irreversible functional and cosmetic damage.

A final word should be said about evaluating the patient with an asymptomatic mass in the neck. Any neck mass in the adult that persists for more than four to six weeks should be suspected as cancerous until proven otherwise, especially in a patient with a history of smoking, drinking, or neck irradiation. The proper evaluation of this particular patient does not consist of immediate open neck biopsy, but should begin with a complete examination of the head and neck followed by a general physical examination. Appropriate blood studies and radiographs as outlined above should be carried out. If complete examination of the head and neck does not reveal a primary lesion, then the patient should undergo endoscopy under general anesthesia, including nasopharyngoscopy, direct laryngoscopy, bronchoscopy, and esophagoscopy. In most instances endoscopy will identify a primary lesion, and appropriate biopsies can be taken. A treatment plan can then be outlined based on the information obtained at endoscopy. In a small percentage of patients, no primary lesion will be grossly evident. Selected random biopsies of the nasopharynx, pyriform sinus, base of tongue, and tonsillar fossa should be performed because previous studies have identified these areas as the most common sites for occult head and neck primary tumors. This careful systematic evaluation will identify the primary tumor in almost all cases. In the small percentage of cases, however, in which no primary lesion is found, exploration of the neck with biopsy of the mass is indicated. Frozen section examination should be performed. If the mass is positive for metastatic squamous cell carcinoma, a radical neck dissection should be carried out. If the biopsy is consistent with adenocarcinoma or lymphoma, then a neck dissection is not indicated and further diagnostic work-up and definitive therapy should be pursued (see Figure 22–16).

Staging

When the primary site of head and neck cancer has been histopathologically confirmed, the extent of disease must be determined; this is clinical staging. Accurate clinical staging is critical for developing the treatment plan. Stage of disease correlates well with prognosis. In cancers of the head and neck the most widely accepted staging system is based on the extent of the primary tumor (T), the degree of nodal involvement (N), and the presence or absence of distant metastases (M). These T, N, and M characteristics are used to define stages I to IV for each site. The most commonly accepted staging system in the United States is that of the American Joint Committee for Cancer Staging and End-Result Reporting (1978). The variables assessed for staging cancers of the head and neck are listed in the accompanying tables (see Tables 22–4 through 22–9). Although anatomic staging in head and neck cancers is very useful, other factors such as tumor differentiation, coexistent illnesses, and nutritional status also markedly affect prognosis and therapy.

Specific and Supportive Management

Specific Therapy for Various Stages of Disease. After a thorough clinical evaluation and histopathologic confirmation of the diagnosis of cancer, consideration of treatment begins. Choice and recommendation of treatment is based on the primary site and histopathology of the tumor, the staging classification of the tumor, the general physical status of the pa-

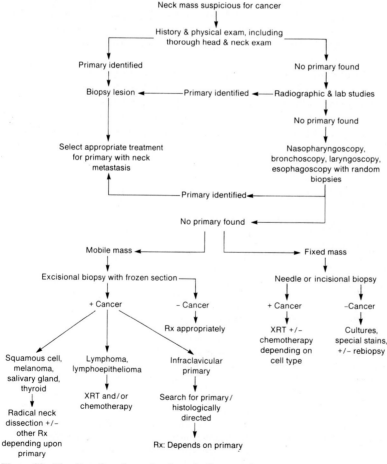

Figure 22–16.   Paradigm for evaluation of solitary neck mass.

Table 22-4. Definition of T Categories for Staging of Cancer of the Oral Cavity and Pharynx

	ORAL CAVITY	NASOPHARYNX	OROPHARYNX	HYPOPHARYNX*
T_1	Tumor 2 cm or less†	Tumor confined to one site or nasopharynx	Tumor less than 2 cm	Tumor confined to site of origin
T_2	Tumor greater than 2 but less than 4 cm	Tumor involving two sites (postero superior) and lateral walls	Tumor greater than 2 cm but less than 4 cm	Extension of tumor to adjacent region or site without fixation of hemilarynx
T_3	Tumor greater than 4 cm	Extension of tumor into nasal cavity or oropharynx	Tumor greater than 4 cm	Extension to adjacent region or site with fixation of hemilarynx
T_4	Massive tumor greater than 4 cm with deep invasion involving antrum pterygoids, base of tongue, or skin of neck	Tumor involvement of skull or cranial nerves	Massive tumor greater than 4 cm with invasion of bone, soft tissue, and neck or root of tongue	Massive tumor involving bone or soft tissues of neck

*Hypopharynx includes pyriform sinus, postcricoid area, and posterior hypopharyngeal wall.
†Greatest diameter.

tient, and the psychosocial condition of the patient at the time of diagnosis. These considerations determine whether treatment is directed at cure, palliation, or simply support. The complex anatomy and physiology of the head and neck interacts with adjacent regions. The structures of the head and neck function whenever the patient breathes, swallows, speaks, or changes facial expression. In light of this, any treatment may affect respiration, deglutition, phonation, and appearance. Treatment often has far-reaching functional and psychologic effects on the patient with head and neck cancer. Therefore, the patient must be an informed and active participant in

treatment decisions throughout the course of therapy. The patient's ultimate decision should be respected at all times. By the same token, the patient should be made aware of the consequences of failing to pursue active treatment.

Although detailed treatment of head and neck cancers is beyond the scope of this chapter, the principles of radiation therapy, surgical therapy, and chemotherapy are presented here. In addition, the benefits and side effects of each treatment modality alone or in combination must be borne in mind. A multidisciplinary approach from the beginning of patient management best accomplishes this

Table 22-5. Definition of T categories for Staging of Cancer of the Larynx

	SUPRAGLOTTIS	GLOTTIS	SUBGLOTTIS
T_1	Tumor confined to site of origin with normal mobility	Tumor confined to glottis with normal mobility	Tumor confined to subglottic region
T_2	Tumor involves adjacent supraglottic site or glottis without fixation	Supraglottic and/or subglottic extension of tumor with normal or impaired mobility of cord	Tumor extension to vocal cords with normal or impaired cord mobility
T_3	Tumor limited to larynx with fixation and/or extension to involve post-cricoid area, medial wall, or pyriform sinus or preepiglottic space	Tumor confined to larynx with cord fixation	Tumor confined to larynx with cord fixation
T_4	Massive tumor extending beyond confines of larynx	Massive tumor with thyroid cartilage destruction and/or extension beyond confines of larynx	Massive tumor with cartilage destruction and/or extension beyond confines of larynx

Table 22-6. Definition of T Categories for Staging of Cancer of the Maxillary Sinus

T_0	No evidence of primary tumor
T_1	Tumor confined to antral mucosa of the infrastructure with no bone erosion or destruction
T_2	Tumor confined to suprastructure mucosa without bone destruction, or the infrastructure with destruction of medial or inferior bony walls only
T_3	More extensive tumor invading skin of cheek, orbit, anterior ethmoid sinuses, pterygoid muscles
T_4	Massive tumor with invasion of cribriform plate, posterior ethmoids, sphenoid, nasopharynx, pterygoid plates, base of skull

rather than referring patients to various consultants after initial treatment is undertaken and a complication or recurrence develops.

The principles of therapy for head and neck cancers directed at cure of the disease try to meet three objectives: (1) to eradicate the neoplasm completely; (2) to give the patient the best functional result by careful planning of the radiation fields or appropriate reconstructive techniques for surgical defects; and (3) to leave the patient with as good a cosmetic result as possible. In certain instances these objectives are met by radiation therapy alone, in others by surgery alone, and in others by combined therapy. One should never choose a modality, however, that may give a good functional and cosmetic result temporarily but might compromise the survival of the patient ultimately.

In cancers deemed unresectable because of local extension or deemed incurable because of diffuse metastatic spread, treatment is directed towards palliation. Palliative treatment

Table 22-7. Definition of N Categories for Staging of Head and Neck Cancer

N_0	No clinically positive nodes
N_1	Single clinically positive homolateral node 3 cm or less in diameter
N_2	Single clinically positive homolateral node more than 3 cm in diameter, or multiple clinically positive homolateral nodes, none more than 6 cm in diameter
N_{2a}	Single clinically positive node more than 3 cm but not more than 6 cm in diameter
N_{2b}	Multiple-clinically positive homolateral nodes, more than 6 cm in diameter
N_3	Massive homolateral node(s), bilateral nodes, or contralateral node(s)
N_{3a}	Clinically positive homolateral node(s), one of which is more than 6 cm in diameter
N_{3b}	Bilateral clinically positive nodes
N_{3c}	Contralateral clinically positive node(s) only

Table 22-8. Definition of M Categories for Staging of Head and Neck Cancer

M_0	No (known) distant metastasis
M_1	Distant metastases present—specify site(s)

may be employed to: (1) control consequences of locally advancing tumor; (2) provide relief from pain, for example, radiotherapy can relieve the extreme pain from bone metastases; (3) provide relief from obstruction, for example, a patient with a far advanced laryngeal tumor may benefit greatly from a tracheostomy to prevent suffocation; and (4) to control excessive bleeding. When considering treatment for palliation, concerns for the patient's quality of life must guide treatment decisions. Treatments with a reasonable prospect of improving quality of life, even though associated with some adverse effects, should be strongly considered. Treatments that may substantially diminish quality of life with only a small chance of benefit should be considered cautiously.

The primary treatment modalities for head and neck cancers involve radiation therapy and surgery applied alone or in combination. At present, the role of chemotherapy in the initial treatment of head and neck cancers is uncertain *(vida infra)*. The choice of treatment modalities depends on: (1) the size and location of the tumor; (2) the gross characteristics of the tumors, that is, exophytic or infiltrative; (3) histopathologic differentiation of the tumor; (4) presence of local bone and muscle involvement; (5) presence or absence of nodal disease; (6) the general medical condition of the patient; (7) socioeconomic condition and occupation of the patient; and (8) the experience of the surgeon and radiotherapist involved. The tools at the disposal of the radiotherapist, the surgeon, and the chemotherapist differ greatly. Only a thorough understanding of the capabilities and limitations of each of these allows selection of the most appropriate modality of treatment.

Table 22-9. Staging Groups Based on the TNM Categories

Stage I	T_1, N_0, M_0
Stage II	T_2, N_0, M_0
Stage III	T_3, N_0, M_0
	$T_1, T_2,$ or $T_3,$ and $N_1,$ and M_0
Stage IV	T_4, N_0 or N_1, M_0
	Any T, N_2 or N_3, M_0
	Any T, Any N, M_1

Radiation Therapy. In general, the tools of the radiation therapist in managing carcinoma of the head and neck are megavoltage radiation with energies of 1,000,000 volts or higher and radioactive isotopes. Megavoltage therapy, when compared to older kilovoltage therapy, provides more homogeneous radiation to the tumor and minimizes damage to surrounding tissues. This has notably reduced the severe problem of radiation dermatitis common with low energy radiation. In institutions without linear accelerators, radiation therapy is generally administered with cobalt 60 units that deliver gamma irradiation with energies in the range of 1.17 to 1.33 megavolts. Major referral centers generally use linear accelerators capable of producing beams of x-rays with energies in the range of four to 35 megavolts. Also, either a linear accelerator or a betatron with energies of six to 20 megavolts or higher can produce electron beams. In addition to external beam therapy, radioactive isotopes are used interstitially, either temporarily or as permanent implants, most often to boost the dose to the primary tumor and spare surrounding tissues. These interstitial sources can be provided by radium 226, iridium 192, gold 198, or iodine 125. Radium and iridium are delivered via needles or after-loading angiocatheter devices. Gold and iodine are provided as interstitial seed implants. External beam therapy is delivered in fractionated doses (usually five/week) over four to six weeks. Curative dosages range from 5500 rads to 6500 rads, depending on the location of the tumor. Small localized areas can be boosted with interstitial implants. Normal tissue in the head and neck region exposed to more than 7000 to 7500 rads, however, can experience substantial radiation damage and the incidence of complications such as osteoradionecrosis, severe fibrosis, carotid artery rupture in necks previously operated upon, and radiation myelitis all increase dramatically. Despite the tremendous advance in technological equipment available to the radiation therapist, including computerized dosimeters, the proper treatment of these lesions with minimal side effects requires an experienced and sophisticated therapist who understands both the nature of these tumors as well as the capabilities and limitations of the equipment.

Surgery. Although the radiation therapist cures the cancer by destroying neoplastic cells within the host, the surgeon relies on gross removal of all involved tissue. Oncologic surgeons attempt to resect the primary tumor in its entirety as well as all involved lymph nodes. After removing the tumor, they make every effort to restore physiologic function and reconstruct all important physiologic and cosmetic defects. In small lesions of the face or oral cavity, wide local excision can often be closed primarily or with a split thickness skin graft, leaving the patient with little or no functional or cosmetic deficit. Superficial lesions of the floor of the mouth or the lateral tongue can often be resected easily and repaired with minimal deficit. Larger lesions, however, which begin to produce some functional deficits, often require extensive resections of physiologically important tissues. In some cases entire organs must be resected to achieve local control, as in laryngectomies for large laryngeal cancers. Advanced lesions of the oral cavity may require partial resections of mandible, palate, tongue, and pharynx, and those of the paranasal sinuses resection of maxilla with orbital exenteration. Any cancer of the head and neck that requires extensive resection may result in alterations of breathing, swallowing, and speech. The degree of the deficit depends on the location of the tumor, the extent of resection, the reconstructive methods employed, and, finally, the patient's motivation and ability to adapt to the alterations imposed by the surgical intervention.

In addition to control of the primary tumor, surgery may be employed to control cervical lymph node metastases. Management of the cervical lymph nodes ultimately depends on the histopathology of the tumor, its location, its propensity to metastasize, as well as the general status of the patient. In general, the patient with small (T_1) lesions and no palpable neck nodes may be treated by removal of the primary tumor only. In patients with moderate sized (T_2 or T_3) lesions and no palpable cervical lymph nodes, treatment may consist of surgical resection of the primary followed by postoperative radiotherapy to the neck. Full-course radiation therapy to the neck can effectively control the development of cervical metastases (Fletcher, 1972). In patients with palpable cervical lymph nodes, however, and patients with large (T_3 or T_4) primary lesions, or in patients with lesions at locations with a high propensity for cervical lymph node metastasis, such as the pyriform sinus or supraglottic larynx, a radical or modifed neck dissection is usually indicated in conjunction with resection of the primary.

When management of cervical lymph nodes is surgical, the operation usually consists of either a classic radical neck dissection or a modified (conservation) neck dissection. Classic radical neck dissection attempts to remove lymphatic channels and surrounding soft tissue *en bloc.* The limits of the dissection are the inferior border of the mandible superiorly, the strap muscles anteriorly, the clavicle inferiorly, and the trapezius muscle posteriorly. Laterally the skin and platysmal muscle are preserved, and medially the dissection is carried to the prevertebral fascia, preserving the scalene and paraspinous muscles. It involves resection of the sternocleidomastoid muscle and omohyoid muscle. The internal and external jugular veins are removed in their course through the neck. Cranial nerve XI is removed, and the sensory cervical nerve roots C_2, C_3, and C_4 are cut as well. The submandibular gland and contents of the submandibular triangle are also resected. The lymph nodes and lymph channels of the upper, middle, and lower jugular chain as well as submental, submaxillary, spinal accessory, parapharyngeal, and supraclavicular lymph nodes are resected without violating major lymphatic channels or lymph node capsules. A neck dissection also involves identifying and preserving the vagus and hypoglossal nerves, sympathetic cervical plexus, phrenic nerve, brachial plexus, and internal and external carotid artery. Radical neck dissection is the time-honored surgical procedure for managing cervical lymph node metastasis (Crile, 1906). Radical neck dissection, however, does result in weakness of the shoulder because of the sacrifice of cranial nerve XI and most patients have a cosmetic deficit secondary to removal of the sternocleidomastoid muscle. In recent years a modified or conservation neck dissection has been developed and advocated in certain instances. A modified or functional neck dissection generally involves dissection of the fascial envelope of lymph node–bearing tissue planes, which results in dissection of the same node–bearing areas as in a classic neck dissection (Bocca and Pignataro, 1967); however, the sternocleidomastoid muscle, internal jugular vein, and cranial nerve XI are preserved. Modified neck dissection may be indicated in patients with a clinically negative neck but who have a great risk of occult nodes. It may also be used in the patient with a single small, freely movable node who is going to receive postoperative radiotherapy (Jesse *et al.,* 1978).

This procedure is indicated in patients with well-differentiated thyroid carcinomas who present with neck metastases. It may be used in patients who are undergoing bilateral neck dissection or who have had one radical neck dissection on the opposite side. Patients with bilateral radical neck dissections may have serious problems with facial edema. It is contraindicated for clinically positive nodes when surgery is the only treatment modality to be used or in a patient who has had a previous modified or regional neck dissection. A modified or functional neck dissection is technically more difficult than a radical neck dissection and therefore only experienced head and neck surgeons should attempt it.

When the primary tumor in the neck has been adequately dealt with, the surgeon is faced with reconstruction of the wound. The primary modalities for reconstruction of a surgical defect are primary closure, skin graft, pedicle flap reconstruction, or free flap reconstruction. The method chosen in any individual case is determined by the size of the defect and should be the one that will provide the best functional result for the patient. In small T_1 and T_2 lesions, primary closure or placement of a split thickness skin graft over mucosal defects often provides excellent functional and cosmetic results. Larger lesions, however, often demand more sophisticated reconstructive techniques involving use of local mucosa, such as tongue or cheek flaps, or the use of more distant pedicle flaps from the forehead, scalp, or deltopectoral area. One of the most promising new developments in head and neck cancer reconstructive work is the use of new musculocutaneous flaps such as the pectoralis major or the trapezius musculocutaneous flap (Ariyan, 1979). These flaps consist of skin, subcutaneous tissue, and muscle with blood supply based on dependable arteries and permit immediate one-stage reconstruction of large surgical defects with rapid, reliable healing and minimal complications (Baek *et al.,* 1982). Free flaps, such as groin flaps transferred to repair head and neck defects, require multiple microvascular anastomoses and have not yet assumed an important role in reconstruction of head and neck defects.

With these basic principles of curative radiation and surgical therapy, a treatment plan for the patient can be outlined. Although final selection of treatment for any given patient is based on a multitude of factors as outlined above, some general guidelines are provided here. Small (T_1) lesions of the mucosal surfaces of the head and neck can be treated by radiation or surgery alone with equally high cure rates (Wang, 1972). The choice of treatment depends on all of the aforementioned factors. Tumors classified T_2 often have better functional and cosmetic results if treated with radiation. The cure rates are not as high as for T_1 lesions, but surgery can still be employed for radiation failures. Larger lesions with a T_3 or T_4 classification often have associated bone or muscle involvement and nodal metastases. These lesions are best treated by a combination of surgery and radiation. Carcinoma of the nasopharynx is best treated by radiation alone, because these tumors are highly radiosensitive and are not easily approached surgically. Radiation therapy is effective for the primary tumor and even for extensive neck disease (Ho, 1978). Small lesions of the lips, oral cavity, oropharynx, and hypopharynx can be treated by radiation or surgery, but large lesions in these areas are best treated by combination therapy. Small T_1 lesions of the vocal cords can be treated by radiation or surgery but radiation gives a much better functional voice, whereas cure rates (85 to 90%) are comparable (Hendrickson *et al.*, 1975). T_2 lesions of the laryngeal glottis are best treated by radiation therapy with surgery reserved for salvage or radiation failures (Jakobsson, 1976). Partial or conservation laryngectomy, however, may be indicated for T_2 lesions depending on their exact location and tumor characteristics. T_3 and T_4 lesions of the larynx require total laryngectomy for adequate control (Miller, 1975).

Although the final decision on modalities is often based on other patient factors, radiation therapy is most effective against less-differentiated actively growing tumors of small size with well-oxygenated cells. Surgery is better suited for well-differentiated slow-growing tumors, tumors with a large amount of radioresistant hypoxic cells, and tumors with gross involvement of cartilage. For extensive T_3 and T_4 lesions or lesions with nodal metastases at initial diagnosis, either modality alone is rarely curative. In these instances combination therapy of radiation and surgery has yielded better results than either one alone.

Although prognosis of cancers in the head and neck depends on differentiation of the tumor, the size of the lesion, and general physical status of the patient, it correlates best with the stage of the disease at the time of diagnosis. In general, patients with stage I and stage II disease respond well to surgery or radiation, with cure rates approaching 60 to 90% depending on the site of origin. In stage III and stage IV disease, cure rates fall precipitously despite combination treatment with surgery, radiation, and chemotherapy. Stage IV carcinoma in many locations of the head and neck has less than 10 to 15% five-year survival. When carcinoma of the lip, for example, is confined to the lip and regional lymph nodes are not involved, the primary lesion can be controlled in 85% of cases. With regional lymph node involvement at initial presentation, control is only 68% (McKay and Seller, 1964). In carcinoma of the tongue, a five-year cure rate varies from 69.2% for patients with stage I disease to 36.6% for those with stage III disease (Spiro and Strong, 1974). Five-year survival rates vary from 63% for stage I tonsil tumors to 21% for stage IV cancers (Jesse and Sugarbaker, 1976). Carcinomas of the hypopharynx including pharyngeal walls, pyriform sinus, postcricoid area, and cervical esophagus are often far advanced when first seen and have predictably poor prognoses. As many as 75% of patients presenting with lesions in these areas have stage III or stage IV disease when first diagnosed. Cancer of the pyriform sinus treated by combination therapy yields only 40 to 50% five-year survival in the best of circumstances and in one series of patients with far-advanced lesions, only 23% were free of disease at two years (Byers *et al.*, 1979; McGavran *et al.*, 1963). Stage I carcinoma of the maxillary sinus has greater than 90% survival rate whereas stage III disease has less than 33% survival rate (Gallagher and Boles, 1970). Poor prognosis for many lesions of the head and neck despite combination therapy is a result of the fact that many head and neck tumors are at stage III or beyond when first diagnosed and have nodal metastases. In addition, certain sites have a higher propensity for cervical metastasis at some point in the course of their disease. These include supraglottic larynx, base of tongue, tonsil, nasopharynx, and hypopharynx (Lindberg, 1972).

For smaller lesions, considerations discussed above do not always indicate radiotherapy as the treatment of choice. Radical radiotherapy with intent to cure is not without morbidity. Treatment course is prolonged and subjects the patient to considerable physiologic stress. Severe mucositis, resulting in dysphagia and impairment of nutrition, is not uncommon. In addition, pain secondary to fibrosis of surrounding tissue and dry thick mucous from radiation may be more distressing than the local deficits of radical surgery.

In patients with large lesions who are selected for combination surgery and radiation therapy the benefits of preoperative versus postoperative radiotherapy are still controversial. The argument over the various combinations is really whether preoperative radiation increases the risk of postoperative complications. Several series suggest that patients receiving high doses of preoperative radiation therapy have increased risk of wound breakdown, fistula formation, flap failure, and carotid blowout. Not all series have corroborated these findings, however. Nevertheless, postoperative complications as a result of preoperative radiation can be substantial and even catastrophic. Therefore, many centers now prefer postoperative radiation therapy. The one disadvantage to postoperative radiation therapy is that patients with wound complications from their primary procedures often have long delays before receiving postoperative radiation therapy. Patients should receive postoperative radiotherapy within three to six weeks following completion of surgery for best results. Preoperative radiotherapy has not been shown superior to postoperative radiotherapy for similarly staged tumors at any site.

Chemotherapy. The chemotherapy of head and neck cancer is the subject of a recent excellent review (Hong and Bromer, 1983). For many years chemotherapy in head and neck cancer was relegated to treating patients with extensive disease or with tumor recurrence following surgery and radiation therapy. Generally, single agents were used and various schedules and techniques of drug administration were manipulated in efforts to improve response rates and durations. Although various drugs produced tumor regression in these groups of patients, complete responses were uncommon, partial responses generally were of short duration, and no major impact was made on survival. Nonetheless, objective tumor regression was occasionally associated with subjective beneficial effects, such as relief of symptoms and improved appetite, with weight gain. Patients previously treated with surgery or radiation therapy responded less often than those with no prior therapy. In addition, severely debilitated patients responded less well than those with good performance statuses. The benefits observed with chemotherapy in some patients with advanced head

and neck cancer, the high failure rate of surgery and radiation therapy in stage III and IV disease at most sites, and the availability of several active drugs provided the impetus for several lines of investigation in recent years. These have included studies of combination chemotherapy, the use of chemotherapy concurrent with radiation therapy in primary treatment, and the administration of chemotherapy prior to surgery and radiation therapy.

SINGLE AGENTS. The most widely studied and most extensively used drug in head and neck cancer is methotrexate (Bertino *et al.,* 1975). Many dose schedules and various routes of administration have been tested, including five-day loading courses (oral or intravenous) (Papac *et al.,* 1963), treatment intravenously every four days to response or toxicity followed by weekly maintenance injections (Lane *et al.,* 1968), weekly intravenous injections (Leone *et al.,* 1968), intravenous high-dose methotrexate and leucovorin rescue (Levitt *et al.,* 1973), and three daily intramuscular injections at three-week intervals (Lehane *et al.,* 1974). In addition, the drug has been given by intra-arterial administration via branches of the carotid artery with intramuscular injection of leucovorin to prevent systemic toxicity (Sullivan *et al.,* 1960). These manipulations have been based on some rationale derived from animal studies, on pharmacokinetic considerations, or they have been empirical.

From all of the reported studies, no program is significantly more effective than another in terms of overall response rate, complete response rate, or survival. In part, this is due to the variations in patient populations studied (number of patients in each study, types of tumors, prior treatment, performance status), definitions of response, degree of adherence to treatment protocols and supportive therapies. A controlled clinical trial, however, that directly compared weekly intravenous methotrexate with high-dose methotrexate and leucovorin rescue failed to establish the superiority of either regimen (DeConti and Schoenfeld, 1981). A study of various high-dose methotrexate regimens with leucovorin rescue failed to show therapeutic benefit that was dose related (Levitt *et al.,* 1973). Response rates to methotrexate in recurrent head and neck cancers vary in the range of 25 to 55 percent. The highest response rates usually occurred in trials with small groups of patients in a single institution. Whether these high response rates reflected closer adherence to a particular protocol or a nonrepresentative favorable patient population on the one hand or more lenient response criteria or investigator bias on the other is difficult to determine. Similarly, in multi-institutional studies with large numbers of patients, which have often yielded low response rates, each investigator's degree of protocol compliance is difficult to know. In addition, patients with poor performance status may predominate in the study. Thus, the "true" response rate to methotrexate is uncertain. The median survival of responders, however, is apparently only in the range of three to five months from the start of therapy. Thus, treatment does not have a large impact on survival even in studies with the highest response rates. Similarly, complete responses are infrequent, which probably accounts for methotrexate therapy's minor effect on survival.

When methotrexate is administered weekly, intravenous doses of 40 to 60 mg/m^2 are generally employed. Assessing renal function prior to administration of this drug is critical, because methotrexate is eliminated exclusively by the kidney. Dosage must be greatly reduced in patients with even moderate reduction in creatinine clearance. If the creatinine clearance is reduced by 50% or more, the drug should be given with extreme caution or not at all. Under these circumstances, plasma methotrexate concentrations should be monitored and leucovorin rescue procedures instituted if methotrexate concentrations are persistently above 10^{-7} mol at 24 hours. Leucovorin dosage is based upon the plasma methotrexate concentration (Bleyer, 1977). Leucovorin may be discontinued when the methotrexate concentration falls to 5×10^{-8} mol.

Studies in our institution demonstrated that three consecutive daily intramuscular injections of methotrexate (12 to 15 mg/kg per day for three days) given at three-week intervals produced a response rate comparable to every fourth-day induction therapy followed by intravenous weekly maintenance. The every-three-week schedule permitted intermittent recovery of immunity, whereas the weekly schedule resulted in continuous immunosuppression (Lehane et al., 1974). This schedule was recently studied by the Southwest Oncology Group. In 106 evaluable patients, the response rate was comparable to that of other large studies of methotrexate, 33%, but the median survival of partial responders was 30 weeks, of complete responders, 84 weeks, and of complete responders and partial responders combined, 46 weeks (Lehane et al., 1980). The recovery of immunocompetence with this schedule of methotrexate therapy may relate to the prolonged responses observed.

Intra-arterial methotrexate therapy is rarely used. The response rates and median survivals of previously treated patients were not significantly superior to intravenous therapy. In addition, the procedure is costly, cumbersome, and associated with complications related to the catheter. Local toxicity to the mucous membranes can be very severe. In certain cases factors relating to the extent of the tumor and its blood supply may also limit the value of intra-arterial therapy.

Other drugs reported active as single agents in head and neck cancer include cisplatin (Wittes et al., 1977), bleomycin (Turrisi et al., 1978), fluorouracil, hydroxyurea, vinblastine, and cyclophosphamide (Livingston and Carter, 1970). None of these appears more effective than methotrexate as a single agent in patients with recurrent disease. Although several studies indicate that cisplatin and methotrexate are equally effective, others suggest some superiority for methotrexate. In addition, nausea, vomiting, nephrotoxicity, and ototoxicity accompany cisplatin therapy, intravenous hydration is required, and the drug is expensive. With these disadvantages most oncologists prefer methotrexate for single-agent therapy in recurrent disease. Renal function must be monitored carefully prior to each course of cisplatin, because each course can potentially inflict nephrotoxicity. Treatment is best withheld if creatinine clearance is reduced substantially. Cisplatin and methotrexate must be used cautiously in combination and with nephrotoxic drugs such as the aminoglycosides. Cisplatin's relatively low hematologic toxicity favors its use in combination chemotherapy. As a single agent, a common dose is 50 mg/m^2 on day one and day eight every four weeks. It has also been administered as 20 mg/m^2 intravenously daily for five days every four weeks and in the same dosage by continuous infusion.

Bleomycin was reported to have a high response rate when studied in Japan, primarily in untreated patients (Ichikawa, 1970). In patients with recurrent disease, however, the response rate is probably in the range of 15 to 20%. As with the other drugs, responses are of short duration. Bleomycin has been incorporated in combination chemotherapy programs because of its minimal hematologic toxicity. The chronic use of bleomycin is limited by cumulative dose-related pulmonary interstitial fibrosis. It is rarely used as a single agent. Bleomycin must be used with caution in patients with chronic lung disease or impaired renal function.

Hydroxyurea, vinblastine, and cyclophosphamide, although noted to be active in some studies, are rarely used because most medical oncologists have been insufficiently impressed with their activity. There is little enthusiasm for their further study alone or in combination for treatment of head and neck neoplasms.

A final word is needed about chemotherapeutic agent evaluations in head and neck cancer. Most of these studies have not been randomized, controlled comparisons and have evaluated only small numbers of patients. The patient groups usually included a mix of primary sites with histologic patterns of squamous cell carcinoma varying widely in degree of differentiation. They often include different proportions of patients with no prior therapy, prior surgery, and/or radiation therapy and even prior chemotherapy. Despite many studies there is no strong evidence that any treatment program produces better response at one primary site than another or that response is related to degree of tumor differentiation. As mentioned earlier, patients with prior surgical or radiation therapy or both usually respond less frequently and with fewer complete responses than patients previously untreated. This becomes evident when comparing results in patients with recurrent disease with those in patients receiving induction chemotherapy prior to planned surgery or radiation treatment.

COMBINATION CHEMOTHERAPY. Methotrexate, cisplatin, bleomycin, vinblastine, fluorouracil and vincristine have been used most commonly in various combination therapies for recurrent head and neck cancers. Although little data support the use of vincristine as a single agent, its use in combinations has been fostered on the basis that it may have vinblastine-like activity without inflicting significant myelosuppression. Regrettably, there is no compelling evidence that combinations have produced greater increases in survival than treatment with methotrexate alone in patients with recurrent advanced head and neck cancer, although higher response rates have been reported (Rowland, K. M. et al., 1984).

CONCURRENT RADIOTHERAPY AND CHEMOTHERAPY. The high failure rate of radiation therapy (inability to control local disease initially, local recurrence, or distant metastases) in patients with far-advanced inoperable disease (stages III and IV) prompted studies of simultaneous chemotherapy and radiation therapy. These studies were undertaken to reduce tumor bulk, to possibly increase the sensitivity of the tumors to radiation, and to kill micrometastases outside the radiation field. Reduction in tumor bulk by chemotherapy theoretically could improve tumor oxygenation and thereby enhance radiation effects. Conversely, reduction of tumor bulk by radiation and/or chemotherapy could recruit cells into cycle and increase the effects of cycle-active agents. Although several chemotherapeutic agents have radiosensitizing properties, these effects are minor. Some studies have suggested improved response rates with such combined treatment (Abe et al., 1978; Ansfield et al., 1970; Gollin et al., 1972; Shanta and Sundaram, 1976), but the largest study available (Fazekas et al., 1980) and others (Stefani et al., 1971; Knowlton et al., 1975) showed no major improvement in patient survival. The concurrent administration of drugs such as hydroxyurea, methotrexate, fluorouracil, and doxorubicin with radiation therapy often results in severe mucositis or cytopenias that require interruption of radiotherapy and supportive measures for nutrition and infection. Radiotherapy treatment delays can negate the possible advantage of radiosensitization. Studies are currently in progress with radiosensitizing agents as well as with drugs that protect normal tissue to determine whether either of these approaches will improve local disease control by radiotherapy.

CHEMOTHERAPY PRIOR TO SURGERY AND/OR RADIATION THERAPY. Interest in administering chemotherapy prior to surgery or radiation therapy in patients with advanced untreated head and neck cancer has recently surged. This has been variously referred to as "adjuvant," "induction," or "neoadjuvant" chemotherapy. It is not adjuvant chemotherapy as the term is commonly used, that is, administration of chemotherapy following debulking by surgery or radiation therapy. The major purposes of this approach are to improve the effects of radiation therapy by reducing tumor bulk prior to irradiation, to increase the proportion of operable patients or improve surgical results by chemotherapy debulking, and to eliminate micrometastases at the earliest possible time. Previously, patients without prior surgery or radiation therapy generally had higher response rates to chemotherapy than those with recurrent disease. This was related to an unaltered vascular supply to the tumor with more effective exposure to chemotherapeutic agents and to the better tolerance of chemotherapy by patients with good performance status. The response rates to induction chemotherapy have been significantly higher with various single and combination drug regimens (Tarpley *et al.,* 1975; Kirkwood *et al.,* 1979; Hong *et al.,* 1980; Spaulding *et al.,* 1980; Al-Sarraf *et al.,* 1981; Ervin *et al.,* 1981), ranging from 50 to over 90 percent, than response rates in recurrent disease. Induction chemotherapy is also associated with more frequent clinically complete remissions. Subsequent surgery or radiation therapy or both has generally been as well tolerated in patients not receiving prior chemotherapy. Patients considered "inoperable" prior to chemotherapy, however, are unlikely to be converted to "operable" status by chemotherapy, because residual tumor is detected microscopically in the surgical specimens of most patients. The surgeon is probably encouraged to operate by the debulking effect of chemotherapy, but the initial margins of the tumor must be respected. Several studies suggest induction therapy followed by definitive surgery and/or radiation promises improved local control. These studies and controlled studies in progress must mature sufficiently to assess the value of this approach to treatment on local control rates and patient survival.

Although optimizing initial treatment approaches to local control is essential, providing adequate adjuvant therapy after local control has been achieved is also essential. Studies are needed to evaluate adjuvant chemotherapy in patients who achieve initial local control in order to determine if such therapy will reduce local and distant recurrences.

Supportive Measures

Cancers of the head and neck occur primarily in patients over 50 years of age who are heavy users of tobacco and alcohol. These patients may have conditions noted in the general population for this age group such as heart disease, hypertension, and diabetes. In addition, they often suffer from coexistent chronic obstructive pulmonary disease, cirrhosis, mal-

nutrition, and poor oral and dental hygiene. In preparation for definitive therapy, these underlying problems must be controlled as much as possible in order to determine the suitability of the patient to undergo general anesthesia and major surgery. The gums and teeth must be given special attention. Full mouth extractions prior to radiation therapy may be necessary when the mandible and maxilla are in the treatment fields. Malnourished patients tolerate chemotherapy, surgery, and radiotherapy more poorly than well-nourished patients. They have a propensity to develop candidiasis and severe mucositis during chemotherapy and radiation therapy, become easily infected, and have impaired wound healing. Every effort should be made to improve nutritional status prior to therapy and to offer nutritional support during treatment orally or enterally when possible or with total parenteral nutrition if necessary. Several studies document reduced complications and improved tolerance of surgery and radiation in malnourished patients treated with total parenteral nutrition (Copeland *et al.,* 1975, 1977, 1979; Dietel *et al.,* 1978). Other necessary medical supportive measures may include blood transfusions to correct severe anemia, antibiotics for the management of infections, maintenance of fluid and electrolyte balance, analgesics for pain, and proper attention to bowel and bladder function, oral hygiene, and skin care. Patients must be urged in the strongest terms to avoid further use of tobacco and alcohol because of their detrimental effects on the epithelium of the upper aerodigestive tract. Psychologic support by the patient's physician and trained psychotherapists, emotional support by family, social workers, and clergy, administration of psychotropic agents, and planned rehabilitation measures are integral aspects of managing patients with head and neck cancers.

Rehabilitation

Rehabilitation is the final phase of the initial management program and will continue for the rest of the patient's life. Rehabilitation takes many forms depending on the location of the patient's tumor, treatment employed, and the complications, if any, encountered. Rehabilitation begins with careful planning of the treatment program initially. The patient should be carefully instructed about alterations of physiologic function and cosmetic appearance that treatment may produce. Any support personnel whose services may be required following treatment, such as maxillofacial prostheticians, dentists, and speech therapists, should consult with the patient prior to treatment for anatomic measurements, extraction, or preoperative counseling. Rehabilitation may simply involve patient reassurance and careful follow-up. More often, however, it involves relearning basic skills such as swallowing and talking. The postoperative laryngectomy patient must relearn how to swallow and then work extensively with a speech therapist to master new forms of communication — esophageal speech, speech via an electrical vibratory device such as an electrolarynx placed under the chin, or a COOPER/RAND instrument placed under the tongue. A third method of vocal rehabilitation is through a BLOM-SINGER prosthesis placed in a surgical pharyngotracheal fistula. Excellent speech is possible since the advent of the newer prostheses. There is still a potential for aspiration through the fistula, however. Patients with extensive oral cavity resections and loss of mandible must relearn to masticate and swallow and the surgical defects may alter the patient's dietary habits for life. Patients with palatal and orbital resection need carefully fitted prostheses to allow swallowing and normal-sounding speech and camouflage of large nasal and orbital defects. After a radical neck dissection the patient may need physical therapy to rehabilitate shoulder weakness. Postoperative rehabilitation may also require the services of an occupational therapist, psychologist, psychiatrist, and others to assist the patient in his recovery and return to a productive life. Ultimately, the patient's rehabilitation is determined by his motivation and ability to adapt to alterations of his anatomic structures and physiologic functions. The extent to which the patient is able to rehabilitate himself is often a function of care and support offered.

Principles of Follow-Up

An integral part of the complete management of the head and neck cancer patient is a rational, systematic follow-up program. The patient's initial response to therapy must be monitored and long-term progress followed. Head and neck cancer patients should be seen on a regular basis for the rest of their lives. The importance of this should be stressed to the patients as part of their initial management. An estimated 75% of all recurrences of head and neck cancer occur in the first year and 90% within the first two years of initial diagnosis and treatment. Therefore, the patient should be seen every two months in the first year, every three months the second and third years, at least every six months in the fourth and fifth years, and yearly thereafter. Follow-up should consist of a complete evaluation of the nutritional, physiologic, physical, and psychologic status of the patient. Complications of therapy, local or regional metastasis, distant metastasis, and development of another primary cancer in the head and neck or the lungs, should be considered and investigated in any patient whose problems persist following initial therapy.

The nutritional status of the patient can be assessed by careful monitoring of the patient's weight and periodic checking of the dietary intake, as well as the caloric and nutritional value of the food consumed. Anorexia, weight loss, anemia, vitamin deficiency, and dehydration are common to patients with head and neck cancers following therapy. Many patients have discomfort on swallowing or altered swallowing after radiotherapy or surgery and are unable to resume eating all of the foods they enjoyed previously. These patients often require blenderized or pureed foods and milk- or soybean-based liquid dietary supplements. Physiologic status, or the patient's ability to chew and swallow, is often directly proportional to the nutritional status the patient is able to maintain. Patients treated for lesions of the oral cavity, pharynx, and larynx commonly have some mild dysphasia after therapy. Most require only reassurance or a change in their diet. A few, however, may require dilatation of a benign stricture and others may occasionally require reinstitution of some type of tube feeding. In all patients symptoms of dysphasia, obstruction, or bleeding should be evaluated for possible tumor recurrence.

The patient should have a thorough physical examination of the head and neck. Ulceration, friable tissue, a mucosal mass in the region of the primary or elsewhere in the upper aerodigestive tract, or the development of cervical lymph nodes should be considered recurrence or a second primary until proven otherwise. Approximately 10 to 15% of patients with carcinoma of the head and neck develop a second primary at some point in their course. Suspected recurrences should be evaluated systematically with appropriate radiographic, endoscopic, and histologic studies. If recurrence is established, then the patient's treatment plan is reevaluated, and consideration given to additional surgery, radiation, or chemotherapy. The ultimate selection of therapy depends on the location, size, and nature of the recurrence or metastasis. Although the key components of follow-up after completion of therapy are a careful history of the patient's progress and meticulous physical examination of the head and neck, a chest roentgenogram should be obtained yearly. Patients with head and neck cancer are at risk for developing pulmonary metastases or a second lung primary. Additional laboratory studies should be reserved for patients who develop symptoms and signs of local or metastatic disease or complications of therapy that warrant further investigation. Laboratory studies will be necessary in patients who develop recurrences and who require further therapy.

Finally, the patient's psychologic status should be assessed. Does he understand and has he accepted his disease? How has he handled his treatment? Has he adapted to alterations in functional habits and cosmetic appearance? Has he returned to work? What adjustments has he made to problems that have developed? Has his family coped with his illness? The answers to these types of questions determine how successful the patient is in dealing with the ramifications of the cancer.

Future Prospects

Because more than 90% of head and neck cancers in the United States are related to excessive consumption of alcohol and tobacco, these cancers are preventable. Curtailment of these social habits would virtually eliminate squamous cell carcinomas of the head and neck. There is some evidence that cigarette smoking is less prevalent in some groups, such as teenagers, and nonsmokers are increasing social pressure to eliminate smoking from public places and emphasizing that this habit is not acceptable to all. Several national expressions of concern regarding the abuse of alcohol have taken place, largely motivated by the obvious relationship between drinking and automobile accidents. In the future, educational efforts emphasizing the advantages of good health and health maintenance must be directed particularly at young people so that they never begin these habits. A successful educational campaign would reduce the incidence of tobacco and alcohol abuse and of head and neck cancers within 50 years. In the interim, other approaches are required.

Vitamin A and other retinoids may have some potential in prevention. Some of these compounds have the capacity *in vitro* to promote differentiation of malignant cells. Deficiency of vitamin A may predispose one to the development of head and neck cancers. Administration of vitamin A or other retinoids on a chronic basis to high-risk groups might be a sound preventive measure. This hypothesis has not been subjected to sufficient trial to assess its merit.

Improvements in radiation therapy promise better local control. Studies of various types of radiation techniques, such as the use of high linear energy transfer radiations (neutrons, pimesons) and dose hyperfractionation, are underway. Other lines of investigation to improve results of radiation therapy involve studies of drugs that either have the ability to radiosensitize cancer cells, such as misonidazole, or, conversely, that can protect normal tissues so that higher doses of radiation may be delivered to cancer tissues.

Controlled studies of chemotherapy prior to surgery or radiation therapy now in progress will provide information on the effect of this approach on local control and survival in stage III and IV disease. Study of adjuvant therapy after surgery and radiation in patients who achieve no evidence of disease status is also needed. More effective drugs will become available in the future and should improve current therapeutic results.

Although there has not been convincing evidence that any form of immunotherapy is helpful in head and neck cancers, this research direction is still open. Some transient responses to leukocyte interferon in patients with head and neck cancer have been reported. Investigations of synthetic interferon are ongoing. Monoclonal antibodies may also have potential for therapy.

REFERENCES

Abe, M.; Shigematsu, Y.; and Kimura, S.: Combined use of bleomycin with radiation in the treatment of cancer. *Recent Results Cancer Res.,* **63**:169–178, 1978.

Al-Sarraf, M.; Drelichman, A.; Jacobs, J.; Kinzie, J.; Hoschner, J.; Loh, J. J.; and Weaver, A.: Adjuvant chemotherapy with cisplatinum, oncovin, bleomycin followed by surgery and/or radiotherapy in patients with advanced previously untreated head and neck cancer: Final report. In Salmon, S., and Jones, S. (eds.):

Adjuvant Therapy of Cancer III. Grune & Stratton, Inc., New York, 1981.

American Joint Committee for Cancer Staging and End-Result Reporting 1978. *Manual for Staging of Cancer.* Whitney Press, Chicago, 1978.

Ansfield, F. J.; Ramirez, G.; Davis, H. L., Jr.; Korbitz, B. C.; Vermund, H.; and Gollin, F. F.: Treatment of advanced cancer of the head and neck. *Cancer,* **25:**78–82, 1970.

Ariyan, S.: The pectoralis major myocutaneous flap. A versatile flap for reconstruction in the head and neck. *Plast. Reconstr. Surg.,* **63:**73–81, 1979.

Baek, S. M.; Lawson, W.; and Biller, H. F.: An analysis of 133 pectoralis major myocutaneous flaps. *Plast. Reconstr. Surg.,* **69:**460–467, 1982.

Baker, S. R., and Krause, C. J.: Cancer of the lip. In Suen, J. W., and Meyers, E. N. (eds.): *Cancer of the Head and Neck.* Churchill Livingstone, Inc., New York, 1981.

Batsakis, J. G.: *Tumors of the Head and Neck. Clinical and Pathological Considerations.* The Williams & Wilkins Company, Baltimore, 1974.

Belsky, J. L.; Tachikawa, K.; Cihak, R. W.; and Yamamoto, T.: Salivary gland tumors in atomic bomb survivors, Hiroshima-Nagasaki, 1957 to 1970. *J.A.M.A.,* **219:**864–868, 1972.

Bertino, J. R.; Boston, B.; and Capizzi, R. L.: The role of chemotherapy in the management of cancer of the head and neck: A review. *Cancer,* **36:**752–757, 1975.

Bleyer, W. A.: Methotrexate: Clinical pharmacology, current status and therapeutic guidelines. *Cancer Treat. Rev.,* **4:**87–101, 1977.

Blot, W. J., and Fraumeni, J. F., Jr.: Geographic patterns of oral cancer in the United States. Etiological implications. *J. Chronic Dis.,* **30:**745–757, 1977.

Bocca, E., and Pignataro, O.: A conservation technique in radical neck dissection. *Ann. Otol. Rhinol. Laryngol.,* **76:**975–987, 1967.

Broders, A. C.: Squamous cell epithelioma of the lip: A study of five hundred and thirty-seven cases. *J.A.M.A.,* **74:**656–664, 1920.

Byers, R. M.; Krueger, W. W.; and Saxton, J.: Use of surgery and postoperative radiation in the treatment of advanced squamous cell carcinoma of the pyriform sinus. *Am. J. Surg.,* **138:**597–599, 1979.

Chan, S. H., and Simons, M. J.: Immunogenetics of nasopharyngeal carcinoma. *Ann. Acad. Med. Singapore,* **6:**342–346, 1977.

Copeland, E. M.; Daly, J. M.; and Dudrick, S. J.: Nutritional concepts in the treatment of head and neck malignancies. *Head Neck Surg.,* **1:**350–363, 1979.

Copeland, E. M.; MacFadyen, B. V., Jr.; MacComb, W. S.; Guillamondegui, O.; Jesse, R. H.; and Dudrick, S. J.: Intravenous hyperalimentation in patients with head and neck cancer. *Cancer,* **35:**606–611, 1975.

Copeland, E. M.; Souchon, E. A.; MacFadyen, B. V., Jr.; Rapp, M. H.; and Dudrick, S. J.: Intravenous hyperalimentation as an adjunct to radiation theapy. *Cancer* **39:**609–616, 1977.

Crile, G. W.: Excision of cancer of head and neck. *J.A.M.A.,* **47:**1780–1786, 1906.

Cutler, S. J., and Young, J. L.: Third national cancer survey: Incidence data. *Natl. Cancer Inst. Monogr.,* **41:**1–454, 1975.

Decker, J., and Goldstein, J. C.: Current concepts in otolaryngology. Risk factors in head and neck cancer. *N. Engl. J. Med.,* **306:**1151–1155, 1982.

De Conti, R. C., and Schoenfeld, D.: A randomized prospective comparison of intermittent methotrexate, methotrexate with leucovorin, and a methotrexate com-bination in head and neck cancer. *Cancer,* **48:**1061–1072, 1981.

Decouflé, P.: Occupation. In Schottenfeld, D., and Fraumeni, J. F., Jr. (eds.): *Cancer Epidemiology and Prevention.* W. B. Saunders Company, Philadelphia, 1982.

de-Thé, G.: The Chinese epidemiological approach of nasopharyngeal carcinoma research and control. *Yale J. Biol. Med.,* **54:**33–39, 1981.

Dietel, M.; Vasic, V.; and Alexander, M. A.: Specialized nutritional support in the cancer patient. Is it worthwhile? *Cancer,* **41:**2359–2363, 1978.

Ebenius, B.: Cancer of the lip. *Acta Radiologica,* [Suppl.] (Stockh.), **48:**1–232, 1945.

Ervin, T. J.; Karp. D. D.; Weichselbaum, R. R.; and Frei, E., III: Adjuvant chemotherapy for squamous carcinoma of the head and neck. In Salmon, S., and Jones, S. (eds.): *Adjuvant Therapy of Cancer III.* Grune & Stratton, Inc., New York, 1981.

Fazekas, J. T.; Sommer, C.; and Kramer, S.: Adjuvant intravenous methotrexate or definitive radiotherapy alone for advanced squamous cancers of the oral cavity, oropharynx, supraglottic larynx or hypopharynx. *Int. J. Radiat. Oncol. Biol. Phys.,* **6:**533–541, 1980.

Fletcher, G. H.: Elective irradiation of subclinical disease in cancers of the head and neck. *Cancer,* **29:**1450–1454, 1972.

Gallagher, T. M., and Boles, R.: Symposium: Treatment of malignancies of paranasal sinuses. Carcinoma of maxillary antrum. *Laryngoscope,* **80:**924–932, 1970.

Gollin, F. F.; Ansfield, F. J.; Brandenburg, J. H.; Ramirez, G.; and Vermund, H.: Combined therapy in advanced head and neck cancer; A randomized study. *Am. J. Roentgenol. Radium Ther. Nucl. Med.,* **114:**83–88, 1972.

Hecht, S. S.; Chen, C. B.; and Hoffman, D.: Tobacco-specific nitrosamines: Occurrence, formation, carcinogenicity, and metabolism. *Occup. Chem. Res.,* **12:**92–98, 1979.

Hendrickson, F. R.; Kline, T. C., Jr.; and Hibbs, G. G.: Primary squamous carcinoma of larynx. *Laryngoscope,* **85:**1650–1666, 1975.

Ho, J. H. C.: An epidemiological and clinical study of nasopharyngeal carcinoma. *Int. J. Radiat. Oncol. Biol. Phys.,* **4:**183–198, 1978.

Hoffman, D.; Schmeltz, I.; Hecht, S.S.; and Wynder, E. L.: Tobacco carcinogenesis. In Gelboin, H., and T'so, P. O. (eds.): *Polycyclic Hydrocarbons and Cancer,* Vol. 1. Academic Press, Inc., New York, 1978.

Hong, W. K.; Bhutani, R.; Shapskay, S. M.; and Strong, M. S.: Induction chemotherapy in advanced previously untreated squamous cell head and neck cancer with cisplatin and bleomycin. In Prestayko, A. W.; Crooke, S. T.; and Carter, S. K. (eds.): *Cisplatin: Current Status and New Developments.* Academic Press, Inc., New York, 1980.

Hong, W. K., and Bromer, R.: Current concepts: Chemotherapy in head and neck cancer. *N. Engl. J. Med.,* **308:**75–79, 1983.

Ichikawa, I.: Clinical effect of bleomycin against squamous cell carcinoma and further development. In *Progress in Antimicrobial and Anticancer Chemotherapy, Proceedings, 6th International Congress of Chemotherapy.* Vol. II. University of Tokyo Press, Tokyo, 1969.

Jakobsson, P. A.: Histological grading of malignancy and prognosis in glottic carcinoma of the larynx. In Alberti, P. W., and Bryce, E. P. (eds.): *Workshops from the Centennial Conference on Laryngeal Cancer,* Appleton-Century-Crofts, New York, 1976.

Jesse, R. H.; Ballantyne, A. J., and Larson, D.: Radical or

modified neck dissection: A therapeutic dilemma. *Am. J. Surg.,* **136:**516–519, 1978.

Jesse, R. H., and Sugarbaker, E. V.: Squamous cell Ca of the oropharynx: Why we fail. *Am. J. Surg.,* **132:**435–438, 1976.

Jørgensen, K.; Elbrond, O.; and Anderson, A. P.: Carcinoma of the lip: A series of 869 cases. *Acta Radiol.* [Oncol.], **12:**177–190, 1973.

King, H., and Haenzel, W.: Cancer mortality among foreign and native born Chinese in the United States. *J. Chronic Dis.,* **26:**623–646, 1973.

Kirkwood, J. M.; Miller, D.; Weichselbaum, R.; and Pitman, S.: Predefinitive and postdefinitive chemotherapy for locally advanced squamous cell carcinoma of the head and neck. *Laryngoscope,* **89:**573–581, 1979.

Knowlton, A. H.; Percarpio, B.; Bobrow, S.; and Fischer, J. L.: Methotrexate and radiation therapy in the treatment of advanced head and neck tumors. *Radiology,* **116:**709–712, 1975.

Lane, M.; Moore, J. E., III; Levin, H.; and Smith, F. E.: Methotrexate therapy for squamous cell carcinomas of the head and neck. *J.A.M.A.,* **204:**561–564, 1968.

Lanier, A. P.; Bender, T. R.; Blot, W. J.; Fraumeni, J. F., Jr.; and Hurlburt, W. B.: Cancer incidence in Alaska natives. *Int. J. Cancer,* **18:**409–412, 1976.

Lehane, D. E.; Lane, M.; and Stuckey, W. J.: A comparison of methotrexate (M) with methyl CCNU (MC) and bleomycin (B) in patients with advanced squamous cell carcinoma of the head and neck (H&N) region: A Southwest Oncology Group Study. *Proc. Am. Soc. Clin. Oncol.,* **21:**331, 1980.

Lehane, D. E.; Lane, M.; and Wardle, M.: Immunocompetence of head and neck cancer patients receiving methotrexate (MTX) by two different schedules. *Proc. Am. Assoc. Cancer Res.,* **15:**190, 1974.

Leone, L. A.; Albala, M. M.; and Rege, V. B.: Treatment of carcinoma of the head and neck with intravenous methotrexate. *Cancer,* **21:**828–837, 1968.

Levitt, M.; Mosher, M. B.; De Conti, R. C.; Farber, L. R.; Skeel, R. T.; Marsh, J. C.; Mitchell, M. S.; Papac, R. J.; Thomas. E. D.; and Bertino, J. R.: Improved therapeutic index of methotrexate with "leucovorin rescue". *Cancer Res.,* **33:**1729–1734, 1973.

Lindberg, R.: Distribution of cervical lymph node metastases from squamous cell carcinoma of upper respiratory and digestive tracts. *Cancer,* **29:**1446–1449, 1972.

Livingston, R. B., and Carter, S. K.: *Single Agents in Cancer Chemotherapy,* Plenum Publishing Corporation, New York, 1970.

Lund, C.; Sogaard, H.; Jørgensen, K.; Elbrond, O.; Hjelm-Hansen, M.; and Anderson, P.: Histological grading of epidermoid carcinomas of the head and neck. *Dan. Med. Bull.,* **24:**162–166, 1977.

McGavran, M. H.; Bauer, W. C.; Spjut, H. J.; and Ogura, J. H.: Carcinoma of pyriform sinus: The results of radical surgery. *Arch. Otolaryngol.,* **78:**826–830, 1963.

McKay, E. N., and Seller, A. H.: A statistical review of Ca of lip. *Can. Med. Assoc. J.,* **90:**670–672, 1964.

Mahboubi, E., and Sayed, G. M.: Oral cavity and pharynx. In Schottenfeld, D., and Fraumeni, J. F., Jr. (eds.): *Cancer Epidemiology and Prevention,* W. B. Saunders Company, Philadelphia, 1982.

Martinez, I.: Factors associated with cancer of the esophagus, mouth and pharynx in Puerto Rico. *J.N.C.I.,* **42:**1069–1094, 1969.

Mashberg, A.; Garfinkel, L.; and Harris, S.: Alcohol as a primary risk factor in oral squamous carcinoma. *Ca,* **31:**146–155, 1981.

Miller, A. B.: The epidemiology of oral cancer. *J. Can. Dent. Assoc.,* **40:**211–217, 1974.

Miller, D.: Management of glottic carcinoma. *Laryngoscope,* **85:**1435–1439, 1975.

Molnár, L.; Rónay, P.; and Tapolcsányi, L.: Carcinoma of the lip: Analysis of the material of 25 years. *Oncology,* **29:**101–121, 1974.

Muir, C. S., and Nectoux, J.: Descriptive epidemiology of malignant neoplasms of nose, nasal cavity, middle ear and accessory sinuses. *J. Clin. Otolaryng. (U.K.),* **5:**195–211, 1980.

Muir, C. S., and Nectoux, J.: International patterns of cancer. In Schottenfeld, D., and Fraumeni, J. F., Jr. (eds.): *Cancer Epidemiology and Prevention.* W. B. Saunders Company, Philadelphia, 1982.

Papac, R.: Jacobs; E.; Foye, L.; and Donohue, D.: Systemic therapy with amethopterin in squamous carcinoma of the head and neck. *Cancer Chemother. Rep.,* **32:**47–54, 1963.

Rowland, K. M.; Taylor, S. G., IV; O'Donnell, M. R.; Spiers, A.; Stott, P. B.; DiConti, R. C.; and Milner, L.: Cisplatin/5-fluorouracil infusion chemotherapy in advanced recurrent cancer of the head and neck. An ECOG pilot study. *Proc. Am. Soc. Clin. Oncol.,* **3:**184, 1984.

Schottenfeld, D.: Alcohol as a co-factor in the etiology of cancer. *Cancer,* **43:**1962–1966, 1979.

Shanmugaratnum, K.: Nasopharynx. In Schottenfeld, D., and Fraumeni, J. F., Jr. (eds.): *Cancer Epidemiology and Prevention.* W. B. Saunders Company, Philadelphia, 1982.

Shanta, V., and Sundaram, K.: The combined therapy of oral cancer. *Gann Monogr. Cancer Res.,* **19:**159–170, 1976.

Silverberg, E.: Cancer statistics, 1983. *Ca,* **33:**9–25, 1983.

Simons, M. J.; Chan, S. H.; Wee, G. B.; Shanmugaratnum, K.; Goh, E. H.; Ho, J. H. C.; Chau, J. C. W.; Darmalingam, S.; Prasad, U.; Betuel, H.; Day, N. E.; and de-Thé, G.: Nasopharyngeal carcinoma and histocompatability antigens. In de-Thé, G., and Ito, Y. (eds.): *Nasopharyngeal Carcinoma: Etiology and Control.* IARC Scientific Publications, Lyon, 1978.

Spaulding, M. B.; Klotch, D.; Grillo, J.; Sanani, S.; and Loré, J. M.: Adjuvant chemotherapy in the treatment of advanced tumors of the head and neck. *Am. J. Surg.,* **140:**538–542, 1980.

Spiro, R. H., and Strong, E. W.: Surgical treatment of cancer of tongue. *Surg. Clin. North Am.,* **54:**759–765, 1974.

Spitzer, W. O.; Hill, G. B.; Chambers, I. W.; Helliwell, B. E.; and Murphy, H. B.: The occupation of fishing as a risk factor in cancer of the lip. *N. Engl. J. Med.,* **293:**419–424, 1975.

Sporn, M. B.: Prevention of epithelial cancer by vitamin A and its synthetic analogs (retinoids). In Hiatt, H. H.; Watson, J. D.; and Winsten, J. A. (eds.): *Origins of Human Cancer.* Cold Spring Harbor Laboratory, Cold Spring Harbor, New York, 1977.

Stefani, S.; Eells, R. W.; and Abbate, J.: Hydroxyurea and radiotherapy in head and neck cancer. Results of prospective controlled study in 126 patients. *Radiology,* **101:**391–396, 1971.

Sullivan, R. D.; Miller, E.; Wood, A. M.; Clifford, P.; Duff, J. K.; Trussell, R.; and Burchenal, J. H.: Continuous infusion cancer chemotherapy in humans—Effects of therapy with intraarterial methotrexate plus intermittent intramuscular citrovorum factor. *Cancer Chemother. Rep.,* **6:**39–44, 1960.

Szpak, C. A.; Stone, M. J.; and Frenkel, E. P.: Some observations concerning the demographic and geographic incidence of carcinoma of the lip and buccal cavity. *Cancer,* **40:**343–348, 1977.

Tarpley, J. L.; Chretien, P. B.; Alexander, J. C.; Hoye, R. C.; Block, J. B.; and Ketcham, A. S.: High dose methotrexate as a preoperative adjuvant in the treatment of epidermoid carcinoma of the head and neck: A feasibility study and clinical trial. *Am. J. Surg.,* **130:**481–486, 1975.

Turrisi, A. T., III; Rosencweig, M.; Von Hoff, D.; Muggia, F. M.: The role of bleomycin in the treatment of advanced head and neck cancer. In Carter, S. K.; Crooke, S. T.; and Umezawa, H. (eds.): *Bleomycin: Current Status and New Developments.* Academic Press, Inc., New York, 1978.

Vogler, W. R.; Lloyd, J. W.; and Milmore, B. K.: A retrospective study of etiological factors in cancer of the mouth, pharynx, and larynx. *Cancer,* **15:**246–258, 1962.

Wang, C. C.: The role of radiation therapy in treatment of carcinoma of oral cavity. *Otolaryngol. Clin. North Am.,* **5:**357–363, 1972.

Waterhouse, J.; Muir, C. S.; Correa, P.; and Powell, J.: *Cancer Incidence in Five Continents,* Vol. III. IARC Scientific Publications, Lyon, 1976.

Winn, D. M.; Blot, W. J.; Shy, C. M.; Pickle, L. W.; Toledo, M. A.; and Fraumeni, J. F., Jr.: Snuff dipping and oral cancer among women in southern United States. *N. Engl. J. Med.,* **304:**745–749, 1981.

Wittes, R. E.; Cvitkovic, E.; Shah, J.; Gerold, F. P.; and Strong, E. W.: Cis-dichlorodiammineplatinum (II) in the treatment of epidermoid carcinoma of the head and neck. *Cancer Treat. Rep.,* **61:**359–366, 1977.

Wynder, E. L.; Bross, I. J.; and Feldman, R. M.: A study of the etiological factors in cancer of the mouth. *Cancer,* **10:**1300–1323, 1957.

Wynder, E. L., and Chan, P. C.: The possible role of riboflavin deficiency in epithelial neoplasia II. Effect on skin tumor development. *Cancer,* **26:**1221–1224, 1970.

Wynder, E. L., and Fryer, J. H.: Etiologic considerations of Plummer-Vinson (Patterson-Kelly) syndrome. *Ann. Intern. Med.,* **49:**1106–1128, 1958.

Wynder, E. L., and Hoffman, D.: Tobacco. In Schottenfeld, D., and Fraumeni, J. F., Jr. (eds.): *Cancer Epidemiology and Prevention.* W. B. Saunders Company, Philadelphia, 1982.

Wynder, E. L.; Mushinski, M. H.; and Spivak, J. C.: Tobacco and alcohol consumption in relation to the development of multiple primary cancers. *Cancer,* **40:**1872–1878, 1977.

Wynder, E. L., and Stellman, S. D.: Comparative epidemiology of tobacco-related cancers. *Cancer Res.,* **37:**4608–4622, 1977.

Young, R.: Asire, A. J.; and Pollcell, E. S.: *SEER Program: Cancer Incidence and Mortality in the United States 1973–1976.* U.S. Government Printing Office, Washington, D.C., 1978.

23

Neoplasms of the Lung

ALBERT H. OWENS, JR., and MARTIN D. ABELOFF

Incidence and Epidemiology

Bronchogenic carcinoma constitutes a major health problem in much of the Western world. In modern times the incidence of this form of cancer has been increasing continuously. In fact, in the United States the age-adjusted death rates for men and women have been doubling about every 15 years.

It is estimated that nearly 140,000 new cases of bronchogenic cancer will be diagnosed in the United States during 1984: Over 96,000 in men and fewer than 44,000 in women. Unfortunately, the number of deaths due to this disorder likely to be recorded is only slightly less (see Table 23–1).

Incidence. The incidence of bronchogenic cancer increases with advancing age, as is the case with many of the common neoplasia of self-renewing epithelial cell systems. Aside from its biologic importance, this circumstance is of practical clinical importance. Physicians managing patients with bronchogenic cancer are often obliged to modify their treatment in accordance with other age-related impairments of major organ systems.

In the United States bronchogenic carcinoma is the most common cause of cancer death in men aged 35 years and older. The death rate due to bronchogenic cancer is more than double the death rate due to cancer of the colon and rectum or cancer of the prostate. Bronchogenic cancer is the second leading cause of cancer death in women of similar age, breast cancer being responsible more frequently. If present trends continue, however, bronchogenic cancer will be the prime cause of cancer deaths in women before the end of this century (see Figure 23–1).

Causal Agents. The increasing incidence of bronchogenic cancer has been associated with urbanization and with industrialization. A variety of environmental agents have been identified as probable causal factors (see Table 23–2). None is as important as cigarette smoking, however, in relation to the increasing frequency of bronchogenic cancer.

Most all of these causal agents are inhaled into the tracheobronchial tree. The size of the particle breathed in has a great deal to do with its penetrance and deposition in the more distal subdivisions of the bronchial tree. Particles 0.5 to 3.0 microns in size are considered the most dangerous because they can gain access to the terminal bronchi and respiratory bronchioles most easily. Naturally, the effect of in-

Table 23–1. Estimated Cancer Deaths in the United States (Males and Females, 1984)

COMMON CANCERS	MALES	FEMALES	TOTAL
Breast	300	37,300	37,600
Colon and rectum	28,800	30,600	59,400
Lung	85,000	36,000	121,000
Prostate	25,000		25,000

Based on data from: *Cancer Facts and Figures, 1984.* American Cancer Society, New York, 1984.

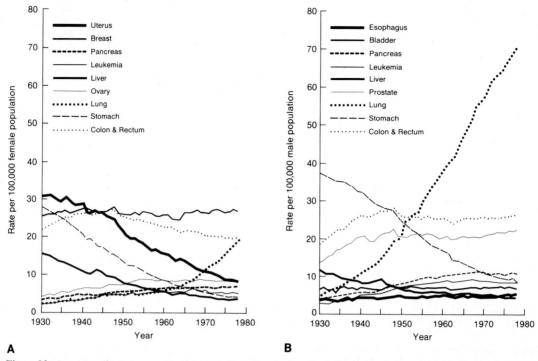

Figure 23–1. Age-adjusted cancer death rates (adjusted to the age distribution of the 1970 U.S. Census Population) for selected sites in females (*A*) and males (*B*) in the United States, 1930–1978. (Sources of data: U.S. National Center for Health Statistics and U.S. Bureau of the Census.) From Silverberg, E.: *Cancer Statistics, 1982.* American Cancer Society, New York, 1982.

Table 23–2. Bronchogenic Carcinoma: Causal Agents

CARCINOGEN	EXPOSURE	ASSOCIATED LESIONS
Arsenic compounds	Pesticide making, smelters	Keratoses (palms and soles
Asbestos	Miners, millers, pipe fitters, shippers	Pulmonary asbestosis, asbestos bodies in sputum, asbestos warts (hands)
Bis(chloromethyl) ether, related compounds	Plastics making, chemical workers	None
Chromate	Smelters	Perforated nasal septum, chronic dermatitis
Hematite (radon?)	Miners	None
Isopropyl oils	Chemical workers	None
Nickel (carbonyl)	Miners, refiners, shippers	Nasal polyps, chronic dermatitis
Radioisotopes (radon)	Miners (uranium), fluorspar, iron ore)	None
Soot, tars, oils	Oil refiners, asphalt plant workers, coke oven workers, chemical workers	Chronic dermatitis and photosensitivity, warts (exposed areas)
Tobacco	Personal use, especially cigarette smoking	Chronic bronchitis, cellular atypia
Vinyl chloride	Chemical workers	None

Based on data from Fraumeni, J. F., Jr.: Respiratory carcinogenesis: An epidemiologic appraisal. *J.N.C.I.*, 55:1039–1046, 1975.

haled noxious agents will be more marked if the respiratory epithelium has been damaged to the point of impairing the normal mucociliary function.

Evidence to the effect that interactions among these noxious inhalants can lead to increases in the development of bronchogenic cancer has been reported. For example, the risk of cancer in workers exposed to asbestos fibers is probably more than doubled if they are cigarette smokers. Whether these adverse outcomes result from intracellular interactions that enhance the carcinogenic process or from damage to the endobronchial epithelium that impairs mucociliary function or both remains to be clarified in most cases.

Etiology and Pathogenesis

Cancers, like most bronchopulmonary disorders, probably result from the deposition and absorption of gaseous and particulate matter on the bronchopulmonary epithelium. The likelihood of cancers developing relates to the integrity of the bronchopulmonary defense

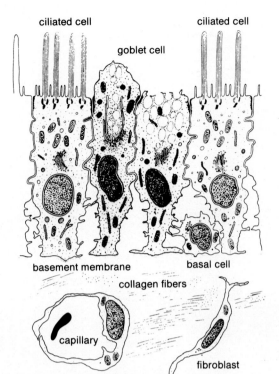

Figure 23–3. Schema of bronchial epithelial cells. From Nagaishi, C.: *Functional Anatomy and Histology of the Lung.* Igaku Shoin Ltd., Tokyo, 1972.

mechanisms and the genetic constitution of the individual as well as to the intensity and duration of exposure to the carcinogenic agent.

The Tracheobronchial Tree. The adult tracheobronchial tree begins at the larynx and is divided into the mainstem, lobar, segmental, and subsegmental bronchi (see Figure 23–2). The tracheobronchial tree is lined by a self-renewing epithelial cell system that presents a pseudostratified appearance on histologic section (see Figure 23–3). The basal cells, which lie in contact with the basement membrane, are capable of proliferation. Presumably they mature into mucus-producing columnar cells that lie along the luminal margin (see Table 23–3). Pale-staining columnar cells with little evidence of maturation are seen rarely. These cells are capable of proliferation and likely have the capacity to differentiate toward mucus-forming cells or toward ciliated cells. In the normal adult bronchial epithelium, mature ciliated cells are the most common type. Usually they are three times more numerous than the mature mucus-producing "goblet" cells.

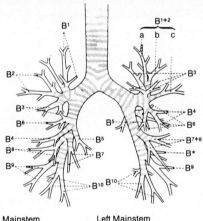

Right Mainstem

Upper Lobe
  RB^1 Apical segment
  RB^2 Posterior
  RB^3 Anterior

Bronchus Intermedius
  Middle lobe
  RB^4 Lateral segment
  RB^5 Medial

Lower Lobe
  RB^6 Superior segment
  RB^7 Mediobasal
  RB^8 Anterior basal
  RB^9 Lateral basal
  RB^{10} Posterior basal

Left Mainstem

Upper Lobe
  Upper Division
    LB^{1+2} Apical-Posterior segment
    LB^3 Anterior

  Lower Division
    LB^4 Sueprior lingular segment
    LB^5 Inferior lingular

Lower Lobe
  LB^6 Superior segment
  LB* Subsuperior
  LB^{7+8} Anterior basal
  LB^9 Lateral basal
  LB^{10} Posterior basal

Figure 23–2. Anatomy of the adult tracheobronchial tree. From Nagaishi, C.: *Functional Anatomy and Histology of the Lung.* Igaku Shoin Ltd., Tokyo, 1972.

Table 23–3. Cellular Components of the Bronchial Epithelium

CELL TYPE	LOCATION		MORPHOLOGIC CHARACTERISTICS					CAPACITY TO		RESPONSE TO INJURY
	Basement Membrane	Lumen	Shape	Microvilli	Mucus	Cilia	Cytoplasm	Proliferate	Differentiate	
Basal cell	+		polyhedral				dark	+	+	hyperplasia
Neurosecretory cell	+	rarely	flask	+			dense granules	+		
Indifferent cell	+	+	columnar	+			clear, pale	+	++	hyperplasia, squamous metaplasia
Mucous cell	+	+	columnar	+	+		mucous granules or large goblets	+	?	hyperplasia, mucous cell metaplasia
Ciliated mucous cell	+	+	columnar	+	+	+				
Ciliated cell	+	+	columnar	+		+	clear, pale			cell loss

Based on data from McDowell, E. M.; Barrett, L. A.; Galvin, F.; Harris, G. C.; and Trump, B. F.: The respiratory epithelium. I. Human bronchus. *J.N.C.I.*, **61**:539–549, 1978, and Trump, B. F.; McDowell, E. M.; Galvin, F.; Barrett, L. A.; Becci, P. I.; Schurch, W.; Kaiser, H. E.; and Harris, C. C.: The respiratory epithelium. III. Histogenesis of epidermoid metaplasia and carcinoma in situ in the human. *J.N.C.I.*, **61**:563–575, 1978.

Argyrophilic cells that contain neurosecretory granules (granular basal cells) are found throughout the epithelium and are capable of synthesizing biogenic amines and polypeptide hormones. Although sparsely distributed in the basal layer of the large bronchi and in the terminal bronchioles, they are most common in the smaller bronchi. The endocrinelike biochemical properties of these cells (Kulchitsky's cells, APUD cells) has led to the suggestion that their embryologic anlagen are distinct from the other cellular elements of the tracheobronchial epithelium. More recent evidence, however, suggests a common cytogenealogy.

The terminal bronchioles are lined by ciliated columnar cells and non-mucus-producing columnar cells (Clara cells). The more distally located alveoli are lined by very thin polygonal cells with a large surface area (type I pneumocytes) and thicker, peglike cells that contain lamellar, surfactant-laden cytoplasmic structures (type II pneumocytes).

Extensive pulmonary and bronchial vascular systems and another distinct vascular system supplying the pleura and chest wall exist (see Figure 23–4). These vascular systems are altered by disease. Neovascularization of cancers, perhaps mediated by tumor cell produced angiogenesis factors, plays an important role in their further development.

A very extensive system of lymphatic vessels draining the lung and tracheobronchial tree is present (see Figure 23–5). With advancing age, the carbon particles deposited in the bronchopulmonary lymph nodes by phagocytic cells provide ample evidence of the atmospheric pollution inhaled by most people. A rich lymphatic flow through the mediastinum is also present (see Figure 23–6). Knowledge of these drainage patterns and their frequent normal variations is important to understanding the spread of bronchogenic carcinoma as well as many other disorders.

Nonrespiratory Tracheobronchial Functions. Air inspired over the moist mucus-

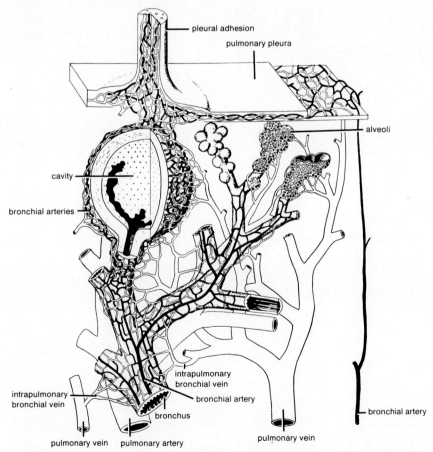

Figure 23–4. Relationship between the pulmonary and bronchial vascular systems. From Nagaishi, C.: *Functional Anatomy and Histology of the Lung.* Igaku Shoin Ltd., Tokyo, 1972.

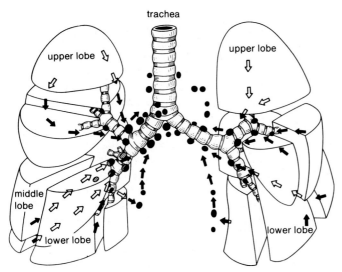

Figure 23–5. Efferent lymph flow of the lung. From Nagaishi, C.: *Functional Anatomy and Histology of the Lung.* Igaku Shoin Ltd., Tokyo, 1972.

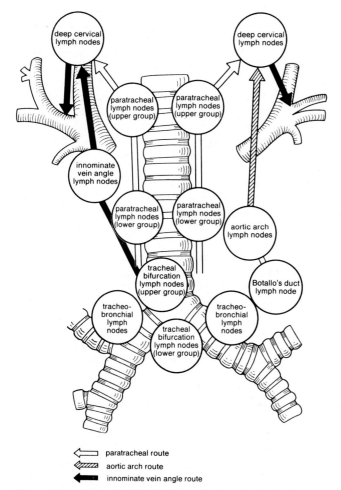

Figure 23–6. Lymphatic flow in the mediastinum. From Nagaishi, C.: *Functional Anatomy and Histology of the Lung.* Igaku Shoin Ltd., Tokyo, 1972.

laden surface of the endobronchial epithelium is warmed rapidly and saturated with water vapor. Soluble gases are absorbed into the body and a portion of the insoluble gases may be adsorbed to some of the components of the mucus that is layered along the epithelial surface. Inhaled particles are caught up in the turbulence and changing velocities as inspired air moves distally in the tracheobronchial passages. Particles 10 microns or larger in size generally fall out on the mucus membranes of the upper air passages. Particles between 0.5 and 3.0 microns in size are usually deposited along the terminal bronchioles. Smaller particles are carried against the respiratory surfaces, but most of them are eventually expired (see Figure 23–7).

Particles deposited along the tracheobronchial epithelium are moved toward the larynx along with the mucous secretions propelled in that direction by ciliary activity. Effective propulsion requires well-hydrated, nonviscid secretions and an intact, vigorous, ciliated epithelium. The epithelium of the terminal bronchioles is densely ciliated. Particles adherent to the respiratory membranes are removed by a variety of phagocytic cells. They tend to collect in the lymphatics along the bronchi and in the hilar lymph nodes.

Damaged Endobronchial Epithelium. Damage to the tracheobronchial epithelium may be caused by a wide variety of infections, systemic disorders, and atmospheric pollutants. Damage due to cigarette smoking is especially widespread.

The epithelium lining the bifurcations of the segmental and subsegmental bronchi is partic-

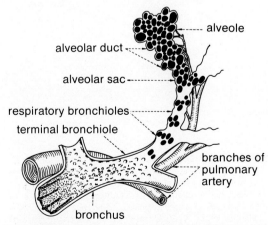

Figure 23–7. Peripheral parts of the bronchial tree and alveolar region. From Nagaishi, C.: *Functional Anatomy and Histology of the Lung.* Igaku Shoin Ltd., Tokyo, 1972.

ularly prone to injury. The basal epithelial cells respond early by proliferating at a greater rate than usual. The number of normally functioning ciliated cells is decreased and there is an increase in the number of "goblet cells" that secrete a viscid mucus. Prolonged and repeated injury leads to even more pronounced changes. The columnar cells are replaced by a metaplastic stratified squamous epithelium (Table 23–3). Eventually the epithelium becomes more disorganized, and marked nuclear atypia and abnormal mitotic patterns are noted, particularly in the basal portions of the mucosa. This process, which may be prolonged over 10 to 20 years, leads to the development of carcinoma *in situ* and frank invasive cancer (Trump *et al.*, 1978).

The morphologic chain of events leading to squamous metaplasia and *in situ* cancer formation has been linked principally to squamous cell (epidermoid) cancer. A similar sequence of events is presumed for small cell cancer based on observations in uranium miners who smoke cigarettes. Adenocarcinomas and large cell carcinomas tend to develop in the more peripheral portions of the tracheobronchial tree, often in association with chronic inflammatory disorders and tissue fibrosis. Foci of adenomatous or metaplastic mucus-producing cells often arise in these areas of progressive tissue damage and repair and are thought to be antecedent to the formation of a frank cancer.

In this setting the physician must remain alert to a higher frequency of bronchogenic cancer and not be lulled into ascribing low-grade symptoms to benign epithelial damage and bronchial inflammation.

Carcinogenesis. In general, bronchogenic cancers appear at the site of the most intense and prolonged exposure to inhaled carcinogens. Usually, a long latency period (of several years) elapses before the neoplastic process becomes clinically manifest. The intracellular processes that lead to neoplastic transformation are complex and not yet completely understood.

A variety of chemical and physical agents are linked to the development of bronchogenic cancer (Table 23–2). The physical agents are essentially those that are radioactive. They are mainly inhaled in particulate form, phagocytized, and lodged in tissues in and about the bronchi, especially in the lymphatics. Over time, the nearby structures are damaged by the irradiation, and cancers may emerge.

Chemical carcinogens affect cells and tissues in various ways. Many years ago it was observed that certain compounds could "initiate" cancer formation, whereas others could promote the process. Some chemical species were "complete carcinogens" in that they could "initiate" and "promote" the neoplastic transformation process. In some instances these actions are related to the intensity of the exposure (in terms of concentration and time) and the developmental status of the cells exposed.

Many chemical carcinogens are not biologically active in the form in which they are inhaled or enter into the bronchial epithelial cells. These "precarcinogens" are metabolized by the mixed function oxidases, hydroxylases, acetylases, and other drug metabolizing enzymes located in the cytoplasm. Some of the metabolic products are biologically inert, whereas others are referred to as the "proximate" or "ultimate" carcinogens because they have been shown to interact with important informational macromolecular compounds within the cell, especially DNA, RNA, and proteins. The changes induced in DNA are thought to be critical to the neoplastic transformation process and to the perpetuation of these characteristics in progeny cells. It is clear that epigenetic factors, however, can also modify the carcinogenic process.

Aside from the intensity of exposure, there are certain factors that contribute to cellular susceptibility to chemical carcinogenesis. Both *in vitro* and *in vivo* experiments indicate that there is an inverse relationship between cellular age and the susceptibility to neoplastic transformation. Thus, younger cells and embryonal cells are more sensitive to the action of carcinogens. In contrast, more mature or more differentiated cells may be disturbed by an exposure to a carcinogen, but neoplastic transformation occurs much less frequently than in the younger cells. The bronchial epithelium that is continually restoring itself following repeated cell damage may be particularly susceptible to carcinogenesis because of the increased number of younger or more immature cells present at the time of exposure. Important heritable differences in the levels of enzyme activities that influence the biologic effects of chemical carcinogens (activation and destruction), may also exist.

Despite the wide variety of the environmental carcinogens that are experienced during daily living and the higher risks of exposure inherent in some occupations, their cumulative contribution to the increasingly high incidence of bronchogenic carcinoma does not approach the magnitude of the effects produced by chronic cigarette smoking. The high prevalence of cigarette smoking among young adults presents a particularly worrisome prospect.

An important point relative to the risks of cigarette smokers for the development of bronchogenic cancer is evident. Smoking cessation will result in a declining cancer risk (see Figure 23–8). This seems to hold even in individuals with a rather long history of heavy smoking.

Oncogenes and Bronchogenic Cancer. In recent years, studies of cancer-causing viruses have revealed at least two dozen genes that are capable of transforming cells in tissue culture (oncogenes). They are related closely to cellular genes (proto-oncogenes) that have been highly conserved through vertebrate evolution

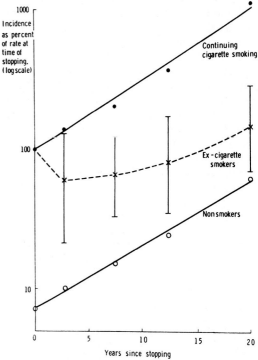

Figure 23–8. Relationship between the incidence of bronchogenic carcinoma and time after cigarette smoking was stopped compared with the relationship in continuing smokers and nonsmokers. Reproduced with permission from Doll, R.: Cancer and aging: The epidemiologic evidence. In Clark, R. L.; Cumley, R. W.; McCay, J. E.; and Copeland, M. M. (eds.): *Tenth International Cancer Congress, Oncology 1970,* vol. V. Copyright © 1971 by Year Book Medical Publishers, Inc., Chicago.

and also exist in certain invertebrates. Proto-oncogenes likely play an important role in the regulation of cell development, although the precise mechanisms remain to be clarified.

Many biologists suspect that a broad range of cancer-causing agents (viruses, radiation, chemicals) act on proto-oncogenes present in normal cells and render them tumorigenic by means of mutation, gene rearrangement, gene amplification, recombination with viruses, and other mechanisms that lead to inappropriate gene expression. The activated oncogenes that result have been detected in many types of human tumors including bronchogenic cancers. They are found, however, in only 20 to 25% of cases or less.

An active mutated oncogene (*ras* family) has been identified in epidermoid (squamous cell) bronchogenic cancer, but not in adjacent normal bronchial epithelium. Chromosomal rearrangement and amplification of the *myc* gene has been found in small cell cancer variant cell lines. Transcription of the *myc* gene has been shown in small cell cancer lines, also, but found lacking in non-small cell lines. Much work is ongoing relative to interactions among oncogenes and the oncogene products (protein kinases, growth factors) that affect malignant cell transformation. More experimentation is needed, however, to clarify the precise role of oncogenes in bronchial carcinogenesis (Griffin and Baylin, 1985).

Behavior of Neoplastic Cells. Neoplastic bronchial epithelial cells display several characteristics common to a variety of malignant cell types. Transformed cells, when placed in culture *(in vitro)*, will proliferate in a relatively unrestrained manner. On growing to confluence, they will continue to divide and pile up on one another in contrast to the behavior of nontransformed cells. Normally, cells growing to confluence will become "contact inhibited" and their proliferative activity will cease.

In vivo neoplastic cells appear to proliferate inappropriately without regard to the normal physiologic inhibitors or the organizing influences of adjacent tissues. Thus, tumors continue to grow in size until they outstrip their blood supply or the availability of suitable nutrients. Neoplastic behavior is recognized by the tumor cells' invasion of surrounding tissues and by their spreading to distant sites through lymphatic channels or through the vascular system. As a result, metastatic tumors form at distant sites.

The properties of tissue invasion and migration to distant parts of the body are not exclusive to malignant (transformed) cells. For example, during embryogenesis cells move from one part of the organism to another and participate in the development of tissues and organs at distant sites. In the adult, B lymphocytes and macrophages wander widely throughout the body in pursuit of their normal functions. In cancer there is a patently inappropriate expression of the properties of tissue invasion and spread to distant sites on the part of the malignant cells.

Tumor Cell Heterogeneity. Although the cellular morphology of many bronchogenic tumors may appear monotonously similar on routine tissue sections stained with hematoxylin and eosin, it is becoming increasingly evident that they express a variety of biologic properties and that they are undergoing continuous change. For example, some of the tumor cells continue to proliferate whereas others may "mature" to a degree. Some of the tumor cells are capable of metastasizing successfully; others are not. Many of the tumor cells may be sensitive to radiation or to chemotherapeutic agents, but those that are resistant may continue to proliferate and spread during the period of active treatment (see Chapter 4).

Genetic Instability. Genetic instability is a property commonly ascribed to cancer cells. This is manifest in the continual changes in chromosomal morphology and number and the high frequency of DNA rearrangements noted in populations of transformed cells. It seems likely that DNA rearrangements and changes in gene expression are responsible for the variations in the biologic behavior of neoplastic cells. For example, DNA rearrangement and gene amplification results in increased cellular resistance to certain anticancer drugs.

Pathology and Natural History

A wide variety of neoplasms arises in the lower respiratory tract. Most of them are malignant. The histologic classification put forward by the World Health Organization will probably serve as the working reference standard for some years to come (see Table 23–4).

Common Histologic Types. Carcinomas arising from the endobronchial epithelium constitute the vast majority (90% or more) of lung cancers (Carter and Eggleston, 1980; Minna *et al.*, 1982). At diagnosis, nearly all bronchogenic cancers are classified into four

Table 23-4. World Health Organization Classification: Cancerous Pleuropulmonary Neoplasms

Epidermoid (squamous cell) carcinoma
Small cell carcinoma
Adenocarcinoma (with or without mucin)
   1. Bronchogenic
   2. Bronchoalveolar
Large cell carcinoma
Combined epidermoid and adenocarcinoma
Carcinoid tumors
Bronchial gland tumors
Papillary tumors of the surface epithelium
Mixed tumors and carcinosarcomas
Sarcomas
Unclassified
Melanoma

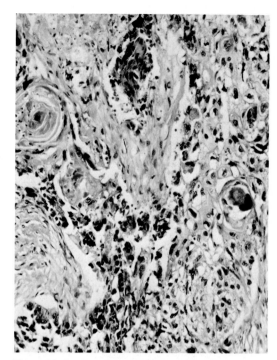

Figure 23-9. Squamous cell (epidermoid) cancer (hematoxylin and eosin × 180).

histopathologic types (see Table 23-5). The precise histogenesis of these cancers is not clear; some researchers feel that they derive from distinct cell lineages, whereas others feel that these cancers represent morphologic variants of a single neoplastic entity.

Squamous cell cancer is more common in males, whereas adenocarcinoma is the most frequent type of cancer encountered in women. The other cell types are seen with equal frequency in both sexes. Squamous cell cancer and small cell cancer occur more frequently in smokers, whereas adenocarcinoma is the predominant tumor in nonsmokers (see Table 23-5).

To comment on changes in the incidence of the several histologic types of bronchogenic cancer is difficult because of the variability associated with the routine process of classification involving large numbers of pathologists. During the past 20 years, however, the relative frequency with which squamous cell cancer is diagnosed seems to be declining, whereas the proportion of adenocarcinoma cases reported is increasing. During the same period, the incidence of lung cancer in women is increasing. Although adenocarcinoma arises most commonly in women, it seems to be occurring more often in men, also.

Squamous Cell Cancer. Squamous cell (epidermoid) cancers are the most common bronchogenic cancers, occurring in nearly 40% of the cases (see Figure 23-9). These tumors usually arise in the larger bronchi and grow toward the main stem bronchus. They develop in areas of damaged bronchial mucosa showing squamous metaplasia, cellular atypia, and dysplasia and intraepithelial cancer. Local tissue invasion and spread to regional lymph nodes occur early in the course of the disease. Lymph node or pleural involvement has been shown in 30 to 40% of resected surgical specimens. Unfortunately, metastatic spread to

Table 23-5. Bronchogenic Carcinoma: Occurrence of Five Major Types in Smokers and Nonsmokers

CELL TYPE	MALE		FEMALE	
	Smoker	Nonsmoker	Smoker	Nonsmoker
Squamous cell	38%	10%	22%	9%
Adenocarcinoma	21	56	35	68
Large cell	17	23	13	10
Small cell	23	6	27	2
Bronchoalveolar	1	5	3	11

Based on data from observations in 2926 cases as reported in Rosenow, E. C., and Carr, D. T.: Bronchogenic carcinoma. *CA*, **29**:233-244, 1979.

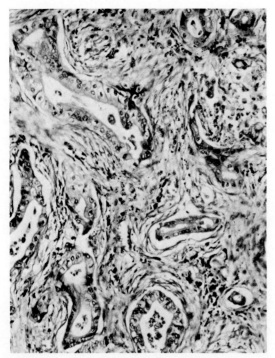

Figure 23–10. Adenocarcinoma (hematoxylin and eosin × 180).

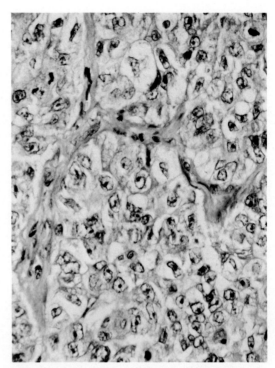

Figure 23–11. Large cell cancer (hematoxylin and eosin × 450).

distant sites is also common. Occasionally, metastatic deposits are responsible for the symptoms that first cause an individual to seek medical advice.

Adenocarcinoma. Adenocarcinomas usually arise in peripheral locations, at times in areas distal to the segmental and subsegmental bronchi (see Figure 23–10). Some extend peripherally, forming subpleural tumors, but more often they grow along the bronchi and narrow their lumina. Pleural involvement appears on presentation in over half of the patients with adenocarcinoma, and regional lymph node involvement is observed less often. At times the glandular structures formed by these cancers have developed to the point that the diagnostician has difficulty distinguishing a primary bronchogenic tumor from metastatic lesions derived from the breast, ovary, colon, or kidney. This is an important distinction to make, especially in view of the treatment implications associated with cancer of the breast or ovary.

Large Cell Carcinoma. Large cell carcinomas usually arise in locations more peripheral than do squamous cell cancers (see Figure 23–11). They may present as rather large subpleural lesions with some tissue necrosis or cavitation. The pleura and regional nodes are involved at presentation in nearly half the cases. Microscopically, large cell cancers may be rather pleomorphic, showing many of the anaplastic features of squamous cell cancer or adenocarcinomas. One variant, the giant cell cancer, is composed of very bizarre cells with giant nuclei and an extensive cytoplasm containing phagocytized materials and mucin vacuoles. Another variant, termed a clear cell cancer, may be confused with metastatic adenocarcinoma of the kidney. Although a primary pulmonary tumor is only rarely composed of nearly all clear cells, up to one-third of squamous cell cancers and adenocarcinomas contain areas of cells with this morphology. The presence of clear cells, however, does not seem to change the outlook for these tumors.

Small Cell Carcinoma. Small cell carcinoma is a rather distinctive bronchogenic cancer (see Figure 23–12). Commonly it begins in the areas of the tracheobronchial tree where the Kulchitsky's cells are most plentiful: The segmental and subsegmental bronchi. Generally, the tumor extends along the submucosa and invades adjacent tissues. Eventually, bronchial obstruction results from extrinsic pressure or, uncommonly, from endo-

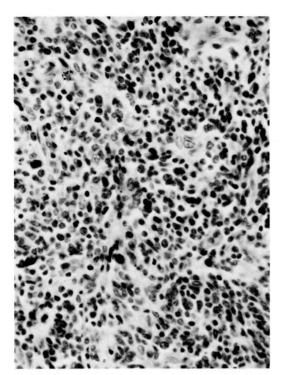

Figure 23-12. Small cell cancer (hematoxylin and eosin × 450).

bronchial tumor growth. Several morphologic variants of small cell cancer exist, but the individual histopathologic types do not seem to have distinctive prognoses. Small cell cancers often contain neurosecretory granules and are capable of synthesizing polypeptide hormones and biogenic amines. Hence, this tumor type often produces paraneoplastic endocrinopathies in affected individuals, and the tumor cells' secretory products may serve as "biomarkers" of the disease.

Small cell cancers are highly metastatic. Even though the tumor cell dissemination remains occult to all current diagnostic methods, widespread involvement is present in all patients at the time of earliest diagnosis.

Bronchoalveolar Carcinoma. Bronchoalveolar carcinoma is a relatively rare tumor, and there exists much uncertainty about its etiology and pathogenesis. That bronchoalveolar cancers may present as single tumors or as multiple nodules has led to the frequent suggestion that they represent multiple primary cancers. The disease in humans bears a striking resemblance to a form of lung cancer in sheep (jagziekte) that is caused by a virus.

Bronchoalveolar cancer usually develops in distal portions of the lung beyond the areas of recognizable bronchi. Some evidence suggests that the pneumocytes may be the cells of origin, because some of the transformed cells display lamellar bodies and surfactant secretions similar to type II pneumocytes. Often the tumor cells appear rather bland, and they tend to spread along the alveolar surfaces.

In many instances, bronchoalveolar cancer develops in association with scars from prior lung disease. The prior lung diseases are varied, including repeated pneumonias, granulomatous inflammation, asbestosis, and systemic sclerosis (scleroderma). Frequently, bronchoalveolar cancers are classified as adenocarcinomas.

Mixed Cell Carcinoma. A small percentage of bronchogenic cancers (1 to 5%) are obviously the mixed cell type at diagnosis. Mixed squamous cell cancers and adenocarcinomas are perhaps most common. Small cell cancers, however, are occasionally seen mixed with squamous cell cancer or adenocarcinoma (see Figure 23-13). Changes in the predominant cancer cell type have been observed in the same patient over time. For example, a patient with a small cell cancer very responsive to treatment may develop an adenocarcinomatous or squamous cell tumor one year or more later (Abeloff *et al.*, 1981).

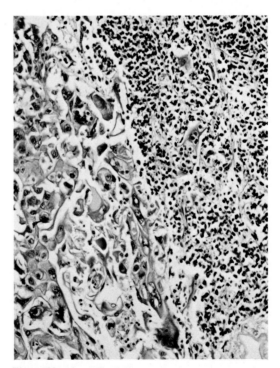

Figure 23-13. Mixed squamous and small cell cancer (hematoxylin and eosin × 180).

The Cytogenealogy of Bronchogenic Cancers. Mounting evidence has been reported that the histologically distinct common forms of bronchogenic cancer are linked by their relationships to the normal processes of cellular proliferation and differentiation that are ongoing in the endobronchial epithelium. For example, morphologic studies of epithelial regeneration following mechanical damage to the human bronchus have identified a large, pluripotent "indifferent cell" that is responsible for the development of the more mature cellular elements of the epithelium. These observations indicate that a common cell type, presumably of endodermal origin, gives rise to the endocrine-type cells as well as the more common "nonendocrine" constituents of the epithelium. Similar morphologic studies also indicate a single cellular origin for small cell and the common forms of non-small-cell bronchogenic cancer (see Figure 23–14).

Small cell cancer is a particularly virulent neoplasm that commonly exhibits neuroendocrine properties. These tumor cells often synthesize biologically active polypeptides and they have the capacity for the synthesis of biogenic amines. Neuron-specific enolase activity may be present in the cytoplasm of these tumor cells as well as the more readily recognizable neurosecretory granules. These characteristics have led to the suggestion that small cell cancers arise from the endocrine cells (Kulchitsky's cells) in the bronchial epithelium and that they are embryologic derivatives of the neural crest. Non-small-cell cancers, on the other hand, were thought to stem from the nonendocrine epithelial cells that were derived originally from the endoderm. One should challenge this concept. Ample evidence is available showing that neuroendocrine properties can be displayed in non-small-cell cancers, although often not to the same degree found in small cell cancers. Biochemical analyses reveal the presence of immunoreactive polypeptide hormones and the enzymes necessary for biogenic amine synthesis in all major histologic types of bronchogenic cancer. Recent studies of several distinctive cell surface

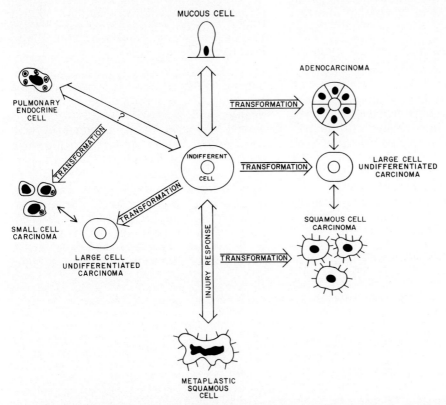

Figure 23–14. Possible developmental relationships among normal and neoplastic cells of the bronchial epithelium. From Baylin, S. B.; Goodwin, G.; and Shaper, J. H.: Analysis of cell surface proteins as a means to study neuroendocrine differentiation in the spectrum of human lung cancers. In Bloom, S. R., and Polak, J. (eds.): *Systemic Role of Regulatory Peptides, 13th Symposia Medica Hoechst.* F. K. Schattauer Verlag, Stuttgart, 1982.

proteins on small cell cancer and non-small-cell cancer clones maintained in long-term culture have provided strong evidence that they are more directly linked through a process of biologic differentiation (Baylin *et al.,* 1982).

Careful morphologic studies have shown that clones of small cell cancer cells maintained in culture lose their neuroendocrine features and change their appearance to resemble large cell undifferentiated cancers. Similar time-related transitions have been observed during successive heterotransplantation passages of small cell cancers in nude mice. Furthermore, morphologic transitions from small cell to non-small-cell cancers coupled with a loss of neuroendocrine properties have been observed in patients.

It seems likely that the direct relationships being demonstrated between common bronchogenic cancers with distinctive cell types somehow reflect the events of cell proliferation and differentiation ongoing in the normal bronchial epithelium. This evidence suggests that neoplasms represent clonal expansions of cells that were transformed at one particular stage of differentiation or another and that tumor cell populations are continually changing as if to mimic maturation processes.

Chromosomal Changes. A variety of abnormalities in chromosomal morphology and number have been reported in association with bronchogenic carcinoma. A number of observations have been made that suggest that the apparent abnormalities change with the passage of time both *in vivo* and *in vitro.* Such changing chromosomal abnormalities are common in a variety of neoplasms, and none seem specific for bronchogenic cancer.

A recent study reports the finding of an acquired chromosomal abnormality, a deletion of 3p, in at least one chromosome 3 in all metaphases examined in 14 patients with small cell cancer. This change was not seen in five non-small-cell lung cancer cell lines, nor was it observed in lymphoblastoid cells derived from two of the patients whose small cell cancers had the 3p (14-23) deletion. Thus, the 3p (14-23) deletion appears specific for this tumor type (Whang-Peng *et al.,* 1982).

Clinical Presentation

Little is known about the constitutional background or the genetic factors that condition the development of bronchogenic cancer. Much more is known about exposures to chemical and physical agents with carcinogenic potential, especially the effects of long-term cigarette smoking. In any event, it is clear that the carcinogenic process is a prolonged one and that the latent period preceding the development of clinical cancer extends over several years.

Bronchogenic cancers often occur in individuals who have pulmonary symptoms, albeit mild ones. Frequently, cigarette smokers develop some cough and sputum production in relation to their chronic bronchitis and impaired mucociliary function and it is difficult to discern the onset of symptoms due to a small endobronchial cancer. On occasion, cancers develop in areas scarred by previous pneumonias, asbestos deposits, and the like. Again it is difficult to detect the early symptoms of the cancer on the background of existing abnormalities.

Well over 80% of patients presenting with bronchogenic cancer are symptomatic when they first seek medical advice (Carter and Eggleston, 1980; Minna *et al.,* 1982). Many of these symptoms may be related to the location of the primary tumor or to the sites of metastatic spread. Some are related to the paraneoplastic effects of the tumor that are mediated by polypeptide hormones and other active tumor cell secretions. In turn, there are some

Table 23-6. Bronchogenic Carcinoma: Origin of Signs and Symptoms on Clinical Presentation

CELL TYPE	PRIMARY TUMOR	REGIONAL SPREAD	DISTANT SPREAD	PARANEOPLASTIC SYNDROMES
Squamous cell	+++	++	+	
Adenocarcinoma	+	+	+++	
Large cell	+++	++	+	
Small cell	++	++	+++	++

Legend: + = occasionally; ++ = frequently; and +++ = very frequently.
Based on data from Cohen, M. H.: Signs and symptoms of bronchogenic carcinoma. In Straus, M. (ed.): *Lung Cancer: Clinical Diagnosis and Treatment.* Grune & Stratton, Inc., New York, 1977.

Table 23-7.   Bronchogenic Carcinoma: Common Chest Radiographic Findings on Clinical Presentation

CELL TYPE	HILAR MASS	PARENCHYMAL		EXTRAPULMONARY	
		Mass	*Obstruction*	*Mediastinum*	*Effusion*
Squamous cell	40%	31%	53%	2%	3%
Adenocarcinoma	17	74	25	6	5
Large cell	32	65	33	11	2
Small cell	78	33	36	17	5

From Rosenow, E. C., and Carr, D. T.: Bronchogenic carcinoma. *CA*, 29:233-244, 1979, © American Cancer Society, Inc., 1979.

general relationships between tumor cell type and clinical symptomatology (see Tables 23-6 and 23-7).

Primary Tumor. The symptoms and signs produced by primary tumors can be related to their location in the tracheobronchial tree (see Table 23-8). Endobronchial tumors cause cough, sputum production, and hemoptysis due to disruption of the epithelial surfaces. Narrowing of the airway may produce stridor and may lead to distal atelectasis and infection, together with their associated signs and symptoms. Occasionally, segmental emphysema may develop distally to an endobronchial obstruction.

Primary tumors located more peripherally may remain clinically silent for some time. At times they become necrotic and infected. Cough, purulent sputum production, and the systemic symptoms associated with pulmonary abscesses result. Hemoptysis may occur as a consequence of blood vessel erosion. Peripheral tumors may also extend to the pleural surfaces and to the chest wall. Pain related to the tumor deposits and dyspnea secondary to pleural effusion may result.

On occasion an apical cancer will extend to the nearby chest wall (superior sulcus) and involve the eighth cervical and first thoracic nerve roots as well as the other structures located in the thoracic inlet. A distinctive clinical picture emerges including pain in the shoulder and arm and a Horner's syndrome due to disruption of the sympathetic chain (Pancoast's tumor).

Regional Spread. Bronchogenic cancers commonly extend to adjacent structures within the mediastinum (see Table 23-9). Rather distinctive clinical patterns often emerge as the first signs of illness. It is also important for the physician to recognize their precise pathogenesis, because these signs and symptoms provide an important commentary concerning the potential of surgical resectability. Among the symptom complexes are those due to extrinsic compression of the esophagus or direct invasion (dysphagia); disruption of the (left) recurrent laryngeal nerve (hoarseness often accompanied by dysphagia); disruption of the phrenic nerve with resulting paralysis of the diaphragm (dyspnea); obstruction of the superior vena cava (edema of the face, neck, arms, and upper torso or venous engorge-

Table 23-8. Bronchogenic Carcinoma: Signs and Symptoms Due to Primary Tumor

Endobronchial (Central) Tumor Growth
   Cough
   Hemoptysis
   Stridor, wheezing respirations
   Dyspnea (obstructive)
   Segmental atelectasis
   Segmental emphysema
   Pneumonia, abscess (fever, sputum production)

Parenchymal (Peripheral) Tumor Growth
   Pain; pleural and chest wall spread
   Cough
   Dyspnea (restrictive)
   Effusion; serous or bloody fluid

Table 23-9. Bronchogenic Carcinoma: Signs and Symptoms Due to Regional Tumor Spread

Mediastinal Involvement
   Dysphagia; esophageal compression or involvement
   Effusion; serous due to lymphatic obstruction, chylous due to thoracic duct involvement

Cardiovascular Involvement
   Facial and cervical edema, prominent venous pattern in neck and arms due to superior vena caval obstruction
   Tamponade, arrhythmia, heart failure due to pericardial involvement (effusion) or cardiac spread

Nerve Involvement
   Horner's syndrome (enophthalmos, meiosis, ptosis) due to interruption of cervical sympathetic chain
   Hoarseness (vocal cord paralysis) and often dysphagia due to (left) recurrent laryngeal nerve damage
   Dyspnea, cough, diaphragmatic paralysis due to phrenic nerve involvement
   Pain in arm and vasomotor signs due to brachial plexus involvement

ment); obstruction of the mediastinal lymphatics (pleural effusion); or invasion of the pericardium or heart (pericardial effusion, tamponade, or cardiac arrhythmia).

Bronchoalveolar Cancer. The clinical presentations of patients with bronchoalveolar carcinoma are varied. Many of the patients, especially those with solitary lesions, are asymptomatic at the time of diagnosis. Up to one-third of patients present complaining of cough that is at times productive of large amounts of mucoid sputum. Because many cases of bronchoalveolar cancer (multinodular or diffuse) involve rather large portions of pulmonary tissue early and because the tumor characteristically spreads along the alveolar surfaces, air exchange can be impeded to a clinically important degree. Reports of extensive arteriovenous shunting in these cancers have been made, also leading to significant arterial oxygen unsaturation.

Distant Metastases. Bronchogenic cancers often metastasize distantly. Although some variation according to cell type can be found, these tumors are very aggressive with respect to their propensity for lymphatic and hematogenous spread to extrathoracic locations. For example, at autopsy, widely metastatic tumors are easily demonstrable in 80 to 100% of cases of small cell cancer, in 50 to 85% of cases of adenocarcinoma or large cell cancer, and in 30 to 55% of cases with squamous cell cancer. Although metastases from all types of bronchogenic carcinoma are generally rather widespread throughout the body, involvement of the central nervous system (brain and meninges), liver, and bones is especially common. Curiously, there is a propensity for metastatic spread to the adrenal regions, less so in squamous cell cancer than in the other types (Matthews *et al.,* 1973; Minna *et al.,* 1982).

Unfortunately, the proportion of patients with bronchogenic cancer having distant metastases at the time of their initial clinical presentation is very large. Many metastases can be identified by current clinical techniques, but many others remain occult despite the physician's best efforts. Several characteristic clinical pictures, however, are frequently encountered (see Table 23–10). As might be expected, supraclavicular lymph node enlargement due to metastatic tumor is relatively common. Some frequently encountered problems related to distant metastatic disease are headache and neurologic deficits due to brain metastases, pain and pathologic fractures due to

Table 23–10. Bronchogenic Carcinoma: Frequent Signs and Symptoms Due to Distant Metastases

Lymphatic Involvement
  Supraclavicular, low cervical node enlargement

Liver Involvement
  Hepatic enlargement, often without failure of function

Bone Involvement
  Pain, fractures, or asymptomatic lytic lesions

Central Nervous System Involvement
  Deficits, seizures, headache, increased intracranial pressure due to brain metastases
  Backache, root pains, spinal cord compression due to meningeal tumor, vascular damage, or vertebral destruction

bony metastases, and painful enlargement and dysfunction of the liver due to extensive involvement. Physicians who occasionally encounter patients with central nervous system deficits or pathologic fractures would do well to remember that these can be the initial signs of bronchogenic cancer, which is a relatively common clinical disorder.

Paraneoplastic Syndromes. In recent years increasing attention has been called to the several paraneoplastic syndromes associated with bronchogenic cancer (see Table 23–11) (see Chapter 6). Increasingly sensitive and specific techniques have enabled the identification and serial measurement of a variety of polypeptides and other physiologically active substances secreted by these tumors, especially small cell cancers. Although the pathogenesis of the hormone-mediated syndromes has been classified, the mechanisms underlying many other paraneoplastic phenomena remain unclear.

It is of practical importance to remember that patients may become symptomatic from these paraneoplastic disorders before their primary tumor becomes clinically apparent. For example, the onset of Cushing's syndrome or polymyositis in individuals who are middle aged or older should suggest the possible presence of bronchogenic cancer. To some extent, tumor-produced secretions (*e.g.,* ACTH and HGH) can serve as a biomarker of tumor activity. Those markers, however, may not be useful guides with the passage of time. Often the cellular makeup of bronchogenic cancers changes to the extent of no longer secreting the marker substance.

Asymptomatic Presentation. Although it is rare for patients with bronchogenic cancer to

Table 23–11. Bronchogenic Carcinoma: Paraneoplastic Syndromes

---

Cutaneous
  Acanthosis nigricans, bullous lesions (erythema multiforme)
  Hyperkeratosis of the palms and soles

Connective Tissue
  Digital clubbing, dermatomyositis, scleroderma

Endocrine-Metabolic
  Hypercalcemia, gynecomastia, hypoglycemia
  Syndromes due to inappropriate secretion of various polypeptide hormones or vasoactive proteins (*e.g.,* ACTH, HGH, vasopressin, calcitonin, bradykinin)

Hemic
  Anemia — marrow hypoplasia, leukoerythroblastosis
  Purpura, bleeding — thrombocytopenia, thrombocytosis, disseminated intravascular coagulation
  Thromboses — migratory thrombophlebitis, marantic endocarditis

Osseous
  Hypertrophic osteoarthropathy

Neuromuscular
  Encephalomyeloneuropathy, especially cerebellar degeneration and peripheral neuropathy
  Myasthenialike (Lambert-Eaton)
  Polymyositis, other myopathies

---

come to medical attention while asymptomatic, it is important that the true nature of their disease be recognized as rapidly as possible when they do. Chest roentgenograms will sometimes detect an unsuspected abnormality that must be evaluated further. About 15% of patients with bronchogenic cancer are first discovered in this manner.

Unfortunately, the true nature of abnormalities due to bronchogenic carcinoma that appear on roentgenograms often is not appreciated immediately. First, similar abnormalities may be caused by non-neoplastic processes, for example, a variety of common infections. Second, bronchogenic cancers often arise in patients with chronic bronchitis or other disorders for which chest roentgenograms frequently appear abnormal. Third, the initial abnormalities caused by cancer may be subtle (for example, segmental emphysema), and no easily discernible tumor mass may be evident. Delineating a small tumor in the hilar area may be quite difficult, especially in patients with long-standing inflammatory disorders. It is important that physicians examine the chest roentgenograms of their patients in conjunction with a radiologist and that appropriate follow-up examinations are completed in a timely fashion.

Prognosis

The clinical course of patients whose bronchogenic cancer was first diagnosed 25 to 30 years ago, before modern radiation therapy and antitumor chemotherapy were applied rather widely, should be examined (Carbone *et al.,* 1970; National Cancer Institute, 1976). Several generalizations about the natural history of these cancers provide useful guides to clinicians:

1. The aggressive nature of bronchogenic cancers and their propensity to metastasize widely before clinical presentation are reflected clearly in the national statistics compiled over the past 30 years (see Table 23–12). Unfortunately, there has been no change in the stage of patients' disease at the time of the initial diagnosis.

2. Over half of all patients with bronchogenic cancer are found to have "inoperable" lesions on completion of their initial clinical evaluation. Ten to 20 years ago, approximately 35% of patients were judged to have resectable lesions at thoracotomy. Even so, nearly half of the surgical specimens showed tumor involvement in regional lymph nodes, and a smaller percentage showed pleural invasion. The extent of this problem can be

Table 23–12. Bronchogenic Carcinoma: Stage at Diagnosis

	1950–54	1955–59	1960–64	1965–69	1970–73
Localized	16%	18%	20%	18%	17%
Regional	25	29	27	22	21
Distant	42	40	43	50	48
Unknown	17	13	11	11	13

Based on data from National Cancer Institute: *SEER Program. Cancer Patient Survival — Report Number 5.* Department of Health, Education and Welfare, Bethesda, Maryland, 1976.

Table 23–13. Bronchogenic Carcinoma: Autopsy Evidence of Persistent Tumor within 30 Days of "Curative" Surgical Resection

CELL TYPE	CASE NUMBER	LOCAL TUMOR ONLY	DISTANT METASTASES
Squamous cell	131	17%	17%
Adenocarcinoma	30	3	40
Large cell	22	0	14
Small cell	19	6	63

From Matthews, M. J.; Kanhouwa, S.; Pickren, J.; and Robinette, D.: Frequency of residual and metastatic tumor in patients undergoing curative surgical resection for lung cancer. *Cancer Chemother. Rep.*, **3**:63–67, 1973.

Table 23–15. Bronchogenic Carcinoma: Five-Year Survival Rate Related to Anatomic and Symptomatic Stages

ANATOMIC STAGE	5-YEAR SURVIVAL	SYMPTOMATIC STAGE	5-YEAR SURVIVAL
		Asymptomatic	18%
I	16%	Primary tumor	12
II	4	Metastatic tumor	0
III	1	Systemic	6
TOTAL	7		7

Based on data from Carbone, P. P.; Frost, J. K.; Feinstein, A. R.; Higgins, G. A.; and Selawry, O. S.: Lung cancer: Perspectives and prospects. *Ann. Intern. Med.*, **73**:1003–1024, 1970.

appreciated from the *post mortem* examinations of patients who died from other causes within one month of a "curative" pulmonary resection (see Table 23–13). The frequency of distant metastatic lesions was especially high in patients with small cell cancer and adenocarcinoma.

Currently, CT scanning and other sensitive imaging techniques have aided significantly in the clinical staging process. As a result, a smaller proportion of lung cancer cases are first found to be "inoperable" at thoracotomy. Similarly, a higher proportion of those patients operated upon have "resectable tumors." Serious limitations remain, however, to the clinician's ability to detect distant metastases of small size.

3. The course of bronchogenic carcinoma is relatively rapid. More than half of the affected individuals die within the first year following their diagnosis. This is especially true of patients with small cell cancers (see Table 23–14).

4. A reasonable relationship between clinical stage at diagnosis and survival has been reported, which is modified somewhat by cell type (see Figure 23–15). Untreated, patients with small cell cancer have a median survival of about four months. In contrast, squamous cell

Table 23–14. Bronchogenic Carcinoma: Two-Year Survival Rates

CELL TYPE	CLINICAL STAGE		
	1	*2*	*3*
Squamous cell	46.6%	39.8%	11.5%
Adenocarcinoma	45.9	14.3	7.9
Large cell	42.8	12.9	12.9
Small cell	6.0	5.0	3.8

From Rosenow, E. C., and Carr, D. T.: Bronchogenic carcinoma. *CA*, **29**:233–244, 1979, American Cancer Society, Inc., 1979.

(epidermoid) cancer may pursue a more indolent course.

5. A relationship has been shown between patients' symptomatic status at the time of their initial clinical presentation and their prognosis for survival (see Table 23–15). The best prognosis was for truly asymptomatic individuals, whereas those with systemic symptoms or symptoms due to metastatic disease fared most poorly. The chronology of symptoms is also of importance. Patients symptomatic for six months or more (indolent disease) had a better outlook for survival than those symptomatic for a shorter time (18% versus 9% five-year survival in the Yale series [Carbone et al., 1970]). This effect seemed independent of anatomic stage.

6. There has been little change in the overall five-year survival experiences in the United States over the past 30 years (see Figure 23–16). The shape of the survival curve reflects the generally fulminant nature of bronchogenic cancer. These statistics, however, do not reflect the more favorable outlook for the few patients treated when their disease is truly localized (40 to 50%, five-year survival). Neither is the very favorable impact of multimodality treatment of small cell cancer experienced during the past few years apparent.

Diagnosis

Cancer Detection in Large Populations. As previously noted, the vast majority of patients with bronchogenic carcinoma present with symptoms. Unfortunately, symptoms secondary to cancer are generally a feature of ad-

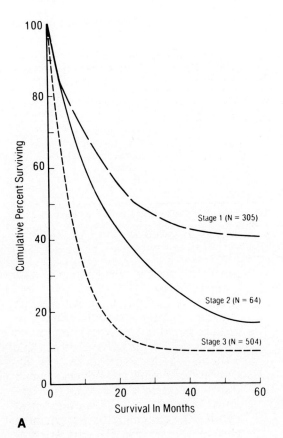

A

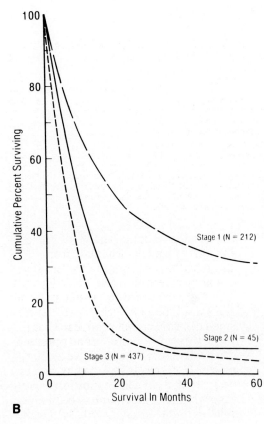

B

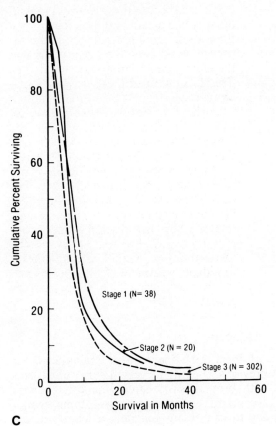

C

Figure 23–15. Survival by clinical stage in patients with squamous cell carcinoma (*A*), adenocarcinoma and large cell carcinoma (*B*), and small cell carcinoma (*C*). From American Joint Committee for Cancer Staging and End-Results Reporting: *Staging of Lung Cancer 1979.* American Joint Committee for Cancer Staging and End-Results Reporting, Chicago, 1979, courtesy of the American Joint Committee on Cancer.

733

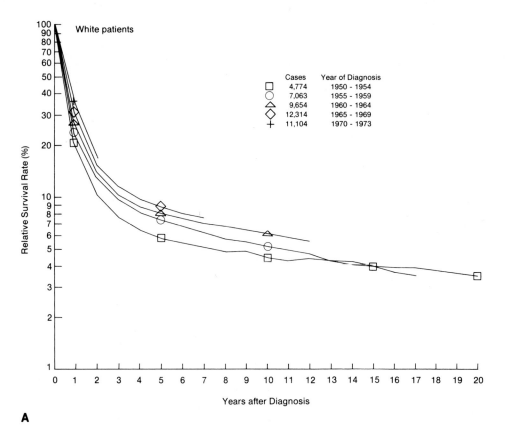

A

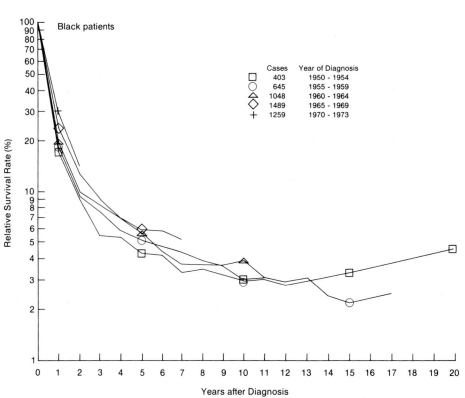

B

Figure 23–16. Bronchogenic carcinoma: Relative survival rates (percent) for all patients (all stages, all cell types) diagnosed from 1950 to 1973. (National Cancer Institute: *SEER Program. Cancer Patient Survival—Report Number 5.* Department of Health, Education and Welfare, Bethesda, Maryland, 1976.)

vanced disease. During the past 30 years only 16 to 20% of newly detected lung cancers have been found to be "localized" (see Table 23–12). Because the therapeutic results in advanced cancer remain disappointing, there has been considerable interest in achieving an "earlier diagnosis" and evaluating its effect on survival. Chest radiography and sputum cytology seemed to be complementary screening techniques. Both can detect centrally located tumors, whereas radiography will more likely show peripheral lesions.

Improvements in exfoliative cytology, chest radiography, and the introduction of the flexible fiberoptic bronchoscope provided the stimulus for a major screening study in the 1970s. The Johns Hopkins Medical Institutions, the Mayo Clinic, and the Memorial Sloan-Kettering Cancer Center organized a cooperative study to determine whether a coordinated program of screening, prompt tumor localization, and therapy was effective in reducing the mortality of bronchogenic cancer. The high-risk population selected for screening consisted of males 45 years of age or older who smoked one pack or more of cigarettes per day. Individuals screened at Johns Hopkins and Sloan-Kettering were divided randomly into two groups: (1) The XC group —yearly chest roentgenograms and sputum cytology and repeat sputum cytology at four-month intervals, and (2) the X group—yearly chest roentgenogram. At the Mayo Clinic, everyone was screened initially by roentgenogram and sputum cytology. Those with no cancer were divided into either a control group that was advised that both tests be performed annually or a study group that was rescreened every four months.

During the past five years intermittent reports have been made of the progress of the study (see Table 23–16). Most of this information concerns the cancer cases discovered during the initial screening activities (prevalence cases). For example, the Johns Hopkins group has recently reported the results of their first screening of 10,387 men (Frost et al., 1984). Thirty-eight cancers were diagnosed in the XC group; 18 (47%) had a positive sputum cytology and 10 (26%) were detected only by cytology. The cases detected by cytologic screening were mainly of squamous cell type. Similarly, 28 (74%) of the 38 XC prevalence cancers had a positive chest roentgenogram and 20 (53%) were detected only by chest roentgenogram. Thus, the detection techniques were complementary; both being positive in only eight of 38 cases (21%). Of the ten detected only by cytology, all were stage I and five of ten were *in situ* cancers.

The prevalence screening detected somewhat more than half the cancers (41/78) at a localized stage, significantly more in the XC (25/38) than in the X group. Sixty-eight percent (26/38) of the XC group were resectable, whereas only 42.5% (17/40) of the X group were—a statistically significant difference. Likewise, the median survival of the XC group (5.6 years) is significantly longer than the X group (one year).

Thus, it appears that the expert use of sputum cytology and chest roentgenograms has enabled each of the institutional study groups to detect a larger than usual proportion of limited stage cancers in a population at high risk. Further, the early survival experience following pulmonary resection is encouraging. Nonetheless, it is not yet possible to make a comprehensive statement concerning the impact of mass screening on mortality due to bronchogenic cancer.

This information, however, does provide some guidance to physicans who are advising selected patients at high risk. The potential benefit of early therapeutic intervention outweighs the cost and inconvenience of chest roentgenograms and sputum cytology studies.

Diagnostic Approach in Individual Patients. The comprehensive evaluation of each patient entails a logical assessment of several factors:

1. The precise identity of the disorder (primary site of cancer and cell type);
2. The extent of the cancer (staging);
3. Functional abnormalities due to cancer, whether directly or indirectly; and
4. Functional deficits due to other disorders.

Table 23–16. Bronchogenic Carcinoma: Results of Cooperative Early Detection Studies Using Chest Radiography and Sputum Cytology

	JHMI	MAYO	MSKCC
Cancer prevalence (cases/1000)	7.6	8.4	7.0
Detection by			
Radiography (%)	53	62	60
Cytology (%)	26	18	33
Both (%)	21	20	7
Curative resection (%)	68	57	69
5-Year Survival (%)	50	40	—

Legend: JHMI = Johns Hopkins Medical Institutions; Mayo = Mayo Clinic; and MSKCC = Memorial Sloan-Kettering Cancer Center.

Table 23–17. Clinical Evaluation Scheme for Patients with Possible Bronchogenic Carcinoma

Initial Survey	History, physical examination, chest roentgenogram, hemogram, liver and bone chemistries				
Initial Diagnostic Groups	PERIPHERAL TUMOR	CENTRAL TUMOR	DISTANT METASTASES	PARANEOPLASTIC SYNDROME	MAJOR ADDED DISEASE
Diagnostic Studies	CT scan Directed biopsy, aspiration or open Pleural fluid exam*	Bronchoscopy, biopsy Gallium scan CT scan Pleural fluid exam* Esophagogram* Venogram*	Biopsy of accessible (palpable) lesion* X-rays* Nuclear scans* CT scans*	Biochemical and physiologic studies*	As appropriate*
Formulations	Tumor. Cell type† Nontumor disease† Etiology obscure Chest wall tumor likely† Chest wall tumor unlikely†	Tumor. Cell type† Nontumor disease† Etiology obscure Mediastinal tumor likely† Mediastinal tumor unlikely†	Areas of possible tumor Tumor. Cell type† Nontumor disease† Etiology obscure	Pathogenesis of syndrome†	Estimate functional impairment, prognosis
Diagnostic Studies	Bronchoscopy, biopsy, special cytology	Mediastinoscopy Limited thoracotomy Esophagoscopy* Directed biopsies	Directed biopsy CNS evaluation*		Pulmonary function tests
Formulations	Tumor. Cell type† Nontumor disease† Etiology obscure Tumor, chest wall† No tumor, chest wall†	Tumor. Cell type† Nontumor disease† Etiology obscure Tumor, mediastinum† No tumor, mediastinum†	Tumor. Cell type† Nontumor disease† Etiology obscure†		Fit for lung resection† Unfit for lung resection†
Diagnostic Studies	Thoracotomy, biopsy	Thoracotomy, biopsy	Evaluate areas of special therapy, *e.g.* CNS*		
Formulations	Tumor. Cell type† Nontumor disease† Extent of disease†	Tumor. Cell type† Nontumor disease† Extent of disease†			

* Diagnostic studies as appropriate to existing signs and symptoms
† Therapeutic decision points: Consider need for further studies before choosing treatments

A thorough understanding of these elements and their likely prognosis is fundamental to the formulation of a sensible therapeutic program.

An initial survey of each patient should include a careful history and physical examination as well as a chest roentgenogram, hemogram, and a panel of blood chemistries to evaluate liver function and abnormalities of bone or calcium metabolism. Other tests appropriate to the patient will likely be ordered; for example, EKG and evaluation of renal and pulmonary function. While performing these studies or evaluating test results the physician must anticipate the data vital to a rational cancer treatment decision. Further, the physician should remember that the history and physical examination generally provide the first (and often best) indications of regional tumor extension or distant metastases. For example, there is no better means of detecting an enlarged supraclavicular lymph node than palpation. After their initial assessments, patients generally can be categorized into one or more diagnostic groups, and their further evaluation can proceed accordingly (see Table 23–17).

Peripheral Tumor. Peripheral bronchogenic cancers usually present as a solitary mass demonstrated on chest roentgenograms. Occasionally these patients are asymptomatic

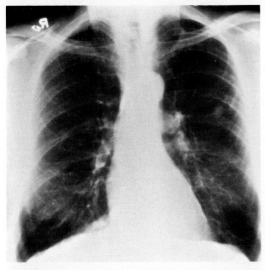

Figure 23–17. A 54-year-old man was found to have this peripheral nodule on a routine chest roentgenogram. A primary adenocarcinoma was removed via a lobectomy; there was no evidence of pelural or mediastinal involvement. His chance for tumor-free five-year survival is about 50%.

(see Figure 23–17). The differential diagnosis is a challenge, because more than 50% of nodules are the result of granulomatous disease, about 30% are due to bronchogenic cancer, and the remaining percentage (less than 20%) result from metastatic cancers, bronchial adenomas, and hamartomas.

Regardless of the characteristics of the nodule, previous radiographs should be reviewed to determine whether or not the mass was previously present and if so, to assess changes in size, if any. Obvious calcium deposited in a focal nonhomogeneous manner within a solitary pulmonary nodule is generally accepted as adequate evidence that the lesion is benign. Gross calcification has been found within less than 1% of primary pulmonary neoplasms.

The detection of homogeneous diffuse calcium within a lesion by conventional chest roentgenograms and tomography is difficult. One study indicated that computed chest tomography (CT) with thin sections (2 to 5 mm) was more sensitive than standard tomography in assessing the density (*i.e.*, the calcification) of pulmonary nodules (Siegelman *et al.*, 1980). A CT measurement of density (the Housenfield unit, abbreviated as H) was calculated for 91 apparently noncalcified pulmonary nodules in 88 patients. The investigators concluded that a CT density number of 164 H or above was sufficient indication of benign disease to follow patients with serial chest radiographs at six-month intervals. A CT number below 146 H is more in keeping with neoplastic disease and is an indication for prompt tissue diagnosis, whereas lesions with a representative CT number of 147 to 163 H are in a borderline category. Patients with such lesions should undergo biopsy or be followed with more frequent chest roentgenograms.

A review of the experience with pulmonary nodules at Johns Hopkins has led to the conclusion that only 2.5% of patients present with a solitary metastatic nodule and a truly occult primary tumor; that is, there is no history of a previous primary tumor, no symptoms or signs suggestive of a primary tumor, and no evidence of blood in urine or stool (Lawhorne *et al.*, 1973). On the basis of this and other studies, a routine upper gastrointestinal series, barium enema, and intravenous pyelogram are not indicated in the evaluation of each patient with a solitary pulmonary nodule.

When a tissue diagnosis of a peripheral pulmonary nodule is deemed necessary, a transthoracic needle aspiration biopsy is the procedure of choice. Chest fluoroscopy and CT scans can be used in guiding a percutaneous needle biopsy. Sputum for cytology should be collected, but only a small percentage of patients will have cancerous cells in their sputum.

If aspiration biopsy is not available or yields negative results, flexible fiberoptic bronchoscopy should be performed. This technique allows examination of the upper and lateral lobes and the more peripheral bronchi in all regions. Further, a variety of cellular samples including biopsies, aspirations, washings, and brushings can be obtained. Even so, it may not be possible to achieve a definitive diagnosis, and in these instances a thoracotomy is often necessary.

Because a high percentage of peripheral cancers invade the pleura or chest wall prior to their clinical presentation, an assessment of this possibility should be completed as well (see Figure 23–18. In this regard, it should be remembered that pleural effusions may result from mediastinal invasion as well as pleural involvement.

Central Tumor. The majority of bronchogenic cancers are centrally located and virtually all patients are symptomatic on presentation. Such lesions give higher diagnostic yields on sputum cytology than do peripheral masses and can be assessed by rigid or fiberoptic bronchoscopy. At times, mediastinoscopy can be useful in establishing the diagnosis.

A very high percentage of patients with centrally located cancers will have tumor involvement of adjacent mediastinal structures when they first seek medical advice. The extent of each patient's disease must be evaluated systematically (staging), because that evaluation is an important determinant of therapy (see Figures 23–19, 23–20, and 23–21).

Distant Metastases. Unfortunately, nearly half of the patients with bronchogenic carcinoma have widely disseminated disease shown during their initial evaluation (see Table 23–12). It is a matter of some practical importance that in nearly every instance clues as to the sites of metastatic involvement can be detected with a careful initial clinical survey (see Tables 23–10 and 23–17). In some cases metastatic sites provide the most sensible source of a tissue diagnosis using, for example, supraclavicular lymph node biopsy, liver biopsy, or bone biopsy.

Paraneoplastic Syndromes. The prompt recognition of a systemic disorder due to an "indirect effect" of cancer is important. When the disorder is life threatening, reversible, and requires prompt therapeutic intervention, this is imperative, as in the case of hypercalcemia. Again, these syndromes are best recognized by an alert physician during the initial clinical evaluation (see Tables 23–11 and 23–17).

Utilizing the sequence of procedures just outlined, the diagnosis of bronchogenic carcinoma can be established prior to thoracotomy

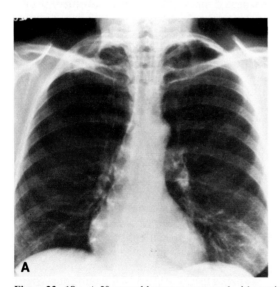 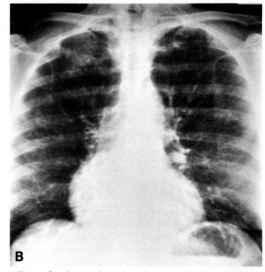

Figure 23–18. A 50-year-old woman presented with persistent discomfort in the right shoulder area. Chest roentgenograms revealed a right apical mass (*A*). A lordotic view reveals the mass more clearly as well as destruction of the second rib (*B*). Biopsy revealed adenocarcinoma. She was treated with radiation therapy.

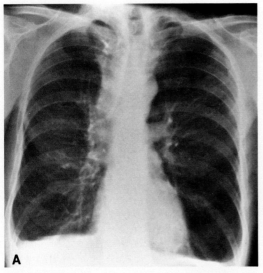
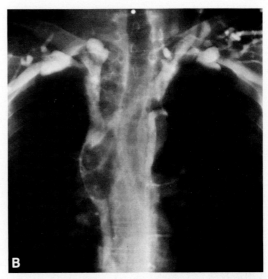

Figure 23-19. A 48-year-old man presented with a centrally located right chest mass (*A*), which was responsible for superior vena caval obstruction (*B*). Sputum cytology revealed small cell cancer. Combination chemotherapy led to a prompt resolution of the caval obstruction and the tumor.

in the majority of cases. The clinician, however, must recognize that the pathologic diagnosis is often made on the basis of small amounts of tissue. The clinician and pathologist must discuss the diagnosis together. If a discrepancy exists between the clinical and pathologic findings, serious consideration should be given to obtaining additional diagnostic material. Major treatment decisions are based not only on distinguishing bronchogenic carcinoma from other cancers but also on distinguishing small cell cancer from the non-small cell types.

Staging

Once a precise pathologic diagnosis has been made, an evaluation of the extent of disease (staging) should be initiated. The staging work-up is best geared to the major therapeutic options that include surgery, radiotherapy, and systemic chemotherapy. In addition, a physiologic evaluation of the patient should be completed promptly. The population of patients with bronchogenic cancer is elderly and has a high incidence of pulmonary disease, arteriosclerotic cardiovascular disease, and other medical problems that must be factored into the risk-benefit analysis of a specific therapy.

General Assessment. The physiologic assessment is directed largely toward determining whether the patient can tolerate either a lobectomy or a pneumonectomy. A thorough history and physical examination can usually identify an important impairment of pulmonary function. If a patient is able to walk up two flights of stairs without distress, it is likely that a major pulmonary resection can be tolerated. Simple tests of pulmonary function, such as spirometry, supplement the clinician's evaluation. For example, the patient's forced expiratory volume in one second (FEV_1) can be used to place the patient into one of three physiologic categories: (1) If the FEV_1 is 2.5 liters or more, the patient can withstand pneumonectomy; (2) if the FEV_1 is less than 1 liter, the patient cannot tolerate lobectomy or pneumonectomy; and (3) if the FEV_1 is between 1.1 and 2.4 liters the risk of resection and type of surgery must be determined by other studies (Mountain, 1977).

Radioisotope ventilation-perfusion scans are useful in patients with a significant impairment and provide information regarding the contribution of various lobes of the lungs to overall pulmonary function. Major resection is contraindicated for patients with pulmonary hypertension, and direct measurements of pulmonary artery pressure with balloon occlusion of the ipsilateral pulmonary artery is probably the most definitive means of assessing the patient's ability to withstand excision of one lung.

The decision regarding the patient's ability to undergo thoracotomy and resection safely is also dependent on the assessment of cardiac

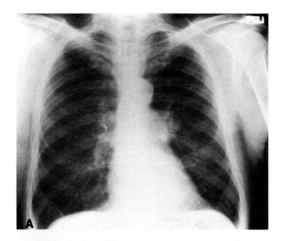

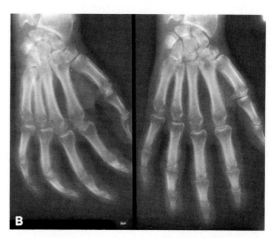

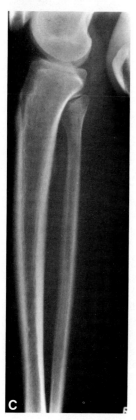

Figure 23–20. A 56-year-old man presented with an apparently resectable squamous cell cancer (*A*), but was referred for consideration of systemic therapy because of a "positive bone scan." Plain films of the hands and wrists (*B*) and legs (*C*) revealed hypertrophic osteoarthropathy. Lobectomy was performed; postsurgical stage II.

function. Operative mortality is increased dramatically in patients with a history of recent myocardial infarction and in patients with severe hypertension, congestive heart failure, and active arrhythmias.

Although the physiologic assessment is designed to evaluate suitability for surgery, these same procedures are useful in planning radiotherapy and/or cytotoxic chemotherapy for patients who have small cell carcinoma (and

are therefore not considered operative candidates), patients who have non-small-cell unresectable carcinoma, or those who refuse surgery. Radiotherapy to the chest and certain chemotherapy agents have pulmonary and cardiac toxicities; therefore a cardiac-pulmonary evaluation is most helpful in planning the details of therapeutic strategy.

Generally, useful information about a patient's overall situation can be conveyed by

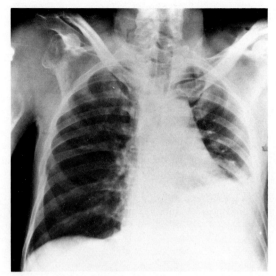

Figure 23-21. A 53-year-old man presented with pain in the right shoulder. Sputum cytology revealed squamous cell cancer. The markedly elevated left diaphragm proved to be paralysed. The proximal end of the right humerus was destroyed by tumor. He was treated with radiation therapy.

means of a systematized performance status score. The one used by the Eastern Cooperative Oncology Group is cited as an example (see Table 23-18). On the whole, these data reflect an individual's ability to tolerate aggressive therapy and indicate an outlook for survival. Most patients with bronchogenic cancer show symptoms and either are fully ambulatory or are in bed less than 50% of the day (PS 1 or 2) at the time of their initial diagnosis.

Staging Systems. Staging systems have been developed to guide clinicians in therapeutic decision making and to achieve uniformity in reporting end results. These systems convey information about the site and size of

the primary tumor, its cell type, and the anatomic extent of the disease. Staging evaluations such as clinical staging determined at the conclusion of the initial diagnostic work-up, surgical staging based on observations at surgery, pathologic (postsurgical) staging, retreatment (clinical) staging, and autopsy staging may be completed at different times in each patient's course.

The American Joint Committee for Cancer Staging and End-Results Reporting developed a staging system for lung cancer based on TNM principles and on a thorough study of more than 2000 cases (Mountain *et al.*, 1974). The data included size and location of each primary tumor, presence of metastases to lymph nodes in the hilar region and in the mediastinum, and the presence of extrapulmonary extension and distant metastases. Complications such as obstructive pneumonitis, atelectasis, and pleural effusion were also recorded. A patient was evaluated only if the cancer had been diagnosed four years or more previously and if follow-up information was available.

The definitions for each category of T, N, and M recommended by the American Joint Committee and the resultant stages of disease are shown in Table 23-19. With the exception of small cell carcinoma, this staging system does provide a basis for selecting patients for resection. In general, patients with stage I and stage II are considered candidates for resection whereas patients with stage III are not.

Staging in Non-Small-Cell Cancer. Because surgical resection offers the best hope of cure to patients with limited stage, non-small-cell cancers, they must be evaluated expeditiously. With this in mind, it is useful to consider the major reasons for judging a patient's tumor to be "inoperable" (see Table 23-20).

Table 23-18. Bronchogenic Carcinoma: Relationship of Performance Status to Survival of Patients with Inoperable Tumors

PERFORMANCE STATUS	DEFINITIONS	MEDIAN SURVIVAL* *(weeks)*
0	Asymptomatic	34
1	Symptomatic, fully ambulatory	24-27
2	Symptomatic, in bed <50% of day	14-21
3	Symptomatic, in bed >50% of day	7-9
4	Bedridden, needs total care	3-5

* Based on data on more than 5,000 men with tumors of all cell types entered into Veteran's Administration protocols (1968-1978).
Based on data from Stanley, K. E.: Prognostic factors for survival in patients with inoperable lung cancer. *J.N.C.I.*, **65**:25-32, 1980.

Table 23-19. Bronchogenic Carcinoma: American Joint Committee Staging System and Definitions of TNM Categories

Primary tumors

T	Primary tumor
T_0	No evidence of primary tumor
T_x	Tumor proven by presence of cancerous cells in bronchopulmonary secretions but not visualized roentgeno-graphically or bronchoscopically
T_{1s}	Carcinoma *in situ*
T_1	Tumor that is 3.0 cm or less at greatest diameter, surrounded by lung or visceral pleura, and without evidence of invasion proximal to a lobar bronchus at bronchoscopy
T_2	Tumor more than 3.0 cm at greatest diameter or tumor of any size that either invades the visceral pleura or has associated atelectasis or obstructive pneumonitis extending to the hilar region. At bronchoscopy the proximal extent of demonstrable tumor must be within a lobar bronchus or at least 2.0 cm distal to the carina. Any associated atelectasis or obstructive pneumonitis must involve less than an entire lung, and there must be no pleural effusion.
T_3	Tumor of any size with direct extension into an adjacent structure such as chest wall, diaphragm, or mediastinum and its contents or tumor demonstrated bronchoscopically to involve a main bronchus less than 2.0 cm distal to the carina; any tumor associated with atelectasis or obstructive pneumonitis of an entire lung or pleural effusion.

Regional lymph nodes

N	Regional lymph nodes
N_0	No demonstrable metastasis to regional lymph nodes
N_1	Metastases to lymph nodes to peribronchial and/or ipsilateral hilar region (including direct extension)
N_2	Metastases to lymph nodes in the mediastinum

Distant metastasis

M	Distant metastases
M_0	No distant metastases
M_1	Distant metastases such as in scalene, cervical, or contralateral hilar lymph nodes, brain, bones, lung, liver, etc.

The above categories of T, N, and M may be combined into the following groups or stages:

Occult carcinoma

$T_x N_0 M_0$	Occult carcinoma with bronchopulmonary secretions containing cancerous cells but without other evidence of the primary tumor or evidence of metastases to the regional lymph nodes or distant metastases

Stage I

$T_{1s} N_0 M_0$	Carcinoma *in situ*
$T_1 N_0 M_0$	Tumor that can be classified T_1 without any metastases or with metastases to the lymph nodes
$T_1 N_1 M_0$	in the peribronchial and/or ipsilateral hilar region only or a tumor that can be classified T_2
$T_2 N_0 M_0$	without any metastasis to nodes or distant metastasis
Note:	$T_x N_1 M_0$ and $T_0 N_1 M_0$ are also theoretically possible, but such a clinical diagnosis would be difficult if not impossible to make. If such a diagnosis is made, it should be included in stage I.

Stage II

$T_2 N_1 M_0$	Tumor classified as T_2 with metastases to the lymph nodes in the ipsilateral hilar region only

Stage III

T_3 with any N or M	Any tumor more extensive than T_2 or any tumor with metastases to the lymph nodes in the
N_2 with any T or M	mediastinum or with distant metastases
M_1 with any T or N	

Based on data from Mountain, C. F.; Carr, D. T.; Martini, N.; Raventos, A.; Stitik, F. P.; and Woolner, L. B.: *Staging of Lung Cancer.* American Joint Committee for Cancer Staging and End-Results Reporting, Chicago, 1979; and Carr, D. T., and Mountain, C. F.: Staging lung cancer. In Straus, M. (ed.): *Lung Cancer: Clinical Diagnosis and Treatment.* Grune & Stratton, Inc., New York, 1977 (reprinted by permission).

Assuming that there are no general contraindications to pulmonary resection because of major associated physiologic disorders, the physician must be certain that the tumor has not spread extensively (Tables 23-17 and 23-21).

Distant Metastases. If no specific clues are discovered during the process of initial clinical evaluation, no justification exists for obtaining bone, liver, or brain scans or other tests designed to uncover evidence of metastatic disease. In one study correlating multiorgan scans

Table 23-20. Bronchogenic Carcinoma: Principal Clinical Indicators of "Inoperability"

Tumor cell type
  Small cell cancer

Tumor involvement of mediastinum
  Great vessel obstruction
    Superior vena caval syndrome
  Nerve entrapment
    Horner's syndrome, paralysis of diaphragm, vocal cord paralysis
  Esophageal obstruction
    Dysphagia, fistula
  Carinal (tracheal) involvement
  Pleural effusion

Tumor involvement of chest wall
  Superior sulcus tumor
  Rib erosion
  Pleural studding (effusion)

Distant metastases

Associated systemic diseases
  Pulmonary insufficiency
  Other major disorders, *e.g.,* cardiovascular or renal

for staging bronchogenic cancer with clinical evaluation, only one of 131 scans performed in patients with no evidence of metastases on general clinical evaluation was truly positive (Ramsdell *et al.,* 1977). Sixteen of 17 positive scans in patients with normal clinical findings were falsely positive (see Figure 23-20). Two of 22 negative scans in patients with abnormal clinical findings were falsely negative. If the clinical evaluation suggests a metastatic site, then appropriate radionuclide scans should be

obtained. A negative scan in this setting does not rule out metastases, and other diagnostic procedures such as sonography, tomography, and perhaps biopsy should be considered.

Chest Wall Extension. General agreement exists that tumor extending to the pleura or involving the chest wall should not be managed by surgical resection alone. In fact, considerable support exists for the use of radiation therapy as the initial treatment of choice. Hence it is important to probe carefully for evidence of tumor extension and document its existence with appropriate biopsies in order to resolve any reasonable doubts (see Figure 23-18 and Tables 23-17 and 23-21).

Mediastinal Extension. It is generally agreed that thoracotomy is not indicated when there exists clinical evidence of mediastinal extension as manifested by recurrent laryngeal nerve palsy, diaphragmatic paralysis, obstruction of superior vena cava or azygos vein, obstruction of right or left main pulmonary artery, or esophageal invasion (see Figures 23-19 and 23-21). A positive carinal biopsy is also a contraindication to surgery.

A number of investigators have advocated the use of gallium 67 citrate scanning in the staging of bronchogenic carcinoma. Gallium citrate is taken up by over 90% of primary lung cancers with no major differences in uptake among the major histologic subtypes. The gallium scan has been reported useful in assessing mediastinal and hilar lymph node metastases, and some investigators have suggested that a negative gallium scan obviates the need for mediastinoscopy. Because gallium is taken up by the other types of cancer and by inflamma-

Table 23-21. Bronchogenic Carcinoma: Primary Utility of Widely Available Staging Studies

DIAGNOSTIC STUDY	PERIPHERAL TUMOR	CHEST WALL EXTENSION	CENTRAL TUMOR	MEDIASTINAL EXTENSION*	DISTANT METASTASES
History, Physical exam		+	+	+	++
Hemogram					++
Liver, bone chemistries					++
Chest roentgenogram	++	+	++	+	+
Gallium scan			+	++	+
CT scan	++	++	+	+	+
Directed biopsy	++	+			++
Bronchoscopy (biopsy)	+		++	+	
Mediastinoscopy (biopsy)			+	++	
Thoracotomy (biopsy)	+		rare	rare	

* Tests such as esophagoscopy (with biopsy) and venography are useful if signs and symptoms are suggestive.

tory tissue as well and because not all bronchogenic cancers concentrate gallium, the gallium 67 scan should not be regarded as a replacement for mediastinoscopy. In general a tissue diagnosis is advisable.

Similar limitations apply to the use of CT scanning in the staging of bronchogenic carcinoma. "Positive" CT scans and radionuclide scans, however, can be helpful in monitoring the course of disease.

If no clinical or radiologic evidence of mediastinal invasion exists, mediastinoscopy should be performed in all patients with central lesions and/or patients with anaplastic carcinomas. Patients with peripheral bronchogenic carcinomas 3 cm in size or smaller (see Figure 23–17) have a very low incidence of mediastinal metastases and should not be routinely subjected to mediastinal exploration (Baker *et al.*, 1979).

Transcervical mediastinoscopy is performed under general or local anesthesia by making a small incision above the manubrium and dissecting down along the trachea initially with the finger and then with the lighted fiberoptic mediastinoscope. Mediastinoscopy is effective for exploring the area around the trachea and major bronchi and for detecting mediastinal lymph node metastases from lesions of the right lung or left lower lobe. The yield of mediastinoscopy is related to the location of the pulmonary tumor and to tumor histology (see Table 23–22) and can be accomplished with very little morbidity and mortality. A review of the complications of mediastinoscopy from published data covering over 7000 patients revealed a morbidity rate of 1.2% and a mortality of 0.038% (Jepson and Rahbek, 1970). The specific complications included bleeding, hemothorax, pneumothorax, wound infection, pneumonia, vocal cord paralysis, esophageal perforation, bradycardia, myocardial infarction, tumor seeding in the suture line, stroke, and air embolus.

Metastatic lesions from the left upper lobe and left main stem bronchus are better detected by a parasternal exploration. Bronchogenic carcinoma arising in the left upper lobe and left main stem bronchus most frequently metastasizes to lymph nodes in the area between the left main pulmonary artery and the arch of the aorta (the aortic-pulmonary window). Although the aortic-pulmonary window is not visualized during the course of a transcervical mediastinoscopy, the area can be examined by a left parasternal exploration. The procedure is performed through a 10-cm incision in the left second intercostal space extending from the lateral border of the sternum. The pleura is entered, the aortic-pulmonary window is palpated and visualized with the mediastinoscope, and biopsies are taken.

Transcervical mediastinoscopy or left parasternal exploration have replaced biopsies of nonpalpable scalene nodes as a means of demonstrating tumor extension. Some controversy regarding the use of mediastinoscopy is based on reports of significant five-year survival rates in patients who had proven involvement of mediastinal lymph nodes and who were treated by pulmonary resection, lymph node dissection, and postoperative radiation therapy (Kirsh *et al.*, 1972; Martini *et al.*, 1980). These patients represent a small subset with well-differentiated squamous cell carcinoma who have lesions confined to ipsilateral lymph nodes without extracapsular spread or fixation to other mediastinal structures.

Staging of Patients with Small Cell Cancer. Staging for patients with small cell carcinoma has different implications than for patients with the other histologic subtypes, because surgical resection is not considered a primary therapeutic option. All patients should receive systemic chemotherapy, perhaps in combination with radiation therapy. Determining the extent of disease in small cell carcinoma, however, is necessary in order to (1) assess the efficacy of the antitumor therapy in individual

Table 23–22. Bronchogenic Carcinoma: Correlation between Mediastinal Lymph Node Involvement and Histology

PATHOLOGY	NUMBER OF PATIENTS	POSITIVE RESULT ON MEDIASTINOSCOPY
All cell types	179	86 (48%)
Well-differentiated squamous cell	64	10 (16%)
Large cell anaplastic	74	47 (68%)
Small cell	23	17 (70%)
Adenocarcinoma	18	12 (66%)

Based on data from Goldberg, E. M.; Glicksman, A. S.; Khan, F. R.; and Nickson, J. J.: Mediastinoscopy for assessing mediastinal spread in clinical staging of carcinoma of the lung. *Cancer,* **25:**347–353, 1970.

patients; (2) determine the need for radiotherapy; (3) prognosticate for the patient; (4) compare the results from different therapeutic trials; and (5) insure uniform reporting of cancer statistics. For example, patients with small cell carcinoma limited to one hemithorax have higher complete response rates and longer survivals than patients with metastases beyond the hemithorax (extensive disease). In addition to receiving systemic chemotherapy, patients with limited disease are candidates for radiotherapy and, in special circumstances, surgery.

Radionuclide scans are routinely utilized in the staging work-up of patients with small cell carcinoma, even in patients who do not have clinical or chemical evidence of organ involvement (Ihde and Hansen, 1981). These studies have higher yields of detecting metastases than in non-small-cell cancer. The results of these scanning procedures are generally not required to plan the treatment for individual patients but are useful for the reasons outlined in the previous paragraph.

Bone scans are positive (*i.e.,* they exhibit multiple focal areas of increased uptake without other clinical or radiographic explanations) in 20 to 40% of patients with small cell cancer at the time of diagnosis. Although patients with positive bone scans frequently have bone pain and/or elevated serum alkaline phosphatase, the scan may be positive in patients with no other clinical or radiographic evidence of bone metastases. Single focal areas of increased uptake of isotope must be regarded with considerable caution. Bone scans are not a good means of following response to therapy, because changes occur very slowly and the changes in number of lesions or intensity of uptake can represent either tumor progression or improvement. Skeletal x-ray surveys are not a sensitive means of detecting bony metastases and should be utilized only to assess the bony architecture at sites of bone pain or positive bone scan.

Bone marrow aspirates and/or biopsies are positive in 20 to 30% of patients at the time of presentation. Aspiration and biopsy are additive in their yield and bilateral aspirates and biopsies increase the yield by 15 to 30%.

A number of radiographic and biopsy techniques are available for detecting liver metastases. These include radionuclide liver scan, CT scan, sonography, and peritoneoscopy with multiple, directed biopsies. A recent study has shown that hepatic metastases occur in 24% of patients at the time of diagnosis and that peritoneoscopy with liver biopsy is the most accurate means of determining their presence (Mulshine *et al.*, 1982). The study, however, also demonstrated that the noninvasive and less costly radionuclide liver scan rarely leads to false staging when other routine procedures are employed concurrently. Hepatomegaly and abnormal liver function tests provide good clues to metastases, but false-positive and negative results are quite common when liver function tests and physical examination are the sole criteria.

Approximately 10% of patients with small cell cancer present with evident central nervous system metastases and 20 to 25% of patients develop signs of such metastases during the course of their disease. Radionuclide brain scans are not a sensitive means of detecting occult intracranial metastases in asymptomatic patients with normal neurologic examinations. In a recent study of 111 untreated patients, CT scans detected brain metastases in seven individuals (6%), all of whom had asymptomatic central nervous system involvement as the only obvious metastatic site (Cruz *et al.,* 1982).

Although the number of sites of metastases and the presence or absence of liver or central nervous system metastases have great impact on survival, it is important to note that the pretreatment performance status and the nutritional status of the patients remain the dominant prognostic factors. Performance status and nutritional status probably relate to tumor burden and disease progression by mechanisms as yet unclear.

Biomarkers. Considerable attention has been directed to identification of biochemical markers that correlate with the extent of disease and response to therapy in patients with small cell carcinoma of the lung. A variety of single biomarkers and batteries of markers have been evaluated, including carcinoembryonic antigen (CEA), polyamines, serum carbohydrates, hormones such as calcitonin, neurophysin, ACTH, ADH, bombesin, β-HCG, and enzymes such as neuron-specific enolase, histaminase, and creatine kinase. Encouraging results have been reported by different investigators, but an adequately sensitive or specific single marker or combination of markers has not been identified. CEA is perhaps the most useful biomarker in bronchogenic cancer. A markedly elevated level is a clue to bone and/or liver metastases in patients with lung cancer. In patients with small cell cancer, CEA may also parallel the course of the tumor and rises in CEA may precede overt clinical relapse by three to four months (Waalkes *et al.,* 1980). Great caution must be exercised in interpreting single levels of CEA; serial determinations must be obtained in order to derive clinically useful information. Tumor cell populations change in time and may no longer produce the biomarker.

Therapy

As mentioned previously, the choice of treatment is based on the site and cell type of the primary tumor, the extent of regional spread, the existence of distant metastases, and the coexistence of important functional abnormalities due to cancer or other disorders. Each patient's status and therapeutic alternatives are reflected in the staging designation (see Tables 23–19 and 23–23).

Non-Small Cell Cancer *Stage I and Stage II Disease.* Definitive resection is the treatment of choice for patients with stage I or II disease (see Figure 23–17 and 23–19). Patients who are not physiologically suitable for major surgery or who refuse surgery are candidates for radiotherapy or cytotoxic chemotherapy and/or experimental therapy.

The selection of the surgical procedure is based on the size and extent of the primary tumor and the physiologic status of the patient. The surgical objective is to insure complete removal of the tumor with minimal loss of normal lung tissue. This goal generally is translated into an operative plan of excising the primary tumor and the lymph nodes surrounding the bronchus associated with the tumor mass. If this can be accomplished by a lobectomy, the curative rate is as good as that following a pneumonectomy. The operative mortality for pneumonectomy, however, is

Table 23–24. Bronchogenic Carcinoma: Survival in Non-Small Cell Cancer Following Apparent Complete Resection by Postsurgical Stage

CELL TYPE	CUMULATIVE PERCENTAGE SURVIVING FIVE YEARS		
	Stage I	*Stage II*	*Stage III*
Squamous cell	54%	36%	22%
Adenocarcinoma and large cell	51%	21%	12%

Reprinted by permission from Mountain, C. F.: Biologic, physiologic, and technical determinants in surgical therapy for lung cancer. In Straus, M. J. (ed.): *Lung Cancer.* Grune & Stratton, Inc., New York, 1977.

approximately 12%—twice that of a lobectomy.

The survival of patients with non-small cell lung cancer who have undergone complete resection may be related to their postsurgical stage (see Table 23–24). Within stage I disease further analysis reveals that the survival of patients who had T_1N_0 lesions is significantly higher than that of patients with T_1N_1 and T_2N_0 tumors. In fact, investigators at the Mayo Clinic have noted that the survival of patients classified as T_1N_0 (91% alive at two years and 80% at five years) is so good that it seems unlikely that currently available adjuvant therapy given to this group could demonstrably improve survival (Williams *et al.,* 1981).

Thoracic surgeons have assessed the results of wedge resections in selected cases. Wedge resections disregard segmental anatomy and may involve a portion of one segment but more commonly transgress segmental planes. In several retrospective analyses of patients with stage I disease (and particularly T_1N_0 lesions), wedge resection resulted in survival rates comparable to those for lobectomy (Hoffman and Ransdell, 1980). Most thoracic surgeons limit the role of wedge resection to patients who have poor pulmonary reserve with peripheral lesions 3 cm or less in diameter. A prospective randomized trial, however,

Table 23–23. Bronchogenic Carcinoma: Principal and Alternative Therapies

TUMOR	SURGICAL RESECTION	RADIATION THERAPY	SYSTEMIC CHEMOTHERAPY	LOCAL CHEMOTHERAPY
Peripheral tumor	++	+		
Chest wall extension	+	++		Effusions
Central tumor	++	+		
Mediastinal extension		++	+	Effusions
Distant metastases		+	+	CNS tumor
Small cell cancer		+	++	
Paraneoplastic syndromes*		+	++	

*With symptomatic therapy, appropriate to pathogenesis
Legend: + = alternative therapy; ++ = principal therapy.

comparing wedge resection and lobectomy in stage I patients has not been performed as yet.

Radiation therapy is a reasonably effective alternative to surgery for patients with stage I and II disease and is especially useful in those for whom surgical procedures are precluded. Five-year survival rates in these circumstances exceed 20%, but it must be remembered that most of this experience has been gained from treating patients not fit enough to undergo surgical resection.

It is clear that surgery and radiation therapy fail to cure the majority of patients, even those with apparently limited-stage disease. These failures stem mainly from the aggressive nature of the tumor and its propensity for regional extension and distant metastases (see Tables 23–12 and 23–13). In general, little evidence is available to suggest that the routine application of regional preoperative or postoperative radiation therapy is useful in the management of patients with stage I or II disease. Although no pertinent data based on formal clinical trials has been reported, it seems reasonable that radiation therapy be given postoperatively to patients with limited-stage disease who turn out to have microscopic tumor in the mediastinal lymph nodes. This same consideration applies to other analogous situations in which the surgical resection was suboptimal or in which a local recurrence of tumor following prior excision occurs.

To date none of the adjuvant chemotherapy trials have yielded consistently encouraging results in the management of disseminated micrometastatic disease. As might be expected there has been considerable interest in enhancing and/or restoring immunologic response in patients as a means of achieving better control of limited-stage bronchogenic cancer. A variety of approaches to immunotherapy have been explored, including systemic active-nonspecific, regional active-nonspecific, immunorestorative, adoptive, and active-specific immunotherapy.

A recent study of regional immunotherapy evaluated the effect of intrapleural BCG (McKneally et al., 1976). This approach was based on earlier observations that postoperative empyema was associated with a good prognosis in patients with operable bronchogenic cancer. Patients with stage I and II non-small-cell cancer were randomized to receive a single dose of BCG intrapleurally during the postoperative period or to receive no immunotherapy. Initially, a greater recurrence rate in the controls with stage I disease than in the immunotherapy group was observed. Follow-up data from McKneally and a larger multi-institutional study, however, have not confirmed these promising early results (Takita, 1984).

Despite a number of other studies that were encouraging in their early phases, there have been no results that conclusively demonstrate a survival benefit for patients treated with immunotherapy. A trial of active-specific immunotherapy utilizing Hollinshead's antigen mixed with complete Freund's adjuvant has been carried out following surgical removal of stage I bronchogenic carcinoma (Stewart et al., 1976). Although the initial survival results looked better than historic controls, it is clear that prospective randomized studies are necessary to identify the efficacy of this or any other form of immunotherapy.

Stage III Disease. Stage III patients are a heterogeneous group whose tumors are generally not "resectable for cure." Within stage III, however, certain patients whose tumors are technically resectable and for whom surgery is a reasonable option when combined with radiation therapy are included. For example, Kirsh and colleagues have reported a five-year survival rate of 29.5% in patients with well-differentiated squamous cell carcinoma with stage III N_2 disease who were treated with mediastinal dissection and postoperative mediastinal irradiation (Kirsh et al., 1972). Thus, "extended pneumonectomy" may be considered where the primary lesion is technically resectable with negative margins and the extent of nodal involvement is limited to the ipsilateral tracheobronchial angle or subcarinal space. In cases with more cephalad extension to the ipsilateral peritracheal nodes, resection would be performed only if the lymph node capsules were intact.

Carcinomas in the superior sulcus appear to be another special subset. These apical tumors are frequently low-grade squamous cell carcinomas that invade the lymphatics in the endothoracic fascia and involve, by direct extension, the lower roots of the brachial plexus, the intercostal nerves, the stellate ganglion, the sympathetic chain, and adjacent ribs and vertebrae producing severe pain and Horner's syndrome. A 34% survival at five years for patients with superior sulcus tumors treated by combined preoperative irradiation and extended resection has been reported (Paulson, 1975). The surgical technique described by

Paulson is an extended *en bloc* resection of the chest wall, usually including posterior portions of the first three ribs, portions of the upper thoracic vertebrae (including the transverse processes), the intercostal nerves, the lower trunk of the brachial plexus, the stellate ganglion, and a portion of the dorsal sympathetic chain together with the involved lung resected by means of either lobectomy or segmental resection. In other peripheral lesions, particularly squamous carcinomas invading the chest wall, *en bloc* resection and appropriate lung resections in association with preoperative radiotherapy have resulted in a five-year survival rate of somewhat less than 20%. Extensive resectional surgery, of course, carries with it an immediate morbidity and mortality as well as significant long-term functional deficits.

Evidence in the literature suggests that carcinomas of the superior pulmonary sulcus can be treated with external irradiation and interstitial implantation of radioactive sources or external irradiation alone with results (20 to 30% survival at five years) equivalent to those for resection with or without preoperative irradiation (Komaki *et al.*, 1981). It has been recommended that the irradiation be given in high doses (6000 rads over a period of six to six and one-half weeks in 180- to 200-rad fractions) to the primary tumor, to the upper and midlevel of the mediastinum, and to the lower cervical and upper thoracic vertebrae.

In addition to assessing relative merits of surgery and radiotherapy on the basis of objective measures of survival, it is important to consider the patients' attitudes toward the risks of therapy and resultant quality of life. One study of risk aversions in patients with operable lung cancer suggests that older patients with life-threatening disease may prefer a treatment with a lesser chance of immediate death even though the prospect of a five-year survival is inferior (McNeil *et al.*, 1978). Therapies should be chosen not only on the basis of survival rates but also on the basis of patient attitudes.

The utilization of radiotherapy in patients with inoperable bronchogenic carcinoma requires a particularly careful risk-benefit evaluation. Obviously, symptomatic patients with far-advanced disease or with an expected survival of only a few months should not be subjected needlessly to a long course of radiotherapy. Radiotherapy in those patients should be directed to sites of acute symptomatology with the goal of achieving relief. This group includes patients with distant metastases, metastases to the opposite thorax or supraclavicular nodes, pleural effusion, recurrent laryngeal nerve paralysis, and superior vena caval syndrome.

How should one manage patients who are minimally symptomatic, but who have inoperable disease limited to the lung of origin with or without hilar and mediastinal adenopathy (see Figure 23–20)? Radiation oncologists agree that such patients should receive immediate aggressive treatment, that is, definitive radiotherapy. This basis for this approach rests on studies that demonstrate a high rate of response and subsequent local control of the cancer (Phillips and Miller, 1978). This leads to an increase in patients' median survival time and a definite but small (6%) chance of five-year survival. In addition, in at least one study the quality of life appears to have been improved. Such radiotherapy (5500 to 6000 rads) resulted in prevention of chest symptoms in a noteworthy percentage (24%) of patients and a marked improvement in symptomatology in those patients who had hemoptysis, dysphagia, local pain, pulmonary infection, dyspnea, and cough.

These potential benefits of radiation therapy must be considered on balance with the complications of the treatment. Radiation skin reaction (alopecia, dermatitis, tanning, subcutaneous fibrosis) and esophagitis do occur, as do radiation pneumonitis, myocarditis or pericarditis, and transverse myelitis. With advances in simulation and treatment-planning techniques, however, higher therapeutic doses can be delivered to the known tumor volume with more effective sparing of adjacent normal tissues. "Hyperfractionation" treatment schedules may also provide added benefits.

Continued interest remains in determining optimal dose and fractionation for the treatment of bronchogenic carcinoma. Many schedules of irradiation have been used, but major attention has been given to the relative effectiveness of split-course therapy versus continuous radiotherapy. Recently, the Radiation Therapy Oncology Group (RTOG) carried out a prospective randomized study of various dose and fractionation schedules in the treatment of inoperable non-small-cell carcinoma (Perez *et al.*, 1980). In this multi-institutional study, the patients were randomized into one of four treatment regimens: A 4000-rad split course (2000 rads in five fractions one week, two weeks rest, and an additional 2000 rads in five fractions in one week), or 4000, 5000, or 6000 rads given in continuous courses, five fractions per week. Preliminary analysis indicated that the continuous regimens resulted in significantly higher complete response rates and longer survivals than the split-course therapy. The patients treated with 5000 or 6000 rads also appeared to have better responses, control of intrathoracic tumor, and survival than those receiving 4000 rads. The survival rate in the continuous irradiation groups is 20 to 25% at two years. A longer follow-up was required, however, to determine the relative efficacy of these different treatment regimens.

Metastatic Disease. In view of the limitations of surgery and radiation therapy, a great deal of effort has been invested in developing effective systemic chemotherapy for bronchogenic carcinoma (Livingston, 1977). A large number of chemotherapeutic agents have been shown to have antitumor activity (see Table 23–25). The response rate to single drugs culled from a number of reports is substantially lower in non-small cell cancer than in small cell cancer. Further, the rapidity and magnitude of the response to single-agent chemotherapy are much more impressive in small cell than in non-small cell cancers. Recent studies have identified newer drugs such as vindesine and cisplatin that have response rates of approximately 25% in non-small cell cancer. Their role in treatment is now receiving a great deal of attention.

In view of the limited efficacy of single-agent chemotherapy, it is not surprising that combination chemotherapy has not made a major impact. In recent years, however, many combination chemotherapy regimens have been evaluated. These studies have produced a variety of conflicting results that has contributed to an increasing uncertainty regarding the role of combination chemotherapy in non-small-cell cancer (Muggia *et al.,* 1984). An analysis of the reasons for these apparent conflicting results is useful for interpreting data from clinical research trials as well as for making therapeutic decisions for individual patients.

One of the recurrent themes in the history of chemotherapy is the initial report of high response rates followed by reports from other institutions or cooperative groups of much lower response rates. An example of a potentially promising new chemotherapeutic regimen in non-small-cell cancer is CAP (cyclophosphamide, doxorubicin, and cisplatin). Response rates of 38% to 48% have been reported with the CAP regimen in two studies at the Mayo Clinic (Eagan *et al.,* 1977, 1979). More recently, several investigators have reported on the efficacy of CAP therapy in large numbers of patients and many trials are in progress. In all of these studies, the overall response rates range from 4% to 48%; the complete response rates have been low (0 to 5%). Responders to CAP generally have a statistically significant survival advantage over nonresponders, but there are other factors independent of drug treatment that determine response and/or survival. In fact, as noted in an excellent review (Aisner and Hansen, 1981), the wide range of response rates is at least partly accounted for by differences among the various study populations in terms of important prognostic factors such as performance status, extent of disease, weight loss, and history of prior therapy. Definitions for evaluation of response and histologic classifications also differ among investigating groups.

Table 23–26 summarizes the results of well-known combination chemotherapeutic regimens in non-small-cell cancer. The low complete response rates and short median survivals are particularly noteworthy. Because of the large number of factors that affect outcome, it has been suggested that the efficacy of combination chemotherapy regimens in non-small-cell cancer can only be determined by well-designed prospective randomized studies that compare a particular chemotherapy regimen to no chemotherapy. Such studies require large patient accrual (hundreds of patients) to achieve adequate statistical evaluation.

It is of practical importance to patient management that systemic cytotoxic chemotherapy does not yield a response rate in non-

Table 23–25. Bronchogenic Carcinoma: Response Rates to Single Chemotherapeutic Agents

	RESPONSE RATE OF SCLC IN %*	RESPONSE RATE NON-SCLC IN %†
Cyclophosphamide (CYTOXAN)	38	10
Doxorubicin (ADRIAMYCIN)	30	18
Methotrexate	30	15
Vincristine (ONCOVIN)	40	17
VP-16-213	50	18

*Small cell lung cancer
†Non-small cell lung cancer

Table 23-26. Summary of Treatment Results with Combination Chemotherapy in Non-Small Cell Cancer

THERAPY	STUDY GROUP	PR (%)*	CR (%)†	MEDIAN SURVIVAL OF ALL PATIENTS
HAM	ECOG	10.4	2.5	22 weeks
CAMP	ECOG	6.5	15.6	19 weeks
FOMi	U. of Texas U. of Arizona	31	5	6 months
CMC	Bowman Gray Piedmont Oncology Association	25	0	5 months

*Partial response
†Complete response
HAM = hexamethylmelamine, doxorubicin, methotrexate
CAMP = cyclophosphamide, doxorubicin, methotrexate, procarbazine
FOMi = 5-fluorouracil, ONCOVIN, mitomycin-C
CMC = cyclophosphamide, methotrexate, CCNU

small-cell cancer adequate for prompt reliable relief of symptoms. That is, complications such as superior vena caval obstruction, bronchial obstruction, and pain due to bone metastasis should be treated with radiotherapy rather than chemotherapy. Radiotherapy can provide at least temporary palliation of symptoms in the majority of patients. For patients who have progressive, widespread metastases that are unlikely to be palliated by radiotherapy, it is reasonable to offer chemotherapy as a treatment option. It is preferable that such patients participate in clinical research protocols so that new knowledge can be gained regarding treatment. Regardless of whether the patients enter into a research protocol or not, they should be well informed regarding the very limited success of chemotherapy and the potential physical, emotional, and economic consequences of their treatment regimen.

Small Cell Cancer. There is remarkable contrast between the efficacy of cytotoxic chemotherapy in small cell cancer and non-small cell cancer. Small cell cancer is so exquisitely sensitive that combination chemotherapy has become the mainstay of treatment (see Figure 23-18).

Only 15 years ago patients with small cell cancer were routinely treated with surgery. From 1962 to 1964, the British Medical Research Council Lung Cancer Working Party conducted its randomized trial comparing surgery to radical radiotherapy (Medical Research Council, 1966). The mean survival achieved with radiotherapy (284 days) was significantly better than that achieved with surgery (199 days). It was equally clear, however, that neither modality altered the course of this widely metastatic cancer.

At approximately the same time that this British study demonstrated the futility of surgery a number of trials indicated that small cell cancer was responsive to a variety of chemotherapeutic agents (see Table 23-25). Single drugs resulted in low complete response rates and the responses were of short duration. Combination chemotherapy regimens similar to those employed in the management of lymphoma, however, led to improved results. The initial trials were conducted mainly in the outpatient setting and few patients required hospitalization. In general, radiotherapy (usually 2500 to 3000 rads) was delivered to the primary tumor in conjunction with the systemic chemotherapy. The overall objective response rates with such regimens exceeded 50%, with a complete response rate of 10 to 20%. It appeared that chemotherapy alone was a reasonable treatment alternative and that complete tumor regression was necessary if noteworthy gains in survival were to be made. It was also shown that patients with localized disease and with a good performance status had the best chances of obtaining a complete response.

With the development of more vigorous combination chemotherapy programs, there has been a definite improvement in therapeutic results. Currently, a response rate of 80% with a complete response of 25 to 50% is achievable with a number of chemotherapy regimens (see Table 23-27). Complications of small cell cancer such as superior vena caval syndrome and bronchial obstruction can be managed successfully with these regimens, again in marked contrast to non-small-cell cancer.

Further intensification of chemotherapy to dose levels similar to those utilized for acute

Table 23-27.   Summary of Treatment Results with Combination Chemotherapy ± Radiotherapy in Small Cell Cancer

STUDY GROUP	THERAPY	STAGE	CR (%)	MEDIAN SURVIVAL OF ALL PATIENTS	1-YEAR SURVIVAL
Southwest Oncology Group	RadioRx + VAC	Localized	41	52 wks	50%
		Extensive	14	26 wks	—
		Total group	22	31 wks	—
Indiana University	RadioRx + VAC	Localized	—	78 wks	26% alive at 26–45+mos
		Extensive	—	36 wks	—
		Total group	41	51 wks	—
Radiation Oncology Branch, NCI	RadioRx + VAC	Localized	79	>2 yrs	—
		Extensive	48	10.5 mos	—
		Total group	66	—	—
NCI-VA Medical Oncology Branch, Washington, D.C.	High-dose CMC	Localized	50	13 mos	75%
		Extensive	26	8.5 mos	21%
		Total group	30	10.5 mos	30%
Baltimore Cancer Research Program, NCI	CAV + alternating non-cross-resistant therapy	Localized	57	11–12 mos	—
		Extensive	29	7.5 mos	—
		Total group	41	—	—
Johns Hopkins	CAV ± RadioRx	Localized	40	65 wks	66%
		Extensive	18	41 wks	42%
		Total group	26	54 wks	51%

NCI = National Cancer Institute; VA = Veterans Administration
CMC = cyclophosphamide, methotrexate, and CCNU; VAC = vincristine, doxorubicin, and cyclophosphamide; CAV = cyclophosphamide, doxorubicin, and VP-16-213
CR = complete response
From Abeloff, M. D.; Ettinger, D. S.; Order, S. E.; Khouri, N.; Mellits, E. D.; Dorschel, N.; and Baumgardner, R.: Intensive induction chemotherapy in 54 patients with small cell carcinoma of the lung. *Cancer Treat. Rep.,* **65:**639–646, 1981.

leukemia are being explored (Markman and Abeloff, 1983). Results with high-dose therapy, however, are not clearly superior to those of less intense regimens, and such treatments cannot be recommended for use outside of experimental settings.

Similarly, the utility of alternating non-cross-resistant chemotherapy regimens is being evaluated. Interest in this approach has been stimulated by Goldie's mathematic model that relates the development of drug resistance in tumor cells to their spontaneous mutation rate (Goldie and Coldman, 1979). This model suggests that alternating effective non-cross-resistant regimens will be more effective than single regimens. Further support for this notion is forthcoming from the encouraging results with alternating MOPP-ABVD in Hodgkin's disease.

The elucidation of the dose-response curve and the optimal sequencing of cytotoxic drugs in small cell cancer continues under active investigation. It is important to note that the intensive chemotherapy regimens were based on high-dose cyclophosphamide because this alkylating agent is very active and can be administered in very high doses (up to 2.4 g/m^2) without irreversible damage to hematopoietic stem cells or dose-limiting extramarrow toxicities. Dose escalation of active nonalkylating agents might provide an important added antitumor effect and such trials are underway with the podophyllotoxin VP-16-213. In addition, the infusion of stored autologous marrow has been used to circumvent severe or even lethal marrow damage. Immunologic and pharmacologic methods of cleansing such marrow of occult tumor cells have added to the interest in autologous marrow rescue techniques.

The role of radiotherapy in small cell cancer is still being defined. Currently there is evidence that irradiation of the primary tumor prolongs survival. Radiotherapy likely improves local control and this may provide an important benefit, particularly to patients with "localized disease."

Cranial radiotherapy has been applied to asymptomatic patients to forestall the development of neurologic deficits due to progressive metastases. Most clinicians now recommend cranial radiotherapy for patients who achieve complete remissions. Radiation therapy of this type, however, will not prevent the progression of leptomeningeal carcinomatosis. Although the administration of chemotherapeutic agents into the cerebrospinal fluid is of some benefit, more effective measures are needed.

In addition to local forms of radiotherapy, "systemic radiotherapy" such as hemibody radiotherapy is being explored for use against small cell cancer. Encouraging results for this modality combined with cytotoxic chemotherapy have been reported recently.

Clearly, impressive therapeutic advances have been made in the management of small cell cancer (Bunn and Ihde, 1981; Greco and Oldham, 1981). The average length of survival for patients treated with modern therapy exceeds one year. Before modern therapy, the average survival time was four months or less. Of greater importance is the fact that patients who attain a complete remission have an average survival of approximately 18 months. Ten percent of patients survive two years or longer without relapse and some of these patients are cured.

Why durable complete responses occur in only the minority of patients is not clear. The antitumor response to combination chemotherapy is generally very dramatic during the first two cycles of treatment but then a plateau in response is noted in the majority of patients. The biologic basis for this plateau in the response curve is actively being investigated in animal models and *in vitro* systems (Gazdar *et al.*, 1981). Morphologic cellular heterogeneity and changes in tumor cell populations have been observed in small cell cancers. Perhaps these changes are related to the mechanisms that underlie the emergence of resistance to therapy (Abeloff and Eggleston, 1981).

Recently, clinical studies have indicated that surgical resection can aid in the management of refractory primary tumors (Comis *et al.*, 1982; Valdivieso *et al.*, 1982). Surgery has been used before chemotherapy in patients with stage I or II disease and after induction chemotherapy in stage III disease. In both approaches, chemotherapy is continued after surgery for one to two years. As yet, the data are insufficient to define the precise role of surgery in this setting but appropriate investigations are continuing. The resection of the primary tumor after chemotherapy also offers an opportunity for detailed pathologic and bi-

ologic studies of the residual tumor. In one study, approximately 40% of patients who underwent resection of residual chest disease that was no longer responsive to chemotherapy had non-small-cell cancer.

Supportive Care

The survival as well as the quality of life of patients with lung cancer is determined not only by specific therapy for the tumor but also by the management of the complications of the disease (Abeloff, 1979). To treat the complications of bronchogenic cancer effectively the clinician must have a working knowledge of the natural history of the tumor and its likely responsiveness to various treatments as well as a good understanding of the physiologic status of the patient.

Complications of bronchogenic cancer and cancer in general can be classified into those related to direct effects of the tumor (see Tables 23–9 and 23–10) and those resulting from indirect effects (see Table 23–11). Examples of some of the common management problems arising from these complications are listed in Table 23–28 and are discussed in the follow section.

Direct Effects of Tumor. *Superior Vena Caval Syndrome.* As noted above, the superior vena caval syndrome results from local-regional spread of cancer to the lymph nodes that surround the superior vena cava. This syndrome occurs most commonly in small cell cancer and squamous cell carcinoma. Lymphomatous involvement of the right anterior mediastinal nodes and the right lateral tracheal nodes as well as distant metastases from breast cancer, colon cancer, and other solid tumors can obstruct the superior vena cava also. Benign causes (such as fibrosing mediastinitis)

Table 23–28. Bronchogenic Cancer: Complications Requiring Special Supportive Care

Direct Effects of Tumor
  Bronchial obstruction
  Superior vena caval obstruction
  Spinal cord compression
  Intracranial metastases
  Leptomeningeal cancer
  Pleural and pericardial effusions
  Bony metastases

Indirect Effects of Tumor
  Endocrine syndromes
  Neuromuscular disorders

account for 5% or less of the cases of superior vena caval syndrome.

The clinical diagnosis is usually obvious from physical findings (most striking are edema of face, neck, arms, upper torso, and prominent venous collaterals) and appropriate historic information. Superior vena caval obstruction in a smoker with a right lung mass on chest roentgenogram is most suggestive of lung cancer but a tissue diagnosis must be established (see Figure 23–18). A precise pathologic diagnosis is essential not only to distinguish bronchogenic carcinoma from other cancerous and benign diseases but also to subclassify bronchogenic carcinoma into small cell or non-small-cell types.

Invasive procedures in a patient with the superior vena caval syndrome must be regarded with caution because disruption of the extensive venous collaterals can result in marked bleeding. Histologic and/or cytologic diagnosis, however, can usually be obtained from sputum or pleural fluid cytology, biopsy of supraclavicular node, or a bronchoscopic procedure. If the patient's hemodynamic status is tenuous or the edema is massive, consideration should be given to delivering radiotherapy to relieve the obstruction prior to performing a biopsy.

The syndrome in a patient with previously untreated small cell cancer can be effectively treated with either combination chemotherapy or radiotherapy (see Figure 23–18). Chemotherapy offers the advantage of providing systemic antitumor effects. Radiotherapy is the treatment of choice in patients with non-small cell cancer or patients with small cell cancer whose condition has worsened during chemotherapy.

Other complications such as airway obstruction and spinal cord compression are generally treated with radiotherapy. Combination chemotherapy, however, is as effective as radiotherapy in relieving bronchial obstruction in newly diagnosed patients with small cell cancer.

Intracranial and Leptomeningeal Metastases. Intracranial metastases are best treated with radiotherapy. Chemotherapy is generally ineffective, in part because of failure of these agents to adequately penetrate the blood-brain barrier. Neither radiotherapy nor systemic chemotherapy is adequate treatment for leptomeningeal metastases. In small cell cancer meningeal carcinomatosis often develops in

association with cranial metastases and spinal cord compression. Intrathecal or, preferably, intraventricular chemotherapy must be integrated with radiotherapy to sites of bulk disease. Unfortunately, the results of treatment of carcinomatous meningitis are generally quite disappointing.

Pleural and Pericardial Effusions. These effusions are generally caused by tumor infiltration of the pleural or pericardial surfaces. In some cases of bronchogenic carcinoma the effusions occur as the result of obstruction of the mediastinal lymphatics or venous circulation. Cancerous effusions can regress as the result of systemic chemotherapy (particularly in small cell cancer) but tube drainage with or without instillation of chemotherapeutic or sclerosing agents is often necessary in order to provide symptomatic relief.

Osteolytic Metastases and Hypercalcemia. Bone metastases are common in bronchogenic cancer, particularly small cell cancer. Although osteolysis may result from a mass of tumor cells growing in the medullary cavity of a bone, it appears that products of tumor cell metabolism that are released into the surrounding area may be most important in promoting bone destruction. Such products include prostaglandin E_2 (PGE_2), osteoclast-activating factor (OAF), parathormonelike substance, and heparin.

Pain secondary to osteolytic metastases is treated most effectively with local radiotherapy. Hypercalcemia is also commonly associated with bone metastases and is best managed by treatment of the underlying neoplasm, ambulation, and hydration. Pharmacologic control of hypercalcemia with drugs such as mithramycin, calcitonin, diphosphonates, or corticosteroids is often necessary and may be lifesaving.

It is interesting to note that hypercalcemia as a complication of small cell cancer is uncommon even though this type of bronchogenic cancer has the greatest incidence of bone metastases. Squamous cell carcinoma has the highest incidence of hypercalcemia and elevated calcium levels often occur in the absence of clinically detectable bone metastases. These data suggest that squamous cell carcinoma has a propensity for synthesizing hypercalcemia-inducing substances whereas small cell cancer lacks this potential.

Indirect Effects of Tumor. *Paraneoplastic Endocrine Syndromes.* As noted above, osteolysis and hypercalcemia can occur as a result of direct and/or indirect effects of bronchogenic cancer. The most common indirect effects are the paraneoplastic endocrine syndromes such as the syndrome of inappropriate ADH secretion (SIADH) and ectopic ACTH production. These ectopic hormone syndromes are generally seen in patients with small cell cancer and are clinically important for a number of reasons. First, these syndromes may be the source of great morbidity. For example, SIADH can result in altered mental status due to hyponatremia and a frank Cushing's syndrome can result from the ectopic production of ACTH. Recognition and treatment of the consequences of ectopic hormone excess may relieve distressing symptoms. Second, the initial clue to the diagnosis of bronchogenic cancer may be the hormone-excess syndrome it induces. For example, hyponatremia (SIADH) may be the first clue to diagnosis of small cell cancer. Third, the presence or reactivation of an ectopic hormone syndrome may provide an indication of the activity of the underlying tumor.

The optimal treatment of the paraneoplastic endocrine syndromes is eradication of the cancer. Often necessary, however, are other measures such as water restriction and demeclocycline in the management of SIADH and drugs such as aminoglutethimide, o'p' DDD, or metyrapone in control of the ectopic ACTH syndrome.

Paraneoplastic Neuromuscular Disorders. A meticulous neurologic examination is essential in the evaluation of patients with bronchogenic cancer because a variety of neurologic problems occur not only as a result of mass lesions but also secondary to paraneoplastic neuromyopathies. Small cell cancer is again the type most commonly associated with these neurologic syndromes.

Treatment of the neoplasm has not generally resulted in improvement of these neurologic symptoms and signs. The development of effective systemic therapy for small cell cancer, however, has resulted in reversal of some of these syndromes. The administration of guanidine provides some relief to patients with the Lambert-Eaton syndrome. Similarly, adrenal corticosteroids are useful in managing polymyositis.

Complications of Therapy. In addition to the complications that result from cancer, the therapies employed can result in noteworthy morbidity and even mortality. The complications of therapy require greater attention as combined modality treatments are used increasingly. In particular, clinicians must be aware of the hematologic, infectious, and neurologic sequelae of combined radiotherapy-chemotherapy treatment programs. As the effectiveness of treatment improves, greater attention will also be directed to the longer-term sequelae of therapy.

Future Prospects

Currently, bronchogenic cancer is a public health problem of major proportions and its incidence continues to increase at a very rapid rate. Abstinence from cigarette smoking would prevent much of this morbidity and mortality. The prospect of appropriate behavioral modification in large and diverse populations, however, does not seem very bright.

Other environmental pollutants are known to cause bronchogenic cancer; nearly all of them are particles of small size or are gases that are inhaled into the tracheobronchial tree. With advances in chemistry and industry, it seems likely that the potential of exposure to carcinogens will increase. It is to be expected that simpler methods will be developed for the early identification of those compounds with the greatest carcinogenic and mutagenic potency and that proper precautions will be taken to avoid undue exposure.

Any process that impairs normal mucociliary function of the epithelial lining of the tracheobronchial tree will lead to an increased risk of bronchogenic cancer. Little is known at present, however, about the specific constitutional factors that determine the susceptibility of the epithelial cells to carcinogenesis. Because there is much promising research in this area, it seems likely that practical biochemical tests that will indicate individual cell vulnerability or resistance to carcinogenesis will be developed within a few years. One can even envision methods of detecting epithelial cells in which the carcinogenic process has been "initiated" but which have not been transformed. Naturally, the implications of such achievements would extend beyond biology and medicine.

The prospects for the earlier detection of lung cancer in large asymptomatic populations using cytologic and radiographic methods similar to those presently available do not seem good. An increasing number of tumor-produced polypeptides and other potential "biomarker" molecules, however, are being identified. Similarly, an increasing number of cell surface proteins and tumor-related antigens are being discovered. Although none thus far are tumor specific, it seems likely that certain of these biomarkers will permit oncologists to monitor the magnitude of the tumor cell burden in individual patients during the course of their disease. Due recognition will have to be given to the ever-changing nature of the tumor cell population and the likelihood that production of the marker molecule may be altered.

Rapid advances are being made in clinical imaging techniques, especially using digital analytic methods. It seems likely that in the near future clinicians will have an increased ability to identify tumors and to determine their volume at sequential intervals. These techniques should lead to improved patient management by enhancing the process of therapeutic decision making. The coupling of physiologic information (e.g., blood flow, oxygenation, and drug uptake) with tumor imaging is an even more exciting prospect that is well within reach.

An especially promising diagnostic imaging technique is based on the use of radiolabeled antibodies directed against tumor-related antigens. For example, radioimmunodetection using anti-CEA antibody appears to be a more sensitive, and possibly more specific, method of revealing at least certain hepatic metastases from bronchogenic cancers and other tumors than any currently available (Goldenberg et al., 1982). It seems likely that this area of work will be pursued vigorously and with good effect.

With rare exceptions, bronchogenic cancers are vexing therapeutic problems. Surgical resection and radiation therapy can achieve cures in the small proportion of patients who truly present with localized tumors. The overall effectiveness of external beam radiation therapy will probably be enhanced by the use of CT scanning and three-dimensional treatment planning. The outlook for patients with small cell cancer has improved markedly in the recent past with the advent of effective multimodality treatment regimens. The progress of the disease, however, in the majority of patients cannot be stemmed totally.

The effectiveness of chemotherapeutic agents can be extended greatly by employing higher doses of drugs to be followed by autologous bone marrow "rescue." Practical in vitro methods are at hand to purge tumor cells from freshly harvested bone marrow and to support patients through relatively short periods of profound aplasia. It is quite possible, also, to achieve a "biologic implant" using antibodies directed against tumor-related antigens to deliver therapeutic doses of radiation. For example, promising degrees of localization have been achieved in bronchogenic cancers using radiolabeled antibodies directed against carcinoembryonic antigen and ferritin. The use of radioimmunoglobulins could possibly be combined with chemotherapeutic agents.

The widespread nature of bronchogenic carcinoma poses a major therapeutic problem. It is possible that radioimmunoglobulin therapy will address distant metastatic disease, but methods will have to be devised to deliver tumoricidal doses of radiation to rather small-sized tumors. Thus far, cytotoxic drugs with broad utility in bronchogenic cancers have not been developed. It is hoped, however, that a greater understanding of the processes of tumor cell proliferation and maturation may yield opportunities for methods of treatment more akin to normal biologic controls.

Chemoprophylaxis for bronchogenic carcinomas offers a challenging prospect. For example, vitamin A deficiency and low blood retinol concentrations have been associated with disordered maturation of the bronchial epithelium, significant cellular atypia, and an apparently increased incidence of cancer. Further, in laboratory model systems it appears that β-carotene, vitamin A, and certain of its analogs as well as vitamin E have anticarcinogenic effects. Studies in humans are few, but the area of chemoprophylaxis would seem to hold great promise, especially for individuals such as cigarette smokers who are at high risk.

REFERENCES

Abeloff, M. D. (ed.): Complications of Cancer. The Johns Hopkins University Press, Baltimore, 1979.

Abeloff, M. D., and Eggleston, J. C.: Morphologic changes following therapy. In Greco, F. A.; Oldham, R. K.; and Bunn, P. A. (eds.): Small Cell Lung Cancer. Grune & Stratton, Inc., New York, 1981.

Abeloff, M. D.; Ettinger, D. S.; Order, S. E.; Khouri, N.; Mellits, E. D.; Dorschel, N.; and Baumgardner, R.: Intensive induction chemotherapy in 54 patients with small cell carcinoma of the lung. Cancer Treat. Rep., 65:639–646, 1981.

Aisner, J., and Hansen, H. H.: Commentary: Current status of chemotherapy for non-small cell lung cancer. *Cancer Treat. Rep.,* **65**:979–986, 1981.

American Cancer Society: *Cancer Facts and Figures, 1984.* American Cancer Society, New York, 1984.

American Joint Committee for Cancer Staging and End-Results Reporting: *Staging of Lung Cancer 1979.* American Joint Committee for Cancer Staging and End-Results Reporting, Chicago, 1979.

Baker, R. R.; Lillemoe, K. D.; and Tockman, M. S.: The indications for transcervical mediastinoscopy in patients with small peripheral bronchogenic carcinomas. *Surg. Gynecol. Obstet.,* **148**:860–862, 1979.

Baylin, S. B.; Goodwin, G.; and Shaper, J. H.: Analysis of cell surface proteins as a means to study neuroendocrine differentiation in the spectrum of human lung cancers. In Bloom, S. R., and Polak, J. (eds.): *Systemic Role of Regulatory Peptides, 13th Symposia Medica Hoechst.* F. K. Schattauer Verlag, Stuttgart, 1982.

Bunn, P. A., and Ihde, D. C.: Small cell bronchogenic carcinoma: A review of therapeutic results. In Livingston, R. B. (ed.): *Lung Cancer.* Martinus Nijhoff Publishers, The Hague, 1981.

Carbone, P. P.; Frost, J. K.; Feinstein, A. R.; Higgins, G. A.; and Selawry, O. S.: Lung cancer: Perspectives and prospects. *Ann. Intern. Med.,* **73**:1003–1024, 1970.

Carr, D. T., and Mountain, C. F.: Staging lung cancer. In Straus, M. (ed.): *Lung Cancer: Clinical Diagnosis and Treatment.* Grune & Stratton, Inc., New York, 1977.

Carter, D., and Eggleston, J. C.: Tumors of the lower respiratory tract. *Atlas of Tumor Pathology.* Armed Forces Institute of Pathology, Washington, D.C., 1980.

Cohen, M. H.: Signs and symptoms of bronchogenic carcinoma. In Straus, M. (ed.): *Lung Cancer: Clinical Diagnosis and Treatment.* Grune & Stratton, Inc., New York, 1977.

Comis, R.; Meyer, J.; Ginsberg, S.; Issell, B.; Gullo, J.; DiFino, S.; Tinsley, R.; Poiesz, B.; and Rudolph, A.: The current results of chemotherapy (CTH) plus adjuvant surgery (AS) in limited small cell anaplastic lung cancer (SCALC). *Proc. ASCO,* **1**:147, 1982.

Cruz, J. M.; Jackson, D. V., Jr.; White, D. R.; Richards, F., II; Muss, H. B.; Stuart, J. J.; Cooper, M. R.; Spurr, C. L.; Pope, E. K.; and Patterson, R. B.: Evaluation of brain metastasis at presentation of small cell carcinoma (SCC) of the lung. *Proc. ASCO,* **1**:142, 1982.

Doll, R.: Cancer and aging: The epidemiologic evidence. In Clark, R. L.; Cumley, R. W.; McCay, J. E.; and Copeland, M. M. (eds.): *Tenth International Cancer Congress, Oncology 1970,* vol. 5. Year Book Medical Publishers, Inc., Chicago, 1971.

Eagan, R. T.; Frytak, S.; Creagan, E. T.; Ingle, J. N.; Kvols, L. K.; and Coles, D. T.: Phase II study of cyclophosphamide, Adriamycin and *cis*-dichlorodiamminoplatinum (II) by infusion in patients with adenocarcinoma and large cell carcinoma of the lung. *Cancer Treat. Rep.,* **63**:1589–1591, 1979.

Eagan, R. T.; Ingle, J. N.; Frytak, S.; Rubin, J.; Kvols, L. K.; Carr, D. T.; Coles, D. T.; and O'Fallon, J. R.: Platinum based polychemotherapy versus dianhydrogalactitol in advanced non-small cell lung cancer. *Cancer Treat. Rep.,* **61**:1339–1345, 1977.

Fraumeni, J. F., Jr.: Respiratory carcinogenesis: An epidemiologic appraisal. *J. N. C. I.,* **55**:1039–1046, 1975.

Frost, J. K.; Ball, W. C., Jr.; Levin, M. L.; Tockman, M. S.; Baker, R. R.; Carter, D.; Eggleston, J. C.; Erozan, Y. S.; Gupta, P. K.; and Khouri, N. F.: Early lung cancer detection: Results of the initial (prevalence) radiologic and cytologic screening in the Johns Hopkins study. *Am. Rev. Respir. Dis.,* **130**:549–554, 1984.

Gazdar, A. F.; Carney, D. N.; Guccin, J. G.; and Baylin, S. B.: Small cell carcinoma of the lung: Cellular origin and relationship to other pulmonary tumors. In Greco, F. A.; Oldham, R. K.; and Bunn, P. A. (eds.): *Small Cell Lung Cancer.* Grune & Stratton, Inc., New York, 1981.

Goldberg, E. M.; Glicksman, A. S.; Khan, F. R.; and Nickson, J. J.: Mediastinoscopy for assessing mediastinal spread in clinical staging of carcinoma of the lung. *Cancer,* **25**:347–353, 1970.

Goldenberg, D. M.; Kim, E. E.; Bennett, S. J.; Shah, U.; Nelson, M. O.; and DeLand, F. H.: A correlative study of carcinoembryonic antigen (CEA) radioimmunodetection (RAID) in the evaluation of hepatic metastases. *Proc. ASCO,* **1**:101, 1982.

Goldie, J. H., and Coldman, A. J.: A mathematical model for relating the drug sensitivity of tumors to their spontaneous mutation rate. *Cancer Treat. Rep.,* **63**:1727–1735, 1979.

Greco, F. A., and Oldham, R. K.: Clinical management of patients with small cell lung cancer. In Greco, F. A.; Oldham, R. K.; and Bunn, P. A. (eds.): *Small Cell Lung Cancer.* Grune & Stratton, Inc., New York, 1981.

Griffin, C. A., and Baylin, S. B.: Expression of the c-myb oncogene in human small cell lung carcinoma. *Cancer Res.,* in press, 1985.

Hoffmann, T. H., and Ransdell, H. T.: Comparison of lobectomy and wedge resection for carcinoma of the lung. *J. Thorac. Cardiovasc. Surg.,* **79**:211–217, 1980.

Ihde, D. C., and Hansen, H. H.: Staging procedures and prognostic factors in small cell carcinoma of the lung. In Greco, F. A.; Oldham, R. K.; and Bunn, P. A. (eds.): *Small Cell Lung Cancer.* Grune & Stratton, Inc., New York, 1981.

Jepson, O., and Rahbek, S. H.: *Mediastinoscopy.* Munksgaard, Copenhagen, 1970.

Kirsh, M. K.; Prior, M. P.; Gago, O.; Moores, W. Y.; Kahn, D. R.; Pellegrino, R. V.; and Sloan, H.: The effect of histological cell type on the prognosis of patients with bronchogenic carcinoma. *Ann. Thorac. Surg.,* **13**:303–310, 1972.

Komaki, R.; Roh, J.; Cox, J. D.; and Lopes da Conceicao, A.: Superior sulcus tumors: Results of irradiation of 36 patients. *Cancer,* **48**:1563–1568, 1981.

Lawhorne, T. W.; Baker, R. R.; and Carter, D.: Adenocarcinoma of the lung presenting as a solitary pulmonary nodule. *Johns Hopk. Med. J.,* **133**:82–87, 1973.

Livingston, R. B.: Combination chemotherapy of bronchogenic carcinoma. I. Non-oat cell. *Cancer Treat. Rev.,* **4**:153–165, 1977.

McDowell, E.M.; Barrett, L. A.; Galvin, F.; Harris, G. C.; and Trump, B. F.: The respiratory epithelium. I. Human bronchus. *J. N. C. I.,* **61**:539–549, 1978.

McKneally, M. F.; Maver, C.; and Kausel, H. W.: Regional immunotherapy of lung cancer with intrapleural BCG. *Lancet,* **1**:377–385, 1976.

McNeil, B. J.; Weichselbaum, R.; and Pauker, S. G.: Fallacy of the five-year survival in lung cancer. *N. Engl. J. Med.,* **299**:1397–1401, 1978.

Markman, M. M., and Abeloff, M. D.: Management of hematologic and infectious complications of intensive induction therapy of small cell carcinoma of the lung. *Am. J. Med.,* **74**:741–746, 1983.

Martini, N.; Flehinger, B. J.; Zaman, M. B.; and Beattie, E. J., Jr.: Prospective study of 445 lung carcinomas with mediastinal lymph node metastases. *J. Thorac. Cardiovasc. Surg.,* **80**:390–399, 1980.

Matthews, M. J.; Kanhouwa, S.; Pickren, J.; and Robinette, D.: Frequency of residual and metastatic tumor in patients undergoing curative surgical resection for lung cancer. *Cancer Chemother. Rep.,* **3:**63–67, 1973.

Medical Research Council: Comparative trial of surgery and radiotherapy for the primary treatment of small celled or oat celled carcinoma of the bronchus. *Lancet,* **2:**979–986, 1966.

Minna, J. D.; Higgins, G. A.; and Glatstein, E. J.: Cancer of the lung. In DeVita, V T.; Hellman, S.; and Rosenberg, S. A. (eds.): *Principles and Practice of Oncology.* J. B. Lippincott Company, Philadelphia, 1982.

Mountain, C. F.: Biologic, physiologic, and technical determinants in surgical therapy for lung cancer. In Straus, M. J. (ed.): *Lung Cancer.* Grune & Stratton, Inc., New York, 1977.

Mountain, C. F.; Carr, D. T.; and Anderson, W. A. D.: A system for the clinical staging of lung cancer. *A. J. R. Radium Ther. Nucl. Med.,* **120:**130–138, 1974.

Mountain, C. F.; Carr, D. T.; Martini, N.; Raventos, A.; Stitik, F. P.; and Woolner, L. B.: *Staging of Lung Cancer.* American Joint Committee for Cancer Staging and End-Results Reporting, Chicago, 1979.

Muggia, F. M.; Blum, R. H.; and Foreman, J. D.: Role of chemotherapy in the treatment of lung cancer: Evolving strategies for non-small-cell histologies. *Int. J. Radiat. Oncol. Biol. Phys.,* **10:**137–145, 1984.

Mulshine, J.; Matthews, M.; Radice, P.; Johnston-Early, A.; Makuch, R.; Ihde, D.; Carney, D.; Cohen, M.; Minna, J.; and Bunn, P. A.: Staging evaluation of the liver in small cell cancer of the lung (SCCL). *Proc. ASCO.* **1:**140, 1982.

Nagaishi, C.: *Functional Anatomy and Histology of the Lung.* University Park Press, Baltimore, 1972.

National Cancer Institute: *SEER Program. Cancer Patient Survival—Report Number 5.* Department of Health, Education and Welfare, Bethesda, Maryland, 1976.

Paulson, D. L.: Carcinomas in the superior pulmonary sulcus. *J. Thorac. Cardiovasc. Surg.,* **70:**1095–1104, 1975.

Perez, C. A.; Stanley, K.; Rubin, P.; Kramer, S.; Brady, L.; Perez-Tamayo, R.; Brown, G. S.; Concannon, J.; Rotman, M.; and Seydel, H. G.: A prospective randomized study of various irradiation doses and fractionation schedules in the treatment of inoperable non-oat-cell carcinoma of the lung. *Cancer,* **45:**2744–2753, 1980.

Phillips, T. L., and Miller, R. J.: Should asymptomatic patients with inoperable bronchogenic carcinoma receive immediate radiotherapy? Yes. *Am. Rev. Respir. Dis.,* **117:**405–410, 1978.

Ramsdell, J. W.; Peters, R. M.; Taylor, A. T.; Alazraki, N. P.; and Tisi, G. M.: Multiorgan scans for staging lung cancer. *J. Thorac. Cardiovasc. Surg.,* **73:**653–659, 1977.

Rosenow, E. C., and Carr, D. T.: Bronchogenic carcinoma. *CA,* **29:**233–244, 1979.

Siegelman, S. S.; Zerhouni, E. A.; Leo, F. P.; Khouri, N. F.; and Stitik, F. P.: CT of the solitary pulmonary nodule. *A. J. R.,* **135:**1–13, 1980.

Stanley, K. E.: Prognostic factors for survival in patients with inoperable lung cancer. *J. N. C. I.,* **65:**25–32, 1980.

Stewart, T. H. M.; Hollinshead, A. C.; Harris, J. E.; Belanger, R.; Crepeau, A.; Hooper, G. D.; Sachs, H. J.; Klassen, D. J.; Hirte, W.; Rapp, E.; Crook, A. F.; Orizaga, M.; Sengar, D. P. S.; and Raman, S.: Immunochemotherapy of lung cancer. *Ann. N.Y. Acad. Sci.,* **277:**436–466, 1976.

Takitas, H.: Surgical adjuvant immunotherapy for lung cancer: A review. *Curr. Surg.,* **41:**254–261, 1984.

Trump, B. F.; McDowell, E. M.; Galvin, F.; Barrett, L. A.; Becci, P. I.; Schurch, W.; Kaiser, H. E.; and Harris, C. C.: The respiratory epithelium. III. Histogenesis of epidermoid metaplasia and carcinoma in situ in the human. *J. N. C. I.,* **61:**563–575, 1978.

Valdivieso, M.; McMurtrey, M. J.; Farha, P.; Frazier, O. H., Jr.; Barkley, H. T.; Paone, J. F.; Spitzer, G.; and Mountain, C. F.: Increasing importance of adjuvant surgery in the therapy of patients with small cell lung cancer. *Proc. ASCO,* **1:**148, 1982.

Waalkes, T. P.; Abeloff, M. D.; Woo, K. B.; Ettinger, D. S.; Ruddon, R. W.; and Aldenderfer, P.: Carcinoembryonic antigen for monitoring patients with small cell carcinoma of the lung during treatment. *Cancer Res.,* **40:**4420–4427, 1980.

Whang-Peng, J.; Kao-Shan, C. S.; Lee, E. C.; Bunn, P. A.; Carney, D. N.; Gazdar, A. F.; and Minna, J.: Specific chromosome defect associated with human small-cell lung cancer. Deletion 3p (14-23). *Science,* **215:**181–182, 1982.

Williams, D. E.; Pairolero, P. C.; Davis, C. S.; Payne, S.; Taylor, W. F.; Uhlenhopp, M. A.; and Fontana, R. S.: Survival of patients surgically treated for stage I lung cancer. *J. Thorac. Cardiovasc. Surg.,* **82:**70–76, 1981.

World Health Organization: *Report on Meeting on the Histological Classification of Lung Tumors.* World Health Organization, Geneva, 1977.

24

Neoplasms of the Mediastinum and Mesothelioma

MICHAEL A. PASSERO and PAUL CALABRESI

TUMORS OF THE MEDIASTINUM

Introduction

Mediastinal masses require a specific diagnosis and treatment, even though half the patients with a mediastinal mass are asymptomatic. In this section, approaches to the diagnosis of mediastinal mass are reviewed, and the more common cancerous tumors of the mediastinum are discussed.

Anatomy

The great anatomists have described the thoracic mediastinum as a sagittal partition that extends from the thoracic outlet superiorly to the diaphragm inferiorly. It is bound by the deep surface of the sternum anteriorly and the thoracic vertebrae posteriorly. The immediate right and left surfaces are formed by the parietal pleura. Although the customary subdivision of the thoracic mediastinum is into four compartments, the superior, anterior, middle, and posterior mediastinum, this is an arbitrary division. Several authors, confronted with the problem of classifying mediastinal lesions by chest roentgenogram, point out the practical difficulties of separating superior from anterior mediastinal masses, and, therefore, they have often combined these two areas into one division. As a result, there is considerable variation in the exact limits of the mediastinal compartments in the current literature, and the reader is cautioned to scrutinize any particular author's scheme for the mediastinal compartments. It is hoped that the application of computerized tomography to mediastinal lesions will help standardize the practical anatomic divisions. This review utilizes the description of the mediastinal compartments found in a widely accepted textbook of chest medicine (Fraser and Pare, 1979). The anterior mediastinum contains the thymus gland, mesenchymal tissue, and the anterior mediastinal lymph nodes. It is bound anteriorly by the sternum and posteriorly by the pericardium, aorta, and brachiocephalic vessels. The middle mediastinum contains the pericardium, the heart, and all the major vessels leaving and entering the heart, plus the trachea, main bronchi, paratracheal and tracheobronchial lymph nodes, phrenic nerves, and the upper portions of the vagus nerves. The posterior mediastinum is bound anteriorly by the pericardium and posteriorly by the vertebral column. The paravertebral zones and posterior gutters are anatomically excluded by this division, but because they contain important structures that may give rise to mediastinal masses, such as the sympathetic nerve chains and peripheral nerves, these areas are usually included with the posterior mediastinum. The posterior mediastinum contains the descending thoracic aorta, the esophagus, the thoracic duct, the lower portion of the vagus nerves, and the posterior mediastinal lymph nodes.

Incidence

In a study from Duke University Medical Center in 1967, the incidence of primary mediastinal tumors and cysts was estimated to be 1 in 3400 admissions (Oldham and Sabiston, 1967). There was no predilection for males or females. In adults, approximately 25% of the mediastinal masses were neoplastic, but in children, the frequency of neoplasia was between 40 and 45% (Hammon and Sabiston, 1979). In a review of 1950 adult patients gleaned from several series on the relative frequency of various primary mediastinal tumors and cysts, the incidence of neurogenic tumor, thymoma, and cysts was about 20% each (Silverman and Sabiston, 1980). The incidence of lymphoma was 13% and of germ cell neoplasms was 11%. Mesenchymal tumors, endocrine tumors, and primary carcinomas were each found in less than 7% of the adult patients. In a review of several series on the frequency of primary mediastinal tumors and cysts occurring in 437 children, neurogenic tumors made up 40% of masses. The incidence of lymphoma was approximately 20%, as was the incidence of all cysts. Germ cell neoplasms contributed about 10% of the lesions as did mesenchymal tumors; primary cancers were much rarer, as were thymomas and endocrine tumors in children. Neurogenic tumors are more common in children under four years of age. In adolescents the frequency of lymphoma increases greatly.

Symptoms and Signs

Approximately 50% of the patients discovered to have a mediastinal mass are asymptomatic. In these patients the mass is discovered by a chest roentgenogram obtained for screening purposes or for another reason. In asymptomatic patients with a mediastinal mass, 90% will have a benign lesion (Rubush *et al.,* 1973; Wychulis *et al.,* 1971). In patients with symptoms, however, 50% will have a neoplasm.

The most common symptoms in patients with mediastinal masses are cough, chest pain, dyspnea, recurrent respiratory infection, and dysphagia (Silverman and Sabiston, 1980).

The symptoms of chest discomfort, fullness, tightness, and pain are the major sensations for the entire region supplied by dermatomes T1 through T6. The upper four dermatomes are supplied by sensory afferent fibers, and in the cord these fibers communicate with one another. All the thoracic viscera are served by sensory fibers in these pathways, including the myocardium, aorta, pericardium, pulmonary

artery, esophagus, and mediastinum. As a result, a mediastinal mass that irritates any of these structures may cause pain that is deep and poorly localized. Often this sensation presents as retrosternal or precordial pain. It may extend into the neck, to the left or right hemithorax, or to the anterior and medial aspects of one or both arms and forearms. Although the dermatomes T5 and T6 comprise fibers from the lower thoracic wall, the diaphragm, the peritoneal surface, the gallbladder, pancreas, duodenum, and stomach, irritation in these structures may also produce pain that is poorly localized and can be confused with pain originating in lesions above the diaphragm.

Compression or invasion of normal mediastinal structures by the mass may also lead to findings such as superior vena caval obstruction, vocal cord paralysis, spinal cord compression, Horner's syndrome, cardiac murmurs, pericarditis, pericardial tamponade, and compression of the right ventricular outflow tract, suggesting primary cardiac disease. Systemic symptoms may also occur. These include nonspecific symptoms such as anorexia, weight loss, and malaise or more specific syndromes such as myasthenia gravis or red cell aplasia, as seen in thymoma, or hypoglycemia, as seen in insulin-producing teratomas.

Approaches to the Mediastinal Mass or Mediastinal Widening

Roentgenographic Techniques. Unfortunately, a decision about whether a mass is benign or cancerous usually cannot be made from a chest roentgenogram, and an invasive procedure may be necessary. Chest roentgenograms and other roentgenographic techniques, however, can provide valuable information about the location, extent, and changes in size of a mediastinal mass (see Table 24–1 and Figure 24–1).

One must first differentiate whether a mass is truly mediastinal or is arising from the adjacent lung or pleura. Because the mediastinum lies outside the pleural sac, a mediastinal mass pressing into the lung parenchyma will have a layer of intact parietal and visceral pleura overlying it. This gives it an extremely convex contour facing the lung. In addition, the pleural lining will often smooth out irregularities of the mass, giving it a well-defined shadow. The upper and lower borders around

Table 24–1. Typical Locations of Mediastinal Masses

ANTERIOR	MIDDLE	POSTERIOR
Thymoma	Lymphomas	Neurogenic neoplasms
Lymphoma	Tracheal neoplasms	Lymphomas
Germinal cell neoplasms	Bronchogenic cysts	Neurenteric cysts
Thyroid and parathyroid masses	Pleuropericardial cysts	Thoracic duct cysts
Mesenchymal neoplasms	Morgagni's hernias	Esophageal tumors, diverticula, and hernia
	Sarcoidosis	Paravertebral abscess
	Dilatation of veins, pulmonary arteries, and aorta	

the mass will taper away from the sharp convex contour of the mass. If a central mass involves the adjacent spine or sternum, it is most likely mediastinal rather than pulmonary in location.

Because intrapulmonary masses move together with adjacent lung markings and mediastinal lesions do not, chest fluoroscopy is an ideal method for differentiating mediastinal from pulmonary lesions. The respiratory movements of mediastinal lesions depend on their locations. Those attached to the esophagus or trachea move with those organs. Lesions involving the nerves or spine seldom move at all. Thymoma and dermoid tumors in the anterior mediastinum either are immobile or move with the heart. Masses elsewhere in the mediastinum may move slightly but usually independently of both the lungs and all the mediastinal structures.

Study of the mediastinal lines may give clues to the origin and location of mediastinal masses. The mediastinal lines include a number of vertical lines visible in the mediastinum, usually seen on well-penetrated chest roentgenograms. These lines have been called the paraesophageal, para-aortic, paraspinal, paracardiac, paravenous, and paratracheal lines. They are usually difficult to distinguish from each other. Deviation of a para- line, however, may indicate the presence of tumor.

One problem in interpreting chest roentgenograms of patients with mediastinal widening is distinguishing between anterior mediastinal

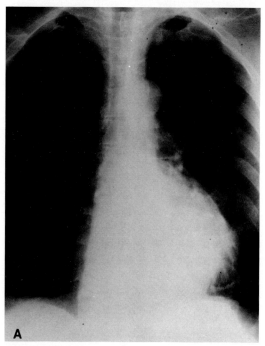
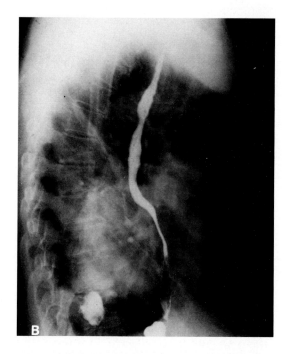

Figure 24–1. (A) Overpenetrated chest roentgenogram suggests a density behind the heart, the "ivory heart" sign. (B) Barium contrast studies reveal anterior displacement of the esophagus by a mass. Oat cell carcinoma invading the mediastinum. (Photos courtesy of Dr. William Colaiace, Roger Williams General Hospital.)

masses and dilatation of the heart or pericardial effusions. The hilum overlay sign is useful in making this distinction (Felson, 1973). In normal individuals, the proximal segment of the visible left pulmonary artery is lateral to the heart and can easily be seen on the chest roentgenogram. With pericardial effusions or cardiac enlargement the left pulmonary artery can still be seen outside the heart border. If a mass is present contiguous to the heart, however, it will also overlap the main pulmonary arteries, which then can be seen within the margins of the mass. Conversely, if a pulmonary artery is seen emerging from the border of an enlarged anterior mediastinal "mass," the "mass" is most likely an enlarged heart or pericardial sac. The hilum convergence sign is used to distinguish between an enlarged pulmonary artery and a juxtahilar mediastinal tumor. If the pulmonary artery branches can be seen converging toward the mass rather than toward the heart, the mass is most likely an enlarged pulmonary artery. If the pulmonary artery branches converge toward the heart itself and not toward the mass, the mass in question is probably a mediastinal mass.

The contents of a mediastinal lesion may be helpful in estimating its nature. The presence of air may suggest a gastroenteric or neurenteric cyst. Calcification is found in several lesions, including thyroid tumors, thymoma, and teratoma. Phleboliths are suggestive of hemangiomas or hemangiosarcomas. Fat in the mediastinum often appears at about the same density of water. The presence of fat suggests teratoma, lipoma, thymolipoma, and mediastinal lipomatosis secondary to steroid therapy. A mass that contains an air bronchogram lies in the pulmonary parenchyma rather than in the mediastinum.

Mediastinal adenopathy is an important roentgenographic finding. Involvement with lymphoma is a common cause of mediastinal lymph node enlargement (Lyons et al., 1959). Mediastinal lymph node enlargement is one of the most common roentgenographic findings in Hodgkin's disease and can be seen on the presenting chest roentgenograms of about 50% of patients (see Figure 24–2). Usually, lymph node involvement is bilateral but asymmetric, with primarily paratracheal and subcarinal nodes being involved more often than the hilar nodes. In both Hodgkin's and non-Hodgkin's lymphomas and leukemias, the nodes often produce a nodular rather than smooth configuration in the mediastinum. Of major importance is the involvement of retrosternal and anterior mediastinal nodes in lymphoma (see Figure 24–3). These are best seen on the lateral chest roentgenogram and computerized tomography. These nodes are almost never involved in sarcoidosis.

One should also be aware of the pattern of mediastinal lymph node involvement in certain infectious and granulomatous diseases. In infectious mononucleosis, both mediastinal and hilar lymph nodes may be involved. In tuberculosis and histoplasmosis, node involvement is usually unilateral. In sarcoidosis, node involvement is often bilateral, symmetric, and usually includes the paratracheal, tracheobronchial, and bronchopulmonary nodes, but, as mentioned above, almost never involves the anterior mediastinal or retrosternal nodes (see Figure 24–4).

Tomography of the mediastinum remains a useful technique for further delineating the extent and sometimes the composition of mediastinal masses. Depending upon the location of the lesion, both frontal and lateral tomography may be useful. In lesions where the hilar areas may be involved, 55° oblique tomography, which provides the best views of the

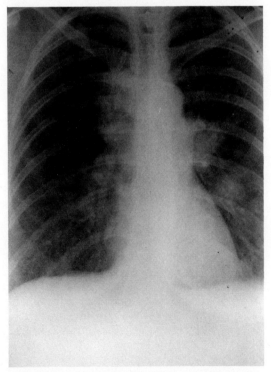

Figure 24–2. Hodgkin's disease with extensive mediastinal and hilar adenopathy. (Photo courtesy of Dr. William Colaiace, Roger Williams General Hospital.)

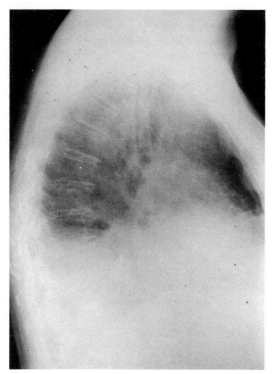

Figure 24-3. Retrosternal node involvement. Histiocytic lymphoma.

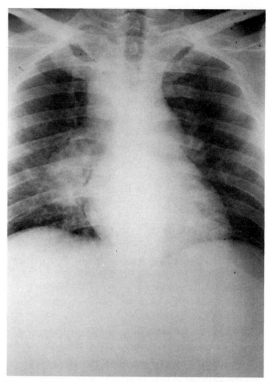

Figure 24-4. A 37-year-old man presented with a large right hilar mass and mediastinal adenopathy. Sarcoidosis was found on scalene node biopsy. (Photo courtesy of Dr. William Colaiace, Roger Williams General Hospital.)

hilum, is the preferred technique. Studies of the local vasculature with aortograms, venograms, pulmonary arteriograms, azygography, and selective thymic venography have been used to separate vascular tumors, aneurysms, and arteriovenous malformations from mediastinal masses. Computerized tomography with contrast studies may replace many of these techniques.

Barium techniques have been used to study masses that either impinge on the esophagus or are intrinsic to the esophagus, such as a posterior hiatal hernia. These studies may also be useful in determining the extent of a mediastinal mass located behind the heart.

Evaluation of potential thyroid masses should include both ultrasound, to identify cystic lesions, and scanning with [131]iodine. [131]Iodine will localize in the thyroid of most patients with mediastinal thyroid tissue. Technetium scanning usually will not be helpful because there is a high background in the blood vessels of the lung and other structures of the chest when using this material. Because goiters are common intrathoracic masses and can be found both in the anterior and posterior mediastinum, these studies will often be rewarding (Irwin *et al.,* 1978).

Computerized Axial Tomography in the Evaluation of Mediastinal Lesions. Computed tomography (CT) has been increasingly important in the evaluation of mediastinal masses. CT provides a transverse cross-sectional image of the mediastinum, separating a mass from normal structures that overlap it as seen by conventional techniques. CT can precisely identify the anatomic extent of mediastinal disease. In addition, the density of the abnormality may allow clues to the differential diagnosis (Kirks and Korobkin, 1981)(see Figure 24-5).

The following general indications for CT of mediastinal abnormalities were proposed after a study to evaluate the ability of computer tomography to delineate the anatomic features of the mediastinum (Heitzman *et al.,* 1977):

1. For evaluation of lesions partially or questionably hidden by mediastinal structures, including lesions of the left lower lobe, where lateral and oblique radiographs are not as helpful as expected;
2. For evaluation of the abnormal or questionably abnormal mediastinum. CT is especially useful to evaluate masses that

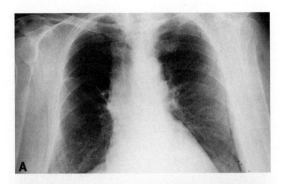

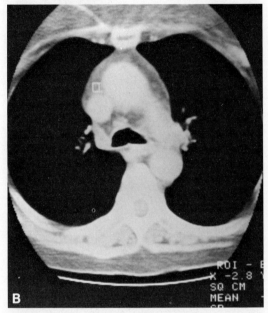

Figure 24-5. (*A*) The chest roentgenogram shows mediastinal widening in an asthmatic patient treated for many years with corticosteroids. (*B*) CT scan. The gray areas around the vessels had the same attenuation values as the subcutaneous fat. Mediastinal lipomatosis. (Photos courtesy of Dr. Harte Crow, Mary Hitchcock Memorial Hospital.)

are small and are partially or completely buried in the mediastinum as seen by conventional techniques. In patients with mediastinal widening caused by fat deposition, the mediastinal structures, especially the vessels, stand out in bold relief against the fat. In older individuals, dilated or tortuous vessels that may be confused with mediastinal pathology can be evaluated by CT;

3. For evaluation of the abnormal or questionably abnormal hilum. Although the hilum is usually not considered a portion of the mediastinum, it is frequently involved by mediastinal disease. CT scanning can distinguish prominent pulmo-

nary vessels from enlarged hilar lymph nodes or neoplastic masses. These studies can be enhanced by the intravenous administration of an iodinated contrast material;

4. For evaluation of the extent and localization of a mediastinal mass; and

5. For evaluation of the contents of mediastinal lesions by determination of their attenuation coefficient. CT scanning can distinguish between blood, fat, air, cerebrospinal fluid, and calcium densities.

Computerized tomography has special application in specific lesions of the mediastinum (see Figure 24-6). For example, CT scanning can identify mediastinal goiter as the cause of a mediastinal abnormality. Features suggesting mediastinal goiter rather than another lesion are: (1) Anatomic continuity with the cervical thyroid; (2) focal calcifications; (3) a relatively high CT number, usually greater than 100 Hounsfield units. This number is higher than that for the soft tissue, such as the muscles of the thoracic cage. In addition, lymphoma or thymoma rarely give a number greater than muscle; (4) a rise in the CT number after bolus administration of iodinated urographic contrast material; and (5) prolonged enhancement after contrast administration (Glazer *et al.*, 1982).

CT can be used to assist fluoroscopically guided aspiration biopsies of central hilar and mediastinal masses. Representative tissue can be obtained and the lesions can be correctly identified as benign or cancerous. A lesion smaller than 1.5 cm and not visible on a lateral chest x-ray can be successfully sampled. Le-

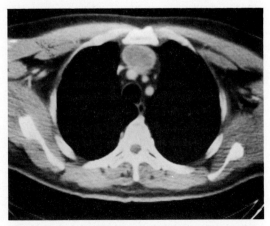

Figure 24-6. CT scan demonstrating a large parathyroid adenoma. (Photo courtesy of Dr. Harte Crow, Mary Hitchcock Memorial Hospital.)

sions that have been diagnosed by cytopathology using this technique include thymomas, adenocarcinomas, germ cell carcinomas, Hodgkin's disease, alveolar cell carcinomas, and a variety of infections including tuberculosis, cryptococcosis, and actinomycosis (Gobien *et al.*, 1981).

Several studies are now available on the use of CT in the evaluation of mediastinal widening. They emphasize that CT can differentiate the vascular from avascular causes of mediastinal widening in about 90% of patients. In 80% of the patients with vascular abnormalities, normal variants, and cystic avascular masses CT provided a specific and correct diagnosis and invasive procedures were avoided. Therefore, several authors now advocate the use of CT as the first procedure after an abnormal chest roentgenogram in the evaluation of mediastinal widening (Baron *et al.*, 1981; Pugatch *et al.*, 1980; Homer *et al.*, 1978).

The combination of CT scanning with contrast techniques is of great value in obtaining further diagnostic information (see Figure 24–7). One recent technique is infusion of a dilute contrast agent through an upper extremity vein. This results in opacification of the superior vena cava and the ipsilateral subclavian and brachiocephalic veins as well as the cranial arteries. This approach is especially useful where the superior vena cava or brachiocephalic vein might be involved by tumor or nodal enlargement. This technique also helps display the azygos veins and any collateral venous circulation that may have developed after obstruction of a major vessel (Kormano *et al.*, 1980).

Computed tomography metrizamide myelography (CTMM) is useful in the preoperative evaluation of posterior mediastinal masses. In this technique, CT is performed following the injection of a small amount of isotonic metrizamide in the subarachnoid space. This allows a simultaneous study of the mediastinal mass, the adjacent mediastinal structures, the pulmonary parenchyma, the spine, and the spinal contents. This technique is helpful in excluding or confirming extradural extension.

The role of computer tomography in evaluating treatment response, to detect relapses, and to assess operability is still being defined. CT has been shown to be superior to conventional radiology, including tomography and lymphography, in detecting pulmonary metastases and mediastinal lymphadenopathy (Husband *et al.*, 1979). Although initial studies of CT in detecting neoplastic involvement

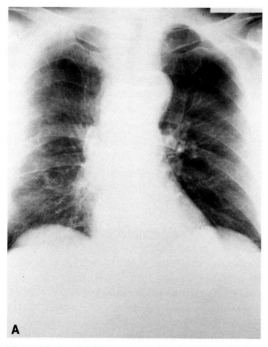

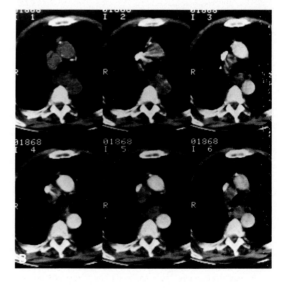

Figure 24–7. (*A*) Chest roentgenogram shows a probable suprahilar mass. (*B*) Dynamic CT scan with contrast. These sections were made at the level of azygos vein and demonstrate enlargement of the azygos node and retrotracheal mass. Lymphoma. (Photo courtesy of Dr. Harte Crow, Mary Hitchcock Memorial Hospital.)

of the mediastinum, particularly involvement of the mediastinal nodes, suggested that CT scanning was not useful, new techniques appear to be changing that conclusion. In one study, in which CT scan impressions were correlated with histologic findings at thoracotomy or mediastinoscopy, the CT scan had a sensitivity of 80% and a specificity of 76% in the detection of neoplastic involvement of the mediastinum. In patients with bronchial carcinoma, the CT scans often showed abnormalities not seen in the chest roentgenograms but in no case did the roentgenograms show abnormalities not demonstrated by the CT scan. Although some have remarked that normal-sized lymph nodes can sometimes contain metastases, in this series all the neoplastic nodes appeared to be greater than 1 cm in diameter and were therefore seen on the CT scan (Rea *et al.*, 1981). The authors concluded that a thoracic CT scan is an essential study in the assessment of the mediastinum in patients with otherwise potentially resectable bronchial carcinoma. It should be noted that in studies with such high-quality definitions of mediastinal structures a two-second scanner is used (Pugatch *et al.*, 1980).

Invasive Procedures. Invasive procedures short of thoracotomy should be considered when there is some clue to the nature or origin of the mediastinal mass and some likelihood that the procedure will provide the diagnosis. If lymphoma is suspected, a bone marrow biopsy may be helpful in yielding the diagnosis. If cervical or supraclavicular nodes are palpable, a biopsy of these should be considered. Bilateral scalene node biopsies in the absence of palpable adenopathy are usually negative and therefore should be avoided. Mediastinoscopy can evaluate right paratracheal adenopathy and in some patients subcarinal adenopathy. The extent of the evaluation depends on the skill of the mediastinoscopist. An anterior mediastinotomy is necessary if biopsy of the left mediastinal lymph nodes is desired. These procedures are worthwhile when the mediastinal mass is suspected to be either a lymphoma, sarcoidosis, other granulomatous disease, or bronchogenic carcinoma.

Bronchoscopy is generally of limited value in the evaluation of mediastinal masses, except when bronchogenic carcinoma is a suspected primary. Esophagoscopy is of value only in mediastinal masses that arise from the esophagus, such as esophageal carcinoma.

Thoracotomy and excision of the mediastinal mass is often necessary for both diagnosis and treatment of the lesion. Material should always be submitted for electron microscopy when possible because several tumors such as seminoma, thymoma, carcinoid, and lymphoma may be difficult to distinguish by light microscopy. In patients who are unable to undergo thoracotomy, an alternative approach is needle biopsy under fluoroscopic guidance or with CT orientation. This procedure is usually performed under local anesthesia. A slotted, 20-gauge, thin-walled needle enables aspiration of large amounts of material. These needles may be as long as seven inches. In lesions immediately adjacent to the major vessels, a 22-gauge, thin-walled needle has been used. In a study of 100 needle aspirates of hilar and mediastinal masses, a positive diagnosis was established in greater than 95% of those subsequently shown to have neoplasms. False-negative results occurred in patients with Hodgkin's disease. Inadvertent puncture of the aorta, superior vena cava, and major pulmonary vessels occurred on numerous occasions but there were no major complications. There was approximately a 12% incidence of pneumothorax; half of these patients required chest tube treatment (Westcott, 1981).

Complications

The major shortcoming of the above diagnostic techniques is that they often fail to differentiate between the many types of tumors found in the mediastinum. Lesions may be missed or their extent not properly demonstrated by these methods. With few exceptions, such as vascular abnormalities, cysts, and lipomatosis, final diagnosis of a mediastinal lesion can be made only by some form of biopsy. The risk of these procedures is usually related to the anesthetic used and the patient's myocardial status.

Systematic Approach to Diagnosis

When evaluating a patient with a mediastinal mass, the physician should integrate the patient's clinical symptoms and findings with anatomic information provided by chest roentgenograms to develop a differential diagnosis of the lesion. This process, particularly precise localization of the lesion, usually leads to additional noninvasive radiographic studies that further define the extent of the lesion or its nature. The physician can then classify the lesion as one of the following:

1. Lesions that do not require surgical intervention for diagnosis, such as mediastinal lipomatosis, calcified lymph nodes, and vascular abnormalities such as aneurysms. These can be adequately diagnosed by CT scans or angiographic studies;

2. Lesions that can be diagnosed by invasive procedures short of thoracotomy. These usually involve lymph nodes and will require mediastinoscopy or mediastinotomy (for left mediastinal nodes). Other procedures that may be valuable are bronchoscopy (in suspected bronchogenic carcinoma), bone marrow biopsy (in lymphoma), and scalene node biopsy (in sarcoidosis); and

3. Lesions that require thoracotomy for diagnoses. These include most primary tumors arising in the mediastinum. A procedure can then be selected that is most likely to yield a diagnosis and lead to appropriate therapy. For patients who cannot undergo thoracotomy or general anesthesia, needle biopsy may provide a diagnosis.

THYMOMAS

Anatomy and Function of the Thymus. The thymus is a lymphoid organ that contains a large number of lymphocytes supported by a reticulum of epithelial cells. In the embryo the epithelial cells arise from the third and fourth branchial clefts and then migrate caudally to the anterior mediastinum to become a bilobed gland. About one-third of normal individuals will have ectopic thoracic or cervical thymic rests. In some areas of the thymus, the epithelial cells aggregate and keratinize to form special structures of unknown function known as Hassall's corpuscles.

The lymphocytes of the thymus are thought to originate from hematopoietic stem cells of the bone marrow and fetal liver prior to birth and from the bone marrow postnatally. Several hormones are produced by the epithelial cells and support differentiation of the lymphocytes, which divide in the cortex. These cells then migrate to the medulla of the gland. They are released to the peripheral circulation as competent T cells, which are responsible for cell-mediated cytotoxicity, suppressor cell activity, and interaction with B-lymphocytes. Active lymphopoiesis may also occur at the cortex. The thymus releases a number of hormones such as thymin, thymosin, and thymopoietin, which are thought to help to maintain T cell competence in peripheral lymphoid tissue. The thymus begins to process precursor cells into T-lymphocytes at about 10 to 12 weeks of gestation. This activity decreases in humans rapidly after birth.

The thymus gradually enlarges until it reaches a size of about 30 to 40 g in late puberty. It then gradually involutes, with the replacement of both the lymphoid and epithelial components by fat. The stress of serious illness or treatment with high doses of glucocorticoids can result in involution of the thymus in several hours.

Incidence and Epidemiology

Thymomas are rare tumors but they represent the most common neoplasm arising in the anterior mediastinum. In a review of several studies encompassing 1950 adult patients with mediastinal masses, 19% had thymomas. These figures probably underestimate the true incidence because only recently has an aggressive approach to the management of myasthenia gravis resulted in the discovery of occult thymomas. Thymomas occur most frequently between the ages of 40 and 60 and rarely occur in children. There is an equal incidence in males and females (LeGolvan and Abell, 1977). It is important to emphasize that the term thymoma indicates a neoplasm of thymic epithelium with a variable degree of lymphocytic elements. Germ cell tumors, Hodgkin's disease, and other lymphomas may arise in the thymus but should not be considered thymomas if a histologic distinction can be made.

Pathology of Thymoma

Grossly, thymomas may have cystic areas or fibrous septi (Rosai and Levine, 1976). The gross appearance at the time of surgery is clinically relevant. The surgeon at operation should determine whether the tumor is encapsulated with no evidence of local invasion or invasive with tumor infiltrating the pericardium, pleura, heart, or great vessels. Studding of the pleura with tumor metastases has also been reported. In particular, the capsule should be studied to determine whether there is discontinuity with local invasion. The capsule should also be examined by frozen section, especially in areas of thick fibrous attachments between the tumor and surrounding structures. This is necessary to determine the invasiveness, which correlates best with the surgical findings rather than the microscopic structure of the tumor.

Several histologic classifications for thymomas have been proposed. One study, from the Mayo Clinic, classified them into four types: Lymphocytic, epithelial, mixed, and spindle cell, which is a variant of the epithelial type (Wychulis *et al.,* 1971). Other authors have combined the lymphocytic and mixed types into a lymphoepithelial group. The lymphocytic tumors consist of a prominent number of lymphocytes against a background of proliferation of epithelial cells. The lymphocytes are small and histologically benign. Lymphoid follicles with defined germinal centers may be present; Hassall's corpuscles may also be seen. In the epithelial tumors, there are sheets, cords, and nests of neoplastic cells, which have large vesicular nuclei, sharply defined nucleoli, indented or folded nuclear membranes, and a generally pale eosinophilic or almost clear cytoplasm. Mitotic figures are not common. Occasionally, pseudorosettes may be seen. In spindle-cell tumors there are cords, sheets, or trabecules of fusiformlike cells with elongated or cigar-shaped nuclei, clumped chromatin, and inconspicuous nucleoli. Lymphocytes may be present at the edges of the tumor and small areas of pseudorosette formation may be seen (LeGolvan and Abell, 1977).

As mentioned above, the neoplastic potential of a thymoma correlates best with the invasion of tissue, as determined during surgery, rather than the histologic appearance of the tumor. The tumor usually directly invades surrounding tissues such as the pericardium, heart, pleura, or great vessels. Very rarely, there are distant metastases to the liver, bone, colon, kidney, brain, and spleen. Some authors believe that the epithelial type is more aggressive and gives rise to distant metastases more frequently than the other histologic types (LeGolvan and Abell, 1977).

At the time of surgery about 65% of thymomas are found to be encapsulated and noninvasive and are therefore considered benign. Approximately 2% of these will recur following resection. On the other hand, of those found to be invasive at the time of surgery, about 20% will recur following resection. In a series from the Mayo Clinic, those patients with an invasive thymoma exhibited a 12.5% long-term survival. In contrast, patients with noninvasive thymoma had survival characteristics similar to those of the general population (Bernatz *et al.,* 1973).

Symptoms and Signs

Approximately two-thirds of patients with thymomas are symptomatic. Although some describe cough, dyspnea, or nonspecific chest pain, as many as 70% have a systemic syndrome associated with the thymoma. The most common illnesses associated with thymoma are myasthenia gravis, which may occur in up to 50% of patients with thymoma, red cell aplasia, hypogammaglobulinemia, collagen vascular disease, megaesophagus, thyroid diseases, and nonthymic cancers. The accompanying table describes the syndromes and diseases that have been associated with thymomas (see Table 24–2).

Myasthenia Gravis.   Myasthenia gravis is

Table 24–2.   Systemic Illness Associated with Primary Mediastinal Masses

Carcinoid of thymus	Cushing's syndrome
Germ cell tumors	Gynecomastia
Pheochromocytomas	Hypertension
Parathyroid adenoma, lymphoma	Hypercalcemia
Intrathoracic goiters	Thyrotoxicosis
Mesothelioma, teratoma, fibrosarcoma, neurosarcoma	Hypoglycemia
Thymoma	Myasthenia gravis, red blood cell aplasia, hypogammaglobulinemia, megaesophagus, myocarditis, dermatomyositis, polymyositis, systemic lupus erythematosis, rheumatoid arthritis, thyroiditis, Sjögren's syndrome, scleroderma, ulcerative colitis, regional enteritis, hyperthyroidism, Cushing's syndrome, Addison's disease, other cancers
Neurofibroma	Osteoarthropathy
Lymphoma	Fever, sweats, pruritus
Neuroblastoma	Opsomyoclonus

an autoimmune disease manifest by rapid exhaustion of voluntary muscles on repetitive contraction, with a delayed return to normal muscular strength. There is strong evidence that myasthenia gravis is caused by the presence of antiacetylcholine-receptor antibodies. These antibodies are directed against the acetylcholine receptors in the end plate or neuromuscular junction of voluntary muscle. The antibodies essentially result in the destruction of these receptors, and postsynaptic function is thus impaired (Drachman, 1978).

Of patients with thymoma, about 70% will be symptomatic, and, of these, about half will have myasthenia gravis. Cancerous thymomas are present in 35 to 40% of the total population of patients with thymoma, whether myasthenia gravis is present or not.

Of patients with myasthenia gravis, about 80% will have an abnormal thymus. The thymic abnormalities fall into two types. Roughly 10 to 30% of patients with myasthenia and abnormal thymic tissue will have either gross or microscopic thymomas. The other patients with myasthenia and an abnormal thymus will have thymic lymphoid follicular hyperplasia, which is a pathologic diagnosis. This process does not necessarily increase the weight or size of the thymus. The pathologic findings include increased numbers of germinal centers in the medullary part of the thymus (Alpert et al., 1971).

In patients with myasthenia gravis, thymectomy will produce improvement in more than 80%. Women younger than 40 seem to have a better response rate to thymectomy than men. After thymectomy, patients with thymoma do not as a group have as great an improvement in muscle strength as those without thymoma. Recent advances in postoperative and long-term medical management of patients with myasthenia gravis, however, suggest that myasthenia gravis is no longer an adverse factor for longevity of patients with thymoma (Wilkens and Castleman, 1979).

A systematic approach for the diagnosis and treatment of patients with myasthenia gravis has been discussed (Drachman, 1978; Wechsler and Olanow, 1980). There is some controversy about the timing of thymectomy. Some prefer to initiate drug therapy and observe the patient for several months, because some patients will have a spontaneous remission. Others favor early thymectomy once generalized myasthenia gravis occurs (Wechsler and Olanow, 1980). Special considerations for

the perioperative management of these patients is beyond the scope of this chapter. The role of preoperative medications, anticholinesterase drugs, the use of corticosteroids, nasotracheal intubation, mechanical ventilation, and high doses of steroids during the perioperative period are discussed in detail elsewhere (Drachman, 1978; Wechsler and Olanow, 1980).

Diagnostic Tests for Myasthenia Gravis. The TENSILON test (edrophonium chloride) is one of the mainstays of the diagnostic panel for myasthenia gravis. TENSILON blocks the hydrolysis of acetylcholine by inhibiting acetylcholine esterase, giving temporary clinical improvement in myasthenia gravis. The test may be found to be positive in up to 90% of patients although it appears to be less so in those who have ocular myasthenia. The TENSILON test should be administered with placebo controls such as saline and nicotinic acid to help eliminate false positives. This test should be performed in a hospital or another place where cardiorespiratory resuscitation can be provided, because deterioration of the patient or allergic reactions to the TENSILON may occur.

Electromyography may support the diagnosis of myasthenia gravis. The Jolly test utilizes repetitive nerve stimulation with observation of the amplitudes of succeeding resultant muscle action potentials. In the normal individual, decrements in amplitude only occur when stimulation frequencies of more than 50/sec are employed. Patients with myasthenia gravis, however, will show decrements of amplitude with stimulation rates of 3/sec. Another test that is employed is the "Jitter" test, which measures the latency between action potentials of two muscle fibers. The latency between two potentials may vary greatly in myasthenia gravis.

Antibody to the acetylcholine esterase receptor can be found in 90% of patients with myasthenia gravis. This can be measured by radioimmunoassay using ^{125}I α-bungarotoxin derived from snake venom. One should remember, however, that the antibody titer, although an important diagnostic tool, does not correlate with the clinical disease state in an individual patient nor are the titers of value in assessing the response to thymectomy.

Diseases that can imitate myasthenia should be considered. These include thyroid disease, multiple sclerosis, myopathic disorders, Lambert-Eaton syndrome, and drug induced phenomenon, such as is seen with penicillamine.

ROENTGENOGRAPHIC FINDINGS AND COMPUTED TOMOGRAPHY IN THE DIAGNOSIS OF THYMIC LESIONS IN PATIENTS WITH MYASTHENIA GRAVIS. The thymus usually is spread out laterally, anterior to the lung and mediastinum and may produce a triangular sail-shaped shadow that can be unilateral or bilateral. This shadow disappears as the thymus involutes. Because the thymus lies against the anterior ribs its lateral borders are often indented by the cartilage and bone, producing a wavy margin on frontal projection. This has been named the thymic wave sign and is absent in thymomas and other anterior mediastinal masses (Mulvey, 1963). Calcifications may be seen in thymomas either at the margins or within the mass.

Several studies address the value of CT scanning for thymoma detection (see Figure 24–8). Studies of the normal thymus by CT scanning indicate that there are great variations in its size, shape, and density. In one study the thymus was identified in 100% of patients under age 30, 73% of patients between 30 to 49 years, and 17% of patients over 49 years of age. The thymus decreased in size with increasing age, but a wide variation was noted in each age group. The density of the thymus was similar to that of muscle in young patients. The attenuation values progressively decreased in older patients and finally became similar to that of fat (Baron et al., 1982; Heiberg et al., 1982).

With increasing experience, radiographers are concluding that mediastinal CT scanning is an appropriate technique for evaluation of thymoma in patients with myasthenia gravis. In one study of 23 patients with myasthenia gravis who underwent thymectomy, four had discrete thymomas. All were detected by CT scanning. Conventional studies were falsely negative in one patient. In the remaining 19 patients, CT scanning was falsely positive in two, but conventional techniques were falsely positive in three (Moore et al., 1982).

In another study, an evaluation of 25 patients with thymic pathology, CT was found useful in suggesting or excluding a diagnosis of thymoma and in distinguishing thymic hyperplasia from thymoma in patients with myasthenia gravis. In that study the thickness of the thymic lobes determined by CT was found to be a more accurate indicator of infiltrating disease than the width. CT was also helpful in differentiating nonthymic cysts from solid tumors and in defining the extent of a thymic neoplasm (Baron et al., 1982). The following guidelines have been recommended for the use of CT in the preoperative detection of thymoma in patients with myasthenia gravis.

1. If thymectomy is clinically mandated independent of thymic pathology (because of symptoms that limit normal activity and that are incompletely relieved by medication), CT should not be routinely performed;

2. Because it is not able to diagnosis mediastinal invasion reliably and because it will only rarely detect unsuspected metastases, CT should not be routinely performed in patients who have a definite anterior mediastinal mass on a chest radiograph (not all radiographers would agree with this recommendation); and

3. In those patients with normal or equivocal chest radiographs and no clinical mandate for thymectomy CT should be routinely performed. In those patients older than 40 years of age and at greater risk for thymoma, CT can sensitively diagnose a neoplasm. In those patients younger than 40, where thymoma occurs less frequently, CT can potentially exclude thymoma although it cannot diagnose it with a high degree of confidence (Fon et al., 1982) because of difficulty in differentiating normal thymus with hyperplasia from thymoma.

Red Cell Aplasia. Pure red cell aplasia is found in about 5% of patients with thymoma, and 30 to 50% of patients with red cell aplasia are thought to have a thymoma. The syndrome usually develops after age 40 and is often associated with the spindle-cell variant of thymoma. Approximately one-third of these patients will respond to thymectomy, adrenal corticosteroids, or immunosuppressive treatment, suggesting an immunologic mechanism for the aplasia. In marrow cultures, serum antibodies and lymphocytes from patients with thymoma and pure red cell aplasia will inhibit erythropoiesis. Antierythropoietin antibodies have been described. Some patients may have a decrease in the numbers of platelets or leukocytes. On bone marrow examination, platelet and leukocyte elements are normal but red cell precursors are not seen (Zeok et al., 1979).

Hypogammaglobulinemia. Hypogammaglobulinemia may be found in about 5% of patients with thymoma. In patients presenting with hypogammaglobulinemia, 10% will have

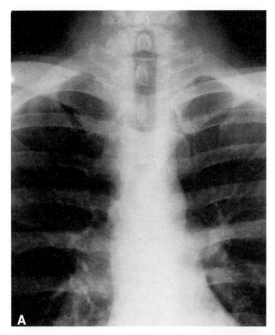

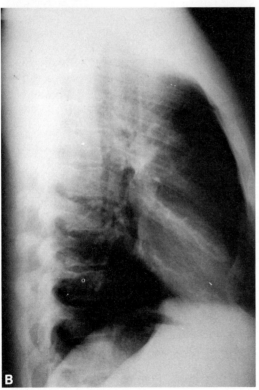

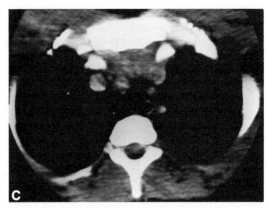

Figure 24–8. A 22-year-old man presented with myasthenia gravis. (*A*) Normal P.A. chest roentgenogram. (*B*) Normal lateral chest roentgenogram. (*C*) CT scan shows a large thymoma. (Photos courtesy of Dr. Harte Crow, Mary Hitchcock Memorial Hospital.)

esis remains to be proven. Hypogammaglobulinemia is also associated with spindle-cell tumors. Thymectomy usually produces little or no response.

Staging

Staging of thymomas is based on the findings at the time of surgery. The capsule should be carefully studied to determine whether local invasion has occurred. Tumors are staged as follows: Stage I: the capsule is intact and there is growth only within the capsule; stage II: there is growth through the capsule into the mediastinal fat tissue, but no additional areas of metastases are found; stage III: there is invasive growth into the surrounding tissue or distant metastases to the pleural surface or elsewhere (Bergh *et al.,* 1978).

Treatment

Nearly all patients who undergo thymectomy will be cured of the tumor if the thymoma is encapsulated and the entire thymus is removed. About 2% of these patients will develop pleural, pericardial, or diaphragmatic metastases at a future date. Thymectomy is indicated if the patient can tolerate the surgery and if the patient has symptoms of myasthenia gravis.

Because thymomas are relatively radiosensitive, radiation therapy should be considered for patients who for other reasons cannot undergo surgery. If a well-encapsulated, noninvasive thymoma is completely removed sur-

a thymoma and one-third of these patients may also have red cell aplasia. Some authors have suggested that the thymoma leads to T cell-mediated suppression of erythropoiesis or immunoglobulin synthesis, but this hypoth-

gically without disturbance of the capsule, postoperative radiotherapy should be deferred. When the thymoma is found to be invasive, an aggressive surgical approach is warranted. As much tumor as possible should be resected when the pericardium, pleura, phrenic nerve, diaphragm, or lung are involved with tumor. These structures should be removed depending upon the patient's ability to tolerate the procedure and the extent of the procedure required. If the heart, trachea, or great vessels are invaded, complete resection may not be possible, but as much tumor as can be safely removed should be resected. The surgeon should define the areas of resected tumor and thymus with radioopaque clips in preparation for radiotherapy. This can usually be administered over a period of three to six weeks in doses of up to 4500 rads. Common complications of radiotherapy include pneumonitis, pericarditis, and, rarely, mediastinitis and myocarditis. If metastases recur, reresection should be considered, because these are usually slow-growing tumors. Special techniques are available for radiation of pleural-based lesions. For patients who fail both radiation and resection, corticosteroids should be employed. Finally, in patients who respond to none of these measures, some success has been observed with chemotherapy with agents such as bleomycin, doxorubicin, cis-platinum, prednisone, and maytansine (Evans et al., 1980; Campbell et al., 1981; Chahihian et al., 1981; Wick et al., 1981).

Although originally it was thought that the prognosis of thymoma was partially dependent upon the presence of myasthenia gravis, improvements in medical management suggest that this is no longer the case (Wilkins and Castleman, 1979). The prognosis at the present appears to be dependent upon the presence of local invasion. The histologic appearance of the tumor has no bearing on prognosis. Patients with invasive thymoma have about a 50% 5-year survival (Batata et al., 1974).

Other Neoplasms of the Thymus. Thymolipoma consists of hyperplastic thymic tissue with large amounts of fat. The mass may be as much as 40 to 50 times the size of a normal thymus. This tumor is asymptomatic, radiolucent, not associated with myasthenia gravis, and does not invade or metastasize. Removal is usually necessary for diagnosis.

Carcinoid tumors of the thymus are derived from the neuroendocrine cells from within the thymus. These tumors have sometimes been confused with thymomas. On removal, the gross appearance may be similar to that of the thymoma. These tumors may be encapsulated but are also invasive and may be metastatic, particularly to bone. Under the light microscope are found sheets of very uniform and round cells that occasionally form an organoid pattern with marked vascularity. Islands of tissue necrosis are seen. Electron microscopy will clearly separate these lesions from thymomas because electron-dense neurosecretory granules can be demonstrated in the cytoplasms of these cells, thereby establishing them as originating in Kulchitsky's or argentaffin cells. The microscopic foci of amorphous necrosis are relatively characteristic of this tumor. Although thymic carcinoids are included in the APUD (amine precursor uptake and decarboxylation) tumors and although they may secrete ACTH, calcitonin, or one of many other hormones, they have never been reported to cause the carcinoid syndrome. Fifty percent of thymic carcinomas, however, will secrete an ACTH-like substance and cause Cushing's syndrome or be associated with multiple endocrine adenomatosis. Because 30% of thymic carcinoids are considered cancerous, treatment includes wide excision of the tumor and thymus, including, if possible, any locally invaded structures. Radiation therapy may help reduce the size of the tumor and palliate symptoms (Felson et al., 1982).

Extragonadal Germ Cell Tumors. The extragonadal germ cell tumors include germinomas or seminomas, teratomas, embryonal carcinoma, teratocarcinoma, choriocarcinoma, and yolk sac tumors (also known as endodermal sinus tumors). Some patients have pure embryonal carcinomas, and others have embryonal carcinomas that contain seminomatous teratocarcinomas, choriocarcinomas, or endodermal sinus elements. The extragonadal germ cell tumors have been divided into seminomatous and nonseminomatous types. Most authors now believe that these tumors are extragonadal in origin rather than being metastases from occult gonadal germ cell tumors (Abell et al., 1965). Seminomas tend to have a much better prognosis and are far more responsive to radiation and chemotherapy than the other neoplastic germ cell tumors. Other sites of origin for these tumors, in addition to the mediastinum and the gonads, are the presacral, sacrococcygeal, and pineal areas.

The histogenesis of extragonadal germ cell tumors is still controversial. Two major theories have gained acceptance: (1) The tumors arise through faulty thymic embryogenesis (Schlumberger, 1946). According to this theory the mediastinal tumors are derived from the thymic anlage that contains germ cells that were dislocated during embryogenesis; and (2) a modified theory has been proposed (Friedman, 1951), according to which the tumors originate from primordial germ cells that migrate to midline structures, including the thymus, during embryogenesis. Two lines of evidence support these theories: (1) Extragonadal mediastinal germ cell tumors are always found adjacent to or within the thymus; and (2) in autopsy studies of patients with germ cell tumors of gonadal origin, metastases to the mediastinum always involve the middle and posterior mediastinal nodes (Martini *et al.*, 1974). The nodes are not necessarily involved when the origin is extragonadal, that is, when they are thymus related.

Teratomas. Teratomas represent the most common germ cell tumor and are composed of multiple tissues not normally found in the thymus or mediastinum. They may contain derivatives of all germ cell layers, although the ectodermal elements are usually most evident. The lesions can be cystic or solid, and occur most frequently in young adults of both sexes. Eighty percent of mediastinal teratomas are benign. Teratomas are frequently calcified and may contain hair and teeth. Although most patients have no symptoms, the most common symptoms are chest pain, cough, or shortness of breath. Occasionally erosion into a bronchus will lead to expectoration of hair and sebaceous material, and an air fluid level may indicate the bronchial communication. Cancerous teratomas may invade adjacent structures, metastasize, and in general cause a poor prognosis (Silverman and Sabiston, 1980).

Seminomas. Seminomas of the mediastinum are most common in men in the age group 20 to 40 years. They may cause symptoms by compression of anterior mediastinal structures, and most patients will have involvement of great vessels at the time of diagnosis.

The histologic differentiation of seminomas from thymomas, lymphomas, and other mediastinal tumors may be difficult. Pathologic features include division of the tumor into numerous islands by fine reticulum fibers, the frequent presence of granulomatous inflammation, cytoplasmic glycogen, and nuclei with coarse chromatin stippling. Electron microscopy may reveal a paucity of desmosomes and absent tonofilaments with complex bizarre nucleoli and short cytoplasmic processes (Polansky *et al.*, 1979). The clinical presentation of seminoma does not differ from that of any slowly invasive or expanding mediastinal tumor. Superior vena caval obstruction may occur with seminoma. Calcification does not occur. Seminoma most commonly spreads throughout the thorax to both the lungs and regional lymph nodes. The next most common sites of metastases are the skeletal system, the liver, spleen, tonsils, thyroid, adrenal, skin, spinal cord, and brain.

Although surgery plays a role in the diagnosis and treatment of seminoma, some authors feel that aggressive surgical resection is not indicated (Silverman and Sabiston, 1980). Radiation therapy is usually very effective in eradicating this tumor, and even when limited skeletal, pulmonary, or nodal metastases are present, combined irradiation and chemotherapy may provide a good chance for either cure or long-term palliation. Although the supraclavicular and low cervical lymph nodes are usually included in the field of radiation, the prophylactic radiation of para-aortic abdominal nodes is not needed. The 5-year survival rate for patients thus treated is approximately 75% (Silverman and Sabiston, 1980). Many authors do not recommend an orchiectomy when the testes are clinically normal (Medini *et al.*, 1979).

Gallium 67 citrate scanning may be helpful in evaluating mediastinal germ cell tumors. This material accumulates in about 75% of metastatic embryonal cell carcinomas, in about half of metastatic seminomas, and in a lower percentage of teratomas (Ayulo *et al.*, 1981).

Nonseminomatous Germ Cell Cancers of the Mediastinum. The nonseminomatous germ cell cancers of the mediastinum include the pure nonseminomatous germ cell tumors and the mixed germ cell carcinomas with embryonal, seminomatous, endodermal sinus, teratomatous, or trophoblastic elements. These are highly cancerous neoplasms of young men that usually present with fulminant symptoms of cough, pain, and dyspnea. There is a high incidence of gynecomastia and hemoptysis. Human chorionic gonadotropin is found in patients with choriocarcinoma;

however, recent reports have shown that β human chorionic gonadotropin levels may also be elevated in embryonal carcinoma, seminoma, and teratocarcinoma (Hainsworth *et al.,* 1982). Alpha fetoprotein is found to be elevated in patients with embryonal carcinoma, teratocarcinoma, and choriocarcinoma and in patients with endodermal sinus tumors. These markers are useful in following the progress of the tumor.

Several studies have demonstrated that patients with Klinefelter's syndrome have a predisposition to the nonseminomatous carcinomas of the mediastinum (Sogge *et al.,* 1979; Curry, *et al.,* 1981; McNeil *et al.,* 1981).

Nonseminomatous carcinomas of the mediastinum are usually lethal within one year in the absence of any treatment. The current treatment plan consists of local resection and intensive cisplatin-containing combination chemotherapy regimens. Although there have been numerous reports that testicular germ cell neoplasms respond better to combination chemotherapy than their mediastinal counterparts, recent studies have demonstrated successful treatment with combination chemotherapy for the mediastinal lesions (Hainsworth *et al.,* 1982). In one study, tumors remaining after chemotherapy were surgically removed if doing so was feasible. Of 31 patients, 21 had a complete remission and the remaining 10 had a partial response. Eighty-nine percent of the patients with complete remission remained free of disease after a median follow-up of 30 months. These response rates are similar to patients with advanced-stage testicular germ cell tumors.

Neurogenic Tumors of the Mediastinum. Neurogenic tumors are the most common mediastinal tumors in children and among the most common mediastinal tumors found in adults. They usually arise in the posterior mediastinum. Many authors divide neurogenic neoplasms into three groups (Fraser and Pare, 1979): (1) Tumors arising from the peripheral nerves. These include the neurilemomas or schwannomas, which arise from the sheath of Schwann, and the neurofibromas, which arise from endoneural tissue. Neoplastic schwannomas, also called neurofibrosarcomas, may arise *de novo* or may result from cancerous degeneration of a neurofibroma. Neurofibromas of the mediastinum may be solitary or they may be associated with von Recklinghausen's disease. Neurofibromas may also degenerate to neurofibrosarcoma; (2) tumors arising

from sympathetic ganglia. These include ganglioneuroma, neuroblastomas, and sympathicoblastomas. The first tumor mentioned is usually benign and easily excised at the time of thoracotomy; and (3) tumors arising from paraganglionic cells. These include the pheochromocytomas and paragangliomas or chemodectomas. These tumors can be benign or neoplastic. The chemodectomas can be locally invasive and may involve the aorta or the pulmonary artery. They can be found anywhere in the mediastinum.

The roentgenographic findings in patients with neurogenic mediastinal masses are of interest. Ganglioneuromas may have an elongated or triangular configuration and less definition than other neurogenic tumors (Wychulis *et al.,* 1971). Calcification is relatively common in these neoplasms although it is not a reliable indicator of benignity. Calcification is usually speckled or punctate although it may be curvilinear or globular.

In a large review of 706 cases of mediastinal neurogenic tumors at the Mayo Clinic, 69 patients had extension through an intervertebral foramen, resulting in the neoplastic mass having the shape of a dumbbell. Ten percent of these tumors were neoplastic. The majority of the 69 patients presented with symptoms of spinal cord compression. More than half the patients had erosion of vertebral pedicles or enlargement of the intervertebral foramen adjacent to the posterior mediastinal mass. The authors recommended myelographic studies to determine whether a dumbbell-shaped tumor is present and recommended a one-stage combined resection carried out by a team of thoracic surgeons and neurosurgeons to remove both the intraspinal and mediastinal component (Akwari *et al.,* 1978).

Although routine myelography may be helpful in determining whether extradural extension has occurred, it is not as definitive as computed tomography with metrizamide myelography. This technique permits visualization of the mediastinal mass, adjacent mediastinal structures, the spine, the spinal contents, and pulmonary parenchyma. Calcifications are more readily identified. This technique can exclude or confirm extradural extension of a paravertebral chest mass. The surgeon therefore has the option of decompressive laminectomy before thoracotomy for definitive removal of the lesion. The initial laminectomy is necessary to reduce neurologic morbidity related to bleeding from residual extradural tumor if the chest approach is used initially (Kirks and Korobkin, 1981).

Mesenchymal Tumors of the Mediastinum. The mesenchymal tumors of the mediastinum include lipomas, liposarcomas, fibromas, hemangiomas, and lymphangiomas or hygromas.

Lipomas tend to occur in the anterior mediastinum. They are easily recognized both by chest roentgenogram and CT scans because their radiographic density is less than that of other soft tissues. Mediastinal lipomas are usually unassociated with symptoms and, because they are soft and pliable, they do not obstruct or compress mediastinal structures. They may resemble pericardial cysts or elevation of a hemidiaphragm. Liposarcomas occur most often in the posterior mediastinum and are often confused with neurogenic tumors.

Mediastinal lipomatosis is the accumulation of fat in the mediastinum that results from Cushing's syndrome or long-term corticosteroid therapy. This tends to produce mediastinal widening and enlarged pleural-pericardial fat pads. Rapid weight gain may also cause this radiographic picture. The fat deposition is asymptomatic and can be readily diagnosed by CT scan.

Hemangiomas are usually found in the anterior mediastinum (Leibovici and Oner, 1962). These masses are usually well-encapsulated and may be multiple. Other associated hemangiomatous malformations may be found in the kidneys, liver, and spleen. One diagnostic sign is a phlebolith.

Lymphangiomas are rare tumors, usually in infants, that may occur in a cystic form that extends into the neck. In older patients, cystic masses may occur in the lower anterior mediastinum. These tumors are usually lined by endothelial cells and are filled with a clear yellow fluid. They are soft and pliable and therefore rarely cause symptoms by compression of adjacent structures.

Angiofollicular Lymphoid Hyperplasia. A group of patients has been described with "large, asymptomatic, benign hyperplastic" mediastinal lymph nodes (Castleman et al., 1956). The nodes contain hyperplastic lymphoid follicles with capillary proliferation and endothelial hyperplasia. The histologic findings may be confused with thymoma and malignant lymphoma. Approximately 200 cases of angiofollicular lymph node hyperplasia have been described and have been divided into the hyaline vascular or plasma cell histologic variants. Most patients have the hyaline vascular type. The enlarged nodes are usually in the mediastinum or appear as a solitary pulmonary nodule although other lymph nodes may be involved. The plasma cell variant has been associated with nephrotic syndrome, anemia, growth failure, fever, hyperglobulinemia, peripheral neuropathy, and hypoalbuminemia.

The diagnosis of angiofollicular lymph node hyperplasia is usually made by direct biopsy of the enlarged node. Ultrasound and thoracic computed tomography have occasionally been used to differentiate these lesions from cystic lesions (Gibbons et al., 1981). Although the lesion is usually solitary, multicentric disease can occur and should be sought once the diagnosis is made, according to the physical findings and the patient's symptoms. Patients have also had retroperitoneal disease with ureteral or urovascular obstruction.

Therapy for angiofollicular lymph node hyperplasia has included surgical resection, radiotherapy, and corticosteroids. In both the hyaline vascular and plasma cell subtypes, surgical removal of isolated lesions is usually curative, particularly when these present as asymptomatic pulmonary masses. Radiation does not appear to be an efficacious form of therapy and chemotherapy appears unwarranted. Case reports have been published that describe improvement of symptoms and regression of lymphadenopathy after several months of high-dose corticosteroids (Hineman et al., 1982).

MESOTHELIOMA

Incidence and Epidemiology

Mesothelioma is a rare lung tumor. With the increasing use of asbestos, the incidence of this tumor appears to be rising. As many as 1100 new cases per year now occur in the United States (Weiss and Muggia, 1979). Over one million men and women were employed as asbestos workers in World War II and the postwar period. Because of the long period between asbestos exposure and the development of mesothelioma, some researchers have estimated that an epidemic of mesothelioma will occur in this country in the next ten to 20 years.

There is still controversy regarding whether or not the presence of mesothelioma of the pleural or peritoneal cavities is pathognomonic of asbestos exposure. For many patients a history of contact with asbestos is not available. Although patients have been reported who have had only casual exposure to asbestos, such as a child whose father is an asbestos worker, casual exposure rarely results in the development of mesothelioma. In workers who have had a heavy exposure for long periods of time, however, a high prevalence of the tumor is found and, in some series, that prevalence has been reported to be as high as 10% (Selikoff, 1976). Most patients with mesotheliomas are men, and the peak incidence is between ages 50 and 70 although case reports describe both children and patients over 80 years of age with mesothelioma. Wives of men who work with asbestos also have an increased risk for the development of pleural mesothelioma.

Etiology and Pathogenesis

The pathogenesis of mesothelioma has attracted considerable interest, and experimental models have recently been developed for study of this problem. The focus of much of this research has been related to the type of asbestos to which an individual has been exposed. Asbestos is a mineral that readily separates into long, flexible fibers, which are classified into chrysotile, which appears as a silky, serpentine fiber, and the amphiboles, which separate into straight, rodlike fibers. Amphiboles differ from chrysotile not only in their physical appearance but also in their chemical composition. The major types of amphiboles are amosite, anthophyllite, and crocidolite. In the United States both types of asbestos are distributed throughout the geologic strata, but mines are active now only in Vermont and Canada. Of the asbestos marketed in this country, more than 90% is chrysotile.

Many studies have explored the differences in the pathogenic potential of these different forms of asbestos. Different mines may produce similar types of asbestos that have different fiber sizes, and because of differences in exposures and differences in techniques of mining and milling the fibers, a determination of the relationships among fiber size, type, composition, and pathogenicity has been difficult. Rates of mesothelioma are different, however, in various exposed populations. In recent studies of mesothelioma, amphiboles were found in lungs of patients with mesothelioma whereas chrysotile was found both in patients with mesothelioma and in similar quantities in controls without mesothelioma (McDonald, 1980; Becklake, 1982). In addition, in studies in Canada, amphiboles were found in the lungs of chrysotile miners although the major airborne dust to which they were exposed was from chrysotile (Rowlands et al., 1982). These studies suggest that there is preferential clearing of the chrysotile fiber as compared with amphiboles, and, for this reason, amphibole exposure may result in mesothelioma.

Particle size and shape may determine clearance, but pathogenic activity may also be related to the time of survival of the particles in the lung before they are cleared. Clearance, of course, is related to the chemical properties of each type of asbestos. Thus, the pathogenic potential of a given fiber may be related to its size and shape as well as to its chemical composition.

In contrast to this hypothesis, recent studies suggest that the dimensions of the fiber and not its chemical properties are the most important factors in determining the development of tumors in rats (Selikoff and Lee, 1978). In these studies, long, thin fibers of a variety of types of asbestos caused tumor growth. This finding is consistent with studies of populations where mesothelioma is found in patients exposed to crocidolite, which is composed of long and thin fibers. Tumors appear to be relatively rare in patients exposed to the blunt, short fibers of such asbestoses as amosite and anthophyllite. Recently, zeolite was reported to be associated with the occurrence of mesothelioma in Turkey (Baris et al., 1981). The fibers of zeolite are structurally similar to crocidolite, but are dissimilar chemically to the asbestos particles.

Little is known of the mechanism of neoplastic transformation of mesothelial cells after exposure to asbestos. This transformation has not occurred in mesothelial cell cultures after exposure to asbestos. The role of cocarcinogens is currently under evaluation.

The mechanism by which asbestos arrives at the peritoneum is unknown. It is thought that the fibers are transported via lymphatics from the lung. Sputum containing asbestos fibers may be coughed and swallowed and fibers may be transported across the mucosa of the gut. Only in patients exposed to amphiboles do peritoneal mesotheliomas occur, perhaps because chrysotile fibers disintegrate in the abdominal tissue.

Pathology

The three major sites of origin of mesothelioma are the pleura, the peritoneum, and the pericardium although rare mesotheliomas of the tunica vaginalis, ovary, uterus, and fallopian tubes have been described. The pleural tumors are by far the most common (Parmley and Woodruff, 1974; Fligiel and Kaneko, 1976; Wood and Bouchelle, 1978).

Mesothelioma metastasizes by direct invasion into nearby tissue although distant metastases may also be seen. Pleural mesothelioma tends to invade the chest wall and then compresses and invades the lung (see Figure 24-9); pleural effusion is usually present. The size of the effusion may decrease over a very short period of time, possibly within weeks, if there is rapid tumor growth, and complete replacement of the hemithorax may result. Diffuse involvement of the pleura at the time of diagnosis usually occurs. In peritoneal mesothelioma, widespread intra-abdominal metastases are common, and serosanguineous ascites is often present. When the primary site is the pleura, distant metastases can include the regional lymph nodes, brain, lungs, adrenal glands, and liver; the diaphragm may also be invaded. With abdominal mesothelioma, frequent sites of metastases are pelvic lymph nodes, liver, lung, pericardium, and pleura. The microscopic appearance of the metastatic cells may differ considerably from that of the cells of the original tumor.

Histology of Mesothelioma. Although mesothelioma can sometimes be diagnosed by needle biopsy, open pleural biopsy is the preferred method for diagnosing the disease. Pleural, pericardial, and peritoneal mesotheliomas do not differ in any major way histologi-

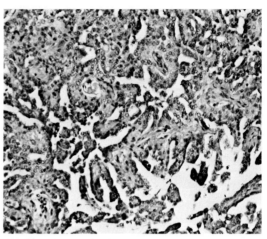

Figure 24-10. Mesothelial mesothelioma with a papillary surface pattern (hematoxylin and eosin ×200).

cally. Most authors classify the tumor into three forms: (1) The epithelial; (2) the fibrous; and (3) the biphasic form, which contains elements of both the epithelial and fibrous varieties (Suzuki, 1980) (see Figures 24-10, 24-11, and 24-12).

Epithelial Form. Several histologic patterns are seen in the epithelial form of mesothelioma. Papillary, tubular, cordlike, and sheetlike arrangements of neoplastic cells are seen. The cells can vary in size and shape, and sometimes two or three patterns can be found in a single biopsy. The sheet-like form must be differentiated from squamous cell carcinoma. In the mesothelioma, however, neither intracellular bridging nor keratinization is found. The papillary and tubular forms may be confused with adenocarcinomas of the lung, ovary, and gastrointestinal tract. The mesothelioma cells may produce intracellular signet-ring-like vacuoles, and, with specific stains, hyaluronic acid can be demonstrated in some of these vacuoles. Glycogen can be found in the cytoplasm although mucin is not found in the mesothelioma cells. The nuclei of the cells of this form are usually round with fine chromatin material. Nuclei are well developed and a high rate of abnormal mitosis is usually not seen.

Fibrous Form. The cells in this form of mesothelioma are reminiscent of the cells of fibrosarcoma. They are often fusiform or spindle shaped, and they often show a parallel arrangement. They may have an ovoid or elongated nucleus and well-developed nucleoli. Pleomorphism is usually not a feature of the histology.

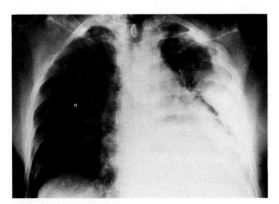

Figure 24-9. Malignant mesothelioma. The tumor mass is surrounding and compressing the left lung.

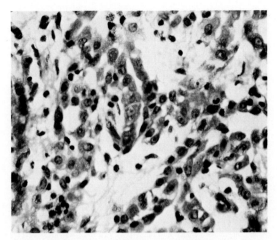

Figure 24–11. Mesothelial mesothelioma showing a papillary and tubular growth pattern, (hematoxylin and eosin ×500).

Biphasic Form. In the biphasic form of mesotheliomas, the epithelial elements can be essentially the same as described above. In addition, in this form, a mesenchymal cell type is usually seen, and frequently cells are found that are at some stage between the two cell types. These have been called "transitional" cells by several authors. The mesenchymal cells appear as elongated or spindle-shaped cells with elongated nuclei and histologic features reminiscent of leiomyosarcoma or fibrosarcoma. The transitional cell is a fusiform cell with characteristics of epithelial cells such as junctional systems or hemidesmosomes. The transitional cells are best viewed by electron microscopy.

Electron Microscopy of Mesothelioma. Transmission electron microscopy is of great

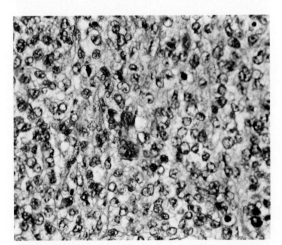

Figure 24–12. Mesothelial mesothelioma, solid grown pattern (×500).

value in the diagnosis of mesothelioma, and all specimens obtained by biopsy from patients suspected of having mesothelioma should be fixed in glutaraldehyde or buffered formalin for electron microscopy. The major role of electron microscopy is for differentiation of mesothelioma from other tumors, particularly from adenocarcinoma (Stoebner *et al.,* 1979; Suzuki, 1980).

Epithelial Form. Electron microscopy of the epithelial form can show a variety of features. In the well-differentiated epithelial form the tumor cell is similar in appearance to hyperplastic mesothelium. Typical structures include microvilli, tonofilaments, and desmosomes, irregularly shaped nuclei with freely dispersed chromatin, and a large nucleolus. Glycogen is usually seen. The features of the epithelial form of mesothelioma that may be helpful in differentiating it from hyperplastic mesothelium include a cell coat of numerous microvillae, a nucleolar alteration with separation of the fibrillar component from the granular one, and a variability in structural differentiation as the tissue is examined. In less well-differentiated epithelial mesotheliomas, some of the epithelial characteristics may be missing, such as with a loss of polarity, loss of microvilli, loss of junctional structures, or discontinuity of the basement membrane. In some epithelial tumors, transitional cells strongly support the diagnosis of mesothelioma. In the epithelial form, cilia, secretory granules containing mucin, and osmiophilic lamellar structures are not found; the presence of these structures implies that the tumor is of another origin.

Fibrous Form. The fibrous form contains cells that lack the characteristics of epithelial cells, such as microvilli, basement membranes, and tonofilaments. These cells appear to be spindle cells or fibroblasts. They frequently exhibit direct cell-to-cell contact. Occasionally, intermediate cells can be identified in the fibrous form of mesothelioma.

The finding of typical or atypical mesothelial cells associated with transitional cells is strong evidence for a diagnosis of mesothelioma. Electron microscopy allows the recognition of these cells and, in the presence of a light microscopic picture of epithelial cells, may allow the discovery of ultrastructural findings consistent with mesothelioma.

Although small foci of cartilage can occasionally be seen in a mesothelioma, two mesotheliomas with unusual histologic features were recently described containing cartilage with foci of calcification and ossification and fibrochondrosarcomatous tissue. These foci were intimately associated with a mesothelioma, which suggested that they formed an integral part of the tumor. One of the tumors contained a cup of cartilage and bone around blood vessels and bronchioles in the lung parenchyma (Goldstein, 1979).

Biphasic Form. Electron microscopy of the biphasic form of mesothelioma can result in the identification of three cell types: The epithelial cell, the intermediate cell, and the mesenchymal cell. The epithelial cells may be quite similar in appearance to those described for the epithelial form of the mesothelioma. The nonepithelial or mesenchymal cell has an appearance similar to a fibroblast; direct contact between cells, however, is often seen. The intermediate or transitional cell has characteristics of both the epithelial and nonepithelial cells. Under the light microscope they may be confused with nonepithelial cells, but electron microscopy usually reveals some ultrastructural features, such as a discontinuous basement membrane, remnants of microvilli, tight junctions, or tonofilaments, that are reminiscent of epithelial cells.

Symptoms and Signs

Presenting clinical symptoms in pleural mesothelioma include dyspnea, chest pain, cough, weight loss, and fever. A few asymptomatic patients can be suspected of having pleural mesothelioma on the basis of an abnormal chest roentgenogram. In peritoneal mesothelioma, abdominal swelling, weight loss, abdominal pain, and anorexia are common complaints (Chahinian *et al.,* 1982). These symptoms usually worsen as the disease progresses. In 25% of patients with pleural mesothelioma in one study, symptoms were present for more than six months before the diagnosis was made. The right side was involved more frequently than the left. Pleural effusion was present at one time or another in 95% of patients. Pleural nodules or thickening, a mass lesion, or an interstitial pattern may be seen, and clubbing may be present. Cardiac findings include pericardial rubs; the murmur of pulmonic stenosis may occur. Echocardiography was positive for pericardial effusion in some patients, but was falsely negative at autopsy or surgery in patients who had pericardial involvement secondary to nodular or diffuse involvement of the pericardium with minimal or no pericardial fluid. Gallium ci-

trate 67 whole body scanning was positive for the primary tumor in nearly 90% of patients (Chahinian *et al.,* 1982).

Initially, pleural fluid may be a problem and may necessitate thoracentesis for symptomatic relief. As the disease progresses the pleural fluid is replaced by tumor. Thoracentesis may yield no fluid at early stages of the disease. Complete involvement of the hemithorax may occur in as short a period as two months.

As the disease advances the patient complains of increasing shortness of breath caused by shunting of blood through the tumor-encased lung. Pain, paraplegia, dysphagia, or respiratory obstruction may occur secondary to the involvement of the vertebral column, esophagus, or trachea, respectively. Superior vena caval obstruction may also occur. The patients usually die of respiratory failure that is often complicated by pneumonia or cardiac arrythmias.

In peritoneal mesothelioma, a physical examination usually reveals a full abdomen in a patient who has been losing weight. Ascites or an obvious abdominal mass is usually present. Peritoneoscopy or laparotomy reveals several large masses along the peritoneum or diffuse studding. These tumors should be biopsied and material submitted for both light and electron microscopy to avoid confusion with metastatic adenocarcinomas, particularly of ovarian origin. Some patients may complain of diarrhea or constipation. Death usually results because of malnutrition and cachexia complicated by small-bowel obstruction.

Routine laboratory studies do not aid in diagnosis of mesothelioma, but several abnormalities may occur. Thrombocytosis may occur at some time during the course of disease, and patients have been reported to have platelet counts above $1,000,000/mm^2$ (Chahinian *et al.,* 1982). Serum carcinoembryonic antigen may be elevated in some patients. Serum immunoelectrophoresis may show an increase in IgG, IgA, or IgM. The reasons for these elevations are not known. Serum alphafetoprotein is usually not elevated.

Diagnosis

Because many tumors can metastasize to the lung or to the peritoneum, a histologic diagnosis is important for distinguishing between mesothelioma and these other tumors (see Figure 24–13). The simplest and most direct approach is usually a needle biopsy of the pleura and examination of pleural fluid cytol-

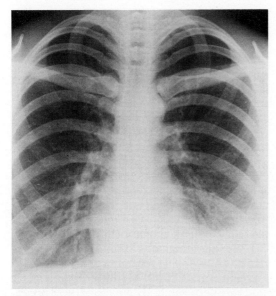

Figure 24-13. A 22-year-old white woman complained of pleuritic chest pain after a tennis game. Thoracentesis revealed bloody exudative pleural fluid. Two weeks later she developed massive bleeding into the pleural cavity. At surgery, a diaphragmatic sarcoma was found invading the pleural space.

ogy. Unfortunately, there is a low yield of positive diagnoses of mesothelioma with this procedure (Antman, 1980; Griffiths *et al.,* 1980) (see Figure 24-14). Because pathologic diagnosis of this tumor is difficult, large amounts of tissue are often necessary for a pathologic examination, which should include light and electron microscopy, in order to make an exact diagnosis. Despite the expertise of the examiner in the fine structure of mesothelioma in one recent series, 33 of 210 mesotheliomas were classified as "probable" after pathologic

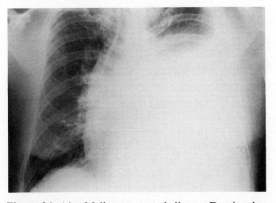

Figure 24-14. Malignant mesothelioma. Despite the appearance consistent with pleural effusion, no fluid could be withdrawn by thoracentesis.

examination (Suzuki, 1980). If needle biopsy and cytologies are negative and mesothelioma is suspected, an open pleural biopsy should be undertaken, and large amounts of tissue should be given to the pathologist for study. For the same reasons that needle biopsy does not yield enough tissue to make a definitive diagnosis, cytologic examination of pleural or peritoneal fluid using both light and electron microscopy of cell blocks continues to have a high false-negative and high false-positive rate (Tao, 1979).

Because of the diversity and complexity of the morphology of mesothelioma, pathologists have sought many methods to ascertain the diagnosis. Routine pleural fluid examination provides no specific information; pleural fluid is usually exudative and bloody, and the glucose concentration varies inversely with the quantity of neoplastic cells (Clarkson, 1964). Although pleural fluid hyaluronic acid levels have been reported to be specific for a diagnosis of mesothelioma when they are greater than 0.8 mg/mL, an overlap can be found with fluid from patients with other causes for pleural effusions. In one study, 12 of 19 patients with mesothelioma had concentrations greater than 0.8 mg/mL. Levels in this range have also been reported for other neoplasms (Rasmussen and Farber, 1967; Legha and Muggia, 1977). In a study by agarose gel electrophoresis of 5359 pleural effusions, hyaluronic acid was detected in 165. Of the patients whose pleural fluid hyaluronic acid was 5 to 50 mg/mL, two-thirds had mesothelioma. In the patients who had levels over 50 mg/mL, 82% had mesothelioma (Boersma *et al.,* 1980). From these studies, it appears that although an elevated hyaluronic acid level in pleural fluid is highly suggestive of mesothelioma, it is not diagnostic. Recent work has suggested that electrophoresis of tumor digests of biopsy specimens in mesothelioma reveals hyaluronic acid, but further studies are needed to confirm this finding (Waxler *et al.,* 1979). A tissue digest of diffuse mesothelioma has been reported to contain elevated concentrations of chondroitin sulfate and only trace amounts of hyaluronic acid, findings that may reveal a biochemical variant of pleural mesothelioma (Iozzo *et al.,* 1981).

Unlike most tumors that metastasize to the pleura, mesothelioma has a tendency to grow along needle tracks and biopsy sites, including thoracotomy scars. Twenty-eight of 327 patients with mesothelioma who had a pleural biopsy, chest tube drainage, or thoracotomy developed a chest wall mass at the site (Elmes and Simpson, 1976). Despite this phenomenon, however, invasive procedures are necessary for both diagnosis and symptomatic relief.

CT Evaluation of Mesothelioma. The CT findings in mesothelioma are not pathognomonic. CT scanning may reveal pleural effusion, rib destruction, pleural plaques or calcifications, intrapulmonary nodules and thickening of pleura, pleural fissures, and paramediastinal structures, especially at the bases and posteriorly (Kreel, 1981). The major value of CT scanning is that it reveals the extent of the tumor, which is usually more widespread than apparent on the chest roentgenogram. CT scanning also demonstrates the tendency of mesothelioma to spread directly into the mediastinum, the chest wall, and the abdomen (Alexander *et al.*, 1981). CT attenuation values have not been helpful in distinguishing between pleural fluid and pleural tumor, probably because the mesotheliomas have variable attenuation values. CT scanning may also reveal the extent of other pulmonary diseases such as asbestosis. These may be a consideration in evaluating the patient for further therapy. CT scanning of the pleural primary tumor may also be of value in following the course taken by patients after chemotherapy or radiation, but further studies are necessary to determine the efficacy of this method.

Systematic Approach. In a patient with a pleural lesion and dyspnea or prolonged chest pain, mesothelioma is a likely diagnosis whether there is a history of asbestos exposure or not. Although there is a low yield of tissue in mesothelioma, thoracentesis and pleural biopsy should usually be performed; if adenocarcinoma of the pleura is present, it can usually be diagnosed by these techniques. If no diagnosis is obtained by pleural biopsy and there are no other sites for biopsy, such as a chest wall mass, open pleural biopsy should be performed, with material submitted for routine and electron microscopy. In peritoneal mesothelioma, direct biopsy of a peritoneal mass is usually the only method for obtaining the diagnosis.

Not all authors agree with this approach. One group of surgeons has concluded that staging of a suspected mesothelioma should take place before any biopsy of the pleural tumor. This approach avoids the possibility of seeding a needle tract or biopsy site until a definitive procedure can take place (Butchart *et al.*, 1981).

Staging

Staging has been recommended by some authors for patients who may undergo radical surgery (Butchart *et al.*, 1981). Their approach is to (1) thoroughly evaluate the anatomic spread of the tumor and (2) at the same time, avoid the risk of seeding tumor into the chest wall by avoiding direct biopsy prior to a definitive evaluation. These authors recommend an evaluation based upon barium studies of the esophagus to determine esophageal compression, bronchoscopy to search for endobronchial lesions, computerized axial tomography to assess chest wall involvement or mediastinal involvement, pneumoperitoneography to evaluate diaphragmatic spread, and, possibly, mediastinoscopy to determine the histology of the cells. In addition, brain, liver, and bone scans are performed. By the use of these procedures, the tumor can be classified into one of the following stages: Stage I—the tumor is confined within the capsule of the parietal pleura; stage II—the tumor is invading the chest wall or is involving mediastinal structures, and/or lymph node involvement inside the chest is seen; stage III—the tumor is penetrating the diaphragm and is involving the peritoneum or the opposite pleural cavity or lymph nodes outside of the chest; and stage IV—distant blood-borne metastases are found.

Obviously, the above procedures are time consuming, costly, and invasive. Several complications can occur such as anesthetic mishaps, pneumonia resulting from bronchoscopy, peritonitis resulting from pneumoperitoneography, and mediastinal hemorrhage related to mediastinoscopy (see Figures 24–15, 24–16, and 24–17). The major value of these procedures is in separating patients for either radical surgery or other treatment.

Specific and Supportive Measures

Surgery. Radical curative surgery has a small role in the treatment of mesothelioma. The tumor is usually widespread at the time of presentation and frequently involves the pleura and the diaphragm. Radical surgery implies removing all the tumor with a wide margin of clearance. Thus, pleuropneumonectomy is performed with excision of the ipsilateral pericardium and hemidiaphragm. Four reports of large series of pleural pneumonectomies have been tabulated (Butchart *et al.*,

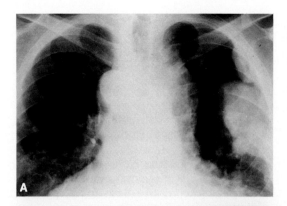

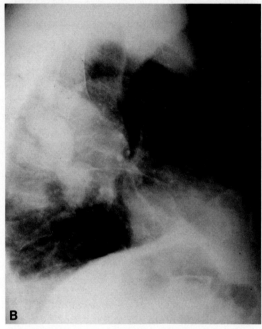

Figure 24-15. (A) P.A. chest roentgenogram shows a large, right-sided mass with mediastinal involvement. (B) Lateral chest roentgenogram. Bronchoscopy revealed tracheal compression. Mediastinoscopy resulted in massive mediastinal hemorrhage and death. Malignant mesothelioma with mediastinal involvement.

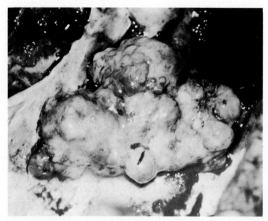

Figure 24-16.   Pathologic specimen from the patient described in Figure 24-15. The site of hemorrhage was the mediastinal aspect of the tumor.

vent recurrent effusions, to reduce discomfort produced by tumor bulk, and to reduce pain caused by invasion of the chest wall. Some authors imply that partial surgical resection leads to an apparent increase in survival following diagnosis, especially when combined with radiotherapy or chemotherapy (Aisner and Wiernik, 1978; Antman *et al.*, 1980). At the present, the role of radical and palliative surgery and their supplementation by radiotherapy or chemotherapy cannot be completely evaluated because of the small number of patients treated and the lack of comparisons with single, alternative therapies. To add to the confusion, in another study patients who had partial resection had longer survival than did patients who had complete resection or biopsy only (Chahinian *et al.*, 1982).

1981), and in these series were found a 10 to 37% two-year survival and a maximum 10% five-year survival. The operative mortalities in two of the series were 23% and 31%. Although some researchers express enthusiasm about removing mesotheliomas in patients with adequate cardiopulmonary and nutritional statuses (Butchart *et al.*, 1981), others remain pessimistic about the role of surgery except for apparent, well-localized lesions (Lewis *et al.*, 1981).

Palliative Surgery. Palliative surgery, usually pleurectomy, has been utilized to pre-

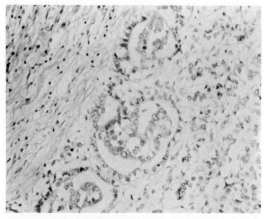

Figure 24-17.   Microscopic section of the tumor shows malignant mesothelioma with glandlike areas in the stroma.

Radiotherapy. Conventional radiotherapy has not been very effective in the treatment of mesothelioma. Temporary control of symptoms has been reported in patients treated with high-dose, high-energy radiotherapy (Chahinian and Holland, 1978; Brady, 1981). Radioactive colloidal compounds, including radioactive colloidal gold and chromic phosphate, have been used in attempts to control recurrent pleural effusions and in small series of patients long-term survival has been effected.

Although some success has been achieved in reducing pain with the use of radiotherapy, the large doses and wide ports required result in radiation pneumonitis; photon therapy with appropriate shielding followed by electron beam therapy helps reduce this problem.

Chemotherapy. Advances in chemotherapy have been hindered by the small number of patients available. Doxorubicin appears to be the most active drug. Cyclophosphamide, methotrexate, 5-fluorouracil, and 5-azacytidine are all thought to have some benefit (Weiss and Muggia, 1979).

Combinations of doxorubicin with other drugs appear more effective than doxorubicin alone or doxorubicin plus radiotherapy (Chahinian et al., 1982). Further studies are necessary to clarify the roles of these agents.

Combined Modality Therapy. Some authors have suggested that the combination of radical surgery or tumor debulking with radiation and/or chemotherapy results in prolongation of survival. No randomized studies are available with which this hypothesis can be evaluated, and it is not clear whether the patients undergoing multimodal therapy who had extensive surgery had other clinical characteristics that were favorable for longer survival (Antman et al., 1980; Chahinian et al., 1982).

Future Prospects

A major step toward the control of a neoplasm is early diagnosis. In one recent study, 25% of patients with mesothelioma were not diagnosed within the first six months after presentation (Chahinian et al., 1982). Further advances in the study of tumor markers and tumor products should help improve this situation.

New trials of combination chemotherapy for combatting mesothelioma are being organized and should lead to better results with chemotherapy. Radiosensitizers and matura-tional agents may have a major role in augmenting chemotherapy animal models, and nude mice bearing mesotheliomas are now available for further drug studies.

Solitary Fibrous Tumors of the Pleura (Benign Mesothelioma). Benign mesotheliomas are discussed because they must be differentiated from malignant mesothelioma. Recent studies have described the clinical and pathologic features of solitary fibrous tumors of the pleura (Scharifker and Kaneko, 1979; Briselli et al., 1981). The origin of the localized fibrous tumor of the pleura remains unknown. The tumor may arise in subpleural areolar tissues (Klemperer and Rabin, 1931), but some researchers have proposed that the mesothelial cell itself is the cell of origin for these tumors. Several authors support the hypothesis that both malignant and benign pleural tumors originate from multipotential cells in submesothelial connective tissue or from both submesothelial fibroblasts and surface mesothelial cells.

Solitary fibrous tumors of the pleura most commonly arise during the fifth and sixth decades of life although they have been reported in children under ten years of age and in octogenarians. No relationship to environmental exposure, including asbestos exposure, has been reported. A slightly higher incidence in women than in men has been noted. The tumor tends to occur equally in the right and left hemithorax, in contrast to malignant mesothelioma, which tends to favor the right hemithorax. The tumor arises more frequently in the visceral rather than the parietal pleura. One-half to three-quarters of the patients are symptomatic, and the most common symptoms are cough, chest pain, dyspnea, pulmonary osteoarthropathy, and fever. Less common symptoms include hemoptysis, chills, night sweats, and weight loss. Pleural effusion and hypoglycemia have been reported.

Most of the solitary fibrous tumors are encapsulated and range in size from 1 to 36 cm, with a mean size of 6 cm. A pedicle is evident on gross examination of most of these tumors. With light microscopic examination, spindle-shaped cells that have minimal nuclear pleomorphism and rare or absent mitoses are visible. There may be areas of necrosis or hyalinization. Variations from these pathologic features have been discussed in the literature (Briselli et al., 1981). Some authors point out that there exists no single histologic feature that allows a definitive prognosis. Favorable prognostic signs, however, are the presence of a pedicle and circumscription of the tumor without invasion into the lung or surrounding structures. Nuclear pleomorphism or a high mitotic rate in the presence of encapsulation does not necessarily imply a poor prognosis. If left untreated, however, these tumors may invade locally and compress vital structures, and the patient will die, usually within two to three years of diagnosis. Resection is usually curative. Although tumor recurrences have been reported, many of those tumors have been successfully removed with repeat resections.

REFERENCES

Abell, M. R.; Fayes, J. V.; and Lampe, I.: Retroperitoneal germinomas (seminomas) without evidence of testicular involvement. *Cancer,* **18:**273–290, 1965.

Aisner, J., and Wiernik, P. H.: Malignant mesothelioma. *Chest,* **74:**438–444, 1978.

Akwari, O. E.; Payne, W. S.; Onofrio, B. N.; Dines, D. E.; and Muhm, J. R.: Dumbbell neurogenic tumors of the mediastinum. *Mayo Clin. Proc.,* **53:**353–358, 1978.

Alexander, E.; Clark, R. A.; Colley, D. P.; and Mitchell, S. E.: CT of malignant pleural mesothelioma. *A.J.R.,* **137:**287–291, 1981.

Alpert, L. I.; Papatestas, A.; Kark, A.; Osserman, R. S.; and Osserman, K.: Histologic reappraisal of the thymus in myasthenia gravis. *Arch. Pathol.,* **91:**55–61, 1971.

Antman, K. H.; Blum, R. H.; Greenberger, J. S.; Flowerdew, G.; Skarin, A. T.; and Canellos, G. P.: Multimodality therapy for malignant mesothelioma based on a study of natural history. *Am. J. Med.,* **68:**356–362, 1980.

Ayulo, M. A.; Dibos, P. E.; Aisner, S. A.; and Moravec, C.L.: Gallium[67] citrate scanning in primary mediastinal seminoma. *J. Nucl. Med.,* **22:**796–797, 1981.

Baris, Y. I.; Saracci, R.; Simonata, L.; Skidmore, J. W.; and Artuioli, M.: Malignant mesothelioma and radiological chest abnormalities in two villages in central Turkey. *Lancet,* **1:**984–987, 1981.

Baron, R. L.; Lee, J. K. T.; Sagel, S. S.; and Levitt, R. G.: Computed tomography of the abnormal thymus. *Radiology,* **142:**127–134, 1982a.

Baron, R. L.; Lee, J. K. T.; Sagel, S. S.; and Peterson, R. R.: Computer tomography of the normal thymus. *Radiology,* **142:**121–125, 1982b.

Baron, R. L.; Levitt, R. G.; Sagel, S. S.; and Stanley, R. J.: Computed tomography evaluation of the mediastinal widening. *Radiology,* **138:**107–113, 1981.

Batata, M. A.; Martini, N.; Huvos, A. G.; Aguilar, R. I.; and Beattie, E. J., Jr.: Thymomas—Clinicopathologic features, therapy and prognosis. *Cancer,* **34:**389–396, 1974.

Becklake, M. R.: Exposure to asbestos and human disease. *N. Engl. J. Med.,* **306:**1480–1481, 1982.

Bergh, N. P.; Gatzinsky, P.; Larsson, S.; Lundin, P.; and Ridell, B.: Tumors of the thymus and thymic region. I. Clinical pathological studies of the thymomas. *Ann. Thorac. Surg.,* **25:**91–98, 1978.

Bernatz, P. E.; Khonsari, S.; Harrison, E. G., Jr.; and Taylor, W. F.: Thymoma. Factors influencing prognosis. *Surg. Clin. North Am.,* **53:**885–892, 1973.

Boersma, A.; Degand, P.; and Biserte, G.: Hyaluronic acid analysis in the diagnosis of pleural mesothelioma. *Bull. Eur. Physiopathol. Respir.,* **16:**41–45, 1980.

Brady, L. W.: Mesothelioma: The role for radiation therapy. *Semin. Oncol.,* **8:**329–334, 1981.

Briselli, M.; Mark, E. J.; and Dickersin, P. R.: Solitary fibrous tumors of the pleura. *Cancer,* **47:**2678–2689, 1981.

Butchart, E. G.; Ashcroft, T.; Barnsley, W. C.; and Holden, M.P.: The role of surgery in diffuse mesothelioma of the pleura. *Semin. Oncol.,* **8:**321–328, 1981.

Campbell, M. D.; Pollard, R.; and Al-Sarraf, M.: A complete response to metastatic malignant thymoma to cisplatinum, doxorubicin and cyclophosphamide, A case report. *Cancer,* **48:**1315–1317, 1981.

Castleman, B.; Iversur, L.; and Menendez, V. P.: Localized mediastinal lymph-node hyperplasia resembling thymoma. *Cancer,* **9:**822–830, 1956.

Chahinian, A. P.; Bhardwaj, S.; Meyer, R. J.; Jaffrey, I. S.; Kirschner, P. A.; and Holland, J. F.: Treatment of invasive and metastatic thymoma. Report of 11 cases. *Cancer,* **47:**1752–1761, 1981.

Chahinian, A. P., and Holland, J. F.: Treatment of diffuse mesothelioma, a review. *Mt. Sinai J. Med. (N.Y.),* **45:**54–67, 1978.

Chahinian, A. P.; Pajac, T. F.; Holland, J. F.; Norton, L.; Ambinder, R. M.; and Mandel, E. M.: Diffuse malignant mesothelioma. *Ann. Intern. Med.,* **96:**746–755, 1982.

Clarkson, B.: Relationship between cell type glucose concentration and response to treatment in neoplastic effusions. *Cancer,* **17:**914–928, 1964.

Curry, W. A.; McKay, C. E.; Richardson, R. L.; and Greco, F. A.: Klinefelter's syndrome and mediastinal germ cell neoplasms. *J. Urol.,* **125:**127–129, 1981.

Davis, J. M. G.: Ultrastructure of the human mesotheliomas. *J.N.C.I.,* **52:**1715–1723, 1974.

Drachman, D. B.: Myasthenia gravis. *N. Engl. J. Med.,* **298:**136, 186, 1978.

Echevarria, R. A., and Arean, V. M.: Ultrastructural evidence of secretory differentiation in a malignant pleural mesothelioma. *Cancer,* **22:**323–332, 1968.

Elmes, P. C., and Simpson, M.: The clinical aspects of mesothelioma. *Q. J. Med.,* **45:**427–449, 1976.

Evans, N.: Mesotheliomas of the uterine and tubal serosa and tunica vaginalis testis. *Am. J. Pathol.,* **19:**1461–1471, 1943.

Evans, W. K.; Thompson, D. M.; Simpson, W. J.; Feld, R.; and Phillips, M. J.: Combination chemotherapy in invasive thymoma. *Cancer,* **46:**1523–1527, 1980.

Felson, B.: *Chest Roentgenology.* W. B. Saunders Company, Philadelphia, 1973.

Felson, B.; Castleman, B.; Levinsohn, E. M.; and Markarian, B.: Cushing's syndrome associated with mediastinal mass. *A.J.R.,* **138:**815–819, 1982.

Fligiel, Z., and Kaneko, M.: Malignant mesothelioma of the tunica vaginalis propria testis in a patient with asbestos exposure. *Cancer,* **37:**1478–1484, 1976.

Fon, G. T.; Bein, M. E.; Mancuso, A. A.; Kessey, J. C.; Lupetin, A. R.; and Wong, W. S.: Computed tomography of the anterior mediastinum in myasthenia gravis. *Radiology,* **142:**135–141, 1982.

Fraser, R. G., and Pare, J. A. P.: *Diagnosis of Diseases of the Chest,* vol. III. W. B. Saunders Company, Philadelphia, 1979.

Friedman, N. B.: The comparative morphogenesis of extragenital and gonadal teratoid tumors. *Cancer,* **4:**265–276, 1951.

Gibbons, J. A.; Rosencrantz, H.; Posey, D. J.; and Watts, M.: Angiofollicular lymphoid hyperplasia resembling a pericardial cyst: Differentiation by computerized tomography. *Ann. Thorac. Surg.,* **32**:193–196, 1981.

Glazer, G. M.; Axel, L.; and Moss, A.: CT diagnosis of mediastinal thyroid. *A.J.R.,* **138**:495–498, 1982.

Gobien, R. P.; Skucas, J.; and Paris, B. S.: CT assisted fluoroscopically guided aspiration biopsy of central hilar and mediastinal masses. *Radiology,* **141**:443–447, 1981.

Goldstein, B.: Two malignant pleura mesotheliomas with unusual histological features. *Thorax,* **34**:375–379, 1979.

Griffiths, M. H.; Riddell, R. J.; and Xipell, J. M.: Malignant mesothelioma: A review of 35 cases with diagnosis and prognosis. *Pathology,* **12**:591–603, 1980.

Hainsworth, J. D.; Einhorn, L. H.; Williams, S. D.; Sewart, M.; and Greco, F. A.: Advanced extragonadal germ cell tumors. *Ann. Intern. Med.,* **97**:7–11, 1982.

Hammon, J. W., Jr., and Sabiston, D. C., Jr.: The mediastinum. In Goldsmith, H. S. (ed.): *Practice of Surgery, Thoracic Surgery.* Harper & Row, Publishers, Inc., Hagerstown, Maryland, 1979.

Heiberg, E.; Wolverson, M. K.; Sundarlam, M.; and Nouri, S.: Normal thymus: CT characteristics in subjects under age 20. *A.J.R.,* **138**:491–494, 1982.

Heitzman, E. R.; Goldwyn, R. L.; and Proto, A. V.: Radiologic analysis of the mediastinum, utilizing computed tomography. *Radiol. Clin. North Am.,* **15**:309–329, 1977.

Hineman, V. L.; Phyliky, R. L.; and Banks, P. M.: Angiofollicular lymph node hyperplasia and peripheral neuropathy. *Mayo Clin. Proc.,* **57**:379–382, 1982.

Homer, M. J.; Wechsler, R. J.; and Carter, B. L. Mediastinal lipomatosis. *Radiology,* **128**:657–661, 1978.

Husband, J. E.; Peckham, M. J.; McDonald, J. S.; and Hendry, W. F.: The role of computed tomography in the management of testicular teratoma. *Clin. Radiol.,* **30**:243–252, 1979.

Iozzo, R. V.; Goldes, J. A.; Chen, W. J.; and Wight, T. N.: Glycosaminoglycans of pleural mesothelioma. A possible biochemical variant containing chondrostin sulfate. *Cancer,* **48**:89–97, 1981.

Irwin, R. S.; Braman, S. S.; Arvanitidis, A. N.; and Hamolsky, M. W.: Thyroid scanning in preoperative diagnosis of mediastinal goiter. *Ann. Intern. Med.,* **89**:73–74, 1978.

Kirks, D. R., and Korobkin, M.: Computed tomography of the chest in infants and children: Techniques and mediastinal evaluation. *Radiol. Clin. North Am.,* **19**:409–419, 1981.

Klemperer, R., and Rabin, C. B. Primary neoplasms of the pleura. *Arch. Pathol.,* **11**:385–412, 1931.

Kormano, M. J.; Dean, P. B.; and Hamlin, D. J.: Upper extremity contrast medium infusion in computer tomography of upper mediastinal masses. *J. Comput. Assist. Tomogr.,* **4**:617–620, 1980.

Kreel, L.: Computer tomography in mesothelioma. *Semin. Oncol.,* **8**:302–312, 1981.

Legha, S., and Muggia, F. M.: Pleural mesothelioma. Clinical features and therapeutic implications. *Ann. Intern. Med.,* **87**:613–621, 1977.

LeGolvan, D. P., and Abell, M. R.: Thymomas. *Cancer,* **39**:2142–2157, 1977.

Leibovici, D., and Oner, V.: Hemangioma of the posterior mediastinum. Review of the literature and report of a case. *Am. Rev. Respir. Dis.,* **86**:415–419, 1962.

Lewis, R. J.; Sisler, G. E.; and MacKenzie, J. W.: Diffuse mixed malignant pleural mesothelioma. *Ann. Thorac. Surg.,* **31**:53–60, 1981.

Lyons, H. A.; Calvey, G. L.; and Sammons, B. P.: The diagnosis and classification of mediastinal masses. *Ann. Intern. Med.,* **51**:897, 1959.

Martini, N.; Golbey, R. B.; Hajdu, S. J.; Whitmore, W. F.; and Beattie, E. J., Jr.: Primary mediastinal germ cell tumors. *Cancer,* **33**:763–769, 1974.

McDonald, J. C.: Asbestos-related disease: An epidemiologic review. In Wagner, J. C. (ed.): *Biological Effects of Mineral Fibers.* International Agency for Research on Cancer, Lyon, 1980.

McNeil, M. M.; Leong, A. S. Y.; and Sage, R. E.: Primary mediastinal embryonal carcinoma in association with Klinefelter's syndrome. *Cancer,* **47**:343–345, 1981.

Medini, E.; Levitt, S. H.; Jones, T. K.; and Rao, Y.: The management of extratesticular seminoma without gonadal involvement. *Cancer,* **44**:2032–2038, 1979.

Moore, A. V.; Korobkin, M.; Powers, B.; Olanow, W.; Ravin, C. E.; Putman, C. E.; Breiman, R. S.; and Ram, P. C.: Thymoma detection by mediastinal CT: Patients with myasthenia gravis. *A.J.R.,* **138**:217–222, 1982.

Mulvey, R. B.: The thymic "wave" sign. *Radiology,* **81**:834–838, 1963.

Oldham, H. N., and Sabiston, D. C., Jr.: Primary tumors and cysts of the mediastinum. *Monogr. Surg. Sci.,* **4**:243–279, 1967.

Pahwa, R.; Ikehara, S.; Pahwa, S. G.; and Good, R. A.: Thymic function in man. *Thymus,* **1**:27, 1979.

Parmley, T. H., and Woodruff, J. D.: The ovarian mesothelioma. *Am. J. Obstet. Gynecol.,* **120**:234–241, 1974.

Polansky, S. M.; Barwick, K. W.; and Ravin, C. E.: Primary mediastinal seminoma. *Am. J. Roentgenol.,* **132**:17–21, 1979.

Pugatch, R. D.; Faling, L. J.; Robbins, A. H.; and Spira, R.: CT diagnosis of benign mediastinal abnormalities. *A.J.R.,* **134**:685–694, 1980.

Rasmussen, K., and Farber, V.: Hyaluronic acid in 247 pleural fluids. *Scand. J. Respir. Dis.,* **48**:366–371, 1967.

Rea, H. H.; Shevland, J. E.; and House, A. J. S.: Accuracy of computed tomographic scanning in assessment of the mediastinum and bronchial carcinoma. *J. Thorac. Cardiovasc. Surg.,* **81**:825–829, 1981.

Rosai, J., and Levine, G. D.: *Tumors of the Thymus. Atlas of Tumor Pathology—Second Series,* Fascicle 13. Armed Forces Institute of Pathology, Washington, D.C., 1976.

Rowlands, N.; Gibbs, G. W.; and McDonald, A. D.: Asbestos fibers in the lungs of chrysotile miners and millers—a preliminary report. *Ann. Occup. Hyg.,* **26**:411–415, 1982.

Rubush, J. L.; Gardiner, I. R.; Boyd, W. C.; and Ehrenhaft, J. L.: Mediastinal tumors: Review of 186 cases. *J. Thorac. Cardiovasc. Surg.,* **65**:216–222, 1973.

Scharifker, D., and Kaneko, M.: Localized fibrous mesothelioma of pleura. *Cancer,* **43**:627–635, 1979.

Schlumberger, H. G.: Teratoma of the anterior mediastinum in the group of military age. A study of 16 cases and a review of theories of genesis. *Arch. Pathol.,* **41**:398–444, 1946.

Schulof, R. S., and Goldstein, A. L.: Thymosin and the endocrine thymus. *Adv. Intern. Med.,* **22**:121–143, 1977.

Selikoff, I. J.: Lung cancer and mesothelioma during prospective surveillance of 1249 asbestos insulation workers 1963–1974. *Ann. N.Y. Acad. Sci.,* **271**:448–56, 1976.

Selikoff, I. J., and Lee, D. H. K. *Asbestos and Disease.* Academic Press, Inc., New York, 1978.

Silverman, N. A., and Sabiston, D. C.: Mediastinal masses. *Surg. Clin. North Am.,* **60:**757–777, 1980.

Sogge, M. R.; McDonald, S. D.; and Cofold, P. B.: The malignant potential of a dysgenetic germ cell in Klinefelter's syndrome. *Am. J. Med.,* **66:**515–518, 1979.

Stoebner, P.; Bernaudin, J. F.; Nebut, M.; and Basset, F.: Contribution of electron microscopy to the diagnosis of pleural mesothelioma. *Ann. N.Y. Acad. Sci.,* **330:**751–760, 1979.

Suzuki, Y.: Pathology of human malignant mesothelioma. *Semin. Oncol.,* **8:**268–282, 1980.

Suzuki, Y.; Churg, J.; and Kannerstein, M.: Ultrastructure of human malignant diffuse mesothelioma. *Am. J. Pathol.,* **85:**241–262, 1976.

Tao, L.: The cytopathology of mesothelioma. *Acta Cytol. (Baltimore),* **23:**209–213, 1979.

Wang, N. S.: Electron microscopy in the diagnosis of pleural mesotheliomas. *Cancer,* **31:**1046–1054, 1973.

Waxler, B.; Eisenstein, R.; and Battifora, H.: Electrophoresis of tissue glycosaminoglycans as an aid in the diagnosis of mesothelioma. *Cancer,* **44:**221–227, 1979.

Wechsler, A. S., and Olanow, C. W.: Myasthenia gravis.

Surg. Clin. North Am., **60:**931–945, 1980.

Weiss, R. B., and Muggia, F. M.: Working conference on mesothelioma treatment trials. *Cancer,* **39:**3799–800, 1979.

Westcott, J. L.: Percutaneous needle aspiration of hilar and mediastinal masses. *Radiology,* **141:**323–329, 1981.

Wick, M. R.; Nichols, W. C.; Ingle, J. N.; Bruckman, J. E.; and Okazaki, H.: Malignant predominantly lymphocytic thymoma with central and peripheral nervous system metastases. *Cancer,* **47:**2036–2043, 1981.

Wilkins, E. W., Jr., and Castleman, B.: Thymoma: A continuing survey at Massachusetts General Hospital. *Ann. Thorac. Surg.,* **28:**252–256, 1979.

Wood, C., and Bouchelle, W. H.: Benign mesothelioma simulating a uterine lyomyoma. *Am. J. Obstet. Gynecol.,* **132:**225–226, 1978.

Wychulis, A. R.; Payne, W. S.; Clagett, O. T.; and Woolner, L. B.: Surgical treatment of mediastinal tumors. A forty year experience. *J. Thorac. Cardiovasc. Surg.,* **62:**379–392, 1971.

Zeok, J. V.; Todd, E. P.; Dillon, M.; DeSimone, P.; and Utley, J. R.: The role of thymectomy in red cell aplasia. *Ann. Thorac. Surg.,* **28:**257–260, 1979.

25

Neoplasms of the Esophagus

MONTAGUE LANE and JOHN C. McKECHNIE

Introduction

Cancer of the esophagus is a disease that at best can be described as dismal. Symptoms occur late in the disease's course and are often initially disregarded by patients and occasionally by physicians. Hence, the disease is usually far advanced at diagnosis. The clinical course of most patients is characterized eventually by starvation and cachexia. Despite technologic advances in diagnosis and therapy, fewer than 5% of patients survive five years.

Incidence and Epidemiology

The incidence of esophageal cancer varies remarkably throughout the world. In the United States it was estimated that there were 8880 new cases of esophageal cancer in 1981 (American Cancer Society, Inc., 1980). This represents approximately 1% of new cancers (excluding nonmelanomatous cancers of the skin and *in situ* carcinomas). The disease is approximately four times more frequent in men than in women (Cutler and Devesa, 1973) and occurs predominantly in individuals 60 years of age and older. It is about three times more common in blacks than in whites (Schoenberg *et al.*, 1971; Cutler and Young, 1975; Garfinkel *et al.*, 1980). The incidence in black men is 13.3/100,000, compared to 3.5/100,000 in white men and 3.4/100,000 in black women, compared to 0.9/100,000 in white women (Garfinkel *et al.*, 1980).

A 105% nationwide increase in mortality from esophageal cancer in black men has occurred in the past 25 years without a corresponding increase in black women or in whites (Schoenberg *et al.*, 1971). It is unknown if this

remarkable change in incidence is the result of increased smoking and alcohol use, urbanization, impoverished socioeconomic conditions, or genetic factors. A study from the Baltimore Veterans Administration Medical Center reports a sudden steep increase in hospital admissions for esophageal cancer in black men in 1978 and 1979 compared to prior years, without a change in numbers of cases among white men (Rogers *et al.*, 1982). An explanation for this phenomenon has not been found despite careful analysis of variables. Whether this observation of a very recent abrupt increase in esophageal cancer in blacks will be representative of a still-worsening national trend or is an isolated occurrence is unknown. Within the United States a higher incidence of esophageal cancer has been recognized in urban areas of the Northeastern states and in Middle Atlantic states, such as South Carolina, compared to other parts of the country (Bates *et al.*, 1971).

The incidence of esophageal cancer varies widely in different regions of the world. Some of the areas of highest incidence include the Caspian littoral, regions adjacent to the Caspian Sea, including the Iranian province of Mazandaran (Kmet and Mahboubi, 1972; Mahboubi *et al.*, 1973), and the Soviet Republics of Kazakstan and Turkmen (Kmet and Mahboubi, 1972), the Transkei region of Cape Province in South Africa (Roussel *et al.*, 1974; Weber and Hecker, 1978), Kenya (Ahmed and Cook, 1969), northern China (British Medical Journal, 1975; Miller, 1978), Curacao (Weber and Hecker, 1978), Puerto Rico (Martinez, 1969), and parts of India (Sanghir *et al.*, 1955) and Ceylon (Stephen and Uragoda, 1970). Regions of high incidence may be separated by a relatively short distance from very low-incidence areas. The countries with high incidence rates include France, Chile, Switzerland, and Japan. The disease occurs with low frequency in Norway, Sweden, Denmark, Israel, and Nigeria (Levin *et al.*, 1974). The incidence in men in the northeast section of Iran is approximately three hundred times that in Nigerian men (Doll and Peto, 1981).

Despite the fact that men are more often afflicted than women, the male/female ratio varies widely in different locales. This ratio is approximately 14:1 in France and 8:1 in Switzerland, as compared to 2 to 3:1 in Norway, Sweden, and the United States, and 1.6:1 in Israel. In the Transkei the male/female ratio in blacks is 9:1 and in whites 4:1. In the Iranian province of Mazandaran the ratio is reversed, 1:1.3 (206/100,000 for men and 262/100,000 for women) (Mahboubi *et al.*, 1973). In many series, carcinoma of the upper third of the esophagus has been more common in women, whereas men more commonly suffer from lesions in the lower two-thirds of the esophagus.

Etiology and Pathogenesis

Epidemiologic evidences of high incidences of esophageal carcinoma in various geographic locales and in different population groups have led to intensive studies of possible etiologic factors, both exogenous and endogenous. Some of the factors that have been most clearly shown to bear some relationship to cancer of the esophagus are listed in Table 25–1. The pathogenesis of esophageal cancer, however, is uncertain, despite these apparent associations.

Social Habits. Excessive use of tobacco and alcohol by patients with esophageal cancer was first reported in 1937 (Ahlbom, 1937). Many studies have since confirmed a strong influence on the incidence of this disease by these factors, singly and together, in various populations. Among smokers the incidence appears to be somewhat higher for those who smoke more than one pack a day than for those smoking less. For alcohol users, the relationship to amount consumed is even more dramatic (Wynder and Bross, 1961). A recent study suggested that although tobacco and alcohol are both important, the amount of alcohol consumed provided a better relationship to esophageal cancer incidence than did the amount of tobacco that was used (Tuyns *et al.*,

Table 25–1. Factors Associated with High Incidence of Esophageal Cancer

FACTOR	COMMENT
Social habits	
Tobacco	Heavy cigarette smoking; chewing; pipe and cigar smoking
Alcohol	Excessive consumption; type of beverage may be a factor
Obstructive lesions	
Benign stricture	Usually secondary to lye; mean age younger
Achalasia	Middle-third lesions
Barrett's esophagus	Adenocarcinomas
Dietary factors	
Plummer-Vinson syndrome	Iron and other nutrient deficiencies; upper-third lesions; females > males
Others	Bracken fern; *Croton flaveus*, dietary deficiencies, nitrosamines
Genetic factors	
Tylosis	Rare
Other primary cancers	Cancers of upper aerodigestive tract

1977). In general, total alcohol intake appears to be more important than type of beverage for esophageal cancer. Certain types of concentrated alcoholic beverages, however, such as pai kan in China (60 to 85% alcohol) (Wynder and Bross, 1961) and apple brandy in Normandy (Tuyns *et al.*, 1979) have been associated with particularly high incidences of esophageal cancer. Both tobacco and alcohol consumption appear to be important factors in the etiology of cancer of the esophagus in the United States, France, Sweden, and Great Britain. In India, tobacco consumption alone (both smoking and chewing, including betel nut admixtures) has been implicated (Joyant, 1977). The very high incidence of esophageal cancer in the Bantu of South Africa has been related to numerous factors, including pipe smoking by men and women and the drinking of home-brewed beer called kaffir, which is often fortified with a brandy (Burrell, 1957).

Obstructive Lesions. Benign stricture of the esophagus has been repeatedly associated with a high incidence of carcinoma (Benedict, 1941; Gerami *et al.*, 1971). Most often these strictures are the result of lye ingestion that has occurred accidentally in children or intentionally by individuals who have unsuccessfully attempted suicide. These cancers occur ten to 30 or more years after lye ingestion, so that the patients are younger than those who develop cancer of the esophagus in the general population. The incidence has been estimated at 3.5 to 5.5% in patients with lye stricture, but may be much higher with longer periods of follow-up. A relationship between benign strictures of other types and carcinoma is less well established (see Figure 25–1B).

Carcinoma of the esophagus has been associated with achalasia in an incidence varying from 0 to 20% (Just-Viera and Haight, 1969). An incidence of 41/100,000 was noted in a group of 1318 patients with achalasia observed for 13 years, which is much above the incidence in the U.S. general population (Wychulis *et al.*, 1971). These cancers may develop anywhere in the esophagus, but the majority occur in the middle third. They are thought to be related to the chronic irritation induced by retained food and secretions.

Barrett's Esophagus. Barrett's esophagus is one in which columnar epithelium has replaced the squamous epithelium of the lower esophagus (see Figure 25–1A) and is thought to be the result of chronic reflux esophagitis.

True adenocarcinomas of the esophagus probably constitute less than 5% of primary esophageal tumors; the vast majority of adenocarcinomas are associated with Barrett's esophagus (Naef *et al.*, 1975; Radigan *et al.*, 1977).

Dietary Factors. The high incidence of esophageal cancer in the Caspian littoral has been related to dietary deficiency of vitamin A and other nutrients (Hormozdiari *et al.*, 1975) secondary to low fruit and vegetable consumption (Cook-Mozaffari *et al.*, 1979). In the Transkei, esophageal cancer has been associated with mineral deficiency in garden plants (Burrell *et al.*, 1966). Deficiency of B vitamins, especially riboflavin, has been suggested as a predisposing factor for esophageal cancer (Wynder, 1979). Sideropenic dysphagia (Plummer-Vinson syndrome; Paterson-Brown-Kelly syndrome) is a syndrome of dysphagia, hypochromic microcytic anemia, mucosal atrophy of the mouth and pharynx, hypoferremia, koilonychia, achlorhydria, and upper esophageal stenosis or web. It evidently is a consequence of nutritional deficiencies of iron and B vitamins, commonly occurs in

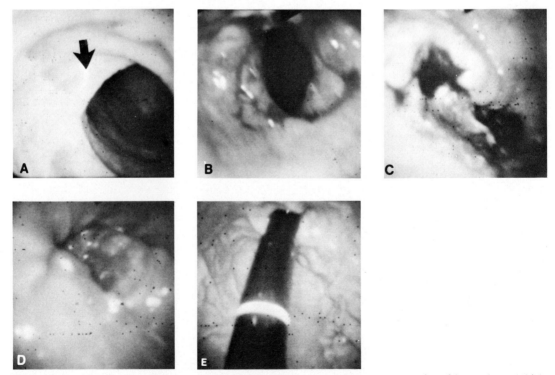

Figure 25–1. (*A*) Barrett's esophagus. Normal squamous epithelium occupies the upper portion of the esophagus, which appears on the left-hand margin and upper margin of the photograph. The columnar epithelium is seen in the central portion of the photograph, invading from below (arrow). (*B*) Benign stricture of the esophagus with polypoid excrescences that simulate tumor. (*C*) Squamous cell carcinoma (noncircumferential) with heaped-up leading edge, ulceration, and luminal narrowing. (*D*) Adenocarcinoma of stomach invading into esophageal submucosa. (*E*) Endoscope in stomach visualizing gastroesophageal junction from below.

Scandinavia and England, and has been related to a high frequency of esophageal cancer, particularly in women, in these countries. These carcinomas generally arise proximal to the webs (Ahlbom, 1936; Lindvall, 1953; Wynder and Fryer, 1958). Japanese who consume bracken fern regularly have three times the risk of developing cancer compared to Japanese who avoid such consumption (Ahmed and Cook, 1969). An excessive incidence of esophageal cancer has been associated with nitrosamines in food in northern China (British Medical Journal, 1975; Miller, 1978) and with ingestion of the juices of *Croton flaveus* in Curacao (Weber and Hecker, 1978).

Genetic Factors. Tylosis is a genetic disorder in which affected individuals have hyperkeratotic changes of the palms and soles and a remarkably high incidence of squamous cell carcinoma of the esophagus. Fortunately, the disease is very rare (Howell-Evans *et al.,* 1958).

Other Primary Cancers. Patients who have had squamous cell cancers of the upper aerodigestive tract are at increased risk for development of carcinoma of the esophagus, presumably because the mucosa of these areas is exposed to the same carcinogenic influences (Goldstein and Zornoza, 1978).

Pathology and Natural History

Approximately 95% of malignant esophageal tumors are squamous cell carcinomas (see Figure 25–12). They vary in degree of differentiation, but generally are moderately or well differentiated tumors. Adenocarcinomas make up the majority of the remainder and may be well or poorly differentiated, or adenoid cystic carcinomas, adenoacanthomas, mucoepidermoid carcinomas, and adenosquamous carcinomas (del Regato and Spjut, 1977). Adenocarcinomas most often arise in the lower esophagus in association with a Barrett's esophagus or in ectopic gastric mucosa (see Figure 25–1D). Rare tumors of the esophagus are those of nonepithelial origin, such as leiomyosarcoma, choriocarcinoma (McKechnie and Fechner, 1971), and rhabdomyosarcoma. In the United States the majority of squamous cell carcinomas arise most often in the middle third and also in the lower third of the esophagus. Upper third lesions are less common, except in Iran and in association with Plummer-Vinson syndrome.

Modes of Spread. The modes of spread of esophageal cancers are best understood after briefly reviewing the structure and anatomic relationships of the esophagus. It is a muscular tube, generally 23 to 25 cm in length, that originates at the lower border of the cricoid cartilage at the level of the C6 vertebra. The upper third of the esophagus includes the cervical esophagus and extends from the pharyngoesophageal junction to the aortic arch; the middle third extends from the aortic arch to the inferior pulmonary vein, some 10 cm above the esophagogastric junction, and the lower third extends from the inferior pulmonary vein to the esophagogastric junction.

Structurally, the esophagus consists of an inner mucosa, a submucosal coat, a muscular coat, and an external fibrous coat. The thick mucous membrane is supplied with blood vessels, nerves, and lymphatics from the submucosa and is perforated by the ducts of excretory glands that empty on its stratified squamous epithelial lining. Longitudinal fibers of muscularis mucosae lie between it and the submucosal layer, which forms a loose connection between the mucosa and the muscular coat, and contains blood vessels, lymphatics, nerves, and the mucous esophageal glands. The muscular coat consists of a layer of thick inner circular fibers and another layer of outer longitudinal fibers. The circular muscle fibers are continuous with the inferior constrictor muscle of the pharynx.

The cervical esophagus descends behind the trachea and recurrent laryngeal nerve and is anterior to the vertebral muscles. It then courses left and is in relation to the thyroid gland and common carotid artery. The esophagus enters the superior mediastinum behind the trachea. The left subclavian artery, thoracic duct, left recurrent laryngeal nerve, and pleura are on its left; the azygos vein and pleura are on its right. It returns to the midline at the level of T5. As it descends in the posterior mediastinum it is behind and to the right of the aortic arch, related in succession anteriorly to the trachea, left mainstem bronchus, pericardium, and diaphragm. Beyond the tracheal bifurcation, the esophagus deviates to the left and anteriorly so that it lies in front of the thoracic aorta, azygos vein, and thoracic duct prior to its passage through the diaphragm at the level of T10. Here it enters the abdomen and joins the stomach at the esophagogastric junction (see Figure 25–1E). The left vagus nerve lies in front and the right lies behind the esophagus below the tracheal bifurcation, and they form a surrounding plexus.

The esophagus receives blood from the inferior thyroidal artery, esophageal branches of the thoracic aorta, the left gastric artery, and the left inferior phrenic. Its venous drainage is to the inferior thyroid, azygos, hemiazygos, and gastric veins, thus being a site of portal-caval anastomoses.

The lymphatics from the mucosa and the submucosa and those from the muscular coats of the esophagus interconnect freely to form an extensive and complex network throughout the length of the organ. These networks eventually form several major lymphatic systems that traverse the outer surface of the esophagus longitudinally, both cephalad and caudad. The systems drain into the cervical, internal jugular, supraclavicular, retrotracheal, paratracheal, subcarinal, paraesophageal, posteromediastinal, para-aortic, and gastric nodes, and connect with the celiac system.

Sites of Metastases. Esophageal carcinomas may extend submucosally in the loose areolar coat for some distance beyond evident mucosal involvement. They tend to metastasize early, involving not only lymph nodes adjacent to the primary site but also those of any of the lymph node groups listed above because of the rich lymphatic connections within and on the surface of the esophagus. Although lesions of the upper esophagus primarily spread to the paratracheal, paraesophageal, and mediastinal nodes, involvement of nodes above the clavicle and below the diaphragm is not unusual. Conversely, middle and lower third lesions most frequently involve mediastinal and abdominal nodes, but may spread cephalad to involve the paraesophageal, paratracheal, supraclavicular, and cervical nodes as well. Cancer may penetrate through the capsules of these nodes into adjacent structures, including nerves, blood vessels, other tissues, and organs. Similarly, esophageal tumors may extend directly to involve the thyroid gland, various arteries and veins, the trachea or bronchus, nerve trunks, and the pleura. Tracheoesophageal and bronchoesophageal fistulas are common complications, as are pleural effusions, recurrent laryngeal and cervical sympathetic paralysis, superior vena caval obstruction, and carotid artery, aortic, pericardial, and left atrial invasion. Fistulous perforation of the aorta is an occasional terminal event. Empyema and mediastinitis may also occur. Clinical manifestations of hematogenous metastases are often overshadowed by the effects of progression of the primary tumor and its local extensions. Nevertheless, such metastases are present in the majority of the patients in autopsy series and most often involve the lungs, liver, bones, and kidneys (del Regato and Spjut, 1977).

Symptoms and Signs. The first symptom of esophageal carcinoma is usually related to mechanical narrowing of the gullet. Although esophageal carcinomas may occasionally present in peculiar ways so far as local invasion, distant metastases, or special paraneoplastic syndromes are concerned, the most common is dysphagia. Initially, dysphagia is noted intermittently for solid food, especially meat and bread, but later for most solid food. Eventually even liquid causes dysphagia as it traverses the narrow esophagus. Dysphagia is a "cardinal symptom" and cannot be ignored. Carcinoma of the esophagus should be the first consideration in a patient older than 40 who presents with dysphagia. Regurgitation and vomiting are other symptoms that may result from obstruction to the passage of food and liquid.

Odynophagia is common in carcinoma of the esophagus after dysphagia is well established. Pain on swallowing, however, may be a presenting symptom in a few patients. Another local effect of tumor is bleeding, which may present as anemia, hematemesis, or melena. When bleeding occurs it usually follows necrosis of the tumor with ulceration. Weight loss rarely is a presenting symptom, but frequently is a late symptom. Although not a presenting complaint, weight loss may well be present by the time the patient complains to his physicians of dysphagia. It is generally accounted for by the decreased food intake secondary to the dysphagia. In advanced metastatic esophageal carcinoma, weight loss also may be related to the metabolic effects of extensive disease.

Since the esophagus has no serosa to contain spread, carcinoma arising in the esophagus commonly spreads to contiguous organs at a very early stage. Pain due to local tumor extension is occasionally encountered prior to dysphagia. The pain is often substernal, but may also be experienced in the posterior thoracic cage. The pain is usually steady and increases with swallowing. Because pain often indicates extension of tumor beyond the esophagus, pain anteceding dysphagia is thought to be bad prognostic sign (Sleisenger and Fordtran, 1978).

Local extension may also produce (1) hoarseness, by invasion of the recurrent laryngeal nerve; (2) coughing after eating or drinking, due to direct aspiration through a tracheoesophageal or bronchoesophageal fistula or overflow from an obstructed esophagus; (3) profuse hemorrhage (either hematemesis or hemoptysis) due to invasion of one of the numerous large vessels within the thorax; (4) facial swelling late in the disease, due to superior vena caval obstruction. Dyspnea may develop secondary to pleural metastases with effusion. Bone pain may occur because of hematogenous bone metastases. Rarely, symptoms of hypercalcemia (somnolence, confusion, thirst, polyuria, nausea, vomiting, constipation, and weakness) may dominate the clinical picture in patients with PTH-producing tumors (Mann and Sachdev, 1977). Ectopic ACTH production and hypertrophic pulmonary osteoarthropathy are other paraneoplastic syndromes that have been reported with esophageal tumors. These disease manifestations are usually found late in the course of esophageal carcinoma.

Physical examination is relatively unhelpful in the patient with carcinoma of the esophagus, because the organ "lies hidden in the thoracic cage." Late in the disease evidence of weight loss, enlarged supraclavicular lymphs nodes, delayed swallowing time, vocal cord paralysis, Horner's syndrome, facial swelling, pleural effusion, or hepatomegaly may be found.

Diagnosis

Although a history is essential for directing attention to the underlying problem, a physical examination is less helpful for diagnosing carcinoma of the esophagus than it is for many other tumors. A chest roentgenogram is an important part of the work-up. It may show a widened mediastinum or a pleural effusion related to the esophageal carcinoma. The chest roentgenogram also may be abnormal in achalasia or lung cancer. Other routine tests are not useful in diagnosis, and specialized methods must be employed.

Method and Yield. The most widely used diagnostic test continues to be an esophagram. If cancer of the esophagus is suspected because of a history of dysphagia, an "upper GI series" should not be ordered alone. An esophagram should be specified, with or without examination of the rest of the upper gastrointestinal tract. The case should be discussed with the radiologist *before* the procedure to enable the radiologist to concentrate on the esophagus and view it both distended and almost empty of barium. All too often "an upper GI" is ordered on a patient with dysphagia and a report comes back to the ordering physician as "normal, except for a hiatal hernia." Hiatal hernia is an extremely common esophageal lesion that is asymptomatic unless complicated by other problems. Dysphagia must not be erroneously ascribed to hiatal hernia, any more than intermittent mild rectal bleeding should be ascribed to diverticula found on barium enema. If the esophagus is normal or shows only a hiatal hernia in a patient with dysphagia, the patient may be given a bolus of bread or a marshmallow, or a cineesophagram may be performed. These procedures help to demonstrate the area in which food hesitates before it is transferred to the stomach (see Figure 25–2). The radiologist may then concentrate on such an area and detect the lesion.

Small cancers frequently are not seen on a routine barium swallow, but these lesions are the ones that may be most amenable to therapy. At best, a barium swallow shows only the location and possibly the extent of the mucosal involvement (see Figure 25–3). Treatment of

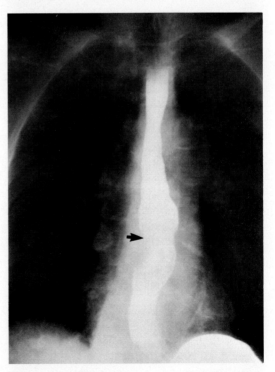

Figure 25–2. Marshmallow swallow illustrating minimal narrowing of esophagus (arrow) in patient with squamous cell carcinoma of esophagus.

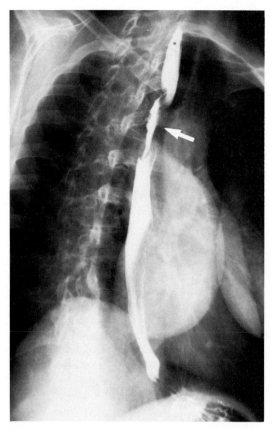

Figure 25–3. Squamous cell carcinoma of upper third of esophagus (arrow).

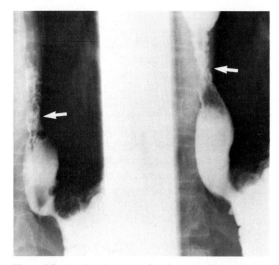

Figure 25–4. Esophagram of patient treated by dilation for "benign stricture" for one year. Patient then had antireflux surgery without benefit. During second operation a squamous cell carcinoma of the esophagus was found (arrows).

carcinoma of the esophagus without a tissue diagnosis is untenable and cannot be provided by roentgenographic means. "Benign" and "neoplastic" strictures may prove to be otherwise (see Figures 25–4 and 25–5). Conditions that may be confused with esophageal carcinoma on an esophagram include benign strictures, achalasia, Schatzki's ring, diffuse esophageal spasm, other primary tumors of the esophagus, extrinsic compression by enlarged lymph nodes, or invasion of the esophagus by a carcinoma of the lung. Occasionally, esophageal carcinoma may be masked by a benign condition, such as lye stricture or achalasia. Some of these radiographic presentations are illustrated in Figures 25–6, 25–7, 25–8, and 25–9.

If a fistula from the esophagus to the tracheobronchial tree is suspected, barium, rather than a radiopaque iodinated solution, should be used to identify it (see Figure 25–10).

Currently, endoscopy is the cornerstone of diagnosis for esophageal lesions (see Figures

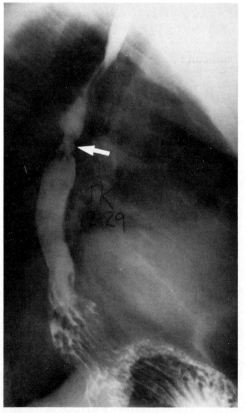

Figure 25–5. Hiatal hernia with Barrett's esophagus and benign stricture (arrow) confirmed surgically.

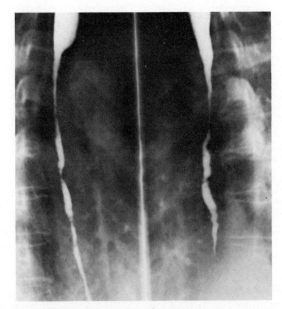

Figure 25-6. Extensive lye stricture.

25-11A and 25-11B). The symptom of dysphagia demands endoscopy. The new, small-diameter, forward-viewing endoscopes permit excellent evaluation of the esophagus with minimal discomfort for the patient. The rigid esophagoscopes used formerly were dangerous, difficult to use, provided poor visualization, and could not be used in patients with

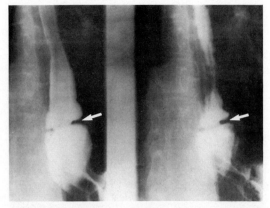

Figure 25-8. Schatzki's ring.

kyphoscoliosis or severe cervical arthritis. With the new, flexible scopes care must be taken to inflate the esophagus and look carefully at all the mucosa. Evaluation of the mucosa is difficult at the cricopharyngeal and, to a lesser extent, at the lower esophageal sphincter, where gastric adenocarcinoma from the cardia of the stomach may invade submucosally into the esophagus. It is important to reverse the endoscope in the stomach and visualize the gastroesophageal junction from below.

Occasionally an esophageal carcinoma may so narrow the lumen that passage of even the

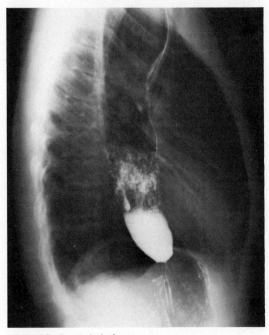

Figure 25-7. Achalasia.

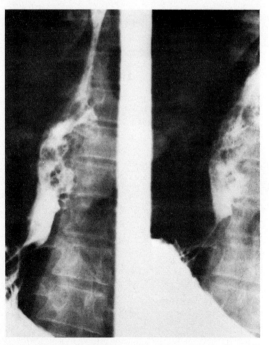

Figure 25-9. Extensive exophytic primary choriocarcinoma of middle and lower third of esophagus.

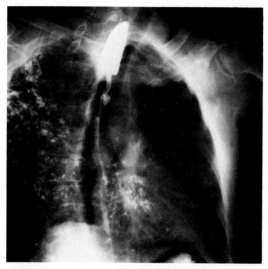

Figure 25–10. Barium swallow in patient with tracheo-esophageal fistula. Note residual barium in lungs.

pediatric endoscope (less than 8 mm in diameter) is impossible. In those circumstances diagnosis must be made by employing the endoscopically directed cytology brush, inserting it into the remaining minimal lumen within the tumor. Similarly, under direct vision, the endoscope may be utilized to place the guide wire into the narrowed lumen for the Eder-Peustow metal olive dilators. After fluoroscopic confirmation that the wire is in the stomach, dilation of the tumor may be undertaken safely. Serial endoscopy may be used to evaluate effects of treatment.

Brush cytology is best obtained by direct visualization during endoscopy rather than by blindly passing the brush through a nasogastric tube to the point of esophageal obstruction. The currently available nonreusable cytology brushes with individual plastic sheathes enable the endoscopist to obtain cytologic brushing at any time during esophagogastroduodenoscopy without removing the scope; brushing,

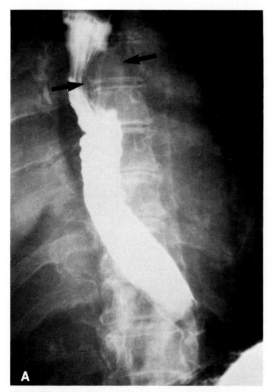

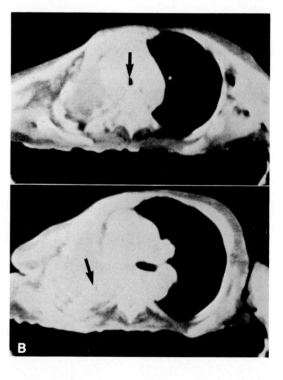

Figure 25–11. (*A*) Esophagram demonstrating carcinoma of the esophagus with extraesophageal extension and compression of left main stem bronchus (tumor occupies region between arrows). (*B*) CT scan demonstrating right upper lobe atelectasis secondary to this tumor, which is obstructing right main stem bronchus. Arrow on upper figure points to trachea. Arrow on lower figure points to narrowed esophagus. Esophagus is displaced to the right and posteriorly by tumor mass extending through its wall and obstructing right main stem bronchus.

therefore, can be done before any hemorrhage results from biopsy or dilation. Brush cytology has been consistently found to be better than biopsy for diagnosis of esophageal carcinoma, its accuracy approaching 100% (Winawer *et al.*, 1975; Halter *et al.*, 1977; Burke *et al.*, 1978).

False-positive cytology of the esophageal area appears to be extremely rare. Several cases initially termed "false-positive" later were found, in fact, to be cases of carcinoma (Maimon *et al.*, 1974). It is not clear what should be done in those cases where a positive brush cytology is obtained without a macroscopically detectable tumor found at endoscopy. It appears, however, that if repeat brush cytologies of a patient's esophagus are interpreted by a competent cytologist as showing squamous cell carcinoma, then consideration must be given to treatment. False-positive esophageal washings, but not direct tumor brushings, have been reported from swallowed sputum containing cancer cells from bronchogenic carcinoma; bronchoscopy may be required to help exclude a bronchogenic carcinoma masquerading as an esophageal carcinoma (Faling *et al.*, 1980).

Endoscopy-directed biopsies are easily obtained, usually after brush cytology. The 2-mm biopsy instrument utilized is so small that perforation or major bleeding rarely occurs. Small, random biopsies of the tumor may show only inflammation or normal mucosa overlying the carcinoma. Although there is a large false-negative rate of 5 to 30% (Winawer *et al.*, 1975), some cases are diagnosed with biopsy when cytology has been negative. To increase the yield of positive biopsies, multiple biopsies should be taken. Even with the small biopsy instrument, biopsies can be relatively deep if repeated biopsies are taken in the same area. Where possible, biopsy should be directed into the middle of the tumor rather than at the leading edge although it is easier to biopsy the leading edge.

Mass screening for carcinoma of the esophagus would not appear to be cost effective due to the relative rarity of the disease, as opposed to screening for gastric cancer in Japan, for example, where that disease is so common. It is not practical to screen all heavy smokers and alcohol drinkers. Screening of selected high-risk groups, such as patients with lye stricture or achalasia, is useful but will only identify a small percentage of patients with carcinoma of the esophagus. These higher risk groups should be screened with brush cytology at endoscopy annually.

Complications. The main shortcoming of radiologic diagnostic methods is failure to detect a lesion of the esophagus. A "normal esophagram" must not be interpreted as proof that there is no carcinoma. Moreover, once a lesion is found it may be misinterpreted. The diagnosis of cancer of the esophagus cannot be made with finality by roentgenogram alone because a tissue diagnosis cannot be made. Other complications include aspiration of barium and constipation from ingestion of barium.

The endoscopy complication rate is very low and appears to be decreasing with the smaller and more flexible endoscopes. Insistence on adequate training for endoscopists will further decrease this complication rate. A nation-wide survey taken in 1974 (Silvis *et al.*, 1976) showed that perforation of the esophagus occurred in less than three of 10,000 cases of esophagogastroduodenoscopy. In dealing with cancer of the esophagus, however, that figure may be increased by introducing a brush biopsy instrument into a nonvisualized lumen, a deep biopsy, or a dilatation. Inflation with air or passage of the instrument may turn an incipient perforation into a serious one. Reaction to medication (that is, local phlebitis, oversedation, or allergic reaction) is the most common complication, occurring in ten of 10,000 cases. These reactions to medication are almost always mild and are rarely a cause of mortality. Endoscopy might miss a lesion, particularly if that lesion is extremely small or if poor technique is utilized. Bleeding may occur from a biopsy. A comparison of endoscopy versus roentgenography is outlined in Table 25–2.

Systematic Approach to Diagnosis. For the four types of patients that present for evaluation of cancer of the esophagus (see Table 25–3), the following approach is recommended:

1. Every patient with dysphagia should properly be evaluated with endoscopy. This evaluation should include biopsy and cytology of any suspicious lesion and should be repeated if necessary after dilation (if dilation proves necessary to visualize the lower part of the lesion). Certainly, a history and physical examination should not be omitted and a chest

Table 25–2. Comparison of Endoscopy and Roentgenography in Diagnosis of Esophageal Carcinoma

ENDOSCOPY	ROENTGENOGRAPHY
Advantages	*Advantages*
1. Tissue diagnosis may be obtained	1. Less costly than endoscopy
2. Better evaluation of intraluminal extent of lesion	2. Better for evaluation of tracheoesophageal and bronchoesophageal fistulas
3. Dilation of narrow lumen, if necessary	3. Evaluation of extraesophageal spread of disease
4. May exclude other diseases of gastrointestinal tract down to second portion of duodenum	
5. May diagnose and treat non-neoplastic causes of dysphagia and an abnormal esophagram	
Disadvantages	*Disadvantages*
1. Invasive	1. Misinterpretation
2. Costly	2. Failure to detect lesion
3. Bleeding	3. No tissue diagnosis
4. Perforation	4. Aspiration of barium into lungs
5. Failure to detect lesion (rare)	5. Constipation

roentgenogram is usually obtained and a barium swallow performed.

2. The patient who, for reasons other than dysphagia, has an esophagram and whose esophagram is abnormal should obviously also have endoscopy with brush cytology and biopsy of the suspicious area.

3. The patients who have certain predisposing factors to esophageal carcinoma, such as achalasia, lye stricture, Barrett's esophagus, tylosis, and possibly benign esophageal stricture, should have endoscopy yearly with cytology. Any suspicious lesions should be biopsied.

4. The patient who has rare presenting symptoms, frequently due to metastases, will need to have those symptoms evaluated by appropriate tests before attention is directed toward the esophagus. Such symptoms might include chest pain, odynophagia, hoarseness, gastrointestinal bleeding, unexplained pulmonary findings, unexplained weight loss, symptoms of hypercalcemia, or bone pain.

Table 25–3. Four Types of Clinical Presentations of Esophageal Carcinoma

1. Dysphagia
2. Abnormal esophagram taken for reasons other than dysphagia
3. Certain predisposing factors with high risk for esophageal cancer
4. Unexplained symptoms

Staging

The purpose of staging is to provide guidelines for therapy and prognosis. Liver function tests, chest roentgenograms, laryngoscopy, CT scan of the chest and upper abdomen, and esophagogastroscopy are diagnostic tests that are necessary for staging. A uniform approach to staging, such as that of the American Joint Committee for Cancer Staging (1978), enables one to compare therapies and outcomes in similar groups of patients (see Table 25–4).

Obtaining numerous invasive tests that are redundant and costly in a disease for which therapy is poor appears not to be cost effective or advantageous to the patient. Determination of operability and staging can usually be accomplished with liver function tests, esophagram, esophagoscopy, chest roentgenogram, vocal cord evaluation, and CT scan. Enlarged supraclavicular or cervical nodes should be biopsied. Bone pain may indicate the need for a bone scan or skeletal survey. A CT scan of the chest and upper abdomen will furnish as much, if not more, information than mediastinography, mediastinoscopy, laparoscopy, laparotomy, whole lung tomograms, liver scan, intravenous pyelogram, azygography, and gallium scan. Radioisotope scanning of esophageal tumors using gallium 67 (Kondo *et al.*, 1979) or cobalt 57-bleomycin (Suzuki *et al.*, 1974) may demarcate the tumor and metastases, but have not yet proven to be superior to CT scan. Because the esophagus is enclosed within the thoracic cage, staging is extremely

Table 25–4. Staging of Carcinoma of the Thoracic Esophagus

TNM Classification
  Primary Tumor (T)
    T_0 No demonstrable tumor in the esophagus
    T_{is} Carcinoma *in situ*
    T_1 Tumor involves 5 cm or less of esophageal length without obstruction, circumfer-
         ential involvement, or extraesophageal spread
    T_2 Tumor involves more than 5 cm of esophageal length without extraesophageal
         spread; or tumor of any size that produces obstruction or involves entire cir-
         cumference without extraesophageal spread
    T_3 Any tumor with evidence of extraesophageal spread
  Nodal Involvement (N)
    N_x (clinical evaluation; lymph nodes cannot be assessed)
    N_0 No positive nodes (surgical evaluation)
    N_1 Positive nodes (surgical evaluation)
  Distant Metastasis (M)
    M_x Not assessed
    M_0 No (known) distant metastasis
    M_1 Distant metastasis present

Staging
  Stage I
    T_{is} N_0 M_0
    T_1 N_0 M_0
    T_1 N_x M_0
  Stage II
    T_2 N_x M_0
    T_2 N_0 M_0
  Stage III
    Any T_3
    Any N_1
    Any M_1

difficult and new techniques are constantly being sought.

Specific and Supportive Management

Specific Therapy for Various Stages of Disease. The primary treatment modalities for cancer of the esophagus are surgery and radiation therapy. Chemotherapy must be considered investigational at the present time.

Surgery. The surgical treatment of esophageal carcinoma has both advocates and adversaries (Ginsberg *et al.,* 1978). Most surgeons write that the only hope for cure must be surgical resection of an early lesion. They further state that patients who survive surgery but who are not cured will have better nutritional status when metastases appear than nonoperated patients (Piccone *et al.,* 1979). Opponents of surgery note that the vast majority of patients with squamous cell carcinoma of the esophagus have unresectable disease at the time of diagnosis. They point out that resection of the esophagus has the highest mortality of any routinely performed surgical procedure (Ginsberg *et al.,* 1978). In fact, the surgical death rate (operative mortality) is more than twice the survival rate.

Evidence of inoperability includes vocal cord paralysis, tracheoesophageal fistula, axis deviation of the esophagus on esophagram, tumor length greater than 5 cm, location of the tumor in the cervical esophagus, sedimentation rate greater than 25 mm/h, evidence of distant metastases or evidence of local spread into vital organs noted on CT scan. In only 20% of patients is the tumor confined to the esophagus at the time of diagnosis (Piccone *et al.,* 1979). Thus, the opportunities for surgical cure are small. For those patients who are taken to surgery and found to have unresectable tumors, bypass surgery may be done. In those patients with resectable lesions, the lower lesions may be removed and the stomach brought into the chest (see Figure 25–12), but colon interposition will be needed for the higher lesions (see Figure 25–13). If the stomach is brought into the chest, pyloroplasty is required because of the high incidence of gastric retention after vagotomy.

In the largest collection of reported series (83,873 patients) one-third of patients with resectable disease died while in the hospital (Earlam and Cunha-Melo, 1980). It was estimated that of any 100 patients, 42 were not eligible for surgery. Of the 58 who went to surgery, 19

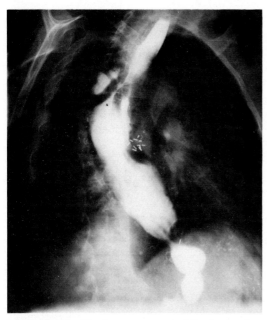

Figure 25-12. Esophagogastrostomy following esophagectomy for carcinoma of the esophagus.

were not resectable. Of the 39 who were resectable, 13 died in the hospital. Twenty-six patients of the original 100 left the hospital after an esophageal resection; 18 lived one year, nine lived two years, and only four were alive five years after the initial hospitalization. This

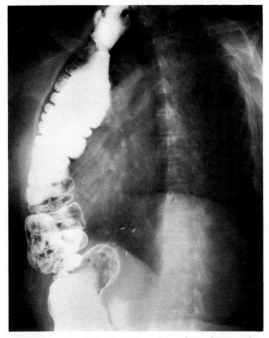

Figure 25-13. Colonic interposition following esophagectomy for carcinoma.

4% five-year survival rate emphasizes that surgery rarely prolongs life in this disorder. Surgery is associated with a high mortality and great expense and yet only improves swallowing and nutrition in the majority of patients so treated. Adenocarcinoma at the gastroesophageal junction responds poorly to radiation therapy and has a much lower mortality for resection than does resection of esophageal squamous cell carcinoma. Surgery appears to be the treatment of choice for this particular entity.

Radiation Therapy. Radiation therapy for carcinoma of the esophagus has been employed (1) with curative intent, (2) preoperatively in an attempt to improve upon surgical results, (3) as palliation in patients considered inoperable due to extent of disease, risks of surgery, and patient refusal of surgery, and (4) as palliation in patients whose disease proves to be nonresectable during surgery or in those with local recurrence following esophagectomy.

Patients selected for therapy with curative intent have pretreatment evaluations that demonstrate lesions less than 10 cm in length, no evident distant metastases, and absence of tracheoesophageal or bronchoesophageal fistulization. Careful pretreatment evaluation, as described previously in this chapter, is essential to establish suitability of patients for attempted curative therapy. Treatment fields must include the demonstrated tumor and sufficient surrounding tissue to encompass possible adjacent, nonevident infiltrative disease without including an excessive volume of normal tissue. The usual dose to tumor is in the range of 5000 to 6000 rads with conventional five-day-a-week fractionation over a six-week interval, most advantageously delivered as megavoltage radiation (6 meV or higher) by a linear accelerator or betatron (Marcial *et al.,* 1966; Appelqvist, 1972; Roussel *et al.,* 1974; Pearson, 1977; Beatty *et al.,* 1979; Earlam and Cunha-Melo, 1980). Equivalent therapy may be administered in shorter intervals using fewer fractions of higher dosage.

Any discussion of therapeutic results in esophageal cancer must take cognizance of the fact that at the time of initial diagnosis only a small percentage of patients are suitable for attempts at curative surgery and a somewhat larger percentage for radiation therapy with curative intent. These percentages may be higher in a referral center. The overall five-year survival of patients with esophageal cancer is 5% or less in large series, irrespective of treatment modalities (Marcial *et al.,* 1966; Appelqvist, 1972; Roussel *et al.,* 1974; Pearson, 1977; Beatty *et al.,* 1979; Earlam and Cunha-Melo, 1980).

Interpretation of even the most optimistic reports of treatment results with surgery, radiation therapy, or a combination of these modalities must be tempered by the realization that the study populations often have been preselected for potential curability. The characteristics of patients in study groups may vary so that direct comparision of results is not possible, that is, gender composition, age distribution, location of lesions, criteria for operability or curative radiotherapy, percentage of patients with residual disease after resection, size distribution of lesions, or extent of work-up to exclude distant metastases may vary. The details of surgical and radiotherapeutic techniques may differ greatly in various reports. In addition, many series do not randomize the assignment of patients to treatment modalities in order to minimize selection variables and many are retrospective studies in which the selection of patients for treatment was performed by different physicians using various criteria over a period of years. Thus, the 17% five-year survival rate with radiotherapy compared to 11% with surgery reported by Pearson (1977) from Edinburgh has not been the general experience.

In a carefully analyzed series from the Princess Margaret Hospital by Beatty *et al.* (1979), patients treated by esophagectomy alone or with preoperative or postoperative radiation therapy have similar survival rates to those treated by radiation with curative intent: 6% at 4.75 years. The *one*-year survival of this group of patients (considered as receiving radical therapy) was 41%, compared to 17% for patients who received palliative radiotherapy only. Women responded better to radiotherapy than did men, as observed in other series. Radiation therapy is preferred in treatment of lesions of the upper third of the esophagus, particularly the cervical esophagus, in which surgical results have been poor and complications are high. In many centers the trend has moved toward radiotherapy in preference to surgery as primary treatment because of the high surgical mortality and the limited survival benefit achieved with either approach.

Preoperative radiotherapy has been used in an effort to improve the results of surgical ther-apy. The purpose of this approach is to increase the percentage of patients resectable for cure by reducing tumor volume and sterilizing peripheral extensions of tumor into adjacent tissues. Although both of these effects have been observed, no conclusive evidence suggests cure rates have been greatly improved. The radiation doses applied have been somewhat lower or in the same range as those used for curative purposes. The different programs of radiation that have been evaluated have produced varying degrees of radiation morbidity and mortality as well as wide variations in postoperative mobidity and mortality (Anabtawi *et al.,* 1964; Nakayama, 1964; Nakayama and Kinoshita, 1974; Marks *et al.,* 1976; Parke and Gregorie, 1976).

Palliative radiation employs doses lower than those usually used with curative intent. Its purpose is to relieve dysphagia and pain, and such treatment does relieve dysphagia in at least 75% of patients (Marcial *et al.,* 1966; El-Mahdi *et al.,* 1971) and often relieves pain as well. Radiation for cure will relieve symptoms in an even higher percentage of patients, particularly in those patients who have stage I disease. The duration of benefit is variable and is often brief. Patients who fail to respond primarily, who relapse, or who develop esophageal strictures will require dilation and other measures to relieve dysphagia and maintain nutrition. In one series (Beatty *et al.,* 1979), 67% of patients receiving radiation for cure developed strictures, and there was overall an 80% failure to control the disease locally. It was estimated that 95% of strictures were associated with persistence of cancer in the esophagus. In a small group of patients with postradiation esophageal obstruction, surgical bypass was associated with much longer survival than were other palliative approaches. The most common side effect of radiation therapy is esophagitis. This generally can be managed through the use of topical anesthetics, pureed or liquid food, and avoidance of hot or cold foods. Occasionally it may be necessary to interrupt the treatment program and provide intravenous hyperalimentation. Less infrequent complications of radiation include tracheoesophageal and bronchoesophageal fistula, hemorrhage, stricture, and radiation pneumonitis.

Chemotherapy. The response of esophageal carcinoma to cancer chemotherapeutic agents has been disappointing. Many agents have had clinical trials, but none have proven to be of major benefit. The majority of these trials have been phase II studies, usually with less than 20 patients and rarely with more than 30. Response rates to specific agents have tended to fall as studies have been repeated and as the size of the study groups has increased. Comparable definitions of response and comparable dosage regimens have not been used in many of these investigations. Determination of magnitude of response at the primary site is difficult to assess, although esophagrams, CT scans, and endoscopy are helpful in this regard. There have been too few studies in patients with easily measurable metastatic disease, largely due to the limited availability of such patients. They constitute a small group and often are unsuitable for study because of their short life expectancy and poor general health. Patients receiving chemotherapy for esophageal cancer, except for some of those being treated prior to surgery or radiation therapy, usually are severely debilitated and die from intercurrent complications of their underlying cancer or from inability to tolerate complications of chemotherapy, such as mucositis and myelosuppression.

Responses to therapy have generally been short (one to three months) or of durations difficult to assess because chemotherapy has been followed by radiation therapy or surgery. The majority of drugs have received limited trials. Bleomycin has been studied more frequently than other agents, consequent to the initial enthusiastic reports that followed its introduction in Japan. Although the drug has some activity, the true response rate is probably about 15% in patients who have received prior radiation therapy. Its attendant major side effects, mucositis and interstitial pneumonitis, also limit its utility in this disease (Yagoda *et al.*, 1972; Blum *et al.*, 1973). Other drugs reported to have some activity are fluorouracil (Livingston and Carter, 1970), methotrexate (Livingston and Carter, 1970), methylglyoxal *bis*-guanylhydrazone (Falkson, 1971), mitomycin, doxorubicin hydrochloride, and cisplatin. Several attempts have been made to improve results by combining two or more of the above agents. Although encouraging response rates have been reported (Kelsen *et al.*, 1978; Hentek *et al.*, 1979; Kolaric *et al.*, 1980; Kelsen *et al.*, 1982), no currently available chemotherapy program has had a significant impact on the survival of patients with esophageal cancer, which is a disappointing 25% at one year from diagnosis. Efforts to improve

treatment results have included the administration of single agents or combinations of drugs prior to, during, and following radiation therapy and in similar programs preoperatively. Although preliminary results in some of these studies are considered encouraging (Kolaric *et al.*, 1980; Coonley *et al.*, 1982; Kelsen *et al.*, 1982), there has been insufficient follow-up to determine the impact of these programs on overall survival.

Perhaps the most encouraging results to date are those of Kelsen *et al.* (1982). In prior studies these workers noted that the combination of cisplatin and bleomycin infusion induced 19% complete plus partial remission in 58 patients with either metastatic or locoregional disease. Studies with vindesine as a single agent resulted in an 18% response rate. In the current program these three drugs are combined. Cisplatin, 3 mg/kg or 120 mg/m^2 (whichever is less), is administered on day one with prehydration and mannitol-induced diuresis. Vindesine, 3 mg/m^2, is given as a rapid intravenous injection on days one, eight, 15, and 22. Bleomycin, 10 units/m^2, is administered as an intravenous loading dose on day three as well as ten units/m^2 as a daily 24-hour infusion for four consecutive days (days three through six). A second cycle is repeated on day 28. In subsequent courses, cisplatin is administered every six weeks and vindesine every two weeks. No additional bleomycin is given after the second course. There is no attenuation schedule for cisplatin or bleomycin. Cisplatin is not administered if the creatinine clearance is <60 cc/min and bleomycin is discontinued if either D_LCO or vital capacity is decreased by 25% of pretreatment values. Vindesine dosage is decreased 50% for white blood cell count (WBC) of 2000 to 2999, platelets of 75,000 to 99,000, or moderate neuropathy. The drug is not administered if there is more severe myelosuppression or if there is severe neuropathy. In 53 evaluable patients, partial remissions occurred in 29 (55%). Seven of 16 patients with metastatic disease had partial remission (44%) with remission duration of two to 18 months (the median was eight months). Partial responses were observed in 22 of 37 patients with locoregional disease. Twenty-three patients with locoregional disease received one course of chemotherapy preoperatively and one course postoperatively; five patients had two courses preoperatively. All patients received 5500 rads of radiation therapy to the involved field in 5.5 to 6.0 weeks starting either two or three weeks after the postoperative chemotherapy or post-operatively in the five patients receiving only preoperative chemotherapy. Twenty-three of 28 patients (82%) had resectable disease, 15 for cure and eight for palliation. There were two operative deaths. Patients with unresectable lesions were all dead within five months. Five of the 23 resectable patients died (two operative deaths, one drug-related death, and two cardiovascular deaths). Median follow-up has been eight months (two to 19 + months). Two resectable patients relapsed. Nephrotoxicity occurred in 19% of the patients and was fatal in one patient who received concomitant gentamicin. Myelosuppression was the dose-limiting toxicity and was related to one death from sepsis. Nausea and vomiting were experienced by 55% of patients and alopecia was almost universal. Neuropathy generally was mild. Although the results of these studies are encouraging, it should be noted that the performance status of this group of patients was high (the median was 70; the range was 30 to 90) and that patients with poor performance status did poorly. This program will have to be studied in a randomized comparison with other therapies, such as surgery or radiotherapy alone, before its efficacy in prolonging survival in locoregional disease can be assessed. Similarly, definitive conclusions cannot be drawn from the study of 16 patients with metastatic disease.

It appears probable that great therapeutic gains will eventually be achieved through a combined modality approach, but only after the discovery of drugs that have much greater intrinsic activity against esophageal cancer than the agents currently available.

Supportive Measures. Patients with esophageal cancer frequently suffer a variety of medical problems. Some of these are a result of heavy tobacco and alcohol use, others are directly due to cancer. Additionally, the majority of these patients are elderly and suffer from unrelated disorders that are common to this age group. Thus, some patients may already have had surgery, radiation therapy, and chemotherapy for prior head and neck cancer. Chronic obstructive pulmonary disease is often present. Impaired liver function or even cirrhosis is not uncommon. As a group, these patients generally suffer from protein-calorie malnutrition and some degree of immunoincompetence. Most have suffered some weight loss and others may be cachectic at the time of diagnosis. Dehydration and electrolyte distur-

bances may be present in varying degrees. Rarely, patients may have hypercalcemia. There may be aspiration of secretions and pneumonitis in cases with severe esophageal obstruction or those with tracheoesophageal or bronchoesophageal fistulas. Coronary artery disease, heart failure, and diabetes may be concomitant medical problems. Efforts should be directed toward repairing nutritional deficits prior to institution of specific therapy.

Nutritional therapy has been reported to reduce surgical complications and to minimize weight loss during radiation therapy and surgery (Copeland et al., 1977a,b, 1979a,b). If there is a reversal of weight loss, patients generally experience diminution of weakness and an increased sense of well-being. Whenever possible, nutritional therapy should be accomplished by enteral feeding. This usually requires the passage of a small-bore nasogastric feeding tube. If obstruction prevents passage of a tube, intravenous hyperalimentation should be instituted. Care must be taken to maintain fluid and electrolyte balance, to correct vitamin deficiencies, and to avoid exacerbation of underlying diabetes or precipitation of cardiac failure secondary to salt and water overloading. Hyperalimentation is often required in the postoperative period until the patient is able to swallow solid foods. It may be needed during radiation therapy and chemotherapy if severe esophagitis is present and until esophageal obstruction is relieved.

Adequate respiratory care before and after surgery must be achieved to promote bronchial cleansing and maximize pulmonary function. Bronchodilators, adrenocorticosteroids, mucolytic agents, ultrasonic nebulizers, heated aerosols, incentive spirometry, and intermittent positive pressure breathing devices may be employed for this purpose. Patients must stop smoking and should be encouraged to breathe deeply and to cough up secretions. Nasotracheal suction may be required to prevent aspiration of secretions. Pulmonary infections should be treated with appropriate antibiotics. Avoidance of pneumonia and maintenance of adequate ventilation are critical for the postoperative patient. Careful attention should be given to the control of diabetes and the treatment of heart failure, hypertension, and other coexistent medical problems during all phases of therapy.

In patients who remain obstructed despite radiation therapy or who develop recurrent obstruction of the esophagus, various approaches have been used to provide nutrition. Esophagectomy with interposition of stomach or colon and esophagogastrostomy as palliative procedures relieve dysphagia, provide a better quality of life, and may prolong survival more satisfactorily than other alimentation procedures. They are, however, associated with a mortality that is considered unacceptably high by many experts in view of the overall short survival of these patients.

Rigid prosthetic tubes have been placed into either the proximal or distal esophagus (Atkinson and Ferguson, 1977; Beckly, 1979). Tubes in the latter location are generally sewn to the stomach to prevent their migration. Rigid tubes are frequently used to prevent food and secretions from entering the lungs when a tracheoesophageal fistula is present. Problems with these tubes include inability to effect their placement because of obstructing tumor, pain, migration of proximal tubes, and reflux of gastric contents with aspiration into the lungs. The tubes have the advantage of allowing the patient to eat. Feeding gastrostomies and jejunostomies are unappealing devices that are poorly accepted by most patients. Long-term nasogastric tube feeding is tolerated by some patients, but is also unpleasant. The continued pressure of even a small-bore tube in the pharynx is intolerable to many patients. When tubes become plugged it may not be possible to pass a replacement successfully. Periodic mechanical dilation of the esophagus may permit patients to maintain oral alimentation for some months (Heit *et al.,* 1978). Home total parenteral nutrition programs can provide satisfactory nutrition for patients unable to eat. Such programs, however, are expensive, require frequent laboratory monitoring, and may be associated with metabolic and catheter complications. The aforementioned techniques may forestall inanition so that patients may succumb more mercifully to some complication of cancer other than starvation. The duration of survival is not increased appreciably by nutritional support or other symptomatic measures. The latter may include oral hygiene, the use of nystatin locally or ketoconazole to control *Candida* infections of the mouth and esophagus, analgesics, drainage and sclerosing agents for pleural effusion, tracheostomy to permit simplified suction of secretions, adequate fluid intake and stool softeners to prevent constipation, and antibiotics for treatment of infections. Utilization of these modes of support may contribute greatly to the patients' comfort, which is a critical consideration in this distressing disease.

Rehabilitation. For the most part, because of the poor prognosis in this disease, patients require supportive therapeutic measures rather than rehabilitation. Primary rehabilitation measures relate to instructions on careful chewing of food and selection of foods and liquids, with respect to quality and quantity as they affect deglutition, such that the patients can adjust to their surgical reconstructions (esophagogastrostomy or esophagocolonostomy). Educational efforts must be directed toward convincing patients to discontinue the habits of cigarette smoking and consumption of alcoholic beverges.

Principles of Follow-Up. After the diagnosis of carcinoma of the esophagus has been established and a treatment plan instituted, the patient requires close follow-up by a physician. That physician must demonstrate to the patient his compassion and interest. When new symptoms arise, they must be evaluated just as if the patient did not have cancer. If the patient leaves the hospital in an adequate nutritional state following surgery, then visits may be as much as a month apart. Symptoms that must be reviewed include dysphagia, pain, regurgitation, cough, evidence of gastrointestinal or upper respiratory bleeding, and bone pain. Pain relief may require focal radiation therapy or narcotics or both later in the course of the disease. Physical examination must include body weight, temperature, and evaluation of nutritional status. Diagnostic studies should be limited. A complete blood count should be done regularly to evaluate anemia and also to detect leukocytosis, which may indicate underlying infection. The patient should be reendoscoped if dysphagia occurs and dilation (Heit *et al.,* 1978) or placement of a prosthesis (Atkinson and Ferguson, 1977; Beckly, 1979) may be attempted at that time. A chest roentgenogram should be obtained if the patient is having cough or fever. Iodinated radiopaque solution should be used for esophagrams if symptoms suggest a tracheoesophageal fistula.

Future Prospects

In the United States, at least 90% of cases of cancer of the esophagus are potentially preventable because it is a disease closely associated with heavy cigarette smoking and alcohol consumption. Experience has shown that heavy users of tobacco and alcohol rarely can be motivated to abstain from these habits. Educational efforts emphasizing the advantages of good health and health maintenance must be directed at young people so that they never begin these habits. A successful educational campaign would result in a marked reduction in the incidence of this disease in 50 years. In the interim, other approaches are required.

The reasons for a poor prognosis in patients with carcinoma of the esophagus are listed in Table 25–5. At present, the prospects for sufficiently early diagnosis of esophageal carcinoma that would have an impact on treatment results are not promising, particularly because the average time to diagnosis from first symptoms is only about four months (Pearson and Le Roux, 1974). This would require a cost-effective and accurate screening technique that could be applied to asymptomatic individuals at high risk. A means for identifying lesions not visible on endoscopy would be highly desirable to be certain that patients detected in some screening procedure truly had carcinoma before they are subjected to therapy. Improvements in local control may derive from the use of high linear energy transfer radiations (neutrons, pi-mesons), from radiosensitizing drugs, or from radioprotective agents. The latter would allow the delivery of higher doses of radiation to tumor without greater injury to normal tissues. Although improved local control no doubt would be beneficial, however, one must bear in mind that death in patients with locally controlled disease is associated with hematogenous and distant lymphatic metastases. It appears probable, therefore, that

Table 25–5. Reasons for a Poor Prognosis in Carcinoma of the Esophagus

1. The long interval during which the tumor is asymptomatic
2. Inaccessibility of tumor to physical examination during asymptomatic interval
3. No serosa to contain the spread of the tumor
4. Unique lymphatic drainage of the esophagus
5. Close proximity to vital organs
6. Dysphagia initially not appreciated as an important symptom by the patient or, occasionally, by the physician
7. Heavy alcohol and cigarette users often have decreased taste appreciation, anorexia, vomiting, and other causes for dysphagia, such as peptic esophagitis
8. Early lesions may be missed on roentgenography

major increases in survival in esophageal cancer must await the development of more effective chemotherapeutic agents. This has been the pattern with other cancers, such as those of the ovary and testicle.

REFERENCES

Ahlbom, H. E.: Simple achlorhydric anemia, Plummer-Vinson syndrome, and carcinoma of the mouth, pharynx, and oesophagus in women: Observation at Radiumhemmet, Stockholm. *Br. Med. J.*, **2**:331–333, 1936.

Ahlbom, H. E.: Prädisponierende Faktoren für Plattenepithelkarzinom in Mund, Hals und Speiseröhre: Eine statistische Untersuchung am Material des Radiumhemmets, Stockholm. *Acta Radiol.*, **18**:163–185, 1937.

Ahmed, N., and Cook, P.: The incidence of cancer of the oesophagus in West Kenya. *Br. J. Cancer*, **23**:302–312, 1969.

American Cancer Society, Inc.: *1981 Cancer Facts and Figures.* American Cancer Society, Inc., New York, 1980.

American Joint Committee for Cancer Staging and End-Results Reporting, 1978: *Manual for Staging of Cancer.* Whitney Press, Chicago, 1978.

Anabtawi, I. N.; Brackney, E. L.; and Ellison, R. G.: Carcinoma of the esophagus treated by combined radiation and surgery. *J. Thorac. Cardiovasc. Surg.*, **48**:205–210, 1964.

Appelqvist, P.: Carcinoma of the esophagus and gastric cardia. *Acta Chir. Scand. [Suppl.]*, **430**:1–86, 1972.

Atkinson, M., and Ferguson, R.: Fiberoptic endoscopic palliative intubation of inoperable oesophagogastric neoplasms. *Br. Med. J.*, **1**:266–267, 1977.

Bates, D. C.; Caston, J. C.; O'Brien, P.; and Sandifer, S. H.: Carcinoma of the esophagus in South Carolina. *J.S.C. Med. Assoc.*, **67**:453–456, 1971.

Beatty, J. D.; De Boer, G.; and Rider, W. D.: Carcinoma of the esophagus. *Cancer*, **43**:2254–2267, 1979.

Beckly, D. E.: Successful endoscopically assisted insertion of Celestin tubes in 2 cases of esophagobronchial fistula. *Gastrointest. Endosc.*, **25**:17–18, 1979.

Benedict, E. B.: Carcinoma of esophagus developing in benign lye stricture. *N. Engl. J. Med.*, **224**:408–412, 1941.

Blum, R. H.; Carter, S. K.; and Agre, K.: A clinical review of bleomycin—a new antineoplastic agent. *Cancer*, **31**:903–914, 1973.

British Medical Journal: Oesophageal cancer in China (editorial). *Br. Med. J.*, **3**:61, 1975.

Burke, E. L.; Sturm, J.; and Williamson, D.: The diagnosis of microscopic carcinoma of the esophagus. *Am. J. Dig. Dis.*, **23**:148–150, 1978.

Burrell, R. J.: Oesophageal cancer in Bantu, *S.Afr. Med. J.*, **31**:401–409, 1957.

Burrell, R. J. W.; Roach, W. A.; and Shadwell, A.: Esophageal cancer in the Bantu of Transkei associated with mineral deficiency in garden plants. *J.N.C.I.*, **36**:201–209, 1966.

Cook-Mozaffari, P. J.; Azordegan, F.; Day, M. E.; Ressicaud, A.; Sabai, C.; and Aranesh, B: Oesophageal cancer studies in the Caspian littoral of Iran: Results of a case-control study. *Br. J. Cancer*, **39**:293–309, 1979.

Coonley, C.; Kelsen, D.; Bains, M.; Hilaris, B; Kaufman,

R.; and Martini N.: Combined modality approach to operable epidermoid carcinoma of the esophagus. *Proc. Am. Soc. Clin. Oncol.,* **1**:95, 1982.

Copeland, E. M., III; Daly, J. M., and Dudrick, S. J.: Nutrition as an adjunct to cancer treatment in the adult. *Cancer Res.,* **37**:2451–2456, 1977a.

Copeland, E. M., III; Daly, J. M.; and Dudrick, S. J.: Nutritional concepts in the treament of head and neck malignancies. *Head Neck Surg.,* **1**:350–363, 1979a.

Copeland, E. M., III; Daly, J. M.; Ota, D. M.; and Dudrick, S. J.: Nutrition, cancer and intravenous hyperalimentation. *Cancer,* **43**:2108–2116, 1979b.

Copeland, E. M., III; Souchou, E. A.; MacFadyen, B. V., Jr.; Rapp, M. H.; and Dudrick, S. J.: Intravenous hyperalimentation as an adjunct to radiation therapy. *Cancer,* **39**:609–616, 1977b.

Cutler, S. J., and Devesa, S. S.: Trends in cancer incidence and mortality in the U.S.A. In Doll, R., and Vodopija, I. (eds.): *Host Environment Interactions in the Etiology of Cancer in Man.* World Heatlth Organization International Agency for Research Cancer, Lyon, France, 1973.

Cutler, S. J., and Young, J. L.: Third National Cancer Survey: Incidence data. *Natl. Cancer Inst. Monogr.,* **41**:1–454, 1975.

del Regato, J. A., and Spjut, H. J.: Cancer of the digestive tract/esophagus. In *Cancer,* 5th ed. The C.V. Mosby Company, St. Louis, 1977.

Doll, R., and Peto, R.: The Causes of cancer: Quantitative estimates of avoidable risks of cancer in the United States today. *J.N.C.I.,* **66**:1192–1308, 1981.

Earlam, R., and Cunha-Melo, J. R.: Oesophageal squamous cell carcinoma: 1. A critical review of surgery. *Br. J. Surg.,* **67**:381–390, 1980.

El-Mahdi, A. M.; Bretz, G. T.; and Lott, S.: Palliative radiation therapy in advanced carcinoma of the esophagus. *Johns Hopk. Med. J.,* **129**:156–162, 1971.

Faling, L. J.; Haesaert, S. P.; and Schimmel, E. M.: Occult bronchogenic carcinoma masquerading as esophageal cancer. *Arch. Intern. Med.,* **140**:489–491, 1980.

Falkson, G.: Methyl-gag (NSC-32946) in the treatment of esophagus cancer. *Cancer Chemother. Rep.,* **55**:209–212, 1971.

Garfinkel, L.; Poindexter, C. E.; and Silverberg, E.: Cancer in black Americans. *CA,* **30**:39–44, 1980.

Gerami, S.; Booth, A.; and Pate, J. W.: Carcinoma of the esophagus engrafted on lye stricture. *Chest,* **59**:226–227, 1971.

Ginsberg, A. L.; Parker, E. F.; and Moertel, C G.: Controversies in gastroenterology. Carcinoma of the esophagus: Is there a role for surgery? *Am. J. Dig. Dis.,* **23**:730–736, 1978.

Goldstein, H. M., and Zornoza, J.: Association of squamous cell carcinoma of the head and neck with cancer of the esophagus. *A J. R.,* **31**:791–794, 1978.

Halter, F.; Witzel, L.; Grétillat, P. A.; Scheurer, U.; and Keller, M.: Diagnostic value of biopsy, guided lavage, and brush cytology in esophagogastroscopy. *Am. J. Dig. Dis.,* **22**:129–131, 1977.

Heit, H. A.; Johnson, L. F.; Siegel, S. R.; and Boyce, H. W., Jr.: Palliative dilation for dysphagia in esophageal carcinoma. *Ann. Intern. Med.,* **89**:629–631, 1978.

Hentek, V.; Vogl, S. E.; Kaplan, B. N.; and Greenwald, E.: Combination chemotherapy of advanced esophageal cancer (ECa) with methotrexate (M), bleomycin (B), and diamminodichloroplatinum (D)—"MBD". *Proc. Am. Soc. Clin. Oncol.,* **20**:400, 1979.

Hirayama, T.: Diet and cancer. *Nutr. Cancer,* **1**:67–81, 1979.

Hormozdiari, H.; Day, N. E.; Aramesh, B.; and Mahboubi, E.: Dietary factors and esophageal cancer in the Caspian littoral of Iran. *Cancer Res.,* **35**:3493–3498, 1975.

Howel-Evans, W.; McConnell, R. B.; Clark, C. A.; and Sheppard, P. M.: Carcinoma of the esophagus with keratosis palmari et plantaris (tylosis): A study of two families. *Q. J. Med.,* **27**:413–429, 1958.

Joyant, K.: Statistical appraisal of the association of smoking and chewing habits to oral and pharyngeal cancers. *Indian J. Cancer,* **14**:293–299, 1977.

Just-Viera, J. O., and Haight, C.: Achalasia and carcinoma of the esophagus. *Surg. Gynecol. Obstet.,* **128**:1081–1095, 1969.

Kelsen, D.; Cvitkovic, E.; Bains, M.; Shils, M.; Howard, J.; Hopfan, S.; and Golbey, R. B.: *cis*-Dichlorodiammineplatinum (II) and bleomycin in the treatment of esophageal carcinoma. *Cancer Treat. Rep.,* **62**:1041–1046, 1978.

Kelsen, D. P.; Bains, M.; Hilaris, B.; Chapman, R.; McCormack, P.; Alexander, J.; Hopfan, S.; and Martini, N.: Combination chemotherapy of esophageal carcinoma using cisplatin, vindesine, and bleomycin. *Cancer,* **49**:1174–1177, 1982.

Kmet, J., and Mahboubi, E.: Esophageal cancer in the Caspian littoral of Iran: Initial studies. *Science,* **175**;846–853, 1972.

Kolaric, K.; Maricic, Z.; Roth, A.; and Dujmovic, I.: Combination of bleomycin and Adriamycin (doxorubicin) with and without radiation in the treatment of inoperable esophageal cancer. *Cancer,* **45**:2265–1273, 1980.

Kondo, M.; Hashimoto, S.; Kubo, A.; Kakegawa, T.; and Ando, N.: ^{67}Ga scanning in the evaluation of esophageal carcinoma. *Radiology,* **131**:723–726, 1979.

Levin, D. L.; Devesa, S. S.; Godwin, J. D., II; and Silverman, D. T.: *Cancer Rates and Risks,* 2nd ed. National Institutes of Health, Washington. D.C., 1974.

Lindvall, N.: Hypopharyngeal carcinoma in sideropenic dysphagia. *Acta Radiol.,* **39**:17–37, 1953.

Livingston, R. B., and Carter, S. K.: *Single Agents in Cancer Chemotherapy.* Plenum Publishing Corporation, New York, 1970.

McKechnie, J. C., and Fechner, R E.: Choriocarcinoma of the esophagus and adenocarcinoma of the esophagus with gonadotropin secretion. *Cancer,* **27**:694–702, 1971.

Mahboubi, E.; Kmet, J.; Cook, P. J.; Day, N. E.; Ghadirian, P.; and Salmasizadeh, S.: Oesophageal cancer studies in the Caspian littoral of Iran: The Caspian Cancer Registry. *Br. J. Cancer,* **28**:197–214, 1973.

Maimon, H. N., Dreskin, R. B., and Cocco, A. E.: Positive esophageal cytology without detectable neoplasm. *Gastrointest. Endosc.,* **20**:156–159, 1974.

Mann, N. S., and Sachdev, A. J.: Carcinoma of the esophagus and hypercalcemia. *Am. J. Gastroenterol.,* **67**:135–140, 1977.

Marcial, V. A.; Tomé, J. M.; Ubiñas, J.; Bosch, A.; and Correa, J. N.: The role of radiation therapy in esophageal cancer. *Radiology,* **87**:231–239, 1966.

Marks, R. D.; Scruggs, J. H.; and Wallace, M.: Pre-operative radiation therapy for carcinoma of the esophagus. *Cancer,* **38**:84–89, 1976.

Martinez, I.: Factors associated with cancer of the esophagus, mouth, and pharynx in Puerto Rico. *J.N.C.I.,* **42**:1069–1094, 1969.

Miller, R. W.: Cancer epidemics in the People's Republic of China. *J.N.C.I.,* **60:**1195–1203, 1978.

Naef, A. P.; Savary, M.; and Ozzello, L.: Columnar-lined lower esophagus: An acquired lesion with malignant predisposition. *J. Thorac. Cardiovasc. Surg.,* **70:**826–835, 1975.

Nakayama, K.: Pre-operative irradiation in the treatment of patients with carcinoma of the esophagus and some other sites. *Clin. Radiol.,* **15:**232–241, 1964.

Nakayama, K., and Kinoshita, Y.: Surgical treatment combined with pre-operative concentrated irradiation. *J.A.M.A.,* **227:**178–181, 1974.

Parke, E. F., and Gregorie, H. B.: Carcinoma of the esophagus; long-term results. *J.A.M.A.,* **235:**1018–1029, 176.

Pearson, J. G.: The present status and future potential of radiotherapy in the management of esophageal cancer. *Cancer,* **39:**882–890, 1977.

Pearson, J. G., and LeRoux, B. T.: Malignant tumors of the esophagus. In Schweigk, H. (ed.): *Handbuch der inneren Medizin: Diseases of the Esophagus.* Springer-Verlag, Berlin, 1974.

Piccone, V. A.; LeVeen, H. H.; Ahmed, N.; and Grosberg, S.: Reappraisal of esophagogastrectomy for esophageal malignancy. *Am. J. Surg.,* **137:**32–38, 1979.

Radigan, L. R.; Glover, J. L.; Shipley, F. E.; and Shoemaker, R. E.: Barrett esophagus. *Arch. Surg.,* **112:**486–491, 1977.

Rogers, E. L.; Goldkind, L.; and Goldkind, S. F.: Increasing frequency of esophageal cancer among black male veterans. *Cancer,* **49:**610–617, 1982.

Rose E. F.: Esophageal cancer in Transkei: 1955–1969. *J.N.C.I.,* **51:**7–16, 1973.

Roussel, A.; Robillard, J.; Souloy, J.; Fourre, D.; and Abbatucci, J. S.: Resultants dans 600 cas de cancer de l'oesophage traités au Centre François-Baclesse de 1964 à 1971. *J. Radiol. Eléctrol. Med. Nucl.,* **55:**485–489, 1974.

Sanghir, L. D.; Rao, K. C. M.; and Khanolkar, V. R.: Smoking and chewing of tobacco in relation to cancer of the upper alimentary tract. *Br. Med. J.,* **1:**1111–1114, 1955.

Schoenberg, B. C.; Bailer, J. C.; and Fraumeni, J. F.: Certain mortality patterns of esophageal cancer in the United States, 1930–1967. *J.N.C.I.,* **46:**63–73, 1971.

Silvis, S. I.; Nebel, O.; Rogers, G.; Sugawa, C.; and Mandelstam, P.: Endoscopic complications. Results of the 1974 American Society for Gastrointestinal Endoscopy Survey. *J.A.M.A.,* **235:**928–930, 1976.

Sleisenger, M. H., and Fordtran, J. S.: *Gastrointestinal Disease,* 2nd Ed. W.B. Saunders Company, Philadelphia, 1978.

Stephen, S. J., and Uragoda, C. G.: Some observations on oesophageal carcinoma in Ceylon, including its relationship to betel chewing. *Br. J. Cancer,* **24:**11–15, 1970.

Suzuki, Y.; Hisada, K.; Hiraki, T.; and Ando, A.: Clinical evaluation of tumor scanning with ^{57}Co-bleomycin. *Radiology,* **113:**139–143, 1974.

Tuyns, A. J.; Péquignot, G.; and Abbatucci, J. S.: Oesophageal cancer and alcohol consumption: Importance of type of beverage. *Int. J. Cancer,* **23:**443–447, 1979.

Tuyns, A. J.; Péquignot, G.; and Jensen, O. M.: Les cancers de l'oesophage en Ille-et-Villaine en fonction des niveaux de consommation d'alcool et de tabac. Des risques qui se multiplient. *Bull. Cancer,* (Paris), **64:**45–60, 1977.

von Zeynek, E. R.: Survey of cancer of the esophagus in relation to other malignant neoplasms. *S. Afr. Med. J.,* **47:**325–331, 1973.

Weber, J., and Hecker, E.: Co-carcinogens of the diterpene ester type from *Croton flaveus L.* and esophageal cancer in Curacao. *Experientia,* **34:**679–682, 1978.

Winawer, S. J.; Sherlock, P.; Belladonna, J. A.; Melamed, M.; and Beattie, E. J., Jr.: Endoscopic brush cytology in esophageal cancer. *J.A.M.A.,* **232:**1358, 1975.

Wychulis, A. R.; Woolam, G. L.; Andersen, H. A.; and Ellis, F. A., Jr.: Achalasia and carcinoma of the esophagus. *J.A.M.A.,* **215:**1638–1641, 1971.

Wynder, E. L.: Dietary habits and cancer epidemiology. *Cancer,* **43:**1955–1961, 1979.

Wynder, E. L., and Bross, I. J.: A study of etiological factors in cancer of the esophagus. *Cancer,* **14:**389–413, 1961.

Wynder, E. L., and Fryer, J. H.: Etiologic considerations of Plummer-Vinson (Patterson-Kelly) syndrome. *Ann. Intern. Med.,* **49:**1106–1128, 1958.

Yagoda, A.; Mukherji, B.; Young, C.; Etcubanas, E.; Lamonte, C.; Smith, J. R.; Tan, C. T. C.; and Krakoff, I. H.: Bleomycin, and antitumor antibiotic: Clinical experience in 274 patients. *Ann. Intern. Med.,* **77:**861–870, 1972.

26

Neoplasms of the Stomach

PHILIP S. SCHEIN and BERNARD LEVIN

GASTRIC CARCINOMA

Incidence and Epidemiology

The incidence of adenocarcinoma of the stomach varies remarkably throughout the world, making it an important model for the study of environmental and genetic etiologic factors for human cancer (Waterhouse, 1981) (see Figure 26–1). The occurrence rates in Japan are 58.4 and 29.9/100,000 for men and women. Although the incidence in Chile is almost as high, the rates in the Dominican Republic and Thailand, in contrast, are roughly 5% that of Japan. In many countries this tumor has demonstrated a continuing reduction in occurrence, most notably in the United States where the incidence in white men has decreased from 29/100,000 to 8/100,000 during the past five decades. It is estimated that approximately 25,000 new cases were diagnosed in the United States in 1984; and the incidence continues to decrease. The average patient is aged 55 to 60 years, and the tumor is twice as common in men as in women.

Etiology and Pathogenesis

Epidemiologic data strongly suggest that environmental and dietary factors make a major contribution to the striking differences in national incidence of this tumor. Studies of Japanese emigrants to Hawaii, and their offspring, have shown a decreasing mortality of gastric cancer compared to native Japanese. This reduction is particularly evident for the intestinal histologic type. The dramatic decrease in occurrence in the United States cannot be explained by a comparable change in the genetic composition of our population, providing further credence for the role of exogenous influences. Occupational risk analyses that have shown an elevated incidence among asbestos and rubber workers, fishermen in Great Britain, Japan, and Canada, and Japanese farmers (Pfeiffer, 1979).

It is suspected that diet plays an important role in the causation of gastric cancer. The possible importance of N-nitroso compounds is supported by the demonstration that N-methyl-N-nitro-nitrosoguanidine (MNNG) is a chemical carcinogen for the stomach of rats and dogs (Endo et al., 1977), and that acetoxy-methyl-methylnitrosamine produces carcinoma in the forestomach of the rat. In man, nitrosamines and nitrosamides can be formed exogenously or endogenously by the nitrosation of secondary amines in food or drugs by nitrites (or nitrate that has been reduced to nitrite) (see Chapter 3B). This reaction may be catalyzed by gastric acid or by bacteria. The finding of bacteria as a catalytic agent may be especially relevant for patients who are regarded to be at increased risk for gastric cancer, such as those with chronic atrophic gastritis and achlorhydria, or those who have recently undergone partial gastric resection for benign ulcer. Under these conditions the stomach can become populated by bacteria that may not only reduce dietary nitrate to nitrite but also accelerate the endogenous formation of nitrosamines (see Figure 26–2). Many drugs have secondary amines within their chemical structure that can be nitrosated by nitrite to form N-nitroso compounds that are either mutagenic in the Ames assay or carcinogenic in animals.

The dietary source highest in nitrites is processed or "cured" meats, in which the chemi-

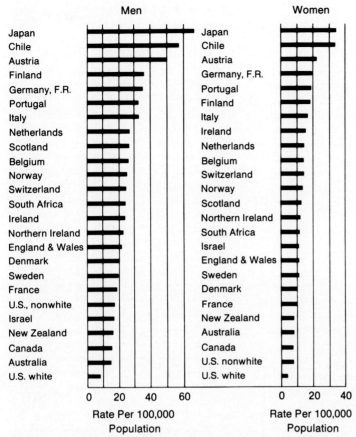

Figure 26–1. International age-adjusted mortality for gastric carcinoma. From U.S. Department of Health, Education and Welfare: *Cancer Rates and Risks.* U.S. Department of Health, Education and Welfare, Bethesda, Maryland, 1974.

cal is directly added to prevent bacterial contamination (and as a coloring agent). Saliva has a high concentration of nitrite as a result of reduction of dietary nitrates by mouth bacteria. The growing concern regarding N-nitroso compounds, ingested or formed endogenously, arises from the recognition that they represent one of the most potent classes of chemical carcinogens in animals (see Chapter 3B).

Although there is no firm evidence that these compounds can cause cancer in man, no animal species has yet been demonstrated to be resistant to their carcinogenic action. At least two indirect correlates have been reported: A high incidence of gastric cancer in Colombia has been recorded in regions with increased nitrate concentration in water and in Chile where the disease has been associated with exposure to nitrogen fertilizers (Tannenbaum *et al.,* 1977). Similarly, the use of crude salt with a high nitrate content to preserve fish has also been offered as a support for the hy-

pothesis. It has been suggested that the decreased incidence of gastric cancer in the United States may be the result of increased use of refrigeration of food, the result of which is a decreased bacterial reduction of nitrate compared to food stored at room temperature, or an increased consumption of dietary ascorbic acid, a vitamin that can inhibit the nitrosation reaction. In addition to nitrites, other food preservation methods, such as pickling and smoking, have been implicated as causal agents of gastric carcinoma. Smoked food may contain carcinogenic hydrocarbons such as 3,4-benzopyrene. Lastly, asbestos has been implicated as a gastric carcinogen (Newhouse, 1981).

Predisposing Factors. Although the etiology of gastric cancer appears intimately related to environmental and dietary factors, a number of important predisposing or "precancerous" conditions have been described. In this regard, it is necessary to define exactly what is meant by the term precancerous. A

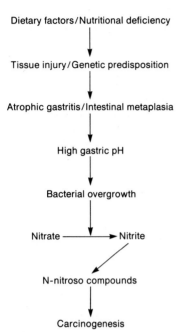

Dietary factors / Nutritional deficiency

Tissue injury / Genetic predisposition

Atrophic gastritis / Intestinal metaplasia

High gastric pH

Bacterial overgrowth

Nitrate ⟶ Nitrite

N-nitroso compounds

Carcinogenesis

Figure 26-2. A possible relationship between atrophic gastritis and nitroso-compound carcinogenesis in the pathogenesis of gastric cancer. From Tannenbaum, S. R.; Archer, M. C.; Wishnok, J. S.; Correa, P.; Cuello, C.; and Haenszel, W.: Nitrate and the etiology of gastric cancer. In Hiatt, H. H.; Watson, J. D.; and Winston, J. A. (eds.): *Origins of Human Cancer.* Cold Spring Harbor Laboratory, Cold Spring Harbor, New York, 1977.

distinction can be made between a precancerous condition and a precancerous lesion. A precancerous condition is a clinical state associated with a greatly increased risk of cancer, whereas a precancerous lesion is a histopathologic abnormality in which cancer is more likely to occur than in an apparently normal counterpart. In the case of gastric carcinoma, attention is being focused on dysplasia as a marker for increased cancer risk. The principal histologic and cytologic features of epithelial dysplasia are cellular atypia, abnormal differentiation, and disorganized mucosal architecture with stratification and loss of polarity of nuclei. These changes can occur in normal gastric (foveolar) epithelium as well as in intestinal metaplasia, both of which may be sources of carcinoma.

Pernicious Anemia. The incidence of gastric cancer in patients with pernicious anemia has been estimated to be approximately 6%, and the age-adjusted incidence of gastric cancer is 10 to 20 times more common in these individuals than in an appropriate control population (Ming, 1974). In addition, multifocal tumor is a more frequent finding. The most common antecedent histologic abnor-

malities include gastric atrophy with intestinal metaplasia (Magnus, 1958). This Type A diffuse form of chronic atrophic gastritis is associated with antiparietal cell antibodies; adenomas are also more frequent in this group than in the general population. Although vitamin B_{12} therapy corrects the hematologic abnormalities and prevents the development of neurologic disease, the gastric mucosal lesions remains, as do the potential for neoplastic transformation. Because of the advanced age of most patients with pernicious anemia, surveillance for cancer in the past has been largely restricted to noninvasive techniques. The cost-effectiveness and tolerance of repeated endoscopic examinations with multiple biopsies continues to be evaluated. After initial findings, the clinical picture and results of current continuing studies will determine the need for further surveillance (Stockbrugger *et al.,* 1983). The presence of severe dysplasia probably is an indication for total gastrectomy.

Atrophic Gastritis. Chronic atrophic gastritis, independent of pernicious anemia (Type B), has been implicated as a predisposing factor for gastric carcinoma. Type B gastritis is more common than Type A and typically starts in the antrum and spreads proximally (Morson *et al.,* 1980). The relationship between this form of atrophic gastritis and gastric cancer is not strong when the high prevalence of atrophic gastritis in some normal populations is considered. The main features are atrophy of gastric glands, a variable degree of inflammation, and associated intestinal metaplasia. The latter consists of replacement of gastric glands by intestinal epithelium containing goblet and Paneth's cells. These changes are most commonly found in the antrum (Morson *et al.,* 1980). In areas of the world where gastric cancer is found in high incidence, the background of atrophic gastritis appears to predispose one to the development of multiple foci of intestinal metaplasia, dysplastic changes, and, eventually, carcinoma (Correa *et al.,* 1970).

Severe epithelial dysplasia is associated with an increased frequency of early and advanced cancer in close proximity, whereas mild to moderate dysplasia is not itself a risk factor; such cases should, nevertheless, be closely monitored. In general, stomach cancer found in association with intestinal metaplasia presents with a well-differentiated histology, whereas the tumor is more likely to be poorly differentiated, with a scirrhous pattern, in cases where metaplasia is not present. The mechanism by which atrophic gastritis predisposes one to carcinoma remains undetermined, but the loss of acid production may allow for population of the stomach by nitrate-reducing bacteria with the intragastric formation of N-nitroso carcinogens (see Figure 26–2).

Adenomas. Polypoid lesions of the stomach can be divided into those with and without a predisposition to neoplastic transformation. Ninety percent are hyperplastic or regenerative polyps and have little neoplastic potential. Less than 5% of the polypoid lesions are true adenomas. These can adopt either a villous or tubulovillous growth pattern, and most are sessile and single. They must be regarded as potential precursors of carcinoma inasmuch as foci of carcinoma have been found in 5 to 50% of these lesions (Ming and Goldman, 1965; Hermanek, 1979). Adenomas, when diagnosed, should be excised because they have a potential for neoplastic change. Hyperplastic polyps may be left in place; coexisting carcinoma elsewhere in the stomach, however, has been reported to occur in 10 to 20% of patients. The diagnosis of a hyperplastic polyp, or adenoma, mandates a careful search for a coexisting early gastric carcinoma.

Hereditary Syndromes: Cancer Families. A threefold greater risk for gastric cancer has been reported among relatives of patients with gastric cancer compared to that in the general population (Woolf, 1956). The cause of this elevated risk is not known. Families with an unexpectedly high incidence of gastric cancers and other cancers have been described; in these cases a definite genetic factor is operational, and all members of the family should be entered into a program of diagnostic surveillance (Lynch and Lynch, 1978).

Postgastrectomy State. The stomach remnant, remaining for 25 or more years after gastrectomy for a benign condition, may be considered a precancerous condition (Morson *et al.,* 1980). In one *post mortem* analysis the incidence of "stump carcinomas" varied from 8.7 to 10.6%, whereas the incidence of gastric cancers in the intact stomach for an age- and sex-matched control group varied from 3.4 to 5.3% (Stalsberg, 1971). Clemencon and co-workers (1976) attempted to avoid the possibility of selection bias by excluding from their analyses hospitalized patients and autopsy material. They studied, by upper endoscopy, 346 ambulatory patients who had undergone a Billroth II gastrojejunostomy. They found 23 gastric stump cancers (6.65%), the majority being located near the anastomoses. No tumors were found in 187 patients for whom the postoperative interval was nine or fewer years. Six carcinomas were diagnosed in 69 cases (8.7%) with an interval of 10 to 19 years, and 15 cancers were found in 70 patients (21.4%) studied 20 or more years after surgery. Overall, 15% of patients had carcinoma in the gastric remnant after a postoperative period of ten or more years. The mean interval between gastric resection and stump cancer was approximately 24 years.

The mechanism by which gastrectomy for benign disease predisposes one to the development of gastric carcinoma remains unknown. Bile reflux over the course of years may result in atrophic gastritis and reduced acid production. Subtotal resection and vagotomy will reduce gastric acid production as well as motility, which may promote the proliferation of nitrate reductase-positive bacteria, thus promoting the intragastric formation of N-nitroso carcinogens.

The five-year survival of patients with stump carcinoma has been reported to be 6% (de Boer *et al.,* 1978); this stresses the need for earlier detection at a curable stage. Prospective endoscopic surveillance in conjunction with multiple biopsies for the detection of dysplasia has shown an approximate cancer incidence of 2 to 3%. Intestinal metaplasia was seen in almost one-half of the patients and showed dysplasia in 13%. Severe dysplasia has been shown to progress to intramucosal carcinoma, but this association is not as well established for mild or moderate changes (Huibregtse *et al.,* 1980).

Cost-benefit analyses are not yet available, and it is not known if this relatively low yield of curable cancers justifies endoscopic surveillance in all postgastrectomy patients. The optimum interval between examinations remains to be determined; as a general guideline, examination every three years may be recommended when dysplastic changes are absent. Annual gastroscopy after a postoperative interval of 20 years, or earlier, is advisable in patients who underwent a gastric resection before their fortieth birthdays. The interval from surgery to cancer is shorter in patients in whom the resection was performed after age 40. Any patient with a subtotal gastric resection and upper abdominal distress should be investigated. The finding of severe dysplasia in itself may be an indication for total gastrectomy.

Gastric Ulcer. The risks for late cancer following "physiologic" surgery such as highly selective vagotomy, or the long term effects of H₂ receptor antagonists, are not known.

The incidence of so-called ulcer cancer, that is, carcinoma developing in a preexisting benign peptic ulcer, has been the subject of considerable controversy. In one series of 664 patients with clinically benign gastric ulcers, cancer was eventually demonstrated in 9% (Larson *et al.*, 1961). It is likely, however, that this is a very rare association (Morson *et al.*, 1980), which in the past was complicated by the difficulties that are encountered in distinguishing benign versus neoplastic ulceration. The present routine use of endoscopic biopsy and cytologic brushing allows for a more definitive diagnosis and, thus, a lower probability of a false-negative interpretation of an ulcerating carcinoma.

Ménétrier's Disease. Texter *et al.* (1953) have reported an increased risk of carcinoma of the stomach as a complication of Ménétrier's disease; the current estimated incidence is approximately 10%. Both intestinal metaplasia and dysplasia have been observed in association with this otherwise benign condition (Morson *et al.*, 1980). In nearly all cases of gastric cancer complicating Ménétrier's disease, the cancer has been diagnosed within 12 months of the diagnosis of the benign disorder.

Blood Groups. Several studies have suggested that gastric cancer is more common in those with blood type A than those with blood type O. The increase in risk is modest, at best, and needs to be better defined (Aird *et al.*, 1953). It has been suggested that the link between blood group and gastric cancer might reside in the nature of the mucopolysaccharide composition of gastric secretions and different susceptibilities to damage by environmental carcinogens (Haas and Schottenfeld, 1978).

Pathology and Staging

Adenocarcinoma of the stomach constitutes approximately 95% of all cancers of this organ. Among the remaining 5% of gastric cancers, over one-half are non-Hodgkin's lymphomas (see Chapter 16). Other lesions include squamous cell carcinoma, carcinoid tumors, leiomyosarcomas, and adenoacanthomas. Several histologic classification systems for the adenocarcinomas are currently being used. In the popular Lauren system, gastric carcinoma is divided into two major groups: Intestinal type and diffuse type (Lauren, 1965). In general,

intestinal-type cancers have a glandular pattern resembling intestinal columnar cells with papillary or solid areas. The tumors tend to have well-defined margins and may demonstrate variation in structure between the center and the periphery. Inflammatory cell infiltration is usually profuse. Diffuse-type carcinomas, in contrast, are composed of separated single cells or small clusters of cells. The growth patterns are not as well defined and exhibit wide and diffuse infiltration; connective tissue proliferation is more marked, and inflammatory cell infiltration is less prominent when compared to the intestinal type. The intestinal metaplasia variety is generally more common than the diffuse, particularly in high-prevalence regions of the world. Patients with gastric cancer with intestinal-type histology, in general, are older than those with the diffuse variety. The histologic classification of the World Health Organization differs from that of the Lauren system in dividing adenocarcinoma of the stomach into papillary, tubular, mucinous, and signet-ring cell types as well as in designating separate categories for adenosquamous, squamous, and undifferentiated carcinoma. The differentiation of the tumor can be further characterized using the Broders classification (1926). Most large series that have analyzed the influence of Broders's grade on the five-year survival of patients with resected gastric cancer have demonstrated that prognosis is markedly influenced by histologic differentiation (Schmitz-Moormann *et al.*, 1979). In the experience of the Mayo Clinic, patients with well-differentiated (grades 1 and 2), unresectable gastric cancer had a median survival of seven months, compared to four months with grade 3 or 4 histology (Moertel *et al.*, 1969), suggesting that Broders's grading has prognostic importance for patients with advanced disease.

Fifty percent of tumors arise from the pyloric and antral regions of the stomach. The body and lesser curvature each bears approximately 20%, the cardia 7%, and the remaining 3% are found in the greater curvature. Tumors arising in the cardiac region are associated with a somewhat poorer prognosis; in addition to the potential for perigastric lymph node metastases, this site also drains to the mediastinal lymph nodes, and surgical resection usually requires a thoracoabdominal approach. Antonioli and Goldman (1982) have described an increase in distal carcinomas containing signet-ring cells in women and an apparent increase in proximal (cardia) lesions in men with a paucity of signet-ring cells.

In regard to gross pathologic features, approximately 75% of gastric carcinomas are ulcerative, 10% are polypoid, and 10% demonstrate either a localized or diffuse desmoplastic reaction (linitis plastica), which is associated with a particularly ominous prognosis (Higgins *et al.*, 1976). The remaining 5% of tumors are characterized as superficial spreading, with sheetlike collections of carcinoma cells replacing the normal gastric mucosa. Many centers report the macroscopic appearance of the gastric cancer using the Borrmann classification: Type 1, circumscribed solitary polypoid cancer without ulceration; type 2, ulcerative carcinoma with elevated borders and sharp limitations; type 3, ulcerative carcinoma with a mixture of elevated borders and diffuse spreading; type 4, diffuse carcinoma (Borrmann, 1926). The prognosis of the latter two types is relatively poor compared to types 1 and 2. It is the opinion of some pathologists that one should not place too much emphasis on these subdivisions because overlap often occurs (Morson and Dawson, 1974).

The modes of dissemination of gastric cancer are presented in Table 26–1. Once established, the tumor may spread into four places: direct and continuous invasion into the greater or lesser omentum, colon, pancreas, esophagus, or liver. The regional lymph nodes are involved early in the disease, and distant metastases to the left supraclavicular (Virchow's node) and the left anterior axillary group are well known. The liver is the most common site for hematogenous metastases, but spread to the lung, including lymphangitic involvement, and bones may also become apparent. Lastly, diffuse implantation of the tumor within the peritoneal cavity is observed in a relatively high percentage of cases and may result in the formation of Blumer's shelf along the rectum or seeding of the ovaries to form a Krukenberg's tumor.

The prognosis of early gastric carcinoma is related to the depth of penetration into the stomach wall and the presence and location of lymph node metastases. These factors have been well accounted for in the design of the staging system by the American Joint Committee (see Table 26–2 and Figure 26–3).

Table 26–1.   Sites of Metastases

Direct Extension
   Gastrohepatic/gastrocolic omenta
   Pancreas
   Diaphragm
   Transverse colon and mesocolon
   Duodenum
   Jejunum and/or its mesentery
   Spleen and gastrosplenic ligament
   Infrahepatic surface of liver
   Superior mesenteric and celiac vessels
   Abdominal wall and kidney

Lymphatic Spread
   Submucosal and subserosal lymphatics
   Gastric and gastroepiploic nodes (along lesser and greater curvatures)
   Celiac axis (porta hepatis, subpyloric, gastroduodenal, splenic-suprapancreatic, retropancreaticoduodenal, and paraesophageal juxtacardiac systems); superior mesenteric, para-aortic chains.
   Left supraclavicular (Virchow's) and left anterior axillary lymph nodes (Irish's)

Hematogenous Spread
   Liver involvement via portal vein
   Secondary involvement from venous systems of other involved organs, principally lungs and bones

Peritoneal Involvement
   Localized involvement (*e.g.*, with lesions on posterior wall and posterior half of the lesser curvature)
   Diffuse peritoneal spread
   Perirectal involvement (Blumer's shelf)
   Ovarian metastases (Krukenberg's tumor)
   Periumbilical metastases

Table 26–2. TNM Classification for Gastric Carcinoma

Primary Tumor (T)

T_X Degree of penetration into stomach wall not determined

T_0 No evidence of primary tumor

T_1 Tumor limited to mucosa and submucosa, regardless of its extent or location

T_2 Tumor involves the mucosa, the submucosa (including the muscularis propria) and extends to or into the serosa but does not penetrate through the serosa

T_3 Tumor penetrates through the serosa without invading contiguous structures

T_4 Tumor penetrates through the serosa and invades the contiguous structures

Nodal Involvement (N)

N_X Metastases to intra-abdominal lymph nodes not determined (*e.g.,* laparotomy not done)

N_0 No metastases to regional lymph nodes

N_1 Involvement of perigastric lymph nodes within 3 cm of the primary tumor along the lesser or greater curvature

N_2 Involvement of the regional lymph nodes more than 3 cm from the primary tumor, which are removed or removable at operation, including those located along the left gastric, splenic, celiac, and common hepatic arteries

N_3 Involvement of other intra-abdominal lymph nodes that are not removable at operation, such as the para-aortic, hepatoduodenal, retropancreatic, and mesenteric nodes

Distant Metastasis (M)

M_X Not assessed

M_0 No (known) distant metastasis

M_1 Distant metastasis present

         Specify _____

         Specify sites according to the following notations:

Peritoneal (PER)	Bone marrow (MAR)
Pulmonary (PUL)	Pleura (PLE)
Osseous (OSS)	Skin (SKI)
Hepatic (HEP)	Eye (EYE)
Brain (BRA)	Other (OTH)
Lymph nodes (LYM) (above diaphragm or nonabdominal)	

Stage Grouping

Stage	Clinical-Diagnostic Staging	Postsurgical Treatment-Pathologic Staging
		$pT_1 N_0 M_0$
I	$cT_1 N_0 M_0$	$pT_2 N_0 M_0$
II	$cT_2 N_0 M_0^*$	$pT_3 N_0 M_0$
	$cT_3 N_0 M_0$	$pT_{1-3} N_1 M_0$
III	$cT_{X-3} N_{1-3}^\dagger M_0$	$pT_{1-3} N_2 M_0$ (resected for cure)
IV	$cT_4 N_{X-3+} M_0$	$pT_{1-3} N_3 M_0$
IV	$cT_4 N_{X-3+} M_0$ (probably not resectable)	$pT_{1-3} N_3 N_0$
		$pT_4 N_{0-3} M_0$ (not resectable)
	$cT_{X-4} N_{X-3} M_1$	pT_{1-4} or pT_X or N_{0-3} or $N_X M_1$

Residual Tumor (R)

R_0 No residual tumor

R_1 Microscopic residual tumor

R_2 Macroscopic residual tumor

         Specify _____

* Not applicable—there is no reliable clinical method of determining the extent of T_2 lesions
† Established by clinical criteria (*e.g.,* echogram, computerized tomography)
From American Joint Committee for Cancer Staging and End-Results
Reporting: *Manual for Staging of Cancer,* 2nd ed. J. B. Lippincott Company, Philadelphia, 1983.

Clinical Presentation

Cancer of the stomach may produce no discernible symptoms for long periods. The initial complaint is usually mild epigastric discomfort, which may present as only a vague sensation of fullness or gas pains or with a typical peptic ulcer pattern partially relieved by antacids. As such, the early symptoms of gastric cancer are often indistinguishable from those of benign upper GI diseases such as peptic ulcer and esophagitis. Eventually the pain

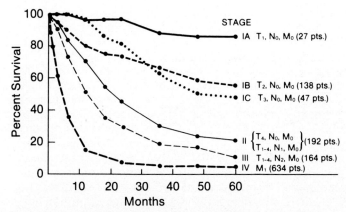

Figure 26–3. The relationship of TNM stage of gastric carcinoma to survival. From Kennedy, B. J.: T-N-M classification for stomach cancer. *Cancer,* **26:**971–980, 1977.

becomes more prominent, bringing the patient to the attention of a physician after the tumor has had an opportunity to grow to the extent that it may no longer be resectable.

Anorexia, early satiety, and distortion of taste and smell all contribute to the common phenomenon of weight loss. Approximately 50% of patients will experience nausea and vomiting, typically with primary tumors of the pylorus, which may progress to partial gastric obstruction. Dysphagia may be the first presenting symptom of a lesion of the cardioesophageal region. Gross hematemesis or melena is uncommon whereas anemia from chronic occult blood loss is a frequent finding.

On physical examination, the left supraclavicular and left anterior axillary lymph node regions must be carefully examined for adenopathy, which may be present in 5% of patients at the time of diagnosis. A minority of patients may have a palpable epigastric mass at the time of presentation. Palpation of the umbilical region may reveal the presence of a subcutaneous nodule. Metastatic disease may manifest itself by a hard nodular liver, the presence of a Blumer's shelf on rectal examination, an enlarged ovary, or the presence of ascites (see Table 26–1).

Gastric cancer has been associated with a variety of paraneoplastic syndromes (Schutt, 1976). Acanthosis nigricans, when it presents as a remote manifestation of neoplastic disease, is found most commonly in association with gastric carcinoma (see Chapter 6D). In addition to the characteristic symmetric, velvety-hyperpigmented lesions over the flexural areas of the body, several additional clinical features suggest the presence of an underlying visceral cancer; these include a patient over 40 years of age, progressive and pruritic hyperkeratotic lesions over the palms and soles, and the presence of papillomatous changes of the mucous membranes.

Dermatomyositis developing in a patient aged 40 to 70 years also raises the possibility of an underlying visceral cancer; gastric carcinoma accounts for the largest number. This collagen-vascular disorder is characterized by weakness and tenderness with inflammation of the proximal muscle groups. The skin rash varies from a subtle violaceous hue on the exposed areas of the face, neck, and trunk to the more classic erythema and edema of the face with heliotrope eyelids secondary to subcutaneous telangiectasis.

A number of hematologic complications have been reported in association with gastric carcinoma (see Chapter 6B). Anemia is common and may be attributed to occult bleeding, chronic disease, rare involvement of the bone marrow by cancer, or the effects of treatment. Microangiopathic hemolytic anemia is a recognized complication of gastric cancer and is characterized by red blood cell fragmentation, a negative Coombs' test, a decreased plasma haptoglobin concentration, elevated LDH_1 and LDH_2 isoenzymes and a reticulocytosis (Sack *et al.,* 1977; Antman *et al.,* 1979). Hemolysis is usually abrupt in onset and of sufficient severity to require repeated transfusions. In some patients an associated thrombocytopenia or evidence of disseminated intravascular coagulation (DIC) occurs. DIC usually occurs in the clinical setting of advanced metastatic disease, where it may be attributed to sepsis or a hemolytic transfusion reaction. Although the coagulopathy is usually widespread, in some patients it may take the form of localized thrombus formation with a clinical picture of either superficial migratory thrombophlebitis (Trousseau's syndrome) or deep vein thrombosis that may antedate the diagnosis of gastric or pancreatic adenocarcinoma by many months. In addition to the possible migratory nature of the phlebitis, the other distinguishing feature is the involvement of unusual sites such as the jugular, cerebral, or chest wall veins. Pulmonary embolization is recognized frequently. An additional manifestation of increased hemostatis is the development of nonbacterial thrombotic vegetations on the mitral and/or aortic heart valves. This syndrome is ordinarily not diagnosed until the patient presents with evidence of embolization to the brain, kidney, spleen, or the coronary artery circulation.

A syndrome with the clinical features of thrombotic thrombocytopenic purpura (TTP) has been described and has been recognized in patients with advanced gastric carcinoma whose tumor has responded to chemotherapy. These patients have manifested the abrupt onset of microangiopathic hemolytic anemia, thrombocytopenia, and progressive renal failure without laboratory evidence of DIC (Kressel et al., 1981). A common feature has been the high titers of circulating plasma immune complexes. Studies are now in progress to determine if there exists an immunologic etiology for the syndrome that is precipitated by tumor-associated antigens or the drugs employed in the treatment of the tumor and mitomycin C in particular (Cantrell et al., 1985). In an anecdotal case, plasmapheresis has been reported to manage successfully the syndrome together with azathioprine as immunosuppressive therapy (Zimmerman et al., 1982).

Diagnosis

The diagnosis of gastric carcinoma needs to be considered in three phases:

1. History and physical examination: The presence of peripheral lymphadenopathy should prompt an investigation employing a biopsy to provide a tissue diagnosis;
2. Barium fluoroscopy of the stomach and endoscopy with biopsy and brushing cytology; and
3. Assessment of extent of spread. Although this may be only definitively made at the time of laparotomy, CT scanning may

provide evidence of extragastric spread such as metastasis to the liver.

Upper Gastrointestinal Radiography. The majority of patients with carcinoma of the stomach present with advanced disease, which is readily diagnosed by conventional barium studies. Nevertheless, approximately 10 to 15% of cancers are not detected and another 15% may be misinterpreted as benign lesions. Benign gastric ulcers characteristically have several distinguishing features, such as projection beyond the contour of the stomach, radiating folds to the ulcer edge, Hampton line, intact surrounding mucosa, and absence of filling defects. These "classic" features may not always be obvious. Cancers in the proximal portion of the stomach are most likely to be overlooked on the conventional single contrast barium study (Laufer, 1979). The double contrast method, with supplementary carbon dioxide or instilled air, increases the sensitivity of the procedure, particularly for the fundus and cardia. The double contrast technique permits more detailed study of the surrounding mucosa, detects nodularity and rigidity, accentuates localized areas of infiltration, and facilitates the differentiation between benign and neoplastic ulcers (see Figure 26–4).

A recent retrospective comparison of single and double contrast studies in the Western literature has indicated that both single and double contrast techniques have a similar sensitivity in the detection of gastric cancers, most of which were presumably advanced (Gelfand and Ott, 1981). In Japan, however, the use of the double contrast technique has facilitated the diagnosis of early gastric cancer. Mass radiologic screening methods coupled with widespread use of endoscopy have led to a rapid increase in the rate of diagnosis of early gastric cancer with corresponding improvement in the overall five-year survival. The frequency of detection of early gastric cancer in Western countries is about 6 to 10% compared to 30% in Japan (Qizilbash and Stevenson, 1979).

Fiberoptic Endoscopy. Most patients with carcinoma of the stomach in the United States are seen late in their courses when the diagnosis is apparent clinically or radiologically. The role of upper gastrointestinal endoscopy in such instances is to provide confirmation of the radiologic diagnosis by obtaining a tissue diagnosis by directed biopsy, which it does with approximately a 90 to 95% accuracy (see

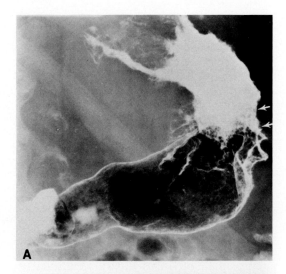

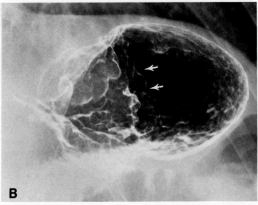

Figure 26–4. Double contrast upper gastrointestinal examination illustrating extensive infiltration of fundus and upper body of stomach.

Table 26–3). Endoscopy with biopsy and cytology is indicated in all patients with a gastric ulcer on barium roentgenogram that has not healed completely in six to 12 weeks. The number of biopsies taken depends on the size and accessibility of the lesion. An exophytic lesion, particularly if it is a soft one such as is seen in the body of the stomach, provides an excellent opportunity for histologic diagnosis whereas a firm lesion in the cardia may be

difficult to biopsy adequately. Most endoscopists favor obtaining a minimum of eight biopsies from suspected neoplasms. Snare cautery has made it possible to obtain suitable material from areas deep from the surface that cannot be reached with the ordinary biopsy forceps. This technique is particularly applicable for neoplasms such as lymphoma or infiltrating adenocarcinoma (for example, linitis plastica), which may be submucosal in location (Bemvenuti *et al.*, 1975).

The procedure of exfoliative cytology of the stomach has evolved from blind washing techniques to directed brushing of a lesion, using a nylon brush passed through the fiberoptic endoscope. If a lesion is not easily accessible to the biopsy forceps, such as a lesion distal to a stricture, brushing cytology is effective. A sheathed brush should always be used because withdrawal of the brush through the biopsy channel leaves some of the cells along the lining of the channel. The cellular material is placed on glass slides and placed in 95% alcohol or sprayed with cytology fixative. The combination of brushing cytology and directed biopsy has increased the accuracy of tissue diagnosis to almost 95% (see Table 26–3).

Computed Tomography. Assessment of the extramucosal extent of the primary neoplasm as well as involvement of other intra-abdominal organs has been facilitated by the use of computed tomography (Moss *et al.*, 1981) (see Figure 26–5). In a recent series of 22 patients, the most common abnormalities were focal gastric wall thickening, ulcerated masses, and diffuse gastric involvement. Computed tomography accurately predicted the operative findings of invasion of the pancreas, esophagus, transverse mesocolon, and spleen. Metastatic involvement of the liver, adrenal glands, and para-aortic lymph nodes was also demonstrated.

In the patient with distant metastases who is not a candidate for palliative resection, computed tomography will reduce the need for operative assessment of the extent of disease. It

Table 26–3. Accuracy of Combined Cytology and Biopsy in the Evaluation of Gastric Cancer

	NUMBER OF PATIENTS IN SAMPLE	CORRECT HISTOLOGY: NO. PATIENTS	CORRECT CYTOLOGY: NO. PATIENTS	RECENT COMBINED CORRECT	REFERENCE
Oxford	84	72	79	93	Boddington, 1978
Chicago	143	74	81	93	Prolla *et al.*, 1977
Oslo	68	53	94	94	Serck-Hanssen *et al.*, 1973
Glasgow	81	67	90	90	Young *et al.*, 1976

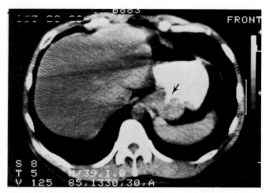

Figure 26–5. CT scan through level of cardia, demonstrating soft tissue mass.

will also direct the attention of the surgeon to areas of possible involvement in order to facilitate accurate staging at the time of palliative or attempted curative resection.

Other Laboratory Techniques. The concentration of serum carcinoembryonic antigen (CEA) has been of little value in the early diagnosis of gastric cancer; it is abnormal in 20 to 60% of patients with advanced cancer but in only 4.5% of patients with early disease (Bunn et al., 1979; Tatsuta et al., 1980). Overall, this technique is not regarded as useful in the follow-up of patients with gastric cancer, as is the case for colorectal carcinoma.

Fetal sulfoglycoprotein antigen has been found in elevated concentration in 91% of those with gastric cancer compared to 54% of patients with benign gastric ulcer, 20% of those with duodenal ulcer, and in 9% of controls (Hakinnen et al., 1980). Like CEA, it is not useful for distinguishing benign and malignant disease.

Screening. The largest experience with screening great numbers of patients has been in Japan, where gastric cancer remains the leading cause of deaths due to cancer. Double contrast upper gastrointestinal radiography, performed in screening centers or in buses equipped with fluoroscopic equipment, has been used as an initial diagnostic measure, providing multiple views of the entire stomach surface. All suspicious findings are further studied with fiberoptic gastroscopy. The result has been a much improved rate of diagnosis of early gastric cancer, with a resultant improvement in five-year survival rates to as high as 80 to 90% for such cases.

Screening large populations in Western society for early gastric cancer is not regarded as cost-effective, in part because of the declining incidence of this tumor in Western society. Efforts at early detection have concentrated on "high risk groups," such as the patient with a gastric remnant or pernicious anemia, where periodic endoscopy with multiple biopsies and brushing cytology of suspicious lesions might be justified.

Early Gastric Cancer. In most reported series outside of Japan, the frequency of early mucosal-submucosal gastric cancer remains under 15% despite an increased awareness of the lesion (Qizilbash et al., 1977). In contrast, studies from Japanese screening centers indicate that up to one-third of all lesions are evaluated early. There appear to be no demonstrable differences in gross or histologic appearance, site, rate of resectability, or the approximate 90% five-year survival rates between early gastric cancer in Japan, and that in the rest of the world. Regardless of the site, the depressed IIc lesion predominates, usually in association with ulceration (IIc + III). These lesions closely simulate peptic ulcers endoscopically and radiologically, and approximately 70% have been found adjacent to benign ulcers with cancer located in the surrounding mucosa and submucosa (Sano, 1921). The endoscopic clues indicating an ulcer's association with early gastric cancer are obtained from a complete examination of its margin. This is best obtained by a side-viewing instrument such as the gastrocamera used by the Japanese in their screening programs.

Early gastric cancer may heal and reulcerate. For this reason, even in the presence of favorable biopsy and cytology reports, follow-up endoscopy should be performed within six weeks to ensure complete healing. If any doubt exists, biopsies and brush cytology should be repeated. Following demonstration of complete healing, endoscopic follow-up should be provided at an interval of six months to one year. More than 50% of benign gastric ulcers recur within one year of complete healing, but this does not imply a carcinomatous condition.

Surgery. The selection of an operative procedure must take into account the stage of disease, the location and size of the primary tumor, as well as possible antecedent surgery for benign disease of the stomach (Lawrence, 1976; Nakajima and Kajitani, 1981) (see Chapter 8). A patient should be regarded as inoperable if evidence is found of disseminated metastases or diffuse peritoneal seeding and ascites. Patients with regional spread of the tumor, however, may benefit from palliative surgery with a resection of the primary tumor. Not only will the potential future complications of gastric obstruction, bleeding, and perforation be reduced, but survival will likely be improved, independent of the form of postoperative treatment that is employed. An operation performed for early gastric cancer must be extensive, ensuring a 5- to 6-cm margin of grossly uninvolved stomach wall, as well as a wide *en bloc* resection of regional lymph nodes. It may include an omentectomy, splenectomy, and a resection in continuity of adjacent organs such as the transverse colon or pancreas if they have become directly invaded by adherent tumor and if the resection is to have curative intent. For lesions of the distal portion of the stomach, the most common surgical approach is a radical partial gastrectomy in which 80 to 90% of the stomach is removed. Primary tumors of the cardia or cardioesophageal region require a radical partial proximal gastrectomy with resection of the lower third of the esophagus through a left thoracoabdominal incision. A total gastrectomy is indicated for linitis plastica, as well as for large, fungating tumors that cannot be widely excised by a subtotal resection or cases with multiple tumors. Additional indications for a total removal of the stomach include gastric carcinoma arising in a patient with pernicious anemia or cancer of the gastric remnant following a previous subtotal gastrectomy for a benign peptic ulcer or tumor.

The procedure for systematic lymph node dissection may include the following: Detachment of the greater omentum from the transverse colon and removal of the anterior leaf of the mesocolon from the omentum; dissection of nodes along the superior mesenteric vein; the pancreatic capsule may be removed as the serous floor of the omental bursa is continuously removed; detachment of the lesser omentum from the undersurface of the left lobe of the liver and dissection of the anterior leaf of the hepatoduodenal ligament; dissection of the lymph nodes behind the pancreas and those in the hepatoduodenal ligament, along the common hepatic artery and around the celiac artery; resection of the left gastropancreatic plica as well as the nodes along the renal artery; and separation of the attachments of the right cardiac to the esophageal hilus and dissection of the lymph nodes of the right cardia. If required, a combined resection of the pancreas and the spleen can be performed for complete removal of nodes along the splenic

vessels or because of tumor invasion of these organs.

Reconstruction after a partial gastrectomy is usually performed by a Billroth I or II anastomosis. Reestablishment of intestinal continuity after a total gastrectomy can be accomplished by several different procedures. The goal is to prevent alkaline reflux and to provide some form of reservoir. In the United States, the Roux-en-Y esophagojejunostomy is widely used to provide flow of bile and pancreatic secretions. In addition, an intestinal pouch can be constructed to serve as a substitute gastric reservoir.

Survival following surgery must be assessed in relationship to the stage of disease at the time of operation. The surgical experience of seven institutions was compiled for the development of the TNM system of the American Joint Committee, and this series serves as a useful analysis of the prognostic importance of specific pathologic presentations (Kennedy, 1977) (see Figure 26–3). For tumors confined to the mucosa (T_1, N_0, M_0) the five-year survival rate was 85%. If the cancer had penetrated into or through the serosa but had not involved the lymph nodes (T_2 or T_3, N_0, M_0), the corresponding survival rate was 47 to 52%. Only 15% of patients with linitis plastica survived. The presence of lymph node metastases markedly reduced the prospects for survival. For a T_2, N_1, M_0 tumor the five-year survival was 25%, and this was further reduced to 8 to 15% if there was involvement of perigastric nodes at a distance from the primary tumor or on both curvatures of the stomach (T_2 or T_3, N_2, M_0). These survival results, correlated with stage, are in basic agreement with those reported from major cancer centers in Japan.

Radiation Therapy. The use of radiation therapy for gastric carcinoma is limited by the tolerance of the organs and tissues of the upper abdomen in relationship to the dose required for effective treatment of the adenocarcinoma. The use of parallel opposed ports, the most commonly employed technique, requires that the extent of irradiation received by kidneys, liver, small intestine, and spinal cord in the field be restricted. Even with careful treatment planning at least one-half of one kidney will be placed into the treatment portal field. The usual tumor dose of 4000 to 5000 rad in four to five weeks exceeds the tolerance of most normal organs in this region.

Radiation therapy for gastric cancer has largely been restricted to the locally unresectable stage of disease. This designation is a generic term that defines those cases in which surgery with curative intent can not be undertaken because of overt or microscopic residual disease in regional lymph nodes or adjacent organs, or where there had been a discontiguous surgical resection. In operational terms, the tumor can be encompassed within a radiation port no larger than 20 cm^2. In retrospective analyses, the use of external beam irradiation alone has provided no survival benefit when compared to matched untreated patients (Moertel and Lavin, 1979). As a consequence, emphasis has been placed on combined modality treatment in which radiation therapy is combined with chemotherapy. In 1965 a comparison of radiation therapy with 5-fluorouracil (5-FU) combined modallity treatment for patients with unresectable tumor was reported (Falkson, 1965). The response rates, defined as subjective or objective improvement, were 0% with irradiation, 17% with 5-FU, and 56% with combined therapy; 12% of patients who received radiotherapy and 5-FU survived 16 to 24 months, whereas with single modality treatment no prolonged survivors were reported.

In 1969, Moertel and colleagues at the Mayo Clinic reported the results of a controlled trial of radiation therapy alone or with 5-FU for locally unresectable gastric cancer (Moertel *et al.*, 1969). Patients were randomized to receive 3500 to 4000 rad (900 to 1200 rad/wk) radiotherapy with either an intravenous isotonic saline placebo or 15 mg/kg 5-FU administered during the first three days of the radiotherapy course. The median survivals for the two treatment groups were roughly equivalent. The analysis of mean survival, however, showed an advantage for combined modality treatment: 13.0 months versus 5.9 months with radiotherapy alone. Three of the 25 patients who received combined treatment were alive at five years, one with recurrent tumor. In contrast, all 23 patients treated with only radiation therapy were dead by 15 months of follow-up. In both this trial and that previously reported by Falkson it is considered likely that 5-FU, administered in such limited dosage, functioned as a radiation sensitizer, a phenomenon well demonstrated in cell culture and *in vivo* rodent tumor models (Vietti *et al.*, 1971).

In 1974, the Gastrointestinal Tumor Study Group designed a controlled trial for locally unresectable gastric cancer in which patients were randomized to either chemotherapy (5-FU plus methyl-CCNU) or combined modality treatment; the latter consisted of 5000 rad delivered in two 2500 rad courses, each of three weeks duration and separated by a two-week rest interval (Gastrointestinal Tumor Study Group, 1982a). 5-FU, 500 mg/m^2, was administered to patients intravenously on the first three days of each split radiotherapy course; these patients were then maintained on the same combination of 5-FU plus methyl-CCNU that had been employed as the sole therapy in the chemotherapy group. Approximately two years into this study and with only 45 patients having been randomized to each treatment arm, a survival advantage was detected for the chemotherapy group (see Figure 26–6). A detailed analysis demonstrated an excess of early deaths with combined treatment during the first ten to 26 weeks of the trials. This resulted from leukopenia-related sepsis and nuritional deficiencies and from tumor progression within the radiotherapy portal during the course of treatment. Continued follow-up over a minimum period of five years has shown that the initial survival advantage with chemotherapy has been lost; and a higher proportion of patients (16% versus 7%) treated with combined radiotherapy are alive and clinically disease free. An analysis of possible prognostic factors that may have influenced this result has demonstrated that patients who had undergone a palliative resection of the primary tumor had a much improved survival, independent of the form of postoperative treatment employed.

Current trials are attempting to improve upon this result with more careful monitoring of hematologic toxicity, the use of enteral and parenteral nutritional support when indicated, and substitution of more effective chemotherapy than 5-FU or methyl-CCNU. The Mid-Atlantic Oncology Program is evaluating a combined modality program in which a single two-month course of FAM chemotherapy (5-FU, doxorubicin, and mitomycin C) is given before radiation therapy to reduce rapidly or stabilize the tumor mass and is followed by continued chemotherapy (Schein *et al.*, 1983).

Chemotherapy. A critical analysis of chemotherapy response rates for gastric cancer from the literature is made difficult by several factors. The majority of past trials have failed to evaluate results in relationship to recognized prognostic factors of the patient population such as age and performance status, nutri-

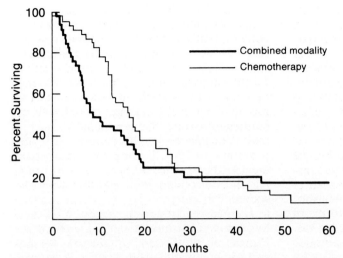

Figure 26-6. Survival of patients with local unresectable gastric carcinoma treated with either chemotherapy alone (5-FU + methyl-CCNU) or combined modality therapy. From Gastrointestinal Tumor Study Group: A comparison of chemotherapy and combined modality therapy for locally advanced gastric carcinoma. *Cancer*, **49**:1771–1777, 1982a.

tional status, histologic grade of the tumor, and sites of metastases. Only when the patients have measurable disease and the trial uses clearly defined criteria of response can response rates be objectively assessed. In many studies these simple requirements have not been fulfilled. Recently designed studies have employed the accepted definitions of complete and partial response. An additional problem has been the inclusion into trials of experimental therapy of patients who were bedridden, cachectic, or jaundiced from hepatic metastases. Patient selection is an essential requirement for a fair assessment of a new treatment, as is carefully avoiding needless toxicity in terminal patients who are more appropriately managed with symptomatic care.

5-FU has been the most extensively studied single agent. Despite over 20 years of clinical use, considerable controversy remains regarding the optimal method of administration of this drug (Comis and Carter, 1974). The most frequently used schedule when 5-FU has been used alone is daily intravenous injections for five consecutive days, the so-called loading course, for which an overall 21% objective response rate, with few complete remissions, has been reported. The duration of response ranges from three to six months.

Mitomycin C, an antibiotic alkylating agent, was developed in Japan where it has been actively used in the treatment of gastric cancer. The initial favorable response rate of 35% reported by Japanese investigators in

Japan could not be duplicated in the early trial in the United States (Frank and Osterberg, 1960). In addition, enthusiasm for this agent was further dampened by reports of serious and persistent depression of bone marrow function when the drug was administered on a daily schedule as well as severe inflammatory reactions following inadvertent extravasation. It became recognized that mitomycin C shares with the chloroethylnitrosoureas the unusual capacity to produce delayed and cumulative hematologic toxicity. Recent trials have employed an intermittent single dose schedule of 10 to 15 mg/m² every six to eight weeks, with greatly improved patient tolerance. The overall reported response rate for gastric cancer treated with mitomycin C in the recent literature is 24% (Baker *et al.,* 1976a; Schein *et al.,* 1978).

The two chloroethylnitrosoureas that have been adequately evaluated in gastric cancer are BCNU and methyl-CCNU (Kovach *et al.,* 1974). BCNU has been reported to produce a 17% response rate when used singly. Methyl-CCNU, the nitrosourea that has been employed in many combination chemotherapy programs, has limited activity as a single agent with a response rate of 8%.

Doxorubicin, an anthracycline antibiotic, has recently been demonstrated to be an important drug for gastric cancer. In controlled trials conducted by the Gastrointestinal Tumor Study Group (GITSG) and the Eastern Cooperative Oncology Group (ECOG) response rates of 22 to 24% for a median duration of four months have been reported for patients with advanced and measurable gastric cancer (Gastrointestinal Tumor Study Group, 1979; Moertel and Lavin, 1979). Doxorubicin has now been incorporated into several active regimens of combination chemotherapy, as will be discussed subsequently.

Recent data from single studies have suggested that triazinate (Baker's antifol) (Bruckner *et al.*, 1982) and *cis*-platinum (La Cave *et al.*, 1983) might have useful therapeutic activity for this disease. In addition, many anticancer agents that have an established place in the management of other forms of human cancer are now being evaluated in gastric cancer. It must be emphasized that despite the finding of modest therapeutic activity with individual drugs, single agent chemotherapy for advanced gastric cancer is an established exercise in futility. The responses last only a few months and such treatment is of little value in improving the survival of patients with this stage of disease involvement.

Combination Chemotherapy. The initial approaches to combination chemotherapy during the past decade have involved the use of 5-FU and the chloroethylnitrosoureas (see Table 26–4). Kovach *et al.* (1974) reported the results of a randomized trial that compared the regimen of BCNU plus 5-FU to each single agent in patients with advanced disease. The combination was reported to produce a 41% response rate, compared to 29% for 5-FU, and 17% for BCNU. No overall survival advantage for the combination was reported when compared to 5-FU and BCNU alone, but at 18 months 25% of the patients treated with the combination were alive, compared to 5 to 10% with the single agents. In an attempt to confirm the activity of this regimen, D'Antona *et al.* (1978) conducted a trial of the same 5-FU and BCNU combination and found a 28% response.

The Mayo Clinic study was soon followed by a similar controlled trial of 5-FU plus nitrosourea chemotherapy conducted by the ECOG, but in this case methyl-CCNU was chosen for study (Moertel *et al.*, 1976). The combination of 5-FU plus methyl-CCNU was reported to produce a 40% response rate, compared to 8% for single agent methyl-CCNU. In addition, a survival advantage was reported for patients who had received the combination, 22-week median versus 10 weeks for methyl-CCNU used alone. In retrospect, this study was flawed by its use of methyl-CCNU as the standard of comparison. The efficacy of this regimen has been placed into further perspective by the results of five additional controlled

Table 26–4. Combination Chemotherapy for Advanced Gastric Cancer: Response Rates and Survivals

REGIMEN	MEASURABLE			NONMEASURABLE		References
	No. of Patients	Response Rate (%)	Median Survival (WKS)	No. of Patients	Median Survival (WKS)	
5-FU + methyl-CCNU						
	55	40	22	—	—	Moertel, 976
	29	21	18	—	—	Baker *et al.*, 1976b
	49	24	16	—	—	Moertel and Lavin, 1979
	18	6	12	—	—	GITSG,* 1982a
				39	27	GITSG,* 1979
5-FU + doxorubicin + mitomycin						
	63	42	28	—	—	Macdonald *et al.*, 1980
	11	55	26	—	—	Bitran *et al.*, 1979
	65	44	25	—	—	Panethiere and Heiburn, 1979
	45	44	28+	—	—	Beretta *et al.*, 1982
	12	25	26	31	37	GITSG,* 1981
	52	39	29.5	—	—	Douglass *et al.*, 1984
5-FU + doxorubicin + methyl-CCNU						
	15	47	23	23	18	GITSG,* 1979
	10	30	30	24	38	GITSG,* 1981
	52	29	24.5	—	—	Douglass *et al.*, 1984
5-FU + doxorubicin + BCNU						
	35	52	—	—	—	Levi *et al.*, 1979

GITSG = Gastrointestinal Tumor Study Group

trials. In a second ECOG program in which the 5-FU and methyl-CCNU combination was compared to 5-FU, the single agent produced a survival equivalent to that achieved with the combination (Moertel and Lavin, 1979). In a third randomized controlled study of the 5-FU plus methyl-CCNU combination by the ECOG, the response rate decreased to 24%, and the corresponding remission rate with 5-FU and mitomycin C was 32% (Moertel and Lavin, 1979). The Gastrointestinal Tumor Study Group (GITSG) also found only modest activity, with only one of 18 patients (6%) achieving an objective response (Gastrointestinal Tumor Study Group, 1979). The Southwest Oncology Group (SWOG) has conducted two controlled trials of this combination with response rates of 21% and 9% (Baker et al., 1976b; Buroker et al., 1979).

Very few data are available on the single agent activity of the antimetabolite cytosine arabinoside in gastric cancer. This drug has been a component of the most commonly used combination in Japan: Mitomycin C, 5-FU, and cytosine arabinoside (MFC) (Ota et al., 1972). The recent Japanese experience with this combination has been reviewed with an overall response rate of 36% (129/356), associated with a mean duration of survival ranging between four and five months (Ogawa, 1978). The GITSG evaluated the same three-drug combination, employing a more intensive schedule; a 17% response rate was recorded, with a nine-week median survival (Gastrointestinal Tumor Study Group, 1979).

In 1974 the Vincent T. Lombardi Cancer Research Center initiated a program to evaluate a combination of 5-fluorouracil, doxorubicin, and mitomycin C (FAM), the three drugs most active against gastric cancer (Schein et al., 1978; Macdonald et al., 1980) (see Figure 26–7). Mitomycin C was given in an intermittent schedule, in recognition of this agent's delayed and cumulative bone marrow toxicity. Twenty-six of 62 patients (42%) achieved a partial remission. The overall median survival was 9.0 months (the range was 2 to 19.5 months), whereas the median survival in responding patients was 12.5 months, with 6 of 26 (25%) responding patients alive for periods in excess of 24 months (see Figure 26–8). Of the 36 patients who failed to respond, the median survival was 3.5 months (ranging from 0.5 to 8.0 months) from the initiation of therapy.

These results have stimulated other investigators to attempt to reproduce these findings. In a nonrandomized trial, Bitran et al. (1979) have reported partial responses in six of eleven (55%) patients with advanced gastric cancer. The overall survival for the eleven patients was 6.5 months, with a projected median survival of 16.5 months for responders. The Southwest Oncology Group (SWOG) has conducted a randomized trial comparing the FAM regimen with the sequential use of the same three drugs (Panethiere and Heiburn, 1979). A 44% response was reported with FAM compared to 27% with sequential therapy. Beretta et al. (1982) have treated 45 patients with measurable gastric cancer and reported a 44% complete response rate, with a median duration of

Drug	Dose (mg/m²)	Route of Administration	Week of Therapy								
			1	2	3	4	5	6	7	8	
5-Fluorouracil	600	Intravenous	x	x			x	x			R
Doxorubicin	30	Intravenous	x				x				E
Mitomycin-C	10	Intravenous	x								P
											E
											A
											T

Dose Attenuation Schedule for
Bone Marrow Depression

Drug dose (%)	Cell count (cells/mm³)	
	WBC	Platelets
100	>3500	>100,000
50	2500-3499	75,000-99,999
None	<2500	< 75,000

Figure 26–7.   The dose, schedule, and dose-reduction scheme of the 5-fluorouracil, doxorubicin, and mitomycin (FAM) chemotherapy regimen for gastric cancer.

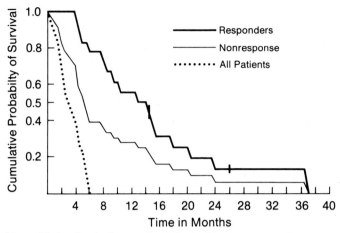

Figure 26–8. Survival curves for patients with advanced gastric cancer who have been treated with the 5-fluorouracil, doxorubicin, and mitomycin (FAM) regimen. From Schein, P. S.; Macdonald, J. S.; Hoth, D.; and Woolley, P. V.: Mitomycin-C: Experience in the United States, with emphasis on gastric cancer. *Cancer Chemother. Pharmacol.,* **1**:73– 75, 1978.

seven months. The mean survival of all cases is in excess of seven months, and 12 months for responding patients. The GITSG (1981) has conducted a controlled trial of a modified FAM regimen (FAMi), in which 5-FU was administered in a loading course. In a series of 12 patients with measurable tumor, the response rate was 25%.

The ECOG has reported the results of a randomized controlled trial in which the original FAM regimen was directly compared to the following combinations: 5-FU, doxorubicin, and methyl-CCNU (FAMe); doxorubicin and mitomycin C (AM); and 5-FU and methyl-CCNU (FUMe) (Douglass *et al.*, 1984). One-hundred ninety-six cases with advanced measurable tumors were evaluable. The objective response rate and median survivals with FAM was 39% and 27 weeks, compared to 29% and 25 weeks with FAMe, 29% and 18 weeks with AM, and 14% and 12 weeks with 5-FUMe. The FAM regimen was associated with the longest median survival, and the largest proportion of patients surviving one year or more. In addition, the FAM program had the lowest rate of severe toxicity. The authors concluded that, based on toxicity and response data, FAM should be considered for future trials as an adjuvant to curative gastric surgery. Several attempts have been made to improve the efficacy of the FAM regimen with the addition of a chloroethylnitrosourea, substitution of ftorafur for 5-FU, or the use of *cis*-platinum for mitomycin (FAP); there has been no increase in therapeutic activity compared to the original FAM combination (Woolley *et al.*, 1981).

Current studies at the Lombardi Cancer Research Center and in the Gastrointestinal Tumor Study Group are now assessing the addition of triazinate to FAM or 5-FU and doxorubicin with appropriate scheduling of this antifol with 5-FU in an attempt to achieve biochemical modulation previously suggested in prior methotrexate and 5-FU regimens.

The Gastrointestinal Tumor Study Group has developed two combinations of 5-FU, doxorubicin, and methyl-CCNU (FAMe). When the original intensive regimen was evaluated in 15 patients with measurable tumors, 47% evidenced an objective response (Gastrointestinal Tumor Study Group, 1981). The median survival of all 30 patients with measurable and nonmeasurable tumor was 12.9 weeks compared to 8.2 weeks using doxorubicin. With the combination drug treatment, 47% of patients evinced noteworthy leukopenia (less than 2000/mm^3), and 21% had sustained thrombocytopenia (less than 50,000/mm^3) during the first course of treatment. In a second trial, the dose of 5-FU was reduced to 325 mg/m^2 during days one through five, methyl-CCNU was administered in a dose of 110 mg/m^2 on day 1, and doxorubicin in a dose of 40 mg/m^2 was given on day 1 (O-Connell and Stablein, 1982). Three of ten patients (30%) with measurable disease responded compared to one of 18 (6%) with 5-FU and methyl-CCNU and three of 13 (23%) with a modification of the FAM regimen (FAMi). The median survival of all patients, with measurable and nonmeasurable tumors, was 38 weeks with FAMe and 37 weeks with FAMi;

both doxorubicin-containing combinations were superior to 5-FU plus methyl-CCNU, the survival rate for which was 27 weeks. In a recently completed trial, FAMe produced a superior survival when compared to the combination of 5-FU plus doxorubicin, but once again severe hematologic toxicity was noted in 47% of patients.

Levi and coworkers (1979) have combined doxorubicin with 5-FU and BCNU (FAB) using a dose and schedule analogous to the FAM regimen. In the initial phase II trial with 35 patients with advanced or unresectable gastric cancer, the complete and partial response rate was 52%. The median survival of responding patients was one year, and 30% were alive at 88 weeks of follow-up. This combination is now being further evaluated in Australia in a phase III advanced disease trial and as a surgical adjuvant treatment.

Adjuvant Therapy. The initial trials of adjuvant chemotherapy for resected gastric cancer in the United States were designed in the late 1950s. Two major controlled trials were carried out concomitantly by the Veteran's Administration Surgical Adjuvant Group (VASAG) and the University Co-Operative Surgical Group, utilizing the alkylating agent thiotepa (Serlin et al., 1969; Dixon et al., 1971). Long-term follow-up has failed to demonstrate any benefit from this treatment, and an increased postoperative mortality was noted in the former study. Following the completion of these studies, the VASAG initiated a controlled trial using fluorodeoxyuridine (FUdR) as a single anticancer agent. Treatment consisted of three daily doses of FUdR immediately following surgery. An extensive analysis of survival data for 459 patients entered into this trial failed to demonstrate a treatment benefit. Because of the high incidence of gastric cancer in Japan, a large number of controlled trials of adjuvant chemotherapy have been initiated in that country. The majority of the studies have utilized either single agent mitomycin C or the MFC combination of mitomycin C, 5-fluorouracil, and cytosine arabinoside (Koyama and Keimura, 1978; Nakajima et al., 1980). Although small differences in survival have been reported for specific histologic subgroups, the possible treatment-related improvements have not been sufficiently consistent such that the regimens could be accepted as a routine postoperative therapy. The Gastrointestinal Tumor Study Group (1982b) reported the results of a controlled trial in which patients with resected gastric cancer were randomized to surgery alone or surgery followed by administration of 5-fluorouracil and methyl-CCNU. Chemotherapy was continued for two years or until a cumulative dose of methyl-CCNU of 1000 mg/m² was attained, or until evidence of tumor relapse appeared. With 142 cases analyzed, an approximate 20% difference in survival at five years favoring the treated group ($P = 0.01$) was reported. No confirmatory data from similarly designed trials have been published.

The emphasis of recently initiated studies of adjuvant chemotherapy has been the use of ADRIAMYCIN-based drug combinations, such as FAM, FAMethyl-CCNU, or FAB. It will take five years of additional patient accrual and follow-up before these controlled trials provide useful data on the effectiveness of this approach to adjuvant management.

Supportive Care. Radical surgical resection of the stomach leaves the patient with a reduced capacity to ingest or absorb essential nutrients. The dumping syndrome is a particularly distressing complication that may limit the volume and types of foods that can be comfortably consumed. It is characterized by immediate postprandial epigastric fullness and cramping, nausea, diarrhea, palpitations, diaphoresis, and lightheadedness. The rapid emptying of the hyperosmolar material from the gastric remnant into the small bowel results in fluid shifts into the jejunum from the intravascular space along the osmotic gradient. Additionally, it has been suggested that the syndrome is mediated in part by the release of serotonin and kinins, which contribute to the hypermotility and vasomotor symptoms. Management of the dumping syndrome includes a regimen of frequent small feedings with a diet high in fat and protein and low in carbohydrates and with fluids restricted at meals. Cyproheptadine, a serotonin antagonist, has been helpful in some patients when administered 30 minutes before meals.

Iron deficiency is the commonest form of anemia following any form of gastric resection. Total gastrectomy or radical partial gastrectomy removes the source of intrinsic factor required for the absorption of vitamin B_{12} in the terminal ileum, and megaloblastic anemia eventually develops after hepatic stores become depleted. In addition, bacterial overgrowth in an efferent loop may compete with the host for the same vitamin. This problem is readily corrected by the administration of parenteral B_{12}, 1000 μg monthly, and the use of oral tetracycline if the vitamin deficiency is recognized as secondary to B_{12} sequestration.

Additional possible chronic complications of gastrectomy include lactase intolerance, osteomalacia, or osteoporosis and malabsorption of fat secondary to a lowered concentration of pancreatic enzymes, impaired biliary tract function, or bacterial deconjugation of bile salts.

Radiation therapy to the upper abdomen produces both anorexia and nausea, both of which may contribute greatly to the patient's already compromised nutritional status. In addition, a transient malabsorption syndrome may be produced as a result of a diffuse damage to the bowel mucosa incorporated in the irradiation field. The late changes of radiation therapy, including inflammation, endarteritis, and fibrosis with possible stricture formation or ulceration, may further compromise the patient's absorptive function.

Chemotherapy is well recognized for its ability to produce anorexia, nausea, and vomiting within the initial 12 to 24 hours of drug administration. Malabsorption has not been described as a treatment-related complication. Prophylactic and symptomatic antiemetic therapy is an essential component of nutritional support to prevent dehydration and to allow for adequate oral food intake during the period of treatment.

The use of combined modality therapy, upper abdominal irradiation and chemotherapy, may severely compromise a patient's ability to take in adequate calories. Unless the nutritional status of the patient is properly monitored, the treatment may result in severe and life-threatening debilitation. In such cases, if therapy cannot be discontinued because it would jeopardize the prospects for tumor control, the patient must receive intensive nutritional support during this period. This may include enteral or parenteral hyperalimentation if oral dietary intake cannot be satisfactorily maintained.

Future Prospects

Gastric carcinoma is the subject of extensive epidemiologic and etiologic investigation. These studies have provided many provocative clues to the cause and possible means of preventing this specific form of cancer. This work continues and should eventually produce guidelines for nutrition and other measures of risk-avoidance that could be validated in prospective studies. The screening programs in Japan have clearly demonstrated the effectiveness of this approach for early diagnosis and improved survival, but unless a cost-effective and specific tumor marker is developed it is unlikely that such an effort will be mounted in Western societies. As a result, we can expect that most patients with gastric carcinoma will be diagnosed when the disease has progressed to a relatively advanced stage, which will require combined modality therapy. The experience of the past eight years of investigation has demonstrated that this tumor is sensitive to drug treatment and that effective palliation, and in some cases prolonged survival, can be achieved. Continued clinical research directed toward the identification of more effective forms of radiation therapy and chemotherapy may eventually result in a greater cure rate for both resected and advanced cases.

REFERENCES

Aird, I.; Benthall, H. H.; and Roberts, J. A. F.: A relationship between cancer of the stomach and the ABO blood groups. *Br. Med. J.,* 1:799–801, 1953.

American Cancer Society: *1984 Cancer Facts and Figures.* American Cancer Society, Inc., New York, 1984.

Antman, K. H.; Skarin, A. T.; Mayer, R. J.; Hargreaves, H. K.; and Cannellos, G. P.: Microangiopathic hemolytic anemia and cancer: A review. *Medicine,* 58:377–384, 1979.

Antoniolo, D. A., and Goldman, H.: Changes in the location and type of gastric adenocarcinoma. *Cancer,* 50:775–781, 1982.

Baker, L. H.; Izbick, D. O.; and Vaitkevicius, V. K.: Phase II study of porfiromycin versus mitomycin-C utilizing acute intermittent schedule. *Med. Pediatr. Oncol.,* 2:207–213, 1976a.

Baker, L. H.; Vaitkevicius, V. K.; and Gehan, E.: Randomized prospective trial comparing 5-fluorouracil (NSC-19893) to 5-fluorouracil and methyl-CCNU (NSC-95411) in advanced gastrointestinal cancer. *Cancer Treat. Rep.,* 60:733–737, 1976b.

Bemvenuti, G. A.; Hattori, K.; Levin, B.; Kirsner, J. B.; and Reilly, R. W.: Endoscopic sampling for tissue diagnosis in gastrointestinal malignancy. *Gastrointest. Endosc.,* 21:159, 1975.

Beretta, G.; Faschini, P.; Labianca, R.; and Luporini, G.: The value of FAM polychemotherapy in advanced gastric carcinoma. *Proc. Am. Soc. Clin. Oncol.,* 1:103, 1982.

Bitran, J. D.; Desser, R. K.; Kozloff, M. F.; Billings, A. A.; and Shapiro, C. M.: Treatment of metastatic pancreatic and gastric adenocarcinoma with fluorouracil, Adriamycin, and mitomycin-C (FAM). *Cancer Treat. Rep.,* 36:2049–2051, 1979.

Boddington, M. M.: Cytological aspects of cancer of the stomach. In Truelove, S. C., and Heyworth, M. D. (eds.): *Topics in Gastroenterology.* Blackwell Scientific Publications, Oxford, England, 1978.

Borrmann, R.: Geschwulate des magens und duodenums. In Henke, F., and Lumbarsch, O. (eds.): *Handbüch der Speziellen Pathologischen Anatomie und Histologie.* Springer, Berlin, 1926.

Broders, A. C.: 1. Carcinoma: Grading & practical application. *Arch. Pathol.,* **2:**376–381, 1926.

Bruckner, H. W.; Lokich, J. J.; and Stablein, D. M.: Studies of triazinate, methotrexate and ICRF-159 in advanced gastric cancer. *Cancer Treat. Rep.,* **66:**1713, 1982.

Bunn, P. A.; Cohen, M. I.; and Widerlite, L.: Simultaneous gastric and plasma carcinoembryonic antigen in 108 patients undergoing gastroscopy. *Gastroenterology,* **76:**734–741, 1979.

Bunn, P. A.; Nugent, J. L.; and Ihde, D. C.: 5-Fluorouracil, methyl-CCNU, Adriamycin, and mitomycin-C in the treatment of advanced gastric cancer. *Cancer Treat. Rep.,* **62:**1287–1289, 1978.

Buroker, T.; Kin, P. N.; and Groppe, C.: 5-FU infusion with mitomycin-C versus 5-FU infusion with methyl-CCNU in treatment of advanced upper gastrointestinal cancer. *Cancer,* **44:**1215–1221, 1979.

Cantrell, J. E.; Phillips, T. M.; and Schein, P. S.: Carcinoma-associated hemolytic-uremia syndrome: A complication of mitomycin-C chemotherapy. *J. Clin. Oncol.,* **3**(5):723–734, 1985.

Clemencon, G.; Baumgartner, R.; Lesethold, E.; Miller, G.; and Neiger, A.: Das Karzinoma des operierten magens *Dtsch. Med. Wochenschr.,* **101:**1015–1020, 1976.

Comis, R. L., and Carter, S. K.: Integration of chemotherapy into combined modality treatment in solid tumors. III. Gastric cancer. *Cancer Treat. Rev.,* **1:**221, 1974.

Correa, P.; Cuello, C.; and Duque, E.: Carcinoma and intestinal metaplasia of the stomach in Colombian migrants. *J.N.C.I.,* **44:**297–306, 1970.

D'Antona, A.; Fraschini, P.; Labianca, R.; and Beretta, G.: Trattamento del carcinoma gastrica in fase avanzata con l'assoriaziona 5-FU + BCNU. *Ruimoni Integrate di Oncologia,* **117,** 1978.

de Boer, J.; Huibregtse, K.; and Tytgat, G. N.: Gastric carcinoma after partial gastrectomy. *Tijdschr. Gastroenterol.,* **3:**157–166, 1978.

Dixon, W. J.; Longmire, W. P.; and Holden, W. D.: Use of thiethylenethiophosphoramide as an adjuvant to the surgical treatment of gastric and colorectal carcinoma: Ten year followups. *Ann. Surg.,* **173:**16, 1971.

Douglass, H.; Lavin, P. T.; Goudsmit, A.; Klaassen, D. J.; and Paul, A. R.: An Eastern Cooperative Oncology Group evaluation of combinations of methyl-CCNU, mitocycin-C, Adriamycin, and 5-fluorouracil in advanced measurable gastric cancer (EST 2277). *J. Clin. Oncol.,* **2:**1372–1381, 1984.

Dunham, L. J., and Bailar, J. C., III: World maps of cancer mortality rate and frequency ratios. *J.N.C.I.,* **41:**155–203, 1968.

Endo, H.; Ishizawa, M.; Endo, T.; Takahashi, K.; Utsunomiya, T.; Kinoshita, N.; Hidaka, K.; and Baba, T.: A possible process of conversion of food components to gastric carcinogens. In Hiatt, H. H.; Watson, J. D.; and Winston, J. A. (eds.): *Origins of Human Cancer.* Cold Spring Harbor Laboratory, Cold Spring Harbor, New York, 1977.

Falkson, G.: Halogenated pyrimidines as radiopotentiators in the treatment of stomach cancer. *Prog. Biochem. Pharmacol.,* **1:**695–700, 1965.

Feldman, F., and Seaman, W. B.: Primary gastric stump cancer. *A.J.R. Radium Ther. Nucl. Med.,* **115:**257–265, 1972.

Fischerman, K., and Koster, K. U.: The augmented histamine test in the differential diagnosis between ulcer and cancer of the stomach. *Gut,* **3:**211–216, 1962.

Frank, W., and Osterberg, A. E.: Mitomycin-C (NSC 26989): An evaluation of the Japanese reports. *Cancer Chemother. Rep.,* **9:**114, 1960.

Gastrointestinal Tumor Study Group. Phase II–III chemotherapy study in advanced gastric cancer. *Cancer Treat. Rep.,* **63:**1871–1876, 1979.

Gastrointestinal Tumor Study Group. A comparative clinical assessment of combination chemotherapy in the management of advanced gastric carcinoma. *Cancer,* **49:**1362–1366, 1981.

Gastrointestinal Tumor Study Group: A comparison of combination of chemotherapy and combined modality therapy for locally advanced gastric carcinoma. *Cancer,* **49:**1771–1777, 1982a.

Gastrointestinal Tumor Study Group: Controlled trial of adjuvant chemotherapy following curative resection for gastric cancer. *Cancer,* **49:**1116–1122, 1982b.

Gelfand, D. W., and Ott, D. J.: Single vs. double contrast gastrointestinal studies: Critical analysis of reported statistics. *A. J. R.,* **137:**523–526, 1981.

Gisselbrecht, C.; Smith, F. P.; Macdonald, J. S.; Korsmeyer, S. J; Boiron, M.; Woolley, P. V. III; and Schein, P. S.: The effect of sequential addition of the nitrosourea, chlorozotocin, to the FAM combination in advanced gastric cancer. *Cancer,* **51:**1792–1794, 1983.

Haas, J. F., and Schottenfeld, D.: Epidemiology of gastric cancer. In Lipkin, M., and Good, R. A. (eds.): *Gastrointestinal Tract Cancer.* Plenum Publishing Corporation, New York. 1978.

Hakinnen, I. P.; Heinonon, R.; Inberg, M. V.; and Viikari, S. J.: The use of oncofetal antigen, FSA in discrimination between benign and malignant gastric ulceration. *Acta Chir. Scand.,* **146:**507–510, 1980.

Hermanek, P.: Gastric polyps & gastric cancer. In Herforth, C., and Schlog, P. (eds.): *Gastric Cancer.* Springer-Verlag, Berlin, 1979.

Higgins, G. A.; Serlin, O.; Amadeo, J. H.; McElhinney, J.; and Keehn, J.: Gastric cancer factors in survival. *Surg. Gastroenterol.,* **10:**393, 1976.

Huibregtse, K.; Offerhaus, J.; Verhoeven, T.; de boer, J.; v. d. Stadt, J.; and Tytgat, G. N.: Endoscopic screening for malignancy in the gastric remnant. *Acta Endosc.,* **11:**171–175, 1980.

Jones, R.: Mitomycin-C. A preliminary report of studies of human pharmacology and initial therapeutic trial. *Cancer Chemother. Rep.,* **2:**3, 1959.

Karlin, D. A.; Mahal, P. S.; and Heifetz, L. J.: Phase I–II study of 5-fluorouracil, Adriamycin, mitomycin-C and methyl-CCNU (FAMMe) chemotherapy for advanced upper gastrointestinal cancer. *Proc. Am. Assoc. Cancer Res.,* **21:**675, 1980.

Kennedy, B. J.: T-N-M classification for stomach cancer. *Cancer,* **26:**971–980, 1977.

Kovach, J. S.; Moertel, C. G.; Schutt, A. J.; Hahn, R. G.; and Reitemeier, R.: A controlled study of combined 1,3-*bis*-(2-chloroethyl)-1-nitrosourea and 5-fluorouracil therapy for advanced gastric and pancreatic cancer. *Cancer,* **33:**563–567, 1974.

Koyama, Y., and Keimura, T.: Controlled clinical trials of chemotherapy as an adjuvant to surgery in gastric carcinoma. *Proc. II Int. Cancer Congr.,* 1–21, 1978.

Kressel, B. R.; Ryan, K. P.; Duong, A. T. T.; Behenberg, J.; and Schein, P. S.: Microangiopathic hemolytic anemia, thrombocytopenia and renal failure in patients treated for adenocarcinoma. *Cancer,* **48:**1738–1745, 1981.

LaCave, A. J.; Izarzugaza, I.; and Anton Aparicio, L. M.:

Phase II clinical trial of cis-dichlorodiammineplatinum in gastric cancer. *Am. J. Clin. Oncol.,* **6:**35–38, 1983.

Larson, N. E.; Cain, J. C.; and Bartholomew, L. G.: Prognosis of the medically treated small gastric ulcer: Comparison of followup data in two series. *N. Engl. J. Med.,* **164:**119, 1961.

Laufer, E.: *Double Contrast Gastrointestinal Radiology.* W.B. Saunders Company, Philadelphia, 1979.

Lauren, P.: The two histological main types of gastric carcinoma: Diffuse and so-called intestinal-type carcinoma. *Acta Pathol. Microbiol. Scand.,* **64:**31, 1965.

Lawrence, W.: Surgical management of gastrointestinal cancer. *Clin. Gastroenterol.,* **5:**703–742, 1976.

Lawson, T. L., and Dodds, W. J.: Infiltrating carcinoma simulating achalasia. *Gastrointest. Radiol.,* **1:**245–251, 1976.

Levi, J. A.; Dalley, D. N.; and Aroney, R. S.: Improved combination chemotherapy in advanced gastric cancer. *Br. Med. J.,* **2:**1471–1473,1979.

Levin, D. L.; Devesa, S. S.; Godwin, J. D.; and Silverman, D. T.: *Cancer Rates and Risks,* 2nd ed. U.S. Department of Health, Education, and Welfare, Bethesda, Maryland, 1974.

Lynch, H. T., and Lynch, P. M.: Heredity and gastrointestinal tract cancer. In Lipkin, M., and Good, R. A. P. (eds.): *Gastrointestinal Tract Cancer.* Plenum Publishing Corporation, New York, 1978.

Macdonald, J. S.; Schein, P. S.; Woolley, P. V.; Boiron, M.; Gisselbrecht, C.; Brunet, R.; and Lagarde, C.: 5-Fluorouracil, doxorubicin, mitomycin-C (FAM) combination chemotherapy for advanced gastric cancer. *Ann. Intern. Med.,* **93:**533–536, 1980.

Magnus, H. A.: A re-assessment of the gastric lesion in pernicious anemia. *J. Clin. Pathol.,* **11:**289–295, 1958.

Ming, S. C.: Histogenesis and premalignant lesions. *J.A.M.A.,* **228:**886–890, 1974.

Ming, S. C., and Goldman, H.: Gastric polyps: A histogenetic classification and its relation to carcinoma. *Cancer,* **18:**7–21, 1965.

Moertel, C. G.: Chemotherapy of gastrointestinal cancer. *Clin. Gastroenterol.,* **5:**777, 1976.

Moertel, C. G.; Childs, D. S.; Rietemeier, R. J.; Colby, M. Y.; and Holdbrook, M. A.: Combined 5-fluorouracil and supravoltage radiation-therapy of locally unresectable gastric cancer. *Lancet,* **2:**865–867, 1969.

Moertel, C. G., and Lavin, P. T.: Phase II–III chemotherapy studies in advanced gastric cancer. *Cancer Treat. Rep.,* **63:**1863–1869, 1979.

Moertel, C. G.; Mittelman, J. A.; Bakemeier, R. F.; Engstrom, P.; and Hanley, J.: Sequential and combination chemotherapy of advanced gastric cancer. *Cancer,* **38:**678–682, 1976.

Morson, B. C., and Dawson, I. M. P.: *Gastrointestinal Pathology.* Blackwell Scientific Publications, Oxford, England, 1974.

Morson, B. C., and Dawson, I. M. P.: *Gastrointestinal Pathology,* 2nd ed. Blackwell Scientific Publications, Oxford, England, 1979.

Morson, B. C.; Sobin, L. H.; Grundman, E.; Johansen, A.; Nagayo, T.; and Serck-Hanssen, A.: Precancerous conditions and epithelial dysplasia in the stomach. *J. Clin. Pathol.,* **33:**711–721, 1980.

Moss, A. A.; Schnyder, P.; Marks, W.; and Margulis, A. R.: Gastric adenocarcinoma: A comparison of the accuracy and economics of staging by computed tomography and surgery. *Gastroenterology,* **80:**45–50, 1981.

Nakajima, T.; Fukami, A.; Takagi, K.; and Kajitani, T.: Adjuvant chemotherapy with mitomycin-C and with a

multi-drug combination of mitomycin-C, 5-fluorouracil and cytosine arabinoside after curative resection of gastric cancer. *Jpn. J. Clin. Oncol.,* **10:**187–194, 1980.

Nakajima, T., and Kajitani, T.: Surgical treatment of gastric cancer with special reference to lymph node dissection. In Friedman, M.; Ogawa, M.; and Kisner, D. (eds.): *Diagnosis and Treatment of Upper Gastrointestinal Tumors.* Excerpta Medica, Amsterdam, 1981.

Newhouse, M.: Epidemiology of asbestos-related tumors. *Sem. Oncol.,* **8:**250–257, 1981.

O'Connell, M. J., and Stablein, D. M.: A prospective clinical trial of 5-fluorouracil, Adriamycin based chemotherapy in unresectable gastric cancer. *Proc. Am. Soc. Clin. Oncol.,* **1:**91, 1982.

Ogawa, M.: A recent overview of chemotherapy for advanced stomach cancer in Japan. *Antibiot. Chemother.,* **24:**149–159, 1978.

Ota, K.; Kurita, S.; and Nishimura, M.: Combination chemotherapy with mitomycin-C, 5-fluorouracil and cytosine arabinoside for advanced cancer in man. *Cancer Chemother. Rep.,* **56:**363–383, 1972.

Panethiere, P. J., and Heiburn, L.: Experience with two treatment schedules in combination chemotherapy of advanced gastric carcinoma. In Carter, S., and Crooke, S. (eds): *Mitomycin-C: Current Status and New Developments.* Academic Press, New York, 1979.

Pfeiffer, C. J.: Exogenous factors in the epidemiology of gastric carcinoma. In Herfarth, C., and Schlag, P. (eds.): *Gastric Cancer,* Springer-Verlag, Berlin, 1979.

Piper, D. W. (ed.): *Stomach Cancer.* Geneva, UICC, 1978.

Prolla, J. C.; Reilly, R. W.; Kirsner, J. B.; and Cockerham, L.: Direct-vision endoscopic cytology and biopsy in the diagnosis of esophageal and gastric tumors: Current experience. *Acta Cytol.* (Baltimore), **21:**399–402, 1977.

Quizilbash, A. H., and Stevenson., G. W.: Early gastric cancer. *Pathol. Annu.,* **1:**317–351, 1979.

Quizilbash, A.; Harnarine, C.; and Castelli, M.: Early gastric carcinoma. *Arch. Pathol. Lab. Med.,* **101:**610–618, 1977.

Sack, G.; Levin, J.; and Bell, W.: Trousseau's syndrome and other manifestations of chronic disseminated coagulopathy in patients with neoplasms. *Medicine,* **56:**1, 1977.

Sano, R.: Pathological analysis of 300 cases of early gastric cancer. In Murakami, T. (ed.): *Early Gastric Cancer.* University of Tokyo Press, Tokyo, 1921.

Schein, P. S.; Macdonald, J. S.; Hoth, D.; and Woolley, P. V.: Mitomycin-C: Experience in the United States; with emphasis on gastric cancer. *Cancer Chemother. Pharmacol.,* **1:**73–75, 1978.

Schein, P. S.; Smith, F. P.; Dritschilo, A.; Stablein, D. M.; and Ahlgren, J. D.: Phase I–II trial of combined modality FAM (5-fluorouracil, Adriamycin and mitomycin-C) plus split course radiation (FAM-RT-FAM) for locally advanced gastric (LAG) and pancreatic (LAP) cancer: A Mid-Atlantic Oncology Program study. *Am. Soc. Clin. Oncol.,* **24:**5, 1983.

Schmitz-Moormann, P.; Heider, A. A.; and Thomas, C.: Cancer of the stomach-prognosis independent of therapy. In Herforth, C., and Schag, P. (eds.): *Gastric Cancer.* Springer-Verlag, Berlin, 1979.

Schutt, A. J.: Paraneoplastic syndromes associated with gastrointestinal cancer. *Clin. Gastroenterol.,* **5:**681–699, 1976.

Serck-Hanssen, A.; Marcussen, J.; and Liawag, I.: The diagnostic value of x-rays, endoscopy, endoscopy brush virology and biology in a consecutive series of 377 patients with gastric disease. In Maltoni, C. (ed.): *Cancer*

Detection and Prevention, Proc. 2nd Int. Symposium of Cancer Detection and Prevention, Bologna. Excerpta Medica, Amsterdam, 1973.

Serlin, O.; Keehn, R. J.; Higgins, G. A.; Harrower, H. W.; and Mendeloff, G. L.: Factors related to survival following resection for gastric carcinoma. *Cancer,* **40**:1318, 1977.

Serlin, O.; Wolkoff, T. S.; Amadeo, J. M.; and Keehn, R. J.: Use of 5-fluorodeoxyuracil as an adjuvant to the surgical management of carcinoma of the stomach. *Cancer,* **24**:223, 1969.

Smith, F. P.; Dritschilo, A.; and Bowers, M. W.: Phase I–II trial of FAM (5-fluorouracil, Adriamycin and mitomycin-C) plus combined modality split course radiation for locally advanced gastric (LAG) and pancreatic (LAP) cancer. *Proc. Am. Soc. Clin. Oncol.,* **1**:97, 1982.

Stalsberg, H. and Taksdal, S.: Stomach cancer following gastric surgery for benign conditions. Lancet, **II**:1175–1177, 1971.

Tannenbaum, S. R.; Archer, M. C.; Wishnok, J. S.; Correa, P.; Cuello, C.; and Haenszel, W.: Nirate and the etiology of gastric cancer. In Hiatt, H. H.; Watson, J. D.; and Winston, J. A. (eds.): *Origins of Human Cancer.* Cold Spring Harbor Laboratory, Cold Spring Harbor, New York, 1977.

Tatsuta, M.; Itoh, T.; and Okura, S.: Carcinoembryonic antigen in gastric juice as an aid in the diagnosis of early gastric cancer. *Cancer,* **46**:2686–2692, 1980.

Texter, E. C.; Legerton, C. W.; Reeves, R. J.; Smith, A. G.; and Ruffin, J. M.: Co-existent carcinoma of the stomach and hypertrophic tastritis. Report of a case with review of the literature. *Gastroenterology,* **24**:579–586, 1953.

Vietti, T.; Eggerding, F.; and Valeriote, F.: Combined effect of X-radiation and 5-fluorouracil on survival of transplanted leukemic cells. *J.N.C.I.,* **47**:865–870, 1971.

Waterhouse, J. A. H.: Epidemiology of upper gastrointestinal tumors. In Friedman, M.; Ogawa, M.; and Kisner, D. (eds.): *Diagnosis and Treatment of Upper Gastrointestinal Tumors.* Excerpta Medica, Amsterdam, 1981.

Woolf, C. M.: A further study on the familial aspects of carcinoma of the stomach. *Am. J. Hum. Genet.,* **8**:102–109, 1956.

Woolley, P. V.; Smith, F. P.; and Estevez, P.: A Phase II trial of 5-FU, Adriamycin and *cis*-platinum (FAP) in advanced cancer. *Proc. Am. Soc. Clin. Oncol.,* **22**:455, 1981.

Young, J. A.; Hughes, H. E.; and McKenzie, J. F.: Report of a pilot study of endoscopic gastric and duodenal cytology. *Acta Cytol.,* **20**:489, 1976.

Zimmerman, S.; Smith, F. P.; Phillips, T. M.; Coffey, R. J.; and Schein, P. S.: Gastric carcinoma and thrombotic thrombocytopenic purpura: Association with plasma immune complex concentrations. *Br. Med. J.,* **284**:1432–1434, 1982.

27

Neoplasms of the Pancreas

PHILIP S. SCHEIN and BERNARD LEVIN

PANCREATIC CARCINOMA

Incidence and Epidemiology

The incidence of pancreatic carcinoma is increasing in the United States (see Figures 3–2 and 3–3). In 1985 an estimated 25,200 cases will be diagnosed, and more than 24,200 people will die from pancreatic carcinoma, the fifth most common form of cancer mortality (American Cancer Society, 1985). Pancreatic cancer is more common in men than in women by a ratio of two to one. The average age at diagnosis is 60 years. The disease has been recognized more frequently in blacks during the past 30 years, and their risks are now calculated to be 30 to 40% greater than whites (Young *et al.,* 1978); blacks in the United States have one of the world's highest rates of pancreatic cancer. Native Hawaiian men are at especially high risk, almost twice that of American white men, whereas the rate for Hawaiian women is not greater than that of their white counterparts. A similar risk has been reported for other groups of Polynesian men (Berg and Connelly, 1979).

Etiology and Pathogenesis

Increasing evidence suggests that pancreatic cancer may result from exposure to chemical carcinogens. The pancreas of rodents is a well-established target for chemically induced neoplasia. The production of pancreatic carcinomas in guinea pigs who received prolonged administration of 1-methyl-1-nitrosourea has been described (Druckrey *et al.,* 1968; Reddy and Rao, 1975). The carcinogenic activity of N-nitroso compounds has been confirmed by studies describing pancreatic adenomas, adenocarcinomas, and acinar cell carcinomas in hamsters exposed to 2, 2'-dihydroxydi-N-propylnitrosamine (Pour *et al.,* 1975). Adenocarcinoma of the rat pancreas has been induced with azaserine.

Several risk factors have been identified. Most epidemiologic studies show an increased incidence of this tumor in the lowest socioeconomic classes and in urban regions (Berg and Connelly, 1979). Analyses of causation in the United States, Canada, and Japan show that individuals of either sex who smoke one to two packs of cigarettes per day have a two- to threefold increased risk of developing pancreatic carcinoma compared to nonsmokers (Berg and Connelly, 1979). The failure to demonstrate an increased rate among pipe and cigar smokers further implicates inhalation of tobacco smoke. Cigarette smoke contains a large number of carcinogens in both the vapor and particulate phases, including nitrosamines, such as those that produce pancreatic tumors in animals (see Chapter 23). Carcinogens metabolized by the liver and secreted into bile may reflux into the proximal portion of the pancreatic duct, which could account for the increased frequency of tumors in the head region of this organ. Further evidence for a chemical causation comes from measurements of increased risk in particular occupational groups, including chemists, coke and gas plant employees, and workers in metal industries. Exposure to β-naphthylamine and benzidine has been specifically implicated (Wynder *et al.,* 1973).

The potential roles of diabetes and pancreatitis in the development of pancreatic carcinoma are controversial. Pancreatic cancer is associated with diabetes, and the discovery of glucose intolerance may antedate the diagnosis of cancer by several months; this may have resulted in an overestimation of the frequency with which diabetics develop pancreatic cancer in some surveys. When recent onset of diabetes was removed from the analysis, one case control study found an apparent sixfold increased risk for diabetic women but not for men (Wynder *et al.,* 1973). Acquired chronic pancreatitis does not predispose one to cancer in this organ; however, a rare familial form of relapsing pancreatitis has been associated with a markedly increased incidence (Moehr *et al.,* 1975).

Recent epidemiologic studies suggest an increased risk associated with coffee drinking and perhaps with decaffeinated coffee (MacMahon *et al.,* 1981). These reports are preliminary and are the subject of continued active investigation. Follow-up of patients with ankylosing spondylitis treated in British radiotherapy clinics, where the estimated dose to the pancreas was 90 rads, has demonstrated an excess of pancreatic cancer (Court-Brown and Doll, 1965). In contrast, no increase in pancreatic cancer is evident in survivors of the atombomb explosions in Japan.

Pathology and Staging

The pathologic features of human pancreatic epithelial neoplasms are described in detail by Cubilla and Fitzgerald (1980) (see Table 27–1). The majority (90%) are adenocarcinomas, with duct cell adenocarcinoma predominating. The site of origin is widely believed to be the pancreatic ductal system. Some evidence, however, from studies in rodents suggests that neoplastic transformation of the

Table 27–1. Classification of Primary Nonendocrine Cancers of the Pancreas

	FREQUENCY
Duct (ductular) cell origin	89%
Duct cell adenocarcinoma	(75%)
Giant cell adenocarcinoma	
Adenosquamous carcinoma	
Cystadenocarcinoma	
Acinar cell adenocarcinoma	1%
Miscellaneous	10%
Mixed type: duct and islet cell	
Connective tissue origin	

Adapted from Cubilla, A. L., and Fitzgerald, P. J.: Surgical pathology of the exocrine pancreas. In Moossa, A. R. (ed.): *Tumors of the Pancreas.* The Williams & Wilkins Company, Baltimore, 1980.

pancreatic acinar cell, after exposure to carcinogens, may cause it to take the appearance of ductal epithelium (Reddy and Rao, 1975). The primary tumor arises in the head region of the pancreas twice as frequently as in the body and tail. Cubilla and Fitzgerald have emphasized that multifocal neoplasia may also be present in the organ in as many as 19% of cases, a fact that has implications for the extent of optimal surgical resection.

In a typical case of duct cell adenocarcinoma, the tumor glands are formed by tall columnar cells with mucin in the cytoplasm, but some are lined with cuboidal cells with little cytoplasm. With well-differentiated histology the cancer cells may resemble the normal epithelium of the biliary and pancreatic duct systems. A desmoplastic response is usually evident with replacement of islets by collagen. Surrounding areas of chronic pancreatitis are common, and hemorrhage, fat necrosis and chronic pancreatitis may also be seen.

Within the generic category of adenocarcinomas a small subset of tumors has the histologic features of cystadenocarcinoma or mucinous cystadenocarcinoma. This entity often presents with an enlarging abdominal mass and frequently contains foci of calcifications that may be seen on plain abdominal roentgenograms. Correct diagnosis of this tumor is important, because it has a better prognosis than the more common duct cell adenocarcinoma (Compagno and Oertel, 1978). Acinar cell carcinoma, representing only 1% of all nonendocrine tumors of the pancreas, is also recognized as a distinct type and affects a younger age group.

Approximately 15% of all newly diagnosed patients have cancer confined to the pancreas, 20% have invasion of regional nodes, and overt distant metastases are evident in the remainder. Tumors in the head of the pancreas are diagnosed earlier because of obstruction of the common bile duct and jaundice, whereas body and tail cancers have a more insidious course and a higher percentage of patients presenting with disseminated disease. Carcinoma of the head of the pancreas frequently involves the second portion of the duodenum, whereas cancer of the body more typically invades the stomach, and cancer of the tail directly involves the spleen and left adrenal gland (see Table 27–2).

The principal sites of local and regional invasion and distant metastases are presented in Table 27–3. Regional lymph nodes are com-

Table 27-2. Organ Directly Invaded (at Autopsy) by Pancreas Duct Cancer in 75 Patients

ANATOMIC SITE INVADED	HEAD %	BODY %	TAIL %
Duodenum	67	24	0
Stomach	25	40	7
Spleen	0	12	36
Left adrenal	0	4	29
Transverse colon	3	12	14
Left kidney	0	4	7
Jejunum	3	4	7
Ureter (right)	3	0	0
Total	48	33	19

Adapted from Cubilla, A. L., and Fitzgerald, P. J.: Metastasis. Pancreatic duct adenocarcinoma. In Day, S.; Myers, L.; Stansly, P.; and Lewis, M. (eds.): *Cancer Invasion and Metastasis.* Raven Press, New York, 1977.

monly involved; in descending order of frequency of metastases they include the posterior pancreaticoduodenal groups, the superior head group, superior body group, inferior head group, and anterior pancreaticoduodenal group (Cubilla and Fitzgerald, 1978). Studies of lymph node involvement at resection indicate that in only 5% of cancers of the head of the pancreas is the disease confined to the organ.

In addition to regional lymph node involvement, the cancer typically invades outside the pancreas to encase and occlude major abdominal vessels such as the portal vein, splenic vein, and superior mesenteric artery. Such involvement is readily diagnosed by arteriography and is a contraindication to curative surgery.

The current TNM staging classification takes into account the known sites of local and

regional spread, as well as distant metastases (see Table 27-4).

Symptoms and Signs

The predominant symptoms of pancreatic cancer result from the direct extension of the tumor into the nerves of the retroperitoneal space, obstruction of the common bile duct, direct invasion of the duodenum as well as other visceral organs, and overt metastatic spread to liver and lungs. These are manifested by pain, anorexia, nausea, weight loss, and epigastric bloating (Moossa *et al.,* 1980) (see Tables 27-5 and 27-6).

Pain is the most common presenting symptom. Initially it may be a vague, poorly localized complaint, but it eventually becomes established as a progressive and persistent problem. Generally, epigastric pain predominates; it may be colicky or dull and steady, with some radiation into the lower back. Less commonly, the pain is confined to the back region, suggesting a possible orthopedic or neurologic condition. Paroxysms may be associated with meals. The pain may be exacerbated at night, and partially relieved by changes in posture, particularly by sitting or bending forward. The prolonged use of heating pads may leave a telltale discoloration of the skin of the abdomen or back. Pain with pancreatic cancer can be largely explained by the encasement of nerve trunks by the tumor and the prominent desmoplastic reaction. Pain is one of the most debilitating features of the disease.

Most patients have a history of recent weight loss, which may be the only sign of the under-

Table 27-3. Sites of Metastases in Carcinoma of the Pancreas—Location of Primary Tumor

SITE OF METASTASIS	HEAD Total Patients: 5233 (%)	BODY AND TAIL Total Patients: 1912 (%)
Regional nodes	75	76
Liver	65	71
Lungs	30	14
Peritoneum	22	38
Duodenum	19	5
Adrenals	13	24
Stomach	11	5
Gallbladder	9	0
Spleen	6	14
Kidney	6	5
Intestines	4	5
Mediastinal nodes	4	5
Other	19	28
No metastasis	13	6

Adapted from Howard, J. M., and Jordan, J. L.: Cancer of the pancreas. *Curr. Probl. Cancer,* 2:1-18, 1977.

Table 27–4.   TNM Classification

Primary Tumor (T)

T_x Minimum requirements cannot be met
T_1 Limited to pancreas, less than 2 cm in diameter
T_2 Limited to pancreas, 2 to 6 cm in diameter
T_3 Over 6 cm in diameter
T_4 Extrapancreatic direct extension to contiguous structures

Nodal Involvement (N)

N_x Minimum requirements cannot be met
N_0 No metastic nodes
N_1 One regional group involved at laparotomy
N_2 Two or more regional groups involved at laparotomy
N_3 Clinical evidence of regional node involvement (no laparotomy)
N_4 Involvement of juxtaregional nodes

Distant Metastasis (M)

M_x Not assessed
M_0 No (known) distant metastasis
M_1 Distant metastasis present: Sites specified according to the following notations:

PUL: pulmonary
OSS: osseous
HEP: hepatic
BRA: brain
LYM: lymph nodes
MAR: bone marrow
PLE: pleura
SKI: skin
EYE: eye
OTH: other

Stage I
$T_1N_0M_0$
$T_1N_xM_0$
$T_2N_0M_0$
$T_2N_xM_0$
$T_xN_0M_0$
$T_xN_xM_0$

Stage II
$T_3N_0M_0$
$T_3N_xM_0$

Stage II
$T_1N_1M_0$
$T_2N_1M_0$
$T_3N_1M_0$
$T_xN_1M_0$

Stage IV
any T, any N, M_1

Table 27–5.   Clinical Features of Cancer of the Pancreas. Primary Site: Head

	% PATIENTS
Symptoms	
Weight loss	92
Jaundice	82
Pain	72
Anorexia	64
Dark urine	63
Light stools	62
Nausea	45
Vomiting	37
Weakness	35
Pruritus	24
Diarrhea	18
Signs	
Jaundice	87
Palpable liver	83
Palpable gallbladder	29
Ascites	14
Abdominal mass	13

Adapted from Howard, J. M., and Jordan, J. L.: Cancer of the pancreas. *Curr. Probl. Cancer,* 2:13, 1977.

Jaundice is an important clinical feature of pancreatic cancer. An estimated 75 to 90% of patients with primary tumors in the head region will become icteric. In most cases jaundice follows a period of abdominal pain. Jaundice, however, may be the first symptom of the disease, resulting from an early occlusion of the common bile duct as it traverses through the head of the pancreas to the ampulla of Vater. This is the subgroup of patients, albeit limited in number, for whom prompt surgery is curative. In contrast, jaundice associated with primary tumors of the body or tail is a late

Table 27–6.   Clinical Features of Cancer of the Pancreas. Primary Site: Body and Tail

	% PATIENTS
Symptoms	
Weight loss	100
Pain	87
Weakness	43
Nausea	43
Vomiting	37
Anorexia	33
Constipation	27
Hematemesis	17
Melena	17
Signs	
Palpable liver	33
Tenderness	27
Abdominal mass	23
Ascites	20
Jaundice	23

Adapted from Howard, J. M., and Jordan, J. L.: Cancer of the pancreas. *Curr. Probl. Cancer,* 2:13, 1977.

lying tumor. This is explained in most cases by a state of anorexia and the poorly understood cachexia that almost universally accompany the disease. Frequently patients describe specific abnormalities in taste sensation and aversions to certain foods, particularly meat. Pancreatic insufficiency with steatorrhea, as well as diabetes (Schwartz *et al.,* 1978), may result from occlusion of the pancreatic duct or direct destruction of the exocrine and endocrine functions of the organ.

finding, usually signifying advanced disease metastatic to the liver or the porta hepatis.

A change in bowel habits is commonly described. With invasion of the duodenum or stomach, there may be symptoms of obstruction, nausea, and vomiting. Frank gastrointestinal bleeding is rare, whereas occult bleeding is detectable in approximately 50% of cases. Thrombophlebitis, classically superficial, migratory, and anticoagulant-resistant, has been shown in some series to occur with increased frequency (see Chapter 6B). It may be the first sign of the disease and has been correlated with tumors of the pancreatic body and tail. Psychiatric disorders have also been described, including depression and anxiety states that may herald the presence of the tumor (Fras *et al.,* 1968).

In many patients symptoms are ill-defined and the physician may not initially consider the diagnosis. In one series the interval between the onset of symptoms and hospital admission was approximately four months (Gullick, 1959; Bragenza and Howat, 1972).

On physical examination there may be signs of generalized cachexia and jaundice, as well as the presence of an enlarged and hard liver. A palpable upper abdominal mass, representing a primary tumor in the tail or body of the pancreas, may be present in 10 to 25% of cases. Obstruction of the splenic vein by tumor encasement can result in splenomegaly with possible hypersplenism, an otherwise uncommon finding with gastrointestinal cancer. A similar occlusion of the portal vein may produce esophageal varices and contribute to the development of ascites. The rare acinar cell carcinoma has been associated with a clinical syndrome of subcutaneous fat necrosis, polyarthralgia, and eosinophilia, as well as elevated serum lipase activity (Robertson and Eeles, 1970).

Diagnosis

Many of the early symptoms of pancreatic cancer are vague and nonspecific and may not arouse suspicion in the patient or physician until the tumor has invaded outside the organ, beyond the limits of curative resection.

Suggested indications (Moossa, 1982) for embarking on investigations include:

1. Recent upper abdominal or back pain or both, consistent with a retroperitoneal origin;
2. Recent vague upper abdominal pain with negative gastrointestinal investigations;
3. Obstructive jaundice;
4. Unexplained weight loss greater than 5% of normal body weight;
5. Pancreatitis in the absence of predisposing factors such as gallstones or alcohol ingestion; and
6. Maturity onset diabetes without a predisposing cause such as family history or obesity.

A large variety of other disorders, benign and neoplastic, may present with signs and symptoms that mimic pancreatic cancer. In a prospective study at the Mayo Clinic (Go *et al.,* 1981), 95 consecutive patients suspected of having pancreatic cancer were investigated prior to laparotomy. A similar study was conducted at the University of Chicago on 186 patients (Moossa and Levin, 1981). The results shown in Table 27–7 demonstrate that in symptomatic patients the presumptive diagnosis was confirmed in 40 to 50% of cases.

Selection of Diagnostic Tests. The approach to diagnosis depends in part on the facilities available. New developments in methods of imaging, such as nuclear magnetic resonance, and the possibility of more sensitive immunologic techniques using monoclonal antibodies may greatly alter our present approach to cancer detection within the next few years. Much of the information in the literature describing the diagnostic yield of specific techniques refers to patients with advanced disease rather than those with early or no symptoms who might benefit most from more prompt diagnosis.

Figure 27–1 presents a schema for evaluat-

Table 27–7. Eventual Diagnosis in Patients Suspected of Having Cancer

	MAYO CLINIC (Go et al., 1981) 95 Patients	UNIVERSITY OF CHICAGO (Moosa and Levin, 1981) 136 Patients
Cancer of the pancreas	50%	40%
Nonpancreatic neoplasms	11%	17%
Chronic pancreatitis	10%	13%
Nonpancreatic, nonneoplastic conditions	29%	30%

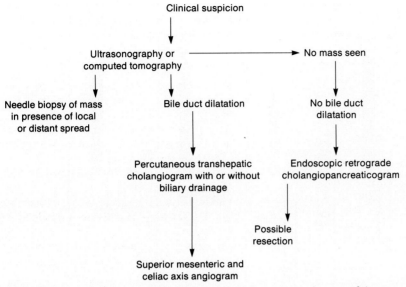

Figure 27–1.   Suggested approach to diagnosis and management of cancer of the pancreas.

ing the patient with suspected cancer. The relative value of specific diagnostic procedures at the University of Chicago is presented in Table 27–8 and Figure 27–2.

Ultrasonography and Computed Tomography (CT).   Noninvasive tests are used in the initial phases of investigation. Institutional preferences and expertise often determine whether ultrasonography or computed tomography (CT) is performed, but they may provide complementary information. They both can indicate enlargement of the pancreas, localized masses, alteration in the contour of the gland, biliary duct dilatation, or the presence of hepatic metastases (see Figures 27–3A, B, and C). Neither test, however, can adequately distinguish pancreatitis from cancer, and there is no effective method to enhance differentially either the tumor or the adjacent benign

pancreatic tissue. In general, ultrasound and CT can detect lesions of the head of the pancreas with equal frequency, whereas body and tail abnormalities are better delineated by CT. The tail of the pancreas is particularly difficult to visualize with ultrasound because of an absence of an acoustic window. Peripancreatic nodal enlargement or vascular invasion can be seen on computed tomography. In the cachectic patient, ultrasonography may be more informative because optimal visualization of the pancreas with CT requires the presence of retroperitoneal fat. By contrast, CT is preferred in the obese patient or when there is a large amount of bowel gas or ascites.

Recently a prospective cooperative study was performed to assess the relative efficacy of computed tomography and ultrasound in detecting and identifying pancreatic lesions

Table 27–8.   Relative Value of Diagnostic Tests in Pancreatic Cancer

| TEST | TECHNICAL FAILURE RATE | PREDICTIVE VALUE | | | |
		Specificity	*Sensitivity*	POSITIVE	NEGATIVE
Ultrasonography	11%	84%	82%	77%	88%
Computed tomography	11%	82%	77%	73%	85%
Pancreatic scan	0%	64%	65%	54%	74%
Duodenal juice analysis for:					
1. low bicarbonate + low volume	9%	99%	10%	94%	63%
2. cytology	9%	99%	68%	99%	83%
ERCP with pancreatography	21%	90%	86%	85%	91%
Cholangiography					
Cytology					
Angiography	0%	72%	73%	63%	81%

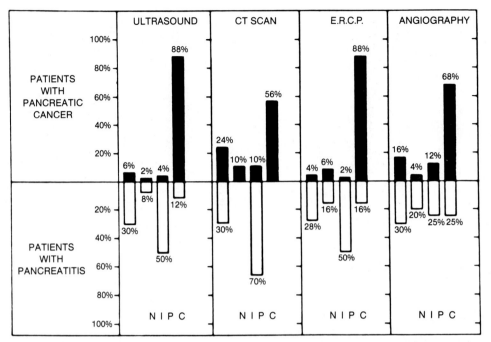

Figure 27–2. Results of four pancreatic imaging tests showing the percentage of pancreatic cancer (solid bars) and chronic pancreatitis (open bars) obtaining each of the following results. N = normal; I = abnormal; P = pancreatitis; C = pancreatic cancer. From Moossa, A. R., and Levin, B.: The diagnosis of "early" pancreatic cancer — The University of Chicago experience. *Cancer* (Suppl.), **47**:1688–1697, 1981.

(Hessel *et al.,* 1982). Of 279 patients, 146 had a normal pancreas and 133 had an abnormal pancreas. Forty-four ultrasound examinations were technically unsatisfactory, a persistent problem with this method. Excluding these suboptimal examinations, CT had a sensitivity of 0.87 and a specificity of 0.90 in detecting an abnormal pancreas. Ultrasound had a sensitivity of 0.69 and a specificity of 0.82. In differentiating between a neoplastic or inflammatory lesion, CT had a sensitivity of 0.84 and ultrasound had a sensitivity of 0.56. Based upon the results of this study, CT appears to be the method of choice for detecting a pancreatic lesion, assessing its extent, and defining its pathology.

Endoscopic Retrograde Cholangiopancreatography (ERCP). The diagnosis of pancreatic cancer by ERCP has been extensively reviewed by Blackstone (1980). To interpret the radiographic images obtained with this procedure, the pathologic events involved must be appreciated. The tumor is usually desmoplastic, and as the mass enlarges it obliterates ductal structures in its path. On reaching the main duct the tumor mass invades or compresses this structure and produces ductal narrowing. Within the tumor mass, necrosis may occur,

which leads to the formation of cystic cavities that may communicate with the main duct. Proximal to the tumor mass an obstructive pancreatitis is produced with inflammation and destruction of the duct (Robbins and Cotran, 1979). A typical radiographic appearance of pancreatic cancer is illustrated in Figure 27–4.

The sensitivity of ERCP for diagnosing pancreatic cancer in experienced centers is 90% (that is, positive studies in patients with cancer) with a specificity of 90% (normal studies in patients without cancer). The complication rate is less than 3%. Material suitable for cytologic analysis can be obtained from the periampullary region by brushing or by aspiration of pancreatic juice; it is positive in up to two-thirds of patients with cancer, thereby providing a definitive diagnosis and is negative in patients with chronic pancreatitis or a normal pancreas.

ERCP has been compared to other methods of diagnosis in pancreatic cancer. In a recent study of 61 patients with suspected pancreatic neoplasms, ERCP results were accurate in 62% of the cases, with 8% false negatives; there was, however, no diagnostic information in 30% because of technical failure. When pancreatic

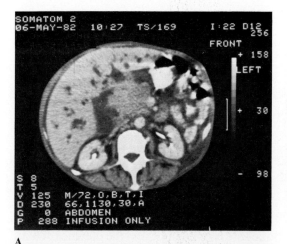

A

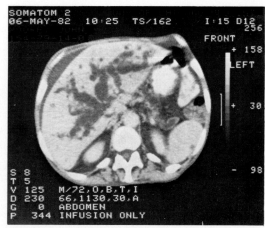

B

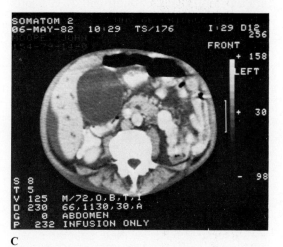

C

Figure 27-3. (*A*) CT scan: Large mass in head of pancreas. (*B*) CT scan: Marked dilatation of intrahepatic bile ducts in pancreatic carcinoma. (*C*) CT scan: Gross distention of gallbladder in pancreatic cancer.

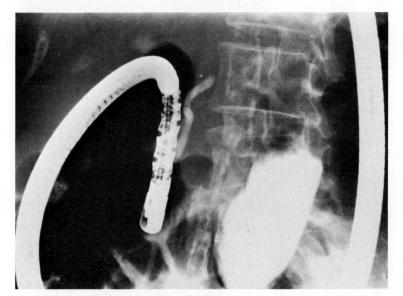

Figure 27-4. ERCP—demonstrating complete obstruction of the pancreatic duct in the midbody of the pancreas.

duct cannulation was successful, the overall accuracy increased to 88%. The results with CT in the same study were 76% correct, 5% false positive, 13% false negatives, and 6% indeterminate. Using ERCP and CT resulted in an accuracy rate of 93%, higher than with either study alone. ERCP and CT examinations are therefore often complementary, and their combined use may produce a more accurate and specific diagnosis (Moss et al., 1980).

In patients with pancreatic neoplasia early diagnosis is vital while the neoplasm is small and amenable to curative surgical resection. Although ERCP facilitates diagnosis, and in particular the detection of periampullary cancers, it does not have the sensitivity to identify cancers in other parts of the pancreas at an early stage (Hall et al., 1978). Tumors in the earliest stages of development are often located peripheral to the larger ductal structures for at least 50% of their natural history (Takashi and Pour, 1975). For human pancreatic cancer there may be a critical size below which ERCP is rarely positive.

Radionuclide Scintigraphy. As a screening test for pancreatic disease ^{75}Se-selenomethionine scanning of the pancreas has generally been discarded. The reasons for this are manyfold: The very high incidence of false-positive scans (estimated to be in the 50% range); the nonspecificity of abnormalities in distinguishing pancreatic cancer from pancreatitis; and the development of ultrasound and CT, which are also noninvasive but considerably more accurate.

Recent efforts have been directed toward ^{11}C-labeled amino acids as radiopharmaceuticals with greater specificity for pancreatic cancer. Preliminary reports on the use of ^{11}C-tryptophan and ^{11}C-methionine in patients with pancreatic disease are available. Scans were performed either on a longitudinal multiplane emission tomographic scanner or, more recently, on positron emission computed tomographic scanners. The results suggest excellent sensitivity and specificity for the detection of pancreatic disease; however, cancer could not be distinguished from pancreatitis. This method has limited general clinical applicability at the moment, in part because the radiopharmaceutical requires a cyclotron for its production and has a very short half-life (Buonocore and Hubner, 1979; Kirschner et al., 1980; Syrota et al., 1982).

Angiography. Since the advent of CT and ultrasound pancreatic angiography is rarely used as a primary diagnostic procedure for symptomatic patients. Rather, it is employed to delineate vascular anatomy, to determine resectability, and occasionally to aid in the differential diagnosis of mass lesions detected by CT or ultrasound. In patients with pancreatic tumors less than 2 cm, or in those that do not enlarge the organ, angiography may still have a selective diagnostic role (Rosch, 1975).

The principal angiographic signs of pancreatic carcinoma include encasement or obstruction of pancreatic or adjacent arteries and narrowing, obstruction, or displacement of the portal, splenic or superior mesenteric veins (see Figure 27–5). Although similar abnormalities can be seen in chronic pancreatitis, they are less frequent, and the presence of both arterial and venous abnormalities is highly suggestive of carcinoma. Most adenocarcinomas of the pancreas generally do not show neovascularity or tumor staining, in contrast to cystadenocarcinomas. A vascular lesion on angiography suggests other diagnoses, such as islet cell tumor, carcinoid, hemangioma, or even peripancreatic lesions such as lymphoma, leiomyosarcoma, or aberrant spleen.

Angiography can be helpful in assessing resectability of pancreatic neoplasm. If there is encasement of only intrapancreatic arteries without involvement of the larger extrapancreatic branches (hepatic, superior mesenteric, gastroduodenal, splenic, etc.), the chance of a resectable lesion is greatly increased and the mean survival time for these patients is also increased (Freeny et al., 1979; Levin et al., 1980).

Cytologic Diagnosis of Pancreatic Cancer. Material from the pancreas for cytologic examination can be obtained in three ways:

1. ERCP: Tumors in the head are diagnosed with greater frequency than those in the body and tail of the pancreas, and the yield is enhanced after secretin stimulation (Blackstone, 1980);
2. Duodenal drainage studies, which, after secretin stimulation, have a sensitivity of about 60%. With cancers of the head of the pancreas, the sensitivity rises to 79%, whereas if the cancer is in the tail the sensitivity drops to 33%. False-positives are unusual, and in one series were reported in four of 1087 patients without pancreatic cancer (Cooper et al., 1978); and
3. Fine-needle aspiration cytology with ultrasound or CT guidance.

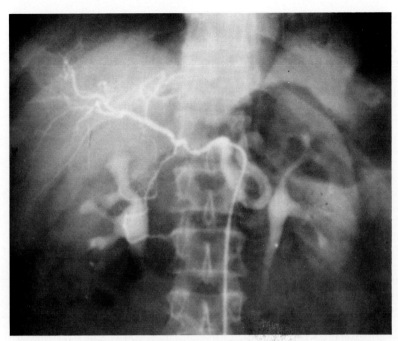

Figure 27–5.   Arteriography: Carcinoma of the head of pancreas encasing common hepatic and gastroduodenal arteries.

Pancreatic Function Studies. These tests involve duodenal intubation and stimulation of pancreatic secretion directly, using intravenous secretin, or indirectly by a test meal. The latter method is not as sensitive in the setting of mild pancreatic insufficiency. The collected pancreatic juice is analyzed for total volume, pH, bicarbonate, and enzyme concentrations. The results of several series indicate a sensitivity of 75 to 90% for pancreatic disease and pancreatic cancer; the specificity is approximately the same (DiMagno *et al.,* 1977).

DiMagno and colleagues used a more sophisticated test employing a constant intravenous infusion of cholecystokinin (CCK) combined with the perfusion of the duodenum and a nonabsorbable marker to allow quantification of enzyme output. In their hands, the test was 88% sensitive and 79% specific for the detection of pancreatic disease (DiMagno *et al.,* 1977). However, a decrease in pancreatic secretion cannot be detected until more than 60% of the total length of the main pancreatic duct has been obstructed (DiMagno *et al.,* 1979).

At the University of Chicago the secretin stimulation test is employed as a semiquantitative test, but it is largely reserved for obtaining material for cytologic examination when endoscopic retrograde cannulation of the pan-creatic duct is unsuccessful (Cooper *et al.,* 1978).

Fine-Needle Aspiration Cytology. Computed tomography or ultrasonography may be used to guide percutaneous fine-needle aspiration to obtain material for cytologic examination (Beazley, 1981). This technique is applicable to tumor masses in the body and tail of the pancreas that are usually unresectable for cure. It is especially useful in the frail patient to avoid a purely diagnostic laparotomy and when surgical bypass is not indicated.

The technique is not advisable in patients with small, potentially resectable cancers, particularly those in the head of the pancreas. Seeding along the aspiration tract is a possible complication (Ferrucci *et al.,* 1979; Smith *et al.,* 1980). The technique should also not be used in patients who require surgical palliation for the relief of jaundice or duodenal obstruction (other than to prepare them for operation by reducing the serum bilirubin concentration).

In a recent study of 53 patients with suspected pancreatic carcinoma, accuracy of fine-needle aspiration cytology was 88.7%, the sensitivity was 86%, and the specificity was 100% (Mitty *et al.,* 1981). In this series, 36 of 37 patients were spared a laparotomy because of the positive biopsy.

Percutaneous Transhepatic Cholangiography. This test is of value in the jaundiced patients with biliary duct dilatation discovered by ultrasonography. It helps to localize the site of obstruction and the same approach can be used to provide percutaneous biliary drainage.

Tumor Markers in Pancreatic Cancer. The serum (systemic and portal venous) levels of various tumor markers have been measured in patients with pancreatic cancer (see Chapter 6A). They include:

1. Oncofetal antigens such as CEA, alphafetoprotein (AFP), and pancreatic oncofetal antigen (POA). Eighty-three percent of pancreatic cancer patients have a CEA level greater than 2.5 ng/mL; however, 65% of patients with other cancers and 45% of those with benign diseases have an elevated plasma concentration (Mackie *et al.,* 1980). These data emphasize the relative lack of sensitivity and specificity of CEA testing. Serial CEA determinations provide a rough clinical estimate of response to therapy. Elevations in plasma CEA level are influenced by two major factors: Total body tumor burden and excretion via the hepatobiliary system. Marked elevations of the CEA in jaundiced patients with extrahepatic obstruction may present a false indication of tumor burden because the CEA may rapidly fall after percutaneous biliary drainage (Zamcheck and Martin, 1981).

   POA is a glycoprotein with a molecular weight between 800,000 and 900,000 (Gelder *et al.,* 1978). It is found in fetal pancreas and pancreatic cancer tissue, but it is not present in the normal adult pancreas. POA is measurable in the sera of most normal individuals but highest serum levels are found in those with carcinoma of the pancreas. Elevated serum levels of POA are also observed in patients with carcinoma of the lung, stomach, colon, biliary tract, and breast as well as in the serum of some pregnant women and others with benign conditions (breast disease, biliary tract stones, and cirrhosis). The usefulness of serial POA levels was analyzed in nine patients with pancreatic cancer who underwent resection of their tumors. In three of the patients, high preoperative serum levels of POA decreased appropriately when the tumors were resected; in one of three patients the POA levels rose again when the tumor recurred. In four other patients whose initial levels were below the upper limit in normal individuals, 14 units, no significant change was found after resection (Gelder *et al.,* 1978).

2. A macrophage leukocyte adherence inhibition (LAI) assay has been studied in pancreatic cancer. The LAI phenomenon is based on the observation that leukocytes from a tumor-bearing host become less adherent to a glass or plastic-coated surface in the presence of a tumor extract of the same histologic type. In one study, the LAI assay detected 100% (5/5) of patients with localized disease without nodal involvement and 85.7% (6/7) of patients with localized disease and spread to peripancreatic lymph nodes (Goldrosen *et al.,* 1981). The test was positive in 66.6% (6/9) of patients with regional lymph node involvement and 55.5% (15/27) of patients with hepatic metastases. However, the assay detected 83.3% (10/12) of pancreatic cancer patients with metastatic disease at locations other than the liver (ascites, peritoneal seeding, lung or bone metastasis). The reported false-positive rate was less than 5% and there was no crossreactivity with pancreatitis. The data are provocative, suggesting that the LAI is particularly useful in early stages of the disease, but further experience in a larger series of patients is required to evaluate this test properly.

3. The concentration of galactosyltransferase isoenzyme II (GI-II) in serum has been compared to CEA, AFP, ultrasonography, CT, and ERCP in the detection of pancreatic cancer. Although the GI-II assay does not distinguish pancreatic carcinoma from other gastrointestinal neoplasms, only ERCP was more sensitive than GI-II in diagnosing pancreatic cancer. Greater sensitivity was achieved when GI-II was combined with ultrasound (92%), CT (88%), and ERCP (100%) (Podolsky *et al.,* 1981). These promising observations remain to be confirmed by other investigators.

4. Other putative markers evaluated include: (1) Hormones (insulin, glucagon, gastrin, calcitonin, parathyroid, hormone, human chorionic gonadotropin);

(2) enzymes (amylase, lipase, trypsin, alkaline phosphatase, 5-nucleotidase, ribonuclease, lactic dehydrogenase, glutamic oxaloacetic transaminase, leucine aminopeptidase; and (3) immunoglobulins such as IgA, IgG, IgM. None of these markers has the sensitivity and specificity necessary for use in pancreatic cancer diagnosis or screening (Moossa, 1982).

Treatment

Surgery. The optimum surgical approach for pancreatic carcinoma must take into account the clinical state of the patient and the anticipated stage of disease, as well as the recognized limitations inherent for this modality (see Chapter 8). Patients with clinically evident advanced metastatic tumor and associated poor performance status (PPS), particularly those with jaundice secondary to hepatic metastases, have little to gain from surgery. For patients with good nutrition and who are ambulatory, palliative surgery for biliary and gastric bypass is associated with a modest improvement in survival, measured in months. The presence of severe jaundice, with serum bilirubin levels in excess of 10 mg/100 mL, is associated with an increased incidence of postoperative complications such as renal failure, hemorrhage, and sepsis in some series, as well as a higher mortality rate (Braasch and Gray, 1977). Decompression of the biliary tract by percutaneous transhepatic drainage or endoscopic placement of a biliary catheter in preparation for surgery has been recommended.

Preoperative staging may demonstrate locally advanced tumor with involvement of a region of bowel or lymph nodes or encasement of an abdominal vessel as revealed by arteriographic evidence. In such cases the surgeon should consult a radiation therapist to consider interstitial or electron beam irradiation as a component of the operative approach. All too often the opportunity for the intraoperative application of these modalities is lost, necessitating a second laparotomy specifically for this purpose.

Only an estimated 15% of patients with pancreatic carcinoma are candidates for a possible pancreaticobiliary resection for cure (Cancer of the Pancreas Task Force, 1981). The presence of disease outside the organ, including involvement of a single regional lymph node, precludes a curative operation. Intraoperative staging, therefore, is an essential requirement

prior to undertaking a Whipple procedure or a total pancreatectomy. In addition, before subjecting the patient to an operation that carries an overall 20% perioperative mortality, the histologic diagnosis of pancreatic cancer should be established if possible. Benign pancreatitis can present as a mass lesion with a consistency that cannot be differentiated from carcinoma even by highly experienced surgeons. Biopsy and frozen section diagnosis should therefore be attempted. Because of obstruction of pancreatic ducts, benign inflammatory tissue surrounds the tumor in almost all instances. A shallow biopsy can result in a false-negative diagnosis of pancreatitis as a result of inadequate sampling, and repeated biopsies may be required. In the past, wedge biopsy has been associated with an unacceptable incidence of fistula formation, abscess, or bleeding. Needle biopsy has largely replaced this technique. For tumors in the head region the needle is passed through the closed or open duodenum so that any resultant fistula will drain into the duodenum (Issacson et al., 1974; Isler et al., 1981). The omentum can be sutured over the needle tract following direct tumor biopsies in the tail and body region. As previously described, thin-needle aspiration biopsy of the pancreas directed by ultrasound or CT scan guidance is associated with a low complication rate.

Radical resection of the pancreas for cure is generally reserved for patients with a small localized tumor in the head region that caused an early obstruction of the common bile duct as it passes through the organ (Moossa and Levin, 1981). Tumors of the body and tail usually present with symptoms that indicate regional or distant spread. The overall five-year survival rate for resected cases is approximately 4%, whereas the risk of a postoperative death far exceeds the probability of cure in most centers (see Table 27-9) (Levin et al., 1978). For this reason many surgeons emphasize the palliative biliary bypass procedures, rather than attempting a pancreatectomy for every potentially resectable case. Table 27-10 presents the data supporting this approach.

The two basic operative procedures with curative intent are the Whipple procedure and the total pancreatectomy. A comparison of survival data from several series is presented in Table 27-11. The classic Whipple procedure consists of resection of the pancreas proximal to the superior mesenteric vein, distal stomach, and duodenum and formation of a gastro-

Table 27–9. Results of Pancreatoduodenal Resection for Carcinoma of the Pancreas

RESEARCHER (LOCATION)	PATIENTS RESECTED	RESECTABILITY	MORTALITY	FIVE-YEAR SURVIVORS
Monge (Mayo)	119	10%	25%	8
Porter (Columbia)	17	9%	11%	0
Morris (Mass. General)	26	21%	34%	2
Glenn (Cornell)	25	9%	24%	1
Jordan (Baylor)	36	—	22%	1
Salmon (Minnesota)	38	18%	33%	1
Lansing (Ochsner)	22	—	27%	3
Park (Pennsylvania)	51	27%	31%	0
Richard (New Orleans)	43	26%	—	2
Leadbetter (Vermont)	6	21%	0	2
Fish (Texas)	16	—	31%	0
Hoffman (Missouri)	13	—	24%	0
Warren (Lahey)	138	—	15%	10
Longmire (California)	39	26%	10%	1
Crile (Cleveland)	28	4%	10%	0
Smith (London)	44	—	20%	2
Hertzberg (Norway)	12	6%	8%	0
Nakase (Japan)	332	18%	25%	6
Total	1005	15%	20%	39 (4%)

Adapted from Levin, B.; ReMine, W. H.; Hermann, R. E.; Schein, P. S.; and Cohn, I.: Panel: Cancer of the pancreas. *Am. J. Surg.*, **135**:185–191, 1978.

jejunostomy and a choledochojejunostomy. Although no data support one technique over the other, several arguments have been advanced in favor of total pancreatectomy (Brooks, 1979). Pancreatic carcinoma is multicentric, with neoplastic changes concurrently present in several regions of the organ in 15 to 20% of cases. This is further complicated by the difficulty in determining the extent of tumor involvement of parenchyma and pancreatic duct so that an adequate margin of normal tissue will be included in the resection. Pathologic examination of resected pancreatic

carcinomas in one series identified tumor at the line of resection after Whipple resection, or cancer in the tail region, in 38% of cases (Brooks, 1979). As a consequence, a Whipple procedure did not achieve local control in a substantial proportion of patients. Although a Whipple procedure leaves a functional portion of pancreatic tissue, the necessary pancreaticojejunostomy raises the risk of an anastomotic leak with attendant complications of postoperative pancreatitis and sepsis as well as death. The total pancreatectomy, however, leaves the patient with a brittle form of dia-

Table 27–10. Comparison of Pancreatoduodenal Resection (PDR) and Biliary Bypass in Potentially Resectable Patients with Carcinoma of the Pancreas

SERIES	NO. OF PATIENTS	MORTALITY	SURVIVAL (MO) *Mean*	SURVIVAL (MO) *Longest*
Crile				
PDR	28	10%	6	22
Bypass	28	8%	12	41
Hertzberg				
PDR	12	8%	17	36
Bypass	12	12.8%	24	50
Monge				
PDR	94	25%	12	60+
Bypass	23	—	12	42
Shapiro				
PDR	24	8%	10.6	22
Bypass	24	4%	8.1	24
Collected series				
PDR	496	21%	13.9	60+

Adapted from Levin, B.; ReMine, W. H.; Hermann, R. E.; Schein, P. S.; and Cohn, I.; Panel: Cancer of the pancreas. *Am. J. Surg.*, **135**:185–191, 1978.

Table 27-11. Comparison of Pancreatoduodenal Resection (PDR) and Total Pancreatectomy in Patients with Carcinoma of Pancreas

RESEARCHER (LOCATION)	PATIENTS RESECTED	MORTALITY	FIVE-YEAR SURVIVORS
Porter (Columbia)			
PDR	27	11%	0
Total	18	28%	0
Warren (Lahey)			
PDR	138	15%	10 (7%)
Total	11	10%	0
Jordan (Baylor)			
PDR	36	22%	1
Total	113	36%	0
Brooks (Peter Bent Brigham)			
PDR	11	21%	0
Total	16	12.5%	3
Nakase (Japan)			
PDR	308	25%	6
Total	45	20%	
ReMine (Mayo)			
PDR	119	25%	8 (7%)
Total	33	21%	2 (6%)

Adapted from Levin, B.; ReMine, W. H.; Hermann, R. E.; Schein, P. S.; and Cohn, I.: Panel: Cancer of the pancreas. *Am. J. Surg.,* **135**:185–191, 1978.

betes as well as an absolute deficiency of exocrine function. More importantly, no conclusive data suggest that this operative approach carries a higher probability of cure (see Table 27-11). Recurrent attacks of ascending cholangitis are common to all procedures involving a biliary bypass, in some cases necessitating chronic oral antibiotic therapy to suppress the growth of bowel flora.

Despite the limitations of surgery for pancreatic cancer, several important forms of palliative treatment can be achieved in carefully selected cases. Biliary and gastric bypass will delay or prevent obstruction of these organs and improve the quality of remaining life. The placement of radio-opaque surgical clips in areas of locally advanced cancer can define a postoperative radiation field that limits the extent of normal tissue toxicity. Specialized forms of intraoperative irradiation can be delivered during the operation. Lastly, splanchnic nerves can be injected with phenol to reduce pain and the narcotic dosage required for its control. Nevertheless, pancreatic carcinoma is a disseminated disease at diagnosis in almost all cases. The current survival rates, independent of stage, will not significantly improve until an effective form of systemic treatment has been developed.

Radiation Therapy. Radiotherapy of pancreatic cancer is largely reserved for patients with locally advanced tumors. A retrospective analysis of results with 3500 rads ^{60}Co irradiation, compared to a group of matched untreated patients, failed to demonstrate either improved survival or useful palliation (Moertel *et al.,* 1969). Subsequently, in 1973, Halsam and coworkers described 6000 rads of radiation therapy using a split course, opposed field, technique in which three 2000 rads increments delivered in two weeks were separated by intervening two-week rest periods (Halsam *et al.,* 1973). The median survival of 23 patients was 7.5 months, with 24% of patients alive at two years. Dobelbower subsequently proposed higher doses of external beam irradiation, employing 45 meV photons and 15 to 40 meV electrons to a maximum tumor dose of 6000 to 7000 rads in seven to nine weeks (Dobelbower, 1979). This study used CT scans, lateral IVP films, and radio-opaque surgical clips to define the irradiated region, as well as field-shaping techniques to spare the spinal cord, kidneys, and liver from excessive dosage. These procedures are recommended for all future studies of external irradiation of the pancreas. The median survival of the 40 patients in this series was approximately one year, and palliation of pain was reported in 22 of 32 cases. Patients who also received chemotherapy demonstrated a somewhat improved survival.

Combined radiation therapy and chemotherapy has now become the standard approach for locally advanced pancreatic cancer. Moertel and colleagues (1969) reported the results of a randomized controlled trial in which patients received 3500 to 4000 rads of external radiotherapy with a saline placebo or combined with intravenous 5-fluorouracil (5-FU), 15 mg/kg on the first three days of the irradiation. Although there was no appreciable difference in median survival, the mean survival for the combined modality treatment group, 10.4 months, was superior to that for the group with radiotherapy alone, 6.3 months ($P = 0.05$). In 1974 the Gastrointestinal Tumor Study Group designed a three-arm trial in which 106 patients were randomly assigned to either 4000 rads split course radiotherapy with 5-FU, 6000 rads split course radiotherapy with 5-FU, or 6000 rads alone (Gastrointestinal Tumor Study Group, 1979). 5-FU was administered intravenously at a dose of 500 mg/m² on the first three days of each 2000-rad split course. The outcome with combined modality treatment was superior to radiotherapy alone with the following median survivals: 4000 rads plus 5-FU, 36 weeks; 6000 rads plus 5-FU, 40 weeks; 6000 rads, 20 weeks (see Figure 27–6). Despite the positive result, few patients survived two years, and local control of the irradiated tumor remained an important clinical

problem, thus emphasizing the need to explore new management approaches for this stage of pancreatic cancer. Recently designed trials employing external beam photon radiotherapy are evaluating three and four field techniques to reduce toxicity for normal tissues, superfractionation, and radiation sensitizers other than 5-FU such as doxorubicin and misonidazole.

Neutron radiotherapy is of considerable interest because of the theoretic advantages of high linear energy transfer (LET) irradiation, reduced requirement for oxygen for cytotoxicity, and the increased relative biologic effect (RBE) compared to photons. Neutron radiotherapy for locally advanced pancreatic cancer was recently evaluated at the Lombardi Cancer Research Center in cooperation with the Mid-Atlantic Neutron Therapy Association (Smith *et al.*, 1981). Nineteen patients were treated with 1716 rads of 15 meV neutrons alone or with 5-FU. The median survival was only six months and, although there was no treatment-related mortality, toxicity was appreciable. Hemorrhagic gastritis, appearing six to nine months after treatment, was described in 25% of patients, along with other

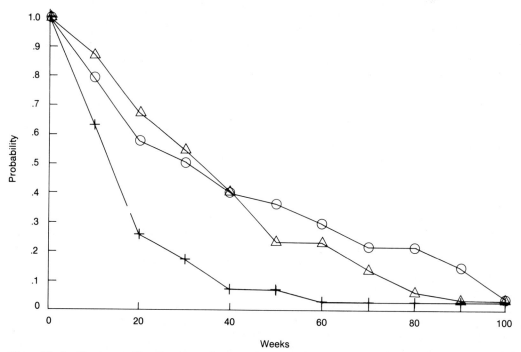

Figure 27–6. Treatment of locally advanced pancreatic cancer with 4000 rads plus 5-fluorouracil (△); 6000 rads alone (+), or 6000 rads plus 5-fluorouracil (○). From Moertel, C. G., *et al.*: Therapy of locally unresectable pancreatic carcinoma: Randomized comparison of high dose (6000 rads) radiation alone, moderate dose radiation (4000 rads + 5-fluorouracil), and high dose radiation + 5-fluorouracil. *Cancer* **48**:1705–1710, 1981.

serious manifestations of gastrointestinal and hepatic toxicity. The conclusion reached was that neutron radiotherapy was no more therapeutic than standard photon irradiation and was appreciably more toxic. Other programs are now evaluating the use of mixed beam (neutron and photon) radiotherapy and helium ions.

Although not a new technique, interstitial radiation therapy has recently attracted increasing attention, particularly the use of ^{125}I because of its physical characteristics. For small tumors that can be adequately implanted, total doses of 15,000 rads can be delivered locally, followed by 4000 to 5000 rads of external photon irradiation. Shipley and colleagues (1980) reported a median survival of 11 months in a series of 12 patients, but despite the achievement of local regional control in 78% of patients, all died within 30 months of follow-up. In addition to the unsuitability of this approach to large regional tumors, the study emphasizes the need for an effective systemic treatment to use in conjunction with all forms of radiotherapy.

A novel approach to intraoperative irradiation is the use of high single doses of electrons: 1000 to 3000 rads (Gunderson *et al.*, 1982). Placing a cone to displace the normal bowel from the field and using an electron energy that penetrates the tumor but not the underlying spinal cord and vasculature make this an attractive technique theoretically. The early results from clinical trials in three centers in the United States, as well as those of Abe and associates (1975) in Japan, do not as yet support the initial enthusiasm for this approach.

The results achieved with radiation therapy and combined modality treatment were placed into better perspective by an analysis of the survival of patients with locally advanced pancreatic cancer treated with chemotherapy (FAM) alone who achieved an equivalent life span (Smith *et al.*, 1983).

Chemotherapy. Few anticancer agents have undergone an adequate trial for activity in patients with advanced measurable pancreatic cancer. This deficiency can be traced to the widely held belief that this tumor has special biologic properties that make it inherently resistant to chemotherapy. This, coupled with the innate difficulties in identifying objective variables for following disease, has dampened the enthusiasm of potential therapeutic investigators. Furthermore, this disease tends to cause rapid debilitation, frequently with pain,

anorexia, weight loss, and malabsorption. So patients are often unsuitable candidates for chemotherapy when they are first seen. Obstructive jaundice and hepatic dysfunction may further impair the effectiveness of administered antineoplastic agents that are primarily removed by biliary excretion.

The literature describing the therapeutic activity of single anticancer agents in pancreatic cancer is of limited value. When response rates are provided, many studies do not include data on response duration or the survival of the patient population. The actual response rates must always be regarded with a great deal of suspicion because pancreatic cancer, even in its advanced states, is often a very difficult disease to measure objectively. Phase II trials, which by definition are an assessment of the activity of a specific treatment, require that the population studied have advanced measurable disease so that the investigator can critically assess tumor response. Most patients with pancreatic cancer that fulfill this criterion have a great tumor burden and an extremely poor performance status, and are unlikely to respond to, or even tolerate, a toxic regimen. The overall position of chemotherapy, therefore, in treating pancreatic cancer remains to be defined and is an almost virgin area of clinical investigation.

The most extensively studied drug for patients with advanced pancreatic cancer is 5-fluorouracil (Carter and Comis, 1975). Surveys of the literature emphasize the wide range of reported response rates, from 0% to 67%, with most current trials of 5-FU chemotherapy reporting responses of 20% or less. This wide range of response data can be attributed to differences in selection of patients, lack of uniformity of objective criteria for response, the difficulty in assessing measurable disease, and the varieties of dosages and scheduling used in the administration of 5-FU. In the past five years the merits of various routes and methods of administration of this drug have been much debated. In particular, the value of oral courses of 5-FU has been studied. Oral 5-FU at 15 mg/kg given once a week was compared to 5-FU at the same dose administered intravenously every week in 30 patients with advanced measurable pancreatic cancer (Stolinsky *et al.*, 1975). The response rate for the group given the drug intravenously was 21%, comparable to previously reported results; none of the patients treated with oral 5-FU responded ($P = 0.04$).

The antibiotic mitomycin-C was reported to have single agent activity comparable to 5-FU, and in collected series from the literature 12 of 44 patients (27%) achieved a response. Initially used in a loading course, this drug was found to cause serious delayed and accumulative myelosuppression resulting in a state of chronic marrow hypoplasia. An intermittent schedule of drug administration analogous to the current use of chloroethylnitrosoureas overcame many of these problems of administration. Mitomycin-C has also been effectively and safely employed in combination regimens (Smith and Schein, 1979).

The literature contains a dearth of information on the activity of classic alkylating agents in pancreatic cancer. A recent study of melphalan produced only a 2% response rate. In an evaluation of the chloroethylnitrosoureas for activity in pancreatic cancer, BCNU was found inactive when used as a single agent in 31 cases studied at the Mayo Clinic (Kovach et al., 1974). Twenty-two of these cases had received no prior chemotherapy. When more recently developed nitrosoureas, CCNU and methyl-CCNU, were tested (Moertel et al., 1969) two of four patients seemed to achieve a response with CCNU. In 15 patients with advanced measurable pancreatic tumor treated with methyl-CCNU, two responded: a 13% rate. The Eastern Cooperative Oncology Group treated a series of 34 patients with methyl-CCNU and found a 9% response rate, with a median survival of 12 weeks (Douglass et al., 1976).

Streptozotocin, a naturally occurring methylnitrosourea, is a potent toxin for the pancreatic islet beta cell in animals, a property that has been exploited clinically in treating islet cell carcinoma. The limited reported experience for adenocarcinoma suggests that this drug also has activity for the major pancreas tumor type. Objective response rates of 31 to 50% were described in small series, a seemingly unrealistic result (Broder and Carter, 1975; Dupriest et al., 1975). Streptozotocin has the advantage of relatively mild myelosuppressive properties. This agent, however, can produce severe nausea and vomiting, and renal tubular toxicity eventually limits treatment.

The Gastrointestinal Tumor Study Group, in an attempt to identify drugs with specific activity for pancreatic carcinoma, undertook a series of phase II studies of individual anticancer agents. Doxorubicin produced a partial response in two of 15 previously untreated patients (13%), whereas methotrexate in conventional doses and actinomycin-D were not active (Schein et al., 1978). Recently responses were observed with hexamethylmelamine in ongoing studies.

Results with combination chemotherapy of pancreatic carcinoma are discouraging; most studies fail to demonstrate survival benefit over 5-FU alone. The number of patients in many pilot studies has been small and, as emphasized, some of the combination regimens contained drugs without any noteworthy single-agent activity in this disease. In addition, many patients entered onto these studies had a poor performance status and, therefore, were less likely to demonstrate benefit from intensive therapies. Recent phase II studies of drug combinations have described enhanced response rates and one-year survivals.

Combination Chemotherapy. Eighty-two randomized patients with advanced pancreatic carcinoma received either 5-FU alone at a dose of 13 mg/kg/day intravenously for five days every five weeks or BCNU alone at 10 mg/kg/day for five days every five weeks (Kovach et al., 1974). A third group of 30 patients received the combination of 5-FU 10 mg/kg/day and BCNU at a dose of 40 mg/m^2/day for five days every five weeks. An objective response was recorded in ten of 30 (33%) patients treated with the combination, an interesting result considering the fact that BCNU demonstrated no single-agent activity in 21 cases. The response rate with single-agent 5-FU was 16%. Despite the increased response rate with the combination there was no survival benefit when compared with either of the single-agent groups. The median duration of survival for all patients was approximately six months.

Two regimens of 5-FU administered by continous intravenous infusion for five days (1000 mg/m^2/24 hours for five days) with either mitomycin-C (20 mg/m^2) or methyl-CCNU (175 mg/m^2) added every eight weeks were compared (Buroker et al., 1978). A total of 144 patients were entered into this randomized trial. The combination of 5-FU and mitomycin-C produced a superior response rate of 30% compared to 17% for 5-FU and methyl-CCNU ($P = 0.03$).

The Vincent T. Lombardi Cancer Research Center initiated a phase II trial of a combination of three drugs, each of which at the time of the study design had reported single-agent activity in pancreatic cancer: Streptozotocin, mitomycin-C, and 5-FU (SMF) (Wiggans et *al.*, 1978). SMF was administered in eight-week cycles, streptozotocin 1 g/m² intravenously and 5-FU 600 mg/m² during weeks one, two, five, and six, and mitomycin-C during week one only; the cycle was repeated on week nine (see Figure 27–7). Twenty-three consecutive cases with advanced measurable pancreatic cancer were entered into this program. Ten of 23 (43%) achieved an objective response, and one patient demonstrated a complete response with regression of biopsy-proved hepatic metastases for over four years. The responders demonstrated a median survival of ten months as compared to three months for the nonresponders, whereas the median survival of all cases was six months (see Figure 27–8). Four of the 23 (17%) cases studied lived one year or longer. An important factor is that the median performance status in this group of patients was 1, that is, the patients were symptomatic but fully ambulatory. This contrasts with other treatment series in which debilitated patients have predominated. Aberhalden and coworkers (1977) and Bukowski and colleagues (1980) obtained results similar to the SMF regimen with their combination of 500 mg/m²/day of 5-FU intravenously for five days, 300 mg/m²/day streptozotocin intravenously for five days with 10 mg/m² mitomycin-C administered intravenously every eight weeks. An objective response was recorded in 5/16 (31%) of the patients treated. A two-drug combination of 5-FU and streptozotocin obtained a 21% response rate in their series. Recently, the Southwest Oncology Group reviewed the early results of a comparative trial of SMF chemotherapy versus mitomycin-C

and 5-fluorouracil alone (Bukowski, 1981). In this SMF regimen 5-FU, 1000 mg/m², was administered as a 24-hour infusion, and streptozotocin, 400 mg/m², was given once every 56 days. A 40% response was reported with SMF compared to 5% with the two-drug combination. The combination of 5-FU and streptozotocin was compared to a combination of streptozotocin and cyclophosphamide by the Eastern Cooperative Oncology Group. A 12% response rate was reported with both regimens.

Following the demonstration that doxorubicin had independent activity for advanced pancreatic cancer, the Lombardi Cancer Research Center initiated a pilot study of the FAM regimen of 5-FU, doxorubicin, and mitomycin-C (Smith *et al.*, 1980). In this regimen 5-FU was administered intravenously during weeks one, two, five, and six; 30 mg/m² of doxorubicin were administered intravenously during weeks one and five; and 10 mg/m² of mitomycin-C were given intravenously in the first week. Of 37 patients with pancreatic cancer treated with this regimen, 25 with advanced measurable disease were available for evaluation of response. The median performance status in this group of patients was 2, with one-fourth of the patients having a performance status of 3 (partially bedridden). Ten of the 25 patients obtained a partial response, with a median survival in excess of nine months for responders. This was followed by a confirmatory trial by Bitran and colleagues that involved a limited number of patients (Bitran *et al.*, 1979).

Adjuvant Therapy.   The Gastrointestinal Tumor Study Group compared the efficacy of

Drug	Dose	Week No.								
		1	2	3	4	5	6	7	8	9
Streptozotocin	1 gm/m² IV	X	X			X	X			R
Mitomycin-C	10 gm/m² IV	X								e
5-Fluorouracil	600 mg/m² IV	X	X			X	X			p
										e
										a
										t

WBC		Platelets	Dose Reduction
Early (2–3 weeks)	2000		5-FU by 25%
Late (4–5 weeks)	1500–2500		MMC by 25%
	1500		MMC by 50%
		50,000–75,000	MMC by 25%
		50,000	MMC by 50%

Figure 27–7.   SMF regimen and dose-attenuation schedule.

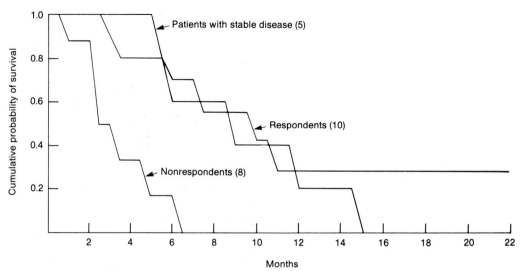

Figure 27–8. Survival of patients with advanced measurable pancreatic cancer treated with the SMF (streptozotocin, mitomycin-C, and 5-fluorouracil) regimen. From Wiggans, R. G.; Woolley, P. V., III; Macdonald, J. S.; Ueno, W.; and Schein, P. S.: Phase II trial of streptozotocin, mitomycin-C and 5-fluorouracil (SMF) in the treatment of advanced pancreatic cancer. *Cancer,* **41**:387–391, 1978.

surgical resection alone versus resection followed by radiotherapy and 5-FU (Kalser *et al.,* 1983). In this small but important trial, 22 patients were randomized to no adjuvant treatment and 21 to combined therapy. A total of 4000 rads, administered in two 2000-rad split courses, was delivered to the region of the pancreas together with 5-FU, 500 mg/m^2 on the first three consecutive days of each course of radiation; 5-FU was continued weekly after radiation therapy for a period of two years or until recurrence. The median survival for the treated group was 20 months, which was superior to that observed for the control group: 11 months ($P = 0.03$). The estimated two-year survival probabilities were 42% for treated and 15% for control groups, respectively. Three patients who received adjuvant therapy lived five years or longer, compared to one treated with surgery alone. This pioneering study is a basis for future trials of adjuvant therapy following curative resection of pancreatic cancer.

Management of Complications. Most patients with pancreatic adenocarcinomas either present with, or soon develop, anorexia and cachexia to the extent that nutritional debilitation is a major factor in causing death. To a variable degree, malnutrition is attributable to pancreatic enzyme deficiency with resultant malabsorption of fat and protein and associated diarrhea. This is particularly true for patients with the tumor located in the head region and with a complete block of the pan-

creatic duct. Therefore, an attempt to restore intestinal lipase and trypsin activity with the use of pancreatic enzymes with meals is essential. Because exposure to the acid conditions of the stomach degrades the oral enzyme preparation, as many as eight tablets may be required, in addition to cimetidine to increase gastric pH. The patient may require supplements in the form of medium chain triglycerides and fat soluble vitamins. Added to this state of exocrine deficiency is the loss of endocrine function, with diabetes mellitus necessitating insulin treatment to insure that ingested glucose is effectively used and that endogenous fat and protein stores are not needlessly consumed. Patients who have undergone a pancreaticoduodenal resection are subject to all the complications resulting from a hemigastrectomy, including the dumping syndrome. The patient is devastated nutritionally by a profound state of anorexia and cachexia that can only be reversed by effective treatment of the underlying neoplasm. For patients considered suitable candidates for active treatment, intensive nutritional support in the form of enteral or intravenous parenteral hyperalimentation may be required until a remission is achieved or anticancer management is deemed futile (see Chapter 45).

Control of pain is an essential component of supportive management, particularly in patients for whom there is no attempt to arrest tumor growth and who are regarded as preterminal. As outlined in Chapter 44, long-act-ing narcotics such as methadone should be used according to a schedule that prevents the perception of pain, if possible. Nerve blocks during initial laparotomy or percutaneously may reduce the narcotic requirement and the attendant complications.

Pancreatic cancer is implicated as a major cause of Trousseau's syndrome, more com-monly found in association with tumors of the tail and body regions. As described in Chapter 6B, this classically takes the form of superficial migratory thrombophlebitis, but deep venous thrombosis and marantic endocarditis are well-recognized complications of this disease. Treatment consists of heparin administration, whereas warfarin sodium (COUMADIN) com-monly fails to control the stage of hypercoagu-lability.

Future Prospects

Despite the recent proliferation of diagnos-tic modalities for pancreatic cancer, there is at present no single test to detect early disease or screen a population at risk. The CT scan is limited by its inability to discern malignant from normal tissue because no method can differentially enhance the density of a tumor. Development of tumor-specific markers is now being emphasized, in an attempt to iden-tify a unique protein in the pancreatic juice of patients with cancer and develop monoclonal antibodies directed against some constituent of the malignant neoplasm.

Several new approaches to the radiothera-peutic management of pancreatic cancer are being evaluated. Although these measures may result in improved local-regional control, the vast majority of patients will nevertheless die of disseminated disease. The management of patients with disease, including the patient whose tumor is resected for cure, requires ef-fective chemotherapy. New drugs with useful therapeutic activity for this tumor must be identified. We are now confined to the use of empirical phase-II trials in patients with ad-vanced measurable tumors. Perhaps the use of clonogenic assays will, in the future, allow more efficient selection of new chemothera-peutic agents for this and other diseases.

Ultimately the most effective approach to this tumor, which has increased in incidence dramatically, is to identify specific risk factors and eliminate them from our environment. Epidemiologic and laboratory studies are being actively pursued to provide a more ex-plicit understanding of the factors that result in the development of this tumor.

PERIAMPULLARY NEOPLASMS

Periampullary neoplasm is a term used to describe a group of cancers that arise from the ampulla of Vater and secondary tissues (see Chapter 28). Generally related are adenocarci-nomas of the terminal part of the duct of Wir-sung, of the smaller ducts near the ampulla of Vater, and the ampulla itself, which is the most common cancer of the terminal common bile duct (Lindenauer *et al.,* 1981).

The precise site of origin of periampullary neoplasms is often impossible to specify. These lesions produce a mass that causes early obstruction of the ampulla and are less fre-quently encountered than neoplasms in the head of the pancreas. Forrest and Longmire (1979) reported 34 periampullary lesions dur-ing 21 years in which they operated upon 245 patients with pancreatic cancer. Men are af-fected more commonly than women (4 : 1), and the average age of presentation is between 50 and 60 years.

The signs and symptoms of periampullary carcinoma are presented in Table 27 – 12. The jaundice is an obvious symptom that causes the patient to seek early medical attention and accounts for a higher proportion of resectable and potentially curable periampullary neo-plasms compared to similar lesions of pancre-atic origin. Forrest and Longmire (1979) re-ported that almost 100% of patients with periampullary neoplasms may have resectable

Table 27 – 12.   Signs and Symptoms of Periampullary Carcinoma

Symptoms	
Jaundice	72–95% (painless in only one-third)
Abdominal pain	35–65%
Weight loss	90%
Anorexia	70%
Nausea	50%
Vomiting	35%
Chills	23%
Charcot's triad (chills, fever, jaundice)	20%
Signs	
Hepatomegaly	25–45%
Fever	35%
Palpable gallbladder	25%
Ascites	6%

tumors compared to only 25% of those with adenocarcinoma of the head of the pancreas. The five-year survival of patients with periampullary lesions undergoing pancreatoduodenectomy was reported between 25 and 50% (Forrest and Longmire, 1979; Lindenaver *et al.*, 1981). A Whipple procedure may be curative, particularly if there is no evidence of local invasion or spread to lymph nodes.

REFERENCES

Abe, M.; Takahaski, M.; Yabumoto, E.; Onoyama, Y.; Torizuka, K.; Tobe, T.; and Mori, K.: Techniques, indications and results of intraoperative radiotherapy of advanced cancers. *Radiology,* **116**:693, 1975.

Aberhalden, R. T.; Bukowski, R. M.; Groppe, C. W.; Hewlett, J. S.; and Weick, J. K.: Streptozotocin and 5-fluorouracil with and without mitomycin in the treatment of pancreatic adenocarcinoma. *Proc. A.S.C.O.,* **18**:301, 1977.

American Cancer Society: *1985 Cancer Facts and Figures.* New York, American Cancer Society, 1985.

Beazley, R. M.: Needle biopsy diagnosis of pancreatic cancer. *Cancer,* **47**:1685–1687, 1981.

Berg, J. W., and Connelly, R. R.: Updating the epidemiologic data on pancreatic cancer. *Semin. Oncol.,* **6**:275–283, 1979.

Bernardino, M. E., and Barnes, P. A.: Imaging the pancreatic neoplasm. *Cancer,* **50**:2681–2688, 1982.

Bitran, J. D.; Desser, R. K.; Kozloff, M. F.; Billings, A. A.; and Shapiro, C. M.: Treatment of metastatic pancreatic and gastric adenocarcinoma with 5-fluorouracil, adriamycin, and mitomycin -C (FAM). *Cancer Treat. Rep.,* **63**:2049–2051, 1979.

Blackstone, M. O.: Endoscopic retrograde cholangio-pancreatography in the diagnosis of pancreatic tumors. In Moossa, A. R. (ed.): *Tumors of the Pancreas.* The Williams & Wilkins Company, Baltimore, 1980.

Braasch, J. W., and Gray, B. N.: Considerations that lower pancreatoduodenectomy morbidity. *Am. J. Pathol.,* **185**:111–115, 1977.

Bragenza, J. M., and Howat, H. T.: Cancer of the exocrine pancreas. *Clin. Gastroenterol.,* **1**:219, 1972.

Broder, L. E., and Carter, S. K.: Streptozotocin: Clinical brochure. National Cancer Institute, Therapy Evaluation Program, Bethesda, Maryland, 1975.

Brooks, J. R.: Operative approach to pancreatic carcinoma. *Semin. Oncol.,* **6**:357–367, 1979.

Bukowski, R. M.: Randomized comparison of 5-FU and mitomycin-C (MF) versus 5-FU, mitomycin-C and stretozotocin (SMF) in pancreatic adenocarcinoma—a Southwest Oncology Group Study. *Proc. Am. Soc. Clin. Oncol.,* **22**:C–472, 1981.

Bukowski, R. M.; Aberhalden, R. T.; Hewlett, J. S.; Weick, J. K.; and Groppe, C. W.: Phase II trial of streptozotocin, mitomycin-C and 5-fluorouracil in adenocarcinoma of the pancreas. *Cancer Clin. Trials,* **3**:321–324, 1980.

Buonocore, E., and Hubner, K. F.: Positron-emission computed tomography of the pancreas: A preliminary study. *Radiology,* **133**:195, 1979.

Buroker, T.; Kim, P. N.; Heilbrun, L.; and Vaitkevicius, V.: 5-FU infusion with mitomycin-C (MMC) vs. 5-FU infusion with methyl-CCNU (Me) in the treatment of advanced upper gastrointestinal cancer. *Proc. Am. Soc. Clin. Oncol.,* **29**:310, 1978.

Cancer of the Pancreas Task Force: Staging of cancer of the pancreas. *Cancer,* **47**:1631–1637, 1981.

Carter, S. K., and Comis, R. L.: The integration of chemotherapy into a combined modality approach for cancer treatment. VI. Pancreatic adenocarcinoma. *Cancer Treat. Rev.,* **2**:193–214, 1975.

Compagno, J., and Oertel, J. E.: Mucinous cystic neoplasms of the pancreas with overt and latent malignancy (cystadenocarcinoma and cystadenoma). A clinicopathologic study of 41 cases. *Am. J. Clin. Pathol.,* **69**:573–580, 1978.

Cooper, M. J.; Moossa, D. E.; Cockerham, L.; Hall, T. J.; Levin, B.; and Moossa, A. R.: The place of duodenal drainage studies in the diagnosis of pancreatic disease. *Surgery,* **84**:457–464, 1978.

Court-Brown, W. M., and Doll, R.: Mortality from cancer and other causes after radiotherapy for alkylosing spondylitis. *Br. Med. J.,* **2**:1327–1332, 1965.

Cubilla, A. L., and Fitzgerald, P. J.: Metastasis. Pancreatic duct adenocarcinoma. In Day, S.; Myers, L.; Stansly, P.; and Lewis, M. (eds.): *Cancer Invasion and Metastasis.* Raven Press, New York, 1977.

Cubilla, A. L., and Fitzgerald, P. J.: Pancreas cancer. Duct adenocarcinoma. A clinical-pathologic study of 380 patients. In *Pathology Annual,* Part 1. Appleton-Century-Crofts, New York, 1978.

Cubilla, A. L., and Fitzgerald, P. J.: Pancreas cancer (non-endocrine). A review. Part I. *Clin. Bull. Mem. Sloan-Kettering Cancer Center,* **8**:144, 1978.

Cubilla, A. L., and Fitzgerald, P. J.: Surgical pathology of the exocrine pancreas. In Moossa, A. R. (ed.): *Tumors of the Pancreas.* The Williams & Wilkins Company, Baltimore, 1980.

Department of Health, Education and Welfare. Biometry Branch, National Cancer Institute: The Third National Cancer Survey: Incidence data. In Cutler, S. J., and Young, J. L. (eds.): *National Cancer Institute Monograph 41.* 1975.

DiMagno, E. P.; Malagelada, J. R.; and Go, V. L. W.: The relationships between pancreatic ductal obstruction and pancreatic secretion in man. *Mayo Clin. Proc.* **54**:157–183, 1979.

DiMagno, E. P.; Malegalada, J. R.; Moertel, C. G.; and Go, V. L. W.: Prospective evaluation of the pancreatic secretion of immuno-active carcinoembryonic antigen, enzyme and bicarbonate in patients suspected of having pancreatic cancer. *Gastroenterology,* **73**:457, 1977.

DiMagno, E. P.; Malegalada, J. R.; Taylor, W. F.; and Go, V. L. W.: A prospective comparison of current diagnostic tests for pancreatic cancer. *N. Engl. J. Med.,* **297**:737, 1977.

Dobelbower, R. R., Jr.: The radiotherapy of pancreatic cancer. *Semin. Oncol.,* **6**:378–389, 1979.

Douglass, H. L., Jr.; Lavin, P. T.; and Moertel, C. G.: Nitrosoureas: Useful agents for treatment of advanced gastrointestinal cancer. *Cancer Treat. Rept.,* **60**:769–780, 1976.

Druckrey, H.; Ivankovic, S.; Bucheler, J.; Preussman, R.; and Thomas, C.: Erzeungung von Magen—und pankreas—krebs beim meerschweinchen durch methyl-nitroso-harnstoff und -urethan. *Krebsforsch.,* **71**:167–182, 1968.

DuPriest, R. W.; Huntington, M. C.; Massey, W. H.; Weiss, A. J.; Wilson, W. L.; and Fletcher, W. S.: Streptozotocin therapy in 22 cancer patients. *Cancer,* **25**:358–367, 1975.

Ferrucci, J. T., Jr.; Wittenberg, J.; Margolis, M. N.; and Carey, R. W.: Malignant seeding of the tract after thin-needle aspiration biopsy. *Radiology,* **130:**345–346, 1979.

Forrest, J. F., and Longmire, W. P., Jr.: Carcinoma of the pancreas and periampullary region. *Ann. Surg.,* **189:**129–138, 1979.

Fras, I.; Litin, E. M.; and Bartholomew, L. G.: Mental symptoms as an aid in the early diagnosis of carcinoma of the pancreas. *Gastroenterology,* **55:**191, 1968.

Freeny, P. C.; Ball, T. J.; and Ryan, J.: Impact of new diagnostic imaging methods on pancreatic angiography. *A.J.R.,* **133:**619, 1979.

Gastrointestinal Tumor Study Group: Comparative therapeutic trial of radiation with or without chemotherapy in pancreatic carcinoma. *Int. J. Radiat. Oncol. Biol. Phys.,* **5:**1643, 1979.

Gelder, F. B.; Reese, C. J.; Moossa, A. R.; Hall, T. J.; and Hunter, R.: Purification, partial characterization and clinical evaluation of a pancreatic oncofetal antigen. *Cancer Res.,* **38:**313–324, 1978.

Go, V. L. W.; Taylor, W. F.; and DiMagno, E. P.: Efforts of early diagnosis of pancreatic cancer: The Mayo Clinic experience. *Cancer,* **47:**1698–1703, 1981.

Goldrosen, M. H.; Dasmahpatra, K.; Jenkins, D.; Howell, J. H.; Arbush, S. G.; Moore, M. C.; and Douglass, H. O.: Microplate leucocyte adherence inhibition (LAI) assay in pancreatic cancer. *Cancer,* **47:**1614–1627, 1981.

Gullick, H. D.: Carcinoma of the pancreas. A review and critical study of 100 cases. *Medicine* (Baltimore), **38:**47, 1959.

Gunderson, L. L.; Shipley, W. U.; Herman, D., Suit, M. D.; Epp, R. E.; Nardi, G.; Wood, W.; Cohen, A.; Nelson, J.; Battit, G.; Biggs, P. J.; Russell, A.; Rockett, A.; and Clark, D.: Intraoperative irradiation: A pilot study combining external beam photon with "boost" dose intraoperative electrons. *Cancer,* **49:**2259–2266, 1982.

Hall, T. J.; Blackstone, M. O.; Cooper, M. J.; Hughes, R. G.; and Moossa, A. R.: Prospective evaluation of endoscopic retrograde cholangiopancreatography in the diagnosis of periampullary cancers. *Ann. Surg.,* **187:**313, 1978.

Halsam, J. B.; Cavanaugh, P. J.; and Stroup, S. L.: Radiation therapy in the treatment of irresectable adenocarcinoma of the pancreas. *Cancer,* **32:**1341–1345, 1973.

Hessel, S. J.; Siegelman, S. S.; McNeil, B. J.; Sanders, R.; Adams, D. F.; Alderson, P. O.; Finberg, H. J.; and Abrams, H. L.: A prospective evaluation of computed tomography and ultrasound of the pancreas. *Radiology,* **143:**129–133, 1982.

Howard, J. M., and Jordan, J. L.: Cancer of the pancreas. *Curr. Probl. Cancer,* **2:**1–18, 1977.

Isaacson, R.; Weiland, L. H.; and McIlrath, D. C.: Biopsy of the pancreas. *Arch. Surg.,* **109:**227, 1974.

Isler, R. J.; Ferrucci, J. T.; Wittenberg, J.; Muller, P.; Simone, J. F.; Van Sonnenberg, E.; and Hall, D. A.: Tissue core biopsy of abdominal tumors with a 22 gauge cutting needle. *A.J.R.,* **136:**725–728, 1981.

Kalser, M.; Ellenberg, S.; Levin, B.; Novak, J.; Ramming, K.; Moertel, C.; Livingstone, A.; Douglas, H.; Mayer, R.; Livston, E.; Leichman, L.; and Schein, P.: Pancreatic cancer: Adjuvant combined radiation and chemotherapy following potentially curative resection. *Proc. Am. Soc. Clin. Oncol.,* **2:**122, 1983.

Kirschner, P. T.; Ryan, J.; Zalutsky, M.; and Harper, P. V.: Positron emission tomography for the evaluation of pancreatic disease. *Semin. Nucl. Med.,* **10:**374, 1980.

Kovach, J. S.; Moertel, C. G.; Schutt, A. J.; Hahn, R. G.; and Reitemeier, R.: A controlled study of combined 1,3-bis (2-chloroethyl)-1-nitrosourea and 5-fluorouracil therapy for advanced gastric and pancreatic cancer. *Cancer,* **33:**563–567, 1974.

Levin, B.; ReMine, W. H.; Hermann, R. E.; Schein, P. S.; and Cohn, I.: Panel: Cancer of the pancreas. *Am. J. Surg.,* **135:**185, 1978.

Levin, D. C.; Wilson, R.; and Abrams, H. L.: The changing role of pancreatic arteriography in the era of computed tomography. *Radiology,* **136:**245, 1980.

Lindenauer, S. M.; Walsh, D. B.; Cronenwett, J. L.; Eckhauser, F.E.; Vahlsing, H. L., and Turcotte, J. G.: Periampullary neoplasms. In Dent, T. L.; Eckhauser, F. E.; Vinik, A. I.; and Turcotte, J. G. (eds.): *Pancreatic Disease.* Grune & Stratton, Inc., New York, 1981.

Mackie, C. R.; Moossa, A. R.; Go, V. L. W.; Noble, G.; Sizemore, G.; Cooper, M. J.; Wood, R. A. B.; Hall, A. W.; Waldmann, T.; Gelder, I.; and Rubenstein, A. H.: Prospective evaluation of some candidate tumor markers in the diagnosis of pancreatic cancer. *Dig. Dis. Sci.,* **25:**161–172, 1980.

MacMahon, B.; Yen, S.; Trichopoulos, D.; Warren, K.; and Nardi, G.: Coffee and cancer of the pancreas. *N. Engl. J. Med.,* **304:**630–633, 1981.

Mitty, H. A.; Efremides, S. C.; and Yeh, H.-C.: Impact of fine needle biopsy on management of patients with carcinoma of the pancreas. *A.J.R.,* **137:**1119–1121, 1981.

Moehr, P.; Ammann, R.; and Lasgiader, F.: Pankreaskarzinom bei chronischer pankreatitis. *Schweiz. Med. Woschenschr.,* **105:**590–592, 1975.

Moertel, C. G.; Childs, D. S.; Reitemeier, R. J.; Colby, M. Y.; and Holbrook, M. A.: Combined 5-fluorouracil and supervoltage radiation therapy of locally unresectable gastrointestinal cancer. *Lancet,* **2:**865–867, 1969.

Moossa, A. R.: Pancreatic cancer: Approach to diagnosis, selection for surgery and choice of operation. *Cancer,* **50:**2689–2698, 1982.

Moossa, A. R., and Levin, B.: Collaborative studies in the diagnosis of pancreatic cancer. *Cancer* (suppl.), **6:**298, 1979.

Moossa, A. R., and Levin, B.: The diagnosis of "early" pancreatic cancer—The University of Chicago experience. *Cancer* (suppl.), **47:**1688–1697, 1981.

Moossa, A. R.; Lewis, M. H.; and Bowie, J. D.: Clinical features and diagnosis of pancreatic cancer. In Moossa, A. R. (ed.): *Tumors of the Pancreas.* The Williams & Wilkins Company, Baltimore, 1980.

Moss, A. A.; Federle, M.; Shapiro, H. A.; Masao, O.; Goldberg, H.; Korobin, M.; and Clemett, A.: The combined use of computed tomography and endoscopic retrograde cholangiopancreatography in the assessment of suspected pancreatic neoplasm: A blind clinical evaluation. *Radiology,* **134:**159–163, 1980.

Podolsky, D. K.; McPhee, M. S.; and Alpert, E.: Galactosyl-transferase isoenzyme II in the detection of pancreatic cancer: Comparison with radiologic, endoscopic and serologic tests. *N. Engl. J. Med.,* **304:**1314–1318, 1981.

Pour, P.; Kruger, F. W.; Althoff, J.; Cardesa, A.; and Mohr, U.: A new approach for induction of pancreatic neoplasms. *Cancer Res.,* **35:**2259–2268, 1975.

Reddy, J. R., and Rao, M. S.: Pancreatic adenocarcinoma in inbred guinea pigs induced by N-methyl-N-nitrosourea. *Cancer Res.,* **35:**2269–2277, 1975.

Robbins, S. C., and Cotran, R. S.: *Pathologic Basis of Disease.* W. B. Saunders Company, Philadelphia, 1979.

Robertson, J. C., and Eeles, G. H.: Syndrome associated

with pancreatic acinar cell carcinoma. *Br. J. Med.,* **2**:709, 1970.

Rosch, J.: Radiological diagnosis of pancreatic cancer. *J. Surg. Oncol.,* **7**:121, 1975.

Schwartz, S. S.; Zeidler, A.; Moossa, A. R.; Kuku, S. F.; and Rubenstein, A. H.: A prospective study of glucose tolerance, insulin, C-peptide and glucagon responses in patients with pancreatic carcinoma. *Am. J. Dig. Dis.,* **23**:1107, 1978.

Shipley W. H.; Nardi, G. L.; Cohen, A. M.; and Ling, C. C.: Iodine-125 implant and external beam irradiation in patients with localized pancreatic carcinoma: A comparative study to surgical resection. *Cancer,* **45**:709, 1980.

Smith, F. P.; Hoth, D. F.; Levin, B.; Karlin, D. A.; Macdonald, J. S.; Woolley, P. V.; and Schein, P. S.: 5-Fluorouracil, adriamycin and mitomycin-C (FAM) chemotherapy in the treatment of a pancreatic carcinoma. *Cancer,* **46**:2014–2018, 1980.

Smith, F. P.; Macdonald, J. S.; Schein, P. S.; and Ornitz, R.: Cutaneous seeding of pancreatic cancer by skinny-needle aspiration biopsy. *Arch. Intern. Med.,* **140**:855, 1980.

Smith, F. P., and Schein, P. S.: Chemotherapy of pancreatic cancer. *Semin. Oncol.,* **6**:368–377, 1979.

Smith, F. P.; Schein, P. S.; Macdonald, J. S.; Woolley, P. V.; Ornitz, R.; and Rogers, C.: Fast neutron irradiation for locally advanced pancreatic cancer. *Int. J. Radiat. Oncol. Phys.,* **7**:1527–1531. 1981.

Smith, F. P.; Woolley, P. V.; Korsmeyer, S.; Byrne, P. J.; Neefe, J. R.; Gullo, J.; Ueno, W.; and Schein, P. S.: Combination chemotherapy with 5-fluorouracil, adriamycin and mitomycin-C (FAM) for locally advanced pancreatic cancer: Equivalence to external beam therapy and implications for future trials. *J. Clin. Oncol.,* **1**:413–415, 1983.

Stolinsky, D. C.; Pugh, R. P.; and Bateman, J. R.: 5-Fluorouracil (NSC-19893) therapy for pancreatic carcinoma: Comparison of oral and intravenous routes. *Cancer Chemother. Rep.,* **59**:1031–1033, 1975.

Syrota, A.; Duquesnoy, N.; Paraf, A.; and Kellershohn, C.: The role of positron emission tomography in the detection of pancreatic disease. *Radiology,* **143**:249, 1982.

Takashi, M., and Pour, P. M.: The results of pancreatography during carcinogenesis. *Am. J. Pathol.,* **91**:57, 1975.

Wiggans, R. G.; Woolley, P. V., III: Macdonald, J. S.; Ueno, W.; and Schein, P. S.: Phase II trial of streptozotocin, mitomycin-C and 5-fluorouracil (SMF) in the treatment of advanced pancreatic cancer. *Cancer,* **41**:387–391, 1978.

Wynder, E. L.; Maabuchi, K.; Maruchi, N.; and Forter, J. G.: Epidemiology of cancer of the pancreas. *J. N. C. I.,* **50**:645–667, 1973.

Young, J. L., Jr.; Asire, A. J.; and Pollack, E. S.: SEER Program. Cancer incidence and mortality in the United States 1973–1976. U.S. Department of Health, Education and Welfare, Bethesda, Maryland, 1978.

Zamcheck, N., and Martin, E. W.: Factors controlling the circulating CEA levels in pancreatic cancer: Some clinical correlations. *Cancer,* **47**:1620–1627, 1981.

28

Neoplasms of the Hepatobiliary System

JAMES D. AHLGREN and PHILIP S. SCHEIN

Introduction

In spite of its relatively low incidence in the United States, the high mortality of hepatobiliary cancer makes it a major problem in both diagnosis and treatment. These diseases frequently remain silent until advanced beyond the point of surgical curability. Diagnosis is imperfect, and confusion with more common benign entities, which present a similar constellation of symptoms, may delay treatment. Proximity to vital structures contributes to relatively low resectability following diagnosis.

BILIARY AND PERIAMPULLARY CARCINOMA

Incidence

It is estimated that currently about 8000 primary cancers of the biliary system are diagnosed in the United States per year or about 4% of all gastrointestinal malignancies (Silverberg, 1983). Of these, primary cancer of the gallbladder is the most common with approximately 5000 new patients yearly, while cholangiocarcinoma and periampullary carcinoma account for the remaining cases.

Etiology and Pathogenesis

Carcinoma of the biliary system is a disease of the older population, with a peak incidence in the sixth to seventh decades. Gallbladder cancer is more common in women (about 67 to 75% of cases), whereas cholangiocarcinoma is somewhat more common in males (60 to 65%) (Strauch, 1960; Fraumeni, 1975; Bedikian et al., 1980).

Numerous etiologic factors and preexisting conditions have been linked with cancers of the biliary system, some of which are listed in Table 28–1. The higher incidence of gallbladder carcinoma in women is thought to reflect the higher rate of cholelithiasis in the female population. Since the early study of Mayo (1903), numerous investigators have confirmed the association between cholelithiasis and cancer of the gallbladder. Calculi have been reported to be present in 54 to 97% of individually collected series of operations performed for carcinoma of the gallbladder; the overall rate of calculi in Strauch's (1960) cumulative series of 867 cases was 72%. Autopsy series of patients with gallbladder cancer have demonstrated an even higher incidence of cholelithiasis. The association of gallstones and carcinoma appears to be independent of age or sex of the patient population studied, suggesting that it serves as a distinct risk factor (Hart et al., 1972b). In contrast, one series of patients with carcinomas from other sites, that metas-

Table 28–1. Some Etiologic Factors in Biliary Cancer

	GALLBLADDER	BILE DUCTS
Cholelithiasis	X	X
Inflammatory bowel disease	X	X
Typhoid carrier state	X	X
Genetic factors	X	X
Chemical carcinogens	X	X
Chronic cholecystitis	X	
Chronic cholangitis		X
Liver fluke infestation		X
Choledochal cysts and dilatations		X
Gardner's syndrome		X
Congenital hepatic fibrosis		X

tasized to the gallbladder, showed only a 16% incidence of gallstones, comparable to the incidence of gallstones in the general population. (Warren and Balch, 1940).

Although these data do not clearly demonstrate a cause-and-effect relationship between cholelithiasis and gallbladder cancer, the concept of prophylactic cholecystectomy upon diagnosis of calculi in the hope of preventing the development of carcinoma (Graham, 1931) is a view still held by some surgeons. This concept has been challenged, however, by Broden and Bengtsson (1980) who evaluated a Swedish population of 213 cases of carcinoma of the gallbladder. Calculi were present in only 42% of their cases, and in only 11% was there evidence for the existence of calculi for more than one year. These authors also noted that a marked reduction in the rate of elective cholecystectomy in Sweden over eight years had failed to affect the incidence of carcinoma. Further, an American study of 123 white patients with silent gallstones (Gracie and Ransohoff, 1982) failed to reveal a single case of gallbladder carcinoma in over 1000 person-years of follow-up.

The association between calculi and cholangiocarcinoma is less clear than with carcinoma of the gallbladder. The average of several series indicates the presence of gallstones with cholangiocarcinoma in approximately one-third of patients (Broe and Cameron, 1981).

Cholangiocarcinoma develops in an estimated 0.4 to 1.4% of patients with ulcerative colitis (Roberts-Thomson et al., 1973; Converse et al., 1971; Ritchie et al., 1974; Akwari et al., 1975) or at a rate almost ten times that of the population at large. Two large series of cholangiocarcinoma (Ross and Braasch, 1973; Bedikian et al., 1980) showed about an 8% rate of antecedent ulcerative colitis. Further, cases of cholangiocarcinoma arising in the ulcerative colitis population do so at a much earlier age than in the general population, comparable to the age at which colorectal carcinoma is diagnosed in the same risk group. The median age of this subgroup of the patients reported by Bedikian and colleagues (1980) was 39. Total proctocolectomy does not appear to protect against subsequent cholangiocarcinoma. Although carcinoma of the gallbladder is not as frequently a complication of ulcerative colitis, it has been reported (Joffe and Antonioli, 1981). An association between Gardner's syndrome and periampullary carcinoma has also been described (Pauli et al., 1980).

Patients with the calcified ("porcelain") gallbladder of end-stage cholecystitis have a substantially increased risk of carcinoma, estimated at 12.5 to 61% (Polk, 1966; Berk et al., 1973). Prophylactic cholecystectomy is probably justified in such patients. Similarly, chronic cholangitis may also be a risk factor for cholangiocarcinoma, although the relationship is much less striking (Donaldson and Guillou, 1979). Typhoid carriers have been found to have a sixfold increased risk of hepatobiliary cancer, further supporting the role of chronic inflammatory disease (Welton et al., 1979).

In some areas of the world, infestation by liver flukes constitutes a major risk factor for cholangiocarcinoma. Clonorchis sinensis, Opisthorchis felineus, and O. viverrini have all been implicated (Bismuth and Malt, 1979). These infections may facilitate the action of specific chemical carcinogens as suggested by studies using Syrian golden hamsters. These animals develop biliary cancer when fed the carcinogen dimethylnitrosamine, but only after they are first infested with O. viverrini (Thamavit et al., 1978). Liver flukes do not appear to increase the risk of gallbladder cancer; the retrospective study of 100 cases of gallbladder carcinoma by Koo et al. (1981) revealed the same rate of Clonorchis infestation as in the general Hong Kong population.

Choledochal cysts and other congenital dilatations of the bile ducts are also recognized to predispose to cholangiocarcinoma. The risk of carcinoma arising in choledochal cysts and congenital dilatations of the bile duct has been estimated variously between 2.5 and 15% (Flanigan, 1977; Todani et al., 1979), with the higher risks associated with Caroli's disease, the more severe congenital form involving segmental intrahepatic ducts (Phinney et al., 1981). Similar problems of bile stasis may contribute to increased risk of carcinoma in congenital hepatic fibrosis (Scott et al., 1980), although most patients with this disease succumb earlier to other causes.

The increased incidence of gallbladder cancer in the Hispanic–American Indian population of the American southwest has been attributed to genetic factors and may not be independent of their concomitant susceptibility to cholelithiasis (Morris et al., 1978; Devor and Buechley, 1980). Other geographic variations sugest possible, as yet undefined, environmental etiologies.

Animal models for chemical induction of

biliary cancers exist, but no human gallbladder carcinogen has been positively identified (Diehl, 1980). Nevertheless, epidemiologic studies have shown a linkage of both gallbladder carcinoma and cholangiocarcinoma to rubber, automotive plant, and wood-finishing workers (Mancuso and Brennan, 1970; Krain, 1972). Links of gallbladder carcinoma with textile and metal-finishing workers, and of cholangiocarcinoma, with chemical and aircraft workers were also identified.

Pathology and Natural History

Histology. Most neoplasms of the gallbladder and biliary tree are malignant, and the most common histology is adenocarcinoma, accounting for approximately 90–95% of gallbladder cancers (Strauch, 1960; Litwin, 1967; Adson, 1973; Arnaud et al., 1979; Shieh et al., 1981). Adenocarcinomas of the gallbladder fall into three main categories: scirrhous (72%), papillary (25%), and colloid (7%) (Arminski, 1949). The papillary histologic subgroup of tumors is characterized by a lesser degree of invasiveness and a somewhat better prognosis (Hart et al., 1972a). Less common histologies include small cell undifferentiated (oat cell) carcinoma (6%), squamous carcinoma (3%), and mixed malignant tumors (2%). Variants of adenocarcinoma exhibiting giant cell histology, intestinal histology, and choriocarcinoma-like areas have also been reported (Black et al., 1978; Bedikian et al., 1980; Albores-Saavedra et al., 1981; Broe and Cameron, 1981). Whereas benign tumors of the gallbladder are usually asymptomatic, in-

cidental findings at cholecystectomy, the rare benign granular cell tumor of the biliary ducts can cause obstructive jaundice, with x-ray findings which mimic cholangiocarcinoma (Farris and Faust, 1979; Jain et al., 1979).

Clinical Presentation. *Gallbladder Cancer.* The early stages of gallbladder cancer, when the disease is most likely to be surgically curable, are unfortunately usually asymptomatic. When the malignancy becomes clinically evident its initial presentation is generally indistinguishable from benign gallbladder disease. In one extensive series, 85% of patients presented with the clinical picture of recurrent cholecystitis (Perpetuo et al., 1978). The most common signs and symptoms of gallbladder cancer are shown in Table 28–2. The majority of patients experience right upper quadrant pain, which may be variously characterized as intermittent or continuous, often aggravated by eating, and often quite localized. Patients with preexisting biliary disease who develop carcinoma are often able to describe a change in the character of their pain, from intermittent and colicky to steady and gnawing. The duration of symptoms is variable, depending upon whether or not there had been preexisting biliary disease. In Strauch's (1960) series the duration of symptoms ranged from one day to four years, with an average of 3.25 months.

Other frequent symptoms are weight loss, anorexia, jaundice, nausea, and fatty food intolerance. As many as 20% of patients may experience chills and fever. These symptoms may be recognized as essentially identical to those of benign gallbladder disease. Since cho-

Table 28–2.   Common Signs and Symptoms in Cancer of the Biliary System

	PERCENTAGE OF PATIENTS WITH GALLBLADDER CANCER*	PERCENTAGE OF PATIENTS WITH CHOLANGIOCARCINOMA†
Pain and/or tenderness	66–97	39–51
Weight loss	50–77	46–95
Hepatomegaly	34–65	39–84
Anorexia	33–52	27–74
Jaundice	44–54	85–97
Nausea and vomiting	8–64	17–30
Palpable GB or RUQ mass	24–40	5–22
Fatty food intolerance	20–33	<10
Chills and/or fever	12–20	<10
Ascites	10–13	<10
Diarrhea	<10	<10
Other‡	<10	<10

* Sources: Strauch, 1960; Litwin, 1967; Robertson and Carlisle, 1967; Keill and DeWeese, 1973; Perpetuo et al., 1978; Arnaud et al., 1979; Koo et al., 1981.
† Sources: Ross et al., 1973; Black et al., 1978; Bedikian et al., 1980; Broe and Cameron, 1981.
‡ Hematemesis, melena, pedal edema, palpable lymph nodes.

lelithiasis and cholecystitis are common problems in the same population, it is not surprising that the majority of gallbladder carcinoma is not recognized until surgery is performed for presumed benign disease. When jaundice occurs with gallbladder carcinoma, it is more frequently related to invasion of liver or bile ducts by carcinoma than to occlusion by a stone, and should, therefore, be considered an unfavorable sign.

Cholangiocarcinoma. Like carcinoma of the gallbladder, cholangiocarcinoma tends to be insidious during its early stages of growth. The most common presenting symptom is jaundice, which results when a major duct is totally occluded by tumor. Concomitant symptoms are listed in Table 28–2, and include essentially the same spectrum of symptoms to be expected with biliary obstruction due to choledocholithiasis or to carcinoma of the head of the pancreas. Preceding clinical jaundice the patient may note pruritus, dark urine, and/or acholic stools. The majority of patients have evidence of advanced disease at the time of diagnosis and may have associated signs of weight loss, hepatomegaly, anorexia, and nausea. If the obstruction is in the common duct, Curvoisier's sign (a palpable distended gallbladder) may also be present. Pain is less common than with gallbladder cancer, but is not infrequent.

A distinct syndrome which can result from tumors at the bifurcation of the hepatic duct has been described by Klatskin (1965). If such a lesion initially obstructs only the left or right hepatic duct, the initial presentation may be mild, with enlargement of the obstructed lobe of the liver and mild pain. Although the serum alkaline phosphatase will be elevated, serum bilirubin may be normal or only mildly increased. If a diagnosis is not established, the patient may actually describe improvement of symptoms as the obstructed hepatic lobe atrophies. Only after the tumor has progressed to obstruct the other duct, or the common hepatic duct, will the patient develop progressive jaundice and the full clinical picture of biliary obstruction.

Occasionally, intraductal growth of hepatocellular carcinoma will give rise to a clinical picture which can be confused with cholangiocarcinoma (Kojiro *et al.,* 1982), but this usually occurs late in the disease.

Periampullary Carcinoma. Like carcinomas of the higher portions of the bile ducts, periampullary carcinomas usually present with jaundice, and the concomitant symptoms of biliary obstruction. Because of their location, they are frequently indistinguishable from carcinomas of the head of the pancreas until surgical exploration. Carcinomas of the ampulla of Vater may exhibit intermittent jaundice, as friable or necrotic tumor breaks off into the duodenum, temporarily relieving biliary obstruction.

Mode of Spread. Both carcinoma of the gallbladder and cholangiocarcinoma can spread via the lymphatics, the blood stream, intraductally, intraperitoneally, and by perineural invasion. Direct extension into the liver is common, and there may be invasion of the stomach, duodenum, and colon. Extension to involve major upper abdominal blood vessels is well recognized and is a major cause for unresectability. Knowledge of the modes of spread is essential in evaluation of the patient for cure or palliation.

The lymphatic drainage of the gallbladder (see Figure 28–1) traverses the cystic node and the pericholedochal nodes (node of the hiatus and superior pancreatoduodenal node). These lymph nodes are commonly involved with tumor, and their enlargement may lead to compression of the common duct and jaundice (Fahim *et al.,* 1962). Lymph drainage from the right side of the gallbladder may bypass the cystic node and pass directly to the node of the hiatus, which also receives drainage from the right lobe of the liver and the common duct; lymphatic obstruction of this system with retrograde flow is probably a major mechanism for tumor spread to the right lobe of the liver. Lymphatics along the hepatic artery do not receive drainage from the gallbladder, but may become involved once the liver has been invaded by tumor. From the superior pancreatoduodenal node, lymphatic drainage may be directly to preaortic nodes around the origin of the celiac artery, or via the pancreatoduodenal chain to nodes around the origin of the superior mesenteric artery.

Veins draining the gallbladder terminate in the liver, where they break up into capillaries and eventually reach the hepatic veins, usually bypassing the portal circulation (see Figure 28–2). Thus, blood-borne metastases can, at least theoretically, be responsible for direct extension to the liver (via the quadrate lobe), as well as for disseminated metastases.

Intraperitoneal spread from gallbladder cancer and cholangiocarcinoma usually takes the form of direct extension to adjacent organs

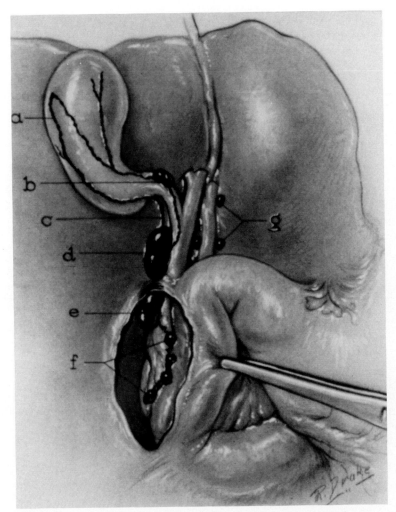

Figure 28–1. Lymphatic drainage of gallbladder. (*a*) Collecting lymphatic trunks on wall of gallbladder; (*b*) cystic node; (*c*) uninterrupted lymph vessels ending in lower nodes; (*d*) node of hiatus; (*e*) superior pancreatoduodenal node; (*f*) posterior pancreatoduodenal nodes; (*g*) nodes along hepatic artery that do not connect with lymphatics from gallbladder. Reproduced from Fahim, R. B.; McDonald, J. R.; Richards, J. C.; and Ferris, D. O.: Carcinoma of the gallbladder: A study of its modes of spread. *Ann. Surg.,* **156:**114–124, 1962, by permission of Lippincott-Harper Publishers.

rather than disseminated carcinomatosis. The organs most frequently involved are the liver, stomach, duodenum, hepatic flexure of the colon, omentum, and the adjacent abdominal wall. Perineural invasion is recorded in about 25% of cases, but its prognostic significance is debated.

Intraductal spread, an often overlooked form of tumor dissemination, is common to both gallbladder cancer and cholangiocarcinoma. This pattern of involvement has been most commonly recognized when ductal obstruction is present, particularly in association with papillary histology (Fahim *et al.,* 1962). Multicentricity, as with other gastrointestinal cancers, is also possible, and difficult to distin-

guish from intraductal seeding. Overall, multisite or diffuse involvement is reported in 3 to 25% of cases in cholangiocarcinoma series.

Diagnosis and Staging

Many of the diagnostic procedures commonly used in evaluation of biliary symptoms offer little or no selectivity between benign and malignant disease. As noted earlier, typically less than 20% of gallbladder cancer is diagnosed before surgery. More common diagnoses are benign biliary disease or carcinoma of the head of the pancreas (Litwin, 1967; Perpetuo *et al.,* 1978; Arnaud *et al.,* 1979). Viewed from a different perspective, gallblad-

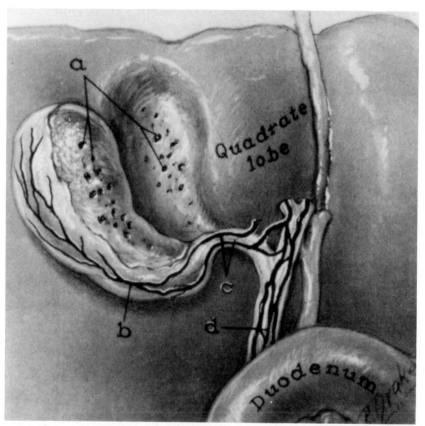

Figure 28-2. Venous drainage of gallbladder. (*a*) Cholecystic veins on hepatic side ending in quadrate lobe; (*b*) cholecystic veins on the peritoneal side communicating with similar veins on neck of gallbladder; (*c*) veins of neck that end directly in quadrate lobe or in plexus around bile ducts, (*d*) which in turn enter quadrate lobe. Reproduced from Fahim, R. B.; McDonald, J. R.; Richards, J. C.; and Ferris, D. O.: Carcinoma of the gallbladder: A study of its modes of spread. *Ann. Surg.*, **156**:114–124, 1962, by permission of Lippincott-Harper Publishers.

der cancer is found in somewhere between 1 and 2% of patients who have biliary tract surgery, usually as an incidental finding (Piehler and Crichlow, 1978). Because of its rarity compared with such entities as cholelithiasis and cholecystitis, the level of suspicion is often low, and otherwise detectable cases are often missed. The 16% of gallbladder cancer patients presenting with the clinical syndrome of acute cholecystitis appear to have less advanced disease with greater resectability and longer survival (Thorbjarnarson, 1960); thus a high index of suspicion in these patients may prevent delay.

Numerous nonspecific laboratory abnormalities may be present with biliary tract cancer. These include anemia, leukocytosis, elevated serum bilirubin, and (most commonly) serum alkaline phosphatase, other abnormal liver function tests, reduced albumin, and an elevated sedimentation rate. The most common roentgenographic examination per-

formed on patients with biliary complaints, the oral cholecystogram, is equally unrewarding. Gallbladders of more than 85% of patients with carcinoma of the gallbladder will fail to visualize, but this will provide no discrimination from benign gallbladder disease. In the few cases where visualization occurs and outlines a filling defect, the cause is much more likely to be a benign deposition of cholesterol (Grieco *et al.*, 1963).

Ultrasonography represents the most useful initial procedure, with CT scanning an alternative. Both of these techniques permit the imaging of the gallbladder, biliary tree, and surrounding structures, irrespective of gallbladder function, and thus provide assistance in discriminating between obstructive and nonobstructive jaundice. Gallbladder wall thickening, which may be hypo- or hyperechogenic, and polypoid wall masses suggest gallbladder cancer (Ruiz *et al.*, 1980). These procedures give an estimate of the degree of tumor extension, as well as providing an assessment of the presence of hepatic metastases.

The identification of dilated bile ducts provides an indication for percutaneous transhepatic cholangiography (see Figure 28-3A). This technique, using the Chiba ("skinny") needle, will almost always define the site of obstruction and frequently will outline the tumor (Michel *et al.*, 1977; Mueller *et al.*, 1982). A dilated ductal system above a "rat tail" constricting lesion in a patient without previous surgery (see Figure 28-3B) is virtually pathognomonic of cholangiocarcinoma (Broe and Cameron, 1981). Extrinsic and intrinsic narrowing of the duct can frequently be distinguished by the shape of the impression. Further, in patients where obstruction is complete, biliary decompression can be effected by cannulation, using the needle as a guide. Preoperative biliary decompression of jaundiced patients may also improve tolerance of subsequent surgery (Wiechel, 1982).

Endoscopic retrograde cholangiopancreatography (ERCP), in the hands of a skilled endoscopist, can be considered as an alternative for visualization of the biliary tree, but does not permit decompression. In addition, ERCP may fail to provide information on the state of the proximal ducts in cases of total obstruction, information which may be critical in determining the optimal surgical approach to management.

Percutaneous transhepatic portography (PTP), as described by Hoevels and Ihse (1979), serves as an additional procedure that may be useful in evaluating patients with cholangiocarcinoma for possible radical surgery. The demonstration of invasion of the portal vein, a common complication, renders the tumor unresectable for cure. Angiography can often provide accurate tumor delineation and may be useful in some cases, especially if tumor is present at or above the bifurcation of the duct, or if hepatoma is a strong consideration. Laparoscopic examination offers a means of diagnosing, obtaining tissue, and assessing resectability, but is not usually performed unless the expectation is that the need for surgery might thereby be obviated.

Although a staging system has been proposed for gallbladder cancer (Nevin *et al.*, 1976), it has not been widely utilized. Tumor

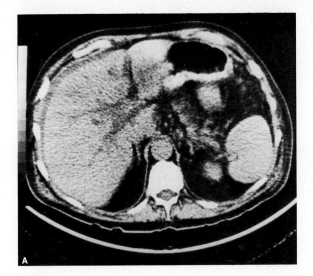
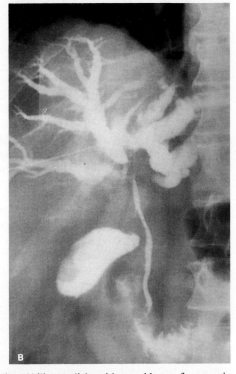

Figure 28-3. (*A*) A 58-year-old man with jaundice. CT scan shows dilated biliary radicles without evidence of pancreatic lesion. (*B*) Percutaneous transhepatic cholangiogram on same patient. Dilated intrahepatic ducts above constricting lesion in region of bifurcation and normal proximal duct and gallbladder suggest cholangiocarcinoma in region of porta hepatis (Klatskin tumor). Courtesy of Clemens Barth, M.D., Department of Radiology, Georgetown University Hospital.

size, extent of local invasion, and extent of nodal and distant metastatic involvement provide a satisfactory descriptive basis for the extent of disease in biliary cancer.

Surgery

Gallbladder Carcinoma. Those patients having carcinoma restricted to the mucosa as an incidental finding during cholecystectomy for cholelithiasis require no further therapy after surgery. Such patients, although only about 5% of total cases, represent a disproportionate majority of long-term survivors (Appleman et al., 1963), 92% in one large review (Vaittinen, 1970).

Patients with advanced disease have a poor prognosis. About 75% of patients will have spread of disease which precludes surgical cure. In the majority of patients in whom this situation has not been identified by preoperative tests, it will be evident at exploration: nodal involvement beyond the limit of lymphadenectomy or tumor extension beyond the feasible range of en bloc resection. Ten percent of patients with cholecystic cancers will have small or noninvasive lesions confined to the gallbladder. The remaining 15% of patients will have early invasive tumors where rational extension of the resection may offer some hope of cure (Adson, 1973; Adson and Farnell, 1981).

Definitive Surgery. Surgery with curative intent is, if we disregard those patients where carcinoma is an incidental finding on microscopic examination, reserved for those 15% or so of patients with early invasive disease. In these cases the service of a pathologist able to perform and interpret frozen sections rapidly is essential. The wall of the gallbladder should be examined microscopically for tumor penetration, and any suspicious areas of the gallbladder fossa should be biopsied and examined. If invasion through the wall and into the fossa is present, a minimum 2.5-cm margin of normal liver tissue should be resected. The cystic and pericholedochal nodes should be excised and examined by frozen section; presence of tumor should lead to lymphadenectomy along the paths of drainage, as earlier described. Adson and Farnell (1981) advocate regional lymphadenectomy in any case, comprising all nodes along the hepatoduodenal ligament, along the hepatic artery, and along the portal rim and common duct to well behind the duodenum and pancreas. Any suspicious nodes should be examined by frozen section.

Choice of technique for obtaining liver margins will depend upon extent of disease. At minimum, wedge resection of the gallbladder bed, starting medial to the fossa and striving for a 2.5-cm, tumor-free margin, is employed. The right hepatic artery, right branch of the portal vein, and right hepatic duct must be identified first. More extensive disease may dictate a so-called middle lobectomy (Adson and Farnell, 1981). On rare occasions an en bloc right hepatic lobectomy may be required, but should be preceded by an adequate examination for involvement of structures such as major vessels, left hepatic duct, or distant nodes, which could render the tumor unresectable.

Unless the surgeon has adequate experience with the full range of techniques which might possibly be required to obtain adequate margins, he should not undertake surgery on a patient with potentially resectable disease, but should refer to an appropriate specialist.

Palliative Surgery. Adequate biopsy specimens, confirmed by frozen-section examination, should be taken to permit a definitive tissue diagnosis. In patients in whom external beam radiation therapy may be considered postoperatively, the tumor margins should be marked with radiopaque surgical clips. If biliary obstruction has not been adequately palliated by percutaneous technique, surgical decompression should be undertaken with the choice of technique depending upon the tumor configuration encountered (see discussion under Cholangiocarcinoma). In unobstructed patients, prophylactic high biliary diversion may have a role in delaying later obstruction and extending the period of symptom-free life. Similarly, gastric diversion should be performed if obstruction is present, or if it may become a manifest problem.

No data are available to indicate that reduction of tumor bulk improves the response of gallbladder carcinoma to radiotherapy or chemotherapy, although debulking does appear to improve response in gastric carcinoma (Gastrointestinal Tumor Study Group, 1982). Thus, if simple cholecystectomy can provide a significant degree of tumor reduction, it has been recommended in most cases.

Cholangiocarcinoma and Periampullary Carcinoma. The principles of surgical evaluation in cholangiocarcinoma are very similar to those in gallbladder cancer. Many unresectable cases can be identified preoperatively and palliated by external or internal transcutaneous drainage. For those patients in whom

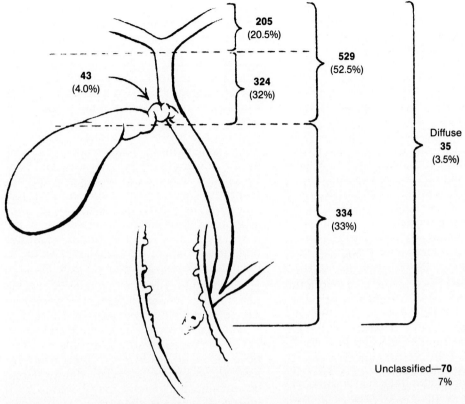

Figure 28-4. Anatomic distribution of primary bile duct tumors throughout the biliary tree among 1011 cases collected from the literature. Reproduced with permission from Broe, P. J., and Cameron, J. L.: The managment of proximal biliary tract tumors. In MacLean, L. D., *et al.,* (eds.): *Advances in Surgery,* Volume 15. Copyright © 1981 by Year Book Medical Publishers, Inc., Chicago.

the decision between palliation and definitive surgery cannot be made before exploration, the surgeon must be prepared for the full range of procedures which might be dictated by the findings at surgery.

Location of Tumors. Surgery for cholangiocarcinoma varies, depending upon location. Four anatomic areas may be considered. Because of inaccessibility, tumors of peripheral intrahepatic ducts must be approached similarly to primary hepatic tumors; techniques applicable to such tumors are discussed elsewhere. Outside the liver, tumors of the upper (bifurcation), middle, and lower (periampullary) duct involve distinct techniques and lead to different resectability rates and prognoses (Adson and Farnell, 1981). The relative distribution of locations of such bile duct tumors is shown in Figure 28-4.

Definitive Surgery. It has been estimated that between 15 and 25% of patients with cholangiocarcinoma may be candidates for a resection with curative intent (Evander *et al.,* 1980; Adson and Farnell, 1981). Operative

mortality is reported between 8 and 15%, while a mean survival of the order of 30 months is commonly reported. In Adson and Farnell's (1981) series of 221 surgical patients, half of the eight five-year survivors had only palliative procedures, suggesting that natural history of the disease contributes as much to extended survival as does aggressive treatment. Nevertheless, strong arguments can be made for attempting definitive surgery in those patients who are resectable, both on the basis of improved quality of life (Evander *et al.,* 1980) and improved prospects based on better diagnosis and surgical technique (Todoroki *et al.,* 1980; Adson and Farnell, 1981).

Even with adequate exposure, the operative evaluation may not be simple. Gross pathologic changes are often subtle and even microscopic differentiation from sclerosing cholangitis may be difficult on frozen examination of small specimens. Indeed, in one series of 45 cases, cholangiocarcinoma was not diagnosed in one-third at the time of initial exploration (Wanebo and Grimes, 1975). Evaluation for operability involves dissection to expose uninvolved duct above and below the tumor. Evidence of distant spread beyond the limits of resection or of lymphadenopathy, or invasion of major blood vessels, will preclude definitive resection. Frozen-section evaluation of resection margins for tumor is essential. Intraductal spread and multicentricity is an underrecognized cause for unresectability; Tompkins and colleagues (1976) have advocated intraoperative endoscopy to rule out additional higher and inaccessible lesions, since such an evaluation may prevent needless radical surgery.

BIFURCATION TUMORS. The extent of sacrifice of liver parenchyma required will depend in part upon the degree of parenchymal invasion. Even more important is vascular involvement that may require lobectomy concomitant with resection of an involved vessel which serves that lobe. Evaluation proceeds by sequentially mobilizing and exploring the portal vein and the hepatic artery, beginning well below the tumor. If neither right nor left vessels are involved, wedge resection may be possible; otherwise lobectomy may be required.

MIDDUCTAL TUMORS. The approach to midductal tumors along the hepatoduodenal ligament again involves isolation of hepatic artery and portal vein. Vascular involvement may dictate sacrifice of one branch with lobectomy. Resection in such cases is similar to that required for gallbladder tumors, with regional lymphadenectomy and *en bloc* resection of tumor and gallbladder, attempting to obtain at least 2.5 cm of tumor-free margin of hepatic parenchyma.

LOWER DUCTAL AND PERIAMPULLARY TUMORS. The approach to lower ductal tumors is the same as for carcinoma of the head of the pancreas: radical pancreatoduodenectomy. Pyloric preservation (Traverso and Longmire, 1980) may be justified in some less aggressive tumors.

HEPATIC TRANSPLANTATION. Total hepatic resection and transplantation, initially thought to hold great promise in cholangiocarcinoma, has largely been abandoned after poor experience with the initial series of patients (Starzl *et al.,* 1979).

Palliative Surgery. Palliation of cholangiocarcinoma almost always involves biliary decompression. The same principles described for gallbladder carcinoma apply: decompression, tissue sampling, use of radiopaque clips to mark tumor margins, and, in some cases, prophylactic gastric outlet bypass. Because cholangiocarcinomas may be slow growing

and slow to metastasize, decompressive technique for extended palliation assumes greater importance.

Where drainage via anastomosis to a defunctionalized Roux limb is feasible, this can be utilized and may be facilitated with stenting (Cameron *et al.,* 1978). Even with hilar tumors where an extrahepatic duct is not available for anastomosis, intrahepatic anastomosis is possible (Bismuth, 1982) and may result in prolonged palliation. In the technique described by Terblanche (1979) a U tube is used that can be replaced in the event of clogging without reopening the abdomen. This is an improvement over T-tube stenting. Basically, after dilatation, a tube is placed via an incision in the lower duct, through the tumor, and out through a peripheral duct and a stab wound in the hepatic capsule. Holes are cut in the tube and positioned above and below the lesion. The two ends of the tube are then externalized, and after drainage to the duodenum is confirmed, are joined externally to form an O. If blockage occurs, the external loop is again opened, and the old tube serves as a guide for replacement percutaneously.

Nonsurgical Management

As noted earlier, the tumors in more than three-fourths of all patients with gallbladder or bile duct carcinoma will be unresectable. Tumors will recur in the majority of patients who undergo definitive surgery. Thus, the great majority of patients with gallbladder cancer or cholangiocarcinoma will at some time be candidates for nonsurgical management. Such management is palliative but may offer major contributions to the patient's quality of life and, in some cases, offer increased survival.

Percutaneous Biliary Decompression. Obstructive jaundice is an almost universal problem in cholangiocarcinoma and occurs frequently in gallbladder cancer as well. Biliary obstruction usually results in significant morbidity including pruritus, infection, pain, nutritional problems, and progressive hepatic failure. These problems have been significant enough to require palliative surgery in many patients.

Klatskin (1965) noted that successful decompression of the biliary tract appears to increase the duration of survival in cholangiocarcinoma. Decompression of only 50% of the liver is adequate to preserve function (Longmire and Tompkins, 1975). Thus, external

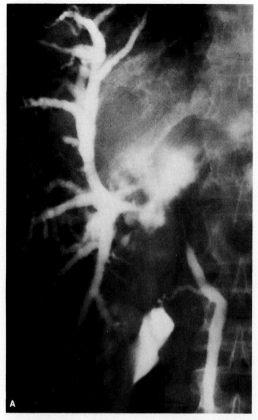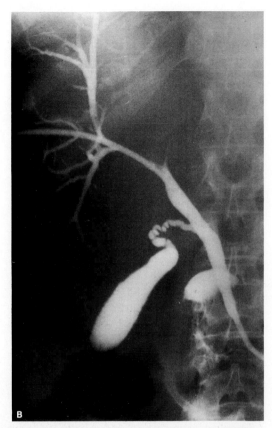

Figure 28–5. (*A*) Klatskin tumor. At percutaneous transhepatic cholangiogram, tumor at bifurcation blocks opacification of left ducts. Some extravasation of dye is seen. (*B*) Same patient: Excellent decompression of right collecting system has been achieved by means of a catheter passed through the tumor to the duodenum via the common duct. Courtesy of Clemens Barth, M.D., Department of Radiology, Georgetown University Hospital.

percutaneous drainage is also a viable palliative technique when internal drainage into the duodenum cannot be achieved, or even where a bifurcation tumor permits access to only the right collecting system. Percutaneous passage of a simple catheter over a fine needle can usually be performed at the time of percutaneous transhepatic cholangiography. The main complication is cholangitis, which eventually occurs in almost every patient maintained on extended drainage (Hansson *et al.*, 1979). Often the decompressing catheter can be passed through the lesion and into the duodenum to provide internal decompression (Figure 28–5). This may be facilitated by using a second percutaneous approach after opacifying the bile ducts via the Chiba needle. Under lateral fluoroscopic guidance a sheathed needle can then be passed into a posterior right duct, resulting in a much better angulation into the common duct.

A similar alternative to surgical decompression is the percutaneous placement of a plastic prosthesis through the lesion, as described by Pereiras *et al.* (1978) and shown in Figure 28–6. The prosthesis, draining to the duodenum, is placed with successive aid of a wire and catheter via a dilated branch of the right hepatic duct. If duodenal drainage is obtained, the catheter is then withdrawn, eliminating the need for external drainage. In the hands of the group reporting the technique, good palliation is obtained with the potential for long-term biliary decompression. The potential drawback is inaccessibility of the prosthesis in the event of later blockage.

Radiation Therapy

Both external beam and intracavitary radiation have been employed in biliary tract cancer. External beam radiotherapy has a major role in palliation, and long survival has been reported in selected groups of radically treated patients (Pilepich and Lambert, 1978).

External Beam Therapy. External beam

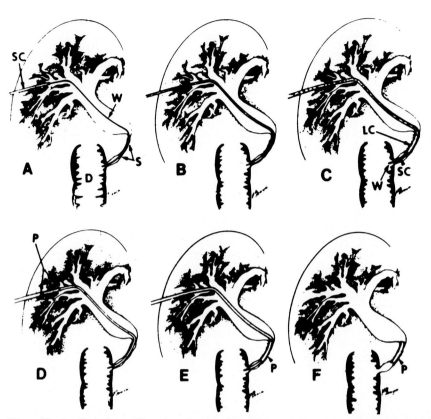

Figure 28–6. Technique of insertion of prosthesis. (*A*) Wire (W) in place through right branch of hepatic biliary tree and through strictured segment (S) into duodenum (D) 8 French catheter (small catheter, SC) being placed over wire. (*B*) Wire and 8 French catheter now in place through level of obstruction. (*C*) Forceful dilatation of stricture segment with 12 French catheter (large catheter, LC) inserted coaxially. (*D*) Large catheter has been removed after dilatation and TEFLON prosthesis (P) is pushed coaxially by the same large catheter. (*E*) Prosthesis at desired level with small catheter distal to it. (*F*) Prosthesis in place; 8 French small catheter and wire have been removed. From Pereiras C. V., Owen J. R., Hutson D., Mejia J., Viamonte M., Chiprut R. O., and Schiff E. R.: Relief of malignant obstructive jaundice by percutaneous insertion of a permanent prosthesis in the biliary tree. *Ann. Intern. Med.,* **89**:589–593, 1978, by permission of American College of Physicians.

radiation therapy to biliary cancer is limited by the tolerance of the major dose-limiting structures: liver, duodenum, stomach, spinal cord, and kidney. The design of fields is greatly improved when limits of the tumor can be accurately delineated by surgical clips placed to define tumor margins at operation. Node-bearing areas are also at risk; these are best delineated by simulation with contrast in the duodenum.

The main dose-limiting structure is the liver. Although radiation hepatitis is reported only rarely in the range of 25 to 30 Gy (Kaplan and Bagshaw, 1968), its incidence approaches 10% in the 30 to 35-Gy range. In the range of 35 to 40 Gy the incidence of radiation hepatitis reaches about 30% and persistent or even fatal cases are reported (Ingold *et al.,* 1965). Limited experience above 40 Gy, a dose that is

ordinarily required for effective control of an adenocarcinoma, is associated with fatal hepatitis in about 50% of cases. Thus, a dose of 30 Gy represents a practical limit for hepatic dosage, and some reduction may be prudent where sensitizing chemotherapy is given in close temporal relationship. Left renal function should be evaluated by IVP before therapy, since fields overlapping most of the right kidney may be required.

Pilepich and Lambert (1978) and Smoron (1977) have described radiotherapy of gallbladder and ductal cancer with doses ranging from 15 to 60 Gy. The lower doses (below 40 Gy in Smoron's series) were reserved for debilitated patients thought unable to tolerate full doses. The combined series totaled 25 patients, approximately equally divided between gallbladder cancer and cholangiocarcinoma.

Anterior and posterior opposing fields from 8 × 8 to 13 × 18 cm were used, with shrinking fields as required to protect liver, spinal cord, and other organs. Good palliation was achieved, even in many of the lower-dose patients, with reduction in pain, jaundice, and T-tube drainage. Among the 17 patients in both series treated with greater than 40 Gy, survival ranged from 1 to 25 + months, with an average of 12 + months. Terblanche (1979) reports results in four patients with cholangiocarcinoma treated by U-tube drainage and 60-Gy external beam radiotherapy, with two of four patients alive at 6 + years and two surviving 2½ and 3 years. Goebel and associates (1979) also discuss local control of gallbladder and bile duct cancer up to 12 months, with shrinking fields and total tumor doses of 40 to 50 Gy.

Intracavitary Radiation. The role of intracavitary radiation in biliary cancer has not yet been well established. Conroy *et al.* (1982) advocate the use of intracatheter radium needles placed via a U tube, as a means of obtaining drainage. They obtained palliation in approximately half of their patients. Ariel and Pack (1960) attempted intracavitary radiation using ^{131}I-labeled rose bengal, a dye rapidly concentrated in the bile. They obtained fair to good palliation in a minority of cases.

Chemotherapy

Because of small numbers of patients, the evaluation of chemotherapeutic protocols in biliary cancer has lagged behind the present state of knowledge in the more common GI malignancies. Single-agent activity has been noted with several of the drugs which are active in other upper GI malignancies (see Table 28–3).

Two combination chemotherapy protocols have been systematically investigated. In cholangiocarcinoma the FAM protocol (described in detail in Chapter 26, neoplasms of the stomach) was administered to 17 consecutive patients with metastatic tumor. Thirteen had objectively measurable disease. A partial response rate of 4/13 (31%) was achieved for a median duration of 8.5 months (Harvey *et al.,* 1984). The median survival was 11.5 months. One patient without measurable disease was alive and apparently disease-free at 72 + months.

The FAB combination (ftorafur 4 gm/m^2 IV days 1 and 22 and 2 gm/m^2 IV days 4 and 26; doxorubicin (ADRIAMYCIN) 60 mg/m^2 IV day 1 and 45 mg/m^2 IV day 22; and BCNU 150 mg/m^2 IV day 1, given in six to eight week cycles) was evaluated by Hall and coworkers (1979). They reported 3/7 (43%) response in a mixed population of gallbladder and bile duct cancer; two complete responses were described. Responders had median survival of 11 months. Ravry and Hester (1979) reported 1/5 partial response with a combination of doxorubicin 60 mg/m^2 IV every three weeks and bleomycin 10 U/m^2 IV every other week.

Chemotherapy delivered via cannulation of the hepatic artery may be more efficacious than when delivered intravenously. Misra and colleagues (1977) reported 9 (69%) responders among 13 patients treated for gallbladder carcinoma metastatic to liver with intra-arterial mitomycin C and 5-FU.

Adjuvant Therapy

By analyzing patterns of failure in 28 patients with biliary tract cancer undergoing curative resection at Massachusetts General Hospital, Kopelson and associates (1981) determined that only 36% developed distant metastases, while local and regional failure

Table 28–3. Drugs with Activity Against Bile Duct or Gallbladder Cancer

DRUG	RESPONSE RATE (PR)	REFERENCE
Mitomycin C	7 : 15 (47%) 0 : 10 (0%) (28% combined)	Crooke and Bradner, 1976 Von Eyben *et al.,* 1980
5-FU	4 : 17 (24%) 3 : 23 (13%) (17% combined)	Haskell, 1980 Davis *et al.,* 1974
BCNU	2 : 4	Haskell, 1980
Doxorubicin (ADRIAMYCIN)	(Anecdotal : 1 CR)	Adolphson and Carpenter, 1982
Neocarzinostatin	(Anecdotal)	Bodey *et al.,* 1981

without distant failure occurred in 52%. The implication is that if postoperative adjuvant radiation therapy could obtain local control, it might be of benefit to more than half of these patients.

No systematic evaluation has been made of adjuvant chemotherapy in biliary carcinoma. Oswalt and Cruz (1977) reported a nonrandomized trial of adjuvant chemotherapy involving 5-FU with or without other drugs in 13 patients with gallbladder cancer. A median survival of 20 weeks versus 8 weeks for untreated patients was claimed; one patient with gross disease after surgery was alive at 6 years on 5-FU. Experience has shown that to achieve statistically significant survival improvement with adjuvant chemotherapy, a regimen having a partial response rate in advanced disease of at least 30% is required. Both the FAM and FAB protocols may be capable of meeting this criterion, but neither has been evaluated in a prospective adjuvant trial.

Future Prospects

Primary carcinoma of the biliary tract still presents major diagnostic and therapeutic problems. Increased diagnostic accuracy and improved surgical technique may result in some improvements, but a wide gap remains. Because failure patterns are frequently local, preoperative, and/or postoperative radiation may contribute significantly and needs to be evaluated in a controlled trial. In this regard the combination of external beam therapy with a local boost from either intracavitary sources or intraoperative radiation may have a role. The further evaluation of chemotherapy for this disease group represents a research objective of high priority.

HEPATOMA

Epidemiology

The incidence of hepatocellular carcinoma demonstrates dramatic geographic variability. It is a relatively rare form of cancer in North America and Western Europe, whereas, in parts of sub-Saharan Africa, Southeast Asia, and Japan, hepatoma takes on increased importance. In some countries it is the single most important cause of cancer death (Higginson and Svoboda, 1970), with the highest incidence reported in Bantu males in Mozambique, a rate almost 500 times greater than that

found in the United States. In the United States, it is estimated that there are approximately 2500 to 3000 deaths per year from hepatoma (Clinical Biometry Section, 1964), and the incidence of this tumor is increasing, particularly in younger individuals and women with noncirrhotic livers (Moertel, 1982).

Etiology and Pathogenesis

The development of hepatoma has been closely correlated with preexisting hepatic cirrhosis. The incidence of associated cirrhosis has varied from 60% (Kew and Geddes, 1982) to as high as 100% (Berman, 1951). Higgins (1970) has estimated that 4% of patients with cirrhosis are destined to develop hepatoma. The risk is regarded as highest in patients with postnecrotic cirrhosis secondary to hepatitis-B infection, and in patients with hemachromatosis (Nissen et al., 1976). Alcoholic cirrhosis is a lesser, but still important, risk factor. The reported frequency of hepatoma in patients with hemachromatosis has ranged from 3 to 27%, the variability perhaps related to the difficulty in differentiating this entity from alcoholic cirrhosis with increased iron stores (Edmondson and Peters, 1982). Because of its high incidence, alcoholic cirrhosis is a major predisposing factor in the United States. Of importance is the failure to find an increased incidence of hepatoma in alcoholics without cirrhosis, and the demonstration that in a patient with established cirrhosis the risk continues with time despite the discontinuation of drinking (Lee, 1966). The cessation of drinking may actually allow the patients to live long enough to develop the tumor. Despite the close correlation between cirrhosis and hepatoma, considerable debate continues as to whether the tumor is a direct complication of the cirrhotic process or whether the two conditions are different end results of the same etiologic factor. Clearly, cirrhosis is not a requirement for the disease, and Okuda and coworkers (1982) have suggested that hepatoma in the noncirrhotic liver is caused by nonviral carcinogens rather than hepatitis-B infection. In a recent study, Bréchot and associates found that some patients who have no serological markers, e.g., HB_sA_g of active HBV infection, nonetheless, do have HBV DNA integrated in hepatocyte genome (Bréchot et al., 1985).

A large number of chemicals have been demonstrated to be direct liver carcinogens in animals, and possibly in man, including mycotoxins, pyrrolizidine alkaloids, cycasin, nitrosamines, and at least 16 different pesticides and herbicides (Christopherson, 1981; Sugar *et al.,* 1979). Particular attention has been given to aflatoxins, a group of food-borne mycotoxins produced by the fungi *Aspergillus flavus* and *A. parasiticus.* Aflatoxin B_1, the most prevalent and toxic member of the family, is a highly potent carcinogen for the liver of rat and rainbow trout after metabolic activation by the microsomal mixed-function oxygenases (Campbell and Hayes, 1976). Cancer of the liver has been demonstrated in monkeys after six years of aflatoxin exposure without associated cirrhosis (Adamson *et al.,* 1973).

Although the relevance of animal data for man is still debated, several clinical epidemiology studies have indicated an association of aflatoxin contamination of food with hepatic cancer. Keen and Martin (1971) correlated the frequency of contamination of peanuts by aflatoxins with hepatoma incidence in three regions of Swaziland and found a definite association. Alpert and colleagues (1971), working in Uganda, were able to demonstrate an association between levels of contamination of beans, maize, and sorghum in provinces with a high incidence of primary hepatic cancer. Linsell and Peers (1977) have carefully analyzed the results of these and other studies and cautiously concluded that the data justify a program of intervention to lower the level of aflatoxin contamination.

Impetus for studies of a possible viral etiology of hepatoma has resulted from the demonstration of a close correlation of this tumor with hepatitis-B virus (HBV). Hepatocellular carcinoma, particularly in endemic regions, occurs frequently in carriers of the hepatitis-B virus surface antigen (HB_sAg), and familial clustering of HBV-associated cancer is frequent in areas where the cancer rate is high (Okuda and Ohnishi, 1982). This may be partly explained by perinatal transmission from mother to infant. HB_sAg has been found with greater frequency in hepatoma patients compared to controls in Africa (Kew *et al.,* 1974), and Japan (Nishioka *et al.,* 1975), as well as in the United States where Yarrish and associates (1980) found circulating HB_sAg in 5 of 34 (15%) patients with hepatoma, compared to none of 139 controls. The control subjects included patients with colonic or lung cancer and healthy blood donors. The frequency of serum HB_sAg in patients with hepatocellular carcinomas in regions of high prevalence has

ranged from 45 to 85% (Kew and Geddes, 1982; Okuda and Ohnishi, 1982). The reported frequency of orcein-positive HB_sAg in hepatic tissue obtained at autopsy is between 15 and 86% (Okuda and Ohnishi, 1982). It is known that hepatitis-B viral DNA can become integrated into the host DNA, and become clonal (see Chapter 3D). In contrast, past infection with hepatitis-A virus has not been correlated with the development of hepatoma (Tabor *et al.,* 1980). Overall, the case for HBV as a carcinogen for the human liver is very strong, and an animal model for viral-induced hepatitis and primary liver carcinoma in *Marmota monax* (woodchucks) gives added support. Interventional studies with the newly developed vaccine in endemic regions of the world will provide the final validation of this hypothesis.

In the past ten years there have been increasing reports of hepatic adenomas in women taking oral contraceptives (Pike *et al.,* 1977). This condition, characterized as a benign lesion composed of vacuolated hepatocytes without portal areas or stellate fibrosis, must be distinguished from focal nodular hyperplasia. In general, women who have taken the preparation for over five years appear to be at greater risk, but the overall incidence of this disorder is still extraordinarily low compared to the millions of women taking these agents (Sherlock, 1975). The clinical features include an asymptomatic or painful mass, but onefourth of the reported patients have presented with sudden life-threatening rupture of the tumor and intra-abdominal hemorrhage. The prognosis is excellent if the adenoma is diagnosed prior to rupture and is resected. The relationship to the estrogen content of the preparation is a subject of further study; estrogen alone has also caused hepatic adenomas (Goldfarb, 1976). In one such tumor the presence of estrogen and progesterone receptors was demonstrated (Macdonald *et al.,* 1978). Of particular concern are reports of hepatic carcinoma in patients taking contraceptive steroids (Davis *et al.,* 1975; Mays *et al.,* 1976), a threat that must be regarded as potentially serious. Hepatocellular carcinoma has also been described in patients receiving androgenic anabolic steroids (Westaby *et al.,* 1977), although the biologic aggressiveness of these tumors has been, in general, quite limited (Christopherson, 1981).

THOROTRAST, containing radioactive thorium dioxide, was used as an agent for biliary imaging between the years 1930 and 1950. The initial cases of hepatic malignancies in which THOROTRAST was implicated were angiosarcomas. Recently, hepatocellular cancer has also been documented (Smoron and Battifora, 1972; Kiely *et al.*, 1973). The abandonment of THOROTRAST as a contrast agent, despite its prolonged half-life in patients already exposed and the long latency of tumorigenesis, will soon make this experience of historical importance only.

Vinyl chloride, now recognized as an important carcinogen for the human liver, induces the development of angiosarcomas. This syndrome was first described by Creech and Johnson (1974), who observed that chemical plant workers exposed to vinyl chloride developed this unusual malignancy of the liver. The initial symptoms included fatigue, weight loss, nausea, abdominal pain, and jaundice, with evidence of hepatomegaly and abnormal liver function. The angiosarcoma usually remains confined to the liver, and death generally results from direct hepatic destruction. The recognition of this industrial hazard and the precautions that have now been instituted have resulted in a marked decrease in incidence of this disorder.

Pathology and Natural History

Gross and Microscopic Pathology. The gross and microscopic pathology of hepatocellular carcinoma can be correlated with the presence or absence of a preexisting cirrhotic condition. In general, a primary cancer arising in a normal liver takes the form of a nodular growth that may be associated with smaller satellites. The tumor may grow to massive proportions and replace much of the normal hepatic parenchyma before symptoms become evident. In the setting of cirrhosis, the tumor may also develop as a well-defined mass, but in smaller groups of patients it will present with a multifocal or a diffuse pattern of multiple small nodules. If the reserve of hepatic function has been compromised by the underlying cirrhosis, replacement of a small proportion of the remaining liver may precipitate early signs of hepatic failure or portal hypertension.

The histologic presentation may vary from a well-differentiated cancer, which may be difficult to distinguish from a regenerating hepatic nodule, to a clear cell pattern, or to one composed of poorly differentiated pleomorphic

cells. The differentiation within any tumor may vary considerably from one area to another (Edmondson and Peters, 1982). In the cirrhotic liver, growth is characterized by nodules with a trabecular cellular pattern, defined by fibrous septi. In the normal liver, the tumor grows as an expanding mass without a capsule. The neoplasm draws its blood supply from the hepatic artery circulation, with flow into the portal veins, which may become occluded by tumor or thrombosis.

Distant metastases are more likely to be found in the noncirrhotic case, perhaps because of the longer survival time, but 50% of patients will still die of progressive liver failure or hemorrhage with no evidence of extrahepatic spread (Linder *et al.*, 1974). The principal sites of metastatic disease include the lung, portal vein, portal lymph nodes, bone, and gallbladder (Edmondson and Peters, 1982).

Clinical Presentation. The principal symptoms (Table 28–4) that bring the patient to medical attention are abdominal pain, a right upper quadrant mass, weight loss, and/or ascites. Less than half of patients are icteric at time of diagnosis and, when present, jaundice is usually mild (Kew, *et al.*, 1971; Ihde *et al.*, 1974). In the patient with an antecedent advanced hepatic cirrhosis, which may in itself be symptomatic, the clinical course may be characterized by progressive deterioration and death within a few months of the diagnosis. In these cases, the patient may evidence jaundice, fever, rapid hepatic enlargement, and bloody ascites as a manifestation of an acute Budd-

Table 28–4. Symptoms and Physical Signs of Hepatoma

	PERCENT
Symptoms	
Abdominal pain	69
Weight loss	71
Weakness, fatigue	23
Anorexia	28
Nausea and vomiting	21
Pruritus	8
Signs	
Hepatomegaly	93
Ascites	61
Splenomegaly	48
Jaundice	44
Fever	24
Arterial bruit	25
Signs of chronic liver disease (spider angiomata, palmar erythema, etc.)	51

Adapted from Kew, M. C.; Geddes, E. W.; Macrab, G. M.; and Bersohn, I.: Hepatitis-B antigen and cirrhosis in Bantu patients with primary liver cancer. *Cancer,* 34:539–541, 1974.

Chiari syndrome and hemorrhage. Acute upper gastrointestinal bleeding may result from portal hypertension. In the noncirrhotic patient with greater initial hepatic reserve, the disease course may be more protracted, but eventually will result in complications of liver failure and/or portal hypertension.

The principal physical findings at time of diagnosis include a palpable liver in almost all cases, which may be nodular and tender. A hepatic friction rub or an arterial bruit may be heard over the liver in 25% of patients (Kew *et al.,* 1971). The spleen is palpable in approximately 25% of the cases. Many patients will also show the physical findings of long-standing chronic liver disease and cirrhosis.

Hepatoma is well recognized for its ability to produce a large number of hormonal syndromes and paraneoplastic phenomena (Gluckman and Turner, 1974). These include erythrocytosis, leukocytosis, dysfibrinogenemia, hypercalcemia, hypoglycemia, porphyria cutanea tarda, carcinoid syndrome, ectopic ACTH production, and others, as shown in Table 28-5. Hepatoma is second to retroperitoneal sarcoma as a cause of extrapancreatic hypoglycemia. The syndrome has been characterized by McFadzean and Yeung (1969) into two distinct types. Type A (87%) develops in patients with poorly differentiated tumor, where the liver does not store glycogen. A low incidence of easily controlled hypoglycemia appears shortly before death. In type B (13%), the patient develops an acquired glycogen storage disease, the result of a deficiency of glucose-6-phosphatase. In this type, the liver contains glycogen but does not respond to the stimulus of hypoglycemia or to glucagon.

Diagnosis

In regions where hepatoma is endemic, a high index of suspicion prevails, and diagnosis is easily made during life. In Western societies, which characteristically have a low incidence of this tumor, a definite diagnosis may be made only at autopsy in as many as 20% of cases (Kew *et al.,* 1971). This is particularly true if the patient has a cirrhotic liver to which the symptoms of hepatoma are ascribed.

Abnormal values in standard liver function tests, such as the alkaline phosphatase, 5'-nucleotidase, and SGOT, are present in approximately 80% of patients and are of little diagnostic value (Ihde *et al.,* 1974). Great emphasis has been placed on the serum concentration of

Table 28-5.   Systemic Manifestations of Hepatoma

TUMOR	SYNDROMES
Hepatoma	Fever, cachexia, and leukocytosis
	Eosinophilia
	Migratory thrombophlebitis
	Vitiligo
	Hypertrophic osteoarthropathy
	Gynecomastia
	Cryofibrinogenemia
	Dysfibrinogenemia
	Hyperlipidemia
	Hypoglycemia
	Hypercalcemia
	Carcinoid syndrome
	Porphyria cutanea tarda
	Abnormal ferritins
	Variant alkaline phosphatase
	Carcinoembryonic antigen
	Alpha-fetoprotein
	Abnormal aldolase
	Polycythemia
Hepatoblastoma	Precocious puberty with tumor production of a gonadotropin
	Hemihypertrophy and cystathioninuria
	Elevated serum levels of alpha-fetoprotein
Hemangiosarcoma	Nephrocalcinosis

Adapted from Gluckman, J. B., and Turner, M. D.: Systemic manifestations of tumors of the small gut and liver. *Ann. N.Y. Acad. Sci.,* **230**:318-331, 1974.

alpha-fetoprotein (AFP) (see Chapter 6A). AFP is an oncofetal antigen, normally synthesized by the liver, yolk sac, and gastrointestinal tract of the human fetus, with a peak output during the twelfth to fifteenth weeks of gestation (Schein, 1982). Serum level usually falls to the normal adult level of less than 40 ng/mL by the sixth to twelfth month following birth. A similar protein was demonstrated in mice bearing a transplantable hepatoma (Abelev *et al.,* 1963), and it was soon found that elevated levels of AFP were present in the serum of patients with hepatocellular carcinoma. It is estimated that 70 to 95% of all patients will present with a serum level in excess of 40 ng/mL (Waldmann and McIntire, 1974). The AFP is not specific for hepatoma, since elevated serum levels are found in approximately 70% of patients with nonseminomatous testicular or extragonadal germ cell cancers, and in as many as 20% of cases of pancreatic and gastric carcinoma. Nor is the test diagnostic of cancer, since modest elevations have been recorded with a wide range of benign liver diseases, including alcoholic cirrhosis and viral hepatitis, and gross elevations (in the hepatoma range) during liver regeneration after fulminant hepatic failure. The finding of a value in excess of 500 ng/mL, while not definitive, strongly supports the suspicion of an underlying neoplasm (Chen and Sung, 1977). The AFP can serve as a useful tumor marker for following a patient after hepatic resection or effective chemotherapy, where AFP should decrease to a normal serum concentration with complete removal, only to rise with evidence of tumor recurrence (McIntyre et al., 1976).

The plain chest roentgenogram may provide diagnostic information, with the presence of an abnormally raised right hemidiaphragm. Hepatic scans, with technetium sulfur colloid and similar imaging materials, will demonstrate the presence of one or more defects in virtually all cases, but cannot distinguish hepatoma from hepatic metastases, cirrhosis, or amebic liver abscess (Ihde et al., 1974; Kew and Geddes, 1982). The latter condition can be identified by the use of ultrasonography. Hepatic computed tomography with enhancement is a valuable tool to assess the extent, number, and location of malignant nodules. Selective hepatic arteriography complements the preceding procedures in the evaluation of resectability and can visualize tumor masses either not visualized or equivocal with the other diagnostic tests. The typical pattern is a tumor with abnormal vasculature, "puddling" of the contrast material, a capillary "blush," delayed clearing of the contrast material, and early filling of the hepatic veins (Kew and Geddes, 1982). One must also attempt to identify invasion of the hepatic veins and inferior vena cava. Ultimately, a histologic confirmation is required, and one of the above diagnostic modalities can be used to direct a biopsy needle into a suspicious abnormality. Percutaneous biopsy, or peritoneoscopy with biopsy, however, should be reserved for lesions which are regarded as unresectable, because of the potential threat of tumor cell seeding of the abdomen.

Treatment

Surgery. Although prompt surgical resection of an isolated hepatoma remains the only modality with curative potential, this approach is limited by several factors. Many patients have extensive cirrhosis and poor hepatic function, which makes them poor candidates for radical surgery. In addition, the presence of a diffuse multicentric pattern of the cancer in the setting of cirrhosis makes re-

section a probable exercise in futility. One must also be careful to exclude patients with evidence of involvement of both lobes or overt evidence of dissemination based upon the results of the preoperative evaluation. This leaves only 20 to 30% of patients who can potentially benefit from radical surgery with curative intent (El-Domeiri et al., 1971; Kappel and Miller, 1972; McBride, 1981). The perioperative mortality following a partial hepatectomy for hepatoma has decreased in the past two decades but has ranged from 4 to 24%. The five-year survival statistics for patients in whom the tumor was regarded as resectable have been disappointing. Adson and Farnell (1981) have described a 36% survival in those patients who survived the resection, but in most other series a survival rate in the range of 16 to 25% is described (El-Domeiri et al., 1971; Linder et al., 1974; McBride, 1981).

Radiotherapy. Radiotherapy of hepatoma is limited by the inherent tolerance of the normal hepatic parenchyma to radiation, as discussed in the previous section on biliary carcinoma. Tolerated doses are likely to be below the threshold required for significant control of primary neoplasms, but a period of symptomatic relief may be achieved (Phillips and Murikami, 1960).

To improve the results with radiotherapy, Friedman and coworkers (1979) combined whole liver irradiation, total dose of 1500 to 2400 rads, with intrahepatic arterial administration of doxorubicin and 5-fluorouracil. 5-Fluorouracil was continuously infused at a dose of 10 mg/kg/day and continued until the radiotherapy course was completed (five to nine days). Doxorubicin was given at a dose of 5 mg/m^2, one to two hours before each radiation treatment, with dosage adjustment for patients with elevated serum bilirubin levels. Thirteen patients were treated; six (46%) evidenced an objective response, and five had apparent stabilization of the disease. Symptomatic improvement was described in 81% of the series. The objective responses had a four-month median duration, with a range of 4 to 15 + months; the median survival of this group of responders was eight months. Hematologic toxicity was mild, and only three patients had a transient deterioration of liver function.

A novel, but still experimental, approach to the radiotherapy of hepatoma is being evaluated by Order and coworkers (1979). Patients are being treated with ^{131}I-labeled antiferritin or anti-CEA antibody in combination with external beam radiation, and with doxorubicin and metronidazole sensitization. With this technique it is hoped that the radiation can be selectively delivered to the tumor while sparing the normal parenchyma to which the antibody has a lesser affinity.

Chemotherapy. Only a limited number of agents have been evaluated in the management of hepatocellular carcinoma. Although 5-fluorouracil had been reported to be highly effective when administered orally, with 50% of a small series having achieved an objective response (Kennedy et al., 1977), this result could not be confirmed in subsequent studies. A more realistic response rate when administered either orally and/or intravenously is 10% or less (Link et al., 1977; Falkson et al., 1978). Falkson and coworkers (1978) failed to demonstrate a single objective response in 43 patients treated with oral 5-FU. The median survival for North American white patients was 7 weeks, for North American blacks was 15 weeks, and for South African blacks was 4 weeks, which appeared, in general, to be inferior to that achieved with doxorubicin in the same randomized controlled trial.

Doxorubicin had been reported to be more effective in hepatoma. Olweny and coworkers (1975) initially described responses in all 11 patients treated in Uganda. Once again, the follow-up studies failed to confirm this initial optimistic report. Idhe et al. (1977) described a 15% response in American patients, and Vogel and coworkers (1977) found a 17% response rate in 41 patients treated in both Zambia and in the United States. In a randomized controlled trial in which doxorubicin had also been administered as a single agent; the overall response rate in 31 previously untreated patients was 10%, whereas 6 of 26 (23%) cases who had received some form of prior chemotherapy responded (Falkson et al., 1978). Of particular interest was the median survival of 60 weeks for the 12 South African black patients, compared to 15 weeks for American whites. This has been interpreted by some as demonstrating that doxorubicin is a superior agent in the African black who may have a different disease because of the higher correlation with hepatitis-B infection or aflatoxin exposure. Nevertheless, because of the small numbers of patients in the study, potential differences in prognostic factors and the failure to demonstrate a difference in the low response rates (13 versus 8% of previously untreated cases), a definite conclusion cannot be drawn.

Neocarzinostatin is a polypeptide antibiotic, isolated from the fermentation of *Strep-tomyces carcinostaticus*. This agent has been evaluated by the Eastern Cooperative Oncology Group in 30 patients who were primarily treated in South Africa (Falkson et al., 1980). Objective responses were reported in seven cases (23%). The median survival of those who achieved a partial response was 17 weeks, compared to six weeks for the entire series.

Only a small number of patients have been treated with standard alkylating agents (including the chloroethylnitrosoureas, streptozotocin, and mitomycin), and with methotrexate, and the vinca alkaloids. The limited data base does not suggest that any of these drugs have important activity for hepatoma.

Despite the limited activity of single agents for this tumor, a number of drug combinations have been evaluated. Moertel (1975) reported the Mayo Clinic experience with the combination of 5-FU and BCNU. Seven of 19 patients (37%) achieved an objective response, and two were maintained for periods in excess of three years. The Eastern Cooperative Oncology Group (Falkson et al., 1978) tested the efficacy of two nitrosourea regimens, oral 5-FU plus streptozotocin, and oral 5-FU plus methyl-CCNU; the response rates were 12 and 5%, respectively.

The Southwest Oncology Group evaluated the combination of 5-FU and doxorubicin and reported that 5 of 38 patients (13%) responded (Baker et al., 1977). In a study limited to 13 patients, 5 (38%) of the patients obtained a remission with the use of 5-FU and mitomycin C (Umsawasdi, et al., 1978). The FAM regimen, which has shown useful activity in cholangiocarcinoma and other upper gastrointestinal sites, has not as yet been evaluated for its effectiveness in hepatoma.

The reported experience with hepatic artery infusions of 5-FU or FUdR consists of a collection of small series, each with less than 20 patients (Haskell, 1980). The overall response rate with intra-arterial fluorinated pyrimidine therapy is estimated to be approximately 40%, compared to the 10% response reported for intravenous administration. In addition, the collective survival of patients treated intra-arterially is 8.5 months, superior to the expected three-month survival with systemic treatment. These results are placed in better perspective if it is recognized that they come from a compilation of 15 different series, with no assessment of prognostic factors such as the presence of cirrhosis, performance status, serum bilirubin concentrations, and so forth. Before any definitive statement regarding the efficacy of intra-arterial treatment can be made, particularly when one considers the potential morbidity of catheter sepsis, thrombosis, and embolization, a properly designed controlled trial is necessary. Of the regimens that have been reported to date, the combined use of external radiotherapy combined with intra-arterial 5-FU and doxorubicin, as previously discussed in the Radiotherapy section (Friedman *et al.,* 1979), appears to be the most promising and should be considered for further study in a controlled trial.

In summary, no form of chemotherapy has demonstrated reproducible therapeutic activity to the extent that it should be considered a standard of treatment for hepatoma. All therapy, in this context, must be regarded as investigational and be the subject of objective assessment for efficacy and toxicity in well-designed clinical trials.

REFERENCES

Abelev, G. I.; Perova, S. D.; Khramkova, N.; Postnikova, Z. A.; and Irlin, I. S.: Production of embryonal-gobulin by transplantable mouse hepatoma. *Transplantation,* 1:174–180, 1963.

Adamson, R. H.; Correa, P.; and Dalgard, D. W.: Brief communication: Occurrence of a primary liver carcinoma in a Rhesus monkey fed aflatoxin B_1. *J.N.C.I.,* 50:549–551, 1973.

Adolphson, C. C., and Carpenter, J. T., Jr.: Response to doxorubicin and mitomycin in cholangiocarcinoma: A case report. *Cancer Treat. Rep.,* 66:209–210, 1982.

Adson, M. A.: Carcinoma of the gallbladder. *Surg. Clin. North Am.,* 53:1203–1216, 1973.

Adson, M. A., and Farnell, M. B.: Hepatobiliary cancer—Surgical considerations. *Mayo Clin. Proc.,* 56:686–699, 1981.

Akwari, O. E.; Van Heerden, J. A.; Foulk, W. T.; and Baggenstoss, A. H.: Cancer of the bile ducts associated with ulcerative colitis. *Ann. Surg.,* 181:303–309, 1975.

Albores-Saavedra, J.; Cruz-Ortiz, H.; Alcantara-Vasques, A.; and Henson, D. E.: Unusual types of gallbladder carcinoma. *Arch. Pathol. Lab. Med.,* 105:287–293, 1981.

Alpert, M. E.; Hutt, M. S. R.; Wogan, G. N.; and Davidson, C. S.: Association between aflatoxin content of food and hepatoma frequency in Uganda. *Cancer,* 28:253–260, 1971.

Appleman, R. M.; Morlock, C. G.; Dahlin, D. C.; and Adson, M. A.: Long-term survival in carcinoma of the gallbladder. *Surg. Gynecol. Obstet.,* 117:459–464, 1963.

Ariel, I. M., and Pack, G. T.: The treatment of inoperable cancer of the biliary system with radioactive (I^{131}) rose bengal. *Am. J. Roentgenol. Radium Ther. Nucl. Med.,* 83:474–490, 1960.

Arminski, T. C.: Primary carcinoma of the gallbladder: A collective review with the addition of twenty-five cases from the Grace Hospital, Detroit, Michigan. *Cancer,* 2:379–398, 1949.

Arnaud, J.-P.; Graf, P.; Gramfort, J.-L.; and Adloff, M.: Primary carcinoma of the gallbladder: Review of 25 cases. *Am. J. Surg.,* 138:403–406, 1979.

Baker, L. H.; Saiki, J. A.; Jones, S. E.; Hewlett, J. S.; Brownlee, R. W.; Stephens, R. L.; and Vaitkevicius, V. K.: Adriamycin and 5-fluorouracil in the treatment of advanced hepatoma: a Southwest Oncology Group Study. *Cancer Treat. Rep.,* 61:1595–1597, 1977.

Bedikian, M.; Valdivieso, M.; DeLaCrus, A.; Martin, R.; Luna, M.; Guinea, V. F.; and Bodey, G. P.: Cancer of the extrahepatic bile ducts. *Med. Pediatr. Oncol.,* 8:53–61, 1980.

Berk, R. N.; Armbuster, T. G.; and Saltzstein, S. L.: Carcinoma in the porcelain gallbladder. *Radiology,* 106:29–31, 1973.

Berman, C.: *Primary Carcinoma of the Liver.* H. K. Lewis and Company, London, 1951.

Bismuth, H.: Surgical therapy of biliary tract cancer. *Proc. 13th Int. Cancer Congress.* Seattle, UICC 1982.

Bismuth, H., and Malt, R. A.: Carcinoma of the biliary tract. *N. Engl. J. Med.,* 301:704–706, 1979.

Black, K.; Hanna, S. S.; Langer, B.; Jirsh, D. W.; and Rider, W. D.: Management of carcinoma of the extrahepatic bile ducts. *Can. J. Surg.,* 21:542–545, 1978.

Bodey, G. P.; Bedikian, A. Y.; Valdivieso, M.; McKelvey, E. M.; and Patt, Y. Z.: Chemotherapeutic management of hepatobiliary and pancreatic cancer. In Stroehlein, J. R., and Romsdahl, M. M. (eds.): *Gastrointestinal Cancer.* Raven Press, New York, 1981.

Broden, G., and Bengtsson, L.: Carcinoma of the gallbladder. Its relation to cholelithiasis and to the concept of prophylactic cholecystectomy. *Acta Chir. Scand.* [Suppl.], 500:15–18, 1980.

Broe, P. J., and Cameron, J. L.: The management of proximal biliary tract tumors. *Adv. Surg.,* 15:47–91, 1981.

Cameron, J. L.; Gayler, B. W.; and Zuidema, G. D.: The use of silastic transhepatic stents in benign and malignant biliary strictures. *Ann. Surg.,* 188:552–561, 1978.

Campbell, T. C., and Hayes, J. R.: The role of aflatoxin metabolism in its toxic lesion. *Toxicol. Appl. Pharmacol.,* 35:199–222, 1976.

Chen, D. S., and Sung, J. L.: Serum alpha-feto protein in hepatocellular carcinoma. *Cancer,* 40:779–783, 1977.

Christopherson, W. M.: Possible etiologic factors for some malignant hepatic tumors. In Stroehlein, J. R., and Romsdahl, M. M. (eds.): *Gastrointestinal Cancer.* Raven Press, New York, 1981.

Clinical Biometry Section: End results in cancer. National Cancer Institute; Report No. 2, Public Health Service, 1964.

Conroy, R. M.: Intracatheter irradiation of biliary tract cancer. *Proc. 13th Int. Cancer Congress,* Seattle, UICC 1982.

Conroy, R. M.; Shahbazian, A. A.; Edwards, K. C.; Moran, E. M.; Swingle, K. F.; Lewis, G. J.; and Pribram, H. F. W.: A new method for treating carcinomatous biliary obstruction with intracatheter radium. *Cancer,* 49:1321–1327, 1982.

Converse, C. F.; Reagan, J. W.; and DeCosse, J. J.: Ulcerative colitis and carcinoma of the bile ducts. *Am. J. Surg.,* 121:39–45, 1971.

Creech, J. L., Jr., and Johnson, M. N.: Angiosarcoma of the liver in the manufacture of polyvinyl chloride. *J. Occup. Med.,* 16:150–151, 1974.

Crooke, S. T., and Bradner, W. T.: Mitomycin-C: A review. *Cancer Treat. Rev.,* 3:121–139, 1976.

Davis, H. L., Jr.; Ramirez, G.; and Ansfield, F. J.: Adenocarcinoma of stomach, pancreas, liver and biliary tracts:

Survival of 328 patients treated with fluoropyrimidine therapy. *Cancer,* **33**:193–197, 1974.

Davis, M.; Portmann, B.; Searle, M.; Wright, R.; and Williams, R.: Histological evidence of carcinoma in a hepatic tumour associated with oral contraceptives. *Br. Med. J. [Clin. Res.],* **4**:496–498, 1975.

Devor, E. J., and Buechley, R. W.: Gallbladder cancer in Hispanic New Mexicans: I. General population, 1957–1977. *Cancer,* **45**:1705–1712, 1980.

Diehl, A. K.: Epidemiology of gallbladder cancer. A synthesis of recent data. *J.N.C.I.,* **65**:1209–1214, 1980.

Donaldson, D. R., and Guillou, P. J.: Extrahepatic cholangiocarcinoma in association with long-standing cholangitis. *Br. J. Clin. Pract.,* **33**:297–300, 1979.

Edmondson, H. A., and Peters, R. L.: Neoplasms of the liver. In Schiff, L., and Schiff, T. R. (eds.): *Diseases of the Liver.* J. B. Lippincott Company, Philadelphia, 1982.

El-Domeiri, A. A.; Havos, A. G.; Goldsmith, H. S.; and Foote, F. W., Jr.: Primary malignant tumors of the liver. *Cancer,* **27**:7–11, 1971.

Evander, A.; Fredlund, P.; Hoevels, J.; Ihse, I.; and Bengmark, S.: Evaluation of aggressive surgery for carcinoma of the extrahepatic bile ducts. *Ann. Surg.,* **191**:23–29, 1980.

Fahim, R. B.; McDonald, J. R.; Richards, J. C.; and Ferris, D. O.: Carcinoma of the gallbladder: A study of its modes of spread. *Ann. Surg.,* **156**:114–124, 1962.

Falkson, G.; Moertel, C. G.; Lavin, P.; Pretorius, F. J.; and Carbone, P. P.: Chemotherapy studies in primary liver cancer. *Cancer,* **42**:2149–2156, 1978.

Falkson, G.; Von Hoff, D.; Klassen, D.; DuPlessis, N.; Van Der Merwe, C. F.; Van Der Merwe, A. M.; and Carbone, P. P.: A phase II study of neocarzinostatin (NSC 157365) in malignant hepatoma. *Cancer Chemother. Pharmacol.,* **4**:33–36, 1980.

Farris, K. B., and Faust, B. F.: Granular cell tumors of biliary ducts. *Arch. Pathol. Lab. Med.,* **103**:510–512, 1979.

Flanigan, D. P.: Biliary carcinoma associated with biliary cysts. *Cancer,* **40**:880–883, 1977.

Fraumeni, J. F.: Cancers of the pancreas and biliary tract: Epidemiological considerations. *Cancer Res.,* **35**:3437–3446, 1975.

Friedman, M. A.; Volkerding, P.; Cassidy, M.; Wasserman, T.; and Phillips, T.: Combined modality nepatic intraarterial (IA) polychemotherapy plus whole liver irradiation (XRT) for patients with neoplasms in the liver. NCOG pilot study. *Proc. Am. Assoc. Cancer Res. Proc. and Am. Soc. Clin. Oncol.,* **20**:307, 1979.

Gastrointestinal Tumor Study Group: A comparison of combination chemotherapy and combined modality therapy for locally advanced gastric carcinoma. *Cancer,* **49**:1771–1777, 1982.

Gluckman, J. B., and Turner, M. D.: Systemic manifestations of tumors of the small gut and liver. *Ann. N.Y. Acad. Sci.,* **230**:318–331, 1974.

Goebel, R. H.; Levene, M. B.; Weichselbaum, R. R.; and Chaffey, J. T.: Techniques for localized radiation of carcinoma of the biliary tree. *Int. J. Radiat. Oncol. Biol. Phys.,* **5**:80, 1979.

Goldfarb, S.: Sex hormones and hepatic neoplasia. *Cancer Res.,* **36**:2584–2584, 1976.

Gracie, W. A., and Ransohoff, D. F.: The natural history of silent gallstones: The innocent gallstone is not a myth. *N. Engl. J. Med.,* **307**:798–800, 1982.

Graham, E. A.: The prevention of carcinoma of the gallbladder. *Ann. Surg.,* **93**:317–322, 1931.

Grieco, R. V.; Bartone, N. F.; and Vasidas, A.: A study of fixed filling defects in the well opacified gallbladder and their evolution. *A.J.R.,* **90**:844–853, 1963.

Hall, S. W.; Benjamin, R. S.; Murphy, W. K.; Valdivieso, M.; and Bodey, G. P.: Adriamycin, BCNU, ftorafur chemotherapy of pancreatic and biliary tract cancer. *Cancer,* **4**:2008–2013, 1979.

Hansson, J. A.; Hoevels, J.; Simert, G.; Tylen, U.; and Vang, J.: Clinical aspects of non-surgical percutaneous transhepatic bile drainage in obstructive lesions of the extrahepatic bile ducts. *Ann. Surg.,* **189**:58–61, 1979.

Hart, J.; Modan, B.; and Hashomer, T.: Factors affecting survival of patients with gallbladder neoplasms. *Arch. Intern. Med.,* **129**:931–934, 1972a.

Hart, J.; Shani, M.; and Modan, B.: Epidemiological aspects of gallbladder and biliary tract neoplasms. *Am. J. Public Health,* **62**:36–39, 1972b.

Harvey, J. H.; Smith, F. P.; and Schein, P. S.: 5-Fluorouracil, mitomycin, and doxorubicin (FAM) in carcinoma of the biliary tract. *J. Clin. Oncol.,* **11**:1245–1248, 1984.

Haskell, C. M.: Cancer of the liver. In Haskell, C. M. (ed.): *Cancer Treatment,* W. B. Saunders Company, Philadelphia, 1980.

Higgins, G. K.: The pathologic anatomy of primary hepatic tumors. In Pack, G. T., and Islami, A. H. (eds.): *Tumors of the Liver. Recent Results in Cancer Research,* Vol. 26. Springer-Verlag New York, Inc., 1970.

Higginson, J., and Svoboda, D. J.: Primary carcinoma of the liver as a pathologist's problem. *Pathol. Annu.,* **5**:61, 1970.

Hoevels, J., and Ihse, I.: Percutaneous transhepatic portography in bile duct carcinoma. Correlation with percutaneous transhepatic cholangiography and angiography. *Fortschr. Geb. Rontgenstr.,* **131**:140–150, 1979.

Ihde, D. C.; Kane, R. C.; Cohen, M. H.; McIntyre, K. R.; and Minna, J. D.: Adriamycin therapy in American patients with hepatocellular carcinoma. *Cancer Treat. Rep.,* **61**:1385–1387, 1977.

Ihde, D. C.; Sherlock, P.; Winawer, S. J.; and Fortner, J. C.: Clinical manifestations of hepatoma. *Am. J. Med.,* **56**:83–91, 1974.

Ingold, J. A.; Reed, G. B.; Kaplan, H. S.; and Bagshaw, M. A.: Radiation hepatitis. *A.J.R.,* **93**:200–208, 1965.

Jain, K. M.; Hastings, O. M.; Rickert, R. R.; Swaminathan, A. P.; and Lazaro, E. J.: Granular cell tumor of the common bile duct: Case report and review of the literature. *Am. J. Gastroenterol.,* **71**:401–407, 1979.

Joffe, N., and Antonioli, D. A.: Primary carcinoma of the gallbladder associated with chronic inflammatory bowel disease. *Clin. Radiol.,* **32**:319–324, 1981.

Kaplan, H. S., and Bagshaw, M. A.: Radiation hepatitis: Possible prevention by combined isotopic and external radiation therapy. *Radiology,* **91**:1214–1220, 1968.

Kappel, D. A., and Miller, D. R.: Primary hepatic carcinoma: A review of thirty-seven patients. *Am. J. Surg.,* **124**:798–802, 1972.

Keen, P., and Martin, P.: Is aflatoxin carcinogenic in man? The evidence in Swaziland. *Trop. Geogr. Med.,* **23**:44–53, 1971.

Keill, R. H., and DeWeese, M. S.: Primary carcinoma of the gallbladder. *Am. J. Surg.,* **125**:726–729, 1973.

Kennedy, P. S.; Lehane, D. E.; Smith, F. E.; and Lane, M.: Oral fluorouracil therapy of hepatoma. *Cancer,* **39**:1930–1935, 1977.

Kew, M. C.; Dos Santos, H. A.; and Sherlock, S.: Diagnosis of primary cancer of the liver. *Br. Med. J. [Clin. Res.],* **4**:408–411, 1971.

Kew, M. C., and Geddes, E. W.: Hepatocellular carcinoma in rural southern African blacks. *Medicine (Baltimore)*, **61**:98–108, 1982.

Kew, M. C.; Geddes, E. W.; Macrab, G. M.; and Bersohn, I.: Hepatitis-B antigen and cirrhosis in Bantu patients with primary liver cancer. *Cancer*, **34**:539–541, 1974.

Kiely, J. M.; Titus, J. L.; and Orvis, A. L.: Thorotrast-induced hepatoma presenting as hyperparathyroidism. *Cancer*, **31**:1312–1314, 1973.

Klatskin, G.: Adenocarcinoma of the hepatic duct at its bifurcation within the porta hepatis: An unusual tumor with distinctive clinical and pathological features. *Am. J. Med.*, **38**:241–256, 1965.

Kojiro, M.; Kawbata, K.; Kawano, Y.; Shirai, F.; Takemoto, N.; and Nakashima, T.: Hepatocellular carcinoma presenting as intrabile duct tumor growth: A clinicopathologic study of 24 cases. *Cancer*, **49**:2144–2147, 1982.

Koo, J.; Wong, J.; Cheng, F. C. Y.; and Ong, G. B.: Carcinoma of the gallbladder. *Br. J. Surg.*, **68**:161–165, 1981.

Kopelson, G.; Galdabini, J.; Warshaw, A. L.; and Gunderson, L. L.: Patterns of failure after curative surgery for extra-hepatic biliary tract carcinoma: Implications for adjuvant therapy. *Int. J. Radiat. Oncol. Biol. Phys.*, **7**:413–417, 1981.

Krain, L. S.: Gallbladder and extrahepatic bile duct carcinoma: Analysis of 1808 cases. *Geriatrics*, **27**:111–117, 1972.

Lee, F. I.: Cirrhosis and hepatoma in alcoholics. *Gut*, **7**:77–85, 1966.

Lees, C. D.; Zapolanski, A.; Cooperman, A. M.; and Hermann, R. E.: Carcinoma of the bile ducts. *Surg. Gynecol. Obstet.*, **151**:193–198, 1980.

Linder, G. T.; Chook, J. N.; and Cohn, I.: Primary liver carcinoma. *Cancer*, **33**:1624–1629, 1974.

Link, J. S.; Bateman, J. R.; Paroly, W. S.; Durkin, W. J.; and Peters, R. L.: 5-fluorouracil in hepatocellular carcinoma: Report of twenty-one cases. *Cancer*, **39**:1936–1939, 1977.

Linsell, C. A., and Peers, F. G.: Field studies on liver cell cancer. In Hiatt, H. H.; Watson, J. D.; and Winston, J. A. (eds.): *Origins of Human Cancer.* Cold Spring Harbor Laboratory, Cold Spring Harbor, New York, 1977.

Litwin, M. S.: Primary carcinoma of the gallbladder: A review of 78 patients. *Arch. Surg.*, **95**:236–240, 1967.

Longmire, W. P., and Tompkins, W. K.: Lesions of the segmental and lobar hepatic ducts. *Ann. Surg.*, **182**:478–493, 1975.

Mancuso, T. F., and Brennan, M. J.: Epidemiological considerations of cancer of the gallbladder, bile ducts and salivary glands in the rubber industry. *J. Occup. Med.*, **12**:333–341, 1970.

Mayo, W. J.: Malignant disease of the common bile duct. *Northwest Med.*, **1**:173–177, 1903.

Mays, E. T.; Christopherson, W. M.; Mahr, M. M.; and Williams, H. C.: Hepatic changes in young women ingesting contraceptive steroids. Hepatic hemorrhage and primary hepatic tumors. *J.A.M.A.*, **235**:730–732, 1976.

Macdonald, J. S.; Lippman, M. E.; Woolley, P. V.; Petrucci, P. P.; and Schein, P. S.: Hepatic estrogen and progesterone receptors in an estrogen-associated hepatic neoplasm. *Cancer Chemother. Pharmacol.*, **1**:135–138, 1978.

McBride, C. M.: Diagnosis and surgical management of primary malignant hepatic tumors. In Stoehlein, J. R., and Romsdahl, M. M. (eds.): *Gastrointestinal Cancer.* Raven Press, New York, 1981.

McFadzean, A. J. S., and Yeung, R. T. T.: Further observations on hypoglycemia in hepatocellular carcinoma. *Am. J. Med.*, **47**:220–227, 1969.

McIntyre, K. R.; Vogel, C. L.; Primack, A.; and Waldmann, T. A.: Effect on surgical and chemotherapeutic treatment on alpha-feto-protein levels in patients with hepatocellular carcinoma. *Cancer*, **37**:677–683, 1976.

Michel, H.; Raynaud, A.; Pomier-Layrargues, G.; Puyeo, J.; DuBois, A.; and Bruel, J. M.: Cholangiographie transparietale laterale: Technique d'Okuda: Reflexions a propos de 111 examens. *Nouv. Presse Med.*, **6**:825–828, 1977.

Misra, N. C.; Jaiswal, M. S. D.; Singh, R. V.; and Das, B.: Intrahepatic arterial infusion of combination of mitomycin-C and 5-fluorouracil in treatment of primary and metastatic liver carcinoma. *Cancer*, **39**:1425–1429, 1977.

Moertel, C. G.: Clinical management of advanced gastrointestinal cancer. *Cancer*, **36**:675–682, 1975.

Moertel, C. G.: Medical management of liver cancer. In Schiff, L., and Schiff, E. R. (eds.): *Diseases of the Liver.* J. B. Lippincott Company, Philadelphia, 1982.

Morris, D. L.; Buechley, R. W.; Key, C. R.; and Morgan, M. V.: Gallbladder disease and gallbladder cancer among American Indians in tricultural New Mexico. *Cancer*, **42**:2472–2477, 1978.

Mueller, P. R.; van Sonnenberg, E.; and Simeone, J. F.: Fine-needle transhepatic cholangiography: Indications and usefulness. *Ann. Intern. Med.*, **97**:567–572, 1982.

Nevin, J. E.; Moran, T. J.; Kay, S.; and King, K.: Primary carcinoma of the gallbladder. *Cancer*, **37**:141–148, 1976.

Nishioka, K.; Levin, A. G.; and Simons, M. J.: Hepatitis B antigen, antigen subtypes, and hepatitis B antibody in normal subjects and patients with liver disease. *Bull. WHO*, **52**:293–300, 1975.

Nissen, E. D.; Kent, O. R.; Nissen, S. E.; and McRae, D. M.: Association of liver tumors with oral contraceptives. *Obstet. Gynecol.*, **48**:49–55, 1976.

Okuda, K.; Nakashima, T.; Sakamoto, K.; Ikari, T.; Kidaka, H.; Kuba, Y.; Sakuma, K.; Motoike, K.; Okuda, H.; and Obata, H.: Hepatocellular carcinoma arising in non-cirrhotic and highly cirrhotic livers. *Cancer*, **49**:450–455, 1982.

Okuda, K., and Ohnishi, K.: Hepatic tumors. In Arias, I. M.; Frenkel, M.; and Wilson, J. H. P. (eds.): *The Liver Annual 2.* Excerpta Medica, Amsterdam, 1982.

Olweny, C. L.; Toya, T.; Katongole-Mbidde, E.; Mugerwe, J.; Kyalwazi, S. K.; and Cohen, H.: Treatment of hepatocellular carcinoma with adriamycin. Preliminary communication. *Cancer*, **36**:1250–1257, 1975.

Order, S. E.; Liebel, S.; Klein, J. L.; Ettinger, D.; Alderson, D.; Siegelman, S.; and Leichner, P.: A phase I–II study of radiolabeled antibody integrated in the treatment of primary hepatic malignancies. *Int. J. Radiat. Oncol. Biol. Phys.*, **6**:703–710, 1979.

Oswalt, C. E., and Cruz, A. B.: Effectiveness of chemotherapy in addition to surgery in treating carcinoma of the gallbladder. *Rev. Surg.*, **34**:436–438, 1977.

Pauli, R. M.; Pauli, M. E.; and Hall, J. G.: Gardner syndrome and periampullary malignancy. *Am. J. Med. Genet.*, **6**:205–219, 1980.

Pereiras, R. J.; Rheingold, O. J.; Hutson, D.; Mejia, J.; Viamonte, M.; Chiprut, R. O.; and Schiff, E. R.: Relief of malignant obstructive jaundice by percutaneous insertion of a permanent prosthesis in the biliary tree. *Ann. Intern. Med.*, **89**:589–593, 1978.

Perpetuo, M. D.; Valdivieso, M.; Heilbrun, L. K.; Nelson, R. S.; Connor, T.; and Bodey, G. P.: Natural history study of gallbladder cancer: A review of 36 years experience at M. D. Anderson Hospital and Tumor Center. *Cancer,* **42**:330–335, 1978.

Phillips, R., and Murikami, K.: Primary neoplasms of the liver. Results of radiation therapy. *Cancer,* **13**:714–720, 1960.

Phinney, P. R.; Auston, G. E.; and Kadell, B. M.: Cholangiocarcinoma arising in Caroli's disease. *Arch. Pathol. Lab. Med.,* **105**:194–197, 1981.

Piehler, J. M., and Crichlow, R. W.: Primary carcinoma of the gallbladder. *Surg. Gynecol. Obstet.,* **147**:929–942, 1978.

Pike, M. C.; Edmondson, H. A.; Benton, B.; and Henderson, B. E.: Liver adenomas and oral contraceptives. In Hiatt, H. H.; Watson, J. D.; and Watson, J. A. (eds.): *Origins of Human Cancer.* Cold Spring Harbor Laboratory, Cold Spring Harbor, New York, 1977.

Pilepich, M. J., and Lambert, P. M.: Radiotherapy of carcinomas of the extrahepatic biliary system. *Radiology,* **127**:767–770, 1978.

Polk, H. C.: Carcinoma of the calcified gallbladder. *Gastroenterology,* **50**:582–585, 1966.

Ravry, M. J. R., and Hester, M.: Phase II study of adriamycin plus bleomycin for the treatment of hepatocellular and biliary tract carcinoma. *Proc. Am. Soc. Clin. Oncol.,* **20**:415, 1979.

Ritchie, J. K.; Allan, R. N.; Macartney, J.; Thompson, H.; Hawley, P. R.; and Cooke, W. T.: Biliary tract carcinoma associated with ulcerative colitis. *Q. J. Med.,* **43**:263–279, 1974.

Roberts-Thomson, I. C.; Strickland, R. G.; and Mackery, I. R.: Bile duct carcinoma in chronic ulcerative colitis. *Aust. N.Z. J. Med.,* **3**:264–267, 1973.

Robertson, W. A., and Carlisle, B. B.: Primary carcinoma of the gallbladder: Review of fifty-two cases. *Am. J. Surg.,* **113**:738–742, 1967.

Ross, A. P., and Braasch, J. W.: Ulcerative colitis and carcinoma of the proximal bile ducts. *Gut,* **14**:94–97, 1973.

Ross, A. P.; Braasch, J. W.; and Warren, K. R.: Carcinoma of the proximal bile ducts. *Surg. Gynecol. Obstet.,* **136**:923–928, 1973.

Ruiz, R.; Teyssou, H.; Fernandez, N.; Carrez, J. P.; Gortchakoff, M.; Manteau, G.; Ter-Davtian, P. M.; and Tessier, J. P.: Ultrasonic diagnosis of primary carcinoma of the gallbladder: A review of 16 cases. *J. Clin. Ultrasound,* **8**:489–495, 1980.

Schein, P. S.: Tumor markers. In Wyngarrden, J. M., and Smith, L. H. (eds.): *Cecil Textbook of Medicine,* 16th ed. W. B. Saunders Company, Philadelphia, 1982.

Scott, J.; Shousa, S.; Thomas, H. C.; and Sherlock, S.: Bile duct carcinoma: A late complication of congenital hepatic fibrosis. *Am. J. Gastroenterol.,* **73**:113–119, 1980.

Sherlock, S.: Hepatic adenomas and oral contraceptives. *Gut,* **16**:753–756, 1975.

Shieh, C. J.; Dunn, E.; and Standard, J. E.: Primary carcinoma of the gallbladder: A review of a 16-year experience at the Waterbury Hospital Health Center. *Cancer,* **47**:996–1004, 1981.

Silverberg, E.: Cancer statistics, 1983. *CA,* **33**:9–25, 1983.

Smoron, G. L.: Radiation therapy of carcinoma of the gallbladder and biliary tract. *Cancer,* **40**:1422–1424, 1977.

Smoron, G. L.; and Battifora, H. A.: Thorotrast-induced hepatoma. *Cancer,* **30**:1252–1259, 1972.

Starzl, T. E.; Koep, L. J.; Halgrimson, C. G.; Hood, J.; Schroter, G. P. J.; Porter, K. A.; and Weil, R.: Fifteen years of clinical liver transplantation. *Gastroenterology,* **77**:375–389, 1979.

Strauch, G. O.: Primary carcinoma of the gallbladder: Presentation of seventy cases from the Rhode Island Hospital and a cumulative review of the last ten years of the American Literature. *Surgery,* **47**:368–383, 1960.

Sugar, J. K.; Toth, K.; Cuska, O.; Gati, E.; and Somfai-Relle, S.: Role of pesticides in hepatocarcinogenesis. In Lapis, K., and Johannessen, J. V. (eds.): *Liver Carcinogenesis.* Hemisphere Publishing Corporation, New York, 1979.

Tabor, I. E.; Trichopoulos, D.; Manousos, Q.; Zaritsanos, X.; Drucker, J. A.; and Gerety, R. J.: Absence of an association between past infection with hepatitis A virus and primary hepatocellular carcinoma. *Int. J. Epidemiol.,* **9**:221–223, 1980.

Terblanche, J.: Carcinoma of the proximal extrahepatic biliary tree. *Surg. Annu.,* **11**:249–265, 1979.

Thamavit, W.; Bhamarapravati, N.; Sahaphong, S.; Vajrasthira, S.; and Angsubhakorn, S.: Effects of dimethylnitrosamine on induction of cholangiocarcinoma in *Opisthorchis viverini*–infected syrian golden hamsters. *Cancer Res.,* **38**:4634–4639, 1978.

Thorbjarnarson, B.: Carcinoma of the gallbladder and acute cholecystitis. *Ann. Surg.,* **151**:241–244, 1960.

Todani, T.; Tabuchi, K.; Watanabe, Y.; and Kobayashi, T.: Carcinoma arising in the wall of congenital bile duct cysts. *Cancer,* **44**:1134–1141, 1979.

Todoroki, T.; Okamura, T.; Fukuo, K.; Nishimura, A.; Otsu, H.; Sato, H.; and Iwasaki, Y.: Gross appearance of carcinoma of the main hepatic duct and its prognosis. *Surg. Gynecol. Obstet.,* **150**:33–40, 1980.

Tompkins, R. K.; Johnson, J.; Storm, F. K.; and Longmire, W. E., Jr.: Operative endoscopy in the management of biliary tract neoplasms. *Am. J. Surg.,* **132**:174–182, 1976.

Traverso, L. W.; and Longmire, W. P., Jr.: Preservation of the pylorus in pancreatoduodenectomy: A follow-up evaluation. *Ann. Surg.,* **192**:306–309, 1980.

Umsawasdi, T.; Chainuvati, T.; and Viranuvatti, V.: Combination chemotherapy of hepatocellular carcinoma with fluorouracil and mitomycin-C (abstr.). *Proc. Am. Assoc. Cancer Res. and A.S.C.O.,* **19**:193, 1978.

Vaittinen, E.: Carcinoma of the gallbladder: A study of 390 cases diagnosed in Finland 1953–1967. *Ann. Chir. Gynaecol.* [59 Suppl.], **168**:7–81, 1970.

Vogel, C. L.; Galey, A. C.; Brooker, R. J.; Anthony, P. P.; and Ziegler, J. L.: A phase II study of adriamycin (NSC 123127) in patients with hepatocellular carcinoma from Zambia and the United States. *Cancer,* **39**:1923–1929, 1977.

Von Eyben, F.; Hellekant, C.; Mattson, M.; Ljungquist, V.; and Jonsson, K.: Mitomycin-C in advanced gallbladder carcinoma. *Acta Radiol. [Oncol.],* **19**:81–84, 1980.

Waldman, T. A., and McIntire, K. R.: The use of radioimmunoassay for alpha-fetoprotein in the diagnosis of malignancy. *Cancer,* **34**:1516, 1974.

Wanebo, H. J., and Grimes, P. F.: Carcinoma of the bile duct: The occult malignancy. *Am. J. Surg.* **130**:262–266, 1975.

Warren, R., and Balch, F. G.: Carcinoma of the gallbladder: The etiological role of gallstones. *Surgery,* **7**:657–666, 1940.

Welton, J. C.; Marr, J. S.; and Friedman, S. M.: Association between hepatobiliary cancer and typhoid carrier state. *Lancet,* **1:**791–794, 1979.

Westaby, D.; Ogle, S. J.; Paradinas, F. J.; Randell, J. B.; and Murray-Lyon, I. M.: Liver damage from long-term methyltestosterone. *Lancet,* **2:**261–263, 1977.

Wiechel, K. L.: Percutaneous transhepatic catheter ther-apy of obstructive jaundice. *Proc. 13th Int. Cancer Congress,* Seattle, UICC 1982.

Yarrish, R. L.; Werner, B. G.; and Blumberg, B. S.: Association of hepatitis B virus with hepatocellular carcinoma in American patients. *Int. J. Cancer,* **26:**711–715, 1980.

29

Neoplasms of the Small Bowel

BERNARD LEVIN

In spite of the length and diversity of structural and cellular elements in the small intestine, benign and malignant tumors are rarely encountered. Only 5% of all gastrointestinal neoplasms arise in the small intestine, and small intestinal cancers account for 1% of all gastrointestinal tract neoplasms (Herbsman *et al.,* 1980). The classification and distribution of primary, benign, and malignant neoplasms of the small intestine are shown in Tables 29–1, 29–2, and 29–3.

Epidemiology

The average age of presentation of both benign and malignant tumors is the fifth and sixth decades of life. A slight predominance of small intestinal neoplasms occurs in men and among blacks. In the United States, the age-adjusted incidence for small bowel tumors per 100,000 for whites is 1.2 for men, and 0.8 for women. The incidence per 100,000 for blacks in the United States is 1.6 for men, and 0.7 for women (Lightdale *et al.,* 1982).

Adenocarcinoma. About half of all small bowel cancers are adenocarcinomas, arising from the intestinal glands. They are usually histologically similar to colonic adenocarcinomas. In the United States, duodenal adenocarcinomas are more common than ileal adenocarcinomas (Silberman *et al.,* 1974).

Risk Factors. REGIONAL ENTERITIS. Crohn's disease is an inflammatory bowel disease of unknown etiology. Several investigators have described an increased incidence of small bowel carcinoma in regional enteritis. A series of 295 patients with regional enteritis was followed for a total of 4,200 person-years (Fielding *et al.,* 1972). Two small bowel adeno-

carcinomas were observed and compared with an expected incidence of 0.02, yielding a relative risk of about 10.

Patients who have had segments of intestine surgically bypassed for Crohn's disease may be at particular risk for developing adenocarcinoma. Areas around fistulous tracts may also form the nidus for the development of adenocarcinoma (Traube *et al.,* 1980).

PEUTZ-JEGHERS SYNDROME. The Peutz-Jeghers syndrome consists of hamartomatous polyps throughout the small and large bowel, and melanin spots on the oral mucosa, lips, and digits. The relative risk of small bowel adenocarcinoma appears to be about 16 times that expected, and the lifetime incidence is 2.4% in patients with this syndrome (Dozois *et al.,* 1969).

FAMILIAL POLYPOSIS COLI. Adenomas of the duodenum have been described in patients with familial polyposis coli. Colon carcinoma occurs in nearly all those who do not undergo colectomy, and they rarely develop periampullary or duodenal adenocarcinoma (Yao *et al.,* 1979). Familial polyposis of the entire gastrointestinal tract has been reported, but small intestinal cancer is very rare (Yonemoto *et al.,* 1969).

GARDNER SYNDROME. Gardner syndrome consists of the following clinical features:

1. Multiple adenomas of the colon and rectum
2. Multiple epidermoid cysts and connective tissue tumors of the skin
3. Multiple osteomas of the skull and mandible; additional lesions include osteomas of the entire skeletal system, postoperative desmoids of the abdominal

Table 29–1. Distribution of Malignant Tumors in the Small Intestine (%)

TYPE OF NEOPLASM	DUODENUM	JEJUNUM	ILEUM
Adenocarcinoma	40	38	22
Carcinoid	6	10	84
Lymphoma	16	48	36
Leiomyosarcoma	10	37	53
Fibrosarcoma and other sarcomas	29	0	71

Adapted from Wilson, J. M.: Melvin, D. B.; and Gray, G. F.: Primary malignancies of the small bowel: A report of 96 cases and review of the literature. *Ann. Surg.*, **180**:175–179, 1974. Loehr, W. J.; Mujahed, Z.; and Zahn, F. D.: Primary lymphoma of the gastrointestinal tract. A review of 100 cases. *Ann. Surg.*, **170**:232–238, 1969.

Table 29–2. Primary Tumors of the Small Intestine (Distribution of Benign Neoplasms in the Small Intestine, Percentage by Region)

TYPE OF NEOPLASM	DUODENUM %	JEJUNUM %	ILEUM %
Adenoma	33	25	42
Fibroma	7	17	76
Hemangioma	8	47	45
Pseudolymphoma	0	17	83
Neurofibroma	19	41	40
Lipoma	24	18	58

Adapted from Wilson, J. M.; Melvin, D. B.; and Gray, G. F.: Primary malignancies of the small bowel: A report of 96 cases and review of the literature. *Ann. Surg.*, **180**:175–179, 1974.

wall, dental abnormalities, carcinoma of the thyroid, and malignant tumors of the central nervous system (Turcot's syndrome)

Small bowel adenomas occur most commonly in the duodenum. Patients with Gardner syndrome have an increased risk for the development of periampullary adenocarcinomas (Schnur and David, 1973).

Carcinoid Tumors. Carcinoid tumors are the second most commonly reported small bowel cancer. These have a predilection for the ileum, probably associated with the higher frequencies of argentaffin cells in ileal glands.

No sex differential has been reported in the incidence of carcinoid tumors. In the Third National Cancer Survey, 119 cases were reported from 1969 to 1971, with 59 men and 60 women, 107 white and 12 black patients (Cutler and Young, 1975). A detailed discussion of these tumors is presented in the Endocrine Neoplasms chapter (see Chapter 32).

Lymphomas. Lymphomas of the gastrointestinal tract are rare, constituting 4.5% of lymphoid neoplasms of all sites, and 1% of all gastrointestinal cancers (Rosenberg *et al.*, 1961; McGovern, 1977). Most intestinal lymphomas are not of primary intestinal origin, but represent a component of systemic disease. Dawson and associates (1981) have suggested the following criteria for considering a lymphoid tumor to be primary in the gastrointestinal tract:

1. Absence of palpable superficial lymphadenopathy
2. Normal total white blood cell count and differential count
3. Absence of enlargement of mediastinal lymph nodes on chest roentgenographs
4. No grossly demonstrable involvement at the time of surgical treatment beyond the involved segment of the intestine and its regional mesenteric lymph nodes
5. Absence of tumor involvement of the liver and spleen

A complete discussion of the natural history and management of these disorders is presented in the chapter dealing with non-Hodgkin's lymphomas (see Chapter 16).

Table 29–3. Classification of Primary Neoplasms of Small Intestine

TISSUE OF ORIGIN	BENIGN	MALIGNANT
Glandular epithelium	Adenoma	Adenocarcinoma
Smooth muscle	Leiomyoma	Leiomyosarcoma
Fibrous tissue	Fibroma	Fibrosarcoma
Lymphoid tissue	Pseudolymphoma	Lymphoma
Vascular tissue	Hemangioma Lymphangioma	Angiosarcoma
Nervous tissue	Neurofibroma	Neurofibrosarcoma
Nerve sheath	Neurilemmoma	Malignant schwannoma
Fat	Lipoma	Liposarcoma
Enterochromaffin tissue		Carcinoid

Adapted from del Regato, J. A., and Spjut, H. J.: *Ackerman and del Regato's Cancer: Diagnosis, Treatment and Prognosis,* 5th ed. The C. V. Mosby Company, St. Louis, 1977.

Factors Suggested to Explain Rarity of Small Bowel Tumors

The rarity of small bowel neoplasms has intrigued many authors. Several hypotheses have been suggested to explain the remarkable disparity in incidence between small and large bowel carcinomas. These include the following (reviewed by Lightdale et al., 1982):

1. Liquid contents of the small intestine may dilute potential carcinogens. Transit time through the small bowel is faster than through the colon, which may reduce exposure of the small intestine to ingested carcinogens.
2. The bacterial population of the colon is much greater than that of the small intestine. The large bowel anaerobes are potentially capable of transforming bile acids into carcinogens.
3. Xenobiotic metabolising enzymes, such as benzypyrene hydroxylase, present in small intestine in high concentration, may detoxify ingested carcinogens. Disease states, such as sprue, associated with an increased risk of intestinal cancer have an associated loss of mucosal benzpyrene hydroxylase (Hoensch et al., 1982).
4. The role of the local immune system has been implicated. The small bowel is an abundant producer of IgA that may act locally to decrease infection by oncogenic viruses.
5. The role of an increased cell turnover remains unclear. Lowenfels (1973) and others have commented that the rapid proliferation of the small intestinal epithelial cells may be a protective phenomenon. In celiac sprue, a markedly increased proliferation rate is observed, but the decreased concentration of benzypyrene hydroxylase may increase the susceptibility of the mucosa to exogenous carcinogens.

Symptoms.   One-half of all benign small bowel tumors remain asymptomatic and may only be discovered incidentally at laparotomy or autopsy. Lack of symptoms is attributable to the liquid contents of the small intestine and the distensibility of the small intestine. Lesions originating in the mucosa grow toward the lumen and may cause proximal or distal mechanical obstruction of the small bowel, producing pain. This presentation is the most common in symptomatic benign tumors (40 to 70%) and is often the result of intussusception (Herbsman et al., 1980). Tumors that develop from the serosa may reach a large size before producing symptoms since they expand into the abdominal cavity. Such tumors may cause a volvulus (Herbsman et al., 1980).

Hemorrhage is the second most common clinical presentation in benign tumors, occurring in 20 to 50% of symptomatic patients. It is caused by mucosal invasion by the neoplasm and, although rarely massive, can produce weakness and anemia (Darling and Welch, 1959).

In contrast to benign tumors, over 70% of malignant small bowel tumors produce symptoms. The most common clinical manifestations are pain and weight loss, followed by nausea and vomiting, hemorrhage, and presence of palpable mass. Pain occurs in 30 to 80% of patients with malignant tumors and is variable, depending on the location of the lesion. It may be described as epigastric burning or diffuse abdominal cramps. Weight loss, while infrequent in benign lesions, is common in malignant tumors and particularly with lymphomas with associated malabsorption syndrome (Herbsman et al., 1980; McGovern, 1977). Symptoms of obstruction are produced by infiltration of the neoplasm and may be intermittent. Massive hemorrhage is a common presenting symptom with sarcomas, but is less common with adenocarcinoma and carcinoids. Sarcomas may also present with acute perforation (Herbsman et al., 1980).

The presence of an abdominal mass is observed in some patients, the result of the large volume of tumor or of dilated intestine proximal to areas of obstruction. Diarrhea and steatorrhea may occur with extensive involvement by lymphoma (Loehr et al., 1969).

Carcinoid tumors can present with evidence of obstruction, malabsorption, or with the carcinoid syndrome in the presence of hepatic metastases.

The initial symptoms of small bowel neoplasms are vague and poorly defined, and the clinician may consider other diagnoses such as cholecystitis, peptic ulcer disease, or diverticulitis. Jaundice may occur with periampullary neoplasms, mimicking biliary tract obstruction or pancreatic cancer.

Signs.   Physical examination may reveal little in patients with benign tumors unless the neoplasms are very large, when a mass may be evident. Abdominal distension, loud borborygmi, and visible peristaltic waves may be present in intestinal obstruction. Intussusception may present with blood in the stool and a tender abdominal mass.

Malignant small bowel neoplasms may show more obvious physical findings. Weight loss, cachexia, an abdominal mass, hepatomegaly, ascites, or evidence of intestinal hemorrhage may be noted. Jaundice may be seen in those with periampullary neoplasms or advanced metastatic disease involving the liver. Peripheral lymphadenopathy may be present in disseminated lymphoma.

Diagnosis

The diagnosis of small intestinal tumors is very difficult because of their nonspecific clinical features. A correct preoperative diagnosis may be anticipated in less than one-third of patients (Ostermiller *et al.,* 1966).

Laboratory Studies. A hypochromic, microcytic anemia may occur as a result of chronic blood loss. Elevation of alkaline phosphatase and bilirubin may occur if the ampulla of Vater is obstructed or if metastases to the liver are present. Elevated levels of plasma serotonin or urinary 5-hydroxy-indole-acetic acid occur in the carcinoid syndrome.

Radiologic Studies. Plain films of the abdomen revealing air-fluid levels and dilated small intestine may confirm the presence of a small bowel obstruction.

Contrast radiography is the most commonly used method of diagnosis of small bowel tumors (Marshak and Lindner, 1970). Adenocarcinoma and lymphoma are the most common tumors to produce ulceration, whereas carcinoid tumors and sarcomas present as intramural masses that grow outward, encroaching on the lumen but not disrupting the mucosa. Intraluminal lesions are often adenomas or, less frequently, leiomyomas.

Hypotonic duodenography using glucagon enhances the diagnostic accuracy of the conventional upper gastrointestinal series by retarding the motion of the duodenum. Subtle mucosal abnormalities may be better visualized by this technique. The small intestine distal to the ligament of Treitz can be evaluated only by meticulously following the barium column to the ileocecal region with interval films. Abnormal areas can be further evaluated by selective nasoenteric intubation (enteroclysis) which permits the introduction of barium and air into a relatively localized segment. The distal ileum is not always well visualized on the

conventional small bowel study; an alternative approach is to reflux barium into the distal ileum at the time of a barium enema.

Mesenteric angiography may be helpful in the localization of vascular tumors such as hemangiomas or carcinoids. Computed tomography is not of value in the diagnosis of lesions confined to the bowel wall, but is of benefit in the definition of the extent of the intra-abdominal neoplasm, such as demonstration of retroperitoneal lymphadenopathy or hepatic metastases.

Endoscopy. Both forward and side-viewing fiberoptic endoscopes are used to examine the entire duodenum. Suspicious lesions can be brushed through the endoscope to provide material for cytologic analysis. Polypoid lesions can be biopsied or, if peduculated, excised using electrosurgical technique. Periampullary lesions can be well visualized; in addition, the pancreatic and biliary trees can be studied by contrast radiography after endoscopic cannulation. The terminal ileum can be viewed retrograde and lesions biopsied in many patients with colonoscopy.

Benign tumors

Adenomas. Adenomas are benign proliferations of epithelium arising from the mucosa or intestinal glands. Most are polypoid and constitute about one-third of all benign small intestinal neoplasms. Adenomas may be subclassified into tubular, tubulovillous, and villous types.

Tubular and tubulovillous adenomas are most commonly located in the duodenum, but are also found in the jejunum and ileum. They are usually single, but multiple adenomas can occur; the entire gastrointestinal tract may be involved in a polyposis syndrome; however, familial polyposis coli does not usually involve the small intestine.

The most common presenting symptom of a benign adenoma is intestinal obstruction due to intussusception; it may reduce spontaneously, and repeated attacks are not unusual. Bleeding may be occult or present as melena.

If intussusception is present, surgical reduction is required, with a careful inspection of the involved portion for signs of vascular compromise requiring segmental resection. Segmental resection will also be necessary for larger sessile lesions, although the majority of adenomas are pedunculated and can be removed by enterotomy and excision.

Villous Adenomas. These are rare lesions which occur predominantly in the duodenum as a broad-based cauliflower-like mass (Steinberg and Shieber, 1971). Symptoms include vague epigastric discomfort or vomiting because of intermittent small bowel obstruction, often present for months before the diagnosis is finally established. Frequently, it is bleeding that finally leads to a thorough investigation. Although most villous adenomas are benign, 40% may have malignant transformation (Shulten *et al.,* 1976).

Diagnosis of villous adenomas can be established by contrast radiography in 75% of patients. Barium coats the interstices of the neoplasm, producing a palisaded or striated pattern. Hypotonic duodenography and endoscopy can also be used to make a diagnosis.

Because of the propensity for malignant transformation, all villous tumors should be excised. This may require segmental resection or, if evidence of malignant change is present, bowel resection with wide margins and removal of the draining lymph nodes. For large duodenal neoplasms, pancreaticoduodenectomy is performed.

Adenoma of Brunner's Glands. These are uncommon, usually solitary, benign polypoid lesions of the duodenum arising from the submucosal Brunner's glands, which secrete a highly viscid alkaline mucus. Since Brunner's glands are most numerous in the first portion of the duodenum, most of these lesions have been reported proximal to the ampulla of Vater. Brunner's gland adenomas can cause bleeding and obstruction and may be confused clinically with peptic ulcer (Herbsman *et al.,* 1980). Double contrast roentgenography, followed by endoscopic biopsy, confirms the diagnosis.

Leiomyomas. These benign neoplasms of smooth muscle are uniformly distributed throughout the small intestine (Ostermiller *et al.,* 1966). Most leiomyomas arise in the muscularis mucosa. Four growth patterns of benign and malignant smooth muscle tumors of the small intestine have been identified: (1) extraluminal (66%); (2) intramural (16%); (3) extraintraluminal (dumbbell-shaped) (11%); and (4) intraluminal (8%). The extraluminal tumors usually attain the largest size and may undergo necrosis and hemorrhage (Starr and Dockerty, 1955).

The usual microscopic picture is that of well-differentiated, spindle-shaped smooth muscle cells arranged in interlacing bundles. Mitoses are absent or rare, and tumors exhibiting more than two mitotic figures per high power field are malignant (Golden and Stout, 1941).

Approximately one-half of these tumors produce bleeding as a result of mucosal ulceration. Radiographic evaluation may be diagnostic if barium lodges in an ulcer crater or cavity in the center of a myoma. Intestinal obstruction may occur in one-quarter of patients with leiomyoma.

Treatment consists of surgical resection, including adequate margins of normal small bowel because it is not always possible at the time of operation to distinguish benign from malignant tumors.

Malignant Tumors

Adenocarcinomas. The most common primary malignant neoplasm of the small bowel is adenocarcinoma, which accounts for about half of the malignant tumors. A male predominance is evident, and the peak incidence is in the sixth and seventh decades (Herbsman *et al.,* 1980). The duodenum is the most frequently affected site (40%). Primary duodenal cancers must be distinguished from those arising from the ampulla of Vater and have been classified as intra-ampullary (57%), periampullary (33%), and supra-ampullary (8%). The supra-ampullary lesions are located in the second portion of the duodenum (Spira *et al.,* 1977).

The next most frequently affected site is the jejunum (38%), and these tumors are usually located within the first 30 cm from the ligament of Treitz (Herbsman *et al.,* 1980).

Adenocarcinomas are either polypoid intraluminal masses or, more frequently, infiltrative annular constricting lesions. These tumors tend to metastasize to regional lymph nodes, as well as distantly to the liver. Histologically, these are often well differentiated and are mucin producing.

Surgical resection is the treatment of choice for small intestinal carcinoma. Adequate margins free of tumor involvement and regional nodes should be included in the resection specimen. In nonresectable lesions, palliative bypass should be performed to relieve symptoms of obstruction.

Duodenal carcinomas close to the pancreas should be treated by pancreaticoduodenal resection (Whipple procedure). In some series this approach has resulted in five-year survivals as high as 50% in selected patients, although the overall survival rate is about 20% (Warren *et al.,* 1975). Patients with metastatic disease or with lesions not amenable to resection have a survival time of about four months (Nakase *et al.,* 1977).

Adequate local excision of the primary tumor, with wide resection of the adjacent mesentery to include regional lymph nodes, is the preferred operation for jejunal or ileal adenocarcinomas. Unfortunately, tumor extensions into the mesentery may involve blood vessels that cannot be resected without sacrificing large segments of the small intestine. The five-year survival rates average approximately 20% (Silberman *et al.,* 1974).

Adjuvant radiation therapy may be of benefit in patients with minimal residual disease after surgical resection, but the tolerance of normal tissues limits the dosage that can be administered. Intraoperative radiation therapy may be more useful since normal tissues can be protected from the beam (Abe *et al.,* 1980).

The use of adjuvant chemotherapy after curative surgical resection has not been recommended. At present, no effective single agent or combination chemotherapy has been established for advanced or metastatic small bowel adenocarcinoma.

Leiomyosarcoma. Leiomyosarcoma is the most frequently occurring malignant connective tissue tumor of the small intestine. Most arise from intestinal smooth muscle, but the tumor may also find its origin from vascular smooth muscle (Herbsman *et al.,* 1980). The male to female ratio is 3 : 1, and most occur in the fifth and sixth decades (Starr and Dockerty, 1955).

Occasionally, the histological differentiation between leiomyoma and leiomyosarcoma may be difficult. Leiomyosarcomas are usually large, and over three-quarters are greater than 5 cm in diameter. These neoplasms are prone to vascular insufficiency which may lead to necrosis, ulceration, and hemorrhage.

Leiomyosarcomas spread by direct extension into adjacent tissues and via the blood stream to the liver, lungs, and bones. Lymph node metastases are unusual.

In more than one-half of patients the chief complaint is hemorrhage, usually in the form of melena produced by ulceration of the overlying mucosa (Starr and Dockerty, 1955). Abdominal discomfort may be caused by the presence of a mass. Intestinal obstruction is unusual because these tumors are usually extraluminal.

Radiographic studies may detect the presence of an ulcerated tumor or displacement of bowel loops. Angiography may show a tumor mass or blush.

Computed tomography may aid in the delineation of an abdominal mass and identify invasion of adjacent organs. Metastatic involvement of retroperitoneal lymph nodes and the liver may also be detected. Endoscopy may be used to visualize and biopsy lesions located in the duodenum or distally within reach of the colonoscope passed retrograde through the ileocecal valve. If the mucosa is not directly invaded, biopsies may be negative if the tumor is intramural.

Surgical excision should be attempted in leiomyosarcoma of the small intestine. This should include wide areas of surrounding tissue, but extensive lymph node dissections are not required since lymphatic metastases are unusual. Five-year survivals as high as 50% have been reported in selected patients after curative resections (Herbsman *et al.,* 1980). In the event of unresectability, palliative segmental excision or bypass should be performed to prevent obstruction.

Based on studies with other sarcomas, radiation therapy may be a useful adjunct after surgical excision (Rosenberg *et al.,* 1961). Doxorubicin in combination with cyclophosphamide, vincristine, and imidazole carboxamide has been reported to produce objective response rates of 65% in advanced sarcomas (Gottlieb, 1974). The role of adjuvant therapy after surgical resection remains to be defined.

Small Intestine Lymphoma. *Etiological Factors.* CELIAC SPRUE. Small intestinal lymphoma may develop in patients with adult celiac sprue, usually after the disease has been present for many years. Harris and associates (1967) analyzed 202 patients with adult celiac disease and found 14 in whom a primary small bowel lymphoma developed later. In 11 patients the tumor occurred while the patient was on a gluten-free diet.

In 1976, Holmes and colleagues reported on an additional ten years of follow-up of Harris's 202 patients and an additional four patients who developed lymphomas involving the small intestine (histiocytic lymphomas). In an additional group of 210 patients with celiac disease, 14 patients were found with lymphomas. The duration of symptoms before the onset of symptoms attributable to lymphoma averaged 26 years. Of the 14 lymphomas, 13 were histiocytic lymphomas involving the small intestine. Interestingly, gastrointestinal carcinomas originating in the esophagus, stomach, and colon, are slightly more frequent than in normal subjects. Other series reviewed by Lightdale support the contention that patients with celiac disease are at an increased risk for small bowel lymphoma (Lightdale *et al.*, 1982).

MEDITERRANEAN ABDOMINAL LYM-PHOMA. (Immunoproliferative Small Intestinal Disease). Malabsorption is a prominent feature in this disorder, which occurs predominantly in young adults. It has been widely reported among Jews and Arabs of Middle Eastern origin, but is rare among Jews of European origin. It is not limited to the Middle East, but occurs sporadically throughout the world, including the black population of the Cape Province, Republic of South Africa (Novis *et al.*, 1971).

Possible etiologic factors have included parasitic infestations associated with poor sanitary conditions in impoverished groups (Ramot and Many, 1972). Small bowel lymphoma is also seen with increased frequency in immune deficiency states (Maurer *et al.*, 1976).

Clinical Features.   Intestinal lymphoma has a bimodal age distribution, with one peak occurring below the age of ten and the other in the sixth decade (Mestel, 1959). Lymphomas are the most common tumors of the gastrointestinal tract in children, particularly between the ages of three and eight years. Male preponderance of two to one has been observed. Most patients with Mediterranean lymphoma are in the third decade, and sex preponderance is not apparent.

Symptoms include anorexia, weight loss, abdominal fullness, and incomplete, chronic obstruction due to narrowing of the lumen by tumor or intussusception. Mucosal ulceration produces bleeding and anemia. An acute abdomen may occur as a result of intestinal perforation. In contrast to the Mediterranean variant, malabsorption is rare. Physical examination may reveal the presence of abdominal masses, ascites, and evidence of intestinal destruction.

These lesions may exhibit several forms (Marshak and Lindner, 1970):

1. Single or multiple metastatic lesions involving primarily the wall of the small bowel
2. Metastatic lesions involving primarily the mesentery, with or without involvement of the adjacent wall of the bowel
3. Multiple metastatic nodules involving both the small bowel and the mesentery. Ascites is particularly common.

Patients frequently present with symptoms indicative of intestinal obstruction, such as pain and increasing abdominal girth or weight loss. Gastrointestinal bleeding may occasionally appear as the first manifestation of metastatic disease. Abdominal examination will usually reveal distention, intra-abdominal masses, or ascites.

Barium contrast studies will demonstrate irregular narrowing of the lumen, occasional evidence of indentation or fixation, and eccentric or concentric fixation. CT scans will help to confirm the presence of extensive intra-abdominal spread or retroperitoneal involvement.

The management of the patient with secondary involvement of the small bowel producing obstruction or hemorrhage should be surgical resection. Appropriate care for the primary tumor may include surgical resection, radiation therapy, or chemotherapy.

The incidence of malignant lymphoma in the intestine varies directly with the amount of lymphoid tissue present. Thus, most lymphomas occur in the ileocecal region and the fewest in the duodenum. In contrast, patients with the Mediterranean variant have a high incidence of proximal involvement.

Dysproteinemia is a typical component of the Mediterranean variant, characterized by the presence of an abnormal fragment of IgA in the serum and urine that is devoid of light chains (Salem *et al.*, 1977), and is related to the Fc portion of the α heavy chain. These abnormal immunoglobulins, however, are not detected in all cases of Mediterranean lymphoma (Seligmann and Rambaud, 1978).

A variety of roentgenologic changes have been described including (1) multiple nodular defects, (2) infiltrating form, (3) polypoid form with intussusception occasionally, (4) endo-exoenteric form with excavation and fistula formation, and (5) predominantly invasive form of the mesentery with large, extraluminal masses or production of a spruelike pattern

Table 29–4. Secondary Involvement of Small Intestine

Segment Involved	Direct Invasion
Duodenum	Colon
	Stomach
	Pancreas
	Kidney
	Retroperitoneum
Jejunum	Colon
	Stomach
	Pancreas
	Kidney
Ileum	Colon
	Pelvic tumors
	Retroperitoneum

(Marshak and Linder, 1970). Computed tomography will be helpful in the definition of retroperitoneal involvement, as well as spread to adjacent organs or the liver.

The therapy of these diseases is discussed in the chapter dealing with non-Hodgkin's lymphomas (see Chapter 16).

Metastatic Tumors. The small intestine may be involved by malignant tumors that originate in adjacent organs and secondarily invade the intestine (see Table 29–4). Extension into the small intestine can produce symptoms of intestinal obstruction or hemorrhage, compression, displacement, or ulceration of the small intestine.

The small intestine may also be involved by metastases arising from other organs. These include malignant melanoma, as well as carcinomas of the cervix, colon, and lung (de Castro *et al.,* 1957).

REFERENCES

Abe, M.; Takahashi, M.; and Yabumoto, E.: Clinical experiences with intraoperative radiotherapy of locally advanced cancers. *Cancer,* **45**:40–48, 1980.

de Castro, C. A.; Dockerty, M. B.; and Mays, C. W.: Metastatic tumors of the small intestine. *Surg. Gynecol. Obstet.,* **105**:159–165, 1957.

Cutler, S. J., and Young, J.: Third National Cancer Survey: Incidence data. *Natl. Cancer Inst. Monogr.,* **41**:1–454, 1975.

Darling, R. C., and Welch, C. E: Tumors of the small intestine. *N. Engl. J. Med.,* **260**:397–408, 1959.

Dawson, I. M. P.; Cornes, J. S.; and Morson, B. C.: Primary malignant lymphoid tumor of the intestinal tract. *Br. J. Surg.,* **47**:80–89, 1981.

Dozois, R. R.; Judd, E. S.; and Dahlin, D. C.: The Peutz-Jeghers syndrome: Is there a predisposition to the development of intestinal malignancy? *Arch. Surg.,* **98**:509–515, 1969.

Fielding, J. R.; Prior, P.; Waterhouse, J. A.; and Cooke, W. T.: Malignancy in Crohn's disease. *Scand. J. Gastroenterol.,* **7**:3–7 1972.

Golden, T., and Stout, A. P.: Smooth muscle tumors of the gastrointestinal tract and retroperitoneal tissues. *Surg. Gynecol. Obstet.,* **73**:784–792, 1941.

Gottlieb, J. A.: Proceedings: Combination chemotherapy of metastatic sarcoma. *Cancer Chemother. Rep.,* **58**:265–270, 1974.

Harris, O. D.; Cooke, W. T.; and Thompson, H.: Malignancy in adult celiac disease and idiopathic steatorrhea. *Am. J. Med.,* **42**:899, 1967.

Herbsman, H.; Wetstein, L.; Rosen, Y.; Orces, H.; Alfonso, A. E.; Iyer, S. K.; and Gardner, B.: Tumors of the small intestine. *Curr. Probl. Surg.,* **17**:3, 1980.

Hoensch, H. P.; Steinhardt, H. J.; and Malchow, H.: Metabolism of xenobiotics in human small intestinal mucosa: Relationship to carcinogenic factors. In Malt, R. A., and Williamson, R. C. (eds.): *Colonic Carcinogenesis.* MTP Press, Lancaster, 1982.

Holmes, G. K. T.; Stokes, P. L.; Sorahan, T. M.; Prior, P.; Waterhouse, J. A. H.; and Cooke, W. T.: Coeliac disease, gluten-free diet and malignancy. *Gut,* **17**:612–619, 1976.

Khojasteh, A.; Haghshenass, M.; and Haghighi, P.: Immunoproliferative small intestinal disease, A "Third-World lesion." *N. Engl. J. Med.,* **33**:1401–1405, 1983.

Kreuning, J.; Bosman, F. T.; Kuiper, G.; Wal, A. M.; and Lindeman, J.: Gastric and duodenal mucosa in "healthy" individuals. An endoscopic and histopathological study of 50 volunteers. *J. Clin. Pathol.,* **31**:69–77, 1978.

Lightdale, C. J.; Koepsell, T. C.; and Sherlock, P.: Small intestinal cancer. In Schottenfeld, D., and Fraumeni, J. (eds.): *Cancer: Epidemiology and Prevention.* W. B. Saunders Company, Philadelphia, 1982.

Loehr, W. J.; Mujahed, Z.; and Zahn, F. D.: Primary lymphoma of the gastrointestinal tract. A review of 100 cases. *Ann. Surg.,* **170**:232–238, 1969.

Lowenfels, A. B.: Why are small bowel tumors so rare? *Lancet,* **1**:24, 1973.

Marshak, R. H., and Lindner, A. E.: *Radiology of the Small Intestine.* W. B. Saunders Company, Philadelphia, 1970.

Maurer, H. S.; Gotoff, S. P.; Allen, L.; and Bolan, J.: Malignant lymphoma of the small intestine in multiple family members: Association with an immunologic deficiency. *Cancer,* **37**:2224–2231, 1976.

McGovern, V. J.: Lymphomas of the gastrointestinal tract. In Yardley, J. H.; Morson, B. C.; and Abell, M. R. (eds.): *The Gastrointestinal Tract.* The Williams and Wilkins, Company, Baltimore, 1977.

Mestel, A. L.: Lymphosarcoma of the small intestine in infancy and childhood. *Ann. Surg.,* **149**:87–94, 1959.

Nakase, A.; Matsumoto, Y.; and Uchida, K.: Surgical treatment of cancer of the pancreas and the periampullary region. Cumulative results in 57 institutions in Japan. *Ann. Surg.,* **185**:52–57, 1977.

Novis, B. H.; Gank, S.; Marks, I. N.; and Selzer, G.: Abdominal lymphoma presenting with malabsorption. *Q. J. Med.,* **40**:521, 1971.

Ostermiller, W.; Joergenson, E. J.; and Weibel, L.: A clinical review of tumors of the small bowel. *Am. J. Surg.,* **111**:403–409, 1966.

Ramot, B., and Many, A.: Primary intestinal lymphoma: Clinical manifestations and possible effect of environmental factors. Recent results. *Cancer Res.,* **39**:193–199, 1972.

del Regato, J. A., and Spjut, H. J.: *Ackerman and del Regato's Cancer: Diagnosis, Treatment and Prognosis,* 5th ed. The C. V. Mosby Company, St. Louis, 1977.

Rosenberg, S. A.; Diamond, H. D.; Jaslowitz, B.; and Crover, L. F.: Lymphosarcoma: A review of 1269 cases. *Medicine, (Baltimore),* **40**:31, 1961.

Salem, P. A., Nassar, V. H., Shahid, M. J., and Hajj, A. A.: "Mediterranean abdominal lymphoma" or immunoproliferative small intestinal disease. Part I: Clinical aspects. *Cancer,* **40**:2941, 1977.

Schnur, P. L., and David, P. Q.: Adenocarcinoma of the duodenum and the Gardner's syndrome. *J.A.M.A.,* **223**:1229–1232, 1973.

Seligman, M., and Rambaud, J. C.: The digestive form of the alpha chain disease. In Lipkin, M., and Good, R. A. (eds.): *Gastrointestinal Tract Cancer.* Plenum Publishing Corporation, New York 1978.

Shulten, M. D.; Oyasu, R.; and Beal, J. M.: Villous adenoma of the duodenum: A case report and review of the literature. *Am. J. Surg.,* **132**:90–96, 1976.

Silberman, H.; Crichlow, R. W.; and Caplan, H. S.: Neoplasms of the small bowel. *Ann. Surg.,* **180**:157–161, 1974.

Spira, I. A.; Ghazi, A.; and Wolff, W.I.: Primary adenocarcinoma of the duodenum. *Cancer,* **39**:1721–1727, 1977.

Starr, G. F., and Dockerty, M. B.: Leiomyomas and leiomyosarcomas of small intestine. *Cancer,* **8**:101–106, 1955.

Steinberg, L. S., and Shieber, W.: Villous adenoma of the small intestine. *Surgery,* **71**:423–430, 1971.

Traube, J.; Simpson, S.; Riddell, R.; Levin, B.; and Kirsner, J. B.: Crohn's disease and adenocarcinoma of the bowel. *Dig. Dis. Sci.,* **25**:939–944, 1980.

Warren, K. W.; Choe, D. S.; and Plaza, J.: Results of radical resection for periampullary cancer. *Ann. Surg.,* **181**:534–540, 1975.

Wilson, J. M.; Melvin, D. B.; and Gray, G. F.: Primary malignancies of the small bowel: A report of 96 cases and review of the literature. *Ann. Surg.,* **180**:175–179, 1974.

Yao, T.; Iida, M.; Ohsato, K.; and Watanabe, H.: Duodenal lesions in familial polyposis of the colon. *Gastroenterology,* **73**:1086–1092, 1979.

Yonemoto, R. H.; Slayback, J. B.; and Byron, R. L.: Familial polyposis of the entire gastrointestinal tract. *Arch. Surg.,* **99**:427–434, 1969.

30

Neoplasms of the Colon

PHILIP S. SCHEIN and BERNARD LEVIN

Incidence and Epidemiology

Carcinoma of the large bowel ranks second to lung cancer in incidence (excluding skin cancer) in the United States. During the year 1985 an estimated 138,000 new cases will be diagnosed, 96,000 arising in the colon and 44,000 in the rectum. Colon cancer in women has a slightly higher frequency compared to that in men, while the reverse is true for rectal cancer. The average age at diagnosis is 60 years, but the disease has been described as early as the second decade of life. Currently, colorectal cancer causes approximately 60,000 deaths per year in the United States, accounting for 13.5% of cancer-related mortality (American Cancer Society, 1985).

This neoplasm demonstrates a marked geographic difference in incidence (see Table 30-1). It is uncommon in southwest Asia and equatorial Africa, but has a high incidence throughout northwestern Europe, the United States, and Canada (Waterhouse, *et al.*, 1976). Colorectal cancers display regional differences within the United States with the highest incidence in the Northeast. Incidence is generally high in countries with high income and high education levels (Blot *et al.*, 1976).

Epidemiologic studies, particularly of migrants, provide strong support for an environmental or dietary etiology. In general, migrants to a geographic region assume the colonic cancer risk of that area. As examples, the mortality rate of colorectal cancer in Japanese immigrants to the United States is three to four times greater than that of Japanese in Japan (Haenzel, *et al.*, 1973). The mortality rate of colon cancer among Puerto Ricans in New York City is higher than in individuals remaining in Puerto Rico (Sherlock, *et al.*, 1975). Cancer of the colon in the black population of the United States has shown increased mortality and now approximates that found in whites. This contrasts with the extremely low incidence of colorectal cancer found among blacks in West Africa (Walker and Burkitt, 1976). According to many investigators, dietary fat intake is significantly lower in Japan and in Puerto Rico when compared to that in the United States, which may be of major etiologic significance. Further support for a dietary influence, as well as for general living habits in the development of colorectal cancer, is derived from studies of Seventh-Day Adventists. They consume little or no meat and less fat than other groups of Americans and have a relatively low rate of colon cancer (Phillips, 1975).

Etiology

Animal models provide ample evidence that colorectal neoplasms can be induced with chemical carcinogens (Reddy, 1976). The finding that the plant product cycasin caused colon cancer in rats led to the identification of related carcinogens, including 1,2-dimethylhydrazine (DMH), azoxymethane, and methylazomethanol. The intrarectal administration of direct-acting N-nitroso alkylating agents, such as N-methyl-N-nitro-N-nitrosoguanidine (MNNG), produced tumors in rats. Lastly, the administration of 3-methyl-4-aminobiphenyl derivatives also induced colon cancer in this species.

Animal models have been used to examine the potential contributing role of diet and environmental factors. Several studies implicated bile acids in promoting colon carcinogenesis. Cholestyramine, a nonabsorbable resin that

Table 30-1. Incidence of Colorectal Cancer (per 100,000 Male Population) in Selected Countries and Regions

	COLON	RECTUM
Connecticut	30.1	18.2
San Francisco Area		
White	28.3	15.2
Black	24.0	10.8
Chinese	23.5	19.5
New Mexico		
White	23.3	12.1
American Indian	1.7	4.9
Canada (British Columbia)	24.1	10.5
Hawaii		
Japanese	22.4	16.3
Chinese	28.7	20.4
Caucasian	23.9	13.5
Filipino	16.8	14.5
Hawaiian	14.1	9.4
New Zealand		
Non-Maori	23.0	15.4
Maori	7.4	4.6
Singapore		
Chinese	11.9	10.0
Malay	3.4	4.7
Warsaw, Poland	10.9	7.7
Nigeria	1.3	1.2

Data from Waterhouse, J.; Muir, C.; Correa, P.; and Powell, J.: *Cancer Incidence in Five Continents,* Vol. 3. International Agency for Research on Cancer, Lyon, 1976; and Stemmerman, G. N.; Nomura, A. M. Y.; Mower, H.; and Glober, G.: Clues (true or false) to the origin of colorectal cancer. In DeCosse, J. J. (ed.): *Large Bowel Cancer.* Churchill Livingstone, Inc., New York, 1981.

increases bile salt excretion, fed to rats enhanced azomethane-induced colon tumors (Nigro *et al.,* 1973). A similar potentiation was observed by surgically diverting bile to the mid-small intestine (Chomchal *et al.,* 1974). This has possible implications for patients undergoing cholecystectomy, as will be described subsequently. Direct evidence that bile acids function as tumor-promoters comes from the studies of Narisawa and Reddy. Rats administered secondary bile acids (taurodeoxycholic acid and lithocholic acid) rectally with MNNG showed an increased number of adenomas, whereas the bile acids themselves did not induce any tumors (Narisawa *et al.,* 1974). Deoxycholic acid increased the numbers of MNNG-induced colon cancers in germ-free rats (Reddy *et al.,* 1976). High-fat diets have similarly increased the number of carcinogen-induced colonic tumors in rats (Reddy, 1976). One proposition is that a high level of fecal bile acids is excreted in this diet, as well as cholesterol metabolites, which may serve as cocarcinogens. Colonic bacterial flora, particularly anaerobic species, have also been implicated by studies in which a marked reduction in car-

cinogen-induced tumors occurred in germ-free or antibiotic-treated rats.

Clinical studies have identified several possible etiologic correlates for colorectal cancer, including the fiber and fat content in diet, as well as the type of colonic bacterial flora. The data have, in specific instances, conflicted, so that definitive conclusions cannot be derived.

Fiber. Burkitt attempted to implicate the Western diet as a major risk factor for this tumor (Walker and Burkitt, 1976). The bowel habits of black African populations was compared to that of those in Western society. In the former group, an increased frequency of defecation, a higher volume of feces voided, a shorter transit time, and a general softer consistency of the stool were reported. In these black Africans the colonic mucosa may be exposed to a fecal carcinogen for a shorter time, and the anaerobic composition of the bowel bacterial flora may differ. Burkitt suggested that the geographic differences in bowel behavior could be related to the increased fiber content of the "low-risk" African diet, compared to the refined sugars and food products in the United States and Great Britain. Other epidemiologic analyses have supported this work. The dietary intake of the low-risk population of Kuopio, Finland, was compared to that of Copenhagen, which had a fourfold greater incidence of colon cancer. The estimated consumption of fat was similar, whereas dietary fiber was higher in Kuopio. A case control study in Israel reported a significantly lower consumption of fiber-rich foods among patients with colon cancer than either hospital or neighborhood controls. No such differences were noted for patients with rectal cancer (Modan, 1977).

Dietary fiber is that part of plant material that resists digestion in the human gastrointestinal tract (Trowell, 1972). It consists of cellulose, hemicellulose, lignin, and pectin, the amounts varying with the type of plant. Many studies have failed to take into account all components of dietary fiber intake. Bingham *et al.* (1979) calculated the average fiber intake by populations in different regions of Britain. They found no significant correlation between total fiber intake and corresponding mortality rates for colon and rectal cancers. The intake of the pentosan fraction of total dietary fiber and of vegetables, other than potatoes, was inversely correlated with mortality from colon cancer. Although placing into doubt the protective role of dietary fiber, these findings suggest that the specific components of fiber rather than crude or total fiber must be studied in investigations of large bowel cancer.

An association of bowel transit time with the risk of colorectal cancer in age- and sex-matched Hawaiian and indigenous Japanese, and Hawaiian caucasians was not confirmed (Glober et al., 1977). The transit time of Hawaiian caucasians was similar to that of indigenous Japanese, in spite of the lower incidence of colorectal cancer in the latter population. Jensen and MacLennan (1979) also were unable to confirm an association between bowel cancer and transit time in Finland and Denmark.

Fat. That the diets of high-risk populations have a greater proportion of fat than those of low-risk populations is generally accepted (Wynder and Reddy, 1977). A high-fat diet was also implicated by case control studies that show a positive association between colorectal cancer and beef intake (Haenzel et al., 1973). Armstrong and Doll (1975) similarly found a strong correlation between dietary meat and fat with incidence and death rate of colorectal cancer. Beef is estimated to contribute 42% of the total fat calories in our population (Reddy, 1976).

A high-fat diet is associated with an increased concentration of fecal bile acids and cholesterol metabolites, as well as of anaerobic bacteria, particularly the nuclear dehydrogenating Clostridia (Hill et al., 1971; Reddy et al., 1978). In controlled studies comparing a high-meat, high-fat Western diet with a no-meat, low-fat diet, the former resulted in a higher level of fecal secondary bile acids and cholesterol metabolites, and increased fecal glucuronidase activity (Reddy, 1976). The fecal constituents of patients with colon cancer, polyps, and ulcerative colitis were also found to have a greater concentration of secondary (microbially derived) bile acids and cholesterol metabolites (Reddy, 1976; Reddy et al., 1978). The activity of fecal bacterial 7-α-dehydroxylase, which converts primary bile acids to their putative carcinogen-promoting secondary forms, was also higher. In contrast, the fecal neutral steroid and bile acid concentrations in patients with familial polyposis were not different from that of controls.

Persons who have had a cholecystectomy have an increased production and turnover of secondary bile acids, primarily deoxycholic acid (Pomare and Heaton, 1973). An association between prior cholecystectomy and increased risk for colon cancer, particularly within the cecum and ascending colon, was reported (Vernick et al., 1980). A more recent study failed to confirm this association (Blanco et al., 1984). The bile salts and neutral steroids are of particular interest because of their steric similarity to the carcinogenic polycyclic aromatic hydrocarbons (Schottenfeld and Winawer, 1982).

Countries with high rates of colorectal cancer also have high rates of atherosclerotic cardiovascular disease. Finland, with a high incidence of coronary heart disease (CHD) and low rates of colorectal cancer, is an exception to this pattern, which may be explained by a high dietary fiber consumption (Waterhouse et al., 1976). In other exceptions, Hawaiians with the highest CHD mortality rates and Filipinos with the most rapid rise in CHD rates have a low risk of colorectal cancer, whereas Chinese with a low CHD risk have the highest incidence of colorectal cancer. The serum cholesterol levels in men who died from CHD and from colorectal cancer in the longitudinal Japan Hawaii Cancer Study differed significantly. The mean cholesterol level was higher in men who died of CHD than among the control group, but those who died of colon cancer had lower blood cholesterol levels than the controls (Stemmerman et al., 1981). A similar finding has been reported from the Framingham Study, where Williams et al. (1981) identified a cohort of men who had relatively low serum cholesterol, therefore a presumably low risk for coronary heart disease, who developed colon cancer. This relationship did not apply to colon cancer in women nor to breast cancer. Weisburger et al. (1982) postulated that these men may have had an extremely effective hepatic conversion of cholesterol to bile acids.

Bacteria. Bacteria comprise about 40% of the fecal mass and humans may have up to 400 species of bacteria in the intestine. Factors such as the composition of the diet, for example, high beef intake, may alter fecal composition. Studies have compared the fecal flora of high- and low-risk populations, including comparisons of Seventh-Day Adventists with nonvegetarian controls, Japanese-Americans on Western and traditional Japanese diets, Hong Kong Chinese at different levels of income, students on meat-free and high-beef diets, elemental diets, diets with different amounts of fat, as well as the fecal bacterial composition of patients with large bowel cancer and nonhereditary large bowel adenomas. The results of these studies have not been consistent and none have succeeded in linking a specific bacterium with colorectal carcinoma (Stemmerman *et al.*, 1981). Although a bacterial role in colonic carcinogenesis is entirely possible, bacterial screens may be incapable of discovering it.

Another approach studied the effect of diet on fecal bacterial enzymes, in particular beta-glucuronidase, nitrosoreductase, and azoreductase, attempting to identify differences in relationship to cancer risk. These bacterial enzymes may be involved in the metabolism of procarcinogens to proximal carcinogens (Mastromarino *et al.*, 1976). A correlation was demonstrated between increased bacterial enzyme activity and diets high in animal protein and fat (Goldin *et al.*, 1981).

Recent evidence suggests that tests for fecal mutagens, such as the Ames assay, may detect important differences between high- and low-risk groups. For example, mutagens for *Salmonella typhimurium*, TA 98, were more common in high-risk Hawaiian-Japanese than in low-risk indigenous Japanese. Transnitrosoase activity was also greater in the feces of Hawaiian-Japanese compared to indigenous Japanese; this enzyme is capable of transferring the nitroso group to an amide acceptor, producing a direct-acting mutagen (Mower *et al.*, 1979).

Although a dogmatic recommendation of dietary measures to prevent cancer may not be possible, a diet low in animal fat and with an ample fiber content is prudent.

Chemopreventive Agents

The possible development of chemopreventive agents that might inhibit or reverse one or more of the recognized stages of carcinogenesis has received increasing interest. Animal models have provided provocative data for a diverse group of preventive agents, such as ascorbic acid, alpha-tocopherol, sodium selenite, and butylated hydroxyanisole (DeCosse, 1982; Wattenberg, 1978).

Selenium effectively inhibits carcinogen-induced tumors in rodents (Jacobs *et al.*, 1977). Selenium may decrease the activity of hydroxylating enzymes that activate procarcinogens, as well as increase the activity of a detoxifying enzyme, glucuronyl transferase. Selenium is a constituent of the enzyme glutathione peroxidase and thereby participates in destroying hydroperoxides and lipoperoxides, thus protecting cells against free radicals.

Jansson *et al.*, (1978) compared cancer mortality rates in the northeastern United States with the corresponding levels of selenium in the water supply. They reported an inverse correlation between mortality from colorectal cancer and selenium levels in the drinking water.

The flavones and indoles are two groups of naturally occurring inducers of increased microsomal mono-oxygenase activity. This microsomal system inactivates such carcinogens as benzopyrene, dimethylbenzanthracene, bracken fern, and aflatoxin. Indole-3 acetonitrile is present in the cruciferous vegetables such as brussels sprouts, cabbage, cauliflower, and broccoli. Graham *et al.* (1978) reported an inverse relationship between the consumption of such vegetables and the relative risk of cancer of the colon.

Bussey *et al.* (1982) reported results of a randomized double-blind trial of ascorbic acid in patients with polyposis coli who had undergone ileorectal anastomosis. The hypothesis was that blocking excessive degradation of fecal steroids by ascorbic acid would inhibit carcinogenesis. They observed a transient reduction in polyp area, as well as a suppression of thymidine uptake by rectal epithelial cells in those patients who received ascorbic acid. These preliminary results regarding the possible protective role of selenium and ascorbic acid, an antioxidant, require further evaluation and confirmation.

Risk Factors (See Table 30-2)

Age Greater than 40 Years. The incidence of colon cancer rises steadily from the age of 40 years in both men and women, doubling every five years to the age of 80 years. Data from the Third National Cancer Survey (U.S.A.) demonstrate that age-specific incidence rates for black and white men and women were similar for colon cancer, particularly from ages 30 to 65. Rectal cancer incidence rates increase slowly after age 70 and decline after 85 years (Schottenfeld and Winawer, 1982).

Inflammatory Bowel Disease. *Ulcerative colitis.* The risk of a patient with a long history of ulcerative colitis developing carcinoma of the large intestine is approximately ten

Table 30-2. Individuals with an Increased Risk for Colorectal Cancer

Environmental (persons over 40 in Western societies)
Familial polyposis syndromes
   Inherited adenomatosis of colon and rectum
   Gardner syndrome
   Turcot syndrome
   Peutz-Jeghers syndrome
Familial cancer syndrome
   Hereditary adenocarcinomatosis
Family history: colon cancer or sporadic colorectal adenomas
Personal history of sporadic colorectal adenomas, colon or rectal cancer, breast or endometrial cancer
Inflammatory bowel disease
   Chronic ulcerative colitis
   Crohn's disease
   Radiation proctocolitis
   Schistosomiasis
   Lymphogranuloma inguinale

times that expected in the general population. The cumulative risk of colorectal cancer during the first ten years after the onset of symptoms is estimated to be 0 to 3%. The probability of colorectal carcinoma increases to 12 to 15% after 20 years and to 50% after 30 years (Leonard-Jones et al., 1977). This highly predisposed group consists of those patients with total or extensive colitis, especially with an early age of onset. Patients with predominantly left-sided disease and long duration of illness are, however, also at increased risk, estimated to be approximately eight times an age- and sex-matched control population (Greenstein et al., 1979). Dysplastic changes in the mucosa increased the probability of developing or having colorectal cancer to 50% in some series. The clinical pathologic features of large bowel cancer arising in the setting of ulcerative colitis include a higher frequency of right and transverse colonic tumors, multicentricity, and undifferentiated and scirrhous histology.

Crohn's Disease. Patients with Crohn's disease of the large bowel with onset before age 21 have a greater risk of developing colorectal cancer than the general population (Weedon et al., 1973). A recent study, not restricted to those whose colitis began under 21 years of age, in which the mean duration of illness was 11 years, found the incidence of colorectal cancer to be about seven times that of age- and sex-matched controls (Greenstein et al., 1981). In both the small and large bowel, the risk of cancer is associated with fistulous disease and bypassed segments (Traube et al., 1980).

History of Colorectal Adenomas. Individuals with a history of colorectal adenomas ap-

pear to have an increased incidence of colorectal cancer. Whereas the incidence of adenomas in the general population is about 5%, 23% of patients with a single colon cancer have associated adenomas (Copeland et al., 1968). There is a 20 to 50% chance of having a second adenoma at the time of the initial diagnosis (synchronous lesion) and approximately a 20 to 30% chance of having a subsequent (metachronous) adenoma. In patients with a second primary large bowel cancer, 50% of synchronous and 60% of metachronous cancers were associated with adenomas (Rider et al., 1959). Overall, these data support the adenoma-carcinoma sequence presented subsequently in this chapter.

History of Colorectal Cancer. In persons with a history of colorectal cancer, the annual incidence of subsequent primary cancer of the large bowel is approximately threefold over that expected in the general population, namely, approximately 3.5 per 1000 patients (Schottenfeld et al., 1969). Overall, there is a 3 to 5% risk for a metachronous tumor.

Association with Other Primary Cancers. Women with colorectal cancers are at increased risk of developing independent primary carcinomas of the breast, uterus, and ovary (Schottenfeld and Winawer, 1982).

Familial Polyposis Syndromes (See Table 30-3). Adenomatosis coli is defined as the condition in which more than 100 adenomas are detected in the large bowel, regardless of familial occurrence. The condition with less than 100 adenomas is termed multiple adenomas. Adenomatosis coli may be subdivided into three groups by the presence and type of extracolonic lesions: simple type (familial polyposis coli), Gardner syndrome, both with

Table 30-3. Classification of Hereditary Gastrointestinal Polyposis

Neoplastic	Adenomatosis of the colon
	Familial polyposis*
	Gardner syndrome
	Turcot syndrome
Hamartomatous	Peutz-Jeghers syndrome†
	Juvenile polyposis of the colon†
	Inflammatory polyposis
	Benign lymphoid hyperplasia
Unclassified polyposis	Metaplastic polyposis
	Cronkite-Canada syndrome

Modified from Utsonomiya, J.; Iwana, T.; and Hirayama, R.: Familial large bowel cancer. In DeCosse, J. J. (ed.): *Large Bowel Cancer.* Churchill Livingstone, Inc., New York, 1981.
* Very high risk of cancer of the large bowel
† Slightly increased risk of cancer of the large bowel

an autosomal dominant form of inheritance, and the Turcot syndrome, a rare syndrome characterized by autosomal recessive inheritance and gastrointestinal polyposis and central nervous system tumors.

The course of adenomatosis coli can be divided into three stages: latent, adenoma, and cancer (Utsonomiya *et al.*, 1981). Half of affected individuals acquire adenomas by late adolescence, and 90% by age 25. In men, the risk for large bowel cancer was 1% by 11 years, 50% by 27 years, and 90% by 43 years of age. In women, the risk for large bowel cancer was 1% by 13 years of age, 50% by 25 years of age, and 90% by 40 years of age. Adenomas of the stomach and duodenum occur in up to 100% in some series, particularly Japan (Utsonomiya *et al.*, 1981).

About 15% of families with a polyposis syndrome will show one or more of the features of the Gardner syndrome. These include desmoid tumors, sebaceous cysts, fibromas, and facial bone osteomas (Gardner, 1962). In addition to large bowel cancer, these patients develop adenomas and adenocarcinomas in the periampullary area.

An autosomal recessive form of inheritance operates in the Turcot syndrome. The manifestations occur at a younger age, with a smaller number of colonic adenomas of larger size and neoplasms of the central nervous system (Turcot *et al.*, 1959).

The incidence of cancer in Peutz-Jeghers syndrome is considerably less than in adenomatosis coli. Multiple hamartomas throughout the gastrointestinal tract are associated with melanin deposition in the buccal mucosa, lips, and other mucocutaneous junctions.

Family History of Large Bowel Cancer. Large bowel cancer in first-degree relatives of a proband with large bowel cancer was increased in several series (Macklin, 1966). The risk is estimated at three or four times the general population. Characteristically, cancers in these patients tended to be located more proximally (Anderson and Romsdahl, 1977) and to appear at an earlier age (Moertel *et al.*, 1958). Whether this represents an inherited predisposition or shared environmental factors is not known.

HEREDITARY COLORECTAL CANCER. This syndrome is characterized by autosomal dominant inheritance, a low mean age (41 years) for the occurrence of colon cancer, and a marked increase in the proximal distribution of cancer. Lynch *et al.* (1977) found 65% of large bowel cancer in the proximal colon (above the sigmoid), whereas only 35% occurred in this portion of the colon in a control population.

CANCER FAMILY SYNDROME. The criteria diagnosing the cancer family syndrome are: (1) an increased incidence of adenocarcinoma, primarily in the colon and endometrium; (2) an increased incidence of multiple primary malignant neoplasms; and (3) early stage of onset and autosomal dominant inheritance. The genetic nature of this syndrome has been confirmed in studies of twins and by HLA typing. Genetic counseling and early detection measures are important here.

Occupational Exposure. Colorectal cancer is generally not viewed as an occupational disease, but some associations are worth noting (Schottenfeld and Winawer, 1982). Groups at increased risk may include individuals involved in metal work, yarn or textiles, and leather goods. The chemical exposures among the metal workers may have included chlorinated cutting oils and cleansing solvents. Acrylonitrile, a substance used in the production of plastics, synthetic rubber, and fibers, was implicated in an excess rate of colonic cancer in textile workers. Epidemiologic studies of woodshop workers have suggested an increased incidence of colon cancer.

Pathology and Patterns of Spread (See Table 30–4)

Embryology and Function. Despite its structural continuity, the colon is anatomically and physiologically composed of separate and distinct halves (Woolley, 1976). In early embryonic life the primitive gut, or archenteron, divides into foregut, midgut, and hindgut. The primitive midgut subsequently gives rise to that portion of the bowel lying between the middescending segment of the duodenum and the midtransverse segment of the colon (Haubrich, 1963). Thus, the right half of the adult colon, up to the middle of the transverse colon, develops embryologically with the small intestine and derives its vascular supply from the superior mesenteric artery. The transverse and sigmoid regions are suspended on a mesentery, absent in the remaining segments of the large bowel. In addition, the rectum lacks a serosal covering, as do the attachment sites of the other portions of the bowel that do not have a freely moving mesentery. Beyond the midtransverse segment, the left

Table 30-4. Patterns of Spread of Colorectal Cancer

Local Routes
    Circularly within bowel wall
    Parallel to bowel wall
    Perpendicular to bowel wall
    Perineural adjacent organs or strictures
Rectal Cancer
    Lymphatic extension
    Perirectal tissue nodes → superior hemorrhoidal vessels
    Aberrant lymphatic vessels → inferior mesenteric artery
    Retrograde lymphatic metastases
Colonic Cancer
    Lymphatic extension → adjacent lymph nodes → distant nodes
Hematogenous Metastases
    Colon to liver → lung
    Rectal to liver
    Rectal to lung
    Rectal to Batson's vertebral venous plexes → vertebral column
Implantation
    Incision
    Anastomotic
    Intrapelvic
    Intraperitoneal

colon and rectum develop from the primitive hindgut; the former is supplied by the inferior mesenteric artery, whereas the rectum is fed by three hemorrhoidal arteries. The upper third of the rectum, between 10 and 15 cm from the anal verge, is supplied by the superior hemorrhoidal artery, which is a branch of the inferior mesenteric artery. The middle and lower thirds of the rectum are supplied by the middle and inferior hemorrhoidal arteries, which are branches of the internal iliac artery. The middle third, which begins at 10 to 12 cm from the anal verge, is defined by the right middle valve of Houston, a landmark for the peritoneal reflection. The lymphatic drainage of the large bowel follows the major arterial system of that region. As a practical consideration, the lymphatic drainage of tumors of the upper third of the rectum travels with the inferior mesenteric artery to its insertion into the aorta at the level of the second lumbar vertebrae. This is important not only for the extent of lymph node dissection required, but also in the design of pre- or postoperative radiation fields. Apart from developmental considerations, the right and left limbs of the colon are anatomically distinguishable. The right side is the larger, having a lumen two to two and one-half times that of the left, and its wall musculature is thinner, making it more compliant and distensible.

Physiologically, the colon is a bifunctional organ that both absorbs water and electrolytes coming from the small intestine and also stores feces (Sleisenger, 1973). The function of the right colon resembles that of the small intestine, with which it shares its development. Absorption involves net influx of sodium in a process that depends upon aldosterone, with a resulting passive reabsorption of water, associated with a loss of potassium to the stool. Normally there is flux of about 55 mEq Na^+ and 500 mL of water per day, but the full capacity of the colon for reabsorption may be six to eight times higher. By contrast, the left colon absorbs only about 10% of the total colonic water and functions predominantly in a storage capacity. The rectum has little absorptive function. Thus, the normal function of the colon is to convert the proximal fecal stream into a semisolid mass that is stored and excreted distally.

Microscopic and Gross Morphologic Features. The most common cancer of the large bowel is an adenocarcinoma, composed of columnar and cuboidal cells, glandular differentiation, and necrosis. The majority produce mucin, while some may secrete large volumes of extracellular mucin (mucoid type), associated with a poor prognosis (Grinnell, 1950). Young patients with colorectal cancer frequently present with signet ring adenocarcinoma, in which mucin accumulates within the cytoplasm, displacing the nucleus; this histologic presentation carries an ominous prognosis. Lastly, a few tumors may present as a scirrhous carcinoma, typically with undifferentiated histology, early lymph node metastases, and a poor prognosis (Woolam *et al.*, 1965).

The gross morphologic features of adenocarcinoma of the colon and rectum vary and can influence symptomatology. Certain morphologic patterns characterize different anatomic locations within the bowel. In particular, the growth of right colonic adenocarcinoma tends to be polypoid, whereas in the left colon it tends to be infiltrative and constrictive (Astler and Coller, 1954). Thus, a typical lesion of the right colon is an intraluminal polypoid mass that occupies only a portion of the wall circumference and is limited in its intramural invasion (Dukes, 1932; Astler and Coller, 1954; Turnbull *et al.,* 1967); annular constriction of the lumen is infrequent. By contrast, neoplastic lesions of the left colon tend to produce obstruction. The more frequent left colon lesion is nodular, sessile, and commonly undergoes ulceration and necrosis. It produces intramural rather than intraluminal growth, with infiltration and thickening of the bowel wall and resultant narrowing of the lumen. Early extension takes place through the muscularis with extramural invasion of contiguous structures. Scirrhous carcinoma, with a predominance of fibrous tissue, is usually found in the left colon, where it is an annular, circumferential lesion. However, the true scirrhous carcinoma—small, stony hard, annular, and containing a desmoplastic component incited by the neoplastic cells—is uncommon; one series had only 29 examples of scirrhous histology out of 12,000 cases of colorectal cancer (Fahl *et al.,* 1960).

The gross morphology of rectal carcinoma is considerably diverse. The lesions include soft, friable, hemorrhagic, mucinous, and papillary adenocarcinomas. Growth may be sessile or polypoid, with or without ulceration, and transmural extension into surrounding structures can lead to involvement of the bladder, prostate gland, or vagina (Astler and Coller, 1954).

Pathologic Features and Their Influence on Survival. Histologic grading correlates with survival (Copeland *et al.,* 1968). Using the Broder's system, Sanfelippo and Beahrs (1972) reviewed 391 cases at the Mayo Clinic and reported five-year survivals of 56% for grades I and II, and 32% for grades III and IV. Dukes, using his own grading system, reported five-year survivals 77% for "low grade" tumors, of 77.3% for "average grade," and 29% for "high grade" cancers (Dukes and Bussey, 1958).

Although histologic grade is an index of prognosis, it can correlate with nodal metastasis, venous involvement, local extension, and distant metastasis (Brown and Warren, 1938; Dukes and Bussey, 1958). Furthermore, criteria used for grading are subjective and the boundaries between grades are not always distinct (Buckwalter and Kent, 1973).

The prognostic significance of tumor size has been analyzed extensively. The preponderance of evidence suggests that size does not correlate with either the frequency of metastasis or survival (Buckwalter and Kent, 1973). Some tumors may remain small, but disseminate quickly and extensively, while others may grow to great size but remain localized (Spratt and Spjut, 1967).

An important biologic characteristic of colon cancer is its tendency to penetrate perpendicularly through the bowel wall rather than by lateral intramural extension beyond the mucosal edge of the tumor. Lateral extension usually progresses no more than 2 cm and only rarely beyond 4 cm (Black and Waugh, 1948). Intramural lymphatic spread is also unusual beyond 1 to 2 cm (Grinnell, 1966). For these reasons, it is standard surgical practice to leave a 5-cm minimum margin between the tumor and point of resection.

The extent of perpendicular penetration of tumor influences prognosis. When tumor is confined to the mucosa without penetration of the muscularis (Astler-Coller stage A), five-year survival ranges from 74 to 100% (Astler and Coller, 1954; Copeland *et al.,* 1968). Once the tumor penetrates into the muscularis (but not through it—stage B_1), the five-year survival diminishes to approximately 65% (Astler and Coller, 1954). Extension completely through the muscularis into the pericolic or mesenteric fat, the original Dukes' stage B (Astler-Coller stage B_2), further reduces the five-year survival. Figures for this stage vary from 25 to 85%, with most series clustering around 40 to 60% (Gilbertsen, 1967; Copeland *et al.,* 1968; Thomas *et al.,* 1969; Turnbull, 1975). Bowel wall penetration may be a strong independent variable. Among all cases studied with involved regional nodes, extension completely through the muscularis resulted in a survival rate (15%) significantly lower than did extension limited to the muscularis (53%) (Copeland *et al.,* 1968).

As proposed by Dukes and coworkers, nodes become involved in an orderly anatomic progression, and skip metastases are unusual (Gabriel *et al.,* 1935). Caudad spread usually occurs only in the presence of blocked lymphatics (Grinnell, 1966), except in the distal 8 cm of the rectum, where the lymphatic anatomy normally allows lateral and distal spread (Jackman and Beahrs, 1968). Lymphatic invasion is a common occurrence, present in over 50% of cases at the time of surgery (Gilbertsen, 1967). Its presence again further reduces the five-year survival to approximately 30%, ranging from 4 to 60% (Thomas et al., 1969; Stearns and Schottenfeld, 1971; Turnbull, 1975).

Both the number and location of involved nodes have been correlated with prognosis. Copeland demonstrated a progressive decrease in survival with increased number of involved nodes; five-year survival for one involved node was 27%, versus 9% for more than five nodes (Copeland et al., 1968). Dukes analyzed his C cases with lymphatic involvement according to location of nodes: those with only paracolic node involvement showed a 40.9% five-year survival, whereas if involvement extended along the lymphovascular pedicle to the highest point of ligature, there was a 13.6% survival (Dukes and Bussey, 1958).

The reported incidence of nodal involvement may be a function of the method and diligence of the pathologic search. Lymph node involvement may be identified either by gross dissection or, much less commonly, by a technique referred to as clearing. In this method, the entire specimen is treated with agents that render the tissue translucent (Pickren, 1975). The percentage of cases with nodal involvement detected by clearing was increased compared to that detected by gross examination, although whether the cases were truly equivalent is uncertain (Coller et al., 1940). Differences in techniques of detection of involved lymph nodes by pathologists may account for some of the wide variation in survival statistics reported in the literature.

Venous invasion has also been associated with decreased survival (Spratt and Spjut, 1967; Copeland et al., 1968; Khankhanian et al., 1976), but studies correlating this phenomenon with the incidence of visceral metastases have produced conflicting results, in part reflecting varying degrees of diligence in detection. With control for involvement of regional lymph nodes, however, the effect is less dramatic. Dukes showed that of all patients with gross evidence of venous invasion, the subgroup with lymphatic metastases had a five-year survival of 25%, whereas the subgroup without lymph node involvement had a five-

year survival of 64% (Dukes and Bussey, 1958). In addition, in patients with Dukes' B lesions, the presence of vascular invasion did not significantly affect either median tumor-free interval or median survival (Khankhanian et al., 1976). Thus, venous invasion does not appear to be an important independent variable.

Although the lymphatic spread from carcinoma of the intraperitoneal colon follows the lymphovascular supply of the mesentery, lymphatic drainage of the rectum deserves special emphasis. The rectum, particularly the upper third, may drain to the inferior mesenteric nodes via the superior hemorrhoidal vessels. In addition, lesions below 8 cm from the anal verge may drain via the middle hemorrhoidal vessels to the internal iliac nodes, while lesions at or below the pectinate line (3 cm) may drain to the inguinal nodes via the perineal lymphatics (Black and Waugh, 1948; Jackman and Beahrs, 1968). This fact may help to explain the poor prognosis that some investigators have associated with rectal carcinomas. Not only may tumor cells gain ready access to nodes beyond the margins of usual resection because of the shorter distance, but the lack of a serosal layer may permit easier involvement of extrarectal tissues. Stearns and Deddish found a 19% incidence of involvement of middle hemorrhoidal, obturator, and internal iliac nodes in patients with Dukes' C rectal cancer undergoing an extended pelvic lymphadenectomy (Stearns and Deddish, 1959).

Distant metastases occur most commonly in the liver and lung (Table 30–4). Reported incidences of liver metastases at the time of initial surgery vary from 15 to 25%, with autopsy figures as high as 64%. Pulmonary metastases occur as a component of metastatic disease in approximately 20 to 30%. This may present as a solitary nodule, raising the question of a primary lung cancer. The dual venous drainage pattern of the lower rectum, the superior hemorrhoidal vein to the inferior vena cava as well as to the portal system and liver, accounts for the relatively high incidence of early pulmonary metastases with tumors arising from this site. Other sites of spread are bone and brain, with extremely variable incidences among different series, but all generally less than 10%. Between 3.4 and 8.0% of cases have ovarian involvement (Burt, 1960; Deddish, 1960), with carcinomas of the left colon and rectum especially likely to metastasize to this organ.

The Evolution and Prognostic Value of Staging Systems (See Figure 30–1).

A rational therapy for colorectal cancer heavily depends upon an understanding of its natural history. Because of this tumor's general tendency to undergo an orderly progression of local-regional invasion (Dukes, 1932), staging systems can meaningfully describe the extent of anatomic involvement. Such systems correlate prognosis with anatomic stage and furthermore may serve as the foundation for selecting specific therapeutic modalities. They also allow appropriate stratification of patients within clinical trials, so that results accurately reflect the effect of the therapy being evaluated.

Within the framework of anatomic staging, various pathologic features of the disease function either as dependent or independent variables with respect to prognosis. These include histology, extent of penetration through bowel wall, venous invasion, and regional lymph node involvement.

In 1932, after an extensive review of over 2000 rectal carcinoma specimens from the St. Mark's Hospital in London, Dukes developed a simple staging system that correlated the degree of penetration of tumor through the colonic wall and the involvement of regional lymph nodes with prognosis (Dukes, 1932). He proposed the following system of classification: stage A, tumor limited to the wall of the rectum; stage B, spread by direct contiguity to extrarectal tissues; and stage C, involvement of regional lymph nodes. Dukes continued his

observations over 30 years and his work confirms the overall validity of these concepts (Dukes and Bussey, 1958). In 1935 Dukes and coworkers proposed that stage C be further divided according to the location of involved nodes: C_1, involved nodes limited to the paracolic region, and C_2, involved nodes to the highest point of ligature of the lymphovascular pedicle. The five-year survival for C_1 cases was 41% compared to 14% for the C_2 category.

Numerous revisions of the original Dukes staging system (Figure 30–1) have been proposed. The results of surgical adjuvant trials have been reported with a heterogeneity of designations, not always carefully defined, which has made interpretation of the surgical therapy reported in the literature extremely difficult. In 1949 Kirklin and coworkers proposed a modification of the Dukes classification in which they distinguished between involvement into but not through the muscularis (designated B_1) and tumor invasion into and through the serosa (designated B_2). This was not a subdivision of the original Dukes stage B, but rather a subdivision of the original Dukes A into A and B_1. Because of the small number of cases in their A and B_1 groups, Kirklin's data did not demonstrate that penetration into the muscularis had an important influence on prognosis. Several investigators, however, have shown a difference in survival between these stages, as discussed below.

Astler and Coller suggested in 1954 that the Kirklin modification be extended to cases with lymph node involvement. They recognized two groups within stage C: C_1, involvement of

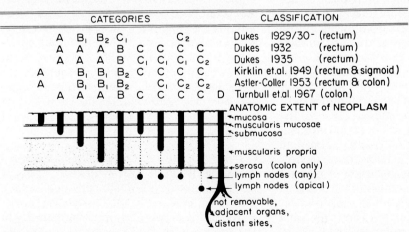

CATEGORIES										CLASSIFICATION
	A	B_1	B_2	C_1			C_2			Dukes 1929/30⁻ (rectum)
	A	A	A	B	C	C	C	C		Dukes 1932 (rectum)
	A	A	A	B	C_1	C_1	C_1	C_2		Dukes 1935 (rectum)
A		B_1	B_1	B_2	C	C	C			Kirklin et.al. 1949 (rectum & sigmoid)
A		B_1	B_1	B_2			C_1	C_2	C_2	Astler-Coller 1953 (rectum & colon)
	A	A	A	B	C	C	C	C	D	Turnbull et.al. 1967 (colon)

Figure 30–1. Evaluation of staging systems for early colorectal cancer. From Donegan W. L., and Decosse, J. J.: Pitfalls and controversies in the staging of colorectal cancer. In Enker, W. E. (ed.) *Cancer of the Colon.* Yearbook Medical Publishers, Chicago, 1978.

regional nodes, plus involvement into but not through the muscularis; and C_2, involvement of regional nodes plus full penetration of the bowel wall. The C_1 category represented only 4% of all cases of early colorectal cancer. In the United States, the Astler-Coller modification is the most widely used.

The Gastrointestinal Tumor Study Group, in designing its adjuvant trials, used a staging system that took into account in prognosis the correlation of Dukes C category with the number of positive lymph nodes (Copeland *et al.,* 1968; Killen *et al.,* 1981; Mittelman *et al.,* 1981). Within these studies, the C_1 designation defines those patients with one to four positive nodes, while C_2 is reserved for those cases with five or more positive nodes.

In 1967 Turnbull and coworkers added another category, stage D, to include cases with adjacent organ invasion, seeding of tumor, and metastases to liver, lung, and bone. This was the first systematic attempt to segregate these cases from the standard Dukes categories, although some authors had distinguished between curative and palliative resections.

ADENOMAS

With the exception of ulcerative colitis, the majority of adenocarcinomas of the large bowel are thought to arise from neoplastic polyps or adenomas.

Prevalence and Distribution

Epidemiologic studies show that adenomas are common, and incidence increases with age in countries with a high or intermediate risk for colorectal cancer. One or more adenomas of the large bowel were present in 58% of men and 47% of women in a survey in the United States (Rickert *et al.,* 1979). Adenomas are uncommon in areas where the incidence of cancer is low; as examples, the prevalence of adenomas varies from almost zero among black South Africans to 10% in Japan and Cali, Colombia (Morson and Day, 1981). The mere presence of adenomas, therefore, does not necessarily convey a high risk, since the propensity for neoplastic transformation is related to size. Only 5% of Japanese adenomas (Muto *et al.,* 1975) and 2% of adenomas in Cali, Colombia (Correa *et al.,* 1972) were greater than 1 cm in diameter. The low incidence of cancer in these two countries can be related to the small number of large adenomas, as well as the total number of adenomas.

Macroscopic and Microscopic Appearances

The classification proposed by the World Health Organization is based on histologic structure and separates adenomas into tubular, villous, and an intermediate tubulovillous type (Morson, 1976).

The typical tubular adenoma is small, spherical, and has a stalk. Its surface is roughly separated into lobules by intercommunicating clefts. In contrast, the villous adenoma may be large and sessile with a velvety surface. Histologically the tubular adenoma consists of closely packed tubular glands that divide and branch. The stalk is formed by normal mucosa and submucosa. In the villous adenoma, fingerlike projections of neoplastic epithelium with a core of normal lamina propria project toward the bowel lumen. The tubulovillous consists of a mixture of tubular and villous adenoma patterns. About 60% of adenomas are tubular, 20 to 30% are tubulovillous, and about 10% are villous (Morson and Day, 1981).

Dysplasia in adenomas may be graded into mild, moderate, or severe. The classification is based on the presence of nuclear changes such as enlargement, pleomorphism, loss of polarity, stratification, and an increase in the number of mitoses. In addition, glandular architectural changes may include irregular budding and a "back-to-back" arrangement. An individual adenoma may exhibit variations in the degree of dysplasia. Severe dysplasia in an adenoma has been described as carcinoma *in situ* but this is an inappropriate term for neoplastic tissue above the level of the muscularis mucosae (Morson and Day, 1981); because of the absence of lymphatics above the level of the muscularis mucosae, such lesions cannot metastasize (Fenoglio *et al.,* 1973).

Development

In the normal adult, the epithelial tissue actively renews itself with a turnover of about three to eight days (McDonald *et al.,* 1964). DNA synthesis is confined to the lower two-thirds of the crypts and occurs principally in the lower one-third. As newly produced cells migrate upward, the probability of entering into a new mitotic cycle declines (Maskens,

1979). The cells eventually become fully mature, desquamate, and die. A variety of modulating factors (neural or hormonal) may modify the dynamics of the epithelial cells and even entire crypts (Tutton and Barkla, 1982).

Using tritiated thymidine, a series of abnormalities were described in the evolution of adenomas. Among these was the presence of immature cells higher up the crypt than normal, associated with unrepressed DNA synthesis, with migration upward from the crypts (Maskens and Deschner, 1971; Deschner 1980). Normally, cell replication and migration are balanced by exfoliation of cells from the mucosal surface. In the adenoma, cell renewal occurs along the surface of the crypt and the entire length of the crypts. DNA-synthesizing cells accumulate on the luminal surface of the mucosa, resulting in an unfolding of the surface epithelium, thus forming new adenomatous tissue.

Neoplastic Potential

Several lines of evidence suggest that adenomas have neoplastic potential. The incidence of coexisting carcinoma and adenoma in the same tumor increases as the tumor size decreases, which may suggest that as cancers increase in size, they destroy the evidence of their origin. In a series of 1961 malignant tumors, Muto *et al.* (1975) found 14% contained varying proportions of adenomatous tissue.

The prevalence of a benign component in carcinomas of the large bowel correlated with their spread through the layers of the bowel wall (Morson, 1966). In tumors confined to the bowel wall, 18% had an adenomatous component, whereas in tumors that had extended into the extramural fat, only 8% showed an adenomatous element (Morson and Day, 1981).

In a study of operative specimens of carcinoma of the colon, one or more adenomas were present in about one-third of patients. In 75% of these, adenomas coexisted with two or more carcinomas, excluding cases of ulcerative colitis and cancer (Morson and Day, 1981).

Epidemiologic evidence from individuals with familial polyposis coli suggests that one or more carcinomas will develop in almost all of those affected if the colon is left in place.

Additional indirect, but persuasive, evidence comes from a 25-year screening study reported by Gilbertsen (1974) from the University of Minnesota Cancer Detection Center. Here, 18,158 patients, 45 years of age or over at the time of initial examination, were followed by annual proctosigmoidoscopy. A total of 103,645 examinations were performed, 85,487 of which consisted of follow-up studies. During this follow-up period, all polyps and adenomas were removed. Eleven adenocarcinomas were found within reach of the sigmoidoscope. Six were confined to the mucosa and four to the mucosa and submucosa, with only one reaching the superficial portion of the muscularis propria. This is in contrast to the 75 to 80 cancers of the distal 25 cm of large bowel predicted to occur in this population.

If carcinomas develop from adenomas, they would be expected to occur in an older age group. Results from cancer detection clinics, where asymptomatic individuals were examined, have shown a difference in average age for adenomas and carcinomas, 50 years versus 58 years, respectively. In familial polyposis coli, carcinomas clearly develop later than the age at which adenomas predominate.

Neoplastic Transformation

Most adenomas do not develop into carcinomas. Considerable evidence suggests that several important factors can be identified in this transition when it occurs:

Size. The neoplastic potential of large adenomas has been shown to be increased compared with small adenomas. In a series of 2489 adenomas from St. Mark's Hospital, those under 1 cm in diameter had a neoplastic rate of 1.3%, those between 1 and 2 cm a rate of 9.5%, whereas with a diameter over 2 cm the rate rose to 46% (Muto *et al.,* 1975).

Histologic Type. The highest malignancy rate is associated with a villous growth pattern. These lesions tend to be larger and exhibit greater cytologic atypia. Invasive neoplasm has been found in 40% of the villous tumors, in less than 5% of the tubular ones, and in 23% of the tubulovillous variety (Muto *et al.,* 1975). In addition, villous lesions may exhibit marked karyotypic abnormalities indicating a further tendency to malignant transformation (Reichmann *et al.,* 1982).

Epithelial dysplasia. The malignant potential of adenomas increases with increasing degrees of dysplasia. Most adenomas smaller than 1 cm usually show only mild dysplasia and have a low malignant potential. With severe dysplasia, the rate of malignant transformation rises to 27% (Morson and Day, 1981).

Practical Aspects of Colon Adenomas

The advent of fiberoptic colonoscopy has facilitated the removal of adenomas throughout the colon. Faced with the resected adenoma containing carcinoma, the gastroenterologist and oncologist must decide upon further management. If the adenoma is totally excised and it has not penetrated the muscularis mucosae, metastases cannot occur. However, once the carcinoma has crossed the muscularis mucosae, the tumor has access to lymphatics. When the infiltrating component is confined to the head of the adenoma, as defined by an imaginary line drawn across the stalk between the points of juncture of adenomatous epithelium with stalk mucosa, metastases are unlikely (Platz, 1978). In deciding whether further surgery is indicated, the oncologist must weigh the operative risks against the possibility that the tumor is already in lymph nodes. The concensus today is that if resection is complete and the carcinoma is well or moderately well differentiated, surgery is not indicated (DeCosse, 1984a,b; Morson *et al.*, 1984).

Tumors that have infiltrated beyond the neck and into the stalk present problems regarding the adequacy of the local excision. Extensive involvement of the stalk, the presence of tumor at the margin of excision, and a poorly differentiated tumor are indications for surgical resection. Approximately 10% of such patients will be found to have nodal metastases (Platz, 1978).

Adenoma Virgule Carcinoma Sequence

In clinical practice, the usual management of colonic polyps is removal, preferably by endoscopic polypectomy. However, observations of a selected group of patients with adenomas who have been followed for varying reasons have confirmed that some adenomas never develop malignant changes. In those that do, the sequence evolves over a long period of time, three to six years, and often as long as 10 to 15 years (Morson and Day, 1981).

Symptoms and Signs

The large bowel is not a homogeneous organ with respect to its normal function, or in the pathologic features of the malignancy that may arise in each anatomic region. This has an important bearing on the constellation of symptoms that tend to characterize tumors of the right colon versus the left colon and rectum (see Table 30–5).

Right Colon. The right colon, including the cecum and ascending portions, is the primary site of large bowel cancer in approximately 15% of cases. The caliber and distensibility of the right colon are sixfold greater than those of the sigmoid region. The tumors arising in the right colon, though large, tend to be soft fungating masses that do not commonly encompass the entire circumference of the bowel. Because of the right colon's functional and pathologic features, tumors are not likely to present with symptoms or signs of obstruction. The possible exceptions are neoplasms that arise in the region immediately adjacent to the ileocecal valve; the resulting symptoms have

Table 30–5. Percentage of Large Bowel Cancer Patients Presenting with Specific Clinical Features Correlated with the Anatomic Location of the Primary Tumor

SERIES	RECTUM					LEFT COLON					RIGHT COLON				
	a	b	c	d	e	a	b	c	d	e	a	b	c	d	e
Abdominal pain	7	24	65	7–26	——	77	77	82	68–82	——	87	65	89	75–90	50†
Bleeding	86	77	80	66–88	77†	46	34	49	49–53	——	9	24	30	8–30	90*
Anemia	——	22	——	——		——	27	——	——	20*	——	76	53	——	50†
Altered bowel habits	79	46	71	69–81		82	56	69	42–82		81	18	54	6–81	
Abdominal mass	——	4.2	0	0		——	33	29	26–46		——	60	69	67–80	43†
Palpable mass on rectal examination	——	66	75	75	80*	——	0	——	——		——	0	——	——	
Obstruction	——	2	7	——		——	28	16	——		——	16	7	——	
Asymptomatic	2	5	——	——		2	0	——	——		3	1	——	——	

References: (a) Swinton *et al.*, 1949; (b) Copeland *et al.*, 1968; (c) Berk and Haubrich, 1963; (d) Moertel, 1973; (e) *De Peyster *et al.*, 1969; †Cattell *et al.*, 1955.

been mistaken for appendicitis in elderly patients. Cecal lesions have presented as appendicitis after obstructing the appendiceal lumen (Sawhney and Kambouris, 1974). Tumors of the right colon are generally insidious in onset. The patient may experience only vague dull abdominal discomfort or colic, which may be misinterpreted as cholecystitis or peptic ulcer. Moreover, by the time the tumor is correctly diagnosed, it may be palpable as an abdominal mass in as many as 75% of cases. Chronic blood loss is a feature of this site of disease. The patient may describe stools that are mahogany red, but all too often the bleeding is diagnosed only by testing for occult blood. For many patients this problem may be sufficiently long-standing to result in symptoms of anemia. Jones and Sleisenger (1973) reported anemia in 65% of patients with tumors of the cecum and ascending colon, and 37% of the anemic patients were symptomatic on that basis. Sawhney and Kambouris (1974) reported that 7% of their patients with cancer of the right colon presented with angina pectoris secondary to anemia.

Left Colon.   Tumors arising in the left colon, including the descending and sigmoid segments, account for approximately 30% of the total. When compared to neoplasms of the right colon, tumors on the left tend to be firm, scirrhous, and circumferential. These factors, coupled with the reduced caliber of the left colon, make acute or chronic symptoms of obstruction an important clinical presentation. Carcinoma is responsible for approximately one-half of acutely obstructed colons, often the initial symptom of the disease. Gius (1948) studied the pathology of the bowel wall in the presence of tumor involvement and noted that luminal stenosis is associated with muscular hypertrophy proximal to the stenosis. He described seven cases of adenocarcinoma of the descending colon and sigmoid that showed moderate to marked thickening of the circular muscle layer and of the longitudinal tineae. Hypertrophic thickening was most marked above the obstruction and increased as the tumor was approached. There was also hypertrophy of the wall below the tumor, albeit to a lesser degree. Such hypertrophy is a compensatory mechanism of the bowel that allows continued function in the presence of partial obstruction. Gius (1948) emphasized that muscular hypertrophy may postpone the onset of obstructive symptoms and delay diagnosis. Presumably, however, an increase in contractility associated with wall thickening may also increase the severity of symptoms once obstruction becomes manifest. Perforation of a diverticulum proximal to a left-sided obstruction may also cause acute onset of pain. More commonly, the clinical manifestations of obstruction are chronic and progressive. The resulting symptoms are protean and include abdominal pain and a change in bowel habits, with constipation at times alternating with diarrhea. The classic description of the pain is that it is aching, cramping or colicky, and present in 60 to 80% of patients (Swinton et al., 1949; Hallstrand, 1954; Cattell et al., 1955). There may be a history of recent need for laxatives or enemas, or decreased caliber of stools. In contrast to the right-sided colonic tumors, bleeding, when present, is more overt, with dark or bright red coating the surface of the stool. The incidence of palpable tumor is less than in the cecum; the literature suggests a range of 25 to 50% of all cases (see Table 30–5).

Rectum.   Carcinomas of the rectum constitute 30% of large bowel tumors, with approximately 75% within the reach of an examining finger. Moertel (1973) has emphasized the need for careful bimanual technique to maximize the yield of digital examination. By massaging the lesion downward with the external hand, neoplasms high in the rectum should be detectable.

The principal symptoms of rectal cancer include bleeding and changes in stool habit. Frequency of stools may increase, accompanied by tenesmus and the urge to defecate in the morning, so-called morning diarrhea. The tumor may produce substantive amounts of mucus, which, if severe, may indicate an underlying large villous adenoma. Because of progressive obstruction of the bowel lumen, the patient may note a decrease in stool caliber. Pain with rectal cancer is regarded as a late and ominous sign since it usually means the tumor has extended into the pararectal tissues and infiltrated nerve trunks. This results in dull, aching perineal or sacral pain that may radiate into the legs. Perineal pain is frequently the first symptom of recurrence of rectal carcinoma. Even in the absence of computed tomographic scan or other objective evidence of relapse, initiation of appropriate antitumor therapy must be considered. Overt bleeding, with red blood coating the stool, is characteristic of rectal cancer with a reported incidence of 65 to 90% (Hallstrand, 1954; Cattell et al.,

1955; Jones and Sleisenger, 1973; Moertel, 1973).

Diagnosis and Screening

The development of screening systems to identify individuals harboring an occult carcinoma or an antecedent premalignant adenoma has received increased interest. The goal is to detect a cancer while asymptomatic, prior to serosal penetration or regional lymph node metastases, with a resultant increase in cure rate with surgery. By the time symptoms initiate diagnostic evaluation, the neoplasm may have already grown to an advanced or incurable stage.

Fecal Occult Blood Test. The development of the guaiac impregnated slide test for the detection of fecal occult blood has stimulated many screening programs for colorectal cancer. In general, these are most successful where attention has been paid to thorough patient education, use of an appropriate red-meat-free diet, and careful follow-up within the health care system.

The technical aspects of performing the test have undergone a number of revisions. A high-fiber, meat-free, low-peroxidase diet is used with six fecal smears prepared over three days. The smear should not be stored but should be tested promptly. Rehydration increases the sensitivity but also the rate of false positivity (Winawer and Sherlock, 1982). The results of current studies are summarized in Table 30–6.

The rate of slide positivity ranges from 1 to 5%, with a predictive value for neoplastic lesions of 20 to 50%. The percentage of patients with positive tests who are ultimately found to have adenomas or cancer increases with the age of the population, ranging from 15% in the age groups of 40 to 49 years to 60% for individuals over 69 years (Winawer and Sherlock,

Table 30–6. Results of Fecal Occult Blood Testing

Patient compliance	
Motivated groups	80%
Unmotivated	15–30
Rate of positive slides	1–5
Predictive value for neoplasia	18–50
Staging of detected cancers	
(Dukes A and B)	60–80
False-positive rate	2
False-negative rate for cancer	9–17
False-negative rate for adenomas	60–75

From Winawer, S. J., and Sherlock, P.: Approach to screening and diagnosis in colorectal cancer. *Semin. Oncol.,* **3:**387–397, 1976.

1982). Approximately one-third of detected neoplastic lesions are carcinomas.

Digital Rectal Examination. Digital rectal examinations should be a part of every screening examination, not only to detect rectal carcinoma, but also prostatic cancer in men. It has several important limitations. The maximum depth of examination is approximately 8 cm. The trend, however, is toward more proximal sites of primary tumors in the large bowel, leading to a decreased yield with this simple procedure.

Sigmoidoscopy. The rectosigmoid can be examined directly by proctosigmoidoscopy. The potential for detecting a substantial number of neoplastic lesions, both adenomas and carcinomas, is high considering the current distribution of more than 50% of these lesions in the most distal 40 cm of bowel. Rigid proctoscopy detects lesions with a high degree of probability in the distal 16 cm of rectosigmoid, but its yield in the range of 16 to 25 cm is less consistent because of technical difficulties. Rigid proctoscopy is not popular among patients and physicians and is generally underused.

Flexible sigmoidoscopy is effective in detecting adenomas and carcinoma of the rectum and sigmoid. With the 65-cm instrument one can visualize about three times the length of bowel viewed with the rigid scope (Winman et al. 1980). A 30-cm instrument recently developed makes this technique to be widely available to primary care physicians after a brief training period. Patient acceptance is much greater than with the rigid instrument.

A double-contrast barium enema should usually be performed prior to fiberoptic colonoscopy because of the small, but definite, false-negative results of colonoscopy, particularly in certain areas: the segments immediately proximal to the hepatic and splenic flexures, the medial aspect of ascending colon, and occasionally the rectosigmoid (see Figure 30–2A, B, C).

In several investigations the double-contrast examination detected an average of 87% of adenomas, compared with 59% detected by the single-contrast method (Gelfand and Ott, 1981). The difference in detection rate was most striking for lesions smaller than 1 cm, of which only one-third were detected by the single-contrast technique. Although the single-contrast has not been compared directly to the double-contrast technique in detecting carcinomas, most radiologists favor the double-

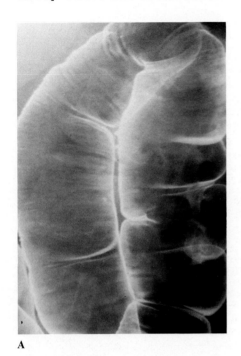

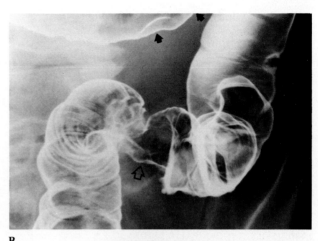

B

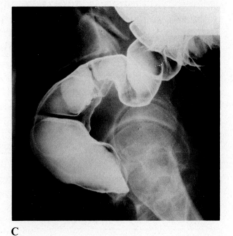

C

Figure 30–2.   Double contrast barium enema. (*A*) Large, pedunculated polyp, in descending colon shown on double contrast barium enema. (*B*) Constricting sigmoid carcinoma (open arrow); serosal metastases from primary sigmoid carcinoma (dark arrows). (*C*) Compression and invasion of rectosigmoid by metastases to pouch of Douglas from primary sigmoid carcinoma.

contrast technique for detecting early neoplasms. Radiologically, advanced colorectal cancers often appear as an annular area of narrowing of the lumen. The transition from normal bowel to neoplasm is usually abrupt and is then referred to as a tumor shelf. Another characteristic appearance is a large polypoid mass formed by intraluminal rather than circumferential growth of the cancer.

Barium enema and colonoscopy are regarded as complementary in that both methods have shortcomings. Colonoscopy may fail to detect a lesion behind a fold or sharply angulated segment of the colon (Miller, 1974). Although colonoscopy can directly view the entire large bowel mucosa, a complete colonoscopy to the cecum can be achieved in only 85 to 90% of patients. The double-contrast barium enema alerts the colonoscopist to the overall anatomy of the colon and the presence of obvious lesions. Both tech-

niques require that the patient be adequately prepared for the study, with appropriate cleansing of the bowel to reduce the incidence of false-negative or -positive examinations.

A biopsy should be routinely performed if colonoscopy detects an obvious carcinoma. Whenever possible, total colonoscopy should follow unless there is an obstructing lesion, since up to 50% of patients may have synchronous adenomas and 1.5 to 5% may have synchronous carcinomas (Winawer, 1981). Adenomas should also be removed for histologic examination.

Plasma Carcinoembryonic Antigen.   This glycoprotein tumor marker is important as a guide to managing colorectal cancer. The preoperative concentration of carcinoembryonic antigen (CEA) had prognostic value, independent of Dukes stage, in some studies. The CEA is the most sensitive and cost-effective test for early detection of recurrent tumor following a complete surgical resection, but a normal level does not completely exclude recurrence. It also has been used to complement standard objective measures for assessing response of overt tumor to chemotherapy and radiotherapy. The utility and limitations of CEA testing are reviewed in detail in the Tumor Markers section of Chapter 6 of this textbook.

Application of Screening Tests. Screening for colorectal cancer should be divided into detection systems directed toward average-risk patients and those addressed to patients with acquired or genetic predispositions (Figures 30–3 and 30–4).

A program of screening for those with an average risk is presented in Figure 30–3. Fecal occult blood testing is done annually and proctosigmoidoscopy, preferably by a flexible method, is performed every three to five years beginning from 40 to 50 years of age. Patients with a history of familial polyposis or Gardner syndrome should have sigmoidoscopy every six months or one year, beginning in early adolescence. Appropriate surgical management should be undertaken if there is evidence of polyposis.

Given a family history of inherited non-polyposis cancer, colonoscopy or double-contrast barium enema, or both, should be

SELECTED HIGH-RISK PATIENTS

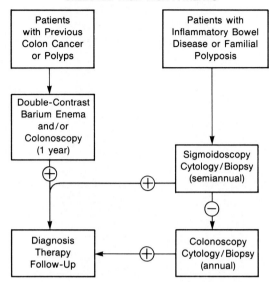

Figure 30–4. Recommended screen program for high-risk patients.

performed every three years, with annual fecal occult blood testing beginning at 20 to 25 years of age. With a suggestive family history, fecal occult blood should be tested annually with flexible proctosigmoidoscopy done every three to five years, beginning at 20 years of age.

Evaluation of Patients Following Colectomy. Patients with prior adenomas or colorectal cancer should have colonoscopy at initial evaluation prior to resection. Subsequently, they should have a colonoscopy or double-contrast enema, or both, every three years. If the patient has had a low anterior resection, flexible sigmoidoscopy can be performed with ease every 12 months. Fecal occult blood tests are also done yearly. Follow-up tests to exclude extracolonic spread include the plasma CEA, chest x-ray films, liver enzyme determinations, and abdominal computed tomography. A National Institute of Health consensus panel concluded that the plasma CEA was the most sensitive test for detecting a recurrent large bowel cancer following surgery. A complete description of the use of CEA in managing early and metastatic colorectal carcinoma is presented in Chapter 6A.

Periodic surveillance is advised for patients with inflammatory bowel disease and a history of pancolitis for seven years or left-sided colitis for 10 to 15 years (see Figure 30–4). This includes annual colonoscopy with multiple biopsies of the colon and rectum. Newly devel-

AVERAGE-RISK PATIENTS

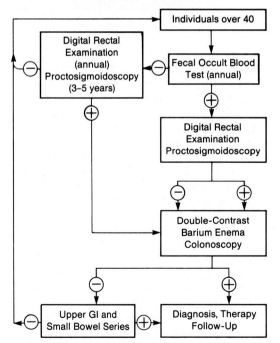

Figure 30–3. Recommended screening program for average-risk patients over the age of 40 years.

oped criteria for dysplasia in biopsies should facilitate clinical management (Riddell *et al.*, 1983). In the presence of a dysplasia-associated lesion or mass, the risk of an underlying carcinoma is extremely high. In one series, this association was found in 7 of 12 patients (Blackstone *et al.*, 1981).

Treatment

Surgery. The essential principles of definitive surgery of the colon and rectum include wide removal of the cancer-bearing bowel segment, allowing at least 6 cm of grossly uninvolved bowel at the distal margin, and the widest feasible excision of draining lymphatics, while minimizing the threat of cancer cell contamination or embolization (Turnbull *et al.*, 1967; Stearns and Schottenfeld, 1971; Turnbull, 1975). Adjacent organs, such as the bladder, posterior vaginal wall, or other intra-abdominal and retroperitoneal organs, are included in the resection wherever contiguous spread or adherence are evident (Enker *et al.*, 1979).

To prevent infection, the bowel is prepared by vigorous mechanical cleansing with enemas, and the patient is placed on preoperative oral antibiotics such as neomycin and erythromycin to reduce bowel flora. If the bowel is partially obstructed and purgation is contraindicated, preparation may include a liquid diet and mild laxatives in addition to antibiotics.

The specific operation depends upon the lymphatic drainage of the region of the large bowel to be resected: the lymphatics of the right and transverse colon are in the mesentery of the organ and follow the vascular tree derived from the superior mesenteric vessels. The lymphatics of the cecal and ascending colon follow the ileocolic and right colic systems to their origin from the superior mesenteric artery. The transverse colon drains along the midcolic artery to the superior mesenteric. The left colon lymphatics, from the splenic flexure, drain downward toward the route of the mesentery as defined by the inferior mesenteric artery. The entire rectum drains along the superior hemorrhoidal artery to the inferior mesenteric artery. Lastly, the lower portion of the rectum, 6 cm from the anal verge, may also drain along the inferior hemorrhoidal arteries or lateral along the middle hemorrhoid. In addition to the varying lymphatic drainage, the lower third of the rectum also has

a dual venous drainage system: the portal system via the superior hemorrhoidal vein and the inferior vena cava from the middle hemorrhoidal veins. This accounts for the higher incidence of early pulmonary metastases with tumors of the lower rectum compared to other regions in the large bowel.

For right colon tumors right hemicolectomy is performed. If the cancer is near the ileocecal valve, a 10- to 12-cm segment of the terminal ileum is also removed, along with its mesentery. Tumors of the hepatic flexure or mid-transverse colon require a right hemicolectomy and a meticulous dissection of the mesentery to the root of the midcolic artery at its origin from the superior mesenteric artery. A left colon cancer is removed with a left hemicolectomy with a dissection to the root of the mesentery defined by the origin of the inferior mesenteric artery. For tumors in the redundant mid- or lower segment region, a segmental resection with dissection to the root of the inferior mesenteric artery is adequate.

Surgery for rectal cancer must take into account the location of the tumor with the possibility of sparing the sphincter without compromising curative effect. For cancers of the distal 5 cm of rectum, where the tumor cannot be mobilized with an adequate margin, a Miles type abdominal perineal resection is performed. The dissection includes the lateral musculoskeletal border and the hypogastric lymph nodes along the lateral pelvic walls, as well as a resection up to the origin of the inferior mesenteric artery. With the exception of poorly differentiated tumors, rectal carcinomas above 11 cm are treated by anterior resection. Cancers located between 6 to 10 cm in the midrectum are also treated by low anterior resection if they are not bulky, have not invaded locally, and are not poorly differentiated. Reconstruction may be performed by hand-sewn anastomosis or the use of stapling devices. Recent attempts at sphincter preservation following low anterior resection have employed the coloanal anastomosis, which may avoid the necessity to divert the fecal stream with a temporary colostomy that is required with many low anterior resections.

Two recently reported series describe the expected results from surgery performed with optimal technique (see Table 30–7). Olson *et al.* (1980) determined the patterns and rate of recurrence after curative resection for colorectal cancer among 281 patients treated at the Peter Bent Brigham Hospital between 1960

Table 30–7. Selected Recent Series Demonstrating Results, by Stage of Disease, with Surgical Resection

Dukes Stage (Astler-Coller Modification)	OLSON ET AL., 1980		ENKER ET AL., 1979	
	No. of Patients	Disease-free Survival(%)	No. of Patients	5-Year Survival(%)
A	26	12	4	100
B$_1$	116	10	34	73.5
B$_2$	60	33	68	64.7
C$_1$	37	35	3	66.7
C$_2$	42	50	62	56.5

and 1971. The overall five-year survival was 49%, and only 10% of patients evidencing tumor recurrence survived for five years. The relapse rate was analyzed in relationship to Dukes stage, using the Astler-Coller modification: A, 12%; B$_1$, 10%; B$_2$, 33%; C$_1$, 35%; and C$_2$, 50%. The initial site of metastases was regional in 33%, distant in 46%, and combined regional-distant in 19%; 65% of patients evidenced an initial distant metastasis.

Enker and colleagues (1979) reported excellent survival results in 216 patients who underwent curative surgery at the University of Chicago. The five-year disease-free survival in relationship to Dukes stage (Astler-Coller) was A, 100%; B$_1$, 74%; B$_2$, 65%; C$_1$, 68%; C$_2$, 57%; and metastatic tumor (Dukes D), 4%.

In some circumstances a patient with a small, low-lying rectal cancer may refuse an abdominal perineal resection, or the patient may not be a candidate for such surgery because of advanced age or debilitation. In these cases, a more conservative approach such as local excision, electrocoagulative fulguration, or endocavitary irradiation may be considered (Baker, 1980). The latter procedure involves inserting an endocavitary contact low-voltage irradiation machine through a treatment proctoscope (Papillon, 1975). Alternatively, the tumor can be implanted with ^{192}Ir in combination with external beam radiotherapy (Sischy and Remington, 1975). These procedures are restricted to accessible small, well-differentiated polypoid lesions involving less than 25% of the rectal circumference.

An important and frequently encountered clinical decision in surgical oncology is whether to resect an isolated hepatic metastasis from colorectal cancer. The reported five-year survival of selected cases with solitary resected metastases ranges from 20 to 42% (Wilson and Adson, 1976; Foster and Berman, 1977; Wanebo et al., 1978b). Foster and Berman (1977) analyzed the outcome of surgery in relation to the diagnosis of the liver metas-

tasis. With synchronous lesions (81 patients), the five-year survival was 18%. This compared well to 25% survival with lesions detected within two years of primary surgery (47 patients) and 25% for metastases diagnosed after two years (50 patients). In the setting of multiple hepatic metastases, the yield of surgical resection is generally less, with Wilson and Adson (1976) reporting a five-year survival of 2%, whereas Foster and Berman (1977) found a 13% survival in 54 cases. In the latter series, there were seven operative deaths. Patient selection requires careful preoperative evaluation for other sites of tumor spread as well as computerized axial tomography and angiography of the celiac axis and superior mesenteric artery to identify the distribution and size of the lesions. Ultimately, resectability can be adequately defined only at surgery (Kim et al., 1975).

The serial measurement of the CEA concentration provides a sensitive and cost-effective means of detecting an early recurrence of colorectal cancer in some cases. Several investigators have examined the role of "second look" laparotomy for asymptomatic patients in whom the only indication of a possible tumor relapse is a consistently rising postoperative level of CEA. The ultimate value of such salvage procedures remains the subject of ongoing clinical research. The results of six reported studies have been recently reviewed (Patterson and Alpert, 1983). Of 117 patients operated on because of an increased plasma CEA, 91% had recurrent tumor. The disease was resectable in 50 patients (43%), but 15 cases had evidence of disseminated cancer. Overall, the local resectability rate was only 30%. In addition, the CEA is not specific for cancer, and elevations due to benign disease could result in needless surgery if an institution's policy is to operate in all cases.

Radiotherapy for Rectal Cancer. Radiotherapy for advanced rectal cancer has largely been restricted to palliation of pain, bleeding, and tenesmus, with objective regression of locally unresectable or recurrent tumor achieved in nearly 80% of patients. Less than 10% of such cases, however, achieve long-term control. One basic approach involves the use of a wide-field dose of 4500 to 5000 rads in five to six weeks, with a boost of 1000 to 1500 rads to a reduced field encompassing the main tumor mass. A common sign of recurrent rectal cancer is perineal pain, which may extend to the lumbar region or the legs. Frequently, a mass is not palpable, nor is there evidence of a mass lesion on CT scan. Almost 90% of such cases receive relief with pelvic irradiation. An additional indication for radiotherapy is to decrease local tumor infiltration to make an unresectable case a candidate for a curative operation. Kligerman (1976) reported a series of 15 selected patients with primary inoperable or nonresectable tumors treated with intensive radiotherapy. Nine were subsequently resected, and 20% remained alive five years or longer. This study suggests that patients with advanced local tumor should be considered for curative surgery if the response to radiotherapy is favorable and there are no signs of distant tumor.

The use of radiation therapy as an adjuvant to surgery for Dukes B_2 and C rectal tumors has received a great deal of study. The analyses support the application of pre- or postoperative pelvic irradiation if sites of relapse are found at reoperation after initial surgery with curative intent. Gunderson and Sosin (1974) reported the reoperation experience at the University of Minnesota. Of 75 patients with Dukes B_2 and C rectal tumors, 52 had recurrent or metastatic disease. Distant metastases as the sole expression of relapse were found in only 8% of cases. Local recurrence and regional lymph node metastases predominated as the only site of failure in 48% and with concurrent distant spread in 92%. This pattern of failure was predictable based upon anatomic factors, specifically the direct extension of the tumor to contiguous tissues and organs, and lymphatic drainage patterns: the upper rectum drains to lymph nodes that follow the superior hemorrhoidal and inferior mesenteric arteries. The latter vessel inserts into the aorta at about the level of L_2. The lower rectum drains inferiorly to the internal iliac nodes. The importance of these observations is that a high percentage of surgical failures in rectal cancer occur in an anatomic distribution that is readily encompassed in a pre- or postoperative radiation field.

In the largest single experience with preoperative radiation as a surgical adjuvant for rectal cancer, between 1937 and 1951, 1276 cases, including 396 Dukes C, were treated preoperatively at dose levels of 1500 to 2000 rads. In a nonrandomized comparison 37% who received radiation therapy were alive at five years, compared to 27% for a nonirradiated group (Quan, 1966). A subsequent randomized study performed at the same institution failed to demonstrate any survival benefit with radiation (Stearns *et al.,* 1975). In addition, it can be seen that in both studies radiation therapy did not alter the relative incidence of Dukes C cases, a claim now made in several other studies.

In 1964 the VA Surgical Adjuvant Group (VASAG) initiated a randomized controlled trial of 2000 rads preoperative radiation to a pelvic port followed by surgery. Patients with low-lying lesions received an additional 500 rads perineal boost. Among the 700 patients in the study (Higgins *et al.,* 1975; Roswit *et al.,* 1975), the operability or resectability rate in the treated and control groups did not differ. For the 453 patients in whom "curative" resection was possible, the five-year survival was 49% for treated versus 39% for controls, a difference not statistically significant. The data were also analyzed for the type of operation performed: 414 patients underwent either a curative or palliative abdominoperineal resection. The five-year survival for those who had received radiation treatment was 41%, compared to 38% for the controls. If the analysis was restricted to curative resection (no gross evidence of residual disease) or Dukes C cases, however, the small difference was no longer statistically valid. In addition, no difference was observed in survival with resections other than the abdominoperineal approach for higher lesions above the peritoneal reflection. The five-year survival of 39% was identical for the treated and the control groups. The VA study did find a reduction in involved lymph nodes in resection in patients who received preoperative radiation therapy—28% Dukes C versus 41% in the control group. Similar data have been reported by Kligerman (1976) using a dose of 4500 rads in five weeks, comparing the integrated incidence of Dukes C cases previously found at Yale–New Haven Hospital and at the University of Oregon using 5000 rads, using historical comparisons.

Both the Memorial Hospital and VASAG trials have been criticized because of the relatively low dose of radiotherapy employed. The

EORTC is now conducting a randomized controlled trial in which one-half of the patients are receiving a pelvic dose of 3450 rads in 19 days. At the present time there is no difference in survival. Thus, despite its general acceptance in many hospitals, there is little evidence that preoperative pelvic irradiation significantly improves the survival of patients who subsequently undergo surgery with curative intent.

Studies of preoperative radiotherapy are beset by important difficulties in analysis. It is impossible to stage the patient accurately, and as a result cases with Dukes A, B_1, and advanced disease will be unnecessarily treated. In addition, total doses of 4000 to 5000 rads require that surgery be delayed for one month after completion of radiotherapy. For these reasons attention is now being directed to postoperative treatment in surgically staged cases with proven Dukes B_2 and C tumors. In 1975, the GITSG initiated a four-arm controlled, randomized trial in postoperative rectal carcinomas of stages B_2 and C. The three treatment arms are (1) radiation therapy with 4000 rads alone; (2) chemotherapy with 5-FU and MeCCNU for 18 months; (3) radiation therapy with 5-FU sensitization followed by 5-FU and MeCCNU. These were compared to surgery alone. With more than four years of median follow-up, 52% of patients treated with surgery alone have had recurrent disease compared to 28% for those who received both postoperative radiation therapy and chemotherapy. Adjuvant chemotherapy or radiotherapy used singly was associated with intermediate recurrence rates of 40%. Statistically significant differences in survival have not as yet been demonstrated. The NSABP is completing a similarly designed controlled trial, testing postoperative chemotherapy or radiation therapy for patients with resected rectal cancer.

Chemotherapy. More than 50% of patients with large-bowel cancer develop disseminated disease and invariably succumb. Despite the application of therapeutic approaches used successfully for other cancers, little progress has been made in the chemotherapeutic management of colorectal carcinoma as reflected in the static survival statistics for the past three decades. No chemotherapy with curative potential is available for the patient with disseminated colon cancer, and palliative chemotherapy to date is characterized by a modest proportion of patients responding, a limited duration of responses, and a marginal impact of response on survival.

Single Anticancer Agents. The development of an effective form of combination chemotherapy requires the identification of drugs active as single agents. Since its development in 1957, 5-fluorouracil (5-FU) has remained the standard chemotherapeutic agent for colon cancer (Heidelberger, 1957). It produced an overall 21% response rate in over 2000 patients compiled by Wasserman *et al.* (1975), but reported response rates show a substantial range (Moertel *et al.,* 1969). A number of studies have addressed the optimal method of administering 5-FU. The original method—the "loading course"—was rapid intravenous injection of 15 mg/kg/day for five days followed by four half doses every other day. This schedule produced substantial toxic effects, with nausea, vomiting, and stomatitis observed in 50 to 90% of patients and bone marrow suppression in more than 70%. Some deaths were attributed to treatment (Moertel, 1975). Recently designed loading courses used a reduced dosage of 12 mg/kg/day for five days, without the additional alternate-day treatment until toxicity.

Other approaches to administration of 5-FU have included oral administration, continuous intravenous infusion lasting 2 to 24 hours or longer, and weekly rapid intravenous injection (Jacobs *et al.,* 1972), the latter correlating with decreased toxicity. Seifert *et al.* (1975) compared a five-day loading course of 12 mg/kg/day with a 96-hour continuous infusion of 30 mg/kg/day. The infusion was associated with more stomatitis but much reduced bone marrow toxicity and a more favorable response rate without improved duration of survival. Other studies have confirmed the advantage of infusion in terms of bone marrow suppression but have failed to confirm an increase in antitumor activity (Leone, 1974). The reduction of myelosuppression has led to the use of 5-FU by infusion in some regimens containing drugs with overlapping myelosuppressive properties.

Oral 5-FU has been employed for advanced colon cancer on the premise that it would be delivered by the portal circulation directly to the liver metastases that commonly occur. In early uncontrolled trials of oral 5-FU, dramatic response rates, especially of hepatic metastases, were reported (Khung *et al.,* 1966; Lahiri *et al.,* 1971; Leone, 1974). The premise was flawed, however, as hepatic metastases draw their blood supply predominantly from the hepatic artery (Bierman *et al.,* 1951–1952; Mann *et al.,* 1953; Healy, 1965; Ackerman *et al.,* 1969). Three controlled trials comparing oral and intravenous 5-FU for colon cancer (Ansfield *et al.,* 1975; Bateman *et al.,* 1975; Hahn *et al.,* 1975; Ansfield *et al.,* 1977) showed a superiority of intravenous administration both in response rate and in response duration, and oral 5-FU was not superior for liver metastases. Inconstant absorption probably accounts for the inferiority of the oral route (Hahn *et al.,* 1975).

The Central Oncology Group compared four basic methods of administering 5-FU in a randomized controlled trial including 141 evaluable patients with advanced measurable adenocarcinoma of the colon (Ansfield *et al.,* 1977). Treatment 1 consisted of five daily intravenous doses of 12 mg/kg followed by half doses every other day to toxicity or to a total of 11 half doses, then weekly maintenance doses of 15 mg/kg. Treatment 2 consisted of weekly intravenous doses of 15 mg/kg. Treatment 3 consisted of 500 mg total dose intravenously for four days followed by 500 mg weekly. Treatment 4 consisted of orally administered 5-FU 15 mg/kg daily for six days, followed by 15 mg/kg once weekly. The analysis showed a statistically superior response rate of 33% for patients who received the loading course (treatment 1), but at the expense of increased toxicity, including severe or life-threatening leukopenia in 18%. Response duration was longer in the patients receiving treatment 1 ($P = 0.0001$), but survival was not prolonged (projected incremental survival four to six months as compared with the other treatment arms), and the difference was not significant ($P = 0.09$). The loading course response rate of 33% was impressive in comparison with the other treatment arms, but this high rate of remission is not in keeping with the accumulated experience with 5-FU as a single agent.

Despite a well-defined response rate and a median remission duration of four to five months in colon cancer patients responding to 5-FU, few studies have proved that a survival benefit attends a response. The Mayo Clinic analysis of the survival of 5-FU responders compared with nonresponders and untreated historical controls showed a definite prolongation of median survival in the responding group (Moertel *et al.,* 1969).

Ftorafur, developed in the Soviet Union, is composed of 5-FU conjugated to a furanyl moiety that is slowly metabolized to the active drug. It was employed as a slow-release form of 5-FU in the hope that its pharmacokinetics might be similar to the continuous infusion method of administration. When administered intravenously, it has shown toxicity to the central nervous system with lethargy and nervousness (Valdivieso, *et al.,* 1976; Buroker *et al.,* 1978). While myelosuppression was minimal relative to 5-FU, there was no apparent benefit when ftorafur was combined with mitomycin-C or methyl-CCNU. A controlled trial of oral ftorafur versus intravenous 5-FU is now in progress.

Many additional cytotoxic drugs have been tested for colon cancer as single agents. Mitomycin C was reported to produce a 12 to 16% response rate (Moertel, 1975), but the response duration was less than three months. The toxic effects of chronic myelosuppression have limited its usefulness. The chloroethylnitrosoureas BCNU, CCNU, and methyl-CCNU have had response rates of 10 to 15% (Moertel, 1975). In one controlled trial methyl-CCNU demonstrated activity equivalent to 5-FU (Moertel, 1973); as a consequence, methyl-CCNU became the favored nitrosourea for colon cancer, which resulted in its use in many drug combinations.

Numerous other drugs, including cyclophosphamide, methotrexate, hexamethylmelamine, melphalan, actinomycin D, doxorubicin and hydroxyurea, have response rates reported as less than 20% (Wasserman *et al.,* 1975) and have not proved useful in colon cancer as single agents. Vincristine, widely used in combinations of drugs for colon cancer, has negligible activity as a single agent (Wasserman *et al.,* 1975). Recent trials of newer agents have included Baker's antifol, which had a 10% response rate (Padilla *et al.,* 1978), as well as metronidazole, chromomycin A, cytembena, pyrazofurin, cytosine arabinoside, and maytansine, all with no responses.

Combination Chemotherapy. Combinations of individually active cytotoxic drugs have produced the greatest advances in cancer chemotherapy. Cancer of the colon has not been a fertile field for the development of drug combinations because of the paucity of drugs with important single-agent activity. Nevertheless, many combinations have been designed and evaluated. Although increased response rates have been reported, no combination has produced a consistent increase in remission rates or survival.

The earliest combinations of 5-FU, BCNU, and mitomycin C produced no better than a 20% response rate (Moertel *et al.,* 1970). In 1974 Falkson *et al.* (1974) compared 5-FU with the combination of 5-FU, BCNU, vincristine, and DTIC in a randomized trial. The combination resulted in tumor regression in 43% of patients, but this was not statistically superior to the 25% response with 5-FU alone. Moertel et al. (1975) subsequently reported a similarly high response rate with the combination of 5-FU, vincristine, and methyl-CCNU, while controls randomized to 5-FU alone had a 19.5% response rate. The success with the combination could not be duplicated by others (Kemeny et al., 1977; Engstrom et al., 1978), and, in the expanded experience at the Mayo Clinic, only 27% of patients overall showed objective tumor regression (Moertel, 1978).

Since vincristine alone is not an active drug for colon cancer, a number of studies have evaluated the two-drug combination of 5-FU and methyl-CCNU. The most favorable result was a 37% response, compared with 7% in randomized controls receiving methyl-CCNU, in a study conducted by the Central Oncology Group (Posey and Morgan, 1977). The Southwest Oncology Group, in a randomized phase III trial of 5-FU, in comparison with 5-FU and methyl-CCNU, reported a 32% response rate for the combination, despite an extremely conservative dose of 5-FU (Baker et al., 1976). Other studies have not confirmed these results with 5-FU and methyl-CCNU, and the overall response rate in 561 patients in eight series is 19% (Baker et al., 1976; Buroker et al., 1977; Lokich et al., 1977; Engstrom et al., 1978; Kane et al., 1978).

The Eastern Cooperative Oncology Group, in addition to evaluating the combination of 5-FU and methyl-CCNU, combined these two drugs with either vincristine or DTIC or both, and also evaluated the combination of 5-FU with hydroxyurea; 5-FU with hydroxyurea achieved the highest response rate of 21% (Engstrom et al., 1978).

Kemeny and coworkers (1983) attempted to increase the efficacy of the combination of 5-FU, methyl-CCNU, and vincristine by adding methyl-nitrosourea streptozotocin (MOF-Strep). Streptozotocin had been reported to have limited therapeutic activity in patients previously treated with 5-FU (Douglass et al., 1976). In a randomized trial (Kemeny et al., 1983) the MOF-streptozotocin combination produced a 32% response rate compared to a 11% response with the base three-drug regimen. This result could not be confirmed by the Gastrointestinal Tumor Study Group (Smith, et al., 1982), where a 16% response rate was found in 40 previously untreated patients.

Recently, Machover et al. (1982) recommended high doses of intravenous leukovorin, 200 mg/m^2/day for five days, in conjunction with 5-FU, 370 to 400 mg/m^2 for five days. Repeated courses were administered every three weeks. The rationale is that for 5-FU to bind covalently to thymidylate synthetase requires the presence of a tetrahydrofolate. A 56% response rate was reported in 16 previously untreated patients, with a 21% response in those with prior chemotherapy. Byrne et al. (1983) were unable to confirm the latter result, but the overall concept is worthy of further evaluation as a first-line treatment.

The use of methotrexate–5-FU combinations to achieve a more effective cytotoxic effect for the fluorinated pyrimidine has also been evaluated in advanced colon cancer. The rationale for possible synergism between the two drugs observed in laboratory models remains a subject of debate. One theory favors an increase in the phosphoribosyl pyrophosphate (PRPP) pool, secondary to methotrexate inhibition of de novo purine synthesis that may result in an increased concentration of ribose metabolites of 5-FU. Cantrell et al. (1982) tested this concept in a clinical trial with no apparent therapeutic benefit.

Hepatic Artery Infusion of Chemotherapy for Hepatic Metastases. An increasingly common approach to managing patients with hepatic metastases is the infusion of 5-FU or its analog 5-FUdR into the hepatic artery. In concept, this technique is supported by two important factors: (1) liver metastases derive most of their blood supply from the hepatic artery, and therefore, very high drug concentrations may be delivered directly to the tumor; (2) the liver is the principal organ for 5-FU catabolism, and therefore, systemic toxicity may be reduced. Ansfield et al. (1975) reported a series of 419 patients in whom a catheter was placed in the hepatic artery, usually from a transbrachial approach; 5-FU was infused continuously at a rate of 20 mg/kg/day for four days and then at 15 mg/kg/day for 17 days, after which weekly intravenous 5-FU was administered. Seventy-five percent of the patients had received prior 5-FU systemically, and 293 patients were considered evaluable. Of these, 55% were considered to have responded with an objective decrease in liver size. Buroker et al. (1976) described a 35% objective response rate with reduction in liver size in 21 colon cancer patients treated with intra-arterial infusions of

5-FUdR. All had failed to respond to adequate trials of systemic 5-FU. In this study, 5-FUdR was administered continuously at 0.3 mg/kg/day via a portable pump connected to a catheter placed in the hepatic artery, through the brachial artery or surgically placed in the abdomen.

The value of intra-arterial 5-FU was directly compared with standard intravenous 5-FU in a randomized study of the Central Oncology Group. Intra-arterial 5-FU was given at a dose of 20 mg/kg/day for 14 days followed by 10 mg/kg/day for seven days. Patients randomized to systemic 5-FU received an intravenous loading course of 12 mg/kg/day for four days and then 6 mg/kg/day every other day for four doses. All patients subsequently received intravenous 5-FU weekly. The response rate was 34% with intra-arterial infusion and 23% with intravenous administration, and the duration of response was somewhat greater with intra-arterial 5-FU. Neither the difference in response rate nor the response duration was statistically significant.

The technology of hepatic artery infusion therapy has substantially advanced with the development of the totally implanted subcutaneous pump. This device consists of two chambers separated by a flexible metal bellows; the more superficial chamber is a drug reservoir which can be easily refilled with the anticancer agent. The second chamber contains a two-phase charging fluid in equilibrium that exerts a constant pressure on the bellows forcing the drug from the reservoir into a catheter selectively placed. When the pump is refilled, the increased volume within the bellows drug chamber causes the fluid vapor in the second chamber to condense to a liquid state, thus restoring energy for the next pumping cycle. This allows for a precise and continuous flow of drug, while reducing the probability of extended hospitalization, physical disability associated with percutaneously placed catheters, as well as the potential of sepsis and catheter perforation.

The initial reported response rates achieved in patients with hepatic arterial chemotherapy for liver metastases have been promising. Ensminger and coworkers (1982) have reported their results in 92 patients with metastatic colorectal cancer, in whom 50 presented with hepatic metastases only. The basic chemotherapeutic regimen consisted of 5-FUdR, 0.3 mg/kg/day for 14 consecutive days, repeated after a two-week rest period. In addition, patients with evidence of extrahepatic disease also received mitomycin C 15 mg/m^2 every six to eight weeks. An 83% response rate was reported for patients without extrahepatic metastases, compared to 74% for those with evidence of tumor outside the liver. Sixty-eight percent of the former group were alive, and the estimated median survival was between 18 to 24 months (see Figure 30–5). Patients with extrahepatic metastases, in contrast, evidenced no apparent survival benefit, with only 35% alive and an estimated median survival of eight to ten months. Despite some early confirmatory results (Cohen *et al.*, 1983), other

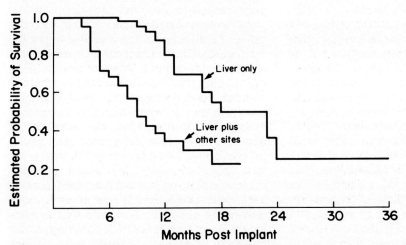

Figure 30–5.   Survival of patients with colorectal cancer with liver metastases treated with hepatic arterial chemotherapy using an implanted pump. From Ensminger, W.; Niederhuber, J.; Gynes, J.; Thrall, W.; Cozz, E.; and Doan, K.: Effective control of liver metastases from colon cancer with an implanted system for hepatic arterial chemotherapy. *Proc. Am. Soc. Clin. Oncol.,* **1:**94, 1982.

centers have as yet been unable to duplicate the result. Toxicity due to hepatic and biliary tract injury and gastroduodenal mucosal ulceration has been noted (Hohn *et al.,* 1985; Faintuch *et al.,* 1984). Before this method is accepted as a standard treatment of patients with metastases confined to the liver, with the necessity of a second laboratory in most instances to place the hepatic artery catheter, a controlled trial against standard intravenous 5-FU is an absolute requirement. The initial results of such a trial conducted by Kemeny and coworkers (1984) suggest that no difference in response rate or survival is achieved.

Adjuvant Chemotherapy of Colon Cancer. The early trials of adjuvant chemotherapy for colon cancer in the United States used alkylating agents, such as thiotepa, without specific rationale or therapeutic success (Dwight *et al.,* 1960). Following the demonstration of independent therapeutic activity of fluorinated pyrimidines, 5-FU and 5-FUdR, for this tumor, subsequent trials incorporated these agents. The Veterans Administration Surgical Adjuvant Group is one of the major investigative groups to evaluate the role of 5-FU as an adjuvant treatment in the United States (Woolley *et al.,* 1979). In the first study of postoperative 5-FU, the patients were men with completely resected adenocarcinoma that had not been diagnosed preoperatively by sigmoidoscopic biopsy. These patients were stratified into three groups: (1) curative resection with no evidence of residual metastasis or tumor at a resection margin, (2) histologic proof that residual tumor was left behind either by biopsy or the finding of tumor at the resection margins, and (3) clinical evidence of tumor, not proven histologically. These groups were randomized separately. Those patients randomized to 5-FU received 12 mg/kg by intravenous injection on five successive days. Group A and group C patients received a second course about seven weeks later, while group B continued to receive the drug courses at six- to eight-week intervals until disease progression or patient death. Of 496 patients entered into this trial, 482 are included in the analysis (235 treated, 247 control). In 338 patients having curative resection, there was a 58.2% five-year survival in the 5-FU group as opposed to 48.0% in the control (see Figure 30–6). In 84 group B patients, there was 35.7% survival at 18 months for those receiving the drug compared to 16.7% in controls. In 60 group C patients, there was 53.6% survival at 18 months

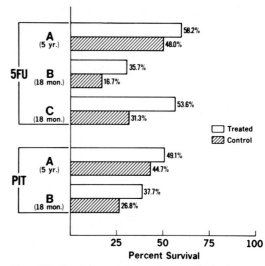

Figure 30–6. Adjuvant chemotherapy of colonic cancer by the Veterans Administration Surgical Adjuvant Group. In the 5-FU trial, two courses of the drug were administered: (*A*) Curative resection. (*B*) Histologic proof of residual tumor. (*C*) Clinical evidence of residual tumor. In the prolonged intermittent treatment (*PIT*) study, patients were treated with 5-FU for 19 months: (*A*) Curative resection. (*B*) Proven residual tumor. From Woolley, P. V.; Higgins, G. A.; and Schein, P. S.: Ongoing trials in the surgical adjuvant management of colorectal cancer. *Recent Results Cancer Res.,* **63:**231–235, 1979.

in those receiving the drug and 31.3% in the control group. None of the results were statistically significant.

In a second study, prolonged intermittent therapy (PIT), patients with large bowel cancer at all sites, including rectum, were eligible. This group contained patients who, upon resection, were found to have one or more unfavorable prognostic indicators: (1) presence of positive lymph nodes, (2) serosal involvement or invasion of perirectal fat, (3) blood vessel or lymphatic invasion, (4) involvement of an organ other than the colon. Patients were then divided into two groups: group A with curative resection and group B with proven residual disease or positive resection margin. The groups were randomized separately to receive or not receive 5-FU. The drug itself was given at a dose of 12 mg/kg/day for five successive days, and these courses were repeated at six- to eight-week intervals. Patients in group A received the drug for 18 months and those in group B until evidence of disease progression or death. In this study 677 patients were eligible for analysis. In the 518 curative patients, survival at five years was 49.1% for patients receiving 5-FU and 44.7% for controls (see Figure 30–6). For 159 patients in group B, survival was 37.7% at 18 months in the 5-FU group and 26.8% in controls.

Optimal response rates for 5-FU in advanced colorectal cancer require that a moderate degree of myelosuppressive toxicity be produced. One of the criticisms of the Veterans Administration's prolonged intermittent therapy study was that relatively few patients developed leukopenia during the 19 months of treatment.

The Central Oncology Group conducted a more intensive trial of 5-FU adjuvant chemotherapy (Grage *et al.*, 1977). Patients undergoing curative or palliative resection were randomized to receive either 5-FU or no further treatment until relapse. 5-FU was administered intravenously using a dose schedule of 12 mg/kg/day for four days followed by 6 mg/kg on alternate days for five additional days. Following a 7- to 14-day rest, weekly maintenance chemotherapy of 12 mg/kg was continued for one year. In contrast to the VA study, 60% of patients developed some degree of leukopenia. On this study 372 patients were entered of which 81% were acceptable for analysis, including 92 patients with Dukes B and 97 patients with Dukes C colorectal cancer who had undergone surgical resection with curative intent. The disease-free interval for the Dukes C curative resection cases approached statistical significance ($P = 0.06$) with a median of 24 months for the chemotherapy group versus 16 months for control. However, this was not translated into an increased survival for the treatment group ($P = 0.18$). In an analysis of the prognostic importance of drug-induced leukopenia, the disease-free interval was significantly longer ($P = 0.004$) for patients in whom the white blood cell count was reduced below 4000 with chemotherapy, but once again there was no significant impact on survival.

In spite of a few isolated, uncontrolled series suggesting benefit with postoperative 5-FU, the consistent conclusions reached by the prospective randomized trials cited make it clear that systemic 5-FU will never be an acceptable standard adjuvant treatment.

Cooperative groups evaluated the efficacy of the combination of 5-FU and methyl-CCNU as an adjuvant treatment for resected colorectal cancer. The results are again consistent, with no apparent reduction in overall recurrence rates. As an example, the Gastrointestinal Tumor Study (Lessner *et al.*, 1982) conducted a controlled trial for B_2 and C colon cancer (> 12 cm from the anal verge) in which 621 patients were randomized to one of the following treatment options: (1) surgery alone, (2) surgery followed by 5-FU plus methyl-CCNU, (3) surgery plus MER (methanol extracted residue of BCG), and (4) surgery plus chemotherapy and immunotherapy. Treatment continued for 70 weeks, and the median postsurgical follow-up was 47 months. One hundred and sixty-five patients (29%) evidenced tumor recurrence, with no significant difference in survival between any of the four treatment arms of the trial. Relapse directly correlated with stage: B_2, 17%; C_1 (one to four nodes), 30%; and C_2 ($>$ five nodes), 55%. Five patients receiving chemotherapy have developed leukemia or preleukemia. Although the recurrence rates were significantly less than anticipated, perhaps reflecting the adequacy of the surgery in the participating institutions, no form of postoperative management influenced either relapse rates or survival.

Taylor *et al.* (1977) designed an innovative approach to the administration of 5-fluorouracil. The drug is given in the portal vein circulation within one week following surgery at a dose of 1000 mg for seven consecutive days. The rationale is that cells seeding the liver from the large bowel will initially draw their blood supply from the portal vein, whereas after they become established as micrometastases they will use the hepatic artery system. Therefore, administration of the drug directly into the portal system when the liver is seeded with tumor cells might be an effective form of treatment. The initial results in this controlled trial appeared promising with improved survival for patients with Dukes B colon cancer and with a significant decrease in hepatic recurrence. There has been no change in the pattern of local or regional recurrence, which has been reflected in a much lesser impact in patients with rectal cancer. A further follow-up of this important trial will soon be available, as will the results of attempts to confirm these results in studies conducted by the Northwest Oncology Group and the Medical Research Council in Great Britain.

The Gastrointestinal Tumor Study Group designed a clinical trial largely directed at the presence of microscopic disease in liver. In this controlled study patients with Dukes B and C colon cancer were randomized to surgery alone or surgery followed by administration of 2100 rads of external radiation to the liver with systemic intravenous 5-fluorouracil, followed by two additional loading courses with the same chemotherapeutic agent. This study has been in progress for only a short period, and there are as yet no reported results.

Recently Gilbert *et al.* (1982) reported the results of a controlled trial in which 176 patients with Dukes B and C colorectal cancer were randomized by surgery alone or surgery plus razoxane (ICRF-159). With a median follow-up of 34 months, the razoxane-treated patients are reported to have a significantly longer disease-free interval than control patients ($P = 0.01$). In regard to survival, 24 of 56 patients in the control group have died (43%) compared to 17 of 64 (27%) in the treated group. This interesting early result requires confirmation in a second randomized trial.

Future Prospects

Despite the improved results with selected series, the mortality from cancer of the large bowel in the United States has remained static for 30 years. For rectal cancer, combined modality postoperative therapy may produce the first tangible increase in survival for this site of disease, but the initial results await maturation and confirmation. Aside from the apparent improved control of hepatic metastases with intra-arterial chemotherapy, drug treatment of colorectal cancer in either the advanced or adjuvant setting has made little progress. Nevertheless, effective treatment of all stages of colorectal cancer depends upon identifying an improved form of systemic therapy. There is, as a consequence, a continued need to evaluate the therapeutic activity of newly developed agents in phase II trials, as well as to develop a predictive *in vitro* assay of drug efficacy to avoid the expense and suffering associated with clinical testing of ineffective agents.

The most direct method for improving the survival statistics for this high-incidence cancer would be to implement a national screening program. The current overall 46% five-year survival could be increased to an estimated 75% with earlier detection of patients who are still asymptomatic. The cost effectiveness of wide-scale fecal occult blood testing, with the necessary follow-up of all positive tests, needs continued study. Ultimately, the etiological factors for colorectal cancer must be identified and the public made aware of the necessity of adjusting life-style and diet, if such measures are proved justified.

REFERENCES

Ackerman, N. B.; Lien, W. M.; Kondi, E. S.; and Silverman, N. A.: The blood supply of experimental liver metastases: 1. The distribution of hepatic artery and portal vein blood to "small" and "large" tumors. *Surgery,* **66:**1067, 1969.

American Cancer Society: *Facts and Figures.* American Cancer Society, New York, 1982.

Anderson, D. E., and Romsdahl, M.: Family history: A criterion for selective screening. In Mulvihill, J. J.; Miller, R. W.; and Fraumeni, J. (eds.): *Genetics of Human Cancer.* Raven Press, New York, 1977.

Ansfield, R.; Klotz, J.; Nealon, T.; Ramirez, G.; Minto, J.; Hill. G.; Wilson, W.; Davis, H.; and Cornell, G.: A phase III study comparing the clinical utility of four regimens of 5-fluorouracil. *Cancer,* **39:**34, 1977.

Ansfield, F. J.; Ramirez, G.; Davis, H. L.; Wirtaneu, G. W.; Johnson, R. O.; Davis, T. E.; Esmaili, M.; Bryan, G. T.; Manolo, F. B.; and Bordeu, E. C.: Further clinical studies with intrahepatic arterial infusion with 5-fluorouracil. *Cancer,* **36:**2413, 1975.

Armstrong, B., and Doll, R.: Development in the epidemiology factors and cancer incidence and mortality in different countries, with special reference to dietary practices. *Int. J. Cancer,* **15:**617–631, 1975.

Astler, U. B., and Coller, F. A.: The prognostic significance of direct extension of carcinoma of the colon and rectum. *Ann. Surg.,* **139:**846-851, 1954.

Baker, A. R.: Local procedures in the management of rectal cancer. *Semin. Oncol.,* **7:**385–391, 1980.

Baker, L. H.; Talley, R. W.; Matter, R.; Lehane, D. E.; Ruffner, B. W.; Jones, S. E.; Morrison, F. S.; Stephens, R. L.; Gehan, E. A.; and Vaitkevicius V. K.: Phase III comparison of the treatment of advanced gastrointestinal cancer with bolus weekly 5-FU vs. methyl-CCNU plus bolus weekly 5-FU: A Southwest Oncology Group Study. *Cancer,* **3:**1, 1976.

Bateman, J.; Irwin, L.; Pugh, R.; Cassidy, F.; and Weiner, J.: Comparison of intravenous and oral administration of 5-fluorouracil for colorectal carcinoma. *Proc. Am. Assoc. Cancer Res. and A.S.C.O.,* **16:**242, 1975.

Berg, J. W., and Howell, M. A.: The geographic pathology of bowel cancer. *Cancer,* **34:**807–815, 1974.

Berk, J. E., and Haubrich, W. S.: Malignant tumors of the colon and rectum, in Bockus, H. L. (ed.): *Gastroenterology,* Vol. 2. W. B. Saunders Company, Philadelphia, 1963.

Bierman, H. R.; Byron, R. L.; Kelley, K. H.; and Grady, A.: Studies on blood supply of tumors in man: III. Vascular patterns of liver by hepatic arteriography in vivo. *J.N.C.I.,* **12:**107–131, 1951.

Bingham, S.; Williams, D. R.; Cole, J. T.; and James, W. P.: Dietary fibre and regional large bowel cancer mortality in Britain. *Br. J. Cancer,* **40:**456–463, 1979.

Black, W. A., and Waugh, J. M.: The intramural extension of carcinoma of the descending colon, sigmoid and rectosigmoid. A pathologic study. *Surg. Gynecol. Obstet.,* **87:**457–464, 1948.

Blackstone, M. O.; Riddell, R. H.; Rogers, B. H. G.; and Levin, B.: Dysplasia-associated lesion or mass (DALM) detected by colonoscopy in long-standing ulcerative colitis: An indication for colectomy. *Gastroenterology,* **80:**366–374, 1981.

Blanco, D.; Ross, N. K.; Paganini-Hill, A.; and Henderson, B. E.: Cholecystectomy and colon cancer. *Dis. Colon Rectum,* **27:**290–292, 1984.

Blot, W. J.; Fraumeni, J. F.; Stone, B. J.; and McKay, F. W.: Geographic patterns of large bowel cancer in the United States. *J.N.C.I.*, **51**:1225–1232, 1976.

Brown, C. E., and Warren, S.: Visceral metastasis from rectal carcinoma. *Surg. Gynecol. Obstet.*, **66**:611–621, 1938.

Buckwalter, J. A., and Kent, T. T.: Prognosis and surgical pathology of carcinoma of the colon. *Surg. Gynecol. Obstet.*, **136**:465–472, 1973.

Bull, A. W,; Soullier, B. K.; Wilson, P. S.; Hayden, M. T.; and Nigro, N. D.: The promotion of azoxymethane induced intestinal cancer by high fat diet in rats. *Cancer Res.*, **39**:4956–4959, 1979.

Burkitt, D.; Walker, A. R.; and Painter, N. S.: Effects of dietary fibre on stools and transit times and its role in the causation of disease. *Lancet*, **2**:1408, 1972.

Buroker, T.; Kim, P. N.; and Heibrun, L.: 5-FU infusion with mitomycin-C vs. 5-FU infusion with methyl-CCNU in the treatment of advanced colon cancer: A phase III study. *Proc. A.S.C.O.*, **18**:271, 1977.

Buroker, T.; Samson, M.; Correa, J.; Fraile, R.; and Vaitkevicius, V. K.: Hepatic artery infusion of 5-FUdR after prior systematic 5 fluorouracil. *Cancer Treat. Rep.*, **60**:1277, 1976.

Buroker, T.; Wojtaszak, B.; Dindogru, A.; DeMattia, M.; Baker, L.; Groth, C.; and Vaitkevicius, V. K.: Phase II trial of ftorafur with mitomycin-C versus ftorafur with methyl-CCNU in untreated colorectal cancer. *Cancer Treat. Rep.*, **62**:689, 1978.

Burt, C. A.: Carcinoma of the ovaries secondary to cancer of the colon and rectum. *Dis. Colon. Rectum*, **3**:352–357, 1960.

Bussey, H. J. R,; De Cosse, J. J.; Deschner, E. E.; Evers, A. A.; Lesser, M. L.; Morson, B. C.; Ritchie, S. M.; Thomson, J. P. S.; and Wadsworth, J.: A randomized trial of ascorbic acid in polyposis coli. *Cancer*, **50**:208–213, 1982.

Byrne, P.; Smith, F.; Treat, J.; Bowers, M. W.; McVie, G.; Huinink, T. B.; and Schein, P. S.: 5-Fluorouracil and higher dose folinic acid treatment of colorectal carcinoma patients. *Proc. Am. Soc. Clin. Oncol.*, **2**:C-474, 1983.

Cantrell, J. E.; Brunet, R.; Lagarde, C.; Schein, P. S.; and Smith, F. P.: Phase II study of sequential methotrexate–5-FU therapy in advance measurable colorectal cancer. *Cancer Treat. Rep.*, **66**:1563–1565, 1982.

Cattell, R. B.; MacKenzie, D. H.; and Colcock, B. P.: Cancer of the colon and rectum. *Surg. Clin. North Am.*, **35**:823–831, 1955.

Chomcahl, C. C.; Bhodracheri, N.; and Nigro, N. D.: The effect of bile on the induction of experimental intestinal tumors in rats. *Dis. Colon Rectum*, **17**:310–312, 1974.

Cohen, A. M.; Greenfield, A.; and Wood, W. C.: Treatment by hepatic arterial chemotherapy using implanted drug pump. *Cancer*, **51**:2013–2019, 1983.

Coller, F. A.; Kay, E. B; and MacIntyre, R. S.: Regional lymphatic metastasis of carcinoma of the rectum. *Surgery*, **8**:294–311, 1940.

Copeland, E. M.; Miller, L. D.; and Jones, R. S.: Prognostic factors in carcinoma of the colon and rectum. *Am. J. Surg.*, **116**:875–881, 1968.

Correa, P.; Duque, E.; Cuello, C.; and Haenzel, W.: Polyps of the colon and rectum in Cali, Colombia. *Int. J. Cancer*, **9**:86–92, 1972.

Crowther, J. S.; Drasar, B. S.; Hill, M. D.; MacLennan, R.; Magnin, D.; Peach, J.; and Teoh-Chan, C. H.: Fecal steroids and bacteria and large bowel cancer in Hong Kong by socioeconomic groups. *Br. J. Cancer*, **34**:191, 1976.

DeCosse, J. J.: Potential for chemoprevention. *Cancer*, **50**:2250–2253, 1982.

DeCosse, J. J.: Are we doing better with large-bowel cancer? *N. Engl. J. Med.*, **310**:782–783, 1984a.

DeCosse, J. J.: Malignant colorectal polyp. *Gut*, **25**:433–436, 1984b.

Deddish, M. R.: Surgical procedures for carcinoma of the left colon and rectum with five year end results following abdominopelvic dissection of lymph nodes. *Am. J. Surg.*, **99**:188–191, 1960.

de Peyster, F. A., and Gilchrist, R. K.: Pathology and manifestation of cancer of the colon and rectum. In Turell, R. (ed.): *Diseases of the Colon and Anorectum*. W. B. Saunders Company, Philadelphia, 1969.

Deschner, E. E.: Relationship of altered proliferation to colonic neoplasia. In Malt, R. A., and Williamson, R. C. N. (eds.): *Colonic Carcinogenesis*. MTP Press, Lancaster, 1980.

Devroede, G.: Risk of cancer in inflammatory bowel disease. In Winawer, S. J.; Schottenfeld, D.; and Sherlock, P. (eds.): *Colorectal Cancer: Prevention, Epidemiology and Screening*. Raven Press, New York, 1980.

Donegan W. L., and DeCosse, J. J.: Pitfalls and controversies in the staging of colorectal cancer. In Enker, W. E. (ed.): *Cancer of the Colon*. Yearbook Medical Publishers, Chicago, 1978.

Douglass, H. O.; Lavin, P. T.; and Moertel, C. G.: Nitrosoureas: Useful agents for the treatment of advanced gastrointestinal cancer. *Cancer Treat. Rep.*, **60**:769, 1976.

Dukes, C. E.: The classification of cancer of the rectum. *J. Pathol. Bacteriol.*, **35**:323–332, 1932.

Dukes, C. E., and Bussey, H. J. R.: The spread of rectal cancer and its effect on prognosis. *Br. J. Cancer*, **12**:309–320, 1958.

Dwight, R. W.; Higgins, G. A., Jr.; and Keehn, R. J.: Factors influencing survival after resection in cancer of the colon and rectum. *Am. J. Surg.*, **117**:512–522, 1960.

Dwight, R. W.; Humphrey, E. W.; and Higgins, G. A.: FUdR as adjuvant to surgery in cancer of the large bowel. *J. Surg. Oncol.*, **5**:243–249, 1973.

Eddy, D. M.: Computer models and the evaluation of colon cancer screening programs. In Winawer, S.; Schottenfeld, D.; and Scherlock, P. (eds.): *Colorectal Cancer: Prevention, Epidemiology and Screening*. Raven Press, New York, 1980.

Eide, T. J., and Stalsberg, H.: Diverticular disease of the large intestine in northern Norway. *Gut*, **20**:609–615, 1979.

Engstrom, P.; MacIntyre, J.; Douglass, H., Jr.; and Carbone, P.: Combination chemotherapy of advanced bowel cancer. *Proc. Am. Assoc. Cancer Res. and A.S.C.O.*, **19**:384, 1978.

Enker, W. E.; Laffer, U. T.; and Block, G. E.: Enhanced survival of patients with colon and rectal cancer is based upon wide anatomic resection. *Ann. Surg.*, **190**:350–357, 1979.

Ensminger, W.; Niederhuber, J.; Gynes, J.; Thrall, W.; Cozzi, E.; and Doan, K.: Effective control of liver metastases from colon cancer with an implanted system for hepatic arterial chemotherapy. *Proc. Am. Soc. Clin. Oncol.*, **1**:94, 1982.

Enterline, H. T.: Polyps and cancer of the large bowel. In Morson, B. C. (ed.): *Current Topics in Pathology*, Vol. 63. *Pathology of the Gastrointestinal Tract*. Sprager, Berlin, 1976.

Fahl, J. C.; Dockerty, M. B.; and Judd, E. S.: Scirrhous carcinoma of the colon and rectum. *Surg. Gynecol. Obstet.*, **3**:759–766, 1960.

Falkson, G.; Van Eden, E. G.; and Falkson, H. C.: Fluorouracil, imidazole carboximide dimethyltriazeno, vincristine and bis-chlorethylnitrosourea in colon cancer. *Cancer,* **33:**1207, 1974.

Fenoglio, C. M.; Kaye, G. I.; and Lane, N.: The distribution of human colonic lymphatics in normal, hyperplastic and adenomatous tissue: Its probable relationship to metastasis from small carcinomas in pedunculated adenomas with two case reports. *Gastroenterology,* **64:**51–66, 1973.

Foster, J. H., and Berman, M. M.: Solid liver tumors. In *Major Problems in Clinical Surgery.* W. B. Saunders Company, Philadelphia, 1977.

Fraumeni, J. F.; Lloyd, W. J.; Smith, E. M.; and Wagoner, J. K.: Cancer mortality among nuns: Role of marital status in etiology of neoplastic disease in women. *J.N.C.I.,* **30:**1781–1795, 1969.

Gabriel, W. B.; Dukes, C. E., and Bussey, H. J. R.: Lymphatic spread in cancer of the rectum. *Br. J. Surg.,* **23:**395–413, 1935.

Gardner, E. J.: Follow-up study of a family group exhibiting dominant inheritance for a syndrome including intestinal polyps, osteomas, fibromas and epidermal cysts. *Am. J. Hum. Genet.,* **14:**376–390, 1962.

Gastrointestinal Tumor Study Group: Adjuvant therapy of colon cancer—Results of a prospectively randomized trial. *N. Engl. J. Med.,* **310:**737–743, 1984.

Gelfand, D. W., and Ott, D. J.: Single vs. double-contrast gastrointestinal studies. *A.J.R.,* **137:**523–528, 1981.

Gilbert, J. M.; Hellmann, K.; Evans, M.; Cassell, P. G.; Stoodley, B.; Ellis, H.; and Wastell, C.: Adjuvant oral razoxane (ICRF-159) in resectable colorectal cancer. *Cancer Chemother. Pharmacol.,* **8:**293–299, 1982.

Gilbertsen, V. A.: Improving the prognosis for patients with intestinal cancer. *Surg. Gynecol. Obstet.,* **124:**1253–1259, 1967.

Gilbertsen, V. A.: Proctosigmoidoscopy and polypectomy in reducing the incidence of rectal cancer. *Cancer,* **34:**936–939, 1974.

Gius, J. A.: The role of hypertrophy of the muscularis in the delayed onset of symptoms in cancer of the colon. *Surgery,* **24:**221–230, 1948.

Glober, G.; Nomura, A.; Kamiyama, S.; Shimada, A.; and Abba, B.: Bowel transit time and stool weight in populations with different colon cancer risks. *Lancet,* **2:**110, 1977.

Goldin, B. R., Lombardi, P.; Mayhew, J.; and Gorbach, S. L.: Factors that affect intestinal bacterial activity: Implications for colon carcinogenesis. In *Gastrointestinal Cancer: Endogenous Factors.* Cold Spring Harbor Laboratory, Cold Spring Harbor, New York, 1981.

Grage, T. B.; Metter, G. E.; Cornell, G. N.; Strawitz, J. G.; Hill, G. J.; Frelick, R. W.; and Moss, S. E.: Adjuvant chemotherapy with 5-fluorouracil after surgical resection of the colorectal carcinoma (COG Protocol 704): A preliminary report. *Am. J. Surg.,* **133:**59–66, 1977.

Grage, T. B.; Shingleton, W. W.; Jubert, A. V.; Elias, E. G.; Aust, J. B.; and Moss, S. E.: Results of a prospective randomized study of hepatic artery infusion with 5-fluorouracil vs. intravenous 5-flourouracil in patients with hepatic metastases from colorectal cancer: A Central Oncology Group Study (COG 7032). *Eur. J. Cancer, Clin. Oncol.* **5:**116, 1979.

Graham, S.; Dayal, H.; Swanson, M.; Nuttleman, A.; and Wilkinson, G.: Diet and the epidemiology of cancer of the colon and rectum. *J.N.C.I.,* **61:**709–715, 1978.

Greenstein, A. J.; Sachar, D. B.; Pucillo, A.; Vassilades, G.; Smith, H.; Kreel, I.; Gelter, S. A.; Janowitz, H. D.; and Aufses, A. H.: Cancer in universal and left-sided ulcerative colitis: Clinical and pathologic features. *Mt. Sinai J. Med. (N.Y.),* **46:**25–32, 1979.

Greenstein, A. J.; Sachar, D. B.; and Smith, H.: A comparison of cancer risk in Crohn's disease and ulcerative colitis. *Cancer,* **48:**2742–2751, 1981.

Grinnell, R. S.: The spread of carcinoma of the colon and rectum. *Cancer,* **3:**641–652, 1950.

Grinnell, R. S.: Lymphatic block with atypical and retrograde metastasis and spread in carcinoma of the colon and rectum. *Ann. Surg.,* **163:**272–279, 1966.

Gunderson, L. L., and Sosin, H.: Areas of failure found at re-operation (second or systematic look) following "curative surgery" for adenocarcinoma of the rectum. *Cancer,* **34:**1278–1292, 1974.

Haenzel, W.; Berg, J. W.; Segi, H.; Kurhara, M.; and Loche, F. B.: Large bowel cancer in Hawaiian Japanese. *J.N.C.I.,* **51:**1765–1776, 1973.

Hahn, R. G.; Moertel, C. G.; Schutt, A. J.; and Bruckner, H. W.: A double-blind comparison of intensive course 5-FU by oral vs. intravenous route in the treatment of colorectal carcinoma. *Cancer,* **35:**1031, 1975.

Hallstrand, D. E.: Carcinoma of the colon and rectum. *Surg. Gynecol. Obstet.,* **99:**234–240, 1954.

Haubrich, W. S.: Embryology of the small and large intestines and anomalies of the small intestine. In Bockrus, H. L. (ed.): *Gastroenterology,* Vol. 2. W. B. Saunders Company, Philadelphia, 1963.

Healey, J. E.: Vascular patterns in human metastatic liver tumors. *Surg. Gynecol. Obstet.,* **120:**1187, 1965.

Heidelberger, C.: Fluorinated pyrimidines, a new class of tumor inhibitory compound. *Nature,* **179:**663, 1957.

Higgins, G. A.; Conn. J. H.; Jordan, P. H.; Humphrey, E. W.; Roswit, B.; and Keehn, R. J.: Preoperative radiotherapy for colorectal cancer. *Ann. Surg.,* **181:**624–631, 1975.

Hill, M. J.; Crowther, J. S.; and Drasar, B. S.: Bacteria and etiology of cancer of the large bowel. *Lancet,* **1:**95–100, 1971.

Jackman, R. J., and Beahrs, O. H.: Surgical anatomic aspects of the colon and rectum and pathways of malignant spread. In *Tumors of the Large Bowel.* W. B. Saunders Company, Philadelphia, 1968.

Jacobs, E. M.; Reeves, W. J.; Wood, D. A.; Pugh, R.; Braunwald, J.; and Bateman, J. R.: Treatment of cancer with weekly intravenous 5-fluorouracil. *Cancer,* **127:**1302, 1972.

Jacobs, M. N.; Jansson, B.; and Griffin, A. C.: Inhibitory effects of selenium on 1,2-dimethylhydrazine and methylazoxymethanol acetate induction of colon tumors. *Cancer Lett.,* **2:**133–138, 1977.

Jansson, B.; Jacobs, M. N.; and Griffin, A. C.: Gastrointestinal cancer: Epidemiology and experimental strides. *Adv. Exp. Med. Biol.,* **91:**305–322, 1978.

Jensen, O. M., and MacLennan, R.: Dietary factors and colorectal cancer in Scandinavia. *Isr. J. Med. Sci.,* **15:**329–335, 1979.

Jones, R. S., and Sleisenger, M. H.: Cancer of the colon and rectum. In Sleisenger, M. H., and Fordtran, J. S. (eds.): *Gastro-intestinal Disease.* W. B. Saunders Company, Philadelphia, 1973.

Kane, R. C.; Cashdollar, M. R.; and Bernath, A. M.: Treatment of advanced colorectal cancer with methyl CCNU plus 5 day 5-fluorouracil infusion, *Cancer Treat. Rep.,* **62:**1521, 1978.

Kemeny, N.; Daly, J.; Oderman, P.; Chun, H.; Petroni, G.; and Geller, N.: Randomized study of intrahepatic vs. systemic infusion of flourodeoxyuridine in patients with liver metastases from colorectal carcinoma. *Proc. Am. Soc. Clin. Oncol.*, **3**:141, 1984.

Kemeny, N.; Yagoda, A.; and Golbey, R.: Randomized study of 2 different schedules of methyl CCNU (MeCCNU), 5-fluorouracil (5-FU), and vincristine (VCR) for metastatic colorectal carcinoma. *Proc. A.S.C.O*, **18**:336, 1977.

Kemeny, N.; Yagoda, A.; and Golbey, R.: Methyl-CCNU, 5-fluorouracil, vincristine and streptozotocin for metastatic colorectal cancer. *Proc. A.S.C.O.*, **19**:354, 1978.

Kemeny, N.; Yagoda, A.; and Golbey, R.: A prospective, randomized study of methyl CCNU, 5-fluorouracil and vincristine (MOF) vs. MOF plus streptozotocin (MOF-STREP). *Cancer*, **51**:20–24, 1983.

Khankhanian, N. K.; Russell, W. O.; and Mavligit, G. M.: Prognostic significance of vascular invasion in colorectal cancer of the Dukes' B class. *Proc. Am. Assoc. Cancer Res. and A.S.C.O.*, **17**:32, 1976.

Khung, C. L.; Hal, T. C.; Piro, A. J.; and Dederick, M. M.: A clinical trial of oral 5-fluorouracil. *Clin. Pharmacol. Ther.*, **7**:527, 1966.

Killen, J. Y.; Holyoke, E. D.; Mittelman, A.; Pickren, J.; Evans, J.; Moertel, C. G.; O'Connell, M. J.; Schutt, A. I.; Rubin, J. R.; McIlrath, D. C.; Lokich, J.; Mayer, R.; Schein, P. S.; Smith, F.; Woolley, P.; Horton, J.; Eckert, C.; Bruckner, H. W.; Aufses, A. A.; Lessner, H. E.; Kalser, M. H.; Kaplan, R. S.; Livingston, A.; Levin, B.; Enker, W.; Bonadonna, G.; Gennari, L.; Castellani, R.; Golbey, R. B.; Stearns, M.; Ramming, K. P.; Van Lancker, J.; Wright, H.; and Ellenberg, S. S.: Adjuvant therapy of adenocarcinoma of the colon following clinically curative resection: An interim report from the gastrointestinal tumor study group (GITSG). *Adjuvant Therapy of Cancer III.* Grune & Stratton, Inc., New York, 1981.

Kim, D. K.; McSweeney, J.; and Yeh, S. D.: Tumours of the liver as demonstrated by angiography, scan and laparotomy. *Surg. Gynecol. Obstet.*, **141**:409–410, 1975.

Kirklin, J. W.; Docherty, M. B.; and Waugh, J. M.: The role of the peritoneal reflection in the prognosis of carcinoma of the rectum and sigmoid colon. *Surg. Gynecol. Obstet.*, **88**:326–331, 1949.

Kligerman, M. M.: Preoperative radiation therapy in rectal cancer. *Cancer*, **36**:691–695, 1975.

Kligerman, M. M.: Radiation therapy for rectal carcinoma. *Semin. Oncol.*, **3**:407–413, 1976.

Lahiri, S. R.; Boileau,; and Hall, T. C.: Treatment of metastatic colorectal carcinoma with 5-fluorouracil by mouth. *Cancer*, **28**:902, 1971.

Leaming, R. H.; Stearns, M. W., Jr.; and Deddish, M. R.: Preoperative irradiation in rectal carcinoma. *Radiology*, **77**:257–263, 1961.

Leonard-Jones, J. E.; Morson, B. C.; Ritchie, J. K.; Shove, D. C.; and Williams, C. B.: Cancer in colitis: Assessment of the individual risk of clinical and histological criteria. *Gastroenterology*, **73**:1280–1289, 1977.

Leone, L. A.: The chemotherapy of colorectal cancer. *Cancer*, **34**:972, 1974.

Lessner, H. E.; Mayer, R. J.; Ellenberg, S.; Holyoke, E. D.; Lokich, J. J.; and Wright, H.: Adjuvant therapy of colon cancer—A prospective randomized trial. *Proc. Am. Soc. Clin. Oncol.*, **1**:91(C-351), 1982.

Lokich, J. J.; Skarin, A. T.; Mayer, R. J.; and Frei, E.: Lack of effectiveness of combined 5-flourouracil and methyl CCNU therapy in advanced colorectal cancer. *Cancer*, **40**:2792, 1977.

Lynch, H. T.; Gurgis, H.; Lynch, J.; Brodley, F. D.; and

MaGee, H.: Cancer of the colon: Socioeconomic varibles in a community. *Am. J. Epidemiol.* **102**:119, 1975.

Lynch, P. M.; Lynch, H. Y.; and Harris, R. E.: Hereditary proximal colon cancer. *Dis. Colon Rectum*, **20**:661–674, 1977.

Machover, L.; Schwarzenberg, L.; Goldschmidt, E.; Toukani, J. M.; Michalski, B.; Hayat, M.; Noreval, T.; Misset, J. L.; Jasmin, C.; Makal, R.; and Mathe, G.: Treatment of advanced colorectal and gastric adenocarcinomous with 5-FU combined with high dose folinic acid. *Cancer Treat. Rep.*, **10**:1803–1809, 1982.

Macklin, M. T.: Inheritance of cancer of the stomach and large intestine. *Am. J. Hum. Genet.*, **10**:42–50, 1966.

Mann, J. D.; Wakim, K. G.; and Baggenstoss, A. H.: The vasculature of the human liver: A study by injection-cast method. *Mayo Clin. Proc.*, **28**:227, 1953.

Maskens, A. P.: Histogenesis of adenomatous polyps in the human large intestine. *Gastroenterology*, **77**:1245–1251, 1979.

Maskens, A. P., and Deschner, E. E.: Tritiated thymidine incorporation into epithelial cells of normal-appearing colorectal mucosa of cancer patients. *J.N.C.I.*, **58**:1221–1224, 1972.

Mastromarino, A.; Reddy, B. S.; and Wynder, E. C.: Metabolic epidemiology of colon cancer enzyme activity of fecal flora. *Am. J. Clin. Nutr.*, **29**:1455–1462, 1976.

McDonald, W. C.; Trer, J. S.; and Everett, N. D.: Cell proliferation and migration in the stomach, duodenum and rectum of man: Radioautographic studies. *Gastroenterology*, **46**:405–417, 1964.

Miller, R. E.: Detection of colon carcinoma and the barium enema. *J.A.M.A.*, **230**:1195–1199, 1974.

Mittelman, A.; Holyoke, E.; Thomas, P. R. M.; Moertel, C. G.; Childs, D. S.; Weiland, L.; Horton, J.; Baxter, D.; Eckert, C.; Levin, B.; Kinzie, J.; Schein, P.; Smith, F.; Dritschilo, A.; Bonadonna, G.; Gennari, L.; Lattuada, A.; Castellani, R.; Golbey, R. B.; Leaming, R.; Kalser, M. H.; Kaplan, R. S.; Lessner, H. E.; Charyulu, K.; Bruckner, H. W.; Aufses, A.; Barba, J.; Mayer, R.; Lokich, J.; Chaffey, J.; Corson, J.; Ramming, K. P.; Langdon, E. A.; Mitchell, M. S.; George, F. W.; Livstone, E. M.; Spiro, H. M.; Knowlton, A.; Novak, J. W.; Ellenberg, S. S.; and Haller, D. G.: Adjuvant chemotherapy and radiotherapy following rectal surgery: An interim report from the Gastrointestinal Tumor Study Group (GITSG). *Adjuvant Therapy of Cancer III.* Grune & Stratton, Inc., New York, 1981.

Modan, B.: Dietary fiber in cancer etiology. *Cancer*, **40**:1887–1891, 1977.

Moertel, C. G.: Large bowel. In Holland, J. F., and Frei, E., III (eds.): *Cancer Medicine.* Lea & Febiger, Philadelphia, 1973.

Moertel, C. G.: Therapy of advanced gastrointestinal cancer with the nitrosoureas. *Cancer Chemother. Rep.* **4**:27, 1973.

Moertel, C. G.: Clinical management of advanced gastrointestinal cancer. *Cancer*, **36**:675, 1975.

Moertel, C. G.: Chemotherapy of gastrointestinal cancer. *N. Engl. J. Med.*, **299**:1049, 1978.

Moertel, C. G.; Bargen, J. A.; and Dockerty, M. B.: Multiple carcinomas of the large intestine: A review of the literature and a study of 261 cases. *Gastroenterology*, **34**:85–98, 1958.

Moertel, C. G.; Reitemeier, R. J.; and Hahn, R. G.: Therapy with the fluorinated pyrimidines. In Moertel, C. G., and Reitemeier, R. J. (eds.): *Advanced Gastrointestinal Cancer.* Hoeber-Harper, New York, 1969.

Moertel, C. G.; Reitemeier, R. J.; and Hahn, R. G.: Combination chemotherapy in advanced gastrointestinal cancer. *Cancer Res.* **30:**1425, 1970.

Moertel, C. G.; Schutt, A. J.; Hahn, R. G.; and Reitemeier, R. J.: Therapy of advanced colorectal cancer with a combination of 5-fluorouracil methyl-1, 3-cis-(2-chlorethyl)-1-nitrosourea and vincristine. *J.N.C.I.,* **54:**69, 1975.

Moore, W. E. C.; Cato, E. P.; Good, I. J.; and Holdeman, L.: The effect of diet on the human fecal flora. Gastrointestinal Cancer: Endogenous Factors. Cold Spring Harbor Laboratory, Cold Spring Harbor, New York, 1981.

Morson, B. C. (in collaboration with Sobin, L.): Histological typing of intestinal tumours. *International Histological Classification of Tumours,* No. 15. World Health Organization, Geneva, 1976.

Morson, B. C.; Bussey, H. J. R.; and Samoorian, S.: Policy of local excision for early cancer of the colorectum. *Gut,* **18:**1045–1050, 1977.

Morson, B. C., and Day, D. W.: Pathology of adenomas and cancer of the large bowel. J. J. De Cosse, (ed.): *Large Bowel Cancer.* Churchill Livingstone, Inc., New York, 1981.

Morson, B. C.; Whiteway, J. E.; Jones, E. A.; Macrae, F. A.; and Williams, C. B.: Histopathology and prognosis of malignant colorectal polyps treated by endoscopic polypectomy. *Gut,* **25:**437–444, 1984.

Mower, H. F.; Ray, R. M.; Shoff, R.; Stemmerman, G. N.; Nomura, A.; and Glober, E.: Fecal bile acids in two Japanese populations with different colon cancer risks. *Cancer Res.,* **39:**28, 1979.

Muto, T.; Bussey, H. J. R.; and Morson, B. C.: The evolution of cancer of the colon and rectum. *Cancer,* **36:**2251–2260, 1975.

Narisawa, T.; Magadia, N. E.; Weisberger, J. H.; and Wynder, E. L.: Promoting effect of bile acids on colon carcinogenesis after intrarectal instillation of N-methyl-N'-nitro-N-nitrosoquanidine in rats. *J.N.C.I.,* **55:**1093–1097, 1974.

Nichols, R. L.; Broido, P.; Condon, R. E.; Gorbach. S. L.; and Nyhus, L. M.: Effect of preoperative neomycin-erythromycin intestinal preparation on the incidence of infectious complications following colon surgery. *Ann. Surg.,* **178:**453, 1973.

Nigro, N. D.; Bhadrachari, N.; and Chomchal, C. D.: A rat model for studying colonic cancer: Effort of cholestyramine on induced tumors. *Dis. Colon Rectum,* **16:**438–443, 1973.

Olson, R. M.; Perencevich, N. P.; Malcolm, A. W.; Chaffey, J. T.; and Wilson, R. E.: Patterns of recurrence following curative resection of adenocarcinomas of the colon and rectum. *Cancer,* **45:**2969–2974, 1980.

Padilla, F.; Correa, J.; Buroker, T.; and Vaitkevicius, V. K.: Phase II study of Baker's antifol in advanced colorectol cancer. *Cancer Treat. Rep.,* **62:**553, 1978.

Painter, N. S., and Burkitt, D. P.: Diverticular disease of the colon: A deficiency disease of Western civilization. *Br. Med. J.,* **2:**450–454, 1971.

Papillon, J.: Intracavitary irradiation of early rectal cancer for cure: A series of 186 cases. *Cancer,* **36:**696–701, 1975.

Patterson, D. S, and Alpert, E.: Tumor markers of the gastrointestinal tract. In Hodgson, H. J. F. and Bloom, S. R. (eds.): *Gastrointestinal and Hepatobiliary Cancer.* Chapman and Hall, London, 1983.

Phillips, R. L.: Role of life-style and dietary habits in risk of

cancer among Seventh-Day Adventists. *Cancer Res.,* **35:**3513–3522, 1975.

Pickren, J. W.: Nodal clearance and detection. *J.A.M.A.,* **231:**969-971, 1975.

Platz, C.: The staging and pathology of colonic carcinomas and adenomas. In Enker, W. E., (ed.): *Carcinoma of the Colon and Rectum.* Year Book Medical Publishers, Inc., Chicago, 1978.

Pomare, E. W., and Heaton, K. W.: Alteration of bile salt metabolism by dietary fibre. *Gut,* **14:**826–832, 1973.

Posey, L., and Morgan, L. R.: Methyl-CCNU vs. methyl-CCNU and 5-fluorouracil in carcinoma of the large bowel. *Cancer Treat. Rep.* **61:**1453, 1977.

Quan, S. H.: Preoperative radiation for carcinoma of the rectum. *N.Y. State J. Med.,* **66:**2243, 1966.

Reddy, B. S.: Dietary factors and cancer of the large bowel. *Semin. Oncol.,* **3:**351–359, 1976.

Reddy, B. S.; Hedges, A. R.; Laakso, K.; and Wynder, E. L.: Metabolic epidemiology of large bowel cancer: Fecal bulk and constituents of high risk North American and low risk Finnish populations. *Cancer,* **42:**2832, 1978.

Reddy, B. S.; Narisawa, T.; Weisburger, J. H.; Narasawa, T.; Weisburger, J. H.; and Wynder, E. L.: Promoting effect of sodium deoxycholate on adenocarcinomas in germ free rats. *J.N.C.I.,* **56:**441–442, 1976.

Reddy, B. S., and Wynder, E. L.: Metabolic epidemiology of colon cancer—Fecal bile acids and neutral steroids in colon cancer patients and patients with adenomatous polyps. *Cancer,* **39:**2533–2539, 1977.

Reichmann, A.; Martin, P.; and Levin, B.: Karyotypic findings in a colonic villous adenoma. *Cancer Genet. Cytogenet.,* **7:**51–57, 1982.

Rickert, R. R.; Auerbach, O.; Garfinkel, L.; Hammond, E. C.; and Frasca, J. M.: Adenomatous lesions of the large bowel. An autopsy study. *Cancer,* **43:**1847–1856, 1979.

Riddell, R. H., *et al.:* Dysplasia in inflammatory bowel disease: Standardized classification with provisional clinical implications. *Hum. Pathol.* **14:**931–968, 1983.

Rider, J. A.; Kirsner, J. B.; and Moeller, H. C.: Polyps of colon and rectum. *J.A.M.A.,* **170:**633–638, 1959.

Roswit, B.; Higgins, G. A.; and Keehn, R. J.: Preoperative irradiation for carcinoma of the rectum and rectosigmoid colon: Report of a national Veterans Administration randomized study. *Cancer,* **35:**1597, 1975.

Sanfelippo, P. M., and Beahrs, O. H.: Factors in the prognosis of adenocarcinoma of the colon and rectum. *Arch. Surg.,* **104:**401–405, 1972.

Sawhney, K. K., and Kambouris, A. A.: Carcinoma of right colon. *Rev. Surg.,* **31:**130–132, 1974.

Schottenfeld, D.; Berg, J. W.; and Vitsky, B.: Incidence of multiple primary cancers. II. Index cancers in the stomach and lower digestive system. *J.N.C.I.,* **43:**77–86, 1969.

Schottenfeld, D., and Haas, J. F.: Epidemiology of colorectal cancer. In Lipkin, M., and Good, R. A. (eds.): *Gastrointestinal Tract Cancer.* Plenum Publishing Corp., New York, 1978.

Schottenfeld, D., and Winawer, S.: Large intestine. In Schottenfeld, D., and Fraumeni, J. (eds.): *Cancer Epidemiology and Prevention.* W. B. Saunders Company, Philadelphia, 1982.

Seifert, P.; Baker, L. H.; Reed, M. L.; and Vaitkevicius, V. K.: Comparison of continuously infused 5-fluorouracil with bolus injection in treatment of patients with colorectal adenocarcinoma. *Cancer,* **36:**123, 1975.

Sherlock, P.; Lipkin, M.; and Winawer, S J.: Predisposing factors in carcinoma of the colon. *Adv. Intern. Med.,* **20:**121–150, 1975.

Sischy, B., and Remington, J. H.: Treatment of carcinoma of the rectum by interstitial irradiation. *Surg. Gynecol. Obstet.,* **141:**562–564, 1975.

Sischy, B.; Remington, J. H.; and Sokel, S. H.: Treatment of rectal carcinomas by means of endocavitary irradiation: A progress report. *Cancer,* **46:**1957–1961, 1980.

Sleisenger, M. H.: Physiology of the colon. In Sleisenger, M. H., and Fordtran, J. S. (eds.): *Gastrointestinal Disease.* W. B. Saunders Company, Philadelphia, 1973.

Smith, F. P.; Ellenberg, S. S.; Mayer, R. J.; Lessner, H. E.; and Horton, J.: Phase II study of MOF strep (methyl-CCNU, vincristine, 5-fluorouracil, streptozotocin) in advanced measurable colorectal carcinoma. *Proc. A.S.C.O.,* **23:**149, 1982.

Spratt, J. S., and Spjut, H. J.: Prevalence and prognosis of individual clinical and pathologic variables associated with colorectal carcinoma. *Cancer,* **20:**1976–1985, 1967.

Stearns, M. W., and Deddish, M. R.: Five year results of abdominopelvic lymph node dissection for carcinoma of the rectum. *Dis. Colon Rectum,* **2:**169–172, 1959.

Stearns, M. W.; Deddish, M. R.; Quan, S. H.; and Leaming, R. H.: Preoperative roentgen therapy for cancer of the rectum and rectosigmoid. *Surg. Gynecol. Obstet.,* **138:**584–586, 1975.

Stearns, M. W., and Schottenfeld, D.: Techniques for the surgical management of colon cancer. *Cancer,* **28:**165–169, 1971.

Stemmerman, G. N.; Nomura, A. M. Y.; Mower, H.; and Glober, G.: Clues (true or false) to the origin of colorectal cancer. In DeCosse, J. J. (ed.): *Large Bowel Cancer.* Churchill Livingstone, Inc., New York, 1981.

Stemmerman, G. N., and Yatani, R.: Diverticulosis and polyps of the large intestine: A necropsy study of Hawaii Japanese. *Cancer,* **31:**1260, 1973.

Swinton, N. W.; Hare, H. F.; and Meissner, W. A.: Diagnosis of cancer in the large bowel. *J.A.M.A.,* **140:**463–469, 1949.

Taylor, I.; Bhooman, P.; and Rowling, J. T.: Adjuvant liver perfusion in colorectal cancer: Initial results of a clinical trial, *Br. Med. J.,* **2:**1320–1322, 1977.

Thomas, W. H.; Larson, R. A.; Wright, H. K.; and Cleveland, J. C.: Analysis of 830 patients with rectal adenocarcinoma. *Surg. Gynecol. Obstet.* **129:**10–14, 1969.

Traube, J.; Simpson, S.; Riddell, R. H.; Levin, B.; and Kirsner, J. B.: Crohn's disease and adenocarcinoma of the bowel. *Dig. Dis. Sci.,* **25:**939–944, 1980.

Trowell, H. C.: Crude fiber, dietary fiber and atherosclerosis. *Atherosclerosis,* **16:**38–46, 1972.

Turcot, J.; Defres, J. P.; and St. Pierre, F.: Malignant tumors of the central nervous system associated with familial polyposis of the colon. *Dis. Colon Rectum.,* **2:**465–468, 1959.

Turnbull, R. A.: The no touch isolation technique of resection. *J.A.M.A.,* **231:**1181–1182, 1975.

Turnbull, R. B.; Kyle, K.; Watson, F. R.; and Spratt J.: Cancer of the colon: The influence of the no-touch isolation technique on survival rates. *Ann. Surg.,* **160:**420–425, 1967.

Tutton, P. J. M., and Barkla, D. H.; Neutral control of cell proliferation in colonic carcinogenesis. In Malt, R. A., and Williamson, R. C. N. (eds.): *Colonic Carcinogenesis.* MTP Press, Lancaster, 1982.

Utsonomiya, J.; Iwana, T.; and Hirayama, R.: Familial large bowel cancer. In DeCosse, J. J. (ed.): *Large Bowel Cancer.* Churchill Livingstone, Inc., New York, 1981.

Valdivieso, M.; Bodey, G. P.; Gottlied, J. B.; and Freireich, E. J.: Clinical evaluation of ftorafur. *Cancer Res.,* **367:**1821, 1976.

Vernick, L. J.; Kuller, L. H.; and Lohsoonthorn, P.: Relationship between cholecystectomy and ascending colon cancer. *Cancer,* **45:**392–395, 1980.

Visiting Faculty Program, Monograph, Winawer, S. J. (exec. ed.): *Colorectal Cancer: Essentials for Primary Care Physicians, 1982.* Office of Continuing Medical Education, Memorial Sloan-Kettering Cancer Center, New York, 1982.

Walker, A. R. P., and Burkitt, D. P.: Colon cancer: epidemiology. *Semin. Oncol.,* **3:**341–350, 1976.

Wanebo, J. H.; Rao, B.; Pinsky, C. M.; Hoffman, R. G.; Stearns, M.; Schwartz, M. K.; and Oettgen, H. F.: Preoperative carcinoembryonic antigen level as a prognostic indicator in colorectal cancer. *N. Engl. J. Med.,* **299:**448, 1978a.

Wanebo, J. H.; Semoglou, C.; and Attiyeh, F.: Surgical management of patients with primary operable colorectal cancer and synchronous liver metastasis. *Am. J. Surg.,* **136:**81–85, 1978b.

Washington, J. A.; Dearing, W. H.; Judd, E. S.; and Elveback, L. R.: Effect of preoperative antibiotic regimen on development of infection after intestinal surgery. *Ann. Surg.,* **180:**567, 1974.

Wasserman, T. H.; Comis, R. L.; Goldsmith, M.; Handelsman, H.; Penta, J. S.; Slavik, M.; Soper, W. T.; and Carter, S. K.: Tabular analysis of the clinical chemotherapy of solid tumors. *Cancer Chemother. Rep.,* **6:**399, 1975.

Waterhouse, J.; Muir, C.; Correa, P.; and Powell, J.: *Cancer Incidence in Five Continents,* Vol. 3. International Agency for Research on Cancer, Lyon, 1976.

Wattenberg, L. W.: Inhibitors of chemical carcinogenesis. *Adv. Cancer Res.,* **26:**197–223, 1978.

Weedon, D. D.; Shorter, R. G.; and Ilstrup, D. M.: Crohn's disease and cancer. *N. Engl. J. Med.,* **289:**1099–1104, 1973.

Weisburger, J. H.; Wynder, E. L.; and Horn, C. L.: Nutritional factors and etiologic mechanisms in the causation of gastrointestinal cancer. *Cancer,* **50:**2541–2549, 1982.

Williams, R. R.; Sorlie, P. D.; Feinleib, M.; McNamara, P. M.; Kannel, W. B.; and Dawber, T. R.: Cancer incidence by levels of cholesterol. *J.A.M.A.,* **245:**247–252, 1981.

Wilson, S. M., and Adson, M. A.: Surgical treatment of hepatic metastases from colorectal cancers. *Arch. Surg.,* **111:**330–334, 1976.

Winawer, S. J.: Colon cancer. In Hunt, R. H., and Waye, J. D. (eds.): *Colonoscopy.* Chapman and Hall, England, 1981.

Winawer, S. J., and Sherlock, P.: Approach to screening and diagnosis in colorectal cancer. *Semin. Oncol.,* **3:**387–397, 1976.

Winawer, S. J., and Sherlock, P.: Surveillance for colorectal cancer in average risk patients, familial high risk groups and in patients with adenomas. *Cancer,* **50:**2609–2614, 1982.

Winman, G.; Berci, G.; and Parish, J.: Superiority of the flexible to the rigid sigmoidoscope. *N. Engl. J. Med.,* **302:**1011–1012, 1980.

Woolam, G. L.; Mackman, R. J.; Ramiriz, R. J.; Beahrs, O. H.; Dockerty, M. B.: Scirrhous carcinoma of the lower intestine. *Surg. Gynecol. Obstet.,* **121:**753–755, 1965.

Woolley, P. V.: Clinical manifestations of cancer of the colon and rectum. *Semin. Oncol.,* **3:**373–376, 1976.

Woolley, P. V.; Higgins, G. A.; and Schein, P. S.: Ongoing trials in the surgical adjuvant managment of colorectal cancer. *Recent Results Cancer Res.,* **63:**231–235, 1979.

Wynder, E. L., and Reddy, B. S.: Metabolic epidemiology of colorectal cancer. *Cancer,* **39:**801–810, 1977.

31

Neoplasms of the Anus

ROBERT J. COFFEY, Jr. and LEONARD L. GUNDERSON

Introduction

Anal carcinoma is an uncommon lesion, comprising 2 to 4% of all carcinomas of the distal 18 cm of the alimentary tract. The heterogeneity of the tissue types and relative rarity of tumors in this region produce confusion in terminology and uncertainty as to optimum treatment. Major clinical reviews note the long duration of symptoms before the diagnosis is made. The clinician should be aware that anal cancer often coexists with other benign conditions of the anorectum. A high index of suspicion with biopsy of abnormal regions is mandatory in patients with anorectal complaints. Figure 31–1 depicts the variety of malignant tumors that occur in this region. This chapter will focus on primary carcinomas of the anal canal.

Incidence and Epidemiology

The Surveillance, Epidemiology, and End Results (SEER) program of the National Cancer Institute obtained cancer incidence data from 1973 to 1977 from ten population centers within the United States, including five states and five large metropolitan areas (Young et al., 1981). The overall age-adjusted incidence of carcinoma of the anus, anal canal, and anorectum was 0.6 per 100,000 population per year. Incidence rates for white men and women were 0.5 and 0.7, and for nonwhite men and women, 0.7 and 0.9, respectively. A higher incidence for women was seen in nine out of ten reporting areas. Most large hospital series from the United States have also noted a higher prevalence of women among their cases. Several series from Great Britain and the

United States have found a higher prevalence of women among those with anal canal cancers, as compared to a predominance of men among the less common anal margin cancers. Reliable incidence data are not available from most other countries.

In the SEER data, age at diagnosis of anal carcinoma ranged from early twenties to over 85 years old. The median age was 65.5 years. The risk of anal cancer increases with age. The incidence of 0.1 per 100,000 per year at age 35 to 39 years increased to 1.9 at ages 60 to 64, 3.5 at 75 to 79, and 4.7 in those 85 and older.

Etiology

There have been many reports of anal carcinoma occurring in patients with a variety of benign anal conditions including fistula, prolapse, fissure, lymphogranuloma venereum, and condyloma acuminata, as well as following local radiation treatment for benign disease in this region (Stearns et al., 1980; Singh et al., 1981; Lee et al., 1981). In some series as many as 60% of patients have a history of longstanding benign anal conditions antedating their anal carcinoma. Because of the frequency of benign anal disease and the rarity of anal carcinoma, it is hard to establish a temporal or causal relationship between the two. The association of the rare mucinous adenocarcinoma with chronic anal fistula is perhaps the most convincing (Getz et al., 1981). More than 130 cases of this association have been reported in the literature, as well as documentation of progression from adenomatous hyperplasia in the fistula to a well-differentiated adenocarcinoma.

917

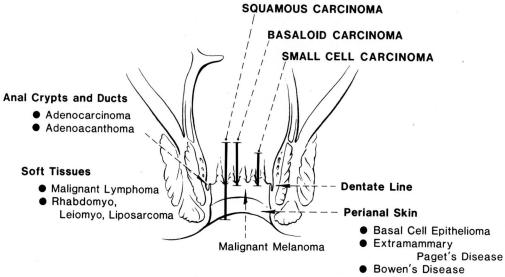

Figure 31–1.   Malignant tumors of the anal region.

Anal cancer has been reported with greater frequency in homosexual men. It has been suggested that anal intercourse may be a risk factor for anal cancer, with infection and/or trauma as the most likely mechanisms. Two additional correlates of homosexual activity in men, an active syphilis serology and never having been married, are related significantly to the incidence of anal cancer (Daling, *et al.,* 1982). Of 189 men between the ages 30 and 79 with anal carcinoma detected by the SEER program, 24% were never married, compared to 7.9% of men with rectal and 7.8% of men with colon cancer. Several large series have noted a high prevalence of multiparous women among their cases of anal cancer. It appears that women with anal carcinoma may have an increased risk of other lower genital tract cancers (Cabrera *et al.,* 1966). The explanation for these associations remains speculative.

Anatomic Considerations and Pathogenesis

Anatomically, the anal canal extends from the anal verge to the dentate line. The surgical anal canal extends more proximally; its proximal limit is the anorectal ring created by the puborectalis muscle. The major anatomic landmarks are noted in Figure 31–2.

As one moves cephalad from the anus, a gradual transition zone is evident between the opaque squamous epithelium below and pink rectal mucosa above. This delicate slighty

darker membrane, derived from the cloaca, and designated the anal transition zone, occurs in the region of the columns of Morgagni, and comprises approximately one-third the length of the anal canal.

The squamous epithelium in the perineal area has characteristic features (sebaceous and sweat glands along with piliary structures), but these dermal appendages are lost as one moves cephalad. The cloaca-derived membrane is composed of transitional epithelium. In addition, anal glands occur in the region of the crypts. The rectal mucosa has typical columnar epithelium. These histologic borders are not sharp; for example, squamous elements often appear above the dentate line, and columnar elements may impinge upon the dentate line.

The sphincter mechanism which surrounds the anal canal is complex. The internal sphincter is a thickening of the circular smooth muscle layer of the rectum; it extends distally to the intersphincteric (Hilton's) line, approximately midway between the dentate line and anal verge. The longitudinal muscle of the rectum continues distally along the anal canal external to the circular muscle and forms the corrugator cutis ani by its fan-shaped insertion into the perianal skin. Encircling these involuntary muscles are two voluntary groups. The puborectalis component of the levator ani group pulls the anorectal angle anteriorly. The external sphincter is thought to be composed of three muscle groups: deep, superficial, and subcutaneous. Currently, however, it is felt

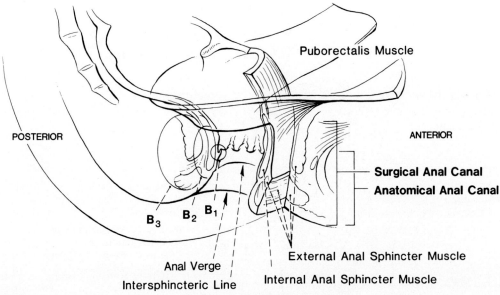

POSTERIOR

Puborectalis Muscle

ANTERIOR

Surgical Anal Canal
Anatomical Anal Canal

B₃   B₂   B₁

External Anal Sphincter Muscle

Anal Verge
Intersphincteric Line

Internal Anal Sphincter Muscle

Figure 31 – 2.   Anatomy of the anal region with modified B staging depicted.

that the three groups act as one continuous muscle mass, which blends with the puborectalis muscle. Lateral to the external sphincter is the fat of the ischiorectal fossa.

The majority of anal carcinomas spread by local extension through the lymphatics. They often spread longitudinally, similar to esophageal carcinoma (Wolfe and Bussey, 1968). Less frequently, they metastasize through the blood stream. The major lymphatic drainage patterns are outlined in Figure 31 – 3. They follow the course of the arterial system. Above the dentate line, the lymphatics drain cephalad via the superior rectal (hemorrhoidal) lymphatics to the inferior mesenteric nodes, and laterally via the middle and inferior rectal vessels to the internal iliac nodes. Below the dentate line, lymph usually drains to the inguinal lymph nodes. Although the location of the primary tumor largely determines the direction of lymphatic spread, exceptions are numerous. It should be emphasized that the lymphatics are rich and the interconnections numerous in the anal region. With obstruction, the usual pattern of spread may be altered. In the experience reported from Memorial Hospital, 6 of 33 patients (18%) with lesions below the dentate line had mesenteric nodal metastasis (Stearn *et al.,* 1980); earlier studies showed that one-third of patients with cancers of the anal margin had mesenteric node involvement (Dillard *et al.,* 1963; Sawyers *et al.,* 1963; Hardy *et al.,* 1969).

The venous drainage pattern is dual, portal, and systemic. The superior rectal (hemorrhoidal) veins drain the upper part of the anal canal into the portal system via the inferior mesenteric vein. The middle rectal veins drain the upper part of the anal canal into the systemic circulation via the internal iliac veins. The inferior rectal veins drain the lower anal canal into the systemic circulation from the internal pudendal veins which empty into the internal iliac veins. Venous invasion results in blood-borne metastasis to liver, lung, bone, and peritoneum in that order of frequency.

Pathology

Because of the differing histologic elements present and the frequent intermixing of such elements in any one tumor, classifications of primary anal tumors have tended to be cumbersome and confusing. The World Health Organization's (WHO) histologic classification of anal carcinomas (Morson and Sobin, 1976) includes:

1. Squamous cell carcinoma
2. Basaloid carcinoma (cloacogenic)
3. Mucoepidermoid carcinoma
4. Adenocarcinoma
5. Undifferentiated carcinoma

Grossly these tumors do not differ in appearance and tend to be ulcerative.

Most reported series focus on squamous cell

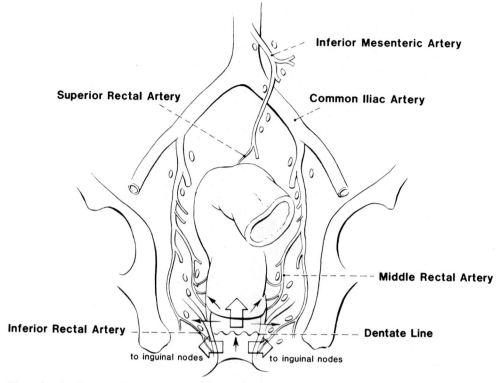

Figure 31–3. Routes of lymphatic spread of anal carcinoma.

and basaloid carcinoma since they are the predominant types. Pathologically, squamous cell and basaloid carcinomas are on a continuum, and an individual tumor often contains elements of both. Squamous cell carcinoma (see Figure 31–4) may occur throughout the length of the anal canal. The lesion tends to be high grade. It grows in strands with islands of tumor cells intermixed. The centers of these islands contain large cells with occasional keratinized cytoplasm. Basaloid carcinoma (see Figure 31–5) is considered a variety of squamous cell carcinoma. The term cloacogenic carcinoma has been used synonymously with basaloid carcinoma, as well as for tumors arising from the cloacogenic zone. Although it is similiar histologically to basal cell carcinoma of the skin with its cohesive growth pattern, well-defined tumor margins, and distinctive palisading of its superficial layer, it differs because of its greater metastatic potential. Basaloid carcinoma arises primarily above the dentate line. The lesion is poorly differentiated in most cases. A number of these lesions will have scattered amounts of keratin present, underlining the overlap with squamous cell carcinoma.

Small cell carcinoma (see Figure 31–6) is a subset of undifferentiated carcinoma by the WHO classification. It is characterized by undifferentiated plump spindling cells that grow in patternless sheets, diffusely infiltrating the surrounding tissue. Small cell carcinoma is of considerable interest because of its probable neuroendocrine origin and aggressive nature (Weatherby *et al.,* 1983).

Mucoepidermoid carcinoma resembles the salivary gland tumor.

Adenocarcinomas comprise three subtypes: rectal type, the most frequent form of adenocarcinoma in the anal canal; anal gland type, a rare tumor composed of small acini and tubules with little mucin production; and those arising in anorectal fistula, which are frequently mucinous.

Staging

The three major staging systems for anal carcinomas are outlined in Table 31–1.

The recent Mayo Clinic series (Boman *et al.,* 1984) used the ABC system. In this series, stage B was modified: B_1, invasion into the internal sphincter; B_2, invasion into the external

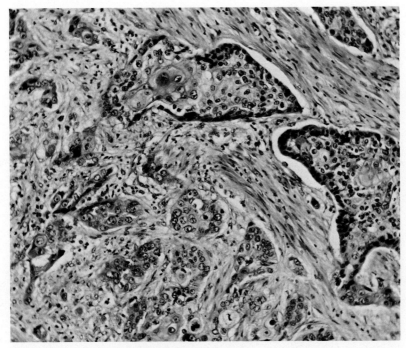

Figure 31–4.   Squamous cell carcinoma of the anus.

sphincter; B_3, invasion into adjacent pelvic tissues (see Figure 31–2). As discussed below, this modification has prognostic significance. Some researchers favor incorporating this modification into the ABC staging system.

Natural History

The Mayo Clinic has recently reported its experience with 189 cases of carcinoma of the anal canal observed between 1950 and 1976

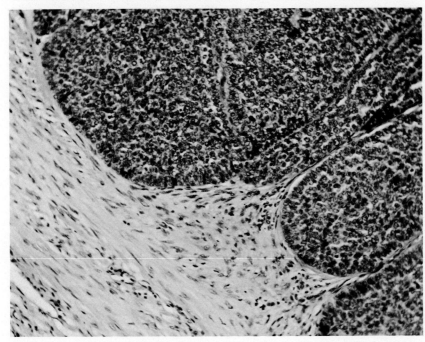

Figure 31–5.   Basaloid carcinoma of the anus.

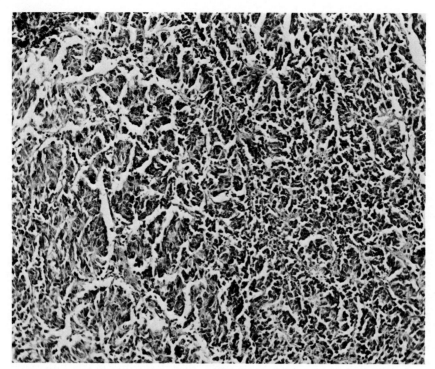

Figure 31–6. Small cell carcinoma of the anus.

(Boman *et al.,* 1984). Squamous cell, basaloid, and small cell carcinoma comprised the major histologic subtypes. Figure 31–7 shows survival by stage for 157 patients with squamous cell and basaloid carcinoma. This includes those who had local excision for superficial lesions (stage A), those who underwent abdominoperineal resection (stage B and C), and those with advanced lesions (stage D). Three patients with early postoperative deaths are excluded from analysis. Because of its more aggressive nature, patients with small-cell carcinoma were analyzed separately. As can be seen, stage is associated with survival. The Kaplan-Meier estimated five-year survival for stage A is 100%; for stage B, 74%; for stage C, 54%; and for stage D, only 6%. The modified B staging was correlated with survival at five years by chi square analysis. An 88% survival was observed for B_1 lesions at five years, compared to a 62% survival for B_3 lesions, with B_2 lesions in an intermediate position with a 79% five-year survival (P < 0.01 by chi square analysis).

No clear consensus has been reported in the literature concerning the natural history of the different histologic types. In the Mayo Clinic series, survival rates were related to tumor histology. Low-grade squamous cell carcinoma was associated with good patient survival, high-grade squamous cell carcinoma and basaloid carcinoma were associated with intermediate survival, and small cell carcinoma was associated with poor survival. The survivorship differences for squamous and basaloid carcinoma were closely related to the stage at which the patient presented, since the tumors of low-grade anaplasia more frequently presented with early-stage lesions. When corrected for stage, these survivorship differences according to histology were not statistically significant (Cox model $P = 0.62$).

Most series have noted an ominous prognosis for patients with inguinal node involvement at the time of initial surgery (Bowman *et al.,* 1984). In the Mayo Clinic series, however, neither the site of nodal involvement (inguinal versus pelvic) nor number of metastatically involved nodes showed prognostic significance.

The prognostic importance of the size of the primary lesion is unclear. Several studies have reported it to be prognostically significant (Stearns *et al.,* 1980), but in the overall Mayo Clinic series it was not an independent prognostic factor.

In most previous series, incidence and patterns of failure have been difficult to ascertain. In two small series from M. D. Anderson Hos-

Table 31–1. Staging Systems for Primary Carcinomas of the Anal Canal

1. ABC Classification (Richards *et al.*, 1962)
   A Tumor confined to anal mucosa and submucosa
   B Invasion into extra-anal tissues without regional lymph node involvement
   C Metastasis into regional lymph nodes

2. Roswell Park Classification (Paradis *et al.*, 1975)
   0 Carcinoma *in situ*
   I Sphincter muscle not involved
   II Sphincter muscle involved
   III Regional metastasis
      A Perirectal nodes only
      B Inguinal nodes
   IV Distant metastasis

3. TNM Pretreatment and Postsurgical Classification (Harmer, 1978)
   T Primary tumor
   T_{is} Preinvasive carcinoma (carcinoma *in situ*)
   T_0 No evidence of primary tumor
   T_1 Tumor occupying not more than one-third of the circumference or length of the canal and not infiltrating the external sphincter muscle
   T_2 Tumor occupying more than one-third of the circumference or length of the anal canal or tumor infiltrating the external sphincter muscle
   T_3 Tumor with extension to rectum or skin but not to other neighboring structures
   T_4 Tumor with extension to neighboring structures
   T_x The minimum requirements to assess the primary tumor cannot be met

   N Regional lymph nodes
   N_0 No evidence of regional lymph node involvement
   N_1 Evidence of involvement of regional lymph nodes
   N_x The minimum requirements to assess the regional lymph nodes cannot be met

   M Distant metastasis
   M_0 No evidence of distant metastasis
   M_1 Evidence of distant metastasis
   M_x The minimum requirements to assess the presence of distant metastasis cannot be met

pital, the risk for local recurrence was analyzed separately for patients with transitional cloacogenic carcinoma (basaloid carcinoma) versus those with squamous cell carcinoma following abdominoperineal resection (Svenson and Montague, 1980; Sugarbaker *et al.*, 1982). For those with transitional cloacogenic carcinoma, surgery alone failed to control local disease in one out of six patients with negative nodes (tumor greater than 2-cm diameter), and six out of nine patients with positive nodes. In a group of 69 patients who underwent curative abdominoperineal resection for squamous cell carcinoma of the anal region between 1948 and 1975, pelvic recurrence occurred in only 1 out of 20 patients (5%), with

tumors less than 3 cm and negative nodes, but markedly increased to 33% in the group with tumors greater than 3 cm and/or with involved nodes. In an analysis from Roswell Park, patterns of failure were analyzed in a more comprehensive fashion (Singh *et al.*, 1981). Incidence and patterns of failure were similar for basaloid and squamous lesions. Local recurrence was more common than distant metastasis; this was related to initial extent of disease and to type of initial treatment. From this analysis, the risk of local recurrence increased once the lesion extended beyond the submucosa into the surrounding muscle. Small patient numbers did not allow differentiation by depth of invasion into the muscular layers.

Of those patients with squamous cell and basaloid carcinoma treated surgically in the Mayo Clinic series, the overall incidence of recurrent disease was 37% (49/134). Of these 49 recurrences, 41 had documented sites of recurrence. The large majority (70%) were local (pelvic) recurrences. A 15% incidence of combined local and distant recurrences was observed, and a 15% incidence of distant-only recurrences. It should be emphasized that the frequency of local recurrences is even higher than that associated with rectal cancer and has important treatment implications.

Table 31–2 and 31–3 show incidence of recurrence by stage and histologic subtype from the Mayo Clinic series. As with survival, stage directly correlated with incidence of local recurrence. Patients with extension only into the internal sphincter had a negligible risk for local recurrence, and it was not until there was extension into the external sphincter that the risk of local recurrence significantly increased. Within histologic subtypes, squamous carcinoma (regardless of grade) and basaloid carcinoma have a similar incidence of recurrence, whereas small cell carcinoma had a significantly higher incidence of recurrence. Once again, this underlines the more aggressive nature of small cell carcinoma, compared to the squamous and basaloid varieties. Conclusions must be tempered by the fact that only seven patients were in the small cell category.

Diagnosis

Bleeding and anal discomfort are the most common symptoms of anal carcinoma. Bleeding occurs at rates of 27 to 60% in reported series (Montague, 1980). Most patients experi-

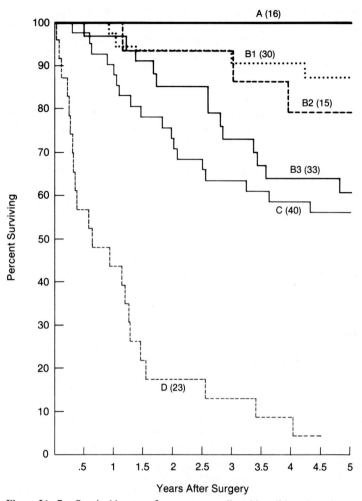

Figure 31–7. Survival by stage for squamous cell and basaloid anal carcinoma.

ence anal discomfort, with 27 to 39% describing this as pain, usually aggravated by a bowel movement. As the tumor advances, the bowel lumen narrows, causing a change in bowel habits. Less common symptoms include awareness of an anal mass or an enlarged inguinal node, pruritus ani, excessive flatus, tenesmus, and anal discharge.

In view of the nonspecific nature of these symptoms, the physician must be vigorous in pursuing anorectal complaints. As discussed above, the physician should recognize that anal cancer often occurs in association with benign conditions of the anus and be aware that homosexuals appear to be a relatively high-risk group.

Early biopsy of suspicious lesions is mandatory. All specimens taken from this area should be subjected to thorough pathologic examination, as a carcinoma will occasionally be

Table 31–2. Recurrence of Squamous Cell and Basaloid Anal Carcinoma by Stage

STAGE	NUMBER OF PATIENTS	NUMBER OF RECURRENCES
A	16	1 (6%)
B_1	30	6 (20%)
B_2	14	3 (21%)
B_3	33	18 (55%)
C	40	21 (53%)

Table 31–3. Recurrence of Anal Carcinoma by Histology

HISTOPATHOLOGY	NUMBER OF PATIENTS	NUMBER OF RECURRENCES
Squamous, grade 1, 2	27	8 (30%)
Squamous, grade 3, 4	57	23 (40%)
Basaloid	49	18 (37%)
Small cell	7	5 (71%)

found in this way. With painful lesions, examination under anesthesia may be necessary to adequately evaluate the local extent of the lesion.

Treatment

Operative Management. In view of the differential behavior of tumors of the anal canal versus those of the anal margin (perineal aspect of the anus), standard surgical treatment is quite different. Lesions of the margin are often localized, exophytic, slightly ulcerative and can be managed, as are other skin cancers, by conservative treatment with local excision (or other sphincter-saving methods such as irradiation) with excellent local control and survival.

Favorable lesions of the anal canal (superficial, less than 2 cm in size, below the dentate line) can be effectively managed by local excision alone. All 12 patients in the Mayo Clinic series fitting this criteria and treated with local excision alone were long-term survivors. Eleven have remained disease-free; one had a local recurrence successfully managed with a subsequent abdominoperineal resection.

With more invasive lesions (large B_2 lesions and beyond), standard treatment is a combined abdominoperineal resection. Some institutions feel that more conservative operative procedures can be combined with radiation or chemotherapy, or both, to yield similar results.

The role of surgery in the management of patients with small cell carcinoma is undefined. Although local disease needs to be controlled, the propensity for systemic spread with this histologic subtype should be recognized. Twelve out of 13 patients with small cell carcinoma in the Mayo Clinic series presented with, or developed, distant metastasis.

Elective groin dissection is of low therapeutic gain and is not utilized in most institutions.

Radiation Therapy. Squamous cell and basaloid carcinomas of the anal canal are generally as radiosensitive as other squamous cell carcinomas. Dose levels achieved with external beam irradiation, however, can be somewhat limited by the problem of perineal reaction, and protracted treatment is required to avoid untoward effects.

Implant and External Beam Irradiation. Historically, irradiation treatment of anal cancer was largely with implantation techniques due to limitations of orthovoltage. Although it achieved cure rates varying from 20 to 53%, it was much maligned as a sole treatment modality due to high complication rates including stricture, infection, necrosis, hemorrhage, and problems of severe postirradiation pain (Montague, 1980; Moertel, 1982). Papillon (1974) reviewed his own series and felt such complications were the result of overdosage or faulty technique (Dalby and Pointon, 1961). He used interstitial irradiation alone, or in combination with external beam methods, in the treatment of 98 patients with selected anal malignancies. Of 64 patients at risk for five years, 44 or 68% were alive and free of disease. If those dying from nonmalignant causes were excluded, the determinant five-year survival rate was 80%. Only 4 of the 98 (4.1%) required radical operative procedures for severe radionecrosis; these occurred within the first two years of treatment. Milder ulceronecrotic reactions occurred in 20 cases which were successfully treated with antibiotic ointment and prednisone.

Papillon attributed his high cure and low necrosis rates to the use of more fractionated schemes. For early lesions, he treated with implant alone, administering two or three implants spaced at intervals of about two months. For advanced lesions, he delivered 3000 rads in three weeks, with supervoltage external irradiation followed in five to eight weeks by an interstitial implant.

External Beam Irradiation (Supervoltage). A number of groups have reported on their experience utilizing carefully fractionated supervoltage external beam irradiation. Results suggest that such techniques, alone or in combination with operation or implants, can achieve good survival and local control, with minimal morbidity (Papillon, 1974; Agar *et al.,* 1979; Green *et al.,* 1980).

The largest series in which supervoltage external beam irradiation was a primary treatment modality was reported by Green and coworkers (1980). They treated a group of 33 patients from 1966 to 1979. Twenty-one of the 33 presented with lesions that were 5 cm or less in diameter (19, anal canal; 2, anal margin). The latter were treated with localized perineal fields, and the rest had inclusion of both the pelvis and perineum. Seventeen of the 21 were treated definitively with irradiation, five after local excision and 12 after biopsy only. The tumor plus nodal areas received 4500 to 5000 rads in 180 to 200 rad fractions, and a boost field to the tumor received an additional

1500 to 2000 rads for a total boost field dose of 6000 to 7500 rads. In the 12 patients treated initially with biopsy and irradiation, no local recurrences have occurred. Three of the 12 did require surgical resection when disease persisted after irradiation. One of the 12 died free of disease at four and one-half years, and the remaining 11 were alive and well from ten months to nine years. Only one patient required anal dilatation for partial stenosis of the anal canal, and no colostomies were required for treatment-related causes.

Preoperative Irradiation and Chemotherapy. A number of institutions have reported favorable results with a combination of preoperative irradiation and concomitant chemotherapy with 5-fluorouracil (5-FU) and mitomycin C. In low-dose irradiation series from Memorial Hospital (Cummings *et al.,* 1982) and from Wayne State University (Newman and Quan, 1976), 3000 rads was given in 15 fractions over three weeks with concomitant chemotherapy. In a higher dose series from Highland Hospital (Nigro *et al.,* 1981), 5000 rads was delivered in 25 fractions over five weeks. In these series, the pathologist was unable to identify residual tumor in a significant percentage of patients who had an abdominoperineal resection after the irradiation (7/12 in the low-dose series from Wayne State; 4/4 in the higher dose series from Highland Hospital).

The Wayne State group favors a more conservative surgical approach following preoperative treatment. Of their total group of 19 patients, 7 of the 15 who had clinical resolution of disease had only wide excision of the area of initial disease after careful examination under anesthesia. In all seven, the specimen was negative on pathologic examination. All seven were free of disease at the time of their report, with six of the seven having been followed for two or more years.

Primary Irradiation and Chemotherapy. In a series from Princess Margaret Hospital (Ager *et al.,* 1979), 13 patients with locally advanced but operable squamous cell carcinoma of the anal canal were treated with radical irradiation (5000 rads in 20 fractions over four weeks), combined with IV mitomycin C (10 mg/m^2), and 5-FU (1000 mg/m^2/24 hours for four days). With a follow-up period of 4 to 34 months, all of the patients had achieved local control and retained anal continence in spite of the fact that seven patients had lesions larger

than 6 cm in maximum diameter. In view of acute (severe perineal reactions in all 13 patients, severe gastrointestinal toxicity in 3) and chronic (moderate perineal resection in all patients) complications, Ager and associates feel modification of their treatment schema is indicated.

Chemotherapy. Scattered reports note activity with a number of chemotherapeutic agents with and without the addition of radiotherapy. These include 5-FU plus mitomycin C (Nigro, *et al.,* 1974; Ager *et al.,* 1979; Bruckner *et al.,* 1979; Sischy *et al.,* 1980; Nigro *et al.,* 1981), vincristine plus bleomycin (Quan *et al.,* 1976), doxorubicin (Livingston *et al.,* 1973), cisplatin (Livingston *et al.,* 1973) and methyl CCNU (Fisher *et al.,* 1978).

Conclusions and Future Prospects

Clinically Resectable Lesions. Recent data suggest that abdominoperineal resection alone may be insufficient local-regional treatment for those patients with extension into the external sphincter or beyond in view of the high incidence of local recurrence (Harmer, 1978; Singh *et al.,* 1981). On the basis of increasing data from other disease sites, the addition of adjuvant irradiation with or without chemotherapy may significantly reduce such risks. Recent experience on the use of adjuvant irradiation for rectal cancer suggests that doses of 4500 to 5000 rads in five to six weeks can be delivered either pre- or postoperatively to the pelvis and perineal tissues with minimal acute and chronic morbidity, provided multiple-field techniques, bladder distention, and so forth, are utilized (Zimm and Wampler, 1981).

Interest has been expressed in the use of sphincter-saving approaches for anal cancer, but it may be difficult to assess the relative efficacy of alternate approaches for a number of reasons. Patient numbers are small. Patients may be unwilling to enter a trial in which they may be randomized to receive an abdominoperineal resection with a colostomy. If preoperative treatment programs are utilized, or primary treatment with irradiation with or without chemotherapy is given, results cannot be easily compared to other treatment options as the extent of disease would be unknown regarding depth of invasion of the primary lesion or nodal involvement.

Although many treatment-related questions

exist, priorities will have to be established in view of the small number of available patients. Studies will have to be organized through existing study groups or through the combined efforts of institutions who see a reasonably large number of such patients. The main surgical questions involve comparison of the presently accepted standard of wide abdominoperineal resection alone, or combined with adjuvant therapy for high-risk groups, versus combinations of sphincter-saving approaches (total excision), or biopsy plus irradiation with or without chemotherapy. Unresolved irradiation questions include primary versus adjuvant treatment, sequencing of adjuvant therapy (pre- versus postoperative versus a combination), dose levels required when used in combination with chemotherapy as either adjuvant or primary treatment, irradiation alone versus in combination with chemotherapy, and external beam alone or in combination with implants when used as primary treatment.

Borderline or Unresectable Lesions. The impressive results of irradiation alone, or used in conjunction with chemotherapy for smaller anal lesions, clearly support a role for such treatment in combination with later surgical resection or implantation of persistent disease. As in an adjuvant setting, important questions remain to be resolved regarding necessary extent of surgery, dose levels techniques of irradiation, and the necessity of concomitant chemotherapy.

For those institutions who utilize combinations of external beam and interstitial irradiation, recent studies demonstrate the marked advantage of doing the implantation procedures with the aid of a perineal template in order to obtain even spacing of the radioactive sources, thereby minimizing underdosing tumor or overdosing normal tissue. When using such combinations, some institutions prefer to deliver 4500 to 5000 rads with external beam techniques (multiple field approaches with or without bladder distention; consider placement of a midline block after 4000 rads in view of the planned implant), followed by a perineal template implant in three to six weeks, and possibly a second such implant three to six weeks after the first.

Advanced Lesions. From a chemotherapeutic standpoint, trials are needed to determine the range of active agents, their optimal delivery schedule, as well as their differing effects on the various histologic subtypes. In particular, the aggressive nature of small cell carcinoma with its systemic spread indicates a need for early institution of chemotherapy.

REFERENCES

Ager, P. ; Samala, E.; Bosworth, J.; Rubin, M.; and Chossein, N. A.: The conservative management of anorectal cancer by radiotherapy. Am. J. Surg., 137:228–230, 1979.

Boman, B. M., Moertel, C. G., O'Connell, M. J., Scott, M. Weiland, L. H., Beart, R. W., Gunderson, L. L., and Spencer, R. J.: Carcinoma of the anal canal—A clinical and pathologic study of 188 cases. Cancer, 54:114–125, 1984.

Bruckner, H. W.; Spigelman, M. K.; Mandel, E.; Cohen, C.; Deppe, G.; Turell, R.; and Schiavone, J.: Carcinoma of the anus treated with a combination of radiotherapy and chemotherapy. Cancer Treat. Rep., 63:395–398, 1979.

Cabrera, A.; Tsukada, Y.; Pickren, J. W.; Moore, R.; and Bross, I. D. J.: Development of lower genital carcinomas in patients with anal carcinoma. Cancer, 19:470–480, 1966.

Cummings, B. J.; Rider, W. D.; Harwood, A. R.; Keane, T. J.; Thomas, G. M.; Erlichman, C.; and Fine, S.: Combined radical radiation therapy and chemotherapy for primary squamous cell carcinoma of the anal canal. Cancer Treat. Rep., 66:489–492, 1982.

Dalby, J. E., and Pointon, J. S.: The treatment of anal carcinoma by interstitial irradiation. A.J.R., 85:515–520, 1961.

Daling, J. R.; Weiss, N. S.; Klopfenstein, L. L.; Cochran, L. E.; Chow, W. H.; and Daifuku, R.: Correlates of homosexual behavior and the incidence of anal carcinoma. J.A.M.A., 247:1988–1990, 1982.

Dillard, B. M.; Spratt, J. S.; Ackerman, L. V.; and Butcher, H. R.: Epidermoid cancer of anal margin and canal. Arch. Surg., 86:100–105, 1963.

Fisher, W. B.; Herbst, K. D.; Sims, J. E.; and Critchfield, C. F.: Metastatic cloacogenic carcinoma of the anus: Sequential responses to adriamycin and cis-dichlorodiammineplatinum. Cancer Treat. Rep., 62:91–97, 1978.

Getz, S. B., Ough, Y. D.; Patterson, R. B.; and Kovalcik, P. J.: Mucinous adenocarcinoma developing in chronic anal fistula: Report of two cases and review of the literature. Dis. Colon Rectum, 24:562–566, 1981.

Green, J. P.; Schaupp, W. C.; Cantril, S. T.; and Schall, G.: Anal carcinoma: Current therapeutic concepts. Am. J. Surg., 140:151–155, 1980.

Hardy, K. J.; Hughes, E. S. R.; and Cuthbertson, A. M.: Squamous cell carcinoma of the anal canal and anal margin. Aust. N. Z. J. Surg., 38:301–305, 1969.

Harmer, M. H.: TNM Classification of Malignant Tumors, 3rd ed. International Union Against Cancer, Geneva, 1978.

Hoskins, B.; Gunderson, L. L.; and Dosoretz, D.: Adjuvant postoperative radiotherapy in carcinoma of the rectum and rectosigmoid. ASTR Proceedings. Int. J. Radiat. Oncol. Biol. Phys., 6:1379, 1980.

Lee, S. H.; McGregor, D. H.; and Kuziez, M. N.: Malignant transformation of perianal condyloma acuminatum: A case report with review of the literature. *Dis. Colon Rectum,* **24**:462–467, 1981.

Livingston, R. B.; Bodey, G. P.; Gottlieb, J. A.; and Frei, E., III: Kinetic scheduling of vincristine and bleomycin in patients with lung cancer and other malignant tumors. *Cancer Chemother. Rep.,* **57**:219–224, 1973.

Moertel, C. G.: The anus. In Holland, J. F., and Frei, E., III (eds.): *Cancer Medicine,* 2nd ed. Lea & Febiger, Philadelphia, 1982.

Montague, E. D.: Squamous cell carcinoma of the anus. In Fletcher, G. H. (ed.): *Textbook of Radiotherapy,* 3rd ed. Lea & Febiger, Philadelphia, 1980.

Morson, B. C., and Sobin, L. H.: Histologic typing of intestinal tumors. *International Histological Classification of Tumors,* No. 15. World Health Organization, Geneva, 1976.

Newman, H. K., and Quan, S. H. O.: Multimodality therapy for epidermoid carcinoma of the anus. *Lancet,* **37**:12–18, 1976.

Nigro, N. D.; Vaitkevicius, V. K.; and Considine, B.: Combined therapy for cancer of the anal canal: A preliminary report. *Dis. Colon Rectum,* **17**:354–356, 1974.

Nigro, N. D.; Vaitkevicuis, V. K.; Buroker, T.; Bradley, G. T.; and Considine, B.: Combined therapy for cancer of the anal canal. *Dis. Colon Rectum,* **24**:73–75, 1981.

Papillon, J.: Radiation therapy in the management of epidermoid carcinoma of the anal region. *Dis. Colon Rectum,* **17**:181–187, 1974.

Paradis, P.; Douglas, H. O.; and Holyoke, E. D.: The clinical implications of a staging system for carcinoma of the anus. *Surg. Gynecol. Obstet.,* **141**:411–416, 1975.

Quan, S. H. O.; Magill, G. B.; Leaming, R. H.; and Hajdu, S. I.: Multidisciplinary preoperative approach to the management of epidermoid carcinoma of the anus and anorectum. *Dis. Colon Rectum,* **20**:89–91, 1978.

Richards, J. C.; Beahrs, D. H.; and Woolner, L. B.: Squamous cell carcinoma of the anus, anal canal and rectum in 109 patients. *Surg. Gynecol. Obstet.,* **114**:475–482, 1962.

Sawyers, J. L.; Herrington, J. L.; and Beachley, F.: Surgical considerations in the treatment of epidermoid carcinoma of the anus. *Ann. Surg.,* **157**:817–824, 1963.

Singh, R.; Nime, F.; and Mittelman, A.: Malignant epithelial tumors of the anal canal. *Cancer,* **48**:411–415, 1981.

Sischy, B.; Remington, J. H.; Sobel, S. H.; and Savlov, E. D.: Treatment of carcinoma of the rectum and squamous carcinoma of the anus by combination chemotherapy, radiotherapy and operation. *Surg. Gynecol. Obstet.,* **151**:369–371, 1980.

Stearns, M. W.; Urmacher, C.; Steinberg, S. S.; Woodruff, J.; and Attiyeh, F.: Cancers of the anal canal. *Curr. Probl. Cancer,* **4**:4–44, 1980.

Sugarbaker, P. H.; Gunderson, L. L.; and Macdonald, J. S.: Cancer of the anal region. In DeVita, V. T.; Hellman, S.; and Rosenberg, S. A. (eds.): *Cancer Principles and Practice of Oncology.* J. B. Lippincott Company, Philadelphia, 1982.

Svenson, E. W., and Montague, E. D.: Results of treatment in cloacogenic carcinoma. *Cancer,* **46**:826–830, 1980.

Weatherby, P.; Wick, M. R.; Kasten, W. R.; and Weiland, L. H.: Small cell undifferentiated (neuroendocrine) carcinoma of the colon and rectum. *Am. J. Clin. Path.* **80**:117–118, 1983.

Wolfe, H. R. I., and Bussey, H. J. R.: Squamous cell carcinoma of the anus. *Br. J. Surg.,* **55**:295–301, 1968.

Young, J. L.; Percy, C. L.; and Asire, A. J.: Surveillance, epidemiology and end results: Incidence and mortality data 1973–1977. *Natl. Cancer Inst. Monogr.,* 57, 1981.

Zimm, S., and Wampler, G. L.: Response of metastatic cloacogenic carcinoma to treatment with semustine. *Cancer,* **48**:2575–2576, 1981.

32

Endocrine Neoplasms

MORTIMER B. LIPSETT

Introduction

Although tumors of the endocrine glands are not common, they present fascinating challenges in pathophysiology, diagnosis, and treatment. The hormone secretion may be the early clue to the existence of a cancer, whose presence must be discerned among the other causes of hypersecretory states of that gland. The excess secretion of a hormone may pose more immediate threats to the patient than does the cancer itself, as with islet cell carcinoma and parathyroid carcinoma. The plasma levels of the hormone may be useful in monitoring the effects of therapy, although specific inhibitors of biosynthesis may have no effect on tumor growth. These points are sufficient to require that the oncologist work in concert with the endocrinologist, and in some cases the gastroenterologist, in the management of patients with functional metastases. Finally, study of patients with secretory cancers of the endocrine glands has given new insights into the biochemistry of gene action and the processing of hormones before they are secreted.

Hormone secretion by cancers of the endocrine glands often has characteristics that distinguish it from normal hormone secretion. In the case of secretion of small molecules, such as cortisol, enzyme biosynthetic activity may not be coordinated, causing increased secretion of intermediates in the biosynthetic sequence. For example, cortisol synthesis by adrenocortical cancer is almost invariably accompanied by an abnormally high secretion of its biosynthetic precursor, 11-deoxycortisol. In the instance of peptide hormone secretion, posttranslational processing may be inaccu-

rate. Thus, insulin is secreted after processing of a larger parent peptide. In insulinomas, enzymatic processing may be defective, giving rise to a variety of molecules in plasma with varying biologic activity. The glycoprotein hormones, such as HCG, may not have the appropriate sugars added after synthesis, again altering physical, chemical, and biologic characteristics. And in the case of hormones composed of two peptide subunits, gene activation may be markedly unequal, resulting in large excesses of a peptide subunit.

Although this chapter will not focus on the inappropriate secretion of hormones by cancers arising from tissues other than the endocrine glands (see Chapter 6F), this occurrence is a fascinating intersection of molecular biology with human disease. The widespread occurrence of HCG and other peptides in many tissues (Odell *et al.,* 1977) makes it seem likely that many genes are "leaky" and continue to express themselves at low levels of activity. With the development of cancer, restraints on gene activation are removed and the cancer can then secrete the hormone. The situation is clearly more complex since some cancers have the propensity for secreting certain peptide hormones, whereas others may secrete a different group. Recently, Roth *et al.* (1982) have proposed that many of the peptide hormones are synthesized by other phyla, including bacteria, and that they may have been intercellular chemical messengers in distant evolutionary time. Thus, the capacity to express their synthesis is maintained through the vertebrates, although specialized tissues can now synthesize and secrete them in large amounts.

In thinking about the origins of many of the

cancers discussed in this chapter, the APUD concept (Pearse, 1969; Schein *et al.,* 1973b; Pearse and Polak, 1978) has heuristic value, even though recent findings cast doubt on the origin of some of the APUD cells. Pearse suggested that many of the hormone-secreting glands have a common neuroectodermal origin and that this could be demonstrated by their common ability for *amine precursor uptake* and *decarboxylation* (APUD). This system is shown in Figure 32–1. Others, however, have shown that not all APUD cells are neuroectodermally derived (Andrew, 1976; Pictet *et al.,* 1976) but that some are derived from the endoderm. Nevertheless, the synthesis of biologically active peptides, both eutop-

ically and ectopically, within the endocrine system is associated with the APUD system. The recent finding of tyrosine hydroxylase, an enzyme identified with catecholamine synthesis, in APUD cells of questionable embryonic origin (Teitelman *et al.,* 1981) again tends to unify the concept. A recent discussion of this concept and its implications may be found in the review by Baylin and Mendelsohn (1980).

The discussion in this chapter will deal only with cancers of the endocrine glands. Functional adenomas are more common, but to cover these areas completely would require a text in endocrinology. References have been selected to emphasize particular points and to present pertinent reviews.

THE APUD SYSTEM

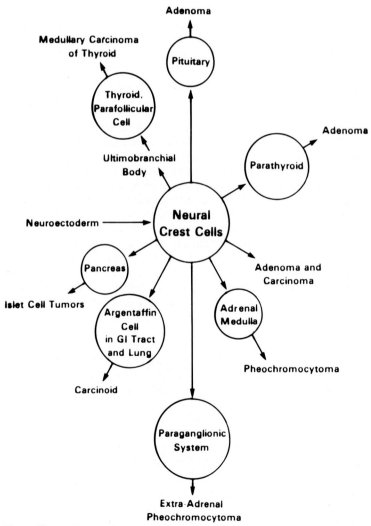

Figure 32–1.   The APUD system.

THYROID CANCER

Thyroid cancer is an uncommon cancer, but of considerable interest for epidemiologic and biologic reasons. Marked differences are evident in the biologic behavior of the cancers manifested by varying growth rates and hormonal activities. The ability to image many of them because of retention of the thyroid's capacity to concentrate iodine is another manifestation of the endocrinologic potential of several of the cancers. A large discrepancy exists between the prevalence of thyroid carcinoma and deaths from it; estimates of prevalence vary from 0.2 to 0.8%, but deaths from thyroid cancer are only 0.006%. Many reasons have been suggested for this, the most important being the low malignancy and slow growth of the most common thyroid cancer, papillary carcinoma.

Etiology

The etiology of thyroid cancer, as that of any other cancer, remains incompletely defined. One of the well-recognized carcinogens, radiation, is of particular importance and will be discussed below. Other proximate carcinogens are unknown, although a chemical carcinogen has induced thyroid cancer in the hypothyroid rat (Doniach, 1950). Many experimental data show that thyroid-stimulating hormone (TSH) is a promoter of carcinogenesis. When rats are rendered hypothyroid by administration of a goitrogen with resulting high TSH levels and epithelial stimulation, radiation is effective in inducing adenomas or carcinomas (Doniach, 1958). Conversely, administration of thyroid hormone to irradiated normal rats markedly reduces tumor formation. The dose of radiation is also significant. Clearly, if the thyroid gland is destroyed, tumors cannot develop. In accord with other experiences with radiation as a carcinogen, even small doses of radiation will increase the incidence of thyroid cancer, particularly in the young.

Radiation-associated thyroid carcinoma is now the most common thyroid cancer. This is a result of the incautious use of radiation for the treatment of supposed thymic hyperplasia, of the tonsil-nasopharynx area, for acne, and tinea capitis. Many of these data have been assembled (DeGroot, 1976).

The latency period for thyroid cancer following irradiation is measured in decades.

Survivors of Hiroshima and Nagasaki who received at least 50 rads had five to ten times the rate of thyroid cancer as did nonirradiated controls, and the peak incidence has probably not yet been reached. Similarly, in 1954, 243 Marshall Islanders were exposed to ^{131}I fallout, and seven of these have developed thyroid cancer with a latency period of 11 to 22 years. The large study by Hempelman et al. (1967) showed that x-radiation of the head and neck during childhood was correlated with the appearance of thyroid nodules and cancer some 20 years later. Thyroid cancer following accidental irradiation of the thyroid in infancy or childhood has been evaluated often (DeGroot, 1976). Most of these cancers have been well-differentiated papillary carcinomas. To summarize the many studies, the incidence of abnormalities of the thyroid gland following radiation in childhood, discovered by either physical examination or scan, is about 20%, and about one-third of these patients or 7% of the population screened had thyroid cancer.

Classification and Prognosis

Although general agreement regarding the classification of these cancers exists, the distribution of cancers is approximate since the results from autopsy series, referral centers, and national surveys are often inconsistent. It is agreed that the most common cancers are papillary carcinoma and mixed papillary and follicular carcinoma (see Table 32–1). For purposes of prognosis and treatment they can be considered as papillary carcinoma. Three clinical subgroups of papillary carcinoma that carry different prognoses have been reported (Woolner et al., 1968). The occult are often found incidentally, and fewer than half of the

Table 32–1. Histologic Classification of Thyroid Tumors and Their Incidence

EPITHELIAL TUMORS	INCIDENCE (%)
Differentiated carcinomas	
Papillary	30
Mixed papillary follicular	34
Follicular	15
Medullary thyroid carcinoma	6
Undifferentiated carcinoma	
Anaplastic	15

Sarcomas
Hemangioendothelioma
Lymphomas
Metastatic tumors

patients have metastatic disease in the lymph nodes. Death from this cancer is rare. The prognosis in the common type, intrathyroidal papillary carcinoma, depends on the size of the tumor; tumors under 5 cm in diameter have an excellent prognosis. Lymph node metastases are more common, but only a small percentage of the patients die of thyroid cancer. When extrathyroidal papillary cancer is discovered, it has penetrated the capsule, usually involves lymph nodes, and recurrence is common. Death is the result of local invasion or extensive metastases; yet over three-quarters of the patients do not die of this disease because of the slow growth rate of the cancer.

Follicular carcinoma has a significantly worse prognosis (Russell *et al.,* 1969). When the disease is apparently confined to the thyroid gland, 5 to 15% of the patients will die of the cancer, although length of survival may be measured in decades. About 50% of follicular cancer demonstrates intrathyroidal spread (Iida *et al.,* 1969), and only 50% of such patients survive six years.

Anaplastic carcinomas usually occur after 40 years of age and are highly malignant. They cause death within a year, either by local invasion or distant metastases. Cures are rare.

In a recent major study (Byar *et al.,* 1979), the significance of several variables on survival was examined. Age, sex, cell type, clinical extent of tumor, lymph node status, and number of metastatic sites had prognostic significance but were not independent variables. The investigators were able to construct a prognostic index that mirrored actual data. Thus, in the best group (see Figure 32–2) the five-year survival was about 95%, whereas in the worst group, containing many of the patients with anaplastic carcinoma, survival was less than 5%. These data are in reasonable agreement with those from many other large series. To achieve some uniformity in assessing results of therapy, the TMN classification and a clinical staging technique are available (see Tables 32–2 and 32–3).

Diagnosis

In spite of extensive experience with thyroid neoplasms, diagnostic recommendations are undergoing change. The history and physical examination still have an important role since a history of radiation to the head and neck or of other family members with thyroid cancers would provide important diagnostic clues. In general, the younger the patient, the greater is the likelihood that a solitary nodule will be cancer. The single nodule has a greater chance of being malignant than does one of several nodules, and a history of recent growth is suggestive. Malignant nodules tend to be harder, and fixation to underlying structures not only strongly suggests cancer, but indicates a poor prognosis as well.

Laboratory Tests. Except for the measurement of calcitonin for the diagnosis of medullary carcinoma, tests of thyroid function have little usefulness in the diagnosis of thyroid cancer. All single nodules or suspicious nod-

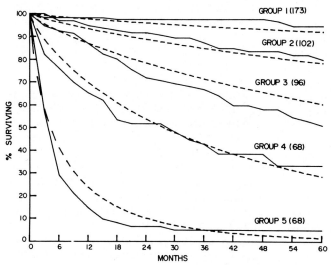

Figure 32–2. Observed (——) and predicted (---) survival curves for the five risk groups.

Table 32–2.   TNM Classification of Malignant Tumors of the Thyroid Gland

Primary tumors

T	Primary tumor
T_0	No palpable tumor.
T_1	Single tumor confined to the gland. No limitation of mobility or deformity* of gland or scanning defect in gland; normal to palpation.
T_2	Multiple tumors or single tumor producing deformity of gland. No limitation of mobility.
T_3	Tumor extension beyond the gland is indicated by fixation or infiltration of surrounding structures.

Regional lymph nodes

N	Regional lymph nodes
N_0	No palpable nodes.
N_1	Movable homolateral nodes.
	N_{1a} Nodes not considered to contain growth.
	N_{1b} Nodes considered to contain growth.
N_2	Movable contralateral or bilateral nodes.
	N_{2a} Nodes not considered to contain growth.
	N_{2b} Nodes considered to contain growth.
N_3	Fixed nodes.

Distant metastases

M	Distant metastases
M_0	No evidence of distant metastases.
M_1	Distant metastases present.

From Harmer, M. T.: Application of the TNM classification rules to malignant tumors of the thyroid gland. *Thyroid Cancer,* pp. 246, UICC Monograph Series, Vol. 12 (reprinted by permission).
* The term *deformity* includes enlargement of the gland.

ules should have a scintigram since hyperfunctional nodules are almost never malignant (Miller and Hamburger, 1965). This does not mean that thyroid cancers will not trap iodine. It is only that they are less efficient at it than is the normal thyroid gland, so that iodine uptake in a thyroid cancer can only be demonstrated after ablating all normal thyroid tissue.

Ultrasonography may be useful in distinguishing among cysts, cystic tumors, and solid tumors (Rosen *et al.,* 1979). Small cysts are unlikely to be cancer, but all cysts should be aspirated and the aspirate examined cytologically. Aspiration of a benign cyst will often suffice for therapy, whereas fluid tends to reaccumulate in a cystic cancer.

Needle biopsy, particularly fine-needle biopsy, has found increasing acceptance as

Table 32–3.   Clinical Staging of Thyroid Cancer

Stage I	Tumors contained within the thyroid gland
Stage II	Tumors with metastases to several nodes without fixation or invasion
Stage III	Local invasion or fixation
Stage IV	Distant metastases

pathologist's skills have improved. When a clearly positive or clearly negative reading has been obtained, the decision about surgery can be made confidently (Gershengorn *et al.,* 1977; Lowhagen *et al.,* 1979; VanHerle *et al.,* 1982).

Although serum thyroglobulin levels may be elevated in thyroid cancer, its measurement does not suffice for diagnosis because similar increases are seen in other thyroid diseases. Serum thyroglobulin levels greater than 10 ng/mL, however, were reliable indicators of metastatic disease (Barsano *et al.,* 1982) and could be used to predict the need for ablative doses of ^{131}I and, when levels were normal, to render unnecessary further imaging studies to detect presumptive metastases.

Treatment

At present, the treatment modalities are surgery, ^{131}I-radiation, and administration of thyroid to suppress thyrotropin. Choice of therapy depends on the cancer type and stage.

As noted above, the relatively benign course of papillary carcinoma, particularly when it is small and solitary, militates against extensive or radical surgery. Thus, lobectomy for a single cancer has produced results similar to those reported by others using more extensive surgery (Buckwalter and Thomas, 1972). Thyroid cancer, however, is often multicentric, and this is certainly true in radiation-induced thyroid cancer. Because of this, a relatively large group of patients with differentiated papillary carcinoma should have near-total thyroidectomy. Lymph node dissection is not indicated. A review of 576 cases of papillary carcinoma (Mazzaferri *et al.,* 1977) showed the importance of this approach.

Follicular cancers are more invasive and metastasize via the blood stream. For these, total thyroidectomy is indicated.

Stage II papillary and follicular cancer is generally managed by total thyroidectomy, modified neck dissection to remove cervical nodes, and administration of ^{131}I to destroy remaining thyroid tissue and preclinical metastases (Mazzaferri *et al.,* 1977). Because of the relative benignity of papillary-follicular carcinoma, even when present in the lymph nodes, the extent of the neck dissection remains an open question.

Stage III cancer is handled similarly, with removal of as much cancer tissue as possible. In stage IV cancer, thyroidectomy or radiation ablation of the thyroid should be performed in order to achieve adequate uptake of ^{131}I into metastases.

Radiation Therapy. This highly specialized topic will be discussed only broadly. If metastatic tumors can be shown to accumulate ^{131}I, then the use of large doses (100 to 200 Ci) of ^{131}I is warranted. This is accomplished by stopping thyroid medication, allowing the patient to become hypothyroid with resultant thyroid stimulating hormone (TSH) stimulation of metastases, and the hope of achieving increased uptake of ^{131}I. One day after administration of ^{131}I, the patients are restarted on thyroid replacement therapy. This cycle can be repeated at three- to four-month intervals. Regression of metastases is seen, but cure is infrequent (Leeper, 1973).

Although radiation effects are normally minimal, some precautions are necessary. The patient should be kept isolated until the body load of ^{131}I is reduced, and provision must be made for the safe disposal of the excreta. Leukemia has been reported after repeated doses of ^{131}I (Pochin, 1960), and pulmonary fibrosis has been seen where there has been extensive uptake in pulmonary metastases with consequent radiation of lung tissue.

Use of Thyroid for Suppression. The use of thyroid preparations to suppress TSH was based on the finding that growth of some differentiated thyroid cancers could be stimulated by TSH. In support of this were reports of regression of metastatic disease by thyroid therapy (Thomas, 1957). Nevertheless, no cures with this modality have been reported, and the procedure of total ablation of the thyroid to induce TSH stimulation of iodine-concentrating ability in the metastases makes the use of thyroid only a late last-ditch maneuver. Cady et al. (1976) claim that thyroid therapy following surgery for differentiated carcinoma caused a decrease in mortality, and many accept this as a recommendation.

Radiation-Induced Thyroid Cancer. Although an epidemic of thyroid cancer in the United States as a result of childhood irradiation of the thyroid is evident (Hempelman et al., 1967), most of the cancers have been papillary. In DeGroot's large experience (1976), 80% of the patients had papillary or mixed follicular-papillary carcinomas. Only rare medullary or anaplastic carcinomas have been seen (Block, 1977).

The natural history of postradiation thyroid carcinoma has been reviewed by Rondebush

and DeGroot (1977). The patients tended to be younger than in the control series (mean age, 28 years) and a higher incidence of multifocal tumors leading to a greater risk of recurrence was reported. Findings of this nature and the many studies of exposed populations (DeGroot, 1976) have led to the following recommendations for persons with known exposure: When palpation of the neck is normal, it is acceptable to follow the patients at yearly intervals. The question of an initial scan of the thyroid gland has not been settled, but the slow growth of these differentiated cancers would seem to make the scan unnecessary in the absence of suspicious findings. When discrete nodules are noted, surgery is indicated unless the nodules are small and the scan is normal. It is then appropriate to try to suppress the thyroid with exogenous thyroid preparations. The enlarged gland with multiple discrete nodules or a single large nodule should be resected. Shimaoka (1977) noted that exogenous thyroid caused shrinkage of the nodules in about 50% of the cases, and Schneider et al. (1978) reported that thyroid suppression after less than total resection reduced the incidence of recurrent disease.

A large surgical experience with postradiation thyroid carcinoma has been reported, and the results have paralleled those noted for similar spontaneous thyroid cancer. Since many of the glands have multifocal disease, the surgeon may not have the luxury of lobectomy for an apparent single nodule. Schneider et al. (1978) showed a 36% chance of nodules developing in the remnant when subtotal thyroidectomy was performed. Recommendations have ranged from lobectomy of a nodule plus hemilobectomy with frozen sections of the apparently uninvolved side to total thyroidectomy if cancer is diagnosed. The risks of total thyroidectomy — damage to the laryngeal nerve and hypoparathyroidism — need to be balanced against the slow growth of papillary carcinoma and the chances of cure. For a complete discussion of this controversy, see DeGroot (1976).

Of incidental interest to the oncologist concerned with the effects of radiation is the report of coexisting thyroid cancer and hyperparathyroidism after neck irradiation (Prinz et al., 1982). In 7 of the 12 patients, a parathyroid adenoma was identified, and hyperplasia was noted in the other five. This finding suggests that the irradiated parathyroid gland undergoes evolution to tumor via hyperplasia, as do the parafollicular cells of the thyroid and the adrenal medulla.

MEDULLARY CARCINOMA OF THE THYROID

Medullary carcinoma of the thyroid (MCT) may be said to be a thyroid cancer on the basis of location only; its cellular origin differs remarkably from other tumors of the thyroid gland. The parafollicular C cells from which the tumor originates (Williams, 1966) are part of the APUD system and differ from the epithelial cells of the thyroid.

Medullary carcinoma comprises about 5 to 10% of all thyroid cancers. The cancer occurs sporadically as part of the syndrome of multiple endocrine neoplasia (MEN) where it is inherited as an autosomal dominant. Although differentiated thyroid cancer occurs more commonly in women than in men, the sex distribution of MCT is about equal. The tumor is bilateral in about half of the sporadic cases, and bilateral and multifocal in most of the familial cases (Hill et al., 1973).

Diagnosis

Any thyroid nodule can be MCT by physical examination, but a family history of pheochromocytoma, hyperparathyroidism, thyroid tumor, or other manifestations of multiple endocrine neoplasia (II) heightens suspicion of MCT. Radiography of the neck may be useful since in one series 35% of the patients had calcifications in the tumor (Keiser et al., 1973). Lymph nodes are frequently involved clinically, and about two-thirds have metastases at surgery (Williams et al., 1966). Amyloid deposited between the spindle-shaped cells of the tumor is characteristic of MCT. Identification of calcitonin mRNA has also been used to diagnose this tumor when the histology was unclear (Chin et al., 1981).

The C cells or parafollicular cells secrete calcitonin, a peptide hormone that inhibits bone resorption in the human. Its secretion is stimulated by an infusion of calcium. MCT retains this physiologic characteristic, and patients with MCT have basal calcitonin levels that are increased over the range of normal (Melvin and Tashjian, 1972). The few that have normal plasma calcitonin levels demonstrate an exaggerated response to calcium or glucagon (Melvin and Tashjian, 1972; Stepansas et al., 1979).

The excessive secretion of calcitonin does not seem to exert any metabolic effect, and the associated parathyroid hyperplasia in the familial form is probably an independent manifestation of the syndrome since it has preceded MCT on occasion (Keiser et al., 1973). The tumor contains large amounts of histaminase (Baylin et al., 1970) and dopa decarboxylase (Atkins et al., 1973), neither of which contributes to the clinical picture. Serum histaminase is increased in many patients with metastatic disease and suggests the presence of metastases (Baylin et al., 1972). The diarrhea that occasionally occurs with this syndrome has been attributed to prostaglandin secretion (Williams, et al., 1968), but others have been unable to relate prostaglandins to the diarrhea (Melvin and Tashjian, 1972).

Treatment

MCT is one cancer in which it is possible to recognize the precancerous state. In the familial form, C-cell hyperplasia has been identified in apparently unaffected members of the kindred (Wolfe et al., 1973). It is thus incumbent upon the physician to measure basal and stimulated calcitonin in all family members. In one family, stimulation tests with calcium or pentagastrin predicted MCT in 12 patients, 11 of whom had no clinical evidence of disease (Miller et al., 1972; Gagel et al., 1975). Similarly, Jones and Sisson (1983) were able to identify eight children whose disease was diagnosed by appropriate testing, since they were members of a family with MEN IIb.

The treatment of MCT is surgical excision. Since the cancer is often multifocal, surgery should include total thyroidectomy and extensive clearance of cervical and parasternal nodes (Chong et al., 1975). As with several other APUD tumors, no chemotherapeutic regimen has substantially influenced the course of metastatic disease. Deftos and Stein (1980) have reported that ^{131}I treatment can occasionally be a useful adjunct to surgery when a calcitonin-secreting remnant is identified following attempts at total thyroidectomy. Doxorubicin has been reported to have activity in patients with advanced stages of disease.

Since pheochromocytomas are part of the MEN II syndrome, it is necessary to ensure that the patient does not have a pheochromocytoma. If one is identified, this should be removed first and recovery permitted before proceeding to excision of the MCT.

The course of a patient with metastatic disease is variable. Death may occur within a few years from metastases to lungs, liver, or bone, or the disease may be relatively indolent with occasional bone or pulmonary metastasis occurring at intervals.

ADRENOCORTICAL CANCER

Adrenocortical cancer is infrequent, difficult to diagnose early, and rarely curable. In one cancer center (Didolkar *et al.,* 1981), the cancer was found in 0.04% of the referred patients. Adrenal carcinoma appears across the age range (Lipsett *et al.,* 1963; Hutter and Kayhoe, 1966), occurring most often in middle age, with a slight predominance in females.

Clinical Pathology

Adrenal carcinomas may be either steroid or nonsteroid producing. Several aspects of the steroid-synthesizing potentials of these cancers may explain many of the anomalous laboratory and clinical features. First, they are relatively inefficient at steroid synthesis. As a result, the tumors must reach a large size before sufficient steroid hormone is secreted to affect clinical findings.

Second, the enzymes of the biosynthetic sequences leading to the synthesis of cortisol, aldosterone, and androstanedione are not coordinated, and there may be relative or absolute blocks in biosynthesis. Thus, steroid hormone precursors may be secreted in excess and have clinical consequences or affect laboratory assays.

Third, under almost every circumstance of steroid biosynthesis, the pathway to C_{19} steroids is intact, causing high urinary 17-ketosteroid (17-KS) excretion in almost all of the syndromes with high steroid secretion.

Fourth, since adult men cannot be "hyper-virilized," excessive androgen synthesis will not be clinically apparent in them unless 17-KS or plasma androgens are measured. Since women are easily virilized, this may account for some of the apparent excess of functional tumors in women.

Table 32–4 lists the hormonal syndromes produced by adrenal cancer and gives an estimate of their frequency. Some specific diagnostic features of these syndromes follow:

Cushing's Syndrome. Plasma 11-deoxy-cortisol and its urinary metabolite, tetrahydro-substances, are always increased due to the rel-

ative 11-β-hydroxylase block (Lipsett *et al.,* 1963). The findings of virilization in association with Cushing's syndrome means adrenal cancer (Bertagna and Orth, 1981). Urinary 17-KS secretion is 100 to 1000 mg daily, considerably higher than secretion with ectopic ACTH-producing tumors.

Virilization. For this clinical syndrome, measurement of urinary 17-KS is warranted to exclude adrenal cancer. Virilization in adrenal cancer is caused by testosterone, which is synthesized peripherally from adrenal androstanedione and dehydroepiandrosterone. It is the excess urinary 17-KS resulting from metabolism of these steroids that distinguishes adrenal cancer from other virilizing syndromes. Rarely, hirsutism may be the only presenting complaint.

Feminization. Plasma androstenedione can be converted peripherally to estrone. This phenomenon produces gynecomastia when excessive androstenedione secretion is present. Feminization is unusual, and the relatively few cases in the world's literature have been summarized by Gabrilove *et al.* (1965). Since rates of aromatization are low, large amounts of androstenedione are required to effect clinically significant plasma estrone concentrations; the major fraction of the androstenedione is metabolized to urinary 17-KS. Thus, measurement of urinary 17-KS will distinguish the feminization caused by adrenal carcinoma from the gynecomastia seen with HCG-producing tumors of the testis and with HCG-producing cancer. Adrenal cancer itself has been reported to produce HCG in amounts large enough to give a positive pregnancy test.

Precocious Puberty. Causes of both masculinization and feminization have been discussed above. Since androgens are the predominant products of adrenal cancer secretion, isosexual precocious puberty usually occurs in boys and virilization in girls. A few cases of feminizing adrenal cancer causing iso-

Table 32–4. Clinical Syndromes Produced by Adrenocortical Cancer

	FREQUENCY (%)
Virilization	25
Virilization and Cushing's syndrome	50
Cushing's syndrome	20
Feminization	< 5
Precocious puberty	< 5
Hypokalemic alkalosis	< 5
Hypoglycemia	< 5

sexual precocious puberty have been reported in girls (Wohltmann et al., 1980).

Sodium Retention and Hypokalemic Alkalosis. These cases are unusual and present with the picture of primary hyperaldosteronism. Carcinomas that secrete aldosterone are rare, however, and the syndrome may be caused by secretion of deoxycorticosterone (Crane and Harris, 1966; Bertagna and Orth, 1981; Grim et al., 1981). Again, urinary 17-KS is high, and the tumor size is incompatible with aldosteroma.

Hypoglycemia. In common with other large mesenchymal tumors in the abdomen and thorax, adrenal cancer may also cause severe hypoglycemia. Plasma insulin levels are low during hypoglycemia, ruling out insulin-secreting tumors. The hypoglycemia has occurred in association with virilization and Cushing's syndrome.

In several series (Lipsett et al., 1963; Hutter and Kayhoe, 1966a), patients with steroid-producing adrenal cancer outnumbered those with nonfunctional tumors. Patients with nonfunctional tumors are usually diagnosed after complaints of pain or presentation of a mass. The retroperitoneal location and the inefficient steroid biosynthesis ensure that the cancer will attain a large size before symptoms caused by the mass or by hormonal secretion begin. Thus, the opportunity to diagnose a small adrenal cancer occurs infrequently, and cure is unlikely (Lipsett et al., 1963; Hutter and Kayhoe, 1966a).

Diagnosis

Extensive discussion of specific diagnostic techniques has been largely superceded by CT scanning or ultrasonography of the abdomen. Large amounts of lipid in the cancer facilitate identification in the CT scan. The scan will also delineate the extent of the cancer and facilitate surgical planning. Iodocholesterol imaging is generally not useful (Schteingart et al., 1981) because, as noted above, tumor steroid synthesis rates are low so that utilization of the cholesterol is inadequate for imaging.

Pathology

Adrenal cancers tend to be large, weighing over 100 g at the time of discovery. Any tumor over 50 g is likely to be cancer. They are pseudoencapsulated and may be locally invasive into kidney, liver, and large blood vessels, the inferior vena cava having been involved on many occasions. Grossly, the tumors are yellow to tan with areas of necrosis and hemorrhage.

Microscopically, it is not always possible to distinguish carcinoma from adenoma. The tumor cells can vary from the spindle-shaped cell in less-differentiated cancers to the large polyhedral cell with abundant eosinophilic cytoplasm. Mitoses may be rare, and some variation in the morphology of the nucleus may be seen in both adenomas and carcinomas. Capsular invasion or blood vessel invasion is the most reliable sign of cancer. The diagnosis of cancer, however, may be made only in retrospect by the finding of metastatic disease many years later. Secretory patterns or even steroid secretion itself cannot be predicted on histologic or histochemical criteria.

Prognosis

Adrenocortical cancer is a highly malignant cancer with a five-year survival rate of 20 to 30%. About half of the patients have metastatic disease at the time of diagnosis. In a small percentage of cases, the course of the disease is slow, metastases recurring over a period of five to ten years. Metastases are to lung, liver, and peritoneum; they rarely involve brain or bone. The survival is clearly different for those patients in whom curative surgery is attempted; this surgery is, of course, an additional index of the extent of disease. The combination of clinical and histologic factors has been used by Hough et al. (1979) to establish prognosis.

Therapy

To achieve cure requires en bloc dissection of the cancer and adjacent structures. First, this requires careful preoperative assessment by angiography and CT scan. It is rare to find a patient in whom surgical cure may be attempted, and this is most often unsuccessful. Nevertheless, surgery is warranted as a debulking procedure on theoretic grounds, although it may not increase the effectiveness of chemotherapy in this situation. In some patients with slowly growing metastases, surgical removal of occasional metastases can provide symptomatic relief.

Adjuvant Therapy. Since metastatic disease exists in most patients at the time of surgery, one important question is the role of adjuvant therapy. Some have advocated radiation of the tumor bed. Although radiation has been considered to be ineffective, the delivery of large enough doses can produce tumor regression. Whether such doses should be delivered to the tumor bed following surgery seems unlikely.

The drug, mitotane (ortho, para prime DDD, o,p'DDD), has been shown to induce regression of metastatic disease (see below). Evidence for effective adjuvant therapy postresection of adrenocortical carcinoma was reported by Schteingart et al. (1982). Twenty-three patients were studied from 1953 to 1981. Six patients had resection of primary disease or local irradiation, or both, and no adjuvant therapy was administered; the mean survival ($\pm$ SD) in this group of patients was 10.3 $\pm$ 8.7 months. Seventeen patients who underwent a curative resection received adjuvant mitotane, with a mean survival of 46.6 $\pm$ 42.7 months. The mean duration of therapy was 28 months (range 4 to 96 months). Confirmation of these effects of mitotane in a randomized prospective trial is required before accepting it as routine postoperative adjuvant therapy. At present, we can only recommend continued surveillance of the patient so that therapy can be instituted promptly. This surveillance should consist of the following: CT scan of abdomen and chest at three- to four-month intervals; measurement of those steroids that were elevated prior to surgery; dexamethasone suppression tests at regular intervals if the tumor had produced cortisol. This last test is necessary since a modest increase of cortisol secretion by a metastatic tumor may not be detected because of the concomitant suppression of the function of the remaining adrenal cortex.

Metastatic Disease

Antihormonal Therapy. Based on the observations that amphenone [3-3-bis (p-aminophenyl)-2-butanone] was an inhibitor of adrenocortical steroid synthesis in laboratory animals, the compound underwent a clinical trial in adrenocortical carcinoma (Hertz et al., 1955). It was demonstrated that amphenone was capable of suppressing the secretion of cortisol in such patients, but the drug proved too toxic for chronic administration (Hertz et al., 1956). Nevertheless, these studies demonstrated the potential effectiveness of this form

of palliative therapy and gave impetus to further clinical research (Tullner, 1964; Lipsett, 1968).

Metyrapone, an inhibitor of 11 β-hydroxylation in cortisol biosynthesis, has been reported useful in the management of individual cases of Cushing's syndrome of adrenal carcinoma; however, it has largely proved ineffective in patients with advanced disease (Daniels et al., 1963). Chemical confirmation of effectiveness requires the direct measurement of plasma cortisol, since its immediate precursor, 11-deoxycortisol, will accumulate and increase its contribution to the Porter-Silber assay for 17-hydroxycorticosteroids (OHCS).

Aminoglutethimide has been used initially for several years as an anticonvulsant; however, with continued use, adrenal insufficiency and goitrous hypothyroidism have been observed. Further studies have demonstrated that the drug produces distinctive histologic changes in the adrenal gland and inhibition of the enzymatic conversion of cholesterol to $\Delta 5$-pregnenolone (Cash et al., 1967). Aminoglutethimide has been shown to be an effective, palliative treatment in Cushing's syndrome secondary to adrenocortical carcinoma, adenoma, and ectopic ACTH production by extra-adrenal carcinomas, with the potential for a rapid and sustained suppression of corticosteroid synthesis (Schteingart et al., 1966; Gorden et al., 1968). Because the drug has the capacity to alter the extra-adrenal metabolism of cortisol, measurement of urinary 17-OHCS excretion alone may overestimate the effectiveness of therapy; plasma cortisol concentrations are a more reliable index of drug effect for this hormone (Fishman et al., 1967). The usual clinical dose is in the range of 1 to 2 g/day; and the important toxicities include anorexia, dermatitis, somnolence, ataxia, and decreased thyroid function.

Anticancer Therapy. Mitotane was shown to induce necrosis of the zonal fasciculi and reticularis in the dog and was subsequently introduced into therapy for adrenocortical carcinoma. Later investigations demonstrated that o,p'DDD was capable of inhibiting steroidogenesis (Nichols and Henniger, 1957; Cueto and Brown, 1958; Vilar and Tullner, 1959). The biochemical mechanism of action was reported to be mediated through the inhibition of the adrenal enzyme, glucose-6-phosphate dehydrogenase. This is the key for the generation of NADPH via the pentose pathway;

NADPH is an essential cofactor in the hydroxylation of cholesterol to 5Δ-pregnenolone (Casorla and Moncloa, 1962).

Between 1960 and 1965, 138 patients with adrenal cancer were treated with o,p′DDD, and the results of this series were reviewed by Hutter and Kayhoe (1966b). Of the patients studied 82% had an initially increased excretion of 17-ketosteroids or 17-hydroxycorticosteroids, or both. A 50% or greater decrease in hormone excretion was achieved in approximately 70% of cases. A minimum of four weeks of therapy was required to ensure an adequate therapeutic trial; of those patients who ultimately responded, only 37% did so by the 21-day period, whereas at 30 days of treatment, 87% of patients demonstrated a reduction in urinary 17-ketosteroid excretion. The average dose required for response was 8.5 g/day, and the median duration of steroid response was approximately nine months.

Not all patients who evidenced a hormonal response achieved a reduction in tumor mass. Of 59 patients with measurable disease, 20, or 34%, demonstrated an objective response, which was accompanied by a decrease in steroid excretion in all cases. The median time to response from start of o,p′DDD treatment was six weeks, with a mean duration of 10.2 months.

In analyzing the clinical features of cases that demonstrated response to treatment, women had higher steroid and objective response rates (76% and 38%) than men (60% and 21%), but age, site of tumor, and location of metastases did not appear to influence the potential benefit from o,p′DDD. Prolongation of life was recorded for patients who obtained an objective tumor regression compared to nonresponders; no difference in survival could be observed based on steroid response alone. The prognosis of women was better than that of the men. Fifty-two percent of women and 38% of men lived four years after diagnosis, with median survivals of 56 and 19 months, respectively (Hutter and Kayhoe, 1966b). Cures of this disease with o,p′DDD in respect to complete absence of tumor, as determined by physical or biochemical measurements, are not known.

An additional 115 patients with adrenal carcinoma have been treated with o,p′DDD between 1965 and 1969, and the data have been reviewed by Lubitz et al. (1973). The measurable disease response in this series was 61%

compared to the previously reported 34%, and the steroid excretion response of 89% demonstrated an improvement over the 72% noted by Hutter and Kayhoe. It was estimated that 54% of patients derived overall benefit from treatment, "clinical response," when the effects of drug toxicity were taken into consideration. The improved response rate is attributed to a shorter median time between diagnosis and treatment with o,p′DDD. Nater et al. (1983) recorded a 19% remission rate in a series of 77 patients.

The majority of patients treated with o,p′DDD have sustained some form of toxicity when dosage was brought up to the therapeutic range of 8 to 10 g/day. In general, it was mild, and commonly consisted of an adverse gastrointestinal reaction with anorexia, nausea, vomiting, or diarrhea. Neuromuscular toxicity has been recorded in 40 to 60% of cases and has usually taken the form of lethargy and somnolence. Dizziness, or vertigo, and dermatologic toxicity are observed in 15% of cases, whereas leukopenia and liver function abnormalities are only rarely a problem (Hutter and Kayhoe, 1966a; Lubitz et al., 1973). Van Slooten et al. (1984) have shown that monitoring plasma o,p′DDD levels will prevent toxicity.

With successful treatment of a functioning tumor, a substantial proportion of patients will develop signs of adrenal insufficiency. This is probably related to the suppressive effect of the long-standing massive steroid excretion of the tumor, to which o,p′DDD may play an additive role. Since o,p′DDD is a chlorinated hydrocarbon, it is a potent inducer of the hepatic P-450 oxygenases. This results in 6-β-hydroxylation of cortisol, rendering the metabolites considerably more polar, thus, not extractable from urine with the usual organic solvents. Thus, a decrease in 17-hydroxycorticoid excretion during mitotane treatment may not mean decreased production of cortisol by the tumor but only a diversion of its urinary metabolites (Bledsoe et al., 1964). Similar effects have been noted in the excretion of the 17-ketosteroids. Since o,p′DDD affects the route, rather than the rate, of removal of steroids from plasma, a decrease in plasma steroids remains a valid index of decreased steroid secretion by the tumor. In patients demonstrating a hormonal response, the need for replacement glucocorticoid therapy should be anticipated.

In summary, objective rates of regression vary around 25% (Lipsett et al., 1963; Hutter and Kayhoe, 1966b), with a median duration of remission of about one year. Some patients have had remissions lasting over three years. Dosage regimens also vary, although most therapists begin with about 10 g daily, reducing this gradually to 1 or 2 g daily as regression is obtained. Diminution in size of metastases on chest x-ray is rarely apparent before six weeks, although laboratory evidence of decreased steroid production may be noted earlier. Prolonged regression has been reported (Lubitz et al., 1973), and an apparent cure was seen with combined use of o,p'DDD and 5-fluorouracil (Ostuni and Roginski, 1975). Recently, cisplatin has been reported to cause regression in four patients, three of whom had previously received o,p'DDD as adjuvant therapy (Tattersall et al., 1980).

PARATHYROID CARCINOMA

Parathyroid carcinoma is one of the rarest of cancers; only 50 cases were accepted by Holmes et al. (1969) in their comprehensive review. The total number of cases now is about 100, and it accounts for only a small percentage of cases of hypercalcemia. Most of the patients with parathyroid carcinoma have had hypercalcemia, and this finding has been considered by some to be necessary for the diagnosis of parathyroid carcinoma.

Data concerning the possible origin of parathyroid carcinoma from preexisting abnormalities are rare. In contrast to medullary carcinoma of the thyroid, a transition to carcinoma from the hyperplastic parathyroid gland of patients with MEN I does not seem to occur. The occurrence of parathyroid carcinoma in two patients with familial hyperparathyroidism (Dinnen et al., 1977), however, suggests that the transition from hyperplasia to cancer can take place.

Diagnosis

Parathyroid carcinoma is usually discovered at surgery for parathyroid disease causing hypercalcemia. No unequivocal diagnostic tests distinguish between adenoma and carcinoma. The plasma calcium concentration tends to be higher with carcinoma than with adenoma or hyperplasia, but a large overlap between the two does exist. Evidence of a neck mass or intraoperative finding of adherence to neck structures suggests cancer.

The histologic picture may be diagnostic of carcinoma when mitoses are seen or where blood vessel invasion occurs. In a comprehensive study, these features and a trabecular pattern with thick fibrous bands were considered characteristic (Schantz and Castlemen, 1973). As with many endocrine tumors, however, an unequivocal diagnosis of cancer is often not possible.

Course

Parathyroid carcinoma usually threatens the patient because of its secretion of parathormone and chronic unremittent severe hypercalcemia, not because of its growth. It is unusual for patients to die as a result of tumor encroachment on vital organs, although this has been reported in one patient with nonfunctional carcinoma. Death usually results from the complications of hypercalcemia: renal disease, cardiac rhythm abnormalities, and hypercalcemic crises. Survival with documented metastatic disease may be prolonged, although the first-year survival rate is less than 50% (Aldinger et al., 1982).

Management

Should the disease be recognized at the time of surgery, most surgeons agree that careful *en bloc* excision of the tumor and involved structures is indicated. This tumor does not generally metastasize via the lymphatics so that radical neck dissection is not warranted. The need for careful dissection without tumor spill is emphasized by documentation of local recurrence following surgery.

If hypercalcemia persists or recurs after surgery, attempts should be made to locate the metastasis using venous catheterization and measurement of parathormone should other diagnostic modalities fail. Prolonged remissions of hypercalcemia have been reported following removal of metastatic deposits.

Medical treatment of the tumor, *qua* cancer, has been unsuccessful. Attempts have been made using a variety of chemotherapies and radiation without success. Because of the slow growth of the tumor, it is in the patient's best interest to direct therapeutic efforts at the hypercalcemia, although measures aimed at this generally have had only transient success.

CARCINOID SYNDROME

The enterochromaffin cell from which carcinoid tumors are derived is part of the APUD system. The carcinoid tumors themselves are heterogeneous with respect to origin, ultrastructure, secretory patterns, and clinical syndromes. Carcinoids arise from components of the primitive embryonic gut. They can occur throughout the gastrointestinal tract, the pancreas, and in the lung. They are rarely found in testis and ovary. Since the pathologist is unable to distinguish between adenoma and carcinoma on the basis of histology, only metastases define carcinoma unequivocally.

Clinical Pathology

To understand the clinical syndromes produced by the common metastatic carcinoid of the ileum, a brief discussion of serotonin synthesis and the kallikrein-bradykinin system is necessary. As shown in Figure 32–3, serotinin (5HT, 5-hydroxytryptamine) is synthesized by the tumor from tryptophan and metabolized to 5-hydroxyindoleacetic acid (5-HIAA) which appears in the urine. The importance of serotonin in the clinical syndromes is still problematic, although the tumor certainly releases serotonin, which is then bound to platelets.

Carcinoid tumors contain and release the enzyme, kallikrein, which acts on an α_2-globulin to split off bradykinin, and its precursor, lysyl-bradykinin, both of which can induce flushing.

The most common sign of the carcinoid syndrome is flushing, followed by diarrhea, heart disease, and edema (see Table 32–5). Earlier recognition of the syndrome has modified slightly the incidence of these signs recorded during the early years of definition of the syndrome.

Flushing. Two types of flush accompany the usual type of metastatic ileal carcinoid. The first is red and diffuse involving the face and upper body. A few minutes in duration, it is provoked by alcohol, excitement, emotional stress, and catecholamines (Robertson *et al.,* 1962).

The second type of flush affects the same areas and, because it is more prolonged, produces venous dilation and a purplish hue. This may result in permanently dilated facial veins and telangiectasia. This flush is more commonly precipitated by alcohol. Infusion of serotonin does not reproduce either flush, but the kinins have been shown to do this, albeit not uniformly (Grahame-Smith, 1972). Since the brief flushes may be due to catecholamine-induced release of kallikrein, α-adrenergic blocking agents have been used successfully (Adamson *et al.,* 1969).

Gastric carcinoids, probably by secreting histamine, produce a patchy, red, and sometimes itchy flush. Roberts *et al.* (1979) have shown that H_1 and H_2 receptor antagonists (diphenhydramine and cimetidine) can inhibit this flushing.

Bronchial carcinoids produce long-lasting flushes (hours to days) that may cover the entire body. Diarrhea may occur or worsen. The etiology is unclear.

Diarrhea. The diarrhea is not necessarily related to the flushing and appears to be related to increasing gut motility, rather than to secretion of fluids as in pancreatic cholera. Since

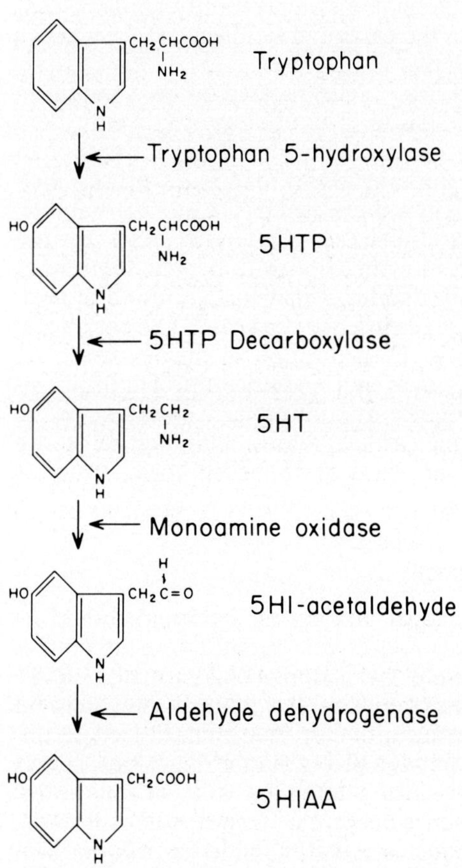

Figure 32–3. Synthesis and metabolism of serotonin.

Table 32–5. Clinical Manifestations of the Carcinoid Syndrome

Total number of cases	79
Men	48
Women	29
Age at presentation	
Men	18–80
Women	33–80
Flushing	74
Diarrhea	68
Asthma	18
Edema	52
Heart disease	41
Dermatitis of pellagra	5
Peptic ulcers	5
Arthralgia	6

From Thorson, A.: *Acta Med. Scand.,* **334** (Suppl. 7):1–132, 1958 (reprinted with permission).

methysergide, a serotonin antagonist, and parachlorophenylalanine, a blocker of sertonin synthesis, are effective singly and in combination in preventing diarrhea, it is presumed that serotonin causes the diarrhea. Evidence has been obtained that infusion of serotonin leads to a pattern of intestinal motility similar to that seen in the carcinoid syndrome (Misiewicz *et al.,* 1966).

Pellagra. Pellagra used to be a common manifestation. The etiology was niacin deficiency caused by the deviation of tryptophan from niacin synthesis to indole synthesis. Pellagra is now prevented by use of nicotinamide.

Heart Disease. Carcinoid heart disease occurs in association with hepatic metastases and presumably a high concentration of serotonin in the inferior vena cava. The pathologic lesion is the deposition of fibrous tissue on heart valves and endothelium. Tricuspid incompetence and pulmonary stenosis are the resulting cardiac lesions. Although serotonin has been thought to be etiologic, proof is lacking.

Treatment

Bronchial and gastric carcinoid should be excised. Reasonable presumption of cure is possible if this is done (Waldenstrom, 1958). Ileal carcinoids rarely produce the carcinoid syndrome until they have metastasized, so unless a mass in present in the ileum that directs the physician's attention to it, or only a few metastases occur, the surgical role is limited. When metastases are confined to only one lobe of the liver, a lobectomy may produce a worthwhile clinical remission (Malafosse, 1974).

Antihormonal Therapy. The serotonin-related symptoms of watery diarrhea, abdominal colic, and malabsorption have received the greatest attention and therapeutic investigation by clinical pharmacologists (Hill, 1971). When mild, these gastrointestinal manifestations may be successfully managed with simple measures, such as opiates and diphenoxylate hydrochloride with atropine for long periods of time. With more severe symptoms, the use of peripheral antagonists of serotonin, methysergide, and cyproheptadine has been effective in controlling diarrhea and, in some cases, malabsorption (Brown *et al.,* 1960; Melmon *et al.,* 1965).

Another avenue of clinical investigation has been the use of agents that are known inhibitors of serotonin synthesis. One of the first to undergo clinical trial was alpha-methyldopa which partially inhibits the decarboxylation of 5-hydroxytryptophan (5-HTP) to serotonin. Results with this compound have been disappointing except for a patient with rare 5-HTP-secreting metastatic carcinoid of gastric origin (Mengel, 1965; Oates and Butler, 1967).

Parachlorophenylalanine (PCPA) is an inhibitor of the enzyme tryptophan 5-hydroxylase involved in the conversion of the amino acid to 5-HTP, the immediate precursor of serotonin. Engelman has demonstrated that PCPA at doses of 2 to 4 g/24 hours can reduce the urinary excretion of 5-hydroxyindoleacetic acid (as in indirect measurement of 5-hydroxyindole synthesis) by 51 to 81% in patients with malignant carcinoid tumors (Engelman and Sjoerdsma, 1966; Sjoerdsma *et al.,* 1970). This was accompanied by good-to-excellent control of diarrhea and other gastrointestinal symptoms. Several toxicities of PCPA have been defined. In addition to lethargy and lightheadedness, chronic administration may be accompanied by such mental aberrations as depression, anxiety, and confusional states. An allergic eosinophilia appearing two to nine weeks after initiation of treatment with PCPA has been observed in 50% of patients. This abnormality is rapidly reversible with withdrawal of the drug, reappears promptly with rechallenge, and is a definite sign for cessation of PCPA therapy. Continued treatment in the presence of eosinophilia has led to the development of urticaria, asthma, and pulmonary infiltrates (Löffler's syndrome) (Sjoerdsma *et al.,* 1970).

It is important to ensure that the patient is not inadvertently placed on a monoamine oxidase inhibitor, such as iproniazid, which might block the degradation of serotonin to its inactive urinary excretion metabolites.

Carcinoid tumors may synthesize and release the proteolytic enzyme, kallikrein, which acts upon a specific α_2-globulin to generate bradykinin, the mediator of the flush (Oates and Sjoerdsma, 1962). Phenothiazines have been shown to antagonize the peripheral action of kinins and have been marginally effective in controlling flushing in some patients (Rocha e Silva and Carcia Lerne, 1963). Corticosteroids have been reported to significantly decrease and prevent the attacks of flushing, particularly in cases of bronchial carcinoid (Ureles et al., 1963; Melmon et al., 1965).

Catecholamines can provoke an attack of flushing, and, on this basis, alpha-adrenergic blocking agents, such as phentolamine, have been proposed as therapeutic agents for patients with this syndrome (Adamson et al., 1969).

As mentioned above, serotonin antagonists such as methysergide and cyproheptadine are often effective in controlling the diarrhea. Since one of the side effects of methysergide treatment in other diseases is cardiac fibrosis, it makes it less likely that serotonin, the agonist, is also responsible for the lesion. More recently, somatostatin has been shown to be effective in inhibiting the flush of the ileal carcinoid (Frolich et al., 1978).

Antineoplastic Therapy. In contrast to the extensive work on the mechanisms and control of carcinoid syndrome, drug treatment of the underlying malignancy until recently has received remarkably little attention. The spectrum of chemotherapeutic agents reported to have activity in this tumor is identical to that of islet cell carcinoma, also of neural crest origin. In a significant proportion of patients, the disease may remain indolent, and active antitumor management may not necessarily be required (Moertel et al., 1961). Some patients with more aggressive tumors will present in time with progressive liver metastases, signs of partial or impending complete intestinal obstruction, ascites, or severe and uncontrollable symptoms. For these patients anticancer therapy is a consideration. Controlled clinical trials of specific chemotherapeutic agents in this disease have been difficult to carry out because of its relative infrequency in any individual medical center; cooperative study group trials have provided objective assessment of the responsiveness of this tumor to a variety of single agents and combinations.

Table 32–6 summarizes examples of the experience with cytotoxic drugs in carcinoid tumors (Mengel and Shaffer, 1973; Moertel, 1975; Legha et al., 1977). Response rates with single agents included: 5-FU, 40%; streptozotocin, 50%; cyclophosphamide, 25%; methotrexate, 17%; phenylalamine mustard, 25%; and doxorubicin, 21%. Combination chemotherapy also proved to be efficacious. The Eastern Cooperative Oncology Group designed a phase III trial comparing streptozotocin plus 5-FU, versus streptozotocin plus cyclophosphamide (Moertel and Hanley, 1979). The combination produced a response rate of

Table 32–6. Chemotherapy for Malignant Carcinoid Tumors

SINGLE AGENT	RESPONDERS/ NO. OF PATIENTS	%	REFERENCE
Phase II trials			
5-Fluorouracil	6/15	40	Moertel, 1975
Streptozotocin	3/6	50	Moertel, 1975
Cyclophosphamide	4/16	25	Mengel and Shaffer, 1973
Methotrexate	1/6	17	Mengel and Shaffer, 1973
Phenylalanine mustard	2/8	25	Mengel and Shaffer, 1973
Doxorubicin	7/33	21	Moertel et al., 1982a
COMBINATION			
Cyclophosphamide/ methotrexate	6/11	55	Mengel and Shaffer, 1973
5-Fluorouracil/ streptozotocin	6/9	67	Moertel et al., 1982a,b
Phase III trials			
5-Fluorouracil/ streptozotocin	14/42	33	Moertel and Hanley, 1979
Cyclophosphamide/ streptozotocin	12/47	26	Moertel and Hanley, 1979

33%, compared to 26% with streptozotocin alone. The authors further demonstrated that response rate and survival were a function of the site of the primary carcinoid tumor (see Table 32–7); patients with small bowel carcinoids had a relatively good prognosis with a response rate of 41% and a median survival of 29 months, while carcinoid tumors of unknown primary had a poor prognosis, with a 17% response rate and median survival of eight months.

Of concern to the clinician caring for the patient with a carcinoid tumor is the rare but potential hazard of precipitating a severe carcinoid crisis with effective cytotoxic therapy. This is particularly worrisome in the patient already manifesting severe carcinoid syndrome and/or excreting greater than 150 mg of 5-HIAA in the 24-hour urine collection. For these patients, the initial dose of cytotoxic therapy should be halved and the patient monitored carefully.

MALIGNANT PHEOCHROMOCYTOMA

As with other endocrine tumors, histologic criteria for malignancy are difficult to establish. The usual criteria of pleomorphism, nuclear atypia, and abundant mitotic figures may be seen in benign tumors (Symington and Goodall, 1953). Capsular invasion is insufficient, although invasion of adjacent tissues does certify malignancy. Malignant pheochromocytomas may be nonfunctional, and extraadrenal tumors have been reported to have a higher incidence of malignancy (Melicow, 1977).

Ten to fifteen percent of pheochromocytomas are malignant (Manger and Gifford, 1977). It is not clear whether familial pheochromocytoma has a higher incidence of malignancy, as noted in one study, since the general experience with patients with multiple endocrine neoplasia has not borne this out. These patients, however, frequently have bilateral tumors, and hyperplasia has been seen as a precursor to the pheochromocytomas (Carney et al., 1975).

Clinical Problems

Functional malignant pheochromocytomas exhibit the same secretory pattern as benign tumors, hence carry the same risks attributable to excessive secretion of epinephrine and norepinephrine: hypertension, stroke, cardiovascular, and renal disease. The manifestations of pheochromocytoma are listed in Table 32–8A and additional features suggestive of pheochromocytoma in Table 32–8B. Any of these may be seen with malignant pheochromocytomas.

Diagnosis

Urinary metanephrines are a good diagnostic measure of functional pheochromocytomas (Van Heerden et al., 1982), but these studies will yield false negatives. Bravo et al. (1979) have demonstrated the value of measuring plasma catecholamines, and in a subse-

Table 32–7. Carcinoid Tumors: Influence of Primary Site on Response and Survival

SITE OF PRIMARY	RESPONSE (%)	MEDIAN SURVIVAL (MO.)
Small bowel	41	29.3
Pancreas	42	21.6
Lung	12	14.9
Colon	——	10.1
Unknown	17	8.0

Adapted from Moertel, C. G., and Hanley, H. A.: Combination chemotherapy trials for metastatic carcinoid tumor and the malignant carcinoid syndrome. *Cancer Clin. Trials,* **2:**327, 1979.

Table 32–8A. Manifestations of Pheochromocytoma

Paroxysmal hypertension
Sustained hypertension with
  Paroxysmal attacks: palpitation, headache, sweating
  Headache
  Sweating and palpitations
  Diabetes
  Postural hypotension or tachycardia
  Hypermetabolism
  Weight loss
  Personality change

Table 32–8B. Other Features Suggestive of Pheochromocytoma

Progressive hypertension
Stable hypertension with diabetes, hypermetabolism
Hypertension in children
Hypertensive response to induction of anesthesia
Neurocutaneous lesions
Hypertensive crises during renal angiogram
Paradoxical response to antihypertensive drugs
Family history of pheochromocytoma, MCT, or hyperparathyroidism

From DeQuattro, V., and Campese, V. M.: Pheochromocytoma: Diagnosis and Therapy. In DeGroot L. J. (ed.): *Endocrinology,* Vol. 2. Grune & Stratton, Inc., New York, 1979 (reprinted by permission).

quent study, they reported that oral clonidine would reduce elevated plasma catecholamines to normal only in patients without tumors (Bravo *et al.*, 1981). Thus, biochemical investigations now have high accuracy in diagnosis of functional tumors of the adrenal medulla. Angiography has been largely superceded by CT scanning. Van Heerden *et al.* (1982) reported high accuracy in localization of the tumor at all sites, thus obviating the need for other diagnostic tools.

Course and Treatment

Malignant pheochromocytomas metastasize to lung, brain, and bone. Metastatic disease may progress very slowly, and the life-threatening complications for many years are caused by the secretory products. Survival for up to 20 years has been noted (Remine *et al.*, 1974), and in a personal experience, one young man with metastatic disease was maintained in good health for 14 years with treatment directed only at symptoms produced by catecholamines.

Therapy of patients with inoperable metastatic disease follows the same principles as those used in preparing a patient for surgery. Blockade of α-adrenergic receptors is accomplished with phentolamine; this may require gradually increasing the dose with progression of disease. Beta-adrenergic blockade may offer additional benefit but should always be used after alpha-adrenergic blockade is established. Otherwise, the removal of the vasodilation effects of the beta-adrenergic receptors may precipitate severe hypertension.

Surgery and radiation have roles in metastatic disease as palliative modalities. Accessible lesions can be treated, often with local and systemic remission. Chemotherapy with streptozotocin has been unsuccessful (Hamilton *et al.*, 1977).

MULTIPLE ENDOCRINE NEOPLASIA (MEN)

The syndromes encountered under this classification overlap with those discussed for pancreatic and adrenal medullary tumors and for medullary carcinoma of the thyroid (MTC). The syndromes are familial, being transmitted as autosomal dominants with high penetrance, variable expressivity, and pleiotropic expression. They link the embryologic origin of these glands with the possibility that a "dysplastic" change or a tendency to develop cancer is determined genetically. The hyperplastic antecedents of MTC (Wolfe *et al.*, 1973) and of pheochromocytoma (Lips *et al.*, 1978) lend credence to the dysplastic hypothesis.

MEN I

Several types of MEN have been delineated, and some additional associations have been noted. In Table 32–9 the manifestations of MEN I, MEN IIa, and MEN IIb are listed. Steiner *et al.* (1968) first characterized types I and II. The MEN I syndrome was defined as a disorder of three glands: parathyroid, pancreatic islet cells, and pituitary.

Parathyroid hyperplasia is the component most frequently noted (Ballard *et al.*, 1964). Next most frequent were the pancreatic islet tumors. Functioning adenomas of the pitui-

Table 32–9. Syndromes of Multiple Endocrine Neoplasia

MEN I	MEN IIA AND IIB
Hyperparathyroidism	Medullary carcinoma of the thyroid
Pancreatic tumors	
Insulinoma	Pheochromocytoma
Somatostatinoma	Hyperparathyroidism (MEN IIa only)
Glucagonoma	
Vipoma	
Pancreatic carcinoid	MEN IIb
Pancreatic polypeptide-secreting tumor	Mucosal neuromas
Pituitary tumors	Marfanoid habitus
Eosinophilic adenoma (acromegaly)	Typical facies
Prolactinoma	Bowel abnormalities
Nonfunctional tumors	
ACTH-secreting tumors	
Adrenal adenomas	
Bronchial carcinoids	
Thyroid nodules	

tary gland occurred in 50% of MEN I, producing pituitary deficiency, hyperprolactinemia, and acromegaly (Eberle and Grun, 1981). From the standpoint of neoplasms, of greatest interest are the neoplasms of the pancreatic islet cells. The causes of death in MEN I (see Table 32–10) (Eberle and Grun, 1981) show that the pancreatic tumors outweigh the other manifestations of MEN I as a threat to the patient's life.

The management of MEN I includes first an awareness of the syndrome. Since almost all patients will eventually become hyperparathyroid (Ballard *et al.,* 1964), continued surveillance of the serum calcium is necessary. Pituitary tumors may make themselves evident in such ways as: amenorrhea with hyperprolactinemia, acromegaly, hypogonadism with cellular destruction, visual field changes, and, rarely, hyperthyroidism caused by tumoral secretion of thyroid-stimulating hormone. Treatment of the parathyroid and pituitary diseases follows the same recommendations as those used in patients without MEN.

The spectrum of secretory patterns of the pancreatic tumors is broad. In the comprehensive review of Eberle and Grun (1981), pancreatic tumors were present in 100 of 122 MEN I patients. The distribution was: gastrinoma, 64%; insulinoma, 24%; glucagonoma, 3%; asymptomatic, 9%. Rare cases of secretion of vasoactive intestinal peptide (VIP) and other peptides occurred. Forty-two percent of the gastrinomas were malignant, and 25% of the insulinomas were malignant. Pancreatic polypeptide, α- and β-HCG, and other peptides such as ACTH may serve as tumor markers.

The adrenal cortex has been involved in about one-third of the cases (Ballard *et al.,* 1964) with adenoma or hyperplasia, although Cushing's syndrome was not present. Bron-

chial carcinoids were present in 4 of 85 patients.

Other associations have been reported. Doumith *et al.* (1982) described the association of adrenal adenomas with hyperaldosteronism and adenomas of stomach and colon with prolactinomas. Berg *et al.* (1976) reported a patient with a growth-hormone–producing pituitary adenoma, bronchial carcinoid, parathyroid hyperplasia, and excess gastric acid secretion associated with hyperplasia of antral and duodenal cells.

MEN II

The differentiation of this group of associated tumors stems from the report of Sipple (1961). Since that time almost 300 patients have been added (Grun and Eberle, 1981). The tumors that constitute MEN II are medullary carcinoma of the thyroid (MCT), pheochromocytoma, and adenoma or hyperplasia of the parathyroid glands. When mucosal neuromas are present as part of a distinctive syndrome, this has been designated MEN IIb. In MEN IIb, parathyroid disease is rare.

MEN IIa is inherited as an autosomal dominant with variable expressivity and high dominance. When the pheochromocytoma is present with MCT, over 70% of cases are bilateral. The functional expression of these pheochromocytomas is identical to that of sporadic pheochromocytoma. The pheochromocytomas may be derived from hyperplastic adrenal medullas (Carney *et al.,* 1975), and even carcinoma has been reported in the same family. This progression from hyperplasia to tumor is similar to the progression noted with medullary carcinoma of the thyroid. This expression of dysplastic change in two of the glands of MEN II suggests a single gene defect in a cell line derived from a common stem cell line. Baylin *et al.* (1976) studied cells from the adrenal and thyroid tumors in a woman mosaic for glucose-6-phosphate dehydrogenase. Since all the tumor cells had the same B pattern, the data are consistent with the hypothesis that the pheochromocytoma and the MCT originated from a common cell line.

In kindreds with MEN II about 50% of the patients have parathyroid disease, and a large fraction of these patients have hypercalcemia. Since the hypercalcemia has preceded MCT, it is probably an independent manifestation of the disorder.

The patients need to be followed carefully,

Table 32–10. Causes of Death in MEN I

		%
Ulcer complications		33
Complications of surgery		27
Stomach/pancreas	19	
Other	8	
Metastatic tumor		11
Hyperparathyroid crisis		11
Pituitary tumor		8
Infection		6
Hypoglycemia		3

Adapted from Eberle, F., and Grun R.: Multiple endocrine neoplasia, type I (MEN I). *Ergeb. Inn. Med. Kinderheilkd.,* **46:**75–150, 1981.

with appropriate measurements of basal and stimulated hormone levels. The high expressivity of the disease is manifested by the finding that whenever parathyroid disease and pheochromocytoma were present, MCT also developed (Keiser *et al.,* 1973). Therefore, serial measurement of calcitonin with stimulation by calcium or pentagastrin at intervals is necessary to detect hyperplasia and neoplastic change.

MEN IIb or MEN III constitutes a distinct diagnostic entity that segregates (Khairi *et al.,* 1975). The patients have multiple neuromas, most easily recognized by "bumpy" lips or eyelids. Marfanoid habitus was present in over 50%. Pheochromocytoma was common, but parathyroid hyperplasia was rare. Other anomalies such as megacolon, diffuse ganglioneuromatosis of the small bowel, and muscle wasting are present to some extent. The facies are characteristic because of the following features: prominent orbital ridges, thick, large lips, coarse features, broad nasal root, heavy gyrate scalp folds, and floppy, low-set ears.

In an extensive review of over 90 patients with this syndrome, the authors pointed out that MCT and pheochromocytoma accounted for deaths of at least 30% of the patients (Carney *et al.,* 1978). With recognition of the syndrome and better diagnostic techniques, pheochromocytoma will be recognized earlier, and the hyperplastic forerunner of MCT will be removed.

CANCERS OF THE PANCREATIC ISLET CELLS

The advent of the radioimmunoassay, immunofluorescence, and a variety of techniques for isolating and identifying peptides has expanded our knowledge of the functional potentials of islet cell tumors and of their prevalence. As of 20 years ago, only islet cell cancer could be diagnosed clinically with reasonable accuracy. Now, five tumors arising from different cell types in the islet have been recognized.

The islet contains the α cells (glucagon), and the β cells (insulin), δ cells (somatostatin), PP cells (human pancreatic polypeptide, HPP), and the enterochromaffin cells (serotinin). These cells are part of the APUD system, and tumors derived from these cells secrete a wide variety of polypeptide hormones.

Diagnosis

The specific syndromes and diagnostic tests will be discussed separately, but some generally applicable principles should be noted. Radioimmunoassay of peptides in the blood obtained by selective venous catheterization is most helpful in the localization of tumors and may reveal metastatic spread. Arterial angiography and CT scanning are useful when the tumor is over 1 cm in diameter; since many of these tumors are small, these are relatively insensitive techniques. Ultrasound has been shown to be of value in detecting hepatic and duodenal metastases. The mainstay of diagnosis is the radioimmunoassay in conjunction with measurements of other peptides secreted by these tumors and the responses to specific stimuli.

Insulinomas

The *sine qua non* of diagnosis is fasting or inappropriate hypoglycemia accompanied by relatively high plasma insulin levels. A variety of other tests for insulinomas have been proposed: a greater than normal response to tolbutamide, the response of serum insulin to an infusion of calcium gluconate, the ratio of proinsulin to insulin, and the presence of precursor forms of insulin in plasma. Each of these tests will sort out patients with insulinomas, but each test has been shown to be inadequate in a small percentage of patients. Carcinomas may be distinguished only after difficulty from adenomas, patients with carcinoma generally having a greater proportion of proinsulin in plasma (Alsever *et al.,* 1975). Additionally, malignant insulinomas secrete HCG-α, HCG-β, or HCG, whereas this has not been found in benign insulinomas (Kahn *et al.,* 1977).

Over 80% of insulinomas are single and benign; malignant insulinomas comprise about 10% of the total (Filipi and Higgins, 1973). The carcinomas may be detected because of hypoglycemia; some of the apparently nonfunctional malignant insulinomas can reach appreciable size and become symptomatic because of local effects.

Since it is seldom possible to distinguish between benign and malignant insulinomas histologically, one can almost never state that a single insulinoma is cancer, even when some of the functional tests discussed above suggest it. Thus, possible cancers are treated as benign insulinomas. When identification of cancers is certain, they have already metastasized locally and to the liver.

Antihormonal Therapy

The recurrent attacks of hypoglycemia that characterize malignant insulinoma can often be palliated during the early stages of the disease with the use of diet and insulin antagonists. Frequent feedings between meals and at bedtime are administered with sufficient glucose to control symptoms. Adjustments in the carbohydrate content of the diet may be required, depending upon the reactivity of the individual tumor, since the stimulus of a large glucose load may lead to an exaggerated release of insulin (Power, 1969). Parenteral glucose supplementation becomes an important adjunct in patients having frequent or sustained hypoglycemia attacks and, during emergencies, rapid injection of 50% glucose may be required and should always be available.

Corticosteroids, human growth hormone, and glucagon have been effective as palliative agents in individual patients (Landau et al., 1958; Mahon et al., 1962; Marks and Rose, 1965; Roth et al., 1966), but because of their overall limited effectiveness, they are best used in combination and with other antihormonal measures. Glucagon is a known stimulant of pancreatic insulin secretion, and it may produce a paradoxical exacerbation of a hypoglycemia episode.

A major advance in the palliation of malignant insulinoma came with the development of diazoxide, an antidiuretic benzothiadiazine. Its potent hyperglycemic properties, originally recognized during its initial use as an antihypertensive agent, have now been extended to the palliation of insulinoma and leucine-sensitive hypoglycemia of infancy (Dollery and Pentecost, 1962; Graber et al., 1966). The mechanisms by which diazoxide produces its hyperglycemic effects are twofold. First, the principal action is a direct inhibition of insulin release, as has been well documented in perfused pancreas preparations (Basabe et al., 1970). The compound is administered orally in divided doses, ranging from 100 to 1000 mg per day. Although a patient's plasma insulin levels, in many cases, can be brought down to asymptomatic concentrations, the tumor will continue to grow and metastasize since diazoxide has no antitumor activity. Edema, on

the basis of renal sodium retention, is an important toxicity. It may be corrected or prevented with the addition of a benzothiadiazine diuretic, such as chlorothiazide or chlormethiazide, which will also serve to synergize the hyperglycemic effects. Additional potential adverse drug reactions include gastric irritation, postural hypotension, supraventricular tachycardia, hyperuricemia, and hirsutism. Palliation of hypoglycemic symptoms can be achieved with diazoxide in cases where the patient refuses surgery, when surgery is dangerous because of advanced patient age or poor general health, or when surgery fails to locate the tumor.

The anticonvulsant diphenylhydantoin, a known hyperglycemic agent in man, has been identified as an inhibitor of insulin release from both the labile and storage beta-cell pools (Levin et al., 1972). Studies in patients with benign insulinomas have shown that the drug can blunt the response to tolbutamide and other provocative stimuli of insulin secretion and suggest that the hyperglycemic properties of this agent may be additive to those of diazoxide. In patients with undiagnosed seizure disorders, however, it is possible that this drug may partially mask both the clinical and diagnostic chemical features of insulinoma. The use of long-acting somatostatin has been noted recently as a way of suppressing insulin secretion.

Glucagonoma

The secretion of glucagon by the pancreatic α cells normally plays an important role in modulating serum glucose concentrations. The unregulated secretion of glucagon by tumors of the α cells produces a distinctive clinical syndrome that was first defined only 16 years ago (McGavran et al., 1966). The cutaneous rash, described as a necrotizing migratory erythema, is the most characteristic feature. Mild insulin-resistant diabetes and weight loss are present, the latter attributed to the catabolic effects of glucagon. The glossitis, cheilosis, and venous thromboses remain without physiologic explanation. Glucagon inhibits intestinal motility; thus, the glucagonoma syndrome often includes ileus and constipation. The diagnostic test is a high plasma glucagon level. The diagnosis of glucagonoma is further suggested by a failure to suppress plasma glucagon with glucose, an abnormal rise in plasma glucagon after infusion of arginine, hypoaminoacidemia, and, if tumor is available, immunoperoxidase staining for glucagon.

In two recent reviews, over 50 cases were reported (Higgins *et al.,* 1979; Stacpoole, 1981). More women than men had the disease, and it occurred predominantly in the fifth and sixth decades. Time to diagnosis has been as long as 15 years, and survival, even with metastatic disease, may be prolonged. Fifty percent of patients with this syndrome present with a primary tumor in the tail or body of the pancreas; 8% have the tumor localized in the head of the pancreas; the remaining patients have diffuse pancreatic involvement. Higgins *et al.,* (1979) noted that in less than one-third of the patients was the tumor potentially curable by excision and that recurrence had occurred in several of these patients. Metastases are mainly to the liver. The occurrence of glucogonoma in association with multiple endocrine neoplasia has been documented (Leichter *et al.,* 1975; Stacpoole *et al.,* 1981).

Somatostatin and some of its analogs have been used successfully to inhibit the secretion of glucagon by the tumor (Kahn *et al.,* 1981). Somatostatin caused a fall in plasma glucose and a decrease in nausea and vomiting that was correlated with the plasma glucagon level. Furthermore, somatostatin injections given twice a day can induce symptomatic improvement, especially in skin lesions, implying a role for glucagon in the manifestation of this aspect

of the syndrome (Paulusma-DeWaal *et al.,* 1982). Limited success has been noted in the treatment of the tumor with DTIC (Straus *et al.,* 1979). Recently, Foley and Lemon (1982) described their experience with DTIC in glucagonomas as illustrated in Table 32–11. These encouraging results with DTIC need further study in a cooperaive group setting. The same group has expanded their experience in the therapy of malignant APUD cell tumors and reported that 9 of 11 patients benefited from DTIC (Kessinger *et al.,* 1983).

Somatostatinoma

Somatostatin was first identified in pituitary cells, and a role in the regulation of growth hormone secretion was ascribed to it. Subsequently, it was recognized as a hormone of the δ cells of the islets; and a full delineation of its physiologic role as a paracrine regulator of insulin and glucagon secretion is pending. It does inhibit the secretion of these hormones, accounting for some of the signs of somatostatinomas. The patients with somatostatin-producing cancers had diabetes, and the majority had steatorrhea and cholecystolithiasis. Metastases to the liver were common (Krejs *et al.,* 1979; Pipeleers *et al.,* 1979).

Somatostatinoma suppresses the secretion of many peptide hormones, including the gastrointestinal hormones: secretin, gastrin, cholecystokinin, and gastric inhibitory peptide. This results in decreased acid secretion with indigestion, steatorrhea, bloating, abdominal distress, and possibly cholelithiasis as a result of hypocontraction of the gallbladder.

Table 32–11. DTIC Therapy for Glucagonomas

ENDOCRINE SYNDROME	RESULTS	DURATION (MONTHS)
Glucagonoma	Complete remission of syndrome	52+
Glucagonoma	Weight gain; glucagon level of 2810 pg/mL fell to 418 pg/mL; improved liver scans	9+
Gastrinoma/ glucagonoma	Gained 10 kg; glucagon level fell from 281 pg/mL to to 125 pg/mL; Karnofsky index increased from 4 to 9	14
Glucagonoma	Decreased pain; normalization of glucagon level; decrease in pancreatic mass	38

Adapted from Foley, J. F., and Lemon, H. M.: DTIC therapy for malignant islet cell tumors. *Proc. A.S.C.O.,* **1**:169, 1969.

Pancreatic Polypeptide-Secreting Islet Cell Tumor

Pancreatic polypeptide (PP) was isolated from insulin preparations and was subsequently localized to a unique cell type in the islet, the PP cell (Larsson *et al.,* 1975). PP has the pharmacologic effects of increasing choledochal tone and inhibiting gallbladder contractility and the exocrine secretions of the pancreas. Floyd *et al.* (1977) noted that PP was increased in patients with insulinomas.

Although the PP cells are located primarily in the head of the pancreas, the few PP-secreting tumors have been located throughout the body of the pancreas. Two cases of tumors comprised primarily of PP cells have been reported; one was associated with the watery diarrhea syndrome and the other with recurrent gastric ulcers in the absence of high plasma gastrin (Schwartz, 1979). PP-secreting cells are components of many of the islet cell tumors and, when present, plasma PP can serve as a tumor marker. A large number of patients with watery diarrhea syndrome and high levels of vasoactive intestinal peptide also have high levels of PP (Bloom, 1978). PP itself has been suggested as a cause of watery diarrhea on the basis of a single case with diarrhea, low VIP levels, and high plasma PP (Larsson et al., 1976).

Ectopic Secretory Islet Cell Tumors

Cells of the pancreatic islets are part of the APUD system, as noted above, and tumors derived from these cells have been shown to contain a variety of peptide hormones. Most of the patients with these tumors will be symptomatic because of the effects of excess peptide hormones rather than tumor invasion of vital organs. Although the tumors will be designated and discussed on the basis of their primary secretory product, a discussion directed at symptom complexes would be equally solid. Thus, peptic ulcer syndrome, diabetes, diarrhea, and dermatitis may be the result of hypersecretion of one of several hormones, combinations of them, or still unidentified factors. Since therapy of metastatic disease is still unsuccessful, only suspicion leading to early diagnosis will improve the opportunity to obtain surgical cure.

Gastrinomas and the Zollinger-Ellison Syndrome

Gastrin, the polypeptide hormone normally secreted by the G cells of the gastric antrum, stimulates gastric secretion. Although G cells may be found in fetal tissue, they are normally not present in the pancreas. Yet, tumors of the G cells in the pancreas are responsible for the Zollinger-Ellison syndrome. If, as hypothesized, these cells are part of the APUD system, then neoplastic dedifferentiation would facilitate the secretion of several peptide hormones such as gastrin, vasoactive intestinal peptide, cholecystokinin, and others. Many of these are present in association with gastrinomas.

Diagnosis

The hallmark of the gastrinoma syndrome is recurrent peptic ulcer in spite of adequate medical or surgical treatment. Intermittent diarrhea, often with steatorrhea, may be present as a result of enzyme inactivation in the small intestine by gastric acid. A history of MEN I has great significance since gastrinoma may be present in up to 50% of these patients (Jensen et al., 1983).

The combination of high gastric acid secretion and hypergastrinemia is strongly suggestive of gastrinoma, but can occur in patients with retained gastric antrum following surgery for peptic ulcer (antrectomy and Billroth II gastric resection) and after gastric outlet obstruction. Gastric rugal hypertrophy, multiple ulcers, or ulceration of the small bowel suggests gastrinoma (Isenberg et al., 1973). Intravenous bombesin did not increase gastrin levels in patients with gastrinoma, although it did in five patients with retained antrum (Basso et al., 1977). Stimulation with secretin may also be helpful since an increase of more than 100 pg/mL of serum gastrin gives a high probability of gastrinoma, although a few false-negative results may be expected (Lamers et al., 1977; Vinik and Glaser, 1981). The calcium infusion test and a standard meal (milk, bread, cheese, and egg) have been used as provocative tests for assessing the gastrin response. The former test has been replaced by the secretin test, whereas the latter is useful in differentiating gastrinomas and other conditions that cause hypergastrinemia and hyperchlorhydria (retained gastric antrum, gastric outlet obstruction, renal failure, antral G-cell hyperplasia, and short bowel syndrome) (Geokas et al., 1982; Jensen et al., 1983).

The localization of the tumors has been discussed extensively (Jensen et al., 1983). Since gastrinomas are so frequently malignant (Zollinger et al., 1980; Bonfils et al., 1981), it is necessary to use every diagnostic modality to rule out metastatic disease before planning surgery. In the few candidates for surgical excision, transhepatic portal-venous gastrin sampling may aid in localization.

Antihormonal Therapy

The most effective treatment of the illness is directed toward the hypersecretion of gastric acid. Before the introduction of the H_2 receptor antagonist, cimetidine, into practice, the only practical way to treat the recurrent duodenal and jejunal ulcers characteristic of gastrinomas was total gastrectomy. Results were disappointing because of the poor operative state of the patients. The use of cimetidine permits recovery and makes surgery easier (Zollinger et al., 1980). Cimetidine with an anticholinergic drug has produced long-term remission of peptic ulcer disease (Jensen et al., 1983).

The antihistaminics, such as diphenylhyramine, commonly used for allergic conditions have chemical structures that do not resemble the hormone they antagonize. Although they are capable of inhibiting histamine-stimulated smooth muscle contraction of the gastrointestinal tract and bronchi, H_1-receptor functions, they have no effect on other H_2 biologic actions of histamine, such as increasing gastric acid secretion, inhibition of uterine contraction, or increasing the rate of atrial contraction.

Structure-activity studies on histamine analogs by Black and coworkers (1972) have resulted in the identification of potent H_2-receptor antagonists, including burimamide, metiamide, and cimetidine. Metiamide, because of its oral formulation, was actively studied and was demonstrated to antagonize histamine and pentagastrin stimulated by meals, and insulin-stimulated gastric acid secretion. In addition, controlled clinical trials in patients with duodenal ulcer disease have shown this agent active in promoting ulcer healing and reduction in ulcer pain. Richardson and Walsh (1976) demonstrated an 85 to 100% inhibition in gastric acid secretion in three patients with the Zollinger-Ellison syndrome. When combined with anticholinergics, this inhibitory effect was markedly prolonged. Chronic therapy for five to ten months was associated with decreased ulcer pain, bleeding, and diarrhea. One case demonstrated tachyphylaxis to the drug, also observed in other series, as demonstrated by a decreased maximum inhibition of acid secretion. Although metiamide has been generally well tolerated, several cases of transient agranulocytosis and one fatality from this complication were recorded (Isenberg, 1976). The methyl thiourea end group of the molecule has been suggested as the probable mediator of this toxicity since similar bone marrow depression was observed with other thiourea-containing drugs. It was because of the bone marrow toxicity of metiamide that cimetidine has become the standard therapy. A recent review described the procedure of management of patients with gastrinoma with this agent (Jensen et al., 1983).

Anticholinergic agents are known to inhibit the secretion of acid from the parietal cell by blockade of the acetylcholine receptor (Soll and Grossman, 1978). As a single agent, anticholinergic agents are seldom effective in reducing gastric acid in the Zollinger-Ellison syndrome. When used in combination with H_2-receptor antagonists, however, they can show increase in and prolong the response of gastric acid secretion compared to the use of H_2-receptor antagonists alone (Collen et al., 1982; McCarthy and Hyman, 1982).

Antineoplastic Therapy

Based on the experience with insulinomas, streptozotocin and streptozotocin in combination with fluorouracil have been used. Although chemotherapy may reduce gastric acid, it is less effective than H_2-receptor antagonists and should probably be used only in an attempt to reduce tumor burden (Jensen et al., 1983). Given the variable course and occasionally prolonged survival of these patients, vigorous chemotherapy should be thoughtfully considered in the light of the amount of metastatic disease and the ease of control of acid secretion.

VIPOMAS

In 1975, Said and Faloona reported high levels of vasoactive intestinal peptide (VIP) in patients with watery diarrhea (pancreatic cholera) and islet cell adenomas. The syndrome is characterized by secretory diarrhea with resulting hypochloremia and hypokalemic alkalosis. When stool fluid is high, several hundred mEq of potassium may be lost (Verner and Morrison, 1974). These patients may also have attacks of flushing reminiscent of the ileal carcinoid syndrome.

It is still uncertain whether the secretory diarrhea associated initially with VIP is always due to VIP. Jaffe et al., (1977) reported that indomethacin, a prostaglandin synthetase inhibitor, was effective in one patient with pancreatic cholera. Several studies (Kahn et al., 1975) noted that the diarrhea, although associated with metastatic tumors, could not be shown to be caused by VIP.

Hutcheon et al. (1979) reported a father and son with MEN I, both of whom had watery diarrhea. Tumors from both contained gastrin and VIP; however, one patient had considerably greater content of VIP than gastrin, and this was reversed in the other.

Treatment of the malignant disease has as its mainstay streptozotocin, as do the other islet cell carcinomas (Kahn *et al.*, 1975). The diarrhea associated with metastatic vipomas can be palliated with prednisone in approximately 50% of patients (Schein *et al.*, 1973b; Fennelly *et al.*, 1982).

Antineoplastic Therapy

The cornerstone of therapy of the islet cell carcinomas is streptozotocin (STZ), a naturally occurring nitrososurea isolated from the fermentation cultures of *Streptomyces achromogenes*. Chemically, the compound is composed of the union of a known anticancer agent, 1-methyl-1-nitrosourea, and glucose (Herr *et al.*, 1967). This antibiotic showed antitumor activity in several screening tests, including the L-1210 and P388 murine leukemias. STZ can selectively destroy the pancreatic islet beta cell and produce experimental diabetes in rodents, dogs, and monkeys (Rakieten *et al.*, 1963). It is not diabetogenic in man. Biochemically, the acute diabetogenic activity of streptozotocin has been related to the compound's ability to be taken up selectively into islets and depress the concentrations of pyridine nucleotides, NAD and NADH; this activity can be prevented in animals with pharmacologic doses of nicotinamide (Schein *et al.*, 1967; Schein *et al.*, 1973; Anderson *et al.*, 1974).

Streptozotocin is administered intravenously at a dose of 500 mg/m²/day for five days at six-week intervals, or alternatively at a weekly dose of 1.0 to 1.5 g/m² (Schein *et al.*, 1974). It has also been used intra-arterially to deliver higher doses directly to the dominant site of metastatic disease (Kahn *et al.*, 1975).

The major side effect of acute toxicity is the severe vomiting that invariably occurs one to four hours after treatment. The efficacy of metoclopramide as an antiemetic has not been fully exlored with this chemotherapeutic agent. STZ produces renal tubular damage, and if warning signs of proteinuria are ignored, there may be severe proximal renal tubular damage (Sadoff, 1970; Schein *et al.*, 1974). The earliest manifestation has been the development of proteinuria in the range of 400 to 1500 mg/24 hours. With more significant nephrotoxicity, excretion of up to 10 g of protein per 24 hours has been documented. If unaccompanied by any other renal function abnormality, proteinuria is usually reversible in two to four weeks. With continued treatment, however, pronounced signs of proximal tubu-

lar damage are produced which include aminoaciduria, phosphaturia, uricosuria, glycosuria, and renal tubular acidosis, all of which are potentially reversible. Two investigators have reported the development of nephrogenic diabetes insipidus after large doses of the drug, and varying degrees of azotemia have been observed (Sadoff, 1970; Murray-Lyon *et al.*, 1971; Smith, 1971). Serious renal toxicity can be avoided by close monitoring of the urine for protein excretion and stopping treatment until full reversal to normal renal function has been documented. In one series of 24 patients receiving STZ, five died of renal failure (Broder and Carter, 1973). The effects of STZ on liver and bone marrow are mild, with a low incidence of neutropenia and elevated hepatic enzyme.

The usefulness of STZ has been examined, and remission rates of 30 to 50% have been reported (Weiss, 1982). It has proved useful in malignant insulinomas with remission rates of 50% and complete regression in 17% (Broder and Carter, 1973; Schein *et al.*, 1973a). Biochemical remission, even when unaccompanied by evidence of tumor regression, may provide useful therapy for the patient. Biochemical remission, in itself, may result in an increase in survival since these cancers, as most endocrine cancers, often kill because of excessive hormonal effects rather than by direct tissue destruction.

Islet cell tumors were noted to respond occasionally to 5-FU (Moertel, 1975). Because STZ had little bone marrow toxicity, the combination of STZ and 5-FU was used in eight patients with a 75% remission rate (Moertel, 1975). In 1972 the Eastern Cooperative Oncology Group initiated a phase III study evaluating streptozotocin alone versus streptozotocin plus 5-fluorouracil (Moertel *et al.*, 1980). Eighty-four patients with islet cell carcinoma, functional and nonfunctional, were randomized to either streptozotocin (500 mg/m²/day for five days) or the combination of streptozotocin (500 mg/m²/day for five days) plus 5-fluorouracil (400 mg/m²/day for five days). Fifteen of 42 patients (36%) treated with streptozotocin alone responded, and 12% achieved a complete remission. Twenty-five of 40 patients treated with the combination streptozotocin plus 5-fluorouracil (63%) responded, and 33% of all responses were complete. No significant difference in duration of response was found for either treatment arm; the median duration of response was 17 months for all responders and 24 months for complete responders. No relationship of response to the functional status of the tumor was noted. Although not statistically significant, patients treated with the combination evidenced survival benefit, 26-month median, compared to 16.5 months for streptozotocin alone. The survival data demonstrate that these patients had an aggressive tumor, with a finite life-span, when compared to the generally perceived indolent nature of islet cell cancers. Both treatment regimens produced major gastrointestinal toxicity (nausea and vomiting) in approximately 80% of patients, which could be directly attributed to the streptozotocin. One-third of patients in both regimens suffered mild and reversible streptozotocin nephrotoxicity. Mild hematologic toxicity was recorded with the combination treatment.

In view of the reduced gastrointestinal toxicity of the glycosylated chlorothylnitrosourea chlorozotocin, the Southwest Oncology Group recently evaluated this drug's use in islet cell carcinomas (Bukowski, 1982). Six of 17 patients responded (2 CR, 4 PR). The median duration of response was four months.

In an Eastern Cooperative Oncology Group trial (Moertel *et al.*, 1982a), doxorubicin (60 mg/m^2 every three to four weeks) was evaluated in 20 patients with a heterogeneity of clinical presentations (no syndrome, gastrin, insulin, PTH, ACTH, glucagon). The response rate was 20%, but only those patients with nonfunctioning tumors benefited from therapy in this study.

REFERENCES

Adamson, A. K.; Grahame-Smith, D. G.; Peart, W. S.; and Starr, M.: Pharmacological blockade of carcinoid flushing provoked by catecholamines and alcohol. *Lancet,* **2**:293–296, 1969.

Aldinger, K. A.; Hickey, R. C.; Ibanez, M. L.; and Samaan, N. A.: Parathyroid carcinoma: A clinical study of seven cases of functioning and two cases of nonfunctioning parathyroid cancer. *Cancer,* **49**:388–397, 1982.

Alsever, R. N.; Roberts, J. P.; Gerber, J. G.; Mako, M. E.; and Rubenstein, A. H.: Insulinoma with low circulating insulin levels: The diagnostic value of proinsulin measurements. *Ann. Intern. Med.,* **82**:347–350, 1975.

Anderson, T.; Schein, P. S.; McMenamin, M. G.; and Cooney, D. A.: Streptozotocin diabetes, correlation with extent of depression of pancreatic islet nicotinamide adenine dinucleotide. *J. Clin. Invest.,* **54**:672–677, 1974.

Andrew, A.: An experimental investigation into the possible neural crest origin of pancreatic APUD (islet) cells. *J. Embryol. Exp. Morphol.,* **35**:577–593, 1976.

Atkins, E.; Beaven, M. A.; and Keiser, J. R.: Dopa decarboxylase in medullary carcinoma of the thyroid. *N. Engl. J. Med.,* **289**:545–548, 1973.

Ayogai, T., and Summerskill, W. H. J.: Gastric secretion with ulcerogenic islet cell tumors. *Arch. Intern. Med.,* **117**:668–672, 1966.

Ballard, H. S.; Frame, B.; and Hartsock, R.: Familial multiple endocrine adenoma–peptic ulcer complex. *Medicine,* **43**:481–516, 1964.

Barsano, C. P.; Skosey, C.; DeGroot, L. J.; and Refetoff, S.: Serum thyroglobulin in the management of patients with thyroid cancer. *Arch. Intern. Med.,* **142**:763–767, 1982.

Basabe, J.; Lopey, N.; Viktora, J.; and Wolff, F.: Studies of insulin secretion in the perfused rat pancreas. *Diabetes,* **19**:271–281, 1970.

Basso, N.; Lezoche, E.; and Giri, S.: Acid and gastrin levels after bombesin and calcium infusion in patients with incomplete antrectomy. *Am. J. Dig. Dis.,* **22**:125–128, 1977.

Baylin, S. B.; Beaven, M. A.; Engelman, K.; and Sjoerdsma, A.: Elevated histaminase activity in medullary carcinoma of the thyroid. *N. Engl. J. Med.,* **283**:1239–1244, 1970.

Baylin, S. B.; Beaven, M. A.; Keiser, H. R.; Tashjian, A. H., Jr.; and Melvin, K. E. W.: Serum histaminase and calcitonin levels in medullary carcinoma of the thyroid. *Lancet,* **1**:455–458, 1972.

Baylin, S. B.; Gann, D. S.; and Hsu, S. H.: Clonal origin of inherited medullary thyroid carcinoma and pheochromocytoma. *Science,* **193**:321–323, 1976.

Baylin, S. B., and Mendelsohn, G.: Ectopic (inappropriate) hormone production by tumors: Mechanism involved and the biological and clinical implications. *Endocr. Rev.,* **1**:45–77, 1980.

Berg, B.; Biorklund, A.; Grimeluis, L.; Ingemansson, S.; Larsson, L.-I.; Stenram, U.; and Akerman, M.: A new pattern of multiple endocrine adenomatosis. *Acta Med. Scand.,* **200**:321–326, 1976.

Bertagna, C., and Orth, D. N.: Clinical and laboratory findings and results of therapy in 58 patients with adrenocortical tumors admitted to a single medical center (1951–1978). *Am. J. Med.,* **71**:855–875, 1981.

Black, J. W.; Duncan, W. A. M.; Durant, C. J.; Ganellin, C. R.; and Parsons, E. M.: Definition and antagonism of histamine H$_2$-receptors. *Nature,* **236**:385–390, 1972.

Bledsoe, T.; Island, D. P.; Ney, R. L.; and Liddle, G. W.: Effect of o,p'DDD on the extraadrenal metabolism or cortisol in man. *J. Clin. Endocrinol. Metab.,* **24**:1303–1311, 1964.

Block, M. A.: Surgery of the irradiated thyroid gland for possible carcinoma criteria, technique, results. In DeGroot, L. J. (ed.): *Radiation-Associated Thyroid Carcinoma.* Grune & Stratton, Inc., New York, 1977.

Bloom, S. R.: VIP and watery diarrhoea VI. In Bloom, S. R. (ed.): *Gut Hormones.* Churchill Livingstone, Inc., Edinburgh, 1978.

Bonfils, S.; Landor, J. H.; Mignon, M.; and Hervir, P.: Results of surgical management in 92 consecutive patients with Zollinger-Ellison syndrome. *Ann. Surg.,* **194**:692–697, 1981.

Bravo, E. L.; Tarazi, R. C.; Grifford, R. W., Jr.; and Stewart, B. H.: Circulating and urinary catecholamines in pheochromocytoma: Diagnostic and pathophysiologic implications. *N. Engl. J. Med.,* **301**:682–686, 1979.

Bravo, E. L.; Tarazi, R. C.; Fouad, F. M.; Vidt, D. G.; Gifford, R. W., Jr,: Clonidine-suppression test: a useful aid in the diagnosis of pheochromocytoma. *N. Eng. J. Med.,* **305**:623–626, 1981.

Broder, L. E., and Carter, S. K.: Results of therapy with streptozotocin in 52 patients. *Ann. Intern. Med.,* **79:**108–118, 1973.

Brown, R. E.; Hill, S. R., Jr.; Berry, K. W.; and Bing, R. J.: Studies on several possible antiserotonin compounds in the functioning carcinoid syndrome. *Clin. Res.,* **8:**61, 1960.

Buckwalter, J. A., and Thomas, C. G.: Selection of surgical treatment for well differentiated thyroid carcinomas. *Ann. Surg.,* **176:**565–577, 1972.

Bukowski, R. M.: Chemotherapy of islet cell carcinoma with chlorozotocin (CLZ): A Southwest Oncology Group Study. *Proc. A.S.C.O.,* **1:**90, 1982.

Byar, D. P.; Green, S. B.; Dor, P.; Williams, E. D.; Colon, J.; VanGilse, H.; Mayer, M.; Sylvester, R. J.; and Van-Globbeke, M.: A prognostic index for thyroid carcinoma. A study of the EORTC thyroid cancer cooperative group. *Eur. J. Cancer Clin. Oncol.,* **15:**1033–1041, 1979.

Cady, B.; Sedwick, C. E.; Meissner, W. A.; Bookwalter, J. R.; Romagosa, V.; and Werber, J.: Changing clinical, pathologic, treatment and survival pattern in differentiated thyroid carcinoma. *Ann. Surg.,* **184:**541–552, 1976.

Carney, A.; Sizemore, G. W.; and Ty, S. G.: Bilateral adrenal medullary hyperplasia in multiple endocrine neoplasia, Type 2. The precursor of bilateral pheochromocytoma. *Mayo Clin. Proc.,* **50:**3–10, 1975.

Carney, J. A.; Sizemore, G. W.; and Hayles, A. B.: Multiple endocrine neoplasia Type 2b. *Pathobiol. Annu.,* **8:**105–153, 1978.

Cash, R.; Brough, A. J.; Cohen, M. N. P.; and Satoh, P. S.: Aminoglutethimide (Elipten-Ciba) as an inhibitor of adrenal steroidogenesis: Mechanism of action and therapeutic trial. *J. Clin. Endocrinol. Metab.,* **27:**1239–1248. 1967.

Casoria, A., and Moncloa, F.: Actions of 1,1-dichloro-2-p-chlorophenyl-2-0-chlorophenylethane on dog adrenal cortex. *Science,* **136:**47, 1962.

Chin, W. W.; Goodman, R. H.; Jacobs, J. W.; Wolfe, H. J.; Daniels, G. H.; and Habener, J. F.: Medullary thyroid carcinoma identified by cell-free translation of tumor messenger ribonucleic acid in a patient with neck mass and syndrome of ectopic adrenocorticotropin. *J. Clin. Endocrinol. Metab.,* **52:**572–574, 1981.

Chong, G. C.; Beahrs, O. H.; Sizemore, G. W.; and Woolner, L. H.: Medullary carcinoma of the thyroid gland. *Cancer,* **35:**695–704, 1975.

Collen, M. J.; Pandol, S. J.; Kaufman, J. P.; Allende, H. D.; Bissonette, B. M.; Jensen, R. T.; and Gardner, J. D.: Beneficial effects of perenzepine, a selective anticholinergic agent, in patients with Zollinger-Ellison syndrome (ZES) (abstract). *Gastroenterology,* **2:**1035, 1982.

Crane, M. G., and Harris, J. J.: Desoxycorticosterone secretion rates in hyperadenocorticism. *J. Clin. Endocrinol. Metab.,* **26:**1135–1143, 1966.

Cueto, C. and Brown, J. H.: Biological studies on an adrenocorticolytic agent and the isolation of the active components. *Endocrinology,* **62:**334–339, 1958.

Daniels, H.; Van Amstel, W. J.; Schopman, W.; and Van Dommelen, C.: Effect of metopirone in a patient with adrenocortical carcinoma. *Acta Endocrinol (Copenh.).,* **44:**346–354, 1963.

Davis, Z.; Moertel, G.; and McIirath, D. C.: The malignant carcinoid syndrome. *Surg. Gynecol. Obstet.,* **137:**637–644, 1973.

Deftos, L. J., and Stein, M. F.: Radioiodine as an adjunct to the surgical treatment of medullary thyroid carcinoma. *J. Clin. Endocrinol. Metab.,* **50:**967–968, 1980.

DeGroot, L. J.: *Radiation-Associated Thyroid Carcinoma.* Grune & Stratton, Inc., New York, 1976.

DeQuattro, V., and Campese, V. M.: Pheochromocytoma: Diagnosis and therapy. In DeGroot L. J. (ed.): *Endocrinology,* Vol. 2. Grune & Stratton, Inc., New York, 1979.

Didolkar, M. S.; Bescher, R. A.; Elias, E. G.; and Moore, R. H.: Natural history of adrenocortical carcinoma. *Cancer,* **47:**2153–2161, 1981.

Dinnen, J. S.; Greenwood, R. H.; Jones, J. H.; Walker, D. A.; and Williams, E. D.: Parathyroid carcinoma in familial hyperparathyroidism. *J. Clin. Pathol.,* **30:**966–975, 1977.

Dollery, C. T., and Pentecost, B.L.: Drug-induced diabetes. *Lancet,* **2:**735–737, 1962.

Doniach, I.: The effect of radioactive iodine alone and in combination with methylthiouracil and acetylaminogluorene upon tumor production in the rat's thyroid gland. *Br. J. Cancer,* **4:**223–234, 1950.

Doniach, I.: Experimental induction of tumors of the thyroid by radiation. *Br. Med. Bull.,* **14:**181–183, 1958.

Doumith, R.; deGennes, J. L.; Cabane, J. P.; and Zygelman, N.: Pituitary prolactinoma, adrenal aldosterone-producing adenomas, gastric schwannoma and colonic polyadenomas: A possible variant of multiple endocrine neoplasia (MEN) type I. *Acta Endocrinol.,* **100:**189–195, 1982.

Eberle, F., and Grun, R.: Multiple endocrine neoplasia, type I (MEN I). *Ergeb. Inn. Med. Kinderheilkd.,* **46:**75–150, 1981.

Ellison, E. H., and Wilson, S. D.: The Zollinger-Ellison syndrome: Reappraisal and evaluation of 260 registered cases. *Ann. Surg.,* **160:**512–530, 1964.

Engelman, K., and Sjoerdsma, A.: Inhibition of catecholamine biosynthesis in man. *Circ. Res.* (Suppl.), **1:**104–109, 1966.

Fennelly, J. J.; Cantwell, B.; Fielding, J. F.; Fitzgerald, O.; and Collins, P. G.: Metastatic pancreatic vipoma: A case report of clinical response following treatment with corticosteroids and actinomycin-D. *Clin. Oncol.,* **8:**167–170, 1982.

Filipi, C. J., and Higgins, G. A.: Diagnosis and management of insulinoma. *Am. J. Surg.,* **125:**231–239, 1973.

Fishman, L. M.; Liddle, G. W.; Island, D. P.; Fleisher, N.; and Kuchel, O.: Effects of aminoglutethimide on adrenal function in man. *J. Clin. Endocrinol. Metab.,* **27:**481–490, 1967.

Floyd, J. C.; Fajan, S. S.; Pek, S.; and Chance, R. E.: A newly recognized pancreatic polypeptide; Plasma levels in health and disease. *Recent Prog. Horm. Res.,* **33:**519–556, 1977.

Foley, J. F., and Lemon, H. M.: DTIC therapy for malignant islet cell tumors. *Proc. A.S.C.O.,* **1:**169, 1982.

Frolich, J. C.; Bloomgarden, Z. T.; Oates, J. A.; McGuigan, J. E.; and Rabinowitz, D.: The carcinoid flush: Provocation by pentagastrin and inhibition by somatostatin. *N. Engl. J. Med.,* **299:**1055–1056, 1978.

Gabrilove, J. L.; Sharma, D. C.; Wotiz, H. H.; and Dorfman, R.: Feminizing adrenal cortical cancers in the male: A review of 52 cases including a case report. *Medicine,* **44:**37–59, 1965.

Gagel, R. F.; Melvin, K. E. W.; Tashjian, A. H., Jr.; Miller, H. H.; Feldman, Z. T.; Wolfe, H. J.; DeLellis, R. A.; Cervi-Skinner, S.; and Reichlin, S.: Natural history of familial medullary thyroid carcinoma — pheochromocytoma syndrome and identification of preneoplastic stages by screening studies: Five year report. *Trans. Assoc. Am. Physicians*, **87**:177–191, 1975.

Geokas, M. C.; Yalow, R. S.; Strauss, E. W.; and Gold, E. M.: Peptide radioimmunoassays in clinical medicine. *Ann. Intern. Med.*, **97**:389–407, 1982.

Gershengorn, M. C.; McClung, M. R.; Chu, E.W.; Hanson, T. A. S.; Weintraub, B. D.; and Robbins, J.: Fine-needle aspiration cytology in the preoperative diagnosis of thyroid nodules. *Ann. Intern. Med.*, **87**:256–269, 1977.

Gorden, P.; Becker, C. E.; Levey, G. S.; and Roth, J.: Efficacy of aminoglutethimide in the ectopic ACTH syndrome. *J. Clin. Endocrinol. Metab.*, **28**:921–923, 1968.

Graber, A. L.; Porte, E., Jr.; and Williams, R. H.: Clinical use of diazoxide and mechanisms for its hyperglycemic effects. *Diabetes*, **15**:143–148, 1966.

Grahame-Smith, D. G.: *The Carcinoid Syndrome*. Heinemann, London, 1972.

Grim, C. E.; Ganguly, A.; Yum, M. N.; Donohue, J. P.; and Weinberger, M. H.: Hyperaldosteronism due to unsuspected adrenal carcinoma: Discovery during investigation of hypertension in a young woman. *J. Urol.*, **126**:783–786, 1981.

Grun, R., and Eberle, F.: Multiple endocrine neoplasia, type II (MEN II). *Ergeb. Inn. Med. Kinderheilkd.*, **46**:152–190, 1981.

Hamilton, F. P. M. Cheikh, E. I.; and Rivera, L. E.: Attempted treatment of inoperable pheochromocytoma with streptozotocin. *Arch. Inter. Med.*, **137**:762–765, 1977.

Hempelman, L. H.; Piper, J. W.; Burke, G. J.; Terry, R.; and Ames, W. R.: Neoplasms in persons treated with x-rays in infancy for thymic enlargement. *J.N.C.I.*, **38**:317–341, 1967.

Herr, R. R.; Jahnke, H. K.; and Argondelis, A. S.: Structure of streptozotocin. *J. Am. Chem. Soc.*, **89**:4808–4809, 1967.

Hertz, R.; Allen, M. J.; Schricker, J. A.; Dhyse, F. G.; and Hallman, L. F.: Studies on amphenone and related compounds. *Recent Prog. Horm. Res.*, **11**:119–147, 1955.

Hertz, R.; Pittman, J. A.; and Graff, M. M.: Amphenone: Toxicity and effects on adrenal and thyroid function in man. *J. Clin. Endocrinol. Metab.*, **16**:705–723, 1956.

Higgins, G. A.; Recant, L.; and Fischman, A. B.: The glucagonoma syndrome: Surgically curable diabetes. *Am. J. Surg.*, **137**:142–148, 1979.

Hill, G. J.: Carcinoid tumors: Pharmacological therapy. *Oncology*, **25**:329–343, 1971.

Hill, C. S., Jr.; Ibanez, M. L.; Samaan, N. A.; Ahearn, M. J.; and Clark, L.: Medullary (solid) carcinoma of the thyroid gland: An analysis of the M.D. Anderson Hospital experience with patients with the tumor, its special features and its histogenesis. *Medicine*, **52**:141–171, 1973.

Holmes, E. C.; Morton, D. L.; and Ketcham, A. S.: Parathyroid carcinoma: Collective review. *Ann. Surg.*, **169**:631–640, 1969.

Hough, A. J.; Hollifield, J. W.; Page, D. L.; Scott, H. W.; and Hartmann, W. H.: Prognostic factors in adrenal cortical tumors. A mathematical analysis of clinical and morphologic data. *Am. J. Clin. Pathol.*, **72**:390–399, 1979.

Hutcheon, D. F.; Bayliss, T. M.; Cameron, J. L.; and Bay-

lin, S. B.: Hormone-mediated watery diarrhea in a family with multiple endocrine neoplasia. *Ann. Intern. Med.*, **90**:932–934, 1979.

Hutter, A. M., and Kayhoe, D. E.: Adrenal cortical carcinoma: Clinical features in 138 patients. *Am. J. Med.*, **41**:572–580, 1966a.

Hutter, A. M., and Kayhoe, D. E.: Adrenal cortical carcinoma: Results of treatment with o,p'DDD in 138 patients. *Am. J. Med.*, **41**:581–592, 1966b.

Iida, F.; Yonekura, M.; and Miyakawa, M.: Study of intraglandular dissemination of thyroid cancer. *Cancer*, **24**:764–771, 1969.

Isenberg, J. I.: H_2-receptor antagonists in the treatment of peptic ulcer. *Ann. Intern. Med.*, **84**:213–214, 1976.

Isenberg, J. I.; Walsh, J. H.; and Grossman, M. I.: Zollinger-Ellison syndrome. *Gastroenterology*, **65**:140–165, 1973.

Jaffe, B. M.; Kopen, D. F.; DeSchryver-Kecskemeti, K.; Gingerich, R. F.; and Grieder, M.: Indomethacin-sensitive pancreatic cholera. *N. Engl. J. Med.*, **287**:817–820, 1977.

Jensen, R. T.; Gardner, J. D.; Raufman, J. P.; Pandol, S. J.; Doppman, J. L.; and Collen, M. J.: Zollinger-Ellison syndrome: Current concepts and management. *Ann. Intern. Med.*, **98**:59–75, 1983.

Jones, B. A., and Sisson, J. E.: Early diagnosis and thyroidectomy in multiple endocrine neoplasia, type 2b. *J. Pediatr.*, **102**:219–223, 1983.

Kahn, C. R.; Bhathera, S. J.; Recant, L.; and Rivier, J.: Use of somatostatin and somatostatin analogs in a patient with glucagonoma. *J. Clin. Endocrinol. Metab.*, **53**:543–549, 1981.

Kahn, C. R.; Levy, A. G.; Gardner, J. D.; Miller, J. V.; Gorden, P.; and Schein, P. S.: Pancreatic cholera: Beneficial effects of streptozotocin. *N. Engl. J. Med.*, **292**:941–945, 1975.

Kahn, C. R.; Rosen, S. W.; Weintraub, B. D.; Fajans, S. S.; and Gorden, P.: Ectopic production of chorionic gonadotropin and its subunits by islet cell tumors. *N. Engl. J. Med.*, **297**:565–569, 1977.

Keiser, H. R.; Beaven, M. A.; Doppman, J.; Wills, S., Jr.; and Buja, L. M.: Sipple's syndrome: Medullary thyroid carcinoma, pheochromocytoma and parathyroid disease. *Ann. Intern. Med.*, **78**:561–579, 1973.

Kessinger, A.; Foley, J. F.; and Lemon, H. M.: Use of DTIC in the malignant carcinoid syndrome. *Cancer Treat. Rep.*, **61**:101–102, 1977.

Kessinger, A., Foley, J. F.; and Lemon, H. M.: Therapy of malignant APUD cell tumors. *Cancer*, **51**:790–794, 1983.

Khairi, M. A.; Dexter, R. N.; Burzynski, N. J.; and Johnston, C. C., Jr.: Mucosal neuroma, pheochromocytoma and medullary thyroid carcinoma, multiple endocrine neoplasia, type 3. *Medicine*, **54**:89–112, 1975.

Kiang, D. T.; Frenning, D. H.; and Bauer, G. E.: Mithramycin for hypoglycemia in malignant insulinoma. *N. Engl. J. Med.*, **299**:134–135, 1978.

Krejs, G. J.; Orci, L.; Conlon, J. M.; Ravazzola, M.; Davis, G. R.; Raskin, P.; Collins, S. M.; McCarthy, D. M.; Baetens, D.; Rubenstein, A.; Aldor, T. A. M.; and Unger, R. H.: Somatostatinoma syndrome. Biochemical, morphologic and clinical features. *N. Engl. J. Med.*, **301**:285–292, 1979.

Lamers, C. B.; Butts, J. T.; and Van Tongeren, J.: Secretin-stimulated serum gastrin levels in hyperparathyroid patients from families with multiple endocrine adenomatosis. *Ann. Intern. Med.*, **86**:719–724, 1977.

Landau, B. R.; Levine, H. J.; and Hertz, R.: Prolonged glucagon administration in a case of hyperinsulinemia due to disseminated islet-cell carcinoma. *N. Engl. J. Med.,* **259**:286–288, 1958.

Larsson, L.-I.; Schwartz, T. W.; Lundquist, G.; Chance, R. E.; Sundler, R.; Rehfeld, J. F.; Grimelius, L.; Fahrenkrug, J.; Schaffalitzky de Muckadell, O. B.; and Moon, N.: Occurrence of human pancreatic polypeptide in pancreatic endocrine tumors. *Am. J. Pathol.,* **85**:675–684, 1976.

Larsson, L.-I.; Sundler, F.; and Hakanson, R.: Immunohistochemical localization of human pancreatic polypeptide (HPP) to a population of islet cells. *Cell Tissue Res.,* **156**:167–171, 1975.

Leeper, R. D.: The effect of ^{131}I therapy on survival of patients with metastatic papillary or follicular thyroid carcinoma. *J. Clin. Endocrinol. Metab.,* **36**:1143–1152, 1973.

Legha, S.S.; Valdivieso, M.; Nelson, R. S.; Benjamin, R. S.; and Bodey, G. P.: Chemotherapy for metastatic carcinoid tumors. Experiences with 32 patients and a review of the literature. *Cancer Treat. Rep.,* **61**:1699–1703, 1977.

Leichter, S. B.; Pagliaraa, A. S.; Grieder, M. H.; Pohl, S.; Rosai, J.; and Kipnis, D. D.: Uncontrolled diabetes mellitus and hyperglucagonemia associated with an islet-cell carcinoma. *Am. J. Med.,* **58**:285–293, 1975.

Levin, S. R.; Grodsky, G. M.; and Hagura, R.: Comparison of the inhibitory effects of diphenylhydantoin and diazoxide upon insulin secretion from the isolated perfused pancreas. *Diabetes,* **21**:856–862, 1972

Lips, C. J. M.; Minder, W. H.; Leo, J. R.; Alleman, A.; and Hackeng, W. H. L.: Evidence of multicentric origin of the multiple endocrine neoplasia syndrome type 2A (Sipple's syndrome) in a large family in the Netherlands. *Am. J. Med.,* **64**:568–578, 1978.

Lipsett, M. G.: Rationale for chemotherapy of Cushing's syndrome. *Clin. Endocrinol.,* **2**:489–497, 1968.

Lipsett, M. G.; Ross, G. T.; and Hertz, R.: Clinical and pathophysiologic aspects of adrenocortical carcinoma. *Am. J. Med.,* **35**:374–383, 1963.

Lowhagen, T.; Granberg, P.-O.; Lundell, G.; Skinnari, P.; Sundblad, R.; and Willems, J. S.: Aspiration biopsy cytology (ABC) in nodules of the thyroid gland suspected to be malignant. *Surg. Clin. North Am.,* **59**:3–18, 1979.

Lubitz, J. A.; Freeman, L.; and Okun, R.: Mitotane use in inoperable adrenal cortical carcinoma. *J.A.M.A.,* **223**:1109–1112, 1973.

Mahon, W. A.; Mitchell, M. L.; Steinke, J.; and Raben, M. S.: Effect of human growth hormone on hypoglycemia states. *N. Engl. J. Med.,* **267**:1179–1183, 1962.

Malafosse, M.: Carcinoid tumours: Surgical problems. *Clin. Gastroenterol.,* **33**:711–719, 1974.

Manger, W. M., and Gifford, R. W., Jr.: *Pheochromocytoma.* Springer-Verlag New York, Inc., New York, 1977.

Marks, V., and Rose, F. C.: *Hypoglycemia.* Blackwell, Oxford, 1965.

Mazzaferri, E. L.; Young, R. L.; Oertel, J. E.; Kemmerer, W. T.; and Page, L. P.: Papillary thyroid carcinoma: The impact of therapy in 576 patients. *Medicine,* **56**:171–196, 1977.

McCarthy, D. M., and Hyman, P. E.: Effect of isopropamide on response to oral cimetidine in patients with Zollinger-Ellison syndrome. *Dig. Dis. Sci.,* **27**:353–359, 1982.

McGavran, M. H.; Ungar, R. R. H.; Recant, L.; Polk, H. C.; Kilo, C.; and Levin, M. E.: A glucagon-secreting

alpha-cell carcinoma of the pancreas. *N. Engl. J. Med.,* **274**:1408–1413, 1966.

Melicow, M. M.: One hundred cases of pheochromocytoma (107 tumors) at the Columbia-Presbyterian Medical Center, 1926–1976. *Cancer,* **40**:1987–2004, 1977.

Melmon, K. L.; Sjoerdsma, A.; and Mason, D. T.: Distinctive clinical and therapeutic aspects of the syndrome associated with bronchial carcinoid tumors. *Am. J. Med.,* **39**:568–581, 1965.

Melmon, K. L.; Sjoerdsma, A.; Oates, J. A.; and Laster, L.: Treatment of malabsorption and diarrhea of the carcinoid syndrome with methylsergide. *Gastroenterology,* **48**:18–24, 1965.

Melvin, K. E. W., and Tashjian, A. H., Jr.: Studies in familial (medullary) thyroid carcinoma. *Recent Prog. Horm. Res.,* **28**:399–470, 1972.

Mengel, C. E.: Therapy of the malignant carcinoid syndrome. *Ann. Intern. Med.,* **62**:587–602, 1965.

Mengel, C. E., and Shaffer, R. D.: The carcinoid syndrome. In Holland, J. F., and Frei, E. (eds.): *Cancer Medicine.* Lea & Febiger, Philadelphia, 1973.

Miller, H. H.; Melvin, K. E. W.; Gibson, J. M.; and Tashjian, A. H., Jr.: Surgical approach to early familial medullary carcinoma of the thyroid. *Am. J. Surg.,* **123**:438–443, 1972.

Miller, J. M., and Hamburger, J. I.: The thyroid scintigram I. The hot nodule. *Radiology,* **84**:66–73, 1965.

Misiewicz, J. J.; Waller, S. L.; and Eisner, M.: Motor response of the human gastrointestinal tract to 5-hydroxytryptamine *in vivo* and *in vitro. Gut,* **7**:208–216, 1966.

Moertel, C. G.: Clinical management of advanced gastrointestinal cancer. *Cancer,* **36**:675–682, 1975.

Moertel, C. G., and Hanley, H. A.: Combination chemotherapy trials for metastatic carcinoid tumor and the malignant carcinoid syndrome. *Cancer Clin. Trials,* **2**:327, 1979.

Moertel, C. G.; Hanley, J. A.; and Johnson, L. A.: Streptozotocin alone compared with streptozotocin plus fluorouracil in the treatment of advanced islet-cell carcinoma. *N. Engl. J. Med.,* **303**:1189–1194, 1980.

Moertel, C. G.; Lavin, P. T.; and Hahn, R. G.: Phase II trial of doxorubicin therapy for advanced islet cell carcinoma. *Cancer Treat. Rep.,* **66**:1567–1569, 1982a.

Moertel, C. G.; Martin, J. K.; O'Connell, M. J.; Rubin, J.; Schutt, A. J.; Hahn, R. G.; Kvols, L. K.; and Reitemeier, R. J.: Phase II trials in the malignant carcinoid tumor and the carcinoid syndrome. *Proc. A.S.C.O.,* **1**:169, 1982b.

Moertel, C. G.; Sauer, W. G.; Dockerty, M. G.; and Baggenstoss, A. H.: Life history of the carcinoid tumor of the small intestine. *Cancer,* **14**:901–912, 1961.

Murray-Lyon, I. M.; Cassar, J.; Coulson, J.; Williams, R.; Ganguli, P. C.; Edwards, J. C.; and Taylor, K. W.: Further studies on streptozotocin therapy for a multiple hormone-producing islet cell carcinoma. *Gut,* **12**:717–720, 1971.

Murray-Lyon, I. M.; Dawson, J. L.; Parsons, V. A.; Rake, M. O.; Blendis, L. M.; Laws, J. W.; and Williams, R.: Treatment of secondary hepatic tumors by ligation of hepatic artery and infusion of cytotoxic drugs. *Lancet,* **2**:172–174, 1970.

Nader, S.; Hickey, R. C.; Sellin, R. V.; and Samaan, N. A.: Adrenol cortical carcinoma. *Cancer,* **52**:707–711, 1983.

Nichols, J., and Henniger, G.: Studies on DDD,2,2-bis (parachlorophenyl)-1,1-dichloroethane. *Exp. Med. Surg.,* **15**:310–316, 1957.

Oates, J. A., and Butler, T. C.: Pharmacologic and endocrine aspects of carcinoid syndrome. *Adv. Pharmacol.,* **5:**109–128, 1967.

Oates, J. A., and Sjoerdsma, A.: A unique syndrome associated with the secretion of 5-hydroxytryptophan by metastatic gastric carcinoids. *Am. J. Med.,* **32:**333–343, 1962.

Odell, W. D.; Wolfsen, A.; Yoshimoto, Y.; Weitzman, R.; Fisher, D.; and Hirose, F.: Ectopic peptide synthesis: A universal concomitant of neoplasia. *Trans. Assoc. Am. Physicians,* **90:**204–225, 1977.

Ostuni, J. A., and Roginski, M. S.: Metastatic adrenal cortical carcinoma: Documented cure with combined chemotherapy. *Arch. Intern. Med.,* **135:**1257–1258, 1975.

Paulusma-DeWaal, J. H.; Bosman, F. T.; Fisher, H. R. A.; Van der Velden, P. D.; and Hackeng, W. H. L.: The glucagonoma syndrome. *Neth. J. Med.,* **25:**127–133, 1982.

Pearse, A. G. E.: The cytochemistry and ultrastructure of polypeptide hormone-producing cells of the APUD series and the embryologic, physiologic, and pathologic implications of the concept. *J. Histochem. Cytochem.,* **12:**303–313, 1969.

Pearse, A. G. E., and Polak, J. M.: The diffuse neuroendocrine system and the APUD concept. In Bloom, S. R. (ed.): *Gut Hormones.* Churchill Livingstone, Edinburgh, 1978.

Pictet, R. L.; Rall, L. B.; Phelps, P.; and Rutter, W. J.: The neural crest and the origin of insulin-producing and other gastrointestinal hormone-producing cells. *Science,* **191:**191–192, 1976.

Pipeleers, D.; Somers, G.; Cepts, W.; DeNutte, N.; and DeVroede, M.: Plasma pancreatic hormones in a case of somatostatinoma: Diagnostic and therapeutic implications. *J. Clin. Endocrinol. Metab.,* **49:**572–579, 1979.

Pochin, E. E.: Leukaemia following radioiodine treatment of thyrotoxicosis. *Br. Med. J.,* **2:**1545–1547, 1960.

Power, L.: A glucose-responsive insulinoma. *J.A.M.A.,* **207:**893–896, 1969.

Prinz, R. A.; Barbato, A. L.; Braithwaite, S. S.; Brooks, M. H.; Laurence, A. M.; and Poloyan, E.: Prior irradiation and the development of coexistent differentiated thyroid cancer and hyperparathyroidism. *Cancer,* **49:**847–877, 1982.

Rakieten, N.; Rakieten, M. L.; and Nadkarni, M. V.: Studies on the diabetogenic action of streptozotocin (NSC-37917). *Cancer Chemother. Rep.,* **29:**91–98, 1963.

Remine, W. H.; Chong, G. C.; VanHeerden, J. A.; Sheps, S. G.; and Harrison, E. G., Jr.: Current management of pheochromocytoma. *Ann. Surg.,* **179:**740–748, 1974.

Richardson, C. T., and Walsh, J. H.: The value of a histamine H_2-receptor antagonist in the management of patients. *N. Engl. J. Med.,* **294:**133–135, 1976.

Roberts, J. L., II.; Marney, S. R., Jr.; and Oates, J. A.: Blockade of the flush associated with metastatic gastric carcinoid by combined histamine H_1 and H_2 receptor antagonists. *N. Engl. J. Med.,* **300:**236–237, 1979.

Robertson, J. I. S.; Peart, W. S.; and Andrews, T. M.: The mechanism of facial flushes in the carcinoid syndrome. *Q. J. Med.,* **31:**103–123, 1962.

Rocha e Silva, M., and Carcia Lerne, J.: Antagonists of bradykinin. *Med. Exp.,* **8:**287–295, 1963.

Rosen, I. B.; Walfish, P. G.; and Miskin, M.: The ultrasound of thyroid masses. *Surg. Clin. North Am.,* **59:**19–33, 1979.

Roth, H.; Thier, S.; and Segal, S.: Zinc glucagon in the management of refractory hypoglycemia due to insulin-producing tumor. *N. Engl. J. Med.,* **274:**493–497, 1966.

Roth, J.; LeRoith, D.; Shiloach, J.; Rosenzweig, J. L.; Lesniak, M. A.; and Havrankova, J.: The evolutionary origins of hormone neurotransmitters and other extracellular chemical messengers. *N. Engl. J. Med.,* **306:**523–527, 1982.

Roundebush, C. P., and DeGroot, L. J.: The natural history of radiation-associated thyroid cancer. In DeGroot, L. J. (ed.): *Radiation-Associated Thyroid Carcinoma.* Grune & Stratton, Inc., New York, 1977.

Rubenstein, A. H.; Kuzuya, H.; and Horwitz, D. L.: Clinical significance of circulating C-peptide in diabetes and hypoglycemic disorders. *Arch. Intern. Med.,* **137:**625–632, 1977.

Russell, W. O.; Ibanex, M. L.; Clark, R. L.; and White, E. C.: Follicular (organoid) carcinoma of the thyroid gland. Report of 84 cases in thyroid cancer. *UICC Monograph Series,* **12:**14–25, 1969.

Sadoff, L.: Nephrotoxicity of streptozotocin (NSC-85998). *Cancer Chemother. Rep.,* **54:**457–459, 1970.

Said, S. I., and Faloona, G. F.: Vasoactive intestinal peptide and watery diarrhea. *N. Engl. J. Med.,* **293:**155–160, 1975.

Schantz, A., and Castleman, B.: Parathyroid carcinoma: A study of 70 cases. *Cancer,* **31:**600–605, 1973.

Schein, P. S.; Cooney, D. A.; McMenamin, M. G.; and Anderson, T.: Streptozotocin diabetes–Further studies on the mechanism of depression of nicotinamide adenine dinucleotide concentrations in mouse pancreatic islets and liver. *Biochem. Pharmacol.,* **22:**2625–2631, 1973.

Schein, P. S.; Cooney, D. A.; and Vernon, M. L.: The use of nicotinamide to modify the toxicity of streptozotocin diabetes without loss of antitumor activity. *Cancer Res.,* **27:**2324–2332, 1967.

Schein, P. S; Kahn, R.; Gorden, P.; Wells, S.; and DeVita, V. T.: Streptozotocin for malignant insulinomas and carcinoid tumors. *Arch. Intern. Med.,* **132:**555–561, 1973a.

Schein, P. S.; LeLellis, R.; Kahn, C. R.; Gorden, P.; and Kraft, A.: Current concepts and management of islet cell tumors. *Ann. Intern. Med.,* **79:**239–257, 1973b.

Schein, P. S.; O'Connell, M. J.; Blom, J.; Hubbard, S.; Magrath, J. T.; Bergevin, P.; Wiernik, P. H.; Ziegler, J. L.; and DeVita, V. T.: Clinical antitumor activity and toxicity of streptozotocin (NSC-85998). *Cancer,* **34:**993–1000, 1974.

Schneider, A. G.; Favus, M. J.; Stachura, M. E.; Arnold, J.; Arnold, M. J.; and Frohman, L. A.: Incidence, prevalence and characteristics of radiation-induced thyroid cancer. *Am. J. Med.,* **64:**243–252, 1978.

Schteingart, D. E.; Cash, R.; and Coon, J. W.: Amino-glutethimide and metastatic adrenal cancer. *J.A.M.A.,* **198:**1007–1010, 1966.

Schteingart, D. E.; Motazed, A.; Noonan, R. A.; and Thompson, N. W.: Treatment of adrenal carcinoma. *Arch. Surg.,* **117:**1142–1146, 1982.

Schteingart, D. E.; Seabold, J. E.; Gross, M. D.; and Swanton, D. P.: Iodocholesterol adrenal tissue uptake and imaging in adrenal neoplasm. *J. Clin. Endocrinol. Metab.,* **52:**1156–1161, 1981.

Schwartz, T. W.: Pancreatic-polypeptide (PP) and endocrine tumours of the pancreas. *Scand. J. Gastroenterol.,* **14:**93–100, 1979.

Shimaoka, K.: Suppressive therapy with thyroid hormones. In DeGroot, L. J. (ed.): *Radiation-Associated*

Thyroid Carcinoma. Grune & Stratton, Inc., New York, 1977.

Sipple, J. H.: The association of pheochromocytoma with carcinoma of the thyroid. *Am. J. Med.,* **31:**163–166, 1961.

Sjoerdsma, A.; Lovenberg, W.; Engelman, K.; Carpenter, W. T.; Wyatt, R. J.; and Gessa, G. L.: Serotonin now: Clinical implications of inhibiting its synthesis with para-chlorophenylalanine. *Ann. Intern. Med.,* **73:**607–629, 1970.

Smith, C. K.: Treatment of malignant insulinoma with streptozotocin. *Diabetologia,* **7:**118–124, 1971.

Soll, A. H., and Grossman, M. J.: Cellular mechanisms in acid secretion. *Annu. Rev. Med.,* **29:**495–507, 1978.

Stacpoole, P. W.: The glucagonoma syndrome: Clinical features, diagnosis and treatment. *Endocr. Rev.,* **2:**347–361, 1981.

Stacpoole, P. W.; Jaspan, J.; Kasselberg, A. G.; Halter, S. A.; Polonsky, K.; Gluck, F. W.; Liljenquist, J. E.; and Rabin, D.: A familial glucagonoma syndrome. Genetic, clinical and biochemical features. *Am. J. Med.,* **70:**1017–1026, 1981.

Steiner, E. L.; Goodman, A. D.; and Powers, R. S.: Study of a kindred with pheochromocytoma, medullary thyroid carcinoma, hyperparathyroidism and Cushing's disease. Multiple endocrine neoplasia, type II. *Medicine,* **47:**371–409, 1968.

Stepanas, A. V.; Samaan, N. A.; Hill, C. S.; and Hickey, R. C.: Medullary thyroid carcinoma. *Cancer,* **43:**825–837, 1979.

Straus, G. M.; Weitzman, S. A.; and Aoki, T. T.: Dimethyltriazenoimidazole carboxamide therapy of malignant glucagonoma. *Ann. Intern. Med.,* **90:**57–58, 1979.

Symington, T., and Goodall, A. L.: Studies in phaeochromocytoma: I. Pathological aspects. *Glasgow Med. J.,* **34:**75–96, 1953.

Tattersall, M. H. N.; Lander, H.; Bain, B.; Stocks, A. E.; Woods, R. L.; Fox, R. M.; Byrne, E.; Trotten, J. R.; and Roos, I.: Cis-platinum treatment of metastatic adrenal carcinoma. *Med. J. Aust.,* **1:**419–421, 1980.

Teitelman, G.; Joh, T. H.; and Reis, D. J.: Transformation of catecholaminergic precursors into glucagon (A) cells in mouse embryonic pancreas. *Proc. Natl. Acad. Sci. U.S.A.,* **78:**5225–5229, 1981.

Thomas, C. G., Jr.: Hormonal treatment of thyroid cancer. *J. Clin. Endocrinol. Metab.,* **17:**232–237, 1957.

Thorson, A.: Studies on carcinoid disease. *Acta Med. Scand.,* **334** (Suppl. 7):1–132, 1958.

Tullner, W.: Nonhormonal inhibitors of adrenocortical steroid biosynthesis. Hormonal steroids, biochemistry, pharmacology and therapeutics. *Proc. First Int. Congr. Horm. Steroids,* pp. 383–395, 1964.

Ureles, A. L.; Murray, M.; and Wolf, R.: Results of pharmacologic treatment in the malignant carcinoid syndrome. *N. Engl. J. Med.,* **269:**435–438, 1963.

Van Heerden, J. A.; Sheps, S. G.; Hamberger, B.; Sheedy, P. F., II.; Poston, J. G.; and ReMine, W. H.: Pheochromocytoma: Current status and changing trends. *Surgery,* **91:**363–373, 1982.

VanHerle, A. J.; Rich, P.; Ljung, B. M.; Ashcraft, M. W.; Solomon, D. H.; and Keeler, E. B.: The thyroid nodule. *Ann. Intern. Med.,* **96:**221–232, 1982.

Van Slooten, H.; Moolenaar, A. J.; Van Seters, A. P.; and Smeenk, D.: The treatment of adrenocortical carcinoma with o,p'DDD: Prognostic simplifications of serum level monitoring. *Eur. J. Cancer Clin. Oncol.,* **20:**47–53, 1984.

Verner, J. V., and Morrison, A. B.: Endocrine pancreatic islet disease with diarrhea: Report of a case due to diffuse hyperplasia of non-beta islet tissue with a review of 54 additional cases. *Arch. Intern. Med.,* **133:**452–500, 1974.

Vilar, P., and Tullner, W. W.: Effects of o,p'DDD on history and 17-hydroxy-cortisteroids output of the dog adrenal cortex. *Endocrinology,* **65:**80–86, 1959.

Vinik, A. I., and Glasser, B.: Pancreatic endocrine tumors. In Dent, T. (ed.): *Pancreatic Disease.* Grune & Stratton, Inc., New York, 1981.

Waldenstrom, J.: Clinical picture of carcinoidosis. *Gastroenterology,* **35:**565–569, 1958.

Walfish, P. G.; Natale, R.; and Chang, C.: Beta adrenergic receptor mechanism in the metabolic-effects of diazoxide in fasted rats. *Diabetes,* **19:**228–233, 1970.

Weiss, R. B.: Streptozotocin: A review of its pharmacology, efficacy and toxicity. *Cancer Treat. Rep.,* **66:**427–438, 1982.

Williams, E. D.: Histogenesis of medullary carcinoma of the thyroid. *J. Clin. Pathol.,* **19:**114–118, 1966.

Williams, E. D.; Brown, C. L.; and Doniach, I.: Pathological and clinical findings in 67 cases of medullary carcinoma of the thyroid. *J. Clin. Pathol.,* **19:**103–113, 1966.

Williams, E. D.; Karim, S. M. M.; and Sandler, M.: Prostaglandin secretion by medullary carcinoma of the thyroid. *Lancet,* **1:**22–23, 1968.

Wohltmann, H.; Mathuri, R. S.; and Williamson, H. P.: Sexual precocity in a female infant due to feminizing adrenal carcinoma. *J. Clin. Endocrinol. Metab.,* **50:**186–189, 1980.

Wolfe, H. J.; Melvin, K. E. W.; Cervi-Skinner, S. J.; Al-Saadi, A. A.; Juliar, J. F.; Jackson, C. E.; and Tashjian, A. H.: C-cell hyperplasia preceding medullary thyroid carcinoma. *N. Engl. J. Med.,* **289:**437–441, 1973.

Woolner, L. B.; Beahrs, O. H.; Black, B. M.; McConahey, W. M.; and Keating, F. R., Jr.: Classification and prognosis of thyroid carcinoma. A study of 885 cases observed in a thirty year period. *Am. J. Surg.,* **102:**354–387, 1961.

Woolner, L. B.; Beahrs, O. H.; Black, B. M.; McConahey, W. M.; and Keating, F. R., Jr.: General considerations and follow-up data on 1181 cases. In Young, S., and Inman, D. R. (eds.): *Thyroid Neoplasia.* Academic Press, Inc., New York, 1968.

Zollinger, R. M.; Ellison, E. C.; Fabri, P. J.; Johnson, J.; Sparks, J.; and Carney, L. C.: Primary peptic ulcerations of the jejunum associated with islet cell tumors: Twenty-five year appraisal. *Ann. Surg.,* **192:**422–430, 1980.

33

Neoplasms of the Breast

GIANNI BONADONNA and PAUL P. CARBONE

Overview

Significant advances have occurred in the understanding of the biology and treatment of breast cancer. New information has challenged previous tenets on many aspects of therapy. Primary therapy is now selected on the basis of biological determinants, as well as clinical examinations. Therapy for advanced disease has become more satisfactory, utilizing combination chemotherapy and biochemical determinants. More information is available on risk assessment for screening and prevention strategies. The involvement of patients in therapeutic and diagnostic decisions is proportionately greater than it was ten years ago. The following chapter will summarize the current state of knowledge in this disease.

Epidemiology and Etiology

In 1982, breast cancer accounted for 26% of all new cases of cancer in women in the United States. This amounts to 112,000 estimated new diagnoses and is contrasted to 77,400 genital, 40,900 respiratory, and 25,500 digestive cancers (Silverberg, 1982). In terms of cancer mortality, breast cancer accounts for the largest number of deaths, approximately 34,000 per annum. In women between the ages of 15 and 74, breast cancer remains the single most common cause of death due to cancer. It is the most significant cause of all deaths in young women under age 50.

Breast cancer incidence varies with age and nationality. In the United States, breast cancer is uncommon before age 30, and the incidence rises rapidly to about age 45 when the peak number of cases occur. In age-specific incidence rates (see Figure 33–1) the rate rises rapidly from under 5/100,000 at age 25 to 150/100,000 at age 50 and then more slowly to over 200/100,000 by age 75. In comparison, the age-adjusted incidence rates for breast cancer in Japanese women are very similar in the premenopausal age groups, but much lower in the postmenopausal age group (Yonemoto, 1980).

Interesting data on breast cancer epidemiology also come from studies of migrant Japanese populations. Over the past three decades a sharp increase in the breast cancer incidence has been reported in Japanese women, mainly in the 45-to-54 age group. The incidence rate in first generation Japanese-American women living in San Francisco, aged 35 to 64, increased three times that of Japanese women living in Japan. The incidence in older (65 to 71 years) first-generation Japanese-American women is almost seven times higher. These marked differences in breast cancer incidence cannot be explained by genetic factors alone, but more likely are influenced by some environmental factors, such as diet. Recent data from Japan indicate that the women who develop breast cancer are taller and heavier than the national average. The effect of "westernization" on cancer incidence is mainly seen in postmenopausal women. The incidence of breast cancer decreased markedly during periods of severe dietary restriction that result in relative amenorrhea and infertility (DeWaard, 1969).

Increased incidence rates of breast cancer occur in Caucasian countries with high socioeconomic levels. The data from Japan, where the overall incidence is low despite a high socioeconomic standard, however, suggest that

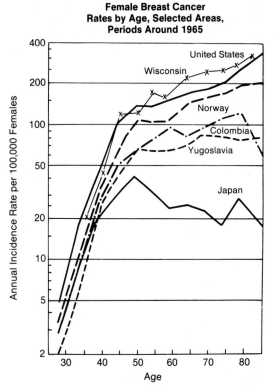

Figure 33–1. Age-specific incidence rates of breast cancer. Modified from Silverberg, E.: Cancer statistics, 1982. *CA,* **32:**15, 1982.

cultural factors such as diet and fertility patterns have more effect on breast cancer incidence than other generalized environmental causes. In Western countries, such as Iceland, there has been a continuous increase in incidence rates in cohorts born between 1870 and 1920 (DeWaard, 1969). It has been suggested that breast cancer incidence may be continuing to rise in certain areas of the world, such as Canada (Grace *et al.,* 1977) and the United States (Cutler *et al.,* 1971).

Risk Factors. Several factors have been shown to relate to a higher risk of developing breast cancer. These include age, nulliparity, late first pregnancy, benign breast disease, family history of breast cancer, and high-fat diet. Reduced risk has been associated with early first pregnancy and early menopause. Other factors have been more controversial and inconsistent. These include obesity, age of menarche, lactation, thyroid disease, hypertension, use of estrogens, and oral contraceptives. The risk of breast cancer is 25% lower in daughters born to young mothers. No relationship to rank of birth has been shown (Rothman *et al.,* 1980).

More recent data suggest that the risk of breast cancer in daughters may be greater if the mother developed breast cancer premenopausally (Wynder *et al.,* 1978). A history of breast cancer in the mother has resulted in greater risk in the daughters for pre- and perimenopausal breast cancer. An interesting report of 160 cases of breast cancer in 151 twins in the Danish Twin Registry addresses the question of genetic factors in cancer (Holm *et al.,* 1980). In five monozygotic and four dizygotic twins, both partners had breast cancer. The hereditability was calculated as 0.30 to 0.40, and the risk of developing breast cancer in the second twin was 6.0 for monozygotic and 2.0 in dizygotic twins. For cancer of other sites, the observed rates were identical for both kinds of twins and were not considered to be as genetically significant. No increased risks for nulliparity or later age of first birth in these twins were reported. Breast cancer usually occurs in the same breast in twins. The authors concluded that genetic factors play a major role in the development of breast cancer in some patients.

A family history of breast cancer in mothers, sisters, and daughters increases the risk of developing breast cancer (Anderson, 1974; Langlands *et al.,* 1976). This risk is related to the age of onset of breast cancer in the relative. The average woman has a 7% chance of developing breast cancer in her lifetime. This risk increases three times if the relative developed breast cancer before menopause. The risk increases dramatically (five times) if the breast cancer is bilateral at any age and nine times if the breast cancer occurred bilaterally and premenopausally (Kelly and Anderson, 1981). These data suggest that bilateral breast cancers are strongly inheritable and that no difference is noted for transmittability through maternal or paternal lines. In a Swedish case-controlled study, the relative risk of familial aggregation in breast cancer was 1.5 to 1.7 for second-degree and first-degree relatives, respectively. If the mother was affected, the daughters' relative risk was 2.0. The authors suggested that even this risk might be biased since women with breast cancer are more likely to recall or find out about relatives with breast cancer (Adami *et al.,* 1980, 1981). Moreover, their data failed to confirm age and bilaterality as significant risk additives, suggesting that environmental factors play a greater role than genetic effects to explain the high risk in United States studies.

In addition to the increased risk in relatives

of patients with breast cancer, clustering of breast cancer with ovarian cancer has been reported (Lynch et al., 1978a), and others have noted associations with gastrointestinal, soft tissue sarcomas (Li and Fraumeni, 1975), brain tumors, and leukemia. Lynch has made some suggestions on genetic counseling of these rare high-risk families, including the use of prophylactic mastectomy (Lynch et al., 1978b).

Rare congenital disorders such as Peutz-Jeghers syndrome (Riley and Swift, 1980), Klinefelter's syndrome, and Cowden's disease (Brownstein et al., 1978) are also associated with increased incidence of cancer of the breast. The latter disease consists of facial benign hair follicle tumors, keratoses, oral papillomas, and fibromas. Among the 21 cases reported in women, 10 have had breast cancer, with a median onset of 36 years.

Radiation and Breast Cancer. The impact of radiation on development of breast cancer is well established for women who have had repeated fluoroscopies (Boice and Monson, 1977), have been treated with x-rays for postpartum mastitis (Shore et al., 1977), or who are survivors of atomic explosions of Hiroshima and Nagasaki (McGregor et al., 1977; Land and McGregor, 1979; Land et al., 1980). The estimate of increased risk was 1.9 excess cases per 10^6 person years for women who were ten years or older at the time of x-radiation. The risk was higher in adolescent women than in older women. The increased risk has been seen in radiated patients under ten as well. The study from the Radiumhemmet in Stockholm, Sweden, reports a rate four times above normal for women receiving radiation for benign conditions (Baral et al., 1977). The average follow-up period was 31.5 years. All of the studies report a linear relationship between dose and development of cancer; however, all these exposures occurred at relatively high doses.

A major controversial issue relates to the effects of very low doses, such as those obtained by repeated mammograms, where the dose might be as low as 0.1 rad or less per exposure. Little increased risk is evident for single or infrequent x-ray examinations of the breasts. The repeated use of mammography under the age of 40 is a theoretical concern that will probably not be resolved by clinical trials.

Hormones and Breast Cancer. The development of breast cancer is probably related to female hormones since it occurs naturally most often in females as compared to males and can be prevented by ovarian castration at an early age. Factors such as parity, age of first pregnancy, age of menarche, and age of menopause are all associated with various changes in risk (MacMahon et al., 1973; Sartwell et al., 1977). The decrease in breast cancer risk with oophorectomy under age 35 is at least 70%, implying an association with ovarian hormones in two-thirds of the women. Despite this obvious association with estrogenic hormones, little information on risk is gained by measuring hormone levels in the urine or blood in normal nonaffected women and following them. Measurements of prolactin and growth hormones, both implicated in breast cancer in animals, have provided no insight for the causation of human breast cancer.

Of major interest is the effect of increased hormone levels during pregnancy and administration of exogenous hormones. Pregnant women with breast cancer represent a small fraction of all breast cancer, ranging between 0.78 and 3% of all cases. Although more procrastination and delay occur in diagnosis in these patients, the prognosis is no less favorable than for other patients when corrected for stage and lymph node status. The effect of pregnancy on subsequent prognosis is surprisingly beneficial. Women who have a coincidental pregnancy and breast cancer seem to have a better prognosis as compared to women who have breast cancer alone (Donegan, 1977). Cytotoxic agents and hormonal therapies have a great impact on fertility, as well as the development of the fetus. The major issue in advising patients who want to become pregnant after treatment for primary breast cancer remains the implication of disease recurrence on the family and the patient. One must also consider the patient's desire to have children.

A more common problem is the role of the administration of exogenous hormones, such as oral birth control pills and estrogens to alleviate menopausal symptoms. No apparent association exists between oral contraceptives and breast cancer. A national survey using SEER data is underway to obtain more definitive information. Likewise, the use of exogenous estrogens in postmenopausal women as a factor in enhanced breast cancer risk has not been defined clearly. One study by Ross, however, showed that women who took estrogens for more than two years, with intact ovaries, had an increased risk of developing breast cancer (Ross et al., 1980). A subsequent study showed a similar risk increase for postoophorectomy patients (Brinton et al., 1981).

In attempting to explain the relationship between breast cancer and hormones, the estrogen window hypothesis has recently been proposed (Korenman, 1980). It is postulated that environmental factors, *i.e.,* carcinogens such as smoking or radiation, are most potent at times when estrogen stimulation is unopposed by progestins. The risk of breast cancer increases as the duration of unopposed estrogens increases. The risk decreases when normal luteal phase – progesterone secretion and pregnancy (estrogen antagonism) occur. Therefore the two most susceptible times are just before menarche and at the onset of menopause. The use of estrogens after menopause prolongs the estrogen-sensitive period. The above facts fit the data from radiation exposure and the effects of age at the time of exposure. A mathematical approach to breast cancer risk was recently published. It attempts to explain breast carcinogenesis on the basis of increased susceptibility related to growth kinetics and the number of susceptible cells (Moolgavkar *et al.,* 1980). This theory predicts a two-step carcinogenesis and suggests that hormones play less of a role, except to cause stimulation and involution of susceptible cells. The carcinogenic factor is not hormones, but rather exogenous substances acting on estrogen-primed cells.

Viruses and Breast Cancer. Viruses have long been associated with murine breast cancer, primarily based on the early work of Bittner who showed that a milk factor from the mother explained the non-Mendelian inheritance of breast cancer. The MMTV has been shown to be a B-type particle. The viruses have been demonstrated in seminal vesicles of males and shown to be transmitted sexually from males. The virus obviously requires other factors to express oncogenicity. B- and C-type particles have been associated with mammary tumors in rats and in rhesus monkeys (Dmochowski, 1973, 1975). In humans, MMTV-like particles have been seen in human milk, breast tumors, pleural effusions, and tissue culture lines. The particles are rare and can be seen best by negative staining techniques. Immunofluorescence studies using MMTV antibodies have demonstrated reactivity in sera from breast cancer patients and some of their relatives. Transfer RNA and reverse transcriptase characteristic of RNA tumor viruses have been demonstrated in the sera of patients with breast cancer. Molecular hybridization studies have also shown homology between human RNA and MMTV. These observations, however, do not prove conclusively that viruses cause human breast cancers. A by-product of this investigation may be the development of specific viral proteins that may prove to be useful in early diagnosis and detection of breast cancer.

Benign Breast Disease and Cancer Risk. Most lesions of the breast removed surgically are caused by benign diseases. These include fibroadenoma, fibrocystic disease, inflammatory disease, and papillomas. The clinical features of these benign diseases and primary management are not pertinent to this chapter. A long association has been observed between these diseases and breast cancer. The expected increase in breast cancer is approximately 1.8 to 2.0 for the combined types of fibrocystic disease (Hutchinson *et al.,* 1980). In women with fibrocystic disease with the various subtypes, the increases in observed cancer as contrasted to expected cancers was 2.45 for those with epithelial hyperplasia or papillomatosis, and no increased risk was seen for cysts, apocrine metaplasia, adenosis, or sclerosing adenosis. Preexisting fibroadenoma or intraductal papilloma was not associated with increased risks.

Pathology

The diagnosis of breast cancer requires histologic proof by biopsy of the primary or secondary tumor, or both. In addition to the diagnosis, the histopathologic and biochemical examinations of the specimens provide information about prognosis, selection of therapy, and the biology of breast cancer.

More than 90% of all cancers of the breast are derived from the epithelial cells of the large and small ducts of the breast. The pattern of the common carcinomas may be infiltrating, papillary, scirrhous, comedo, or medullary. Often in the same cancer one may see several types. The most common diagnostic category of cancer is the *infiltrating ductal,* accounting for 70% of all breast cancers (see Figure 33 – 2A and B). On section, the tumors are hard, gritty, and contain necrotic foci. A scirrhous reaction is associated with these tumors and gives the hard character to the tumor on sectioning. Microscopically, these tumors show invasion by closely packed epithelial cells into the cleftlike spaces surrounding the normal breast tissue. The infiltrating cells may be threadlike and are described as single filing. Invasion of the Cooper's ligaments causes dimpling of the overlying skin.

The next largest numbers of cancers arise

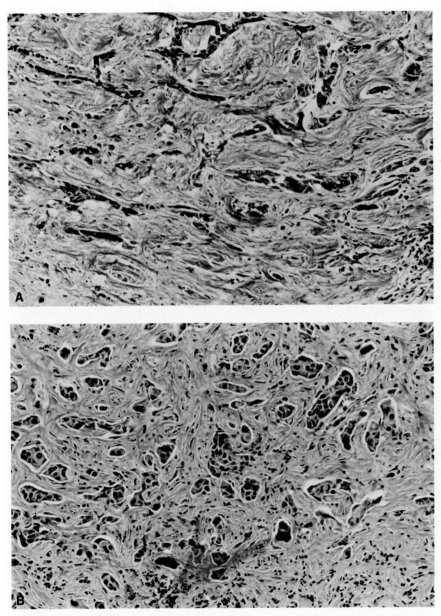

Figure 33 – 2. (*A*) Scirrhous carcinoma of the breast composed of chain cells of infiltrating tumor cells in a fibrous stroma. (*B*) Scirrhous carcinoma with relative anaplastic cells in a fibrous stroma. (Courtesy of Dr. Kennedy Gilchrist, University of Wisconsin.)

from large ducts and are called *ductal carcinomas. Medullary carcinoma* comprises one subset of large duct cancers (Ridolfi *et al.,* 1977). Characteristically, the tumors are large, with relatively noninfiltrative or pushing margins, and contain large numbers of inflammatory cells, especially lymphocytes. The tumors rarely show skin dimpling or ulceration. Despite its very aggressive histologic appearance of large, ovoid cells with vesicular nuclei, this tumor has a relatively good prognosis and has a

lower metastatic potential. Other types of large ductal cancer include *tubular* and *mucinous colloid carcinoma*. In the tubular variety the cells are highly undifferentiated and arranged in large tubular patterns with or without central necrosis (Eusebi *et al.,* 1979). The former are called comedo, and the latter ductal or tubular carcinomas. The tumors are usually small and may be associated with lobular carcinoma *in situ* (see Figure 33 – 3). Mucinous carcinoma may become quite large and is

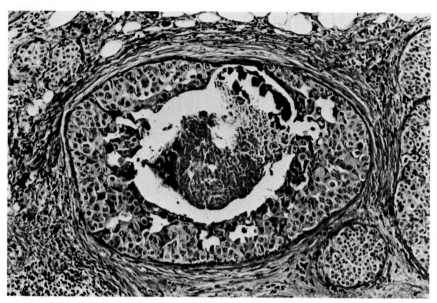

Figure 33–3. Intraductal carcinoma with central necrosis. (Courtesy of Dr. Kennedy Gilchrist, University of Wisconsin.)

characterized by mucin-containing epithelial cancer cells. These tumors may resemble mixed tumor of the parotid.

A tumor of the smaller terminal lobules of the breast is named *lobular carcinoma* and comprises about 3% of cases (Gaton and Czernobilsky, 1974). The cancer cells may be strictly intralobular and be *in situ* or noninvasive or infiltrating much like a ductal carcinoma (see Figure 33–4A and B). The cells are small in size and uniform, with cytoplasm that is foamy. Usually associated areas of lobular carcinoma *in situ* are present in other parts of the specimen. The patients are usually a decade younger than patients with other cancer. Lymph node invasion occurs in about 50% of cases. A major feature of this disease is that it may be bilateral in as many as 42% of the patients. Elctive random biopsies of the opposite breast reveal either lobular carcinoma *in situ* or invasive cancer in 0 to 20% of the cases (Donegan and Perez-Mesa, 1972). Mammography of the breast may be normal in 40% of patients who show histologic features of cancer.

Signet Cell Carcinoma. Signet cell carcinomas of the breast are relatively rare tumors characterized by a clear cytoplasm and a compressed nucleus (Merion and Livolski, 1981). The tumor is associated in lobular carcinoma *in situ* or infiltrating lobular carcinoma in all cases and has been considered a variant of that

disease rather than a mucinous carcinoma. The cells are mucin-positive. Curiously, these tumors metastasize with high frequency to the abdomen and infiltrate the gastrointestinal tract, adrenals, and ureters. The severe desmoplastic reaction in the abdomen may cause ureteral or intestinal obstruction.

Papillary Adenocarcinoma. Papillary adenocarcinoma has its origin in the large central ducts, and occurs in less than 1% of cases. It tends to grow slowly and attains a large size. The tumor occurs in younger women and is associated with a bloody nipple discharge. Under the microscope, the cells are arranged in a dendritic, papillary pattern. Lymphocytes invading the edges of the tumor and cellular invasion at the attachment of the papillary structure are features of malignancy. These tumors rarely metastasize. The tumor must be distinguished from the benign intraductal papilloma. Treatment consists of surgical excision with mastectomy.

Paget's Disease of the Breast. Paget's disease, first described in 1874, is characterized as chronic eczematoid inflammation of the nipple that precedes development of a carcinoma of the breast. Usually the patient notices the eczematoid skin reaction, itchiness, and soreness of the nipple and does not feel a specific lump. The overall incidence is about 1 to 3% of all cancers (Nance *et al.,* 1970). The lesion, limited to the nipple, is felt to be an intraepi-

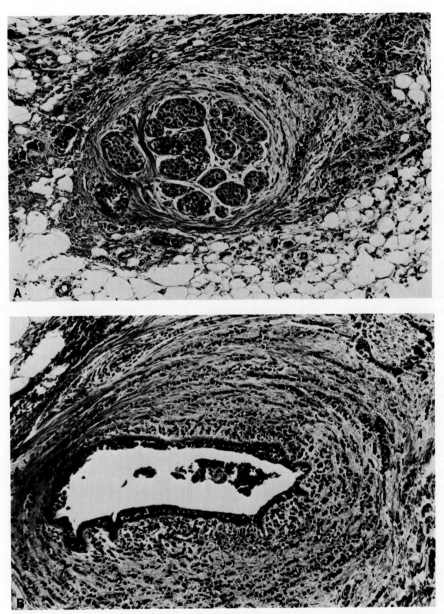

Figure 33 – 4.   (*A*) Breast lobule distended by lobular carcinoma *in situ* and infiltrating lobular carcinoma in surrounding adipose tissue. (*B*) Targetoid growth pattern of infiltrating lobular carcinoma with cancer cells in single file formation around breast duct. (Courtesy of Dr. Kennedy Gilchrist, University of Wisconsin.)

thelial extension of the underlying cancer. Examination for the underlying cancer using mammography and duct instillation of contrast media is extremely important. The prognosis is excellent unless lymph node invasion has taken place. In one series, 32 of 53 patients (61%) had an underlying mass (Nance *et al.,* 1970). The average age was 55, similar to that of other patients with breast cancer, and the duration of symptoms was about one year. In

women without masses, by extensive sectioning the pathologists could demonstrate an underlying noninvasive or malignant intraductal cancer. The prognosis was directly related to involvement of axillary nodes.

Cystosarcoma Phyllodes.   Cystosarcoma phyllodes was first described in 1838 by Mueller as a fibroepithelial tumor with a relatively benign clinical behavior. The gross appearance is that of a large, gray, cauliflowerlike lesion, with mucoid and nonhomogeneous features that are hard, gritty, cystic, or fleshy. Microscopically, the tumor is allied to a fibroadenoma and has increased cellularity. The differentiation between benign and malignant lesions is based on the appearance of the stroma and not the epithelial component. The malignant changes in the stroma consist of focal cellularity, severe nuclear atypia, frequent atypical mitoses, and pleomorphism in cell shape.

The usual clinical presentation is a small breast mass that starts to grow rapidly. The tumor grows large, but does not invade the skin or ulcerate. Diagnosis is established by biopsy. Metastases, occurring in less than 10%, are usually blood borne and are usually detected within the first three years. Other sarcomas of the breast may occur such as fibrosarcomas, liposarcomas, angiosarcomas, leio-, and rhabdomyosarcomas (Lattes, 1978). These appear not to arise from underlying fibroadenomas or cystosarcomas. The tumors behave clinically as their counterparts in other tissues.

Lymphomas of the Breast. Primary lymphomas may be seen in the breast, although characteristically the tumor in the breast is associated with other evidence of disease in lymph nodes or visceral organs (Mambo *et al.,* 1977). The histologic features most often are those of the non-Hodgkin's lymphoma. Hodgkin's disease of the breast is much less common. These patients should be evaluated as if they had primary lymphoma. Burkitt's tumor of the breast has also been reported, particularly in Africa.

Lymphangiosarcoma. Most patients with this disease have had chronic lymphedema following radical mastectomy and less frequently with other causes of lymphedema. The lymphedema duration is usually 7 to 23 years before onset of the sarcoma. Postoperative radiation was used in 22 of 34 patients reported by Sordillo and colleagues (1981). The patients usually develop repeated local recurrences and eventually metastases to the lungs. Limb amputation as a treatment, while drastic, seems to be less frequently associated with metastases. The median survival of patients was 31 months after diagnosis.

Metastatic Cancers. Cancers metastatic to the breast can occur from any organ, although in women the most commonly seen tumors are melanomas and bronchus cancers (McIntosh *et al.,* 1976). In men, one can see prostate

cancer metastatic to the hypertrophic gland stimulated by estrogens. The tumors usually appear discrete, smooth, or multinodular and are confused with benign tumors except for their rapid growth.

Prognostic Pathologic Parameters. *Nuclear and Cellular Grade.* In addition to the pathologic patterns and cell types, prognosis in breast cancer is clearly related to histologic and nuclear grading. More than 90% of cancers, however, are moderately or poorly differentiated, and relatively few (10%) are well differentiated either in cellular or nuclear morphology. Agreement among various pathologists is difficult on replicate evaluations. Therefore, this parameter is not consistently used in predicting prognosis with any degree of confidence on a routine basis (Cutler *et al.,* 1966; Maynard *et al.,* 1978).

The features of the tumor associated with nodal metastases and high treatment failure rate have been reviewed by Fisher (see Table 33–1) (Fisher *et al.,* 1976; Fisher and Fisher, 1977). These, in general, are similar and expected: large tumors, anaplastic nuclear and histologic grade, blood vessel and nerve invasion, nipple involvement, and capsular extension of tumor. Conversely, favorable parameters are those associated with well-differentiated tumors that are slow growing. The histologic appearance of the regional lymph nodes as a parameter of prognosis re-

Table 33–1. Pathologic Features Associated with Early Treatment Failures

---

Pathologically positive axillary nodes
Noncircumscribed tumor (macro- and microscopic)
Histologic type — N_{OS}; N_{OS} + lobular > N_{OS} + tubular; medullary;
    Lobular invasive; N_{OS} + mucinous > N_{OS} + pap.; N_{OS} + lobular + tubular > mucinous; tubular
Nuclear grade — $1 > 2 > 3$
Histologic grade — $3 > 2 > 1$
Tumor necrosis
Lymphatic invasion
Blood vessel invasion
Cell reaction to tumor
Mucin — absent/slight > moderate > marked
Intraductal component of cancer — comedo > solid or papillary > adenocystic or combinations
Microscopic involvement of skin overlying tumor
Nipple involvement
Capsular extension of nodal metastases
Intralymphatic extension in quadrants remote from primary tumor

---

Modified from Fisher, E. R., and Fisher, B.: Relationship of pathologic and some clinical discriminants to the spread of breast cancer. *Int. J. Radiat. Oncol. Biol. Phys.,* **2:**747–750, 1977.

sulted in contradictory reports (Bell *et al.,* 1969; Champion *et al.,* 1972; DiPaola *et al.,* 1974; Flores *et al.,* 1974).

Tumor Size. Tumor size is related to prognosis and survival. Tumor size, whether measured clinically or in the pathology laboratory, however, is not an independent variable in the presence of nodal involvement. Larger tumors tend to have more axillary metastases than smaller tumors.

Other histologic parameters, such as inflammatory reaction in the tumor or the lymph nodes, and lymphatic or blood vessel invasion have been correlated with prognosis. Interobserver variation and the dominance of lymph node invasion, however, diminish their clinical significance.

More recently, measurement of the tumor estrogen receptor (ER) content has been shown to be related to recurrence, independent of nodal status (Knight *et al.,* 1977; Cooke *et al.,* 1979). These studies, confirmed by others, indicated the recurrence of breast cancer after primary surgery can be more rapid in ER-negative patients than in ER-positive individuals. This relationship appears to be related to the degree of tumor differentiation. Others have shown this relationship diminishes in importance if one segregates tumors on the basis of histologic grade (Maynard *et al.,* 1978). Nevertheless, the measurement of ER can be quantitated readily and is being tested in clinical trials as an independent parameter for using adjunctive therapy. Uncertainty continues as to whether ER status predicts for the rate of recurrence or for the overall recurrence rate.

Nodal Status. The most useful parameter of prognosis in the past 20 years for selection of adjunctive therapy is that based on the number of lymph nodes involved. Data from the NSABP, and subsequently confirmed by others, have clearly shown the value of lymph node involvement on prognosis (see Table 33–2) (Fisher *et al.,* 1975; Valagussa *et al.,* 1978). This parameter seems to be independent of the number of nodes examined. Even when only a single node is positive, the prognosis is significantly worse than when the single node removed is negative. Examining increasingly larger numbers of nodes for prognosis is of no value. Those with few nodes removed (less than ten), who had negative nodes, clearly had the same prognosis as those who had 25 to 30 nodes negative (Fisher *et al.,* 1970). Studies done by the Kings/Cambridge Trial (Cancer Research Campaign Working Party, 1980), as well as the NSABP (Fisher, 1981), show that the removal of glands or treatment with x-ray did not influence overall prognosis and survival.

The clinical evaluation of axillae for lymph node involvement is also fraught with problems. The palpation of the axillae and finding no lymph nodes was associated with 39% positive on pathologic examination. Likewise, palpable nodes do not contain cancer 25% of the time. Palpable, fixed or mobile, nodes in the axilla are associated with a poor prognosis.

Noninvasive Cancer of the Breast. The two major types of noninvasive cancer of the breast are intraductal carcinoma and lobular carcinoma *in situ* (Patchefsky *et al.,* 1977; Schwartz *et al.,* 1978; Rosen *et al.,* 1979). The intraduc-

Table 33–2. Average 10-Year Results After Mastectomy Alone (All Data Are in Percent)

AXILLARY NODES			T_1	T_2	T_{3a}
Positive	Relapse-free survival	25	50	25	17
	1–3 nodes	33			
	>3 nodes	15			
	Local-regional recurrence*	18			
	Total survival	40	65	40	20
	1–3 nodes	54			
	>3 nodes	25			
Negative	Relapse-free survival	75	80	70	70
	Local-regional recurrence*	6			
	Total survival	82	90	80	80

All above-mentioned results are not significantly different between pre- and postmenopausal women. In patients with ER+ tumors the five-year relapse-free and total survival rates are superior compared to patients with ER− tumors.

* As first sign of primary treatment failure.

tal carcinoma is characterized by proliferation of ductal lining with a malignant appearance, but it does not invade through the duct (Carter, 1977). Studies have suggested that many patients may have evidence of invasion on further sectioning. About 70% of patients who do not show invasion are alive at 15 years. The recommended treatment is mastectomy.

Lobular carcinoma *in situ* is usually nonpalpable disease clinically. The incidence varies, but may be as high as 2% of all biopsies. The average age is usually 44, five years younger than patients with invasive lobular carcinoma, and ten years younger than those with infiltrating ductal cancer. The lesion may feel like fibrocystic disease if palpable and may be multicentric or bilateral. In 25 to 60% of patients the lesion is associated with an infiltrating carcinoma. This *in situ* lesion treated by local excision results in frank cancer subsequently in 15% of patients by 15 years (Rosen *et al.*, 1979).

Clinically Nonpalpable Lesions of the Breast. As x-ray examination of the breast has become widespread, radiographic abnormalities in the breast without clinically palpable lesions have become valid indications for biopsy. Techniques for localizing the lesion, such as needle placement and subsequent verification of the biopsy by radiographic examination, have become routine. The lesions recommended for biopsy usually involve abnormal breast calcifications, stellate-shaped masses with ill-defined borders, large smooth lesions, or areas of distorted breast architecture. As many as 70% of these lesions will be benign. The rest are invasive or noninvasive cancers. The latter include *in situ* ductal or lobular carcinomas (Schwartz *et al.*, 1978). Of the cancers, about 20% will have nodal or disseminated metastases. In another large series reported by Patchefsky *et al.* (1977), 42% of 149 cancers detected at a mass screening center were nonpalpable. Only 5 of 62 were associated with positive nodes, in contrast to 34 of 87 with palpable lesions. Rosen *et al.* (1979), reviewing data at Sloan-Kettering Memorial Hospital, reported their findings in 122 biopsies of minimal cancers and their implications for therapy. They recommend that all patients with *in situ* ductal cancer should have a total mastectomy and low axillary node dissection, because 40% of the time residual cancer or progressive cancer will occur. For lobular *in situ* cancer, the risk of occult invasive cancer is low; however, because of multicentricity, the recommendation is also for mastectomy.

Bilateral Breast Cancer. The frequency of bilateral breast cancer has been estimated to be 0.7 to 1% per year (Devitt, 1971; Finney *et al.*, 1972; Wilson and Alberty, 1973; Watanetittan and Ram, 1974; Kesseler *et al.*, 1976; Martin *et al.*, 1982). Slack's reporting for the NSABP indicates that of 2734 patients followed for six years 1.9% developed cancer in the second breast (Slack *et al.*, 1973). Synchronous breast cancer is particularly lethal and is associated with a 15-year survival (2.5%) with a median survival of 52.5 months. Bilateral nonsynchronous cancers have a better prognosis, with 20% of patients alive at 15 years, and a median survival of 96 months. The cancer in the second breast is often similar to the first in location, histology, and axillary node involvement (Prior and Waterhouse, 1978). Researchers have shown that patients who develop cancers in the second breast are likely to be younger, less fertile, and have a strong family history of breast cancer. The risk of developing the second cancer has suggested the use of random biopsies of the opposite breast in a mirror-image location. This practice may identify more pathologic diagnoses, but may not be associated with better overall results (King *et al.*, 1976). The use of mammography to detect the second cancer has allowed the detection of smaller lesions and fewer nodal invasive tumors (Egan, 1976).

Natural History

Breast cancer can be considered a chronic disease in most women, with a continuing mortality up to 20 years or more. Langlands *et al.*, reporting from Edinburg on a survey of 3878 patients noted that mortality due to breast cancer in stage I and II patients was increased up to 20 years. The excess in mortality was 58%, and they reported excess deaths in the period 15 to 20 years postmastectomy (Langlands *et al.*, 1979). A cohort of 1458 patients treated with mastectomy was followed for up to 30 years with only 99 patients lost to follow-up (Adair *et al.*, 1974). Approximately 13% were known to be alive, and the actuarial survival was 38%. Of the 1185 known deaths, 836 (70.5%) were caused by cancer, and 349 (29.5%) were the result of other causes. The risk of cancer mortality from the first cancer was 4%, and risk from a new second cancer was 21% in the 20- to 30-year group. In a study of cancer mortality, it was noted that all patients died with metastatic disease, primarily the result of organ failure (lungs, heart, liver) (Hagemeister *et al.,* 1980). Infection was a major cause of death in 24%. Leukopenia secondary to chemotherapy was not related to infection. Thus, the major problems in the control of breast cancer are primarily the local control of disease, the treatment of occult metastases, and the prevention of a second breast cancer. These factors must be taken into account at the time of primary therapy and considered for the long-term follow-up that must extend for two or three decades.

Growth Rates of Cancer. In experimental tumors, the specific measurements of cell cycle times, growth fraction, doubling times, and cell loss factors can be calculated (Post *et al.,* 1977). The major findings indicate that tumor volume and tumor weight do not correlate with cell kinetic parameters, except that the slowest growing tumors have low labeling indices and high cell loss factors. Marked variations are noted in cell cycle parameters in the spontaneous tumors, not unlike human tumors (Braunschweiger *et al.,* 1977). In human tumors less than 4% of cells are engaged in DNA synthesis, and measurements of S phase indicate that this is approximately 24 hours long. Post (1977) identified a wide range of intermitotic times. Other investigators have attempted to look at labeling indices (LI) as a parameter for estimating response to chemotherapy. In one study, decreases in labeling indices *in vivo* postchemotherapy correlated with response to chemotherapy (Murphy *et al.,* 1975). Other investigators have shown enhancement of LI *in vitro* by FU and FUDR. LI was not correlated with tumor size or metastases (Meyer and Facher, 1977). Although DNA synthesis times do not vary from one patient to another, marked variation occurs in LI and growth fraction. Few differences in growth parameters were noted between primary and metastatic tumors (Schiffer *et al.,* 1979).

Estimates of breast cancer doubling times (DT) have been made using mammograms (Heuser *et al.,* 1979), mastectomy scar recurrences (Pearlman, 1976), and nodules (Philippe and Le Gal, 1968; Boyd *et al.,* 1981). All demonstrate a wide variation in DT from 3 to 944 days, with averages of 42 to 311 days. Some have suggested a bimodal distribution of 25 to 93 days. Correlations with clinical prognosis and DT have been consistent only if one defines a short versus a long time (Spratt *et al.,* 1977).

Tumor Immunity. Prognosis in breast cancer can be related to host factors as well as tumor factors. Host factors that influence resistance to tumors can only be measured indirectly and have been shown to be related to pathologic features, specific immune measurements, and estimations of general immune competence. Correlations exist between tumor lymphocyte infiltration, lymph node hyperplasia, circulating lymphocyte levels (Papatestas *et al.,* 1976), skin test reactivity (Wanebo *et al.,* 1976) both nonspecific and using breast cancer cells (extracts), and lymphocyte reactivity and survivals. Nonspecific host factors and therapy influence these same parameters. In general, advanced disease and previous heavy therapy result in more immune impairment (Stjernsward *et al.,* 1972). Whether these parameters are specific for host-tumor interaction, as contrasted to postdisease or treatment, needs to be demonstrated. The importance of routine assessment of immune competence, except as a research tool, remains speculative. An interesting study of the prognosis after the second cancer identified no major difference in clinical course, suggesting the immune stimulation of the host by the first cancer did not protect the patient (Khafagy *et al.,* 1975).

The attempt to enhance therapeutic effects by immune stimulants has been investigated (Black and Leis, 1971; Alford *et al.,* 1973; Fossati *et al.,* 1979). BCG (Cochran *et al.,* 1974; Stolfi *et al.* 1974; Sparks *et al.,* 1977), *Corynebacterium parvum* (Fisher *et al.,* 1975), T antigen (Springer *et al.,* 1980), and levamisole (Rojas *et al.,* 1976) have been used in various clinical trials. Although one can demonstrate changes in immune measurements, true clinical effectiveness has been limited to only one controlled study using levamisole (Rojas *et al.,* 1976) and animal experiments (Fisher *et al.,* 1975).

Prognosis of Clinical Parameters in Women with Disease. Recently, information that identifies clinical parameters relating to prognosis and the subsequent development of breast cancer has become available. Increased body weight, defined as more than 60 to 64 kg, as compared to women under 60 kg, has been shown to affect prognosis adversely, independent of nodal and histologic parameters (Donegan *et al.,* 1978; Boyd *et al.,* 1981). Other authors have suggested that early age of menarche (≤ 11 years) is an adverse factor related to survival (Juret *et al.,* 1976). Optimal survival occurred in women whose menarche occurred at age 15. It has been reported that parous women had significantly better five-year survivals (60%) versus nulliparous (46%) (Papatestas *et al.,* 1980). In some studies the effect of parity has been associated with decreased risk of tumor induction, primarily in younger women, whereas parity influenced prognosis in women of all ages. In another study, low serum cholesterol and low body weight had a favorable effect on five-year disease-free recurrence rates, as compared to high serum cholesterol and high body weight. The differences were 68% and 32% ($P = .0004$) (Tartter *et al.,* 1981).

Diagnosis

Current diagnosis of primary breast cancer includes a sequential approach that utilizes physical examination, mammography, needle aspiration cytology, and biopsy. This sequential approach has essentially replaced the former urgent admission for excision biopsy and diagnosis by rapid histopathologic frozen section while the patient remained anesthetized. As a consequence, the doctor-patient relationship has considerably improved since it allows women to participate in the discussion of their illness and to be consulted on the methods of treatment once a diagnosis is made.

Physical Evaluation. The early detection and effective primary treatment of all breast cancer remain the ultimate goal of clinical research. Most patients, however, still present with a specific complaint of a lump or pain in the breast. The woman may describe a thickening rather than a lump. This lump may be affected by changes in hormone levels associated with the events of the menstrual cycle. In addition to the lump in the breast, a woman may complain of a nipple discharge which may have a wide range of characteristics, including milky, watery, and bloody. The bloody discharge is not always associated with a cancer, but may result from other causes such as a benign papilloma.

On physical examination, one should carefully inspect the breast, supraclavicular fossae, and the axillae with the arm in various positions. The arms should be on the hips first and then raised over the head. The comparison of symmetry of the breasts must be done and the skin examined for irregularities such as edema, dimpling, retraction, redness, excoriation, nodularity, and so forth. The position of the nipple should be examined, looking for retraction, inversion, or deviation.

With the patient in both the upright and supine position, one should examine both axillae and supraclavicular areas looking for nodes. The breast is best examined with the patient lying down with a pillow under the appropriate shoulder. The breasts should be systematically examined with the flat of the second, third, and fourth fingers by palpation. The examiner needs to look for changes in consistency, nodularity, or pain. The shape of the lesion as well as the size needs to be recorded. Often a picture drawn on the chart will be a better record than a written description. Most masses are benign. A lesion, however, that has obvious irregularity in size, associated with retraction of the skin, or is fixed to the chest wall muscles is highly suspicious. It is important to teach the patient to examine herself by feeling her own breasts and to show her what is normal to palpation.

Careful examination of the abdomen also must be done, looking for liver enlargement. Examination of the lungs by percussion and auscultation should be carried out, looking for evidence of an effusion. Percussion over the spine, clavicles, and ribs may elicit pain secondary to bony metastases. Suspicious lesions of the breast should be examined with a mammogram, particularly if a previous mammogram is available and the woman is over 40. In any patient, but especially the younger patient (less than 40 years), a mammogram may be misleading. One must use clinical judgment as well as x-ray examination.

Deciding whether to follow a lesion, obtain a roentgenogram, or aspirate it is a difficult process to outline. Factors such as age of the patient, previous biopsies and aspirations, and mammography are all involved in the process, as well as the physical characteristics of the lesion. In general, one needs to have an experienced physician, preferably a surgeon, and an experienced mammographer involved in the process.

If the lesion is suggestive of malignancy either by clinical or x-ray study, however, needle or open biopsy should be attempted. The needle aspiration biopsy is very useful because the procedure can be an outpatient one, and the results obtained quickly. The physician can then involve the patient in the final therapeutic decision early. When the lesion is either nonpalpable or small, or if the physician is not sure, an open biopsy should be done. A second definitive operation may be required to complete the therapy.

Mammography. In clinical practice, bilateral mammography (or xeromammography, a radiographic process resulting in the enhancement of the edges of anatomic and pathologic structures through "harder" x-rays) has an established role and should be performed at any age in the preoperative evaluation when physical findings indicate a significant suspicion of cancer. The mammographic examination should be performed with modern techniques utilizing < 1 rad. This average dose to the breast carries a minimal risk of developing breast cancer. Xeromammography and film-screen mammography, although excellent methods of breast cancer detection, both have their advantages and drawbacks. For example, relative soft-tissue densities are sometimes more reliably evaluated in film-screen images, whereas calcifications are sometimes more evident in xeromammographic images. Film-screen mammography tends to record fatty or fibrofatty breast more reliably than xeromammography, and the latter tends to record dense, dysplastic breast tissue more reliably than the former. With both methods, breast compression is an important factor in enhancing details.

In interpreting the radiologic report, clinicians should keep in mind a few basic rules.

1. Mammography should not replace a physical examination, nor the physical examination replace mammography.
2. A negative mammogram or negative physical examination should never deter a biopsy of a suspicious lesion that has been detected by either method.
3. Mammography cannot be relied upon to invariably differentiate benign from malignant disease; therefore, biopsy is the only method of providing reliable criteria for determining malignancy.
4. Clustered, finely stippled, angular, lacy, or branching calcifications are characteristics of carcinoma. Cancer, in fact, exhibits mammographic evidence of calcification in approximately 50% of cases. Fat necrosis, however, a benign disorder, may manifest *identical* calcifications. Sclerosing adenosis, a commonly occurring benign disorder, may contain finely stippled calcifications which are usually more scattered in distribution. Intraductal papillomas may contain a rosette pattern of several small calcifications that may resemble that of malignancy. Scat-tered, ring-shaped, or coarse linear calcifications reflect calcified inspissated cellular and lipid debris of benign secretory disease. All suspicious clusters of calcifications should be biopsied, and in the presence of nonpalpable lesions specimen radiography is highly advisable.
5. In breasts that are dense, without much fat, such as those of young, nulliparous, pregnant, and lactating women, or those manifesting severe mammary dysplasia, even a large carcinoma may be obscured by the dense tissue that surrounds it.
6. If the cancer is too small to be palpable, the associated mammographic signs include, beside calcifications, a segmental prominence of one or more ducts and a localized distortion of breast architecture.
7. In infiltrating duct carcinomas, which represent the large majority of breast malignancies, the key mammographic feature distinguishing carcinoma from most benign breast masses is the irregular margin of the mass. The irregularity reflects spicules of fibrous connective tissue and cords of tumor cells aggressively infiltrating the surrounding tissue. In contrast, the great majority of discrete benign masses (cysts and fibroadenomas) appear sharply circumscribed.
8. Lobular carcinoma, a less common variety, is difficult to detect mammographically because it is found most commonly in dysplastic breasts and tends not to form a distinct mass.
9. Comedocarcinoma frequently results in a characteristic branching pattern of calcifications.

Other radiologic techniques for diagnosis and evaluation of breast disease include mammary duct injection and computer-assisted tomographic mammography. The prime indication for duct injection is a bloody discharge from the nipple. Injection of radiopaque contrast medium into the discharging duct with subsequent radiography not only localizes the causative lesion, but reveals the involved duct anatomy as well. Papillomas, duct hyperplasia, and some intraductal and infiltrative carcinomas may be visualized in this manner. Duct aspiration for cytology before the injection of contrast material also can be performed. Computerized tomography appears to be superior to mammography for detecting cancers in dense, premenopausal dysplastic breasts and for recognizing precancerous high-risk lesions. Computed tomography should not replace conventional mammography in routine breast examinations, but it affords a definite diagnostic tool when the mammographic and/or physical examination are inconclusive (Chang *et al.*, 1980).

Among the nonradiologic techniques, thermography and ultrasound (Lapayowker and Revesz, 1980) should be mentioned. Thermography is a reproducible noninvasive test that involves the visual display of infrared emission and depicts minimal temperature variations at the skin surface. The resultant pattern primarily reflects the heat of blood in superficial veins, the blood being conveyed into these veins from the deep mammary veins by way of intermediary subareolar venous plexus. The major shortcomings of thermography are its acknowledged deficiencies in diagnostic specificity and sensitivity. This procedure has not proven to be of significant value in detecting early breast cancer. In selected cases, however, it may be useful in combination with other factors to reduce the number of women who should receive routine mammograms for screening purposes. In its present state ultrasound mammography can be utilized to distinguish between cystic and solid palpable masses, especially in nodular breasts that are difficult to evaluate clinically and mammographically. New techniques allow for sectional analysis of breast tissue much like computerized tomography. The application of computerized ultrasound tomography may become more widespread as its utility is determined.

Aspiration Cytology. Needle aspiration of a palpable breast mass (Zajicek, 1979; Rilke, 1982) has almost replaced needle incision biopsy because it is less distressing and equally effective for tumor diagnosis. It can be used to confirm clinical diagnosis of malignancy, to ascertain the malignancy in clinically benign-appearing lesions, and to contribute to a more accurate definition of the preoperative diagnosis.

The purpose of the technique is to aspirate a small amount of tumor juice that can be smeared onto a slide and stained. The recommended procedure is to use a 10-mL syringe and a 21- or 22-gauge needle. The tumor is fixed between the left index finger and thumb in a right-handed person and the needle inserted into the center of the tissue, about 2 cc of air having first been drawn into the syringe

barrel. The texture of the tumor can be assessed during needling and, if the tumor is a cyst, fluid will be drawn up into the syringe when the plunger is withdrawn. When needling solid tumors, it is important to put the needle tip into the middle of the nodule, and then aspirate with much force while moving the tip of the needle about, sampling different areas of the tumor. The small volume of air drawn into the syringe before needling is now used to expirate the material sucked out of the tumor onto glass slides. The tissue on the slide is smeared immediately in a similar way to a blood film or marrow aspirate; the cells are air dried and stained with May Grünwald Giemsa, or wet fixed in alcohol and stained with the Papanicolaou modification of the hematoxylin and eosin stain.

The appearance of the cells ranges from infrequent clusters and single small cells that are found in fibrotic benign mammary dysplastic lesions to numerous, loosely cohesive, large cells with pleomorphic nuclei and irregular chromatin patterns seen in carcinomas. Between these extremes is a variety of appearances in which the diagnostic criteria may be difficult to apply (Zajicek, 1979). The rate of accuracy of malignant lesions ranges from 70 to 98%, that for benign lesions from 90 to 96%.

Based on thousands of aspirates of palpable mammary nodules, the sensitivity (0.67) and the specificity (0.98) of fine-needle aspiration cytology was reported. The predictive value for positive results was 0.97 and for negative results 0.68 (Rilke, 1982). The sensitivity and the predictive value for negative results reflected the fairly high incidence of inadequate smears due to small numbers of malignant cells in the smears. This can range between 15 and 25% and can be decreased about 50% by combining the Millipore method with fine-needle aspiration cytology. At the present time, it is felt that in an institution without an experienced cytopathologist, and where aspiration biopsies are taken for the most part by residents, a definitive cytology diagnosis of epithelial malignancy can be made in about 50% of cases with palpable mammary cancer, thus avoiding frozen sections. In an additional 20% of positive cases, the cytologic diagnosis indicates the need for a biopsy with histologic examination. When the total number of biopsies performed on the basis of cytologic indication is considered, the yield of positive findings is 93% (Rilke, 1982).

Screening Modalities. Screening programs for the early detection of breast cancer have not been as successful as was expected. Breast cancer screening at younger ages has been of no apparent benefit, a certain radiation hazard is involved in repeated mammograms, and the long-term health costs outweigh the long-term health benefits for a large proportion of potential screens.

Mass Screening Programs. The rationale behind screening for breast cancer is *secondary prevention; i.e.,* detection and treatment of an early stage may be the only means of controlling this disease since *primary prevention* remains impossible as long as the causative factors remain obscure. Mammography has proven to be the most effective available method for early detection. The question of whether the mortality of breast cancer can be significantly reduced by screening an asymptomatic population with mammography alone can be answered only by performing a prospective randomized controlled study on a sufficiently large population, using mammography as the only screening method. Such a study would also enable a precise benefit/risk analysis of mammography screening.

The early results of such studies initiated in Sweden in 1977 (Tabar and Dean, 1982) indicated that mammography screening has resulted in the treatment of a large number of breast cancers at an earlier stage(s). In fact, 40% of the screening-detected tumors were either *in situ* or had infiltrative carcinoma ≤ 10 mm, and only 19% of all screening-detected cancers had axillary lymph node metastases. The number of cases without lymph node metastases was significantly higher in both the screened population and the total study population as compared to the control group. The screening process appears to have a positive educational effect, resulting in a new pattern of stage distribution of breast cancer (Strax, 1980). Thus, in screening centers using modern mammographic techniques about 40% of the cancers discovered are ≤ 10 mm in diameter and 50 to 70% of all detected lesions are nonpalpable. The well-known study of the Health Insurance Plan (HIP) of Greater New York showed that through annual screening by a combination of modalities (medical history, physical examination, and mammography), 79% of those cancers found on mammography had no node involvement, and 75% of those cancers found on palpation alone were localized (Strax, 1980). This program reduced mortality from breast cancer in almost 40% of women over the age of 50. In contrast, no mortality reduction occurred in younger women,

probably because the denser breasts in this age group made radiologic examination more difficult.

During the late 1970s controversy and probably a disproportionate amount of attention was focused on the hypothetical risk of breast cancer induced by screening programs (Upton *et al.,* 1977). This led to a considerable reduction in the radiation dose used in mammography. Since the risk of radiation-induced breast cancer is age-dependent, the theoretical risk of exposure to 1 rad after the age of 30 is 3.5 induced cancers per one million women-years. With modern low-dose mammographic technique (mean breast dose of 0.3 rad per examination), the risk might result in one excess breast cancer per one million women-years exposed after the age of 30, with a latent period of 15 years (Tabar and Dean, 1982).

From the practical point of view, and until the mortality data from ongoing prospective randomized trials become available, it seems reasonable to screen women over 50 years of age with a combination of physical examination and low-dose mammography. Women under 50 years may continue to be screened by physical examination, but should be screened with mammography only if they have had breast cancer, or if they are between the ages of 40 and 49 and have a mother or sister who has had cancer of the breast (Thier, 1977). The recommendations of the American Cancer Society and comments are shown in Table 33–3.

Self-Examination of the Breast. It is well known that women may find their own cancer. The self-examination of the breast has been advocated for many years as a screening modality for detection of breast cancer. The basic steps in self-examination of the breast can be summarized as follows. At monthly intervals, and if premenopausal after the completion of a menstrual period, the woman views her breasts in front of a mirror, first with arms down and then with arms elevated. She should look for irregularity of the size of the breast and for new abnormality in appearance (asymmetry, flattening, dimpling, changes in the nipple). Then the woman lies supine with a small pillow or folded towel under the shoulder of the side to be examined, and raises her arm on that side above the head. Palpation is performed with the flat of the fingers of the opposite hand in a methodical fashion to include the entire breast. The full procedure is subsequently performed for the other side.

The method is simple, inexpensive, and safe but emotional problems may be enhanced by

Table 33-3. Breast Cancer Detection for Asymptomatic Women

GUIDELINES OF THE AMERICAN CANCER SOCIETY 1982	COMMENTS
1. Breast self-examination should be done monthly in women over age 20.	1. Women should be taught how to do the examination and how the menstrual cycle may affect the gland consistency.
2. Women over 40 should have breast physical examination by physicians every year. Between the ages of 20 and 40, examination should be every three years.	2. About 13% of breast cancer lesions in younger women may be detected only by physical examination and are missed on mammogram. Overall, about 90% will be picked up by physical examination.
3. A baseline mammogram should be done around age 40.	3. This single mammogram should not increase the risk of developing more cancers.
4. Women over 50 should have a mammogram yearly if feasible.	4. Yearly mammograms after age 50 have been shown to decrease mortality. The problem is that no one knows how often to repeat mammograms if the examination is negative for five or more years.
5. Women with strong family histories of breast cancer may need more frequent examinations.	5. Familial history, particularly for bilateral breast cancer occurring before age 50, constitutes a high risk, and intervention procedures need to be considered much earlier than age 40 or 50.

monthly apprehension about breast cancer. Particularly in high-risk groups, self-examination seems to result in detection of presumably earlier breast cancers, although clear, supportive evidence of the efficacy of self-examination is still lacking (Moore, 1978).

Staging

The vast majority of patients with breast cancer will die from disseminated disease because local-regional treatments alone have failed to lengthen survival. Therefore, the crucial problem in staging is to define those patients whose lengths of survival following diagnosis are short since no further therapy will be required for these patients. The two methods utilized include (1) examination of the primary tumor and regional nodes for any relevant prognostic factors, and (2) an attempt to identify metastases that may eventually cause symptoms.

Methods and Yield. The classic method for clinical staging combines physical examination with the appropriate imaging tests of the organs that represent the common sites for metastases. Since the most common sites for distant metastases are bone, lung, and liver, staging tests are oriented around these three organs. Less common sites of disease are brain, bone marrow, abdominal cavity, and distant lymph nodes. Therefore, they should be explored in specific clinical situations.

The best objective clinical assessment of the primary tumor combines palpation with mammography and describes the findings uti-

lizing the terminology of the TNM system (International Union Against Cancer, 1978). Palpation is definitely less accurate in the assessment of regional nodes. When axillary nodes are palpable, histologic evidence of metastatic disease is not found in approximately 25% of cases. Conversely, when axillary nodes are not palpable, histologic involvement is detected in approximately 30% of cases. Thus, the best assessment of axillary nodes is by accurate histologic examination following complete axillary dissection. A limited axillary dissection with removal of relatively few nodes can be considered adequate to determine whether a patient has positive (N+) or negative (N−) axillary nodes. Only full dissection, rather than node sampling, increases the probability that more than three involved nodes will be detected even if the Halstedian axillary dissection does not affect the incidence of distant disease or the ultimate survival of patients. The above-mentioned statements are supported by the findings reported in a recent analysis of NSABP (Fisher *et al.,* 1981). In fact, 17% of all clinically negative node patients had > 3 nodes histologically positive and as many as 15%; 6% of all patients with negative nodes by palpation had ≥ 3 nodes histologically positive and as many as 15%; 6% of all patients with negative nodes by palpation had *10* positive nodes. The extent of axillary node involvement must be known in determining prognosis and in selecting appropriate adjuvant therapy.

For the purpose of analysis, the pathologic staging of the axillary nodes is divided into three levels. *Level I:* nodes are located inferiorly to the lower border of the pectoralis minor muscle; *level II:* nodes are located beneath the pectoralis minor muscle; *level III:* nodes are located at the apex of the axilla. Prognosis seems more related to the total number of nodes involved rather than the level of involvement.

Since extended radical mastectomy has become an obsolete surgical procedure, the internal mammary nodes are not available regularly for pathologic examination. In recent years, internal mammary lymphoscintigraphy has been utilized to permit visualization of approximately seven nodes from the xiphoid level to the supraclavicular area. The procedure is performed by injecting 0.2 mL (approximately 0.5 to 1.0 MCi) of ^{99m}Tc-antimony sulfide colloid into the posterior rectus sheath (Harris and Hellman, 1983). Abnormal lymphoscintiscans are manifested as a decrease in the relative radiocolloid within the lymph node. They may be performed in patients at high risk of occult internal mammary lymph node metastases before planning radiation therapy.

Today, our ability to detect micrometastases is still poor. Monoclonal antibody probes may become important in the near future in the detection of micrometastases by physical or radioimmunoassay techniques and also in yielding classifications with therapeutic value. Among the other humoral tumor markers, only CEA has been extensively studied. Unfortunately, it is not tumor-specific, therefore, a number of positive findings can be observed in the presence of other concomitant diseases in the colon, liver, and pancreas. The most important use of CEA may be in the detection of recurrence.

Asymptomatic osseous metastases are found on roentgenograms in less than 2% of routine studies. Since nearly 50% of a given bone segment can be destroyed by tumor before osteolytic, sclerotic, or a mixed pattern of osseous metastases becomes clearly evident through x-ray examination, bone scans have often replaced bone roentgenograms. Bone scans, in fact, permit bony metastases to be detected while still asymptomatic and as early as 12 months before they can be seen on roentgenograms (Citrin *et al.,* 1975; Gerber *et al.,* 1977; British Breast Group, 1978; Clark *et al.,* 1978). Unfortunately, bone scans are not specific, and other lesions associated with osteoblastic activity (*e.g.,* arthritis, old fractures, Paget's disease) cause abnormalities that can

be differentiated only with roentgenograms. Furthermore, although a suspicious scan portends a poor prognosis, contrary to expectation, it is not associated with a high rate of initial treatment failure in bone ($<15\%$). As the sole indication of dissemination, an abnormality on a bone scan, particularly in the absence of bone pain, should be confirmed with convincing radiographs (tomograms) or a biopsy before concluding that distant metastases are present. Urinary hydroxyproline/creatinine ratio combined with an abnormal serum alkaline phosphatase can represent a sensitive index of the presence of occult skeletal metastases. A high rate of false-negative findings still occurs, therefore, the above-mentioned biochemical tests become crucial in the presence of an abnormal scan.

Asymptomatic lung metastases occasionally can be found on routine radiographs. Insufficient information is available on the value of routine whole-lung tomography. An isolated parenchymal density should prompt tomograms followed by needle biopsy if additional nodules are not apparent. Since pulmonary scintigraphy is probably no more accurate than lung tomograms, both tests are not indicated as routine staging procedures. Computerized tomography of the lung may be used in place of standard tomography.

The early diagnosis of hepatic metastases is extremely difficult. Generally, physical examination for metastatic involvement of the liver is not helpful. About 50% of livers are impalpable even when gross involvement is present since the organ size often does not enlarge with metastatic disease. Liver scans are not helpful unless the metatases are in excess of 2 cm in diameter. Today, liver scans are often replaced by echotomography to screen for metastatic disease, and in the presence of suspicious findings this test must be supplemented by computerized tomography. Among the biochemical tests, alkaline phosphatase and γ-glutamyl transpeptidase seem most useful. When both elevated tests are combined with computerized tomography showing multiple lesions, the diagnosis of hepatic metastases is practically certain. In selected patients, *e.g.,* those showing an isolated defect at tomography, laparoscopy with liver biopsy is indicated.

Cerebral metastases in a patient with apparently early mammary carcinoma are exceedingly rare. Therefore, in these patients routine screening of cerebral metastases is not indicated. Even in the presence of recurrent breast cancer, brain scans of patients without symptoms are abnormal in only 1% of cases. When a patient develops symptoms or signs of intracranial metastases, however, computerized brain tomography is essential. In women with persisting anemia, particularly of leukoerythroblastic type, and in the absence of abnormal bone scan, bilateral needle bone marrow core biopsy from both posterior iliac crests may reveal the presence of marrow extrinsic cells. Special screening of the less common sites of metastatic involvement is not indicated unless the patient shows symptoms or signs suggesting this involvement.

The postsurgical histopathologic classification (p TNM) is less often utilized on a routine basis, although for prognostic purposes and postsurgical decisions, pathologic staging, particularly of N, is more important than clinical staging. Thus, in practice, for final stage (1) the size of T will be that measured by a calliper once the surgical specimen is removed and cleared of the surrounding fat; (2) the status of N will be defined by the number of involved nodes over the total number of nodes examined histologically. To ensure an adequate pathologic examination of the axillary lymph nodes, an average of 18 to 25 nodes should be thoroughly and carefully examined. Their distribution level should be reported. The surgical pathology report should also specify whether the neoplasia was unicentric or microscopically multicentric and whether neoplastic invasion of veins, intratumoral and peritumoral lymphatics, and fat tissue was present or absent.

Classification of the TNM system achieves reasonably precise description and recording of the apparent anatomic extent of disease. A tumor with four degrees of T, four degrees of N, and two degrees of M will have 32 TNM categories (see Table 33–4). For purposes of tabulation and analysis, except in very large series, it is necessary to condense these categories into a convenient number of TNM stagegroups as reported below.

Stage Grouping

Stage I	T_{1a}, T_{1b}	N_0, N_{1a}	M_0
Stage II	T_0, T_{1a}, T_{1b}	N_{1b}	M_0
T_{2a}, T_{2b}	N_0, N_{1a}	M_0	
T_{2a}, T_{2b}	N_{1b}	M_0	
Stage IIIa	T_{3a}, T_{3b}	N_0, N_1	M_0
$T_{1a,b}, T_{2a,b}, T_{3a,b}$	N_2	M_0	
Stage IIIb	$T_{1a,b}, T_{2a,b}, T_{3a,b}$	N_3	M_0
$T_{4a,b,c}$	Any N	M_0	
Stage IV	Any T	Any N	M_1

In patients with disseminated disease, the results are often expressed by categories of "dominant site of involvement" for they bear prognostic relevance particularly in patients treated with endocrine manipulations. Patients are classified into the *soft tissue category* when only cutaneous, subcutaneous, mammary, or superficial lymphatic structures are involved, the *osseous category* when skeletal lesions exist without visceral involvement, and into *visceral category* when there are visceral lesions (with or without soft tissue and/or osseous involvement).

Systematic Approach. The following staging approach is indicated in patients presenting to the clinic with breast cancer, confirmed by aspiration cytology and/or mammography.

$T_1-T_2-T_{3a}$
1. Complete physical examination
2. Chest roentgenogram
3. Isotropic bone scan
4. Liver function tests
    If scan shows abnormalities or bone pain is present, ray tomogram of the involved area(s) and urinary hydroxyproline/creatinine ratio should be obtained. If liver function tests are abnormal or liver is palpable, liver scan or ultrasound should be obtained. If either is abnormal, computerized liver tomography and/or laparoscopy should be performed.
5. Internal mammary lymphoscintigraphy may be performed in patients with inner quadrant primary.

$T_{3b}-T_4$
1 to 4: as above
6. Liver scan or ultrasound. If either is abnormal, computerized tomography and/or laparoscopy should be performed.

Any T, M_1
1 to 6: as above
    If pleural effusion is evident, thoracentesis with cytology should be performed.
    If neurologic symptoms or signs are present, computerized brain tomography should be obtained.
    Additional roentgenograms and/or biopsies (*e.g.*, needle bone marrow biopsies, lumbar puncture) should be performed in accordance to specific clinical situations.

Specific and Supportive Management

The choice of optimal management for all stages of breast cancer has challenged over the decades the skill and the experience of numerous clinicians. Today, the critical reevaluation of natural history and the advent of effective systemic therapy have modified considerably the conventional strategic approach, at least in

Table 33–4.   Staging Classification

The most widely used pretreatment clinical staging classification for breast cancer is that adopted by both the International Union Against Cancer (UICC) and the American Joint Commission (AJC) in Cancer Staging and End Result Reporting (International Union Against Cancer, 1978). It is based on the TNM system (T: tumor, N: node, M: metastasis) and is reproduced below.

Primary tumor

T	Primary tumor
T_{is}	Preinvasive carcinoma (carcinoma *in situ*), noninfiltrating intraductal carcinoma, or Paget's disease, of the nipple with no demonstrable tumor
Note:	Paget's disease associated with a demonstrable tumor is classified according to the size of the tumor.
T_0	No evidence of primary tumor
Note:	Dimpling of the skin, nipple retraction or any other skin changes, except those in T_4, may occur in T_1, T_2 or T_3 without affecting the classification.
T_1	Tumor of 2 cm or less in its greatest dimension
T_{1a}	With no fixation to underlying pectoral fascia and/or muscle
T_{1b}	With fixation to underlying pectoral fascia and/or muscle
T_2	Tumor more than 2 cm but not more than 5 cm in its greatest dimension
T_{2a}	With no fixation to underlying pectoral fascia and/or muscle
T_{2b}	With fixation to underlying pectoral fascia and/or muscle
T_3	Tumor more than 5 cm in its greatest dimension
T_{3a}	With no fixation to underlying pectoral fascia and/or muscle
T_{3b}	With fixation to underlying pectoral fascia and/or muscle
T_4	Tumor of any size with direct extension to chest wall or skin
Note:	Chest wall includes ribs, intercostal muscles, and serratus anterior muscle, but not pectoral muscle.
T_{4a}	With fixation to chest wall
T_{4b}	With edema, infiltration, or ulceration of skin of breast (including peau d'orange), or satellite skin nodules confined to the same breast
T_{4c}	Both of above
Note:	Cases of inflammatory carcinoma should be reported as a separate group.
T_X	The minimum requirements to assess the primary tumor cannot be met

Regional lymph nodes

N	Regional lymph nodes
N_0	No palpable homolateral axillary lymph nodes
N_1	Movable homolateral axillary lymph nodes
N_{1a}	Nodes not considered to contain growth
N_{1b}	Nodes considered to contain growth
N_2	Homolateral axillary lymph nodes fixed to one another, or to other structures, and considered to contain growth
N_3	Homolateral supraclavicular or infraclavicular lymph nodes considered to contain growth or edema of the arm
Note:	Edema of the arm may be caused by lymphatic obstruction: lymph nodes may not then be palpable.
N_X	The minimum requirements to assess the regional lymph nodes cannot be met

Distant metastases

M	Distant metastases
M_0	No evidence of distant metastases
M_1	Evidence of distant metastases
M_x	The minimum requirements to assess the presence of distant metastases cannot be met

The category M_1 may be subdivided according to the following notation:

PUL = Pulmonary	MAR = Bone marrow
OSS = Osseous	PLE = Pleura
HEP = Hepatic	SKI = Skin
BRA = Brain	EYE = Eye
LYM = Lymph nodes	OTH = Other

given subsets. As a consequence of changing strategy, treatment selection tends to be based more on biological considerations than on anatomic principles. More recently, considerable attention has been focused on quality of life in terms of cosmetic results and psychological reactions for operable women, as well as on acute and late toxic effects for patients subjected to chemotherapy. Successful therapy of mammary cancer begins with local control. Recent findings have indicated that improvements in survival will require the addition of effective systemic therapy to achieve local control. The management of advanced disease consists of a sequential use of hormonal manipulations and cytotoxic chemotherapy designed to meet the needs of individual patients. Controlled clinical trials have contributed greatly to the medical progress achieved in breast cancer. Research efforts are still required to improve current approaches to management and treatment.

Local-Regional Therapy. The local-regional control of breast cancer involves a range of treatment options, and the specific choice remains only partially resolved by the study of available clinical research information (Carter, 1982).

Surgery. For many years halstedian concepts based on anatomic principles have rigidly guided the local-regional therapy of resectable breast cancer (Fisher and Gebhardt, 1978). The classic *radical mastectomy* consists of removal of the entire breast and pectoralis major and minor muscles along with *en bloc* complete dissection of axillary lymph nodes and fat. The apogee of the Halstedian approach was represented by the *extended radical mastectomy* in which the *en bloc* lymph node dissection was enlarged to include the internal mammary node chain. In recent years, the most common operation performed in many centers all over the world has been the so-called *modified radical mastectomy* in which axillary dissection is performed with preservation of the pectoralis major muscle. Other surgical procedures utilized, often on the basis of a surgeon's personal convictions, are *total* or *simple mastectomy* in which the breast is removed along with either full axillary dissection or only sampling of level I and II axillary lymph nodes (see Chapter 8).

The National Cancer Institute Consensus Conference on "The Treatment of Primary Breast Cancer: Management of Local Disease" held in 1979 concluded that for women with T_1–T_2–T_{3a}, N_{0-1}, M_0 disease, relapse-free and total survival results were comparable, regardless of the surgical procedure (see Table 33–2). Furthermore, the inefficacy of internal mammary node dissection in breast cancer surgery was confirmed (Veronesi and Valagussa, 1981). Thus, total mastectomy with complete axillary dissection performed for the purpose of staging, as well as for therapeutic benefit, is recognized as the current standard treatment for stage I and II disease. These conclusions and the frequent systemic nature of apparent localized breast cancer, particularly when the axillary lymph nodes are histologically involved (Fisher and Gebhardt, 1978), prompted a redefinition of the rationale for primary breast cancer treatment. Consequently, a more flexible and biologic approach is now being applied in many patients, although the results of current trials should not

be considered as definitive without more follow-up. In women with small primary tumors (T_1 and selected T_2 N_{0-1}), lesser surgical breast procedures have become attractive alternatives, whereas in subsets at high risk of distant micrometastases, adjuvant systemic therapy is being administered.

The definition of conservative surgery for small breast tumors should be limited to procedures preserving the form of the breast. They include *quadrantectomy, segmental resection, tylectomy, lumpectomy,* and *excisional biopsy.* As proposed by Veronesi *et al.* (1981) quadrantectomy comprises the resection of an entire quadrant of the breast, together with the overlying skin and the corresponding portion of the fascial sheet of the pectoralis major muscle. Whenever possible, as in tumors located in the upper quadrants, the full axillary dissection is performed *en bloc* and in continuity with the breast quadrantectomy. For tumors of the lower quadrants, the axillary dissection is performed with a separate incision. The eight-year results of the randomized Milan trial indicate that Halsted radical mastectomy and quadrantectomy plus postoperative irradiation yielded identical survival results (see Figure 33–5A and B). Segmental mastectomy, as carried out in the NSABP trial for T_1–T_2 (≤ 4 cm) N_1 M_0 breast cancer (Fisher and Gebhardt, 1978), is a similar type of surgical procedure; whereas tylectomy, lumpectomy, and excisional biopsy are lesser procedures and should involve axillary dissection or sampling of axillary nodes.

After any of the conservative surgical procedures mentioned above, postoperative irradiation to control occult tumor in the residual breast is usually administered. Radiotherapy may not be needed when quadrantectomy or segmental resection is performed. The clinical relevance of tumor multicentricity in women subjected to conservative surgery will be resolved only by the long-term analysis of ongoing prospective randomized trials, that is, with and without postoperative irradiation (Fisher and Gebhardt, 1978).

In summary, the debate on the selection of surgical treatment for primary breast cancer should first consider the natural history of the disease as well as available data (Carter, 1982). Whenever technically feasible, the choice for the extent of surgery should also take into account the problem of cosmetic results. Women having tumors ≥ 3 cm, provided the breasts are not too small, will find conservative proce-

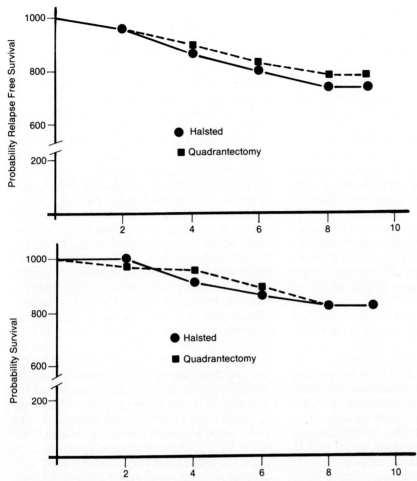

Figure 33-5. Comparison of Halsted radical mastectomy and quadrantectomy plus postoperative radiation therapy. From Veronesi, U., *et al.:* Comparing radical mastectomy with quadranectomy axillary dissection, and radiotherapy in patients with small cancers of the breast. *N. Engl. J. Med.,* **305**:6–11, 1981.

dures acceptable. Thus, the knowledge of the heterogeneity of breast cancer should teach physicians and patients that no universally accepted treatment can be applied to all patients with primary breast cancer (Valagussa *et al.,* 1983).

Radiotherapy. The role of radiotherapy in the management of breast cancer has changed drastically during the past few years (Fisher and Gebhardt, 1978; Fisher *et al.,* 1981). Utilized for many decades as postoperative treatment following radical surgery, radiation therapy today in experienced hands, and with appropriately selected patients, can be successfully integrated with limited surgery in the curative treatment of primary breast cancer, representing an alternative to mastectomy (Brady, 1982; Harris and Hellman, 1983).

Postoperative Radiotherapy. Postoperative

radiotherapy is defined as irradiation that follows Halsted or modified radical mastectomy or simple mastectomy performed with curative intent within two to four weeks. The rationale of postoperative radiotherapy is the eradication of residual microscopic disease, thus preventing the subsequent development of local-regional recurrences and distant spread. Although field arrangement as well as tumor doses have varied greatly over the years and among different centers, the modern treatment plan schematically consists of the irradiation of the anterior chest wall to include the mastectomy scar and the ipsilateral internal mammary nodes, the apex of axilla and the supraclavicular node area, utilizing supervoltage equipment and a tumor dose of 4000 to 5000 rads in four to five weeks.

Although a significant reduction of local-regional failures has been documented in patients given postoperative radiotherapy compared to patients treated only with mastectomy, the probability of distant treatment failure and mortality has not decreased. The addition of postoperative irradiation to the internal mammary nodes also fails to alter the probability of a distant tumor failure or death (Fisher *et al.,* 1981; Nevin *et al.,* 1982). Furthermore, in women receiving adjuvant treatment the concomitant or sequential delivery of radiotherapy with chemotherapy often prevents, with no additional therapeutic benefit, the optimal administration of intensive drug doses (Harris and Hellman, 1983). The possibility that postsurgical irradition is detrimental to patients' survival because of significant lymphocyte depression and loss of immunocompetence remains controversial and has raised innumerable questions (Stjernsward *et al.,* 1972; Brady, 1982). Recent observations, however, would support the concept of deleterious effect in N− women whose five- and ten-year survival rates were 20% less when given postoperative irradiation following radical mastectomy (Nevin *et al.,* 1982). For these reasons, the routine use of postoperative radiotherapy is not indicated in women subjected to mastectomy for T_1–T_2–T_{3a} breast cancer.

Radiotherapy and Primary Management. A more logical extension of the use of postoperative radiotherapy is represented by primary irradiation as an alternative to mastectomy to achieve equivalent local-regional tumor control without the disfigurement produced by extensive surgery. The conservative management of breast cancer utilizing radical irradiation, either along with or following gross removal of the primary tumor by excisional biopsy, was pioneered by Baclesse more than 40 years ago. Since the early European and Canadian studies, reports on the efficacy of radiotherapy without mastectomy in the primary management of breast cancer have appeared in the medical literature with increasing frequency, particularly from French and North American investigators (Hellman *et al.,* 1980; Brady, 1982; Harris and Hellman, 1983).

Current principles of radical radiotherapy for primary breast cancer can be summarized as follows: (1) the gross tumor mass should be surgically removed, along with sampling of the axillary nodes for staging purposes; (2) the treatment volume includes the entire breast, as well as the axillary, supraclavicular, and inter-nal mammary nodes; (3) the supervoltage equipment is utilized, and treatment should be carefully planned by experienced radiation therapists; (4) the dose consists of 4500 to 5000 rads to the areas of subclinical disease plus an optional boost of 1000 to 2000 rads to the tumor area. Some radiation therapists utilize implants with iridium 92 instead of the boost technique with external beam (Hellman *et al.,* 1980; Harris and Hellman, 1983). Larger radiation doses ($\geq$6000 rads) are required for the local control of bulky tumors.

The results from the most representative European and American series are encouraging. In spite of different policies utilized in patient selection, staging procedures, and radiation techniques, the outcomes are remarkably consistent, and for primary tumors less then 3 cm in diameter, total survival appears comparable to that obtained with Halsted or modified radical mastectomy. All radiation therapists stress the prognostic importance of tumor size. For tumors larger than 3 cm and/or in the presence of clinical or pathologic axillary nodes, survival rates are lower as compared to less advanced cases. In these groups the results, however, even within a combined modality setting, are comparable to those reported by conventional surgery. For tumors less than 3 cm, the incidence of local recurrence is less than 10%, and no obvious correlation exists with the radiation techniques (with and without boost, with and without iridium-92 implant. The rate of women requiring salvage mastectomy for recurrent residual disease was higher in the initial European series compared to recent North American series (< 10%). Salvage mastectomy may be required more often if the primary tumor is large and not surgically removed before radiation.

Cosmetic results following curative radiotherapy are good to excellent in more than 75% of patients and are influenced by the location and extent of the biopsy procedures, the time-dose factors of radiation therapy, and the technique of radiation. In experienced hands, radiation sequelae are rare (< 10%) and consist primarily of rib fractures, radiation pneumonitis, excessive skin and subcutaneous fibrosis, limitation of arm motion and brachial plexus injury (sensory). In women who are to receive adjuvant chemotherapy, the medical oncologists may encounter some difficulty in delivering optimal doses because of frequent myelosuppression during the initial cycles (Harris and Hellman, 1983).

The results of modern primary radiotherapy strongly suggest that this modality in experienced hands, with appropriately selected patients, and following the removal of primary tumor and axillary nodes can be considered an alternative to mastectomy. Thus, the potential of primary radiotherapy should not be ignored, and the alternative to primary surgery should be discussed with the patient. Both physicians and patients, however, should be aware that further clinical research is required to better define patient selection, extent of conservative surgery (*e.g.,* excisional biopsy versus quadrantectomy or segmental resection, node sampling versus full axillary dissection), and technique of irradiation (*e.g.,* boost with extenal beam versus iridium implantation). Last but not least, clinicians should be aware that, at the present moment, the correct application of modern radiotherapeutic technique is still limited to major centers.

Primary radiotherapy is also indicated in the presence of locally advanced (T_{3b}–T_4) breast cancer. Since most patients present with bulky tumors, high radiation doses (5000 to 6000 rads) are required. Local control can be achieved in 40 to 70% of women with inoperable breast cancer. The achievement of local control is primarily a function of tumor size, dose of radiation, and of the ability to perform total excision of the bulky tumor. In spite of control of local-regional disease, the cancer is seldom totally erradicated by optimal irradiation since the majority of women will develop distant metastases. Thus, with radiotherapy alone the prognosis is usually poor (five-year survival, 25 to 30%), particularly in the presence of palpable regional adenopathy (five-year survival, 15 to 20%) or inflammatory carcinoma (median survival, 14 to 16 months). By combining chemotherapy followed by radiotherapy in patients with no inflammatory carcinoma, local-regional control can be achieved in 75% of patients, but the five-year survival has not greatly improved over radiotherapy alone. Better results were recently reported (Valagussa *et al.,* 1982) by the sequence utilizing chemotherapy plus mastectomy plus chemotherapy (local-regional control, 82%; five-year survival, 50%). Clearly, today, the treatment of choice is not yet characterized. The current results suggest that more aggressive multimodal treatment (including endocrine therapy if estrogen receptors (ER) are positive) is required. With the exception of inflammatory carcinoma, treatment should probably begin with cytoreductive surgery followed by postoperative irradiation followed by systemic chemotherapy.

Palliative Radiotherapy. Radiation therapy still maintains its important role in the palliative treatment of numerous clinical sequellae of cancer. It can replace surgical castration when surgery is interdicted or refused; it should be utilized in the presence of various neurologic syndromes, such as brain metastases, epidural compression, large supraclavicular adenopathy producing compression on the brachial plexus; it is indicated in the presence of painful osseous lesions refractory to medical treatment or when a high risk of bone fracture is present. In these situations, the tumor dose varies from 2500 to 4000 rads, and the palliative effect is achieved in at least 66% of the patients.

Systemic Therapy. Systemic therapy for breast cancer has evolved from a dependence on hormonal therapy as applied before 1970 to primary combination chemotherapy, not only for disseminated disease and locally advanced tumors but also for the control of micrometastases. This evolution led to the development of a sequential schema for endocrine manipulations and cytotoxic chemotherapy for various groups of patients. Improved clinical benefit has been achieved in most subgroups. In the presence of advanced disease, the choice of initial therapeutic approach is based on the sites of metastatic disease, its rapidity of growth, the menopausal status of the patient, and the ER status. In primary tumors for which definitive local-regional therapy (surgery, radiotherapy, or the combination of both) is indicated, the decision of applying adjuvant therapy is based upon the presence of established prognostic parameters such as the histologic involvement of axillary nodes.

A vast literature on systemic therapy for breast carcinoma has been accumulated during the past decade (Henderson, 1982; Powles, 1982), and a thorough analysis of each treatment option will probably confuse rather than facilitate the discussion. Therefore, only the principal operational guidelines to properly manage the most common clinical situations are provided in this chapter.

Endocrine Therapy. Current endocrine therapy includes castration, antiestrogens, progestational agents, and aminoglutethimide. The mechanisms of action of these agents are described in Chapter 10. Estrogens, androgens, corticosteroids, and prolactin inhibitors are utilized less often, and adrenalectomy, as well as all forms of hypophysectomy, is practically obsolete. Endocrine manipulations are utilized in the presence of advanced breast cancer, but their use as adjuvant treatment, with or without chemotherapy, remains, at present, experimental.

Hormonal therapy is the conceptual approach of choice, if the pattern of metastasis is not life threatening, precluding waiting 8 to 12 weeks for therapeutic benefit. Endocrine management is avoided in patients with lymphangitic pulmonary metastasis, liver metastasis, hepatic dysfunction, brain metastasis, and recurrent pleural effusions. If hormonal therapy is not precluded by the urgency of serious disease, then the next critical variable is the ER status. If the ER assay is negative (*i.e.,* < 5 femtomole/mg cytosol protein), the response rate after hormonal therapy is less than 10%, and cytotoxic chemotherapy represents the treatment of choice. If the patient is ER positive or ER was not determined, the choice of hormonal therapy depends on menopausal status. If the woman is premenopausal or the cessation of menses was less than 12 months ago, then surgical castration is the standard option. If the woman is postmenopausal, the initial choice is between the antiestrogen, tamoxifen, and oral estrogens. Tamoxifen is becoming increasingly the first choice because of its comparative lower toxicity and similar response rate. Secondary therapy is dependent upon the response to initial hormonal treatment as well as to metastatic pattern of disease. If the patient has shown objective tumor response to an initial endocrine manipulation, the treatment of choice is another hormonal attack, such as aminoglutethimide, progestational agents, and androgens. If the initial hormonal therapy has not achieved a significant response, chemotherapy becomes the treatment of choice.

Table 33–5 summarizes the regimens and the principal side effects for the hormonal compounds most often utilized. The effect of endocrine treatment may take up to three months before clinical documentation of the initial response. Therefore, additive hormonal therapy should be continued until the clinical and/or radiologic evidence of tumor progression is unquestionable. In the absence of ER, the response rate is about 25 to 30%, highest for tamoxifen (35 to 40%) and lowest for androgens (15 to 20%). The probability of achieving tumor response is rather high (≥ 50%) for women with disease-free interval > 2 years or age > 60 years, and/or with limited soft tissue involvement. In patients with ER-positive tumors the chance to achieve hormonal response is directly proportional to the level of ER. Also women with both ER and PgR positive achieve a higher response rate (60 to 80%). In patients with favorable parameters, complete tumor disappearance is not a rare finding; it can be observed in up to 25% of cases, particularly if they present with limited, slow-growing disease in soft tissue or bone. In most patients the median duration of response exceeds six months, and in a few cases it may last for years.

Hormone therapy plus chemotherapy for advanced breast cancer has yielded, in general, a higher response rate compared to either single modality. The median duration of response as well as the median survival, however, was not significantly improved. Thus, this combined approach has limited indications, with the possible exception of women with low ER values (5 to 10 fmol) and rapidly growing tumor. In an adjuvant situation the results are still preliminary (see Adjuvant Therapy section of this chapter). The concomitant administration of two hormones has yielded inconclusive results.

Chemotherapy. The chemotherapy of advanced breast cancer in the decade of the 1980s is predominantly cyclical combination chemotherapy that in most reported studies appears superior to sequential single-agent chemotherapy. Initial combination chemotherapy can be administered in a wide range of situations that are not comparable as to prognosis for response and survival. These include aggressive visceral dominant disease, inflammatory carcinoma, ER− tumors, hormonal failures, and hormonal responders with aggressive visceral dominant disease after two hormonal approaches. This is one of the main reasons, along with the criteria of response utilized and the data-reporting technique, that chemotherapy results vary so often in the medical literature.

The standard combination of choice has not yet been identified. In fact, all tested regimens provide comparable response rates, ranging from 50 to 75% regardless of ER status, with a probable higher incidence for regimens containing doxorubicin (60 to 75%). The most commonly used drug combinations employ cyclophosphamide and/or doxorubicin, often in association with fluorouracil and metho-

Table 33-5. Conventional Dose Regimens and Principal Side Effects of Hormonal Compounds Most Often Utilized in the Treatment of Breast Cancer

HORMONE	DOSE REGIMEN	MAJOR SIDE EFFECTS
Androgens		
Testosterone propionate	100 mg × 3/wk, IM	Hirsutism, deepening of the voice, acne, increase in libido, frontal balding, clitoral hypertrophy, salt and water retention, and occult or manifest edema
Testolactone	100 mg × 3/wk, IM	
Fluoxymesterone	20–30 mg daily, PO	
Calusterone	200 mg daily, PO	
Estrogens		
Diethylstilbestrol	5 mg × 3 daily, PO	Nausea and vomiting, salt and water retention, urinary incontinence, vaginal bleeding, vaginitis, nipple pigmentation, flare of bone pain, hypercalcemia
Ethinyl estradiol	1 mg × 3 daily, PO	
Antiestrogens		
Tamoxifen	10 mg × 2–3 daily, PO	Nausea, dizziness, cutaneous rash, leukopenia and thrombocytopenia (very rare), flare of bone pain (rare), hypercalcemia
Progestins		
Medroxyprogesterone acetate	500 mg daily, IM × 30 days, then twice weekly	Water retention, muscle cramps, vaginal bleeding, moon face, increased body weight, thrombophlebitis, gluteal abscess (all after medroxyprogesterone acetate)
Megestrol acetate	20 mg × 3 daily, PO	
Norethinedrone	40–80 mg daily, PO	
Hydrolase inhibitors		
Aminoglutethimide	250 mg twice a day with hydrocortisone 100 mg/day for two weeks, then 250 mg twice a day with 40 mg hydrocortisone	Lethargy, skin rash, weakness

trexate. They are reported, along with the average response rates, in Table 33-6. One of the disappointments in the chemotherapy of breast cancer has been the failure to achieve a high degree of complete responders, which usually do not exceed 20%. The median duration of complete plus partial remission is six to eight months. The median survival is between one and two years, occasionally as long as 2.5 to 3 years from the initiation of chemotherapy. Responders survive significantly longer than nonresponders.

Responses to chemotherapy are seen in almost all metastatic sites with the possible exception of the central nervous system; their incidence is often higher in women with soft tissue or lung disease as compared to multiple visceral sites or bone lesions. Performance status, weight loss, and extensive prior radiotherapy seem to have a major influence on the response rate (see section on Prognostic Factors). In most responsive patients the time to initial tumor regression is usually two to four weeks, with the exception of osteolytic bone lesions which may take several weeks or months before showing partial or complete re-

calcification. A slow response also can be observed with liver involvement, and this emphasizes the importance of not abandoning a treatment regimen for at least three months unless unequivocal evidence of tumor progression is present. It is possible that some patients have a transient progression during the first six to eight weeks before response, especially when bone scans or serum CEA are used to monitor the disease. Patients with no objective evidence of tumor response may have a subjective response as a result of a placebo effect or as a reflection of the fact that an objective measure of response derives from both tumor cell kill and subsequent healing, such as bone recalcification after eradication of tumor.

Second-line or salvage chemotherapy usually yields an objective response rate that is lower (20 to 35%) than with the initial drug regimen and a complete remission rate of <10%. It is generally advisable to utilize as secondary therapy drugs that are potentially non-cross-resistant to those utilized as initial treatment. For example, in women failing on CMFVP or CMF, doxorubicin (50 to 75 mg/m² IV every three to four weeks), or mito-

Table 33-6. Most Common Drug Combinations in the Treatment of Breast Cancer

REGIMEN	DRUG DOSAGE AND SCHEDULE	
CMFVP	Cyclophosphamide	80 mg/m² PO daily
	Methotrexate	20 mg/m² IV weekly
	Fluorouracil	500 mg/m² IV weekly
	Vincristine	1.0 mg/m² IV weekly
	Prednisone	30 mg/m² PO daily × 15 (then taper)
CMF	Cyclophosphamide	100 mg/m² PO days 1–14
	Methotrexate	60 mg/m² IV days 1 & 8
	5-Fluorouracil	600 mg/m² IV days 1 & 8
	(repeat cycles every 4 wk)	
AC	Doxorubicin	40 mg/m² IV day 1
	Cyclophosphamide	200 mg/m² PO days 3–6
	(repeat cycles every 3–4 wk)	
CAF	Cyclophosphamide	100 mg/m² PO days 1–14
	Doxorubicin	30 mg/m² IV days 1 & 8
	Fluorouracil	500 mg/m² IV days 1 & 8
	(repeat cycles every 4 wk)	
FAC	Fluorouracil	500 mg/m² IV days 1 & 8
	Doxorubicin	50 mg/m² IV day 1
	Cyclophosphamide	500 mg/m² IV day 1
	(repeat cycles every 4 wk)	
DAV	Dibromodulcitol	150 mg/m² PO days 1–10
	Doxorubicin	45 mg/m² IV day 1
	Vincristine	1.2 mg/m² IV day 1
	(repeat cycles every 4 wk)	

mycin (10 to 15 mg/m² every six weeks), or a combination of both (doxorubicin 40 to 50 mg/m² IV every three weeks and mitomycin 10 mg/m² IV every six weeks) can represent the most appropriate treatment. In women resistant to AC or FAC, either mitomycin alone or in combination with vinblastine (4 to 6 mg/m² IV every 10 to 15 days) can be utilized. A number of single drugs and current drugs undergoing phase II evaluation may be tried. The judicious administration of conventional doses of vindesine, VP-16, mitoxantrone may induce response in 15 to 20% of patients.

When treating breast cancer with chemotherapy, especially with a multiple-drug regimen, physicians should follow the classic rules: (1) patients must have adequate bone marrow reserve (white blood cells ≥ 3500/mm³, platelets ≥ 100.000/mm³). (2) If doxorubicin is part of the drug combination, there should not be a past history of significant heart disease or severe myocardial damage. Liver function tests should be within normal limits. (3) If methotrexate is included in the combination, blood urea nitrogen, serum creatinine, and creatinine clearance should be within normal limits. (4) There should be no pulmonary fibrosis before starting therapy with nitrosourea derivatives or mitomycin. Whenever technically feasible, cyclical combination chemotherapy should be administered at full doses, for available data suggest that response may be dose related. Thus, in the presence of myelotoxicity it may be necessary to delay the subsequent dose until full marrow recovery occurs rather than continue therapy utilizing dose reductions. The optimal duration of treatment in the absence of tumor progression remains controversial. In fact, in the majority of patients the maximum tumor regression (usually partial) occurs within the first four to six months with no further cytoreductive effect observed in spite of continuous undiminished drug administration. Therefore, the real need for prolonged drug administration, particularly when minimal tumor response and/or diminished quality of life because of severe side effects is evident, remains questionable.

Toxic manifestations from the various poly drug regimens utilized in the treatment of breast cancer are those of compounds included in the combinations extensively described in Chapter 10 of this book. Bone marrow suppression almost always represents the dose-limiting factor, and the cumulative dose of doxorubicin should not exceed 550 mg/m² because of potential life-threatening heart failure.

Adjuvant Treatment. Modern adjuvant treatment for breast cancer was initiated in 1972. The goal is the eradication of micrometastases that lie outside the range of local-regional control modalities (Carter, 1980; Bonadonna and Valagussa, 1982). The concept of distant micrometastases at the time of initial diagnosis is supported by the high rate of metastatic failure despite optimal local therapy. The most potent prognostic indicator of potential distant metastases is the presence of involved axillary lymph nodes. Other prognostic factors include the size of the tumor and the ER content of the primary tumor. An extensive data base exists supporting the view that metastatic failure is higher, in both node-positive and node-negative women, in ER-poor primary tumors compared to ER-rich primaries.

The strategy of using adjuvant chemotherapy is derived from the tenets of cell kinetics and tumor cell kill hypotheses: micrometastases will contain a low cell number and will also have a high growth fraction, making them more vulnerable to the effects of cytotoxic drugs, particularly cell cycle–specific agents. In this situation, utilizing the maximally tolerated doses, it is theoretically possible to achieve total tumor cell eradication.

The relevant concepts derived from animal tumor models and empirical clinical experience are the following: (1) systemic treatment is indicated in the subgroup of patients at high risk for treatment failure after local-regional modality (N+ and/or ER− women); (2) systemic treatment should be initiated as soon as possible, that is, within two to four weeks, after surgery and/or radiotherapy; (3) the administration of adjuvant therapy should be intensive, utilizing full or nearly full doses, and prolonged in duration since solid tumors may contain a fraction of cells that have temporarily entered a nonproliferative state (G_0 cells); (4) combinations of drugs are usually more effective than single agents; (5) optimal scheduling is critical, and drug response of the primary tumor may not reliably predict the sensitivity of micrometastases to cell cycle–specific drugs, nor may the response of clinically advanced tumors predict optimal scheduling of the same drugs against micrometastatic foci.

The choice of drugs, as well as drug dosage and schedule, for use as adjuvant treatment has been derived from the empirical experience achieved in clinically evident metastatic disease. It is assumed that the cell kill potential of a therapy that is effective as palliative management of a bulky tumor might be sufficient to eradicate smaller micrometastatic deposits.

The current results of several important trials of adjuvant therapy are summarized in Table 33–7 (Salmon and Jones, 1981). None

of the available data should be considered as definitive, and as a consequence recommendations cannot as yet be made for patients treated outside of prospective clinical studies. A few important concepts can be derived from those studies, particularly the randomized trials, and the following conclusions can be applied in changing the treatment strategy of high-risk patients.

Five-Year Relapse-Free Survival. This has been significantly improved in women subjected to combination chemotherapy, CMF, CMFVP, AC, FAC, compared to those treated only with surgery. The results are more favorable in women with 1 to 3 compared to > 3 axillary nodes positive.

Menopausal Status. The results dealing with relapse-free survival related to menopausal status are somewhat contradictory, for in some studies (CMF program in Milan) the findings in premenopausal women appear superior compared to postmenopausal women, whereas with other regimens (CMFVP, AC, FAC) no difference was observed at five years between the two menopausal categories.

Five-Year Survival. A significant improvement has not been clearly demonstrated in all subsets given adjuvant chemotherapy. The trend is always in favor of multimodal approach, and the first CMF program (Bonadonna and Valagussa, 1982) has shown an unquestionable significant survival advantage up to seven years from mastectomy in premenopausal women.

Number of Drugs and Dose Levels. Both relapse-free and total survival rates are superior in women treated with combination chemotherapy compared to single agents such as PAM or cyclophosphamide, as well as in patients who received full-dose regimen compared to less intensive doses (Bonadonna and Valagussa, 1981).

Treatment Duration. The optimal duration of adjuvant therapy has not been elucidated. Recent findings (Bonadonna and Valagussa, 1982) have indicated that six cycles of CMF yielded at five years the same results as 12 cycles (see Figure 33–6). This indicates that the maximum tumor cytoreduction is achieved during the first few months, and by utilizing the same drug regimen, prolonging therapy beyond the sixth month is unnecessary.

ER Status. Within an adjuvant setting ER status does not appear to predict the response to chemotherapy, for the five-year relapse-

Table 33–7. Essential Five-Year Results Available in 1982 from Representative Adjuvant Studies (Data Refer to Node-Positive Women Operated on with Radical or Modified Radical Mastectomy)

INSTITUTION OR GROUP	ADJUVANT TREATMENT	ESSENTIAL RESULTS
Milan Cancer Institute	CMF for 12 cycles	RFS: 59% (1–3: 69%, >3: 40%), SURV: 78% For comparative dose levels no significant difference between pre- and postmenopause Superiority of CMF vs CTR confirmed at 7 years (RFS: 49%, CTR: 35%). SURV: difference significant only in premenopausal women (CMF: 78%, CTR: 61%)
	CMF 12 vs 6 cycles	No difference in RFS and survival No difference in RFS between ER+ and ER− tumors
Memorial Center	CMF 12 vs 24 cycles ± levamisole	No difference in RFS and survival No benefit from levamisole
NSABP	PAM for 2 years	Improved RFS after PAM in premenopause with 1–3 nodes (80%) vs CTR (55%)
	PAM + FU vs PAM for 18 months	Superiority of PAM + FU vs PAM in RFS and SURV Best results observed in postmenopause >3 nodes
SWOG	CMFVP vs PAM for 2 years	Superiority of CMFVP vs PAM in RFS and SURV in all major subgroups No difference between pre- and postmenopausal women
Arizona University	CA for 8 cycles ± RT	RFS: 1–3: 77%, >3: 50%. No difference between pre- and postmenopause. No benefit from RT
M. D. Anderson Hospital	FAC + BCG ± RT for 2 years	RFS: 62% (1–3: 75%, >3: 65%), SURV: 70% Best results with full dose regimen No difference between pre- and postmenopause No benefit from RT or BCG

CTR = Control group (surgery only)
RFS = Relapse-free survival
RT = Postoperative radiotherapy
SURV = Survival

free survival was similar between ER+ and ER− tumors in the CMF program (Salmon and Jones, 1981; Bonadonna and Valagussa, 1982). Total survival may be longer in ER+ tumors compared to ER− tumors, probably as a consequence of tumor response to endocrine manipulations utilized at the time of primary treatment failure.

Salvage Therapy. The use of chemotherapy in patients with a recurrence following breast cancer treatment with a local-regional modality is simply palliative, and essentially all such patients can be expected to succumb to the disease. In women with recurrent neoplasms receiving adjuvant chemotherapy, second-line treatment should include non-cross-resistant drugs and/or endocrine therapy in patients with ER+ tumors. Even in women who had drug-induced amenorrhea, castration

can produce a 25 to 35% response rate. The results achieved by retreating the patients with the same initial regimen are not definitive. Preliminary findings, however, would suggest that a 30 to 40% response rate can be obtained in women whose disease-free interval from the last dose of adjuvant chemotherapy was longer than 12 months.

Chemotherapy Plus Hormones. The results of combined treatment utilizing adjuvant chemohormonal therapy are still premature. Preliminary results (Fisher et al., 1981; Hubay et al., 1981) would suggest improved relapse-free and total survival in ER+ patients given combination chemotherapy and tamoxifen. For the time being, this approach remains experimental.

Chemotherapy Plus Immunotherapy. All randomized trials testing the value of immu-

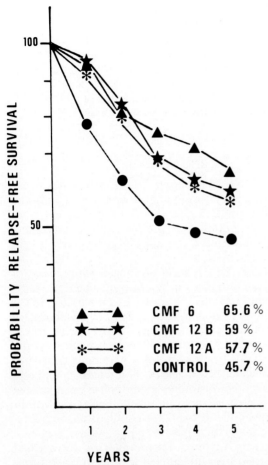

Figure 33–6. Comparison of 6-month versus 12-month CMF adjuvant chemotherapy for stage II breast cancer. CMF 12A versus control represents the original randomized trial. CMF 12B versus CMF 6 represents the second randomized trial, specifically evaluating the relapse-free survival with the reduced period of treatment. From Bonadonna, G., and Valagussa, P.: Chemotherapy of breast cancer: Current views and results. *Int. J. Radiat. Oncol. Biol. Phys.*, 9:279–297, 1983.

notherapy (BCG, levamisole, tumor cell vaccine) combined with chemotherapy have failed to improve the results over adjuvant chemotherapy alone (Salmon and Jones, 1981; Bonadonna and Valagussa, 1982). An interesting positive result utilizing adjuvant poly A : poly U was reported by a French group (Lacour *et al.,* 1980), but the findings remain to be confirmed at five years and should be the subject of confirmation by other investigators before they are accepted as a standard postoperative approach.

Chemotherapy Plus Radiotherapy. The value of the classic postoperative irradiation within a combined modality setting in patients subjected to mastectomy appears negative. In fact, available results from one study would indicate that one might negate an improved relapse-free and total survival rate by the addition of postoperative irradiation (Bonadonna and Valagussa, 1982). Furthermore, the concomitant adjuvant radiotherapy and chemotherapy may prevent the administration of full drug doses during the crucial first six months of treatment because of myelosuppression. In N+ women following breast-saving procedures, relapse-free and total survival results appear superimposable to those reported after mastectomy plus adjuvant chemotherapy. If full axillary dissection is performed and irradiation is limited solely to the breast, only 12 to 15% of patients will experience severe myelosuppression by combined radiotherapy and chemotherapy (Harris and Hellman, 1983).

Node Negative Patients. Patients with N−, ER− tumors, particularly those who are premenopausal, have a poor relapse-free survival, that is, almost superimposable to that of all N+ patients (Salmon and Jones, 1981; Bonadonna and Valagussa, 1982). Controlled trials are now in progress to determine the role of adjuvant chemotherapy in this subgroup.

Early Versus Late Toxicity. Acute toxicity from adjuvant chemotherapy is not substantially different from that observed in patients treated for advanced disease. Utilizing CMF, frank alopecia does not occur in more than 10% of women, whereas with doxorubicin-containing regimens the incidence of this side effect increases to 70 to 80%. FAC or AC chemotherapy has been reported to produce congestive heart failure in a limited number of cases. Therefore, in an adjuvant situation, the cumulative dose of doxorubicin should not exceed 280 to 300 mg/m^2. Although transient elevation of SGOT, SGPT, and LDH with or without associated increased bilirubin can occur in a small fraction of patients receiving CMF or CMFVP chemotherapy, requiring a temporary discontinuation of methotrexate, hepatic fibrosis does not appear, at present, to be an important problem. From current reports (Salmon and Jones, 1981; Bonadonna and Valagussa, 1982) evidence that prolonged adjuvant chemotherapy containing PAM or cyclophosphamide has increased the incidence of second tumors in breast cancer patients is not available. In particular, no patient developed acute leukemia when treated with the CMF program.

It should be recognized that available data

are still too recent to provide meaningful conclusions in terms of drug-induced carcinogenesis.

In summary, present results would suggest that adjuvant combination chemotherapy can be recommended at least in all N+ premenopausal women. In postmenopausal patients the recommendation for routine systemic therapy is less firm, mainly because of apparent contradictory reports in the medical literature. Ideally, adjuvant treatment should be started within two to four weeks from surgery and given in full doses for about six months. Thus, in the presence of treatment-induced myelosuppression it is advisable to delay therapy rather than using a dose attenuation schedule. Unless given within the context of a research trial, a doxorubicin-containing regimen should be limited today to women with > 3 involved nodes. Continuing research is directed toward clarifying unresolved problems such as the relative efficacy of sequential versus alternating non-cross-resistant regimens, the usefulness of different drug schedules, the role of endocrine therapy, the optimal treatment duration, the cost-benefit ratio, and a definition of which patients should receive adjuvant therapy.

While recognizing the limitations imposed by persisting uncertainties regarding the optimal treatment for various disease subsets, the suggested guidelines are listed in Table 33–8.

Management of Selected Complications

Disseminated breast cancer often gives rise to a number of clinical complications. Their prompt recognition is vital to provide effective treatment.

Skeletal Metastases. In addition to being painful, extensive osteolytic lesions in weight-bearing regions such as the femora and humeri are highly susceptible to fractures. Irradiation to doses in the range of 3000 to 4000 rads results in effective pain relief and some bone healing. The optimal management of impending or actual fracture of the femur, however, usually involves stabilization by internal fixation or replacement of anatomic structures with prosthetic parts (Fidler, 1973). This allows the patient to become ambulatory, thus decreasing the risks associated with immobilization that include hypercalcemia, bronchopneumonia, and venous thrombosis. The presence of multiple lesions is not a contraindication to orthopedic surgery, and surgical

management of bilateral femoral fractures is not uncommon.

A frequent complication is also pathologic fracture of a vertebra or epidural involvement. Muscle weakness, nerve root pain, paresthesias, and urinary retention are common clinical features. One should not hesitate to perform a myelogram when neurologic symptoms and signs are suspicious. The optimal local treatment is usually radiotherapy (3000 to 4000 rads) and, in selected cases, surgical decompression.

CNS Metastases. Brain metastases occur in 25 to 50% of patients with overt metastatic disease (DiStefano et al., 1979). In a few cases they manifest as the first sign of metastatic breast cancer; this appears particularly true in women subjected to adjuvant chemotherapy (5%). This reflects prolonged suppression of systemic disease by adjuvant chemotherapy, with less effect in controlling metastases in the brain (Paterson et al., 1982). Leptomeningeal metastases are also increasingly being recognized (Little et al., 1974; Wasserstrom et al., 1982). Brain symptoms and signs consist of headache, changes in the mental status (lethargy, confusion, or memory loss), generalized or focal seizures, persistent nausea and vomiting, difficulty walking, papilledema, and occasionally diabetes insipidus. When the neoplasm involves retro-orbital or intraorbital structures, the clinical features include proptosis and visual impairment. Among cranial nerve symptoms and signs, the most common features are diplopia, ocular muscle paresis (III, IV, VI), hearing loss, and visual loss. Spinal symptoms may include weakness, usually affecting the legs, paresthesias in one or more extremities, radicular pain, and bladder and bowel dysfunction. A cauda equina syndrome is a relatively common complaint.

The presence of brain involvement can be confirmed by computerized tomography, while the most important diagnostic tests for leptomeningeal metastasis are examination of CSF for cytology and chemistry as well as a lumbar myelogram to demonstrate irregular filling of the subarachnoid space.

Radiation therapy to the whole brain (3000 to 4000 rads) combined with dexamethasone (8 to 16 mg/day) represents the standard treatment of brain metastases, both retro-orbital and intraorbital involvement. Irradiation directed to the site(s) of major clinical involvement is also recommended in the presence of meningeal carcinomatosis and is usually com-

Table 33–8. Suggested Guidelines for Therapy

Local-regional therapy

T_1N_{0-1} Quadrantectomy or segmental resection or excisional biopsy
+ Axillary dissection
+ Radiotherapy to residual breast

T_2N_{0-1} Total mastectomy
+ Axillary dissection, or
In selected patients (T < 4 cm) as for T_1 tumors

$T_{3a}N_{0-1}$ Total or modified radical mastectomy

Combined treatment

N+ Local-regional therapy as above
+ Combination chemotherapy for 6 to 12 months in ER+ and ER− tumors
Doxorubicin-containing regimens only if N+ > 3 nodes
Chemotherapy plus tamoxifen may be considered in ER+ patients

N− Adjuvant chemotherapy remains experimental
Combination chemotherapy for 6 months may be considered in premenopausal
patients with ER− or peritumoral or intratumoral lymphatic emboli

$T_{3b}-T_4N_{0-2}$ Total or modified radical mastectomy
+ Postoperative radiotherapy
+ Combination chemotherapy for 6 months
± Endocrine therapy depending on ER status

$T_{3b}-T_4N_3$ Combination chemotherapy for 2–3 cycles
↓
Intensive local-regional radiotherapy
↓
Further chemotherapy for 3–5 cycles
± Endocrine therapy depending on ER status

Inflammatory Cancer

Combination chemotherapy for 2–3 cycles
± Endocrine therapy depending on ER status
↓
Radiotherapy if at least good PR is achieved
↓
Further chemotherapy (3–5 cycles) if local control is achieved

Systemic therapy in advanced disease

Premenopausal patients

ER− Progression ER+
Polychemotherapy Castration CR or PR
↓ ↓
Non-cross-resistant drugs Tamoxifen or estrogens or aminogluthethimide
↓ ↓ CR or PR
New drugs Progestins or androgens
Progression

Postmenopausal patients

ER− ER+
Polychemotherapy Progression Tamoxifen or estrogens
CR or PR
↓
Non-cross-resistant drugs Aminogluthethimide
CR or PR
↓
↓ Progestins
New drugs
Progression

---

bined with intrathecal administration of methotrexate (10 mg/m²), cytosine arabinoside (25 to 30 mg/m²), or thiotepa (2 to 3 mg/m²) every three to six days, depending on myelotoxicity, until the CSF becomes free of neoplastic cells. Drugs can also be instilled through a ventricular cannula attached to a subcutaneous reservoir (Ommaya device). By pursuing vigorous therapy, improvement of symptoms and signs can be obtained in at least 60% of patients.

Local Recurrences. The appearance of metastases many years after primary treatment is not rare, and the long latency period after the primary treatment remains unexplained. Fifty-seven patients who developed recurrences five years after primary surgery were reported and compared to 66 patients who recurred one to two years after treatment (Pap-aioannou *et al.,* 1967). For the later relapses the mean time to recurrence was 10.4 years. Despite this long latent period, the mean survival time was 1.9 months. Thus, the authors conclude that the local recurrence is associated with early deaths, and because the recurrence is local does not imply a benign course. This same conclusion was suggested by Dao and Nemoto (1963) who also reported that skin recurrence was shortly followed by systemic metastases. These studies and others clearly indicate the need for investigation and treatment for systemic metastases when skin recurrence occurs.

Although radiation therapy decreases the local recurrence rate, it is not absolute in its ability to prevent this complication. The management of local recurrences in irradiated areas is a problem that may require careful superficial x-ray therapy or local excision and skin grafting of necrotic and bleeding areas (Elkort *et al.,* 1980).

Bone Marrow Involvement. Bone involvement occurs in the majority of patients with metastases. Bone metastases can be suspected by clinical history evaluation and confirmed by bone x-rays or scans. Bone marrow examination, including a biopsy, may be positive in about 40% of patients with known bone metastases on x-ray or scan. Only 4% (1/24 patients) with negative x-rays and scans were positive for tumor cells in the bone marrow (Ingle *et al.,* 1978). In another study using only x-rays, aspiration biopsies produced positive cells in only 1.6% of patients with negative x-rays (Ridell and Landys, 1979). Peripheral blood parameters did not predict for bone marrow involvement.

Hypercalcemia. Breast cancer is the malignancy most commonly associated with hypercalcemia (see Chapters 6F and 40). The etiologic factor in breast cancer is clearly metastatic bone disease in the vast majority of patients. Other possible mechanisms include primary hyperparathyroidism, estrogen or tamoxifen flare, and ectopic-PTH production or pseudohyperparathyroidism. In a large series reported by Hickey *et al.* (1982), 19% of elevated serum calciums in a large cancer center were in 1311 patients with breast cancer. Of these, three were believed to be caused by primary hyperparathyroidism. In another three patients the cause of the increased calcium was believed to be the result of ectopic PTH production suggested by bioacti-

vity for PTH from the tumor tissue itself, with normal parathyroid tissue at histologic evaluation.

The management of hypercalcemia (levels over 12 mg/mL) includes the administration of intravenous normal saline and furosemide every six hours. Supplemental potassium administration must be done to counteract K^+ loss in the urine. Mithramycin 25 μg/kg can be given IV to lower calcium levels rapidly, and repeated doses every three to four days may be necessary. Other measures to lower serum calcium include prostaglandin inhibitors, calcitonin (Deftos and First, 1981; Hickey *et al.,* 1982), and corticosteroids (Binstock and Mundy, 1980). Recently, a new experimental approach using etidronate, a diphosphonate similar to compounds used in Paget's disease and bone scanning, has been shown to diminish serum calcium due to metastatic disease when given orally and systemically (Frijlink *et al.,* 1979; Cohen *et al.,* 1981; Jacobs *et al.,* 1981).

Abdominal Metastases. The evaluation of patients for intra-abdominal metastases has led at least one investigator to perform diagnostic staging laparotomies. In a series of 43 patients with metastatic disease, 6 were suspected of having abdominal metastases, and laparotomy revealed 16 to have intra-abdominal metastases (Meirion-Thomas *et al.,* 1978). Most often the tumor involvement was in multiple areas, with liver metastases and ovarian and/or adrenal metastases the principal sites of involvement.

Pulmonary Metastases. Metastatic breast cancer involving the lungs is common. Usually the nodules are multiple and grossly visible by x-ray. However, lymphangitic invasion of the lungs may occur with relatively normal-looking x-rays or films that may be confused with pulmonary fibrosis. Biopsy of the lung, transcutaneously or transbronchially, may be required to establish the diagnosis. Patients with breast cancer receiving mitomycin and long-term alkylating agents may develop interstitial infiltrates secondary to drug toxicity that can be confused with lymphangitic spread or infectious causes. Occasionally patients will present with a cough and a normal chest x-ray. Bronchoscopy may indicate the presence of intrabronchial tumors. Another pulmonary problem presents itself in the patient with an isolated nodule in the lung. Cahan and Castro (1975) reported a series of 72 patients with breast cancer at Memorial Hospital who developed a synchronous or metachronous solitary lung shadow. Forty-three had primary lung cancers, and 23 had breast cancer metastases; 6 had benign lesions, indicating the necessity of an aggressive diagnostic approach in these patients with isolated pulmonary nodules.

Pleural Effusions. Pleural effusions are relatively common in patients with breast cancer and may cause serious respiratory insufficiency. In a series of 105 cases reported from Guy's Hospital in London, the median time from diagnosis to clinically detectable pleural effusions was 41.5 months with a range of 0 to 246 months (Fentiman *et al.,* 1981). About 50% of the effusions were on the same side as the original cancer, and 10% were bilateral. Important factors in the natural history of these patients were medial or central breast lesions and stage III disease, but the development of pleural effusions was not related to the size of the tumor or histologic differentiation. Forty-five patients (43%) had pleural effusion as the first manifestation, and 60% of the patients already had other evidence for metastatic disease. The median survival after the effusion was 13 months. Despite a variety of treatment approaches, only 17% achieved local control, and the worst treatment approach was with aspiration alone.

In an earlier study of 50 patients, high protein (exudate), low sugar, and blood cells were usually diagnostic of a malignant effusion (Rosato *et al.* 1974). In their series, 60% of the pleural fluid cytologies were positive for malignant cells. Recently, others have suggested that an elevated CEA (> 12 ng/mL) was characteristic of malignant effusion. Rittgers *et al.* (1978) found that of 70 effusions in patients with malignant disease, 40% were positive for malignant cells, and 34% had a CEA of greater than 12 ng/mL. They suggest that the increased CEA is highly supportive of a malignant effusion.

The approach to an effusion associated with malignant cells depends on the extent of the symptoms and the systemic treatment options available. If the effusions are small and relatively asymptomatic, systemic administration of drugs as treatment should be done. If the effusion is symptomatic and/or the patient has had prior therapy, thoracostomy tube drainage and instillation of tetracycline (0.5 g) is performed. External drainage is continued for 12 to 24 more hours, and then the tube is pulled. An aspiration alone is rarely successful. The use of special pleuroperitoneal shunts that can be pumped is a new promising technique, more likely to be successful if the effusions are not excessively bloody (Weese and Schouten, 1982). The shunts contain heparin in the tube wall that may help keep the tube patent.

Other Metastatic Manifestations. Extrahepatic biliary tract metastases with involvement of the large biliary ducts, resulting in jaundice, must be differentiated from jaundice caused by intrahepatic metastases. In a series from the Massachusetts General Hospital, 49 patients with breast cancer presented with jaundice and had documented extrabiliary metastases (Kopelson *et al.,* 1980). Of these, 21 patients were discovered at autopsy, and 28 were diagnosed *ante mortem.* Therapy was instituted with bypass surgery or cannulation percutaneously followed by radition therapy. Significant benefit occurred in two-thirds of the patients. The main biliary duct was the primary site of obstruction, the result of neoplastic nodes, although intraductal metastases could be seen. These patients had a much better prognosis than those with intrahepatic involvement.

Ureteral obstruction is another uncommon manifestation of breast cancer (Feun *et al.,* 1979). Retroperitoneal disease seems to be a complication of long-standing breast cancer and may be a more specific site of recurrence for patients with the signet cell cancer of the breast (Merion and Livolsi, 1981). These patients may present with renal failure and large kidneys, and the abnormality may be first detected on a bone scan. Hormonal agents and XRT to the ureters may produce an excellent response. The diagnosis may clinically be considered retroperitoneal fibrosis because the ureters appear to be obstructed at multiple areas characteristic of this disease.

Breast Cancer Presenting as an Axillary Mass. Discrete axillary adenopathy in women with no obvious infectious lesion may be the first sign of either a lymphoma or breast cancer. This presentation represents about 0.4 to 1% of all breast cancers (Vezzoni *et al.,* 1979). Characteristically, these patients have no palpable disease in the breast. In a series reported from Milan of 49 patients, 31 of whom had mammograms, only 14 were believed to have a suspicious or abnormal mammogram. Of the 44 patients treated with mastectomy, 11 patients had no microscopic neoplasm in the breast, and 23 of the 33 patients with cancer had lesions < 1.0 cm. The five-year survival was 85% for the 33 patients with cancer and 100% for the 11 without cancer in the breast. In two other series from Memorial Hospital, the findings indicate similar excellent prognosis (Ashikari *et al.,* 1976; Rosen, 1980). In a series of eight patients, only preinvasive cancer was found. Thus, these patients after a thorough search for metastatic disease should undergo a mastectomy.

Criteria of Tumor Response

The definition of tumor response is important to continue or change treatment and represents a critical variable in the data analysis. In advanced disease, criteria of response are not uniform, and a number of different systems for recording response have been developed. The rules formulated by UICC and the NCI are, in all important details, identical (Hayward *et al.,* 1979).

Definition of Response. The measurable lesions or a representative number of them should be measured at each assessment. In the case of bidimensional lesions, regression is defined as when all lesions disappear or when each individual lesion or those selected for clinical judgment or study decrease by 50% or more, with no lesions increasing in size. In each case, no new lesions should appear.

For unidimensional lesions, in the case of regression the same rules apply as in bidimensional lesions, except that regression is taken as a decrease of 50% or more in one measurement.

Evaluable but nonmeasurable lesions include osseous metastases, pulmonary infiltration, skin infiltration, and pleural effusion. Serial evidence of appreciable change must be documented by radiography or photography. Neither the development nor healing of ulcers within skin metastases should be taken as sole evidence of change of status. Pathologic fractures or vertebral collapse is not necessarily evidence of progressive disease. Osteoblastic metastases are not valuable for purposes of assessing response to treatment.

Categories of Response. *Complete Response.* Complete response is defined as the disappearance of all lesions determined by two observations, not less than four weeks apart. In the case of lytic bone metastases, radiologic examination must show them to have calcified.

Partial Response. Partial response is defined as 50% or greater decrease in measurable lesions and unequivocal improvement in evaluable but nonmeasurable lesions determined by two observations, not less than four weeks apart. It is not necessary for every lesion to have regressed to qualify for partial response, but no lesion should have progressed.

No Change. Lesions are unchanged if there is < 50% decrease or < 25% increase in size of measurable lesions.

Progressive Disease. (1) Mixed: some lesions regress, while others progress or new lesions appear. (2) Failure: progression of some or all lesions and/or appearance of new lesions, while no lesions regress.

Principles of Follow-up

After Primary Treatment. Patients should be examined at regular intervals (*e.g.,* every three months) and in particular during the first three years after surgery and/or radiotherapy since this is the period of highest incidence of tumor recurrence. As a general guideline, roentgenograms of chest, serum alkaline phosphatase, plasma CEA, and bone scans should be performed, in the absence of signs and symptoms, every six months for the first three years and then once a year. The performance of radioisotopic studies of the liver on a routine basis remains somewhat controversial and in many centers has been supplanted by measures of serum liver function tests that, if abnormal, are followed by hepatic nuclear medicine or CT scan. Since bone scans can provide a number of false-positive findings, suspicious lesions in the absence of bone pain should also be studied with appropriate x-rays and/or biopsies. Similar considerations apply to the liver scan where suspicious radioisotopic findings in the absence of enlarged liver should preferably be confirmed histologically. In the absence of neurologic complaints, a brain scan is not routinely performed during follow-up.

In patients treated with breast-saving procedures, as well as in those given radiotherapy because of inoperable disease, bilateral mammography should be obtained every six months for the first three years from completion of treatment, and then once a year. Whenever a suspicious nodule is visible on mammogram or becomes palpable, excisional biopsy must be performed. In patients subjected to mastectomy, repeat mammography of contralateral breast may be performed at 12-month intervals, unless suspicious nodules become palpable.

Whenever technically feasible, primary treatment failure should also be confirmed by excisional biopsy. Biopsy of the involved areas or organ could be of primary importance, especially in patients with "late" recurrence, since the histopathologic examination of the lesion may reveal the presence of a second primary neoplasm.

During adjuvant chemotherapy, women should be examined at least once a month to monitor drug-induced toxicity. Unless treatment produces frequent and prolonged myelosuppression, routine blood counts beyond the day of intravenous drug administration (*e.g.,* on day 1 and 8 of each CMF or FAC course) are not necessary. As previously stressed, in the presence of myelosuppression, it is advisable to delay the subsequent course for one to two weeks rather than utilize a reduced dose schedule. Suggested biochemical tests comprise routine blood chemistry to include serum creatinine every three to six months when methotrexate is part of the combination. In the presence of treatment failure, other biochemical tests can be carried out, and the choice usually depends upon the clinical situation (*e.g.,* serum and urine calcium levels if bone metastases are detected, complete liver function tests if hepatic involvement is evident or suspected). During treatment with doxorubicin measurements of systolic time interval and ejection fraction should be reserved for patients with a history of preexisting cardiac disease, and when the total accumulative dose approaches 400 mg/m^2.

During Systemic Therapy for Advanced Disease. Women receiving endocrine treatment can be examined every six to eight weeks, and appropriate x-ray examinations performed approximately every three months, unless symptoms and signs of disease progression become evident. It is important to recall that in many patients receiving additive hormonal therapy the initial objective response may require two to three months of treatment.

During cytotoxic chemotherapy, peripheral blood counts should be checked, following the same rules outlined for women undergoing adjuvant chemotherapy. Bone marrow biopsy or aspiration is almost never required unless to explain persistent myelosuppression or a leukoerythroblastic peripheral blood picture. The assessment of the measurable tumor mass should be made, initially, at monthly intervals, and subsequently every three months using the appropriate diagnostic modality: chest x-ray, nuclear scan, CT scan or bone scan, and relevant x rays to document the degree and duration of response.

Rehabilitation

The successful rehabilitation of a patient with breast cancer must include attention to optimum psychological as well as physical adjustment. This applies particularly to women subjected to mastectomy, as well as those undergoing adjuvant chemotherapy. Most of the physical and emotional consequences of mutilating surgery and/or prolonged cytotoxic therapy can be managed satisfactorily with the assistance of an informed, concerned physician. In fact, one of the most important psychological defenses patients have in fighting their disease or the side effects of treatment is hope, and physicians and supporting staff can provide meaningful information concerning the cure rate or the chance for a longer life.

Restoration After Surgery. After recovery from anesthesia in patients subjected to mastectomy and axillary dissection, the arm-abducted position should be maximized and the patient encouraged to start using the arm. Before discharge, she should be given written instructions concerning motor exercise for shoulder adduction, forward flexion, and internal and external rotation. In selected patients the exercises can be performed with the help of a rehabilitation therapist. No one can predict how soon after mastectomy the patient can be ready for a prosthesis. Various factors enter into making this decision (*e.g.,* wound healing and relative degree of sensitivity of the chest). Several types of prostheses are available: those filled with silicone gel, liquid/air, or polyester fiber, or those made of weighted or unweighted foam rubber.

Breast Reconstruction. Today, a number of alternative methods to breast reconstruction are available, and most women consider reconstruction approximately six months after the mastectomy (Snyderman, 1980). The most important methods include correction of the scar, reduction of the remaining breast, insertion of a special prosthesis, and formation of the areolar-nipple complex. The current use of a musculocutaneous flap differs from the previous technique in that the muscle underlying the skin is included, and the entire unit is rotated on a single vascular pedicle. The three most common musculocutaneous flaps in use are those utilizing the latissimus dorsi, the pectoralis major, and the rectus abdominis. The recent availability of the musculocutaneous flap has given a new dimension also to the reconstruction of chest wall defects produced by wide excision in women with local recurrent cancer, radiation necrosis, and tumor lysis with ulceration.

Edema of the Arm. Almost all mastectomy patients will have some postoperative edema in the upper arm, and swelling will subside in most women in a matter of weeks or months. The causative factors of edema include extent of axillary dissection, obesity, grade of cancer growth, surgical methods, postoperative complications (notably infection, skin necrosis, and prolonged collection of axillary fluids), and postoperative irradiation. To prevent postoperative edema, patients should be advised to elevate the arm when casually sitting and to use the arm as much as possible for routine activities. Women should avoid injury to the arm. With the modified mastectomy, without postoperative radiation, many of the past complications of arm edema and weakness associated with the radical mastectomy are much less frequent.

Women who have significant discomfort from an edematous arm may be helped by treatment with compression pumping. Women with recurrent edema successfully treated by pumping can purchase an electrically or manually operated pump and sleeve for home use. Some patients are helped by the continuous compression produced by an elastic sleeve. Women with significant circulatory block in the axilla (*e.g.,* by postoperative radiation) may benefit by creation of a lymphatic-venous anastomosis.

Psychological Adjustment. The systematic study of the many psychological reactions of women to breast cancer is still in its early stages (Sanger and Reznikoff, 1981). Therefore, at present, only general guidelines can be provided. Adaptation to breast cancer depends on two parameters: one derived from the patient and one from the disease. The latter includes the extent of tumor spread, surgical operability, need for adjuvant therapy, the full application of rehabilitative measures, that is, plastic reconstruction when appropriate, and the psychological management by the oncologist in the doctor-patient relationship (Moris, 1979; Holland and Mastrovito, 1980).

Stress syndromes in breast cancer occur most often at certain key points: around the time of mastectomy (perioperative syndromes), in the rehabilitative phases, during drug adjuvant treatment, and at the time of disseminated disease, particularly at the time of first relapse. The stress responses are usually characterized by situational anxiety and depression. Psychological stress is often produced in women undergoing adjuvant chemotherapy and frequent follow-up examinations because they represent evidence of a continuing threat to life as well as body integrity. Patients subjected to prolonged adjuvant chemotherapy have a tendency to overeat and thus increase their body weight. They may suddenly refuse to complete treatment. Stress responses are best managed by counseling and support from nurses, social workers, mental health professionals, or other patients with cancer, depending on the severity of symptoms and complicating factors. In the more severe cases, antidepressants are often of value, particularly when insomnia is a prominent symptom. Amitriptyline or imipramine, beginning at 50 mg at bedtime and increased to a therapeutic trial of 150 mg, may significantly improve mood and activity within two to three weeks.

Male Breast Cancer

Male breast cancer accounts for less than 1% of all breast cancers (Crichlow, 1972, 1976; Meyskens *et al.,* 1976). In the United States, the annual estimate of new cases is approximately 700. The histologic pattern is similar to that of women, except that lobular carcinoma has not been reported in men. The median age of onset is approximately 60. Male breast cancer tends to occur in countries that have a high incidence of liver cancer, presumably related to hepatic metabolism of hormones. Exogenous hormone administration may increase the incidence of male breast cancer when used in large, long-term doses as in transsexuals. Estrogen administration in men with prostate cancer may lead to gynecomastia but not an increased incidence of breast cancer. Testicular abnormalities, such as orchitis, atrophic testicles and Kleinfelter's syndrome, have been associated with men developing breast cancer (Roswit and Edlis, 1978). Radiation has been shown to increase the incidence of breast cancer in men as well as women.

Most cancers in men present as a painless

mass. Because of a longer duration of symptoms, the tumor is often found with more advanced manifestations such as skin involvement, muscle invasion, or even systemic metastases. The differential diagnosis must include other causes for gynecomastia. Most cancers are unilateral, hard, irregular, and eccentric. Bilateral, smooth, well-defined masses not involving the skin are associated with benign causes. About 40% of patients with cancer will have microscopic gynecomastia (Heller *et al.,* 1978).

Therapy for male breast cancer is similar to that for women for comparable stages. Management of disseminated lesions begins with orchiectomy, where the chances of response are high, 45 to 88% (Neifeld *et al.,* 1976). A correlation between estrogen receptors and response is not evident. ER-negative patients will often respond to hormonal therapies. Other ablative procedures such as adrenalectomy and hypophysectomy may give excellent second responses. After these procedures additive hormonal therapy with estrogens, androgens, and progestins is not helpful. Tamoxifen has been able to induce responses in 48% of male patients (Hortobagyi *et al.,* 1979; Patterson *et al.,* 1980). Recently, an antiandrogen, cyproterone acetate, has been shown to induce clinical responses in three of three patients (Lopez and Barduagni, 1982). Chemotherapy response appears to be similar in character to that of women. Survival is reported to be less in men than women, particularly after ten years with comparable stages (Crichlow, 1976), although some studies report similar results (Heller *et al.,* 1978; Yap *et al.,* 1979).

Prognostic Factors

Various parameters have been recognized to be of prognostic value in the treatment of primary and advanced breast cancer, and eventually in the patient survival. Most of these parameters can be visualized as clinical expressions of the growth rate of the tumor and its tendency to spread. Until very recently, most studies have evaluated only one factor at a time for its prognostic significance. In recent years, the development of multivariate methodology using logistic regression to assess the effect of covariates on prognosis has become a productive area of statistical research. Computer programs are now available for many of these methods, and applications are beginning to appear in the medical literature.

Primary Disease.   *Clinical Findings.*   Clinical findings include clinical history, age and menopausal status, and clinical stage (Rozencweig and Heuson, 1975; Stewart and Rubens, 1982).

Although it is generally believed that early diagnosis improves treatment outcome as delay is often associated with large tumors and high incidence of axillary involvement, several observations have reaffirmed the lack of consistent relationship between delay and survival. Since prognosis is affected unfavorably by rapid tumor growth, long delays in diagnosis could be associated with slowly growing tumors. This plausible explanation is confirmed, in part, by the results of the Health Insurance Plan (HIP) for Greater New York (Strax, 1980). The findings of this project indicated that the screening procedure may detect cancers with an extremely favorable prognosis, both in terms of nodal status and survival, that is, with an inherently good prognosis. The influence of age and menopausal status on survival may depend to some extent on other variables such as stage. Patients less than 35 years of age have frequently been reported to show a poorer survival than older women, possibly the result of a comparatively higher incidence of positive axillary nodes. Following radical mastectomy, the ten-year relapse-free and total survival rates are similar between pre- and postmenopausal women, the difference being related only to nodal status (N+ versus N−). Pregnancy does not considerably alter the prognosis of breast cancer, whether occurring at the same time as the disease or after its primary treatment.

Clinical staging indicates a progressively worse prognosis with increasing T, N, and M values. The presence of clinically palpable lymph nodes also influences prognosis (adversely), particularly in the presence of supraclavicular adenopathy (N_3). Since the error in correct lymph node evaluation is approximately 35%, the prognostic influence of axillary nodes will be analyzed in detail when the importance of pathologic stage is described. Fixation of the primary tumor to the skin or the underlying structures (T_{3b}–T_4) and fixation of the axillary nodes to one another or to other anatomic structures (N_2) greatly lower the survival results. In contrast, location of the tumor in the breast does not affect the five- and ten-year results of mastectomy.

Histopathologic Findings.   Gross and microscopic structural features of breast carcinoma provide a more meaningful assessment of the prognosis than clinical staging alone.

The axillary node status and particularly the number of axillary nodes involved currently represent the most simple, reproducible, and important prognostic indicator in patients with resectable breast cancer (that is, ten-year relapse-free survival following Halsted mastectomy: N−, 75%; N+, 25%; N+ 1−3 nodes, 35%; N+ >3 nodes, 13−15%). The worst prognosis has been observed in women with concomitant involvement of axillary and internal mammary nodes. Relapse-free and total survival rates are related to the extent of axillary adenopathy also in patients subjected to adjuvant therapy. Small metastatic deposits in axillary nodes appear to be correlated with longer survival than extensive metastatic involvement. The prognostic significance of level of axillary involvement remains uncertain and both relapse-free and total survival rates appear to be more correlated to the number of positive nodes than to their anatomic level of involvement. Extranodal invasion is associated with poor prognosis, but this pathologic finding is often encountered in women with >3 nodes.

Other Prognostic Factors. Other prognostic factors primarily concern the influence of steroid receptors, tumor growth fraction, and other biologic markers (Buckman *et al.,* 1982; Stewart and Rubens, 1982).

Although a general consensus on the influence of ER on prognosis of early breast cancer has not yet been reached, the vast majority of published reports have supported the original observation that the ER status affects the relapse-free survival in women with both involved and uninvolved axillary nodes (McGuire, 1978). In fact, regardless of stage and menopausal status, patients with ER+ tumors have a significantly lower recurrence rate than patients whose tumors were ER−. Preliminary results on patients receiving adjuvant chemotherapy, however, showed the five-year relapse-free survival was not significantly affected by the ER status. This finding is in accord with a general observation made in disseminated breast cancer that ER status is not predictive of response to chemotherapy (Bonadonna *et al.,* 1980). This observation could also help in the selection of node-negative women who could be candidates for adjuvant chemotherapy (five-year relapse-free survival: ER+ ≥80%, ER− ≤45%). Less

information exists on the use of PgR as a prognostic aid. The five-year relapse-free survival of operable women with ER+ PgR+ tumors, however, was reported to be 100% compared to about 80% for women with ER+ PgR− tumors. Growth characteristics of invasive mammary tumors estimated by the labeling index (LI) have yielded conflicting views on the relevance of LI as an independent prognostic factor, because as tumor type becomes more undifferentiated (that is, with high LI), an increase in the proportion of ER− tumors occurs. Recent findings have indicated that the proliferative activity of primary breast cancer is always higher in ER− tumors than in ER+ tumors within the same menopausal group, and a decrease in proliferative activity was observed from pre- to postmenopausal women within ER+ and ER− tumors (Bertuzzi *et al.,* 1981).

Beside steroid hormone receptors, other biologic markers have been studied as prognostic factors. They are milk-specific proteins (α-lactalbumin), epithelial components (carcinoembryonic antigen, lectin concanavalin A), as well as contractile and structural components (myosin and actin, lamina and collagen, fibronectin). A major problem of using biologic markers to assess human carcinomas is the heterogeneity of their expression found within tumors. This feature has been highlighted recently with the use of monoclonal antibodies to breast antigens. It may be that studies of antigen distribution will be more instructive about tumor biology than prognostication in a clinical setting.

Locally Advanced Disease. When $T_{3b}-T_4$ breast cancer is treated with radiotherapy alone, median survival is about two years and only about 15% of patients survive more than five years. Survival is particularly poor in those patients with symptoms of less than six months before presentation, as well as in those with large primary tumors and regional node involvement. In contrast, small localized primary tumors (<4 cm) and deep fixation to the chest wall are often associated with good response and long survival following radiotherapy. In patients treated with a combined modality approach, both freedom from progression and total survival are affected by nodal status and tumor size (Valagussa *et al.,* 1983). In selected patients, that is, those with no supraclavicular adenopathy or inflammatory carcinoma, radical surgery preceded and followed by chemotherapy can yield a five-year survival of about 50%. ER status and menopausal status do not appear to be prognostic factors in primary locally advanced breast cancer.

Tumors with dermal lymphatic infiltration (inflammatory carcinoma), with or without regional adenopathy, invariably carry a very poor prognosis. Few women treated with combined chemotherapy and irradiation remain alive after five years.

Disseminated Disease. In disseminated disease several prognostic factors are usually involved. The single most important factor consists of the objective tumor response for, as previously described, all responders show a longer median survival compared to nonresponders. The established variables influencing response, and consequently survival, are also related to the type of first systemic treatment—endocrine therapy or chemotherapy (see Table 33–9). Today, many patients with recurrent or clinically overt metastatic breast cancer receive various forms of endocrine therapy and chemotherapy before death because ER are either positive or undetermined. Therefore, prognosis is ultimately affected by a combination of variables that are mainly represented by the tumor cell burden at the start of systemic therapy, as well as by its metastatic and growth patterns.

Established prognostic factors (Rozencweig and Heuson, 1975; Stewart and Rubens, 1982) can be summarized as follows. The free interval (time elapsed from primary treatment to first relapse) is a prognostic variable of paramount importance. Free intervals longer than two years are distinctly associated with higher rates of long survival, probably because long free intervals reflect slow-growing tumors and tend to respond favorably to endocrine treatment. The opposite finding that a short free interval is associated to high response to poly-chemotherapy has not been confirmed by all investigators. The influence of site of metastatic disease on both survival and response to various treatment modalities is important in two ways. First, involvement of certain vital organs such as liver, brain, spinal cord, and lungs (diffuse lymphangitis type of spread) results in a poor treatment response and prognosis. Second, the extent of metastases is significant because both endocrine treatment and chemotherapy usually have limited efficacy in the presence of high tumor cell burden. Therefore, prognosis is inversely related to the number of sites involved, the degree of organ involvement, and the size of metastases. In this context, extensive prior radiotherapy, low performance status, and weight loss are all strongly related to low response rates and short survival times. The site of the dominant lesion affects both survival and response to endocrine and cytotoxic treatments in such a way that soft tissue categories have a more favorable outcome than the osseous categories, and the latter more favorable than visceral categories. With modern combination chemotherapy the lowest response rate and the poorest survival are associated with the concomitant involvement of visceral, osseous, and soft tissue metastases. Age and menopausal status have a distinct prognostic value. Patients below age 35 appear to respond poorly to castration (they often have ER− tumors), and women two years postmenopause have a poorer response to endocrine and often to cytotoxic therapy, as well as short survival. Finally, a remission with the first endocrine treatment distinctly increases the likelihood of a subsequent response to other hormonal manipulations. The results of hormonal therapy are of no predictive value on the effectiveness of subsequent cytotoxic chemotherapy, although previous endocrine therapy may unfavorably affect the rate of response when compared to no prior therapy. Prior chemotherapy invariably affects unfavorably the results of second-line chemotherapy.

Future Prospects

The ultimate objective of treatment of any neoplasm is to minimize morbidity and mortality to the point where the disease is either prevented or treated with very high degrees of success with low toxicity. Other parameters that must be considered are the economic costs

Table 33–9. Conventional Prognostic Variables Affecting Treatment Response and Survival of Disseminated Breast Cancer

AFTER ENDOCRINE THERAPY	AFTER CHEMOTHERAPY
Estrogen receptor level	Performance status and weight loss
Prior response to therapy	Extensive prior irradiation
Free interval	Multiple organ involvement
Dominant site of lesion	Impaired organ function
Menopausal status	Prior chemotherapy

of treatment approaches. Even minimal surgery and radiation therapy are time consuming and costly to the patient. Adjuvant therapy still needs to be proven to show a major impact on survival in most patients beyond five years.

What are some of the future areas of research that offer potential? Some of the major areas to explore in the future are ways of preventing the cancer and detecting or treating the cancer in the subclinical stage. The prevention of cancer using retinoids or growth modulators still remains experimental (Sachs, 1978). The use of dibutyryl cyclic AMP (Cho-Chung *et al.,* 1981), retinoids (Schroder and Black, 1980), and embryonic mammary mesenchyme (DeCosse *et al.,* 1973) have all been shown in experimental systems to inhibit tumor growth. Their clinical application remains to be done. The use of prophylactic mastectomy to prevent cancer in the opposite breast is a very radical way to diminish cancer incidence.

Several approaches diminish host toxicity. Breast reconstruction is a very effective way of mitigating the disfigurement of radical surgery (McColl, 1979; Woods, 1980). A potential method to diminish toxicity caused by chemotherapy would include the pretherapeutic testing of the cancer for resistance and sensitivity to chemotherapy. Various techniques have been proposed including *in vitro* testing (Volm *et al.,* 1979), clonogenic assays (Asano and Mandel, 1981), xenografts in nude mice (Shafie and Grantham, 1981), and the estrogen receptor test. All of these, except the latter, have not proven to be clinically useful, although further work needs to be done. Not only are we to be concerned about the immediate toxicity of cancer treatments, but we must be aware that many of our drugs and even radiation therapy are associated with long-term effects such as leukemia (Rosner *et al.,* 1978), pulmonary fibrosis, and heart falure. These long-term effects must be factored into the cost-benefit ratio of the treatment decision.

Finally, the use of biological markers to detect tumor cell numbers has been extremely useful in the therapy of choriocarcinoma and testicular cancers. These markers can be used to detect subclinical disease as well as to monitor therapy. In breast cancer, a variety of disease activity markers have been found (Woo *et al.,* 1978). Whether these can be used to predict failure or response needs to be determined. The ultimate marker would be one detected in the blood or urine, that is not necessarily specific for breast cancer, but that does correlate with tumor cell numbers.

REFERENCES

Adair, F.; Berg, J.; Joubert, L.; and Robbins, G. F.: Long-term followup of breast cancer patients: The 30-year report. *Cancer,* 33:1145–1150, 1974.

Adami, H. O.; Hansen, J.; Jung, B.; and Rimsten, A.: Familiality in breast cancer: A case-control study in a Swedish population. *Br. J. Cancer,* 42:71–77, 1980.

Adami, H. O.; Hansen, J.; Jung, B.; and Rimsten, A.: Characteristics of familial breast cancer in Sweden: Absence of relation to age and unilateral versus bilateral disease. *Cancer,* 43:1688–1695, 1981.

Alford, C.; Hollinshead, A. C.; and Herberman, R. B.: Delayed cutaneous hypersensitivity reactions to extracts of malignant and normal human breast cells. *Ann. Surg.,* 178:20–24, 1973.

Anderson, D. E.: Genetic study of breast cancer: Identification of a high risk group. *Cancer,* 34:1090–1097, 1974.

Asano, S., and Mandel, T. E.: Colonies formed in agar from human breast cancer and their identification as T-lymphocytes. *J.N.C.I.,* 67:25–32, 1981.

Ashikari, R.; Rosen, P. P.; Urban, J. A.; and Senoo, T.: Breast cancer presenting as an axillary mass. *Ann. Surg.,* 183:415–417, 1976.

Baral, E.; Larsson, L. E.; and Mattsson, B.: Breast cancer following irradiation of the breast. *Cancer,* 40:2905–2910, 1977.

Bell, J. R.; Friedell, G.; and Goldenberg, I. S.: Prognostic significance of pathologic findings in human breast carcinoma. *Surg. Gynecol. Obstet.,* 129:258–262, 1969.

Bertuzzi, A.; Daidone, M. G.; Di Fonzo, G.; and Silvestrini, R.: Relationship among estrogen receptors, proliferative activity and menopausal status in breast cancer. *Breast Cancer Res. Treat.,* 1:253–262, 1981.

Binstock, M. L., and Mundy, G. R.: Effect of calcitonin and glucocorticoids in combination on the hypercalcemia of malignancy. *Ann. Intern. Med.,* 93:269–272, 1980.

Black, M. M., and Leis, H. P., Jr.: Cellular responses to autologous breast cancer tissue—Correlation with stage and lymphoreticuloendothelial reactive. *Cancer,* 28:263–273, 1971.

Boice, J. D., Jr., and Monson, R. R.: Breast cancer in women after repeated fluoroscopic examinations of the chest. *J.N.C.I.,* 59:823–832, 1977.

Bonadonna, G., and Valagussa, P.: Dose-response effect of adjuvant chemotherapy in breast cancer. *N. Engl. J. Med.,* 304:10–15, 1981.

Bonadonna, G., and Valagussa, P.: Chemotherapy of breast cancer: Current views and results. *Int. J. Radiat. Oncol. Biol. Phys.,* 9:279–297, 1983.

Bonadonna, G.; Valagussa, P.; Tancini, G.; and DeFronzo, G.: Estrogen receptor status and response to chemotherapy in early and advanced breast cancer. *Cancer Chemother. Pharmacol.,* 4:37–41, 1980.

Boyd, N. F.; Campbell, J. E.; Germanson, T.; Thomson, D. B.; Sutherland, D. J.; and Meakin, J. W.: Body weight and prognosis in breast cancer. *J.N.C.I.,* 67:785–789, 1981.

Boyd, N. F.; Meakin, J. W.; Hayward, J. L.; and Brown,

T. C.: Clinical estimation of the growth rate of breast cancer. *Cancer,* **48:**1037–1042, 1981.

Brady, L.: The changing role of radiotherapy. In Bonadonna, G. (ed.): *Breast Cancer: Recent Advances in Diagnosis and Treatment.* John Wiley & Sons, Ltd., London, 1982.

Braunschweiger, P. G.; Poulakos, L.; and Schiffer, L. M.: Cell kinetics *in vivo* and *in vitro* for C3H/He spontaneous mammary tumors. *J.N.C.I.,* **59:**1197–1204, 1977.

Brinton, L. A.; Hooever, R. N.; Szklo, M.; and Fraumeni, J. F., Jr.: Menopausal estrogen use and risk of breast cancer. *Cancer,* **47:**2517–2522, 1981.

British Breast Group: Bone scanning in breast cancer. *Br. Med. J.,* **2:**180–181, 1978.

Brownstein, M. H.; Wolf, M.; and Bikowski, J. B.: Cowden's disease—A cutaneous marker of breast cancer. *Cancer,* **41:**2393–2398, 1978.

Buckman, R.; Coombs, R. C.; Dearnaley, D. P.; *et al.:* Some clinical use of biological markers. In Bonadonna, G. (ed.): *Breast Cancer: Recent Advances in Diagnosis and Treatment.* John Wiley & Sons, Ltd., London, 1982.

Cahan, W. G., and Castro, E. B.: Significance of a solitary lung shadow in patients with breast cancer. *Ann. Surg.,* **181:**137–143, 1975.

Cancer Research Campaign Working Party: Cancer Research Campaign (King's/Cambridge trial for early breast cancer). *Lancet,* **2:**55–60, 1980.

Carter, D.: Intraductal papillary tumors of the breast—A study of 78 cases. *Cancer,* **39:**1689–1692, 1977.

Carter, S. K.: Surgery plus adjuvant chemotherapy. A review of therapeutic implications. I. Breast cancer. *Cancer Chemother. Pharmacol.,* **4:**147–163, 1980.

Carter, S. K.: The dilemma of local control therapy of breast cancer. *West. J. Med.,* **136:**336–338, 1982.

Champion, H. R.; Wallace, I. W. J.; and Prescott, R. J.: Histology in breast cancer prognosis. *Br. J. Cancer,* **26:**129–138, 1972.

Chang, J.; Sibala, J. L.; Fritz, S. L.; Dwyer, S. J.; Templeton, A. W.; Fritz, L.; and Jewell, W. R.: Computed tomography in detection and diagnosis of breast cancer. *Cancer* (Suppl.), **46:**939–946, 1980.

Cho-Chung, Y. S.; Clair, T.; Bodwin, J. S.; and Berghoffer, B. A.: Growth arrest and morphological change of human breast cancer cells by dibutyryl cyclic AM and L-arginine. *Science,* **214:**77–79, 1981.

Citrin, D. L.; Bessent, R. G.; Greig, W. R.; McKellar, N. J.; Furnival, C.; and Blumgart, L. H.: The application of the Tc phosphate bone scan to the study of breast cancer. *Br. J. Surg.,* **62:**201–204, 1975.

Clark, D. G.; Painter, R. W.; and Sziklas, J. J.: Indications for bone scans in preoperative evaluation of breast cancer. *Am. J. Surg.,* **135:**667–670, 1978.

Cochran, A. J.; Grant, R. M.; Spilg, W. G.; Mackie, R. M.; Ross, C. E.; Hoyle, D. E.; and Russell, J. M.: Sensitization to tumour-associated antigens in human breast carcinoma. *Int. J. Cancer,* **14:**19–25, 1974.

Cohen, A. I.; Koeller, J.; Davis, T. E.; and Citrin, D. L.: IV dichloromethylene diphosphonate in cancer-associated hypercalcemia: A phase I–II evaluation. *Cancer Treat. Rep.,* **65:**651–653, 1981.

Cooke, T.; George, D.; Shields, R.; Maynard, P.; and Griffiths, K.: Oestrogen receptors and prognosis in early breast cancer. *Lancet,* **1:**995–997, 1979.

Crichlow, R. W.: Carcinoma of the male breast. *Surg. Gynecol. Obstet.,* **134:**1011–1019, 1972.

Crichlow, R. W.: Breast cancer in males. *Breast,* **2:**12–16, 1976.

Cutler, S. J.; Black, M. M.; Friedell, G. H.; Vidone, R. A.; and Goldenberg, I. S.: Prognostic factors in cancer of the female breast—II. Reproducibility of histopathologic classification. *Cancer,* **19:**75–82, 1966.

Cutler, S. J.; Christine, B.; and Barclay, T. H. C.: Increasing incidence and decreasing mortality rates for breast cancer. *Cancer,* **28:**1376–1380, 1971.

Dao, T. L., and Nemoto, T.: The clinical significance of skin recurrence after radical mastectomy in women with cancer of the breast. *Surg. Gynecol. Obstet.,* **177:**447–453, 1963.

DeCosse, J. J.; Gossens, C. L.; Kuzma, J. F.; and Unsworth, B. R.: Breast cancer: Induction of differentiation by embryonic tissue. *Science,* **181:**1057–1058, 1973.

Deftos, L. J., and First, B. P.: Calcitonin as a drug. *Ann. Intern. Med.,* **95:**192–197, 1981.

Devitt, J. E.: Bilateral mammary cancer. *Ann. Surg.,* **174:**774–778, 1971.

DeWaard, F.: The epidemiology of breast cancer: Review and prospects. *Int. J. Cancer,* **4:**577–586, 1969.

DiPaola, M.; Angelini, L.; Bertolotti, A.; and Colizza, S.: Host resistance in relation to survival in breast cancer. *Br. Med. J.,* **4:**268–270. 1974.

DiStefano, A.; Yap, H. Y.; Hortonbagyi, G. N.; and Blumenschein, G. R.: The natural history of breast cancer patients with brain metastases. *Cancer,* **44:**1913–1918, 1979.

Dmochowski, L.: The viral factor in the genesis of breast cancer: Present evidence. *Triangle,* **12:**37–47, 1973.

Dmochowski, L.: Viruses and human breast cancer. *Breast,* **1:**16–19, 1975.

Donegan, W. L.: Breast cancer and pregnancy. *Obstet. Gynecol.,* **50:**244–252, 1977.

Donegan, W. L.; Hartz, A. J.; and Rimm, A. A.: The association of body weight with recurrent cancer of the breast. *Cancer,* **41:**1590–1595, 1978.

Donegan, W. L., and Perez-Mesa, C. M.: Lobular carcinoma—An indication for elective biopsy of the second breast. *Ann. Surg.,* **176:**178–187, 1972.

Dowden, R. V.; McCraw, J. B.; and Dibbell, D. G.: The breast reconstruction patient and her health insurance carrier. *J.A.M.A.,* **242:**2779–2782, 1979.

Egan, R. L.: Bilateral breast carcinomas—Role of mammography. *Cancer,* **38:**931–938, 1976.

Elkort, R. J.; Kelly, W.; Mozden, P. J.; and Feldman, M. I.: A combined treatment program for the management of locally recurrent breast cancer following chest wall irradiation. *Cancer,* **46:**647–653, 1980.

Eusebi, V.; Betts, C. M.; and Bussolati, G.: Tubular carcinoma: A variant of secretory breast carcinoma. *Histopathology,* **3:**407–419, 1979.

Everson, R. B.; Lippman, M. E.; Thompson, E. B.; McGuire, W. L.; Wittliff, J. L.; DeSombre, E. R.; Jensen, E. V.; Singhakowinta, A.; Brooks, S. C., Jr.; and Neifeld, J. P.: Clinical correlations of steroid receptors and male breast cancer. *Cancer Res.,* **40:**991–997, 1980.

Fentiman, I. S.; Millis, R.; Sexton, S.; and Hayward, J. L.: Pleural effusion in breast cancer: A review of 105 cases. *Cancer,* **47:**2087–2092, 1981.

Feun, L. G.; Drelichman, A.; Singhakowinta, A.; and Vaitkevicius, V. K.: Ureteral obstruction secondary to metastatic breast carcinoma. *Cancer,* **46:**1164–1171, 1979.

Fidler, M.: Prophylactic internal fixation of secondary

neoplastic deposits in long bones. *Br. Med. J.,* **1**:341–343, 1973.

Finney, G. G., Jr.; Finney, G. G.; Montague, A. C. W.; Stonesifer, G. L., Jr.; and Brown, C. C.: Bilateral breast cancer, clinical and pathological review. *Ann. Surg.,* **175**:635–646, 1972.

Fisher, B.: A commentary on the role of the surgeon in primary breast cancer. *Breast Cancer Res. Treat.,* **1**:17–26, 1981.

Fisher, B., and Gebhardt, M. C.: The evolution of breast cancer surgery: Past, present, and future. *Semin. Oncol.,* **5**:385–394, 1978.

Fisher, B.; Redmond, C.; Brown, A.; Wolmark, N.; Wittliff, J.; Fisher, E. R.; Plotkin, D.; Bowman, D.; Sachs, S.; Wolter, J.; Frelick, R.; Desser, R.; LiCalzi, N.; Geggie, P.; Campbell, T.; Elias, E. G.; Prager, D.; Koontz, P.; Volk, H.; Dimitrov, N.; Gardner, B.; Lerner, H.; and Shibata, H.: Treatment of primary breast cancer with chemotherapy and tamoxifen. *N. Engl. J. Med.,* **305**:1–6, 1981.

Fisher, B.; Slack, N. H.; and Cooperating Investigators: Number of lymph nodes examined and the prognosis of breast cancer. *Surg. Gynecol. Obstet.,* **131**:79, 1970.

Fisher, B.; Slack, N.; Katrych, D.; and Wolmark, N.: Ten year followup of breast cancer patients in a cooperative clinical trial evaluating surgical adjuvant chemotherapy. *Surg. Gynecol. Obstet.,* **140**:528–534, 1975.

Fisher, B.; Wolmark, N.; Bauer, M.; Redmond, C.; and Gebhardt, M.: The accuracy of clinical nodal staging and of limited axillary dissection as a determinant of histologic nodal status in carcinoma of the breast. *Surg. Gynecol. Obstet.,* **152**:765–772, 1981.

Fisher, B.; Wolmark, N.; Redmond, C.; Deutsch, M.; Fisher, E. R.; and participating NSABP investigators: Findings from NSABP Protocol No. B-04: Comparison of radical mastectomy with alternative treatments. II. The clinical and biological significance of medial-central breast cancers. *Cancer,* **48**:1863–1872, 1981.

Fisher, B.; Wolmark, N.; Saffer, E.; and Fisher, E. R.: Inhibitory effect of prolonged *Corynebacterium parvum* and cyclophosphamide administration on the growth of established tumors. *Cancer,* **35**:134–143, 1975.

Fisher, E. R., and Fisher, B.: Relationship of pathologic and some clinical discriminants to the spread of breast cancer. *Int. J. Radiat. Oncol. Biol. Phys.,* **2**:747–750, 1977.

Fisher, E. R.; Gregorio, R.; Redmond, C.; Dekker, A.; and Fisher, B.: Pathologic findings from the national surgical adjuvant breast project (protocol No. 4). *Am. J. Clin. Pathol.,* **65**:21–30, 1976.

Flores, L.; Arlen, M.; Elguezabal, A.; Livingston, S. F.; and Levowitz, B. S.: Host tumor relationships in medullary carcinoma of the breast. *Surg. Gynecol. Obstet.,* **139**:683–688, 1974.

Fossati, G.; Canevari, S.; Pierotti, M. A.; Vezzoni, P.; Della Porta, G.; and Vaglini, M.: Delayed cutaneous hypersensitivity reactions to extracts of breast cancer and melanoma tissue in cancer patients. *J.N.C.I.,* **62**:1381–1385, 1979.

Frijlink, W. B.; Velde, J. T.; Bijvoet, O. L. M.; and Heynen, G.: Treatment of Paget's disease with (3-amino-1-hydroxypropylidine)-1,1-bisphosphonate (A.P.D.). *Lancet,* **1**:800–803, 1979.

Gaton, E., and Czernobilsky, B.: Lobular carcinoma *in situ* of the breast—A retrospective study from a general hospital in Israel. *Isr. J. Med. Sci.,* **10**:1106–1111, 1974.

Gerber, F. H.; Goodreau, J. J.; Kirchner, P. T.; and Fouty, W. J.: Efficacy of preoperative and postoperative bone

scanning in the management of breast carcinoma. *N. Engl. J. Med.,* **297**:300–303, 1977.

Grace, M.; Gaudette, L. A.; and Burns, P. E.: The increasing incidence of breast cancer in Alberta 1953–1973. *Cancer,* **40**:358–363, 1977.

Hagemeister, F. B., Jr.; Buzdar, A. U.; Luna, M. A.; and Blumenschein, G. R.: Causes of death in breast cancer—A clinicopathologic study. *Cancer,* **46**:162–167, 1980.

Harris, J. R., and Hellman, S. (eds.): *Alternatives to Mastectomy.* J. B. Lippincott Company, Philadelphia, 1983.

Hayward, J. L.; Carbone, P. P.; Rubens, R.D.; Heuson, J. C.; Kumaoka, S.; Segaloff, A.: Assessment of response to therapy in advanced breast cancer. *Br. J. Cancer,* **38**:201, 1978.

Heller, K. S.; Rosen, P. P.; Schottenfeld, D.; Ashikari, R.; and Kinne, D. W.: Male breast cancer: A clinicopathologic study of 97 cases. *Ann. Surg.,* **188**:60–65, 1978.

Hellman, S.; Harris, J. R.; and Leven, M. B.: Radiation therapy of early carcinoma of the breast without mastectomy. *Cancer,* **46**:988–994, 1980.

Henderson, C.: Chemotherapy for advanced disease. In Bonadonna, G. (ed.): *Breast Cancer: Recent Advances in Diagnosis and Treatment.* John Wiley & Sons, Ltd., London, 1982.

Heuser, L.; Spratt, J. S.; and Polk, H. C., Jr.: Growth rates of primary breast cancers. *Cancer,* **43**:1888–1894, 1979.

Hickey, R. C.; Samaan, N. A.; and Jackson, G. L.: Hypercalcemia in patients with breast cancer—Osseous metastases, hyperplastic parathyroid tissue, or pseudohyperparathyroidism? *Arch. Surg.,* **116**:545–552, 1982.

Holland, J. C., and Mastrovito, R.: Psychologic adaptation to breast cancer. *Cancer,* **46**:1045–1052, 1980.

Holm, N. V.; Hauge, M.; and Harvald, B.: Etiologic factors of breast cancer elucidated by a study of unselected twins. *J.N.C.I.,* **65**:285–298, 1980.

Hortobagyi, G. N.; DiStefano, A.; Legha, S. S.; Buzdar, A. U.; and Blumenschein, G. R.: Hormonal therapy with tamoxifen in male breast cancer. *Cancer Treat. Rep.,* **63**:539–541, 1979.

Hubay, C. A.; Pearson, O. H.; Marshall, J. S.; Stellato, T. A.; Rhodes, R. S.; Debanne, S. M.; Rosenblatt, J.; Mansour, E. G.; Hermann, R. E.; Jones, J. C.; Flynn, W. J.; Eckert, C.; and McGuire, W. L.: Adjuvant therapy of stage II breast cancer: 48-month follow-up of a prospective randomized trial. *Breast Cancer Res. Treat.,* **1**:77–82, 1981.

Hutchinson, W. B.; Thomas, D. B.; Hamlin, W. B.; Roth, G. J.; Peterson, A. V.; and Williams, B.: Risk of breast cancer in women with benign breast disease. *J.N.C.I.,* **65**:13–20, 1980.

Ingle, J. N.; Tormey, D. C.; and Tan, H. K.: The bone marrow examination in breast cancer. *Cancer,* **41**:670–674, 1978.

International Union Against Cancer: *TNM Classification of Malignant Tumors,* 3rd ed. International Union Against Cancer, Geneva, 1978.

Jacobs, T. P.; Siris, E. S.; Bilezikian, J. P.; Baquiran, D. C.; Shane, E.; and Canfield, R. E.: Hypercalcemia of malignancy: Treatment with intravenous dichloromethylene diphosphonate. *Ann. Intern. Med.,* **94**:312–316, 1981.

Juret, P.; Couette, J. E.; Mandard, A. M.; Carré, A.; Delozier, T.; Brune, D.; and Vernhes, J. C.: Age at menarche as a prognostic factor in human breast cancer. *Eur. J. Cancer,* **12**:701–704, 1976.

Kelly, P. T., and Anderson, D. E.: Familial breast cancer:

New data show lower risks for some sisters and daughters. *Your Patient & Cancer,* **1:**25–32, 1981.

Kesseler, H. J.; Grier, R. N.; Seidman, I.; and McIlveen, S. J.: Bilateral primary breast cancer. *J.A.M.A.,* **236:**278–280, 1976.

Khafagy, M. M.; Schottenfeld, D.; and Robbins, G. F.: Prognosis of the second breast cancer—The role of previous exposure to the first primary. *Cancer,* **35:**596–599, 1975.

King, R. E.; Terz, J. J.; and Lawrence, W., Jr.: Experience with opposite breast biopsy in patients with operable breast cancer. *Cancer,* **37:**43–45, 1976.

Knight, W. A.; Livingston, R. B.; Gregory, E. J.; and McGuire, W. L.: Estrogen receptor as an independent prognostic factor in breast cancer. *Cancer Res.,* **37:**4669–4671, 1977.

Kopelson, G.; Chu, A. M.; Doucette, J. A.; and Gunderson, L. L.: Extra-hepatic biliary tract metastases from breast cancer. *Int. J. Radiat. Oncol. Biol. Phys.,* **6:**497–504, 1980.

Korenman, S. G.: Oestrogen window hypothesis of the aetiology of breast cancer. *Lancet,* **1:**700–701, 1980.

Lacour, J.; Lacour, F.; Spira, A.; Petit, J. Y.; Sarrazin, D.; Mickelson, M.; DeLage, G.; and Contesso, G.; and Viguier, J.: Adjuvant treatment with polyadenylic-polyuridylic acid (Poly A-Poly U) in operable breast cancer. *Lancet,* **2:**161–164, 1980.

Land, C. E.; Boice, J. D., Jr.; Shore, R. E.; Norman, J. E.; and Tokunaga, M.: Breast cancer risk from low-dose exposures to ionizing radiation: Results of parallel analysis of three exposed populations of women. *J.N.C.I.,* **65:**353–376, 1980.

Land, C. E., and McGregor, D. H.: Breast cancer incidence among atomic bomb survivors: Implications for radiobiologic risk at low doses. *J.N.C.I.,* **62:**17–21, 1979.

Langlands, A. O.; Kerr, G. R.; and Bloomer, S. M.: Familial breast cancer. *Clin. Oncol.,* **2:**41–45, 1976.

Langlands, A. O.; Pocock, S. J.; Kerr, G. R.; and Gore, S. M.: Long-term survival of patients with breast cancer: A study of the curability of the disease *Br. Med. J.,* **2:**1247–1251, 1979.

Lapayowker, M. S., and Revesz G.: Thermography and ultrasound in detection and diagnosis of breast cancer. *Cancer,* **46**(Suppl.):933–938, 1980.

Lattes, R.: Sarcomas of the breast. *Int. J. Radiat. Oncol. Biol. Phys.,* **4:**705–708, 1978.

Li, F. P., and Fraumeni, J. F.: Familial breast cancer, soft-tissue sarcomas, and other neoplasms. *Ann. Intern. Med.,* **83:**833–834, 1975.

Little, J. R.; Dale, A. J. D.; and Okazaki, H.: Meningeal carcinomatosis. *Arch. Neurol.,* **30:**138–143, 1974.

Lopez, M., and Barduagni, A.: Cyproterone acetate in advanced male breast cancer. *Cancer,* **49:**9–11, 1982.

Lynch, H. T.; Harris, R. E.; Guirgis, H. A.; Malone, K.; Carmody, L. L.; and Lynch, J. F.: Familial association of breast/ovarian carcinoma. *Cancer,* **41:**1543–1549, 1978a.

Lynch, H. T.; Harris, R. E.; Organ, C. H., Jr.; and Lynch, J. F.: Management of familial breast cancer. *Arch. Surg.,* **113:**1053–1058, 1978b.

MacMahon, B.; Cole, P.; and Brown, J.: Etiology of human breast cancer: A review. *J.N.C.I.,* **59:**21–42, 1973.

Mambo, N. C.; Burke, J. S.; and Butler, J. J.: Primary malignant lymphomas of the breast. *Cancer,* **39:**2033–2040, 1977.

Martin, J. K., Jr.; VanHeerden, J. A.; and Gaffey, T. A.: Synchronous and metachronous carcinoma of the breast. *Surgery,* **1:**12–16, 1982.

Maynard, P. V.; Davies, C. J.; Blamey, R. W.; Elston, C. W.; Johnson, J.; and Griffiths, K.: Relationship between oestrogen receptor content and histologic grade in human primary breast cancer. *Br. J. Cancer,* **38:**745–748, 1978.

McColl, I.: Reconstruction of the breast with omentum after subcutaneous mastectomy. *Lancet,* **1:**134–135, 1979.

McGregor, D. H.; Land, C. E.; Choi, K.; Tokuoka, S.; Liu, P. I.; Wakabayashi, T.; and Beebe, G. W.: Breast cancer incidence among atomic bomb survivors, Hiroshima and Nagasaki, 1950–69. *J.N.C.I.,* **59:**799–811, 1977.

McGuire, W. L.: Hormone receptors: Their role in predicting prognosis and response to endocrine therapy. *Semin. Oncol.,* **5:**428–433, 1978.

McIntosh, I. H., Hooper, A. A., Millis, R. R., and Greening, W. P.: Metastatic carcinoma within the breast. *Clin. Oncol.,* **2:**393–401, 1976.

Meirion-Thomas, J.; Redding, W. H.; Coombes, R. C.; Sloane, J. P.; Ford, H. T.; Gazet, J-C.; and Powles, T. J.: Failure to detect intraabdominal metastases from breast cancer: A case for staging laparotomy. *Br. Med. J.,* **2:**157–159, 1978.

Merion, M. J., and Livolsi, V. A.: Signet ring carcinoma of the female breast: A clinicopathologic analysis of 24 cases. *Cancer,* **48:**1830–1837, 1981.

Meyer, J. S., and Facher, R.: Thymidine labeling index of human breast carcinoma—Enhancement of *in vitro* labeling by 5-fluorouracil and 5-fluoro-2′-deoxyuridine. *Cancer,* **39:**2524–2532, 1977.

Meyskens, F. L., Jr.; Tormey, D. C.; and Neifeld, J. P.: Male breast cancer: a review. *Cancer Treat. Rev.,* **3:**83–93, 1976.

Moolgavkar, S. H.; Day, N. E.; and Stevens, R. G.: Two-stage model for carcinogenesis: Epidemiology of breast cancer in females. *J.N.C.I.,* **65:**559–569, 1980.

Moore, F. D.: Breast self-examination. *N. Engl. J. Med.,* **299:**304–305, 1978.

Moris, T.: Psychologic adjustment to mastectomy. *Cancer Treat. Rev.,* **6:**41–61, 1979.

Murphy, W. K.; Livingston, R. B.; Ruiz, V. G.; Gercovich, F. G.; George, S. L.; Hart, J. S.; and Freireich, E. J.: Serial labeling index determination as a predictor of response in human solid tumors. *Cancer Res.,* **35:**1438–1444, 1975.

Nance, F. C.; DeLoach, D. H.; Welsh, R. A.; and Becker, W. F.: Paget's disease of the breast. *Ann. Surg.,* **171:**864–874, 1970.

Neifeld, J. P.; Meyskens, F.; Tormey, D. C.; and Javadpour, N.: The role of orchiectomy in the management of advanced male breast cancer. *Cancer,* **37:**992–995, 1976.

Nevin, J. E.; Baggerly, J. T.; and Laird, T. K.: Radiotherapy as an adjuvant in the treatment of carcinoma of the breast. *Cancer,* **49:**1194–1200, 1982.

Papaioannou, A. N.; Tanz, F. J.; and Volk, H.: Fate of patients with recurrent carcinoma of the breast—Recurrence five or more years after initial treatment. *Cancer,* **20:**371–376, 1967.

Papatestas, A. E.; Lesnick, G. J.; Genkins, G.; and Aufses, A. H., Jr.: The prognostic significance of peripheral lymphocyte counts in patients with breast carcinoma. *Cancer,* **37:**164–168, 1976.

Papatestas, A. E.; Mulvihill, M.; Josi, C.; Ioannovich, J.; Lesnick, G.; and Aufses, A. H., Jr.: Parity and prognosis in breast cancer. *Cancer,* **45:**191–194, 1980.

Patchefsky, A. S.; Shaber, G. S.; Schwartz, G. F.; Feig, S. A.; and Nerlinger, R. E.: The pathology of breast cancer detected by mass population screening. *Cancer,* **40**:1659–1670, 1977.

Paterson, A. H. G.; Agarwal, M.; Lees, A.; Hanson, J.; and Szafran, O.: Brain metastases in breast cancer patients receiving adjuvant chemotherapy. *Cancer,* **49**:651–654, 1982.

Patterson, J. S.; Battersby, L. A.; and Bach, B. K.: Use of tamoxifen in advanced male breast cancer. *Cancer Treat. Rep.,* **64**:801–804, 1980.

Pearlman, A. W.: Breast cancer—Influence of growth rate on prognosis and treatment evaluation—A study based on mastectomy scar recurrences. *Cancer,* **38**:1826–1833, 1976.

Philippe, E., and Le Gal, Y.: Growth of seventy-eight recurrent mammary cancers—Quantitative study. *Cancer,* **21**:461–467, 1968.

Post, J.; Sklarew, R. J.; and Hoffman, J.: The proliferative patterns of human breast cancer cells *in vivo. Cancer,* **39**:1500–1507, 1977.

Powles, T. J.: Present role of hormonal therapy. In Bonadonna, G. (ed.): *Breast Cancer: Recent Advances in Diagnosis and Treatment.* John Wiley & Sons, Ltd., London, 1982.

Prior, P., and Waterhouse, J. A. H.: Incidence of bilateral tumours in a population-based series of breast-cancer patients. I. Two approaches to an epidemiological analysis. *Br. J. Cancer,* **37**:620–634, 1978.

Ridell, B., and Landys, K.: Incidence and histopathology of metastases of mammary carcinoma in biopsies from the posterior iliac crest. *Cancer,* **44**:1782–1788, 1979.

Ridolfi, R. L.; Rosen, P. P.; Port, A.; Kinne, D.; and Mike, V.: Medullary carcinoma of the breast—A clinicopathologic study with 10 year follow-up. *Cancer,* **40**:1365–1385, 1977.

Riley, E., and Swift, M.: A family with Peutz-Jeghers syndrome and bilateral breast cancer. *Cancer,* **46**:815–817, 1980.

Rilke, F.: Influence of pathologic factors in management. In Bonadonna, G. (ed.): *Breast Cancer: Recent Advances in Diagnosis and Treatment.* John Wiley & Sons, Ltd., London, 1982.

Rittgers, R. A.; Loewenstein, M. S.; Feinerman, A. E.; Kupchik, H. Z.; Marcel, B. R.; Koff, R. S.; and Zamcheck, N.: Carcinoembryonic antigen levels in benign and malignant pleural effusions. *Ann. Intern. Med.,* **88**:631–634, 1978.

Rojas, A. F.; Mickiewicz, E.; Feierstein, J. N.; Glait, H.; and Olivari, A. J.: Levamisole in advanced human breast cancer. *Lancet,* **1**:211–215, 1976.

Rosato, F. E.; Wallach, M. W.; and Rosato, E. F.: The management of malignant effusions from breast cancer. *J. Surg. Oncol.,* **6**:441–449, 1974.

Rosen, P. P.: Axillary lymph node metastases in patients with occult noninvasive breast carcinoma. *Cancer,* **46**:1298–1306, 1980.

Rosen, P. P.; Senie, R.; Schottenfeld, D.; and Ashikari, R.: Noninvasive breast carcinoma—Frequency of unsuspected invasion and implications for treatment. *Ann. Surg.,* **189**:337–382, 1979.

Rosner, F.; Carey, R. W.; and Zarrabi, M. H.: Breast cancer and acute leukemia: Report of 24 cases and review of the literature. *Am. J. Hematol.,* **4**:151–172, 1978.

Ross, R. K.; Paganini-Hill, A.; Gerkins, V. C.; Mack, T. M.; Pfeffer, R.; Author, M.; and Henderson, B. E.: A case-control study of menopausal estrogen therapy and breast cancer. *J.A.M.A.,* **243**:1635–1639, 1980.

Roswit, B., and Edlis, H.: Carcinoma of the male breast: A thirty year experience and literature review. *Int. J. Radiat. Oncol. Biol. Phys.,* **4**:711–715, 1978.

Rothman, K. J.; MacMahon, B.; Lin, T. M.; Lowe, C. R.; Mirra, A. P.; Ravnihar, B.; Salber, E. J.; Trichopoulos, D.; and Yuasa, S.: Maternal age and birth rank of women with breast cancer. *J.N.C. I.,* **65**:719–722, 1980.

Rozencweig, M., and Heuson, J. C.: Breast cancer: Prognostic factors and clinical evaluation. In Staquet, M. J. (ed.): *Cancer Therapy: Prognostic Factors and Criteria of Response.* Raven Press, New York, 1975.

Sachs, L.: Control of normal cell differentiation and the phenotypic reversion of malignancy in myeloid leukaemia. *Nature,* **274**:535–539, 1978.

Salmon, S. E., and Jones, S. E. (eds.): *Adjuvant Therapy of Cancer,* Vol. III. Grune & Stratton, Inc., New York, 1981.

Sanger, C. K. and Reznikoff, M.: A comparison of the psychologic effects of breast-saving procedures with the modified radical mastectomy. *Cancer,* **48**:2341–2346, 1981.

Sartwell, P. E.; Arthes, F. G.; and Tonascia, J. A.: Exogenous hormones, reproductive history, and breast cancer. *J.A.M.A.,* **59**:1589–1592, 1977.

Schiffer, L. M.; Braunschweiger, P. G.; Stragand, J. J.; and Poulakos, L.: The cell kinetics of human mammary cancers. *Cancer,* **43**:1707–1719, 1979.

Schroder, E. W., and Black, P. H.: Retinoids: Tumor preventors or tumor enhancers? *J.N.C.I.,* **65**:671–674, 1980.

Schwartz, G. F.; Feig, S. A.; and Patchefsky, A. S.: Clinicopathologic correlations and significance of clinically occult mammary lesions. *Cancer,* **41**:1147–1153, 1978.

Shafie, S. M., and Grantham, F. H.: Role of hormones in the growth and regression of human breast cancer cells (MCF-7) transplanted into athymic nude mice. *J.N.C.I.,* **67**:51–56, 1981.

Shore, R. E.; Hempelmann, L. H.; Kowaluk, E.; Mansur, P. S.; Pasternack, B. S.; Albert, R. E.; and Haughie, G. E.: Breast neoplasms in women treated with x-rays for acute postpartum mastitis. *J.N.C.I.* **59**:813–822, 1977.

Silverberg, E.: Cancer statistics, 1982. *CA,* **32**:15, 1982.

Slack, N. H.; Bross, I. D. J.; Nemoto, T.; and Fisher, B.: Experiences with bilateral primary carcinoma of the breast. *Surg. Gynecol. Obstet.,* **136**:433–440, 1973.

Snyderman, R. K.: Alternatives in reconstructive surgery after mastectomy. *Cancer,* **46**:1053–1058, 1980.

Sordillo, P. P.; Chapman, R.; Hajdu, S. T.; Magill, G. B.; and Golbey, R. B.: Lymphangiosarcoma. *Cancer,* **48**:1647–1679, 1981.

Sparks, F. C.; Albert, N. E.; Andreone, P. A.; and Breeding, J. H.: Effect of bacillus Calmette-Guérin on immunosuppression from cyclophosphamide, methotrexate, and 5-fluorouracil. *Cancer Res.,* **37**:2560–2564, 1977.

Spratt, J. S., Jr.; Kaltenbach, M. L.; and Spratt, J. A.: Cytokinetic definition of acute and chronic breast cancer. *Cancer Res.,* **37**:226–230, 1977.

Springer, G. F.; Murthy, M. S.; Desai, P. R.; and Scanlon, E. F.: Breast cancer patient's cell-mediated immune response to Thomsen-Friedenreich (T) antigen. *Cancer,* **45**:2949–2954, 1980.

Stewart, J. F., and Rubens, R. D.: General prognostic factors. In Bonadonna, G. (ed.): *Breast Cancer: Recent Advances in Diagnosis and Treatment.* John Wiley & Sons, Ltd., London, 1982.

Stjernsward, J.; Jondal, M.; Vanky, F.; Wigzell, H.; and Sealy, R.: Lymphopenia and change in distribution of human B and T lymphocytes in peripheral blood induced by irradiation for mammary carcinoma. *Lancet,* **6:**1352–1356, 1972.

Stolfi, R. L.; Fugmann, R. A.; Stolfi, L. M.; and Martin, D. S.: Synergism between host antitumor immunity and combined modality therapy against murine breast cancer. *Int. J. Cancer,* **13:**389–403, 1974.

Strax, P.: Strategy (motivation) for detection of early breast cancer. *Cancer,* **46**(Suppl.):926–929, 1980.

Sugarbaker, P. H.; Beard, J. O.; and Drum, D. E.: Detection of hepatic metastases from cancer of the breast. *Am. J. Surg.,* **133:**531–535, 1977.

Tabar, L., and Dean, P. B.: Risks and benefits of mammography in population screening for breast cancer. In Bonadonna, G. (ed.): *Breast Cancer: Recent Advances in Diagnosis and Treatment.* John Wiley & Sons, Ltd., London, 1982.

Tartter, P.; Papatesttas, A.; Ioannovich, J.; Mulvihill, M. N.; Lesnick, G.; and Aufses, A. H.: Cholesterol and obesity as prognostic factors in breast cancer. *Cancer,* **47:**2222–2227, 1981.

Thier, S. O.: Breast cancer screening: A view from outside the controversy. *N. Engl. J. Med.,* **297:**1063–1065, 1977.

Upton, A. C.; Beebe, G. W.; Brown, J. M.; Quimby, E. H.; and Shellabarger, C.: Report of NCI ad hoc working group on the risks associated with mammography in mass screening for the detection of breast cancer. *J.N.C.I.,* **59:**481–493, 1977.

Valagussa, P.; Bonadonna, G.; and Veronesi, U.: Patterns of relapse and survival in operable breast cancer with positive and negative axillary nodes. *Tumori,* **64:**241–558, 1978.

Valagussa, P.; Harris, J. R.; and Hellman, S. (eds.): *Alternatives to Mastectomy.* J.B. Lippincott Company, Philadelphia, 1983.

Valagussa, P.; Zambetti, M.; Bignami, P.; *et al.*: $T_{3b} - T_4$ breast cancer: Factors affecting results in combining modality treatments. *Clin. Exp. Metastasis,* **1:**191–202, 1983.

Veronesi, U.; Saccozzi, R.; DelVecchio, M.; Banfi, A.; Clemente, C.; DeLena, M.; Gallus, G.; Graco, M.; Luini, A.; Marubini, E.; Muscolino, G.; Rilke, F.; Salvadori, B.; Zecchini, A.; and Zucali, R.: Comparing radi-

cal mastectomy with quadrantectomy axillary dissection, and radiotherapy in patients with small cancers of the breast. *N. Engl. J. Med.,* **305:**6–11, 1981.

Veronesi, U., and Valagussa, P.: Inefficacy of internal mammary nodes dissection in breast cancer surgery. *Cancer,* **47:**170–175, 1981.

Vezzoni, P.; Balestrazzi, A.; Bignami, P.; Concolino, F.; Gennari, L.; and Veronesi, U.: Axillary lymph node metastases from occult carcinoma of the breast. *Tumori,* **65:**87–91, 1979.

Volm, M.; Wayss, K.; Kaufmann, M.; and Mattern, J.: Pretherapeutic detection of tumour resistance and the results of tumour chemotherapy. *Eur. J. Cancer,* **15:**983–993, 1979.

Wanebo, H. J.; Rosen, P. P.; Thaler, T.; Urban, J. A.; and Oettgen, H. F.: Immunobiology of operable breast cancer: An assessment of biologic risk by immunoparameters. *Ann. Surg.,* **184:**258–267, 1976.

Wasserstrom, W. R.; Glass, J. P.; and Posner, J. B.: Diagnosis and treatment of leptomeningeal metastases: Experience with 90 patients. *Cancer,* **49:**759–772, 1982.

Watanatittan, S., and Ram, M. D.: Non-simultaneous bilateral breast carcinoma. *Surgery,* **75:**740–745, 1974.

Weese, J. L., and Schouten, J. T.: Pleural peritoneal shunts for the treatment of malignant pleural effusions. *Surg. Gynecol. Obstet.,* **154:**391–392, 1982.

Wilson, N. D., and Alberty, R. E.: Bilateral carcinoma of the breast. *Am. J. Surg.,* **126:**244–248, 1973.

Woo, K. B.; Waalkes, T. P.; Ahmann, D. L.; Tormey, D. C.; Gehrke, C. W.; and Oliverio, V. T.: A quantitative approach to determining disease response during therapy using multiple biologic markers—Application to carcinoma of the breast. *Cancer,* **46:**1685–1703, 1978.

Woods, J. E.: Breast reconstruction after mastectomy. *Surg. Gynecol. Obstet.,* **150:**869–874, 1980.

Wynder, E. L.; MacCornack, F. A.; and Stellman, S. D.: The epidemiology of breast cancer in 785 United States caucasian women. *Cancer,* **41:**2341–2354, 1978.

Yap, H. Y.; Tashima, C. K.; Blumenschein, G. R.; and Eckles, N. E.: Male breast cancer: A natural history study. *Cancer,* **44:**748–754, 1979.

Yonemoto, R. H.: Breast cancer in Japan and the United States—Epidemiology, hormone receptors, pathology, and survival. *Arch. Surg.,* **115:**1056–1062, 1980.

Zajicek, J.: The aspiration biopsy smear. In Koss, L. G. (ed.): *Diagnostic Cytology and its Histopathologic Bases.* J. B. Lippincott Company, Philadelphia, 1979.

34

Gynecologic Neoplasms

JOHN R. DURANT and GEORGE A. OMURA

Introduction

The impact of cancers of the genital tract on American women has changed dramatically over the past 50 years. In 1930, uterine cancer, primarily cancer of the cervix, was the leading cause of cancer death among women. At that time, it had an age-adjusted death rate of 30/100,000 women. It is now responsible for a death rate of less than 8/100,000, causing only 5% of cancer deaths. By way of contrast, during this same half century, breast cancer mortality has altered only slightly, remaining between 25 and 28/100,000. Among gynecologic cancers, endometrial cancer kills about one-half as many women as cervical cancer. Today, ovarian cancer is estimated to be responsible for more deaths among American women (11,400) than uterine cancer of all types (10,100), and uterine cervix in particular (7100) (Silverberg, 1982). Other sources estimate even fewer deaths from cervical cancer (U.S. Department of Health Education, and Welfare, 1976). Ovarian cancer is rapidly becoming the most important public health hazard among these cancers. As will be noted, there has also been an increase in endometrial cancers, probably the result of exogenous estrogen ingestion; however, most of these are curable cancers.

CANCER OF THE CERVIX

Epidemiology

The dramatic decrease in deaths from invasive cancer of the cervix is often attributed to the widespread application of screening using the Pap test. This may not be an entirely ade-

quate explanation. The decline in death due to invasive cervical cancer began about 1935, long before the introduction of the Pap smear. In fact, it was not until 1948 that the American Cancer Society sponsored the first interdisciplinary conference on the Pap smear (American Cancer Society, 1976). Nevertheless, since its introduction, there has been general acceptance by the American public of the value of screening using the Pap smear. By 1976, at least one Pap test had been conducted in 82% of American women between the ages of 18 and 34 (Gallup Omnibus, 1977).

Despite the decline in death rate, the precursor pathophysiologic and etiologic factors potentially leading to invasive carcinoma of the cervix have not decreased so dramatically. Screening procedures for cervical cancer generally reveal about six *in situ* cancers for each invasive cancer (American Cancer Society, 1976). If *in situ* cancer is a precursor of invasive cancer (see Table 34 – 1), the total number of potential new cases of invasive cancer of the cervix anticipated in 1982 is approximately 100,000. Among women, only breast cancer (112,000 new cases) is more frequent (Silverberg, 1982).

The dispute surrounding the changing epidemiology of invasive cancer of the cervix is based on a number of observations and their possible causes. First, during the same half century in which invasive cancer of the cervix was decreasing as a cause of death, so were cancers of two other sites, stomach and liver (Silverberg, 1982), at a rate almost equal to that of the cervix. Although the decline in deaths from cancer of the liver might be attributed to better reporting of primary sites, that from cancer of the stomach cannot be sim-

Table 34-1. Studies Showing Progression of *In Situ* to Invasive Carcinoma of the Cervix

AUTHOR	PATIENT (NO.)	PRO-GRESSION (%)	FOLLOW-UP (YEARS)
Peterson, 1955, 1956	127	30 40*	10
Kottmeier, 1953	14	57	10+
Kottmeier, 1961	31	71	12+
Koss, *et al.*, 1963	67	75†	3+

* As revised by Clemmesen and Poulsen, 1971.
† Did not regress.

ilarly explained. No widespread effective screening technique was applied to cancer of the stomach. Had such a screening technique been utilized, the improved survival from this cause might have been falsely ascribed to the screening test introduced.

Second, although severe dysplasia and *in situ* cancer are pathologic lesions generally considered to be precursors of invasive cancer, follow-up studies of patients identified as having such lesions indicate that many do not progress to invasive cancer during follow-up periods of up to nine years (Foltz and Kelsey, 1978). Some return to normal, suggesting either spontaneous regression or inaccurate diagnosis. For example, several decades ago, among a group of 127 Danish women with untreated *in situ* cancer, only 33% developed invasive cancer within nine years (Peterson, 1956). Subsequently, two other studies traced women with smears positive for *in situ* or invasive cancer who refused biopsy and treatment. Among 60 of these women who were followed for at least five years, one-third had negative smears (Kinlen and Spriggs, 1978). Similar data exist regarding severe dysplasia, indicating that only 12 to 29% of untreated women followed for 1 to 14 years subsequently develop *in situ* cervical cancer (Stern and Neely, 1963; Hall and Walton, 1968). Therefore, it is not possible to extrapolate with accuracy the potential future incidence of invasive cervical cancer from that of severe dysplasia and *in situ* cancer since the biologic potential of the precursor lesion cannot be determined.

Consequently, the improved survival from cancer of the cervix appears not to be solely a function of improved early cancer detection as a result of widespread screening with the Pap smear. Another possibility could be a reduction in those risk factors that favor the probability of precursor lesions becoming invasive

cancer. Indeed, the widespread discovery of *in situ* cancer and the declining mortality from invasive cancer have even provoked the question: "Is cured early cancer truly cancer?" (Hutter, 1982). At any rate, epidemiologists no longer include *in situ* cancer of the cervix in general cancer-incidence statistics.

The marked decrease in the mortality rate from cancer of the cervix in American women has not been uniform throughout all populations or regions (Silverberg, 1982). Death from cancer of the cervix accounts for 5% of cancer mortality in Puerto Rico, 3.7% of those in the District of Columbia, and 3.1% in Alabama. At the other extreme, less than 2% of deaths from cancer in Connecticut are the result of cervical cancer. Cancer death rates for cancer of the uterus (largely, cancer of the cervix) vary widely around the world. Paraguay is first with 36.3 deaths/100,000, followed by Venezuela with 33.3/100,000, and Costa Rica with 24.4/100,000. Nicaragua has the lowest death rate of 42 countries surveyed by the American Cancer Society with 1.4/100,000. The United States ranks thirtieth with 8.9/100,000. Some of these differences may be ascribed to variability in accuracy of reporting, but surely not all of them are. For instance, among developed countries, the death rate varies from 11.8/100,000 in Japan (seventeenth) to 5.8/100,000 in Israel (thirty-ninth).

Cancer of the cervix has many of the characteristics of a venereal disease. It is associated with both poor socioeconomic status and increased sexual exposure. Most studies indicate a correlation between carcinoma of the cervix and early onset of sexual activity, multiple sexual partners, and frequent pregnancy (Higginson and Muir, 1973). A low incidence among those with discriminating or celebate sexual habits, such as the Amish and Roman Catholic nuns, is cited as further evidence to support the thesis that this disease is venereal (Melnick, 1981). Some believe that the low incidence of the disease in those of Jewish origin supports the notion that a carcinogenic agent is present in the smegma of uncircumcised males (Rawls *et al.*, 1968).

Etiology and Carcinogenesis

The above considerations have led a number of investigators to search for an infectious agent that could produce a venereal cancer. Recently, Rapp reviewed the evidence that HSV-2, a DNA virus usually transmitted by genital contact, was the prime candidate for such an etiologic agent (Rapp, 1981) (see Chapter 3D). As epidemiologic evidence for veneral spread, he cited a prospective study by Kessler conducted over a 20-year period (Kessler, 1977). The second wives of white men whose first wives had had cervical cancer were traced. The study group had almost two and one-half-fold increased incidence of carcinoma *in situ* compared to controls, and twice as many had abnormal cervical cytology. Twenty-nine such marital clusters were found, when only 11.6 would have been predicted. These differences were statistically significant. Studies of anti-HSV-2 antibodies among women with cervical carcinoma show both a greater frequency of positive tests and a higher titer (Thomas and Rawls, 1978; Nahmias *et al.*, 1973; Christenson and Espmark, 1977). More convincing is evidence showing that HSV-2-specific antigens can be found in exfoliated human cervical cells, particularly those of cervical cancer. Jones *et al.* (1978) found that 60% of human cervical cancers have HSV-2 RNA, whereas very few normal human cervical cells do. Tissue culture studies have shown HSV-2-induced host chromosomal damage and subsequent DNA synthesis, as well as induction of host DNA repair enzymes. The observation that the virus could transform hamster cells *in vitro* (Roizman and Frenkel, 1967) was the first clue to the pathogenesis of the disease. Subsequently, this was shown to be a common phenomenon in nature, being demonstrated for chicken, guinea pig, rat, and human cells. Introduction of the virus into the cervix of monkeys and vagina of mice induces dysplasia in monkeys and carcinomas in mice (Rapp, 1981). Finally, in women, cervical dysplasias and carcinoma *in situ* were found in 106/598 (17%) women who had genital herpes, compared to a frequency of only 25/299 (8%) in those without it (Nahmias *et al.*, 1970). Thus, this evidence links HSV-2 to cancer of the cervix, and indicates that the virus could be an important etiologic agent. It is not possible to fulfill Koch's postulates, but for the moment, HSV-2 appears to be a frequent, important, although not always essential, component of the etiologic cascade leading to cancer of the cervix. HSV-2 is the cause of a major epidemic of benign veneral disease in the United States. If it is also an etiologic factor in carcinoma of the cervix, it is plausible to suggest that carcinoma of the cervix could once again become a serious public health problem.

Current Screening Policy

These epidemiologic and biologic considerations led to a reevaluation of the American Cancer Society's long-standing policy of recommending an annual Pap smear for every woman every year. Part of the impetus for this stemmed from a paper by Foltz and Kelsey (1978), entitled "The Annual Pap Test: A Dubious Policy Success." In 1980, the American Cancer Society published revised recommendations advising less frequent screening (American Cancer Society, 1980). This caused considerable controversy for a number of reasons.

First, many recognized the pitfalls inherent in interpreting the data, but believed that screening was an important factor responsible for the declining incidence of invasive cancer of the cervix (see Table 34–2). The Walton Report (1976) and a study by Miller *et al.* (1976) related the intensity of screening to the declining mortality from invasive cervix cancer. Johannesson *et al.* (1978) reported from Iceland, where 85% of women were screened at least once and where good records were available, that six years after opening a widely used clinic in the capital of Reykjavik the death rate from invasive cancer of the cervix fell from 32.1/100,000 to 14.6/100,000. The frequency of late-stage tumors at initial diagnosis also diminished.

The American Cancer Society's revised recommendations do not deny that screening is useful, only that it should be done less frequently. The recommendations are that all asymptomatic women over 20 and sexually active symptomatic women under 20 have two annual Pap smears. If negative, a Pap smear every three years until age 65 is recommended, along with a physical examination. After age 40, a pelvic examination is recommended annually, but the Pap smear only every three

Table 34–2. Studies Comparing Incidence of Invasive Carcinoma of Cervix in Screened and Unscreened Women

AUTHOR	YEAR	SITE	RATE	AGE
Fidler *et al.*, 1968	1968	British Columbia	Screened: 5/100,000 Unscreened: 20/100,000	>20
Figge *et al.*, 1970	1970	Scotland	Screened: 55/100,000 Unscreened: 310/100,000	>30

years. The less frequent examinations recommended were based on the following rationale (American Cancer Society, 1980):

1. The minimal average duration of carcinoma *in situ* is eight years.
2. Dysplasia precedes carcinoma *in situ* by five to ten years.
3. Regression of abnormal smears usually occurs within one year, making two smears a year apart excellent indicators of spontaneous regression.
4. Most screening plans associated with reduced mortality used screening intervals greater than one year.
5. Screening every three years accounts for 97% of the decreased mortality.
6. An econometric model showed little cost benefit either in low- or high-risk women for screening conducted more frequently than every three years.
7. A conservative recommendation of screening every three years is made because of concern about the false-negative rate, estimated to be about 30%. Actually, with a lead time from dysplasia to invasive cancer of more than ten years, successful rescreening could be less frequent than every three years.
8. Costs of rescreening: Fidler *et al.* (1968) estimated likely positives in those rescreened to be 1/75,000 when performed at a frequency of every three or more years. Even the study estimating the highest case-detection rate as a result of rescreening (Figge *et al.,* 1970) predicts only 1/3,682 when screening is done annually. Overall, the American Cancer Society estimates that annual rescreening produces one cancer for every 50,000 women examined.
9. In high-risk women under 40, screening every three years should permit early detection of cervical cancer.
10. A similar policy is practiced in Great Britain, Canada, and Finland.

The American Cancer Society's recommendations dismiss the residual value of an annual pelvic examination as a screen for ovarian carcinoma in those under 40. Because ovarian cancer is so rare at that age, the detection rate would be 1/10,000 women examined if all incident new cases were detected. These recommendations precipitated intense controversy and an NIH consensus conference which failed to resolve the issue (NIH, 1980).

The accepted scientific evidence indicates that, except in high-risk populations who normally do not seek medical care, no benefit is provided in having a Pap smear more frequently than every three years after two negative smears taken a year apart.

One of the factors leading to the emphasis on screening at greater intervals is the biologic uncertainty of a positive smear finding the cancer *in situ.* As noted earlier, it may be unnecessary for a significant number of women with severe dysplasia and *in situ* cancer who will undergo spontaneous regressions. The usual treatment for cancer *in situ* is a simple hysterectomy after cold cone biopsy. In addition to exposing the patient to a small, but real, risk of harm from operative mortality, nonfatal complications are possible (Hatch *et al.,* 1981). The treatment may be unduly aggressive and produce both unnecessary cost and sacrifice a desired future capacity for childbearing. Less aggressive and much cheaper alternatives such as cryo (Hatch *et al.,* 1981) or laser surgery (Masterson *et al.,* 1981), as well as topical 5-FU (Petrilli *et al.,* 1980) are now available. Thus, the need for a major operation solely because of an abnormal cytologic finding may be diminishing.

The real problem in public health policy for carcinoma of the cervix is not, however, the direct and indirect cost of a screening program. It is how to reduce further the mortality from this relatively rare cause of death. The ideal solution would be to reach the 15 to 20% of women who have never had a Pap smear because they are the ones at highest risk. A recent experience in Alabama, a high-risk area in this country, illustrates how difficult this is to accomplish (Lehman *et al.,* unpublished data). From 1974 to 1978, 51,193 women, primarily from rural areas, were screened by public health nurses. Two-thirds were over the age of 35, and 70% were white. Of these women, 5505 were considered to be at high risk for endometrial cancer and also had a jet wash performed, permitting the estimate of a minimum false-negative rate for the Pap smear. Sixty-four women with either severe dysplasia, *in situ,* or invasive cancer were identified in this high-risk group. Of these, the Pap smear missed nine isolated by the jet wash, producing a minimum 14% false-negative rate. The Pap smear identified a total of 212 confirmed dysplasias and cancers in the entire group of women screened. Of these, 25 were invasive, and 114 were *in situ* cancers. The remaining 73 were dysplasias.

The cost of the program for the Pap smear alone in these 51,193 women was $1,764,415. The cost per abnormality was more than $8,300. If the cancers alone are considered, the relative cost was almost $12,500 per case discovered. It should be noted that only 15/25 women with invasive cancer never had a Pap smear before. In two cases, the prior Pap smear was positive. Eighty of 114 women with *in situ* cancer had been tested previously and, of these, 13 had a previous positive smear. Thus, 90/139 (65%) of the women with proven histologic malignancies in this program had been screened before, and 15/139 (11%) had previous positive findings for which follow-up care had not been provided.

Diagnosis

The diagnosis of carcinoma of the cervix now is generally made by routine screening of asymptomatic women. Pap smears may be reported as class I to V or according to the characteristics of exfoliated cells from an otherwise apparently normal cervix. These are generally reported as follows:

Class I   Negative or normal
Class II   Inflammation, mild dysplasia
Class III Moderate to severe dysplasia
Class IV   Carcinoma *in situ*
Class V   Invasive carcinoma

Recommendations for managing these conditions are shown in Table 34–3 and Figure 34–1 (Austin, 1975).

Colposcopy with cryosurgery is an increas-ingly important alternative to the usual practice of cold surgical cone biopsy of the cervix as a diagnostic approach to smears showing moderate to severe dysplasia or carcinoma *in situ* (see Figure 34–2). Gynecologists who are experienced with this procedure should be able to obtain an accurate diagnosis without conization in about 85% of patients (Stafl and Mattingly, 1973). The colposcopist examines the cervix using a special microscope with low magnification. Using a green filter, the vasculature of the cervix can be visualized, photographs taken, and biopsies obtained from areas of abnormality (see Figure 34–3). The lesions identified can then be treated with cryosurgery. When this is done, between 18 and 34% of patients will subsequently have a negative smear and require only routine follow-up with repeat cytology. Of patients with positive smears, 1 to 3% will be found to have invasive cancer and can have treatment planned without the need for conization. The remainder will have dysplastic or *in situ* lesions (cervical intraepithelial neoplasia [CIN]) (Figure 34–4) and can be followed without additional therapy if the following criteria are met:

1. Preservation of fertility desired.
2. All lesions are on the ectocervix and can be completely visualized.
3. The entire transition zone from cervix to endocervix is visualized.
4. Colposcopic biopsy is equivalent histologically to the cytologic diagnosis.
5. No invasive cancer is found.
6. Endocervical curettage for those with *in situ* carcinoma is negative.

Table 34–3.   Pap Smear Findings and Evaluation

		CLASSIC	MODERN
Class I	Negative	Repeat regularly	
Class II	Inflammation — mild dysplasia	Treat infection and repeat in 3 months	Treat infection and repeat in 3 months. If still abnormal, colposcopy
Class III	Moderate — severe dysplasia	Conization of cervix if no gross lesion to biopsy by Schiller's staining	Colposcopy and use flow sheet for evaluation and treatment (see Figure 34–1)
Class IV	Carcinoma *in situ*		
Class V	Invasive carcinoma		

From Austin, J. M.: The abnormal Pap smear and its evaluation — The modern approach. *J. Med. Assoc. State Ala.,* **44:**418, 1975 (reprinted with permission).

PAP SMEARS FINDINGS AND EVALUATION

		(Classical)	*(Modern)*
Class I	(Negative)	Repeat regularly	
Class II	(Inflammation-mild dysplasia	Treat infection and repeat in 3 months	Treat infection and repeat in 3 months - If still abnormal, colposcopy
Class III	(Moderate-severe dysplasia)	Conization of cervix if no gross lesion to biopsy by Schiller's staining	Colposcopy and use flow sheet for evaluation and treatment. (See Figure 34-2.)
Class IV	(Carcinoma in situ)		
Class V	(Invasive carcinoma)		

Figure 34–1. Comparison of classical and modern recommendations for management of Pap smears according to old and new classification of abnormalities. From Austin, J. M.: The abnormal Pap smear and its evaluation—The modern approach. *J. Med. Assoc. State Ala.,* **44:**418, 1975.

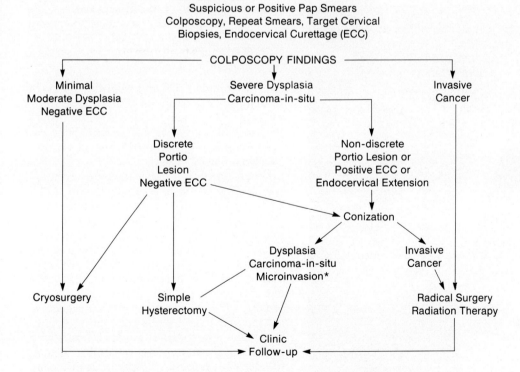

MANAGEMENT OF ATYPICAL SMEARS
Suspicious or Positive Pap Smears
Colposcopy, Repeat Smears, Target Cervical
Biopsies, Endocervical Curettage (ECC)

——— COLPOSCOPY FINDINGS ———

Minimal Moderate Dysplasia Negative ECC

Severe Dysplasia Carcinoma-in-situ

Invasive Cancer

Discrete Portio Lesion Negative ECC

Non-discrete Portio Lesion or Positive ECC or Endocervical Extension

Conization

Dysplasia Carcinoma-in-situ Microinvasion*

Invasive Cancer

Cryosurgery

Simple Hysterectomy

Radical Surgery Radiation Therapy

Clinic Follow-up

*Microinvasion—See text for details of definition and guidelines for management.

Figure 34–2. Wire diagram illustrating decision tree for management of CIN (cervical intraepithelial neoplasia). From Austin, J. M.: The abnormal Pap smear and its evaluation—The modern approach. *J. Med. Assoc. State Ala.,* **44:**418, 1975.

7. The patient can be relied upon to return for follow-up.

A cytologic diagnosis of *in situ* carcinoma is an indication for an endocervical curettage. Other indications include (1) a visualized lesion which extends into the endocervical canal, (2) inability to visualize the entire transition zone, (3) the absence of a lesion, or (4) differing histologic and cytologic diagnoses (Scott *et al.,* 1981).

The importance of patient reliability in follow-up is stressed by the observation that among nearly 1000 women treated by cryosurgery at the University of Alabama in Birmingham since 1970, almost one-fourth did not return. One reevaluation patient subsequently developed an invasive carcinoma but was successfully treated with radiotherapy. Among the patients who did return for follow-up and who had at least two smears, persistance of the cytologic abnormality occurred in 10%. Some of these required hysterectomy. Recurrent cytologic abnormalities were noted in 2 to 3%. Of the women with the most advanced cytologic abnormalities, persistent dis-

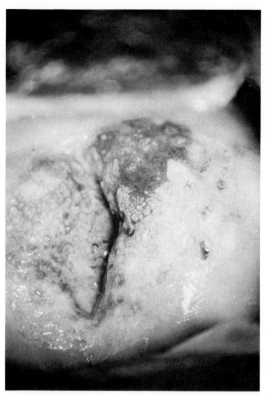

Figure 34–4. The cervix of a patient with carcinoma in situ. The lesion at 1 o'clock is obvious. Biopsy is done, and the lesion is destroyed by the cryostat unless there are indications for further evaluations.

ease was found in 20% and recurrent disease in nearly 4%. These patients were all successfully managed. No patient in this series is known to have died of cancer. Similar, or perhaps better, results can also be obtained using a CO_2 laser (Masterson *et al.,* 1981).

When conization rather than hysterectomy was performed on 1500 patients with frank carcinoma *in situ* reported by Bjerre *et al.* (1976; Bjerre, 1978), 12.8% failed to return for follow-up between 5 and 15 years. In another series of 1219 patients with carcinoma *in situ* who had conization only, 6.8% had persistent disease and 3.4% recurrent carcinoma *in situ* after many years of follow-up (Burghardt and Holzer, 1980). The results with less aggressive treatment than cryosurgery or conization indicate that colposcopically guided biopsies with endocervical curettage are preferable because the alternatives require hospitalization and are nine times as expensive (Scott *et al.,* 1981). The alternatives constitute sufficient treatment for most women with cytologically abnormal cervical smears that do not show

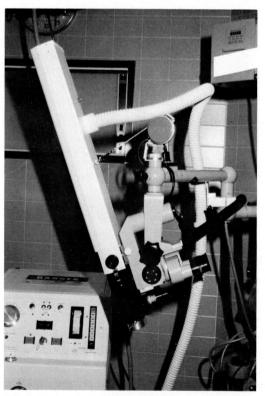

Figure 34–3. Colposcope with cryostat. The eyepiece is used to magnify the cervix and permit visualization of the pattern of cervical blood vessels.

frankly invasive carcinoma. Despite an annual increase in the number of abnormal Pap smears referred to these physicians, the number of conizations decreased from 38 per year to less than 10. Furthermore, before colposcopy, only 64% of the cones found the most advanced lesion of CIN versus 81% after it was instituted. This resulted in an annual savings in health-care costs of more than $50,000 per year and the elimination each year of two or three severe complications from conization. Not a single patient in this program has yet developed an invasive carcinoma of the cervix.

These data demonstrate that conization is no longer needed for most patients with severe dysplasia or carcinoma *in situ* and that these lesions can usually be treated with a simple one-hour office procedure.

Thus, only a few women with biologically unusual and very aggressive cancers, or those who completely neglect their health, should succumb to invasive cancer of the cervix.

Patients with invasive cancer of the cervix, as contrasted to those with *in situ* disease, are usually symptomatic. Symptoms include abnormal vaginal bleeding, either postcoital or menometrorrhagia. Some, particularly those with large, necrotic tumors, will have foul-smelling discharge, and as the disease progresses, pelvic or low-back pain may occur.

Examination of the cervix may show ulceration. Sometimes the growth is exophytic with large, ulcerated polypoid lesions. Diffuse infiltration may produce an enlarged, hard cervix. The diagnosis is easily established by a punch biopsy. The remainder of the work-up is designed to provide accurate staging in order to determine treatment and prognosis. The work-up includes the following:

Complete blood count, including platelet count
Blood chemistries, particularly to assess renal and liver function
X-rays and other studies as follows:

1. A chest X-ray and IVP are recommended for all patients. Cystoscopy is done in all those with disease at least as advanced as clinical stage IIb.
2. Barium enema and rectosigmoidoscopy are done for all patients with rectal complaints and in those with clinical stage III or more advanced disease in order to assess possible rectal involvement.
3. Lymphography is relied upon in some institutions. Clear-cut positives are use-

ful, but false negatives have led to the investigation of operative staging *(vida infra)*. Some use the skinny-needle biopsy to confirm positive x-ray findings (Tao *et al.,* 1980).

Staging of Carcinoma of the Cervix

Preinvasive carcinoma
Stage 0	Carcinoma *in situ,* intraepithelial carcinoma.

Invasive carcinoma
Stage I	Carcinoma strictly confined to the cervix (extension to the corpus should be disregarded).
Stage IA	The cancer cannot be diagnosed by clinical examination; (1) early stromal invasion and (2) occult cancer.
Stage IB	All other cases of stage I.
Stage II	The carcinoma extends beyond the cervix but has not extended onto the pelvic wall. The carcinoma involves the vagina, but not the lower third.
Stage IIA	No obvious parametrial involvement.
Stage IIB	Obvious parametrial involvement.
Stage III	The carcinoma has extended onto the pelvic wall. On rectal examination, there is no cancer-free space between the tumor and the pelvic wall. The tumor involves the lower third of the vagina.
Stage IIIA	No extension onto the pelvic wall.
Stage IIIB	Extension onto the pelvic wall.
Stage IV	The carcinoma has extended beyond the true pelvis or has involved the mucosa of the bladder or rectum. Bullous edema as the only finding does not mean that the patient is stage IV.

A gynecologist and a radiation oncologist should both examine the patient under anesthesia at the time of a fractional dilatation and curettage of the endocervical canal and endometrium. This is done to provide an accurate examination to determine the upper extent of the tumor and to design a program of treatment. Staging, therefore, is primarily clinical, with the only pathologic assessment being that of the uterus itself.

Because of dissatisfaction with clinical staging, even when lymphography is done, studies evaluating laparotomy have been conducted. Results of these studies have indicated significant discrepancy between clinical and pathologic staging, with the most important finding being the presence of unsuspected, involved para-aortic nodes. Since these are not treated in the usual program, they could be an important cause of treatment failure. Combining the series of five different groups investigating laparotomy as a staging procedure, the risk of para-aortic node involvement rises with advancing clinical stage as follows (Nelson *et al.*, 1974; Piver and Barlow, 1977; Wharton *et al.*, 1977; Sudarsanam *et al.*, 1978; Lagasse *et al.*, 1980; Tao *et al.*, 1980:

CLINICAL STAGE	% PATIENTS WITH POSITIVE PARA-AORTIC NODES	
IB	19/319	(6%)
IIA	7/53	(13%)
IIB	42/214	(19%)
IIIA–IV	74/216	(34%)

Thus, clinical staging failed to reveal an extent of disease sufficient at the time of diagnosis to account for treatment failure in 142/802 (16%).

The important question, however, is not whether staging is more accurate when laparotomy is done, but whether (with minimal risk) it will, as in Hodgkin's disease, result in altered treatment that improves the survival. To date, this question has not been answered. A selective review of the literature by Lagasse *et al.* (1980) found that of those who had a laparotomy with treatment altered so as to include involved para-aortic nodes, 30/124 survived free of disease for up to three years. They believed the expected prognosis for these patients to be much poorer. Complications thought to be the result of larger radiation portals utilizing high doses were greatly increased. Further problems with routine staging laparotomy are suggested by a small series in which 34.8% of the patients with positive para-aortic nodes had positive scalene node biopsy making the findings on laparotomy almost irrelevant (Buchsbaum, 1979). Despite this, routine scalene node biopsy in another study was a totally unproductive pursuit (Perez-Mesa and Spratt, 1976). Accordingly, for the moment, laparotomy as a staging tool in carcinoma of the cervix remains questionable.

Pathology

The histologic types of invasive cancer of the cervix include squamous cell, adenocarcinoma, clear cell, and undifferentiated. The vast majority of cancers are of squamous cell origin, repesenting 89% of 290 consecutive cases in the Gynecologic Oncology Group (GOG) (Lagasse *et al.*, 1980) and 88% of 1390 cases seen over 11 years at the University of Alabama in Birmingham (Shingleton *et al.*, 1981). The great majority of the remainder are

adenocarcinoma. There has been some dispute as to the meaning of the pathologic distinction between squamous cell carcinoma and adenocarcinoma. For instance, in the GOG study, 75% of a small number of patients with positive aortic nodes who were clinically stage IB had adenocarcinoma. Shingleton's review of the world's largest continuous series of cases of adenocarcinoma of the cervix showed no important differences in staging, treatment, or prognosis, when compared to squamous cell carcinoma.

Treatment

Stage 0. The treatment of stage 0 carcinoma of the cervix was discussed in the section on diagnosis and screening.

Stage IA. (Microinvasive Carcinoma). This stage of disease is uncommon. Among 861 carefully evaluated cases of all stages of invasive squamous cell cancer of the cervix, only 51 (6%) were stage IA when the diagnosis was restricted to those with 5 mm or less invasion of the stroma (Shingleton *et al.*, 1979).

Precise criteria for the diagnosis of this stage have not, however, been clearly set down. As indicated above, it is an occult cancer with early stromal invasion and requires, therefore, careful pathologic evaluation. In an attempt to define this entity further, the Gynecologic Oncology Group initiated a multi-institutional clinical-pathologic study which permitted treatment according to institutional preference (Sedlis *et al.*, 1979). Acceptable treatment choices included conization, simple or radical hysterectomy, or radiation therapy. The study was analyzed after 265 patients had been entered and pathologic review of the cones and/ or hysterectomy specimens completed. Almost 50% on reexamination of the pathologic specimens did not have microinvasive (stage IA) cervical cancer. In 75% of these cases, the correct diagnosis was intraepithelial cancer *(in situ)*, and in 14%, it was invasive cancer (stage IB). The remaining 11% were excluded for other reasons. Thus, overdiagnosis was common and probably resulted in overtreatment since simple hysterectomy was the least aggressive treatment permitted, and, as noted before, conization or even cryo or laser surgery would have been satisfactory for many patients with this stage of disease. The failure to recognize more advanced disease occurred in 6.8% of the cases, leading to the possibility of undertreatment. The fact that microinvasive cancer is not a benign disorder is evidenced by the fact that 2 of the 133 patients who met the pathologic criteria, and who were treated with simple hysterectomy, experienced a recurrence and died. As a result of this experience, the diagnosis of stage IA carcinoma of the cervix should not be taken lightly, and careful pathologic examination and consultation should be undertaken in this circumstance. Individualization of treatment is important. Simple hysterectomy is appropriate for minimal stage IA disease, but if the invasion is more than 2 mm deep or 4 mm wide, or invasion of the capillarylike spaces is visualized, radical surgery or radiation therapy is the appropriate treatment.

Treatment of Stage IB Through IIIB. Patients in this group are usually treated with radiation therapy. Radical surgery is an acceptable, but seldom used, alternative. The goal is cure. The principles of management include:

1. Accurate dosimetry so that radiation can be delivered to the cancer according to its actual anatomic location. This requires the services of a radiation physicist as well as careful review of port films.
2. A proper combination of internal (intracavitary or interstitial) and external megavoltage (^{60}CO or linear accelerator) radiation so as to reduce the tumor bulk and prevent excessive doses to the bladder (> 5000 rads) and rectum (> 4500 rads).

Generally, the radiation therapist attempts to deliver approximately 7000 rads to a point 2 cm lateral to the midline of the uterine cavity at a point 2 cm from the cervical os (point A) and 6000 rads to a point 3 cm lateral to point A (point B). The details of these programs depend upon the bulk of the lesion (large tumors require later intracavitary insertions), the extent of the tumor (more advanced stages require larger ports), and the anatomy of the individual patient.

No study shows an advantage of surgery over radiation therapy, and no study suggests that both modalities together are necessary or beneficial.

Stage IV. As noted previously, stage IV cancer of the cervix is increasingly rare. Indeed, since 1967, only 5% of patients presented with disease this advanced (Shingleton et al., 1979), and little change in this percentage of patients has occurred during the past decade.

Few patients with disease this advanced can be cured either by radiation or radical surgery. A few patients whose disease is locally advanced by virtue of invasion of the rectum or bladder can be cured either by radical, exenterative surgery or aggressive radiation therapy. The exenterative procedure removes the disease, the regional nodes, and the involved rectum or bladder, or both. Those who have disease that extends beyond these areas are not candidates for cure.

Treatment of Recurrent Disease. *Salvage Therapy.* Salvage therapy with curative intent for persistent or recurrent disease can be accomplished in selected patients who have local or regional disease only. The five-year actuarial survival, in a series of 141 patients treated with a Wertheim hysterectomy at the Mayo Clinic between 1956 and 1975, was nearly 60%. At 14 years, it was about 50%. The operative complications of this procedure are considerable but not prohibitive, with 38% of all patients having experienced operative complication. Interstitial fistulae (4.3%), urinary fistulae (13.0), and pelvic abscesses (7.8%) were particularly likely in patients who had failed radiotherapy (Webb and Symmonds, 1979). Radiotherapeutic salvage of patients with IA through IIB disease, who have been primarily treated with surgery, can be achieved occasionally. In one series, salvage therapy of primary treatment failures, regardless of whether surgery or radiation was initially used, has been successfully accomplished in only 13/67 (19%) of those in which it was attempted during the past decade (Shingleton et al., 1982).

Chemotherapy. Investigation of drugs effective in carcinoma of the cervix has been limited by the relatively small numbers of patients who relapse and die of their disease. Further limitations to the evaluation of these agents include the fact that many patients have urinary obstruction, producing compromised renal function and consequent poor marrow function, and perhaps altered metabolism of the agents. Most patients have had major prior radiotherapy which reduces marrow reserve and may reduce drug delivery to the tumor secondary to reduced blood flow to the pelvis. Finally, the coincidence of fibrosis, tumor, and infection may make it extremely difficult to evaluate accurately the effectiveness of a given agent. Responses, when they occur, are almost invariably partial and of short duration (Thigpen et al., 1981b). Some investigators have the impression that extrapelvic lesions may be more responsive (Omura *et al.,* 1978). To date, although a number of drugs have been found to have occasional or marginal activity in cancer of the cervix (Omura, 1973; Omura and Roberts, 1973; Omura *et al.,* 1978; Omura *et al.,* 1981b), only cisplatin has consistently produced responses. As a single agent, when evaluated in a cooperative group, 95/381 (24.9%) previously untreated patients receiving cisplatin every three weeks had an objective response. Forty (10.5%) were complete responses. The survival of the responders was significantly ($P = .001$) increased when compared to nonresponders (Bonomi *et al.,* 1982). The Southwest Oncology Group has reported a response rate as high as 60% for a combination of bleomycin, vincristine, and mitomycin C, but the median duration of response was less than three months (Baker and Opipari, 1977), raising questions regarding the significance of the responses reported. Current studies are evaluating infusions of cisplatin, combinations of marginally active drugs, and cisplatin as an adjuvant (Thigpen *et al.,* 1981a).

Prognosis

Survival in carcinoma of the cervix can be closely correlated with stage and substage. Approximately 75% of all stage I patients survived five or more years, but only 2/26 patients with stage IA died compared to 36/283 with IB; this difference is not statistically significant owing to the small numbers of IA patients. Shingleton *et al.* (1982) have recently analyzed this material and pointed out the additional importance of the size of the primary tumor in stage IB, with smaller lesions (<2 cm) being more favorable.

Overall, approximate five-year survival by stage is as follows (Shingleton *et al.,* 1979):

STAGE	PERCENT	SUBSTAGE	PERCENT	PERCENT OF ALL PATIENTS
I	75	A	92	53
		B	73	
II	55	A	70	30
		B	45	
III	21	A	80	
		B	0	12.3
IV	25			4.7

In stage II, however, only 15/65 patients with-

out parametrial involvement (substage A) have died versus 55/158 with parametrial disease (substage B), a difference which is highly significant ($P = 0.02$). Indeed, virtually no difference in survival exists between those with IB and IIA disease. There have been few patients with stage IIIA disease (8/869), but their survival is as good as those with stage IB disease. These data suggest the need for a new staging system.

No patient with stage IIIB disease has survived three years, and few patients with stage IV disease survive more than a year. These data indicate that extension of the disease laterally is both more common and more detrimental than anterior or posterior spread.

These data are approximately comparable to results in many series. It is not possible, however, to compare directly one series with another because of differences in age, staging procedures, and referral patterns.

Prospects for the Future

To further reduce the mortality from cancer of the cervix, earlier detection is necessary to identify patients before they present with extensive parametrial involvement or the presence of para-aortic node metastases. Whether this is possible is questionable. As noted earlier, public education and screening may have accomplished as much as is feasible. Adjuvant programs that could make initial radiotherapy or surgery more effective are now being conducted. One such study involves the use of cisplatin (Thigpen *et al.,* 1981a), another approach involves the use of radiosensitizers such as hydroxyurea (Hreshchyshyn *et al.,* 1976), misonidazole, and radioprotectors (Phillips, 1981). Since cisplatin provides a response rate of up to 50%, with some complete remissions, this approach is worthy of consideration (Durant, 1981). Studies in this area are underway, but have not yet yielded clinically useful information. Results from misonidazole and radioprotector (Yuhas *et al.,* 1980) studies are not sufficiently mature to be evaluated. One positive study utilizing hydroxyurea, ineffective by itself as a chemotherapeutic agent but a probable radiosensitizer, has been reported. The Gynecologic Oncology Group compared 51 previously untreated stage IIIB and IVA patients given radiotherapy and hydroxyurea with 46 women given the same radiotherapy and a placebo. Superior complete response rates, disease-free survival, and survival were reported for those given hydroxyurea. These patients also experienced greater toxicity (Hreshchyshyn *et al.,* 1976). Potential flaws in the study included the use of clinical staging only, a high inevaluability rate, and greater toxicity for those given hydroxyurea. Such results need to be confirmed and attempts made to improve local control.

Ultimately, the control of advanced disease will require not only better local therapy, but also a truly effective adjuvant program for those who have unsuspected but more widespread disease.

CARCINOMA OF THE VAGINA

Epidemiology

Although cancer of the vagina is extremely rare, it constitutes 1 to 2% of all cancer of the female genital tract. At the University of Alabama in Birmingham over the past ten years, 105/2187 (5%) of all gynecologic cancers have been vaginal primaries (Shingleton *et al.,* 1979). This is much higher than the natural prevalence of this disease as determined from the Third National Cancer Survey, which indicated that about 2% of the gynecologic cancers originated in the vagina (Cutler and Young, 1975).

Squamous Cell Carcinoma. Since the discovery of *in situ* carcinoma of the cervix and the ease of diagnosis with the Pap smear, it has become apparent that women successfully treated for either dysplasia, *in situ,* or invasive carcinoma of the cervix are at high risk for epithelial carcinoma of the vagina, particularly the upper vagina. Although the appearance of an invasive epithelial cancer of the vagina after therapy for invasive cancer of the cervix might be considered a recurrence, or persistence, of a previous inadequately treated cervical cancer, it is apparent this is not the explanation for many cases. Marcus (1961) postulated a "field effect" as an explanation for multiple squamous cell cancers of the genital tract. This hypothesis states that in some women, the genital tract is at high risk for epithelial cancers, particularly in the upper vagina, although they may occur anywhere in the lower genital tract.

In a 15-year review of vaginal cancer reported by Marchant *et al.* (1974), 157 cases of vaginal cancer were identified. Of these, approximately two-thirds occurred within three years of the cervical cancer and had pathologic and cytologic similarities with each other, suggesting an identical disease process. In another one-third, however, the two cancers were more widely separated in time and, in each instance, although there were histologic similarities, easily recognized cytologic distinctions between the two cancers were noted. Of the 37 primary cases of vaginal cancer so identified, 27 were invasive epidermoid, 3 were invasive adenocarcinomas, and only 7 *in situ.* Ten of 27 died within an average of a year. Previous radiation therapy was not the etiologic event in these cases, since they occurred with equal frequency whether radiation or hysterectomy was the treatment of the first cancer.

More recently, carcinoma *in situ* of the vagina has been recognized more frequently, especially after hysterectomy or conization as successful treatment for *in situ* carcinoma. Fourteen such patients were identified by Barclay (1979) and 23 by Hernandez-Linares *et al.* (1980). The interval between the two *in situ* cancers was as long as 19 years. Only 6 of a total of 33 *in situ* vaginal cancers occurred in women who had not had prior therapy for cervical cancer.

These data indicate that women treated successfully for *in situ* and invasive cancer of the cervix require regular follow-up, not only to facilitate early detection of recurrences, but in order to screen for a subsequent cancer of the vagina. Although the incidence of this phenomenon is generally estimated to be only 1 to 3%, Kolstad and Klem (1976) estimate that 20% of these will become invasive with a lethal potential.

The diagnosis of carcinoma *in situ* is usually made by Pap smear. Thereafter, colposcopy is done in order to localize the lesion, obtain a biopsy, and plan treatment. Treatment itself depends upon the clinical circumstances. Options include (1) irradiation, particularly with intravaginal sources; (2) surgical resection, which may vary from local excision to total vaginectomy with skin grafting; and (3) local destruction, *i.e.,* cautery, cryosurgery, laser surgery, or topical 5-FU (Hernandez-Linares *et al.,* 1980).

Invasive carcinoma of the vagina requires consultation between gynecologist and radiotherapist. The factors influencing the selection of therapy depend upon whether the patient has had radiotherapy, her age, sexual activity, and so forth. No effective systemic therapy is available for this disease.

At the University of Alabama in Birmingham, when invasive cancer of the vagina was confined to that organ (stage I), all of the patients were cured, as were three with microinvasion. When invasion into subvaginal tissue (stage II) was evident, only about 40% could be cured, and no patient with more extensive disease survived more than a year and a half (Shingleton et al., 1979).

Clear Cell Cancer of the Vagina. This is a second important type of cancer occurring primarily in the vagina of girls and young women and is associated with maternal ingestion of diethylstilbestrol (DES). It was first described in 1971 by Herbst and colleagues (1971). The data on all cases of this type occurring in women born since 1940 have been collected in a special registry. Herbst (1981) has recently reviewed the subject and made recommendations regarding its diagnosis and management. As of June, 1980, 389/429 cases had adequate histories to determine whether maternal exposure to DES and its analogs had occurred. Of these, 63% had positive histories of exposure to the conjugated estrogens, dienestrol, hexestrol, or DES. The peak incidence of the disease occurred in the mid-1970s since fewer cases have been reported since that time. The youngest reported patient was seven years old, the oldest, 30. Ninety-five percent occurred in those 14 and older. Fifty-eight percent were stage I. Eighty percent of all patients, regardless of stage, appear to be cured, probably because of early diagnosis.

Clear cell adenocarcinoma is an uncommon complication of much more common sequelae of maternal conjugated estrogen use. These include vaginal adenosis, often with squamous metaplasia, cervical collars, cervical erosion, cervical hypoplasia, cockscomb cervix, transverse ridges, and other developmental uterine abnormalities (Bibbo et al., 1977; Kaufman et al., 1977; Haney et al., 1979; Herbst et al., 1979; O'Brien et al, 1979; Robboy et al., 1979). In addition, genitourinary developmental abnormalities in men have been reported, including cryptorchidism and testicular hypoplasia (Bibbo et al., 1977; Gill et al., 1979). Male infertility may be a sequela. No increased risk of cancer in male offspring or the mothers of these patients has been unequivocally demonstrated (Glebatis and Janerich, 1981). About one-third of exposed female offspring will have such changes, which can usually be well delineated with the colposcope.

Concern over the future for exposed populations has been sufficiently great that one state (New York) has established a publicly supported registry and voluntary program for both sons and daughters of those exposed, as well as their mothers. Estimates of exposure rates for those born between 1941 and 1970 are slightly more than 1%. This is less than estimated by the DES task force (Bibbo et al., 1978) but still substantial. In 1978, it was estimated that between 200,000 and 360,000 residents of New York State and between four and five million residents of the United States were at risk.

Patients who have a history of maternal DES exposure should be referred to a gynecologist experienced in colposcopy. Regular examination should begin at the menarche or at age 14, whichever occurs first. Thereafter, twice yearly follow-up is recommended for those without lesions (Herbst, 1981). Specific measures for those with lesions should be carried out at the discretion of the appropriate gynecologist.

Most DES-exposed women will have no abnormality. Those who have lesions will usually have a benign course, and those with neoplasm can usually be cured by the appropriate surgical procedure. Since the practice of DES administration to prevent spontaneous abortion has been abandoned, it is likely this entity will gradually disappear (Glebatis and Janerich, 1981). This is the only human neoplasm known to be the result of intrauterine exposure to conjugated estrogen, but, as noted in the section on carcinoma of the uterine corpus, it is not the only gynecologic cancer associated with this biochemical structure.

MISCELLANEOUS CANCERS OF THE VAGINA

Occasionally, other cancers will originate in the vagina. Recently, Chung et al., (1980) isolated 19 cases of primary melanoma of the vagina identified in a review of records for 40 years at Memorial Sloan Kettering Cancer Center and the Connecticut Tumor Registry. Management and prognosis in these patients are the same as for melanoma in general (Balch et al., and 1978).

Malignant tumors rarely occur in the vagina of children (Barber and Graber, 1973) with only 3% of all pediatric cancers being gynecologic. Such cancers include endodermal sinus cancers (Beller et al., 1979), embryonal rhabdomyosarcoma (Barber and Graber, 1973), and botryoid sarcoma (Barber and Graber, 1973). These patients should be referred to a pediatric cancer center where a team of specialists is available.

VULVAR CANCER

Vulvar cancer, like vaginal cancer, is unusual. In the Third National Cancer Survey, it comprised 3% of all gynecologic cancers and was three times as prevalent as vaginal cancer (Cutler and Young, 1975). Over the most recent ten-year period at the University of Alabama in Birmingham (Shingleton *et al.*, 1979), 155 cases were diagnosed. Of these, the majority (53.5%) were invasive squamous cell cancers. The majority of the remainder (30%) were *in situ.* A number of rare tumors, such as melanoma, comprised the remainder.

Unfortunately, most of the patients presenting with invasive cancer had relatively advanced disease. When the cancer was confined to the vulva and was less than 2 cm in diameter (stage I), the prognosis was good, and more than 80% have been cured. With more extensive involvement (stages II through IV), the five-year survival is between 40 and 50%. Treatment of carcinoma *in situ* and stage I disease is usually surgical. The usual operation is a radical vulvectomy with limited dissection of regional lymph nodes. Treatment of patients with more advanced stages requires a more extensive operation, including a radical dissection of regional groin nodes and *en bloc* removal of other tissues, depending upon the location and extent of the disease. The GOG is currently studying the value of node irradiation in those with positive groin nodes. No known effective drugs have been identified for this disease.

OVARIAN CANCER

Incidence and Epidemiology

Currently, about 18,000 new cases of ovarian cancer are reported per year in the United States, with 11,400 deaths (Silverberg, 1982). It is the fourth leading cause of cancer death among women in this country and is responsible for 47% of all gynecologic cancer deaths. The symptoms of early cancer are nonspecific, hence, the majority (66%) present with advanced (stage III and IV) disease (Shingleton *et al.*, 1979). The incidence of the usual epithelial types increases with age; the median age at diagnosis is about 57 years, with a range from the twenties to the eighties. Ovarian cancer is much less common in Japan than in the United States, but the incidence increases in Japanese who move to this country. Carcinomas are more common in single women and nulliparous married women. Tumors of germ cell origin are seen in children and teenagers.

Ovarian cancer has rarely been reported to affect members of a family (Lurain and Piver, 1979). The genetic implications of the few reported familial clusters are unclear. Women with breast cancer have an increased incidence of ovarian cancer. Rubella infection during the peripuerperal period also appears to increase the risk (McGowan *et al.*, 1979). Risk factors may differ for the serous and endometrioid cell types; for the latter histology, association has been shown with hypertension and obesity (Szamborski *et al.*, 1981). The use of oral contraceptives, however, does not increase the risk (Willett *et al.*, 1981).

Pathology and Natural History

The pathology of ovarian tumors is complex. This subject is reviewed in detail elsewhere (Scully, 1970, 1977). Tumors, benign or malignant, can arise from the surface epithelium, germ cells, stromal tissue, or other mesenchymal elements of the ovary. An abbreviated classification is presented in Table 34-4. This incomplete list emphasizes the common cell types and/or those where chemotherapy has been adequately evaluated. Metastases to the ovary (Webb *et al.*, 1975; Metz *et al.*, 1980), especially from cancers of the colon, stomach, uterus or breast, comprise 4 to 8% of ovarian cancers (Scully, 1970) and underscore the need for adequate diagnosis and staging (Omura, 1981). Occasionally, no primary site can be found (Metz *et al.*, 1980; Roth and Ehrlich, 1977). Psammoma bodies have typically been associated with ovarian cancer but are not diagnostic (LiVolsi, 1977). Borderline tumors (carcinomas of low malignant potential) are an especially troublesome problem in management; such tumors may be associated with peritoneal implants and metastases, but still have a benign course (Scully, 1977). This seems to emphasize that the grade or degree of differentiation of malignant tumors has important prognostic value

Table 34-4. Abbreviated Classification of Ovarian Tumors

I. Epithelial tumors
   A. Benign
   B. Borderline
   C. Malignant

II. Germ cell tumors
   A. Dysgerminoma
   B. Carcinoma (embryonal, chorio-, terato-)*
   C. Endodermal sinus tumor*
   D. Other

III. Stromal tumors
   A. Granulosa cell*
   B. Sertoli's cell
   C. Other

IV. Sarcomas*

V. Other ovarian tumors

VI. Metastatic to ovary

* Drugs are known to be active and may be indicated.

(Scully, 1977; Ozols *et al.,* 1980a; Omura *et al.,* 1983a). Approximately 90% of ovarian cancers are of epithelial origin. They may be solid, cystic, or both and are often bilateral.

A typical distribution of histologic types has been reported from the Gynecologic Oncology Group: serous, 55% (endometrioid 12%); mucinous, 6%; clear cell, 5%; undifferentiated, 5%; mixed epithelial, 4%; and other 13% (Omura *et al.,* 1983a). The rare Brenner tumor (Yoonessi and Abell, 1979; Woodruff *et al.,* 1981) is also included within the category of epithelial ovarian tumors.

Modes of Spread and Sites of Metastasis

Direct extension to other pelvic structures, intraperitoneal seeding, and lymphatic spread to para-aortic and pelvic nodes are common. Clinically significant hematogenous spread, in contrast, is rare in epithelial ovarian cancers. Involvement of the diaphragm may occur early (Rosenoff *et al.,* 1975) and is especially important because of its impact on staging and management. The serosa of the liver is more frequently involved than the parenchyma. Omental involvement, when present, may be gross or may involve only a few microscopic deposits.

Signs and Symptoms

Vague pelvic and/or abdominal discomfort and indigestion are common but nonspecific symptoms. Urinary frequency or abnormal vaginal bleeding or/and abdominal swelling may be a presenting complaint, but the latter generally reflects advanced disease and/or ascites. Nevertheless, some of the largest tumors are benign. A palpable ovary in a postmenopausal woman is highly suspect for carcinoma (Barber and Graber, 1971). With more advanced disease, large pelvic or abdominal mass may be noted, or ascites or pleural effusion may be present.

Diagnosis and Staging

In most cases, early diagnosis is accidental. No satisfactory screening method is known. Routine pelvic examination identifies few cases. In patients with a suspected or proven diagnosis, culdocentesis for cytologic study of peritoneal fluid has been advocated (McGowan and Bunnag, 1976). It has not been widely employed because of patient discomfort, false negatives, and failure to demonstrate improved survival. In contrast to the other gynecologic cancers, the staging system for ovarian cancer requires surgery in most instances to determine the extent to which the peritoneal surfaces and contents are involved. The staging system is shown in Table 34-5. For the common epithelial cancers of the ovary, a total abdominal hysterectomy and bilateral salpingo-oophorectomy are usually indicated, even in the face of advanced disease. Omentectomy or omental biopsy, thorough exploration of all the peritoneal surfaces, including biopsy of the undersurface of the diaphragm, and peritoneal washings for cytology are indicated. The complications of surgical staging include the risk of anesthesia, the risk of bleeding from node sampling, and biopsy of peritoneum and diaphragm. There may be a slight increase in postoperative adhesions. Pneumothorax is a possible risk of diaphragmatic biopsy. Injury to the bowel and bladder is possible. In one series of 26 patients where a major effort at "debulking" was undertaken, two episodes of sepsis but no postoperative deaths were reported (Griffith *et al.,* 1979).

Lymphangiography (Fuks, 1975) and peritoneoscopy (Rosenoff *et al.,* 1975) have been advocated as components of staging, but these techniques have limited use when removal of the primary lesion and debulking surgery are contemplated.

Treatment

Surgical removal of as much tumor as possible should be attempted. Patients with a small volume of disease after surgery (largest resid-

Table 34–5.   FIGO Classification of Ovarian Carcinoma

Stage I	Growth limited to the ovaries.
IA	Growth limited to one ovary; no ascites.
	i. No tumor on the external surface; capsule intact.
	ii. Tumor present on the external surface and/or capsule ruptured.
IB	Growth limited to both ovaries; no ascites.
	i. No tumor on the external surface; capsule intact.
	ii. Tumor present on the external surface and/or capsule(s) ruptured.
IC	Tumor either stage IA or stage IB, but with ascites* present or positive peritoneal washings.
Stage II	Growth involving one or both ovaries with pelvic extension.
IIA	Extension and/or metastases to the uterus and/or tubes.
IIB	Extension to other pelvic tissues.
IIC	Tumor either stage IIA or stage IIB, but with ascites* present or positive peritoneal washings.
Stage III	Growth involving one or both ovaries with intraperitoneal metastases outside the pelvis and/or positive retroperitoneal nodes. Tumor limited to the true pelvis with histologically proven malignant extension to small bowel or omentum.
Stage IV	Growth involving one or both ovaries with distant metastases. If pleural effusion is present, there must be positive cytology to allot a case to stage IV. Parenchymal liver metastases equals stage IV.
Special Category	Unexplored cases which are thought to be ovarian carcinoma.

* Ascites is peritoneal effusion which in the opinion of the surgeon is pathologic and/or clearly exceeds normal amounts.

ual nodules equal to or less than 1 cm) demonstrate an improved response to chemotherapy as well as longer survival than those with a greater extent of disease (Griffith *et al.,* 1979; Smith and Day, 1979; Wharton and Herson, 1981). If at the time of initial treatment planning the patient has not been adequately diagnosed, staged, or undergone adequate surgical removal, reexploration of bulk tumor must be considered. Postsurgical treatment depends on the stage.

Stage I.   In patients with stage IAi, grade 1 lesion, the likelihood of surgical cure is at least 90 to 95% (Webb *et al.,* 1973; Hreshchyshyn *et al.,* 1980). Occasional patients in this good prognosis category may be treated with unilateral oophorectomy. The value of postsurgical treatment in this circumstance is unclear, but some investigators recommend melphalan or intraperitoneal radioactive phosphorus. The Gynecologic Oncology Group and Ovarian Cancer Study Group are currently comparing melphalan versus observation in stage IAi and IBi cases, and with moderately differentiated histology. The survival of poorly differentiated stage I cases may be as low as 50% (Webb *et al.,* 1973; Hreshchyshyn *et al.,* 1980), mandating that additional therapy be considered. In one study, adjunctive melphalan appeared superior to external radiotherapy (Hreshchyshyn *et al.,* 1980). Alternatively, ^{32}P can be considered if there are no adhesions or other technical problems preventing the safe use of this isotope. Since meticulous staging is a relatively recent practice, and carefully controlled stud-

ies in stage I are difficult to establish, the value of adjuvant treatment is not entirely clear; improvement in survival to 80% may occur with isotope treatment (Decker *et al.,* 1973; Buchsbaum *et al.,* 1975). The Gynecologic Oncology Group and Ovarian Cancer Study Group compared melphalan versus ^{32}P in stage IC, IAii, and IBii as well as stage II cases. Stage I borderline tumors were adequately managed with surgery alone (Creasman *et al.,* 1982).

Stage II.   In the past, surgery with or without radiotherapy has produced variable results; recurrence rates ranged from 20 to 50% for well-differentiated lesions with no apparent residual disease, to 67 to 100% for less well-differentiated lesions, or when there is residual disease after surgery (Fuks, 1975; Malkasian *et al.,* 1975). These variations are related to how diligently surgical staging is conducted. With more thorough assessment of extent of disease, very few stage II cases (disease limited to the pelvis) are identified (Rosenoff *et al.,* 1975); Piver *et al.,* 1978a).

Stage III and IV.   Virtually every patient with advanced disease is destined to have a recurrence if surgery alone is performed. Mustard-type alkylating agent therapy has been used in the treatment of ovarian cancer (reviewed by Katz *et al.,* 1981; Willson *et al.,* 1981). Variable but definite benefits result from cyclophosphamide, melphalan, chlorambucil, or thiotepa. A small proportion of patients appear to have been cured with such postoperative treatment (Smith *et al.,* 1976). Three other drugs have emerged as having significant activity in ovarian carcinoma: hexamethylmelamine, doxorubicin, and cisplatin. The effectiveness of the latter is at least comparable to that of the mustards (Bruckner et al., 1981; Gershenson et al., 1981). The Gynecologic Oncology Group has screened several other agents such as CCNU, methyl CCNU (Omura et al., 1977), piperazinedione (Delgado et al., 1978), VP-16 (Slayton et al., 1979), and dianhydrogalactitol (Blom et al., 1980) without promising results. Some of the standard anticancer drugs have not been adequately evaluated (DeVita et al., 1976). Recently, the tumor stem cell assay has identified vinblastine and bleomycin as potentially useful agents in selected patients, but these have not been systemically tested for activity (Alberts et al., 1981).

Despite a compelling rationale for combination chemotherapy, it has been surprisingly difficult to show that drug combinations were actually superior to melphalan alone in ovarian cancer. Table 34–6 summarizes several regimens. Recently, it was reported that hexamethylmelamine, cyclophosphamide, methotrexate, and fluorouracil were superior to melphalan (Young et al., 1978). These results have not been confirmed (Carmo-Pereira et al., 1981). The Gynecologic Oncology Group compared melphalan plus 5-FU plus or minus actinomycin versus actinomycin plus 5-FU plus cyclophosphamide (ACFUCY) versus melphalan alone. None of these combinations identified any advantage (Park et al., 1980). A subsequent study comparing melphalan alone, versus melphalan plus hexamethylmelamine, versus doxorubicin plus cyclophos-

phamide showed an advantage for the doxorubicin combination in response rate. This did not, however, improve the progression-free interval or survival (Omura et al., 1983b). A more recent study comparing doxorubicin plus cyclophosphamide with or without cisplatin indicates a significant improvement in complete remission rate and remission duration for the cisplatin combination. There also appears to be a favorable impact of the cisplatin plus doxorubicin plus cyclophosphamide regimen on the frequency of negative second-look laparotomies (Omura et al., 1982). Edmonson et al., (1979) compared cyclophosphamide versus cyclophosphamide plus doxorubicin. In patients with bulk disease, the regimens were equivalent; in patients with minimal residual disease, the combination had a slight advantage. Doxorubicin plus cisplatin was found superior to cisplatin alone, albeit in small groups of patients (Bruckner et al., 1981). A current study of the GOG is comparing cyclophosphamide plus cisplatin, versus cyclophosphamide plus doxorubicin plus cisplatin in minimal residual disease which should better define the role of doxorubicin in ovarian cancer (Omura et al., unpublished data). If combination chemotherapy is to be introduced into the treatment of earlier stage disease, the combination with the best risk-benefit ratio needs to be identified. A recent report of improved results by varying the time of drug administration within the circadian cycle is of great interest, but requires confirmation (Hrushesky et al., 1981).

Second-line chemotherapy for ovarian carcinoma is unsatisfactory. Hexamethylmela-

Table 34–6.   Some Drug Combinations in Advanced Ovarian Carcinoma

REGIMEN	PATIENT (NUMBER)	CLINICAL COMPLETE RESPONSE (%)	NEGATIVE SECOND LOOK	MEDIAN SURVIVAL (MONTHS)	REFERENCE
H-PAM	97	28	9/22	13.5	Omura et al., 1983b
AC	173	25	6/30	14–15	Omura et al., 1983b
AP	15	40	——	19	Bruckner et al., 1981
CAP	91	44	9/20	15+	Omura et al., 1982
HCMF	40	——	13/40	29*	Young et al., 1978
CHAP	60	40	——	15	Vogl et al., 1981
HCAP	43	53	3/29	——	Greco et al., 1981
CHFP	51	41	5/37	18	Young et al., 1981

  H = Hexamethylmelamine
PAM = Melphalan
  A = Doxorubicin
  C = Cyclophosphamide
  P = Cisplatin
  M = Methotrexate
  F = Fluorouracil

* Patients with small-volume disease were included.

mine has very limited value in this setting (Omura et al., 1981a). In fact, the only "salvage" therapy worth emphasizing at present is cisplatin, and only if the patient has not previously received this drug (Piver et al., 1978b).

Intraperitoneal chemotherapy (Ozols et al., 1980b; Speyer et al. 1980) is of considerable interest since ovarian carcinoma is primarily a disease of the peritoneal surfaces. Drug penetration into tumor masses using this approach is limited, however, suggesting that this technique may apply to a select group of patients with minimal residual disease.

Radiotherapy. The role of radiotherapy in stage III disease is controversial. Since the entire peritoneum and its contents are often involved, the abdomen and pelvis must be treated, including both kidneys, the liver, and diaphragm. The tumoricidal dose for ovarian carcinoma is not well established, but presumably is in excess of the 3000-rad fractionated dose usually administered to the kidneys and liver (Fuks, 1975). Thus, some locations within the abdominal cavity may be undertreated when these organs are shielded. Most studies of radiotherapy in ovarian cancer antedate meticulous surgical staging. The toxicity of whole abdominal radiation to bowel, kidneys, and liver, along with the large volume of bone marrow irradiated, may compromise the patient's tolerance for subsequent chemotherapy. Despite these obstacles, favorable results have been reported with postoperative radiation alone, or in combination with chlorambucil (Dembo et al., 1979). Because of the therapeutic benefits produced by platinum-based combination chemotherapy, radiotherapy is not routinely used in many institutions as part of the primary treatment of stage III disease.

Immunotherapy. Interim analysis of a randomized trial suggests that BCG vaccination added to doxorubicin plus cyclophosphamide improves survival in advanced ovarian cancer (Alberts et al., 1979). The Southwest Oncology Group and the GOG are currently attempting to confirm this observation in randomized studies, but using a different strain of BCG and adding cisplatin to each arm. Interferon had modest antitumor effects in a small group of patients (Einhorn et al., 1982).

Endocrine Therapy of Ovarian Cancer. At least two hormonal agents have been tried in advanced ovarian cancer. Anecdotal reports of benefit from progestins prompted Slayton et al. (1981) to administer medroxyprogesterone acetate to 19 patients with ovarian cancers of many types. With unselected histology, no objective responses were observed in this group. Myers et al. (1981) described objective responses (1 CR and 2 PR) in three patients with serous carcinomas treated with tamoxifen.

Management of Ascites. Both intraperitoneal chemotherapy and irradiation using ^{32}P have been advocated when systemic chemotherapy fails to control ascites. Unfortunately, they are frequently unsuccessful, especially if large tumor masses are present. Repeated paracenteses in such patients do not significantly lower serum protein levels and may be used for symptomatic relief as necessary (Lifshitz and Buchsbaum, 1976).

Second-Look Laparotomy

Reexploration after achievement of a clinically complete response frequently reveals residual cancer. It is very encouraging that some patients have no evidence of disease when reexplored, have prolonged remissions, and may be cured (Smith et al., 1976). For a few patients with localized residual disease amenable to resection, a partial to a complete response may be observed. In such a case, a prolonged remission is not likely, but occasional patients did benefit from this type of surgical resection (Smith et al., 1976). The currently available salvage therapy is not predictably useful, but external radiotherapy, intraperitoneal ^{32}P, or intraperitoneal chemotherapy might be considered if small-volume tumor masses are left after second-look surgery. Thus, second-look laparotomy is often a consideration in the management of this disease. The current indications for such a procedure include documentation of complete response (at which point chemotherapy can presumably be stopped), resection of isolated residual lesions, and debulking prior to retreatment with some other regional or systemic therapy. The appropriate time for second-look surgery has not been established. Smith et al. (1976) recommended at least ten cycles of monthly melphalan before reexploration. Patients who were explored earlier were less likely to have a sustained remission, despite negative findings, than if treatment continued for a longer time. With combination chemotherapy, complete pathologic remission may occur more rapidly. Currently, some studies include second-look surgery after six months of treatment (Omura et al., 1982). A controlled trial randomizing the duration of treatment prior to second-look operations for clinical complete remissions needs to be considered.

UNCOMMON CELL TYPES

Treatment

A wide variety of rare tumors is included under the rubric of nonepithelial ovarian tumors. Only those with current implications regarding management with chemotherapy will be discussed here.

Ovarian Sarcomas. These rare cancers are currently being treated with 75 mg/m² of doxorubicin every three weeks in a GOG study. Vincristine plus actinomycin and concomitant irradiation were ineffective in an earlier trial (C. P. Morrow, unpublished data).

Germ Cell Tumors. These lesions are more commonly seen in children and adolescents. They include dysgerminoma, endodermal sinus tumor, teratoma, choriocarcinoma, and embryonal carcinoma (Kurman and Norris, 1976; Creasman et al., 1979; Brodeur, 1981).

Malignant Teratoma. Postoperative treatment with vincristine, actinomycin, and cyclophosphamide may improve survival in this rare cancer (Curry et al., 1978; Slayton et al., 1978). Recent studies have investigated the effect of vinblastine, bleomycin, and cisplatin when used for testicular cancer.

Endodermal Sinus Tumor (Yolk Sac Tumor; Teilum's Tumor). This lesion is a particularly aggressive type of germ cell tumor that may arise in extragonadal sites (Pileri et al., 1980). Postoperative combination chemotherapy has had a major impact on the prognosis in this disease. Serum alpha fetoprotein determined by radioimmune assay serves as a monitor of response to treatment (Gallion et al., 1979; Romero and Schwartz, 1981; Ishiguro et al., 1981). Vincristine, actinomycin, and cyclophosphamide (VAC) are effective in combination and have been advocated as adjuvant therapy, even in stage I cases (Slayton et al., 1978; Gallion et al., 1979). It may be curative in about half of these patients. More recently, vinblastine, bleomycin, and cisplatin in combination have been successfully used in advanced disease and in some patients failing VAC (Julian et al., 1980). The current GOG protocol in stage III and IV recurrent germ cell tumors employs vinblastine, bleomycin, and cisplatin (Williams et al., 1981).

Dysgerminoma. This tumor is analogous to the male seminoma and shares its marked radiosensitivity. Thus, even advanced disease is managed with irradiation. Patients with stage IA pure dysgerminoma had an excellent (95%) five-year survival in one series when unilateral adnexectomy was the only therapy (Gordon et al., 1981).

Other Germ Cell Tumors. Primary choriocarcinoma of the ovary is quite rare and is more resistant to chemotherapy than gestational trophoblastic neoplasia. Nevertheless, with aggressive surgery and combination chemotherapy, cure is possible in perhaps half of such patients (Gerbie et al., 1975).

Granulosa Cell Tumors. These are ovarian stromal tumors of relatively low malignant potential, but sometimes associated with very late recurrence (Evans et al., 1980). In at least one series, the prognosis was poor at an advanced clinical stage with tumor rupture or pronounced nuclear atypia (Bjorkholm and Silfversward, 1981). Prognosis may be better in premenarchal girls (Lack et al., 1981). With rare exceptions, total abdominal hysterectomy and bilateral salpingo-oophorectomy should be done (Evans et al., 1980; Bjorkholm and Silfversward, 1981). Postoperative radiotherapy is frequently employed, especially if the tumor is ruptured, or for small volumes of residual disease, but its value has not been thoroughly documented (Schwartz and Smith, 1976). Granulosa-theca cell tumors are managed in the same way as granulosa cell tumors. Pure thecomas should be regarded separately in the treatment of granulosa cell tumors (Stenwig et al., 1979).

Several drugs have been used with variable success. Two patients with stage III disease treated with actinomycin plus fluorouracil plus cyclophosphamide had sustained remissions; none of nine treated with melphalan had a complete response (Schwartz and Smith, 1976). The VAC combination has also been used. In view of the relative rarity of recurrent or advanced disease, it is difficult to set up a controlled clinical trial, and the effectiveness of adjuvant radiotherapy or chemotherapy in these tumors must await prolonged follow-up. Currently, the GOG is testing VAC in stage II, III, IV, and recurrent cases and is employing doxorubicin in patients refractory to the combination.

Complications of Treatment. The risks of surgery, radiotherapy, and chemotherapy in ovarian cancer include the complications of abdominal exploration, irradiation of radiosensitive abdominal organs and tissues, and the side effects of the individual anticancer drugs. One issue of great concern is the onco-genic potential of alkylating agent treatment, especially when used as adjuvants for early stage disease. A significantly increased inci-dence of acute myelogenous leukemia (AML) in patients with ovarian cancer who were treated with mustard-type alkylating agents has been reported (Reimer *et al.,* 1977). The risk of AML approached 10% in women who have prolonged survival after extensive alky-lating agent treatment (Messerschmidt *et al.,* 1981). Thus, the decision to use such agents in adjuvant therapy of early stage ovarian cancer at relatively low risk of recurrence must be balanced against the risk of fatal bone marrow toxicity and of serious late effects.

Follow-up

Clinical evaluation and laboratory tests such as computed tomography are inaccurate means of follow-up in ovarian cancer. Lapa-roscopy and second-look laparotomy are very helpful, but repeated use of such interventions is not practical. Culdocentesis has been advo-cated but is not widely practiced (McGowan and Bunnag, 1976; Villa Santa and Jovan-ovski, 1980). The possibility of specific sero-logic markers for ovarian cancer and the search for tumor-associated antigens have been investigated by several groups. A murine monoclonal antibody has been described that reacts with cell lines and tumor tissue from ovarian cancer patients (Bast *et al.,* 1981). An ovarian tumor-associated antigen with fea-tures distinguishing it from carcinoembryonic antigen (CEA) has also been studied (Knauf and Urbach, 1978). It is apparently more sen-sitive than CEA in detecting the presence of ovarian cancer. An amylase that is seemingly characteristic of serous ovarian neoplasms has been identified (Van Kley *et al.,* 1981). To date, none of these serologic approaches has had practical application. Presently, patients with ovarian cancer require prolonged follow-up, including pelvic and general physical ex-aminations and sonar scans because of the risk of late recurrence or the late effects of treat-ment, especially oncogenesis.

Future Prospects

Prevention without first defining etiology seems illogical, especially in a disease as infre-quent as ovarian cancer. A serologic test for early ovarian cancer or minimal residual dis-ease would be a major advance, but presently, no methods appear likely to accomplish this goal. Other screening approaches are either not promising or not practical. Currently available drug combinations will cure some, but not all patients. New drugs and more skill-ful use of current drugs are needed for epithe-lial cancers. Combining radiotherapy with drugs such as cisplatin or with radiation-sensi-tizing agents is another avenue which may be productive.

NEOPLASMS OF THE FALLOPIAN TUBE

Primary cancer of the fallopian tube is rare. Secondary involvement of these structures from uterine or ovarian cancer is more com-mon. The cause of tubal cancer is unknown. Most cases are carcinomas, but sarcomas and choriocarcinoma have been reported. Spread usually follows a pattern similar to that of ovarian cancer, initially involving pelvic struc-tures and peritoneal surfaces. The average age has been 54 to 58 (range, 33 to 82) in various series (Kinzel, 1976; Benedet *et al.,* 1977; Her-shey *et al.,* 1981; Tamimi and Figge, 1981). Common symptoms are postmenopausal bleeding, pelvic pain, vaginal discharge, and/ or abdominal distention. The pain may be col-icky. Early diagnosis is difficult, and when the diagnosis is made, it is often because of an adnexal mass which has been found. Ascites may be present in more advanced cases. The combination of vaginal bleeding and/or posi-tive Pap smear without evidence of cervical cancer and a negative endometrial biopsy is very suggestive of the diagnosis. Definitive diagnosis requires laparotomy. No standard staging system is available, but is usually pat-terned after that used in ovarian cancer. An-other system based on the premise that the fallopian tube is a hollow viscus has been pro-posed (Schiller and Silverberg, 1971).

Treatment

Total abdominal hysterectomy and bilateral salpingo-oophorectomy, with careful explora-tion and biopsy of the omentum and perito-neal surfaces as well as cytologic washings, are indicated as in ovarian cancer. The value of postoperative radioactive phosphorus instilla-tion is uncertain, but is frequently recom-mended when all bulk disease can be removed (Benedet *et al.,* 1977). External pelvic radia-tion has been used in some cases. Six of eight (75%) patients with disease limited to the tube and without serosal penetration were free of disease at five years, while only 3 of 15 (20%) were free of disease if spread beyond the ovary or uterus had occurred (Benedet *et al.*, 1977). Occasional patients survive despite more advanced spread, but the relative contributions of radiotherapy and chemotherapy to these anecdotal good results are unclear. Drug regimens similar to those used in ovarian cancer have been employed, but have not been successful. A review of the literature reported one complete response with melphalan plus a progestin (Boronow, 1973). Deppe *et al.* (1980a) observed a complete response in two patients treated with cisplatin, doxorubicin, and a progestin (MEGACE or PROVERA); one patient also received cyclophosphamide. The progestin was added in these cases because of the known effects of such agents on normal tubal epithelium and its similarity to endometrial tissue. Unfortunately, the rarity of this cancer virtually precludes any randomized therapeutic trials.

ENDOMETRIAL AND OTHER NEOPLASMS OF THE UTERUS

Incidence and Epidemiology

For 1982, the estimated number of new cases of corpus cancer in this country was 39,000 (Silverberg, 1982), making it the most common invasive gynecologic cancer. The incidence appears to be increasing, at least in part because of increasing numbers of older women in the population, but also because of widespread use of conjugated estrogens to treat menopausal symptoms.

The median age at diagnosis for adenocarcinoma is about 62 years. Fifteen to 25% of patients are premenopausal; in one series, 4.3% were under age 40 (Shingleton *et al.*, 1979). Among the premenopausal cases, many have polycystic ovaries with anovulatory menstrual cycles. Obesity, nulliparity, late menopause, and diabetes are associated with an increased risk of endometrial carcinoma (McMahon, 1974). A family history of this cancer is sometimes noted. There appears to be a lower incidence in Japanese and a higher incidence in Jewish women.

Etiology and Pathogenesis

The cause of corpus cancer is unknown, but a substantial association with both endoge-

nous and exogenous estrogens does exist. The epidemiologic characteristics noted above are largely explained in terms of prolonged exposure to estrogens (especially when unopposed by progestins) and possible abnormal metabolism of steroid precursors (Schindler *et al.*, 1972; Siiteri *et al.*, 1974). Patients with feminizing ovarian tumors also have an increased risk. Adenomatous endometrial hyperplasia is usually associated with prolonged estrogen stimulation and is regarded as a premalignant lesion, albeit only a small minority of such patients develop overt cancer (Gusberg and Kaplan, 1963).

Several retrospective studies have associated exogenous estrogen use with an increased risk of endometrial carcinoma. Although these studies have been criticized on methodologic grounds (Horwitz *et al.*, 1981), the conclusion is generally accepted (Judd *et al.*, 1981). The risk is reduced when estrogen therapy is stopped (Walker and Jick, 1980).

Pathology and Natural History

Primary malignant lesions of the corpus are usually adenocarcinoma (86%) arising in the endometrium. Squamous elements are occasionally present (adenoacanthoma and adenosquamous carcinoma). Sarcomas are much less common, whereas primary squamous carcinoma represents a rare disease with a poor prognosis (Melan *et al.*, 1979). Metastases to the corpus may occur from primary cancers in other pelvic organs or from distant sites such as ovary or endocervix. This may result in considerable confusion on the origin of the malignancy.

Adenocarcinoma may be well differentiated (grade 1), moderately well differentiated (grade 2), or poorly differentiated (grade 3). The grade has a significant correlation with prognosis (Wade *et al.*, 1967). Although the size of the uterine cavity may vary for other reasons, enlargement as judged by sounding of the uterine cavity does correlate with a poorer prognosis. Endometrial cancer initially invades into the myometrium or becomes diffuse in the endometrial cavity where it may spread down to involve the cervix. Either deep myometrial invasion or endocervical involvement adversely affects survival. The tumor may also spread by direct extension into the tubes and ovaries. About 10% of clinical stage I cases will have node involvement, more commonly in the pelvic than in the para-aortic region (Creasman *et al.*, 1976). The lymphatic drainage of the upper part of the fundus is to the para-aortic and common iliac nodes. With endocervical involvement, the drainage is to the obturator, hypogastric, and external iliac nodes. Vaginal involvement at initial diagnosis is rare, but vaginal cuff recurrence after hysterectomy has been described in 5 to 10% of cases (Wade *et al.,* 1967; Graham, 1971; Morrow *et al.,* 1976).

Contamination of the peritoneal cavity by tumor cells may occur either by serosal penetration or spread up through the fallopian tubes (Creasman *et al.,* 1981). Subsequent involvement of other abdominal organs, hematogenous spread to lungs, and less commonly to bone, liver, pleura and other sites, may be seen early or late. Lung metastases are usually multiple, and in one report of four patients with solitary lung lesions, there were concurrent metastases in other distant sites (Ballon *et al.,* 1979). In that series, however, only 2.3% of cases with endometrial carcinoma developed pulmonary metastases (in striking contrast to uterine sarcomas), reflecting the relatively high cure rate in early stage disease and the likelihood of pelvic and abdominal spread rather than hematogenous spread in those who fail primary treatment. Recurrences are usually apparent within the first two or three years; late recurrences are uncommon (Wade *et al.,* 1967).

Signs and Symptoms

Abnormal vaginal bleeding or spotting is usually the first manifestation of endometrial carcinoma. Especially significant is postmenopausal bleeding. In premenopausal and perimenopausal women, irregular periods and/or excessive bleeding may be noted. Pelvic or low-back pain may reflect more advanced disease or may be secondary to coexistent benign pelvic lesions. Symptoms related to distant metastasis are occasionally present. The typical patient is obese, hypertensive, and diabetic. Uterine enlargement or infiltration and thickening of the cervix and adjacent pelvic structures should be identified if present.

Diagnosis and Screening

Routine Pap smears have only limited value in detecting endometrial cancer because of inadequate numbers of cells in the typical specimens. Endocervical and intrauterine aspirations improve the yield, but one must be prepared to perform endometrial biopsy or fractional curettage if the patient's history is suggestive and lesser procedures are negative. There has been considerable interest in the so-called jet washer and other endometrial sampling techniques (Koss *et al.,* 1981) which do not require formal biopsy for diagnosing endometrial cancer. False-negative results remain a problem (Richart *et al.,* 1979). Endometrial biopsy can be done as an office procedure, but the more definitive fractional dilatation and curettage requires anesthesia. A procedure such as fractional curettage with separate sampling of the cervix, endocervix, and uterine cavity is essential in evaluating cervical involvement; such involvement changes the stage, management, and prognosis. Sounding of the uterine cavity is done as part of the procedure in order to measure uterine size. Currently, screening of asymptomatic women with pelvic examination, Pap smears, and endometrial sampling has a low yield and high cost; more emphasis on obese patients who have used exogenous estrogens may improve the yield (Koss *et al.,* 1981; Lehman *et al.,* unpublished data). On the other hand, patients with abnormal bleeding must be evaluated in detail.

The risk of the diagnostic evaluation is largely confined to the potential for perforating the uterus during instrumentation, excessive bleeding from biopsy sites, and the risk of anesthesia. Discomfort and pain from manipulating and instrumenting the cervix are not a significant problem except perhaps in the screening situation, where such symptoms may deter some women from repeated screening.

Staging

Currently, endometrial carcinoma is staged by a combination of clinical findings, uterine sounding, and grade of histologic differentiation of tumor. The work-up must include appropriate tests to evaluate possible involvement of the bladder or rectum. Operative findings are not included although increasing interest has been expressed in surgical staging of selected patients. Table 34–7 shows the FIGO staging system; carcinoma *in situ* equals stage 0. In one study, 78% were stage I; 11%, stage II; 5%, stage III; and 6%, stage IV (Shingleton *et al.,* 1979).

As suggested earlier, pelvic examination for staging is frequently combined with a fractional D & C done under anesthesia. The uterine size, parametrial involvement, and

Table 34–7. FIGO Classification of Endometrial Carcinoma

Stage I   Confined to the corpus (G_1, G_2, G_3)
   IA   The length of the uterine cavity is 8 cm or less
   IB   The length of the uterine cavity is more than 8 cm
     G_1 (well differentiated)–G_3 (poorly differentiated)
Stage II   Involvement of corpus and cervix
Stage III   Extension outside corpus but not outside true pelvis
Stage IV   Involvement of bladder or rectum or extension outside pelvis

possible vaginal involvement are evaluated. Cystoscopy, barium enema, and proctoscopy are usually indicated. Hysterography has been advocated, and pelvic sonar scans, lymphangiograms, and isotope scans are useful in selected patients (Schwartz *et al.,* 1975). Blood counts, liver and kidney function tests, chest x-rays, and an intravenous pyelogram are all part of the preoperative evaluation.

In addition to the importance of histologic differentiation, findings on pelvic examination, and uterine size, three other factors have prognostic importance in the woman without distant metastases. These include the depth of myometrial invasion, presence or absence of tumor cells in peritoneal washings, and lymph node metastasis. All potentially influence selection of treatment. If the tumor extended to within 5 mm of the serosal surface of the uterus, the five-year survival was 65%, compared with 97% if the tumor was more than 10 mm from the serosa (Lutz *et al.,* 1978). A 15.5% incidence of a positive peritoneal cytology in clinical stage I cases was found (Creasman *et al.,* 1981). Of 13 patients with this finding, but no other evidence of cancer outside the uterus, six subsequently died of abdominal carcinomatosis. Morrow *et al.* (1973) and Creasman *et al.* (1976) have observed that about 11% of stage I cases have pelvic node metastases and that the majority of such patients failed to be cured despite the use of postoperative radiation. With higher grade or stage or deeper myometrial invasion, node metastases become more common (Creasman *et al.,* 1976). Thus, there has been a trend in recent years toward surgical staging coupled with primary surgical treatment for stage I cases, reserving radiation therapy for specific situations.

Treatment

Stage I. Several different approaches to treatment are currently advocated. If the tumor can be encompassed by a radiation port which permits adequate doses, many patients can be cured without surgery (thus providing an alternative for medically inoperable patients), but this approach in stage I is generally inferior to surgery alone. The possibility of improving results by combining surgery and irradiation has led to programs of preoperative intracavitary radiation and pre- or postoperative external radiation. A prospective trial in stage I was reported where all patients underwent a hysterectomy and bilateral salpingo-oophorectomy, followed by vaginal radium application (to reduce vaginal cuff recurrences (Aalders *et al.,* 1980). No specific evaluation of node involvement or peritoneal cytology was described. Then patients were randomly assigned to no further treatment or to 4000 rads of external pelvic radiation over four weeks. The group receiving external radiation had a statistically significant reduction in vaginal and pelvic recurrences (1.9 versus 6.9%), but developed more distant metastases than the control group. The net result was no survival advantage for the more extensively treated group (92% versus 89% at five years). Why this group had more distant metastases was unclear. The patients who benefited most from external therapy were those who had both a grade 3 lesion and deep myometrial invasion. Such patients had a reduction in vaginal and pelvic recurrences from 19.6 to 4.5% and a decrease in cancer deaths from 27.5 to 18.2%.

In stage I, grade 1, patients, preoperative internal or external radiation has not been shown to improve the excellent results (90 to 96% five-year survival) from surgery alone (Salazar *et al.,* 1978c; Glasburn, 1981; Lewis and Bundy, 1981). Moreover, vaginal cuff recurrence is sufficiently infrequent that vaginal radium treatment can be omitted (Prem *et al.,* 1979). Thus, most such patients can be treated with surgery alone.

Postoperative radiation is used if the operative findings are unfavorable. Radioactive phosphorus (^{32}P) has been advocated if the peritoneal cytology is positive. A reduction in recurrence rate from 38 to 13% was observed with intraperitoneal instillation of ^{32}P in a small historically controlled study (Creasman *et al.*, 1981). With deep myometrial invasion, cervical involvement, or extension outside the uterus or positive nodes, external pelvic radiation is used. If the para-aortic nodes are involved, para-aortic radiation is also advocated, despite the increased risk of complications from large treatment volumes.

With stage I, grades 2 and 3, surgical cure was achieved in 62 to 88% of cases in one report (Salazar *et al.*, 1978c). Preoperative radiotherapy may improve these results slightly (Salazar *et al.*, 1978c; Surwit *et al.*, 1981), although this approach has not been confirmed in a randomized study. As noted above (Aalders *et al.*, 1980), postoperative radiation did increase the cure rate in grade 3 cases and pathologic staging allows more individualized treatment based on the operative findings.

Patients with grade 2 or 3 lesions but no other unfavorable prognostic factors are usually treated postoperatively with vaginal "mold" irradiation that appears to reduce the vaginal cuff recurrence rate from 10 to 3% (Wade *et al.*, 1967; Graham, 1971). Survival is not clearly improved by treating this area, but the risk of such treatment is minimal, and vaginal recurrence can be troublesome.

Stage II. Since fewer than 15% of endometrial cancers are clinical stage II, randomized controlled therapeutic trials have been difficult to organize. Thus, most results of treatment in stage II have been evaluated historically. The cervical involvement may be occult or gross, superficial or invading the stroma of the cervix. In one series (Homesley *et al.*, 1977), when the only spread beyond the corpus was to the cervix, occult involvement was associated with a better survival (89%) than gross spread (57%). The incidence of nodal involvement in this series was similar in the two groups (21 versus 25%). The possibility of false-positive results (endometrial curettings thought to be cervical) was not, however, rigorously excluded. In one report, stromal invasion of the cervix reduced survival to 30 versus 67% without such invasion ($P < .05$) (Surwit *et al.*, 1978). In another series, a significant difference in survival between gross (56%) and microscopic (95%) involvement was observed (Kinsella *et al.*, 1980). The variation in results from series to series may relate in part to how the extent of involvement is defined. Kinsella *et al.* (1980) also found a failure rate with grade 3 histology of 42% compared with 6% in grade 1 and 5% in grade 2 ($P < .01$).

Preoperative external radiation plus intracavitary radiation followed by a total hysterectomy and salpingo-oophorectomy has yielded a 70 to 80% survival (Prem *et al.*, 1979; Kinsella *et al.*, 1980; Surwit *et al.*, 1981). The overall survival in stage II cases of only 51% (Morrow *et al.*, 1973) includes additional patients receiving only radiotherapy because of inoperability related to medical factors. The results with radiation alone are generally inferior to a combined approach. As with stage I, proponents suggest performing surgery first, with "tailored" radiation subsequently (Morrow *et al.*, 1973). This would allow more precise staging and may improve results in early stage disease since upstaged patients with a worse prognosis are not included in the analysis.

Stage III. By clinical staging, less than 10% of cases are in this category, and survival is in the range of 26 to 31%. Many institutions use intracavitary plus external radiation without surgery (Antoniades *et al.*, 1976). Clinical staging, however, does not account for three different subsets of patients with differing prognosis for whom different approaches may be needed. One group consists of those tumors that are stage clinical I or II, but with positive nodes. A second group has extrauterine disease limited to the ovary and/or tube. The third group presents with tumors spread beyond these organs to vagina, parametrium, peritoneum, or nodes. Relapse-free survival of 80% for the second group and 15% ($P = 0.01$) for the last has been reported (Bruckman *et al.*, 1980). Most patients in that series were treated with intracavitary radium, surgery, and postoperative external pelvic irradiation. These results suggest an even less favorable prognosis than generally quoted for stage III, but a much better prognosis in those stage III patients with only adnexal spread.

Stage IV. Only 5 to 6% of cases present as stage IV, and the cure rate is less than 10% (Beck, 1979). As with earlier stages, the existence of subsets of patients (involvement of bladder or rectum versus more distant spread) needs to be considered as well as the possibility that occasional patients in the former group can be salvaged by aggressive internal and external radiation and/or exenterative surgery. A standard treatment plan has not emerged for this relatively rare problem. Some institutions advocate chemotherapy or progestin therapy in such cases, but to date, there is no proof that such treatment is of use in the adjuvant setting in endometrial cancer. A recent report (Bokhman *et al.,* 1981) of improved survival using adjuvant progestins needs to be confirmed.

Distant Spread and Recurrent Disease

Recurrences in the pelvis should be evaluated for possible further surgical and/or radiotherapeutic approaches. When systemic treatment is indicated, progestins are the initial choice because of their favorable therapeutic index. The intramuscular preparations have been supplanted in some centers by megestrol acetate, a potent oral agent. Only 30% of patients show an objective response to progestins (Reifenstein, 1971) and in one series, only 16% of patients responded (Piver *et al.,* 1980). In general, responders have neoplasms that are better differentiated, but this is not necessarily the case, at least in regard to lung metastases (Ballon *et al.,* 1979). Following the recognition that some endometrial cancers have steroid hormone receptors, there has been a recent effort to select potential candidates for progestin therapy based on the presence of estrogen and progesterone receptors (Creasman *et al.,* 1980; Hunter *et al.,* 1980; Gurpide, 1981). Preliminary studies (Hunter *et al.,* 1980) indicate that 50 to 70% of patients are receptor positive, almost twice the response rate. Patients without receptors, however, are unlikely to respond (Creasman *et al.,* 1980). Correlation between tumor grade and receptor level in initial studies has been variable (Creasman *et al.,* 1980; Hunter *et al.,* 1980; Gurpide, 1981). Further progress in standardizing assays and larger scale clinicolaboratory correlations should define the role of receptor assays in planning treatment.

As with other endocrine-responsive cancers, a response to progestin therapy may be slow in onset. An observation period of at least two or three months is necessary before concluding that a patient is unresponsive. Occasional responses have been quite prolonged, and in one series, the average response duration was 20 months (Reifenstein, 1971). In preliminary studies, the antiestrogen, tamoxifen, has been effective after an initial progesterone response (Bonte *et al.,* 1981).

Very few cytotoxic agents have been systematically evaluated in endometrial cancer. This is, in part, the result of the long tradition of progestin therapy which has spanned most of the modern chemotherapy era. Furthermore, such patients are frequently elderly and have a poor performance status, so many drugs have not been evaluated in this disease. The previous custom of conducting broad phase II trials of new drugs meant that most gynecologic cancers were not systematically evaluated. Of those drugs that have been studied, doxorubicin appears to be most active [11 CR + 5 PR of 32 patients (37%) treated with 60 mg/m² every three weeks] (Thigpen *et al.,* 1979). Cumulative experience with cyclophosphamide (7/33) and 5-FU (10/43) (DeVita *et al.,* 1976) implies some activity for those drugs as well.

A randomized trial conducted by the GOG compared 5-FU, megestrol, doxorubicin, and cyclophosphamide versus 5 FU, megestrol, and melphalan. Both regimens produced objective responses in 37% of cases, but the melphalan combination that was administered at a relatively high dose caused more severe marrow toxicity (Cohen *et al.,* 1984). Thus, initial reports of 15/20 responses to doxorubicin, cyclophosphamide, 5-FU, plus megestrol (Bruckner and Deppe, 1977) and 14/15 responses to melphalan, 5-FU, plus megestrol (Cohen *et al.,* 1977) were not confirmed. It is still not clear whether combination regimens are superior to doxorubicin alone, and a randomized study of doxorubicin with or without cyclophosphamide is being conducted by the GOG. The need for such a study is supported by a phase II study in which doxorubicin plus cyclophosphamide yielded only 31% partial responses (Seski *et al.,* 1981).

High-dose cisplatin therapy may also have some activity in this cancer; Deppe *et al.* (1980b) observed responses in 4/13 patients who had failed to respond to other drug regimens. Seski *et al.* (1982) also found this drug to be active. When administering 50 mg/m² every three weeks, however, the GOG observed only 1/25 responses (Thigpen *et al.,* 1981b).

Follow-up

Since almost 90% of recurrences are apparent within the first three years (Wade *et al.,* 1967), and since half involve pelvic structures, close follow-up with periodic pelvic examinations is appropriate during this period, especially in those with unfavorable prognostic factors. Particular attention is paid to the possibility of vaginal cuff recurrence. The most cost-effective approach has not been defined. A recent GOG protocol for high-risk stage I patients has employed clinical follow-up every three months for the first three years and then every six months. A chest x-ray and intravenous pyelogram is obtained every six months for two years and then yearly.

Prospects for the Future

Although screening for this type of cancer has serious limitations, further education of women and family physicians about the importance of evaluating postmenopausal bleeding should increase the percentage of cases diagnosed at stage I. Tailoring therapy to subsets of patients with different prognostic factors should improve results while reducing complications. Although there have been efforts to conduct randomized studies of surgery and/or irradiation in endometrial cancer, they are difficult to execute because of the considerable success already achieved in stage I and the paucity of more advanced cases. A clearer definition of what can be accomplished with irradiation when the nodes are involved could increase the salvage rate in such cases. The adjunctive role of radiation sensitizers such as misonidazole needs to be evaluated. The role of chemotherapy, both in advanced disease and as an adjunct in early stage high-risk patients, is just beginning to be evaluated. If hormone receptor status can identify those patients who will not benefit from progestins, these patients can be entered into first-line chemotherapy trials, rather than waiting until they have failed hormonal therapy, at which point their performance status is likely to have deteriorated, and a response to any therapy is unlikely. At the same time, if those who are highly responsive to progestins can be accurately identified, further study of the adjunctive role of progestins may be indicated.

UTERINE SARCOMAS

These cancers, although differing among themselves, are sufficiently different in clinical behavior, prognosis, and treatment from endometrial carcinoma that they require separate discussion. Sarcomas are said to comprise from 5 to 10% of corpus cancers (Salazar *et al.*, 1978a; Shingleton *et al.*, 1979). The relative incidence of the four major types is better defined. Salazar *et al.* (1978a) found mixed mesodermal sarcomas to comprise 60%, leiomyosarcoma 28%, endometrial stromal sarcoma 8%, and others 4% of cases. The GOG experi-

ence has been similar, with mixed mesodermal sarcomas equally divided between heterologous and homologous types. This distribution is different from that of Vardi and Tovell (1980) who stated that 50 to 70% are leiomyosarcoma. A review of 147 cases at a single referral center found 48% to be leiomyosarcoma, 20% stromal sarcoma, and 16% homologous mixed mesodermal tumors (Badib *et al.*, 1969). Of stage I and II cases, the distribution reported subsequently from the same institution (Vongtama *et al.*, 1976) was 22/104 leiomyosarcoma, 25/104 stromal sarcoma, 30/104 heterologous, 27/104 heterologous, and 27/104 homologous mixed mesodermal sarcomas. Varying criteria for diagnosis for leiomyosarcoma versus cellular leiomyoma (Silverberg, 1971; Christopherson *et al.*, 1972) and varying referral patterns for different subtypes may explain these differences.

Epidemiology and Etiology

The median age was 60 years (range, 27 to 84) (Omura *et al.*, 1983a); in some series, the median age for leiomyosarcoma is a decade younger than for other cell types. Previous therapeutic radiation is frequently mentioned as a causative factor in bone and soft tissue sarcomas. If that is true, many women who have previously had pelvic radiotherapy without hysterectomy primarily for cervix cancer are at risk. A small population irradiated for benign disease might also be at risk. Norris and Taylor (1965) note a history of prior radiation exposure in uterine sarcomas in 12% of cases, but Silverberg (1971) notes that less than 5% of leiomyosarcoma cases have such a history. In fact, a review of the literature (Messerschmidt *et al.*, 1981) suggests no significant increase in such lesions. Patients with a prior history of cancer were excluded from the GOG studies, so no relevant information is available from that source. As noted in the section on cervical cancer, such patients are more likely to have vaginal cancer secondary to the so called "field effect."

Malignant degeneration of myomas has been thought to be a source of leiomyosarcoma. Although the likelihood of such change is low, Silverberg (1971) observed that 11 of 34 leiomyosarcomas originated in a benign myoma. Endogenous or exogenous estrogen exposure does not appear to play a role in the genesis of uterine sarcomas, but it is of interest that premenopausal patients with leiomyosarcoma, and without vascular invasion, appear to have a better prognosis than postmenopausal patients (Silverberg, 1971).

Pathology and Natural History

As with other soft tissue sarcomas, the pathologic classification of the uterine sarcomas is complex (Ober, 1959) and subject to dispute. The classification developed by the GOG is based upon whether the derivation of the sarcoma is primarily from uterine smooth muscle, or from the glands and stroma. Leiomyosarcoma, endometrial stromal sarcoma, and mixed mesodermal tumors are the major histologic types; the latter are further subclassified as homologous (carcinosarcoma), if all the elements in the tumor have normal counterparts in the uterus, and heterologous if they do not (for example, cartilage or striated muscle). A variety of other types of sarcomas, such as rhabdomyosarcoma and lymphoma, are reported with a much lower frequency.

It should be mentioned that leiomyosarcoma must be differentiated from cellular leiomyoma and bizarre leiomyoma (Christopherson et al., 1972), as well as the entity of benign metastasizing leiomyoma (Banner et al., 1981). Endometrial stromal sarcoma must be distinguished from endolymphatic stromal myosis (Yoonessi and Hart, 1977).

Vascular invasion and early spread to distant sites, especially the lungs, are common. Spread within the pelvis is also prominent, as evidenced by many cases with local extension or pelvic recurrence. One study indicated that 36% of mixed mesodermal tumors presented with involved pelvic nodes (DiSaia et al., 1973). A prospective GOG study of stage I and II sarcoma is comparing the pattern of recurrence in leiomyosarcomas compared with mixed mesodermal sarcomas; of 44 leiomyosarcomas, 16 (36%) have recurred, with 10/16 (63%) developing pulmonary metastases. Of 88 mixed mesodermal sarcomas, 35 (40%) have recurred, with 16/35 (46%) involving pelvis or vagina, and only 11/35 (31%) recurring in the lungs (Omura et al., personal communication).

Signs and Symptoms

Salazar et al. (1978a) reported that 86% of patients presented with abnormal vaginal bleeding, 19% with abdominal pain, and 15% with an abdominal mass. In another series of leiomyosarcomas, 59% had bleeding, and 38% had abdominal distention or a mass (Vardi and Tovell, 1980). In mixed mesodermal sarcomas postmenopausal bleeding was prominent, but abdominal pain was uncommon (DiSaia et al., 1973). All seven patients with stromal sarcoma reported by Yoonessi and Hart (1977) presented with abnormal vaginal bleeding.

In addition to bleeding, some patients present with a friable polypoid mass protruding from the cervix. An enlarged irregular uterus is common and frequently may mimic uterine fibroids, which is not surprising since leiomyosarcoma may be found within a fibroid (Silverberg, 1971). A rapidly enlarging uterus is sometimes noted, and with more advanced disease, involvement of other pelvic structures and/or distant sites may be apparent.

Diagnosis

If tumor fragments are present on vaginal examination, these should be examined histologically, but endometrial biopsy or dilatation and curettage is usually required. In some cases, especially if a lesion is submucosal or within a benign fibroid, a definite preoperative diagnosis may not be possible. No effective screening techniques are available.

Staging

No official staging system for uterine sarcomas is available, but most centers use a modification of the endometrial carcinoma staging. Grade of tumor is not included in the criteria for stage I. Prognostic value regarding the size of the uterine cavity is not clear. Prompted by the previous observation that pelvic and aortic node involvement in stage I and II cases was relatively common (DiSaia et al., 1973), the GOG is currently conducting a study of surgical staging of uterine sarcomas. Better definition of pelvic spread patterns should allow better pelvic control of disease. Careful radiographic evaluation of the chest for evidence of lung metastases is indicated.

Treatment

Total abdominal hysterectomy and salpingo-oophorectomy should be done unless the patient is medically inoperable or has obvious metastatic disease. The value of pelvic lymphadenectomy as a therapeutic endeavor is unclear. Adjunctive pelvic radiation may improve local control (Salazar *et al.,* 1978b) but this has not been proven. Badib *et al.* (1969) retrospectively reported improvement in survival (from 50 to 81%) in stage I cases with adjunctive radiotherapy. It is of interest that 4 of 9 stage I patients treated with radiation alone (one in each cell type) survived, indicating that some of these tumors may be radio-responsive and may benefit from radiation if the entire extent of the disease can be encompassed. Badib's findings were supported by Gilbert *et al.* (1975) and by DiSaia *et al.* (1973) for mixed mesodermal tumors, but not for leiomyosarcoma. Vongtama *et al.* (1976) expanded on the series reported by Badib and concluded that radiotherapy was of adjunctive value in stage I in the major cell types except leiomyosarcoma. The current GOG experience, mentioned above, shows a higher rate of pulmonary recurrences in leiomyosarcoma and helps to explain why pelvic radiotherapy does not improve survival in such patients. Clearly, controlled trials of adjunctive radiation in early stage mixed mesodermal tumors are needed.

When adjusted for stage, the prognosis for the different cell types is similar, with five-year survival in stage I of 50% for mixed mesodermal sarcomas, 56% for leiomyosarcoma, and 55% for stromal sarcomas. Eleven percent of cases more advanced than stage I survive five years, independent of cell type (Salazar *et al.,* 1978a).

Chemotherapy of Uterine Sarcomas

For some years, the assumption was made that success in treating soft tissue sarcomas in children could be extrapolated to adults. It is now clear that adults must be evaluated and studied independently. Another common assumption is that most soft tissue sarcomas have similar response rates to doxorubicin combinations. Recent GOG experience suggests that this may not apply to all uterine sarcomas. According to the literature, the response rate for most adult soft tissue sarcomas is about 27% using doxorubicin alone and in the range of 45 to 68% for combinations including this drug (Blum *et al.,* 1980; Rivkin *et al.,* 1980; Yap *et al.,* 1980). Few controlled trials in soft tissue sarcomas have been made. Rosenbaum and Schoenfield (1977) found that doxorubicin alone at 70 mg/m^2 per dose

was more effective than doxorubicin at 50 mg/m^2 plus cytoxan plus vincristine or vincristine plus actinomycin plus cytoxan (VAC). No responses to methyl CCNU among 11 cases were found and no responses in 17 patients treated with doxorubicin or actinomycin combinations (Creagan *et al.,* 1976). Only a 13.5% response rate was observed using vincristine, actinomycin, cyclophosphamide, doxorubicin, and methotrexate in soft tissue sarcomas (Bryant and Wiltshaw, 1980). Leiomyosarcomas arising from various sites appear to be at least as responsive (32%) as the entire group of soft tissue sarcomas (27%) to doxorubicin (Pinedo and Kenis, 1977). DTIC alone (Pinedo and Kenis, 1977) seemed more effective in leiomyosarcomas (6/24 or 25%) than in the general group of soft tissue sarcomas (16%). A complete response in three of six uterine leiomyosarcomas treated with doxorubicin plus DTIC plus vincristine was reported (Aziza *et al.,* 1979).

The role of cisplatin in treatment of sarcomas is unclear. Karakousis *et al.* (1979) reported two complete remissions and one partial remission among 13 metastatic sarcomas, but Sampson *et al.* (1979) observed only one partial remission among 16 leiomyosarcomas. Bramwell *et al.* (1979) reported no responses in 17 sarcoma patients, including three leiomyosarcomas. All of these patients had had extensive prior treatment.

High-dose methotrexate achieved only one response in 18 patients with soft tissue sarcomas (Karakousis *et al.,* 1980). Fluorouracil has not been systematically evaluated in recent years, although Malkasian *et al.* (1967) reported responses in gynecologic sarcomas. One of seven leiomyosarcomas had a partial response to hexamethylmelamine (Borden *et al.,* 1977).

Although most reports have indicated similar response rates for various types of sarcomas, mixed mesodermal sarcomas are seldom separately identified in these reports. A recent study by the GOG (Omura *et al.,* 1983a) compared doxorubicin with or without DTIC in advanced or recurrent uterine sarcomas. Of 85 patients with measurable disease treated with doxorubicin alone, 5 (5.9%) had a complete response, and 10 (11.8%) had a partial response. Of 70 patients with measurable disease randomized to doxorubicin plus DTIC, 7 (10%) had a complete response, and 10 (14.3%) had a partial response. These results were not significantly different. When the individual cell types were examined, the response rate (CR + PR) for leiomyosarcoma was 27% for one drug and 29% for both drugs. In the case of homologous mixed mesodermal tumors, both regimens produced only a 9% response rate. In the category of heterologous tumors, doxorubicin alone produced a response in 2 of 22 patients (9%), compared with 6 out of 22 (29%) for the combination. These differences were not significant, but the combination regimen produced significantly more gastrointestinal and hematologic toxicity. Lung metastases responded more frequently to combination therapy (8 responses of 21 cases, compared with 2 responses of 20 cases, $P = 0.04$), but there was no survival advantage in this group. The apparent advantage of the combination in treating lung metastases must be tempered by the observation that equally toxic dose regimens were not evaluated. Leiomyosarcomas had a significantly longer survival than other cell types (12.4 months versus 6 months), regardless of the regimen. The results in leiomyosarcoma are similar to what has previously been described for doxorubicin alone. The most striking observation was the very poor results in mixed mesodermal tumors: 11/77 (14%) responses.

The combination of vincristine plus actinomycin plus cyclophosphamide (VAC), previously popular for the treatment of soft tissue sarcomas, was evaluated in 41 patients with uterine sarcomas after failing doxorubicin with or without DTIC; there were no responses in that group (Omura et al., 1983a). New agents will be needed if further progress is to be made in the management of uterine sarcomas.

Finally, since early stage patients are at substantial risk of recurrence after initial surgery, a prospective randomized trial is being conducted by the GOG which is evaluating adjuvant doxorubicin against no further treatment. Although no conclusions can be drawn as yet, a striking improvement in relapse-free survival is not apparent. This is not surprising given the rather modest level of activity of doxorubicin in advanced disease.

GESTATIONAL TROPHOBLASTIC NEOPLASIA

Incidence and Epidemiology

The term gestational trophoblastic neoplasia (GTN) encompasses hydatidiform mole,

invasive mole (chorioadenoma destruens), and gestational choriocarcinoma. These are tumors of placental tissues. They represent the first type of cancer cured with chemotherapy and provide a model for the successful interdisciplinary management of cancer employing several modes of treatment, as well as a sensitive marker for detection of minimal residual disease. Remarkable responsiveness to several drugs was needed to optimize results. These elements properly employed produce a high cure rate, even in the face of widespread metastasis.

In the United States, the reported incidence of hydatidiform mole ranges from 1 in 1000 to 1 in 2000 pregnancies. In other parts of the world, however, especially southeast Asia, a tenfold greater incidence has been reported (Teoh et al., 1971). Higher incidence has been associated with low socioeconomic status and/ or poor nutrition. The incidence of gestational choriocarcinoma is 10 to 20 times less than that of mole.

Most patients with moles are in the 20 to 29-year-old group, paralleling the high frequency of pregnancy in this group. The risk is significantly increased (fourfold) in pregnant women over age 39 (Bagshawe, 1976).

Etiology and Pathogenesis

The cause is unknown, but as already suggested, gestational trophoblastic neoplasia is associated with pregnancy (normal, ectopic, aborted, or molar pregnancy). GTN may not be recognized for months or even years after the pregnancy. Most (80 to 85%) patients with a hydatidiform mole will have a spontaneous and permanent regression of the process after evacuation of the mole. This suggests either a low level of neoplastic potential, or that host factors are important in its control. Trophoblastic cells derived from the blastocyst stage of the embryo have both paternal and maternal genes. It has been assumed that the same is true of GTN and that it could be regarded as an allogeneic graft (Tomoda et al., 1976). This cannot be proven because HLA antigens are not generally expressed in trophoblastic cells or choriocarcinoma cells (Jones and Bodner, 1980). This may, however, merely be a reflection of in vitro resistance of trophoblast cells to lymphocyte-mediated cytotoxicity, possibly because of a surface coating of acid mucoprotein (August et al., 1979).

Recent evidence suggests that moles originate in most cases from fertilization by a haploid sperm with loss of the maternal nuclear component. Three choriocarcinoma cases studied by Wake *et al.* (1981) showed heterozygosity, suggesting a lack of common lineage with moles and thus that choriocarcinoma does not actually arise from a preceding molar pregnancy. They suggest that defective ova may be the basis of both choriocarcinoma and preceding moles. In addition, in moles, the duplication of a paternal haploid set appears to contribute to pathogenesis (Wake *et al.*, 1981).

Pathology and Natural History

A mole classically has the gross appearance of a cluster of small grapes, which represent numerous dilated chorionic villi. Microscopically, cytotrophoblast and syncytiotrophoblast are seen in varying proportions. "Hydropic" swelling and absence of blood vessels are also present. Invasive mole is diagnosed when the villous structure is maintained, but the tumor invades myometrial blood vessels or dissects between muscle bundles. Choriocarcinoma is apt to be grossly hemorrhagic, friable, and necrotic. Microscopically, there are interlacing strands of cytotrophoblast and syncytiotrophoblast but a loss of the villous structures (Gore and Hertig, 1976).

In one series of 38 patients with metastatic trophoblastic disease, 50% had lung involvement, 26% had spread in the pelvis, 16% had liver involvement, 13% brain metastases, and 8% had vaginal metastases (Goldstein, 1972).

Signs and Symptoms

In a mole, the initial manifestations are usually those of a pregnancy. As the process evolves, abnormal uterine bleeding, excessive uterine size, early toxemia of pregnancy, absent fetal heart sounds, and absence of a fetal skeleton are very suggestive of the diagnosis. Hyperthyroidism from thyrotropin production by the trophoblastic cells has been described (Hershman, 1972). Trophoblastic pulmonary embolism has also been reported (Twigs *et al.*, 1979; Orr *et al.*, 1980; Smith *et al.*, 1981).

Theca lutein cysts of the ovaries may be present temporarily, secondary to stimulation by HCG. Passage of molar tissue is common and may be available for histologic examination. Metastatic disease may be asymptomatic or may produce signs and symptoms related to the particular site of metastasis. On occasion, a "stroke" from a hemorrhagic cerebral lesion is the presenting manifestation (Gurwitt *et al.*, 1975).

Diagnosis and Staging

Hydatidiform Mole. A patient who is initially thought to be pregnant but who has vaginal bleeding, an excessive elevation of HCG, and/or uterine enlargement excessive for the duration of the pregnancy (especially in association with bilateral ovarian enlargement) may be suspected of having a mole. Sonar scanning produces a characteristic echo pattern giving the appearance of a snow storm (Fleischer *et al.*, 1978). Radio-opaque contrast material can be injected into the uterus and produces a honeycomb pattern on x-ray. If molar tissue has been passed, it should be examined histologically.

The great majority (80%) of moles (Curry *et al.*, 1975) will regress spontaneously after evacuation, usually by suction curettage. Weekly HCG titers are followed for six to eight weeks with the expectation that the titer will rapidly normalize in two months and remain normal over the next year. If the titer plateaus or rises, chemotherapy is indicated (Schlaerth *et al.*, 1981). Evidence of metastatic disease is also an indication for treatment. If choriocarcinoma is identified in the curettage material, spontaneous regression is unlikely, so treatment is initiated, as in the case of persistent disease.

Persistent Disease. After evacuation of a mole, older patients, those with ovarian enlargement, "large-for-date" uteri, or transient pulmonary symptoms (Twigs *et al.*, 1979; Orr *et al.*, 1980) are more likely to have persistent disease. It has been reported that "partial" moles (associated with a fetus, cord, and/or amniotic membrane) (Jones, 1981) do not give rise to persistent disease, whereas "complete" moles, lacking those features but showing marked trophoblastic hyperplasia and anaplasia, are associated with a risk of sequelae. From a practical management standpoint, the distinction to be made is between metastatic versus nonmetastatic (confined to the uterus) trophoblastic disease, and between good prognosis (low risk) versus poor prognosis (high risk) cases (Hammond *et al.*, 1973). These considerations are more important in management than a pathologic classification into mole, invasive mole, or choriocarcinoma, although histologic distinctions are still of note

(Deligdisch *et al.*, 1978). A recent addition to the list of high-risk factors is an antecedent term pregnancy; such cases are more likely to present with other poor prognostic factors, but seem to have an additional risk, perhaps related to impaired host immunity (Miller *et al.*, 1979).

The history of a prior mole is not always obvious, and the patient may present without gynecologic complaints and without pelvic abnormalities. A history of a previous ectopic or term pregnancy, or irregular vaginal bleeding in conjunction with pulmonary, hepatic, or brain lesions, should always prompt the measurement of an HCG titer. Work-up should include history, physical and pelvic examinations, chest x-ray, intravenous pyelogram, scans of the head and liver, hepatic and renal function tests, and an HCG.

In patients with persistent HCG elevation, but no obvious site of disease, pelvic arteriography may be helpful. Recently, the use of radiolabeled antibody to HCG has been used on an investigational basis to localize disease that could not otherwise be detected (Hatch *et al.*, 1980a).

HCG

A major deficiency in the follow-up of most types of cancer is the inability to detect accurately minimal residual disease. In trophoblastic disease, however, the serial measurement of human chorionic gonadotropin allows the detection of minute amounts of residual tumor. In general, there appears to be a direct relationship between the HCG level and the amount of tumor present. Previous assays did not distinguish between HCG and pituitary luteinizing hormone, but the beta subunit assay (Vaitukaitis *et al.*, 1972) generally does. It has been estimated that normal trophoblastic tissue secretes 1.4×10^{-2} IU of HCG per cell per day and that a choriocarcinoma produces 5×10^{-5} IU per cell per day (Braunstein *et al.*, 1973). No more than 10,000 cells (approximately 10 μg of tumor) are required to give a positive result (Surwit and Hammond, 1980). Pregnancy tests are not sufficiently sensitive to properly manage trophoblastic disease.

In general, after three weekly negative serum beta-HCG titers, a permanent remission is seen, but occasional recurrences in the first year do occur, and late relapses have rarely been described (McComb and Yuen, 1980; Vaughn *et al.*, 1980). Assay of the alpha subunit of HCG may be a useful adjunct in identifying patients who are prone to recurrence and require more intensive follow-up after apparently successful treatment (Quigley *et al.*, 1980).

Urinary HCG determinations have been largely supplanted by serum determinations for routine management. Wehmann *et al.* (1981) report, however, that a highly sensitive assay for urinary HCG extracted from 24-hour urine collections improves the ability to detect persistent disease in certain patients whose serum titers have become undetectable.

In the radioimmunoassay for beta-HCG, cross-reactivity between beta-HCG and pituitary LH is not ordinarily found, but cross-reactivity with high levels of LH has been reported and is a potential source of a false-positive error in the follow-up of oophorectomized patients with choriocarcinoma (Hatch *et al.*, 1980c). Other types of cancer sometimes secrete HCG (Braunstein *et al.*, 1973). In fact, a case has recently been seen (Hatch *et al.*, 1980b) in which a patient cured of trophoblastic disease appeared to have a late relapse, but actually had developed a second neoplasm, an HCG-secreting lung cancer.

Treatment

The early history in recognizing the value of chemotherapy for trophoblastic disease has been reviewed by Li (1979). In general, current management is so successful that innovations in treatment must be made with great care, lest any compromise in the cure rate occur. Nevertheless, high-risk groups of patients in whom therapy is not routinely successful and progress in treatment is needed have been identified. In addition, simplifying treatment schedules and reducing toxicity wherever possible are needed.

Prophylactic Chemotherapy. This approach has sometimes been advocated after evacuation of a mole, especially where appropriate follow-up cannot be assured. It is not recommended for routine use in view of the small percentage of patients who actually require chemotherapy and the risk of toxicity.

Nonmetastatic Trophoblastic Disease. If persistent nonmetastatic disease is diagnosed and no further childbearing is planned, hysterectomy in conjunction with the first course of single-agent chemotherapy (methotrexate or actinomycin D) should be curative and appears to reduce the duration and total dose of chemotherapy required (Hammond *et al.,* 1980). Careful follow-up is indicated, however.

If reproductive potential is to be preserved and if renal and hepatic function are normal, repeated courses of methotrexate can be used. Previously, 15 to 25 mg of methotrexate as a single daily dose for five days was employed. This often produced marrow toxicity and stomatitis. More recently, Berkowitz and Goldstein (1979) and Hammond *et al.* (1980) have used 1 mg/kg of methotrexate intramuscularly on days 1, 3, 5, and 7, with citrovorum factor 0.1 mg/kg intramuscularly on days 2, 4, 6, and 8. This regimen is repeated at seven-day intervals as long as the titer is elevated. They report that toxicity is markedly reduced if the schedule is followed carefully. If the response to methotrexate is incomplete, actinomycin D 10 to 13 μg/kg daily for five days can be used. If toxicity is not excessive, courses are repeated at 14-day intervals after a seven-day rest period. It is unclear whether these dose schedules and cycle times are optimal, but they have been highly successful.

In one series of 122 patients treated primarily with chemotherapy, 106 (87%) achieved cure with chemotherapy alone (Hammond *et al.,* 1980), while only 16 required secondary treatment (pelvic infusion chemotherapy and/ or hysterectomy). Some patients need multiple courses of the initial drug regimen, and occasional neoplasms demonstrate resistance to the first agent and require alternate chemotherapy before being cured.

Using methotrexate plus citrovorum factor, 36 of 41 patients (88%) required only one course of treatment, while one patient was not cured until actinomycin was given. If the titer fell progressively, further treatment was delayed. A tenfold decrease of the titer within 18 days indicated additional therapy was not needed (Berkowitz and Goldstein, 1979).

Metastatic Disease (Good Prognosis). These patients were treated initially with a single drug as described above. Of 40 patients, 35 (88%) achieved remission with chemotherapy alone, whereas five subsequently required hysterectomy (Hammond *et al.,* 1980). Three patients (5.4%) had a relapse and were successfully retreated with chemotherapy. Even though the titer may rapidly normalize, pul-

monary lesions may take months to disappear. Thus, if serial titers indicate sustained remission, additional courses or surgical intervention can be deferred while the evolution of the case is observed. The ultimate cure rate in good-prognosis metastatic disease should be 100%, but requires a flexible approach and careful follow-up.

Metastatic Disease (High Risk). This group of patients (see Table 34 – 8) continues to be a therapeutic challenge. Triple therapy (actinomycin plus methotrexate plus an alkylating agent, either cyclophosphamide or chlorambucil) has been advocated for a number of years, having initially been proposed by Li (1979) for testicular cancer. Of 34 patients treated by Hammond's group, 20 (59%) achieved remission with combination chemotherapy. Some of these patients also received cerebral or hepatic radiation. Of the other 14, 11 required subsequent surgery for resistant foci of disease. Another 29 patients had surgery initially as part of a combined treatment program. Of the total of 40 patients operated on, 22 (55%) achieved remission, while 18 died. Considering all cases, 42 of 63 (67%) achieved remission. The majority of this group responded to additional treatment; 21% subsequently relapsed. More recently, the remission rate for poor-prognosis patients at the Southeastern Trophoblastic Disease Center has approached 90% (Hammond *et al.,* 1980). In some cases, a more elaborate multiagent regimen or vinblastine plus bleomycin plus cisplatin has been used (Surwit and Hammond, 1980). It is unclear whether these regimens have advantages over the MAC regimen, but more effective regimens should be developed. In particular, in a case where a patient has

Table 34 – 8. Metastatic Trophoblastic Disease

Good prognosis (low risk)
Duration less than 4 months
Low serum HCG titer (after curettage): less than 40,000 milli IU per mL
No liver or brain involvement
Poor prognosis (high risk)
Long duration of symptoms
High titer
Brain or liver metastasis
Unsuccessful prior chemotherapy
Antecedent term gestation

Adapted from Hammond, C.; Borchert, L.; Tyrey, L.; Creasman, W. T.; and Parker, R. T.: Treatment of metastatic trophoblastic disease: Good and poor prognosis. *Am. J. Obstet. Gynecol.,* **115:**451–457, 1973.

already failed single-agent treatment with actinomycin or methotrexate, using that agent in combination again must be questioned.

In addition to actinomycin, methotrexate and mustard-type alkylating agents, vinblastine, vincristine, mercaptopurine, doxorubicin, cisplatin, VP-16, and diazo-oxo-norleucine (DON) have had some activity as single agents (Bagshawe, 1969; Jones, 1981; Willson *et al.,* 1981), but definitive response rates have not been established. Given the high level of success with current regimens, it is difficult to evaluate new agents except as third- or fourth-line treatments. It is possible that drug screening against choriocarcinoma transplanted to nude mice (Hayashi *et al.,* 1978) may be helpful in developing new regimens.

Brain involvement is a serious but not hopeless complication. Weed and Hammond (1980) reported 14 patients with brain metastases; all had prior or concurrent pulmonary metastases; 4 presented without any neurologic signs or symptoms. Whole-brain radiation in doses up to 3000 rads in ten days was given along with triple chemotherapy. Seven patients (50%) were cured. Four of the patients also had craniotomies for removal of tumor. Of these, three survived. Thus, four had brain metastases cured without surgery. Bagshawe's experience with treating brain metastases was less favorable (9 cures among 41 patients). Of 20 patients who developed brain metastases during treatment, none survived (Bagshawe and Harland, 1976).

Tashima *et al.,* (1965) and Bagshawe and Harland (1976) advocated the measurement of spinal fluid HCG titers, but Weed and Hammond (1980) and Berkowitz *et al.* (1981b) did not find this to be of consistent help diagnostically. The value of intrathecal chemotherapy is unclear (Surwit and Hammond, 1980).

Liver involvement has been associated with a poor prognosis in the Duke experience. Only 15% of such patients survive. When this hepatic involvement is diagnosed, 2000 rads in ten days to the whole liver is recommended, along with triple chemotherapy. Recently, selective hepatic artery occlusion has been advocated (Grumbine *et al.,* 1980), but its value is unclear.

In view of the relatively high recurrence rate (21%) in patients with high-risk metastatic disease, additional courses of chemotherapy after the HGC titer has normalized are advocated by most groups. The optimal number of additional treatments has not been determined, but two extra courses are probably sufficient.

Rehabilitation

Gestational trophoblastic disease is notable for its high degree of curability, the preservation of reproductive function in most patients, and the avoidance of complications of cancer and cancer chemotherapy. Thus, rehabilitation is complete in most patients. Follow-up of subsequent pregnancies has indicated no increase in fetal wastage, congenital abnormalities, complicated pregnancies, or an increased incidence of other cancers (Lewis, 1980).

Follow-up

As indicated, serial HCG titers are a critical part of follow-up of trophoblastic disease. As with any laboratory test, the HCG determination is subject to error, so that isolated titers that are unexpectedly high or low should be repeated before changing current management. After evacuation of a mole and spontaneous remission demonstrated by three normal weekly titers, clinical follow-up and additional titers should be done every two months for the next year. During this time, contraception should be practiced, since a new pregnancy would confuse the follow-up. Oral contraceptives appear to be safe for this purpose (Berkowitz *et al.,* 1981a). A similar plan is used after chemotherapy of nonmetastatic disease, but an additional one or two years of follow-up with titers every four to six months is appropriate in view of the rare instances of late recurrence (Vaughn *et al.,* 1980). In patients with metastatic disease, some centers have obtained six-month titers indefinitely after the first year of remission (Surwit and Hammond, 1980). Periodic chest x-rays, physical and pelvic examinations, and assessment of known metastatic sites should be done along with the titers. As noted above, the clinician should be aware that nonviable mass lesions sometimes take months to disappear.

Future Prospects

Lewis (1980) mentions the treatment of resistant disease and brain and liver metastases, etiologic studies, immunobiologic advances, new HCG assays, and further evaluation of long-term effects of combination chemotherapy as areas for future study and additional progress. In addition, the optimal drug use and selection of multidrug regimens that have largely been on a empiric basis can be clinically evaluated.

REFERENCES

Aalders, J.; Abeler, V.; Kolstad, P.; and Onsrud, M: Postoperative external irradiation and prognostic parameters in stage I endometrial carcinoma, clinical and histopathologic study of 540 patients. *Obstet. Gynecol.,* **56:**419–426, 1980.

Alberts, D.; Chen, H.; Salmon, S.; Surwit, E.; Young, L.; Moon, T.; and Meyskens, F.: Chemotherapy of ovarian cancer directed by the human tumor stem cell assay. *Cancer Chemother. Pharmacol.* **6:**279–285, 1981.

Alberts, D.; Moon, T.; Stephens, R.; Willson, H.; Oishi, N.; Hilgers, R.; O'Toole, R.; and Thigpen, T.: Randomized study of chemoimmunotherapy for advanced ovarian carcinoma: A preliminary report of a Southwest Oncology Group Study. *Cancer Treat. Rep.* **63:**325–331, 1979.

American Cancer Society: Cancer of the cervix. *CA,* **30:**215–223, 1980.

American Cancer Society, Connecticut Division: *Cytology Services in Connecticut, 1970–1974.* American Cancer Society, Woodbridge, Connecticut, 1976.

Antoniades, J.; Brady, L.; and Lewis, G.: The management of stage III carcinoma of the endometrium. *Cancer,* **38:**1838–1842, 1976.

August, C.; Cox, S.; and Naughton, M.: Interaction of choriocarcinoma cells and human peripheral blood lymphocytes, resistance of cultured choriocarcinoma cells to cell mediated cytotoxicity by mitogen activated lymphocytes. *J. Clin. Invest.,* **63:**428–436, 1979.

Austin, J. M.: The abnormal Pap smear and its evaluation — The modern approach. *J. Med. Assoc. State Ala.,* **44:**417–419, 1975.

Aziza, F.; Bitran, J.; Javehari, G.; and Herbst, A. L.: Remission of uterine leiomyosarcomas treated with vincristine, adriamycin and dimethyl triazeno imidazole carboxamide. *Am. J. Obstet. Gynecol.,* **133:**379–381, 1979.

Badib, A.; Vongtama, V.; Kurohara, S.; and Webster, J.: Radiotherapy in the treatment of sarcomas of the corpus uteri. *Cancer,* **24:**724–729, 1969.

Bagshawe, K.: *Choriocarcinoma.* The Williams & Wilkins Company, Baltimore, 1969.

Bagshawe, K.: Risk and prognostic factors in trophoblastic neoplasia. *Cancer,* **38:**1373–1385, 1976.

Bagshawe, K. D., and Harland, S.: Immunodiagnosis and monitoring of gonadotropin-producing metastases in the central nervous system. *Cancer,* **38:**112–118, 1976.

Baker, L., and Opipari, M.: Mitomycin-C vincristine and bleomycin in disseminated squamous cell cancer of the uterine cervix. *Proc. Am. Soc. Clin. Oncol.,* **18:**272, 1977.

Balch, C. M.; Murad, T. M.; Soong, S-J.; Ingalls, A. L.; Halpern, N.; and Maddox, W. A.: A multifactorial analysis of melanoma — Prognostic histopathologic features comparing Clark's and Breslow's staging methods. *Ann. Surg.,* **188:**732–742, 1978.

Ballon, S.; Burman, M.; Donaldson, R.; Growdon, W.; and Lagasse, L.: Pulmonary metastatis of endometrial carcinoma. *Gynecol. Oncol.* **7:**56–65, 1979.

Banner, A.; Carrington, C.; Emory, W.; Kittle, F.; Leonard, G.; Ringus, J.; Taylor, P.; and Addington, W.: Efficacy of oophorectomy in lymphangioleiomyomatosis and benign metastasizing leiomyoma. *N. Engl. J. Med.,* **305:**204–209, 1981.

Barber, H., and Graber, E.: The PMPO Syndrome. *Obstet. Gynecol.,* **38:**921–23, 1971.

Barber, H. R. K., and Graber, E. A.: Gynecological tumors in childhood and adolescent tumors. *Obstet. Gynecol. Surv.,* **28:**357–381, 1973.

Barclay, D. L.: Carcinoma of the vagina after hysterectomy for severe dysplasia or carcinoma in situ of the cervix. *Gynecol. Oncol.,* **8:**1–11, 1979.

Barlow, J., Piver, M., and Lele, S.: High dose methotrexate with rescue plus cyclophosphamide as initial chemotherapy in ovarian adenocarcinoma. *Cancer,* **46:**1333–1338, 1980.

Bast, R.; Fenney, M.; Lazarus, H.; Nadler, L.; Colvin, R.; and Knapp, R.: Reactivity of a monoclonal antibody with human ovarian carcinoma. *J. Clin. Invest.,* **68:**1331–1337, 1981.

Beck, R.: Experience in treating 288 patients with endometrial carcinoma from 1968 to 1972. *Am. J. Obstet. Gynecol.,* **133:**260–267, 1979.

Beller, F. K.; Neinhaus, H.; Schmudt, V.; Gizycki, B.; Schellong, T.; Bunte, H.; and Schandt, W.: Endodermal germ cell carcinoma (endodermal sinus tumor) of the vagina in infant girls. *J. Cancer Res. Clin. Oncol.,* **94:**295–306, 1979.

Benedet, J.; White, G.; Fairey, R.; and Boyes, D.: Adenocarcinoma of the fallopian tube, experience with 41 patients. *Obstet. Gynecol.,* **50:**654–657, 1977.

Berkowitz, R., and Goldstein, D.: Methotrexate with citrovorum factor rescue for non-metastatic gestational trophoblastic neoplasms. *Obstet. Gynecol.,* **54:**725–728, 1979.

Berkowitz, R.; Goldstein, D.; Marean, A.; and Bernstein, M.: Oral contraceptives and post molar trophoblastic disease. *Obstet. Gynecol.,* **58:**474–477, 1981a.

Berkowitz, R.; Osathanondh, R.; Goldstein, D.; Martin, P.; and Mallampati, Datta S.: Cerebrospinal fluid HCG levels in normal pregnancy and choriocarcinoma. *Surg. Gynecol. Obstet.,* **153:**687–689, 1981b.

Bibbo, M.; Gill, W. B.; Azizi, F.; Blough, R.; Fang, P.; Rosenfield, R.; Sehumacher, G.; Sleeper, K.; Sonek, M.; and Wied, G.: Follow-up study of male and female offspring of DES-exposed mothers. *Obstet. Gynecol.,* **49:**1–8, 1977.

Bibbo, M.; Haenszel, W. M.; Wied, G. L.; Hubby, M.; and Herbst, A. L.: A twenty-five year follow-up study of women exposed to diethylstilbestrol during pregnancy. *N. Engl. J. Med.,* **298:**763–767, 1978.

Bjerre, B.: Further treatment after conization. *J. Reprod. Med.,* **21:**232, 1978.

Bjerre, B.; Eliasson, G.; Linell, F.; Soderberg, H.; and Sjoberg, N.: Conization as only treatment of carcinoma in situ of the uterine cervix. *Am. J. Obstet. Gynecol.,* **125:**143–152, 1976.

Bjorkholm, E., and Silfversward, C.: Prognostic factors in granulosa cell tumors. *Gynecol. Oncol.,* **11:**262–274, 1981.

Blom, J.: Blessing, J.; Mladineo, J.; Mangan, C.; Ehrlich, C.; and Homesley, H.: Dianhydrogalactitol (DAG) in the treatment of advanced gynecologic malignancies.

Proc. Am. Assoc. Cancer Res. and A.S.C.O., **21**:416, (Abstr. C384), 1980.

Blum, R.; Croson, J.; Wilson, R.; Greenberger, J.; Canellos, G.; and Frei, E., III: Successful treatment of metastatic sarcomas with cyclophosphamide, adriamycin and DTIC. *Cancer,* **46**:1722–1726, 1980.

Bokhman, J.; Chepick, O.; Volkova, A.; and Vishnevsky, A.: Adjuvant hormone therapy of primary endometrial carcinoma with oxyprogesterone caproate. *Gynecol. Oncol.,* **11**:371–378, 1981.

Bonomi, P.; Bruckner, H.; Cohen, C.; Marshall, R.; Blessing, J.; and Slayton, R.: A randomized trial of three cisplatin regimens in squamous cell carcinoma of the cervix. *Proc. A.S.C.O.,* **1**:110 (abstr. #425), 1982.

Bonte, J.; Ide, P.; Billiet, G.; and Wagnants, P.: Tamoxifen as a possible chemotherapeutic agent in endometrial adenocarcinoma. *Gynecol. Oncol.,* **11**:140–161, 1981.

Borden, E.; Larson, P.; Ansfield, F.; Bryan, G.; Johnson, R.; Ramirez, G.; and Wilson, W. L.: Hexamethylmelamine treatment of sarcomas and lymphomas. *Med. Pediatr. Oncol.,* **3**:401–406, 1977.

Boronow, R.: Chemotherapy for disseminated tubal cancer. *Obstet. Gynecol.,* **42**:62–65, 1973.

Bramwell, V.; Brugarolas, A.; Mouridsen, H.; Cheix, F.; DeJager, R.; Van Oosterom, A.; Vendrik, C.; Pinedo, H.; and DePauw, M.: EORTC phase II study of *cis*-platin in CYVADIC-resistant soft tissue sarcoma. *Eur. J. Cancer,* **15**:1511–1513, 1979.

Braunstein, G.; Grodin, J.; Vaitukaitis, J.; and Ross, G.: Secretory rates of human chorionic gonadotropin by normal trophoblasts. *Am. J. Obstet. Gynecol.,* **115**:447–450, 1973.

Brodeur, G.; Howarth, C.; Pratt, C.; Caces, J.; and Hustu, H.: Malignant germ cell tumors in 57 children and adolescents. *Cancer,* **48**:1890–1898, 1981.

Bruckman, J.; Bloomer, W.; Marck, A.; Ehrmann, R.; and Knapp, R.: Stage II adenocarcinoma of the endometrium: Two prognostic groups. *Gynecol. Oncol.,* **9**:12–17, 1980.

Bruckner, H.; Cohen, C.; Goldberg, J.; Kabakow, B.; Wallach, R.; Deppe, G.; Greenspan, E.; Gusberg, S.; and Holland, J.: Improved chemotherapy for ovarian cancer with cisdiaminedichloroplatinum and adriamycin. *Cancer,* **47**:2288–2294, 1981.

Bruckner, H., and Deppe, G.: Combination chemotherapy of advanced endometrial adenocarcinoma with adriamycin, cyclophosphamide, 5-fluorouracil and medroxyprogesterone acetate. *Obstet. Gynecol.,* **50**: 10S–12S, 1977.

Bryant, B., and Wiltshaw, E.: Results of the Royal Marsden Hospital: Second soft tissue sarcoma schedule chemotherapy regimen in the management of advanced sarcoma. *Cancer Treat. Rep.,* **64**:689–692, 1980.

Buchsbaum, H. J.: Extrapelvic lymph node metastases in cervical carcinoma. *Am. J. Obstet. Gynecol.,* **133**:814, 1979.

Buchsbaum, H.; Keetel, W.; and Latourette, H.: The role of radioisotopes as adjunct therapy of localized ovarian cancer. *Semin. Oncol.,* **2**:247–252, 1975.

Burghardt, E., and Holzer, E.: Treatment of carcinoma in situ: Evaluation of 1609 cases. *Obstet. Gynecol.,* **5**:55, 1980.

Carmo-Pereira, J.; Costa, F.; Henriques, E.; and Ricardo, J.: Advanced ovarian carcinoma: A prospective and randomized clinical trial of cyclophosphamide versus combination cytotoxic chemotherapy (HEXA-CAF). *Cancer,* **48**:1947–1951, 1981.

Christenson, B., and Espmark, A.: Long-term follow-up studies on herpes simplex antibodies in the course of cervical cancer: Patterns of neutralizing antibodies. *Am. J. Epidemiol.,* **105**:296, 1977.

Christopherson, W.; Williamson, E.; and Gray, L.: Leiomyosarcoma of the uterus. *Cancer,* **115**(29):1512–1517, 1972.

Chung, A. F.; Casey, M. J.; Flannery, J. T.; Woodruff, J. M.; and Lewis, J. L.: Malignant melanoma of the vagina—Report of 19 cases. *Obstet. Gynecol.,* **55**:720–727, 1980.

Clemmensen, J., and Poulsen, H.: *Report of the Ministry of the Interior,* Document 3. Copenhagen, 1971.

Cohen, C. J.; Bruckner, H. W.; Deppe, G.; Blessing J. A.; Homesley, H.; Lee, J. H.; and Watring, W.: Multidrug treatment of advanced and recurrent endometrial carcinoma: A Gynecologic Oncology Group study. *Obstet. Gynecol.,* **63**:719–726, 1984.

Cohen, C.; Deppe, G.; and Bruckner, H.: Treatment of advanced adenocarcinoma of the endometrium with melphalan, 5-fluorouracil and medroxy progesterone acetate: A preliminary study. *Obstet. Gynecol.* **50**:415–417, 1977.

Creagan, E.; Hahn, R.; Ahmann, D.; Edmondson, J.; Bisel, H.; and Eagan, R.: A comparative clinical trial evaluating the combination of adriamycin, DTIC, and vincristine, the combination of actinomycin, cyclophosphamide and vincristine and a single agent, methyl CCNU in advanced sarcomas. *Cancer Treat. Rep.,* **60**:1385–1387, 1976.

Creasman, W.; Boronow, R.; Morrow, C.; DiSaia, P.; and Blessing, J.: Adenocarcinoma of the endometrium: Its metastatic lymph node potential: A preliminary report. *Gynecol. Oncol.,* **4**:239–243, 1976.

Creasman, W.; DiSaia, P.; Blessing, J.; Wilkisen, R.; Johnston, W.; and Week, J.: Prognostic significance of peritoneal cytology in patients with endometrial cancer and preliminary data concerning therapy with intraperitoneal radiopharmaceuticals. *Am. J. Obstet. Gynecol.,* **141**,921–929, 1981.

Creasman, W.; Fetter, B.; Hammond, C.; and Parker, R.: Germ cell malignancies of the ovary. *Obstet. Gynecol.,* **53**:226–230, 1979.

Creasman, W.; McCarty, K., Sr.; Barton, T.; and McCarty, K., Jr.: Clinical correlates of estrogen and progesterone binding proteins in human endometrial adenocarcinoma. *Obstet. Gynecol.,* **55**:363–370, 1980.

Creasman, W.; Park, R.; Norris, H.; DiSaia, P. J.; Morrow, C. P.; and Hreshchyshyn, M.: Stage I borderline tumors of the ovary. *Obstet. Gynecol.,* **59**:93–96, 1982.

Curry, S.; Hammond, C.; Tyrey, L.; Creasman, W.; and Parker, R.: Hydatidiform mole, diagnosis, management and long term follow-up of 347 patients. *Obstet. Gynecol.,* **45**:1–8, 1975.

Curry, S.; Smith, J.; and Gallagher, H.: Malignant teratoma of the ovary: Prognostic factors and treatment. *Am. J. Obstet. Gynecol.,* **131**:845–849, 1978.

Cutler, S. J., and Young, J. L.: *Third National Cancer Survey: Incidence Data.* Natl. Cancer Inst. Monogr. 41. March, 1975.

Decker, D.; Webb, M.; and Holbrook, M.: Radiogold treatment of epithelial cancer of ovary: Late results. *Am. J. Obstet. Gynecol.,* **115**:751–758, 1973.

Delgado, G.; Thigpen, T.; Dolan, T.; and Morrison, F.: Phase II trial of piperazinidine in treatment of advanced ovarian adenocarcinoma. *Proc. Am. Assoc. Cancer Res. and A.S.C.O.,* **19**:332 (abstr. C101), 1978.

Deligdisch, L.; Driscoll, S.; and Goldstein, D.: Gestational trophoblastic neoplasms: Morphologic correlates of therapeutic response. *Am. J. Obstet. Gynecol.,* **130:**801–806, 1978.

Dembo, A.; Bush, R.; Beale, F.; Bena, H.; Pringle, J.; Sturgeon, J.; and Reid, J.: Ovarian carcinoma: Improved survival following abdominopelvic irradiation in patients with a completed pelvic operation. *Am. J. Obstet. Gynecol.,* **134:**793–800, 1979.

Deppe, G.; Bruckner, H.; and Cohen, C.: Combination chemotherapy for advanced carcinoma of the fallopian tube. *Obstet. Gynecol.,* **56:**530–532, 1980a.

Deppe, G.; Cohen, C.; and Bruckner, H.: Treatment of advanced endometrial adenocarcinoma with cis-dichlorodiammineplatinum after intensive prior therapy. *Gynecol. Oncol.,* **10:**51–54, 1980b.

DeVita, V.; Wasserman, T.; Young, R.; and Carter, S.: Perspectives on research in gynecologic oncology: Treatment protocols. *Cancer,* **38:**509–525, 1976.

DiSaia, P.; Castro, J.; and Rutledge, F.: Mixed mesodermal sarcoma of the uterus. *A.J.R.,* **117:**632–636, 1973.

Durant, J. R.: Future of combined modality therapy. *Int. J. Radiat. Oncol. Biol. Phys.,* **7:**783–790, 1981.

Edmonson, J.; Fleming, T.; Decker, D.; Malkasian, G.; Jorgensen, E.; Gefferies, J.; Webb, M.; and Kvols, L.: Different chemotherapeutic sensitivities and host factors affecting prognosis in advanced ovarian carcinoma versus minimal residual disease. *Cancer Treat. Rep.,* **63:**241–247, 1979.

Einhorn, N.; Cantell, K.; Einhorn, S.; and Strander, H.: Human leukocyte interferon therapy for advanced ovarian carcinoma. *Am. J. Clin. Oncol.,* **5:**167–172, 1982.

Evans, A.; Gaffey, T.; Malkasian, G.; and Annegers, J.: Clinicopathologic review of 118 granulosa and 82 theca cell tumors. *Obstet. Gynecol.,* **55:**231–238, 1980.

Fidler, H. K.; Boyes, D. A.; and Worth, A. J.: Cervical cancer detection in British Columbia. *J. Obstet. Gynaecol. Brit. Comm.,* **75:**392–404, 1968.

Figge, D. C.; Bennington, J. L.; and Scheveid, A. I.: Cervical cancer, after initial negative and atypical vaginal cytology. *Am. J. Obstet. Gynecol.,* **108:**422–428, 1970.

Fleischer, A.; James, A.; Krause, D.; and Millis, J.: Sonographic patterns in trophoblastic diseases. *Radiology,* **126:**215–220, 1978.

Foltz, A. M., and Kelsey, J. L.: The annual Pap test: A dubious policy success.. *Milbank Mem. Fund Q.,* **56:**426–462, 1978.

Fuks, Z.: External radiotherapy of ovarian cancer: Standard approaches and new frontiers. *Semin. Oncol.,* **2:**253–266, 1975.

Gallion, H.; VanNagell, J.; Powell, D.; Donaldson, E.; and Hanson, M.: Therapy of endodermal sinus tumor of the ovary. *Am. J. Obstet. Gynecol.,* **135:**447–451, 1979.

Gallup Omnibus: *A Survey Concerning Cigarette Smoking, Health Check-ups, Cancer Detection Tests. A Summary of the Findings.* Conducted for the American Cancer Society, Inc. The Gallup Organization, Inc., GO 7695T, 1977.

Gerbie, M.; Brewer, J.; and Tamimi, H.: Primary choriocarcinoma of the ovary. *Obstet. Gynecol.,* **46:**720–723, 1975.

Gershenson, D.; Wharton, J.; Herson, J.; Edwards, C.; and Rutledge, F.: Single agent cisplatin therapy for advanced ovarian cancer. *Obstet. Gynecol.,* **58:**487–496, 1981.

Gilbert, H. A.; Kagan, A. R.; Lagasse, L.; Jacobs, M. R.; and Tawa, K.: The value of radiation therapy in uterine sarcoma. *Obstet. Gynecol.,* **45:**84–88, 1975.

Gill, W. B.; Schumacher, G. F. B.; Bibbo, M.; Straus,

F. H., II; and Schoenberg, H. W.: Association of diethylstilbestrol exposure in utero with cryptorchidism, testicular hypoplasia and semen abnormalities. *J. Urol.,* **122:**36–39, 1979.

Glassburn, J.: Carcinoma of the endometrium. *Cancer,* **48:**575–581, 1981.

Glebatis, D. M., and Janerich, D. T.: A statewide approach to diethylstilbestrol—The New York Program. *N. Engl. J. Med.,* **304:**47–50, 1981.

Goldstein, D.: The chemotherapy of gestational trophoblastic disease, principles of clinical management. *J.A.M.A.,* **220:**209–213, 1972.

Gordon, A.; Lippman, D.; and Woodruff, J.: Dysgerminoma: A review of 158 cases from the Emil Novak Ovarian Tumor Registry. *Obstet. Gynecol.,* **58:**497–504, 1981.

Gore, H., and Hertig, A.: Trophoblastic lesions. In Nealon, T. (ed.): *Management of the Patient with Cancer,* 2nd ed. W. B. Saunders Company, Philadelphia, 1976.

Graham, J.: The value of pre-operative or post-operative treatment by radium for carcinoma of the uterine body. *Surg. Gynecol. Obstet.,* **132:**855–860, 1971.

Greco, F.; Julian, C.; Richardson, R.; Burnett, L.; Hande, K.; and Oldham, R.: Advanced ovarian cancer: Brief intensive combination chemotherapy and second-look operation. *Obstet. Gynecol.,* **58:**199–205, 1981.

Griffith, C.; Parker, L.; and Fuller, A.: Role of cytoreductive surgical treatment in the management of advanced ovarian cancer. *Cancer Treat. Rep.,* **63:**235–240, 1979.

Grumbine, F.; Rosenshein, N.; Brereton, H.; and Kalfman, S.: Management of liver metastasis from gestational trophoblastic neoplasia. *Am. J. Obstet. Gynecol.,* **137:**959–961, 1980.

Gurpide, E.: Hormone receptors in endometrial cancer. *Cancer,* **48:**638–641, 1981.

Gurwitt, L.; Long, J.; and Clark, R.: Cerebral metastatic choriocarcinoma. A postpartum cause of stroke. *Obstet. Gynecol.,* **45:**583–588, 1975.

Gusberg, S., and Kaplan, A.: Precursors of corpus cancer IV. Adenomatous hyperplasia as stage 0 carcinoma of the endometrium. *Am. J. Obstet. Gynecol.,* **87:**662–678, 1963.

Hall, J. E., and Walton, L.: Dysplasia of the cervix. *Am. J. Obstet. Gynecol.,* **100:**662–671, 1968.

Hammond, C.; Borchert, L.; Tyrey, L.; Creasman, W. T.; and Parker, R. T.: Treatment of metastatic trophoblastic disease: Good and poor prognosis. *Am. J. Obstet. Gynecol.,* **115:**451–457, 1973.

Hammond, C.; Weed, J.; and Currie, J.: The role of operation in the current therapy of gestational trophoblastic disease. *Am. J. Obstet. Gynecol.,* **136:**844–858, 1980.

Haney, A. F.; Hammond, D. B.; Soules, M. R.; and Creasman, W. T.: Diethylstilbestrol induced upper genital tract abnormalities. *Fertil. Steril.,* **31:**142–146, 1979.

Hatch, K.; Mann, W.; Boots, L.; Tauxe, W.; Shingleton, H.; and Buchina, E.: Localization of choriocarcinoma by 131-I-beta HCG antibody. *Gynecol. Oncol.,* **10:**253–261, 1980a.

Hatch, K. D.; Shingleton, H. M.; Austin, J. M.; Soong, S.-J.; and Bradley, D. H.: Cryosurgery of cervical intraepithelial neoplasia. *Obstet. Gynecol.,* **57:**692–698, 1981.

Hatch, K.; Shingleton, H.; Gore, H.; Younger, B.; and Boots L.: Human chorionic gonadotropin secreting large cell carcinoma of the lung detected during follow-up of a patient previously treated for gestational trophoblastic disease. *Gynecol. Oncol.,* **10:**98–104, 1980b.

Hatch, K.; Shingleton, H.; Younger, J.; and Boots, L.: Elevated beta HCG titers in oophorectomized women being treated for trophoblastic disease. *Am. J. Obstet. Gynecol.,* **137:**122, 1980c.

Hayashi, H.; Kameya, T.; Shimosato, Y.; and Mukojima, T.: Chemotherapy of human choriocarcinoma transplanted to nude mice. *Am. J. Obstet. Gynecol.,* **131:**548–554, 1978.

Herbst, A. L.: Clear cell adenocarcinoma and the current status of DES-exposed females. *Cancer,* **48:**484–488, 1981.

Herbst, A. L.; Scully, K. E.; and Robboy, S. J.: Prenatal diethylstilbestrol exposure and human genital tract abnormalities. *Natl. Cancer Instit. Monogr.,* **51:**25–35, 1979.

Herbst, A. L.; Ulfelder, H.; and Poskanzer, D. C.: Adenocarcinoma of the vagina: Association of maternal stilbestrol therapy with tumor appearance in young women. *N. Engl. J. Med.,* **284:**878–881, 1971.

Hernandez-Linares, W.; Puthawala, A.; Nolan, J. F.; Jernstrom, P. H.; and Morrow, C. P.: Carcinoma in situ of the vagina: Past and present management. *Obstet. Gynecol.,* **56:**356–360, 1980.

Hershey, D.; Fennell, R.; and Major, F.: Primary carcinoma of the fallopian tube. *Obstet. Gynecol.,* **57:**367–370, 1981.

Hershman, J.: Hyperthyroidism induced by trophoblastic thyrotropin. *Mayo Clin. Proc.,* **47:**913–918, 1972.

Higginson, J., and Muir, C. S.: Epidemiology. In Holland, J. F., and Frei, E. (eds.): *Cancer Medicine.* Lea & Febiger, Philadelphia, 1973.

Homesley, H.; Boronow, R.; and Lewis, J.: Stage II endometrial adenocarcinoma, Memorial Hospital for Cancer, 1949–1965. *Obstet. Gynecol.,* **49:**604–608, 1977.

Horwitz, R.; Feinstein, A.; Horwitz, S.; and Robboy, S.: Necropsy diagnosis of endometrial cancer and detection bias in case control studies. *Lancet,* **2:**66–68, 1981.

Hreshchyshyn, M.; Aron, B.; Boronow, R.; Franklin, E.; Shingleton, H.; and Blessing, J.: Hydroxyurea or placebo combined with radiation to treat stage IIIB and IV cervical cancer confined to the pelvis. *Int. J. Radiat. Oncol. Biol. Phys.,* **5:**317–322, 1976.

Hreshchyshyn, M.; Park, R.; Blessing, J.; Norris, H.; Levy, D.; Lagasse, L.; and Creasman, W.: The role of adjuvant therapy in stage I ovarian cancer. *Am. J. Obstet. Gynecol.,* **138:**139–145, 1980.

Hrushesky, W.; Levi, F.; Kennedy, B.; Theologides, A.; and Frenning, D.: Results of circadian time qualified chemotherapy in patients with advanced ovarian cancer. *Proc. Am. Assoc. Cancer Res. and ASCO,* **22:**472 (abstr. C546), 1981.

Hunter, R.; Longcope, C.; and Jordan, V.: Steroid hormone receptors in adenocarcoma of the endometrium. *Gynecol. Oncol.,* **10:**152–161, 1980.

Hutter, R. V. P.: Is cured early cancer truly cancer? *CA,* **32:**2–9, 1982.

Ishiguro, T.; Yoshida, Y.; Tenzaki, T.; Ohshima, M.; and Suzuki, H.: AFP in yolk sac tumor and solid teratoma of the ovary: Significance of postoperative serum AFP. *Cancer,* **48:**2480–2484, 1981.

Johannesson, G.; Geirsson, G.; and Day, N.: The effect of mass screening in Iceland, 1965–1974, on the incidence and mortality of cervical carcinoma. *Int. J. Cancer,* **21:**418–425, 1978.

Jones, E., and Bodner, W.: Lack of expression of HLA antigens on choriocarcinoma cell lines. *Tissue Antigens,* **16:**195–202, 1980.

Jones, K. W.; Tenoglir, C. M.; Shevchuk-Chaban, M.; Maitland, N. J.; and McDougall, J. K.: Detection of herpes simplex virus type 2 mRNA in human cervical biopsies by in situ cytological hybridization. In de-The, G.; Henle, W.; and Rapp, F. (eds.): *Oncogenesis and Herpesviruses III.* IARC, Lyon, France, 1978.

Jones, W.: Trophoblastic tumors—Prognostic factors. *Cancer,* **48:**602–607, 1981.

Judd, H.; Cleary, R.; Creasman, W.; Figge, D.; Kase, N.; Rosenwaks, Z.; and Tagatz, G.: Endocrine replacement therapy. *Obstet. Gynecol.,* **58:**267–275, 1981.

Julian, C.; Barrett, J.; Richardson, R.; and Greco, F.: Bleomycin, vinblastine and cis-platinum in the treatment of advanced endodermal sinus tumor. *Obstet. Gynecol.,* **56:**396–401, 1980.

Karakousis, C.; Holtermann, O.; and Holyoke, E.: Cisdichlorodiamineplatinum in metastatic soft tissue sarcomas. *Cancer Treat. Rep.,* **63:**2071–2075, 1979.

Karakousis, C.; Rao, U.; and Carlson, M.: High dose methotrexate and secondary chemotherapy in metastatic soft tissue sarcomas. *Cancer,* **46:**1345–1358, 1980.

Katz, M.; Schwartz, P.; Kapp, D.; and Luikart, S.: Epithelial carcinoma of the ovary: Current strategies. *Ann. Intern. Med.,* **95:**98–111, 1981.

Kaufman, R. H.; Binder, G. L.; Gray, P. M., Jr.; and Adam, E.: Upper genital tract changes associated with exposure in utero to diethylstilbestrol. *Am. J. Obstet. Gynecol.,* **128:**51–59, 1977.

Kessler, I. I.: Venereal factors in human cervical cancer: Evidence from marital clusters. *Cancer,* **39:**1912–1919, 1977.

Kinlen, L. J., and Spriggs, A. I.: Women with positive cervical smears but without surgical intervention. *Lancet,* **2:**463–465, 1978.

Kinsella, T.; Bloomer, W.; Lavin, P.; and Knapp, R.: Stage II endometrial carcinoma: Ten year follow-up of combined radiation and surgical treatment. *Gynecol. Oncol.,* **10:**290–297, 1980.

Kinzel, G.: Primary carcinoma of the fallopian tube. *Am. J. Obstet. Gynecol.,* **125:**816–820, 1976.

Knauf, S., and Urbach, G.: The development of a double antibody radioimmunoassay for detecting ovarian tumor associated antigen fraction OCA in plasma. *Am. J. Obstet. Gynecol.,* **131:**780–788, 1976.

Kolstad, P., and Klem, V.: Long-term follow-up of 1121 cases of carcinoma in situ. *Obstet. Gynecol.,* **48:**125–129, 1976.

Koss, L.; Schreiber, K.; Oberlander, S.; Moukhtar, M.; Levine, H.; and Moussouris, H.: Screening of asymptomatic women for endometrial cancer. *Cancer,* **31:**300–317, 1981.

Koss, L. G.; Stewart, F. W.; Foote, F. W.; Jordan, M. J.; Bader, G. M.; and Day, E.: Some histological aspects of behavior of epidermoid carcinoma in situ and related lesions of the uterine cervix. *Cancer,* **16:**1160–1211, 1963.

Kottmeier, H. L.: *Carcinoma of the Female Genitalia.* The Williams & Wilkins Company, Baltimore, 1953.

Kottmeier, H. L.: Evolution et traitement des epitheliomas. *Rev. Fr. Gynecol. Obstet.,* **56:**821–826, 1961.

Kurman, R., and Norris, H.: Malignant mixed germ cell tumors of the ovary. A clinical and pathologic analysis of 30 cases. *Obstet. Gynecol.,* **48:**579–589, 1976.

Lack, E.; Perez-Atayde, A.; Murthy, A.; Goldstein, D.; Crigler, J.; and Vawter, G.: Granulosa theca cell tumors in premenarchal girls: A clinical and pathologic study of 10 cases. *Cancer,* **48:**1846–1854, 1981.

Lagasse, L. D.; Creasman, W. T.; Shingleton, H. M.; Ford, J. H.; and Blessing, J. A.: Results and complications of operative staging in cervical cancer: Experience of the Gynecologic Oncology Group. *Gynecol. Oncol.,* **9:**90–98, 1980.

Lehman, H. F.; Cain, M. G.; Wolf, F. S.; Satterwhite, W.; Charles, E. D.; Ames, C. W.; and Greely, L. G.: A comparison of the results of the Papanicolaou test and Garvler jet wash on asymptomatic women. (Unpublished data.)

Lewis, G., and Bundy, B.: Surgery for endometrial cancer. *Cancer,* **48:**568–574, 1981.

Lewis, J.: Treatment of metastatic gestational trophoblastic neoplasms. A brief review of developments in the years 1968 to 1978. *Am. J. Obstet. Gynecol.,* **136:**163–172, 1980.

Li, M.: The historical background of successful chemotherapy for advanced gestational trophoblastic tumors. *Am. J. Obstet. Gynecol.,* **135:**266–272, 1979.

Lifshitz, S., and Buchsbaum, H.: The effect of paracentesis on serum proteins. *Gynecol. Oncol.,* **4:**347–353, 1976.

LiVolshi, V.: Adenocarcinoma of the endometrium with psammoma bodies. *Obstet. Gynecol.,* **50:**725–728, 1977.

Lurain, J., and Piver, M.: Familial ovarian cancer. *Gynecol. Oncol.,* **8:**185–192, 1979.

Lutz, M.; Underwood, P.; Kreutner, A.; and Miller, M.: Endometrial carcinoma: A new method of classification of therapeutic and prognostic significance. *Gynecol. Oncol.,* **6:**83–94, 1978.

Malkasian, G.; Decker, D.; and Webb, M.: Histology of epithelial tumors of the ovary: Clinical usefulness and prognostic significance of the histologic classification and grading. *Semin. Oncol.,* **2:**191–201, 1975.

Malkasian, G.; Mussey, E.; Decker, D.; and Johnson, C. E.: Chemotherapy of gynecologic sarcomas. *Cancer Chemother. Rep.,* **51:**507–516, 1967.

Marcus, S. L.: Multiple squamous cell carcinomas involving the cervix, vagina, and vulva. *Am.. J. Obstet. Gynecol.,* **80:**802–812, 1961.

Masterson, B. J.; Krantz, E. E.; Calkins, J. W.; Magrina, J. F.; and Carter, R. P.: The carbon dioxide laser in cervical intraepithelial neoplasia: A five-year experience in treating 230 patients. *Am. J. Obstet. Gynecol.,* **139:**565–567, 1981.

McComb, T., and Yuen, B.: Recurrence of metastatic trophoblastic disease after negative plasma human chorionic gonadotropin beta sub-unit assay. *Gynecol. Oncol.,* **9:**114–116, 1980.

McGowan, L.; Berent, L.; Lendar, W.; and Norris, H.: The woman at risk for developing ovarian cancer. *Gynecol. Oncol.,* **7:**325–344, 1979.

McGowan, L., and Bunnag, B.: The evaluation of therapy for ovarian cancer. *Gynecol. Oncol.,* **4:**375–383, 1976.

McMahon, B.: Risk factors for endometrial cancer. *Gynecol. Oncol.,* **2:**122, 1974.

Melan, J.; Wanner, L.; Schulz, D.; and Cassel, E.: Primary squamous cell carcinoma of the endometrium. *Obstet. Gynecol.,* **53:**115–119, 1979.

Melnick, J. L.: Preface. *Curr. Probl. Cancer,* **6:**3–4, 1981.

Merchant, S.; Murad, T. M.; Dowling, E. A.; and Durant, J. R.: Diagnosis of vaginal carcinoma from cytologic material. *Acta Cytol. (Baltimore),* **18:**494–502, 1974.

Messerschmidt, G.; Hoover, R,; and Young, R.: Gynecologic cancer treatment: Risk factors for therapeutically induced neoplasia. *Cancer,* **48:**442–450, 1981.

Metz, S.; Karnei, Veach, S.; and Hoskins, W.: Krukenberg carcinoma of the ovary with bone marrow involvement.

Report of two cases and review of the literature. *Obstet. Gynecol.,* **55:**99–104, 1980.

Miller, A. B.; Lindsey, J.; and Hill, G. B.: Mortality from cancer of the uterus in Canada and its relationship to screening for cancer of the cervix. *Int. J. Cancer,* **17:**602–612, 1976.

Miller, J.; Surwit, E.; and Hammond, C.: Choriocarcinoma following term pregnancy. *Obstet. Gynecol.,* **53:**207–212, 1979.

Morrow, C.; DiSaia, P.; and Townsend, D.: Current management of endometrial carcinoma. *Obstet. Gynecol.,* **42:**399–406, 1973.

Morrow, C.; DiSaia, P.; and Townsend, D.: The role of post-operative irradiation in the management of stage I adenocarcinoma of the endometrium. *A.J.R.,* **127:**325–329, 1976.

Myers, A.; Moore, G.; and Major, F.: Advanced ovarian carcinoma: Response to anti-estrogen therapy. *Cancer,* **48:**2368–2370, 1981.

Nahmias, A. J.; Josey, W. E.; Naib, Z. M.; Luce, C. F.; and Guest, B. A.: Antibodies to herpes virus hominis type 1 and 2 in human: II. Women with cervical cancer. *Am. J. Epidemiol.,* **91:**547, 1970.

Nahmias, A. J.; Naib, Z. M.; Josey, W. E.; Franklin, E.; and Jenkins, R.: Prospective studies of the association of genital herpes simplex injection and cervical anaplasia. *Cancer Res.,* **33:**1491–1497, 1973.

Nelson, J. H., Jr.; Macasaet, M. A.; Lu, T.; Bohoquez, J. F.; Smart, G. E.; Nicastri, A. D.; and Walton, L. A.: The incidence and significance of para-aortic lymph node metastases in late invasive carcinoma of the cervix. *Am. J. Obstet. Gynecol.,* **118:**749, 1974.

NIH Consensus Development Conference on Cervical Cancer Screening: *The Pap Smear.* National Institutes of Health, Bethesda, Maryland, 1980.

Norris, H., and Taylor, H.: Post-irradiation sarcomas of the uterus. *Obstet. Gynecol.,* **26:**689–694, 1965.

Ober, W.: Uterine sarcomas: Histogenesis and taxonomy. *Ann. N.Y. Acad. Sci.,* **75:**568–585, 1959.

O'Brien, P. C.; Noller, K. L.; Robboy, S. J.; Barnes, A. B.; Kaufman, R. H.; Tilley, B. C.; and Townsend, D. E.: Vaginal epithelial changes in young women enrolled in the National Cooperative Diethylstilbestrol Adenosis (DESAD) Project. *Obstet. Gynecol.,* **53:**300–308, 1979.

Omura, G. A.: Chemotherapy and hormone therapy in gynecologic cancer. *South. Med. J.,* **66:**689–692, 1973.

Omura, G.: Are all stage III cancers of the ovary really ovarian cancers? *Cancer Clin. Trials,* **4:**219–220, 1981.

Omura, G.; DiSaia, P.; Blessing, J.; Boronow, R.; Hreshchyshyn, M.; and Park, R.: Chemotherapy for mustard-resistant ovarian adenocarcinoma: A randomized trial of CCNU and methyl-CCNU. *Cancer Treat. Rep.,* **61:**1533–1535, 1977.

Omura, G.; Ehrlich, C.; and Blessing, J.: A randomized trial of cyclophosphamide plus adriamycin with or without cis-platinum in ovarian carcinoma. *Proc. Am. Assoc. Cancer Res. and A.S.C.O.,* **1:**104 (abstr. #403), 1982.

Omura, G.; Greco, F.; and Birch, R.: Hexamethylmelamine in mustard-resistant ovarian adenocarcinoma. *Cancer Treat. Rep.,* **65:**530–531, 1981a.

Omura, G. A.; Major, F. J.; Blessing, J. A.; Sedlacek, T. V.; Thigpen, J. T.; Creasman, W. T.; and Zino, R. J.: A randomized study of adriamycin with and without dimethyl triazenoimidazole carboxamide in advanced uterine sarcomas. *Cancer* **52:**626–632, 1983a.

Omura, G.; Morrow, C.; Blessing, J.; Miller, A.; Buchsbaum, H.; Homesley, H.; and Leone, L.: A randomized comparison of melphalan versus melphalan plus hexamethylmelamine versus adriamycin plus cyclophosphamide in ovarian adenocarcinoma. *Cancer* **51**:783–789, 1983b.

Omura, G. A., and Roberts, G. A.: Combination therapy of solid tumors using 1,3-bis(2-chloroethyl)-1-nitrosourea (BCNU), vincristine, methotrexate, and 5-fluorouracil. *Cancer,* **31**:1374–1381, 1973.

Omura, G. A.; Shingleton, H. M.; Creasman, W. T.; Blessing, J. A.; and Boronow, R. C.: Chemotherapy of gynecologic cancer with nitrosoureas: A randomized trial of CCNU and methyl-CCNU in cancers of the cervix, corpus, vagina and vulva. *Cancer Treat. Rep.,* **62**:833–835, 1978.

Omura, G. A.; Velez-Garcia, E.; and Birch, R.: Phase II randomized study of doxorubicin, vincristine, and 5-FU versus cyclophosphamide in advanced squamous cell carcinoma of the cervix. *Cancer Treat. Rep.,* **65**:901–903, 1981b.

Orr, J.; Austin, J.; Hatch, K.; Shingleton, H.; Younger, J.: and Boots, L.: Acute pulmonary edema associated with molar pregnancies: A high risk factor for development of persistent trophoblastic disease. *Am. J. Obstet. Gynecol.,* **136**:412–415, 1980.

Ozols, R.; Garvin, A.; Costa, J.; Simon, R.; and Young, R. C.: Advanced ovarian cancer: Correlation of histologic grade with response to therapy and survival. *Cancer,* **45**:572–581, 1980a.

Ozols, R.; Willson, J.; Weltz, M.; Krotzinger, K.; Myers, C.; and Young, R.: Inhibition of human ovarian cancer colony formation by adriamycin and its major metabolites. *Cancer Res.,* **40**:4109–4112, 1980b.

Park, R.; Blom, J.; DiSaia, P.; Lagasse, L.; and Blessing, J.: Treatment of women with disseminated or recurrent advanced ovarian cancer with melphalan alone or in combination with 5-fluorouracil and dactinomycin or with the combination of cytoxan, 5-fluorouracil and dactinomycin. *Cancer,* **45**:2529–2542, 1980.

Parker, L.; Griffith, C.; Yankee, R.; Knapp, R.; and Canellos, G.: High dose methotrexate with leucovorin rescue in ovarian cancer: A phase II study. *Cancer Treat. Rep.,* **63**:275–279, 1979.

Perez-Mesa, C., and Spratt, J. S.: Scalene node biopsy in the pretreatment staging of carcinoma of the cervix uteri. *Am. J. Obstet. Gynecol.,* **125**:93–95, 1976.

Peterson, O.: Precancerous changes of the cervical epithelium in relation to manifest cervical carcinoma. *Acta Radiol. [Suppl.] (Stockh.),* 127, 1955.

Peterson, O.: Spontaneous course of cervical precancerous condition. *Am. J. Obstet. Gynecol.,* **72**:1063–1071, 1956.

Petrilli, E. S.; Townsend, D. E.; Morrow, C. P.; and Nakao, C. Y.: Vaginal intraepithelial neoplasia: Biologic aspects and treatment with topical 5-fluorouracil and the carbon dioxide laser. *Am. J. Obstet. Gynecol.,* **138**:321–328, 1981.

Phillips, T. L.: Sensitizers and protectors in clinical oncology. *Semin. Oncol.,* **8**:65–82, 1981.

Pileri, S.; Martinelli, G.; Serra, L.; and Bazzocchi, F.: Endodermal sinus tumor arising in the endometrium. *Obstet. Gynecol.,* **56**:391–396, 1980.

Pinedo, H., and Kenis, Y.: Chemotherapy of advanced soft tissue sarcomas in adults. *Cancer Treat. Rev.,* **4**:67–86, 1977.

Piver, M. S., and Barlow, J. J.: High doses irradiation to biopsy confirmed aortic node metastases from carcinoma of the uterine cervix. *Cancer,* **39**:1243–1246, 1977.

Piver, M.; Barlow, J.; and Lele, S.: Incidence of sub-clinical metastasis in stage I and II ovarian carcinoma. *Obstet. Gynecol.,* **52**:100–104, 1078a.

Piver, M.; Barlow, J.; Lele, S.; and Higby, D.: Cisdichlorodiamine platinum as third line chemotherapy in advanced ovarian adenocarcinoma. *Cancer Treat. Rep.,* **62**:559, 1978b.

Piver, M.; Barlow, J.; Lurain, J.; and Blumenson, L.: Medroxyprogestrone acetate (depo-orovera) vs. hydroxyprogestrone caproate (delalutin) in women with metastatic endometrial adenocarcinoma. *Cancer,* **45**:268–272, 1980.

Prem, K.; Adcock, L.; Okagaki, T.; and Jones, T.: The evolution of a treatment program for adenocarcinoma of the endometrium. *Am. J. Obstet. Gynecol.,* **133**:803–813, 1979.

Quigley, M.; Tyrey, L.; and Hammond, C.: Utility of assay of alpha sub-unit of human chorionic gonadotropin in management of gestational trophoblastic malignancies. *Am. J. Obstet. Gynecol.,* **138**:545–549, 1980.

Rapp, F.: Herpes simplex virus type 2 and cervical cancer. *Curr. Probl. Cancer,* **6**:5–18, 1981.

Rawls, W. E.; Laurel, D.; Melnick, J. L.; Glicksman, J. M.; and Kaufman, R. H.: A search for viruses in smegma, premalignant, and early malignant cervical tissues: The isolation of herpes-viruses with distinct antigenic properties. *Am. J. Epidemiol.,* **87**:647, 1968.

Reifenstein, E.: Hydroxyprogesterone caproate therapy in advanced endometrial cancer. *Cancer,* **27**:485–502, 1971.

Reimer, R.; Hoover, R.; Fraumeni, J.; and Young, R.: Acute leukemia after alkylating agent therapy of ovarian cancer. *N. Engl. J. Med.,* **297**:177–181, 1977.

Richart, R.; Marchbein, H.; and Sherman, A.: Studies of the Gravelee jet washer in the detection of endometrial neoplasia. *Gynecol. Oncol.,* **8**:49–59, 1979.

Rivkin, S.; Gottlieb, J.; Thigpen, T.; Mawla, N. G.; Saiki, J.; and Dixon, D. O.: Methyl-CCNU and adriamycin for patients with metastatic sarcomas. *Cancer,* **46**:446–451, 1980.

Robboy, S. J.; Kaufman, R. H.; Prat, J.; Welch, W. R.; Gaffey, T.; Scully, R. E.; Richart, R.; Fenoglio, C. M.; Virata, R.; and Tilley, B.: Pathologic findings in young women enrolled in the National Cooperative Diethylstilbestrol Adenosis (DESAD) Project. *Obstet. Gynecol.,* **53**:309–317, 1979.

Roizman, B., and Frenkel, N.: Does genital herpes cause cancer? A midway assessment. In Caterall, R. D., and Nicol, C. S. (eds.): *Sexually Transmitted Disease.* Academic Press, Inc., New York, 1967.

Romero, R., and Schwartz, P.: Alpha feto-protein determinations in the management of endodermal sinus tumors and mixed germ cells tumors of the ovary. *Am. J. Obstet. Gynecol.,* **141**:126–131, 1981.

Rosenbaum, C., and Schoenfield, D.: Treatment of advanced soft tissue sarcomas. *Proc. Am. Assoc. Cancer Res. and A.S.C.O.,* **18**:287, 1977.

Rosenoff, S.; Young, R.; Anderson, T.; Bagley, C.; Chabner, B.; Schein, P.; Hubbard, S.; and DeVita, V.: Peritoneoscopy: A valuable staging tool in ovarian carcinoma. *Ann. Intern. Med.,* **83**:36–41, 1975.

Roth, L., and Ehrlich, C.: Mucinous cysadenocarcinoma of the retroperitoneum. *Obstet. Gynecol.,* **49**:486–488, 1977.

Salazar, O.; Bonfiglio, T.; Patten, S.; Keller, B.; Fieldstein, M.; Dunne, M.; and Rudolph, J.: Uterine sarcomas, natural history, treatment and prognosis. *Cancer,* **42**:1152–1160, 1978a.

Salazar, O.; Bonfiglio, T.; Patten, S.; Keller, B.; Fieldstein, M.; Dunne, M.; and Rudolph, J.: Uterine sarcomas, analysis of failures with special emphasis on the use of adjuvant radiation therapy. *Cancer,* **42:**1161–1170, 1978b.

Salazar, O.; Feldstein, M.; DePapp, E.; Bonfiglio, T. A.; Keller, B. E.; Rubin, P.; and Randolph, J. H.: The management of clinical stage I endometrial carcinoma. *Cancer,* **41:**1016–1026, 1978c.

Sampson, M.; Baker, L.; Benjamin, R.; Lane, M.; and Plager, C.: Cis-dichlorodiamineplatinum in advanced soft tissue and bony sarcomas: A Southwest Oncology Group Study. *Cancer Treat. Rep.,* **63:**2027–2029, 1979.

Sampson, R. J.; Hisao, O.; Key, C. R.; Buncher, C. R.; and Iijima, S.: Metastases from occult thyroid carcinoma: An autopsy study from Hiroshima and Nagasaki, Japan. *Cancer,* **25:**803–811, 1970.

Schiller, H., and Silverberg, S.: Staging and prognosis in primary carcinoma of the fallopian tube. *Cancer,* **28:**389–395, 1971.

Schindler, A.; Ebert, A.; and Friedrich, E.: Conversion of androstenedione to estrone by human fat tissue. *J. Clin. Endocrinol. Metab.,* **35:**627–630, 1972.

Schlaerth, J.; Morrow, C.; Kletzky, O.; Nalick, R.; and D'Ablaing, G.: Prognostic characteristics of serum human chorionic gonadotropin titer regression following molar pregnancy. *Obstet. Gynecol.,* **58:**478–482, 1981.

Schwartz, P.; Kohorn, E.; Knowlton, A.; and Morris, J.: Routine use of hysterography in endometrial carcinoma and postmenopausal bleeding. *Obstet. Gynecol.,* **45:**378–384, 1975.

Schwartz, P., and Smith, J.: Treatment of ovarian stromal tumors. *Am. J. Obstet. Gynecol.,* **125:**402–411, 1976.

Scott, L. K.; Shingleton, H. M.; Hatch, K. D.; and Maisiak, R. S.: Impact of a colposcopy satellite clinic. *South. Med. J.,* **74:**513–519, 1981.

Scully, R.: Recent progress in ovarian cancer. *Hum. Pathol.,* **1:**73–98, 1970.

Scully, R.: Ovarian tumors, a review. *Am. J. Pathol.,* **87:**686–720, 1977.

Sedlis, A.; Sall, S.; Tsukada, Y.; Park, R.; Manyan, C.; Shingleton, H. M.; and Blessing, J. A.: Microinvasive carcinoma of the uterine cervix: A clinical pathologic study. *Am. J. Obstet. Gynecol.,* **133:**64–74, 1979.

Seski, J.; Edwards, C.; Gershenson, D.; and Copeland, L.: Doxorubicin and cyclophosphamide chemotherapy for disseminated endometrial cancer. *Obstet. Gynecol.,* **58:**88–91, 1981.

Seski, J.; Edwards, C.; Herson, J.; and Rutledge, F.: Cisplatin chemotherapy for disseminated endometrial cancer. *Obstet. Gynecol.,* **59:**225–228, 1982.

Shingleton, H. M.; Gore, H.; Bradley, D. H.; and Soong, S-J.: Adenocarcinoma of the cervix. I. Clinical evaluation and pathologic features. *Am. J. Obstet. Gynecol.,* **139:**799–814, 1981.

Shingleton, H. M.; Gore, H.; Soong, S-J.; Hatch, K. D.; Orr, J. W.; and Austin, J. M.: Tumor recurrence and survival in stage IB cancer of the cervix. Presented at the Annual Meeting of the American Radium Society, March 14–16, San Antonio, Texas, 1982.

Shingleton, H. M.; Soong, S-J.; and Bradley, D. H.: Gynecologic oncology admissions: A ten-year report (1969–1979). Comprehensive Cancer Center, University of Alabama in Birmingham, November, 1979.

Siiteri, P.; Schwarz, B.; and MacDonald, P.: Estrogen receptors and the estrone hypothesis in relation to endometrial and breast cancer. *Gynecol. Oncol.,* **2:**228–238, 1974.

Silverberg, E.: Cancer statistics. *CA,* **32:**15–31, 1982.

Silverberg, S.: Leiomyosarcoma of the uterus. A clinical pathologic study. *Obstet. Gynecol.,* **38:**613–627, 1971.

Slayton, R.; Hreshchyshyn, M.; Silverberg, S.; Shingleton, H.; Park, R.; DiSaia, P.; and Blessing, J.: Treatment of malignant ovarian germ cell tumors: Response to vincristine, dactinomycin and cyclophosphamide (preliminary report). *Cancer,* **43:**390–398, 1978.

Slayton, R.; Petty, W.; and Blessing, J.: Phase II trial of VP16 in treatment of advanced ovarian adenocarcinoma. *Proc. Am. Assoc. Cancer Res. and A.S.C.O.,* **20:**190 (abstr. 768), 1979.

Slayton, R.; Ragano, M.; and Creech, R.: Progestin therapy for advanced ovarian cancer: A phase III Eastern Cooperative Oncology Group trial. *Cancer Treat. Rep.,* **65:**895–896, 1981.

Smith, J.; Alsuleiman, S.; Bishop, H.; Kassar, N.; and Jonas, H.: Trophoblastic pulmonary embolism. *South. Med. J.,* **74:**916–919, 1981.

Smith, J. P., and Day, T. G., Jr.: Review of ovarian cancer at the University of Texas System Cancer Center, M. D. Anderson Hospital and Tumor Institute. *Am. J. Obstet. Gynecol.,* **135:**984–990, 1979.

Smith, J.; Delgado, G.; and Rutledge, F.: Second look operation in ovarian carcinoma, post chemotherapy. *Cancer,* **38:**1438–1442, 1976.

Speyer, J.; Collins, J.; Dedrick, R.; Brennan, M.; Buckpitt, A.; Londer, H.; Devita, V.; and Myers, C.: Phase I and pharmacological studies of 5-fluorouracil administered intraperitoneally. *Cancer Res.,* **40:**467–472, 1980.

Stafl, A., and Mattingly, R.: Colposcopic diagnosis of cervical neoplasia. *Obstet. Gynecol.,* **41:**168–176, 1973.

Stenwig, J.; Hazekamp, J.; and Beecham, J.: Granulosa cell tumors of the ovary. A clinicopathological study of 118 cases with long-term follow-up. *Gynecol. Oncol.,* **7:**136–152, 1979.

Stern, E., and Neely, P. M.: Carcinoma and dysplasia of the cervix: A comparison of rates for new and returning population. *Acta Cytol. (Baltimore),* **7:**357–361, 1963.

Sudarsanam, A.; Komanduri, C.; Belinson, J.; Averette, H.; Goldberg, M.; Hintz, B.; Thirumala, M.; and Ford, J.: Influence of exploratory celiotomy on the management of carcinoma of the cervix. A preliminary report. *Cancer,* **41:**1049–1053, 1978.

Surwit, E.; Fowler, W.; and Rogoff, E.: Stage II carcinoma of the endometrium, and analysis of treatment. *Obstet. Gynecol.,* **52:**97–99, 1978.

Surwit, E., and Hammond, C.: Treatment of metastatic trophoblastic disease with poor prognosis. *Obstet. Gynecol.,* **55:**565–570, 1980.

Surwit, E.; Joelsson, I.; and Einhorn, N.: Adjunctive radiation therapy in the management of stage I cancer of the endometrium. *Obstet. Gynecol.,* **58:**590–595, 1981.

Szamborski, J.; Czerwinski, W.; Gadomska, H.; Kowalski, M.; and Wacher-Pujdak, B: Case control study of high risk factors in ovarian carcinomas. *Gynecol. Oncol.,* **11:**8–16, 1981.

Tamimi, H., and Figge, D: Adenocarcinoma of the uterine tube: Potential for lymph node metastasis. *Am. J. Obstet. Gynecol.,* **141:**132–137, 1981.

Tao, L. C.; Pearson, F. G.; Delarue, N. C.; Langer, B.; and Sanders, D. E.: Percutaneous fine-needle aspiration biopsy. I. Its value to clinical practice. *Cancer,* **45:**1480–1485, 1980.

Tashima, C.; Timberger, R.; and Burdick, R.: Cerebral spinal fluid titer of chorionic gonadotropin in patients with intra-cranial metastatic choriocarcinoma. *J. Clin. Endocrinol. Metab.,* **25:**1493–1495, 1965.

Teoh, E.; Dawood, M.; and Ratnam, S.: Epidemiology of hydatidiform mole in Singapore. *Am. J. Obstet. Gynecol.,* **110:**415–420, 1971.

Thigpen, T.; Buchsbaum, H.; Mangan, C.; and Blessing, J.: Phase II trial of adriamycin in the treatment of advanced or recurrent endometrial carcinoma: A Gynecologic Oncology Group Study. *Cancer Treat. Rep.,* **63:**21–27, 1979.

Thigpen, T.; Shingleton, H.; Homsley, H.; Lagasse, L.; and Blessing, J.: Cisplatinum in treatment of advanced or recurrent squamous cell carcinoma of the cervix: A phase II study of the Gynecologic Oncology Group. *Cancer,* **48:**899–903, 1981a.

Thigpen, T.; Vance, R. B.; Balducci, L.; and Blessing, J.: Chemotherapy in the management of advanced or recurrent cervical and endometrial carcinoma. *Cancer,* **48:**658–665, 1981b.

Thomas, D. B, and Rawls, W. E.: Relationship of herpes simplex virus type-2 antibodies and squamous dysplasia to cervical carcinoma in situ. *Cancer,* **42:**2716–2725, 1978.

Tomoda, Y.; Fuma, M.; Saiki, N.; Ishizuka, N.; and Akaza, T.: Immunologic studies in patients with trophoblastic neoplasia. *Am. J. Obstet. Gynecol.,* **126:**661–667, 1976.

Twigs, L.; Morrow, C.; and Schlaerth, J.: Acute pulmonary complications of molar pregnancy. *Am. J. Obstet. Gynecol.,* **135:**189–194, 1979.

U.S. Department of Health, Education, and Welfare: *U.S. Vital Statistics: Mortality.* Unpublished Data: Trend C, Tables 292 and 292A, Death and Death Rates, United States. U.S. D.H.E.W., Washington, D.C., 1976.

Vaitukaitis, J.; Braunstein, G.; and Ross, G.: A radioimmunoassay which specifically measures human chorionic gonadotropin in the presence of human luteinizing hormone. *Am. J. Obstet. Gynecol.,* **113:**751–758, 1972.

Van Kley, H.; Cramer, S.; and Bruns, D.: Serous ovarian neoplastic amylase (SONA): A potentially useful market for serous ovarian tumors. *Cancer,* **48:**1444–1449, 1981.

Vardi, J., and Tovell, H.: Leiomyosarcoma of the uterus: Clinical pathologic study. *Obstet. Gynecol.,* **56:**428–434, 1980.

Vaughn, T.; Surwit, E.; and Hammond, C.: Late recurrences of gestational trophoblastic neoplasia. *Am. J. Obstet. Gynecol.,* **138:**73–76, 1980.

Villa Santa, U., and Jovanovski, D.: Follow-up study of ovarian carcinoma by cytology of cul-de-sac aspirates. *Gynecol. Oncol.,* **10:**58–62, 1980.

Vogl, S.; Pagano, M.; and Kaplan, B.: Cyclophosphamide, hexamethylmelamine, adriamycin and diamminedichloroplatinum versus melphalan for advanced ovarian cancer. A randomized prospective trial of the Eastern Cooperative Oncology Group. *Proc. Am. Assoc. Cancer Res. and A.S.C.O.,* **22:**473 (abstr. C548), 1981.

Vongtama, V.; Karlen, J.; Piver, S.; Tsukada, Y.; and Moore, R.: Treatment results and prognostic factors in stage I and II sarcomas of the corpus uteri. *A.J.R.,* **126:**139–147, 1976.

Wade, M.; Kohorn, E.; and Morris, J.: Adenocarcinoma of the endometrium: Evaluation of pre-operative irradiation and factors influencing prognosis. *Am. J. Obstet. Gynecol.,* **99:**869–876, 1967.

Wake, N.; Tanaka, K.; Chapman, V.; Matsui, S.; and

Sandberg, A.: Chromosomes and cellular origins of choriocarcinoma. *Cancer Res.,* **41:**3137–3143, 1981.

Walker, A., and Jick, H.: Declining rates of endometrial cancer. *Obstet. Gynecol.,* **56:**733–736, 1980.

Walton Report, The: Cervical cancer screening programs. *Can. Med. Assoc. J.,* **114:**1003–1031, 1976.

Webb, M.; Decker, D.; and Mussey, E.: Cancer metastatic to the ovary. Factors influencing survival. *Obstet. Gynecol.,* **45:**391–396, 1975.

Webb, M.; Decker, D.; Mussey, E.; and Williams, T.: Factors influencing survival in stage I ovarian cancer. *Am. J. Obstet. Gynecol.,* **116:**222–228, 1973.

Webb, M. J., and Symmonds, R. E.: Wertheim hysterectomy: A reappraisal. *Obstet. Gynecol.,* **54:**140–145, 1979.

Weed, J., and Hammond, C.: Cerebral metastatic choriocarcinoma: Intensive therapy and prognosis. *Obstet. Gynecol.,* **55:**89–94, 1980.

Wehmann, R.; Ayala, A.; Birken, S.; Canfield, R.; and Nisula, B.: Improved monitoring of gestational trophoblastic neoplasia using a highly sensitive assay for urinary human chorionic gonadotropin. *Am. J. Obstet. Gynecol.,* **140:**753–757, 1981.

Wharton, J., and Herson, J.: Surgery for common epithelial tumors of the ovary. *Cancer,* **48:**582–589, 1981.

Wharton, J. T.; Jones, H. W., III; Day, T. G.; Rutledge, F. N.; and Fletcher, G. H.: Preirradiation celiotomy and extended field irradiation for invasive carcinoma of the cervix. *Obstet. Gynecol.,* **49:**333, 1977.

Willett, W.; Bain, C.; Hennekens, C.; Rosner, B.; and Speizer, F.: Oral contraceptives and risk of ovarian cancer. *Cancer,* **48:**1684–1687, 1981.

Williams, S.; Slayton, R.; Silverberg, S.; Ehrlich, C.; Einhorn, L.; and Blessing, J.: Response of malignant ovarian germ cell tumors to cisplatinum, vinblastine and bleomycin. *Proc. Am. Assoc. Cancer Res. and A.S.C.O.,* **22:**463 (abstr. C509), 1981.

Willson, J.; Ozols, R.; Lewis, B.; and Young, R.: Current status of therapeutic modalities for treatment of gynecologic malignancies with emphasis on chemotherapy. *Am. J. Obstet. Gynecol.,* **141:**81–98, 1981.

Woodruff, J.; Dietrich, D.; Genadry, R.; and Parmley, T.: Proliferative and malignant Brenner tumors, review of 49 cases. *Am. J. Obstet. Gynecol.,* **141:**118–125, 1981.

Yap, B.; Baker, L.; Sinkovics, J.; Rivkin, S. E.; Bottomley, R.; Thigpen, T.; Burgess, M. A.; Benjamin, R.; and Bodey, G.: Cyclophosphamide, vincristine, adriamycin and DTIC combination chemotherapy for the treatment of advanced sarcomas. *Cancer,* **46:**446–451, 1980.

Yoonessi, M., and Abell, M.: Brenner tumors of the ovary. *Obstet. Gynecol.,* **54:**90–96, 1979.

Yoonessi, M., and Hart, W. R.: Endometrial stromal sarcomas. *Cancer,* **40:**898–906, 1977.

Young, R.; Chabner, B.; Hubbard, S.; Fisher, R.; Bender, R.; Anderson, T.; Simon, R.; Canellos, G.; and DeVita, V.: Advanced ovarian adenocarcinoma. A prospective clinical trial of melphalan versus combination chemotherapy. *N. Engl. J. Med.,* **299:**1261–1266, 1978.

Young, R.; Howser, D.; Myers, C.; Ozols, R.; Fisher, R.; Wesley, M.; and Chabner, B.: Combination chemotherapy (Chex-up) with intraperitoneal maintenance in advanced ovarian adenocarcinoma. *Proc. Am. Assoc. Cancer Res. and A.S.C.O.,* **22:**465 (abstr. C518), 1981.

Yuhas, J. M.; Spellman, J. M.; and Culo, F.: The role of WR-2721 in radiotherapy and/or chemotherapy. *Cancer Clin. Trials,* **3:**211–216, 1980.

35

Neoplasms of the Kidney, Bladder, and Prostate

HARRY W. HERR and ALAN YAGODA

Introduction

Carcinoma of the kidney, urinary bladder, and prostate comprises a unique spectrum of neoplasia. In the United States, prostatic adenocarcinoma is the third most frequent cancer in men. It occurs primarily in an older population, has a serum biologic marker which can be followed, and is a hormonally sensitive tumor. Transitional cell carcinoma of the urinary tract, thought to be a carcinogen-induced cancer, is, to some degree, responsive to radiotherapy and chemotherapy. By contrast, renal cell cancer afflicts a younger age group, is relatively insensitive to irradiation and chemotherapy, produces various hormonal substances resulting in unusual paraneoplastic syndromes, and is one of the rare neoplasms to exhibit spontaneous tumor regression.

This chapter will describe diagnostic criteria, the type of work-up required for therapeutic decisions, and the accepted management approaches to each disease. An attempt will be made to delineate the problems relating to the accepted therapeutic protocols.

NEOPLASMS OF THE KIDNEY

Incidence and Epidemiology

Malignant neoplasms of the kidney account for 3% of human cancers, and renal adenocarcinoma, or renal cell carcinoma, comprises 85% of all renal tumors. In 1985, approximately 19,700 patients with renal carcinoma will be newly diagnosed in the United States, with an estimated 8,900 deaths. (Silverberg, 1985).

Although most of these tumors occur sporadically, familial cases have been reported. Patients usually present between the ages of 50 and 70, with the disease being two to three times more common in men than in women. The incidence of renal cancer appears to be increasing, particularly among men.

Initially, renal cell carcinoma was thought to develop from embryonic nests of adrenal tissue, hence the name hypernephroma. Although the etiology is unknown, about one-third of renal adenocarcinomas in men have been related to tobacco use. The risk of developing this tumor is estimated to increase five-fold in men who are heavy cigarette smokers. A similar increased risk is observed in cigar smokers and in men who chew tobacco. Obesity in women and diets rich in animal fats and cholesterol in both men and women seem to increase the risk of kidney cancer. In the male golden hamster, stilbestrol pellets can induce renal carcinomas, thus hormonal imbalance has been suggested as a possible etiology in humans (Kirkman, 1959). About 30% of patients with von Hippel-Lindau disease develop clinically apparent renal adenocarcinoma, which, in half, is metastatic at diagnosis (Wynder et al., 1974). Recently, Cohen et al., (1979) have described a reciprocal translocation between chromosomes 3 and 8 (t[3;8] [p 14;q24]) in a family with a 60% incidence of bilateral renal cancer in three generations. In most human tumors, however, inconsistent karyotypic changes (translocation, hypodiploidy, deletion, and so forth) have been described.

Pathology

Renal tumors are solid, usually pseudoencapsulated masses, with satellite tumor nodules occurring in 10 to 16% of patients. They show no preference as to intrarenal site and occur bilaterally in 1% of patients. Evidence suggests that the proximal tubular epithelial cell is the major cell of origin of renal adenocarcinoma. This portion of the renal tubular epithelium develops embryologically from the metanephric tubule and duct (wolffian), which induces surrounding mesoderm to form the uriniferous tubules. Some cancers develop from the distal tubules and the short papillary ducts of Bellini. The typical angiographic findings of renal cancer can be absent in the former, and histologic stains for mucin may be positive in the latter (Aufderheide and Streitz, 1974). Based on cytoplasmic appearance, four distinct patterns of tumor have been identified: clear in approximately 25% of cases, granular in 12%, mixed in 50%, and spindle-sarcomatoid in 14% (Skinner *et al.,* 1971). Patterns of tumor growth include papillary, trabecular, tubular, cystic, and solid. Papillary adenocarcinomas, which represent 5 to 15% of all renal carcinomas, are relatively avascular and are associated with a five-year survival rate of 85%, compared with 52% for nonpapillary carcinomas. Granular cell and sarcomatoid varieties may have a less favorable prognosis than the clear and mixed cell types (Prout, 1973).

Natural History

At nephrectomy, these tumors have an average diameter of 7.5 cm, which, assuming no cell loss, represents over 90% of a tumor's kinetic life history. Early growth of renal adenocarcinoma is typically asymptomatic, and diagnosis is usually made relatively late in its natural history (de Kernion *et al.,* 1978). In a Memorial Sloan-Kettering Cancer Center series of 383 cases, 42% of asymptomatic patients had metastases at initial presentation. Of the patients who were symptomatic for less than two months, 31% had metastases, compared with 69% of cases who had symptoms for two months or longer. These data suggest that early renal carcinomas represent a malignancy of low grade. Metastases occur in 8% of pa-

tients with tumors of 5 cm or less in diameter, but in 80% of those with lesions greater than 10 cm. Reports of metastases from tumors as small as 0.5 cm in diameter, however, indicate that tumor size is not a reliable index of metastatic potential.

In the Memorial Hospital series of 262 men and 121 women with renal cell cancer, the median survival from diagnosis was 17.4 months, with a wide range of 16 to 239 months. Certain features of the natural history of renal cell cancer determine the rationale for treatment and provide an understanding of treatment failure. As indicated, a long period of local expansile growth precedes the infiltration and metastases which characterize the malignant process. Anecdotal clinical evidence indicates that this period may be as long as 30 years, but the average interval is uncertain.

Modes of Spread. The disease spreads by direct extension either to adjacent structures or to distant sites via lymphatic, hematogenous, or lymphohematogenous pathways. In 45% of cases, the tumor may involve the perinephric fatty tissue. Local extension beyond Gerota's fascia involving adjacent viscera may occur, and metastases to the ipsilateral adrenal gland are observed in up to 10% of patients who are clinically free of other evidence of disease. This is related to the high frequency of invasion of the perinephric fat. Renal vein invasion is found in 30% of patients, and extension of thrombus into the inferior vena cava has been found in up to 10% of patients. Such extension occurs predominantly in men. It usually originates in the right kidney and, in 25% of cases, is associated with nonvisualization of the involved kidney on intravenous pyelography (IVP). The adverse prognostic significance of main renal vein invasion may have been exaggerated, and venous invasion alone, in the absence of nodal or other spread, may have no significant adverse effect on prognosis. It should not deter an attempt at curative nephrectomy. Regional lymph node involvement is found at nephrectomy in approximately 10 to 30% of patients without evidence of other metastases, and the subsequent incidence of distant metastases is 50% greater in such cases. Thus, renal cancer seems to spread systemically at or about the same time as regional nodal involvement, a surgically discouraging observation when considering the value of a regional lymph node dissection along with nephrectomy.

Sites of Metastases. Distant metastases, either synchronous or metachronous, remain the primary cause of therapeutic failure. Approximately one-fourth to one-third of patients have metastases at the time of diagnosis, and of these, 70% are limited to only one organ: 40% involving the lungs, 22% in bone, and 8% in other organs. In 30% of patients with synchronous metastases, multiple organ sites are often involved. Approximately 60% of patients have metastases to the lungs, 30% to bone, and 30% to the liver. No area is inviolate, and the capacity of kidney cancer to metastasize to bizarre sites is well known. Table 35–1 summarizes 107 patients without evidence of metastases and 152 patients who had metastases at the time of diagnosis. Generally, patients with malignant hepatomegaly and CNS or spinal cord involvement have a short survival, whereas those with only pulmonary or nodal involvement live much longer. Patients presenting with brain metastases survived only six months from diagnosis. In 1 to 3% of patients, an apparently solitary metastasis was found at diagnosis, chiefly in the lung or proximal long bone, either the humerus or femur.

Of those patients who die as a result of recurrent renal adenocarcinoma, 5% have local recurrence, and 95% have distant metastases. Patients considered inoperable by virtue of advanced local disease and/or metastases have a limited life expectancy. In a series of 443 cases of renal cell cancer (Riches, 1964), only 4.4% survived three years, and 1.7% five years. In a study of 141 patients who presented with metastatic disease, Middleton (1967) had no survivors at two years. Other investigators (Katz and Davis, 1977; de Kernion *et al.,* 1978) have reported a 42 to 82% death rate at one year in patients with metastastic disease. The Memorial Hospital experience indicates that approximately half of such patients succumb within one year, and more than 75% within three years. Fewer than 10% survive five years or more.

The demonstrably long natural history of renal cell cancer, the appearance of metastases or local recurrence 20 or more years following an apparently curative nephrectomy, the frequency of local vascular invasion, probable systemic tumor embolization, and the occurrence of "spontaneous regressions" have long stimulated the concept that tumor-host interrelations are important, especially in the clinical behavior of renal adenocarcinoma (Katz and Schapira, 1982).

Clinical Presentation

Signs and Symptoms. Seventy-five percent of patients with renal adenocarcinoma seek medical care because of urologic symptoms. Thirty percent have clinical evidence of metastases at diagnosis, and 10% have symptoms referable to metastatic lesions. In up to 6% of cases, the tumor is discovered incidentally (Skinner *et al.,* 1971).

Table 35–1.   Metastatic Relapse in 257 Cases of Renal Cell Cancer at Memorial Hospital

INITIAL RELAPSE SITE	INCIDENCE (%)	DIAGNOSIS TO RELAPSE (MONTHS)	RELAPSE TO DEATH (MONTHS)	DIAGNOSIS TO DEATH (MONTHS)
Metachronous (N = 107)				
Lung	35	19	14	39
Bone	31	22	13	32
Local-regional*	14	7	13	17
Kidney	6	65	26	98
Spinal cord	5	9	6	15
Liver	4	8	4	11
Nodes	4	49	15	75
Synchronous (N = 152)				
Lung	41	3	4	9
Bone	24	2	8	10
Local-regional*	6	10	6	6
Kidney	——	——	——	——
Spinal cord	4	2	8	10
Liver	8	6	6	3
Nodes	——	——	——	——

* Perinephric soft tissue, renal fossa, and hilar lymph nodes.

Presenting urologic symptoms, alone or in combination, include gross or microscopic hematuria in two-thirds of patients, flank or abdominal pain in 40%, and a palpable mass in 30 to 45%. The classic triad of hematuria, a mass, and pain occurs in only 9% (Skinner et al., 1971). As the sole presenting manifestation of renal adenocarcinoma, hematuria occurs in 40% of patients, flank pain in 10%, abdominal mass in 6%, and fever in 2 to 7%.

At diagnosis, approximately one-fourth of cases have nonhemolytic anemia and weight loss, and 20%, low-grade fever. A triad of fever, anemia, and haptoglobinemia has been noted. Paraneoplastic syndromes have been associated with the elaboration of various hormones. For example, elevated erythropoietin levels, particularly with new radioimmunoassay (RIA) techniques (Sherwood and Goldwasser, 1979), have been reported in up to 50% of patients, although erythrocytosis occurs in only 5 to 10%. Hypertension may be present in as many as 20% of patients. Hypercalcemia, which occurs in 3 to 5% of patients, is commonly the result of bone metastases, but may result from ectopic or even primary hyperparathyroidism, or production of prostaglandins by the tumor. In the absence of liver metastases, hepatic dysfunction, so-called "hypernephroma hepatopathy," occurs in approximately 19 to 40% of patients. These abnormalities usually resolve promptly after nephrectomy if all tumor has been removed. In a recent series of 81 cases (Fletcher et al., 1981), 42% had some abnormality in liver function tests, and 19% had at least three or more abnormal tests without radographic or clinical evidence of extrahepatic disease. Frequently, the serum alkaline phosphatase and glutamyl transferase levels are elevated. Hepatopathy may recur, however, with the appearance of extrahepatic metastases, as may other generalized symptoms associated with the tumor, such as exacerbation of fever, night sweats, anorexia, weight loss, and elevated ESR. When symptoms of hypernephroma hepatopathy disappear after surgery, prognosis is good (35 months), but when they persist, it generally indicates residual disease and early death.

Diagnosis

The diagnosis of renal adenocarcinoma depends largely on radiologic techniques (Clay-men et al., 1979). Although urinalysis is important, hematuria is absent in up to 35% of patients. Proteinuria has been described in 90% of patients, but, like urinary levels of lactic dehydrogenase, it is a relatively poor screening technique. Intravenous pyelography (IVP) is the principal triage examination for identifying renal masses, although small masses, less than 4 cm in diameter, are not consistently visualized. This fact, combined with the inherent risk and cost-effective considerations, make IVP impractical as a screening test for renal cancer. The development of a more practical screening test and/or definition of a high-risk population in which available screening techniques might logically be applied are clearly needed.

Radiologic evidence of calcification is observed in 4% of renal mass lesions, 2% of benign cysts, and in up to 13% of renal adenocarcinomas. The location and pattern of calcification within a renal mass are significant. Of renal masses containing amorphous or punctuate, nonperipheral calcification, 87% are malignant, as are 20% of those showing only peripheral curvilinear calcification, and 38% showing both peripheral and nonperipheral calcification.

Ultrasonography can differentiate solid from cystic masses with 95% accuracy, although lesions smaller than 2 to 3 cm are below the limits of sonographic resolution. The IVP and sonography in combination have a reported accuracy of 88 to 98% in diagnosing renal cysts and a 86% rate in diagnosing carcinoma. Excellent correlation has been reported between surgical or autopsy findings and sonographic detection of tumor in the renal vein and inferior vena cava. In fact, real-time ultrasonography is replacing inferior venacavography in assessing patency of that vein.

Computed tomography (CT scan) diagnoses renal adenocarcinoma with an accuracy rate of 95% and a false-positive rate of only 1 to 2%. The technique identifies perinephric extension with an approximate 80% accuracy. It detects tumor extension into the main renal vein in 79% of cases and tumor infiltration in the inferior vena cava in 91% of patients. Although CT scan does identify enlarged regional lymph nodes better than high-dose angiography, it is unable to differentiate hyperplasia from carcinoma (Weyman et al., 1980). The detection of hepatic and other visceral metastases, as well as local tumor recurrences, is another important use for CT scans.

When the IVP with tomography, ultrasonography, and/or CT scans cannot unequivocally exclude carcinoma, then aspiration of fluid via cyst puncture is a common practice. Presence of a solid mass, malignant cells on cytology, or a bloody aspirate indicates a possible carcinoma. When findings from sonography, cyst puncture, and cyst fluid analysis all indicate a benign cyst, the diagnosis is accurate in 97% of cases. Cystic degeneration of a malignant tumor, association of a simple cyst with an adjacent carcinoma or one involving the cyst wall, or a multilocular cyst still accounts for a 3% false-positive rate.

Selective renal angiography correctly diagnoses 97% of renal adenocarcinomas. A false-positive rate of 3% is largely the result of localized inflammatory diseases of the kidney or other rare tumors. Renal adenocarcinoma is typically hypervascular, although 10 to 15% of tumors may be relatively hypovascular because of tumor necrosis, a papillary tumor pattern, or, rarely, the occurrence of a tumor within a cyst.

Visualization of a renal vein tumor thrombus during renal arteriography is a reliable sign of tumor extension into the renal vein. An absence or delayed visualization of the renal vein suggests tumor thrombus obstructing venous return, whereas early visualization of the main renal vein, the result of arteriovenous shunting, is generally a reliable sign of the absence of significant obstruction of the renal vein. Venacavography is indicated when tumor thrombus is suspected and probably should be employed in all large right-sided tumors that may significantly compress, invade, or extend into and up the lumen of the inferior vena cava. Real-time ultrasonography

can also be used. Angiography is helpful in identifying visceral, vertebral, contralateral renal, and retroperitoneal, or lumbar metastases. Celiac angiography may detect hepatic lesions as small as 0.75 cm in diameter. Arteriography is also a useful guide for the surgeon in planning his approach in especially large renal tumors.

Bone scanning, using 99^m technetium diphosphonate or pyrophosphate, is the most sensitive method for detecting osseous metastases and can detect 98% of such lesions. In selected patients, such as those with sarcomatoid renal cancer, radionuclide scans do not seem to detect osteolytic lesions, and skeletal surveys must be periodically performed. Skeletal radiographs are relatively insensitive for detecting early bone lesions, since 40% or more of bone calcium must be replaced by tumor before it can be observed on a plane film. In the absence of symptoms referable to metastatic deposits, bone and hepatic scintiscans are recommended to detect metastases in these areas only if biochemical abnormalities, such as an elevated alkaline phosphatase determination, are present.

Staging

Systems of histologic grading and staging of renal cell cancers have established relevance to prognosis (Boxer *et al.,* 1979). Tumor stage reflects the extent to which the biologic potential or grade of a tumor has been realized and offers the best insight into prognosis. The staging systems generally used are those of Robson and colleagues (1969) and the TNM classification which are outlined and compared in Table 35–2. Using Robson's pathologic staging system, approximately 33% of all patients

Table 35–2. Staging of Renal Carcinoma

TNM STAGING			
Clinical	*Pathologic*	EXTENT OF DISEASE	ROBSON STAGE
T_1	P_1	Tumor within capsule ($<$2 cm)	I
T_2	P_2	Tumor within capsule ($>$2 cm)	
T_3	P_3	Tumor in perinephric fat	II
T_3	P_3	Tumor in renal vein	
N_1–N_3	PN_1–PN_3	Tumor in regional nodes	III
	V_2	Tumor in inferior vena cava	
T_4	P_4	Adjacent organ invasion	
N_4	PN_4	Tumor in juxtaregional lymph nodes	IV
M_1	PM_1	Distant metastases	

present with stage I lesions, 7 to 12% with stage II, 24 to 36% with stage III, and 25 to 31% with stage IV (Skinner *et al.,* 1972). Tumor grade and stage are related. Only 8% of low-grade tumors present as stage IV lesions, compared to more than 60% with high-grade lesions. Anaplastic and sarcomatoid tumors are three times more likely to be metastatic at presentation and twice as likely to metastasize subsequently. Since the prognostic significance of lymph node metastases is more ominous than that of renal vein invasion alone, the inclusion of both major renal vein and regional lymph node involvement in a common category is a significant limitation of the current staging system.

Treatment

Surgery. Renal adenocarcinoma is a lethal disease, with survival rates for untreated patients approximating 36% at one year, 4% at three years, and 2% at five years. Nephrectomy with a surgical mortality of 2 to 5% is the principal therapy for renal cell carcinoma. Nephrectomy is a potentially curative procedure in patients with stage I or II (five-year survival of 66%), and III (five-year survival of 42%) neoplasms. Occasionally, selected patients with stage IV are cured when definitive surgical therapy includes local extensions or metastases. Unfortunately, pre- or postoperative irradiation is ineffective in controlling local recurrences or improving survival (van der Werf-Messing, 1973).

Since renal tumors often extend into perirenal tissues, radical or extended nephrectomy is employed. Surgery includes adequate exposure to permit the widest and safest excision with minimal tumor manipulation, preliminary ligation of the main renal artery and vein, intact removal of Gerota's fascia, with its contained kidney, perinephric fat, and adrenal gland, systematic regional lymph node dissection, and excision of as much of the ureter as is accessible through the operative exposure.

The average and best reported survival results with radical nephrectomy according to stage are presented in Table 35–3. Few reports have been published in which a precise technique of radical nephrectomy has been described, the pathologic stage of renal cancer indicated, and the overall five- and ten-year survival rates provided. Published results indicate that tumor stage correlates with prognosis, although the difference between stages I and II

Table 35–3. Survival of Patients with Renal Cell Carcinoma after Nephrectomy

ROBSON STAGE	5-YEAR (%)	10-YEAR (%)
I	59–80*	39–70
II	51–64	17–66
III	34–48	20–38
IV	5	2

* Average best reported survival by Robson *et al.,* 1969; Skinner *et al.,* 1971; and Boxer *et al.,* 1979.

is not impressive. Patients alive and tumor-free ten years after nephrectomy are believed to be cured, but recurrences after this time are not uncommon. Assuming that ten-year survival rates are equivalent to cure rates, it is possible to calculate the potential curability of patients who present with localized renal adenocarcinoma. Only 43% of all patients are curable at the time of initial diagnosis. Only 60% of patients with potentially curable lesions, that is, stage I, II, or III disease, who undergo a radical nephrectomy and regional lymph node dissection are actually cured. Despite apparent local or regional disease at diagnosis, renal carcinoma is often already systemic and is the ultimate cause of treatment failure in most patients. Thirty percent of patients with stage I disease, 33% with stage II disease, and 62% with stage III disease already have micrometastases at the time of nephrectomy.

The role of radical nephrectomy for patients with stage IV disease is controversial (Montie *et al.,* 1977). Occasionally, radical nephrectomy for potential cure of stage IV disease may be performed in conjunction with definitive treatment, usually by surgical excision of one or more coexisting metastases in the lung or bone, and in sites amenable to surgical excision (*i.e.,* scapula, long bones, and so forth). In selective cases, definitive resection of a solitary metastatic deposit in conjunction with nephrectomy for the primary tumor yields five-year survival rates in the 30 to 35% range. Some investigators will perform a resection of a solitary lesion if there has been no growth or no doubling of the lesion within three to six months. At this time, no available method to define the patient population that would be helped by radical resection of an isolated metastasis is available. Radical nephrectomy for potential cure may also be performed in patients with stage IV neoplasms that have contiguous structures directly involved. Such resections have involved removal of the spleen and portions of the liver, colon, and pancreas. Five-year survival rates following such extended resections are rarely more than 10%. Local nonresectability may result from direct tumor invasion of the diaphragm, paravertebral musculature, or adjacent great vessels or from massive hilar regional lymph node involvement.

Partial nephrectomy is usually selected for the management of renal cancer in patients with small (less than 3 cm) cortical and localized, low-grade neoplasms, bilateral tumors, or a tumor in a solitary kidney. Selective renal angiography has facilitated both case selection and the surgical procedure itself. Techniques for *in vivo* perfusion of the kidney and *ex vivo* renal "bench" surgery, with or without autotransplantation, have encouraged more aggressive approaches in this area. If an adequate margin of perinephric fat and an adequate margin of surrounding kidney parenchyma are excised with the tumor, then partial excision provides a perfectly suitable cancer operation. Surgical mortality and morbidity are low.

Radical nephrectomy has been utilized in patients with metastatic stage IV neoplasms for relief of local pain, anemia, and hematuria and for relief of such systemic symptoms as malaise, fever, and weight loss that may be attributed to the bulk of the patient's neoplasm. All of these indications for nephrectomy, however, may also be accomplished in some patients by means of renal artery embolization and infarction, a procedure that is recommended if the risk and morbidity inherent in an extended nephrectomy for a large, bulky tumor are unacceptably high. Sometimes, angioinfarction reduces a bulky lesion sufficiently to permit surgical excision.

Radical nephrectomy has been advocated in patients with distant metastases in order to induce a spontaneous regression. Although data are lacking, there seems to be little doubt that the surgical mortality of nephrectomy, especially in the palliative situation, exceeds the probability of obtaining a spontaneous regression. Furthermore, most, but not all, reported spontaneous regressions have followed nephrectomy. Spontaneous regressions, when present, are generally of short duration, and no clear improvement in survival following nephrectomy has been reported (Katz and Shipira, 1982).

Embolization. Transcatheter embolization (angioinfarction) of renal adenocarcinoma is used as palliative therapy in patients with disseminated disease. In patients with localized disease, it is used as an adjunct to nephrectomy or, possibly, to modify previously unresectable tumors. A variety of materials have been used as embolizing agents, including gel foam, muscle, and autologous blood clot, although recently, the Gianturco coil has been favored. Complications of angioinfarction include embolization of other organs, renal failure secondary to the use of excessive contrast material, and a self-limiting postinfarction syndrome manifested by flank pain, fever, and an elevated lactic dehydrogenase level. Preoperative angioinfarction in patients with distant metastases, followed by nephrectomy and progesterone treatment, has produced an objective response rate of 28% and stabilization of disease in 21% (Swanson, 1979). Responses were observed only in patients with pulmonary metastases. Such responses may simply reflect the natural history of the disease, rather than an effective treatment. A randomized trial has been undertaken to evaluate this procedure.

Radiotherapy. Although initial reports were optimistic, controlled prospective studies have shown no survival benefit from pre- or postoperative radiotherapy. In fact, irradiation was found to be detrimental in one prospective randomized trial (Finney, 1973). On occasion, radiation therapy may control local symptoms such as pain or bleeding in patients not otherwise candidates for nephrectomy. The effectiveness of angioinfarction for this purpose, however, suggests that radiotherapy may no longer be appropriate. Radiation modifiers and sensitizers, neutron and heavy-charged particle radiotherapy, intraoperative electron beam therapy, and hyperthermia for treatment of this tumor must be considered experimental at this time.

A major role for radiotherapy in this disease is to control or palliate spinal cord lesions, osseous disease, and central nervous system metastases. Since these tumors frequently metastasize to the brain and spinal cord, clinicians must be alert to any signs relating to such lesions. Any change in gait, mentation, pain, headache, or, in particular, personality should lead to further neurologic investigations. CT scans are most helpful in defining metastases. When lesions are suspected, high doses of corticosteroids should be administered immediately (*i.e.,* dexamethasone, 50 to 100 mg, with subsequent tapering). Radiation therapy should not be administered to a known osteolytic vertebral lesion without proper evaluation of neurologic symptoms, particularly in the thoracic area. The possibility of extradural disease should be considered. Pain, either over the affected vertebrae or radicular in nature, may indicate spinal cord disease. Relatively asymptomatic patients have been seen who, on myelography, show a complete spinal cord block. If a block is present, a cisternal myelogram is needed to confirm its cephalad extent. In these cases, corticosteroids and irradiation are required. A careful history documenting subtle signs, such as pain in the thoracic vertebrae induced by coughing or straining at the time of defecation, or pain while putting on a heavy overcoat, should lead to further neurologic examination. After confirmation of disease, appropriate radiation therapy should be administered, and 6 to 12 weeks later, a re-fluoromyelogram should be performed. Another area that requires early radiation therapy is an osteolytic lesion in a weight-bearing area.

Generally, minor signs and symptoms in patients with renal cell carcinoma should not be dismissed since often metastases or paraneoplastic effects of the disease are discovered.

Chemotherapy. Since the initial reports proving that renal tumors can be induced in Syrian golden hamsters with the prolonged use of estrogens, hormonal dependency of renal adenocarcinomas has been investigated (Kirkman, 1959). Antiandrogens, antiestrogens, androgens, and progestins have all been utilized. Bloom (1973) has reported a 15 to 20% objective response rate (21% in men, 8% in women), and up to 35 to 40% improvement or stabilization of disease with medroxyprogesterone acetate, 100 mg, PO daily, or 800 to 1000 mg, IM weekly in a depo preparation, and/or testosterone proprionate, 100 mg daily or 400 mg weekly. Recent evidence in a large number of trials describes a response rate of < 1 to 2% (Hrushesky and Murphy, 1977; Yagoda et al., 1982). The few responses that do occur are observed within four to six weeks after initiating therapy, primarily in soft tissue masses and almost never in osseous metastases. Firm evidence indicating significant hormone binding sites for hypernephroma is lacking, and receptor studies have not correlated with response (Concolino et al., 1978). Although some patients respond, and hormonal manipulation induces minimal toxicity and permits an active therapeutic approach to the patient, alternative agents and modalities of therapy are lacking.

Unfortunately, chemotherapy has also been ineffective. More than 30 drugs, and many more combination regimens, have been tried without significant clinical benefit. Recent trials (see Table 35–4) have found no objective tumor regression greater than 10 to 15% with vinblastine sulfate, semustine, carmustine, triazinate, dactinomycin, 4'epidoxorubicin, vindesine, chlorozotocin, cisplatin, bisantrene, hydroxyurea, 4'-demethoxydaunorubicin, m-AMSA, gallium nitrate, and methyl guanylhydrazone (methyl G) singly and in combination with vinblastine sulfate (Hahn et al., 1981; Stolbach et al., 1981; Yagoda et al., 1982).

The delay in metastases and reports of spontaneous regression have led to an immunologic approach. Currently, no evidence has been presented indicating clinical benefit with

Table 35–4. Selected Chemotherapy Trials for Hypernephroma

DRUG	NO. CASES	% CR + PR
AMSA*	21	0
Androgens	170	3
Bisantrene	53	4
Bleomycin	20	0
Chlorambucil	24	16
Chlorozotocin (DCNU)	21	0
Cisplatin	49	0
Cyclophosphamide	98	7
Dactinomycin	89	1
4'-Demethoxydaunorubicin	12	8
Dianhydrogalactitol	56	0
Doxorubicin	31	0
4'-Epidoxorubicin	29	10
Etiopside	53	2
5-Fluorouracil	90	8
Flutamide	25	4
Gallium nitrate	11	0
Lomustine (CCNU)	59	7
Mercaptopurine	29	7
Methyl-G	83	11
Methyl-G + vinblastine	15	0
Mitomycin C	23	11
Naloxidine	20	5
PALA†	15	0
Piperazenedione	23	0
Progestins	695	5
Semustine (MeCCNU)	57	7
Tamoxifen	137	7
Triazinate	59	5
Vinblastine	199	8–25‡
Vinblastine + CCNU	89	12
Vindesine	28	0

Summation of results in the literature by Hruschesky and Murphy, 1977; Al-Sarraf et al., 1981; Hahn et al., 1981; Stolbach et al., 1981; and Yagoda et al., 1982; and recent data from trials at Memorial Hospital.
* AMSA = Acrindinylamino-methanesulfon-m-anisidie.
† PALA = N-(phosphonacetyl)-L-aspartic acid.
‡ High and low percentages from two separate reviews, but with additional data from randomized trials, a lower rate of 8 to 15% is more credible.

immune ribonucleic acid, BCG, transfer factor, poly IC:LC, interferon, or autologous tumor vaccines. Although complete and partial remissions have occasionally been observed in a small number of cases, there have been no large phase II or randomized phase III studies. One study has shown no benefit compared to the poor results obtained with hormones alone (Montie *et al.,* 1981).

Standard therapy is considered to be progestins, vinblastine sulfate, 4–6 mg/m^2 IV weekly, or a nitrosourea. Many oncologists have suggested new investigational drugs obtained for phase II evaluation.

Without significant response rates, any use of cytotoxic or hormonal agents, or irradiation for prophylaxis is not recommended.

Future Prospects

Although important advances in the understanding and treatment of renal cell carcinoma have been made, signficant challenges remain. The clinical history of this tumor suggests that growth is relatively silent until late in its natural history, and, in most cases, the disease is already systemic at diagnosis. The maximum benefit of surgical treatment appears to have been reached. Enhanced survival will require the development and application of adjunctive therapies, both for occult metastases, and for manifestly advanced disease. Further studies of the epidemiology, etiology, biochemistry, and immunology may provide new insights, as well as the development of earlier detection modalities and newer chemotherapeutic agents, and will result in some progress in this rather bleak area of oncology.

BLADDER CANCER

Incidence and Epidemiology

Carcinoma of the bladder is recognized as a spectrum of clinical pathologic entities with widely varying biologic behavior. It ranges from relatively benign papillary growths that usually express an indolent course with multiple recurrences to highly malignant anaplastic tumors that are deeply invasive, widely metastasizing, and rapidly lethal. About 90% of bladder carcinomas are transitional cell carcinomas, 6 to 7% are squamous cell carcinomas, and 1 to 2% are adenocarcinomas. Foci of squamous cell carcinoma and adenomatous

features may be present in as high as 20% of infiltrating transitional cell carcinomas (Mostofi, 1968).

Bladder cancer will account for approximately 40,000 new cases in 1985, and will be responsible for 11,000 deaths (Silverberg, 1985). Men are affected three times more frequently than women. Evidence suggests the incidence rate of bladder cancer may be increasing in men, although the age-adjusted mortality has remained nearly constant in both sexes over the past 45 years.

Studies of the epidemiology of bladder cancer have provided important insights into the potential causes for this disease (Wynder and Goldsmith, 1977). Many possible etiologic factors have been identified, including (1) occupation (chemical, dye stuff, leather processing, rubber, and plastic industries), (2) habits (smoking and perhaps coffee drinking), (3) diet (bracken fern, nitrosamines, tryptophan metabolites, and nonnutritive sweeteners), medications (phenacetin, and cyclophosphamide), and (4) chronic bladder infections (bilharzial cystitis or prolonged catheter drainage in paraplegics). Although bladder cancer may represent a spectrum of diseases with different causes, the complexity of the problem of causation has been increased by evidence that bladder carcinogenesis may be a multistage process of initiating and promoting factors. Initiation may follow a single exposure to a carcinogen at a dose level that is too low to induce manifest cancer. Promotion may then follow a varying period of exposure to a noncarcinogenic agent. Initiation is regarded as irreversible, but promotion may be prevented or inhibited before the development of an autonomous tumor. The recognition that initiation may be irreversible necessitates the exclusion of carcinogenic drugs from the workplace and human environment, while chemoprevention agents (*i.e., cis*-retinoic acid, vitamin-A derivatives) may be useful in modulating promoting factors.

Diagnosis

The diagnosis is usually made when the disease is still limited to the bladder and pelvis. Bladder tumors commonly produce symptoms when they still can be treated. Hematuria is the presenting symptom in approximately 80% of patients. Urinary frequency, urgency, and dysuria may also alert the patient to seek medical attention. At times, symptoms of vesicle irritability may be quite severe and resemble interstitial cystitis. Since this is rare in men, such symptoms should alert the physician to the possibility of bladder cancer. Occasionally, patients may present with weight loss and bone pain resulting from distant metastases.

Bladder tumors may be superficial, papillary, and relatively benign, despite a high recurrence rate, or they may present initially as a solid, infiltrating, more aggressive cancer. The aggressive natural history of high-grade and high-stage bladder cancer is confirmed by the disappointing survival rates achieved over the past 30 years, regardless of treatment. Aggressive bladder tumors spread by local infiltration of the bladder wall, followed by lymphatic and vascular invasion, usually in direct proportion to, but not entirely dependent upon, the depth of local bladder penetration. Regional lymph node metastases and distant dissemination may then occur sequentially or independently of one another.

The diagnosis is usually made with urinary cytologic examination, cystoendoscopy, and transurethral biopsy. Once the diagnosis is established by the pathologic findings, before any treatment decision is made, it is essential to define the extent or stage of the disease.

Staging

Stage, grade, multicentricity, location, and size, are the principal tumor features that affect the selection of treatment for patients with bladder cancer. Tumor grade provides a practical indication of growth potential since, at the time of treatment, most high-grade tumors (III and IV) are found to be deeply infiltrating, whereas most low-grade tumors (I and II) are found to be in situ or superficially infiltrating. Tumor stage is a direct indication of the extent to which growth potential has been realized. Multicentricity in time and space (polychronotropism) is still an unquantified variable of bladder tumor behavior that limits the applicability of some treatment options (Whitmore, 1979).

Although a variety of tumor and host factors influence selection of treatment, clinical staging is currently the most important in deciding between a conservative or a radical approach to management. Clinical staging may be defined as the clinician's effort to determine the pathologic extent of the disease. Moreover, staging identifies the upper limits of curability

by the extent of surgical excision. The logic of staging as a guide in efforts to control locoregional disease by means of extended surgery or irradiation was provided by the landmark autopsy study of Jewett and Strong (1946), who discovered that the depth of bladder wall invasion correlated with the incidence of metastases in regional lymph nodes and distant sites. This study and that of Marshall (1952) have served as an impetus to establish local tumor control by various techniques selected on the basis of staging.

Pretreatment evaluation should include the following: (1) a complete history with regard to previous urothelial tumors, (2) intravenous urography to define multicentricity within the upper urinary tracts and document the presence or absence of ureteral obstruction, and (3) cystoendoscopy and biopsy under general anesthesia. The bladder should be examined endoscopically to determine the location, number, and gross pathologic characteristics of the tumor(s), appearance of the adjacent and entire bladder mucosa, and presence of tumor at the ureteral orifices, in the bladder neck and urethra. The tumor should be characterized as papillary, sessile, broad-based, pedunculated, solid, or ulcerated. If the tumor or tumors are small, they should be completely resected. If the tumor is extensive, sufficient biopsy material should be obtained to reveal the cell type and grade, the depth of invasion, and the presence of lymphatic and vascular involvement. Biopsy of suspicious areas of bladder mucosa adjacent to, and peripheral to, the primary lesion is also performed, as well as selected site biopsies of the bladder neck and prostatic urethra to document the presence of in situ carcinoma. Continued presence of diffuse in situ lesions may favor radical therapy over conservative therapy, as well as determine its extent. (4) Bimanual examination under anesthesia before and after resection aids in estimating the depth of infiltration, completeness of resection, and fixation to adjacent organs or pelvic side wall. Most important, bimanual examination helps determine the operability of a given neoplasm. (5) Voided urine or saline bladder washing for cytologic examination is useful in the detection and especially the follow-up after treatment in patients with bladder cancer. (6) A complete blood count, as well as tests of renal and liver function, should also be part of the pretreatment evaluation.

Other examinations, such as CT scans, lymphangiography, and bone or liver scans, have not generally been included in the regular assessment unless specific indications warrant such studies. Lymphangiography has not been useful since obturator and other local-regional nodes are rarely visualized, and minimal nodal invasion cannot be accurately determined. CT scans are much more useful, but still fail to predict sufficiently the extent of bladder wall tumor invasion or delineate local-regional involvement. Stage D_2 lesions are more readily documented. Transrectal sonography has major limitations, but the new technique of transurethral ultrasonography may permit a better assessment of not only bladder wall invasion (stage B), but also, local-regional involvement (stage C). Presently recognized clinical stages of bladder cancer are shown in Table 35–5.

Clinical staging is imprecise. Limitations of clinical staging, based upon correlations with the pathologic stage after cystectomy and pelvic lymph node dissection, are readily apparent. Understaging is far more common than overstaging, with one-third of patients having clinically B_1 lesions (tumors superficially invading muscle) reclassified pathologically as stage B_2 or C. The clinical staging error increases with the depth of bladder wall penetration found pathologically. Patients with deeply infiltrating (B, C) carcinomas frequently (37%) show invasion of contiguous viscera or metastases in the regional lymph nodes or beyond. Staging accuracy exceeds 80% in distinguishing between low-stage neoplasms that may be treated conservatively from apparently localized lesions of more advanced stages that require aggressive therapy. An exception is that group of patients who have failed full-course irradiation.

Treatment

An appropriate assessment of the patient and of the disease relative to tumor stage, histologic grade, tumor size, and multiplicity precedes any treatment. Such assessment involves evaluation of the patient's physical and mental capacities to tolerate therapy, clinical staging to select the therapy that offers the optimal balance between tumor control and functional preservation, and plans for appropriate rehabilitation and follow-up. Any therapeutic decision involves consideration of surgery, irradiation, and, more recently in advanced disease, both modalities coupled with chemotherapy. Local treatment is defined as that treatment limited to a part or parts of the bladder, and radical or aggressive treatment as that treatment directed to the entire bladder.

Carcinoma *in situ* (T_{IS}, T_0). Carcinoma *in situ* represents flat, usually high-grade lesions confined to the bladder mucosa, which may be focal or diffuse, and often account for severe symptoms of frequency, urgency, and dysuria. Since T_{IS} was first described in 1952 (Melicow, 1952), this clinicopathologic entity is being recognized with increasing frequency. Although every epithelial (transitional cell) cancer has an *in situ* phase, a lesion does not have to be invasive to be designated as "cancer." Potential for invasion is implicit in this designation. Most invasive bladder cancer likely evolves from *in situ* lesions. The fre-

Table 35–5. Bladder Cancer Staging

JEWETT-MARSHALL		TNM	
		Clinical	*Pathologic*
0	No tumor-definitive specimen	T_0	P_0
	Carcinoma *in situ*	T_{IS}	P_{IS}
	Papillary tumor invasion		
		T_1	P_1
A	Invasion of lamina propria		
B_1	Superficial	T_2	P_2
	Muscle invasion		
B_2	Deep	T_{3a}	
			P_3
C	Invasion of perivesical fat	T_{3b}	
D_1	Invasion of contiguous viscera	T_{4a}	P_4
	Pelvic nodes	N_{1-3}	
D_2	Distant metastases	M_1	
	Nodes above aortic bifurcation	N_4	

quency of this critical event and the interval in which such evolution occurs are unpredictable. The poorly defined natural history and biologic behavior of *in situ* carcinoma provide no firm basis for categorical treatment recommendations. Multicentricity in space and time and the presence or absence of associated solid or papillary tumors are factors currently influencing management of flat carcinoma *in situ*. Since such lesions are confined to the bladder mucosa, T_{IS} is considered potentially curable by local means.

In situ carcinoma (positive urinary cytology and negative cystoendoscopy) may have a long preclinical course, with minimal or no symptomatic change. Eventually such lesions may evolve into a focal variety, with or without associated papillary tumors. A pathologic distinction must be made between a benign papilloma, frequently called grade I transitional cell carcinoma, and a true carcinoma. Benign papillomas do recur. Patients presenting initially with one papilloma have a 30% recurrence rate, while those with two or more papillomas have a greater than 70% recurrence rate. They are not invasive, and only 4 to 13% of patients will eventually have carcinoma *in situ*. Endoscopic destruction is the initial approach to treatment of focal lesions and is generally successful in eradicating such tumors, although persistence and/or recurrence is the rule. In 50 to 80% of cases, diffuse *in situ* cancers, clinically characterized by a history of progressive and often severe symptoms of vesicle irritability, are associated with a subsequent development of infiltrating cancers. They represent a clinically ominous extreme in the *in situ* cancer spectrum for which cystectomy as cure may be indicated. Clearly, endoscopic fulguration becomes impractical for the more diffuse variety, but more recently, intravesical immunotherapy with BCG and chemotherapy with thiophosphoramide (thiotepa), doxorubicin, mitomycin C, and epidyl (ethoglucid) have demonstrated a positive effect in erdicating *in situ* lesions and, in some instances, preventing recurrences for periods greater than one year. Recent data (Herr, 1982) indicate that BCG has prevented recurrences for up to two years, and relapse is more frequent in the ureters and prostatic ducts, areas which do not have contact with intravesically administered BCG. Cystectomy is generally advised for diffuse *in situ* cancers when a six-month course of intravesical therapy fails and for lesions that are associated with severe bladder symptoms, diminished bladder capacity, or involve the bladder neck, prostatic urethra, or prostate gland.

An important consideration is the ability of the urologist to follow adequately suspected areas of relapse. Since the prostatic ducts can never be fully visualized endoscopically and thereby properly evaluated for recurrence, radical surgery for such lesions is recommended frequently.

Stage T_1 (A). Most small, superficial papillary, low-grade tumors can be treated successfully by transurethral resection and fulguration of the bladder (TURB). Lesions suitable for this procedure must be readily accessible to the resectoscope and must have distinct margins. The entire tumor, together with a small portion of underlying muscle, is removed from the bladder wall. New tumors can develop in the same area or elsewhere in the bladder mucosa in up to 85% of patients, and subsequent invasion may eventually develop in 30% of patients. Patients with bladder carcinoma treated conservatively with TURB must be followed closely with cystoscopy and cytologic examination every three months initially, and at longer intervals if no new tumors develop after one year. The five-year survival of patients with low-stage bladder tumors treated with TURB approaches 80%. This may improve with the wider use of adjunctive intravesical therapy.

Intravesical therapy has proven to be of both therapeutic and prophylactic benefit in reducing the recurrence rate of superficial bladder tumors (Soloway, 1980). Intravesical instillation of thiophosphoramide, 60 mg/60 mL distilled water weekly for six weeks, has been used most widely in this country. A second course, weekly for four consecutive weeks, is administered if a partial response is documented at follow-up cystoscopy. Approximately one-fourth to one-third of all tumors will show complete regression, and another one-third will achieve a partial remission. Since the molecular weight of thiophosphoramide is low, systemic absorption occurs, and the major toxicity is transient myelosuppression (leukopenia and thrombocytopenia). Recovery usually occurs in two to four weeks. The long-term value of intravesical thiophosphoramide as prophylaxis against recurrence or development of new tumors remains in doubt, and its efficacy against diffuse *in situ* carcinoma is marginal. Although the overall complete and partial remission rates with thiophosphoramide intravesically are approximately 25% and 24 to 38%, respectively, the effectiveness may depend on the type of disease being treated. In many earlier studies, results included patients with benign papillomas and not true T_1 lesions. Burnand and associates (1976), who compared a single dose of 90 mg of thiophosphoramide with placebo administered immediately after transurethral resection, describe a statistically significant decrease in the "reimplantation rate" of tumor cells, 44% versus 3%, respectively. When thiotepa is instilled for prophylaxis three days to one month after eradication of all visible disease, improvement in the disease-free interval and in the recurrence rate is marginal when compared to a control group, 40 to 49% for thiotepa versus 52 to 60% for the control group. When thiotepa is employed as active therapy for existing low-stage lesions, tumor recurrence rates decrease, and disease-free intervals increase, particularly if continued prophylaxis is maintained in responders. Other drugs that have been used for intravesical therapy are listed in Table 35–6.

In Europe, epodyl (ethoglucid, triethylene glycol diglycidyl ether) has been utilized in patients with bladder cancer, although no comparative trials have been attempted in the United States. Preliminary results of recent prospective trials of mitomycin C (molecular weight, 334) and BCG (bacillus Galmette-Guérin) indicate both to be very effective agents. Approximately 50% of patients obtained a complete response, and another one-third showed a partial remission. These agents may well replace thiotepa as standard therapy (Soloway, 1982). Allergic reactions (desquamation), limited to the hands or perineal area, have been described in patients given mitomycin C intravesically. This toxic side effect is the

result of a contact dermatitis, which can be avoided with meticulous cleansing of all areas of potential drug contact.

Radiation therapy for such tumors is ineffective in eradicating the existing tumor. Evidence that radiation therapy prevents new tumor occurrence is not available.

Stage T_2 (B_1). Tumors with superficial muscle invasion may be of low to high grade and are associated with a significant incidence of lymph node metastases (25%). Many of these tumors may be controlled by TURB, the limitation being that, once in muscle, tumor cells have access to lymphatic and vascular channels which may permit their rapid spread. In fact, approximately 50% of such patients will eventually die of metastatic disease despite adequate control of the primary neoplasm. Partial or total cystectomy, however, does not improve the control of a superficially infiltrating, low-grade tumor better than TURB with adequate margins. More aggressive or extensive therapy is generally required for tumors infiltrating muscle or for a solitary invasive neoplasm that cannot be resected endoscopically, safely and reliably. The decision to abandon conservative approaches in favor of more radical treatment requires considerable experience and judgment.

An occasional patient with a solitary tumor of limited size, located sufficiently distant from the bladder base and neck to allow inclusion of a 2-cm margin of normal bladder wall peripheral to the lesion, may be a candidate for partial cystectomy (Utz *et al.,* 1973). A previous history of bladder tumor elsewhere or concomitant multifocal lesions on random biopsy are contraindications to segmental resection. The multicentric nature of bladder tumors limits the applicability of partial cystectomy but, in the selected patient, offers five-year survival rates comparable to those of total cystectomy (see Table 35–7).

External radiotherapy is often advised for muscle-infiltrating bladder cancers (van der Werf-Messing, 1975). Irradiation has the advantage of preservation of bladder and sexual function, and a lower morbidity and mortality rate. It can be used for patients who are not surgical candidates because of advanced age or medical contraindications. If external radiotherapy fails to control the tumor, salvage cystectomy may still be possible, with an anticipated 30% five-year survival for patients who fail irradiation (Wallace *et al.,* 1976; Smith and Whitmore, 1981a).

Table 35–6.   Intravesical Chemotherapy

Doxorubicin	50 mg/50 mL NS twice a week for one week, then monthly for 12 months 40 mg/20 mL NS twice a week 80 mg/40 mL NS monthly
Epodyl	100 mL of 1% solution weekly for twelve weeks, then every other week for three months, and once every three months thereafter
Thiotepa	60 mg/60 mL sterile water once a week for four weeks, then monthly
Mitomycin C	40 mg/40 mL once a week for eight weeks.
BCG	120 mg/50 mL NS, once a week for six weeks

Table 35-7. Bladder Cancer: Five-Year Survival Following Surgical Treatment at Memorial Sloan-Kettering Cancer Center

METHOD	STAGE (%)					
	T_{is}	T_1	T_2	T_{3a}	T_{3b}	T_4
TUR	71	62-77	57-59	23	2-7	0
Segmental resection	75-80	57-80	43-58	16-33	6-29	0-20
Cystectomy	50-77	35-50	45-50	29-40	10-18	0-4

Radiation therapy with megavoltage equipment usually involves administration of 6000 to 7000 rads to the bladder and 4000 to 5000 rads to the regional lymph nodes over a six- to seven-week period. Patients treated with radiation therapy usually experience dysuria, urgency, frequency, and diarrhea, but symptoms usually subside a few weeks after completion of therapy. Severe complications, such as contracted bladder, hemorrhage, and radiation cystitis or proctitis, develop in 4 to 14% of patients. The local failure rate following radiation therapy is about 50%, and survival rates diminish as tumor stage increases. Radiotherapy may be anticipated to cure only 20% of deeply infiltrating tumors (Goffinet *et al.*, 1975).

The apparent control of some tumors, patient acceptance, and survival rates that are not vastly different from those achieved with surgical treatment of tumors of similar stage help sustain an active role for radiation treatment of bladder cancer. The capacity to control a tumor, and yet preserve function, has encouraged efforts to identify those patients (or neoplasms) for whom radiation therapy would be the optimal treatment and to encourage clinical and radiobiologic research directed at improving the therapeutic ratio between antitumor effect and radiation complications.

In otherwise healthy patients, radical cystectomy, with or without preoperative irradiation, is usually advised for muscle-infiltrating tumors that are multicentric and unsuitable for segmental resection (Smith *et al.*, 1982). Radical cystectomy involves removal of bladder and prostate in men, bladder, urethra, anterior vaginal wall, and genital organs in women, and urinary diversion, usually an ileal conduit. It includes excision of perivesical fat, urachus, and overlying peritoneum in both sexes. The plane of dissection is adjacent to the muscular and bony walls of the pelvis. Often, a pelvic lymph node dissection is included. Incontinuity excision of the entire male urethra is performed for multifocal tumors located at or near the bladder neck or involving the pros-

tatic urethra. Cystectomy is a major surgical procedure, entailing a significant morbidity (30%) and sacrifice of normal urinary and sexual functions. In recent years, surgical mortality has been significantly reduced to less than 2%.

Radical cystectomy achieves approximately a 60% five-year survival rate in patients with superficially infiltrating tumors. The pelvic local recurrence rate alone is less that 10%, with 40% of patients failing as a result of systemic disease owing to unrecognized preexisting metastases.

Stage T_3 (B_2 and C). Deeply infiltrating bladder cancers are generally not amenable to any form of conservative therapy and require more aggressive treatment, either radiation therapy or total cystectomy. Either modality used alone for such lesions results in no more than a 20% five-year survival (Whitmore, 1979). Because of the poor results after either treatment modality used alone, radiation therapy (2000 rads in five days, or 4000 rads or more at 1000 rads per week) has been employed preoperatively as an adjunct to radical cystectomy in an effort to reduce tumor spillage and iatrogenic dissemination at surgery (Wallace and Bloom, 1976; Miller, 1977; Whitmore *et al.*, 1977a). Several randomized and nonrandomized series have shown improved survival with the combined treatment compared to radical cystectomy or external radiation therapy alone (see Table 35-8). Five-year survival in patients with the T_3 lesions has approximately doubled with the use of preoperative irradiation and cystectomy (40 to 50%) compared to radical cystectomy alone (20 to 25%). Improved survival is particularly evident in patients whose tumors are downstaged by irradiation, as demonstrated by a pathologic (P) stage less than the initial clinical (T) stage. Stage reduction after preoperative radiation therapy is observed in approximately one-third of cases. The favorable effects of preoperative irradiation have also contributed to a reduction in pelvic recurrences and, to some extent, to eliminating relapse due to distant

Table 35–8. Bladder Cancer: Preoperative Radiation Therapy and Cystectomy in Clinical Stage T_3 Disease

	RADS/ WEEK(S)	NO.	TOTAL 5-YEAR SURVIVAL	$P \leq T$		P_0	
				INCIDENCE	5-YEAR SURVIVAL	INCIDENCE	5-YEAR SURVIVAL
Whitmore, 1981*	2000/1	104	40%	27/104 (26%)	49%	2/104 (2%)	50%
Whitmore et al., 1977a, b	4000/4	50	34%	22/50 (44%)	44%	7/50 (14%)	57%
Wallace and Bloom, 1976	4000/4	77	42%	36/77 (47%)	51%	23/77 (30%)	NA
van der Werf-Messing, 1981	4000/4	141	45%	96/141 (68%)	46–76%	42/141 (30%)	59%
Slack et al., 1977	4500/4.5	67	36%	38/66 (58%)	53%	21/66 (32%)	57%
Miller, 1977	5000/5	30	53%	22/30 (73%)	59%	13/30 (43%)	69%

NA = Not available.

* Includes Whitmore et al., 1977a,b; Whitmore, 1980; Smith et al., 1981a,b; 1982; and Whitmore, 1981.

dissemination. Properly used, preoperative irradiation has not increased the complication rate, nor has it made cystectomy more difficult.

Stage T_4N_+ (D). Patients with adjacent organ involvement or regional pelvic lymph node metastases have a poor prognosis, despite control of the primary neoplasm with integrated irradiation and cystectomy. Pelvic lymph node involvement is observed in 44% of such patients with T_4 lesions. Approximately 50% of patients with positive pelvic nodes die within ten months, 70% within one year, and 90% within two years. Less than 5% live five years (see Figure 35–1) (Smith and Whitmore,

1981b). Such dismal survival rates in patients with local-regional disease, coupled with the observation that 50 to 60% of the patients with T_3 or T_4 lesions will eventually die of their disease, supports the need for adjuvant or preadjuvant chemotherapy trials in an effort to reduce the rate of systemic treatment failure.

Chemotherapy of Advanced Disease

Major chemotherapeutic advances have been made in the treatment of patients with urothelial tract tumors (renal pelvis, ureter, urethra, urinary bladder, and prostatic ducts). The most efficacious agents are cisplatin and

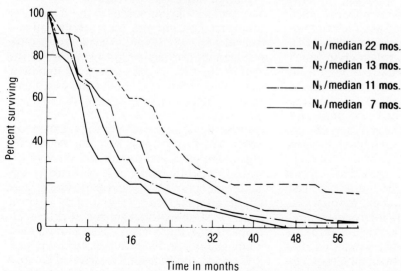

Figure 35–1. Survival curves of 134 patients with bladder cancer at Memorial Hospital undergoing radical cystectomy and lymph node dissection with a urinary diversion stratified for extent of nodal (N) disease. Median survival for N_1 patients was 22 months, N_2 13 months, N_3 11 months, and N_4 7 months.

methotrexate and, to a lesser extent, doxorubicin, vinblastine sulfate, and mitomycin C (Yagoda, 1980; Yagoda et al., 1982). Although various combination regimens of these agents seem to offer additional benefit clinically, new active agents still need to be defined.

Currently, cisplatin is the most active single agent, with a response rate of approximately 30%. The usual dose of cisplatin is 70 mg/m^2 IV every three weeks. Other schedules — 50 mg/m^2 IV every three weeks, 1 mg/kg IV weekly for six consecutive weeks, or 20 mg/m^2 IV for five consecutive days every four weeks — achieve similar response rates. The number of remissions is higher in selected patients with metastases to soft tissue sites, such as liver, lung, subcutaneous, and nodal areas (40%), and lower for local-regional and osseous sites (Yagoda, 1980; Oliver, 1981). Objective tumor regression is evidenced in four to six weeks, or after two doses, but may result in a response within 7 to 21 days. Although the average duration of remission is only five months, responders do live significantly longer than nonresponders, 64 versus 22 weeks, respectively ($P = 0.00001$). A few patients have achieved complete unmaintained remission for one to five years. Recently, the role of maintenance cisplatin therapy has been questioned (Herr, 1980). Cisplatin, intravesically and intravenously, is ineffective for stage 0 and A lesions, but may be of some value when combined with preoperative radiotherapy (Needles, et al., 1982b; Blumenreich et al., 1982). Tumor downstaging occurs in 38% (9/24) of cases with P$_0$ in 21% (5/24) given cisplatin and irradiation, versus a nonrandomized (a patient during the same time interval who refused cisplatin) control group in which downstaging occurs in 20% (8/39) with P$_0$ in only 5% (2/39) (Herr et al., 1983). Preliminary results of a randomized trial of adjuvant cisplatin therapy after radical cystectomy for stage B and C disease have been disappointing, but most patients never completed the prescribed schedule.

Methotrexate is another agent that exhibits good antitumor activity for transitional cell carcinoma, particularly in local-regional disease (Hall and Turner, 1980; Natale et al., 1981; Oliver, 1981; Turner, 1981a, 1981b). In a recent update, Turner (1981b) reports a 50% remission rate in 64 cases, with 44% responding in metastatic disease sites compared to 16% with local-regional tumors. In a smaller series of cases, the investigator noted responses in

metastases in 33%, versus 25% in the primary tumor (Oliver, in press). In a report by Natale et al. (1981), 26% of cases, most of whom were previously treated with other cytotoxic agents, achieved a complete or partial remission with doses of 30–40 mg/m^2 IV weekly. Almost all responses occurred after two to six doses and persisted approximately five months. Responders lived significantly longer than nonresponders, 52 versus 28 weeks, respectively ($P < 0.01$). The British, who have explored various doses and schedules of methotrexate, utilize three different schedules: 50 mg IV, 100 mg IV with and without folinic acid, and 200 mg IM with 21 mg IM of folinic acid at 6, 12, and 24 hours every two weeks. Response occurs in 35 to 50% of cases, with a significant number of cases with T$_3$ or T$_4$ lesions showing tumor regression. Methotrexate is inactive (7%) in bilharzial bladder cancer. Recently, prospective randomized adjuvant chemotherapy trials with methotrexate, pre- and postoperative, have been initiated in patients at high risk for recurrence (Oliver, 1981; Socquet, 1981). In addition, methotrexate orally may be effective against stage A disease (Hall et al., 1981).

Doxorubicin, vinblastine sulfate, and mitomycin C are slightly less effective agents, with response rates of 15 to 20% (Yagoda, 1980; Yagoda et al., 1982). With doxorubicin, response begins after two to three once-every-three-weeks doses, with vinblastine sulfate after four to six weekly doses, and with mitomycin C, after one to two once-every-six-weeks doses. There seems to be a dose-response relationship with doxorubicin. Patients receiving 60–75 mg/m^2 had a higher response rate than those receiving 30–45 mg/m^2. When all three agents are used singly, the duration of response is short, three to five months, but a small number of cases did achieve complete remission.

Other single agents have been evaluated (see Table 35–9), but most lack significant efficacy. Although older studies of 5-fluorouracil and cyclophosphamide, both used singly, suggest some activity, more recent results have not been impressive.

Many combination regimens have been attempted (see Table 35–9), incorporating cisplatin and doxorubicin and, recently, vinblastine and methotrexate derivatives. Few randomized trials have been performed. Although the remission rate with cisplatin singly is 30%, combination cisplatin regimens report

Table 35-9. Chemotherapy of Bladder Cancer

DRUG(S)	MSKCC ALL PATIENTS		UNTREATED		LITERATURE ALL PATIENTS	
	N	%CR/PR	N	%CR/PR	N	%CR/PR
Cisplatin	56	30	38	40	320	30
+cyclophosphamide	34	44	27	44	102	26
+doxorubicin	34	59	27	56	72	46
+doxorubicin + cyclophosphamide	28	46	22	41	202	46
+doxorubicin + 5-fluorouracil					44	44
Doxorubicin	44	16	20	20	223	18
+cyclophosphamide	18	17	12	17	37	18
+cyclophosphamide + 5-fluoroura- cil					24	21
+5-fluorouracil					103	39
+cyclophosphamide + methotrexate					26	38
+cyclophosphamide + bleomycin					23	35
+VM-26*					24	19
Methotrexate	42	26	16	38	103	39
+vinblastine	36	38	34	38	36	38
Vinblastine	28	18	19	17	38	16
Neocarzinostatin	19	5			19	5
AMSA	19	11			19	11
Methyl glyoxalhydrazone	3	0			3	0
Bisantrene	13	0			13	0
PALA	12	0			12	0
Etiopside					29	0
VM-26					108	16
Bleomycin					79	5
Mitomycin C					42	13

* 4'-demethyl-epipodophyllotoxin 9-(4,6-0-2-thenylidene)-β-d-gylcopyranside.

rates of 40 to 50%. There may be some additive effect in the combination of cisplatin and doxorubicin in increasing responses and the overall survival rates, but the number of complete remissions have not increased, and no evidence of synergism has been documented. The most popular combination is cisplatin and doxorubicin, with or without cyclophosphamide (CISCA or CAP). In the M. D. Anderson trial (Samuels *et al.*, 1980), a 50% (25/50 cases) remission rate is reported, while in the Memorial Hospital trial (Schwartz *et al.*, in press), 46% (13/28 cases) had complete or partial remissions. In addition, in the latter trial, responders lived significantly $(P = <0.001)$ longer than nonresponders, 91 versus 38 weeks, respectively (see Figure 35-2). At Memorial Hospital, when cisplatin is compared to the three-drug combination (CAP) in previously untreated, selected patients, there is no significant difference in response rates (40% in 38 cases versus 46% in 26 cases). When all reported cases are compared, however, the response rate for cisplatin in 273 cases is 31% (95% confidence limits 26 to 36%), versus 46% (95% confidence limits 39 to 53%) in 202 cases given the CAP $(P = <0.002)$.

The most frequently employed drug combi-

nation is cisplatin, 70 mg/m^2, and doxorubicin, 45 mg/m^2 IV, every three to four weeks with or without >250 mg/m^2 of cyclophosphamide. There have been prospective randomized trials utilizing cisplatin versus three- and two-drug combinations; and in one such trial, cisplatin and cyclophosphamide was slightly inferior to cisplatin alone; whereas in another trial, the three-drug combination was more effective than cisplatin alone (Yagoda *et al.*, 1982). Many other drug combinations have been tried, but none seem to increase significantly the number of remissions, the complete response rate, or the duration of remission (Yagoda, 1980). A more recent drug combination that has been explored is the use of cisplatin and methotrexate or a derivative, dichloromethotrexate.

One combination that has minimal toxicity yet appears to be effective is methotrexate and vinblastine sulfate. The dose of methotrexate is 40 mg/m^2 and that of vinblastine sulfate, 4 mg/m^2 IV every week. The response rate in 38 patients was 44%, with a median duration of greater than five months, range, >2 to 12 months (Needles *et al.*, 1982).

The most active first and second-line chemotherapeutic agents have been combined

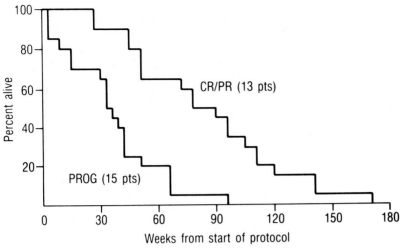

Figure 35–2. Survival of 28 patients with metastatic, bidimensionally measurable bladder cancer treated at Memorial Hospital with cisplatin, cyclophosphamide, and doxorubicin.

into the M-VAC regimen and used to treat advanced urothelial cancer. M-VAC (monthly cycles of methotrexate, 30 mg/m², followed 24 hours later by vinblastine, 3 mg/m², doxorubicin, 30 mg/m², and cisplatin, 70 mg/m², with vinblastine and methotrexate repeated on days 15 and 22) given to 25 patients with transitional cell carcinoma of the urothelial tract induced significant tumor regression in 71%. Complete remission, clinically (CR$_c$), was observed in 12 out of 24 patients (50%; 95% confidence limits 30 to 70%) with bidimensionally measurable "indicator" lesions, six of whom have been confirmed pathologically (CR$_p$). Four patients, after surgical exploration, required downstaging to a partial remission (PR$_p$). The median duration of response has not yet been reached at 9.5+ months, range 4.5+ to 16+. Five (21%) patients had a PR$_c$ for 4 to 8+ months, one had a minor response for four months, and one had stable disease for 11+ months. All metastatic sites have responded including bone (6/8 cases), liver (3/5), local-regional (12/17) and intravesical (6/7) disease. M-VAC toxicity included moderately severe myelosuppresion that resulted in nadir sepsis in four patients and a drug-related death in one, mild to moderate anorexia, vomiting, alopecia, and renal dysfunction.

These preliminary results suggest M-VAC is extremely effective against local-regional and disseminated urothelial tract tumors with the expectation (95% confidence limits) of inducing objective (CR$_c$ + PR$_c$) tumor regression in 53 to 89% of cases.

Adjunct chemotherapy trials utilizing cisplatin singly, methotrexate singly, doxorubicin and 5-fluorouracil, and cisplatin, cyclophosphamide, and doxorubicin have produced response rates of 25 to 30%. Results of such trials should become available in the next two years, but, at this time, adjuvant chemotherapy is still experimental.

Future Prospects

The major advances in the management of bladder cancer in the past 35 years have included an appreciation of its natural history and the identification of subgroups of patients at high risk for disease recurrence. In low-grade and early-stage tumors, the tendency for multiple recurrences or development of new tumors, the recognition of the potentially ominous nature of *in situ* carcinoma, the dedifferentiation of superficial tumors with subsequent recurrences, and the development of more aggressive invasive tumors in some patients remain therapeutic challenges. Simple, but reliable, methods for the early detection of recurrences and the identification of biologic factors that would predict subsequent clinical behavior of these tumors need to be developed. Investigations in this regard include the detection of AB (H) antigens, flowcytometry to monitor response and malignant changes, chromosomal analysis and tumor karyotypes, as well as the exploration of other tumor markers. If high-risk patients can be identified, more aggressive and optimal treatment can be initiated earlier, producing an improved prognosis.

Although some improvement in survival of patients with deeply invasive carcinoma of the bladder has been achieved with combined pre-operative radiotherapy and cystectomy, more than 50% of such patients succumb to distant metastases. In this group, it is necessary to attempt to improve the local control rate, perhaps by the use of hypoxic cell radiosensitizers and adjuvant chemotherapy in addition to radiotherapy and cystectomy, and, to control distant metastases by use of adjuvant systemic chemotherapy and/or immunotherapy.

PROSTATE CANCER

Incidence and Epidemiology

Prostatic carcinoma is the second most common malignant neoplasm occurring in men, surpassed in frequency only by carcinoma of the lung. At birth, American men have approximately a 5% risk of developing cancer of the prostate and a 2% risk of dying from it. It is estimated that 86,000 new cases of carcinoma of the prostate will be recognized in the United States this year and that more than 25,000 will die of the disease (Silverberg, 1985). In the past four decades, both the frequency and mortality rates of prostatic cancer have been increasing. Despite the clinical importance of this major oncologic problem, the optimal therapy has yet to be defined. Legitimate questions have been raised regarding the contributions of treatment to the cure and survival of these patients. The frequency with which physicians encounter the disease and the variety of manifestations reinforce the need to understand more about clinical presentations and diagnosis to allow earlier detection and therapy.

In the United States, the most striking feature of the epidemiology of prostatic carcinoma is the marked difference in incidence and mortality rates between whites and blacks (Ernster *et al.,* 1978). The age-adjusted mortality rate for carcinoma of the prostate is 23/100,000 per year, but for the black population the mortality rate is almost twice that figure, 41/100,000. The incidence rate for the black population is about 50% greater than that of the total population. Attempts to explain these differences on the basis of socioeconomic class differences have failed.

The risk of prostatic cancer increases with advancing age. Although uncommon before the age of 50, it increases rapidly in incidence from 20.8/100,000 men in the age group 50 to 54, sometimes doubling in incidence with each successive five-year age group, to reach an incidence approximating 1000/100,000, or 1% per year, in the age group 85 and above. This discrepancy in the incidence of clinical and latent carcinoma of the prostate suggests a quiescent period of several decades between malignant transformation and the appearance of clinical symptoms. The existence of this latency period between transformation and expression has led to the conclusion that prostatic carcinoma in the elderly has a favorable prognosis, which is not necessarily true. Although evidence to support a poor prognosis in men younger than age 50 has been contradictory, the younger the patient at the time of diagnosis, the greater the probability that the cancer *per se* will adversely affect life expectancy.

Studies have suggested that men who develop prostatic cancer have been sexually more active than other men, as indicated by the following findings: greater number of sexual partners, more frequent coitus, greater incidence of venereal disease, and less satisfaction with the frequency of intercourse (Higgins, 1975). Epidemiologic studies have failed to demonstrate differences between groups with cancer and control groups in socioeconomic status, education level, alcohol habits, or cigarette smoking.

The etiology of prostatic cancer is unknown. A hormonal basis for the disease has been supported by the experimental and clinical demonstration of regression following castration or estrogen therapy. Abnormal androgen and estrogen profiles in patients with prostatic cancer relative to age-adjusted normal controls have also been noted (Winkelstein, 1979). Additional support is suggested by the absence of the disease in eunuchs, infrequent presentation in patients with bilateral testicular atrophy (paraplegics), and the infrequency in patients with cirrhosis of the liver, where estrogen levels are high.

The relationship between benign prostatic hyperplasia (BPH) and cancer of the prostate remains speculative. No firm evidence links BPH as a possible precursor of prostatic cancer. The frequency with which BPH and cancer of the prostate coincide provides no definitive basis for any form of prophylactic surgery in BPH patients.

Diagnosis

Adenocarcinoma of the prostate gland is recognized as a slowly growing tumor, displaying an extremely variable rate and pattern of disease progression. Rather than progressing from a latent or focal tumor (stage A) to a clinically detectable nodule, or from disease confined within the capsule of the gland (stage B) to an extracapsular disease infiltrating locally (stage C), then finally progressing to widespread metastases (stage D), any or all of the possibilities shown in Figure 35–3 may and do occur (Whitmore, 1973). The rate and pattern of disease progression are unpredictable *in any individual patient,* and, in some instances, the neoplasm may remain essentially unchanged during the lifetime of the patient. In the absence of sensitive indicators of biologic behavior, other than serial observations of prostatic size over time, important clinical data are the findings at the last digital rectal examination of the prostate gland.

Since early disease is asymptomatic, early diagnosis of prostatic carcinoma is uncommon. Regular digital rectal examination, especially after 50 years of age, should be stressed. The majority of patients present with either locally advanced disease (35 to 40%) or evidence of metastases (40 to 45%). Since adenocarcinoma arises in the periphery of the gland, local symptoms are usually absent until the disease progresses to obstruct the urethra or the bladder neck, producing symptoms of urinary hesitancy, frequency, nocturia, incomplete emptying, or dysuria. Such symptoms have been reported in more than 60% of cases. Gross hematuria is uncommon and, when present, suggests tumor invasion of the bladder neck or trigone. Patients may present with symptoms of metastases, such as bone pain, weight loss, anorexia, and malaise. On occasion, rectal obstruction may produce abdominal pain, constipation, and rectal bleeding. Rarely, a patient presents with hematospermia (Catalona and Scott, 1978).

The single most important factor in diagnosing prostatic cancer is a properly performed digital rectal examination. The sensitivity and specificity of a rectal examination is 0.69 and 0.89, respectively, with an accuracy (efficiency) of 85%. The predictive value of a positive test is 67% and, for a negative test, 91% (Guinan *et al.,* 1980). Prostatic acid phosphatase by radioimmunoassay (RIA-PAP) or counterimmunoelectrophoresis (CIEP) is a very poor substitute for the gloved finger (Watson and Tang, 1980). Any area of asymmetry, firmness, or induration should be considered suspicious for carcinoma. A classic finding is a hard nodule within the prostate, clearly of a different consistency than the remainder of the gland. With local progression, loss of the median and lateral sulcus occurs, as well as upward and outward growth, which may involve the seminal vesicles. The tumor eventually invades the bladder base and fixes the prostate to the lateral pelvic side walls. At that stage, the prostate may be diffusely hard, irregular, nodular, and poorly defined on examination.

Approximately one-half of prostatic nodules are malignant, and the other half are benign—a hyperplastic nodule, an infarcted area, a calculus, or granulomatous disease. A histologic diagnosis is mandatory and readily accomplished by needle biopsy of the palpably suspicious area. Needle biopsy has an accuracy rate of 90 to 95%, but a negative biopsy or presence of normal prostatic tissue with persistence of a palpably abnormal area on digital rectal examination should warrant consideration of repeated biopsies.

Staging

The presently accepted staging system is shown in Figure 35–4. Stage A prostatic

Prostatic Cancer

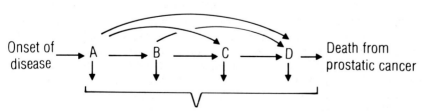

Figure 35–3. Progression of prostatic cancer by stage.

STAGE A
LATENT PROSTATIC CANCER

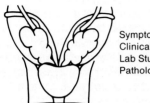

Symptoms: None
Clinical Findings: Negative
Lab Studies: Negative
Pathology: Carcinoma

STAGE B
EARLY PROSTATIC CANCER

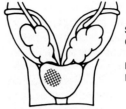

Symptoms: None
Clinical Findings:
    Prostatic Nodule
Lab Studies: Negative
Pathology: Carcinoma

STAGE C
ADVANCED PROSTATIC CANCER
WITHOUT METASTASES

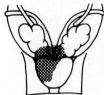

Symptoms: ? Urinary or None
Clinical Findings: Extensive
    Prostatic Induration
Lab Studies: ? Ureteral Obstruction
    ?   Acid Phosphatase
Pathology: Carcinoma

STAGE D
ADVANCED PROSTATIC CANCER WITH METASTASES

Symptoms: ? Bone Pain, Urinary
    Symptoms
Clinical Findings: Variable Prostatic
    Induration: Metastases
Lab Studies: Metastases
    ?   Acid Phosphatase
    ?   Alkaline Phosphatase

Figure 35–4.   Stages of prostatic cancer.

cancer is unsuspected malignant disease found incidentally in a prostatectomy specimen after surgery performed for clinically benign disease. When three or less microscopic foci of well-differentiated tumor are found, the lesion is assigned to an A_1 category, while more than three microscopic foci or presence of a high-grade tumor is classified as an A_2 neoplasm. Stage B cancer of the prostate is disease confined clinically within the prostatic capsule. This may involve a discrete 1.5-cm, or less, nodular tumor termed stage B_1 or a neoplasm that may occupy most or all of one lobe (stage B_2) or both lobes (stage B_3). Approximately 10 to 15% of cases present with stage B disease. One-fourth will die of prostatic cancer within 15 years. Patients with high-grade and large lesions have an increase in nodal metastases and earlier mortality (Barnes and Ninan, 1972). Clinical stage C prostatic cancer invades the prostatic capsule, lateral sulcus, or the seminal vesicles. Subclassifications of the C category have been proposed, based on the tumor size. Pathologic staging, however, indicates that more than one-half of all cases are truly stage D. Therefore, interpretation of published clinical trials of patients with stage C disease is difficult (Freiha *et al.*, 1979). Stage D cancer of the prostate is metastatic disease that may involve pelvic lymph nodes (stage D_1) or distant nodal, bony, or visceral metastases

(stage D_2). Five-year survival of untreated cases is less than 20%.

Once the diagnosis of prostatic carcinoma has been established pathologically, an accurate assessment or staging of the extent of disease is required. All patients should have histologic grading of the prostatic tumor, a radionuclide bone scan with selected bone x-rays to investigate abnormalities, if any, a serum acid and alkaline phosphatase level, and a chest x-ray. At this time, the value of the creatinine phosphokinase (CPK), isoenzyme BB, lactic dehydrogenase, and radioimmunoassay techniques for acid phosphatase levels is uncertain. Selected patients may also require a bipedal lymphangiogram (especially useful in the detection of retroperitoneal metastases), a pelvic and perhaps an abdominal CT scan, an intravenous pyelogram, especially with large local lesions in which ureteral obstruction is suspected, a barium enema in patients with rectal or other large bowel symptoms, and, on occasion, a myelogram in patients with bony metastases and neurologic symptoms suggesting impending spinal cord compression.

The inability of lymphangiography and CT scans to document local tumor extension and local-regional nodal involvement has led to other relatively noninvasive techniques, such as transrectal and transureteral sonography and percutaneous CT scan or sonogram-guided thin-needle aspiration biopsy of suspected tumor areas. Prostatic contour and density, and extraprostatic tumor extension into the soft tissue, fat planes, and the seminal vesicles (particularly the angle) can be evaluated, but, at times, tissue attenuation among normal, hyperplastic, and neoplastic masses is unreliable (Resnick, 1981).

Since clinical staging is so inaccurate, a number of urologists recommend a staging pelvic lymph node dissection before assigning therapy. Lymph node metastases are found in approximately 10% of patients with stage A disease, 10 to 25% with stage B, and 30 to 60% with stage C neoplasms. The incidence of lymph node metastases increases with high-grade tumors: fewer than 22% for grade I, 54% for grade II, and 77% for grade III; or 14%, 32%, and 50 to 100% for Gleason's grades 2 – 5, 6, and 7 – 10, respectively. Understaging occurs in at least one-third of cases, but when careful pathologic review with multiple thin serial sections of the prostatic gland is performed, the percentage increases markedly in tumors greater than 35 g (40 to 50% versus 5 to 18%) and in specimens where greater than 35% of the prostate shows tumor involvement (Flocks *et al.,* 1959; Grossman *et al.,* 1980; Paulson *et al.,* 1980). In a Memorial Hospital series of 300 cases with apparently localized prostatic cancer, 40% were found to have lymph node involvement and, of these, 29% had a solitary node. Metastases were found in the surgical specimen in 7% of patients clinically stage B_1, 43% stage B_2, and 60% stage C (Fowler and Whitmore, 1981). The morbidity in a staging lymph node dissection is high, and the information gained is rarely of pivotal significance since no form of therapy in the face of positive pelvic nodes has been shown to alter either the rate or pattern of disease progression. In fact, lymph node dissection for prostatic cancer should be considered as simply a staging procedure and nontherapeutic. Pelvic lymph node dissection may be warranted only in selected patients who are considered candidates for radical prostatectomy, since complications (impotence, incontinence, and so forth) are sufficiently great to contraindicate routine use in face of positive nodes. Pelvic lymph node dissection is often employed when interstitial irradiation is used because the procedure does not increase morbidity yet provides information of prognostic significance for individual patients. Pelvic lymphadenectomy delays the initiation of external irradiation and may significantly increase its complication rate without altering therapy.

Prostatic cancer may spread both by lymphatic and hematogenous routes, although, in the majority of cases, regional lymph node spread seems to be the earliest mode of metastases. Osseous metastases, usually involving the axial skeleton, possibly via Batson's plexus, are the next most frequent development. Radiographically, the metastatic pattern is classically osteoblastic in 80% of cases, osteolytic in 5%, and a mixed pattern in 15%. A radionuclide bone scan is the most sensitive modality for detecting bony metastases. Such lesions are readily visualized; but suspicious, poorly defined, or localized lesions may need to be confirmed by needle aspiration or bone biopsy. Prostatic metastases have been documented by biopsy in Paget lesions of the bone. Bone marrow acid phosphatase has not proven to be of value. The more common sites of visceral metastases are the lungs, usually with a lymphangitic pattern, liver, and adrenal glands, which may be involved in up to 20 or 25% of patients with advanced disease.

Treatment

No universally accepted therapy is available for patients with prostatic cancer. With all the data available during the past 40 years, and since the introduction of hormonal manipulation, recommendations for treatment are usually based on stage and grade of the primary lesion, age and general medical condition of the patient, the anticipated side effects imposed by such therapy, and, most significantly, the experience and philosophy of the physician. Various treatment possibilities exist for apparently localized disease, including radical prostatectomy, irradiation (either external beam or interstitial irradiation), and endocrine manipulation. In selected patients, observation, with treatment only as necessary, may be appropriate. The absence of controlled studies with surgical staging and the varied and unpredictable natural history of prostatic cancer, especially in an elderly population, make categorical treatment recommendations impractical. A logical approach to management is to advise the patient of the varied therapeutic options that have been utilized for management of prostatic cancer and then follow with a specific recommendation.

Stage A. Stage A disease is found in 10% of all prostatectomy specimens. Focal stage A_1

adenocarcinoma may represent no significant threat to the patient, since the anticipated survival is similar to an age-matched control population without cancer of the prostate. Thus, no specific therapy is warranted, except careful observation. A compilation of data from various studies conducted by the Veterans Administration Cooperative Urologic Research Group found that only 5 (1.9%) of 262 patients with focal stage A disease die as a result of prostatic cancer (Byar et al., 1972). If through screening and educational programs, more patients are discovered with stage I disease (37% in the study by Donohue et al. 1979), the need for a curative therapy becomes crucial. The present data show that only 2.5% of 400 patients die of prostatic cancer, whether given diethylstilbestrol, a radical prostatectomy, or no treatment. Perhaps only the subgroup of stage A_2 patients may benefit (Smith, 1981).

Management of the more diffuse, or high-grade stage A_2, adenocarcinoma is controversial. Although clinically benign on digital rectal examination, the grade and diffuse nature of such lesions indicate that some are biologically more aggressive than detectable early stage B tumors. At the time of diagnosis, up to 33% of patients with A_2 disease already have regional lymph node metastases. The surgery to relieve prostatic obstruction precipitates more hazardous complications in subsequent radical surgery and, in some instances, radiation therapy. For example, interstitial irradiation using iodine-125 seeds (^{125}I) is usually not administered to these patients because insufficient residual prostatic tissue remains to implant. Some urologists advise radical prostatectomy, but most believe patients are best treated with external megavoltage radiation therapy, beginning six to eight weeks after prostatectomy to permit healing and minimize local complications.

Stage B. Selecting the most appropriate therapy for a patient with disease confined to the prostate remains an enigma for many urologists. Modalities that may potentially cure the disease include radical prostatectomy and radiation therapy. Radical surgery is associated with almost universal sexual impotence and, on occasion, total or partial urinary incontinence. This has dissuaded urologists and patients from its routine use, despite the fact that this modality has achieved the most consistent disease-free 15-year survival rates (Walsh and Jewitt, 1980). Development of improved megavoltage radiation therapy has resulted in a resurgence of irradiation in an attempt to eradicate or control localized disease. On a practical basis, radical surgery is generally reserved only for patients with stage B_1 localized nodules (Jewett, 1975), with larger stage B tumors, either treated by external megavoltage (Walsh and Jewitt, 1980), radiation therapy (Bagshaw et al., 1975), interstitial irradiation with iodine-125 (Whitmore, 1980), or a combined method employing interstitial gold-198, followed by supplemental external irradiation (Carlton et al., 1972). Advantages and disadvantages of each modality primarily involve side effects of treatment, although all are associated with local failure rates of approximately 10%. Most treatment failures result from unrecognized, or recognized, regional and/or distant metastases. Survival rates achieved in patients treated with radical prostatectomy or external megavoltage radiation therapy are approximately 60 to 80% at five years, 50% at ten years, and 20 to 30% at 15 years. Ten- and 15-year survival rates are not yet available for interstitial irradiation techniques.

Very few patients (8%) are candidates for radical prostatectomy. These patients should have stage B_1 disease clinically; a moderately well-differentiated tumor pathologically; a negative work-up for distant metastases; a normal serum prostatic acid phosphatase determination; and an expected natural life survival of at least ten years. In a patient 70 years of age or less, without other severe illness, one-third will still die within 15 years of prostatic cancer and perhaps only 2% will be cured with radical excision. More disappointing is the finding of Byar (1980), who noted a marginal difference in progression rates, without significant improvement in survival in patients with stage I disease treated by placebo, radical prostatectomy, or diethylstilbestrol (DES) and prostatectomy.

Stage C. Hormonal therapy is the usual treatment for patients with large, bulky, stage C neoplasms producing bladder outlet obstruction or ureteral obstruction. These symptoms can be relieved in up to 80% of all cases. Such lesions frequently have already metastasized to the pelvic nodes or bone. The current recommendation is 1 to 3 mg of DES daily, with monitoring of serum testosterone to assure that treatment induces a castrate level of less than 50 ng%. Therapy with DES is not curative, and almost all symptomatic patients, even after a response, will relapse within one to two years. Time to progression of disease and overall survival are not affected by hormonal manipulation, whether begun prophylactically to prevent progression or therapeutically at the time of symptoms (Byar *et al.,* 1979).

Patients with smaller and more well-defined stage C tumors and minimal or no lower urinary tract symptoms may be considered for curative radiation therapy, either interstitial or external. Local control rates and survival after therapy for stage C disease are not comparable to those of similar treatment applied to stage B disease, although selected patients benefit by appropriately applied radiation therapy. In a recent update of the Memorial Hospital experience, in the first 100 cases treated with interstitial irradiation for clinical stage C disease, 33 (76%) of 42 patients survived five years, of whom only 9 (23%) were tumor-free. The dissemination rate was 34% at five years, even for patients with negative nodes at lymphadenectomy (see Figures 35–5, and 35–6). At nine years, 52% were alive, some having subsequently received hormonal therapy, 87% of cases with benign nodes versus only 14% with positive nodes. Initially, 28 cases had nodal involvement microscopically and therefore were stage D pathologically. For most patients with stage C neoplasms, external radiotherapy appears to offer the best chance for total tumor eradication. A curative dose of radiation ther-

apy is generally in the range of 6000 to 7000 rads, delivered over a six- to seven-week interval to the prostate, paraprostatic tissue, and sometimes, using a lower dose, to regional pelvic lymph nodes. Complications, which vary with the size of the port, include nausea, anorexia, diarrhea, occasional rectal pain and bleeding, and lower extremity and genital lymphedema. Severe rectal or urinary complications lasting six or more months may occur in as many as 10% of patients. Treatment for radiation failure, manifested as local progression, has included total prostatectomy, full-dose interstitial irradiation, or hormonal manipulation. Although the latter treatment is generally preferred, optimal management in this group of patients has not been defined.

Advanced Disease (Stage D)

Response Criteria. Since the vast majority of patients have only osseous disease and any assessment of remission is almost impossible in this metastatic site, other response parameters have been sought. Subjective changes in weight, performance status, work habits, pain, analgesic requirements, and sense of well-being have been frequently incorporated into a scoring system or response schema. Changes in bone scans, x-rays, hydroxyproline excre-

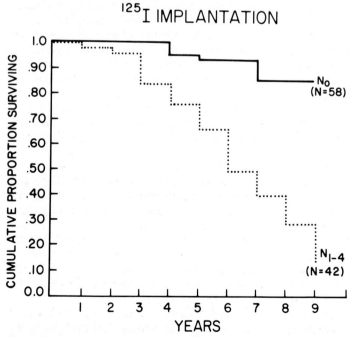

^{125}I IMPLANTATION

Figure 35–5. Survival of 100 patients with clinical Stages B_1, B_2, and C prostatic cancer treated with ^{125}I interstitial radiotherapy, 42 of whom were found to have lymph node involvement (N_{1-4}), pathologically.

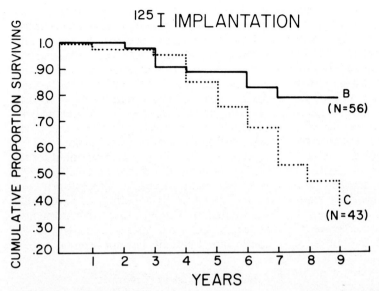

Figure 35–6. Survival of 100 patients with clinical stages B_1, B_2, and C prostatic cancer treated with ^{125}I interstitial radiotherapy.

tion rates, lymph and scrotal edema, intravenous pyelograms, bone marrow and serum acid phosphatase levels, and CPK-BB values have all proven to be either inaccurate or too insensitive (Yagoda, 1973, Yagoda *et al.*, 1979). Although patients with only bidimensionally measurable disease parameters (standard phase II patient selection criteria) have been selected for clinical trials by some investigators, such cases may represent an advanced, thus, possibly, a poorly responsive group. Reliance on survival alone for defining response may be inappropriate without relating changes in patient survival to the natural history (*i.e.*, time from symptoms to diagnosis, diagnosis to protocol, and protocol to death/follow-up).

Few patients achieve a complete or partial remission. Most have stabilization of disease (Yagoda *et al.*, 1979; Torti and Carter, 1980; Yagoda *et al.*, 1982). The National Prostatic Cancer Project (NPCP) has coined a new terminology, "objective regression," which is equivalent to a complete or partial remission, while "objective response" includes stabilization of disease. Most oncologists still employ the term "objective response" to indicate only patients who achieve a complete or partial remission. The critical factor seems to be the inability to document the effects of cytotoxic chemotherapy in osseous metastases and in a nonhomogeneous cell population. Mixed responses do occur, and without sensitive biologic markers to monitor the nonhomogen-

eous cell population, response may be underestimated or, at times, grossly overestimated. The NPCP criteria attempt to recognize such differences. A significant decrease in the serum acid phosphatase value is used to denote tumor regression, whereas a subsequent "increase in acid and alkaline phosphatase alone is not considered an indication of progression; these should be used in conjunction with other criteria" (Schmidt, 1980). Since the determinants of response in patients with advanced prostatic cancer are imprecise, survival, subjective changes in symptoms, and unidimensional disease parameters comprise the majority of measurements.

Hormones. Currently, hormonal manipulation is the most effective therapy to decrease androgen level. As shown in Figure 35–7, various hormones affect the production of testicular derived androgens. Since prostatic adenocarcinoma starts in an androgen milieu, the primary form of attack is to modulate androgen levels by castration, hypophysectomy, exogenous antiandrogens, or estrogens. The use of androgens singly, at any time in this disease, is to be discouraged, since up to 87% of patients will have exacerbation of subjective and objective disease parameters (Fowler and Whitmore, 1982).

Diethylstilbestrol, 1 mg daily, is the most frequently employed drug, and no other agent is more efficacious. Although stilbestrol dosage will not suppress plasma testosterone levels

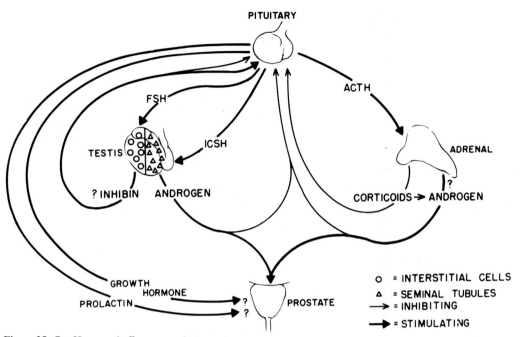

PITUITARY

ACTH

FSH

ICSH

TESTIS

ADRENAL

? INHIBIN   ANDROGEN

CORTICOIDS → ANDROGEN

?

GROWTH
HORMONE

PROLACTIN

?
?   PROSTATE

o = INTERSTITIAL CELLS
Δ = SEMINAL TUBULES
→ = INHIBITING
➤ = STIMULATING

Figure 35–7. Hormonal effects on testicular androgen production.

completely, it is generally sufficient to control the disease subjectively in 50 to 80% of cases, and objectively in 20 to 50%. Stilbestrol in a dose of 1 mg every eight hours will suppress the plasma testosterone level to <50 ng%, irrespective of response. Within six months, most patients will exhibit a small, yet significant, increase in testosterone levels (Robinson and Thomas, 1971). Increasing doses of stilbestrol or the use of diethylstilbestrol diphosphate, 1000 mg IV daily for five consecutive days, induces no additional benefit, but does increase the incidence of cardiovascular complications. Hormonal manipulation is not innocuous. Deep vein thrombosis, phlebitis, pulmonary emboli, myocardial infarction, and cerebrovascular accidents occur with increasing frequency when high doses of estrogens are used (Byar *et al.*, 1979). In a recent study by Glashan and Robinson (1981), 29% of cases given stilbestrol, 3 mg daily, and 25% estramustine, 560 mg daily, had cardiovascular complications with a drug-related mortality of 16% for both groups. Only 8% of cases who underwent an orchiectomy alone had any complications and only 3% died. Of greater significance, in the latter study, seven of nine deaths occurred in 29 patients with local disease where no other deaths were due to carcinoma. Orchiectomy has none of the side effects of estrogens, such as gynecomastia,

feminization, and cardiovascular complications, and is as effective in controlling disease, either as initial or delayed therapy, in previously untreated patients.

Response to hormonal manipulation in the majority of cases is extremely rapid, with some patients having relief of pain immediately after orchiectomy, or within 24 hours after starting stilbestrol. Response may be delayed for as long as six weeks, thus, therapy must be continued for six to eight weeks before being considered a failure. Generally, patients are continued on oral estrogens because of the fear of enhancing the development of hormonally insensitive cells, as yet an unproven hypothesis. Although response may persist for one month to more than 12 years, the average duration is usually 9 to 12 months, with survival after hormonal failure of approximately 6 to 12 months. Although orchiectomy is performed frequently following hormonal failure, subjective response is uncommon, and objective tumor regression is rare.

The important question for physicians is when to start hormonal therapy. All available data, including those of randomized, prospective trials, indicate hormonal manipulation does not prolong survival, although it may delay the onset of symptoms. When patients were randomized to placebo, 5 mg of diethylstilbestrol daily, orchiectomy, or stilbestrol and orchiectomy, no significant difference was observed, except for an increase in complications and mortality due to cardiovascular disease, usually within one year of starting therapy. Doses of stilbestrol of 0.2 mg, 1.0 mg, and 5.0 mg versus placebo were also evaluated. The 1-mg dose was superior with fewer cardiovascular complications, whereas the placebo and the 0.2-mg dose were ineffective. The 1.0- and 5.0-mg doses of diethylstilbestrol produced similar results in controlling symptoms and in controlling the disease (Byar *et al.,* 1979). Diethylstilbestrol, 1 mg daily, was found to be better than, or equally effective as, another estrogen, PREMARIN 2.5 mg daily, a progestational agent, PROVERA (medroxyprogesterone acetate), 30 mg daily, and PROVERA and diethylstilbestrol (Byar, 1980). In another trial, in 167 cases (EORTC protocol #30761), diethylstilbestrol was more effective than PROVERA or ANDROCUR (cyproterone acetate). Relapse occurred in 19% versus 41 and 33%, respectively. When diethylstilbestrol was compared with estramustine in 204 cases (EORTC protocol #39762), 11% of cases relapsed with the former versus 15% with the latter. Cardiovascular complications were 8 versus 5%, respectively (Smith, 1981).

New hormonal agents have been tried, including various decapeptide analogs of the hypothalamic releasing factors. Such decapeptides release both LH (luteinizing hormone) and/or FSH (follicle-stimulating hormone) from the pituitary gland. Various synthetic analogs (LHRH, luteinizing hormone – releasing factor, and Gn-RH, gonadotropin-releasing hormone) have recently been entered into clinical trials (Jacobi and Wenderoth, 1982). The major drawback of such compounds is the requirement for subcutaneous or per nasal administraton. Preliminary data on leuprolide and buserelin show that both synthetic analogs are effective in unpretreated cases, but are, as expected, relatively ineffective in previously treated patients. Adrenalectomy, medical or surgical, hypophysectomy, cyproterone acetate (ANDROCUR), and flutamide (4'-nitro-3'-trifluoromethyl isobutyranilide) have also been relatively ineffective in previously treated cases. This conclusion is not unexpected, since hormonally sensitive cells probably disappear with initial hormonal manipulation and remaining cells are hormonally insensitive.

Flutamide is a nonsteroidal, pure antiandrogen devoid of direct hormonal activity, yet it increases LH and testosterone levels in the

Table 35–10. Chemotherapy of Advanced Prostatic Cancer

	NO. PATIENTS	%PR	%PR + STAB.
AMSA	28	0	7
Carmustine	10	—	40
Cisplatin	100	24	32*
Cyclophosphamide	171	2	28
Dacarbazine	64	3	23
Doxorubicin	127	15	22
Estramustine	168	8	27
5-Fluorouracil	106	15	43
Hydroxyurea	35	48	57†
Melphalan	35	0	—
Mitotane	12	0	14
Neocarzinostatin	20	0	0
Prednimustine	70	1	20
Procarbazine	58	2	10
Semustine	33	3	—
Streptozotocin	38	0	32
Vincristine	36	6	18
Doxorubicin			
+ cisplatin	40	13	50
+ cyclophosphamide	62	16	39
+ cyclophosphamide + 5-fluorouracil	52	25	56
+ cyclophosphamide + carmustine	27	26	48
+ cyclophosphamide + cisplatin	33	21	61
+ mitomycin C + 5-fluorouracil	55	22	35
Cyclophosphamide + cisplatin + prednisone	22	0	45
5-Fluorouracil + cyclophosphamide + methotrexate	15	7	47
+ methotrexate + vincristine + melphalan + prednisone	84	7	89

* Majority of responses from one series (17/54) which markedly increases the overall rate.
† Hydroxyurea was combined with a hormone. NPCP is evaluating hydroxyurea used singly.

noncastrated male and probably has a direct effect on prostatic cells. In the initial report by Sogani and Whitmore (1979), flutamide induced a similar rate, quality, and duration (10.5 months) of response as did diethylstilbestrol. A prospective randomized trial comparing flutamide with diethylstilbestrol showed similar response rates, yet, at this time, cardiovascular complications have been less frequent with the former agent. Other new drugs include estramustine, a *nor*-nitrogen mustard attached to estradiol, and prednimustine, chlorambucil attached to prednisolone. It had been hoped that such compounds would permit the rapid introduction of cytotoxic agents directly into the cytoplasm or nucleus, via hormone-binding sites on tumor cell membranes. Estramustine seems to work primarily as a hormone, however, and induces no myelosuppression. Therefore, it has no advantage over diethylstilbestrol. Prednimustine has been found to be ineffective and has no role for prostatic cancer.

Since the efficacy of hormonal manipulation is limited, other modalities are needed. Radiation therapy should be utilized to control local symptoms and for relief of osseous or pelvic pain in patients with advanced disease. Androgens or thyrocalcitonin, with intravenously administered radioactive bone-seeking radioisotopes, has generally been ineffective. Currently, immunotherapy with BCG, interferon, or other immunologic modulators provides unproven therapeutic options. Interest in cytotoxic chemotherapeutic agents for treatment of advanced prostatic cancer began in 1973, and, more recently, such agents have been combined with hormones in patients with early disease.

Chemotherapy. Prior to 1973, few chemotherapeutic agents had been studied systematically (Yagoda, 1973). Recently, a large number of trials have been initiated, mostly phase II, but some randomized phase III studies, to evaluate single agents and combination drug regimens. The most thoroughly studied agent is cyclophosphamide. Table 35–10 lists many single and combination cytotoxic drugs that have had clinical trials. Although the review includes drug trials that employed varied doses and schedules, and patient selection and response criteria, the overall results are disappointing when only complete and partial remissions are considered. When stabilization of disease is incorporated into the response rate, the number of so-called "objective responses" increases dramatically. For example, in the National Prostatic Cancer Project (NPCP) trials #100 and #300, the complete and partial remission rate with cyclophosphamide is 0 to 7%, while with stabilization, the rate increases to 26 to 46%. Responders lived longer than nonresponders, 45+ versus <20 weeks. Physicians must remain somewhat skeptical when responses in various reviews list rates of 37, 7, and 2% for cyclophosphamide, and 23, 16, and 5% for doxorubicin (Torti and Carter, 1980; Smith, 1981; Yagoda *et al.,* 1982). The NPCP

concludes from their data that cyclophosphamide, which was better than 5-fluorouracil, 46 versus 36%, respectively, should be considered the standard drug.

Doxorubicin has had extensive trials, some suggesting a dose-response relationship: high doses induce more responses. In a trial recently completed at Memorial Hospital, in patients with soft tissue lesions, only 2 (5%) of 39 cases responded, while 3 additional patients had a minor response, 1 stabilized, and 5 had a mixed response. Other single-agent therapies have not been efficacious. Recently, vindesine has been reported to induce remission in 5 of 21 cases, and methyl-G had a 17% remission rate in 18 adequately treated cases with bidimensionally measurable disease. The latter agent is interesting because it interferes with polyamine synthesis and, with difluoromethyl ornithine, dramatically inhibits prostatic cancer in rats (Heston *et al.,* 1982).

With the promising reports of positive antitumor activity with some single agents, combination regimens were started in unpretreated and previously treated patients in hope of obtaining, if no synergism, at least an additive effect. The most popular combinations are doxorubicin and cyclophosphamide, cyclophosphamide and 5-fluorouracil, and all three drugs together, with or without prednisone and melphalan. Another combination is mitomycin C, with doxorubicin and 5-fluorouracil. It is important to recognize that with all such drug combinations, doses in patients with advanced prostatic cancer may have to be modified because of extensive prior irradiation to bone marrow-containing areas and myelophthisis resulting from tumor infiltration. At best, using various combination regimens, remissions, excluding stabilization, are described in only 15 to 25% of cases. Response rates increase again when stabilization of disease is treated as a remission. Obviously, some patients do respond. For most patients, however, little clinical benefit is obtained, except for a positive approach to the patient's disease. New drugs, new drug combinations, and new methodologies for measuring response are needed.

General. Corticosteroids are frequently very effective (greater than 50%) in controlling symptoms of pain, malaise, and weight loss. At Memorial Hospital, many patients are given prednisone, 40 to 60 mg daily for five consecutive days. Subjective improvement always will occur within one to five days, and if benefit is obtained, the dose is decreased by 5 mg weekly to a minimal dose, generally 15 to 20 mg daily. If no improvement is observed within five days, prednisone is stopped. Patients must have no prior history which precludes the use of steroids. All aspirin-containing compounds must be avoided. If symptoms are persistent, adequate analgesics and irradiation to the troublesome areas are given. Not all pain, however, is simply secondary to osseous disease, and physicians must be aware of the potential for extradural disease and spinal cord compression, not uncommon in patients with prostatic cancer. Myelography may be required.

Another complication of prostatic adenocarcinoma is disseminated intravascular coagulation (DIC), which can be acute or chronic. Treatment consists of heparin and, in unpretreated cases, estrogens. AMICAR (epsilon aminocaproic acid) should not be used. In previously treated cases, DIC is usually a terminal event, although chemotherapy may be attempted to induce a response. Patients frequently present with dyspnea, which can be secondary to lymphangitic tumor in lung, pulmonary emboli, and/or tumor emboli. Symptomatic treatment should be administered but generally is of marginal success, unless the underlying problem is embolization secondary to a pelvic mass. Nonbacterial thrombotic endocarditis has also been described in this patient population and is generally a terminal event. Meningeal carcinomatosis and base of brain involvement are troublesome sequelae of advanced disease. The latter is untreatable, although full spinal axis irradiation and chemotherapy via an Ommaya shunt have been attempted. For the latter problem, radiation therapy to the base of the skull has been generally helpful in ameliorating symptoms (Greenberg *et al.*, 1981).

Future Prospects

After 40 years of utilizing various therapeutic modalities, the most effective treatment of cancer of the prostate has still not been defined. What is needed is the identification of those patients who require an aggressive approach, as well as clarification of those cases who should receive minimal ornotherapy. "Appropriate treatment implies that therapy be applied neither to those for whom it is unnecessary nor to those for whom it will prove ineffective" (Whitmore, 1973). New markers such as urinary hydroxyproline excretion rates, prostacyclines, and polyamines, and the development of an accurate methodology for androgen-binding sites in prostatic tumor cells may be of assistance. The roles of hyperthermia, new biologic markers, monoclonal antibodies, new radiotherapy methods, and immunologic maneuvers all need to be defined. Although standard therapy can be offered to patients, physicians must be aware of clinical trials of new investigational, or even experimental, agents that may, in the long run, offer more hope and progress in controlling this disease.

REFERENCES

Al-Sarraf, M.; Bonnet, E. J.; Saiki, J.; Gagliano, R.; Pugh, R.; Lehane, D.; Dixon, D.; and Bottomley, R.: Study of tamoxifen in metastatic renal cell carcinoma and the influence of certain prognostic factors: a Southwest Oncology Group study. *Cancer Treat. Rep.*, **65**:447–451, 1981.

Aufderheide, A. C., and Streitz, J. M.: Mucinous adenocarcinoma of the renal pelvis: Report of two cases. *Cancer*, **33**:167–173, 1974.

Bagshaw, M. A.; Ray, G. R.; Pistenma, D. A.; Castellino, R. A.; and Meares, E. M., Jr.: External beam radiation therapy of primary carcinoma of the prostate. *Cancer*, **36**:723–728, 1975.

Barnes, R. W., and Ninan, C. A.: Carcinoma of the prostate—Biopsy and conservative therapy. *J. Urol.*, **108**:887–900, 1972.

Bloom, H. J. B.: Hormone induced and spontaneous regression of metastatic renal cancer. *Cancer*, **32**:1066–1071, 1973.

Blumenreich, M. S.; Needles, B.; Yagoda, A.; Sogani, P. C.; Grabstald., H., and Whitmore, W. F., Jr.: Intravesical cisplatin for superficial bladder tumors. *Cancer*, **50**:863–865, 1982.

Boxer, R. J.; Waisman, J.; Lieber, M. M.; Mampaso, F. M.; and Skinner, D. G.: Renal carcinoma: Computer analysis of 96 patients treated by nephrectomy. *J. Urol.*, **122**:598–601, 1979.

Burnand, K. G.; Boyd, P. J. R.; Mayo, M. E.; Shuttleworth, K. E. D.; and Lloyd-Davies, R. W.: Single dose intravesical thio-tepa as an adjuvant to cystodiathermy in the treatment of transitional cell bladder carcinoma. *Br. J. Urol.*, **48**:55–59, 1976.

Byar, D. P.: Review of the Veterans Administration studies of cancer of the prostate and new results concerning treatment of stage I and II tumors. In Pavone-Macaluso, M.; Smith, P. H.; and Edsmyr, F. (eds.): *Bladder Tumors and Other Topics in Urological Oncology*, Plenum Publishing Corporation, New York, 1980.

Byar, D. P., and The Veterans Administration Co-operative Urologic Research Group: Survival of patients with incidentally found microscopic cancer of the prostate: Results of a clinical trial of conservative treatment. *J. Urol.*, **108**:908–913, 1972.

Byar, D. P., and The Veterans Administration Co-operative Urologic Research Group: Studies of carcinoma of the prostate. *Cancer*, **32**:1126–2230, 1979.

Carlton, C. E., Jr.; Dawoud, F.; Hudgins, P.; and Scott, R.,

Jr.: Irradiation treatment of carcinoma of the prostate: A preliminary report based on 8 years experience. *J. Urol.,* **108:**924–927, 1972.

Catalona, W. J., and Scott, W. W.: Carcinoma of the prostate. *J. Urol.,* **119:**1–8, 1978.

Claymen, R. V.; Williams, R. D.; and Fraley, E. E.: The pursuit of the renal mass. *N. Engl. J. Med.,* **300:**72–74, 1979.

Cohen, A. J.; Li, F. P.; Berg, S.; Marchetto, D. J.; Tsai, S.; Jacobs, S. C.; and Brown, R. S.: Hereditary renal cell carcinoma associated with a chromosomal translocation. *N. Engl. J. Med.,* **301:**592–595, 1979.

Concolino, G.; Marocchi, A.; Conti, C.; Tenaglia, R.; DiSilverio, F.; and Bracci, U.: Human renal cell carcinoma and hormone dependent tumor. *Cancer Res.,* **38:**4340–4344, 1978.

de Kernion, J. B.; Ramming, K. P.; and Smith, R. B.: The natural history of metastatic renal cell carcinoma: A computer analysis. *J. Urol.,* **120:**148–152, 1978.

Donohue, R. E.; Fauver, H. E.; Whitesal, J. A.; and Pfister, R. R.: Staging prostatic cancer: A different distribution. *J. Urol.,* **122:**327–329, 1979.

Ernster, V. L.; Seluin, S.; and Sacks, S. T.: Prostatic cancer: Mortality and incidence rates by race and social class. *Am. J. Epidemiol.,* **107:**311–319, 1978.

Finney, R.: The value of radiotherapy in the treatment of hypernephroma—A clinical trial. *Br. J. Urol.,* **45:**258–269, 1973.

Fletcher, M. S.; Packham, D. A.; Pryor, J. P.; and Yates-Bell, A. J.: Hepatic dysfunction in renal carcinoma. *Br. J. Urol.,* **53:**533–536, 1981.

Flocks, R. H.; Culp, D. A.; and Porto, R.: Lymphatic spread from prostatic cancer. *J. Urol.,* **81:**194–196, 1959.

Fowler, J. E., Jr., and Whitmore, W. F., Jr.: The incidence and extent of pelvic lymph node metastases in apparently localized prostatic cancer. *Cancer,* **47:**2941–2945, 1981.

Fowler, J. E., Jr., and Whitmore, W. F., Jr.: Considerations for the use of testosterone with systemic chemotherapy in prostatic cancer. *Cancer,* **50:**1373–1377, 1982.

Freiha, F. S.; Pistenma, D. A.; and Bagshaw, M. A.: Pelvic lymphadenectomy for staging prostate carcinoma: Is it always necessary? *J. Urol.,* **122:**176–177, 1979.

Glashan, R. W., and Robinson, M. R. G.: Cardiovascular complications in the treatment of prostatic carcinoma. *Br. J. Urol.,* **53:**624–627, 1981.

Goffinet, D. R.; Schneider, M. J.; Glatstein, E. J.; Ludwig, H.; Ray, G. R.; Dunnick, N. R.; and Bagshaw, M. A.: Bladder cancer results of radiation therapy in 384 patients. *Radiology,* **117:**149–153, 1975.

Greenberg, H. S.; Deck, M. D. F.; Vikram, B.; Chu, F. C. H.; and Posner, J. B.: Metastasis to the base of the skull; clinical findings in 43 patients. *Neurology (N.Y.),* **31:**530–537, 1981.

Grossman, I. C.; Carpiniello, V.; Greenberg, S. H.; Malloy, T. R.; and Wein, A. J.: Staging pelvic lymphadenectomy for carcinoma of the prostate: Review of 91 cases. *J. Urol.,* **124:**632–634, 1980.

Guinan, P.; Bush, I.; Ray, V.; Vieth, R.; Rao, R.; and Bhatti, R.: The accuracy of the rectal examination in the diagnosis of prostate carcinoma. *N. Engl. J. Med.,* **303:**499–503, 1980.

Hahn, R. B.; Begg, C. B.; and Davis, T.: Phase II study of vinblastine, CCNU, triazinate and dactinomycin in advanced renal cell cancer. *Cancer Treat. Rep.,* **65:**711–713, 1981.

Hall, R. R.; Herring, D. W.; McGill, A. C.; and Gibb, I.:

Oral methotrexate therapy for multiple superficial bladder carcinoma. *Cancer Treat. Rep.,* **65:**175–178, 1981.

Hall, R. R., and Turner, A. G.: Methotrexate treatment for advanced bladder cancer: A review after 6 years. *Br. J. Urol.,* **52:**403, 1980.

Herr, H. W.: Cis-diamminedichloride platinum II in the treatment of advanced bladder cancer. *J. Urol.,* **123:**853–855, 1980.

Herr, H. W.; Pinsky, C. M.; Whitmore, W. F., Jr.; Oettgen, H.; and Melamed, M. R.: Effect of intravesical BCG in carcinoma in situ of the bladder. *Cancer,* **51:**1323–1326, 1983.

Herr, H. W.; Yagoda, A.; Batata, M.; Sogani, P. C.; and Whitmore, W. F., Jr.: Planned pre-operative cisplatin and radiation therapy for locally advanced bladder cancer. *Cancer,* **52:**2205–2208, 1983.

Heston, W. D. W.; Kadmon, D.; Lazan, D. W.; and Fair, W. R.: Copenhagen rat prostatic tumor ornithine decarboxylase activity (ODC) and the effect of ODC inhibitor alpha-difluoromethylonithine. *Prostate,* **3:**383–389, 1982.

Higgins, I. T. T.: The epidemiology of cancer of the prostate. *J. Chronic Dis.,* **28:**343–348, 1975.

Hrushesky, W. J., and Murphy, G. P.: Current status of the therapy of advanced renal carcinoma. *J. Surg. Oncol.,* **9:**277–288, 1977.

Jacobi, G. H., and Wenderoth, U. K.: Gonadotropin-releasing hormones analogues for prostate cancer: Untoward side effects of high-dose regimens acquire a therapeutical dimension. *Eur. Urol.,* **8:**129–134, 1982.

Jewett, H. J.: The present status of radical prostatectomy for stages A and B prostatic cancer. *Urol. Clin. North Am.,* **2:**105–124, 1975.

Jewett, H. J., and Strong, G. H.: Infiltrating carcinoma of the bladder—Relation of depth of penetration of the bladder wall to incidence of local extension and metastasis. *J. Urol.,* **55:**366–372, 1946.

Katz, S. A., and Davis, J. E.: Renal adenocarcinoma. Prognostics and treatment reflected by survival. *Urology,* **10:**10–11, 1977.

Katz, S. A., and Schapira, H. S.: Spontaneous regression of genitourinary cancer—An update. *J. Urol.,* **128:**1–4, 1982.

Kirkman, H.: Estrogen-induced tumors of the kidney in the Syrian hamster. *Natl. Cancer Inst. Monogr.,* **1:**1–37, 1959.

Klein, L. A.: Prostatic carcinoma. *N. Engl. J. Med.,* **300:**824–833, 1979.

Marshall, V. F.: The relation of the preoperative estimate to the pathologic demonstration of the extent of vesical neoplasms. *J. Urol.,* **68:**714–718, 1952.

Melicow, M. N.: Histological study of vesical urothelium intervening between gross neoplasm in total cystectomy. *J. Urol.,* **68:**261, 1952.

Middleton, R. G.: Surgery for metastatic renal cell carcinoma. *J. Urol.,* **97:**973–977, 1967.

Miller, L. S.: Bladder cancer: Superiority of preoperative irradiation and cystectomy in clinical stages B_2 and C. *Cancer,* **39:**973–980, 1977.

Montie, J. E.; Burkowski, R. M.; James, R. E.; Straffon, R. A.; and Stewart, B. H.: A critical review of immunotherapy of disseminated renal adenocarcinoma. Read at the Annual Meeting of the American Urological Association, Boston, May 10–14, 1981.

Montie, J. E.; Stewart, B. H.; Straffon, R. A.; Banowsky, L. H. W.; Hewitt, C. B.; and Montague, D. R.: The role of adjunctive nephrectomy in patients with metastatic renal cell carcinoma. *J. Urol.,* **117:**272–275, 1977.

Mostofi, F. K.: Pathological aspects and spread of carcinoma of the bladder. *J.A.M.A.,* **206:**1764–1769, 1968.

Natale, R. B.; Yagoda, A.; Watson, R. C.; Whitmore, W. F., Jr.; Bluemenreich, M.; and Braun, D. W., Jr.: Methotrexate: An active drug in bladder cancer. *Cancer,* **47:**1246–1250, 1981.

Needles, B.; Ahmed, T.; Blumenreich, M.; Yagoda, A.; and Watson, R. C.: Phase II trial of vinblastine and methotrexate in urothelial tract tumors. *Proc. Am. Assoc. Cancer. Res.,* **23:**113, 1982.

Needles, B.; Yagoda, A.; Sogani, P. C.; Grabstald, H.; and Whitmore, W. F., Jr.: Intravenous cisplatin for superficial bladder tumors. *Cancer,* **50:**1722–1723, 1982b.

Oliver, R. T. D.: Effect of chemotherapy on locally recurrent invasive bladder tumors. In Oliver, R. T. D.; Hendry, W. F.; Bloom, H. J. G., (eds): *Bladder Cancer.* Butterworth, London, 1981.

Oliver, R. T. D.; England, H. R.; Risdon, R. A.; Blandy, J. P.: Methotrexate in the treatment of metastatic and recurrent primary transitional cell carcinoma. *J. Urol.,* **131:**483–485, 1984.

Paulson, D. F.; Piserchia, P. V.; and Gardner, W.: Predictors of lymphatic spread in prostatic adenocarcinoma. Uro-Oncology Research Group Study. *J. Urol.,* **123:**697–699, 1980.

Prout, G. R.: The kidney and ureter. In Holland, J. F., and Frei, E. (eds.): *Cancer Medicine.* Lea & Febiger, Philadelphia, 1973.

Resnick, M. E.: Non-invasive techniques in evaluating patients with carcinoma of the prostate. *J. Urol.,* **17:**25–30, 1981.

Riches, E.: The natural history of renal tumors. In *Tumors of the Kidney and Ureter.* E. & S. Livingston, Ltd., Edinburgh, 1964.

Robinson, C. J., and Thomas, B. S.: Effect of hormonal therapy on plasma testosterone levels in prostate cancer. *Br. Med. J.,* **4:**391–394, 1971.

Robson, C. J.; Churchill, B. M.; and Anderson, W.: The results of radical nephrectomy for renal cell carcinoma. *J. Urol.,* **101:**297–301, 1969.

Samuels, M. L.; Logothetis, C.; Trindade, A.; and Johnson, D. E.: Cytoxan, adriamycin, and cisplatinum (CISCA) in metastatic bladder cancer. *Proc. Am. Assoc. Cancer Res.,* **21:**137, 1980.

Schmidt, J. D.: Chemotherapy of hormone-resistant stage D prostate cancer. *J. Urol.,* **123:**797–805, 1980.

Schwartz, S.; Yagoda, A.; Natale, R. B.; Watson, R. C.; Whitmore, W.; and Lesser, M.: Phase II trial of sequentialy administered cisplatin, cyclophosphamide and adriamycin for urothelial tract tumors. *J. Urol.* (in press).

Sherwood, J. B., and Goldwasser, E. A.: Radioimmunoassay for erythropoietin. *Blood,* **54:**885–893, 1979.

Silverberg, E.: Cancer statistics, 1982. *CA,* **32:**15–23, 1985.

Skinner, D. G.; Colvin, R. B.; Vermillion, C. D.; Pfister, R. C.; and Leadbetter, W. F.: Diagnosis and management of renal cell carcinoma. A clinical and pathologic study of 309 cases. *Cancer,* **28:**1165–117, 1971.

Skinner, D. G.; Vermillion, C. D.; and Colvin, R. B.: The surgical management of renal cell carcinoma. *J. Urol.,* **107:**705–710, 1972.

Slack, N. A.; Bross, I. D. J.; and Prout, G. R., Jr.: Five year follow-up results of a collaborative study of therapies for carcinoma of the bladder. *J. Surg. Oncol.,* **9:**393–405, 1977.

Smith, J. A., Jr.; Batata, M.; Grabstald, H.; Sogani, P. C.; Herr, H. W.; and Whitmore, W. F., Jr.: Preoperative irradiation and cystectomy for bladder cancer. *Cancer,* **48:**869–876, 1982.

Smith, J. A., Jr., and Whitmore, W. F., Jr.: Salvage cystectomy for bladder cancer after failure of definitive irradiation. *J. Urol.,* **125:**643–646, 1981a.

Smith, J. A., Jr., and Whitmore, W. F., Jr.: Regional lymph node metastasis from bladder cancer. *J. Urol.,* **126:**591–593, 1981b.

Smith, P. H.: Endocrine and cytotoxic therapy. In Duncan, W. (ed.): *Prostate Cancer. Recent Results in Cancer Research.* Springer-Verlag, Berlin, 1981.

Socquet, Y.: Surgery and adjuvant chemotherapy with high-dose methotrexate and folinic acid rescue for infiltrating tumors of the bladder. *Cancer Treat. Rep.,* **65:**187–189, 1981.

Sogani, P. C., and Whitmore, W. F., Jr.: Experience with flutamide in previously untreated patients with advanced prostatic cancer. *J. Urol.,* **122:**640–643, 1979.

Soloway, M. S.: Rationale for intensive intravesical chemotherapy for superficial bladder cancer. *J. Urol.,* **123:**461–466, 1980.

Soloway, M. S.: Intravesical chemotherapy in superficial bladder cancer. In Spiers, A. S. D. (ed.): *Chemotherapy and Urological Malignancy.* Springer-Verlag, New York, 1982.

Stolbach, L. L.; Berg, C. B.; Hall, T.; and Horton, J.: Treatment of renal carcinoma: A phase III randomized trial of oral medroxyprogesterone (Provera), hydroxyurea and nafoxidine. *Cancer Treat. Rep.,* **65:**689–692, 1981.

Steinberg, C.; Yagoda, A.; Scher, H.; Hollander, P.; Watson, R. C.; Ahmed, T.: Methotrexate, vinblastine, adriamycin, and cisplatin for transitional cell carcinoma. *Proc. Am. Soc. Clin. Oncol.,* **3:**156, 1983.

Swanson, D. A.: The current immunologic status of renal carcinoma. *Bull. Cancer (Paris),* **31:**36–39, 1979.

Torti, F. M., and Carter, S. K.: The chemotherapy of prostate adenocarcinoma. *Ann. Intern. Med.,* **92:**681–689, 1980.

Turner, A. G.: Methotrexate. In Oliver, R. T. D.; Hendry, W. F.; and Bloom, H. J. G. (eds.): *Bladder Cancer.* Butterworth, London, 1981a.

Turner, A. G.: Methotrexate in advanced bladder cancer. *Cancer Treat. Rep.,* **65:**183–186, 1981b.

Utz, D. C.; Scmitz, S. E.; Fugelso, P. D.; and Farrow, G. U.: A clinicopathologic evaluation of partial cystectomy for carcinoma of the urinary bladder. *Cancer,* **32:**1075–1077, 1973.

van der Werf-Messing, B.: Carcinoma of the kidney. *Cancer,* **32:**1056–1061, 1973.

van der Werf-Messing, B.: Carcinoma of the bladder $T_3N_xM_0$ treated by preoperative irradiation followed by cystectomy. *Cancer,* **36:**718–722, 1975.

van der Werf-Messing, B.: Combined modality treatment of bladder cancer at the Rotterdam Radiotherapy Institute. In Connelly, J. G. (ed.): *Carcinoma of the Bladder.* Raven Press, New York, 1981.

Wallace, D. M., and Bloom, J. H. G.: The management of deeply infiltrating (T3) bladder carcinoma: Controlled trial of radical radiotherapy versus preoperative radiotherapy and radical cystectomy. *Br. J. Urol.,* **48:**587–594, 1976.

Walsh, P. C., and Jewett, H. J.: Radical surgery for prostatic cancer. *Cancer,* **45:**1906–1911, 1980.

Watson, R. A., and Tang, D. B.: The predictive value of prostatic acid phosphatase as a screening procedure for prostatic cancer. *N. Engl. J. Med.,* **303:**497–499, 1980.

Weyman, P. J.; McClennan, B. L.; Stanley, R. J.; Levitt, R. G.; and Sagel, S. S.: Comparison of computer tomography and angiography in the evaluation of renal carcinoma. *Radiology,* **137:**417–424, 1980.

Whitmore, W. F., Jr.: The natural history of prostatic cancer. *Cancer,* **32:**1104–1112, 1973.

Whitmore, W. F., Jr.: Management of bladder cancer. *Curr. Probl. Cancer,* **4:**3–48, 1979.

Whitmore, W. F., Jr.: Interstitial radiation therapy for carcinoma of the prostate. *Prostate,* **1:**157–168, 1980.

Whitmore, W. F., Jr.: Integrated irradiation and cystectomy in bladder cancer. In Connolly, J. G. (ed.): *Carcinoma of the Bladder.* Raven Press, New York, 1981.

Whitmore, W. F., Jr.: Batata, M. A.; Ghoneim, M. A.; Grabstald, H.; and Unal, A..: Radical cystectomy with or without prior irradiation in the treatment of bladder cancer. *J. Urol.,* **108:**184–189, 1977a.

Whitmore, W. F., Jr.; Batata, M. A.; Hilaris, B. S.; Reddy, G. N.; Unal, A.; Ghoneim, M. A.; Grabstald, H.; and Chu, F.: A comparative study of two preoperative regimens with cystectomy for bladder cancer. *Cancer,* **40:**1077–1086, 1977b.

Winkelstein, W., Jr., and Ernster, U. L.: Epidemiology and etiology. In Murphy, G. (ed.): *Prostatic*

Cancer, PSG Publishing Company, Inc., Littleton, Massachusetts, 1979.

Wynder, E. L., and Goldsmith, R.: The epidemiology of bladder cancer—A second look. *Cancer,* **40:**1246–1268, 1977.

Wynder, E. L.; Mabuchi, K.; and Whitmore, W. F., Jr.: Epidemiology of adenocarcinoma of the kidney. *J.N.C.I.,* **53:**1619–1634, 1974.

Yagoda, A.: Non-hormonal cytotoxic agents in the treatment of prostate adenocarcinoma. *Cancer,* **32:**1131–1140, 1973.

Yagoda, A.: Chemotherapy of metastatic bladder cancer. *Cancer,* **45:**1879–1888, 1980.

Yagoda, A.; Bosl, G.; and Scher, H.: Advances in chemotherapy. In Javadpour, N. (ed.): *Recent Advances in Urologic Cancer.* The Williams & Wilkins Company, Baltimore, 1982.

Yagoda, A.; Watson, R. C.; Natale, R. B.; Barzell, W. E.; Sogani, P. C.; Grabstald, H.; and Whitmore, W. F., Jr.: A critical analysis of response criteria in patients with prostate cancer treated with cisdiamminedichloride platinum II. *Cancer,* **44:**1553–1559, 1979.

36

Neoplasms of the Testis

STEPHEN D. WILLIAMS and LAWRENCE H. EINHORN

Introduction

Testicular cancer is a relatively rare disease, accounting for 1% of all male neoplasms. Approximately 5000 new cases per year have been reported. This contrasts sharply with lung, breast, and colorectal cancer, each comprising over 100,000 new cases per year. Despite its low incidence, testis cancer is an extremely important disease for several reasons:

1. It occurs in a relatively young age group. Germ cell tumors are the most common carcinoma in males, ages 15 to 35, and the average age of newly diagnosed patients is 25 years.
2. Testicular cancer is one of the few neoplastic diseases to have serum markers that enable the clinician to document the course of the disease and make important therapeutic decisions.
3. Testicular cancer is a fascinating biologic disease, as successful therapy is apparently capable of changing the histology from a highly virulent, rapidly metastasizing carcinoma to a more indolent, nonmetastasizing mature teratoma.
4. Most important, testicular cancer has become a landmark cancer because it is a highly curable solid tumor.

Incidence and Epidemiology

The incidence of testicular cancer is 4 per 100,000 in the United States and rising slightly. Worldwide, Denmark has the highest incidence of germ cell tumors. The disease is less common in black and orientals than Caucasians. It is more commonly found in higher socioeconomic strata. The reported 1 to 2%

incidence of a second primary testicular cancer is probably surreptitiously low in the 1980s because of the improved survival of such patients. Although late relapses following successful surgery or chemotherapy are rare, the incidence of new contralateral primary tumors warrants prolonged follow-up. The etiology of testicular carcinoma is largely unknown. Certain pathologic conditions are associated with an increased incidence, the most important of these being cryptorchidism. Orchidopexy performed after puberty is associated with a substantial risk of subsequent malignant degeneration. An inherent germinal defect may be responsible for both cryptorchidism and tumor formation. An increased incidence of dysgenetic tissue has been identified in the cryptorchid testis, and this may account for the increased susceptibility to subsequent malignant degeneration. Patients with a unilateral undescended testis should be at increased risk for cancer in the contralateral testis, if dysgenesis is a factor in tumor formation. It has been shown that 20% of tumors developing in patients with an antecedent history of cryptorchidism arose in the contralateral apparently normal testis.

Other clinical conditions associated with an increased incidence of testicular cancer are less well defined. There appears to be an increased incidence in subfertile men, although cause-and-effect relationships are not clear. An increased incidence of testicular tumors in the atrophic testis is likely.

Pathology and Natural History

Histology. Tumors of germinal cell origin comprise over 90% of all testicular neoplasms.

Nongerminal tumors such as Leydig cell tumors, sarcomas, or lymphomas are exceedingly rare and will not be discussed in this chapter.

Four major types of testicular cancer are seen: seminoma, embryonal carcinoma, mature or immature teratoma, and choriocarcinoma. A fifth type, endodermal sinus, or yolk sac carcinoma, is more common in children or as a primary mediastinal germ cell tumor. It is very rare as a pure form in the adult. Each basic cell type can be seen alone or in combination in the orchiectomy specimen. Teratocarcinoma is basically a combination of teratoma plus embryonal carcinoma. The most commonly used classification system is shown in Table 36–1.

The histogenesis and interrelationship of testicular germ cell tumors are quite controversial. Perhaps the best explanation is that proposed by Teilum. In this, germ cell tumors may be divided into those that are unipotential (seminoma) and those that are undifferentiated and multipotential. The latter, for whatever reason, may differentiate toward extraembryonic (endodermal sinus) or embryonic (teratoma) structures (Roth and Gillespie, 1980). This theory seems to explain the frequent observation of more than one cell type in the primary tumor and the occasional discrepancy in histology between the primary and metastatic deposits. As will be discussed in subsequent sections, however, from the clinicians' point of view, the major distinction is between pure seminoma tumors and tumors containing any other elements, the nonseminomatous germ cell tumors (NSGCT).

Pure seminoma accounts for about 40% of testicular germ cell tumors and tends to occur in somewhat older patients. Pathologically they are subdivided into typical, anaplastic, and spermatocytic subtypes, although many feel the distinction between the first two types is arbitrary and not clinically relevant. Seminoma pathologically must be distinguished from embryonal carcinoma, metastatic tumors, and lymphoma. Seminoma is characterized by large uniform cells separated by delicate fibrous septa with variable components of lymphocytic infiltration and fibrosis and with infrequent mitotic figures.

About 15 to 20% of testis tumors are embryonal carcinoma, characterized by large cells with a primitive epithelial appearance and abundant mitotic figures, and areas of hemorrhage and necrosis.

Teratomas are complex neoplasms containing elements from two or more germ cell layers. They may have varying degrees of maturity, but no grading system exists as is available for ovarian teratomas. In fact, even the most benign-appearing teratoma may be associated with the development of metastases.

Pure choriocarcinomas are rare, but such elements are frequently found associated with other cell types. Choriocarcinoma is composed of syncytiotrophoblasts and cytotrophoblasts. In pure form, the primary tumor is frequently small, but associated with the early development of widespread metastases and very high gonadotropin levels. Necrosis and hemorrhage are prominent.

Pure endodermal sinus tumor is almost always seen in childhood. Histologically, Schillar-Duval bodies are prominent, and alpha-fetoprotein production is universal.

Most intriguing is the rare occurrence of true extragonadal germ cell tumors. These are pathologically and clinically similar to their testicular counterparts. They usually occur in midline areas, the retroperitoneum and mediastinum, and presumably originate from embryonic nests of germ cell tissue.

Modes of Spread. Testicular cancer may remain localized intrascrotally for significant periods of time. There have been anecdotal reports of patients with massive testicular swelling present over a period of several years with no evidence of lymphatic or hematogenous spread.

Testicular cancer spreads lymphatically to the retroperitoneal nodes, although inguinal node involvement may be seen in patients with prior scrotal or inguinal surgery which has disrupted the usual lymphatic drainage. Hematogenous spread is primarily to the lungs. At the time of initial diagnosis, 40% of nonseminomatous germ cell tumors are stage I limited to the testis; 40% stage II pathologically positive retroperitoneal nodes; and 20% stage III disease elsewhere, usually pulmonary. Occasionally, metastases to liver, brain, or elsewhere are seen, but bone metastases are unusual except in seminoma. Once a patient

Table 36–1. Dixon Moore Pathologic Classification

    I Pure seminoma
   II Embryonal, with or without seminoma
  III Teratoma
   IV Teratocarcinoma with embryonal, teratoma, or choriocarcinoma
    V Choriocarcinoma

develops hematogenous dissemination, rapid progression of metastases may ensue. Seminoma is more likely to remain localized, as 70% are clinical stage I at presentation. Ten to twenty percent of clinical stage I patients would likely be pathologic stage II if subjected to a retroperitoneal lymphadenectomy. This procedure is unnecessary because seminoma is exquisitely radiosensitive.

Signs and Symptoms. Typically, a patient with testicular cancer is asymptomatic except for unilateral, nontender testicular enlargement, although pain may be reported. The enlargement may be episodic, abrupt, or may wax and wane. Some patients have flank pain or back pain due to retroperitoneal node metastases. Gonadotropin production may lead to tender gynecomastia. Mediastinal or pulmonary metastases may cause chest pain and/or dyspnea, but these symptoms are not seen in the absence of far-advanced disease. Symptomatic liver or brain metastases are unusual but seen occasionally.

Physical examination is usually normal except for a firm scrotal mass that cannot be separated from the testis and does not transilluminate (i.e., not a hydrocele). On occasion, patients will have a palpable abdominal mass from retroperitoneal nodal metastases. Likewise, cervical or supraclavicular lymphadenopathy will be noted occasionally.

Patients with extragonadal tumors usually present with signs and symptoms of a mediastinal or retroperitoneal mass. Accordingly, advanced disease is usually present at diagnosis.

Diagnosis

Too often, major delays by the patient or physician occur before the proper diagnosis is ascertained. A three- to six-month period from the first testicular symptom to the time of diagnosis is usual. Greater than 50% of patients with testis cancer are initially misdiagnosed as having epididymitis. Other causes of scrotal mass would include hernia, torsion, hydrocele, or other primary or metastatic tumors. Important considerations are the ability to transilluminate the mass and the ability by careful palpation to separate the testis from the mass and epididymal and cord structures posteriorly.

Whenever a scrotal mass is found that does not transilluminate and is not separable from the epididymis and cord, the diagnosis of testicular cancer should be considered, and an inguinal exploration should follow. Testicular biopsy or scrotal orchiectomy must not be performed, as these procedures potentially contaminate the scrotum and alter the normal testicular lymphatics. At the time of inguinal exploration, if the possibility of malignancy exists, the orchiectomy should be completed. This procedure will confirm the diagnosis and also initiate therapy.

As discussed in a subsequent section, serum marker determinations are not very useful in the diagnosis of a scrotal mass. If positive, cancer exists, but many patients with early stage NSGCT and most seminoma patients will have normal markers.

Finally, it should be mentioned that a frequently misinterpreted symptom in such patients is back pain. Patients may not notice or mention a scrotal mass, but consult the physician because of back pain, a symptom whose significance may not be appreciated in a young healthy-appearing patient.

Staging

Once a diagnosis of testicular cancer is established, a staging evaluation is initiated to determine the extent of disease. Staging determines proper initial therapy and also documents response to such treatment.

The most commonly used staging classifications for seminoma and NSGCT are shown in Tables 36–2 and 36–3. Staging evaluation should include serum markers, liver function studies, LDH, chest radiograph and whole-lung tomograms or computerized tomography (CT), and some evaluation of retroperitoneal involvement. No totally reliable method of accomplishing the latter is available; lymphangiography, computerized tomography, and ultrasonography all have significant errors, both false positives and negatives (Rowland *et. al.,* 1982). Early-stage NSGCT patients are usually treated with retroperitoneal lymphadenectomy. Thus, the only staging distinction of importance in the absence of stage III disease in

Table 36–2. Staging of Seminoma

Stage I	Testis only
Stage IIA	Positive retroperitoneal nodes on lymphangiogram or abdominal CT scan
Stage IIB	Palpable abdominal mass
Stage III	Supradiaphragmatic adenopathy—mediastinal and/or cervical
Stage IV	Visceral metastases—lung, bone, liver, and/or brain

Table 36–3. Staging of NSGCT

Stage I	Testis only
Stage IIA	Positive retroperitoneal nodes at lymphadenectomy, but less than six in number and not grossly positive
Stage IIB	Grossly positive retroperitoneal nodes and/or greater than five nodes positive
Stage IIC	Palpable abdominal mass
Stage III	Supradiaphragmatic spread — usually pulmonary metastases

these patients is to exclude surgically unresectable retroperitoneal involvement. CT scanning performs this function adequately, therefore, many favor omitting the more invasive lymphangiogram. The situation for seminoma is less clear, as these patients will not have surgical staging of the retroperitoneum. It is doubtful, however, that lymphangiography adds enough to accurate staging to warrant this procedure. Many radiotherapists, however, use the results of this procedure for treatment planning. Whole-lung tomograms or chest CT scans are important in the initial staging of an NSGCT patient with a normal PA and lateral chest x-ray. Between 5 and 10% of such cases will have positive tomography, thereby changing the stage from locoregional, requiring lymphadenectomy, to disseminated, requiring chemotherapy.

Markers

One of the major improvements in the management of testis tumor patients is the understanding and general availability of radioimmunoassay determinations of human chorionic gonadotropin (HCG) and alpha-fetoprotein (AFP). AFP is a glycoprotein that is a major serum protein of the human fetus. It is often elevated in patients with hepatoma or NSGCT, and rarely in patients with enteric adenocarcinomas and patients recovering from severe hepatitis. Thus, it tends to be a highly specific finding for hepatoma or NSGCT. It has a metabolic half-time of about five days.

HCG is another glycoprotein normally secreted by the human placenta. It is composed of alpha and beta subunits; the former is immunologically similar to lutenizing hormone (LH), and the latter theoretically immunologically distinct. Thus, most assays now measure the beta subunit. A serum HCG of greater than 1000 (normal <3 ng/mL) will be associated with a positive pregnancy test. Elevated HCG is seen in pregnancy and in some patients with other neoplasms such as lung and bladder cancer. It has a metabolic half-time of 18 to 24 hours. One recognized cause of a false-positive HCG is poor antibody specificity in the assay. A markedly elevated LH level as seen in hypogonadism may cross-react with the HCG assay. This may become a problem in an occasional testis tumor patient after intensive chemotherapy and surgery. If doubt exists, the distinction can easily be identified by repeating the HCG a few days after an injection of testosterone cypionate.

Serum markers are particularly useful in the following situations: (1) evaluation of the patient with seminoma, (2) following the patient after chemotherapy, radiotherapy, or surgery for seminoma or NSGCT, and (3) evaluating the critically ill patient suspected of having a germ cell tumor.

Theoretically, patients with seminoma should have a normal HCG and AFP. An elevated AFP in such a patient connotes the presence of NSGCT, and traditionally these patients have done less well than seminoma patients with normal AFPs. Generally, it is agreed that the seminoma patient with an elevated AFP should be treated as having NSGCT. The implications of an elevated HCG are less well defined. The evidence now implies, however, that an elevated HCG without pathologic evidence of NSGCT does not affect prognosis or require different therapy.

Markers are also a sensitive indicator of response to chemotherapy or surgery. They should fall in a predictable fashion after lymphadenectomy for early-stage disease according to their known half-time. They should also fall rapidly during treatment with systemic chemotherapy for metastatic disease. In both situations, serial marker determinations after chemotherapy or surgery may be a sensitive early indicator of relapse. About one-third of patients who relapse after lymphadenectomy will have an elevated marker as their first manifestation of disease. This finding is specific and the patient must be treated, even in the absence of radiographic abnormalities. It must be remembered, however, that about 10% of patients with metastatic disease, and a much larger number of patients with stage I or II disease, will have normal markers. Thus, normal markers in no way exclude the presence of active disease.

Finally, extragonadal germ cell tumors are being recognized much more frequently

(Richardson *et al.,* 1981). This diagnosis should be considered in any patient with a midline tumor; however, they may be interpreted pathologically as undifferentiated carcinoma. An elevated marker will provide presumptive evidence of a germ cell origin. In a critically ill patient, a positive pregnancy test will suffice and may even make a tissue diagnosis unnecessary.

Treatment: Seminoma

As discussed in earlier sections, the diagnosis of pure seminoma requires that no other elements be present in the primary tumor and that serum AFP is normal. At least modest elevations of the serum HCG, however, do not preclude this diagnosis.

The mainstay of therapy for patients with seminoma is external radiation. As discussed previously, about 70% of such patients will be in clinical stage I at the time of diagnosis. The possibility of staging error is obvious, however, and it has been standard practice to irradiate the regional lymphatics prophylactically. Seminoma is exquisitely radiosensitive; a dosage of 2500 to 3000 rads is adequate for control in such a situation. Table 36–4 shows the results of therapy compiled from five published series (Doornbos *et al.,* 1975; Calman *et al.,* 1979; Jackson *et al.,* 1980; Dosoretz *et al.,* 1981; Thomas *et al.,* 1982). Only 24/768 (3%) clinical stage I patients died of seminoma. Many of these patients would have been classified as stage II, but modern staging procedures were not routinely employed.

Clinical stage II has traditionally been subdivided into two subgroups, although investigators have differed in the criteria employed to differentiate the two (palpable versus nonpalpable or an arbitrary size distinction on lymphangiography). Whatever the distinction employed, patients in stage IIA (variously

Table 36–4. Radiotherapy of Seminoma*

STAGE†	NUMBER	DIED OF SEMINOMA
I	768	24 (3%)
IIA	151	15 (10%)
IIB	107	33 (31%)
III and IV	67	41 (61%)

* Pooled data from Thomas *et al.,* 1982; Doombos *et al.,* 1975; Calman *et al.,* 1979; Jackson *et al.,* 1980; and Dosoretz *et al.,* 1981.
† Stage I = clinically negative retroperitoneal nodes; IIA = positive nodes variously defined ranging from <5 cm to nonpalpable; IIB = variously defined greater than IIA; III = positive supradiaphragmatic nodes; IV = visceral metastases.

defined) enjoy excellent prospects for cure with radiation. Patients in stage IIB; however, have a significant likelihood of treatment failure. Likewise, radiation is unlikely to control the occasional patient with supradiaphragmatic seminoma at presentation. In these latter two groups significant controversy exists regarding proper management, the role of chemotherapy of advanced seminoma, and the proper extent of radiation portals in stage II patients.

Chemotherapy of testicular cancer will be discussed in a subsequent section. At Indiana University, patients with recurrent seminoma and those presenting initially with stage III and IV disease have routinely been treated according to the same chemotherapy protocols as their nonseminomatous counterparts. These regimens involved various combinations of cisplatin plus vinblastine plus bleomycin with or without doxorubicin (PVB ± A). Of the 31 seminoma patients treated with this protocol, 21 were complete responders. Twelve of these patients had received no previous irradiation, and ten attained complete remission (CR) (Williams and Einhorn, 1985).

It has been the opinion of radiation oncologists that prophylactic treatment of the mediastinum is required for all stage II patients. This concept, however, has not been tested in a controlled clinical trial, and a recent publication has challenged this concept (Thomas *et al.,* 1982). In this series from the Princess Margaret Hospital, prophylactic treatment of the mediastinum was not given. No isolated failures in the mediastinum were reported in 40 stage IIA patients. Ten of the 46 stage IIB patients failed in the mediastinum; yet seven were salvaged by subsequent irradiation. A more detailed review of the subject may be found in the above-mentioned reference. In the absence of a controlled clinical trial, no evidence suggests that prophylactic treatment of the mediastinum is indicated; the overwhelming majority of patients will be receiving unnecessary treatment.

Considering these data, it seems that the proper initial management for patients with supradiaphragmatic or visceral metastases from seminoma at diagnosis is chemotherapy. Patients with stage IIA disease would appear to be optimally managed with infradiaphragmatic irradiation only. Management of patients with bulky stage II seminoma is controversial. One approach would be irradiation to the whole abdomen, with careful subsequent observation, and combination chemotherapy promptly at relapse. This strategy would spare many patients chemotherapy, and timely treatment of relapsing patients should yield high cure rates without major chemotherapy-related morbidity in patients spared mediastinal irradiation. Initial chemotherapy has its proponents, however, and would appear to be a reasonable option in the absence of a controlled trial.

Treatment: NSGCT

Disseminated Disease. Perhaps the most striking advance in the decade of the 1970s was the improvement in the results of chemotherapeutic management of disseminated testicular cancer. In the 1960s, standard treatment of advanced disease was actinomycin D with or without methotrexate and chlorambucil. Results of treatment were quite respectable with an objective response rate of 40 to 50% and a complete remission rate of 10 to 20%. Most impressive was that approximately one-half of the complete responders never relapsed. If recurrence was destined to occur, it would do so within the first two years.

In the latter 1960s and early 1970s the single-agent activity of vinblastine and bleomycin was documented. Subsequently, studies at M. D. Anderson Hospital provided clinical evidence of the previously postulated synergism of these two agents (Samuels *et al.*, 1976). Finally, in the early 1970s the striking single-agent activity of cisplatin was recognized (Higby *et al.*, 1974). Subsequent studies at several institutions employed various combinations of cisplatin, vinblastine, bleomycin, with or without other agents.

The evolution in the last decade of chemotherapy regimens for advanced disease is illustrated by sequential studies done at Indiana University. In the original study, done between 1974 and 1976, 27 of 47 evaluable patients were disease-free survivors for more than five years (Einhorn and Donohue, 1977). This original treatment regimen is shown in Table 36–5. Of note, the vinblastine dose was 0.4 mg-kg, patients received a fourth course only if they had not yet attained CR, and all patients received maintenance vinblastine.

The major toxicity of this regimen was neutropenia. The second study, between 1976 and 1978, was a random prospective trial evaluating a reduced vinblastine dose (0.3 mg/kg) (Einhorn and Williams, 1980). The third arm

Table 36–5. Original PVB Regimen*

Cisplatin	20 mg/M² IV daily for 5 days
Vinblastine	0.2 mg/kg IV days 1 & 2
Bleomycin	30 units IV days 2, 9, 16

* Courses repeated every three weeks (total courses, three or four).

evaluated the value of the addition of a fourth drug, doxorubicin. The results of therapy were identical, and 57/78 patients were long disease-free survivors.

Most recently, a study done by Indiana University and the Southeastern Cancer Study Group further evaluated the usefulness of doxorubicin and the value of maintenance therapy in patients in CR or disease-free after resection of teratoma (Einhorn *et al.*, 1981b). No differences in induction arms and no demonstrable value of maintenance vinblastine were noted. Overall, of 181 Indiana patients, 138 were disease-free with follow-up of 16 to 59 months (Williams *et al.*, 1983).

Studies at Memorial Hospital have given similar results. Their most recent regimen (VAB-6) is shown in Table 36–6. With fairly short follow-up, 21/25 patients were disease-free (Vugrin *et al.*, 1981).

Numerous other institutions and cooperative groups have duplicated these results. One study of note is the one of the Southwest Oncology Group (Samson *et al.*, 1981). They have apparently demonstrated a dose response curve for cisplatin. CR rate and survival for a regimen including high-dose cisplatin (120 mg/M²) was superior to that of a low-dose regimen (15 mg/M² daily for 5 days).

Response to chemotherapy is usually quite prompt. Symptoms and potentially difficult problems, such as obstructive uropathy, are relieved promptly, and no management is required other than chemotherapy. Figure 36–1A and B illustrates the rapidity of response usually seen.

In summary, about 80% of patients with disseminated disease treated with cisplatin-based chemotherapy will achieve disease-free status. Relapse rate will be approximately 10%, and

Table 36–6. VAB VI

Day 1:	Cyclophosphamide	600 mg/M² IV
	Bleomycin	30 units IV
	Actinomycin D	1 mg/M² IV
	Vinblastine	4 mg/M² IV
Day 1–3:	Bleomycin	20 units/M²/day by continuous infusion
Day 4:	Cisplatin	120 mg/M²

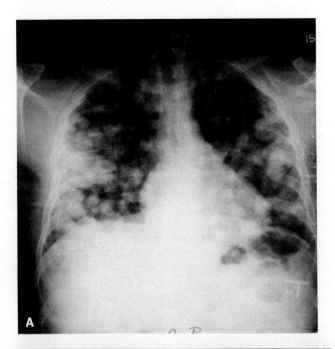

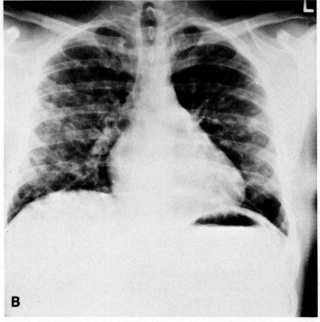

Figure 36–1. (*A*) Advanced pulmonary metastases of embryonal carcinoma. (*B*) Same patient three weeks after initiation of chemotherapy.

nearly 70% will be long survivors. Maintenance therapy is not required for patients in CR; maximum benefit from initial chemotherapy will be attained in 9 to 12 weeks. The addition of other active drugs to regimens containing cisplatin, vinblastine, and bleomycin has no proven value.

An additional drug with single agent activity is VP-16 (etoposide). Several investigators have noted objective responses in drug-refractory patients. These are partial and not of major clinical benefit. This agent, however, is of considerable value when combined with cisplatin in patients failing to attain CR or relapsing from complete remission, but not refractory to cisplatin. The salvage regimen used at Indiana University is shown in Table 36-7. Approximately 25% of patients in the groups

Table 36-7. Salvage Therapy

Cisplatin	20 mg/M² daily for 5 days
VP — 16	100 mg/M² daily × 4 — 5
	±
Bleomycin	30 units weekly

mentioned above who fail to be cured with first treatment will experience durable CR with salvage treatment (Williams and Einhorn, 1982b). Important prognostic factors are initial response and time to progression.

Some additional points regarding the management of these patients should be discussed. In the literature disagreement exists regarding the independent variables affecting prognosis. Tumor bulk, however, is clearly related to outcome. Because germ cell tumors proliferate rapidly, chemotherapy should be instituted as soon as feasible after the diagnosis is established, chemotherapy courses should be closely spaced, and dose reductions should not be made unless clearly warranted (*i.e.*, granulocytopenic fever). The tolerance of aggressive chemotherapy by these young healthy patients is quite striking.

A special subgroup of patients are those with brain metastases. This finding will be present occasionally in newly diagnosed patients, and will occur in a few others during therapy. Brain metastases being the sole cause of death is very unusual, occurring in only 2/276 consecutive Indiana patients. Moreover, in this same group of 276 patients, 5/19 patients with CNS involvement are long-term disease-free survivors. All five received cranial irradiation, but craniotomy was done in only one. All received at least two courses of cisplatin-based therapy after CNS treatment. Although numbers were small in this trial, the data suggest that such patients should receive chemotherapy after CNS treatment.

Postchemotherapy surgery is a complex issue. It has been the practice at most major centers to surgically excise any masses radiographically apparent that persist postchemotherapy. The usual procedure is a retroperitoneal lymph node dissection (RPLND), with or without excision of residual pulmonary or mediastinal masses. On many occasions, a combined thoracoabdominal procedure can be accomplished. Pathologic findings of surgery will be fibrosis/necrosis in one-third mature or immature teratoma in one-third, and carcinoma in one-third. The latter patients clearly benefit from surgery, as the ma-

jority will remain disease-free if they receive postoperative chemotherapy, whereas earlier experience had shown a high relapse rate if no chemotherapy is given.

More complex is the role of excision of residual teratoma. It does appear that some patients with unresected teratoma are at risk of local growth of the residual mass with potential for compression of adjacent structures. Likewise, few patients have been seen with recurrent carcinoma four to ten years after initial treatment. It is possible that late recurrences arise in previously unresected teratoma.

In a recent review of the Indiana University experience, 52 patients with resected teratoma underwent blinded retrospective pathology review (Loehrer *et al.*, 1983). In this group, nine patients experienced recurrent teratoma and nine carcinoma. Some of the patients with recurrent teratoma, generally manifested as a slowly enlarging local mass with normal markers, were successfully treated with further surgery. Risk of recurrence of either teratoma or carcinoma did not correlate with the histologic grade of teratoma. It was more frequent in patients who had bulky disease resected earlier and also in a subgroup of seven patients whose pathologic diagnosis at initial surgery was sarcoma.

In summary, it is impossible to define preoperatively which patients will pathologically exhibit only fibrosis/necrosis versus teratoma or carcinoma. Patients who are drug refractory (*i.e.*, rising markers) do not benefit from surgery. Patients with normal markers and persistent teratoma or carcinoma, however, do appear to benefit from complete excision of residual masses. Evidence that exploratory surgery is required in patients who have normal chest and abdominal radiographic studies after completion of chemotherapy has not been substantiated (Einhorn *et al.*, 1981a; Vugrin *et al.*, 1981; Bracken *et al.*, 1983).

Of concern in a population with such a high probability for long survival are the potential long-term effects of treatment. The most common short-term toxic effect of treatment is myelosuppression. Cisplatin nephrotoxicity and bleomycin lung disease are occasionally seen. Evidence that progressive dysfunction of either of these organ systems will ensue after completion of treatment has not been identified.

One troublesome late effect of treatment well described has been Raynaud's phenomenon (Vogelzang *et al.*, 1981). Precise etiologic factors are unclear. It has been reported in patients treated with vinblastine plus bleomycin alone, as well as the PVB regimen; in the latter group it may be seen in 30 to 35% of patients. It is more prevalent in cigarette smokers and may only be partially reversible over long periods of time. Management is not very successful, but should at least include cessation of smoking, as well as other therapeutic methods for this condition.

Second neoplasms to date have not been a major complication, although the period of observation of PVB patients may not yet be sufficient to define the ultimate risk. To date, only one nontesticular second cancer has been seen at Indiana University. This pathologically was a widely disseminated angiosarcoma in a patient who had also had radiation therapy. Second neoplasms may be more often seen in patients receiving classic alkylating agents in addition to PVB. A 1% incidence of new primary tumors occurs in the contralateral testis in successfully treated patients.

Finally, reproductive effects of chemotherapy on gonadal function must be considered. In prospective and retrospective studies at Indiana University (Drasga et al., 1983), it has been documented that the majority of patients with disseminated disease are oligospermic or azospermic at diagnosis before any treatment other than unilateral orchiectomy. Most are not suitable candidates for semen cryopreservation. Initial effects of chemotherapy are the development of azospermia in most patients. With the passage of time however, a remarkable recovery occurs, so that approximately 50% of patients had normal semen analysis at a median follow-up of 40 months after initiation of treatment. Effects on levels of follicle-stimulating and lutenizing hormones and testosterone were not consistent. Thus, reproductive effects of PVB appear to be substantially less than those seen in patients with Hodgkin's disease and lymphoma treated with regimens containing alkylating agents and procarbazine. Although no data are available, presumably alkylating agents contained in VAB-type regimens will have similar deleterious effects as those seen in lymphoma. To date, no information on increased risk of fetal abnormality in children fathered by treated patients has been identified. Several Indiana patients have fathered children with no obvious excess fetal wastage or congenital abnormality.

Relevant areas for future investigations include definition of a highly favorable patient population who might achieve equally good results with less treatment. For patients with bulky presentations, innovative treatment may be considered. Initial cytoreductive surgery has not benefitted such patients (Javadpour et al., 1982). High-dose chemotherapy with or without autologous marrow rescue, fixed alternating combinations, and the earlier use of VP-16 are all under investigation currently.

Early-Stage Disease. About 80% of patients with NSGCT will have stage I (testis alone) or stage II (testis plus retroperitoneal nodes) disease at diagnosis. Staging and initial management (orchiectomy) are discussed in an earlier section. Additional considerations requiring comment are management of retroperitoneal nodes and the use of adjuvant chemotherapy.

Traditional treatment of retroperitoneal lymphatics has been either retroperitoneal lymph node dissection (RPLND) or radiation therapy. In the United States, RPLND has been the standard procedure in clinical stage I and II testicular cancer. This procedure involves radical resection of retroperitoneal lymph nodes from the renal hilus to the bifurcation of the iliac arteries, may be unilateral or bilateral, and may or may not involve suprahilar dissection. This procedure allows precise pathologic staging, as 15 to 35% of clinical stage I patients in reality will be pathologic stage II. It is a formidable surgical procedure, but in experienced hands has acceptable short-term morbidity and an operative mortality that approaches zero. The major complication is interruption of sympathetic nerves that control ejaculation, resulting in a dry ejaculate and infertility; sexual function is unaltered.

Several centers have reported results of RPLND (Skinner and Scardino, 1980; Williams and Einhorn, 1982a). Similar findings have been observed: namely, about 10% of patients who are pathologic stage I will develop pulmonary metastases, and resected stage II patients who do not receive adjuvant chemotherapy have a 35 to 50% risk of relapse.

It is conceivable that in the modern chemotherapy era, radiation may give equivalent results, although to date no such documentation has been made. It is acknowledged that radiation is not likely to control disease greater than 2 cm (Tyrrell and Peckham, 1976). The late consequences are not well defined, but at Indiana complications have included repetitive small bowel obstruction and lumbar radiculopathy at the doses required for NSGCT, which are considerably higher than that necessary for treatment of seminoma. Risk of sterility is not clear, but some patients do retain fertility. Tolerance of subsequent chemotherapy, if necessary, is reduced. With these considerations in mind and until results are available from radiotherapy series that are equivalent to those numerous studies involving RPLND, radiotherapy must be considered inferior to surgery.

A controversial issue in patients treated with RPLND is the role of adjuvant chemotherapy. Traditionally, it was recommended in all stage II patients, and many clinicians also treated stage I patients. This approach has been reevaluated in the modern chemotherapy era. Although for all stage III patients treated with PVB, the CR rate is 70 to 80%, it is 98 to 99% in patients with minimal metastatic disease. Thus, an alternate approach would be to withhold adjuvant chemotherapy in completely resected stage II patients and follow them closely with monthly markers and chest x-rays, giving prompt treatment at relapse.

Table 36–8 outlines the results of the treatment of early-stage disease at Indiana University from 1974 to 1980. It would appear that observation after RPLND is a valid option as there has been only one cancer death in 68 stage II patients treated with ineffective adjuvant therapy (actinomycin D) or observation.

If adjuvant chemotherapy is employed, however, it appears that short-term therapy should include cisplatin. In patients so treated, the risk of relapse is essentially zero. Currently, a large intergroup study is in progress to determine, among other things, the role of adjuvant chemotherapy. In this study, pathologic stage I patients are registered and followed. Stage II patients randomly postoperatively receive a brief course of cisplatin-containing chemotherapy or are observed. Additional aspects of the study include central pathology and radiology review. Until results of this study are available, it would appear that either option is reasonable for stage II patients.

The reproductive consequences of RPLND deserve further comment. About 25% of newly diagnosed testis tumor patients with no other treatment than unilateral orchiectomy will be subfertile or infertile. It is unknown whether the defect is transient or permanent, and the reasons for these findings are not known. In any case, patients having a full bilateral RPLND will almost universally be infertile. Most urologists, however, will limit the inferior extent of the contralateral dissection in patients who intraoperatively appear to have no nodal involvement. Many of these patients will maintain ejaculatory competence. Finally, another group of patients may have suitable ejaculations when treated with imipramine or sympathomimetic agents. Thus, the reproductive consequences of RPLND may be overemphasized.

Recently, the necessity of treatment of regional lymphatics has been questioned for patients who have no evidence of retroperitoneal metastases by serologic and radiographic studies. It is acknowledged that a significant staging error exists, and presumably patients with untreated retroperitoneal disease will develop disease progression and ultimately require therapy. With the early and appropriate use of chemotherapy, however, the overwhelming majority of these patients should be salvaged.

Early results of three clinical trials have been published (see Table 36–9) (Peckham *et al.,* 1982; Sogani *et al.,* 1983; Sturgeon *et al.,* 1983). Short periods of follow-up prevent definitive conclusions. Patients were carefully selected and initial staging was rigorous, including both lymphangiography and computerized tomography. Likewise, patients had monthly markers, and chest x-rays, and computerized tomography every two to three months after orchiectomy. Treatment at relapse was basically chemotherapy, although in the Princess Margaret series radiotherapy was given to patients who had definite retroperitoneal progression; four of six such patients required subsequent chemotherapy.

It appears that orchiectomy alone may be

Table 36–8. Early-Stage Disease: Indiana Experience

Stage I
  No adjuvant therapy
    Number: 78
    Relapse: 8 (10%)
    Presently NED: 77 (99%)
    Minimum follow-up = 3 years
Stage II
  Adjuvant actinomycin- D
    Number: 30
    Relapse: 14 (47%)
    Presently NED: 29 (97%)
    Minimum follow-up = 6 years
  Adjuvant PVB
    Number: 18
    Relapse: 0
  No adjuvant therapy
    Number: 38
    Relapse: 17 (45%)
    Presently NED: 37 (97%)
    Minimum followup = 38 months

Table 36–9.   Orchiectomy Alone in Clinical Stage I Disease

INSTITUTION	NUMBER	PATIENT POPULATION AND STAGING	RECURRENCE	DISEASE-FREE	FOLLOW-UP	REFERENCE
Royal Marsden	53	No tumor at cut end of cord; normal LAG,* IVP, CT, ultrasound, markers	9 (17%)	53	6–40 months (median = 15)	Peckham et al., 1982
Princess Margaret	20	Normal LAG, CT, markers	8 (40%)	20	14 months median	Sturegeon et al., 1983
Memorial	36	T_1 primary; normal LAG, markers, CT, IVP	7 (19%)	36	14 months median	Sogani et al., 1983

* Lymphangiogram.

adequate management for these patients, but the selected value and meticulous follow-up of these patients must be kept in mind before these results are applied in a widespread manner. Moreover, RPLND gives accurate staging and a 99% cure rate, with avoidance of chemotherapy in the majority of patients. Treatment mortality approaches zero, and the only serious complication is ejaculation dysfunction. Such successful cancer treatment should not be discarded lightly.

Extragonadal Neoplasms

Clinical manifestations and diagnosis of extragonadal germ cell tumors have been discussed previously. In general, these neoplasms are not amenable to complete surgical extirpation, and even when complete resection is possible, survival with surgery alone is poor.

The same general principles that apply to testicular cancer also apply to extragonadal tumors. The mainstay of treatment for nonseminomatous tumors is cisplatin-based chemotherapy, and surgical resection of residual disease is frequently required. These patients tend to fare less well than their testicular counterparts, but the differences are often related to extent of disease at diagnosis rather than intrinsic biologic differences; these patients tend to have very bulky disease.

Extragonadal pure seminomas are rare occurrences. They have the radiosensitivity of their testicular counterparts. Patients with locally advanced and metastatic disease have a significant failure rate and probably should be treated initially with chemotherapy.

Extragonadal tumors occur more frequently than previously recognized. The group at Vanderbilt University have reported a series of 12 patients initially thought to have poorly differentiated epithelial tumors of uncertain primary (Richardson et al., 1981). The germ cell origin of these neoplasms was later confirmed by marker determination, pathology review, immunoperoxidase staining for HCG or AFP, or subsequent clinical course, for example, response to PVB. Five patients attained durable CR with appropriate treatment. A potential germ cell origin should be considered in any patient, man or woman, with a poorly differentiated tumor of uncertain origin, particularly in a young patient with a mediastinal or retroperitoneal mass.

It should be noted that in these patients a gonadal origin must be excluded. A careful physical examination plus testicular ultrasonography will suffice. In a series of 19 patients at Indiana University who had orchiectomy after chemotherapy, 3 patients in complete remission had potentially serious pathology in the testis (teratoma or carcinoma) (Greist et al., 1983). Thus, it appears that the testis may be a drug sanctuary, at least in some patients, and that orchiectomy should eventually be performed if a testis primary is expected.

Summary

Testicular cancer is a landmark adult solid tumor. Through a logical period of evolution, chemotherapeutic regimens have developed with a high propensity for cure in disseminated disease. Subsequently, the roles of surgery and radiotherapy have not diminished in importance, but are being redefined. Greater than 90% of all patients (both NSGCT and seminoma) can be cured with an acceptable level of treatment-related morbidity. Certain other adult solid tumors (particularly ovarian and small cell lung carcinoma) should follow a similar pattern in the future.

REFERENCES

Bracken, R. B.; Johnson, D. E.; Frazier, O. H.; Logothetis, C. J.; Trindade, A.; and Samuels, M. L.: The role of surgery following chemotherapy in stage III germ cell neoplasms. *J. Urol.,* **129:**39–43, 1983.

Calman, F. M. B.; Peckham, M. H.; and Hendry, W. F.: The pattern of spread and treatment of metastases in testicular seminoma. *Br. J. Urol.,* **51:**154–160, 1979.

Doornbos, J. F.; Hussey, D. H.; and Johnson, D. E.: Radiotherapy for pure seminoma of the testis. *Radiology,* **116:**401–404, 1975.

Dosoretz, D. E.; Shipley, W. U.; Blitzer, P. H.; Gilbert, S.; Prat, J.; Parkhurst, E.; and Wang, C. C.: Megavoltage irradiation for pure testicular seminoma: Results and patterns of failure. *Cancer,* **42:**2184–2190, 1981.

Drasga, R. E.; Einhorn, L. H.; Williams, S. D.; Patel, D. N.; and Stevens, E. E.: Fertility after chemotherapy for testicular cancer. *J. Clin. Oncol.,* **1:**179–183, 1983.

Einhorn, L. H., and Donohue, J. P.: *Cis*-diamminedichloroplatinum, vinblastine, and bleomycin combination chemotherapy in disseminated testicular cancer. *Ann. Intern. Med.,* **87:**293–298, 1977.

Einhorn, L. H., and Williams, S. D.: Chemotherapy of disseminated testicular cancer. *Cancer,* **46:**1339–1344, 1980.

Einhorn, L. H.; Williams, S. D.; Mandelbaum, I.; and Donohue, J. P.: Surgical resection in disseminated testicular cancer following chemotherapeutic cytoreduction. *Cancer,* **48:**904–908, 1981a.

Einhorn, L. H.; Williams, S. D.; Troner, M.; Birch, R.; and Greco, F. A.: The role of maintenance therapy in disseminated testicular cancer. *N. Engl. J. Med.,* **305:**727–721, 1981b.

Greist, A.; Williams, S. D.; Einhorn, L. H.; Donohue, J. P.; Rowland, R. G.; and Estes, N.: Pathologic findings at orchiectomy following chemotherapy for disseminated testicular cancer. *Proc. Am. Soc. Clin. Oncol.,* **2:**139, 1983.

Higby, D. J.; Wallace, J. H.; Albert, D.; and Holland, J. F.: Diamminodichloroplatinum in the chemotherapy of testicular tumors. *J. Urol.,* **112:**100–104, 1974.

Jackson, S. M.; Olivotto, L.; McLoughlin, M. G.; and Coy, P.: Radiation therapy for seminoma of the testis: Results in British Columbia. *Can. Med. Assoc. J.,* **123:**507–512, 1980.

Javadpour, N.; Ozols, R. F.; Anderson, T.; Barlock, A. B.; Wesley, R.; and Young, R. C.: A randomized trial of cytoreductive surgery followed by chemotherapy versus chemotherapy alone in bulky stage III testicular cancer with poor prognostic features. *Cancer,* **50:**2004–2010, 1982.

Loehrer, P. J.; Williams, S. D.; Clark, S. D.; Einhorn, L. H.; Donohue, J. P.; Mandelbaum, I.; and Rohn, R. J.: Teratoma following chemotherapy for non-seminomatous germ cell tumor (NSGCT: A clinicopathologic coorelation). *Proc. Am. Soc. Clin. Oncol.,* **2:**139, 1983.

Peckham, M. J.; Husband, J. E.; Barrett, A.; Hendry, W. F.: Orchidectomy alone in testicular stage I non-seminomatous germ-cell tumours. *Lancet,* **2:**678–680, 1982.

Richardson, R. L.; Schoumacher, R. A.; Fer, M. F.; Hande, K. R.; Forbes, J. T.; Oldham, R. K.; and Greco, F. A.: The unrecognized extragonadal germ cell cancer syndrome. *Ann. Intern. Med.,* **94:**181–186, 1981.

Roth, L. M., and Gillespie, J. J.: Pathology and ultrasound of germinal neoplasms of the testis. In Einhorn, L. H. (ed.): *Testicular Tumors: Management and Treatment.* Masson Publishing U.S.A., Inc., New York, 1980.

Rowland, R. G.; Weisman, D.; Williams, S. D.; Einhorn, L. H.; Klatte, E. C.; and Donohue, J. P.: Accuracy of preoperative staging in stages A and B non-seminomatous germ cell testis tumors. *J. Urol.,* **127:**718–720, 1982.

Samson, M. K.; Stephens, R. L.; and Klugo, R. C.: Positive dose-response of high vs. low dose cisplatin, vinblastine and bleomycin in disseminated germ cell neoplasm of the testis. *Proc. Am. Soc. Clin. Oncol.,* **22:**470, 1981.

Samuels, M. L.; Lanzotti, V. J.; Holoye, P. Y.; Boyle, L. E.; Smith, T. L.; and Johnson, D. E.: Combination chemotherapy in germinal cell tumors. *Cancer Treat. Rev.,* **3:**185–204, 1976.

Skinner, D. G., and Scardino, P. T.: Relevance of biochemical tumor markers and lymphadenectomy in management in non-seminomatous testis tumors: Current perspective. *J. Urol.,* **123:**378–382, 1980.

Sogani, P. C.; Whitmore, W. F.; Herr, H.; Bosl, G.; Golbey, R.; Watson, R.; and DeCosse, J.: Orchiectomy alone in treatment of clinical stage I non-seminomatous germ cell tumor of testis (NSGCTT). *Proc. Am. Soc. Clin. Oncol.,* **2:**140, 1983.

Sturgeon, J. F. G.; Herman, J. G.; Jewett, M. A. S.; Alison, R. E.; Gospodarowicz, M. K.; and Comisarow, R.: A policy of surveillance alone after Orchidectomy for clinical stage I non-seminomatous testis tumours. *Proc. Am. Soc. Clin. Oncol.,* **2:**142, 1983.

Thomas, G. M.; Rider, W. D.; Dembo, A. J.; Cummings, B. J.; Gospodarowicz, M.; Hawkins, N. V.; Herman, J. G.; and Keen, C. W.: Seminoma of the testis: Results of treatment and patterns of failure after radiation therapy. *Int. J. Radiat. Oncol. Biol. Phys.,* **8:**165–174, 1982.

Tyrrell, C. J., and Peckham, M. J.: The response of lymph node metastases of testicular teratoma to radiation therapy. *Br. J. Urol.,* **48:**363–370, 1976.

Vogelzang, N. J.; Bosl, G. J.; Johnson, K.; and Kennedy, B. J.: Raynaud's phenomenon: A common toxicity after combination chemotherapy for testicular cancer. *Ann. Intern. Med.,* **95:**288–292, 1981.

Vugrin, D.; Herr, H. W.; Whitmore, W. F.; Sogani, P. C.; and Golbey, R. B.: VAB-6 combination chemotherapy in disseminated cancer of the testis. *Ann. Intern. Med.,* **95:**59–61, 1981.

Vugrin, D.; Whitmore, W. F.; Sogani, P. C.; Bains, M.; Herr, H. W.; and Golbey, R. B.: Combined chemotherapy and surgery in treatment of advanced germ-cell tumors. *Cancer,* **47:**2228–2231, 1981.

Williams, S. D., and Einhorn, L. H.: Clinical stage I testis tumors: The medical oncologist's view. *Cancer Treat. Rep.,* **66:**15–18, 1982a.

Williams, S. D., and Einhorn, L.H.: Etoposide salvage therapy for refractory germ cell tumors: An update. *Cancer Treat. Rev.,* **9**(Suppl. A):67–71, 1982b.

Williams, S. D., and Einhorn, L. H.: Treatment of seminoma. In Garnick, M. B. (ed.): *Genitourinary Cancer,* Churchill Livingstone, New York, 1985.

Williams, S. D.; Turner, S.; Loehrer, P. J.; and Einhorn, L. H.: Testicular cancer: Results of reinduction therapy. *Proc. Am. Soc. Clin. Oncol.,* **2:**137, 1983.

37

Tumors of the Central Nervous System

EDWARD H. OLDFIELD, BARRY H. SMITH,
and PAUL L. KORNBLITH

INTRODUCTION

Tumors of the brain and spinal cord comprise a remarkably diverse group of neoplastic and nonneoplastic conditions that may occur at any site within the central nervous system (CNS) and in patients of any age. They may be conveniently grouped into (1) intrinsic tumors of the brain and its coverings, (2) metastatic tumors of the brain, (3) intrinsic tumors of the spinal cord, and (4) metastatic tumors of the spine.

Lesions within any of these groups are characterized by unique features that must be considered for optimal patient management: (1) The brain and spinal cord are confined within the unyielding skull and spinal canal; a mass lesion may, therefore, cause symptoms and signs by displacing (without destroying) normal tissue, by invading neural tissue, or by increasing intracranial pressure. (2) The precise localization of function, combined with the failure of central nervous system tissue to regenerate, underlies the production of devastating and irreversible neurologic deficits by relatively small, but critically placed lesions. (3) This combination of focal differentiation of function, inability to regenerate, and inability of other neural areas to take on the lost function of a damaged area frequently restricts the surgeon's excision of a neoplasm to one that is incomplete. (4) Malignant CNS tumors infiltrate adjacent normal tissue but rarely spread by metastasis. (5) Many chemotherapeutic agents, after raising expectations of success with solid tumors of other organs, penetrate the blood-brain barrier poorly and, therefore, have limited access to brain and spinal tumors.

The modern era of brain tumor therapy began in the late nineteenth century. In 1879, William Macewan performed the first known cranial operation for neoplasm (Bucy, 1979). His patient survived for several years following the procedure. In June of 1887, Victor Horsley performed the first removal of an intraspinal tumor under the supervision of the leading neurologist of the time, William Gowers (Walker, 1959). It was the appointment of Mr. Horsley as surgeon to The National Hospital for the Paralyzed and Epileptic, Queen Square, in 1896 that initiated the surgical speciality whose primary effort was to advance the understanding and treatment of central nervous system mass lesions. It remained for Harvey Cushing to introduce a system for the successful care of brain tumor patients (Cushing, 1931). Cushing, after caring for over 2000 patients with brain tumors, described the behavior, histology, and classification of the lesions and designed successful strategies for their surgical removal and patient pre- and postoperative care (Cushing, 1932). This pioneering period of surgery of the nervous system was followed by the development of improved anesthesia and the introduction of neuroradiologic contrast procedures, particularly the ventriculogram in 1918 and the pneumoencephalogram in 1919 by Walter E. Dandy (Dandy, 1918, 1919) and the cerebral arteriogram in 1927 by Egas Moniz (Moniz, 1934).

Following World War II, tremendous advances were seen in technical surgery and anesthetic support and it became possible routinely to remove benign, accessible brain and spinal cord tumors. Coincidentally, technical improvement in radiation therapy, especially the development of megavoltage equipment, made precisely delivered, high-dose treatment possible. Malignant lesions, frustrating to the neurosurgeon because of their invasiveness, usual unresectability, and propensity for subarachnoid spread, could then be effectively irradiated in many instances. Radiation therapy became the first measure to make a significant difference in the outcome of histologically malignant lesions, especially in children and young adults (Walker *et al.,* 1976). Improved skill in radiation therapy has brought continued enhancement of response.

In 1971, the first computerized tomographic scan of the brain was demonstrated and the machinery introduced to clinical medicine. This remarkable technique has virtually eliminated the routine use of invasive diagnostic studies, such as pneumoencephalography and angiography.

The current era of brain and spinal tumor therapy has seen a remarkable advance in microsurgical techniques for the treatment of difficult and inaccessible lesions. The treatment of malignant tumors with chemotherapeutic agents, especially the nitrosoureas, combined with surgery and irradiation, has also been shown to produce some improvement in survival (Walker *et al.,* 1980).

In this chapter, the biologic, anatomic, and pathologic considerations of primary CNS neoplasms will be discussed, and the clinical pictures of the tumors as a group will be described. Inasmuch as multimodal therapy is often required for each of the tumor types, the discussions of therapy will include radiation and chemotherapy. The most speculative aspect, "New Developments and Future Prospects," will conclude the chapter.

PRIMARY INTRACRANIAL NEOPLASMS

Overview

Classification. The classification of tumors of the nervous system is based on the presumed cell of origin, the degree of differentiation, and distinctive clinical behavior. They may be primary neoplasms in all degrees of differentiation derived from any of the multiple normal cellular constituents of this organ, or they may be nonneoplastic but tumorous conditions derived from normal constituents. They may be tumorous conditions or true neoplasms derived from embryologically misplaced tissues, or they may be metastatic neo-

plasms from any primary site outside the brain.

Initial attempts at classification were based on the histologic resemblance of the tumor cells to the embryologic developmental stages of normal glial and neuronal elements. In 1926, Bailey and Cushing proposed "A Classification of the Tumours of the Glioma Groups on a Histogenetic Basis with a Correlated Study of Prognosis" and created a classification of clinical value by correlating the types of tumor with survival times (Bailey and Cushing, 1926). Their original scheme, after decades of gradual alteration and much controversy, is the basis of the classification most accepted in the United States, that devised by Russell and Rubinstein (Russell and Rubinstein, 1977). The World Health Organization Brain Tumor Classification is outlined in Table 37–1.

This chapter is organized along both "cell of origin" and regional or anatomic lines. For

Table 37–1. World Health Organization Brain Tumor Classification

Tumors of Neuroepithelial Tissue
  Astrocytic tumors
    Astrocytoma
      Fibrillary
      Protoplasmic
      Gemistocytic
    Pilocytic astrocytoma
    Subependymal giant cell astrocytoma (ventricular tumor of tuberous sclerosis)
    Astroblastoma
    Anaplastic astrocytoma
  Oligodendroglial tumors
    Oligodendroglioma
    Mixed oligoastrocytoma
    Anaplastic oligodendroglioma
  Ependymal and choroid plexus tumors
    Ependymoma
      Variants
        Myxopapillary ependymoma
        Papillary ependymoma
        Subependymoma
    Anaplastic ependymoma
    Choroid plexus papilloma
    Anaplastic choroid plexus papilloma
  Pineal cell tumors
    Pineocytoma
    Pineoblastoma
  Neuronal tumors
    Gangliocytoma
    Ganglioglioma
    Ganglioneuroblastoma
    Anaplastic gangliocytoma and ganglioglioma
    Neuroblastoma
  Poorly differentiated and embryonal tumors
    Glioblastoma
      Variants
        Glioblastoma with sarcomatous component
        Giant cell glioblastoma

Table 37-1.   *(Continued)*

Medulloblastoma
  Variants
  Desmoplastic
  Medullomyoblastoma
Medulloepithelioma
Primitive polar spongioblastoma
Gliomatosis cerebri
Tumors of Nerve Sheath Cells
Neurilemmoma
Anaplastic neurilemmoma
Neurofibroma
Anaplastic neurofibroma
Tumors of Meningeal and Related Tissue
Meningioma
Meningeal sarcoma
Xanthomatous tumors
Primary melanotic tumors
Others
Primary Malignant Lymphomas
Tumors of Blood Vessel Origin
Hemangioblastoma
Monstrocellular sarcoma
Germ Cell Tumors
Germinoma
Embryonal carcinoma
Choriocarcinoma
Teratoma
Other Malformative Tumors and Tumorlike Lesions
Craniopharyngioma
Rathke's cleft cyst
Epidermoid cyst
Dermoid cyst
Colloid cyst of the third ventricle
Enterogenous cyst
Other cysts
Lipoma
Choristoma
Hypothalamic neuronal hamartoma
Nasal glial heterotopia
Vascular Malformations
Capillary telangiectasia
Cavernous angioma
Arteriovenous malformation
Venous malformation
Sturge-Weber disease
Tumors of the Anterior Pituitary
Pituitary adenomas
Pituitary adenocarcinoma
Local Extension from Regional Tumors
Glomus jugulare tumors
Chordoma
Chondroma
Chondrosarcoma
Olfactory neuroblastoma
Adenoid cystic carcinoma
Other
Metastatic Tumor
Unclassified Tumors

instance, intracranial ependymomas are discussed as a unit considering only their cell of origin since their morphology and biologic behavior are independent of location. On the other hand, we review the astrocytic neoplasms both geographically and by cell of ori-

gin because their morphology and clinical behavior are often dependent upon location.

In assessing the malignant potential of a brain tumor, it is important to understand the difference between cytologic and biologic malignancy. Cytologic malignancy is a morphologic assessment of anaplasia based upon cytologic and nuclear pleomorphism, cellularity, necrosis, mitoses, and invasiveness. Biologic malignancy is the likelihood that a tumor will kill the patient. Most cytologically malignant brain tumors are also biologically malignant, despite treatment presently available. Various factors, including the brain's exquisite sensitivity to increased internal pressure, dictate that certain cytologically benign tumors can be biologically malignant.

It is common to find both differentiated and anaplastic cells in different areas of the same tumor. Since the most malignant portion mandates the patient's clinical course, it is the portion for which the neuropathologist conventionally names the tumor.

Epidemiology.   *Incidence.*   Primary tumors of the central nervous system and its coverings account for 1.2% of all autopsy deaths and for 9.2% of all primary neoplasms. Eighty-five percent of these tumors arise within the cranial cavity, and 15% are spinal in origin (Russell and Rubinstein, 1977). The incidence of brain tumors at all ages is 4 to 13/100,000 inhabitants (Behrend, 1974). The majority of brain tumors occur in two age peaks, one in childhood (3 to 12 years), the other in later life (50 to 70 years) (see Figure 37-1).

Central nervous system tumors comprise the most common group of solid tumors in the young, accounting for 20% of all pediatric neoplasms. The pediatric tumors are quite different in histology, topography, and behavior from those of adult life. Figure 37-2 depicts the topographic distribution of intracranial tumors in children and adults, and Figure 37-3 shows the age distribution of the major types of brain tumors. About 70% of pediatric brain tumors arise in the posterior fossa (brainstem or cerebellum), whereas, in adults, 70% are supratentorial, the majority arising within the cerebral hemispheres.

Genetics.   Most central nervous system tumors lack genetic predisposition and occur randomly in the population, although the phakomatoses, discussed below, clearly demonstrate a hereditary component.

Neurofibromatosis (von Recklinghausen's disease) represents a genetic condition, with autosomal dominant inheritance in approxi-

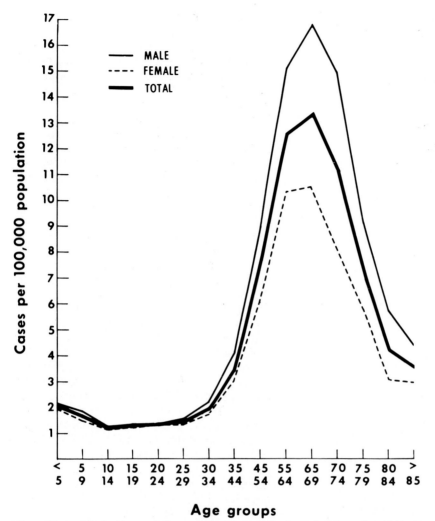

Figure 37–1. The incidence of all types of brain tumors in the United States in 1966 is shown by five-year age groups. Note the male predominance in adults. Data from U. S. Department of Health, Education and Welfare—Public Health Service: *Vital Statistics Rates in the United States 1940–1960.* Washington, D.C., 1968.

mately 50% of cases. These patients develop tumors of the central and the peripheral nervous systems, derived from neural crest anlage (neurofibroma, schwannoma, pheochromocytoma) or the derivatives of the neural tube (astrocytoma, ependymoma). Twenty percent to over 50% of patients with optic glioma have coexisting von Recklinghausen's disease.

Tuberous sclerosis, characterized by the triad of skin lesions, epilepsy, and mental retardation, is a hereditary condition with an uncertain mode of transmission. The intracranial tubers may be intracerebral or subependymal in location and can undergo malignant transformation.

Lindau disease, inherited in an autosomal dominant manner, includes hemangioblastoma of the cerebellum, spinal cord, or retina.

In human meningiomas, chromosome 22 has frequent abnormalities, usually in the form of dislocations, translocations, and deletions (Zankl and Zang, 1972). In Turcot syndrome, familial polyposis of the colon is associated with malignant gliomas.

Chemical. Although it is estimated that 80 to 90% of human cancer is caused by chemicals (Boyland, 1969; Higginson, 1972), at present there is little definitive evidence linking CNS tumors to environmental carcinogens. Chemical induction of human brain tumors, however, has been suggested in epidemiologic studies relating increased incidence of primary CNS neoplasms to employment in the rubber industry (Mancuso, 1963; Selikoff and Hammond, 1982).

Viral. There is no evidence in humans for a

TOPOGRAPHIC DISTRIBUTION OF INTRACRANIAL TUMORS IN CHILDHOOD

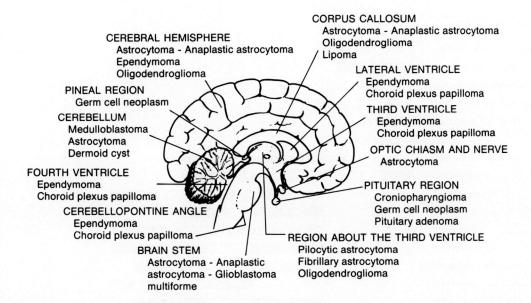

CORPUS CALLOSUM
Astrocytoma - Anaplastic astrocytoma
Oligodendroglioma
Lipoma

CEREBRAL HEMISPHERE
Astrocytoma - Anaplastic astrocytoma
Ependymoma
Oligodendroglioma

LATERAL VENTRICLE
Ependymoma
Choroid plexus papilloma

THIRD VENTRICLE
Ependymoma
Choroid plexus papilloma

PINEAL REGION
Germ cell neoplasm

CEREBELLUM
Medulloblastoma
Astrocytoma
Dermoid cyst

OPTIC CHIASM AND NERVE
Astrocytoma

FOURTH VENTRICLE
Ependymoma
Choroid plexus papilloma

PITUITARY REGION
Croniopharyngioma
Germ cell neoplasm
Pituitary adenoma

CEREBELLOPONTINE ANGLE
Ependymoma
Choroid plexus papilloma

REGION ABOUT THE THIRD VENTRICLE
Pilocytic astrocytoma
Fibrillary astrocytoma
Oligodendroglioma

BRAIN STEM
Astrocytoma - Anaplastic
astrocytoma - Glioblastoma
multiforme

TOPOGRAPHIC DISTRIBUTION OF INTRACRANIAL TUMORS IN ADULTHOOD

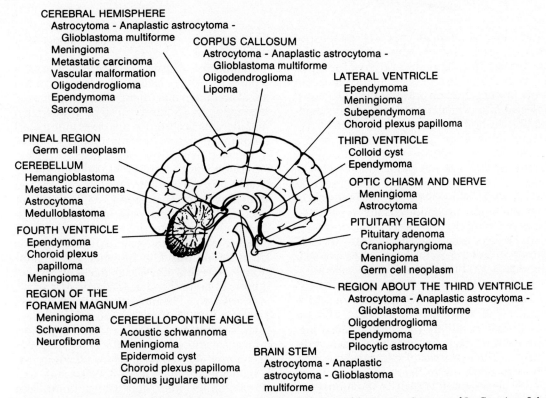

CEREBRAL HEMISPHERE
Astrocytoma - Anaplastic astrocytoma -
  Glioblastoma multiforme
Meningioma
Metastatic carcinoma
Vascular malformation
Oligodendroglioma
Ependymoma
Sarcoma

CORPUS CALLOSUM
Astrocytoma - Anaplastic astrocytoma -
  Glioblastoma multiforme
Oligodendroglioma
Lipoma

LATERAL VENTRICLE
Ependymoma
Meningioma
Subependymoma
Choroid plexus papilloma

PINEAL REGION
Germ cell neoplasm

CEREBELLUM
Hemangioblastoma
Metastatic carcinoma
Astrocytoma
Medulloblastoma

THIRD VENTRICLE
Colloid cyst
Ependymoma

OPTIC CHIASM AND NERVE
Meningioma
Astrocytoma

PITUITARY REGION
Pituitary adenoma
Craniopharyngioma
Meningioma
Germ cell neoplasm

FOURTH VENTRICLE
Ependymoma
Choroid plexus
  papilloma
Meningioma

**REGION OF THE
FOREMEN MAGNUM**
Meningioma
Schwannoma
Neurofibroma

REGION ABOUT THE THIRD VENTRICLE
Astrocytoma - Anaplastic astrocytoma -
  Glioblastoma multiforme
Oligodendroglioma
Ependymoma
Pilocytic astrocytoma

CEREBELLOPONTINE ANGLE
Acoustic schwannoma
Meningioma
Epidermoid cyst
Choroid plexus papilloma
Glomus jugulare tumor

BRAIN STEM
Astrocytoma - Anaplastic
astrocytoma - Glioblastoma
multiforme

Figure 37-2.   From Burger, P. C., and Vogel, F. S.: *Surgical Pathology of the Nervous System and Its Coverings.* John Wiley & Sons, Inc., New York, 1976, p. 192.

INCIDENCE OF BRAIN TUMORS ACCORDING TO AGE

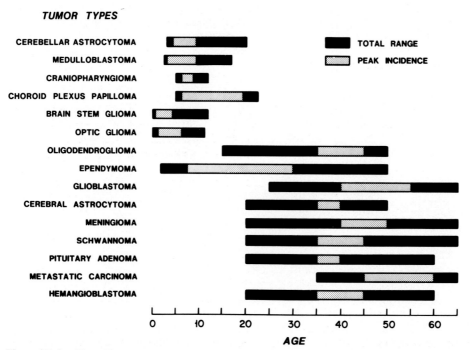

Figure 37–3.   From Youmans, J. R. (ed.): *Neurological Surgery,* Vol. III, W. B. Saunders Co., Philadelphia, 1973, p. 1321.

viral etiology, although it is well established that viruses can induce brain tumors after intracerebral inoculation in a variety of animals. Perhaps the most striking evidence is recent work in which human polyomavirus (JC virus) injected into primates produced tumors comparable to human astrocytomas after an 18-month incubation period (London *et al.,* 1978). This type of slow virus effect may account for some of the problems in isolating viruses from human tumors. The study of Farwell *et al.* (1979) suggests that the inadvertent contamination of polio vaccine with SV40 virus in Connecticut between 1956 and 1962 may be responsible for the increase in CNS tumors in children in that state in the five-year interval 1960–1965, particularly medulloblastoma.

Trauma.   Evidence that trauma can lead to human CNS neoplasia has not been substantiated. The possibility that head trauma predisposes to intracranial neoplasia was investigated in 2953 patients of Olmstead County, Minnesota, who were followed for a total of 29,859 person-years. The observed number of subsequent brain tumors (4) did not differ

from the expected number (4.1) (Annegers *et al.,* 1979).

Radiation.   Almost all intracranial tumors reported to have developed after irradiation are of mesenchymal origin, either sarcomas or meningiomas (Soloway, 1966). Intracranial meningioma occurred in five cases many years following radiation therapy of the scalp for tinea capitis (ringworm of the scalp) (Munk *et al.,* 1969). In a study of 11,000 children in Israel who were irradiated for tinea capitis and studied retrospectively for 12 to 23 years, intracranial neoplasms were increased in irradiated children compared to siblings and to matched groups of the general population. The latent period was 7 to 21 years, and meningiomas were four times as frequent as "other" tumors of brain (Modan *et al.,* 1974).

Hormonal.   The incidence of most tumors increases with age, with the exception of those tumors dependent upon production of hormones (ovary, testes, pituitary). Sexual predilection is well established for glioblastoma, hemangioblastoma, medulloblastoma, and pinealoma in men and schwannoma and meningioma in women (Zülch and Mennel,

1974). In patients with a nervous system neoplasm and a second primary malignancy, only with the combination of breast cancer and meningioma does the number of observed cases exceed the number expected (Schoenberg et al., 1975). Meningiomas occasionally enlarge rapidly during pregnancy (Michelsen and New, 1969). The significance of the presence of estrogen-binding receptor protein in the cytoplasmic fraction of meningiomas (Donnell et al., 1979; Martuza et al., 1981) is as yet undetermined.

Other. The development of primary CNS lymphoma in immunosuppressed patients far exceeds the general population incidence (Schneck and Penn, 1971). The combination of the "immunologically privileged CNS" and the suppression of the immune surveillance system has been the proposed mechanism of origin of these lesions.

Biologic Characteristics. The development of CNS tumors can be considered in relationship to two variables: the kinetics of tumor growth and the local evolution. Growth is by tumor expansion, infiltration, or metastasis. Distant metastases are sufficiently rare so that this is not a major consideration.

Kinetics. The kinetics of each class of CNS tumor vary. Marked variations are evident in the growth rates of tumors within each class. The overall growth kinetics of both intracranial and spinal tumors are slow. A low growth fraction even in the highly malignant tumors has been reported (Hoshino et al., 1975a). Because of the confined nature of both intracranial and spinal regions, even a slow-growing tumor can have devastating effects. In the slow-growing lesions of the brain, gradual compression of surrounding structures allows them to adapt better to the pressure. Long histories of vague symptomatology often accompany lesions, such as olfactory groove meningiomas. In tissue culture studies, there is variability of growth rate among individual tumors which appears to predict their clinical outcome (Brooks et al., 1975).

Local Evolution. The local evolution of CNS tumor growth depends largely on the degree of tumor invasiveness. The malignant potential is measured primarily on the ability of the tumor to infiltrate normal neural or bony tissues. Benign tumors cause effects primarily by pressure, whereas the malignant or invasive lesions act by both pressure and actual tissue destruction.

The pressure effects of CNS tumors can be grouped as displacement, herniations, ventricular obstructions, and vascular compressions. Displacement of normal CNS structures is the most common feature of growth and is often the finding in contrast radiography which demonstrates the mass lesion's presence. Herniation occurs when either the uncus of the medial temporal lobe is displaced medially against the midbrain or the cerebellar tonsils are forced against the medulla. Either can result in death. Ventricular obstruction can occur with any tumor in proximity to the ventricles but is particularly common with tumors in the region of the third and fourth ventricles. Such obstruction then results in hydrocephalus, in which continued cerebrospinal fluid (CSF) production causes increasing pressure on brain substance.

Patterns of Spread. The patterns of spread of CNS tumors are quite distinct from those of other tumors. No lymphatic system is present within the CNS. Hematogenous spread does occur, but is rare. A factor often associated with hematogenous spread is operative intervention. It is not clear whether the relative infrequency of hematogenous spread relates to the relative immunologically privileged status of the CNS, or whether the short life expectancy with the highly malignant tumors merely does not allow sufficient time for systemic metastases to become manifest.

The major patterns of spread, therefore, involve local invasion and CSF seeding. These tumors, in particular the intracranial astrocytomas, have cells with the capability of invading normal brain to a remarkable degree. The cells can be found at points distant from the primary focus, even 6 cm or more distant. This distant spread has led many to question whether the lesions have multifocal origins or if abnormal cells migrate within the brain tissue to distant sites. In a systematic study of the growth of gliomas, Scherer (1940) found collections of glioma cells surrounding neurons, in the perivascular spaces, and in the subpial layer of the cortex at sites noncontiguous with the main tumor mass. His *post mortem* studies also demonstrated tumor involvement of the contralateral hemisphere in many patients. Some basis for this invasiveness can be appreciated from astrocytoma tissue cultures which display remarkable cellular motility and from a recent study by Scott et al. (1978) in which malignant astrocytoma cells were able to find, penetrate, and grow through a 1-mm opening in a nucleopore filter.

The spread of tumors by local or distal seeding by way of CSF pathways is another significant concern. Tumor characteristics important for dissemination in this manner are proximity of tumor cells to the cerebrospinal fluid, paucity of tumor stroma, and decreased adhesiveness of tumor cells. Meningiomas, pituitary tumors, and chordomas rarely seed, whereas medulloblastomas and pineal dysgerminomas seed frequently. The seeding of these latter two occurs both by spread into the intracranial subarachnoid space along the surface of the brain to local sites and by the so-called drop metastases which fall via the CSF to the spinal subarachnoid space and then form secondary tumors.

This process of CSF seeding is an extremely important part of the pathogenesis of these two tumor types, and treatment must include consideration of this problem. The secondary seedings grow on nerve roots (causing pain in a root distribution) or on the coverings of the spinal cord (resulting in cord compression). All levels of the spinal axis can be involved, but the lumbosacral area is the most frequent site. Ependymomas also occasionally spread by the CSF. Our experience, based on autopsy studies, indicates that glioblastomas are spread in this manner more frequently than previously recognized.

Tumor dissemination to the bloodstream by ventriculovenous shunting operations or to the peritoneal or pleural space by ventriculoperitoneal or pleural shunting procedures to relieve hydrocephalus has also been reported.

Although systemic spread by the hematogenous route is rare, specific instances of extracranial metastasis of malignant astrocytomas, ependymomas, medulloblastomas, and malignant meningiomas have been reported (Shuangshoti et al., 1970). On rare occasions, an intracranial malignant tumor may even present first by its extracranial metastasis. Most patients with systemic metastases have undergone surgical intervention, but there are reports of metastases prior to surgery (Labitzke, 1962).

Tumor cells penetrating the vessel wall and within the lumen of blood vessels in glioblastoma have been demonstrated with light and electron microscopy (Labitzke, 1962; Kung et al., 1969). Why do patients with glioblastoma suffer such a low incidence of metastasis outside the CNS? Carcinogen-induced glial tumors in animals grow without difficulty when transplanted to subcutaneous tissue but do not metastasize (Zimmerman and Arnold, 1943). Patients with glioblastoma have been given subcutaneous inoculations of their own tumor, with two of six producing neoplastic proliferation (Grace et al., 1961).

With improvements in the treatment of patients with malignant astrocytoma, and therefore longer survivals, more metastases will become manifest.

Symptoms and Signs. It must be stated at the outset that no constellation of symptoms and physical findings is pathognomonic for an intracranial tumor and that tumors of the brain may exist with hardly any symptoms.

The diagnosis of an intracranial tumor should be considered in the patient who develops persistent or recurrent headaches to which he is unaccustomed, or when focal neurologic symptoms develop slowly and gradually increase in severity.

The signs and symptoms most frequently encountered are headache, seizures, abnormal states of consciousness, mental symptoms, changes in vision, and progressive motor deficit. These will be discussed here and specific clinical syndromes associated with particular tumors will be covered in later sections of the chapter.

Headache. Headaches are early complaints in about one-third of tumor patients and are quite variable in character. They cannot be differentiated either by their nature or their location from headaches of other causes. Severe recurrent headaches in a person previously free of them or headaches awakening the patient early in the morning should put one on guard. The headache is usually of no localizing significance, however, tumors above the tentorium are more likely to cause pain in the frontal or temporal areas, and tumors below the tentorium tend to cause retroauricular or suboccipital pain. The mechanism of the headache is not known, but presumably is a consequence of traction or pressure on the pain-producing intracranial structures (dura, blood vessels, or nerves). With elevated intracranial pressure, bifrontal and bitemporal headache is the rule, regardless of the location of the tumor.

Seizures. Focal or generalized seizures are common in patients with tumors of the cerebral hemispheres, but are rare with tumors in the brain stem or posterior fossa. In various series, 20 to 60% of all patients with cerebral tumors have seizures, either as the initial symptom or occurring before tumor diagnosis.

The focal seizures occurring with tumors cannot be distinguished by their characteristics from those occurring from other organic causes, nor do the generalized seizures differ from those of idiopathic epilepsy. Focal or generalized seizures may precede other symptoms of an intracranial neoplasm by weeks, by months, or, in cases of slowly growing tumor, such as oligodendroglioma or meningioma, by several years.

Generalized seizures have no localizing value. Seizures with an olfactory or gustatory aura localize the tumor to the temporal lobe, as do seizures with hallucinations of formed images and psychomotor seizures. Visual phenomena of unformed images, such as flashes of light, implicate an occipital lobe lesion. Jacksonian and focal sensory seizures originate from the motor and sensory gyri anterior and posterior to the rolandic fissure. The onset of seizures after early childhood must be evaluated with at least an EEG and CT scan with contrast enhancement, in addition to the neurologic history and physical examination.

Mental Symptoms. Changes in mental function may occur with any of the intracranial tumors in any location, although they are more common with tumors in the anterior portions of the cerebral hemispheres. The patient initially develops a change in behavior hardly perceptible to the family, such as forgetfulness, loss of attention to detail, blunting of initiative, or subtle loss of intellectual sharpness. Initially family members or peers believe the patient is depressed or worried, but within a few weeks or months these symptoms become more prominent. The patient may develop indifference to common social practices, such as unconcern about the act of voiding urine in public.

Physical Examination. Significant findings on examination which point to a diagnosis of an intracranial tumor are signs of increased intracranial pressure and focal neurologic deficit.

Optic disc edema (papilledema), with blurring of the disc margins, venous engorgement, and retinal hemorrhages, is a common finding in patients with intracranial tumor but may be present in other conditions, such as pseudotumor cerebri, hydrocephalus, and anything else that causes intracranial hypertension. False localizing signs in the presence of increased intracranial pressure, such as unilateral or bilateral external rectus palsy, may be misleading to the uninitiated.

When focal neurologic signs are present, the intracranial tumors can be localized. Deficits in speech production or comprehension indicate a lesion in the posterior frontal operculum (Broca's area) or the posterior aspect of the superior temporal gyrus (Wernicke's area), respectively. Visual field defects result from temporal, parietal, or occipital lobe injury or from distortion or invasion of the optic nerves, chiasm, or tracts. Localization of involvement in the visual system can be determined from analysis of the visual field deficit (see Figure 37–4). Damage or displacement of the posterior frontal lobe or the anterior parietal lobe causes paralysis or sensory loss of the contralateral face, arm, or leg, depending on the precise location along the cerebral convexity (see Figures 37–5 and 37–6).

Special diagnostic studies confirm the suspected diagnosis, aid in precise localization, implicate a particular tumor type, and outline the anatomic relationship of the tumor mass to the cerebral blood vessels and the ventricular system.

Diagnostic Procedures. The intimation of an intracranial tumor by symptoms of headache, seizure, or focal neurologic dysfunction obligates the physician to obtain further diagnostic studies. The neurologic examination enables one to determine the patient's overall neurologic status and to judge the degree of urgency in proceeding with the evaluation process. Moreover, the degree of urgency may influence the choice of diagnostic studies to include only those that are essential for immediate management decisions. For example, a patient with a posterior fossa cerebellopontine angle tumor whose life is endangered by acute obstructive hydrocephalus needs a CT scan and CSF shunting procedure prior to in-depth analysis of auditory and vestibular function.

Quantitative Techniques Adjunctive to the Neurologic Examination. TANGENT SCREEN AND PERIMETRY. In the evaluation of the visual fields, the finding of deficits on confrontation requires more precise appraisal. With these techniques, the extent of the deficits, the margins and degree of congruity (concordance of the deficit comparing the fields of the eyes tested separately) of the defects can be determined. Subtle changes not discovered by confrontation testing will often become apparent. Examinations before and after therapy provide a means of quantifying the effects of the tumor and the treatment on the status of the

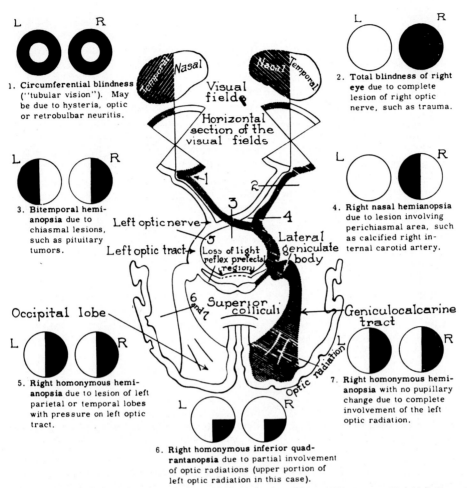

1. **Circumferential blindness** ("tubular vision"). May be due to hysteria, optic or retrobulbar neuritis.

2. **Total blindness of right eye** due to complete lesion of right optic nerve, such as trauma.

Visual field

Horizontal section of the visual fields

3. **Bitemporal hemi-anopsia** due to chiasmal lesions, such as pituitary tumors.

4. **Right nasal hemianopsia** due to lesion involving perichiasmal area, such as calcified right internal carotid artery.

Left optic nerve

Left optic tract

Lateral geniculate body

Loss of light reflex prefectal region

Occipital lobe

Superior colliculi

Geniculocalcarine tract

Optic radiation

5. **Right homonymous hemi-anopsia** due to lesion of left parietal or temporal lobes with pressure on left optic tract.

7. **Right homonymous hemi-anopsia** with no pupillary change due to complete involvement of the left optic radiation.

6. **Right homonymous inferior quad-rantanopsia** due to partial involvement of optic radiations (upper portion of left optic radiation in this case).

Figure 37–4.   Visual field deficits and their relationship to the optic pathways. From Chusid, J. G., and McDonald, J. J.: *Correlative Neuroanatomy and Functional Neurology,* 13th ed. Lange Medical Publications, Los Altos, CA, 1967, p. 85.

visual pathways. The specific type of visual field abnormality correlated with the site of injury along the optic pathways is depicted in Figure 37–4.

CALORIC TESTING.   Stimulation of the semicircular canal with cold or warm water allows assessment of the vestibular nerve and the integrity of the neural pathways within the brain stem connecting the vestibular system with the nuclei of the abducens and oculomotor nerves. In the normal patient, cold caloric stimulation results in nystagmus, with the fast component away from the side of stimulation. In the comatose patient, up to 120 mL of ice water is slowly irrigated into the external auditory canal with a small catheter and the response of extraocular movement observed. Smaller amounts of water are used in the alert patient being tested to assess vestibular nerve status. Abnormal movements or nystagmus

that is increased or decreased in amplitude or duration can help to indicate the degree and site of pathology.

Lumbar Puncture.   Discussion of lumbar puncture (LP) in the diagnosis of intracranial tumors should begin with the caution that this procedure holds significant dangers for certain categories of patients. Those who have elevated intracranial pressure (ICP), as indicated by lethargy and the finding of papilledema, are at particular risk, as are those patients with lesions of the temporal lobe and cerebellum. The danger consists of the alteration in pressure relationships between the intracranial compartments, and between the intracranial and spinal compartments, that can occur when CSF is withdrawn from the lumbar space.

In the great majority of intracranial tumors, little can be gained by lumbar puncture and

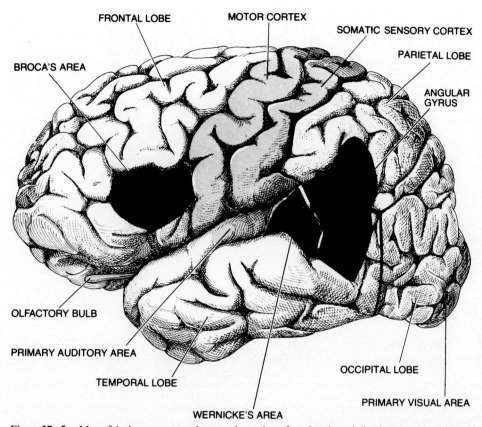

Figure 37–5. Map of the human cortex shows regions whose functional specializations have been identified. Much of the cortex is given over to comparatively elementary functions: the generation of movement and the primary analysis of sensations. These areas, which include the motor and somatic sensory regions and the primary visual, auditory, and olfactory areas, are present in all species that have a well-developed cortex, and are called on in the course of many activities. Several other regions (dark color) are more narrowly specialized. Broca's area and Wernicke's area are involved in the production and comprehension of language. The angular gyrus is thought to mediate between visual and auditory forms of information. These functional specializations have been detected only on the left side of the brain; the corresponding areas of the right hemisphere do not have the same linguistic competence. The right hemisphere, which is not shown, has its own specialized abilities, including the analysis of some aspects of music and of complex visual patterns. The anatomical regions associated with these faculties, however, are not as well defined as the language areas. Even in the left hemisphere the assignment of functions to sites in the cortex is only approximate; some areas may have functions in addition to those indicated, and some functions may be carried out in more than one place. From Geschwind, N.: Specializations of the human brain. *Scientific American* **241**(3):186, 1979.

analysis of the CSF collected. In certain tumor types, however, such as medulloblastoma, pineal region tumors, and ependymomas, one acquires information pertinent to patient management. In these patients, the lumbar puncture is performed only after special diagnostic studies have given the clinician information which can be used to assess the potential risks and benefits of the procedure. When the decision has been made to proceed, the risk can be minimized by the use of a small-caliber needle, slow withdrawal of a minimal amount of CSF, and, in some cases, pretreatment with steroids or mannitol.

The pertinent measurements include CSF pressure dynamics, color, protein, sugar, cell count, bacterial culture, gram stain, millipore filtration, cytocentrifugation, and tissue culture for malignant cells.

The procedure is performed with the patient in the lateral position, preferably at the L4–5 interspace, using a 22-gauge spinal needle. Assurance that one is in the subarachnoid space can be made by observing the movement of CSF with respiration. Initially, the evaluation of ICP is performed using a manometer. Findings of over 150 mm of H_2O are of concern, although not always abnormal. A pressure over 200 mm of H_2O in a relaxed patient suggests true raised ICP and supports the diag-

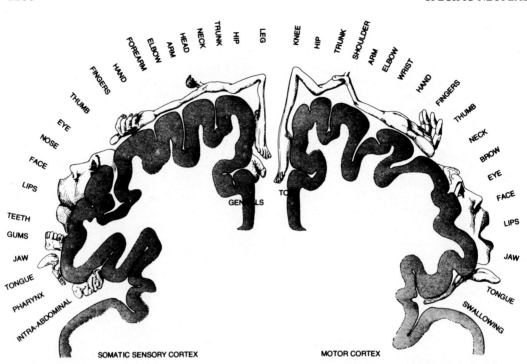

Figure 37–6. Somatic sensory and motor regions of the cerebral cortex are specialized in the sense that every site in these regions can be associated with some part of the body. In other words, most of the body can be mapped onto the cortex, yielding two distorted homunculi. The distortions come about because the area of the cortex dedicated to a part of the body is proportional not to that part's actual size, but to the precision with which it must be controlled. In man the motor and somatic sensory regions given over to the face and to the hands are greatly exaggerated. Only half of each cortical region is shown: the left somatic sensory area (which receives sensations primarily from the right side of the body) and the right motor cortex (which exercises control over movement in the left half of the body). From Geschwind, N.: Specializations of the human brain. *Scientific American,* **241**(3):182, 1979.

nosis of a mass lesion. At levels above 200 mm, only minimal CSF amounts should be withdrawn and the needle removed promptly.

The CSF dynamics can be observed by asking the patient to breathe deeply and watching the CSF excursions in the manometer. Valsalva's maneuver is not a part of the evaluation of intracranial mass lesions.

The color and appearance of the CSF can aid in determining whether bleeding, high protein, or infection is present. Reddish fluid suggests recent hemorrhage; yellowish (xanthochromic) fluid indicates old bleeding or high-protein content. A viscous appearance may occur with either high protein or infection. Turbidity suggests infection.

Cerebrospinal fluid protein content has classically been one of the most useful biochemical parameters indicating tumor presence. Elevation of CSF protein above 40 mg/100 mL is suggestive of tumor. Increased protein, however, can be produced by blood or infection in the CSF, and less frequently by cerebrovascular occlusive disease. Numerous

efforts have been made to characterize the CSF proteins. For example, α-fetaprotein, human chorionic gonadotropin, and carcinoembryonic antigen have been found in patients with intracranial germ cell tumors. CSF sugar below 50 mg/mL is suggestive of an infectious process, such as meningitis or viral encephalitis. Tumors may also lower CSF sugar, especially in diffuse leukemia or carcinomatous meningitis.

Millipore filtration and, more recently, CSF tissue culture can be very useful diagnostic adjuncts. These techniques find their greatest utility in tumors originating near or reaching out to the brain surface, such as metastatic tumors, and in cases of CSF seeding, as with medulloblastoma, where exfoliated tumor cells may be identified. Millipore study can detect nuclear abnormalities in some detail and thus indicate malignancy, but little if any cytoplasmic detail is evident.

CSF tissue culture improves the ability to evaluate size, shape, and cell process formation. In recent studies, an almost twofold higher rate of tumor detection by CSF culture compared with millipore filtration was found (Kajikawa *et al.*, 1977; Black *et al.*, 1978). Combining millipore and culture techniques, better results can be obtained. The use of CSF cell identification techniques should be considered a routine adjunct in patients with CNS tumors likely to have CSF seeding.

Electroencephalogram. The electroencephalogram (EEG) allows demonstration of either increased or diminished electrical activity of the brain. In general, brain tumors produce a regional slowing of electrical activity. When a specific seizure focus is present, spikes or spike and wave foci can occur in relation to a tumor. The EEG is often normal in patients with brain tumors and thus has limited value as a screening device.

Radiographic Examination. Computerized tomographic scanning has largely replaced plain skull x-rays, radioisotope brain scanning, angiography, pneumoencephalography, and ventriculography in the diagnosis of brain tumors. These investigations, however, can still be helpful in specific instances.

SKULL FILMS. Abnormalities seen on plain skull x-rays of patients with brain tumors include calcification, bony erosions, and hyperostoses.

In general, calcifications represent slow tumor growth and thus suggest a benign lesion. Many vascular lesions, such as arteriovenous malformation, also calcify. Oligodendrogliomas, craniopharyngiomas, astrocytomas, and meningiomas calcify more frequently than the other tumors of the central nervous system. Although the incidence of calcification in the glial neoplasms is much less in the astrocytomas than the oligodendrogliomas, the greater frequency of the astrocytomas allows them to represent the greatest fraction of calcifying intracranial neoplasms. Approximately 20% of astrocytomas have calcification, whereas 50% of oligodendrogliomas display areas of calcification on skull x-rays (Russell and Rubinstein, 1977). Large areas of diffuse calcification, appearing as fluffy white patches, are seen with oligodendrogliomas, although no pathognomonic features discriminate the specific glial tumors.

Seventy percent to eighty percent of craniopharyngiomas calcify (duBoulay and Trickey, 1962). The sellar or suprasellar location and the curvilinear, thin calcifications following the contours of the tumor capsule allow presumptive diagnosis. Aneurysms in the parasellar area, however, may look identical. Calcification occurs with much greater frequency in pediatric patients with craniopharyngiomas than in adults.

Meningiomas vary in their tendency to calcify and in the type of calcification produced. Five to 10% have visible calcifications. These may be small, speckled flecks or a dense area of bony calcification. The psammomatous varieties are most likely to calcify (Taveras and Wood, 1976).

In contrast to these specific abnormal calcifications, normal calcifications may occur in the pineal gland, habenula, choroid plexus, dura, intracranial ligaments, and vessel walls. The normal calcification of the pineal gland in most patients (55%) allows a reference point to detect shift of this midline structure as a result of tumors or other intracranial mass lesions (Chambers *et al.*, 1976).

Erosion of normally calcified structures results from long-standing increased intracranial pressure or from direct lytic activity of adjacent tumors. The lamina dura and clinoid processes of the sella turcica are often eroded in patients with intracranial hypertension. In children, chronic pressure erosion of the inner table of the skull can lead to the "beaten silver" appearance. Meningiomas can cause local bone erosion or hyperostosis and occasionally can be diagnosed on plain skull films by hyperostosis in a typical location, such as the planum sphenoidale, tuberculum sella, or sphenoid wing.

TOMOGRAPHY. This technique is now used most frequently for the evaluation of bone changes produced by tumors at the skull base. Hypocycloidal polytomography, as contrasted to linear tomography, markedly decreases streaking artifacts and is the preferred technique. Common applications include detailed study of focal erosion of the sella floor by microadenomas, enlargement of the internal auditory meatus by acoustic neuromas, and widening of the optic canal by optic nerve gliomas.

RADIOISOTOPE BRAIN SCAN. Brain scanning with radioisotopes, previously an important technique in tumor diagnosis, now assumes a less prominent role owing to the development of the CT scan. Alderson *et al.* (1977), in a compilation of reports, found a 94% overall detection rate for the CT scan, as compared with 85% for the brain scan in brain tumors. The detection of intracranial tumors by brain scanning ranges from more than 90% with meningiomas, anaplastic astrocytomas, glioblastoma multiforme, and medulloblastomas to little greater than 50% for pituitary adenomas.

In cost effectiveness and diagnostic efficacy, the CT scan is preferable to the brain scan where facilities for both are available (Evans and Jost, 1977).

The enthusiasm for the CT scan should not obscure the complementary role of the radionuclide study, however. It is often helpful in correct preoperative localization of tumors high on the cerebral convexity and the parasagittal and vertex areas, areas where CT localization may be misleading.

CT SCAN. In no discipline has the introduction of the CT scan been more noteworthy than the study of the brain. Since its introduction into clinical medicine in 1972, it has virtually replaced all other diagnostic studies in the investigation of patients suspected of harboring intracranial mass lesions. In this technique, computerized tomographic cuts allow a detailed analysis of density changes to be made with precision. It distinguishes between CSF, blood, edema, tumor, and normal brain tissue by means of quantitative density differences.

Greater than 90% success in diagnosis of presence or absence of tumors has been noted with intraparenchymal lesions (Greitz, 1975). Low-grade, well-differentiated astrocytomas still present a problem, with detection rates as low as 70% being reported. Late-model CT scanners can detect lesions as small as 0.5 cm and allow greater discrimination of subtle soft tissue density gradients. They will undoubtedly improve the already impressive detection rates.

Detection results from observation of deformity of the ventricular system, the subarachnoid space, the presence of a hypodense area of brain edema or tumor tissue, or abnormal calcification within a lesion (calcification which may not have been seen on routine x-rays). The use of contrast enhancement (that is, computed tomography after intravenous injection of iodine-containing contrast medium) can markedly sharpen the tumor delineation and is especially helpful in the posterior fossa, where small tumors may be more difficult to visualize owing to the proximity of the surrounding bone.

Of equal importance to detection is the ability to analyze brain masses with the scan images. A lesion can be definitively localized by its contrast enhancement in the midst of a mass effect, and the character of lesions can often be assessed. For instance, one can separate meningiomas from gliomas and with some accuracy differentiate low-grade from high-grade astrocytomas.

CT scanning in the coronal plane and coronal and sagittal reconstruction images aid in surgical localization, in addition to giving details of the relationship of the tumor to the ventricular system and the dural septa (falx and tentorium). Metrizamide CT cisternography (CT scanning following the lumbar instillation of water-soluble contrast into the CSF) greatly helps in the assessment of basal tumors impinging upon the subarachnoid space, such as acoustic neuromas, pituitary adenomas, foramen magnum tumors, and lesions of the optic chiasm.

If the history and neurologic findings are suggestive of a brain tumor, the performance of a CT scan is the next logical step.

ANGIOGRAPHY. For a period of about 20 years (1955 to 1975), angiography was crucial in cerebral tumor diagnosis. It now represents a valuable diagnostic and preoperative adjunct, although it is no longer used as a primary screening technique as it was prior to the CT scan.

Presently, the majority of angiograms are performed by the retrograde femoral route, using a catheter to inject x-ray opaque contrast material into either the carotid or vertebral arteries. For most studies, a common carotid injection is used but selective internal or external injections have special uses, such as an external carotid injection for visualizing a meningioma. Angiography does carry risks, including stroke, embolism, and hemorrhage (the last two at the local site of injection and intracerebrally). Some patients may have allergic or idiosyncratic reactions to iodine-containing contrast material.

For current indications for angiography in brain tumor patients, see Table 37–2. Most of these represent preoperative study for planning surgical strategy, but diagnostic data are obtained as well.

Among the findings of diagnostic importance evident on angiography are tumor blush, displacement of vessels from their normal position, and the temporal sequence of the filling pattern of arteries and veins in the tumor area. For example, early filling of veins draining a tumor intrinsic to the cerebral hemispheres implicates the neovascularity present in a glioblastoma multiforme.

PNEUMOENCEPHALOGRAPHY AND VEN-

Table 37-2. Indications for Angiography in Brain Tumor Patients

1. To detect a possible vascular lesion producing a mass effect, *i.e.*, an AVM, giant arterial aneurysm, or vein of Galen aneurysm
2. Preoperative evaluation of tumor vasculature (especially useful in large meningiomas and glomus jugulare tumors)
3. Preoperative assessment of a hormonally inactive pituitary macroadenoma with suprasellar extension (to eliminate the chances of entering a carotid aneurysm at transsphenoidal surgery)
4. To outline preoperatively the course of important cerebral vessels adjacent to a tumor so that their injury during surgery is less likely
5. To determine preoperatively the patency of the dural venous sinuses and collateral venous flow in meningiomas adjacent to or invading the dural sinuses.

TRICULOGRAPHY. The air contrast studies developed by Walter E. Dandy (1918, 1919) revolutionized the diagnostic approach to intracranial mass lesions. Before their introduction, only the neurologic examination and the occasional finding on the skull films were available for either tumor screening or localization. These techniques involve patient risk and discomfort. With the exception of the investigation of the empty-sella syndrome, they are rarely indicated. Even in this special circumstance, metrizamide CT cisternography is now preferred in most centers.

Systematic Diagnostic Assessment. Special studies cannot replace the careful history and physical examination in the evaluation of the brain tumor suspect. Many neurologic disorders, such as pseudotumor cerebri, and viral encephalitides, simulate intracranial neoplastic masses. The general physical examination is valuable in formulating a differential diagnosis and in evaluating the patient's ability to tolerate surgery. Chest radiograms may disclose primary lung carcinoma, previously undiagnosed, in a patient whose clinical presentation stems from cerebral metastases. After these basic steps, the CT scan seems the most dependable, safest, and highest yield diagnostic study for brain tumors.

Table 37-3 reviews the recommended sequence of clinical evaluation of the brain tumor suspect, and Table 37-4 outlines the indications for the use of the major diagnostic techniques which have been described.

General Physiologic Principles Affecting Management. Certain pathophysiologic mechanisms account for the clinical difficulties of patients with brain tumors. Optimal patient care requires understanding these mechanisms.

Intracranial Volume-Pressure Relationship. Brain tissue, blood, and cerebrospinal fluid are the normal constituents of the body space surrounded by the unyielding skull, the intracranial cavity. These elements are incompressible, and the degree of rigidity of the adult skull is such that an increase in the volume of one element must occur at the expense of one or both of the others. During the gradual expansion of a mass lesion, the volume displaced from the intracranial space may be CSF, blood, or brain tissue fluid. As the mass enlarges, the volume of CSF within the skull is reduced by increased absorption by the arachnoid villi and by displacement of CSF into the spinal subarachnoid space (Langfitt, 1982). The blood volume of the brain diminishes as the capacitance venous vessels reduce their content. Without these compensatory mechanisms, the addition of volumes less than a fraction of a milliliter to the normal intracranial contents would elevate the intracranial pressure to levels greatly exceeding the systemic arterial pressure.

As Figure 37-7 demonstrates, regardless of this initial compensation, as a mass progressively increases in size, the limits of these adjustments are surpassed. A small incremental volume added to the intracranial space at this time will dangerously elevate intracranial pressure. When a patient's partially compensated status is on the steep segment of the volume-pressure curve, an increase in intracranial blood volume induced by respiratory change, a small increment in tumor growth, or an advancement of the degree of hydrocephalus may have profound clinical consequences.

Autoregulation of Cerebral Blood Flow. Under normal circumstances, a constant cerebral blood flow is maintained despite changes in systemic arterial pressure between 50 and 150 mm Hg (Lassen, 1959). Figure 37-8 demonstrates the effect of alteration of mean arterial pressure on cerebral blood flow. The phenomenon of varying the resistance of the cerebral vessels to maintain constant flow, re-

Table 37–3. Outline of Clinical Evaluation for Brain Tumor Patients

A. Clinical history (general symptoms for intracranial tumors)	
1. Headache	
2. Seizures	
3. Progressively increasing weakness or sensory loss	
4. Visual loss	Blurring of field of vision or diplopia
5. Hearing loss	Tinnitus or decreased acuity
6. Vomiting	
7. Gait disturbance	
B. Neurologic examination	
1. Mental status	Decreased alertness and decline in intellectual function with increased intracranial pressure in frontal, temporal, and parietal lesions
2. Cranial nerves	
CN I. Anosmia	Suggestive of anterior fossa tumors, especially olfactory groove meningioma
CN II. Papilledema	Increased intracranial pressure
Visual field defects	Localize lesion depending on portion of pathways affected
CN III, IV, VI. Decreased ocular motility	Owing to increased pressure or tumors affecting brain stem
CN V. Facial sensation loss and corneal reflex loss	Tumors of cerebellopontine angle
CN VII. Facial movement loss	Tumors of cerebellopontine angle
CN VIII. Hearing loss — balance problems	Tumors of cerebellopontine angle
CN IX, X. Difficulty in swallowing	Tumors at base of brain
CN XI. Asymmetry in shoulder shrugging	Tumors at base of brain
CN XII. Asymmetry in protruding tongue	Tumors deviate tongue to side of lesion
3. Motor function	Weakness of hemiplegic type with spasticity in lesions of motor cortex and descending corticospinal pathways
4. Reflex dysfunction	Hyperactive reflexes and abnormal reflexes (Babinski)
5. Sensory loss	Corresponding to area of sensory cortex or ascending pathways involved
6. Coordination deficits	Ataxia, dysmetria in cerebellar and some brain stem lesions
C. Radiologic studies	
1. Skull films	Shifts in calcified structures, hyperostosis, bone erosion, abnormal calcification
2. CT scan	Masses, location, edema, character of lesion
3. Isotope scan	Location of masses
4. Angiography	For feeding vessels, sequence of vessel filling, and preoperative anatomy relationships
5. Metrizamide CT cisternography	
D. Ancillary studies for diagnosis	
1. Audiometric examination	For lesions of cerebellopontine angle
2. Tangent screen and perimetry	Detailed visual field documentation
3. Lumbar puncture	When concerned about possibility of infectious process or tumor that spreads by CSF seeding

Based on Kornblith, P. L.; Walker, M. D.; and Cassady, J. R.: Neoplasms of the central nervous system. In DeVita, V. T.; Hellman, S.; and Rosenberg, S. A. (eds.): *Principles and Practice of Oncology.* J. B. Lippincott Company, Philadelphia, 1982.

gardless of alterations in perfusion pressure, is known as autoregulation. The cerebral perfusion pressure (CPP) is the difference between systemic arterial pressure and intracranial pressure. When intracranial pressure increases such that the cerebral perfusion pressure is below the limits of autoregulation, the cerebral blood flow varies linearly with the cerebral perfusion pressure; as intracranial pressure approaches systemic arterial pressure, the blood flow to the brain is compromised, and ischemic brain injury results. That a transient period of hypotension during a period of such compromise would have devastating influence on the patient's neurologic condition is easily understood.

Hypoxia, trauma, cerebral infarction, and anesthesia alter or prevent autoregulation of flow, removing the element of variable cerebrovascular resistance; and cerebral blood

Table 37–4. Role of Diagnostic Techniques in Evaluation of Brain Tumor Patients

TECHNIQUE	INDICATIONS
History	All patients
Neurologic examination	All patients
General medical and metabolic evaluation	All patients
Skull x-ray	All patients
CT scan	All patients with history and examination suggestive of brain tumor
EEG	Patients with seizure disorders
Isotope scan	Preoperative tumor localization, patients allergic to iodine with nondiagnostic CT scan without contrast
Angiography	As outlined in Table 37–2
Metrizamide CT Cisternogram	Basal tumors (acoustic neuroma not demonstrated by routine CT scan, foramen magnum tumors, optic chiasm lesions) and empty-sella syndrome
Lumbar puncture	Differentiating tumor from infection, CSF analysis for tumor marker proteins (HCG, CEA, AFP), detection of CSF seeding of tumor cells (medulloblastoma, ependymoma, pinealoma)

Based on Kornblith, P. L.; Walker, M. D.; and Cassady, J. R.: Neoplasms of the central nervous system. In DeVita, V. T.; Hellman, S.; and Rosenberg, S. A. (eds.): *Principles and Practice of Oncology.* J. B. Lippincott Company, Philadelphia, 1982.

flow varies directly with perfusion pressure. Intracranial blood volume increases as cerebral blood flow increases. For the reasons outlined in the discussion of the volume-pressure relationship, the patient who has approached the limits of compensation for an intracranial mass may be critically influenced by alterations in blood pressure, hypoxia, hypercapnia, and volatile anesthetic agents (see Figure 37–9A).

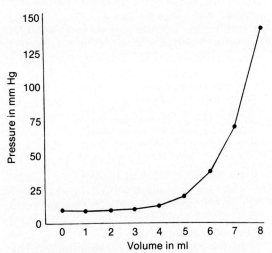

Figure 37–7. Volume–pressure graph demonstrating intracranial pressure in millimeters of mercury as an extradural balloon is inflated at a rate of 1 ml/hr in a Rhesus monkey. From Langfitt, T. W., Weinstein, J. D., and Kassell, N. F., in Caveness, W. F., and Walker, A. E. (eds.): *Head Injury: Conference Proceedings, 1966.* J. B. Lippincott Co., Philadelphia, 1966.

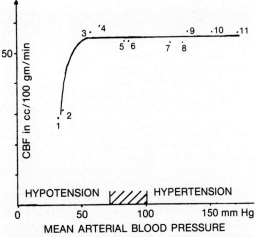

Figure 37–8. Diagram showing relationship of mean arterial blood pressure and cerebral blood flow of 11 patients with different acute and chronic conditions. The conditions represented by the numbers are 1–4, drug-induced hypotension, 5–6, normal pregnant women and normal young men, 7–11, drug-induced and essential hypertension. From Lassen, N.: Cerebral blood flow and oxygen uptake. *Acta Neurol. Scand.* **39:**197, 1959.

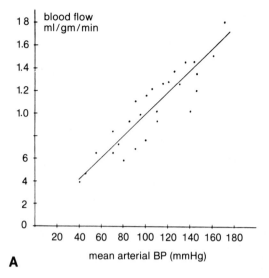

A

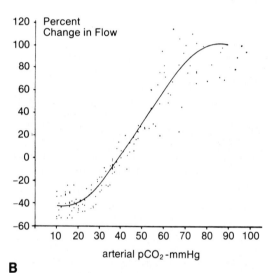

B

Figure 37–9. Influence of P_{CO_2} and blood pressure on cerebral blood flow in the dog. (*A*) Changes of blood flow with alterations of mean arterial blood pressure during hypercapnea. (*B*) Changes of cerebral blood flow as P_{CO_2} is varied during normotension. From Harper, A. M.: The inter-relationship between $2P_{CO_2}$ and blood pressure in the regulation of blood flow through the cerebral cortex. *Acta Neurol. Scand.,* **41**(Suppl. 14):96, 1965.

Chemoregulation of Cerebral Blood Flow. Carbon dioxide is the most potent cerebrovascular dilator that is known. The relaxation of the smooth muscle of the cerebral arterioles diminishes cerebrovascular resistance, increasing cerebral blood flow and intracranial blood volume (see Figure 37–9B). Within the range of 30 to 60 mm Hg CO_2 tension, there is a 2.5% change in blood flow as the P_{CO_2} increases or decreases 1 mm Hg.

Knowledge of this physiologic effect has practical importance. Hyperventilation reduces elevated intracranial pressure more rapidly than any other therapeutic maneuver. Therefore, endotracheal intubation and hyperventilation may be life-saving for the patient *in extremis* undergoing transtentorial or tonsillar herniation from an intracranial mass lesion. Respiratory failure with hypercapnia abolishes cerebral autoregulation and causes vasodilatation, increasing cerebral blood flow (see Figure 37–9A) and intracranial blood volume, with potential catastrophic consequences in the brain tumor victim with partially compromised volume-pressure dynamics.

Brain Edema. Edema is an important effect on adjacent neural tissue by primary and metastatic cerebral tumors. Brain edema has been classified into three categories: vasogenic edema, cytotoxic edema, and interstitial edema (Fishman, 1975). Brain tumors produce vasogenic edema in the vicinity of tumor growth and will be the only type considered here. Increased permeability of the capillary endothelium allows plasma to enter the extracellular spaces. This increased permeability is a result of defects in the tight endothelial cell junctions of tumor neovascularity and of increased vesicular transport across the endothelial cells. The accumulation of plasma filtrate, with its high-protein content, in the extracellular spaces and between layers of myelin augments the intracranial space occupation of the tumor mass and alters the ionic balance of nerve fibers, impairing their function. Once pressure is raised in a particular region of the brain, it begins to cause displacement and herniation of brain tissue (Fishman, 1975).

Brain Herniations. The cranial cavity is divided into three compartments by the rigid dural folds of the falx cerebri and the tentorium. The local pressure from a mass within one compartment is not evenly distributed, but causes shift or herniations of brain tissue from one compartment to another.

The two clinically important herniations are transtentorial herniation (central and uncal types) and cerebellar tonsil–foramen magnum herniation.

In the uncal type of transtentorial herniation, as a laterally placed lesion displaces the medial aspect of the temporal lobe (the uncus) through the oval-shaped tentorial opening, the subadjacent oculomotor nerve and the brain stem are compressed. Pupillary dilatation, ptosis, and ophthalmoplegia on the involved side are followed by altered consciousness, respiratory changes (Cheyne-Stokes breathing, central neurogenic hyperventilation, and so forth), and posturing abnormalities (decorticate and decerebrate posturing).

The central type of transtentorial herniation is usually the result of a more medially located mass producing rostral-caudal displacement of the brain stem and an advancing zone of ischemia of the brain stem in a rostral-caudal direction. Clinically, this type is characterized by early stupor, change in respiratory pattern, and small pupils giving way to coma and decorticate and decerebrate posturing as the syndrome progresses. In both the uncal and central types of transtentorial herniation, the level of neurologic function proceeds in a stepwise manner from the diencephalon to midbrain, pons, and medulla as the patient's deterioration progresses.

The lethal effect of the cerebellar tonsil – foramen magnum herniation is caused by compression of the medulla. Early signs are head tilt, stiff neck, and arching of the neck, presumably owing to extension of the cerebellar tonsils into the foramen magnum. Later, the typical signs of tonic extensor spasms of the extremities, respiratory disturbances, pulse irregularities, and loss of consciousness occur. Herniation of this type may occur with tumors in the supra- or infratentorial compartment.

Steroid Therapy. Since their introduction into the clinical management of cerebral neoplasms in 1961, steroids have been used extensively in a wide variety of pathologic conditions affecting the nervous system (Galicich and French, 1961). High-dose glucocorticoid therapy may dramatically reduce the focal and general signs of primary and metastatic brain tumor, signs which may be caused more by peritumoral edema than by the tumor itself.

The usual starting dose is 10 mg dexamethasone, and 4 mg every six hours thereafter, or an equivalent dose of methylprednisolone. Although an occasional patient may improve within a few hours of steroid administration, most require therapy for at least 24 hours before a change in clinical performance appears. Experimental work studying cold-induced edema (the most dramatic experimental model for vasogenic edema) demonstrated that objective laboratory findings of the beneficial effect of steroids were not measurable until the second 24-hour interval after injury; and then the reduction in edema was progressive (Pappius and McCann, 1969). Steroid therapy cannot be relied upon to reverse the rapidly deteriorating neurologic condition of the seriously ill patient. More rapidly effective measures are required.

Hypertonic Solutions. The reduction of intracranial pressure by osmotherapy was introduced by Weed and McKibben in 1919. Since that time, many osmotically active agents have been employed to combat cerebral edema, including magnesium sulfate, sodium chloride, sucrose, glucose, urea, isosorbide, succinate, sodium lactate, mannitol, and glycerol. The principle governing their use has been the creation of an effective osmotic gradient between the intravascular compartment and the brain interstitial and intracellular compartments so that tissue water will pass from edematous and normal tissue into the bloodstream. The effectiveness of this therapy depends upon the unique blood-brain permeability barrier to water-soluble materials. Areas in which this physiologic barrier is disrupted, *i.e.,* areas of vasogenic edema, will not have a reduction in bulk by administration of hypertonic solution. Thus, the parts of the brain most likely to shrink are the areas of normal brain where the capillary endothelial bed is intact. The clinical effectiveness of this reduction in intracranial tissue bulk can be related to the patient's intracranial volume-pressure status, as previously discussed.

Intravenous mannitol is the current agent of choice in a concentration of 20 to 25% administered rapidly to allow maximum osmotic gradient to develop. The recommended dose is 0.25 to 1.50 mg/kg. The lower doses are equal in effectiveness to the previously standard 1.0 to 1.5 mg/kg dose and are less likely to result in problems with systemic hyperosmolarity after repeated use (Marshall *et al.,* 1978). Intracranial pressure falls within 10 to 20 minutes of infusion and may be sustained at lower levels for several hours. Therefore, the patient requiring immediate reduction of intracranial pressure in order to gain time for diagnostic study or operative intervention may be managed by a rapid intravenous bolus of mannitol or by endotracheal intubation and controlled ventilation, or both.

Glial Tumors

Astrocytic Tumors. *Epidemiology.* Tumors of glial origin comprise about 60% of all primary CNS tumors. Of the five types of glial cells (astrocytes, oligodendroglia, ependymal cells, microglial cells, and more primitive precursor cells), the astrocytic series (including glioblastoma) gives rise to the most frequent glial-derived brain tumors, whereas in the spinal cord, where gliomas are less common, tumors of ependymal glial origin are preponderant. From the Russell and Rubinstein series, comprising 496 cases collected from 1928 to 1939 and 1946 to 1955, the percentage incidence of the principal types of gliomas was glioblastoma multiforme, 55%; astrocytoma, 20.5%; ependymoma, 6%; medulloblastoma, 6%; and oligodendroglioma, 5%; choroid plexus papillomas, colloid cysts, and other less common tumors account for the remaining 7%. Whether microglia have the same common embryonic origin, *i.e.,* neuroectodermal, is questionable (McKeever and Balentine, 1978); and it is not clear that they should be included in the glioma tumor series.

Based on the Survey of Intracranial Neoplasms (National Institute of Neurological and Communicative Disorders and Stroke, 1977), a conservative estimate of the incidence of all intracranial tumors is approximately 17/100,000, with primary malignant intracranial tumors having an incidence of approximately 2.5/100,000. From the studies of Kurland (1958) and Percy *et al.* (1972), there were 12.6/100,000 primary cerebral tumors, with 28% of these being astrocytic. Noting a rise in the incidence of cerebral tumors from 1 to 75 years of age, they found a final rate of 25/100,000, although other authors (Cushing, 1932; Merritt, 1959; Jänisch *et al.*, 1967) showed a drop after age 45.

Age is an important consideration in gliomas, with several studies (Cushing 1930, 1931, 1932; Bailey, 1933; Zülch, 1940; Bailey *et al.*, 1948; Zülch and Borck, 1952) showing age-dependent preponderance of a particular intracranial tumor type and location. Cerebellar astrocytomas have their peak incidence in individuals under 20 years of age (ages 3 to 12) (Farwell *et al.*, 1977). In the third and fourth decades, astrocytic tumors are most common and are located in cerebral hemispheres. By the fifth to sixth decades, malignant astrocytomas and/or glioblastomas, along with metastatic lesions, are more common; and it is these decades that show the second glial tumor incidence peak (Youmans, 1973; Farwell *et al.*, 1977).

Sex distribution of glial tumors is another issue. Overall, one sees a slight preponderance of men (55.6%) to women (44.4%) (Zülch, 1965) with glioma series tumors, whereas women show a preponderance for meningiomas and neurinomas. McKeran and Thomas (1980) have pointed out that sex differences they have seen were most marked in grade II and III astrocytomas, anaplastic astrocytomas, and oligodendrogliomas, whereas no sex differences were apparent in well-differentiated astrocytomas. Overall, however, from studies of Percy *et al.* (1972), it would appear that sex differences in glial tumor incidence are not great.

Etiology and Pathogenesis. From an etiologic point of view, studies to date indicate that most of the glial series tumors are spontaneous (Russell and Rubinstein, 1977). Genetic predisposition seems likely in relatively few cases (Koch, 1954; Zülch, 1956; Hauge and Harvald, 1960; Kjellin *et al.*, 1960; Blattner *et al.*, 1979). Neurofibromatosis is of particular interest in this respect because of its autosomal dominant pattern of inheritance and because of the association of optic gliomas, as well as other glial tumors (Schenkein *et al.*, 1974). Tuberous sclerosis (Bourneville's disease) is yet another example of a syndrome associated with glial tumors that has a genetic basis, as is Turcot syndrome (Adams and Victor, 1977). The clear inheritance pattern in at least some retinoblastomas (Knudson, 1971) lends added weight to the notion that some glial tumors may have an origin in genetic inheritance.

Having looked at the inheritance data, however, it is clear that only a relative minority of glial tumors so far appear to have a genetic etiology. The possibility that nests of glial cells with a high mitotic potential remain as remnants of an abnormal developmental process is another etiologic mechanism of some interest. This seems likely to account for some neural tumors in infancy (Kadin *et al.*, 1970). Since such embryonic cell nests are found only rarely in human brains after four months of age (Friede, 1973), however, it seems unlikely that they can explain the origin of all adult-onset tumors (Weller, 1980).

The possibility that astrocytic tumors may have a viral etiology has long been of interest. Although glial tumors can be produced in animals by the injection of both RNA and DNA viruses, there has been no evidence to date implicating viruses in the etiology of human brain tumors (Copeland and Bigner, 1978; Bigner *et al.*, 1981). Curiously, infections with known oncogenic virus occur in the human brain. Papovaviruses of the JC strain are found in the brains of patients with progressive multifocal leukoencephalopathy (Padgett *et al.*,

1971; Narayan *et al.*, 1973), and groups of bizarre astrocytes found in the demyelinating lesions resemble those of malignant gliomas (Castaigne *et al.*, 1974). In addition, JC virus injected into newborn hamster brains produced malignant tumors in 83% of the animals (Walker, 1973; ZuRhein and Varakis, 1975). More recently, London *et al.* (1978) have been able to produce gliomas in primates utilizing human JC virus. The latency of tumor development is approximately 18 months. Avian and murine sarcoma virus in puppies (Bigner *et al.*, 1969; Wodinski *et al.*, 1969), in mice, and in rats (Yung *et al.*, 1976; Copeland and Bigner, 1978) have also been used to produce malignant astrocytoma models.

Chemical carcinogens are another potential etiologic factor; but, as for the viruses, the bulk of evidence relates to experimental tumor models in animals. Occasional clusters of malignant tumors have appeared in particular work situations. The most recent was in association with petrochemical workers in Texas. The evidence directly implicating exposure to chemicals has been reviewed without a definitive answer (Selikoff and Hammond, 1982).

In animal models, administration of 2-acetylaminofluorene, with and without lead subacetate (Vazquez-Lopez, 1945; Hoch-Ligeti and Russell, 1950; Oyasu *et al.*, 1970), and most notably N-nitroso compounds, such as methylnitrosourea (MNU) and ethylnitrosourea (ENU) (for reviews, see Wechsler *et al.*, 1969; Zimmerman, 1969; Benda *et al.*, 1971; Druckrey *et al.*, 1972; Koestner *et al.*, 1972 Wechsler, 1972; Jänisch and Schreiber, 1974; Russell and Rubinstein, 1977), produce nervous system tumors. The central nervous system tumors are almost all gliomas, with periventricular subependymal growths being most frequent, oligodendrogliomas second, and astrocytomas third after ENU administration (Sipe *et al.*, 1974). Glioblastomas are, interestingly enough, uncommon.

Trauma has also been suggested to be a cause of brain tumors, but the evidence is only circumstantial and rather weak for astrocytomas (Russell and Rubinstein, 1977).

Pathology and Natural History. Astrocytomas are most commonly classified today by the Kernohan system (Kernohan *et al.*, 1949), which provides for four tumor grades (*i.e.*, 1, 2, 3, 4), with 1 being the most benign and 4 the most malignant, or glioblastoma multiforme. This simplification of previous classification schemes, such as those of Bailey and Cushing (1926) and Cox (1933), has proven to be a very useful and practical one. It may not, however, provide fully for the classification of pure astroblastomas and polar spongioblastomas (see Russell and Rubinstein, 1977).

Russell and Rubinstein (1977) have proposed the subdivision of astrocytomas into five subtypes:

1. Protoplasmic
2. Fibrillary
3. Pilocytic
4. Gemistocytic
5. Anaplastic

There has been controversy as to how glioblastoma multiforme should be classified (*i.e.*, as anaplastic or as a separate category).

No one classification scheme is entirely satisfactory for glial tumors. As Bucy and Gustafson put it (1939), "Classification must be regarded as providing merely arbitrary pockets into which we can place tumors in order that they may be more easily considered. No two gliomas are identical." Recognizing the limitations of any classification attempt, consideration of the principal subtypes is nonetheless worthwhile for the insights it offers into the biologic variety of glial neoplasms. Important, too, is recognizing that the various subtypes of glial tumor cells vary according to the location of the tumor in the central nervous system.

Protoplasmic astrocytomas are a rare form of astrocytic tumor and are restricted to the cerebral hemispheres, although protoplasmic tumor cells can also be seen in cerebellar tumors. The cells resemble protoplasmic astrocytes, but they are generally more swollen and have fewer, shorter processes. No neuroglial fibrils are present. Because of a poor blood supply, these tumors frequently show microcystic degeneration.

Fibrillary astrocytomas represent a more common subtype, showing neuroglial fibrils in contrast to the protoplasmic tumors. Infiltration of normal brain, especially fiber tracts, is a notable tendency, as is cystic degeneration with the formation of eosinophilic hyaline granules. Tumors with a predominant fibrillary histologic cell type can arise at several sites in the CNS of individuals at any age. In the adult, they are most common in the cerebral hemispheres, whereas cerebellar, brain stem, and hypothalamic sites are more common in childhood and adolescence.

Pilocytic astrocytomas are classified as either the adult or juvenile form. The former are located in the cerebral hemispheres, as closely packed bundles of broad bipolar cells without a tendency to microcystic degeneration. The latter, as indicated by the name, are found in children, predominantly in the hypothalamus and cerebellum. Although they may show features consistent with malignant change, including vascular endothelial cell proliferation, these subtypes are associated with better survival than other astrocytoma types.

The subclass of gemistocytic astrocytomas is restricted to the cerebral hemispheres and, as a pure tumor, is rare (Sherer, 1940; Elvidge and Martinez-Coll,1956). Russell and Rubinstein (1977) indicate that this tumor subtype may be a precursor for glioblastoma multiforme since, from their experience, 80% actually show such a conversion. The cells making up these tumors are quite distinctive, with large globose cell bodies with hyaline and eosinophilic cytoplasm. Also showing distinctive, large, hyaline cytoplasm are the neoplastic glial cells of the subependymal astrocytomas of tuberous sclerosis.

Anaplasia is a tendency of astrocytomas, reflecting less a histologic subtype than a loss of differentiated cell properties. Studying a series of 98 astrocytomas, Russell and Rubinstein noted that 72 had undergone malignant change and that almost half of these (34) would be classified as glioblastomas. If only the diffuse cerebral astrocytomas are considered (*i.e.,* leaving out cerebellar tumors as well as the pilocytic tumors), then better than 90% appear to dedifferentiate to more malignant forms (Russell and Rubinstein, 1977).

Several features herald the onset of anaplasia (which, in the Kernohan grading system, corresponds to grade 3 and 4, whereas the benign tumors are in grade 1 and 2). At the macroscopic level, these include necrosis and hemorrhage, as well as evident vascular proliferation. At the microscopic level, prominent features are increased cellularity, pleomorphic tumor cells and cell nuclei, mitoses, and vascular proliferation, as well as endothelial cell proliferation and a marked infiltrative tendency (see Figures 37–10 through 37–14). These features are, of course, those of the glioblastoma multiforme. There has been substantial controversy in the literature as to whether anaplastic astrocytomas should be differentiated from glioblastoma multiforme in the sense that the former represents the staged development of anaplasia, whereas the latter may arise

as a malignancy without a precursor, more differentiated state. The evidence is not clear; and it is more than reasonable at this point to consider the two together, while leaving open the possibility that there is a distinct subclass of highly malignant, rapidly progressive tumors that may arise as *de novo* malignancies. Certainly this would fit some cases we have encountered clinically.

With the marked vascular proliferation characteristic of these tumors, there is the possibility of sarcomatous change, which has been estimated by Morantz *et al.* (1976) to occur in 8% of all cases of glioblastoma. Yet another feature, noted above, is the infiltrative nature of these tumors. Infiltration of the ependyma of the lateral and third ventricles is frequent. Once through the ependyma, metastatic spread of the tumor cells within the cerebrospinal fluid spaces (so-called "drop metastases") occurs. Remote extracranial metastasis is also possible and has been documented with increasing frequency (Ehrenreich and Devlin, 1958; Feigin *et al.,* 1958; Garret, 1958; Labitzke, 1962; Wisiol *et al.,* 1962; Rubinstein, 1967; Smith *et al.,* 1969).

The malignant glial tumors have a maximal incidence between ages 45 and 55. As noted earlier, there is a slight male preponderance. Sites of intracranial incidence, as determined from a 20-year survey of all gliomas (malignant and benign) by McKeran and Thomas (1980) are shown in Figure 37–15. The preponderance of frontal and temporal tumors is of interest. Table 37–5 shows the preponderance of intermediate and anaplastic tumors in this 20-year survey (1955–1975).

The natural history of the astrocytic tumors is as diverse as the pathology. For the more benign (*i.e.,* lower-grade) tumors, a long, slow course extending over several years is the rule, unless the particular tumor location leads to secondary effects, such as obstructive hydrocephalus or simply massive tumor and brain herniation at advanced stages. Substantial neurologic deficits can, of course, occur at any time and can make such relatively benign lesions malignant by virtue of their neurologic effects.

Even within the more anaplastic tumors, the growth rates of the tumors vary markedly. Although the overall rate of growth of astrocytic tumors is low, with a low growth fraction in even the most malignant tumors (Hoshino *et al.,* 1975b), any significant growth within the rigid cavity that is provided by the skull can

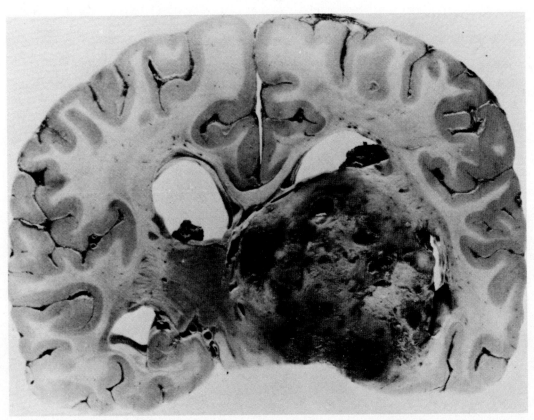

Figure 37-10. Coronal section of brain showing a glioblastoma involving the basal ganglia. Areas of viable tumor, hemorrhage, and necrosis can be seen grossly. Midline shift is substantial. From Russell, D. C., and Rubinstein, L. J.: *Pathology of Tumors of the Nervous System.* Williams & Wilkins Co., Baltimore, 1977, p. 229.

lead to rapidly increasing intracranial pressure with the displacement and compromise of vital brain structures, such as the brain stem (*i.e.,* herniation). Both the benign and malignant astrocytic tumors are characterized by the ability for local invasion. In the case of the malignant astrocytic tumors, whose growth is more rapid, destruction of normal tissue occurs, whereas the slower growth of the benign tumors can permit displacement of the normal tissue, hence greater structural and functional preservation.

The variability of tumor growth kinetics, location of the tumor, age of the patient, vascularity of the tumor, and a variety of less well-understood factors must then be taken into account if one is to talk about natural history (Gehan and Walker, 1977). For the low-grade tumors, survivals of five or more years are not unusual. For the more malignant tumors, survivals in untreated patients are a few months from the time of diagnosis. Generally, the clinical history is correspondingly short as well.

Clinical Presentation. The natural history of astrocytic tumors would suggest that both headaches and seizures would be likely to be early symptoms. Overall, headache appears to be the most common initial symptom (see Tables 37-6 and 37-7); although, as can be seen from a comparison of the data from the Toronto General Hospital (Morley, 1973) and the National Hospitals, London (McKeran and Thomas, 1980), it is not always clear-cut that headache is more common than seizures. By the time of first assessment, headache is quite clearly the dominant symptom. Headache, of course, reflects the raised intracranial pressure resulting from the tumor mass; the seizures reflect disordered neuronal and glial structure and function. As can be seen from Tables 37-6 and 37-7, mental change and hemiparesis were the most common presenting signs after headache and epilepsy. For focal signs, the location of the lesion is critical; but for the diffuse signs, such as headache, no notable correlation with lesion location has been identified.

The onset of symptoms may be either acute

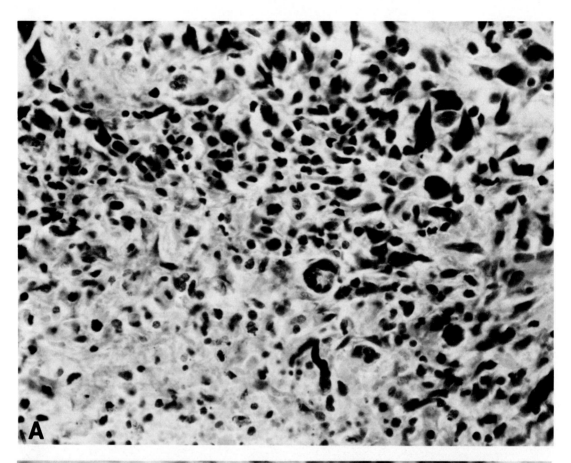

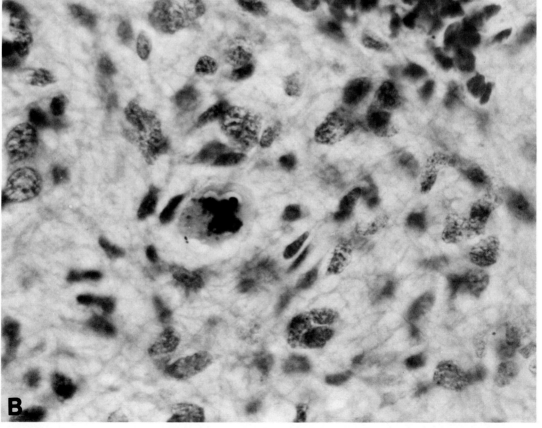

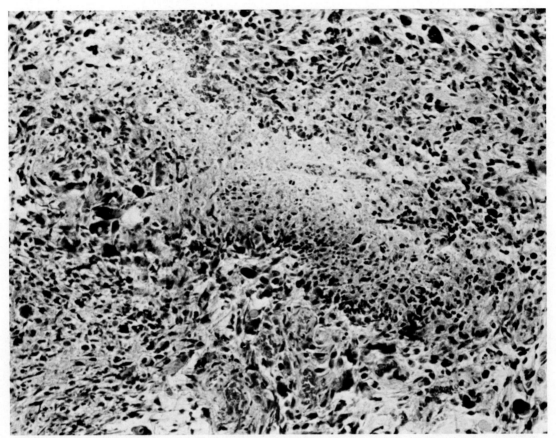

Figure 37–12. Glioblastoma showing regional necrosis and pseudopalisades formation. ×190. (Courtesy of Dr. Paul McKeever.)

or gradual. The occurrence of seizure activity in an adult is of acute onset by definition, but an additional 9 to 10% of patients presenting with other first symptoms also present acutely. In these, a possible vascular problem, such as a stroke, may be considered. The remaining patients have a more gradual onset, with more symptoms becoming apparent with time, whatever the initial problem. Progression of symptoms is the hallmark of glial tumors. Not surprisingly, gradual decline in neurologic function is most often associated with low-grade relatively benign astrocytomas, whereas more rapid, stepwise deterioration is found with anaplastic astrocytomas. In the National Hospitals, London, series, only 1 of 615 cerebral glioma cases failed to show clinical progression, suggestive of compressive or infiltrative lesion. Gehan and Walker (1977), in a

comprehensive study of prognostic factors relative to presenting symptoms, found that both seizures and cranial nerve symptoms were associated with a more favorable prognosis, whereas the presence or absence of headaches, personality changes, motor symptoms, speech abnormalities, and sensory problems made little difference (see Table 37–8).

With respect to clinical signs at first clinical assessment, hemiparesis (see Table 37–9) was the most common finding (61.7%) in the National Hospitals series. Cranial nerve palsy, mental deterioration, and papilledema all followed closely (52 to 54%). Hemianesthesia (34.6%), hemianopia (32.8%), dysphasia (28%), and visual failure (21.3%) complete the list.

From the Gehan and Walker study (1977), age is clearly an important factor, with the

Figure 37–11. (*A*) Region of glioblastoma showing features of hypercellularity of nuclear pleomorphism. ×479. (*B*) Abnormal mitosis in malignant glial tumor. The number of mitoses seen in any given field is indicative of degree of malignancy. ×723. (Courtesy of Dr. Paul McKeever.)

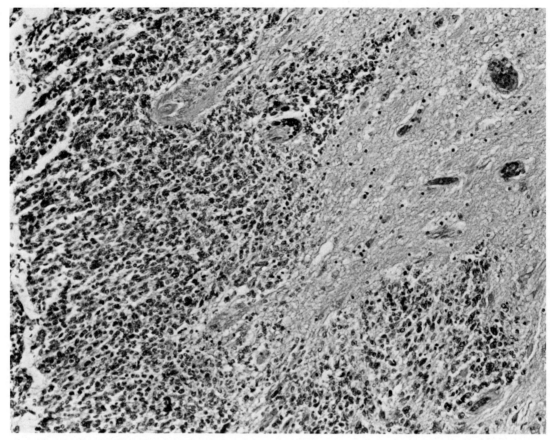

Figure 37–13. Invasive margin of glioblastoma. The local infiltrative nature of these tumors makes complete surgical resection extremely unlikely. ×190. (Courtesy of Dr. Paul McKeever.)

younger population faring significantly better than those over 60 years. Also, signs suggestive of a parietal lobe tumor indicate a less favorable prognosis. Cranial nerve signs again are favorable (see Table 37–8).

Investigation. A sequence for evaluation of the patient with an astrocytic tumor, or for that matter any brain tumor patient, is shown in Table 38–3, which is modified from Kornblith *et al.* (1982b).

The goals of any such assessment are several. These include (1) detection of any lesion, (2) localization and assessment of its extent, (3) ascertainment of its specific type and degree of malignancy, and (4) at times, if surgery is indicated, determination of the details of the arterial and venous vascular supply (Kendall, 1980).

The computerized tomographic (CT) scan, made possible by the work of Hounsfield and his colleagues (see Di Chiro and Brooks, 1979), has revolutionized glioma tumor diagnosis and follow-up, allowing high-resolution, non-

invasive determination of tumor and normal brain structure. Relying on the differential absorption of x-rays by different molecular constituents, the CT scanner distinguishes between cerebrospinal fluid, edema, normal brain (white and gray matter), as well as tumor tissue. With the addition of intravenous iodine-containing contrast, additional information as to the vascularity and, to some extent, the permeability of the tumor vasculature can be obtained. With the latest scanners providing for not only the traditional horizontal tomographic brain slices, but also coronal cuts and three-dimensional reconstructions, it has become the most accurate single diagnostic procedure available. A better than 95% success rate for the determination of the presence or absence of tumors has been noted with intraparenchymal lesions (Greitz, 1975; Gonzalez *et al.,* 1976), although low-grade gliomas are less reliably detected.

Most glial-derived tumors, and particularly the astrocytomas with which this section is

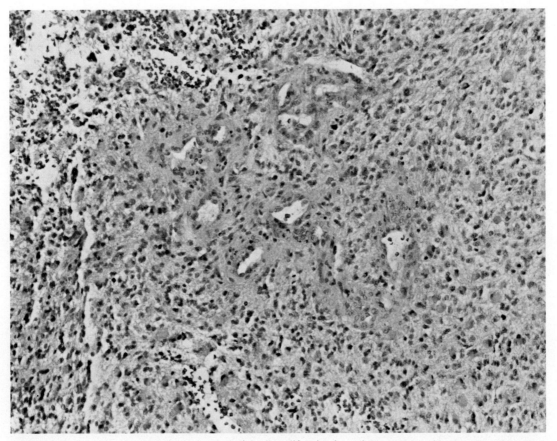

Figure 37-14. Increased vascularity and endothelial cell proliferation in a glioblastoma. ×190. (Courtesy of Dr. Paul McKeever.)

concerned, appear as areas of abnormal, mixed attenuation, much of which is in the nearly normal range. White matter edema is common surrounding the tumor, especially in the more malignant tumors. Calcification is seen in approximately 18% of glial tumors, is most common in the more benign tumors (30%), and is least common in the high-grade lesions (10%) (see Figure 37-16 through 37-18). Ninety-eight percent of malignant astrocytomas show contrast enhancement (see Figure 37-19A, B); but, as pointed out by Kendall (1980), it is not always of high intensity. The enhancement is generally irregular, frequently yielding a ring. Homogeneous enhancement occurs in about 20% of malignant astrocytomas, making them difficult to distinguish from meningiomas, metastatic lesions, and a variety of other tumor and nontumor lesions.

Grade I astrocytomas are of lower or isodense attenuation, show calcification in about one-third of cases, and have little or no asso-

ciated edema. They show little, if any, contrast enhancement. Grade II astrocytomas generally fall in between these characteristics and those of the more malignant tumors.

Isotope (gamma) encephalography, generally with pertechnetate, may be useful but is less reliable than CT and provides less differential diagnostic information. The appearance of the so-called butterfly glioma, which is an infiltrating tumor of the corpus callosum, is characteristic. New isotopic techniques, especially those of positron emission computed tomographic scanning, appear very promising for revealing functional, metabolic, as well as other dynamic aspects of astrocytic tumor (Di Chiro *et al.,* 1982; see "New Developments and Future Prospects" at the end of this chapter).

Angiography, usually performed by the retrograde transfemoral route and no longer a screening procedure because of the effectiveness of CT scanning, nonetheless remains useful. Preoperative angiography details the surgi-

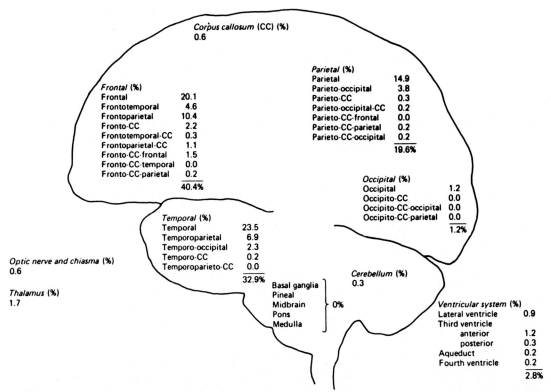

Figure 37–15. The incidence of gliomas at different cerebral sites, investigated at the National Hospitals, London (1955–1975). CC, corpus callosum. From McKeran, R. O., and Thomas, D. G. T.: The clinical study of gliomas. In Thomas, D. G. T., and Graham, D. I. (eds.): *Brain Tumors. Scientific Basis, Clinical Investigation and Current Therapy.* Butterworth, Boston, 1980, p. 200.

cally relevant tumor vasculature, giving useful landmarks for the resection. The appearance of early draining veins is associated with the more malignant astrocytomas. Angiography will also indicate the presence of highly vascular lesions, such as arteriovenous malformations and aneurysms, and may increase resolution and localization in the posterior fossa. Because angiography is an invasive technique, significant complications can occur, including stroke, embolism, and hemorrhage.

Therapy and Management. Just as for other tumors, three therapeutic avenues are open in the treatment of astrocytomas: surgery, radiation, and chemotherapy. Several general points in relationship to therapy need to be made. Because of their origin in the parenchyma of the brain, astrocytomas are, by their very nature and the functions served by the brain around them, difficult to remove by surgery, whether they are benign or malignant. Although the lower-grade astrocytomas are associated with longer survivals, they nonetheless present difficulties in excision that are

greater or lesser dependent on their location in the brain. For the more malignant tumors (*i.e.,* astrocytomas of grade III or IV), with their marked propensity for local invasion, the problems are even more significant. It is those factors that have made astrocytomas, particularly of the malignant type, so difficult to treat and notorious for poor survival. Perhaps more than for tumors in other body locations, the availability of effective therapy adjunctive to surgical excision is critical.

SURGICAL TREATMENT. The role of surgery in astrocytic tumors of the central nervous system is severalfold. Perhaps the most important aspect is the establishment of a diagnosis. Although the CT scan has a high degree of accuracy, the pathologic examination of tissue obtained at surgery conveys very specific and sometimes unexpected information (such as abscess as opposed to glioma). Yet another facet is the decompression of normal brain tissue, with its accompanying relief of such symptoms as headache, deterioration in mental status, or loss of visual acuity, all of which

Table 37–5. Distribution of Different Histologic Types of Glioma, Investigated at the National Hospitals, London (1955–1975)

TYPE OF TUMOR		FRONTAL	TEMPORAL	PARIETAL	OCCIPITAL	CORPUS CALLOSUM	THALAMUS	CERE-BELLUM	LATERAL VENTRICLE	AQUEDUCT	THIRD VENTRICLE	FOURTH VENTRICLE	OPTIC NERVE
Well differentiated	Count	N=22	N=15	N=7	N=0	N=0	N=1	N=0	N=0	N=0	N=2	N=0	N=1
	Row %	45.8	31.3	14.6	0	0	2.1	0	0	0	4.2	0	2.1
	Column %	9.0	7.4	5.6	0	0	10.0	0	0	0	25.0	0	50.0
	Total %	3.6	2.4	1.1	0	0	0.2	0	0	0	0.3	0	0.2
Intermediate		N=139	N=120	N=58	N=4	N=1	N=8	N=2	N=3	N=1	N=6	N=1	N=1
		40.4	34.9	16.9	1.2	0.3	2.3	0.6	0.9	0.3	1.7	0.3	0.3
		56.7	58.8	47.5	50.0	25.0	80.0	100.0	50.0	100.0	75.0	100.0	50.0
		22.7	19.6	9.5	0.7	0.2	1.3	0.3	0.5	0.2	1.0	0.2	0.2
Anaplastic		N=66	N=61	N=45	N=4	N=3	N=1	N=0	N=0	N=0	N=0	N=0	N=0
		36.7	33.9	25.0	2.2	1.7	0.6	0	0	0	0	0	0
		26.9	29.9	36.9	50.0	75.0	10.0	0	0	0	0	0	0
		10.8	10.0	7.3	0.7	0.5	0.2	0	0	0	0	0	0
Oligodendroglioma		N=17	N=7	N=11	N=0	N=0	N=0	N=0	N=1	N=0	N=0	N=0	N=0
		47.2	19.4	30.6	0	0	0	0	2.8	0	0	0	0
		6.9	3.4	9.0	0	0	0	0	16.7	0	0	0	0
		2.8	1.1	1.8	0	0	0	0	0.2	0	0	0	0
Ependymoma		N=0	N=1	N=1	N=0	N=0	N=0	N=0	N=2	N=0	N=0	N=0	N=0
		0	25.0	25.0	0	0	0	0	50.0	0	0	0	0
		0	0.5	0.8	0	0	0	0	33.3	0	0	0	0
		0	0.2	0.2	0	0	0	0	0.3	0	0	0	0
Astrocytosis (nonspecific gliosis on autopsy)		N=1	N=0	N=0	N=0	N=0	N=0	N=0	N=0	N=0	N=0	N=0	N=0
		100.0	0	0	0	0	0	0	0	0	0	0	0
		0.4	0	0	0	0	0	0	0	0	0	0	0
		0.2	0	0	0	0	0	0	0	0	0	0	0

Reprinted by permission from McKeran, P. O., and Thomas, D. G. T.: The clinical study of gliomas. In Thomas, D. G. T., and Graham, D. I. (eds.): *Brain Tumours: Scientific Basis, Clinical Investigation and Current Therapy.* Butterworth, Boston, 1980.

The first figure in each box indicates the total number of cases, the second the percentage of the horizontal row, the third the percentage in the vertical row with that particular physical sign, and the fourth the overall percentage of a specific tumor type with a particular physical sign in the total population of tumors. (Total number of cases: 615.)

Table 37-6.   The Frequency of Symptoms at Presentation Compared to that at Assessment and Diagnosis in Cerebral Gliomas Investigated at the National Hospitals, London (1955–1975)

SYMPTOM	RELATIVE FREQUENCY AS INITIAL SYMPTOM (%)	RELATIVE FREQUENCY AT ASSESSMENT AND DIAGNOSIS (%)
Epilepsy	38.3	53.9
Grand mal	15.9	20.4
Focal	14.7	22.8
Temporal lobe	7.2	8.6
Minor absence	0.5	2.1
No epilepsy	61.7	46.1
Headache	35.2	71.4
Mental change	16.5	52.2
Hemiparesis	10.3	43.3
Vomiting	7.5	31.5
Dysphasia	6.9	27.0
Impaired consciousness	4.6	24.8
Visual failure	4.3	17.9
Hemianesthesia	3.4	13.6
Hemianopia	1.8	8.1
Cranial nerve palsy	1.8	10.9
Miscellaneous	2.3	7.0

Reprinted by permission from McKeran, R. O.; and Thomas, D. G. T.: The clinical study of gliomas. In Thomas, D. G. T.; and Graham, D. I. (eds.): *Brain Tumours. Scientific Basis, Clinical Investigation and Current Therapy.* Butterworth, Boston, 1980, p. 202.)

may or may not be relieved by the administration of corticosteroids. Substantial removal of tumor burden (for example, 90% in extensive procedures) should, in addition, make adjunctive therapies theoretically more effective. Surgery is, however, unlikely to remove an established focal neurologic deficit, unless it is a remote pressure effect.

Surgical procedures for astrocytomas can take the form of biopsy, partial resection, gross total tumor removal, and partial or complete lobectomy in the case of tumors in certain frontal, occipital, temporal, and cerebellar locations. More extensive surgical attempts (*i.e.,* hemispherectomy) have been reported (Bell and Karnosh, 1949), but not widely adopted.

Biopsy, by either needle or open techniques, can be useful in cases of otherwise inaccessible lesions (dominant parietal lobe, thalamus) or for patients unable to tolerate a craniotomy and resection. Jelsma and Bucy (1969) suggested biopsy as an approach to all gliomas, but the data of others subsequently suggested that the relatively high rate of inconclusive diagnosis (30%) may limit the utility of the biopsy by itself (Rossi *et al.,* 1979). In addition, risk of hemorrhage and postbiopsy edema add to the limitations. CT-directed stereotactic biopsy, however, seems quite useful for difficult-to-reach areas.

The practicality of more extensive surgical resections (partial resection, gross total tumor removal, partial or total lobectomy) depends on the location and extent of infiltration of the tumor, whether benign or malignant. The locally invasive properties of the malignant tumors make gross total removal difficult, if not quite unlikely. As noted by Garfield (1980), reports of the effects upon survival of subtotal or partial removal of supratentorial malignant gliomas have not been consistent (Frankel and German, 1958; Roth and Elvidge, 1960; Hitchcock and Sato, 1964; Jelsma and Bucy, 1967; Weir, 1973.) This inconsistency is not surprising in that the advent of high-resolution CT scanning has demonstrated that gross total tumor removal is almost never that, but, in fact, a partial resection.

The benefits of resection, although they may vary from patient to patient, are, nonetheless, clear. With operative mortality less than 1%, and with careful surgical technique, it is possible to offer the patient considerable benefit, if even for a limited time, especially when tumor bulk *per se* is the problem. Where advanced neurologic deficits exist and are unlikely to improve, diagnosis and at least some decompression may still be helpful. Of course, the decision as to how much to attempt must be individualized. For the more benign forms of the astrocytomas, particularly those of childhood, resection with or without radiation therapy may be associated with long survivals (Gol and McKissock, 1959; Gol, 1961, 1962).

In some cases, it is possible to consider reoperation for recurrent malignant glial

Table 37–7. Correlation of First Symptom with Pathology of Intracranial Gliomas (Toronto General Hospital)

PATHOLOGIC DIAGNOSIS	HEADACHE	EPILEPSY (UNSPECIFIED)	GRAND MAL EPILEPSY	FOCAL EPILEPSY	MOTOR, SENSORY, VISUAL, SPEECH IMPAIRMENT	MENTAL OR PERSONALITY CHANGE	OTHER	NOT KNOWN	
Glioblastoma	278	10	72	45	160	136	50	2	753
Astrocytoma (malignant)	131	18	70	31	56	32	37	1	376
Astrocytoma (fibrillary)	14	3	9	3	3	1	8		41
Oligodendroglioma	13	0	10	2	4	3	0		32
Mixed gliomas	16	4	8	7	5	4	2		46
Glioma (unspecified)	14	0	7	1	6	2	5		35
Ependymoma	27	0	1	4	4	3	8		47
Microgliomatosis	6	0	0	0	1	2	0		9
Medulloblastoma	11	0	0	0	4	1	3		19
Other	7	0	1	1	3	2	2		16
Total	517	35	178	94	246	186	115	3	1374

Reprinted by permission from Morley, T. P.: Intrinsic tumors of the cerebral hemispheres. In Youmans, J. R. (ed.): *Neurological Surgery*, Vol. 3. W. B. Saunders Company, Philadelphia, 1973, p. 1355.

Table 37–8. Correlation Between Early Symptoms and Prognosis of Brain Tumors

PATIENT CHARACTERISTIC	NUMBER OF PATIENTS	NUMBER OF DEATHS	MEDIAN SURVIVAL RATES	P
Age (yr)				
0–49	61	54	40	
50–59	76	75	29	0.005
60 and over	88	86	18	
Diagnosis				
Glioblastoma multiforme and malignant glioma	191	184	25	
Malignant astrocytoma	18	16	33	0.19
All others	16	15	36	
Sex				
Male	143	135	27	
Female	82	80	25	0.24
Location				
Cerebellum	3	3	18	
BG thalamus	2	2	14	
Frontal	72	67	25	
Occipital	15	14	43	0.15
Parietal	59	59	21	
Temporal	74	70	27	
Tumor characteristics				
Hypovascular				
No	207	199	25	
Yes	18	16	40	0.03
Invasive				
No	98	9	25	
Yes	127	12	27	0.78
Solid				
No	161	156	27	
Yes	64	59	22	0.44
Necrotic				
No	110	102	24	
Yes	115	113	27	0.95
Soft				
No	115	111	24	
Yes	110	104	28	0.33
Friable				
No	195	187	24	
Yes	30	28	35	0.055
Cystic				
No	174	165	27	
Yes	51	50	25	0.21
Hard				
No	200	191	28	
Yes	25	24	14	0.13
Vascular				
No	153	147	25	
Yes	72	68	28	0.45
Encapsulated				
No	212	203	26	
Yes	13	12	26	0.28
Symptoms				
Headache				
No	97	94	28	
Yes	128	121	25	0.56
Personality change				
No	144	137	27	
Yes	81	78	25	0.85
Motor symptoms				
No	111	105	27	
Yes	114	110	26	0.37
Seizure				
No	163	160	24	
Yes	62	55	31	0.05

Table 37–8.   *(Continued)*

PATIENT CHARACTERISTIC	NUMBER OF PATIENTS	NUMBER OF DEATHS	MEDIAN SURVIVAL RATES	P
Speech				
No	166	157	27	0.43
Yes	59	58	25	
General complaints				
No	209	199	26	0.68
Yes	16	16	27	
Sensory				
No	194	186	27	0.70
Yes	31	29	23	
Cranial nerves, II, III, IV, VI				
No	208	198	25	0.13
Yes	17	17	34	
Rapid unconsciousness				
No	212	202	26	0.82
Yes	13	13	26	
Cranial nerves other				
No	217	207	26	0.62
Yes	8	8	27	
Cerebellar				
No	222	212	27	0.77
Yes	3	3	12	
Other				
No	182	173	27	0.32
Yes	43	42	21	
Time from symptoms to operation (wk)				
0–25	200	191	27	
26–51	12	12	19	0.85
52 or more	13	12	22	
Left or right				
Left	102	99	22	0.13
Right	123	116	28	
Type of operation				
Biopsy only	12	12	14	0.1
Partial or total resection	213	203	27	
All Patients	225	215	26	

Reprinted by permission from Gehan, E. A., and Walker, M. D.: Prognostic factors for patients with brain tumors. *Natl. Cancer Inst. Monogr.,* **46:**189–195, 1977.

Table 37–9.   The Frequency of Signs at Assessment and Diagnosis in Cerebral Gliomas, Investigated at the National Hospitals, London (1955–1975)

SIGNS	ABSOLUTE NUMBER OF CASES	RELATIVE FREQUENCY (%)
Hemiparesis	403	61.7
Cranial nerve palsy	354	54.2
Mental deterioration	349	53.4
Papilledema	340	52.1
Hemianesthesia	226	34.6
Hemianopia	214	32.8
Dysphasia	183	28.0
Visual failure	139	21.3

Reprinted by permission from McKeran, R. O.; and Thomas, D. G. T.: The clinical study of gliomas. In Thomas, D. G. T., and Graham, D. I. (eds.): *Brain Tumors. Scientific Basis, Clinical Investigation and Current Therapy.* Butterworth, Boston, 1980.

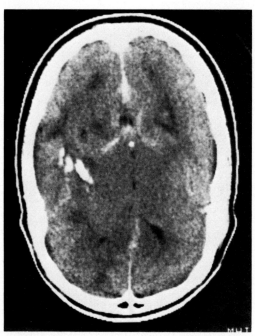

Figure 37–16. CT scan showing right parietal low-grade astrocytoma with calcification. Contrast has been used for this scan, but tumor itself shows little or no enhancement.

tumors, especially where tumor bulk is the problem. In selected cases, this may be associated with prolonged survival. In an analysis of the indications for reoperation, Young *et al.* (1981) found that reoperation is most likely to

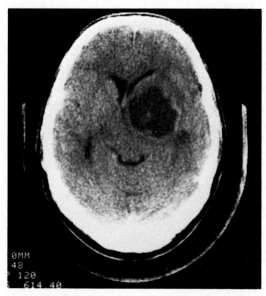

Figure 37–17. CT scan showing malignant astrocytoma in left frontoparietal area. The low-density area is indicative of tumor. No contrast has been used for this scan.

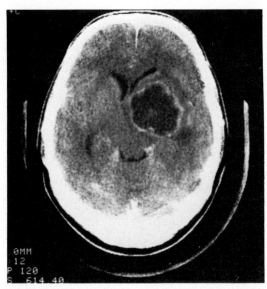

Figure 37–18. Contrast has been used and the tumor rim is clearly enhancing. The central area may include a sizable necrotic component.

produce good results when the Karnofsky rating is at least 60, and the interval between operations is more than six months.

RADIATION THERAPY. The data of the Brain Tumor Study Group (BTSG) (Gehan and Walker, 1977; Walker *et al.,* 1978) suggest that radiation therapy has a clear role in the treatment of malignant gliomas. In these studies, all patients received surgery and were randomized to control group (no further treatment), x-ray therapy, 1,3-*bis*(2-chlorethyl)-1-nitrosourea (BCNU), and BCNU plus x-ray therapy. The percentiles of survival time by treatment group (see Table 37–10) indicate the substantial contribution of radiation therapy to survival. These data are in agreement with the other studies in the literature, even though the lack of uniformity in selection and treatment of patients makes precise comparisons difficult. Despite these beneficial effects early in the postoperative course, however, the radiated patients eventually succumb to the disease process, indicating that radiation therapy is not the final answer to malignant astrocytomas. All curves (as noted by Salcman, 1980) converge at 18 to 24 months, irrespective of treatment (see Figure 37–20).

Its eventual failure is recognized, but radiation therapy is clearly warranted after surgery. The total dose of radiation that provides both optimal effectiveness and least risk of radiation necrosis or other radiation-related complications is generally felt to be between 5000

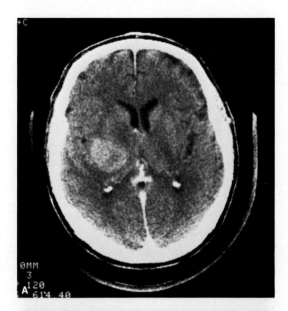

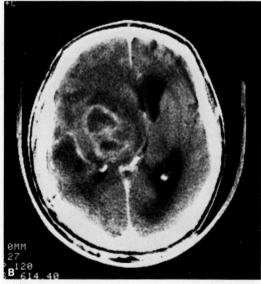

Figure 37-19. (*A*) and (*B*) CT scans in a patient with progressive glioblastoma. Contrast has been used. The progressive and rapid destruction of normal brain tissue is evident in the scan. The scans were done only seven weeks apart.

and 6000 rads, with the major portion (70 to 75%) of this dose being delivered as whole-brain irradiation and the rest to the operative site alone. Some authors disagree with this (see Scanlon and Taylor, 1979). Doses of radiation above 6000 to 7000 rads appear to be associated with an unacceptable risk of radiation necrosis, although improvement in survival is suggested with higher doses (up to 8000 rads) to the local tumor site (Salazar *et al.,* 1979;

Kornblith *et al.,* 1982b). Cobalt-60 megavoltage irradiation is considered standard inasmuch as it has a small penumbra (margin outside the main energy beam) and better absorption of energy at a greater depth. Shaw *et al.* (1978) and Catterall *et al.* (1980) have attempted to utilize fast neutron beam irradiation. Although extensive coagulative necrosis of much of the tumor mass was noted in 13 patients who came to autopsy (out of a total of 34), the length and quality of survival of these patients did not show any improvement.

Common practice is to use multiple fields and fractionated doses. The use of multiple fields ensures even delivery to the tumor and avoidance of hot spots or areas of overirradiation of normal tissue. (See Capra, 1980, for review.) Fractionation (200 rads/day over six to seven weeks, with weekend breaks) is utilized to take advantage of recovery of cells from sublethal damage, reoxygenation of the tumor, and repair of normal tissue, as well as growing tumor. Efforts have been and are currently underway with misonidazole and metronidazole as radiosensitizers to enhance glial tumor cell killing (Urtasun *et al.,* 1976, 1977; Bleehen, 1980; Carabell *et al.,* 1981; Wasserman *et al.,* 1981). Bromodeoxyurine has been and is also being utilized (Sano *et al.,* 1968; see also Bloom, 1975), as is hyperoxygenation (Chang *et al.,* 1975).

Overall results for patients with malignant astrocytomas (grade IV, glioblastoma multiforme) receiving conventional megavoltage radiation therapy include 25 to 50% with one-year survival, 10% with two-year survival, and 0 to 3% with five-year survivals (Kornblith *et al.,* 1982b). Survivals for patients with grade III lesions are better, with up to 70% surviving for one year, 40% for two years, and 10 to 20% for five or more years (Stage and Stein, 1974; Bloom, 1975; Sheline, 1975, 1976; Walsh *et al.* 1975; Salazar *et al.,* 1979). As has been noted in many studies now (and very carefully in the BTSG work), age is an important factor, with patients younger than 20 years faring significantly better than older patients, especially those 50 years and older (Marsa *et al.,* 1973; Stage and Stein, 1974; Gehan and Walker, 1977; Salazar *et al.,* 1979).

The value of radiation therapy in patients with low-grade gliomas (grades I and II) has been more controversial. Where the tumor has been completely excised, it does not appear to be of benefit (Leibel *et al.,* 1975). Where removal is incomplete, the data, although not as

Table 37–10. Percentiles of Survival Time by Treatment and Other Classifications of Patients in the Valid Study Group

PATIENT CHARACTERISTIC	PATIENTS (NO.)	DEATHS (NO.)	PERCENTILES OF SURVIVAL TIME, (WK)			
			75	*50*	*25*	*P*
Treatment						
Control	31	31	9	14	21	
XRT*	70	65	18	36	50	<0.001
BCNU†	51	51	9	18	28	
BCNU + XRT	73	68	16	34	60	
Adequate treatment						
No	58	56	4	9	26	=0.002
Yes	167	159	18	30	49	
Total	225	215	13	26	48	
Protocol violations	78	72	9	33	49	=0.70

Reprinted by permission from Gehan, E. A., and Walker, M. D.: Prognostic factors for patients with brain tumors. *Natl. Cancer Inst. Monogr.,* **46**:189–195, 1977.
* x-ray therapy
† 1,3-*bis*(2-chloroethyl)-1-nitrosourea

good as one would like them to be, indicate that localized radiation therapy is of benefit, a benefit which seems to increase with longer follow-up (Bouchard and Peirce, 1960; Marsa *et al.,* 1973, 1975; Bloom, 1975; Bloom and Walsh, 1975; Leibel *et al.,* 1975; Sheline, 1975; Fazekas, 1977; Griffin *et al.,* 1979; Kim *et al.,* 1980). Leibel *et al.* (1975), for example, have shown a five-year survival of 46 percent versus 19 percent in irradiated and non-irradiated pa-

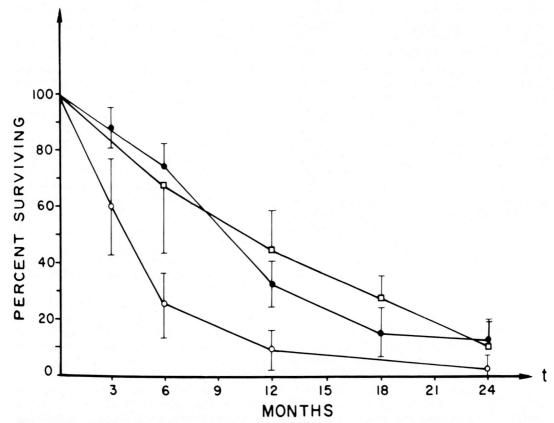

Figure 37–20. Percentage of glioblastoma patients surviving as a function of time and treatment. The means ± 1 SD are plotted to demonstrate the variability in survival rates reported for different groups of patients treated by operation alone (○, 6 studies, 349 cases), operation + radiotherapy (●, 11 studies, 568 cases), and operation + radiotherapy + drug (□, 5 studies, 146 cases). Note the convergence of all survival curves at 18 to 24 months. From Salcman, M.: Survival in glioblastoma: Historical perspective. *Neurosurgery,* **7**(5):437, 1980.

tients, respectively (see also Dibden, 1962; Gol, 1962; Kramer, 1973).

In general, then, radiation therapy as an adjunct to incomplete surgical excision for low-grade astrocytomas appears warranted with a regime similar to that for the more malignant astrocytic lesions. For children, careful thought is required as radiation may be more damaging to the central nervous system, as well as to body development in general (Onoyama *et al.*, 1975). Radiation is not indicated, as a general rule, for microcystic astrocytomas of the cerebellum in young children.

CHEMOTHERAPY. Although surgery and radiation therapy are of benefit for patients with astrocytomas, additional therapy is required. Chemotherapy for such tumors is an obvious possibility, and various chemotherapeutic agents have been tested singly or in combination since the late 1950s. The localization of these tumors and their relative lack of propensity to metastasize would seem to make them ideal candidates for chemotherapy.

Several features complicate the chemotherapy of brain tumors. They include (1) heterogeneity of biologic properties despite indistinguishable histology; (2) the presence of the blood-brain barrier to limit, or at least complicate, drug delivery; (3) poorly understood tumor cell kinetics (Hoshino *et al.*, 1975a; Hoshino, 1977); (4) variations in vasculature and tumor structure, blood flow, oxygen supply, permeability, blood-to-brain transport, and necrosis that cannot be predicted on the basis of any simple model; and (5) significant variability in course and survival with tumor location in the brain (Levin and Edwards, 1980; Balsberg *et al.*, 1983; Horowitz *et al.*, 1983; Kornblith *et al.*, 1982b; Molnar *et al.*, 1983). As has been pointed out, as the distance from the capillary to the tumor cell becomes greater (*i.e.*, as the tumor enlarges), the less likely it is that adequate drug concentrations will reach the tumor because of the concentration gradients, diffusional limits, and chemical and biotransformation of the agent (Levin *et al.*, 1976). In addition, the drug concentrations achieved may be sufficient only to induce resistance, not to produce any significant cytotoxicity.

These difficulties, together with the problems of adequate, properly randomized, and controlled studies conducted in a setting where both surgery and radiation therapy have also been carried out, have made progress with brain tumor chemotherapy slow. A summary of the clinical trials to date is given in Table

37–11 from Kornblith *et al.* (1982b). Another representation of the data, taken from Levin and Edwards (1980), is given in Table 37–12.

The frequency of nitrosourea use (CCNU or BCNU) in the various trials conducted to date attests to the interest and effort exerted on these agents over the last 20 years. The nitrosoureas seem particularly suited to brain tumor therapy because they are highly lipid soluble, thereby having the capability of penetrating the blood-brain barrier. Early phase II studies (Walker and Hurwitz, 1970; Wilson *et al.*, 1970) showed improvement in almost 50% of patients on an 80 to 100 mg/m^2/day for three days every six to eight weeks schedule, and thus encouraged more studies. More precise answers as to the effectiveness of BCNU, however, came with the Brain Tumor Study Group controlled prospective randomized trials (Walker *et al.*, 1978) which showed that, although radiation therapy increased median survival by 150%, BCNU only added 30% to median survival. However, at 18 months, approximately 20% of the patients who received both BCNU and radiation therapy were still alive, while less than half as many patients who received only one therapeutic modality were alive.

CCNU (1-(2-chloroethyl)-3—cyclohexyl-1-nitrosourea) can be taken orally and, therefore, has been easy to deliver. Evaluated by the E.O.R.T.C. Brain Tumor Group in a well-controlled trial, it was concluded that CCNU prolongs total survival time and yields objective remission in 30% of patients, but that it should be administered only after relapse (for patients who have a progression-free interval) (E.O.R.T.C., 1978). Other studies, however, have not demonstrated CCNU's value (Reagan *et al.*, 1976; Weir *et al.*, 1976; Garrett *et al.*, 1978).

Procarbazine has been reported to be active against brain tumors (Kumar *et al.*, 1974) and has been utilized in combination with CCNU and vincristine by Shapiro and Young (1976), with a median survival of 50 weeks. Gutin *et al.* (1975) and Levin *et al.* (1980) used the procarbazine-CCNU-vincristine treatment for patients with recurrent malignant brain tumors, with 42% showing disease stabilization, a median time to progression of 26 weeks, and 30% survival without tumor progression at one year. The combination of BCNU and hydroxyurea with radiation may also be of value (Levin *et al.*, 1979). Other nonrandomized studies have also looked at various combinations of chemotherapy agents, but the data

Table 37–11. Summary of Chemotherapy Trials

AUTHOR	STUDY DESIGN	TUMOR TYPE* AND PERCENT	NUMBER (EVALUABLE/ENTERED)	PRETREATMENT CONDITIONS	TREATMENT GROUPS	RESULTS† MTP	RESULTS† MST	COMMENTS
Levin	Randomized	GBM 62 Non-GBM 37	99/130	Surgery	RadTH & BCNU RadTh, BCNU & hydroxyurea	31 wk 42		Significant at $P = 0.04$
Sweet	Randomized	Astrocytoma III & IV 21		Surgery & RadTh	BCNU BCNU & VM-26	61 wk 94		Difference not statistically significant
Salero	Randomized	GBM 100	102/105	Surgery Randomize in 2 wk	RadTh RadTh & BCNU RadTh & CCNU	38 wk 45 52	45 wk 52 69	RadTh & CCNU only significantly better than RadTh alone. $P = 0.05$
Jellinger	Consecutive Historic Selective	GBM 66 MA 44	116	Surgery	Supportive care RadTh COMP‡ RadTh & COMP	16 wk 29 29 30	23 wk 46 46 58	Uncontrolled, consecutive and selected patients. Any therapy better than supportive care alone
Garrett	Randomized	GBM 68 MA 29 Other 3	69/74	Biopsy	RadTh RadTh & CCNU		35 wk 56	Not statistically significant
Heiss	Consecutive & Historic	GBM 100	77	Surgery Some RadTh	Control CCNU Polychemotherapy COMP	11 wk 15 20 39	27 wk 28 35 46	Combined retrospective and previous series. Not stratified by RadTh. COMP appeared better
EORTC-BTG (Hildebrand) 1. Randomized		GBM 40 Astro. III & IV 31	81/111	Surgery & RadTh Good performance status, no steroids	CCNU (after surgery) CCNU (after prog.)	34.5 wk 31	43 wk } 62	Significant $P = 0.05$
2. Randomized		Other 29	22/111	Surgery & RadTh Poor performance status, steroids required	Control CCNU		21.5 wk } 31	Significant $P = 0.01$
Walker	Randomized	GBM 90 MA 9 Other 1	222/303	Surgery & randomize in 2 wk	Control BCNU RadTh BCNU & RadTh	14 wk 18.5 35.0 34.5		RadTh and RadTh & BCNU statistically significant from control $P = 0.001$
Shapiro	Randomized	Malignant glioma 33	33	Surgery	BCNU & RadTh BCNU & VCR BCNU, VCR, & RadTh	30.0 wk 44.5		No significant difference demonstrated

Author	Design	Tumor type	%	N	Protocol	Treatment	MTP	MST	Comments
Reagan	Randomized	Astrocytoma III & IV		63 / 72	Surgery; Randomize in 2 wk	RadTh / CCNU / RadTh & CCNU	30 wk / 17 / 30	49 wk / 28 / 52	Suboptimal RadTh (5000 rads). Stopped treating upon recurrence. CCNU inferior to other treatments $P = 0.02$
Walker	Randomized	GBM / MA / Other	84 / 11 / 5	358 / 467	Surgery; Randomize in 2 wk	MeCCNU / RadTH / RadTh & MeCCNU / RadTh & BCNU	24 wk / 36 / 42 / 51		RadTH and BCNU vs. RadTh, $P = 0.072$; MCNU vs RadTh, $P = 0.048$
Weir	Randomized & crossover	Astrocytoma III & IV / Other	97 / 7	40	Surgery; Randomize in 2 wk	RadTh / CCNU / RadTh & CCNU	23 wk / 14 / 31	27 wk / 37 / 36	7 RadTh crossed to CCNU; 10 CCNU crossed to RadTh. Those who had combination treatment survived longer
Seiler	Consecutive vs. historic	GBM / MA	63 / 37	52	Surgery; RadTh	CCNU / Procarbazine / Bleomycin / Control	56 wk		No significant difference
Eagan	Randomized	GBM / MA	71 / 29	42 / 43	Surgery; RadTh; Randomize in 2 wk	Dianhydrogalactitol / Control	51 wk / 67 wk / 35		Split course RadTh given to half the patients. DAG vs. control, $P = 0.02$

* GBM = Glioblastoma multiformi; MA = malignant astrocytoma;
† MTP = median time to progression; MST = median survival time.
‡ "COMP" = CCNU, vincristine, methotrexate, and procarbazine.

(Levin, V. A.; Wilson, C. B.; Davis, R.; et al.: A phase III comparison of BCNU, hydroxyurea, and radiation therapy to BCNU and radiation therapy for treatment of primary malignant gliomas. J. Neurosurg., 51:526–532, 1979; Sweet, D. L.; Hendler, F. J.; Hanlon, K.; et al.: Treatment of grade III and IV astrocytomas with BCNU alone and in combination with VM-26 following surgery and radiation therapy. Cancer Treat. Rep., 63:1707–1711, 1979; Salero, C. L.; Monfardini, S.; Brambilla, C.; et al.: Controlled study with BCNU vs. CCNU as adjuvant chemotherapy following surgery plus radiotherapy for gliomas. Acta Neurochir. (Wien.), 51:243–48, 1979; Jellinger, K.; Kothbauer, P.; Volc, D.; et al.: Combination chemotherapy (COMP protocol) and radiotherapy of anaplastic supratentorial gliomas. Acta Neurochir. (Wien.), 51:1–13, 1979; Garrett, M. J.; Hughes, H. J.; and Freedman, L. S.: A comparison of radiotherapy alone with radiotherapy and CCNU in cerebral glioma. Clin. Oncol. 4:71–76, 1978; Heiss, W. D.: Chemotherapy of malignant gliomas: Comparison of the effect of polychemo- and CCNU-therapy. Acta Neurochir. (Wien.), 42:109–115, 1978; E.O.R.T.C. Brain Tumor Group: Effect of CCNU on survival rate of objective remission and duration of free interval in patients with malignant brain glioma—Final evaluation. Eur. J. Cancer, 14:851–856, 1978; Walker, M.D.; Alexander, F., Jr.; Hunt, W. E.; et al.: An evaluation of BCNU and/or radiotherapy in the treatment of anaplastic gliomas. (A cooperative clinical trial for the Brain Tumor Study Group.) J. Neurosurg., 49:333–343, 1978; Shapiro, W. R., and Young, D. F.: Chemotherapy of malignant glioma with BCNU and vincristine. Neurology, 24:380, 1974; Reagan, T. J.; Bisel, H. J.; Childs, D. S.; et al.: Controlled study of CCNU and radiation therapy in malignant astrocytoma. J. Neurosurg. 44:186–190, 1976; Walker, M. D.; Green, S. B.; Byar, D. P.; et al.: Randomized comparisons of radiotherapy and nitrosoureas for malignant glioma after surgery. N. Engl. J. Med., 303:1323–1329, 1980; Weir, B.; Band, P.; Urtasun, R.; et al.: Radiotherapy and BCNU in the treatment of high-grade supratentorial astrocytomas. J. Neurosurg., 45:129–134, 1976; Seiler, R. W.; Greiner, P. H.; Zimmerman, A.; et al.: Radiotherapy combined with procarbazine, bleomycin, and CCNU in the treatment of high-grade supratentorial astrocytomas. J. Neurosurg. 48:861–865, 1978; and Eagan, R. T.; Childs, D. S., Jr.; Layton, D. D., Jr.; et al.: Dianhydrogalactitol and radiation therapy. Treatment of supratentorial glioma. J.A.M.A. 241:2046–2050, 1979.)

Table 37–12. Relative Efficacy of Chemotherapy in Primary
Malignant Gliomas

DRUG	PRIMARY CHEMOTHERAPY	ADJUVANT CHEMOTHERAPY
BCNU	+++	+
Bleomycin	NE	+
BIC	+	NE
BUDR	NE	++
CCNU	++	+
DTIC	NE	NE
Dianhydrogalactitol	∅	+
Epodyl	NE	NE
FU	NE	∅
HU	NE	+
MeCCNU	+	∅
MTX	+	∅
Metronidazole	NE	+
Mithramycin	+	∅
Nitrogen mustard	+	NE
PCB	++	∅
Thiotepa	∅	NE
Vinblastine	+	NE
VCR	+	NE
VM-26	+	NE
ADR-VM-26-CCNU	++	NE
BCNU-FU	+++	NE
BCNU-MTX-VCR	NE	+
BCNU-PCB	+++	NE
BCNU-VCR	+	∅
BCNU-VM-26	+	∅
CCNU-PCB-VCR	NE	++
CCNU-VCR-MTX	++	∅
DTIC-MeCCNU (or CCNU)	NE	NE
MeCCNU-VM-26	NE	∅
PCB-CCNU-VCR-(PCV No. 3)	+++	NE
BCNU-HU	NE	++

NE = Nonevaluable because of incomplete information, less than six patients with similar tumors, method of evaluation not defined, or no study reported.
∅ = No evidence of activity when evaluated as a primary form of chemotherapy, or no
better than irradiation alone when evaluated in adjuvant chemotherapy studies.
+ = slight activity; ++ = moderate activity; +++ = good activity defined as a median
increase in survival time or time to tumor progression of six to nine months for primary
chemotherapy; an increase in survival time or time to tumor progression of two to four
months for adjuvant chemotherapy, or doubling of long-term survivors over irradiation
alone.
ADR = ADRIAMYCIN (doxorubicin); BCNU = 1,3-*bis*(2-chloroethyl)-1-nitrosourea;
BIC = *bis*(2-chloroethyl-1-triazeno)imidazole-4-carboxamide; BUDR = bromode-
oxyuridine riboside; CCNU = 1-(2-chloroethyl)-3-cyclohexyl-1-nitrosourea; DTIC =
5-(3,3-dimethyl-1-triazeno)imidazole-4-carboxamide; MeCCNU = 1-(2-chloroethyl)-
3-(4-methylcyclohexyl)-1-nitrosourea; MTX = methotrexate; PCB = procarbazine =
N-isopropyl-(2-methylhydrazino)-p-toluamide monohydrochloride; Thiotepa =
triethylene thiophosphoamide; VCR = vincristine; VM-26 = epipodophyllotoxin.
Reprinted by permission from Levin, V. A., and Edwards, M. S.: Chemotherapy of
primary malignant gliomas. In Thomas, D. G. T., and Graham, D. I. (eds.): *Brain
Tumors.* Scientific Basis, Clinical Investigation and Current Therapy. Butterworth, Boston, 1980.

are not yet convincing as to their utility (Shapiro and Young, 1974; Heiss, 1978; Seiler *et
al.,* 1978; Avellanosa *et al.,* 1979; Jellinger *et
al.,* 1979). Intra-arterial chemotherapy (especially with BCNU) may be another approach
and is currently undergoing trials in several
centers. A major advantage is the approximately three- to fivefold or greater increase in
concentration of the drug delivered to the
tumor. Other new agents, including aziridinylbenzoquinone (AZQ), cisplatin, and deriva-
tions thereof, are also under study (see final
section of this chapter).

For malignant astrocytic tumors, BCNU,
CCNU, and perhaps procarbazine-CCNU and
vincristine, are currently felt to be useful pal-

liative adjunctive agents. For low-grade astrocytomas, it appears best to withhold all chemotherapy until recurrence occurs, at which time some tumors have actually progressed to a more malignant form.

The toxicities of chemotherapy are important factors limiting the treatment. Nitrosoureas are known to cause significant bone marrow toxicity and, with prolonged therapy, pulmonary fibrosis, hepatic toxicity, renal failure, as well as other tumors (Cohen *et al.,* 1976) are known to occur. Other undesirable effects, including interaction with radiation therapy, may also become apparent as patients survive longer. Burger *et al.* (1979) found late-delayed radiation necrosis in 4 patients in a series of 17 who had received 5000 to 6000 rads. Two of these had received BCNU. Two additional patients showed focal necrosis. Clearly, we have a way to go before optimal, effective antiglioma chemotherapy is available.

Oligodendroglioma. Oligodendroglia are derived from neuroectoderm, as are astrocytes and ependymal cells. They lie in contact with the axons and neurons, occur primarily in the white matter, and produce the myelin sheath that surrounds axons within the brain and spinal cord.

Epidemiology. Oligodendrogliomas constitute 5% of intracranial gliomas (Russell and Rubinstein, 1977). Predominantly a tumor of adult life, their peak incidence is between the ages of 40 and 50 years (Zülch, 1964).

Pathology. It is not surprising that these lesions have a predilection for the white matter of the cerebral hemispheres in proportion to the tissue mass of each lobe, with the frontal lobes being the most common location.

In the purely oligodendroglial lesion, the tumor margins are well defined, both grossly and microscopically. A high incidence of calcification is evident. The lesion occasionally penetrates the cerebral cortex and adheres to the dura, or may encroach upon or grow into the ventricular system.

These neoplasms are sheets of small round cells of uniform diameter traversed by a delicate capillary network. An important, but artifactual, diagnostic feature of oligodendrogliomas is the presence of perinuclear halos, or fried-egg appearance. This is the result of the pronounced propensity of these cells to undergo degeneration with the appearance of acute swelling, which happens with such consistency it is of diagnostic importance. Sub-

mission of a small piece of adjacent normal brain tissue for comparable histologic processing along with the tumor tissue is often helpful to the neuropathologist since normal tissue does not undergo acute swelling, but may show similar histologic changes with improper fixation.

The histologic purity of many oligodendrogliomas is disrupted by the presence of areas of neoplastic astrocytes or ependymal cells. Some of these areas have the appearance of islands of normal or reactive astrocytes surrounded by the oligodendroglioma, while others are distinctly neoplastic and may comprise a significant portion of the neoplastic mass. When the latter occurs, the tumor is designated a mixed glioma or an oligoastrocytoma, although it is not clear that the prognosis is altered. Weir and Elvidge (1968) found little influence of nuclear pleomorphism, endothelial proliferation, or frequent mitoses on the survival interval from the onset of symptoms or postoperatively in a series of 63 patients with oligodendrogliomas.

Sufficient evidence demonstrates that the oligodendroglial or an astrocytic component may undergo malignant transformation to the histologic and biologic characteristics of a glioblastoma multiforme after years of behaving as an indolent benign tumor (Zülch, 1964; Barnard, 1968).

Clinical Presentation. Epilepsy is the most common initial symptom and may antedate the diagnosis of intracranial tumor by several years. Tumors near the midline disrupt CSF flow by compression or invasion of the ventricular system and typically produce symptoms of increased intracranial pressure earlier than lesions in the lobes of the cerebral hemispheres.

Investigation. Plain skull x-rays disclose calcification in 50 to 60% of oligodendrogliomas (Earnest *et al.,* 1950; Weir and Elvidge, 1968). Electroencephalography, performed for the evaluation of seizures, is abnormal in as many as 89% of oligodendroglioma patients (Weir and Elvidge, 1968). CT scanning demonstrates calcification in 90% of patients and tumor enhancement with contrast in 66% (Vonofakos *et al.,* 1979). Angiography reveals an avascular mass, but demonstrates no characteristics diagnostic of tumor type.

Therapy and Management. When pure, these tumors are benign and extremely slow-growing. For a purely oligodendroglial lesion, surgical extirpation is usually possible with good, short-term results and a favorable long-term prognosis. Complete excision is not possible in the majority of cases, however, due to microscopic infiltration of adjacent functionally important brain tissue.

Indications for use of radiation therapy, radiation dose, and techniques recommended generally parallel those for astrocytomas. Series comparing results achieved with postoperative irradiation to those with surgery alone show an advantage for the irradiated group (Roberts and German, 1966; Chin *et al.,* 1980). Sheline (1975) demonstrated improvement in survival at five years (85 versus 31%) and this continued at ten years (55 versus 25%). Similar results have been achieved by Bouchard and Peirce (1960); and Chin *et al.,* (1980) have demonstrated a reduction in clinical recurrences, from 55% with surgery alone to 21% with surgery followed by radiation therapy. The value of radiotherapy is not definitive, however, Weir and Elvidge (1968) reported the mean survival of patients undergoing surgery and radiation therapy for oligodendroglioma to be 4 years, compared with 6.4 years with surgery alone.

Two major facets of this cerebral tumor render its biologic behavior and management more complex. These tumors are frequently composed of both astrocytic and oligodendroglial elements and thus are rarely pure. The second problem is represented by the relatively rare malignant oligodendroglioma.

In the case of the mixed oligoastrocytoma, the treatment plan is dependent on which cell type predominates. The presence of oligodendroglia in the midst of an astrocytoma is a good prognostic sign, but the presence of malignant astrocytes in an oligodendroglia is unfavorable. It is important to sample the pathologic material thoroughly to see whether foci of either type are present. These mixed tumors, therefore, are difficult to describe as a group because of the spectrum of malignancy they encompass, depending on the make-up of the mix.

The malignant pure oligodendroglioma behaves in much the same way as an infiltrating astrocytoma, and the management is similar. These lesions have been noted to develop subarachnoid seeding deposits with greater regularity than astrocytomas, however, especially when periventricular in location or when histologically less well differentiated.

Oligodendrogliomas account for only 1.5% of all brain tumors and, therefore, are not seen frequently enough to have significant chemotherapy study data. Upon recurrence and reoperation, however, progressive dedifferentiation is frequently seen; and the tumor takes on more of the characteristics of a malignant glioma or glioblastoma multiforme (Roberts and German, 1966). Following the demonstration of such changes, the patients should receive radiotherapy, if not previously administered, and consideration should be given to chemotherapy as utilized for malignant glioma.

Ependymoma. *Epidemiology.* The ependymal cells are of neuroectodermal origin and are found lining the ventricles and the central canal of the spinal cord. They are distinguished by their cilia, which aid in CSF movement.

Ependymomas are indolent and slow-growing glial neoplasms of ependymal cells and constitute 6% of intracranial gliomas (Russell and Rubinstein, 1977). They occur with a slightly higher frequency in males than females, with an average age of 16 to 20 years at diagnosis. Between 50 and 60% occur in children less than 15 years old (Kricheff *et al.,* 1964b; Barone and Elvidge, 1970). Twenty-five percent of tumors in and around the fourth ventricle are ependymomas.

Pathology. Ependymal neoplasms are regarded as one of the more benign glial neoplasms. Of the gliomas, despite the absence of a tumor capsule, these tumors are grossly the most demarcated from the surrounding brain. Microscopically, the sharply circumscribed tumor margin may be helpful in histologic diagnosis.

Ependymomas are classified into two groups: typical ependymomas and anaplastic ependymomas. Both groups may be identified by angulated cells, oval nuclei with pinpoint chromatin, true ependymal rosettes (see Figure 37–21), perivascular pseudorosettes, or the finding of blepharoplasts, which are a structural anlage for the attachment of cilia. Anaplastic ependymomas contain areas of pleomorphism, including multinucleation, giant cells, mitotic figures, vascular changes, and necrotic areas, although the general pattern still indicates the original cell type.

Two-thirds of intracranial ependymal neoplasms originate in the infratentorial space within the fourth ventricle, and one-third supratentorially. The supratentorial lesions are characterized by the following: (1) one-half arise from the ventricular lining, extending into the ventricle or the cerebral white matter;

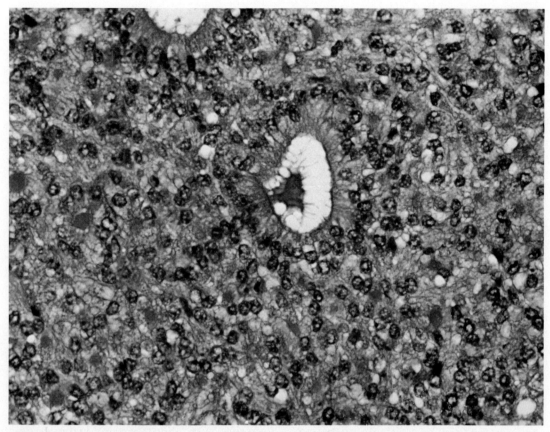

Figure 37–21.   The true ependymal rosette, a formation of columnar cells radially oriented around a distinct central lumen, is pathognomonic of an ependymoma. ×450.

(2) one-half are within the cerebral hemispheres, entirely separate from the ependymal surface, possibly originating from embryonic cell nests within the hemisphere (Mørk and Løken, 1977); (3) 40% are partially cystic; (4) about 75% of those arising from the ependymal lining are adjacent to or within the lateral ventricles and 25% adjacent to or within the third ventricle; (5) there is a higher percentage of anaplastic ependymomas in children and adults in the supratentorial compartment when compared to infratentorial ependymomas (Dohrmann *et al.,* 1976; Mørk and Løken, 1977).

The infratentorial ependymomas all arise within the fourth ventricle, the dominant location of ependymomas in childhood. Those arising in this location have a lower incidence of anaplasia and a longer average postoperative patient survival, but a greater risk of spread via CSF seeding to distant sites within the intrathecal space. They have commonly spread by contiguous growth into the basal cis-

terns of the posterior fossa, via the foramen of Magendie into the cisterna magna, via the foramen of Luschka into the prepontine cistern, or into the rostral cervical spine at the time of diagnosis. Spread to the ventral aspect of the brain stem or spinal canal limits the surgical excision to one which is incomplete.

Little information is available on the clinical course of untreated ependymomas. In the 101 cases reported by Mørk and Løken in 1977, 11 patients with symptomatic intracranial ependymomas received no therapy. After the onset of symptoms, 50% survived one year, and no patient lived longer than three years (Mørk and Løken, 1977).

Clinical Presentation.   Presenting symptoms are related to the location of the neoplasm rather than its histologic type. The most common symptoms manifest increased intracranial pressure resulting from obstruction of CSF flow by intraventricular tumor and include headache, nausea, vomiting, and papilledema. Symptoms of local involvement serve to differentiate the two tumor locations; paresis and seizures predominate in the supratentorial group, and ataxia, vertigo, and meningismus in those located infratentorially.

Investigation. Skull x-rays occasionally reveal evidence of increased intracranial pressure, and abnormal calcification can be identified in 20% of patients with supratentorial ependymomas.

Computed tomography has replaced ventriculography and angiography for diagnosis and localization. The differentiation between tumors of the brain stem and tumors of the fourth ventricle may still be difficult.

Detection of seeding of tumor into the spinal subarachnoid space requires CSF cytology or myelography. To reduce the risk of herniation, lumbar puncture should be avoided until after therapy of the tumor mass or hydrocephalus.

Therapy and Management. All intracranial ependymomas should be treated by surgical removal, followed by radiation therapy. The routine administration of irradiation to the craniospinal axis is controversial, and the potential of chemotherapy has been inadequately investigated. The rationale of these therapies is discussed below.

SURGICAL TREATMENT. In the series of 65 patients reported by Kricheff and his associates (1964a), although all of the 52 infratentorial tumors arose in the fourth ventricle, only 4 were limited to the fourth ventricle at the time of initial exploration. Thirty-six (69%) had grown into the cisterna magna; and, of these, 16 (31%) extended below the foramen magnum into the cervical subarachnoid space. Three had grown into the cerebellopontine cisterns, and 18 tumors invaded the cerebellar hemispheres, or vermis (13) or the brain stem (5). The supratentorial lesions are located deep within the hemispheres and are often quite large. For these reasons, complete operative removal is uncommon. Operative decompression reduces tumor burden, allows relief of CSF flow obstruction and reduction in compression of the surrounding brain, permits histopathologic diagnosis and determination of the degree of anaplasia, and confirms the presence of a neoplasm that is likely to be sensitive to radiation therapy. The operative mortality rates in early series varied from 20 to 50%; but with current techniques, this rate should be in the range of 5% or less. An area of controversy is routine preoperative CSF shunting procedures in those patients with hydrocephalus. As

with medulloblastomas, such shunts place protected sites at risk for tumor spread and should not be used unless clearly necessary. If CSF drainage is required preoperatively, we prefer a temporary, external drainage system.

RADIATION THERAPY. Virtually all studies demonstrate that postoperative irradiation considerably improves survival for both children and adults with ependymoma. A 20 to 30% increase in survival at five years was found with intracranial lesions (Mørk and Løken, 1977). Similar results have been shown by others (Fokes and Earle, 1969; Barone and Elvidge, 1970). Radiation doses in excess of 4500 rads achieved improved results compared with lower doses (Phillips *et al.,* 1964; Kim and Fayos, 1977).

Numerous studies demonstrate the considerable incidence of subarachnoid seeding with ependymomas (Kricheff *et al.,* 1964a; Sagerman *et al.,* 1965; Shuman *et al.,* 1975). *Post mortem* evaluation demonstrates this risk to average 20 to 30% in most series. Clinically, symptomatic seeding occurs less frequently, although several recent papers focus attention on this problem (Sagerman *et al.,* 1965; Bloom and Walsh, 1975; Salazar *et al.,* 1975; Kim and Fayos, 1977). Factors tending to increase this risk include infratentorial location, proximity to the ventricular lining, and higher grade of malignancy (Salazar *et al.,* 1975; Dohrmann *et al.,* 1976; Kim and Fayos, 1977). Based on this information, irradiation of the craniospinal axis is recommended for posterior fossa lesions or high-grade tumors at any site. Such treatment for supratentorial, lower-grade lesions that are somewhat removed from the ventricular lining does not seem warranted.

Radiation in excess of 5000 rads delivered over 5.5 to 6 weeks is recommended for the primary lesion; and when craniospinal treatment is necessary, doses of 3000 to 3500 rads are delivered over 3.5 to 4 weeks.

From 40 to 60% of patients with intracranial ependymomas survive five years. As with other relatively benign neoplasms of the CNS, the prognosis is as dependent upon the location of the lesion as it is upon the histologic grade. Local recurrence rather than distal spread limits survival. Whether histologic grade has prognostic significance is a matter of contention. Although earlier series demonstrated no correlation between the histologic varieties of ependymoma and their biologic behavior (Mabon *et al.,* 1949; Ringertz and Reymond, 1949; Kricheff *et al.,* 1964a, Barone and Elvidge, 1970), more recent reports indicate that patients with anaplastic ependymomas fare considerably less well than those with lower-grade lesions (Salazar *et al.,* 1975; Dohrmann *et al.,* 1976; Kim and Fayos, 1977; Mørk and Løken, 1977).

CHEMOTHERAPY. Although ependymomas are highly responsive to surgery and radiotherapy, and a prolonged high quality of life can be anticipated, recurrence eventually takes place. Chemotherapy has been carried out only occasionally in late-stage recurrent tumors. In Cangir's study utilizing MOPP, one recurrent patient was treated with no response (Cangir *et al.,* 1978). Four out of six late-recurrent ependymomas treated with the nitrosoureas were noted to have a positive response (Shapiro, 1975).

The major study that will provide basic information on the treatment of ependymoblastoma is being carried out by the Children's Cancer Study Group (CCSG) in conjunction with the medulloblastoma study discussed below. As a separate stratification, patients with ependymoblastomas will receive standard prescribed courses of radiotherapy and will be randomized to no additional therapy or to receive CCNU, vincristine, and prednisone. More than 40 patients have been entered into this study; however, it is too early for results to be meaningful.

The survival curve of patients who have ependymomas is generally biphasic, in which the first half succumb rather promptly to their disease, with a median survival of approximately one year, regardless of the supra- or infratentorial location of the tumor. After five years, the slope of the survival curve has markedly flattened out, with approximately 40 to 60% of patients alive. Clearly, these patients comprise a different biologic entity than those seen in the earlier portion of the survival curve and deserve vigorous investigation as to what characteristics might account for their increased survival.

Choroid Plexus Papilloma. Embryologically, the choroid plexus originates by the protrusion of a rich network of blood vessels into the ependymal covering of the brain cavities, the ventricles. The tufted extensions, comprised of connective tissue and vascular stroma covered by cuboidal or columnar epithelium derived from ependyma, form the choroid plexuses.

Tumors of the choroid plexus, papillomas, comprise about 0.5% of all intracranial neoplasms (Cushing, 1932). They occur with greater frequency in children, accounting for 2.3 to 3% of intracranial tumors in patients less than 12 years of age (Matson, 1969; Hawkins, 1980).

The macroscopic appearance of these papillomas is a globular, irregular mass with a rough surface resembling cauliflower. Their texture is soft to gritty, and they are quite vascular, a characteristic that has greatly influenced the operative results for this benign tumor.

Microscopically, the tumor closely resembles normal choroid plexus. A core of vascularized connective tissue stroma is covered by a single layer of epithelium. Malignant forms are rare and can usually be easily identified by invasion of adjacent neural structures, loss of papillary architecture, and cytologically malignant features with numerous mitoses and anaplasia. Cerebrospinal fluid seeding occurs in the benign and malignant forms, but, as expected, is seen more frequently with malignant lesions. The electron microscopic characteristics typical of fluid-transporting epithelium support oversecretion of cerebrospinal fluid as the cause of the communicating hydrocephalus which commonly accompanies these tumors (Carter *et al.,* 1972). Another possibility is partial occlusion of the CSF absorptive pathways by leakage of blood into the CSF or by the high-protein content of the CSF associated with choroid plexus papillomas (Russell and Rubinstein, 1977). The intraventricular location of these lesions can also partially obstruct the flow of CSF within the ventricular system, resulting in obstructive hydrocephalus.

About 50% of these tumors occur in the fourth ventricle, a site more likely to be involved in adults. The trigone of the lateral ventricles is more commonly affected in children (Matson, 1969; Hawkins, 1980).

The clinical presentation typically suggests only raised intracranial pressure. In children, this is indicated by increasing head circumference and vomiting. Adults complain of headache, nausea, and vomiting. Nystagmus and ataxia are more common with a fourth ventricular location.

Investigation consists of plain skull roentgenography, computed tomography, and arteriography. The plain x-rays reveal changes due to hydrocephalus and increased intracranial pressure: split sutures in infants and sellar erosion in older children. A small fraction contain sufficient calcium to be visualized on regular x-rays. The CT scan is diagnostic. A lobulated intraventricular mass, with or without foci of calcification or hemorrhage that dramatically enhances following contrast infusion, is seen uniformly. The pattern of ventricular dilatation is also apparent with this technique (Zimmerman and Bilaniuk, 1979; Hawkins, 1980).

Angiography discloses hypertrophy of the choroidal artery supplying the tumor and a capillary blush of the tumor mass. With choroid plexus papillomas, this study is now used more for preoperative analysis of the tumor's blood supply than as a diagnostic aid.

Treatment is surgical excision, with special attention to isolation and section of the arterial feeding vessels prior to manipulation of the tumor mass. Failure to adhere to this principle results in excessive hemorrhage and high operative mortality (Matson, 1969; Raimondi and Guiterrez, 1975; Hawkins, 1980). This maneuver facilitates the remainder of the operation by reducing the tumor size, in addition to diminishing operative bleeding into the ventricles and CSF.

Radiation and chemotherapy offer little of value with choroid plexus papillomas. Postoperative radiation therapy is advised if histologic features of anaplasia are present. If such features exist, inspection of the CSF by cytology and tissue culture is indicated. Cerebrospinal fluid dissemination of an anaplastic choroid plexus papilloma merits consideration of craniospinal axis radiation and chemotherapy, although these modalities are unproven for this particular circumstance.

Medulloblastoma. *Epidemiology.* This tumor represents the most common malignant CNS tumor of childhood, with maximal incidence in the second five years of the first decade of life. Fifty percent occur in the first decade, and almost all are diagnosed before the age of 30 years (Zülch and Mennel, 1974). Males are affected more often than females by a ratio of 4 to 3 (Russell and Rubinstein, 1977).

Pathology. The precursor cell of the medulloblastoma is the multipotential neuroepithelial cell of the inferior medullary velum, which migrates laterally over the cerebellar hemispheres during embryonic development to become the external granular cell layer. This superficial layer of small cells can be seen throughout the cerebellar cortex at birth. During the first year of life, these cells either migrate into the definitive granular cell layer or differentiate into the cortical neuroglia of the cerebellum. These facts logically explain the preponderant location of this tumor in the roof of the fourth ventricle in childhood and the less common adult tumor found laterally and superficially in the cerebellar hemispheres. Kadin *et al.* (1970) reported a neonate with midline tumor of the cerebellar vermis merging laterally with the histologically similar fetal external granular cell layer. The concept of the congenital character of these lesions is strengthened by the report of cerebellar medulloblastomas in two sets of identical twins, aged 8 and 11 weeks (Griepentrog and Pauly, 1957).

Recent ultrastructural, immunohistochemical, and tissue culture studies support combinations of a tendency toward astroglial and neuronal differentiation of these tumors. Ermel and Brucher (1974) observed neuronal dense-core vesicles and rudimentary synaptic structures with the electron microscope, implicating the neuroblastic cell. Examples of astrocytic differentiation have also been established ultrastructurally (Rubinstein *et al.*, 1974). In addition, tissue culture studies support the bipotentiality of the medulloblastoma cell for both neuronal and glial differentiation (Liss, 1969; Lumsden, 1974). Astrocytic differentiation in 11 of 13 cases of medulloblastoma was shown by immunoperoxidase staining for glial fibrillary acidic protein, an antigen found only in glial cells, by Palmer *et al.* (1981).

Most medulloblastomas are relatively discrete, homogeneous masses of soft consistency in the cerebellar vermis, with variable extension between the tonsils into the cisterna magna or into the fourth ventricular floor. A tendency to more lateral placement in the cerebellar hemispheres is often noted in the older age groups, where the lesions are usually firmer and have a greater propensity to involve the meninges (Chatty and Earle, 1971).

This tumor tends to grow aggressively and is always histologically malignant. The tumor is invasive and is not encapsulated. The cells have an elongated carrot shape, and a field of cells is distinctively homogeneous. The cells and nuclei stain very darkly, with unrelieved sheets of anaplastic cells characterizing the common lesion. One occasionally encounters rosettes structured of anaplastic cells perpendicularly placed around an eosinophilic core (the Homer Wright rosette), evidence of neuroblastic origin (Burger and Vogel, 1976). The laterally placed lesions of the cerebellar hemispheres, when superficial, may elicit a mesenchymal reaction of the overlying leptomeninges with inclusion of collagen and reticulin into the tumor mass, the desmoplastic medulloblastoma. Fundamental to this term is the concept that the collagen and reticulin arise from meningeal infiltration and reaction and are not indicators of a mesenchymal origin of the neoplasm.

Medulloblastomas may spread by way of CSF pathways into the cervical, thoracic, or lumbar subarachnoid areas, the ventricular system, or the intracranial subarachnoid space. When dissemination occurs outside the central nervous system, it preferentially involves bone and cervical lymph nodes.

Clinical Presentation. As an embryonic tumor, a medulloblastoma's biologic aggressiveness produces symptoms that progress rapidly after its onset. Obstruction of CSF circulation, by partial occlusion of the cerebral aqueduct or the fourth ventricle, causes hydrocephalus with increased intracranial pressure, nausea, projectile vomiting, and papilledema in children older than 18 months. In infants, open cranial sutures initially decompress increased pressure by cranial growth. Usually there is truncal ataxia with frequent falls. Visual and brain stem symptoms and signs appear. Head tilt and neck stiffness may be present as an effort to relieve suboccipital pain from downward displacement of the cerebellar tonsils or extension of tumor into the upper cervical canal.

Investigation. Routine skull films may disclose separation of the cranial sutures if the child is less than ten years old. A similar finding in an older child indicates a long-standing increase in intracranial pressure beginning prior to the normal age of suture closure and is more likely to be found with a benign tumor.

Other studies add little to the information gained from CT scanning, which demonstrates the presence and degree of associated hydrocephalus, as well as localizing the tumor sufficiently for planning surgery (see Figure 37–22A, B). Patients with increased intracranial pressure requiring sedation for CT scanning should be monitored closely because a sudden increase in intracranial pressure can result in abrupt neurologic deterioration requiring emergency management. Diagnosis is aided by cytologic or tissue culture examination of the cerebrospinal fluid. Since irradiation of the craniospinal axis is standard therapy in all patients with medulloblastoma, and lumbar puncture can precipitate tonsillar herniation and death, it is not recommended preoperatively in these patients.

Therapy and Management. PREOPERA-

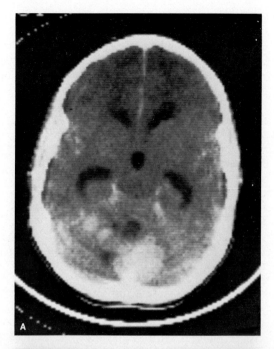

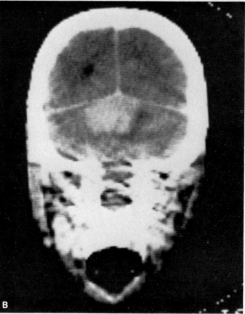

Figure 37–22. Axial (*A*) and coronal (*B*) CT scan demonstrating medulloblastoma in the superior cerebellar vermis. The enhancing tumor lies posterior to the fourth ventrical in *A* and inferior to the tentorium in *B*. By partially occluding the fourth ventricle, the tumor is causing moderate hydrocephalus.

TIVE PREPARATION. Corticosteroid therapy decreases peritumor edema and restores partial patency of obstructed CSF circulation. Dramatic clinical improvement ensues almost without exception.

Preoperative CSF diversion procedures may spread tumor to extraneural sites or may be complicated by infection and should be reserved for patients refractory to a trial of steroid therapy or those in immediate jeopardy from increased intracranial pressure.

SURGERY. There seems to be little doubt that, with medulloblastoma, the more radical the tumor resection, the better the postoperative survival. This was initially emphasized by Harvey Cushing in 1930, but later studies revealed no difference in survival of patients who underwent biopsy and irradiation compared to those who underwent radical removal and irradiation (Berger and Elvidge, 1963). Standard therapy became irradiation following surgical removal of sufficient tumor to allow reestablishment of CSF flow. Compelling evidence now indicates better prognosis in those patients with complete tumor excision. In a series of patients treated by the same staff and with similar irradiation therapy, the percentage of patients with relapse-free survival at four years was 38% in those patients treated in the five-year period in which partial resection was performed and 84% in the patients treated over a similar period but with total resection (Norris *et al.*, 1981). Similar experience has been documented by others (Gerosa *et al.*, 1980). The use of the binocular microscope, with improved depth perception and magnifi-

cation, allows more extensive resection of these lesions, some of which invade the brain stem at the floor of the fourth ventricle. Circumstances prohibiting total tumor removal include pontine, medullary, or cerebellar peduncle infiltration in a manner which could cause devastating neurologic deficit if complete removal were attempted. However, there is no place for *planned* subtotal removal.

RADIATION THERAPY. After surgery and a suitable interval for recovery, radiation therapy, with or without chemotherapy, should begin. Rarely, a patient presents with symptoms of spinal cord compromise from a subarachnoid deposit, and evaluation reveals a primary lesion in the posterior fossa. Virtually all lesions arise in the cerebellum.

Surgical treatment alone is never sufficient therapy for this tumor, as Cushing (1930) aptly demonstrated. Radiation therapy represents the only currently available modality that offers the potential of cure. Early studies demonstrated the necessity for treatment of the entire neuraxis by irradiation. Subsequent studies have supported this (see Figure 37–23). A technically demanding treatment plan must be followed to permit maximum efficacy with acceptable morbidity. Dosimetric aspects have been described by Van Dyk and colleagues (1977). During treatment of the tumor site, concurrent treatment of the entire neuraxis,

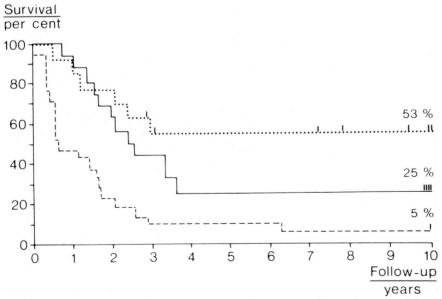

Figure 37-23. Survival (Kaplan-Meier) for patients with medulloblastoma who received whole CNS (···) (*N* = 13), posterior fossa and spinal (——) (*N* = 16), or posterior fossa (---) (*N* = 21) irradiation therapy. From Landberg, T. G., *et al.*: Improvements in the radiotherapy of medulloblastoma, 1946–1975. *Cancer*, **45**:676, 1980.

rather than sequential treatment of separate geographic regions, is essential. This is done to minimize the risk of cells migrating from untreated areas (Harisiadis and Chang, 1977). Many studies suggest that irradiation of the posterior fossa primary site to doses approaching 5500 rads, with 180-rad daily fractions in six to seven weeks, is preferable to lower-dose treatment, especially for locally more advanced or prognostically unfavorable lesions (Bloom *et al.,* 1969; Chang *et al.,* 1969; Bloom, 1975; Bloom and Walsh, 1975; Sheline, 1975; Harisiadis and Chang, 1977).

Although radiation doses of 3500 rads or more are usually recommended for treatment of subclinical spinal subarachnoid disease and more than 4000 rads for the remainder of the brain, data confirming these recommended dose levels are scant. Bloom and colleagues, using lower doses in the past, achieved substantial survival improvement and long-term control in approximately 25% of treated patients (Aron, 1969; Bloom *et al.,* 1969; Hope-Stone, 1970). Virtually all failures in patients receiving neuraxis treatment are at the primary, posterior fossa site. The overwhelming primary relapse site has been the posterior fossa in patients treated with appropriate neuraxis irradiation and receiving more than 2500 rads to prophylactic sites. The issue of dose to these sites of potential subclinical disease is of considerable importance, as a major portion of the radiation-related morbidity occurs outside the posterior fossa and is clearly dose related.

In contrast to the absence of clear dose-response data for these subclinical sites, evidence has accumulated demonstrating improved local and overall control following posterior fossa doses in excess of 5000 rads. Harisiadis and Chang (1979), studying equally staged lesions, were able to demonstrate significant control improvement with higher doses. Several other recent series confirm this view.

Improvement in equipment and in technical aspects of treatment, combined with administration of higher radiation doses to the posterior fossa, has resulted in a substantial improvement in results. In particular, three-year survival has improved, with more than 60% of irradiated patients living at this interval. Although a substantial increase in the time to relapse has occurred, late relapses decrease the overall differences at five years. Bloom and others have shown the value of the Collin's risk period (age at diagnosis plus nine months) in

predicting an accurate risk period for recurrence (Bloom *et al.,* 1969; Wilson, 1970; Quest *et al.,* 1978). Relapse beyond this period is rare in patients with medulloblastoma. With better local control and longer survival, a larger percentage of patients now demonstrate systemic (extra-CNS) metastases, especially to bones, where a characteristic diffuse blastic appearance is produced. The placement of a shunt to the pleural or peritoneal cavity increases the risk of tumor seeding to these locations. Such shunts have also been credited with increasing systemic dissemination to other sites. The latter is controversial, however, and a shunt is certainly not necessary for this occurrence, as there have been several instances without prior shunting.

The prognosis for older patients (over 15 years) with medulloblastoma has been stated to be better than that for younger children. In fact, although three-year survival appears to be superior for older patients, at five years survival for younger patients is superior and shows the advantage of longer follow-up.

Should tumor recurrence develop several years after initial treatment and be limited to the posterior fossa, a second course of irradiation (limited) can provide prolonged survival and, on rare occasions, apparent cure.

The clinical benefit of such retreatment clearly outweighs the increased risk of brain necrosis. The increasing frequency of late relapses heightens interest in the combined use of systemic chemotherapy with irradiation.

CHEMOTHERAPY. Since medulloblastoma accounts for one-fourth of all pediatric brain tumors, a significant number of patients may be accrued for therapeutic trials. Carefully planned maximal dose radiotherapy has resulted in a median survival of patients with medulloblastoma of four to five years. As previously stated, most tumors recur at their original site. Therefore, chemotherapeutic trials are appropriate. Unfortunately, most reports contain less than a half-dozen cases who have been treated on a comparatively *ad hoc* basis at the time they become symptomatic.

It is generally accepted that medulloblastomas are chemosensitive, as well as radiosensitive, although the duration of response is frequently brief or unreported. Only preliminary information is available on two major prospective randomized studies currently underway (Bloom, 1979; Evans *et al.,* 1979). Both studies require the patient to have had a surgical biopsy and both compare radiotherapy to radiotherapy plus CCNU and vincristine. In addition, the study carried out by Evans and co-workers (1979) adds prednisone. Preliminary analysis of a study being carried out by the International Society of Pediatric Oncology indicates a slightly greater median time to progression for patients receiving radiotherapy and chemotherapy in comparison with those who receive radiotherapy alone. It is too early to determine if the preliminary analysis will continue to show the same trend or if selective and prognostic factors will account for the difference. These studies will form a basis for controlled clinical trials in the treatment of children with medulloblastoma.

Although vincristine has been reported as being useful for the treatment of gliomas, it has rarely been used alone. A response in three out of four patients with recurrent medulloblastomas has been reported (Rosenstock et al., 1976). A wide variety of other phase II studies of patients with recurrent or progressive tumor have added vincristine to other drugs, such as the nitrosoureas, procarbazine, nitrogen mustard, and methotrexate. Cangir had an impressive 80% response rate, with a median duration of response of 11 months, in ten patients who received MOPP (Cangir et al., 1978). Thomas et al., (1980) had a 100% response rate in eight patients with recurrent medulloblastoma treated with vincristine, BCNU, dexamethasone, intravenous methotrexate, and intrathecal methotrexate. Severe toxicity was seen, with four early deaths in nine patients treated immediately postoperatively in combination with radiotherapy (Thomas et al., 1980). They attributed the toxicity to delivery of intrathecal methotrexate and to BCNU delivery during radiotherapy. When they were discontinued while radiotherapy was being delivered, considerably less toxicity was seen.

The long life span these patients enjoy includes a long therapeutic period that complicates the design of a therapeutic study of medulloblastoma. Radiotherapy, chemotherapy, and their combination can affect endocrine and mental functions of children. These factors must be considered when designing therapeutic studies.

Tumors of Neuronal Cells or Their Precursors

Neural tumors of the CNS are rare. The most common tumor of this group is the neuroblastoma, a peripheral nervous system tumor which only extremely rarely originates within the brain. Of the CNS neural tumors, the ganglion cell tumors, gangliocytoma and ganglioglioma, are most representative. Although it is generally agreed that medulloblastomas are neuroepithelial tumors, existing evidence does not allow one to confidently categorize them into either the glial or neuronal set.

Gangliocytoma and Ganglioglioma. These are tumors containing authentic ganglion cells in their composition. The gangliocytoma is composed of abnormal ganglion cells with a nonneoplastic glial stroma. In the ganglioglioma, both the ganglion cells and the glial stroma are neoplastic. The tumor behavior depends upon the degree of anaplasia of the glial component.

Gangliocytomas and ganglioglioma are tumors of the frontal or temporal lobes or the region surrounding the third ventricle. They occur most commonly between 10 and 30 years of age, but may arise in infancy or in later life. Benign lesions are usually small and well circumscribed. This histology is distinctive and usually easily recognized. Large, neuron-like ganglion cells stain for Nissl substance with cresyl violet. The degree of glial cell differentiation parallels that of the ganglion cells and, in most cases, is similar to that of an astrocytoma. As in the low-grade astrocytomas, however, anaplastic change may develop. Russell and Rubinstein (1962) have reported a patient with progression to glioblastoma 23 years after partial removal of a ganglioglioma of the left frontal lobe.

Glomus Jugulare Tumors. These tumors, which arise from paraganglionic cells in the adventitia of the jugular bulb or nearby, are often brought to clinical attention because of slowly progressive aural symptoms (deafness, tinnitus, vertigo, external canal bleeding) or neurologic symptoms (swallowing or phonation difficulties). Histologically, they have been grouped with the other nonchromaffin paragangliomas or chemodectomas, such as carotid body tumors. Women are most commonly affected. Although lymph node and, rarely, distant metastases have been noted, they are most commonly locally progressive.

Because of their vascular nature and location, surgical management is often accompanied by major blood loss, morbidity, and mortality. Complete extirpation, despite these complications, is occasionally possible (Rosenwasser, 1952; Bradley and Maxwell, 1954;

Hawkins, 1961; Newman *et al.*, 1973). In view of this, radiation therapy after biopsy or attempted removal has been increasingly recommended.

These lesions were formerly considered to be radioresistant. This mistaken conclusion was probably the result of lower maximum tumor doses, possibly using only orthovoltage equipment, as well as the protracted regression commonly seen after irradiation of slowly progressive lesions. With newer megavoltage techniques, several recent reports document irradiation control of glomus tumors (van Miert, 1964; Newman *et al.*, 1973). A tumor dose of approximately 5000 to 5500 rads in six to seven weeks produces superior results when compared with lower doses (van Miert, 1964; Grubb and Lampe, 1965; Maruyama *et al.*, 1971; Hudgins, 1972; Newman *et al.*, 1973). Chemotherapy has not been utilized in glomus jugulare tumors.

Tumors of Mesodermal Tissues

Meningioma.   *Epidemiology.*   Meningiomas rank second only to gliomas in incidence of primary intracranial tumors, comprising 15 to 18% of such lesions. Although they may occur at any age, they are most commonly present in the later decades of middle life. The ratio of females to males is 2 to 1 for intracranial tumors and 4 to 1 for intraspinal meningiomas. They account for about 3 to 4% of intracranial tumors in those less than 20 years old. In children, there is no sex predilection for meningiomas; the posterior fossa and intraventricular locations are represented in greater frequency than in adults; and they are apt to behave more aggressively than adult meningiomas (Russell and Rubinstein 1977; Deen *et al.*, 1982).

Etiology and Pathogenesis.   Although some controversy still exists, it is generally agreed that the meningothelial cell is the cell of origin of meningiomas and that the distribution of meningiomas is related to the great abundance of these cells in the arachnoid villi. Such cells are also found scattered diffusely in the intracranial and intraspinal arachnoid membranes and occasionally in the choroid plexus and tela choroidea.

Divergent opinions have long existed over the potential of head trauma to predispose to meningioma formation. Annegers *et al.* (1979), in retrospective analysis of a community population of 2953 patients followed for a total of 29,859 person-years, found no difference in the observed number of brain tumors (4) from the expected number (4.1).

Radiation therapy and hormonal influences have been implicated in the etiology and progression of meningiomas and have been previously discussed in this chapter. There is a 2-to-1 female-to-male ratio, a greater than expected association of meningioma and breast cancer (Schoenberg, 1977), an occasional rapid enlargement of a meningioma during pregnancy (Michelsen and New, 1969), and presence of estradiol-binding receptor protein in the cytoplasmic fraction of meningiomas (Donnell *et al.*, 1979; Martuza *et al.*, 1981). In one series, 13 of 15 patients with multiple meningiomas were women (Lusins and Nakagawa, 1981).

Pathology.   As a group, meningiomas are considered relatively benign lesions, but can become malignant; and two subclasses appear to be invasive from the start. Except for the invasive types, the majority of benign meningiomas are encapsulated and are well demarcated from surrounding tissues. Their sites of predilection within the intracranial region can be seen in Table 37–13. Sites of surgical importance include the sphenoid wing, tuberculum sellae, parasagittal region, olfactory groove, clivus, foramen magnum, and convexity. Certain of these lesions have anatomic features that make the tumor's behavior "malignant," although the histology may be benign. Sphenoid wing meningiomas in the medial portion, which can invade the cavernous sinus or encircle the carotid artery, represent this behavior most clearly.

A somewhat simplified classification of meningiomas is used here combining features of the schemes of Rubinstein (1972) and Burger and Vogel (1976). By considering the primary cell type, one can divide meningiomas into fibroblastic, syncytial (meningothelial), angioblastic, papillary, and sarcomatous varieties. Combinations may be present in any tumor. Combinations of fibroblastic and syncytial meningiomas, called transitional meningiomas, are particularly common (see Figure 37–24). The fibroblastic and syncytial varieties are self-descriptive and are benign, slow-growing tumors. An important diagnostic feature of most meningiomas is a circular nest of cells that tends to form a whorl. These whorls are the probable source of psammoma bodies when they eventually become calcified. These bodies connote a slow-

Table 37–13. Sites of Predilection, Relative Frequency, and Common Clinical Presentation of Intracranial Meningiomas

SITE	PERCENT	SYMPTOMS
Parasagittal and falx	24	Focal epilepsy of lower extremity, paraparesis if tumor on both sides of midline, headaches and mental changes if anterior, hemianopia if posterior
Convexity	18	Epilepsy and focal neurologic deficit
Sphenoid ridge Inner ⅓		Visual loss, field defect on one or both eyes, optic atrophy, ophthalmoplegia, hypesthesia in distribution of first division of trigeminal nerve
Outer ⅔		Focal motor or temporal lobe seizures, headaches, increased intracranial pressure
Olfactory groove	10	Foster Kennedy syndrome (ipsilateral optic atrophy and anosmia and contralateral papilledema), mental deterioration
Suprasellar	10	Visual loss unilateral or bilateral, bitemporal hemianopia.
Posterior fossa	9	Ataxia, hydrocephalus, hearing loss, trigeminal distribution sensory loss or pain, hemifacial spasm

Derived from Quest, D. O.: Meningiomas: An update. *Neurosurgery,* **3**:219–225, 1978.

growing, benign subclass, called the psammomatous meningioma, when present in great abundance.

The pathologic diagnosis of a meningioma is usually not difficult given dural attachment, globular shape, typical whorled meningothelial cells, and psammoma bodies. Furthermore, the scrupulous categorization of a particular tumor within the benign varieties (fibroblastic, syncytial, transitional, and psam-

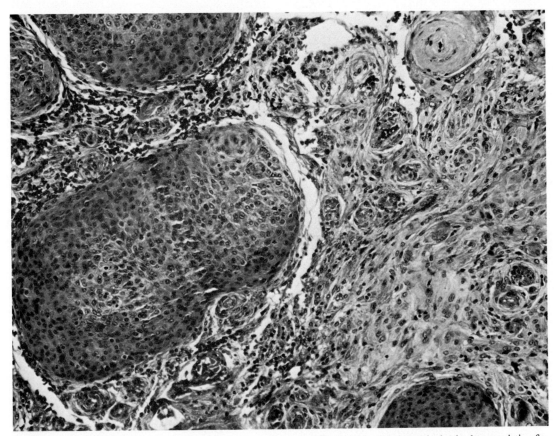

Figure 37–24. Meningothelial cells with indistinct margins are aggregated into lobules and whorls characteristic of a meningioma. ×200.

momatous) has little practical significance because the biologic characteristics, location, prognosis, and tendency to recur are similar among these groups. Marked nuclear pleomorphism, numerous mitoses, extensive necrosis, and macroscopic or microscopic evidence of invasion are indications of rapid growth and predict more aggressive behavior (Burger and Vogel, 1976).

The angioblastic, papillary, and sarcomatous types constitute most of the malignant meningiomas and occur rarely. Angioblastic meningiomas are divided into two groups. The tumors of one group are histologically similar to the cerebellar hemangioblastomas, and those of the other group are the hemangiopericytomas. The hemangiopericytomas and the papillary meningiomas are invariably associated with other histologic features of malignancy and display aggressive clinical behavior marked by a high rate of local recurrence or the development of distant metastases (Ludwin *et al.*, 1975; Goellner *et al.*, 1978).

Clinical Presentation. Like other extra-axial, intracranial tumors, meningiomas elicit symptoms by compression and displacement of adjacent brain tissue or cranial nerves. Because they tend to arise in certain locations, the clinical presentation of each tumor can be best described in reference to its anatomic position. Table 37–13 depicts the major sites of predilection of the intracranial meningiomas, the relative frequency among all intracranial meningiomas, and the most common manner of presentation of a meningioma at a particular site.

Investigation. Plain films of the skull are diagnostic for meningioma in 30 to 60% of cases (Taveras and Wood, 1976). Direct evidence for intracranial meningioma includes hyperostosis, increased vascular markings of the normal meningeal arteries, tumor calcification (see Figure 37–25A, B), and bone destruction.

Computed tomography (CT) has replaced radioisotope scanning, pneumoencephalography, and arteriography in the diagnosis of these lesions. The later generation CT scanners allow detection of lesions as small as 0.5 cm in size and often permit a positive diagnosis of meningioma. The typical appearance is a homogeneous high-density mass with distinct borders and striking contrast enhancement.

Angiography, although an excellent diagnostic study for meningiomas, is now employed primarily to reveal the relationship of the adjacent intracranial arteries and the vas-cular supply (see Figure 37–26) of the tumor in planning the operation. Occasionally, it is used as a confirmatory study, if the diagnosis is still in question following a CT scan. Arteriography is especially helpful in evaluating basal, parasagittal, and posterior fossa meningiomas. Plain skull films and CT scan will generally suffice for the convexity tumors.

Therapy and Management. Meningiomas are considered benign tumors with a favorable prognosis. It is best to group these tumors into three general therapeutic groups: (1) accessible (resectable) benign lesions, (2) inaccessible (only partially resectable) benign lesions, and (3) malignant meningiomas.

The concept of resectability, as it applies to meningiomas, depends to a large part on the anatomic location of the lesion; but other factors, including the size of the lesion and the age and health of the patient, need to be taken into account. This is particularly true since even the accessible lesions often require long and strenuous operations. In general, meningiomas located in the convexity, in the olfactory groove region, and those intraparenchymally in the cortex can be removed in their entirety.

When these tumors are in the parasagittal region, concerns about the sagittal sinus can often lead to leaving a portion of the tumor adherent to the sinus. The risks of ligating and removing a portion of the sinus with the tumor are greatest in posterior falx lesions and less in anterior ones. On many occasions, a partial resection of the involved portion of the wall of the sinus, followed by venous grafting or oversewing of the sinus, will maintain patency of the sinus and tumor removal can be completed. If the sagittal sinus is completely resected, especially in the posterior two-thirds of its course, cerebral swelling, venous engorgement, and venous infarction with intracerebral hemorrhage can produce significant morbidity and mortality. If the sinus has been slowly and totally occluded by the tumor, allowing collateral flow to develop around the area of tumor involvement, the occluded segment may be safely removed with the tumor. In the older patient, if the sinus is patent but the lateral wall has been invaded by the tumor, the tumor is partially resected, leaving the small portion invading the sinus. The potential of subsequent clinical recurrence that may have to be treated with reoperation is accepted in such an instance.

Meningiomas of the sphenoid wing have been divided into two groups, lateral and me-

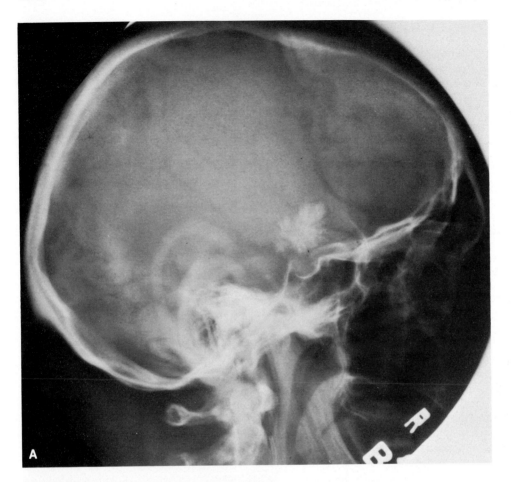

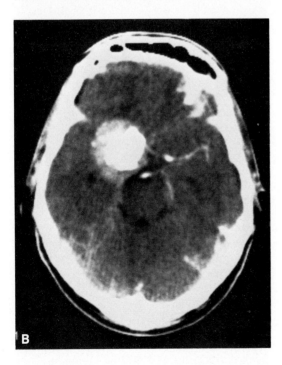

Figure 37–25. (*A*) Dense calcification within medial sphenoid wing meningioma seen on plain lateral skull x-ray. (*B*) Same patient. CT scan following intravenous contrast administration shows central calcification surrounded by tumor soft tissue enhancement.

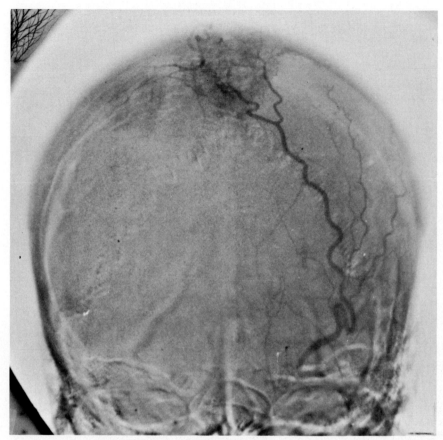

Figure 37–26. Selective external carotid arteriogram of a parasagittal meningioma. Enlarged occipital artery supplies tumor (midline tumor blush at vertex) transcranially.

dial. The lateral lesions are both lateral and anterior, can present with proptosis, and may be first seen and managed by ophthalmic surgeons. These lesions may be mistaken for fibrous dysplasia and followed for years before their true neoplastic origin is clear. Total removal should be planned for young, healthy patients. These lesions often are in the sphenoid bone, expanding the bone itself, and extensive bony removal may be difficult. Special techniques for bone removal using an air drill with steel and diamond burrs enable this bony removal to be accomplished.

Medial sphenoid wing lesions often involve the carotid artery and cavernous sinus and, although benign, can invade or be extremely adherent to these structures, preventing complete removal. Microneurosurgical techniques are mandatory in the excision of these lesions and the other basal meningiomas.

The likelihood of local recurrence of benign meningiomas depends on the completeness of the surgical removal. It is important to remove even the smallest points of tumor attachment if safely possible, as these foci allow tumor recurrence (Simpson, 1957; Earle and Richany, 1969).

Intracranial meningiomas recur in 10% of patients after complete surgical removal of the tumor and the dura at the site of tumor attachment. In those cases with macroscopically complete tumor removal and cauterization of the site of dural attachment, 16% recur, whereas with complete removal, there is a clinical recurrence rate of 40% (Simpson, 1957).

In the benign lesion, consideration of the age of the patient is an important factor in surgical planning. In an elderly patient with a slow-growing tumor, debulking and decompression of the tumor may be safer than total removal. In the younger patients, for benign tumors that are not totally removed, consideration should be given to radiotherapy.

Radiation Therapy. Even after apparent complete removal, a small number of patients will suffer recurrence. Incomplete removal of larger tumors is particularly common in certain locations, including the posterior two-thirds of the central venous sinus, the clivus, and Meckel's cave–middle cranial fossa region (Quest, 1978). Plaquelike tumors of the inner portion of the sphenoid wing are relatively common, usually very slow growing, quite extensive, and occasionally impossible to resect completely (Castellano *et al.*, 1952).

Reports documenting the efficacy of irradiation for incompletely resected or recurrent meningiomas are sparse (Friedman, 1977). Perhaps most encouraging is the report of Wara and colleagues (1975b). Of 104 patients with incompletely resected meningiomas, 43 of 58 (74%) patients not receiving postoperative irradiation developed clinical recurrence, as opposed to 10 of 34 (29%) patients receiving postoperative irradiation. Supporting data have been reported by King and colleagues (1966), and similar data are available for children (Leibel *et al.*, 1976).

Therefore, radiation therapy after attempted initial surgical resection is recommended where minimal residual disease remains in an attempt to delay or decrease the overall incidence of clinical recurrence. A radiation dose in excess of 4500 to 5000 rads, delivered in five to six weeks in 150-rad to 280-rad fractions, appears to be needed.

Finally, it must be emphasized that ultimate clinical control requires nearly complete or complete resection, as attempts to deliver radiation doses in excess of 5000 rads are limited in deep-seated lesions by the frequent proximity and radiation tolerance of normal brain or brain stem. The necessity for careful treatment planning, with multiple fields of irradiation to permit maximum tumor dose homogeneity and optimum sparing of surrounding normal brain, is evident. If there is evidence of the angioblastic, papillary, or hemangiopericytoma types of tumor, then a more extensive operative procedure, including lobectomy if the tumor is situated in an appropriate site, may be indicated.

The survival curves for patients with malignant and benign meningiomas are shown in Figure 37–27. The role of radiation therapy in malignant, angioblastic, and papillary meningiomas or hemangiopericytomas is not yet clarified; but because of their known tendency to invade adjacent brain and dura, to recur, and to develop metastases, radiation therapy is recommended as a routine measure following complete or incomplete excision of one of these histologic types.

Meningeal sarcomas are essentially primary malignant tumors of the brain that may develop metastases to the lung or other sites. These tumors are rarely resectable; but when anatomy permits, tumor removal is indicated. Treatment techniques and general rationale discussed previously for less aggressive lesions pertain. Radiation doses should be carried to tolerance levels of the adjacent normal brain, even when only microscopic residual tumor remains. For most sites, radiation doses of 5500 to 6500 rads in six to seven weeks will be possible.

Although the primary treatment of meningioma is surgical, adjuvant chemotherapy should be considered in those cases where the tumor has regrown after multiple procedures and has failed to respond to radiotherapy. Under these circumstances, the tumor frequently undergoes progressive neoplastic degeneration and may take on a sarcomatous appearance. In such cases, chemotherapeutic regimens for sarcomas might be considered.

Hemangioblastoma. These are benign vascular tumors which usually arise in the cerebellum of adults and frequently produce a large cyst. They occur solely within the neuraxis.

Epidemiology. Hemangioblastomas comprise 1.5 to 2.0% of brain tumors and 7 to 12% of posterior fossa tumors (Russell and Rubinstein, 1977). Young adults are predominantly afflicted, with an average age of 30 to 40 years in most series.

In 1926, Lindau described the association of hemangioblastoma of the cerebellum with vascular tumors of the retina (previously reported by von Hippel in 1904) and with tumors and cysts at other sites. The lesions currently recognized as being occasionally associated with cerebellar hemangioblastoma include retinal hemangioblastoma, renal cell carcinoma, epididymal papillary cystadenoma, pheochromocytoma, and visceral cysts of the kidney, liver, and pancreas. Multiple cerebellar hemangioblastomas, or the association of cerebellar hemangioblastoma with the previously listed lesions, is known as Lindau's disease. Twenty percent of patients with a cerebellar hemangioblastoma have multiple CNS hemangioblastomas or have a family history of hemangioblastoma. This complex may be familial or occur sporadically. The familial type

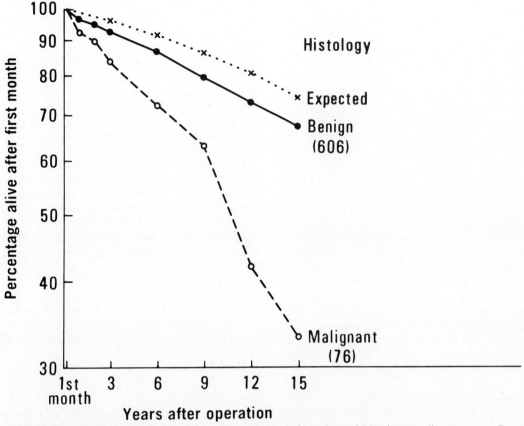

Figure 37-27.   Survival curves from one month postoperatively for patients with benign or malignant tumors. Expected survival curve is also shown. From MacCarty, C. S., *et al.*: Meningeal tumors of the brain. In Youmans, J. R. (ed): *Neurological Surgery,* Volume 5. W. B. Saunders Co., Philadelphia, 1982, p. 2965.

is transmitted in an autosomal dominant pattern. Patients with a family history of, or actually affected with, von Hippel-Lindau complex present at a younger age. The average age at presentation was 30 years, compared to 42 years for other cases in Jeffreys' series (1975a).

Pathology. These benign tumors primarily affect the cerebellar hemispheres. Hemangioblastomas involving the cerebral hemispheres, brain stem, and spinal cord make up less than 20%. The cerebellar lesions are usually well demarcated, bright-red mural nodules in the wall of an adjacent cyst filled with proteinaceous, xanthochromic fluid.

Microscopically, the hemangioblastoma contains a peculiar mix of two distinct cell types. A proliferation of plump, vesicular endothelial cells surrounding irregular vascular spaces is separated by dark, chromatin-staining stromal cells. The endothelial origin of the perivascular cells has been demonstrated im-

munologically (Kawamura *et al.,* 1973). Perivascular histiocytes, mesenchymal precursors of endothelial cells, and leptomeningeal derivatives have been the implicated, but unproven, histogenitors of the stromal cell.

In the series of Jeffreys (1975a) the cystic component of cerebellar hemangioblastomas averaged 33 mL in volume and contained an average protein content of 3.7 g/100 mL. Cumings (1950) found the cystic fluid to be similar to blood with respect to amino acid nitrogen, mucoprotein, and alkaline phosphatase. He suggested that the cyst fluid arose by diffusion from the blood through the abnormal vasculature of the mural nodule.

The secretion of erythropoietin by the stromal cells of these tumors results in polycythemia in 10 to 20% of patients (Cramer and Kinsey, 1952; Palmer, 1972). The erythropoietin is found within the cyst fluid and in the plasma. Forty-two percent of Jeffreys' (1975b) patients had hemoglobin levels exceeding 16 g/dL. Cytoplasmic secretory granules of the stromal cells detected by electron microscopy (EM) have been implicated as the source of erythropoietin (Ishwar *et al.,* 1971).

Clinical Presentation. The initial disturbance is almost uniformly generalized or suboccipital headache. At diagnosis, ataxia, nystagmus, and papilledema are usually present. A minority of patients experience subarachnoid or intraparenchymal hemorrhage as the initial symptom. Generally, the clinical presentation is similar to other slowly growing mass lesions of the cerebellar hemispheres.

Ophthalmic examination may reveal retinal hemangioblastomas. In an adult patient with neurologic findings originating in the posterior fossa and retinal hemangioblastoma or polycythemia, the diagnosis of cerebellar hemangioblastoma should be considered.

Investigation. Localization and identification of the tumor require angiography or computed tomography. Radioisotope scanning demonstrates most of these lesions, but may miss those that are cystic and does not help in the assessment of tumor type.

Contrast-enhanced CT demonstrates the cystic and solid types of tumors and reflects pathologic characteristics, but may not distinguish solid hemangioblastomas from other cerebellar neoplasms. The tumor density is similar to brain density on the unenhanced scans; but following contrast injection, it is enhanced prominently. The cyst, adjacent to most tumors, has a low attenuation coefficient (see Figure 37–28A).

Arteriography is particularly rewarding. Tumors stain homogeneously in the capillary phase of the arteriogram with a characteristic blush, allowing an accurate preoperative diagnosis (see Figure 37–28B). Multiple tumors may be overlooked by CT scanning, but are rarely missed by angiography. For this reason, CT scanning and angiography are recommended for all patients undergoing evaluation for a suspected hemangioblastoma.

Therapy and Management. These neoplasms are among the most favorable of intrinsic tumors of the nervous system for surgical excision. After entering the cyst cavity, the mural nodule is removed by dissecting around its periphery. Recurrence occurs in only 3 to 10% with complete removal of the mural nodule (Palmer, 1972; Jeffreys, 1975a). Aspiration of the cyst without excision of the tumor results in improvement in less than 20% of cases

for greater than 48 hours (Palmer, 1972; Jeffreys, 1975a). In patients with incomplete tumor removal, more than 50% die of tumor recurrence.

The solid tumors present a more difficult task for removal, largely owing to the increased risk of brain stem location and greater tendency to bleed with surgical manipulation.

Survival rates are 90% at five years and 80% at ten years in patients surviving the initial operation (Palmer, 1972).

Documented reduction of tumor size and diminished angiographic vascularity with radiation therapy have appeared in case reports (Helle *et al.,* 1980; Richardson *et al.,* 1980), but radiation generally does not reduce or eliminate tumor, prevent tumor regrowth, or suppress erythropoietic activity (Palmer, 1972; Jeffreys, 1975a).

Long-term management of hemangioblastoma patients requires consideration of the potential for separate foci of new growths, which tend to develop into tumors in a serial fashion and for which continued outpatient observation is mandatory.

Primary Lymphoma. Primary CNS lymphomas have received increasing attention because they occur more frequently in patients who have received immunosuppressive therapy for transplantation. These tumors have caused confusion about the cell of origin. That primary CNS lymphomas contain intracellular or surface immunoglobulin suggests that they are of lymphoreticular origin, not neuroepithelial origin, as was once believed (Garvin *et al.,* 1976; Varadachari *et al.,* 1978). The tumors are composed of mononuclear cells with anaplastic nuclei that invade the neural parenchyma and have predilection for the perivascular space (McKeever and Balentine, 1978). The picture can be confused with encephalitis. These neoplasms tend to be cortical in location and contain fibrous stroma or reticulin networks which stain with reticulin stains.

These CNS lymphomas are malignant tumors, invade locally, and may develop subarachnoid seeding. When other lymphoma sites are found, the CNS tumor is considered part of the systemic disease and not a primary site. Metastatic tumors are usually meningeal in location and not focal within the brain.

Without therapy, the average survival after diagnosis is less than one month. Surgical excision alone improves survival by only a few weeks. These neoplasms are dramatically ra-

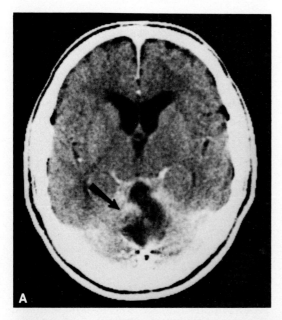

Figure 37–28. (*A*) CT scan demonstrating hemangioblastoma of superior cerebellar vermis. An enhancing mural nodule (arrow) lies in the wall of the associated cerebellar cyst. (*B*) Same patient. Vertebral arteriogram reveals "blush" of mural nodule in superior cerebellar vermis.

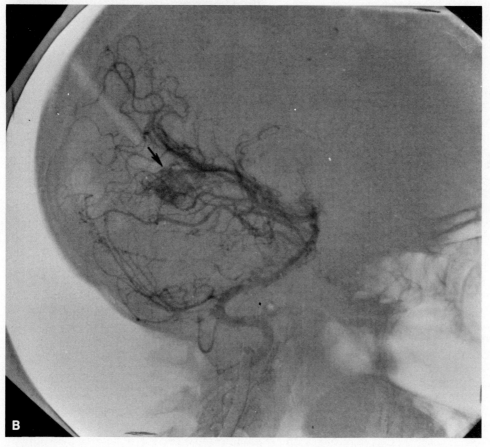

diosensitive. Patients receiving radiation therapy have 17 to 48 months average survival (Jellinger *et al.,* 1975; Schoenberg *et al.,* 1975; Zimmerman, 1975). Therefore, the goal of operative therapy is to establish a diagnosis, and it is unnecessary if cytologic analysis of the CSF is diagnostic. Whole-brain irradiation with 4500 rads is followed by focal therapy of 500 to 1000 rads to the tumor area (Littman and Wang, 1975). Lymphoma cells in the spinal fluid or clinical evidence of spinal involvement occurs frequently in these tumors; and if present, treatment should include spinal axis irradiation.

Tumors of Nerve Sheath Cells

Acoustic Neuroma (Acoustic Schwannoma). Schwann's cells sheathe the axons of the peripheral nerves from the point of penetration of the pia mater to the nerve terminal and are responsible for the myelin sheath of the peripheral and cranial nerves. They are regarded as homologous with the oligodendroglia of the central nervous system. The embryologic origin of the Schwann's cell is the neural crest, *i.e.,* neuroectodermal.

Epidemiology. Intracranial tumors of Schwann's cell origin are called schwannomas or neuromas. Sensory nerves are primarily affected. The great majority of intracranial nerve sheath tumors occur in cerebellopontine angle, originating from the vestibular portion of the eighth cranial nerve, the acoustic neuroma.

Acoustic neuromas comprise from 2 to 8% of all intracranial tumors (Schoenberg *et al.,* 1976; Russell and Rubinstein, 1977.) They are usually discovered in the later decades of middle life, with two-thirds of patients older than 40 years. The lesions occur predominantly in women, 54 to 76% of most series (Kasantikul *et al.,* 1980). Because most of the larger tumors appear in women (Kasantikul *et al.,* 1980) and because of reports of accelerated growth during pregnancy (Cushing, 1917), a hormonal effect is also implicated.

Increased risk of acoustic neuroma has been observed in patients with von Recklinghausen's disease. The tumors in these patients tend to be larger, occur earlier, grow more rapidly, are more cellular, and are often associated with other tumors (Kasantikul *et al.,* 1980; Martuza and Ojemann, 1982).

Bilateral acoustic neuromas have been considered a manifestation of a particular variant of von Recklinghausen's disease, even in the absence of other manifestations. They are transmitted as autosomal dominant. A family of six affected generations has been reported (Gardner and Turner, 1940).

Pathology. The acoustic neuroma is a benign, well-encapsulated tumor taking origin from the vestibular portion of the eighth cranial nerve at the transition zone where the Schwann's cells replace the oligodendroglia near the internal auditory meatus. The tumor frequently begins its growth within the auditory canal, imparting a conical shape to the most lateral segment of tumor compared to the more rounded component within the cerebellopontine angle. The facial nerve becomes stretched over the lobulated surface of the tumor, whereas the acoustic nerve may be splayed within the tumor capsule or within the tumor mass.

In histologic study, two types of tissue are seen in many tumors, Antoni type A and B tissue. In type A areas, the cells form a highly distinctive palisading pattern; whereas in areas of type B, a reticular pattern predominates. Electron microscopy demonstrates a lamellar pattern of elongated cell processes covered by basement membranes, corresponding to Antoni type A tissue. In areas of Antoni type B tissue, the cells, which also have basement membranes, contain large numbers of organelles and vacuoles compatible with a high degree of metabolic activity (Russell and Rubinstein, 1977). In tissue culture, two distinct tumor cell types, corresponding to the two tissue types of Antoni, are seen in early passages.

Specific estradiol binding in the cytoplasmic fraction of schwannomas (acoustic neuromas) has been demonstrated by Martuza *et al.,* (1981) in 7 of 16 tumors. Intravenously administered radioactive estrogen in rats localizes in the sensory ganglia of the cranial and spinal nerves, loci where Schwann's cell tumors develop. These facts, in conjunction with the previously described epidemiologic tendencies of acoustic neuromas, support a hormonal influence in their pathogenesis and growth.

Clinical Presentation. This is greatly dependent upon the size of the tumor. The earliest symptom of acoustic neuroma is usually hearing loss of gradual onset, often associated with tinnitus. The loss of hearing may initially appear as poor speech discrimination, especially when the patient is using the telephone with the affected ear. Episodes of vertigo and gait unsteadiness may occur, in addition to hearing disturbance, when the tumor is still small. As the tumor increases in size, the facial nerve, trigeminal nerve, and brain stem are compressed, causing the patient to experience disturbance in balance, alteration of taste, and suboccipital headache. Paresthesia or pain in the face, nystagmus, dysmetria, and diminished corneal sensation may be found in patients with large lesions. Rarely, altered mentation and gait disturbance are the initial symptoms referable to an acoustic neuroma with associated hydrocephalus.

Investigation. The diagnostic evaluation of the patient suspected of suffering an acoustic neuroma consists of auditory, vestibular, and radiographic studies. Testing begins with otologic evaluation.

In patients with unilateral progressive hearing loss, about 10% will have an acoustic neuroma. Since the majority of acoustic tumor suspects have symptoms or signs of cochlear nerve dysfunction, audiometry should be done in all suspects to define better this complaint.

Several of the traditional audiometric tests, such as Békésy audiometry, the short-increment sensitivity index (SISI), and the alternate binaural loudness balance test (ABLB), have been abandoned in recent years in favor of more reliable screening methods. These methods distinguish conductive from sensorineural hearing loss and discriminate cochlear from nerve deficit. Pure tone audiograms show an early high-frequency hearing loss. Testing of speech discrimination gives an indication of both the degree of useful hearing that is present and the retrocochlear location of the lesion. Threshold tone decay, acoustic reflex testing, and brain stem auditory evoked responses are also useful diagnostic measures.

In vestibular examination, the most reliable test of an eighth nerve lesion is reduced caloric response to cold water, measured by electronystagmography. Patients with smaller tumors show vestibular abnormalities in only 40 to 50% of cases. For this reason, some authors have questioned the applicability of this study as a screening procedure (Hart and Davenport, 1981).

Definitive diagnosis of tumor is not made from auditory and vestibular testing, but the results of these studies, combined with the clinical history, lead to a decision regarding special x-ray studies.

Seventy to 90% of acoustic tumors cause abnormalities on either routine skull films with special views (Stenvers, slit perorbital) or with tomograms of the petrous pyramids. Radiographic abnormalities include erosion of the superior margin of the internal auditory canal, flaring of the internal auditory meatus, and asymmetric (more than 1 mm) widening of the internal auditory canal (Hart and Davenport, 1981).

Computed tomography is quite helpful in the evaluation of these patients (see Figure 37–29). Tumors of 1.5 cm or larger will be seen on most scans, and lesions with diameters as small as 0.5 cm can be detected with the later CT models with higher resolution. Tumors with diameters less than 1.5 cm may be missed on any machine, however. CT data manipulation to display structures of bone density can be used to evaluate the internal auditory canal and meatus. Acoustic neuromas are distinguished from meningiomas (which are more dense than brain and stain strongly with contrast enhancement) and from cholesteatomas (which are hypodense compared to normal brain tissues and enhance poorly). Metrizamide and air CT cisternography to evaluate the cerebellopontine angle can demonstrate small tumors at or within the canal not seen by routine CT methods and will probably prove useful in evaluating the smaller lesions.

When the CT scan is positive and the internal auditory canal is abnormal, no other study is required, unless the large size of the lesion

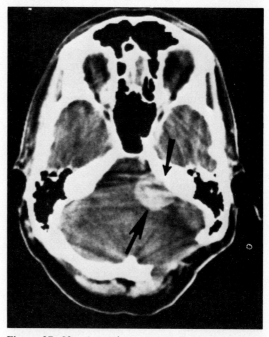

Figure 37–29. Acoustic neuroma. Enhancing tumor mass in left cerebellopontine angle. Smaller arrow indicates internal auditory meatus. Tumor has regrown following previous surgery.

merits angiography to evaluate the relationship of the posterior fossa vasculature to the tumor.

In the evaluation of the smaller lesions, posterior fossa myelography is the standard by which other diagnostic procedures must be evaluated. Positive contrast is manipulated into the cerebellopontine angle under fluoroscopic control, with the auditory canal of interest in the dependent position. Intracanalicular tumors cause incomplete filling of the canal. This study is abnormal in more than 98% of patients with acoustic tumor. False-positive results occur in less than 1% (Hart and Davenport, 1981). Expense, patient discomfort, and the rare complication of arachnoiditis may allow metrizamide or air CT cisternography to replace posterior fossa myelography if it proves to be as accurate.

Arteriography has no place in the preoperative evaluation of small lesions with an abnormal internal auditory meatus or canal. If the canal meatus is normal and a mass has been demonstrated in the cerebellopontine angle, angiography of the vertebral-basilar circulation is done to investigate the possibility of the presence of an aneurysm, arteriovenous malformation, or vascular tumor. Angiography is frequently used with the larger tumors, not primarily as a diagnostic study, but to outline the relation of the anterior and posterior inferior cerebellar arteries to the tumor for aid in intraoperative preservation of these important vessels.

Therapy and Management. The development of sophisticated audiometric and neuroradiologic techniques allows early diagnosis, and the binocular operating microscope and microsurgical technique have found a major application with these tumors. Today, mortality rates are less than 1% for all but those with very large tumors with poor preoperative neurologic status (Yasargil and Fox, 1974; Malis, 1975; Ojemann, 1978; Rand et al., 1982).

The otologic surgeons, already acquainted with the benefits of the operating microscope, were the first to report the use of the microscope for the removal of acoustic tumors (House, 1961). Their approach was a translabyrinthine operation for smaller tumors and a combined translabyrinthine-petrosal approach for the larger lesions in which the medial margin of the tumor could not be dissected from the adjacent brain stem under direct visualization with the limited access of the translabyrinthine approach.

Rand and Kurze (1965) subsequently incorporated modern microneurosurgical techniques into the unilateral suboccipital craniectomy and transmeatal approach developed by Walter Dandy at Johns Hopkins Hospital in the 1920s (Dandy, 1941). This surgical procedure results in total tumor removal, with preservation of facial nerve function in almost 100% of patients with tumors less than 2.0 cm in size and 70 to 85% of patients with tumors greater than 2.0 cm in size (Yasargil and Fox, 1974; Ojemann, 1978; Rand et al., 1982). Several reports have documented the preservation of useful hearing after removal of acoustic neuromas of up to 2.0 cm in diameter.

Many physicians are convinced that the suboccipital transmeatal excision of these tumors is preferred to any procedure which uses the translabyrinthine approach for several reasons. These include (1) hearing is sacrificed by the translabyrinthine route, but it may be maintained occasionally by the suboccipital route; (2) tumors of any size can be removed with the exposure achieved by the suboccipital approach, requiring the surgeon to develop depth of experience in a single procedure rather than selecting different operations dependent on tumor size; and (3) in any tumor that is extracanalicular, separation of tumor from the brain stem is dangerous with the limited exposure of the translabyrinthine approach.

Consideration must be given to whether the small intracanalicular tumors should be removed at all. The study of Kasantikul et al., (1980) indicates that the smaller tumors may be slower-growing lesions, with different biologic behavior than the larger ones. It is unlikely that removal of these tumors provides an improvement in hearing. The growth (or lack of growth) of these small lesions may be adequately monitored with metrizamide or air CT cisternography, or posterior fossa myelography at intervals. This is especially true for late middle-aged or older patients. A young patient with good cochlear nerve function on the affected side would be the exception in which an early operation is recommended to attempt to preserve functional hearing. Intraoperative brain stem auditory evoked responses allow continuous monitoring of cochlear nerve function.

At this time, radiation therapy or chemotherapy in the treatment of acoustic neuroma is not clearly indicated. In a new therapeutic model, Hirsh et al. (1979) have reported using focused beam irradiation with highly collimated beams from multiple gamma-emitting 60 sources of stereotactic delivery in nine patients with acoustic neuromas. Arrest of growth or shrinkage of tumor was seen in eight of nine cases.

Pineal Region Neoplasms

The discussion of the pineal region neoplasms as a group is justified by their common symptomatology, location, and distinctive histologic appearance. Most of these tumors originate from displaced embryonic tissue or from the parenchymatous elements of the normal pineal gland. The classification of the remarkable diversity of neoplasms found in this area is shown in Table 37–14.

Epidemiology. Tumors of the pineal gland as a group comprise 0.4 to 1.0% of all intracranial tumors, but account for 3 to 8% of pediatric intracranial tumors. More than 50% of these tumors occur in patients less than 20 years of age. The germ cell tumors occur predominantly in males; the pineocytomas, pineoblastomas, glial tumors, and cysts are distributed equally between the sexes. In Japan, the reported incidence of intracranial germ cell

Table 37–14. Pathologic Classification of Tumors in the Pineal Region

---

 I. Tumors of germ cell origin
   A. Typical teratomas and teratoid tumors
      Teratoma (including dermoid and epidermoid)
      Embryonal carcinoma (endodermal sinus
        tumor)
      Choriocarcinoma
      Rhabdomyosarcoma
   B. Germinoma (atypical teratoma, pinealoma)
      Pineal
      Ectopic (suprasellar)
 II. Tumors of pineal parenchymal cell origin
   A. Pineoblastoma
   B. Pineocytoma
III. Glial and other forms
   A. Astrocytoma
   B. Glioblastoma
   C. Ependymoma
   D. Choroid plexus papilloma
   E. Meningioma, hemangiopericytoma
IV. Cysts
   A. Epidermoid and dermoid cysts
   B. Nonneoplastic cysts and vascular lesions
      Arachnoid cysts
      Arteriovenous malformations
      Vein of Galen aneurysms

Derived from Russell, D. C.; and Rubinstein, L. J.: *Pathology of Tumors of the Nervous System,* 4th ed. Williams & Wilkins Company, Baltimore, 1977.

tumors has been as high as 5.1% of intracranial neoplasms.

Pathology. Teratomas (tumors composed of two or more tissues foreign to the organ of origin) of the pineal region exhibit a diversity of histologic appearances owing to the multitude of potential constituents and the degree of differentiation of each. They may contain cartilage, bone, teeth, squamous epithelium, or less-mature components, such as foci resembling endodermal sinus tumors of the gonads, chorioepithelioma, or other teratoid elements.

Also included with the tumors of germ cell origin is the germinoma, the most common form of growth at the site of the pineal gland. In the Childrens Cancer Study Group, of 118 patients, 36 of the 57 cases (64%) of pineal area tumors with biopsy had germinoma (Wara *et al.,* 1979). The typical microscopic appearance, as in germinomas of the mediastinum or gonads, consists of large spherical eosinophilic cells mixed with a smaller number of small cells identical in appearance to lymphocytes. Indeed, immunologic techniques demonstrate that they are T lymphocytes and probably are not a neoplastic element of the tumor, but a response to it.

The ectopic pinealoma is a neoplasm histopathologically identical to germinomas of the pineal region, but located in the hypothalamus or pituitary. Rarely, an ectopic pinealoma of the hypothalamus and a germinoma of the pineal gland occur in the same patient.

The pineocytoma and pineoblastoma originate from cells of the pineal gland and are quite rare. The pineocytoma is a fully differentiated neoplasm of slow evolution, whereas pineoblastoma designates a more malignant tumor which has a proclivity to CSF seeding and, microscopically, may be indistinguishable from a medulloblastoma.

A variety of gliomas (listed in Table 37–14) originate in the pineal body, as may dermoid and epidermoid tumors and arachnoid cysts.

Clinical Presentation. Symptomatology reflects the anatomic structures affected by these tumors. Because of their strategic location adjacent to the aqueduct of Sylvius, obstructive hydrocephalus, with increased intracranial pressure, nausea, vomiting, and papilledema, is common. Truncal or limb ataxia results from compression of the superior cerebellar peduncles or the superior portion of the vermis. Deficits in extraocular motility and pupillary function result from in of the area of the superior colliculus and the nu clei of the oculomotor nerves. Among these are limitation of upward conjugate gaze, mydriasis and inequality of the pupils, diminished or absent pupillary light reflex, and loss of the pupillary accommodation response (Rand and Lemmen, 1952).

Precocious puberty, when present, invariably occurs in the male. When occurring in patients with pineal area tumors, this syndrome is hypothesized to be caused by obliteration of the normally occurring secretion of melatonin by the pineal gland. Melatonin inhibits gonadal maturation.

Patients with germ cell tumors of the suprasellar area (ectopic pinealoma, suprasellar atypical teratoma) present with the triad of diabetes insipidus, hypopituitarism, and visual disturbance. These symptoms, however, can result from tumors of similar histopathology in the pineal region metastasizing anteriorly or causing obstructive hydrocephalus and dilatation of the third ventricle (Camins and Mount, 1974).

Investigation. Radiographic investigation of these patients includes skull x-ray, CT scan, and (in selected instances) angiography.

Plain skull x-rays may demonstrate abnormal areas of calcification or premature calcification in the region of the pineal gland. Pineal calcification greater than 10 mm in diameter is abnormal and prepubertal pineal calcification is sufficiently uncommon to lead to the suspicion of a pineal tumor (Rand and Lemmen, 1952). The presence or character of abnormal pineal calcification, however, does not correlate with tumor type.

The CT scan has supplanted the ventriculogram, pneumoencephalogram, and the arteriogram in the diagnosis of pineal region lesions. The CT scan defines the limits of the tumor and its relationship with the third ventricle, midbrain, and quadrigeminal cistern, and displays the presence or absence of cysts, low-density fluid, and fat density within the mass. It remains to be seen whether the diagnosis of a particular tumor type and the presence or absence of malignancy can be distinguished by this technique (Zimmerman et al., 1980; Futrell et al., 1981).

For tumors in this location, angiography serves two purposes. It distinguishes vascular lesions (such as aneurysms of the vein of Galen or arteriovenous malformations) from true neoplasms if the CT scan is inconclusive. If surgery for excision or biopsy is planned, it outlines the position of the vessels that must be

preserved and their relationship to the tumor in the operative field. This is important information in planning the surgical approach and in intraoperative orientation.

Elevated plasma and CSF concentrations of human chorionic gonadotropin, alpha-fetoprotein, and carcinoembryonic antigen have been reported with germ cell tumors of the pineal area and the suprasellar area (Arita et al., 1980; Jordan et al., 1980; Suzuki and Tanaka, 1980). The detection of these substances in abnormal amounts may prove useful in the preoperative prediction of tumor type when deciding if surgery should be recommended.

Therapy and Management. Before 1970, the operative mortality after surgical excision or biopsy of pineal area neoplasms was as high as 70% (Rand and Lemmen, 1952). Since most of these tumors are germinomas, highly sensitive radiocurable tumors, the standard therapy was a CSF shunting procedure followed by radiation therapy. As refinements in radiotherapy evolved, survival and recurrence-free intervals improved with five-year survival of 60 to 88% (Jenkin et al., 1978; Sung et al., 1978; Wara et al., 1979; Abay et al., 1981; Griffin et al., 1981; Rao et al., 1981).

In the pineal area, 35 to 50% of tumors are not germinomas. They are a heterogeneous group, consisting of tumors that are not radiosensitive but are surgically excisable (such as teratomas, epidermoid and dermoid cysts, and other cysts), as well as tumors that may respond to selective chemotherapy (such as endodermal sinus tumors, recurrent germinomas, pineoblastomas, and so forth). Histologic confirmation of tumor type is of paramount importance in the selection of, and in evaluating the response to, therapy for each of the many types of tumors in this area.

Two relatively recent developments allow reconsideration of therapeutic strategies. The advent of the use of the operating microscope and microneurosurgical techniques has made surgical procedures in the pineal region practical, with operative mortality now less than 5% and minimal morbidity (Suzuki and Iwabuchi, 1965; Sano, 1976; Stein, 1979). The CT scan enables certain lesions, such as cysts, epidermoid and dermoid tumors, and teratomas, to be accurately identified (Zimmerman et al., 1980). As previously stated, these lesions are radioresistant, have no tendency for CSF seeding, and can potentially be totally excised.

The CT scan does not allow distinction between the solid malignant tumors: germinoma, malignant teratoma, astrocytoma, pineocytoma, pineoblastoma, and the rarer tumors. The infiltrative character of these tumors does not allow surgical cure, and surgery increases the risk of CSF dissemination of tumor. Sung *et al.,* (1978) reported that 8 of 22 patients with histologically verified tumors had spinal metastases, compared to 3 of 50 patients with tumors without surgery. Of the germinomas exposed surgically and biopsied or undergoing partial resection, 57% metastasized to the cerebral or spinal subarachnoid space. In the report from the Children Cancer Study Group, 14% of biopsy-proven germinomas had spinal metastases versus 1.7% in the no-biopsy group (Wara *et al.,* 1979).

A ventricular CSF shunting procedure should be the initial therapy for those individuals with obstructive hydrocephalus and increased intracranial pressure.

If the CT scan demonstrates a cystic, benign tumor, surgical exposure (either with an occipital interhemispheric or a supracerebellar infratentorial approach) and attempted complete removal comprise the treatment of choice.

A solid tumor with no CT characteristics of a radioresistant, benign tumor should be treated initially with radiation therapy. The rapidity of response of tumors on serial CT scans following radiation should give some ideas about the histology of the lesion. A repeat CT scan should be performed at 3000 rads and compared to the scan taken prior to radiotherapy. If the scan at 3000 rads shows complete resolution of disease or prominent reduction in size, the tumor is assumed to be a radiosensitive lesion; and radiation therapy is completed to a total dose of whole-brain irradiation of 4000 to 4500 rads and a ventricular or tumor field boost to 5000 to 5500 rads. If the scan at 3000 rads leads one to suspect a radioresistant tumor, histologic diagnosis is obtained by surgical biopsy or excision. There is no evidence that prior shunting and radiation therapy compromise the result of a direct surgical attack.

The decision to irradiate the spinal axis must be based upon the level of suspicion of CSF seeding. Routine prophylactic spinal irradiation is not recommended. The incidence of spinal subarachnoid involvement in patients with simultaneous pineal and hypothalamic lesions, surgically manipulated germinomas, and patients with positive CSF cytology warrants spinal irradiation. Routine cytology is not sufficiently sensitive to the presence of disseminating tumor to be relied upon (Chapman and Linggood, 1980). Millipore filtered CSF tissue culture techniques appear to increase the sensitivity of CSF examinations (Black *et al.,* 1978). Sano (1976) has reported 60% positive diagnosis with this method.

Positive results of plasma or CSF human chorionic gonadotropin, carcinoembryonic antigen, or alpha-fetoprotein indicate a germ cell tumor and probable radiosensitivity.

Germinoma of the pineal gland is identical to seminoma of the testicle in its pathology and radiosensitivity (Friedman, 1947). No study has determined if the lower therapeutic doses customarily used to treat testicular seminomas would successfully cure these histologically similar tumors in the pineal and suprasellar areas.

Tumors of Developmental Origin

Craniopharyngioma. The anterior lobe and pars intermedia of the pituitary gland develop by maturity of an embryonic diverticulum of the stomodeum, Rathke's pouch. Current theories attribute the cellular origin of craniopharyngiomas to Rathke's pouch remnants, metaplasia of the adenohypophysis, or from the squamous cell nests adjacent to the pituitary gland and stalk found incidentally at autopsy in many adults. Presumably, the latter are also the remnants of Rathke's pouch.

Epidemiology. Craniopharyngiomas are the most common intracranial tumor of childhood not derived from neuroepithelium. They make up 7% of primary childhood intracranial tumors and about 2 to 3% of brain tumors of all age groups. The peak incidence in childhood (40 to 50%) occurs before the age of 20 years and is followed by a relatively stable occurrence in the decades of adulthood (Russell and Rubinstein, 1977).

Pathology. Most craniopharyngiomas arise in the suprasellar subarachnoid space just posterior to, beneath, or anterior to the optic chiasm. In this location, they frequently adhere to the tuber cinereum of the hypothalamus. Intrasellar and third ventricular tumors occur less frequently.

Macroscopically, craniopharyngiomas appear well defined at the brain tumor interface but may be strongly adherent to the optic nerves and chiasm, the carotid arteries, and the hypothalamus, especially in tumors previously treated with operation or radiation therapy.

These are usually heterogeneous tumors with cystic and solid components, although completely cystic and completely solid craniopharyngiomas are not rare. Size varies from small asymptomatic tumors found at autopsy of less than 0.5 cm in diameter to over 10-cm lesions, with extension into the anterior, middle, or posterior fossa.

These lesions are distinguished from epidermoid tumors, not by histologic dissimilarities, but by their proclivity to the suprasellar and intrasellar areas and their characteristic clinical features. The solid portions consist of a peripheral layer of cuboidal or columnar epithelium surrounding a central area of stratified squamous epithelium and foci of cystic degeneration and keratinization. The cyst fluid is typically dark in color, viscous, and rich in cholesterol crystals. It can be irritating to CNS tissue and has caused aseptic meningitis and communicating hydrocephalus after spilling into the cerebrospinal fluid.

The margin of tumor contiguous with neural tissue may elicit an intense glial reaction of the subadjacent glia, with proliferation and alterations in morphology of the glial cells, that is, gliosis. This gliotic reaction resembles, and can be confused with, anaplastic change of the tumor, which rarely occurs with craniopharyngiomas. A small percentage of tumors do have an atypical, histologic pattern with increased mitoses and dense cellularity. In tissue culture, these atypical lesions have a rapidly growing cell population, malignant ultrastructural features, and the ability to form cholesterol crystals. Typical tumors do not exhibit these characteristics (Liszczak et al., 1978).

Clinical Presentation. The symptoms and physical findings in the patient with craniopharyngioma emerge from direct tumor compression of the many potentially symptomatic central nervous system structures surrounding the suprasellar and sellar areas. These include the optic nerves and chiasm, the hypothalamus, the pituitary, and the third ventricle.

The most frequent complaint is visual failure. Children tend not to appreciate visual loss as early as adults. In many cases, children are nearly blind by the time of recognition. Therefore, visual field defects are more common in adults, and optic atrophy is seen much more frequently in children. Obstruction of the third ventricle at the foramen of Monro by a large tumor effects a rise in intracranial pressure, with vomiting and papilledema in about one-third of affected children. This is less common in adults, where a similar obstruction more frequently results in dementia.

Hypothalamic and pituitary distortion produce endocrine deficiency. In the older patients, this manifests initially as hypogonadism, with amenorrhea or loss of sexual potency. Children suffer delayed pubescence, growth failure, or obesity. Hypothalamic involvement may produce somnolence and diabetes insipidus at any age.

Investigation. In order to outline more precisely the visual deficit, a formal visual field analysis and neuro-ophthalmology consultation are obtained.

Symptoms of endocrine dysfunction indicate a complete evaluation of pituitary function. Preoperative and postoperative assessments by an interested endocrinologist are particularly critical in children.

Craniopharyngiomas are one of the few intracranial tumors in which a tissue diagnosis can be made with reasonable confidence by plain skull x-rays. More than 90% of children and 50% of adults with a craniopharyngioma have suprasellar or intrasellar calcification or an enlarged sella.

The CT scan is abnormal in almost all cases. Small amounts of calcification not seen on plain x-rays may be detected. Contrast enhancement accentuates the density of the solid component. Cystic areas display more densely than CSF, but less densely than brain tissue. Coronal CT scanning may aid the definition of intrasellar or intraventricular extension (Naidich et al., 1976; Fitz et al., 1978) (see Figure 37–30).

Ideally, the relationships of the solid and cystic tumor components to the optic chiasm, the vessels in the parasellar area, and the ventricular system are determined by the preoperative radiologic studies. Angiography may be required, but pneumoencephalography and ventriculography add little to the information obtained with modern CT scanning and are of sufficient risk to discourage their use.

Treatment and Results. Critique of the various treatments of craniopharyngiomas requires consideration of several factors. The natural history may vary significantly from patient to patient. In seven untreated patients with long histories reported by Bartlett (1971b), six were alive and well an average of 20.5 years after the onset of symptoms. This tendency seems to be greater in the older patients (Ross-Russell and Pennybacker, 1961).

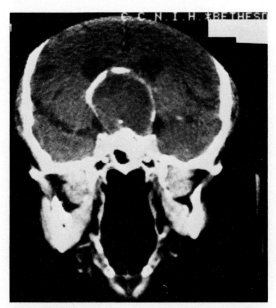

Figure 37-30. Coronal CT scan of large suprasellar craniopharyngioma. Tumor occludes the foramen of Monro by its superior extension. Partially calcified tumor capsule encloses cystic interior with attenuation coefficient between that of brain tissue and CSF.

It is the exception, rather than the norm, in either age group, however; and a long history of symptoms before treatment probably indicates a slowly growing tumor in both the young and old.

Clinical recurrence of tumor 20 symptom-free years after complete excision has been reported (Bartlett, 1971b). Therefore, new therapies, such as application of microneurosurgical techniques and injection of beta-emitting isotopes into the cystic portion, require an extended observation period after treatment for meaningful analysis.

Early attempts at total excision of these lesions was associated with prohibitive mortality until perioperative glucocorticoid administration was introduced. Total excision, when it can be safely accomplished, yields the best results and is the treatment of choice (Matson and Crigler, 1969; Bartlett, 1971b; Hoff and Patterson, 1972; Katz, 1975; Sweet, 1976; Hoffman *et al.,* 1977). The experienced surgeon can accomplish this in most patients who have not been treated previously with surgery or radiation therapy. Hoffman *et al.,* (1977) have reported 87% survival at 6.4 years after total excision, with no recurrence at an average of five years after surgery. Eight patients, who had the operating microscope used during their surgery for total tumor removal, experienced no operative morbidity and were alive at the time of his report, with no evidence of recurrence. Operative mortality of 0 to 2% has been achieved, even in the era prior to the use of the operating microscope (Matson and Crigler, 1969; Hoff and Patterson, 1972).

After incomplete tumor removal, radiation therapy delays recurrence and prolongs survival (Bartlett, 1971b; Hoff and Patterson 1972; Onoyama *et al.,* 1977). Radiation therapy as primary therapy has also been recommended after initial biopsy and cyst decompression (Kramer *et al.,* 1968; Bloom, 1973). Because of the considerable surgical morbidity and mortality, especially prior to the availability of corticosteroids, Kramer initiated an attempt at the Royal Marsden Hospital to control this lesion with irradiation after conservative surgery. Initially, using radiation doses of 6000 to 7000 rads in seven to eight weeks by a multiple field or rotational technique, almost uniform control was obtained. A recent update of this series, with radiation dose reduction to 5500 rads in six weeks shows five-year and ten-year survival rates of 85 and 72%, respectively. Thirty-eight patients receiving uniform 6 MEV megavoltage treatment had a five-year survival rate in excess of 90%. Similar results have been obtained in a series of patients treated at the Jefferson Medical School by Kramer and by the group at the Joint Center for Radiotherapy. Virtually uniform local control has been obtained in children treated with conservative surgery followed by multiple field or rotational megavoltage irradiation totaling 5500 rads in six weeks using 180-rad fractions daily. Similar results, especially with children, have recently been reported by Onoyama and others (1977). This initial response to radiation therapy has been temporary in other series, only delaying eventual tumor recurrence (Hoff and Patterson, 1972; Hoffman *et al.,* 1977; Shapiro *et al.,* 1979). The tumor recurred in 50% of children treated with cyst aspiration and radiation at an average of 4.4 years in the series of Shapiro *et al.* (1979). The response cannot always be attributed to radiotherapy since many patients have experienced long-term survival after cyst decompression and biopsy alone (Bartlett, 1971a, 1971b; Hoff and Patterson, 1972; Hoffman *et al.,* 1977). Overall disease-free survival is reduced when adult patients have been treated or lower doses of radiation have been used.

In conclusion, in recent years, the better endocrinologic management of craniopharyngioma patients and the reduced operative morbidity with the operating microscope have allowed a much higher incidence of complete and safe excision of these tumors. If tumor adherence to important parasellar structures, such as the carotid arteries, does not allow total excision, one may elect to use radiation therapy (5000 to 6000 rads over five to six weeks) or to postpone irradiation until evidence of tumor progression occurs on follow-up CT scanning.

Cystic recurrence after radiation therapy may be treated by intermittent aspiration stereotactically or by surgically placing a catheter within the tumor cyst and connecting it to a reservoir beneath the scalp for intermittent percutaneous aspiration. Purely intrasellar craniopharyngiomas should be removed completely using the operating microscope and transsphenoidal approach.

Colloid Cyst. During embryogenesis of the third ventricle, a folded evagination of the ventricular wall neuroepithelium (the paraphysis) is formed; later, in fetal development, it degenerates. The choroid plexus, ependyma, and paraphysis are all derived from neuroepithelium. Abnormal folding of the neuroepithelium in this region during embryonic development forms a colloid cyst of the anterior third ventricle, with attachment just posterior to the foramen of Monro. Shuangshoti *et al.,* (1965) have correlated the different histology of the wall and contents of the cysts in this region to origin by evagination or invagination of the neuroepithelium. They emphasize that, although the most common location of these neuroepithelial cysts is at the anterior segment of the roof of the third ventricle, cysts with similar histology and mechanism of origin are found in other ventricular or paraventricular locations.

These tumors are typically 1 to 3 cm in diameter and smooth, spherical cysts with a wall of cuboidal, columnar, or squamous cells. The soft, gelatinous contents of the cysts are formed by secretory products, desquamated cells, and hemorrhages from the thin membranous cyst wall.

Although they arise with less than 2% of the incidence of gliomas, the pendulous attachment at the foramen of Monro may give rise to symptomatology sufficiently unique to permit a presumptive diagnosis by the history alone. Intermittent ventricular obstruction, with sudden ventricular expansion, precipitates episodes of headache, vomiting, loss of consciousness, and leg weakness. These symptoms were relieved in 8 of 29 patients in one series by a change in position, presumably allowing the cyst to swing away from its obstructing position (Kelly, 1951). Sudden deterioration and death due to acute ventricular obstruction may take place spontaneously or follow lumbar puncture (Kelly, 1951; Little and MacCarty, 1974).

The most common manner of presentation, however, is less striking and without localization. These latter patients present with headache and papilledema or with dementia and gait disturbance without evidence of papilledema. They may be misdiagnosed initially as having pseudotumor cerebri or normal pressure hydrocephalus.

The diagnosis of colloid cysts has been simplified by the CT scan. A spherical mass in the anterior third ventricle at the foramen of Monro, of equal or greater radiographic density than that of the brain, establishes the diagnosis. Enlargement of the lateral ventricles is common. The mass of the colloid cyst may increase its absorption coefficient after intravascular injection of contrast material (Sackett *et al.,* 1975; Sage *et al.,* 1975).

The treatment recommended is surgical removal. Transcortical or transcallosal exposure of the interventricular foramen allows delivery of the collapsed tumor into the lateral ventricle after aspiration of the cyst contents. Then, transection of the pedicle and removal of the mass are easily accomplished (Greenwood, 1949; McKissock, 1951).

Pituitary Tumors

Epidemiology. Microadenomas (tumors less than 10-mm diameter) of the pituitary gland are found in as many as 27% of subjects in unselected autopsy series of asymptomatic persons (Borrow *et al.,* 1981). Clinically evident pituitary tumors comprise 3.4 to 17.8% of all primary intracranial tumors (Russell and Rubinstein, 1977). Therefore, most pituitary adenomas are not clinically important, or at least do not produce recognized symptomatology. Those that cause hypersecretion of one or more hormones of the adenohypophysis (the endocrine-active adenomas) or that cause symptoms by compressing the normal pituitary or adjacent neural structures (the endocrine-inactive and the endocrine-active adenomas) represent the pituitary tumors requiring medical management (see also Chapter 32).

The relative incidence of the symptomatic pituitary tumors has been difficult to determine because of the tendency of patients to be attracted to centers establishing a reputation with a particular tumor type. Landolt and Wilson (1982), in their review of tumors of the sella and parasellar area, estimated the following frequencies: (1) endocrine-inactive tumors, 20%; (2) growth hormone–secreting adenomas (acromegaly, gigantism), 25%; (3) prolactinomas, 35%; (4) corticotropic adenomas (Cushing's, Nelson's syndromes), 5%; and (5) adenomas producing more than one hormone, 10%.

Pathology. Pituitary tumors were formerly classified by conventional staining techniques into chromophobe, eosinophilic, and basophilic adenomas. This scheme, however, does not consistently correlate with the clinical syndromes or endocrine data. For example, chromophobe adenomas may be endocrinologically inactive or may secrete adrenocorticotropic hormone (ACTH), growth hormone (GH), or prolactin (PRL). What is required is that the histologic classification reflect the different clinical syndromes and the characteristic laboratory data found in each syndrome. A classification based upon the results of immunofluorescent staining of the cytoplasmic secretory granules, which contain the specific releasing hormones, is evolving.

Gross pathologic distinction of adenomas from the normal pituitary can frequently be accomplished by differences in texture and color. Small tumors are more difficult to recognize than larger tumors. The orange-yellow color and firm consistency of the normal anterior pituitary gland contrasts with the soft, grayish-white tissue of most well-defined microadenomas.

As the tumor enlarges, it expands the sella, focally erodes the bone of the sellar floor, or grows upward, stretching the diaphragma sellae superiorly. As further progression occurs, it may invade the subadjacent sphenoid sinus, expand into the suprasellar area, compressing the optic nerves or chiasm, or compress or invade the cavernous sinus laterally.

Microscopically, pituitary adenomas are homogeneous with monotonous sheets of epithelial cells of uniform size. The tumor architecture may be diffuse cellular, sinusoidal, or papillary. All three types conspicuously lack the stromal connective tissue septae surrounding the lobules of the normal pituitary gland. Occasionally, microscopic features of malignancy, such as cellular pleomorphism, multinucleated cells, and mitoses, are seen. These are often unrelated to duration of symptoms, response to therapy, and survival.

Electron microscopic studies show electron-dense secretory granules in the cells of virtually all pituitary adenomas, regardless of whether or not the patient has signs of endocrine hyperfunction (Tomiyasu *et al.,* 1973; Lewis and Van Noorden, 1974). The release of the secretory granule's contents into the intercellular space by fusion of the membrane of the hormone granule with the cell membrane (exocytosis) is visible in most cases (Farquhar, 1961).

Recent histologic studies, utilizing immunofluorescent and immunoperoxidase staining techniques, have defined the nature of the cytoplasmic secretory granules of the normal pituitary gland and pituitary adenomas.

Clinical Presentation and Laboratory Examination. Pituitary adenomas come to the physician's attention because of endocrine disturbances or visual disorders. Visual disturbance results from suprasellar extension of tumor compressing the optic nerve or chiasm. The patient experiences diminished visual acuity in one or both eyes, or may gradually develop complete or partial bitemporal hemianopia. After long-standing compression of an optic nerve or the optic chiasm, optic nerve head atrophy occurs, and pallor of the optic disc can be seen by funduscopic examination. Compression or invasion of the cavernous sinus causes ocular palsies. Extensive suprasellar growth can obstruct the foramen of Monro, resulting in obstructive hydrocephalus or compression of the hypothalamus, leading to diabetes insipidus, somnolence, or hypothermia. The development of radioimmunoassays for measurement of pituitary hormones has made possible the detection of adenomas at an early stage and the delineation of several endocrine syndromes.

Hyperprolactinemia (Amenorrhea-Galactorrhea Syndrome). The most common type of pituitary tumors are those that secrete prolactin (PRL), hyperprolactinemia being reported in 70% in one series of patients with pituitary tumors (Antunes *et al.,* 1977). This syndrome usually becomes manifest during the childbearing years, when a patient desirous of becoming pregnant consults the gynecologist with complaints of amenorrhea and galactorrhea. Infertility, without alteration of the normal menstrual cycle, or amenorrhea, without galactorrhea, may also result from hyperprolactinemia. Serum prolactin levels are usually in excess of 100 ng/mL (Kleinberg *et al.*, 1977).

Males with prolactin-secreting tumors generally present with larger tumors and complaints of headache, impotence, and visual abnormalities. Galactorrhea is rare.

In tumors, basal levels of prolactin are elevated above the normal level of 25 ng/mL. Many other conditions are associated with hyperprolactinemia, such as hypothyroidism, progesterone therapy, and phenothiazine and tricyclic antidepressant therapy. These must also be considered in the patient with elevated serum prolactin.

Prolactin levels normally fluctuate diurnally, with a two- to three-fold rise during sleep between 2:00 and 4:00 A.M. The response of a normal patient to chlorpromazine is a sustained rise in serum PRL of at least double the basal value one to two hours after the drug is given. Thyrotropin-releasing hormone produces a three- to fivefold rise of PRL 20 to 30 minutes after administration. Patients harboring prolactin tumors do not respond to these stimuli with elevation of serum PRL.

Acromegaly. Overproduction of growth hormone (GH) produces acromegaly. Prior to puberty, excess secretion of GH results in gigantism. The characteristic clinical changes, alteration of facial features, and increasing glove and shoe size progress insidiously over months or years before the diagnosis is made. In addition, many patients suffer from diabetes mellitus, osteoarthritic-like changes in bones and joints, cardiomegaly, and congestive heart failure. Signs of compression of the anterior visual system are often present. Untreated acromegaly is associated with decreased life expectancy; as many as one-half of patients will die before the age of 50 if untreated (Wright *et al.*, 1970). Mortality is usually a result of cardiovascular disease.

The diagnosis is made on the basis of the characteristic clinical changes and elevation of serum GH values (> 10 ng/mL for females and > 5 ng/mL for males), with abnormal response to glucose. Occasionally, the patient's basal GH level may be normal despite the clinical picture of acromegaly. However, during a glucose tolerance test, growth hormone values will not be depressed. In normal persons with GH values in the basal range, the GH decreases to 0, or less than 1 ng per mL within 30 to 60 minutes after the beginning of a glucose tolerance test. In active acromegaly, the response of GH during glucose stimulation remains unchanged, falls toward, but not to, normal, or rises (Daughaday and Cryer, 1980).

Some patients with acromegaly also have hyperprolactinemia and galactorrhea. Whether the pathogenesis of the elevated serum PRL is caused by autonomous secretion by tumor cells distinct from the GH-producing tumor cells or by restriction of delivery of a prolactin inhibitory factor to the normal pituitary gland by the tumor presence, has not been fully worked out.

As many as one-third of patients with active acromegaly have carpal tunnel syndrome in one or both hands. The symptoms of this syndrome generally disappear within several days of removal of the pituitary adenoma (O'Duffy *et al.*, 1973).

Cushing's Syndrome and Nelson's Syndrome. Cushing's syndrome is the result of elevated serum levels of adrenal corticosteroids, which cause truncal obesity, hypertension, weakness, amenorrhea, hirsutism, abdominal striae, glycosuria, osteoporosis, and, in some cases, a characteristic psychosis. The incidence in the female is three times that in the male. The syndrome may be caused by a pituitary tumor, an adrenal tumor, or an ectopic ACTH-producing neoplasm. Most patients with Cushing's syndrome harbor ACTH-secreting pituitary microadenomas. These patients (1) have elevated serum levels of cortisol and urinary-free cortisol, or lack normal diurnal variation in serum cortisol levels; (2) have elevated or normal ACTH; (3) have a lack of cortisol suppression, with 0.5 mg of dexamethasone given every six hours; and (4) show suppression of cortisol and ACTH, with 2 mg of dexamethasone given every six hours. Low values of serum ACTH imply an adrenal tumor, and levels greater than 300 pg/mL (normal, 20 to 100 pg/mL) lead one to suspect an ACTH-producing ectopic neoplasm. Failure to suppress excess cortisol or ACTH secretion with the high-dose dexamethasone suppression test indicates either an adrenal tumor or an ectopic ACTH-producing tumor. Space does not permit an in-depth review of the typical signs, symptoms, and laboratory measurements in Cushing's disease. These are readily available in standard endocrine texts (see Williams, 1982).

Nelson's syndrome is the development of hyperpigmentation and an ACTH-secreting pituitary tumor following bilateral adrenalectomy (Nelson *et al.,* 1958). Initially, it was believed that the pituitary tumor resulted from the bilateral adrenalectomy. It is now evident that most of these patients had unrecognized ACTH-secreting pituitary tumors prior to adrenalectomy, which became recognized only after months or years of further growth after the operation. These pituitary tumors may be particularly aggressive, invasive of adjacent structures, and difficult to treat successfully.

Radiologic Investigation. The clinical presentation and endocrine testing establish the presence of a hypersecreting pituitary adenoma; the neuroradiologic examination permits assessment of tumor size and location of potential extrasellar extension of endocrine-active and endocrine-inactive adenomas and, in addition, confirms the diagnosis of endocrine-inactive pituitary adenomas.

Skull Radiographs and Tomograms. Plain skull films and frontal and lateral tomograms at 1- to 2-mm intervals are recommended in all patients suspected of harboring pituitary tumors. Microadenomas may produce no abnormality in either of these studies, or they may focally erode the sella floor or result in lateral sloping of the sella floor. However, these changes have been noted in *post mortem* studies in persons without pituitary tumors and cannot be relied upon either to confirm the presence of or confidently localize a microadenoma (Borrow *et al.,* 1981).

As the tumor grows, destruction of the dorsum sella occurs, and the sella exceeds its normal dimensions (240 to 1092 mm^3) (Di Chiro and Nelson, 1962). Tumor growth often erodes the sella floor and expands into the sphenoid sinus.

Computed Tomography. CT scanning (Figure 37–31A, B) demonstrates tumors with extrasellar extension but does not permit visualization of most microadenomas (Banna *et al.,* 1980). Superior extension encroaches upon the suprasellar cistern and can be further recognized by homogeneous or mottled contrast enhancement. Coronal scanning outlines the suprasellar expansion and its compression of the third ventricle. The superior image quality of the latest model scanners has allowed this study to replace pneumoencephalography for the examination of these tumors.

Arteriography. Until recently, carotid arteriography was considered part of the routine preoperative evaluation of pituitary ade-

nomas. Now, arteriograms need to be obtained only when evaluating endocrine-inactive tumors, because, in these cases, it is essential to rule out the presence of an intrasellar carotid artery aneurysm. Digital subtraction arteriography will probably replace carotid arteriography for this purpose, as the development and refinement of the technique evolves.

Therapy. The ideal therapy of pituitary tumors has four objectives: (1) complete eradication of the pituitary adenoma; (2) decompression of the nervous structures, particularly the visual pathways; (3) return to a normal, stable hormonal status; and (4) minimum of associated therapeutic morbidity and no mortality. No treatment achieves these ideal objectives in every case. Therefore, a combination of various forms of treatment may be required for the optimal result in any given patient. Basically, three different methods of treatment can be used, alone or in combination. These include operative procedures (transcranial or transsphenoidal excision); radiotherapy with proton-beam, cobalt-60, or high-voltage irradiation; and medical treatment with antisecretory drugs, such as bromocriptine. Specific indications for a transcranial operative approach are suprasellar growth laterally into the temporal fossa, posteriorly behind the clivus, and anteriorly beneath the frontal lobes. With the endocrine-active and endocrine-inactive adenomas, therapeutic success has been better with tumors limited to the sella.

Prolactinomas. At this time, the treatment of prolactin-producing pituitary tumors is transsphenoidal removal or by transcranial excision, possibly combined with the transsphenoidal approach, if there is lateral extension or extensive suprasellar extension. Tumor size greater than 1 cm in diameter and serum prolactin values greater than 200 ng/mL have been poor prognostic factors for the results of operations in most series. Normalization of prolactin levels and menses after transsphenoidal surgery in patients whose preoperative prolactin levels are less than 200 ng/mL occurs in 70 to 80% of patients, whereas those patients with preoperative prolactin levels greater than 200 ng/mL have an approximately 35 to 50% incidence of normal postoperative prolactin values and return of normal menses (Antunes *et al.,* 1977; Chang *et al.,* 1977; Hardy *et al.,* 1978; Aubourg *et al.,* 1980; Faria and Tindall, 1982). Treatment with high-voltage radiation therapy, cobalt-60, or the linear accelerator usually reduces serum prolactin, but not to

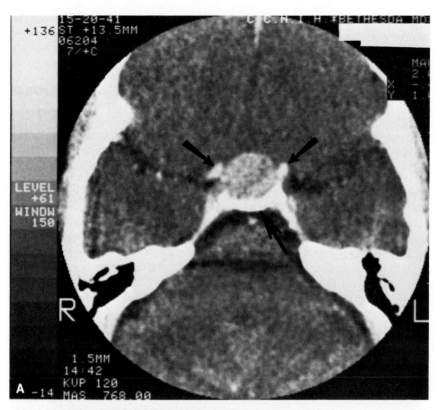

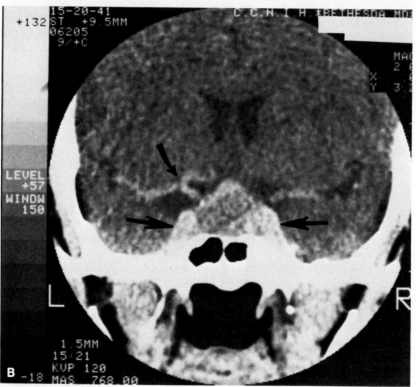

normal levels; and it takes months to years for this limited response to become manifest.

Bromocriptine, a dopamine agonist, is frequently successful in reducing circulating prolactin to normal, restoring menses and fertility, and in reducing tumor size (George et al., 1979; Thorner et al., 1980; Chiodini et al., 1981; Wollesen et al., 1982). However, current evidence indicates that, although bromocriptine can reduce the tumor size and slow the rate of secretion, it cannot effect a cure. Several cases have been reported of rapid recurrence of prolactinoma volume, elevated prolactin levels, and visual compression within days of discontinuing prolonged therapy with bromocriptine (Thorner et al., 1981).

Combinations of surgery, bromocriptine, and irradiation therapy may be required to improve the therapy of these tumors, especially macroadenomas and tumors associated with serum prolactin levels exceeding 200 ng/mL.

Growth Hormone–Secreting Adenomas. Because of the chronic morbidity and early mortality associated with acromegaly, an aggressive approach to therapy can be justified. Two of the widely used modalities for the treatment of growth hormone–secreting tumors of the pituitary include surgery and irradiation.

In more than three-fourths of patients undergoing transsphenoidal operations for acromegaly, growth hormone levels revert to normal within 24 hours. Clinical improvement is often striking and prompt, with disappearance of arthritic pain, early regression of soft tissue changes, and weight loss (Hardy, 1973; Baskin et al., 1982). About 5 to 10% of patients lose some degree of pituitary function and require hormonal replacement (Hardy, 1973; Baskin et al., 1982). Incomplete responses and therapeutic failures are more frequent with suprasellar extension of tumor, preoperative GH greater than 40 ng/mL, or diffuse destruction of the sella floor (Baskin et al., 1982).

For the alternative approach, irradiation, both conventional and proton-beam irradiation have been employed. Conventional irradiation, with 4000 to 6000 rads delivered during a period of 5 to 7.5 weeks, has been an accepted treatment for many years. Normal growth hormone levels can be expected in about 70% of patients (Eastman et al., 1979). Such reductions can be extremely and unacceptably delayed, sometimes requiring four to six years to accomplish. Partial or complete hypopituitarism induced by therapy is frequently seen (Aloia and Archambeau, 1978).

With proton-beam therapy, a focused beam of 12,000 to 15,000 rads can be delivered to the pituitary tumor. The beam is aligned so that the Bragg peak is centered in the anterior portion of the sella. Under these conditions, 75 to 90% of the anterior lobe will be destroyed by radionecrosis. The fall in growth hormone occurs slowly—growth hormone levels in 30% of patients falling to less than 5 ng/mL within two years and 68% within six years of treatment (Lawrence et al., 1975). There are, however, considerable numbers of patients with hypopituitarism (20 to 35%), visual field defects, and extraocular nerve palsies (up to 29%) (Kjellberg et al., 1968; Dawson and Dingman, 1970; Kjellberg and Kliman, 1971; Daughaday and Cryer, 1980). Furthermore, patients with extrasellar extension of tumor cannot be treated. This form of therapy is available in only two centers in the United States.

If the serum GH remains elevated after transsphenoidal surgery, conventional radiation therapy almost uniformly results in a return to normal values. When both transsphenoidal excision and irradiation are required for remission, the incidence of hypopituitarism exceeds 50% (Baskin et al., 1982).

ACTH-Secreting Pituitary Adenomas. Before initiating therapy for Cushing's syndrome, the diagnosis of an ACTH-secreting pituitary tumor must be firmly established. Since most of these tumors are too small to cause sella changes or to be detected by special radiographic procedures, the clinician reaches the diagnosis by the previously described laboratory tests.

When the diagnosis of a pituitary tumor as

Figure 37–31. (*A*) Enhanced CT scan demonstrating ACTH-secreting pituitary adenoma in two patients with previous bilateral adrenalectomy for Cushing's disease (Nelson's syndrome). Contrast-containing internal carotid arteries (small arrows) lie at lateral margins of spherical tumor.

(*B*) Coronal CT scan following intravenous infusion of contrast. Same patient as *A*. Pituitary adenoma is between more densely enhancing right and left cavernous sinuses (large arrows). Location of intracranial bifurcation of left internal carotid artery into middle cerebral artery and anterior cerebral artery is shown by small arrow. Note obliteration of chiasmatic cistern by suprasellar tumor extension.

the cause of hypercortisolism can be made, transsphenoidal operation is the treatment of choice. More than 90% of patients with intrasellar tumors reverse the clinical manifestations of hypercortisolism, and adrenocorticotropin (ACTH) and cortisol levels return to normal (Salassa *et al.*, 1978; Tyrrell *et al.*, 1978; Boggan *et al.*, 1982). Transsphenoidal surgery induced long-term remission in 12 of 23 patients harboring adenomas, with extrasellar extension reported by Boggan *et al.* (1982). Despite precise assays for cortisol and ACTH, a small fraction of patients will prove not to have pituitary adenomas. Instead, either ectopic secretion of ACTH will subsequently be demonstrated or diffuse hyperplasia of the anterior pituitary will be found.

Conventional megavoltage pituitary irradiation (4000 to 5000 rads) was administered to 51 patients reported by Orth and Liddle (1971). Although such treatment did not result in restoration of normal diurnal rhythm in plasma cortisol or normal responses to dexamethasone suppression tests in patients considered cured, 23 of 51 patients improved enough to require no further therapy. Subsidence of the disease after successful irradiation takes at least several months, however, and the patient with advanced Cushing's syndrome may have complications of the disease before responding. Kjellberg and Kliman (1975) effected total remissions in 63% of patients treated with proton-beam irradiation.

PRIMARY SPINAL NEOPLASMS

Overview

Tumors of the spinal canal are conveniently grouped into extradural, intradural-extramedullary, and intramedullary tumors. This classification has diagnostic importance. The extradural lesions (those arising outside the dural covering of the spinal cord) are almost all metastatic and will not be discussed in this chapter. The intradural-extramedullary lesions (those arising outside the spinal cord, but within the dura) are usually benign tumors that can be surgically cured, whereas the intramedullary lesions (those arising within the spinal cord substance) are well defined and accessible to surgical excision (ependymomas) or infiltrative with little chance of total removal (astrocytomas) (see Figure 37–32).

Biological Characteristics. The spinal cord is an ovoid neural structure that lies within the spinal canal, extending from the foramen magnum to the intervertebral level between L_1 and L_2. The lower limit of the spinal cord extends to L_3 at birth; but as the vertebral column grows in childhood, the relationship of the vertebral and neural segments changes. Therefore, the adult thoracic and upper lumbar cord levels are located two to three levels higher than the corresponding vertebral body. For instance, the L_1 spinal cord segment lies opposite the T_{11} vertebral body.

The first pair of spinal nerves exits the vertebral column between the atlas and the skull. The remaining cervical roots exit above the vertebral body of corresponding number, except for the eighth cervical root, which leaves below the C_7 vertebra. The remaining spinal roots exit below the vertebra of their number.

Spinal tumor symptoms and signs stem from compression or invasion of the nerve roots, long tracts, or central gray of the spinal cord. They may also result from vascular compression. Clinical manifestations of nerve root or central gray damage are segmental in distribution, whereas expression of long tract involvement is usually half the body below the lesion level. Corticospinal tract or posterior column functional interruption produces ipsilateral loss of motor or vibratory and position sense, respectively. Damage to the spinothalamic tract, a crossed spinal tract, results in suppression of pain and temperature sensation on the opposite body half below the damaged level. When extramedullary tumors impinge on the spinal cord from a lateral direction, pain and temperature loss contralateral to the maximum motor weakness may occur (Brown-Séquard syndrome) and are frequently seen with spinal meningiomas and neurofibromas.

Epidemiology. In the Mayo Clinic series of 8784 primary tumors of the central nervous system and its sheath elements, only 15% were intraspinal (Sloof *et al.*, 1964). Although primary spinal tumors have the same cellular origins as those arising in the brain, the relative incidences of the various cell types differ remarkably from those harbored by the cranial cavity; the majority of intraspinal neoplasms are benign and produce symptoms by spinal cord compression rather than invasion. The incidence of primary spinal tumors is shown in Figure 37–33A, and the relative incidence of the intramedullary spinal cord gliomas is shown in Figure 37–33B.

Fifty-five percent of intraspinal tumors arise

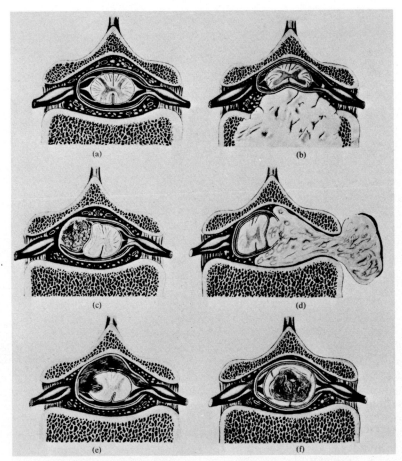

Figure 37–32.   Relationship of different types of spinal cord tumor to the spinal cord: (*a*) normal relationship; (*b*) extradural, extramedullary tumor (usually metastasis); (*c*) intradural, extramedullary tumor, e.g., meningioma; (*d*) extradural and intradural tumor, e.g., neurofibroma, meningioma; (*e*) intradural, extramedullary and intramedullary tumor, e.g., neurofibroma; (*f*) intradural, intramedullary astrocytoma, ependymoma. From Shafer, E. R.: Chirurgie des Gehirns und Rückenmarks im Kindes- und Jugendalter. Bushe, K. A., and Glees, P. (eds.), Hippokrates-Verlag, Stuttgart, 1968, p. 1159.

from the covering of the spinal cord (meningiomas) or a nerve root (schwannomas). The sex distribution of intraspinal meningiomas indicates a female-to-male preponderance of 4 : 1, compared to a 2 : 1 female-to-male ratio in intracranial meningiomas (Sloof *et al.,* 1964). Neurofibromas are equally distributed between the sexes.

Symptoms and Signs.   Spinal canal tumors must be distinguished from other diseases that cause radicular (nerve root) or myelopathic (spinal cord) symptoms. The differential diagnosis frequently includes disorders (such as demyelinating or degenerative diseases) that currently have no effective therapy. Therefore, in patients whose complaints suggest the possibility of a space-occupying lesion of the spinal canal, even if the likelihood is small, the diag-

nostic approach should be to eliminate that possibility.

Patients with spinal cord tumors usually have one of three clinical pictures: (1) a painful radicular-spinal cord syndrome, (2) a pure sensorimotor spinal tract syndrome, or (3) an intramedullary syndrome (Adams and Victor, 1981).

Radicular-Spinal Cord Syndrome.   The vast majority of intradural-extramedullary tumors are meningiomas or neurofibromas — benign tumors with slow growth rates which compress rather than invade the spinal cord and produce neurologic syndromes that progress very slowly. Because these tumors originate within or adjacent to a nerve root, radicular pain (pain in the distribution of a sensory nerve root) and spinal pain are often initial

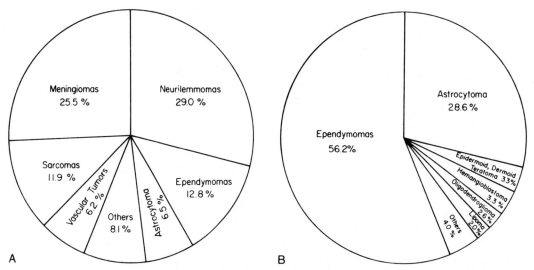

Figure 37–33. (*A*) Relative incidence of intramedullary spinal cord tumors. (*B*) Relative incidence of tumors of the spinal cord, based on a review of 1322 spinal cord tumors reported from the Mayo Clinic. From Connolly, E. S.: Spinal cord tumors in adults. In Youmans, J. R. (ed.): *Neurological Surgery*, Vol. 5. W. B. Saunders Co., Philadelphia, 1982, p. 3197.

symptoms. The pain may be knifelike or a dull ache with superimposed sharp pains that are intensified by cough, sneeze, or strain. Segmental sensory changes, such as paresthesias or numbness, often precede the manifestations of spinal cord compression by months or years. The latter consist of an asymmetric spastic weakness of the legs, a sensory level on the trunk below which perception of pain and temperature is reduced or lost, posterior column signs, and a spastic bladder under weak voluntary control. Gait disturbance and urinary urgency or incontinence proceed at a variable pace. The slowly evolving neurologic syndrome frequently is misdiagnosed as diabetic neuropathy, primary lateral sclerosis, or cervical spondylosis. The radicular pain and the sensory level are critical in determining the level of the lesion.

Sensorimotor Spinal Tract Syndromes. In these, the predominant clinical picture stems from compression and (less often) from invasion and destruction of spinal cord tracts. The onset is gradual and the course progressive over months. The initial disturbance is likely to be motor and the distribution asymmetric. With thoracic lesions, weakness and stiffness of one leg are followed by symptoms in the other one. Tingling paresthesias may arise from dorsal column involvement. Pain and temperature are affected more frequently than the other sensory modalities, and initial loss is contralateral to the maximum motor weakness (Brown-Séquard syndrome).

Bladder and, less frequently, bowel paralysis occur late in the progression of the syndrome, usually with coincident motor paralysis of the legs. If the compression is relieved, symptoms recover in reverse order of their onset, with the first part affected usually the last to recover.

Intramedullary Syndrome. Intramedullary tumors, originating within the spinal cord, commonly progress insidiously and painlessly. The syndrome is characterized by segmental weakness and atrophy of the hands and arms, with loss of tendon reflexes and segmental anesthesia of dissociated type (loss of pain and temperature sense and preservation of sense of position and touch). The dissociated sensory loss is caused by cavitation and destruction of the decussating pain and temperature fibers, with sparing of the uncrossed fibers for touch and proprioception. The restriction of the lesion to one area of the spinal cord accounts for the cape distribution or suspended sensory loss. The segmental distribution of muscle atrophy results from destruction of the anterior horn central gray neurons. As the intramedullary mass enlarges, the longitudinal spinal cord tracts become involved, the lower extremities develop spastic paresis, and difficulty with urinary continence emerges.

Many patients' histories and physical examinations do not place them clearly into one of the above syndromes; occasionally, a pure intramedullary syndrome is caused by an extramedullary tumor or even an extradural tumor. Rarely, an intramedullary tumor exhibits the symptoms and signs of a typically extramedullary syndrome. Therefore, the syndromes listed above are generally helpful, but cannot be relied upon for a specific diagnosis without additional special diagnostic investigation.

Diagnostic Procedures. Special diagnostic techniques precisely localize the primary spinal tumor and delineate the rostral and caudal extent. In many instances, a preoperative diagnosis of tumor type can be made. Plain spinal x-rays, tomograms, myelography, angiography, and CT scanning represent the special diagnostic tests for spinal cord tumors.

Plain X-Rays. This is the initial study ordered after the history and physical examination. The anteroposterior (AP) view should be inspected for evidence of widening of the interpeduncular distance, indicating a long-standing compression on the medial cortex of the pedicles. This most often occurs with intradural lesions and tumors of disordered embryogenesis. Extradural malignant lesions produce loss of a pedicle, focal lytic or blastic areas of bone destruction, and vertebral body collapse. Intervertebral foramina widening and scalloping of the vertebral bodies occur more frequently with benign tumors.

Children with congenital tumors, such as lipomas, dermoids, and teratomas, have coincident developmental anomalies of the bony spinal column. Among these anomalies are hemivertebrae, spina bifida, diastematomyelia, and fused vertebrae.

Myelography. This is the most important special procedure in the investigation of spinal cord tumors. Generally, the myelogram distinguishes extradural, intramedullary, or intradural-extramedullary tumor location.

Cerebrospinal fluid collection is best postponed until myelography if a spinal tumor is suspected. In the presence of a total block, a pressure differential between the spinal subarachnoid space above and below the lesion can be accentuated by lumbar puncture and fluid removal. A sudden shift in the relationship of the tumor mass and spinal cord can ensue, evoking a deterioration in the patient's neurologic status, possibly causing paraplegia. Therefore, if one suspects a total block, a fine spinal needle (22 gauge) is employed, and no fluid is removed. The myelographer then injects 2 mL of contrast and, under fluoroscopy, inspects for a complete block to the flow of the contrast material. If such an obstruction exists, the needle is removed and a lateral C_1–C_2 puncture is performed to outline the superior limit of the lesion. In the absence of a complete block, injection of additional contrast material allows full visualization of the area of suspicion.

The typical appearance of an extradural lesion is the "paintbrush" ending at the level of total myelographic block. Displacement of the dura away from the spinal canal periphery narrows the subarachnoid space adjacent to the tumor, resulting in a gradual tapering above and below the point of maximal encroachment.

Intradural-extramedullary tumors are identified by a characteristic cup or capping defect outlining the smooth surface of a meningioma or neurofibroma. More than 80% of these lesions also cause spinal cord displacement. The deviation of the myelographic cord shadow in the anteroposterior (AP) view and the lateral view pinpoints the location of the tumor in relation to the spinal cord (Shapiro *et al.*, 1961).

Intramedullary tumors enlarge the spinal cord from within and cause a fusiform enlargement of the spinal cord shadow (see Figure 37–34). The ratio of the transverse dimension of the cord shadow to the transverse diameter

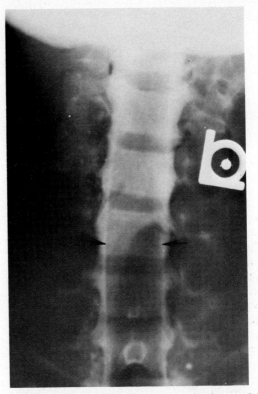

Figure 37–34. Myelogram demonstrating intramedullary spinal cord ependymoma. The lateral margins of the widened cord shadow are indicated by arrows.

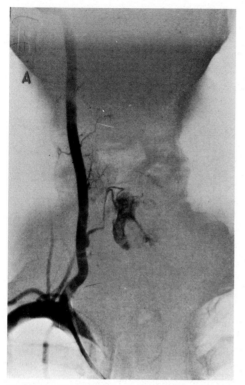

Figure 37–35. Dense vascularity of spinal cord hemangioblastoma is revealed by subclavian arteriogram. Primary feeding vessel originates from right vertebral artery. Subtraction technique.

of the subarachnoid space using the AP view is normally no greater than 0.8. If this ratio is increased, one must suspect an intramedullary cord tumor. A centrally placed extradural or intradural-extramedullary lesion compressing the spinal cord from an anterior direction, such as an extradural osteophyte, however, may also enlarge the cord shadow and, on superficial examination, be misdiagnosed as an intramedullary spinal cord tumor.

Spinal Angiography. Occasionally, myelography demonstrates the shadow of dilated, tortuous vessels on the spinal cord surface and the differential diagnosis of an intramedullary tumor, with increased blood supply and venous drainage, versus a spinal arteriovenous malformation arises. Selective spinal angiography by injection of contrast into the individual intercoastal arteries establishes the diagnosis and delineates the arterial feeding vessels. With this procedure, spinal hemangioblastomas display a well-circumscribed and dense capillary blush that is diagnostic (see Figure 37–35).

CT Scanning. Although this study does not have an established role in the assessment of patients with spinal cord tumors, it is frequently a useful adjunct to the studies cited above, especially after injection of water-soluble contrast material into the CSF. Spinal column alterations such as bone changes, osteophytes of degenerative disk disease, and bony impingement upon the spinal canal by vertebral body collapse due to metastatic neoplasm, are particularly well visualized.

Intradural-Extramedullary Tumors

The two primary tumors in this compartment are the neurilemmoma (schwannoma) and the meningioma. Combined, they make up 55% of all spinal tumors, excluding metastatic deposits.

Neurilemmoma (Schwannoma). About 1 mm from the surface of the spinal cord, the transition from the oligodendroglial investment of the axis cylinders of the spinal nerve roots to Schwann's cells occurs. Schwannomas arise along these sensory roots and share anatomic and histopathologic features with their intracranial counterparts, the acoustic neuromas, and their peripheral nerve counterparts, the peripheral schwannomas.

In the series reported by Sloof *et al.* (1964), schwannomas constituted 29% of all primary intraspinal tumors, exceeding the meningiomas and the gliomas in frequency. They have no predilection for a specific segment of the spine, occurring with equal frequency along the nerve roots from the cervical to the sacral divisions. Despite the higher incidence in patients with von Recklinghausen's disease for both single and multiple schwannomas, most of these tumors occur as solitary lesions in patients without the stigmata of neurofibromatosis. Some extend through the intervertebral foramen, producing a tumor with a constricted segment connecting the lobular intradural and paraspinal components, the dumbbell or hourglass neurilemmoma.

Related to their origin from the sensory nerve roots and extramedullary location are the radicular and myelopathic sequelae of their growth. Afflicted patients most commonly present with a radicular-spinal canal syndrome (previously discussed).

The treatment of these lesions is surgical. They are virtually always benign, discrete tumors that are well encapsulated and accessible to total excision using microneurosurgical techniques.

Meningioma. Meningiomas comprise 25% of all spinal cord tumors. They primarily affect women in the fourth through the sixth decades of life. Their partiality for women exceeds that of the intracranial meningiomas, with 80% of spinal meningiomas occurring in women (Sloof *et al.,* 1964).

Meningiomas may occur anywhere within the spinal canal, but two-thirds originate in the thoracic region. The high incidence of meningiomas in the proximity of the sensory nerve roots has been attributed to their origin from clusters of meningothelial cells concentrated in villous structures near the dorsal root ganglia (Burger and Vogel, 1976).

Spinal meningiomas have a globular shape and are histologically identical to those arising intracranially. Clinical presentation begins with symptoms of either nerve root or spinal cord compression and progresses to exhibit long tract involvement in all patients as tumor growth proceeds.

Surgical excision is the only proven treatment of these lesions. If complete removal can be accomplished, including all attachments of the tumor to dura and removal of the dura at the region of tumor origin, recurrence is rare.

Should removal of a neurilemmoma or meningioma be incomplete, consideration should be given to radiation therapy. This reasoning is not based on documented success with spinal neurofibromas or meningiomas, but on the response of histologically identical intracranial tumors.

Intramedullary Tumors

The primary tumors in this category are the glial tumors, astrocytomas, and ependymomas, and hemangioblastomas. As in the brain, the majority of intrinsic spinal cord tumors are gliomas, although similar types of gliomas are not found in the same proportions in the spinal cord as the brain. For instance, ependymomas comprised 56% of the intramedullary spinal tumors in the series investigated by Sloof *et al.,* and 64% of the spinal cord gliomas, compared to 6% of intracranial gliomas (Sloof *et al.,* 1964; Russell and Rubinstein, 1977).

Ependymoma. These intrinsic tumors arise at any point in the spinal cord from ependymal cells lining the central canal. The cauda equina and conus medullaris are particularly affected and account for more than 50% of cases. The peak incidence is in the fourth and fifth decades. Pain or weakness of a limb usually initiates the clinical onset of symptoms. Advancement of tumor size results in the ultimate development of an intramedullary syndrome or sensorimotor spinal tract syndrome. As previously discussed, myelography exhibits a fusiform enlargement of the involved spinal cord segment, or, in the case of a cauda equina ependymoma, a lobulated mass displacing the roots of the cauda equina.

These tumors are usually benign histologically, with well-circumscribed margins, allowing total tumor removal without increasing neurologic deficit in most cases (Fischer and Mansuy, 1980; Guidetti *et al.,* 1981). Optimal results require use of the operating microscope and attention to the details of meticulous microsurgical technique.

When one is confronted with an infiltrating ependymoma and complete removal is impossible, radiotherapy should be delivered postoperatively. Somewhat greater experience with irradiation is available for ependymomas of the spinal cord, as compared with astrocytomas. Almost all reports attest to the considerable efficacy of such treatment, with the great majority of patients surviving for protracted time periods without evidence of recurrent disease when adequate radiation doses and fields have been used. Surprisingly, low radiation doses have been reported to result in long-term symptom control when gross residual disease has been irradiated (Scott, 1974). In the series of Guidetti *et al.* (1981), those patients undergoing partial removal or myelotomy only followed by radiation therapy survived an average of 103 months and 98 months, respectively, compared to 125 months after total removal. The beneficial effects of irradiation on functional recovery and survival after incomplete tumor removal have also been demonstrated by others (Wood *et al.,* 1954; Barone and Elvidge, 1970; Schwade *et al.,* 1978). In evaluating the effects of any therapy, the natural course of spinal cord gliomas without treatment is an important, although unknown, entity. In the Mayo Clinic series of Woltman *et al.* (1951), the average postoperative survival of 34 patients who received no further therapy was six years. Obviously, to assess adequately therapeutic efficacy, long-term study will be required.

A radiation dose of 5000 rads, delivered in 150-rad to 180-rad fractions during six weeks, has been well tolerated and effective. Radiation fields should have generous superior and inferior margins of at least 2 cm to 3 cm around known disease or radiographic abnormality.

Astrocytoma. Spinal astrocytomas occur less frequently than ependymomas. They constitute about 30% of spinal cord gliomas. The relative incidence of these gliomas in the cervical, thoracic, lumbar, and sacral cord segments is proportional to the length of each cord segment. The peak incidence, as in the ependymomas, is in the fourth through fifth decades.

These tumors vary considerably in their histologic differentiation. In contrast to the intracranial astrocytic tumors, the majority of spinal astrocytomas show greater differentiation, with less than 5% displaying anaplastic features.

The clinical presentation of spinal astrocytomas is similar to that of ependymomas. Myelography does not allow discrimination between intramedullary ependymomas and astrocytomas. Both cause the characteristic segmental fusiform spinal cord enlargement.

The determining factor in their surgical treatment is the degree of tumor infiltration of the surrounding cord. When the tumor is both histologically benign and well demarcated from the cord, surgical removal provides successful treatment. Benign lesions that invade the cord structure and malignant tumors can rarely be removed surgically. The absence of a cleavage plane at the tumor margin in the great majority of these lesions limits tumor removal. In the operative series of 53 astrocytomas reported by Guidetti et al. (1981), the average survival after partial tumor removal and radiation therapy was more than two years greater than patients treated by myelotomy and radiotherapy. Attempts at extensive tumor removal cannot be justified if the potential of precipitating additional neurologic deficit is increased. In these cases, the therapeutic plan is to perform a posterior myelotomy extending the full length of the tumor, to extract the tumor that is clearly demarcated from the normal tissue and, in the surgeon's judgment, can be removed without increasing disability, and then to treat with radiation therapy.

As a result of the relative rarity of these tumors, few reports are available detailing the results after radiation therapy of spinal cord astrocytomas. Available information indicates that it enhances functional recovery after surgical treatment of spinal gliomas, as well as prolonging survival and improving the symptom-free interval (Wood et al., 1954; Schwade et al., 1978). Reports of responses in patients with tumor recurrence, who were treated with radiation therapy alone, strongly support the primary effect of radiation therapy on these tumors (Wood et al., 1954; Kopelson et al., 1980).

A tumor dose of approximately 5000 rads, delivered in 150- to 180-rad fractions during six weeks, appears safe and relatively effective (Wood et al., 1954; Marsa et al., 1975; Schwade et al., 1978). Substantially higher radiation doses given for spinal cord tumors have produced a significant incidence of radiation myelitis (Wara et al., 1975a). Three of 15 patients treated with a mean dose of 5700 rads (range: 5000 to 6700 rads) developed late complications (Marsa et al., 1975). It would appear that the optimum dose range lies between 4500 and 5500 rads, delivered in a relatively protracted fashion.

Hemangioblastoma. Approximately 3 to 4% of intramedullary spinal cord tumors are hemangioblastomas (Sloof et al., 1964). These tumors may occur extradurally (11%), and may be either extramedullary (25%) or intramedullary (63%) within the dura (Yasargil et al., 1976). They are identical to intracranial hemangioblastomas histologically and, like their intracranial counterparts, are well-defined lesions with circumscribed tumor margins, allowing surgical cure. The intramedullary examples are nearly all situated in the dorsal part of the spinal cord behind the central canal, a thankful circumstance for the neurosurgeon. Syringomyelia is present in about two-thirds of cases and Lindau's disease in one-third. Simultaneous posterior fossa and spinal hemangioblastomas are quite common and occurred in 8 of 12 cases in one series (Yasargil et al., 1976). The diagnosis is established by spinal angiography, which is diagnostic (see Figure 37–35) after the myelogram reveals venous varicosities on the cord surface.

Treatment is total removal. This can be accomplished without increasing the neural deficit in almost all patients by using the operative microscope and microsurgical techniques. Radiation therapy offers questionable benefit in the treatment of these lesions.

The high incidence of retinal and cerebellar hemangioblastomas, renal tumors and cysts, and pheochromocytomas dictates a screening evaluation of at least an intravenous pyelogram (IVP), CT scan of the posterior fossa, and retinal neuro-opthalmologic examination in these patients, even if they have no symptoms referable to involvement by these commonly associated lesions.

Tumors of Developmental Origin

Chordoma. Chordomas make up 1% of all spinal cord tumors. These tumors arise from remnants of the embryonic notochord. Evidence of notochordal origin is based upon the characteristic axial location of these tumors adjacent to the dura in a ventral extradural position and the light and electron microscopic features common to this tumor and the notochord (Murad and Murthy, 1970).

Men predominate, with a male-to-female ratio of 2:1 to 3:1. Lesions of the clivus represent 40% of the reported cases of chordoma, the others arising on the spine with a strong proclivity for the sacrococcygeal region. Most affected individuals are in the third to seventh decade of life. Chordomas are lobulated, slow-growing masses eliciting symptoms by local expansion rather than metastasis. Microscopically, their characteristic mucin-producing and physaliphorous cells permit immediate diagnosis.

Chordomas erode the adjacent bone of the clivus, sacrum, or spine and produce both lytic and sclerotic foci of abnormality on plain x-rays. Myelography, polytomograms, and CT scan further define the soft and hard tissue involvement and extent of encroachment upon the nervous system.

All reported series demonstrate the importance of surgery as primary therapy. Extensive and, when necessary, repeated surgical removal may be of great benefit. Surgery is rarely totally successful however, and the overwhelming majority of tumors recur. The location of these lesions and their extensive and insidious growth are primarily responsible for local failure.

Radiation therapy regularly produces tumor regression, and this response may persist for years. Very high radiation doses, in excess of 5000 rads in five weeks, however, are necessary to produce a significant response duration, and local failure nearly always occurs. Suit and Rich (1982) recommended radiation doses exceeding 6000 rads, with supplementation by proton-beam therapy for an additional 1000 rads or more. Data from Pearlman and Friedman (1970) demonstrate that the five-year sur-vival incidence increases considerably with doses above 6000 rads. Based on the almost routine development of local failure after surgery, postoperative radiation therapy is recommended for all patients (Pearlman and Friedman, 1970; Phillips and Newman, 1974; Steckler and Martin, 1974; Twefik et al., 1977; Suit and Rich, 1982).

When the lesion is inferior to the spinal cord, the risk of central nervous system damage is eliminated. Long-term survival is more common with the sacrococcygeal lesions, where higher doses of irradiation can be given by techniques that minimize bowel irradiation. When disease extent permits, a radiation dose of 7000 rads in 7.5 to 8 weeks delivered by suitably directed fields is suggested (Steckler and Martin, 1974).

Epidermoid, Dermoid, and Teratoma. These tumors comprise 1 to 2% of spinal cord tumors. Although they occasionally occur in other segments of the spine, most occur in the lower lumbar and sacral areas, where they cause low-back pain, weakness of the legs, and urinary incontinence. These congenital tumors are usually associated with other lumbar developmental defects unveiled by physical examination (hypertrichosis, cutaneous angioma, dermal sinus) or by plain spinal x-rays (spina bifida). Children are primarily affected.

These are benign lesions (except for the occasional malignant teratoma) and can usually be totally excised. Dense adherence of the tumor capsule to the conus medullaris may prohibit total resection and permit clinical recurrence later. At that time, further operative intervention may be required. Chemotherapy and radiation therapy have not been used in the treatment of these lesions, except for the malignant teratomas, which may require both forms of therapy, depending upon the adequacy of surgical removal.

Other intrinsic tumors of the spine and spinal cord are less common and less distinctive. The management of these tumors follows the general principles that have been discussed.

NEW DEVELOPMENTS AND FUTURE PROSPECTS

Much work remains to be done if the therapy of central nervous system tumors is to be improved. The fact remains that the prognosis for patients with malignant CNS tumors is poor despite advances in surgery, radiation, and chemotherapy. Even with combined therapy using all three modalities, life expectancy for the average patient with a glioblastoma multiforme is less than one year. For patients with metastatic cerebral disease, the life expectancy is only three to four months. A major problem for the treatment of malignant primary CNS tumors is that they are invasive, moving into normal brain tissue that is not subject to surgical resection without causing the patient significant neurologic deficit. Radiation therapy, chemotherapy, and perhaps immunotherapy seem the logical adjunctive therapies to seek out and destroy these invasive tumor cells; but the survival statistics indicate that truly effective techniques do not yet exist for any one of these modalities. Radiation therapy, although the single most effective modality to date (when combined with surgery), has been limited because the differential sensitivity between normal and abnormal brain cells is relatively slim, and the complication of radiation necrosis is serious. For chemotherapy, limitations have included (1) the availability of only one class of cytotoxic agents—the nitrosoureas (Walker *et al.,* 1978), (2) the relatively small growth fraction of malignant brain tumors (Hoshino *et al.,* 1972, 1975a, 1975b), (3) the effects of the agents used on bone marrow and other organs, (4) the difficulties of delivery of the drug to all areas of the tumor, and (5) the evident resistance of many tumors to the available chemotherapy agents. For immunotherapy, the effects of various trials to date have been weak, if any, and these effects have been achieved only with minimal tumor burden (Trouillas, 1980). It would appear that immunotherapy must be used in conjunction with the other modalities above to be of value.

Several issues loom as critical for both present and future malignant brain tumor research. (1) For a therapy program to be successful, it appears that (at least for the near future) it will have to be multimodal; some combination of all four current modalities (surgery, radiation therapy, chemotherapy, and immunotherapy) will have to be available. The aim at any one time, of course, is the maintenance, if not removal, of a minimal tumor burden. (2) Because of patient tumor variability or heterogeneity, multimodal, individualized therapy based on a knowledge of the biologic characteristics of each tumor

seems essential. (3) Improved diagnostic techniques are required to permit early diagnosis of the original tumor, as well as of recurrence and/or treatment failure. A better measure of the extent of local invasion needs to be identified. (4) Improved surgical tools for maximum resection with minimal neurologic morbidity, combined possibly with local intraoperative immunologic and/or cytotoxic agent therapy, are needed. (5) Enhancement of tumor, as opposed to normal brain, sensitivity to radiation therapy needs further development. (6) Availability of more chemotherapeutic agents with differing molecular mechanisms of cytotoxicity, as well as cell cycle specificity and more combination chemotherapy trials, is essential. (7) Better understanding of both the cellular and serologic immune factors in glioma patients is needed.

In addition, it is imperative that we look again at each element of our therapeutic armamentarium, including steroids and anticonvulsants, to determine the advantages and disadvantages of the various combinations of treatment. Some combinations may actually be working against the patient's best interests by producing, for example, immune suppression.

Promising approaches representing different levels of attack of the problems are currently underway in several centers, both in the United States and Europe. It is useful to examine some of these approaches for the hopeful perspective they provide as to the directions in which central nervous system tumor research and clinical trials are evolving.

Diagnostic Techniques

The introduction of the CT scan in 1971 was a revolutionary advance for the diagnosis and follow-up of brain tumors. Detecting density differences in normal and abnormal brain tissue, the CT scan gives structural information, as well as (with infusion of contrast) a crude measure of the vascularity of tumors. Sequential CT scans provide evidence of progression or regression of tumors, help to identify the need for alternative, adjunctive treatment or reoperation, and point to causes of deterioration other than those related directly to the tumor (Norman *et al.,* 1976; Pay *et al.,* 1976; Marks and Gado, 1977; Salcman *et al.,* 1981).

The techniques of tomographic imaging, the key to the success of the transmission CT scan, have now been applied to radionuclide scanning, enabling the development of new approaches to visualization of brain function, as well as brain structure. Emission computerized tomographic scanning provides what is, in effect, an *in vivo* autoradiogram, indicating brain and tumor biochemistry (Ell *et al.*, 1980).

Positron emission computed tomography (PET) has been used at the National Institutes of Health to measure local cerebral glucose utilization by the 2-[^{18}F]fluoro-2-deoxyglucose (FDG) technique in 23 cases of verified or suspected primary cerebral tumors. The data indicate a positive correlation between glycolysis and the degree of malignancy in these tumors, with low-grade astrocytomas (grade I and II) showing an average glucose consumption of 4.0 ± 1.8 mg/100 g/min, whereas tumors of grade III and IV show a rate of 8.3 ± 3.8 mg/100 g/min. Figures 37–36A, B and 37–37A, B provide a visual comparison of high- and low-grade tumors as seen in the PET scan and CT scan. From these same studies, it also appears that PET, utilizing the deoxyglucose technique, may be able to detect recurrence earlier than transmission CT scanning.

Oxidative metabolism in gliomas has also been evaluated with the PET scanner in Britain. Frackowiak and coworkers (1982), using $^{15}O_2$ and having found low oxidative metabolism in high-grade gliomas, suggest that combined studies utilizing both FDG and $^{15}O_2$ may be helpful in differentiating the glycolytic activity of normal gray matter from that of tumors.

These studies represent only a beginning for PET scanning. Positron-emitting radionuclides can be coupled with many substances to examine different aspects of tumor metabolism. An extremely important area of application may be the quantification of the state of the blood-brain barrier in individual tumors and the consequent implications for delivery of chemotherapeutic agents (Vick, 1980). In addition, the delivery of chemotherapeutic agents to brain or spinal cord tumors can be followed by PET techniques. With the availability (in the not-too-distant future) of monoclonal antiglioma antibody, detection of the original, residual, or recurrent tumor may be enhanced. Such chemotherapeutic and immunologic studies open the possibility that both diagnostic and therapeutic modalities may one day be combined in PET techniques.

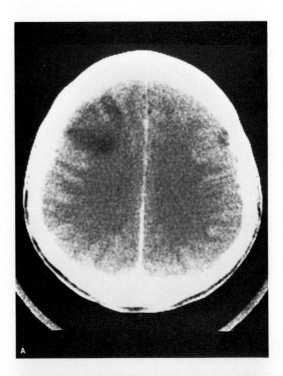

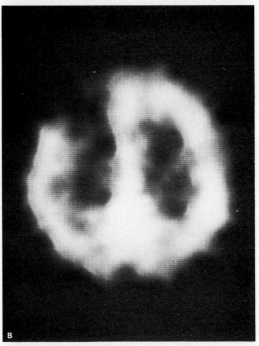

Figure 37–36. (*A*) CT scan with contrast of low-grade frontal astrocytoma. Note the absence of enchancement. (*B*) Positron emission tomographic scan with ^{18}F-2-deoxyglucose. A low metabolic rate is evident in the tumor area (dark) compared to normal cortex (white). A low metabolic rate as determined by ^{18}F-2DG uptake is characteristic of low-grade tumors (see text). (Courtesy of Drs. Giovanni DeChiro, Rodney Brooks, and Nicholas Patronas.)

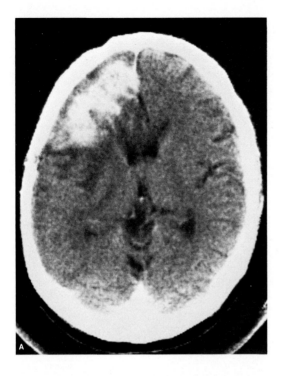

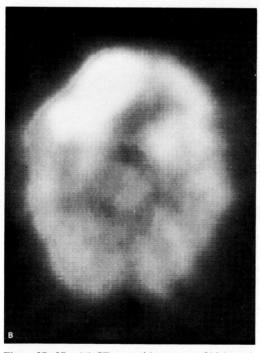

Figure 37–37. (*A*) CT scan with contrast of high-grade (malignant) frontal astrocytoma. Positive contrast enhancement is present. (*B*) PET scan with [18]F-2DG shows high metabolic rate typical of high-grade gliomas (see text). Courtesy of Drs. Giovanni DiChiro, Rodney Brooks, and Nicholas Patronas.

One limitation of PET, as compared to standard transmission CT scanning, has been its relatively poor resolution: 1 mm for CT, as opposed to 15 mm for PET. Brooks *et al.* (1981) have recently developed the so-called Neuro-PET which, utilizing a much greater number of detectors, has improved the PET resolution to approximately 7 mm.

Another new technique that seems to hold substantial promise for brain tumor imaging is tomographic nuclear magnetic resonance (NMR). This technique, based as it is on excitation of hydrogen nuclei, does not require injection of any materials. A striking feature of the NMR images obtained to date is the clear differentiation between gray and white matter. The clearer differentiation results from the hydrogen in gray matter being associated with water and in white matter being associated with fats (Doyle *et al.*, 1981). The glioblastoma multiforme shown in Figure 37–38 (both CT scan and NMR view) illustrates clear loss of white matter in the NMR view.

Quite a different approach to diagnosis and follow-up evaluation for recurrence is represented by biochemical evaluations utilizing tumor markers or indicators in blood or CSF. For certain types of CNS tumors, such markers are well known and reliable. For pituitary tumors, the respective hormones are also clear guides to type and recurrence of the tumor. In the case of malignant primary brain or spinal cord tumors, polyamines have been evaluated extensively by Fulton *et al.* (1980). Proteins and lipids, such as alpha-fetoprotein, human chorionic gonadotropin, and carcinoembryonic antigen, may also be valuable, although not necessarily specific (Grossi-Paoletti *et al.*, 1971). The need to examine CSF is a limitation of any such technique since, in patients with raised intracranial pressure, a lumbar puncture may result in herniation. Ventricular reservoirs are not always available or desirable. Where intracranial pressure is not a problem, the use of CSF tissue culture and immunofluorescent labeling in combination with millipore filtration may aid in the diagnosis of tumors seeding the CSF pathways (Black *et al.*, 1978).

In vitro assays to characterize the cell biologic properties of individual patient glioma cells, to determine their sensitivity to specific chemotherapeutic agents, and to determine the patient's own immunologic responses to the tumor are appealing theoretically because they may provide a basis for improved therapy

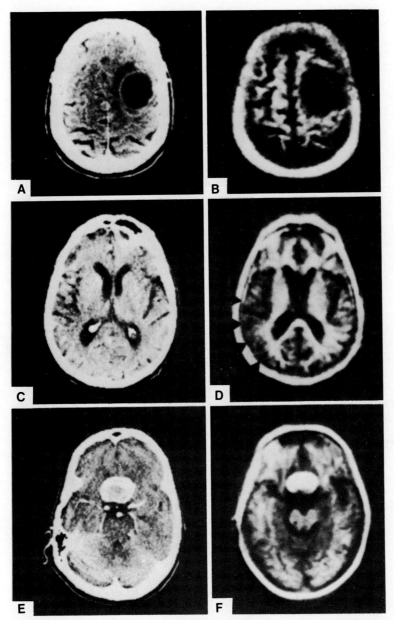

Figure 37–38.   (*A* and *B*) Glioblastoma multiforme. The tumor is seen as a central low attenuation region with rim enhancement on CT (*A*). The NMR scan shows the tumor with greater contrast and demonstrates the loss of white matter within the tumor (*B*).

(*C* and *D*) Cerebral infarction. Minimal evidence of a low attenuation lesion and widening of the cerebral sulci are seen in the region of the posterior operculum on CT (*C*). Loss of white matter over a more extensive region is demonstrated on NMR (arrows) (*D*).

(*E* and *F*) Aneurysm. The lesion and intracranial blood vessels are demonstrated with contrast enhanced CT. The NMR scan shows a white region within the lesion representing clotted blood.

From Doyle, F. H., *et al.*: Imaging of the brain by nuclear magnetic resonance. *Lancet*, 2:56, 1981.

and a prediction of clinical course without adding any patient risk. An important result of these studies has been the appreciation of the heterogeneity of CNS tumors, both within a given tumor class and grade, as well as within an individual's own tumor (Bigner *et al.,* 1981, Kornblith *et al.,* 1981). This heterogeneity indicates that successful therapy will undoubtedly have to be individualized, if such therapy is ever to have a rational basis for improvement. Thus, *in vitro* assays of individual patient tumor cells obtained at surgery and used immediately or grown in tissue culture appear to be important for the future of glioma therapy.

Various *in vitro* models have been utilized in recent years for both chemotherapy and immunology testing in glioma patients (Holmes and Little, 1974; Kornblith *et al.,* 1974, 1979, 1982a; Rosenblum *et al.,* 1977; Kornblith and Szypko, 1978; Salmon *et al.,* 1978; Coakham and Kornblith, 1979; Kornblith, 1980). The practicality and reliability of such *in vitro* colony formation and microcytotoxicity have been amply shown. The microcytotoxicity assay utilized in our laboratory has demonstrated significant variation in responsiveness of cultured individual patient glioma cell lines to 1,3-*bis*(2-chloroethyl)-1-nitorosurea (BCNU), with more than 100 lines now tested (Kornblith and Szypko, 1978; Kornblith *et al.,* 1981). Sensitivity or resistance in these populations appears to correlate with DNA interstrand crosslink formation (Kohn, 1977; Erikson *et al.,* 1978), as well as membrane and cytoplasmic factors not as yet fully characterized (Fornace *et al.,* 1978; Smith *et al.,* 1982). Whatever the mechanism, these data have enabled separation of *in vitro* glioma BCNU-sensitive and insensitive populations; and this *in vitro* separation appears to have a clinical correlation (Kornblith *et al.,* 1981).

Taking a different approach, Rosenblum and colleagues (1977, 1978) have developed an *in vitro* colony formation assay that is thought to study the cells most likely to proliferate in the *in vivo* tumor, that is, those with ability to form clones. They have found greater clonogenic capacity for malignant gliomas than for grade I and II astrocytomas. Salmon *et al.* (1978) are also using a colony formation assay to determine *in vitro* sensitivity to chemotherapeutic drugs (and have attempted to correlate their *in vitro* data with clinical response). Tumor cells from individual patients are prepared as suspensions, treated with each drug, and plated in agar. Drug effect is measured as reduction of colonies relative to control colonies. These investigators and their collaborators have studied the chemotherapeutic sensitivities of a wide range of human solid tumors. Clinical correlation studies have indicated that patients who show resistance *in vitro* do not show *in vivo* responses to the clinical agent.

Several agents are currently under study in the various *in vitro* chemotherapy test systems.

In the microcytotoxicity assay in our laboratories, aziridinylbenzoquinone (AZQ) and cisplatin both look promising, compared to BCNU. Since the mechanisms of each of these three agents vary, they may well provide an augmented chemotherapeutic armamentarium for malignant gliomas. Early data for AZQ (20 mg/m^2 on day 1 and day 8, 28-day treatment cycle) indicate a 25 to 30% response rate in malignant glioma patients who have failed other therapeutic modalities (Curt *et al.,* 1981). Trials with cisplatin and CBDCA (a less toxic platinum derivative) are also underway.

With regard to immunologic responses, allogeneic and autologous microcytotoxicity testing and an immune adherence assay have indicated that a significant proportion of brain tumor patients have a humoral immune response to their tumors. This humoral immune response appears to involve IgG and IgM for the observed cytotoxicity, and primarily IgM for the immune adherence (Kornblith *et al.,* 1979). In a series of 42 glioma patients, 45% of patients had detectable cytotoxic antibodies directed against their own cultured tumor cells. When tumor grade was correlated with immune response, 15 of 20 patients with grade I, II, or III astrocytomas had antigens detectable in autologous sera, whereas only 5 of 22 patients with grade IV astrocytomas had such responses. This cytotoxicity appears to be restricted to tumor cells, suggesting tumor antigenic specificity. Perhaps more important, these immune responses are highly correlated with survival in primary malignant brain tumor patients (Kornblith *et al.,* 1983). Also correlating with increased survival are age, tumor grade, functional status, and duration of symptoms at the time of diagnosis (Walker *et al.,* 1980). The autologous cytotoxic humoral response thus appears to be an example of an immunologic response that can serve as a biologic predictive factor in survival of adult glioma patients. Such predictive value has been sought, but not confirmed, in tests of general immune responsiveness, such as immunoglobulin and lymphocyte levels, lymphocyte subpopulation assays, recall antigen skin testing, and serum blocking activity (Brooks and Roszman, 1980). Although the cytotoxic antibody assay does not appear to offer significant advantages over clinical and histologic predictive factors at the time of diagnosis, it does appear to be able to provide information regarding immunocompetence in patient follow-up.

The intimate relationship of cytotoxic antibody incidence with clinical course and the findings of a correlation between degree of differentiation and the immune response suggest that humoral factors may be important in the development of approaches to alter the immune status of tumor patients to therapeutic advantage. For example, considerable evidence is available indicating that circulating immune complexes play a role in abrogating antitumor immunity and adversely affect prognosis (Theofilopoulos and Dixon, 1979; Robins and Baldwin, 1978). Antibody sequestration in complexes or in tumor-bound form may be the explanation for our findings in patients with glioma. Consistent with this possibility is the fact that Martin-Archard *et al.* (1980) have reported that IgG binding activity is significantly elevated in high- as compared to low-grade glial tumors, and that this is associated with decreased patient survival. It may be of interest to try staph-A-treated plasmapheresis protocols in malignant CNS tumors to see if these effects can be reversed. Work on the isolation of the antigens is also proceeding (Birkmayer and Stass, 1980).

From the point of view of cellular immune parameters, various authors have reported mixed results with some assays, such as intradermal tests showing apparent immune suppression and others (graft rejection, lymphocyte, transformation test; and lymphocyte cytotoxicity *in vitro*), indicating a variably responsive cellular immune system in glioma patients (Bloom *et al.*, 1960; Grace *et al.*, 1961; Ciembroniewicz and Kolar, 1967; Stjernsward, 1971; Brooks *et al.*, 1972, 1974; Trouillas, 1973; Young *et al.*, 1976a, b; Mahaley *et al.*, 1977; Levy, 1978).

Recent studies by Gately *et al.* (1982) have shown normal or near normal capability of glioma patients' lymphocytes to respond to mitogens and to generate cytolytic lymphocyte responses to allogeneic lymphocytes *in vitro.* Despite this, these patients have not been able to make strong cytolytic lymphocyte responses to their own tumors *in vivo.* For example, five of eight glioma lines were unable to stimulate allogeneic cytolytic T-lymphocyte (CTL) responses in mixed lymphocyte tumor cultures *in vitro.* Analysis of the reasons for the failure of these lines to induce CTL generation revealed three separate mechanisms of importance. In the case of two of the nonstimulatory glioma lines, CTL specific for the gliomas could be generated if responding lymphocytes

were cultured with glioma cells in the presence of irradiated lymphocytes from a third individual. Hence, these two lines possessed a defect in immunogenicity that could be overcome by help from an allogeneic mixed lymphocyte reaction (Gately *et al.*, 1982). The nature of this help is under further study. One glioma, when added to a mixture of lymphocytes from two allogeneic individuals, inhibited the mixed lymphocyte reaction that would have occurred otherwise. Inhibition was shown to be caused by the secretion of a macromolecular, nonspecific immunosuppressive substance(s). Two of the nonstimulatory gliomas were shown to secrete a thick coat of mucopolysaccharide, which impeded contact between lymphocytes and glioma cells. In the case of one glioma line that was studied extensively, removing this coat with the enzyme hyaluronidase permitted increased generation of CTL specific for the glioma. Such CTL generation, however, required the presence of both responder lymphocytes and irradiated lymphocytes from a third individual. Hence, the inability of this glioma line to elicit cytolytic lymphocyte responses represented the combined effects of both the presence of a protective mucopolysaccharide coat and a separate defect in immunogenicity.

Thus, the five glioma lines that failed to stimulate allogeneic CTL responses each possessed one or more of the following escape mechanisms: (1) an intrinsic defect in immunogenicity, the nature of which is as yet poorly defined, but which may involve a defect in the ability to stimulate helper T cells; (2) the secretion of nonspecific immunosuppressive substance(s); and (3) the production of a protective mucopolysaccharide coat. It is thus apparent that further studies of how these escape mechanisms operate and by what means they may be overcome are likely to be of central importance to the successful use of immunotherapy in glioma patients. In addition, characterization of the ability of individual glioma lines to interact with the cellular immune system *in vitro* may contribute to the planning of individualized immunotherapeutic regimens. The ability to elicit allogeneic cytolytic lymphocyte responses *in vitro* suggests that efforts to modify these tumors to increase their immunogenicity, while blocking the production of immunosuppressive factors and of mucopolysaccharide coats, may be important if immunotherapy is to be successful. One such effort *in vitro,* using dibutyrl cAMP and dimethylformamide, already shows promise

(Gumerlock *et al.,* 1981). The cellular immune mechanisms beginning to be elucidated hold substantial promise of providing new immunotherapeutic modalities.

Surgical Innovations

Surgical approaches to benign and malignant central nervous system (CNS) tumors have been a mainstay of therapy since Cushing's time. Useful for both diagnosis and decompression, surgery nonetheless has not solved the problem of malignant brain tumors, such as glioblastoma multiforme, because of (1) limitations of the extent of resection, secondary to proximity of critical brain areas; (2) the local invasive properties of such tumors, which prevent resolution of clear-cut margins: (3) the inaccessibility of deep-seated or brain stem tumor locations; and (4) the poor regenerative properties of brain and spinal cord neural tissue. Despite these limitations, surgery and radiation therapy, as noted above, have been the two most effective modalities for malignant brain tumor therapy.

Several new tools and techniques promise to improve the effectiveness and safety of surgical approaches. Improvements in neuroanesthesia techniques, as well as the long-established benefits of corticosteroids, have helped to lower overall morbidity. The advent of microneurosurgical techniques has added to the safety of resection of a variety of CNS tumors, such as those located in the cerebellopontine angle, at the base of the skull, sphenoid ridge, or the spinal canal or cord. Ultrasonic resection, by means of devices such as the CAVI-TRON, permits removal of tumor from difficult areas without traction on normal brain tissue. The CO_2 and argon lasers add fine resection control and coagulation capabilities enabling, for example, the removal of small tumor remnants adherent to important cerebral or spinal cord vessels or cranial nerves. Combined with other modalities, such as the use of tumor-selective and wavelength-specific absorptive materials (such as hematoporphyrin), the laser may find even more utility as a means of selective tumor cell destruction (Laws *et al.,* 1981), enabling wider resection with less damage to normal CNS structures. CT-assisted stereotactic biopsy (Heilbrun, *et al.,* 1983) and resection of deep-seated tumors (such as thalamic lesions) (Kelly *et al.,* 1982) also added to the surgical armamentarium. Another new technique uses microwave probes implanted in the brain to destroy malignant tumors (Salcman and Samaras, 1981). This, too, promises to be useful for difficult-to-reach, as well as more accessible, lesions.

Intraoperative monitoring of averaged evoked potential activity, now becoming more widely available, is of particular value for assurance of functional integrity during surgery (as well as for diagnosis and postoperative follow-up). Depending upon the location of surgery, visual evoked potentials, brain stem auditory evoked potentials, and somatosensory evoked potentials can be utilized. Brain stem evoked responses, for example, measure auditory system integrity and are thus useful in the resection of cerebellopontine angle tumors, whereas somatosensory potentials are of particular value for spinal cord tumor resections (for review, see Chiappa and Ropper, 1982.)

For the malignant and locally invasive tumors, such as glioblastoma multiforme, surgery remains limited in seeking out and destroying the tumor cells among the neurons and normal glia. Unfortunately, because any remaining tumor cells continue to have potential for uncontrolled growth, adjunctive therapy (including radiation therapy, chemotherapy, and perhaps immunotherapy) will continue to be required for the foreseeable future. Not to be minimized, however, is the value of not only the primary surgery, but also the possibility of reoperations, at least in selected cases, such as those restricted to one frontal lobe. In a recent study, Young *et al.* (1981) suggested that reoperation is most likely to produce good results when the Karnofsky rating is at least 60 and the interval between operations is longer than six months. Location of the tumor and age were not clearly related to the outcome.

Radiation Therapy

Current or recent experimental approaches to radiation therapy include (1) altered radiation delivery schedules, (2) attempts to utilize different radiation modalities, (3) radiation sensitizers, (4) combinations of conventional radiation therapy and chemotherapy, and (5) interstitial radiation. As malignant brain tumor patients survive longer because of improved combinations of surgery, radiation therapy, and chemotherapy, undesirable side effects of conventional high-dose radiation therapy (4500 to 6000 rads) are appearing with somewhat greater frequency, resulting in increased research emphasis on enhancing the sensitivity differential between normal and malignant neural tissue.

Generally accepted delivery of conventional radiation therapy is approximately 200 rads per day during a six-week period, to a total dose of up to 6000 rads. Douglas (1977) has utilized superfractionation (three fractions per day of 100 rads separated by 3 to 3.5 hours, for a total of 45 to 60 fractions, with a 1000-rad boost during five days to the tumor itself) with some slight improvement in results. The long-term results of this therapy are not known.

Fast neutron irradiation has been utilized by Shaw et al. (1978) (8MV) and Catterall et al. (1980) (7.5 MV), with median survival of approximately five months from completion of treatment—a survival not significantly different from that with standard radiation therapy. Furthermore, in the Shaw et al. study, the cause of death appeared to be related to brain effects of the fast neutron irradiation.

The use of radiosensitizers is theoretically appealing because of the possibilities for increased tumor, rather than normal brain, damage. One radiosensitizer, a halogenated thymidine analog, 5-bromodeoxyuridine (BUDR), is incorporated by dividing tumor cells but not quiescent normal brain cells. Given via intra-arterial infusion in combination with 5000 to 6000 rads, BUDR therapy resulted in 21% and 7% three-year survivals in patients with moderately and highly malignant tumors, respectively (Sano et al., 1968). New trials of intravenous BUDR in conjunction with irradiation are currently underway as a collaborative effort involving the National Institute of Neurological and Communicative Disorders and Stroke and the NCI of the National Institutes of Health, as well as other institutions. One trial of hyperbaric oxygen with irradiation (Chang et al., 1975) showed statistically significant increases in one- and two-year survivals. The hypoxic cell sensitizer, metronidazole, has shown some enhancement for glioblastoma when combined with irradiation (Urtasun et al., 1976, 1977), but toxic effects of the agent and a need to compare the data with standard irradiation dosages remain as problems.

Combined chemotherapy (nitrosoureas) and radiation therapy has been tested. Wheeler et al. (1977) found that radiation damage was potentiated when BCNU was given 15 hours prior to irradiation in in vitro experiments with the 9L rat tumor line. The Brain Tumor Study Group (BTSG), in a randomized patient trial

(Walker, 1973, 1975; Walker and Gehan, 1972), showed a median survival gain of only weeks with this method. There is also some evidence that hydroxyurea combined with radiation therapy gives better results than radiation therapy alone (Irwin et al., 1975; Lerner, 1975; Levin and Edwards, 1980).

Finally, interstitial radiation with radioisotope-containing seeds placed into the actual tumor bed (Hosobuchi et al., 1980; Bernstein and Gutin, 1981) is still another promising avenue of clinical research. It will, however, still be some time before this approach can be fully evaluated.

Chemotherapy

Problems and prospects in the area of chemotherapy are several. As pointed out by Levin and Edwards (1980), although chemotherapy agents have so far produced only modest increases in survival rates, they currently offer the greatest hope for extending the lives of brain tumor patients. Critical issues include (1) the invasive nature of malignant glial tumors, (2) the heterogeneity of the state of the blood-brain barrier in different zones of the tumor, (3) the relative burden of well-vascularized or poorly-vascularized cell zones, (4) tumor cell population heterogeneity with respect to chemotherapy agent sensitivity, and (5) the potential for chromosomal or phenotypic drift and the emergence of resistant subpopulations.

From a clinical point of view, these biologic issues come together in two major problems: the need for improved delivery and the availability of several agents dependent on differing mechanisms so that resistance to one does not limit therapy. In vitro evidence derived from the sensitivity of glioma cells in culture to BCNU (Kornblith and Szypko, 1978) has suggested that virtually all glioma cells are sensitive to BCNU if the ambient concentration is sufficiently high.

A significant problem related to drug delivery is the state of the blood-brain barrier within the tumor. In one view, the tumor can be divided into a central core with necrosis, poor perfusion, and a small viable tumor fraction, and an outer shell of viable tumor and good perfusion, but a leaky blood-brain barrier. For the scattered invasive cells beyond this shell of tumor, perhaps the third zone, the vasculature and blood-brain barrier are normal (Levin and Edwards, 1980). Vick (1980), as well as Blasberg *et al.* (1983), Horowitz *et al.* (1983), and Molnar *et al.* (1982), has shown that the situation is yet more complicated, with the state of the blood-brain barrier varying even within the hypothetical zones outlined above. Such heterogeneity makes the question of drug delivery even more complicated than previously thought. The advent of positron emission computed tomographic (PET) scanning should make it possible to study individual tumors *in vivo* and thus help to determine the best mode of drug delivery for a given patient's tumor based on a direct assessment of the blood-brain barrier characteristics. As previously noted, metabolic studies utilizing ^{18}F-2-deoxyglucose have already proven helpful in grading gliomas.

Although it is important to gain more information about the blood-brain barrier in individual glioma patients, increased drug delivery to as much of the tumor as possible would still seem to be of value. Two recent approaches to this problem are of interest. The first, the delivery of BCNU by local, intra-arterial perfusion, is capable of increasing the concentration of BCNU delivered to the tumor by a factor of three- to fivefold. This should be sufficient to increase cell kill, but the final appraisal of this technique must await the collection of sufficient follow-up data to determine the true gain in patient survival and quality of life. This technique is now being utilized in several centers.

A different approach is being taken by Neuwelt *et al.* (1981) Reasoning that the blood-brain barrier is a major limitation to more effective antibrain tumor therapy, especially for nonlipophilic drugs, Neuwelt has produced disruption of the blood-brain barrier using mannitol and found manyfold increases in the delivery of methotrexate, a nonlipophilic drug. For BCNU, of course, little advantage to blood-brain barrier breakdown is possible, since its penetration is rapid. Much work remains to be done to determine not only the safety of this technique, but also its value in a range of tumors, some of which already have extensive blood-brain barrier breakdown. A critical point for any drug-delivery modality is that individual drug pharmacokinetics must be considered before choosing one as opposed to another method. For a drug with a low extraction ratio, for example, intra-arterial perfusion may offer no advantages.

Apart from the delivery problem are the issues of tumor cell heterogeneity and the need for a battery of cytotoxic drugs with differing molecular mechanisms of action. The size of the tumor, its growth fraction, and previous therapeutic history in the case of recurrence are all critical elements. Overall, the nitrosoureas have proven to be the single most useful drug class for gliomas. Unfortunately, BCNU and CCNU have proven to add relatively little to overall malignant glioma patient survival, making a difference of only a few weeks of survival in the BTSG data (Walker *et al.,* 1980). As noted earlier, other drugs utilized include procarbazine and vincristine, which, when given together with CCNU as the PCV combination (Shapiro and Young, 1976; Levin *et al.,* 1980), may be the most effective combination yet. The superiority, however, is merely a matter of additional weeks of survival.

New agents, aziridinylbenzoquinone (AZQ), cisplatin, and CBDCA (a platinum derivative), are currently in early clinical trials for brain tumors as primary treatment and for adjuvant therapy. Early data with AZQ from M. D. Anderson Hospital, the Mayo Clinic, and the National Institutes of Health (Curt *et al.,* 1982) indicate a 25% response rate in patients who have failed other therapies.

Whichever drugs, or combinations thereof, ultimately prove to be most useful in treating brain tumors, it appears from the biologic evidence available to date that the optimum therapy for each patient's tumor will have to be individualized. That is to say, each tumor's pattern of sensitivity is different. It is clearly not desirable to give a patient a toxic drug that is not effective against the patient's tumor. Encouraging evidence that tissue culture systems are relevant to the process of predicting tumor response to a battery of cytotoxic agents is accumulating. Various assays (Kornblith and Szypko, 1978; Rosenblum *et al.,* 1978; Thomas *et al.,* 1979; Erikson *et al.,* 1980) have been utilized for gliomas. Both the microtiter and clonogenic assays appear to predict resistance with 90 to 100% accuracy when correlated with clinical results. Sensitive cells are less reliable indicators of clinical response, being correct in approximately 60% of cases (Salmon *et al.,* 1978; Kornblith *et al.,* 1981). The ability to automate these assays using image analysis techniques makes them even more attractive (Smith and Liszczak, 1980). Another very promising assay is the alkaline-elution assay for DNA interstrand cross-links developed by Erikson *et al.* (1980, 1982). The clinical predictive accuracy of this assay is in the process of being established. Its precision and reliability, especially as applied to acutely dissociated tumor specimens (thus determining the population sensitivity without the selective factors of tissue culture), make this a very attractive approach.

Having determined that both sensitive and resistant populations are in the tissue culture, the various *in vitro* assays outlined are useful for the studies of mechanisms of sensitivity or resistance (Smith *et al.*, 1983; Erikson *et al.*, 1980, 1982). It is hoped that new and better therapeutic regimens can be derived from such studies. Although much more work remains to be done, the possibilities of individualized testing, the existence of new and active chemotherapeutic agents, the availability of new delivery techniques, and the availability of cell biologic systems for the study of glioma cell drug sensitivity all combine to make the prospects for significant improvements in brain tumor chemotherapy good.

Immunology and Immunotherapy

Theoretically, a very appealing approach to cerebral tumors, immunotherapy, has yet to be established as a useful treatment modality for cerebral tumors. Substantial progress in understanding both the cellular and serologic responses to CNS tumors is being made. Although the central nervous system may be an "immunologically privileged" site, as suggested by Medawar (1948), it is not, of course, immunologically isolated. Production of antibodies to apparent glial tumor antigens has been detected in glioma patients and correlates with an improved survival (Kornblith *et al.*, 1982a). Similarly, cellular immunologic studies, such as those by Brooks *et al.* (1972), Young *et al.* (1976a, b), and Gately *et al.* (1982), have shown impaired lymphocyte responsiveness to glial tumors. Thus, although several studies have shown lymphocytic infiltration of gliomas (Berstrand and Mannen, 1960; Ridley and Cavanagh, 1971; Schiffer *et al.*, 1974; Takeuchi and Barnard, 1976), the lymphocyte response is not providing much therapeutic benefit. These studies implicate a soluble factor or factors elaborated by the malignant tumor cells that suppress immunologic reactivity. Dick *et al.* (1983), in addition, have shown that a mucopolysaccharide matrix secreted by some tumor cells can prevent cytolytic attack by lymphocytes. Finally, there may be the phenomenon of immunologically dependent tumor enhancement, which Trouillas (1980) has suggested for the failure of the Bloom *et al.* (1973) human glioma immunotherapy trial, in which survival in the treated group was actually reduced compared to that of the untreated group.

Immunotherapy protocols in glioma patients have taken several forms. Takakura *et al.* (1972) utilized histocompatible nontumor donors to provide bone marrow transplants for intravenous injection or white blood cells for tumor cavity injection in 18 glioblastoma patients and achieved a 60% two-year survival. Trouillas and Lapras (1969) grafted the patient's own tumor into the thigh and later catheterized the thoracic duct repeatedly to obtain lymphocytes for injection into the tumor bed in three cases and noted only a limited efficiency for this technique. Young *et al.* (1977) used repeated intratumor injection of mixed autologous lymphocytes and leukocytes, with 8 of 17 glioblastoma patients showing improvement. The effects of the immunotherapy alone, however, were difficult to separate from other therapeutic effects. Intrathecal autologous lymphocyte infusions with lymphocyte invasion of the tumor bed have also been studied (Neuwelt and Hill, 1980).

Attempting specific active immunotherapy, Trouillas (1971, 1973) injected autologous tumor extracts with Freund's complete adjuvant weekly in low-grade and malignant glioma patients with an increase in survival in the latter group of up to two months. Bloom *et al.* (1973) were able to show no significant difference in survival between patients injected with their own irradiated tumor cells. More recent efforts to stimulate the immune system have similarly not reported success, although it is early in the process. Combined stimulation with BCG, PPD, and autologous tumor cells treated with neuraminidase has also been tested in glioma patients without significant benefit (Ommaya, 1976). Plasmapheresis with reinfusion of staphylococcus protein-A plasma or other bacterial wall components treated to remove antigen-antibody complexes is also being tested.

Monoclonal antibody techniques now available suggest new approaches to immunotherapy. With specific antiglioma antibodies, it should be possible both to improve diagnostic localization studies and, for therapeutic purposes, gain either a direct cytotoxic effect or, more likely, use these antibodies with bound isotope or cytotoxic drugs to achieve antitumor efficacy.

Further exploration of the interactions of glioma cells with antibodies and the cellular immune system should ultimately lead to effective immunotherapy, whether as primary therapy or, more likely, adjuvant therapy. Keeping tumor bulk to a minimum appears to be critical to successful immunotherapy.

Biologic Modification Therapy

One final area of interest for future therapy of brain tumors is the use of biologic agents to modify glioma cell growth or alter antigenic expression to differentiate glioma cells. Central to this potential mode of therapy is the utilization of biologic or nontoxic agents to transform tumor cells either into a more radio-, immuno-, or chemosensitive state or into a low-, or terminal-growth phase. Agents of interest include interferon, 3':5'-cyclic adenosine monophosphate (cAMP), and polar solvents (such as dimethylformamide sodium butyrate). The differentiation of glioma cells by dibutyrl cyclic AMP (db-cAMP) (and for some butyric acid itself), has been known for some time (Sato *et al.,* 1975; Steinbach and Schubert, 1975; Stavron *et al.,* 1979; Smith and Liszczak, 1980). Alterations in cytotoxic sensitivity after both db-cAMP and DMF exposure have been reported (Gumerlock *et al.,* 1981), supporting the possibility of biologic tumor modification. Human fibroblast interferon, as well as glioma cell interferon (stimulated by superinduction techniques), can result in reduced growth rates and morphologic changes in some, but not all, glioma-derived cell lines. Control of vascular proliferation by blocking glial tumor angiogenesis factor production of the effects is yet another possibility (Folkman and Haudenschild, 1980). Early clinical trials involving interferon inducer, poly IC and poly ICLC (Shitara *et al.,* 1979; Nakamura *et al.,* 1982), as well as fibroblast and leukocyte interferon (Medenica, 1981; Osther *et al.,* 1981), have indicated some promise for these approaches, but more data will be needed to evaluate their places in the antiglioma clinical armamentarium.

Conclusions

Central nervous system tumors continue to present a major challenge for neurologists, neurosurgeons, and neuro-oncologists. In part, this results from the interference of such tumors with normal CNS structure and function, as well as the locally invasive qualities of malignant glial tumors. Although both surgery and radiation therapy are effective in reducing tumor burden and lead to prolonged survival, the average glioma patient's life expectancy is still less than a year. The full potential of adjunctive chemotherapy or immunotherapy has not been realized. Substantial advances in basic biologic understanding of CNS tumors, as well as new diagnostic techniques and predictive *in vitro* chemotherapeutic and immunologic assays, promise therapeutic progress in the near future. The heterogeneous nature of malignant brain tumor cell populations, both from tumor to tumor and within a given tumor, demands individualization of therapy. New techniques should help to provide this therapy. Improved survival will probably depend on multicomponent primary and adjuvant therapy.

REFERENCES

Abay, E. O.; Laws, E. R., Jr.; Grado, G. L.; Bruckman, J. E.; Forbes, G. S.; Gomez, M. R.; and Scott, M.: Pineal tumors in children and adolescents. *J. Neurosurg.,* **55:**889–895, 1981.

Adams, R. D., and Victor, M.: *Principles of Neurology.* McGraw-Hill, Inc., New York, 1977.

Adams, R. D., and Victor, M.: *Principles of Neurology,* 2nd ed. McGraw-Hill, Inc., New York, 1981.

Alderson, P. O.; Gado, M. H.; and Siegal, B. B.: Computerized cranial tomography and radionuclide imaging in the detection of intracranial mass lesions. *Semin. Nucl. Med.,* **7:**161–173, 1977.

Aloia, J. F., and Archambeau, J. O.: Hypopituitarism following pituitary irradiation for acromegaly. *Horm. Res.,* **9:**201–207, 1978.

Annegers, J. F.; Laws, E. R.; Kurland, L. T.; and Grabow, J. D.: Head trauma and subsequent brain tumors. *Neurosurgery,* **4:**203–206, 1979.

Antunes, J. L.; Housepian, E. M.; Frantz, A. G.; Holub, D. A.; Hui, R. M.; Carmel, P. W.; and Quest, D. O.: Prolactin-secreting pituitary tumors. *Ann. Neurol.,* **2:**148–153, 1977.

Arafah, B. M.; Brodkey, J. S.; Kaufman, B.; Velasco, M.; Manni, A.; and Pearson, O. H.: Transsphenoidal microsurgery in the treatment of acromegaly and gigantism. *J. Clin. Endocrinol. Metab.,* **50:**578–585, 1980.

Arita, N.; Bitoh, S.; Ushio, Y.; Hayakawa, T.; Hasegawa, H.; Fujiwara, M.; Ozaki, K.; Par-Khen, L.; and Takesada, M.: Primary pineal endodermal sinus tumor with elevated serum and CSF alphafetoprotein levels. Case report. *J. Neurosurg.,* **53:**244–248, 1980.

Aron, B. S.: Twenty years' experience with radiation therapy of medulloblastoma. *A. J. R.,* **105:**37–42, 1969.

Aubourg, P. R.; Derome, P. J.; Peillon, F.; Jedynak, C. P.; Visot, A.; LeGentil, P.; Balagura, S.; and Guiot, G.: Endocrine outcome after transsphenoidal adenomectomy for prolactinoma: Prolactin levels and tumor size as predicting factors. *Surg. Neurol.,* **14:**141–143, 1980.

Avellanosa, A. M.; West, C. R.; Tsukada, Y.; Higby, D. J.;

Bakshi, S.; Reese, P. A.; and Jennings, E.: Chemotherapy of nonirradiated malignant gliomas. Phase II. Study of the combination of methyl-CCNU, vincristine, and procarbazine. *Cancer,* **44:**839–846, 1979.

Bailey, P.: *Intracranial Tumors.* Charles C Thomas, Publisher, Springfield, Illinois, 1933.

Bailey, P.; Buchanan, D. N.; and Bucy, P. C.: *Intracranial Tumors of Infancy and Childhood,* 2nd ed. University of Chicago Press, Chicago, 1948.

Bailey, P., and Cushing, H.: *A Classification of the Tumours of the Glioma Group on a Histogenetic Basis with a Correlated Study of Prognosis.* J. B. Lippincott Company, Philadelphia, 1926.

Banna, M.; Baker, H. L., Jr.; and Houser, O. W.: Pituitary and parapituitary tumours on computed tomography—A review article based on 230 cases. *Br. J. Radiol.,* **53:**1123–1143, 1980.

Barnard, R. O.: The development of malignancy in oligodendrogliomas. *J. Pathol.,* **96:**113–123, 1968.

Barone, B. M., and Elvidge, A. R.: Ependymomas. A clinical survey. *J. Neurosurg.,* **33:**428–438, 1970.

Bartlett, J. R.: Craniopharyngiomas: An analysis of some aspects of symptomatology, radiology and histology. *Brain,* **94:**725–732, 1971a.

Bartlett, J. R.: Craniopharyngiomas—A summary of 85 cases. *J. Neurol. Neurosurg. Psychiatry,* **34:**37–41, 1971b.

Baskin, D. S.; Boggan, J. E.; and Wilson, C. B.: Transsphenoidal microsurgical removal of growth hormone–secreting pituitary adenomas—A review of 137 cases. *J. Neurosurg.,* **56:**634–641, 1982.

Behrend, R. C. H.: Epidemiology of brain tumours. In Vinken, P. J., and Bruyn, G. W. (eds.): *Handbook of Clinical Neurology. Tumours of the Brain and Skull. Part I.* American Elsevier Publishers, Inc., New York, 1974.

Bell, E., Jr., and Karnosh, L. J.: Cerebral hemispherectomy. Report of a case ten years after operation. *J. Neurosurg.,* **6:**285–293, 1949.

Benda, P.; Someda, K.; Messer, J.; and Sweet, W. H.: Morphological and immunochemical studies of rat glial tumors and clonal strains propagated in culture. *J. Neurosurg.,* **34:**310–323, 1971.

Berger, E. C., and Elvidge, A. R.: Medulloblastomas and cerebellar sarcomas. A clinical survey. *J. Neurosurg.,* **20:**139–144, 1963.

Bernstein, M., and Gutin, P. H.: Interstitial irradiation of brain tumors: A review. *Neurosurgery,* **9:**741–750, 1981.

Bertrand, I., and Mannen, H.: Étude des réactions vasculaires dans les astrocytomes. *Rev. Neurol (Paris),* **102:**3–19, 1960.

Bigner, D. D.; Bigner, S. H.; Pontén, J.; Westermark, B.; Mahaley, M. S.; Ruoslahti, E.; Herschman, H.; Eng, L. F.; and Wikstrand, C. J.: Heterogeneity of genotypic and phenotypic characteristics of fifteen permanent cell lines derived from human gliomas. *J. Neuropathol. Exp. Neurol.,* **40:**201–229, 1981.

Bigner, D. D.; Fritz, R. B.; and Day, E. D.: Cerebral physiology in dogs after brain tumor induction with Schmidt-Ruppin Rous sarcoma virus: Experiences with radioiodinated normal and antiviral immunoglobulin. *J.N.C.I.,* **43:**565–573, 1969.

Birkmayer, G. D., and Stass, H. P.: Humoral immune response in glioma patients: A solubilized glioma-associated membrane antigen as a tool for detecting circulating antibodies. *Int. J. Cancer,* **25:**445–452, 1980.

Black, P. M.; Callahan, L. V.; and Kornblith, P. L.: Tissue cultures from cerebrospinal fluid specimens in the study of human brain tumors. *J. Neurosurg.,* **49:**697–704, 1978.

Blasberg, R.; Molnar, P.; Horowitz, M.; Kornblith, P. L.; Pleasants, R.; and Fenstermacher, J.: Quantitative autoradiographic measurements of regional blood flow in the RT-9 brain tumor model. *J. Neurosurg.,* **58:**863–873, 1983.

Blattner, W. A.; McGuire, D. B.; Mulvihill, J. J.; Lampkin, B. C., Hananian, J.; and Fraumeni, J. F., Jr.: Genealogy of cancer in a family. *J.A.M.A.,* **241:**259–261, 1979.

Bleehen, N. M.: The Cambridge glioma trial of misonidazole and radiation therapy with associated pharmacokinetic studies. *Cancer Clin. Trials,* **3:**267–273, 1980.

Bloom, H. J. G.: Radiotherapy of pituitary tumors. In Jenkins, J. S. (ed.): *Pituitary Tumors.* Butterworth, London, 1973.

Bloom, H. J. G.: Combined modality therapy for intracranial tumors. *Cancer,* **35:**111–120, 1975.

Bloom, H. J. G.: Prospects for increasing survival in children with medulloblastoma: Present and future studies. *Neurooncology,* **1:**245–260, 1979.

Bloom, H. J. G.; Peckham, M. J.; Richardson, A. E.; Alexander, P. A.; and Payne, P. M.: Glioblastoma multiforme: A controlled trial to assess the value of specific active immunotherapy in patients treated by radical surgery and radiotherapy. *Br. J. Cancer,* **27:**253–267, 1973.

Bloom, H. J. G.; Wallace, E. W. K.; and Henk, J. M.: The treatment and prognosis of medulloblastoma in children. A study of 82 verified cases. *A. J. R.,* **105:**43–62, 1969.

Bloom, H. J. G., and Walsh, L. S.: Tumors of the central nervous system. In Bloom, H. J. G.; Lemerle, J.; and Neidhardt, M. K. (eds.): *Cancer in Children. Clinical Management.* Springer Verlag New York, Inc., New York, 1975.

Bloom, W. H.; Carstairs, K. C.; Crompton, M. R.; and McKissock, W.: Autologous glioma transplantation. *Lancet,* **2:**77–78, 1960.

Boggan, J. E.; Tyrrell, J. B.; and Wilson, C. B.: Transsphenoidal management of Cushing's disease: Report of 100 cases. Presented at the 1982 Annual Meeting of the American Association of Neurological Surgeons. Honolulu, Hawaii, 1982.

Borrow, G. N.; Wortzman, G.; Rewcastle, N. B.; Holgate, R. C.; and Kovacs, K.: Microadenomas of the pituitary and abnormal sellar tomograms in an unselected autopsy series. *N. Engl. J. Med.,* **304:**156–158, 1981.

Bouchard, J., and Peirce, C. B.: Radiation therapy in the management of neoplasms of the central nervous system, with a special note in regard to children: Twenty years' experience, 1939–1958. *A. J. R.,* **84:**610–628, 1960.

Boyland, E.: The correlation of experimental carcinogenesis and cancer in man. *Prog. Exp. Tumor Res.,* **11:**222–234, 1969.

Bradley, W. H., and Maxwell, J. H.: Neoplasms of middle ear and mastoid: Report of 54 cases. *Laryngoscope,* **64:**533–556, 1954.

Brooks, B. R.; Hochberg, F.; Kornblith, P. L.; Quindlen, E.; and Richardson, E. P., Jr.: Morphologic and kinetic analysis of explant cultures of 100 CNS biopsy specimens. *J. Neuropathol. Exp. Neurol.,* **34:**112 (Abstr. #122), 1975.

Brooks, R. A.; Sank, V. J.; Friauf, W. S.; Leighton, S. B.; Cascio, H. E.; and DiChiro, G.: Design considerations for positron emission tomography. *IEEE Trans. Biomed. Eng.,* **BME-28:**158–177, 1981.

Brooks, W. H.; Caldwell, H. D.; and Mortara, R. H.: Immune responses in patients with gliomas. *Surg. Neurol.,* **2:**419–423, 1974.

Brooks, W. H.; Netsky, M. G.; Normansell, D. E.; and Horwitz, D. A.: Depressed cell-mediated immunity in patients with primary intracranial tumors. Characterization of a humoral immunosuppressive factor. *J. Exp. Med.,* **136:**1631–1647, 1972.

Brooks, W. H., and Roszman, T. L.: Cellular immune responsiveness of patients with primary intracranial tumors. In Thomas, D. G. T., and Graham, D. I. (eds.): *Brain Tumours: Scientific Basis, Clinical Investigation and Current Therapy.* Butterworth, London, 1980.

Bucy, P. C.: Research on brain tumors. In Paoletti, P.; Walker, M. D.; Butti, G.; and Knerich, R. (eds.): *Neurooncology—Volume I. Multidisciplinary Aspects of Brain Tumor Therapy.* Elsevier/North-Holland Biomedical Press, Amsterdam, 1979.

Bucy, P. C., and Gustafson, W. A.: Structure, nature and classification of cerebellar astrocytomas. *Am. J. Cancer,* **35:**327–353, 1939.

Burger, P. C.; Mahaley, M. S., Jr.; Dudka, L.; and Vogel, F. S.: The morphologic effects of radiation administered therapeutically for intracranial gliomas. A postmortem study of 25 cases. *Cancer,* **44:**1256–1272, 1979.

Burger, P. C., and Vogel, F. S.: *Surgical Pathology of the Nervous System and Its Coverings.* John Wiley & Sons, Inc., New York, 1976.

Butler, A. B.; Brooks, W. H.; and Netsky, M. G.: Classification and biology of brain tumors. In Youmans, J. R. (ed.): *Clinical Neurosurgery.* W. B. Saunders Company, Philadelphia, 1982.

Camins, M. B., and Mount, L. A.: Primary suprasellar atypical teratoma. *Brain,* **97:**447–456, 1974.

Cangir, A.; VanEys, J.; Berry, D. H.; Huizdala, E.; and Morgan, S. K.: Combination chemotherapy with MOPP in children with recurrent brain tumors. *Med. Pediatr. Oncol.,* **4:**253–261, 1978.

Capra, L. G.: Radiotherapy of cerebral gliomas. In Thomas, D. G. T., and Graham, D. I. (eds.): *Brain Tumours. Scientific Basis, Clinical Investigation, and Current Therapy.* Butterworth, Boston, 1980.

Carabell, S. C.; Bruno, L. A.; Weinstein, A. S.; Richter, M. P.; Chang, C. H.; Weiler, C. B.; and Goodman, R. L.: Misonidazole and radiotherapy to treat malignant glioma: A phase II trial of the Radiation Therapy Oncology Group. *Int. J. Radiat. Oncol. Biol. Phys.,* **7:**71–77, 1981.

Carter, L. P.; Beggs, J.; and Waggener, J. D.: Ultrastructure of three choroid plexus papillomas. *Cancer,* **30:**1130–1136, 1972.

Castaigne, P.; Rondot, P.; Escourolle, R.; Ribadeau-Dumas, J-L.; Cathala, F.; and Hauw, J. J.: Leucoencephalopathie multifocale progressive et 'gliomes' multiples. *Rev. Neurol. (Paris),* **130:**379–392, 1974.

Castellano, F.; Guidetti, B.; and Olivecrona, H.: Pterional meningiomas "en plaque." *J. Neurosurg.,* **9:**188–196, 1952.

Catterall, M.; Bloom, H. J. G.; Ash, D. V.; Walsh, L.; Richardson, A.; Uttley, D.; Gowing, N. F. C.; Lewis, P.; and Chaucer, B.: Fast neutrons compared with megavoltage x-rays in the treatment of patients with supratentorial glioblastoma: A controlled pilot study. *Int. J. Radiat. Oncol. Biol. Phys.,* **6:**261–266, 1980.

Chambers, A. A.; Lukin, R.; and Tsunekawa, N.: Calcification in a chromophobe adenoma. Case report. *J. Neurosurg.,* **44:**623–625, 1976.

Chang, C. H.; Housepian, E. M.; and Herbert, C. Jr.: An operative staging system and a megavoltage radiotherapeutic technique for cerebellar medulloblastomas. *Radiology,* **93:**1351–1359, 1969.

Chang, C. H.; Housepian, E. M.; Sciarra, D.; and Herbert, C. M.: Hyperbaric oxygen and radiation therapy for malignant gliomas. In Seydel, H. G. (ed.): *Tumors of the Nervous System.* John Wiley & Sons, Inc., New York, 1975.

Chang, R. J.; Keye, W. R., Jr.; Young, J. R.; Wilson, C. B.; and Jaffe, R. B.: Detection, evaluation, and treatment of pituitary microadenomas in patients with galactorrhea and amenorrhea. *Am. J. Obstet. Gynecol.,* **128:**356–363, 1977.

Chapman, P. H., and Linggood, R. M.: The management of pineal area tumors: A recent reappraisal. *Cancer,* **46:**1253–1257, 1980.

Chatty, E. M., and Earle, K. M.: Medulloblastoma. A report of 201 cases with emphasis on the relationship of histologic variants to survival. *Cancer,* **28:**977–983, 1971.

Chiappa, K. H., and Ropper, A. H.: Evoked potentials in clinical medicine (Parts one and two). *N. Engl. J. Med.,* **306:**1140–1150, 1982; **306:**1205–1211, 1982.

Chin, H. W.; Hazel, J. J.; Kim, T. H.; and Webster, J. H.: Oligodendrogliomas. I. A clinical study of cerebral oligodendrogliomas. *Cancer,* **45:**1458–1466, 1980.

Chiodini, P.; Liuzzi, A.; Cozzi, R.; Verde, G.; Oppizzi, G.; Dallabonzana, D.; Spelta, B.; Silvestrini, F.; Borghi, G.; Luccarelli, G.; Rainer, E.; and Horowski, R.: Size reduction of macroprolactinomas by bromocriptine or lisuride treatment. *J. Clin. Endocrinol. Metab.,* **53:**737–743, 1981.

Ciembroniewicz, J., and Kolar, O.: Eosinophilic response in glioblastoma tissue culture after addition of autologous lymphocytes. *Science,* **157:**1054–1055, 1967.

Coakham, H. B., and Kornblith, P. L.: The humoral immune response of patients to their gliomas. *Acta Neurochir. [Suppl.],* **28:**475–479, 1979.

Cohen, R. J.; Wiernik, P. H.; and Walker, M. D.: Acute nonlymphocytic leukemia associated with nitrosourea chemotherapy: Report of two cases. *Cancer Treat. Rep.,* **60:**1257–1261, 1976.

Copeland, D. D., and Bigner, D. D.: Glial-mesenchymal tropism of *in vivo* avian sarcoma virus neuro-oncogenesis in rats. *Acta Neuropathol. (Berl.),* **41:**23–25, 1978.

Cox, L. B.: The cytology of the glioma group; with special reference to the inclusion of cells derived from the invaded tissue. *Am. J. Pathol.,* **9:**839–898, 1933.

Cramer, F., and Kinsey, M. W.: The cerebellar hemangioblastomas. Review of fifty-three cases, with special reference to cerebellar cysts and the association of polycythemia. *Arch. Neurol. Psychiatr.,* **67:**237–252, 1952.

Cumings, J. N.: The chemistry of cerebral cysts. *Brain,* **73:**244–250, 1950.

Curt, G. A.; Schilsky, R.; Kufta, C.; Smith, B. H.; Thomas, C.; and Young, R.: A phase II study of AZQ in high-grade gliomas. *Proc. Am. Soc. Clin. Oncol.,* **1:**13 (Abstr. #C-52), 1982.

Cushing, H.: *Tumors of the Nervus Acusticus and the Syndrome of the Cerebellopontine Angle.* W. B. Saunders Company, Philadelphia, 1917.

Cushing, H.: Experiences with cerebellar medulloblastomas: A critical review. *Acta Pathol. Microbiol. Scand.,* **7:**1–86, 1930.

Cushing, H.: Experiences with cerebellar astrocytomas—A critical review of 76 cases. *Surg. Gynecol. Obstet.,* **52:**129–204, 1931.

Cushing, H.: *Intracranial Tumors. Notes Upon a Series of*

Two Thousand Verified Cases with Surgical-Mortality Percentages Pertaining Thereto. Charles C Thomas, Publisher, Springfield, Illinois, 1932.

Dandy, W. E.: Ventriculography following the injection of air into the cerebral ventricles. *Ann. Surg.,* **68:**5–11, 1918.

Dandy, W. E.: Röentgenography of the brain after injection of air into the spinal canal. *Ann. Surg.,* **70:**397–403, 1919.

Dandy, W. E.: Results of removal of acoustic tumors by the unilateral approach. *Arch. Surg.,* **42:**1026–1033, 1941.

Daughaday, W. H., and Cryer, P. E.: Growth hormone hypersecretion and acromegaly. In Krieger, D. T. (ed.): *Neuroendocrinology.* Sinauer Associates, Sunderland, Massachusetts, 1980.

Dawson, D. M., and Dingman, J. F.: Hazards of proton-beam pituitary irradiation. *N. Engl. J. Med.,* **282:**1434, 1970.

Deen, G. D., Jr.; Scheithaur, B. W.; and Ebersold, M. J.: Clinical and pathological study of meningiomas of the first two decades of life. *J. Neurosurg.,* **56:**317–322, 1982.

Dibden, F. A.: Radiotherapy of brain tumors. *Australas. Radiol.,* **6:**122–129, 1962.

Di Chiro, G., and Brooks, R. A.: The 1979 Nobel prize in physiology or medicine. *Science,* **260:**1060–1062, 1979.

Di Chiro, G.; De La Paz, R. L.; Brooks, R. A.; Sokoloff, L.; Kornblith, P. L.; Smith, B. H.; Petronas, N. J.; Kufta, C. V.; Kessler, R. M.; Johnston, G. S.; Manning, R. G.; and Wolf, A. P.: Glucose utilization of cerebral gliomas measured by (18F) fluorodeoxyglucose and positron emission tomography. *Neurology,* **32:**1323–1329, 1982.

Di Chiro, G., and Nelson, K. B.: The volume of the sella turcica. *A. J. R.* **87:**989–1008, 1962.

Dick, S. J.; Macchi, B.,; Papazoglou, S.; Oldfield, E. H.; Kornblith, P. L.; Smith, B. H.; Gately, M. K.: Lymphoid cell-glioma cell interaction enhances cell coat production by human gliomas: Novel suppresor mechanism. *Science,* **220:**739–742, 1983.

Dohrmann, G. J.; Farwell, J. R.; and Flannery, J. T.: Ependymomas and ependymoblastomas in children. *J. Neurosurg.,* **45:**273–283, 1976.

Donnell, M. S.; Meyer, G. A.; and Donegan, W. L.: Estrogen-receptor protein in intracranial meningiomas. *J. Neurosurg.,* **50:**499–502, 1979.

Douglas, B. G.: Preliminary results using superfractionation in the treatment of glioblastoma multiforme. *J. Can. Assoc. Radiol.,* **28:**106–110, 1977.

Doyle, F. H.; Gore, J. C.; Pennock, J. M.; Bydder, G. M.; Orr, J. S.; Steiner, R. E.; Young, I. R.; Burl, M.; Clow, H.; Gilderdale, D. J.; Bailes, D. R.; and Walters, P. E.: Imaging of the brain by nuclear magnetic resonance. *Lancet,* **2:**53–57, 1981.

Druckrey, H.; Ivankovic, S.; Preussmann, R.; Zülch, K. J.; and Mennel, H. D.: Selective induction of malignant tumors of the nervous system by resorptive carcinogens. In Kirsch, W. M.; Grossi-Paoletti, E.; and Paoletti, P. (eds.): *The Experimental Biology of Brain Tumors.* Charles C Thomas, Publisher, Springfield, Illinois, 1972.

duBoulay, G. H., and Trickey, S. F.: Case reports. Calcifications in chromophobe adenoma. *Br. J. Radiol.,* **35:**793–795, 1962.

Earle, K. M., and Richany, S. F.: Meningiomas: A study of the histology, incidence and biologic behavior of 243 cases from the Frazier-Grant collection of brain tumors. *Med. Ann. D.C.,* **38:**353–358, 1969.

Earnest, F.; Kernohan, J. W.; and Craig, W. M.: Oligodendrogliomas: A review of two hundred cases. *Arch. Neurol. Psychiatr.,* **63:**964–976, 1950.

Eastman, R. C.; Gorden, P.; and Roth, J.: Conventional supervoltage irradiation is an effective treatment for acromegaly. *J. Clin. Endocrinol. Metab.,* **48:**931–940, 1979.

Ehrenreich, T., and Devlin, J. F.: A complex of glioblastoma and spindle-cell sarcoma with pulmonary metastasis. *Arch. Pathol.,* **66:**536–549, 1958.

Ell, P. J.; Deacon, J. M.; Ducassou, D.; and Brendel, A.: Emission and transmission brain tomography. *Br. Med. J.,* **280:**438–440, 1980.

Elvidge, A. R., and Martinez-Coll, A.: Long-term follow-up of 106 cases of astrocytoma, 1928–1939. *J. Neurosurg.,* **13:**318–331, 1956.

E.O.R.T.C. Brain Tumor Group: Effect of CCNU on survival rate of objective remission and duration of free interval in patients with malignant brain glioma—Final evaluation. *Eur. J. Cancer,* **14:**851–856, 1978.

Erikson, L. C.; Bradley, M. O.; and Kohn, K. W.: Differential inhibition of the rejoining of x-ray induced DNA strand breaks in normal and transformed human fibroblasts treated with 1,3-*bis*(2-chloroethyl)-1-nitrosourea *in vitro. Cancer Res.,* **38:**672–677, 1978.

Erikson, L. C.; Laurent, G.; Sharkey, N. A.; and Kohn, K. W.: DNA cross-linking and monoadduct repair in nitrosourea-treated human tumor cells. *Nature,* **288:**727–729, 1980.

Erikson, L. C.; Sariban, E.; Zlotogorski, C.; Laurent, G.; Kohn, K. W.; Smith, B. H.; and Kornblith, P. L.: Differences in chloroethylnitrosoureas (CNS)-induced DNA interstrand cross-linking among cell lines derived from malignant gliomas. *Proc. Am. Assoc. Cancer Res.,* **23:**163 (Abstr. #641), 1982.

Ermel, A. E., and Brucher, J. M.: Arguments ultrastructuraux en faveur de l'appartenance du médulloblastome à la lignée neuronale. *Acta Neurol. Belg.,* **74:**208–220, 1974.

Evans, A. E.; Anderson, J.; Chang, C., Jenkin, R. D. T.; Kramer, S.; Schoenfeld, D.; and Wilson, C.: Adjuvant chemotherapy for medulloblastoma and ependymoma. *Neurooncology,* **1:**219–222, 1979.

Evans, R. G., and Jost, R. G.: The clinical efficacy and cost analysis of cranial computed tomography and the radionuclide brain scan. *Semin. Nucl. Med.,* **7:**129–136, 1977.

Faria, M. A., Jr., and Tindall, G. T.: Transsphenoidal microsurgery for prolactin-secreting pituitary adenomas. Results in 100 women with the amenorrhea-galactorrhea syndrome. *J. Neurosurg.,* **56:**33–43, 1982.

Farquhar, M. G.: Origin and fate of secretory granules in cells of the anterior pituitary gland. *Trans. N.Y. Acad. Sci.,* **23:**346–351, 1961.

Farwell, J. R.; Dohrmann, G. J.; and Flannery, J. T.: Central nervous system tumors in children. *Cancer,* **40:**3123–3132, 1977.

Farwell, J. R.; Dohrmann, G. J.; Marrett, L. D.; and Meigs, J. W.: Effect of SV40 virus-contaminated polio vaccine on the incidence and type of CNS neoplasms in children: A population-based study. *Ann. Neurol.,* **6:**166–167, 1979.

Fazekas, J. T.: Treatment of grades I and II brain astrocytomas. The role of radiotherapy. *Int. J. Radiat. Oncol. Biol. Phys.,* **2:**661–666, 1977.

Feigin, I.; Allen, L. B.; Lipkin, L.; and Gross, S. W.: The

endothelial hyperplasia of the cerebral blood vessels with brain tumors, and its sarcomatous transformation. *Cancer,* **2:**264–277, 1958.

Fischer, G., and Mansuy, L.: Total removal of intramedullary ependymomas: Follow-up study of 16 cases. *Surg. Neurol.,* **14:**243–249, 1980.

Fishman, R. A.: Brain edema. *N. Engl. J. Med.,* **293:**706–711, 1975.

Fitz, C. R.; Wortzman, G.; Harwood-Nash, D. C.; Holgate, R. C.; Barry, J. F.; and Bolt, D. W.: Computed tomography in craniopharyngiomas. *Radiology,* **127:**687–691, 1978.

Fokes, E. C., Jr., and Earle, K. M.: Ependymomas: Clinical and pathological aspects. *J. Neurosurg.,* **30:**585–594, 1969.

Folkman, J., and Haudenschild, C.: Angiogenesis *in vitro. Nature,* **288:**551–556, 1980.

Fornace, A. J., Jr.; Kohn, K. W.; and Kann, H. E., Jr.: Inhibition of the ligase step of excision repair by 2-chloroethyl isocyanate, a decomposition product of 1,3-*bis*(2-chloroethyl)-1-nitrosourea. *Cancer Res.,* **38:**1064–1069, 1978.

Frackowiak, R. S.: Personal communication, 1982.

Frankel, S. A., and German, W. J.: Glioblastoma multiforme. Review of 214 cases with regard to natural history, pathology, diagnostic methods and treatment. *J. Neurosurg.,* **15:**489–503, 1958.

Friede, R. L.: Dating the development of human cerebellum. *Acta Neuropathol. (Berl.),* **23:**48–58, 1973.

Friedman, M.: Irradiation of meningioma: A prototype circumscribed tumor for planning high-dose irradiation of the brain. *Int. J. Radiat. Oncol. Biol. Phys.,* **2:**949–958, 1977.

Friedman, N. B.: Germinoma of the pineal. Its identity with germinoma ("seminoma") of the testis. *Cancer Res.,* **7:**363–368, 1947.

Fulton, D. S.; Levin, V. A.; Lubich, W. P.: Wilson, C. B.; and Marton, L. J.: Cerebrospinal fluid polyamines in patients with glioblastoma multiforme and anaplastic astrocytoma. *Cancer Res.,* **40:**3293–3296, 1980.

Futrell, N. N.; Osborn, A. G.; and Cheson, B. D.: Pineal region tumors: Computed tomographic-pathologic spectrum. *A.J.R.,* **137:**951–956, 1981.

Galicich, J. H., and French, L. A.: Use of dexamethasone in the treatment of cerebral edema resulting from brain tumors and brain surgery. *Am. Pract. Dig. Treat.,* **12:**169–174, 1961.

Garner, W. J., and Turner, O.: Bilateral acoustic neurofibromas. Further clinical and pathologic data on hereditary deafness and Recklinhausen's disease. *Arch. Neurol. Psychiatr.,* **13:**76–99, 1940.

Garfield, J.: Surgery of cerebral gliomas. In Thomas, D. G. T., and Graham, D. I. (eds.): *Brain Tumours. Scientific Basis, Clinical Investigation and Current Therapy.* Butterworth, Boston, 1980.

Garret, R.: Glioblastoma and fibrosarcoma of the brain with extracranial metastases. *Cancer,* **2:**888–894, 1958.

Garrett, M. J.; Hughes, H. J.; and Freedman, L. S.: A comparison of radiotherapy alone with radiotherapy and CCNU in cerebral glioma. *Clin. Oncol.,* **4:**71–76, 1978.

Garvin, A. J.; Spicer, S. S.; and McKeever, P. F.: The cytochemical demonstration of intracellular immunoglobulin in neoplasms of lymphoreticular tissue. *Am. J. Pathol.,* **82:**457–478, 1976.

Gately, M. K.; Glaser, M.; Dick, S. J.; Mettetal, R. W., Jr.; and Kornblith, P. L.: *In vitro* studies on cell-mediated immune response to human brain tumors. I. Require-

ment for third party stimulator lymphocytes in the induction of cell-mediated cytotoxic responses to allogeneic cultured gliomas. *J.N.C.I.,* **69:**1245–1254, 1982.

Gehan, E. A., and Walker, M. D.: Prognostic factors for patients with brain tumors. *Natl. Cancer Inst. Monogr.,* **46:**189–195, 1977.

George, S. R.; Burrow, G. N.; Zinman, B.; and Ezrin, C.: Regression of pituitary tumors, a possible effect of bromergocryptine. *Am. J. Med.,* **66:**697–702, 1979.

Gerosa, M.; DiStefano, E.; Carli, M.; and Iraci, G.: Combined treatment of pediatric medulloblastoma—A review of an integrated program (two-arm chemotherapy trial). *Childs Brain,* **6:**262–273, 1980.

Goellner, J. R.; Laws, E. R., Jr.; Soule, E. H.; and Okazaki, H.: Hemangiopericytoma of the meninges: Mayo Clinic experience. *Am. J. Clin. Pathol.,* **70:**375–380, 1978.

Gol, A.: The relatively benign astrocytomas of the cerebrum—A clinical study of 194 verified cases. *J. Neurosurg.,* **18:**501–506, 1961.

Gol, A.: Cerebral astrocytomas in childhood. A clinical study. *J. Neurosurg.,* **19:**577–582, 1962.

Gol, A., and McKissock, W.: The cerebellar astrocytomas. A report on 98 verified cases. *J. Neurosurg.,* **16:**287–296, 1959.

Gonzalez, C. F.; Grossman, C. B.; and Palacios, E.: *Computed Brain and Orbital Tomography.* John Wiley & Sons, Inc., New York, 1976.

Grace, J. T.; Perese, D. M.; Metzgar, R. S.; Sasabe, T.; and Holdridge, B.: Tumour autograft responses in patients with glioblastoma multiforme. *J. Neurosurg.,* **18:**159–167, 1961.

Greenwood, J.: Paraphyseal cysts of the third ventricle: With report of eight cases. *J. Neurosurg.,* **6:**153–159, 1949.

Greitz, T.: Computer tomography for diagnosis of intracranial tumours compared with other neuroradiologic procedures. *Acta Radiol. [Suppl.] (Stockh.),* **346:**14–20, 1975.

Griepentrog, F., and Pauly, H.: Intra- und extrakranielle, frühmanifeste medulloblastome bei erbgleichen zwillingen. *Zentralbl. Neurochir.,* **17:**129–140, 1957.

Griffin, B. R.; Griffin, T. W.; Tong, D. Y. K.; Russell, A. H.; Kurtz, J.; Laramore, G. E.; and Groudine, M.: Pineal region tumors: Results of radiation therapy and indications for elective spinal irradiation. *Int. J. Radiat. Oncol. Biol. Phys.,* **7:**605–608, 1981.

Griffin, T. W.; Beaufait, D.; and Blasko, J. C.: Cystic cerebellar astrocytomas in childhood. *Cancer,* **44:**276–280, 1979.

Grossi-Paoletti, E.; Paoletti, P.; and Fumagalli, R.: Lipids in brain tumors. *J. Neurosurg.,* **34:**454–455, 1971.

Grubb, W. B., Jr., and Lampe, I.: Role of radiation therapy in treatment of chemodectomas of glomus jugulare. *Laryngoscope,* **75:**1861–1871, 1965.

Guidetti, B.; Mercuri, S.; and Vagnozzi, R.: Long-term results of the surgical treatment of 129 intramedullary spinal gliomas. *J. Neurosurg.,* **54:**323–330, 1981.

Gumerlock, M. K.; Smith, B. H.; Pollock, L. A.; and Kornblith, P. L.: Chemical differentiation of cultured human glioma cells: Morphologic and immunologic effects. *Surg. Forum,* **32:**475–477, 1981.

Gutin, P. H.; Wilson, C. B.; Kumar, A. R. V.; Boldrey, E. B.; Levin, V.; Powell, M.; and Enot, K. J.: Phase II study of procarbazine, CCNU and vincristine combination chemotherapy in the treatment of malignant brain tumors. *Cancer,* **35:**1398–1404, 1975.

Hardy, J.: Transsphenoidal surgery of hypersecreting pituitary tumors. In Kohler, P. O., and Ross, G. T. (eds.):

Diagnosis and Treatment of Pituitary Tumors. International Congress Series 303. American Elsevier Publishers, Inc., New York, 1973.

Hardy, J.; Beauregard, H.; and Robert, F.: Prolactin-secreting pituitary adenomas: Transsphenoidal microsurgical treatment. In Robyn, C., and Harter, M. (eds.): *Progress in Prolactin Physiology and Pathology.* Elsevier North-Holland, Inc., New York, 1978.

Harisiadis, L., and Chang, C. H.: Medulloblastoma in children: A correlation between staging and results of treatment. *Int. J. Radiat. Oncol. Biol. Phys.,* **2:**833–841, 1977.

Hart, R. G., and Davenport, J.: Diagnosis of acoustic neuroma. *Neurosurgery,* **9:**450–463, 1981.

Hauge, M., and Harvald, B.: Studies in the etiology of intracranial tumours. *Acta Psychiatr. Scand.,* **35:**163–170, 1960.

Hawkins, J. C., III.: Treatment of choroid plexus papillomas in children: A brief analysis of twenty years' experience. *Neurosurgery,* **6:**380–384, 1980.

Hawkins, T. D.: Glomus jugulare and carotid body tumours. *Clin. Radiol.,* **12:**199–213, 1961.

Heilbrun, M. P.; Roberts, T. S.; Apuzzo, M. L. J.; Wells, T. H., Jr.; Sabshin, J. K.: Preliminary experience with Brown-Roberts-Wells (BRW) computerized tomography stereotactic guidance system. *J. Neurosurg.,* **59:**217–222, 1983

Heiss, W. D.: Chemotherapy of malignant gliomas: Comparison of the effect of polychemo- and CCNU-therapy. *Acta Neurochir. (Wein),* **42:**109–115, 1978.

Helle, T. L.; Conley, F. K.; and Britt, R. H.: Effect of radiation therapy on hemangioblastoma: A case report and review of the literature. *Neurosurgery,* **6:**82–86, 1980.

Higginson, J.: The role of geographical pathology in environmental carcinogenesis. In *Environment and Cancer. 24th Symposium on Fundamental Cancer Research.* The Williams & Wilkins Company, Baltimore, 1972.

Hitchcock, E., and Sato, F.: Treatment of malignant gliomata. *J. Neurosurg.,* **21:**497–506, 1964.

Hoch-Ligeti, C., and Russell, D. S.: Primary tumors of the brains and meninges in rats fed with 2-acetylaminofluorene. *Acta Un. Int. Cancr.,* **7:**126–129, 1950.

Hoff, J. T., and Patterson, R. H.: Craniopharyngiomas in children and adults. *J. Neurosurg.,* **36:**299–302, 1972.

Hoffman, H. J.; Hendrick, E. B.; Humphreys, R. P.; Buncie, J. R.; Armstrong, D. L.; and Jenkin, D. T.: Management of craniopharyngioma in children. *J. Neurosurg.,* **47:**218–227, 1977.

Holmes, H. L., and Little, J. M.: Tissue-culture microtest for predicting response of human cancer to chemotherapy. *Lancet,* **2:**985–987, 1974.

Hope-Stone, H. F.: Results of treatment of medulloblastomas. *J. Neurosurg.,* **32:**83–88, 1970.

Horowitz, M.; Blasberg, R.; Molnar, P.; Strong, J.; Kornblith, P. L.; Pleasants, R.; and Fenstermacher, J.: Regional [^{14}C]misonidazole distribution in experimental RT-9 brain tumors. *Cancer Res.,* **43:**3800–3807, 1983.

Hoshino, T.: Therapeutic implications of brain tumor cell kinetics. *Natl. Cancer Inst. Monogr.,* **46:**29–35, 1977.

Hoshino, T.; Barker, M.; and Wilson, C. B.: The kinetics of cultured human glioma cells. Autoradiographic studies. *Acta Neuropathol. (Berl.),* **32:**235–244, 1975a.

Hoshino, T.; Barker, M.; Wilson, C. B.; Boldrey, E. B.; and Fewer, D.: Cell kinetics of human gliomas. *J. Neurosurg.,* **37:**15–26, 1972.

Hoshino, T.; Wilson, C. B.; Rosenblum, M. L.; and Barker, M.: Chemotherapeutic implications of growth fraction and cell cycle time in glioblastomas. *J. Neurosurg.,* **43:**127–135, 1975b.

Hosobuchi, Y.; Phillips, T. L.; Stupar, T. A.; and Gutin, P. H.: Interstitial brachytherapy of primary brain tumors. *J. Neurosurg.,* **53:**613–617, 1980.

House, W. F.: Surgical exposure of the internal auditory canal and its contents through the middle, cranial fossa. *Laryngoscope,* **71:**1363–1385, 1961.

Hudgins, P. T.: Radiotherapy for extensive glomus jugulare tumors. *Radiology,* **103:**427–429, 1972.

Irwin, L.; George, F.; Pitts, F.; and Davis, R.: Hydroxyurea (HU) + radiation therapy (RT) in primary intra-cranial malignant glial tumors. *Proc. Am. Assoc. Cancer Res. and A.S.C.O.,* **16:**243 (Abstr. #1088), 1975.

Ishwar, S.; Taniguchi, R. M.; and Vogel, F. S.: Multiple supratentorial hemangioblastomas: Case study and ultrastructural characteristics. *J. Neurosurg.,* **35:**396–405, 1971.

Jänisch, W.; Fennwarth, B.; and Lagemann, A.: Zur epidemiologie der Geschwülste des zentralnervensystems. *Dtsch. Z. Nervenheilk.,* **191:**80–90, 1967.

Jänisch, W., and Schreiber, D.: Experimental brain tumours. In Vinken, P. J., and Bruyn, G. W. (eds.): *Handbook of Clinical Neurology. Tumours of the Brain and Skull.* Elsevier North-Holland, Inc., New York, 1974.

Jeffreys, R. V.: Clinical and surgical aspects of posterior fossa haemangioblastomata. *J. Neurol. Neurosurg. Psychiatry,* **38:**105–111, 1975a.

Jeffreys, R. V.: Pathological and haematological aspects of posterior fossa haemangioblastomata. *J. Neurol. Neurosurg. Psychiatry,* **38:**112–119, 1975b.

Jellinger, K.; Kothbauer, P.; Volc, D.; Vollmer, R.; and Weib, R.: Combination chemotherapy (COMP protocol) and radiotherapy of anaplastic supratentorial gliomas. *Acta Neurochir. (Wien),* **51:**1–13, 1979.

Jellinger, K.; Radaskiewicz, T.; and Slowik, F.: Primary malignant lymphomas of the central nervous system in man. *Acta Neuropathol. [Suppl.] (Berl.),* **6:**95–102, 1975.

Jelsma, R., and Bucy, P. C.: The treatment of glioblastoma multiforme of the brain. *J. Neurosurg.,* **27:**388–400, 1967.

Jelsma, R., and Bucy, P. C.: Glioblastoma multiforme. Its treatment and some factors effecting survival. *Arch. Neurol.,* **20:**161–171, 1969.

Jenkin, R. D. T.; Simpson, W. J. K.; and Keen, C. W.: Pineal and suprasellar germinomas—Results of radiation treatment. *J. Neurosurg.,* **48:**99–107, 1978.

Jordan, R. M.; Kendall, J. W.; McClung, M.; and Kammer, H.: Concentration of human chorionic gonadotropin in the cerebrospinal fluid of patients with germinal cell hypothalamic tumors. *Pediatrics,* **65:**121–124, 1980.

Kadin, M. E.; Rubinstein, L. J.; and Nelson, J. S.: Neonatal cerebellar medulloblastoma originating from the fetal external granular layer. *J. Neuropathol. Exp. Neurol.,* **29:**583–600, 1970.

Kajikawa, H.; Ohta, T.; Ohshiro, H.; Harada, K.; Ishikawa, S.; Uozumi, T.; Kodama, M.; and Okada, T.: Cerebrospinal fluid cytology in patients with brain tumours: A simple method using the cell culture technique. *Acta Cytol. (Baltimore),* **21:**162–167, 1977.

Kasantikul, V.; Netsky, M. G.; Glasscock, M. E., III.; and Hays, J. W.: Acoustic neurilemmoma. Clinicoanatomical study of 103 patients. *J. Neurosurg.,* **52:**28–35, 1980.

Katz, E. L.: Late results of radical excision of craniopharyngiomas in children. *J. Neurosurg.,* **42:**86–90, 1975.

Kawamura, J.; Garcia, A. H.; and Kamijyo, Y.: Cerebellar hemangioblastoma: Histogenesis of stromal cells. *Cancer,* **31:**1528–1540, 1973.

Kelly, P. J.; Alker, G. J.; and Goerss, S.: Computer-assisted stereotactic laser microsurgery for the treatment of intracranial neoplasms. *Neurosurgery,* **10:**324–331, 1982.

Kelly, R.: Colloid cysts of the third ventricle. Analysis of twenty-nine cases. *Brain,* **74:**23–65, 1951.

Kendall, B.: Neuroradiology. In Thomas, D. G. T., and Graham, D. I. (eds.): *Brain Tumours. Scientific Basis, Clinical Investigation, and Current Therapy.* Butterworth, Boston, 1980.

Kernohan, J. W.; Mabon, R. F.; Svien, H. J.; and Adson, A. W.: A simplified classification of the gliomas. *Mayo Clin. Proc.,* **24:**71–75, 1949.

Kim, T. H.; Chin, H. W.; Pollan, S.; Hazel, J. H.; and Webster, J. H.: Radiotherapy of primary brain stem tumors. *Int. J. Radiat. Oncol. Biol. Phys.,* **6:**51–57, 1980.

Kim, Y. H., and Fayos, J. V.: Intracranial ependymomas. *Radiology,* **124:**805–808, 1977.

King, D. L.; Chang, C. H.; and Pool, J. L.: Radiotherapy in the management of meningiomas. *Acta Radiol. [Ther.] (Stockh.)* **5:**26–33, 1966.

Kjellberg, R. N., and Kliman, B.: Proton beam therapy. *N. Engl. J. Med.,* **284:**333, 1971.

Kjellberg, R. N., and Kliman, B.: Bragg peak proton hypophysectomy for hyperpituitarism and neoplasms. *Prog. Neurol. Surg.,* **6:**295–325, 1975.

Kjellberg, R. N.; Shintani, A.; Frantz, A. G.; and Kliman, B.: Proton-beam therapy in acromegaly. *N. Engl. J. Med.,* **278:**689–695, 1968.

Kjellin, K.; Müller, R.; and Aström, K. E.: The occurrence of brain tumors in several members of a family. *J. Neuropathol. Exp. Neurol.,* **19:**528–537, 1960.

Kleinberg, D. L.; Noel, G. L.; and Franz, A. G.: Galactorrhea: A study of 235 cases including 48 with pituitary tumors. *N. Engl. J. Med.,* **296:**589–600, 1977.

Knudson, A. G., Jr.: Mutation and cancer: Statistical study of retinoblastoma. *Proc. Natl. Acad. Sci. U.S.A.,* **68:**820–828, 1971.

Koch, G.: Beitrag zur erblichkeit der hirngeschwülste. *Acta Genet. Med. Gemellol. (Roma),* **3:**170–191, 1954.

Koestner, A.; Swenberg, J. A.; and Wechsler, W.: Experimental tumors of the nervous system induced by resorptive N-nitrosourea compounds. *Prog. Exp. Tumor Res.,* **17:**9–30, 1972.

Kohn, K. W.: Interstrand cross-linking of DNA by 1,3-*bis*(2-chloroethyl)-1-nitrosourea and other 1-(2-haloethyl)-1-nitrosoureas. *Cancer Res.,* **37:**1450–1454, 1977.

Kopelson, G.; Linggood, R. M.; Kleinman, G. M.; Doucette, J.; and Wang, C. C.: Management of intramedullary spinal cord tumors. *Radiology,* **135:**473–479, 1980.

Kornblith, P. L.: Humoral immunity. In Thomas, D. G. T., and Graham, D. I. (eds.): *Brain Tumours. Scientific Basis, Clinical Investigation, and Current Therapy.* Butterworth, Boston, 1980.

Kornblith, P. L.; Coakham, H. B.; Pollock, L.; Wood, W. C.; Green, S. B.; and Smith, B. H.: Autologous serological responses in glioma patients: Correlation with tumor grade and survival. *Cancer,* **52:**2230–2235, 1983.

Kornblith, P. L.; Dohan, F. C., Jr.; Wood, W. C.; and Whitman, B. O.: Human astrocytoma: Serum-mediated immunologic response. *Cancer,* **33:**1512–1519, 1974.

Kornblith, P. L.; Pollock, L. A.; Coakham, H. B.; Quindlen, E. A.; and Wood, W. C.: Cytotoxic antibody responses in astrocytoma patients—An improved allogenic assay. *J. Neurosurg.,* **51:**47–52, 1979.

Kornblith, P. L.; Smith, B. H.; and Leonard, L. A.: Response of cultured human brain tumors to nitrosoureas: Correlation with clinical data. *Cancer,* **47:**255–265, 1981.

Kornblith, P. L., and Szypko, P. E.: Variations in response of human brain tumors to BCNU *in vitro. J. Neurosurg.,* **48:**580–586, 1978.

Kornblith, P. L.; Walker, M. D.; and Cassady, J. R.: Neoplasms of the central nervous system. In DeVita, V. T., Jr.; Hellman, S.; and Rosenberg, S. A. (eds.): *Cancer— Principles and Practice of Oncology.* J. B. Lippincott Company, Philadelphia, 1982b.

Kramer, S.: Cancer of the central nervous system— Radiation therapy in the management of malignant gliomas. In *Seventh National Cancer Conference Proceedings.* J. B. Lippincott Company, Philadelphia, 1973.

Kramer, S.; Southard, M.; and Mansfield, C. M.: Radiotherapy in the management of craniopharyngiomas. Further experiences and late results. *A.J.R.,* **103:**44–52, 1968.

Kricheff, I. I.; Becker, M.; Schneck, S. A.; and Taveras, J. M.: Intracranial ependymomas. A study of survival in 65 cases treated by surgery and irradiation. *A.J.R.,* **91:**167–175, 1964a.

Kricheff, I. I.; Becker, M.; Schneck, S. A.; and Taveras, J. M.: Intracranial ependymomas: Factors influencing prognosis. *J. Neurosurg.,* **2:**7–14, 1964b.

Kumar, A. R. V.; Renaudin, J.; Wilson, C. B.; Boldrey, E. B.; Enot, K. J.; and Levin, V. A.: Procarbazine hydrochloride in the treatment of brain tumors. Phase 2 study. *J. Neurosurg.,* **40:**365–371, 1974.

Kung, P. C.; Lee, J. C.; and Bakay, L.: Vascular invasion by glioma cells in man: An electron microscope study. *J. Neurosurg.,* **31:**339–345, 1969.

Kurland, L. T.: The frequency of intracranial and intraspinal neoplasms in the resident population of Rochester, Minnesota. *J. Neurosurg.,* **15:**627–641, 1958.

Labitzke, H. G.: Glioblastoma multiforme with remote extracranial metastases. *Arch. Pathol.,* **73:**223–229, 1962.

Landolt, A. M., and Wilson, C. B.: Tumors of the sella and parasellar area in adults. In Youmans, J. R. (ed.): *Neurological Surgery, 2nd ed.* W. B. Saunders Company, Philadelphia, 1982.

Langfitt, T. W.: Increased intracranial pressure and the cerebral circulation. In Youmans, J. R. (ed.): *Neurological Surgery, 2nd ed.* W. B. Saunders Company, Philadelphia, 1982.

Lassen, N. A.: Cerebral blood flow and oxygen consumption in man. *Physiol. Rev.,* **39:**183–238, 1959.

Lawrence, J. H.; Linfoot, J. A.; Born, J. L.; Tobias, C. A.; Chong, C. Y.; Okerlund, M. O.; Manuvgian, E.; Garcia, J. F.; and Connell, G. M.: Heavy particle irradiation of the pituitary. *Prog. Neurol. Surg.,* **6:**272–294, 1975.

Laws, E. R., Jr.; Cortese, D. A.; Kinsey, J. H.; Eagan, R. T.; and Anderson, R. E.: Photoradiation therapy in the treatment of malignant brain tumors: A phase I (feasibility) study. *Neurosurgery,* **9:**672–678, 1981.

Leibel, S. A.; Sheline, G. E.; Wara, W. M.; Boldrey, E. B.; and Nielsen, S. L.: The role of radiation therapy in the treatment of astrocytomas. *Cancer,* **35:**1551–1557, 1975.

Leibel, S. A.; Wara, W. M.; Sheline, G. E.; Townsend, J. J.;

and Boldrey, E. B.: The treatment of meningiomas in childhood. *Cancer,* **37**:2709–2712, 1976.

Lerner, H. J.: Hydroxyurea and irradiation in the treatment of astrocytomas. *Proc. Am. Assoc. Cancer Res. and A.S.C.O.,* **16**:5 (Abstr. #20), 1975.

Levin, V. A., and Edwards, M. S.: Chemotherapy of primary malignant gliomas. In Thomas, D. G. T., and Graham, D. I. (eds.): *Brain Tumours. Scientific Basis, Clinical Investigation, and Current Therapy.* Butterworth, Boston, 1980.

Levin, V. A.; Edwards, M. S.; Wright, D. C.; Seager, M. L.; Schimberg, T. P.; Townsend, J. J.; and Wilson, C. B.: Modified procarbazine, CCNU, and vincristine (PCV3) combination chemotherapy in the treatment of malignant brain tumors. *Cancer Treat. Rep.,* **64**:237–241, 1980.

Levin, V. A.; Landahl, H.; and Patlak, C. S.: Considerations in selecting effective brain tumor agents: Capillary permeability and sequestered cell populations. *Proc. Am. Assoc. Cancer Res. and A.S.C.O.,* **17**:202 (Abstr. #806), 1976.

Levin, V. A.; Wilson, C. B.; Davis, R.; Wara, W. M.; Pischer, T. L.; and Irwin, L.: A phase III comparison of BCNU, hydroxyurea, and radiation therapy to BCNU and radiation therapy for treatment of primary malignant gliomas. *J. Neurosurg.,* **51**:526–532, 1979.

Levy, N. L.: Specificity of lymphocyte-mediated cytotoxicity in patients with primary intracranial tumors. *J. Immunol.,* **121**:903–915, 1978.

Lewis, P. D., and Van Noorden, S.: "Nonfunctioning" pituitary tumors. A light and electron microscopical study. *Arch. Pathol.,* **97**:178–182, 1974.

Lindau, A.: Studien über kleinhirncysten bau, pathogeneses und beziehungen zur angiomatosis retinae. *Acta Pathol. Microbiol. Scand. [Suppl.],* **1**:1–128, 1926.

Liss, L.: Glial and parenchymal neoplasms in tissue culture. In Scharenberg, K., and Liss, L. (eds.): *Neuroectodermal Tumors of the Central and Peripheral Nervous System.* The Williams & Wilkins Company, Baltimore, 1969.

Liszczak, T.; Richardson, E. P.: Phillips, J. P.; Jacobson, S.; and Kornblith, P. L.: Morphological, biochemical, ultrastructural, tissue culture and clinical observations of typical and aggressive craniopharyngiomas. *Acta Neuropathol. (Berl.),* **43**:191–203, 1978.

Little, J. R., and MacCarty, C. S.: Colloid cysts of the third ventricle. *J. Neurosurg.,* **39**:230–235, 1974.

Littman, P., and Wang, C. C.: Reticulum cell sarcoma of the brain: A review of the literature and a study of 19 cases. *Cancer,* **35**:1412–1420, 1975.

London, W. T.; Houff, S. A.; Madden, D. L.; Fuccillo, D. A.; Gravell, M.; Wallen, W. C.; Palmer, A. E.; and Sever, J. L.: Brain tumors in owl monkeys inoculated with a human polyomavirus (JC virus). *Science,* **201**:1246–1249, 1978.

Ludwin, S. K.; Rubinstein, L. J.; and Russell, D. S.: Papillary meningioma: A malignant variant of meningioma. *Cancer,* **36**:1363–1373, 1975.

Lumsden, C. E.: Tissue culture of brain tumours. In Vinken, P. J., and Bruyn, G. W. (eds.): *Handbook of Clinical Neurology,* Vol. 17. Elsevier North-Holland Publishing Company, Amsterdam, 1974.

Lusins, J. O., and Nakagawa, H.: Multiple meningiomas evaluated by computed tomography. *Neurosurgery,* **9**:137–141, 1981.

Mabon, R. F.; Svien, H. J.; Kernohan, J. W.; and Craig, W. M.: Ependymomas. *Mayo Clin. Proc.,* **24**:65–70, 1949.

Mahaley, M. S.; Brooks, W. H.; Roszman, T. J. L.; Bigner,

D. D.; Dudka, L.; and Richardson, S.: Immunobiology of primary intracranial tumors. I. Studies of the cellular and humoral general immune competence of brain tumor patients. *J. Neurosurg.,* **46**:467–476, 1977.

Malis, L. I.: Microsurgical treatment of acoustic neurinomas. In Handa, H. (ed.): *Microneurosurgery. International Symposium on Microneurosurgery, Kyoto, October 1973.* University Park Press, Baltimore, 1975.

Mancuso, T. F.: Tumors of the central nervous system. Industrial considerations. *Acta Unio Int. Contra Cancrum,* **19**:488–489, 1963.

Marks, J. E.; and Gado, M.: Serial computed tomography of primary brain tumors following surgery, irradiation, and chemotherapy. *Radiology,* **125**:119–125, 1977.

Marsa, G. W.; Goffinet, D. R.; Rubinstein, L. J.; and Bagshaw, M. A.: Megavoltage irradiation in the treatment of gliomas of the brain and spinal cord. *Cancer,* **36**:1681–1689, 1975.

Marsa, G. W.; Probert, J. C.; Rubinstein, L. J.; and Bagshaw, M. A.: Radiation therapy in the treatment of childhood astrocytic gliomas. *Cancer,* **32**:646–655, 1973.

Marshall, L. F.; Smith, R. W.; Rauscher, L. A.; and Shapiro, H. M.: Mannitol dose requirements in brain-injured patients. *J. Neurosurg.,* **48**:169–172, 1978.

Martin-Archard, A.; de Tribolet, N.; Louis, J. A.; and Zander, E.: Immune complexes associated with brain tumors: Correlated with prognosis. *Surg. Neurol.,* **13**:161–164, 1980.

Martuza, R. L.; MacLaughlin, D. T.; and Ojemann, R. G.: Specific estradiol binding in schwannomas, meningiomas, and neurofibromas. *Neurosurgery,* **9**:665–671, 1981.

Martuza, R. L., and Ojemann, R. G.: Bilateral acoustic neuromas: Clinical aspects, pathogenesis, and treatment. *Neurosurgery,* **10**:1–12, 1982.

Maruyama, Y.; Gold, L. H. A.; and Kieffer, S. A.: Clinical and angiographic evaluation of radiotherapeutic response of glomus jugulare tumors. *Radiology,* **101**:397–399, 1971.

Matson, D. D.: Tumors of the choroid plexus. In *Neurosurgery of Infancy and Childhood,* 2nd ed. Charles C Thomas, Publisher, Springfield, Illinois, 1969.

Matson, D. D., and Crigler, J. F.: Management of craniopharyngioma in childhood. *J. Neurosurg.,* **30**:377–390, 1969.

McKeever, P. E., and Balentine, J. D.: Macrophage migration through the brain parenchyma to the perivascular space following particle ingestion. *Am. J. Pathol.,* **93**:153–164, 1978.

McKeran, R. O., and Thomas, D. G. T.: The clinical study of gliomas. In Thomas, D. G. T., and Graham, D. I. (eds.): *Brain Tumours. Scientific Basis, Clinical Investigation and Current Therapy.* Butterworth, Boston, 1980.

McKissock, W.: The surgical treatment of colloid cyst of the third ventricle. *Brain,* **74**:1–9, 1951.

Medawar, P. B.: Immunity to homologous grated skin. III. The fate of skin homografts transplanted to the brain, to subcutaneous tissue and to the anterior chamber of the eye. *Br. J. Exp. Pathol.,* **29**:58–69, 1948.

Medenica, O. O.: Personal communication, 1981.

Merritt, H. H.: *A Textbook of Neurology,* 2nd ed. Lea & Febiger, Philadelphia, 1959.

Michelsen, J. J., and New, P. F. J.: Brain tumor and pregnancy. *J. Neurol. Neurosurg. Psychiatry,* **32**:305–307, 1969.

Modan, B.; Baidatz, D.; Mart, H.; Steinitz, R.; and Levin,

S. G.: Radiation-induced head and neck tumors. *Lancet,* **1:**277–279, 1974.

Molnar, P.; Blasberg, R.; Horowitz, M.; Smith, B. H.; and Fenstermacher, J.: Regional blood-to-brain transport in RT-9 brain tumors. *J. Neurosurg.,* **58:**874–884, 1983.

Moniz, E.: *L'Angiographie Cerebrale: Ses Applications et Résultats en Anatomie, Physiologie, et Clinique.* Masson, Paris, 1934.

Morantz, R. A.; Feigin, I.; and Ransohoff, J.: Clinical and pathological study of 24 cases of gliosarcoma. *J. Neurosurg.,* **45:**398–408, 1976.

Mørk, S. J., and Løken, A. C.: Ependymoma—A follow-up study of 101 cases. *Cancer,* **40:**907–915, 1977.

Morley, T. P.: Tumors of the cranial meninges. In Youmans, J. R. (ed.): *Neurological Surgery,* Vol. 3. W. B. Saunders Company, Philadelphia, 1973.

Munk, J.; Peyser, E.; and Gruszkiewicz, J.: Radiation-induced intracranial neoplasms. *Clin. Radiol.,* **20:**90–94, 1969.

Murad, T. M., and Murthy, M. S. N.: Ultrastructure of a chordoma. *Cancer,* **25:**1204–1215, 1970.

Naidich, T. P.; Pinto, R. S.; Kushner, M. J.; Lin, J. P.; Kricheff, I. I.; Leeds, N. E.; and Chase, N. E.: Evaluation of sellar and parasellar masses by computed tomography. *Radiology,* **120:**91–99, 1976.

Nakamura, O.; Shitara, N.; Matsutani, M.; Takakura, K.; and Machida, H.: Phase I–II trials of poly(ICLC) in malignant brain tumor patients. *J. Interferon Res.,* **2:**1–4, 1982.

Narayan, O.; Penney, J. B.; Johnson, R. T.; Herndon, R. M.; and Weiner, L. P.: Etiology of progressive multifocal leukoencephalopathy: Identification of papovavirus. *N. Engl. J. Med.,* **289:**1278–1282, 1973.

National Institute of Neurological and Communicative Disorders and Stroke, Office of Biometry and Field Studies: *Survey of Intracranial Neoplasms. Final Report.* Contract No. NO1-NS-4-2336, Bethesda, Maryland, 1977.

Nelson, D. H.; Meakin, J. W.; Dealy, J. B., Jr.: Matson, D. D.; Emerson, K., Jr.; and Thorn, G. W.: ACTH-producing tumor of the pituitary gland. *N. Engl. J. Med.,* **259:**161–164, 1958.

Neuwelt, E. A.; Glasberg, M.; Diehl, J. T.; Frenkel, E. P.; and Barnett, P.: Osmotic blood-brain barrier disruption in the posterior fossa of the dog. *J. Neurosurg.,* **55:**742–748, 1981.

Neuwelt, E. A., and Hill, S. A.: Intrathecal lymphocyte infusions. In Wood, J. H. (ed.): *Neurobiology of Cerebrospinal Fluid.* Plenum Publishing Corporation, New York, 1980.

Newman, H.; Rowe, J. F., Jr.; and Phillips, T. L.: Radiation therapy of the glomus jugulare tumor. *A. J. R.,* **118:**663–669, 1973.

Norman, D.; Enzmann, D.; Levin, V. A.; Wilson, C. B.; and Newton, T. H.: Computed tomography in the evaluation of malignant glioma before and after therapy. *Radiology,* **121:**85–88, 1976.

Norris, D. G.; Bruce, D. A.; Byrd, R. L.; Schut, L.; Littman, P.; Bilaniuk, L. T.; Zimmerman, R. A.; and Capp, R.: Improved relapse-free survival in medulloblastoma utilizing modern techniques. *Neurosurgery,* **9:**661–664, 1981.

O'Duffy, J. D.; Randall, R. V.; and MacCarty, C. S.: Neuropathy (carpal-tunnel syndrome) in acromegaly: A sign of endocrine overactivity. *Ann. Intern. Med.,* **78:**379–383, 1973.

Ojemann, R. G.: Microsurgical suboccipital approach to cerebellopontine angle tumors. *Clin. Neurosurg.,* **25:**461–479, 1978.

Ommaya, A. K.: Immunotherapy of gliomas: A review. *Adv. Neurol.,* **15:**337–359, 1976.

Onoyama, Y.; Abe, M.; Takahashi, M.; Yabumoto, E.; and Sakamoto, T.: Radiation therapy of brain tumors in children. *Radiology,* **115:**687–693, 1975.

Onoyama, Y.; Ono, K.; Yabumoto, E.; and Takeuchi, J.: Radiation therapy of craniopharyngioma. *Radiology,* **125:**799–803, 1977.

Orth, D. N., and Liddle, G. W.: Results of treatment in 108 patients with Cushing's syndrome. *N. Engl. J. Med.,* **285:**243–247, 1971.

Osther, K.; Salford, L. G.; Hornmark-Stenstam, B.; Flodgren, P.; Christophersen, I. S.; Magnusson, K.; and the Southern Sweden Neuro-Oncology Group: Local versus systemic human leukocyte interferon treatment. In DeMaeyer, E.; Galasso, G.; and Schellekens, H. (eds.): *The Biology of the Interferon System.* Elsevier North Holland, Inc., New York, 1981.

Oyasu, R.; Battifora, H. A.; Clasen, R. A.; McDonald, J. H.; and Hass, G. M.: Induction of cerebral gliomas in rats with dietary lead subacetate and 2-acetylaminofluorene. *Cancer Res.,* **30:**1248–1261, 1970.

Padgett, B. L.; Walker, D. L.; ZuRhein, G. M.; and Eckroade, R. J.: Cultivation of papova-like virus from human brain with progressive multifocal leucoencephalopathy. *Lancet,* **1:**1257–1260, 1971.

Palmer, J. J.: Hemangioblastomas: A review of eighty-one cases. *Acta Neurochir. (Wien),* **27:**125–148, 1972.

Palmer, J. O.; Kasselberg, A. G.; and Netsky, M. G.: Differentiation of medulloblastoma: Studies including immunohistochemical localization of glial fibrillary acid protein. *J. Neurosurg.,* **55:**161–169, 1981.

Pappius, H. M., and McCann, W. P.: Effects of steroids on cerebral edema in cats. *Arch. Neurol.,* **20:**207–216, 1969.

Pay, N. T.; Carella, R. J.; Lin, J. P.; and Kricheff, I. I.: The usefulness of computed tomography during and after radiation therapy in patients with brain tumors. *Radiology,* **121:**79–83, 1976.

Pearlman, A. W., and Friedman, M.: Radical radiation therapy of chordoma. *A.J.R.,* **108:**333–341, 1970.

Percy, A. K.; Elveback, L. R.; Okazaki, H.; and Kurland, L. T.: Neoplasms of the central nervous system: Epidemiologic considerations. *Neurology,* **22:**40–48, 1972.

Phillips, T. L., and Newman, H.: Chordoma. In Deeley, T. J. (ed.): *Modern Radiotherapy and Oncology: Central Nervous System Tumours.* Butterworth, London, 1974.

Phillips, T. L.; Sheline, G. E.; and Boldrey, E.: Therapeutic considerations in tumors affecting the central nervous system: Ependymomas. *Radiology,* **83:**98–105, 1964.

Pistenma, D. A.; Goffinet, D. R.; Bagshaw, M. A.; Hanbery, J. W.; and Eltringham, J. R.: Treatment of acromegaly with megavoltage radiation therapy. *Int. J. Radiat. Oncol. Biol. Phys.,* **1:**885–893, 1976.

Quest, D. O.: Meningiomas: An update. *Neurosurgery,* **3:**219–225, 1978.

Quest, D. O.; Brisman, R.; Antunes, J. L.; and Housepian, E. M.: Period of risk for recurrence in medulloblastoma. *J. Neurosurg.,* **48:**159–163, 1978.

Raimondi, A. J., and Guiterrez, F. A.: Diagnosis and surgical treatment of choroid plexus papillomas. *Childs Brain,* **1:**81–115, 1975.

Rall, D. P., and Zubrod, C. G.: Mechanisms of drug absorption and excretion. Passage of drugs in and out of the central nervous system. *Annu. Rev. Pharmacol.,* 2:109–128, 1962.

Rand, R. W.; Dirks, D. D.; Morgan, D. D.; and Bentson, D. R.: Acoustic neuromas. In Youmans, J. R. (ed.): *Neurological Surgery.* W. B. Saunders Company, Philadelphia, 1982.

Rand, R. W., and Kurze, T. L.: Facial nerve preservation by posterior fossa transmeatal microdissection in total removal of acoustic tumors. *J. Neurol. Neurosurg. Psychiatry,* 28:311–316, 1965.

Rand, R. W., and Lemmen, L. J.: Tumors of the posterior portion of the third ventricle. *J. Neurosurg.,* 10:1–18, 1952.

Rao, Y. T.; Medini, E.; Haselow, R. E.; Jones, T. K., Jr.; and Levitt, S. H.: Pineal and ectopic pineal tumors: The role of radiation therapy. *Cancer,* 48:708–713, 1981.

Reagan, T. J.; Bisel, H. F.; Childs, D. S., Jr.; Layton, D. D.; Rhoton, A. L., Jr.; and Taylor, W. F.: Controlled study of CCNU and radiation therapy in malignant astrocytoma. *J. Neurosurg.,* 44:186–190, 1976.

Richardson, R. G.; Griffin, T. W.; and Parker, R. G.: Intramedullary hemangioblastoma of the spinal cord. *Cancer,* 45:49–50, 1980.

Ridley, A., and Cavanagh, J. B.: Lymphocytic infiltration in gliomas: Evidence of possible host resistance. *Brain,* 94:117–124, 1971.

Ringertz, N., and Reymond, A.: Ependymomas and choroid plexus papillomas. *J. Neuropathol. Exp. Neurol.,* 8:355–380, 1949.

Roberts, M., and German, W. J.: A long term study of patients with oligodendrogliomas. Follow-up of 50 cases, including Dr. Harvey Cushing's series. *J. Neurosurg.,* 24:697–700, 1966.

Robins, R. A., and Baldwin, R. W.: Immune complexes in cancer. *Cancer Immunol. Immunother.,* 4:1–3, 1978.

Rosenblum, M. L.; Knebel, K. D.; Vasquez, D. A.; and Wilson, C. B.: Brain tumor therapy, quantitative analysis using a model system. *J. Neurosurg.,* 46:145–154, 1977.

Rosenblum, M. L.; Vasquez, D. A.; Hoshino, T.; and Wilson, C. B.: Development of a clonogenic cell assay for human brain tumors. *Cancer,* 41:2305–2314, 1978.

Rosenstock, J. G.; Evans, A. E.; and Schut, L.: Response to vincristine of recurrent brain tumors in children. *J. Neurosurg.,* 45:135–140, 1976.

Rosenwasser, H.: Glomus jugularis tumor of the middle ear. (Carotid body tumor, tympanic body tumor, nonchromaffin paraganglioma.) *Laryngoscope,* 62:623–633, 1952.

Rossi, G. F.; Feoli, F.; Fernandez, E.; Meglio, M.; Mazzone, P.; and Pissolato, P.: The role of surgery in the treatment of supratentorial brain gliomas. In Paoletti, P.; Walker, M. D.; Butti, G.; and Knerich, R. (eds.): *Neurooncology, Volume I. Multidisciplinary Aspects of Brain Tumor Therapy.* Elsevier North-Holland, Inc., Amsterdam, 1979.

Ross-Russell, R. W., and Pennybacker, J. B.: Craniopharyngioma in the elderly. *J. Neurol. Neurosurg. Psychiatry,* 24:1–13, 1961.

Roth, J. G., and Elvidge, A. R.: Glioblastoma multiforme — A clinical survey. *J. Neurosurg.,* 17:736–750, 1960.

Rubinstein, L. J.: Development of extracranial metastases from a malignant astrocytoma in the absence of previous craniotomy. *J. Neurosurg.,* 26:542–547, 1967.

Rubinstein, L. J.: *Tumors of the Central Nervous System. Atlas of Tumor Pathology,* Fasc. 6. Armed Forces Institute of Pathology, Washington, D.C., 1972.

Rubinstein, L. J.; Herman, M. M.; and Hanberry, J. W.: The relationship between differentiating medulloblastoma and dedifferentiating diffuse cerebellar astrocytoma. Light, electron microscopic, tissue, and organ culture observations. *Cancer,* 33:675–690, 1974.

Russell, D. S., and Rubinstein, L. J.: Ganglioglioma: A case with long history and malignant evolution. *J. Neuropathol. Exp. Neurol.,* 21:185–193, 1962.

Russell, D. S., and Rubinstein, L. J.: *Pathology of Tumours of the Nervous System,* 4th ed. The Williams & Wilkins Company, Baltimore, 1977.

Sackett, J. F.; Messina, A. V.; and Petito, C. K.: Computed tomography and magnification vertebral angiotomography in the diagnosis of colloid cysts of the third ventricle. *Radiology,* 116:95–100, 1975.

Sage, M. R.; McAllister, V. L.; Kendall, B. E.; Bull, J. W. D.; and Moseley, I. F.: Radiology in the diagnosis of colloid cysts of the third ventricle. *Br. J. Radiol.,* 48:708–723, 1975.

Sagerman, R. H.; Bagshaw, M. A.; and Hanberg, J.: Considerations in the treatment of ependymomas. *Radiology,* 84:401–408, 1965.

Salassa, R. M.; Laws, E. R., Jr.; Carpenter, P. C.; and Northcutt, R. C.: Transsphenoidal removal of pituitary microadenoma in Cushing's disease. *Mayo Clin. Proc.,* 53:24–28, 1978.

Salazar, O. M.; Rubin, P.; Bassano, D.; and Marcial, V. A.: Improved survival of patients with intracranial ependymomas by irradiation: Dose selection and field extension. *Cancer,* 35:1563–1573, 1975.

Salazar, O. M.; Rubin, P.; Feldstein, M. L.; and Pizzutiello, R.: High dose radiation therapy in the treatment of malignant gliomas: Final report. *Int. J. Radiat. Oncol. Biol. Phys.,* 5:1733–1740, 1979.

Salcman, M.: Survival in glioblastoma: Historical perspective. *Neurosurgery,* 7:435–439, 1980.

Salcman, M.; Levine, H.; and Rao, K.: Value of sequential computed tomography in the multimodality treatment of glioblastoma multiforme. *Neurosurgery,* 8:15–19, 1981.

Salcman, M., and Samaras, G. M.: Hyperthermia for brain tumors: Biophysical rationale. *Neurosurgery,* 9:327–335, 1981.

Salmon, S. E.; Hamburger, A. W.; Soehnlen, B.; Durie, B. G. M.; Alberts, D. S.; and Moon, T. E.: Quantitation of differential sensitivity of human-tumor stem cells to anticancer drugs. *N. Engl. J. Med.,* 298:1321–1327, 1978.

Sano, K.: Diagnosis and treatment of tumors in the pineal region. *Acta Neurochir. (Wien),* 34:153–157, 1976.

Sano, K.; Hoshino, T.; and Nagai, M.: Radiosensitization of brain tumor cells with a thymidine analogue (bromouridine). *J. Neurosurg.,* 28:530–538, 1968.

Sato, S.; Sugimura, T.; Yoda, K.; and Fujimura, S.: Morphological differentiation of cultured mouse glioblastoma cells induced by dibutyryl cyclic adenosine monophosphate. *Cancer Res.,* 35:2494–2499, 1975.

Scanlon, P. W.; and Taylor, W. F.: Radiotherapy of intracranial astrocytomas: Analysis of 417 cases treated from 1960 through 1969. *Neurosurgery,* 5:301–308, 1979.

Schenkein, I.; Bueker, E. D.; Helson, L.; Axelrod, F.; and Dancis, J.: Increased nerve-growth-stimulating activity in disseminated neurofibromatosis. *N. Engl. J. Med.,* 290:613–614, 1974.

Scherer, H. J.: The forms of growth in gliomas and their practical significance. *Brain,* 63:1–112, 1940.

Schiffer, D.; Croveri, G.; and Pautasso, C.: Frequenza e

significato degli infiltrati linfo-plasmacellulari nei gliomi umani. *Tumori,* **60:**177–184, 1974.

Schneck, S. A., and Penn, I.: De-novo brain tumor in renal-transplant recipients. *Lancet,* **1:**983–986, 1971.

Schoenberg, B. S.: Multiple primary neoplasms and the nervous system. *Cancer,* **40:**1961–1967, 1977.

Schoenberg, B. S.; Christine, B. W.; and Whisnant, J. P.: Nervous system neoplasms and primary malignancies of other sites. *Neurology,* **25:**705–712, 1975.

Schoenberg, B. S.; Christine, B. W.; and Whisnant, J. P.: The descriptive epidemiology of primary intracranial neoplasms: The Connecticut experience. *Am. J. Epidemiol.,* **104:**499–510, 1976.

Schwade, J. G.; Wara, W. M.; Sheline, G. E.; Sorgen, S.; and Wilson, C. B.: Management of primary spinal cord tumors. *Int. J. Radiat. Oncol. Biol. Phys.,* **4:**389–393, 1978.

Scott, M.: Infiltrating ependymomas of the cauda equina. Treatment by conservative surgery plus radiotherapy. *J. Neurosurg.,* **41:**446–448, 1974.

Scott, R. M.; Liszczak, T. M.; and Kornblith, P. L.: "Invasiveness" in tissue culture: A technique for study of gliomas. *Surg. Forum,* **29:**531–533, 1978.

Seiler, R. W.; Greiner, R. H.; Zimmerman, A.; and Markwalder, H.: Radiotherapy combined with procarbazine, bleomycin, and CCNU in the treatment of high-grade supratentorial astrocytomas. *J. Neurosurg.,* **48:**861–865, 1978.

Selikoff, I. J., and Hammond, E. C. (eds.): Brain tumors in the chemical industry. *Ann. N.Y. Acad. Sci.,* **381:**1–364, 1982.

Shapiro, J. H.; Och, M.; and Jacobson, H. G.: Differential diagnosis of intradural (extramedullary) and extradural spinal canal tumors. *Radiology,* **76:**718–732, 1961.

Shapiro, K.; Till, K.; and Grant, D. N.: Craniopharyngioma in childhood: A rational approach to treatment. *J. Neurosurg.,* **50:**617–623, 1979.

Shapiro, W. R.: Chemotherapy of primary malignant brain tumors in children. *Cancer,* **35:**965–972, 1975.

Shapiro, W. R., and Young, D. F.: Chemotherapy of malignant glioma with BCNU and vincristine sulfate. *Neurology (New York),* **24:**380 (Abstr. #GS45), 1974.

Shapiro, W. R., and Young, D. F.: Chemotherapy of malignant glioma with CCNU alone and CCNU combined with vincristine sulfate and procarbazine hydrochloride. *Trans. Am. Neurol. Assoc.,* **101:**217–220, 1976.

Shaw, C.-M.; Sumi, S. M.; Alvord, E. C., Jr.; Gerdes, A. J.; Spence, A.; and Parker, R. G.: Fast-neuron irradiation of glioblastoma multiforme—Neuropathological analysis. *J. Neurosurg.,* **49:**1–12, 1978.

Sheline, G. E.: Radiation therapy of primary tumors. *Semin. Oncol.,* **2:**29–42, 1975.

Sheline, G. E.: The importance of distinguishing tumor grade in malignant gliomas: Treatment and prognosis. *Int. J. Radiat. Oncol. Biol. Phys.,* **1:**781–786, 1976.

Sherer, H. J.: The forms of growth in gliomas and their practical significance. *Brain,* **63:**1–35, 1940.

Shitara, N.; Takakura, K.; and Sano, K.: Interferon and its implication for malignant brain tumor. *Neurol. Surg. (Japan),* **7:**645–652, 1979.

Shuangshoti, S.; Hongsaprabhas, C.; and Netsky, M. G.: Metastasizing meningioma. *Cancer,* **26:**832–841, 1970.

Shuangshoti, S.; Roberts, M. P.; and Netsky, M. G.: Neuroepithelial (colloid) cysts. Pathogenesis and relation to choroid plexus and ependyma. *Arch. Pathol.,* **80:**214–224, 1965.

Shuman, R. M.; Alvord, E. C., Jr.; and Leech, R. W.: The biology of childhood ependymomas. *Arch. Neurol.,* **32:**731–739, 1975.

Simpson, D.: The recurrence of intracranial meningiomas after surgical treatment. *J. Neurol. Neurosurg. Psychiatry,* **20:**22–39, 1957.

Sipe, J. C.; Rubinstein, L. J.; Herman, M. M.; and Bignami, A.: Ethylnitrosourea-induced astrocytomas. Morphologic observations on rat tumors maintained in tissue and organ culture systems. *Lab. Invest.,* **31:**571–579, 1974.

Sloof, J. L.; Kernohan, J. W.; and MacCarty, C. S.: *Primary Intramedullary Tumors of the Spinal Cord and Filum Terminale.* W. B. Saunders Company, Philadelphia, 1964.

Smith, B. H., and Liszczak, T.: Target cell factors in the detection of humoral immune responses to human brain tumors. In Rosenberg, S. (ed.): *Serologic Analysis of Solid Tumor Antigens.* Academic Press, Inc., New York, 1980.

Smith, B. H.; Vaughan, M.; Greenwood, M. A.; Kornblith, P. L.; Robinson, A.; Shitara, N.; and McKeever, P. E.: Membrane and cytoplasmic changes in 1,3-bis(2-chloroethyl)-1-nitrosurea (BCNU)-sensitive and resistant human malignant glioma-derived cell lines. *J. Neuro Oncology,* **1:**237–248, 1983.

Smith, D. R.; Hardman, J. M.; and Earle, K. M.: Metastasizing neuroectodermal tumors of the central nervous system. *J. Neurosurg.,* **31:**50–58, 1969.

Soloway, H. B.: Radiation-induced neoplasms following curative therapy for retinoblastoma. *Cancer,* **19:**1984–1988, 1966.

Stage, W., and Stein, J.: Treatment of malignant astrocytomas. *A.J.R.,* **120:**7–18, 1974.

Stavron, D.; Zünkes, K.; and Anzil, A. P.: Morphological, immunocytochemical and biological characteristics of experimental rabbit brain tumors in tissue culture. *J. Neurol. Sci.,* **42:**365–379, 1979.

Steckler, R. M., and Martin, R. G.: Sacrococcygeal chordoma. *Ann. Surg.,* **40:**579–581, 1974.

Stein, B. M.: Supracerebellar-infratentorial approach to pineal tumors. *Surg. Neurol.,* **11:**331–337, 1979.

Steinbach, J. H., and Schubert, D.: Multiple modes of dibutyrl cyclic AMP-induced process formation by clonal nerve and glial cells. *Exp. Cell Res.,* **91:**449–453, 1975.

Stjernswärd, J.: Immunity to tumors in man and the possibility of immunotherapy. Communication at the Congress "Immunity and Cancer," Paris, October 13–14, 1971.

Suit, H., and Rich, T.: Personal communication, 1982.

Sung, D. I.; Harisiadis, L.; and Chang, C. H.: Midline pineal tumors and suprasellar germinomas: Highly curable by irradiation. *Radiology,* **128:**745–751, 1978.

Suzuki, J., and Iwabuchi, T.: Surgical removal of pineal tumors (pinealomas and teratomas). Experience in a series of 19 cases. *J. Neurosurg.,* **23:**565–571, 1965.

Suzuki, Y., and Tanaka, R.: Carcinoembryonic antigen in patients with intracranial tumors. *J. Neurosurg.,* **53:**355–360, 1980.

Sweet, W. H.: Radical surgical treatment of craniopharyngioma. *Clin. Neurosurg.,* **23:**52–79, 1976.

Takakura, K.; Miki, Y.; Kubo, O.; Owaga, N.; Matsutani, M.; and Sano, K.: Adjuvant immunotherapy for malignant brain tumors. *Jpn. J. Clin. Oncol.,* **2:**109–120, 1972.

Takeuchi, J., and Barnard, R. O.: Perivascular lymphocytic cuffing in astrocytomas. *Acta Neuropathol. (Berl.),* **35:**265–271, 1976.

Taveras, J. M., and Wood, E. H.: *Diagnostic Neuroradiology*, 2nd ed. Vols. 1 and 2. The Williams & Wilkins Company, Baltimore, 1976.

Tewfik, H. H.; McGinnis, W. L.; Nordstrom, D. G.; and Latourette, H. B.: Chordoma. Evaluation of clinical behavior and treatment modalities. *Int. J. Radiat. Oncol. Biol. Phys.,* **2**:959–962, 1977.

Theofilopoulos, A. N., and Dixon, F. J.: Immune complexes associated with neoplasia. In Herberman, R. B., and McIntire, K. R.: (eds.): *Immunodiagnosis of Cancer,* Part 2. Marcel Dekker, Inc., New York, 1979.

Thomas, D. G. T.; Darling, J. L.; Freshney, R. I.; and Morgan, D.: *In vitro* chemosensitivity assay of human gliomas by scintillation autofluorography. In Paoletti, P.; Walker, M. D.; Butte, G.; and Knerich, R. (eds.): *Multidisciplinary Aspects of Brain Tumor Therapy.* Elsevier North-Holland Biomedical Press, Amsterdam, 1979.

Thomas, P. R. M.; Duffner, P. K.; Cohen, M. E.; Sinks, L. F.; Tebbi, C.; and Freeman, A. I.: Multimodality therapy for medulloblastoma. *Cancer,* **45**:666–669, 1980.

Thorner, M. O.; Martin, W. H.; Rogol, A. D.; Morris, J. L.; Perryman, R. L.; Conway, B. P.; Howards, S. S.; Wolfman, M. G.; and MacLeod, R. M.: Rapid regression of pituitary prolactinomas during bromocriptine treatment. *J. Clin. Endocrinol. Metab.,* **51**:438–445, 1980.

Thorner, M. O.; Perryman, R. L.; Rogol, A. D.; Conway, B. P.; MacLeod, R. M.; Login, I. S.; and Morris, J. L.: Rapid changes of prolactinoma volume after withdrawal and reinstitution of bromocriptine. *J. Clin. Endocrinol. Metab.,* **53**:480–483, 1981.

Tomiyasu, U.; Hirano, H.; and Zimmerman, H. M.: Fine structure of human pituitary adenoma. *Arch. Pathol.,* **95**:287–292, 1973.

Trouillas, P.: Carcino-fetal antigen in glial tumours. *Lancet,* **2**:552, 1971.

Trouillas, P.: Immunologie et immunothérapie des tumeurs cérébrales. Etat actuel. *Rev. Neurol. (Paris),* **128**:23–38, 1973.

Trouillas, P.: Immunotherapy of cerebral tumours. In Thomas, D. G. T., and Graham, D. I. (eds.): *Brain Tumours: Scientific Basis, Clinical Investigation and Current Therapy.* Butterworth, Boston, 1980.

Trouillas, P., and Lapras, C.: L'immunothérapie cellulaire des glioblastomes cérébraux. A propos de deux résultats. *J. Med. Lyon,* **50**:1269–1291, 1969.

Tyrrell, J. B.; Brooks, R. M.; Fitzgerald, P. A.; Cofoid, P. B.; Forsham, P. H.; and Wilson, C. B.: Cushing's disease: Selective transsphenoidal resection of pituitary microadenomas. *N. Engl. J. Med.,* **298**:753–758, 1978.

Urtasun, R. C.; Band, P. R.; Chapman, J. D.; and Feldstein, M. L.: Radiation plus metronidazole for glioblastoma. *N. Engl. J. Med.,* **296**:757, 1977.

Urtasun, R. C.; Band, P. R.; Chapman, J. D.; Feldstein, M. L.; Mielke, B.; and Fryer, C.: Radiation and high-dose metronidazole in supratentorial glioblastomas. *N. Engl. J. Med.,* **294**:1364–1367, 1976.

Van Dyk, J.; Jenkin, R. D. T.; Leung, P. M. K.; and Cunningham, J. R.: Medulloblastoma: Treatment technique and radiation dosimetry. *Int. J. Radiat. Oncol. Biol. Phys.,* **2**:993–1005, 1977.

van Miert, P. J.: The treatment of chemodectomas by radiotherapy. *Proc. R. Soc. Lond. (Biol.),* **57**:946–951, 1964.

Varadachari, C.; Palutke, M.; Climie, A. R. W.; Weise, R. W.; and Chason, J. L.: Immunoblastic sarcoma (histiocytic lymphoma) of the brain with B-cell markers. Case report. *J. Neurosurg.,* **49**:887–892, 1978.

Vazquez-Lopez, E.: Glioma in a rat fed with 2-acetylaminofluorene. *Nature,* **156**:296–297, 1945.

Vick, N. A.: Brain tumor microvasculature. In Weiss, L.; Gilbert, H. A.; and Posner, J. B. (eds.): *Brain Metastasis,* Vol. II. G. K. Hall & Company, Boston, 1980.

von Hippel, E.: Über eine setir seltene erkrankung der netzhaut: Klinische Beobachtungen. *Graefes Arch. Ophthalmol.,* **59**:83–106, 1904.

Vonofakos, D.; Marcu, H.; and Hacker, H.: Oligodendrogliomas: CT patterns with emphasis on features indicating malignancy. *J. Comput. Assist. Tomogr.,* **3**:783–788, 1979.

Walker, A. B.: The dawn of neurosurgery. *Clin. Neurosurg.,* **6**:1–38, 1959.

Walker, M. D.: Nitrosoureas in central nervous system tumors. *Cancer Chemother. Rep.,* Part 3, **4**:21–26, 1973.

Walker, M. D.: Chemotherapy: Adjuvant to surgery and radiation therapy. *Semin. Oncol.,* **2**:69–72, 1975.

Walker, M. D.; Alexander, E., Jr.; Hunt, W. E.; Leventhal, C. M.; Mahaley, M. S., Jr.; Mealey, J.; Norrell, H. A.; Owens, G.; Ransohoff, J.; Wilson, C. B.; and Gehan, E. A.: Evaluation of mithramycin in the treatment of anaplastic gliomas. *J. Neurosurg.,* **44**:655–667, 1976.

Walker, M. D.; Alexander, E., Jr.; Hunt, W. E.; MacCarty, C. S.; Mahaley, M S.; Mealey, J., Jr.; Norrell, H. A.; Owens, G.; Ransohoff, J.; Wilson, C. B.; Gehan, E. A.; and Strike, T. A.: Evaluation of BCNU and/or radiotherapy in the treatment of anaplastic gliomas. A cooperative clinical trial. *J. Neurosurg.,* **49**:333–343, 1978.

Walker, M. D., and Gehan, E.: An evaluation of 1-3-*bis*(2-chloroethyl)-1-nitrosourea (BCNU) and irradiation alone and in combination for the treatment of malignant glioma. *Proc. Am. Assoc. Cancer Res.,* **13**:67 (Abstract #267), 1972.

Walker, M. D.; Green, S. B.; Byar, D. P.; Alexander, E., Jr.; Batzdorf, U.; Brooks, W. H.; Hunt, W. E.; MacCarty, C. S.; Mahaley, M. S., Jr.; Mealey, J., Jr.; Owens, G.; Ransohoff, J., II, Robertson, J. T.; Shapiro, W. R.; Smith, K. R., Jr.; Wilson, C. B.; and Strike, T. A.: Randomized comparisons of radiotherapy and nitrosoureas for the treatment of malignant glioma after surgery. *N. Engl. J. Med.,* **303**:1323–1329, 1980.

Walker, M. D., and Hurwitz, B. S.: BCNU 1,3-*bis*(2-chloroethyl)-1-nitrosourea (NSC 409962) in the treatment of malignant brain tumor—A preliminary report. *Cancer Chemother. Rep.,* **54**:263–271, 1970.

Walsh, J. M.; Cassady, J. R.; Frei, E., III, Kornblith, P. L.; and Welch, K.: Recent advances in the treatment of primary brain tumors. A seminar. *Arch. Surg.,* **110**:696–702, 1975.

Wara, W. M.; Jenkin, R. D. T.; Evans, A.; Ertel, I.; Hittle, R.; Ortega, J.; Wilson, C. B.; and Hammond, D.: Tumors of the pineal and suprasellar region: Childrens Cancer Study Group treatment results 1960–1975—A report from Childrens Cancer Study Group. *Cancer,* **43**:698–701, 1979.

Wara, W. M.; Phillips, T. L.; Sheline, G. E.; and Schwade, J. G.: Radiation tolerance of the spinal cord. *Cancer,* **35**:1558–1562, 1975a.

Wara, W. M.; Sheline, G. E.; Newman, H.; Townsend, J. J.; and Boldrey, E. B.: Radiation therapy of meningiomas. *A.J.R.,* **123**:453–458, 1975b.

Wasserman, T. H.; Stetz, J.; and Phillips, T. L.: Radiation Therapy Oncology Group clinical trials with misonidazole. *Cancer,* **47**:2382–2390, 1981.

Wechsler, W.: Old and new concepts of oncogenesis in the

nervous system of man and animals. *Prog. Exp. Tumor Res.,* **17:**219–278, 1972.

Wechsler, W.; Kleihues, P.; Matsumoto, D.; Zülch, K. J.; Ivankovic, S.; Preussmann, R.; and Druckrey, H.: Pathology of experimental neurogenic tumors chemically induced during prenatal and postnatal life. *Ann. N.Y. Acad. Sci.,* **159:**360–408, 1969.

Weed, L. H., and McKibben, P. S.: Pressure changes in cerebrospinal fluid following intravenous injection of solutions of various concentrations. *Am. J. Physiol.,* **48:**512–530, 1919.

Weir, B.: The relative significance of factors affecting postoperative survival in astrocytomas, grades 3 and 4. *J. Neurosurg.,* **38:**448–452, 1973.

Weir, B.; Band, P.; Urtasun, R.; Blain, G.; McLean, D.; Wilson, F.; Mielke, B.; and Grace, M.: Radiotherapy and CCNU in the treatment of high-grade supratentorial astrocytomas. *J. Neurosurg.,* **45:**129–134, 1976.

Weir, B., and Elvidge, A. R.: Oligodendrogliomas. An analysis of 63 cases. *J. Neurosurg.,* **29:**500–505, 1968.

Weller, R. O.: Perspectives in neuro-oncology. In Thomas, D. G. T., and Graham, D. I. (eds.): *Brain Tumours. Scientific Basis, Clinical Investigation and Current Therapy.* Butterworth, Boston, 1980.

Wheeler, K. T.; Deen, D. F.; Wilson, C. B.; Williams, M. E.; and Sheppard, S.: BCNU-modification of the *in vitro* radiation response in 9L brain tumor cells of rats. *Int. J. Radiat. Oncol. Biol. Phys.,* **2:**79–88, 1977.

Williams, R. H. (ed.): *Textbook of Endocrinology,* 5th ed. W. B. Saunders Company, Philadelphia, 1982.

Wilson, C. B.: Medulloblastoma: current views regarding the tumor and its treatment. *Oncology,* **24:**273–290, 1970.

Wilson, C. B.; Boldrey, F. B.; and Enot K. J.: 1,3-*bis*(2-chloroethyl)-1-nitrosourea (NSC 409962) in the treatment of brain tumors. *Cancer Chemother. Rep.,* **54:**273–281, 1970.

Wisiol, E. S.; Handler, S.; and French, L. A.: Extracranial metastases of a glioblastoma multiforme. *J. Neurosurg.,* **19:**186–194, 1962.

Wodinski, I.; Kensler, C. J.; and Rall, D. P.: The induction and transplantation of brain tumors in neonate beagles. *Proc. Am. Assoc. Cancer Res.,* **10:**99 (Abstr. 394), 1969.

Wollesen, F.; Andersen, T.; and Karle, A.: Size reduction of extrasellar pituitary tumors during bromocriptine treatment—Quantitation of effect on different types of tumors. *Ann. Intern. Med.,* **96:**281–286, 1982.

Woltman, H. W.; Kernohan, J. W.; Adson, A. W.; and Craig, W. M.: Intramedullary tumors of the spinal cord and gliomas of intradural portion of filum terminale. Fate of patients who have these tumors. *Arch. Neurol. Psychiatry,* **65:**387–393, 1951.

Wood, E. H.; Berne, A. S.; and Taveras, J. M.: The value of radiation therapy in the management of intrinsic tumors of the spinal cord. *Radiology,* **63:**11–22, 1954.

Wright, A. D.; Hill, D. M.; Lowy, C.; and Fraser, T. R.: Mortality in acromegaly. *Q. J. Med.,* **39:**1–16, 1970.

Yasargil, M. G.; Antic, J.; Laciga, R.; de Preux, J.; Fideler, R. W.; and Boone, S. C.: The microsurgical removal of intramedullary spinal hemangioblastomas. *Surg. Neurol.,* **6:**141–148, 1976.

Yasargil, M. G., and Fox, J. L.: The microsurgical approach to acoustic neuromas. *Surg. Neurol.,* **2:**393–398, 1974.

Youmans, J. R.: *Neurological Surgery,* Vol. III. W. B. Saunders Company, Philadelphia, 1973.

Young, B.; Oldfield, E. H.; Marksbery, W. R.; Haack, D.; Tibbs, P. A.; McCombs, P.; Chin, H. W.; Maruyama, Y.; and Meacham, W. F.: Reoperation for glioblastoma. *J. Neurosurg.,* **55:**917–921, 1981.

Young, H. F.; Kaplan, A. M.; and Regelson, W.: Immunotherapy with autologous white cell infusions ("lymphocytes") in the treatment of recurrent glioblastoma multiforme. *Cancer,* **40:**1037–1044, 1977.

Young, H. F.; Sakalas, R.; and Kaplan, A. M.: Inhibition of cell-mediated immunity in patients with brain tumors. *Surg. Neurol.,* **5:**19–23, 1976a.

Young, H. F.; Sakalas, R.; and Kaplan, A. M.: Immunologic depression in cerebral gliomas. *Adv. Neurol.,* **15:**327–335, 1976b.

Yung, W. K.; Blank, N. K.; and Vick, N. A.: "Glioblastoma." Induction of a reproducible autochthonous tumor in rats with murine sarcoma virus. *Neurology,* **26:**76–83, 1976.

Zankl, H., and Zang, K. D.: Cytological and cytogenetical studies on brain tumors. IV. Identification of the missing G chromosome in human meningiomas as No. 22 by fluorescence technique. *Hum. Genet.,* **14:**167–169, 1972.

Zimmerman, H. M.: Brain tumors: Their incidence and classification in man and their experimental production. *Ann. N.Y. Acad. Sci.,* **159:**337–359, 1969.

Zimmerman, H. M.: Malignant lymphomas of the nervous system. *Acta Neuropathol. [Suppl.] (Berl.),* **6:**69–74, 1975.

Zimmerman, H. M., and Arnold, H.: Chemical carcinogens and animal species as factors—Experimental brain tumors. *J. Neuropathol. Exp. Neurol.,* **2:**416–417, 1943.

Zimmerman, R. A., and Bilaniuk, L. T.: Computed tomography of choroid plexus lesions. *CT,* **3:**93–103, 1979.

Zimmerman, R. A.; Bilaniuk, L. T.; Wood, J. H.; Bruce, D. A.; and Schut, L.: Computed tomography of pineal, parapineal, and histologically related tumors. *Radiology,* **137:**669–677, 1980.

Zülch, K. J.: Über das 'sogenannte' kleinhirnastrocytom. *Virchows Arch. [Pathol. Anat.],* **307:**222–252, 1940.

Zülch, K. J.: Biologie und pathologie der hirngeschwülste. In Olivecrona, H., and Tönnis, W. (eds.): *Handbuch der Neurochirurgie,* Vol. 3. Springer, Berlin, 1956.

Zülch, K. J.: On the definition of the polymorphous oligodendroglioma. *Acta Neurochir. [Suppl.] (Wien),* **10:**166–172, 1964.

Zülch, K. J.: *Brain Tumours, Their Biology and Their Pathology,* 2nd ed. Springer-Verlag New York, Inc., New York, 1965.

Zülch, K. J., and Borck, W. F.: Tafeln über die relative häufigkeit der hirngeschwülste in verschiedenen altersklassen. *Zentralbl. Neurochir.,* **12:**93–97, 1952.

Zülch, K. J., and Mennel, H. D.: The biology of brain tumours. In Vinken, P. J., and Bruyn, G. W. (eds.): *Handbook of Clinical Neurology,* Vol. 16. North-Holland Publishing Company, Amsterdam, 1974.

ZuRhein, G. M., and Varakis, J.: Morphology of brain tumors induced in Syrian hamsters after inoculation with JC virus, a new human papova-virus. in Környey, St.; Tariska, St.; and Gosztonyi, G. (eds.): *Proceedings of VIIth International Congress of Neuropathology,* Vol. 1. Excerpta Medica, Amsterdam, 1975.

38

Sarcomas

STEVEN I. HAJDU and GERALD ROSEN

In the past decade the role of combination therapy, surgery, irradiation, and chemotherapy in increasing the cure rate of malignant neoplasms such as mammary carcinoma, germ cell tumors, osteogenic sarcoma and Ewing's sarcoma has been documented (Gottlieb *et al.,* 1972; Jaffe, 1972; Rosen *et al.,* 1974; Burchenal, 1975; DeVita *et al.,* 1975). Little progress has been made, however, in the treatment of most soft tissue sarcomas. The difficulty is partly owing to the fact that the term "soft tissue sarcoma" implies in its definition a heterogeneity of over 50 types of neoplasms. In addition to the many different types of neoplasms, the term "soft tissue sarcoma" also refers to a wide variety of neoplasms at distinct stages with various metastasizing potentials. Many recent studies are inadequate because all sarcomas are grouped together, regardless of their histogenesis, histologic type, site of origin, or clinical stage.

Histologic Type and Grade of Sarcoma

To appreciate the role of various modalities of therapy in the treatment of soft tissue and bone sarcomas, it is necessary to know the histologic type of the sarcoma, the size, site, histologic grade, and stage of disease. In each case, it must be determined whether surgery alone is sufficient, or, whether irradiation and chemotherapy should be considered in combination with surgery (Dahlin and Conventry, 1967; Rosenberg *et al.,* 1978; Hajdu, 1979, 1981, 1982; Enneking *et al.,* 1980).

The first consideration for the initiation of the most appropriate therapy in the treatment of sarcomas should be the histologic type and grade of sarcoma (Hajdu, 1979; Huvos, 1979).

Histogenetically sarcomas may arise from diverse connective tissue elements (see Figure 38-1) and are named after the dominant cell type (see Table 38-1). Although for practical purposes, such a classification is useful, some overlapping between various categories exists. For example, peripheral nerve may give rise to fibrous histiocytoma, bone may be the site of fibrosarcoma, and osteogenic sarcoma may originate in soft tissues (Hajdu and Hajdu, 1976; Hajdu, 1980; Fine *et al.,* 1982).

The majority of sarcomas can occur in both low-grade and high-grade histologic forms. In general, histologic grading is assigned after histologic typing (Russell *et al.,* 1981) (see Table 38-2). Although the subclassification of soft tissue and bone sarcomas according to the scheme presented in Tables 38-3, 38-4, and 38-5 is not universally accepted, it is a practical working classification. It has a built-in flexibility and permits combined consideration of soft tissue and bone sarcomas according to their histogenesis and histologic grade (Hajdu, 1982).

Malignant fibroblastic fibrous histiocytoma is perhaps one of the best-known forms of malignant fibrous histiocytomas (see Figure 38-2). When it presents in subcutaneous tissues, it is commonly referred to as *dermatofibrosarcoma protuberans.* The majority of these neoplasms are located on either the trunk or the shoulder (see Table 38-3). They are often bulky and multinodular growths of several years' duration. Studies of superficial malignant fibroblastic fibrous histiocytoma indicate that 64 (53%) of 119 tumors treated by wide excision recurred, most of them within one year, and nine of the ten patients who had metastatic disease died with pulmonary me-

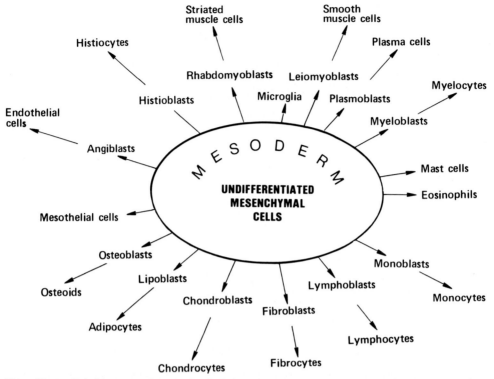

Figure 38-1. Primitive mesenchymal cells of soft tissue and bone may produce any of these forms, and mature cells may dedifferentiate to undifferentiated or poorly differentiated elements. From Hajdu, S. I.: *Pathology of Soft Tissue Tumors.* Lea & Febiger, Philadelphia, 1979.

tastases (Hajdu, 1979; Zaatari, in preparation). The primary treatment of malignant fibroblastic fibrous histiocytoma should be surgical resection, with generous and tumor-free margins (Shiu *et al.*, 1975; Shiu and Hajdu, 1981).

Desmoid tumors are divided according to their clinical presentation into abdominal and extra-abdominal forms. The abdominal desmoids are usually limited to the anterior abdominal wall and are primarily a disease of young adult women (Shiu *et al.*, 1980). In contrast, the so-called extra-abdominal desmoid is primarily a disease of men in the third and fourth decades. Grossly and microscopically extra-abdominal desmoids are identical to abdominal desmoids. Desmoids are, in general, solitary well-defined neoplasms ranging in size from a few centimeters to several inches (see Figure 38-3). The primary treatment should be to prevent recurrence by complete excision with generous and tumor free margins. Death

Table 38-1. Histogenetic Classification of Sarcomas

TISSUE OF ORIGIN	TYPE OF SARCOMA
Fibrous tissue	Fibrous histiocytoma
	Fibrosarcoma
Tendosynovial tissue	Tendosynovial sarcoma
Adipose tissue	Liposarcoma
Muscle	Leiomyosarcoma
	Rhabdomyosarcoma
Vessels	Lymphangiosarcoma
	Hemangiosarcoma
Peripheral nerve	Malignant peripheral nerve tumor
Bone	Osteogenic sarcoma
	Chondrosarcoma
	Ewing's sarcoma
	Chordoma
Miscellaneous tissue	Malignant granular cell tumor
	Alveolar soft part sarcoma
	Malignant mesenchymoma

Table 38-2. Histologic Grade of Sarcomas

LOW GRADE	HIGH GRADE
Hypocellular	Hypercellular
Good maturation	Poor maturation
Much stroma	Minimal stroma
Hypovascular	Hypervascular
Minimal necrosis	Much necrosis
Less than 5 mitoses per 10 high-power fields	More than 5 mitoses per 10 high-power fields

Table 38–3. Low-Grade Sarcomas

HISTOLOGIC TYPE	AVE. AGE	SEX PREVALENCE	MOST COMMON SITE	MOST COMMON PRESENTATION	AVE. SIZE (CM)	HISTOLOGIC PATTERN	DOMINANT CELL TYPE	MOST COMMON STAGE	AVE. 5-YR SURVIVAL (%)
Malignant fibroblastic fibrous histiocytoma*	45	Male	Trunk	Superficial	5	Arranged	Fibrillar spindle	I	85
Desmoid tumor	25	Male	Arm and thigh	Deep	5	Spreading	Plump spindle	I	95
Chordoid sarcoma	40	Male	Hand	Superficial	2	Lacy	Granular epithelioid	0	75
Well-differentiated liposarcoma*	45	Male	Trunk	—	5	Lacy	Fibrillar spindle	I	95
Myxoid liposarcoma	40	Male	Thigh	Deep	10	Lacy	Fibrillar spindle	II	95
Kaposi's sarcoma	55	Male	Leg	Superficial	2	Alveolar	Fibrillar spindle	0	60
Adamantinoma	30	—	Tibia	Deep	2	Epithelioid	Granular epithelioid	I	90

* Can be primary in soft tissues or in bone.

Table 38–4. High-Grade Sarcomas

HISTOLOGIC TYPE	AVE. AGE	SEX PREVALENCE	MOST COMMON SITE	MOST COMMON PRESENTATION	AVE. SIZE (CM)	HISTOLOGIC PATTERN	DOMINANT CELL TYPE	MOST COMMON STAGE	AVE. 5-YR SURVIVAL (%)
Pleomorphic fibrosarcoma*	50	Male	Thigh	Deep	15	Disarranged	Plump spindle	III	35
Monophasic tendosynovial sarcoma	25	Male	Thigh	Deep	15	Spreading	Fibrillar spindle	III	30
Epithelioid sarcoma	25	Male	Forearm	Superficial	2	Epithelioid	Granular epithelioid	I	65
Clear cell sarcoma	30	Male	Leg	Deep	5	Epithelioid	Clear epithelioid	II	55
Lipoblastic liposarcoma	45	Male	Thigh	Deep	10	Epithelioid	Granular epithelioid	III	50
Pleomorphic liposarcoma	55	Male	Thigh	Deep	15	Disarranged	Pleomorphic giant	III	45
Rhabdomyoblastoma	20	Male	—	Deep	5	Epithelioid	Isomorphic giant	II	40
Embryonal rhabdomyosarcoma	10	Male	Thigh	Deep	10	Spreading	Fibrillar spindle	III	65
Pleomorphic rhabdomyosarcoma	50	Male	Thigh	Deep	15	Disarranged	Pleomorphic giant	III	25
Lymphangiosarcoma	50	Female	Arm	—	5	Alveolar	Granular epithelioid	III	10
Primitive neuroectodermal tumor	25	Male	Trunk	Deep	5	Epithelioid	Granular epithelioid	III	30
Intraskeletal osteogenic sarcoma	15	Male	Tibia Humerus	Deep	5	Disarranged	Pleomorphic giant	III	50
Extraskeletal osteogenic sarcoma	50	Male	—	Deep	10	Disarranged	Pleomorphic giant	III	15
Ewing's sarcoma†	20	Male	Tibia Humerus	Deep	5	Epithelioid	Granular epithelioid	III	75
Chordoma	50	—	Sacrum	Deep	10	Alveolar	Epithelioid	III	55
Granulocytic sarcoma	20	Male	—	Deep	5	Epithelioid	Granular epithelioid	III	5

* Can be primary in bone.
† Can be primary in soft tissues.

Table 38–5. Sarcomas That Are Either Low Grade or High Grade

HISTOLOGIC TYPE	AVE. AGE	SEX PREVALENCE	MOST COMMON SITE	MOST COMMON PRESENTATION	AVE. SIZE (CM)	HISTOLOGIC PATTERN	DOMINANT CELL TYPE	MOST COMMON STAGE	AVE. 5-YR SURVIVAL (%)
Malignant histiocytic fibrous histiocytoma*	35	Male	Tibia Femur	Deep	10	Epithelioid	Isomorphic giant	II	55
Malignant pleomorphic fibrous histiocytoma†	50	Male	Buttock Arm	Deep	5	Disarranged	Pleomorphic giant	III	50
Fibroblastic fibrosarcoma†	45	Male	Thigh	Deep	10	Arranged	Plump spindle	III	45
Biphasic tendosynovial sarcoma	35	Male	Knee	Deep	10	Epithelioid	Granular epithelioid	II	65
Fibroblastic liposarcoma	45	Male	Thigh	Deep	10	Arranged	Fibrillar spindle	III	60
Leiomyoblastoma	50	Female	—	Deep	5	Epithelioid	Clear epithelioid	II	60
Leiomyosarcoma	55	Female	Leg	—	5	Spreading	Plump spindle	II	60
Hemangiosarcoma†	45	Male	Trunk	—	5	Alveolar	Granular epithelioid	III	35
Hemangiopericytoma†	40	Male	—	Deep	10	Alveolar	Fibrillar spindle	II	60
Malignant peripheral nerve tumor	40	Female	Thigh	Deep	10	Spreading	Fibrillar spindle	II	60
Chondrosarcoma*	45	Male	Thigh	Deep	10	Lacy	Clear epithelioid	II	60
Mesenchymal chondrosarcoma*	25	—	—	Deep	5	Spreading	Fibrillar spindle	III	60
Malignant granular cell tumor	45	Female	—	Superficial	5	Epithelioid	—	II	75
Alveolar soft part sarcoma	35	Female	Thigh	Deep	10	Alveolar	Pleomorphic giant	III	50
Plasmacytoma†	50	—	—	Deep	10	Epithelioid	Granular epithelioid	III	45
Malignant mesenchymoma	45	—	—	Deep	10	—	—	—	—
Undifferentiated soft tissue sarcoma	—	—	—	—	—	—	—	—	—

* Can be primary in soft tissues.
† Can be primary in bone.

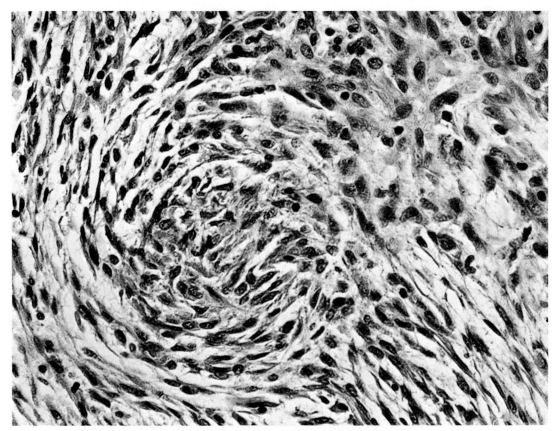

Figure 38-2. Malignant fibroblastic fibrous histiocytoma exhibiting storiform pattern (H & E ×420).

from local extension of desmoid tumors into vital structures is rare (see Figure 35-4) (see Table 38-3), and metastasis is almost unheard of (Hajdu, 1979).

Chordoid sarcoma (Hajdu *et al.,* 1977) is a very rare form of tendosynovial sarcoma found most commonly in the palm of the hand and wrist of middle-aged men. Chordoid sarcomas are slowly growing, locally recurring neoplasms and should be treated by surgical excision (see Table 38-3).

Well-differentiated liposarcoma is an uncommon neoplasm and believed to be a nonmetastasizing tumor. It usually presents as a pseudoencapsulated tumor in the deep subcutis or fascial tissues. The pathologist must microscopically distinguish these low-grade malignant neoplasms from cellular or atypical lipomas. Local surgical excision is considered as the treatment of choice (see Table 38-3).

Myxoid liposarcoma is the most common type of liposarcoma (Hajdu, 1979, 1982) (see Figure 38-5). It occurs commonly in the thigh, groin, trunk and popliteal areas. Usually

bulky pseudoencapsulated neoplasms, they occur most commonly in middle-aged men (see Table 38-3). They seldom recur after excision with clear margins, and metastatic spread without more malignant transformation is uncommon. Irradiation may play a role in the treatment of myxoid liposarcomas that are not managable by surgery alone (Suit *et al.,* 1975, 1981; Fine *et al.,* 1982; Hilaris *et al.,* 1982).

Kaposi's sarcoma is usually listed as a form of vascular neoplasm. The recent epidemic outbreak of this disease in male homosexuals, however, reinforced the nonendothelial, nonvascular theories of origin (Hajdu, 1979; Thomsen *et al.,* 1981; Lobenthal *et al.,* 1983; Urmacher *et al.,* 1982). Kaposi's sarcomas in nongays occur more commonly in elderly men, Jews and Italians, and those of Eastern European and Russian extraction. It is also common in certain parts of Africa. They are also associated with malignant lymphoreticular neoplasms. An estimated one-third of the patients with Kaposi's sarcoma die of a second

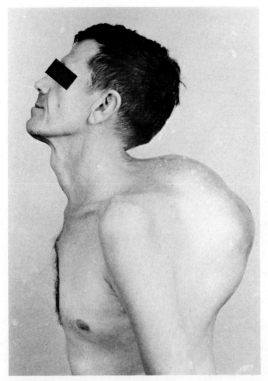

Figure 38–3. Bulky desmoid tumor.

primary neoplasm (Hajdu, 1979). Although the etiology and histogenesis of Kaposi's sarcoma remain uncertain, recently accumulated information indicates that deficient immune responsiveness in combination with viral infection plays an important role in the chain of events that leads to the appearance of Kaposi's sarcoma (Lobenthal *et al.,* 1983; Urmacher *et al.,* 1982).

Adamantinoma of long bone is a very rare

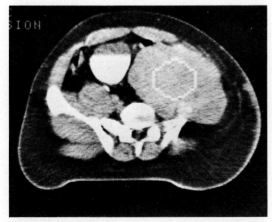

Figure 38–4. Desmoid tumor of the pelvis showing invasion of right ilium.

neoplasm that develops in the tibia of adults (see Table 38–3). It is a radiographically well-defined lesion with central lytic and sclerotic marginal zones. Despite its characteristic histologic, epithelioid appearance, the histogenesis remains controversial. Most agree that *en bloc* excision followed by endoprosthesis is the most appropriate modality of therapy of this low-grade malignant neoplasm (Huvos, 1979).

Pleomorphic fibrosarcoma is usually a high-grade soft tissue sarcoma, but it may be primary in bone (see Table 38–4). Grossly, and in clinical presentation, fully malignant fibrosarcomas are not very different from low-grade fibrosarcomas. Most patients have a history of long duration and enlargement of a painless mass. Pleomorphic fibrosarcoma may contain, in addition to the usual fibroblastic neoplastic elements, bizarre mononuclear and multinodular tumor giant cells (see Figure 38–6). High-grade fibrosarcomas must be excised with clear surgical margins when they are first encountered. Amputation should be the treatment of choice if any possibility exists that excision or resection will fail. These neoplasms are not sensitive to radiation and durable chemotherapy responses are seldom observed (Shiu *et al.,* 1975; Sordillo *et al.,* 1981c; Gerson *et al.,* 1982).

Monophasic tendosynovial sarcoma is the most common form of tendosynovial sarcomas (see Figure 38–7). The Memorial experience (Hajdu *et al.,* 1977) with these high-grade sarcomas indicates that only 26% of the 59 patients with this tumor survived for five years. Approximately 50% of the patients have pulmonary metastases at the time of initial diagnosis. Most of the monophasic tenosynovial sarcomas are greater than 5 cm, but small, sclerosing histopathologic lesions are not uncommon (Lee *et al.,* 1974; Hajdu, 1979; Krall *et al.,* 1981). They are found most commonly in the deep soft tissues of the thigh, foot, and shoulder. Treatment should be directed at complete removal of the primary, with or without mutilating surgery, and initiating optimal chemotherapy as soon as possible. Irradiation has limited value in the treatment of these neoplasms (Hajdu *et al.,* 1977; Shiu *et al.,* 1979; Smith and Hajdu, 1979; Sordillo *et al.,* 1981c).

Epithelioid sarcoma is an uncommon form of tendosynovial sarcoma. The name indicates its histologic resemblance to malignant epithelial neoplasms, carcinomas (see Figure 38–8). These neoplasms usually occur in young men

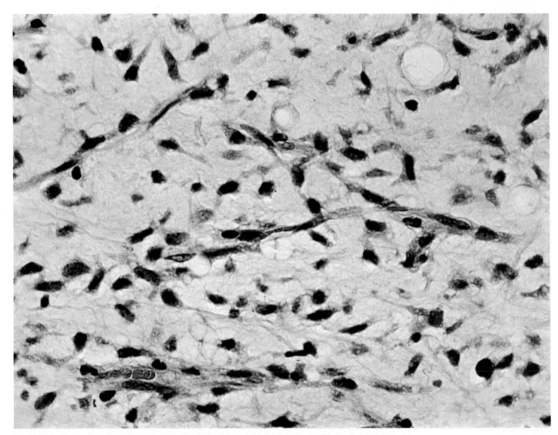

Figure 38–5. Myxoid liposarcoma showing rich capillary network (H & E ×420).

and are most commonly located in the fore-arms, palmar aspect of the hand (see Figure 38–9), leg, or plantar regions of the foot (see Table 38–4). In approximately one-third of the cases these neoplasms are multifocal in presentation along tendons and fascial-apo-neurotic structures of the same anatomic re-gion. Epithelioid sarcoma has a tendency to metastasize to regional lymph nodes more fre-quently than any other soft tissue sarcoma, ex-cept embryonal rhabdomyosarcoma (Pat-chefsky *et al.,* 1977; Hajdu, 1979, 1985).

Clear cell sarcoma in the pure form is a very rare variety of tendosynovial sarcoma. It often appears, however, in combination with other histopathologic forms, *e.g.,* epithelioid sar-coma. Clear cell sarcomas are fully malignant high-grade neoplasms (Hajdu *et al.,* 1977). They may occur at any site of the body, but they have particular predilection for the ten-dinous and aponeurotic areas of the extremi-ties. They should be treated by a combination of surgery and chemotherapy (Shiu *et al.,* 1979).

Lipoblastic liposarcoma is a high-grade neo-plasm of adipose tissue composed predomi-nantly of lipoblasts, precursors of mature fat cells. They are usually deeply seated neo-plasms with an indolent course. Studies of these neoplasms show that 67% recurred after surgical excision, and more than 50% of the patients died with metastatic disease in less than five years after initial diagnosis (Hajdu, 1979, 1985). Owing to the primitive adipose nature of these relatively uncommon neo-plasms, significant responses to irradiation and chemotherapy may be possible (Sordillo *et al.,* 1981c; Suit *et al.,* 1981; Hilaris *et al.,* 1982).

Pleomorphic liposarcoma is the most malig-nant form of liposarcoma. It usually has an insidious and indolent onset with an acceler-ated downhill course soon after the diagnosis. Approximately 20% of pleomorphic liposar-comas have at an earlier stage of the disease demonstrated myoid, lipoblastic, or fibro-blastic growth patterns (see Figure 38–10). Pleomorphic liposarcomas are highly malig-

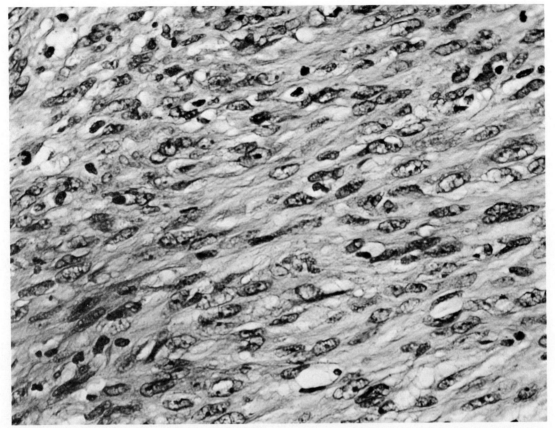

Figure 38-6. Fibrosarcoma, high grade, composed of mononucleated and multinucleated fibroblastic cells (H & E ×420).

nant neoplasms with a 56% rate of recurrence and an overall mortality rate of 77% (Hajdu, 1979; Cody *et al.,* 1981; Fortner *et al.,* 1981).

Rhabdomyoblastoma is a primitive, blastic form of rhabdomyosarcoma (Hajdu, 1979). It has a very distinct microscopic appearance and stains positive for myoglobin (Hajdu, 1979, 1985; Mukai *et al.,* 1979). It is a very uncommon high-grade malignant neoplasm, and all available modalities of treatment have limited value.

Embryonal rhabdomyosarcoma may appear in a number of histologic forms (Lloyd *et al.,* 1983). The most common types are known as botryoid (myxoid), alveolar, spreading (spindle cell), and epithelioid (round cell) (see Figure 38-11). Most embryonal rhabdomyosarcomas, if adequately sampled, have an admixture of the various histologic types. Embryonal rhabdomyosarcoma is the most common soft tissue sarcoma in children. The age incidence of children with embryonal rhabdomyosarcoma varies according to the

primary site of the tumor. The paradox of embryonal rhabdomyosarcoma is that it often occurs in anatomic structures where striated muscle is not usually found, *e.g.,* bile duct, urinary bladder, vagina, spermatic cord, and prostate (Hajdu and Hajdu, 1976; Hajdu, 1980). There have been major recent advances in the management of embryonal rhabdomyosarcoma. Combined treatment with surgery, irradiation therapy, and chemotherapy is the standard current management (Sutow *et al.,* 1966; Heyn *et al.,* 1974; Wilbur, 1974). As a result of combined therapy, surgery, irradiation, and chemotherapy, more than 60% of patients survive beyond five years. The case fatality rate of embryonal rhabdomyosarcoma in adults, however, is well over 60% (Lloyd *et al.,* 1983).

Pleomorphic rhabdomyosarcoma is a disease of adults (see Table 38-4). It is most prevalent in the fifth and sixth decades, and men and women are affected in almost equal proportion (Hajdu, 1979). These neoplasms are

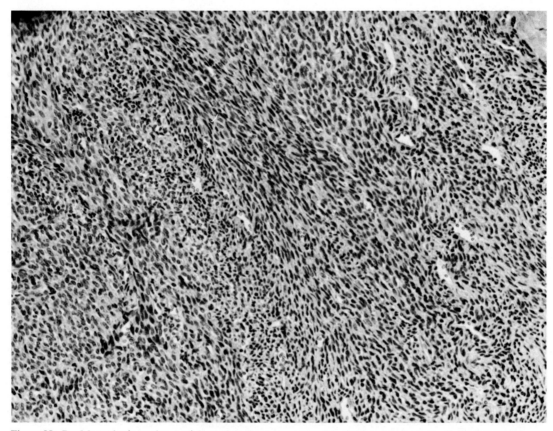

Figure 38-7. Monophasic tendosynovial sarcoma shows monomorphic tightly packed small cells (H & E ×420).

always high grade histologically, and most reach a considerable size prior to diagnosis. Many of the pleomorphic rhabdomyosarcomas can be traced to inter- or intramuscular fascial tissues as the most probable source of origin. They appear most commonly in the thigh, shoulder, and upper arm (Hajdu, 1979, 1985). In most cases, diligent search with the electron microscope reveals characteristic arrangements of thin and thick myofilaments (see Figure 38-12). In the majority of the cases, immunochemical stain for myoglobin is at least focally positive. Pleomorphic rhabdomyosarcoma is one of the most malignant forms of soft tissue sarcoma, and, at present, irradiation and chemotherapy are not effective.

Lymphangiosarcomas are often found in association with long-standing acquired or congenital lymphedema (Hajdu, 1979; Sordillo *et al.,* 1981a). The pathogenesis of lymphangiosarcoma is poorly understood. Clinically, the first sign of lymphangiosarcoma is the appearance of macular skin lesions, which, in time,

become confluent with areas of erosion and ulceration. The results of treatment are disappointing, but all patients with this disease must be considered as candidates for multimodality therapy (Sordillo *et al.,* 1981a,c).

Primitive neuroectodermal tumor, or so-called adult neuroblastoma, is a disease of young adults. It may appear in any region of the body and should be considered as a high-grade neoplasm that resists all known modalities of therapy (Hajdu, 1979).

Intraskeletal osteogenic sarcoma is the most common primary bone tumor of children and young adults (see Table 38-4). It is about three times more common than Ewing's sarcoma, and about twice as frequent as chondrosarcoma. It is a malignant spindle cell tumor in which the neoplastic cells produce osteoid or immature bone (see Figure 38-13). The rate of tumor growth, the degree of differentiation, and the symptoms vary widely. Osteogenic sarcomas are found most commonly in the long bones of the extremities. The distal femur is the primary site in more than one-third of

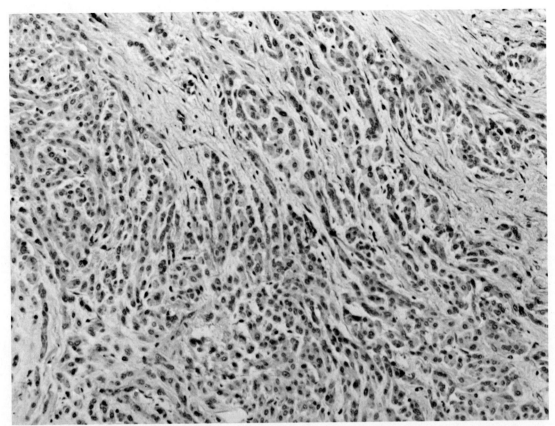

Figure 38-8.   Epithelioid sarcoma composed of oval or cuboidal cells in cords and clusters (H & E ×420).

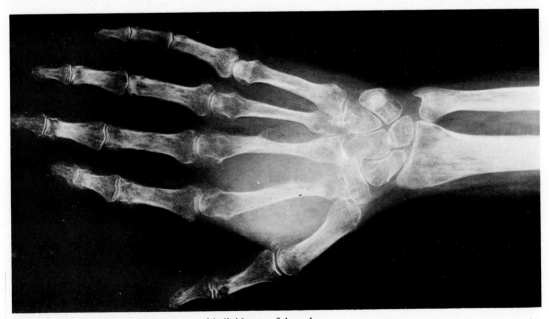

Figure 38-9.   Tendosynovial sarcoma, epithelioid type of the palm.

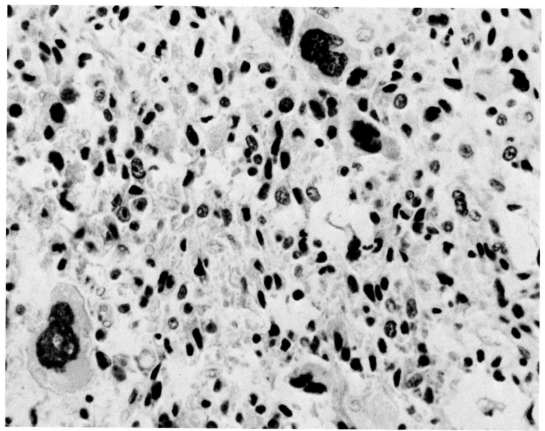

Figure 38-10. Pleomorphic liposarcoma exhibits a combination of small, undifferentiated and large bizarre and multinucleated neoplastic cells.

the cases. The proximal humerus and proximal tibia, combined, are the site of another third of osteogenic sarcomas. Radiographic and histologic findings can establish the diagnosis in the majority of the cases (Dahlin and Conventry, 1967; Farr *et al.*, 1974; Hajdu and Hajdu, 1976; Huvos, 1979). Determination of the serum alkaline phosphatase plays an important role in determining prognosis. Elevated or increasing values indicate the presence or spreading of osteogenic sarcoma. The primary concern in the treatment of osteogenic sarcomas is the complete control of the primary lesion. This can be achieved by amputation, or by preoperative and postoperative multidrug chemotherapy in combination with *en bloc* resection of the primary tumor (see Figures 38-14 and 38-15). Chemotherapy may control and diminish metastatic disease. Surgical excision of metastases, especially pulmonary metastases, has been shown to prolong survival (Gottlieb *et al.*, 1975; Jaffe *et al.*,

1977; Rosen *et al.*, 1978, 1979; Huvos, 1979; Campanacci *et al.*, 1981).

Extraskeletal osteogenic sarcoma is seldom seen under the age of 40. It may appear in any part of the body. No effective therapy is known for this uncommon, but highly malignant neoplasm (Sordillo *et al.*, 1983).

Ewing's sarcoma is an undifferentiated malignant mesenchymal tumor that is often found in the midshaft of long bones, *e.g.*, femur, tibia, humerus, and fibula, and flat bones such as ilium and ribs (see Figure 38-16). Radiographically, most of the Ewing's sarcomas have a typical appearance, exhibiting symmetric, fusiform outline, irregular bone destruction and parallel, onionskin, periosteal reaction (see Figure 38-17). Until recently, the treatment of Ewing's sarcoma has been primarily amputation, and the prognosis was regarded as guarded. At present, for most patients with Ewing's sarcomas, complete resection by excision or amputation of the pri-

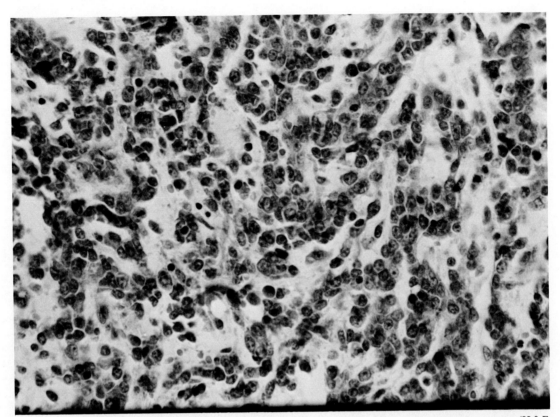

Figure 38–11. Embryonal rhabdomyosarcoma forming nests, cords, and tubules in a partly myxomatous stroma (H & E ×500).

mary lesion is recommended. It is advised that whenever feasible, preoperative irradiation with a dose of 6000 to 7000 rads in combination with chemotherapy should be initiated (Rosen *et al.,* 1974, 1978; Rosen, 1978).

Chordoma of the sacrococcygeal area is most commonly seen during the fifth and sixth decades (see Table 38–4). The less common form of spheno-occipital chordoma is seen in the teenage group and young adults. Chordomas are usually well demarcated, lobulated, and partially translucent neoplasms which usually extend into adjacent soft tissues. The treatment of chordomas is primarily surgical. Irradiation and chemotherapy seem to have little beneficial effect (Dahlin and MacCarty, 1952; Hajdu and Hajdu, 1976; Huvos, 1979).

Granulocytic sarcoma or chloroma is a disease of young adults (see Table 38–4). It is a dangerous hematopoietic neoplasm mimicking soft tissue sarcoma. Its periosteal location should alert clinician and pathologist to this neoplasm. In the majority of cases, usually within a year, the nature of the disease be-

comes apparent in the form of acute myelocytic leukemia (Hajdu, 1979).

Malignant histiocytic fibrous histiocytoma, or so-called malignant giant cell tumor, can be primary in bone as well as in soft tissues (see Table 38–5). It is a disease of young adults. The intraskeletal form is found most often in the distal femur and proximal part of the tibia. The thigh and upper arm are the most frequent soft tissue sites that may develop into histologically characteristic neoplasms. Whether they are low- or high-grade lesions, must be determined by the pathologist after careful consideration of the balance between stromal and giant cell elements (Hajdu, 1979; Huvos, 1979).

Malignant pleomorphic fibrous histiocytoma is seldom observed in bone. In soft tissues, the most common sites are buttock, thigh, arm, and neck (Hajdu, 1979; Soule and Enriquez, 1972). They are deeply seated and infiltrative lesions. Histologically, they may occasionally appear low grade, but most often they are highly malignant neoplasms with

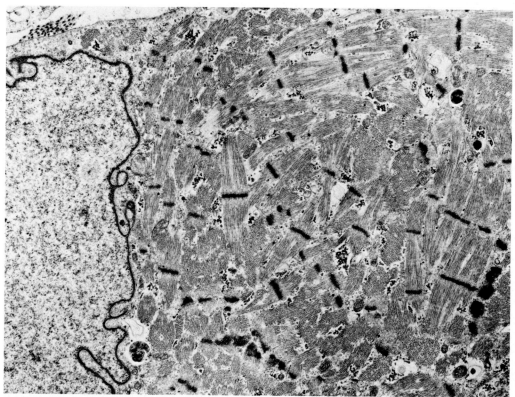

Figure 38–12. Ultrastructural appearance of rhabdomyosarcoma. Arranged thin and thick filaments are Z bands (×10,000).

a disarranged growth pattern (see Figure 38–18).

Fibroblastic fibrosarcoma is another neoplasm that occurs most often in soft tissues and in bones. It is usually a bulky lesion with infiltrative edges, and the thigh is the most common site. Histologically, pathologists are able to diagnose fibroblastic fibrosarcomas with relative ease because of their characteristic herringbone appearance. Grading of these sarcomas depends on thorough assessment of cellularity, number of cells in mitosis, and other features (Castro *et al.,* 1973; Chung and Enzinger, 1976; Soule and Pritchard, 1976).

Biphasic tenosynovial sarcomas are neoplasms of soft tissues and found most commonly in the proximity of major joints (Hajdu *et al.,* 1977; Hajdu, 1979). It is a disease of young men. *En bloc* or muscle group resection is the primary treatment. If, according to the pathologist's evaluation, the lesion is high grade, excision should be followed by appropriate chemotherapy (Sordillo *et al.,* 1981c).

Fibroblastic liposarcoma, or spindle cell li-

posarcoma, is more often high grade than low (Hajdu, 1979). It is found mainly in the thigh and is usually bulky in appearance. It is a spindle cell neoplasm with a rich branching capillary network. Treatment for the high-grade lesions should combine surgery, pre- or postoperative irradiation, and chemotherapy (Sordillo *et al.,* 1981c).

Leiomyoblastoma, or round cell smooth muscle sarcoma, is seldom seen in soft tissues, but almost 50% of visceral and parenchymal smooth muscle sarcomas are microscopically leiomyoblastomas (Shiu *et al.,* 1982). Grading of such neoplasms must be based on a number of cytologic and histologic features. Treatment should be planned according to site, size, and grade of the neoplasm.

Leiomyosarcomas are ubiquitous in the human body. In soft tissue, they often appear subcutaneously and are seldom found in deep tissues. Histologic grade, size, and location will dictate therapy. Low-grade forms can be successfully treated by appropriate local surgery. Fully malignant leiomyosarcomas require

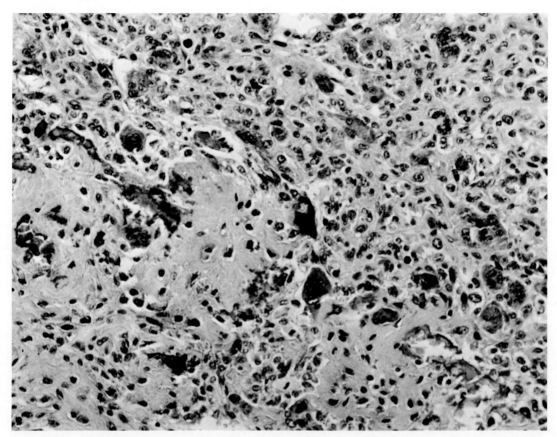

Figure 38–13.   Osteogenic sarcoma shows deposits of malignant osteoid and high grade cellular elements (H & E × 300).

chemotherapy similar to that for rhabdomyo-sarcomas (Sordillo *et al.*, 1981c).

Hemangiosarcoma of bone as well as soft tissues is relatively uncommon. In most cases, hemangiosarcomas are high-grade neoplasms and affect middle-aged men and women with almost equal frequency. If a hemangiosar-coma is diagnosed as high grade, the lesion requires optimal surgery and chemotherapy (see Figure 38 – 19) (Sordillo *et al.*, 1981c).

Hemangiopericytoma is another vascular neoplasm that can be histologically low as well as high grade. It is predominantly a disease of young men and can be found at any site (Hajdu, 1979).

Malignant peripheral nerve tumors are very complex neoplasms in their presentation as well as in histologic appearance (see Table 38 – 5). Histologic grading, however, can be done by pathologists in most cases without much difficulty. Prognostication and therapeutic planning, however, must be done in considera-tion of whether the neoplasm is small or large,

and whether it is solitary or multifocal. One of the paradoxic features of these neoplasms is that even low-grade forms can be life-threaten-ing if they are found in association with von Recklinghausen's disease. It is mandatory that each patient be studied with full knowledge of the clinical and family history. Malignant pe-ripheral nerve neoplasms that present in com-bination with neurofibromatosis, or appear histologically high grade, should be treated by surgical resection and appropriate chemother-apy (Sordillo *et al.*, 1981b).

Chondrosarcomas can be high- or low-grade neoplasms. They are found most commonly intraskeletally in middle-aged men. They ap-pear almost exclusively in soft tissues in el-derly men (Hajdu, 1982). Histologic grading plays an important role in their management. Low-grade chondrosarcomas, despite full size, seldom require more than good local sur-gery (Dahlin and Salvador, 1974; Huvos, 1979). High-grade forms require well-planned chemotherapy, in addition to optimal surgery.

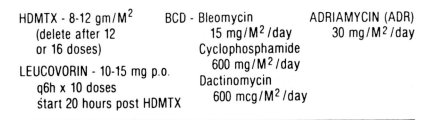

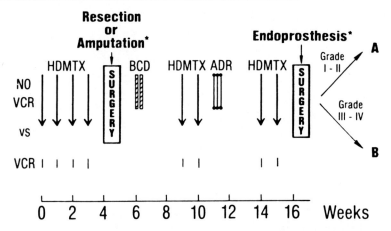

*Patients who are to undergo resection or amputation will have surgery at approximately four weeks; patients who are to undergo endoprosthetic replacement will have surgery at approximately 16 weeks.

Figure 38-14. Preoperative chemotherapy given to all patients with primary osteogenic sarcoma of an extremity. All patients receive the entire 16 weeks of induction chemotherapy, regardless of the time of surgery, prior to the selection of further adjuvant chemotherapy and upon the histologic response of primary tumor.

Mesenchymal chondrosarcomas are predominantly seen in young adults in bone or in soft tissues (see Figure 38–20). They are high-grade neoplasms, in most cases, and should be treated accordingly.

Malignant granular cell tumor and alveolar soft part sarcoma are very uncommon neoplasms (Hajdu, 1979). Both lesions affect adult women more commonly than men and can have a protracted clinical course. Treatment should be designed with consideration of size, location, cellularity, and duration of the neoplasm. Because of the rare occurrence of these neoplasms, no accurate information is available as to the best modality of therapy.

Plasmacytomas are seldom solitary in bone and present most often in soft tissue. Local treatment should be planned after systemic involvement with the disease has been ruled out (Hajdu, 1979).

Malignant mesenchymoma of soft tissues is extremely rare, and it is doubtful that it occurs intraskeletally.

Undifferentiated soft tissue sarcomas do not permit subclassification owing to their non-specific histologic features. Approximately 5%

of soft tissue sarcomas and less than 1% of bone sarcomas belong to this category (Hajdu, 1979). Sarcomas without recognizable histologic features should be graded based on cellularity, number of mitoses, and so forth for therapeutic purposes and reconsidered for definitive classification when additional material is available for examination (see Table 38–5).

Aspiration cytology, because of limited sampling and marked cytologic resemblance of reactive, benign neoplastic and malignant neoplastic lesions, only has a limited role in the primary diagnosis of soft tissue and bone sarcomas. In assessment of surgical margins, recurrences, and metastases it can be very informative (Hajdu and Melamed, 1973; Hajdu and Hajdu, 1976; Geisinger *et al.,* 1984; Hajdu, 1985).

Staging

Armed with the knowledge of the size, less than 5 cm or more than 5 cm, and the site, superficial or deep, and histologic grade, low or high grade, the neoplasm's staging can be

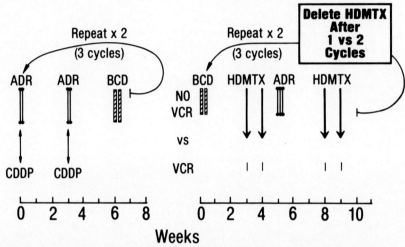

Histologic Response of Primary Tumor

GRADE I - II
(T - 10A)

ADR 30 mg/m^2/day
CDDP 120 mg/m^2 or 3 mg/kg

GRADE III - IV
(T - 10B)

Bleomycin 15 mg/m^2/day
Cyclophosphamide 600 mg/m^2/day
Dactinomycin 600 mcg/m^2/day

Repeat x 2
(3 cycles)

ADR   ADR   BCD

CDDP   CDDP

Repeat x 2
(3 cycles)

BCD   HDMTX   ADR   HDMTX
NO
VCR

vs

VCR

Delete HDMTX
After
1 vs 2
Cycles

0   2   4   6   8   0   2   4   6   8   10
Weeks

Figure 38–15.   Maintenance chemotherapy for osteogenic sarcoma. In regimen A, a three-week rest is usually required following the ADRIAMYCIN–cisplatinum combination chemotherapy, and a 2 to 3 week rest is required following the BCD chemotherapy. In regimen B, chemotherapy is resumed one week after each high-dose methotrexate treatment, but a three-week rest is usually required following the ADRIAMYCIN. Every other high-dose methotrexate treatment is deleted in young children receiving regimen B when the methotrexate dose of 12 g/m^2 calculates to more than 450 mg/kg.

achieved by considering three favorable and three poor prognostic signs in combination (see Table 38–6). A stage 0 sarcoma has three favorable prognostic indicators, a stage I neoplasm only two favorable prognostic indicators, a stage II tumor only one good prognostic sign, a stage III sarcoma three unfavorable prognostic indicators, and stage IV neoplasms present with metastases (see Figure 38–21). By this design, all neoplasms beyond the superficial fascia, including all bone sarcomas, are considered deep lesions.

In reviewing more than 1000 primary soft tissue sarcomas according to histologic type and stage of the sarcoma (see Table 38–7) it was found that 17 patients who had stage 0 sarcoma were all alive and well following local surgery alone. Sixteen of 189 patients (8%) with stage I sarcomas died of disease, and 179 of 501 patients (36%) with stage II tumors have died of their disease. Almost 80% of patients with stage III soft tissue sarcomas (505 of 641 patients) have died of disease (see Table 38–7).

Therefore, it is generally recommended that all patients with stage III soft tissue sarcomas should be given adjuvant chemotherapy. With an overall mortality rate of approximately 36% it is also desirable to treat patients with stage II sarcomas with adjuvant chemotherapy in addition to surgery; however, stage II patients would have to be evaluated separately from stage III patients when one is examining the efficacy of a particular adjuvant chemotherapy protocol for the treatment of soft tissue sarcoma.

Treatment

Surgery.   Adequate surgery is the best local treatment for sarcomas, and if the sarcoma is not easily resectable without amputation, irradiation, in the form of external radiation or brachytherapy, should be employed (Castro *et al.,* 1973; Hajdu, 1979; Suite *et al.,* 1981; Fine *et al.,* 1982; Hilaris *et al.,* 1982).

Surgical excision, simple or wide, should be

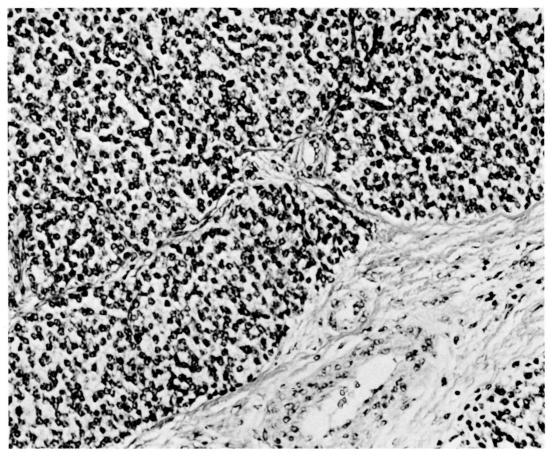

Figure 38-16. Ewing's sarcoma composed of small cells in lacy arrangement (H & E ×300).

limited to neoplasms with defined surgical borders. The infiltrative nature of sarcomas beyond visible borders calls for *monobloc* resection. This technique is suitable for the majority of sarcomas, especially soft tissue sarcomas. In a series of 75 previously untreated sarcomas treated by *monobloc* resection, the neoplasm recurred in only 15% of the patients (Hajdu, 1979).

For many years amputation has been regarded as the treatment of choice for sarcomas. Currently, amputation should be resorted to only when the neoplasm cannot be removed by less mutilating surgery. Despite the low risk of local recurrence, treatment by amputation does not offer a significant improvement in survival. The failure of amputative procedures to offer improved survival rates has led to the replacement of amputation with function-saving surgical techniques.

Radiotherapy. Radiotherapy has an important role in the primary management of sarcomas such as liposarcoma, embryonal rhabdomyosarcoma, and Ewing's sarcoma. Despite innovation in techniques and equipment, recurrences are encountered even after seemingly adequate treatment. Questions about the optimal timing of radiotherapy in relation to surgery and chemotherapy, methods of dosage fraction, and sensitivity of individual sarcomas remain to be answered. Several prospective studies are underway to clarify the role of conservative surgery, external beam radiation, and chemotherapy for various types of sarcomas.

It seems that perioperative brachytherapy, with immediate postoperative application of radioactive (^{192}Ir) seeds by delivering high-dose irradiation to the tumor bed assures local control of the disease in the majority of soft tissue sarcomas (Hilaris *et al.,* 1982).

Chemotherapy. In the case of chemotherapy, the activity of various single agents, as well as the role of combination chemotherapy,

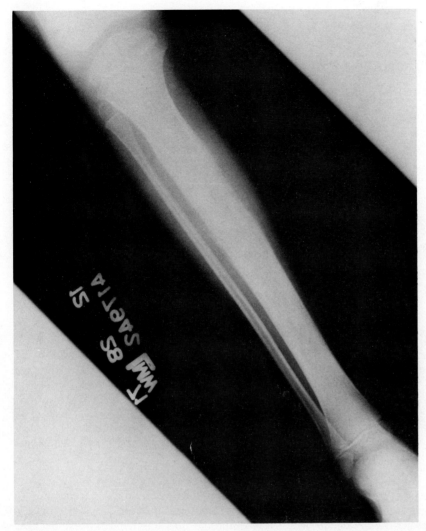

Figure 38-17. Ewing's sarcoma of the tibia showing cortical defect and periosteal thickening.

its desirability, and superiority of single-agent chemotherapy, must be evaluated and understood. Chemotherapy should not be advocated postoperatively in an attempt to enhance the effect of noncurative local therapy. Chemotherapy may be employed preoperatively, however, in an effort to shrink inoperable sarcomas so that either they become operable or, by shrinkage of the sarcoma, the surgery performed can still be adequate while sparing more normal tissue. This may make it easier for the surgeon to perform a radical procedure or reduce the radiation damage to normal tissues.

Adjuvant chemotherapy is indicated in all patients who have a finite possibility of developing metastases following surgery. These pa-

tients include all patients with high-grade (see Table 38-4) or stage III sarcomas (see Table 38-7). Sarcomas that might be in the stage II category and have demonstrated mortality given the known metastases in more than 25% of patients (see Table 38-7) should also be treated with adjuvant chemotherapy.

One of the first drugs shown to be effective in the treatment of solid tumors was dactinomycin. In 1959, Tan *et al.* reported on the efficacy of dactinomycin in solid tumors in childhood. She observed objective regression of tumor in 6 of 16 patients with Wilms' tumor, 1 of 5 patients with embryonal rhabdomyosarcoma, and 3 of 7 patients with neuroblastoma. The subsequent use of dactinomycin in the treatment of solid tumors has primarily been in

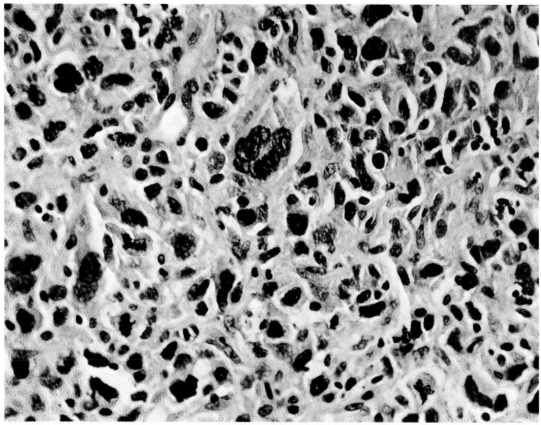

Figure 38–18. Malignant pleomorphic fibrous histiocytoma, histologically high grade, shows the presence of mononucleated and multinucleated neoplastic elements (H & E ×420).

combinations with other drugs. The efficacy of dactinomycin in the treatment of Ewing's sarcoma has been evaluated (Rosen *et al.,* 1974). In that study, objective evidence of regression of pulmonary metastases was observed following dactinomycin in four of five patients being treated for metastatic Ewing's sarcoma. A review of the literature of the use of dactinomycin as a single agent indicates that of 21 patients with adult sarcomas reported, only 14 have had evaluable disease. Four of these 14 patients (28%) had objective evidence of tumor regression, indicating that dactinomycin may be of potential value in the treatment of adult soft tissue sarcomas (see Table 38–8).

Vincristine sulfate was originally shown to be effective in the treatment of metastatic Wilms' tumor. Studies by Sutow *et al.* (1966) demonstrated a high response rate of evaluable patients to vincristine so that this agent has become one of the first-line drugs for this tumor. Single-agent vincristine has also been

shown to be effective in the treatment of Ewing's sarcoma (Sutow *et al.,* 1966), rhabdomyosarcoma, and leiomyosarcoma. Because of the relative lack of myelosuppressive toxicity, vincristine sulfate has become an agent that has frequently been incorporated into combination chemotherapy regimens.

Of all the alkylating agents, cyclophosphamide has received the most attention in the treatment of soft tissue sarcomas. The reason for the popularity of cyclophosphamide is that it produces a predictable myelosuppression approximately one week from the administration of a single intravenous dose, making it a more predictable drug than, for instance, nitrogen mustard. Nitrogen mustard may result in prolonged delays in the resumption of chemotherapy, since manifestations of bone marrow depression can occur four to six weeks following the administration of a single dose. Cyclophosphamide has been studied extensively as a single agent in the treatment of soft

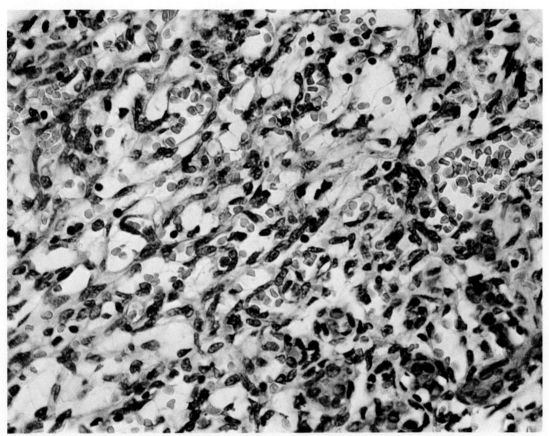

Figure 38–19.   High grade hemangiosarcoma showing neoplastic endothelial cells forming vascular channels (H & E ×420).

tissue sarcomas in children. In reviewing the literature, Livingston and Carter (1970) found 33 objective responses among 56 patients with rhabdomyosarcoma. The highest response rates were reported in series where the drug was given intravenously at the dose of 30 mg/kg weekly, or 10 mg/kg daily until a nadir white blood count of 1500 (or lower) occurred. In addition to the responses obtained in rhabdomyosarcoma, Ewing's sarcoma had response rates in patients being treated with evaluable disease. In osteogenic sarcoma, in 16 evaluable patients only two responded, however, the doses of cyclophosphamide employed in the various studies in the treatment of osteogenic sarcoma were not optimal. No responses were reported in 11 patients who received an oral dose of 5 mg/kg. One of two patients treated with 10 mg/kg per day until the white blood cell count fell to 1500 or below had an objective response to this treatment. The activity of cyclophosphamide against pe-

diatric sarcomas and its predictable toxicity have made it a valuable drug for incorporation into multidrug protocols for the treatment of sarcomas.

Methotrexate is a drug that has been used primarily in the treatment of leukemia. The use of methotrexate as a single agent in the treatment of soft tissue and bone sarcomas is limited. A series of 41 patients with soft tissue sarcomas who received single-agent methotrexate was described (Wiltshaw, 1967; Subramainian and Wiltshaw, 1978). The doses varied from daily oral methotrexate to intravenous methotrexate in doses from 50 mg to 500 mg infused over 18 to 36 hours. The majority of patients treated in this series were adults and had high-grade sarcomas. The majority of responding patients had either leiomyosarcoma or fibrosarcoma. They recorded a complete response rate of 15% (six patients), with nine additional patients having partial remissions, for an overall response rate of 37% to metho-

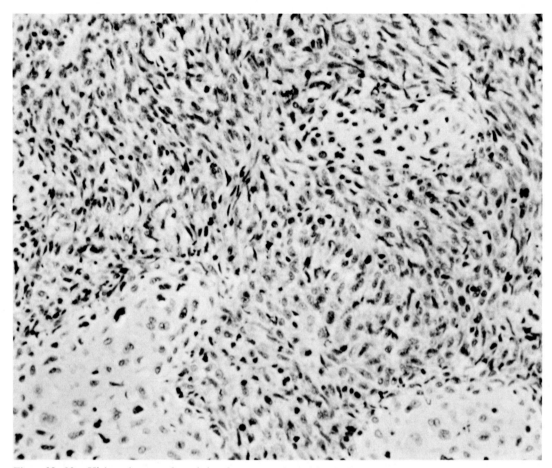

Figure 38-20. High grade mesenchymal chondrosarcoma shows islands of malignant chondrocytes and immature and slender mesenchymal cells (H & E ×300).

trexate as a single agent. These same authors used methotrexate at the dose of 200 mg as an intravenous infusion over 24 hours combined with dactinomycin, vincristine, 5-fluorouracil, and cyclophosphamide. Folinic acid rescue was utilized following the 200 mg methotrexate infusion. Although it is difficult to evaluate the additive effect of methotrexate in this group of patients, they achieved a positive response rate of 67% in 12 patients so treated, with 25% complete responses. Two of the three complete responders were alive five years after treatment.

High-dose methotrexate at a dose of 8 to 12 gm/m² with folinic acid rescue has been reported to be effective as a single agent in the treatment of osteogenic sarcoma (Jaffe, 1972; Jaffe *et al.,* 1977), with response rates as high as 70% in patients with evaluable disease (Rosen *et al.,* 1979). Because it is an extremely effective agent in the treatment of osteogenic sar-

coma, there has been a great deal of speculation as to its effectiveness in the treatment of other high-grade sarcomas, and more trials of high-dose methotrexate with folinic acid rescue in evaluable soft tissue sarcomas is strongly indicated (Isacoff *et al.,* 1978). Although very effective in the treatment of osteogenic sarcoma, the experience at Memorial Sloan-Kettering Cancer Center has been that this treatment modality does not produce meaningful remissions in patients with the small cell sar-

Table 38-6. Factors Influencing Prognosis of Sarcomas

SARCOMA	FAVORABLE PROGNOSTIC SIGNS	UNFAVORABLE PROGNOSTIC SIGNS
Size	Small	Big
Site	Superficial	Deep
Histologic grade	Low	High

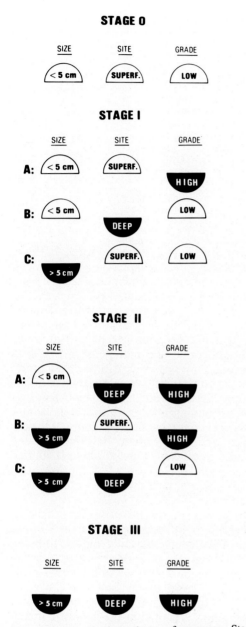

STAGE 0

SIZE | SITE | GRADE
< 5 cm | SUPERF. | LOW

STAGE I

SIZE | SITE | GRADE

A: < 5 cm | SUPERF. | HIGH

B: < 5 cm | DEEP | LOW

C: > 5 cm | SUPERF. | LOW

STAGE II

SIZE | SITE | GRADE

A: < 5 cm | DEEP | HIGH

B: > 5 cm | SUPERF. | HIGH

C: > 5 cm | DEEP | LOW

STAGE III

SIZE | SITE | GRADE

> 5 cm | DEEP | HIGH

Figure 38–21. Staging scheme of sarcomas. Stage 0 tumor = three favorable prognostic signs; Stage I tumor = two favorable prognostic signs and one unfavorable prognostic sign; Stage II tumor = one favorable prognostic sign and two unfavorable prognostic signs; Stage III tumor = three unfavorable signs; and Stage IV tumor = evidence of metastasis.

comas such as Ewing's sarcoma and embryonal rhabdomyosarcoma.

Doxorubicin was first shown to have a wide spectrum of activity against solid tumors in the early 1970s. Researchers reported on the use of doxorubicin and its efficacy in evaluable rhabdomyosarcomas and Ewing's sarcomas

(Sutow, 1968; Tan *et al.,* 1973). The results of these studies demonstrated that the addition of doxorubicin to other agents such as cyclophosphamide, dactinomycin, and vincristine significantly increased response rates and disease-free survival rates above those obtainable with other drug protocols not utilizing doxorubicin. In the more resistant high-grade sarcomas, doxorubicin was first shown to be effective in the treatment of evaluable osteogenic sarcoma. Cortes not only demonstrated the efficacy of doxorubicin in the treatment of osteogenic sarcoma, but demonstrated that a dose-response curve indicated that the highest responses were obtained when the drug was utilized at the dose of 30 mg/m² per day for three days (total 90 mg/m² per course) (Cortes *et al.,* 1972). Although 90 mg/m² per course produces the highest response rate, many patients cannot tolerate this dose of doxorubicin, and indeed when doxorubicin is used in combination with other agents, the dose is usually limited to 50 to 75 mg/m² to prevent severe myelosuppression. Doxorubicin was shown to produce an objective response rate of 31% in 49 adult patients treated in the Southwest Oncology Group (Gottlieb *et al.,* 1972, 1975). In that phase II study of doxorubicin, the drug was administered at the dose of 75 mg/m² per course. In subsequent studies, doxorubicin was combined with other agents to produce still higher response rates; however, the dose of doxorubicin in those combination chemotherapy trials was gradually reduced to 50 mg/m² (Gottlieb, 1974; Gottlieb *et al.,* 1972, 1975).

Dacarbazine [5-(3,3-dimethyl-1-triazeno) imidazole-4-carboxamide, DTIC)] is an agent primarily useful in the treatment of malignant melanoma. Phase II studies with this agent in sarcomas are limited. In evaluable soft tissue sarcomas, 15% to 20% response rates have been reported (Luce *et al.,* 1980). The dose schedule used in obtaining these responses was 250 mg/m² per day for five days. A response of less than 20% would not seem to indicate that this agent was very effective in the treatment of soft tissue sarcomas. Its use in drug combinations by the Southwest Oncology Group, however, in combination with doxorubicin to achieve a response rate of 42% (Gottlieb *et al.,* 1972) has increased its acceptance in many centers in the treatment of sarcomas. Responses observed in some patients with neurofibrosarcoma and tendosynovial sarcoma with this combination of agents suggest that there is

Table 38-7. Mortality of Common Soft Tissue Sarcomas by Tissue Type and Stage of the Primary Lesion

HISTOLOGIC TYPE	I	(%)	II	(%)	III	(%)	TOTAL	(%)
Malignant fibrous histiocytoma	1/93	(1)	20/77	(26)	83/109	(76)	104/279	(37)
Liposarcoma	1/9	(11)	26/98	(27)	75/113	(66)	102/220	(46)
Fibrosarcoma	1/4	(25)	16/42	(38)	52/68	(76)	69/114	(60)
Synovial sarcoma	1/3	(33)	26/66	(39)	48/51	(94)	75/120	(62)
Pleomorphic rhabdomyosarcoma	——	——	12/21	(57)	62/67	(93)	74/88	(84)
Embryonal rhabdomyosarcoma	——	——	35/58	(60)	137/182	(75)	172/240	(72)
Leiomyosarcoma*	——	——	——	——	——	——	16/22	(73)
Angiosarcoma	9/16	(56)	7/8	(88)	15/16	(94)	23/30	(77)
Malignant schwannoma	9/16	(56)	22/29	(76)	33/35	(94)	64/80	(80)
Total	14/131	(11)	164/399	(41)	505/641	(79)	698/1193	(59)

Reprinted by permission from Hajdu, S. I.: *Pathology of Soft Tissue Tumors.* Lea & Febiger, Philadelphia, 1979.
* Nonuterine extremity leiomyosarcomas presumably of vascular origin.

indeed synergy between doxorubicin and DTIC (Goldman, *et al.*, 1977).

Cisplatin is a compound with alkylating activity that has been shown to be effective in the treatment of a variety of human neoplasms, both as a single agent and in combination. The efficacy of cisplatin in advanced osteogenic sarcoma has been reported (Ochs *et al.*, 1978). Five responses in nine patients with advanced evaluable disease were observed. The majority of patients having responses did so with the use of cisplatin in doses of 90 to 120 mg/m^2 per course. In a larger series of Memorial Sloan-Kettering Cancer Center patients with evaluable osteogenic sarcoma, a response rate of 20% using a dose of 120 mg/m^2 with mannitol diuresis was observed. Although a 20% response rate is considered minimal evidence of activity of a single agent, the efficacy of cisplatin in the treatment of osteogenic sarcoma was particularly impressive in that the majority of the patients treated were previously resistant to alkylating agents (cyclophosphamide at a dose of 1200 mg/m^2). Moreover, the majority of the responses observed were clinically significant responses. In a study of the Southwest Oncology Group, it was concluded that cisplatin has minimal activity in treating advanced soft tissue and bony sarcomas (Samson *et al.*, 1979). It should be noted that the dose schedule used in that study was 15 mg/m^2 for five consecutive days. In another study, one complete response was reported in a patient with embryonal rhabdomyosarcoma treated at a low dose of 1 mg/kg per week for four consecutive weeks (Karakousis *et al.*, 1979). An additional two responses (one complete and one partial) in two patients with spindle cell sarcomas (leiomyosarcoma and malignant fibrous histiocytoma) treated with cisplatin at a dose of 100 mg/m^2 were reported. Both of these patients had relapsed after treatment with the combination cyclophosphamide, vincristine, doxorubicin, and DTIC. Using the dose of cisplatin of 120 mg/m^2 with mannitol diuresis, responses in previously treated patients with fibrosarcoma, rhabdomyosarcoma, leiomyosarcoma, and malignant fibrous histiocytoma were observed. Although the number of patients at this time is too small to quote response rates, the initial trial of high-dose cisplatin with mannitol diuresis in soft tissue sarcomas is encouraging because many of the responses observed seem to be dramatic and clinically significant. Further phase II studies with high-dose cisplatin (120 mg/m^2 or 3 mg/kg) with mannitol diuresis seem to be indicated (Table 38-8).

The literature is replete with reports of many combinations of drugs used to treat various types of malignancies. Only those combinations of drugs that have been proven to be effective in patients with sarcomas will be considered (see Table 38-9).

The history of combination chemotherapy for sarcomas is rooted in the pediatric literature when, in 1971, Wilbur demonstrated that significant responses in children with advanced embryonal rhabdomyosarcoma could be obtained through the use of a combination of vincristine, dactinomycin, and cyclophosphamide (VAC) (Heyn *et al.*, 1974; Wilbur, 1974). In this regimen, the best responses were noted when cyclophosphamide was used at the intravenous dose of 10 mg/kg daily for seven to ten days given in combination with dactinomycin and vincristine. Indeed this combination chemotherapy was effective not only in embryonal rhabdomyosarcoma in children, but showed evidence of activity in the treat-

Table 38-8.   Single-Agent Chemotherapy in Evaluable Soft Tissue Sarcomas

DRUG	USUAL DOSAGE (mg/m^2)	SMALL CELL SARCOMAS	SPINDLE CELL SARCOMAS	COMMENT
Dactinomycin	0.450 × 5 every 2-3 weeks	++	+/−*	Active in combination
Vincristine	1.5-2.0 weekly	++	+/−*	Active in combination
Cyclophosphamide	500-1200 every 2-3 weeks	+++	+/−*	Active in combination
Methotrexate	50-350 every 2-3 weeks	−*	++	Active in combination
Methotrexate (with folinic acid)	1500-10,000 every 1-3 weeks	+/−*	+/−*	+++ in osteogenic sarcoma May be active in combination
DTIC	250 × 5 every 3 weeks	+/−*	++	Active in combination
Doxorubicin	60-80 every 2-3 weeks	+++	+++	Active in combination
Cisplatin (with mannitol diuresis)	90-100 every 2-3 weeks	++	+++	More data needed, degree of responses seen has been significant

* Minimal data available, needs further investigation.

ment of metastatic Ewing's sarcoma. When dealing with the adult sarcomas, however, the results of VAC chemotherapy were disappointing (Gottlieb *et al.,* 1972, 1975). At about this time, doxorubicin had proven efficacy in the treatment of sarcomas such as leiomyosarcoma, liposarcoma, and osteogenic sarcoma. The Southwest Oncology Group decided to use doxorubicin as the cornerstone of combination chemotherapy in the treatment of adult sarcomas (Gottlieb *et al.,* 1975). DTIC, when combined with doxorubicin, increased the response rate of sarcomas from 31 to 41%. Al-

though this is a small increment, the numbers of patients were large enough to demonstrate that this was a significant increase in the response rate to this combination of drugs. The further addition of vincristine and cyclophosphamide increased the response rate of adult soft tissue sarcomas to 55% in 136 patients (Yap *et al.,* 1980). The combination of cyclophosphamide, vincristine, doxorubicin, and DTIC (CYVADIC) required the dose of doxorubicin to be reduced to 50 mg/m^2, and that of cyclophosphamide to 500 mg/m^2. This regimen has been widely accepted and has shown

Table 38-9.   Current Combination Chemotherapy Regimens for Adult Soft Tissue Sarcomas

INVESTIGATOR (INSTITUTE)	AGENT	DOSE	SCHEDULE	FREQUENCY
Yap *et al.,* 1980 (MDA—SWOG) CYVADIC	Cytoxan	500 mg/M^2	Day 1	3 weeks
	Vincristine	2 mg	Days 1 & 5	
	Doxorubicin	50 mg/M^2	Day 1	
	DTIC	250 mg/M^2	Days 1-5	
Benjamin *et al.,* 1977a,b (MDA—SWOG) CYVADACT	Cytoxan	500 mg/M^2	Day 1	3 weeks
	Vincristine	2 mg	Days 1 & 5	
	Doxorubicin	50 mg/M^2	Day 1	
	Dactinomycin	00 μg/M^2	Day	
Rivkin *et al.,* 1980 (SHMC—SWOG) MAD	Methyl-CCNU	150 mg/M^2	Day 1	6 weeks
	Doxorubicin	60 mg/M^2	Day 1	
	Doxorubicin	45 mg/M^2	Day 22	
Rosen *et al.,* 1974 (MSKCC) T-11	Cytoxan	1200 mg/M^2	Day 1, day 42	9 weeks
	Doxorubicin	30 mg/M^2	Days 1 & 2, 42 & 43	
	Methotrexate	18 mg/M^2	Days 1 & 2, 42 & 43	
	Vincristine	2 mg	Days 1, 7, 14 & 21	
	Bleomycin	15 mg/M^2	Days 21 & 22	
	Cytoxan	600 mg/M^2	Days 21 & 22	
	Dactinomycin	600 μg/M^2	Days 21 & 22	

MDA = M.D. Anderson Hospital and Tumor Institute
SWOG = Southwest Oncology Group
SHMC = Swedish Hospital Medical Center
MSKCC = Memorial Sloan-Kettering Cancer Center

responses (Leite *et al.*, 1977) and increased survival when used in an adjuvant chemotherapy study in patients with a variety of sarcomas, notably liposarcoma, leiomyosarcoma, rhabdomyosarcoma, malignant fibrous histiocytoma, tendosynovial sarcoma, malignant peripheral nerve tumor, and fibrosarcoma.

The addition of high-dose methotrexate to protocols for soft tissue sarcomas other than osteogenic sarcoma is of questionable value since no adequate phase II data regarding the role of high-dose methotrexate with folinic acid rescue in soft tissue sarcomas have been reported. Nevertheless, higher survival rates in a group of 49 patients treated with doxorubicin, cyclophosphamide, and high-dose methotrexate plus immunotherapy with *Corynebacterium parvum* have been demonstrated (Rosenberg *et al.*, 1978).

At Memorial Sloan-Kettering Cancer Center, doxorubicin was incorporated into the treatment of pediatric sarcomas at an earlier date and combined with vincristine, dactinomycin and cyclophosphamide in an adjuvant chemotherapy protocol in 1970. Because of this experience, this same sequential chemotherapy protocol was used in some of the more common adult sarcomas and showed activity (Rosen *et al*, 1974). Two patients with tendosynovial sarcoma are alive and free of disease eight years following their treatment. One patient had an incompletely excised tumor in the head and neck area, and one patient had pulmonary metastases which completely responded to chemotherapy.

In 1975, chemotherapy with the combination of vincristine, doxorubicin, cyclophosphamide, and methotrexate, as well as the combination of bleomycin, cyclophosphamide, and dactinomycin, had evolved for the treatment of sarcomas such as embryonal rhabdomyosarcoma and Ewing's sarcoma (Parente *et al.*, 1978). These combinations seemed to be particularly effective, and indeed 12 of 13 patients with evaluable Ewing's sarcoma responded to initial treatment with the combination of bleomycin, cyclophosphamide, and dactinomycin, Twenty of 21 patients with evaluable Ewing's sarcoma responded to the initial treatment with cyclophosphamide, doxorubicin, and methotrexate. This very high response rate in the malignant small cell sarcomas has prompted the use of these combinations for the adjuvant treatment of all patients with soft tissue sarcomas. Agents are combined and adminis-

tered in maximal dosage. Thus, cyclophosphamide is given at a dose of 1200 mg/m^2 with doxorubicin at a dose of 60 mg/m^2, and methotrexate at a dose of 36 mg/m^2 over a period of two days. The combination of bleomycin, cyclophosphamide, and dactinomycin (BCD) is utilized again with cyclophosphamide 1200 mg/m^2, bleomycin 30 mg/m^2, and dactinomycin 1.2 mg/m^2 given over two days. These schedules of drugs represents a combination given at maximally tolerated doses and are not without potent side effects. The majority of patients being treated on this protocol require brief hospitalizations for the treatment of suspected sepsis during periods of leukopenia and packed cell transfusions for anemia that develops approximately two weeks following the initiation of treatment (see Figure 38–20).

The combination of bleomycin and cyclophosphamide has also been shown to be effective in the treatment of evaluable high-grade sarcomas such as osteogenic sarcoma (Mosende *et al.*, 1977). In an initial study, responses were noted in 8 of 13 patients with osteogenic sarcoma, and a follow-up study has shown that 17 of 22 patients with evaluable primary osteogenic sarcoma had initial responses to this combination chemotherapy which was given as the first treatment in a multidrug chemotherapy protocol. Its activity in this resistant sarcoma is an indication that this combination may be active in the treatment of other sarcomas. Indeed, three of four patients with evaluable malignant fibrous histiocytoma showed significant responses to BCD chemotherapy.

These chemotherapy combinations represent the maximally tolerable doses of known effective agents in the treatment of sarcomas; DTIC is not recommended since current regimens utilizing this agent call for five-day courses of treatment, which is inefficient and probably ineffective. In addition, the lack of DTIC in the treatment protocol allows the use of approximately twice the dose of cyclophosphamide as is used in the CYVADIC protocol. This, it is believed, is responsible for the higher response rate observed with this protocol as compared to CYVADIC, where it can be compared in the treatment of the small cell sarcomas such as Ewing's sarcoma.

Combination chemotherapy protocols in current use are enumerated in Table 38–9, and the response rates noted by various investigators of both small cell sarcomas and spindle cell sarcomas are shown in Table 38–10.

Table 38–10. Combination Chemotherapy in the Treatment of Evaluable Sarcomas—Total (Complete and Partial) Response Rates

PROTOCOL (See Table 38–9)	SMALL CELL SARCOMAS* # Pts.	(% Response)	SPINDLE CELL SARCOMAS† # Pts.	(% Response)	ALL SARCOMAS # Pts.	(% Response)
CYVADIC	18/34	(53%)	45/52	(45%)	63/126	(50)
CYVADIC + PE	N/A		N/A+		11/14	(79)
CYVADACT	N/A		N/A+		64/224	(36)
MAD	12/22	(55%)	11/27	(41%)	23/49	(47)
T-11	81/93	(87%)‡	11/18	(61%)#	92/111	(82)

PE = Protected environment used with drug escalations of 20% per course of CYVADIC.
N/A = Published data not available.
* Small cell sarcomas include angiosarcoma, Ewing's sarcoma, rhabdomyosarcoma, mesenchymal sarcomas and undifferentiated small cell sarcomas, Kaposi's sarcoma, and mesothelioma.
† Spindle cell sarcomas include fibrosarcoma, malignant fibrous histiocytoma, osteogenic sarcoma, liposarcoma, leiomyosarcoma, chondrosarcoma, neurofibroma, and synovial sarcoma.
‡ T-11 chemotherapy calls for drugs to be given in two-day courses every three weeks. These data include patients treated with the same drug combinations and total doses over five- and three-day courses in prior protocols as well as in two-day courses in the current protocol. Response rates for all three regimens were identical.
# Includes responses in 8/13 patients with osteogenic sarcoma who responded to the bleomycin, cyclophosphamide, dactinomycin phase of the T-11 protocol.

Patients treated for leiomyosarcoma had a better response rate than has been reported with other drug regimens in the CYVADIC protocol. This is probably attributed to the inclusion of DTIC in the CYVADIC regimen (Parente *et al.*, 1978). DTIC has shown only a 12% response rate in the treatment of most sarcomas, while, approximately 25% of patients with leiomyosarcoma treated with DTIC as a single agent responded to this drug. In addition to the Southwest Oncology Group study with CYVADIC noted in Table 38–10, this drug regimen was originally studied at the M. D. Anderson Hospital where the overall response rate was 59% (Luce *et al.*, 1970; Gottlieb *et al.*, 1972; Azizi *et al.*, 1979; Benjamin *et al.*, 1977a,b; Yap *et al.*, 1980).

Recently, Rivkin *et al.* (1980) reported a similar response (approximately 45%) to a regimen which included methyl-CCNU and doxorubicin (MAD). They concluded that this regimen was as good as CYVADIC in producing the same response rate in sarcoma patients, but was much easier to administer and was better tolerated than CYVADIC. Indeed, they pointed out that the overall survival of patients with evaluable metastatic sarcomas was similar for the MAD regimen as it was for both CYVADIC and CYVADACT.

The Southwest Oncology Group conducted a study comparing CYVADIC and CYVADACT, where DTIC was replaced with dactinomycin (the latter has shown to be effective in the treatment of pediatric sarcomas) (Tan, 1959; Wilbur, 1974). After treating approximately 200 patients with each regimen, it was concluded that the overall response rate to

CYVADIC (48%) was superior to that obtained with CYVADACT, where the overall response rate was 39%. Twelve complete responses were reported in each group. CYVADIC was significantly more successful in treating patients with fibrosarcoma, leiomyosarcoma, and tendosynovial sarcoma. In addition, the median duration of response in the CYVADIC regimen was longer than that obtained with the CYVADACT regimen (Benjamin *et al.*, 1977a,b).

In the original phase II studies of doxorubicin in the treatment of solid tumors, a dose-response curve was noted that showed doxorubicin was more effective in higher doses. Indeed, a 20% response rate in patients given 45 mg/m^2 of doxorubicin, a 29% response rate in patients receiving 60 mg/m^2, and a 36% response rate in patients receiving 75 mg/m^2 were noted (Benjamin *et al.*, 1977a,b). This confirmed earlier work done in the treatment of osteogenic sarcoma, where it was shown that 75 mg/m^2 produced a higher response rate than 60 mg/m^2 of doxorubicin, and the highest response rate in the spindle cell sarcoma, osteogenic sarcoma, was achieved with the dose of 90 mg/m^2. As a result, initial studies were done at the M. D. Anderson Hospital where the dose of doxorubicin, as well as that of cyclophosphamide and DTIC, was escalated by increments of 20%, and patients were placed in a protective environment to try to avoid the severe complications of profound leukopenia. In that pilot study, a 79% response rate of CYVADIC was documented. Patients treated in this protocol must be meticulously followed, however, and given supportive care to prevent mortality from overwhelming sepsis (Benjamin *et al.,* 1977a,b).

Similarly, patients treated at Memorial Sloan-Kettering Cancer Center have achieved a very high response rate to combination chemotherapy as depicted in the T-11 chemotherapy protocol (see Figure 38–22). The high response rates obtained with this chemotherapy protocol in the treatment of sarcomas is overstated because this protocol originated in the pediatric and adolescent unit where the majority of patients had small cell sarcomas such as Ewing's sarcoma and rhabdomyosarcoma. These sarcomas are notoriously more responsive to chemotherapy than are the adult sarcomas, and again the high response rate is probably the result of the large dose of cyclophosphamide used in each course of chemotherapy (1200 mg/m²). These high response rates, however, have been duplicated in patients with adult sarcomas including Ewing's sarcoma, pleomorphic rhabdomyosarcoma,

malignant fibrous histiocytoma, and mesenchymal chondrosarcoma. Again, with the T-11 chemotherapy protocol, the doses described are rather high, and approximately 50% of the patients require frequent brief hospitalizations for supportive therapy during periods of leukopenia accompanied by fever. If this occurs more than once, subsequent doses of cyclophosphamide are reduced by 30% for the next course of chemotherapy. With the use of this protocol, patients must be followed meticulously to detect periods during which supportive therapy is required.

Thus, by utilizing chemotherapy regimens where the maximum doses of each single agent are employed, higher overall response rates of disease can be obtained, and it is likely that these regimens will yield higher disease-free survival rates when used as adjuvants. These regimens should only be used at centers where the surveillance and necessary supportive therapy is constantly available, and used only in

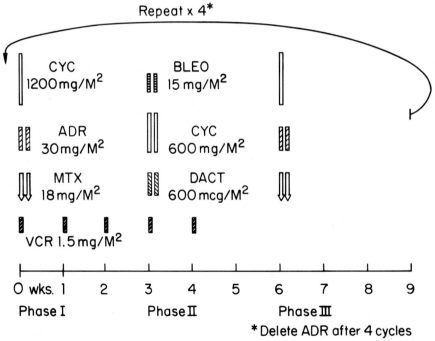

Figure 38–22. T-11 combination chemotherapy utilized at Memorial Sloan-Kettering Cancer Center. Drug combinations are given over a period of two days, approximately every three weeks. Cyclophosphamide is given at the dose of 1,200 mg/m² on day 1 of the first and third phase of chemotherapy, and at the dose of 600 mg/m² on days 1 and 2 of the second phase of chemotherapy. ADRIAMYCIN is given at the dose of 30 mg/m² daily for two days, methotrexate at the dose of 18 mg/m² daily for two days, bleomycin at the dose of 15 mg/m² daily for two days, and dactinomycin at the dose of 600 mg/m² daily for two days. Vincristine is given at the dose of 1.5 mg/m² with a maximum dose of 2.0 mg. If patients require admission in the hospital for supportive care following profound leukopenia and fever as a result of any given phase of this chemotherapy, the dose of cyclophosphamide is reduced by 30% in future administrations of that phase of chemotherapy. A majority of patients enumerated in the table, who have responded to this chemotherapy with small-cell sarcomas, are patients with Ewing's sarcoma whose evaluable disease included the primary tumor which was not given local therapy until after approximately three complete cycles of T-11 chemotherapy. Twenty of 20 patients with evaluable metastatic Ewing's sarcoma responded to this chemotherapy protocol.

patients who are at a very high risk of succumbing to metastatic disease, or in adjuvant chemotherapy settings where the recurrence rate for that particular patient's disease is expected to be high.

An extensive experience in the treatment of two common bone sarcomas, Ewing's sarcoma and osteogenic sarcoma, has led to the conclusion that when patients present with a primary tumor, it is advantageous to initiate systemic chemotherapy before local surgery or radiation therapy (see Figure 38–14) (Rosen *et al.,* 1979, 1982).

If a patient presents with a tumor that can be completely and radically excised at the time of the biopsy, it is preferable to have the surgery performed first. In the majority of patients, however, open biopsies usually precede definitive surgery. In this case preoperative chemotherapy is preferable. This has several advantages. Preoperative chemotherapy allows the patients to receive early systemic chemotherapy for the eradication of microfoci of disease which are usually already present in the majority of patients at presentation with highly malignant sarcomas. No delay is necessary in starting chemotherapy owing to postoperative complications. Preoperative chemotherapy can frequently shrink a primary tumor, making possible less ablative surgery. Of course, surgery must be radical at all times with the need for negative microscopic margins of resection. Shrinkage of a large tumor, particularly in an extremity, however, frequently redefines normal planes and eradicates tumor vascularity along with tumor, making the surgery easier to perform. The same is true for chemotherapy given before radiation therapy to spare more normal tissue at the time of local therapy. In addition, shrinking of a large tumor mass may eliminate hypoxic necrotic areas within the center of the tumor, making it more resistant to local radiation therapy. Of course, if one is to administer chemotherapy prior to local therapy, that chemotherapy must be aggressive enough to actually reduce the size of the primary tumor and prevent it from growing in the majority of patients.

This approach gives an indication of the effectiveness of chemotherapy in the patient. It allows the development of further data on the response rate of primary sarcomas to the chemotherapy protocol being utilized. It has been found in the treatment of osteogenic sarcoma that the minority of patients whose primary tumor does not respond immediately and satisfactorily to chemotherapy are indeed the patients at risk for relapsing when that same chemotherapy is continued as adjuvant chemotherapy. Therefore, alternative chemotherapy protocols are being developed for patients who do not show a satisfactory response of their primary tumor to initial chemotherapy. Of course, patients must be monitored very carefully while on preoperative chemotherapy, not allowing the primary tumor to become inoperable at any point. This necessitates very careful observation of the patient and frequent documentation of the patient's primary tumor disease state. The use of nuclear imaging and CT scans at frequent intervals can ensure that the patient is responding to preoperative chemotherapy, and allow documentation of the response.

Only through the latter approach can it be hoped to obtain sufficient data on all of the different types of sarcomas and their sensitivity to various chemotherapeutic agents. Not only is this important for clinical investigation, but it benefits the patient in that if chemotherapy is proven not to be effective in a particular patient, it would be in the patient's best interest to use a different chemotherapy protocol in the postoperative period. The experience with osteogenic sarcoma has demonstrated that 100% of patients showing a good response to preoperative chemotherapy are disease-free survivors when continued on that same chemotherapy protocol postoperatively (see Figure 38–15). Approximately 60% of the patients who do not respond favorably, however, go on to relapse following the continuation of the same chemotherapy protocol. We have recently added cisplatin to the chemotherapy protocol for patients who do not have a favorable response of their primary tumor when postoperative chemotherapy is commenced. Initial results are extremely encouraging and should serve as a model for the treatment of other sarcomas.

With consideration of all available modalities of therapy, the following conclusions can be made:

1. *Patients presenting for treatment following ablative surgery of their high-grade sarcoma:* These patients should be placed on adjuvant combination chemotherapy. Their disease-free interval should be evaluated with reference to the stage of primary tumor involved.
2. *Patients presenting with a primary malignant sarcoma following biopsy:* These patients should undergo intensive com-

bination chemotherapy preoperatively. The response of the primary tumor should be continued if there is a favorable histologic response; if the primary tumor has not responded to preoperative chemotherapy, a different chemotherapy regimen should be substituted following local therapy.

3. *Patients presenting with tumor and distant metastases:* These patients should also be treated with preoperative combination chemotherapy. Local therapy should be delayed from two to four months until the distant metastases can be objectively controlled with combination chemotherapy. Following the successful control of distant metastases, the primary tumor may receive local therapy; in addition, areas that contain metastatic deposits require local therapy. Radiation therapy is given to the lungs for sarcomas such as embryonal rhabdomyosarcoma and Ewing's sarcoma even though pulmonary metastases may have responded completely to chemotherapy. In cases of high-grade sarcomas such as pleomorphic liposarcoma, fibrosarcoma, fibrous histiocytoma, pleomorphic rhabdomyosarcoma, and osteogenic sarcoma, surgical removal of residual nodules following surgery for the primary tumor is indicated. Postoperatively, adjuvant chemotherapy is continued with the same regimen. In patients who fail to respond to combination chemotherapy, the phase II agents with expected activity in the treatment of that particular disease should be tried, either alone or in combination, following failure of the first-line combination chemotherapy protocol. Examples of agents currently under investigation are high-dose methotrexate with folinic acid rescue, high-dose cisplatin with mannitol diuresis, and high-dose cisplatin in combination with doxorubicin. Should any of these agents be effective in treating the patient who has failed to respond to conventional combination chemotherapy, they should be continued in the postoperative setting.

4. *Patients presenting following primary surgery with distant metastases:* These patients should be treated the same as patients in group 2. With the investigational approach to each individual patient, more data can be generated on the role of both combination chemotherapy and new phase II agents in the treatment of these rare sarcomas. This approach allows modification of protocols and continued observation of an increase in the response rate by treating patients with evaluable disease. The investigative approach does not preclude excellent medical care for the patient, since it is in the patient's best interest that the role of effective chemotherapy in the treatment of his sarcoma be documented. Those few patients who are not responsive are identified as those who will be at a high risk to relapse even if continued on the same adjuvant chemotherapy. Other drugs can then be utilized which may be more effective for that particular patient in an attempt to achieve prolonged disease-free survival. The best hope to achieve the highest cure rates in treatment of any soft tissue or bone sarcoma is, of course, to try to keep the patient free of disease. Once metastases develop, the chance of patient salvage has diminished. In addition, the majority of patients receiving preoperative chemotherapy also benefit by the ability to use less aggressive local therapy following chemotherapy. Local therapy must stand on its own merits, but it is well known that the smaller the size of the primary tumor, the easier it is to achieve permanent local control.

Future Prospects

The progress made in the treatment of soft tissue and bone sarcomas during the last decade is encouraging. It is hoped that better understanding of the biologic behavior (Hajdu and Fogh, 1978; Hajdu et al., 1981; Kissane et al., 1981), growth patterns (Erlandson, 1981; Newman and Hajdu, in preparation), and cytochemistry (Hajdu, 1985) of sarcomas will lead to more meaningful classification and subdivision of sarcomas that are geared to therapeutic plans. Continuous cooperation of pathologists, surgeons, radiation therapists, and medical oncologists will further our understanding of these relatively rare but very complex malignant neoplasms.

REFERENCES

Azizi, F.; Bitran, J.; Javehari, G.; and Herbst, A. L.: Remission of uterine leiomyosarcomas treated with vincristine, ADRIAMYCIN and dimethyltriazeno-imidazole carboximide. *Am. J. Obstet. Gynecol.,* **133:**379, 1979.

Benjamin, R. S.; Baker, L. H.; O'Bryan, R. M.; Moon, T. E.; and Gottlieb, J. A.: Advances in the chemotherapy of soft tissue sarcomas. *Med. Clin. North Am.,* **61:**1039, 1977a.

Benjamin, R. S.; Baker, L. H.; Rodriguez, V.; O'Bryan, R. M.; Stephens, R. L.; Sinkovics, J. G.; Thigpen, T.; King, G. W.; Bottomley, R.; Groppe, C. W., Jr.; Bodey, G. P.; and Gottlieb, J. A.: The chemotherapy of soft tissue sarcomas in adults. In: *Management of Primary Bone and Soft Tissue Tumors.* Year Book Medical Publishers, Inc., Chicago, 1977b.

Burchenal, J. H.: From wild fowl to stalking horses. Alchemy in chemotherapy. *Cancer,* **35:**1121, 1975.

Campanacci, M.; Bacci, G.; Bertoni, F.; Picci, P.; Minutillo, A.; and Franceschi, C.: The treatment of osteosarcoma of the extremities. *Cancer,* **48:**1569, 1981.

Castro, E. B.; Hajdu, S. I.; and Fortner, J. G.: Surgical therapy of fibrosarcoma of extremities. *Arch. Surg.,* **107:**284, 1973.

Chung, E. B., and Enzinger, F. M.: Infantile fibrosarcoma. *Cancer,* **38:**729, 1976.

Cody, H. S.; Turnbull, A. D.; Fortner, J. G.; and Hajdu, S. I.: The continuing challenge of retroperitoneal sarcomas. *Cancer,* **47:**2147, 1981.

Cortes, E. P.; Holland, J. F.; Wang, J. J; and Sinks, L. F.: Doxorubicin in disseminated osteosarcoma. *J.A.M.A.,* **221:**1132, 1972.

Dahlin, D. C., and Conventry, M. B.: Osteogenic sarcoma. A study of 600 cases. *J. Bone Joint Surg. [Am]* **49:**101, 1967.

Dahlin, D. C., and MacCarty, C. S.: Chordoma. A study of fifty-nine cases. *Cancer,* **5:**1170, 1952.

Dahlin, D. C., and Salvador, A. H.: Chondrosarcomas of bones of the hands and feet. A study of 30 cases. *Cancer,* **34:**755, 1974.

DeVita, V. T.; Young, R. C.; and Canellos, G. P.: Combination versus single agent chemotherapy. A review of the basis for selection of drug treatment of cancer. *Cancer,* **35:**98, 1975.

Enneking, W. F.; Spanier, S. S.; and Goodman, M. A.: The surgical staging of musculoskeletal sarcoma. *J. Bone Joint Surg. [Am.],* **62A:**1027, 1980.

Erlandson, R. A.: *Diagnosing Transmission Electron Microscopy of Human Tumors. The Interpretation of Submicroscopic Structures in Human Neoplastic Cells.* Masson Publishing U.S.A., Inc., New York, 1981.

Farr, G. H.; Huvos, A. G.; Marcove, R.; Higinbotham, N. L.; and Foote, F. W.: Telangiectatic osteogenic sarcoma: A review of 28 cases. *Cancer,* **34:**1150, 1974.

Fine, G.; Hajdu, S. I.; Morton, D. L.; Eilber, F. R.; Suit, H. D.; and Weiss, S. W.: Soft tissue sarcoma. Classification and treatment (a symposium). In Sommers, S. S., and Rosen, P. P. (eds.): *Pathology Annual,* Part 1, Vol. 17. Appleton-Century-Crofts, New York, 1982.

Fortner, J. G.; Martin, S.; Hajdu S. I.; and Turnbull, A.: Primary sarcoma of the retroperitoneum. *Semin. Oncol.,* **8:**180, 1981.

Geisinger, K. R.; Hajdu, S. I.; and Miller, D. R.: Exfoliative cytology of nonlymphoreticular neoplasms in children. *Acta Cytologica,* **28:**16, 1984.

Gerson, R.; Shiu, M. H.; and Hajdu, S. I.: Sarcoma of the buttock: A trend toward limb-saving resection. *J. Surg. Oncol.,* **19:**238, 1982.

Goldman, R. L.; Jones, S. E.; and Heusinkveld, R. S.: Combination chemotherapy of metastatic malignant schwannoma with vincristine, ADRIAMYCIN, cyclo-

phosphamide and imidazole carboxamide. *Cancer,* **39:**1955, 1977.

Gottlieb, J. A.: Combination chemotherapy for metastatic sarcoma. *Cancer Chemother. Rep.,* **58:**265, 1974.

Gottlieb, J. A.; Baker, L. H.; O'Bryan, R. M.; Sinkovics, J. G.; Hoogstraten, B.; Quagliana, J. M.; Rivkin, S. E.; Bodey, G. P., Sr.; Rodriguez, V. T.; Blumenschein, G. R.; Saiki, J. H.; Coltman, C., Jr.; Burgess, M. A.; Sullivan, P.; Thigpen, T.; Bottomley, R.; Balcerzak, S.; and Moon, T. E.: ADRIAMYCIN (NSC-123127) used alone and in combination for soft tissue and bony sarcomas. *Cancer Chemother. Rep.,* part 3, **6:**271, 1975.

Gottlieb, J. A.; Baker, L. H.; Quagliana, J. M.; Luce, J. K.; Whitecar, J. P., Jr.; Sinkovics, J. G.; Rivkin, S. E.; Brownlee, R.; and Frei, E., III: Chemotherapy of sarcomas with a combination of ADRIAMYCIN and di-methyl-triazeno-imidazole carboxamide. *Cancer,* **30:**1632, 1972.

Hajdu, S. I.: *Pathology of Soft Tissue Tumors.* Lea & Febiger, Philadelphia, 1979.

Hajdu, S. I.: The paradox of sarcomas. *Acta Cytol. (Baltimore),* **24:**373, 1980.

Hajdu, S. I.: Soft tissue sarcoma. Classification and natural history. *CA,* **31:**271, 1981.

Hajdu, S. I.: *Differential Diagnosis of Soft Tissue and Bone Tumors.* Lea & Febiger, Philadelphia, 1985.

Hajdu, S. I., and Fogh, J.: The nude mouse as a diagnostic tool in human tumor cell research. In Fogh, J., and Giovanella, B. C. (eds.): *The Nude Mouse in Experimental and Clinical Research.* Academic Press, Inc., New York, 1978.

Hajdu, S. I., and Hajdu, E. O.: *Cytopathology of Sarcomas and Other Nonepithelial Malignant Tumors.* W. B. Saunders Company, Philadelphia, 1976.

Hajdu, S. I.; Lemos, L. B.; Kozakewich, H.; and Beattie, E. J.: Growth pattern and differentiation of human soft tissue sarcomas in nude mice. *Cancer,* **47:**90, 1981.

Hajdu, S. I., and Melamed, M. R.: The diagnostic value of aspiration smears. *Am. J. Clin. Pathol.,* **59:**350, 1973.

Hajdu, S. I.; Shiu, M. H.; and Fortner, J. G.: Tendosynovial sarcoma: A clinicopathological study of 136 cases. *Cancer,* **39:**1201, 1977.

Hajdu, S. I.; Shiu, M. H.; and Sordillo, P.: Extraskeletal chondrosarcoma. *Cancer,* In Press.

Heyn, R. M.; Holland, R.,; Newton, W. A.; Tefft, M.,; Breslow, N.; and Hartman, J. R.: The role of combined chemotherapy in the treatment of rhabdomyosarcoma in children. *Cancer,* **34:**2128, 1974.

Hilaris, B. S.; Shiu, M. H.; Nori, N.; Batata, M. A.; Hopfan, S.; Anderson, L. R.; Hajdu, S. I.; and Turnbull, A. D.: Perioperative brachytherapy and surgery in soft tissue sarcomas. In Hilaris, B. S., and Nori, D. (eds.): *Brachytherapy Oncology — 1982.* Memorial Sloan-Kettering Cancer Center, New York, 1982.

Huvos, A. G.: *Bone Tumors: Diagnosis, Treatment and Prognosis.* W. B. Saunders Company, Philadelphia, 1979.

Isacoff, W. H.; Eilber, F.; Tabbarah, H.; Klein, P.; Dollinger, M.; Lemkin, S.; Sheehy, P.; Cone, L.; Rosenloom, B.; Sieger, L.; and Block, J. B.: Phase II clinical trial with high dose methotrexate therapy and citrovorum factor rescue. *Cancer Treat. Rep.,* **62:**1295, 1978.

Jaffe, N.: Recent advances in the chemotherapy of metastatic osteogenic sarcoma. *Cancer,* **20:**1627, 1972.

Jaffe, N.; Frei, E.; Traggis, D.; and Watta, H.: Weekly high dose methotrexate-citrovorum factor in osteogenic sarcoma. *Cancer,* **39:**45, 1977.

Karakousis, C. P.; Holtermann, O. A.; and Holyoke, E. D.: *Cis*-dichlorodiammineplatinum (II) in metastatic soft tissue sarcomas. *Cancer Treat. Rep.,* **63**:2071, 1979.

Kissane, J. M.; Askin, F. B.; Nesbit, M. E., Jr.; Vietti, T. J.; Burgert, E. D., Jr.; Cangir, A.; Gehan, E. A.; Perez, C. A.; Pritchard, D. J.; and Tefft, M.: Sarcomas of bone in childhood: Pathologic aspects. *Natl. Cancer Inst. Monogr.* **56**:29-41, 1981.

Krall, R. A.; Kostianovsky, M.; and Patchefsky, A. S.: Synovial sarcoma. A clinical, pathological and ultrastructural study of 26 cases supporting the recognition of monophasic variant. *Am. J. Surg. Pathol.,* **5**:137, 1981.

Lee, S. M.; Hajdu, S. I.; and Exelby, P. R.: Synovial sarcoma in children. *Surg. Gynecol. Obstet.,* **138**:701, 1974.

Leite, C.; Goodwin, J. W.; Sinkovics, J. G.; Baker, L. H.; and Benjamin, T.: Chemotherapy of malignant fibrous histiocytoma. *Cancer,* **40**:2019, 1977.

Livingston, R. B., and Carter, S. K.: *Single Agents in Cancer Chemotherapy.* Plenum Publishing Corporation, New York, 1970.

Lloyd, R. V.; Hajdu, S. I.; and Knapper, W. H.: Embryonal rhabdomyosarcoma in adults. *Cancer,* **51**:557, 1983.

Lobenthal, S.; Hajdu, S. I.; and Urmacher, C.: Cytologic findings in homosexual males. *Acta Cytol.,* **27**:597, 1983.

Luce, J. K.; Thurman, W. G.; Isaacs, B. L.; and Talley, R. W.: Clinical trials with the antitumor agent 5(3,3-dimethyl-1-triazeno)imidazole-4-carboxamide (NSC-45388). *Cancer Chemother. Rep.,* **54**:119, 1970.

Mosende, C.; Gutierrez, M.; Caparros, B; and Rosen, G.: Combination chemotherapy with bleomycin, cyclophosphamide and dactinomycin for the treatment of osteogenic sarcoma. *Cancer,* **40**:2779, 1977.

Mukai, K.; Rosai, J.; and Hallaway, B. E.: Localization of myoglobin in normal and neoplastic skeletal muscle cells using an immunoperoxidase method. *Am. J. Surg. Pathol.,* **3**:375, 1979.

Newman, H., and Hajdu, S. I.: Growth rate and differentiation of human soft tissue and bone neoplasms in athymic mice. In preparation.

Ochs, J. J.; Freeman, A. I.; Douglass, H. O., Jr.; Higby, D. S.; Mindell, E. R.; and Sinks, L. F.: *Cis*-dichlorodiammineplatinum (II) in advanced osteogenic sarcoma. *Cancer Treat. Rep.,* **62**:239, 1978.

Parente, J. T.; Axelrod, M. R.; Levy, J. L.; and Chiang, C. E.: Leiomyosarcoma of the uterus with pulmonary metastases: A favorable response to operation and chemotherapy in a patient monitored with serial carcinoembryonic antigen. *Am. J. Obstet. Gynecol.* (Communications in Brief), **131**:812, 1978.

Patchefsky, A. S.; Soriano, R.; and Kostianovsky, M: Epithelioid sarcoma: Ultrastructural similarity to nodular synovitis. *Cancer,* **39**:143, 1977.

Rivkin, S. E.; Gottlieb, J. A.; Thigpen, T.; El Mawla, N. G.; Saiki, J.; and Dixon, D. O.: Methyl CCNU and ADRIAMYCIN for patients with metastatic sarcomas: A Southwest Oncology Group study. *Cancer,* **46**:446, 1980.

Rosen, G.: Primary Ewing's sarcoma: The multidisciplinary lesion. *Int. J. Radiat. Oncol. Biol. Phys.,* **4**:527, 1978.

Rosen, G.; Huvos, A. G.; Mosende, C.; Beattie, E. J., Jr.; Exelby, P. R.; Capparos, B.; and Marcove, R. C.: Chemotherapy and thoracotomy for metastatic osteogenic sarcoma: A model for adjuvant chemotherapy and the rationale for the timing of thoracic surgery. *Cancer,* **41**:841, 1978.

Rosen, G.; Juergens, H.; Caparros, B.; Nirenberg, A.; Huvos, A. G.; and Marcove, R. C.: Combination chemotherapy (T-6) in the multidisciplinary treatment of Ewing's sarcoma. *Natl. Cancer Inst. Monogr.,* **56**:213-220, 1981.

Rosen, G.; Marcove, R. C.; and Caparros, B.: Primary osteogenic sarcoma: The rationale for preoperative chemotherapy and delayed surgery. *Cancer,* **43**:2163, 1979.

Rosen, G.; Wollner, N.; Tan, C.; Wu, S. J.; Hajdu, S. I.; Cham, W.; D'Angio, G. J.; and Murphy, M. L.: Disease-free survival in children with Ewing's sarcoma treated with radiation therapy and adjuvant four-drug sequential chemotherapy. *Cancer,* **33**:384, 1974.

Rosenberg, S. A.; Kent, H.; Costa, J.; Webber, B. L.; Young, R.; Chabner, B.; Baker, A. R.; Brennan, M. F.; Chretien, P. B.; Cohen, M. H.; de Moss, E. V.; Sears, H. F.; Seipp, C.; and Simon, R.: Prospective randomized evaluation of the role of limb-sparing surgery, radiation therapy and adjuvant chemoimmunotherapy in the treatment of adult soft tissue sarcomas. *Surgery,* **84**:62, 1978.

Russell, W. O.; Cohen, J.; Edomson, J. H.; Enzinger, F.; Hajdu, S. I.; Heise, H.; Martin, R. G.; Miller, W. T.; Schmitz, R. L.; and Suit, H. D.: Staging system for soft tissue sarcomas. *Semin. Oncol.,* **8**:156, 1981.

Samson, M. K.; Baker, L. H.; Bentamin, R. S.; Lane, M.; and Plager, C.: *Cis*-dichlorodiammine-platinum (II) in advanced soft tissue and bone sarcomas. *Cancer Treat. Rep.,* **63**:2027, 1979.

Shiu, M. H.; Castro, E. B.; Hajdu, S. I.; and Fortner, J. G.: Surgical treatment of 297 soft tissue sarcomas of the lower extremity. *Ann. Surg.,* **182**:597, 1975.

Shiu, M. H.; Farr, G. H.; Papachristou, D. N.; and Hajdu, S. I.: Myosarcomas of the stomach: Natural history, prognostic factors and management. *Cancer,* **49**:177, 1982.

Shiu, M. H.; Flacbaum, L.; Hajdu, S. I.; and Fortner, J. G.: Malignant soft tissue tumors of the anterior abdominal wall. *Arch. Surg.,* **115**:152, 1980.

Shiu, M. H., and Hajdu, S. I.: Management of soft tissue sarcoma of the extremity. *Semin. Oncol.,* **8**:172, 1981.

Shiu, M. H.; McCormack, P. M.; Hajdu, S. I.; and Fortner, J. G.: Surgical treatment of tendosynovial sarcoma. *Cancer,* **43**:889, 1979.

Smith, J., and Hajdu, S. I.: Blastic bone metastases from tendosynovial sarcoma. *Clin. Bull. MSKCC,* **9**:130, 1979.

Sordillo, P. P.; Chapman, R.; Hajdu, S. I.; Magill, G. B.; and Golbey, R. B.: Lymphangiosarcoma. *Cancer,* **48**:1674, 1981a.

Sordillo, P. P.; Helson, L.; Hajdu, S. I.; Magill, G. B.; Kosloff, C.; Golbey, R. B.; and Beattie, E. J.: Malignant schwannoma. Clinical characteristics, survival and response to therapy. *Cancer,* **47**:2503, 1981b.

Sordillo, P. P.; Magill, G. B.; Shiu, M. H.; Lesser, M., Hajdu, S. I.; and Golbey, R. B.: Adjuvant chemotherapy of soft-part sarcomas with ALMOD (S4). *J. Surg. Oncol.,* **18**:345, 1981c.

Sordillo, P. P.; Hajdu, S. I.; Magill, G. B.; and Golbey, R. B.: Extraosseous osteogenic sarcoma. Review of 48 patients. *Cancer,* **51**:727, 1983.

Soule, E. H., and Enriquez, P.: Atypical fibrous histiocytoma, malignant fibrous histiocytoma, malignant histiocytoma and epithelioid sarcoma. A comparative study of sixty-five tumors. *Cancer,* **30**:128, 1972.

Soule, E. H., and Pritchard, D. J.: Fibrosarcoma in infants and children. *Cancer,* **40**:1711, 1976.

Subramanian, S., and Wiltshaw, E.: Chemotherapy of sarcomas: A comparison of three regimens. *Lancet,* 1:683, 1978.

Suit, H. D.; Proppe, K. H.; Mankin, H. J.; and Wood, W. C.: Preoperative radiation therapy for sarcoma of soft tissue. *Cancer,* 47:2269, 1981.

Suit, H.; Russell, W. O. and Martin, R. G.: Sarcoma of soft tissue: Clinical and histopathologic parameters and response to treatment. *Cancer,* 35:1478, 1975.

Sutow, W. W.: Vincristine (NSC-67574) therapy for malignant solid tumors in children (except Wilms' tumor). *Cancer Chemother. Rep.,* 52:485, 1968.

Sutow, W. W.; Berry, D. H.; Haddy, T. B.; Sullivan, M. P.; Watkins, W. L.; and Windmiller, J.: Vincristine sulfate therapy in children with metastatic soft tissue sarcoma. *Pediatrics,* 38:465, 1966.

Tan, C. T. C.; Dargeon, H. W.; and Burchenal, J. H.: The effect of actinomycin D on cancer in childhood. *Pediatrics,* 24:544, 1959.

Tan, C.; Etcubanas, E.; Wollner, N.; Rosen, G.; Gilladoga, A.; Showel, J.; Murphy, M. L.; and Krakoff, I. H.: Adriamycin—an antitumor antibiotic in the treatment of neoplastic diseases. *Cancer,* 32:9, 1973.

Thomsen, H. K.; Jacobsen, M.; and Malchow-Miller, A.: Kaposi's sarcoma among homosexual men in Europe. *Lancet,* 2:688, 1981.

Urmacher, C.; Myskowski, P.; Ochoa, M.; Kris, M.; and Safai, B.: Outbreak of Kaposi's sarcoma with cytomegalovirus infection in young homosexual males. *Am. J. Med.,* 72:569, 1982.

Wilbur, J. R.: Combination chemotherapy for embryonal rhabdomyosarcoma. *Cancer Chemother. Rep.,* 58:281, 1974.

Wiltshaw, E.: Methotrexate in treatment of sarcomata. *Br. J. Med.,* 2:142, 1967.

Yap, B. S.; Baker, L. H.; Sinkovics, J. G.; Rivkin, S. E.; Bottomley, R.; Thigpen, T.; Burgess, M. A.; Benjamin, R. S.; and Bodey, G. P.: Cyclophosphamide, vincristine, ADRIAMYCIN and DTIC (CYVADIC) combination chemotherapy for the treatment of advanced sarcomas. *Cancer Treat. Rep.,* 64:93, 1980.

Zaatari, G.; Hajdu, S. I.; and Shiu, M. H.: Soft tissue sarcomas of the trunk., In preparation.

39

Pediatric Neoplasms

DONALD PINKEL and CATHRYN B. HOWARTH

EPIDEMIOLOGY AND ETIOLOGY

Cancer is the most frequent cause of death from disease in American children over 1 year of age. The death rate of 4.4 per 100,000 population among children aged 1 through 14 is almost one-half of the incidence rate of 11 per 100,000 (Silverberg, 1982). Acute leukemia is the most frequent type of cancer, followed by brain tumors, lymphomas, and neuroblastoma (see Table 39–1).

The types and frequencies of pediatric neoplasms vary with age, sex, ethnicity, socioeconomic status, and geographic location. For example, neuroblastoma is most frequent in the first four years of life, whereas bone sarcomas typically occur in adolescents and young adults. Thymic lymphoma and leukemia occur more often in boys than girls (Sen and Borella, 1975). Ewing's sarcoma is a disease of white children, not black (Fraumeni, 1982). Acute lymphocytic leukemia affects middle-class children more frequently than poor children (Pinkel and Nefzger, 1959). B-lymphoblastic lymphoma (Burkitt's tumor) strikes African children more often than American or European children (Epstein and Achong, 1979). These variations suggest differences in etiology and indicate the importance of genetic, developmental, sexual, and environmental factors in the pathogenesis of childhood cancer.

Some pediatric neoplasms clearly demonstrate genetic etiology. For example, bilateral retinoblastoma is transmitted from parent to child as an autosomal dominant trait. Other neoplasms develop in children with hereditary preneoplastic developmental disorders, such as multiple neurofibromatosis, xeroderma

pigmentosum, Fanconi's aplastic anemia, Wiskott-Aldrich syndrome, and Beckwith-Weideman syndrome (Fraumeni, 1982). In still other instances of familial cancer, whether genetic or environmental factors or both are causative is not clear. For example, instances of childhood rhabdomyosarcoma in siblings have been associated with increased frequency of breast cancer in their mothers and female relatives (Fraumeni, 1982).

Three types of environmental agents have been associated with pathogenesis of childhood cancer: ionizing radiation, drugs, and viruses (Miller, 1978). Children exposed to atomic-bomb radiation have an increased incidence of leukemia. Thymic irradiation in early infancy leads to high rates of thyroid carcinoma and leukemia. Therapeutic radiation is often followed by second tumors in the radiated areas.

The only drug demonstrated to cause cancer in children is stilbestrol. The female children of mothers who received this hormone during pregnancy are at risk of adenocarcinoma of the vagina during late adolescence (Miller, 1978). Careful clinical observation may identify other drug-related cancers in children.

Viruses have long been suspect in the causation of pediatric neoplasms, particularly acute leukemia. The two-to-six-year age peak in frequency of acute lymphocytic leukemia, the higher incidence in upper socioeconomic groups, and the reports of temporal spatial aggregation of cases may suggest a widespread infectious agent with a low rate of clinical expression (Pinkel and Nefzger, 1959). However, many studies have failed to confirm significant case aggregation, and intensive investigation has failed to reveal candidate viruses. The only

Table 39-1. Cancer Incidence by Site (For Children Under 15, SEER Program, 1973-1976)

RANK	SITE	NUMBER OF CASES	PERCENT OF TOTAL	RATE PER 1,000,000 CHILDREN
1.	Leukemia	664	30.2	33.6
2.	Central nervous system	409	18.6	20.7
3.	Lymphomas	298	13.6	15.1
4.	Sympathetic nervous system	170	7.7	8.6
5.	Soft tissue	141	6.5	7.1
6.	Kidney	135	6.1	6.8
7.	Bone	101	4.6	5.1
8.	Retinoblastoma	58	2.6	3.0
9.	Liver	26	1.2	1.3
	All others	195	8.9	9.9
	All sites	2,197	100.0	111.1

Source: SEER Program, National Cancer Institute
Reproduced by permission of the American Cancer Society from Silverberg, E.: Cancer statistics, 1982. *CA,* **32:**15-31, 1982.

virus identified with a childhood cancer is Epstein-Barr virus (EBV), which is associated with B-lymphoblastic lymphoma (Burkitt's tumor) as it occurs in African children (Epstein and Achong, 1979). Since these children sometimes develop acute B-cell lymphocytic leukemia, EBV is also leukemia-associated. Whether a safe, effective vaccine against EBV will be developed and whether it will prevent B-lymphoblastic lymphoma and leukemia in African children are yet to be determined (Epstein, 1979).

DIFFERENCES BETWEEN CHILDHOOD AND ADULT CANCER

Cancer is much less frequent in children than adults. However, taking into account the years of productive life, saving a two-year-old child from cancer may have many times the value of saving a 50-year-old adult. The significance of childhood cancer in human terms is thus at least as great as that of adult cancer.

Children have different types of cancer from adults. Leukemias and sarcomas predominate in children, whereas carcinomas form the bulk of adult neoplasms. Two-thirds of childhood neoplasms arise from lymphohematopoietic and nervous tissues and 90% of adult cancer is epithelial (Silverberg, 1982). Typical childhood neoplasms such as neuroblastoma and Wilms' tumors are rare in adults, while typical adult cancers are either rare in children, as intestinal carcinoma, or not reported, as bronchogenic carcinoma.

The pathogenesis of cancer in children and adults is different. Adult cancers are largely related to chemical carcinogenesis, often environmental. Cigarette smoking alone accounts for 30% of adult cancer. On the other hand children's cancers seem more often related to genetic factors and developmental disorders. Childhood rhabdomyosarcoma, for example, appears to consist of anaplastic mesenchymal cells differentiating toward primitive skeletal muscle cells, whereas adult rhabdomyosarcoma is a neoplasm of skeletal muscle cells themselves.

Pediatric neoplasms usually grow more rapidly than adult neoplasms. Growth fractions are greater, mitoses more frequent, and local extension and metastases occur earlier. On the other hand, the risk periods for relapse and metastases tend to be shorter. For example, most children with Wilms' tumor who remain free of cancer for two years are cured (Lemerle *et al.,* 1975).

The patterns of metastatic spread tend to differ between childhood and adult neoplasms. Pediatric neoplasms more often metastasize by venous channels and appear early in lungs and long bones. Adult cancers more commonly metastasize by lymphatic channels.

Pediatric neoplasms generally are more responsive to anticancer drugs than adult cancers. The development of effective cancer chemotherapy and its integration into multidisciplinary evaluation and treatment have produced a tenfold decline in childhood cancer mortality over the past 25 years (Pinkel, 1978). Except for a relatively small percentage of cancers, cancer chemotherapy has not appreciably influenced adult cancer mortality.

For the majority of pediatric neoplasms, chemotherapy is now first-line treatment, supplemented by surgery and radiation therapy as required. For most adult neoplasms, surgery and radiation therapy are the primary modalities of treatment, and chemotherapy remains adjuvant or palliative.

Last, and perhaps most important, children are dynamic, growing, developing, differentiating persons, whereas adults have already reached maturity. While attempting to cure children of cancer, oncologists must be constantly aware of their developmental needs and the importance of preserving and promoting their capacity for normal growth and development: physical, functional, and social.

GENERAL PRINCIPLES OF CARING FOR CHILDREN WITH CANCER

Promptness in evaluation and treatment is important in caring for children with cancer. Tumor growth and progression can be rapid, and disease stage can advance from a good prognosis to a poor prognosis within a few days. In the case of thymic lymphoblastic lymphoma, a child admitted ambulatory in the morning can be strangling by midnight. Surgeons, pathologists, and radiologists who work with children must be willing to work through nights and weekends to establish accurate diagnosis and staging quickly so that the oncologist can initiate specific and timely treatment.

Histopathologic and cytologic diagnosis of pediatric neoplasms can be difficult because they are frequently so anaplastic. For this reason initial aspiration, biopsy, or resection of children's cancers need to be conducted in a children's cancer center where morphologists have continuous intensive experience with pediatric neoplasms and are prepared to use electron microscopy, cytochemistry, cell surface marker, immunofluorescence, and tissue culture methods. To do otherwise is to risk unwarranted delay in diagnosis or, worse, inaccurate or incomplete diagnosis.

Because pediatric neoplasms constitute only 1% of all cancer, most surgeons, radiotherapists, and chemotherapists have little continuing experience with them. As a result, their knowledge of current practices and their skills in pediatric cancer tend to be rusty despite good training as residents and fellows. The physician who first suspects that a child has cancer best fulfills a golden opportunity to assure the child the best chance for cure by referring the child to a children's cancer center.

The initial approach to all pediatric neoplasms should be *curative,* regardless of stage. There are three reasons for this principle. First, many children can recover from advanced cancer. For example, approximately one-half of patients with Wilms' tumor metastatic to the lungs are cured with combination chemotherapy and low-dose pulmonary irradiation (Wara *et al.,* 1974). Infants with bone marrow metastases of neuroblastoma are often cured (Jaffe, 1976). Second, palliative methods usually give brief respite in children's neoplasms because of rapid growth rates and tendency to early relapses when tumor is not completely eradicated. Third, curing a child preserves a whole lifetime with all its potentials, not merely extends twilight years.

Treatment of children with cancer needs to be *comprehensive* and *coordinated* from the day the diagnosis is suspected. The medical team of pediatric oncologist, pathologist, diagnostic radiologist, surgeon, and radiation oncologist must work as one to assure optimal management. In addition, nurses, rehabilitationists, dentists, dietitians, psychologists, and social workers are part of the team to enhance the total care of the patient. Most important, the child and the family need a trusted primary physician in the community or the cancer center with whom they can plan treatment and learn how to cope with the disease and its management. This primary physician is the child's advocate, the fulcrum for balancing treatment options with patient needs, and the final arbiter of health care decisions.

Honesty with the child as well as the family is an important principle. The children must be told their diagnoses and their questions answered truthfully, with tact, sensitivity, and regard for their developmental level. Diagnosis and treatment options are best discussed in family conferences that include the patient. Signed permission for treatment should be obtained from all children who can write their names.

SUPPORTIVE CARE

Prompt bacteriocidal antibiotic therapy for suspected sepsis and timely platelet transfusions for serious thrombocytopenic bleeding often extend life so that specific measures can exert their effect. However, some supportive modalities must be carefully weighed against their risks and their value critically questioned. In this category are reverse isolation systems, particularly "life islands," parenteral hyperalimentation, granulocyte transfusions, and prophylactic antibacterials.

Life-island isolation and parenteral hyperalimentation may allow administration of higher doses of antineoplastic drugs that produce immunosuppression, granulocytopenia, and nutritional disturbances. Therapeutic margins of antineoplastic drugs, however, are generally narrow and no proof exists that the additional dosage achieved in this way affects the course of neoplasms. Second, the superiority of life-island isolation over ordinary handwash and room isolation or home care is not established. Finally, such measures work against the objective of normalizing life for the child with cancer because they extend hospitalization, disrupt school attendance and customary play, and interfere with the usual social bonds of family and friends.

Because of recent advances in home health services, parenteral hyperalimentation can now be safely and conveniently administered during the night at home by parents. The advantage of good nutrition can be attained without the liability of hospitalization.

Although granulocyte transfusions have been used for 20 years in patients with granulocytopenia and serious infection, their value remains equivocal (Strauss et al., 1981). The risks of sensitization and pulmonary compromise by leukocyte sequestration are evident.

In a comparative study in children with leukemia at exceptionally high risk of Pneumocystis carinii pneumonia, co-trimoxazole was effective in its prevention (Hughes et al., 1977). Co-trimoxazole can produce megaloblastic anemia, leukopenia, and thrombocytopenia (Asmar et al., 1979; Kobrinski and Ramsay, 1981). Whether it reduces tolerance to cancer chemotherapy, contributes to methotrexate-associated encephalopathy, or provides sufficient protection against bacterial infections to justify its prophylactic administration to patients not at high risk of Pneumocystis pneumonia is not determined.

FOLLOW-UP CARE

Children with cancer are at high risk of numerous sequelae of their neoplasms and their treatment (Jaffe, 1979). For this reason, they need to be evaluated regularly throughout the rest of their lives.

Late recurrences of pediatric neoplasms are not unusual, particularly with medulloblastoma and Ewing's sarcoma. In addition, children cured of one cancer are at excessive risk of a second neoplasm (Li, 1977; Pratt et al., 1981a). Some second cancers are distinct from the first, such as osteogenic sarcoma of the limbs in children cured of retinoblastoma. Some appear to be related, such as Hodgkin's disease or acute myelocytic leukemia in patients in remission of acute lymphocytic leukemia. Others are caused by the treatment, such as fibrosarcoma at the site of prior radiation therapy. Early detection and prompt treatment of second neoplasms improve chances of cure.

Endocrinopathy following cancer therapy has been well described (Jaffe, 1979). Hypothyroidism, hypopituitarism, and hypogonadism are particularly important side effects in children because they can interfere with normal growth and development, social and sexual as well as physical and emotional. Early detection, timely counseling, and hormonal substitution can profoundly improve the quality of survival.

Virtually all organ systems can demonstrate sequelae of cancer therapy. Muscle atrophy in former radiation portals can result in muscle weakness and muscle imbalance. Children who have received radiation for Wilms' tumor often develop scoliosis (Riseborough et al., 1976). Radiotherapy can retard or arrest bone growth. Extremity radiation can be followed by unequal length, and lumbar spine irradiation can lead to lordosis. At high radiation doses aseptic necrosis of bone and destruction of joints can result in severe disability (Jaffe, 1979).

Cardiomyopathy after anthracycline therapy, leukoencephalopathy and hepatic fibrosis after methotrexate, pulmonary fibrosis after bleomycin, urinary bladder fibrosis and carcinoma after cyclophosphamide, peripheral neuropathy after vincristine, and auditory loss after cisplatin are described in Chapter 10 of this text. Whether these agents are producing more subtle changes in growing and developing organ systems that will emerge as major pathology with the increased demands of full growth and maturation is a pertinent question. In order to answer this question, careful observations over the years are needed with specific testing of organ systems that are candidates for dysfunction.

Children cured of cancer are often left with handicaps—physical, psychological, and social. Follow-up care must make certain that the patients receive the necessary educational, social, rehabilitation, and psychological services.

Finally, for children with neoplasms that are hereditable or associated with hereditable disorders, genetic counseling is an essential component of follow-up care.

THE CHILD WHO DIES OF CANCER

Despite the remarkable improvements in curing children of cancer, approximately one-half of patients still die. The child eventually reaches a point where the cancer can no longer be controlled. At this time, the health care team needs to change its focus to the conduct of dying. Gentle, tactful, honest discussion with the child and family together so that all hear what the others hear is paramount. This encourages truthful relations between the patient and family and promotes their closeness and intimacy, the most effective prophylaxis against alienation and terror.

When the child is dying, the bonds forged between the primary physician-advocate and his team and the child and family become most valuable. The family who is confident of the competence and caring of their child's physician and colleagues is usually able to cope peacefully with the child's impending death. Although sedatives, narcotics, and palliative irradiation can be useful, the most important supportive measure is continued concern, trust, respect, and caring.

Children with cancer should die at home in a familiar environment with their families (Martinson, 1979). This helps prevent unwarranted medical interventions and promotes the child's comfort and the family's mourning. Conduct of death at home requires family counseling about the practical as well as emotional aspects of death and a dedicated home health service. House calls by a familiar nurse practitioner or the primary nurse and the primary physician greatly benefit the patient and family and are rewarding to the nurse and physician. Intravenous fluid and narcotic therapy are often ably handled by parents and siblings with instruction and supervision by nurse or physician. Death in peace and with dignity is as ancient and as worthy a goal of medicine as cure of cancer.

CHILDHOOD LEUKEMIA AND NON-HODGKIN'S LYMPHOMA

Definitions

Because of their close relationship in children, leukemia and non-Hodgkin's lymphoma are considered together (Pinkel *et al.,* 1975; Crist *et al.,* 1981). These malignant neoplasms of lymphopoietic and hematopoietic tissues most often originate in bone marrow but frequently arise from thymus, lymph nodes, and lymphatic tissue of the nasopharynx and gastrointestinal tract. In children they tend to spread readily to all organs and tissues and to populate the peripheral blood. In this discussion, current concepts of the biology of leukemia and lymphoma are used to categorize and describe this group of neoplasms.

Common Acute Lymphocytic Leukemia

Biology and Clinical Features. Common acute lymphocytic leukemia (ALL) is the most frequent of the leukemia-lymphoma neoplasms in American and European children, representing approximately 70% of childhood ALL (Greaves *et al.,* 1981a). Characteristically, it is found in children between ages two and six years and accounts for the peak incidence of ALL in this age group. It is seen equally in boys and girls, more frequently in white children than black, and more often among the socioeconomically privileged than the underprivileged. It generally arises from bone marrow but occasionally can develop in lymph nodes as a lymphoblastic lymphoma without leukemia (Bernard *et al.,* 1979). These children often present initially with severe anemia, granulocytopenia, and thrombocytopenia. Peripheral blood lymphoblast and lymphocyte counts tend to be low initially but can reach high levels as the disease evolves.

Morphologically, the cells of common ALL range from small, benign-appearing lymphocytes to large lymphoblasts and primitive undifferentiated cells of bizarre morphology. Relative proportions of these cell types and the degree of monotony among the cells vary from patient to patient and sometimes in the same patient at different times. Cytochemical studies of common ALL cells often demonstrate periodic-acid Schiff (PAS)–positive granules and terminal deoxynucleotide transferase (TdT) activity. With immunofluorescence techniques the cell surfaces demonstrate Ia antigen and common ALL antigen. In some cases intracytoplasmic immunoglobulin is also demonstrated, a characteristic of the pre-B lymphocyte (Vogler *et al.*, 1978), leading to a belief that common ALL is a neoplasm of B-lymphocyte lineage.

Common ALL cells tend to have a slower rate of replication than other forms of ALL, as suggested by leukemia cell labeling studies, as well as clinical observation (Murphy *et al.*, 1977). However, patients with common ALL who present with very high initial lymphocyte/lymphoblast counts in the peripheral blood may have higher labeling indices and more rapid clinical courses, resembling those of thymic ALL (Dow *et al.*, 1982). These observations correlate with the finding that children with common ALL and lower initial leukemia cell counts treated with modern therapy tend to have a gradual relapse rate during four to five years. This probably reflects the relatively slow replication rates of the leukemia cells that escape eradication by therapy. On the other hand, children with initial leukemia cell levels over 100,000 mm³ tend to have a rapid relapse rate for approximately one and a half years. Those remaining in continuous remission for two years have little or no risk of later relapse (Mauer, 1980). This probably reflects the rapid replication rate of the leukemia cells not destroyed by treatment.

Children with low initial leukemia cell counts, however, have a much higher cure rate than those with high counts, despite the longer duration of their risk of relapse. Perhaps most treatment plans are better suited for eradication of slowly replicating rather than rapidly replicating leukemia cells. The treatment results of the Berlin group hint that this may be the case (Henze *et al.*, 1981). Highly intensive chemotherapy early in the course of ALL was followed by less intensive therapy for three years. No difference between the remission experience of children with initially high leukemia cell levels as compared to those with low levels was reported.

The clinical symptoms and signs of common ALL are the result of pancytopenia and invasion of normal organs and tissues by leukemia cells. Anemia results in pallor, fatigue, and anorexia. Granulocytopenia is manifest by severe, intractable infection, and thrombocytopenia by bleeding. Splenomegaly, hepatomegaly, and lymphadenomegaly are variable. Periosteal and synovial infiltration can result in bone pain and arthralgia, renal infiltration in nephromegaly, hematuria, polyuria, and hypertension. In rare instances children can present with congestive heart failure owing to cardiac involvement or increased intracranial pressure caused by meningeal infiltration.

Diagnosis of common ALL is made by study of aspirated bone marrow. Replacement of normal hematopoiesis by leukemic lymphoblasts, lymphocytes, and primitive cells that demonstrate Ia antigen and common ALL antigen indicates common ALL.

Treatment of Common Acute Lymphocytic Leukemia. *Remission Induction and Continuation.* With modern treatment approximately 60% of children with common ALL survive free of leukemia, off therapy, at minimal risk of relapse, and presumably cured (Pinkel, 1979). The objective of treatment is therefore cure, not palliation, and success is measured by cure rate and not by complete remission duration or survival (see Figure 39–1).

Management can be divided into several phases. First is immediate, thorough evaluation for extent of disease, organ system infiltration, bleeding problems, infection, and psychosocial features of the child and family. Next, the educational process of child and family is initiated, supportive measures such as blood component therapy and antibiotics are inaugurated as required, and remission induction with chemotherapy is started. The combination of prednisone, 40 mg/m²/day, vincristine, 1.5 mg/m²/week, and L-asparaginase, 6000 units/m² three times weekly induces complete clinical and hematologic remission in most patients within four weeks (Miller *et al.*, 1981). For children with large masses of neoplastic tissues or high initial leukemia cell counts, intravenous fluid, sodium bicarbonate, and allopurinol therapy precede chemotherapy and are continued for the first three to four days in order to avoid hyperuricemia and urate nephropathy.

Once complete hematologic remission is ascertained from bone marrow examination, continuation chemotherapy is initiated with the objective of eradicating systemic leukemia.

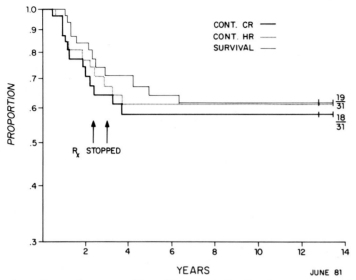

Figure 39–1. Complete and hematologic remission duration and survival of children with ALL treated with combination chemotherapy and preventive meningeal irradiation at St. Jude Children's Research Hospital in a 1967–68 study. The plateau of continuous complete remission suggests the curability of ALL.

Most pediatric hematologist/oncologists agree that daily mercaptopurine, 50 to 75 mg/m², and weekly methotrexate, 20 to 25 mg/m², are highly valuable (Aur *et al.,* 1978). Beyond that considerable uncertainty and contradictory evidence exists about the value of "early intensive" chemotherapy, "rotating combinations," and "reinduction pulses" throughout the course of continuation chemotherapy. The value of drugs such as cyclophosphamide, the anthracyclines, and arabinosyl cytosine in common ALL is questionable. Whether periodic courses of prednisone, vincristine, and L-asparaginase improve cure rate is not established. At some cancer centers intravenous infusions of "intermediate high" doses of methotrexate are administered during remission with the goal of achieving higher and possibly more effective levels of the drug in all tissues (Moe *et al.,* 1981). Others are using sequential pairs of drugs that are considered effective in prolonging remission.

Treatment of common ALL is evolving but slowly. Six or seven years of follow-up are required to evaluate the efficacy of treatment regimens.

Prevention and Treatment of Meningeal Relapse. When effective combination chemotherapy was developed in the 1960s and hema-tologic remissions were lengthened, the arachnoid meninges became the most frequent site of initial clinical relapse. Meningeal relapse was usually followed by hematologic relapse or chronic meningeal leukemia with neurologic disability and eventual death (see Figure 39–2). Two factors were primarily responsible for meningeal relapse. First, leukemic infiltration of the arachnoid tissue is generally present at diagnosis of ALL. The degree of infiltration, especially in the deep perivascular arachnoid, is greater with the more florid leukemia associated with high initial leukemia cell counts. Second, some antileukemia drugs, such as methotrexate and mercaptopurine, diffuse poorly into cerebrospinal fluid (CSF) so that levels are too low to be effective against arachnoid leukemia (Pinkel, 1979).

A highly effective method of preventing meningeal relapse is cranial meningeal irradiation accompanied by several weekly doses of intrathecal methotrexate and followed by repeated intrathecal injections of methotrexate every 8 to 12 weeks for three years (Sallan *et al.,* 1978). There are two objections to this method. First, many children can remain free of meningeal relapse without cranial irradiation. Second, cranial irradiation, particularly

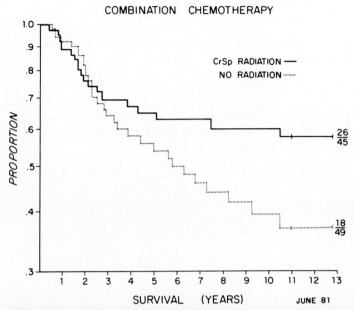

Figure 39 – 2.   Influence of preventive meningeal therapy on survival of patients with ALL. In this St. Jude study one half of patients received craniospinal irradiation early in remission while the other half received craniospinal irradiation at meningeal relapse or at the end of three years of continuous complete remission. Eleven years later the early irradiation group demonstrates significantly better survival.

in preschool children, often produces a fever-somnolence syndrome six weeks later, apparently increases the risk of methotrexate encephalopathy, may by itself be responsible for later learning disorders, and carries the risk of carcinogenesis for decades afterward (D'Angio, 1978).

For children with common ALL and low initial leukemia cell counts, intrathecal chemotherapy during remission induction and periodically throughout continuation chemotherapy seems to be adequate. A triple-drug regimen, consisting of methotrexate, arabinosyl cytosine, and hydrocortisone, appears to be the most effective (Sullivan *et al.,* 1981).

Treatment of initial meningeal relapse consists of craniospinal meningeal irradiation, weekly intrathecal injections with methotrexate and arabinosyl cytosine for six weeks, and monthly intrathecal chemotherapy for at least one year. Systemic chemotherapy is continued, as long as hematologic remission remains, for a minimum of one year from the date of meningeal relapse. If the patient has already received cranial irradiation, the irradiation is usually postponed until after termination of all chemotherapy. Many children with initial

meningeal relapse treated in this manner subsequently remain in complete remission for many years, and some are apparently cured (Pinkel *et al.,* 1977).

Testicular Relapse.   Although meningeal relapse occurs more frequently during the first three years of remission, initial testicular relapse tends to occur later, often after chemotherapy is stopped. Incidence ranges from less than 5% to as high as 40% of boys in various reports (Byrd, 1981).

The evidence favors the hypothesis that testicular relapse reflects inadequate systemic control of leukemia rather than some unique feature of the testes. Experimental studies have demonstrated that several antileukemia drugs perfuse testicular interstitial tissue well (Forrest *et al.,* 1981). Since this is the site of testicular relapse, poor drug perfusion cannot be held accountable. Second, children treated by intensive and mostly intravenous chemotherapy appear to have a lower frequency of initial testicular relapse than those treated with less vigorous oral regimens. Third, testicular relapse is often followed by hematologic relapse within a few months despite testicular irradiation, particularly when it occurs during systemic chemotherapy. Finally, a recent investigation revealed that one-half of boys with clinically isolated testicular relapse had intra-abdominal leukemia at exploratory laparotomy (Byrd, 1981).

In order to prevent testicular relapse, attention needs to be focused on more adequate systemic chemotherapy rather than on other measures.

Treatment of Hematologic Relapse. When bone marrow relapse occurs during combination chemotherapy, the outlook for cure becomes dim. Usually complete remission can be reinduced and sometimes will continue for six months to two years on a different drug combination or schedule. However, death with resistant leukemia or intercurrent infection is the usual outcome (Mauer, 1980). For this reason, bone marrow ablation with total-body irradiation and high-dose systemic chemotherapy followed by histocompatible marrow transplantation is currently used in children with ALL in second remission whose relapses occurred while on chemotherapy or within six months after it was stopped (Thomas *et al.*, 1979).

Bone marrow relapses that occur six months or more after cessation of therapy are more responsive to drug treatment. Many of these patients remain in lengthy remission after two to three years of combination chemotherapy (Riveria *et al.*, 1979).

Cessation of Therapy. Treatment is usually stopped after two and a half to three years of continuous complete remission if bone marrow, cerebrospinal fluid, and, in boys, testicular biopsy are free of leukemia. There is no proof that further chemotherapy with its continued risk of serious toxicity adds to the eventual cure rate (Mauer, 1980). In the months following cessation of therapy, hematopoiesis returns to normal, appetite and growth rate often increase, and the children become more active and energetic (see Figure 39–3). An "immunologic rebound" often occurs with bone marrow lymphoblastosis and lymphocytosis that may be confused with hematologic relapse (Simone *et al.*, 1978).

The risk of relapse is approximately 20% after cessation of chemotherapy, higher in boys and lower in girls. Most relapses occur in the first two years after discontinuation. Children who remain free of leukemia for three years afterward appear to have only a slight risk of relapse and can generally be considered cured (Mauer, 1980).

Thymic Lymphoblastic Lymphoma and Thymic Acute Lymphocytic Leukemia

Biology and Clinical Features. These disorders are different stages of the same neoplasm (Dow *et al.*, 1977; Crist *et al.*, 1981). Thymic lymphocytic cancer arises from thymus and possibly lymph nodes, spreads to adjacent tissues and distant lymph nodes, infiltrates the bone marrow, and eventually invades most organs and tissues, including the arachnoid meninges and testes.

The cells are largely primitive lymphoblasts with large nuclei containing one to two nucleoli and scant basophilic cytoplasm. In tissue sections normal-appearing histiocytes are scattered among the lymphoblasts. Cytochemically, the lymphoblasts are positive for terminal deoxynucleotidyl transferase and for acid phosphatase and often demonstrate coarse glycogen particles on PAS stain.

Immunologically, the lymphoblasts usually form heat-stable rosettes and demonstrate thymic surface antigens. Cells of localized lymphoma tend to display thymic antigens associated with more mature normal thymocytes, whereas those of thymic ALL usually have antigenic profiles in keeping with less mature thymocytes (Greaves *et al.*, 1981b). This finding is consistent with other pediatric neoplasms, such as Wilms' tumor, where the less differentiated tumors tend to metastasize earlier, and the more differentiated tumors tend to be localized.

Thymic leukemia and lymphoma cells tend to replicate faster than common ALL cells. This is reflected by higher labeling indices of the cells and rapid clinical progression of the disease (Murphy *et al.*, 1977, 1979).

Thymic lymphoma-ALL occurs most frequently in boys over six years of age, less frequently in girls, and infrequently in preschool children. Approximately one-half of patients present with a large thymic mass, often sufficient to cause respiratory obstruction and superior vena cava syndrome. When bone marrow infiltration has occurred, the peripheral lymphoblast count rises rapidly, reaching levels over 100,000 mm^3. At presentation, however, the hemoglobin, granulocyte, and platelet levels may be within normal limits, despite high lymphoblast counts.

Thymic ALL represents approximately 15 to 20% of ALL in children and adolescents.

Serious metabolic disturbances often accompany thymic lymphoma-ALL. Among

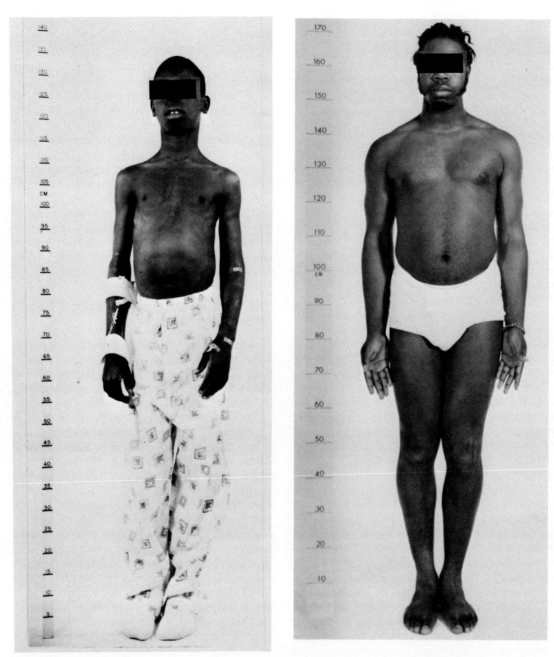

Figure 39–3. This patient illustrates cure of ALL. Admitted at age 11 years with an initial white blood cell count of 225,000 and marked hepatosplenomegaly, he is now 25 years old, free of leukemia for 14 years, and off treatment 12 years.

them are hyperuricemia, hyperkalemia, hypercalcemia, and hyperphosphatemia.

Treatment of Thymic Lymphoblastic Lymphoma-ALL. Treatment of patients with thymic lymphoma-ALL who have a large obstructive anterior mediastinal mass is one of the few medical emergencies in oncology (see Figure 39–4). Rapid diagnosis by marrow aspiration,

node biopsy, or, if there is no other way, by mediastinoscopy, is essential. Occasionally, intravenous hydrocortisone prior to diagnosis is necessary as both emergency relief and a diagnostic test.

Two combination chemotherapy programs have successfully cured most patients whose disease has not yet involved the marrow and

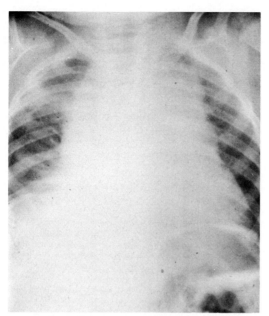

Figure 39–4. Thymic mass in child with thymic lymphoma-acute lymphocytic leukemia.

peripheral blood. The LSA-L2 regimen of Memorial Sloan-Kettering Cancer Center and the Sidney Farber Cancer Institute program both involve multiple antineoplastic drugs administered intravenously, orally, and intrathecally (Weinstein *et al.,* 1979; Wollner *et al.,* 1979). The Farber program also includes cranial irradiation to prevent meningeal relapse. Mediastinal irradiation probably does not add to the efficacy of treatment and can be omitted.

The same regimens are less successful for thymic ALL (Sallan *et al.,* 1978). This experience is again consistent with other pediatric neoplasms. When gross metastases are present at diagnosis, the prognosis is less favorable. However, many children, especially those with lower initial blood lymphoblast levels, are cured. With increasing knowledge of the specific features of thymic lymphoma-leukemia cell physiology, drug selection and drug schedules are being tailored more specifically for thymic lymphoma-ALL. For example, adenosine deaminase activity is especially high in thymic lymphoblasts (Ganeshaguru *et al.,* 1981). An inhibitor of this enzyme, deoxycoformycin, was reported to produce remissions in 7 out of 12 patients with thymic ALL but in none with other types (Prentice *et al.,* 1981). Labeling indices of thymic ALL cells tend to be higher than those of common ALL cells (Dow

et al., 1982). This suggests that more intensive, continuous chemotherapy early in the course of treatment might be more effective for thymic ALL. A recent exploratory study seems to support this suggestion (Henze *et al.,* 1981).

In treating thymic lymphoma-ALL, abundant parenteral hydration, urine alkalinization, and allopurinol administration must accompany and, if possible, precede antileukemia chemotherapy. Frequent blood chemistry determination and cardiac monitoring are also advisable for the first two to four days of chemotherapy.

Children with thymic lymphoma-ALL relapse early or not at all. Usually those who remain disease-free for two years have little or no risk of relapse thereafter (Sallan *et al.,* 1980).

B-Lymphoblastic Lymphoma and B-Cell Acute Lymphocytic Leukemia

Biology and Clinical Features. B-lymphoblastic lymphoma, or Burkitt-like lymphoma, and B-cell ALL are similar neoplasms in children (Preud'homme *et al.,* 1981). They consist of highly anaplastic, large round cells with uniform appearance. The nuclei are large with primitive chromatin pattern and distinct nucleoli. The cytoplasm is more abundant and more basophilic than in thymic lymphoma-ALL or common ALL cells, tends to contain large vacuoles, and stains with methyl green pyronin. The cell membranes demonstrate monoclonal immunoglobulin and contain Ia antigen and common ALL antigen. Tissue sections reveal numerous benign-appearing histiocytes among the B lymphoblasts, more than in sections of thymic lymphoma-ALL.

In African children, evidence of Epstein-Barr (EB) virus infection is commonly found in the neoplastic B lymphoblasts by virus isolation in cell culture, immunofluorescent staining for EB virus antigen, or DNA hybridization techniques (Epstein and Achong, 1979). In Europe and the United States, most B-lymphoblastic lymphomas do not show EB virus infection. Since Burkitt originally described this tumor in African children, here the term Burkitt's lymphoma is reserved for the EB virus-associated B-lymphoblastic lymphoma of African children.

B-lymphoblastic lymphoma and ALL cells tend to be the most rapidly replicating of all lymphoma-leukemia cells. Mitotic figures are very frequent, and labelling indices are high (Murphy *et al.,* 1979). On cytogenetic study the cells demonstrate a chromosomal translocation, t (8q− ; 14q+) most frequently, but in some cases t (2p+; 8q−) or t (8q−; 22q+) (Epstein and Achong, 1979).

B-lymphoblastic lymphoma arises from lymphoid tissue of the nasopharynx, sinuses, orbit, gastrointestinal tract, lymph nodes, and possibly at times from the bone marrow. A characteristic syndrome in the United States is acute intussusception in the school-age child caused by ileocecal lymphoma. In African children, the disease often presents in the facial bones. In both American and African children, the first signs can be enlarged peripheral lymph nodes or diffuse adbominal swelling with enlargement of kidneys, ovaries, liver, spleen, and testes as well as bowel involvement. Rapid progression is the rule, tumor masses often increasing remarkably from day to day. Meningeal invasion can occur early, often by direct extension from nasopharyngeal lymphomas (Ziegler, 1981).

When the disease involves bone marrow and peripheral blood, it is called B cell or "Burkitt cell" acute lymphocytic leukemia (Magrath and Ziegler, 1979). Only about 2% of children with ALL in the United States present in this manner, but many others first diagnosed at the lymphoma stage eventually develop this clinical situation. Occasionally, children with B-cell ALL do not have large lymphomatous masses at diagnosis, suggesting that their disease may arise from the marrow.

Treatment and Prognosis. As with other pediatric neoplasms, treatment and prognosis depend on the stage at diagnosis. The majority of children with localized B-lymphoblastic lymphoma of the terminal ileum and cecum can be cured by surgical excision and antineoplastic chemotherapy with or without abdominal irradiation. Many children with tumors localized to the head and neck can also be cured by chemotherapy. Children with diffuse abdominal involvement have a less favorable prognosis. Those with bone marrow, blood, and meningeal disease rarely survive more than a few months (Ziegler, 1981).

Cyclophosphamide and arabinosyl cytosine appear to be the most effective agents, but methotrexate, vincristine, doxorubicin, and prednisone also produce responses. Because of the rapid replication rate and high growth fraction of B-lymphoblastic lymphoma-ALL cells,

early, highly intensive, continuous chemotherapy seems to be the best approach. Patients with head and neck or generalized tumor need some form of preventive meningeal therapy. As with thymic lymphoma-ALL, hydration, alkalinization, and allopurinol administration are necessary during the initial few days of treatment. Most children who remain in complete remission for one year have little risk of later relapse. The high mortality of children with widespread B-lymphoblastic lymphoma-ALL emphasizes the need for innovative approaches in drug selection, combination, and schedules (Nkrumah *et al.,* 1977; Ziegler, 1981).

As implied, for all lymphatic lymphomas and ALLs, mass of neoplasm at diagnosis and replication rates of lymphoma-ALL cells seem to be related in an important way to the intensity, continuity, and duration of chemotherapy required for cure.

Patients with low initial tumor burdens and slow neoplastic cell replication seem to require less intensive chemotherapy more intermittently for longer times. Patients with high initial tumor burdens and rapid neoplastic cell replication seem to require more intensive chemotherapy more continuously for shorter periods. Although B-lymphoblastic lymphoma-ALL cells tend to replicate more rapidly than thymic, and thymic more rapidly than common, there is considerable overlap. Replication rate rather than immunologic cell type probably predicates the intensity, continuity, and duration of chemotherapy.

On the other hand, there is evidence that immunologic cell type is important in selecting drugs and drug combinations (Holcenberg and Camitta, 1981). This probably reflects differences among the cell types in cell membrane composition, enzyme activities, and metabolism. Choice of agents and combinations is reasonably predicated on whether the lymphoma-ALL cells are common, thymic, or B type.

"Null Cell" Acute Lymphocytic Leukemia

Less is known about null cell or undifferentiated ALL than about the other lymphocyte neoplasms described here. Cell morphology and cytochemistry do not distinguish it from common ALL. The cell type is defined solely by immunologic studies, which fail to demonstrate common ALL or thymic antigens or surface immunoglobulin (Greaves *et al.,* 1981a). The presence of cell membrane Ia antigen in many cases suggests that the cells are derived from bone marrow lymphocytes. Whether the neoplasm may present as a localized or regional lymphoma in lymphatic tissue or lymph nodes outside of the bone marrow is not clear.

Null cell ALL cells replicate more rapidly than those of common ALL, and initial leukemia cell counts tend to be higher (Dow *et al.,* 1982). The disease is more frequently seen in infants less than one year old, adolescents, and adults. Response to chemotherapy, duration of remission, and cure rate are less than in common ALL (Greaves *et al.,* 1981a). Care must be taken to differentiate null cell ALL from highly anaplastic forms of acute nonlymphocytic leukemia.

Null cell ALL is usually treated like common ALL. However, some centers are using acute nonlymphocytic leukemia treatment regimens as well. Some are providing bone marrow transplantation in first remission for the adolescents and adults who have histocompatible donors.

Diffuse Histiocytic Lymphoma – Acute Histiocytic Leukemia

Formerly called reticulum cell sarcoma and now termed large cell lymphoma, the origin and nature of this neoplasm appear to be heterogeneous (Berard *et al.,* 1978). However, it can arise in lymph nodes, skin, viscera, and bone marrow of children, particularly adolescents. The cells are large and often have folded nuclei and abundant cytoplasm with cytoplasmic processes. When bone marrow and blood are involved, either initially or as the neoplasm progresses, the term acute histiocytic leukemia is used (Pinkel *et al.,* 1975). In the leukemic patients erythrophagocytosis and pinocytosis can be observed with accompanying hemolytic anemia and hypoalbuminemia. As with thymic lymphoblastic lymphoma, meningeal infiltration can ensue independently of leukemia.

Treatment for histiocytic lymphoma is combination chemotherapy, sometimes accompanied by radiation therapy to local tumor masses. We use a modified version of the COMLA regimen, adding doxorubicin to the cyclophosphamide portion of the program (Sweet *et al.,* 1980). A 50% cure rate for ad-

vanced histiocytic lymphoma is reported for adults; recent data for children are not available.

Acute histiocytic leukemia is usually treated like other forms of acute nonlymphocytic leukemia. Survival rates are generally low.

Histiocytic medullary reticulosis or malignant histiocytosis is rarely observed in children. It has a rapidly progressive, fatal course. We have treated one child successfully with the modified COMLA regimen.

Acute Nonlymphocytic Leukemia (ANLL) in Children

Approximately 20% of acute leukemia in children is nonlymphocytic (Choi and Simone, 1976). The incidence rate is fairly constant throughout infancy, childhood, and adolescence. Acute myelocytic leukemia is most frequent, followed by acute myelomonocytic, acute histiocytic, acute promyelocytic, acute monocytic, and acute erythroleukemia. Morphology, cytochemistry, biology, and clinical features are similar to those in adult ANLL as described in Chapter 18 of this text.

Treatment of childhood ANLL presently consists of remission induction with daunorubicin and arabinosyl cytosine, followed by bone marrow ablation with total-body irradiation and intensive chemotherapy and subsequent bone marrow transplantation from a histocompatible sibling (Sanders *et al.,* 1981). With this regimen, over one-half of children survive free of leukemia and are apparently cured. Hematologic relapse is unusual. Deaths are usually caused by pneumonia, sepsis, or graft-versus-host disease within four months of transplantation.

Children who do not have a histocompatible donor receive continued chemotherapy with daunorubicin, arabinosyl cytosine, mercaptopurine, or thioguanine. Intrathecal methotrexate and arabinosyl cytosine are administered monthly to prevent meningeal relapse. A recent highly intensive treatment program with the acronym VAPA includes several other drugs as well (Weinstein *et al.,* 1980). Approximately 40% of children entered into this program remain leukemia-free after cessation of treatment. Unlike adults in the program, they appear to be free of relapse risk after two years of complete remission. The results suggest that a high proportion of children with ANLL may be curable with chemotherapy.

Chronic Granulocytic Leukemia in Children

Adult-type chronic granulocytic leukemia with t(9q+; 22q−) chromosomal translocation occurs in older children and adolescents. Its biology, clinical features, treatment, and course are similar to those of adults (Smith and Johnson, 1974). Infants and preschool children develop a form of chronic granulocytic leukemia that has no consistent chromosomal translocation (Brodeur *et al.*, 1979). The disease apparently originates in bone marrow and is characterized by myeloid and erythroid hyperplasia and reduced megakaryocytes. Soft-agar cloning suggests that the leukemic cells are derived from granulocyte-monocyte progenitors (Barak *et al.*, 1981). The peripheral blood demonstrates anemia, myelocytosis, monocytosis, and thrombocytopenia. Fetal hemoglobin is often increased and leukocyte alkaline phosphatase reduced. Clinical features are fever, malnutrition, growth failure, marked splenomegaly, skin eruptions, and bleeding. The median survival is less than a year. The disease must be carefully differentiated from chronic infection with cytomegalovirus, rubella, *Toxoplasma,* mycobacteria, or *Histoplasma.*

Treatment of juvenile chronic granulocytic leukemia with antineoplastic drugs produces transient reduction in splenomegaly and leukocytosis. Remissions following splenectomy have been reported (Smith and Johnson, 1974).

HODGKIN'S DISEASE

Epidemiologic differences have been reported in Hodgkin's disease in younger patients. In underdeveloped countries, Hodgkin's disease occurs at an earlier age than in more developed parts of the world. Male predominance is more marked in younger patients. The lymphocyte-predominant histologic variant is seen more frequently and the lymphocyte-depleted form less often than in adults. However, there is no evidence that Hodgkin's disease in childhood and adolescence responds less favorably to treatment than in adults.

Certain considerations regarding the morbidity of treatment are more pertinent in children and adolescents. In patients with early-stage disease, *e.g.,* stage I and IIa with small mediastinal masses, the least toxic treatment is probably radiation therapy in conventional doses. In more advanced disease, when radiotherapy is combined with chemotherapy, reduced doses of radiation have been used without adversely affecting disease-free survival (Murphy and Donaldson, 1982). (See Chapter 15.)

BRAIN TUMORS

Primary brain tumors are the most common solid tumors of childhood, comprising one-fifth of all malignant disease in children less than 15 years of age (Young and Miller, 1975). Although congenital tumors do occur, most series show highest incidence in the latter part of the first decade (Bloom and Walsh, 1975; Gjerris, 1976; Yates *et al.,* 1979). Brain tumors in childhood tend to occur centrally along the neural axis. Two-thirds arise in the posterior fossa, the predominant histologic type being gliomas (see Table 39–2). Metastatic tumors are infrequent and usually associated with widespread tumor dissemination.

The most frequent presenting symptoms and signs result from raised intracranial pressure secondary to obstructive hydrocephalus (enlarging head, headache, vomiting, neck pain, torticollis, blurring of vision). Disturbances in cerebellar and brain stem function with ataxia, nystagmus and cranial nerve palsies are also seen. Focal seizures and weakness attributable to cortical involvement are rare. In most children the diagnosis of primary brain tumor can be made on CT scan without invasive studies. Although surgery can be curative for the low-grade cerebellar astrocytoma, in most cases only biopsy or incomplete resection is possible. In tumors of the brain stem or thalamus, biopsy is often not feasible and the diagnosis is made without histologic confirmation. Treatment of most brain tumors is primarily radiation therapy with variation in field according to tumor type (see below). Survival rates vary with histology, site, and extent of tumor (see Chapter 37).

Astrocytoma

Astrocytoma is the most common primary brain or spinal cord tumor of childhood. In contrast to adults, the majority are of low-grade malignancy. *Glioblastoma multiforme*

Table 39–2. Incidence of Intracranial Tumors at All Ages and in Children Under 15 Years

TUMOR	ALL AGES (%)	CHILDREN (%)
Glioma	45	70
Astrocytoma	15	30
Glioblastoma	15	5
Oligodendroglioma	8	1
Medulloblastoma	4	20
Ependymoma	4	10
Meningioma	15	1
Neurinoma	6	<0.5
Pituitary adenoma	6	1
Metastases	5–20	<0.5
Craniopharyngioma	3	10
Choroid plexus papilloma	0.5	3
Pinealoma	1	2
Hemangioma	3	1
Epidermoids	2	0.5
Dermoids-teratomas	<0.5	3
Sarcoma	2	4
Optic gliomas	1	4

Approximate figures based on collected reports from literature. Reprinted by permission from Bloom, H. J. G., and Walsh, L. S.: Tumours of the central nervous system. In Bloom, H. J. G.; Lemerle, J.; Neidhardt, M. K.; and Voute, P. A. (eds.): *Cancer in Children.* Springer-Verlag, Berlin, 1975.

constitutes less than 10% of childhood brain tumors (Bloom and Walsh, 1975; Gjerris, 1976). When cerebellar astrocytomas are cystic, surgical removal often results in cure. In the less common cerebral tumors, partial resection is followed by radiation therapy, and five-year survival rates are approximately 50%. With midline tumors of the brain stem and thalamus, survival rates of 20 to 50%, respectively, are reported (Bloom and Walsh, 1975).

Medulloblastoma

Medulloblastoma occurs almost exclusively in children and constitutes 20% of their primary brain tumors. It arises in the posterior fossa, predominantly in the roof of the fourth ventricle, though occupying a more lateral position in older patients. Histologically, medulloblastoma shares similarities with neuroblastoma and retinoblastoma in the formation of tumor cell rosettes. A characteristic feature is the tendency to disseminate and proliferate by the cerebrospinal fluid (CSF) pathways with involvement of distant cranial and spinal meninges. Complete removal is seldom possible, but surgery is necessary to document histology, determine the extent of the tumor, and reestablish the flow of cerebrospinal fluid ei-

ther by removal of tumor or insertion of a ventricular shunt. Radiation therapy is the primary modality of tumor control and, because of the CSF dissemination, it is directed to the entire neural axis. Recurrent medulloblastoma will respond to chemotherapy with either single agents, such as vincristine or procarbazine, or combined regimens (Howarth, 1982). Unfortunately, adjuvant chemotherapy has not yet influenced disease-free survival. Although in the best series five-year survival rates after surgery and irradiation approach 50%, relapses continue to occur for many years.

Ependymoma

Two-thirds of intracranial ependymomas occur in patients less than 15 years of age. The tumors are derived from cells lining the ventricular system, and in children they arise most frequently in the posterior fossa in the floor of the fourth ventricle. Prognosis is related to proximity to vital midline structures, as well as to histologic grade. Although they may appear well circumscribed, surgery is not curative. Radiation therapy is the primary modality of treatment. Subarachnoid seeding has been reported in approximately 13% of cases and is most frequently (50%) seen in patients with posterior fossa tumors (Fokes and Earle, 1969; Bloom and Walsh, 1975). Consequently, neural axis irradiation is recommended for tumors arising in the posterior fossa as well as for high-grade supratentorial tumors. The five-year survival rate is approximately 40% (Bloom and Walsh, 1975). Some ependymomas are responsive to systemic chemotherapy, but no data indicate that chemotherapy contributes to cure rate.

Hypothalamic Tumors

Hypothalamic tumors are a rare group of brain tumors with unusual clinical features. They are seen predominantly in infancy and childhood. The diencephalic syndrome presents before three years of age with failure to gain weight and wasting in an otherwise healthy child. A low-grade astrocytoma in the anterior floor of the third ventricle or anterior hypothalamus is usually found, and irradiation leads to dramatic improvement (Bloom and Walsh, 1975).

Precocious puberty may be associated with tumors in the hypothalamic region. These may be gliomas, teratomas, craniopharyngiomas, or extension from pinealomas. Surgery followed by irradiation is the usual management, and prognosis is dependent on the histologic type.

Sequelae

Survivors of brain tumors in childhood often experience considerable morbidity. Gross neurologic or mental impairment may be attributable to the direct or indirect effects of the tumor or surgery. Conventional radiotherapy does not cause gross brain damage, but the immature nervous system is more sensitive to radiation, and subtle changes have been noted in survivors of acute lymphatic leukemia who received low-dose irradiation for CNS prophylaxis. Recently, endocrine deficiencies were also discovered following radiotherapy. Growth-hormone deficiency was found within one year of treatment in 50% of children receiving 2700 rads (Shalet et al., 1978). With high doses, other pituitary deficiencies may be seen (Richards et al., 1976). Survivors of brain tumors should be observed prospectively for these remediable handicaps.

SARCOMAS

Soft Tissue Sarcomas

Soft tissue sarcomas account for approximately 1% of all neoplastic disease. However, in children they constitute a larger proportion of all solid tumors, between 6 and 6.5% (Young and Miller, 1975; Birch et al., 1980). Rhabdomyosarcoma is the most common soft tissue sarcoma in childhood. The less common forms, such as liposarcoma, angiosarcoma, synovial sarcoma, and fibrosarcoma, are exceedingly rare. Except for the fibromatoses (see below), their behavior in children is the same as in adults. As a group these tumors are less responsive to chemotherapy and irradiation than rhabdomyosarcoma. The general concern of pediatric oncology — to limit the morbidity of treatment — applies especially to these patients.

Rhabdomyosarcoma. Embryonal rhabdomyosarcoma is the most common soft tissue sarcoma of childhood (Young and Miller, 1975; Birch et al., 1982). It is often misdiagnosed, but less now than in the past. The tumor has slight male predominance but no racial variation. It shows a bimodal age distribution with a peak in the first five years of life owing to the frequency of head and neck and genitourinary tumors and a peak in late adolescence owing to extremity and male genitourinary tumors (Miller, 1981; Pinkel and Pratt, 1982). The tumor arises from embryonic mesenchyme and shows histologic and ultrastructural evidence of varying stages of embryonic muscle differentiation (Mierau and Favara, 1980). Electron microscopy is important for establishing cytologic diagnosis. Grossly, the tumors may appear encapsulated, but they are notorious for infiltrating along tissue planes well outside the evident tumor limits. When the tumor arises from a submucosal location, it assumes a grapelike form, the so-called sarcoma botryoides. Such tumors are characteristic in the nasopharynx, vagina, and bladder. Metastases chiefly occur via hematogenous dissemination, but lymph node involvement may also be important. One-third to one-fifth of patients have metastases at presentation, most commonly involving the lungs, lymph nodes, bones, bone marrow, and liver.

The three histologic variants seen in childhood are embryonal or compact, botryoid, and alveolar. The more differentiated pleomorphic rhabdomyosarcoma of adults is seldom seen in children. The histologic pattern is largely related to the site of the tumor. The alveolar pattern is associated with tumors of the extremities, whereas the botyroid pattern is observed in submucosal sites (Horn and Enterline, 1959). Invasive and metastatic behavior is related to the degree of anaplasia of the tumor cells.

Approximately one-third of all primary tumors occur in the head and neck regions (Pratt et al., 1981b). They are seen mainly in the first decade and are often misdiagnosed, with a median time to diagnosis of two months. Ten percent arise in the orbit and present with proptosis, loss of vision, or a fungating mass. Nasopharyngeal tumors may present with epistaxis, nasal polyp, trismus, or nasal speech, and middle ear tumors with otorrhea, a polypoid mass, or cranial nerve palsies. CT scanning is useful in evaluating the extent of tumor and detecting intracranial invasion. The so-called parameningeal sites — nasopharynx, nasal sinuses, middle ear, and orbit — are associated with a 35% incidence of intracranial extension (Teft et al., 1978).

The next most common site is the genitourinary tract. In younger patients the vagina, prostate, and bladder are involved. Older males tend to have paratesticular primaries. Presenting symptoms are difficulty with micturition, bleeding, polypoid mass, or painless scrotal swelling.

Extremity tumors constitute approximately one-sixth of the total and a greater proportion of these patients have metastases at presentation (Gehan et al., 1981). Less commonly, primary tumors arise on the trunk in sites such as the retroperitoneum, perineum, the perianal region, and the chest wall without age-specific association. The tendency for particular sites to be associated with certain age groups is unexplained.

Only one in six tumors can be excised completely, either because of location or extensive infiltration (Pratt et al., 1981b; Gehan et al., 1981). Metastatic evaluation should include chest x-ray films, bone scan, liver-spleen scan, and bone marrow aspiration. CT scan is essential in evaluating head and neck, retroperitoneal, and pelvic tumors. It may also be useful in determining the outer limits of extremity tumors or the presence of pelvic or retroperitoneal nodes in lower extremity tumors. Some authors advocate routine lymphangiography for staging of lower extremity tumors. The spinal fluid in patients with tumors in parameningeal sites should be examined.

Those patients in whom complete resection has been achieved receive adjuvant chemotherapy with vincristine, cyclophosphamide, and dactinomycin. Radiation therapy is not required for local control (Hays, 1980). In patients with unresectable tumors, chemotherapy with vincristine, cyclophosphamide, and dactinomycin with or without doxorubicin results in tumor regression in approximately 75% of patients. With the addition of radiotherapy, complete clinical regressions can be achieved in approximately 70% (Hays, 1980; Pratt et al., 1981b). Following chemotherapy with or without radiotherapy, initially unresectable tumors can often be resected. However, when microscopic residual disease remains, radiation therapy is unavoidable despite its morbidity for future growth and development.

In the management of orbital tumors, the earlier practice of exenteration has been replaced by irradiation and systemic chemotherapy with equally good results. In tumors of parameningeal sites, even without evidence of extension into the cranium, irradiation of the adjacent cranial meninges with a 2-cm margin is recommended (Teft et al., 1978). In patients with demonstrable intracranial extension, cranial irradiation is added when the cerebrospinal fluid contains rhabdomyosarcoma cells.

Historically, most relapses of rhabdomyosarcoma occurred within two years of diagnosis, and for this reason a two-year duration of adjuvant chemotherapy was recommended. More recently 12 or 18 months of chemotherapy have been used, depending on the stage of the tumor. Patients must be followed for metastases with frequent chest x-rays, bone scans, and bone marrow aspirations. All abnormal studies at diagnosis should be repeated at least every three months after remission is achieved and continued for at least two years after treatment is stopped.

The prognosis for survival is directly related to stage at diagnosis and degree of tumor cell anaplasia (Gehan et al., 1981; Pratt et al., 1981b) (see Figure 39–5). For patients with completely resected tumors, the two-year disease-free survival is 83% and for those with incompletely resected local tumors 72%. Patients with nonresectable and metastatic tumors fare less well (Gehan et al., 1981). The site of the primary tumor is also prognostically

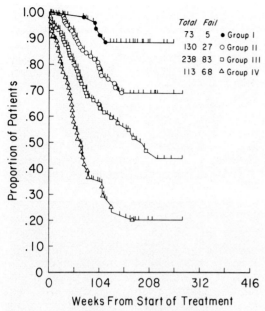

Figure 39–5. Childhood rhabdomyosarcoma—effect of initial stage (group) on survival. From Gehan, E. A., *et al.*: Prognostic factors in children with rhabdomyosarcoma. *Natl. Cancer Inst. Monogr.,* **56**:193–199, 1981.

significant. Patients with genitourinary and orbital primaries have a more favorable outlook. Extremity and retroperitoneal tumors have the worst prognosis, while head and neck sites are intermediate.

Complications of treatment can be severe and even fatal. Combinations of radiation and chemotherapy may lead to severe bladder fibrosis, death from gastrointestinal obstruction, and severe skeletal deformities. Blindness may result from either exenteration of the orbit or radiation-induced cataracts or phthisis bulbi. Radical surgical procedures such as amputation or pelvic exenteration have obvious morbidity. As with other pediatric neoplasms, the long-term toxic effects of chemotherapy are as yet uncertain, but the risks of sterility and of second neoplasms following irradiation are apparent.

Fibrosarcoma and Fibromatoses. These entities are discussed together since the histology of one blends indistinguishably with the other (Stout, 1962; Chung and Enzinger, 1976). They differ from adult fibrosarcoma in their relatively benign behavior. In adults the metastatic rate approaches 50%, whereas in childhood the rate is only 7 to 8%. Fibrosarcomas show a predilection for distal extremities. They may also occur on the head and neck as well as on the trunk, particularly in the

paraspinal region. The incidence in males is about twice that in females. Most tumors present within the first five years of life and can occasionally be congenital. The main clinical feature is painless swelling, which may enlarge rapidly or cause problems by local invasion. Histologically, the tumors are poorly encapsulated and infiltrate widely into the surrounding tissues. Treatment is by wide excision, which in some locations may necessitate amputation. Local recurrence may ensue in 17% of patients (Chung and Enzinger, 1976). The long-term survival rate, however, is greater than 80%. Some fibromatoses have been known to undergo spontaneous regression. Unfortunately, histologic grading has not proven predictive of tumor recurrence (Stout, 1962).

Ewing's Sarcoma

Ewing's sarcoma is a pediatric neoplasm in that the incidence is greatest in the first two decades of life (Pritchard *et al.,* 1975), and its biologic behavior is similar to that of other embryonal tumors. Ewing postulated that the tumor originated from mesenchymal cells of the bone marrow (Ewing, 1921). The diagnosis is based on clinical and radiologic features, as well as histology and cytology.

Initial evaluation of the patient should include computerized scan of the tumor site for extent of soft tissue involvement, a chest x-ray film with tomograms or computerized tomography to exclude pulmonary metastases, a bone scan, and bone marrow aspiration. Ewing's sarcoma usually responds well to radiotherapy and chemotherapy (see Figure 39–6). With combination chemotherapy using cyclophosphamide and doxorubicin, almost all patients have rapid tumor regression and a significant proportion experience complete regression within three months of diagnosis (Hayes *et al.,* 1981b; Rosen *et al.,* 1981a). At this time, resection of the original tumor-bearing bone, for example, clavicle, rib, scapula, ilium, fibula, or metatarsal bones, is attempted. Radiation therapy is reserved for microscopic or bulky residual disease. Two current treatment programs use only 3000 rads for incompletely resected tumors that demonstrate only microscopic residual tumor following chemotherapy (Hayes *et al.,* 1981b; Rosen *et al.,* 1981a). Chemotherapy is usually continued for a total of one year.

Although most patients have complete

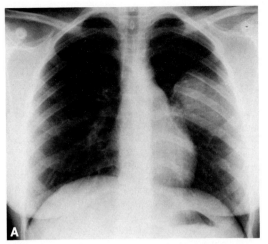

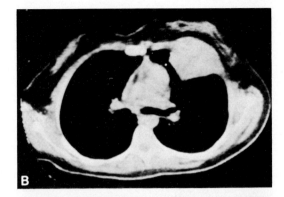

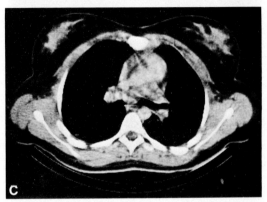

Figure 39–6. Response of Ewing's sarcoma to chemotherapy. (*A*) Chest roentgenogram demonstrating left fourth rib tumor. (*B*) Computerized tomogram demonstrating same tumor. (*C*) Computerized tomogram after 12 weeks of treatment with cyclophosphamide and doxorubicin.

tumor regression with radiation therapy and chemotherapy, patients in past treatment programs have shown continued risk of relapse for many years. In one series, 25% of relapses occurred after three years of disease-free survival (Jereb *et al.*, 1980).

Considerable morbidity is associated with the use of radiation therapy and combination chemotherapy, including growth deformity, pathologic fractures, and second neoplasms (Rosen *et al.*, 1981a). Current treatment of Ewing's sarcoma places less reliance on radiation therapy for local control. Primary amputation is often used in young children with tumors of distal lower extremities. As indicated above, surgical resection of the primary tumor is attempted after initial chemotherapy, and radiation therapy is given only to those with residual disease (Hayes *et al.*, 1981; Rosen *et al.*, 1981a).

Osteosarcoma

Osteosarcoma is predominantly a tumor of the second and third decades of life (Uribe-Botero *et al.*, 1977; Miller, 1981). Tumors of the humerus occur earlier than tumors of the lower femur and upper tibia. After 13 years of age, when male growth rate exceeds that of females, osteosarcoma is more frequent in males than females. Animal studies have found that giant breeds of dogs have 300 times the incidence of osteosarcoma than standard breeds (Miller, 1981). The association with bone healing, such as in osteomyelitis and Paget's disease, is seldom seen in the pediatric age group. Familial occurrence of osteosarcoma and association with brain tumor, adrenocortical carcinoma, and rhabdomyosarcoma have been reported. Patients with the dominantly inherited form of retinoblastoma and with Gardner's syndrome have increased incidence of osteosarcoma and other tumors. Multifocal tumors, which occur rarely, also suggest a genetic predisposition.

Osteogenic sarcoma usually arises in a metaphysis. Hematogenous dissemination is the usual route, and the lungs are the main site of metastases. Bone metastases are reported in 10% or less of patients in most clinical series but were found in 37% of an autopsy series (Uribe-Botero, *et al.*, 1977). Since less than 20% of patients treated by amputation alone survive free of metastases, 80% are assumed to have distant microscopic disease at diagnosis. Detection of metastases is now more sensitive with CT scanning.

In the last 15 years, improved survival has been demonstrated by several centers (Sutow *et al.*, 1976; Campanacci *et al.*, 1981; Gilchrist *et al.*, 1981; Harvei and Solheim, 1981; Jaffe *et al.*, 1981; Rosen *et al.*, 1981b). This reflects several factors. Close surveillance for and an aggressive surgical approach to pulmonary metastases when detected probably account for greater overall survival. However, chemotherapy using methotrexate and doxorubicin with or without other agents probably has altered the course of osteosarcoma, as indicated by the decreased numbers of patients developing metastases, increased time to the development of metastases, and the reduced number of metastases per patient. All these factors also make salvage of such patients by surgery more effective. No evidence shows that the biology of the tumor has changed during this period (Campanacci *et al.*, 1981).

Another recent development is the use of limb salvage procedures. This is not available for all patients, limiting factors being location and extent of tumor as well as the patient's age and growth potential. The end result is not a normal leg, but one that is functional with orthopedic support and cosmetically satisfactory. Such procedures have demonstrated the effectiveness of preoperative chemotherapy and have also led to a predictable correlation of tumor response with long-term prognosis (Rosen *et al.*, 1981b).

The prognosis of patients with unresectable osteogenic sarcoma remains poor, and various experimental methods have failed to improve it substantially. Osteosarcoma remains a difficult therapeutic problem that demands rational and carefully planned prospective trials.

NEUROBLASTOMA

Neuroblastoma is the most common extracranial solid tumor in childhood, constituting 6.5% of pediatric neoplasms (Birch *et al.*, 1980). The tumor arises from neuroectoderm and consists of anaplastic sympathetic ganglion cells. Approximately 50% of tumors originate in the adrenal medulla, but may occur anywhere along the sympathetic chain (Jaffe, 1976). Neuroblastoma affects predominantly preschool-aged children; one-half are less than two years of age at diagnosis. Approximately

60% of patients have disseminated tumor at presentation, usually involving the bones, bone marrow, liver, or skin. Pulmonary metastases are unusual. The presenting symptoms may be related to the primary tumor (abdominal mass, spinal cord compression secondary to intraspinal extension, Horner's syndrome), to metastatic tumor (bone pain, proptosis), or to the metabolic effects of catecholamines or vasoactive polypeptides secreted by the tumor (hypertension, diarrhea). Most children with neuroblastoma have constitutional symptoms at presentation. The tumor is frequently calcified, and 80% of the patients have elevated levels of catecholamines, chiefly homovanillic acid (HVA) and vanillylmandelic acid (VMA) (LaBrosse *et al.*, 1980). Bone marrow aspirates show typical neuroblastoma clusters or rosettes in the majority of patients with disseminated disease (Green *et al.*, 1981). Consequently, biopsy of the primary tumor is often unnecessary.

Treatment consists of surgery and chemotherapy, with radiation therapy reserved for incomplete tumor responses or palliation of pain. Prognosis is related to stage of disease and age of patient. Localized tumors, whether totally or incompletely resectable, may be cured in 70 to 100% of cases, but almost 80% of patients with metastatic disease die despite multiagent chemotherapy. In a recently published study using sequential cyclophosphamide and doxorubicin in a cyclic regimen for metastatic neuroblastoma, complete responses were produced in 52% of patients and median survival was 22 months (Green *et al.*, 1981). Another effective drug combination, cisplatin and epipodophyllotoxin (VM-26), produced complete responses in 27% of patients, including some whose tumors were resistant to the cyclophosphamide-doxorubicin combination (Hayes *et al.*, 1981a). Current cooperative protocols are testing the benefits of combining both regimens.

Patients less than one year of age at diagnosis have a better prognosis with all stages of tumors. Survival under one year approaches 70%, but in older children survival rate is 20% or less (Jaffe, 1976). This disparity is related to differing biologic behavior. Rarely, spontaneous regression of disseminated neuroblastoma has occurred in infants less than six months old (Jaffe, 1976). Autopsies on infants who died from other causes show an incidence of focal neuroblastoma 50 times the rate of clinical neuroblastoma, suggesting that many of these tumors undergo spontaneous maturation or regression (Beckwith and Perrin, 1963). Whether neuroblastoma under one year has a better prognosis because of host factors or whether it represents a multifocal benign condition is unknown (Knudson and Meadows, 1980). However, prior to the advent of chemotherapy most infants with disseminated neuroblastoma died (Gross *et al.*, 1959). Infants with neuroblastoma require treatment, but the good prognosis for this group of patients and the morbidity of treatment at this age dictate the minimum therapy necessary for tumor control.

Neuroblastoma was one of the first tumors in which serologic antibodies to the tumor were reported. Surface antigens on tumor cells are nonspecific and are found also in brain. Antisera to neuroblastoma antigens are being tested for detecting small numbers of tumor cells in bone marrow specimens (Lauer *et al.*, 1978). Some interesting clinical observations may have immunologic implications. In the syndrome of opsomyoclonus and neuroblastoma, the symptoms may result from an antibody to neuroblastoma cells cross-reacting with cerebellar cells. These patients have a better prognosis, but this is probably related to lower stage at diagnosis and more mature histology. A common observation at second-look surgery following chemotherapy or radiotherapy is conversion of neuroblastoma to ganglioneuroblastoma. This probably represents selective destruction of the more anaplastic cells by treatment rather than maturation or some immunologic phenomenon. Some observers have noted lymphocytic infiltration of regressing neuroblastoma, but its significance is not defined.

Retrospective analysis has shown improved prognosis in patients whose tumors exhibited more mature features (Hughes *et al.*, 1974). Biochemical maturation as determined by an elevated VMA/HVA ratio has also been associated with better survival rates (LaBrosse *et al.*, 1980). *In vitro* differentiation has been reported with nerve growth factor and with maneuvers that increase intracellular cyclic AMP (ganglioneuroma and mature ganglion cells have higher levels of cyclic AMP than neuroblastoma cells). Therapeutic attempts along these lines, however, have been unsuccessful thus far.

Although rare, familial occurrence of neuroblastoma has been reported in several kindred (Knudson and Meadows, 1980). Karyotypic analysis of tumor cells has not demonstrated a consistent abnormality, although a recent study revealed association with deletion in the short arm of chromosome 1 (Brodeur *et al.*, 1981a). Recent reports suggest an association of neuroblastoma with the fetal hydantoin syndrome. Obviously, such patients, as well as those with a family history of neuroblastoma, should be followed prospectively, perhaps with serial estimates of catecholamines.

WILMS' TUMOR

Wilms' tumor occurs predominantly in preschool-age children. It is curable in more than 80% of those presenting with localized tumor and in approximately one-half of those with metastatic disease (D'Angio *et al.*, 1981). This success has increased the need to reduce the morbidity of treatment without compromising its effectiveness.

Wilms' tumor accounts for more than 5% of all childhood neoplasms (Birch *et al.*, 1980). Increased frequency has been noted in association with hemihypertrophy and Beckwith-Wiedemann syndrome (Tank and Kay, 1979). A rare syndrome of Wilms' tumor, bilateral aniridia, and mental retardation are associated with a specific chromosomal defect — deletion of the short arm of chromosome 11 (Yunis and Ramsay, 1980). Approximately 10% of patients have bilateral tumors (Bond, 1975; Malcolm *et al.*, 1980). Several instances of familial Wilms' tumor have been reported both with and without associated abnormalities. These observations suggest a genetic component in the origin of Wilms' tumor (Knudson and Strong, 1972).

The majority of Wilms' tumors show a predominantly epithelial pattern with formation of pseudotubules and glomeruli in a mesenchymal stroma. Occasionally, ectopic mesenchymal differentiation can be seen with cartilage and muscle formation. Initially confined to the kidney and well encapsulated, the tumor often extends to blood vessels and regional lymph nodes. Metastatic disease is present in approximately 10 to 20% of patients at diagnosis, predominantly in the lung. Liver and, less commonly, bone and brain metastases can occur (see Table 39–3).

The most frequent presenting feature is painless flank swelling. Hematuria occurs in approximately 25% of patients and hypertension in 12%. By contrast with neuroblastoma,

Table 39-3. Wilms' Tumor: Group (or Stage) and Prognosis

		2 YR DFS*
Group I	Tumor limited to kidney Completely excised	88%
Group II	Tumor extends beyond kidney Completely excised	78%
Group III	Residual nonhematogenous tumor confined to abdomen	70%
Group IV	Hematogenous metastasis (liver, lung, bone, brain)	49%
Group V	Bilateral renal tumors	63%†

Reprinted by permission from D'Angio, G. J.; Evans, A.; Breslow, N.; Beckwith, B.; Bishop, H.; Farewell, V.; Goodwin, W.; Leape, L.; Palmer, N.; Sinks, L.; Sutow, W.; Teft, M.; and Wolff, J.: The treatment of Wilms' tumor: Results of the second National Wilms' Tumor Study Group. *Cancer*, **47**:2302–2311, 1981.
* DFS = Disease-free survival
† From Malcolm *et al.,* 1981.

constitutional disturbances are unusual, and calcification of the primary tumor is uncommon. The diagnosis is usually suggested by intravenous pyelography and confirmed by abdominal ultrasound or CT scan.

Treatment consists of nephrectomy by way of a transabdominal approach with examination of the contralateral kidney and sampling of hilar and periaortic nodes. The replacement of the flank incision by the transabdominal approach is credited with improving the survival from 15 to 32% (Gross and Neuhauser, 1950). Postoperative irradiation to the tumor bed increased survival to almost 50%. The introduction of dactinomycin, vincristine, and doxorubicin, initially as single agents, improved survival further and allowed treatment of disseminated disease (Aron, 1974). Approximately 50% of patients with metastatic tumor can now be cured (Wara *et al.,* 1974; D'Angio *et al.,* 1981). The survival of patients with gross residual tumor after surgery and bilateral tumors has also significantly improved. Radiotherapy is not required in patients with localized stage I tumors who receive chemotherapy. However, among these patients are the historic 15 to 30% who survive after nephrectomy alone. They have yet to be segregated as a subgroup who require neither chemotherapy nor radiotherapy after surgery.

Analysis of several prospective studies has identified certain adverse prognostic features. In the past, size of tumor, capsular invasion, renal vein invasion, and lymph node involvement were shown to increase the risk of metastasis and recurrence (Jereb and Sandstedt, 1973; Kumar *et al.,* 1975). More recently, ear-

lier observations that epithelial differentiation was associated with greater survival have been extended (Jereb and Sandstedt, 1973). Anaplastic and sarcomatous variants with great risk of recurrence and metastases are now recognized to occur in approximately 11.5% of patients (Beckwith and Palmer, 1978).

In the 10% of patients with bilateral tumors, two-thirds of the tumors are synchronous, and in one-third the second tumor develops after an interval of months to several years. With modern therapy 60% of these children survive. Removal of the more affected kidney and partial resection or biopsy of the less affected kidney are usually performed, and chemotherapy is administered. If residual tumor remains, either radiation therapy or a second surgical approach after therapy may be used. The age of patients with bilateral tumors tends to be younger than the average of all patients with Wilms' tumor, histologic examination often shows foci of nodular renal blastema, and the incidence of associated congenital malformation is higher. These three associations suggest a genetic etiology for bilateral Wilms' tumor (Knudson and Strong, 1972).

Kidney tumors occurring in infants in the first weeks of life used to be classified as Wilms' tumor, although they differed considerably in histologic appearance and behavior (Bolande, 1974). Congenital mesoblastic nephroma usually presents in the first few weeks of life as an abdominal mass. These are fully encapsulated tumors composed of mesenchymal tissue. Surgical excision is usually the only treatment required. Nephroblastomatosis occurs less frequently and may be bilateral. The relationship with Wilms' tumor is unclear, but there are patients reported in whom invasive tumor subsequently developed. Focal areas of nodular renal blastema have been observed in association with Wilms' tumor, more commonly with bilateral tumors, suggesting a causal relationship or common origin (Bolande, 1974). Nephroblastomatosis and nodular renal blastema are also frequently associated with Beckwith-Weidemann syndrome and hemihypertrophy.

Based on these observations, a group of children with high risk of developing Wilms' tumor can be identified. This includes children with hemihypertrophy and Beckwith-Weidemann syndrome, with sporadic bilateral aniridia, with nephroblastomatosis, and congenital mesoblastic nephroma, and siblings and offspring of patients with bilateral tumors. Physicians need to monitor such children closely for the development of tumor without adding unnecessary medical risks or psychological burdens to them and their families. Physical examination every three months with pyelography every six months until age seven years has been suggested (Tank and Kay, 1979), although ultrasonography might be a potentially less harmful method of surveillance.

The morbidity associated with treatment becomes increasingly important as cure rate of patients with localized Wilms' tumor increases. Radiation has been associated with muscle atrophy, impaired bone growth, spinal shortening and deformity, and second cancers within the radiation fields (Jaffe et al., 1980). Chemotherapy potentiates these toxic effects and adds others. Only careful studies such as those which demonstrated that radiotherapy was not necessary in the management of stage I tumors will determine the minimal effective treatment necessary to cure each stage and histologic variety of Wilms' tumor. All available patients should be enrolled in studies designed to answer these questions.

GERM CELL TUMORS OF INFANTS AND CHILDREN

Germ cell tumors constitute 3% of all pediatric cancer. They are thought to arise from primordial germ cells and may arise anywhere along the migratory pathway of the developing gonad. The common origin of these tumors is evidenced by finding similar histologic types, albeit in different proportions, at sites as diverse as the ovary and testis, and the presacral, retroperitoneal, anterior mediastinal, cervical, and intracranial regions. Tumors may contain mixtures of the five cell types—germinoma (dysgerminoma or seminoma), choriocarcinoma, embryonal carcinoma, endodermal sinus tumor, and teratoma. Certain sites are associated with a particular age. Thus, sacrococcygeal tumors are almost entirely limited to the first five years of life with a female predominance, while mediastinal tumors occur late in the second and in the third decades and mostly in males. Although the prognosis for survival correlates with the stage at diagnosis (Brodeur et al., 1981b), certain differences in pathophysiology relate to site, age, and histology. Most series report a better survival with germinoma, largely because of its marked radiosensitivity. The pure form is rarely seen in fe-

males and tends to occur in the ovaries early in the second decade, whereas in males it is one of the more common tumors and occurs late in the second and third decades. Metastases are chiefly to lymph nodes (Mostofi, 1973). Choriocarcinoma occurs rarely in the pure form and is notorious for its rapid hematogenous dissemination. Brain metastases are seen most frequently with this type but are not uncommon following pulmonary metastases from endodermal sinus tumor or embryonal carcinoma. Teratomas contain elements of all three fetal layers, and the degree of malignancy is related to the presence of embryonal carcinoma, endodermal sinus tumor, or choriocarcinoma.

Certain features are common to germ cell tumors of all types. Thus the production of chemical markers detectable in the serum—alpha-fetoprotein, the beta subunit of human chorionic gonadotropin, and carcinoembryonic antigen—may aid in identifying the tumor type and monitoring the response to treatment. Immunohistochemical stains allow detection of these substances in histologic specimens. Another feature is the apparent differentiation of disseminated tumors reported with both testicular and ovarian tumors. Whether this is a differential effect of drugs in destroying the more anaplastic elements or whether it represents maturation of immature cell types is not clear. This feature has not been observed for tumors originating in the sacrococcygeal region.

The varying behavior of these tumors in particular sites is described below together with the relation of age to location.

Germ Cell Tumors of the Ovaries

In childhood and early adolescence 60% of ovarian tumors are of germ cell origin (Abell et al., 1965). The benign cystic teratoma accounts for two thirds of these, although the proportion of malignant germ cell tumor approaches 50% in premenarchal girls. The malignant tumors are comprised of almost equal proportions of germinoma, endodermal sinus tumor, and malignant teratoma; embryonal carcinoma of the type seen in the adult testis is less common. Patients with dysgerminoma tend to be older, whereas endodermal sinus tumors occur in younger patients. Only the benign cystic teratoma has a high bilateral incidence. In the remainder the incidence is less than 10%. Patients with tumors localized to the ovary without capsular invasion have a good prognosis. Intra-abdominal extension frequently precedes hematogenous dissemination. The common presenting feature is an abdominal mass, although pain may sometimes be a feature. Endocrine abnormalities are unusual in these patients.

Treatment consists of oophorectomy or attempted excision of more extensive disease, together with chemotherapy and possibly a second attempt at resection. Radiation is given for unresectable disease. In dysgerminoma, simple oophorectomy will suffice with radiotherapy for residual tumor; chemotherapy is not routinely indicated.

Testicular Germ Cell Tumors

The incidence of testicular tumors in childhood shows a biphasic pattern, most cases occurring in the first three years or after puberty (Mostofi, 1973; Exelby, 1980). Three cell types predominate: endodermal sinus tumor (orchioblastoma, yolk sac carcinoma or infantile embryonal carcinoma), embryonal carcinoma, and teratoma. Seminoma and choriocarcinoma are almost never seen in childhood.

In children less than three years of age, the tumors are predominantly endodermal sinus tumors, and metastases are primarily to the lung. Retroperitoneal lymph node involvement is unusual. The frequency of metastases in apparently localized tumor approaches 20%, and salvage rate of these patients is poor. For this reason, adjuvant chemotherapy with vincristine, cyclophosphamide, and dactinomycin is usually given for six months after inguinal orchiectomy. The cure rate of infantile endodermal sinus tumor of the testis is 80%. Occasionally, the adult embryonal carcinoma or teratoma is found in a testicular tumor in this age group. These few patients should probably have exploratory laparotomy and lymph node examination.

In postpubertal patients, testicular tumors are usually embryonal carcinoma or teratoma, and their management is the same as that in adults.

Extragonadal Germ Cell Tumors

The most frequent extragonadal site for germ cell tumors in infancy and childhood is the sacrococcygeal region. These tumors are thought to arise from Hensen's node or the primitive knot. Females are affected four times

as often as males (Gross, 1951; Valdisseri and Yunis, 1981); this may be related to later maturing of the female gonad (Gross, 1951). The majority of sacrococcygeal tumors are teratomas involving elements of all three germ layers. Although mostly composed of mature elements, immature tissues are present in 10 to 20% and most commonly consist of neuroepithelial elements. Calcification is present in approximately one-third. In the histologic examination of these tumors, wide sampling of the material must be carried out in order to exclude a malignant element. Benign immature tissue must also be distinguished from the frankly malignant. The malignant element is frequently endodermal sinus tumor and occasionally embryonal carcinoma. Dysgerminoma and choriocarcinoma are not seen in this location. Metastases are composed almost entirely of embryonal carcinoma and endodermal sinus tumor.

In the neonate the tumors usually present as visible swellings in the region of the coccyx. They may achieve considerable size, but 90% are benign. The coccyx is usually attached to the tumor. Complete excision is usually possible without damage to the pelvic viscera. The coccyx must be removed since failure to do so is associated with a high risk of local recurrence, particularly with malignant tumors.

In older infants sacrococcygeal teratomas are most often malignant. Frequently, the tumors are not visible externally, and the patients present with symptoms of pelvic obstruction. Occasionally, the tumors present as buttock swellings. Characteristically, they invade the surrounding tissues and are unresectable. Despite radiation therapy and combination chemotherapy, the outlook is poor with almost no survivors. In a minority of these patients, a swelling is visible at birth which becomes larger prior to diagnosis. Whether this represents malignant change in a previously benign teratoma is not known, but all such tumors should be excised with the coccyx in the neonatal period.

Retroperitoneal germ cell tumors occur later in the first decade of life. The majority are teratomas, but only 10% are malignant. The prognosis depends on their amenability to surgical excision. Teratomas in the anterior mediastinum may occur throughout childhood. They are predominantly benign, and the prognosis depends on resectability. Malignant germ cell tumors in this location occur predominantly in men late in the second and in the third decades with seminomas comprising approximately one-third of them. The remainder are of mixed-cell type, although occasionally a pure endodermal sinus tumor is seen. Although a response to chemotherapy, irradiation, or both is frequently obtained, the only long-term survivors among patients with unresectable malignant germ cell tumors of the mediastinum are those with seminoma.

RETINOBLASTOMA

Retinoblastoma is the most frequent malignant tumor of the eye in children. The incidence rate in American children under age five years is 11.2 per million. The cure rate in the United States now exceeds 90%. Since some of the survivors have the genetically dominant form of this tumor, an increased incidence may be expected in the future. All patients with bilateral tumors, whether sporadic or familial, and 10% of those with unilateral tumors are believed to have the autosomal dominant gene for this tumor. The eyes of both parents must be examined since an estimated 1% of retinoblastomas may undergo spontaneous regression leaving a detectable scar on the retina (Shields and Augsburger, 1981). Several patients with the D-deletion syndrome have been noted to have retinoblastoma. More recently, improved techniques in karyotypic analysis have showed a specific deletion in the long arm of chromosome 13 (13ql.4) in somatic cells of a few patients with bilateral retinoblastoma and in some of the tumors themselves (Gallie, 1980).

Patients with familial or bilateral retinoblastoma have an increased incidence of other primary tumors, particularly osteosarcoma, which may or may not be within the radiation port (Chapter 3E). In one such family the patient had multifocal osteosarcoma.

Although retinoblastoma at birth is unusual, it may become apparent within a few weeks of life. Bilaterally affected patients present earlier than unilateral patients and are seldom first discovered after three years of age (Pendergrass and Davis, 1980). Retinoblastoma arises from the fetal retinal layer and grows either forward into the vitreous or dissects off the retina. Involvement of the optic nerve may be present in 25% of patients, and extension into the brain may result if tumor has extended beyond the cut end of the optic

nerve (Howarth *et al.*, 1980). Tumor cells in the optic nerve may also gain access to the subarachnoid space some 12 mm behind the globe. Hematogenous dissemination is associated with involvement of the vascular choroid or the emissary vessels, or with extension through the sclera. Preauricular and cervical lymph node involvement is usually associated with orbital disease. Distant metastases tend to involve the bone and bone marrow. As with neuroblastoma, lung metastases are exceedingly rare.

Presentation is usually with leukokoria — a white pupillary reflex. Strabismus or squint is not uncommon and probably results from interference with vision and fixation reflexes. Other findings may include heterochromia of the iris, pain and congestion from secondary glaucoma, orbital inflammation simulating endophthalmitis, and tumor cells in the anterior chamber simulating hypopyon. Most unilateral tumors are more advanced at presentation than bilateral tumors, and in bilateral tumors it is usual for the eyes to be asymmetrically involved. Multifocal disease is not uncommon even in unilateral tumors.

The diagnosis is based on the history and ophthalmologic examination using binocular, indirect ophthalmoscopy. This, together with ultrasonography, will differentiate most other causes of leukokoria including retrolental fibroplasia, persistent primary vitreous, Coats' disease, and nematode ophthalmitis (Bishop and Madson, 1975; Shields and Augsburger, 1981). Clinical evaluation should also include skull and orbital x-ray films, CT scan of head and orbit to detect optic nerve involvement or gross intracranial disease, spinal fluid examination, and bone marrow aspiration. A bone scan is useful as a baseline study in advanced disease.

Treatment historically has been by enucleation. Presently, vision may be preserved if less than 50% of the retina is involved by tumor. Enucleation is reserved for patients with advanced unilateral disease or for the worst affected eye of bilateral tumors.

Radiation therapy has been used to treat nonenucleated eyes in bilateral disease and eyes with tumor involving less than 50% of the retina where an attempt is being made to preserve vision. It is also used where small tumors involve the fovea or are adjacent to the disc. Conventional practice is to give 3800 to 4500 rads via an anterior and lateral port over three to four weeks. For smaller, more peripherally located tumors, local measures are used. These include cobalt plaques, photocoagulation, and cryotherapy.

Chemotherapy is indicated in most patients at risk for hematogenous dissemination, *i.e.*, those with extrabulbar disease (orbital involvement, lymph node involvement) or extensive choroidal or emissary vein infiltration. Most experience has been with vincristine and cyclophosphamide, which often produce therapeutic responses in patients with measurable disease (Howarth *et al.*, 1980). Similarity of retinoblastoma with neuroblastoma suggests that doxorubicin might also be effective. Intracranial extension is usually treated with a combination of radiotherapy and chemotherapy but is almost invariably fatal.

In Western countries where the majority of patients have tumors confined to the globe at presentation, the mortality rate is now less than 10%. This is attributable to earlier stage at diagnosis. Improved methods of treatment may result in a better quality of survival with better preservation of vision. In Third World countries, children present with advanced disease, and mortality rates exceed 75% (Gaitan-Yanguas, 1978; Howarth *et al.*, 1980).

Unfortunately, despite advances in cytogenetic technology, the asymptomatic carrier of the retinoblastoma gene cannot yet be detected. Genetic counseling of all affected patients and families is mandatory, however. In sporadic cases presenting with bilateral disease, the child's progeny have a 40% risk of retinoblastoma. The risk to siblings of the patient is approximately 8%. In unilateral sporadic disease the risk to siblings is 1%, and the risk to the progeny of the patient 5%. Patients with bilateral tumors should be followed carefully for the development of other secondary malignancies.

HISTIOCYTOSIS X

The term histiocytosis X is currently used to represent three related disorders of infants, children, and adolescents: eosinophilic granuloma, Hand-Schüller-Christian disease, and Letterer-Siwe disease. All three are characterized by proliferation of benign-appearing histiocytes, with a greater or lesser degree of macrophage and giant cell formation combined with infiltration by normal-appearing eosino-

phils, lymphocytes, and fibrocytes. Etiology is unknown. Staging systems have been proposed but not generally agreed on (Greenberger *et al.*, 1981).

Eosinophilic granuloma usually presents as a sharply defined osteolytic bone lesion in any flat or long bone. In older children it tends to remain localized, but in young infants it is usually a bellwether for Letterer-Siwe disease and in toddlers for Hand-Schüller-Christian disease. Solitary eosinophilic granuloma is best treated by surgical curettage. If this is not possible, small doses of radiotherapy may be followed by resolution. When multiple bones are sequentially or simultaneously involved, systemic chemotherapy may be indicated.

Hand-Schüller-Christian disease is characterized by multiple bone lesions, particularly cranial, and involvement of lymph nodes, liver, spleen, gingiva, and sometimes lung. Hypothalamic infiltration is frequent and leads to diabetes insipidus and retarded linear growth. The disease tends to occur in the toddler and to have a protracted, generally nonfatal, but often permanently disabling course. Chemotherapy is usually effective in producing regression of the lesions and can favorably alter the eventual outcome. Low-dose radiotherapy is reported to correct the hypothalamic disease if administered at first signs of diabetes insipidus (Nesbit and Krivit, 1975).

Letterer-Siwe disease primarily affects young infants. The babies have cranial lesions and widespread skin infiltrations that can mimic seborrheic dermatitis or be mistaken for petechiae. Liver, spleen, and lymph nodes are usually involved, and the disease tends to progress rapidly to involve lungs and bone marrow. Pancytopenia, bleeding, infection, pulmonary insufficiency, marasmus, and death commonly ensue. Chemotherapy usually causes regression of disease and often results in cure.

Since these disorders are reactive rather than neoplastic, chemotherapy is designed to inhibit the histiocytic reaction rather than to destroy all histiocytes. For this reason, single-drug treatment at a dosage no higher than that required to induce and maintain clinical remission is favored. Prednisone is most consistent in producing regression so it is reserved for induction of initial and subsequent remissions. Weekly doses of methotrexate, vinblastine, or cyclophosphamide or daily chlorambucil or mercaptopurine are introduced during remission induction and then continued to maintain remission. A thymic extract is being used experimentally in one center (Osband *et al.,* 1981). Treatment is usually stopped after the patient has been disease-free for two years.

MALIGNANT NEOPLASMS OF ADULTS IN CHILDREN

Carcinoma

Carcinoma is extremely rare in children. When diagnosed, a search should be made for genetic predisposition and environmental influences.

The infrequency of colorectal carcinoma in children is responsible for delay in diagnosis, with the result that many of these children present with advanced disease (Pratt *et al.,* 1977). Children with colorectal carcinoma differ from adults in that the anatomic predilection for the rectosigmoid area seen in adults is not observed, and mucinous adenocarcinoma, which is relatively infrequent in adults, constitutes a greater proportion of tumor types. Predisposing factors include ulcerative colitis, familial polyposis, and Gardner's syndrome (see Chapter 3E). However, environmental influences cannot be excluded even in these patients, and a search should be made in all.

An association with environmental agents was found with clear cell adenocarcinoma of the vagina of young women, now recognized as caused by diethylstilbestrol given to their mothers in the first trimester (Miller, 1978). Recently, carcinoma of the cervix was observed in a young woman who had received cyclophosphamide, suggesting that carcinomas may be induced by alkylating agents.

Hepatocellular carcinoma and benign hepatoma are associated with the administration of androgens. Most of these patients had been treated for aplastic anemia, but some had nonhematologic disorders (Miller, 1978). Other predisposing factors in hepatic carcinoma include cirrhosis, perhaps induced by metabolic disorders, hepatitis B, and possibly exposure to aflatoxin.

Radiation has been associated with the development of carcinomas also. The best-recognized association is with thyroid carcinoma in children irradiated for enlarged tonsils or thymus. In recent years the proportion of children with thyroid carcinoma with a history of prior irradiation has declined, but it should always be sought in each patient. Most thyroid carcinomas in childhood are of the papillary type and have a good prognosis, even in those patients with pulmonary metastases. Carcinoma of the breast and carcinoma of the colon have been reported occurring within previous radiation ports. The frequency may increase with longer survival of patients successfully treated for pediatric cancer.

Squamous cell carcinoma of the skin is exceedingly rare in childhood, except in association with xeroderma pigmentosum. This inherited condition occurs more often among people of North Africa (Miller, 1978).

Melanoma

Melanoma has rarely been reported in childhood. It may develop from nevi present at birth. In adults it is associated with exposure to sunlight, and the most frequent sites are on exposed skin (Pratt *et al.,* 1981b). The incidence of melanoma may have recently increased, perhaps related to changes in socioeconomic factors in the Northern Hemisphere.

Lymphoepithelioma

Nasopharyngeal carcinoma or lymphoepithelioma occurs predominantly in adolescents and young adults. It shows striking racial and geographic variations and is associated with evidence of Epstein-Barr virus infection in all patients. Viral DNA can often be detected in tumor cells by hybridization techniques. Measurements of serum antibody correlate with tumor burden and with response to treatment or recurrence of disease. This may become the first cancer preventable by immunization (Ablashi *et al.,* 1981).

BENIGN TUMORS PECULIAR TO INFANTS AND CHILDREN

Certain congenital malformations, hamartomas, and other benign tumors occurring in infancy and early childhood are sometimes alarming in appearance but only rarely cause serious clinical problems. Some resolve spontaneously. Treatment should be limited to those instances where medically indicated, and modalities with the least long-term morbidity should be used.

Vascular tumors exhibit a wide variety of appearances. The nevus flammeus or port-wine stain is usually present at birth and only infrequently disappears spontaneously. Although often extensive, these tumors are usually flat, and the most common problem is cosmetic. Occasionally, lesions on the face may be associated with intracranial vascular anomalies in the Sturge-Weber syndrome.

Tuberous or strawberry hemangiomas are not usually present at birth but appear within the first few weeks of life and are frequently multiple. The cutaneous variety seldom causes any problems and generally regresses spontaneously before the child is five years old. Surgery and radiation therapy should be avoided, even though the tumors appear alarming in size and location. More deeply seated hemangiomas may be less likely to regress spontaneously.

Giant hemangiomas in infancy that involve the trunk or extremities may be associated with thrombocytopenia, microangiopathic hemolytic anemia, consumption coagulopathy, and high-output cardiac failure. Occasionally, spontaneous thrombosis and involution may occur. In patients with symptomatic lesions, treatment has included corticosteroids, freezing, sclerosing injections, excision, and radiotherapy. Response has been variable, and some patients die despite treatment.

Lymphangiomas are often present at birth and usually develop within the first year of life. They are believed to develop from sequestered elements of primitive lymphatic sacs and most commonly involve the neck and axilla. The most frequent site in the neck is the posterior triangle. In the anterior triangle the mass may communicate with the floor of the mouth and be associated with airway obstruction. The chief complication is infection which in the past led to the death of the patient or occasionally spontaneous regression. Treatment is by complete surgical excision.

The phakomatoses include polyostotic fibrous dysplasia, tuberous sclerosis, and multiple neurofibromatoses. The last disease can be associated not only with neurofibrosarcoma but with a wide variety of neoplasms.

Angiofibroma

Angiofibroma is a benign tumor occurring in boys during the adrenarche. It arises from vascular tissue of the nasopharynx and presents as a vascular mass which may invade the nasal sinuses or the base of the skull. The most frequent manifestation is severe epistaxis. These tumors may respond to estrogens, and after shrinkage they are surgically removed. Radiotherapy should be avoided. Sarcomatous changes have rarely been reported.

DISEASES THAT MIMIC CANCER IN CHILDREN

One of the most challenging tasks of the pediatric oncologist and colleagues in pediatric pathology and radiology is to differentiate benign disorders from malignant neoplasms in children. The stakes are high because of the need for prompt, specific treatment of childhood cancer and the necessity of avoiding the hazards of unwarranted cancer therapy.

Infectious diseases are the most frequent imitators of cancer in children (Dorfman and Warnke, 1974). Pertussis can elicit remarkable peripheral lymphocytosis resembling acute lymphocytic leukemia. Mycobacterial, *Histoplasma,* cytomegalovirus, and Epstein-Barr virus infections can result in histiocytosis and myelomonocytosis resembling neoplastic disease. Cat-scratch disease or coccidioidomycosis can be confused with Hodgkin's disease or histiocytic lymphoma, North American blastomycosis with eosinophilic granuloma, and partially treated osteomyelitis with Ewing's sarcoma or osteogenic sarcoma.

Genetic disorders can also be mistaken for cancer. Infants with Down's syndrome may demonstrate self-limited hematoproliferations resembling acute or chronic myelocytic leukemia, erythremia, or acute lymphocytic leukemia (Engel *et al.,* 1964). In fact, the lymphoblastosis of normal newborn marrow may seem neoplastic to the inexperienced. Infants and children with severe immunodeficiency disorders, congenital agranulocytosis, and chronic granulomatous disease are sometimes misdiagnosed as having malignant histiocytosis or acute monocytic leukemia (Nesbit and Krivit, 1975).

Healing bone fractures, particularly in abused children where history of trauma is concealed, can appear similar to primary or metastatic bone tumors. The anticonvulsant phenytoin can produce lymphoid hyperplasia resembling lymphoma (Miller, 1978).

REFERENCES

Abell, M. R.; Johnson, V. J.; and Holtz, F.: Ovarian neoplasms in childhood and adolescence. *Am. J. Obstet. Gynecol.,* **92:**1059–1081, 1965.

Ablashi, D. V.; Krueger, G. R.; and Grundmann, E.: International symposium on nasopharyngeal carcinoma — Basic research as applied to diagnosis and treatment. *Cancer Res.,* **41:**2014–2016, 1981.

Aron, B. S.: Wilms' tumor — A clinical study of eighty-one patients. *Cancer,* **33:**637–646, 1974.

Asmar, B. I.; Maqbool, S.; and Dajani, A. S.: Hematologic abnormalities after oral trimethoprim-sulfamethoxazole therapy in children. *Am. J. Dis. Child.,* **135:**1100–1103, 1979.

Aur, R. J. A.; Simone, J. V.; Verzosa, M. S.; Hustu, H. O.; Barker, L. F.; Pinkel, D. P.; Rivera, G.; Dahl, G. V.; Wood, A.; Stagner, S.; and Mason, C.: Childhood acute lymphocytic leukemia: Study VIII. *Cancer,* **42:**2123–2134, 1978.

Barak, Y.; Levin, S.; Vogel, R.; Cohen, I. J.; Wallach, B.; Nir, E.; and Zaizov, R.: Juvenile and adult types of chronic granulocytic leukemia of childhood: Growth patterns and characteristics of granulocyte-macrophage colony forming cells. *Am. J. Hematol.,* **10:**269–275, 1981.

Beckwith, J. B., and Palmer, N. F.: Histology and prognosis of Wilms' tumor. Results from the First National Wilms' Study. *Cancer,* **41:**1937–1948, 1978.

Beckwith, J. B., and Perrin, E. V.: *In situ* neuroblastomas. A contribution to the natural history of neural crest tumors. *Am. J. Pathol.,* **43:**1089–1100, 1963.

Berard, C. W.; Jaffe, E. S.; Braylan, R. C.; Mann, R. B.; and Nanba, K.: Immunologic aspects and pathology of the malignant lymphomas. *Cancer,* **42:**911–921, 1978.

Bernard, A.; Boumsell, L.; Bayle, C.; Richard, Y.; Coppin, H.; Penit, C.; Rouget, P.; Micheau, C.; Clausse, B.; Gerard-Marchant, R.; Dausset, J.; and Lemerle, J.: Subsets of malignant lymphomas in children related to the cell phenotype. *Blood,* **54:**1058–1068, 1979.

Birch, J. M.; Marsden, H. B.; and Swindell, R.: Incidence of malignant disease in childhood. A 24 year review of the Manchester Childrens Tumor Registry data. *Br. J. Cancer,* **42:**215–223, 1980.

Bishop, J. O., and Madson, E. C.: Retinoblastoma: Review of current status. *Surv. Ophthalmol.,* **19:**342–366, 1975.

Bloom, H. J. G., and Walsh, L. S.: Tumours of the central nervous system. In Bloom, H. J. G.; Lemerle, J.; Neidhardt, M. K.; and Voute, P. A. (eds.): *Cancer in Children.* Springer-Verlag, Berlin, 1975.

Bolande, R. P.: Congenital and infantile neoplasia of the kidney. *Lancet,* **2:**1497–1499, 1974.

Bond, J. V.: Bilateral Wilms' tumor. Age at diagnosis associated congenital anomalies and possible pattern of inheritance. *Lancet,* **2:**482–484, 1975.

Brodeur, G. M.; Dow, L. W.; and Williams, D. L.: Cytogenetic features of juvenile chronic myelogenous leukemia. *Blood,* **53:**812–819, 1979.

Brodeur, G. M.; Green, A. A.; Hayes, F. A.; Williams, K. J.; Williams, D. L.; and Tsiatis, A. A.: Cytogenetic features of human neuroblastomas and cell lines. *Cancer Res.,* **41:**4678–4684, 1981a.

Brodeur, G. M.; Howarth, C. B.; Pratt, C. B.; Caces, J.; and Hustu, H. O.: Malignant germ cell tumors in 57 children and adolescents. *Cancer,* **48:**1890–1898, 1981b.

Byrd, R. L.: Testicular leukemia: Incidence and management results. *Med. Pediatr. Oncol.,* **9:**493–500, 1981.

Campanacci, M.; Bacci, G.; Bertoni, F.; Picci, P.; Minutillo, A.; and Franceschi, C.: The treatment of osteosarcoma of the extremities. *Cancer,* **48:**1569–1581, 1981.

Choi, S.-I., and Simone, J. V.: Acute nonlymphocytic leukemia in 171 children. *Med. Pediatr. Oncol.,* **2:**119–146, 1976.

Chung, E. B., and Enzinger, F. M.: Infantile fibrosarcoma. *Cancer,* **38:**729–739, 1976.

Crist, W. M.; Kelly, D. R.; Ragab, A. H.; Roper, M.; Dearth, J. C.; Castelberry, R. P.; and Flint, A.: Predictive ability of Lukes-Collins classification for immunologic phenotypes of childhood non-Hodgkin lymphoma. *Cancer,* **48:**2070–2075, 1981.

D'Angio, G. J.: Complications of treatment encountered in lymphoma-leukemia long-term survivors. *Cancer,* **42:**1015–1025, 1978.

D'Angio, G. J.; Evans, A.; Breslow, N.; Beckwith, B.; Bishop, H.; Farewell, V.; Goodwin, W.; Leape, L.; Palmer, N.; Sinks, L.; Sutow, W.; Teft, M.; and Wolff, J.: The treatment of Wilms' tumor: Results of the second National Wilms' Tumor Study Group. *Cancer,* **47:**2302–2311, 1981.

Dorfman, R. F., and Warnke, R.: Lymphadenopathy simulating the malignant lymphomas. *Hum. Pathol.,* **5:**519–550, 1974.

Dow, L. W.; Borella, L.; Sen, L.; Aur, R. J. A.; George, S. L.; Mauer, A. M.; and Simone, J. V.: Initial prognostic factors and lymphoblast-erythrocyte rosette formation in 109 children with acute lymphoblastic leukemia. *Blood,* **50:**671–682, 1977.

Dow, L. W.; Chang, L. J. A.; Tsiatis, A. A.; Melvin, S. L.; and Bowman, W. P.: Relationship of pretreatment lymphoblast proliferative activity and prognosis in 97 children with acute lymphoblastic leukemia. *Blood,* **59:**1197–1202, 1982.

Engel, R. R.; Hammond, D.; Eitzman, D. V.; Pearson, H.; and Krivit, W.: Transient congenital leukemia in seven infants with mongolism. *J. Pediatr.,* **65:**303–305, 1964.

Epstein, M. A.: Vaccine control of EB virus-associated tumors. In Epstein, M. A., and Achong, B. G. (eds.): *The Epstein-Barr Virus.* Springer-Verlag, New York, Inc., New York, 1979.

Epstein, M. A., and Achong, B. G.: The relationship of the virus to Burkitt's lymphoma. In Epstein, M. A., and Achong, B. G. (eds.): *The Epstein-Barr Virus.* Springer-Verlag, New York, Inc., New York, 1979.

Ewing, J.: Diffuse endothelioma of bone. *Proc. N.Y. Pathol. Soc.,* **21:**17–24, 1921.

Exelby, P. R.: Testicular cancer in children. *Cancer,* **45:**1803–1809, 1980.

Fokes, E. C., and Earle, K. M.: Ependymomas: Clinical and pathological aspects. *J. Neurosurg.,* **30:**585–594, 1969.

Forrest, J. B.; Turner, T. T.; and Howards, S. S.: Cyclophosphamide, vincristine, and the blood testis barrier. *Invest. Urol.,* **18:**443–444, 1981.

Fraumeni, J. F., Jr.: Genetic factors. In Holland, J. F., and Frei, E., III (eds.): *Cancer Medicine.* Lea & Febiger, Philadelphia, 1982.

Gaitan-Yanguas, M.: Retinoblastoma: Analysis of 235 cases. *Int. J. Radiat. Oncol. Biol. Phys.,* **4:**359–365, 1978.

Gallie, B. L.: Gene carrier detection in retinoblastoma. *Ophthalmology (Rochester),* **87:**591–594, 1980.

Ganeshaguru, K.; Lee, N.; Llewellin, P.; Prentice, H. G.; Hoffbrand, A. V.; Catovsky, D.; Habeshaw, J. A., Robinson, J.; and Greaves, M. F.: Adenosine deaminase concentrations in leukaemia and lymphoma: Relation to cell phenotypes. *Leuk. Res.,* **5:**215–222, 1981.

Gehan, E. A.; Glover, F. N.; Maurer, H. M.; Sutow, W. W.; Hays, D. M.; Lawrence, W.; Newton, W. A.; and Soule, E. H.: Prognostic factors in children with rhabdomyosarcoma. *Natl. Cancer Inst. Monogr.,* **56:**83–92, 1981.

Gilchrist, G. S.; Pritchard, D. J.; Dahlin, D. C.; Ivins, J. C.; Taylor, W. F.; and Edmonson, J. H.: Management of osteosarcoma. A perspective based on the Mayo Clinic experience. *Natl. Cancer Inst. Monogr.,* **56:**193–199, 1981.

Gjerris, F.: Clinical aspects and long term prognosis of intracranial tumors in infancy and childhood. *Dev. Med. Child Neurol.,* **18:**145–159, 1976.

Greaves M. F.; Janossy, G.; Peto, J.; and Kay, H.: Immunologically defined subclasses of acute lymphoblastic leukaemia in children: Their relationship to presentation features and prognosis. *Br. J. Haematol.,* **48:**179–197, 1981a.

Greaves, M. F.; Rao, J.; Hariri, G.; Verbi, W.; Catovsky, D.; Kung, P.; and Goldstein, G.: Phenotypic heterogeneity and cellular origins of T cell malignancies. *Leuk. Res.,* **5:**281–299, 1981b.

Green, A. A.; Hayes, F. A.; and Hustu, H. O.: Sequential cyclophosphamide and doxorubicin for induction of complete remission in children with disseminated neuroblastoma. *Cancer,* **48:**2310–2317, 1981.

Greenberger, J. S.; Crocker, A. C.; Vawter, G.; Jaffe, N.; and Cassady, J. R.: Results of treatment of 127 patients with systemic histiocytosis (Letterer-Siwe syndrome, Schuller-Christian syndrome and multifocal eosinophilic granuloma). *Medicine,* **60:**311–337, 1981.

Gross, R. E.; Clatworthy, H. W.; and Meeker, I. A.: Sacrococcygeal teratomas in infants and children. *Surg. Gynecol. Obstet.,* **92:**341–354, 1951.

Gross, R. E.; Farber, S.; and Martin, L. W.: Neuroblastoma sympatheticum. *Pediatrics,* **23:**1179–1191, 1959.

Gross, R. E., and Neuhauser, E. B. D.: Treatment of mixed tumors of the kidney in childhood. *Pediatrics,* **6:**841–852, 1950.

Harvei, S., and Solheim, O.: The prognosis in osteosarcoma; Norwegian national data. *Cancer,* **48:**1719–1723, 1981.

Hayes, F. A.; Green, A. A.; Casper, J.; Cornet, J.; and Evans, E. W.: Clinical evaluation of sequentially scheduled cisplatin and VM26 in neuroblastoma. *Cancer,* **48:**1715–1718, 1981a.

Hayes, F. A.; Thompson, E. I.; Hustu, H. O.; and Kumar, M.: Chemotherapeutic induction of remission in Ewings sarcoma. *Proc. Am Assoc. Cancer Res.,* **22:**150, 1981b.

Hays, D. M.: The management of rhabdomyosarcoma in children and young adults. *World J. Surg.,* **4:**15–28, 1980.

Henze, G.; Langermann, H.-J.; Ritter, J.; Schellong, G.; and Reihm, H.: Treatment strategy for different risk groups in childhood acute lymphoblastic leukemia: A report from the BFM Study Group. In Neth, R.; Gallo, R. C.; Graf, T.; Mannweiler, K.; and Winkler, K. (eds.): *Modern Trends in Human Leukemia IV.* Springer-Verlag New York, Inc., New York, 1981.

Holcenberg, J. S., and Camitta, B. M.: Recent approaches to the treatment of acute lymphocytic leukemia in childhood. *Annu. Rev. Pharmacol. Toxicol.,* **21:**231–249, 1981.

Horn, R. C., and Enterline, H. T.: Rhabdomyosarcoma: A

clinicopathological study and classification of 39 cases. *Cancer,* **11:**181–199, 1959.

Howarth, C.; Meyer, D.; Hustu, H. O.; Johnson, W. W.; Shanks, E.; and Pratt, C.: Stage related combined modality treatment of retinoblastoma: Results of a prospective study. *Cancer,* **45:**851–858, 1980.

Howarth, C. B.: Medulloblastoma. In Carter, S. K.; Glatstein, E.; and Livingston, R. B. (eds.): *Principles of Cancer Treatment.* McGraw-Hill, Inc., New York, 1982.

Hughes, M.; Marsden, H. B.; and Palmer, M. K.: Histologic patterns of neuroblastoma related to prognosis and clinical staging. *Cancer,* **34:**1706–1711, 1974.

Hughes, W. T.; Kuhn, S.; Chaudhary, S.; Feldman, S.; Verzosa, M.; Aur, R. J. A.; Pratt, C.; and George, S. L.: Successful chemoprophylaxis for *Pneumocystis carinii* pneumonitis. *N. Engl. J. Med.,* **297:**1419–1426, 1977.

Jaffe, N.: Neuroblastoma: Review of the literature and an examination of factors contributing to its enigmatic character. *Cancer Treat. Rev.,* **3:**61–82, 1976.

Jaffe, N.: Pediatric cancer—Delayed sequelae of treatment. *ACS Proceedings of National Conference on Care of Children with Cancer.* American Cancer Society, Boston, 1978.

Jaffe, N.; Link, M. P.; Cohen, D.; Traggis, D.; Frei, E.; Watts, H.; Beardsley, G. P.; and Abelson, H. T.: High dose methotrexate in osteogenic sarcoma. *Natl. Cancer Inst. Monogr.,* **56:**201–206, 1981.

Jaffe, N.; McNeese, M.; Mayfield, J. K.; and Riseborough, E. J.: Childhood urologic cancer therapy related sequelae and their impact on management. *Cancer,* **45:**1815–1822, 1980.

Jereb, B.; Brody, B.; Rosen, G.; and Nisce, L. Z.: Ewing sarcoma—Analysis of 100 cases. *Proc. Am. Assoc. Cancer Res.,* **21:**387, 1980.

Jereb, B., and Sandstedt, B.: Structure and size versus prognosis in nephroblastoma. *Cancer,* **31:**1473–1481, 1973.

Knudson, A. G., and Meadows, A. T.: Regression of neuroblastoma IV-S: A genetic hypothesis. *N. Engl. J. Med.,* **302:**1254–1256, 1980.

Knudson, A. G., and Strong, L. C.: Mutation and cancer. A model for Wilms' tumor of the kidney. *J.N.C.I.,* **48:**313–324, 1972.

Kobrinsky, N. L., and Ramsay, N. K. C.: Acute megaloblastic anemia induced by high-dose trimethoprim-sulfamethoxazole. *Ann. Intern. Med.,* **94:**780–781, 1981.

Kumar, A. P. M.; Hustu, O.; Fleming, I. D.; Wrenn, E. L.; Pratt, C. B.; Johnson, W.; and Pinkel, D.: Capsular and vascular invasion: important prognostic factors in Wilms' tumor. *J. Pediatr. Surg.,* **10:**301–309, 1975.

LaBrosse, E. H.; Com-Nougue, C.; Zucker, J.-M.; Comoy, E.; Bohoun, C.; Lemerle, J.; and Schweisguth, O.: Urinary excretion of 3 methoxy-4-hydroxymandelic acid and 3-methoxy-4-hydroxyphenylacetic acid by 288 patients with neuroblastoma and related neural crest tumors. *Cancer Res.,* **40:**1995–2001, 1980.

Lauer, S. J.; Casper, J. T.; and Borella, L.: The use of antibody-dependent cell mediated cytotoxicity (ADCC) assay to identify neuroblasts in human bone marrow. *J. Clin. Lab. Immunol.,* **1:**77–82, 1978.

Lemerle, J.; Tournade, M. F.; Sarrazin, D.; and Valayer, J.: Tumours of the Kidney. In Bloom, H. J. G.; Lemerle, J.; Neidhardt, M. K.; and Voute, P. A. (eds.): *Cancer in Children: Clinical Management.* Springer-Verlag New York, Inc., New York, 1975.

Li, F. P.: Second malignant tumors after cancer in childhood. *Cancer,* **40:**1899–1902, 1977.

Magrath, I. T., and Ziegler, J. L.: Bone marrow involvement in Burkitt's lymphoma and its relationship to acute B-cell leukemia. *Leuk. Res.,* **4**:33–59, 1979.

Malcolm, A. W.; Jaffe, N.; Folkman, M. J.; and Cassady, J. R.: Bilateral Wilms' tumor. *Int. J. Radiat. Oncol. Biol. Phys.,* **6**:167–174, 1980.

Martinson, I. M.: Home care for the child with cancer. *ACS Proceedings of National Conference on Care of Children with Cancer,* American Cancer Society, Boston, 1978.

Mauer, A. M.: Therapy of acute lymphoblastic leukemia in childhood. *Blood,* **56**:1–10, 1980.

Mierau, G. W., and Favara, B. E.: Rhabdomyosarcoma in children. Ultrastructural study of 31 cases. *Cancer,* **46**:2035–2040, 1980.

Miller, D. R.; Leikin, S.; Albo, V.; Sather, H.; Karon, M.; and Hammond, D.: Intensive therapy and prognostic factors in acute lymphoblastic leukemia of childhood: CCG 141. In Neth, R.; Gallo, R. C.; Graf, T.; Mannweiler, K.; and Winkler, K (eds.): *Modern Trends in Human Leukemia IV.* Springer-Verlag New York, Inc., New York, 1981.

Miller, R. W.: Environmental causes of cancer in childhood. In Barness, L. A.: (ed.): *Advances in Pediatrics.* Year Book Medical Publishers, Inc., Chicago, 1978.

Miller, R. W.: Contrasting epidemiology of childhood osteosarcoma, Ewings tumor and rhabdomyosarcoma. Sarcomas of soft tissue and bone. *Natl. Cancer Inst. Monogr.,* **56**:9–14, 1981.

Moe, P. J.; Seip, M.; and Finne, P. H.: Intermediate dose methotrexate (IDM) in childhood acute lymphocytic leukemia in Norway. *Acta Paediatr. Scand.,* **70**:73–79, 1981.

Mostofi, F. K.: Testicular tumors. *Cancer,* **32**:1186–1201, 1973.

Murphy, S. B.; Aur, R. J. A.; Simone, J. V.; George, S.; and Mauer, A. M.: Pretreatment cytokinetic studies in 94 children with acute leukemia. Relationship to other variables at diagnosis and to outcome of standard treatment. *Blood,* **49**:683–691, 1977.

Murphy, S. B., and Donaldson, S. S.: Pediatric lymphoma. In Carter, S. K.; Glatstein, E.; and Livingston, R. B. (eds.): *Principles of Cancer Treatment.* McGraw-Hill, Inc., New York, 1982.

Murphy, S. B.; Melvin, S. L.; and Mauer, A. M.: Correlation of tumor cell kinetic studies with surface marker results in childhood non-Hodgkin's lymphoma. *Cancer Res.,* **39**:1534–1538, 1979.

Nesbit, M. E., Jr., and Krivit, W.: Histiocytosis. In Bloom, H. J. G.; Lemerle, J.; Neidhardt, M. K.; and Voute, P. A. (eds.): *Cancer in Children: Clinical Management.* Springer-Verlag New York, Inc., New York, 1975.

Nkrumah, F. K.; Perkins, I. V.; Hyg, Ms.; and Biggar, R. J.: Combination chemotherapy in abdominal Burkitt's lymphoma. *Cancer,* **40**:1410–1416, 1977.

Osband, M. E.; Lipton, J. M.; Lavin, P.; Levey, R.; Vawter, G.; Greenberger, J. S.; McCaffrey, R. P.; and Parkman, R.: Histiocytosis-X: Demonstration of abnormal immunity, T-cell histamine H2-receptor deficiency, and successful treatment with thymic extract. *N. Engl. J. Med.,* **304**:146–153, 1981.

Pendergrass, T. W., and Davis, S.: Incidence of retinoblastoma in the United States. *Arch. Ophthalmol.,* **98**:1204–1210, 1980.

Pinkel, D.: Cure of the child with cancer—Definition and prospective. *ACS Proceedings of National Conference on Care of Child with Cancer.* American Cancer Society, Boston, 1978.

Pinkel, D.: The Ninth Annual David Karnofsky Lecture: Treatment of acute lymphocytic leukemia. *Cancer,* **43**:1128–1137, 1979.

Pinkel, D.; Hustu, H. O.; Aur, R. J. A.; Smith, K.; Borella, L. D.; and Simone, J.: Radiotherapy in leukemia and lymphoma of children. *Cancer,* **39**:817–824, 1977.

Pinkel, D.; Johnson, W.; and Aur, R. J. A.: Non-Hodgkin's lymphoma in children. *Br. J. Cancer,* **31**:298–323, 1975.

Pinkel, D., and Nefzger, D.: Some epidemiological features of childhood leukemia in the Buffalo, N.Y. area. *Cancer,* **12**:351–358, 1959.

Pinkel, D., and Pratt, C.: Embryonal rhabdomyosarcoma. In Holland, J. F. and Frei, E., III (eds.): *Cancer Medicine.* Lea & Febiger, Philadelphia, 1982.

Pratt, C. B., and George, S. L.: Second malignant neoplasms among children and adolescents treated for cancer. *Proc. Am. Assoc. Cancer Res.,* **22**:151, 1981.

Pratt, C. B.; Hustu, H. O.; Kumar, M.; Johnson, W. W.; Ransom, J. L.; Howarth, C. B.; and George, S. L.: Treatment of childhood rhabdomyosarcoma at St. Jude Childrens' Research Hospital 1962–1978. *Natl. Cancer Inst. Monogr.,* **56**:93–101, 1981a.

Pratt C. B.; Palmer, M. K.; Thatcher, N.; and Crowther, D.: Malignant melanoma in children and adolescents. *Cancer,* **47**:392–397, 1981b.

Pratt, C. B.; Rivera, G.; Shanks, E.; Johnson, W. W.; Howarth, C.; Terrell, W.; and Kumar, A. P. M.: Colorectal carcinoma in adolescents; implications regarding etiology. *Cancer,* **40**:2464–2472, 1977.

Prentice, H. G.; Lee, N.; Blacklock, H.; Smyth, J. F.; Russell, N. H.; Ganeshaguru, K.; Piga, A.; and Hoffbrand, A. V.: Therapeutic selectivity of and prediction of response to 2'-deoxycoformycin in acute leukaemia. *Lancet,* **2**:1250–1254, 1981.

Preud'homme, J.-L.; Brouet, J.-C.; Danon, F.; Flandrin, G.; and Schaison, G.: Acute lymphoblastic leukemia with Burkitt's lymphoma cells: Membrane markers and serum immunoglobulin. *J.N.C.I.,* **66**:261–264, 1981.

Pritchard, D. J.; Dahlin, D. C.; Dauphine, R. T.; Taylor, W. F.; and Beabout, J. W.: Ewings sarcoma: A clinicopathological and statistical analysis of patients surviving five years or longer. *J. Bone Joint Surg.,* **57A**:10–16, 1975.

Richards, G. E.; Wara, W. M.; Grumbach, M. M.; Kaplan, S. L.; Sheline, G. E.; and Conte, F. A.: Delayed onset of hypopituitarism: Sequelae of therapeutic irradiation of central nervous system eye and middle ear tumors. *J. Pediatr.,* **89**:553–559, 1976.

Riseborough, E. J.; Grabias, S. L.; Burton, R. I.; and Jaffe, N.: Skeletal alterations following irradiation for Wilms' tumor. *J. Bone Joint Surg.,* **58A**:526–536, 1976.

Rivera, G.; Aur, R. J. A.; Dahl, G. V.; Pratt, C. B.; Hustu, H. O.; George, S. L.; and Mauer, A. M.: Second cessation of therapy in childhood lymphocytic leukemia. *Blood,* **53**:1114–1120, 1979.

Rosen, G.; Caparros, B.; Nirenberg, A.; Marcove, R. C.; Huvos, A. G.; Kosloff, C.; Lane, J.; and Murphy, M. L.: Ewings sarcoma: Ten-year experience with adjuvant chemotherapy. *Cancer,* **47**:2204–2213, 1981a.

Rosen, G.; Nirenberg, A.; Caparros, B.; Juergens, H.; Kosloff, C.; Mehta, B. M.; Marcove, R. C.; and Huvos, A. G.: Osteogenic sarcoma: Eighty percent three year disease free survival with combination chemotherapy. *Natl. Cancer Inst. Monogr.,* **56**:213–220, 1981b.

Rosenberg, S. A.; Flye, M. W.; Conkle, D.; Seipp, C. A.; Levine, A. S.; and Simon, R. M.: Treatment of osteogenic sarcoma. (II) Aggressive resection of pulmonary metastases. *Cancer Treat. Rep.,* **63**:753–756, 1979.

Sallan, S. E.; Camitta, B. M.; Cassady, J. R.; Nathan, D.

G.; and Frei, E., III: Intermittent combination chemotherapy with Adriamycin for childhood acute lymphoblastic leukemia: Clinical results. *Blood,* **51:**425–433, 1978.

Sallan, S. E.; Ritz, J.; Pesando, J.; Gelber, R.; O'Brien, C.; Hitchcock, S.; Coral, F.; and Schlossman, S. F.: Cell surface antigens: Prognostic implications in childhood acute lymphoblastic leukemia. *Blood,* **55:**395–402, 1980.

Sanders, J. E.; Thomas, E. D.; and the Seattle Marrow Transplant Group: Marrow transplantation for children with acute leukemia in first remission. *Med. Pediatr. Oncol.,* **9:**423–427, 1981.

Sen, L., and Borella, L.: Clinical importance of lymphoblasts with T markers in childhood acute leukemia. *N. Engl. J. Med.,* **292:**828–832, 1975.

Shalet, S. M.; Beardwell, C. G.; Aaron, B. M.; Pearson, D.; and Morris-Jones, P. H.: Growth impairment in children treated for brain tumors. *Arch. Dis. Child.,* **53:**491–494, 1978.

Shields, J. A., and Augsburger, J. J.: Current approaches to the diagnosis and management of retinoblastoma. *Surv. Ophthalmol.,* **25:**347–372, 1981.

Silverberg, E.: Cancer statistics, 1982. *CA,* **32:**15–31, 1982.

Simone, J. V.; Aur, R. J. A.; Hustu, H. O.; Verzosa, M. S.; and Pinkel, D.: Three to ten years after cessation of therapy in children with leukemia. *Cancer,* **42:**839–844, 1978.

Smith, K. L., and Johnson, W.: Classification of chronic myelocytic leukemia in children. *Cancer,* **34:**670–679, 1974.

Stout, A. P.: Fibrosarcoma in infants and children. *Cancer,* **15:**1028–1040, 1962.

Strauss, R. G.; Connett, J. E.; Gale, R. P.; Bloomfield, C. D.; Herzig, G. P.; McCullough, J.; Maguire, L. C.; Winston, D. J.; Ho, W.; Stump, D. C.; Miller, W. V.; and Koepke, J. A.: A controlled trial of prophylactic granulocyte transfusions during initial induction chemotherapy for acute myelogenous leukemia. *N. Engl. J. Med.,* **305:**597–602, 1981.

Sullivan, M. P.; Dyment, P.; Hvizdala, E.; Steuber, P.; and Chen, T.: Favorable comparison of ALL Out #2 with "total" therapy in the treatment of childhood acute leukemia: The equivalence of intrathecal chemotherapy and radiotherapy as CNS prophylaxis. *Proc. Am. Assoc. Cancer Res.,* **22:**170, 1981.

Sutow, W. W.; Gehan, E. A.; Vietti, T. J.; Frias, A. E.; and Dyment, P. G.: Multidrug chemotherapy in primary treatment of osteosarcoma. *J. Bone Joint Surg.,* **58:**629–635, 1976.

Sweet, D. L.; Golomb, H. M.; Ultmann, J. E.; Miller, J. B.;

Stein, R. S.; Lester, E. P.; Mintz, U.; Bitran, J. D.; Streuli, R. A.; Daly, K.; and Roth, N. O.: Cyclophosphamide, vincristine, methotrexate with leucovorin rescue, and cytarabine (COMLA) combination sequential chemotherapy for advanced diffuse histiocytic lymphoma. *Ann. Intern. Med.,* **92:**785–790, 1980.

Tank, E. S., and Kay, R.: Neoplasms associated with hemihypertrophy, Beckwith-Wiedemann syndrome and aniridia. *J. Urol.,* **124:**266–268, 1979.

Teft, M.; Fernandez, C.; Donaldson, M.; Newton, W.; and Moon, T. E.: Incidence of meningeal involvement by rhabdomyosarcoma of the head and neck in children. *Cancer,* **42:**253–258, 1978.

Thomas, E. D.; Sanders, J. E.; Flournoy, N.; Johnson, F. L.; Buckner, C. D.; Clift, R. A.; Fefer, A.; Goodell, B. W.; Storb, R.; and Weiden, P. L.: Marrow transplantation for patients with acute lymphoblastic leukemia in remission. *Blood,* **54:**468–476, 1979.

Uribe-Botero, G.; Russell, W. O.; Sutow, W. W.; and Martin, R. G.: Primary osteosarcoma of bone: A clinicopathologic investigation of 243 cases, with necropsy studies in 54. *Am. J. Clin. Pathol.,* **67:**427–435, 1977.

Valdiserri, R. O., and Yunis, E. J.: Sacrococcygeal teratomas; A review of 68 cases. *Cancer,* **48:**217–221, 1981.

Vogler, L. B.; Crist, W. M.; Brockman, D. E.; Pearl, E. R.; Lawton, A. R.; and Cooper, M. D..: Pre-B cell leukemia: A new phenotype of childhood lymphoblastic leukemia. *N. Engl. J. Med.,* **298:**872–878, 1978.

Wara, W. M.; Margolis, L. W.; Smith, W. B.; Kushner, J. H.; and de Lorimier, A. A.: Treatment of metastatic Wilms' tumor. *Radiology,* **112:**695–697, 1974.

Weinstein, H. J.; Mayer, R. J.; Rosenthal, D. S.; Camitta, B. M.; Coral, F. S.; Nathan, D. G.; and Frei, E., III: Treatment of acute myelogenous leukemia in children and adults. *N. Engl. J. Med.,* **303:**473–478, 1980.

Weinstein, H. J.; Vance, Z. B.; Jaffe, N.; Buell, D.; Cassady, J. R.; and Nathan, D. G.: Improved prognosis for patients with mediastinal lymphoblastic lymphoma. *Blood,* **53:**687–694, 1979.

Wollner, N.; Exelby, P. R.; and Lieberman, P. H.: Non-Hodgkin's lymphoma in children: A progress report on the original patients treated with the LAS₂-L₂ protocol. *Cancer,* **44:**1990–1999, 1979.

Yates, A. J.; Becker, L. E.; and Sachs, L. A.: Brain tumors in childhood. *Childs Brain,* **5:**31–39, 1979.

Young, J. L., and Miller, R. W.: Incidence of malignant tumors in U.S. children. *J. Pediatr.,* **86:**254–258, 1975.

Yunis, J. J., and Ramsay, N. K. C.: Familial occurrence of the aniridia-Wilms' tumor syndrome with deletion 11p 13–14.1. *J. Pediatr.,* **96:**1027–1030, 1980.

Ziegler, J. L.: Burkitt's lymphoma. *N. Engl. J. Med.,* **305:**735–745, 1981.

Section Three
Supportive Care

40

Oncologic Emergencies and Special Complications

DONNA J. GLOVER and JOHN H. GLICK

MANAGEMENT CONSIDERATIONS

Oncologic emergencies are commonly encountered problems in the practice of medicine, both for the general internist and medical oncologist. As patients with neoplastic disease survive longer owing to a wide variety of therapeutic modalities and improved supportive care, complications of the underlying malignancy and of the treatment itself are more frequently observed. Table 40–1 summarizes important management considerations for patients presenting with an oncologic emergency. Although each of these points will be discussed separately, the physician must rapidly integrate these variables into a thoughtful plan for either treating or preventing an emergent complication. Due regard for the multiple variables facilitates the decision of whether to institute any treatment at all, how aggressive the treatment should be, and, most important, what are the goals of any therapeutic intervention.

The presenting symptoms and tempo of symptom development are the initial considerations faced by most clinicians. Are the symptoms secondary to a structural or metabolic complication of the tumor itself (*e.g.*, superior vena caval obstruction or inappropriate antidiuretic hormone (ADH) secretion in lung cancer); or are the symptoms secondary to complications of antineoplastic therapy (*e.g.*, hypercalcemia in a patient with metastatic breast carcinoma recently started on tamoxifen)? How rapidly are the symptoms progressing and what is the tempo of the underlying malignancy are questions that must be considered promptly in assessing a patient with a presumed oncologic emergency. Not all patients who present with early signs of superior vena caval obstruction require emergency radiotherapy. Conversely, an expanding mass lesion in the brain with increased intracranial pressure requires emergency corticosteroids and radiotherapy.

The particular point in the natural history of the underlying tumor at which the patient presents with the oncologic emergency is a major ingredient in formulating an appropriate plan. If no previous histologic diagnosis of malignancy has been established, the physician is occasionally faced with the dilemma of initiating emergency treatment for life-threatening symptoms in a cancer patient without tissue confirmation. Once the serious symptomatology is reversed, a more complete workup can be initiated, including histologic confirmation and staging. In a patient with a known preexisting malignancy, the interval between the diagnosis and treatment of the primary lesion and the development of the oncologic emergency is important. For example, a patient with renal cell carcinoma who presents with a solitary brain metastasis many years after nephrectomy might be a candidate for surgical resection of the mass lesion in the brain.

The status of other metastatic sites and the state of control of the primary provide valuable information. A woman with a painful lytic metastasis through 50% of the cortex of the femur may be a candidate for internal fixa-

Table 40–1. Management Considerations for Patients Presenting with an Oncologic Emergency

1. Symptoms
    a. Secondary to the tumor
    b. Secondary to complications of therapy
2. Tempo of symptoms and disease progression
3. Natural history of the specific tumor
    a. Problem of the undiagnosed primary
    b. Interval between treatment of the primary lesion and development of metastases and/or the oncologic emergency
    c. Status of the primary and other metastatic sites
    d. End-stage disease
4. Responsiveness to available antineoplastic therapy
    a. Previously untreated versus prior therapy
    b. Treatment of the underlying malignancy
    c. Treatment of the complication itself
    d. Prevention of complications
5. General medical condition
    a. Age
    b. Nutrition
    c. Performance status
    d. Concurrent medical problems
    e. Psychologic status
6. Goals of therapy
    a. Palliative versus curative
    b. Quality of life
    c. Objectives of the patient and family
    d. Toxicity of treatment

tion prior to radiotherapy. The same patient with dyspnea secondary to lymphangitic pulmonary metastases, who has previously exhausted conventional chemohormonal therapy, is more appropriately treated with immobilization and radiotherapy to the femur. Does the patient have end-stage metastatic disease? In this situation, treatment of the oncologic complication may needlessly prolong survival and render the patient susceptible to even more debilitating symptoms of the underlying neoplasm.

In the emergency situation the clinician must consider the responsiveness of the underlying tumor to antineoplastic therapy. Is the patient previously untreated, or have all available therapeutic modalities been exhausted? The general approach to the therapy of an oncologic emergency is to treat the underlying tumor itself. This implies, however, that effective therapy is available. Hyponatremia, secondary to inappropriate ADH secretion in small cell lung cancer, responds promptly to combination chemotherapy. Therapy may be directed at relieving the complication itself rather than treating the unrlying tumor. Malignant and rapidly progressive pleural effusions secondary to adenocarcinoma of the lung require emergency thoracentesis or insertion of a chest tube fol-

lowed by instillation of a sclerosing agent. Prevention of complications often provides the best medical care. Uric acid nephropathy in a patient with a hematologic malignancy can be prevented by vigorous hydration, urinary alkalinization, and allopurinol prior to cytotoxic chemotherapy.

The general medical condition of the patient must be factored into the decision of how vigorously to treat the oncologic emergency. It is rare for a young adult with acute myelogenous leukemia refractory to all chemotherapeutic agents not to be given aggressive antibiotic and hematologic support, even in the final days of the terminal illness. Moreover, elderly patients with small cell lung carcinoma may be denied vigorous initial therapy, although their chance for prolonged survival is good. Such facts notwithstanding, advanced age is frequently a justifiable reason for withholding emergency therapy and sparing the terminal patient toxicity for marginal gain. The patient's nutritional and performance status must be evaluated since these are major determinants of prognosis and tolerance to treatment. Do concurrent medical problems pose a major limitation on the quality of life and tolerance to the planned therapeutic intervention? Severe congestive heart failure or intrinsic renal disease may limit the type and intensity of chemotherapy and may contraindicate any treatment at all.

The psychologic status of the patient and the family frequently affects the physician's judgment about aggressive management of a complication in the terminally ill patient. It is a natural tendency to react negatively to the thought of surgical intervention for bowel obstruction in a severely depressed, withdrawn patient with far-advanced abdominal carcinomatosis. Conversely, one may be tempted to initiate an inappropriately aggressive therapeutic plan in a patient with the same disease who remains cheerful, hopeful, and apparently well adjusted to the diagnosis.

The goal of therapy must be carefully weighed before therapeutic intervention is initiated. Debilitating symptoms secondary to an acute metabolic abnormality may constitute an immediate life-threatening emergency. These disturbances can occasionally lead the physician to believe erroneously that the tumor has irreversibly progressed. Treatment of the complication may reverse the metabolic abnormality, however, allowing the patient to be treated aggressively for long-term palliation or even cure. When the goal is potential cure, the degree of acceptable risk can be quite high, and a radical treatment plan involving aggressive and hazardous therapy may be warranted. Is the goal long-term palliation with significant prolongation of survival rather than cure? It may be argued that additional survival at the cost of morbidity from the underlying treatment is hardly worthwhile if the patient will die despite therapy. However, additional time may be valuable to the patient and the family in achieving their own personal objectives. The major aim of emergency treatment in advanced malignant disease remains symptom relief, even if life expectancy is limited. Restoration of the patient to a reasonable functional status is often the goal of emergency treatment leading to improved quality of life. The risk-versus-benefit ratio of any therapeutic plan must be evaluated for each individual, using the management considerations in Table 40–1. The primary physician must always remember the option of not treating the emergent complication. No treatment is often the most appropriate choice for the patient with widespead, terminal malignancy that is not responsive to systemic therapy.

This chapter will review common structural and metabolic emergencies and special complications faced by patients with neoplastic disease. Attention will be focused on the differential diagnosis among underlying malignancy, complications of treatment, or benign etiologies seen in the patient with cancer. The pathophysiology, clinical presentation, diagnostic evaluation, and therapy for each complication will be presented. Management of the most commonly encountered oncologic complication, that of fever and infection in the immunosuppressed, myelosuppressed host, will be covered separately in Chapter 41.

STRUCTURAL EMERGENCIES

Pericardial Effusions and Neoplastic Cardiac Tamponade

Pericardial effusions and cardiac metastases are frequently seen in far-advanced malignant disease. At autopsy, between 0.1 to 21% of all patients with metastatic cancer have cardiac or pericardial metastases (Scott and Garvin, 1939; Bisel et al., 1953; Goodie, 1955; Theologides, 1978). The clinical importance of this oncologic emergency is illustrated by

Thurber's autopsy series in which pericardial metastases were the primary cause of death in approximately 35% of cases and were contributory to death in 50% (Thurber et al., 1962). Benign pericardial or mediastinal tumors, such as fibromas, teratomas, or angiomas, rarely cause neoplastic pericarditis (Marsten et al., 1966; Theologides, 1978). The most common metastatic tumors involving the pericardium are carcinoma of the lung and breast followed by lymphoma, leukemia, melanoma, gastrointestinal primaries, and sarcomas. Malignant tumors arising in adjacent structures, including lung or esophageal carcinoma, directly invade the pericardium, while more distant primaries metastasize to the pericardium by hematogenous spread (DeLoach and Haynes, 1953; Cohen et al., 1955; Goodie, 1955; Thurber et al., 1962; Martini et al., 1977). Metastatic tumors are significantly more common than the rare primary malignancies of the pericardium, including mesothelioma and rhabdomyosarcomas. These tumors frequently are associated with rapid accumulation of massive amounts of hemorrhagic fluid, resulting in cardiac tamponade (Sytman et al., 1971; Theologides, 1978).

Malignant pericardial effusions are the most common cause of cardiac tamponade, although occasional patients present with tamponade secondary to tumor encasing the heart (Spodick and Kumar, 1968) or to postirradiation pericarditis (Hurst, 1959; Applefeld et al., 1981). Cardiac tamponade presents as a medical emergency with clinical signs of circulatory collapse appearing abruptly, even though the cause of the effusion or constriction may develop slowly over a period of months to years (Theologides, 1978).

Pathophysiology. Malignant pericardial effusions are usually secondary to multiple metastases involving the parietal rather than visceral pericardium (Gassman et al., 1955; Theologides, 1978). In an autopsy series of more than 100 patients with pericardial metastases, 50% had direct invasion of the pericardium by an adjacent mediastinal malignancy, 30% had diffuse neoplastic infiltration and thickening of the pericardium, and 10% had pericardial studding with isolated tumor nodules. Rarely, a single localized pericardial metastasis will be responsible for the effusion. Patients with extensive pericardial disease often have contiguous epicardial or myocardial metastases (Gassman et al., 1955).

Neoplastic cardiac tamponade results from

either accumulation of malignant fluid within the pericardial sac, pericardial constriction by tumor, or radiation pericarditis with a thickened, fibrotic, noncompliant pericardium and associated effusion (Williams and Soutter, 1954; Applefeld et al., 1981). The severity of tamponade depends on how rapidly the pericardial fluid develops and the volume of fluid accumulated. When pericardial fluid accumulates slowly, the pericardium stretches and cardiac contractility is not significantly compromised. When the pericardium is thickened by tumor or radiation fibrosis, a small pericardial effusion produces significant cardiac compression (Williams and Soutter, 1954; Spodick and Kumar, 1968; Pories and Gaudiani, 1975). With time, increased pericardial pressure interferes with ventricular expansion and diastolic filling, resulting in decreased stroke volume. As the ventricular diastolic pressure increases, the atrioventricular valves close prematurely and the myocardial fibers shorten. Stroke volume decreases, leading to hypotension and compensatory tachycardia. As ventricular pressures rise, the mean left atrial, pulmonary arterial, venous, right atrial, and vena caval pressures rise and eventually equalize (Spodick and Kumar, 1968; Pories and Gaudiani, 1975). Tachycardia and peripheral vasoconstriction develop in an attempt to maintain arterial pressure, increase blood volume, and improve venous return. Eventually, compensatory mechanisms cannot prevent circulatory collapse (Spodick and Kumar, 1968; Pories and Gaudiana, 1975).

Clinical Presentation. Patients with malignant pericardial effusions, but without tamponade, are commonly asymptomatic, or have symptoms attributed to general manifestations of metastatic disease. In a large autopsy series, less than 30% of patients with pericardial effusions had cardiac symptoms prior to death, and in less than 10% were pericardial metastases diagnosed prior to death (Thurber et al., 1962; Theologides, 1978). Clinical symptoms are similar to those of pericarditis from other causes. The most common symptoms include dyspnea, thoracic pain, orthopnea, cyanosis, and dysphagia. Physical examination often reveals cardiac enlargement and pleural effusion, but is otherwise rarely helpful unless signs of cardiac tamponade are present.

Patients with tamponade or constriction complain of dyspnea, cough, and oppressive retrosternal chest pain which is relieved by leaning forward. Occasionally, patients describe hoarseness, hiccups, nausea, vomiting, and epigastric pain. Decreased cerebral perfusion produces seizures and alterations in consciousness, ranging from mild confusion to coma (Theologides, 1978). Physical examination may reveal an acutely anxious, diaphoretic patient with peripheral cyanosis, engorged neck veins, facial plethora, and neck swelling. Systolic and pulse pressures are decreased. Pulsus paradoxus and inspiratory neck vein swelling are often present. Carotid and peripheral pulses are weak, and heart sounds are generally distant. An early diastolic sound may be heard with constrictive pericarditis. As venous pressure increases, edema, ascites, hepatosplenomegaly, and hepatojugular reflux develop (Theologides, 1978).

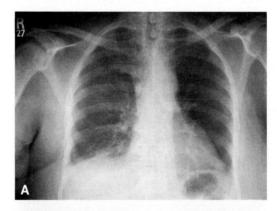

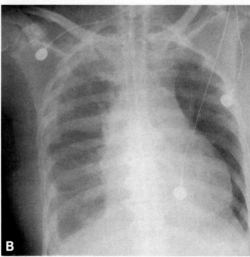

Figure 40-1. Pericardial tamponade. Chest radiographs of a 57-year-old woman with metastatic breast carcinoma admitted with pericardial tamponade. (*A*) Six months prior to admission the heart is of normal size. (*B*) Globular symmetric enlargement of the cardiac silhouette is caused by a large pericardial effusion. Bulging of the cardiac borders obliterates the cardiophrenic angles.

Diagnostic Evaluation. Clinical signs and symptoms of pericardial disease secondary to malignancy may be subtle and the diagnosis difficult to establish. Chest radiographs reveal abnormalities in more than 50% of patients, including cardiac enlargement, mediastinal widening or hilar adenopathy (see Figure 40–1). However, cardiac size may be normal with constriction from tumor or radiation fibrosis (Spodick and Kumar, 1968; Hancock, 1975; Martin *et al.,* 1975). Pericardial metastases may rarely produce nodular, irregular heart borders. Patients with large pericardial effusions typically have a globular cardiac silhouette caused by shortening and widening of the mediastinum and loss of the normal arcuate borders (Spodick and Kumar, 1968; Niarchos, 1975).

The electrocardiogram may reveal minimal changes (Thurber *et al.,* 1962) or typical changes associated with pericardial effusions, including low QRS voltage in the limb leads, sinus tachycardia, elevations of the ST segment, and T-wave changes (Spodick and Kumar, 1968). Ventricular alternans is less specific than total electrical alternans with alterations of both the P wave and the QRS-T complex (Niarchos, 1975). After a small amount of pericardial fluid is removed by pericardiocentesis, electrical alternans may disappear. However, electrical alternans may also resolve with clinical stability or worsening of tamponade and is, therefore, not a reliable diagnostic parameter (Lawrence and Cronin, 1963). Electrocardiographic signs of neoplastic constrictive pericarditis are nonspecific, but include deformed P waves, low QRS complexes, and flat, inverted T waves (Hancock, 1975).

Echocardiography is the most specific and sensitive noninvasive method for diagnosing pericardial effusions (D'Cruz *et al.,* 1972; Pories and Gaudiani, 1975; Morris, 1976; Millman *et al.,* 1977). With posterior pericardial effusions, two distinct echoes are seen, one from the effusion and one from the posterior heart border. The region between these areas indicates the size of the effusion or thickness of the pericardium (see Figure 40–2). Pericardial metastases may appear as sonolucent spaces posterior to the left ventricular epicardium (Hancock, 1975; Millman *et al.,* 1977). Specific abnormalities of anterior mitral valve motion are diagnostic for tamponade (D'Cruz *et al.,* 1972).

Pericardial tamponade, constriction, and congestive cardiomyopathies may be accompanied by pericardial effusion. Physical examination and noninvasive studies frequently will not provide adequate information to differentiate between pericardial and myocardial disease. When this differentiation is important, right heart catheterization is a useful diagnostic maneuver. In pericardial tamponade or constriction, intracardiac diastolic pressures are typically elevated above 14 mm Hg (Spodick, 1967). Pulmonary wedge, pulmonary artery diastolic, right ventricular end-diastolic, mean right atrial, and superior vena caval pressures equalize. Similar pressure tracings have been reported with infiltrative cardiomyopathies.

Table 40–2 lists important hemodynamic differences associated with tamponade, constriction, and cardiomyopathies. In constrictive pericarditis, cardiac catheterization demonstrates elevations in mean right atrial and biventricular end-diastolic pressures, an M pattern to the right atrial pulse pressure, and an early diastolic dip in both ventricles. Cardiac output is better maintained in constriction and paradoxic pulse less pronounced. In tamponade, vena caval pressure tracings reveal a single nadir, the x descent, which corresponds to atrial filling during ventricular systole. In constriction, a second brief period of rapid early ventricular diastolic filling produces a deep y descent in caval pressures and the classic diastolic dip in ventricular pressures. Cardiac output is markedly depressed with significant tamponade, but improves immediately following pericardiocentesis. This rapid hemodynamic improvement is pathognomonic for tamponade and may be the most definitive factor in differential diagnosis (Shabetai *et al.,* 1970; Fowler, 1978; Hudson, 1978).

Pericardiocentesis should always be performed for diagnostic and therapeutic purposes when a significant pericardial effusion is present in a patient with neoplastic disease. Pericardiocentesis may not be necessary, however, when an asymptomatic moderate effusion develops following mediastinal radiation (*e.g.,* Hodgkin's disease). Fifty percent of malignant pericardial effusions are hemorrhagic and 40% serosanguinous. Hemorrhagic pericardial fluid rarely clots and typically has a lower hematocrit than systemic blood (Martini *et al.,* 1977; Hankins *et al.,* 1980). Pericardial fluid should be analyzed for culture, cell count, and cytologic examination. Pericardial fluid cytology is quite accurate in diagnosing

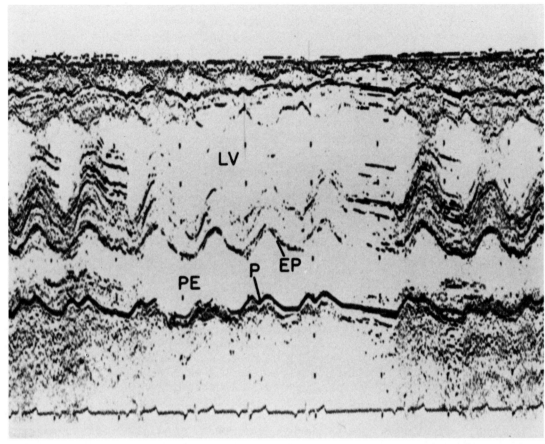

Figure 40–2. Echocardiogram of pericardial effusion. The effusion corresponds to the sonolucent space between the ventricular wall and pericardium.

Table 40–2. Hemodynamics of Myocardial and Pericardial Disease

	PERICARDIAL TAMPONADE	PERICARDIAL CONSTRICTION	CARDIOMYOPATHY
Left atrial pressure	Equals RAP	Equals RAP	10 to 20 mm Hg > RAP
Right atrial pressure	≥15 mm Hg	≥15 mm Hg usually with prominent y trough	Usually ≤15 mm if PWP is normal
Cardiac output	Decreased	Usually normal with normal AV difference	Decreased
RVP	No diastolic dip	Consistent early	Early diastolic dip may disappear with therapy
RVDP	≤⅓ systolic BP	≥⅓ systolic RVP	≤⅓ systolic RVP
PAP	Systolic PAP often ≤40 mm Hg	Systolic PAP < 40 mm Hg	Systolic PAP often ≥45–65 mm Hg
Respiratory variation in pressures	Usually present	Absent	Usually present
Diastolic pressure plateau	RAP = RVDP = PADP = PWP	RAP = RVDP = PADP = PWP	PWP < RAP

Derived from Shabetai *et al.,* 1970; Fowler, 1978; Hudson, 1978.
RAP = right atrial pressure; AV = arteriovenous; RVDP = right ventricular diastolic pressure; PADP = pulmonary arterial diastolic pressure; PWP = pulmonary wedge pressure; RVP = right ventricular pressure; PAP = pulmonary artery pressure.

metastatic carcinoma to the pericardium; however, false-negative cytologies are frequently noted with lymphomas and mesotheliomas (Zipf and Johnston, 1972; Martini *et al.*, 1977; Krikorian and Hancock, 1978; Theologides, 1978). If cytologic examination of a large amount of pericardial fluid is negative, and a histologic diagnosis is deemed important to future management, a pericardial biopsy may be obtained under local anesthesia using the subxiphoid approach. With this approach, tumor nodules are observed or palpated in approximately 50% of patients (Hankins *et al.*, 1980). Using a left anterior thoracotomy, a higher percentage of positive biopsies are obtained, but with increased morbidity secondary to complications from general anesthesia (Williams and Soutter, 1954; Hill and Cohen, 1970; Hankins *et al.*, 1980).

Therapy. Patients with malignant pericardial effusions often require emergency pericardiocentesis before definitive local therapy is initiated to prevent recurrent tamponade. Pericardiocentesis should be preceded by echocardiography. Patients with either small effusions or effusions posterior to the left ventricle rarely have tamponade and have a significantly greater risk of complications from pericardiocentesis. When small effusions are present or pericardial constriction without hemodynamic compromise is established, therapy is directed to local modalities. These include pericardial window, radiotherapy, pericardiectomy, sclerosing agents, and effective systemic antineoplastic agents (Krikorian and Hancock, 1978).

Definitive treatment of pericardial metastases depends on the sensitivity of the primary tumor to systemic therapy or radiotherapy, prior treatment, and life expectancy. Patients with neoplastic tamponade from metastatic breast cancer may be effectively palliated with pericardiocentesis followed by systemic chemotherapy, and additive hormonal manipulation if indicated. Lymphomas usually can be managed by a combination of pericardiocentesis, local radiotherapy, and systemic chemotherapy. Pericardial metastases from non-small cell lung carcinoma can be treated with pericardial drainage, sclerosing agents, and local radiotherapy. Pericardiectomy is required for radiation-induced pericardial constriction, but should generally be avoided with extensive pericardial metastases (Theologides, 1978).

When clinical signs and symptoms suggest cardiac tamponade, pericardiocentesis should be performed as an emergency procedure. Absolute indications for emergency pericardiocentesis include (1) the presence of cyanosis, dyspnea, shock, or impaired conciousness, (2) peripheral venous pressure greater than 130 mm Hg, (3) pulsus paradoxus greater than 50% of the pulse pressure, or (4) a decrease in pulse pressure by greater than 20 mm Hg. Pericardiocentesis should be done with blood pressure and electrocardiographic monitoring, preferably in an intensive care unit (Spodick, 1967). Dramatic clinical improvement, with decrease in peripheral venous pressure and disappearance of electrical alternans and pulsus paradoxus, frequently follows removal of as little as 50 mL of pericardial fluid (Kilpatrick and Chapman, 1965; Cassell and Dullum, 1967; Spodick, 1967; Hill and Cohen, 1970). Complications of pericardiocentesis include (1) trauma to the myocardium which may produce arrhythmias or hemorrhage, (2) laceration of the heart, coronary arteries, or internal mammary artery, (3) penetration of the pleural cavity, and (4) sudden death (Cassell and Dullum, 1967).

If dyspnea or cyanosis is present, supplemental oxygen should be given. Positive pressure breathing is contraindicated because of increased intrapleural and intrapericardial pressures that decrease venous return (Kilpatrick and Chapman, 1965; Spodick, 1967; Pories and Gaudiani, 1975; Theologides, 1978). Prior to emergency pericardiocentesis, attempts should be made to improve cardiac contractility and filling with isoproterenol and blood volume expansion (Theologides, 1978).

Unless definitive local therapeutic modalities to prevent recurrent tamponade are initiated, tamponade generally recurs within 24 to 48 hours following pericardiocentesis. It is difficult to compare therapeutic results with pericardial windows, different sclerosing agents, or radiotherapy since responses are not based on objective criteria. Generally, a procedure is considered effective if (1) the pericardial effusion decreases or disappears for over 30 days, (2) no symptoms of tamponade develop for over 30 days, and (3) there is no requirement for repeated pericardiocentesis. The duration of response and overall survival are also influenced by the extent of metastatic disease, tumor type, and response to concurrent systemic hormonal or chemotherapy (Hill and Cohen, 1970; Terry and Kligerman, 1970; Rubinson and Bolooki, 1972; Cham *et al.*,

1975; Lajos et al., 1975; Martini et al., 1977; Davis et al., 1978; Hankins et al., 1980).

Indwelling pericardial cathethers are used to administer intrapericardial sclerosing agents. These drugs induce an inflammatory response, fibrosis, and obliteration of the pericardial space, which prevent pericardial fluid reaccumulation. After symptoms of tamponade are relieved with pericardiocentesis, an indwelling catheter is left in place. The sclerosing agent is then instilled until there is no further pericardial drainage. A variety of sclerosing agents and radioisotopes have been used. It is difficult to evaluate the duration of response with different agents since other treatment modalities are often used concurrently. The most popular sclerosing agent is tetracycline (Rubinson and Bolooki, 1972; Davis et al., 1978). Following pericardial drainage, 500 to 1000 mg of tetracycline are instilled through pericardial cannulas and flushed with normal saline. The catheter remains in place, and the procedure is repeated every two to three days until sclerosis is complete, as demonstrated by no drainage during the preceding 24 hours. In one small series reported by Rubinson, all patients had resolution of symptoms for three to ten months following tetracycline sclerosis. Mild temperature elevations and local pain are common mild complications (Rubinson and Bolooki, 1972; Davis et al., 1978; Tattersall, 1980). Quinacrine and talc have been used with good success, but with more toxicity (Lokich, 1973; Flannery et al., 1975; Smith et al., 1978). Chemotherapeutic agents such as nitrogen mustard, 5-fluorouracil, methotrexate, and thiotepa have been used with variable results, but complications are more frequently reported. These common complications include bone marrow suppression which interferes with systemic chemotherapy. Sudden death following the injection of intrapericardial nitrogen mustard has been reported (Theologides, 1978). Encouraging results were noted in early series with the use of radioactive phosphorus, yttrium, and gold (Martini et al., 1977; Theologides, 1978). Using intrapericardial radioactive isotopes, excellent responses were obtained in 70% of patients, with a three-month median survival in patients with distant metastases and a 15-month survival with localized disease at presentation (Martini et al., 1977).

Approximately 50% of patients with neoplastic pericardial disease will respond to radiotherapy, depending on the origin of the primary (Terry and Kligerman, 1970; Lokich, 1973; Cham et al., 1975). The radiation dose depends on the radiosensitivity of the tumor. Usually, 150 to 200 rads per day are delivered to a total dose of 2500 to 3500 rads over a three- to four-week period. Patients with leukemia or lymphoma respond to lower doses, 1500 to 2000 rads over one and a half to two weeks. It is difficult to quantitate objective responses, but most investigators define response as relief of cardiac symptoms and improvement in radiologic and electrocardiographic abnormalities. Using these criteria, responses with external radiotherapy occur in over 70% of patients with breast cancer, 25% with lung cancer, and 85% with leukemia or lymphoma (Terry and Kligerman, 1970; Cham et al., 1975). Response and duration of palliation depend on the radiosensitivity of the tumor.

In recent series, pleural-pericardial windows provided prolonged palliation with little morbidity (Williams and Soutter, 1954; Hill and Cohen, 1970; Fredrickson et al., 1971; Lajos et al., 1975). Hill and Cohen (1970) reported that symptoms were relieved from 3.5 to 13 months following this procedure. The favored surgical technique is inferior pericardiotomy using the subxiphoid approach. Under local anesthesia, inferior pericardiotomy provides immediate relief of cardiac compression, with complication rates ranging from 0 to 2%, and only one death in a series of 180 patients (Williams and Soutter, 1954; Rose, 1962; Hankins et al., 1980). Symptoms of tamponade and effusion recur in less than 5% of patients (Hankins et al., 1980). Thus, overall survival is determined primarily by the extent of distant metastases.

The window may be created by left anterior thoracotomy when additional tissue is required for diagnosis or there is extensive tumor encasement. The left anterior thoracotomy approach, however, requires general anesthesia and is associated with higher morbidity and mortality rates. This approach is also successful in 70% of cases (Williams and Soutter, 1954; Hill and Cohen, 1970). In Lajos' series of patients treated with inferior pleural-pericardial windows and instillation of intrapericardial chemotherapy, all patients responded with no recurrences prior to death (Lajos et al., 1975). In a retrospective review of the literature, Smith et al., (1974) found no significant differences in survival or palliation with pleural-pericardial windows compared to conservative therapy using pericardiocentesis, intrapericardial and/or systemic chemotherapy, or hormonal therapy. Unfortunately, controlled trials comparing different treatment modalities are not available.

Pericardiectomy is the therapy of choice for radiation-induced pericardial disease that does not respond to more conservative medical therapy, including corticosteroids. Pericardiectomy generally should not be attempted with extensive metastases to the pericardium because of the relatively short life expectancy and difficult surgical technique with associated high morbidity (Theologides, 1978).

If effective systemic therapy is available, it should be administered either concurrently with local therapy or as soon as the patient is clinically stable. Following emergency pericardiocentesis, the type of definitive local therapy depends on the sensitivity of the primary tumor to chemotherapy or hormonal manipulation, prior treatment, extent of metastatic disease, medical condition of the patient, and life expectancy. Early diagnosis and treatment of neoplastic pericardial disease, however, often provide excellent palliation and prolonged survival.

Pleural Effusions

Symptomatic malignant pleural effusions are a commonly encountered clinical problem for the medical oncologist. Pleural effusions compress lung tissue, resulting in reduced lung volumes, respiratory compromise, atelectasis, and infection. The most common malignancies associated with pleural effusions are carcinoma of the lung, breast, ovary, and lymphoma (Austin and Flye, 1979). In a series of 601 women with metastatic breast cancer, 48% developed malignant effusions and 25% required intracavitary therapy (Fracchia et al., 1970). At autopsy or during the course of their disease, 30 to 33% of patients with lung cancer, 6 to 17% with ovarian cancer, 16 to 23% with Hodgkin's disease, and 20 to 33% with non-Hodgkin's lymphoma have pleural effusions documented (Farber, 1954; Westling, 1965; Austin and Flye, 1979; Kaplan, 1980). Following the development of a malignant effusion, survival depends on the extent of metastatic disease and probability of response to both local and systemic therapy. Patients with pleural effusions secondary to breast carcinoma, lymphoma, and mesothelioma generally have the longest survivals following defin-

itive local treatments (Ariel et al., 1966; Weick et al., 1973; Rosato et al., 1974; Martini et al., 1975).

Pathophysiology. The pleural space normally contains less than 5 mL of fluid. Protein-free fluid is filtered from systemic capillaries in the parietal pleura into the pleural space and reabsorbed by the pulmonary capillaries in the visceral pleura. Lymphatics reabsorb the minimal amount of protein that enters the pleural space from the pleural surfaces. Thus, the normal pleural fluid dynamic equilibrium is controlled by hydrostatic and colloidal osmotic pressures, capillary permeability, and lymphatic drainage. If this balance is upset, pleural fluid will accumulate until a new equilibrium is established (Austin and Flye, 1979).

The most common cause of malignant effusions is direct neoplastic pleural involvement. Small tumor implants within the pleura increase capillary permeability. Hemorrhagic effusions result from local erosion of blood vessels within the pleura. Large tumor implants may cause lymphatic obstruction, which further impairs reabsorption of pleural fluid (Friedman and Slater, 1978). Neoplastic involvement of mediastinal lymph nodes impairs pleural lymphatic drainage. These exudative effusions usually have negative cytologies, unless pleural metastases are also present.

The pathophysiology of malignant effusions without serosal implants has been investigated in the animal model by injecting tumor cell suspensions into the pleural space. The free-floating malignant cells produce a local inflammatory response which appears to alter capillary permeability and irritate the serosal surfaces, resulting in exudative effusions. This situation may occur clinically in patients with exudative effusions and 2000 to 4000 malignant cells/mm^3 without obvious serosal implants (Friedman and Slater, 1978).

Pleural effusions may occur in association with the superior vena cava (SVC) syndrome or pericardial constriction and tamponade owing to increased venous pressure. This results in decreased reabsorption of fluid by both capillaries and lymphatics. Less than 30% of patients with the SVC syndrome, pericardial constriction, or tamponade, however, have elevation in venous pressure sufficient to cause pleural effusions. Effusions secondary to obstructive pneumonitis result from obstruction of pulmonary veins and lymphatics, which increases capillary hydrostatic pressures and impairs absorption of proteinaceous pleural fluid (Friedman and Slater, 1978).

Clinical Presentation and Diagnostic Evaluation. Patients most often present with dyspnea, which is typically worse in the supine position. A dry cough is frequently present and ranges in intensity from mild to debilitating. Even with large effusions, pleuritic pain may be absent, unless there are associated pleural implants. Physical examination reveals dullness to percussion and decreased breath sounds over the effusion. A pleural friction rub may be audible over areas of neoplastic pleural involvement (Austin and Flye, 1979; Kaplan, 1980). Effusions are seen on routine upright posteroanterior (PA) and lateral chest films when at least 300 mL of pleural fluid are present. As little as 100 mL of fluid may be detected on decubitus films, which should be performed on all patients to determine if the fluid layers out or is loculated (Rigler, 1931; Kaunitz, 1939).

Thoracentesis should be performed for diagnosis and relief of symptoms. Gravity pleural fluid drainage is the preferred method for fluid collection with thoracentesis. Vacuum bottles should be avoided since the increased pressure results in an increased risk of pneumothorax. Ultrasound may be necessary to differentiate loculated fluid from solid tumor nodules, fibrosis, or underlying lung, and to localize the appropriate site for thoracentesis. Pleural fluid should be sent for appropriate cultures, cell count, cytology, protein, lactic dehydrogenase (LDH), glucose, and, in selected cases, carcinoembryonic antigen levels (CEA), amylase, and cytogenetic analysis (Austin and Flye, 1979). The gross appearance of most malignant effusions is often similar to that of benign effusions. A hemorrhagic effusion ($\geq$ 100,000 red blood cells/mm^3) suggests tumor, trauma, tuberculosis, or pulmonary infarction. Empyema fluid is usually viscous, malodorous, and produces a clear supernatant after centrifugation. Chylous effusions, secondary to thoracic duct obstruction, are odorless and do not separate after centrifugation (Austin and Flye, 1979).

A useful initial step in determining the etiology of the effusion is separation of effusions into exudates and transudates. Exudative effusions have an increased amount of protein in the pleural space. All malignant effusions, except those caused by lymphatic obstruction, are exudates; however, exudative effusions are also characteristic of tuberculosis, pulmonary

infarction, pneumonia, trauma, and collagen vascular diseases. To separate exudates from transudates accurately, simultaneous measurement of serum and pleural fluid protein and LDH should be performed. Pleural effusions are characterized as exudates if the pleural fluid protein to serum protein ratio is greater than 0.5, the pleural fluid LDH to serum LDH ratio is greater than 0.6, or the pleural fluid LDH is greater than 200 mg/dL (Light et al., 1972).

Cell counts are usually increased with a predominance of mononuclear cells, especially in cases with positive cytologies. Pleural fluid cytology is diagnostic in 65 to 73% of all malignant effusions when a large amount of heparinized pleural fluid is obtained for examination. Routine cytologic examination should include examination of the cell block after fixation and sectioning. Occasionally, repeated thoracenteses are required before malignant cells are detected. In large series of patients with neoplastic effusions, positive cytologies were obtained in 42 to 53%, 64, 69, and 73% after the first, second, third, and fourth pleural fluid analyses, respectively (Jarvi et al., 1972; Salyer et al., 1975). Effusions caused by mediastinal lymphatic obstruction are relatively acellular. Since most effusions in patients with lymphoma result from lymphatic obstruction rather than direct pleural involvement, cytologies are rarely positive. Pleural infiltration is most common with diffuse histiocytic lymphoma and least common with Hodgkin's disease (Melamed, 1963).

If the diagnosis cannot be obtained by thoracentesis, pleural biopsy with either a Cope needle or thoracostomy is diagnostic in 49 to 56% of malignant effusions. By combining pleural biopsy and cytology, over 90% of neoplastic effusions are diagnosed (Salyer et al., 1975). Effusions with negative cytologies and biopsies usually are secondary to mechanisms other than pleural metastases, such as lymphatic obstruction, bronchial obstruction, or elevation in venous pressures (Salyer et al., 1975; Austin and Flye, 1979). Glucose levels may be low in inflammatory effusions secondary to infection or malignancy. Pleural fluid amylase may be elevated with pancreatic cancer or acute pancreatitis. Elevated CEA levels occur in 34 to 55% of malignant effusions and are rarely associated with a benign process.

Therapy. Control of recurrent malignant effusions will provide significant palliation for most patients. Neoplasms that are responsive to chemotherapy or hormonal therapy should be treated with thoracentesis and systemic therapy, reserving local therapy for nonresponders. This is particularly evident with metastatic breast carcinoma. Patients with effusions caused by mediastinal lymphatic obstruction, most commonly from lymphoma, may be treated effectively with mediastinal radiotherapy or chemotherapy. The choice of whether to use systemic or local therapy depends on the probability of a significant response to systemic therapy, prior treatment, the etiology of the effusion, and the general medical condition of the patient.

Thoracentesis is invariably utilized for initial palliation and diagnosis. In the majority of patients with solid tumors, the pleural fluid will reaccumulate rapidly. In Anderson's series of 97 patients treated with an initial therapeutic thoracentesis, all but four patients demonstrated reaccumulation of fluid within one month. The median time to recurrence, requiring further therapy, was 4.2 days (Anderson et al., 1974). Frequent thoracenteses should be avoided, as they are complicated by pneumothorax, fluid loculation, empyema, and hypoproteinemia.

The efficacy of different local therapeutic modalities is difficult to evaluate and compare. Most investigators define responders as those patients not requiring thoracentesis for at least two months following therapy. However, patients may have received concurrent systemic hormonal therapy, chemotherapy, or radiotherapy. Other series include patients who have been previously treated with intrapleural therapy. These patients have little chance of responding to additional intracavitary therapy because of significant pleural fibrosis and loculation (Austin and Flye, 1979).

Thoracostomy tube drainage alone controls effusions with response rates ranging from 0 to 86%. The instillation of intrapleural sclerosing agents appears to improve response rates; however, adequate controlled trials are not available (Lambert et al., 1967; Anderson et al., 1974; Izbicki et al., 1975). With intrapleural tetracycline, quinacrine, talc, radioisotopes, or nitrogen mustard, most patients achieve excellent palliation. Following intrapleural therapy, the visceral and parietal pleura are fused with a dense fibroblastic reaction which prevents fluid reaccumulation. The efficacy of these intrapleural agents is felt to be related to this obliterative pleuritis, rather than a direct antineoplastic effect, since at autopsy most patients have tumor implants within the fused pleura (Kniseley and Andrews, 1953; Mark et al., 1964; Leininger et al., 1969).

Over 50% of malignant effusions are effectively controlled with thoracostomy tube drainage and intrapleural therapy. Following local anesthesia, a 24 French thoracic catheter is inserted in the eighth intercostal space at the midaxillary line. The effusion is then drained using a water-seal suction device. Daily chest films should be obtained to evaluate the chest-tube position and amount of residual pleural fluid. The sclerosing agent is injected intrapleurally after all the fluid is removed, the lung expanded, and the chest-tube drainage has generally decreased to 100 to 200 mL per day. After the agent is allowed to distribute over the pleural space, the chest tube is clamped. If fluid reaccumulates, additional intrapleural therapy on a daily basis may be required before the chest tube is removed (Rubinson and Bolooki, 1972).

The choice of which agent to instill into the pleural cavity is controversial. Excellent palliation is achieved with intrapleural tetracycline, talc, quinacrine, nitrogen mustard, or radioisotopes. Currently, the most popular sclerosing agent is tetracycline, which controls 80 to 83% of effusions with few side effects. Pleuritic pain and transient fever are easily managed with mild analgesics and antipyretics. Usually only one tetracycline injection is required. If the effusion is not controlled after three instillations, however, other local modalities should be considered.

Although it is rarely used today, Alder reported that with intrapleural talc suspensions, 93% of recurrent malignant pleural effusions were successfully controlled. When talc instillation is performed with general anesthesia and thoracotomy, a high perioperative mortality rate occurs. Currently, with thoracostomy drainage and intrapleural instillation of a talc suspension, morbidity is limited to transient pleuritic pain. This pain is adequately controlled with analgesics (Adler and Sayek, 1976).

Intrapleural quinacrine controls 80% of malignant effusions, but toxicity is significant. Fifty to 90% of patients develop fever, 23-78% pleuritic pain, 14% transient hypotension, and 10% central nervous system manifestations, including hallucinations, and seizures (Ultmann et al., 1963; Dollinger et al., 1967; Borja and Pugh, 1973; Kisner et al., 1977). In the early 1950s intrapleural radioisotopes were the most frequently used technique to control large effusions. Radioactive ^{198}Au or the less expensive ^{32}Cr phosphate produced responses in 55 to 61% of patients. Toxicity was minimal, with nausea and vomiting occurring in 20 to 25% of patients (Austin and Flye, 1979).

Nitrogen mustard was the first chemotherapeutic agent injected intrapleurally. Over 50% of patients had good palliation with intracavitary nitrogen mustard. Responses were seen in 66% of patients with lung cancer, 73% with ovarian cancer, and 37% with lymphoma. Intracavitary nitrogen mustard is now rarely used owing to its relatively high incidence of side effects. Many patients experience moderately severe pleuritic pain, fever, nausea, and vomiting. Owing to systemic absorption of nitrogen mustard, unpredictable myelosuppression limits the use of concurrent systemic chemotherapy (Mark et al., 1964; Austin and Flye, 1979). Intrapleural doxorubicin and bleomycin have been reported to control 78 to 89% of malignant effusions with minimal toxicity (Paladine et al., 1976; Keffort et al., 1980). Less impressive results have been obtained with other intracavitary chemotherapeutic drugs, including 5-fluorouracil and thiotepa (Austin and Flye, 1979; Trotter et al., 1979).

Although pleurectomy controls 99% of malignant effusions, it is rarely employed today. Pleurectomy is associated with high morbidity and mortality rates of 23% and 6 to 10%, respectively (Jensik et al., 1963; Martini et al., 1975). Since the more conservative treatment approaches previously described offer excellent palliation, invasive surgical procedures are rarely required.

Radiotherapy has also been utilized as a palliative modality. Strober provided effective palliation for 70% of patients with radiotherapy using a moving strip technique and supervoltage therapy (Strober et al., 1973). Radiation therapy is most effective, however, when the effusion develops secondary to neoplastic obstruction of mediastinal lymphatics. Approximately, 90% of patients with lymphoma have complete resolution of pleural effusions following mediastinal irradiation (Bruneau and Rubin, 1965; Carmel and Kaplan, 1973). Even when no obvious mediastinal adenopathy is present, up to 70% of patients with lymphoma and negative pleural cytologies may have resolution of effusions following mediastinal irradiation (Bruneau and Rubin, 1965; Austin and Flye, 1979).

Superior Vena Caval Syndrome

Malignant neoplasms are responsible for at least 80% of cases of superior vena caval (SVC) obstruction. Tumor arising in or invading the mediastinum impairs venous drainage of the head, neck, and upper thoracic area (Perez et al., 1978; Shimm et al., 1981). As shown in Table 40–3, bronchogenic carcinoma, most notably the small cell anaplastic and squamous cell subtypes, accounts for at least 75% of malignant SVC syndromes (Rubin et al., 1963; Davenport et al., 1978; Perez et al., 1978; Shimm et al., 1981). Five to 15% of patients

Table 40–3. Neoplastic Causes of Superior Vena Caval Syndrome

DIAGNOSIS	PEREZ	DAVENPORT	SCHRAUFNAGEL
Bronchogenic carcinoma	67	25	67
Small cell anaplastic	31	20	19
Epidermoid	17	5	24
Large cell	10		1
Adenocarcinoma	8	1	6
Not specified	1		17
Lymphoma	14	2	10
Other neoplasms	3	8	13
Breast carcinoma	1	2	6
Germ cell	1		2
Kaposi's sarcoma	1		1
Mesothelioma			1
Thymoma			1
Thyroid		1	
Cervix		1	
Ovary		1	
Total	84	35	90

Derived from Davenport et al., 1978; Perez et al., 1978, Schraufnagel et al., 1981.

with lung cancer develop SVC obstruction during the course of their disease. SVC syndrome is a frequent presenting sign of small cell carcinomas, occurring in 30% with limited disease (Dombernowsky and Hanson, 1978). Ten to 15% of neoplastic SVC obstructions are secondary to lymphoma, most commonly diffuse large cell (histiocytic) lymphoma (Perez *et al.*, 1978). Superior vena caval syndrome has also been reported with other malignancies arising in or metastasizing to the mediastinum, including thymoma, carcinoma of the breast, ovary, cervix, thyroid, larynx, and, rarely, testicular neoplasms and Kaposi's sarcoma. In the older literature up to 40% of cases of superior vena caval syndrome were the result of benign causes, including granulomatous or sclerosing mediastinitis, tuberculosis or syphilitic aneurysms (Schechter, 1954). In recent series, less than 15% of SVC syndromes are secondary to the nonmalignant causes listed in Table 40–4 (Mahajan *et al.*, 1975; Perez *et al.*, 1978; Nogiere *et al.*, 1979; Schraufnagel *et al.*, 1981; Van Houtte and Fruhling, 1981).

Pathophysiology.   Superior vena caval syndrome results from compression or obstruction of the superior cava and its associated tributaries by the primary tumor or nodal metastases. Because of low intravascular pressure, the vena cava is easily compressed by adjacent expanding masses. If the azygos or other collateral veins are patent, the superior vena caval syndrome may not result, despite blockage of this major tributary. The superior vena cava extends from the junction of the brachiocephalic veins to the right atrium, a distance of approximately 7 cm. Adjacent structures including the trachea, right mainstem bronchus, pulmonary artery, aorta, brachiocephalic artery, paratracheal nodes, and thymus allow little room for tumor growth within this compartment without SVC compression (Roswit *et al.*, 1953; Perez *et al.*, 1978).

SVC obstruction reduces venous return from the head, neck, thorax, and upper ex-

Table 40–4.   Nonmalignant Causes of Superior Vena Caval Syndrome

Number of patients with SVC syndrome		107
Number of patients with benign etiology		16
Mediastinal fibrosis	8	
Thrombosis	3	
Goiter	3	
Aneurysm	1	
Radiation fibrosis	1	

Derived from Schraufnagel *et al.*, 1981.

Table 40–5.   Superior Vena Caval Syndrome: Symptoms and Signs

FINDING	NO.	PERCENT
Total no. of patients	84	
Thorax vein distention	56	67
Neck vein distention	49	59
Edema of face	47	56
Tachypnea	34	40
Plethora of face	16	19
Cyanosis	13	15
Edema of upper extremities	8	9.5

Derived from Perez *et al.*, 1978.

tremities. Elevated venous pressures lead to facial and upper extremity edema, pleural and pericardial effusions, and tracheal edema. Cardiac output declines with decreased venous return to the heart. Alterations in consciousness and other cerebral signs may be secondary to brain edema and low cardiac output.

Clinical Presentation.   The severity of clinical findings depends on the extent of SVC compression and rapidity of tumor progression. Patients may have an indolent course if gradual SVC compression allows time for collateral circulation to develop. Table 40–5 lists the clinical symptoms and signs of SVC syndrome. Facial, cervical, thoracic, and upper extremity venous dilatation and edema are common symptoms at presentation. Cardiopulmonary symptoms including dyspnea, fatigue, and cough occur later in the course of SVC obstruction and are typically worse in the supine position. Cough may be present earlier if lung carcinoma is the underlying etiology. Approximately 20% have associated chest pain or dysphagia at diagnosis. Rarely, laryngeal or bronchial edema or obstruction results in stridor. Depending on the extent of disease, 2 to 22% of patients will have neurologic symptoms including headache, altered consciousness, or decreased visual acuity. Early physical findings include neck vein distention, cervicofacial edema, and dilated retinal, thoracic, conjunctival, and subglossal veins. Tachypena is often present. Emergency treatment is indicated when physical examination suggests cerebral dysfunction, reduced cardiac function, or upper airway edema (Perez *et al.*, 1978; Schraufnagel *et al.*, 1981).

Diagnostic Evaluation.   The full-blown syndrome is easy to recognize, but SVC obstruction may be difficult to diagnose when clinical signs are subtle or insidious in onset. Old photographs should be obtained to com-

firm cervicofacial swelling. In cases where the diagnosis of superior vena caval syndrome is equivocal, radionuclide scans and venography are safe and efficient diagnostic tests (see Figure 40–3). These studies also may be useful in defining the anatomy of venous drainage, localizing the obstruction, and planning radiotherapy portals (Howard, 1967; Gollub *et al.*, 1980; Van Houtte and Fruhling, 1981). Bilateral injection of a radionuclide allows better visualization of collateral circulation and major veins (Van Houtte and Fruhling, 1981). Follow-up radionuclide studies may be obtained to assess response to treatment, although serial physical examination and chest radiographs are usually sufficient (Gollub *et al.*, 1980).

Once the diagnosis of SVC syndrome is established, the etiology must be determined. Most patients with neoplastic SVC syndrome require histologic confirmation of malignancy before appropriate treatment can be initiated. In the life-threatening situation, emergency radiotherapy may be started before a histologic diagnosis is obtained. Shimm reported that only 22% of patients with newly diagnosed SVC syndrome had a previous history of known malignancy (Shimm *et al.*, 1981). The majority of patients have a superior mediastinal mass on chest radiography. Fifty percent have associated pulmonary parenchymal lesions or hilar adenopathy and 20 to 25% a right-sided pleural effusion (Perez *et al.*, 1978). Table 40–6 lists diagnostic procedures that have been utilized to obtain pathology prior to

initiating therapy. An attempt to establish the diagnosis by cytologic or histologic confirmation should be made by the least invasive technique available. Sputum cytology, bronchoscopy with bronchial biopsies and washings, and biopsy of palpable lymphadenopathy provide the correct diagnosis in 70% of cases (Perez *et al.*, 1978). The primary diagnosis may be established by bone marrow biopsies in patients with small cell lung carcinoma or lymphoma. If less aggressive attempts have failed to make a definitive diagnosis, invasive procedures, including thoracotomy or mediastinoscopy can be performed safely if tracheal obstruction is not present. In the past, invasive procedures were postponed until radiation was initiated to avoid cardiopulmonary complications and bleeding (Ahmann, 1984). Once radiotherapy is initiated, diagnostic procedures should not be delayed beyond 72 hours, otherwise a definitive diagnosis may not be established owing to tissue necrosis (Shim *et al.*, 1981).

Therapy. Radiotherapy is the primary therapy for most cases of malignant SVC syndrome. Radiotherapy is frequently given to the mediastinum alone to achieve rapid resolution of symptoms. Most carcinomas are treated with initial high daily fractions (400 rads for three to four days), followed by dose reduction to 150 to 200 rads per day for a total dose of 3000 to 5000 rads. The total dose of radiotherapy depends on tumor size, radioresponsiveness, and probability of response to systemic antineoplastic therapy (Rubin *et al.*, 1963;

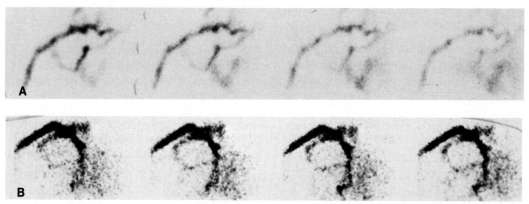

Figure 40–3. Dynamic radionuclide imaging: superior vena caval syndrome. Radionuclide scans are performed by injecting ^{99m}Tc-labeled microspheres into a vein in the upper extremity with impaired venous return. This technique visualizes the major veins and collateral circulation and identifies areas with impaired venous flow. (*A*) A 60-year-old man with complete obstruction of the superior vena cava secondary to small cell lung carcinoma. (*B*) A 55-year-old woman with partial obstruction of the superior vena cava secondary to squamous cell carcinoma of the lung. The arrows indicate the site of obstruction.

Table 40-6. Superior Vena Caval Syndrome: Methods of Diagnosis

METHOD	TOTAL NO. PATIENTS	POSITIVE DIAGNOSIS No. Patients	%
Thoracotomy and biopsy	19	19	100
Mediastinoscopy and biopsy	11	9	81
Bronchoscopy and biopsy	45	28	62
Lymph node biopsy			
Scalene	22	11	50
Supraclavicular (palpable)	19	16	84
Cytology			
Sputum	24	15	63
Bronchial washings	12	6	50
Pleural effusion	4	4	100

Derived from Perez *et al.,* 1978.

Davenport *et al.,* 1978, Perez *et al.,* 1978). Patients with lymphoma generally are treated with 2000 to 4000 rads, while non-small cell bronchogenic carcinomas require 5000 to 7000 rads over a five- to seven-week period (Rubin *et al.,* 1963; Rubin and Ciccio, 1971; Davenport *et al.,* 1978; Perez *et al.,* 1978).

The radiation portal should include at least a 2-cm margin around the tumor. Patients with limited non-small cell lung cancer have the portal expanded to include mediastinal, hilar, and supraclavicular lymph nodes, and any adjacent pulmonary parenchymal lesions. Mantle irradiation may be preferable to mediastinal irradiation in selected cases of Hodgkin's disease or malignant lymphoma (Davenport *et al.,* 1978; Perez *et al.,* 1978).

Radiation responses are evaluated using subjective and objective criteria. Improvement in dyspnea and clearing of mental status are considered subjective responses to radiation therapy, while objective responses are evaluated by decreased venous dilatation and edema and improvement on chest radiographs. Table 40-7 lists the subjective and objective radiation responses observed by Davenport. Subjective improvement typically precedes objective signs of response by three to seven days (Davenport *et al.,* 1978). Over 70% of patients with bronchogenic carcinoma and over 95% with lymphoma have resolution of SVC syndrome following radiotherapy. Patients with small cell anaplastic carcinoma or lymphoma generally have more complete and prompt responses (Howard, 1967; Perez *et al.,* 1978).

SVC syndrome secondary to either small cell lung carcinoma or non-Hodgkin's lymphoma may also respond rapidly to systemic chemotherapy. Kane *et al.* and Dombernowsky reported that all patients presenting with SVC syndrome secondary to small cell lung cancer responded within seven days to combination chemotherapy (Kane *et al.,* 1976; Dombernowsky and Hanson, 1978). If cerebral or cardiopulmonary signs are present, chemotherapy should be combined with a modest dose of radiotherapy (1000 to 2000 rads) (Perez *et al.,* 1978). Sclerosing agents should not be injected into dilated upper extremity veins under high pressure. Several investigators have observed more rapid responses when anticoagulants or fibrinolytic agents were used in conjunction with radiotherapy or chemotherapy (Salsali and Cliffton, 1965; Ghosh and Cliffton, 1973). Although Ghosh reported that patients treated with anticoagulants had more rapid improvement and shorter hospitalizations, there was no difference in overall survival (Ghosh and Cliffton, 1973). Since large controlled trials are lacking, antithrombotic therapy may be associated with more risk than benefit in neoplastic SVC syndrome. Corticosteroids transiently de-

Table 40-7. Subjective and Objective Response of Superior Vena Caval Obstruction to Radiation Therapy

	RESPONSE OF SVC SYNDROME No. of Patients	Days	%
Total number	35		
Subjective	27	3-4	77
	32	7	91
Objective	23	7	66
	31	14	89

Derived from Davenport *et al.,* 1978.

crease edema and inflammatory reactions associated with tumor necrosis and irradiation, but generally are not administered for more than three to seven days.

High morbidity and mortality rates have been reported with surgical procedures to relieve superior vena caval obstruction. Surgical bypass procedures should be reserved for the rare patient in good physical condition, who has a reasonable life expectancy, but has received maximal prior radiotherapy with little chance of response to chemotherapy (Effeney *et al.,* 1973; Avasthi and Moghissi, 1977; Yoshimura *et al.,* 1979; Bass *et al.,* 1980).

Airway Obstruction

Tracheal and endobronchial tumors that occlude a significant portion of the airway lumen must be treated promptly before infection, respiratory distress, or irreversible obstruction occurs. The majority of cancer patients who develop bronchial obstruction have endobronchial tumor (Sise and Crichlow, 1978), whereas tracheal obstruction is more often the result of benign causes, including tracheal stenosis following prolonged intubation, tracheomalacia, or tracheal edema from infection or recent radiotherapy (Weisel *et al.,* 1961; Grillo, 1973). Patients with tumors of the hypopharynx and larynx rarely present with signs of upper airway obstruction, as most patients undergo elective tracheostomy before significant airway compromise develops (Sise and Crichlow, 1978).

Bronchial obstruction is usually caused by primary lung carcinoma. At presentation, signs of bronchial obstruction are evident on chest radiographs in 53% of patients with squamous cell lung carcinoma, 25% with adenocarcinoma, 33% with large cell carcinoma, and 38% with small cell carcinoma (Miller, 1977). In Brewer's series, 70% of patients operated on for primary lung cancer had endobronchial tumor. Twenty percent had an endobronchial lesion in a mainstem bronchus and 50% in a lobar bronchus (Brewer, 1977). Endobronchial metastases from sources other than lung primaries are rare. The incidence of significant endobronchial metastases is less than 2% at autopsy. If patients with microscopic endobronchial metastases are included, however, the incidence ranges from 25 to 50% (King and Castleman, 1943; Rosenblatt *et al.,* 1966; Braman and Whitcomb, 1975; Baumgartner and Mark, 1980). Breast, colon, and renal cell carcinomas are the most common histologies associated with endobronchial metastases, although endobronchial spread also has been reported with sarcomas, melanomas, and ovarian cancers (Braman and Whitcomb, 1975; Fitzgerald, 1977).

Clinical Presentation. Symptoms suggestive of intermittent upper airway obstruction may be present 6 to 15 months before a tracheal neoplasm is discovered (Houston *et al.,* 1969; Weber and Grillo, 1978a,b). Most patients are relatively asymptomatic until at least 75% of the lumen is occluded (Sise and Crichlow, 1978; Weber and Grillo, 1978a). Presenting symptoms include dyspnea, orthopnea, cough, wheezing, stridor, hoarseness, hemoptysis, tracheoesophageal fistula, and aspiration pneumonia (Belen and Rotman, 1977; Sise and Crichlow, 1978; Weber and Grillo, 1978a). Bronchial obstruction usually produces cough, hemoptysis, wheezing, and eventually postobstructive pneumonia (Baumgartner and Mark, 1980).

It is often difficult to differentiate bronchial from tracheal obstruction on physical examination. High-pitched breathing or stridor indicates a high degree of laryngeal or tracheal obstruction. Inspiratory movements are prolonged with extreme retraction of the intercostal spaces. Localized wheezing or rhonchi may be heard over the partially obstructed airway. If inspiratory rhonchi are audible over both hemithoraces, palpable rhonchi may be appreciated over the site of obstruction. With significant bronchial narrowing, the trachea deviates toward the affected side during inspiration, and away from it during expiration. Signs of consolidation are characteristically present over obstructed pulmonary segments. Symptoms and signs of bacterial pneumonia may be found with postobstructive infection.

Diagnostic Evaluation. The severity of symptoms and tempo of symptom progression dictate the thoroughness of diagnostic evaluation. All patients with symptoms of tracheal obstruction should have radiographic studies performed. Lateral neck films with soft tissue technique provide the best views of the upper third of the trachea. The diagnosis may be detected on routine chest roentgenogram if significant tracheal narrowing or an associated mediastinal mass is seen. Bilateral oblique chest films may be sufficient to assess the tracheal contours. Before initiating therapy, overpenetrated tracheal films, tomography (including oblique and lateral views), tracheal fluoroscopy, and barium swallow should be obtained (Weber and Grillo, 1978a,b). CT scans may better define the extent and degree of tracheal obstruction. These radiographic studies often aid in defining the histology prior to biopsy. The extent of intra- and extratracheal involvement influences subsequent treatment plans. Benign tracheal tumors commonly are well circumscribed or lobulated masses usually less than 2 cm in diameter. Calcification may be seen in benign tracheal chondromas (Weber and Grillo, 1978b).

Tracheal sarcomas appear as large, broad-based polypoid endotracheal masses with irregular margins. Most tracheal neoplasms extend from 2 to 10 cm along the tracheal lumen. The tracheal mucosa is irregular and ulcerated. Significant narrowing of the lumen occurs with far-advanced lesions. Mediastinal widening or extrinsic compression or invasion of the esophagus, superior vena cava, or bronchi suggests extratracheal extension. If the tracheal tumor involves a mainstem bronchus, chest radiographs may reveal air trapping, atelectasis, and postobstructive pneumonia (Weber and Grillo, 1978b).

Definitive histologic diagnosis requires tracheoscopy and directed biopsy, but these invasive procedures can precipitate complete obstruction. If radiologic studies are nondiagnostic, upper airway obstruction may be confirmed using flow-volume loops with the patient breathing a mixture of 80% helium and 20% oxygen (Miller and Hyatt, 1973; Belen and Rotman, 1977).

Bronchial obstruction is associated with radiographic abnormalities, including atelectasis, segmental consolidation, or a triangular pleural density. Routine chest films demonstrate signs of obstructive pneumonitis in 75% of patients with significant bronchial obstruction. Tomography or expiratory films may be helpful in establishing the diagnosis of early endobronchial neoplasms in symptomatic patients with normal chest radiographs. Previous chest films should be reviewed to determine the duration of obstructive pneumonitis (see Figure 40–4). Appropriate cultures should be obtained if fever or other signs of infection are present. A definitive diagnosis is made with fiberoptic bronchoscopy, biopsy, and sputum cytology (Weber and Grillo, 1978a; Baumgartner and Mark, 1980).

Therapy. Patients presenting with symptoms of impending upper airway obstruction must be treated immediately to avoid severe respiratory insufficiency and death. If the obstructing lesion is located in the hypopharynx, larynx, or upper one-third of the trachea, a low tracheostomy should be performed using a transverse incision if curative surgery is anticipated. Long tracheostomy tubes should be inserted after tracheal dilation if the obstructing lesion is in the lower trachea (Silver, 1977; Sise and Crichlow, 1978).

Most patients are treated with emergency radiotherapy after an airway is established. High doses of dexamethasone, 10 to 16 mg a day, are begun prior to radiotherapy to reduce edema and are gradually tapered as symptoms

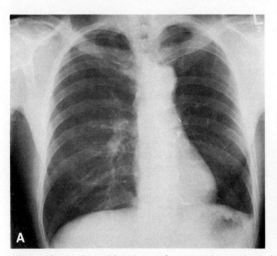
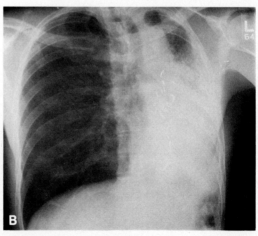

Figure 40–4. Bronchial obstruction secondary to bronchogenic carcinoma. (*A*) Chest film of a 51-year-old man with previous lobectomy for poorly differentiated squamous cell lung cancer. (*B*) Eight months later, atelectasis of the left lung has developed secondary to an obstructing endobronchial tumor.

subside. Tracheal tumors are generally treated with daily 180- to 200-rad fractions. Radiosensitive tumors, including lymphoma and small cell anaplastic carcinoma, can be effectively treated to a total dose of 4000 to 5000 rads. More radioresistant tumors, such as squamous cell carcinoma, generally require 6000 to 7000 rads, with spinal cord blocks after 4000 to 4500 rads (Percarpio et al., 1978; Rostrom and Morgan, 1978; Sise and Crichlow, 1978). Rostrom and Morgan (1978) reported that 75% of patients with obstruction secondary to extratracheal extension had objective responses to radiotherapy. Radiation therapy is generally well tolerated, with side effects limited to mild dysphagia, skin erythema, and tracheal stenosis, occurring in 43, 41, and 10% of patients, respectively (Rostrom and Morgan, 1978).

Thirty to 50% of tracheal tumors are resectable (Grillo, 1973; Sise and Crichlow, 1978). Patients should be considered for surgery if there is no evidence of extratracheal metastases and less than 50 to 60% of the tracheal length is infiltrated with tumor. The goals of surgery are to relieve airway obstruction and to offer the possibility of cure. Patients with slow-growing tracheal metastases, such as thyroid carcinoma, should also be considered for tracheal resection and reconstruction, if survival is not limited by systemic metastases. Limited squamous cell and adenoid cystic carcinomas should be treated with surgical resection and postoperative radiotherapy. Surgery also provides excellent palliation and a high chance of cure with benign and low-grade tracheal malignancies. If technically possible, tracheal resection and reconstruction should be done as a single procedure (Grillo, 1978).

Patients with primary lung cancer obstructing a major bronchus are rarely curable with surgery (Brewer, 1977). If curative radiotherapy is planned for inoperable, localized obstructing non-small cell carcinoma, the tumor volume should receive a midplane dose of 5500 to 6000 rads. Initially, it is difficult to delineate the margins of the tumor from obstructive pneumonitis. Radiation portals should be reduced as atelectasis resolves. Smaller radiation doses (from 2000 rads in one week to 3500 rads in 3.5 weeks) are employed when the goal is palliation (Caldwell and Bagshaw, 1968; Line and Deeley, 1972; Lee, 1977). External radiotherapy offers prompt palliation if the obstruction is of recent onset. Bronchial obstruction from small cell anaplas-

tic lung cancer is promptly relieved with either combination chemotherapy or a combination of radiotherapy and chemotherapy (Cox et al., 1979; Greco et al., 1979).

If the patient was refractory to prior radiotherapy, palliation may be obtained with implantation of iridium seeds, laser beam therapy, or cryosurgery (Laforet et al., 1976; Rostrom and Morgan, 1978; Sise and Crichlow, 1978; Sanderson et al., 1981). Bronchoscopic cryosurgery provides effective palliation if the obstructing lesion has a small surface area and is situated in either the trachea, mainstem bronchi, or lower lobe bronchus. Deeply invasive or peribronchial tumors are unlikely to respond to cryosurgery, because the depth of penetration from freezing is limited to a few millimeters. If cryosurgery is used with bulky tumors, either the tumor can be debrided with subsequent freezing of the tumor base, or the cryoprobe can be used to thrombose the tumor followed by debridement (Sanderson et al., 1981).

Brain Metastases

Patients who present with signs of increased intracranial pressure, cerebellar herniation, or intracranial hemorrhage secondary to brain metastases require immediate treatment. Even with insidious neurologic deterioration, however, treatment should be initiated promptly when brain metastases are diagnosed in order to prevent permanent neurologic dysfunction. Owing to prolongation of survival with chemotherapy and radiotherapy, brain metastases are a commonly encountered problem for the oncologist. Patients develop brain metastases in the clinical setting of terminal illness and in the absence of progressive metastatic disease outside the central nervous system (CNS). The latter phenomenon is not surprising since most chemotherapeutic drugs fail to penetrate the blood-brain barrier (Shapiro et al., 1975a,b, 1977). For example, Bunn reported that 10% of patients with small cell lung carcinoma are found to have brain metastases at presentation. Of patients with the same tumor surviving two years, 80% develop brain metastases if they do not receive prophylactic cranial irradiation (Bunn et al., 1978; Nugent et al., 1979). The incidence of CNS metastases also appears to be increasing among women with metastatic breast carcinoma. Yap reported that between 10 and 34% of patients with metastatic breast cancer have brain metastases at autopsy (Yap *et al.,* 1978). These data have been confirmed by Posner who observed that 18% of patients with terminal neoplastic disease had intracranial metastases at autopsy (Posner, 1977). Table 40–8 lists the malignancies most commonly associated with brain metastases.

Although brain metastases are responsible for the majority of neurologic deficits in patients with metastatic cancer, benign etiologies must be excluded. Cerebrovascular thrombosis or intracranial hemorrhage should be suspected when there is a history of hypertensive cardiovascular disease. Elderly patients may develop focal neurologic signs secondary to metabolic disturbances commonly associated with malignancy, including hyponatremia, hypercalcemia, and hypoglycemia. Brain abscesses and meningitis are more prevalent among immunosuppressed cancer patients. Spinal cord compression should be considered in the differential diagnosis of neurologic dysfunction, if neither cerebral nor cranial nerve signs are present. When neurologic signs recur following whole-brain radiation for metastatic disease, it may be difficult to differentiate recurrent tumor from postirradiation brain necrosis.

Pathophysiology and Clinical Presentation. Intracranial metastases may be anatomically located in the extradural and subdural spaces, but more frequently are intracerebral. Extradural and subdural metastases produce focal neurologic signs by extrinisic compression of the brain, whereas intracerebral lesions compress and directly invade the brain parenchyma. Posner reported that over 60% of patients with intracranial mass lesions have multiple metastases at autopsy (Posner *et al.,* 1977). Brain metastases most frequently occur by hematogenous spread. In adults, 90% of brain metastases are located in the cerebrum,

8% in the cerebellum, and 2% in the brain stem (Veith and Odom, 1965).

Neurologic symptoms from brain metastases generally progress rapidly over one to three weeks. Clinical signs vary, depending on the anatomic location of the metastasis, extent of peritumoral edema, and intracranial pressure (Veith and Odom, 1965; Shehata *et al.,* 1974; Posner, 1977). A detailed neurologic examination often detects more extensive neurologic dysfunction than is suggested by the history obtained from the patient or family members. Frontal lobe metastases frequently present with mental status changes, ranging from lethargy and memory loss to coma. Hemiparesis, unilateral sensory loss, and aphasia suggest a parietal lesion. Visual disturbances may be seen with occipital, pituitary, or brain stem metastases. Cerebellar signs include ataxia, dysmetria, and broad-based gait.

Increased intracranial pressure may be secondary to extensive peritumoral edema or ventricular obstruction by tumor. Dilatation of one or both pupils denotes a sudden increase in intracranial pressure. Increased intracranial pressure from an intracerebral mass lesion produces bradycardia and hypertension, while cerebellar masses often produce tachycardia and hypotension. As intracranial pressure increases, retinal veins become engorged and dilated leading to swelling of the optic discs. In a recent series of patients with brain metastases, 25% had papilledema at presentation (Posner *et al.,* 1977). Deterioration in mental status (ranging from somnolence to coma), headache, seizures, and nausea or vomiting are characteristic symptoms associated with increased intracranial pressure.

Seizures occur in approximately 15% of cases, but are more frequent among patients with melanoma, associated carcinomatous meningitis, or increased intracranial pressure.

Table 40–8. Primary Origin of Neoplasms Metastatic to Brain

TUMOR	VEITH AND ODOM, 1965 No. of Cases (%)		BORGELT *et al.,* 1980 No. of Cases (%)		SHEHATA *et al.,* 1974 No. of Cases (%)	
Lung	86	(28)	1067	(59)	40	(49)
Breast	51	(16)	312	(17)	15	(18.5)
Melanoma	49	(16)	60	(3)		
Unknown	44	(14)			4	(5)
GU tract	22	(7)			3	(4)
Colon	16	(5)			6	(7.5)
Skin and sinuses	14	(4)				
Sarcoma	8	(3)				
Other	23	(7)	373	(21)	13	(16)
Total	313		1812		81	

At presentation, more than 50% of patients complain of headache, usually mild but gradually progressive. The headache is present upon awakening, before arising from bed, and generally improves within 30 minutes after arising (Shehata *et al.*, 1974; Posner *et al.*, 1977).

Diagnostic Evaluation. Computerized transaxial tomography (CT) is the safest and most accurate diagnostic test and should be obtained as an emergency procedure in all patients with a suspected mass lesion in the brain (see Figure 40–5). When CT scans are performed with and without RENOGRAFIN contrast, tumors greater than 1 cm in diameter are rarely not detected. In addition to defining the size, number, and location of the mass lesion(s), CT scans also demonstrate peritumoral edema, ventricular size, hemorrhage, shift of midline structures, and changes suggestive of carcinomatous meningitis (Posner, 1977; Amundsen *et al.*, 1978). Nuclear brain scans are less sensitive, but approximately 70% of patients with CNS metastases on CT scan have positive brain scans (Shehata *et al.*, 1974).

Electroencephalograms and skull films are rarely helpful. Radiographic changes of increased intracranial pressure or pineal shift were seen in only 6% in Posner's series. Skull films may be helpful in the rare patient with increased intracranial pressure caused by a skull metastasis overlying and occluding the sagittal sinus. Occasionally, arteriography may be indicated in localizing the lesion and in determining the tumor's vascular pattern if a surgical approach is contemplated (Posner, 1977).

Therapy. Without treatment, the median survival from brain metastases is one month. The goal of palliative therapy is to reverse promptly the neurologic deficit and to restore the patient to functional status. Immediate administration of corticosteroids and prompt radiotherapy consultation should be obtained when patients present with symptoms or signs of increased intracranial pressure or rapid deterioration in neurologic status (Posner, 1977).

Corticosteroids reduce peritumoral edema and improve neurologic function in 60 to 75% of patients. Symptoms associated with increased intracranial pressure, including headache and alteration in consciousness, respond more promptly, but focal motor and sensory deficits may also improve. Steroids provide temporary benefit, but if more definitive therapy is not initiated, survival is only prolonged for a few weeks (Young *et al.*, 1974; Kramer *et al.*, 1977; Posner *et al.*, 1977).

The initial corticosteroid dose is usually equivalent to 16 mg of dexamethasone a day in divided doses. If symptoms fail to improve, a trial of higher dose steroids, up to 100 mg of dexamethasone, should be employed for several days. Once more definitive therapy is initiated, the steroid dose is gradually decreased to the lowest effective dose and discontinued, if possible. If neurologic deterioration occurs with tapering steroids, the dose may have to be temporarily increased. Patients with minor neurologic deficits may not require corticosteroids. Controlled trials have demonstrated that corticosteroids hasten neurologic recovery, but do not improve response rates or survival four weeks after radiotherapy is initiated (Young *et al.*, 1974; Kramer *et al.*, 1977; Posner *et al.*, 1977).

If intracranial pressure does not promptly respond to corticosteroids, mannitol or glycerol is required promptly to reverse acute neurologic decompensation. Mannitol is given intravenously as a 50-g bolus or as a 20% infusion. Glycerol, given 1 g/kg intravenously or orally every four hours, produces less electrolyte imbalance and less volume depletion than mannitol, but also has a shorter duration of action. If increased intracranial pressure

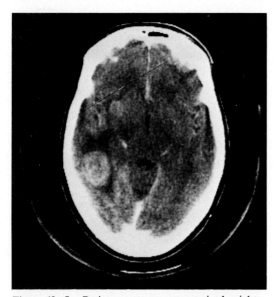

Figure 40–5. Brain metastases: computerized axial tomography. A 45-year-old woman with small cell lung carcinoma. A computed tomography scan shows the typical appearance of a metastatic lesion with surrounding edema.

fails to respond to steroids, osmotic therapy, and radiation, temporary emergency procedures may be required to relieve pressure. These emergency procedures include insertion of a #16 ventricular needle or Scott cannula through a frontal or occipital burr hole, ventriculoperitoneal shunts, or, rarely, decompression by removal of the frontal or temporal bone.

Anticonvulsants should be administered in all patients presenting with seizures, but are not routinely prescribed. If diphenylhydantoin is used in conjunction with corticosteroids, frequent dose adjustments are necessary since the duration of action of both drugs will be decreased (Posner *et al.,* 1977).

Radiotherapy is the primary palliative modality for patients with brain metastases and should be initiated promptly. The whole brain is usually treated, since 36 to 85% of patients with brain metastases have multiple lesions at autopsy (Ask-Upmark, 1956; Pool *et al.,* 1957; Harr and Patterson, 1972; Shehata *et al.,* 1974; Posner, 1977). Radiation doses range from 1000 rads in one fraction to 4000 to 5000 rads over four to five weeks. The Radiation Therapy Oncology Group (RTOG) compared different dose and fractionation schedules to define the optimal palliative treatment for brain metastases. Over 1000 patients were entered in the first trial which compared 4000 rads over three or four weeks to 3000 rads over two or three weeks. The most favorable results in terms of response and survival were seen with 3000 rads over two weeks or 4000 rads over three weeks (Kramer *et al.,* 1977).

To decrease treatment time, hospitalization, and medical costs, Shehata treated 80 patients with 1000 rads in a single dose. Thirty-five percent had excellent neurologic recovery with an overall median survival of 150 days. In two series of over 130 patients treated with the same schedule, functional improvement occurred in 65 to 75% (Hindo *et al.,* 1970; Shehata *et al.,* 1974). However, Young reported that patients with increased intracranial pressure had a 50% decrease in duration of survival with high-dose, short-fractionation therapy, when retrospectively compared to more conventional protracted treatment regimens (Young *et al.,* 1974).

To further define the optimal radiation schedule, the second RTOG brain metastases study compared the conventional 3000 rads over two weeks or 4000 rads over three weeks to either 2000 rads in one week or 1200 rads in

two days. The shorter treatment courses were associated with a decreased median survial of 70 days compared to 140 days with 3000 rads over two weeks. The latter treatment plan is now considered the treatment schedule of choice for multiple brain metastases (Kramer *et al.,* 1977).

Approximately 40 to 69% of patients will have neurologic improvement and 35 to 41% major functional improvement following whole-brain radiotherapy (Hindo *et al.,* 1970; Deutsh *et al.,* 1974; Shehata *et al.,* 1974; Kramer *et al.,* 1977; Borgelt *et al.,* 1980). In the second RTOG study, 69 to 86% had improvement in specific neurologic symptoms, and 32 to 66% had complete resolution of neurologic deficits. Covariate analysis revealed three factors that favorably influenced functional neurologic improvement: ambulatory status at presentation, absence of systemic metastases, and an unknown primary source. Despite initial improvement, 30 to 50% of patients die with recurrent brain metastases (Borgelt *et al.,* 1980). Patients may benefit from retreatment if neurologic deterioration occurs. Shehata has observed benefit in 68% of patients from a second course of radiation given as a single 1000-rad dose, 50% from a third course, and 66% from a fourth course (Shehata *et al.,* 1974). One to two months after radiotherapy is complete, patients may develop lethargy, somnolence, and confusion. This postirradiation syndrome is effectively treated with a short course of steroids, but is often difficult to distinguish from tumor recurrence (Posner, 1977).

Surgical therapy is indicated when the diagnosis of brain metastases is uncertain, particularly in patients without a previous diagnosis of malignancy or in a patient without widespread systemic disease. Emergency surgical intervention is also indicated in patients with hydrocephalus caused by ventricular obstruction or with temporal or cerebellar masses not responding to medical management and radiotherapy. In these settings, surgical decompression is associated with high mortality rates. Unfortunately, the margins of tumor rarely can be defined, so that a complete resection is impossible. It is controversial whether surgery or radiotherapy provides better palliation for (1) a solitary brain lesion with a relatively long interval between initial diagnosis and treatment of the primary cancer and the appearance of a brain metastasis; (2) slowly growing relatively radioresistant tumors (*e.g.,* alveolar soft part sarcoma); or (3) when neurologic dysfunction progresses rapidly owing to increased intracranial pressure despite osmotic therapy and corticosteroids (Posner, 1977; Winston *et al.,* 1980).

Surgery relieves increased intracranial pressure and improves neurologic function by removing the mass lesion, decreasing edema, and removing the cause of obstruction to cerebrospinal fluid flow (Winston *et al.,* 1980). With surgery, approximately 50% of patients have functional improvement, and 25% have full neurologic recovery (Winston *et al.,* 1980). Thirty-day mortality rates range from 10 to 30%, with increased surgical morbidity and mortality rates occurring among debilitated patients with cardiopulmonary insufficiency or increased intracranial pressure (Ransohoff, 1975; Posner, 1977; Winston *et al.,* 1980). In earlier surgical series, 7 to 17% required reoperation for hematoma or infection (Posner, 1977). With surgical removal of a solitary brain metastasis, median survival ranges from 5 to 12 months (Veith and Odom, 1965; Ransohoff, 1975; Posner, 1977; Galicich *et al.,* 1980; Winston *et al.,* 1980). One- and two-year survival rates range from 22 to 48% and 10 to 13%, respectively (Ransohoff, 1975; Winston *et al.,* 1980). The percentage of patients surviving for one year according to tumor type is shown in Table 40–9. These impressive survival statistics are undoubtedly the result of patient selection in these surgical series (Winston *et al.,* 1980). Winston identified important prognostic factors that predicted prolonged survival after neurosurgery, including minor preoperative neurologic dysfunction, a long interval between the diagnosis of the primary malignancy and brain metastasis (range, 8 to 36 months), gross tumor removal, and postoperative radiotherapy (Winston *et al.,* 1980).

Prospective controlled trials comparing surgery, radiotherapy, or combined modality treatment are not available. Until controlled

Table 40–9. One-Year Survival After Surgical Resection of Solitary Brain Metastasis

	%
Breast cancer	48
Unknown primary	34
Melanoma	32
Renal cell	27
Lung cancer	19

Derived from Winston *et al.,* 1980.

Table 40–10. Criteria for Surgical Resection of Brain Metastases

1. Solitary brain metastasis
2. Metastasis located in an easily accessible area, such that surgical resection will not increase neurologic deficit
3. Ambulatory status preoperatively
4. No evidence of a primary neoplasm
5. Systemic metastases are well controlled or no threat to a reasonable life expectancy
6. Tumor is relatively radioresistant

studies demonstrate improved functional results or survival with surgical intervention, surgery should be reserved for the select group of patients listed in Table 40–10. The majority of patients with brain metastases respond to palliative radiotherapy and medical management. Surgical resection is rarely performed in clinical practice.

Carcinomatous Meningitis

Carcinomatous meningitis is an oncologic emergency which is increasing in frequency owing to prolongation of survival with systemic therapy and an increased awareness of this problem among clinicians. In a recent large autopsy series, 4% of patients with terminal cancer had diffuse, widespread seeding of the leptomeninges by metastases (Posner *et al.,* 1977; Shapiro *et al.,* 1977; Wasserstrom *et al.,* 1982). As an example of the importance of this problem clinically, Yap reported that 10% of patients with metastatic breast cancer have leptomeningeal metastases at autopsy (Yap *et al.,* 1978). The incidence of leptomeningeal spread also appears to be increasing among patients with lymphoma, sarcoma, small cell lung cancer, and ovarian carcinoma (Mayer *et al.,* 1978; Yap *et al.,* 1978; Nugent *et al.,* 1979; Bunn *et al.,* 1981; Wasserstrom *et al.,,* 1982). Adenocarcinomas appear to have a propensity for leptomeningeal spread compared to squamous cell carcinomas or sarcomas (Little *et al.,* 1974; Olsen *et al.,* 1974; Young *et al.,* 1975; Posner *et al.,* 1977; Shapiro *et al.,* 1977; Levitt *et al.,* 1980; Wasserstrom *et al.,* 1982). Table 40–11 lists the common solid tumors associated with carcinomatous meningitis. The diagnosis and treatment of leukemic meningitis is described in Chapter 18.

Carcinomatous meningitis may develop in the absence of progressive metastatic disease outside the central nervous system, since most chemotherapeutic agents fail to penetrate the blood-brain barrier (Shapiro *et al.,* 1975a;

Table 40-11. Solid Tumors Associated with Carcinomatous Meningitis

PRIMARY TUMOR	NO. OF PATIENTS	%
Breast	46	51
Lung	23	26
Adenocarcinoma	13	
Oat cell	6	
Epidermoid	3	
Large cell	1	
Melanoma	11	12
Genitourinary	5	5
Head and neck	2	2
Breast and colon	1	1
Adenocarcinoma— unknown primary	2	2
Total number	90	

Derived from Wasserstrom *et al.*, 1982.

Shapiro *et al.*, 1977). In Yap's series at the time of diagnosis of leptomeningeal metastases, only 36% of patients with metastatic breast cancer had progressive systemic disease. Sixteen percent presented with carcinomatous meningitis as the first sign of recurrent breast cancer, and 30% were otherwise in systemic remission on chemotherapy when carcinomatous meningitis was first diagnosed (Yap *et al.*, 1978).

Pathophysiology. A variety of mechanisms have been proposed to explain the development of leptomeningeal carcinomatosis. *Post mortem* studies have demonstrated that malignant cells enter the central nervous system via thin-walled microscopic veins in the arachnoid membrane (Price and Johnson, 1973). Rupture of parenchymal brain or choroidal plexus metastases may introduce malignant cells into the cerebrospinal fluid. Paravertebral tumors, such as lymphomas, grow along nerve roots and directly involve the spinal subarachnoid space through the neural foramina. However, since the majority of patients with carcinomatous meningitis do not have associated parenchymal brain, choroidal, or paravertebral metastases at autopsy, the most common etiology for leptomeningeal metastasis appears to be via the hematogenous route (Price and Johnson, 1973; Wasserstrom *et al.*, 1982).

At autopsy two pathologic patterns are frequently noted. The brain and spinal surfaces may be diffusely covered by a thin layer of malignant cells; whereas metastases to the cauda equina, spinal, and cranial nerves commonly grow in a nodular, multifocal pattern. Additional histologic findings may include in-

creased fibrosis caused by an enhanced inflammatory reaction and neovascularization. New blood vessels, which lack properties common to the blood-brain barrier, allow increased absorption of chemotherapy and intravenous contrast used in computerized tomography. The tumor may also invade cranial and spinal nerves as they pass through the subarachnoid space. As the tumor progresses, it infiltrates penetrating vessels of the brain and spinal cord and occasionally ruptures through the pial membrane with subsequent invasion of the brain or spinal parenchyma. Malignant cells tend to settle in the basal cisterns, interfering with cerebrospinal fluid flow and absorption, and eventually leading to obstructive hydrocephalus (Gonzalez-Vitale and Garcia-Bunuel, 1976; Wasserstrom *et al.*, 1982).

Clinical Presentation. The diagnosis of neoplastic meningitis should always be suspected when there are symptoms or signs involving more than one structural area of the neuroaxis. Clinical symptoms are divided into three categories, depending on whether leptomeningeal tumor involves the brain, cranial nerves, and/or spinal cord. Wasserstrom *et al.*, (1982) recently reported that over 75% of patients presented with neurologic abnormalities in more than one area of the neuroaxis. Neurologic symptoms are generally present for less than three months prior to diagnosis, but occasionally subtle neurologic signs may progress over three to six months. At presentation, patients may have few neurologic complaints, but a detailed neurologic examination often suggests more widespread meningeal involvement (Olsen *et al.*, 1974; Yap *et al.*, 1978; Wasserstrom *et al.*, 1982).

The incidence of cerebral, cranial nerve, and spinal cord abnormalities noted in three recent series of patients with carcinomatous meningitis are summarized in Tables 40-12, 40-13, and 40-14. Headache is often severe and associated with persistent nausea, vomiting, and lightheadedness. Patients or family members may note mental status changes with lethargy, confusion, or memory loss being commonly reported. In addition, 40% of patients initially complain of symptoms caused by cranial nerve dysfunction. Diplopia, hearing loss, facial numbness, and decreased visual acuity are the most common presenting brain stem symptoms. Over 70% of patients with carcinomatous meningitis present with spinal cord metastases. Common initial complaints include weakness in the extremities, paresthe-

Table 40–12. Frequency of Cerebral Symptoms and Signs in Patients with Carcinomatous Meningitis

	%
Symptoms	
Headache	38–52
Change in mental status	17–48
Persistent nausea or vomiting	8–14
Dizziness or lightheadedness	12–16
Transient loss of consciousness	3–6
Aphasia	2
Diabetes insipidus	2
Signs	
Abnormal mental status examination	31–56
Positive Babinski sign	32–50
Papilledema	6–20
Ataxic gait	13
Hemiparesis	2

Derived from Olsen *et al.*, 1974; Yap *et al.*, 1978; Wasserstrom *et al.*, 1982.

Table 40–14. Frequency of Spinal Cord Symptoms and Signs in Patients with Carcinomatous Meningitis

	%
Symptoms	
Weakness	33
Paresthesias	31
Back pain	25
Radicular pain	19
Bowel/bladder dysfunction	13
Signs	
Reflex asymmetry	67
Weakness	64
Cauda equina syndrome	33
Sensory loss	31
Straight-leg raising	13
Decreased rectal tone	12
Nuchal rigidity	11

Derived from Olsen *et al.*, 1974; Yap *et al.*, 1978; Wasserstrom *et al.*, 1982.

sias, localized back pain, and, rarely, bladder and bowel dysfunction. (Olsen *et al.*, 1974; Posner *et al.*, 1977; Yap *et al.*, 1978; Wasserstrom *et al.*, 1982).

Diagnostic Evaluation. A high index of suspicion is critical to the early diagnosis of carcinomatous or lymphomatous meningitis. The diagnosis is established by cerebrospinal fluid cytologic examination. Cell count and differential cytocentrifugation of CSF may provide a prompt diagnosis on review of Wright-Giemsa smear. Additional CSF should be ana-

Table 40–13. Frequency of Cranial Nerve Dysfunction in Patients with Carcinomatous Meningitis at Presentation

	%
Symptoms	
Diplopia	8–24
Hearing loss	6–24
Facial numbness	6
Decreased visual acuity	6–36
Blindness	3
Dysarthria	0–8
Loss of taste	3
Tinnitus	2–8
Hoarseness	2
Dysphagia	2
Vertigo	1–2
Signs	
Ocular muscle paresis	20–46
Facial weakness	17–42
Hearing loss	10–30
Visual loss—optic neuritis	2–6
Trigeminal neuropathy	6–12
Hypoglossal neuropathy	6–8
Blindness	0–4
Decreased gag reflex	4–16

Derived from Olsen *et al.*, 1974; Yap *et al.*, 1978; Wasserstrom *et al.*, 1982.

lyzed for glucose and protein with simultaneous serum determinations. Routine cultures are also performed when indicated. At least 5 mL of CSF should be sent for cytology. If carcinomatous meningitis is suspected clinically, and there are CSF abnormalities (high opening pressure, leukocytosis, elevated protein, or low glucose), but the cytology remains negative, repeated lumbar punctures are required to confirm the diagnosis. In three recent series of patients subsequently found to have carcinomatous meningitis, malignant cells were seen on cytologic examination after the first, second, and third lumbar punctures in 42 to 66%, 60 to 87%, and 68 to 96%, respectively (Olsen *et al.*, 1974; Kirkwood and Bankole, 1981; Wasserstrom *et al.*, 1982). Occasionally, patients will have repeatedly negative lumbar CSF cytologies, but positive cytologies in cisternal or ventricular fluid. Less than 10% of patients with leptomeningeal metastases will have persistently negative cytologies when the tumor is strongly adherent to the meninges (Olsen *et al.*, 1974; Kirkwood and Bankole, 1981; Wasserstrom *et al.*, 1982).

Table 40–15 lists the frequency of associated cerebrospinal fluid abnormalities in three large series with carcinomatous meningitis. More than half the patients have one or more of the following CSF abnormalities: opening pressures above 160 mm of water; increased white cell counts, commonly with a reactive lymphocytosis; and CSF protein elevation. Decreased CSF glucose occurs in 40% at presentation and in over 70% prior to death (Olsen *et al.*, 1974; Yap *et al.*, 1978; Wasserman *et al.*, 1982).

Table 40–15. Characteristics of Cerebrospinal Fluid at Presentation in Patients with Carcinomatous Meningitis

	% ABNORMAL	RANGE
Opening pressure	50	60–450
White cell count	52	0–1800
Glucose	31–38	0–244
Protein	29–81	24–2485
Initial cytology	42–69	

Derived from Olsen *et al.*, 1974; Yap *et al.*, 1978; Wasserstrom *et al.*, 1982.

Biochemical tumor markers in cerebrospinal fluid may be helpful in diagnosis when cytologies are persistently negative. CSF B-glucouronidase levels above 80 μmU/L, CEA levels above 1 ng/mL, and LDH enzyme 5:1 ratios greater than 15% strongly suggest carcinomatous meningitis. However, the present data are too preliminary to rely only on these biochemical markers for diagnostic purposes (Brain and Karr, 1955; Schold *et al.*, 1980; Shuttleworth and Allen, 1980; Wasserstrom *et al.*, 1982).

Computerized axial tomography is helpful in confirming the diagnosis of leptomeningeal carcinomatosis and is important to rule out concomitant brain metastases, which are present in over 20% of patients. Hydrocephalus and contrast enhancement in the meninges and periventricular area suggest leptomeningeal disease. Ventricular enlargement occurs in approximately 30% of cases. Even without an obstructing mass lesion, hydrocephalus may occur secondary to blockage of the subarachnoid absorptive pathways by malignant cells. In the absence of infectious meningitis, contrast enhancement in the basal cisterns or cerebral sulci suggests malignancy. In Wasserstrom's series, the CT scan was normal in only 20 of 68 patients with carcinomatous meningitis. Sixteen of these patients had brain metastases and three subdural effusions (Olsen *et al.*, 1974; Yap *et al.*, 1978; Wasserman *et al.*, 1982). Thus, CT scanning should be performed in all patients with solid tumors who are suspected of having carcinomatous meningitis.

Patients with symptoms or signs suggestive of metastases to the spinal cord or cauda equina should have emergency myelography prior to radiation (see Figure 40–6). Wasserstrom *et al.* (1982) reported that over 50% of patients who had myelograms performed for suspected leptomeningeal spinal metastases had either spinal epidural lesions or thickening

and nodularity of nerve roots in the subarachnoid space. All epidural metastases and symptomatic nerve root metastases must be included in radiation portals, as discussed in the section on spinal cord metastases.

Therapy. Treatment of carcinomatous meningitis is directed at prolonging survival and stabilizing or improving neurologic dysfunction. Without treatment, most patients die within four to six weeks owing to progressive neurologic deterioration (Little *et al.*, 1974; Olsen *et al.*, 1974). Most patients are effectively palliated with a combination of intrathecal chemotherapy and local radiotherapy to symptomatic leptomeningeal metastases.

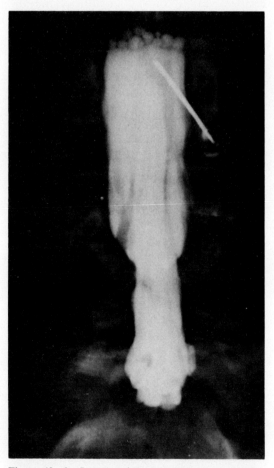

Figure 40–6. Leptomeningeal metastases. A 48-year-old woman with carcinomatous meningitis and brain metastases secondary to metastatic breast cancer. Three months after presenting with brain metastases, she developed lower extremity weakness. Cerebrospinal fluid cytology revealed malignant cells and a myelogram demonstrated multiple defects caused by nodular tumor implants along the spinal cord and nerve roots.

When cerebral signs are present, whole-brain radiotherapy is required to eradicate tumor in the cerebral sulci which are not reached by intrathecal chemotherapy (Blasberg et al., 1977; Shapiro et al., 1977). When cranial nerve abnormalities are apparent, the radiation port must also encompass the brain stem. Myelography should be performed in patients with spinal cord or nerve root symptoms so that appropriate radiation ports can be planned. Generally, 2400 to 3000 rads are administered to the whole brain over two weeks, whereas the dose to spinal metastases is frequently higher (3000 to 4000 rads), depending on the radiosensitivity of the primary tumor. Local radiotherapy is combined with intrathecal chemotherapy to prevent reseeding and to eradicate asymptomatic metastases not included in the radiation field (Blasberg et al., 1977; Shapiro et al., 1977; Wasserstrom et al., 1982).

Therapeutic drug levels are generally not achieved in the CSF with parenteral administration, therefore, chemotherapy must be given intrathecally by lumbar puncture or intraventricularly after placement of an Ommaya reservoir (Shapiro et al., 1977; Yap et al., 1978; Bleyer and Poplack, 1979; Wasserstrom et al., 1982).

Intraventricular therapy has three advantages over lumbar injections. (1) Intraventricular injection assures optimal CSF chemotherapeutic drug concentrations, as drugs administered by lumbar puncture may only reach the subdural or epidural spaces. Even with injection into the lumbar subarachnoid space, therapeutic drug concentrations are rarely achieved in the ventricles. (2) Intraventricular injection allows chemotherapeutic agents to follow the normal pathways of CSF flow so that all parts of the meninges are treated. (3) Patients frequently prefer intraventricular injections via the Ommaya reservoir, as these injections are usually painless (Galicich and Guido, 1974; Shapiro et al.,

1975a; Shapiro et al., 1977; Bleyer and Poplack, 1979).

In carcinomatous meningitis, controlled trials have not been done to compare the efficacy of ventricular chemotherapy via the Ommaya reservoir to lumbar puncture intrathecal chemotherapy. Compared to retrospective series, recent reports suggest that increased response rates of longer duration are obtained when intraventricular chemotherapy is combined with radiotherapy to areas of symptomatic neurologic disease. Trump (1981) reported 15 responses among 16 patients with leptomeningeal metastases treated with a combination of intraventricular methotrexate and thiotepa, in addition to local radiotherapy. In Yap's series, using biweekly intraventricular methotrexate with radiotherapy, 67% of patients with carcinomatous meningitis secondary to breast cancer achieved normalization of CSF and neurologic improvement or stabilization. The median survival of responders was 6.5 months compared to one month for nonresponders. These results were considerably better than the two-month median survival in a similar series of patients treated with less aggressive intrathecal therapy (Yap et al., 1978). Excellent results were reported in 90 patients with leptomeningeal metastases treated with intraventricular chemotherapy and local radiotherapy. Over 60% with breast cancer, 100% with lymphomas, 50% with lung cancer, and 40% with melanoma and carcinomatous meningitis improved or stabilized while on therapy. The median and range of survival according to tumor type in this series are summarized in Table 40–16 (Wasserstrom et al., 1982). Comparative studies in leukemic meningitis suggest that intraventricular therapy is more effective than lumbar injections, in terms of improved response rates and longer durations of response (Shapiro et al., 1977; Bleyer and Poplack, 1979).

Using the transoccipital approach and intraoperative fluoroscopy, Ommaya reservoirs

Table 40–16. Leptomeningeal Metastases from Solid Tumors: Results of Treatment in 90 Patients

PRIMARY TUMOR	NO. (INCOMPLETE) FOLLOW-UP		IMPROVED	STABILIZED	% STABILIZED OR IMPROVED	RELAPSE PRIOR TO DEATH	MEDIAN SURVIVAL (MONTHS)	
Breast	46	(4)	12	16	61	13	7.2	(1–29)
Lung	23	(2)	4	5	39	4	4.0	(1–10)
Melanoma	11	(1)	2	0	18	2	3.6	(1–12)
Other	10	(1)	3	0	30	3	6.3	(2–12)
Total	90		21	21	47	22	5.8	(1–29)

Derived from Wasserstrom et al., 1982.

can be inserted with less than 2% morbidity and no perioperative mortality (Galicich and Guido, 1974). When Ommaya reservoirs are placed in patients with increased intracranial pressure, large subgaleal collections of CSF may develop when ventricular fluid flows back along the catheter through the dura. Generally, Ommaya reservoirs are contraindicated in patients with increased intracranial pressure. It has been reported, however, that Ommaya devices can safely be placed in patients with hydrocephalus if the device is connected to a ventriculoperitoneal shunt. Using an on-off valve, the shunt is closed for four hours after intraventricular chemotherapy administration to allow optimal drug delivery (Wasserstrom et al., 1982).

The decision to place an intraventricular device depends on tumor type, radioresponsiveness, patient's life expectancy, and anatomic considerations, including hydrocephalus or multiple brain metastases. Aggressive intraventricular therapy is indicated in carcinomatous meningitis from breast cancer in the absence of progressive systemic disease or major neurologic deficits. Intraventricular therapy does not appear to improve the poor prognosis for patients with leptomeningeal metastases from melanoma or lung cancer or for those with progressive systemic disease (Yap et al., 1978; Wasserstrom et al., 1982). However, lymphomatous meningitis responds promptly to initial intrathecal therapy by lumbar injection and local radiotherapy. Lymphomatous meningitis is generally diagnosed in the setting of systemic relapse, poor prognosis histology, and limited survival (Shapiro et al., 1977; Lokich and Garbo, 1981).

Methotrexate is the most frequently used intrathecal agent, administered alone or in combination with thiotepa or cytosine arabinoside (Rubinstein et al., 1975; Shapiro et al., 1977; Yap et al., 1978; Bleyer and Poplack, 1979; Bunn et al., 1981; Trump, 1981). Citrovorum factor decreases methotrexate's systemic toxicity without altering its antitumor efficacy in the central nervous system. Since citrovorum does not cross the blood-brain barrier, it may be administered immediately after methotrexate (Lokich and Garbo, 1981). A dose of 10 mg of citrovorum factor orally or parenterally is prescribed every six hours for two to six doses following intrathecal methotrexate to prevent hematologic toxicity and oral mucositis. Excellent results are reported with intrathecal thiotepa, but owing to its relatively short half-life, other agents are usually chosen as first-line therapy (Gutin et al., 1976). Cytosine arabinoside is effective alone or in combination with methotrexate in leukemic and some cases of lymphomatous meningitis; but unfortunately, the drug has little activity in most solid tumors (Wang and Pratt, 1970; Ziegler et al., 1972; Band et al., 1973; Shapiro et al., 1975b).

Initially, intrathecal chemotherapy is given twice a week until symptoms improve or stabilize and CSF abnormalities resolve. After negative cytologies are obtained and there is neurologic stabilization, consolidation intrathecal chemotherapy is frequently administered weekly and gradually spaced out to monthly injections. If malignant cells remain in the CSF or there is neurologic progression on the first regimen, alternative agents may be effective either alone or in combination (Yap et al., 1978; Wasserstrom et al., 1982). The standard intrathecal doses for each agent are listed in Table 40–17.

Prolonged palliation may be achieved in 50 to 90% of patients with lymphomatous meningitis. Intrathecal methotrexate or Ara-C is frequently combined with radiotherapy. Although most lymphomas are responsive to alkylating agents, trials should be done to establish whether the addition of intrathecal thiotepa improves the duration and rate of response in lymphomatous meningitis (Griffin et al., 1971; Olsen et al., 1974; Bunn et al., 1981; Lokich and Garbo, 1981). Lymphomatous meningitis differs in one respect from that observed in solid tumor patients in that systemic chemotherapy may be effective in the treatment of meningeal involvement. Zuckerman reported neurologic improvement in over 80% of patients with lymphomatous meningitis following high-dose systemic methotrexate and leucovorin rescue; 50% had complete disappearance of malignant cells on follow-up cytologic examination (Zuckerman et al., 1971).

Prophylactic intrathecal chemotherapy and whole-brain radiation to prevent leptomeningeal relapse are routinely administered to patients with acute lymphocytic leukemia, acute

Table 40–17. Intrathecal Chemotherapy Doses

DRUG	LUMBAR INJECTION	INTRAVENTRICULAR INJECTION
Methotrexate	12–15 mg	10–12 mg
Cytosine arabinoside	45 mg	30–45 mg
Thiotepa	15 mg	10 mg

lymphoblastic lymphoma, and Burkitt's lymphoma. As survival is prolonged in patients with solid tumors, (e.g., small cell lung cancer), patients at high risk for central nervous system relapse might be considered for prophylactic therapy to prevent neoplastic meningitis. Future investigative efforts should be directed toward prevention, earlier diagnosis to prevent neurologic disability, and more effective methods of treatment. Limited success has been seen with the lipid-soluble nitrosoureas in the treatment of meningeal leukemia, but other lipid-soluble investigational drugs, including VP-16, might be evaluated (Lokich and Garbo, 1981).

Spinal Cord Compression

Spinal cord compression from metastases to the epidural space results in irreversible neurologic damage unless emergency treatment is promptly initiated. Autopsy studies have revealed that 5% of all patients with systemic cancer have tumor involving the epidural space (Posner et al., 1977). More than 95% of spinal cord metastases are extramedullary, while 1 to 3% are intramedullary (Del Regato, 1977; Gilbert et al., 1978b; Rodriguez and Dinapoli, 1980). The majority of metastatic epidural tumors arise within the vertebral body and invade the epidural space anterior to the spinal cord (Gilbert et al., 1978a). Carcinoma of the lung, breast, and prostate, multiple myeloma, and lymphoma are the most common tumors associated with spinal cord compression.

The thoracic spine is the most frequent site of epidural metastases, accounting for 68 to 75% of lesions. Metastatic breast and lung carcinomas are the primary tumors most commonly associated with thoracic cord compression. Lumbosacral cord or nerve root compression accounts for 16 to 20% of epidural metastases, with gastrointestinal primaries having the highest predilection for this region (Bruckman and Bloomer, 1978; Gilbert et al., 1978b). Patients with lymphoma may develop epidural metastases when tumor extends from retroperitoneal, mediastinal, or paraspinal nodes through the intravertebral foramina.

Pathophysiology. Spinal cord and nerve root compression may be secondary to epidural tumor or vertebral collapse from destructive osseous metastases. Neurologic dysfunction also occurs if vascular compromise produces spinal cord ischemia and hemorrhage (Bruckman and Bloomer, 1978; Rodriguez and Dinapoli, 1980). The majority of epidural metastases arise from adjacent vertebral metastases. The tumor directly invades the extradural space and eventually extends along the spinal canal. Paraspinal tumors (e.g., lymphoma) also enter the extradural space through intervertebral foramina, while pelvic malignancies frequently metastasize to the extradural space by hematogenous spread through the paravertebral venous plexus (Bruckman and Bloomer, 1978).

When neurologic signs of spinal cord compression are apparent, most patients have extensive epidural tumor. Rarely is there a localized, circumscribed mass of tumor which might be removed surgically. The majority of patients have a diffuse plaque of tumor on one aspect of the dura (usually anteriorly) or concentrically constricting the dura. Patients with widespread vertebral metastases or extensive retroperitoneal adenopathy may have multiple noncontiguous spinal cord metastases (Brice and McKissock, 1965). Pain associated with spinal cord compression may be secondary to neoplastic vertebral collapse, stretching of the periosteum, or nerve root compression (Rodriguez and Dinapoli, 1980). Experimental models of cord compression suggest that the earliest neurologic deficit is motor dysfunction followed by loss of temperature and light touch. The last sensory modalities to be affected are pain and pinprick (Bruckman and Bloomer, 1978). Autonomic bladder or bowel dysfunction is a late and unfavorable sign. If cord compression is not treated immediately, infarction and permanent neurologic dysfunction result.

Clinical Presentation. Symptoms suggestive of spinal cord compression are frequently present one to six months prior to definitive diagnosis. Over 95% of patients present initially with symptoms of progressive pain (Gilbert et al., 1978b). Pain is characteristically central in location, but may have a radicular component. Central pain is localized over the epidural lesion, but may occur a distance from the site of cord compression if there are multiple vertebral metastases. Pain is aggravated by recumbency, weight-bearing, coughing, sneezing, or the Valsalva maneuver and is relieved by sitting. Radicular pain frequently is associated with cervical or lumbar involvement (Wild and Parker, 1963). Radicular thoracic pain may be mistaken for pleurisy, pancreatitis, or cholecystitis. Classically, radicular thoracic pain is bilateral and localized to one or two vertebral segments below the area of cord compression (Brice and McKissock, 1965; Rubin *et al.*, 1969; White *et al.*, 1971; Marshall and Langfitt, 1977; Gilbert *et al.*, 1978b).

Muscle weakness is rarely the first symptom suggestive of cord compression (Gilbert *et al.*, 1978b). The incidence of motor abnormalities has decreased in recent series owing to earlier diagnosis. Cervical spinal cord compression results in upper extremity and respiratory muscle paralysis, while lower extremity weakness may be associated with cord compression at any level.

At presentation, over half the patients have sensory changes, including numbness, tingling, coldness, or paresthesias. Bladder or bowel dysfunction is rarely the first sign of cord compression. Patients typically describe symptoms of urinary retention and constipation progressing to bladder and bowel incontinence. The majority of patients with symptoms of autonomic dysfunction either present with or rapidly develop paralysis (Gilbert *et al.*, 1978b; Rodriguez and Dinapoli, 1980). Metastases to the cauda equina produce saddle anesthesia, impaired urethral, vaginal, and rectal sensation, bladder dysfunction, and decreased sensation in the lumbosacral dermatomes (Bruckman and Bloomer, 1978).

Physical examination may help localize the level of epidural compression, but is not a substitute for myelography. Pain, which is elicited by straight-leg raising, neck flexion, or vertebral percussion, is helpful in identifying the level of cord compression. The upper limit of the sensory level is often one or two vertebral bodies below the site of compression. The degree of motor weakness should be assessed at least on a daily basis. More frequent neurologic examinations are required in the patient with rapidly progressive symptoms. Patients with symptoms of autonomic dysfunction frequently present with signs of decreased rectal tone and decreased perineal sensation. Deep tendon reflexes may be brisk with cord compression and absent with nerve root compression. Abnormalities in gait are usually the result of paresis or proprioceptive sensory loss. Gilbert noted that severe gait ataxia may occur without other cerebellar signs (Posner *et al.*, 1977; Gilbert *et al.*, 1978b).

Diagnostic Evaluation. Spinal cord compression is always an emergency, especially when neurologic signs are progressing rapidly. Once the patient becomes paraplegic, there is little chance of regaining function. Seventy to 90% of patients with epidural tumor have evidence of vertebral metastases on spine films. Generally, the osseous metastases are located at the level of cord compression. Appropriate radiographs may reveal vertebral collapse, osteolytic lesions, pedicle erosion, or, rarely, a paraspinal mass (Wild and Parker, 1963; Bruckman and Bloomer, 1978; Gilbert *et al.*, 1978b; Rodriguez and Dinapoli, 1980; Rodichuk *et al.*, 1981). Normal radiographs are more common in patients with lymphoma or retroperitoneal tumors (Torma, 1957).

Rodichuk *et al.* (1981) initiated a prospective clinical trial designed to diagnose early spinal cord metastases before irreversible neurologic damage occurred. Table 40–18

Table 40–18. Diagnostic Value of Roentgenograms of the Spine

		ABNORMAL ROENTGENOGRAM*		NORMAL ROENTGENOGRAM	
GROUP	NO.	Positive Myelogram	Negative Myelogram	Positive Myelogram	Negative Myelogram
Patients with abnormalities on neurologic examination					
I Myelopathy	18	13	1	1	3
II Radiculopathy	28	14	2	3	9
III Plexopathy	5	0	0	0	2
Patients with no abnormalities on neurologic examination					
IV Abnormal radiology	25	15	7	0	3
V Normal radiology	17	0	0	0	7
Total	93	42	10	4	24

Reprinted with permission from Rodichuk, L. D.; Harper, G. R.; Ruckdeschel, J. C.; Roberson, G.; Barron, K. D.; and Horton J.: Early diagnosis of spinal epidural metastases. *Am. J. Med.*, **70:**1181–1188, 1981.
* Roentgenograms of the spine were considered abnormal when they showed evidence of vertebral metastases in the symptomatic area and normal when they showed no abnormality. Myelograms were considered positive when they showed evidence of extramedullary metastatic tumor and negative when they did not.

illustrates the diagnostic value of spine films performed for suspected cord compression. They demonstrated that abnormalities on plain films often predicted the presence of epidural tumor in cancer patients presenting with back pain or a myelopathy. Ninety-three percent of patients with neurologic signs secondary to cord compression had radiographic evidence of vertebral metastases on plain films. Appropriate radiographs correctly predicted the presence or absence of epidural tumor in 82% of patients with radiculopathy and 72% with central back pain without myelopathy. Osseous metastases were detected at the level of the block in 88% of patients with radiculopathy and 68% with central back pain. Epidural metastases were documented by myelography in 81% with roentgenographic abnormalities and 14% with negative bone films regardless of neurologic deficits. Although bone scans are more sensitive in detecting early osseous metastases, they are less accurate in predicting spinal cord compression. Rodichuk reported that none of the patients with positive nuclear scans and normal radiographs had abnormalities on myelography (Rodichuk *et al.*, 1981).

The most important and definitive study is the myelogram. This should be performed immediately in all patients with suspected cord compression to determine the proximal and distal extent of the tumor mass and to determine if multiple lesions are present (see Figure 40–7). Generally, iophendylate contrast is injected into the subarachnoid space by lumbar puncture. Metrizamide, a water-soluble contrast material, may better differentiate spinal stenosis from a complete block, but often produces a mild arachnoiditis. Also, since water-soluble contrast is reabsorbed, follow-up films cannot be performed to assess therapeutic response. If a complete block is present, the upper limit of the block must be defined. Cisternal or lateral cervical punctures are required if the upper limit cannot be defined by air injection following lumbar iophendylate myelography (Levine and Olmstead, 1979; Katz *et al.*, 1981).

Cerebrospinal fluid should not be removed if a complete block is demonstrated. If CSF can be obtained safely, fluid should be sent for glucose, protein, cell count, cytology, and appropriate stains and cultures if infection is suspected. Protein elevation usually correlates with the degree of subarachnoid block (Rodriguez and Dinapoli, 1980). Unless infection or carcinomatosis meningitis is suspected, CSF

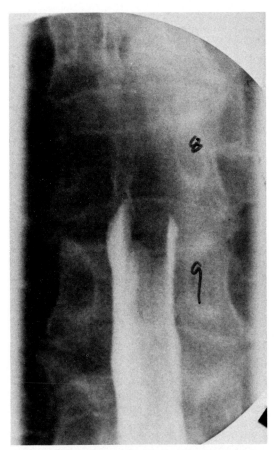

Figure 40–7. Myelogram demonstrating extradural thoracic spinal cord compression secondary to metastatic lung carcinoma. Complete block of the subarachnoid space has occurred in the midthoracic spine.

examination is generally nondiagnostic. If a myelogram cannot be performed, a metrizamide CT scan may delineate the subarachnoid space and define the area of block. CT scans of the spine, spinal canal, vertebral foramina, and paravertebral soft tissues may also identify abnormalities that are not seen on plain films or myelography. CT scans are particularly helpful in patients with abdominal or pelvic neoplasms. They commonly have neurologic deficits from cauda equina metastases or sacral root compression secondary to pelvic or retroperitoneal adenopathy (Rodriguez and Dinapoli, 1980).

Therapy. Prompt radiotherapy and neurosurgical consultation must be obtained when spinal cord compression is suspected. Prospective randomized trials have not been performed to determine in which clinical situations surgery, radiotherapy, or combined modality treatment should be utilized. Treatment decisions must be based on tumor type, clinical expertise, the level of spinal cord compression, tempo of symptom progression, and prior therapy.

Radiotherapy is the primary treatment for most patients with epidural metastases and should be initiated immediately after the diagnosis is made. Patients with slowly progressive disease or epidural metastases to the cauda equina should be managed with radiotherapy alone. When surgical decompression and postoperative radiotherapy were retrospectively compared to radiation alone in a nonrandomized trial, there was no significant difference in the percentage of patients remaining ambulatory at the completion of therapy (Gilbert et al., 1978b). Radiation portals should include the entire area of block and two vertebral bodies above and below the block (Rubin, 1969; Rodriguez and Dinapoli, 1980). Radiation doses range from 3000 to 4000 rads over two to three weeks. Four-hundred-rads fractions are generally administered for three days, followed by daily 180- to 200-rad fractions to a total dose of 4000 rads (Rubin, 1969; Rubin et al., 1969). These doses of radiotherapy are not associated with increased edema or neurologic deterioration if corticosteroids are administered.

Patients with radioresponsive tumors including seminoma, lymphoma, multiple myeloma, or Ewing's sarcoma have higher response rates to radiotherapy than patients with more radioresistant tumors, including soft tissue sarcoma or melanoma (Rubin, 1969; Sahn and Robinson, 1978; Rodriguez and Dinapoli, 1980). Gilbert et al. (1978a,b) reported that over 50% of patients with rapid neurologic deterioration improved with radiotherapy. Patients with autonomic dysfunction or paraplegia rarely respond to either surgery or radiotherapy (Wild and Parker, 1963; White et al., 1971; Posner, 1977).

Historically, laminectomy provides prompt decompression of the spinal cord and nerve roots, but the majority of the tumor can rarely be removed (Rodriguez and Dinapoli, 1980). Most epidural metastases arise anterior to the spinal cord, making it extremely difficult to remove tumor by a posterior approach without damaging the cord. A posterior laminectomy frequently produces an unstable spine. The posterior elements of the spine must be surgically removed, leaving the anterior supporting elements destroyed by tumor. Brice

and McKissock (1965) reported that with posterior laminectomy 47% of patients with posterior epidural metastases and 17% with anterior metastases had neurologic recovery. Although perioperative mortality rates have decreased from a high of 13% to approximately 5% in recent series, 10 to 33% of patients have more extensive neurologic abnormalities postoperatively (Torma, 1957; Brice and McKissock, 1965; White et al., 1971; Bruckman and Bloomer, 1978; Gilbert et al., 1978b).

Ambulatory patients may benefit from surgical decompression. Livingston also reported that 25% of patients who were paraplegic preoperatively had functional improvement with surgery. However, most neurosurgical series report that only 5% of paraplegic patients have any neurologic recovery with surgical decompression (Bruckman and Bloomer, 1978; Livingston and Perrin, 1978). Surgery is generally contraindicated when there are multiple areas of cord compression.

Absolute indications for surgery include patients with an uncertain diagnosis, particularly those without a previous histologic diagnosis of malignancy, or in cases where infection or epidural hematoma must be ruled out. High cervical cord lesions result in death from respiratory paralysis unless decompression is accomplished. When neurologic signs progress over 48 to 72 hours despite steroids and radiotherapy, emergency decompression should be attempted. Operative results, however, are generally poor in this group of patients. Patients with recurrent cord compression after a long interval following radiotherapy might also benefit from surgery if they are in otherwise good general condition. Most of the tumor cannot be removed at surgery in the majority of patients. Therefore, following decompression, postoperative radiotherapy should be given to decrease residual tumor, prevent tumor regrowth, and improve pain and functional status (Wild and Parker, 1963). Unfortunately, less than half of patients treated with surgery and postoperative radiotherapy are ambulatory at the completion of therapy (Wild and Parker, 1963; Rodriguez and Dinapoli, 1980).

Corticosteroids may temporarily reduce peritumoral edema and improve neurologic function. Although steroids are generally prescribed, prospective randomized trials have not been performed to confirm their therapeutic efficacy. The initial steroid dose is equivalent to 16 mg of dexamethasone a day in divided doses. The optimal corticosteroid dose has not been established for cord compression. In Posner's series, dexamethasone, 100 mg a day, was administered concurrently with high-fraction radiotherapy for three days. High-dose steroids were more effective in relieving pain, but were not statistically superior to more conventional therapy in terms of improvement in functional status (Posner, 1977).

Chemotherapy rarely has a major therapeutic role in spinal cord compression. If the tumor is responsive to chemotherapy and the patient is not refractory to active drugs, however, this modality should be administered in conjunction with or soon after radiotherapy or surgery (Murphy and Bilge, 1964; Silverberg and Jacobs, 1971; Ushio et al., 1977a,b). For example, patients with lymphoma or metastatic breast cancer might benefit from combination chemotherapy if not refractory to prior treatment with these modalities.

Pathologic Fractures and Bone Metastases

Bone metastases are rarely life threatening, but frequently cause significant disability for patients with advanced malignancy. Relief of pain and prevention of pathologic fracture are the major therapeutic objectives. Once a pathologic fracture has occurred, the major goals are stabilization, pain relief, and regaining functional status. Long bones, particularly the femur or humerus, are common sites of pathologic fractures. Lytic bone metastases arise in the medullary canal and eventually involve the bony cortex. Lytic metastases, which involve cortical bone, are more likely to fracture than blastic metastases in the same location. Once cortical bone is weakened, minimal stress may precipitate a pathologic fracture. Weight-bearing may precipitate femoral, humeral, pelvic, or vertebral compression fractures, while rib fractures may develop following prolonged coughing. The most common primary neoplasms metastasizing to bone are carcinomas of the breast, lung, and prostate, followed by multiple myeloma, hypernephromas, thyroid carcinoma, and tumors of unknown primary (Vaughn and Brindley, 1979).

Pathophysiology and Clinical Presentation. Osseous metastases usually result from hematogenous, rather than lymphatic, spread. Both lytic and blastic metastases disrupt normal bony architecture. Blastic lesions are surrounded by a margin of reactive new-bone formation, which may protect against pathologic fracture. Osteolytic lesions arise in the medullary canal and commonly erode the cortex, which increases the risk of pathologic fracture.

Patients with bone metastases typically present with localized pain that is gradual in onset, progressive over a period of weeks to months, and is more severe at night. Pain is caused by periosteal stretching, either secondary to direct pressure from the tumor or by weakening of the bone, producing mechanical stress at the tumor site (Hendrickson and Steinkop, 1975). Osseous metastases in the lower extremities or pelvis are painful primarily on weight-bearing. A sudden dramatic increase in pain suggests a pathologic fracture and should be evaluated promptly with appropriate radiographs and orthopedic consultation. Percussion tenderness at the site of bony involvement is a highly reliable clinical sign (Hendrickson and Steinkop, 1975). Neurologic deficits may be present secondary to either nerve entrapment or spinal cord compression from vertebral metastases; therefore, a careful neurologic examination is essential. Pathologic fractures may result from radiation-induced osteonecrosis, rather than metastases. Radiation decreases the bone's vascular supply and osteocyte activity, ultimately resulting in osteoporosis and reactive sclerosis. Radiation osteonecrosis usually occurs in adults who have been treated with over 5000 rads to the involved site (Libshitz and Southard, 1974; Levene et al., 1977).

Diagnostic Evaluation. Appropriate radiographs of symptomatic areas should be obtained to define the extent of lytic or blastic lesions, to evaluate the structural integrity of the bone, and to identify the potential risk for pathologic fracture. Bone films will not detect small metastases unless they are greater than 1 cm with at least 30 to 50% of bony demineralization. Radiographically, osseous metastases may have lytic, blastic, or a mixed lytic-blastic appearance. Osteolytic lesions appear as irregular areas of decreased radiodensity, the result of extensive bone destruction; whereas blastic metastases have increased density owing to increased medullary bone formation. Lytic metastases involving over 25% of the cortex demand prophylactic treatment to prevent pathologic fracture (see Figure 40–8). If radiographs demonstrate mixed lytic and blastic lesions in previously irradiated bone, radiation osteonecrosis must be considered in the differential diagnosis. Radiation portals and doses should be reviewed since radiation osteitis is

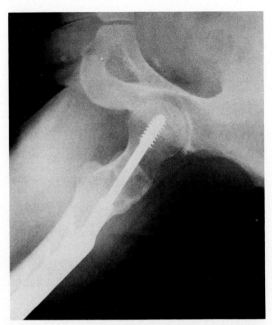

Figure 40-8. A large osteolytic metastasis in a 50-year-old man with adenocarcinoma of the lung. Prophylactic internal fixation and postoperative radiotherapy were performed to reduce the risk of pathologic fracture.

limited to the treatment field and rarely occurs unless high radiation doses were delivered (Howland *et al.,* 1975).

Neoplastic bony involvement frequently is present beyond the radiographic abnormality and may be detected by bone scan (Teplick and Haskin, 1971). Technetium-99^m-labeled phosphate bone scans are more sensitive in detecting early bone metastases than plain radiographs (Pistenma *et al.,* 1975). Bone lesions appear as increased areas of uptake on scan when there is adequate blood flow and reactive new-bone formation. False-negative scans occur with pure lytic destructive metastases; whereas blastic metastases avidly concentrate the radionuclide caused by medullary bone formation (Blair and McAfee, 1976; McNeil, 1978). Bone scans are excellent screening tests, but are certainly not specific for neoplastic disease. Radiographs of any suspicious areas should be obtained to exclude benign causes including trauma, infection, arthritis, or Paget's disease. Skeletal surveys are generally more sensitive than bone scans in patients with lytic metastases (*e.g.,* multiple myeloma). Blair and McAfee (1976) reported that 2 to 8% of patients with lytic osseous metastases had negative scans. Tomography may be necessary to document cortical destruction and to assess

therapeutic response. If surgery or radiotherapy is contemplated, the adjacent bone should be evaluated by bone scan and radiographs, so that contiguous metastases are included in treatment planning.

Therapy. Pathologic fractures are a devastating consequence of osseous metastases. Prophylactic treatment of incipient pathologic fractures prevents intractable pain, immobility, and associated complications including hypercalcemia, decubitus ulcers, and infection. Most osteolytic metastases involving over 25% of the cortex in a major weight-bearing bone should be prophylactically treated. Preventive therapy may include radiation, internal fixation, external stabilization, systemic hormonal or chemotherapy, or a combination of these modalities. The goal of therapy is to relieve pain, improve function, and prevent pathologic fracture. Therapeutic decisions must be individualized according to the radiosensitivity of the tumor, response rates to hormonal or systemic chemotherapy, extent of metastatic disease, tempo of symptoms, physical status of the patient, and life expectancy.

Local radiotherapy relieves pain from bone metastases in 73 to 96% of patients and affords effective palliation for 55 to 78% of patients for over one year or until death (Allen *et al.,* 1976; Gilbert *et al.,* 1977; Nussbaum *et al.,* 1977; Garmatis and Chu, 1978). Pain relief is usually superior in nonweight-bearing bones without large lytic lesions (Gilbert *et al.,* 1977). A high proportion of patients with radiosensitive tumors, including breast cancer, multiple myeloma, lymphoma, and occasionally lung cancer, have excellent, prolonged subjective responses (Allen *et al.,* 1976; Nussbaum *et al.,* 1977; Garmatis and Chu, 1978). Garmatis and Chu (1978) reported that 96% of women with metastatic breast cancer had adequate pain relief and 20% complete pain relief for an average of 12 months following radiotherapy. In order to obtain significant palliation with more radioresistant tumors (*e.g.,* renal cell or prostate), larger doses of radiotherapy may be required (Allen *et al.,* 1976; Gilbert *et al.,* 1977; Garmatis and Chu, 1978).

The maximum daily dose of radiotherapy depends on normal tissue tolerance. Greater than 300- to 400-rad fractions should not be used in treatment of vertebral metastases, nor should large fields that include portions of the bowel. Cervical or thoracic spine metastases should be treated with 3000- to 4000-rad total dose over a 2.5- to 4-week period to achieve long-term control and prophylaxis against fracture or spinal cord compression (Allen *et al.*, 1976). Low-dose (500 to 2000 rads), short-fractionation (one to five fractions) radiotherapy may provide effective long-term palliation comparable to more prolonged treatment courses (Allen *et al.*, 1976; Penn, 1976; Nussbaum *et al.*, 1977). Unfortunately, the duration of response is difficult to evaluate owing to the short median survival in most series. Many radiotherapists recommend more protracted radiotherapy (3000 to 4000 rads delivered over 2.5 to 4 weeks) for patients with potential prolonged survival, as is frequently seen in advanced breast cancer or solitary bone metastases (Allen *et al.*, 1976). Short-course, low-dose therapy is obviously advantageous for patients with a short life expectancy.

The radiation field should include the area of painful bony involvement with an adjacent margin of uninvolved asymptomatic bone. Patients with multiple vertebral metastases may benefit from total spinal radiation if there is little hope of response to systemic antitumor therapy and the entire vertebral column is involved. In a series of patients with vertebral metastases treated with localized vertebral radiotherapy, over 40% required a second course of radiotherapy to the axial skeleton, and 9% a third course prior to death (Bagshaw, 1971; Eisen *et al.*, 1973; Nussbaum *et al.*, 1977). Total spinal radiotherapy is rarely used owing to significant myelosuppression, which, in turn, interferes with future chemotherapy.

A second course of radiotherapy to the same site should be administered for palliation of recurrent bone pain if the first course of radiation provided excellent palliation for at least 6 to 12 months. Obviously, normal tissue tolerance must be considered in administering a second course of therapy (Nussbaum *et al.*, 1977). This is particularly important in preventing radiation osteitis or myelitis. Despite excellent subjective response rates to local radiotherapy, only a fraction of lytic metastases show signs of reossification (Ryan *et al.*, 1976). Up to 70% of radiosensitive bone metastases (*e.g.*, breast cancer) show signs of recalcification following radiotherapy, although radiographic signs of healing are rarely observed with more radioresistant malignancies. Comparative studies are needed to define the optimal radiotherapy dose and fractionation schedule to prevent pathologic fractures. Penn reported no significant difference in the number of pathologic fractures in major weight-bearing bones irradiated with either a single, high-dose of radiation or the standard 3000 rads over a two-week period (Penn, 1976).

Most patients with incipient pathologic fractures in major weight-bearing bones are managed with internal fixation and postoperative radiotherapy. Many of the surgical procedures and management decisions used to treat pathologic fractures also pertain to the patient with an incipient fracture who requires prophylactic stabilization. Once a pathologic fracture occurs, the goals of treatment are stabilization, pain relief, functional improvement, and prompt ambulation if possible. Operative internal fixation relieves pain in 85 to 90% of patients. Without internal fixation, radiotherapy will relieve pain in 55 to 65% with pathologic fracture, but does not provide immediate stabilization (Douglas *et al.*, 1976; Vaughn and Brindley, 1979). After internal fixation, 61 to 78% of patients are either ambulatory or functional, whereas only 23% treated by other methods of stabilization (*e.g.*, casting or braces) obtained a functional status (Douglas *et al.*, 1976; Ryan *et al.*, 1976; Nussbaum *et al.*, 1977; Vaughn and Brindley, 1979).

Depending on the patient's general status and projected survival, several methods of stabilization should be considered in management of pathologic fractures. The best results are obtained with operative metallic fixation or joint replacement (Douglas *et al.*, 1976; Nussbaum *et al.*, 1977). Good-quality radiographs of the entire bone must be obtained preoperatively. Internal fixation is usually unsuccessful if the integrity of adjacent bone is weakened by osteoporosis or multiple metastases (Nussbaum *et al.*, 1977). If a second metastatic lesion is found, metallic devices used for internal fixation must be placed so that excessive stress is not concentrated in the second weakened area. Internal fixation provides effective prophylaxis against lateral fractures caused by tension stress, but does not prevent compression fracture.

Prior to surgery, perioperative complications should be anticipated. Patients immobilized with hypercalcemia or significant osteoporosis rarely regain function postoperatively. Hemorrhagic complications should be anticipated with osseous metastases from renal, breast, or thyroid carcinoma. Preoperatively, coagulopathies and thrombocytopenia should be corrected with factor replacement and platelet transfusions (Nussbaum *et al.*, 1977).

If a large tumor cavity follows curettage, the

bony defect should be filled with methyl methacrylate. Methyl methacrylate facilitates fracture fixation and stabilizes osteoporotic or weakened tumorous bone with minimal side effects. These include rare hypersensitivity reactions, fragmentation, and late osteomyelitis (Douglas *et al.,* 1976; Ryan *et al.,* 1976; Nussbaum *et al.,* 1977).

The most common site of pathologic fractures is the shaft of the femur or femoral neck. When the metastasis involves only a small portion of bone, the fracture may be treated as a nonneoplastic fracture of the same area followed by radiotherapy to facilitate healing. This conservative approach should not be utilized with femoral neck fractures which often fail to heal even following aggressive surgical therapy (Douglas *et al.,* 1976; Nussbaum *et al.,* 1977). Fractures of the femoral head and neck are generally treated by replacement hemiarthroplasty. With extensive involvement of the acetabulum, patients commonly have continuing pain and little chance of ambulation despite hemiarthroplasty (Perez *et al.,* 1972; Nussbaum *et al.,* 1977; Vaughn and Brindley, 1979). Femoral shaft fractures are treated with Schneider rods (Ryan *et al.,* 1976; Nussbaum *et al.,* 1977; Vaughn and Brindley, 1979). If a femoral shaft metastasis is over 2.5 cm in diameter, involves the cortex, or is associated with significant pain, prophylactic intramedullary nailing should be considered.

Most humeral fractures are located in the mid- or proximal one-third of the shaft (Douglas *et al.,* 1976). Depending on the prognosis of the patient, these fractures can be treated aggressively with intramedullary Rush rods or conservatively with simple slings (Douglas *et al.,* 1976; Nussbaum *et al.,* 1977; Vaughn and Brindley, 1979). Internal fixation improves function and relieves pain in over 90% of patients (Douglas *et al.,* 1976; Vaughn and Brindley, 1976). Schneider intramedullary rods are used for operative fixation of forearm fractures, while a forearm cast or fiberglass splint should be considered in patients with short life expectancies (Nussbaum *et al.,* 1977; Vaughn and Brindley, 1979). If the patient's projected survival is short, external fixation should be considered using traction, casts, splints, braces, or slings (Nussbaum *et al.,* 1977).

Thoracic lumbar spine metastases are usually stabilized with corset and brace fixation if no neurologic deficits are evident (Nussbaum *et al.,* 1977). If signs of neurologic compromise are present, emergency treatment for spinal cord compression is indicated.

If radiotherapy was not given before surgery, radiotherapy is usually given postoperatively, preferably in a rapid course of approximately 2000 rads over five days. Postoperative radiotherapy may help sterilize the remaining tumor and enhance bony union (Nussbaum *et al.,* 1977).

Obstructive Uropathy

Neoplastic obstructive uropathy is often complicated by infection, renal calculi, and ultimately hydronephrosis with irreversible renal tubular damage, culminating in renal failure and death (Garnick and Mayer, 1978). Urinary diversion or effective antineoplastic therapy may relieve obstruction, but in the terminal patient, aggressive measures to reverse obstruction should be avoided. Obstructive uropathy is divided into two broad categories: bladder outlet and ureteral obstruction. Bladder outlet obstruction is frequently secondary to prostatic cancer or benign prostate hypertrophy. Ureteral obstruction is seen most commonly with intra-abdominal and retroperitoneal tumors, including sarcoma, non-Hodgkin's lymphomas, and carcinomas of the cervix, bladder, prostate, ovary, and rectum (Goldstein, 1967; Geller and Lin, 1975; Van Dyke and Van Nagell, 1975; Williams and Peet, 1976; Michigan and Catalano, 1977; Garnick and Mayer, 1978).

Pathophysiology. Ureteral obstruction is the most common cause of obstructive uropathy. Tumor may directly invade the ureter, but more frequently produces extrinsic compression (Richmond *et al.,* 1962; Abeloff and Lenhard, 1974; Koziol, 1974; Garnick and Mayer, 1978; Herwig, 1980). Although recurrent tumor is the leading cause of ureteral obstruction in the cancer patient, nonneoplastic etiologies must be considered in the differential diagnosis. Patients with pelvic and retroperitoneal neoplasms may develop ureteral strictures secondary to fibrosis and adhesions from prior radiotherapy or surgery. Renal calculi are seen with chronic hypercalciuria, hyperuricemia, or urinary tract infection. Retroperitoneal surgery may be complicated by abscesses or hematomas which may compress the ureters. Acute hyperuricemic nephropathy is generally secondary to uric acid deposition in the renal tubules. Ureteral obstruction from uric acid crystals, however, has been reported in association with hematologic cancer both before and after chemotherapy (Kjellstrand *et al.*, 1974).

Bladder outlet obstruction typically leads to progressive bladder enlargement, bilateral ureteral dilatation, and hydronephrosis. Chronic partial urethral obstruction produces hypertrophy of the bladder wall musculature and diverticuli. Bladder outlet obstruction may be secondary to mechanical factors, as seen with prostatic and cervical carcinoma or urethral strictures from radiation fibrosis or cyclophosphamide cystitis. The central nervous system controls bladder evacuation by relaxing striated muscle and contracting the smooth muscle in the bladder wall. Thus, urinary retention may occur with brain, spinal cord, sacral root, or bladder metastases, or with medications that depress the central or autonomic nervous system (Herwig, 1980; Gutman and Boxer, 1982).

Regardless of the etiology of urinary tract obstruction, the pathologic changes in the dilated structures proximal to the site of obstruction are identical. Initially with acute obstruction, renal tubular pressure rises, and glomerular filtration rates markedly decrease. Within the first 24 hours, renal blood flow, glomerular filtration rate, tubular secretion, concentrating ability, and ureteral pressure begin to decline (Gutman and Boxer, 1982). When bilateral urinary obstruction is relieved before there is significant irreversible renal damage, a postobstructive diuresis occurs (Wilson, 1977; Gillenwater, 1979; Wright and Howard, 1981). A significant diuresis following release of unilateral renal obstruction is rarely observed. Experimental data suggest that the etiology of postobstructive diuresis includes (1) retention of urea and other unidentified substances; (2) relative sparing of juxtamedullary nephrons, so that the filtration rate following relief of obstruction exceeds the tubular capacity for salt and water reabsorption; or (3) greater tubular pressures in bilateral obstruction (Gutman and Boxer, 1982).

Clinical Presentation. Patients with advanced pelvic or retroperitoneal neoplasms commonly present with obstructive uropathy. Obstruction may be found in the initial staging evaluation or may be suspected in the patient with urinary retention, flank pain, hematuria, or signs of urinary tract infection. Unfortunately, ureteral obstruction is often not diagnosed until renal damage results in uremic obtundation, seizures, volume overload, and an-

uria (Goldstein, 1967; Pillay and Dunea, 1971; Garnick and Mayer, 1978; Herwig, 1980). Prostatic urethral obstruction is recognized earlier and is usually preceded by symptoms of hesitancy, urgency, nocturia, frequency, decreased force of the urinary stream, and dribbling. However, a neurogenic bladder secondary to brain or spinal cord metastases may present with similar symptoms (Pillay and Dunea, 1971; Garnick and Mayer, 1978; Herwig, 1980; Gutman and Boxer, 1982).

Polyuria, occasionally alternating with oliguria, suggests tubular dysfunction from partial bilateral obstruction (Gutman and Boxer, 1982). Severe flank pain is typically associated with acute obstruction of the ureter or renal pelvis. The intensity of pain is proportional to the rate of ureteral dilatation rather than the degree of dilatation or hyperperistalsis (Wright and Howard, 1981). Nausea, vomiting, and, rarely, ileus are also associated with acute obstruction or uremia from chronic obstruction (Kelalis, 1976).

Physical examination may reveal prostatic, bladder, or renal enlargement, or a mass in the pelvis, flank, or rectum (Herwig, 1980). Costovertebral angle pain suggests acute obstruction or infection. Associated neurologic signs, including decreased anal sphincter tone or abnormal bulbocavernosus reflexes, are suggestive of a neurogenic bladder. Urethral strictures are found at the time of bladder catheterization.

Diagnostic Evaluation. Obstructive uropathy can be readily diagnosed by intravenous pyelography (IVP), renal ultrasound, renal nuclear scan, or computerized tomography (CT) of the retroperitoneum. Urethral obstruction should be excluded by catheterization. A normal urine analysis does not exclude obstructive uropathy, although nonspecific abnormalities, including proteinuria, inappropriately low urine osmolality, hematuria, renal tubular cells, or pyuria, are often seen. The presence of white cells and bacteria suggests infection behind an obstruction, which requires immediate drainage and parenteral antibiotics. In the absence of infection, a fasting urine pH greater than 6 is suggestive of a renal acidifying defect, an early sign of tubular obstruction. Nephrolithiasis should be suspected with crystalluria. Routine serum chemistries, including creatinine, electrolytes, blood urea nitrogen, calcium, phosphorus, uric acid, and the hematologic profile, should be monitored carefully.

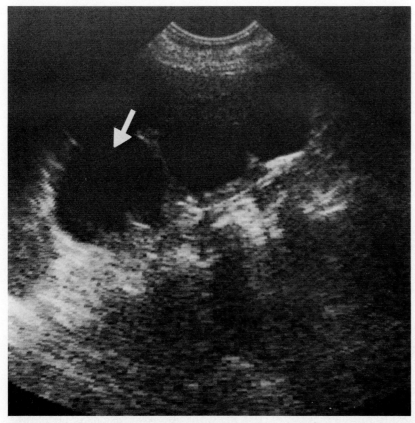

Figure 40–9. Renal ultrasound: hydronephrosis. A 72-year-old woman with bilateral hydronephrosis secondary to locally advanced rectal carcinoma. The pelvic calyceal system (arrows) is markedly dilated due to bilateral ureteral obstruction.

Before initiating appropriate therapy, the site of complete or partial obstruction must be accurately determined (Pillay and Dunea, 1971; Smith and Bartrum, 1976; Garnick and Mayer, 1978; Herwig, 1980). When obstructive uropathy is suspected, hydronephrosis should be confirmed with renal ultrasound, especially when the risks of contrast-induced nephrotoxicity are high (see Figure 40–9). Ultrasound may also demonstrate pelvic or retroperitoneal masses, ureteral dilatation, and calculi. The residual renal cortex can be assessed by renal ultrasound. If adequate cortical tissue is present, renal failure is often reversible following relief of obstruction (Russell and Resnick, 1979). Unless dye allergy or severe renal damage is present, intravenous urograms usually define the site of blockage (see Figure 40–10). To avoid dye-induced nephrotoxicity, patients must be well hydrated prior to examination. Even with complete obstruction, some contrast is concentrated so that delayed films (up to 36 hours) are helpful in the

diagnosis of hydronephrosis. The site of obstruction is identified by IVP in approximately 80% of patients with acute urinary obstruction (Bretland et al., 1972). Since a dilated collecting system does not necessarily imply obstruction, a repeat injection of contrast or a radionuclide study following hydration and intravenous diuretics may be necessary (Carvallo et al., 1978; O'Reilly et al., 1978; Koff et al., 1979).

Radionuclide scans are safer than IVP studies because nephrotoxic contrast is avoided. In the dilated nonobstructed kidney, furosemide, 0.3 mg/kg, produces an obvious decrease in renal ^{99m}Tc-DTPA, which does not occur with obstruction (Koff et al., 1979). Radionuclide renal scans quantitate the emptying rates for each kidney and collecting system and are extremely helpful in unusual types of obstruction, including ureteral stenosis from urinary diversion or previous surgery (Feun et al., 1979). Renal scans are also useful in predicting recovery of renal function. If technetium-99

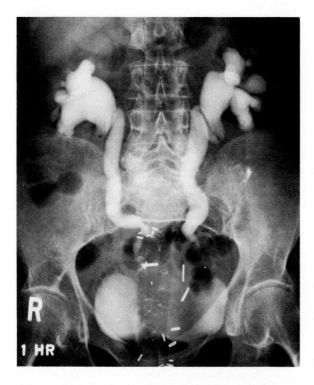

Figure 40-10. Obstructive uropathy: bilateral hydronephrosis. A 47-year-old woman with recurrent adenocarcinoma of the sigmoid invading the bladder, resulting in bilateral hydronephrosis. The kidneys, renal calyceal system, and ureters are extremely dilated. A large mass is invading the bladder and obstructing both ureters.

flow and static imaging scans demonstrate good renal perfusion and concentration, excellent results are obtained following relief of obstruction (Lome *et al.,* 1979).

Computerized tomography is more expensive than ultrasound and less specific than scans or dye studies, but occasionally is useful in differentiating hydronephrosis from cystic renal disease and in identifying masses that might be obstructing the collecting system (McClennan and Fair, 1979).

In the past, retrograde pyelography was often necessary to define the site of obstruction. With the current use of percutaneous antegrade pyelography, obstruction can be diagnosed and relieved without the risks of anesthesia. Under ultrasound guidance, a catheter is placed in the dilated renal pelvis, aspirated urine is analyzed and cultured, and contrast injected to localize the obstruction. An attempt is made to advance the catheter through the obstruction to restore internal ureteral drainage. If this is unsuccessful, obstruction may be relieved with external drainage. In partial obstruction an antegrade catheter may be necessary to obtain pressure measurements. Retroperitoneal bleeding and infection are potential complications, but rarely occur (Barbaric, 1979; Gerber *et al.,* 1981).

Transurethral or suprapubic cystoscopy is necessary to diagnose bladder outlet obstruction from prostatic hypertrophy or neoplasms, urethral stricture, and bladder neck contracture. The ureteral orifices should be well visualized and urinary flow confirmed from each orifice. Appropriate biopsies and cytologies should be obtained. If ureteral obstruction is diagnosed at cystoscopy, percutaneous antegrade pyelography should be instituted to relieve obstruction. With this technique, retrograde catheterization is rarely required (Gutman and Boxer, 1982). Urodynamic studies and urethrocystography are helpful in differentiating bladder dysfunction secondary to neuromuscular or mechanical causes (Herwig, 1980).

Therapy. Permanent renal damage and death from uremia will result unless urinary obstruction is relieved. Infection, hyperkalemia, and acidosis must be treated promptly. Renal obstruction may be relieved by effective antineoplastic therapy, bladder catheterization, or urinary diversion, but if obstruction occurs in the terminally ill patient, only supportive care should be offered. The decision to relieve an obstructing lesion must be carefully considered, as patient survival, but not comfort, may be prolonged.

Lower urinary tract obstruction is temporarily relieved by an indwelling urethral catheter. If bladder outlet obstruction is not relieved by this conservative approach, suprapubic cystotomy or cutaneous vesicostomy is required. If the cause of bladder outlet obstruction cannot be promptly corrected, suprapubic cystotomy is preferable to an indwelling urethral catheter. Suprapubic cystostomies are more comfortable and associated with fewer urinary and epididymal infections. Suprapubic bladder decompression also avoids prostatic swelling from urethral catheterization and allows urethral voiding capacity to be assessed easily without recatheterization (Herwig, 1980).

In partially denervated bladders, parasympathomimetic drugs (e.g., bethanechol) may strengthen bladder musculature and prevent overflow incontinence. Low-pressure incontinence can be improved by adrenergic agonists (e.g., ephedrine). Anticholinergics (e.g., probanthine) help uninhibited or reflex neurogenic bladders (Herwig, 1980).

Prostatic urethral obstruction is generally treated with transurethral resection. Obstruction caused by advanced prostate cancer may be relieved by orchiectomy or estrogens within several days if the tumor is hormonally responsive. In several small series, radiation relieved prostatic obstruction, with response rates varying from 25 to 90% following 4000 to 7500 rads. As maximal benefit from radiation is often delayed, transurethral resection or a temporary procedure for urinary diversion should be performed prior to radiotherapy (Carlton et al., 1972; Kraus et al., 1972; Green et al., 1974; Megalli et al., 1974; Michigan and Catalano, 1977).

Most ureteral obstructions can be relieved by percutaneous antegrade catheterization or nephrostomy. These procedures avoid the risks of anesthesia and surgery associated with retrograde pyelography and placement of ureteral stents (Loenning et al., 1974; Brin et al., 1975; Michigan and Catalano, 1977; Barbaric, 1979; Pfister and Newhouse, 1979; Kohler et al., 1980; Gerber et al., 1981). Percutaneous antegrade pyelography is now the preferred procedure for diagnosis and treatment of neoplastic ureteral obstruction. Internal drainage can be accomplished if the ureteral catheter is advanced through the obstruction (Barbaric, 1979; Gerber et al., 1981). If these methods are ineffective, an attempt is made to place indwelling ureteral stents, if the ureteral orifices can be identified with cystoscopy and retrograde pyelography (Gibbons et al., 1976; Hepperlen et al., 1978; Smith et al., 1978).

When less invasive methods fail to relieve obstruction, surgery is indicated if the patient has a reasonable life expectancy and irreversible renal damage has not already occurred. The site(s) of obstruction must be determined preoperatively, especially with pelvic malignancies when both urethral and ureteral obstruction may coexist. Unilateral obstruction can be treated surgically with permanent nephrostomy, percutaneous ureterostomy, or, rarely in selected patients, with transureteroureterostomy. Bilateral nephrostomies, ureterostomies, ureteroileostomy, or ureteral implantation into the bladder dome provide permanent palliation for bilateral ureteral obstruction (McNamara and Butkus, 1980; Meyer et al., 1980).

Ureteropyelostomy or the more recent techniques of ureteral implantation offer effective long-term palliation with extremely low morbidity. In a recent review, it was reported that late ureteral obstruction occurred in less than 2% of patients following ureteropyelostomy; and fewer than 10% developed postoperative fistula or early ureterovesical obstruction (Greenberg et al., 1977). Ileal loops are associated with high complication rates, ranging from 30 to 70%. Surgical revision is frequently necessary because of reobstruction or fistula formation. Enteritis, fibrosis, and adhesions from previous pelvic surgery or radiotherapy have led to the use of jejunal conduits, which avoid areas with a high probability of tumor recurrence or adhesions from previous surgery and radiotherapy (Norton and Javapour, 1977). Ureterosigmoidostomy is rarely performed because of the high incidence of infection from reflux of colonic bacteria. Cancer patients are rarely candidates for chronic dialysis programs, but acute dialysis may be indicated until renal function is restored.

Radiation therapy effectively relieves neoplastic ureteral obstruction secondary to radioresponsive tumors, including breast carcinoma and lymphoma, but chemotherapy may be equally effective (Abeloff and Lenhard, 1974; Loening et al., 1974; Williams and Peet, 1976; Kopelson et al., 1981). Appropriate dose adjustments must be made for renal insufficiency and nephrotoxic drugs (e.g., cisplatin, methotrexate, and streptozocin) should be avoided. Severe inflammation of the uroepithelium occurs after prolonged exposure to the active urinary metabolites of cyclophosphamide, and this drug should be avoided when urinary obstruction is suspected.

Appropriate intravenous fluids should be administered for at least 24 to 48 hours after relief of bilateral obstruction. Serum creatinine, electrolytes, magnesium, and calcium should be measured daily for the first three to ten days if massive diuresis occurs. Repeated attempts to discontinue vigorous hydration should be made beginning 48 hours after obstruction is relieved (Gutman and Boxer, 1982). If obstructive uropathy is diagnosed and effectively treated before irreversible renal damage occurs, renal function should be restored with little morbidity or mortality.

Gastrointestinal Obstruction

Gastrointestinal obstruction is a common complication of advanced intra-abdominal malignancy. Unless appropriate therapy is promptly initiated, volume depletion and metabolic alkalosis will develop secondary to loss of fluids and electrolytes from vomiting and intraluminal sequestration. Perforation caused by increased intraluminal pressure is an infrequent complication of untreated obstruction (Harken et al., 1975).

Esophageal obstruction is usually secondary to tumor, but inflammation and edema from infection, radiation, or chemotherapy should be excluded by endoscopy and biopsy. Gastric outlet obstruction may also be secondary to benign etiologies, for example, peptic ulcer disease, rather than antral gastric carcinoma.

Recurrent tumor is the primary cause of small bowel obstruction in the cancer patient, but obstruction may also result from hernias, intussusception, and adhesions from previous surgery or radiotherapy. Primary tumors of the small bowel are rare and more frequently present with hemorrhage. Metastases to the small bowel may result from direct invasion by adjacent primary neoplasms, submucosal metastases, or abdominal carcinomatosis. Multiple tumor implants frequently produce studding of the bowel and peritoneal surfaces. Intraluminal metastases commonly present with hemorrhage rather than with malignant intestinal obstruction or intussusception. Table 40–19 lists the primary malignancies most frequently associated with metastatic small bowel obstruction (De Castro et al., 1957; Ngan, 1970; Ellis et al., 1972; Veen et al., 1976; Herbsman et al., 1980).

Osteen reported that one-third of intestinal

Table 40–19. Primary Malignancies Commonly Associated with Small Bowel Metastases and Obstruction

ABDOMINAL CARCINOMATOSIS	DIRECT INVASION	SUBMUCOSAL METASTASES
Ovary	Ovary	Ovary
Pancreas	Pancreas	Breast
Colon	Colon	Lung
Stomach	Stomach	Melanoma
	Retroperitoneal sarcoma	Cervix
	Kidney	Esophagus

Derived from de Castro et al., 1957; Ngan, 1970; Ellis et al., 1972; Veen et al., 1976; Herbsman et al., 1980.

obstructions associated with known malignancy were the result of benign causes. Prior radiotherapy or surgery is frequently complicated by adhesions and intermittent bowel obstruction. Narcotic analgesics, hypercalcemia, hypokalemia, and immobilization decrease colonic motility and may precipitate fecal impaction. However, neoplastic disease is more frequently the cause of bowel obstruction. Table 40–20 lists the clinical factors that increase the probability that the obstruction is secondary to malignancy (Osteen et al., 1980). Colonic obstruction is often the presenting sign of colorectal carcinoma. Colon cancer patients presenting with bowel obstruction have higher surgical morbidity and mortality rates and a poorer prognosis regardless of lymph node status. (Hickey and Hyde, 1965; Minister, 1969; Watters, 1969; Glenn and McSherry, 1971; Ragland et al., 1971; Ulin et al., 1971; Welch and Donaldson, 1974; Clark et al., 1975).

Clinical Presentation. Patients with esophageal obstruction usually present with progressive dysphagia, pain, and weight loss. Perforation, tracheoesphageal fistula, and aspiration pneumonia should be suspected if fever or cough develops in the setting of esophageal obstruction. Patients with gastric outlet obstruction usually complain of progressive early satiety, postprandial epigastric pain, and intermittent nausea and vomiting. Projectile vom-

Table 40–20. Factors Predisposing Toward the Diagnosis of Bowel Obstruction Secondary to Malignancy

1. A diagnosis of colorectal cancer
2. Known metastatic disease at presentation
3. An advanced primary carcinoma at initial diagnosis
4. A short time interval between the diagnosis of the primary tumor and intestinal obstruction.

Derived from Osteen et al., 1980.

iting typically occurs with complete antral obstruction. Unless there is a history suggestive of peptic ulcer disease prior to gastric obstruction, the etiology is rarely the result of a benign cause (Gunnlaugsson *et al.*, 1970).

Intestinal obstruction produces vomiting, abdominal distention, obstipation, and intermittent, nonlocalizing, crampy abdominal pain. Proximal small bowel obstruction is associated with frequent vomiting without severe pain or distention unless perforation or strangulation occurs. Obstipation, marked abdominal distention, and severe colicky abdominal pain are characteristic features of complete large bowel obstruction. Fever and signs of vasomotor collapse in association with abdominal rigidity, distention, and rebound tenderness suggest perforation or infarction. Bowel sounds are generally high pitched and active in early intestinal obstruction, but ileus is typical following prolonged obstruction. A careful abdominal, rectal, and pelvic examination must be performed (Lo *et al.*, 1966; Faulconer *et al.*, 1971; Glenn and McSherry, 1971; Ulin *et al.*, 1971; Glass and LeDuc, 1973; Welch and Donaldson, 1974; Sise and Crichlow, 1978).

Diagnostic Evaluation. When clinical features suggest gastrointestinal obstruction, initial studies should include routine complete blood counts, serum electrolytes, amylase, SMA-12, and urine analysis. Chest radiographs may reveal a mediastinal mass, pneumonitis, or proximal esophageal dilatation from obstruction. In acute obstruction, four-way abdominal films characteristically demonstrate air-fluid levels in the dilated bowel loops proximal to the obstructed bowel. A uniform gas pattern is seen with ileus. Free air under the diaphragm or in the mediastinum suggests perforation. Infarction or intraluminal hemorrhage should be suspected when radiographs reveal thickened bowel wall and "thumbprinting." If clinical features suggest intra-abdominal perforation, meglumine diatrizoate contrast should be used to define the site of obstruction or perforation. Upper gastrointestinal barium studies are contraindicated, unless the obstruction is proximal to the gastric antrum. An upper gastrointestinal series should be performed if esophageal or gastric obstruction is suspected. If esophageal perforation is suspected, barium should be used to avoid pulmonary complications from meglumine diatrizoate. Patients with intestinal obstruction should be followed with serial

flat plate and upright abdominal films to assess the response to medical therapy. Proctoscopy, barium enema, and, occasionally, a small bowel enema are required to localize the site of intestinal obstruction. Barium enemas must be performed without bowel preparation or excessive pressure to avoid perforation (Faulconer *et al.*, 1971; Ulin *et al.*, 1971; Sise and Crichlow, 1978). Small bowel enemas are often required to localize the site of partial small bowel obstruction before surgery. Small bowel enemas are frequently helpful in differentiating neoplastic obstruction from benign etiologies. Radiation produces mucosal atrophy, ulceration, and narrowed, nondistensible bowel. Adhesions may be seen from prior surgery or radiotherapy. Contrast may leak through the site of perforation associated with obstruction. Endoscopy and biopsy should be performed if the etiology of esophageal, gastric, or colonic obstruction is not obvious by noninvasive studies (Sise and Crichlow, 1978).

Computerized tomography may detect large retroperitoneal, pelvic, or mesenteric masses extrinsically compressing the bowel. In addition, CT scans are helpful in identifying an intra-abdominal abscess associated with perforation or ascites. Ascites is frequently observed with bowel infarction and perforation. Owing to abdominal distention, paracentesis should be performed under ultrasound guidance to avoid penetration of distended bowel loops. With perforation, the peritoneal fluid is often serosanguineous, foul smelling, with high granulocyte counts, and elevated amylase levels. Colonic bacteria are often cultured when signs of peritonitis are present.

Therapy. The therapeutic approach to gastrointestinal obstruction depends on the site and etiology of the obstruction, and the patient's general physical condition and projected survival. The terminal patient with diffuse abdominal carcinomatosis should be managed supportively with analgesics and decompression, whereas a patient initially presenting with an obstructing colorectal carcinoma might be a candidate for curative resection. Treatment is divided into five broad categories: correction of metabolic abnormalities, supportive medical care, surgery, local radiotherapy, and systemic antitumor therapy. Patients with gastrointestinal obstruction require intravenous fluid and electrolyte replacement to correct volume contraction and metabolic disturbances. Metabolic alkalosis is common when there is significant loss of gastric acid following prolonged vomiting or nasogastric decompression (Harken *et al.,* 1975). Correction of hypokalemia or hypercalcemia improves bowel motility. If gastrointestinal obstruction is prolonged or surgery is anticipated, intravenous hyperalimentation should be initiated to improve nutritional status. Nasogastric or small intestinal decompression must be instituted to decrease vomiting, abdominal distention, and prevent aspiration. Antibiotics are indicated if perforation or infarction is suspected.

Radiotherapy frequently provides effective palliation for esophageal obstruction secondary to primary esophageal tumors or metastases. Dysphagia is relieved in approximately 80% of patients. A significant proportion of patients, however, develop recurrent obstructive symptoms within three to six months (Marcial *et al.,* 1966; Wara *et al.,* 1976; Elkon *et al.,* 1978). Patients with complete esophageal obstruction are rarely candidates for curative resection. Surgery relieves obstruction, however, in over 90% of patients with esophageal carcinoma. If surgical resection is not feasible, the site of obstruction can be bypassed with esophagogastrostomy or colonic interposition (Orringer and Sloan, 1975; Steiger *et al.,* 1978).

Endoesophageal intubation, esophageal dilatation, or cervical esophagostomy and gastrostomy are additional methods utilized in specific patients for temporary palliation. Esophageal intubation should be utilized when additional radiation cannot be delivered, and the patient is not an operative candidate. If the site of obstruction is limited to the upper esophagus, a Mackler or Souttar tube can be blindly pushed through the obstruction. Celestin tubes are more frequently used since most patients have a long area of obstruction in the distal esophagus. The Celestin tube is inserted in the proximal esophagus, positioned in the distal esophagus using a guidewire, and sutured to the stomach. Perioperative mortality is high (10 to 40%), however, because of perforation and mediastinitis (Duvoisin *et al.,* 1967; Thomas, 1974; Cukingham and Carey, 1978). If complete obstruction has not occurred, esophageal dilation alone or in combination with local radiotherapy provides temporary palliation with minimal morbidity (Heit *et al.,* 1978).

Localized antral gastric carcinoma should be treated by radical subtotal gastrectomy. If distant metastases or extensive perigastric lymph node involvement is evident, a less radical subtotal palliative gastrectomy should be performed. When the stomach is diffusely involved with tumor, total gastrectomy should be performed if technically feasible. Gastric outlet obstruction caused by advanced pancreatic or biliary carcinoma can be temporarily palliated with a side-to-side gastrojejunostomy. If extensive omental involvement is anticipated, a posterior retrocolic gastroenterostomy should be performed (Sise and Crichlow, 1978).

Intestinal obstruction from adhesions secondary to prior surgery is initially treated with small intestinal intubation and decompression. Acute radiation enteritis may respond to parenteral steroids and decompression. However, patients presenting with bowel obstruction secondary to neoplastic causes have less than a 25% chance of response to medical decompression (Glass and LeDuc, 1973; Osteen *et al.,* 1980). Patients responding to medical therapy will usually improve within three days of decompression. More than 40% of these patients, however, require surgery for recurrent obstruction at a later date (Osteen, *et al.,* 1980). The majority of patients with small bowel obstruction have multiple tumor implants and rarely respond to intestinal intubation (Glass and LeDuc, 1973; Pathak *et al.,* 1980). Placement of a Miller-Abbott or other long intestinal tube will alleviate the risk of perforation, relieve pain and vomiting, and aid in identifying the site of obstruction. When obstruction is complicated by perforation, strangulation, or bowel infarction, emergency surgical intervention is required. Partial bowel obstruction may respond to several days' decompression. If surgery is postponed with complete obstruction, however, the bowel segment may strangulate or perforate. If a single, easily resectable bowel metastasis is present, resection should be attempted. Most obstructing metastatic lesions, however, are treated with a side-to-side bypass to the transverse colon or ileum. Enterostomy catheters and intra-abdominal drainage tubes should be avoided as they may be associated with tumor growth along their tracts.

Colorectal obstruction requires emergency treatment to avoid perforation and strangulation (Glenn and McSherry, 1971; Ulin *et al.,* 1971; Welch and Donaldson, 1974). A diverting cecostomy or colostomy may be performed under general or local anesthesia using an intercostal block. This temporary procedure is followed in 10 to 14 days by elective bowel resection and reanastomosis. Rectal obstruction is associated with far-advanced rectal carcinomas, which frequently require radiation and diverting colostomy before resection (Welch and Donaldson, 1974; Sise and Crichlow, 1978).

Primary radiotherapy or systemic chemotherapy may relieve obstruction caused by responsive neoplasms (e.g., lymphoma and carcinomas of the breast, ovary, and stomach). Tumor shrinkage and relief of obstruction with either of these modalities, however, may be complicated by an increased risk of infection, perforation, and hemorrhage.

METABOLIC EMERGENCIES

Hypercalcemia

Hypercalcemia is the most common life-threatening metabolic emergency encountered by the medical oncologist. Cancer patients usually develop hypercalcemia when the rate of calcium mobilization from bone exceeds the renal threshold for calcium excretion. The incidence of hypercalcemia in the general population ranges from 0.5 to 3.6% in hospitalized patients and from 0.1 to 0.6% among outpatients. Hyperparathyroidism is the most common etiology for hypercalcemia in the outpatient population, whereas cancer is the leading cause of hypercalcemia among inpatients (Gordon et al., 1966; McLellan et al., 1968; Besarb and Caro, 1978; Mezzaferri et al., 1978; Frisken et al., 1981). Although 40 to 50% of hypercalcemic patients have an underlying malignancy, hypercalcemia is rarely a presenting sign of neoplastic disease (Mazzaferri et al., 1978; Frisken et al., 1981).

The most common neoplasms associated with hypercalcemia are carcinoma of the breast and lung, followed by hypernephroma, multiple myeloma, and carcinoma of the head and neck, esophagus, and thyroid (Jessiman et al., 1963; Mannheimer, 1965; Mazzaferri et al., 1978; Murray et al., 1978; Frisken et al., 1981). During the natural history of their disease, hypercalcemia occurs in 33% of patients with myeloma, and in 4 to 6% of patients with solid tumors (Frisken et al., 1981). More than 75% of patients with hypercalcemia of malignancy have metastatic disease and over 86% have bone metastases (Myers, 1973; Bockman, 1980). Forty to fifty percent of women with bone metastases secondary to breast carcinoma develop hypercalcemia, which is often aggravated by hormonal therapy (Myers, 1973; Murray et al., 1978). Although the majority of patients have osseous metastases, the extent of bony metastatic disease does not correlate with the level of hypercalcemia (Murray et al., 1978; Sherwood, 1980). Despite the high prevalence of bone marrow and bone involvement in advanced lymphoma and leukemia, hypercalcemia is rarely reported (Myers, 1973; Bockman, 1980; Skrabanek et al., 1980). In vitro studies suggest that myeloma patients develop hypercalcemia secondary to the osteolytic effects of osteoclast activating factor, rather than direct neoplastic bone resorption (Mundy et al., 1974b; Sherwood, 1980).

Fifteen to twenty percent of solid tumors associated with hypercalcemia have no evidence of osseous spread. Humoral substances, including parathyroid hormone or osteolytic prostaglandins, may be secreted by tumor cells. Ectopic hormone production occurs most often with epidermoid or large cell anaplastic lung cancer and hypernephroma (Murray et al., 1978).

Pathophysiology. Increased bone resorption is the primary etiology of hypercalcemia associated with malignancy. Osteoclast activity and proliferation may be stimulated directly by osseous metastases or indirectly by ectopic humoral substances (Besarb and Caro, 1978; Mundy, 1978). Bone metastases are frequently surrounded by a zone of osteoclasts. It is unclear whether increased calcium mobilization is secondary to direct neoplastic bony destruction or release of osteolytic substances by the tumor (Tashjian et al., 1972; Powell et al., 1973; Mundy et al., 1974a,b; Mundy and Raisz, 1977; Besarb and Caro, 1978). Selected neoplastic cell lines are capable of direct bone resorption without increased osteoclast activity. Most human tumor cell lines are incapable of osteolysis, however, without stimulation of osteoclast proliferation or activity (Haddad et al., 1970; Murray et al., 1978).

Ectopic secretion of parathyroid hormone or parathyrotropic substances produces a clinical syndrome indistinguishable from hyperparathyroidism. Laboratory studies demonstrate increased levels of immunoreactive PTH in association with hypercalcemia, hypophosphatemia, increased urinary cAMP excretion, and elevations in bone alkaline phosphatase (Sherwood, 1980). Hypercalcemia from ectopic parathyroid hormone secretion is reported most frequently with hypernephromas, hepatomas, pheochromocytomas, ovarian tumors, and squamous cell carcinoma of the lung, head and neck, or esophagus (Besarb and Caro, 1978; Murray et al., 1978; Skrabanek et al., 1980). In many patients appropriate data are not available to support excessive neoplastic PTH production (Murray et al., 1978; Skrabanek et al., 1980).

Recent evidence suggests that ectopic PTH may be a less important cause of hypercalcemia than previously reported. Hypercalcemia and concurrent PTH elevation do not necessarily imply that ectopic hormone secretion is the major etiology of hypercalcemia. Using four different immunoassays, there was no clear correlation between increased serum calcium and parathormone levels in hypercalcemic cancer patients (Benson et al., 1974; Raisz et al., 1979; Bockman, 1980). Other investigators have reported immunochemical differences in parathyroid hormone among patients with neoplasms and those with primary hyperparathyroidism (Benson et al., 1974; Buckle, 1974; Murray et al., 1978). Since both high and low molecular weight PTH-like substances have been identified in oncology patients, osteolysis and resultant hypercalcemia could be caused by excessive release of pro-PTH or C-terminal fragments rather than intact hormone (Murray et al., 1978). Primary hyperparathyroidism is rarely excluded by finding normal or atrophic parathyroid glands at surgery or autopsy, or by selective venous catheterization studies (Besarb and Caro, 1978; Murray et al., 1978; Skrabanek et al., 1980). Skrabanek reported that surgical exploration of the neck revealed parathyroid adenomas or hyperplasia in 34 of 170 cancer patients with a preoperative diagnosis of ectopic PTH secretion (Skrabanek et al., 1980). In many patients ectopic PTH secretion is not well established by either documented neoplastic arteriovenous PTH differences or temporal reductions in PTH and calcium with tumor regression. Extractable PTH is rarely demonstrated in malignant tissue. In general, well-documented cases of ectopic PTH secretion account for a small fraction of tumor-induced hypercalcemia.

Less than 50% of hypercalcemic cancer patients without bone metastases have elevated immunoactive PTH levels. In the animal model, early studies inferred that prostaglandins might be the primary osteolytic factor in tumor-induced hypercalcemia (Tashjian et al.,

1974; Voelkel et al., 1975). Osteolytic prostaglandins, such as PGE_2 and 15-keto-13,14-dihydro-PGE_2, have been extracted from tumor tissue in vitro (Tashjian et al., 1974; Murray et al., 1978). Elevated levels of serum and urinary prostaglandins have been measured in hypercalcemic patients with cancer of the lung, kidney, and ovary (Brereton et al., 1974; Tashjian et al., 1974; Seyberth et al., 1975; Josse et al., 1981). Inhibitors of prostaglandin synthesis, including aspirin, indomethacin, and glucocorticoids, are occasionally successful in controlling hypercalcemia, but clinical results are generally less impressive than in vitro data (Tashjian et al., 1974; Seyberth et al., 1975; Tashjian, 1975; Murray et al., 1978). Although animal models and in vitro studies suggest that excessive secretion of osteolytic prostaglandins by tumor cells might produce hypercalcemia, few human data support a major role for ectopic prostaglandins in tumor-induced hypercalcemia (Tashjian et al., 1972; Josse et al., 1981).

In hematologic malignancies bone resorption is mediated by osteoclast activating factor (OAF), a potent osteolytic peptide. In tissue culture, selected hematologic malignancies, including multiple myeloma, lymphosarcoma cell leukemia, and Burkitt's lymphoma, appear to elaborate OAF (Mundy et al., 1974a,b; Besarb and Caro, 1978; Murray et al., 1978; Bockman, 1980). OAF stimulates osteoclast proliferation, bone resorption, and osteoclast release of lyzosomal enzymes and collagenase (Eilon and Raisz, 1978). Despite in vitro osteolytic activity, elevated levels of OAF do not always correlate with hypercalcemia.

Other theoretical mechanisms for tumor-induced hypercalcemia have been reported. Several groups have reported small series of hypercalcemic patients with increased urinary 3,5-cyclic monophosphate levels without elevations in serum PTH or prostaglandin levels. However, no humoral mediator responsible for the associated hypercalcemia has been identified (Seyberth et al., 1976; Murray et al., 1978; Bockman, 1980; Stewart et al., 1980). Increased concentrations of osteolytic vitamin D-like phytosterols have been identified in breast cancers from hypercalcemic women, but serum phytosterols also may be increased in normal healthy women or normocalcemic women with breast cancer (Gordon et al., 1966; Haddad et al., 1970; Bockman, 1980).

Clinical Presentation and Diagnostic Evaluation. Hypercalcemia is rarely a presenting sign of malignancy. Gastrointestinal, renal, and neurologic abnormalities are the earliest symptoms of hypercalcemia in the cancer patient. The severity of symptoms depends on the degree of hypercalcemia, the rate at which hypercalcemia develops, the general physical condition of the patient, and other associated metabolic disorders (Lee et al., 1978).

The earliest symptoms include nonspecific complaints of fatigue, anorexia, nausea, polyuria, polydipsia, and constipation, which are followed by intractable vomiting and obstipation as the calcium level rises. Mild hypercalcemia is frequently associated with vague neurologic findings, including muscle weakness, lethargy, apathy, and hyporeflexia. Polyuria, polydipsia, and nocturia are early signs of hypercalcemic renal tubular dysfunction, which mimics nephrogenic diabetes insipidus. Renal tubular acidosis, glycosuria, aminoaciduria, and hyperphosphaturia suggest irreversible tubular damage from prolonged hypercalcuria (Epstein, 1968; Mazzaferri et al., 1978). Polyuria, vomiting, and anorexia result in profound volume depletion. With hypovolemia, glomerular filtration rate decreases, calcium increases, and ultimately renal failure and acidosis compound the metabolic derangements. Severe hypercalcemia produces alterations in mental status, psychotic behavior, seizures, stupor, coma, and ultimately death.

Acute rises in calcium may cause sudden death from cardiac arrhythmias, ventricular systole, or bradycardia (Voss and Drake, 1967; Shiner et al., 1969; Besarb and Caro, 1978). Without treatment, hypercalcemic cancer patients rarely live long enough to develop the signs of chronic hypercalcemia, which are frequently associated with primary hyperparathyroidism. Soft tissue and vascular calcification, pruritus, renal stones, peptic ulcer disease, and band keratopathy are rarely reported complications of hypercalcemia of malignancy (Besarb and Caro, 1978).

Laboratory studies should include serial serum calcium determinations, phosphate, alkaline phosphatase, electrolytes, BUN, and creatinine. Immunoreactive PTH levels may be helpful when hypophosphatemia suggests ectopic secretion. Ionized calcium levels are occasionally useful, since the clinical manifestations of hypercalcemia correlate with increased ionized, rather than protein-bound, calcium. Patients with hyperproteinemia associated with myeloma may have elevated serum calciums caused by abnormal paraprotein

binding without elevation in ionized calcium. Patients with hypoalbuminemia may have mild symptoms of hypercalcemia with normal calcium serum levels. Significant hypercalcemia is often associated with electrocardiographic abnormalities including shortening of the QT interval, widening of the T wave, bradycardia, PR prolongation, and various arrhythmias (Voss and Drake, 1967).

Therapy. The therapeutic approach depends on the etiology of hypercalcemia, severity of associated clinical signs, and probability of response to effective antitumor therapy. Mild hypercalcemia is often corrected with intravenous hydration. Although hypercalcemia typically improves with effective antineoplastic therapy (Connors and Howard, 1956; Plimpton and Gellhorn, 1956), most hypercalcemic cancer patients require additional therapy directed at decreasing the serum calcium level. Therapeutic goals must be redirected to alter the metabolic balance by directly decreasing calcium resorption from bone, increasing urinary excretion, or decreasing calcium intake. Immobilization leading to increased osteolysis must be avoided. Constipation should be corrected with enemas, laxatives, and, if necessary, disimpaction. Medications that may potentiate hypercalcemia (e.g., thiazide diuretics or vitamins A and D) should be discontinued immediately. When mild hypercalcemia is precipitated by hormonal therapy for metastatic breast cancer, the hormone frequently can be continued without undue risk. Until the mild hypercalcemia resolves, patients should be treated with hydration, steroids, and, if necessary, mithramycin. When severe, life-threatening hypercalcemia occurs after hormonal therapy for breast cancer, the hormone should be discontinued immediately.

Intravascular volume must be increased to promote urinary calcium excretion (Segaloff, 1981). Aggressive saline hydration increases urinary sodium, hence, calcium excretion, as the urinary clearance rates for calcium parallel sodium excretion (Murray et al., 1978; Segaloff, 1981). Patients with mild hypercalcemia respond to intravenous hydration with either normal saline or 5% dextrose, 0.45% normal saline. Severe hypercalcemia should be treated with aggressive hydration (e.g., 250 to 300 mL/hr) and intravenous furosemide to further decrease renal tubular reabsorption of both sodium and calcium (Bockman, 1980; Segaloff, 1981). If furosemide is used to potentiate urinary calcium excretion, the rate of hydration must be increased accordingly to prevent dehydration. In life-threatening situations, more aggressive hydration in combination with furosemide, 80 to 100 mg every two hours, will temporarily decrease calcium levels to an acceptable range (Suki et al., 1970).

Glucocorticoids are effective in controlling hypercalcemia associated with hematologic cancers, including multiple myeloma, lymphoma, and leukemia. Steroids are also effective in hypercalcemic patients with breast cancer, especially when hypercalcemia follows hormonal therapy. However, glucocorticoids are rarely beneficial in other solid tumors associated with hypercalcemia (Jessiman et al., 1963; Lazor and Rosenberg, 1964; Mannheimer, 1965; Muggia and Heinemann, 1970). Steroids have numerous metabolic effects, which may explain their mechanism of action. Raisz reported that corticosteroids block bone resorption secondary to osteoclast activating factor (Raisz et al., 1979). In pharmacologic doses, steroids may also lower serum calcium by increasing urinary calcium excretion, decreasing intestinal absorption, and after chronic administration, producing negative calcium balance in bone (Laake, 1960; Kimberg et al., 1971; Jowsey and Balasubramaniam, 1972). Inhibition of prostaglandin synthesis and antitumor effects in steroid-sensitive tumors may also contribute to their hypocalcemic effects (Lazor and Rosenberg, 1964; Bockman, 1980). High doses of corticosteroids, prednisone, 40 to 100 mg, or cortisol, 100 to 300 mg daily, are generally required for several days before serum calcium falls (Bockman, 1980; Segaloff, 1981).

Mithramycin inhibits DNA-directed RNA synthesis and bone resorption by decreasing the number and activity of osteoclasts. These hypocalcemic effects occur even without bone metastases (Perlia et al., 1970; Elias and Evans, 1972). Although mithramycin is frequently administered over four hours, it is our current practice to administer this agent as an intravenous bolus through a freshly inserted IV line. Extravasation of mithramycin must be avoided, as this would produce severe local tissue necrosis. Mithramycin (15 to 25 μg/kg) begins to correct hypercalcemia within 6 to 48 hours. Hypocalcemic effects generally last for three to seven days. Hypercalcemic patients often require one or two injections per week, unless other effective therapy is initiated. If no response occurs within the first 48 hours, a second dose should be administered (Perlia et al., 1970; Elias and Evans, 1972; Bockman, 1980; Segaloff, 1981). Side effects of mithramycin in the intermittent, low-dose schedule employed for hypercalcemia are unusual. They include dose-related thrombocytopenia, coagulopathy, postural hypotension, hepatocellular dysfunction, and renal dysfunction with proteinuria (Kennedy, 1970; Perlia et al., 1970; Elias and Evans, 1972).

Inhibitors of prostaglandin synthesis are occasionally effective in managing hypercalcemia associated with high serum prostaglandin levels. Initial studies demonstrated beneficial effects in a small group of hypercalcemia cancer patients with increased immunoactive prostaglandin levels. However, subsequent trials using either indomethacin, 25 mg every six hours, or acetylsalicylic acid have failed to substantiate the initial therapeutic claims (Tashjian et al., 1974; Robertson et al., 1976; Besarb and Caro, 1978; Bockman, 1980).

Calcitonin is a potent hypocalcemic hormone which is secreted by the parafollicular cells in the thyroid gland. By inhibiting bone resorption, calcitonin produces a prompt fall in serum calcium (ranging from 1 to 4 mg/dL) within hours of administration (Krane et al., 1973; Vaughn and Vaitkevigius, 1974; Binstock and Mundy, 1980). Hypercalcemic patients with active bone resorption or hematologic cancer have the most impressive responses, but beneficial results have occurred in most solid tumors as well (Binstock and Mundy, 1980). Salmon calcitonin is given in daily doses [3 to 6 Medical Research Council (MRC) units/kg] intravenously or twice daily by intramuscular or subcutaneous injections (100 to 400 MRC) (Habener et al., 1972; Segaloff, 1981). However, the beneficial effects of calcitonin are short-lived, unless glucocorticoid therapy is given with calcitonin. Clinical studies have shown that with concurrent prednisone, the hypocalcemic effects of calcitonin may be maintained for significantly longer periods. When hypercalcemia recurs, temporary discontinuation and subsequent reinstitution of calcitonin will occasionally produce a second response within 48 hours.

Diphosphonates, which suppress both calcium-phosphate deposition and bone resorption, have effectively controlled hypercalcemia secondary to Paget's disease. Preliminary clinical trials using dichloromethylene diphosphonate (2.5 to 5.0 mg/kg per day for up to seven days) have shown encouraging results, primarily in patients with breast cancer and myeloma (Chapuy et al., 1980; Jacobs et al.,

1981). Jacobs reported that mean serum calcium fell by 4 mg/dL, while urinary calcium and hydroxyproline excretion decreased by 50 to 60% (Jacobs *et al.,* 1981).

Intravenous phosphate should only be given to control life-threatening hypercalcemia that is refractory to the more conventional measures described above. Although intravenous phosphate produces a rapid fall in serum calcium, it is rarely used owing to associated side effects, including hypotension, hypocalcemia, renal failure, and death (Goldsmith and Ingbar, 1966; Breuer and LeBauer, 1967; Dudley and Blackburn, 1970). Serum calcium decreases within minutes following a phosphate infusion, but the maximal hypocalcemic effect is typically delayed for up to five days. A 50-mmol infusion of mono- or dibasic anhydrous KPO_4 is administered over six to eight hours and is not repeated more frequently than every 24 hours (Goldsmith and Ingbar, 1967). Although oral phosphates (1 to 3 g sodium acid phosphate) are an effective, relatively safe method of controlling mild hypercalcemia, they are rarely used today owing to associated nausea and diarrhea (Bockman, 1980).

Life-threatening hypercalcemia can also be managed with dialysis if other measures fail. Most hypercalcemic cancer patients are effectively managed with hydration, mobilization, effective antitumor therapy, and gradually tapering doses of either mithramycin, calcitonin, or corticosteroids. If effective systemic antineoplastic therapy is not available, a maintenance program must be initiated to keep the serum calcium near normal levels. Serum calcium and phosphate should be monitored two times per week. Adequate hydration and ambulation should be encouraged. If corticosteroids are used, the dose should be gradually tapered to the lowest effective therapeutic dose. If mithramycin is utilized chronically, the interval between injections is gradually lengthened. The same principle applies when calcitonin is used. The interval between calcitonin injections may be increased from 12 to 24 hours. If normal calcium levels are then maintained, the daily calcitonin dosage can then be reduced by one-half. Further dose reductions and ultimate discontinuation of hypocalcemic therapy depend on achieving a significant antitumor resonse (Segaloff, 1981).

Uric Acid Nephropathy

Acute nephropathy occurs when increased uric acid production results in hyperuricemia and deposition of uric acid crystals in the urinary tract. Although uric acid nephropathy may occur spontaneously, it is most frequently reported as a complication following cytotoxic chemotherapy, radiotherapy, or prednisone in hematologic cancer (Kjellstrand *et al.,* 1974; Klinenberg *et al.,* 1975; Garnick and Mayer, 1978). It is also a common feature of the tumor lysis syndrome, most often associated with Burkitt's lymphoma. Spontaneous hyperuricemic nephropathy is more frequent among patients with lymphoma than leukemia (Kjellstrand *et al.,* 1974). Hyperuricemia is most commonly associated with cancers that have increased rates of cell turnover. The high mitotic activity and marked cytoreduction following effective antitumor therapy increase purine metabolism and potentiate hyperuricemia (Kjellstrand *et al.,* 1974). Previously untreated leukemics have increased urate excretion compared to normal controls. The frequency and degree of hyperuricemia appear to correlate better with the cytologic type of leukemia, than with the degree of leukocytosis. For example, urate excretion is higher in "aleukemic" acute myelocytic leukemia than in chronic lymphocytic leukemia with elevated peripheral lymphocyte counts (Sandberg *et al.,* 1956; Garnick and Mayer, 1978).

Prophylactic treatment with allopurinol, intravenous hydration, and alkalinization of urine has decreased the incidence, and perhaps the severity of acute hyperuricemic nephropathy. Mortality rates in older series ranged from 47 to 100%, but now with more aggressive medical therapy and hemodialysis, renal function returns to baseline within a few days after the serum uric acid falls below 10 to 20 mg/dL (Kjellstrand *et al.,* 1974).

Hyperuricemia may also contribute to renal failure in chronic myeloproliferative syndromes, multiple myeloma, and squamous cell carcinomas of the head and neck, but uric acid nephropathy has rarely been reported with solid tumors (Kjellstrand *et al.,* 1974; Crittenden and Ackerman, 1977; Boss and Seegmiller, 1979).

Pathophysiology. Uric acid is filtered by the glomeruli and subsequently reabsorbed and secreted in the renal tubules. The highest concentration of uric acid occurs in the distal tubules and collecting ducts where urine acidification occurs, thus potentiating precipitation. Early investigators postulated that most cases of acute hyperuricemic nephropathy occurred secondary to uric acid crystals blocking the distal tubules and collecting ducts. However, with appropriate treatment there is rapid improvement in renal function, which would not be seen with irreversible glomerular or tubular damage (Rieselbach et al., 1964; Kjellstrand et al., 1974; Robinson and Yarger, 1977). This hypothesis is further supported by both human renal biopsy and autopsy studies (Kanwar and Manaligod, 1975; Klinenberg et al., 1975; Spencer et al., 1976; Crittenden and Ackerman, 1977). On histologic section, loosely organized urate crystal deposits are seen in the collecting ducts and distal tubules. In the animal model, similar histologic changes are seen in association with increased intraluminal hydrostatic pressure proximal to the site of tubular obstruction.

In early reports hyperuricemic cancer patients often presented with classic symptoms of ureteral stones. Diagnostic studies demonstrated ureteral obstruction secondary to uric acid deposits in 30 to 100% of cases. However, in more recent series less than 10% of patients had intraureteral uric acid deposits. Uric acid calculi appear to be more common in patients with chronic moderate hyperuricemia, particularly with chronic myeloproliferative syndromes (e.g., polycythemia) (Rieselbach et al., 1964; Gutman and Yu, 1968, 1972; Kjellstrand et al., 1974; Spencer et al., 1976; Robinson and Yarger, 1977). Chronic hyperuricemia may also cause vascular inflammation and nephrosclerosis, but these features are probably of minor importance in acute uric acid nephropathy (Kanwar and Manaligod, 1975; Garnick and Mayer, 1978).

Clinical Presentation and Diagnostic Evaluation. Owing to the relatively low incidence of ureteral obstruction, flank pain and gross hematuria are rarely observed (Kjellstrand et al., 1974). Patients generally present with nausea, vomiting, lethargy, oliguria, and other signs of uremia (Kjellstrand et al., 1974; Klinenberg et al., 1975; Boss and Seegmiller, 1979).

It is important to recognize acute hyperuricemic renal failure before anuria occurs. With early appropriate treatment, there is an excellent chance of reversing renal dysfunction (Kjellstrand et al., 1974; Robinson and Yarger, 1977; Kelton et al., 1978). Unless there is severe hyperuricemia, it is often difficult to differentiate acute hyperuricemic nephropathy from other causes of acute renal failure with secondary hyperuricemia. In recent series the mean serum uric acid level at presentation was 20.1 mg/dl (ranging from 9.2 to 92 mg/dl) (Kjellstrand et al., 1974; Warren et al., 1975; Kelton et al., 1978).

If clinical signs suggest extrarenal obstruction, appropriate studies described in the section on obstructive uropathy should be performed to exclude ureteral blockage (Kjellstrand et al., 1974). Intravenous contrast should be avoided, since hyperuricemia potentiates dye-induced nephrotoxicity. Serum electrolytes, blood urea nitrogen, creatinine, calcium, phosphorus, and uric acid must be followed closely. Hyperphosphatemia and hypocalcemia may occur out of proportion to the degree of uremia, especially with rapid tumor lysis (Kjellstrand et al., 1974). Hyperuricemic nephropathy cannot be differentiated from other causes of acute renal failure by serum creatinine, BUN, or uric acid ratios (Warren et al., 1975; Kelton et al., 1978).

Urine analysis is helpful if uric acid crystals are seen, but a normal urine analysis does not exclude the diagnosis, since crystalluria and hematuria may occur only in the acute phase (Kjellstrand et al., 1974; Klinenberg et al., 1975). A urine sample should be analyzed for uric acid and creatinine, since Kelton has observed that a urinary uric acid to creatinine ratio greater than one is relatively specific for hyperuricemic nephropathy (Kelton et al., 1978).

Therapy. Prevention of hyperuricemic nephropathy is the most appropriate therapy. Patients at high risk for hyperuricemic renal failure should be treated with allopurinol, vigorous hydration, and urine alkalinization for at least 48 hours prior to cytotoxic therapy. Drugs that block tubular reabsorption of uric acid, including aspirin, radiographic contrast, probenecid, and thiazide diuretics should be avoided (Klinenberg et al., 1975). Patients at risk for uric acid nephropathy should have antineoplastic therapy delayed, if possible, until serum uric acid is normalized, urine pH is maintained above 7, and intravenous hydration is initiated to ensure a urine volume of ≥ 3 liters per day (Holland and Holland, 1968; Kjellstrand et al., 1974; Robinson and Yarger, 1977; Garnick and Mayer, 1978; Boss and Seegmiller, 1979).

Urinary alkalinization is accomplished with either daily acetazolamide, 1 g in divided doses, or intravenous sodium bicarbonate, 100 mEq/m² daily. Uric acid solubility decreases markedly when urine pH falls below 6, while solubility is maximal with a pH > 7.5. Thus, attempts to increase urinary pH above 7.5 are not necessary and may complicate the clinical situation by producing a significant metabolic alkalosis (Kjellstrand et al., 1974; Klinenberg *et al.*, 1975; Robinson and Yarger, 1977; Garnick and Mayer, 1978; Boss and Seegmiller, 1979). Potassium and magnesium levels must be followed closely and replacement therapy initiated to avoid metabolic complications. Allopurinol, in doses up to 800 mg per day, acts primarily by decreasing uric acid production by competitively inhibiting xanthine oxidase (Klinenberg *et al.*, 1975; Robinson and Yarger, 1977; Garnick and Mayer, 1978; Boss and Seegmiller, 1979). Theoretically, high xanthine levels may produce xanthine stones, but his has not been reported in this clinical setting (Band *et al.*, 1973; Klinenberg *et al.*, 1975). Allopurinol also decreases uric acid production by decreasing 4-phosphoribosyl-pyrophosphate aminotransferase, which results in decreased purine synthesis (Rastegar and Thier, 1972). Precipitation of acute gouty arthropathy is rare, and prophylactic colchicine is not necessary when allopurinol is administered.

This prophylactic treatment plan may be adequate for mild nonoliguric hyperuricemic nephropathy. If oliguria or anuria occurs, ureteral obstruction should be excluded by renal ultrasound or antegrade or retrograde pyelography, since nephrotoxic contrast should be avoided. Once hydronephrosis is excluded, mannitol or high-dose intravenous furosemide should be administered in an attempt to restore urine flow. A urethral catheter should be inserted to accurately measure hourly urine output. If a prompt diuresis does not occur within a few hours, emergency hemodialysis is indicated (Kjellstrand *et al.*, 1974).

If dialysis is required, a hollow fiber kidney apparatus will correct hyperuricemia more quickly than either peritoneal or coil hemodialysis (Steinberg *et al.*, 1975; Garnick and Mayer, 1978). Hemodialysis appears to improve morbidity and mortality. All patients in Kjellstrand's series had rapid return of renal function and prompt diuresis when the serum uric acid level fell below 10 to 20 mg/dL. Uric acid levels fall by 50% following six hours of hemodialysis. The majority of patients require approximately six days (range, 4 to 11 days) of dialysis before hyperuricemia resolves and renal function returns to normal (Kjellstrand *et al.*, 1974).

Most patients who require hemodialysis have elevated calcium-phosphate products above 70. To prevent calcium-phosphate precipitation, which theoretically increases nephrotoxicity, a low calcium dialysate should be used. Aluminum hydroxide may also be beneficial to decrease gastrointestinal phosphate absorption (Kjellstrand *et al.*, 1974). If hemodialysis is contraindicated, uric acid clearance can be improved by adding albumin to the peritoneal dialysis fluid to increase urate protein binding and removal (Klinenberg *et al.*, 1975). Alkalinizing the dialysate to neutral pH with sodium bicarbonate also enhances uric acid clearance (Knochel and Mason, 1966). With aggressive modern therapy, acute hyperuricemic nephropathy is associated with extremely low morbidity and mortality (Kjellstrand *et al.*, 1974; Steinberg *et al.*, 1975).

Hyponatremia

When serum sodium falls abruptly or reaches levels below 115 mg/dL, brain edema and increased intracranial pressure produce neurologic dysfunction. Alteration in mental status, seizures, coma, and ultimately death result unless emergency treatment is initiated (Segaloff, 1981).

The common causes of hyponatremia in the cancer patient are listed in Table 40–21. The syndrome of inappropriate antidiuretic hormone (SIADH) secretion occurs in 1 to 2% of

Table 40–21. Etiology of Hyponatremia in the Cancer Patient

A. Chronic hyponatremia
  1. Syndrome of inappropriate ADH secretion
  2. Reset osmostat
  3. Glucocorticoid deficiency
    a. Anterior hypopituitarism
    b. Adrenal insufficiency
    c. Abrupt withdrawal of glucocorticoid drug therapy
  4. Chronic renal disease
B. Acute water intoxication
  1. Acute hypovolemia (*e.g.*, hemorrhage)
  2. During the early postoperative period
C. Extrarenal sodium loss
  1. Gastrointestinal losses
    a. Vomiting
    b. Diarrhea
  2. Third-space effects
    a. Ascites
    b. Ileus
D. Renal losses
  1. Diuretics
  2. Adrenal insufficiency with mineralocorticoid deficiency
  3. Sodium-renal diseases
E. Pseudohyponatremia
  1. Hyperproteinemia (*e.g.*, paraproteins)
  2. Hyperlipidemia (*e.g.*, intravenous hyperalimentation)
F. Water redistribution
  1. Mannitol infusions
  2. Hyperglycemia

patients with cancer (Azzopardi *et al.,* 1970). Hyponatremia secondary to excessive ADH secretion is usually asymptomatic at presentation unless the serum sodium concentration falls rapidly. Despite hypotonic plasma, the urine is inappropriately concentrated with high sodium concentrations. Renal, thyroid, and adrenal function must be normal to confirm the diagnosis of SIADH (DeFronzo and Thier, 1980; Goldberg, 1981; Trump, 1981). Although SIADH is a relatively common paraneoplastic syndrome, ectopic antidiuretic hormone secretion has only been reported with bronchogenic carcinoma (Moses *et al.,* 1976; Comis *et al.,* 1980). Small cell carcinoma of the lung is the most common malignancy associated with ectopic ADH secretion (Hantman *et al.,* 1973; North *et al.,* 1979; Comis *et al.,* 1980; Kelly and Morton 1980). Over 50% of patients with small cell lung cancer have subclinical signs of SIADH following a water-load, but only 8 to 10% have clinically significant hyponatremia caused by SIADH (Hantman *et al.,* 1973). SIADH has also been reported with cancer of the prostate, adrenal cortex, esophagus, pancreas, colon, head and neck, carcinoid, thymoma, lymphoma, and mesothelioma (Bartter and Schwartz, 1967; Cassileth and Trotman, 1975; Perks *et al.,* 1979; Trump *et al.,* 1980). SIADH is more frequently seen secondary to pulmonary or CNS metastases or medications, including morphine, vincristine, and cyclophosphamide (DeFronzo and Thier, 1980; Goldberg, 1981).

Hyponatremia with chronic debilitating diseases, such as cancer, may also be secondary to a "reset osmostat." Hyponatremia is usually mild, not progressive, and resolves with effective antitumor therapy. Adrenal insufficiency, secondary to abrupt withdrawal of glucocorticoids or metastases to the pituitary or adrenal glands, is often complicated by mild hyponatremia caused by volume contraction and mineralocorticoid deficiency (Agus and Goldberg, 1971; DeFronzo and Thier, 1980; Goldberg, 1981). Dilutional hyponatremia may be seen in severe hepatic disease, congestive heart failure, or acute renal failure complicating advanced neoplastic disease (DeFronzo and Thier, 1980; Goldberg, 1981). Oncology patients frequently develop hyponatremia secondary to volume contraction from vomiting, diarrhea, ascites, pancreatitis, diuretics, or corticosteroid insufficiency (Goldberg, 1981).

Factitious or pseudohyponatremia occurs with hyperlipidemia, hyperproteinemia, and mannitol infusions used with high-dose platinum (Aviram *et al.,* 1967; Murray *et al.,* 1975; DeFronzo and Thier, 1980).

Pathophysiology. SIADH secretion produces excessive water reabsorption in the collecting ducts. Increased water reabsorption enhances distal sodium delivery by producing a mild increase in intravascular volume. Volume expansion increases renal perfusion, decreases proximal tubular reabsorption of sodium, and decreases aldosterone effect (DeFronzo and Thier, 1980). ADH is secreted either by the posterior pituitary or by malignant cells in patients with small cell lung carcinoma (Kelly and Morton, 1980). SIADH has been associated with a variety of benign pulmonary and central nervous system disorders which may occur in the setting of malignancy (Moses *et al.,* 1976). The differential diagnosis of SIADH is summarized in Table 40–22.

Volume-overloaded patients with congestive heart failure, liver failure, or acute renal failure develop dilutional hyponatremia. Despite increased total body sodium and water content, the "effective" circulating plasma volume is reduced. Decreased renal perfusion produces greater back diffusion of water in the collecting duct and increased ADH secretion, resulting in dilutional hyponatremia (DeFronzo and Thier, 1980).

Total body salt and water content is decreased in volume contraction. Renal perfu-

---

Table 40–22. Differential Diagnosis of the Syndrome of Inappropriate ADH Secretion

A. SIADH in malignancy
   1. Ectopic production (*e.g.,* small cell anaplastic lung cancer)
   2. Excessive ADH release
B. Pulmonary diseases
   1. Infection (*e.g.,* pneumonia, lung abscess)
   2. Tumor (not associated with ectopic production)
C. CNS disorders
   1. Metastases
   2. Seizures
   3. Infection (*e.g.,* meningitis, encephalitis, abscess)
   4. Intracranial hemorrhage (*e.g.,* subdural or subarachnoid hemorrhage)
D. Addison's disease
E. Hypothyroidism
F. Drugs (*e.g.,* opiates, cyclophosphamide, vincristine, barbiturates, thiazides, β-adrenergic agonists, chlorpropamide)
G. Exogenous administration
H. Delirium tremens
 I. Porphyria

Derived from DeFronzo and Thier, 1980; Goldberg, 1981.

sion decreases and ADH secretion is stimulated. If there is an associated renal loss of sodium secondary to diuretics, interstitial disease, or mineralocortocoid deficiency, more profound hyponatremia results.

Pseudohyponatremia occurs when large concentrations of macromolecules (*e.g.,* lipids or paraproteins) are present in plasma. Plasma sodium concentration is measured as the sodium concentration per unit of plasma. If the plasma contains macromolecules, the percentage of water in plasma is decreased. A low sodium concentration is reported by the laboratory, despite a normal sodium concentration in water (DeFronzo and Thier, 1980). If the serum concentration of an impermeable solute (*e.g.,* mannitol or glucose) increases, an osmotic gradient is produced, allowing water to move from the intra- to extracellular space (Aviram *et al.,* 1967; Katz, 1973; Feig and McCurdy, 1977).

Clinical Presentation. Patients with mild hyponatremia initially present with nonspecific symptoms, including anorexia, nausea, vomiting, muscle cramps, and bloating. Neurologic symptoms may be subtle. Fatigue, headache, decreased memory, irritability, and somnolence are frequently reported. A rapid decrease in serum sodium or a value below 115 mg/dL results in alterations in mental status ranging from lethargy and confusion to coma, seizures, and psychotic behavior (Trump *et al.,* 1980; Goldberg, 1981). Physical examination is typically unrevealing unless hyponatremia is severe or sudden in onset. Alterations in mental status, pathologic reflexes, papilledema, and, rarely, focal neurologic signs may be elicited (Goldberg, 1981; Trump, 1981).

Diagnostic Evaluation. Prior to initiating therapy, the etiology of hyponatremia must be defined. Serum protein electrophoresis, lipids, and glucose levels are determined in patients with suspected pseudohyponatremia secondary to hyperproteinemia, hyperlipidemia, or hyperglycemia. Medications must be carefully reviewed. Chemotherapeutic agents (*e.g.,* vincristine or cyclophosphamide), mannitol, morphine, diuretics, and steroid withdrawal may contribute to hyponatremia. The diagnostic workup is simplified by accurately assessing the patient's volume status as shown in Table 40–23. The history, physical examination, and review of fluid intake and output aid in determining whether the patient is hyper-, hypo-, or euvolemic. Serum and urine electrolytes and osmolality, in addition to renal function, are measured. Patients with SIADH have an inappropriately concentrated urine for the level of hyponatremia. Urine osmolality is usually greater than plasma osmolality, but is never maximally diluted (less than 100 mosm). Despite a concentrated urine, the blood urea nitrogen is usually low owing to mild volume expansion. Serum uric acid and phosphate levels are typically depressed secondary to decreased proximal tubular reabsorption (DeFronzo *et al.,* 1976; DeFronzo and Thier, 1980; Goldberg, 1981).

If laboratory studies suggest SIADH, thyroid and adrenal dysfunction must be excluded, as severe hypothyroidism or corticosteroid deficiency produces similar abnormalities. Chest x-rays and CT scans should be obtained if there are associated pulmonary or neurologic symptoms because the most effective therapy for SIADH is treatment of the underlying cause.

Therapy. The optimal treatment is correction of the pathologic process responsible for hyponatremia. The most effective treatment for SIADH is to correct the underlying cause of excessive antidiuretic hormone production. Serum sodium normalizes when patients with small cell lung carcinoma respond to combi-

Table 40–23. Pathophysiologic Approach to the Diagnosis of Hyponatremia

VOLUME STATUS	URINE SODIUM	URINE OSMOLALITY	BUN	TREATMENT
Normal extracellular fluid SIADH	↑	↑	↓	Treat underlying disease, water restriction, demeclocycline
Reset osmostat	Variable	Variable	Normal	Treat underlying disease
Increased extracellular fluid (heart failure, nephrosis, cirrhosis)	↓	↑ → Isotonic	Normal → ↑	Sodium and water restriction
Decreased extracellular fluid Nonrenal losses	↓	↑ → Isotonic	Normal → ↑	Isotonic NaCl
Renal losses	↑	Isotonic	Normal → ↑	Treat underlying disease

Derived from DeFronzo and Thier, 1980.

nation chemotherapy or radiotherapy. Radiotherapy for brain metastases may alleviate SIADH. If the etiology is drug-induced SIADH (*e.g.,* morphine or barbiturates), hyponatremia will resolve promptly once the offending agent is discontinued (Cohen *et al.,* 1978; North *et al.,* 1979).

If the cause of excessive ADH secretion cannot be corrected, the initial approach for symptomatic SIADH with a serum sodium below 125 mg/dL is water restriction. If free-water intake is restricted to 500 to 1000 mL per day, a gradual negative free-water balance will correct hyponatremia over seven to ten days (Thomas *et al.,* 1978; DeFronzo and Thier, 1980; Goldberg, 1981; Segaloff, 1981; Trump, 1981). If water restriction is ineffective and there is little chance of obtaining a significant antitumor response, demeclocycline can correct hyponatremia by inhibiting ADH's stimulus for free-water reabsorption in the collecting duct (Singer and Rotenberg, 1973; DeFronzo and Thier, 1980; Geheb and Cox, 1980; Goldberg, 1981). Lithium also corrects hyponatremia by antagonizing ADH's effects in the distal nephron, but demeclocycline appears to be more effective by producing a dose-dependent reversible nephrogenic diabetes insipidus (DeTroyer and Demanet, 1975; Forrest *et al.,* 1978; Geheb and Cox, 1980; Trump, 1981).

Trump reported that patients with SIADH secondary to cancer or aplastic anemia had excellent responses to demeclocycline. Despite receiving large volumes of fluid, the average pretreatment serum sodium (121 mEq/L) uniformly rose above 130 mEq/L within 3.5 days of initiating therapy (Trump, 1981). Reversible nephrotoxicity is the only significant toxicity of demeclocycline (Miller *et al.,* 1980; Trump, 1981). Approximately 35% of the patients in Trump's series developed elevations in BUN above 25 mg/dL with an average maximum creatinine of 2.4 mg/dL. All patients with nephrotoxicity were receiving other nephrotoxic drugs or higher doses of demeclocycline. Renal function returned to normal in three patients after discontinuing demeclocycline and other nephrotoxic drugs, but three other patients died of widespread metastases and sepsis with moderately severe renal failure (BUN, 116 to 198 mg/dL, and creatinine, 2.2 to 4.8 mg/dL prior to death) (Trump, 1981).

Renal toxicity appears to correlate with elevated plasma drug levels (Miller *et al.,* 1980; Trump, 1981). Since demeclocycline is excreted in the urine and bile, patients with renal or hepatic dysfunction have an increased risk of nephrotoxicity (Cherill *et al.,* 1975; Carrilho *et al.,* 1977; Forrest *et al.,* 1978; Geheb and Cox, 1980; Trump, 1981). Demeclocycline is given orally in divided doses ranging from 600 to 1200 mg daily. The initial daily dose is 600 mg. However, lower doses should be used with significant liver or renal disease or in patients concurrently receiving other nephrotoxic drugs (Miller *et al.,* 1980).

Severely hyponatremic patients with seizures or coma from SIADH should be treated with 3% hypertonic saline or isotonic saline and IV furosemide, 1 mg/kg. This regimen produces an isotonic diuresis (Hantman *et al.,* 1973). Once serum sodium rises above a critical level, other measures previously described should be instituted to gradually correct hyponatremia. An attempt is made in volume-expanded patients to improve associated cardiac, renal, or liver dysfunction. Volume-contracted states are managed with intravenous fluids (usually isotonic saline) and correction of associated acid-base disturbances (DeFronzo and Thier, 1980; Goldberg, 1981).

Hypoglycemia

Insulinomas and other islet cell tumors of the pancreas are the most common neoplasms associated with fasting hypoglycemia. Excessive insulin secretion is characteristic of islet cell tumor–induced hypoglycemia, but has not been reported with sarcomas, hepatomas, or other nonislet cell neoplasms (Marks and Rose, 1965; Laurent *et al.,* 1971; Fajans and Floyd, 1976; Kahn, 1980). The most common nonislet cell neoplasms associated with hypoglycemia are listed in Table 40–24. The majority of these tumors are massive (up to 10 to 20 kg) mesenchymal tumors, including fibrosarcomas, mesotheliomas, and spindle cell sarcomas (Papaioannou, 1966; Laurent *et al.,*

Table 40–24. Non-Islet Cell Tumors Associated with Hypoglycemia

TUMOR TYPE	%
Mesenchymal	45
Hepatoma	23
Adrenocortical carcinoma	10
Gastrointestinal tumors	8
Lymphoma-leukemia	6
Others (hypernephroma, pheochromocytomas, anaplastic carcinomas, pseudomyoma)	8

Derived from Kahn, 1980.

1971; Marks, 1976; Millard *et al.,* 1976; Skrabanek and Powell, 1978; Anderson and Lokich, 1979; Kahn, 1980). Less than 25% of patients with hepatoma develop hypoglycemia during the course of their disease. Hypoglycemia is primarily associated with the more well-differentiated, slowly growing hepatocellular tumors (McFadzean and Yeung, 1969). Hypoglycemia also has been reported in association with every common tumor, but rarely with carcinomas of the lung or breast (Kahn, 1980).

Pathophysiology. Glucose homeostasis is controlled by a balance of adequate caloric intake, gluconeogenesis, glycogenolysis, and appropriate hormonal regulation of these processes (Kahn, 1980). Tumor-induced hypoglycemia is thought to be caused by the following factors: (1) secretion of insulin or an insulinlike substance, (2) excessive glucose utilization by the tumor, and (3) failure of compensatory mechanisms, including inhibition of gluconeogenesis or glycogenolysis, hepatic failure, or suppression of counterregulatory hormones (Papaioannou, 1966; Unger, 1966; Laurent *et al.,* 1971; Marks, 1976; Skrabanek and Powell, 1978; Kahn, 1980).

Excessive ectopic insulin secretion has been reported only with islet cell tumors (Skrabanek and Powell, 1978). However, using different bioassays, increased insulinlike activity has been measured in serum from patients with hypoglycemia and nonislet tumors. These substances are now referred to as nonsuppressible insulinlike activity (NSILA), since only 5 to 10% of this insulinlike activity can be neutralized with anti-insulin antibodies.

NSILA is a combination of a high molecular weight glycoproteins and low molecular weight insulinlike growth factors, IGF and IGF2, and somatomedins A and C. NSILA shares the growth-promoting and metabolic effects of insulin. Compared to insulin, the growth-promoting effects of low molecular weight NSILA are fiftyfold greater, but its metabolic effects are only 1 to 2% as potent (Hall *et al.,* 1975; Zapf *et al.,* 1978a,b). High molecular weight NSILA shares insulin's metabolic properties, but lacks growth-promoting capabilities (Jakob *et al.,* 1967; Hall *et al.,* 1975; Van Wyck *et al.,* 1975; Poffenbarger and Boully 1976; Rinderknecht and Humbel 1976, 1978; Ginsberg *et al.,* 1979).

Increased levels of low molecular weight NSILA have been detected in nonislet cell tumors associated with hypoglycemia by radioreceptor and bioassays (Megyusi *et al.,*

1974; Hyodo *et al.,* 1977; Kahn, 1980; Gordan *et al.,* 1981). High serum levels of low molecular weight NSILA have been reported with hemangiopericytomas, hepatomas, pheochromocytomas, adrenocortical carcinomas, and other mesenchymal tumors; while other malignancies associated with hypoglycemia (*e.g.,* leukemia, lymphoma, and gastrointestinal tumors) have low to normal NSILA (Kahn, 1980; Gordan *et al.,* 1981). Eighty percent of patients with fibrosarcomas and hypoglycemia have elevated serum levels of high molecular weight NSILA, but quantities of these metabolically active glycoproteins have not been measured in tumor extracts (Poffenbarger and Boully 1976; Prine and Poffenbarger, 1978; Plovnick *et al.,* 1979).

Normally, glucocorticoid, growth hormone, glucagon, and ACTH secretion increase in response to a rapid reduction in serum glucose. Although low values of these counterregulatory hormones have been measured in selected patients with tumor-induced hypoglycemia, the fall in glucose is usually not enough to produce an increase in these hormones. Presently, data are not available to implicate decreased secretion of these counterregulatory hormones as a major etiologic factor of this paraneoplastic process (Kahn, 1980).

Most neoplasms have increased rates of glycolysis and anaerobic metabolism. Increased glucose utilization was originally one of the more popular theoretical explanations for hypoglycemia associated with large sarcomas. However, glycogenolysis and gluconeogenesis should compensate for increased rates of glycolysis, unless these compensatory mechanisms are inhibited. Oncology patients appear to have reduced rates of gluconeogenesis, (Chandalia and Boshell, 1972; Silbert *et al.,* 1976), diminished gluconeogenic and glucogenolytic responses to epinephrine or glucagon (Shapiro *et al.,* 1966; Jakob *et al.,* 1967; Chandalia and Boshell, 1972), and elevated hepatic glycogen levels secondary to reduced glycogenolysis (Laurent *et al.,* 1971; Marks, 1976). A small percentage of cancer patients have elevated tryptophan levels, which inhibit phosphoenol pyruvate carboxykinase, a major gluconeogenic enzyme (Silbert *et al.,* 1976). These preliminary observations tend to support a role for impaired glucose homeostasis in tumor-induced hypoglycemia, but are far from conclusive.

Clinical Presentation. Most patients present with neuropsychiatric symptoms of hypoglycemia, including excessive fatigue, weakness, dizziness, confusion, or somnolence. Symptoms of reactive hypoglycemia are rare. These symptoms may be subtle and may be attributed to depression, systemic therapy, or to the neoplastic process in general. Symptoms tend to occur after fasting in the early morning or late afternoon. When the blood glucose level falls below 40 to 45 mg/dL for prolonged periods, seizures and coma may occur. Elderly patients with significant cerebrovascular disease often develop focal neurologic signs (Kahn, 1980). A high index of suspicion is necessary to prevent irreversible neurologic dysfunction.

Diagnostic Evaluation. Hypoglycemia associated with malignancy is characteristically associated with fasting. Blood glucose levels should be obtained at the first suspicion of symptomatic hypoglycemia. Fasting blood sugar determinations, as well as late-afternoon values, are most helpful in making the diagnosis. Increased insulin levels and fasting glucose levels below 50 mg/dL are characteristic of insulinomas and other insulin-secreting islet cell tumors. Patients with nonislet cell tumors have normal-to-low insulin levels during periods of hypoglycemia (Stefanini et al., 1974; Kahn, 1980). Before hypoglycemia is attributed to a paraneoplastic process, one must exclude common causes of severe hypoglycemia, which include exogenous insulin, oral hypoglycemic agents, alcohol abuse, severe malnutrition, and sepsis. Glucocorticoid insufficiency, caused by adrenal or pituitary metastases or steroid withdrawal, must be included in the differential diagnosis (Kahn, 1980; Miller et al., 1980). Artificial hypoglycemia also occurs in patients with high leukocyte counts when blood remains in collection tubes for prolonged periods prior to separation (Field et al., 1961).

Patients with suspected insulinomas or islet cell tumors should have simultaneous fasting glucose and insulin levels. Proinsulin levels and proinsulin : insulin ratios are usually elevated in insulinomas. Rubenstein has reported that malignant insulinomas appear to have the highest proinsulin levels (Rubenstein et al., 1977). Provocative glucagon or tolbutamide tests are rarely necessary to confirm the diagnosis of insulinoma (Kahn, 1980). If laboratory tests suggest an insulinoma, preoperative studies directed at tumor localization are selected from a wide range of radiographic procedures, including CT scans, ultrasound, selective arteriography, transhepatic selective venous catheterization for insulin determination, and occasionally endoscopic retrograde cholangiopancreatography. Sixty-six to ninety-one percent of islet cell tumors are diagnosed and localized by arteriography preoperatively (Stefanini et al., 1974; Van Heerden et al., 1979). If technically feasible, insulinlike plasma factors should be measured by bioassay, or radioreceptor technique in patients with hypoglycemia associated with nonislet cell tumors.

Therapy. Neurologic symptoms secondary to hypoglycemia are rapidly corrected with intravenous injections of 50% dextrose followed by continuous infusions of 10% dextrose. Localized insulinomas are frequently cured by surgery. Excellent results are obtained with simple enucleation or subtotal pancreatectomy; total pancreatectomy is generally unnecessary (Stefanini et al., 1974). The rare patient with metastatic or inoperable insulinoma can be effectively palliated with chemotherapy or diazoxide, as described in Chapter 10.

Hypoglycemia associated with nonislet cell tumors responds to effective antineoplastic therapy. For example, hypoglycemia resolves following surgical resection of fibrosarcomas. A combination of radiotherapy and doxorubicin-based chemotherapy may relieve hypoglycemia secondary to mesothelioma (Papaioannou, 1966; Kahn, 1980). Patients should be instructed to have frequent between-meal and bedtime snacks and occasionally must be awakened from sleep to prevent nocturnal hypoglycemia. Glucocorticoids, growth hormone, or glucagon may provide temporary palliation (Papaioannou, 1966), but unless there is a significant antitumor response, progressive hypoglycemia may be the cause of neurologic disability and death.

REFERENCES

Abeloff, M. D., and Lenhard, R. E.: Clinical management of uretheral obstruction secondary to malignant lymphoma. *Johns Hopkins Med. J.,* **134:**34–42, 1974.

Adler, R. H., and Sayek, I.: Treatment of malignant pleural effusion: A method using tube thoracostomy and talc. *Ann. Thorac. Surg.,* **22:**8–15, 1976.

Agus, Z. S., and Goldberg, M.: Role of antidiuretic hormone in the abnormal water diuresis of anterior hypopituitarism in man. *J. Clin. Invest.,* **50:**1478–1479, 1971.

Ahmann, F. R.: A reassessment of the clinical implications of the superior vena caval syndrome. *J. Clin. Oncol.,* **2:**961–969, 1984.

Allen, K. L.; Johnson, T. W.; and Hibbs, G. G.: Effective bone palliation as related to various treatment regimens. *Cancer*, 37:984–987, 1976.

Amundsen, P.; Dugstad, G.; and Syvertsen, A. H.: The reliability of computer tomography for the diagnosis and differential diagnosis of meningiomas, gliomas, and brain metastases. *Acta Neurochir. (Wien)*, 41:177–190, 1978.

Anderson, C. B.; Philpott, G. W.; and Ferguson, T. B.: The treatment of malignant pleural effusions. *Cancer*, 33:916–922, 1974.

Anderson, N., and Lokich, J. J.: Mesenchymal tumors associated with hypoglycemia: Case report and review of the literature. *Cancer*, 44:785–790, 1979.

Applefeld, M. M.; Slawson, R. G.; Hall-Criags, M.; Green, D. C.; Singleton, R. T.; and Wiernik, P. H.: Delayed pericardial disease after radiotherapy. *Am. J. Cardiol.*, 47:210–213, 1981.

Ariel, I. M.; Oruperza, R.; and Pack, G. T.: Intracavitary administration of radioactive isotopes in the control of effusions due to cancer. *Cancer*, 19:1096–1102, 1966.

Ask-Upmark, E.: Metastatic tumors of the brain and their localization. *Acta Med. Scand.*, 154:1–9, 1956.

Au, W. Y. W.: Calcitonin treatment of hypercalcemia due to parathyroid carcinoma: Synergistic effects of prednisone on long-term treatment of hypercalcemia. *Arch. Intern. Med.*, 135:1594–1597, 1975.

Austin, E. H., and Flye, M. W.: The treatment of recurrent malignant pleural effusion. *Ann. Thorac. Surg.*, 28:190–203, 1979.

Avasthi, R. B., and Moghissi, K.: Malignant obstruction of the superior vena cava and its palliation. *J. Thorac. Cardiovasc. Surg.*, 74:244–248, 1977.

Aviram, A.; Pean, A.; Czackzes, J. W.; and Ullman, T. D.: Hyperosmolality with hyponatremia caused by inappropriate administration of mannitol *Am. J. Med.*, 42:648–650, 1967.

Azzopardi, J. G.; Freeman, E.; and Poole, G.: Endocrine and metabolic disorders in bronchial carcinoma. *Br. Med. J.*, 4:528–529, 1970.

Bagshaw, M. A.: Presumptive palliative irradiation in metastatic carcinoma of the breast. *Cancer*, 28:1692–1694, 1971.

Band, P. R.; Holland, J. F.; Bernard, J.; Weil, M.; Walker, M.; and Rall, D.: Treatment of central nervous system leukemia with intrathecal cytosine arabinoside. *Cancer*, 32:743–744, 1973.

Band, P. R.; Silverberg, D. S.; Henderson, J. F.; Ulan, R. A.; Wensel, R. H.; Banerjee, T. K.; and Little, A. S.: Xanthine nephropathy in a patient with lymphosarcoma treated with allopurinol. *N. Engl. J. Med.*, 283:354, 1970.

Barbaric, Z. L.: Interventional uroradiography. *Radiol. Clin. North Am.*, 17:413–433, 1979.

Barry, H.; Parker, R.; and Gerdes, A.: Irradiation of brain metastases. *Acta Radiol.*, 13:535–544, 1974.

Bartter, F. C., and Schwartz, W. B.: The syndrome of inappropriate secretion of antidiuretic hormone. *Am. J. Med.*, 42:790–805, 1967.

Bass, J.; Pan, H. C.; and Gottesman, L.: Superior vena cava syndrome: Report of a new operative technique. *J. Natl. Med. Assoc.*, 72:1105–1109, 1980.

Baumgartner, W. A., and Mark, J. B. D.: Metastatic malignancies from distant sites to the tracheobronchial tree. *J. Thorac. Cardiovasc. Surg.*, 79:499–503, 1980.

Belen, J. E., and Rotman, H. H.: Primary carcinoma of the trachea. Physiologic diagnosis and review of the literature. *Chest*, 72:675–676, 1977.

Bender, R. A., and Hansen, H.: Hypercalcemia in bronchogenic carcinoma: A prospective study of 200 patients. *Ann. Intern. Med.*, 80:205–208, 1974.

Benson, R. C., Jr.; Riggs, B. L.; Pickard, B. M.; and Arnaud, C. D.: Radioimmunoassay of parathyroid hormone in hypercalcemic patients with malignant disease. *Am. J. Med.*, 56:821–826, 1974.

Berry, E. M.; Guta, M. M.; Turner, S. J.; and Burns, R. R.: Variation in plasma calcium with induced changes in plasma specific gravity, total protein, and albumin. *Br. Med. J.*, 4:640–643, 1973.

Besarb, A., and Caro, J. F.: Mechanisms of hypercalcemia in malignancy. *Cancer*, 41:2276–2285, 1978.

Binstock, M. L., and Mundy, G. R.: Effect of calcitonin and glucocorticoids in combination on the hypercalcemia of malignancy. *Ann. Intern. Med.*, 93:269–272, 1980.

Bisel, H. F.; Worblewski, F.; and LaDue, J. S.: Incidence and clinical manifestations of cardiac metastases. *J.A.M.A.*, 153:712–715, 1953.

Black, L. F.: The pleural space and pleural fluid. *Mayo Clin. Proc.*, 47:493–506, 1972.

Blackman, M. R.; Rosen, S. W.; and Weintraub, B. D.: Ectopic hormones. *Adv. Intern. Med.*, 23:85–113, 1978.

Blair, R. J., and McAfee, J. G.: Radiological detection of skeletal metastases: Radiographics vs. scans. *Int. J. Radiat. Oncol. Biol. Phys.*, 1:1201, 1976.

Blasberg, R. G.; Patlak, C. S.; and Shapiro, W. R.: Distribution of methotrexate in the cerebral spinal fluid and brain after interventricular administration. *Cancer Treat. Rep.*, 61:633–641, 1977.

Bleyer, W. A., and Poplack, D. G.: Intraventricular versus intralumbar methotrexate for central nervous system leukemia: Prolonged remission with the Ommaya reservoir. *Med. Pediatr. Oncol.*, 6:207–213, 1979.

Bockman, R. S.: Hypercalcemia in malignancy. *Clin. Endocrinol. Metab.*, 9:317–333, 1980.

Borgelt, B.; Gelber, R.; Kramer, S.; Brady, L. W.; Chang, C. H.; Davis, L. W.; Perez, C. A.; and Hendrickson, F. R.: The palliation of brain metastases: Final results of the first two studies by the Radiation Therapy Oncology Group. *Int. J. Radiat. Oncol. Biol. Phys.*, 6:1–9, 1980.

Borja, E. R., and Pugh, R. P.: Single-dose quinacrine (Atabrine) and thoracostomy in the control of pleural effusion in patients with neoplastic diseases. *Cancer*, 31:899–902, 1973.

Boss, G. R., and Seegmiller, J. E.: Hyperuricemia and gout: Classification, complications, and management. *N. Engl. J. Med.*, 300:1459–1468, 1979.

Brady, L. W.; O'Neill, E. A.; and Farber, S. H.: Unusual sites of metastases. *Semin. Oncol.*, 4:59–64, 1977.

Brain, G. O., and Karr, J. P.: Diffuse leptomeningeal carcinomatosis. Clinical and pathologic characteristics. *Neurology*, 5:706–722, 1955.

Braman, S. S., and Whitcomb, M. E.: Endobronchial metastasis. *Arch. Intern. Med.*, 135:543–547, 1975.

Brautbar, N., and Luboshitzky, R.: Combined calcitonin and oral phosphate treatment for hypercalcemia in multiple myeloma. *Arch. Intern. Med.*, 137:914–916, 1977.

Brereton, H. D.; Halushka, P. V.; Alexander, R. W.; Mason, D. M.; Keiser, H. R.; and DeVita, V. T.: Indomethacin-responsive hypercalcemia in a patient with renal-cell adenocarcinoma. *N. Engl. J. Med.*, 291:83–85, 1974.

Bretland, P. M.: *Acute Ureteric Obstruction—A Clinical and Radiological Study*. Butterworth, London, 1972.

Breuer, R. I., and LeBauer, J.: Caution in the use of phosphates in the treatment of severe hypercalcemia. *J. Clin. Endocrinol. Metab.,* **27**:695–698, 1967.

Brewer, L. A.: Patterns of survival in lung cancer. *Chest,* **71**:644–650, 1977.

Brice, J., and McKissock, W.: Surgical treatment of malignant extradural spinal tumors. *Br. Med. J.,* **2**:1341–1344, 1965.

Bricout, P. B.; Modur, R. S.; and Feldman, M. I.: Importance of myelography in early diagnosis of spinal epidural disease. *J.A.M.A.,* **73**:543–546, 1981.

Brin, E. N.; Schiff, M.; and Weiss, R. M.: Palliative urinary diversion for pelvic malignancy. *J. Urol.,* **113**:619–622, 1975.

Bruckman, J. E., and Bloomer, W. D.: Management of spinal cord compression. *Semin. Oncol.,* **5**:135–140, 1978.

Bruneau, R., and Rubin, P.: The management of pleural effusions and chylothorax in lymphoma. *Radiology,* **85**:1085–1095, 1965.

Buckle, R.: Ectopic PTH syndrome, pseudohyperparathyroidism: Hypercalcemia of malignancy. *Clin. Endocrinol. Metab.,* **3**:237–251, 1974.

Bunn, P. A., Jr.; Nugent, J. L.; and Matthews, M. J.: Central nervous system metastases in small cell bronchogenic carcinoma. *Semin. Oncol.,* **5**:314–322, 1978.

Bunn, P.; Rosen, S.; Aisner, J.; Matthews, M.; Glatstein, E.; and Wiernick, P.: Carcinomatous leptomeningitis in patients with small cell lung cancer: A frequent, treatable complication. *Proc. Am. Assoc. Cancer Res., and A.S.C.O.,* **21**:641 (Abstr. C-39), 1981.

Bunn, P. A., Jr.; Schein, P. S.; Banks, P. M.; and DeVita, V. T., Jr.: Central nervous system complications in patients with diffuse histocytic and undifferentiated lymphoma and leukemia revisited. *Blood,* **41**:3–10, 1976.

Cadman, E., and Bertino, J. R.: Chemotherapy of skeletal metastasis. *Int. J. Radiat. Oncol. Biol. Phys.,* **1**:121, 1976.

Caldwell, W. L., and Bagshaw, M. A.: Indications for and results of irradiation of carcinoma of the lung. *Cancer,* **22**:999–1004, 1968.

Carey, R. W.; Schmidt, G. W.; Kopald, H. H.; and Kantrowitz, P. A.: Massive extraskeletal calcification during phosphate treatment of hypercalcemia. *Arch. Intern. Med.,* **122**:150–155, 1968.

Carlton, C. E., Jr.; Dawoud, F.; Hudgins, P.; and Scott, R., Jr.: Irradiation treatment of carcinoma of the prostate: A preliminary report based on 8 years of experience. *J. Urol.,* **108**:924–927, 1972.

Carmel, R. J., and Kaplan, H. S.: Mantle irradiation in Hodgkin's disease. *Cancer,* **37**:2813–2825, 1973.

Carrilho, F.; Bosch, J.; Arroyo, V.; Mas, A.; Viver, J.; and Rocles, J.: Renal failure associated with demeclocycline in cirrhosis. *Ann. Intern. Med.,* **87**:195–197, 1977.

Carvallo, A.; Rakowski, T. A.; Argy, W. P., Jr.; and Schreiner, G. E.: Acute renal failure following drip infusion pyelography. *Am. J. Med.,* **65**:38, 1978.

Cassell, P., and Dullum, P.: The management of cardiac tamponade: Drainage of pericardial effusions. *Br. J. Surg.,* **54**:620–626, 1967.

Cassileth, P. A., and Trotman, B. W.: Inappropriate antidiuretic hormone in Hodgkin's disease. *Am. J. Med. Sci.,* **265**:233–235, 1975.

Castellino, R. A.; Glatstein, E.; Turbow, M. M.; Rosenberg, S.; and Kaplan, H. S.: Latent radiation injury of lungs or heart activated by steroid withdrawal. *Ann. Intern. Med.,* **80**:593–599, 1974.

Cham, W. C.; Freiman, A. H.; Carstens, P. H. B.; and Chu,

F. C. H.: Radiation therapy of cardiac and pericardial metastases. *Radiology,* **114**:701–704, 1975.

Chan, P. Y., and Norman, A.: Hyperthermia effects of methyl methacrylate in bone metastases. *Proc. Am. Assoc. Cancer Res.,* **20**:299, 1979.

Chandalia, H. B., and Boshell, B. R.: Hypoglycemia associated with extrapancreatic tumors. *Arch. Intern. Med.,* **129**:447–456, 1972.

Chapuy, M. C.; Meunier, P. J.; Alexandre, C. M.; and Vignon, E. P.: Effects of disodium dichloromethylene diphosphonate on hypercalcemia produced by bone metastases. *J. Clin. Invest.,* **65**:1243–1247, 1980.

Cherrill, D. A.; Stote, R. M.; Birge, J. R.; and Singer, I.: Demeclocycline treatment in the syndrome of inappropriate antidiuretic hormone secretion. *Ann. Intern. Med.,* **83**:654–656, 1975.

Clark, J.; Hall, A. W.; and Moosa, A. R.: Treatment of obstructing cancer of the colon and rectum. *Surg. Gynecol. Obstet.,* **141**:541–544, 1975.

Clarkson, B.: Relationship between cell type, glucose concentration, and response to treatment in neoplastic effusions. *Cancer,* **17**:914–928, 1964.

Cohen, G. U.; Perry, T. M.; and Evans, J. M.: Neoplastic invasion of the heart and pericardium. *Ann. Intern. Med.,* **42**:1238–1245, 1955.

Cohen, M. H.; Bunn, P. A., Jr.; Ihde, D. C.; Fossieck, B. E., Jr.; and Minna, J. D.: Chemotherapy rather than demeclocycline for inappropriate secretion of antidiuretic hormone. *N. Engl. J. Med.,* **298**:1423, 1978.

Cohn, K. E.; Stewart, J. R.; Fajardo, L. F.; and Hancock, E. W.: Heart disease following radiation. *Medicine,* **46**:281–298, 1967.

Collins, J. D.; Bassett, L.; Main, G. D.; and Kagan, C.: Percutaneous biopsy following positive bone scans. *Radiology,* **132**:439–442, 1979.

Comis, R. L.; Miller, M.; and Ginsburg, S. J.: Abnormalities in water homeostasis in small cell anaplastic lung cancer. *Cancer,* **45**:2414–2421, 1980.

Connors, T. B., and Howard, J. F.: The etiology of hypercalcemia associated with lung carcinoma. *J. Clin. Invest.,* **35**:697–698, 1956.

Cox, J. D.; Byhardt, R.; Komaki, R.; Wilson, J. F.; Libnoch, J. A.; and Hansen, R.: Interaction of thoracic irradiation and chemotherapy on local control and survival in small cell carcinoma of the lung. *Cancer Treat. Rep.,* **63**:1251–1255, 1979.

Crittenden, D. R., and Ackerman, G. L.: Hyperuricemic acute renal failure in disseminated carcinoma. *Arch. Intern. Med.,* **137**:97–99, 1977.

Cukingham, R. A., and Carey, J. S.: Carcinoma of the esophagus. *Ann. Thorac. Surg.,* **26**:274–286, 1978.

Das Gupta, T. K., and Brasfield, R. D.: Metastatic melanoma of the gastrointestinal tract. *Arch. Surg.,* **88**:969–973, 1964.

Davenport, D.; Ferree, C.; Blake, D.; and Raben, M.: Radiation therapy in treatment of superior vena caval obstruction. *Cancer,* **42**:2600–2603, 1978.

Davis, S.; Sharma, S. M.; Blumberg, E. D.; and Kim, C. S.: Intrapericardial tetracycline for the management of cardiac tamponade secondary to maglignant pericardial effusion. *N. Engl. J. Med.,* **299**:1113–1114, 1978.

D'Cruz, I. A.; Cohen, H. C.; Prabhu, R.; and Glick, G.: Diagnoses of cardiac tamponade by echocardiography: Changes in mitral valve motion and ventricular dimensions with special reference to paradoxical pulse. *Circulation,* **52**:460–465, 1972.

de Castro, C. A.; Dockerty, M. B.; and Mays, C. W.: Metastatic tumors of the small intestines. *Surg. Gynecol. Obstet.,* **106:**159–165, 1957.

Decaux, G.; Brimiovlle, S.; Genette, F.; and Mockel, J.: Treatment of the syndrome of inappropriate secretion of antidiuretic hormone by urea. *Am. J. Med.,* **69:**99–106, 1980.

DeFronzo, R. A.; Goldberg, M.; and Agus, Z. S.: Normal diluting capacity in hyponatremic patients. *Ann. Intern. Med.,* **84:**538–542, 1976.

DeFronzo, R. A., and Thier, S. O.: Pathophysiologic approach to hyponatremia. *Arch. Intern. Med.,* **140:**897–902, 1980.

DeLoach, J. F., and Haynes, J. W.: Secondary tumors of the heart and pericardium: Review of the subject and report of one hundred thirty-seven cases. *Arch. Intern. Med.,* **91:**224–249, 1953.

DelRegato, J.: Pathways of metastatic spread of malignant tumors. *Semin. Oncol.,* **4:**33–38, 1977.

Demers, L. M.; Allegra, J. C.; Harvey, H. A.; Lipton, A.; Luderer, J. R.; Moertel, R.; and Brenner, D. E.: Plasma prostaglandins in hypercalcemic patients with neoplastic disease. *Cancer,* **39:**1559–1562, 1977.

DeTroyer, A., and Demanet, J. C.: Correction of antidiuresis by demeclocycline. *N. Engl. J. Med.,* **293:**915–918, 1975.

Deutsch, M.; Parsons, J.; and Mercado, R.: Radiotherapy for intracranial metastases. *Cancer,* **34:**1607–1611, 1974.

Dollinger, M. R.; Krakoff, I. H.; and Karnofsky, D. A.: Quinacrine (Atabrine) in the treatment of neoplastic effusions. *Ann. Intern. Med.,* **66:**249–257, 1967.

Dombernowsky, P., and Hanson, H.: Combination chemotherapy in the management of superior vena caval obstruction in small-cell anaplastic carcinoma of the lung. *Acta Med. Scand.,* **204:**513–516, 1978.

Douglas, H. O.; Shukla, S. K.; and Mindell, E.: Treatment of pathological fractures of long bones excluding those due to breast cancer. *J. Bone Joint Surg.,* **58A:**1055–1061, 1976.

Dudley, F. J., and Blackburn, C. R. B.: Extraskeletal calcification complicating oral neutral-phosphate therapy. *Lancet,* **2:**628–630, 1970.

Duvoisin, G. E.; Ellis, F. H.; and Payne, W. S.: The value of palliative prostheses in malignant lesions of the esophagus. *Surg. Clin. North Am.,* **47:**827, 1967.

Earll, J. M.; Kurtzman, N. A.; and Moser, R. H.: Hypercalcemia and hypertension. *Ann. Intern. Med.,* **64:**378–381, 1966.

Edelson, R. N.; Deck, M. D. F.; and Posner, J. B.: Intramedullary spinal cord metastases: Clinical and radiographic findings in nine cases. *Neurology,* **22:**1222–1231, 1972.

Effeney, D. J.; Windsor, H. M.; and Shanahan, M. K.: Superior vena caval obstruction: Resection and bypass for malignant lesions. *Aust. N.Z. J. Surg.,* **42:**231–237, 1973.

Eilon, G., and Raisz, L. G.: Comparison of the effects of stimulators and inhibitors of resorption on the release of lysosomal enzymes and radioactive factor from fetal bone in organ culture. *Endocrinology,* **103:**1969–1975, 1978.

Eisen, H. M.; Bosworth, J. L.; and Ghossein, N. A.: The rationale for whole-spine irradiation in metastatic breast cancer. *Radiology,* **108:**417–418, 1973.

Eisenberg, E.: Effect of intravenous phosphate, serum strontium, and calcium. *N. Engl. J. Med.,* **282:**889–892, 1970.

Elias, E. G., and Evans, J. T.: Hypercalcemic crises in neoplastic diseases: Management with mithramycin. *Surgery,* **71:**631–635, 1972.

Elkon, D.; Lee, M. S.; and Hendrickson, F. R.: Carcinoma of the esophagus—Sites of recurrence and palliative benefits after definitive radiotherapy. *Int. J. Radiat. Oncol. Biol. Phys.,* **4:**615, 1978.

Ellis, H.; Morgan, M. N.; and Watsell, C.: "Curative" surgery in carcinoma of the colon involving the duodenum. A report of 6 cases. *Br. J. Surg.,* **59:**932–935, 1972.

Epstein, F. M.: Calcium and the kidney. *Am. J. Med.,* **45:**700–714, 1968.

Fajans, S., and Floyd, J. C.: Fasting hypoglycemia in adults. *N. Engl. J. Med.,* **294:**766–770, 1976.

Farber, S. M.: *Lung Cancer.* Charles C Thomas, Publisher, Springfield, Illinois, 1954.

Faulconer, H. T.; Ferguson, J. A.; and Van Zwalenburg, B. R.: The surgical significance of complete retrograde obstruction of the colon. *Dis. Colon Rectum,* **14:**428–430, 1971.

Feig, P. U., and McCurdy, D. K.: The hypertonic state. *N. Engl. J. Med.,* **297:**1444–1454, 1977.

Feun, L. G.; Drelichman, A.; Singhakowinta, A.; and Vaitkevicius, V. K.: Ureteral obstruction secondary to metastatic breast carcinoma. *Cancer,* **44:**1164–1171, 1979.

Field, J. B., and Williams, H. E.: Artifactual hypoglycemia associated with leukemia. *N. Engl. J. Med.,* **265:**946–948, 1961.

Fitzgerald, R. H.: Endobroncheal metastases. *South Med. J.,* **70:**440–441, 1977.

Flannery, E. P.; Gregoratos, G.; and Corder, M. P.: Pericardial effusions in patients with malignant diseases. *Arch. Intern. Med.,* **135:**976–977, 1975.

Forrest, J. N., Jr.; Cox, M.; Hong, C.; Morrison, G.; Bia, M.; and Singer, I.: Superiority of demeclocycline over lithium in the treatment of chronic syndrome of inappropriate secretion of antidiuretic hormone. *N. Engl. J. Med.,* **298:**173–177, 1978.

Fowler, N. O.: Diseases of the pericardium. *Curr. Probl. Cardiol.,* **2:**38, 1978.

Fracchia, A. A.; Knapper, W. H.; Carey, J. T.; and Farrow, J. H.: Intrapleural chemotherapy for effusion from metastatic breast carcinoma. *Cancer,* **26:**626–629, 1970.

Fredrickson, R. T.; Cohen, L. S.; and Mullens, G. B.: Pericardial windows or pericardiocentesis for pericardial effusions. *Am. Heart J.,* **82:**158–162, 1971.

Friedman, M. A., and Slater, E.: Malignant pleural effusions. *Cancer Treat. Rev.,* **5:**49–66, 1978.

Frisken, R. A.; Heath, D. A.; and Bord, A. M.: Hypercalcemia—A hospital survey. *Q. J. Med.,* **196:**405–418, 1980.

Frisken, R. A.; Heath, D. A.; Somers, S.; and Bold, A. M.: Hypercalcemia in hospital patients. *Lancet,* **1:**202–207, 1981.

Fulmer, D. H.; Dimich, A. B.; Rothschild, E. O.; and Myers, W. P. L.: Treatment of hypercalcemia: Comparison of intravenously administered phosphate, sulfate, and hydrocortisone. *Arch. Intern. Med.,* **129:**923–930, 1972.

Galicich, J. H., and Guido, L. J.: Ommaya device in carcinomatous and leukemic meningitis: Surgical experience in 45 cases. *Surg. Clin. North Am.,* **54:**915–922, 1974.

Galicich, J. H.; Sundaresan, V.; and Thaler, H. T.: Surgical treatment of single brain metastases. *J. Neurosurg.,* **53:**63–67, 1980.

Garmatis, L. J., and Chu, F. C. H.: The effectiveness of radiation therapy in the treatment of bone metastases from breast cancer. *Radiology* **126:**235–237, 1978.

Garnick, M. B., and Mayer, R. J.: Acute renal failure associated with neoplastic disease and its treatment. *Semin. Oncol.,* **5:**156–165, 1978.

Gassman, H. D.; Meadows, R., Jr.; and Baker, L. A.: Metastatic tumors of the heart. *Am. J. Med.,* **19:**357–365, 1955.

Geheb, M., and Cox, M.: Renal effects of demeclocycline. *J.A.M.A.,* **243:**2519–2520, 1980.

Geller, S. A., and Lin, C. S.: Ureteral obstruction from metastatic breast carcinoma. *Arch. Pathol.,* **99:**476–478, 1975.

Gerber, W. L.; Brown, R. C.; and Culp, D. A.: Percutaneous nephrostomy with immediate dilation. *J. Urol.,* **125:**169–171, 1981.

Ghosh, B. C., and Cliffton, E. E.: Malignant tumors with superior vena cava obstruction. *N.Y. State J. Med.,* **73:**283–289, 1973.

Gibbons, R. P.; Correa, R. J., Jr.; Cummings, K. B.; and Mason, T.: Experience with indwelling ureteral stent catheters. *J. Urol.,* **115:**22–26, 1976.

Gilbert, H.; Apuzzo, M., Marshall, L.; Kagan, A. R.; Crue, B.; Wagner, J.; Fuchs, K.; Rush, J.; Rao, A.; Nussbaum, H.; and Cham, P.: Neoplastic epidural spinal cord compression: A current perspective. *J.A.M.A.,* **240:**2771–2773, 1978a.

Gilbert, H. A.; Kagan, A. R.; Nussbaum, H.; Rao, A. R.; Satzman, J.; Chan, P.; and Forsythe, A.: Evaluation of radiation therapy for bone metastases: Pain relief and quality of life. *A. J. R.,* **129:**1095–1096, 1977.

Gilbert, R. W.; Kim, J. H.; and Posner, J. B.: Epidural spinal cord compression from metastatic tumor: Diagnosis and treatment. *Ann. Neurol.,* **3:**40–51, 1978b.

Gillenwater, J. Y.: The pathophysiology of urinary obstruction. In Harrison, J. H.; Gittes, R. F.; Perlmutter, A. D.; Stamey, T. A.; and Walsh, P. C. (eds.): *Campbell's Urology,* 4th ed. W. B. Saunders Company, Philadelphia, 1979.

Ginsberg, B. H.; Kahn, C. R.; Roth, J.; Megyesi, K.; and Baumann, G.: Identification and high-yield purification of insulin-like growth factors (NSILA-s and somatomedins) from human plasma by use of endogenous binding proteins. *J. Clin. Endocrinol. Metab.,* **48:**43–49, 1979.

Glass, R. L., and LeDuc, R. J.: Small intestinal obstruction from peritoneal carcinomatosis. *Am. J. Surg.,* **125:**316–317, 1973.

Glenn, F., and McSherry, C. K.: Obstruction and perforation in colorectal cancer. *Ann. Surg.,* **173:**983–992, 1971.

Goldberg, M.: Hyponatremia. *Med. Clin. North Am.,* **65:**251–269, 1981.

Goldsmith, R. S., and Ingbar, S. H.: Inorganic phosphate treatment of hypercalcemia of diverse etiologies. *N. Engl. J. Med.,* **274:**1–7, 1966.

Goldsmith, R. S., and Ingbar, S. H.: Phosphate, sulphate, and hypercalcemia. *Ann. Med.,* **67:**463–464, 1967.

Goldstein, A. G.: Metastatic carcinoma to the bladder. *J. Urol.,* **98:**209–215, 1967.

Gollub, S.; Hirose, T.; and Klauher, J.: Scintigraphic sequelae of superior vena caval obstruction. *Clin. Nucl. Med.,* **5:**89–93, 1980.

Goltzman, D.; Stewart, A. F.; and Broadus, A. E.: Malignancy-associated hypercalcemia: Evaluation with bio-chemical bioassay for parathyroid hormone. *J. Clin. Endocrinol. Metab.,* **53:**899–904, 1981.

Gomes, M. N., and Hufnagel, C. A.: Superior vena caval obstruction. *Ann. Thorac. Surg.,* **20:**344–359, 1975.

Gonzalez-Vitale, J. C., and Garcia-Bunuel, R.: Meningeal carcinomatosis. *Cancer,* **37:**2906–2911, 1976.

Goodie, R. B.: Secondary tumors of the heart and pericardium. *Br. Heart J.,* **17:**183–188, 1955.

Gordan, P.; Hendricks, C. M.; Kahn, C. R.; Megyesi, K.; and Roth J.: Hypoglycemia associated with non-islet cell tumor and insulin-like growth factors. *N. Engl. J. Med.,* **305:**1452–1455, 1981.

Gordon, G. S.; Canring, T. J.; Erhardt, L.; Hansen, J.; and Lubich, W.: Osteolytic sterol in human breast cancer. *Science,* **151:**1216–1228, 1966.

Gordon, G. S.; Eisenberg, E.; Loken, H. F.; Gardner, B.; and Hayashida, T.: Clinical endocrinology of parathyroid hormone excess. *Recent Prog. Horm. Res.,* **18:**297–336, 1962.

Gorter, K.: Results of laminectomy in spinal cord compression due to tumors. *Acta Neurochir. (Wien),* **42:**177–187, 1978.

Greco, F. A.; Richardson, R. L.; Snell, J. D.; Stroup, S. L.; and Oldham, R. K.: Small cell lung cancer: Complete remission and improved survival. *Am. J. Med.,* **66:**625–630, 1979.

Green, N.; Melbye, R. W.; George, F. W., III; and Morrow, J.: Radiation therapy of inoperable localized prostatic carcinoma: An assessment of tumor response and complications. *J. Urol.,* **3:**662–664, 1974.

Greenberg, H. S.; Kim, J.; and Posner, J. B.: Epidural spinal cord compression from metastatic tumor: Results with a new treatment protocol. *Ann. Neurol.,* **8:**361–366, 1980.

Greenberg, S. H.; Wein, A. J.; Perloff, L. J.; and Barker, C. F.: Ureteropyelostomy and ureteroneocystostomy in renal transplantation: Postoperative urological complications. *J. Urol.,* **118:**17–19, 1977.

Griffin, J. W.; Thompson, R. W.; Mitchinson, M. J.; de-Keiweit, J. C.; and Welland, F. H.: Lymphomatous leptomeningitis. *Am. J. Med.,* **51:**200–208, 1971.

Grillo, H. C.: Obstructing lesions of the trachea. *Ann. Otol. Rhinol. Laryngol.,* **82:**770–777, 1973.

Grillo, H. C.: Tracheal tumors: Surgical management. *Ann. Thorac. Surg.,* **26:**112–124, 1978.

Gunnlaugsson, G. H.; Wychulis, A. R.; Roland, C.; and Ellis, F. H.: Analysis of the records of 1,657 patients with cancer of the esophagus and cardia of the stomach. *Surg. Gynecol. Obstet.,* **130:**977–1005, 1970.

Gutin, P. H.; Weiss, H. D.; Wiernik, P. H.; and Walker, M. D.: Intrathecal thiotepa in the treatment of malignant meningeal disease. *Cancer,* **38:**1471–1475, 1976.

Gutman, A. B., and Yu, T. F.: Uric acid nephrolithiasis. *Am. J. Med.,* **45:**756–779, 1968.

Gutman, A. B., and Yu, T. F.: Renal mechanisms for regulation of uric acid excretion, with special reference to normal and gouty man. *Semin. Arthritis Rheum.,* **2:**1–46, 1972.

Gutman, F. D., and Boxer, R. J.: Neoplasms involving the kidney or producing renal failure via urinary obstruction. In Rieselbach, R. E., and Garnick, M. B. (eds.): *Cancer and the Kidney.* Lea & Febiger, Philadelphia, 1982.

Habener, J. R.; Singer, F. R.; Deltos, L. J.; and Potts, J. T., Jr.: Immunological stability of calcitonin in plasma. *Endocrinology,* **90:**952–960, 1972.

Haddad, J. G., Jr.; Couranz, S. J.; and Avioli, L. V.: Circulating phylosterols in normal females, lactating mothers, and breast cancer patients. *J. Clin. Endocrinol. Metab.,* **30:**174–180, 1970.

Hall, A. J., and Mackay, N. N. S.: The results of laminectomy for compression of the cord and cauda equina by extradural malignant tumor. *J. Bone Joint Surg.,* **55B:**497–505, 1973.

Hall, K.; Takano, K.; Fryklund, L.; and Sievertsson, H.: Somatomedins. *Adv. Metab. Disord.,* **8:**19–46, 1975.

Hancock, E. W.: Constrictive pericarditis: Clinical clues to diagnosis. *J.A.M.A.,* **232:**176–177, 1975.

Hankins, J. R.; Scatterfield, J. R.; Aisner, J.; Wiernik, P. H.; and McLaughlin, J. R.: Pericardial window for malignant pericardial effusion. *Ann. Thorac. Surg.,* **30:**465–471, 1980.

Hantman, O.; Rossier, B.; Zohlman, R.; and Schrier, R.: Rapid correction of hyponatremia in the syndrome of inappropriate-secretion of antidiuretic hormone. *Ann. Intern. Med.,* **78:**870–875, 1973.

Harken, A. H.; Gabel, R. A.; Fencis, V.; and Moore, F. D.: Hydrochloric acid in the correction of metabolic acidosis. *Arch. Surg.,* **110:**819–821, 1975.

Harr, F., and Patterson, R. H.: Surgery for metastatic intracranial neoplasm. *Cancer,* **38:**1241–1245, 1972.

Harrington, K. D.; Sim, F. H.; Enis, J. F.; Johnston, J. A.; Dick, H. M.; and Gristino, A. G.: Methylmethacrylate as an adjunct in internal fixation of pathologic fractures. *J. Bone Joint Surg.,* **58A:**1047–1055, 1976.

Hayward, M. L.; Howell, D. A.; O'Donnell, J. F.; and Maurer, L. H.: Hypercalcemia complicating small cell carcinoma. *Cancer,* **48:**1643–1646, 1981.

Heit, H. A.; Johnson, L. F.; Siegel, S. R.; and Boyce, H. W., Jr.: Palliative dilatation for dysphagia in esophageal carcinoma. *Ann. Intern. Med.,* **89:**629–631, 1978.

Hendrickson, F. R.: Radiation therapy of metastatic tumors. *Semin. Oncol.,* **2:**43–46, 1975.

Hendrickson, F. R.: The optimum schedule for palliative radiotherapy for metastatic brain cancer. *Int. J. Radiat. Oncol. Biol. Phys.,* **2:**165–168, 1977.

Hendrickson, F. R.; Shehata, W. M.; and Kirchner, H. B.: Radiation therapy for osseous metastasis. *Int. J. Radiat. Oncol. Biol. Phys.,* **1:**275–278, 1976.

Hendrickson, F. R., and Steinkop, M. B.: Management of osseous metastases. *Semin. Oncol.,* **2:**399–404, 1975.

Hepperlen, T. W.; Mardis, H. R.; and Kammandel, H.: Self-retained internal ureteral stents: A new approach. *J. Urol.,* **119:**731, 1978.

Herbert, L. A.; Lemann, J., Jr.; Petersen, J. R.; and Lennon, E. J.: Studies of the mechanism by which phosphate infusion lowers serum calcium concentration. *J. Clin. Invest.,* **45:**1886–1894, 1966.

Herbsman, H.; Wetstein, L.; Rosen, Y.; Orces, H.; Alfonso, A. E.; Iyer, S. K.; and Gardner, B.: Tumors of the small intestine. *Curr. Probl. Surg.,* **17:**121–182, 1980.

Herwig, K. R.: Management of urinary incontinence and retention in the patient with advanced cancer. *J.A.M.A.,* **244:**2203–2204, 1980.

Hickey, R. C., and Hyde, H. P.: Neoplastic obstruction of the large bowel. *Surg. Clin. North Am.,* **45:**1157–1163, 1965.

Hill, G. J., II, and Cohen, B. I.: Pleural pericardial window for palliation of cardiac tamponade due to cancer. *Cancer,* **26:**81–93, 1970.

Hindo, W. A., DeTrane, F. A., Lee, M. S.; and Hendrickson, F. R.: Large dose increment irradiation in treatment of cerebral metastasis. *Cancer,* **26:**138–141, 1970.

Holland, P., and Holland, N. H.: Prevention and management of acute hyperuricemia in childhood leukemia. *J. Pediatr.,* **72:**358–366, 1968.

Houston, H. E.; Rayne, W. S.; Harrison, E. G.; and Olsen, A. M.: Primary cancers of the trachea. *Arch. Surg.,* **99:**132–140, 1969.

Howard, N.: Mediastinal obstruction. In *Lung Cancer.* E. & S. Livingstone, London, 1967.

Howland, W.; Loeffler, R.; Starchman, D.; and Johnson, R.: Post-irradiation atrophic changes of bone and related complications. *Radiology,* **117:**677–685, 1975.

Hudson, R. E. B.: Diseases of the pericardium. In Hurst, J. W.; Logue, R. B.; Schlant, R. C.; and Wenger, N. K. (eds.): *The Heart,* 4th ed. McGraw-Hill, Inc., New York, 1978.

Hurst, W.: Radiation fibrosis of pericardium with cardiac tamponade: Case report with post-mortem studies and a review of the literature. *Can. Med. Assoc. J.,* **81:**377–380, 1959.

Husto, H. O.; Aur, R. J.; Verzosa, M. S.; Simone, J. V.; and Pinkel, D.: Prevention of central nervous system leukemia by irradiation. *Cancer,* **32:**585–597, 1973.

Hyodo, T.; Megyesi, K.; Kahn, C. R.; Roth, J.; and Friesen, H.: Adrenocortical carcinoma and hypoglycemia: Evidence for production of nonsuppressible insulin-like activity by the tumour. *J. Clin. Endocrinol. Metab.,* **44:**1175–1184, 1977.

Izbicki, R.; Weyhing, B. T., III; and Baker, L.: Pleural effusion in cancer patients—A prospective randomized study of pleural drainage with the addition of radioactive phosphorus to the pleural space vs. pleural drainage alone. *Cancer,* **36:**1511–1518, 1975.

Jacob, A.; Hauri, C.; and Froesch, E. R.: Nonsuppressible insulin-like activity in human serum. III. Differentiation of two distinct molecules with nonsuppressible ILA. *J. Clin. Invest.,* **47:**2678–2688, 1968.

Jacobs, T. P.; Siris, E. S.; Bilezikian, J. P.; Bacquiran, D. C.; Shane, E.; and Canfield, R. E.: Hypercalcemia of malignancy: Treatment with intravenous dichloromethylene diphosphorate. *Ann. Intern. Med.,* **94:**312–316, 1981.

Jakob, A.; Meyer, V. A.; Flury, A.; Ziegler, W. H.; Labhart, A.; and Froesch, E. R.: The pathogenesis of tumor hypoglycemia. Blocks of hepatic glucose release and of adipose tissue lipolysis. *Diabetologia,* **3:**506–514, 1967.

Jarvi, O. H.; Kunnas, R. J.; and Laitio, M. T.: The accuracy and significance of cytologic cancer diagnosis of pleural effusions. *Acta Cytol. (Baltimore),* **16:**152, 1972.

Jensen, N. H., and Roesdahl, K.: Single dose irradiation of bone metastasis. *Acta Radiol. Ther. Phys. Biol.,* **15:**337, 1976.

Jensen, T. M.; Dillon, W. L.; and Reckling, F. W.: Changing concepts in the management of pathological and impending pathological fractures. *J. Trauma,* **16:**496–502, 1976.

Jensik, R.; Cagle, J. E., Jr.; Milloy, F.; Perlia, C.; Taylor, S.; Kofman, S.; and Beattie, E. J.: Pleurectomy in the treatment of pleural effusion due to metastatic malignancy. *J. Thorac. Cardiovasc. Surg.,* **46:**322–330, 1963.

Jessiman, A. B.; Emerson, K. J.; Shah, R. C.; and Moore, F. D.: Hypercalcemia in carcinoma of the breast. *Ann. Surg.,* **157:**377–393, 1963.

Johnson, A. D.: Pathology of metastatic tumors of bone. *Clin. Orthop.,* **73:**8, 1970.

Josse, R. G; Wilson, D. R.; Heersche, J. N. M.; Mills, J. R. F.; and Murray, T. M.: Hypercalcemia with ovarian carcinoma: Evidence of a pathogenetic role for prostaglandins. *Cancer,* **48:**1233–1241, 1981.

Jowsey, J.: Quantitative microradiography. A new approach in the evaluation of metabolic bone disease. *Am. J. Med.,* **40:**485–491, 1966.

Jowsey, J., and Balasubramaniam, P.: Effect of phosphate supplements on soft tissue calcification and bone turnover. *Clin. Sci.,* **42:**289–299, 1972.

Kahn, C. R.: The riddle of tumour hypoglycemia revisited. *Clin. Endocrinol. Metab.,* **9:**335–360, 1980.

Kane, R. C.; Cohen, M. H.; Broder, L. E.; and Bull, M. J.: Superior vena cava obstruction due to small cell anaplastic lung carcinoma. *J.A.M.A.,* **235:**1717–1719, 1976.

Kanwar, Y. S., and Manaligod, J. D.: Leukemic urate nephropathy. *Arch. Pathol.,* **99:**467–472, 1975.

Kaplan, H. S.: *Hodgkin's Disease,* 2nd ed. Harvard University Press, Cambridge, Massachusetts, 1980.

Katz, M. A.: Hyperglycemia-induced hyponatremia — Calculation of expected serum sodium depression. *N. Engl. J. Med.,* **289:**843–844, 1973.

Katz, P. B.; Lee, Y.; Wallace, S.; and Ray, R. D.: Myelography of spinal block from epidural tumor: A new approach *A.J.R.,* **136:**945–947, 1981.

Kaunitz, J.: Landmarks in simple pleural effusions. *J.A.M.A.,* **113:**1312, 1939.

Keffort, R. F.; Woods, R. L.; Fox, R. M.; and Tattersall, M. H. N.: Intracavitary Adriamycin, nitrogen mustard, and tetracycline in the control of malignant effusions. *Med. J. Aust.,* **8:**447–448, 1980.

Kelalis, P. P.: Ureteropelvic junction. In Kelalis, P. P., and King, L. R. (eds.): *Clinical Pediatric Urology.* W. B. Saunders Company, Philadelphia, 1976.

Kelly, P., and Morton, J. J.: Antidiuretic hormone immunoactivity in tumor tissue from patients with bronchogenic carcinoma: With and without hyponaremia. *Br. Med. J.,* **12:**99–101, 1980.

Kelton, J.; Kelley, W. N.; and Holmes, E. W.: A rapid method for the diagnosis of acute uric acid nephropathy. *Arch. Intern. Med.,* **138:**612–615, 1978.

Kennedy, B. J.: Metabolic and toxic effects of mithramycin during tumor therapy. *Am. J. Med.,* **49:**494–503, 1970.

Kilpatrick, Z. M., and Chapman, C. B.: On pericardiocentesis. *Am. J. Cardiol.,* **16:**722–728, 1965.

Kimberg, D. V.; Berg, R. D.; Gershon, E.; and Graudusius, R. T.: Effect of cortisone treatment on the active transport of calcium by the small intestine. *J. Clin. Invest.,* **50:**1309–1321, 1971.

King, D. S., and Castleman, B.: Bronchial involvement in metastatic pulmonary malignancy. *J. Thorac. Surg.,* **12:**305–315, 1943.

Kinsey, D. L.; Carter, D.; and Klassen, K. P.: Simplified management of malignant pleural effusion. *Arch. Surg.,* **89:**389–391, 1964.

Kirkwood, J. M., and Bankole, D. O.: Carcinomatous meningitis at Yale 1970–1980. *Proc. Am. Assoc. Cancer Res. and A.S.C.O.,* **22:**633, 1981.

Kisner, D.; Bayly, T.; Sybert, A.; Macdonald, J.; Tsou, E.; Shnider, B.; and Schein, P.: Tetracycline and quinacrine in the control of malignant pleural effusion: a randomized clinical trial. *Proc. Am. Assoc. Cancer Res. and A.S.C.O.* **18:**290, 1977.

Kjellstrand, C. M.; Campbell, D. C., II; Von Hartitzsch, B.; and Buselmeier, T. J.: Hyperuricemic acute renal failure. *Arch. Intern. Med.,* **133:**349–359, 1974.

Klinenberg, J. R.; Kippen, I.; and Bluestone, R.: Hyperuricemic nephropathy: Pathologic features and factors influencing urate deposition. *Nephron,* **14:**99–115, 1975.

Kniseley, R. M., and Andrews, G. A.: Pathological changes following intracavitary therapy with colloidal Au-198. *Cancer,* **6:**303, 1953.

Knochel, J. P., and Mason, A. D.: Effect of alkalinization on peritoneal diffusion of uric acid. *Am. J. Physiol.,* **210:**1160, 1966.

Koff, S. A.; Thrall, J. H.; and Keyes, J. W.: Diuretic radionuclide urography: A non-invasive method for evaluating nephroureteral dilatation. *J. Urol.,* **122:**451–454, 1979.

Kohler, J. P.; Lyon, E. S.; and Schoenberg, H. W.: Reassessment of circle tube nephrostomy in advanced malignancy. *J. Urol.,* **123:**17–18, 1980.

Kopelson, G.; Munzenrider, J. E.; Kelley, R. M.; and Shiply, W. U.: Radiation therapy for ureteral metastases from breast carcinoma. *Cancer,* **47:**1976–1979, 1981.

Koziol, I.: Reticulum cell sarcoma: Unusual cause of ureteral obstruction. *Urology,* **4:**456–458, 1974.

Kramer, S.; Hendrickson, F.; and Zelen, M.: Therapeutic trials in the management of metastatic brain tumors by different time/dose fractionation schemes of radiation therapy. *Nat. Cancer Inst. Monogr.,* **46:**213–221, 1977.

Krane, S. M.; Harris, E. D., Jr.; Singer, F. R.; and Potts, J. T.: Acute effects of calcitonin on bone formation in man. *Metabolism,* **22:**51–58, 1973.

Kraus, P. A.; Lytton, B.; Weiss, R. M.; and Prosnitz, L. R.: Radiation therapy for local palliative treatment of prostatic cancer. *J. Urol.,* **108:**612–614, 1972.

Krikorian, J. G., and Hancock, E. W.: Pericardiocentesis. *Am. J. Med.,* **65:**808–814, 1978.

Laake, H.: The action of corticosteriods in the renal absorption of calcium. *Acta Endocrinol.,* **34:**60–64, 1960.

Laforet, E.; Berger, R.; and Vaughan, C.: Carcinoma obstructing the trachea. Treatment by laser resection. *N. Engl. J. Med.,* **295:**1579–1584, 1976.

Lajos, T. Z.; Black, H. E.; Cooper, R. G.; and Wanka, J.: Pericardial decompression. *Ann. Thorac. Surg.,* **19:**47–53, 1975.

Lambert, C. J.; Shah, H. H.; Urschel, H. C., Jr.; and Paulson, D. L.: The treatment of malignant pleural effusions by closed trocar tube drainage. *Ann. Thorac. Surg.,* **3:**1–5, 1967.

Laurent, J.; Derby, G.; and Floquet, J.: Hypoglycemic tumors. *Excerpta Medica,* Amsterdam, 1971.

Lawrence, L. T., and Cronin, J. F.: Electrical alternans and pericardial tamponade. *Arch. Intern. Med.,* **112:**415–418, 1963.

Lazor, M. Z., and Rosenberg, L. E.: Mechanisms of adrenal-steroid reversal of hypercalcemia in multiple myeloma. *N. Engl. J. Med.,* **270:**749–755, 1964.

Lee, D. B. N.; Zawada, E. T.; and Kleeman, C. R.: The pathophysiology and clinical aspects of hypercalcemic disorders. *West. J. Med.,* **129:**278–320, 1978.

Lee, R. E.: Radiotherapy for Lung Cancer. In Straus, M. J. (ed.): *Lung Cancer: Clinical Diagnosis and Treatment.* Grune & Stratton, Inc., New York, 1977.

Leff, A.; Hopewell, P. C., and Costello, J.: Pleural effusion from malignancy. *Ann. Intern. Med.,* **88:**532–537, 1978.

Leininger, B. J.; Barker, W. L.; and Langston, H. T.: A simplified method for management of malignant pleural effusion. *J. Thorac. Cardiovasc. Surg.,* **58:**758–763, 1969.

Levene, M.; Harris, J.; and Hellman, S.: Treatment of carcinoma of the breast by radiation therapy. *Cancer,* **39:**2840–2845, 1977.

Levine, H. L., and Olmstead, E. J.: Myelographic evaluation of nontraumatic spinal canal obstruction: A new approach. *A.J.R.,* **133:**715–718, 1979.

Levitt, L. J.; Dawson, D. M.; Rosenthal, D. S.; and Moloney, W. C.: CNS involvement in the non-Hodgkin's lymphomas. *Cancer,* **45**:545–552, 1980.

Lewit, T.; Karman, S.; Terracina, S.; and Beemer, A. M.: Malignant tumor of the trachea. *Chest,* **60**:498–499, 1971.

Libshitz, H., and Southard, M.: Complications of radiotherapy: The thorax. *Semin. Roentgenol.,* **9**:41–49, 1974.

Light, R. W.; MacGregor, M. I.; and Luchsinger, P. C.: Pleural effusions: The diagnostic separation of transudates and exudates. *Ann. Intern. Med.,* **77**:507–513, 1972.

Line, D., and Deeley, T. J.: Palliative therapy. In Deeley, T. J. (ed.): *Carcinoma of the Bronchus.* Appleton-Century-Crofts, New York, 1972.

Little, J. R.; Dale, A. J. D.; and Okazaki, H.: Meningeal carcinomatosis: Clinical manifestations. *Arch. Neurol.,* **30**:138–143, 1974.

Livingston, K. E., and Perrin, R. G.: The neurosurgical management of spinal metastasis causing cord and cauda equina compression. *J. Neurosurg.,* **49**:839–843, 1978.

Lo, A. M.; Evans, W. C.; and Carey, L. C.: Review of small bowel obstruction at Milwaukee County General Hospital. *Am. J. Surg.,* **111**:884–887, 1966.

Loening, S.; Carson, C. C.; and Faxon, D. P.: Ureteral obstruction associated with Hodgkin's disease. *J. Urol.,* **111**:345–349, 1974.

Lokich, J. J.: The management of malignant pericardial effusions. *J.A.M.A.,* **224**:1401–1404, 1973.

Lokich, J., and Garbo, C.: Leptomeningeal lymphoma: Perspectives on management. *Cancer Treat. Rev.,* **8**:102–110, 1981.

Lokich, J. J., and Goodman, R.: Superior vena cava syndrome. *J.A.M.A.,* **231**:58–61, 1965.

Lome, L. G.; Pinsky, S.; and Levy, L.: Dynamic renal scan in the non-visualizing kidney. *J. Urol.,* **121**:148–152, 1979.

Mahajan, V.; Strimlan, V.; Van Ordstrand, H. S.; and Loop, F. D.: Benign superior vena caval syndrome. *Chest,* **68**:32–35, 1975.

Mannheimer, I. H.: Hypercalcemia of breast cancer. *Cancer,* **18**:679–691, 1965.

Marcial, V. A.; Tome, J. M.; Ubinas, J.; Bosch, A.; and Correa, J. N.: The role of radiation therapy in esophageal cancer. *Radiology,* **87**:231, 1966.

Mark, J. B. D.; Goldberg, I. S.; and Montague, A. C.: Intrapleural mechlorethamine hydrochloride therapy for malignant pleural effusion. *J.A.M.A.,* **187**:858, 1964.

Marks, V.: Hypoglycemia: Other causes. *Clin. Endocrinol. Metab.,* **5**:769–782, 1976.

Marks, V., and Rose, F. C.: *Hypoglycemia.* Blackwell, Oxford, 1965.

Marsa, G. W., and Johnson, R. E.: Altered patterns of metastasis following treatment of Ewings sarcoma with radiotherapy and adjuvant chemotherapy. *Cancer,* **27**:1051–1054, 1971.

Marshall, L. F., and Langfitt, T. W.: Combined therapy for metastatic extradural tumors of the spine. *Cancer,* **40**:2067–2070, 1977.

Marsten, J. L.; Cooper, A. G.; and Ankeney, J. L.: Acute cardiac tamponade due to perforation of a benign mediastinal teratoma into the pericardial sac: Review of cardiovascular manifestations of mediastinal teratomas. *J. Thorac. Cardiovasc. Surg.,* **51**:700–707, 1966.

Martin, R. G.; Ruckdeschel, J. C.; Chang, P.; Byhardt, R.;

Bouchard, R. J.; and Wiernik, P. H.: Radiation-related pericarditis. *Am. J. Cardiol.,* **35**:216–220, 1975.

Martini, N.; Bains, M. S.; and Beattie, E. J., Jr.: Indications for pleurectomy in malignant effusion. *Cancer,* **35**:734–738, 1975.

Martini, N.; Freiman, A. H.; Watson, R. C.; and Harris, B. S.: Intrapericardial instillation of radioactive chromic phosphate in malignant pericardial effusion. *A.J.R.,* **128**:639–641, 1977.

Masland, D. S.; Rotz, C. T., Jr.; and Harris, J. H.: Post-radiation pericarditis with chronic pericardial effusion. *Ann. Intern. Med.,* **68**:97–102, 1968.

Mayer, G. P.; Keaton, J. A.; Hurst, J. G.; and Habener, J. F.: Effects of plasma calcium concentration on the relative proportion of hormonic and carboxyl fragments in parathyroid venous blood. *Endocrinology,* **104**:1778–1784, 1979.

Mayer, R. J.; Berkowitz, R. S.; and Griffiths, C. T.: Central nervous system involvement by ovarian carcinoma: A complication of prolonged survival with metastatic disease. *Proc. Am. Assoc. Cancer Res. and A.S.C.O.,* **19**:318, 1978.

Mazzaferri, E. L.; O'Dorisio, T. M.; and LaBuglio, A. F.: Treatment of hypercalcemia associated with malignancy. *Semin. Oncol.,* **5**:141–153, 1978.

McClennan, B. L., and Fair, W. F.: CT scanning in urology. *Urol. Clin. North Am.,* **6**:343–374, 1979.

McFadzean, A. J. S., and Yeung, R. T. T.: Further observations on hypoglycemia in hepatocellular carcinoma. *Am. J. Med.,* **47**:220–235, 1969.

McLellan, G.; Baird, C. W.; and Melick, R.: Hypercalcemia in an Australian hospital adult population. *Med. J. Aust.,* **2**:354–356, 1968.

McNamara, T. E., and Butkus, D. E.: Nephrostomy in patients with ureteral obstruction secondary to non-urologic malignancy. *Arch. Intern. Med.,* **140**:494–497, 1980.

McNeil, B. J.: Rationale for the use of bone scans in selected metastatic and primary bone tumors. *Semin. Nucl. Med.,* **8**:336–345, 1978.

Megalli, M. R.; Gursel, E. O.; Demirag, H.; Veenema, R. J.; and Guttman, R.: External radiotherapy in ureteral obstruction secondary to locally invasive prostatic cancer. *Urology,* **3**:562–564, 1974.

Megyesi, K.; Kahn, C. R.; Roth, J.; Froesch, E. R.; Humbel, R. E.; Zapf, J.; and Neville, D. M., Jr.: Insulin and nonsuppressible insulin-like activity: Evidence for separate plasma membrane receptor sites. *Biochem. Biophys. Res. Commun.,* **57**:307–315, 1974.

Melamed, M. R.: The cytologic presentation of malignant lymphomas and related diseases in effusions. *Cancer,* **16**:413–431, 1963.

Meyer, J. E.; Yatsuhashi, M., and Green, T. H., Jr.: Palliative urinary diversion in patients with advanced pelvic malignancy. *Cancer,* **45**:2698–2701, 1980.

Michigan, S., and Catalano, W. J.: Ureteral obstruction from prostatic carcinoma: Response to endocrine and radiation therapy. *J. Urol.,* **118**:733–738, 1977.

Millard, P. R.; Jerrome, D. W.; and Millward-Sadler, G. H.: Spindle-cell tumors and hypoglycemia. *J. Clin. Pathol.,* **29**:520–529, 1976.

Miller, P. D.; Linas, S. L.; and Schirer, R. W.: Plasma demeclocycline levels and nephrotoxicity, correlation in hyponatremic cirrhotic patients. *J.A.M.A.,* **243**:2513–2515, 1980.

Miller, R. D., and Hyatt, R. E.: Evaluation of obstructing lesions of the trachea and larynx by flow-volume loops. *Am. Rev. Respir. Dis.,* **108**:475–481, 1973.

Miller, S. I.; Wallace, R. J., Jr.; Mushner, D. M.; Septimus, E. J.; Kohl, S.; and Baughn, R. E.: Hypoglycemia as a manifestation of sepsis. *Am. J. Med.*, **68**:649–653, 1980.

Miller, W. E.: Roentgenographic manifestations of lung cancer. In Straus, M. J. (ed.): *Lung Cancer: Clinical Diagnosis and Treatment.* Grune & Stratton, New York, 1977.

Millman, A.; Meller, J.; Motro, M.; Blank, H. S.; Horowitz, I.; Herman, M.; and Teichholz, L. E.: Pericardial tumor or fibrosis mimicking pericardial effusion by echocardiography. *Ann. Intern. Med.*, **86**:434–436, 1977.

Minister, J. J.: Comparison of obstructing and nonobstructing carcinoma of the colon. *Cancer,* **17**:242–247, 1969.

Moertel, C. G.: Clinical management of advanced gastrointestinal cancer. *Cancer,* **36**:675–682, 1975.

Montana, G. S.; Meachum, W. F.; and Caldwell, W. L.: Brain irradiation for metastatic disease of lung origin. *Cancer,* **29**:1477–1480, 1972.

Morris, A. L.: Echo evaluation of tamponade. *Circulation,* **53**:746–747, 1976.

Moses, A. M.; Miller M.; and Streeten, D. H. P.: Pathophysiologic and pharmacologic alterations in the release and action of ADH. *Metabolism,* **25**:697–721, 1976.

Muggia, F. M., and Cassileth, P. A.: Constrictive pericarditis following irradiation therapy. *Am. J. Med.*, **44**:116–123, 1968.

Muggia, F. M., and Heinemann, H. O.: Hypercalcemia associated with neoplastic disease. *Arch. Intern. Med.*, **73**:281–290, 1970.

Mullan, J., and Evans, J. P.: Neoplastic disease of the spinal extradural space. *Arch. Surg.,* **74**:900–907, 1957.

Mundy, G. R.: Calcium and cancer. *Life Sci.,* **23**:1735–1744, 1978.

Mundy, G. R.; Luben, R. A.; Raisz, L. G.; Oppenheim, J. J.; and Buell, D. N.: Bone-resorbing activity in supernatants from lymphoid cell lines. *N. Engl. J. Med.,* **290**:867–871, 1974a.

Mundy, G. R., and Raisz, L. G.: Big and little forms of osteoclast activating factor. *J. Clin. Invest.,* **60**:122–128, 1977.

Mundy, G. R.; Raisz, L. G.; Cooper, R. A.; Schechter, G. P.; and Salmon, S. E.: Evidence for the secretion of an osteoclast stimulating factor in myeloma. *N. Engl. J. Med.,* **291**:1041–1046, 1974b.

Murphy, W. T., and Bilge, N.: Compression of the spinal cord in patients with malignant lymphoma. *Radiology,* **82**:495–500, 1964.

Murray, T. M.; Josse, R. G.; and Heersche, J. N. M.: Hypercalcemia and cancer: An update. *Can. Med. Assoc. J.,* **119**:915–920, 1978.

Murray, T.; Long, W.; and Narins, R. G.: Multiple myeloma and the anion gap. *N. Engl. J. Med.,* **292**:574–575, 1975.

Myers, W. P. L.: Hypercalcemia associated with malignant diseases. In *Endocrine and Nonendocrine Hormone-producing tumors.* Yearbook Medical Publishers, Inc., Chicago, 1973.

Neer, R.; Singer, F.; Habener, J.; Peacock, M.; and Murray, T.: Escape from calcitonin during therapy of hypercalcemia. *Clin. Res.,* **18**:676, 1970.

Ngan, H.: Involvement of the duodenum by metastases from tumors of the genital tract. *Br. J. Radiol.,* **43**:701–705, 1970.

Niarchos, A. P.: Electrical alternans in cardiac tamponade. *Thorax,* **30**:228–233, 1975.

Nisce, L. Z.; Hilaris, B. S.; and Chu, F. C. H.: A review of experience with irradiation of brain metastases *A.J.R.,* **111**:329–333, 1971.

Nogiere, C.; Mincer, F.; and Botstein, C.: The survival in patients with bronchogenic carcinoma complicated by superior vena caval obstruction. *Chest,* **75**:325–329, 1979.

North, W. G.; Maurer, H.; and O'Donnell, J. F.: Human neurophysins and small cell carcinoma. *Clin. Res.,* **27**:390A, 1979.

Norton, J. A., and Javapour, N.: Jejunal loop interposition in patients with ileal loop conduit failure after pelvic exenteration. *Am. J. Surg.,* **134**:404–407, 1977.

Nugent, J. L.; Bunn, P. A., Jr.; Matthews, M. J.; Ihde, D. C.; Cohen, M. H.; Gazdar, A.; and Minna, J. D.: CNS metastases in small cell bronchogenic carcinoma. Increasing frequency and changing pattern with lengthening survival. *Cancer,* **44**:1885–1893, 1979.

Nussbaum, H.; Allen B.; Kagan, R.; Gilbert, H. A.; Rao, A.; and Chan, P.: Management of bone metastases—Multidiscinplinary approach. *Semin. Oncol.,* **4**:93–97, 1977.

Odell, W. D., and Wolfsen, A. R.: Humoral syndromes associated with cancer. *Annu. Rev. Med.,* **29**:379–406, 1978.

Olsen, M. E.; Chernik, N. L.; and Posner, J. B.: Infiltration of the leptomeninges by systemic cancer. *Arch. Neurol.,* **30**:122–137, 1974.

O'Reilly, P. H.; Lawson, R. S.; Shields, R. A.; Testa, H. J.; Edwards, E. C.; and Carroll, R. N.: Diuresis renography in equivocal urinary tract obstruction. *Br. J. Urol.,* **50**:76–80, 1978.

Orringer, M. B., and Sloan, H.: Substernal gastric bypass of the excluded thoracic esophagus for palliation of esophageal carcinoma. *J. Thorac. Cardiovasc. Surg.,* **70**:836–851, 1975.

Osteen, R. T.; Guyton, S.; Steele, G., Jr.; and Wilson, R. E.: Malignant intestinal obstruction. *Surgery,* **87**:611–615, 1980.

Paladine, W.; Cunningham, T. J.; Sponzo, R.; Donavan, M.; Olson, K.; and Horton, J.: Intracavitary bleomycin in the management of malignant effusions. *Cancer,* **38**:1903–1908, 1976.

Papaioannou, A. N.: Tumors other than insulinomas associated with hypoglycemia. *Surg. Gynecol. Obstet.,* **123**:1093–1109, 1966.

Parrish, F. F., and Murray, J. A.: Surgical treatment for secondary neoplastic fractures. A retrospective study of 96 patients. *J. Bone Joint Surg.,* **52**:665–686, 1970.

Pathak, V.; Swaminathan, A. P.; Shuman, S. S.; Raina, S.; and Rush, B. F.: Intestinal obstruction in carcinomatosis. *Am. Surg.,* **46**:691–693, 1980.

Penn, C. R. H.: Single dose and fractionated palliative irradiation for osseous metastasis. *Clin Radiol.,* **27**:405–408, 1976.

Percarpio, B.; Price, J. C.; and Murphy, P.: Endotracheal irradiation of adenoid cystic carcinoma of the trachea. *Ther. Radiol.,* **128**:209–210, 1978.

Perez, C. A.; Bradfield, J. S.; and Morgan, H. C.: Management of pathologic fractures. *Cancer,* **29**:684–693, 1972.

Perez, C. A.; Presant, C. A.; and Van Amburg, A. L., III: Management of superior vena cava syndrome. *Semin. Oncol.,* **5**:123–134, 1978.

Perks, M. H.; Stanhope, R.; and Green, M.: Hyponatremia and mesothelioma. *Br. J. Dis. Chest,* **73**:89–91, 1979.

Perlia, C. P.; Gubisch, N. J.; Wolter, J.; Edelberg, D., Dederick, M. M., and Taylor, S. G.: Mithramycin treatment of hypercalcemia. *Cancer,* **25**:389–394, 1970.

Pfister, R. C., and Newhouse, J. H.: Interventional percutaneous nephrostomy and other procedures. *Radiol. Clin. North Am.,* **17**:351–363, 1979.

Pillay, V. K. G., and Dunea, G.: Clinical aspects of obstructive uropathy. *Med. Clin. North Am.,* **55**:1417–1427, 1971.

Pistenma, D. A.; McDougall, I. R.; and Kriss, J. P.: Screening for bone metastasis. *J.A.M.A.,* **231**:46–50, 1975.

Plimpton, C. H., and Gellhorn, A.: Hypercalcemia in malignant disease without evidence of bone destruction. *Am. J. Med.,* **21**:750–759, 1956.

Plovnick, H.; Ruderman, N. B.; Aoki, T.; Chideckel, E. W.; and Poffenbarger, P. L.: Non-B-cell tumor hypoglycemia associated with increased nonsuppressible insulin-like protein. *Am. J. Med.,* **66**:154–159, 1979.

Poffenbarger, P. L., and Boully, A.: Development of an immunoassay for human serum nonsuppressible insulin-like protein (NSILP). In James, V. H.: (ed.): *Proceedings of the 5th International Congress Endocrinology.* Elsevier, Hamburg, 1976.

Pool, J. L.; Ransohoff, J.; and Tornell, J. W.: The treatment of malignant brain tumors primary and metastatic. *N.Y. State J. Med.,* **57**:3983, 1957.

Pories, W. J., and Gaudiani, V. A.: Cardiac tamponade. *Surg. Clin. North Am.,* **55**:573–589, 1975.

Posner, J. B.: Management of central nervous system metastases. *Semin. Oncol.,* **4**:81–91, 1977.

Posner, J. B., and Chernik, N. L.: Intracranial metastases from systemic cancer. *Adv. Neurol.,* **19**:579–592, 1978.

Posner, J. B.; Howeison J.; and Cvitkovic, E.: Disappearing spinal cord compression: Oncologic effect of corticosteroids (and other chemotherapeutic agents) on epidural metastases. *Ann. Neurol.,* **2**:409–413, 1977.

Powell, D.; Singer, F. R.; Murray, T. M.; Minkin, C.; and Potts, J. T., Jr.: Non-parathyroid humoral hypercalcemia in patients with neoplastic diseases. *N. Engl. J. Med.,* **289**:176–181, 1973.

Powles, T. J.; Dowsch, M.; and Easty, G. C.: Breast cancer osteolysis, bone metastases, and antiosteolytic effect of aspirin. *Lancet,* **1**:608–610, 1976.

Price, R. A., and Johnson, W. W.: The central nervous system in childhood leukemia. *Cancer,* **31**:520–533, 1973.

Prine, M. J., and Poffenbarger, P. L.: Elevated serum nonsuppressible insulin-like protein levels in cancer patients. *Clin. Res.,* **26**:424A, 1978.

Ragland, J. J.; Londe, A. M.; and Spratt, J. S.: Correlation of the prognosis of obstructing colorectal carcinoma with clinical and pathologic variables. *Am J. Surg.,* **121**:552–556, 1971.

Raisz, L. G., and Niemann, I.: Effect of phosphate, calcium and magnesium on bone resorption and hormonal responses in tissue culture. *Endocrinology,* **85**:446–452, 1969.

Raisz, L. G.; Yajnik, C. H.; Bockman, R. S.; and Bower, B. B.: Comparison of commercially-available parathyroid hormone immunoassays in the differential diagnosis of hypercalcemia due to primary hyperparathryoidism or malignancy. *Ann. Med.,* **91**:739–740, 1979.

Ransohoff, J.: Surgical management of metastatic tumors. *Semin. Oncol.,* **2**:21–18, 1975.

Rastegar, A., and Thier, S. O.: The physiologic approach to hyperuricemia. *N. Engl. J. Med.,* **286**:470–476, 1972.

Richmond, J.; Sherman, R. S.; Diamond, H. D.; and

Craver, L. F.: Renal lesions associated with malignant lymphomas. *Am. J. Med.,* **32**:184–207, 1962.

Rieselbach, R. E.; Bentzel, C. J.; Cotlove, E.; Frei, E.; and Freireich, E. J.: Uric acid excretion and renal function in the acute hyperuricemia of leukemia. *Am. J. Med.,* **37**:872–884, 1964.

Rieselbach, R. E.; DeChiro, B.; Freireich, E. J.; and Rall, D. P.: Subarachnoid distribution of drugs after lumbar injection. *N. Engl. J. Med.,* **267**:1237–1278, 1962.

Rigler, L. G.: Roentgen diagnosis of small pleural effusions: New roentgenographic position. *J.A.M.A.,* **96**:104, 1931.

Rinderknecht, E., and Humbel, R. E.: Polypeptides with nonsuppressible insulin-like and cell growth–promoting activities in human serum: Isolation, chemical characterization, and some biological properties of forms I and II. *Proc. Natl. Acad. Sci. USA,* **73**:2365–2369, 1976.

Rinderknecht, E., and Humbel, R. E.: The amino acid sequence of human insulin-like growth factor and its structural homology with proinsulin. *J. Biol. Chem.,* **253**:2769–2776, 1978.

Robertson, R. P.; Baylink, D. J.; Metz, S. A.; and Cummings, K. B.: Plasma prostaglandin-E in patients with cancer with and without hypercalcemia. *J. Clin. Endocrinol. Metab.,* **43**:1330–1335, 1976.

Robinson, R. R., and Yarger, W. E.: Acute uric acid nephropathy. *Arch. Intern. Med.,* **137**:839–840, 1977.

Rodichok, L. D.; Harper, G. R.; Ruckdeschel, J. C.; Roberson, G.; Barron, K. D.; and Horton, J.: Early diagnosis of spinal epidural metastases. *Am. J. Med.,* **70**:1181–1188, 1981.

Rodriguez, M., and Dinapoli, R. P.: Spinal cord compression with special reference to metastatic epidural tumors. *Mayo Clin. Proc.,* **55**:442–448, 1980.

Rosato, F. E.; Wallach, M. W.; and Rosato, E. F.: The management of malignant effusions from breast cancer. *J. Surg. Oncol.,* **6**:441–449, 1974.

Rose, R. G.: Intracavitary radioactive colloidal gold: Results in 257 cancer patients. *J. Nucl. Med.,* **3**:323–331, 1962.

Rosenblatt, M. B.; Lisa, J. R.; and Trinidad, S.: Pitfalls in the clinical and histologic diagnosis of bronchogenic carcinoma. *Dis. Chest,* **40**:296–404, 1966.

Rostrom, A. Y., and Morgan, R. L.: Results of treating primary tumours of the trachea by irradiation. *Thorax,* **33**:387–393, 1978.

Roswit, B.; Kaplan, G.; and Jacobsen, H. G.: The superior vena cava obstruction syndrome in bronchogenic carcinoma. *Radiology,* **61**:722–737, 1953.

Rubenstein, A. H.; Kuzuya, H.; and Horwitz, D. L.: Clinical significance of circulating C-peptide in diabetes and hypoglycemia disorders. *Arch. Med.,* **137**:625, 1977.

Rubenstein, L. J.; Herman, M. M.; Long, T. F.; and Wilbur, J. R.: Disseminated necrotizing leukoencephalopathy: A complication of treated central nervous system leukemia and lymphoma. *Cancer,* **35**:291–305, 1975.

Rubin, P.: Extradural spinal cord compression by tumor. Part I: Experimental production and treatment trials. *Radiology,* **93**:1243–1248, 1969.

Rubin, P., and Ciccio, S.: High daily dose for rapid decompression. In Deeley, T. J. (ed.): *Modern Radiotherapy: Carcinoma of the Bronchus.* Appleton-Century-Crofts, New York, 1971.

Rubin, P.; Green, J.; Holzwasher, G.; and Gerle, R.: Superior vena caval syndrome. Slow low dose versus rapid high dose schedules. *Radiology,* **81**:388–401, 1963.

Rubin, P.; Mayer, E.; and Poulter, C.: Extradural spinal

cord decompression by tumor. Part I: High daily dose experience without laminectomy. *Radiology,* **93:**1248 – 1260, 1969.

Rubinson, R. M., and Bolooki, H.: Intrapleural tetracycline for control of malignant pleural effusion: A preliminary report. *South. Med. J.,* **65:**847 – 849, 1972.

Russell, J. M., and Resnick, M. I.: Ultrasound in urology. *Urol. Clin. North Am.,* **6:**445 – 468, 1979.

Ryan, J. R.; Rowe, D. E.; and Salciccioli, G. G.: Prophylactic internal fixation of the femur for neoplastic lesions. *J. Bone Joint Surg.,* **58A:**1071 – 1074, 1976.

Sahn, E. E., and Robinson, W. A.: Spinal cord compression in lymphoma. *Am. J. Med. Sci.,* **276:**93 – 98, 1978.

Salsali, M., and Cliffton, E. E.: Superior vena caval obstruction with carcinoma of the lung. *Surg. Gynecol. Obstet.,* **121:**783 – 788, 1965.

Salyer, W. R.; Eggleston, J. C.; and Erozan, Y. S.: Efficacy of pleural needle biopsy and pleural fluid cytopathology in the diagnosis of malignant neoplasm involving the pleura. *Chest,* **67:**536 – 539, 1975.

Samaan, N. A.; Hickey, R. C.; Sethi, M. R.; Yang, K. P.; and Wallace, S.: Hypercalcemia in patients with known malignant disease. *Surgery,* **80:**382 – 389, 1976.

Sandberg, A. A.; Cartwright, G. E.; and Wintrobe, M. M.: Studies on Leukemia. I. Uric acid excretion. *Blood,* **11:**154 – 166, 1956.

Sanderson, D. R.; Neel, H. B.; and Fontana, R. S.: Bronchoscopic cryotherapy. *Ann. Otol. Rhinol. Laryngol.,* **90:**354 – 358, 1981.

Schechter, M. M.: The superior vena cava syndrome. *Am. J. Med. Sci.,* **227:**46 – 56, 1954.

Schold, S. C.; Wasserstrom, W. R.; Fleisher, M.; Schwartz, M.; and Posner, J. B.: Cerebrospinal fluid biochemical markers of central nervous system metastasis. *Ann. Neurol.,* **8:**597 – 604, 1980.

Schraufnagel, D. F.; Hill, B.; Leech, J. A.; and Pare, A. P.: Superior vena caval obstruction. Is it a medical emergency? *Am. J. Med.,* **70:**1169 – 1174, 1981.

Scott, R. W., and Garvin, C. F.: Tumors of the heart and pericardium. *Am. Heart J.,* **17:**431 – 436, 1939.

Segaloff, A.: Managing endocrine and metabolic problems in the patient with advanced cancer. *J.A.M.A.,* **245:**177 – 179, 1981.

Seyberth, H. W.; Segre, G. V.; Morgan, J. L.; Sweetman, B. J.; Potts, J. T., Jr.; and Oates, J. A.: Prostaglandins as mediators of hypercalcemia associated with certain types of cancer. *N. Engl. J. Med.,* **293:**1278 – 1283, 1975.

Shabetai, R.; Fowler, N. O.; and Guntheroth, W. B.: The hemodynamics of cardiac tamponade and constrictive pericarditis. *Am. J. Cardiol.,* **26:**480 – 489, 1970.

Shapiro, M.; Simcha, A.; Rosenmunn, E.; and Shafir, E.: Hypoglycemia associated with neonatal neuroblastoma and abnormal responses of serum glucose and free fatty acids to epinephrine injection. *Isr. J. Med. Sci.,* **2:**705 – 714, 1966.

Shapiro, W. R.; Chernik, N. L.: and Posner, J. B.: Necrotizing encephalopathy following intraventricular instillation of methotrexate. *Arch. Neurol.,* **28:**96 – 102, 1973.

Shapiro, W. R.; Posner, J. B.; Ushio, Y.; Chernik, N. L.; and Young, D. F.: Treatment of meningeal neoplasms. *Cancer Treat. Rep.,* **61:**733 – 743, 1977.

Shapiro, W. R.; Young, D. F.: and Mehta, B. M.: Methotrexate: Distribution in cerebrospinal fluid after intravenous, ventricular and lumbar injection. *N. Engl. J. Med.,* **293:**161 – 166, 1975a.

Shapiro, W. R.; Young, D. F.; and Posner, J. B.: Treatment of leptomeningeal neoplasm with intraventricular

methotrexate and ARA-C. *Proc. Am. Assoc. Cancer Res. and A.S.C.O.,* **16:**190, 1975b.

Shehata, W. M.; Hendrickson, F. R.; and Hindo, W. A.: Rapid fractionation technique and re-treatment of cerebral metastases by irradiation. *Cancer,* **34:**257 – 261, 1974.

Sherwood, L. M.; O'Riordan, J. L. H.; Aurback, G. D.; and Potts, J. T.: Production of parathyroid tumor. *J. Clin. Endocrinol. Metab.,* **27:**140 – 146, 1967.

Sherwood, L. W.: The multiple causes of hypercalcemia in malignant disease. *N. Engl. J. Med.,* **303:**1412 – 1413, 1980.

Shimm, D. S.; Logue, G. L.; and Rigsby, L. C.: Evaluating the superior vena cava syndrome. *J.A.M.A.,* **245:**951 – 953, 1981.

Shiner, P. T.; Harris, W. S.; and Weissler, A. M.: Effects of acute changes in serum calcium levels on the systolic time intervals in man. *Am. J. Cardiol.,* **24:**42 – 48, 1969.

Shuttleworth, E., and Allen, N.: CSF B-glucuronidase assay in the diagnosis of neoplastic meningitis. *Arch. Neurol.,* **37:**684 – 687, 1980.

Silbert, S. K.; Rossini, A.; Ghazvinian, S.; Widrich, W. C.; Marks, L. J.; and Sawin, C. T.: Tumor hypoglycemia. Deficient splanchnic output and deficient glucagon secretion. *Diabetes,* **25:**202 – 206, 1976.

Silver, C. E.: Surgical management of neoplasms of the larynx, hypopharynx, and cervical esophagus. *Curr. Probl. Surg.,* **14:**9, 1977.

Silverberg, I. J., and Jacobs, E. M.: Treatment of spinal cord compression in Hodgkin's disease. *Cancer,* **27:**308 – 313, 1971.

Singer, I., and Rotenberg, D.: Demeclocycline-induced nephrogenic diabetes insipidus. *Ann. Intern. Med.,* **79:**679 – 683, 1973.

Sise, J. G., and Crichlow, R. W.: Obstruction due to malignant tumors. *Semin. Oncol.,* **5:**213 – 224, 1978.

Skrabanek, P.; McPartlin, J.; and Powell, D.: Tumor hypercalcemia and "ectopic hyperparathyroidism." *Medicine,* **59:**262 – 282, 1980.

Skrabanek, P., and Powell, D.: Ectopic insulin and Occam's razor: Reappraisal of the riddle of tumor hypoglycemia. *Clin. Endocrinol.,* **9:**141 – 154, 1978.

Smith, A. D.; Lange, P. H.; Miller, R. P.; and Reinke, D. R.: Introduction of the Gibbons ureteral stent facilitated by antecedent percutaneous nephrostomy. *J. Urol.,* **120:**543 – 544, 1978.

Smith, E. H., and Bartrum, R. J.: Ultrasound and renal failure. In Griffiths, H. J. (ed.): *Radiology of Renal Failure.* W. B. Saunders Company, Philadelphia, 1976.

Smith, F. E.; Lane, M.; and Hudgins, P. T.: Conservative management of malignant pericardial effusions. *Cancer,* **33:**47 – 57, 1974.

Spaulding, S. W., and Walser, M.: Treatment of experimental hypercalcemia with oral phosphate. *J. Clin. Endocrinol. Metab.,* **31:**531 – 538, 1970.

Spencer, H. W.; Yarger, W. E.; and Robinson, R. E.: Alterations of renal function during dietary-induced hyperuricemia in the rat. *Kidney Int.,* **9:**489 – 500, 1976.

Spodick, D. H.: Acute cardiac tamponade: Pathologic physiology, diagnosis, and management. *Prog. Cardiovasc. Dis.,* **10:**64 – 96, 1967.

Spodick, D. H., and Kumar, S.: Subacute constrictive pericarditis with cardiac tamponade. *Dis. Chest,* **54:**62 – 66, 1968.

Stefanini, P.; Carboni, M.; Patrassi, N.; and Basoli, A.: Beta islet cell tumors of the pancreas: Results of a study on 1067 cases. *Surgery,* **75:**597 – 609, 1974.

Steiger, Z.; Nickel, W. D.; Wilson, R. F.; and Arbuw, A.:

Improved surgical palliation of advanced carcinoma of the esophagus. *Am J. Surg.,* **135**:782–784, 1978.

Steinberg, I.: Effusive-constrictive radiation pericarditis. Two cases illustrating value of angiocardiography in diagnosis. *Am. J. Cardiol.,* **19**:434–439, 1976.

Steinberg, S. M.; Galen, M. A.; Lazarus, J. M.; Lowrie, E. G.; Hampers, C. L.; and Jaffe, N.: Hemodialysis for acute uric acid nephropathy. *Am. J. Dis. Child.,* **129**:956–958, 1975.

Stewart, A.; Horst, R.; Deftos, L.; Cadman, E.; Lang, R.; Rasmussen, H.; and Broadus, A.: A non-PTH renotropic factor in humoral hypercalcemia of malignancy. *Clin. Res.,* **27**:377 (abstr.), 1979.

Stewart, A. F.; Horst, R.; Deftos, L. J.; Cadman, E. C.; Lang, R.; and Broadus, A. E.: Biochemical evaluation of patients with cancer-associated hypercalcemia. *N. Engl. J. Med.,* **303**:1377–1383, 1980.

Stewart, J. R.; Cohn, K. E.; Fajardo, F.; Hancock, E. W.; and Kaplan, H. S.: Radiation induced heart disease. A study of twenty-five patients. *Radiology,* **89**:302–310, 1967.

Stewart, W. R.; Gelberman, R. H.; Harrelson, J. M.; and Seigler, H. F.: Skeletal metastases of melanoma. *J. Bone Joint Surg.,* **60A**:645–649, 1978.

Strober, S. J.; Klotz, E.; Kuperman, A.; and Ghossein, N. A.: Malignant pleural disease—A radiotherapeutic approach to the problem. *J.A.M.A.,* **226**:296–299, 1973.

Suki, W. N.; Yium, J. J.; and Von Minden, M.: Acute treatment of hypercalcemia with furosemide. *N. Engl. J. Med.,* **283**:836–842, 1970.

Sytman, A. L., and Mac Alpin, R. N.: Primary pericardial mesothelioma: Report of two cases and review of the literature. *Am. Heart J.,* **81**:760–769, 1971.

Tashjian, A. H.: Prostaglandins, hypercalcemia, and cancer. *N. Engl. J. Med.,* **293**:1317–1318, 1975.

Tashjian, A. H. Jr.; Voelkel, E. F.; Goldhaber, P.; and Levine, L.: Prostaglandins, calcium metabolism and cancer. *Fed. Proc.,* **33**:81–86, 1974.

Tashjian, A. H.; Voelkel, E. F.; Levine, L.; and Goldhaber, P.: Evidence that the bone resorption-stimulating factor produced by mouse fibrosarcoma cells is prostaglandin E_2: A new model for the hypercalcemia of cancer. *J. Exp. Med.,* **136**:1329–1343, 1972.

Tattersall, M. H. N.: Intracavitary adriamycin, nitrogen mustard, and tetracycline in the control of malignant effusions. *Med. J. Aust.,* **2**:447–448, 1980.

Teplick, J. G., and Haskin, M. E.: Diseases of the bone. In Teplick, J. G., and Haskin, M. E. (eds.): *Roentgenologic Diagnosis.* W. B. Saunders Company, Philadelphia, 1971.

Terry, L. N., and Kligerman, M. M.: Pericardial and myocardial involvement by lymphomas and leukemias: The role of radiotherapy. *Cancer,* **25**:1003–1008, 1970.

Theologides, A.: Neoplastic cardiac tamponade. *Semin. Oncol.,* **5**:181–192, 1978.

Thomas, A. N.: Treatment of malignant esophageal obstruction by endoesophageal intubation. *Am. J. Surg.,* **128**:306–314, 1974.

Thomas, T. H.; Morgan, D. B.; and Swaminathan, R.: Severe hyponatremia: A study of 17 patients. *Lancet,* **1**:621–624, 1978.

Thurber, D. L.; Edwards, J. E.: and Achoe, R. W. P.: Secondary malignant tumors of the pericardium. *Circulation,* **26**:228–241, 1962.

Torma, T.: Malignant tumors of the spine and the spinal extradural space: A study based on 250 histologically verified cases. *Acta Chir. Scand. [Suppl.]* **225**:1–176, 1957.

Trotter, J. M.; Stuart, J. E. B.; MacBeath, F.; McVie, J. G.; and Calman, K. C.: The management of malignant effusions with bleomycin. *Br. J. Cancer,* **40**:316, 1979.

Trump, D. L.: Serious hyponatremia in patients with cancer. *Cancer,* **47**:2908–2912, 1981.

Trump, D. L.; Abeloff, M. D.; and Baylin, S. B.: Studies of water and cortisol metabolism in patients with small cell bronchogenic carcinoma and other neoplasms. *Proc. Am. Soc. Clin. Oncol.,* **21**:320, 1980.

Ulin, A. W.; Declement, F. A.; and James, P. M.: Large bowel obstruction due to carcinoma. *Am. Fam. Physician,* **3**:79–84, 1971.

Ulin, A. W., and Ehrlich, E. W.: Current views related to management of large bowel obstruction caused by carcinoma of the colon. *Am. J. Surg.,* **104**:463–467, 1962.

Ultman, J. E.: Diagnosis and treatment of neoplastic effusions. *Cancer,* **12**:42–50, 1962.

Ultman, J. E.; Gellhorn, A.; Osnos, M.; and Hirschberg, E.: The effect of quinacrine on neoplastic effusions and certain of their enzymes. *Cancer,* **16**:283–288, 1963.

Unger, J. D.; Chiang, L. C.; and Unger, G. F.: Apparent reformation of the base of the skull following radiotherapy for nasopharyngeal carcinoma. *Radiology,* **126**:779–782, 1978.

Unger, R. H.: The riddle of tumor hypoglycemia. *Am. J. Med.,* **40**:325–330, 1966.

Ushio, Y.; Posner, R.; Kim, J. H.; Shapiro, W. R.; and Posner, J. B.: Treatment of experimental spinal cord compression by epidural neoplasms. *J. Neurosurg.,* **37**:380–390, 1977a.

Ushio, Y.; Posner, R.; Posner, J. B.; and Shapiro, W. R.: Experimental spinal cord compression by epidural neoplasms. *Neurology,* **27**:422–429, 1977b.

Van Dyke, A. H., and van Nagell, J. R.: The prognostic significance of ureteral obstruction in patients with recurrent carcinoma of the cervix uteri. *Surg. Gynecol. Obstet.,* **141**:371–373, 1975.

Van Heerden, J. A.; Edis, A. J.; and Service, F. J.: The surgical aspects of insulinomas. *Ann. Surg.,* **189**:677–682, 1979.

Van Houtte, P.; DeJager, R.; Lustman-Maréchal, J.; and Kenis, Y.: Prognostic value of the superior vena cava syndrome as the presenting sign of small cell anaplastic carcinoma of the lung. *Eur. J. Cancer,* **16**:1447–1450, 1980.

Van Houtte, P., and Fruhling, J.: Radionuclide venography in the evaluation of superior vena cava syndrome. *Clin. Nucl. Med.,* **6**:177–183, 1981.

Van Wyck, J. J.; Underwood, L. E.; Baseman, J. B.; Hintz, R. L.; Clemmons, D. R.; and Marshall, R. N.: Exploration of the insulin-like and growth promoting properties of somatomedin by membrane receptor assays. *Adv. Metab. Disord.,* **8**:128–150, 1975.

Vaughn, C. B., and Vaitkevigius, V. K.: The effects of calcitonin in hypercalcemia in patients with malignancy. *Cancer,* **34**:1268–1271, 1974.

Vaughn, P. B., and Brindley, H. H.: Pathologic fractures of long bones. *South. Med. J.,* **72**:788–794, 1979.

Veen, H. F.; Oscarson, J. E. A.; and Malt, R. A.: Alien cancers of the duodenum. *Surg. Gynecol. Obstet.,* **143**:39–42, 1976.

Veith, R. G., and Odom, G. L.: Intracranial metastases and their neurosurgical treatment. *J. Neurosurg.,* **23**:375–383, 1965.

Voelkel, E. F.; Tashjian, A. H., Jr.; Franklin, R.; Wasserman, E.; and Levine, L.: Hypercalcemia and tumor-prostaglandins: The VX 2 carcinoma model in the rabbit. *Metabolism,* **24**:973–986, 1975.

Voss, D. M., and Drake, E. H.: Cardiac manifestations of hyperparathyroidism with presentation of a previously unreported arrhythmia. *Am. Heart J.,* **73:**235–239, 1967.

Wang, J. J., and Pratt, C. B.: Intrathecal arabinosyl cytosine in meningeal leukemia. *Cancer,* **25:**531–534, 1970.

Wara, W. M.; Mauch, P. M.; Thomas, A. N.; and Phillips, T. L.: Palliation for carcinoma of the esophagus. *Radiology,* **121:**717–720, 1976.

Warren, F. J.; Leitch, A. G.; and Leggett, R. J.: Hyperuricemic acute renal failure after epileptic seizures. *Lancet,* **2:**385–387, 1975.

Washington, J. A.; Holland, J. M.; and Ketchum, A. S.: Return of renal function following diversion of the obstructed ureter. *Cancer,* **18:**1457–1461, 1965.

Wasserstrom, W. R.; Glass, J. P.; and Posner, J. B.: Diagnosis and treatment of leptomeningeal metastases from solid tumors: Experience with 90 patients. *Cancer,* **49:**759–772, 1982.

Watters, N. A.: Survival after obstruction of the colon by carcinoma. *Can. J. Surg.,* **12:**124–128, 1969.

Weber, A. L., and Grillo, H. C.: Tracheal tumors: Radiological, clinical and pathological evaluation. *Adv. Otorhinolaryngol.,* **24:**170–176, 1978a.

Weber, A. L., and Grillo, H. C.: Tracheal tumors: A radiological, clinical and pathological evaluation of 84 cases: *Radiol. Clin. North Am.,* **16:**227–246, 1978b.

Weick, J. K.; Kiely, J. M.; Harrison, E. G.; Carr, D. T.; and Scanlon, P. W.: Pleural effusion in lymphoma. *Cancer,* **31:**848–853, 1973.

Weisberger, A. S.; Levine, B.; and Storaasli, J. P.: Use of nitrogen mustard in treatment of serous effusions of neoplastic origin. *J.A.M.A.,* **159:**1704–1707, 1955.

Weisel, W.; Lepley, D., Jr.; and Watson, R. R.: Respiratory tract adenomas. A ten year survey. *Ann. Surg.,* **154:**898–902, 1961.

Welch, J. P., and Donaldson, G. A.: Management of severe obstruction of the large bowel due to malignant disease. *Am. J. Surg.,* **127:**492–499, 1974.

Wengraf, C.: Oat cell carcinoma of the trachea. *J. Laryngol,* **84:**267–274, 1970.

West, J., and Moor, M.: Intracranial metastases: Behavioral patterns related to primary site and results of treatment by whole brain irradiation. *Int. J. Radiat. Oncol. Biol. Phys.,* **6:**11–15, 1980.

Westling, P.: Studies of the prognosis in Hodgkin's disease. *Acta Radiol.* [suppl.] *(Stockh.),* **245:**5–125, 1965.

White, W. A.; Patterson, R. H.; and Bergland, R. M.: Role of surgery in the treatment of spinal cord compression by metastatic neoplasm. *Cancer,* **27:**558–561, 1971.

Wild, W. O., and Parker, R. W.: Metastatic epidural tumor of the spine. A study of 45 cases. *Arch. Surg.,* **87:**137–142, 1963.

Williams, G., and Peet, T. N. D.: Bilateral ureteral ob-

struction due to malignant lymphoma. *Urology,* **7:**649–651, 1976.

Williams, G., and Soutter, L.: Pericardial tamponade. *Arch. Intern. Med.,* **94:**571–584, 1954.

Wilson, C. B.: Brain metastases: The basis for surgical selection. *Int. J. Radiat. Oncol. Biol. Phys.,* **2:**169–172, 1977.

Wilson, D. R.: Pathophysiology of obstructive nephropathy. *Kidney Int.,* **18:**281–292, 1980.

Winston, K. R.; Walsh, J. W.; and Fisher, E. G.: Results of operative treatment of intracranial metastatic tumors. *Cancer,* **45:**2639–2645, 1980.

Woods, P.: Chronic constrictive pericarditis. *Am. J. Cardiol.,* **7:**48–61, 1961.

Wright, F. S., and Howard, S. S.: Obstructive injury. In Brenner, B. M., and Rector, F. C., Jr. (eds.): *The Kidney,* 2nd ed. W. B. Saunders Company, Philadelphia, 1981.

Yap, H. Y.; Yap, B. S.; Tashima, C. K.; DiStefano, A.; and Blumenschein, G. R.: Meningeal carcinomatosis in breast cancer. *Cancer,* **42:**283–286, 1978.

Yoshimura, H.; Kazama, S.; Asari, H.; Itoh, H.; Tominaga, S.; and Ishihara, A.: Lung cancer involving the superior vena cava: Pneumonectomy with concomitant partial resection of the superior vena cava. *J. Thorac. Cardiovasc. Surg.,* **77:**83–86, 1979.

Young, D.; Posner, J.; Chu, F.; and Neisce, F.: Rapid course radiation therapy of cerebral metastases: Results and complications. *Cancer,* **34:**1069–1076, 1974.

Young, D. F.; Shapiro, W. R.; and Posner, J. B.: Treatment of leptomeningeal cancer. *Neurology,* **25:**370, 1975.

Zapf, J.; Rinderknecht, E.; Humbel, R. E.; and Froesch, E. R.: Nonsuppressible, insulin-like activity from human serum: Recent accomplishments and their physiologic implications. *Metabolism,* **27:**1803–1828, 1978a.

Zapf, J.; Schoenle, E.; and Froesch, E. R.: Insulin-like growth factors I and II: Some biological actions and receptor binding characteristics of two purified constituents of nonsuppressible insulin-like activity of human serum. *Eur. J. Biochem.,* **87:**285–296, 1978b.

Ziegler, J. L.; Blumming, A. S.; Fass, L.; and Morrow, R. H., Jr.: Relapse patterns in Burkitt's lymphoma. *Cancer Res.,* **32:**1267–1272, 1972.

Ziegler, J. L.; Morrow, R. H.; Fass, L.; Kyalwazi, S. K.; and Carbone, P. P.: Treatment of Burkitt's tumor with cyclophosphamide. *Cancer,* **26:**474–484, 1970.

Zipf, R. E., Jr., and Johnston, W. W.: The role of cytology in the evaluation of pericardial effusions. *Chest,* **62:**593–596, 1972.

Zuckerman, K. S.; Skarin, A. T.; Pitman, S. W.; Rosenthal, D. S.; and Canellos, G. P.: High-dose methotrexate with citrovorum factor in the treatment of advanced non-Hodgkin's lymphoma including CNS involvement. *Blood,* **48:**983, 1971.

41

Infectious Considerations in Cancer

STEPHEN H. ZINNER and JEAN KLASTERSKY

Patients with neoplastic disorders are at increased risk of infection, either because of their underlying disease, the treatment for their underlying disease, or as a result of prolonged hospitalization. The underlying disease in many cases dictates the type of antitumor therapy which, in turn, influences the degree of increased risk for infection. The type of infection likely to occur in patients with cancer is fairly predictable and, in a large part, these infections are potentially preventable and often treatable. For a comprehensive understanding of this problem, it is important to review the mechanisms of acquisition of infections in patients with cancer, some of the specific immune defects induced by cancer and its treatment, the clinical manifestations of infection, an approach to treatment of infection in these patients, and, finally, the preventive measures shown to be useful in reducing infections in patients with neoplastic disease.

MECHANISM OF ACQUISITION OF INFECTIONS

Changes in Endogenous Microflora

Much of the risk of infection in patients with cancer is associated with prolonged hospitalization and suppression of normal host defenses resulting from chemotherapy (see Table 41–1). Approximately half of these infections are the result of endogenous microflora present on admission to the hospital. The remainder are from organisms acquired during the hospital stay. These organisms colonize various mucosal and skin sites and are likely to be more virulent and resistant to more anti-microbial agents than the organisms present on admission (Schimpff *et al.,* 1972b). Organisms responsible for bacteremia in profoundly neutropenic patients may be found colonizing various body sites before development of bacteremia. Colonization of the nasopharynx with potentially pathogenic gram-negative rods directly correlates with severity of illness (Johanson *et al.,* 1969). Colonization with *Candida tropicalis* but not *Candida albicans* is predictive of subsequent invasive fungal infection (Sandford *et al.,* 1980).

Local Effects of Tumor Growth

Primary skin tumors (*e.g.,* squamous cell carcinoma, mycosis fungoides) or secondary skin lesions produce erosive or ulcerative lesions which may predispose to local infection and bacteremia with *Staphylococcus aureus* or group A *β*-hemolytic streptococcus. In the oral cavity and nasopharynx, ulcerating carcinomas may predispose to local infection with streptococci, pneumococci, or *Haemophilus* species. Mixed anaerobic necrotizing infections may begin in the mouth, nose, or throat and may invade facial bones with subsequent osteomyelitis, or may spread to the meninges with subsequent meningitis, and/or paramen-ingeal, or intracerebral abscess formation. Ulceration along the gastrointestinal tract may occur with locally invasive neoplasms or as a result of therapy for acute leukemia. These rents in the mucosal barrier may result in local abscess formation, actinomycosis, or gram-negative rod bacteremia. Invasive organisms may enter the circulation from skin or mucous membrane sites damaged by radiation to adja-

Table 41–1. Some Likely Pathogens in Patients with Cancer

PREDISPOSING CONDITION	ORGANISMS
Skin lesions	*Staphylococcus aureus* *Staphylococcus epidermis* *Streptococcus pyogenes*
Oral cavity lesions Nasopharyngeal carci- noma	Streptococci *Streptococcus pneumoniae* (pneumococcus) *Haemophilus* species Anaerobes
Gastrointestinal ulcer- ation	*Actinomyces* species Gram-negative rods
Bronchial obstruction	Anaerobes Streptococci Gram-negative rods
Intestinal obstruction	*Bacteroides fragilis et al.*
Acute lymphocytic leu- kemia Altered T-cell function Hodgkin's disease	*Mycobacterium tuberculosis* *Listeria monocytogenes* *Salmonella* species *Cryptococcus neoformans* *Nocardia asteroides* *Candida* species *Torulopsis glabrata* *Aspergillus* species *Mucor* species *Pneumocystis carinii* *Toxoplasma gondii* Cytomegalovirus Herpes simplex virus Varicella-zoster virus
Splenectomy Myeloma Waldenström's *macroglobulinemia*	*Streptococcus pneumoniae* *Haemophilus influenzae* *Neisseria meningitidis* *Klebsiella pneumoniae*
Neutropenia Acute leukemia	*Staphylococcus aureus* *Staphylococcus epidermidis* *Escherichia coli* *Klebsiella pneumoniae* *Pseudomonas aeruginosa* *Candida* species *Aspergillus* species

cent tumors. Ulcerating neoplasms of the female genital tract may result in invasive infection caused by enterococci, anaerobic or aerobic gram-negative rods, or *Clostridia* species.

Another local effect of tumor growth is obstruction at various sites. Tumor-related obstruction of a bronchus or a bronchiolar segment results in the retention of mucous secretions and subsequent infection distal to the obstruction. Pneumonia and lung abscess may develop caused by proliferation of normally commensal mouth flora including streptococci, *Bacteroides* species, *Fusobacte-rium,* or spirochetes. *Streptococcus pneumoniae* (pneumococcus) may produce this infection if acquired outside the hospital, although pathogenic gram-negative rods such as *Klebsiella* and *Pseudomonas aeruginosa* are likely pathogens in hospitalized patients. Patients with esophageal obstruction or dysfunction secondary to neoplasia are prone to aspiration of bacteria-laden oral secretions with subsequent development of necrotizing pneumonitis, lung abscess, and bronchopleural fistula with purulent empyema. Frequent aspiration is often a consequence of laryngeal and posterior nasopharyngeal carcinoma.

Invasive and obstructing lesions in the gastrointestinal tract often result in bowel perforation with subsequent peritonitis and intra-abdominal abscess formation. Anaerobic organisms normally present in the fecal flora, such as *Actinomyces,* may proliferate at a site of tumor-induced necrosis along the gastrointestinal tract. Suppurative actinomycosis may result, with typical draining sinuses to the abdominal wall.

Tumors that obstruct the structures of the genitourinary tract produce hydronephrosis or pyonephrosis. Carcinomas of the lower urinary tract and bladder, and pelvic tumors that obstruct urinary outflow, result in increased amounts of residual urine which, in turn, fosters the development of persistent or recurrent urinary tract infections. Normally, micturition protects against infection by removing introduced bacteria. This protection is lost with significant obstruction or dysfunction. Similarly, tumors obstructing vascular beds in the pelvic region, or elsewhere, may result in thrombophlebitis, which may become secondarily infected. Bacteremia resulting from obstruction often reflects the location of the primary lesion. For example, intestinal obstruction is associated with *Bacteroides fragilis* bacteremia; urinary tract obstruction is associated with *Escherichia coli* or other facultative gram-negative rod bacteremia.

Metastatic tumor to bone marrow may be associated with a general increased risk of infection as a result of myelophthisis, thus impairing normal bone marrow elements. Myeloid metaplasia and myelofibrosis may result from widespread bone marrow metastasis. Myelophthisic marrows occur most frequently with metastatic carcinoma of breast, prostate, lung, kidney, adrenal, thyroid, or in malignant melanoma. Severe bone marrow involvement may occur with Hodgkin's disease and more often with other lymphomas, with resulting neutropenia.

Immunologic Effects of Neoplastic Disease

Patients with advanced neoplasms of any type are likely to have nonspecific defects in both humoral and cellular immunity which may contribute to their increased risk of serious infection. More specific defects in T-cell – or B-cell – mediated immune function may be present inherently in a variety of untreated neoplastic disorders.

Abnormalities in the cellular-mediated immune system have been described as inherent features of some untreated neoplasms. Patients with untreated Hodgkin's disease have decreased delayed hypersensitivity responses to recall antigens such as mumps, histoplasmin, Candida, and PPD. Not all such patients manifest these defects, and they may be rather subtle in untreated stage I or stage II Hodgkin's disease. The number of circulating T- lymphocytes may be normal when determined by anti-T cell antibodies, although the ability to form E rosettes is decreased in advanced Hodgkin's disease and may be slightly depressed in patients with early disease. Some evidence suggests that this latter defect may be caused by a serum-inhibiting factor. The T-lymphocyte response to phytohemagglutinin and the ability to proliferate in mixed lymphocyte cultures, however, are depressed in these patients. Patients with tumors of the head and neck may also manifest some defects of cell-mediated immunity.

Acute lymphoblastic leukemia (ALL) in childhood of the usual non-B, non-T type is not associated with definite abnormalities in T-cell function prior to chemotherapy. Some studies have suggested that delayed hypersensitivity to recall antigens is abnormal in these patients. Normal children, however, also may not respond to these antigens. Depressed cell-mediated immunity in untreated patients with ALL has been reported. Certainly, cell-mediated immunity is severely depressed during intensive chemotherapy for this and other neoplasms.

Patients whose primary immune defect is altered cell-mediated immunity are at increased risk of disseminated infections with intracellular bacteria such as *Mycobacterium tuberculosis, Listeria monocytogenes, Salmonella* species, and *Brucella* species. These patients are also at special risk of contracting DNA-viral infections such as cytomegalovirus, herpes simplex virus, and varicella-zoster virus. Patients with T-cell defects also are at risk of acquiring yeast infections and, in particular, meningitis and pulmonary infection with *Cryptococcus neoformans,* and disseminated infection with *Candida* species, *Torulopsis glabrata, Mucor,* and *Aspergillus* species. Specific alterations in T-cell function, such as altered ratio of T-helper to T-suppressor lymphocytes, have been associated with increased risk of pneumonia from *Pneumocystis carinii.* Other organisms, such as *Toxoplasma gondii* and *Nocardia asteroides,* also may cause disseminated infection in these patients.

A new form of immunodeficiency was described in 1981. The acquired immunodeficiency syndrome (AIDS) has been seen primarily in young homosexually active men, intravenous drug addicts, Haitian refugees, and patients with hemophilia. A few cases have occurred in recipients of blood transfusions and in sexual contacts of high-risk persons. These patients present with Kaposi's sarcoma (see Chapter 20) and/or opportunistic infections caused by *Pneumocystis carinii,* herpesvirus hominis, cytomegalovirus, *Candida albicans, Cryptococcus neoformans, Mycobacterium tuberculosis, Mycobacterium avium intracellulare, Cryptosporidium* species, *Isospora belli, Toxoplasma gondii,* and so forth. Cerebral and other lymphomas have been described. The syndrome is associated with anergy to recall and new skin test antigens, lymphopenia, with reduced numbers and depressed function of the T4 subset of T lymphocytes (recently designated as T4+, Leu 8+, TQ1+ by the monoclonal antibodies recognizing these lymphocytes). In vitro, lymphocytes from patients with AIDS show decreased responsiveness to mitogens and antigens, as well as diminished release of interleukin-2. B-cell activity is increased, hypergammaglobulinemia may be present, and these patients show a reduced ability to synthesize antibody in response to new antigens. The syndrome is due to a lymphotrophic retrovirus designated as human T-lymphotrophic virus III (HTLV-III), AIDS-associated virus (AAV) and lymphadenopathy-associated virus (LAV). Currently, no treatment is available and the mortality rate is more than 40%, and is higher in patients with opportunistic infections.

Alteration in B-lymphocyte immune function is likely to occur in patients with untreated chronic lymphocytic leukemia, multiple myeloma, and Waldenström's macroglobulinemia. Patients with acute myelocytic leukemia and acute lymphocytic leukemia before treatment and patients with Hodgkin's disease before splenectomy, irradiation, or chemotherapy have intact B-cell immunity, although the numbers of normal B cells may be reduced in some individuals with lymphocytic leukemia. Since B-cell immunity mediates humoral or antibody-related immunity, immunoglobulin antibody levels may be decreased, and these patients may exhibit decreased responsiveness to antigenic stimulation.

Patients with multiple myeloma have increased levels of immunoglobulin which does not react with bacterial antigens and does not protect against infection. These patients, as well as those with Waldenström's macroglobulinemia, have decreased polyclonal immunoglobulin response to bacterial antigens.

Patients with defects in humoral antibody are most susceptible to infection with encapsulated bacteria such as *Streptococcus pneumoniae, Haemophilus influenzae, Neisseria meningitidis,* and *Klebsiella pneumoniae.*

Effects of Treatment for Neoplastic Disease

Many chemotherapeutic agents (see Chapter 10) induce bone marrow suppression with neutropenia. Neutropenia may also occur after total-body irradiation. Some cytotoxic drugs inhibit neutrophil function, such as migration and chemotaxis, and large doses of corticosteroids may inhibit neutrophil killing activity.

Bacteremia is the ultimate result of granulocytopenia or impaired neutrophil function. Nearly all patients who remain profoundly neutropenic (<100 circulating neutrophils per mL^3) become infected by the third week of neutropenia, or earlier. Patients with lesser degrees of neutropenia have a somewhat lower frequency of bacterial infection, but this risk is increased with the duration of granulocyte depression (Bodey *et al.*, 1966). Bacteremia in severely neutropenic patients is most often caused by *Escherichia coli, Klebsiella pneumoniae, Pseudomonas aeruginosa,* or *Staphylococcus aureus.* The distribution of these infections may depend upon local hospital flora, as well as the colonization of the gastrointestinal tract and other body sites before onset of bacteremia. Other organisms including *Serratia marcescens, Enterobacter, Aeromonas,* *Proteus* species, and *Acinetobacter* species may also cause bacteremia in neutropenic patients. *Bacteroides fragilis* bacteremia occurs, but is relatively uncommon in neutropenic patients with leukemia, unless there is associated invasive or obstructive disease of the gastrointestinal or genitourinary tracts. Invasive fungal infections caused by *Aspergillus fumigatus, Candida albicans, Candida tropicalis, Mucor* species, and other agents may occur in severely neutropenic patients. These infections may occur simultaneously with bacterial infections or may develop during antibiotic therapy for a primary bacterial infection. Cellular immune factors are also involved in the defense against fungi.

Patients with profound neutropenia may have defective leukocyte mobilization, and they may not be able to limit bacterial invasion locally. Thus, they show few of the usual signs of inflammation, such as swelling, tenderness and heat over the affected area. Abscess formation may be limited. Local infection may appear more subtle and be more easily overlooked than that in otherwise normal hosts. Radiologic findings of pneumonia, for example, may not be present at the onset of infection, and a radiologic infiltrate may not appear until several days after pneumonitis has developed. Frequent X-ray films of the chest should be obtained in neutropenic patients with fever in order to identify pneumonia as a possible source.

Many chemotherapeutic agents (see Chapter 10) may produce severe ulcerations in the mucous membranes of the oropharynx and the esophagus, as well as the small and large bowel. These ulcers may be the site of invasion and eventual bacteremia or fungemia secondary to locally contaminating gram-negative bacteria or fungi. These lesions may also lead to anorectal abscesses. Chemotherapeutic agents that irritate the venous endothelium may produce phlebitis and subsequent bacteremia.

Radiation therapy, as well as corticosteroids and several chemotherapeutic agents, may produce cellular immune defects by means of lympholytic or other actions. Splenectomy patients may have deficient complement production and may also have limited ability to opsonize and clear bacterial pathogens (Ravy *et al.*, 1972). Combination of chemotherapy, splenectomy, and radiation therapy may predispose patients to overwhelming infection with encapsulated bacterial pathogens, such as

S. pneumoniae and *H. influenzae.* Extensive surgery, often necessary for advanced invasive tumors, may predispose to infection by removing large areas of otherwise protective tissue.

Iatrogenic Factors

All hospitalized patients are at risk of acquiring potentially pathogenic organisms during their confinement. Several procedures that bypass the ordinary host defenses are associated with an increased risk of infection in hospitalized patients. Plastic intravenous catheters have been implicated as a major source of nosocomial bacteremia, and the risk of this infection increases with the duration of catheterization. Antibiotic and antiseptic agents applied to the catheter site have not produced significant reductions in rates of bacteremia. Plastic catheters should not be used during prolonged periods of granulocytopenia; steel venous needles or short butterfly-type needles are preferable. Some centers routinely use Hickman or Broviak cannulae, which are inserted surgically. The intravenous tubing and the administered fluid itself should be treated with utmost care and changed every two days.

Infections associated with the use of respiratory ventilators and tracheostomy are not uncommon in patients with cancer, especially in the immediate postoperative period. Nosocomial pneumonia may develop from colonization of various parts of the respiratory therapy apparatus, and pathogenic organisms may be spread from patient to patient by the hands of hospital personnel.

Urinary bladder catheters are well-known sources of bacteremic infection in all hospitalized patients. The use of these devices should be severely limited in patients with cancer who are at increased risk of infection, and careful maintenance of closed sterile drainage with daily meatal care is essential.

CLINICAL MANIFESTATIONS OF INFECTIONS

The clinical presentations of infection in patients with cancer may be influenced by the condition of the host. Although an attempt is made to separate infections in neutropenic patients from those in immunosuppressed patients, some patients with cancer may be both neutropenic and immunosuppressed, and

some of these infections may occur in both types of patients. Patients with cancer may also present with infection at more than one site and with more than one infecting organism at any given site.

Neutropenic Patients

Fever. Fever is extremely common in compromised patients and may be a presenting sign of many neoplastic diseases. The clinician must decide whether fever reflects the presence of infection or is the result of another process. Prolonged and sophisticated evaluation of fever, however, is rarely possible in these patients since infection in the compromised or neutropenic host often has a rapidly unfavorable course in the absence of prompt and appropriate therapy.

In a neutropenic patient, fever should be considered to indicate the presence of infection, unless proven otherwise (see Table 41 – 2). This important principle in managing these patients implies that therapy must often be undertaken without knowledge of the precise microbiologic nature of the infecting organisms. Such empiric therapy is particularly indicated in neutropenic patients and in those with humoral immune deficiencies who often present with disseminated bacterial infection. Empiric therapy should be directed at the most likely microbiologic possibilities and should be undertaken as soon as bacteriologic specimens are obtained. As a general rule, microbiologic documentation of febrile episodes will be obtained in about 40% of neutropenic patients; in half of these, bacteremia will be documented. In the remaining febrile neutropenic patients, no precise microbiologic documentation of infection can be established, although many will respond clinically to empiric treatment with broad-spectrum antibiotics (E.O.R.T.C., International Antimicrobial Therapy Project Group, 1978).

Table 41 – 2. Probability of Infection in Neutropenic Patients with Fever

	%
Microbiologically documented	16 – 20
Bacteremia	20 – 21
Clinically documented	20 – 21
Possible infection	17 – 20
Infection doubted	17 – 26

Modified from the E.O.R.T.C. International Antimicrobial Therapy Project Group, 1978, 1983b.

Long-standing fever without obvious cause may be present in 1% of patients admitted to a cancer service (Klastersky *et al.,* 1973). In most of these patients, fever is ultimately proven to be caused by infection, but, occasionally, it may be attributed to the neoplastic process in patients with acute leukemia, lymphoma, and extensive cancer, especially if hepatic metastases are present. Infection of hepatic tumor by anaerobic bacteria is often suspected, but not always proven. Other noninfectious diseases, such as thrombophlebitis with pulmonary embolism, and various iatrogenic procedures, such as blood-product transfusion, administration of pyrogenic medications (*e.g.,* bleomycin), or allergic reactions should be considered. When such noninfectious causes can be recognized readily, empiric therapy of presumed infection is not necessary.

Bacteremia. Many studies, including large cooperative trials (E.O.R.T.C. International Antimicrobial Therapy Project Group, 1978), have established that bacteremia can be demonstrated in about 20% of neutropenic patients presenting with fever. During the past few years, however, preventive measures such as reduction of organism acquisition, microbial suppression, and prompt use of empiric antibiotics, have markedly reduced the frequency of bacteremia. The organisms most frequently isolated are *S. aureus* and gramnegative bacilli, such as *P. aeruginosa, E. coli,* and *Klebsiella* sp. Infections caused by *Staphylococcus epidermidis* are increasing.

The common primary sources of bacteremia include pneumonia, anal lesions, and pharyngitis. Urinary bladder and venous catheters are also frequently associated with bacteremia. Notwithstanding the benign appearance of lesions at these sites, they are major sources for bacteremia in neutropenic patients. Fever may be the only sign of bacteremia in neutropenic patients because of inadequate neutrophil-mediated response, which may obscure the clinical signs and symptoms of local infection.

Vasomotor failure (septic shock) may occur in neutropenic patients as a result of bacteremia, even if empiric therapy is undertaken rapidly. In this situation, often either the underlying neoplastic disease has progressed beyond any reasonable curative or palliative therapy, or the empiric antimicrobial therapy was inadequate.

Fungemia occurs in neutropenic leukemic patients and is frequently accompanied by bacteremia. *Candida tropicalis* fungemia with widespread tissue invasion has been reported with increasing frequency (Edwards *et al.,* 1978; Jones, 1981) (see Figure 41–1). Fungemia caused by *Candida* species may be present with fungal endophthalmitis, often before positive blood cultures. Orbital pain, decreased visual acuity, clouding of the vitreous with white, or fluffy exudates in the vitreous or retina may be noted.

Pneumonia. Pneumonia is common in both neutropenic and immunosuppressed patients. In more than 75% of neutropenic patients with pneumonia, the infection is caused by gram-negative bacilli (*Pseudomonas aeruginosa, Escherichia coli, Klebsiella* species) and *Staphylococcus aureus.* The remaining infections are caused by viruses, *Nocardia,* or fungal pathogens, among which, *Aspergillus* species or *Candida* species are implicated most commonly. Pulmonary pathogens, such as *Streptococcus pneumoniae,* influenza virus, *Cryptococcus neoformans,* cytomegalovirus, *Toxoplasma gondii* or *Pneumocystis carinii* which often cause pneumonia in patients with solid tumors or in immunocompromised hosts, tend to produce pneumonia less commonly in neutropenic patients. Similarly, *Mycoplasma* species, *Legionella* species, and *Mycobacterium tuberculosis* are not frequent causes of primary pneumonia in neutropenic patients, but any of these organisms may cause infection in the presence of immunosuppressive drugs such as corticosteroids.

Because of the poor inflammatory response associated with severe granulocytopenia, few or no physical findings are present at first examination, and the chest x-ray film may be normal. Minimal physical findings usually become apparent within a few days, however, and usually an infiltrate eventually develops on the chest x-ray film. Both the physical examination and radiography must be repeated daily to ensure adequate detection of pneumonia in the neutropenic patient with fever (Sickles *et al.,* 1975).

Sputum production is usually minimal and consists of nonpurulent material. It may be of little diagnostic value because the pharynx of many hospitalized patients is colonized with gram-negative bacilli. To what extent the culture of potential bacterial or fungal pathogens from the upper respiratory tract is indicative of the causative agent of pneumonia has not yet been established. The gram-stained sputum

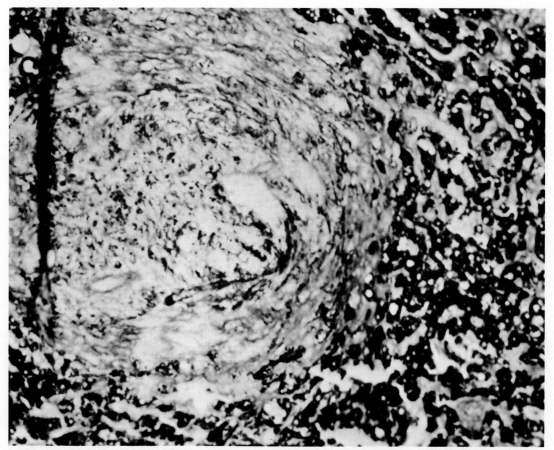

Figure 41–1. Gomori's methenamine silver stain of liver from a patient with acute myelocytic leukemia and disseminated *Candida tropicalis* infection. (Courtesy of Dr. Lewis Johnson, Roger Williams General Hospital.)

smear may be misleading because polymorphonuclear leukocytes are present only in small numbers. Respiratory epithelial cells and mixed oral-tracheal flora may confuse the interpretation of the smear. More sophisticated diagnostic procedures, such as transtracheal aspiration, transtracheal selective bronchial brushing, percutaneous lung aspirate, or lung biopsy, are often required in order to establish an etiologic diagnosis. These invasive procedures, however, are difficult to perform in severely ill and thrombocytopenic patients requiring prompt antimicrobial therapy. When pneumonia is caused by bacterial pathogens in a neutropenic patient, the blood cultures are positive in as many as 60% of cases. Multiple blood cultures should be obtained in neutropenic patients with pneumonia.

The differential diagnosis of pneumonitis in the neutropenic patient is often difficult. Specific etiologies may not be determined if blood cultures are negative, and more defin-

itive biopsies are not possible. Noninfectious causes, such as radiation pneumonitis, pulmonary embolism, leukoagglutinin reaction, spread of tumor, or leukemic infiltration, and chemotherapy-related pneumonitis (*e.g.,* bleomycin, cyclophosphamide, busulfan, methotrexate) should be considered.

Diagnostic clues may be available. Patients in remission or receiving maintenance chemotherapy who acquire infections outside the hospital may be infected with *S. pneumoniae* or influenza virus. The likelihood of developing gram-negative bacterial or staphylococcal pneumonia increases with the duration of hospitalization and is usually associated with relapse or induction chemotherapy in the case of leukemia. The specific organism acquired in the hospital and its antibiotic susceptibility may vary with the local hospital environment.

The onset of pulmonary infection secondary to bacterial pathogens is usually acute and rapid, whereas that caused by fungi, *Nocardia,*

Mycobacteria, and *Pneumocystis carinii* is more gradual. Patients with overwhelming bacterial or viral pneumonitis are frequently hypoxemic (with arterial $Po_2 < 65$ mm Hg), whereas those with fungal, tuberculous, or nocardial infection are well oxygenated (Rubin and Greene, 1981). Bacterial pneumonitis is more likely to spread rapidly than pneumonia resulting from other types of pathogens.

The radiologic appearance of a lung infiltrate is rarely diagnostic, but may help limit the range of diagnostic possibilities in both neutropenic and immunosuppressed patients. Table 41–2 outlines some of the clinical and roentgenologic features of infection with the major opportunistic pulmonary pathogens in both neutropenic and immunosuppressed patients. No single finding is specific, and additional measures are necessary to confirm the diagnosis (see below).

In one series of patients with hematologic neoplasms (Pennington and Feldman, 1977), localized consolidation or cavitation was most frequent with bacterial infections, followed by fungal infection, whereas *P. carinii* and viral pneumonias more often presented as diffuse interstitial infiltrates. Multiple abscesses and infected pneumatoceles may be formed with *Staphylococcus aureus* infections. *Klebsiella pneumoniae* may produce a necrotizing lobar pneumonitis with cavitation and swelling of the lobe, and *Pseudomonas aeruginosa* may cause a bacteremic pneumonitis, in the neutropenic patient. In this infection, necrotizing vasculitis and nodular infarcts may occur in the pulmonary parenchyma (Williams *et al.,* 1976). *Nocardia asteroides, Mycobacteria* species, *Legionella* species, and DNA viruses are more likely to cause infection in immunosuppressed hosts rather than in neutropenic patients.

Aspergillus or *Mucor* pneumonia may produce increasing areas of consolidation with hemorrhagic infarction, pleuritic pain, and hemoptysis, often suggesting a diagnosis of pulmonary embolism. Early in the course of aspergillus infection in neutropenic patients, few clinical or radiologic findings may be present. Pulmonary infiltrates may develop after days or weeks of infection and may imply

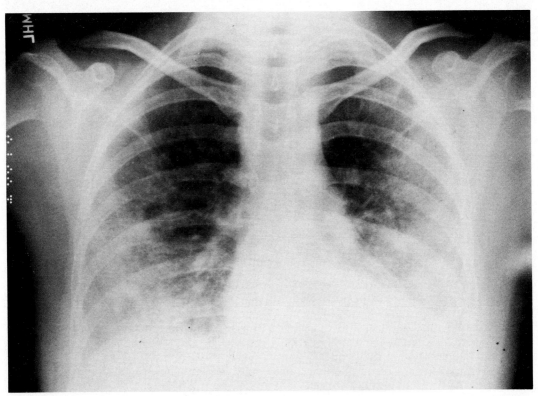

Figure 41–2. Chest X-ray from a patient with *Pneumocystis carinii* pneumonia. (Courtesy of Dr. Sidney Braman, Rhode Island Hospital.)

imminent death. Early therapy with amphotericin, possibly initiated empirically, may
prove necessary.

Candida albicans and *C. tropicalis* may
produce miliary abscesses or lobar infiltrates in
neutropenic patients, often following treatment for a bacterial pneumonia. As with
aspergillosis, early findings may be limited,
and the diagnosis is often made at *post mortem*
examination. *Cryptococcus neoformans* may
cause solitary or multiple nodules, lobar consolidation, or diffuse pneumonitis, and infection may disseminate to the meninges and
elsewhere, even with relatively minimal pulmonary lesions. Other fungi including *Histoplasma capsulatum, Coccidioides immitis,* or
Blastomyces dermatitidis may cause interstitial, alveolar, or nodular infiltrates.

Pneumocystis carinii, a probable protozoan
agent, produces pneumonia in patients with
acute lymphocytic leukemia, chronic lymphocytic leukemia, and immunosuppressed individuals with a variety of underlying diseases
(see Figures 41 – 2, 41 – 3). Fever, hypoxia, and
cyanosis with early bilateral perihilar interstitial infiltrates are common. Spread of infiltrate
to the peripheral lung fields develops later, but
consolidation with mediastinal sparing, with
or without pleural effusions, also has been described. Prophylactic trimethoprim-sulfamethoxazole successfully prevents this infection in children with acute lymphocytic
leukemia (Hughes *et al.,* 1977).

Oral and Pharyngeal Infections. Infection
of the oropharynx may be the first sign of acute
leukemia or granulocytopenia, but this infection more commonly follows the administration of cytotoxic chemotherapy. With bacterial, fungal, or viral pharyngitis, the patient
complains of severe pharyngeal pain, difficulty
in swallowing, fever, and chills. The throat is
erythematous, but without exudate; cervical

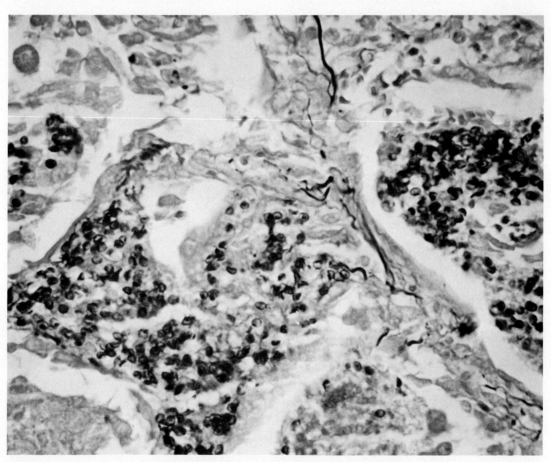

Figure 41 – 3. Biopsy of lung from a patient with *Pneumocystis carinii* pnemonia stained with Gomori's methenamine silver.

adenopathy is not always present, although the patient may complain of tenderness on palpation. Because of the poor inflammatory response, most of these cases of pharyngitis initially appear remarkably benign.

Throat cultures yield multiple organisms, such as gram-negative bacilli and *Staphylococcus aureus.* In the absence of positive blood cultures, it is difficult to decide which organism is actually responsible for the pharyngitis. As in pneumonia, an initial viral or mycoplasma infection may be followed by invasion of bacterial pathogens. When the oropharyngeal mucosa presents with the characteristic white ulcerative lesions of candidiasis, the etiology is obvious. *Candida* species frequently cause pharyngitis and may seriously limit swallowing. Uncomplicated *Candida* stomatitis or pharyngitis rarely results in candidemia.

Sinusitis is not very common in neutropenic patients. When present, however, identifying the responsible pathogenic agent is essential, although invasive diagnostic procedures may be hazardous because of accompanying thrombocytopenia. Although most viruses, *S. pneumoniae, Staphylococcus aureus,* and gram-negative bacilli cause most cases, the presence of acute sinusitis in a neutropenic patient should raise the suspicion of mucormycosis or aspergillosis.

Skin and Soft Tissue Infections. These infections are very often iatrogenic and related to sites of trauma by venipunctures, bone marrow aspiration, or surgical wounds. Areas of ecchymosis can also become superinfected. Spontaneous skin infection also occurs, and minor axillary or groin folliculitis may progress to large abscesses with bloodstream dissemination.

Most of these infections are caused by *Staphylococcus aureus,* but gram-negative rods, including *Pseudomonas aeruginosa,* may be involved, especially in periorbital or perianal cellulitis. Viral infection of the skin is relatively uncommon in the neutropenic patient. When present, however, varicella-zoster and herpes simplex virus infections may be-

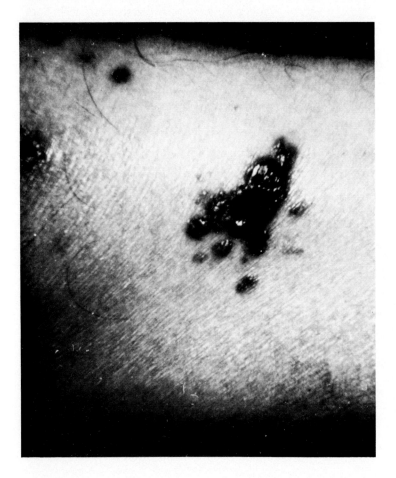

Figure 41–4. Ecthyma gangrenosum. Widely spaced necrotic skin lesions in a neutropenic patient with *Pseudomonas aeruginosa* bacteremia.

come superinfected by bacterial pathogens and develop extensive secondary cellulitis. In neutropenic patients, the skin is also a secondary site of many infections, for example, ecthyma gangrenosum in *Pseudomonas aeruginosa* bacteremia (see Figure 41–4), papular lesions in disseminated candidiasis, or the lesions of cryptococcosis (Figure 41–5) and nocardiosis.

The skin also can be the site of neoplasms, especially in leukemia and lymphomas, as well as of nonspecific manifestations of neoplastic disease (*e.g.*, pyoderma gangrenosum). These noninfectious lesions can be difficult to distinguish from skin infections and usually require biopsy to establish the precise diagnosis.

Anorectal Infections.   Infection of the anorectal area typically occurs in leukemic granulocytopenic patients, especially those with acute monocytic or myelomonocytic leukemia. True abscesses are uncommon, since most infections present as anal fissures or inflamed hemorrhoids. Extensive perineal cellulitis may develop, and hemorrhagic necrotic material, but rarely frank pus, is aspirated from the lesions. These lesions are extremely

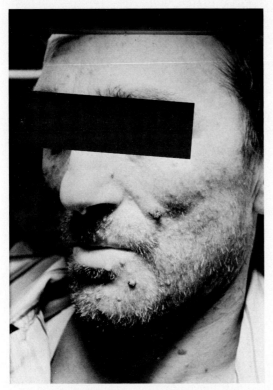

Figure 41–5.   Cutaneous involvement in a patient with disseminated *Cryptococcus neoformans* infection.

painful at examination or during bowel movements. Even when they appear relatively benign, they can result in bacteremia.

Pseudomonas aeruginosa and, less commonly, *E. coli* and *Klebsiella* species are usually responsible for anorectal infections in neutropenic patients. Aspiration of the cellulitis may also yield gram-positive cocci and anaerobic gram-negative rods, such as *Bacteroides* species. Bacteremia from this site is usually caused by *P. aeruginosa* and, to a lesser extent, *E. coli* or *Klebsiella* species. Infections in the perirectal area are frequently overlooked. Daily rectal examinations should be performed in febrile neutropenic patients without any obvious site of infection. The use of prophylactic, oral, nonabsorbable antibiotics may have decreased the incidence of perianal and perirectal lesions in granulocytopenic patients. Radiation therapy to the leukemic infiltrates underlying these infected sites may be associated with improved outcome.

Esophagitis and Colitis.   The esophagus is an important site of infection in neutropenic patients, because the combination of cytotoxic mucosal alteration and gastric acid reflux predisposes to microbial invasion. Most cases are caused by *Candida* species; however, early esophagoscopy with biopsy frequently implicates herpes simplex virus or gram-negative bacilli. Esophagitis presents with burning substernal pain or dysphagia or both. The diagnosis should be confirmed by esophagoscopy with biopsy. Barium swallow reveals a ragged mucosa, but does not differentiate fungal from viral or bacterial esophagitis.

Necrotizing lesions of the colon occur frequently in patients with neoplasia. These lesions have been identified chiefly in autopsy studies and may be pseudomembranous, necrotic, or ischemic. Most of these patients die from bacteremia caused by intestinal flora. Patients with necrotizing colitis are most often granulocytopenic and have received antineoplastic and antimicrobial therapy during the weeks preceding their terminal illness. Stomatitis and necrotizing pharyngitis, as well as abdominal pain and distention, are associated with this type of colitis. Whether these lesions are primarily infectious or represent superinfection of preexisting lesions is unclear. Regardless of etiology, they permit access of bacteria from the large bowel into the bloodstream.

Urinary Tract Infection.   Urinary tract infection is relatively uncommon in neutropenic patients with leukemia. Most often a specific predisposing factor is present, such as a catheter or other form of instrumentation, obstruction of the urinary tract, or recurrent urinary tract infection. When present in a neutropenic patient, the infection often results in bacteremia. Strict adherence to a catheter care program is the best protection against sepsis from the urinary tract and results in a marked reduction of urinary tract infections in neutropenic patients. As with other sites, the minimal inflammatory response limits the diagnostic value of dysuria and pyuria. Diagnosis depends on examination of the urinary sediment and quantitative urine cultures.

Immunosuppressed Patients

Patients with neoplastic disorders may be immunosuppressed for a few days to several weeks or months, depending on the nature of therapy directed at the primary disease. A variety of opportunistic infections may occur, and there is some overlap with infections occurring in neutropenic patients. More than one organism may cause infection at the same or separate sites in immunosuppressed patients.

Pneumonitis. Pulmonary infiltrates are extremely common in febrile immunosup-

pressed patients. *Mycobacterium tuberculosis,* atypical *Mycobacteria, Nocardia asteroides, Legionella pneumophila* and other species, *Candida* species, *Phycomycetes, Cryptococcus neoformans, Histoplasma capsulatum, Coccidioides immitis,* herpes simplex virus, cytomegalovirus, varicella-zoster, *Pneumocystis carinii, Toxoplasma gondii,* and *Strongyloides stercoralis* may produce pneumonitis in these patients (Table 41–3). Few specific diagnostic clinical or radiologic clues exist. Fever and nonproductive cough are usually present with all of these infections. Significant early hypoxia is most suggestive of *Pneumocystis carinii* infection, but this may also occur with cytomegalovirus, varicella-zoster, *Legionella* species, and other bacterial infections. As outlined in Table 41–3, x-ray film findings are rarely diagnostic, but certain patterns are suggestive. Lobar or bronchopneumonic infiltrates are consistent with bacterial pneumonia and infection with *Candida* species, *Aspergillus* species, and the *Phycomycetes.* Interstitial infiltrates are usually observed with viral and protozoan infections. Cavitation occurs with mycobacterial and nocardial infections, but also may be seen with *Aspergillus, Cryptococcus, Phycomycetes,* and, rarely, with *Legionella* infections. Nodular infiltrates may

Table 41–3. Suggestive Clinical and Radiologic Clues to the Presence of Pulmonary Infection in Patients with Cancer

ORGANISM	USUAL SETTING	CLINICAL FEATURES	RADIOLOGIC FINDINGS
I. Bacteria			
a. *Staphylococcus aureus*	Neutropenia, antibiotic therapy, hospital associated, postinfluenza	Fever, chills, cough and sputum	Bronchopneumonia, rapid spread, pneumatoceles, multiple abscesses
b. *Klebsiella pneumoniae*	Neutropenia, hospital associated, antibiotic therapy	Fever, chills, cough dyspnea, thick sputum, hemoptysis	Lobar infiltrate, swollen edematous lobe with bulging fissure
c. *Pseudomonas aeruginosa*	Neutropenia, antibiotic therapy, hospital associated	Fever, chills, cough, hemoptysis	Bronchopneumonia, nodular infiltrates; congestion, edema, necrotizing process
d. *Legionella pneumophila* and related sp. *(L. micdadei)*	Immunosuppression, corticosteroids, hospital associated	Fever, cough, chills, dyspnea, hypoxemia, ↑ liver function tests, hypophosphatemia, renal failure	Patchy infiltrates, progressing to multilobar consolidation; cavitation and pleural effusions occasionally
e. *Mycobacterium tuberculosis*	Hodgkin's disease, lymphosarcoma, reticulum cell sarcoma, sarcoma of lung, corticosteroids	Fever, weight loss, night sweats, fulminant tuberculous, pneumonia	Apical foci, pleural effusions, miliary nodules, diffuse infiltrates, cavities
f. Atypical mycobacteria	Lymphoma, corticosteroids, acquired immunodeficiency syndrome (AIDS)	Fever, weight loss, night sweats, cough, other organ dissemination	Upper lobe apical foci, nodular infiltrates, and pleural effusions
g. *Nocardia asteroides*	Immunosuppression, corticosteroids	Fever, dry cough, pleuritis, pain, also malaise, may be asymptomatic early	Localized lobar or segmental infiltrates, single or multiple nodular densities, thick-walled abscess cavities

Table 41–3.   *(continued)*

ORGANISM	USUAL SETTING	CLINICAL FEATURES	RADIOLOGIC FINDINGS
II. Fungi			
a. *Candida albicans* and other sp.	Neutropenia, acute leukemia, immunosuppression, diabetes, antibiotics	Fever, chills, nonspecific symptoms, minimal clinical findings early	Extensive multilobar bronchopneumonia (often follows treatment for bacterial pneumonia), may show miliary abscesses
b. *Aspergillus* sp.	Neutropenia, leukemia	Cough, fever, dyspnea, pleuritic pain, hemoptysis	Necrotizing bronchopneumonia, hemorrhagic infarction, patchy infiltrates, nodular densities, cavitation, may be negative early
c. *Phycomycetes* (*Mucor, Rhizopus* sp.)	Neutropenia, leukemia, lymphoma, diabetes	Fever, cough, nonspecific symptoms, hemoptysis, pleural rub	Patchy infiltrates, bronchopneumonia, consolidation, cavity formation
d. *Cryptococcus neoformans*	Lymphoma, immunosuppression, Hodgkin's disease, leukemia	Cough, chest pain, low-grade fever, may be asymptomatic	Single-mass lesion ± cavity, multiple small nodules, lobar, segmental, consolidation, diffuse pneumonitis
III. Viruses			
a. Herpes simplex	Immunosuppression	Tracheobronchitis, pneumonitis associated with oral or esophageal lesions	Focal or disseminated infiltrates
b. Varicella-zoster	Hodgkin's disease, lymphoma, immunosuppression, acute leukemia	Dyspnea, dry cough, wheezing, rash, eruption	Bilateral peribronchiolar, nodular infiltrates, apical sparing
c. Cytomegalovirus	Leukemia, Hodgkin's disease, immunosuppression, bone marrow transplants	Fever, dry cough, dyspnea, hypoxemia	Interstitial infiltrates, bilateral small nodular densities
IV. Other organisms			
a. *Pneumocystis carinii*	Acute leukemia, lymphoma, chronic leukemia, immunosuppression, AIDS	Fever, dyspnea, dry cough, hypoxemia, cyanosis	Interstitial infiltrate, perihilar, may spare periphery early, rare nodular densities, and pleural effusions
b. *Toxoplasma gondii*	Immunosuppression, Hodgkin's disease, other neoplasms after chemotherapy	Chills, fever, malaise, dry cough, dyspnea, respiratory failure	Interstitial pneumonitis, edema, bronchopneumonia
c. *Strongyloides stercoralis*	Cancer (intestinal), chemotherapy, corticosteroids (travel history)	Associated gastrointestinal disease (peritonitis)	Diffuse alveolar or nodular infiltrates

occur with *Mycobacteria, Nocardia, Aspergillus, Cryptococcus,* varicella-zoster, cytomegalovirus, *Strongyloides,* and, rarely, with *Pneumocystis carinii* (Bode *et al.,* 1974; Williams *et al.,* 1976).

In most series, bilateral diffuse interstitial infiltrates in the immunosuppressed patient are caused by *Pneumocystis carinii,* but other entities such as cytomegalovirus infection, herpes virus infection, leukemic infiltration, lymphoma, drug-induced pneumonitis may exist. Lung biopsy is almost always necessary to establish the diagnosis in diffuse interstitial pneumonitis (see Figures 41–2, 41–3). The open-chest technique probably produces the best diagnostic yield and the lowest frequency of complications (Greenman *et al.,* 1975; Leight and Michaelis, 1978). In a recent study (Jaffe *et al.,* 1981) of immunosuppressed patients with diffuse bilateral pneumonitis, an open-chest biopsy was diagnostic in 81% of the patients. Of these specimens, *Pneumocystis carinii* was found in 38%; other infections in 24%, and the underlying neoplastic disease in 19%. Complications associated with open-lung biopsy occur in 7 to 19% of patients and include hemorrhage, pneumothorax, pneumonia, wound dehiscence, and hemoptysis.

Biopsy of affected lung can also be obtained via the transbronchial approach through the fiberoptic bronchoscope. Diagnostic material is obtained in 76 to 84% of specimens, although nonspecific interstitial pneumonitis is diagnosed frequently. Pneumocystis, fungal, and viral pneumonia are also diagnosable and false-negative results for *P. carinii* infection are rare (Feldman *et al.,* 1977; Matthay *et al.,* 1977). Complications of this procedure include hemorrhage, pneumothorax, pneumonia, and mild hemoptysis. The diagnostic yield of the transbronchial approach is lower than that of open-lung biopsy in some centers, probably because of the smaller sample of tissue obtained.

Needle aspiration, needle biopsy, and trephine needle biopsy are also used to diagnose pulmonary infections in these patients. In most series, however, the diagnostic yield is lower and the complication rates are higher than with open or transbronchial biopsies.

Tuberculosis. Tuberculosis is an infrequent disease in patients with neoplasia, but it becomes an important consideration when these patients are immunosuppressed. Primary infection with *Mycobacterium tuberculosis* provides the host with persisting resistance to exogenous reinfection, but viable dormant bacilli are harbored within tubercles in activated macrophages. Factors that depress cell-mediated immunity favor endogenous reinfection. A review of tuberculosis among cancer patients (Kaplan *et al.,* 1974) described two patterns of infection. In patients with pulmonary or head and neck tumors, the infection is usually present when the neoplasm is diagnosed. In patients with cellular immune deficits such as lymphoma, tuberculosis develops during, or shortly after, antineoplastic treatment. The severity of the infection correlates with the degree of immunosuppressive therapy. Disseminated tuberculosis is most frequent in patients treated with radiation, steroids, or cytotoxic agents. Overall, tuberculosis occurs in about 1% of patients with cancer. Disseminated tuberculosis is associated with a 90% mortality rate.

The clinical diagnosis is often difficult, since at least 20% of the patients have no previous history of tuberculosis and may lack the usual signs of tuberculosis. Fever and hematologic abnormalities are nonspecific, and chest films are nondiagnostic in 50% of the cases. Skin test reaction to tuberculin may be negative, especially in heavily immunosuppressed patients. Liver biopsy is recommended to demonstrate this infection since almost all patients with disseminated tuberculosis have granulomas in the liver. A liver biopsy should be performed in patients with fever and elevated liver alkaline phosphatase, unless these abnormal findings are otherwise explained. Bone marrow biopsy, pleural biopsy, or open-lung biopsy may reveal diagnostic granuloma, which may be positive for acid-fast bacilli on smear or culture.

Prophylactic isoniazid should be given to all patients with a positive tuberculin skin test when prolonged immunosuppressive therapy is contemplated. Any suspicion of active tuberculosis in these patients should be treated more aggressively with two or more antituberculosis drugs. In geographic areas where atypical mycobacterial species are responsible for clinical disease, these mycobacteria cause infection in cancer patients as frequently as does *M. tuberculosis. Mycobacterium kansasii* and *M. fortuitum* are the most commonly isolated organisms, the majority of which involve the lung (Feld *et al.,* 1976).

Central Nervous System Infection. Central nervous system (CNS) infections represent only about 0.2% of admissions to large cancer centers. These infections are most frequent in patients with lymphomas, neurosurgical tumors, neutropenia, and after splenectomy. CNS infections in cancer patients present as meningitis in approximately two-thirds of cases, and as cerebral abscess in approximately 25% (Chernik *et al.,* 1973, 1977). Viral encephalitis and encephalomyelitis account for the other cases and are found chiefly in immunosuppressed patients (see Table 41–4).

Meningitis. Meningitis in the neutropenic patient occasionally may result from the usual bacteria such as *S. pneumoniae, Neisseria meningitidis* (especially in the splenectomized patient), but more often this infection is caused by *Pseudomonas aeruginosa* or other gram-negative enteric bacilli. *Bacillus* species, *Candida, Aspergillus,* or *Mucor* species may infect the meninges of neutropenic patients. Meningitis in neutropenic patients may follow bacteremia or fungemia. These patients present with high fever but may have only minimal, or extremely subtle, neurologic findings. Headache and minimal changes in mentation or level of consciousness should prompt lumbar or cisternal puncture in order to obtain cerebrospinal fluid. Pleocytosis may be severely limited in the face of profound neutropenia, but the organisms are usually visible on gram stain or potassium hydroxide (KOH) preparations (for fungi) and, almost always,

Table 41–4.   Central Nervous System Infection in Patients with Cancer

INFECTION/ USUAL CAUSATIVE AGENTS	CLINICAL CLUES	LABORATORY FINDINGS
Meningitis*		
Streptococcus pneumoniae	Neutropenia, splenectomy, fever, ± nuchal rigidity, headache postsurgery (head and neck)	Minimal pleocytosis if neutropenic, gram-positive diplococci on smear, positive culture, positive CIE in CSF or urine, blood cultures positive, CSF protein ↑, glucose ↓
N. meningitidis	Neutropenia, splenectomy, fever, rash, headache, arthralgias, ± nuchal rigidity, rapid progression	Minimal pleocytosis, gram-negative diplococci on smear, positive culture, CIE positive in CSF, blood cultures positive, CSF protein ↑, glucose ↓
Pseudomonas aeruginosa Enterobacteriaceae	Neutropenia, leukemia, fever, headache, minimal neurologic findings, minimal defects in mentation or level of consciousness, ecthyma gangrenosum	Minimal pleocytosis, gram-negative rods on smear, positive cultures of CSF and blood
Listeria monocytogenes	Immunosuppression, T-lymphocyte defects, ± CNS signs, fever, headache, ± nuchal rigidity, minimal personality change, cranial nerve palsy	Mononuclear or polymorphonuclear pleocytosis, CSF protein ↑, glucose ↓, or normal + gram stain of CSF sediment (30%), positive CSF culture
Cryptococcus neoformans	Immunosuppression, low-grade fever, minimal nuchal rigidity, mild headache, ± cranial nerve palsy, personality change, insidious onset	Lymphocytic pleocytosis, positive CSF gram stain or India ink preparation, positive culture (large volumes), positive latex agglutination in CSF or serum
Meningoencephalitis		
Toxoplasma gondii	Immunosuppression, lymphoma, meningoencephalitic ± focal signs, multiple organ involvement, rapid progression	Minimal pleocytosis (lymphocytes), IgM-IFA specific antibody rise, Sabin Feldman dye test ≥ 1:1000
Varicella-zoster virus Herpes simplex virus	Immunosuppression, skin lesions	Brain biopsy positive, positive vesicle culture
Brain abscess†		
Aspergillus species Mucor	Neutropenia, immunosuppression, nasopharyngeal involvement, ± brain abscess, sudden onset of major neurologic findings, postneurosurgery, pulmonary infection	Mild lymphocytic pleocytosis, CSF protein, glucose, ± culture
Nocardia asteroides	Immunosuppression, T-lymphocyte defects, pulmonary infection, subcutaneous abscesses, focal neurologic signs	†Biopsy of brain abscess, †culture at other sites of infection

* Other organisms can cause meningitis in these patients: *Staphylococcus aureus*, *Legionella* sp., *Corynebacterium* sp., *Haemophilus influenzae*, *Bacillus* sp., *Candida* sp., *Histoplasma capsulatum*, *Coccidioides imitis*, and so on.
† Brain abscesses can also be caused by *Cryptococcus neoformans*, *Candida* sp., *S. epidermidis*, *S. aureus*, and so forth.

are cultured from the cerebrospinal fluid (Chernik *et al.*, 1977; Armstrong, 1981).

Immunocompromised patients develop meningitis caused by a different spectrum of organisms. *Listeria monocytogenes* is the most frequent bacterial agent in this setting. These patients may have sepsis and bacteremia but minimal CNS findings, or they may present with low-grade fever, headache, and personality change. Still other patients present with fulminant meningitis with nuchal rigidity, seizures, dyskinesis, and coma. The cerebro-spinal fluid shows an increased number of polymorphonuclear or mononuclear infiltrates (rarely up to 10,000/cu mm); protein is usually elevated and glucose depressed. The density of organisms may be low, so that gram stains are only positive for gram-positive bacilli in approximately 30% of cases. Culture of cerebrospinal fluid, and often blood, will be positive for *L. monocytogenes*.

Cryptococcus neoformans, a yeastlike fungus, is a common cause of meningitis in immunosuppressed patients, especially in those with Hodgkin's and other lymphomas. This infection may be extremely subtle, with low-grade fever and mild headache, but rarely with nuchal rigidity. Subtle cranial nerve findings may be present and diplopia, pupillary abnormalities, mild extraocular muscle dysfunction, blurred vision, facial paralysis, hearing loss, or disturbed taste sensation, may be the only neurologic findings. Mild or minimal personality change, confusion, but rarely coma, may occur. The onset of this infection is gradual, over several weeks or months. Cryptococci may also cause lesions in the lung and on the skin (see Figure 41–5).

Lumbar puncture is usually diagnostic, but as much as 10 mL of cerebrospinal fluid may be required to demonstrate the organisms on culture because of their low density in the lumbar spinal fluid. Organisms may be seen on gram-stained or India ink preparations of centrifuged spinal fluid. If the organism is not cultivated on first attempt, another lumbar puncture, with filtration of the cerebrospinal fluid through a millipore filter and subsequent culture of the filter, can increase the diagnostic yield. A lymphocytic pleocytosis (10 to 500/μL), depressed cerebrospinal fluid glucose, and elevated cerebrospinal fluid proteins are usually present. Latex agglutination tests for cryptococcal antigen are usually positive in cerebrospinal fluid and occasionally in serum.

Varicella-zoster and herpes simplex virus may cause meningitis in the immunocompromised patient with cancer. When varicella-zoster virus disseminates from a thoracic or abdominal dermatome, CNS involvement is unusual. With cranial nerve zoster, however, spread to the meninges and brain cortex is not uncommon. The cerebrospinal fluid findings are not specific, although a lymphocytic pleocytosis is usual. Cerebrospinal fluid glucose is normal, and the virus is rarely cultured from spinal fluid, but can often be isolated from brain biopsy specimens. Diagnosis is usually apparent from the associated skin vesicles, smears of which reveal multinucleated giant cells and intranuclear inclusion bodies when slide preparations of lesion scrapings are stained with Wright or Giemsa stains.

Toxoplasma gondii may produce a necrotizing meningitis or meningoencephalitis in the immunosuppressed patient. This may result from reactivation of latent cysts in nervous tissue at the time of immunosuppression. Fever, altered consciousness, headache, and seizures may occur, but some patients may be asymptomatic. Diagnosis rests on serologic documentation of a change in antibody titers.

Other agents, such as *Legionella pneumophila, Bacillus* species, *Strongyloides stercoralis, Mucor, Candida* species, may produce meningitis in immunosuppressed patients, and tuberculous meningitis also may occur. Many of the organisms mentioned above may also produce an encephalitic picture, clinically. Patients with neurosurgical tumors may develop meningitis postoperatively as a result of gram-negative bacilli, including *Pseudomonas aeruginosa* and *Klebsiella pneumoniae,* or from *Staphylococcus aureus, S. epidermidis,* diphtheroids, *Candida tropicalis, Candida albicans, Aspergillus* species.

Brain Abscess. Brain abscess, either single or multiple, may be caused by mixed anaerobic, aerobic, gram-negative, and gram-positive flora in the neutropenic patient, or by *Nocardia asteroides, Cryptococcus neoformans, Aspergillus* species, and occasionally other organisms.

Nocardia are gram-positive branching rods, that stain weakly acid-fast with dilute sulfuric acid used as the decolorizing agent. Brain abscess is usually associated with involvement of the pulmonary parenchyma, and isolation of the organism from the sputum of a patient with localizing CNS findings is presumptive evidence of nocardial brain abscess. Other infections may coexist, and the diagnosis is confirmed by brain biopsy (with subsequent drainage if abscess is confirmed).

Skin Infections. Infectious skin lesions in patients with cancer can result from dissemination of various infections *(Pseudomonas aeruginosa* [see Figure 41–4], *Candida* species, *Cryptococcus neoformans* [see Figure 41–5]). The differential diagnosis between skin manifestations caused by infection and those related directly to neoplastic disease is often difficult and frequently requires biopsy.

In immunocompromised patients, varicella-zoster is probably responsible for most skin infections (see Figure 41–6). Herpes simplex virus frequently produces vesicular lesions in the perilabial area (see Figure 41–7). The severely immunocompromised patient may present with generalized disseminated lesions (Kaposi's varicelliform eruption). Zoster occurs presumably as a result of reactivation of the virus believed to be dormant in the nervous system ganglia, although controversies exist with regard to the occurrence of zoster as a primary infection. In one series of patients

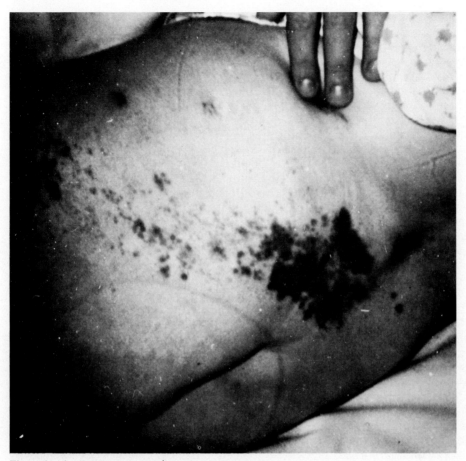

Figure 41–6. Dermatomal eruption of varicella-zoster.

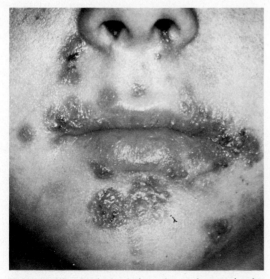

Figure 41–7. Vesicular lesions due to herpes simplex virus.

with cancer, 25% of the cases of zoster occurred in patients with Hodgkin's disease. Atypical generalized zoster and disseminated varicella-zoster infection occurred in 30% of patients. (Schimpff *et al.,* 1972a). The major predisposing factors for zoster include anergy, recent irradiation, and immunosuppression with corticosteroids or chemotherapy. Most cases of zoster develop within 6 to 12 months after completion of radiation therapy. Varicella-zoster infection often involves irradiated or tumor-involved dermatomes.

Clinically, zoster begins with burning dermatomal pain, followed by the appearance of vesicles which progress to crusted pustules (see Figure 41–6). New lesions appear for as long as seven days, and their crusts may persist four weeks. Dissemination may occur at sites distant from the primary dermatome. Mortality from zoster is low, even with dissemination, although considerable morbidity results from neuralgia, superinfection, and neurologic complications. Visceral dissemination may occur.

Hepatitis and Enteric Infections. Hepatitis is a frequent problem in patients with cancer, especially when multiple blood transfusions are required. Viral hepatitis is usually less evident clinically in immunosuppressed patients than in normal patients. In addition to hepatitis caused by viruses B and A, other viruses, most of which are not yet clearly identified, can cause a similar disease. Most cases of transfusion associated hepatitis are due to the recently identified non-A, non-B hepatitis virus. Neutropenic and immunosuppressed patients may also have bacterial and fungal hepatitis, including that caused by *Candida tropicalis* (see Figure 41-1). The differential diagnosis requires liver biopsy and adequate microbiologic investigation since the clinical and laboratory presentation is not specific. It may be difficult to differentiate B and A viral hepatitis from that caused by cytomegalovirus or from *Toxoplasma gondii*. Cytomegalovirus is rarely associated with adenopathy, whereas with toxoplasmosis it is almost the rule. Secondary hepatitis may be a direct consequence of disseminated bacteria, fungal, viral or parasitic infection.

Enteritis in cancer patients can be caused by bacterial and viral pathogens. Patients who develop bacteremia with *Salmonella* species often have an underlying illness such as lymphoma, carcinoma, or hemolytic disease. Only 20% of these patients have associated gastrointestinal complaints, whereas symptomatic salmonellosis is more common in patients with no underlying disease. This suggests that immunosuppressed patients can become bacteremic during salmonella infection, even in the absence of overt alimentary abnormalities. In a major cancer center, salmonella infection occurred most frequently in patients with lymphoma and lymphocytic leukemia (Wolfe *et al.*, 1971). These patients developed infection with *Salmonella typhimurium* and *Salmonella derby* most frequently, and 35% had associated bacteremia. Most of the bacteremic cases had recently received corticosteroids, radiation therapy, or cytotoxic therapy.

Enteritis secondary to herpes simplex virus or cytomegalovirus most often takes the form of esophagitis or colitis. Both of these infections are frequently polymicrobial. *Strongyloides stercoralis* causes enteritis with severe crampy pain, abdominal distention, fever, shock, and neurologic signs. In severely immunosuppressed patients, this infection is often accompanied by bacteremia with multiple organisms of intestinal origin and concurrent pneumonitis. Duodenal aspirates will yield the organism, which may also be identified occasionally in the sputum.

Diagnosis and Diagnostic Procedures

The neutropenic patient is predisposed to bloodstream invasion by bacterial and other pathogens. The initial focus of infection may be clinically unremarkable because of the lack of inflammatory reaction. Blood cultures are often the only means to an etiologic diagnosis. When local infection occurs, aspiration of these sites may provide a microbiologic diagnosis.

Since bacterial and fungal colonization of many body sites is extremely common in these patients, however, such cultures may be contaminated. Correlation of gram-stain readings with culture of aspirated material and blood cultures provides more secure diagnoses. Whenever possible, biopsy of local lesions should be performed and examined by special stains to reveal bacteria, fungi, or pneumocysts. Cultures of urine, pleural fluid, abscess cavities, ascitic fluid are usually positive with infection at these sites.

Whenever pneumonitis is documented by chest films, an aggressive approach to the specific etiologic diagnosis is recommended. Invasive procedures, discussed above, can be performed with supportive platelet transfusions, if required. In major cancer centers, a coordinated approach involving a team of oncologists, thoracic surgeons, hematologists, infectious disease specialists, pathologists, and microbiologists can optimize the diagnostic yield in these clinical situations. A recent report has questioned the risk-benefit ratio of this procedure in neutropenic patients (McCabe *et al.*, 1984).

Patients with neurologic infection also require an aggressive diagnostic approach. Lumbar puncture is essential in patients with any suggestive central nervous system signs or symptoms, which may be very subtle in patients with limited inflammatory response. Caution should be used in patients with space-occupying mass lesions or obvious increased intracranial pressure. Brain scans and computerized axial tomographic scans should be obtained before lumbar puncture in patients with predominant focal neurologic signs.

Lumbar spinal fluid should be examined for cellular reaction (both the number and type of cells should be described). Spinal fluid glucose and protein should be determined and the centrifuged sediment examined by gram stain, India ink, and KOH preparations. Since the density of organisms responsible for some meningitides may be quite low *(e.g., Crypto-coccus neoformans, Mycobacterium tuberculosis, Listeria monocytogenes)*, large volumes of cerebrospinal fluid (as much as 10 mL) should be obtained and cultured. Occasionally, in the face of spinal canal obstruction, cisternal puncture may be required to yield a diagnosis.

Serologic demonstration of opportunistic infection in the immunocompromised patient has not been uniformly successful, possibly as a result of the relatively poor antibody response in some of these patients. Methods have been developed for the detection of microbial antigens, however, and are quite useful diagnostic tools. For example, countercurrent immunoelectrophoresis (CIE) of spinal fluid can demonstrate the presence of antigens of *S. pneumoniae, Haemophilus influenzae,* and *N. meningitidis.* Latex agglutination tests will demonstrate cryptococcal antigens in spinal fluid and serum of infected patients. *Aspergillus* antigens may be detected in serum by radioimmunoassay, and a variety of techniques have been described for detecting *Candida* antigens, including serum precipitins, CIE, passive hemagglutination inhibition, gas liquid chromatography, and the enzyme-linked immunosorbant assay (ELISA). The availability of these tests varies widely, and the reliability of any individual test in a given laboratory should be known.

The diagnosis of viral infection in patients with cancer requires biopsy of lesions or affected tissue *(e.g.,* in encephalitis), with subsequent culture. Skin lesions in patients with herpes virus infections typically reveal multinucleated giant cells with intranuclear inclusions when the base of these lesions is scraped and stained with Wright's Giemsa, or other trichrome stains. These cells may be seen in biopsy specimens from other sites and occasionally in sputum cells from patients with varicella-zoster pneumonitis. Direct immunofluorescent antibody tests may also be useful when applied to cells or tissue specimens. Cytomegalovirus may be identified in cultures within two to three weeks, and viremia or viruria can thus be detected.

Protozoan infections are difficult to diagnose without tissue specimens. *Pneumocystis carinii* can be identified in tissue and bronchial washing specimens stained with Gomori's methenamine silver (see Figure 41–3). Other stains, such as Giemsa, Gram-Weigert, or toluidine blue, may be useful rapid stains but should not replace silver stains for definitive diagnosis. Trophozoites of *Toxoplasma gondii* may be identified in tissues, but the usual diagnosis of toxoplasmosis is made serologically. Although a high titer (with the Sabin-Feldman dye test, indirect immunofluorescent antibody, or indirect hemagglutinating antibody) may persist for years after infection, a fourfold or greater change in acute and convalescent sera is usually diagnostic. Some humoral response occurs even in immunosuppressed infected patients. Although a brain biopsy is optimal in the presence of a mass lesion, most consultants would treat presumptively for CNS toxoplasmosis in the presence of strong serologic evidence.

In general, untreated infection with any organism is likely to progress rapidly in the patient with cancer, especially in the presence of neutropenia, immunosuppression, or obstruction. The more aggressive diagnostic approach permits prompt institution of specific therapy with the greatest chance of cure.

TREATMENT OF INFECTION

When the infecting organism is identified by smear, culture, or other technique, therapy should be instituted promptly in high doses, intravenously whenever possible. Intrathecal or intraventricular antimicrobial agents may be necessary in some CNS bacterial or fungal infections. The drugs of choice for the usual infecting organisms are listed in Table 41–5. A textbook of infectious diseases can provide more details on antimicrobial therapy. The following discussion provides guidelines to managing of infections in patients with cancer, both when the organism has been identified and when therapy must be instituted for presumed infection with bacteria, fungi, protozoa, or viruses.

Bacterial Infections

Empiric Antibiotic Therapy. Most infectious disease experts recommend treatment of severe bacterial infections based on microbio-

Table 41–5. Treatment of Infections in Patients with Cancer

CONDITION OR ORGANISM	SUGGESTED AGENTS
Neutropenia, fever	Broad-spectrum beta-lactam* plus aminoglycoside†
Methicillin-resistant *Staphylococcus*	Vancomycin ± rifampin
Klebsiella pneumoniae	Cephalosporin or broad-spectrum beta-lactam* plus aminoglycoside†
Pseudomonas aeruginosa	Carbenicillin, ticarcillin, azlocillin, mezlocillin or piperacillin plus aminoglycoside†
Legionella pneumophila	Erythromycin, rifampin
Listeria monocytogenes	Ampicillin ± aminoglycoside, erythromycin, others
Mycobacterium tuberculosis	Isoniazid, rifampin, ethambutol, streptomycin
Nocardia asteroides	Sulfonamides, trimethoprim-sulfamethoxazole
Candida species	Oral: nystatin; ketoconazole Systemic: amphotericin B
Aspergillus species	Amphotericin B
Mucor, Rhizopus	Amphotericin B
Cryptococcus neoformans	Amphotericin B
Varicella-zoster virus, herpes simplex virus	Vidarabine, acyclovir
Pneumocystis carinii	Trimethoprim-sulfamethoxazole, pentamidine isethionate
Toxoplasma gondii	Pyrimethamine and sulfonamide
Strongyloides stercoralis	Thiabendazole

* Such as ticarcillin, carbenicillin, piperacillin, azlocillin, mezlocillin, moxalactam, cefotaxime, cefoperazone, ceftriaxone, ceftizoxime, cefmenoxime, ceftazidime.
† Gentamicin, tobramycin, netilmicin, amikacin often active against strains resistant to other aminoglycosides.

logic data obtained from the infected patient. In neutropenic patients, however, infections can present without typical signs and symptoms. The lack of granulocytes limits the inflammatory response and, despite the absence of a conspicuous infected site, an infection may pursue a relentless fulminant course unless treated promptly (Sickles *et al.,* 1975). The mortality rate for *Pseudomonas aeruginosa* infection in neutropenic patients exceeds 50% within 48 hours of the onset of fever. The rapid

progression of infection in untreated neutropenic patients and the high likelihood of bacterial infections as the cause of fever in these individuals have led to the concept of empiric antimicrobial therapy.

Neutropenic patients should receive antimicrobial therapy as soon as fever is documented, unless the febrile episode is obviously related to anticancer drugs or to other causes, such as transfusion of blood products. Empiric antimicrobial therapy is probably largely responsible for the improvement of the prognosis of infection in these patients (Schimpff *et al.,* 1971).

As indicated in Table 41–2, bacterial infection is implicated as the cause of fever in neutropenic patients in more than 60% of cases and most of these patients are infected with *Staphylococcus aureus* or gram-negative bacteria, such as *P. aeruginosa, Escherichia coli,* or *Klebsiella pneumoniae* (E.O.R.T.C. International Antimicrobial Therapy Project Group, 1978). Localized *Candida* infection is also common, but fungemia is present in only 5% of bacteremic or septicemic patients.

Any antimicrobial regimen used empirically in neutropenic febrile patients should provide adequate coverage against the most frequently isolated bacterial pathogens. Among the useful antibiotics in these situations, aminoglycosides, such as gentamicin, tobramycin, or amikacin have a suitable antimicrobial spectrum, although many centers report increasing resistance to the former two agents.

Initial clinical experience with aminoglycosides alone as empiric therapy in neutropenic patients, however, was disappointing. The narrow margin between the effective dose and the toxic dose of aminoglycosides, as well as the variable serum levels obtained with the usual doses, is probably responsible for frequent undertreatment of these patients, even though these antibiotics are extremely effective *in vitro* against most pathogens isolated from neutropenic patients. Several studies reviewed recently (Klastersky and Zinner, 1982) suggest that the addition of an expanded spectrum penicillin, or cephalosporin, to aminoglycosides is associated with significantly better results in neutropenic patients whose offending pathogens are fully sensitive to the aminoglycoside alone.

The new generation cephalosporins and related compounds (cefoperazone, cefmenoxime, cefotaxime, moxalactam, ceftizoxime, ceftriaxone, ceftazidime, imipenem) are effective *in vitro* against gram-negative organisms isolated from febrile neutropenic patients with the probable exception of *P. aeruginosa* for some agents. Clinical experience with the use of these antibiotics alone, however, is still extremely limited. Whether these antibiotics may be effective for empiric therapy in neutropenic patients when used as a single agent, or whether they should still be administered in combination with other antimicrobial drugs, drugs, such as the aminoglycosides, remains to be determined. Their potential use in this clinical situation most likely depends on the rate of emergence of resistant organisms. Since the rate of emergence of strains resistant to the aminoglycosides is still low, successful empiric therapy of febrile neutropenic patients is most likely with combinations of antibiotics that include an aminoglycoside. The new quinolone antibiotics (e.g., enoxacin, ciprofloxacin, pefloxacin, etc.) have not been studied extensively in these patients.

Combinations of beta-lactam antibiotics (such as carbenicillin plus cephalothin, azlocillin plus cefotaxime, piperacillin plus moxalactam), or of trimethoprim-sulfamethoxazole with broad-spectrum penicillins, have been suggested for treating febrile neutropenic patients. The potential for antibiotic antagonism and the likelihood of resistant strains emerging, however, will condition the future usefulness of these regimens.

Antimicrobial synergism is another consideration in using antibiotic combinations in these patients. Synergism is the interaction of two or more antimicrobial agents, in which their effect in combination is greater than their individual effects when used alone. Although there are no standardized methods to evaluate synergism *in vitro,* the results obtained by the checkerboard and time-kill methods can be correlated with increased bactericidal activity in the serum of patients receiving combinations of antibiotics that are synergistic by these *in vitro* techniques (Young, 1982).

Synergism can result in considerable potentiation of one antimicrobial by the other *in vitro.* In view of this, high levels of antimicrobial activity in serum, and presumably at the site of infection, obtained in patients treated with synergistic combinations are not surprising. High serum bactericidal activity is predictive of a favorable outcome in gram-negative bacillary infection (Levy and Klastersky, 1982). In a review of several published studies,

the success rate treating of Gram-negative bacterial infections was 74% in patients treated with synergistic combinations, compared with only 42% in those patients who received nonsynergistic antibiotic combinations (Klastersky and Zinner, 1982). Most of these patients were neutropenic or had underlying neoplastic disease.

The basic requirements for empiric antibiotic therapy for febrile neutropenic patients include a broad antimicrobial spectrum and the potential for synergistic interaction. Of the many different combinations of antibiotics used in an attempt to achieve this goal (Klastersky, 1979a), the combination of carbenicillin or ticarcillin with an aminoglycoside probably represents optimal therapy. Overall, 70% of neutropenic patients treated empirically with this type of combination will respond satisfactorily. Better clinical results may possibly be achieved by further modification of the presently available antimicrobial regimens. Most failures of empiric antimicrobial therapy can be attributed to nonbacterial infection or unremitting underlying neoplastic disease. As bacterial strains resistant to these antibiotics emerge, other antimicrobials may have to be considered. The new ureidopenicillins such as azlocillin, mezlocillin, or piperacillin, and the latest cephalosporins may prove to be as effective as the current regimens.

The duration of empiric therapy depends on whether granulocytopenia subsides during the course of treatment. When granulocytopenia resolves, the outcome is generally favorable, and antibiotic therapy should not be prolonged beyond the ten days usually employed to treat gram-negative rod bacteremia in non-neutropenic patients. When granulocytopenia persists, however, antibiotics should probably be continued until the granulocyte count returns to levels above $500/\mu L$, even with a favorable clinical response to empiric therapy.

Early discontinuation of empiric antibiotics in persistently neutropenic patients may result in recurrent febrile episodes, sometimes associated with fatal microbiologically documented infections (Pizzo *et al.,* 1979). Although prolonged antimicrobial therapy in neutropenic patients might result in an increased rate of superinfections, granulocytopenia is the more important factor predisposing to infection.

Granulocyte Transfusions. About 30% of febrile neutropenic patients treated with empiric antibiotics fail to respond. Some of these patients die as a result of profound granulocytopenia related to uncontrolled underlying neoplastic disease. In others, infection will persist, in spite of antibiotics. If the infection can be documented microbiologically, antibiotic therapy should be adjusted according to the *in vitro* susceptibility of the offending pathogen. Antibiotics should be selected to achieve high bactericidal activity in the serum (equal to or greater than 1:16). If bacteremia persists or local infection progresses, an undrained focus of infection should be sought carefully. Computerized tomography and isotopic scans performed with labeled granulocytes may be helpful.

Granulocyte transfusions are indicated in granulocytopenic patients with nonresponsive bacterial sepsis. Several clinical trials have established the effectiveness of transfusions of granulocytes in patients with neutropenia and bacteremia, especially when the latter results from localized undrained infection (Klastersky, 1979b). Granulocyte transfusion is most effective in patients with persisting profound bone marrow aplasia and microbiologically documented infections. Empiric early use of granulocyte transfusions in high-risk febrile neutropenic patients is probably not indicated (E.O.R.T.C. International Antimicrobial Therapy Project Group, 1982a). More detailed information on granulocyte transfusions may be found in Chapter 42.

Lithium Carbonate. Lithium carbonate has been found to produce a leukocytosis when administered to psychotic patients. Although not without some toxicity, lithium may help reduce the neutropenia, as well as subsequent fever and infection associated with cancer chemotherapy (Stein *et al.,* 1977; Lyman *et al.,* 1980). These studies have involved patients with lung and other solid tumors; further studies are needed to demonstrate beneficial effects in leukemic patients.

Empiric Antifungal Therapy. Neutropenic patients may also fail to respond to empiric antimicrobial therapy because of fungal infection. In general, fungal infection is not microbiologically documented early in the febrile episode, but can be suspected occasionally from surveillance cultures. Disseminated fungal infection has been documented in patients with hematologic neoplasms and neutropenia who die from febrile illnesses despite the administration of broad-spectrum antibiotics. The frequency of fungal infections at autopsy in these patients approaches 30%.

Preliminary studies suggest that early treatment of fungal infection is associated with improved outcome (Pizzo *et al.,* 1982). Early therapy with amphotericin B may prove appropriate in neutropenic patients with fever but without microbiologically documented infection who do not respond to a short course of empiric antimicrobial therapy. Further clinical trials are needed to test this concept of empiric antifungal therapy and to evaluate new antifungal agents. Until the results of such trials are available, amphotericin remains the standard antifungal agent for empiric administration in this clinical situation.

Immunotherapy for Infection. The overall mortality from gram-negative bacteremia remains unacceptably high despite new combinations of active antibiotics. A better understanding of the pathogenesis of shock and sophisticated supportive care in patients with altered host defense mechanisms are necessary. In these infections, endotoxinemia may contribute to the development of coagulation abnormalities, shock, and death, even with appropriate antimicrobial therapy. Antiserum to shared antigenic components of endotoxin (lipopolysaccharide) from gram-negative rods can protect against the local and generalized Schwartzman reaction in experimental animals. These antibodies to bacterial core glycolipids are also protective against the lethal consequences of gram-negative rod bacteremia in neutropenic and nonneutropenic animals (McCabe, 1972; Ziegler *et al.,* 1975).

Recently, human antiserum to the J5 mutant of *E. coli* 0111 (whose cell wall contains lipid and sugar moieties shared by most gram-negative rods) was given to patients with gram-negative rod bacteremia in a double-blind controlled study with preimmune normal human plasma. These patients also received optimal supportive therapy. This study showed a decrease in mortality in recipients of the hyperimmune plasma, especially in patients with shock (Glauser *et al.,* 1982; Ziegler *et al.,* 1982). However, these effects were not as pronounced in neutropenic patients. In addition, prophylactic administration of hyperimmune core glycolipid plasma reduced the incidence of febrile episodes in a small study of neutropenic patients with cancer (Wolf *et al.,* 1980) but did not prevent gram-negative infections when given in a single dose (McCutchan *et al.,* 1983). Further studies of the effectiveness of shared passive antibody therapy are needed to establish the role of immunotherapy in treating bacterial infections in this patient population.

Fungal Infections

Autopsy studies have indicated that disseminated fungal disease occurs in about 30% of patients with neoplasms. Disseminated infections caused by *Candida* species or *Aspergillus* species can be treated adequately if antifungal therapy is initiated early. These observations are the basis for the use of empiric antifungal therapy, the value of which remains to be proven in suitably controlled studies. Currently, only amphotericin B is effective as antifungal therapy in this patient group. It is administered parenterally and is active against *Aspergillus* and most strains of *Candida,* as well as other fungi. Despite its activity against these fungal pathogens, the clinical experience with amphotericin B has been disappointing. It is toxic to the kidney and red blood cells, and prolonged treatment is necessary. Moreover, unless therapy is started early, often before the diagnosis is proven, cure rates are low. During recent years, combinations of antifungal agents have been studied with the hope of lowering the morbidity and mortality rates caused by fungal infections in compromised patients (as well as the incidence of adverse effects of amphotericin B). The use of combinations of antifungal agents for systemic mycotic diseases has recently been reviewed (Meunier-Carpentier, 1982).

For candidiasis and cryptococcosis, a combination of amphotericin B and 5-fluorocytosine (5-FC) is optimal therapy. The efficacy of the combination may be related to antifungal synergism and/or prevention, by amphotericin B, of emergence of *Candida* sp. strains resistant to 5-FC. In a controlled study of patients with cryptococcal meningitis comparing amphotericin B and the combination of lower dose amphotericin B and 5-FC, the combination cured, or improved, more patients, produced fewer failures or relapses, and provided more rapid sterilization of the cerebrospinal fluid with less nephrotoxicity than did amphotericin B alone (Bennett *et al.,* 1979). Whether intraventricular amphotericin B might have some benefit during the initial stage of cryptococcal meningitis remains to be studied.

Preliminary data in patients with cancer and candidiasis indicate that combined therapy with amphotericin B and miconazole may be less effective than amphotericin alone. This combination should not be used routinely, pending further evaluation.

Amphotericin B is the treatment of choice for aspergillosis. Results are disappointing, however, unless antifungal therapy is undertaken very early during the course of the disease. Since infection with *Aspergillus* species in patients with cancer is usually a late complication, occurring with unremitting underlying neoplastic disease, the poor results may not be solely the result of amphotericin failure. The combination of amphotericin B with either 5-FC or rifampin may be successful in selected patients. No controlled trials of these combinations compared with amphotericin B alone are available, however, and these combinations of drugs cannot now be recommended as standard therapy in suspected or demonstrated aspergillosis in patients with cancer.

Two new imidazole compounds, miconazole and ketoconazole, are available for the treatment of fungal infections. The latter compound is administered orally. These drugs are active *in vitro* against *Candida* species, the dermatophytes, *Coccidioides immitis, Cryptococcus neoformans, Blastomyces dermatidis, Histoplasma capsulatum,* and many others.

In patients with cancer and fungal infections, ketaconazole is useful for treating of Candida esophagitis or stomatopharyngitis (thrush), and topical miconazole therapy is effective in genital and cutaneous candidiasis. Amphotericin B, however, remains the drug of choice in invasive or systemic candidiasis.

Cryptococcal infections, including meningitis unresponsive to amphotericin B plus 5-fluorocytosine, may be treated with miconazole, but the number of successfully treated cases is low. Ketoconazole is effective therapy for coccidioidomycosis, but in the immunocompromised patient amphotericin B remains the drug of choice. The imidazoles are not useful in treating aspergillosis or mucormycosis.

Whether granulocyte transfusions are useful in treating fungal infections in neutropenic patients is unclear. Since neutropenia is the basic defect predisposing to fungal infection, and since granulocyte transfusions have been useful in animal models of fungal infections, granulocytes might be important in the management of disseminated fungal disease. Severe pulmonary reactions, however, have been reported with the combined use of amphotericin B and granulocyte transfusions. Although these observations were made primarily in patients with gram-negative bacterial infections, caution should be exercised when granulocyte transfusions and amphotericin B are used together.

Parasitic Infections

The combination of trimethoprim and sulfamethoxazole (co-trimoxazole) has been proven effective in the prevention of *Pneumocystis carinii* in children with acute leukemia (Hughes *et al.,* 1977). Co-trimoxazole has also been used for oral therapy for this infection, at a total daily dose of 100 mg/kg of sulfamethoxazole and 20 mg/kg of trimethoprim. Intravenous therapy is preferred, and the usual adult dose is two ampuls (each ampul contains 80 mg trimethoprim and 400 mg sulfamethoxazole) every six hours (Sattler and Remington, 1981). If administered early, treatment with co-trimoxazole results in a favorable response in 50 to 80% of patients. Therapy should be continued for 10 to 14 days. Pentamidine isethionate (4 mg/kg once daily intramuscularly or intravenously) is also effective therapy for *Pneumocystis carinii* pneumonia. Adverse reactions include sterile abscesses at the inoculation site, azotemia, hypoglycemia, and hypotension. Combining co-trimoxazole with pentamidine does not seem to improve the clinical results.

For disseminated toxoplasmosis, the combination of pyrimethamine and a sulfonamide is effective therapy. The sulfonamide, preferably sulfadiazine, should be administered (6 to 8 g/day) with particular attention to hydration in order to prevent renal tubular precipitation. Pyrimethamine (50 to 75 mg/day) should be administered with folinic acid (6 mg/day). A similar regimen has been used occasionally with success in *Pneumocystis carinii* pneumonia. In central nervous system infections caused by *Toxoplasma gondii,* pyrimethamine has been administered by the intraventricular route since it does not cross the bloodbrain barrier. Other parasitic diseases are rare in patients with cancer. *Strongyloides stercoralis* infection may be controlled by thiabendazole (25 mg/kg every 12 hr) and a decrease in the dose of corticosteroids, if applicable. Giardiasis, malaria, and amebic infections are exceedingly rare in patients with cancer and should be treated by conventional methods.

Viral Infections

No treatment offers proven effectiveness for viral infections in patients with cancer, with the exception of infections caused by herpes simplex and varicella-zoster. Zoster immune globulin ameliorates varicella when given to susceptible hosts during the incubation period. Its role in treating disseminated or localized varicella-zoster infection is not established.

For both varicella-zoster and herpes simplex infections, the administration of adenine arabinoside (vidarabine) has resulted in favorable clinical responses. The dosage recommended is 50 mg/kg of body weight per day, given intravenously over 12 hours for 10 days. If administered early in the course of herpetic encephalitis, the drug results in a higher rate of recovery and a lower incidence of serious debilitating complications than placebo. Its effectiveness in cutaneous or esophageal herpes simplex infections has not been studied in controlled trials. In varicella-zoster, the administration of adenine arabinoside has been reported to reduce extension of skin lesions.

Acyclovir (acycloguanosine) is also effective in the treatment of disseminated varicella-zoster and herpes simplex infection in immunocompromised patients with cancer. It is given as an intravenous infusion at 5 mg/kg or 250 mg/m² every 8 hours for 5 to 7 days. Acyclovir may also be used to treat localized zoster in these patients to minimize visceral dissemination. The use of interferon requires further laboratory and clinical studies before it can be recommended as routine therapy for these infections. Infections caused by herpes simplex and varicella-zoster are the most responsive to antiviral agents (Hirsch, 1982). No adequate treatment is available for cytomegalovirus infection.

THE PREVENTION OF INFECTION

Prevention of Infection During Granulocytopenia

General Measures. Most important are attempts to improve the patient's underlying condition, in order to reverse granulocytopenia as promptly as possible. During profound neutropenia, avoiding invasive traumatic procedures may prevent many infectious complications. All intravenous medications should be given by small needles that are changed at least every 48 hours. Catheter site dressings should be changed daily, and intravenous tubing should be changed every 48 to 72 hours. Plastic catheters should be avoided since the risk of infection increases with their duration. Pressure should be exerted following venipuncture and bone marrow aspiration to reduce occurrence of hematomas, that may become infected. Shaving should produce as little trauma as possible, and occlusive antiperspirants should not be used.

It is difficult to prevent completely the acquisition of new organisms. Patients should be housed in rooms with individual bathrooms, however, rather than in large open wards. All medical and paramedical personnel should be carefully trained in personal hygiene, of which thorough and frequent handwashing is most important. The patient should be instructed in personal hygiene, including daily bathing and shampooing with antimicrobial compounds, such as chlorhexidine or povidone-iodine.

Food is a common source for acquiring potential pathogens, but a completely sterile diet is difficult to prepare and is usually poorly tolerated. A diet of low microbial content (cooked food diet) can be prepared without difficulty, and all uncooked foods, such as salads, should be eliminated (Remington and Schimpff, 1981). Canned foods and pasteurized products are generally sterile, or nearly so. Drinking and bathing water should be evaluated intermittently. Sterile bottled water may be necessary if the water is contaminated.

Effective housekeeping in the patient's room should include the use of a disinfectant, the double-bucket system for mopping, and daily cleaning of all horizontal surfaces and bathroom structures with a phenolic disinfectant. Mouth care, including daily brushing and flossing will reduce dental plaque and may prevent acute periodontal infection. Dental consultation should be obtained before the initiation of myelosuppressive therapy.

Disinfectant or antibiotic-containing ointment, applied to the axillae three times a day has been shown to decrease substantially the frequency of axillary infection. Similar prophylaxis can be used to clean the perianal and the vulvar regions. Attempts to obtain microbial suppression are described below. A review concerning prevention of infection in granulocytopenic patients has been published (Schimpff, 1980).

Granulocyte Replacement. Since granulocytopenia is the major factor predisposing to bacterial and fungal infection, stimulation of endogenous granulocyte production or granulocyte transfusion prophylactically may reduce the frequency and severity of infection. Preliminary observations indicate that lithium carbonate, which induces reversible leukocy-

tosis when given to psychiatric patients, may ameliorate leukopenia associated with cancer chemotherapy. Moderate reduction in severe febrile episodes and infection-related deaths has been observed in some, but not all, patients treated with lithium. Whether lithium carbonate may be effective during prolonged periods of granulocytopenia is not clear. Lithium is associated with toxic side effects, such as nausea, vomiting, mucositis, lethargy, and tremor (Lyman *et al.,* 1980; Stein *et al.,* 1977).

Corticosteroids and etiocholanolone stimulate production and/or release of granulocytes. These techniques however, have not been investigated fully for the prevention of infection in granulocytopenic patients. The potential benefit of corticoid-induced granulocytosis must be counterbalanced by the immunosuppressive and anti-inflammatory effects of corticosteroids. Granulocyte replacement by transfusion is a more direct approach to supportive treatment for the neutropenic patient. The prophylactic use of granulocyte transfusions was effective in preventing infection in at least one large controlled clinical trial. The principal effect of granulocyte transfusion in these patients was the prevention of severe episodes of infection, including bacteremia. Overall survival, however, was identical in transfused and nontransfused patients (Klastersky, 1979b). Among several major complications of prophylactic granulocyte transfusions reported are the frequent development of lymphocytotoxic antibodies and refractoriness to further granulocyte and platelet transfusions. Because of this high incidence of alloimmunization, prophylactic granulocytes should be transfused only from HLA-compatible donors. Diffuse pneumonitis and disseminated cytomegalovirus infection have been reported with prophylactic granulocyte transfusions.

If appropriate combinations of antibiotics are administered early during infection and supplemented by therapeutic transfusions of granulocytes when bone marrow failure is severe, mortality from infection in neutropenic patients is relatively low. Death from infection usually occurs only when the underlying neoplastic disease is unremitting or when severe noninfectious complications from anticancer therapy have occurred. Therefore, with the present state of technology, it is difficult to recommend routine and systematic prophylactic granulocyte transfusions.

Protective Environment and Prophylactic Antibiotics. In order to protect patients during periods of high risk for infection, several programs have been designed to provide isolation from nosocomial flora and to suppress potentially pathogenic endogenous flora. The use of protected environments (PE) and microbial suppression with orally administered prophylactic antibiotics (PA) has been extensively studied and reviewed (Buckner et al., 1978; Klastersky, 1979c). Protective environments plus prophylactic antibiotics (PEPA) have reduced the frequency of infection in neutropenic patients. PA alone was as effective as PEPA in reducing infection in some controlled studies, and less effective than PEPA in others. Reports of the efficacy of PA alone, compared to standard ward care without isolation and microbial suppression, are also conflicting. PE alone, that is, without microbial suppression, has been evaluated in only two studies (Yates and Holland, 1973; Dietrich et al., 1977). Both found PE as effective as PEPA, and more effective than standard care, in preventing infections in neutropenic patients with acute nonlymphocytic leukemia. PE and PEPA may be particularly effective in preventing pulmonary infections.

Prophylactic Antibiotics. A variety of antibiotic combinations for oral administration have been recommended as effective prophylaxis against infection in neutropenic patients. Results differ in different centers, and no one regimen is universally indicated. A retrospective analysis recently showed that all infections, including bacteremia, were significantly reduced in neutropenic patients receiving some oral prophylactic antibiotic regimen, compared with similar patients not receiving these drugs (E.O.R.T.C. International Antimicrobial Therapy Project Group, 1983b). These regimens can be divided to three groups: (1) aminoglycoside containing, (2) trimethoprim-sulfamethoxazole, and (3) selective or partial antibiotic decontamination.

AMINOGLYCOSIDE-CONTAINING REGIMENS. The combination of gentamicin (200 mg), vancomycin (250 to 500 mg), and nystatin (tablets or suspension 500,000 to 600,000 units) orally (GVN) given every four to six hours was studied extensively (Bodey et al., 1971; Levi et al., 1973; Levine et al., 1973; Schimpff et al., 1975). Most studies demonstrated a reduction in stool pathogens, as well as the incidence of severe infection, in GVN recipients compared with untreated controls, although the effect of laminar air flow isolators cannot always be separated. The major disadvantage of this regimen is its high cost and the

unpleasant taste that requires intensive supportive care in order to overcome nausea.

Other investigators have used framycetin, colistin, and nystatin (FRACON) with some success (Storring et al., 1977). Bacteremia was reduced in recipients, and this regimen was given every six hours with less nausea.

Gentamicin plus nystatin (GN) is recently compared to GVN in a randomized trial (Bender et al., 1979). GN was tolerated somewhat better than GVN, and the incidence of infection and bacteremia was similar in both groups. Other regimens, including rotating oral or intravenous antibiotics, have been studied and, although they may be as effective as other procedures, they cannot be strongly recommended (Rodriguez et al., 1978).

Complications of these regimens include colonization and subsequent infection with aminoglycoside-resistant organisms. These patients may serve as reservoirs of antibiotic-resistant bacteria which may spread to other patients. In addition, if used, they should be continued for the duration of granulocytopenia, since the risk of infection may be increased when these drugs are discontinued (Hahn et al., 1978).

TRIMETHOPRIM-SULFAMETHOXAZOLE (TMP-SMX; CO-TRIMOXAZOLE). When co-trimoxazole was used to reduce infections with *P. carinii* in leukemic children, a reduction in gram-positive and gram-negative bacterial infections was also noted (Hughes et al., 1977). In a subsequent study of adult neutropenic patients, two tablets every 12 hours of TMP-SMX reduced the incidence of urinary infections and bacteremia compared to that in nonrecipients (Gurwith et al., 1979). These results, however, have not been reproduced in all other studies. The E.O.R.T.C. International Antimicrobial Therapy Project Group (1984) studied 342 patients, randomized to receive TMP-SMX or placebo. Patients were allowed to receive GN or GVN, if this was the practice of the participating institution, although no beneficial effect of TMP-SMX prophyloxis was found in patients with acute nonlymphocytic leukemia, infection and bacteremia were reduced in other neutropenic patients who received TMP-SMX.

Recently, TMP-SMX plus nystatin was compared to GN in neutropenic patients with leukemia (Wade et al., 1981). Compliance was better and cost was considerably lower with the former regimen, and the rates of overall infection and infection-related deaths were equal in the two treatment groups. Differences in the sites and types of infection did occur, with more gram-positive organisms isolated from the TMP-SMX group and more gram-negative rods from the GN group.

SELECTIVE OR PARTIAL ANTIBIOTIC DECONTAMINATION. The concept of colonization resistance has been introduced to describe the protective activity of the gastrointestinal flora, perhaps related to the presence of anaerobes (Van der Waaij et al., 1972). By selectively modulating the gastrointestinal flora in neutropenic patients with antibiotics that preserve colonization resistance (such as co-trimoxazole, nalidixic acid, polymyxins, neomycin, amphotericin B), reduction in infection has been reported (Sleijfer et al., 1979; Guiot et al., 1981, 1983). This approach has not been studied in a randomized trial against the above-mentioned oral antibiotic regimens.

The ultimate goal for prevention of infection in patients with leukemia is to achieve improved rates of complete remission and prolonged survival. In only one study has an improved rate of remission been demonstrated in association with PEPA, but without prolonged survival (Schimpff et al., 1975). When all available studies are summarized, the rate of complete remission in acute leukemias treated with PEPA was 59%, compared with 44% in non-PEPA controls. The ultimate survival rate, however, was identical in both groups.

Oral Antifungal Agents. Most patients who receive decontamination regimens also receive orally nonabsorbable antifungal agents since the incidence of fungal infection in neutropenic patients is extremely high. Until recently, no clear data were available on the frequency of systemic fungal infections. Oral amphotericin B is effective in decreasing the incidence of systemic *Candida* infection in patients with hematologic neoplasms who received antibiotics within two weeks of death (Ezdinli et al., 1979). Miconazole may also be effective as prophylaxis against local *Candida* infection when administered orally. A recent study (Meunier-Carpentier et al., 1983a,b) suggests miconazole and ketoconazole, administered orally, are equally effective in preventing *Candida* species colonization and possibly infection in neutropenic patients. Antimicrobial prophylaxis against *Aspergillus* infection has not been as successful, and laminar air flow isolation may be the best protection against this air-borne fungus.

Bacterial Vaccines. Patients with acute leukemia are best vaccinated with pneumococcal vaccine when they are in remission since their antibody response is limited during chemotherapy. Other active bacterial vaccines may not be active during relapse or chemotherapy. A vaccine against *Pseudomonas aeruginosa* has been studied in patients with leukemia. These patients are able to mount only a short-lived antibody response (Young et al., 1973). Protection against death and some reduction in *Pseudomonas* bacteremia was reported, but significant fever and soreness of the vaccinated arm have limited the use of this vaccine. Studies of the possible use of antibodies to *Pseudomonas* exotoxins are in progress in experimental animals.

Passive immunization with core glycolipid antibody, discussed in a previous section, and active cross-reactive immunization against gram-negative rod bacteremias remain investigational procedures.

Prevention of Infection in Immunosuppressed Patients

Tuberculosis and Other Mycobacterial Infections. Therapy for infection with disseminated tuberculosis in patients with cellular immune deficiency is not universally effective, and diagnosis is often difficult. Tuberculin testing provides the best method to define those patients at risk for tuberculosis, and skin tests should be performed on all patients with neoplastic diseases. Patients with positive tuberculin reactions who have evidence of previous clinical tuberculosis should be treated with isoniazid prophylactically (300 mg/day), especially if they are scheduled to receive immunosuppressive agents. Although there are no data clearly supporting these recommendations, and in spite of the potential toxicity of isoniazid, it is reasonable to continue prophylaxis for as long as the patient remains immunosuppressed.

Bacterial and Fungal Infections. Splenectomized patients, especially those with Hodgkin's disease, are at increased risk of serious, life-threatening infections. Pneumococcal and other encapsulated bacteria have been implicated most frequently. Polyvalent pneumococcal vaccine has been introduced to prevent this type of infection. All pneumococcal serotypes, however, are not represented in the vaccine, and the response varies with the immunologic capability of the host. Pneumococcal vaccine should be given before splenectomy. Penicillin prophylaxis may be useful in splenectomized children.

Infections with *Salmonella* species are frequent in patients with leukemia or lymphoma. Very little is known about the prevention of salmonellosis in patients with neoplastic disease. Vaccination is probably of limited usefulness, not only because of the large variety of infecting *Salmonella* species, but also because of the poor response to antigenic challenge. In immunosuppressed patients with recurrent *Salmonella* infection, continuous administration of ampicillin may be effective.

No specific prophylaxis is available for *Listeria monocytogenes, Nocardia asteroides,* and *Legionella pneumophila.* Similarly, the prevention of fungal diseases in immunocompromised hosts is limited to the use of gastrointestinal decontamination with antifungal agents and effective isolation to prevent air-borne infection. Oral antifungal prophylaxis has not been proven to be thoroughly effective in preventing systemic fungal infections. A high index of suspicion, rapid invasive diagnostic efforts, and early empiric therapy may be most effective in minimizing death from invasive fungal disease.

Viral Infections. Immunocompromised patients are not more susceptible than the general population to common viral infections, including influenza. Most patients with cancer can be effectively vaccinated against influenza. Immunosuppression, however, definitely predisposes to severe infections caused by varicella-zoster virus, herpes simplex, and cytomegalovirus. Zoster immune globulin will reduce the incidence and severity of varicella when administered to leukemic children after presumed exposure. The isolation of patients with contagious varicella-zoster infections is especially important in cancer hospitals.

Prophylactic interferon and transfer factor to prevent cytomegalovirus and herpes simplex virus infections have been studied recently in patients after renal transplantation. Interferon delayed shedding of cytomegalovirus and decreased the incidence of viremia after transplantation, but did not alter shedding of herpes simplex virus and, moreover, did not affect long-term survival. Human leukocyte interferon has been used in treating varicella-zoster in patients with cancer. High doses of interferon appeared to limit cutaneous dissemination, visceral complications, and progression distant from the primary dermatome. Intravenous acyclovir (5 mg/kg, q8h) may limit progression and visceral dissemination of varicella-zoster. Vaccination with a live

cytomegalovirus has been evaluated recently in patients after renal transplantation. The vaccine increased cellular and humoral immunity, was associated with minimal morbidity, and appeared not to reactivate cytomegalovirus infections in intensely immunosuppressed patients. Further studies are needed in patients with cancer.

The recently introduced hepatitis B vaccine is effective in preventing hepatitis in persons at high risk of exposure to hepatitis B virus. The vaccine must be given intramuscularly in three injections, initially, at one month, and at six months. The antibody response of patients with leukemia and other immunosuppressing neoplasms is much lower than in normal hosts. Vaccination should be attempted early in the course of the illness or when the patient is in remission, especially for individuals expected to require large numbers of transfusions with blood or blood products. The efficacy of hepatitis B vaccine has not been fully evaluated in patients with neoplastic disorders.

Protozoan Infections. No chemoprophylaxis or immunoprophylaxis is available for toxoplasmosis. The infection is acquired from cats and by ingesting raw meat. Susceptible patients who lack antibodies should avoid these sources of possible contamination.

Effective prophylaxis is available for *Pneumocystis carinii* infections (Hughes *et al.,* 1977). Treatment with trimethoprim-sulfamethoxazole eliminated *Pneumocystis carinii* pneumonia in children with acute lymphoblastic leukemia. Co-trimoxazole (two regular strength tablets, or one double-strength tablet twice a day) should be administered to patients at high risk of acquiring *Pneumocystis carinii* pneumonia, such as those undergoing maintenance therapy for acute lymphoblastic leukemia, patients who have undergone organ or bone marrow transplantation, and those who are treated for prolonged periods with immunosuppressive drugs. Although further studies are needed, co-trimoxazole also may decrease the frequency of other infections in these patients, such as pneumococcal pneumonia and infections of the urinary tract.

REFERENCES

Armstrong, D.: Central nervous system infections in the compromised host. In Rubin, R. H., and Young L. S. (eds): *Clinical Approach to Infections in the Compromised Host.* Plenum Medical Book Company, New York, 1981.

Bender, J. F.; Schimpff, S. C.; Young, V. M.; Fortner, C. L.; Brouillet, M. D.; Love, L. J.; and Wiernik, P. H.: Role of vancomycin as a component of oral nonabsorbable antibiotics for microbial suppression in leukemic patients. *Antimicrob. Agents Chemother.,* **15**:455–460, 1979.

Bennett, J. E.; Dismukes, W. E.; Duma, R. J.; Medoff, G.; Sande, M. A.; Gallis, H.; Leonard, J.; Fields, B. T.; Bradshaw, M.; Haywood, H.; McGee, Z. A.; Cate, T. R.; Cobbs, C. G.; Warner, J. F.; and Alling, D. W.: A comparison of amphotericin B alone and combined with flucytosine in the treatment of cryptococcal meningitis. *N. Engl. J. Med.,* **301**:126–131, 1979.

Bode, F. R.; Paré, J. A. P.; and Fraser, R. G.: Pulmonary diseases in the compromised host. *Medicine,* **53**:255–293, 1974.

Bodey, G. P.; Buckley, M.; Sathe, Y. S.; and Freireich, E. J.: Quantitative relationship between circulating leukocytes and infections in patients with acute leukemia. *Ann. Intern. Med.,* **64**:328–340, 1966.

Bodey, G. P.; Gehan, E. A.; Freireich, E. J.; and Frei, E., III: Protected environment–prophylactic antibiotic program in the chemotherapy of acute leukemia. *Am. J. Med. Sci.,* **262**:138–151, 1971.

Buckner, C. D.; Clift, R. A.; Sanders, J. E.; Meyers, J. D.; Counts, G. W.; Farewell, V. T.; and Thomas, E. D.: Protective environment for marrow transplant recipients. A prospective study. *Ann. Intern. Med.,* **89**:893–901, 1978.

Chernik, N. L.; Armstrong, D.; and Posner, J. B.: Central nervous system infections in patients with cancer. *Medicine,* **52**:563–581, 1973.

Chernik, N. L.; Armstrong, D.; and Posner, J. B.: Central nervous system infections in patients with cancer: Changing patterns. *Cancer,* **40**:268–274, 1977.

Dietrich, M.; Gaus, W.; Vossen, J.; van der Waiij, D.; and Wendt, F.: Protective isolation and antimicrobial decontamination in patients with high susceptibility to infection. *Infection,* **5**:107–114, 1977.

Edwards, J. E. Jr.; Lehrer, R. I.; Stiehm, S. R.; Fischer, J. J.; and Young, L. S.: Severe candidal infections, clinical perspective, immune defense mechanisms and current concepts of therapy. *Ann. Intern. Med.,* **89**:91–106, 1978.

E.O.R.T.C. International Antimicrobial Therapy Project Group: Three antibiotic regimens in the treatment of infection in febrile granulocytopenic patients with cancer. *J. Infect. Dis.,* **137**:14–29, 1978.

E.O.R.T.C. International Antimicrobial Therapy Project Group: Early granulocyte transfusion in high risk febrile neutropenic patients. *Schweiz. Med. Wochenschr.,* (Suppl.) **14**:46–48, 1983a.

E.O.R.T.C. International Antimicrobial Therapy Project Group: Combination of amikacin and carbenicillin with or without cefazolin as empirical treatment of febrile neutropenic patients. *J. Clin. Oncol.,* **1**:597–603, 1983b.

E.O.R.T.C. International Antimicrobial Therapy Project Group: Trimethoprim-sulfamethoxazole in the prevention of infection in neutropenic patients. *J. Infect. Dis.,* **150**:372–379, 1984.

Ezdinli, E. Z.; O'Sullivan, D. D.; Wasser, L. P.; Kim, U.; and Stutzman, L.: Oral amphotericin B for candidiasis in patients with hematologic neoplasm. An autopsy study. *J.A.M.A.,* **242**:258–260, 1979.

Feld, R.; Bodey, G. P.; and Groschel, D.: Mycobacteriosis in patients with malignant disease. *Arch. Intern. Med.,* **136**:67–70, 1976.

Feldman, N. J.; Pennington, J. E.; and Ehrie, M. G.: Transbronchial lung biopsy in the compromised host. *J.A.M.A.,* **238**:1377–1379, 1977.

Glauser, M. P.; McCutchan J. A.; Ziegler, E. J.; and Braude, A.: Adjuvant therapy for severe infections. In Klastersky, J., and Staquet, M. J. (eds.): *Combination Antibiotic Therapy in the Compromised Host.* Raven Press, New York, 1982.

Greenman, R. L.; Goodall, P. T.; and King, D.: Lung biopsy in immunocompromised hosts. *Am. J. Med.,* **59**:488–496, 1975.

Guiot, H. F. L.; van den Broek, P. J.; van der Meer, J. W. M.; and vanFurth, R.: Selective antimicrobial modulation of the intestinal flora of patients with acute non-lymphocytic leukemia: A double-blind, placebo-controlled study. *J. Infect. Dis.,* **147**:615–623, 1983.

Guiot, H. F. L.; van der Meer, J. W. M.; and van Furth, R.: Selective antimicrobial modulation of human microbial flora: Infection prevention in patients with decreased host defense mechanisms by selective elimination of potentially pathogenic bacteria. *J. Infect. Dis.,* **143**:644–654, 1981.

Gurwith, M. J.; Brunton, J. L.; Lank, B. A.; Harding, G. K. M.; and Ronald, A. R.: A prospective controlled investigation of prophylactic trimethoprim/sulfamethoxazole in hospitalized granulocytopenic patients. *Am. J. Med.,* **66**:248–256, 1979.

Hahn, D. M.; Schimpff, S. C.; Fortner, C. C.; Smyth, A. C.; Young, V. M.; and Wiernik, P. H.: Infection in acute leukemia patients receiving oral nonabsorbable antibiotics. *Antimicrob. Agents Chemother.,* **13**:958–964, 1978.

Hirsch, M. S.: Chemotherapy and immunotherapy of opportunistic viral infections. In Klastersky, J. (ed.): *Infections in Cancer Patients.* Raven Press, New York, 1982.

Hughes, W. T.; Kuhn, S.; Chaudary, S.; Feldman, S.; Verzosa, M.; Aur, J. A. R.; Pratt, C.; and George, S. L.: Successful chemoprophylaxis for *Pneumocystis carinii* pneumonitis. *N. Engl. J. Med.,* **297**:1419–1426, 1977.

Jaffe, J. P., and Maki, D. G.: Lung biopsy in immunocompromised patients. One institution's experience and an approach to management of pulmonary disease in the compromised host. *Cancer,* **48**:1144–1153, 1981.

Johanson, W. G.; Peirce, A. K.; and Sanford, J. P.: Changing pharyngeal bacterial flora of hospitalized patients. Emergence of gram-negative bacilli. *N. Engl. J. Med.,* **281**:1137–1140, 1969.

Jones, J. M.: Granulomatous hapatitis due to *Candida albicans* in patients with acute leukemia. *Ann. Intern. Med.,* **94**:475–477, 1981.

Kaplan, M. H.; Armstrong, D.; and Rosen, P.: Tuberculosis complicating neoplastic disease. A review of 201 cases. *Cancer,* **33**:850–858, 1974.

Klastersky, J.: Combinations of antibiotics for therapy of severe infections in cancer patients. In Glauser, M., and Klastersky, J. (eds.): Proceedings of a symposium on therapy and prevention of infections in cancer patients. *Eur. J. Cancer,* **15**(Suppl.):3–13, 1979a.

Klastersky, J.: Granulocyte transfusions as a therapy and a prophylaxis of infection in neutropenic patients. In Glauser, M., and Klastersky, J. (eds.): Proceedings of a symposium on therapy and prevention of infections in cancer patients. *Eur. J. Cancer,* **15**(Suppl.):15–22, 1979b.

Klastersky, J.: Protected environment and prophylactic antibiotics as an adjunct to cancer chemotherapy: How useful? In Tagnon, H., and Staquet, M. (eds.): *Controversies in Cancer. Design of Trials and Treatment,*

14:121–127. Masson Publishing U.S.A., Inc., New York, 1979c.

Klastersky, J.; Weerts, D.; Hensgens, C.; and Debusscher, L.: Fever of unexplained origin in patients with cancer. *Eur. J. Cancer,* 9:649–656, 1973.

Klastersky, J., and Zinner, S. H.: Synergistic combinations of antibiotics in Gram-negative bacillary infections. *Rev. Infect. Dis.,* 4:294–301, 1982.

Leight, G. S., and Michaelis, L. L.: Open lung biopsy for the diagnosis of acute, diffuse pulmonary infiltrates in the immunosuppressed patient. *Chest,* 73:477–480, 1978.

Levi, J. A.; Vincent, P. C.; Jennis, F.; Lind, D. E.; and Gunz, F. W.: Prophylactic oral antibiotics in the management of acute leukemia. *Med. J. Aust.,* 1:1025–1029, 1973.

Levine, A. S.; Siegel, S. E.; Schreiber, A. D.; Hauser, J.; Preisler, H.; Goldstein, I. M.; Seidler, F.; Simon, R.; Perry, S.; Bennett, J. E.; and Henderson, E. S.: Protected environments and prophylactic antibiotics: A prospective controlled study of their utility in the therapy of acute leukemia. *N. Engl. J. Med.,* 288:477–483, 1973.

Levy, J., and Klastersky, J.: Serum bactericidal test: A review with emphasis on its role in the evaluation of antibiotic combinations. In Klastersky, J., and Staquet, M. J. (eds.): *Combination Antibiotic Therapy in the Compromised Host.* Raven Press, New York, 1982.

Lyman, G. H.; Williams, C. C.; and Preston, D.: The use of lithium carbonate to reduce infection and leukopenia during systemic chemotherapy. *N. Engl. J. Med.,* 302:257–260, 1980.

Mathay, R. A.; Farmer, W. C.; and Odeno, D.: Diagnostic fiberoptic bronchoscopy in the immunocompromised host with pulmonary infiltrates. *Thorax,* 32:539–545, 1977.

McCabe, R. E.; Brooks, R. G.; and Remington, J.S.: Is open lung biopsy for pulmonary infiltrate justified in patients with acute leukemia? Abstracts of the Third International Symposium on Infections in the Immunocompromised Host, Toronto, June, 1984.

McCabe, W. R.: Immunization with R mutants of *S. minnesota.* I. Protection against challenge with heterologous Gram-negative bacilli. *J. Immunol.,* 108:601–610, 1972.

McCutchan, J. A.; Wolf, J. L.; Ziegler, E. J.; and Brande, A. I.: Ineffectiveness of single dose human antiserum to core glycolipid (*E. coli* J 5) for prophylaxis of bacteremic gram negative infections in patients with prolonged neutropenia. *Swiss Medical J.,* 113(Suppl. 14):40–45, 1983.

Meunier-Carpentier, F.: Combination of antifungal agents for systemic mycotic diseases. In Klastersky, J., and Staquet, J. J. (eds.): *Combination Antibiotic Therapy in the Compromised Host.* Raven Press, New York, 1982a.

Meunier-Carpentier, F.; Cruciani, M.; and Klastersky, J.: Oral prophylaxis with miconazole or ketoconazole of invasive fungal disease in neutropenic cancer patients. *Eur. J. Cancer and Clin. Oncol.,* 19:43–48, 1983a.

Meunier-Carpentier, F.; Snoek, R.; and Klastersky, J.: Fungal surveillance cultures in neutropenic patients receiving prophylactically ketoconazole, amphotericin B or a placebo. In *Proceedings of the Second International Symposium on Infections in the Immunocompromised Host,* Easmon, C. S. F.; and Gaya, H. eds., London, Academic Press, 356–358, 1983b.

Pennington, N. E., and Feldman, J. T.: Pulmonary infiltrates and fever in patients with hematologic malig-

nancy: Assessment of transbronchial biopsy. *Am. J. Med.,* 62:581–587, 1977.

Pizzo, P. A.; Robichaud, K. J.; Gill, F. A.; Witebsky, F. G.; Levine, A. S.; Deisseroth, A. B.; Glaubiger, D. L.; Maclowry, J. D.; Magrath, I. T.; Poplack, D. G.; and Simon, R. M.: Duration of empiric antibiotic therapy in granulocytopenic patients with cancer. *Am. J. Med.,* 67:194–200, 1979.

Pizzo, P. A.; Robichaud, K. J.; Gill, F. A.; and Witebsky, F.G.: Empiric antibiotic and antifungal therapy for cancer patients with prolonged fever and granulocytopenia. *Am. J. Med.,* 72:101–111, 1982.

Ravy, M.; Maldonado, N.; Velez-Garcia, E.; Montalvo, J.; and Santiago, P. J.: Serious infection after splenectomy for the staging of Hodgkin's disease. *Ann. Intern. Med.,* 77:11–14, 1972.

Remington, J. S., and Schimpff, S. C.: Please don't eat the salads. *N. Engl. J. Med.,* 304:433–435, 1981.

Rodriguez, V.; Bodey, G. P.; Freireich, E. J.; McCredie, K. B.; Gutterman, J. U.; Keating, M. J.; Smith, T. L.; and Gehan, E. A.: Randomized trial of protected environment-prophylactic antibiotics in 145 adults with acute leukemia. *Medicine,* 57:253–266, 1978.

Rubin, R. H., and Greene, R.: Etiology and management of the compromised patient with fever and pulmonary infiltrates. In Rubin, R. H., and Young, L. S. (eds.): *Clinical Approach to Infection in the Compromised Host.* Plenum Medical Book Company, New York, 1981.

Sandford, G. R.; Merz, W. G.; Wingard, J. R.; Charache, P.; and Saral, R.: The value of fungal surveillance cultures as predictors of systemic fungal infections. *J. Infect. Dis.,* 192:503–509, 1980.

Sattler, F. R., and Remington, J. S.: Intravenous trimethoprim-sulfamethoxazole therapy for *Pneumocystis carinii* pneumonia. *Am. J. Med.,* 70:1215–1221, 1981.

Schimpff, S. C.: Infection prevention during granulocytopenia. In Remington, J. S., and Swartz, M. N. (eds.): *Current Clinical Topics in Infectious Diseases.* McGraw-Hill, Inc., New York, 1980.

Schimpff, S. C.; Green, W. H.; Young, V. M.; Fortner, C. L.; Jepsen, L.; Cusack, N.; Block, J. B.; and Wiernik, P. H.: Infection prevention in acute non-lymphocytic leukemia: Laminar flow room reverse isolation with oral, nonabsorbable antibiotic prophylaxis. *Ann. Intern. Med.,* 82:351–358, 1975.

Schimpff, S. C.; Satterlee, W.; Young, V. M.; and Serpick, A.: Empiric therapy with carbenicillin and gentamicin for febrile patients with cancer and granulocytopenia. *N. Engl. J. Med.,* 284:1061–1066, 1971.

Schimpff, S. C.; Serpick, A. A.; Stoler, B.; Rumack, B.; Mellin, H.; Joseph, J. M.; and Block, J.: Varicella zoster infection in patients with cancer. *Ann. Intern. Med.,* 76:241–254, 1972a.

Schimpff, S. C.; Young, V. M.; Greene, W. H.; Vermeulen, G. D.; Moody, M. R.; and Wiernik, P. H.: Origin of infection in acute non-lymphocytic leukemia. Significance of hospital acquisition of potential pathogens. *Ann. Intern. Med.,* 77:707–714, 1972b.

Sickles, E. A.; Greene, W. H.; and Wiernik, P. H.: Clinical presentation of infection in granulocytopenic patients. *Arch. Intern. Med.,* 135:715–719, 1975.

Sleijfer, D. T.; Mulder, N. H.; de Vries-Hospers, H. G.; Fidler, V.; Nieweg, H. O.; van der Waaij, D.; and van Saene, H. K. F: Infection prevention in granulocytopenic patients by selective decontamination of the digestive tract. In van der Waaij, D., and Verhoef, J. (eds.): *New Criteria for Antimicrobial Therapy: Maintenance of Digestive Tract Colonization Resistance.* Excerpta Medica, Amsterdam, 1979.

Stein, R. S.; Beaman, C.; Ali, M. Y.; Hansen, R.; Jenkins, D. D.; and Jumean, H. G.: Lithium carbonate attenuation of chemotherapy induced neutropenia. *N. Engl. J. Med.,* **297:**430–431, 1977.

Storring, R. A.; Jameson, B.; McElwain, T. J.; Wiltshaw, E.; Spiers, A. D. S.; and Gaya, H.: Oral non-absorbed antibiotics prevent infection in acute non-lymphoblastic leukemia. *Lancet,* **2:**837–840, 1977.

van der Waaij, D.; Berghuis, J. M.; and Lekkerkerk, J. E. C.: Colonization resistance of the digestive tract of mice during systemic antibiotic treatment. *J. Hyg. (Lond.),* **70:**605–610, 1972.

Wade, J. C.; Schimpff, S. C.; Hargadon, M. T.; Fortner, C. L.; Young, V. M.; and Wiernik, P. H.: A comparison of trimethoprim-sulfamethoxazole plus nystatin with gentamicin plus nystatin in the prevention of infections in acute leukemia. *N. Engl. J. Med.,* **304:**1057–1062, 1981.

Williams, D. M.; Krick, J. A.; and Remington, J. S.: Pulmonary infection in the compromised host. *Am. Rev. Respir. Dis.,* **114:**359–394, 593–627, 1976.

Wolf, J. L.; McCutchan, J. A.; Ziegler, E. J.; and Braude, A. I.: Prophylactic-antibody to core lipopolysaccharide in neutropenia. In *Current Chemotherapy and Infectious Diseases.* American Society of Microbiology, Washington, D.C., 1980.

Wolfe, M. S.; Armstrong, D.; Louria, D. B.; and Blevins, A.: Salmonellosis in patients with neoplastic disease. *Arch. Intern. Med.,* **128:**546–554, 1971.

Yates, J. W., and Holland, J. F.: A controlled study of isolation and endogenous microbial suppression in acute myelocytic leukemia patients. *Cancer,* **32:**1490–1498, 1973.

Young, L. S.: Significance of *in vitro* tests. In Klastersky, J., and Staquet, M. J. (eds.): *Combination Antibiotic Therapy in the Compromised Host.* Raven Press, New York, 1982.

Young, L. S.; Meyer, R. D.; and Armstrong, D.: *Pseudomonas aeruginosa* vaccine in cancer patients. *Ann. Intern. Med.,* **79:**518–527, 1973.

Ziegler, E. J.; McCutchan, J. A.; Douglas, H.; and Braude, A. I.: Prevention of lethal *Pseudomonas bacteremia* with epimerase deficient *E. coli* antiserum, *Trans. Assoc. Am. Physicians,* **88:**101–108, 1975.

Ziegler, E. J.; McCutchan, J. A.; Fierer, J.; Glauser, M. P.; Sadoff, J. C.; Douglas, H.; and Braude, A. I.: Treatment of gram-negative bacteremia and shock with human antiserum to a mutant *Escherichia coli, N. Engl. J. Med.,* **307:**1225–1230, 1982.

42

Hematologic Considerations in Cancer

CHARLES A. SCHIFFER and PETER H. WIERNIK

Infection and hemorrhage are the major limiting, life-threatening toxicities occurring during the standard therapy for patients with leukemia and the intensive treatment of patients with solid tumors. In this chapter we will review the current approach to the use of red blood cell, platelet, and granulocyte transfusions.

RED BLOOD CELL (RBC) TRANSFUSION

Most patients with cancer and virtually all patients with leukemia require RBC transfusions at some stage during their illness. In most patients RBC are given because of symptomatic, slowly developing anemia caused by impaired marrow production. Whole blood is needed only when massive hemorrhage has occurred, and all patients should initially receive packed red blood cells. Fresh whole blood is rarely, if ever, indicated. Red cells are well preserved in stored blood, coagulation factors are best derived from fresh frozen plasma, and there are not enough granulocytes or platelets in fresh blood to make a difference. The use of leukocyte-depleted RBC preparations should be reserved for the minority of patients who have transfusion reactions secondary to the development of antibodies against leukocytes present in the packed RBC or those who will require long-term chronic transfusion, such as patients with aplastic anemia. Either saline-washed or RBC that have been buffy-coat depleted by centrifugation should be used initially in such alloimmunized patients. Frozen, deglycerolized RBC, which are considerably more expensive and time consuming to prepare, should be used in the

small number of patients in whom reactions persist despite premedication and the use of washed RBC. More than 95% of the white blood cells are removed when blood is frozen. It should be noted that all of the methods of leukocyte depletion result in some (10 to 20%) loss of RBC so that the rise in hematocrit may be somewhat lower than with standard units of packed RBC.

Autologous transfusion can be accomplished with blood that has been frozen or kept liquid. Newer additives now permit liquid storage of RBC for 49 days. This procedure is sometimes used for patients with cancer undergoing elective surgery (staging laparotomy) in an effort to prevent alloimmunization, hepatitis, and other transfusion-related problems. This procedure, however, has not been common practice.

The complications of red cell transfusion must be fully appreciated by the oncologist. Hemolytic transfusion reactions are the most serious complication, and the reader is urged to refer to standard hematology texts for a full understanding of the diagnosis and management of this problem. Leukoagglutinins in the blood of the recipient may cause febrile and even hypotensive reactions. Flushing may occur almost at once when the transfusion is begun. Fever may be delayed for an hour or more. Additional transfusions to such patients should be accomplished with leukocyte-poor blood as discussed above. Immediate anaphylactoid hypersensitivity reactions characterized by urticaria can result from an interaction between transfused IgA and recipient anti-IgA in the occasional IgA deficient recipient (incidence approximately 1/750 patients). Such reactions can be serious and cannot be predicted.

Further transfusions should consist of extensively washed RBC to eliminate residual donor plasma. Vasoconstrictive substances may be released from banked red cells but they rarely cause clinical problems. Citrate toxicity, caused by a fall in ionized calcium, is rarely a problem in adults unless rapid and massive transfusion with citrated blood has occurred in a patient with significant impairment of liver function.

The most frequent significant problem associated with blood transfusion in patients with cancer is the transmission of viral hepatitis and other infections. Despite improved methods of detection of donors likely to transmit hepatitis, some cancer centers report an increasing incidence of posttransfusion hepatitis, especially in leukemia patients. Several studies have disclosed an enhanced remission duration and survival in leukemia patients who experience posttransfusion hepatitis, and this curious observation is under study in many laboratories.

Lymphocytes in transfused blood can cause a graft-versus-host reaction, and granulocytes can cause febrile reactions and pulmonary insufficiency. They are rarely of clinical impact after red cell or whole blood transfusion.

Blood should always be administered at room temperature unless the patient is known to have a specific indication that dictates otherwise, such as cold agglutinins.

PLATELET TRANSFUSION THERAPY

Platelet Collection

Most platelets for transfusion are prepared as a byproduct of whole blood donation. A single platelet concentrate (PC) or platelet unit should contain about 0.7 to 0.9×10^{11} platelets or approximately 75 to 80% of the platelets contained in the original unit of blood. Until recently, storage of platelets was limited to 72 hours. A number of studies have demonstrated that when storage is done properly, stored platelets maintain near-normal posttransfusion recovery, survival, and hemostatic effectiveness (Murphy and Gardner, 1971; Slichter and Harker, 1976; Filip and Aster, 1978; Holme et al., 1978). Current regulations permit storage of PC for up to seven days before transfusion (Hogge and Schiffer, 1983). The development of new plastic bags with increased permeability to oxygen permitted this extension of shelf life which should, in turn,

increase platelet availability, particularly on weekends. Platelet preparation and storage vary considerably, however, among blood centers. Additional deleterious effects that can occur during transport from blood centers to hospitals are possible. Current mandated quality control testing is minimal and probably inadequate to detect moderate degrees of damage that may occur during collection and storage owing to practices in individual blood banks. It is therefore important that clinicians provide careful posttransfusion follow-up so that any possible difficulties caused by platelet storage can be detected and corrected (Schiffer, 1981).

The dose of platelets required varies according to the size of the recipient and the desired elevation in platelet count. To raise the platelet count to the normal range in order to achieve hemostasis is normally not required, and an appropriate goal for most patients is a platelet count of 50,000 to 70,000/μL one hour after transfusion. Although the number of platelets per unit of PC can vary considerably, as an estimate, this posttransfusion level can be achieved by transfusion of 1 unit of PC/10 kg of lean body weight. A transfusion to an average, uncomplicated adult should contain 6 to 8 units of PC and result in an increment of approximately 10,000/μL/unit shortly after transfusion.

In addition to pooled preparations of PC from multiple donors, multiple units of platelets can also be obtained from single donors using a variety of cytopheresis machines or by repeated manual centrifugation techniques (Aisner et al., 1976; Hester et al., 1979a,b; Dutcher et al., 1981; Katz et al., 1981). To date most single-donor collections have been used to provide histocompatible platelets from selected donors for alloimmunized patients. Single-donor platelets are a more expensive product than the more readily available pooled PC and should not be used as a standard platelet transfusion product in preference to pooled PC (Schiffer and Slichter, 1982).

Indications for Platelet Transfusions

The likelihood of hemorrhage in a given patient is related to the platelet count, the functional quality of the circulating platelets, the etiology of the thrombocytopenia, and the presence of other clinical factors such as coagulation disorders, infection, and potential bleeding sites. The decision to administer platelet transfusions depends on an assessment of all these factors. Thus, the platelet count alone should not serve as the sole criterion for platelet transfusion. Patients with normal marrow function and thrombocytopenia caused by peripheral platelet destruction infrequently require, and probably usually do not benefit from, platelet transfusion because the transfused platelets are removed rapidly by the same mechanisms that destroy the patient's own platelets. This is particularly true in patients with immune (antibody)-mediated platelet destruction. Platelet transfusions are therefore usually reserved for patients with evidence of decreased platelet production. Platelet transfusions can be administered both to prevent hemorrhage and to ameliorate or stop already established bleeding. Spontaneous hemorrhage usually occurs in mucocutaneous sites and only rarely at platelet counts above 15,000 to 20,000/μL despite the marked prolongation of bleeding time at these levels (Roy et al., 1973; Belt et al., 1978). Strictly prophylactic platelet transfusions to otherwise stable recipients are usually administered to patients with leukemia and severe (less than 15,000 to 20,000/μL) thrombocytopenia who are expected to remain aplastic for weeks following therapy (Schiffer, 1978). Transfusions are administered at the 10,000 to 20,000/μL range because it is known that the platelet count is likely to fall further in these intensively treated patients. In addition, these patients are usually concurrently granulocytopenic and at risk for infection or have mucosal damage as a result of chemotherapy. Prophylactic transfusions are required less frequently in patients with solid tumors because of the shorter periods of marrow aplasia that accompany the treatment of these disorders and should not be utilized in stable patients with aplastic anemia because of the indefinite duration of transfusion support that may be required. Although some debate the frequency with which prophylactic transfusions may be required, most centers in the United States utilize platelets prophylactically in patients with leukemia receiving or recovering from induction therapy (Higby et al., 1974; Schiffer, 1978; Schiffer, et al., 1978b). Recently, it has been demonstrated in patients with leukemia that the incidence of alloimmunization, the most troublesome side effect of platelet transfusion, is unrelated to the number of platelet transfusions the patient receives. This observation suggests that prophylactic transfusions should not be withheld to prevent alloimmunization (Dutcher et al., 1980).

Table 42–1. Factors Increasing the Risk of Hemorrhage in Thrombocytopenic Patients

1. Coagulation abnormalities
2. Infection
3. Preexisting bleeding sites (mucositis, sites of tumor)
4. Hepatic, renal disease
5. Increased intracranial pressure (protracted coughing or vomiting)
6. Rapid falls in platelet count
7. Diagnostic or therapeutic procedures
8. Drugs affecting platelet function

Other clinical factors that contribute to hemorrhage in thrombocytopenic patients are listed in Table 42–1. In seriously ill patients with these or other active medical problems, it is advisable to maintain the platelet count in at least the 20,000 to 30,000/μL range. Patients receiving heparin for disseminated intravascular coagulation occurring during leukemia treatment or patients with high blast counts undergoing treatment with resulting rapid cytolysis should probably have platelet counts of 40,000 to 50,000/μL during the few days of active therapy when their risk of bleeding is highest.

Although invasive procedures should be minimized in thrombocytopenic patients, many tests (bone marrow aspirates and biopsies, lumbar punctures) must be done either at diagnosis or during treatment. No comprehensive data provide guidelines as to the platelet count at which various procedures can be administered safely. Some procedures, when it is possible to apply direct pressure to the puncture site, such as radial arterial punctures or bone marrow aspirates, can clearly be done without undue hazard at counts less than 20,000/μL. Lumbar punctures can also probably be done safely with platelet counts in the 20,000 to 30,000/μL range, although it is preferable to do this procedure, if possible, at a time when the patient would otherwise be scheduled to receive platelet transfusions. Other procedures, such as bronchoscopy with biopsies, in which even a small amount of bleeding can be catastrophic, are more problematic. In general, however, it has been our experience that larger procedures, including major surgery, can be done safely with platelet counts in the 40,000 to 50,000/μL range in the absence of other coagulation abnormalities. Indeed, should bleeding occur or continue at platelet counts greater than 50,000 to 60,000/μL, one should be concerned that other, nonplatelet etiologies (coagulopathy, anatomic causes) are the major cause of the continued hemorrhage. Major procedures should never be done unless an adequate supply of platelets is readily available, and unless it has been demonstrated that platelet counts of this level can be consistently achieved and maintained.

Side Effects of Platelet Transfusion

A number of side effects may occur following platelet transfusions, some of which can be ameliorated or prevented by close cooperation between the blood bank and the clinician (see Table 42–2).

1. *Transfusion reactions* following platelet transfusion can be caused by sensitization to histocompatibility antigens, RBC antigens, or plasma proteins. Transfusion reactions are usually mild, consisting of a sensation of chilliness and 1 to 2° F rises in temperature with or without urticaria. Alloimmunization to HLA or leukocyte antigens is the most common cause of reactions. In some patients, reactions can be prevented by centrifugation of the pooled platelet concentrates at 180 × g for three minutes, which removes the majority of contaminating leukocytes (Herzig *et al.,* 1975).

2. *Circulatory congestion,* particularly in children or elderly recipients, can occur because a pool of 6 to 8 units of PC represents a volume load of 300 to 400 mL of plasma. If necessary, the volume of plasma can be reduced before infusion by an additional centrifugation of the pooled concentrates with resuspension of the platelet button in a smaller volume. These concentrated transfusions should be administered immediately after preparation because of marked decreases in platelet viability after storage at high-platelet concentrations.

3. *Transmission of infectious diseases* is a well-known complication of blood transfusion and can be a particular problem in immunosuppressed patients. Although type B hepatitis is relatively uncommon because of improved donor screening tests, non-A, non-B hepatitis

remains a problem in recipients exposed to large numbers of units of blood (Alter *et al.,* 1972). Toxoplasmosis, cytomegalovirus, Salmonella, and, rarely, malaria infections have been described in recipients of platelets and other blood products (Rhame *et al.,* 1973; Garfield *et al.,* 1978). Another unusual but more acute problem is the transfusion of bacteria which have proliferated in platelet concentrates stored at room temperature (Buchholz *et al.,* 1971). If a severe febrile reaction occurs shortly after the infusion is begun, the transfusion should be discontinued, appropriate cultures done, and antibiotic therapy should be considered in granulocytopenic recipients. Fortunately, experience with room-temperature storage has shown that the transmission of bacterial infection is exceedingly uncommon (Silver *et al.,* 1970).

4. *Graft-versus-host disease* (GVHD) can occur in heavily immunosuppressed patients because of the presence of significant numbers of viable lymphocytes in platelet concentrates. This is a very rare problem in adult patients with solid tumors or acute leukemia, and blood products for these patients need not be irradiated prior to transfusion.

5. *Hemolysis of recipient red cells:* Transfusion of large volumes of plasma increases the probability of producing a direct Coombs test in the recipient if ABO-incompatible platelets are administered. Because most transfusions consist of the plasma from many different donors, few of whom can be expected to have high-titer antibodies, the risk of significant recipient hemolysis is very low.

6. *Sensitization to Rh_o (D) and other RBC antigens* can occur in recipients of multiple transfusions because of the small number of RBCs present in essentially all platelet preparations. This infrequently results in clinically important future difficulties in obtaining compatible RBCs for transfusion.

7. *Alloimmunization* to histocompatibility antigens occurs in the majority of recipients of multiple random-donor platelet transfusions and represents the most important long-term complication of platelet transfusion. Estimates of the frequency of alloimmunization following random-donor platelet transfusion vary from approximately 50 to 100%, depending in part on the patient population being studied and the intensity of cytotoxic and immunosuppressive therapy being administered (Tejada *et al.,* 1973; Green *et al.,* 1976; Schiffer *et al.,* 1976a; Howard and Perkins, 1978; Dutcher *et al.,* 1980, 1981a). The management

---

Table 42–2.   Hazards of Platelet Transfusion

1. Transfusion reactions
2. Circulatory congestion
3. Transmission of blood-borne infectious diseases
4. Graft-versus-host disease (GVHD)
5. Transfusion of red cell alloantibodies in incompatible plasma
6. Sensitization to RBC antigens
7. Alloimmunization

of alloimmunized patients is one of the most difficult problems in platelet transfusion and will be discussed in detail.

Management of Alloimmunization

Diagnosis. Alloimmunization should be suspected in patients who fail to achieve adequate platelet count increments after transfusion. Although a wide variety of clinical factors (see Table 42–3) can modify posttransfusion kinetics, in most circumstances platelet survival is affected more profoundly than platelet recovery. Thus, even patients with severe infection or disseminated intravascular coagulation (DIC) can have relatively normal immediate posttransfusion recoveries accompanied by much shortened platelet survivals. Massive splenomegaly, shock, and perhaps massive hemorrhage represent exceptions to this observation. In contrast, alloimmunized patients tend to have both markedly shortened platelet recoveries and survivals. It is, therefore, usually possible to distinguish alloimmunization from other complicating medical factors by measurement of platelet count increments one hour after transfusion. If poor increments are achieved at 24 hours after transfusion, all such patients should have one-hour counts done following their next transfusion. One-hour posttransfusion increments of less than 4,000 per unit are highly suggestive of alloimmunization in the absence of splenomegaly, overwhelming infection, or bleeding (Daly *et al.,* 1980). The one-hour increment should be done using fresh platelets because it is possible, in some patients, that the poor increments could be the result of transfusion of platelets damaged by improper storage. Measurement of lymphocytotoxic antibody (anti-HLA) can help confirm the diagnosis and indicate the need for single-donor histocompatible platelets (Hogge *et al.,* 1983a). Immune platelet destruction can also be the result of drug-related antibodies. Drug-directed antibodies can destroy platelets either by initial coating of the

Table 42–3. Factors Affecting the Recovery and Survival of Transfused Platelets

1. Alloimmunization
2. Hepatosplenomegaly
3. Disseminated intravascular coagulation
4. Infection, fever
5. Drug-associated antibody
6. Duration and method of platelet storage
7. Circulating immune complexes (?)

platelet by the drug or by absorption of the drug-antibody complex to the surface of the platelet with subsequent clearing by the reticuloendothelial system. Although this phenomenon has been described with a large number of drugs, quinidine, antibiotics (penicillins, sulfa drugs), and diuretics are the most common offenders (Karpatkin, 1971; Schiffer *et al.,* 1976b; Cimo *et al.,* 1977). The diagnosis should be suspected in patients who remain thrombocytopenic with megakaryocytes in the marrow or in whom well-matched platelet transfusions are unsuccessful. All medications should be discontinued or switched in such patients. Recently, it has also been suggested that circulating immune complexes, often detectable in patients with leukemia, may promote nonspecific platelet clearance and therefore decreased posttransfusion recovery (Kutti *et al.,* 1981). These observations remain to be confirmed by further studies.

Donor Selection. Platelets have HLA antigens that are shared with all other tissues and tested for most easily on lymphocytes, as well as platelet-specific antigens expressed on their surface (Schiffer, 1980). Although antibodies against platelet-specific antigens account for refractoriness in a small percentage of patients (Brand *et al.,* 1978; Schiffer, 1980), most alloimmunized patients can be successfully supported with platelets matched at the HLA and B loci (Yankee *et al.,* 1969; Lohrmann *et al.,* 1974; Duquesnoy *et al.,* 1977; Aster, 1978; Brand *et al.,* 1978; Gmur *et al.,* 1978). Most alloimmunized patients develop multispecific antibody (*i.e.,* directed against large numbers of HLA antigens), and because of this, they are less likely to respond successfully to platelets that are partially matched, but also mismatched for other HLA antigens. Thus, if HLA typing is not immediately available and one attempts to use family members as donors, it is best to utilize sibling donors first because, in most cases, parent-to-child or child-to-parent combinations include potential mismatches of the two HLA antigens contributed by the other parent.

Many blood centers have recruited large numbers of HLA-typed donors whose HLA types are stored in computer files that are searched when a particular recipient requires HLA-matched platelets (Graw *et al.,* 1977). Because of the large number of HLA antigens, however, it is sometimes necessary to screen more than 1000 to 2000 donors to find a single HLA-identical donor for a particular patient

(Duquesnoy *et al.,* 1977; Graw *et al.,* 1977). If perfectly matched platelets are not available, it is sometimes possible to successfully utilize platelets that are mismatched for antigens that are serologically cross-reactive (*i.e.,* antigenically similar) to the recipient's antigens (Duquesnoy *et al.,* 1977). Although the success of this approach is highly variable from patient to patient, in many patients the cross-reactive antigen will not be recognized as foreign and good posttransfusion count increments can occur. Certain other HLA antigens, such as the HLA, B44, B45 group are only weakly expressed on platelets in some donors (Liebert and Aster, 1977). Therefore, it is sometimes possible to mismatch for these antigens as well. As with random-donor platelets, the effect of HLA-matched platelets should be measured by careful assessment of increments 1 and 24 hours after transfusion.

When no histocompatible donors are available, the management of alloimmunized patients is difficult. It is inadvisable to continue to administer prophylactic transfusion to such patients. Bleeding in these patients can occasionally be managed by administration of large numbers of units of random-donor platelets either in a bolus or by prolonged continuous infusion. Although most patients do not respond to this approach, an occasional response will be seen that may be related to temporary removal of antibody by infusion of incompatible platelets, allowing subsequently administered platelets to have a short, but nonetheless increased, survival (Nagasawa *et al.,* 1978). In addition, when many units of platelets are given, it is possible that a fortuitously histocompatible unit will be selected that can exert some hemostatic effect.

Another approach to the management of alloimmunized patients is the provision of autologous platelets obtained at the time of remission of the patient's disease and transfused subsequently during periods of thrombocytopenia. Platelets can be frozen using dimethylsulfoxide as a cryoprotective agent for at least three years at liquid-nitrogen temperatures with preservation of morphology and the capacity to circulate and function hemostatically posttransfusion (Schiffer *et al.,* 1978a; Daly *et al.,* 1979a). Presently, this technology is available only in research settings, although the cryopreservation and the thawing procedures are relatively simple and should be available on a more widespread basis within the next few years. In addition, it is possible to freeze plate-

lets from donors known to be compatible with particular patients, thereby guaranteeing the availability of histocompatible platelets on short notice.

GRANULOCYTE TRANSFUSION THERAPY

A series of controlled trials in human beings (Higby *et al.,* 1975; Alavi *et al.,* 1977; Herzig *et al.,* 1977; Vogler and Winton, 1977) and animals (Epstein *et al.,* 1974; Dale *et al.,* 1976), as well as multiple, well-described observations of the benefits in other groups of patients (Graw *et al.,* 1972; McCredie *et al.,* 1973; Schiffer *et al.,* 1975b; Aisner *et al.,* 1978), has resulted in acceptance of the utility of therapeutic granulocyte transfusions in selected circumstances. A detailed analysis of the strengths and limitations of the available studies is beyond the scope of this chapter, and the reader is referred to several recent, comprehensive reviews (Boggs, 1974; Higby and Burnett, 1980; Schiffer and Aisner, 1980).

Granulocyte Collection

Granulocytes have approximately the same buoyant density as lighter red blood cells so that, in contrast to platelets, it is difficult to separate granulocytes from whole blood for transfusion by simple manual centrifugation. The same cytopheresis machines that are suitable for platelet collection by differential centrifugation from single donors can be used, with some modifications, for granulocyte collection (McCredie *et al.,* 1974; Mishler *et al.,* 1974; Huestis *et al.,* 1975; Hester *et al.,* 1979b; Aisner *et al.,* 1981; Kalmin and Grindon, 1981). Although these collection procedures have an excellent safety record, a number of medications, including corticosteroids and hydroxyethyl starch, are administered to donors to maximize the granulocyte yields. Because of these medications, as well as the inconvenience and the discomfort of multiple venipunctures, careful consideration should be given before initiating granulocyte transfusions, particularly since some donors are asked to donate on multiple occasions because of histocompatibility considerations. Filtration leukopheresis (FL), a collection method used in many centers in the early 1970s, is now rarely used in the United States because of concern about untoward side effects in donors (Dahlke *et al.,* 1979), possibly related to activation of the complement system during donation (Schiffer *et al.*, 1975a; Nusbacher *et al.*, 1978). In addition, transfusion of granulocytes obtained by this method is associated with an increased incidence of severe recipient reactions (Aisner *et al.*, 1978) owing to cell damage during the collection procedure (Wright *et al.*, 1978; Klock *et al.*, 1979) compared to cells obtained by differential centrifugation.

Although there have been major improvements in cytopheresis technology, the number of granulocytes that can be obtained from normal donors is far less than the number normal individuals mobilize to fight infection. Occasionally, it is possible to obtain more than one transfusion per day from two or more donors for severely infected individuals (Higby *et al.*, 1976). An alternate approach is to utilize patients with chronic myelogenous leukemia (CML) with high white counts in order to harvest near-physiologic numbers of leukocytes for transfusion. In addition, because early myeloid precursors are also administered, one often notes sustained production of granulocytes for a number of days following one or two transfusions of nonirradiated CML leukocytes (Schwarzenberg *et al.*, 1967; Eyre *et al.*, 1970; Schiffer *et al.*, 1982). In contrast, few circulating granulocytes remain the day after transfusion from normal donors. Although data indicate that granulocytes can be stored for up to 24 hours after collection, function appears to deteriorate with increasing storage, particularly after 24 hours (Glasser, 1977; Price and Dale, 1978; McCullough, 1980). Thus, all granulocyte transfusions should be administered as soon as possible after collection through an ordinary blood filter over a one-and-a-half- to three-hour period of time (approximately 10^{10} cells/hour).

Indications for Granulocyte Transfusions

At least 75 to 80% of infected granulocytopenic patients improve when treated with appropriate antibiotic therapy (E.O.R.T.C., 1978; Keating *et al.*, 1979; Klastersky, 1979; Love *et al.*, 1979, 1980). Granulocyte transfusions, therefore, should be used only for patients who either are failing to respond to antibiotic therapy or are likely to do more poorly because of certain clinical factors. Virtually all large antibiotic trials in granulocytopenic patients have shown that the most important prognostic factor (aside from the choice of appropriate antibiotics) is the recovery of the pa-

tient's bone marrow with production of endogenous granulocytes (E.O.R.T.C., 1978; Love *et al.*, 1979). Rises in granulocyte count of as little as $100/\mu L$ within four to seven days of the onset of infection are associated with response rates of greater than 90 to 95% in most studies. Thus, granulocyte transfusions are rarely indicated in the absence of profound (less than $100/mm^3$) granulocytopenia. Prior to initiating granulocyte transfusion, it is often helpful to perform bone marrow examinations because transfusions frequently can be withheld in patients in whom bone marrow recovery is imminent.

The site of infection, the type of organism, and the presence of bacteremia are additional important prognostic factors. Morbidity and mortality are higher for parenchymal infections, particularly pneumonia, than for more localized infections such as cellulitis. Infections with gram-negative organisms are generally more serious than gram-positive-organism infections, particularly when associated with bacteremia. Mortality is further increased when infection is caused by antibiotic-resistant organisms and, obviously, all infections are more poorly tolerated by older patients with preexisting cardiac, renal, or hepatic dysfunction.

Because of the dosage problems imposed by the limitations of collection technology, it is preferable to begin granulocyte transfusions when clinical suspicion suggests that antibiotic therapy is ineffective. Poorer risk patients can be identified using the guidelines presented above, and tentative arrangements for granulocyte transfusion can be made with identification and scheduling of suitable donors. If the patient improves or if marrow recovery occurs, donations can be cancelled. In general, decisions about the need for granulocyte transfusions can be made in most patients within 24 to 36 hours of the onset of infection.

Once the decision is made to provide granulocyte transfusions, the transfusions should be given at least daily, using collection equipment that provides the highest possible yields. When granulocytes from normal donors are used, most patients require at least three to four daily transfusions before maximal clinical responses are seen. The duration of granulocyte transfusion therapy is determined by the clinical response, and in some patients can present a difficult clinical decision. Clearly, patients who recover endogenous marrow function do not require further transfusions. In responding patients, without marrow recovery, transfusions are usually continued until the more serious signs and symptoms of infection have abated.

More problematic are decisions in patients in whom severe transfusion reactions occur or a poor clinical response is evident. In general, if fresh, appropriately prepared granulocytes are used, severe reactions are indicative of donor-recipient histoincompatibility and suggest that different donors be utilized. In patients in whom infections progress or at best stabilize, a rigorous search for secondary infections with new bacterial or, more commonly, fungal organisms is indicated so that new antibiotics can be begun or doses increased. Patients receiving appropriate antibiotics whose condition continues to worsen are unlikely to benefit from further granulocyte transfusions. In practice, marrow recovery, clinical improvement, alloimmunization with limitation of the number of available donors, or patient death occurs within two weeks of the onset of transfusion so that it is uncommon to administer granulocyte transfusions for longer than this period of time.

Relatively little has been published dealing with the treatment of fungal infections with granulocyte transfusions. Clinically, it is well recognized that serious systemic fungal infections in nonimmunosuppressed patients develop almost exclusively in the setting of severe granulocytopenia. Similarly, clinical improvement with eradication of fungal infection often occurs promptly with marrow regeneration. In a dog model of systemic *Candida* infection, evidence suggests that granulocyte transfusions can decrease the severity of fungal infections, although insufficient transfusions were administered to demonstrate cures of the infections (Chow *et al.*, 1980). These observations suggest that granulocyte transfusions could theoretically be effective in fungal infections. It is likely that dosage considerations are of greater importance than with bacterial infections, since considerable delays in diagnosis and institution of amphotericin B often occur, and infections are far advanced when transfusions are begun.

Side Effects of Granulocyte Transfusion

If appropriate donors are used and the granulocytes are collected and prepared properly and administered slowly, there should be no major change in the patient's condition during or after the granulocyte infusion. Severe pyro-

genic reactions can and often do occur, however, and should be regarded as a sign that a problem in donor-recipient histocompatibility or in the quality of the granulocyte preparation itself has occurred. These more severe febrile reactions are usually accompanied by shaking chills and can be associated with tachycardia, anxiety, dyspnea, and blood pressure changes. Cessation of the transfusion with or without the administration of acetaminophen or antihistamines generally ameliorates the reactions within a short period of time.

A variety of pulmonary signs and symptoms can also occur during or after the granulocyte transfusion. Worsening pulmonary status can be the result of progressive pneumonia, volume overload, an immunologic reaction to the transfused granulocytes, increased inflammation owing to migration of granulocytes to an area of pneumonitis, or, in patients receiving amphotericin B, related to possible interaction with the drug resulting in trapping of the granulocytes in the pulmonary vasculature (Boxer *et al.*, 1981; Wright *et al.*, 1981). It is often difficult to distinguish among these possibilities, and additional transfusions should be given with great care.

Last, an increased incidence of cytomegalovirus (CMV) infections has been described in bone marrow transplant patients receiving granulocyte transfusions (Winston *et al.*, 1980; Hersman *et al.*, 1982). These CMV infections occurred predominantly in recipients without serologic evidence of prior exposure to CMV and was associated with an increased incidence of interstitial pneumonia. Although there may also be an increase in CMV acquisition in nonmarrow transplant patients with acute leukemia receiving granulocyte transfusions (Winston *et al.*, 1980), the infections in these patients are usually less severe and more often subclinical.

Histocompatibility Testing

It is well known that the vast majority of febrile reactions following red blood cell transfusions are caused by recipient antibody directed against leukocytes administered with the whole blood or packed RBCs. It was not surprising, therefore, given the larger number of cells administered with leukocyte transfusions, that often severe febrile, allergic reactions were described in many recipients in the early granulocyte transfusion literature (Graw *et al.*, 1970; Goldstein *et al.*, 1971). Until recently, however, most centers did not consider possible histocompatibility barriers when selecting donors for granulocyte transfusion.

In granulocytopenic animal models, it has been demonstrated that random-donor granulocytes do not migrate to sites of infection in alloimmunized dogs. In these studies posttransfusion granulocyte recovery and migration to skin windows (Appelbaum et al., 1977) or to the cerebrospinal fluid in dogs with induced meningitis (Chow et al., 1980) were markedly reduced in alloimmunized animals compared to nonimmunized controls. In another model in which bacteremia was induced in granulocytopenic dogs, survival was also impaired in alloimmunized granulocyte transfusion recipients (Westrick et al., 1977). It is difficult to perform comparable experiments in human beings, and because of the large number of variables that affect ultimate clinical response in these complex, seriously ill patients, it has been difficult to correlate in vitro histocompatibility tests with any posttransfusion clinical parameter (Ungerleider et al., 1979). In particular, posttransfusion recovery of transfused granulocytes is usually quite low, with absolute posttransfusion increments in the 100 to $300/\mu L$ range and infrequently greater than $1000/\mu L$. Because of inaccuracies of counts and differentials at these WBC levels, posttransfusion increments have been an unsatisfactory means of assessing the results of granulocyte transfusion.

The recent use of the radioisotope indium-111 as a granulocyte label has enabled experiments to be done in human beings that have provided parallel results to those noted in animals. Two studies have been done in which granulocytopenic patients with discrete areas of infection received indium-111-labeled granulocytes from nonmatched donors with follow-up scans done over the sites of infection (Dutcher et al., 1983; McCullough et al., 1981). Migration of granulocytes to infected sites as early as 30 minutes after injection was noted in nonalloimmunized patients (Dutcher et al., 1981). These observations indicate that careful pretransfusion cross-matching and donor screening is unnecessary for nonimmunized recipients. In contrast, with few exceptions, scans were negative in alloimmunized patients, indicating an absence of granulocyte migration and suggesting that nonmatched granulocyte transfusions administered to such patients would be ineffective.

It is the question of what constitutes a matched transfusion that remains problematic. Granulocytes have a number of different types of antigens on their surfaces, including antigens unique to granulocytes (granulocyte-specific antigens) as well as antigens shared with other cells (Lalezari, 1977a,b). Granulocyte-specific antigens are inherited independently of HLA antigens and have gene frequencies of 30 to 70%, so that it is likely that donors will be mismatched for some of these antigens. Further complicating matters is the difficulty in reproducibly and rapidly performing granulocyte-antibody testing and cross-matching in vitro.

Neither of the indium-111 studies permits conclusions to be made about whether granulocyte-specific or HLA antigens are most important for cross-matching purposes. Examples are available in both studies of successful migration in spite of either positive lymphocytotoxic or leukoagglutinin cross-matches. Nonetheless, both studies indicate that in view of the expense, likelihood of recipient side effects, minimum chance of efficacy, and the risk, albeit small, of donor side effects, alloimmunized patients should not receive granulocyte transfusions from random donors. Our center attempts to utilize compatible platelet donors as granulocyte donors with a preference for family members, in the hope that the granulocyte-specific antigens, which cannot be typed easily, are more likely to be identifiable in the family setting. In some patients it is helpful to monitor the platelet-count increments after mixed platelet-granulocyte transfusions as an indirect marker for compatibility. If significant transfusion reactions occur, new donors are used, and if no closely matched donors are available, transfusions are discontinued. It is unusual to be able to identify large numbers of potentially compatible donors for alloimmunized patients. Therefore, donors are often requested to donate repetitively for such patients. This may present a significant burden for some donors and should be considered when a course of transfusions is initiated.

It has been noted that recipients of granulocyte transfusions frequently become alloimmunized and develop transfusion reactions toward the end of a series of granulocyte transfusions (Thompson et al., 1977; Schiffer et al., 1979). This is a particular problem in patients receiving prophylactic granulocyte transfusion in an attempt to prevent infection in granulocytopenic patients (Mannoni et al., 1977; Schiffer et al., 1979; Strauss et al., 1981). Although such transfusions probably are successful in decreasing the acquisition of infection, no improvement in survival has been seen, presumably because the acquired infections could be treated successfully with antibiotics (Mannoni *et al.,* 1977; Clift *et al.,* 1978; Strauss *et al.,* 1981). Because of the cost (Rosenshein *et al.,* 1980), high rate of alloimmunization and transfusion reactions, and donor considerations, prophylactic granulocyte transfusions should be used only in investigational settings, if at all (Schiffer, 1982).

It has been suggested that lithium carbonate administered to patients receiving intensive chemotherapy may reduce the incidence and duration of severe granulocytopenia, therefore reducing or eliminating the need for granulocyte transfusions. Leukocytosis has been well documented as an effect of lithium therapy in psychiatric patients. This leukocytosis is accompanied by enhanced proliferation of human granulocyte colonies *in vitro* (Tisman *et al.,* 1973) and enhanced production of colony-stimulating activity by cultured human leukocytes (Joyce and Chervenick, 1975). Evidence suggests that a primary effect of lithium may be stimulation of the pluripotent stem cell (Levitt and Quesenberry, 1980), and this observation has led to some concern about the use of lithium in acute leukemia patients. Lithium has been used as an adjunct to intensive therapy in a variety of neoplastic disorders without a significant advantage for lithium-treated patients being clearly demonstrated. In one small recent controlled study, oat cell carcinoma patients treated with combination chemotherapy had fewer infections and shorter hospitalizations if they also received lithium compared to controls who did not (Lyman *et al.,* 1980). Lithium-treated patients had a higher incidence of other problems which require frequent lithium-dose modification or discontinuation of the drug. In addition, while lithium may shorten the period of moderate granulocytopenia (100–500/mL), there is no change in the duration of severe (<100/mL) granulocytopenia. Thus, lithium is of little clinical value in controlling drug-induced bone marrow suppression patients receiving intensive myelosuppressive therapy.

REFERENCES

Aisner, J.; Schiffer, C. A.; Daly, P. A.; and Buchholz, D. H.: Evaluation of gravity leukapheresis and comparison with intermittent centrifugation leukapheresis. *Transfusion,* 21:100–106, 1981.

Aisner, J.; Schiffer, C. A.; and Wiernik, P. H.: Granulocyte transfusions: Evaluation of factors influencing results and a comparison of filtration and intermittent centrifugation leukapheresis. *Br. J. Haematol.,* 38:121–129, 1978.

Aisner, J.; Schiffer, C. A.; and Wolff, J. H.: A standardized technique for efficient platelet and leukocyte collection using the Model 30 Blood Processor. *Transfusion,* 16:437–445, 1976.

Alavi, J. B.; Root, R. K.; and Djerassi, I.; Evans, A. E.; Gluckman, S. J.; MacGregor, R. R.; Guerry, D.; Schreiber, A. D.; Shaw, J. M.; Koch, P., and Cooper, R. A.: A randomized clinical trial of granulocyte transfusions for infection in acute leukemia. *N. Engl. J. Med.,* 296:706–711, 1977.

Alter, H. J.; Holland, P. V.; and Purcell, R. H.: Posttransfusion hepatitis after exclusion of commercial and hepatitis-B antigen-positive donors. *Ann. Intern. Med.,* 77:691, 1972.

Appelbaum, F. R.; Trapani, R. J.; and Graw, R. G., Jr.: Consequences of prior alloimmunization during granulocyte transfusion. *Transfusion,* 17:460–464, 1977.

Aster, R. H.: Matching of blood platelets for transfusion. *Am. J. Hematol.,* 5:373–378, 1978.

Belt, R. J.; Leite, C.; Haas, C. D.; and Stephens, R. L.: Incidence of hemorrhagic complications in patients with cancer. *J.A.M.A.,* 239:2571–2574, 1978.

Boggs, D. R.: Transfusion of neutrophils as prevention or treatment of infection in patients with neutropenia. *N. Engl. J. Med.,* 290:1055–1062, 1974.

Boxer, L. A.; Ingraham, L. M.; Allen, J.: Oseas, R. S.; and Baehner, R. L.: Amphotericin-B promotes leukocyte aggregation of nylon-wool-fiber-treated polymorphonuclear leukocytes. *Blood,* 58:518–522, 1981.

Brand, A.; van Leeuwen, A.; Eernisse, J. G.; and van Rood, J. J.: Platelet transfusion therapy. Optimal donor selection with a combination of lymphocytotoxicity and platelet fluorescence tests. *Blood,* 51:781–788, 1978.

Buchholz, D. H.; Young, V. M.; and Friedman, N. R.: Bacterial proliferation in platelet products stored at room temperature. *N. Engl. J. Med.,* 285:429, 1971.

Chow, H. S.; Sarpel, S. C.; and Epstein, R. B.: Pathophysiology of *Candida albicans* meningitis in normal, neutropenic, and granulocyte-transfused dogs. *Blood,* 55:546–551, 1980.

Cimo, P. L.; Pisciotta, A. V.; and Desai, R. G.: Detection of drug-dependent antibodies by the ⁵¹Cr platelet lysis test: Documentation of immune thrombocytopenia induced by diphenylhydantoin, diazepam, and sulfisoxazole. *Am. J. Hematol.,* 2:65–72, 1977.

Clift, R. A.; Saunders, J. E.; Thomas, E. D.; Williams, B.; and Buckner, C. D.: Granulocyte tranfusions for the prevention of infection in patients receiving bone-marrow transplants. *N. Engl. J. Med.,* 298:1052–1057, 1978.

Dahlke, M. B.; Shah, S. L.; Sherwood, W. C.; Shafer, A. W., and Brownstein, P. K.: Priapism during filtration leukapheresis. *Transfusion,* 19:482–486, 1979.

Dale, D. C.; Reynolds, H. Y.; and Pennington, J. E.: Experimental pseudomonas pneumonia in leukopenic dogs: Comparison of therapy with antibiotics and granulocyte transfusions. *Blood,* 47:869–876, 1976.

Daly, P. A.; Schiffer, C. A.; Aisner, J.; and Wiernik, P. H.: Successful transfusion of platelets cryopreserved for more than 3 years. *Blood,* 54:1023–1027, 1979a.

Daly, P. A.; Schiffer, C. A.; Aisner, J.; and Wiernik, P. H.: A comparison of platelets prepared by the Haemonetics Model 30 and multiunit bag plateletpheresis. *Transfusion,* 19:778–781, 1979b.

Daly, P. A.; Schiffer, C. A.; Aisner, J.; and Wiernik, P. H.: Platelet transfusion therapy—One hour post-transfusion increments are valuable in predicting the need for HLA-matched preparations. *J.A.M.A., 243*:435–438, 1980.

Duquesnoy, R. J.; Filip, D. J.; and Rodey, G. E.: Successful transfusion of platelets "mismatched" for HLA antigens to alloimmunized thrombocytopenic patients. *Am. J. Hematol., 2*:219–226, 1977.

Dutcher, J. P.; Schiffer, C. A.; Aisner, J.; and Wiernik, P. H.: Alloimmunization following platelet transfusion: The absence of a dose response relationship. *Blood, 57*:395–398, 1980.

Dutcher, J. P.; Schiffer, C. A.; Aisner, J.; and Wiernik, P. H.: Long term followup of patients with leukemia receiving platelet transfusions: Identification of a large group of patients who do not become alloimmunized. *Blood, 58*:1007–1011, 1981a.

Dutcher, J. P.; Schiffer, C. A.; and Johnston, G. S.: Rapid migration of ¹¹¹Indium-labeled granulocytes to sites of infection. *N. Engl. J. Med., 304*:586–589, 1981b.

Dutcher, J. P.; Schiffer, C. A.; Johnston, G. S.; Papenberg, D.; Daly, P. A.; Aisner, J.; and Wiernik, P. H.: Alloimmunization prevents the migration of transfused ¹¹¹Indium-labeled granulocytes to sites of infection. *Blood, 62*:815–820, 1983.

E.O.R.T.C. International Antimicrobial Therapy Project Group: Three antibiotic regimens in the treatment of infection in febrile granulocytopenic patients with cancer. *J. Infect. Dis., 137*:14–29, 1978.

Epstein, R. B.; Waxman, F. J.; and Bennett, B. T.: Pseudomonas septicemia in neutropenic dogs. I. Treatment with granulocyte transfusions. *Transfusion, 14*:51–57, 1974.

Eyre, J. H.; Goldstein, I. M.; and Perry, S.: Leukocyte transfusions: Function of transfused granulocytes from donors with chronic myelocytic leukemia. *Blood, 36*:432–442, 1970.

Fahey, J. L.; Scoggins, R.; Utz, J. P.; and Szwed, C. F.: Infection, antibody response and gamma globulin components in multiple myeloma and macroglobulinemia. *Am. J. Med., 35*:698–707, 1963.

Filip, D. J., and Aster, R. H.: Relative hemostatic effectiveness of human platelets stored at 4° and 22°C. *J. Lab. Clin. Med., 91*:618–624, 1978.

Garfield, M. D.; Ershler, W. B.; and Maki, D. G.: Malaria transmission by platelet concentrate transfusion. *J.A.M.A., 240*:2285, 1978.

Glasser, L.: Effect of storage on normal neutrophils collected by discontinuous-flow centrifugation leukapheresis. *Blood, 50*:1145–1150, 1977.

Gmur, J.; von Felten, A.; and Frick, P.: Platelet support in polysensitized patients: Role of HLA specificities and crossmatch testing for donor selection. *Blood, 51*:903–909, 1978.

Goldstein, I. M.; Eyre, H. J.; and Terasaki, P. I.: Leukocyte transfusions: Role of leukocyte alloantibodies in determining transfusion response. *Transfusion, 11*:19–24, 1971.

Graw, R. G.; Goldstein, I. M.; Eyre, H. J.; and Terasaki, P. I.: Histocompatibility testing for leukocyte transfusion. *Lancet, 1*:77–78, 1970.

Graw, R. G.; Herzig, R. H.; and Langston, M. G.: National donor registry and computer transfusion programs for platelet transfusions. *Transplant. Proc., 9*:225–227, 1977.

Graw, R. G.; Herzig, G.; and Perry, S.: Normal granulocyte transfusion therapy. Treatment of septicemia due to gram-negative bacteria. *N. Engl. J. Med., 287*:367–371, 1972.

Green, D.; Tiro, A.; and Basiliere, J.: Cytotoxic antibody complicating platelet support in acute leukemia. *J.A.M.A., 236*:1044, 1976.

Gurwith, M. J.; Brunton, J. L.; Lank, B. A.; Harding, G. K. M.; and Ronald, A. R.: A prospective controlled investigation of prophylactic trimethoprim/sulfamethoxazole in hospitalized granulocytopenic patients. *Am. J. Med., 66*:248–256, 1979.

Hersman, J.; Meyers, J. D.; Thomas, E. D.; Buckner, C. D.; and Clift, R.: The effect of granulocyte transfusions on the incidence of cytomegalovirus infection after allogeneic marrow transplantation. *Ann. Intern. Med., 96*:149–152, 1982.

Herzig, R. H.; Herzig, G. P.; and Bull, M. I.: Correction of poor platelet transfusion responses with leukocyte poor HLA-matched platelet concentrates. *Blood, 46*:743, 1975.

Herzig, B. H.; Herzig, G. P.; Graw, R. G., Jr.; Bull, M. I.; and Ray, K. K.: Granulocyte transfusion therapy for gram-negative septicemia. *N. Engl. J. Med., 296*:701–705, 1977.

Hester, J. P.; Kellogg, R. M.; Mulzet, A. P.; Kruger, V. R.; McCredie, K. B.; and Freireich, E. J.: Variable anticoagulant (AC) flow rates for plateletpheresis in the dual stage disposable channel. *Blood, 54*(Suppl. 1):124a, 1979a.

Hester, J. P.; Kellogg, R. M.; Mulzet, A. P.; Kruger, V. R.; McCredie, K. B.; and Freireich, E. J.: Principles of blood separation and component extraction in a disposable continuous-flow single-stage channel. *Blood, 54*:254–268, 1979b.

Higby, D. J., and Burnett, D.: Granulocyte transfusions: Current status. *Blood, 55*:2–8, 1980.

Higby, D. J.; Cohen, E.; Holland, J. F.; and Sinks, L.: The prophylactic treatment of thrombocytopenic leukemic patients with platelets: A double blind study. *Transfusion, 14*:440–446, 1974.

Higby, D. J.; Freeman, A.; and Henderson, E. S.: Granulocyte transfusions in children using filter-collected cells. *Cancer, 38*:1407–1413, 1976.

Higby, D. J.; Yates, J. W.; Henderson, E. S.; and Holland J. F.: Filtration leukapheresis for granulocyte transfusion therapy. *N. Engl. J. Med., 292*:761–766, 1975.

Hogge, D. E.; Dutcher, J. P.; Aisner, J.; and Schiffer, C. A.: Lymphocytotoxic antibody is a predicter of response to random donor platelet transfusion. *Am. J. Hematol., 14*:363–370, 1983a.

Hogge, D. E., and Schiffer, C. A.: Seven day platelet storage in second generation CLX blood bags. *Blood 62*(suppl. 1):234a, 1983b.

Holme, S.; Vaidja, K.; and Murphy, S.: Platelet storage at 22°C: Effect of type of agitation on morphology, viability, and function *in vitro. Blood, 52*:425–436, 1978.

Howard, J. E., and Perkins, H. A.: The natural history of alloimmunization to platelets. *Transfusion, 18*:496, 1978.

Huestis, D. W.; White, R. F.; Price, M. J.; and Inman, M.: Use of hydroxyethyl starch to improve granulocyte collection in the Latham blood processor. *Transfusion, 15*:559–564, 1975.

Joyce, R. A., and Chervenick, P. A.: Effect of lithium on the release of colony stimulating activity (CSA) from blood leukocytes. *Proc. Am. Soc. Hematol., 18*:126, 1975.

Kalmin, N. E., and Grindon, A. J.: Pheresis with the IBM 2997. *Transfusion, 21*:325–329, 1981.

Karpatkin, S.: Drug-induced thrombocytopenia. *Am. J. Med. Sci.,* **262**:69–78, 1971.

Katz, A. J.; Genco, P. V.; Blumberg, N.; Snyder, E. L.; Camp, B.; and Morse, E. E.: Platelet collection and transfusion using the Fenwal CS-3000 cell separator. *Transfusion,* **21**:560–563, 1981.

Keating, M. J.; Bodey, G. P.; Valdivieso, M.; and Rodriguez, V.: A randomized comparative trial of three aminoglycosides—comparison of continuous infusions of gentamicin, amikacin and sisomicin combined with carbenicillin in the treatment of infections in neutropenic patients with malignancies. *Medicine,* **58**:159–170, 1979.

Klastersky, J.: Combinations of antibiotics for therapy of severe infections in cancer patients. *Eur. J. Cancer,* **15**:3–13, 1979.

Klastersky, J.; Cappel, R.; and Daneau, D.: Clinical significance of *in vitro* synergism between antibiotics in gram-negative infections. *Antimicrob. Agents Chemother.,* **2**:470–475, 1972.

Klock, J. C.; Boyles, J.; Bainton, D. F.; and Stossel, T. P.: Nylon-fiber-induced neutrophil fragmentation. *Blood,* **54**:1216–1229, 1979.

Kutti, J.; Zaroulis, C. G.; Safai-Kutti, S.; Dinsmore, R. E.; Day, N. K.; and Good, R. A.: Evidence that circulating immune complexes remove transfused platelets from the circulation. *Am. J. Hematol.,* **11**:255–259, 1981.

Lalezari, P.: Neutrophil antigens: immunology and clinical implications. In Greenwalt, T. J., and Jamison, G. A. (eds.): *The Granulocyte: Function and Clinical Utilization.* Alan R. Liss, Inc., New York, 1977a.

Lalezari, P.: Neutrophil-specific antigens: Their relationship to neonatal and acquired neutropenias with comments on the possible role of organ-specific alloantigens in organ transplantation. *Transplant. Proc.,* **9**:1881–1886, 1977b.

Levitt, L. J. and Quesenberry, P. J.: Effect of lithium on murine hematopoiesis in a liquid culture system. *N. Engl. J. Med.,* **302**:713–719, 1980.

Liebert, M., and Aster, R. H.: Expression of HLA-B12 on platelets, on lymphocytes and in serum: A quantitative study. *Tissue Antigens,* **9**:199–208, 1977.

Lohrmann, H. P.; Bull, M. I.; and Decter, J. A.: Platelet transfusions from HL-A compatible unrelated donors to alloimmunized patients. *Ann. Intern. Med.,* **80**:9–14, 1974.

Love, L. J.; Schimpff, S. C.; Hahn, D. M.; Young, V. M.; Standiford H. C.; Bender, J. F.; Fortner, C. L.; and Wiernik, P. H.: Randomized trial of empiric antibiotic therapy with ticarcillin in combinaton with gentamicin, amikacin or netilmicin in febrile patients with granulocytopenia and cancer. *Am. J. Med.,* **66**:603–610, 1979.

Love, L. J., Schimpff, S. C.; Schiffer, C. A.; and Wiernik, P. H.: Improved prognosis for granulocytopenic patients with gram-negative bacteremia. *Am. J. Med.,* **68**:643–648, 1980.

Lyman, G. H.; Williams, C. G.; and Preston, D.: The use of lithium carbonate to reduce infection and leukopenia during systemic chemotherapy. *N. Engl. J. Med.,* **302**:257–260, 1980.

Mannoni, P.; Rodet, M.; and Radeau, E.: Granulocyte transfusion: Efficiency of prophylactic granulocyte transfusions in care of patients with acute leukemia. In Hogman, C. S.; Lindahl-Kiessling, K.; and Wigzell, H. (eds.): *Blood Leukocytes: Function and Use in Therapy.* Almquist and Wiksell International, Stockholm, 1977.

McCredie, K. B.; Freireich, E. J.; Hester, J. P.; and Vallejos, C.: Leukocyte transfusion therapy for patients with host-defense failure. *Transplant. Proc.,* **5**:1285–1289, 1973.

McCredie, K. B.; Freireich, E. J.; Hester, J. P.; and Vallejos, C.: Increased granulocyte collection with the blood cell separator and the addition of etiocholanolone and hydroxyethyl starch. *Transfusion,* **14**:357–364, 1974.

McCullough, J.: Liquid preservation of granulocytes. *Transfusion,* **20**:129–137, 1980.

McCullough, J.; Weiblen, B. J.; Clay, M. E.; and Forstrom, L.: Effect of leukocyte antibodies on the fate *in vivo* of indium-111-labeled granulocytes. *Blood,* **58**:164–170, 1981.

Mishler, J. M.; Higby, D. J.; and Rhomberg, W.: Hydroxyethyl starch and dexamethasone as an adjunct to leukocyte separation with the IBM blood cell separator. *Transfusion,* **14**:352–356, 1974.

Murphy, S., and Gardner, F. H.: Platelet storage at 22°C; metabolic, morphologic and functional studies. *J. Clin. Invest.,* **50**:370–377, 1971.

Murphy, S., and Simon, T.: Characteristics of prolonged platelet storage in a new container. *Transfusion,* **21**:637, 1981.

Nagasawa, T.; Kim, B. K.; and Baldini, M. G.: Temporary suppression of circulating platelet antiplatelet alloantibodies by the massive infusion of fresh, stored or lyophilized platelets. *Transfusion,* **18**:429, 1978.

Nusbacher, J.; Rosenfeld, S. I.; MacPherson, J. L.; Thiem, P. A.; and Leddy, J. P.: Nylon fiber leukapheresis: Associated complement component changes and granulocytopenia. *Blood,* **51**:359–365, 1978.

Price, T. H., and Dale, D. C.: Neutrophil transfusion: Effect of storage and of collection method on neutrophil blood kinetics. *Blood,* **51**:789–798, 1978.

Rhame, F. S.; Root, R. K.; and MacLowry, J. D.: Salmonella septicemia from platelet transfusions. Study of an outbreak traced to a hematogenous carrier of *Salmonella cholerae-suis. Ann. Intern. Med.,* **78**:633, 1973.

Rosenshein, M. S.; Farewell, V. T.; Price, T. H.; Larson, E. B.; and Dale, D. C.: The cost effectiveness of therapeutic and prophylactic leukocyte transfusion. *N. Engl. J. Med.,* **302**:1058–1062, 1980.

Roy, A. J.; Jaffe, N.; and Djerassi, I.: Prophylactic platelet transfusions in children with acute leukemia: A dose response study. *Transfusion,* **13**:283–290, 1973.

Schiffer, C. A.: Principles of granulocyte transfusion therapy. *Med. Clin. North Am.,* **61**:1119–1131, 1977.

Schiffer, C. A.: Annotation: Some aspects of recent advances in the use of blood cell components. *Br. J. Haematol.,* **39**:289–294, 1978.

Schiffer, C. A.: Clinical importance of antiplatelet antibody testing for the blood bank. In Bell, C. A. (ed.): *A Seminar on Antigens on Blood Cells and Body Fluids.* American Association of Blood Banks, Washington, D.C., 1980.

Schiffer, C. A.: International Forum: What are the parameters to be controlled in platelet concentrates in order that they may be offered to the medical profession as a standardized product with specific properties? *Vox Sang.,* **40**:122–124, 1981.

Schiffer, C. A.: Is prophylactic granulocyte transfusion in the best interest of the patient? In Wiernik, P. H. (ed.): *Controversies in Oncology.* John Wiley & Sons, Inc., New York, 1982.

Schiffer, C. A., and Aisner, J.: Rational approach to granulocyte transfusion therapy. In LoBue, J., and Silber, R. (eds.): *Contemporary Hematology/Oncology.* Plenum Publishing Corporation, New York, 1980.

Schiffer, C. A.; Aisner, J.; Daly, P. A.; Schimpff, S. C.; and Wiernik, P. H.: Alloimmunization following prophylactic granulocyte transfusion. *Blood,* **54:**766–775, 1979.

Schiffer, C. A.; Aisner, J.; Dutcher, J.; and Wiernik, P. H.: Sustained post transfusion granulocyte count increments following transfusion of leukocytes obtained from patients with chronic myelogenous leukemia. *Am. J. Hematol.,* **15:**65–74, 1982.

Schiffer, C. A.; Aisner, J.; and Wiernik, P. H.: Frozen autologous platelet transfusion for patients with leukemia. *N. Engl. J. Med.,* **299:**7–12, 1978a.

Schiffer, C. A.; Aisner, J.; and Wiernik, P. H.: Platelet transfusion therapy for patients with leukemia. In Greenwalt, T. J., and Jamieson, G. A. (eds.): *The Blood Platelet in Transfusion Therapy.* Alan R. Liss, Inc., New York, 1978b.

Schiffer, C. A.; Aisner, J.; and Wiernik, P. H.: Transient neutropenia induced by transfusion of blood exposed to nylon fiber filters. *Blood,* **45:**141–146, 1975a.

Schiffer, C. A.; Buchholz, D. H.; Aisner, J.; Betts, S. W.; and Wiernik, P. H.: Clinical experience with transfusion of granulocytes obtained by continuous flow filtration leukopheresis. *Am. J. Med.,* **58:**373–381, 1975b.

Schiffer, C. A.; Lichtenfeld, J. L.; and Wiernik, P. H.: Antibody response in patients with acute non-lymphocytic leukemia. *Cancer,* **37:**2177–2182, 1976a.

Schiffer, C. A., and Slichter, S. J.: Platelet transfusions from single donors. *N. Engl. J. Med.,* **307:**245–248, 1982.

Schiffer, C. A.; Weinstein, H. J.; and Wiernik, P. H.: Methicillin-associated thrombocytopenia. *Ann. Intern. Med.,* **85:**3, 1976b.

Schwarzenberg, L.; Mathe, G.; and Amiel, J. L.: Study of factors determining the usefulness and complications of leukocyte transfusions. *Am. J. Med.,* **43:**206–213, 1967.

Silver, H.; Sonnenwirth, A. C.; and Beisser, L. D.: Bacteriologic study of platelet concentrates prepared and stored without refrigeration. *Transfusion,* **10:**315, 1970.

Slichter, S. J.: Efficacy of platelets collected by semi-continuous flow centrifugation (Haemonetics Model 30). *Br. J. Haematol.,* **38:**131–140, 1978.

Slichter, S. J., and Harker, L. A.: Preparation and storage of platelet concentrates: II. Storage variables influencing platelet viability and function. *Br. J. Haematol.,* **34:**403–418, 1976.

Strauss, R. G.; Connett, J. E.; Gale, R. P.; Bloomfield, C. D.; Herzig, G. P.; McCullough, J.; Maguire, L. C.; Winston, D. J.; Ho, W.; Stump, D. C.; Miller, W. V.; and Koepke, J. A.: A controlled trial of prophylactic granulocyte transfusions during initial induction chemotherapy for acute myelogenous leukemia. *N. Engl. J. Med.,* **305:**597–603, 1981.

Tejada, F.; Bias, W. B.; and Santos, G. W.: Immunologic response of patients with acute leukemia to platelet transfusions. *Blood,* **42:**405, 1973.

Thompson, J. S.; Burns, C. P.; and Herbick, J. M.: Stimulation of granulocyte antibodies by granulocyte transfusion. *Blood,* **50:**303, 1977.

Tisman, G.; Herbert, V.; and Rosenblatt, S.: Evidence that lithium induces human granulocyte proliferation: Elevated serum vitamin B_{12} binding capacity *in vivo. Br. J. Haematol.,* **24:**767–771, 1973.

Ungerleider, R. S.; Appelbaum, F. R.; Trapani, R. J.; and Diesseroth, A. B.: Lack of predictive value of antileukocyte antibody screening in granulocyte transfusion therapy. *Transfusion,* **19:**90–94, 1979.

Vogler, W. R., and Winton, E. F.: A controlled study of the efficacy of granulocyte transfusions in patients with neutropenia. *Am. J. Med.,* **63:**548–554, 1977.

Westrick, M. A.; Debelak-Fehir, K. M.; and Epstein, R. B.: The effect of prior whole blood transfusion on subsequent granulocyte support in leukopenic dogs. *Transfusion,* **17:**611–614, 1977.

Winston, D. J.; Ho, W. G.; Howell, C. L.; Miller, M. J.; Mickey, R.; Martin, W. J.; Lin, C. H.; and Gale, R. P.: Cytomegalovirus infections associated with leukocyte transfusions. *Ann. Intern. Med.,* **93:**671–675, 1980.

Wright, D. G.; Kauffmann, J. C.; Terpstra, G. K.; Graw, R. G.; Diesseroth, A. B.; and Gallin, J. I.: Mobilization and exocytosis of specific (secondary) granules by human neutrophils during adherence to nylon wool in filtration leukapheresis (FL). *Blood,* **52:**770–782, 1978.

Wright, D. G.; Robichaud, K. J.; Pizzo, P. A.; and Deisseroth, A. B.: Lethal pulmonary reactions associated with the combined use of amphotericin B and leukocyte transfusions. *N. Engl. J. Med.,* **304:**1185–1189, 1981.

Yankee, R. A.; Grumet, F. C.; and Rogentine, G. N.: Platelet transfusion therapy. The selection of compatible platelet donors for refractory patients by lymphocyte HL-A typing. *N. Engl. J. Med.,* **281:**1208–1212, 1969.

43

Bone Marrow Transplantation for Cancer

ALEXANDER FEFER

Bone marrow transplantation represents the ultimate in supportive care of the pancytopenic and immunologically compromised patient. Following early unsuccessful experiences with bone marrow transplantation, advances in knowledge of human histocompatibility typing, immunosuppression, supportive care during pancytopenia, and fundamental transplantation immunology have created a resurgence of interest in this procedure. Consequently, bone marrow transplantation is now used widely to treat patients with severe combined immunodeficiency disease, aplastic anemia, acute leukemia and other hematologic neoplasms, and, more rarely, nonhematologic neoplasms and nonneoplastic hematologic diseases. The results have clearly identified patients for whom bone marrow transplantation now is the treatment of choice. This experience has also identified the principal problems to be resolved in order to increase the success rate and applicability of bone marrow transplantation. Thus, bone marrow transplantation, formerly reserved for patients *in extremis,* can greatly benefit and sometimes cure selected patients with neoplastic and nonneoplastic diseases.

The role of bone marrow transplantation in antitumor therapy is based on the following assumptions: (1) antitumor chemotherapeutic agents or radiation or both, if given in sufficient doses, can totally eradicate a given tumor, (2) the dose of antitumor agents is limited largely by their toxicity to the patient's normal marrow, and, (3) if normal bone marrow is available for transplantation, higher and potentially curative antitumor doses of drugs or radiation or both can be administered, and

the donor marrow can save the patient from iatrogenic death.

A marrow transplant from a genetically identical twin is known as "syngeneic," marrow from a donor not an identical twin is "allogeneic," and the patient's own marrow is "autologous." This chapter focuses on using allogeneic marrow from HLA-matched sibling donors to treat neoplastic disease. However, to appreciate the results obtained and the immunologic and neoplastic problems observed, the results of allogeneic marrow transplantation for aplastic anemia are first reviewed. These results highlight the largely immunologic problems presented by marrow transplantation in the absence of neoplasia. The results of syngeneic marrow transplantations to treat neoplasia are then reviewed, so as to emphasize the problems presented by the need to eradicate the tumor without the complications posed by transplantation immunology. The potential of autologous marrow in treating hematologic and nonhematologic neoplasms is then briefly reviewed.

TECHNIQUE OF MARROW ASPIRATION

The technique of marrow aspiration and infusion is simple and poses no important problems for donor or host (Thomas *et al.,* 1975). In the operating room, under spinal or general anaesthesia, 100 to 150 marrow aspirations are performed on the anterior and posterior iliac crests of the donor. About 200 to 800 mL of marrow mixed with blood is collected in heparin, screened to remove large particles, transferred to a transfusion bag, and administered to the patient intravenously. The marrow stem cells pass through the pulmonary circulation and settle and reconstitute all marrow function almost solely in the medullary cavities. Several days before marrow aspiration, a unit of blood is drawn from the donor and is returned to the donor during the aspiration, thereby avoiding exposing the marrow donor to unrelated blood. The donor is usually hospitalized for one to two nights but has no ill effects other than several days of local soreness. Although the precise number of donor cells required for engraftment is not known, the recipient usually receives about 10^8 to 10^9 nucleated cells per kilogram body weight.

HISTOCOMPATIBILITY

The human major histocompatibility complex is designated human leukocyte antigen (HLA). The HLA gene complex consists of a series of closely linked loci on chromosome 6 designated HLA-A, -B, -C, and -D. The chromosomal region is known as a haplotype. Each individual inherits one haplotype from the mother and one from the father. The antigens located at HLA-A, -B, and -C subloci are defined serologically, and those at the HLA-D locus (HLA-DW antigens) are detected by the mixed leukocyte culture test. A locus identical with or closely related to HLA-D, called DR (D-related), can be serologically typed by using B lymphocytes. Since the HLA-A, -B, and -C loci are closely linked to HLA-D, siblings who are HLA-A, -B, and -C identical are likely to be HLA-D identical. Despite this complexity, within any given family there can be only four haplotypes. Therefore, for any given patient each sibling has one chance in four of being HLA-identical with the patient. The overwhelming majority of bone marrow transplants have been performed between HLA-identical siblings.

SYNGENEIC BONE MARROW TRANSPLANTATION FOR APLASTIC ANEMIA

Genetically identical twins are obviously identical not only for HLA but for *all* genetic loci and should therefore readily accept each other's tissues and organs. Theoretically, patients with severe aplastic anemia should be cured merely by simple infusion of marrow from their genetically identical normal twins without other therapy. However, only about half the patients thus treated have promptly recovered hematologic function. Perhaps the aplastic anemia in patients who did not respond reflected an abnormal microenvironment or an autoimmune destruction of marrow. Accordingly, some of these unresponding patients totally recovered normal function after immunosuppression by cyclophosphamide (50 mg/kg body weight per day for four days) and a second infusion of twin marrow (Appelbaum and Fefer, 1981). Therefore, all patients with aplastic anemia should be asked whether they have a normal genetically identical twin and, if they do, they should receive a simple marrow infusion. If no engraftment occurs within three weeks, cyclophosphamide and a second twin marrow infusion are indicated.

ALLOGENEIC BONE MARROW TRANSPLANTATION FOR SEVERE APLASTIC ANEMIA

Severe aplastic anemia is most often of unknown etiology and is almost always fatal. On the basis of evidence for an immunologic mechanism for the underlying disease (Appelbaum and Fefer, 1981), various immunosuppressive therapies were attempted with variable but generally unsatisfactory results. The most effective treatment is bone marrow transplantation (Camitta *et al.,* 1982).

Simple infusion of marrow from an HLA-identical sibling is always rejected. Despite optimal HLA-matching between donor and patient, the patient must be immunologically suppressed to permit marrow engraftment. The most widely used regimen for HLA-matched sibling marrow grafting for aplastic anemia is immunosuppression by cyclophosphamide 50 mg/kg for four days, followed 36 hours later by the infusion of donor marrow. Engraftment, reflected histologically and by peripheral blood counts, usually occurs 10 to 20 days later.

In contrast to transplantation of other foreign organs, the immunologic barrier in bone marrow transplantation is *bi*directional, *i.e.,* not only can the host reject the marrow graft but, since the infused donor marrow contains lymphocytes potentially immunologically reactive against the recipient, the graft can reject the host and cause graft-versus-host disease. In an effort to prevent or alleviate graft-versus-host disease, most recipients of HLA-identical sibling marrow receive a three-month regimen of immunosuppressive methotrexate after marrow infusion. In the past, 40 to 50% of all patients with severe aplastic anemia thus treated with bone marrow transplantation experienced complete engraftment and long-term survival beyond five years after transplantation. A prospectively randomized study of patients with severe aplastic anemia showed that allogeneic bone marrow transplantation was significantly more effective than conventional therapy (Camitta *et al.,* 1982).

The principal impediments to greater success of allogeneic marrow transplantation for aplastic anemia are graft-versus-host disease, interstitial pneumonia, and graft rejection (Camitta *et al.,* 1982). Graft-versus-host disease is an immunologic reaction of engrafted T cells against host tissue, especially skin, gut, and liver. Despite optimal HLA-matching and prophylaxis with methotrexate, 25 to 30% of aplastic anemia patients receiving allogeneic marrow transplants suffer moderate to severe acute graft-versus-host disease. About 10% of the deaths are attributable to graft-versus-host disease, especially to the severe immunologic deficiency that accompanies it and promotes fatal infections.

Of patients who survive beyond six months after bone marrow transplantation, 20 to 30% develop *chronic* graft-versus-host disease, which consists of clinical syndromes suggestive of autoimmune diseases involving skin, liver, gut, and mucous membranes. Chronic graft-versus-host disease causes substantial morbidity but usually responds to treatment with combination chemotherapy and rarely causes death. Graft-versus-host disease is uncommon in children and young adults but increases dramatically in incidence and severity in patients over 30 years of age.

Although transplant recipients can develop bacterial or fungal pneumonias, the principal and critical pneumonia they suffer is a non-bacterial, nonfungal interstitial pneumonitis occurring in 16% of patients with aplastic anemia treated with cyclophosphamide and allogeneic marrow. The pneumonitis tends to occur within four months after marrow transplantation. Approximately 50% of patients who develop interstitial pneumonitis die from it. The interstitial pneumonitis is attributed to cytomegalovirus infection in about 50% of af-

fected patients, but the cause remains unknown in the balance of patients. The prophylactic use of trimethoprim sulfamethoxazole has abolished the problem of *Pneumocystis carinii* pneumonia.

By far the principal cause of death in patients with severe aplastic anemia who received cyclophosphamide and HLA-matched sibling marrow was graft rejection, which used to occur in 30 to 70% of the recipients. This problem is now effectively resolved (Camitta *et al.,* 1982). A major factor that predisposed aplastic patients to marrow graft rejection was found to be exposure to blood products via transfusions prior to the cyclophosphamide conditioning — especially, but not necessarily, from family members. Such transfusions possibly sensitize the patient to cross-reacting "minor" histocompatibility antigens and cause subsequent rejection of the donor marrow. Avoiding such transfusions proved highly beneficial. Indeed, over 80% of patients with aplastic anemia who received a marrow transplant *before* receiving any blood transfusions are long-term survivors.

Graft rejection was also more likely in patients who received the smallest number of marrow cells. Accordingly, in a recent study (Camitta *et al.,* 1982), patients with severe aplastic anemia who had been exposed to multiple transfusions and were, therefore, likely to reject a marrow graft, received viable donor buffy coat cells — as a source of additional hematopoietic stem cells — after the same marrow transplantation regimen. The incidence of graft rejection decreased markedly to only 14%. However, the incidence of chronic graft-versus-host disease rose concurrently to 50%. Nevertheless, 70% of the entire patient group became long-term survivors.

In summary, the results clearly demonstrate that allogeneic bone marrow transplantation is the treatment of choice for children and young adults with severe aplastic anemia and that the probability of success is greatest in those patients not given transfusions before marrow transplantation. Therefore, every patient with severe aplastic anemia should undergo histocompatibility testing with siblings and parents as soon as the diagnosis is made. All patients under 30 with an HLA-matched sibling should be referred to a marrow transplant center for marrow transplantation before exposure to blood products. Older patients and patients without what is now known as an appropriate marrow donor may still be considered for bone marrow transplantation at some centers with different conditioning regimens for marrow transplantation, such as total lymphoid irradiation, or other immunosuppressive regimens, such as antithymocyte globulin (Camitta et al., 1982).

SYNGENEIC BONE MARROW TRANSPLANTATION FOR NEOPLASIA

The rare patient with neoplasia who has a normal monozygotic identical twin offers a unique opportunity to study the antitumor efficacy of a given supralethal dose of chemotherapy and radiation as well as its toxicity to normal tissues. In this setting transplantation immunology is not a serious problem — the principal problem is the presence of the tumor. The feasibility of this approach was first reported in 1959 (Thomas et al., 1959). Two patients with acute lymphocytic leukemia were treated with supralethal doses of total body irradiation and infusion of twin marrow. Although the leukemia recurred within three months, the results showed that normal marrow function could be reconstituted by bone marrow transplantation. A decade later the same approach began to be reexplored. Since then, the Seattle team has treated over 140 patients for a variety of hematologic neoplasms with a combination of chemotherapy, total body irradiation, and transplantation of marrow from a normal monozygotic genetically identical twin. The basic chemoradiotherapy regimen consists of cyclophosphamide intravenously 60 mg/kg on two successive days and, two to four days later, a supralethal dose of total body irradiation from two opposing cobalt-60 sources for a midline tissue dose of 1000 rads delivered at 5.6 to 8.0 rads per minute. Marrow is infused within 24 hours after total body irradiation. Some of the patients received additional chemotherapeutic agents shortly before the standard conditioning regimen was administered.

Syngeneic Bone Marrow Transplantation for Acute Leukemia

As with any experimental procedure, this approach was first tried in patients whose disease was refractory to conventional therapy and who were often in unusually poor clinical condition. Thirty-four patients ages 4 to 67 years with refractory acute leukemia were

treated with chemoradiotherapy and twin bone marrow transplantation (Fefer et al., 1981). Eight patients (three with acute lymphocytic leukemia, five with acute nonlymphocytic leukemia) remain in complete unmaintained remission four to ten years after bone marrow transplantation and are considered cured.

Treatment-related deaths, in the absence of detectable leukemia, were rare. The main problem was resistance of leukemia to the therapy as reflected by persistence of detectable leukemia or recurrence after a complete remission of only a few months. Additional chemotherapy immediately prior to the chemoradiotherapy conditioning regimen had no important effect on the likelihood of leukemic relapse nor did the use of fractionated radiation for a larger cumulative dose of total-body irradiation. Attempts are in progress to decrease the leukemic recurrence by performing bone marrow transplantation when the patients are in a chemotherapy-induced complete — but probably short — remission. Preliminary results are quite encouraging (Fefer et al., 1983).

Syngeneic Bone Marrow Transplantation for Refractory Lymphoma

Eight patients with disseminated non-Hodgkin's lymphoma who failed conventional therapy were treated with high-dose chemotherapy, supralethal total-body irradiation, and syngeneic marrow (Appelbaum et al., 1981). Four, aged 19 to 51 years, remain in complete unmaintained remission 26 to 140 months after bone marrow transplantation. One patient died in complete remission of Pseudomonas pneumonia six months after marrow transplantation. In the other three patients the lymphoma persisted or relapsed after marrow transplantation. The results show that even end-stage non-Hodgkin's lymphoma is potentially curable by supralethal chemoradiotherapy and twin bone marrow transplantation. The challenge continues to be how to increase the antitumor effect by altering antitumor therapy before and after marrow transplant.

Syngeneic Bone Marrow Transplantation for Chronic Granulocytic Leukemia

Given the dismal prognosis of patients with chronic granulocytic leukemia in blast crisis on conventional therapy, the Seattle team treated ten patients in the terminal phase of their disease — most in very poor clinical condition — with supralethal chemoradiotherapy and transplantation of normal twin marrow (Fefer et al., 1982b). The results were quite poor. Only one patient is alive. She relapsed 11 months after marrow transplantation, was retreated with chemoradiotherapy and another twin marrow transplant, and remains in complete remission 4 years after the second transplant.

Since most patients with chronic granulocytic leukemia die within two to four years after diagnosis, investigators have explored the use of aggressive chemotherapy during the *chronic* phase of chronic granulocytic leukemia in an effort to eradicate the abnormal Philadelphia (Ph[1])-positive clone and thus prevent blast crisis. The results are disappointing because cytogenetic conversion is uncommon, incomplete, and usually transient. In view of the possibility that the doses of antitumor agents used by others were limited by myelosuppression, supralethal chemoradiotherapy with transplantation of marrow from a normal twin was used to treat 16 patients in the chronic phase (Fefer et al., 1982b, 1984). All experienced a hematologic and cytogenetic complete remission with disappearance of all Ph[1]-positive cells. Two patients died of interstitial idiopathic pneumonitis while in complete remission. Three patients relapsed 13 to 24 months after marrow transplantation and remain in the chronic phase of chronic granulocytic leukemia at 4 to 6 years after bone marrow transplantation. Eleven patients remain in hematologic and cytogenetic complete remission 28 to 104 months after marrow transplantation (median 64) (Fefer et al., 1984). Assuming the lowest rates of transformation to blast crisis and death among the many series of patients reviewed by Sokal (1976), the probability of obtaining our results after a marrow transplant is <0.0001. Thus the Ph[1]-positive clone can be ablated and blast crisis delayed or prevented by this approach.

Syngeneic Bone Marrow Transplantation for Other Neoplasms

The rationale for syngeneic bone marrow transplantation as an adjunct to supralethal chemoradiotherapy should apply to patients with other hematologic neoplasms. For example, one patient with multiple myeloma responsive to therapy (Osserman et al., 1982) and another refractory to conventional therapy (Fefer et al., 1982c) benefited greatly from treatment with cyclophosphamide and total-body irradiation. All symptoms and all hematologic abnormalities disappeared, and the paraprotein decreased markedly. One patient showed progression of the disease one and one-half years after marrow transplantation (Osserman et al., 1982), while the other shows no progression 64 months after transplantation (Fefer et al., 1982c). Moreover, one patient with hairy cell leukemia who relapsed after responding to splenectomy underwent chemoradiotherapy and twin bone marrow transplantation and remains in complete unmaintained remission six years after transplantation (Cheever et al., 1982). Additional patients are being studied to determine the efficacy of this approach.

Syngeneic marrow transplantation does not have to be restricted to treating hematologic neoplasms or even to those that involve the marrow. Syngeneic marrow transplantation could conceivably be beneficial in other nonhematologic neoplasms such as neuroblastoma, oat cell carcinoma of the lung, carcinoma of the prostate, breast, and ovary and others that may or may not involve the bone marrow. Such neoplasms are sufficiently sensitive to conventional doses of chemotherapy or radiotherapy or both to suggest that, if larger treatment doses could be safely administered because exogeneous normal marrow was available, a far greater and potentially curative antitumor effect might be induced. Moreover, this rationale, coupled with the low incidence of death attributable to the chemoradiotherapy and twin marrow transplantation *per se,* justifies exploring this approach even in patients whose nonhematologic neoplasms are not especially responsive to available forms of therapy but who are young and willing to accept the risks of experimental treatment. Accordingly, all patients with virtually *any* neoplasms should be asked whether they have a genetically identical twin so that twin marrow transplantation can be considered at the optimal point in the clinical course of the disease.

Toxicities and Complications

Variable but potentially substantial morbidity is associated with the chemoradiotherapy for syngeneic bone marrow transplantation (Fefer et al., 1981, 1982b). Acutely, cyclophosphamide causes variable gastrointestinal toxicity, cystitis, and potential fluid retention. Acute toxicity is associated with total-body irradiation—fever, parotitis, nausea, vomiting, and diarrhea of variable severity and duration. Engraftment is usually detectable two to three weeks after bone marrow transplantation. Until safe blood counts are attained, appropriate supportive measures are essential. These include broad-spectrum antibiotics for fever of unknown origin associated with neutropenia and platelet transfusion from random donors, matched donors, and, if necessary, twin donors. Infections are not common. The most common problem is mucositis, most often complicated by infection with herpes simplex. Most patients are discharged from the hospital within four to six weeks after marrow transplantation when they approach hematologic normalcy and can eat enough to maintain weight.

Within the first four months after marrow transplantation, the patients are at risk from interstitial pneumonitis. On open-lung biopsy, such interstitial pneumonitis is usually found to be idiopathic, presumably caused by radiation (Appelbaum *et al.,* 1982). Interstitial pneumonitis is more common in patients over 50 and in those who receive additional chemotherapy prior to the cyclophosphamide and total body irradiation. Overall, death caused by treatment—without detectable neoplasm —is rare. The long-term complications associated with or attributable to radiation include cataracts that occur several years after marrow transplantation and are surgically correctable, mild growth retardation in children, some delay in the development of secondary sex characteristics, and amenorrhea and aspermia. However, the vast majority of patients who are in remission from their neoplasm after syngeneic bone marrow transplantation eventually lead normal lives.

ALLOGENEIC BONE MARROW TRANSPLANTATION FOR NEOPLASIA

Most human bone marrow transplants were done to treat acute leukemia and involved supralethal chemoradiotherapy plus marrow from HLA-matched sibling donors (Gale, 1982; Thomas, 1982). The results reflect some of the same problems of transplantation immunology as noted above for allogeneic marrow transplantation for aplastic anemia, as

well as problems posed by the need to eradicate tumor cells, as observed with syngeneic marrow transplantation for acute leukemia.

Preparation of the Recipient

The pretransplant conditioning regimen must be sufficiently immunosuppressive to prevent host rejection of the donor marrow and sufficiently cytotoxic to eradicate the leukemia. Various conditioning regimens have been employed, depending on the transplant center and the nature and stage of the disease to be treated. However, almost all regimens include a supralethal dose of total-body irradiation because radiation is capable of eradicating leukemia cells and penetrating the privileged sites of leukemia not accessible to chemotherapeutic agents. The most widely used conditioning regimen for allogeneic bone marrow transplantation is essentially the same as that described above for syngeneic marrow transplantation for leukemia, namely, cyclophosphamide, 60 mg/kg per day for two days, followed by 1000-rad total-body irradiation. In addition, intrathecal methotrexate is administered prior to marrow infusion as prophylaxis against leukemia in the central nervous system, and a three-month regimen of immunosuppressive methotrexate is used as prophylaxis against graft-versus-host disease. The complexity of the combination of immunologic and neoplastic problems in allogeneic marrow transplantation for acute leukemia and the treatment-associated morbidity and mortality justifies this approach only with the objective of cure, not merely a temporary complete remission.

Supportive Care

The conditioning regimen normally causes total marrow aplasia. The donor marrow, infused within hours after total body irradiation, normally requires two to four weeks for engraftment and hematopoietic reconstitution and somewhat longer to produce adequate numbers of granulocytes and platelets.

In contrast to marrow rejection by aplastic anemia patients, patients transplanted with marrow as treatment for leukemia rarely reject donor marrow, even if they had blood transfusions prior to referral for marrow transplantation. The lack of rejection may reflect immunosuppression by the leukemia, greater immunosuppression by the pregrafting irradiation, or lack of sensitization by pregrafting transfusions in patients on immunosuppressive antileukemic chemotherapy.

During the pancytopenic period, supportive care is similar to that required for any other severely immunologically compromised patient treated with aggressive chemotherapy. Although ultraisolation techniques including laminar-airflow-room isolation with skin sterilization, sterile diet, and gut sterilizaton by oral nonabsorbable antibiotics can prevent some infections and fevers, no clear-cut advantage has been demonstrated in terms of ultimate survival (Buckner *er al.,* 1978a). Consequently, most patients are treated with routine hospital isolation with masks and handwashing. The antibiotic coverge for neutropenic patients who are febrile is essentially the same as that used for nontransplant neutropenic immunologically compromised leukemic patients on combination chemotherapy.

Prophylactic granulocyte transfusions may be given to patients whose granulocyte count falls below $200/mm^2$, and therapeutic granulocyte transfusions are appropriate for neutropenic patients with bacterial or fungal infections. A platelet count of about $20,000/mm^2$ is usually maintained by platelet transfusions from random donors. If the patient becomes refractory to those platelets, platelets are obtained from haploidentical family members, *i.e.,* members who share with the patient one genetically identical haplotype but not the other haplotype. The HLA-identical marrow donor must often supply platelet transfusions if no other donors are available or effective. Granulocytes, platelets, or packed red blood cells, when administered to the transplant recipient, are all irradiated *in vitro* with 1500 rads to inactivate lymphocytes that might produce graft-versus-host disease.

Finally, a major advance in supportive care of these patients is the Hickman modification of the Broviac catheter (Hickman *et al.,* 1979). It is used to draw the necessary blood samples, administer intravenous medications, and provide hyperalimentation to maintain adequate nutrition in patients who probably have mucositis, gastrointestinal toxicity, and inability to eat for a substantial period of time. The catheter is threaded through the cephalic vein to the upper part of the right atrium and is then tunneled subcutaneously, eventually emerging as a small rubber tube sticking through the skin of the thorax. The catheter is usually in place for about three months but can remain even longer and is easily removed when no longer needed or if it becomes infected, which rarely happens.

Allogeneic Bone Marrow Transplantation for Acute Leukemia in Relapse

As in any experimental procedure with potential morbidity and mortality, allogeneic marrow transplantation was first tried in leukemic patients with a dismal prognosis considered to be in the terminal stage of their disease, and often in extremely poor condition. Of 100 patients with end-stage acute lymphocytic leukemia or acute nonlymphocytic leukemia thus transplanted, 13% remain in complete unmaintained remission six to ten years after transplantation and are considered cured (Thomas *et al.,* 1977). About 50% of the patients died within the first three months largely the result of graft-versus-host disease, opportunistic infections, interstitial pneumonitis, and veno-occlusive disease of the liver. Of patients who survived these calamities, leukemia recurred in most within two years after transplantation. An actuarial analysis indicates that, in the absence of other causes of death, about 65% of the patients would relapse. Thus, the chief problem preventing a higher cure and survival rate with allogeneic marrow transplantation for refractory acute leukemia is *not* rejection, which occurs in less than 5% of leukemic patients given this conditioning regimen, but leukemic recurrence, interstitial pneumonitis—idiopathic or attributed to cytomegalovirus—acute and/or chronic graft-versus-host disease, and veno-occlusive disease of the liver. Administering more intensive chemotherapy or radiotherapy or both before transplantation of marrow to patients in relapse has not increased the percentage of long-term, tumor-free survivors after transplantation (Gale, 1982; Thomas, 1982).

Allogenic Bone Marrow Transplantation for Acute Lymphocytic Leukemia in Complete Remission

Some of the problems encountered in patients who underwent marrow transplantation when their leukemia was grossly detectable might be decreased by transplanting marrow to patients in chemotherapy-induced complete remission. Their tumor burden at the time of transplantation would be far smaller and potentially more readily eradicated by supralethal chemoradiotherapy. Moreover, the patient in remission should be better able to tolerate the complications of marrow transplantation. Therfore, HLA-matched sibling donor marrow transplantation was attempted in patients with acute leukemia who were in complete remission but whose remission was anticipated to be short. Patients with acute lymphocytic leukemia in second or subsequent remissions were selected because once a relapse occurs after the first complete remission, the patients have a poor prognosis with a short median survival time. Of 22 patients thus transplanted and reported (Thomas et al., 1979b), 6 remain in complete unmaintained remission three to five years after transplantation. Three patients died of interstitial pneumonitis within three months after transplantation. However, the principal problem remained leukemic relapse, which occured in 12 patients. The decrease in the nonleukemic deaths is encouraging, although the persistence of leukemic recurrence remains a challenging problem and requires new approaches to tumor eradication.

Allogeneic Bone Marrow Transplantation for Acute Nonlymphocytic Leukemia in First Complete Remission

The same rationale was used to justify marrow transplantation to treat acute nonlymphocytic leukemia in remission. Patients in their first remission, however, were used because they tend to relapse in a median time of about 12 to 18 months and less than 20% of such remissions last for three years. Of an initial series of 19 patients thus treated in their first remission (Thomas et al., 1979a), 11 patients remain in continuous unmaintained complete remission four to six years after marrow transplantation. The deaths were the result of graft-versus-host disease or interstitial pneumonitis, whereas leukemia rarely recurred.

This approach has now been used in the same center on more than 100 patients with acute nonlymphocytic leukemia in first complete remission (Thomas, 1982). The results confirm those of the original series and have been confirmed by other transplant centers (Gale, 1982). An actuarial analysis indicated about a 10% probability of leukemic relapse after transplantation. Since transplantation-

related problems, other than leukemic relapse, still exist, the overall end results of allogeneic marrow transplantation for acute nonlymphocytic leukemia in first complete remission show approximately 40 to 70% long-term, tumor-free survival five years after marrow transplantation. The percentage is largely a function of patient age — patients under 30 do significantly better than those over 30 years. A recent prospectively randomized study of patients with acute nonlymphocytic leukemia transplanted in first complete remission with HLA-identical sibling marrow after conditioning with cyclophosphamide plus either 1000 rads at a single sitting or 200 rads per day for six consecutive days confirmed the decreased leukemic recurrence and revealed a statistically significant improvement in overall survival of patients treated with fractionated radiation (Thomas et al., 1982). Moreover, a prospective comparative study showed that more patients with acute myelogeneous leukemia (AML) in first complete remission were cured by marrow transplantation than by additional chemotherapy (Appelbaum et al., 1984).

Allogeneic Bone Marrow Transplantation for Chronic Granulocytic Leukemia

Patients with chronic granulocytic leukemia in the accelerated phase or in blast crisis received marrow transplants from HLA-identical siblings. Most recipients died soon after transplantation, but about 15% became long-term tumor-free survivors. Attempts are in progress to assess the efficacy of marrow transplantation in treating the rare patients who achieve a chemotherapy-induced remission from blast crisis.

Many centers are now reporting encouraging results with transplantation of HLA-identical sibling marrow during the *chronic* phase of chronic granulocytic leukemia. This approach was stimulated by the long-lasting cytogenetic and hematologic complete remissions obtained with marrow from normal identical twins (Fefer et al., 1982b) and by the encouraging experience with allogeneic marrow transplantation for acute nonlymphocytic leukemia in first remission (Thomas et al., 1982). Of the first ten patients recently reported (Clift et al., 1982) who received HLA-matched sibling marrow during the chronic phase of chronic granulocytic leukemia and were followed for at least one year after transplantation, six remain in complete clinical hematologic and cytogenetic remission 13 to 37 months after transplantation. A preliminary retrospective analysis on many more patients transplanted during the chronic accelerated or blastic phase of the disease confirms the very encouraging results obtained in the chronic phase and the disappointing results obtained in the later phases (Fefer, *et al.,* 1984).

Role of ABO Antigens in Bone Marrow Transplantation

Although major ABO incompatibility between marrow donor and recipient can cause a significant hemolytic reaction when marrow cells are infused, no evidence suggests that hematopoietic stem cells express ABO antigens. Plasma exchange can reduce the titer of the patient's antibody to donor red cells. When this approach was used in 17 patients who received a marrow transplant across a major ABO incompatibility, 16 achieved successful marrow reconstitution (Buckner *et al.,* 1978b). ABO incompatibility does not substantially increase the risk of marrow graft rejection or the incidence or severity of graft-versus-host disease.

The Use of Donors Other than HLA-Identical Siblings for Bone Marrow Transplantation in Acute Leukemia

Since less than 40% of patients with acute leukemia in the United States are likely to have an HLA-identical sibling, extension of marrow transplantation to other donor-recipient combinations is being explored. HLA and mixed leukocyte culture (MLC) tests are performed on all family members to try to identify parents or siblings who are one haplotype-identical with the patient and who, by chance, share with the patient some additional antigens on the other haplotype. Such donors and recipients are genotypically HLA-identical for one haplotype and have a well-defined phenotypic identity for one or more of the other HLA loci on the other haplotype. A partial compatibility between patient and parent donor may exist when the parent is homozygous for HLA, when both parents share two or more HLA antigens, or when HLA recombination has occurred.

Marrow from donors other than HLA-matched siblings was transplanted into 27 patients who had acute lymphocytic or nonlymphocytic leukemia in relapse or remission. The results show that the stage and type of disease and clinical status of the patient principally determine the prognosis or end result of marrow transplantation, not the particular degree of histoincompatibility between donor and host (Clift *et al.,* 1981). Time to engraftment and the incidence and severity of graft-versus-host disease did not differ significantly between patients receiving marrow from a haploidentical parent or sibling donor mismatched for one or more HLA antigens and patients receiving HLA-matched sibling marrow. Indeed, even incompatibility for the D-locus did not preclude successful marrow engraftment. However, the series of patients is too small to analyze whether results were a function of the particular family relationship of the donor to the patient or of the particular HLA locus at which a mismatch occurred.

Thus, the results for patients receiving marrow from HLA-incompatible donors do not differ significantly from those for patients receiving marrow from genotypically HLA-identical siblings. Indeed, since identity for HLA-A, -B, and -DR can now be documented serologically, the possibility of finding an *unrelated* donor who may share those antigens with the patient, especially the patient who has one of the more common HLA haplotypes, is very real if a large panel of potential donors becomes available. In one patient with acute lymphocytic leukemia transplanted in second remission with marrow from an unrelated donor phenotypically identical at HLA-A, -B, -D, and -DR, no particular posttransplantation complications, no graft-versus-host disease, and long-term, tumor-free survival were reported (Hansen *et al.,* 1980). Clearly, in the near future, a marrow donor for patients with common haplotypes may be routinely selected from a large, possibly national, panel of unrelated people.

Who Should Be Referred for Allogeneic Marrow Transplantation for Neoplasia?

Every patient with a hematologic neoplasm should undergo HLA typing with siblings and family as early as possible after diagnosis. The mortality for patients undergoing allogeneic marrow transplantation after the age of 50 is at this writing too high to justify the transplant. Patients under 50 who have an appropriate marrow donor should be considered for marrow transplantation at some time in the course of their disease. Acute leukemia unresponsive to chemotherapy should be treated with marrow transplantation because there is a 15 to 20% chance of cure with marrow transplantation and no chance with conventional therapy.

Whenever possible, marrow transplantation should be performed when the patient is in complete remission. Although patients with acute lymphocytic leukemia exhibit a high degree of leukemic recurrence even when marrow transplantation is performed in remission, allogeneic marrow transplantation should still be performed for adults with acute lymphocytic leukemia in first complete remission, for children with bad-risk acute lymphocytic leukemia in first complete remission, and in children with good-risk acute lymphocytic leukemia in their second complete remission. This recommendation is based on the poor results obtained in those conditions with conventional therapy as compared with better results obtained with marrow transplantation. Patients with acute nonlymphocytic leukemia in first complete remission are the best candidates for allogeneic marrow transplantation. The results to date are especially impressive for patients under age 30. Since the transplant risks are greater for patients over 30, it may be better to use conventional chemotherapy and to postpone the transplant until the earliest evidence of relapse.

The results of allogeneic marrow transplantation for chronic granulocytic leukemia are preliminary but encouraging and suggest that such patients be treated with marrow transplantation at some time in the course of their disease. The results strongly suggest, but do not yet prove, that marrow transplantation should be performed during the chronic phase of chronic granulocytic leukemia rather than during the accelerated phase or blast crisis. The principal basis for this recommendation is the very beneficial results obtained with identical twin marrow transplantation during the chronic phase of chronic granulocytic leukemia, in contrast to the poor results obtained with twin marrow transplantation during blast crisis. The ethical problem of subjecting patients, especially those over 30 years of age, who may remain in chronic-phase chronic granulocytic leukemia for several years to a

procedure associated with substantial treatment-related mortality cannot be minimized. Allogeneic marrow transplantation in the chronic phase of chronic granulocytic leukemia is most appropriate for patients under 30 years of age and less likely to die of transplant-related causes. Patients over 30 can be allowed to remain on conventional therapy, postponing marrow transplantation until the first sign of a change to the accelerated phase.

Finally, allogeneic marrow transplantation should be explored in diseases other than the leukemias. The results of identical twin marrow transplants strongly suggest that selected young patients with lymphomas, multiple myeloma, or hairy cell leukemia who have an appropriate marrow donor should be referred for possible allogeneic marrow transplantation when they have become refractory to conventional treatment.

Impediments to Success in Allogeneic Marrow Transplantation for Hematologic Neoplasms

The principal problems limiting the success of allogeneic marrow transplantation for acute leukemia are leukemic relapse, interstitial pneumonitis, veno-occlusive disease of the liver, and graft-versus-host disease.

Recurrence of Neoplasms. The incidence of leukemic relapse in acute nonlymphocytic leukemia has been dramatically reduced by performing the transplant when the patients are in their first chemotherapy-induced complete remission. Approaches to decreasing posttransplant leukemic relapses in patients with acute lymphocytic leukemia or with acute leukemia not amenable to chemotherapy-induced complete remission will probably involve additional chemotherapy as part of a conditioning regimen, additional chemotherapy in the form of consolidation, and intensification or maintenance therapy after marrow transplantation.

Leukemic recurrences stem from progeny of the original host-type leukemic cells that escaped eradiction by the chemoradiotherapy. Indeed, appropriate cytogenetic markers showed that the recurrent leukemia after marrow transplantation usually represented recurrence in the host-type cell. However, in two female patients with acute lymphocytic leukemia treated with only supralethal total-body irradiation and marrow from an HLA-matched brother, the recurrence was in donor-type cells. This was demonstrated by karyotype analysis of the chromosomes and by the demonstration of fluorescent Y bodies in the interphase leukemic cells (Thomas, 1982). Others have reported three additional recurrences (one acute lymphocytic leukemia, two acute nonlymphocytic leukemia) in what appeared to be donor-type cells (Gale, 1982). In addition, an immunoblastic sarcoma of donor type was reported to have developed in a patient transplanted for acute nonlymphocytic leukemia (Thomas, 1982). Several theoretical explanations for these results have been offered (Thomas, 1982) but cannot yet be tested. The vast majority of relapses that could be characterized, however, turned out to be of host type. Obviously, relapses that occur in syngeneic marrow transplant recipients cannot be characterized.

Interstitial Pneumonitis. The interstitial pneumonitis, a major problem in allogeneic marrow transplant recipients, is caused by cytomegalovirus in about half of the patients and is idiopathic on open-lung biopsy in the other half (Meyers and Thomas, 1981). It tends to occur within the first four months after transplantation and is usually fatal.

Cytomegalovirus pneumonitis has thus far not responded to any therapy. Acyclovir, interferon, and hyperimmune globulin are being tested, thus far without significant effect. Many cases of idiopathic interstitial pneumonitis are thought to reflect damage by therapy, especially radiation. Total-body irradiation is now being administered in fractionated doses over six or seven days rather than at a single sitting in the hope that it will be less toxic to the lungs and decrease the incidence of fatal interstitial pneumonitis (Thomas *et al.,* 1982).

Veno-occlusive Disease. Veno-occlusive disease of the liver can occur after chemotherapy and radiation even without bone marrow transplantation (Shulman *et al.,* 1980). In a prospective study of 255 consecutive patients transplanted with marrow for leukemia, 21% had veno-occlusive disease pathologically or clinically or both. Patients are diagnosed as having veno-occlusive disease when at least two of the following features are present: jaundice, hepatomegaly, ascites or unexplained weight gain, and no other known cause for liver disease. Of the patients with veno-occlusive disease, one-third died partly the result of the veno-occlusive disease; another 13% ex-hibited signs of veno-occlusive disease which persisted throughout their hospital course but did not contribute to death; and 53% showed complete resolution of clinical veno-occlusive disease. Patients with an elevated SGOT at transplantation or who received additional chemotherapy immediately preceding cyclophosphamide and irradiation were especially likely to develop veno-occlusive disease.

Graft-Versus-Host Disease. Graft-versus-host disease, both acute and chronic, remains a formidable problem. Acute graft-versus-host disease varies greatly in severity, from a mild rash to a massive desquamation with a burn-like picture. Gastrointestinal involvement may be reflected by mild nausea or severe vomiting, diarrhea, pain, and ileus. Hepatic dysfunction is mostly characterized by elevations in bilirubin, SGOT, and alkaline phosphatase. Graft-versus-host disease in patients given marrow from HLA-matched donors probably reflects a reaction of donor T cells to "minor" histocompatibility antigens on host cells that present techniques that cannot readily recognize.

Attempts to prevent the development of severe graft-versus-host disease largely involve using methotrexate or cyclophosphamide prophylactically. One does not seem to be more or less effective than the other. Prednisone and antithymocyte globulin have not been significantly effective either prophylactically or in treating established graft-versus-host disease, especially as measured by the number of long-term survivors. Thus, despite optimal histocompatibility matching between donor and recipient and the most widely used prophylactic therapy, approximately 40% of patients transplanted for acute leukemia develop moderate to severe graft-versus-host disease and about a third of those patients die from the disease.

Chronic graft-versus-host disease now occurs in 20 to 25% of patients who survive 100 days after marrow transplantation. The principal manifestations include skin disease that may progress to scleroderma, severe buccal mucositis, keratoconjunctivitis, chronic hepatic disease, development of esophageal strictures, and involvement of small and large intestine with resultant cachexia. The patients suffer severe immunologic deficiency and are susceptible to recurrent and occasionally fatal bacterial infections. Chronic graft-versus-host disease, which may or may not be preceded by acute graft-versus-host disease, appears to be amenable to treatment with a combination of azathioprine and prednisone in about 80% of the patients (Thomas, 1982).

Recipients of allogeneic marrow exhibit defects in immunologic reactivity for the first several weeks after transplantation, recovering after several months to a year. The immunologic deficiency is more marked in the presence of graft-versus-host disease. The patients are likely to develop opportunistic infections until immunologic reactivity is restored (Thomas, 1982). Patients who do not develop graft-versus-host disease recover immunologic competence more rapidly and are far less susceptible to infections. Evidence suggests that graft-versus-host disease reflects a defect in immunologic regulation and that changes in the balance between different T-cell subsets, i.e., cytoxic cells, suppressor cells, helper cells, and perhaps other regulatory lymphocytes, may determine whether graft-versus-host disease and general immunologic deficiency will occur.

Of various approaches being investigated to prevent, treat, or ameliorate graft-versus-host disease, cyclosporin A, a promising new immunosuppressive agent, has yielded some preliminary encouraging results. The greatest emphasis, however, is on eliminating from the marrow the T cells that cause graft-versus-host disease. Various physical separation techniques have been tried. Most attention, however, is now on using monoclonal antibodies directed against human T cells for treating donor marrow *in vitro* to reduce the number of T cells, decrease the incidence of graft-versus-host disease, and, to a lesser extent, to test the utility of such antibodies when administered *in vivo* to the patients.

Attempts to decrease or abolish graft-versus-host disease are complicated by the observation that, as might be anticipated from various animal studies, graft-versus-host disease may exert a significant antileukemic effect in humans (Weiden *et al.,* 1979). The rate of leukemic relapse in patients transplanted for refractory acute leukemia was significantly lower in those who developed graft-versus-host disease after allogeneic marrow transplantation than in those who did not or in those who could not develop graft-versus-host disease because they received marrow from an identical twin. Therefore, it might be best to control rather than prevent graft-versus-host disease, to modulate its severity and duration, and to use it for its antileukemic effect. The ultimate goal would be to render donor T cells preferentially or specifically more effective against the leukemia cells than against normal host tissue (Fefer *et al.,* 1982a).

AUTOLOGOUS MARROW TRANSPLANTATION

The possibility of obtaining a patient's own marrow, freezing it, then reinfusing it after the patient has been treated with intensive antitumor chemoradiotherapy has long been entertained. Viable marrow can be cryopreserved and maintained for long periods of time, and transplantation of normal marrow obtained from genetically identical twins has yielded extremely encouraging results. In fact, unless autologous marrow is postulated to be capable of a greater antitumor effect than that of twin marrow, identical twin marrow transplantation may represent the best results that one can expect with transplantation of autologous marrow.

In order for autologous marrow transplantation to be an effective therapeutic modality against neoplasms, several assumptions must be made: (1) the tumor being treated must be significantly more sensitive to a supralethal dose of chemoradiotherapy than to conventional doses; (2) the autologous marrow must reconstitute the hematopoietic function of the recipient after marrow aplasia induced by supralethal chemoradiotherapy; and (3) the infused marrow must be free of tumor cells. The validity of the first assumption is supported largely by the results of identical twin marrow transplants. The validity of the second assumption is strongly supported by reports in which stored autologous marrow infused after chemoradiotherapy successfully reconstituted hematopoietic function. The validity of the third assumption has not yet been substantiated and is difficult to prove.

Patients with acute leukemia have been treated with chemoradiotherapy and autologous marrow obtained and cryopreserved when the patients were in complete remission and no tumor cells were detectable in the marrow by available techniques. The results were generally poor in that leukemia recurred within a few weeks to months. Although results in several patients with lymphomas similarly treated are somewhat more encouraging, the reasons for the successes and failures remain unclear. Nevertheless, on the assumption that tumor cell contamination of infused marrow is indeed a critical deleterious factor, much effort is being expended in purging tumor cells from the marrow by a variety of physical, pharmacologic, or immunologic methods, especially by using monoclonal antibodies with preferential specificity against the tumor cells. The studies must continue before any conclusions can be drawn (Gale, 1982).

FUTURE OF MARROW TRANSPLANTATION FOR NEOPLASIA

Marrow transplantation is clearly beneficial and even curative in a substantial number of patients with an ever-increasing number of conditions. However, it is still experimental and fraught with major problems. Its therapeutic usefulness and application will greatly expand when the principal problems that limit its success today (see Table 43–1) are resolved, when additional evidence substantiates the view that an HLA-identical donor is not absolutely essential, and when effective chemoradiotherapy regimens are identified from studies of marrow transplantation in identical twins and then applied to autologous marrow transplantation. Experienced specialized centers should continue to perform marrow transplantation so that the major problems of transplantation immunology and tumor eradication (which require the study of large num-

bers of patients) can be most efficiently investigated. At the rate of progress in this field, the role of marrow transplantation in oncology is likely to increase greatly in the near future and will eventually be offered to patients outside specialized centers (Fefer, 1982).

REFERENCES

Applebaum, F. R.; Dahlberg, S.; Thomas, D.; Buckner, D.; Cheever, M. A.; Clift, R. A.; Crowley, J.; Deeg, H. J.; Fefer, A.; Greenberg, P. D,; Kadin, M.; Smith, W.; Stewart, P.; Sullivan, K.; Storb, R.; and Weiden, P.: Bone marrow transplantation or chemotherapy after remission induction for adults with acute nonlymphoblastic leukemia. *Ann. Intern. Med.,* **101**:581–588, 1984.

Appelbaum, F. R., and Fefer, A.: The pathogenesis of aplastic anemia. *Semin. Hematol.,* **18**:241–257, 1981.

Appelbaum, F. R.; Fefer, A.; Cheever, M. A.; Buckner, C. D.; Greenberg, P. D.; Kaplan, H. G.; Storb, R.; and Thomas, E. D.: Treatment of non-Hodgkin's lymphoma with marrow transplantation in identical twins. *Blood,* **58**:509–513, 1981.

Appelbaum, F. R.; Meyers, J. D., Fefer, A.; Flournoy, N.; Cheever, M. A.; Greenberg, P. D.; Hackman, R.; and Thomas, E. D.: Nonbacterial nonfungal pneumonia following marrow transplantation in 100 identical twins. *Transplantation,* **33**:265–268, 1982.

Buckner, C. D.; Clift, R. A.; Sanders, J. E.; Meyers, J. D.; Counts, G. W.; Farwell, V. T.; Thomas, E. D.; and the Seattle Marrow Transplant Team: Protective environment for marrow transplantation recipients. A prospective study. *Ann. Intern. Med.,* **89**:893–901, 1978a.

Buckner, C. D.; Clift, R. A.; Sanders, J. E.; Williams, B.; Gray, M.; Storb, R.; and Thomas, E. D.: ABO-incompatible marrow transplants. *Transplantation,* **26**:233–238, 1978b.

Camitta, B. M.; Storb, R.; and Thomas, E. D.: Aplastic anemia. Pathogenesis, diagnosis, treatment and prognosis. *N. Engl. J. Med.,* **306**:645–652, 712–718, 1982.

Cheever, M. A.; Fefer, A.; Greenberg, P. D.; Appelbaum, F. R.; Armitage, J. O.; Buckner, C. D.; Sale, G. E.; Storb, R.; Witherspoon, R. P.; and Thomas, E. D.: Treatment of hairy cell leukemia with chemoradiotherapy and identical twin bone marrow transplantation. *N. Engl. J. Med.,* **2**:621–624, 1982.

Clift, R. A.; Buckner, C. D.; Thomas, E. D.; Doney, K.; Fefer, A.; Neiman, P. E.; Singer, J.; Sanders, J.; Stewart, P.; Sullivan, K.M.; Deeg, J.; and Storb, R.: The treatment of chronic granulocytic leukemia in chronic phase by allogeneic marrow transplantation. *Lancet,* in press.

Clift, R. A.; Hansen, J. A.; and Thomas, E. D.: The role of HLA in marrow transplantation. *Transplant. Proc.,* **13**:234–236, 1981.

Fefer, A.: Future of bone marrow transplantation in oncology. *Int. J. Radiat. Oncol. Biol. Phys.,* **8**:949–950, 1982.

Fefer, A.; Cheever, M. A.; and Greenberg, P. D.: Overview of prospects and problems of lymphocyte transfer for cancer therapy. In Fefer, A., and Goldstein, A. L. (eds.): *The Potential Role of T Cells in Cancer Therapy.* Raven Press, New York, 1982a.

Fefer, A.; Cheever, M. A.; Greenberg, P. D.; Appelbaum, F. R.; Boyd, C. N.; Buckner, C. D.; Kaplan, H. G.; Ram-

Table 43–1.   Problems of Bone Marrow Transplant

TYPE OF BONE MARROW TRANSPLANTATION	CHIEF PROBLEMS THAT LIMIT SUCCESS
Syngeneic, for acute leukemia	Leukemic relapse
Allogeneic, for aplastic anemia	Graft rejection Graft-versus-host disease Interstitial pneumonitis
Allogeneic, for acute leukemia in relapse or in second or later complete remission	Leukemic relapse Graft-versus-host disease Interstitial pneumonitis Veno-occlusive disease of the liver
Allogeneic, for acute non-lymphocytic leukemia in first complete remission	Graft-versus-host disease Interstitial pneumonits Leukemic relapse
Autologous, for hematologic malignancies	Resistance of tumor to chemoradiotherapy ? Presence of tumor in infused bone marrow
Autologous, for malignancies that do not involve marrow	Resistance of tumor to chemoradiotherapy

berg, R.; Sanders, J. E.; Storb, R.; and Thomas, E. D.: Treatment of chronic granulocytic leukemia with chemoradiotherapy and transplantation of marrow from identical twins. *N. Engl. J. Med.,* **306**:63–68, 1982b.

Fefer, A.; Cheever, M. A.; Greenberg, P. D.; Appelbaum, F. R.; Buckner, C. D.; Clift, R. A.; Sanders, J.; Storb, R.; and Thomas, E. C.: Bone marrow transplantation for acute leukemia in patients with identical twins: improved results with BMT in complete remission. *Proc. Am. Soc. Clin. Oncol.,* **2**:182, 1983.

Fefer, A.; Cheever, M. A.; Thomas, E. D.; Appelbaum, F. R.; Buckner, C. D.; Clift, R. A.; Glucksberg, H.; Greenberg, P. D.; Johnson, F. L.; Kaplan, H. G.; Sanders, J. E.; Storb, R.; and Weiden, P. L.: Bone marrow transplantation for refractory acute leukemia in 34 patients with identical twins. *Blood,* **57**:421–430, 1981.

Fefer, A.; Clift, R. A.; Doney, K.; Appelbaum, F. R.; Buckner, C. D.; Cheever, M. A.; Deeg, N. J.; Greenberg, P. D.; Sanders, J.; Storb, R.; and Thomas, E. C.: Syngeneic and allogeneic bone marrow transplantation for chronic granulocytic leukemia. *Proc. Am. Soc. Clin. Oncol.,* **3**:205, 1984.

Fefer, A.; Greenberg, P. D.; Cheever, M. A.; Appelbaum, F. R.; Bluming, A. Z.; Storb, R.; and Thomas, E. D.: Treatment of multiple myeloma with chemoradiotherapy and identical twin bone marrow transplantation. *Proc. Am. Soc. Clin. Oncol.,* **1**:188, (Abstr.), 1982c.

Gale, R. P.: Progress in bone marrow transplantation in man. *Surv. Immunol. Res.,* **1**:40–66, 1982.

Hansen, J. A.; Clift, R. A.; Thomas, E. D.; Buckner, C. D.; Storb, R.; Giblett, E. R.: Transplantation of marrow from an unrelated donor to a patient with acute leukemia. *N. Engl. J. Med.,* **303**:565–567, 1980.

Hickman, R. O.; Buckner, C. D.; Clift, R. A.; Sanders, J. E.; Stewart, P.; and Thomas, E. D.: A modified right atrial catheter for access to the venous system in marrow transplant recipients. *Surgery,* **148**:871–875, 1979.

Meyers, J. D., and Thomas, E. D. Infection complicating bone marrow transplantation. In Young, L. S., and Rubin, R. H. (eds.): *Clinical Approach to Infection in the Immunocompromised Host.* Plenum Press, New York, 1981.

Osserman, E. F.; DiRe, L. B.; DiRe, J.; Sherman, W. H.; Hersman, J. A.; and Storb, R.: Identical twin marrow transplantation in multiple myeloma. *Acta Haematol.,* **68**:215–223, 1982.

Shulman, H. M.; McDonald, G. B.; Matthews, D.; Doney, K. C.; Kopecky, K. J.; Gauvreau, J. M.; and Thomas, E. D.: An analysis of hepatic venocclusive disease and centrilobular hepatic degeneration following bone marrow transplantation. *Gastroenterology,* **79**:1178–1191, 1980.

Sokal, J. E.: Evaluation of survival data for chronic myelocytic leukemia. *Am. J. Hematol.,* **1**:493–500, 1976.

Thomas, E. D.: The role of marrow transplantation in the eradication of malignant disease. *Cancer,* **49**:1963–1969, 1982.

Thomas, E. D.; Buckner, C. D.; Banaji, M.; Clift, R. A.; Fefer, A.; Flournoy, N.; Goodell, B. W.; Hickman, R. O.; Lerner, K. G.; Neiman, P. E.; Sale, G. E.; Sanders, J. E.; Singer, J.; Stevens, M.; Storb, R.; and Weiden, P. L.: One hundred patients with acute leukemia treated by chemotherapy, total body irradiation, and allogeneic marrow transplantation. *Blood,* **49**:511–533, 1977.

Thomas, E. D.; Buckner, C. D.; Clift, R. A.; Fefer, A.; Johnson, F. L.; Neiman, P. E.; Sale, G. E.; Sanders, J. E.; Singer, J. W.; Shulman, H.; Storb, R.; and Weiden, P. L.: Marrow transplantation for acute nonlymphoblastic leukemia in first remission. *N. Engl. J. Med.,* **301**:597–599, 1979a.

Thomas, E. D.; Clift, R. A.; Hersman, J.; Sanders, J. E.; Stewart, P.; Buckner, C. D.; Fefer, A.; McGuffin, R.; Smith, J. W.; and Storb, R.: Marrow transplantation for acute nonlymphoblastic leukemia in first remission using fractionated or single-dose irradiation. *Int. J. Radiat. Oncol.* **8**:817–822, 1982.

Thomas, E. D.; Lochte, H. L., Jr.; Cannon, J. H.; Sahler, O. D.; and Ferrebee, J. W.: Supralethal whole body irradiation and isologous marrow transplantation in man. *J. Clin. Invest.,* **38**:1709–1716, 1959.

Thomas, E. D.; Sanders, J. E.; Flournoy, N.; Johnson, F. L.; Buckner, C. D.; Clift, R. A.; Fefer, A.; Goodell, B. W.; Storb, R.; and Weiden, P. L.: Marrow transplantation for patients with acute lymphoblastic leukemia in remission. *Blood,* **54**:468–476, 1979b.

Thomas, E. D.; Storb, R.; Clift, R. A.; Fefer, A.; Johnson, F. L.; Neiman, P. E.; Lerner, K. G.; Glucksberg, H.; and Buckner, C. D.: Bone marrow transplantation. *N. Engl. J. Med.,* **292**:832–843, 895–902, 1975.

Weiden, P. L.; Flournoy, N.; Thomas, E. D.; Prentice, R.; Fefer, A.; Buckner, C. D.; and Storb, R.: Antileukemic effect of graft-versus-host disease in human recipients of allogeneic-marrow grafts. *N. Engl. J. Med.,* **300**:1068–1073, 1979.

44

Control of Pain in Cancer

KATHLEEN M. FOLEY

Pain, an invariable complication of cancer, is among the most feared of its consequences. Since pain in the patient with cancer may be caused by any of the pathophysiologic alterations that affect the general population, its presence does not necessarily imply recurrent or persistent disease. The clinical assessment of pain in patients with cancer requires a specific expertise, culled from a clear understanding of the nature of the pain and its underlying pathophysiology. Detailed analyses of patients with cancer and pain demonstrate a series of common specific pain syndromes unique to this disease process. These pain syndromes are often misdiagnosed because they are unfamiliar to general physicians (Bonica, 1953; Foley, 1979a). More importantly, several causes of pain may coexist in a single patient (Twycross, 1982). Therefore, a detailed diagnostic evaluation with a clear definition of the clinical pain syndrome helps to assure appropriate use of available therapeutic procedures.

EPIDEMIOLOGY

Of patients with cancer in terminal care facilities, 50 to 60% have pain (Bonica, 1979). Of both adult and pediatric patients receiving active therapy, 30 to 40% have pain (Foley, 1979a). From studies at Memorial Sloan-Kettering Cancer Center (MSKCC) certain tumors are associated with a higher incidence of pain, that is, 85% of patients with primary bone tumors and 52% of patients with carcinoma of the breast had pain, in contrast with only 5% of patients with leukemia. Pain can vary according to primary site and progression of the disease (Daut and Cleeland, 1982). In this study, pain caused by cancer interfered with activity and enjoyment of life to a greater extent than that from any other cause. This observation emphasizes the fact that when evaluating pain in the patient with cancer, the "pain complaint" must be recognized as only a symptom, not a diagnosis. Pain perception then is not simply a function of the amount of physical injury sustained by the patient.

Patients with cancer can readily be divided into those with acute pain and those with chronic pain. The exact point at which acute pain becomes chronic is not known, but pain lasting for longer than six months is usually considered to be a chronic pain. The management of patients and their response to treatment are often different for each of these groups. Patients with acute pain have a well-defined temporal pattern of pain onset, usually associated with subjective and objective physical signs and signs of a hyperactive autonomic nervous system. In contrast, chronic pain is persistent, with a less well-defined temporal onset, the signs of autonomic nervous system hyperactivity are absent, and psychologic and social factors may color the clinical symptomatology. Evaluating pain in any patient is difficult because the physician has limited objective signs by which to determine the severity of pain.

SPECIFIC PAIN SYNDROMES

The common pain syndromes in patients with cancer are divided into three major categories (see Table 44-1). The first and most important category is pain associated with direct tumor involvement. Seventy-eight per-

Table 44-1. Specific Pain Syndromes in Patients with Cancer

I. Pain syndromes associated with direct tumor infiltration
  A. Tumor infiltration of bone
    1. Metastases to base of skull syndromes
      a. Jugular foramen metastases
      b. Clivus metastases
      c. Sphenoid sinus metastases
    2. Metastases to vertebral bodies
      a. Odontoid fractures
      b. C_7, T_1 metastases
      c. L_1 metastases
      d. Sacral metastases
  B. Tumor infiltration of nerve, plexus, root, meninges, spinal cord
    1. Peripheral neuropathy
    2. Brachial plexopathy
    3. Lumbosacral plexopathy
    4. Leptomeningeal metastases
    5. Epidural spinal cord compression
  C. Tumor infiltration of hollow viscus

II. Pain syndromes associated with cancer therapy
  A. Postsurgical pain syndromes
    1. Postmastectomy syndrome
    2. Postthoracotomy syndrome
    3. Postradical neck syndrome
    4. Phantom limb syndrome
  B. Postchemotherapy pain syndromes
    1. Peripheral neuropathy
    2. Aseptic necrosis of the femoral head
    3. Steroid pseudorheumatism
    4. Postherpetic neuralgia
  C. Postradiation pain syndromes
    1. Radiation fibrosis of brachial and lumbosacral plexus
    2. Radiation myelopathy
    3. Radiation-induced peripheral nerve tumors

III. Pain syndromes unassociated with cancer or cancer therapy
  A. Cervical and lumbar osteoarthritis
  B. Osteoporosis
  C. Thoracic and abdominal aneurysms
  D. Diabetic neuropathy

---

cent of pain problems seen in the MSKCC inpatient population were in this category. Metastatic bone disease (50%), nerve compression or infiltration (25%), and hollow viscus involvement (15%) were the most common causes of pain from direct tumor involvement. This percentage drops to 62% when assessing pain in an outpatient cancer population (Kanner *et al.,* 1981b). These patients generally present with acute pain that, when appropriately diagnosed and treated, dramatically resolves. When pain from nerve compression or infiltration from tumor is associated with significant neurologic deficits, however, chronic pain often persists even when the primary tumor has been eradicated.

Such patients represent difficult pain management problems.

The second category includes pain syndromes associated with cancer therapy: surgery, chemotherapy, or radiation therapy. This group accounted for approximately 19% of pain problems in hospitalized cancer patients and 28% of pain problems seen in an outpatient cancer pain clinic. Each of these primary therapy modalities is associated with a series of specific pain syndromes with a characteristic pain pattern and clinical presentation. The pain is more commonly chronic, although acute pain syndromes also occur. Similarly, managing these patients is difficult because treatment of the cause of pain is limited by our current inability to repair injured nerve, reverse radiation injury, or prevent the complications of chemotherapy. However, recognition of pain not directly related to tumor growth is imperative since it markedly alters the patient's therapy, prognosis, and psychologic state.

The third major category of pain syndromes includes those unrelated to the cancer or the cancer therapy. Approximately 3% of inpatients and approximately 10% of outpatients have pain unrelated to their cancer or cancer therapy. For example, these pain syndromes include osteomyelitis, osteoporosis, diabetic neuropathy, rheumatoid arthritis, and aortic aneurysm. Obviously, accurate diagnosis in this group of patients clearly alters therapy and prognosis.

The distribution of the types of pain syndromes varies with the setting in which patients are evaluated. Outpatient pain evaluation tends to show a higher incidence of chronic pain syndromes, either as complications of cancer therapy or independent of the cancer or the cancer therapy. This observation further supports the need for a sophisticated evaluation of pain in patients with cancer and an accurate diagnosis of their specific pain syndromes.

Certain general principles should be followed in evaluating pain in patients with cancer in order to avoid misdiagnosis of the specific pain syndrome (Foley, 1982a).

GENERAL PRINCIPLES

Elicit a Clear History

The physician must assess multiple factors including age, sex, cultural and environmental influences, and psychologic factors to direct appropriate diagnostic and therapeutic approaches. In our experience with patients with cancer, the complaint of pain can rarely, if ever, be assigned to psychologic influences alone. In almost all instances pain eventually proves to have an organic basis. Certain characteristic descriptions associated with the clinical pain syndromes can help define the nature of the complaint. Noting the onset of pain, its characteristics, its referral patterns, the exacerbating and relieving factors, and associated signs and symptoms can often lead to the diagnosis. For example, in a patient complaining of severe elbow pain, exacerbated by coughing, the finding of Horner's syndrome indicates paraspinal involvement of tumor at the T_1 level. In patients with signs and symptoms involving the brachial plexus, the characteristics of pain can distinguish patients with tumor infiltration of the plexus from those with radiation fibrosis of the plexus (Kori *et al.,* 1981a). In patients with Pancoast's tumor the progression of pain is closely associated with the development of epidural spinal cord compression, often with a normal neurologic examination (Kanner *et al.,* 1982b). Last, back pain may be the only complaint in up to 20% of patients with epidural spinal cord compression preceding objective changes in either neurologic signs or symptoms (Rodichok *et al.,* 1981).

Referral patterns of pain are also particularly important. Referred pain in the arm or leg is often the first presentation of tumor infiltration of the brachial or lumbar plexus. This symptom is often misinterpreted for weeks or months because of the absence of objective neurologic signs suggesting proximal plexus involvement. Referred pain sites are usually tender to palpation, and the pain is often misinterpreted as suggesting local pathology. A common pattern in patients with cancer is pain referred to both iliac crests in disease involving the L_1 vertebral body (Kellgren, 1939).

After a careful history of the details of the pain complaint and associated medical and neurologic symptoms, a careful psychosocial history provides information about how pain influences the patient's day-to-day living and psychologic and social functioning. To what degree does anxiety or depression play a role in the patient's pain complaint? To what degree does fear or the significance of pain alter the patient's complaint of pain? Does the complaint represent a "cry for help" in a patient with a masked depression? Does the patient have a previous history of psychiatric disease

or chronic pain? A structured psychiatric interview can assess all these factors. The information obtained is invaluable in determining the "suffering" component of the pain complaint (Bond, 1979). In patients with previous psychiatric disease or a history of chronic pain, the presence of pain may make them decompensate or function at a much lower level than would be predicted from their medical illness. No matter how anxious or depressed the patient, how bizarre the symptomatology or how significant the past history of the chronic pain state, however, the symptoms must be carefully evaluated to establish or rule out the presence or absence of recurrent disease. Since metastatic disease is insidious and protean, pain may precede objective physical, neurologic, or radiologic findings for several weeks to months. The physician must then rely on the patient's verbal report of pain which is clearly colored by previous pain experience and premorbid psychiatric state. To date, no battery of psychologic tests can provide more useful information than that obtained from a structured psychiatric interview. The standard battery of psychologic tests, such as the Minnesota Multiphasic Personality test, could not distinguish cancer patients with chronic pain from patients with chronic pain of a nonneoplastic nature (Pasternak, 1980).

Examine the Site of Pain

If the physical and neurologic examinations are normal, clinical history should direct further assessment. Certain types of pain syndromes in this population of patients suggest possible causes of pain and direct early diagnostic intervention. This is of particular value in patients with tumor infiltration of nerve or spinal cord in whom early diagnosis and treatment can markedly improve their ability to function.

Use the Appropriate Diagnostic Tools

The limitations of available diagnostic procedures in diagnosing metastatic disease should be recognized by those ordering them. Similarly, diagnostic procedures should be personally reviewed with the specialist interpreting them to ensure adequate visualization of the area under study. Normal plain x-ray films should not overrule a strong clinical impression of bony metastases. Plain films cannot assess certain areas of the body where bone shadows overlap, such as the base of skull and the vertebral bodies, specifically the C_2 area, the C_7 area, and the sacrum. The bone scan is more sensitive for demonstrating abnormalities, often three to four months before changes appear on plain films. Again, a positive bone scan does not establish the diagnosis of metastatic disease since patients with osteoporosis and collapsed vertebrae may have positive scans. Similarly, infections and disuse atrophy are associated with positive bone scans. A negative scan does not rule out bony metastatic disease. For example, when bony metastatic disease occurs in a previously irradiated site, the bone scan is often negative. Also an increasing number of patients have proven bony disease and negative bone scans in cancer of the lung (Pistenma *et al.*, 1975; Thrupkaew *et al.*, 1975; Kelly *et al.*, 1979; Kori *et al.*, 1981b). Hypocycloidal tomography can provide further definition of bony abnormalities. Computerized transaxial tomography has dramatically helped the diagnostic evaluation of the patient with cancer.

When patients with metastases to bone are evaluated, specifically metastases involving the spine, the differential diagnosis includes degenerative disk disease, osteoporosis, and epidural spinal cord compression. Osteoporosis often mimics the signs and symptoms of metastatic bone disease. Radiographic differentiation of these two entities can also be difficult. Tomography and CT scanning are more useful in delineating the nature of the collapse. Tomography in osteoporotic vertebral body disease reveals intact vertebral body bony plates and symmetric bony collapse, in contrast to metastatic disease where the vertebral sites are eroded with associated pedicle destruction and asymmetric collapse of the vertebral body (Kori *et al.*, 1981b). To rule out epidural disease, myelography or CT scanning with metrizamide in the subarachnoid space is necessary. If the radiologic studies are not helpful, needle biopsy or surgical exploration of the area should be done to establish a tissue diagnosis.

Treat the Pain Early

Persistent pain debilitates the patient physically and psychologically. Early treatment of pain while investigating its source will markedly improve the patient's ability to participate in the necessary diagnostic procedures. No patient should be inadequately evaluated because of his pain. No evidence supports withholding analgesics while establishing the nature of the pain.

PAIN SYNDROMES ASSOCIATED WITH DIRECT TUMOR INFILTRATION

Tumor Infiltration of Bone

Pain from invasion of bone by either primary or metastatic tumors is the most common cause of pain in both adults and children with cancer. The underlying neurophysiologic and neuropharmacologic mechanisms of bone pain are poorly understood. Anatomic studies reveal that both myelinated and occasionally unmyelinated nerve fibers are present in bone, most dense in the region of compact bones (Bonica, 1953). The periosteum and all the components of joints, except the articular cartilage, are pain-sensitive structures, whereas the cortex and bone marrow are considered to be pain-insensitive bone structures (Kellgren, 1939; Cooper *et al.*, 1966). The vascular supply to bone has its own nerve fiber network, but the role these nerves play in the generation of pain remains unstudied. Peripherally, nociceptors in bone can be activated by both mechanical and chemical stimulation. Pathologically, metastatic tumor in bone is associated with two processes: (1) active bone destruction and (2) new bone formation. Current hypotheses for the origin of bone pain relate to the role of prostaglandins in the metastatic process and come from several lines of evidence since prostaglandins are important in both the osteolytic and osteoclastic effects of bone metastases (Galasko, 1976). For example, the prostaglandins E_1 and E_2 are potent agents producing hyperalgesia (Ferreira *et al.*, 1978). Drugs that inhibit prostaglandin synthesis inhibit pain and, in some instances, tumor growth in both clinical and experimental studies (Stoll, 1973; Brodie, 1974). In patients with multiple myeloma, osteoclast activity factor (OAF) (Horton *et al.*, 1972), a nonprostaglandin substance, is thought to be the pain-producing substance. Other factors may also influence or control the appearance of pain in patients with metastatic bone disease but have not been fully assessed, including the role of bone macrophages, changes in host cells, circulating factors such as calcitonin, variations in calcium metabolism, and hormone receptor status of the metastatic tumor (Bockman and Myers, 1977). From the clinical point of view, metastatic tumor involvement of bone produces pain in one of two ways: (1) by direct involvement of the bone and activation of the nociceptors locally, or (2) by compression of adjacent nerves, soft tissue, or vascular structures. A detailed description of pain and metastatic bone disease is beyond the scope of this chapter. Several important pain syndromes involving bone are often misdiagnosed, however, because physicians are unfamiliar with the characteristic signs and symptoms.

Metastases to the Base of the Skull. The syndromes associated with metastases to the base of the skull have been reviewed in detail (Greenberg *et al.*, 1981). Such metastases are more common in patients with nasopharyngeal tumors but can occur with any tumor type that metastasizes to bone. The syndromes in this group all share two common features: (1) pain is the earliest complaint, often preceding neurologic signs and symptoms by several weeks to months, and (2) documentation by plain x-ray films is often difficult, requiring the use of tomography and CT scanning. CT scans appear superior to all radiologic diagnostic studies in evaluating tumor involvement in this region.

Jugular Foramen Syndrome. Occipital pain referred to the vertex of the head and ipsilateral shoulder and arm is an early presenting symptom. Head movement often exacerbates the pain, with associated local tenderness over the occipital condyle. The patient's signs and symptoms vary with the cranial nerve involved but can include hoarseness, dysarthria, dysphasia, neck and shoulder weakness, and ptosis. Neurologic examination can help localize the lesion by determining the function of the ninth, tenth, eleventh, and twelfth cranial nerves. Involvement of all four of these nerves suggests jugular foramen and hypoglossal canal involvement with secondary nerve dysfunction. Horner's syndrome suggests sympathetic involvement extracranially but in close proximity to the jugular foramen.

Clivus Metastases. Pain characterized by vertex headache exacerbated by neck flexion is a common mode of presentation. Lower cranial nerve dysfunction (sixth to twelfth) usually begins unilaterally but often progresses to bilateral lower cranial nerve dysfunction.

Sphenoid Sinus Metastases. Severe bifrontal headache radiating to both temples with intermittent retro-orbital pain suggests this entity. The patient often complains of nasal stuffiness or a sense of fullness in the head with concomitant diplopia. The neurologic sign of unilateral or bilateral sixth nerve palsy further suggests the diagnosis.

Metastases to Vertebral Bodies. These syndromes share two common features: (1) pain is an early symptom preceding neurologic signs and symptoms, and (2) if the nature of the pain is not accurately diagnosed, irreversible neurologic deficits including paraplegia and quadriplegia may develop. In a recent series, 85% of patients with epidural spinal cord compression had vertebral body metastases, and in 10% of patients with cord compression pain was the only complaint in the absence of any neurologic finding (Gilbert *et al.*, 1978). Some typical pain syndromes are described below.

Odontoid Fractures. Pain in this region can result from pathologic fracture and secondary subluxation with resulting spinal cord or brain stem compression. Fractures of the odontoid process in patients with cancer are most often secondary to destruction of the atlas and are an important group of vertebral metastases from systemic cancer (Sundaresan *et al.*, 1981). Of 18 patients with odontoid fracture, 17 had severe neck pain and neck stiffness, while signs of cord compression were noted in only 4 patients. The pain characteristically radiates over the posterior aspect of the skull to the vertex and is exacerbated by neck movement, particularly neck flexion. Neurologic signs include progressive sensory and motor findings beginning in the upper extremities with associated autonomic dysfunction, but pain is the earliest symptom. Neck manipulation in these patients is dangerous, and tomography is necessary to confirm the diagnosis. Early diagnosis of tumor in the vertebral body before subluxation or fracture allows therapy to be directed at the control of tumor growth, *e.g.,* radiation therapy, before misalignment becomes evident.

C_7–T_1 *Vertebral Metastases.* This is a common site for metastatic disease originating from lung, breast, and lymphoma. Pain originating from metastatic disease to the C_7–T_1 vertebral bodies is usually localized to the adjacent paraspinal area and characterized by a constant, dull aching pain radiating bilaterally to both shoulders. Percussion may elicit tenderness over the spinous process at this level. With nerve root compression, radicular pain in the C_7, C_8, T_1 distribution is most often unilaterally in the posterior arm, elbow, and ulnar aspect of the hand. The neurologic symptoms include paresthesias and numbness in the fourth and fifth fingers with progressive hand and triceps weakness. Horner's syndrome suggests paravertebral sympathetic involvement. Metastatic bone disease at this level results from either hematogenous spread to bone or more commonly from tumor originating in the brachial plexus or paravertebral space spreading along the nerves to the contiguous vertebral body and epidural space. Plain x-ray films of the cervical and thoracic spine do not adequately visualize the C_7, T_1 area because of overlapping cardiac and bony structures. CT scan is the diagnostic procedure of choice to define the presence of metastatic disease (Kori *et al.,* 1981a; Cascino *et al.,* 1983). In patients with bilateral radicular symptoms or signs of spinal cord dysfunction, myelography should be performed to rule out an associated epidural spinal cord compression.

Lumbar Metastases—L_1. Dull, aching midback pain exacerbated by lying or sitting and relieved by standing is the usual presenting complaint. Movement exacerbates the pain, particularly when the patient goes from the recumbent to the standing position. The pain is often referred bilaterally to the sacroiliac regions or radicular to the superior iliac crests unilaterally or bilaterally. Lack of knowledge of these referred points for L_1 disease often confuses the diagnostic workup.

Sacral Metastases. Aching pain beginning insidiously in the lower back or coccygeal region exacerbated by lying or sitting and relieved by walking is the common clinical complaint for tumor infiltration of the sacrum. Increasing pain with neurologic signs and symptoms of perianal sensory loss, bowel and bladder dysfunction, and impotence help localize the site of the disease. Some patients may complain of specific tenderness over the sciatic notch and radicular symptoms in the sciatic nerve distribution associated with nerve compression from local bony changes in the sacrum. CT scan is the most useful diagnostic procedure; plain x-ray films are usually inadequate to assess this region fully. In certain instances, barium enema, IVP, and/or lymphangiogram may help define the presence of presacral tumors.

Tumor Infiltration of Nerve, Plexus, Meninges, and Spinal Cord

The pain syndromes in this group are caused by either direct tumor infiltration of nerve, by progressive compression of nerve structures, or by sudden compression by metastatic fractures of bone adjacent to nerves or nerve roots. The neuropathology of these lesions has not been correlated with the nature of pain, but neurophysiologic evidence suggests that persistent mechanical and noxious stimulation of nociceptors combined with the partial damage of axons and nerve membranes may account for the types of pain seen in this group of syndromes.

Tumor Infiltration of Peripheral Nerve. Constant burning pain with hypesthesia and dysesthesia in the area of sensory loss is the usual clinical presentation. The most common cause of infiltration of the peripheral nerve is from tumors that invade the paravertebral or retroperitoneal space. The pain is commonly radicular and unilateral and a careful sensory examination can often delineate the site of nerve compression. The most common example of infiltration of peripheral nerve is metastatic tumor involvement of rib, producing intercostal nerve entrapment. These syndromes can be diagnosed clinically with confirmation by CT scanning to document the anatomic region of nerve compression.

Tumor Infiltration of the Brachial Plexus. Pain in the shoulder or arm is the earliest presenting symptom of tumor infiltration of the brachial plexus. The lower plexus (C_7-T_1) is the most common site for tumor infiltration, but the site may vary with the tumor type. For example, in patients with breast cancer and lymphoma, infiltration of the upper plexus in the C_{5-6} distributions commonly occurs. In contrast, in patients with carcinoma of the lung, infiltration of the lower brachial plexus predominates. The patterns of pain also vary with the site of plexus involvement. Tumor infiltration of the upper plexus is usually associated with pain in the paraspinal space as far down as lateral to the T_4 vertebral body, with radicular pain in the shoulder and anterior aspect of the upper arm. Pain from lower plexus involvement is characterized by referred pain to the infrascapular area, the posterior aspect of the arm and elbow. The neurologic symptoms of pain and paresthesias in the fourth and fifth fingers may precede objective clinical signs for several weeks to months. Typically, pain precedes motor or sensory changes; objective motor signs occur before distinct sensory signs. The supraclavicular and axillary regions may be normal on examination, particularly in those patients with a lower plexopathy. Horner's syndrome suggests sympathetic involvement in the paravertebral space and is commonly associated with involvement of the lower plexus. Tumor in the brachial plexus commonly spreads along the nerve root into the epidural space. From studies in patients with breast cancer and lung cancer, the incidence of epidural spinal cord compression associated with brachial plexus infiltration is as high as 20 to 50% (Kori et al., 1981a; Kanner et al., 1982b). In a study of pain in patients with Pancoast's tumors, of 30 patients presenting with a superior pulmonary sulcus tumor, 28 had pain, and 27 of the 28 patients were diagnosed initially as having osteoarthritis of the spine or bursitis of the shoulder for up to 12 months before the tumor was diagnosed. Pain, the most common presenting symptom in brachial plexus disease, is also the most reliable indication of initial, recurrent, or progressive disease. In patients who obtained initial pain relief, recurrence of pain was the first and at times the only sign of recurrent disease.

A second problem in evaluating patients with pain in the distribution of the brachial plexus arises in the patient who received radiation therapy. In this case, the differential diagnosis must include radiation fibrosis of the plexus. Table 44–2 describes the characteristics of the pain symptomatology. Studies in patients with brachial plexus lesions indicate that careful attention to the pattern of pain and

neurologic deficit combined with CT scans of the plexus can provide sufficient information to diagnose tumor infiltrations from radiation fibrosis and obviate the need for surgical explorations or needle biopsy. Other differential diagnoses include brachial neuritis, rotator cuff tear at the shoulder joint, and cervical disk disease. These common pain syndromes are often misdiagnosed in patients who have brachial plexus tumor infiltration. Each of these syndromes has characteristic neurologic signs and symptoms, previously well described.

Tumor Infiltration of the Lumbosacral Plexus. This entity is most common in patients with genitourinary, gynecologic, and colonic cancers but can occur from any tumor that metastasizes to this anatomic region. Local tumor extension into adjacent lymph nodes and bone produces pain, which varies with the site of plexus involvement. In a review of 85 patients with lumbosacral plexopathy, 67% of patients had direct tumor extension; in 22% it was from metastatic disease and in 11% the primary site of tumor was unknown. Pain was the presenting symptom in 91% of patients, with weakness in 60% and numbness in 42%. The pain is of two types: local pain in the sacrum or sacroiliac joint, low back, or groin, and radicular pain in the lateral, posterior, or anterior leg (Jaeckle et al., 1985). CT scanning is the most useful diagnostic study to define the

Table 44–2. Characteristics of Pain in 100 Patients with Brachial Plexopathy

	TUMOR GROUP (78 PTS.)	RADIATION GROUP (22 PTS.)
Presenting symptoms	82%	18%
Location	Shoulder, upper arm, elbow Radiates to fourth and fifth fingers	Shoulder, wrist, hand
Nature	Dull aching in shoulder Lancinating pain in elbow and ulnar aspect of hand Occasional dysesthesias, burning, freezing sensations	Aching pain in shoulder Tightness and heaviness in arm and hand Paresthesias in $C_{5,6}$ distribution in hand
Severity	Moderate—severe 98% severe	Mild—moderate 35% severe
Course	Progressive neurologic dysfunction, atrophy, weakness, C_7–T_1 distribution Pain persistent	Progressive weakness in $C_{5,6}$ distribution Pain stabilizes or improves with appearance of weakness

Reprinted by permission from Foley, K. M.: Clinical assessment of cancer pain. *Acta Anaesthesiol. (Scand.) [Suppl.]*, **74:**91–96, 1982.

soft tissue masses or bony abnormalities in the lumbosacral and pelvic regions. Specific studies like lymphangiography and certain radionuclide scans, or gallium scans in patients with Hodgkin's disease, may add information to suggest the presence of tumor in adjacent lymph tissue. The differential diagnosis includes lumbar neuritis, postsurgical lumbar plexopathy, radiation fibrosis, and lumbar disk disease. Again, each of these entities has a characteristic neurologic presentation and should be differentiated from tumor infiltration of the lumbar plexus.

Leptomeningeal Metastases. In this clinical entity tumor infiltrates the cerebrospinal leptomeninges with or without concomitant invasion of the parenchyma of the nervous system (Olson *et al.,* 1978). Pain occurs in 40% of patients and is generally of two types: (1) headache, with or without neck stiffness, characterized by constant pain, and (2) back pain, most commonly localized to the low back and buttock regions. Pain results from traction on tumor-infiltrated nerves and meninges. Lumbar puncture is the procedure of choice to detect neoplastic cells in the cerebrospinal fluid (CSF) of these patients. An elevated CSF protein and low glucose concentration are often associated findings. In patients with low-back and buttock pain, myelography can help delineate tumor nodules along the nerves and the cauda equina. The differential diagnosis varies with the site of neurologic involvement. However, in patients with known cancer, signs and symptoms of neurologic dysfunction at several levels of the neuraxis should suggest this diagnosis. Alternative considerations may include fungal meningitis, cauda equina epidural tumor, and arachnoiditis.

Epidural Spinal Cord Compression. Severe neck and back pain is the hallmark of this entity. Gilbert *et al.* (1978) reviewed 130 patients with epidural spinal cord compression and found that pain was the initial symptom in 96% of patients and in 10% was the only symptom. The pain occurs from local bone or root compression of generally two types: (1) local pain over the involved vertebral body or (2) radicular pain unilaterally in patients with cervical or lumbosacral compression and bilaterally in those with thoracic cord compression. The neurologic symptoms vary with the site of epidural disease and commonly include motor weakness progressing to paraplegia, a level of sensory loss of bowel and bladder function. Eighty-five percent of patients had associated vertebral body tumor. Plain x-ray films of the spine do not delineate the integrity of the epidural space, and lumbar and cisternal myelography are necessary to delineate the extent of the epidural block. CT scanning with metrizamide in the subarachnoid space can also delineate the degree of epidural block. The full extent of epidural tumor must be defined to provide appropriate treatment. Patients with cancer may also have multiple levels of epidural cord compression, and these observations support the need for full lumbar and cervical myelography.

PAIN SYNDROMES ASSOCIATED WITH CANCER THERAPY

Clinical pain syndromes occur in the course of, or subsequent to, treatment of cancer patients with surgery, chemotherapy, or radiation therapy. These syndromes are of two types. The first type occurs acutely, within weeks, after the specific therapy, such as immediate postoperative pain syndromes, the mucositis of chemotherapy, and the radiation-induced esophagitis. These syndromes are readily recognized, and the associated pain is self-limited. The second type occurs several weeks to months and, in certain instances, years later and presents the clinical problem — is the pain a complication of therapy or recurrent disease? The incidence of these late pain syndromes is not known, but they represent an important aspect of the differential diagnosis of the pain complaint for both the patient and physician.

Postsurgical Pain Syndromes

Postmastectomy Pain Syndrome. Four to 10 percent of women having any surgical procedure on the breast from lumpectomy to radical mastectomy develop this syndrome. The pain can occur immediately or up to several months following surgery and is characterized as a tight, constricting, burning pain in the posterior arm, axilla, and anterior chest wall. Often a trigger-point area in the axilla recreates the pain on palpation. Movement exacerbates the pain and patients often posture their arms in a flexed position close to the chest wall. This posturing leads to the development of a frozen shoulder and secondary pain from disuse atrophy of the arm and shoulder muscles.

Postmastectomy pain results from the interruption of the intercostal brachial nerve, a sensory cutaneous branch of T_1-T_2, and subsequent formation of a traumatic neuroma at the end of the severed nerve. Neuroanatomic studies reveal that the size and distribution of this nerve vary widely, which may account for its varied clinical appearance (Wood, 1978; Granek *et al.*, 1983). The syndrome can be clearly distinguished from tumor infiltration of the brachial plexus. Physical therapy to prevent shoulder immobilization, local rubbing of the area, nerve blocks of the trigger point with local anesthetics, and small doses of amitriptyline have had some limited success. Breast reconstruction does not lessen the pain nor the sensation of tightness in the anterior chest wall.

Postthoracotomy Pain Syndrome. The clinical features include pain in the distribution of the intercostal brachial nerve following surgical injury or interruption. The pain is of two types: (1) the immediate postoperative pain, which clears in 75% of patients by three months and is associated with sensory loss in the area of the scar, and (2) persistent postoperative pain for longer than three months or the recurrence of pain in the surgical area following resolution of the initial postoperative pain. Studies (Kanner *et al.*, 1982a) suggest that this latter type of pain has a statistically high association with recurrent tumor or infiltration in the chest wall, paraspinal, or epidural space. The CT scan, rather than the chest x-ray film, is the diagnostic procedure to assess this particular pain problem. In less than 5 to 10% of patients on follow-up did the development of a traumatic neuroma or nerve injury cause this clinical pain syndrome. In patients with recurrent tumor, therapy directed at the tumor is the treatment of choice for the pain. For patients with nerve injury only, local rubbing, transcutaneous nerve stimulation, and amitriptyline have been used with varied success.

Postradical Neck Pain Syndromes. One type of pain syndrome following radical neck dissection may be associated with surgical injury or interruption of the cervical nerves and is characterized by a constant burning sensation in the area of sensory loss. Dysesthesias and intermittent shocklike pain may also be present. Carbamazepine is particularly useful in this group of patients for managing the dysesthetic component of the pain. The second type of pain syndrome in patients with radical neck dissection includes a series of musculo-skeletal pain problems resulting from surgical injury to motor nerves that innervate the shoulder and upper arm. These syndromes are characterized by aching pain in the shoulder and neck, often exacerbated by sitting up and walking around and relieved by lying down. They usually include the suprascapular nerve entrapment syndrome and pain secondary to thoracic outlet compression. Local nerve blocks and support slings can markedly relieve these muscle tension complaints and prevent progressive motor and sensory symptoms and signs.

Phantom Limb and Stump Pain. Pain following surgical amputation of a limb is of two types: stump pain and phantom limb pain. These painful clinical entities are distinct from phantom limb sensation that all patients experience following limb amputation. The phantom limb pain is usually characterized by a burning, cramping pain in the phantom limb, often identical in nature and location to the preoperative pain. Stump pain can be triggered by local pressure on the stump and is associated with the presence of a traumatic neuroma. Stump pain is exacerbated by movement and pressure and relieved by rest, in contrast to phantom limb pain which is unaffected by any mechanical stimuli. The underlying mechanisms of such pain are controversial (Carlin *et al.*, 1978). Phantom limb pain frequently clears within two months of the surgical procedure. Its recurrence may be the first sign of disease recurrence in a proximal nerve root, mimicking the original phantom limb pain. Carbamazepine to suppress the acute shocklike pain often associated with stump pain, local transcutaneous electrical stimulation, and amitriptyline in small doses are all reported to be of some value in managing this group of pain syndromes.

Postchemotherapy Pain Syndromes

Peripheral Neuropathy. The painful dysesthesias following treatment with the vinca-alkaloid drugs are part of a symmetric polyneuropathy. They are usually localized to the hands and feet and characterized as a burning pain exacerbated by superficial stimuli. In children a more diffuse syndrome occurs, characterized by generalized myalgias and arthralgias, often beginning with jaw pain and progressing to a symmetric polyneuropathy including cranial nerve dysfunction. The syndrome is self-limited, usually lasting from four to six weeks. Pain resolution is associated with partial resolution of nerve function. Amitriptyline is particularly useful in managing this group of pain syndromes.

Steroid Pseudorheumatism. This entity occurs after both rapid and slow withdrawal of steroid medication in patients taking these drugs for any length of time (Rotstein and Good, 1957). The syndrome consists of prominent diffuse myalgias and arthralgias with muscle and joint tenderness on palpation but without objective inflammatory signs. Generalized malaise and fatigue are common features of this entity. The signs and symptoms revert with reinstitution of the steroid medication. This pain syndrome is common in patients who are being pulsed with steroids as part of their chemotherapy regimen. Steroid withdrawal often markedly exacerbates pain from bony metastases or epidural cord compression.

Aseptic Necrosis of Bone. Aseptic necrosis of the humeral and, more commonly, the femoral head are known complications of cancer therapy, specifically chronic steroid therapy (Ihde and DeVita, 1975). Pain in the shoulder or knee and leg is the common presenting complaint, with x-ray film changes occurring several weeks to months after the onset of pain. Limitation of joint movements with progressive inability to use the arm or hip functionally is the natural history of this illness. It is most common in patients with Hodgkin's disease but can occur in any patient on chronic steroid therapy. The bone scan is the most useful diagnostic procedure and is usually positive before changes in plain films appear. The appropriate treatment is replacement of the diseased area, which dramatically resolves the pain complaint.

Postherpetic Neuralgia. This well-described clinical entity is characterized by persistent pain after cutaneous eruptions from herpes zoster infection have cleared. In patients with cancer, herpes zoster infection commonly occurs in the area of tumor pathology or in the port of previous radiation therapy. The true incidence of postherpetic neuralgia in patients with cancer is unknown, but it appears to be more common in patients who develop the infection after the age of 50. There are generally three types of pain: (1) continuous burning pain in the area of sensory loss, (2) painful dysesthesias, and (3) intermittent shocklike pain. The management of patients with postherpetic neuralgia has been recently reviewed (Price, 1982). The current approach includes mild analgesics, amitriptyline in low doses, and carbamazepine to manage the intermittent shocklike pain. Although the site of the postherpetic neuralgia pain does not necessarily correspond to the site of previous tumor in patients, the presence of the pain often obscures underlying pathology. Again, careful attention to the patient's complaint and to the motor and sensory examination is imperative. If the sensory loss is more extensive than the scarring or if the motor findings are out of the distribution of the nerves involved, further workup of the patient may be necessary to rule out some other cause, such as metastatic disease in bone, paraspinal space, or epidural space.

Postradiation Therapy Pain Syndromes

Radiation Fibrosis of the Brachial Plexus. Pain in the distribution of the brachial plexus following radiation therapy is caused by fibrosis of the surrounding connective tissue and secondary injury to nerve. It may appear as early as 6 months or as late as 20 years following radiation treatment (Stoll and Andrews, 1966). Differentiating radiation fibrosis from recurrent tumor is a difficult diagnostic problem (Kori *et al.,* 1981a). The clinical symptoms include complaints of numbness or paresthesias in the hand, usually in a C_{5-6} distribution. Pain occurs later in the course of the clinical entity and is often characterized as diffuse arm pain. Lymphedema in the arm, radiation skin changes, and induration of the supraclavicular and axillary areas are often present. The neurologic signs include sensory changes in the C_{5-6} distribution and motor weakness in the deltoid and biceps muscles. These signs progress to the development of a painful, useless, swollen extremity. Table 44–2 summarizes the clinical presentation and characteristics of pain. No specific pain therapy is effective in this very difficult management problem. Forequarter amputation of the limb, high cervical cordotomy, and multiple rhizotomies have all had very limited success. This is a most distressing pain syndrome in patients whose disease appears to be cured.

Radiation Fibrosis of the Lumbosacral Plexus. Radiation fibrosis of the lumbosacral plexus is much less common than radiation fibrosis of the brachial plexus (Thomas *et al.,*

1985). The low incidence appears related to the tumor type which does not have the comparable long survival times of breast cancer. Pain in the leg or perineum from radiation fibrosis of the lumbar plexus represents a difficult diagnostic problem. A history of radiation treatment and local skin changes or lymphedema of the leg with x-ray film changes demonstrating radiation necrosis of hip or sacrum help establish the diagnosis. The diagnostic workup must differentiate fibrosis from tumor infiltration and should include plain x-ray films of the area and CT scanning. The prognosis for this particular disorder is bleak. Commonly, pain progresses, leading to disability and paraplegia secondary to loss of motor and sensory function.

Radiation Myelopathy. Pain is an early symptom in 15% of patients with this entity (Jellinger and Sturm, 1971). The pain may be localized to the area of spinal cord damage or may be referred with dysesthesias below the level of injury. Clinically, the neurologic symptoms and signs are those of a Brown-Séquard syndrome characterized by an ipsilateral motor paresis with a contralateral sensory loss at the cervicothoracic level. The syndrome progresses to a complete transverse myelopathy. Careful plain x-ray films of the spine and myelography should be taken and are commonly normal. Occasionally, widening of the cord at the injured area may be noted. The differential diagnosis includes intramedullary tumor, epidural spinal cord compression, arteriovenous malformation, or a transverse myelitis, but the clinical history taken with the neurologic findings usually yields the diagnosis. Management of the pain with carbamazepine may be of some value, but no effective therapies are available.

Radiation-Induced Peripheral Nerve Tumors. A painful enlarging mass in an area of previous irradiation suggests this entity. Seven of nine patients who developed radiation-induced nerve tumors presented with pain, progressive neurologic deficit, and a palpable mass involving either the brachial or lumbar plexus. These tumors developed 4 to 20 years following radiation therapy when patients were cured of their original tumor (Foley et al., 1979c). This experience emphasizes the need to assess the patient with recurrent pain and an atypical presentation, perhaps late in the course of an illness. Needle biopsy or surgical exploration may be necessary to define the nature of the tumor.

PAIN SYNDROMES UNASSOCIATED WITH CANCER OR CANCER THERAPY

Common pain syndromes that occur in the general population include pain from cervical and lumbar osteoarthritis, osteoporosis and collapsed vertebral bodies, thoracic and abdominal aneurysms, and diabetic neuropathy. Three percent of inpatients and 10% of outpatients seen by the MSKCC Pain Service fall in this category. This group stresses the need for a clear definition of the pain complaint.

THERAPEUTIC APPROACHES TO CANCER PAIN

The methods of pain management and the goals of therapy vary with each individual patient. For patients undergoing active therapy or diagnosis for cancer, pain control should help them tolerate the necessary diagnostic and therapeutic approaches and allow them to function. In patients with terminal illness, pain control should provide adequate relief to allow them to function at a reasonable level, but this level may be limited more by their tumor than by their pain. A series of medical and surgical approaches to the management of cancer pain have been defined. Their use often depends upon the clinical expertise available, but evidence suggests that patients with cancer pain are managed most effectively by a multidisciplinary approach, including the oncologist, neurologist, anesthesiologist, clinical pharmacologist, and neurosurgeon (Foley, 1979b). Certain approaches to managing pain, however, should be within the armamentarium of any physician, and these generally fall within the category of drug therapy.

Medical Therapy

Drug Therapy. Analgesic drugs are the mainstay of therapy for acute cancer pain and are also important in managing patients with chronic cancer pain problems. Analgesic drug therapy may be divided into three groups of medications: group I: the nonnarcotic analgesics such as aspirin and the nonsteroidal antiinflammatory drugs (NSAID); group II: the narcotic agonists and antagonists; group III: the adjuvant analgesic drugs. This latter group includes a series of different categories of drugs that produce analgesia in certain pain states by mechanisms not clearly established and not directly related to the opiate receptor or prostaglandin system.

Nonnarcotic Analgesics. Nonnarcotic analgesics are a heterogeneous group of substances differing in chemical structure and pharmacologic action including aspirin, acetaminophen, and the nonsteroidal anti-inflammatory drugs (NSAID). These drugs have varied roles as analgesic, anti-inflammatory, and antipyretic drugs. Aspirin is the prototypical drug and the most commonly used. These drugs are commonly administered orally and used in treating mild to moderate pain. In contrast to the opioid or narcotic analgesics, tolerance and physical dependence do not develop. Their mechanisms of action are controversial. The current hypothesis is that aspirin and the nonsteroidal anti-inflammatory drugs reduce or prevent the sensitization of pain receptors to nociceptive stimuli by preventing prostaglandin release peripherally and in some cases centrally (Ferreira, 1979). In the cancer patient with bone metastases these drugs may play a special role because of their ability to inhibit prostaglandin synthetase. Since the development of bone metastases is associated with prostaglandin function, the ability of these drugs to inhibit prostaglandin synthetase may explain their ability to produce enhanced pain relief in this population of patients. Studies by Galasko (1976) suggest that aspirin has antitumor properties as well. These drugs are the first-line medications for managing cancer pain.

The choice and use of the nonnarcotic analgesic must be individualized for each patient by adequate trials of one nonnarcotic analgesic before switching to alternative agents (Beaver, 1965; Gerbershagen, 1979). The drug should be administered at regular intervals to maximum levels. If one drug produces inadequate analgesia, one of the other NSAID drugs should be tried. Physicians tend to overprescribe nonnarcotic analgesics and underprescribe narcotic analgesics. If pain control is ineffective with a nonnarcotic analgesic, narcotic analgesics alone or in combination with the nonnarcotic should be considered.

Narcotic Analgesics. Patients with severe pain and terminal illness can be adequately managed with narcotic analgesics in up to 95% of cases. The effective use of this group of drugs balances the desirable effect of pain relief against the undesirable effects of excessive sedation, constipation, tolerance, and physical dependence. Tolerance means that on repeated administration increasing doses of the drug are necessary to produce the desired analgesic effect. Physical dependence follows the chronic administration of narcotic drugs when signs of withdrawal occur with abrupt cessation of the drug. Both tolerance and physical dependence are pharmacologic effects of chronic narcotic administration but are distinct from addiction—psychologic dependence. Addiction means a concomitant behavioral pattern of drug abuse in which the individual craves the drug for other than pain relief and becomes overwhelmingly involved in using the drug and securing its supply. Because of the potential for abuse with these drugs and the misconception by both clinicians and patients that physical dependence and addiction are interchangeable, narcotic analgesics have not been most beneficially used in patients with cancer and chronic pain (Marks and Sachar, 1973; Foley, 1981). This reluctance to use narcotics is further increased by careful monitoring by federal and state governments and physicians in prescribing them. In addition, pharmacists dispensing such prescriptions must follow strict regulations in handling these drugs. The practical use of these drugs has been previously reviewed (Houde, 1979; Twycross and Ventafridda, 1980; Foley, 1982b; Inturrisi, 1982), but many clinicians remain ignorant about their applied pharmacology.

GENERAL PHARMACOLOGIC PRINCIPLES. Some important clinical pharmacologic principles that must be followed to use the narcotic analgesics effectively are considered here briefly. For mild pain, a nonnarcotic analgesic like aspirin or acetaminophen, or the narcotic analgesics like propoxyphene and codeine, are the drugs of choice. For moderate pain, codeine, meperidine, and oxycodone are commonly used, whereas morphine, hydromorphone, methadone, and levorphanol are reserved for severe pain. Table 44–3 lists the equianalgesic doses for the commonly used narcotics and nonnarcotics. Relative potencies of the analgesics are based on single-dose studies (Houde, 1979). Table 44–3 also includes the available pharmacokinetic data on the drugs commonly used which are essential to ensure appropriate drug use. Lack of attention to these equianalgesic doses when switching from one medication to another or from one route of administration to another often causes unnecessary recurrence of pain. Lack of

Table 44–3. Oral Nonnarcotic and Narcotic Analgesics for Mild to Moderate Pain

ANALGESIC	ROUTE	EQUIANALGESIC DOSE*	DURATION	PLASMA HALF-LIFE (HR)	COMMENTS
Aspirin	PO	650	4–6	3–5	Standard for nonnarcotic comparison; GI and hematologic effects limit use in cancer patients
Acetaminophen	PO	650	4–6	1–4	Weak anti-inflammatory effects; safer than aspirin
Propoxyphene	PO	65	4–6	12	Biotransformed to potentially toxic metabolite norpropoxyphene; used in combination with nonnarcotic analgesics
Codeine	PO	32	4–6	3	Biotransformed to morphine; available in combinations with nonnarcotic analgesics
Meperidine	PO	50	4–6	3–4	Biotransformed to active toxic metabolite normeperidine, produces myoclonus seizures
Pentazocine	PO	30	4–6	2–3	Psychotomimetic effects with escalation of dose; only available in combinations with naloxone or aspirin

Oral and Parenteral Narcotic Analgesics for Severe Pain

Narcotic Agonists

ANALGESIC	ROUTE	EQUIANALGESIC DOSE*	DURATION	PLASMA HALF-LIFE (HR)	COMMENTS
Morphine	IM PO	10 60	4–6 4–7	2–3.5	Standard for comparison; available in slow-release tablets
Codeine	IM PO	130 200†	4–6 4–6	3	Biotransformed to morphine; useful as initial narcotic analgesic
Oxycodone	IM PO	15 30	 3–5	—	Short-acting; available as 5-mg dose in combination with aspirin and acetaminophen
Heroin	IM PO	5 (60)	4–5 4–5	0.5	Illegal in U.S.; high solubility for parenteral administration
Levorphanol (LEVODROMORAN)	IM PO	2 4	4–6 4–7	12–16	Good oral potency, requires careful titration in initial dosing because of drug accumulation, more soluble than morphine
Hydromorphone (DILAUDID)	IM PO	1.5 7.5	4–5 4–6	2–3	Available in high potency injectable form (10 mg/ml) for cachetic patient and rectal suppositories
Oxymorphone (NUMORPHAN)	IM PR	1 10	4–6 4–6	2–3	Available in parenteral and rectal suppository forms only
Meperidine (DEMEROL)	IM PO	75 300†	4–5 4–6	3–4 Normeperidine 12–16	Contraindicated in patients with renal disease, accumulation of active toxic metabolite normeperidine, produces CNS excitation
Methadone (DOLOPHINE)	IM PO	10 20		15–30	Good oral potency, requires careful titration in initial dosing to avoid drug accumulation

continued

Table 44–3. *(Continued)*

ANALGESIC	ROUTE	EQUIANALGESIC DOSE*	DURATION	PLASMA HALF-LIFE (HR)	COMMENTS
Mixed-Agonist Antagonists					
Pentazocine (TALWIN)	IM PO	60 180†	4–6 4–7	2–3	Limited use in cancer pain; psychotomimetic effects with dose escalation, available only in combination with naloxone, aspirin or acetaminophen; may precipitate withdrawal in tolerant patients
Nalbuphine (NUBAIN)	IM PO	10 —	4–6	5	Not available orally; less psychotomimetic effects than pentazocine; may precipitate withdrawal in tolerant patient
Butorphanol (STADOL)	IM PO	2 —	4–6	2.5–3.5	Not available orally; psychotomimetic effects; may precipitate withdrawal in tolerant patients
Partial Agonists					
Buprenorphine (TEMGESIC)	IM IL	0.4 0.8	4–6 5–6	?	Not available in U.S.; no psychotomimetic effects; may precipitate withdrawal in tolerant patients

* Equianalgesic dose = (1) relative potency of drugs compared to aspirin for mild to moderate pain; (2) based on single-dose studies in which an intramuscular dose of each drug listed was compared to morphine to establish relative potency for severe pain. Oral doses are those recommended when changing from parenteral to oral routes.
† Initial oral doses of these drugs are listed under mild to moderate pain. From Foley, K. M.: The treatment of cancer pain. *N. Engl. J. Med.,* **313**(2), 1985.

attention to pharmacokinetic parameters can lead to using drugs whose accumulation could cause excessive side effects. Drugs such as methadone and levorphanol which are effective analgesics in managing cancer pain have particularly long plasma half-lives (Sawe *et al.,* 1981). Their repeated administration, particularly in patients not previously exposed to narcotics and therefore nontolerant, may lead to excessive sedation and respiratory depression (Ettinger *et al.,* 1979; Dixon *et al.,* 1980). These side effects can be easily avoided by adjusting the dose of drug at intervals and by anticipating such effects. More important, the plasma half-life of the analgesic is not directly related to its analgesic efficacy. Both of these drugs with long plasma half-lives produce analgesia for only four to six hours.

When switching from one medication to another in the patient tolerant to narcotic analgesics, the calculated equianalgesic dose should be reduced to one-third or one-half of this amount and used as a test dose at a regular fixed interval. This empiric dose adjustment is based on current clinical pharmacologic stud-ies demonstrating that the relative potency of drugs changes with repeated administration. Detailed studies are not available at this time. Before a narcotic analgesic is accepted as ineffective in an individual patient, the drug should be given regularly at intervals based on the duration of effect. In general, this approach keeps the patient's pain at a tolerable level and limits the patient's anxiety about medication (Fordyce *et al.,* 1973).

Using combinations of drugs may be more effective on controlling a patient's pain. Combining a narcotic with a nonnarcotic and certain adjuvant analgesic drugs often produces additive analgesia. The physician can thus enhance the patient's analgesia without escalating the narcotic dose. Drugs such as the nonnarcotic analgesics and hydroxyzine appear to enhance the analgesia of the narcotic analgesics, while drugs such as diazepam and chlorpromazine enhance the sedative effects of the narcotic analgesics without additive analgesia. In some instances, these sedative effects may limit the amount of narcotic analgesic used. This is often a disservice to the patient who is oversedated with drugs that are not primarily analgesics.

The route of administration varies with the patient's needs. Orally administered drugs have a slower onset of action than parenterally administered drugs. In the patient who requires immediate relief, parenteral administration, either intramuscularly or intravenously, is the route of choice. The rectal route is available for patients who cannot take oral drugs or in whom parenteral administration is contraindicated. Continuous subcutaneous and intravenous infusions of narcotics may be appropriate for patients with certain chronic states, specifically those with a terminal illness. Such infusions maintain smooth analgesic control, avoiding erratic oral absorption, particularly in patients with gastrointestinal disturbances. The starting intravenous dose varies with the drug but is approximately equal to the parenteral dose determined by prior narcotic experience of the patient and adjusted by need. Recently, epidural and intrathecal administration of narcotics has been also reported to be effective (Max *et al.,* 1981).

Since the side effects of narcotic analgesics often limit their effective use, careful attention to managing them is essential. In all patients taking narcotic drugs chronically, tolerance occurs within days of starting drug therapy. The earliest sign of tolerance is the patient's complaint that the duration of effective analgesia has decreased. Increasing the frequency of drug administration or increasing the amount of drug at each dose is necessary to overcome tolerance. Since cross-tolerance among the narcotic analgesics is not complete, switching from one narcotic drug to another often improves the analgesic effect. Constipation and sedation can be avoided by cathartics and stimulants.

Abrupt withdrawal of narcotic analgesics in patients receiving them chronically produces agitation, tremors, insomnia, fever, and marked autonomic nervous system hyperexcitability. Slowly tapering the dose of the narcotic analgesic prevents such withdrawal symptoms. The appearance of abstinence symptoms from the time of drug withdrawal is related to the elimination curve of the particular drug. Reinstituting the drug in doses of 25% of the previous daily dose suppresses these symptoms.

All attempts should be made to optimize therapy for the patient. The metabolism of narcotic drugs is so variable that individual variations in analgesia and side effects commonly have a pharmacologic basis rather than a psychologic basis (Inturrisi *et al.,* 1981). The psychologic state of the patient, however, is of paramount importance in effectively treating cancer pain. When analgesic therapy is not effective, even when pushed to excessive side effects, psychologic factors may play a role and drugs directed at anxiety and depression may be necessary to provide adequate pain control.

Adjuvant Analgesic Drugs. The clinical interest in using these drugs in cancer pain management developed from a greater understanding of the neuropharmacology of pain. Recognition of the important role of neurotransmitters in central pain modulation (Mayer and Price, 1976) and the ability of the adjuvant analgesic drugs to enhance or block neurotransmitter function led to trials in clinical pain states. Although the role and the clinical use of these drugs in cancer pain are not well established, they are predominantly used as coanalgesics. Efficacy studies for the coanalgesic or analgesic properties of these drugs are lacking. Their appropriate use to enhance analgesia or to treat side effects depends on the careful assessment of the clinical signs and symptoms. The choice of the adjuvant drug should be individualized to provide the simplest and most potent combination of drugs. Some of the commonly used adjuvant analgesics are reviewed briefly.

ANTICONVULSANTS. Phenytoin and carbamazepine suppress spontaneous neuronal firing. They are the drugs of choice for treating trigeminal neuralgia and have been reported anecdotally to be useful in certain chronic pain states, such as diabetic neuropathy and postherpetic neuralgia. In patients with cancer pain, carbamazepine has been specifically helpful in managing acute shocklike neuralgia pain of cranial and high cervical distribution in pain syndromes caused by tumor infiltration or traumatic neuroma. In patients with phantom limb pain secondary to traumatic neuroma, carbamazepine has also been anecdotally reported to be useful. Leukopenia is an idiosyncratic side effect of the use of carbamazepine and, in our experience, cancer patients are at greater risk to develop this complication because of compromised bone marrow from previous cancer therapy. This drug should therefore be used carefully in this population of patients.

PHENOTHIAZINES. Methotrimeprazine is the phenothiazine drug with the most prominent analgesic properties (Lasagna and Dekornfeld, 1961). The drug also has antiemetic and antianxiety properties and is useful to manage cancer pain in special circumstances such as the patient tolerant to narcotic analgesics. It offers an alternative method to produce analgesia in the patient with bowel obstruction and pain since it obviates the constipatory effects of narcotics. Its side effects include postural hypotension, excessive sedation, and extrapyramidal side effects. The long-term effects of the drug have not been studied.

Chlorpromazine. This phenothiazine is widely used in treating patients with terminal illness and cancer pain (Sadove et al., 1954; Gordon and Campbell, 1956; Lipman, 1975; Twycross, 1977; Halpern, 1979). The only controlled study (Houde and Wallenstein, 1955) reported no significant difference in pain relief in 34 patients with cancer taking morphine alone versus morphine in combination with 25 mg of chlorpromazine. Twycross suggests that in terminal cancer the main indication for phenothiazine is as an antiemetic but also that in patients with an appreciable psychologic component to their pain, chlorpromazine in conjunction with oral morphine often yields better results than a higher dose of morphine alone.

Prochlorperazine. This drug has mild analgesic properties, but its main indication is as an antiemetic. In combination with the narcotic analgesics, it counteracts their emetic properties, but whether it produces sedative analgesia is unknown.

Fluphenazine. This phenothiazine, when compared to nine phenothiazines, was noted to have mild analgesic properties. More recently, the drug has been used in combination with the tricyclic antidepressants to treat certain partial deafferentation syndromes (Taub, 1973).

BUTYROPHENONES. Haloperidol. This drug is most widely used in managing major psychiatric disorders. Its usefulness in managing cancer pain is anecdotal. Several authors have reported its clinical usefulness in patients with cancer pain, suggesting that it works as a coanalgesic allowing for reduction of the narcotic dose (Shimm et al., 1979). Breivik and Rennemo (1982) retrospectively studied the use of psychotropic drugs in 56 patients receiving methadone for control of cancer pain. They suggested that haloperidol was useful both as a coanalgesic and to treat side effects in patients receiving methadone. At the present time, haloperidol is the first-line drug in managing acute psychosis and delirium in patients with cancer, but its role in pain management is less clear.

ANTIDEPRESSANTS. Amitriptyline. The tricyclic antidepressants may be the most useful group of psychotropic drugs presently used in pain management. Their analgesic effects are mediated by enhancing serotonin activity within the central nervous system. In clinical trials amitriptyline ameliorates tension and migraine headaches and has analgesic effects independent of its antidepressant effects in patients with postherpetic neuralgia (Watson et al., 1982). In patients with cancer pain amitriptyline plays a major role in managing neuropathic pain and phantom limb sensation. It is also used as a hypnotic to eliminate the insomnia associated with chronic cancer pain. These effects occur at doses far below those required to treat depression.

ANTIHISTAMINES. Hydroxyzine. This drug is a minor tranquilizer with antihistaminic, antispasmodic, and antiemetic activity. Hyroxyzine has potent analgesic activity that, when combined with morphine, produces additive analgesic effects. The sedative effects of this combination were only slightly greater than that of morphine alone (Beaver, 1976).

AMPHETAMINES. Dextroamphetamine. This drug in doses of 10 mg intramuscularly is reported to produce additive analgesic effects when compared with morphine in single-dose studies of postoperative pain (Forrest et al., 1977). Amphetamines counteract the sedation in a patient receiving adequate analgesia but incapacitated by the sedative effects. Small doses (2.5 to 5 mg orally) of dextroamphetamine once or twice a day reduce the sedative effects of the narcotic analgesics. The clinical usefulness of this observation with repeated doses has not been studied.

STEROIDS. Corticosteroids are reported to have both specific and nonspecific benefits in managing acute and chronic cancer pain. The ability to produce euphoria, increased appetite, and weight gain contributes greatly to the patient's sense of well-being in terminal illness. Steroids may reduce pain of metastatic bone origin and are used as oncolytic agents in certain types of tumors. Several studies demonstrate prolonged survival time and reduced narcotic doses to control pain in terminal cancer patients receiving corticosteroids (Schell, 1966, 1972). Steroids produce dramatic pain relief in patients with epidural cord compression and tumor infiltration of the brachial and lumbosacral plexus (Gilbert *et al.,* 1978).

CANNABINOIDS.   Studies of delta-9-tetrahydrocannabinol have demonstrated that it produces euphoric, analgesic, appetite-stimulant, and antiemetic effects. Harris (1979) reviewed the use of cannabinoids as analgesics citing four well-controlled studies in which good analgesic activity was accompanied by a high incidence of side effects including drowsiness, hypotension, and bradycardia. At the present time, the major use of these drugs in cancer pain management remains untested.

COCAINE.   Snow (1897) initially reported this drug as effective in combination with opium in treating pain associated with neoplasms. No controlled studies assess cocaine as an analgesic alone or as a coanalgesic. Twycross (1977) evaluated the role of cocaine in the Brompton cocktail and noted that in 10-mg increments per dose cocaine resulted in a small but statistically significant increase in alertness, but that discontinuing it had no detectable effect. On the basis of this study cocaine has been withdrawn from the standard Brompton cocktail.

LEVODOPA.   Several reports describe the successful use of levodopa in relieving pain in patients with carcinoma of the breast and prostate, hypernephroma, and lymphoma (Minton, 1974; Tolis, 1975). In one patient with carcinoma of the prostate, pain relief was achieved despite radiographic evidence of tumor progression. Minton's study (1974) included a series of 30 patients with bony metastases from breast carcinoma who were treated with a two-day course of levadopa in 250- to 500-mg doses every four hours. Ten of 30 patients had dramatic pain relief. In nine of the ten patients prolactin levels were suppressed to 50% of normal. The dramatic pain relief may be related to prolactin suppression in patients with hormone-dependent metastatic breast tumors (Minton, 1974). Whether the analgesic effects of levodopa are mediated by peripheral mechanisms, by hormonal suppression, or by a central mechanism is unknown. This approach in cancer patients with pain is more experimental than therapeutic at this time.

Alternative Therapies for Cancer Pain

A series of pain management modalities are commonly used in combination with drug therapy. Each of these techniques requires specific expertise to be applied successfully. Although these procedures are widely used clinically, controlled studies of their effectiveness are lacking.

Nerve Block.   Nerve blocks, temporary and permanent, are rarely the sole approach to managing cancer pain syndromes. They are most useful in treating patients with areas of well-localized pain. The procedures can be divided into four major types: (1) myofascial trigger-point injections, (2) peripheral nerve blocks, (3) autonomic nerve blocks, and (4) intrathecal nerve blocks (Bonica, 1953; Brechner, 1977). Standard textbooks describe in detail the various techniques for each of these procedures, which are considered briefly here.

Trigger-Point Injections.   These are office procedures using either saline or a short-acting local anesthetic injected into the trigger point of pain, dramatically relieving muscle spasm pain.

Peripheral Nerve Blocks.   Peripheral nerve blocks are used both diagnostically to localize the nerve distribution of pain and therapeutically to interrupt pain transmission within a determined nerve distribution. Such blocks provide temporary pain relief, but the technique is limited to areas of the body where interruption of both motor and sensory function does not interfere with the patient's functional status. They are most useful in the acute management of pain in the distribution of the intercostal nerves.

Autonomic Nerve Blocks.   Autonomic nerve blocks to relieve pain associated with brachial plexus and lumbar plexus tumor infiltration are described, but quantitative assessment of their success rates is not available, except for celiac plexus blocks in treating patients with carcinoma of the pancreas. Convincing data suggest that bilateral alcohol injections of the celiac plexus are very effective in treating midabdominal pain associated with intra-abdominal tumors. Good results have been reported in 60 to 80% of patients treated (Brechner *et al.,* 1977).

Both short- and long-acting anesthetics are used for temporary peripheral nerve and autonomic block, whereas phenol and alcohol are the common chemical neurolytic agents for permanent blocks. Their use is controversial, and the role of permanent blocks in managing cancer pain is not fully established (Wood, 1978b). When permanent nerve blocks are used, patients must be informed that pain relief is associated with both motor and sensory dysfunction. In any patient undergoing chemical neurolysis peripherally or intrathecally, temporary blocks should be done first several times to determine the exact nerve distribution of the pain and to allow the patient to perceive the numbness that follows the procedure. In some instances, patients would rather tolerate the pain than the persistent numbness associated with blocks. In cases of intrathecal cauda equina blocks for perineal pain, myelography should be performed to rule out tumor infiltration producing an epidural block.

Transcutaneous Electrical Nerve Stimulation (TENS). TENS involves applying low- and high-intensity stimulation to peripheral nerves to activate selectively the large diameter fibers and "close the gate" to pain perception centrally. This technique is based on the gate theory of pain (Melzack and Wall, 1965) which called attention to the potential use of electrical stimulation to manage painful states. TENS is reported effective in 75 to 80% of patients with acute pain. TENS appears useful in managing neuropathic pain associated with tumor infiltration of the brachial plexus and postsurgical neuropathic pain (Ventafridda et al., 1979). TENS is a safe noninvasive method with minimal risk and side effects. The analgesia, however, if it occurs, is transient, and the effective use of TENS demands close patient supervision by trained personnel. The high cost of individual stimulators and its limited efficacy limit widespread use of this technique.

Acupuncture. Acupuncture in managing cancer pain has not been adequately tested. In a series of patients evaluated at MSKCC, 13 of 39 patients reported good or fair results with acupuncture, but the effects were transient. Experimental data suggest that acupuncture effects the endogenous mechanisms of pain since its analgesic effects can be partially reversed by naloxone administration (Mayer et al., 1977).

Hypnosis. Hypnosis in managing cancer pain has received increasing attention (Cangello, 1962; Sacerdote, 1970). Studies suggest its usefulness in reducing pain and anxiety as well as improving organ function. The clinical literature is based predominantly on case reports purporting that 50% of cancer patients can obtain some relief from hypnosis. Controlled clinical studies are lacking, but the anecdotal evidence is sufficient to suggest its usefulness as an adjunctive method of pain control. The analgesia produced by hypnosis is not reversed by naloxone, suggesting that its mechanism of action is different from those of acupuncture and TENS (Mayer et al., 1976).

Surgical Approaches to Cancer Pain

The neurosurgical approach to managing cancer pain includes two major categories of procedures. In neuroablative procedures surgical or radiofrequency lesions are made along pain pathways. In neurostimulatory procedures electrodes are stereotactically placed to activate pain inhibitory pathways. Both approaches are extensively reviewed (White and Sweet, 1969; Onofrio and Campa, 1972; Friedberg, 1975).

The use of neurosurgical procedures in the cancer patient represents a dilemma to both patients and physicians. Historically, neurosurgical procedures for cancer pain were performed late in the course of the patient's illness, often in debilitated patients. The development of overriding medical problems thwarted full evaluation of their effectiveness and duration of action. In contrast, patients with cancer and their physicians are often unwilling to consider neuroablative or neurostimulatory procedures and their concomitant risks before trying the primary modalities and analgesic regimen. Thus neurosurgical procedures are often a last resort, making evaluation of their effectiveness difficult at best. The appropriate patient and procedure must be selected according to the specific pain problem. Guidelines in using these procedures include an adequate prior trial of conventional methods for pain relief, i.e., radiation therapy, chemotherapy, and drug therapy, a thorough evaluation of the patient's medical and neurologic status to evaluate prognosis, and full patient awareness of the potential risks and benefits of the planned procedure.

At the current time, two surgical procedures have demonstrated value in managing patients with cancer and pain. The first is cordotomy which involves sectioning of the spinothalamic tract in the anterolateral spinal cord (Nathan, 1963). The second is hypophysectomy, either surgically by removal of the pituitary gland or chemically by injection of alcohol into the pituitary gland.

Cordotomy. Sectioning the spinothalamic track can be done in a variety of ways, but high cervical percutaneous cordotomy is the procedure of choice to relieve unilateral pain below the midthoracic region. In an awake and cooperative patient, a needle electrode is inserted into the cord at the C_{1-2} levels. Electrical stimulation before and clinical monitoring during the procedure allow adequate evaluation of the size of the lesion. Patients with midline or bilateral pain need bilateral cordotomy. It must be carried out at different levels to obviate respiratory difficulties, specifically phrenic nerve paralysis that may occur with high cervical lesions. For patients requiring bilateral cordotomy, high cervical percutaneous cardotomy is done on one side and open high thoracic cordotomy on the other. In patients with upper extremity pain, high cervical cordotomy is particularly effective. The advantage of a percutaneous cordotomy is that it avoids general anesthesia and a prolonged period of recuperation, while allowing careful monitoring of the effects of the lesion in an awake patient. Major complications include ipsilateral motor weakness in 10 to 20% of patients and disturbances in bowel and bladder function after bilateral cordotomy — usually transient but possibly permanent. Unfortunately, 7 to 10% of patients undergoing these procedures develop pain in a mirror site opposite the cordotomy. Even more distressing, a comparable number of patients develop pain previously unrecognized in another site which becomes as intractable as the pain for which the cordotomy was performed. This emphasizes the usefulness of the technique in patients with localized disease (Kanner et al., 1981a).

Hypophysectomy. Pituitary ablation was first introduced as part of the hormonal therapy for treating hormone-dependent tumors, specifically carcinoma of the breast and prostate (Luft and Olivecrona, 1957). Objective remission or lack of progression occurs in as many as 30 to 40% of patients after this procedure. Dramatic pain relief independent of marked antitumor effect has also been described following both surgical hypophysectomy (transsphenoidal route) (Tindall et al., 1977) and, more recently, chemical hypophysectomy (alcohol injection) in patients with diffuse pain from widespread bony metastases. Several authors have reported dramatic pain relief using alcohol injection directly into the sella turcica in patients with intractable pain and malignant disease (Moricca, 1974; Katz and Levin, 1977; Lipton et al., 1978). More patients received pain relief than actually achieved tumor regression with either surgical removal or alcohol injection of the pituitary gland. These findings suggest that the endo-

crine alterations following hypophysectomy are not directly responsible for the pain relief. To support this point, endocrine evaluation following transsphenoidal hypophysectomy in 15 patients with metastatic breast cancer revealed that only 1 of 15 showed evidence of total pituitary ablation, whereas, in all 15 patients bone pain diminished or disappeared within 24 hours of operation (LaRossa et al., 1978). Such data suggest that interruption of hormonal control does not mediate the analgesic effects. Chemical hypophysectomy does not appear technically superior to transsphenoidal hypophysectomy in relieving pain, and the incidence of diabetes insipidus, 10 to 20%, is the same for both procedures. Some authors criticize the use of hypophysectomy solely as a pain procedure, making its use controversial at best (Brodkey et al., 1978). Additional clinical studies should help clarify this controversy.

REFERENCES

Beaver, W. T.: Mild analgesics: A review of their clinical pharmacology. Am. J. Med. Sci., **251**:576–599, 1965.

Beaver, W. T.: Comparison of analgesic effects of morphine sulfate, hydroxyzine and their combination in patients with postoperative pain. In Bonica, J. J., and Ventafridda, V. (eds.): Advances in Pain Research and Therapy. Raven Press, New York, 1976.

Bockman, R. S., and Myers, W. P. L.: Osteotropism in human breast cancer. In Day, S. B.; Stansly, P.; Myers, W. P. L.; and Garattini, S. (eds.): Cancer Invasion and Metastases: Biologic Mechanisms and Therapy. Raven Press, New York, 1977.

Bond, M. R.: Psychologic and psychiatric techniques for relief of advanced cancer pain. In Bonica, J. J., and Ventafridda, V. (eds.): Advances in Pain Research and Therapy, Vol. 2. Raven Press, New York, 1979.

Bonica, J. J.: The Management of Pain. Lea & Febiger, Philadelphia, 1953.

Bonica, J. J.: Importance of the problem. In Bonica, J. J., and Ventafridda, V. (eds.): Advances in Pain Research and Therapy, Vol. 2. Raven Press, New York, 1979.

Brechner, V. L.; Ferrer-Brechner, T.; and Allen G. D.: Anesthetic measures in management of pain associated with malignancy. Semin. Oncol., **4**:99–108, 1977.

Breivik, H., and Rennemo, F.: Clinical evaluation of combined treatment with methadone and psychotropic drugs in cancer patients. Acta Anaesthesiol. Scand. [Suppl.], **74**:135–140, 1982.

Brodie, G. N.: Indomethacin and bone pain. Lancet, **1**:1160, 1974.

Brodkey, J. S.; Pearson, O. H.; and Manni, A.: Hypophysectomy for relief of bone pain in breast cancer. N. Engl. J. Med., **299**:1016, 1978.

Cangello, V. W.: Hypnosis for the patient with cancer. Am. J. Clin. Hypn., **4**:215–226, 1962.

Carlin, P. L.; Wall, P. D.; Nadvorna, H.; and Steinbach, T.: Phantom limbs and related phenomena in recent traumatic amputations. Neurology, **28**:211–217, 1978.

Cascino, T. L.; Kori, S.; Krol, G.; and Foley, K. M.: CT

scanning of the brachial plexus in patients with cancer. *Neurology,* **33:**1553–1557, 1983.

Cooper, P. R.; Milgram, J. W.; and Robinson, R. A.: Morphology of the osteum. *J. Bone Joint Surg.,* **48:**1239–1271, 1966.

Daut, R. L., and Cleeland, C. S.: The prevalence and severity of pain in cancer. *Cancer,* **50:**1913–1918, 1982.

Dixon, R.; Crews, T.; Mohacsi, C.; Inturrisi, C. E.; and Foley, K. M.: Levorphanol: Radioimmunoassay and plasma concentration profiles in dog and man. *Res. Commun. Chem. Pathol. Pharmacol.,* **29:**535–548, 1980.

Ettinger, D. S.; Vitale, P. J.; and Trump, D. C.: Important clinical pharmacologic considerations in the use of methadone in cancer patients. *Cancer Treat. Rep.,* **63:**457–459, 1979.

Ferreira, S.: Site of analgesic action of aspirin-like drugs and opioids. In Beers, R. F., and Basset, E. G. (eds.): *Mechanisms of Pain and Analgesic Compounds.* Raven Press, New York, 1979.

Ferreira, S. H.; Nakamura, M.; and Castro, M. S. A.: The hyperalgesic effects of prostacyclin and prostaglandin E_2. *Prostaglandins,* **16:**31–37, 1978.

Foley, K. M.: Pain syndromes in patients with cancer. In Bonica, J. J., and Ventafridda, V. (eds.): *Advances in Pain Research and Therapy,* Vol. 2. Raven Press, New York, 1979a.

Foley, K. M.: The management of pain of malignant origin. In Tyler, H. R., and Dawson, D. M. (eds.): *Current Neurology,* Vol. 2. Houghton Mifflin Company, Boston, 1979b.

Foley, K. M.: Current controversies in the management of cancer pain. *Natl. Inst. Drug Abuse Res. Monogr. Ser.,* **36:**169–181, 1981.

Foley, K. M.: Clinical assessment of pain. *Acta Anaesthesiol. Scand. [Suppl.],* **74:**91–96, 1982a.

Foley, K. M.: The practical use of narcotic analgesics. In Reidenberg, M. M. (ed.): *Med. Clin. North Am.,* **66:**1091–1104, 1982b.

Foley, K. M.: The treatment of cancer pain. *N. Engl. J. Med.,* **313**(2), 1985.

Foley, K. M.; Woodruff, J.; Ellis, F.; and Posner, J. B.: Radiation-induced malignant and atypical schwannomas. *Ann. Neurol,* **7:**311–318, 1979c.

Fordyce, W. E.; Fowles, R. S.; Lehmann, J.; *et al.*: Operant conditioning in the treatment of chronic pain. *Arch. Phys. Med. Rehabil.,* **54:**399–408, 1973.

Forrest, W. H.; Brown, B. W.; Brown, C. R.; DeFalque, R.; Gold, M.; Gordon, H. E.; James, K. E.; Katz, J.; Mahler, D. L.; Schroff, P.; and Teutsch, G.: Dextroamphetamine with morphine for the treatment of postoperative pain. *N. Engl. J. Med.,* **296:**712–715, 1977.

Friedberg, S.: Neurosurgical treatment of pain caused by cancer. *Med. Clin. North Am.,* **59:**481–485, 1975.

Galasko, C. S. B.: Mechanisms of bone destruction in the development of skeletal metastases. *Nature,* **263:**507–510, 1976.

Gerbershagen, H. U.: Non-narcotic analgesics. In Bonica, J. J., and Ventafridda, V. (eds.): *Advances in Pain Research and Therapy,* Vol. 2. Raven Press, New York, 1979.

Gilbert, R. W.; Kim, J.-H.; and Posner, J. B.: Epidural spinal cord compression from metastatic tumor: Diagnosis and treatment. *Ann. Neurol.,* **3:**40–51, 1978.

Gordon, R. A., and Campbell, M.: The use of chlorpromazine in intractable pain associated with terminal carcinoma. *Can. Med. Assoc. J.,* **75:**420–424, 1956.

Granek, I.; Ashikari, R.; and Foley, K. M.: Postmastectomy pain syndrome: Clinical and anatomical correlates. *Proc. A.S.C.O.,* **3:**122, 1983.

Greenberg, J. S.; Deck, M. D. F.; Vikram, B.; Chu, F. C. H.; and Posner, J. B.: Metastasis to the base of the skull: Clinical findings in 43 patients. *Neurology,* **31:**530–537, 1981.

Greenberg, J. S.; Kim, J. H.; and Posner, J. B.: Epidural spinal cord compression from metastatic tumor: Results with a new treatment protocol. *Ann. Neurol.,* **8:**361–366, 1980.

Halpern, L. W.: Psychotropics, ataractics and related drugs. In Bonica, J. J., and Ventafridda, V. (eds.): *Advances in Pain Research ad Therapy,* Vol. 2. Raven Press, New York, 1979.

Harris, L. S.: Cannabioids as analgesics. In Beers, R. F., and Basset, E. G. (eds.): *Mechanisms of Pain and Analgesic Compounds.* Raven Press, New York, 1979.

Horton, J. E.; Raisz, L. G.; Simmons, H. A.; Oppenheim, J. J.; and Mergenhagen, S. E.: Bone resorbing activity on supernatant fluid from cultured human peripheral blood leukocytes. *Science,* **177:**793–795, 1972.

Houde, R. W.: Systemic analgesics and related drugs: Narcotic analgesics. In Bonica, J. J., and Ventafridda, V. (eds.): *Advances in Pain Research and Therapy,* Vol. 2. Raven Press, New York, 1979.

Houde, R. W., and Wallenstein, S. L.: Analgesic power of chlorpromazine alone and in combination with morphine. *Fed. Proc.,* **14:**353, 1955 (Abstr.).

Ihde, D. C., and DeVita, V. T.: Osteonecrosis of the femoral head in patients with lymphoma treated with intermittent combination chemotherapy (including corticosteroids). *Cancer,* **36:**1585–1588, 1975.

Inturrisi, C. E.: Narcotic drugs. In Reidenberg, M. M. (ed.): *Med. Clin. North Am.,* **66:**1061–1071, 1982.

Inturrisi, C. E.; Foley, K. M.; Kaiko, R. F.; and Houde, R. W.: Disposition and effects of intravenous (IV) methadone (MET) in cancer patients. *Proceedings of the Third World Congress on Pain of the International Association for the Study of Pain.* Edinburgh, Scotland, Suppl. 1, 1981.

Jaeckle, K. A.; Young, D. F.; and Foley, K. M.: The natural history of lumbosacral plexopathy in cancer. *Neurology,* **35:**8–15, 1985.

Jellinger, K., and Sturm, K. W.: Delayed radiation myelopathy in man. *J. Neurol. Sci.,* **14:**389–408, 1971.

Kanner, R. M., and Foley, K. M.: Patterns of narcotic drug use in a cancer pain clinic. *Ann. N.Y. Acad. Sci.,* **362:**161–172, 1981b.

Kanner, R. M.; Foley, K. M.; and Galicich, J.: Patient selection for cordotomy in patients with cancer. *Neurology,* **31:**45, 1981a.

Kanner, R. M.; Martini, N.; and Foley, K. M.: Nature and incidence of post-thoracotomy pain. *Proc. A.S.C.O.,* **1:**152, 1982a.

Kanner, R. M.; Martini, N.; and Foley, K. M.: Incidence of pain and other clinical manifestations of superior pulmonary sulcus tumor (Pancoast's tumors). In Bonica, J. J., and Ventafridda, V. (eds.): *Advances in Pain Research and Therapy,* Vol. 4. Raven Press, New York, 1982b.

Katz, J., and Levin, A. B.: Treatment of diffuse metastatic cancer pain by instillation of alcohol into the sella turcica. *Anesthesiology,* **46:**115–121, 1977.

Kellgren, J. G.: On the distribution of pain arising from deep somatic structures with charts of segmental pain areas. *Clin. Sci,* **435:**303–323, 1939.

Kelly, R. J.; Cowan, R. J.; Ferree, C. B.; Raben, M.; and Maynard, D.: Efficacy of radionuclide scanning in patients with lung cancer. *J.A.M.A.*, **242**:2855–2857, 1979.

Kori, S. H.; Foley, K. M.; and Posner, J. B.: Brachial plexus lesions in patients with cancer: Clinical findings in 100 cases. *Neurology*, **31**:45–50, 1981a.

Kori, S. H.; Krol, G.; and Foley, K. M.: Computed tomographic evaluation of bone and soft tissue metastases. In Weiss, L., and Gilbert, H. A. (eds.): *Bone Metastases, Metastases Monograph Series*, Vol. 3, G. K. Hall & Company, Boston, 1981b.

LaRossa, J. T.; Strong, S.; and Melby, J. C.: Endocrinologically incomplete transethnoidal transsphenoidal hypophysectomy with relief of bone pain in breast cancer. *N. Engl. J. Med.*, **298**:1332–1335, 1978.

Lasagna, L., and Dekornfeld, T. J.: Methotrimeprazine, a new phenothiazine derivative with analgesic properties. *J.A.M.A.*, **178**:119–122, 1961.

Lipman, A.: Drug therapy in terminally ill patients. *Am. J. Hosp. Pharm.*, **32**:270–276, 1975.

Lipton, S.; Miles, J. B.; Williams, N.; and Bark-Jones, N.: Pituitary alcohol injection for the relief of pain. *Pain*, **5**:73–82, 1978.

Luft, R., and Olivecrona, H.: Hypophysectomy in the treatment of malignant tumors. *Cancer*, **10**:789–794, 1957.

Marks, R. M., and Sachar, E. J.: Undertreatment of medical inpatients with narcotic analgesics. *Ann. Intern. Med.*, **78**:173–181, 1973.

Max, M. B.; Inturrisi, C. E.; Grabinski, P.; Kaiko, R. F.; and Foley, K. M.: Epidural opiates: Plasma and cerebrospinal fluid (CSF) pharmacokinetics of morphine, methadone, and beta-endorphin. *Neurology*, **31**:95, 1981.

Mayer, D. J., and Price, D. D.: Central nervous system mechanisms of analgesia. *Pain*, **2**:379–404, 1976.

Mayer, D. J.; Price, D. D.; and Rafu, A.: Antagonism of acupuncture analgesia in man by the narcotic antagonist naloxone. *Brain Res.*, **121**:368–372, 1977.

Melzack, R., and Wall, P. D.: Pain mechanisms: A new theory. *Science*, **150**:971–974, 1965.

Minton, J. P.: The response of breast cancer patients with bone pain to L-dopa. *Cancer*, **33**:358–363, 1974.

Moricca, G.: Chemical hypophysectomy for cancer pain. In Bonica, J. J. (ed.): *Advances in Neurology*, Vol. 4. Raven Press, New York, 1974.

Nathan, P. W.: Results of antero-lateral cordotomy for pain in cancer. *J. Neurol. Neurosurg. Psychiatry*, **26**:353–362, 1963.

Olson, M. E.; Chernik, N. L.; and Posner, J. B.: Infiltration of the leptomeninges by systemic cancer: A clinical and pathological study. *Arch. Neurol.*, **30**:122–137, 1978.

Onofrio, B. M., and Campa, H. K.: Evaluation of rhizotomy. Review of 12 years' experience. *J. Neurosurg.*, **36**:751–755, 1972.

Pasternak, S.: Personality traits and cognitive style in chronic pain patients. Doctoral dissertation. Columbia University Graduate School of Arts and Sciences, New York, 1980.

Pistenma, D. A.; McDougall, I. R.; and Kress, J. P.: Screening for bone metastases: Are only scans necessary? *J.A.M.A.*, **231**:46–50, 1975.

Price, R. W.: Herpes zoster: An approach to systemic therapy. In Reidenberg, M. M. (ed.): *Med. Clin. North Am.*, **66**:1105–1118, 1982.

Rodichok, L. D.; Harper, G. R.; Ruckdeschel, J. C.; Price, A.; Roberson, G.; Barron, K. D.; Horton, J.: Early diagnosis of spinal epidural metastases. *Am. J. Med.*, **70**:1181–1188, 1981.

Rotstein, J., and Good, R. A.: Steroid pseudorheumatism. *Arch. Intern. Med.*, **99**:545–555, 1957.

Sacerdote, P.: Theory and practice of pain control in malignancy and other protracted or recurring painful illnesses. *Int. J. Clin. Exp. Hypn.*, **18**:160–180, 1970.

Sadove, M. S.; Levin, M. J.; Rose, R. F.; Schwartz, L.; and Witt, F. W.: Chlorpromazine and narcotics in the management of pain of malignant lesions. *J.A.M.A.*, **155**:625–629, 1954.

Sawe, J.; Hansen, J.; Ginman, C.; Hartvig, P.; Jakobsson, P. A.; Milsson, M.-I.; Rane, A.; and Anggard, E.: Patient-controlled dose regimen of methadone for chronic cancer pain. *Br. Med. J.*, **282**:771–773, 1981.

Schell, H. W.: The risk of adrenal corticosteroid therapy in far advanced cancer. *Am. J. Med. Sci.*, **252**:641–644, 1966.

Schell, H. W.: Adrenal corticosteroid therapy in far advanced cancer. *Geriatrics*, **27**:131–141, 1972.

Shimm, D. S.; Logue, G. L.; Maltbie, A. A.; and Dugan, S.: Medical management of chronic cancer pain. *J.A.M.A.*, **241**:2408–2412, 1979.

Snow, H: The opium–cocaine treatment of malignant disease. *Br. Med. J.*, **1**:1019–1020, 1897.

Stoll, B. A.: Indomethacin in breast cancer. *Lancet*, **2**:384, 1973.

Stoll, B. A., and Andrews, J. T.: Radiation-induced peripheral neuropathy. *Br. Med. J.*, **1**:834–837, 1966.

Sundaresan, N.; Galicich, J. H.; Lane, J.: Treatment of odontoid fractures in cancer patients. *J. Neurosurg.*, **54**:468–472, 1981.

Taub, A.: Relief of post-herpetic neuralgia with psychotropic drugs. *J. Neurosurg.*, **39**:235–241, 1973.

Thomas, J. E.; Cascino, T. E.; and Earle, J. D.: Differential diagnosis between radiation and tumor plexopathy of the pelvis. *Neurology*, **35**:1–7, 1985.

Thrupkaew, A.; Henken, R.; and Quinl, J. L.: False negative bone scans in disseminated metastatic diseases. *Radiology*, **113**:383–386, 1975.

Tindall, G. T.; Nixon, D. W.; Christy, J. H.; and Neill, J. D.: Pain relief in metastatic cancer other than breast and prostate gland following transsphenoidal hypophysectomy. *J. Neurosurg.*, **47**:659–662, 1977.

Tolis, G. J.: L-dopa for pain from bone metastases. *N. Engl. J. Med.*, **292**:1353–1354, 1975.

Twycross, R. G.: Value of cocaine in opiate containing elixers. *Br. Med. J.*, **2**:1348, 1977.

Twycross, R. G.: Pain in far advanced cancer. *Pain*, **14**:303–310, 1982.

Twycross, R. G., and Ventafridda, V. G. (eds.): *The Continuing Care of Terminal Cancer Patients.* Pergamon Press, Inc., Oxford, 1980.

Ventafridda, V.; Sganzerla, E. P.; Fochi, C.; Pozzi, G.; and Cordini, G.: Transcutaneous nerve stimulation in cancer pain. In Bonica, J. J. (ed.): *Advances in Cancer Pain.* Raven Press, New York, 1979.

Watson, C. P.; Evans, R. J.; Reid, K.; Merskey, H.; Goldsmith, L.; and Warsh, J.: Amitriptyline vs. placebo in postherpetic neuralgia. *Neurology*, **32**:671–673, 1982.

White, J. C., and Sweet, W. H.: *Pain and the Neurosurgeon.* Charles C Thomas, Publisher, Springfield, Illinois, 1969.

Wood, K. M.: Intercostobrachial nerve entrapment syndrome. *South Med. J.*, **76**:662–663, 1978a.

Wood, K. M.: The use of phenol as a neurolytic agent: A review. *Pain*, **5**:205–229, 1978b.

45

Nutritional Factors in Cancer

GEORGE L. BLACKBURN, MARIJEAN M. MILLER, and
ALBERT BOTHE, JR.

Nutritional status is a major factor in the clinical course and outcome of the patient with cancer. Loss of appetite and anorexia can deplete the patient's strength independent of the effects of medical care. Nutritional depletion may interfere with oncologic therapy and prolong the morbidity of therapeutic complications. Although malnutrition is generally accepted as prevalent in patients with cancer, a great deal of controversy surrounds the formulation of guidelines for nutritional support.

In providing nutritional support for the patient with cancer common questions are:

1. How does nutritional support benefit the patient with cancer?
2. What are the risks of nutritional support, especially in relation to tumor growth?
3. What guidelines exist for administering nutritional support in the patient with cancer?

These questions are the major points of discussion among nutritionists and oncologists investigating the utility of nutritional support in the patient with cancer. Tentative answers are presented in this chapter.

Nutritional support can often improve the quality of life of the patient receiving cancer therapy. Improved nutritional status, immune response, and response to oncologic therapy are observed in patients with cancer receiving nutritional support as an adjunct to oncologic therapy. Little evidence currently suggests, however, that nutritional support has a role in treating patients who can no longer benefit from oncologic therapy.

Risk of disproportionately stimulating cancer growth through nutritional support is minimal when properly selected patients receive the therapy. Animal studies report both increases in tumor growth and no tumor growth when tumor-bearing rats received nutritional support (Cameron and Paviat, 1976; Daly et al., 1978) . Until recently, developing human nutritional support guidelines, or even clinical investigative protocols, based on these animal studies has been difficult since their shortcomings have often been as obvious as a failure to interpret tumor weight in proportion to host body weight.

The most extensive clinical work on nutritional support in patients with cancer is that of Copeland (Copeland, et al., 1979). In clinical experience with over 1500 patients with cancer he observed no increase in tumor growth that could be attributed to nutritional support. Future controlled trial studies are necessary to elucidate the most beneficial means of administering nutritional support. The questions to be answered include: does cancer type affect the magnitude of a malnourished patient's response to nutritional support, and when during a course radiotherapy or chemotherapy should nutritional support be administered for maximum benefit? These questions have only vague answers at this time.

Nutritional support is of proven benefit to selected patients with cancer, however, and is associated clinically with few risks when administered according to the guidelines below.

1. In patients with cancer unable to benefit from oncologic therapy, intensive nutri-

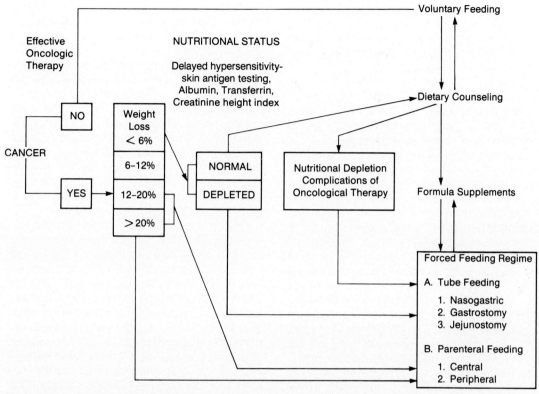

Figure 45 – 1.   Decision tree for nutritional support in the cancer patient. From Blackburn, G. L., DiScala, C.; Miller, M. M.; Champagne, C; Lahey, M.; Bothe, A., Jr.; and Bistrian, B. R.: Preliminary report on collaborative study for home parenteral nutrition patients. Second Bermuda Symposium on Clinical Nutrition, 1982.

tional support (*e.g.,* hyperalimentation) is *not* indicated.

2. In patients with mild to moderate nutritional deficits (*i.e.,* weight loss, very low serum proteins), supportive feeding is indicated. When possible, nutritional support may be provided in the form of oral supplementation. When required, enteral or parenteral support or both may be administered. Figure 45 – 1 is a therapeutic decision tree for nutritional support in the patient with cancer.

SUPPORTING EVIDENCE

Malnutrition

Malnutrition in the patient with cancer is common and is associated with varying stages of most cancers and with the treatment modalities. Studies of the nutritional status of hospitalized medical and surgical patients have found that patients with cancer are in the group with the highest prevalence of malnutri-

tion (Hill *et al.,* 1975; Bistrian *et al.,* 1976). In fact, protein malnutrition is the most common secondary diagnosis in patients with cancer (Harvey *et al.,* 1979). A few cancer types are associated with specific nutritional deficits (Copeland *et al.,* 1977; Shils, 1977b), but generally, where both the tumor/host interaction and the treatment affect nutritional status, the exact etiology of malnutrition is difficult to determine. Changes in body composition (Warnold *et al.,* 1978), anthropometric indices (Mullen *et al.,* 1980), creatinine-height ratios (Nixon *et al.,* 1980), and immune competence (Copeland *et al.,* 1977; Harvey *et al.,* 1979) are all documented in patients with cancer.

Cachexia

Cachexia in the patient with cancer is characterized by weakness, loss of appetite, depleted or altered host body compartments, hormonal aberrations, and, in the terminal stage, progressive loss of vital function. In most cases, cachexia is best understood as the net result of various metabolic stresses. Anorexia, specific tumor effects, and nutritional injury during cancer therapy may all contribute to the onset of cancer cachexia (see Figure 45–2).

Anorexia.   Anorexia accompanies most neoplasms and is a major contributing factor in the development of the cachexic state. Often, loss of appetite is an important initial symptom of an underlying neoplasm.

In a comprehensive analysis of the multiple variables involved in the pathophysiology of anorexia in patients with cancer (DeWys, 1974), a clinical picture of "loss of appetite" is suggested as the net result of tumor, host, and treatment variables. Obstruction, change in taste perception, depression, or an acquired food aversion caused by a tumor often leads to reduced appetite, as discussed in more detail later. Anorexia, however, is only one of the factors contributing to the development of cachexia since some patients have reported weight loss without loss of appetite (Brennan, 1977; Pollard and the Pancreatic Cancer Task Force, 1981) (see Figure 45–2). Specific tumor effects and nutritional injury during oncologic therapy also contribute to the onset of cachexia.

Taste Abnormalities.   Taste abnormalities are reported in some patients with cancer. Previously enjoyed foods become unappealing when they take on distorted flavors, often strongly bitter or sour. For example, a chocolate candy bar may taste like Baker's chocolate. As a result, patients avoid many foods, leading to reduced intake and an unbalanced diet.

The causes of taste abnormalities are unknown, although they are attributed to the disease process and injury during oncologic therapy. Learned food aversions during oncologic treatment may also cause a patient to avoid some foods (Berstein, 1978). In children, an aversion may develop to a food eaten prior to gastrointestinal toxic chemotherapy.

Objective tests of taste perception in patients with cancer show patients have varied taste perceptions. A reduced threshold for sucrose and urea is associated with reduced caloric intake (DeWys, 1974; DeWys and Walters, 1975; DeWys, 1977). DeWys correlated this reduced oral threshold for urea with an aversion for red meat, which is high in urea content. In contrast, Settle *et al.,* (1979) reported higher taste recognition thresholds in patients with cancer. Patients with lung cancer may have reduced thresholds for sour tastes (Williams and Cohen, 1978). Although differences between patients with cancer and controls

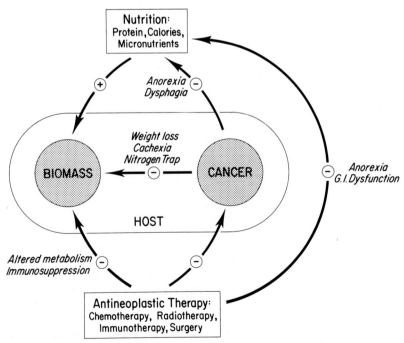

Figure 45–2.   The malnutrition prevalent in cancer patients is of multiple etiology. From Blackburn, G. L., and Bothe, A. F.: Assessment of malnutrition in cancer patients. *Cancer Bull.,* **30:**88–93, 1978.

were not significant for bitter, sweet, or salt tastes, patients with cancer showed more variation in taste sensitivity than controls. Thus some patients may have heightened taste perception, whereas others have a diminished taste sense.

Williams suggests patients keep individual dietary histories to identify food aversions. Foods can then be modified to ensure that nutritional requirements are met. The Yale Comprehensive Cancer Care Center has published a helpful book for patients with cancer offering tips and recipes to make nutritious foods more palatable (Morra *et al.*, 1982).

Depression. Depression and associated reduced physical activity often result in appetite decrease. Reduced activity results in reduced caloric requirements. With less caloric intake, the patient is likely to take part in fewer activities, thus a cycle begins with a net result of weight loss caused by inadequate intake (Young, 1977).

Patients' depression related to the cancer disease process can be relieved and treated. Chapter 50 discusses approaches for dealing with depression in patients with cancer.

Tumor Effects. Specific tumor effects may induce shifts in host metabolism that also contribute to the onset of cancer cachexia. Host protein anabolism and energy metabolism have been found to be less efficient in patients with cancer. Tumor effects on host metabolism may be great in patients who lose substantial weight in the absence of anorexia. For ex-

ample, the Pancreatic Cancer Task Force reported 80% of 924 patients with pancreatic cancer had weight loss prior to diagnosis (Pollard and the Pancreatic Cancer Task Force, 1981). Fifty percent of the patients with pancreatic cancer studied had experienced weight loss for longer than two months prior to diagnosis, whereas only 26% of these patients reported anorexia during this period. Thus no anorexia was reported in half of the patients with pancreatic cancer with long-term weight loss. Numerous theories attempt to account for the weight loss which is so common in malignant disease.

Protein Metabolism. Protein metabolism is central to the normal functioning of major organs and the host immune response. Several possible means by which the growing neoplasm may affect the etiology of protein-calorie malnutrition (marasmus) have been investigated. A tumor may cause several alterations in protein and energy metabolism which are summarized in Table 45–1.

Many studies support the hypothesis that tumors can alter host protein homeostasis and induce a net loss of host tissue. Additional studies reveal 30 to 100% of patients with cancer are in negative nitrogen balance (Watkin, 1961), although other investigations show equivocal nitrogen balance in cancer patients (Müller, *et al.*, 1982). Lundholm *et al.* (1978a) demonstrated a net efflux of amino acids from skeletal muscle in patients with cancer. Some authors suggest that tumors cause peripheral tissue wasting in hypocaloric states similar to that seen in states of stress or injury and hypothesize that this is an extension of the normally adaptive response of fat and skeletal protein mobilization while sparing visceral protein (Munro, 1964).

Animal studies conducted in our Nutrition/ Metabolism Laboratory suggest that growing neoplasms inappropriately alter the metabolism of host protein. Protein synthetic rates were significantly reduced in the skeletal muscle of tumor-bearing animals, while rates of whole-body protein degradation were elevated. In contrast to rat tissue, fractional rates of tumor protein breakdown were decreased suggesting that, relative to lean body mass, the tumor did "trap" nitrogen (Kawamura *et al.*, 1982). Without nutritional support, host protein became depleted.

Changes in body glucose metabolism have also been reported in patients with cancer. An attenuated response in blood glucose to insulin

Table 45–1. Tumor-Induced Alterations in Protein and Energy Metabolism

Reduced protein synthesis	Blackburn *et al*, 1977
Altered carbohydrate tolerance leading to a diabetic-like state	Schein *et al*, 1975
Specific anorectic effect	DeWys, 1977
Mechanical intestinal obstruction	Shils, 1977b
Less efficient utilization of energy and nitrogen in the host	Warnold *et al*, 1978
Reduced ability to adapt to the starved state resulting in an inability to conserve vital body mass	Brennan, 1977; Burt *et al*, 1980; Norton *et al*, 1980
Increase in whole-body glucose recycling	Waterhouse, 1974
Increase in gluconeogenesis from alanine	Waterhouse *et al*, 1979
Insulin resistance	Lundholm *et al*, 1978b
Increased turnover of glucose	Lundholm *et al*, 1978a

challenge in patients with cancer has been observed compared to controls (Lundholm *et al.,* 1978b). Results suggest insulin resistance in the liver and skeletal muscles in patients with cancer. An increase in whole-body glucose-recycling rate in patients with cancer through pyruvate and lactate was reported (Waterhouse, 1974). More recently, gluconeogenesis from alanine was found to increase in patients with advanced cancer (Waterhouse *et al.,* 1979). Gluconeogenesis suppression with small amounts of glucose was still possible in these patients with cancer, however, similar to controls. The importance of gluconeogenesis and Cori cycle activity in the increased energy expenditure in patients with cancer is unknown since neither appears to contribute to daily energy expenditures (Holroyde *et al.,* 1975; Young, 1977).

Radiation Injury. Several forms of radiation injury threaten the nutritional status of the patient with cancer. Factors influencing the severity of nutritional injury include the site of radiation, dose, and duration of therapy. Nutritional injury is associated with both the acute and late effects of radiation therapy. Table 45–2 summarizes the nutritional complications commonly experienced. The effects of radiation therapy on nutritional status have been discussed thoroughly (Donaldson, 1977, 1981; Donaldson and Lenon, 1979).

Table 45–2. Localized Effects of Radiation Therapy on Patients' Nutritional Status

REGION	ACUTE	CHRONIC
Oral cavity and pharynx	Sore throat	Ulcer
	Dysphagia	Xerostomia
	Xerostomia	Dental caries
	Mucositis	Osteoradionecrosis
	Anorexia	Trismus
	Alteration in smell	Altered taste
	Loss of taste	
Esophagus	Dysphagia	Fibrosis
		Stenosis
		Fistula
Stomach, small and large intestine	Anorexia	Ulcer
	Nausea	Malabsorption
	Vomiting	Diarrhea
	Diarrhea	Chronic enteritis
	Acute enteritis	Chronic colitis
	Acute colitis	
Liver and pancreas	Anorexia	Ascites
	Nausea	Jaundice
	Vomiting	

Reprinted by permission from Donaldson, S. S.: Nutrition problems associated with radiation therapy. In Newell, G. R., and Ellison, N. M. (eds.): *Nutrition and Cancer: Etiology and Treatment.* Raven Press, New York, 1981.

Loss of taste seriously affects patients receiving radiation of the oral cavity and pharynx. Patients experience both heightened and suppressed taste sensations. Loss of taste is exponential and rapid after oral pharyngeal irradiation as measured by quantitative tests of taste sensitivity to quinine, sucrose, and hydrochloric acid (Longer, 1973). Preirradiation taste sensitivity is often regained 60 to 120 days after therapy is completed. Based on this study, dietary intake should be monitored for the duration of radiation therapy and for four to six months following the treatment period to ensure balanced dietary intake.

In animal studies, the olfactory system, in particular the peripheral olfactory apparatus, appears sensitive to irradiation (Cooper, 1968). The human olfactory response to radiation has received little study.

Salivation may decrease as a result of irradiation to the head and neck, leading to altered eating habits. Patients may also experience increased sensitivity of their teeth to extremes in temperature and sweets. In a study of weight change during a six- to eight-week course of external beam therapy to the head and neck regions, 93% of 114 patients lost weight. The average loss was 3.7 kg. Approximately 9% lost more than 10% of their body weight between initiation and completion of their courses of radiotherapy (Donaldson, 1981).

Radiation to the stomach and small and large intestine is associated with various complications that affect patients' nutritional status. Low-dose gastric irradiation reduces gastric acidity, whereas high doses can induce ulcer formation. Radiation to the small and large bowel commonly produce nausea, vomiting, and diarrhea. At any time following high-dose gastrointestinal irradiation, patients may develop radiation-induced enteritis in the form of chronic diarrhea or bowel obstruction.

Upper abdominal radiation to the liver can produce temporary "radiation hepatitis," characterized by anorexia, nausea and vomiting, and abdominal distention. Radiation to the pancreas similarly may result acutely in anorexia, nausea, and vomiting.

Chemotherapy. Chemotherapy affects host tissue as well as the targeted neoplasms, thus can affect the nutritional status of the host. Table 45–3 summarizes several of the most common chemotherapy drugs affecting dietary intake.

Practically every major class of compounds used in chemotherapy and immunotherapy produces nausea and vomiting (Ohnuma and Holland, 1977), accompanied by anorexia. Patients often have reduced dietary intake, electrolyte imbalance, weakness, and progressive weight loss.

Antiemetic therapy in some cases reduces or completely alleviates nausea and vomiting. Recent double-blind studies of delta-9-tetrahydrocannabinal (THC), the major ingredient of marijuana, showed that THC frequently produced complete or partial alleviation of nausea and vomiting (Dow and Meyers, 1981). In addition, the antiemetic activity of THC is correlated with increasing THC plasma concentrations. Other antiemetic agents are chlorpromazine, prochlorperazine, thiethylperazine, droperidol, and haloperidol. These agents have sedative and extrapyramidal side effects, however, that do not correlate with drug antiemetic activity. See Mitchell and Schein (1982) for a more extensive discussion of the present antiemetic therapies.

Some chemotherapeutic agents commonly produce mucosal toxicities including oral ulceration, cheilosis, glossitis, and pharyngitis. Actinomycin D, cytarabine, 5-fluorouracil, hydroxyurea, and methotrexate all can produce ulceration. Although chemotherapy can diminish the nutritional status of the patient, thereby aggravating the effect of tumor-related malabsorption syndromes, chemotherapy treatment may not induce malabsorption (Mitchell and Schein, 1982). No changes in small intestine absorptive function with either a single-agent or combination chemotherapy were observed.

In cases where chemotherapy results in prolonged and uncontrolled diarrhea, dehydration, electrolyte imbalance, inanition, and accelerated malnutrition occur. Supportive nutritional care is indicated to maintain host tissue.

Chemotherapeutic agents affect major organ systems and may result in decreased efficiency of metabolism. The liver is especially vulnerable. Hepatic injury is commonly associated with anorexia. Hypoalbuminemia follows diffuse hepatocellular damage. Renal dysfunction may occur with agents such as hydroxyurea. Cardiac toxicity may present as congestive heart failure with water retention and electrolyte imbalance. Ohnuma and Holland (1977) and more recently Carter (1981) provide comprehensive discussions of the nutritional consequences of chemotherapy and immunotherapy.

Surgical Injury. Surgical injury also causes the nutritional depletion so often found in patients with cancer. For the general surgical population, nutritional support is clearly a powerful tool. A patient with good nutritional status has fewer postoperative complications. If nutritional assessment reveals malnutrition, elective surgery should be delayed until nutritional status improves (Blackburn and Harvey, 1981). The patient with cancer requiring surgery often suffers the nutritional consequences of the disease state as well as depletion associated with chemotherapy, immunotherapy, or radiation therapy. These patients should receive nutritional assessment prior to surgery and nutritional support when necessary.

Several surgical procedures result in conditions requiring nutritional intervention. Radical resection of the oropharyngeal area often necessitates tube feeding. Conditions associated with esophagectomy and esophageal reconstruction may include gastric stasis secondary to vagotomy, malabsorption, and the development of fistula or stenosis. Gastric surgery may result in a dumping syndrome, malabsorption, or hypoglycemia.

Intestinal resection can result in a variety of nutritional complications depending on the site and extent of resection. Resection of the jejunum may decrease efficiency of absorption of many nutrients. Resection of the ileum commonly results in vitamin B_{12} deficiency and bile salt losses. With massive bowel resection, malabsorption leading to malnutrition is common as reported in jejunoileal bypass for morbid obesity (Bray, 1976). Abnormalities of salt and water balance are commonly associated with ileostomy and colostomy. Bypass procedures can also result in a blind loop syndrome with specific nutritional deficiencies that can only be diagnosed through nutritional assessment.

Patients with pancreatic cancer should receive nutritional assessment, since prior to surgery they are often jaundiced and have lost weight. For those undergoing pancreatectomy, malabsorption, endocrine, and exocrine insufficiency are common postsurgical problems.

Patients with cancer undergoing ureterosigmoidostomy may experience hyperchloremic acidosis and potassium depletion in addition to common postoperative problems.

Both the disease process and the treatment will challenge the nutritional status of the patient with cancer. For these reasons, periodic

Table 45–3. Agents Affecting Dietary Intake

	CATEGORY OF DRUG	TOXICITY					OTHER EFFECTS
		STOMATITIS	ANOREXIA	VOMITING	NAUSEA	DIARRHEA	
Chemotherapeutic agents							
Bleomycin	Antibiotic	x	x	x	x		Fever, pulmonary toxicity
Cyclophosphamide	Alkylating agent		x	x	x		Hemorrhagic cystitis
Cytarabine	Antimetabolite		x	x	x	x	Oral inflammation and/or ulcerations, abdominal pain
Cisplatin	DNA intercolating agent			x	x	x	Thrombocytopenia
Dactinomycin	Antibiotic	x	x	x	x	x	Oral ulcerations
Doxorubicin	Antibiotic	x	x	x	x	x	Cardiac toxicity, red urine
5-Fluorouracil	Antimetabolite	x	x	x	x	x	Oral ulcerations
Hydroxyurea	Antimetabolite	x	x	x	x	x	Constipation, ulceration of buccal mucosa, renal dysfunction
Melphalan	Alkylating agent			x	x		
6-Mercaptopurine	Antimetabolite	x	x	x	x		Fever, liver dysfunction
Methotrexate	Antimetabolite	x	x	x	x	x	Hepatic toxicity, oral ulcerations, gingivitis

Drug	Classification							Side effects
Nitrogen mustard (mechlorethamine)	Alkylating agent	x	x			x		Metallic taste in mouth following injection, headache, fever
Nitrosoureas (CCNU), (methyl CCNU)			x		x			Prolonged anorexia
Vinblastine	Vinca alkaloid	x	x		x		x	Constipation, abdominal pain, glossitis, numbness in extremities
Vincristine	Vinca alkaloid		x		x			Constipation, abdominal pain, numbness in extremities
Immunotherapy								
Corynebacterium parvum	Macrophage stimulator		x	x	x			Fever, abdominal cramping
Interferon	Macrophage stimulator		x		x			Fever, abdominal cramping
Hormonal Agents								
Prednisone	Steroid				x			Increases white blood cell count
Megestrol	Progesterone		x		x			Cramping

nutritional assessments are necessary with nutritional support when indicated.

Benefits and Risks from Nutritional Support

Obviously, many sources produce the malnutrition commonly observed in patients with cancer. Whether nutritional depletion is insidious in onset or marked by a rapid decline, the consequences can be severe if the patient does not receive nutritional support. Evidence that nutritional support is of benefit to this patient population comes from several areas of research.

Improved Response to Therapy. Improved response to oncologic therapy is documented in patients with cancer undergoing curative-goal antineoplastic therapy.

Adjunct to Radiation Therapy. As an adjunct to radiation therapy, nutritional support is beneficial to certain patients with cancer. Kinsella *et al.* (1981) examined nutritional support prospectively during pelvic irradiation. Thirty-two patients receiving either curative or palliative radiation therapy were randomized to receive intravenous hyperalimentation or to be maintained on their regular oral diet.

Curative-goal hyperalimentation patients tolerated therapy well according to both functional and nutritional measures. The planned course of external beam therapy was completed without treatment break, and patients were fully active posttherapy. In comparison with the curative-goal control-fed patients, the hyperalimentation patients had a significant weight gain averaging 4 kg. Also, curative-goal intravenously fed patients had significant increases in serum transferrin, reflecting improved visceral protein status, as well as positive delayed skin hypersensitivity skin tests at completion of the radiation course, reflecting improved immune competence.

Adjunct to Chemotherapy. Issell *et al.* (1978) conducted a prospective randomized trial of nutritional support in 26 patients with extensive histologically proven squamous cell lung cancer. The chemoimmunotherapeutic agents were *Corynebacterium parvum,* isophosphamide, and doxorubicin. Thirteen patients received intravenous hyperalimentation for 31 days, while a control group was maintained on its regular oral diet. Patients were evenly distributed in each group according to weight loss prior to therapy, performance status, and schedule of *C. parvum* administration.

The patients receiving intravenous hyperalimentation experienced significant weight gain as compared to orally fed controls. Weight gain was predominantly the result of an increase in lean body mass since arm muscle circumference increased significantly. Fat stores, as measured by triceps skinfold, remained unchanged. In addition, the duration of nausea and vomiting associated with the administration of chemotherapy was reduced in the intravenous hyperalimentation group. When the intravenous hyperalimentation group was placed back on oral diets during a second course of chemotherapy, the significant reductions in nausea and vomiting and increased weight and lean body mass were not maintained.

Adjunct to Surgery. Müller *et al.* (1982) reported on the influence of ten days of preoperative parenteral nutrition in 125 patients undergoing surgery to treat gastrointestinal carcinoma. In this prospective clinical trial, patients were stratified by tumor site and nutritional status and then randomized to receive parenteral nutrition or the regular hospital diet. The 66 patients receiving parenteral nutrition had significantly fewer major complications and a reduced mortality rate. Significance resulted from both an improvement in the status of the parenteral group and a deterioration of the status of the control group.

In these controlled prospective studies, therefore, intravenous hyperalimentation improved patient tolerance to oncologic therapy (radiation, chemotherapy, or surgery) as well as nutritional status.

Evidence for Improved Immune Competence and Nutritional Status. Harvey *et al.* (1979) reported on 161 patients with cancer who received nutritional support. Of the 32 patients initially anergic, 27 became immunocompetent with nutritional therapy and only three died, while all five who remained anergic died. Patients discharged after completion of therapy had higher initial serum albumin and transferrin levels. In those patients who remained on nutritional support for three or more weeks, serum transferrin increased significantly during the course of nutritional support.

Harvey *et al.* (1979) reported that patients with cancer with better visceral protein status prior to therapy (measured by serum albumin and transferrin) were more likely to be discharged from the hospital after oncologic therapy. Those patients who responded to nutritional support and oncologic therapy with reversal of anergy were approximately 90% more likely to survive their hospital stay than those who remained anergic. Whether reversal of anergy in such studies is the result of nutritional support or the combined effect of nutritional support and oncologic therapy is not yet determined. However, nutritional support alone is documented to reverse anergy in the stressed malnourished hospitalized patient (Mullen *et al.*, 1980). Daly *et al.* (1980) also found intravenous hyperalimentation to be associated with restored skin test reactivity in 51% of the malnourished patients with cancer studied who were receiving intravenous hyperalimentation.

Risks and Nutritional Support. Providers of oncologic therapy often ask two questions: (1) Can nutritional support induce tumor growth? (2) If parenteral nutrition is indicated (enteral is not possible), do the risks of catheter and other complications outweigh any benefit from nutritional support?

The first question has been answered by both published clinical experience and animal studies. Copeland *et al.* (1977) report that in treating over 1500 patients with cancer undergoing oncologic therapy, no clinical evidence is seen that nutritional support alone can stimulate tumor growth or speed disease progression. *They emphasize, however, that therapies such as total parenteral nutrition should be reserved for those patients with cancer who have a realistic expectation of responding to oncologic therapy.*

In certain animal models, cancer growth was noted during nutritional support (Cameron and Paviat, 1976). Further animal studies have had varied results. For instance, Daly *et al.* (1978) reported that although tumors in nutritionally repleted animals were larger, tumor-weight-to-body-weight ratios were not significantly different between nutritionally repleted and control animals. Studies such as this emphasize the difficulties of applying risk/benefit analyses from animal models to clinical application of nutritional support. Further prospective clinical studies of tumor metabolism are necessary.

A recent animal study of tumor amino acid kinetics during tumor growth reports net host tissue catabolism (Kawamura *et al.*, 1982). Rat whole-body rates of protein degradation were elevated, and protein synthetic rates were reduced in skeletal muscle. However, the fractional rates of tumor protein breakdown were reduced. Thus relative to lean body mass, the net effect was one of the tumor "trapping"

nitrogen. These results suggest that without nutritional support host protein depletion occurs.

Regarding complications associated with total parenteral nutrition, evidence supports the safety of nutritional support in the patient with cancer, even in the presence of considerable immunodeficiency or severe complicating illnesses. Right atrial silastic catheters were used in 25 adult patients with acute leukemia undergoing intensive chemotherapy (Abraham *et al.*, 1979). Despite the fact that all of these patients suffered from granulocytopenia, some from thrombocytopenia, and others had bacteremia or fungemia, catheters remained in place for a median of four weeks with minimal complications. Of the 15 patients with systemic infections, in only one case was the catheter tip itself infected requiring removal. Autopsies were conducted in 8 of 15 patients who died with the catheter in place. No infection, thrombus, or abnormalities of the heart, blood, or pulmonary vessels were observed.

Copeland *et al.* (1979) also reported few complications in use of the parenteral technique in over 1000 patients with cancer. Sepsis related to indwelling subclavian vein feeding was minimal, and other complications (*i.e.*, leaks) were limited and easily corrected (Copeland *et al.*, 1974). Catheter complications are infrequent in the hands of trained clinicians and are of the same type found in general medical/surgical populations receiving total parenteral nutrition. A subclavian vein catheter was recently used to provide continuous intravenous infusion of chemotherapeutic agents (Lokich *et al.*, 1981). Home chemotherapy programs have also been devised that parallel the techniques used in home total parenteral nutrition (Harrison and Glenesk, 1981).

Parenteral nutrition techniques are discussed extensively with modes of nutritional intervention later in this chapter.

Future Research Needs in Nutrition/Oncology. A recent panel put forth recommendations for future research on nutritional support in patients with cancer (Brennan and Copeland, 1981). Carefully controlled, randomized, prospective studies are urgently needed to answer questions such as which patients benefit most from nutritional support and what is the optimal time and duration for nutritional support in conjunction with a course of oncologic therapy. Future research must also elucidate the nature of tumor metabolism.

Clearly, large multicenter studies are required to examine the benefit of nutritional support therapies in those patients with cancer who can potentially respond to antineoplastic therapy, but whose response is limited or absent as a result of malnutrition. Given the magnitude of individual variation, even among patients with the same type of cancer, several hundred if not several thousand patients must be studied to evaluate precisely the risks and benefits associated with nutritional support during antineoplastic therapy. Randomized trials are difficult to conduct, since many interacting variables are present in those patients with cancer in need of hyperalimentation. Often patients have had cancer for many months and have received or are receiving varying courses of chemotherapy. Such variables as histologic type, tumor stage, and extent of metastases also affect body metabolism.

Guidelines for Nutritional Support

Despite the controversies surrounding nutritional support in the patient with cancer, accumulated evidence makes it clear that total parenteral nutrition is "a major tool in the management of cancer" (Brennan and Copeland, 1981). Copeland (1981) put forth the following statement on the indications for total parenteral nutrition in the patient with cancer.

A candidate for total parenteral nutrition is a malnourished patient who cannot be renourished enterally, (*i.e.,* GI tract dysfunction) who has a potentially responsive tumor, and who cannot receive an adequate trial of anticancer therapy because of the possibility of complications secondary to the combined effects of malnutrition and oncologic therapy.

Evaluation of Nutritional Status. Implementation of nutritional support requires adequate nutritional assessment. Three simple assessment techniques are used initially to screen for protein-calorie malnutrition: *weight/height, percentage of regular weight lost,* and *serum albumin* levels. These assessment measures are sensitive enough to identify most patients with major protein-calorie malnutrition. Energy and protein needs are the primary concern since they are the most difficult to provide owing to the large volume required to deliver these nutrients daily. Of the over 30 nutrients required by humans, most can be easily administered through daily oral supplements or in supplements added to intravenous solutions.

Weight/Height. Since a patient's height is

essentially constant, the weight/height parameter is an individualized measure of nutritional status. The weight/height index is the ratio of the patient's present weight to the ideal value for the same height and gender (Metropolitan Life Insurance Company [see Table 45 – 4]). A weight/height index less than 90% of standard should be interpreted as moderate nutritional depletion. A weight/height index less that 80% of standard indicates severe depletion.

In some cases, water retention or loss is the source of weight change rather than real changes in body cell mass or protein content. Thus, other assessment parameters should be used in conjunction with the weight/height index, *i.e.,* serum albumin levels, to ensure accurate evaluation of a patient's protein nutritional status.

Percent of Weight Lost (Rate). The patient's weight history should also be interpreted in terms of percentage of regular weight lost (see Table 45 – 5). Rate of weight loss gives some indication of severity of nutritional depletion. For instance, a loss of 5% of body weight in one month or 10% weight loss in six months indicates severe weight loss (Blackburn *et al.,* 1982).

Water retention may also affect the accuracy of percent of weight lost. Another limitation of

Table 45–4. Fogarty International Center Conference on Obesity Recommended Weight in Relation to Height*

HEIGHT	MEN		WOMEN	
Inches	Average	Range	Average	Range
58	——	——	102	92–119
59	——	——	104	94–112
60	——	——	107	96–125
61	——	——	110	99–128
62	123	112–141	113	102–131
63	127	115–144	116	105–134
64	130	118–148	120	108–138
65	133	121–152	123	111–142
66	136	124–156	128	114–146
67	140	128–161	132	118–150
68	145	132–166	136	122–154
69	149	136–170	140	126–158
70	153	140–174	144	130–163
71	158	144–179	148	134–168
72	162	148–184	152	138–173
73	166	152–189	——	——
74	171	156–194	——	——
75	176	160–199	——	——
76	181	164–204	——	——

* Height without shoes, weight without clothes.
Reprinted by permission from Bray, G. A.: *Obesity in Perspective,* Vol. 2, Part 1, Appendix III, Table 1a. Department of Health, Education, and Welfare (NIH) 75–708, 1975. (Adapted from the Table of the Metropolitan Life Insurance Co.)

Table 45–5. Evaluation of Weight Change

	SIGNIFICANT WEIGHT LOSS (%)	SEVERE WEIGHT LOSS (%)
1 week	1–2*	>2
1 month	5	>5
3 months	7.5	>7.5
6 months	10	>10

Reprinted by permission from Blackburn, G. L.; DiScala, C.; Miller, M. M.; Champagne, C.; Lahey, M.; Bothe, A., Jr.; and Bistrian, B. R.: Preliminary report on collaborative study for home parenteral nutrition patients. Second Bermuda Symposium on Clinical Nutrition, 1982.

* Percent weight change =

$$\frac{(\text{Usual weight} - \text{Actual weight})}{(\text{Usual weight})} \times 100$$

this parameter is that the amount of weight loss alone cannot identify the nature of the weight loss. Weight loss can range from predominantly fat loss, as is found in the dieting obese consuming a high-protein diet (Bistrian et al., 1977), to lean tissue loss in states of semistarvation or after injury (Duke et al., 1970; Runcie and Hilditch, 1974). Thus, these two weight-loss parameters, weight/height and percent weight loss, should be evaluated in conjunction with measures of visceral protein status.

Serum Albumin. Serum albumin is used most frequently in measuring visceral protein function. A serum albumin < 3.0 g/dL represents medically important depletion. As Table 45–6 shows for the hospitalized patient, low albumin levels are associated with malnutrition (anergy) and conditions with increased morbidity (sepsis) and increased mortality rates. An albumin < 3.5 g/dL suggests the possibility of protein-calorie malnutrition and indicates the need for a more comprehensive nutritional assessment.

Hypoalbuminemia, however, is not always the direct result of protein-calorie malnutrition. Depressed serum albumin levels may also follow surgery, infections, or injury in

Table 45–6. Probability Estimates Using Serum Albumin

	<10%	<25%	50%	>75%	>90%
Anergy	5.2	4.2	3.2	2.2	1.2
Sepsis	4.3	3.7	3.1	2.5	1.9
Death	4.9	4.0	3.2	2.3	1.5

Reprinted by permission from Harvey, K. B.; Moldawer, L. L.; Bistrian, B. R.; and Blackburn, G. L.: Biological measures for the formulation of a hospital prognostic index. *Am. J. Clin. Nutr.,* **34:**2013–2022, 1981.

which the proportion of albumin in the extravascular compartment is decreased owing to wound edema, reduced lymphatic return, or sodium retention. To maximize the validity of serum albumin as a measure of nutritional status, diagnosis should be made on the basis of either preoperative or ten-day postoperative measures, when possible. Nephrotic syndromes, protein-losing enteropathies, or liver disease may also result in depressed albumin levels independent of nutrient intake.

Bistrian (1981) discussed the value and limitations of serum albumin levels as a measure of protein nutritional status. Serum albumin does not respond promptly, within two weeks, to nutritional support intervention in cases where stress is long term from sepsis or severe injury since the half-life of albumin is 18 to 20 days. For evaluation of nutritional status during ongoing nutritional support, the clinician depends more heavily on serum transferrin levels. The half-life of transferrin is substantially shorter, seven days, making transferrin levels more responsive to effective nutritional support.

Despite this limitation, albumin levels are an important tool in initial nutritional assessment for several reasons. First, in conjunction with easily obtained weight/height index and measure of percent of weight loss, albumin levels can give the clinician a clear idea whether protein malnutrition is present, and so justify administration of the full battery of nutritional assessment tests. Albumin levels also allow the clinician to distinguish the marasmic patient from the hypoalbuminemic (kwashiorkor) patient, an important role of nutritional assessment.

In the marasmic patient, body weight (fat and muscle), triceps skinfold (fat), and arm muscle circumferences (skeletal muscle) are depleted, whereas visceral protein status, serum albumin, and immune competence remain within normal range. Thus low albumin levels can alert the clinician to the possibility of a kwashiorkor-like situation.

Under the increased stress of injury or infection, marasmic patients often develop the more severe kwashiorkor-like syndrome associated with dramatic increases in morbidity and mortality. In the stressed patient with cancer, the kwashiorkor-like syndrome can be devastating. The value of identifying marasmic individuals is to intervene with nutritional support prior to the development of the kwashiorkor-like syndrome which is highly probable if any additional stress, *i.e.,* infection, occurs.

If any abnormal values among weight/height index, calculation of percent body weight loss, and serum albumin levels are found, a more comprehensive assessment including the following measures should be done to determine the appropriate nutritional support therapy (see Table 45–7).

Triceps Skinfold Measurement. Triceps skinfold measurement (TSF) assesses body fat mass and is easily done using large calipers at the upper left arm. The more valuable arm muscle circumference (AMC) is derived using TSF:

AMC = Arm circumference − (TSF)

Table 45–7. Nutritional Assessment Parameters

	STANDARDS
Initial evaluation	
Weight/height (kg/cm)	Table 45–4
Rate weight loss (% weight loss/time)	Table 45–5
Serum albumin (g/dL)	≥ 3.5 g/dL
Complete evaluation to include also	
A. Anthropometrics	
Triceps skinfold (mm)	Table 45–8
Arm muscle circumference	Table 45–8
B. Biochemical indices	
Urine	
Creatinine height index	Table 45–9
Urine urea nitrogen	6–7 g/24°
Nitrogen balance*	0–+1 g/24°
Catabolic index*	See text
Serum	
Transferrin g/dL*	≥ 170 g/dL
Total lymphocyte count	≥ 1500 cells/mm³
T₄	4–12 μg/dL
Plasma	
Sodium	134–145 mEq/L
Potassium	3.5–5.5 mEq/L
Free fatty acids	.340–.725 mEq/L
Butyrate	0.06–0.17 mmol/L
Glucose	65–120 mg%
Insulin	6–34 μIU/mL
C. Immune function: delayed hypersensitivity	
Skin tests	
Candida*	≥ 5 mm induration
Mumps*	≥ 5 mm erythema/induration
Tetanus toxoid	≥ 5 mm induration
D. Prognostic indices	
Prognostic nutritional index (risk of complications)	High ≥ 50%
	Moderate 40–49%
	Low <40%
Hospital Nutritional Index (HNI) (risk of mortality during hospital stay)	High < −1
	Moderate +1 to −1
	Low > +1

* In addition to initial assessment, these measures are sensitive enough to be used in the evaluation of patient benefit from a particular nutritional support regime.

The AMC is a sensitive measure of protein nutritional status. Both the AMC and TSF are severely depleted when below the fifth percentile (Bistrian, 1980) (see Table 45–8). In edematous states or in amputees where weights are inaccurate indicators of malnutrition, the AMC is particularly useful (Bistrian, 1980).

Creatinine Height Index. Since creatinine is a product of muscle metabolism, the excretion of creatinine in the urine is proportional to the amount of lean body mass. The patient's 24 hour urine creatinine excretion is compared to normal table values based on sex, age, and height characteristics. Standards of the creatinine/height index values correlate best with lean body mass, surface area, and body weight when 24-hour urine collections are done over a period of several days. The short-term response of creatinine excretion to nutritional support is of little use owing to the variability in completeness of urine collection in the clinical setting. Although creatinine excretion can be estimated on a 12-hour collection, collections for several days are necessary to ensure accuracy. To measure response to therapy, creatinine urine collections should be continued for several weeks. Standards for creatinine excretion based on height are shown in Table 45–9.

Transferrin Levels. Transferrin levels < 170 g/dL reflect visceral protein depletion. As mentioned previously, transferrin is more likely than albumin to reflect any improve-

Table 45–8. Percentiles for Triceps Skinfold for Whites of the United States Health and Nutrition Examination Survey I of 1971 to 1974

AGE GROUP	TRICEPS SKINFOLD PERCENTILES (MM)							
	n	5	10	25	50	75	90	95
Males								
18–18.9	91	4	5	6	9	13	20	24
19–24.9	531	4	5	7	10	15	20	22
25–34.9	971	5	6	8	12	16	20	24
35–44.9	806	5	6	8	12	16	20	23
45–54.9	898	6	6	8	12	15	20	25
55–64.9	734	5	6	8	11	14	19	22
65–74.9	1503	4	6	8	11	15	19	22
Females								
18–18.9	109	10	12	15	18	22	26	30
19–24.9	1060	10	11	14	18	24	30	34
25–34.9	1987	10	12	16	21	27	34	37
35–44.9	1614	12	14	18	23	29	35	38
45–54.9	1047	12	16	20	25	30	36	40
55–64.9	809	12	16	20	25	31	36	38
65–74.9	1670	12	14	18	24	29	34	36

Reprinted by permission from Frisancho, A. R.: Triceps skinfold and upper arm muscle size norms for assessment of nutritional status. *Am. J. Clin. Nutr.,* 27:1052–1059, 1974.

Table 45–9. Ideal Urinary Creatinine Values

MEN		WOMEN	
Height (cm)	*Ideal Creatinine (mg)*	*Height (cm)*	*Ideal Creatinine (mg)*
157.5	1288	147.3	830
160.0	1325	149.9	851
162.6	1359	152.4	875
165.1	1386	154.9	900
167.6	1426	157.5	925
170.2	1467	160.0	949
172.2	1513	162.6	977
175.3	1555	165.1	1006
177.8	1596	167.6	1044
180.3	1642	170.2	1076
182.9	1691	172.7	1109
185.4	1739	175.3	1141
188.0	1785	177.8	1174
190.5	1831	180.3	1206
193.0	1891	182.9	1240

ments in patient nutritional status during nutritional therapy. However, transferrin measurements have two major disadvantages. Transferrin also reflects iron status. Iron-deficient patients show high levels, whereas iron-loaded patients show depressed levels as compared to other patients with similar degrees of malnutrition. In addition, multiple transfusions will lower serum transferrin levels (Bistrian, 1981).

Immune Function Tests. Immunodeficiency is often closely coupled with protein/calorie malnutrition. Immunodeficiency in conjunction with abnormalities in any three of the initial assessment measures signals the need for nutritional support. Cellular immunity is most sensitive to malnutrition, although protein deficiency also affects leukocyte function.

The recall antigens used by the nutrition support service at the New England Deaconess Hospital to detect anergy are *Candida* (Hollister-Stier), mumps skin test antigen (Lilly), and dermatophyten (Hollister-Stier), or tetanus toxoid (Wyeth). The preparations are as follows: 0.1 mL of a solution of *Candida* allergic extract (1 : 10 w/v in 50% glycerin) is diluted 1 : 100 with normal saline and 01.1 mL of the mumps skin test antigen is used. These antigens are placed intradermally on the flexor surface of the forearm. Any induration of more than 5 mm after 24 and 48 hours is considered a positive response.

Prognostic Indices. The Prognostic Nutritional Index (PNI) (Mullen *et al.,* 1980) and the Hospital Prognostic Index (HPN) (Harvey *et al.,* 1981) may be used in initial assessment to predict probability of complications and of

survival, respectively. These formulas are as follows:

PNI = 158% − 16.6 (albumin) − 0.78 (triceps skinfold)
    − 0.2 (transferrin) − 5.8 (delayed hypersensitivity)

Key: anergy = 1, immunocompetence = 2

Interpretation: risk of complication:
  high = ≥ 50%, moderate = 40–49%, low = < 40%.

HPN = .91 (albumin) − 1.00 (delayed hypersensitivity)
    − 1.44 (sepsis) + 0.98 (diagnosis) − 1.09

Key: immunocompetence = 1, anergy = 2
  no sepsis = 1, sepsis = 2
  cancer = 1, no cancer = 2

Interpretation: probability of mortality:
  high = < −1, moderate = −1 to +1, low = > +1

In both indices, serum albumin levels are the most sensitive single variable for predicting outcome during subsequent hospital course. For this reason, these indices are limited, like serum albumin, as dynamic measures of patient benefit from nutritional support. These prognostic indices are useful for the initial assessment and can be reevaluated after a minimum of three weeks on nutritional support.

Bistrian (1984) includes a comprehensive critique and update on the nutritional assessment techniques discussed here. The paper also reviews the less routine techniques not commonly used owing to expense or difficulties in administration.

Evaluation of Ongoing Nutritional Support. During administration of nutritional support several nutritional assessment parameters are repeated routinely to evaluate patient benefit as well to tailor daily nutritional support to the patient's requirements.

Serum albumin, arm muscle circumference, and the creatinine height index are not sensitive enough to monitor the effects of nutritional support over the short term. Serum transferrin responds quickly if stress is limited. In initially anergic patients, immune competence should return after seven to ten days of nutritional therapy even when stress is present. Failure to reverse anergy after two weeks of nutritional support generally signals a poor prognosis. Nitrogen balance calculation is perhaps the simplest way to assess the interaction between nutritional therapy and the patient's nutritional status daily.

The clinician must carefully differentiate weight change caused by retained fluid from lean body mass weight gain. Malnourished patients can develop increased intravascular volumes and congestive heart failure (Heymsfield *et al.,* 1978) or refeeding edema (Keys *et al.,*

1950). During nutritional support, improvements in lean body mass are slow and are measurable after approximately six weeks. An increase in weight during the first one or two weeks of nutritional support suggests water retention. Thus, in the initial weeks of nutritional support, nitrogen balance is the dependable measure to determine the influence of nutritional support on lean body mass.

Nitrogen Balance. Nitrogen balance indicates a patient's protein balance, thus reflects changes in lean body mass. The formula is:

$$\text{Nitrogen balance} = \frac{\text{protein intake (g)}}{6.25}$$
$$- (24\text{-hr urine urea nitrogen} + 4 \text{ g})$$

Urine urea nitrogen is easily measured and is the principal form of urine nitrogen. Urea corresponds to protein breakdown. The other forms of nitrogen excreted, nonurea urine nitrogen, fecal, and integumental nitrogen, are lost at a fairly stable rate except when diarrhea is present. The 4 g are added to the last term to estimate fecal and integumental losses.

Catabolic Index. Another important variable in designing nutritional therapy is the degree of catabolic stress the patient is experiencing. The efficiency of dietary protein use is reduced by stress which leads to an increased conversion of dietary and endogenous protein to glucose and urea via gluconeogenesis. When the diet is low in or devoid of protein, such as when hospitalized patients are maintained on dextrose or electrolyte solutions intravenously, the urinary nitrogen excretion can be used as an index of protein catabolic rates. In cases where dietary protein intake is in excess of 20 g/day, urinary nitrogen excretion is increased, thus urinary nitrogen excretion is a poor index of protein catabolic rate. To compensate, the catabolic index is used (Bistrian, 1981):

Catabolic index =
24-hour urine nitrogen excretion − [½ dietary nitrogen (g) intake + 3]

Interpretation:
0 = no significant stress
1–5 = mild stress
5 = moderate to severe stress

This formula is based on the premise that approximately 50% of dietary protein is converted to urea in mild to moderately stressed individuals and that 3 g of urea nitrogen are produced even in the absence of dietary protein.

Patient Requirements. *The Marasmic Patient.* The marasmic patient without significant stress requires 30 to 40 Kcal/kg and 1.5 g protein/kg of ideal body weight (see Figure 45–3). Such support should lead to slow weight gain and positive nitrogen balance of 2 to 6 g nitrogen. This nitrogen balance reflects a gain of 60 to 180 g lean tissue/day normally matched by an equivalent amount of fat. When weight gain exceeds 360 g/day the patient is probably retaining an excess amount of water.

The Hypoalbuminemic Patient. The above nutritional regime leads to weight gain in the hypoalbuminemic patient in similar proportions. Serum transferrin should increase in seven to ten days, whereas serum albumin may not increase for at least two weeks.

With concomitant stress, nitrogen retention in the hypoalbuminemic patient is limited, and only simple nitrogen balance may be obtained until the stress, *i.e.,* infection, is relieved. Since nitrogen retention is limited in the hypoalbuminemic patient, weight gain is even more likely to reflect fat or water gain or both rather than substantial lean body mass gain. Patient weight gain and nitrogen balance must be carefully monitored until stress is relieved. In the patient with cancer with either of these states of malnutrition, nutritional support therapy must be continuously evaluated.

Enteral Feeding. When the intestinal tract is intact, liquid formula diets are recommended. Numerous products exist and fall into four major categories: dietary supplements, meal replacements, defined formula diets, and feeding modules. Dietary supplements include a broad range of products designed to be added to regular meal feedings to provide specific nutritional requirements. Meal replacements can provide all of the patient's nutritional requirements as a substitute for daily dietary intake. Particular problems of nutrient absorption can be met using the defined formula diets. Feeding modules provide individual food group components, *i.e.,* protein, carbohydrate, or fat. The historic background, physiology, delivery techniques, and cost of such formulas are detailed by Bothe *et al.* (1981). Some commonly used formulas are shown in Table 45–10.

Patients with cancer who can tolerate oral feeding may prefer the bland meal replacement, ISOCAL. This diet does not require chewing, has acceptable taste, and allows the patient to quantify intake easily. Eating can be

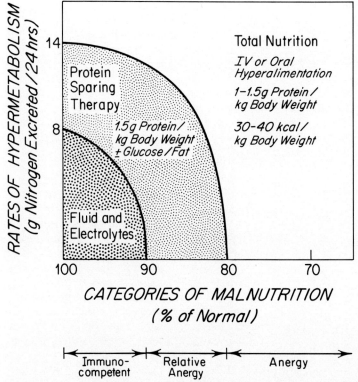

Figure 45–3. Nutritional support should be tailored to the requirements of the patient with cancer. From Bistrian, B. R., and Bothe, A., Jr.: Nutritional management of the patient with cancer. In Lokich, J. (ed.): *Clinical Cancer Medicine.* G. K. Hall & Company, Boston, 1980.

spread out over a long period. Few risks are involved. Osmotic diarrhea may develop owing to the hyperosmolar nature of the diets, or steatorrhea and diarrhea owing to diet fat content, especially in patients with pancreatic dysfunction. These formulas tend to be low in sodium, although they are often high in potassium.

Tube Feeding. When voluntary oral feeding is insufficient, tube feeding or parenteral feeding may be used. A decision tree for patient selection for tube feeding is shown in Figure 45–4. When the gastrointestinal tract is functional, but oral intake is insufficient, tube feeding should be used rather than parenteral feeding.

Patients are best fed continuously by gravity drip or by infusion pump through silastic feeding tubes (small, 7–9 French). The HEDECO design has the added advantage of a weighted mercury tip. Flow rates are initiated at 40 to 50 mL/hr and then increased slowly to full flow rates over several days. Often, formulas are begun at half dilution and later administered undiluted. The rate should be increased first, then solution strength increased to the

desired concentration. Nasogastric or naso-duodenal feeding is most practical. With these techniques, the patient's head should be maintained at a 30-degree elevation to avoid aspiration. For chronic management, surgical insertion of a gastrostomy or jejunostomy tube may be necessary.

Parenteral Nutrition. Complete parenteral nutrition can be administered temporarily by peripheral vein. Peripheral administration is possible for several combinations of slightly hypertonic solutions, such as a 3% amino acid solution or 5% dextrose accompanied by 10% fat emulsion. Such a diet maintains moderately catabolic patients and repletes malnourished patients only slowly owing to the volume limitation in total calories and protein that can be delivered. Solutions are shown in Table 45–11.

Complications are few, but the amino acid–dextrose component of a peripheral feeding system can cause phlebitis. Administering fat emulsion and the amino acid–glucose mixture together through a Y connector minimizes this complication.

Central vein intravenous hyperalimenta-

Table 45–10. Enteral Formulas

	cal/mL	Osmolarity (mosm)	% cal Protein	% cal CHO	% cal Fat	N:cal	Protein Source	CHO Source	Fat Source	mEq Na/L	Function
1. SUPPLEMENTS											
CARNATION INSTANT BREAKFAST and whole milk (Carnation)	1.05	NA	22	51	27	1:88	Whole-milk, nonfat dry milk, sodium caseinate, soy protein isolate	Sucrose, corn syrup solids, lactose	Whole-milk fat	40.4	High-protein supplement; oral or tube feeding
CITROTEIN (Doyle)	0.66	500	24	73	0.5	1:178	Pasteurized egg white solids	Sucrose, maltodextrins	Vegetable oil	31	Minimal fat, high-protein supplement
LANOLAC (Mead-Johnson)	0.67	NA	21	30	49	1:93	Casein	Lactose	Coconut oil	1.1	Low-sodium protein beverage
LOLACTENE (Doyle)	0.8	670	26	53	21	1:70	Low-lactose nonfat dry milk, sodium caseinate	Corn syrup solids, sucrose	Vegetable oil	38	99.6% lactose-free supplement
MERETINE LIQUID (Doyle)	1.0	560–617	24	46	30	1:79	Concentrated sweet skim milk, sodium, caseinate	Corn syrup solids, sucrose	Vegetable oil	40	High-protein supplement for oral or tube feeding
MERITINE POWDER and whole milk (Doyle)	1.06	690	26	45	29	1:71	Processed nonfat dry milk	Corn syrup solids	Cows' milk fat	41.8	High protein supplement for oral or tube feeding
SUSTACAL LIQUID (Mead-Johnson)	1.0	625	24	55	21	1:79	Calcium caseinate, soy protein isolate	Sucrose, corn syrup	Partially hydrogenated soy oil	40	Lactose-free, high-protein supplement
SUSTACAL POWDER and whole milk (Mead-Johnson)	1.3	756	24	54	22	1:79	Nonfat dry milk	Sucrose, corn syrup	Cows' milk, fat	30.7	High-protein supplement. When mixed with milk contains 114 g lactose
SUSTACAL PUDDING (per 5- oz, 37-g can) (Mead-Johnson)	0.6/g	NA	11.3	53.2	35.5	1:196	Nonfat milk	Sucrose, starch	Hydrogenated soy oil	5.2	High-calorie supplement Offers change in consistency
SUSTAGEN POWDER (Mead-Johnson)	0.7	721	24	68	8	1:79	Nonfat milk, powdered whole milk, calcium caseinates	Corn syrup solids, dextrose	Cows' milk, fat	54	High-calorie (mainly from CHO), high-protein, low-fat formula for oral use or tube feeding

1422

2. MEAL REPLACEMENTS

Product							Protein source	Carbohydrate source	Fat source		Comments
COMPLEAT "B" (Doyle)	1.0	517	16	48	36	1:131	Puree beef, nonfat dry milk	Maltodextrin, vegetable and fruit purees, sucrose	Corn oil, beef fat	55.1	Blenderized house diet for tube feeding
ENSURE (Ross)	1.06	450	14	54.5	31.5	1:153	Sodium and calcium caseinates, soy protein isolate	Corn syrup solids, sucrose	Corn oil	32.2	Lactose-free meal replacement formula for oral or tube. Flavored
ENSURE PLUS (Ross)	1.5	600*	14.6	53	32	1:146	Sodium and calcium caseinates, soy protein isolate	Corn syrup solids, sucrose	Corn oil	46	Calorically dense formula for oral or tube feeding
FORMULA 2 (Cutter)	1.0	435–510	15	49	36	1:142	Skim milk, beef, egg yolk	Sucrose, vegetables, orange juice, wheat flour	Corn oil, egg yolk, beef fat	26	Blenderized tube feeding, nutritionally complete
ISOCAL (Mead-Johnson)	1.06	300	13	50	37	1:168	Calcium and sodium caseinates, soy protein isolate	Glucose oligosaccharides	Soy oil (80%), MCT (20%)	23	Unflavored tube feeding formula, lactose-free
MAGNACAL (Organon)	2.0	590*	14	50	36	1:154	Calcium caseinate, sodium caseinate	Maltodextrin, corn syrup solids, sucrose	Soy oil monoglycerides	43.5	High-calorie formula, nutritionally complete tube or oral feeding
NUTRI-1000 LF (Cutter)	1.06	304	15.1	46.7	38.2	1:141	Skim milk	Sucrose, lactose, dextrin-maltose, dextrose	Corn oil	22.9	Lactose-free meal replacement formula for oral or tube feeding
OSMOLITE (Ross)	1.06	300	14	54.6	31.4	1:157	Sodium and calcium caseinates, soy protein isolate	Corn syrup solids	MCT (20%), corn oil, soy oil	23	Unflavored tube feeding formula, lactose-free
PORTAGEN (Mead-Johnson)	1.0	354	14	46	40	1:154	Sodium caseinate	Corn syrup solids, sucrose	MCT (86%), corn oil (14%)	20.4	Intended for use with those patients who malabsorb long-chain fats, essentially lactose-free (<0.3 g lactose/960 mL)

continued

Table 45-10. *(continued)*

	cal/mL	Osmolarity (mosm)	% cal Protein	% cal CHO	% cal Fat	N:cal	Protein Source	CHO Source	Fat Source	mEq Na/L	Function
PRECISION ISOTONIC (Doyle)	0.96		12	60	28	1:184	Pasteurized egg white solids	Glucose oligosaccharides, sucrose	Soy oil	33	Isotonic formula for oral or tube feeding
RENU (Organon)	1.01	330*	13	51	36	1:166	Sodium and calcium caseinates	Maltodextrin, corn syrup, corn and malt syrup	Soy oil, monodiglycerides	21.7	Tube or oral feeding, low sodium
TRAVASORB WHOLE-PROTEIN LIQUID (Travenol)	1.06	450*	14	54.5	31.5	1:154	Sodium and calcium caseinates, soy protein isolate	Sucrose, corn syrup solids	Corn oil, soy oil (partially hydrogenated)	32	Lactose-free tube or oral feeding
VITANEED (Organon)	1.02	400*	14	51	35	1:157	Puree beef, calcium caseinate	Corn syrup solids, maltodextrin, puree fruit/vegetable	Soy oil, monodiglycerides	23.9	Blenderized tube feeding, nutritionally complete
3. DEFINED FORMULA DIETS											
FLEXICAL (Mead-Johnson)	1.0	550*	9	61	30	1:253	Hydrolyzed casein and methionine, tyrosine, tryptophan,	Corn syrup solids, dextrioligosaccharides	MCT (20%), partially hydrogenated soy oil (80%)	15.2	Protein source is 70% free amino acids, 30% small peptides. Usually for tube feeding; flavored packs available
PRECISION-LR (Doyle)	1.08	600	9.5	89.9	1.3	1:239	Pasteurized egg white solids	Maltodextrin sucrose	Soy oil, MCT	30.5	Low-residue minimal fat formula for oral or tube feeding. Protein source requires digestion
PRECISION-HN (Doyle)	1.1	580	16.6	82.6	1.1	1:125	Pasteurized egg white solids	Maltodextrin sucrose	Soy oil, MCT	42.6	High-nitrogen, low-residue, minimal fat formula for oral or tube feeding. Protein source requires digestion

Product (Manufacturer)	kcal/ml	Osmolality				Ratio	Protein source	Carbohydrate source	Fat source		Comments
TRAVASORB STANDARD (Travenol)	1.0	450*	12	76	12	1:202	Oligopeptides of fortified lactalbumin	Glucose oligosaccharides	MCT (40%), sunflower oil (60%)	40	"Elemental" oligopeptide. Protein source of high biologic value. Although easily absorbed, some digestive capacity required. Minimal residue. Unflavored, flavored packs available (increase osmolarity)
TRAVASORB HN (Travenol)	1.0	450*	18	70	12	1:126	Oligopeptides of fortified lactalbumin	Glucose, oligosaccharides	MCT (40%), sunflower oil (60%)	40	"Elemental" oligopeptide. High nitrogen. Although easily absorbed, some digestive capacity required. Minimal residue, unflavored, flavored packets available (increase osmolarity)
TRAVASORB MCT (Travenol)	1.0	250*	20	50	30	1:100	Lactalbumin, potassium caseinate	Corn syrup solids	MCT, sunflower oil	15	Protein source requires digestion; high-protein content. Low osmolarity. Low sodium, 80% of fat calories from MCT, unflavored
VIPEP (Cutter)	1.0	520*	10	68	22	1:228	Enzymatically hydrolyzed whole-fish protein concentrate	Corn syrup solids, glucose potassium gluconate, corn starch	MCT oil, corn oil	32.6	19.6% free amino acids; 72.5% di-, tetrapeptides; 7.9% 4–14 amino acid chain; 18% fat calories as MCT; 4% as corn oil

continued

Table 45–10. *(continued)*

	cal/mL	Osmolarity (mosm)	% cal Protein	% cal CHO	% cal Fat	N:cal	Protein Source	CHO Source	Fat Source	mEq Na/L	Function
VITAL (Ross)	1.0	450*	16.7	74	9.3	1:125	Enzymatically hydrolyzed soy, whey, meat, free amino acids	Glucose oligo- and polysaccarides, sucrose	Safflower oil, MCT-oil	17	Hydrolyzed protein source, (owing to tetrapeptides for oral or tube feeding)
VIVONEX STANDARD (unflavored) (flavored) (Morton-Norwich)	1.0	550 610–678	8.2	90.5	1.3	1:281	Crystalline amino acids	Glucose, oligosaccharides	Safflower oil	20	Minimal fat, low-residue formula, easily absorbed protein source
VIVONEX HN (unflavored) (flavored) (Morton-Norwich)	1.0	810 850–920	17.7	81.5	0.8	1:125	Crystalline amino acids	Glucose, oligosaccharides	Safflower oil	23	Minimal fat, low-residue, high-protein formula. Easily absorbed protein source
AMIN-AID (McGaw)	1.95	850*	4	74.8	21.2	1:638	Essential amino acids	Maltodextrines, sugar, citric acid	Partially hydrogenated soy oil, mono- and di-glycerides	14.7	Provides high-calorie, low-protein diet of essential amino acids only. For use in renal failure. Contains no vitamins. Limited electrolytes
HEPATIC-AID (McGaw)	1.6	900	10.4	69.8	19.8	1:225	Essential and nonessential amino acids; BCAA enriched	Maltodextrins, sucrose	Soybean oil, mono- and di-glycerides	None	Provides high-calorie BCAA-enriched formula; theoretically useful in treatment of hepatic encephalopathy. No vitamins or minerals

4. FEEDING MODULES

	cal/mL	Osmolarity (mosm)	% cal Protein	% cal CHO	% cal Fat	N:cal	Protein Source	CHO Source	Fat Source	mEq Na/L	Function
CASEC (powder) (per 100 g) (Mead-Johnson)	3.6/g	—	95	0	4.8		Calcium caseinate	None	Butter fat	6	Concentrated protein source

Product							Carbohydrate source	Fat source		Description
CONTROLYTE (powder) (Doyle)	5.0/g	—	Negligible	57	43	Trace	Polysaccharides of deionized partial hydrolysate of corn starch	Vegetable oil	0.65/100 g	Provides calorie source
MCT OIL (per 100 mL) (Mead-Johnson)	7.7	—	0	0	100	—	None	MCT	0	Special dietary supplement for patients malabsorbing long-chain fat
MICROLIPID (Organon)	4.5	32*	0	0	100	None	None	Safflower oil, mono-, diglycerides	0	A 50% fat emulsion used to increase caloric density of enteral feedings
POLYCOSE (liquid) (Ross)	2.0	570*	0	96	0	None	Hydrolyzed corn starch	None	26.2	—
POLYCOSE (powder) (Ross)	4 cal/min	—	0	96	0	None	Hydrolyzed corn starch	None	4.7/100 g	Provides calorie source, low osmolarity. Tasteless
PRO-MIX (Nubro)	3.7	—	80	4.2	3.9	Whey	Lactose	Milk fat	6.5/100 g	Concentrated protein source
SUMACAL (Organon)	2.0	680*	100	0	0	None	Maltodextrin, glucose, syrup solids	None	8.7	Liquid carbohydrate source used to increase caloric density of enteral feedings
SUMACAL PLUS (Organon)	2.5	890*	100	0	0	None	Maltodextrin, glucose, syrup solids	None	9.1	Liquid carbohydrate source used to increase caloric density of enteral feedings

NA = not available
* mosm/kg H_2O
BCA = branched-chain amino acids
MCT = medium-chain triglycerides
From Bothe, A., Jr.; Wade, J. E.; and Blackburn, G. L.: Enteral nutrition. An overview. In Hill, G. L. (ed.): *Nutrition and the Surgical Patient.* Churchill Livingstone, Inc., New York, 1981.

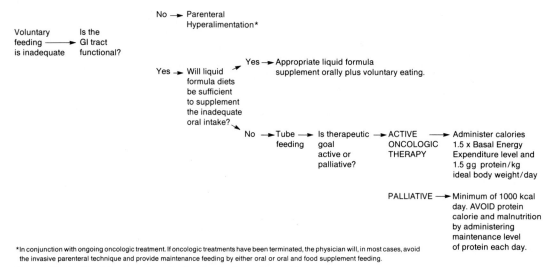

*In conjunction with ongoing oncologic treatment. If oncologic treatments have been terminated, the physician will, in most cases, avoid the invasive parenteral technique and provide maintenance feeding by either oral or oral and food supplement feeding.

Figure 45–4. Decision tree for tube feeding in the patient with cancer.

tion is an effective and more flexible means of nutritional support. Solutions are hyperosmolar (1800 to 2400 mosm/L). A central vein is used for infusion to prevent damage to the peripheral vein. In the usual procedure, a polyvinyl or silastic catheter is threaded percutaneously into the subclavian or external jugular vein and directed to the superior vena cava. Before administration of hyperosmolar solutions, the placement of the catheter must be verified radiographically. Strict aseptic techniques are required including mechanical cleaning to disinfect and defat the skin as well as the application of a povidone-iodine ointment to the skin surrounding the catheter site. After placement, a completely occlusive sterile dressing should be applied and changed every two to three days (Blackburn and Harvey, 1981). Recently, this central vein hyperalimentation technique was used for continuous infusion chemotherapy (Lokich *et al.,* 1981) since agents, such as 5-FU, that have short half-lives *in vivo* may be more effectively administered continuously.

Moosman (1973) described the anatomy of infraclavicular subclavian vein catheterization. Catheter-associated complications are few in the hands of a trained clinician (Hopkins, 1982). Two catheter-related complications can occur: pneumothorax and thrombosis of the subclavian vein (Padberg *et al.,* 1981). Pneumothorax can be diagnosed early (Hopkins, 1982). To minimize the second complication, 6000 to 8000 units of heparin per day can be included in the solutions, if not contraindicated.

With central vein hyperalimentation, patients can receive continuous infusion of pro-

Table 45–11. Crystalline Amino Acid Infusions for Peripheral Use

	FREAMINE III 3% w/electrolytes (McGaw)	AMINOSYN 3.5% M (Abbott)	3.5% TRAVASOL M w/ electrolytes 45 (Travenol)
Protein concentration (%)	3.0	3.5	3.5
Nitrogen (1 g/100 mL)	0.46	0.55	0.59
Electrolytes (mEq/L)			
Sodium	35	47	25
Potassium	24.5	13	15
Magnesium	5	3	5
Chloride	40	40	25
Acetate	44	52	54
Phosphate	3.5	3.5	7.5
Osmolarity (mosm/L)	405	470	450
pH	6.8	6.0	—
Supplied in (mL)	1000	1000	500 1000

Table 45–12.   Parenteral Crystalline Amino Acid Solutions
(g/100 g Total Amino Acids Present)

Essential	AMINOSYN 5% AMINOSYN 7% AMINOSYN 10%	FREAMINE II 8.5% (II)	FREAMINE III 8.5% (III)	TRAVASOL 5.5% TRAVASOL 8.5% TRAVASOL 10% (5.5/8.5%)	(10%)
L-Isoleucine	7.3	6.9	5.9	4.8	6.0
L-Leucine	9.5	9.1	7.7	6.2	7.3
L-Lysine	7.3*	10.2*	8.7*	5.8	5.8‡
L-Methionine	4.0	5.3†	4.5	5.8	4.0
L-Phenylalanine	4.4	5.6	4.8	6.2	5.6
L-Threonine	5.3	4.0	3.4	4.2	4.2
L-Tryptophan	1.7	1.5	1.3	1.8	1.8
L-Valine	8.0	6.6	5.6	4.5	5.8
	47.5	49.2	41.9	39.3	40.5
Nonessential	BCAA = 24.8%	22.6%	26.2%	15.5%	19.1%
L-Tyrosine	0.6	——	——	0.4	0.4
L-Alanine	12.9	7.1	6.0	20.7	20.7
L-Arginine	10.0	3.6	8.1	10.3	11.5
L-Histidine	3.0	2.8	2.4	4.4	4.8
L-Proline	8.8	11.2	9.5	4.2	6.8
L-Serine	4.3	5.9	5.0		5.0
L-Glycine	12.9	20.0	——	20.7	10.3
L-Cysteine HCl	——	0.2	0.2		
L-Aspartic Acid	——	——	——		——
L-Glutamic Acid	——	——	——	——	——
	52.5	50.8	31.2	60.7	59.5

This chart is designed to provide information on amino acid composition only. For full formula and prescribing information, consult product literature.

* Provided as acetate salt.
† Provided as D-L methionine.
‡ Provided as the HCl salt.

tein, fat, and carbohydrate for extended periods. The clinical biochemistry which is the basis for hyperalimentation has been extensively discussed (Blackburn and Harvey, 1981). Solution concentrations of 4.25 to 5% amino acids in 25% dextrose are customary. Feedings should provide caloric intake no greater than 130% of the patient's calculated basal energy expenditure. Commonly, this translates into 2000 to 2400 Kcal/day to meet the requirements of most postsurgical, critical care, or moderately injured patients.

The compositions of available solutions are presented in Table 45–12. Nonprotein calories may be supplied by glucose and fat. Lipid emulsions, 10 and 20%, can be piggybacked into the hyperalimentation solution of amino acids and glucose to allow administration via the central line. Alternatively, since emulsified fat does not exert an osmotic pressure and the caloric content is twice that of dextrose, 1500 to 2500 Kcal of lipids in 2 to 3 L can be administered through a peripheral vein.

Solution additives are shown in Table 45–

13. Special attention should be paid to potassium, magnesium, and phosphate since serious deficiencies in these nutrients can occur in several days if supplies are inadequate. Vitamin K, folic acid, and vitamin B_{12} should be provided initially and then at one-week intervals. Iron may be added daily. Owing to the

Table 45–13.   Additives

Sodium chloride (60 to 150 mEq per day)
Potassium chloride (60 to 100 mEq per day)
Calcium gluceptate (9.0 mEq per day)
Magnesium sulfate (8.1 mEq per day)
Potassium phosphate (30 to 45 mEq per day)
Sodium acetate (40 mEq per day)
Potassium acetate (as required)
Sodium phosphate (as required)
Trace minerals: Cu, Zn, Mn, Cr, and I (40 mL per day)
Ampul vitamins B and C (Tuesday through Saturday)
Vial multivitamins (MVI) (Monday)
Folic acid (0.5 to 1.5 g per week, Monday)
Vitamin B_{12} (50 to 100 μg per week, Monday)
Iron (1.0 to 2.0 mg per day)
Units heparin (6000 to 8000 units per day)
Units *per liter* regular insulin

high carbohydrate content of the hyperalimentation solution, fat-soluble vitamins are provided daily. At routine intervals, a trace mineral solution containing zinc, copper, manganese, chromium, and iodine should be administered, following the American Medical Association's recommendations for zinc, copper, chromium, and manganese in parenteral solutions (American Medical Association, 1979). The members of the nutrition support team should be familiar with the clinical signs and symptoms of trace mineral deficiency syndromes.

Hypertonic intravenous solutions are administered at slow rates initially (for example, 50 mL/hr for the first 24 hours) to allow adaptation to the glucose load. Full feeding rates can be achieved after two to three days. When insulin is necessary, routine six to eight hourly capillary blood glucose levels should be taken to regulate the insulin dose continuously as the glucose load is changed. A monitoring protocol should be designed including BUN, creatinine, and UUN values on a weekly basis. Routine laboratory work including serum electrolytes should be done Monday, Wednesday, and Friday of the first week and subsequently once or twice a week. Complete blood cell count, serum albumin, liver function tests, calcium, phosphorus, and magnesium levels are tested once weekly or biweekly. Medications should not routinely be administered piggyback via the central line as this increases the risk of infection and leaks.

When the patient receiving hyperalimentation can tolerate tube or oral feeding, or when no further oncologic treatment is planned, the patient is ordinarily weaned from parenteral hyperalimentation. Since rapid withdrawal of hyperalimentation can result in hypoglycemia, weaning should be gradual and patient blood sugar levels monitored.

Alternatively, if long-term parenteral nutritional support is required to sustain the patient with cancer, home total parenteral nutrition therapy may be indicated. Patients with gastrointestinal disability can successfully administer their solutions at home at about one-third the cost of hospital care (Blackburn et al., 1982). Patients with short bowel syndrome secondary to cancer resection or with radiation enteritis requiring prolonged nutritional support are candidates for home hyperalimentation.

Weiss et al. (1982) applied home total parenteral nutrition to carefully selected patients with recurrent incurable cancer for whom oral or tube feeding was impossible. Six of the nine patients studied benefited from a more normal life-style at home for three or more months rather than spending their final months confined to a hospital room.

The home technique is basically the same as the hospital technique except that, at home, the patient or the family takes responsibility for solution administration (Bothe et al., 1979). For long-term parenteral hyperalimentation, a Hickman catheter is recommended since this silastic catheter has two DACRON cuffs that help secure placement and also reduce the chance of ascending bacterial infection. At home, some patients can receive their entire volume of solution overnight allowing complete mobility during the day. Outpatient contact with the hospital nutrition support team continues during home total parenteral nutrition.

Total parenteral nutrition therapy is best administered and monitored by a team consisting of a physician, nurse, pharmacist, and dietitian. A group effort ensures that the therapy is successfully and safely administered in a fashion tailored to each patient's nutritional requirements (Nehme, 1980).

REFERENCES

Abrahm, J.; Mullen, J. L.; Jacobson, N.; and Polomano, R.: Continuous central venous access in patients with acute leukemia. Cancer Treat. Rep., 63:2099–2100, 1979.

American Medical Association, Department of Foods and Nutrition: Guidelines for essential trace element preparations for parenteral use. J.A.M.A., 241:2051, 1979.

Berstein, I. L.: Learned taste aversion in children receiving chemotherapy. Science, 200:1302–1303, 1978.

Bistrian, B. R.: Anthropometric norms used in assessment of hospitalized patients. Am. J. Clin. Nutr., 33:2211–2214, 1980.

Bistrian, B. R.: Assessment of hospital protein-calorie malnutrition. In Hill, G. (ed.): Nutrition and the Surgical Patient. Churchill Livingstone, Inc., Edinburgh, 1981.

Bistrian, B. R.: Nutritional assessment of the hospitalized patient: A critique and an update. In Wright, R. A., and Heymsfield, S. (eds.): Nutritional Assessment. Blackwell Scientific Publications, Inc., Boston, 1978.

Bistrian, B. R.; Blackburn, G. L.; Vitale, J.; Cochran, D.; and Naylor, J.: Prevalence of malnutrition in general medical patients. J.A.M.A., 235:1567–1570, 1976.

Bistrian, B. R., and Bothe, A., Jr.: Nutritional management of the patient with cancer. In Lokich, J. (ed.): Clinical Cancer Medicine. G. K. Hall & Company, Boston, 1980.

Bistrian, B. R.; Winterer, J.; Blackburn, G. L.; Young, V. R.; and Sherman, M.: Effect of a protein sparing diet and brief fast on nitrogen metabolism in mildly obese subjects. J. Lab. Clin. Med., 89:1030–1035, 1977.

Blackburn, G. L., and Bothe, A. F.: Assessment of malnutrition in cancer patients. *Cancer Bull.,* **30:**88–93, 1978.

Blackburn, G. L.; DiScala, C.; Miller, M. M.; Champagne, C.; Lahey, M.; Bothe, A., Jr.; and Bistrian, B. R.: Preliminary report on collaborative study for home parenteral nutrition patients. Second Bermuda Symposium on Clinical Nutrition, 1982.

Blackburn, G. L., and Harvey, K. B.: Nutrition in surgical patients. In Hardy, J. D. (ed.): *Surgery, Basic Principles and Practice.* J. B. Lippincott Company, New York, 1981.

Blackburn, G. L., and Harvey, K. B.: Nutritional assessment as a routine in clinical medicine. *Postgrad. Med.,* **71:**46–63, 1982.

Blackburn, G. L.; Maini, B. S.; Bistrian, B. R.; and McDermott, W. V., Jr.: The effect of cancer on nitrogen, electrolyte, and mineral metabolism. *Cancer Res.,* **37:**2348–2353, 1977.

Blackburn, G. L., and Wolfe, R. R.: Clinical biochemistry and intravenous hyperalimentation. In Alberti, K. G. M. M., and Price, C. P. (eds.): *Recent Advances in Biochemistry.* Churchhill Livingstone, Inc., Edinburgh, 1981.

Bothe, A., Jr.; Orr, G.; Bistrian, B. R.; and Blackburn, G. L.: Home hyperalimentation. *Compr. Ther.* **5:**54–61, 1979.

Bothe, A., Jr.; Wade, J. E.; and Blackburn, G. L.: Enteral nutrition. An overview. In Hill, G. L. (ed.): *Nutrition and the Surgical Patient.* Churchill Livingstone, Inc., New York, 1981.

Bray, G. A.: *Obesity in Perspective,* Vol. 2, Part 1, App. II, Table 1a. Department of Health, Education and Welfare, (NIH) 1975, p. 72.

Bray, G. A.: Intestinal bypass operation as a treatment for obesity. *Ann. Intern. Med.,* **85:**97–109, 1976.

Brennan, M. F.: Uncomplicated starvation versus cancer cachexia. *Cancer Res.,* **37:**2359–2364, 1977.

Brennan, M. F., and Copeland, E. M.: Panel report in nutritional support of patients with cancer. *Am. J. Clin. Nutr.,* **34:**1199–1205, 1981.

Burt, M. E.; Norton, J. A.; and Brennan, M. F.: The human tumor-bearing limit: An ex-vivo model. *Surgery,* **87:**128–132, 1980.

Cameron, I. L., and Paviat, W. A.: Stimulation of growth of a transplantable hepatoma in rats by parenteral nutrition. *J.N.C.I.,* **56:**597–601, 1976.

Carter, S. K.: Nutritional problems associated with cancer chemotherapy. In Newell, G. R., and Ellison, N. M. (eds.): *Nutrition and Cancer: Etiology and Treatment.* Raven Press, New York, 1981.

Conger, A. D.: Loss and recovery of taste acuity in patients irradiated to the oral cavity. *Radiat. Res.,* **53:**338–347, 1973.

Cooper, G. P.: Receptor origin of the olfactory bulb response to ionizing radiation. *Am. J. Physiol.,* **215:**803–806, 1968.

Copeland, E. M.: Total parenteral nutrition in cancer. *N. Engl. J. Med.,* **305:**1589, 1981.

Copeland, E. M.; Daly, J. M.; Ota, D. M.; and Dudrick, S. J.: Nutrition, cancer, and intravenous hyperalimentation, *Cancer,* **43:**2108–2116, 1979.

Copeland, E. M.; MacFadyen, B. V.; MacComb, W. S.; Guillamondegui, O.; Jesse, R. H.; and Dudrick, S. J.: Intravenous hyperalimentation in patients with head and neck cancer. *Cancer,* **35:**606–611, 1975.

Copeland, E. M.; MacFadyen, B. V. Jr.; McGown, C.; and Dudrick, S. J.: The use of hyperalimentation in patients with potential sepsis. *Surg. Gynecol. Obstet.,* **138:**377–380, 1974.

Copeland, E. M.; Souchon, E. A.; MacFadyen, B. V.; Rapp, M. A.; and Dudrick, S. J.: Intravenous hyperalimentation as an adjunct to radiation therapy. *Cancer,* **59:**608–616, 1977.

Daly, J. M.; Dudrick, S. J.; and Copeland, E. M.: Intravenous hyperalimentation: Effect of delayed cutaneous hypersensitivity in cancer patients. *Ann. Surg.,* **192:**587–592, 1980.

Daly, J. M.; Reynolds, H. M.; Rowland, B. J.; Baguero, G.; Dudrick, S. J.; and Copeland, E. M.: Nutritional manipulation of tumor-bearing animals: Effects on body weight, serum protein levels, and tumor growth. *Surg. Forum,* **29:**143–144, 1978.

DeWys, W. D.: Abnormalities of taste as a remote effect of a neoplasm. *Ann. N.Y. Acad. Sci.,* **230:**427–434, 1974.

DeWys, W. D., and Walters, K.: Abnormalities of taste sensation in cancer patients. *Cancer,* **36:**1888–1896, 1975.

Donaldson, S. S.: Nutritional consequences of radiotherapy. *Cancer Res.,* **37:**2407–2413, 1977.

Donaldson, S. S.: Nutritional problems associated with radiation therapy. In Newell, G. R., and Ellison, N. M. (eds.): *Nutrition and Cancer: Etiology and Treatment.* Raven Press, New York, 1981.

Donaldson, S. S., and Lenon, R. A.: Alterations of nutritional status. Impact of chemotherapy and radiation therapy. *Cancer,* **43:**2036–2052, 1979.

Dow, G. J., and Meyers, F. H.: The California Program for the investigational use of THC and marihuana in heterogeneous populations experiencing nausea and vomiting from anticancer therapy. *J. Clin. Pharmacol.,* 21(Suppl. 8–9):128S–132S, 1981.

Duke, J. H.; Jorgensen, S. B.; Broel, J. R.; Long, C. L.; and Kinney, J. M.: Contribution of protein to calorie expenditure following injury. *Surgery,* **68:**168–174, 1970.

Frisancho, A. R.: Triceps skinfold and upper arm muscle size norms for assessment of nutritional status. *Am. J. Clin. Nutr.,* **27:**1052–1059, 1974.

Gates, C., and Hans, P.: Psychologic complications of malignancy. In Lokich, J. (ed.): *Clinical Cancer Medicine Treatment Tactics.* G. K. Hall & Company, Boston, 1980.

Harrison, B. R., and Clenesk, P. T.: Continuous infusion — 5-fluorouracil via portable infusion pump. *Am. J. IV Ther. Clin. Nutr.,* **8:**51–62, 1981.

Harvey, K. B.; Bothe, A., Jr.; and Blackburn, G. L.: Nutritional assessment and patient outcome during oncologic therapy. *Cancer (Suppl.),* **43:**2065–2069, 1979.

Harvey, K. B.; Moldawer, L. L.; Bistrian, B. R.; and Blackburn, G. L.: Biological measures for the formulation of a hospital prognostic index. *Am. J. Clin. Nutr.,* **34:**2013–2022, 1981.

Heymsfield, S. B.; Bethel, R. A.; Ansley, J. D.; Gibbs, D. M.; Felner, J. M.; and Nutter, D. D.: Cardiac abnormalities in cachectic patients before and during nutritional repletion. *Am. Heart J.,* **95:**584–594, 1978.

Hill, G. L.; Blackett, R. L.; Pickford, J.; Burkinshaw, L.; Young, G. A.; Warren, J.; Schorah, C. J.; and Morgan, D. B.: Malnutrition in surgical patients: An unrecognized problem, *Lancet,* **1:**689–692, 1975.

Holroyde, C. P.; Gabuzda, T. G.; Putnam, R. C.; Paul, P.; and Reichard, G. A.: Altered glucose metabolism in metastatic carcinoma. *Cancer Res.,* **35:**3710–3714, 1975.

Hopkins, B. S.: Diagnosing bacterial complications of temporary central venous catheters. *Clin. Consult. Nutr. Supp.,* **2:**14–15, 1982.

Issell, B. F.; Valdivieso, M.; Zaren, H. A.; Dudrick, S. J.; Freireich, E.; Copeland, E. W.; and Bodey, G. P.: Protection against chemotherapy toxicity by IV hyperalimentation. *Cancer Treat. Rep.,* **62:**1139–1143, 1978.

Jelliffee, D. B.: *The Assessment of the Nutritional Status of the Community.* W.H.O., Geneva, 1966.

Kawamura, I.; Moldawer, L. L.; Keenan, R. A.; Batist, G.; Bothe, A., Jr.; Bistrian, B. R.; and Blackburn, G. L.: Altered amino acid kinetics in rats with progressive tumor growth. *Cancer Res.,* **42:**824–829, 1982.

Keys, A.; Brozek, J.; Henschel, A.; Mickelson, O.; and Taylor, H. L.: *The Biology of Human Starvation.* University of Minnesota Press, Minneapolis, 1950.

Kinsella, T. J.; Malcolm, A. W.; Bothe, A., Jr.; Valerio, D.; and Blackburn, G. L.: Prospective study of nutritional support during pelvic irradiation. *Int. J. Radiat. Oncol. Biol. Phys.,* **7:**543–548, 1981.

Lokich, J.; Bothe, A.; Fine, N.; and Perri, J.: Phase I study of protacted venous infusion of 5-fluorouracil. *Cancer,* **48:**2565–2568, 1981.

Lundholm, K.; Edstrom, S.; Ekman, L.; Karlberg, I.; Bylund, A. C.; and Schersten, T.: A comparative study of the influence of malignant tumor on host metabolism in mice and man. *Cancer,* **42:**453–461, 1978a.

Lundholm, K.; Holm, G.; and Schersten, T.: Insulin resistance in patients with cancer. *Cancer Res.,* **38:**4665–4670, 1978b.

Mitchell, E. P., and Schein, P. S.: Gastrointestinal toxicity of chemotherapeutic agents. *Semin. Oncol.,* **9:**52–64, 1982.

Moosman, D. A.: The anatomy of infraclavicular subclavian vein catheterization and its complications. *Surg. Gynecol. Obstet.,* **136:**71–74, 1973.

Morra, M. E.; Suski, N.; and Johnson, B. L.: *Recipes and Tips for Better Nutrition During Cancer Treatment.* United States Department of Public Health Services, Bethesda, Maryland, 1982.

Mullen, J. L.; Buzby, G. P.; Matthews, D. C.; Smale, B. F.; and Rosato, E. F.: Reduction of operative morbidity and mortality by combined preoperative and postoperative nutritional support. *Ann. Surg.,* **192:**604–613, 1980.

Müller, J. M.; Brenner, U.; Dienst C.; Pichlmaier, H.: Preoperative parenteral feeding in patients with gastrointestinal carcinoma. *Lancet,* **1:**68–71, 1982.

Munro, H. N.: A general survey of pathological changes in protein metabolism. In Munro, H. N., and Allison, J. B. (eds.): *Mammalian Protein Metabolism,* Vol. 2. Academic Press, Inc., New York, 1964.

Nehme, A. E.: Nutritional support of the hospitalized patient. *J.A.M.A.,* **243:**1906–1908, 1980.

Nixon, D. W.; Heymsfield, S. B.; Cohen, A. E.; Kutner, M.

H.; Ansley, J.; Lawson, D. H.; and Rudman, D.: Protein calorie malnutrition in hospitalized cancer patients. *Am. J. Med.,* **68:**683–690, 1980.

Norton, J. A.; Burt, M. E.; and Brennan, M. F.: In vivo utilization of substrate by human sarcoma-bearing limbs. *Cancer,* **45:**2934–2939, 1980.

Ohnuma, T., and Holland, J. F.: Nutritional consequences of cancer chemotherapy and immunotherapy. *Cancer Res.,* **37:**2395–2406, 1977.

Padberg, F. T.; Ruggiero, J. A.; and Blackburn, G. L.: Central venous catheterization for parenteral nutrition. *Ann. Surg.,* **193:**264–270, 1981.

Pollard, H. M. and the Pancreatic Cancer Task Force: Staging of cancer of the pancreas. *Cancer,* **47:**1631–1637, 1981.

Runcie, J., and Hilditch, T. E.: Energy provision, tissue utilization, and weight loss in prolonged starvation. *Br. Med. J.,* **2:**352–356, 1974.

Schein, P. S.; MacDonald, J. S.; Waters, C.; and Hardak, D.: Nutritional complications of cancer and its treatment. *Semin. Oncol.,* **2:**337–347, 1975.

Settle, R. G.; Quinn, M. R.; Brand, J. Q.; Kane, M. R.; Mullen, J. L.; and Brown, R.: Gustatory evaluation of cancer patients. In van Eys, J.; Seelig, M. S.; and Nichols, B. L. (eds.): *Nutrition and Cancer.* SP Medical and Scientific Books, New York, 1979.

Shils, M. E.: Effects on nutrition of surgery of the liver, pancreas, and genitourinary tract. *Cancer Res.,* **37:**2387–2394, 1977a.

Shils, M. E.: Nutritional problems associated with gastrointestinal and genitourinary cancer. *Cancer Res.,* **37:**2366–2372, 1977b.

Warnold, I.; Lundholm, K.; and Schersten, T.: Energy balance and body composition in cancer patients. *Cancer Res.,* **38:**1801–1807, 1978.

Waterhouse, C.: Lactate metabolism in patients with cancer. *Cancer,* **33:**66–71, 1974.

Waterhouse, C.; Jeanpretre, N.; and Keilson, J.: Gluconeogenesis from alanine in patients with progressive malignant disease. *Cancer Res.,* **39:**1968–1972, 1979.

Watkin, D. M.: Nitrogen balance as affected by neoplastic disease and its therapy. *Am. J. Clin. Nutr.,* **9:**446–460, 1961.

Weiss, S. M.; Worthington, P. H.; Prioleau, M.; and Rosato, F. E.: Home total parenteral nutrition on cancer patients. *Cancer,* **50:**1210–1213, 1982.

Williams, L. R., and Cohen, M. H.: Altered taste thresholds in lung cancer. *Am. J. Clin. Nutr.,* **31:**122–125, 1978.

Young, V. R.: Energy metabolism and requirements in the cancer patient. *Cancer Res.,* **37:**2336–2347, 1977.

46

Specific Considerations for the Geriatric Patient with Cancer

B. J. KENNEDY

Among the health, social, and economic problems older persons face, the complexities of medical care assume major importance. Cancer is among the more serious diseases affecting the elderly. With advancing age, the probability of developing cancer increases rapidly. Approximately 50% of all cancers occur in people over 65 years of age (Cutler and Young, 1975).

The probability of developing cancer between the ages of 20 and 40 is 1% for men and 1.5% for women, but between the ages of 65 and 85 it increases to 17% for women and 23% for men (Seidman *et al.,* 1978). The probability of developing cancer within the next five-year period is approximately 1 in 700 at the age of 25, but 1 in 14 at the age of 65 (Peto *et al.,* 1975).

Not only does cancer affect the older age group in our society disproportionately, but the nation's number of older persons is increasing and will constitute a larger percentage of the future population. In 1900 the over-65 age group represented 4.1% of the entire population. In 1975 this same age group represented 10% of the population. The number of persons over 65 years of age is estimated to more than double in the next 50 years, continuing to make cancer a major health problem among elderly Americans. People over 75 frequently have multiple diseases; this age population consumes five times more drugs per capita than do younger segments of the population. Recognizing that cancer is a common cause of disability and death in the elderly, specific diagnostic and therapeutic approaches and problems of clinical judgment are being emphasized in this chapter.

The incidence of most cancers increases with age, but appears to decline after 85 to 90 years of age (Lew, 1978). A few primary sites — stomach, colon and rectum, prostate in men, and breast in women — account for more than 40% of the invasive cancers in patients over 60 years of age (Cutler and Eisenberg, 1964). Lung cancer, common in elderly men, is becoming increasingly common in women and is projected to exceed the incidence of breast cancer by 1985. As physicians evaluate older patients, they must direct attention to areas where cancer most commonly occurs.

Past medical research has emphasized the treatment of neoplasms in the younger population and produced major accomplishments in curing acute leukemia in children, testis cancer, and Hodgkin's disease. Little systematic work has focused on older cancer patients with respect to diagnosis, behavior, and management. Many clinical studies excluded the aged patient by setting arbitrary age limitations. In recognition of this defect in the health care system, a recent directive of the National Institutes of Health removed age limits on research protocols it sponsors.

Studies of cancer and aging share many disciplines and resources. Clearly, cancer research may help to elucidate problems of aging and, conversely, research on aging may aid in understanding cancers (Butler and Gastel, 1979).

If all common causes of death in humans

were to be eliminated, their life-span would still be fixed at about 90 or 100 years (Hayflick, 1976). If the causes of death attributable to major cardiovascular and renal diseases were eliminated, a person born today would gain 11.8 years in life expectation. A 65-year-old would gain 11.4 years. Total elimination of cancer would result in an additional 2.5 years of life expectation for a newborn and 1.4 years for a 65-year-old person. The best approximation for the maximum human life-span is slightly over 100 years (Hayflick, 1980).

BIOLOGIC CHARACTERISTICS

It is uncertain whether age-related changes lead to cancer, whether aging and cancer result from a common process, or whether the two phenomena are the result of the lengthy period both require to develop (Butler and Gastel, 1979).

The same types of cancer exhibit different characteristics in the old and young. Cancers of the colon and breast, for example, are less aggressive in the elderly, whereas cancers of the cervix and thyroid behave in an opposite manner. Information-containing molecules in the genetic apparatus may induce the aging process (Hayflick, 1980). Similar hypotheses attempt to explain the development of cancer. The role of aging in the evolution of cancer involves many factors, including malignant transformation caused by various environmental carcinogens, alterations in hormonal regulation of various enzyme levels (Pitot, 1977), errors in stem cell maturation, and viral infection.

Cell-mediated immunity may play a major role in protecting against cancer. Immunologic surveillance seems to be inefficient for the elderly, thereby increasing susceptibility to malignant transformation (Penn, 1974). Experimental transplanted tumors in aged mice have revealed an increased take of tumor growth, a reduced latent period, accelerated growth rate, and increased therapy resistance.

The age-related decline in immune function may be the basis of aging and may contribute to the increased incidence of cancer with age (Kay, 1978). Age-associated decreases in immune function seem to accompany increases in tumor susceptibility (Butler and Gastel, 1979), although this concept is not accepted by all. People receiving immunosuppressive agents and those who suffer from immunode-

ficiency syndromes are at risk for developing certain types of cancers, particularly the lymphoproliferative neoplasms. Many of the age-associated increases in cancer incidence are the result of cumulative effects of environmental insult over a period of time. Age-related changes in immune function may have implications for results of therapy.

The animal tumor model is basic to the study of aging and cancer. Considerable standardization of animal use is necessary. Hollander (1973) emphasized the importance of specifying the maximum age and 50% survival time of the strain of animals used, rather than describing them as old when they reached a particular age. Spontaneous cancers in aged animals may be more valid models of human tumors than those induced by carcinogenic agents (Burton, 1977).

When benzpyrene was applied to the skin of mice at various ages, the increase in tumor incidence with age reflected the duration of exposure and was independent of age at the start of exposure (Peto et al., 1975). Other studies suggest that aging may increase the susceptibility of tissues to carcinogens (Ebbesen, 1973).

Epidemiologic studies have elucidated common mechanisms of aging and carcinogens. Sunlight is associated with both aging and cancer of the skin (Willis, 1978). Lung cancer, strongly associated with a history of smoking, is less prominent in elderly nonsmokers. Postmenopausal estrogen therapy, prescribed to alleviate age-associated changes, increased the risk of endometrial cancer (Antunes et al., 1979). Studies of elderly groups have demonstrated the lag time between exposure to carcinogens, such as asbestos and industrial chemicals, and the development of cancer. More extensive studies of cell biology, biochemistry, genetics, and epidemiology are needed to elucidate the relationship of aging and cancer (Butler and Gastel, 1979).

MANAGEMENT OF SPECIFIC NEOPLASMS

Most elderly patients benefit from careful consideration of specific, comprehensive management plans to defeat a cancer. Major cancer surgery in the elderly is justified when procedures are well planned and patients are carefully selected (Peterson and Kennedy, 1979). Most elderly patients will tolerate chemotherapy when used with appropriate caution. Other health problems must be considered in the management of a cancer in the aged patient. A nonmalignant disease may be of overriding importance and make the treatment of the cancer comparatively trivial. The patient's general health and the individual cancer are more important in cancer management than the patient's specific age. Radiotherapy may be an excellent alternative, especially in patients at risk from anesthesia.

Breast Cancer

In women, breast cancer is the most common cancer and the leading cause of death from cancer (Silverberg, 1985). The incidence increases with age; one-half of all patients with breast cancer are over 65 years (Haagensen, 1971). During the past 50 years, the mortality rate has remained relatively unchanged, giving rise to frequent claims that no progress has been made in treating this disease. Yet, with appropriate hormonal and chemotherapies, survival has been prolonged. Older women seem to have a slower growing disease process and a more indolent clinical course with metastatic disease. For untreated breast cancer, the average survival is 40 months for women between 45 and 75 years of age from the time of diagnosis (Haagensen, 1971). Survival after diagnosis and treatment seems to be improving among women over 75 years (Brian *et al.,* 1980), associated with a decline in the proportion of women with regional lymph node involvement or distant metastases on initial diagnosis, reflecting efforts to detect the disease earlier. Screening for breast cancer by mammography has recently been shown to result in earlier detection of breast cancer, hence improved survival in older women.

Surgery. As a primary treatment of breast cancer, surgery is as successful in the elderly as in younger patients. In women over 70 years of age, the overall five- and ten-year absolute survival rates of 54 and 41%, respectively, did not differ significantly from the survival rates of younger patients (Herbsman *et al.,* 1981). There is little justification for avoiding conventional operative treatment in elderly patients with breast cancer solely on the basis of advanced age, especially in view of the trend toward less aggressive surgery with decreased risk.

Radiation Therapy. Local excision of tumor with axillary node sampling and external beam radiation therapy has produced a survival rate comparable to that for radical mastectomy (Harris *et al.,* 1978; Veronesi *et al.,* 1981). Radiotherapy may be very appropriate for older women in whom aggressive surgery would be hazardous. Because long-term survival figures in the United States are not available, it is yet to be determined whether radiotherapy will supplement surgical procedures for the elderly patient.

The data regarding survival in older patients must be considered in light of the information regarding estrogen receptors. Patients with estrogen receptor-rich tumors have less recurrence following surgery than those with estrogen receptor-poor tumors. The incidence of estrogen-rich tumors increases with age, accounting for the favorable response in the elderly.

Adjuvant Chemotherapy. With the demonstration of antitumor effects of combination chemotherapy in metastatic breast cancer, chemotherapy as an adjuvant to surgery or radiotherapy is indicated. In patients with axillary node involvement on initial diagnosis (stage II), adjuvant chemotherapy in premenopausal women is well established. The rate of recurrence was decreased by one-half, and at seven years the survival time was increased. Postmenopausal women who received adjuvant chemotherapy did not seem to show the advantage (Bonadonna *et al.,* 1978). A more recent analysis of the same data, however, demonstrated that postmenopausal women who received a major portion of the calculated dose were benefited — evidence of significant dose relationship (Bonadonna and Valagussa, 1980). Few studies have included women over 65 or 70 years of age, hence, the role of adjuvant chemotherapy and the tolerance of more intensive chemotherapies in the elderly are undetermined.

Hormonal Therapy. The incidence of tumor regression with estrogen therapy steadily increases with age in postmenopausal women (Nathanson, 1951). Regression of metastatic breast cancer occurred in 18% of women under 60 years, 32% of women 60 to 69 years, 39% of women 70 to 79 years, and 59% of those 80 years of age and over ($P < 0.01$) (Stoll, 1973).

The older the postmenopausal patient, the greater amount of periductal elastic tissue hyperplasia is noted in untreated breast cancer. Those women undergoing regression of primary inoperable breast cancers during hormone therapy have a tenfold augmentation of this reactive process (Emerson *et al.,* 1953). In postmenopausal women tumors particularly susceptible to hormone-induced regression were characterized by abundant sclerosis and periductal elastic tissue hyperplasia.

A further explanation of this increased response rate is the higher incidence of estrogen receptor-containing tumors. In premenopausal women, only 40% had estrogen receptor-rich tumors, whereas, the incidence exceeded over 75% in women over 75 years of age (McGuire *et al.,* 1975). Approximately 55% of patients with estrogen-rich tumors respond to hormonal therapies.

Women more than ten years postmenopausal (56%) have responded at significantly higher rates to an estrogen antagonist than those less than ten years beyond the menopause (41%) (Manni *et al.,* 1979). The response rate is even greater if the patient had an estrogen receptor-rich tumor responsive to initial estrogen therapy. The elderly patient with other subsequent hormonal therapies continues to show a higher incidence of response to hormonal manipulation. Those patients initially responding to estrogen therapy are more likely to respond to hypophysectomy, adrenalectomy, or aminoglutethimide (Kennedy, 1981).

Hormonal therapy is of proven benefit in elderly women with metastatic breast cancer and may control the disease for an extended period of time. Increasing knowledge of the biologic characteristics of breast cancer in the elderly patient may produce selective and successive hormonal therapies to control the disease. In women with estrogen receptor-rich primary tumors, hormonal therapy may be the initial therapy.

Cytotoxic Chemotherapy. The response of breast cancer to cyclophosphamide does not vary appreciably with age, although response to 5-fluorouracil may decrease progressively (Broder and Tormey, 1974). Older patients with metastatic disease respond less than do younger patients to both phenylalanine mustard and the standard combination of cyclophosphamide, methotrexate, and 5-fluorouracil (Canellos *et al.,* 1976). Doxorubicin seems to be especially effective in older patients (Broder and Tormey, 1974) and in combination chemotherapy (Tranum *et al.,* 1978). Frequently, doses of chemotherapeutic agents are reduced in the elderly because of fear of inducing severe myelosuppression, perhaps inhibiting desired therapeutic effects. Estrogen recep-

tor-rich tumors have shown greater response to cytotoxic chemotherapy than estrogen receptor-poor tumors (Kiang *et al.,* 1978). Because of this observation, hormone therapy (diethylstilbestrol) and chemotherapy (5-fluorouracil plus cyclophosphamide) have been administered in combination. Although the response rate to the combination is similar to that when each modality is used in succession, survival rate seems greater in those receiving the treatments in combination (Kiang *et al.,* 1981).

Lung Cancer

Cancer of the lung occurs more frequently than any other cancer in men over the age of 75 and is the chief cause of cancer death. In the past 45 years, the death rate in men from lung cancer has increased 25-fold. The death rate is also increasing steadily in women and is projected to surpass that of breast cancer by 1985. Since most pulmonary cancers are related to the carcinogens in tobacco smoke, the duration of regular exposure correlates best with the incidence in a given population. Since a number of years must elapse before the onset of the disease, the population that places itself at risk will become apparent with the onset of the cancer in the older ages. Lung cancer probably is not a direct result of the aging process, but reflects the long period of time necessary to induce lung cancer from tobacco.

Surgery. The clinical course of unresected lung cancer in the elderly is as dismal as in younger patients, with 22% surviving at 6 months and 7% at 12 months (Evans, 1973). A careful assessment of cardiopulmonary function and a search for metastatic disease help select suitable candidates for thoracotomy. The operative mortality for pneumectomy and lobectomy in patients over 65 years of age is approximately twice that observed in younger patients with lung cancer (Evans, 1973). Approximately 15 to 30% of patients have resectable tumors, and of these 12 to 40% survive four or five years. This represents a very small proportion of all elderly patients with lung cancer. Nevertheless, they survive considerably longer than patients with tumors that cannot be resected. Surgery remains a primary therapeutic modality for those patients with resectable tumors. In the non-small cell carcinomas, the procedures required for curative resection carry considerable risk, and there is a general reluctance to subject aged patients to such procedures. Recently, the effectiveness of chemotherapy in small cell carcinoma has eliminated surgery as the primary treatment of this specific histologic type.

Radiotherapy. For unresectable lung cancers, radiotherapy may be effective (Lee, 1974). The patient must have adequate respiratory reserve to accommodate the loss of functional capacity with high-dose radiotherapy. Radiotherapy is advocated for limited disease, that is, disease confined to one side of the chest. Palliative radiotherapy to reduce bulky masses may correct bronchial obstruction and prevent secondary infections of the lung.

Chemotherapy. In small cell carcinoma of the lung, combination chemotherapy regimens regularly prove effective. Median survival has improved from 2 months to more than 12 months with intensive therapy (Livingstone *et al.,* 1978). A few patients have survived several years without therapy and appear to be cured. The fundamental agents currently employed include cyclophosphamide, doxorubicin, vincristine, cisplatin, nitrosoureas, and VP-16 (epipodophyllotoxin). Up to 91% of patients have responded to combination therapies (Greco *et al.,* 1979). Because of these excellent responses, surgery and radiotherapy have been reduced to supportive positions.

In non-small cell carcinoma, results of chemotherapy regimens are far from satisfactory. Although the current trend is to employ combination chemotherapy, phase I and phase II drugs are employed in investigative programs before using more standard agents that have little to offer.

The elderly patient with lung cancer invariably has emphysema and poor ventilatory function. These patients are more susceptible to pulmonary infection and rapidly become debilitated. Supportive therapies in nutrition, early use of antibiotics, and in some instances adrenocorticosteroids are essential to maintaining the well-being of the patient. The vast majority of elderly individuals with lung cancer will die of this disease.

Prostate Cancer

Cancer of the prostate is a disease of aging. In most patients, the disease is advanced when diagnosed, although routine examinations can detect it early.

Physical examination or autopsy reveals cancer of the prostate in 40 to 57% of men over 70 years of age (Waisman and Mott, 1978). The incidence of prostate cancer has increased more than 20% in the past 25 years and may reflect an increase in the older population. Survival in prostate cancer bears no relationship to the age at diagnosis, but correlates well with the extent of the disease at diagnosis (Corrieri *et al.,* 1970). No difference exists in the distribution of histologic grades when considering the age of diagnosis.

Local Management. Definitive or palliative surgical removal or radiotherapy or both are used to control local prostate cancer. Radical prostatectomy has been the accepted treatment for carcinoma of the prostate gland defined within the prostatic capsule. This procedure, however, results in impotence in all patients and incontinence in 10 to 15% (Mathes and Page, 1978). In the elderly age group, intercurrent illness and risk restrict the use of surgery. Instead, external beam irradiation has been of value (Bagshaw *et al.,* 1965). Iodine-125 implantation combined with pelvic lymphadenectomy has produced fewer side effects. The management of prostatic carcinoma in the elderly demands an interdisciplinary consideration of the various modalities.

Advanced Prostate Cancer. Advanced prostate cancer is successfully managed by bilateral orchiectomy or administration of estrogenic hormones. The benefits of estrogen therapy are attended by risk of cardiovascular complications (Blackard *et al.,* 1970; Byar, 1973). In this Veterans Administration study of patients over 55 years of age treated with estrogens, the mortality from cardiovascular events increased with age regardless of the presence or absence of identifiable underlying cardiovascular disease. Patients with preexisting cardiovascular disease were at nearly double the risk of dying compared to those of the same age without known cardiovascular disease. In subsequent studies the risk from cardiovascular disease decreased with reduction of the dose of estrogenic hormones. Considering the risk of estrogen therapy at the modified dose and death from cancer, estrogenic hormone in symptomatic patients is valid. The Veterans Administration's study showed that it was not necessary to treat a patient with advanced prostate cancer until the disease was symptomatic — there was no difference in survival rate.

Chemotherapy. With failure of hormonal manipulations, cytotoxic chemotherapy agents may be efficacious. Included among these are doxorubicin, cisplatin, 5-fluorouracil, and cyclophosphamide. Some of these have major toxic effects involving the cardiovascular and renal systems. In elderly patients, preexisting disease limits their use.

Leukemia

Chronic Lymphocytic Leukemia. Chronic lymphocytic leukemia accounts for one of every four cases of leukemia and is one of the principal hematologic neoplastic diseases of the elderly. A monoclonal accumulation of malignant B-cell lymphocytes, the disease is often considered indolent because the median survival is approximately six or more years. The increase in routine blood tests will enhance the likelihood of detecting chronic lymphocytic leukemia at an early stage in the elderly. During the course of the illness, the serum IgM tends to be low and the IgG progressively decreases. Ultimately, the patient becomes immunodeficient. One-third of these patients die of causes unrelated to the leukemia (Boggs *et al.*, 1966).

Chronic lymphocytic leukemia has a less favorable prognosis in the elderly with a median survival in patients over 60 to 70 years of age of 58 and 30 months, respectively (Boggs *et al.*, 1966; Zippin *et al.*, 1973), a shorter survival rate than for younger patients. The relatively poor median survival of patients over 70 years of age may be the result of the fact that the disease is more advanced at diagnosis in older individuals (Boggs *et al.*, 1966; Rai *et al.*, 1975). It is not established that chronic lymphocytic leukemia is more aggressive in the elderly.

Because of the broad clinical manifestations of chronic lymphocytic leukemia, a five-tiered clinical staging system has been proposed based on the prognostic significance in the accumulation of malignant lymphocytes over time (Rai *et al.*, 1975). Patients presenting only with lymphocytosis below 40,000 had median survival of more than 12 years. As the accumulation of lymphocytes increases, splenomegaly and hepatomegaly develop — unfavorable prognostic signs. When anemia and thrombocytopenia appear, median life expectancy is only 19 months. The prognostic significance of the staging system was apparently more important than such factors as age and sex (Silber, 1982). Age was statistically insignificant in prognosis.

Because of the long survival in patients with early detected chronic lymphocytic leukemia, the impact of specific therapy is difficult to measure, especially in patients over the age of 70. Many years are required to assess comparative treatment programs, and such studies are complicated by deaths from unrelated causes as the patient groups age. Treatment is usually initiated when specific signs and symptoms occur. Whether chemotherapy contributes to prolongation of survival is still to be proven, but benefit is implied.

Since patients with chronic lymphocytic leukemia are immunosuppressed, they are more susceptible to developing second primary neoplasms. The incidence of a second cancer is approximately 15% and especially occurs in patients with abnormal electrophoretic patterns (Gunz and Angur, 1965). The specific lesions include skin cancers, colorectal cancer, lung cancer, and multiple myeloma. A patient with chronic lymphocytic leukemia should be thoroughly screened at least every two years for other neoplasms. Once second cancers are detected, treatment should be as aggressive as in a patient without chronic lymphocytic leukemia.

Acute Nonlymphocytic Leukemia. Approximately 40% of acute nonlymphocytic leukemia occurs in patients over 60 years of age, and the incidence appears to be rising (Gunz and Hough, 1956; Cutler *et al.*, 1967). Advancing age adversely affects prognosis (Peterson, 1982) and continues to influence the philosophy of treatment of older patients with acute leukemia. The fact that the population of the United States is proportionally growing older with a striking increase in the incidence of leukemia in the elderly makes this disease in aged persons a significant health problem. Of all of the adults with leukemia encountered, 35 to 40% are over 60 years of age (Cutler *et al.*, 1967). The elderly constitute a major segment of patients afflicted by acute leukemia and are characterized by at least one adverse prognostic variable, which is age. Some types of acute nonlymphocytic leukemia in elderly patients may be clinically and biologically different from that seen in younger patients. A significant difference has not been observed according to morphologic subtypes (Bloomfield and Theologides, 1973).

Equivalent proportions of older and younger patients seem sensitive to the cytotoxic effects of the drugs (Peterson, 1982). The major reason for the poorer prognosis in the elderly is that they tolerate the rigors of having leukemia and the effects of chemotherapeutic intervention less well than do younger patients; hence, the elderly have a larger proportion of treatment-related deaths.

The aging process affects a variety of organs and tissues. The impairment of these systems may not be apparent until the particular system or the entire host is placed under stress. Under these new conditions, the aged patient with leukemia may be unable to meet the additional demands caused by the disease and therapy and the decompensation that ensues.

The physiology of aging produces important alterations in the pharmacologic absorption, metabolism, and excretion of chemotherapeutic agents, antiemetics, and antibiotics. Because of the underlying status of coronary circulation and the myocardium, the heart may not withstand the stress presented by hemorrhage, anemia, and infection as well as the potential cardiotoxic effects of the anthracycline antibiotics.

A major factor in an older person's ability to withstand or recover from treatment is the resiliency or regenerative capacity of the aging marrow after intensive chemotherapy. Elderly patients tolerate myelosuppressive and other toxic effects of chemotherapy less well than do younger patients. However, the time it takes for marrow to regenerate after treatment does not differ between younger and older individuals (Rai et al., 1981), therefore, this factor may not account for the lower response rate to treatment. It is the ability to survive the period of myelosuppression that compromises the elderly (Peterson, 1982). Another factor is that renal function deteriorates approximately three times more often in the elderly than in young patients being treated specifically for acute leukemia.

The untreated elderly patient with acute leukemia is more susceptible to early death than treated elderly patients. When the elderly die after intensive chemotherapy, it is the result of toxicity and complications rather than from persistence of the leukemia. Even before therapy, the elderly patients have a higher incidence of infection (Rai et al., 1981).

Since attaining remission is the primary factor in determining life expectancy for all patients regardless of age, induction chemotherapy has become the focus of investigation for managing acute nonlymphocytic leukemia. Neither advances in supportive care nor the most efficacious drugs used as single agents provided an adequate opportunity for the elderly to achieve remissions, so the philosophy arose not to treat patients in the older age group. The introduction of cytosine arabinoside and daunorubicin accomplished complete remission in 25 to 50% of younger patients, but the response in elderly patients was substantially lower. These combinations of chemotherapies did imply that more intensive chemotherapy would be effective.

In a 1973 study, elderly patients who achieved complete remission benefited as greatly as younger patients in duration of remission and prolonged length of survival (Bloomfield and Theologides, 1973). In a subsequent study of intensive chemotherapy, the complete remission rate in patients 60 to 70 years of age was 50%, similar to that in younger patients (Peterson and Bloomfield, 1977). The overall survival of patients 60 to 70 years of age was comparable to that seen in young patients. Only 8% of patients over 70 years of age, however, achieved remission. Combination chemotherapy in other studies produced complete remissions exceeding 60% in adults under 50 years, 55% in patients 50 to 65 years, and 30% or more in those over 65 years of age (Rai et al., 1981; Keating et al., 1981). An increasingly high percentage of elderly patients are now undergoing complete remission. The elderly are also among the patients who are long-term disease-free survivors and in whom cure is implied (Peterson et al., 1980).

The new advances in treating elderly leukemia patients have resulted from raising the doses of individual drugs, improving the dosage schedule, adding new effective agents to the therapeutic regimens, and providing comprehensive supportive care. The latter includes antibiotic therapy, leukapheresis, and leukocyte and platelet transfusions. Elderly patients now have a better opportunity to benefit from intensive induction treatment, and their management must reflect this improved prognosis.

Lymphoma

Age is an important factor in studying the biology of Hodgkin's disease and non-Hodgkin's lymphomas. During the past ten years a major change has occurred in the understanding of malignant lymphomas and their management.

Hodgkin's Disease. Hodgkin's disease accounts for only 1% of all new cancers in the United States. It has a bimodal age-incidence curve peaking in the late twenties, then declining to age 45 after which the incidence increases steadily with age (Cutler and Young, 1975). The combination chemotherapies have had a major impact on survival of patients with advanced Hodgkin's disease. A major prognostic factor influencing complete response, response duration, and survival is age. For patients over 60 years of age, few data are available regarding the course of Hodgkin's disease. The Southwest Oncology Group (Coltman, 1980), using MOPP alone, produced a lower fail rate in young patients than in older patients. Moreover, the survival rate was better for those under 40 years than over that age. However, the group over 60 years had a better survival than those 40 to 60 years of age.

The Cancer and Leukemia Group B assessed its results in 385 patients with multidrug combination chemotherapies in advanced Hodgkin's disease according to age (Peterson et al., 1982). The response rate was 70% in 205 patients less than 40 years of age, 66% in 107 patients between 40 and 59 years, and 40% in 73 patients greater than 60 years of age. The difference in the complete response rate between patients of less than 60 years and those greater than 60 years of age was significant ($P = 0.0001$). Age at the time of diagnosis was the predominant factor affecting response. The response rate was not significantly higher in those older patients who received full doses of chemotherapy.

Age was also associated with an increased frequency of serious leukopenia and thrombocytopenia. Once in complete remission, patients over 60 years of age experience the shortest median time to recurrence — 33 months. The low complete response rate and the short duration of remission in the patients greater than 60 years of age resulted in a median survival time of 18 months.

Dose and adherence to time schedules during early MOPP chemotherapy may influence the frequency of response. On the other hand, when the analysis was restricted to older patients who received greater than 90% of the projected drug doses, the complete remission rate, the median time to recurrence (20 months), and the duration of survival (27 months) were much shorter than in younger patients.

The frequency of toxicity and complications and the absence of an identifiable effect of dose on response suggest that different combinations of drugs or alternative treatment schedules are needed for older patients. Perhaps durable remissions are observed less frequently as age increases because of the distinct biologic behavior of Hodgkin's disease in older adults or because of modifications in host factors associated with aging (Peterson et al., 1982). A careful analysis of therapy results will aid in developing more adequate treatment programs for the elderly.

Non-Hodgkin's Lymphocytic Lymphoma. Stage III and stage IV of non-Hodgkin's lymphocytic lymphoma are not curable by any known therapy (Rosenberg, 1979). Yet they are responsive to chemotherapy and tend to have an indolent course. Patients over 50 years of age with minimal disease can be observed over a period of months before a treatment program is recommended. A few elderly patients may never require treatment (Rosenberg, 1979). Other elderly patients may have a striking objective regression of bulky tumor, but never attain a complete remission. Foci of lymphoma cells may remain in the bone marrow. Even patients with a good but incomplete remission may not require maintenance chemotherapy.

Other Cancers

Colorectal Cancer. Cancer of the colon and rectum is the second most common form of cancer in men and women. Cancers of the entire gastrointestinal tract comprise between 25 and 44% of all cancers occurring after 75 years of age (Cutler and Eisenberg, 1964).

Early detection can result in management by surgery, with 85% of patients with stage I disease surviving five years. Unfortunately, in many elderly patients the diagnosis of colorectal cancer is made in the late phase of the disease because the elderly do not obtain routine health examinations. This precludes any chance for cure by surgery. The role of radiotherapy in managing colorectal cancer in the elderly remains unanswered. In some elderly patients, when surgery is a risk, fulguration may be the primary treatment for small cancers less than 10 cm from the anus. Polypoid lesions at any site are also treatable by this method.

For advanced disease, the effectiveness of chemotherapy is limited. In patients 49 to 60 years of age, 19% obtain objective regression with 5-fluorouracil. In those over 70 years of age, ony 8% have achieved regression (Moertel and Reitemeier, 1969). This may reflect the reluctance of physicians to use intensive doses of chemotherapeutic agents in older patients. A cooperative group study, however, had a response rate of 10% for patients less than 70 and 9% for those greater than 70 (Begg and Carbone, 1983).

Skin Cancer. So-called aged skin is a result not of the natural aging process, but primarily of exposure to sunlight. Elastotic degeneration of sun-exposed skin begins in early adult life, and each prolonged exposure to the sun irreversibly damages the skin. This cumulative damage characterizes the appearance of the skin in the elderly.

The vast majority of skin cancers, especially in men, are caused by overexposure to the sun. Farmers, fishermen, and those living at high altitudes are especially prone to this disease; hence long-term exposure to the toxin, sun, results in increasing occurrence of cancer in the elderly. In 25% of persons with senile or actinic keratoses, squamous cell cancer ultimately develops in one or more lesions (Willis, 1978). Sun screen agents can protect against the harmful effects of sunlight. Once the damage has occurred, however, benign and premalignant keratoses and superficial malignancies should be removed by the methods available.

Glioblastoma. After radiation therapy and chemotherapy for malignant glioblastoma multiforme, patients under 50 years of age survive longer than patients over 50. Without treatment, these age groups have similar survival times (Rosenblum *et al.,* 1982). In a study of *in vitro* sensitivity testing of clonogenic cells obtained from biopsy specimens, seven of eight patients under the age of 50 were sensitive to CCNU compared with only one of eight older patients. Patient age was inversely correlated with *in vitro* cell kill, and patients with sensitive cells were significantly younger than those with resistant cells. Influence of age on survival after treatment is probably the result of an inherent difference in the sensitivity of clonogenic cells to radiation or chemotherapeutic agents or both (Rosenblum *et al.,* 1982).

In 625 patients with surgically resected malignant glioblastoma multiforme, the median survival was 21 months for patients less than 40 years of age, 9 months for patients aged 40 to 60, and 6 months for those over 60 (Horton *et al.,* 1982). It was concluded that the addition of chemotherapy with BCNU or MeCCNU plus DTIC to radiotherapy provided significant long-term survival benefit for patients under 60, but no benefit for patients over that age. In the older age group no patient survived beyond two years.

Adverse Drug Reactions in the Elderly

Approximately 25% of the prescription drugs sold in this country are taken by 11% of the population — those over 65 years of age. Seventy percent of drugs taken by the elderly are nonprescription. When social drugs such as alcohol, caffeine, and nicotine are added, the nation's elderly use an average of 5.6 different drugs each day. Senility is sometimes the mistaken diagnosis for a person suffering only from confusion or other conditions related to too much medicine. When the elderly do seek help, they often see a number of different physicians for their ailments. Deteriorating eyesight, hearing, or memory may also contribute to errors in self-medication among the elderly (Pharmacopeial Convention, 1982).

Increased frequency of adverse drug reactions with a variety of agents is associated with increasing age. In many commonly used agents, age itself cannot be isolated as the sole biologic factor explaining the association of toxicity with age. Age is closely related to increased severity and duration of disease, which themselves lead to more frequent toxicity (Greenblatt *et al.,* 1982).

Older patients often have been excluded from chemotherapy clinical trials in order to avoid adverse effects. In adjuvant chemotherapy studies of stage II breast cancer, most patients over age 70 were excluded. Yet this same age group has an increasing incidence of that disease. Given the therapeutic effectiveness of chemotherapy in several tumor systems, the elderly should be included in clinical studies with special emphasis on developing appropriate treatment regimens.

Although the bone marrow in an elderly patient is less functional, it has the ability to recover from myelosuppressive chemotherapy. Unexpected neutropenia or thrombocytopenia can occur. With agents that impair cardiac or pulmonary function, the elderly patient requires special monitoring since cardiac and pulmonary reserve may be limited. With adequate caution, elderly patients can tolerate full doses of chemotherapy. The apparent increased frequency of adverse reactions to certain drugs in the elderly, the clinical impressions of increased drug sensitivity in old age, and the limitations in treating the elderly with chemotherapy have stimulated research focusing on the biologic mechanisms of drug toxicity in the elderly.

Drug Distribution. Changes in body composition with age may influence drug distribution. On the average, in the aging person lean body mass declines and adipose tissue mass increases in relation to total body weight. The distribution of extensively protein-bound drugs may also be influenced by changes in the extent of binding to plasma protein. An age-related decline in plasma albumin concentrations has been consistently reported. Changes in the function of the gastrointestinal tract in old age include a reduction in gastric parietal cell function leading to impaired acid secretion and an elevation in gastric pH (Geokas and Haverback, 1969). Reduced rates of gastric emptying have been described. Yet, essentially no available evidence supports impaired drug absorption in old age or that the extent of gastrointestinal absorption is importantly altered (Greenblatt *et al.,* 1982).

Drug Clearance. The mechanisms of hepatic excretion of drugs and their alteration with old age are complex. Hepatic function tests do not necessarily reflect drug-metabolizing capacity. The function of hepatic microsomal enzymes for oxidative drug metabolism may be impaired in old age leading to reduced drug clearance. Hepatic blood flow is a major determinant of total clearance in a number of commonly used drugs. An estimated 40 to 45% reduction in total liver blood flow may be observed in elderly persons as compared to young adults (Geokas and Haverback, 1969).

The glomerular filtration rate declines predictably in old age with a mean 35% reduction in the elderly as compared with the young. The decline in renal function in the elderly (Rowe *et al.,* 1976) may not cause a meaningful elevation in serum creatinine concentration. Creatinine clearance is a more reliable indicator of renal function. The renal function as measured by creatinine clearance is impaired in the elderly. Because of this, older patients have been excluded from studies using cisplatin because of its renal toxic effect.

In a study of creatinine clearance during cisplatin therapy, there was an 8 mL/minute loss of creatinine clearance per course for patients under 40, and a 2.4 mL/minute loss for patients over 60. The conclusion was that nephrotoxicity of cisplatin does not worsen with advancing age. In fact, older patients may have less nephrotoxicity than younger patients; hence, the older patient should be treated as aggressively as a younger patient (Hrushesky *et al.,* 1984).

The susceptibility of patients over 70 years of age to cancer chemotherapy was compared to patients less than 70 years (Begg and Carbone, 1983). In general, elderly patients have rates of severe toxicity identical to their younger counterparts. In a few of the studies, a greater hematologic reaction was noted with methotrexate and methyl CCNU. Not treating elderly patients as aggressively as younger patients or excluding elderly patients from protocols is not justified. Rather, exclusions should be based on physiologic functional parameters and not on an arbitrary age limit. This supports the recent directive from the National Cancer Institute prohibiting age restriction in clinical studies of cancer chemotherapy.

Cardiac Toxicity. Doxorubicin is associated with the development of cardiomyopathy with an overall incidence of doxorubicin-induced congestive heart failure of 2.2%. This toxicity is related to the total dose of doxorubicin administered with a continuum of increasing risk. Age is a risk factor for developing doxorubicin-induced congestive heart failure, which occurred in patients older than 60 at three times the rate of those younger. The degree of disparity increases as the total dose of doxorubicin increases (Praga *et al.,* 1979).

Quackery. Older patients are more susceptible to hustlers of cancer remedies. Speedy cures, secret tests and drugs, special diets, and faith healers attract the elderly. In many instances the elderly may choose these types of remedies instead of following the potential curative therapies of the medical care system. Moreover, even the children of elderly patients may succumb to the appeals of quackery.

Coping

The problems of supportive management in elderly patients with cancer are complex. Management of pain, nausea, and drug interreactions, as well as the patient's emotional, social, and economic needs, must be emphasized. The elderly may decline diagnostic and therapeutic procedures because they do not understand recent advances in medical care and believe that cancer is hopeless. The family should participate in decisions about therapy, which frequently involve socioeconomic aspects of care. Patient-group counseling programs, family counseling, and home health care services can provide supportive care.

The incidence of cancer increases with advancing age. The complications of the disease, as well as the complications of therapies, add stress to a biologic system already decompensating as the result of the process of aging. By focusing attention on the elderly, concepts of therapy appropriate for that age group are being developed. Decisions on diagnosis and treatment can be made based on an individual need (Kennedy, 1983).

REFERENCES

Antunes, C. M. F.; Stolley, P. D.; Rosenshein, N. B.; Davies, J. L.; Tonascia, J. A.; Brown, C.; Burnett, L.; Rutledge, A.; Pokempner, M.; and Garcia, R.: Endometrial cancer and estrogen use. Report of a large case-control study. *N. Engl. J. Med.,* **300:**9–13, 1979.

Bagshaw, M. A.; Kaplan, H. S.; and Sagerman, R. H.: Linear accelerator supervoltage radiotherapy. VII. Carcinoma of the prostate. *Radiology,* **85:**121–129, 1965.

Begg, C. B., and Carbone, P. P.: Clinical trials and drug toxicity in the elderly: The experience of the Eastern Cooperative Oncology Group. *Cancer,* **52:**1986–1992, 1983.

Blackard, C. E.; Doe, R. P.; Mellinger, G. T.; and Byar, D. P.: Incidence of cardiovascular disease and death in patients receiving diethylstilbestrol for carcinoma of the prostate. *Cancer,* **26:**249–256, 1970.

Bloomfield, C. D., and Theologides, A.: Acute granulocytic leukemia in elderly patients. *J.A.M.A.,* **226:**1190–1193, 1973.

Boggs, D. R.; Sofferman, S. A.; Wintrobe, M. M.; and Cartwright, G. E.: Factors influencing the duration of survival of patients with chronic lymphocytic leukemia. *Am. J. Med.,* **40:**243–254, 1966.

Bonadonna, G., and Valagussa, P.: Dose response effect of CMF in breast cancer. *Proc. Am. Soc. Clin. Oncol.,* **21:**413, 1980.

Bonadonna, G.; Valagussa, P.; Rossi, A.; Zucali, R.; Tancini, G.; Bajetta, E.; Brambilla, C.; De Lena, M.; Di Fronzo, G.; Banfi, A.; Rilke, F.; and Veronesi, U.: Are surgical adjuvant trials altering the course of breast cancer? *Semin. Oncol.,* **5:**450–464, 1978.

Brian, D. D.; Melton, L. J., III; Goellner, J. R.; Williams, R. L.; and O'Fallon, W. M.: Breast cancer incidence, prevalence, mortality and survivorship in Rochester, Minnesota, 1935 to 1974. *Mayo Clin. Proc.,* **55:**355–359, 1980.

Broder, L. E., and Tormey, D. C.: Combination chemotherapy of carcinoma of the breast. *Cancer Treat. Rev.,* **1:**183–203, 1974.

Burton, A. C.: Why do human cancer death rates increase with age? A new method of analysis of the biology of cancer. *Perspect. Biol. Med.,* **20:**327–344, 1977.

Butler, R. N., and Gastel, B.: Aging and cancer management. Part II: Research perspectives. *CA,* **29:**333–340, 1979.

Byar, D. P.: Proceedings: The Veterans Administration Cooperative Urological Research Group's studies of cancer of the prostate. *Cancer,* **32:**1126–1130, 1973.

Canellos, G. P.; Pocock, S. J.; Taylor, S. G., III; Sears, M. E.; Klaasen, D. J.; and Band, P. R.: Combination chemotherapy for metastatic breast carcinoma. Prospective comparison of multiple drug therapy with L-phenylalanine mustard. *Cancer,* **38:**1882–1886, 1976.

Coltman, J. A., Jr.: Chemotherapy of advanced Hodgkin's disease. *Semin. Oncol.,* **7:**155–173, 1980.

Corrieri, J. N., Jr.; Cornog, J. L.; and Murphy, J. J.: Prognosis in patients with carcinoma of the prostate. *Cancer,* **25:**911–918, 1970.

Cutler, S. J., and Eisenberg, H.: Cancer in the aged. *Ann. N.Y. Acad. Sci.,* **114:**771–781, 1964.

Cutler, S. J., and Young, J. L. (eds.): Third National Cancer Survey: Incidence Data, *Natl. Cancer Inst. Monogr.,* **41,** 1975.

Cutler, S. J.; Axtell, L.; and Heise H.: Ten thousand cases of leukemia: 1940–1962. *J.N.C.I.,* **39:**993–1026, 1967.

Ebbesen, P.: Papilloma induction in different aged skin grafts to young recipients. *Nature,* **241:**280–281, 1973.

Emerson, W. J.; Kennedy, B. J.; Graham, J. M.; and Nathanson, I. T.: Pathology of primary and recurrent carcinoma of the tumor breast after administration of steroid hormones. *Cancer,* **6:**641–670, 1953.

Evans, E. W.: Resection for bronchial carcinoma in the elderly. *Thorax,* **28:**86–88, 1973.

Geokas, M. C., and Haverback, B. J.: The aging gastrointestinal tract. *Am. J. Surg.,* **117:**881–982, 1969.

Greco, F. A.; Richardson, R. L.; Snell, J. P.; Stroup, S. L.; and Oldham, R. K.: Small cell lung cancer complete remission and improved survival. *Am. J. Med.,* **66:**625–630, 1979.

Greenblatt, D. J.; Sellers, E. M.; and Shader, R. I.: Drug disposition in old age. *N. Engl. J. Med.,* **306:**1081–1088, 1982.

Gunz, F. W., and Angur, H. B.: Leukemia and cancer in the same patient. *Cancer,* **18:**145–152, 1965.

Gunz, F. W., and Hough, R. F.: Acute leukemia over the age of fifty: A study of its incidence and natural history. *Blood,* **11:**882–901, 1956.

Haagensen, C. D.: *Diseases of the Breast,* 2nd ed. W. B. Saunders Company, Philadelphia, 1971.

Harris, J. R.; Levene, M. B.; and Hellman, S.: The role of radiation therapy in the primary treatment of carcinoma of the breast. *Semin. Oncol.,* **5:**403–416, 1978.

Hayflick, L.: Biology of aging. *N. Engl. J. Med.,* **295:**1302–1308, 1976.

Hayflick, L.: The cell biology of human aging. *Roche Seminars on Aging,* **2:**3–11, 1980.

Herbsman, H.; Feldman, J.; Seldera, J.; Gardner, B.; and Alfonson, A. E.: Survival following breast cancer surgery in the elderly. *Cancer,* **47:**2358–2363, 1981.

Hollander, C. F.: Animal models for aging and cancer research. *J.N.C.I.,* **51:**3–5, 1973.

Horton, J.; Chang, C.; and Schoenfield, D.: Influence of age on effectiveness of multi-model treatment for malignant brain glioma. *Proc. Am. Assoc. Cancer Res.,* **23:**119, 1982.

Hrushesky, W. J. M.; Shimp, W.; and Kennedy, B. J.: Lack of age-dependent cisplatin nephrotoxicity. *Am. J. Med.,* **76:**579–584, 1984.

Kay, M. M. B.: The effects of aging on immune function. In Walters, H. (ed.): *The Handbook of Cancer Immunology,* Vol. I. Garland Publishing, Inc., New York, 1978.

Keating, M. J.; Smith, T. L.; Gehan, E. A.; McCredie, K. B.; Bodey, G. P.; Spitzer, G.; Hersh, E.; Gutterman, J.; and Freireich, E. J.: Factors related to length of complete remission in adult acute leukemia. *Cancer,* **45:**2017–2029, 1980.

Keating, M. J.; Smith, T. L.; McCredie, K. B.; Bodey, G. P.; Hersh, E. M.; Gutterman, J. U.; Gehan E.; and Freireich, E. J.: A four-year experience with anthracycline, cytosine, arabinoside, vincristine, and prednisone combination chemotherapy in 325 adults with acute leukemia. *Cancer,* **47:**2779–2788, 1981.

Kennedy, B. J.: Endocrine extirpation, estrogen antagonists, and adrenal gland inhibitors in the hormonal management of postmenopausal women with breast cancer. In Harris, J. (ed.): *Reviews on Endocrine-Related Cancer.* Imperial Chemical, Wilmington, Delaware, 1981.

Kennedy, B. J.: Clinical oncology focus on the elderly. In Yaneik, R. (ed): *Perspectives on Prevention and Treatment of Cancer in the Elderly.* Raven Press, New York, 1983.

Kiang, D. T.; Frenning, D. H.; Gay, J.; Goldman, A. I. and Kennedy, B. J.: Combination therapy of hormone and cytotoxic agents in advanced breast cancer. *Cancer,* **47:**452–456, 1981.

Kiang, D. T.; Frenning, D. H.; Goldman, A. I.; Ascensao, V. F.; and Kennedy, B. J.: Estrogen receptors and responses to chemotherapy and hormonal therapy in advanced breast cancer. *N. Engl. J. Med.,* **299:**1330–1334, 1978.

Lee, R. E.: Radiotherapy of bronchogenic carcinoma. *Semin. Oncol,* **1:**245–252, 1974.

Lew, E. A.: Cancer in old age. *CA,* **28:**2–6, 1978.

Livingston, R. B.; Moore, T. N.; Heilbrun, L.; Bottomley, R.; Lehane, D.; Rivkin, S. E.; and Thigpen, T.: Small-cell carcinoma of the lung: Combined chemotherapy and radiation. A Southwest Oncology Group Study. *Ann. Intern. Med.,* **88:**194–199, 1978.

Manni, A.; Trujillo, J. E.; Marshall, J. S.; Brodkey, J.; and Pearson, O. H.: Antihormone treatment of stage IV breast cancer. *Cancer,* **43:**444–450, 1979.

Mathes, G. L., and Page, R. C.: An alternative to radical surgery for cancer of the prostate. *Geriatrics,* **33:**53–54, 1978.

McGuire, W. L.; Pearson, O. H.; and Segaloff, A.: Predicting hormone responsiveness in human breast cancer. In McGuire, W. L.; Carbone, P. P.; and Vollmer, E. P. (eds.): *Estrogen Receptors in Human Breast Cancer.* Raven Press, New York, 1975.

Moertel, C. G., and Reitemeier, R. J.: Clinical features influencing therapeutic response to fluorinated pyrimidines. In Moertel, C. G., and Reitemeier, R. (eds.): *Advanced Gastrointestinal Cancer: Clinical Management and Chemotherapy.* Hoeber, New York, 1969.

Nathanson, I. T.: Sex hormones and castration in advanced breast cancer. *Radiology,* **56:**535–552, 1951.

Penn, I.: Occurrence of cancer in immune deficiencies. *Cancer,* **34:**858–866, 1974.

Peterson, B. A.: Acute nonlymphocytic leukemia in the elderly: Biology and treatment. In Bloomfield, C. D. (ed.): *Adult Leukemia.* Martinus Nijhoff Publishers, The Hague, Netherlands, 1982.

Peterson, B. A., and Bloomfield, C. D.: Treatment of acute nonlymphocytic leukemia in elderly patients: A prospective study of intensive chemotherapy. *Cancer,* **40:**647–652, 1977.

Peterson, B. A., and Kennedy, B. J.: Aging and cancer management. Part I: Clinical observations. *CA,* **29:**322–332, 1979.

Peterson, B. A.; Bloomfield, C. D.; Bosl, G. J.; Gibbs, G.; and Malloy, M.: Intensive five-drug combination chemotherapy for adult acute nonlymphocytic leukemia. *Cancer,* **46:**663–668, 1980.

Peterson, B. A.; Pajak, T. F.; Cooper, M. R.; Nissen, N. I.; Glidewell, O. J.; Holland, J. F.; Bloomfield, C. D.; and Gottlieb, A. J.: Effect of age on therapeutic response and survival in advanced Hodgkin's disease. *Cancer Treat. Rep.,* **66:**889–898, 1982.

Peto, R.; Roe, F. J. C.; Lee, P. N.; Levy, L.; and Clack, J.: Cancer and ageing in mice and men. *Br. J. Cancer,* **32:**411–426, 1975.

Pharmacopeial Convention: Adverse drug reactions in the elderly. *About Your Medicines,* **2:**1–2, 1982.

Pitot, H. C.: Carcinogenesis and aging—two related phenomena? A review. *Am. J. Pathol.,* **87:**444–472, 1977.

Praga, C.; Beretta, G.; Vigo, P. L.; Lenaz, G. R.; Pollini, C.; Bonadonna, G.; Canetta, R.; Castellani, R.; Villa E.; Gallagher, C. G.; von Melchner, H.; Hayat, M.; Ribaud, P.; De Wasch, G.; Mattsson, W.; Heinz, R.; Waldner, R.; Kolaric, K.; Buehner, R.; Ten Bokkel-Huyninck, W.; Perevodchikova, N. I.; Manzuik, L. A.; Senn, H. J.; and Mayr, A. C.: Adriamycin cardiotoxicity: A survey of 1273 patients (834). *Cancer Treat. Rep.,* **63:**827–834, 1979.

Rai, K. R.; Glidewell, O.; Wienberg, V.; and Holland, J. F.: Long time remission in acute myelocytic leukemia (AMC): Report of a multi-institutional cooperative study. *Proc. Am. Soc. Clin. Oncol.,* **22:**481, 1981.

Rai, K. R.; Sawitsky, A.; Cronkite, E. P.; Chanana, A. D.; Levy, R. N.; and Pasternack, B. S.: Clinical staging of chronic lymphocytic leukemia. *Blood,* **46:**219–234, 1975.

Rosenberg, S. A.: Non-Hodgkin's lymphoma—selection of treatment on the basis of histologic type. *N. Engl. J. Med.,* **301:**924–928, 1979.

Rosenblum, M. L.; Dougherty, D. V.; Barger, G. R.; Levin, V. A.; Gerosa, M.; Reese, C.; Davis, R. L.; and Wilson, C. B.: Age-related chemosensitivity of stem cells from human malignant brain tumors. *Lancet,* **1:**885–887, 1982.

Rowe, J. W.; Andres, R.; Tobin, J. D., Norris, A. H.; and Shock, N. W.: The effects of age on creatinine clearance in man: A cross-sectional and longitudinal study. *J. Gerontol.,* **31:**155–163, 1976.

Seidman, H.; Silverberg, E.; and Bodden, A.: Probabilities of eventually developing and of dying of cancer (risk among persons previously undiagnosed with cancer). *Cancer,* **28:**33–46, 1978.

Silber, R.: Chronic lymphocytic leukemia in the elderly. *Hosp. Pract.,* **19:**131–141, 1982.

Silverberg, E.: Cancer Statistics, 1985. *CA,* **35:**19–35, 1985.

Stoll, B. A.: Hypothesis: Breast cancer regression under oestrogen therapy. *Br. Med. J.,* **3:**446–450, 1973.

Tranum, B.; Hoogstraten, B.; Kennedy, A.; Vaughn, C. B.; Samal, B.; Thigpen, T.; Rivkin, S.; Smith, F.; Palmer, R. L.; Costanzi, J.; Tucker, W. G.; Wilson, H.; and Maloney, T. R.: Adriamycin in combination for the treatment of breast cancer: A Southwest Oncology Group Study. *Cancer,* **41:**2078–2083, 1978.

Veronesi, U.; Saccozzi, R.; DelVecchio, M.; Banfi, A.; Clemente, C.; DeLena, M.; Gallus, G.; Greco, M; Luini, A.; Marubini, E.; Muscolino, G.; Rilke, F.; Salvadori, B.; Zecchini, A.; and Zucali, R.: Comparing radical mastectomy with quadrantectomy, axillary dissection, and radiotherapy in patients with small cancers of the breast. *N. Engl. J. Med.,* **305:**6–11, 1981.

Waisman, J., and Mott, L. J. M.: Pathology of neoplasms of the prostate gland. In Skinner, D. G., and deKernion, J. B. (eds.): *Genitourinary Cancer.* W. B. Saunders Company, Philadelphia, 1978.

Willis, I.: Sunlight, aging, and skin cancer. *Geriatrics,* **33:**33–36, 1978.

Zippin, C.; Cutler, S. J.; Reeves, W. J., Jr.; and Lum, D.: Survival in chronic lymphocytic leukemia. *Blood,* **42:**367–376, 1973.

47

Nursing Considerations in Cancer

LAURA J. HILDERLEY

Among all those involved in the care of the cancer patient, the oncology nurse may be best suited to provide the total support and continuity of care so needed by the patient and family. As Henke (1980a) points out, the oncology nurse has an essential role in all facets of care for patients with cancer. The nurse can provide screening and detection, nutritional management, psychosocial support, patient and family education, treatment, and follow-up, in addition to direct physical care.

Emphasis on the multifaceted role of the oncology nurse is not meant to minimize the contribution of others who give care. The team approach to management of the patient with cancer is certainly the ideal, and teams are in place in many institutions and settings. In many other locations ranging from urban medical centers to small community hospitals, however, the nurse is the one constant to whom the patient with cancer can turn.

THE ONCOLOGY NURSE

The Nursing Section of the Cancer Control Branch of the National Cancer Institute established the first formal education program for oncology nursing in 1948. This program strengthened the undergraduate cancer curriculum by providing intensive courses for graduate students and faculty. The passage of the National Cancer Act in 1971 gave cancer nursing education a substantial boost. Oncology nursing as a specialty grew dramatically during the 1970s and continues to grow into the 1980s. The Oncology Nursing Society, incorporated in 1975 with around 200 charter members, had over 8000 members in 1985. Thus oncology nursing is a distinct and recognizable specialty with a major impact on the care and treatment of cancer patients.

Oncology Nursing Roles

The nursing role in oncology is as varied as the treatment modalities employed. Oncology nurses have subspecialized in areas such as medical and surgical oncology, nursing education, radiation oncology, research, administration, and hospice care (Henke, 1980; Hubbard, 1981; Stromborg, 1981; Scogna and Schoenberger, 1982).

Chemotherapy Nurse. Most oncology nurses practice in a chemotherapy or medical oncology setting, and their primary responsibility lies in the careful administration of chemotherapeutic agents. This nurse must be skilled in venipuncture, knowledgeable about each agent being used, aware of protocol requirements, alert for toxicities and most important, sensitive to the many needs of the patient and family. Technical skills and detailed knowledge of treatment regimens are important, of course, to the efficient operation of the clinic, office, or hospital unit. However, it is the nurse's holistic approach to patient care that distinguishes the nursing role from others in the same setting. Few oncology nurses would view themselves as "medication nurses." Rather, their role is to assess, treat, comfort, care, listen, teach, provide, observe, refer, support, and counsel the patient and the family.

The nurse in medical oncology carries out a variety of responsibilities and functions (Croft,

1976; Scholin *et al.,* 1978; Coburn, 1979; Maxwell, 1979; Hunter and Johnson, 1980; Jones *et al.,* 1981; Spross *et al.,* 1982). Roles vary with the setting and the geographic location. Oncology nursing in a major medical center differs from that in a community hospital. Likewise, the oncology nurse on an inpatient unit will have functions outside of the realm of the office nurse, although both may administer chemotherapy.

Research Nurse. Some of the first oncology nurses were protocol nurses whose functions included data management, as well as administration of agents being used in clinical trials. These responsibilities required organizational skills, clinical expertise, and interpersonal communication skills of the highest level. Today, in many clinical research settings, the nurse is often the only constant in a milieu of variables as residents, fellows, and house staff rotate through the oncology service. The nurse's familiarity with both the protocol and the patient provides the continuity lacking from any other source. Patient compliance, so vital to the collection of evaluable data, is often a direct result of how the patient and family perceive the nursing support.

The nurse in a research setting can serve as a patient advocate, helping to assure the patient's rights to full information about the disease and its treatment. Although the physician must obtain informed consent, the nurse is frequently in the best position to observe whether or not the patient truly understands and accepts the investigational nature of the treatment protocol. The patient's anxiety level when informed consent is obtained may preclude true informed consent. Because of the close nurse-patient relationship and the frequency of contact, nurses can assess the patient's level of understanding and fill in information gaps that may interfere with patient acceptance of a treatment regimen.

Radiation Oncology Nurse. One of the newest areas of subspecialization within oncology nursing is in the care of patients receiving radiation therapy. Patients referred to the radiotherapist may leave those who give them their primary care and support for periods ranging from ten days to several months. Some patients may take up residence near a treatment facility miles from home. The radiation oncology nurse can provide the consistency and support these patients need throughout treatment and follow-up care.

Radiation therapy is probably the least well-understood treatment modality among the lay population as well as medical professionals. Nurses should provide ongoing education for the patient about the treatment and its effects. Nurses can relieve anxiety about the unknown by teaching patients what not to expect as well as the likely side effects. One very common anxiety-producing misconception is that radiation treatment will cause nausea, vomiting, and hair loss. These reactions are site-specific, however, and the oncology nurse can give accurate information to the patient regarding side effects of a particular treatment.

Teaching extends beyond the patient and family to include nursing peers and other professionals (Hilderley, 1980). A course of radiation therapy usually occupies but a small portion of the cancer patient's total disease course. Physicians and nurses who will see the patient on an ongoing basis must be provided with full information about the patient's treatment, including not only the observed effects, but delayed or late effects of radiation treatment. Nurse-to-nurse communication and teaching can help realize continuity of care.

Oncology Nursing Educator. The specific teaching responsibilities of the nurse in medical and radiation oncology, as well as in a research setting, have been mentioned. There is, however, another role for nurses prepared at the master's or doctoral level, that of nursing educator. The oncology nursing educator teaches that portion of the undergraduate curriculum covering oncology nursing, provides continuing education courses in oncology nursing for registered nurses, or teaches in an oncology master's program or in an oncology track in a medical-surgical nursing program. Obviously, the oncology nursing educator must be an experienced oncology nurse as well as a well-prepared educator.

Given (1980) outlines a framework for a cancer nursing curriculum, stressing the need for a *fundamental* level of preparation as well as *advanced* preparation for the oncology nursing specialist.

NURSING CARE OF THE ONCOLOGY PATIENT

Assessing the Patient

As the oncology nurses' role was defined and accepted by their medical colleagues, patient problems and concerns were identified that were amenable to interventions of professional nursing practice. Nursing diagnoses as the result of assessment had been discussed in the nursing literature since the early 1960s (Abdellah, 1961; Chambers, 1962; Komorita, 1965). Assessment tools were developed in the 1960s and 1970s (McCain, 1965; Smith, 1968). It was not until 1973, however, that a formal attempt was made to establish some degree of standardization of the language at the First National Conference on the Classification of Nursing Diagnoses (Gebbie and Lavin, 1974). These events were particularly important to oncology nursing practice as it emerged as a distinct specialty during that same period. A variety of assessment tools have now been developed, and each has applicability in a given setting. Assessment tools help establish a data base upon which to develop a plan of care.

Assessment is not a one-time process. Oncology patients experience remissions and exacerbations in their disease condition. Chemotherapeutic agents have varied effects on the tumor and side effects on the patient. As the drugs are changed, patient education must change. Assessment of the patient newly diagnosed with colorectal cancer differs from that obtained when this same patient returns to the outpatient department for the first postoperative visit. As Donley (1978) points out, "Assessment is a process that is begun when the nurse first meets the patient and continues each time there is a nurse-patient interaction, no matter how brief the interaction may be." A nursing assessment form developed by Welch et al. (1982) is readily adaptable and expandable to suit a variety of oncology care settings (see Figure 47–1).

Table 47–1 presents an overview of chemotherapeutic agents and is meant to be used in conjunction with specific product information regarding dosage, administration, and precautions. A detailed discussion of chemotherapeutic agents can be found in Chapter 10. Most institutions have specific guidelines for the administration of chemotherapy by qualified nurses. Policies may vary regarding the nursing protocols in the event of extravasation or in routines for premedicating with antiemetics. The Oncology Nursing Society has published an excellent teaching tool that can be incorporated easily into any setting where nurses administer chemotherapy (Miller et al., 1984).

Guidelines for Care of Specific Manifestations of Disease and Treatment

Nursing care of the cancer patient is an extension of basic care of any patient experiencing an alteration in normal bodily function or life-style. With advances in treatment, many patients live longer and face the problems of chronicity. Nursing care should focus on the management of chronic problems, as well as on the acute and sometimes self-limiting manifestations of cancer and its treatment.

Pain Management. Nurses must face the pain experienced by the patient with cancer to realize holistic patient care. Whether somatic or psychogenic, pain of varying degrees is going to challenge the patient, the family, and the nurse at some time during the illness of many cancer patients. Those providing care should explore alternative drugs and methods for pain control rather than be discouraged by the inability to resolve pain to the point of distancing themselves from this patient (see Chapter 44).

In no area of nursing practice is there more opportunity for independent action based on sound application of knowledge than in discovering the patient's particular needs for pain relief, in revealing the measures that work best for him, and in solving the problem of pain. And I submit that in no area have we overlooked our responsibilities more (Jarrett, 1965).

Fortunately, times have changed and the continually expanding role of nurses in cancer patient management has addressed Jarrett's concern in 1965. Nurses now work collaboratively with physicians in pain management. Much has been written on the use of narcotics and analgesics in cancer pain management (McCaffery, 1979; Lipman, 1980; Pierce and Ya Deau, 1980; Jacox and Rogers, 1981). In many settings, the physician prescribes but relies on the nurse to suggest the appropriate drug, dosage, and schedule. The experienced nurse evaluates the effectiveness of the particular analgesics, recommends adjustments in dosage, and suggests alternative medications if indicated.

The etiology of pain is not always clear, therefore pain cannot always be treated by removing the cause. However, when a clear cause-and-effect relationship can be identified, removing the cause may require surgical procedures to relieve compression or obstruction,

ONCOLOGY NURSING ASSESSMENT TOOL

DATE OF ASSESSMENT _____   **PATIENT IDENTIFICATION**

INFORMANT _____   NAME _____

NEXT OF KIN _____   ADDRESS _____

ADDRESS _____   _____

_____   _____

PHONE _____   PHONE _____

                                        DOB _____

I. IMPORTANT DATA

    Age/Sex _____   Vital Signs   T _____ P _____ R _____

    Marital Status _____   Allergies _____

    Height _____   Responsible Doctors: _____

    Weight _____   _____

II. CHIEF COMPLAINT:

III. PAST HISTORY:

    A. Other Major Illnesses or Health Problems:
       Problem: Date of Diagnosis: Treatment:

    B. Cancer History:

TREATMENT	TYPE	WHEN	WHERE	SIDE EFFECTS
SURGERY				
RADIATION				
CHEMOTHERAPY				
IMMUNOTHERAPY				

Figure 47–1.   Adapted with permission from Welch, D.; Follo, J.; and Nelson, E.: The development of a specialized nursing assessment tool for cancer patients. *Oncology Nursing Forum,* **9**(1):37–44, 1982.

neurosurgical interventions such as laminectomy, rhizotomy, nerve blocks, or other techniques for interrupting sensory nerve pathways. Radiation therapy for pain control in bony metastases is usually very effective. Although these interventions may produce excellent results, there is still need for analgesic management in the interim and for those in whom the results are less satisfactory.

Assessment.   The subjective nature of pain

IV.   REVIEW OF SYSTEMS

	Subjective (Patient Reports)	Objective (Nurse Observes)
A. Eyes		
B. Ears		
C. Mouth/Throat		
D. Gastrointestinal		
1) Nutrition		
2) Elimination		
E. Respiration		
F. Circulation		
G. Genitourinary		
H. Skin		
I. Neuromuscular		
1) Sleep		
2) Mobility		
3) Pain		

V.   PERSONAL-SOCIAL HISTORY

    A. Birthplace:

    B. Education:

    C. Occupation:

    D. Religion:

    E. Finances:

    F. Living Arrangements:

VI.   FAMILY HISTORY AND RELATIONSHIPS

    A. Disease History:

    B. Family Members/Supportive Others:

    C. Family's Perception of Illness (via patient):

    D. Family's Perception of Illness (via family):

Figure 47–1.   *(continued)*

makes assessment a continuing challenge calling for keen observation and evaluation of verbal and nonverbal cues. Patients will display individual tolerance and pain threshholds, as well as cultural differences in expressing pain. Self-limiting pain (postoperative) needs to be considered for its relative intensity and brevity as compared to the chronic pain with which some cancer patients must live.

Selection of Analgesics and Adjusting Dosage. Individual differences among patients preclude standard management of pain. Of the many analgesics and synthetic substitutes available today, only one or a few may be ef-

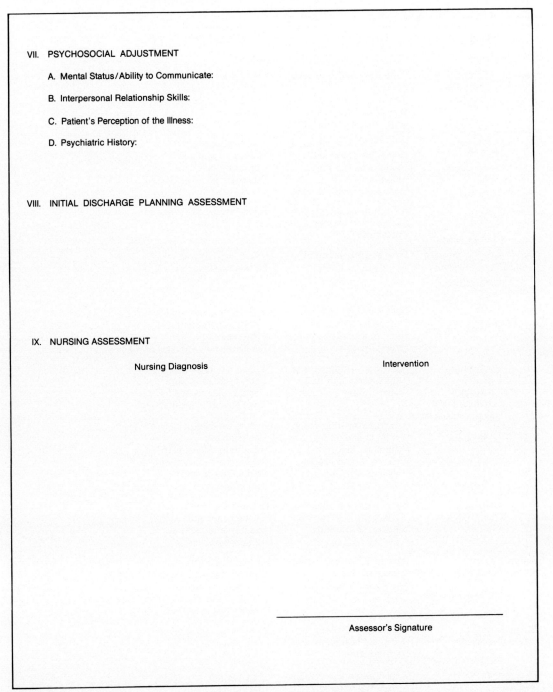

VII. PSYCHOSOCIAL ADJUSTMENT

    A. Mental Status/Ability to Communicate:

    B. Interpersonal Relationship Skills:

    C. Patient's Perception of the Illness:

    D. Psychiatric History:

VIII. INITIAL DISCHARGE PLANNING ASSESSMENT

IX. NURSING ASSESSMENT

               Nursing Diagnosis   Intervention

_____

Assessor's Signature

Figure 47–1. *(concluded)*

fective for any given patient. Although a medication should be given an adequate trial before it is discontinued, sometimes numerous attempts are made before finding the most effective pain-reliever. Likewise, it is not uncommon that a previously adequate drug and dosage are no longer effective and need to be replaced.

It is generally agreed that escalating dosage to the optimum level is better than starting with maximum amounts. If high levels of analgesics are successful in controlling pain from

Table 47-1. Chemotherapeutic Agents—Nursing Implications

DRUGS	MAJOR TOXICITIES	NURSING IMPLICATIONS
Alkylating Agents		
Mechlorethamine (MUSTARGEN, HN₂, nitrogen mustard)	Bone marrow suppression Vesicant Nausea and vomiting Skin rash, fever, chills, Amenorrhea, sterility	Administer via running IV Avoid skin contact Give antiemetics prior to treatment
Cyclophosphamide (CTX, CYT, CYTOXAN, ENDOXAN)	Bone marrow suppression Hemorrhagic cystitis Nausea and vomiting Alopecia Stomatitis, hepatotoxicity	Ensure hydration Monitor output and electrolytes Tablets are not to be chewed
Chlorambucil (LEUKERAN)	Bone marrow suppression Nausea and vomiting Amenorrhea	Tablets are not to be chewed
L-Phenylalanine mustard (L-Pam, melphalan, ALKERAN, L-sarcolysin)	Bone marrow suppression Sterility	Usually well tolerated Tablets are not to be chewed
Busulfan (MYLERAN)	Bone marrow suppression Pulmonary fibrosis Gynecomastia and sterility Hyperpigmentation	Assess pulmonary status prior to treatment and throughout Tablets are not to be chewed
Triethylenemelamine (TEM, thiotepa, TSPA, triethylene, thiophosphoramide)	Bone marrow suppression Nausea and vomiting at higher doses	When used for intracavitary instillation, turn patient side to side for one hour after instillation
Carmustine (BCNU, BiCNU)	Bone marrow suppression Nausea and vomiting Pulmonary fibrosis CNS, renal, and hepatic toxicity	Premedicate with antiemetics May produce local pain and generalized flushing caused by diluent (alcohol)
Lomustine (CCNU, CeeNU)	Bone marrow suppression (delayed) Nausea and vomiting	Premedicate with antiemetics and sedative Administer at night on empty stomach
Semustine (Methyl-CCNU)	Bone marrow suppression (delayed) Nausea and vomiting	Premedicate with antiemetics and sedative Administer at night on empty stomach Do not confuse with CCNU
Streptozocin (Streptozotocin)	Nausea and vomiting Renal and hepatic toxicity Hyperglycemia	Monitor urinary proteins and glucose
Dacarbazine (DTIC)	Bone marrow suppression Nausea and vomiting	Extravasation may cause thrombophlebitis Protect powder from light
Mitomycin (mitomycin C, MUTAMYCIN)	Bone marrow suppression Nausea and vomiting, diarrhea Fever, malaise Renal toxicity Vesicant	Give directly into tubing of established IV Premedicate with antiemetics Myelosuppression is cumulative

continued

Table 47–1. *(continued)*

DRUGS	MAJOR TOXICITIES	NURSING IMPLICATIONS
Antimetabolites		
Methotrexate (amethopterin, MTX)	Bone marrow suppression Nausea and vomiting Alopecia Mucositis Renal toxicity at high doses Hepatotoxic Neurotoxicity and arachnoiditis with intrathecal administration	At high doses requires rescue with citrovorum factor Thorough hydration (IV) and premedication with antiemetics Rigorous oral hygiene measures Avoid salicylates, sulfonamides, chloramphenicol, tetracyclines, and phenytoin (MTX may be displaced from plasma proteins by these agents) Monitor renal output and renal function
Fluorouracil (5-FU, 5-fluorouracil)	Bone marrow suppression Nausea, diarrhea, and vomiting Stomatitis, ataxia, alopecia Photosensitivity	Rigorous oral hygiene measures Very low therapeutic index requires careful monitoring Avoid exposure to sun
Mercaptopurine (6-MP, 6-mercaptopurine, PURINETHOL)	Bone marrow suppression Nausea and vomiting Hepatotoxicity with jaundice	Reduce doses for patients with impaired hepatic or renal function Allopurinol enhances toxicity as well as therapeutic effect
Thioguanine (TG, 6-thioguanine)	Moderate bone marrow suppression Nausea and vomiting possible Stomatitis, diarrhea	Reduce doses for patients with impaired hepatic or renal function Oral hygiene measures
Cytosine arabinoside (ara-C, cytarabine, arabinosyl cytosine, CYTOSAR)	Bone marrow suppression Nausea and vomiting, stomatitis, diarrhea Alopecia Hepatotoxicity	Oral hygiene measures Monitor hepatic function
Hydroxyurea (HYDREA)	Bone marrow suppression Nausea and vomiting Dermatologic reactions	Assure patient's understanding of dosage schedule
Vinca Alkaloids Vincristine sulfate (ONCOVIN, VCR)	Paresthesias, muscle weakness, foot drop, wrist drop, loss of deep tendon reflexes, constipation, paralytic ileus, hoarseness, jaw pain Vesicant	Observe carefully for signs of neurotoxicity Administer laxatives, stool softeners Give directly into tubing of established IV
Vinblastine sulfate (VELBAN, VBL)	Bone marrow suppression Nausea and vomiting, stomatitis, alopecia Neurotoxicity similar to that of vincristine, plus depression, headache, convulsions, psychoses Vesicant	Observe for signs of neurotoxicity Administer laxatives, stool softeners Give directly into tubing of established IV

continued

Table 47–1. *(continued)*

DRUGS	MAJOR TOXICITIES	NURSING IMPLICATIONS
Etoposide (VP-16)	Bone marrow suppression Alopecia Anorexia Possible bronchial spasm and hypotension may be associated with rapid infusion	Administer antihistamines for bronchospasm Administer slowly
Antibiotics		
Dactinomycin (actinomycin D, COSMEGEN)	Bone marrow suppression Nausea and vomiting, diarrhea Stomatitis, glossitis Alopecia Radiosensitization Radiation recall Vesicant	Premedicate with antiemetics Give directly into tubing of established IV Oral hygiene measures
Bleomycin sulfate (BLENOXANE, BLEO)	Anaphylaxis Bronchial spasm Hypotension Alopecia Mucocutaneous reactions such as pruritus, vesiculation, ulceration Stomatitis Pulmonary fibrosis Fever	Use test dose Observe for signs of anaphylaxis and have antidotes ready Observe for mucocutaneous reactions, especially over pressure points
Mithramycin (MITHRACIN)	Bone marrow suppression Clotting disorders Nausea and vomiting Vesicant Stomatitis Renal and hepatic toxicity	Careful monitoring for hemorrhagic signs Premedicate with antiemetics Monitor renal and liver functions Oral hygiene measures
Doxorubicin hydrochloride (ADRIAMYCIN, ADM)	Bone marrow suppression Nausea and vomiting Alopecia Hepatic toxicity Cardiac toxicity Vesicant Radiation recall	Given directly into tubing of established IV Oral hygiene measures Causes red discoloration of urine Cumulative dose limited to 550 mg/m^2 Observe for signs of congestive heart failure
Daunorubicin (daunomycin, rubidomycin, CERUBIDINE, DAUNOBLASTINA, DNR)	Bone marrow suppression Hepatic toxicity Cardiac toxicity Nausea and vomiting Vesicant Alopecia	Same as for doxorubicin except cumulative dose limited to 450–500 mg/m^2
Miscellaneous Agents		
L-Asparaginase (L-asparagine amidohydrolase, ELSPAR)	Anaphylaxis Hepatic, renal, pancreatic, and CNS toxicities Fever, chills, urticaria	Observe for signs of anaphylaxis and have antidotes ready Observe for signs of hyperglycemia, bleeding, CNS dysfunction (depression, impaired sensorium, coma)

continued

Table 47–1. *(continued)*

DRUGS	MAJOR TOXICITIES	NURSING IMPLICATIONS
Procarbazine hydrochloride (MATULANE)	Bone marrow suppression Nausea and vomiting Psychic disturbances CNS effects	Avoid concomitant use of CNS depressants Alcohol ingestion causes warmth and reddening of the face and headache Hypertension may result from use of sympatho-mimetics, tricyclic antidepressants, and foods rich in tyramine
Cisplatin (PLATINOL, DDP)	Nausea and vomiting Renal toxicity Ototoxicity Neuropathies Anaphylactic-like reactions Hypomagnesemia	Administer antiemetics and IV hydration before, during, and for 24 hours after treatment Monitor urine output Observe for facial edema, bronchoconstriction tachycardia, hypotension Do not use aluminum needles or IV equipment

the outset, it may never be known whether lesser doses would be equally effective. Thus the patient receives more medication than needed and has nothing in reserve when pain intensifies.

Similarly, the relative potency of analgesics should be considered, selecting those of lower potency first and gradually moving to stronger preparations as the patient's pain intensifies. Many published tables list the equianalgesic quality of narcotic and nonnarcotic analgesics. Although discrepancies exist, and personal experience in pain management will influence the selection of an agent, most sources agree generally on the relative potency of common analgesics (McCaffery, 1979; Jaffe and Martin, 1980; Jacox and Rogers, 1981).

Analgesics and Their Relationship to Other Medications. When prescribing analgesics, all other medications the patient may be taking must be considered. Sedatives, hypnotics, and tranquilizers are sometimes prescribed for cancer patients, perhaps before pain becomes a problem or as a means of minimizing pain. High-potency narcotics administered concomitantly can produce dangerous levels of sedation and deepen depression. Controlling pain often eliminates the need for sedatives and tranquilizers.

Analgesics containing aspirin should be avoided in patients receiving steroid therapy because of the gastric toxicity of both aspirin and steroids.

In patients with impaired renal or liver function, selection of medications should take

into account any potential for further damage to these organs. With the variety of analgesics available, a suitable and safe choice can usually be made.

Personalities and individual tolerance influence the pain experience. Cancer patients with pain need caring and supportive nursing management.

One of the major hurdles to overcome is the fear of addiction that many individuals harbor. Unfortunately, this fear also influences nurses and physicians in their management of pain. When pain is real, analgesics are needed. If the source of pain can be removed, pain medications can be decreased. When pain becomes chronic and intractable, patients may need to be on narcotic analgesics for long periods. A patient may become tolerant to a particular narcotic and addiction may be suspected. However, changing to another agent may provide pain control once again.

The evaluation of dose becomes more difficult for outpatients and requires frequent telephone contact by the nurse to reassure both patient and family. Prescribing "one or two tablets every four to six hours" gives some individuals too much choice. They take only one tablet, wait a full six hours as the pain worsens, and by the time they take a second tablet, it is ineffective because of the level of pain. For the inexperienced patient or family member, specific directions are often better.

Another common error made by patients is to "hold off" until they are in severe pain before taking their medication. These individuals need to be made at ease in taking their analgesics regularly during waking hours, rather than sporadically. Most analgesics require a sufficient and steady dosage to attain blood levels that are effective in pain control. Here again, the nurse has an important role in teaching and supporting the patient.

Pain may be linked with fatigue, anxiety, guilt, depression, insomnia, and other distressing factors. Relieving the pain may also relieve some of these other problems. On the other hand, until the psychologic factors are addressed with appropriate interventions, pain may not be amenable to standard forms of treatment.

Comfort Measures for Pain Relief. In efforts to find the perfect analgesic for the cancer patient, basic nursing comfort measures may be forgotten. Pain may be caused by constipation, malnourishment, poor circulation, edema, pressure, immobility, position, inflammation, or ulceration.

Positioning and good body alignment are sometimes all that is needed to bring comfort to the patient with bone metastases. Frequent position changes for the nonambulatory patient are important not only for comfort, but to improve circulation. Ischemic pain may be eased through applying heat, unless otherwise contraindicated (when the patient is being irradiated to the painful site). Support with a sling can help relieve bone pain. Similarly, a cane or walker may help relieve pain in weight-bearing areas.

When edema causes discomfort and pain, efforts should be made to determine the source of edema and provide appropriate relief. Simple elevation of the dependent edematous part may ease pain. Exercise can also help to relieve edema through muscle contraction, which assists in promoting return of lymphatic fluid through the lymphatic vessels.

Support hose (in both men and women) is helpful in leg edema but must fit properly avoiding tight elastic bands on hosiery or undergarments at all times. To help prevent dependent edema, support hose and garments should be put on either while the patient is lying in bed or immediately after arising in the morning before edema worsens.

For patients who have undergone radical surgical procedures involving dissection of inguinal lymph nodes, edema of the legs, labia, scrotum, or entire perineal area may cause major discomfort and disability. Axillary dissection with or without mastectomy can also produce painful lymphedema. In these cases

ordinary support garments are usually not sufficient. A physical therapist can fit appropriately therapeutic products such as Jobst support garments. The usual procedure involves consecutive treatments of the edematous limb with a pump mechanism to push fluid back into the central circulation. Measurements are taken before and after treatment, and when the edematous part no longer decreases in size, the appropriate garment is fitted. Treatments may need to continue periodically, and the patient should be encouraged to wear the support garment consistently.

One other means of promoting lymphatic return from the lower extremities is elevation of the foot of the bed. Patients often think that sleeping with their feet on a pillow is sufficient. However, to accomplish true gravity return, the foot of the bed should be elevated on 6-inch blocks.

Adequate rest and sleep not only are important to general health, but take on even greater significance in terms of pain management. Patients are sometimes able to manage well during the waking hours, controlling pain with mild analgesics and through the diversion of daytime activities. During the quiet and sometimes lonely nighttime hours, pain seems to intensify, when, in fact, it may be the *awareness* of pain that has intensified. As patients lose sleep, they are less able to cope with the stresses (including pain) that they previously were able to handle. Tiredness can lead to loss of appetite and to the need for sleep during the daytime. This cycle of sleeplessness at night, pain, anorexia, and napping during the day can become a real management problem. The patient's presenting complaint may be increased pain, leading to the prescribing of more and stronger analgesics. However, a closer look at the situation can uncover the problems of sleeplessness — fear, loneliness, and heightened awareness, all of which the patient identifies as pain. Before making any major changes in analgesia, a sedative or hypnotic should be tried at bedtime. In addition, daytime napping should be discouraged so that the patient is truly ready for a good night's sleep.

Some individuals do need additional rest and sleep in the daytime. Again, several short naps are not as beneficial as settling into bed for several hours of real sleep. To this end, the patient should be encouraged to go to bed or at least to avoid dozing off in a chair in the midst of a busy household.

When the patient is hospitalized, providing

restful and sleep-inducing conditions is usually more difficult than in the home. Nurses can be instrumental in scheduling necessary procedures that will least disturb the patient and in helping visitors to understand the patient's need for rest, while also ascertaining the patient's wishes regarding visitors.

Some consider relaxation through guided imagery a very useful technique for controlling not only pain, but nausea and stress as well (McCaffery, 1979; Donovan, 1980). Because it is a system of noninvasive pain management, it is sometimes more acceptable to the patient than other alternatives. The techniques for learning guided imagery are fairly simple and, for the motivated patient, can be helpful. McCaffery summarizes the application in pain management as follows:

Thus, guided imagery for the purpose of pain relief involves using one's imagination to develop sensory images that decrease the intensity of pain or that becomes a pleasant or nonpainful substitute for pain. In other words, guided imagery may act as an analgesic or anesthetic (McCaffery, 1979, p. 159).

Patients using guided imagery should do so with the responsible physician's understanding. Rarely does this technique become the sole method of pain control, but it may be a supplement or tentative alternative to more conventional methods of pain management.

Nutritional Needs. Nutrition problems among patients with cancer may require the greatest patience and ingenuity. Many factors are implicated in the development of cancer cachexia, ranging from the depletion of fat and protein stores to the anorexia that is a common side effect of treatment. The problem of maintaining nutrition may last only as long as does the treatment. In some patients with cancer, however, even when treatment ceases, the problems of nutritional management continue.

No single dietary plan is appropriate for all patients, but the eager patient or family member may demand a prescribed dietary regime to aid in the treatment of the specific cancer. There is something magical about food in the minds of many, who believe that if they could just eat enough of the right things they will somehow help to conquer this cancer. This is especially true in the well-meaning spouse who tries in vain to select and prepare foods from which the patient will derive therapeutic benefit.

Optimal nutrition is important, however, and helping to ensure that nutritional needs are met is a function of the nurse, whether in the hospital, clinic, office, or community setting.

The physiology of nutrition in cancer is complex and in some instances not fully understood. Numerous texts and articles address the nutritional needs of the cancer patient. Chapter 45 in this text, Fedak, 1981, and Moritz *et al.* (in press), provide comprehensive discussions of nutritional management.

A variety of public and private organizations publish helpful nutrition information for patients and families in the form of booklets, pamphlets, and brochures. A list of nutrition information resources designed particularly for cancer patients is included at the end of this chapter. The nurse, physician, or dietitian should always accompany any literature with personal support, individualizing the printed materials to patients.

Some basic ideas that can be incorporated into nutrition teaching include:

Stimulating the Appetite

Eat in the company of family or friends.

Have a glass of wine or an aperitif before meals.

Serve food in an attractive manner.

A flower and a pretty placement can brighten even a bedside tray.

Try to eat on a regular basis.

Serve small portions to avoid overwhelming the patient with the prospect of a big meal.

Serve meals in a room other than that in which they are prepared. Cooking odors are sometimes disagreeable.

Five or six small meals may be tolerated more easily than the usual three.

Ways to Make Eating Easier

Sitting up at a table is best. Use pillows and other supports as necessary.

Choose favorite foods; indulge the patient.

Keep meals interesting and varied.

Have a variety of nutritious snacks readily available.

Avoid distractions such as TV or reading at mealtime.

When Chewing or Swallowing Is Difficult

Select naturally soft foods such as cottage cheese, fish, potatoes, custards.

Chop, grind, or puree foods.

Prepared foods for infants can be substituted for those requiring chewing.

High-protein, high-carbohydrate drinks (eggnog, ice-cream shakes, instant liquid meals, commercial nutritional supplements) can be used between meals or substituted for regular foods if necessary.

When Taste Sensations Change

Use a variety of spices and seasonings to enhance flavor (use with caution if mouth is sore).

Warm foods usually have more flavor than cold.

Sweets may taste too sweet, so decrease sugar content.

Good oral hygiene before meals can help improve taste sensation.

If meat seems unappealing, substitute cheese, milk products, legumes, and eggs for protein sources. Highly flavored meats such as hot dogs, sausage, ham, or bacon may be palatable.

Hyperalimentation and total parenteral nutrition (TPN) are useful for meeting nutritional requirements in some situations (Dudrick and Rhoads, 1971; Shils, 1972; Copeland *et al.* 1978). Nursing care of patients receiving TPN requires skill and thorough understanding of the principles involved. *Hyperalimentation Standards of Practice* of the National Intravenous Therapy Association, Inc. (NITA), provides excellent guidelines for holistic management of the patient on hyperalimentation (Colley *et al.,* 1981). In addition to the standards, this publication addresses:

Patient assessment
Infusates
Catheter placement
Catheter site care and dressing change
Intravenous administration set change
Infection control
Metabolic aspects
Catheter removal

Other special dietary adjustments include low-residue diet for control of diarrhea, high-residue for constipation, and tyramine-limited during administration of procarbazine. Residue-adjusted diets are fairly standard, and the dietitian in most institutions can provide them. Such diets should be thoroughly explained to the patient, emphasizing their temporal nature, and the need to make adjustments as the condition warrants. For example, patients receiving pelvic irradiation may require a low-residue diet to help control treatment-induced diarrhea (Hilderley, in press). For most of these patients, symptoms subside

in a week to ten days after treatment ends, and they can gradually resume a normal diet. Unless patients are carefully instructed as to the nature and purpose of the low-residue diet, they may inadvertently continue it to the point of inducing constipation.

Dietary adjustments necessitated by constipation include increasing the fiber content and assuring that plenty of fluids are included. Foods emphasized are fruits, vegetables, and bran or whole-grain bread and cereal products. Printed instructions for specific foods to add or delete should be used along with personal instruction. Health professionals sometimes assume that simply telling a patient to "increase the bulk in your diet" will bring about the desired change. Especially in nutrition teaching, one needs to evaluate carefully the patient's level of understanding and proceed accordingly.

A tyramine-restricted diet is based on the fact that procarbazine is a monoamine oxidase inhibitor. Pressor amines such as tyramine are normally detoxified in the gastrointestinal tract by monoamine oxidase. In the presence of procarbazine, however, detoxification is blocked and varying degrees of sympathomimetic activity can occur. Some patients experience hypertension, palpitations, headache, and facial flushing after eating foods with high tyramine content.

Although individual response varies, and "food-drug interactions with procarbazine are rare, anecdotal and of minor clinical significance" (Maxwell, 1980), it is well to inform the patient of potential problems.

Foods to be avoided, or at least taken with caution, include:

Cheddar and other ripe cheeses
Alcoholic beverages and Chianti wine in
  particular
Pickled herring
Chicken livers
Sausages
Chocolate
Yoghurt

As with all special or restricted diets, it is important to individualize restrictions, considering the potential for risk versus depriving the patient of a favorite food.

Nausea, Vomiting, Anorexia. Cancer and its treatment can produce varying degrees of appetite disturbance, ranging from slight anorexia to actual vomiting. Maintaining adequate nutrition in the presence of such altered intake can be very difficult. When nausea is treatment-induced and self-limiting (a few hours' to a few days' duration), there may be no problem with nutritional status if normal eating patterns are resumed between therapy cycles. During nausea and anorexia, fluids should be encouraged, but intake of solid foods may not be feasible.

For the patient receiving radiation therapy to large areas of the abdomen and to the epigastric region, nausea and vomiting can occur, generally most intensely within three to four hours following treatment. The diet should be light for several hours prior to treatment, and only clear fluids taken for a few hours afterward. Vomiting will usually subside, allowing the patient to eat reasonably well approximately six to eight hours after treatment. For this reason, radiation treatment should be scheduled by midmorning so that patients can take an evening meal with relative ease.

Medications to help control nausea and vomiting may be necessary when the problem is persistent and severe. An antacid product may be advisable for even a mild degree of constant nausea.

Antiemetics are available in preparations for oral, injectable, or rectal administration, and a suitable route should be determined for each situation. Anticipatory antiemetic administration may be necessary when oral medication is vomited before absorption. If nausea and vomiting are already well established, parenteral or rectal preparations can be used until the patient can retain oral medications.

Patients experiencing treatment-induced nausea and vomiting should be taught to take their antiemetic regularly as long as treatment continues. Sometimes, when nausea has been controlled, patients feel that the antiemetic has done its job and is no longer needed. Stopping medication then leads to the onset of symptoms, and it may take several days of escalating dosage or varied routes of administration to get nausea under control once again. Many antiemetics cause drowsiness and the appropriate precautions should be observed.

Suggestions for the Cancer Patient with Nausea or Vomiting

Eat small amounts, slowly and frequently.
Sip liquids (or ice chips), during the day, but not at mealtime.
Try crackers or dry toast first thing in the morning.
If mornings are the best time of day, use this opportunity for a high-calorie, high-protein breakfast.
Avoid foods that are very sweet, spicy, or fatty. Fried foods are particularly difficult to digest.
Cool or cold foods may be tolerated better than warm.
Food preparation odors may add to nausea.
Rest after eating, but do not lie flat.
Fresh air and loose-fitting clothing can help.
Don't eat special or favorite foods when nauseated, since these foods may then become associated with the feeling of nausea.

When vomiting continues for extended periods, monitor patients carefully for symptoms and signs of electrolyte imbalance. Particular attention should be paid to difficulty in ambulation, muscular weakness and imbalance, numbness and other paresthesias, decreasing levels of consciousness, and rapid pulse. Signs of dehydration will usually precede laboratory changes and include dryness of oral mucosa, dryness and decreased skin turgor, small amounts of concentrated urine, and listlessness.

Patient monitoring and fluid replacement for the inpatient should be routine. The outpatient, however, is particularly susceptible to serious dehydration unless closely monitored. Here again, nursing plays a vital role in maintaining telephone contact with patient and family between clinic or office visits and arranging visiting nurse follow-up when indicated. Patients or responsible family members can be taught to watch for signs of dehydration as well as how to increase fluid intake.

Suggestions for Increasing Oral Fluid Intake

Eat fruits with high-water content such as watermelon, honeydew melon, cantaloupe.
Try broth, gelatin, and sherbet.
Suck on popsicles and ice chips.
Tea, carbonated drinks, and fruit juices are usually well tolerated.

Constipation.   One of the most distressing problems patients with cancer encounter is constipation. Several factors can contribute to the onset of constipation, including diet, activity, and medication.

Dietary changes necessitated by either the disease or its treatment can produce constipation in patients with cancer. Fiber content and fluids are the most important dietary contributions to maintaining normal stool bulk and intestinal stimulation. When appetites fail or when patients are placed on special diets such as soft, liquid, or bland, the natural fiber content is markedly decreased. Similarly, if nausea occurs, the concomitant decreased intake can lead to constipation. Prolonged constipation can lead to a cycle of loss of appetite, followed by constipation, causing further appetite loss.

Decreased activity can lead to constipation, as particularly seen in the bedridden patient. When a patient decreases some of the normal activities of daily living, such as climbing stairs, housework, or yardwork, however, constipation can also develop. Coupled with decreased physical activity, sometimes a change in daily routine interferes with the usual pattern of elimination.

Possibly the most frequent cause of constipation in patients with cancer is medication. Narcotics and neurotoxic chemotherapeutic agents (primarily vincristine and vinblastine) inhibit or reduce peristalsis causing stool to move very slowly through the small and large bowel. Longer transit time allows more water to be absorbed, which leads to hard stools and constipation.

Assessing the patient with cancer for possible complications like constipation should become a routine part of nursing care. Preventive or prophylactic treatment should be instituted for any patient receiving narcotic analgesics or neurotoxic chemotherapeutic agents. Generally, a stool softener given once or twice daily should be prescribed when starting these drugs. A mild bowel stimulant (available in combination with softeners) may also be needed. Adding fiber to the diet with bran and whole-grain cereal products when feasible is also recommended. Fluid should be increased to help compensate for the increased intestinal absorption, and a hot drink before breakfast is sometimes helpful.

Exercise should be encouraged within individual limitations. If patients are simply told to get more exercise, they may interpret this as meaning calisthenics, impossible for many. Instead, encourage walking, along with an attempt to establish a regular time for elimination. Providing privacy is most important.

If constipation is already established, stool softeners, fiber, and fluids are not usually effective. Enemas or glycerin suppositories may be needed to facilitate evacuation, after which a prophylactic program can be instituted.

When an impaction has occurred, liquid stool passing around it may be mistaken for diarrhea. Careful assessment will reveal lack of bowel movements for a number of days prior to the onset of liquid stools. Manual disimpaction followed by cleansing enemas will help to resolve the problem.

Preventing Infection. Many cancer patients are at high risk for developing infections owing to the nature of the disease itself and because of the effects of treatment. Infection is the leading cause of morbidity, as well as mortality, in the cancer patient.

Neoplasms of the hematopoietic and reticuloendothelial system are characterized by immunologic deficiencies. The immunosuppressive effects of intensive therapy can lead to opportunistic infections by previously nonpathogenic organisms.

Careful monitoring of blood counts and awareness of the nadir period for chemotherapeutic agents will help in the nursing management of patients at risk for infection. In addition, awareness of possible sites for the invasion of infectious organisms should facilitate nursing care and foster preventive care and teaching. Yasko and Lauffer (1981) have proposed a comprehensive teaching plan for preventing or minimizing the possibility of infection in cancer patients. Other sources discuss the specific problems of granulocytopenia and concomitant nursing care (Graham and Rubal, 1980; Patterson, 1980; Bates and Orton, 1981; Fox, 1981). Leukapheresis and granulocyte transfusion requiring specific facilities and expertise are also presented by Graham and Patterson.

The following general points should be observed in caring for the compromised host and preventing possible infection:

Be aware of routes of entry for pathogens including the skin, respiratory tract, genitourinary tract, bloodstream, and gastrointestinal tract.

Provide meticulous skin care to maintain skin integrity.

Avoid injections whenever possible.

Maintain scrupulous technique in caring for continuous infusion sites, especially central lines.

Perineal care should be performed regularly by the nurse or patient, with attention to breaks in the skin, mucosal irritation, itching, or burning on urination.

Prevent rectal fissures and abscess; avoid

rectal thermometers, enemas, rectal medications.

Observe for characteristic odor and appearance of monilial infection, especially in the oral cavity and upper gastrointestinal tract.

Avoid unnecessary catheterization. Use scrupulous technique and avoid trauma to urethra when catheterizing. Maintain sterility of closed drainage systems.

Observe for signs and symptoms of respiratory infection. Promote adequate ventilation, especially in the bedridden patient through frequent turning, coughing, and deep-breathing.

Suction with care to avoid tissue trauma. Use sterile technique in caring for new tracheostomies. Medical asepsis should be maintained in caring for established tracheostomies.

Maintain optimal nutrition to promote healing and aid in combating infection.

Oral Care. Stomatitis, mucositis and xerostomia occur with distressing frequency in cancer patients. Certain chemotherapeutic agents, as well as radiation therapy to the head and neck area, produce some of the most severe side effects in terms of patient comfort and tolerance. Stomatitis and mucositis are used interchangeably to describe inflammation and ulceration in the oral cavity and oropharynx. Confluent areas of white or yellowish membrane form on the tongue, as well as on the gingival and buccal surfaces. Pain, discomfort, and decreased intake usually accompany this reaction. Xerostomia describes the dryness that occurs when radiation therapy causes a decrease in saliva production. This condition may be either temporary or permanent, depending on the dose received and the percentage of salivary glands irradiated.

A series of articles by Daeffler reviews both medical and nursing literature on oral hygiene (1980a,b, 1981). Agents for oral care and instruments for providing oral hygiene are presented and compared. Two other recent publications provide comprehensive guidelines for oral care and patient teaching (Beck, 1981; Yasko, 1982).

The following guidelines are the basis for oral care of the patient with cancer:

Inspect and assess the integrity of the oral mucosa daily. Observe for inflammation, ulceration, candidiasis, moisture content, and state of hygiene.

Provide gentle but thorough oral care for patients unable to do self-care.

Teach patients to care for oral tissues according to institutional standards.

Avoid astringent solutions and those with an alcohol base. Hydrogen peroxide, if used, should always be diluted with 2 parts water to 1 part H_2O_2.

Use a soft bristle toothbrush or gauze squares to avoid traumatizing tissues.

Do not try to remove the confluent plaques that form in mucositis. This will cause pain and possible bleeding.

Evaluate oral intake and suggest appropriate diet for chewing or swallowing problems.

Teach patient to avoid highly spiced foods as well as very hot or very cold foods. Encourage intake of high-calorie, high-protein diet.

Alcohol consumption and smoking of any kind should be discontinued.

Obtain orders for appropriate antibiotics when infection is present.

CONCLUSION

Supportive care of the person with cancer calls for the special skills of a team of care givers. Physicians, nutritionists, social workers, nurses, and others provide the services needed to help ease the effects of cancer and its treatment.

Among these disciplines, nursing is unique in its role, in that nursing practice requires knowledge and skills drawn from all other health professions. Treatment of side effects, administration of chemotherapeutic agents, nutritional support, counseling and teaching, all are a part of nursing practice. This broad range of therapeutic and supportive contributions can be provided by nurses, assuring coordination and continuity of care for the person with cancer and the family.

NUTRITION INFORMATION FOR PATIENTS

1. *Eating Hints — Recipes and Tips for Better Nutrition During Cancer Treatment.* U.S. Department of Health and Human Services. NIH Publication No. 82-2079, 1982.
2. *Diet and Nutrition — A Resource for Parents of Children with Cancer.* U.S. Department of Health and Human Services. NIH Publication No. 81-2038, 1981.
   Eating Hints and *Diet and Nutrition* are both available free of charge by writing to:

Office of Cancer Communications
National Cancer Institute
Building 31, Room 10 A 18
Bethesda, MD 20205

3. Seagren, J.: *Joy of Eating.* This colorful, well-organized pamphlet may be purchased in quantity by writing for a price list to:
Jill Seagren, R.D., M.S.
5413 Avenida Fiesta
La Jolla, CA 92037

4. *Nutrition for Patients Receiving Chemotherapy and Radiation Treatment.* American Cancer Society, New York, 1974. Available from most units and divisions of the American Cancer Society.

REFERENCES

Abdellah, F.: Meeting patient needs—an approach to teaching. Paper presented at biennial convention of the National League for Nursing, Cleveland, Ohio, April 10–14, 1961.

Bates, M., and Orton, M.: Infection control in clients with acute leukemia. In Marino, L. (ed.): *Cancer Nursing.* The C. V. Mosby Company, St. Louis, 1981.

Beck, S.: Teaching to prevent stomatitis. In Donovan, M. (ed.): *Cancer Care: A Guide for Patient Education.* Appleton-Century-Crofts, New York, 1981.

Chambers, W.: Nursing Diagnosis. *Am. J. Nurs.,* **62:**102–104, 1962.

Coburn, K.: Oncology nursing in the local community. *Cancer Nurs.,* **2:**287–295, 1979.

Colley, R.; Appleby, L.; Ayello, E.; Garner, J.; Gough, J.; and Maher, M.: Hyperalimentation standards of practice of the National Intravenous Therapy Association, Inc. *NITA,* 4:105–107, 1981.

Copeland, E. M.; MacFayden, B. V.; and Dudrick, S. J.: Intravenous hyperalimentation in cancer patients. *J. Surg. Res.,* **16:**241–247, 1978.

Croft, C.: Nursing practice in a cancer clinic. In Peterson, B., and Kellog, E. (eds.): *Current Practice in Oncologic Nursing,* Vol. 1. The C. V. Mosby Company, St. Louis, 1976.

Cullen, M.: Current interventions for doxorubicin extravasation. *Oncol. Nurs. Forum,* 9:52–53, 1982.

Daeffler, R.: Oral hygiene measures for patients with cancer. I. *Cancer Nurs.,* **3:**347–356, 1980a.

Daeffler, R.: Oral hygiene measures for patients with cancer. II. *Cancer Nurs.,* **3:**427–432, 1980b.

Daeffler, R.: Oral hygiene measures for patients with cancer. III. *Cancer Nurs.,* **4:**29–35, 1981.

Donley, D.: Nursing assessment of the oncology patient. In Burkhalter, P., and Donley, D. (eds.): *Dynamics of Oncology Nursing.* McGraw-Hill, Inc., New York, 1978.

Donovan, M.: Relaxation with guided imagery: A useful technique. *Cancer Nurs.,* **3:**27–32, 1980.

Dudrick, S. J., and Rhoads, J. E.: New horizons for intravenous feeding. *J.A.M.A.,* **215:**939–949, 1971.

Eustace, P.: History and development of cisplatin in the management of malignant disease. *Cancer Nurs.,* **3:**373–378, 1980.

Fedak, M.: Nutrition and cancer. In Donovan, M. (ed.): *Cancer Care: A Guide for Patient Education.* Appleton-Century-Crofts, New York, 1981.

Fox, L.: Granulocytopenia in the adult cancer patient. *Cancer Nurs.,* **4:**459–466, 1981.

Gebbie, K., and Lavin, M.: Classifying nursing diagnoses. *Am. J. Nurs.,* **74:**250–253, 1974.

Given, B.: Education of the oncology nurse: The key to excellent patient care. *Semin. Oncol.,* **7:**71–79, 1980.

Graham, V., and Rubal, B.: Recipient and donor response to granulocyte transfusion and leukapheresis. *Cancer Nurs.,* **3:**97–100, 1980.

Henke, C.: Emerging roles of the nurse in oncology. *Semin. Oncol.,* **7:**4–8, 1980a.

Henke, C. (ed.): The nurse oncologist. *Semin. Oncol.,* **7:**4–8, 1980b.

Hilderley, L.: The role of the nurse in radiation oncology. *Semin. Oncol.,* **7:**39–47, 1980.

Hilderley, L.: Radiotherapy. In Groenwald, S. (ed.): *Cancer Nursing: Principles and Practice.* Wadsworth Health Sciences Division, Belmont, California (in press).

Hubbard, S.: Chemotherapy and the cancer nurse. In Marino, L. (ed.): *Cancer Nursing.* The C. V. Mosby Company, St. Louis, 1981.

Hunter, G., and Johnson, S.: Physical support systems for the homebound oncology patient. *Oncol. Nurs. Forum,* 7:21–23, 1980.

Jacox, A., and Rogers, A.: The nursing management of pain. In Marino, L. (ed.): *Cancer Nursing.* The C. V. Mosby Company, St. Louis, 1981.

Jaffe, J., and Martin, W.: Opioid analgesics and antagonists. In Gilman, A. G.; Goodman, L.; and Gilman, A. (eds.): *The Pharmacological Basis of Therapeutics,* 6th ed. Macmillan, Inc., New York, 1980.

Jarrett, V.: The keeper of the keys. *Am. J. Nurs.,* **65:**69, 1965.

Jones, L.; Miller, N.; and Wegmann, J.: Organizing cancer inpatient care: Scattered-bed versus oncology unit approach. *Oncol. Nurs. Forum,* 8:31–36, 1981.

Komorita, N.: Nursing diagnosis. *Am. J. Nurs.,* **63:**83–86, 1965.

Kreamer, K.: Anaphylaxis resulting from chemotherapy. *Oncol. Nurs. Forum,* 8:13–16, 1981.

Levitt, D.: Use of the heparin lock on an outpatient basis. *Cancer Nurs.,* **4:**115–119, 1981.

Lipman, A.: Drug therapy in cancer pain. *Cancer Nurs.,* **3:**39–46, 1980.

Maxwell, M.: Nurse practitioner chemotherapy clinic. *Cancer Nurs.,* **2:**211–218, 1979.

Maxwell, M.: Reexamining the dietary restrictions with procarbazine (an MAOI). *Cancer Nurs.,* **3:**451–457, 1980.

McCaffery, M.: *Nursing Management of the Patient with Pain,* 2nd ed. J. B. Lippincott, Company, Philadelphia, 1979.

McCain, R.: Nursing by assessment—Not intuition. *Am. J. Nurs.,* **65:**82–84, 1965.

Miller, S.; Dodd, M.; Goodman, M.; and Pluth, N.: *Cancer Chemotherapy: Guidelines and Recommendations for Nursing Education and Practice,* Oncology Nursing Society, Pittsburgh, 1984.

Moritz, D.; Suski, N.; and Dixon, J.: Malnutrition. In Groenwald, S. (ed.): *Cancer Nursing: Principles and Practice.* Wadsworth Health Sciences Division, Belmont, California (in press).

Owen, H.; Klove, C.; and Cotanch, P.: Bone marrow harvesting and high-dose BCNU therapy: Nursing implications. *Cancer Nurs.,* **4:**199–205, 1981.

Patterson, P.: Granulocyte transfusion: Nursing considerations. *Cancer Nurs.,* **3:**101–104, 1980.

Pierce, J., and YaDeau, R.: Methadone for pain relief in

disseminated malignant disease. *Oncol. Nurs. Forum,* **7**:14–17, 1980.

Satterwhite, B.; Pryor, A.; and Harris, M.: Development and evaluation of chemotherapy fact sheets. *Cancer Nurs.,* **3**:277–283, 1980.

Scholin, M.; Murray, J.; Wharton, J.; and Rutledge, F.: The gynecology chemotherapy nurse specialist. *Cancer Nurs.,* **1**:456–462, 1978.

Scogna, D., and Schoenberger, C.: Biological response modifiers: An overview and nursing implications. *Oncol. Nurs. Forum,* **9**:45–59, 1982.

Shils, M. E.: Guidelines for total parenteral nutrition. *J.A.M.A.,* **220**:1721–1729, 1972.

Smith, D.: A clinical nursing tool. *Am. J. Nurs.,* **68**:2384–2388, 1968.

Spross, J.; Grand, M.; Cullen, M.; Stuart, M.; and Frogge, M.: Issues in chemotherapy administration. Oncol. Nurs. Forum, **9**:50–54, 1982.

Stromborg, M.: Nursing's contribution to case finding and the early detection of cancer. In Marino, L. (ed.): *Cancer Nursing.* The C. V. Mosby Company, St. Louis, 1981.

Welch, D.; Follo, J.; and Nelson, E.: The development of a specialized nursing assessment tool for cancer patients. *Oncol. Nurs. Forum,* **9**:37–44, 1982.

Yasko, J.: *Care of the Client Receiving External Radiation Therapy.* Reston Publishing Company, Inc., Reston, Virginia, 1982.

Yasko, J., and Lauffer, B.: Infection in the cancer patient. In Donovan, M. (ed.): *Cancer Care, A Guide for Patient Education.* Appleton-Century-Crofts, New York, 1981.

48

Hospice Care for the Patient with Cancer

JACK M. ZIMMERMAN

In spite of the numerous modalities available for the treatment of malignant tumors, for many patients, at some point, cure becomes impossible. The problems faced by dying patients deserve the earnest attention of physicians. A suitable means of organizing and delivering that specific form of care is the subject of this chapter. It must be emphasized that such emphasis on terminal care in no way detracts from the critical importance of prevention, early detection, appropriate curative treatment, and vigorous rehabilitation of cancer patients.

FUNDAMENTAL CONSIDERATIONS IN THE CARE OF THE TERMINALLY ILL

Terminally ill patients and their families face a variety of problems. These are very familiar to physicians who care for such patients and have been the subject of considerable interest and study (Mount, 1976a; Ryder and Ross, 1977). They fall into several categories.

Some of the problems are related to the patient's illness and its complications. Symptoms such as pain, weakness, anorexia, dyspnea, and others can be a source of great suffering both to patients and their loved ones. In the wake of serious illness come a variety of preexisting and new physical and psychosocial problems, often compounded by financial difficulties (Garland, 1978).

In addition, the patient and family must deal with the fact of impending death (Trillin, 1981). They may cope with approaching loss and separation in a number of ways, including denial. Whatever techniques the patient and the family use, there are significant psycho-logic, emotional, and spiritual matters that press in upon all who are involved.

Those involved with the care of dying patients recognize that such care has often been less than optimal. At times, in an effort to "do something," patients with incurable cancer have been provided with useless antitumor therapy which they and their family and friends perceive as contributing to their suffering rather than relieving it. On the other hand a "nothing further can be done" attitude has sometimes compounded the desperation, isolation, and loneliness the dying patient experiences. So, frequently our efforts to cope with the multitude of difficulties faced by patient and family seem feeble.

Many factors have contributed to suboptimal care for the terminally ill. These include increased specialization and consequent fragmentation in medical practice, the tendency to institutionalize anyone seriously ill from any cause, and overuse of readily available sophisticated diagnostic and therapeutic measures. Prevalent attitudes toward the dying process and death also play a role. All these factors have created some impediments to appropriate care of the dying patient.

In approaching the matter of improving the care of the terminally ill, it is wise to begin with the difficult task of articulating the objectives of such care. The overall goal is to make the dying process as comfortable as possible. This includes attention to both the *quantity* and the *quality* of life. To achieve this goal a number of specific objectives for a program for the care of the terminally ill can be identified (Zimmerman, 1981). Such a program should provide the finest available medical management for the patient's physical problems. It should provide patients and their families an appropriate understanding of the nature of the patient's situation. It should make available to patient and family suitable psychosocial, spiritual, and financial assistance. All patient care should be rendered in the optimal setting for the patient's physical status. Care should be comprehensive and available at all times. Such a program must be financially feasible. Ideally it should have a positive impact on the remainder of the health care system and should provide for ongoing research and education in the care of the terminally ill.

ORIGINS OF HOSPICE CARE

In recent years a semiorganized response to the problems of the care of the terminally ill has developed in the form of hospices. Although its origins extend far back in history and to the finest traditions of medicine and nursing, the modern hospice care movement arose in very large measure from the efforts of Dr. Ciceley Saunders. After preliminary work in other settings, Dr. Saunders opened St. Christopher's Hospice in Syndenham, England, in 1967, specifically for the care of the terminally ill. Since that time numerous other programs have developed, initially throughout the United Kingdom, and in the last several years in Canada, the United States (Comptroller General, 1979), and other parts of the world. For a number of reasons, the spread of hospice care has been characterized as a "movement."

The term *hospice* of course dates back to medieval times when it was used to designate a way station for travelers. Over the years it has had a variety of different meanings and still does. As applied to the care of the dying, however, it has come to identify a method of approach to terminal illness.

ORGANIZING AND FINANCING OF HOSPICE PROGRAMS

Innovation, flexibility, and diversity have characterized the development of hospices. One of the healthiest aspects of hospice care has been the capacity of individual programs to adapt to specific local circumstances (Buckingham and Lupa, 1982). The many different models have made it difficult to categorize them clearly.

St. Christopher's and most of the English programs are best characterized as *free-standing* hospices. They are located in buildings that are separate from and, for the most part, unassociated with hospitals or other institutions. Some programs in the United States such as Hospice, Inc., in Connecticut and the Hospice of Marin in California have employed this model.

In the United States and Canada *hospital-based* programs have been developed. In some instances the inpatient facility is a separate identifiable unit as it is at the Royal Victoria Hospital in Montreal. Elsewhere, such as at Church Hospital in Baltimore, all of the inpatients are on a single nursing unit but are mixed in with other patients in "swing beds." A third variation of this model is that at St. Luke's Hospital in New York, where a symptom-relief team visits patients in "scatter beds" throughout the hospital. Most free-standing and hospital-based programs also offer home care.

Certain programs are essentially *outpatient* ones without an inpatient component and usually aim to develop the capacity for continuity with inpatient management through one or more hospitals or other institutions.

The administrative structure of a hospice program can be adapted to local circumstances. For free-standing hospices there must be, of course, a governing board with overall responsibility. For hospital-based hospices the hospital governing board can serve this function, and the hospice operation can be handled in much the same fashion as are other interdisciplinary programs such as hyperalimentation. It is often helpful to have the program under the direction of a medical staff committee. Feasibility studies, potential patient loads, criteria and procedures for admission, and staffing patterns must be established. Operating policy must be set and, from time to time, altered. The precise mechanism for this can be designed to suit the individual circumstances within which the hospice is to function (Cameron, 1981).

Almost all hospice programs have utilized a multidisciplinary team. The composition of the team has varied depending upon local circumstances. Physician involvement is vital because, to be truly effective, hospice care must be a medically based program. Such physician participation can be accomplished in a number of ways. In some programs all patients entered are placed under the care of a hospice physician. In other programs the referring physician continues to serve as the patient's attending physician. In some, such as the one at Church Hospital, the referring physician is offered the option of continuing to attend the patient or of placing the patient under the care of a hospice physician.

Excellent nursing care is an essential ingredient of hospice care. In many programs nurses serve as overall program coordinators. Social workers, chaplains, dietitians, pharmacists, physical therapists, and speech therapists are full-fledged members of the team.

In most hospice programs volunteers have played a critical role. They have been of immense value both with inpatients and in the home care setting. The volunteer offers a perspective that is different from that of the professional and, when properly trained, can offer invaluable service to patients in a variety of ways. The use of volunteers has made some hospice programs financially feasible.

Hospice team members must be carefully selected. Confidence, compassion, sensitivity, integrity, and maturity are essential characteristics of the hospice worker. Once selected, hospice team members must be thoroughly trained to provide hospice care and must be given continuing education. Their performance must be evaluated. Staff stress, so-called burnout, in those working with the terminally ill has been noted. Some measures have proven useful in minimizing, detecting, and treating such stress (Zimmerman, 1981).

Ideally, a hospice program should be able to provide continuity of care to each patient in the location the patient's status demands: hospital, intermediate care facility, or home. In actuality, few hospice programs have achieved this ideal. As noted, the organizational structure of most programs is such that continuity is to some extent lost in one or two of these settings.

For inpatient hospital care, standing hospital policies and procedures can and should be relaxed somewhat for hospice patients. It has been shown it is possible to do this without detriment to the care of the hospice or other hospital patients. Visitors may be permitted around the clock, pets may be allowed to visit, and connubial visits can be arranged. Although all of the facilities of inhospital care are available, the nature of hospice care is such that little use is made of highly technical diagnostic and therapeutic methods.

For a number of reasons, terminally ill patients should be at home as much as possible. Once the patient and the family understand the situation and are provided with the necessary techniques to make care at home comfortable, the patient and family want to have home care (Wilkes, 1973). Certain requirements must be met before home care is possible. The mechanisms of symptom control must be manageable at home. At least one person in the home must be able and willing to provide the care necessary. A well-trained home care staff that includes many members of the hospice team must be available. Suitable equipment and supplies are necessary in the home. Ready accessibility to a higher level of care is also necessary.

The vast majority of patients can be managed either in the hospital or at home. For a few patients, however, an intermediate care facility of some type is essential. Most frequently, such care is necessitated by the lack of an able and willing care-giver in the home. Occasionally, the nature of the patient's symptoms combined with life expectancy makes neither acute hospital care nor home care feasible.

Financing of hospice care has two dimensions, each of which is important. The first is encompassed in the question, "How expensive is hospice care?" The answer to this question is somewhat complex. For example, one must begin by comparing the expense of hospice care with the expense of alternatives. Compared to no care at all, hospice care is more costly. When measured against conventional care including periodic sophisticated laboratory studies, the use of intravenous feeding, chemotherapy, and radiation, hospice care compares favorably in expense.

While a hospice patient is in the hospital, relatively little use is made of technologically sophisticated diagnostic and therapeutic measures. On the other hand, hospice care is labor-intensive. A substantial portion of this attention, however, can be provided by volunteers and by family. The net result of this low-technology, labor-intensive care is that the average inpatient cost per patient day for hospice patients is probably somewhat less than that for terminally ill patients managed outside the hospice setting (Breindel and Gravely, 1980).

Furthermore, the availability of excellent home care makes it possible for the hospice patient to spend a larger proportion of the terminal illness at home. Because it is somewhat more sophisticated and organized, home care costs are doubtless somewhat higher, as a rule, for hospice than for nonhospice patients.

Data are still being gathered on this matter, but on the basis of the information available to date, it would appear that somewhat lower daily inpatient costs and shorter hospital stays combined with somewhat higher home care costs and longer outpatient stays result in hospice care being an economically attractive alternative to traditional terminal care.

The other dimension of the financial aspect of hospice care is defined by the question "How does one get reimbursed for hospice care?" For inpatients in an acute hospital, reimbursement is essentially the same as for nonhospice patients. The patient hospitalized under a hospice program would generally require hospitalization if not in the program. Therefore, third-party payers reimburse for such patients in much the same fashion as they would for any other hospitalized patient.

Reimbursement for outpatient care is somewhat more complex and less complete. Health insurance developed in the United States largely as *hospitalization* insurance, and the consequences of this approach still exist. Many patients do not have a home care provision in their health insurance. For such patients limited reimbursement is available from third-party payers for home care. Increasingly, insurers are recognizing the advantages of outpatient care in reducing overall health care costs. Consequently, some patients do possess home care coverage, and many services are reimbursed. Even for these patients, however, certain features of coverage are not suitable for hospice care. For example, frequently stipulations state that the patient must have had a prior period of hospitalization or that the patient must be homebound. Home care visits for hospice patients are usually longer than those for patients on other types of home care. Bereavement follow-up for the family, which is a part of hospice care, is usually not covered by health insurance. Therefore, for many aspects of hospice home care, reimbursement is presently incomplete.

For free-standing hospices the reimbursement problem may be even more severe. In some areas such institutions are not recognized as a part of the health care system and are not reimbursed at all.

The problem of reimbursement for hospice care is being addressed in a number of ways. Demonstration projects sponsored by federal and state government and insurance carriers are experimenting with liberalized reimbursement formulas. Legislation mandating the inclusion of hospice care in health insurance options offered has been passed in several states. There are many problems yet to be solved, but there have been some encouraging developments.

GENERAL FEATURES OF HOSPICE CARE

One of the most prominent features of hospice programs as they have developed has been their diversity. This has been most evident in the organization and administration of patient care. Therefore, it is difficult to provide a precise definition of hospice care. Certain common elements, however, are woven through care in various hospices so consistently that they can be defined as cardinal principles of such care.

Symptom Control

Care is directed primarily at symptom control rather than at control of the disease process. This does not mean that in patients with cancer antitumor therapy has no part. It does mean that such therapy plays a secondary role because it is administered only to control symptoms. The techniques used to relieve symptoms, for the most part, avoid sophisticated technologic methods. They emphasize intense personal attention.

The Patient and the Family as the Unit of Care

Although true to some extent of all medical care, for the terminally ill it is particularly important that the family as well as the patient receive attention. The family can be regarded as having a dual role in hospice care. In part they are the *recipients* of care, including such psychologic, social, and financial support as may be appropriate. One aspect of this care is the development of some insight into the patient's illness, prognosis, and management. Once this level of understanding is achieved, family members can, in a real sense, become *providers* of care to the patient.

Care Provided in the Most Appropriate Setting

At all times during their terminal illness patients should be in the setting most appropriate to their needs. This may be at home, in the hospital, or in some type of intermediate care facility. Hospice care is usually designed to provide continuity as the patient's condition dictates change from one setting to another. Ideally, then, hospices are programs not places.

Care Provided by a Multidisciplinary Team

As noted, terminally ill patients and their families face a variety of difficulties of different origins and types, including problems related to disease or impending death, and those that were preexisting before the patient became terminally ill. Problems may be physical, psychologic, social, financial, legal, and/or spiritual. A team approach is best suited to deal with them, and coordination of this effort is of critical importance.

Each hospice program decides for itself the definition of "terminal illness" that will make a patient eligible for entry into the program. Most hospices are directed primarily or exclusively at patients in terminal stages of cancer. Others will admit patients with other forms of terminal disease such as the progressive neurologic disorders like multiple sclerosis. Whatever the nature of disease accepted, each program must set criteria and establish procedures for entry into the program.

Terminal illness can be defined in a number of ways. For patients with cancer it is usually defined as the existence of a neoplasm for which treatment does not offer a reasonable possibility of cure or significant palliation. For many patients it is easy to recognize when this criterion is met, whereas in other cases there may be less clear-cut agreement. In such instances the use of consultation or a tumor board can be helpful. The decision to consider a patient incurable is obviously a momentous one and must be made with great care. But for terminally ill patients, it is usually to their advantage that the situation be forthrightly defined and acted upon. Hospice care then opens the potential to make dying more comfortable.

Most hospice programs establish additional criteria for entry. These will depend upon local circumstances, particularly if they incorporate home care. The available facilities for home care, for example, may be such that the patient must live within a defined geographic area. If no intermediate care facility is available, the hospice program may accept only patients with an identifiable care-giver in the home. The procedure for enrollment of patients will also vary from one hospice program to another depending upon individual circumstances.

In terminal illness, patient and family comprehension and acceptance of the diagnosis and prognosis are important, complicated, and controversial problems. Hospice care includes attention to this matter.

Terminally ill patients and their families vary considerably in their capacity to comprehend and accept their situation. For the most part, dying patients suspect or even "know" that they are terminally ill relatively early in their course. Denial does occur in most patients at some time and in an occasional patient is persistent. Nonetheless, surveys of terminally ill patients have usually demonstrated, from a variety of sources, that most have perceived the nature of their problem and furthermore that they wish candid discussion with their physician and others involved in their management (Saunders, 1965; Mount, 1976a).

Once the decision has been made that a patient is terminally ill, one of the first matters to be dealt with is patient and family understanding of the situation. The approach must be highly individualized. As noted, different levels of understanding are appropriate for different patients and families. Furthermore, one must be prepared to accept widely varying levels of understanding in the same patient from day to day. Therefore, coping with patient and family comprehension and acceptance of diagnosis and prognosis is not something done only once. It must receive continuing attention.

It is equally important that *listening* should precede *telling*. One must perceive where the patient and the family are in their understanding before one can begin to provide advice and assistance. One cannot tell a patient and family what they are not ready to hear. To attempt to do so will result in either frustration for the "teller" or disruption for the patient. Conversely, one cannot successfully withhold what the patient already knows. In order to avoid these problems, it is imperative that the care-giver listen carefully.

In listening and telling, nonverbal communication in both directions is of immense importance. Body movements, eye contact, and touch are often as important as the spoken word.

One may inform a patient about the illness and prognosis in many different ways. As a general rule, the truth presented in kindly fashion, at an appropriate time, and in a suitable setting can open channels that will be most useful to the patient and the family throughout the terminal illness.

SYMPTOM CONTROL IN THE DYING PATIENT

In identifying symptom control as one of the cardinal principles of hospice care, the term *symptom* is defined broadly to include family, social, financial, and other problems. In this section, however, the term is used more narrowly to mean physical symptoms.

Principles of Symptom Control

General Considerations. It is important to recognize that no standard, approved, hospice technique is available for dealing with any individual symptom. Underlying the approach to symptom management, however, are certain principles consistently adopted by hospice programs.

In general, physical symptoms must be relieved first. The patient who is in severe pain is unable to cope with social and financial problems very effectively, let alone deal with the spiritual aspects of facing death. Intense nausea and vomiting preclude meaningful thought and dialogue. Psychosocial problems, however, can aggravate physical symptoms. Support in coping with them can simplify symptom management.

Adequate communication with the patient regarding the symptoms is essential to their relief. Those caring for the patient must elicit information regarding the presence, nature, and severity of symptoms. This requires that care-givers provide both time and a receptive attitude. Without this, effective symptom relief is impossible.

Meticulous follow-up with appropriate adjustment of therapy is essential. Effectiveness of therapeutic measures must be monitored and ineffective treatment discontinued or replaced. When the primary focus is symptom relief, it is very easy to permit useless medications and treatments to accumulate.

Because symptoms are by their nature subjective, it is difficult to measure and convey in concrete terms the degree of success achieved in symptom relief. The impression of those who have worked in hospice programs is one of variable success with different symptoms. Pain control has for the most part been very successful. For other symptoms, such as weakness and anorexia, relief has been less striking and consistent.

Special Problems. In symptom relief for the terminally ill a number of issues have often raised serious problems.

Aggressive Therapy. Whether to employ intensive treatment, either antitumor therapy or other active measures, can in some instances be a difficult decision. Treatment in the form of surgery, radiation, and/or chemotherapy is used in hospice care only insofar as it contributes to symptom relief. Even within this dimension, however, it is not always possible to find agreement as to a particular modality's prospect of contributing to symptom relief. Furthermore, the value of other invasive techniques in palliative care is often conjectural. Whether to place an intramedullary nail or an intraluminal esophageal tube to relieve symptoms may be difficult to decide. Skillful clinical judgment is required and usually makes use of adequate consultation and careful discussion with the patient and the family.

Prophylactic Palliation. Prevention of potential symptoms may create some difficult choices, for example, whether or not to administer antitumor therapy for a minimally symptomatic neoplasm that may cause serious problems in the future. In patients with vertebral metastasis manifested only by pain, the question often arises as to whether early myelogram and surgical decompression of the spinal cord should be carried out before symptoms of neurologic deficit develop (Onfrio, 1980).

Treatment of Symptom Versus Search for the Cause of Symptom. Should one simply treat a symptom or search carefully for its cause with the prospect that specific treatment of the cause may be more effective than treatment of the symptom? Nausea, for example, may be caused by a wide variety of underlying problems ranging from medication to intestinal obstruction. Sometimes the cause of a symptom is easy to recognize, but in other cases may require an exhaustive diagnostic evaluation. Individualization is essential. Although complex technical methods of diagnosis and treatment are deemphasized, common sense and experience sometimes dictate the performance of selected laboratory tests where the potential yield in terms of practical help is substantial.

Treatment of Intercurrent Disorders. Patients with advanced malignant neoplasms are prone to develop certain intercurrent problems such as pneumonia and are not immune from others such as myocardial infarction. Once again, individualization is essential. Pneumonia occurring as a truly terminal event in a patient with widely disseminated metastatic tumor may best be left untreated. Myocardial infarction in a comfortable patient with incurable neoplasm and a life expectancy of several months, however, is usually best dealt with as it would be in a patient without cancer.

Techniques of Symptom Control

The following material outlines techniques that have proven useful in handling some of the specific symptoms commonly seen in patients dying of cancer. More detailed descriptions of the approaches employed in various hospice programs are available (Mount, 1976b; Saunders, 1978; Zimmerman, 1981). Abeloff (1979) has provided a comprehensive review of symptoms in cancer patients. The methods of symptom control utilized in hospice care will be recognized, for the most part, as conventional therapy. In dealing with certain problems, such as low-grade intestinal obstruction in the severely ill patient, however, unconventional approaches may be employed.

Pain. Although not uniformly present, pain is a common symptom in patients terminally ill from cancer. In fact, in the minds of many patients and families death from cancer is equated with pain. This sets the stage for the pain-fear cycle which must be interrupted for this symptom to be well controlled. The companion fear possessed by most patients is of being heavily drugged with narcotics so that life loses all meaning and dignity. For those patients with pain, this symptom must be relieved first before other problems can be dealt with, otherwise it is a barrier to all purposeful activity.

In the terminally ill patient with cancer, pain can be caused by either the tumor itself or other factors. Pain caused by hemorrhoids, fecal impaction, or dental caries can be a source of discomfort in the terminally ill and should be treated appropriately. For pain caused by tumor, first thought should be given to appropriate therapy: surgical excision, radiation, chemotherapy, or other measures. If antitumor therapy is impractical, fails to provide relief, or its effect is to be delayed, alternative approaches must be employed, such as analgesics, nerve blocks, transcutaneous electrical stimulation, neurosurgical procedures (Long, 1980), hypnosis, and acupuncture. Although each of these measures has its place, drugs have been the key technique used in hospice care.

In using analgesics, the mildest effective agent should be selected. The oral route should be used if possible. Because they are easier to swallow and dosage can be adjusted more readily, liquids are usually preferable to pills and capsules. When the oral route cannot be used, rectal suppositories are quite suitable. The schedule of administration of analgesics and narcotics is most important. Whereas PRN use of medications is very useful in handling acute pain, it is seldom indicated for the tumor pain of the terminally ill patient.

One may view pain relief by drugs in the terminally ill as a spectrum. At one end is unrelieved pain and at the opposite end is stupor from drug overdose. Fortunately, for most agents a rather broad central area of the spectrum in which the patient is pain-free but awake and alert is available. The objective is to titrate the patient into that portion of the spectrum and to maintain that level of pain control. To accomplish this, *regular* administration of analgesic is essential. The precise dosage of pain medication necessary to get and keep the patient in the pain-free/alert portion of the spectrum depends upon a number of variables and is a highly individual matter at any given point in time.

In approaching the terminally ill patient with chronic pain the first step is to provide assurance that pain can be relieved and alertness maintained. The next step is to titrate the patient into that central portion of the spectrum. For patients with mild pain it is generally suitable to begin with small doses and gradually increase them until the pain is relieved. For patients with more severe pain it is often preferable to first provide a good night's rest with adequate analgesic and then to decrease the dose gradually.

As indicated, the mildest effective agent should be used. Although at one time a mixture of heroin or morphine with cocaine and alcohol (Brompton's mixture) was employed in many hospice programs, recently single agents, such as aqueous morphine, have been administered when potent analgesics are required. Aqueous morphine is quite soluble and can be mixed with virtually any flavoring vehicle desired. When the rectal route must be used, hydromorphone suppositories are a good choice.

In the terminally ill, addiction is of course not a consideration. In addition, when narcotics are given for control of physical pain, dependency does not develop in the same fashion as it does when the drug is taken primarily for its euphoric effect. This has been demonstrated in patients for whom potent narcotics are used as a temporary measure while antitumor therapy, such as radiation, is employed for longer lasting pain control. Such patients are able to discontinue their narcotic rather readily once antitumor therapy has taken effect. Although increasing dosage of narcotic may be necessary to keep the patient pain-free as tumor advances, the nature of the development of drug tolerance is such that as dosage requirement increases, so does resistance to side effects of the drug. Therefore, drowsiness does not appear. Late in the course of advancing malignancy, however, debility tends to narrow the pain-free/alert portion of the spectrum. Consequently, in the few days before the death of a feeble patient the only choice may be between intense pain and markedly diminished level of consciousness.

Bone pain from osseous metastases is one of the most intense and resistant forms of pain. The addition of nonsteroidal antiinflammatory agents such as aspirin, ibuprofen, phenylbutazone or indomethacin may produce dramatic effect. Steroid preparations such as dexamethasone or prednisone can be used, particularly when pain is caused by nerve compression or by tumor in a confined space such as the head or pelvis.

As pain is controlled by pharmacologic means, it is important to remember that narcotics produce nausea and anxiety potentiates pain. Prochlorperazine is often helpful for its antiemetic and tranquilizing effects.

Constipation is also a problem with most potent analgesics, and ample stool softener should be administered with them.

Weakness. Weakness occurs in various forms in the terminally ill. For most patients it is a part of the final common pathway to death as tumor advances. In this form it cannot be

ameliorated. Sometimes weakness is a distressing symptom out of proportion to the patient's tumor load, however, and in this circumstance it deserves attention.

The first step in dealing with such weakness is to search for and deal appropriately with specific causes such as anemia, hypokalemia, and hypercalcemia. The patient should be encouraged in activity, and formal physical therapy can be very helpful. The use of corticosteroids or a testosterone preparation is often helpful. At times a central nervous system stimulant such as methylphenidate can be used with good effect.

Thirst. Thirst and dry mouth can be very distressing symptoms and are aggravated by dehydration, mouth breathing, and the use of narcotics. Careful attention to mouth care, frequent small sips of fluid, and sucking on ice chips can provide relief. An artificial saliva containing methycellulose and glycerin is also useful.

Hemorrhage. In the terminally ill patient bleeding, ranging from trivial to exsanguinating, can originate from a number of sources. The primary tumor, whether it is located on the body surface or in the viscera, may bleed. Hemorrhage can also occur from nontumor sources such as erosive gastritis or epistaxis. Coagulation disorders may play a role.

Minor bleeding usually requires no treatment, although it must be remembered that even slight bleeding can be a frightening experience for the patient and family. Accordingly, explanation and reassurance are an important part of treatment. When bleeding is more severe, it can present a difficult dilemma. In determining whether aggressive efforts should be undertaken to identify the source of bleeding, to control hemorrhage, and to maintain adequate blood volume, a number of factors must be considered. These include the patient's general condition, the extent and distribution of tumor, the presence of intercurrent conditions, and the cause of bleeding. The wishes of the patient and family should be sought. There must be no hesitancy in using consultation. It is best to make a clear and forthright decision for or against aggressive management in this situation.

Anorexia. Anorexia can be caused by a number of factors in the patient with advanced malignancy. At times, it simply seems to be caused by the presence of extensive tumor. In other instances, it may be the result of drugs, hypercalcemia, depression, or other factors.

Sometimes no reasonable explanation is found. Easily correctable causes should be dealt with appropriately.

Anorexia occurring early in a patient's terminal course may result in acceleration of malnutrition which can compromise both the quantity and quality of the patient's remaining life. In such instances it is worthwhile to try to encourage the intake of adequate nutrition. Corticosteroids and testosterone preparations can be administered as well as tricyclic antidepressants such as doxepin. Alcoholic beverages stimulate appetite. Dietary supplements can be helpful. Generally speaking, elemental diets and intravenous hyperalimentation have very limited use in the terminally ill.

For patients in the late stages of their disease, nutritional replenishment is of little importance. In this circumstance anorexia is usually more distressing to the family than to the patient. Close relatives tend to present the patient with large quantities of nutritious food with exhortations to eat, all of which aggravates the anorexia. This is one of those areas in which understanding by family members is of critical importance. They should be encouraged to accept that emphasis must now shift from maintenance of nutritional status to enhancement of the patient's comfort through the provision of small, appetizing meals. Careful meal planning is of utmost importance.

Dysphagia. Difficulty swallowing can originate from a number of sources in the terminally ill. One should determine its cause. Dysphagia caused by pain from radiation-induced pharyngitis or esophagitis is often improved by the use of viscous lidocaine. *Candida* infection should be treated with nystatin suspension.

Tumor obstruction in the hypopharynx and esophagus is, of course, a common cause of dysphagia. Relatively early in the course of the disease, feeding tubes or the insertion of intraluminal esophageal tubes, such as the Celestin, may be helpful (Hankins *et al.*, 1979).

In the late stages of disease, adequate hydration and nutrition can usually be maintained by frequently and patiently providing small feedings of liquids. Gastrostomy and the use of intravenous fluids contribute to palliation in patients with advanced malignancy only in certain special circumstances (King and Zimmerman, 1965).

Nausea and Vomiting. Specific treatable causes of nausea and vomiting such as digitalis intoxication should be dealt with appropriately. Intestinal obstruction is a common and sometimes vexing source. When the underly-

ing cause of nausea and vomiting cannot be corrected, the liberal use of antiemetics such as prochlorperazine can provide relief.

Constipation. Many factors, such as decreased food bulk, prolonged inactivity, and narcotic use, contribute to the development of constipation in terminally ill patients. High doses of docusate sodium plus a senna pod laxative usually keep the bowels moving relatively well. It must be remembered that fecal impaction is common in dying patients; if it occurs, manual disimpaction is usually necessary.

Diarrhea. Underlying causes of diarrhea such as medication and fecal impaction should be treated appropriately. Diphenoxylate with atropine and loperamide are useful when no treatable cause of diarrhea can be found.

Intestinal Obstruction. The handling of intestinal obstruction in terminally ill patients must be individualized. Account should be taken of the patient's general condition and the extent of the tumor, as well as the level and degree of obstruction (Osteen *et al.*, 1980). Complete distal colonic obstruction in a patient with relatively limited disease is usually best dealt with by the performance of colostomy. For the patient with widely disseminated intraperitoneal tumor producing partial or low-grade small bowel obstruction, however, nonoperative treatment without the use of nasogastric tube or intravenous fluids may be effective. Pain can be controlled with adequate analgesics and nausea with large doses of antiemetics. Stool softeners are liberally administered, and the patient is allowed to eat and drink. Although the patient will be free of pain and nausea, vomiting will occur periodically. Vomiting in the absence of pain and nausea has been described by some patients as similar to the sensation of voiding or defecating. Such an approach often permits the patient more comfortable final days than does the use of nasogastric tube and intravenous fluids or the performance of a futile laparotomy in the setting of abdominal carcinomatosis.

Cough. Treatable sources of cough such as postnasal drip should be sought and treated in the usual fashion. In addition, measures directed at treatment of the cough itself should be undertaken. The air should be adequately humidified. Expectorants such as potassium iodide and guaifenesin should be used if the sputum is thick. Codeine, either alone or in other preparations, is an excellent cough suppressant, as are the more potent narcotics.

Dyspnea. Remediable causes of dyspnea such as pleural accumulations should be drained and bronchospasm relieved with bronchodilators. When such measures do not produce relief, the use of oxygen, sedation, and careful positioning of the patient can provide considerable comfort. When dyspnea is associated with wheezing, dexamethasone often proves useful.

Depression. The first step in dealing with depression is the provision of simple psychologic support by members of the hospice care team. This, combined with relief of pain and the easing of some of the patient's socioeconomic burdens, can often improve the patient's mood. Tricyclic antidepressants such as doxepin are very helpful, and short-term benefit is sometimes achieved with the use of methylphenidate. Cocaine produces euphoria, but its side effects can be bothersome, particularly in elderly patients who may become quite confused on small doses. Psychiatric consultation is usually not necessary except as it may be required for the management of a psychiatric condition that antedated the terminal illness.

Insomnia. Sleeplessness in a terminally ill patient can range from a minor complaint to a devastating problem. Severe insomnia can contribute to the patient's overall debility and can have a profound impact on the family, in some circumstances making home care impossible and necessitating hospitalization.

When insomnia is mild, it is helpful for the patient and family to understand that loss of sleep is common and not harmful. Nighttime activities such as reading, watching television, and painting should be made available to the patient. One must be certain that pain is adequately relieved. When more severe insomnia occurs, a tricyclic antidepressant given at bedtime may be useful. Barbiturates and benzodiazepines frequently contribute to depression and are unlikely to be very helpful for severe insomnia in the terminally ill.

Dementia. Treatable causes of dementia such as excessive medication or correctable metabolic disturbances should be sought and dealt with appropriately. If hypoxia is a factor, oxygen should be given. When no reversible cause of dementia is present, primary attention should be directed at combating restlessness and agitation and to the support of close family members for whom this is a particularly distressing symptom. Chlorpromazine can be used in an effort to control agitation. For dementia with limited agitation, haloperidol may be helpful.

Paralysis. Individualization is essential for the palliative care of paralysis of all types and degrees. The major factors in determining the optimal approach are the site and cause of paralysis, the extent of tumor, and life expectancy. Physical therapy should be employed in patients with established paralysis if there is reason to believe that aggressive measures will restore function for a time. For most terminally ill patients with paralysis, however, rehabilitation is not feasible. In such circumstances attention should be directed primarily to the provision of comfort and the avoidance of skin breakdown.

Decubitus Ulcers. For decubitus ulcers in the terminally ill, as for other patients, prevention is more effective than treatment. In addition, the earlier a decubitus ulcer is detected, the more satisfactorily it can be handled. Therefore in the course of the terminally ill patient's routine daily care, one must be aware of the susceptibility to the development of decubitus ulcers. Alertness to the potential for the development of decubitus ulcers, the provision of good nursing care for their prevention, and prompt detection is of the utmost importance.

Fungating Growths, Draining Fistulae and Similar Lesions. In the management of an ulcerated, fungating mass on the skin, the objectives are to keep the exposed growth clean, dry, and odor-free while avoiding the development of frank infection and hemorrhage. Hydrogen peroxide solutions and other mild oxidizing agents can be quite helpful. Acetic acid and some of the preparations utilized for burn therapy such as mafenide acetate have been suggested (Wood, 1980). When bloody oozing does occur, the topical application of a vasoconstrictor such as epinephrine or a hemostatic agent such as absorbable gelatin sponge may be useful. Antitumor therapy including excision, cryotherapy, electrocoagulation, radiotherapy, and systemic treatment such as chemotherapy should be considered. The decision should be made on the basis of the individual circumstances. On the extremities, excisional therapy, including amputation, may in some situations be a most rewarding palliative maneuver.

Fistulae from various sites such as the intestine, urinary tract, and bronchus can be the source of considerable discomfort. The usual measures of collecting drainage and providing good skin care are important. Fistulae in the perianal area originating either from the urinary tract or intestinal tract can be particularly bothersome. When these occur, a choice must be made between local care, which is likely to be rather unsatisfactory, and the performance of a urinary or fecal diversion procedure.

CONCLUSION

Hospice care is not a unified entity that can be precisely defined. Nonetheless, the common features of most hospice programs offer an opportunity to improve the way in which dying patients and their families cope with the problems of terminal illness. They do this through focus on symptom relief, using a multidisciplinary team which can address the physical, psychosocial, financial, and spiritual problems faced by the patient and the family. This care can be comprehensive and can be offered continuously in whatever setting is most appropriate for the patient: hospital, intermediate facility, or home.

Although the experience of many hospice programs in many locations offers strong evidence of the success of the techniques employed, hospice care is still evolving. There is much yet to be learned and much to be taught about the care of the dying patient.

Vigorous and careful clinical research is necessary. The development of standards and accreditation of hospice programs are still needed, but it is hoped they will protect and preserve the flexibility and innovation that have characterized hospice. Hospice care must remain within the mainstream of medical practice. This is essential for the success of hospice, but also because it is through this avenue that hospice programs can enrich all medical care.

REFERENCES

Abeloff, M. D.: *Complications of Cancer: Diagnosis and Management.* The Johns Hopkins University Press, Baltimore, 1979.

Breindel, C. L., and Gravely, G. E.: Costs of Providing a Mixed-Unit Hospice Program. Working paper, Department of Health Administration, Medical College of Virginia, Richmond, 1980.

Buckingham, R. W., and Lupa, D.: A Comparative Study of hospice services in the United States. *Am. J. Public Health,* 72:455–463, 1982.

Cameron, G. R.: Administration of a hospice program. In Zimmerman, J. M. (ed.): *Hospice: Complete Care for the Terminally Ill.,* Urban & Schwarzenberg, Inc., Baltimore, 1981.

Comptroller General: Report to the Congress of the United States. HRD 79–50, General Accounting Office, March 6, 1979.

Garland, C. A.: *Psychosocial Care of the Dying Patient.* McGraw-Hill, Inc., New York, 1978.

Hankins, J. F.; Cole, F. N.; Attar, S.; Satterfield, J. R.; and McLaughlin, J. S.: Palliation of esophageal Carcinoma with intraluminal tubes—Experience with thirty patients. *Ann. Thorac. Surg.,* 28:224, 1979.

King, T. C., and Zimmerman, J. M.: Gastrostomies in patients with incurable cancer. *Am. Surg.,* 31:251, 1965.

Long, D. M.: Relief of cancer pain by surgical and nerve blocking procedures. *J.A.M.A.,* 244:2759, 1980.

Mount, B. M.: The problem of caring for the dying in a general hospital; the palliative care unit as a possible solution. *Can. Med. Assoc. J.,* 115:119, 1976a.

Mount, B. M.: Palliative care service: October 1976 report. Montreal Royal Victoria Hospital/McGill University, Montreal, 1976b.

Onfrio, B. M.: Metastatic disease to the spine, *Mayo Clin. Proc.,* 55:460, 1980.

Osteen, R. T.; Guyton, S.; Steele, G.; and Wilson, R. E.: Malignant intestinal obstruction. *Surgery,* 87:611, 1980.

Ryder, C. F., and Ross, D. M.: Terminal care—Issues and alternatives. *Public Health Rep.,* 92:20, 1977.

Saunders, C. M.: Telling Patients. *District Nursing,* 8:149, 1965.

Saunders, C. M.: *The Management of Terminal Illness.* Edward Arnold Ltd., London, 1978.

Trillin, A. S.: Of dragons and garden peas: A cancer patient talks to doctors. *N. Engl. J. Med.,* 304:699, 1981.

Wilkes, S.: How to provide effective home care for the terminally ill. *Geriatrics,* 28:93, 1973.

Wood, D. K.: The draining malignant ulceration. *J.A.M.A.,* 244:820, 1980.

Zimmerman, J. M.: *Hospice: Complete Care for the Terminally Ill.* Urban and Schwarzenberg, Baltimore, 1981.

49

Psychosocial Aspects of Terminal Care

CHARLES R. TARTAGLIA and MILA TECALA

Although advances in detection and treatment of neoplastic disorders draw attention to the need for assisting patients to live with cancer as fully and functionally as possible, the grim fact remains that most of these patients have a shortened life expectancy and will, sooner or later, succumb to the disease. The problems of patients in the terminal phase of illness and how they can be helped require concern. A textbook on medical oncology properly devotes space to the psychosocial issues of terminal care.

DEFINITION OF TERMINALITY

Conversations in medical and paramedical circles, as well as the literature in the field, are replete with references to "terminal care" and "terminal illness"; yet definitions of terminality and delineation of the terminal phase of illness are difficult to find.

The inevitability of dying is a generality to which a person may assent intellectually without acknowledging its reality in one's own life. A serious illness, potentially fatal, brings that reality home, eventually overcoming the individual's effort to deny it. The knowledge, partial or complete, of impending death seriously alters the person's perception of the *death trajectory* (Pattison, 1977), that is, the view ahead to the end of life.

In a person newly aware of mortality, there is an initial *crisis period* that is marked by heightened anxiety with, like any crisis, the dual potential for integrative or disintegrative resolution. This period of crisis gives way to a *chronic living-dying phase* of highly variable duration when the person confronts the implications of the illness and impending death, and adapts, well or badly, to associated problems and fears. In successful adaptation, the individual can maintain some degree of autonomy, complete unfinished business, retain self-respect, and resist the pull of regression until physical decline brings on the *terminal phase.* The terminal period is characterized by withdrawal from others, self-absorption, conservation of energies, growing apathy, decreased anxiety with increase in depression, and relinquishing personal autonomy and control to others.

As in all evolutionary schemata of a person's passage through the life cycle, there is no sharp demarcation between one stage and another. Rather the stages merge with one another and, at times, blend imperceptibly. It is impossible, therefore, to specify precisely when a person's terminal phase begins. By bearing in mind the characteristics just enumerated and being alert to their appearance in the course of illness, those caring for the patient are able to recognize this stage readily when it does clearly emerge.

How a person resolves the initial crisis of awareness of death in the foreseeable future determines the psychologic state in which the person confronts the implications of that fact. Similarly, how family members deal with these issues contributes to the nature and extent of the problems encountered in the chronic living-dying phase. Finally, how patients and families handle these preliminary phases and the relationships established and maintained with the medical personnel determine the character of the terminal phase.

INFORMING THE PATIENT

Integral to the quality of the relationships of patients and families with health care personnel is the quality of communication. Among the more important issues they must discuss is the patient's ongoing status, with the various ethical and clinical dilemmas that this raises.

Ethical Considerations

Informing patients with respect to diagnosis and prognosis in terminal illness is one of the most controversial issues in medical ethics. In its simplest terms, the conflict lies between the basic moral principle of veracity, as well as the patient's right to make informed choices, and the physician's obligation to do no harm — *primum non nocere.* Although moral philosophers disagree, truth is preferable, with deception requiring justification as an exception. Yet, most philosophers and physicians agree that, at times, the truth must be tempered by consideration of the harm that it may bring (Bok, 1978).

Persons may balance truth against potential harm in different ways, depending upon what ethical principle they are following, for example, protecting the patient's comfort *versus* protecting the right to know, and upon their assessment of the harm or gain that might result.

In a review of nine studies (Veatch, 1978), laymen consistently, and by margins varying from 60 to 98%, indicated they wished to be told of a diagnosis of terminal illness. On the other hand, physicians, by margins of 70 to 88%, said they would usually not, or never, tell a patient about a terminal diagnosis.

Of interest is a study (Noyes *et al.,* 1977) indicating a 50% increase between 1971 and 1976 in numbers of physicians and medical students willing always, or frequently, to tell patients their prognoses, representing about three-quarters of the medical personnel surveyed. This and other work (Novack *et al.,* 1979) may imply a trend toward consensus between physicians and laymen regarding this important matter of truthfulness and openness in communication. For the present, however, legitimate ethical differences exist, and each person is responsible for abiding by relevant ethical principles in the matter of information disclosure.

Clinical Issues

If one accepts that satisfactory relationships among patients, families, and health care personnel depend heavily upon trust and mutual respect, and that truthfulness is fundamental to the existence of that trust, then certain clinical considerations become relevant.

An important consideration is that communication is a two-way street. The physician, or other health care professional, does not simply tell patients various things about their conditions. Rather, the process is a collaboration in which professional, patient, and family members exchange information relevant to their ongoing dealings. The clinical management of this process of communication can be discussed under several headings: whether to tell, when to tell, what to tell, and how to tell.

Whether to Tell. From a practical standpoint, there are relevant data on the subject of whether to tell a patient about a terminal diagnosis and prognosis. Patients from whom the truth has been withheld often know, or strongly suspect, their prognoses. In one study (Hinton, 1980), more than 75% of the patients surveyed recognized that they were dying of cancer and communicated that knowledge to staff members who displayed an open attitude. These patients said they preferred frank communication and were happier when such openness prevailed.

Another report (Klagsbrun, 1971) describes several cases exemplifying patients' efforts, in the absence of direct and open communication, to use indirect and disguised requests for information — most often directed to nursing staff. The report further suggests that successful rehabilitation of a patient with cancer, terminal or not, depends on the health professional's sensitivity to these muted communications.

Finally, in practice it is virtually impossible to prevent patients' learning about their status, a situation attributable to the fact that information from the media about their disease is readily available, and everyone faces an increased threat of litigation in the areas of freedom of information and informed consent (Freireich, 1979; Novack *et al.,* 1979).

Given all this, physicians and other health professionals are prudent to adopt a general policy of frank and open exchange of information with patients. A few patients will not want to know, and scarcely anyone will want to know everything all the time, but it is wise to let patients inform their care-givers of that fact as part of their participation in the communication process.

When and What to Tell. Succinctly, patients and families should get whatever information they want, whenever they want or need it. Openness must begin in the first contact, often at the time of the initial diagnostic workup, and should continue throughout the course of the illness.

Openness can be properly thought of as a climate of communication. It need not involve a constant recounting of every detail of a person's condition and course. Patients and their families vary, in both the amount and frequency of information they require. Some patients may wish to know every detail of their conditions, even when that news is grim and painful. At the other extreme, others may wish to know only what is required for them to cooperate with their treatment and nothing more. Most people fall somewhere between these two extremes and will invariably offer clues to which medical professionals must be attentive to determine when and how much information to impart.

Patients and family members should feel that the physicians and others will offer needed information and will respond directly and frankly to whatever questions are asked. Medical professionals establish their availability and willingness to listen and tolerate whatever information the patient and the family need or wish to convey, without criticizing or withdrawing.

Patients and families need to know what is wrong, in at least a general way, in order to make some sense of the treatment program proposed. They need to know what is to be done about the disease and be assured that the physician will attend them and stand by them. Moreover, they need to know something of what is expected of them. They also need to have this information updated, refined, and reiterated, as new developments occur.

Finally, they and medical personnel need to know what cannot be known. Prognosis is an apt example. Statistical ranges and averages offer relatively little information about the course of any particular individual's disease. The rare, but nonetheless occasional, spontaneous remission must give one pause in predicting an individual's course, as does the occasional unexpected relapse and decline

(Brauer, 1960). Patients and families also need to be aware of the limitations of the professionals' knowledge and skills.

How to Tell. There is no "right" or "best" way to die. Human beings display a host of differing attitudes, values, perceptions, and ways of coping. Patients may differ from family members, as well as from health professionals. For this reason, there is no convenient recipe, either for helping patients die or for determining precisely how to speak and act with them and their families. One must ask the patient and family how and what can be of greatest assistance and to listen to the response — not only what is explicitly done and said, but also what is implied.

Crucial to such an inquiring and receptive approach is the success of the medical personnels' efforts to come to terms with their own attitudes and feelings about dying (Weisman, 1972; Pearson, 1979). Peculiarly high levels of death anxiety among physicians have been noted (Feifel, 1965), but such anxiety is certainly not confined to physicians. A considerable amount of energy and personal discipline are required to confront these issues and to develop the degree of familiarity and mastery necessary to carry out a professional role with the terminally ill patient.

Although no comprehensive list of do's and don'ts is possible for conducting these complex and variable relationships between caregivers and the recipients of that care, a few common-sense practices can be mentioned.

Conversations about grave matters are generally best conducted sitting down, face to face, and in private, in order to provide a personal and supportive environment. Most patients are intimidated by someone standing over them, especially by a whole congregation of professionals, as is the usual case on ward rounds. Eye contact diminishes the patient's sense of isolation, as do the privacy and intimacy of a one-on-one situation.

Avoiding technical terms, or explaining such terms if they must be used, is extremely important, both to ensure that the patient and family member understand the information and to enhance the sense of collaboration between them and the caregiver.

It is best to be brief. Too much information in one dose can confuse and befuddle, as much as too little.

Rehearsing what has to be said can allow it to be delivered with greater calm and in a lucid and tactful manner designed to encourage further dialogue (Cassem, 1974).

The care-giver should allow some amount of time, perhaps as little as a few minutes, to await a response from the patient or family member — either to ask a question or to react to the information provided. Unpleasant information, especially if unanticipated, may leave the recipient stunned and momentarily speechless. Interrupting a meeting at such a point can destroy a relationship with the patient. Silence, or a gentle inquiry with respect to the person's thoughts and feelings, is advisable if there is no immediate response.

The patient is often comforted by being touched. A number of authors (Cassem, 1974; Pearson, 1979) emphasize the imortance of touch in establishing a feeling of contact and in communicating a sense of recognition and worth.

Finally, information offered on one occasion can be reiterated at the next meeting or perhaps on several subsequent occasions. Unfamiliar data, especially if also distressing, can be very difficult to absorb and respond to in the usually brief contacts between care-givers and patients or family members. The repeated opportunities allow patients and family to digest the information, formulate and ask questions, and express their evolving concerns. The repetition also allows the care-givers in observing these responses to ascertain the state of adaptation of patient and family member, for example, whether and how much denial is operating, the degree of openness, and the character of their thinking and feeling about the issue, as a guide to further intervention and management.

PATIENTS' REACTIONS TO THEIR TERMINAL STATES

The effort to catalogue patients' reactions to the information that they have a fatal, or potentially fatal, illness has led to a number of published descriptions of reactions and several proposed schemata for their sequence.

Elizabeth Kübler-Ross (1969) has detailed five stages: denial, anger, depression, bargaining, and acceptance corresponding to the patients' responses of initial incredulity (Who, me?), anger or despair (Why me?), equivocal acceptance (Yes, me but . . .), and benign resignation (Yes, me).

Avery Weisman has emphasized the evolution of patients' awareness of their mortality when presented with a fatal diagnosis, from absolute denial, through a stage of "middle knowledge," to a stage of acceptance as death draws near (Weisman, 1972). He further describes several orders of denial: *first-order denial,* involving a disavowal of the primary facts of illness, *second-order denial,* in which the patient ignores the dire implications of the disease, and *third-order denial,* in which the patient accepts the diagnosis and its implications, but continues to resist the idea that death will result.

Weisman goes on to propose three psychosocial stages in the course of terminal illness. The first of these, *denial and postponement,* is characterized by first-order denial, and the patient's behavior is marked by avoidance and delay in seeking diagnosis for symptoms that are rationalized as innocuous and insignificant.

The second stage, *mitigation and displacement,* sees first-order denial give way to second-order denial and middle knowledge. As the diagnosis is confirmed and the initial anxiety of the crisis period swells, patients, unable to ignore the grim facts of their situation, may feel remorse or outrage. An attitude of blaming develops; self-blame for their condition is associated with shame, guilt, and depression, while blaming others takes the form of angry criticism and accusations of real, or imagined, failings in others, including family and medical personnel. A paranoid mentality in which the patient feels victimized is common (Brauer, 1960). Some patients equivocate, still hoping to forestall the inevitable: "I know I must die," they say, "but I want to finish one last bit of work, attend one last function, see one last birthday," and so on. These responses of residual denial, anger, depression, and bargaining correspond roughly to Kübler-Ross's first four stages and the phase of chronic living-dying (Pattison, 1977) mentioned earlier.

A curious interweaving or alternation of depression and denial has been noted (Abrams, 1970, particularly as the terminal phase approaches. The patients attempt to maintain an acceptable image of themselves during a time of bewilderment, confusion, and painful realization that they are no longer their usual self. The elements of middle knowledge in the patient, at one moment acknowledging death and manifesting profound grief and despair, at another denying this prospect and even talking about plans for the remote future, present a confusing picture, and one that sorely taxes the endurance of family members and care-givers alike. Indeed, this period in the course of the illness seriously threatens the relationship of patient and care-giver, at times leading the latter to regard the patient as ungrateful and unappreciative, and the former to feel isolated and criticized by the care-giver.

As the illness progresses and unmistakable signs of decline emerge, patients may resume denial, repudiating things that have already been acknowledged. This attitude signals the approach to the terminal phase, what Weisman calls the third psychosocial stage, *counter-control and cessation.* With physical condition deteriorating and symptoms becoming more persistent and unresponsive, the patient is increasingly less able to maintain a functional autonomy and must relinquish more and more control to the caregivers. If the relationship with care-givers has been maintained, and open communication has permitted trust to develop along with some harmony of goals, this process can occur with a minimum of disruption and distress.

Eventually, it is hoped that the patient will regress to a self-absorbed state, increasingly detached from even closest companions, concerned only with the avoidance of suffering, and retreat into a kind of "limbo of living" until death comes. In this stage, concern with the disease is properly supplanted by concern with the patient and the effort to relieve or, at least, minimize pain and suffering.

Four types of death can be defined at this juncture (Pattison, 1977): *sociologic death,* when the survivors detach themselves from the patient; *psychic death,* when the patient capitulates and regresses into the self; *biologic death,* when consciousness ceases; and *physiologic death,* when the vital organs stop functioning.

At times, these occur out of phase. Survivors may give up on patients before they are ready to die, exposing them to the tragedy of abandonment, perhaps the greatest fear of the dying patient. At times, a patient may capitulate long before the survivors do, and before biologic death and physiologic death are at hand, creating a kind of living death. In the best circumstances, with proper care and attention, these four types of death occur in close temporal proximity and allow the patient to experience a so-called "good" death.

Variations in Responses

The reactions described are the general human responses to a universal fear of dying. Mankind tries to confront, contend with, and, it is hoped, attenuate that fear, in order to allow for a death that is peaceful and free of suffering. These responses, however, vary strikingly among individuals, both in character and intensity, and one must look to the individual patient for an explanation.

Psychiatrists have grouped individuals into personality types on the basis of similarities in their coping styles: dependent personality, obsessional personality, histrionic personality, and so forth. Each member of a type shares certain sensitivities and preoccupations, for example, attachment in the dependent personality, control in the obsessional personality, and physical attactiveness in the histrionic personality (Kahana, 1964).

Moreover, the fear of dying is not a unitary fear but an aggregate of fears: fears of separation, of loss of control, and of disfigurement, to name a few. If care-givers can identify one or several of these component fears and their association with the peculiar vulnerability of a certain personality type, they can gain better understanding of patients' responses.

Individual differences in response among terminally ill persons also depend on where they are in their life cycle. Erikson (1950) has identified eight stages of personal development, designated by the psychosocial task of each stage. Accordingly, the young adult, concerned with establishing a close and enduring relationship with another, is most troubled by the interpersonal isolation caused by serious illness. The adult in the middle years is more concerned with a legacy to the next generation, and the major preoccupation in the face of terminal illness is likely to be that of providing for the family, especially the children. The older adult, on the other hand, is concerned that life goals have been achieved satisfactorily, if not completely, and faces dying with equanimity or despair, depending upon the perceived success or failure in that regard.

Children's Reactions to Terminal Illness

With a dying child, the situation is at once more tragic and more complex. The death of a child is always untimely and tragic—a life ended before it has come to flower. The differing levels of understanding possible at different ages make efforts to ease the process more complicated.

The factors influencing a child's response to death have been enumerated (Gullo, 1973): *the nature of the disease and its effects,* involving frequency and intensity of symptoms with different types and sites of cancer and the degree of disability; *the modes of treatment required,* at times the noxious effects of the treatment may be more uncomfortable and handicapping than the disease itself; *the nature of the child's relationship with parents,* involving the psychologic impact of "the only child," "the unwanted child," "the wished-for child"; *the nature of the support from medical personnel,* the child's adaptation to the "other family"—the hospital staff; *the communication patterns between the dying child and the family,* emphasizing the importance of dealing honestly with the child in support of a sense of trust, which will color the way the child views the world; *the child's integration and manifestation of the strengths and weaknesses developed in the course of living,* particularly the child's techniques for relating to others, frequently modeled on those of the parents; and *the child's level of understanding,* the nature of the child's developing concept of death and dying.

Regarding this last factor, four levels of understanding can be identified beginning with one year of age. The infant, the severely retarded person, or one whose consciousness is significantly impaired has little or no understanding of death.

For the toddler (age one to three years) illness and dying are largely a matter of physical discomfort and separation from parents, or others to whom the child may be attached. For a child this age, attachment to parents is critical to a sense of self and security. Illness threatens that security, and intense separation anxiety is characteristic of this phase (Pattison, 1977).

The preschool child (age four to six years) has developed a primitive awareness of death. Death and sleep, or lack of motion, tend to be equated, and death is seen as reversible. Magic and fantasy are dominant elements in the preschooler's egocentric world; accordingly, the child is apt to view illness as punishment for real or imagined actions. Hospitalization may be regarded as abandonment by parents, whose sorrow the child interprets as disapproval and disappointment.

Schoolage children (age six to ten years) are able to reason and reflect and have a beginning

recognition that death is universal and final. They tend, however, to personify and externalize death (the angel of death, grim reaper), perhaps allowing them to believe that personal death might be avoided (Nagy, 1948). Pain and mutilation from illness or medical procedures are the most prominent fears at this age.

Preadolescent and adolescent children (age ten years and older) have a concept of death similar to that of the adult. The child is also intensely preoccupied with self-image and with the effort to establish independence from the parents. Physical beauty and strength are prized as at no other time in one's life cycle. Dying negates all this since the adolescent endures regression, loss of control, and an altered body image. The result is a sense of shame and fury, the latter often directed at parents and medical staff (Schowalter, 1970). Death anxiety, similar to that of the adult, is clearly apparent.

FAMILIES' REACTIONS TO THE TERMINAL STATE OF A FAMILY MEMBER

Although all people die their own deaths, dying is also a family experience, and the anguish, fears, sadness, and guilt for a terminally ill loved one reverberate throughout the family network. Established roles and tasks shift, and the entire family must go through a period of readjustment and reequilibration in order to achieve a balance appropriate to the situation (Goldberg, 1973). The dying and death of a family member can be viewed as a major life crisis and, like any crisis, have the potential for settling previously unresolved issues by mobilizing new patterns of solving problems, which can lead to growth and maturity (Parad and Caplan, 1965).

Assessing a family's responses when a member is dying necessitates attention to several factors: (1) their previous adjustment to stress and the types of coping mechanisms used; (2) their previous marital or parent-child relationships; (3) the realistic impact of the illness and loss; and (4) the psychologic meaning attached to the illness and loss.

Each family member undergoes a set of responses similar to those experienced by the patient—denial, outrage, depression, equivocal acceptance, and, if all goes well, a final state of resignation that allows the wound in the family, created by the loss of a loved one, to heal, and the family to reintegrate and resume its functioning.

Several issues and situations deserve special note. These are not specific to families nor inherent in the terminal stage, but are experienced by patients and staff as well and may occur throughout the course of illness.

Alienation/Isolation

Just as patients at times withdraw from interpersonal contact, there may be mutual alienation between patient and family. Family members commonly feel overwhelmed by the disease and inadequate to give support to the dying family member. Withdrawal and isolation are sometimes the consequence of their fears of rejection and failure, a situation further complicated by the resulting lack of communication.

Response to Disfigurement and Mutilation

This refers not only to surgical deformity, but also to changes resulting from radiation and chemotherapy. Since their accepted role is to provide support and nurture, family members are often afraid to look at scars, ostomies and so forth, lest they betray their revulsion and cause the patient to feel rejected. Families lacking an opportunity to express their feelings uncensored may come eventually to find this situation intolerable.

Helplessness and Vulnerability

In the terminal stage patients lose control over bodily functioning and over making decisions and feel generally hopeless and helpless; families are often also immobilized by such feelings. Their fear that nothing they can do will alter the situation, coupled with their failed attempts, reinforce their feelings of insecurity. It is not uncommon to hear a wife or mother say, "It would have been easier for me if I were the one dying."

Reactions to Mortality

Cancer precipitates an unavoidable confrontation with mortality, the fear of dying, and all that it implies. For the family, particularly in the terminal stage of illness, a painful ambivalence exists between wanting to keep the dying person alive as long as possible and the wish to ease the suffering and burden, both for the patient and for themselves.

Family Behavior Patterns. Certain behavior patterns are observed in families, which are forms of coping, but tend to create problems for the patient, the health team, and sometimes for the family as well. These include the overreactive family, the overprotective family, the manipulative family, and the masochistic family.

The overreactive family is one whose responses to a diagnosis or prognosis, or any slight changes of routine, are exaggerated. They tend to engulf or smother the patient and to complain excessively about seemingly insignificant issues. The patient in such a family is often passive and withdrawn.

In the overprotective family, family members, without consulting the patient, take control over making decisions because they believe the patient is incapable, or too emotionally upset, to make decisions. In many situations, this may be a projection of the family members' feelings of inadequacy. Often, the overprotective family is also overreactive, and the patient is not only passive and withdrawn, but exhibits a muted rage.

The manipulative family is characterized by the conscious, or unconscious, attempt of one or more family members to set one person against another to achieve control. These persons tend to be suspicious, perhaps the underlying reason for the manipulativeness. Such family members may manipulate the medical team in order to direct treatment for their own convenience, using anger against the staff and threats of litigation to intimidate and obtain their own way. Such behavior is among the most difficult to manage.

The masochistic family manifests a strong need to suffer in what is appropriately termed the "martyr syndrome." For example, the wife may devotedly care for her husband, all the while complaining of the sacrifice entailed, blaming her failing health on strains, and lamenting that no one cares. She rejects offers of help, however, because they never meet her unrealistic and unattainable standards. Understandably, the patient in such a family is often guilt-ridden for being such a burden to his loved ones.

Stages of Reaction

The legitimate tasks of a family dealing with the terminal illness of one of its members include becoming aware of the impending loss, maintaining support for the dying member, accepting the final fatal outcome, and grieving.

Anticipatory grief is the first phase of a process of reaction and adaptation to illness when death is expected. Grieving begins as soon as the patient and family are faced with the reality of imminent loss (Weisman, 1972). This type of grief, however, differs from postdeath grief in that an element of uncertainty is inherent, grief increases as death approaches, and anticipatory grief is limited by time, ending with the death of the patient (Lebow, 1976). When there is effective, open communication between patient and family member, this time can be used to complete unfinished business, to heal relationships, and, with the patient's blessing, for the family to begin to rearrange their lives.

With the patient's death, the family must complete its mourning and heal its psychologic wounds. The symptomatology of this experience (Lindemann, 1944) involves intense periods of mental and physical distress, usually in waves lasting anywhere from 20 minutes up to an hour in time. Deep sadness, a lump in the throat, deep, sighing respirations, an empty feeling in the stomach associated with decreased appetite, lack of strength, and feelings of exhaustion are universal at this stage. There are often insomnia, a curious sense of unreality, and an increased emotional distance from others, who may be treated with irritability and anger. Warmth in relationships with other people often suffers, and the grieving are intensely preoccupied with whatever they have lost. Nightmares about the loss may occur as well. Survivors frequently feel guilty as if, had they done what they might or should have, the loss could have been averted. They may be restless and engage in aimless activity, but at the same time, have a great deal of difficulty in initiating and following through with any sort of patterned or organized activity.

The duration of this period largely depends on the success of the grief-work — that is, the ability of people to free themselves from what has been lost, to adjust to an environment without the loved one, and to initiate new interests, activities, and relationships. During several weeks to a few months, the various symptoms will gradually lessen, and the survivors will become more interested in going on with life.

MANAGEMENT OF PATIENTS AND FAMILIES

The multiplicity of problems and responses of terminally ill patients and their families can be reduced to a handful of specific conflicts to

which health professionals can apply their efforts.

Perhaps the most obvious problem is the physical ravages of the illness and treatment. Another is the steady diminution of personal autonomy, with a growing, and often repugnant, dependence upon others. A related issue is the struggle to maintain some sense of mastery and control in the face of a growing helplessness. Many patients feel a heightened sense of urgency to make their shrinking time for living productive. Another problem is to resist the undermining effect of illness on their sense of identity, as they are confronted with the progressive and often radical changes in appearance, comfort, and functioning. Underlying all of these problems is the basic struggle to maintain a feeling of personal worth and self-esteem.

Patients exhibit a set of noxious responses corresponding to these issues and problems, including denial when resisting awareness, anxiety and anger as awareness dawns, and depression and hopelessness when full realization occurs.

Denial

Denial is not *per se* a problem. Indeed, it may spare the patient and the family enormous suffering. Denial can be a problem, however, when it prevents a patient from accepting and cooperating with the treatment regimen, when it interferes with attending to important personal business such as preparing a will, and when it puts the individual out of phase with loved ones. Similarly, denial among family members can interfere with their availability to the patient and impede their responsiveness.

Denial should never be encouraged, but it need only be challenged when it outlives its usefulness. Then the challenge should be selective, aimed only at the areas and issues where denial is an impediment, and only to the extent necessary to reduce or relieve that impediment. Even then, denial can be a very sturdy defense and resist the most vigorous challenges. This resistance can be a signal to retreat, before frustration alienates one from the patient or family members. Should reassessment suggest sufficient cause or a weakening of resistance, then renew the challenge.

Only when denial sufficiently abates can professionals assist patient and family to address their unfinished business with one another and make the patient's remaining time as meaningful as possible. In this regard, whether patients are clearly terminal or not, once they acknowledge the possibility of dying, it can be useful to inquire tactfully how they would wish to spend their time and what goals they might wish to set. Patients may focus on the struggle to survive as long as possible or exclusively on the quality of that survival. What is important is that patient and family be helped to find compatible goals.

Anxiety

Anxiety is another troubling emotion. One of the first orders of business is to attempt to differentiate anxiety from fear. In the most simplistic formulation, fear is a response to an identifiable threat, while anxiety is a response to a perceived but unidentified threat. Since their clinical manifestations may not be easily distinguishable, it is important to begin by inquiring about the patient's or family member's perception of the nature of what frightens them or makes them anxious. If the source of the feeling can be identified, a number of possibilities may exist.

Often fear is based on lack of information — about what is happening or is about to happen, and about what resources exist for dealing with the threat. In these situations, supplying whatever information possible can go a long way toward reducing the fear. This effort addresses the issue of diminished control and mastery and offers patient and family an opportunity for intellectual mastery, even when they cannot directly control events themselves.

When the nature of the threat cannot be readily identified, consultation with a mental health professional may produce a clearer picture of the threatening issues.

Whether anxiety or fear is the problem, an important component of the emotion is that one feels not only helpless, but alone. Knowing that others realize the situation, are interested and available, and appreciate what the individual is experiencing can often attenuate patient's distress in a remarkable way.

In addition, antianxiety medications can be used judiciously as an adjunct to personal effort, as can specialized techniques, such as progressive relaxation, biofeedback, and the like.

Physical Suffering

Physical suffering, especially pain, was addressed in detail in Chapter 44. Emotion — anxiety, depression, and so forth — greatly contributes to physical discomfort. Reducing the emotional component of suffering can often diminish the perceived physical distress as well, perhaps decreasing the need for medications with their own potential for discomfort.

Anger

Anger may be the most difficult emotion to deal with, particularly if it is directed at medical personnel, because the implicit adversarial attitude tends to invite an adversarial response. Caregivers may feel cut off from the patient or family members, as well as defensive and antagonistic toward those they are trying to help. Yet they should try to look past the angry facade and appreciate the overwhelming fear and helplessness that prompt it, for which the anger is an attempt to compensate. Anger must be understood and tolerated, without censuring or patronizing. It should be handled in a matter-of-fact manner, acknowledging from where the anger stems and reminding the patient to focus on the real enemy.

On occasion, medical personnel do, in fact, inadvertently hurt or offend those in their care, and they need to be ready, without undue breast-beating or hostile defensiveness, to admit their mistakes and modify their approach accordingly. In so doing, they acknowledge the patient's integrity as a person, as someone of consequence, to be taken seriously and able to exercise in this way some capacity to take care of himself.

Depression

Depression is another emotion that at some point all patients, and virtually all family members, will experience. Depression is a general term, used these days to describe everything from normal grief and mourning to profound morbid states. The degree of depression may be difficult to distinguish clinically, but when faced with seriously diminished self-esteem and a global sense of helplessness, medical personnel should assume that they are dealing with a morbid situation and take appropriate action.

In less morbid depressive states, self-esteem can respond favorably to the support of caregivers, professional and nonprofessional alike. The key elements are the continued regard and respect with which care-givers treat the depressed person. This may include warmth and compassion, but also firmness and clearly articulated expectations, based on the person's capacities. A realistically based expectation voiced by a trusted care-giver implicitly acknowledges the other's ability to meet it and can be a potent reassurance to someone obsessed with self-doubts about abilities.

Similarly, in less serious depressive states medical personnel can effectively handle hopelessness. The hope most often thought of is the hope for survival. Realistically, in terminal illness the time comes when there is little substance to such hope. Hope is the necessary preventive to despair, but hopes other than for longevity can serve well in that regard. Care-givers can help a terminal patient or family member recognize that fact and look for alternative sources of hope, for example, hope for minimal pain or hope for continued attachment to loved ones until death. In more serious morbid depression, these efforts by care-givers will very likely be unsuccessful, and formal psychiatric intervention is indicated, including biologic treatment (antidepressant medication or electroconvulsive therapy) in addition to psychotherapeutic approaches.

Problem Behaviors of Family

For the problem behaviors of families described earlier, a few guidelines are in order. First, when discussing prognosis, changes in treatment, types of medication, and so forth, speak initially with the patient alone so that he or she can absorb the information and make decisions without being engulfed, overprotected, or manipulated by the family. A subsequent meeting with family members to keep them informed and to offer opportunities for questions and explanations can help reduce the family's anxiety and need for complaint.

Second, in dealing with a manipulative family, differences of opinion among the professionals must be resolved among themselves in order to present a unified front to the family. A wise move is to identify a staff spokesperson and insist that all communications with family be channeled through that person. The necessary conditions for treatment must be clearly identified by the professionals and articulated to patient and family, and appropriate limits must be enforced.

Finally, in dealing with the masochistic families, remember that complaints are often a plea for appreciation of their suffering, not for relief. For such persons, suffering fulfills a psychologic need, and they will invariably thwart efforts to improve the situation. Therefore, it is best to simply acknowledge the masochistic family members' discomfort and encourage them to go on.

Ultimately, it will probably be the professionals' role to accept an increased responsibility for the symptomatic care of the patients, to relinquish gradually their ties with them as they regress into the final decline, to witness their death, grieve their loss, and endeavor to assist the family to grieve theirs.

Multidisciplinary Approach

Assisting patients and their families through a terminal illness is a multidisciplinary exercise upon which the expertise of a number of professionals can be brought to bear. A common core group might include primary physician, nurse, psychiatrist, psychologist, social worker, and clergyman.

The primary physician has the central role throughout the course of illness and, in the terminal stage, has the critical task of controlling pain and other symptoms. In the midst of the fear and anguish of a terminal illness, the physician's presence and understanding offer continuity and enormous reassurance. The nurse offers physical care to the dying patient —dressing wounds, administering medications—and provides most of the patient's human contact. By their "laying on of hands" —always a healing symbol—nurses can soothe a tense and anxious patient, providing support and nurturing.

The psychiatrist offers psychotherapeutic intervention, pharmacologic guidance in the use of antidepressant and anxiolytic agents, and consults with the treatment team in order to develop patient management strategies, control staff anxiety, and reduce "burnout." The psychologist serves a similar function, often with special expertise in hypnosis, biofeedback, relaxation techniques, and other behavioral interventions. The social worker's role is also multifaceted: mobilizing community resources to aid the patient and family, providing counseling, especially in intrafamilial and interpersonal conflict, and, at times, collaborating with psychiatrist and psychologist in consultation with the rest of the team. Finally, the clergy have for centuries been entrusted with the soul. In recent years, they have developed their role as pastoral counselors, offering spiritual comfort to dying patients and their families. This multidisciplinary approach has been particularly well developed in the hospice setting as discussed in Chapter 48.

REACTIONS OF HEALTH CARE PROFESSIONALS

Health care professionals also experience a variety of emotional responses, similar to those of the patients and family members, in dealing with terminal illness. Physicians and nurses daily witness the traumatic course of fatal illness. They share the anguish of feeling simultaneously responsible and helpless, and labor under the burden of often excessive expectations from their patients, the patients' families, and themselves.

Most gravely ill people tend to attribute excessive power to the health professional, especially the physician, as they feel their own diminishing. The family may share this view also. For their own parts, physicians have a large element of the "hero" in their self-concept (Artiss and Levine, 1973) that leads them to expect a larger-than-life performance from themselves. This phenomenon, coupled with physicians' usually overdeveloped sense of responsibility, makes them exceedingly vulnerable to the implicit accusation of inadequacy and failure that their dying patients personify.

Physicians try to deal with this threat to their professional self-esteem by a number of coping techniques: denial, emotional isolation, intellectualization, projection, displacement, avoidance, and rationalization.

Denial is usually short-lived as a technique for dealing with terminal cancer patients, but more common is a selective isolation from consciousness of feelings, while maintaining an overintellectualized awareness of the facts of the patients' condition. This emotional isolation is exceedingly difficult to sustain, however, in the face of strong displays of anger, accusation, and despair by patients whose own protective denial ebbs as their condition worsens. At this point, holding themselves responsible, no matter how unrealistically, physicians are apt to feel guilty and ashamed.

In general, physicians tolerate the sense of inadequacy and helplessness poorly, antithetical as it is to their self-image, and a feeling of indignation and fury is likely to supplant it. They may blame the patient for their professional frustration as patients and family members may blame physicians for not curing the disease. Failure is projected to the patient, or displaced to family, fellow professionals, and so on. The attendant resentment threatens the relationship with patient and family, who are regarded as adversaries rather than collaborators. Physicians who recognize the inappropriateness of this reaction are at risk of becoming greatly depressed.

The continued pain of ongoing contact with fatally ill patients, particularly in the terminal phase, leads some physicians to withdraw and avoid the patient. Other persons — psychiatrist, social worker, minister — will be sent in their stead, while physicians rationalize their avoidance — "I haven't time." "There's nothing more I can do." "The mental health specialist has more expertise." — giving a certain legitimacy to their retreat.

For nurses, a similar pattern unfolds (see Chapter 47). More concerned with comforting than curing, they are faced with patients who are most unlikely to be comfortable, no matter how diligent and expert their ministrations. Nurses, too, may withdraw their emotions and become absorbed with the more technical, depersonalized aspects of care. This may include a rigid emphasis on getting patients to die in "the prescribed manner," for example, marching lockstep and on schedule through Kübler-Ross's five stages.

Nurses generally have trouble maintaining emotional aloofness, running counter as it does to the professional ideal of compassionate, caring attention. As a result, they encounter frustration, personal limitation, sadness, and loss that, when the nurse's tolerance is exceeded, gives rise to a panoply of responses: irritability, suspiciousness, contemptuousness, apathy, rigidity, depression, indifference, and emotional impenetrability, called "the burnout syndrome" (Maslach, 1976).

All of the phenomena just described can be viewed as the health professionals' encounter with their own "mortality" in its constituent problems: concerns over separation, competence, vulnerability, identity, personal worth, and so forth. This encounter properly handled, not simply evaded or negated, has the potential of helping health professionals accept their mortality, that is, their human limitations and foibles, and to equip them better for their role in terminal care.

HELP FOR THE HELPERS

As indicated above, the considerable stress for health care professionals threatens their effectiveness, as well as their comfort. Virtually no systematic studies, however, quantitate this stress or document the effects on the personal and professional lives of these individuals.

Several published reports recount efforts to help health care personnel handle the stresses better (Artiss and Levine, 1973; Richards and Schmale, 1974; Vachon et al., 1978). The reports strongly suggest the effectiveness of these helping efforts, which can be generally grouped into formal and informal exercises.

Formal exercises include conferences, seminars, and support groups. They are directed at students, trainees, practicing physicians, and working nurses, as well as clergymen, social workers, and other paramedical professionals. Although format and primary agenda vary, the common goals of such exercises are to express and discuss feelings and attitudes toward dealing with the terminally ill and their families and to provide support through realizing that one does not labor alone.

Informal exercises often take the form of conversations in the work setting among members of a common discipline or among members of different disciplines. Mental health consultants, for example, the consultation-liaison psychiatrist or psychologist, can stimulate and focus such conversations. These conversations provide consensual validation for one's observations and impressions, offer opportunities for practical problem-solving and realistic monitoring of expectations, and, above all, reduce the sense of personal isolation that intensifies the inherent stressfulness of the work.

Not everyone is inclined and equipped to participate in these sorts of group activities. For this latter group, it is especially important to have ready access to referral resources, usually mental health specialists such as psychiatrists, medical psychologists, social workers, and pastoral counselors.

REFERENCES

Abrams, R. D.: Denial and depression in the terminal cancer patient. *Psychiatr. Q.* **45:**1–11, 1970.

Artiss, K. L., and Levine, A. S.: Doctor-patient relation in severe illness: A seminar for oncology fellows. *N. Engl. J. Med.,* **288:**1210–1214, 1973.

Bok, S.: Truth-telling. II. Ethical aspects. In Reich, W. T. (ed.): *Encyclopedia of Bioethics.* Macmillan, Inc., New York, 1978.

Brauer, P. H.: Should the patient be told the truth? *Nurs.*

Outlook, **8:**672–676, 1960.

Cassem, N. H.: What you can do for dying patients. *Med. Dimensions,* **2:**29–34, 1974.

Erikson, E. H.: *Childhood and Society.* W. W. Norton & Co., Inc., New York, 1950.

Feifel, H.: The function of attitudes toward death: Attitudes of patient and doctor. *G.A.P.,* **5:**632–641, 1965.

Freireich, E.: Should the patient know? *J.A.M.A.,* **241:**928, 1979.

Glaser, B. G., and Strauss, A. C.: *Awareness of Dying.* Aldine Publishing Co., Chicago, 1966.

Goldberg, S.: Family tasks and reactions in the crisis of death. *Soc. Casework,* **54:**406–411, 1973.

Gullo, S. V.: Games children play when they're dying. *Med. Dimensions,* **2:**23–28, 1973.

Hinton, J.: Whom do dying patients tell? *Br. Med. J.,* **281:**1328–1330, 1980.

Kahana, R. J.: Personality types in medical practice. In Zinberg, N. E. (ed.): *Psychiatry and Medical Practice in a General Hospital.* International Universities Press, Inc., New York, 1964.

Klagsbrun, S. C.: Communications in the treatment of cancer. *Am. J. Nurs.,* **71:** 944–948, 1971.

Kübler-Ross, E.: *On Death and Dying.* Macmillan, Inc., New York, 1969.

Lebow, G. H.: Facilitating adaptation in anticipatory mourning. *Soc. Casework,* **57:**458–465, 1976.

Lindemann, E.: Symptomatology and management of acute grief. *Am. J. Psychiatry,* **101:**141–148, 1944.

Maslach, C.: Burned-out. *Hum. Behavior,* **5:**17–22, 1976.

Nagy, M.: The child's theories concerning death. *J. Genet. Psychol.,* **73:**3–27, 1948.

Novack, D. H.; Plumer, R.; Smith, R. L.; Ochitill, H.; Morrow, G. R.; and Bennett, J. M.: Changes in physicians' attitudes toward telling the cancer patient. *J.A.M.A.,* **241:**897–900, 1979.

Noyes, R.; Jochimsen, P. R.; and Travis, T. A.: The changing attitudes of physcians toward prolonging life. *J. Am. Geriatr. Soc.,* **25:**470–474, 1977.

Parad, H. J., and Caplan, G.: A framework for studying families in crisis. In Parad, H. J. (ed.): *Crisis Intervention: Selected Readings.* Family Services Association of America, New York, 1965.

Pattison, E. M.: *The Experience of Dying.* Prentice-Hall, Inc., Englewood Cliffs, New Jersey, 1977.

Pearson, P. W.: The dying patient with oral malignant disease. *Otolaryngol. Clin. North Am.,* **12:**241–244, 1979.

Richards, A. I., and Schmale, A. H.: Psychosocial conferences in medical oncology: Role in a training program. *Ann. Intern. Med.,* **80:**541–545, 1974.

Schowalter, J. E.: The child's reactions to his own terminal illness. In Schoenberg, B.; Carr, A. C.; Peretz, D.; and Kutscher, A. H. (eds.): *Loss and Grief: Psychological Management in Medical Practice.* Columbia University Press, New York, 1970.

Vachon, M. L. S.; Lyall, W. A. L., and Freeman, S. J. J.: Measurement and management of stress in health professionals working with advanced cancer patients. *Death Educ.,* **1:**365–375, 1978.

Veatch, R. M.: Truth-telling. I. Attitudes. In Reich, W. T. (ed.): *Encyclopedia of Bioethics.* Macmillan, Inc., New York, 1978.

Weisman, A. D.: *On Dying and Denying: A Psychiatric Study of Terminality.* Behavioral Publications, Inc., New York, 1972.

50

Psychosocial Aspects of Coping with Cancer

RICHARD J. GOLDBERG and ANDREW E. SLABY

Men that look no further than outside think health an appurtenance unto life and quarrel with our constitution for being sick.

But I who have looked at the innermost parts of man and knowe what tender filaments that fabric hangs on oft wonder that we are not always so

And considering the thousand doors that lead to death do thank my God that I can die but once.

Thomas Browne
Religio Medici
Norwich, England
1643

Cancer, more than any other disease, carries a stigma. The diagnosis echoes in the souls of patients for years, even unto death from other causes. Cancer can occur at any time, and no one is selectively spared. A young person, a "good" person, a talented person, a hardened criminal, a rich and powerful person — all may be invited to death by cancer. Even in the absence of risk factors, cancer strikes.

The picture today is by no means hopeless. In fact, persons with a number of neoplastic illnesses may seriously court hope of remission with cure. Nevertheless, those afflicted still feel hopeless, cheated, and that life somehow has been removed from their control. It is unfathomable that cells within one's own body can devour it. An infection is usually caused by something outside one's body. The person with cancer cannot look beyond for the insult except to genetic predisposition, or risk factors, such as ingestion of carcinogenic agents, exposure to radiation, or smoking. Absenting these, the reality is that something went wrong with one's own cells. Victims are helpless ob-

servers of a phenomenon outside their control. They do not know when the cancer began, even sometimes where in the body it originated. In some instances, such as with acute myelogenous leukemia, nothing can or could have been done to prevent the disease. Not preventive consultation with the most clinically skilled and technically adept physicians, infinite amounts of money and power, nor a life free of carcinogenic vices can prevent the disease.

Although it is an illusion ever to assume we can truly control our own lives, the awful awareness of on "what tender filaments" that fabric of life hangs creates in most patients with cancer a crisis — a turning point. The trite phrase that no one lives forever becomes a personal reality for the victims of cancer and their family, lovers, friends, health care providers, and community. For some, the attitude and reaction of those about them are more difficult to experience than their own feelings about life-threatening illness. One adolescent girl afflicted with leukemia at age 15 succinctly stated:

My mom needs to have it one way or the other. Either I am going to live, or I am going to die. When she heard about the new malignancy, she started working toward I am going to die. I can't accept that. I'm alive. I feel good right now . . . well, at least pretty good, and I am still doing things I like to do (Slaby *et al.*, submitted for publication).

Another child, a 17-year-old boy with the same illness, reflected:

It is good to talk, to get it out . . . just to tell how I feel. I used to think I would live forever. Now I realize I am pretty close to dying. I am not afraid to talk about it. I didn't want to avoid it because it is a fact. It is just the way it is. I am sorry if anyone feels depressed by it. I don't want that to happen (Slaby *et al.*, submitted for publication).

The unexpectedness of human tragedy even in the absence of so-called risk-factors, the uncertainty of recurrence even decades later, and the deterioration and pain that may accompany death terrify, focus, and mature persons in ways those not affected may never experience. Coping with cancer is possible. Most people afflicted with it and their loved ones do, but it is never easy.

The "tender filaments" that interweave to create the person in sickness and in health are biologic, psychologic, sociologic, and existential. These factors interact in predictable ways to help individuals adapt to internal and external threats to their beings. Internal threats to the person's integrity are not only of an intrapsychic conflictual nature; altered biologic homeostasis determines how people feel, perceive their environment, and how they function (Slaby *et al.*, 1981). Some people are more vulnerable to certain alterations in physiologic functioning because of genetic predisposition, current illness, or stress. Family histories may be replete with cardiovascular disease, diabetes, or unipolar affective illness. Less fortunate individuals may be constitutionally prone to more than one disease. Biologic illness may occur without a genetic predisposition. Mood, thought, or behavior may be altered by disease processes directly affecting the brain, as well as by any illness that alters the metabolism or physiologic functioning of the body as a whole. Some cancers alter endocrine functioning. Others, such as pancreatic carcinoma, may cause a mood change by mechanisms still not fully understood. A neoplastic process or its treatment may so alter the body's immune response that infection may occur, for example, fungal growths within the brain. Some therapeutic interventions, such as steroids, may alter personality as a direct toxic effect, and predispose individuals to infections that alter how they feel and act. Diseases like leukemia may cause widespread alterations in the physiologic homeostasis such that disease occurs that alters behavior, for example, leukemic infiltration of the brain, infection, or intracerebral hemorrhage.

Psychologic factors influence how a person adapts to internal physiologic changes associated with having cancer, as well as how they adapt to the treatments required, to the response of others, to the fact they have cancer, and to the isolation, loss of autonomy, and physical morbidity. Individual defenses vary and are based both on constitutional factors and adaptive responses learned early in childhood. Some persons are constitutionally hypomanic and tend to view the world through pink-tinted glasses. Even when struck with cancer, they seize upon tragedy as an opportunity to grow and savor life more richly, even when their days are numbered. Others are constitutionally predisposed to viewing the world through blue-tinted glasses. They may be haunted for years by the fact that they once had a positive Pap smear, even if cancer does not ensue. If cancer does occur, their worst fears are corroborated, and they retreat from life, making rehabilitation difficult. Others can adapt to stress under normal conditions very well, but when confronted with a life-threatening illness, their defenses fail them, or they become so rigid in their response that normal functioning is seriously impaired.

Social factors influence response to cancer in many ways. Individuals with strong social supports, in terms of family, friends, and lovers, respond differently to the diagnosis of life-threatening illness, as well as to the effects of chemotherapy, radiation, and surgery, than those with little or no support. The latter feel a sense of aloneness and loss of autonomy more acutely as they confront a disease that alters their ability to function and may lead to a lingering death. How a community, and especially a family and intimate friends, feel about the diagnosis of cancer influences how patients themselves feel about it, how well they fight it, and how well they tolerate treatment. For some nonafflicted individuals, the diagnosis of cancer is tantamount to that of leprosy in biblical times. They withdraw from people with it for fear they too will become either afflicted or depressed by the daily confrontation with someone who is deteriorating before them.

Existential factors are those ineffable philosophical or religious themes that influence how an individual confronts the inevitable realities of life. Some individuals, when confronted with a disease that is beyond their control and may bring about premature death, give up and die. Others, with bodies riddled with disease, fight with a will to live that defies empiric description. They want to go on to see a child marry or to celebrate one more birthday. This will to go on enables some individuals to live for longer than predicted or than objective evidence of disease spread would explain.

The following sections elaborate on how biologic, psychologic, social, and existential variables interact to alter mood, thought, or behavior in individuals with cancer, and how an understanding of these factors enables a care-giver to improve a patient's ability to cope with cancer.

BIOLOGIC FACTORS

Although major physical illness is stressful and disruptive, altered mood or behavior in cancer patients should not be automatically labeled a "psychologic" reaction. Biologic impairment of brain function can produce conditions that on the surface are indistinguishable from a wide variety of psychologic disorders. The development of a systematic approach to psychosocial problems in patients with cancer has been hampered by the scientifically unsupported view that psychologic distress, such as depression, is an inevitable aspect of the disease. For example, "Wouldn't you be depressed if you had cancer?" frequently is a disclaimer discouraging closer evaluation of the problem. Psychiatric symptoms are analogous to fever, jaundice, or anemia, and require differential diagnostic evaluation. Several common biologic factors contribute to patient disabilities which are often mistakenly presumed to be "psychogenic."

Organic Mental Disorders (OMD) in Cancer Patients

Complex medical problems are so prevalent in patients with cancer that organically induced mental disorders *should be the first consideration in evaluating any patient who develops impaired mood, thought, or behavior.* Many medical disorders impair neural function in the central nervous system (CNS), the final common denominator in all OMDs. The symptoms of CNS impairment depend on the region affected and severity of the insult. Generalized metabolic impairment often leads to delirium, referred to by Engel and Romano (1959) as a "syndrome of cerebral insufficiency." Delirium, often fluctuating in its clinical cause, is characterized by:

1. Difficulty sustaining attention
2. Disorientation and memory impairment

3. Perceptual distortion (along a continuum from misperceptions to hallucinations)
4. Increased or decreased psychomotor activity
5. Insomnia or daytime drowsiness

In its most dramatic form, delirium is easily recognized. The patient is obviously confused, agitated, and may have frightening or disturbing sensory distortions. In less severe cases, OMD may be recognized only by challenging the person with specific questions about mental status (Folstein and McHugh, 1975), since many patients mask their confusion by appearing quiet, depressed, or anxious. Behavioral changes in medical patients often are the outcome of underlying cognitive impairment.

Case Study. A 52-year-old married mother of two children had assisted her husband in his insurance business until two years ago when carcinoma of the breast was diagnosed. After a mastectomy and radiation treatment she did well for approximately one year when her personality began to change. She became irritable at home and short-tempered with her family and friends. People became uncomfortable around her and wondered what had happened to this formerly pleasant and sociable woman with no previous nervous disorders. Friends and family suggested a variety of hypotheses. Some thought that the first anniversary of her breast surgery brought back painful feelings that influenced her behavior. Others felt that she was "keeping too much inside" and was refusing to confront the serious nature of her illness. Still others speculated that she was purposely driving people away to ease the emotional pain for everyone involved. The patient suddenly developed a seizure disorder, however, was admitted to the hospital, and metastases to the brain from the original breast cancer was diagnosed. In retrospect, the location of this tumor probably accounted for her personality change, not an unusual initial presentation of tumor involvement of the brain (Posner, 1971). The patient was treated with further irradiation and placed on steroids to control cerebral edema. Approximately one week after initiation of steroid therapy, her personality underwent another shift. She became phenomenally energetic, euphoric, and talkative. The family was encouraged by this remarkable change in her outlook and felt that she was very encouraged by the successful management of her symptoms. Within a few days, however, her speech became more inappropriate and somewhat incoherent; she began to describe frightening apparitions in her room. At this point, the family felt the emotional strain had "driven her crazy." Her doctor, however, recognized the psychotic symptoms as a direct secondary result of steroid treatment, an effect that occurs in a small percentage of patients (Carroll, 1977; Ling et al., 1981). The addition of another medication, haloperidol, resulted in normalization of her mood and speech, and disappearance of hallucinations. In addition to euphoria or psychosis, steroids can produce symptoms of depression, which can confuse both the patient and the physician. Psychiatric symptoms can occur when the dose of steroids is increased, when it is maintained, or when it is tapered. Although steroids are commonly implicated in psychiatric symptoms, it is not often easy to separate the relative contribution of the steroid from the underlying medical condition.

Recognizing brain impairment that results in an organic mental disorder is important because it often has a specific cause and direct treatment; failure to treat may lead to permanent deficits and unnecessary suffering. It is estimated that 28% of hopitalized medical patients have serious cognitive impairment (Cavanaugh, 1983), and delirium is frequently misdiagnosed as a behavioral problem (Levine et al., 1978). The following impairments, common in patients with cancer, are often overlooked when they present as a "psychiatric" symptom.

Metabolic Encephalopathies

Metabolic encephalopathy is the most common neurologic complication in hospitalized patients with cancer (Posner, 1971) and accounts for a significant number of problems misdiagnosed as psychiatric. The most common metabolic consequence of neoplastic disease is *hypercalcemia* (Segaloff, 1981). Hypercalcemia is most frequent in breast cancer patients, although it also occurs in association with bronchogenic carcinoma and other neoplasms. In addition to the current interest in the medical dimensions of this disorder (Sherwood, 1980; Stewart et al., 1980), the psychiatric implications of hypercalcemia are important. In one study of 12 patients with cancer and hypercalcemia, 7 had psychiatric symptoms, including depression, anxiety, paranoid psychosis, or delirium (Weizman et al., 1979).

Liver failure frequently complicates any cancer that metastasizes to that organ and produces changes in brain functions (Shafer and Jones, 1982), resulting in fluctuating confusion, restlessness, and emotional lability. *Hyponatremia* can result from tumors that produce the syndrome of inappropriate secretion of antidiuretic hormone, such as carcinoma of the lung. In addition to neurologic symptoms such as headache, increased intracranial pressure, ataxia, and seizures, low sodium can lead to cognitive impairment and confusion, which may affect behavior and mood, although primary mood distubance *per se* has not been attributed to this abnormality (Gehi et al., 1981). Vomiting or diarrhea and long-term diuretic therapy can lead to *hypomagnesemia.* Psychiatric symptoms may be the first manifestation of magnesium imbalance and may persist for several days after the magnesium level has returned to normal (Webb and Gehi, 1981). Symptoms include personality change, nervousness, irritability, and restlessness. Depression can be a later sequela (Hall and Joffe, 1973). When a patient with pulmonary impairment exhibits any sudden change in mood, thought, or behavior, the clinician should check blood gases to determine whether oxygen level has substantially decreased. *Endocrine imbalances,* including hypothyroidism and disturbances in *cortisol metabolism,* may be responsible for depressive symptoms. In addition, a series of ectopically produced psychoactive hormonal substances, including parathormone, vasopressin, methionine enkephalin, and beta-endorphin, are increasingly being recognized as possibly responsible for changes of mental status in some patients (Pullan et al., 1980).

Central Nervous System Tumors and Metastases

Central nervous system tumors or metastases can present as psychiatric symptoms (Malamud, 1967). Cerebral metastases are frequently complications of various cancers. Although few clinicians would mistake the generalized tonic-clonic activity of a grand mal seizure, the wide variety of psychiatric disturbances that can be the concomitant of seizure activity are not well appreciated. In one review of 68 cases of cerebral metastases, 30% had behavioral or mental changes as the presenting symptom (Posner, 1971). Subjective emotional symptoms include feelings of intense depression, euphoria, paranoia, or severe anxiety with a sense of impending doom. Anxiety is the most common ictal emotional state associated with temporal lobe epilepsy (Weil, 1959), although it can be directly caused by a variety of medical disorders (Goldberg, 1982).

Nonbacterial Thrombotic Endocarditis

Patients with cancer may be prone to developing nonbacterial thrombotic endocarditis, which may lead to cerebral embolism (Bryan, 1969; MacKenzie and Popkin, 1980). This is not a rare disorder. An estimated 10% of all cerebral embolic events arise from it (Barron *et al.*, 1976). Eighty percent of cases of nonbacterial thrombotic endocarditis are associated with known or occult carcinoma, most often from the pancreas, colon, or lung (Rosen and Armstrong, 1973). According to one study, 30% of the resulting symptoms are without focal neurologic signs (Reagan and Okazaki, 1974) and present instead with abrupt onset of delirium or selective cognitive impairment. A stepwise progression of symptoms of organic mental disorder should raise the question of ongoing embolization associated with this disorder. Cranial CT scans are the definitive noninvasive diagnostic test for cerebral tumors, although some false-negative studies may result from older machines with low resolution.

Cerebral Carcinomatosis

Some leukemias (most commonly, acute lymphoblastic leukemia) and carcinoma of the breast, lung, pancreas, stomach, or prostate are associated with cerebral carcinomatosis, which may present as a mental disorder (Posner, 1971). Obviously, all patients with changes in mood, thought, or behavior should have a careful neurologic examination to search for associated signs of central nervous system involvement.

Infections

Patients with cancer are predisposed to central nervous system infections (Armstrong *et al.*, 1971) because of altered host resistance, the tumor itself, chemotherapy, and the hospital environment. A number of bacteria can be involved in addition to fungal and viral agents. Although a central nervous system infection can present as an overwhelming medical catastrophe, at other times it may run a subacute

course, with symptoms of attention or behavioral disturbances waxing and waning. For this reason, patients with presumed psychiatric disturbances should be examined for fever and infection. Finally, effects of cancer in the central nervous system have been reported without the presence of metastases. These *remote effects* of carcinoma (Shapiro, 1976) probably do occur, although most often they can be diagnosed only by exclusion.

Medication

Patients with life-threatening illness regularly receive many medications with potential psychiatric consequences. In the medical setting, the unrecognized effects of drugs probably account for a substantial number of problems mistaken as psychologic in nature. Reviews of the prescribing practices of physicians treating patients with cancer indicate that patients usually receive more than one medication that affects the central nervous system (Derogatis *et al.*, 1979; Goldberg *et al.*, 1985). In fact, three drugs among the most commonly prescribed in the United States today, cimetidine, propranolol, and diazepam, are well known to produce a variety of disorders of mood, thought, and behavior including psychosis, confusion, depression, or irritability. As the number of medications increases, drug interactions rise geometrically, making an adverse psychiatric effect more likely.

Recent reviews have compiled the large number of medications associated with psychiatric consequences (Abromowicz, 1981). Antihypertensives, including methyldopa, reserpine, propranolol, and prazosin, are associated with clinically notable depression, as well as fatigue, confusion, and impotence (Paykel *et al.* 1982). Digitalis toxicity can lead to irritability, agitation, and hallucinations (Greenblatt and Shader, 1972; Shear and Sacks, 1978). Levodopa may result in a wide variety of symptoms including depression, mania, hallucinations, or confusion (Goodwin, 1972). Finally, cimetidine, used for the treatment of peptic ulcer, can produce confusion, depression, paranoia, and other psychiatric states (Finkelstein and Isselbacher, 1978; Crowder and Pate, 1980; Weddington, *et al.*, 1981).

In addition to other adverse effects, certain chemotherapeutic agents are associated with unique psychiatric consequences. L-Asparaginase can produce confusion, depression, paranoia, or bizarre behavior (Holland et al., 1974). Vincristine is well known to produce alterations in sensation, muscle function, and autonomic functions. The earliest signs of such neuropathic changes include depression of the Achilles tendon reflex at the ankle, followed by tingling sensations in the fingers and toes, leading to weakness, muscle pain, and sensory loss in the extremities. Impairment of the autonomic nervous system can result in constipation or more severe loss of bowel function leading to obstruction. Most symptoms remit after the drug is discontinued, but the weakness may be irreversible and should not be erroneously ascribed to some psychiatric condition such as depression or loss of motivation.

Among alkylating agents, mechlorethamine has been reported to produce a toxic encephalopathy, presenting with a wide variety of psychiatric symptoms and rapidly leading to changes in level of consciousness and delirium (Bethlenfalvay and Bergin, 1972; Calabresi and Parks, 1985). Similar, but transient, impairment of brain function may occasionally result from the alkylating agent cyclophosphamide (Tashima, 1975). Among the antimetabolites, methotrexate, when used intrathecally, occasionally produces dementia (Bleyer, 1977; Proceedings, 1977). One group reported a significantly higher incidence of anxiety and depression in patients with breast cancer receiving cyclophosphamide, methotrexate, and 5-fluorouracil (CMF) compared to patients treated with melphalan (Maguire et al., 1980).

Given the large number of chemotherapeutic agents available and their pervasive systemic effects, it is remarkable that the central nervous system alterations leading to loss of cognitive ability or the development of psychiatric symptoms are so few. Sorting out direct toxic drug effects from some of the indirect effects on the central nervous system secondary to altered function of major organs such as lungs, liver, or kidney is very difficult. Although patients with cancer receiving chemotherapy seem to have a high incidence of cognitive impairment, systemic metabolic factors other than chemotherapy probably account for such impairments in memory, concentration, and attention (Silberfarb et al., 1980). It has been demonstrated, however, that vincristine use is associated with depressive symptoms (Peterson and Popkin, 1980; Silberfarb et al., 1983).

Steroids can cause profound psychiatric side

effects soon after the drug is initiated, while it is maintained, or when it is being tapered. The effects may include symptoms of depression, irritability, euphoria, or psychosis (Carroll, 1977; Ling et al., 1981).

Some of the side effects of *radiotherapy* are associated with presumed, or actual, psychiatric consequences (Allen, 1978). Early reactions, although self-limiting, during or immediately after radiation therapy include loss of appetite, nausea, vomiting, or diarrhea, which can create a sense of debilitation with secondary effects on mood and attitude. The long-term effects of brain irradiation on mental functioning have been studied recently (Moss et al., 1981). Long-term follow-up of children who received prophylactic cranial irradiation has demonstrated some decreased intellectual capacity compared to children with similar disease who did not receive such irradiation. There has not yet been documentation of intellectual impairment in adults.

Psychiatric Consultation

Psychiatric consultation is important in diagnosing an underlying organic mental disorder, assisting in its differential evaluation (including its separation from other psychiatric syndromes such as depression), and planning treatment. Unfortunately, patients, families, and some medical professionals attach an unnecessary stigma to psychiatric consultation. Failure to recognize and treat an organic mental disorder can unnecessarily alienate the patient from friends and environment, as well as result in premature loss of functional status. A psychiatric referral is often misperceived as implying that the patient's difficulties are "all in his head," or that the patient is a "mental case." On the contrary, psychiatric consultation is an important dimension of medical care, insofar as the psychiatrist is trained to evaluate and diagnose those biomedical disorders that mimic psychologic or psychosocial disturbances. Primary treatment consists of identifying and correcting the underlying medical abnormality. In addition, certain adjunctive treatment measures are helpful. Small doses of neuroleptic medication, such as haloperidol, may help control the agitation of a confused patient. Environmental manipulations are often overlooked despite their important impact on minimizing patient confusion. Confused patients often can improve remarkably if they are provided with large, readable calendars and clocks, along with night lights, familiar objects from home, and frequent orientation by staff and family. Clear, straightforward, and consistent communication from the staff and family also helps the patients organize their experiences.

Because the care of patients with life-threatening illness is so emotionally charged, premature assumptions are often made about psychologic factors being the cause of their disturbances. In addition, failure to be completely aware of the spectrum of presentations of organic mental disorders and the prevalence of these disorders in patients with life-threatening illness probably accounts for other mistaken diagnoses.

The Biology of Depression in Patients with Cancer

Much of the difficulty in understanding depression arises from the fact that the same word is used to describe a variety of situations. For instance, depression is used to refer to the transient disappointments everyone feels following some minor failure or loss. Such brief reactive states can hardly be considered an illness. Such situations are more accurately called adjustment problems, characterized by depressive features. Uncomplicated grief or bereavement can be mistakenly called depression. Most people, however, experience a grieving process that is self-limited and culturally sanctioned. Depression can also describe some individuals with chronically negative outlooks. Depression can describe a collection of the somatic sequelae of physical illness, such as fatigue, loss of appetite, and difficulty in sleeping or in concentrating. Such depressions are actually secondary to the systemic consequences of medical illness or may be associated with an organic mental disorder, as discussed in the previous section. Finally, depression can be a severe and disabling constellation of physical and psychologic symptoms that appear to have an underlying biologic basis. This latter type of depression is now referred to by a number of terms, including primary or major depression (or affective disorder).

How many patients with cancer develop a major depressive episode? Until recently, estimates depended on the anecdotal impressions of clinicians. During the past ten years, a clinical and research liaison between psychiatry and oncology programs has begun to produce formal research data gathered systematically. The prevalence of depression in patients with cancer has been widely reported to range from 37% (Peck, 1972) to 50% (Hinton, 1972), and even 75% (Craig and Abeloff, 1974) of hospitalized patients with neoplastic disorders referred to psychiatry. Such figures, however, are generally inflated by studies restricted to samples not representative of the general population of patients with cancer. Furthermore, the evaluative questionnaires used to assess depression can be misleading because many of the somatic symptoms of cancer and its treatment can artificially inflate the overall score, indicating depression when the patient actually is not suffering from the kind of pessimism and self-deprecatory thoughts that characterize patients with actual depression. When the psychologic symptoms are carefully separated from those that are illness-related, approximately 20% of patients with advanced cancer have at least moderately severe depression (Plumb and Holland, 1981; Bukberg et al., 1984). In the case of the patient with cancer, a wide variety of medical complications can create symptoms that mislead the patient and clinician into assuming that depression exists; similarly, many signs and symptoms can be mistakenly ascribed to depression, when they are actually the result of the medical illness. All the medical conditions associated with organic mental disorders, described previously, must be routinely considered when evaluating depressive symptoms in a patient with cancer.

Symptoms mimicking depression, when accounted for by an underlying medical disorder, are sometimes called secondary depressions to distinguish them from primary major depression, in which there is no such medically identifiable cause. Depression is especially difficult to diagnose in the face of pain. Depression often disappears when pain is adequately treated. The primary treatment of all secondary depression involves correcting the underlying medical condition. Such secondary depression can be clinically indistinguishable from a primary psychiatric depressive disorder. For example, in the midst of depression secondary to hypothyroidism, the patient may feel worthless, excessively guilty for past behavior, and will reveal, during a psychiatric interview, important childhood and developmental events that could logically contribute to the depressive condition. In fact, such patients commonly participate in psychotherapy for long periods of time, while both the patient and therapist are convinced that the depression has a psychologic basis. Correction of the underlying medical disorder, once it is recognized, will often resolve the symptoms, and the negative preoccupation with disturbing past events disappears. Of course in patients with medically based depressive symptoms, emotional and personal concerns and experience must always be considered. If patients with secondary depression, such as associated with potassium deficiency, are not truly depressed to begin with, their self-esteem and interpersonal relationships are likely to suffer if the symptoms remain untreated long enough.

Much of the current understanding of the biology of depression rests on observations made more than 30 years ago that patients receiving reserpine for treatment of hypertension developed a constellation of symptoms identical to those of severely depressed psychiatric patients. Because reserpine was known to exert its antihypertensive effects by depleting catecholamines, it was hypothesized that depression also resulted from a lack of these neurotransmitters. Since that time, a wealth of data has supported the notion that biogenic amine neurotransmitters play a major role in vulnerability to, and onset of, major depression. Recently, a significant portion of psychiatric patients with major depression were reported to have abnormalities in response to several tests of neuroendocrine function, notably the dexamethasone suppression test (Carroll et al., 1981) and the TRH stimulation test (Loosen and Prange, 1982). Other indicators of biologic brain impairment in major depression include abnormalities in sleep physiology documented by special sleep studies (McCarley, 1982; Sitaram et al., 1982). Furthermore, vulnerability to depression clearly has a genetic basis (Weitkamp, et al., 1981). Although the general population's risk of developing a major depressive episode is somewhat less than 2%, in the first-degree relatives of those who have had major depression, it rises to approximately 16%. Identifying major depression is important since it means that antidepressant medication should be considered as an adjunctive component of treatment.

Despite the rapid progress in our understanding of the biology of depression, a simple laboratory test cannot yet diagnose major depression in medical patients. Basically, diagnosis depends on identifying a constellation of clinical signs and symptoms in the patient. Recently, a set of criteria for making the diagnosis of a major depressive episode has been agreed upon and published in a standardized *Diagnostic and Statistical Manual of Mental Disorders* of the American Psychiatric Assocation (1980). In order to meet the criteria for the diagnosis of a major depressive episode, the patient must have a prominently and persistently depressed mood, not simply sad feelings from time to time lasting only hours to a few days. Other symptoms include loss of interest or pleasure in usual activities, feelings of worthlessness, self-reproach or excessive guilt, impaired concentration or thinking, suicidal ideation or being speeded up or slowed down in thinking or movement. Symptoms such as sleep and appetite disturbance or fatigue are less useful in physically ill patients.

Antidepressants in Cancer Patients

Despite the recognition that depression is prevalent in patients with cancer, antidepressants in this population account for only about 1% of the psychotropic drugs prescribed (Derogatis et al., 1979; Goldberg et al., 1985). In general, oncologists are not familiar with the use of antidepressants and tend to prescribe tranquilizers whenever a person seems distressed (Derogatis et al., 1979). Unfortunately, tranquilizers, such as diazepam, in depressed patients usually only result in a deepening of the depression and possibly the unnecessary superimposition of confusion.

To date, no published studies have documented the efficacy of antidepressants specifically in patients with cancer. Without such research, what type of patients, with what symptoms, will respond to antidepressants cannot be predicted. Nevertheless, on clinical grounds, antidepressants are generally effective in many depressed patients with cancer. A trial of antidepressant medication is warranted for patients disabled by depressive symptoms, including sleep or appetite disturbance, fatigue, lack of concentration, excessive pessimism, guilt, or self-doubt. If patients have had a previous episode of depression, or if there is a strong family history of depression, depressive symptoms are more likely to represent a true episode of major depression. Psychotropic medications cannot change underlying personality problems or the harsh realities of misfortune; however, they often can alleviate symptoms that impair patients' innate coping resources, allowing them to grapple more effectively with adverse circumstances. The management of depression in the patient with cancer involves attention to a combination of underlying medical and psychosocial issues (Goldberg, 1981). The details for prescribing antidepressant drugs are generally available (Hollister, 1978a,b; Kessler, 1978).

The first step in the evaluation of a presumed psychiatric symptom in patients with advanced cancer should be a review of underlying medical factors. In many cases, symptoms will resolve after the identification and correction of the underlying medical abnormality. In other cases, no clear medical cause will be found, or the symptoms will continue even after the medical factors are treated as fully as possible. The next step, therefore, is to address the major psychosocial issues that are commonly associated with the problems experienced by this group of patients.

STRESS AND CANCER

Cancer was once naively thought (and still is in some unsophisticated medical and social circles) to be simply a biologic disease. Stress is generally recognized to play a role in depression, heart attacks, and ulcers. Tumors, however, were an example of how even the well-balanced may fall prey to illness. Everyone experiences stress. Few illnesses can be explained totally by a model that does not include psychosocial factors among the predictive variables. Even accidents are more frequent among a selected few, labeled appropriately the "accident prone." Several studies of tuberculosis clearly demonstrate the relationship of stress to the development of infection by the *Mycobacterium tuberculosis,* a ubiquitous microorganism in some populations. In one study in a large metropolitan area several years ago, the incidence of tuberculosis was greatest in the black population in the highest quality housing. These findings suggest that being part of a minority group living in a wealthy, predominantly white community would be a psychologic stress not ameliorated by the physical or economic comfort of the area. Others have found the incidence of tuberculosis higher in those who live alone, in those who have never married, in those who are divorced, and in those with greater job and housing mobility (McCollum, 1969).

Comparable research (Reiser, 1975) in psychoneuroendocrinology and developmental psychophysiology shows that endocrine functioning alters in animals confronted with a stress and influences their resistance to a variety of pathogenic organisms as well as the rate of growth of neoplastic tissue (Adler, 1967; La Barba, 1970). Central neurophysiologic mechanisms are believed to mediate the effects of stress on host resistance by influencing immunologic reactions, including the levels of circulatory antibodies and tissue sensitivity to histamine (Przbylski, 1969; Stein *et al.,* 1969). A number of hormones, separately or in combination, appear to be involved, not only in hormone-dependent diseases but also in neoplastic and infectious diseases (Mason, 1975). Several animal models of disease susceptibility demonstrate the effects of manipulation of infantile environments, for example, crowded or solitary conditions of rearing, and later adult resistance or susceptibility to pathogenic challenges with viruses, as well as to behavioral manipulations known to be stressful (Adler, 1967; Adler and Plaut, 1968; Friedman *et al.,* 1969). These, and other studies, form the experimental basis for understanding how stress in early life may predispose individuals to be less able to resist either external psychosocial stress or internal and external biologic stress in later life, as well as how stress in adult life may lead to a number of psychologic and medical illnesses and decrease the ability to impede the progress of disease within their own bodies.

A key factor in managing patients with cancer is an awareness of how marital and interpersonal stress may work against the patient's best efforts to combat an illness. A patient in an unhappy or tense marriage may be so concerned about struggling with the marital conflict that little energy is left to fight the disease. A depressed person may become more so when cancer occurs and is thereby more vulnerable to the ravages of the disease, its treatments, and its complications. The crisis created by a husband who walks out on a wife after she has a mastectomy, or the silent withdrawal of family members or friends of a patient wasting away with a terminal cancer, impedes whatever biologic successes may be anticipated with radiotherapy, chemotherapy, or surgery.

A patient with cancer is confronted by many stresses that are unique to the disease. These include loss of autonomy, beauty, potency, friends and family, alienation, fear of death, mutilation, treatment morbidity, limited functioning, change in body image, pain, greater dependence on others for care, failing financial resources, uncertain prognosis, medical complications of the illness, mood change, and cognitive deterioration. Despite a common assumption that the distress associated with cancer is accounted for by physical morbidity, in fact, at least half is caused by psychosocial factors (Goldberg, 1981).

PSYCHOLOGIC FACTORS

Loss, and fear of further loss, is a pervasive feeling in many patients with cancer. Their autonomy is threatened as they find themselves attempting to cope with a disease that appears beyond their or the physician's control. Neither the most skilled medical care providers nor unlimited financial resources can deter the course of some forms of the illness. Ironically, the body is destroying itself from within. In addition, chemotherapy and radiotherapy have consequences that are also not easily controlled. They may indeed destroy neoplastic cells but, in addition, affect other rapidly proliferating cells, resulting in such unpleasant effects as loss of hair and diarrhea. Palliative surgery may leave a person without a limb, without the ability to talk, without a breast, or with a colostomy. Both patients, especially the young and sexually active, and those around them feel a loss and a threat of further loss. Family, friends, and care-givers, especially if they are the same age or if they have other loved ones of the same age, feel all too immediately the transience of life and may attempt to avoid confronting an individual, the patient, who has been mutilated either by disease or the treatment process and may deteriorate into death.

The effect of loss of autonomy or control varies with age. For adolescents, control is both a developmental task and a treatment issue. The loss of control in both children and adults may lead to anger, panic, anxiety, or depression, which may interfere with therapy.

Elizabeth Kübler-Ross has generically portrayed the stages by which individuals and those closest to them come to terms with a life-threatening illness and the unanticipated reality of loss of life—denial and isolation, anger, bargaining, depression, and acceptance.

Noncompliance and antitherapeutic behavior are attempts, albeit self-destructive, to regain some control (Goldberg, 1983). Suicide is an effort to gain control over life, ironically by electing to end it before a malignant disease ends it, as if the only thing the person can control is exit from life. Dying patients cannot prevent death, but they can prevent the further deterioration of their bodies, further pain, and further loss of functioning by choosing to die. In those with a genetic predisposition to affective illness, or an early childhood characterized by frustration of needs and loss, the depression that accompanies loss of autonomy is often magnified.

Patients *need* the opportunity to exercise some control by participating in selection of their treatment and treatment environment (Goldberg, 1983). Patients retain a sense of control by continued involvement in financial issues, learning behavioral methods, such as self-relaxation to decrease side effects of drugs and pain, even by selecting the vein for an intravenous line. Intellectual mastery is a means of asserting control over the feared and incompletely understood disease process and therapeutic interventions. Members of the oncology health care team can provide information and engage patients and those closest to them as allies by sharing the results of diagnostic investigations and suggesting that a patient keep track of medication and other therapeutic interventions in a journal. Most, *but not all,* patients prefer to know their diagnoses rather than be kept in ignorance (Goldberg, 1984). Withholding a diagnosis deprives a patient of the opportunity to take responsibility, and a patient may interpret this as loss of all control. For a few, denial is part of coping with both illness and therapy. Confronting the reality of impending death may lead to immobilizing depression, for some an abdication of life—"the giving up syndrome."

Finally, patients may overcome the loss of control by altruistic behavior. Patients may be taught to serve as role models for other patients in how to cope with adverse effects of drugs, such as nausea and loss of hair, how to adapt to mutilative surgery, such as colostomies, mastectomies, and amputations. Self-help and pre- and postmastectomy groups, amputee groups, and ostomy groups are an integral part of many oncology services.

SOCIAL FACTORS

Social and environmental factors influence how patients, those closest to them, and the clinical staff cope with a life-threatening illness. Social factors are important, both in the onset of illness, as well as in adaptation to symptoms of illness (Dohrenwend and Dohrenwend, 1981; Mechanic, 1982). The diagnosis of cancer still carries a stigma, and those affected fear abandonment by relatives, friends, and care-givers. Confronting dying patients and patients with illnesses with poor prognoses is difficult, not only for the lay public, but also for care-givers. Support groups for patients and their relatives allow them to voice the fear of abandonment and discuss ways of coping with responses of others at work or school.

Staff find comfort in staff support groups, in sharing responses to making the diagnosis of a life-threatening illness, and their own frustrations in treating illnesses that are often incurable. Burnout is diminished and anger and irritability mollified when staff can talk about their deep feelings and find that others share and understand them. Nothing helps one understand as much as to be understood. Many hospice programs provide an environment that allows patients, families, and staff to talk about a process that is not easily understood nor easily rationalized. This support can result in greater tolerance of pain and of limited physical functioning. It can assuage depression and reduce anxiety. The physical presence of others reduces the sense of alienation by encouraging communication in words and gestures. Clasped hands convey more than learned treatises on disengagement at time of death.

Practical issues of social support include assistance in homemaking, transportation to medical care, and provision of a physical environment that is distracting and pleasant. Television, radios with earphones, and computer games can distract patients receiving chemotherapy. Nausea, originally caused by cytotoxic agents, can become a conditioned response to a medical oncologic clinic. Stimuli producing incompatible responses can, in some instances, ward off untoward conditioned symptoms of necessary therapeutic interventions.

Cancer brings with it a loss of social desirability when individuals most intensely need others to make them feel accepted and part of something greater than themselves. Family, lovers, friends, and employers withdraw. Some assume cancer is contagious; others are afraid that they will cry or say something insensitive. Some feel guilty for not having been more available to the afflicted persons before they were ill. Others cannot bear an existential confrontation with their own vulnerability to illness and misfortune. Those most intimate with the patient may feel angry that the patient will die and leave them alone to raise a family, to fend economically for themselves, and to face the world without comfort and support. Educational material and a comprehensive source book have been made available through the National Cancer Institute (National Institutes of Health, 1980).

The alterations in body image and sense of well-being impede patients and spouses, lovers, or friends from providing physically the external corroboration of tenderness for those who value physical intimacy. Couples may need to be helped to learn new ways of feeling comfortable with and of physically pleasing each other. Touch, rather than consummated intercourse, may become the primary mode of relatedness.

The crisis precipitated by an unexpected physical illness provides an opportunity for a quality of communication that would have not otherwise existed. If handled poorly, it can lead to behavior that can destroy a relationship when support is most needed. A marriage may dissolve or a family may disintegrate. The key to working with patients in crisis is to take advantage of their vulnerability and to help patients and those around them grow through having experienced human tragedy.

EXISTENTIAL FACTORS

Many with cancer face the question of the degree to which quality of life may be compromised before death. Care-givers and family members are often confronted by a patient dying or in great pain asking, "Why should I go on?" The answer for each person is different. To some, suicide, as discussed earlier, is an exercise of the ultimate control. We cannot control entry into the world, nor can we control when and how we will depart from it, unless we elect to take our own life.

The problem with a totally permissive posture regarding the right of individuals to take their own lives is that perceptions of their choices at a time of great pain and depression may be distorted. Patients may be suicidal because of metabolic aberrations or endogenous depression, and not because they rationally feel they have the right to decide how they are to live and die. An individual's right to take his or her own life is an ethical issue that has not, and will never be, easily resolved. Psychiatric consultation is indicated where suicidal ideation is present in order to ascertain the intensity of the feelings and obtain an understanding of its basis. If a patient's mood or perception is being altered by some biologic process, he or she has the right to have appropriate treatment.

If a depression is alleviated, a patient may find that to share the remaining moments with children, spouse, lover, or friends may be preferable to death. Some find that the nearness of death brings about a change in the quality of life and a freedom from mundane concerns. The presence of family, friends, lovers, clergy, and hospice workers may help patients discover within themselves reasons to live. Walker Percy speaks of this in *The Second Coming* (Percy, 1980):

Not once had he been present for his life
So his life had passed like a dream.
Is it possible for people to miss their lives in the same way everyone misses a plane?
And how is it that death, the
nearness of death can restore a missed life?

The restoration of a missed life is an ironic reward for a lingering death, but for many a prize they will never obtain if spared this human tragedy.

REFERENCES

Abromowicz, M. (ed.): Drugs that cause psychiatric symptoms. *Med. Letter,* **23:**9–12, 1982.

Ader, R.: The influences of psychological factors on disease susceptibility in animals. In Conalty, M. L. (ed.): *Husbandry of Laboratory Animals.* Academic Press, Inc., London, 1967.

Ader, R., and Plaut, S. M.: Effects of prenatal maternal handling and differential housing on offspring emotionality, plasma corticosterone levels, and susceptibility to gastric erosions. *Psychosom. Med.,* **30:**277–286, 1968.

Allen, J. C.: The effects of cancer therapy on the nervous system. *J. Pediatr.,* **93:**903–909, 1978.

Armstrong, D.; Young, L. S.; Meyer, R. D.; and Blevins, A. H.: Infectious complications of neoplastic disease. *Med. Clin. North Am.,* **55:**729–745, 1971.

Barron, K. D.; Sigueira, E.; and Hirano, A.: Cerebral embolism caused by nonbacterial thrombotic endocarditis. *Neurology,* **10:**391–397, 1976.

Bethlenfalvay, N. C., and Bergin, J. J.: Severe cerebral toxicity after intravenous nitrogen mustard therapy. *Cancer,* **29:**366, 1972.

Bleyer, W. A.: Methotrexate: Clinical pharmacology current status and therapeutic guidelines. *Cancer Treat. Rev.,* **4:**87, 1977.

Bryan, C. S.: Nonbacterial thrombotic endocarditis with malignant tumors. *Am. J. Med.,* **47:**787–793, 1969.

Bukberg J.; Penman, D.; and Holland, J. C.: Depression in

hospitalized cancer patients. *Psychosom. Med.,* **46:**199–212, 1984.

Calabresi, P. and Parks, R. E., Jr.: Alkylating agents, antimetabolites, hormones, and other antiproliferative agents. In Goodman, L. S., and Gilman, A. (eds.): *The Pharmacological Basis of Therapeutics,* 7th ed. Macmillan, Inc., New York, 1985.

Carroll, B. J.; Feinberg, M.; Greden, J. F.; Tarika, J.; Albala, A. A.; Haskett, R. F.; James, N. M.; Kronfol, Z.; Lohr, N.; Steiner, M.; de Vigne, J. P.; and Young, E.: A specific laboratory test for the diagnosis of melancholia. Standardization, validation and clinical utility. *Arch. Gen. Psychiatry,* **38:**15–22, 1981.

Carroll, B. J.: Psychiatric disorders and steriods. In Usdin, E.; Hamburg, D. A.; and Barchas, J. D. (eds.): *Neuroregulators and Psychiatric Disorders.* Oxford University Press, Oxford, 1977.

Cavanaugh, S. V. A.: The prevalence of emotional and cognitive dysfunction in a general medical population: using the MMSE, GHQ, and BDI. *Gen. Hosp. Psychiatry,* **5:**15–24, 1983.

Craig, T. J., and Abeloff, M. D.: Psychiatric symptomatology among hospitalized cancer patients. *Am. J. Psychiatry,* **131:**1323–1327, 1974.

Crowder, M. K., and Pate, J. K.: A case report of cimetidine-induced depressive syndrome. *Am. J. Psychiatry,* **137:**11, 1980.

Derogatis, L. R.; Feldstein, M.; Morrow, G.; Schnale, A.; Schmitt, M.; Gates, C.; Murawski, B.; Holland, J.; Penman, D.; Melisaratos, N.; Enelow, A. J.; and Adler, L. M.: A survey of psychotropic drug prescriptions in an oncology population. *Cancer,* **44:**1919–1929, 1979.

Diagnostic and Statistical Manual of Mental Disorders, 3rd ed. American Psychiatric Association, Washington, D.C., 1980.

Dohrenwend, B. S., and Dohrenwend, B. P.: Stressful life events and their contexts. In Locke, B. Z., and Slaby, A. E. (series eds.): *Monographs in Psychosocial Epidemiology,* Vol.2. Neale Watson Academic Publications, Inc., New York, 1981.

Drugs that cause psychiatric symptoms. *The Medical Letter,* **23:**9–12, Feb. 6, 1981.

Engel, G. L., and Romano, J.: Delirium, a syndrome of cerebral insufficiency. *J. Chronic Dis.,* **9:**260–276, 1959.

Finkelstein, W., and Isselbacher, K. J.: Drug therapy: Cimetidine. *N. Engl. J. Med.,* **299:**992–996, 1978.

Folstein, M., and McHugh, P.: "Mini-mental state." A practical method for grading the cognitive state of patients for the clinician, *J. Psychiatr. Res.,* **12:**189–198, 1975.

Friedman, S.; Glasgow, L. B., and Adler, R.: Psychosocial factors modifying host resistance to experimental infections. *Ann. N.Y. Acad. Sci.,* **164:**381–393, 1969.

Gehi, M. H.; Rosenthal, R. H.; Fizette, N. B.; Crowe, L. R.; and Webb, W. L.: Psychiatric manifestations of hyponatremia. *Psychosomatics,* **22:**739–743, 1981.

Goldberg, R. J.: Management of depression in the patient with advanced cancer. *J.A.M.A.,* **246:**373–376, 1981.

Goldberg, R. J.: *Anxiety: A Guide to Biobehavioral Diagnosis and Therapy for Physicians and Mental Health Clinicians.* Medical Examination Publishing Co., Inc., Garden City, New York, 1982.

Goldberg, R. J.: Systematic understanding of cancer patients who refuse treatment. *Psychother. Psychosom.,* **39:**180–189, 1983.

Goldberg, R. J.: Disclosure of information to adult cancer patients: issues and update. *J. Clin. Oncol.,* **2:**948–955, 1984.

Goldberg, R. J., and Mor, V.: Psychotropic drug use in terminal cancer patients. *Psychosomatics,* in press, 1985.

Goodwin, F. K.: Behavioral effects of L–DOPA in man. In Shader, R. I. (ed.): *Psychiatric Complications of Medical Drugs.* Raven Press, New York, 1972.

Greenblatt, D. J., and Shader, R. I.: Digitalis toxicity. In Shader, R. I. (ed.): *Psychiatric Complications of Medical Drugs.* Raven Press, New York, 1972.

Hall, R. C. W., and Joffe, J. R.: Hypomagnesemia: Physical and psychiatric symptoms. *J.A.M.A.,* **224:**1749– 1751, 1973.

Hinton, J.: The psychiatry of terminal illness in adults and children. *Proc. R. Soc. Med.,* **65:**1035–1040, 1972.

Holland, J.; Fasanello, S.; and Ohnuma, T.: Psychiatric symptoms associated with L-asparaginase administration. *J. Psychiatr. Res.,* **10:**150–113, 1974.

Hollister, L. E.: Tricyclic antidepressants (first of two parts), *N. Engl. J. Med.,* **299:**1106–1110, 1978a.

Hollister, L. E.: Tricyclic antidepressants (second of two parts). *N Engl. J. Med.,* **299:**1168–1172, 1978b.

Kessler, K. A.: Tricyclic antidepressants: Mode of action and clinical use. In Lipton, M. A.; DiMascio, A.; and Killam, K. F. (eds.): *Psychopharmacology: A Generation of Progress.* Raven Press, New York, 1978.

Knights, E. B. and Folstein, M. S.: Unsuspected emotional and cognitive disturbance in medical patients. *Ann. Intern. Med.,* **87:**723–724, 1977.

Kübler-Ross, E.: *On Death and Dying.* Macmillan, Inc., New York, 1970.

La Barba, R. C. Experimental and environmental factors in cancer; A review of research with animals. *Psychosom. Med.,* **32:**259–274, 1970.

Levine, P. M.; Silberfarb, P. M.; and Lipowski, Z. J.: Mental disorders in cancer patients. A study of 100 psychiatric referrals. *Cancer,* **42:**1385–1391, 1978.

Ling, M. H. M.; Perry, P. J.; and Tsuang, M. T.: Side effects of corticosteroid therapy. *Arch. Gen. Psychiatry,* **38:**471–477, 1981.

Loosen, P. T., and Prange, A. J.: Serum thyrotropin response to thyrotropin-releasing hormone in psychiatric patients: A review. *Am. J. Psychiatry,* **139:**405–416, 1982.

McCarley, R. W.: REM sleep and depression: Common neurobiological control mechanisms. *Am. J. Psychiatry,* **139:**565–570, 1982.

McCollum, R. W.: Epidemiology lecture notes. With acknowledgements to R. J. Cassell (Public Health Concepts in Social Work). Yale University, New Haven, 1969.

MacKenzie, T. B., and Popkin, M. K.: Psychological manifestations of nonbacterial thrombotic endocarditis. *Am. J. Psychiatry,* **137:**8, 1980.

Maguire, G. P.; Tait, A.; Brooke, M.; and Thomas, C.: Psychiatric morbidity and physical toxicity associated with adjuvant chemotherapy after mastectomy. *Br. Med. Jr.,* **281:**1179–1180, 1980.

Malamud, N.: Psychiatric disorder with intracranial tumors of the limbic system. *Arch. Neurol.,* **17:**113– 128, 1967.

Mason, V. W.: Clinical psychophysiology, psychoendocrine mechanisms. In *American Handbook of Psychiatry.* Basic Books, Inc., Publishers, New York, 1975.

Mechanic D.: Symptoms, illness, behavior, and help-seeking. In Locke, B. Z., and Slaby, A. E. (eds.): *Monographs in Psychosocial Epidemiology,* Vol. 3. Neale Watson Academic Publications, Inc., New York, 1982.

Moss, H. A.; Nannis, E. D.; and Poplack, D. G.: The effects of prophylactic treatment of the central nervous system on the intellectual functioning of children with acute lymphocytic leukemia. *Am. J. Med.,* **71:**47–52, 1981.

National Institutes of Health. *Coping With Cancer.* Publication No. 80–2199. U.S. Department of Health, Education, and Welfare, Washington, D.C., 1980.

Paykel, E. S.; Pleminger, R.; and Watson, J. P.: Psychiatric side effects of antihypertensive drugs other than reserpine. *J. Clin. Psychopharmacol.,* **2:**14–39, 1982.

Peck, A.: Emotional reactions to having cancer. *J. Roentgenol. Radium Ther. Nucl. Med.,* **114:**591–599, 1972.

Percy, W.: *The Second Coming.* Farrar Strauss & Giroux, Inc., New York, 1980.

Peterson, L. G., and Popkin, M. K.: Neuropsychiatric effects on chemotherapeutic agents for cancer. *Psychosomatics,* **21:**141–153, 1980.

Plumb, M. M., and Holland, J.: Comparative studies of psychological function in patients with advanced cancer. I. Self-reported depressive symptoms. *Psychosom. Med.,* **39:**264–276, 1977.

Plumb, M., and Holland, J.: Comparative studies of psychological function in patients with advanced cancer: II. Interviewer-rated current and past psychological symptoms. *Psychosom. Med.,* **43:**243–254, 1981.

Posner, J. B.: Neurological complications of systemic cancer. *Med. Clin. North Am.,* **55:**625–646, 1971.

Proceedings of the Workshop on Antimetabolites and the Central Nervous System. *Cancer Treat. Rep.* **61:**505, 1977.

Przbylski, A.: Effect of stimulation and coagulation of the midbrain reticular formation in the bronchial musculature: A modification of histamine susceptibility. *J. Neuro-Visc. Rel.,* **31:**171–188, 1969.

Pullan, P. T.; Clement-Jones, V.; Corder, R.; Lowry, P. J.; Pees, G. M.; Rees, L. H.; Besser, G. M.; Macedo, M. M.; Galvao-Teles, A.: Ectopic production of methionine enkephalin and beta-endorphin. *Br. Med. J.,* **1:**758–759, 1980.

Reagan, T. J., and Okazaki, H.: The thrombotic syndrome associated with carcinoma. *Arch. Neurol.,* **31:**390–395, 1974.

Reiser, M.: Changing theoretical concepts in psychosomatic medicine. In Arieti, S. (ed.): *American Handbook of Psychiatry,* Vol. IV. Basic Books, Inc., Publishers, New York, 1975.

Rosen, P. R., and Armstrong, D.: Nonbacterial thrombotic endocarditis in patients with malignant neoplastic diseases. *Am. J. Med.,* **54:**23–29, 1973.

Schafer, D. F., and Jones, E. A.: Hepatic encephalopathy and the y-aminobutyric-acid neurotransmitter system. *Lancet,* **1:**18–20, 1982.

Segaloff, A.: Managing endocrine and metabolic problems in the patient with advanced cancer. *J.A.M.A.,* **245:**177–179, 1981.

Shapiro, W. R.: Remote effects of neoplasm on central nervous system encephalopathy. In Thompson, R. A., and Green, J. R. (eds.): *Advances in Neurology,* Vol. 15. Raven Press, New York, 1976.

Shear, M. K., and Sacks, M.: Digitalis delirium: Psychiatric considerations. *Int. J. Psychiatry Med.,* **8:**371–380, 1977–1978.

Sherwood, L. M.: The multiple causes of hypercalcemia in malignant disease. *N. Engl. J. Med.,* **303:**1412–1413, 1980.

Silberfarb, P. M.; Holland, J.; Anbar, D.; Bahna, G.; Maurer, L. H.; Chahinian, A. P.; and Comis, R.: Psychological response of patients receiving two drug regimens for lung carcinoma. *Am. J. Psychiatry,* **140:**110– 111, 1983.

Silberfarb, P. M.; Philibert, D.; and Levine, P. M.: Psychosocial aspects of neoplastic disease: II. Affective and cognitive effects of chemotherapy in cancer patients. *Am. J. Psychiatry,* **137:**597–601, 1980.

Sitaram, N.; Nurnberger, J. I.; Gershon, E. S.; and Gillin, J. C.: Cholinergic regulation of mood and REM sleep: Potential model and marker of vulnerability to affective disorder. *Am. J. Psychiatry,* **139:**571–576, 1982.

Slaby, A. E., LaFarge, S.; and Tull, R.: *Videotaping Dying Children* (Submitted for publication).

Slaby, A. E.; Tancredi, L. R.; and Liet, J.: *Clinical Psychiatric Medicine.* Harper & Row, Publishers, Inc., New York, 1981.

Stein, M.; Schiavi, R. C.; and Luparello, T. J.: The hypothalamus and immune process. *Ann. N.Y. Acad. Sci.,* **164:**464–472, 1969.

Stewart, A. F.; Horst, R.; Deftos, L. J.; Cadman, E. C.; Lang, R.; and Broadus, A. E.: Biochemical evaluation of patients with cancer-associated hypercalcemia. *N. Engl. J. Med.,* **303:**1377–1383, 1980.

Tashima, C. K.: Immediate cerebral symptoms during rapid intravenous administration of cyclophosphamide. *Cancer Chemother. Rep. Part I,* **59:**441, 1975.

Webb, W. L., and Gehi, M.: Electrolyte and fluid imbalance: neuropsychiatric manifestations. *Psychosomatics,* **22:**199–203, 1981.

Weddington, W. W.; Muelling, A. E.; Moosa, H. H.; Kimball, C. P.; and Rowlett, R. R.: Cimetidine toxic reactions masquerading as delirium tremens. *J.A.M.A.,* **245:**1058–1059, 1981.

Weill, A. A.: Ictal emotions occurring in temporal lobe dysfunction. *Arch. Neurol.,* **1:**87–97, 1959.

Weitkamp, L. R.; Stancer, H. C.; Persad, E.; Flood, C.; and Guttormsen, S.: Depressive disorders and HLA: A gene on chromosome 6 that can affect behavior. *N. Engl. J. Med.,* **305:**1301–1306, 1981.

Weizman, A.; Eldar, M.; Schoenfeld, Y.; Hirschoin, M.; Wissenbeck, H.; and Pinkhas, J.: Hypercalcemia-induced psychopathology in malignant diseases. *Br. J. Psychiatry,* **135:**363–366, 1979.

51

Rehabilitation of the Patient with Cancer

J. HERBERT DIETZ, JR.

OVERVIEW

General Concepts

The annual incidence of new cases of cancer in the United States today is over 850,000. Each year, however, an increase in the number of patients whose disease is either cured or better controlled is evident. Recent figures indicate that 47% or more will be cured, and most of the remainder can expect to have the benefits of prolonged survival. Therefore, more and more patients resume their day-to-day lives, subject only to whatever disabilities they may have developed as a result of their disease or the treatment rendered. This impacts on concepts of caring for the cancer patient: how best can we help these patients "readapt" to society?

Philosophy

The philosophy or strategy of management for the patient with cancer is to try to predict not only the outcome of the disease and its therapy, but the future course. Practically the entire classification of disabilities is found in the population of patients with cancer. The disabilities created by the present modalities of therapy are apt to be more disabling than those resulting from therapeutic procedures for non-neoplastic conditions.

Rehabilitation techniques are of proven value in the comprehensive care of the patient with cancer. Readaptation, defined as accommodation or adjustment to personal needs for survival and maximum function, is considered the synonym for rehabilitation. Rehabilitation should be provided to enhance the quality of survival, regardless of life expectancy. The objectives are achievement of maximal physical, psychosocial, emotional, and, when possible, vocational rehabilitation of patients and development of training programs for medical and other personnel involved in such rehabilitation.

The benefits of adaptive rehabilitation should be made available to as many patients with cancer as possible. In the past, rehabilitation was begun only after completion of all other treatments, when the disability alone was left for consideration. Efforts were concentrated on patients in whom the disease or handicap had stabilized, and in whom the financial investment of rehabilitation would be justified by future productivity. Often patients with cancer did not reach this category until much valuable time had been lost. Eligibility rules excluded many patients with residual disease, thus overlooking the special human needs of the patient with an uncertain future. An early approach to rehabilitation is not difficult. Basic information needed to plan a program includes age, sex, some index of family setting, and type of employment. These factors provide guidance toward clarifying the most effective program for the individual, as well as toward helping plan for short- or long-term efforts directed at a particular disability.

Rehabilitation is the responsibility of the patient's personal physician with the help of every member of the medical team taking care of the patient, the rehabilitation staff, as well as the various community organizations that can provide additional assistance. The physician needs to make an initial assessment of potential as well as actual disability upon which an appropriate rehabilitation program can be based. The patient's rehabilitation needs can be met by referring the patient to the rehabilitation service for direct attention. The sooner rehabilitation efforts are begun, the more effective the results are going to be.

Each patient has highly individual needs that negate any predetermined, rigid programming. Individual consideration and planning are essential for success. The patient's total illness includes the disability and its effect on emotional and social status. The illness is a result of the combination of the cancer, the treatment, personal characteristics, and the life setting. The extent of rehabilitation provided each patient with cancer depends, therefore, on individual need.

Pediatric rehabilitation requires special consideration because of the special needs of the child. Educational level, experience, and degree of independence distinguish each child. Development of parental understanding and support requires input from the hospital staff. Communication is particularly important in helping children. Parents should be included in training sessions to teach them how to carry out instruction and assistance for their child at times when the staff cannot be with the patient. Teaching routines for the patient are both individual and group and so engender the benefits of mutual encouragement, competition, acceptance, and motivation. The child has different attitudes about the need for privacy than the adult.

Methodology

An early start enables the rehabilitation staff to provide initial services at the bedside, coinciding and concomitant with definitive clinical care. When referred, hospitalized patients should be examined initially by the rehabilitation staff at the bedside. This makes it possible to arrange for prompt individual programs based on the findings of the physical examination, consideration of the type and extent of neoplastic disease, the possibility of additional coexisting disease or disability, the patient's age, occupational history, and previous treatment.

The importance of this early approach to rehabilitation is demonstrated by patients on bed rest who are not involved in any structured bed activity program. Inactivity on bed rest can result in a loss of up to 3% of physical strength per day, and any additional handicap owing to age or preexisting weakness or dysfunction may carry patients beyond an independent ability to get out of bed and try to function. Emotional disability may result from prolonged inactivity of any kind. The patient's physical strength and endurance are interdependent. When physical endurance has become depleted, attempts at rehabilitation are slowed or even severely jeopardized, and may fail.

Some patients can accept their diagnosis or a changed physical status more readily than others; many, perhaps the majority, believe they will be unable to resume a normal existence in a job, at home, or in their community. Supportive communication and counseling are essential for these patients.

Patients with cancer often feel they have no future to look forward to. These feelings are aggravated by the fact that many physicians, nurses, social workers, counselors, and most allied health care personnel themselves do not have confidence in the future of a patient with cancer. The common concept is that the patient with cancer is fundamentally very sick and is probably not going to get better.

Communication breakdowns often occur when the physician is unable to examine his or her own feelings and, therefore, avoids the issue and communication with the patient. The sooner the patient can begin to talk about the problem, the sooner the adaptive rehabilitation adjustment becomes established.

Goals

Adaptive rehabilitation must ensure an appropriate and obtainable goal toward which treatment is directed. The goal for each patient is determined by an aggregate of factors relevant to the individual. These include age, type and stage of neoplastic disease, other concomitant diseases, other unrelated disabilities, inherent physical ability, social background, basic education, and job or work experience. The patients' home circumstances must be taken into account: do they live alone or in the midst of a supportive family, are there stairs or other barriers to mobility, what are the distances to and from work, and is public transportation available?

Classification of the goals includes:

Preventive   **Supportive**
Restorative   **Palliative**

In order to define the adaptations necessary for a patient to meet physical and personal needs, one of these approaches should be considered: *preventive,* when the disability can be predicted and appropriate training can prevent or reduce the severity of its effect; *restorative,* if no residual or only minimal handicap can be forseen; *supportive,* if ongoing disease or persistent disability must be tolerated, but appropriate care can offer some control of problems and improvements of day-to-day performance; or *palliative,* if disease is advanced and basic disability cannot be corrected, but where training can aid performance, pain can be reduced, hygienic problems lessened, decubitus ulcers treated or prevented, and maintenance of whatever independent functions the patient can assume for the remainder of life can be secured. Only a small percentage of patients have been identified who are not candidates for any program of adaptive care, owing to such factors as severe disease-related inability or refusal to submit to a program.

Predictable disability for the medical patient occurs, for example, when reactions can be expected to chemotherapy, to prolonged bed rest, to isolation requirements, to nutritional deficits, to emotional stress and reaction, to pain, and to anger, depression, and fear. Neurologic dysfunction may be predicted and its impact and handicap lessened when a therapy program is provided, including appropriate assisting apparatus for the patient. Respiratory distress and insufficiency can be reduced by the preventive teaching of proper techniques of coughing, breathing, and control of physical activity. Additional benefit is gained for patients having preexisting chronic pulmonary disease by respiratory physical therapy procedures.

The obvious disabilities found among patients with cancer vary and are related to the site of the disease or organ system involved, either regional or generalized. The more subtle disabilities, not so physically obvious, are the emotional, psychologic, and interpersonal effects of disease and treatment. Prompt recognition by the clinician of existing disability or reactive problem along with early referral for appropriate treatment enhances optimum patient compliance and response.

Tabulation of some of the needs and prescriptions for care according to the above general goals is as follows:

PURPOSE OR NEED	REHABILITATION MEASURES
Restoration of maximal ROM (range of motion), motor power, and function for head and neck, extremities, and trunk disabilities	Active and resistive exercises, specific activity routines (as appropriate to focal disability), active and assisted range of motion
Mobilization— ambulation and elevation activities for lower limb functional deficit (or absence)	Ambulation and elevation training, trapeze provision, orthosis, and planning for prostheses (as indicated)
Increase in efficiency and independence for upper extremity function deficit	Occupational therapy and physical therapy measures for upper extremity and hand function, strength, and dexterity
Wheelchair use and independence for patients unable to ambulate	Transfer training and wheelchair activities of daily living (ADL) instruction. Prescription of appropriate wheelchair for home use, as indicated
Lymphedema, when present	Elevation, support, exercises, elastic sleeve, intermittent pneumatic compression (if not contraindicated), instruction in care and prevention routines
Respiratory function support and effective coughing	Instruction and assistance in voluntary respiratory function, deep breathing, diaphragmatic breathing, regional costal expansion, coughing (with postural drainage, cupping, vibration, as indicated, when no contraindications exist). Addition of devices for moisturization of inspired air (ultrasonic nebulizer), incentive spirometer, respiratory volume improvement (intermittent positive pressure breathing apparatus), as indicated
Restoration of emotional control and stability	Supportive care by rehabilitation staff, nursing staff, social work staff, psychologist, psychiatrist (if indicated), clergy, family, union representative, and employer

continued

PURPOSE OR NEED	REHABILITATION MEASURES
Restoration of comfort (including back-pain relief)	Back-sparing training and ADL, postural alignment instruction, ROM (active and assisted)
	Bed ADL instructions, proper positioning, cushioning, bolstering, turning, and prevention of formation or worsening of decubitus ulcers
	Hydrocollator packs, where no contraindication exists
	Ongoing back and activity programs should be given to the patient for continuing use in the hospital or at home.
	Consultation by pain control team for occasional patients with residual pain not responding to standard analgesics
Restoration of vocational and social status	Involvement of patient with family, vocational counselor, union representative, community agencies, employer

Phases of Care

Adaptive rehabilitation is best conducted with consideration for the various phases of care in the course of the patient's treatment. The phases of care are:

Initial diagnosis with pretreatment
Definitive therapy
Convalescence
Transition

The *pretreatment phase* has a preventive aspect. Disabilities can be reduced or prevented if training and instruction given in advance of predictable handicap caused by disease or its treatment are followed, including chemotherapeutic agents, pain medications, restrictions imposed by catheters, drainage tubes, central venous pressure lines, and other lines or infusions. Patients may have preexisting lung disease such as bronchiectasis, fibrosis and emphysema, asthma, or reduced pulmonary functional efficiency secondary to pre-

vious thoracic surgery. They need training in the proper techniques of voluntary control of breathing mechanics and adequate coughing to promote clearing of secretions.

During the *definitive therapy phase* immediate reactions and restrictions imposed by treatment may nauseate or otherwise sicken the patient. The treatment may also depress or frighten the patient. Supportive attitudes and understanding listening may reduce the severity of the patient's reactions. Programs of physical activity will preserve strength, aid motivation, and prevent vascular and deteriorative complications, such as thrombosis, decubitus ulcers, and pulmonary hypostatic congestion. Such physical activity includes muscle-setting exercises without breath-holding, scheduled deep breathing with periodic sighing, and bed-position changes. As frequently as permissible, out-of-bed periods should be arranged with ambulation, if possible, and standing or sitting, if not. Upright position drops the diaphragm and expands the lower lobes of the lungs, as well as stimulating general circulation.

Direct follow-through is mandatory through the *convalescent phase* in order for the rehabilitation process to achieve success. Daily supervised activity and supportive care are required to prevent deterioration of both physical and emotional stamina and motivation. All patients should have at least an active exercise program to be performed either in bed, in a chair, or about their rooms or hallway, as each case may permit. Ropes, dumbbells, and exercise rods add an element of purpose and interest in exercise performance. The hospital recreation service can offer help with poorly motivated patients and children. For all patients the recreation service provides change, added interest and motivation, and a source of pleasant distraction.

The medical staff should have knowledge and understanding of the availability and content or purpose of the program to be delivered by the rehabilitation service. This involves application of measures directed at adaptation by the patient throughout the phases of medical care and in accordance with a realistic goal set for each individual.

Von Doeltz (1971) has noted that, "People will react to a diagnosis of cancer within the framework of the meaning that the illness has to them and with their usual modes of reacting to stress." Illness that may have a lethal prognosis and may be protracted and severe is a source of stress that poses major adjustment problems for the patient and the involved family. Kaplan and the Stanford University group have found that family organization may be injured or destroyed by stress that is mishandled. Coping responses, whether adaptive or maladaptive, are manifested during the early weeks following confirmation of a diagnosis of cancer. This early period is felt to be the time when response to intervention has its greatest potential since coping patterns have not become fixed and unyielding.

Direct, consistent advice and emotional support of the patient by the staff will prevent the confusion, distrust, and lack of compliance that follow misinformation and unrealistic goal-setting. Generally, the patient will pass through stages of depression, anger, denial, and frustration, but will eventually come to accept and comply when given appropriate interdisciplinary support. Staff intercommunication and mutual awareness of the patient's status are based on such an effort.

Unfortunately for both the patient and the staff of physicians and nurses, much of cancer treatment can be unpleasant and difficult to tolerate. Only some of the treatment is understood by most patients. Programs of activity should be directed toward teaching patients to achieve maximum satisfaction in activities performed daily to meet their needs. Motivation must be maintained in order to secure and ensure the compliance of the patient. If patients are or become unable to help themselves or tolerate treatment, consultation and treatment from the clinical psychologist or psychiatrist should be sought.

During the *transition phase* special attention should be given to securing each patient's maximal functional independence and satisfactory levels of self-care. Physical and occupational therapy programs need to be directed at resumption of the habitual behavior and activities of daily living for the individual patient. Domanski and colleagues (1979) have underscored the need to develop a collaborative process to ensure continuity of care as patients move between hospital and community. This involves multidisciplinary and interagency effort. Medical, psychologic, and vocational components are interdependent, and failure to overcome psychosocial problems may nullify otherwise successful treatment. The total psychosocial problems include:

1. The attitude of the individual to the disease and/or disability
2. The relationship between the individual and the family
3. The attitude of the family toward the sick or disabled individual and the family input toward care and support
4. The attitude of the local community, including voluntary organizations, toward the sick or disabled individual and its availability to and inclusion of the patient
5. The role of social programs of the state and public authorities relating to the patient

A primary concern of the social phase of rehabilitation is the relationship of the individual to the environment. Success or failure in rehabilitation is usually determined by patients' ability to adjust to the environment. An objective of comprehensive care is to increase the patient's competence to deal effectively with the environment, economically, vocationally, and socially. Adjustment to disease, disability, environment, and the rehabilitation process by the patient is made easier by the social worker's efforts to alter appropriately the patient's physical and social setting, if necessary.

As soon as discharge from the hospital can be considered and the patient has reached the transition stage, *discharge planning* should begin. Facing the future becomes paramount for the patient, and efforts by the hospital staff must be increased to provide information, to allow the patient opportunities for practicing self-care skills, and eliminating or reducing the fears of leaving the protective environment of the hospital. Patient orientation in this phase of care changes from self to self-in-relation-to-others.

The posthospital period for the patient is characterized by (1) recovery of physical well-being, (2) perfecting self-care, (3) resumption of social roles, including return to employment, if applicable. Failure in the first results in physical disability, failure in the second causes handicap, and failure in the third is failure to be rehabilitated. The rehabilitation process can fail when the patients are taught to function and take care of themselves only in the supportive hospital environment, and are discharged without a home care plan or possibly needed referral to an outpatient facility.

Learned skills and development of community contacts and assistance are not automatically transposed into the postdischarge setting. The home and community environment must become an ongoing supportive reality. Work or vocational return for the patient, with assessment, training, and involvement, becomes essential for all eligible individuals.

Discharge planning should start as soon as the patient's course will allow. The patient's diagnosis and response to care will govern the formulation of a plan. The physician, social worker, or a responsible nurse should discuss future social and vocational possibilities with both the patient and family. Only realistic expectations should be held and offered for the patient's consideration. Discharge planning should be supplemented by specific instructions covering individual patient needs or medication, activity level, and, if applicable, wound care, orthopedic and daily living functions and problems, and stomal care.

The patient may need guidance concerning the facilities and characteristics of home. Architectural barriers may be present or modifications may be needed of bathrooms and kitchens, doorway widths, and bannisters or railings may be needed in hallways. Arrangements may have to be made for transportation to and from work or to rehabilitation or other health care facilities. Proper devices and equipment should be ordered or supplied, or the patient should be instructed where they can be obtained. Summaries of care must be given and a listing of predicted needs should be written for any facility to which the patient is transferred.

When the patient is to be discharged home, a written activity and appropriate medication and treatment schedule should be provided to ensure proper continued performance at home. If home nursing, home health aides, meal delivery, or other services are indicated, arrangements for these are best made in advance of discharge. A schedule for medical follow-up should be given to the patient before leaving the hospital. Speech therapists, occupational and physical therapists, nurses, and psychologists should all be available for appropriate care at home or after discharge. Ongoing care may need to be arranged with a physician or dentist, the latter being extremely important for head and neck cancer patients. Welfare help and Medicare and Medicaid assistance may need to be obtained to give support to the patient. The social worker is the best-trained person on the staff for this service.

The social worker should be involved with discharge planning and should be called in as soon as discharge is contemplated to allow adequate time to meet the patient's needs, particularly in obtaining help from outside agencies in the community. These include:

1. Visiting Nurse Association
2. American Cancer Society
3. Special education programs (especially for young patients)
4. Sheltered workshops
5. Special services — employment and placement
6. Meals-on-Wheels

Insurance support may help defray costs of training and equipment. If the patient is a member of a labor union, a union counselor may provide direction and assistance. Discharge planning should recommend the help of voluntary health agencies, such as the services of the American Cancer Society for advice, assistance, and the provision of direct help for eligible patients.

Outpatient care should be available to all patients whose rehabilitation would improve if continuation of treatment followed discharge from the hospital. This applies particularly to amputees who are awaiting a prosthesis and to patients who need speech therapy, vocational counseling, or psychologic assistance. Special education is particularly useful for some children.

Retraining may be necessary for handicapped individuals to permit them to return to work. Contact with the individual patient's employer (with the patient's signed permission) relevant to return to work may become necessary in discharge planning, as well as in outpatient care and follow-up. Employers frequently entertain grave doubts as to the wisdom of having a person with a history of cancer return to work for a variety of reasons including feared absenteeism, inefficiency of work performance, insurance problems, and fundamental fear of the disease, including ideas of contagion.

Home Care

Home care for patients is usually a sequel of hospital care, but occasionally it can be considered as an alternative. Estimates have been made that indicate expert home care costs are one-half to two-thirds the cost of care in most hospitals and less than half that in specialized large centers. Home care may also enhance the quality of life for the patient who will remain ill and confined.

Home care should provide high-quality, individualized care to selected patients. Eligibility for home care should be approved by the patient's physician, and it should be something the patient wants. It is not suitable for patients who live alone, or whose families cannot take care of them between visits of the professional staff. Preferably patients should be independently mobile in their activities of daily living. Bedridden patients have greater problems.

A major share in the ongoing responsibility of adaptive home care programs frequently rests with the patient's family, but their involvement is often neglected. It should be an integral part of rehabilitation management by the patient care team. The social worker should be called upon to determine the best use of home and community agency assistance.

Home care is not always easy, and some patients may need special procedures that require transportation to medical facilities. The services provided by ideal home health care include home visits by a physician, visiting nurse, social worker, home health aide, homemaker services, and provision and maintenance of prosthetic and orthopedic devices, medical equipment, transportation to medical facilities and clinics, food-service delivery (if needed), and hospital-based home care services.

Criteria for judging the suitability of the individual home have been suggested and include:

Quiet
Stairs, outside or inside
Privacy
Doorway and hall space to accommodate a
  wheelchair
Presence of small children
Available adult day and night
Access to a telephone

Patients discharged home from the hospital who are in need of ongoing rehabilitation care must be given individual home programs with details of exercises and daily living functions that have been learned in the hospital. They may need to attend outpatient rehabilitation service training at their hospital or a facility nearer their home. Accordingly, referrals to the appropriate service should be made promptly with adequate details of diagnosis, prognosis, disability description, and program suggestions.

The Terminal Patient

Patients with advanced cancer are not going to respond progressively or well to treatment and are likely to die before discharge. These terminal patients are important candidates for the adaptive concept of rehabilitation. They have realistic goals of either support, at best, or palliation. They must be helped, in accordance with their individual potential, to maintain maximum independence in physical function and daily living activities. They need maximum support in emotional control and in the reduction of pain or other complications. The program selected for each individual should consider the disability in light of the prognosis and the time-for-life probability, with a realistic attempt to attain performance levels that can be maintained for the longest periods of time. For example, the patient with metastatic disease causing cord compression and paraparesis should not have physical therapy restricted only to improving residual performance in ambulation, which at best might be of short duration, but should be instructed in independence in wheelchair use in activities of daily living.

The stabilizing effects of a dependable schedule of modified performance and emotional support therapy prevent these advanced-disease patients from feeling forsaken during the remainder of the life that they will live.

Hospice

The hospice program (described in more detail in Chapter 48) is intended to act as an impetus in support of home care. It complements existing care centers and methods, rather than competing with them, and utilizes the patient's physician as a member of the caring team. Quality hospice programs have an appropriate place and role in the care of the terminally ill cancer patient and should, therefore, receive the support of allied health professions, not only for their humanitarian social worth, but for their contribution in reducing the potential catastrophic economic impact upon the individual and the family.

PROBLEMS IN ASSOCIATION WITH NONSURGICAL CANCER TREATMENT

General Support

Nurses are important members of the rehabilitation team. Their understanding and support are essential to the success of each patient's program. Without their assistance in motivation and repetition, the patient may fail.

They see the patient both first and last, and with training, they can coordinate many phases of the program. In the pretreatment phase, after the physician's diagnostic interview and examination, the nurse can talk to the patient, providing direction about the future, and offering standard nursing advice as well as giving the patient the opportunity for emotional ventilation.

The nurses' impressions of the patient should be made available to the physician and to the hospital team including the patient's attitudes and any evidence of emotional insecurity, dependency, or immaturity. In addition, they can pinpoint social and economic problems. They can ascertain whether the patient lives alone, with spouse and family, or with parents. They can identify the need for obtaining the services of a homemaker, if anyone else is sick at home, or if other home problems are posed by the patient's hospitalization.

Economic problems can also be evaluated by the nurse. For example, should the medical social worker investigate temporary community-agency-assistance possibilities or welfare support? Will return to previous work or rehire be difficult? Should the medical social worker explain to the employer that the patient can return to full productive work?

The nursing personnel must understand and practice rehabilitation techniques in order to provide effective care and assistance to the disabled patient. The approaches apply to various disabilities and include bed and chair positioning and transfer of patients, posture and body mechanics, basic nursing procedures for skin care and decubitus ulcer prevention and care, activities of daily living (including feeding, bathing, and toileting), use of the tilt table, application of prescribed slings, corsets, collars, braces, orthoses, and prostheses, ambulation assistance, and osteomy care.

Rehabilitation nursing is a specific approach. The patient's course is improved if knowledgeable nursing supportive care is available. Nursing personnel should carry out and repeat the training initiated by the physical or occupational therapist. They should support the counsel and direction of the social worker. This input will eliminate fragmentation of care and allow the patient with disability to practice and learn performance that will improve independence.

Rubin (1971) believes the related ongoing objectives of nursing care are to:

1. Communicate effectively with the patient, the family, and other team members
2. Provide physical and psychologic comfort for the patient and family
3. Help to protect the patient from complications associated with the disease, the treatment, the patient's infirmities, hazards in the environment, and decreased mobility
4. Help the patient deal with anxiety and maintain hope
5. Teach the patient and family skills needed to achieve reasonable independence for the patient
6. Assist the patient to learn to live with disability, if necessary, which involves teaching techniques of self-care
7. Assist the terminally ill patient to die with dignity

Rehabilitation measures must often be instituted in patients undergoing specific treatment. Those that must be instituted for postsurgical patients are beyond the scope of this chapter, but the interested reader is referred to the author's text on rehabilitation oncology (Dietz, 1981). Posttreatment measures of direct interest to medical oncologists are considered below.

Chemotherapy

It is well known that the toxicity of chemotherapeutic agents is not confined to the cancer cell. Patients are sickened by the reactions of their normal tissues and organ systems. Some of the symptoms and signs include cheilitis, glossitis, leukopenia and infection, thrombocytopenia and bleeding, anemia, nausea, vomiting, anorexia, diarrhea, interstitial pulmonary fibrosis, alopecia, skin pigmentation, fatigue, muscular weakness, and weight loss.

This long list merely emphasizes that the patient's treatment should not stop with administration of the chemotherapy, but should include recognition and consideration of the problems generated, with all possible appropriate measures taken to modify the impact on endurance and independent performance.

Nausea may be reduced if the patient is given small, frequent feedings and if antiemetics are used before meals and at bedtime. Medication can be given parenterally, if vomiting is persistent. At times, administration of chemotherapeutic agents at night may reduce nausea. This is helped by preceding the medication with a sedative and phenothiazine. Marked malnutrition may occur. For the definition and treatment of nutritional deficit the reader is referred to Chapter 45.

Stomatitis and pharyngitis are aggravated by foods that contain irritating substances such as citric acid. Occasionally, painful ulcers and persistent oral problems will need analgesics such as lidocaine, 2% viscous solution, held in the mouth for relief.

Patients who have developed thrombocytopenia should never be subjected to any manipulation that could cause tissue injury by contusion, tear, or stretching, and so result in bleeding.

Hair loss varies and occurs frequently. It is more extensive in high-dose regimens and creates cosmetic problems. It has been suggested that the use of a tourniquet about the forehead, temples, and occiput to isolate the scalp temporarily can reduce or prevent hair loss. This should only be done if occult disease is not likely in the scalp or skull. Hair will usually regrow, but in the meantime wigs for both sexes and all ages should be considered for the individual patient.

Radiation Therapy

One-quarter to one-third of all patients with cancer will receive radiation therapy during the course of their disease. Radiation therapy may be a primary therapeutic agent, or it may be used in combination with surgery or chemotherapy to facilitate effective treatment and to lessen the amount of the other modality.

Radiation therapy causes changes in normal tissues, and resulting symptoms may limit levels of function. Fibrosis may occur in the lungs leading to respiratory problems. Voluntary respiratory patterns and control and paced breathing may limit dyspnea on exertion. Affected joints need gentle active and assisted range-of-motion exercises. Any forceful stretching is contraindicated. Radiation therapy may cause skin reactions such as erythema, telangiectasia, and thinning. Burns are seldom seen, but pigmentation may develop. Postradiation-therapy skin protection should include gentle handling, protection from trauma, application of petrolatum-based, bland ointment, and avoidance of chronic irritation from pressure or rubbing by clothing. Sunburn, of course, should be avoided.

Radiation necrosis of soft tissue is rare, but interference with wound healing in previously irradiated tissue may be encountered, as well as decrease in the resistance of such areas to stress or trauma. Measures of physical therapy must be gentle in such cases. Passive strength or force should never be used. Instead, the patient should be encouraged to use active input in performing his own range of motion. The buoyancy of underwater support in the therapeutic pool is often beneficial, and the patient's skin should be protected from the water by light applications of petrolatum or vitamin A and D ointment. Massage should be avoided on skin exposed to radiation therapy, and application of heat or hot packs in any form is contraindicated.

Reaction of the head and neck to radiation therapy may be severe. Treatment by adaptive measures has been detailed by Dietz (1981). These patients should be advised to stop smoking and to avoid alcohol consumption. Nutritional problems often arise and must be addressed.

The nervous system is relatively resistant to radiation, although pathological changes have been reported. Perineural fibrosis of tissues surrounding peripheral nerves may occur with resulting entrapment, and the symptoms are mainly painful, with associated hypersensitivity and a burning type of discomfort. Treatment is mainly supportive and symptomatic, with protection of the area (such as the chest wall) by light-weight, soft covering to avoid irritation by contact and temperature change, application of nonallergenic, emollient lotions or creams to protect the skin from dryness and chapping, and gentle maintenance of range of motion of regional joints to prevent skin contracture.

Time is the patient's ally, and each patient should be encouraged that the pain is not expected to persist, but will slowly and gradually become less in severity. So much of chronic pain is attitudinally aggravated that early supportive reassurance is mandatory.

Postradiation therapy reactions of the gastrointestinal tract include nausea, pharyngitis, esophagitis, diarrhea, and intestinal obstruction with resultant nutritional problems. Radiation therapy to the bladder and perineum may be followed by dysuria. All these symptoms require medical rather than rehabilitation care for control. Hair loss with radiation therapy to the head may be permanent, but an appropriate wig may restore the patient's appearance and tolerance.

Radiation exposure of bone may be followed by aseptic radiation necrosis. Certain types of bone destruction may benefit from orthopedic consultation with consideration for possible joint replacement. Skeletal changes and bone-growth deficits in children from tumor irradiation are related in part to the age of the patient at the time of radiation therapy, and in follow-up they should be watched for and treated wherever possible.

Altered Immune States and Bone Marrow Transplantation

Attempts to stimulate immunity factors in the deficient patient may temporarily sicken and weaken the patient, and if confined during this period to inactive bed rest, deterioration in strength and endurance will occur. Adaptive rehabilitation requires an appropriate bed or room program to prevent some, if not all, of this deterioration.

Immune deficiency may preexist or may be a result of treatment. Susceptibility to infection is increased, and the patient must be protected from exposure. The associated use of laminar flow and reverse isolation requires that recommended activity programs be provided in isolation and limited space areas, and by properly trained personnel. This isolation and confinement can reduce both physical and emotional stamina if appropriate individual programs of activity and support are not added to the patient's regimen of care.

Immunosuppression by corticosteroids may be associated with poor wound healing and with osteoporosis. These conditions require adaptive reduction of stress in activity, reduction of weight bearing in the presence of femoral head necrosis, and provision to the patient of whatever orthopedic support might be indicated.

A patient with immunodeficiency may exhibit no measurable physical disability, or may be host to a variety of problems. Handicaps will differ with the individual complex of disease and unrelated problems. If the platelets are low, the patient may have to be protected from all injury. Stress may add to the problems. Adaptation to treatment and living must be instructed and assisted for each organ system, according to needs and findings. Measures directed at patient adaptation include instruction and training in general conditioning, exercise, and provision of useful equipment which can be left with the patient, such as dumbbells and leg exercisers.

Such programs are to be started and instructed in the preisolation phase, whenever possible, as better personal contact can be made then with the therapist. Games and other diversions provided by the recreation therapy service will ease the boredom of isolation and provide emotional support. Appropriate exercise routines for the restricted and confined patient will slow up deterioration of strength and endurance. Specific instructions should be given in performance to reduce or circumvent handicaps in mobility and range of joint movement.

The therapist treating the patient with immunodeficiency should pay careful attention to rules of isolation to avoid exposing the patient to personal infections that may be transmissible. These include colds and sore throats and herpes simplex infections, as well as body surface infections, especially of the hands.

Maneuvers of care such as percussion, massage, chest vibration, or any vigorous handling would be contraindicated in the presence of coagulopathy and easy bleeding. Instruction and support in voluntary respiratory function will help promote improved ventilation and mobilization of tracheobronchial secretions. Postural drainage instruction will assist patients in maintaining a clear airway. Voluntary control of respiratory function is a constant need, and help and instruction should be available to the patient throughout the day. It is essential that the nursing staff consistently support and continue the instruction given at regular intervals by the rehabilitation staff. Patients with reduced vigor and endurance will do best with frequently repeated, short periods of instruction and performance.

Equipment provided to a patient for use during reverse isolation or in laminar flow units must be sterilized before being offered.

Such equipment is then left with the patient, rather than shifting it to another person for use.

The patient may need frequent supportive encouragement, and occasionally the psychiatrist or clinical psychologist will need to be called in to help support the patient and encouraging compliance with treatment.

Patients who are candidates for bone marrow transplantation fall into the immunodeficiency category. Preparation for transplant acceptance can involve placement of the patient in reverse isolation for relatively long periods of time. This creates physical and emotional restrictions. The physical problems routinely include generalized, progressive weakness and decreased endurance. The emotional problems produced by relative isolation are aggravated by inactivity and boredom. Fear and dismay are increased by the patient's inability to exert and practice any positive effort for his own benefit.

Adaptive treatment should be started before isolation and transplant, with training in independent performance of active range of motion of limbs and spine, isometric exercises, the use of the bicycle, weights, and dumbbells. These exercises can be continued, as appropriate, during the isolation period.

Flexion contractures, especially at hips and knees, develop quite promptly in patients who must stay in bed, especially if they are given pillows under their knees for comfort. Such pillow support should not be allowed. Patients also should be encouraged to lie prone for 20- to 50-minute periods several times a day. This will also correct knee and hip flexion which occurs with side-lying positions.

Decubitus ulcers occur in patients on bed rest, and more rapidly when they have anemia and depleted subcutaneous fat. The area most frequently involved is sacral. Side-lying, prone positioning, and frequent turning in bed will reduce such instances. A good preventive measure generally, and certainly if any redness occurs over pressure points, is the use of a gelfoam flotation pad, resting in a cut-out, foam, leveling mattress. The gel pad should be centrally positioned to protect both sacrum and trochanters. Studies of decubitus-ulcer prevention have also shown that a camping-type, air mattress filled with povidone-iodine in water, rather than air, has proven convenient and effective.

The physical therapy program should include:

A. Preisolation (and pretransplant)
   1. Conditioning exercises against resistance — for arms and legs
   2. Trunk exercises
   3. Specific exercises to prevent shortening of the hip flexors and hamstrings
   4. Respiratory function training — including deep breathing and coughing
B. Isolation (posttransplant)
   1. Continuation of all exercises or institution of program, if not previously started
   2. Gelfoam pad with leveling mattress
   3. Bed positioning and turning instruction
   4. Ambulation training, as appropriate, with or without assistive devices, to increase endurance and improve respiratory function
   5. Continued respiratory function instruction
   6. Recreation therapy to provide diversion, variety, motivation, and emotional support
C. Postisolation
   1. Gradually increased physical exercises and activity upon termination of isolation to increase strength and endurance
   2. Continued respiratory function instruction
   3. Restoration to home and community activity

Hemodialysis

Patients undergoing dialysis present a variety of problems which tend more to psychologic and emotional handicap than to physical. Patients' adaptation to their status is aided by supportive efforts in counseling, active exercises, diversional activities, and prevocational evaluation. Assistance may be needed in the activities of daily living.

Day-to-day fluctuation in patient symptoms requires a daily assessment of each patient's status in order to avoid inappropriate care programs. At times the patient feels well and wishes to work on an activity, while at other times he only wants to talk or just to sleep. Dialysis patients have been noted to become passive from need to comply with medical orders and should be given an opportunity to act upon something, rather than being acted upon, by engaging in pursuits which are self-directed and allow emotionally satisfying control. Crafts and activities should have some element of aggression, and many must be adaptable for one-handed use. Rug punching, copper tooling, weaving with raffia, and leather lacing are examples of these. Games such as dart throwing (there are such available in which darts adhere with VELCRO rather than sharp points) are also possible. Patients who have sore arms for periods and can use only one limb can be taught one-handed techniques for independence in self-care activities.

Interesting activity performance makes time on the dialysis machine seem shorter and diverts attention from preoccupation with physical symptoms. If there is a group of patients, positive socialization allows sharing common interests other than illness. Individual activities support self-concepts of identity and are useful at home during periods of insomnia. Some patients have reported that a mechanical, repetitive activity lulls them back to sleep, while others have stated that working on a project makes the sleepless nights more bearable.

Maintaining contact with families, and keeping them informed about available rehabilitation equipment and sources for it, helps ease life at home. Patients who take activities home often reveal information about family dynamics when discussing these activities with the staff. This information can be valuable to the staff. Home projects may get an entire family working together and sharing a new interest, allowing combined family-patient participation.

Patients who may at some time return to work can occupy themselves with projects that have meaning to them and that help overcome self-doubts about their abilities. Vocational possibilities should always be kept in mind and patients should be encouraged and helped to work in that direction.

Critical Care Unit and Life-Sustaining Devices

Periods of treatment in the critical care unit and reactions to, or tolerance of, life-sustaining devices and treatment create severe patient reactions. Difficulty in coping generates denial, avoidance, and isolation. Patients may become afraid of the machine they are attached to, suspicious of its competence and its dependability. They will not sleep and distrust becomes depression. Their problems are aggravated by the medical and nursing staff when

they read and adjust the equipment and pay minimal attention, if any, to the patient.

Understanding and help for these patients are of great importance to allow their recovery and rehabilitation. Appropriate personal solicitude, communications, timely explanation and advice, and attention to patients' concerns and questions will support their hopes and allay their anxieties.

SPECIAL CONSIDERATIONS IN REHABILITATION OF THE CANCER PATIENT

Pain

When pain is the patient's complaint, a search should be made for its cause. The control of pain is an important factor to consider in rehabilitation. There should be assessment of the psychologic factors capable of influencing pain and suffering. The causes of pain may be related to direct effects of the tumor or the treatment, or to some unrelated cause. Tumor may cause painful invasion, compression, or blockage. Viscera, bones, nerve roots or plexuses, or cord may become involved, with generation of pain. Treatment by chemotherapy may cause peripheral neuropathies or painful local infiltrations with necrosis. Steroids can cause painful osteoporosis and myopathy. Radiation therapy may have early or late painful effects of osteonecrosis, plexopathy, or myelopathy. Surgery may have resulted in transection of nerves with development of painful neuromas, phantom pain, or pain from suture ligation. For a more complete discussion of the management of pain, see Chapter 44.

Relief of Pain. Physical therapy measures that can be useful in pain relief or control include instruction to the patient who has back pain in back-sparing activities both in bed and in daily living. Splints and slings may provide relief for upper extremity problems, and elevation may relieve lower extremity pain. Simultaneous "exercising" of both the normal limb and a phantom limb may help to relieve phantom pain. Exercise for other types of pain may create aggravation rather than relief. A positive approach with personal attention and assistance improves the patients' tolerance of pain and can appear to provide relief. Pain treatment by heat from a moist hot pack or radiant unit is not really useful, except as a diversionary approach, and can be harmful if the associated increased reflex circulation can cause either bleeding, metastasis, or increase in lymphedema.

The uses of acupuncture and transcutaneous electrical neurostimulation have been extensively investigated, but dependable, reproducible responses have not been documented. Selected patients, especially those with suitable psychologic characteristics, may respond to those modalities. Otherwise, they are reported to rank with placebos. Radiation therapy may promptly decrease the size and pressure or blocking effect of a tumor, and this can promptly relieve pain.

Causalgia and paresthesia are occasionally relieved by the application of hot packs or cold packs and by gentle massage. Sympathectomy may also help. It has been recommended in some centers that for the persistent, uncontrollable case of pain or causalgia, hypnosis, administered by an accredited professional, may be helpful.

Nervous System Involvement by Tumor

Motor and sensory deficits and coordination loss may be direct effects of involvement by cancer of the brain, spinal cord, or peripheral nerves. Destructive or toxic changes may cause functional deficits as a result of surgical, medical, or radiation procedures and treatments. Cancer, particularly when it involves the lung or when it is diffuse, may have varied, remote effects on the neuromuscular system.

Rehabilitation of the patient with nervous system involvement requires prompt recognition of the disability. If the neurologic disability can be identified based on the knowledge of the sequellae of planned treatment, advance preventive training can lessen the handicap. Otherwise, rehabilitation measures should begin as soon as the disability is diagnosed in order to minimize weakness caused by inactivity or disease and to maintain proprioceptive and sensory stimuli. The patient with a poor prognosis, yet capable of adaptation, deserves all appropriate care.

The entire spectrum of plegias and neuropathies may be encountered. The general treatment may be the standard recognized care programs for such disabilities. Unless otherwise contraindicated, treatment should be started on this basis.

Neuropathy. Peripheral neuropathy in the medical patient may be caused by the toxic effects of drugs or by invasive disease. Although the disability is primarily caused by the

resultant muscle weakness and sensory loss, superimposed contractures and trophic changes may complicate the situation. Involvement may be diffuse and bilateral, or focal following single-nerve or plexus involvement.

The rehabilitation program for the patient with peripheral nerve involvement is often of long duration. The initial treatment stages are preventive. Passive motions are utilized to prevent joint contractures and the development of adhesions between tendons and their sheaths. These maneuvers may retard, but cannot prevent, reduction in muscle volume and tone. Electrical stimulation is also useful for prevention of muscle atrophy, but in no way appears to influence the rate of neuron regeneration. Special splints, casts, or braces may be necessary to prevent overstretching of the involved muscle by its intact antagonist or by gravity. If these devices are used, they should be designed to allow removal for daily passive movements of the involved joints.

When voluntary motion begins to return, the program is supplemented by intensive muscle reeducation procedures. At first these are performed with gravity eliminated, but they are gradually increased until progressive resistive exercises can be utilized.

Paraparesis, Paraplegia, Quadriplegia. Prescription of a program of adaptive measures for patients with bilateral lower extremity functional deficit depends on each individual's upper extremity functional power and the degree of lower extremity motor loss. If the patient also has nonfunctional power in one or both upper extremities, program consideration should be for quadriparesis or quadriplegia. If current function cannot be maintained or improved, then concentration on training for this alone is unrealistic, and orders must be written to teach the patient to compensate for his increasing future disability.

Appropriate bracing, if necessary for support, and ambulation training should be given with the use of a walker or crutches if there can be expectation of appreciable survival time with preservation of function. If life expectancy is short for the patient, or if disability is expected to progress rapidly, then efforts should be on transfer training and independence in wheelchair activities for daily living.

Exercises to preserve strength of the upper extremities and of residual lower extremity control are important for all patients. Loss of abdominal muscle power may require prescription of a sitting corset, and patients who have high thoracic level lesions will benefit from instruction in adequate respiratory function. A corset may improve their ability to cough and clear respiratory secretions.

Bladder function impairment may need catheter control or an external collection device. Bowel function impairment may necessitate assistance and training.

The patient with paraplegia or quadriplegia needs a coordinated program designed (1) to prevent ducubitus ulcers, (2) to maintain range of motion, (3) to prevent contractures, (4) to improve the power of those muscles that are intact, (5) to strengthen weakened muscles to their maximal capacity, (6) to establish a satisfactory bowel and bladder program, and (7) to reestablish independence in activities of daily living.

Other Neurologic Deficits. Problems related to sensory losses of touch, pain, and temperature are not responsive to direct therapy. The patient can be assisted, however, by training and substitution of other sensory modalities, or patterns of activity, to minimize the effect of the loss. Ataxia may be related to tumor or surgical effects directly on posterior-column and cerebellar function and from cerebellar degeneration secondary to remote effects of cancer. Ambulation training between parallel bars, Frenkel's exercises, and mirror self-observation all can be of value for the patient. Such therapy may also help those patients with cerebellar and cerebral hemisphere changes who have bizarre concepts of self-position in space. Visual field defects and diplopia need appropriate understanding and training for compensation.

Remote Effects of Cancer on the Nervous System. The presence of cancer may produce clinical syndromes that are the evidence of remote or secondary effects. These remote effects of cancer on the nervous system produce varying clinical syndromes. Symptoms may develop after those of the neoplasm, or they may precede other evidence of the neoplastic disease. Muscular weakness and wasting occur, with weakness most frequently in the limb girdle and proximal muscles, rather than distally. Pain may accompany the weakness. Symptoms vary in severity or remit for long or short periods without regard to the course of the tumor or its treatment. See Chapter 37 for a more complete discussion.

In addition to, or apart from, the remote effects of cancer on the nervous system and the muscles are similar effects of medications such as steroids and cancer chemotherapeutic agents. Supervoltage radiation therapy also may create malfunction in the nervous system. After irradiation, peripheral nerve dysfunction tends to be late in appearance and may not occur until a year or longer after the radiation therapy has been administered, whereas effects on the central nervous system are earlier and are directly related to the degree of change within the cells of the central nervous system itself.

The rehabilitation program is the same as for findings that are directly tumor or treatment related. It is important to teach the patient active moving and static muscle-setting exercises as preventive measures against the changes resulting from disuse and lack of range of motion. Impairment of motor coordination may be improved by special training in eye-hand coordination exercises and special gait training and practice. Occupational therapy, in addition to physical therapy, assists the patient with upper extremity problems.

Care of the Paraplegic

Maintenance of Range of Joint Motion. All joints of the affected extremities should be taken through a complete range of motion twice daily. Patients who have residual muscle power but with some weakness should be encouraged to carry through their range of motion actively, as far as possible, and the therapist should then complete the range of motion passively. Prevention of contractures is important for both the care and comfort of the patient.

Therapeutic Exercise. For the paraparetic or paraplegic patient, general conditioning exercises should be designed to strengthen the shoulder depressors and the muscle extensor groups of the upper extremities, as well as any muscles of trunk, abdomen, and lower extremities that the patient can power. The patient should also be taught sitting balance and transfer techniques back and forth from bed to chair.

Early standing with temporary bracing, if necessary, or the use of a tilt table improves circulation and respiratory function, retards osteoporosis, and is frequently emotionally satisfying to the patient. Patients with cancer with quadriplegia are usually not candidates for bracing and ambulation. These patients often need the care of an attendant.

Activities of Daily Living. The program in activities of daily living includes training in bed activities, toilet functions, eating, dressing and undressing, hand, and wheelchair activities.

Skin Care and Decubitus Ulcer Control. The paraplegic patient must be turned at least every two hours, day and night, in order to prevent decubitus-ulcer formation. Nurses should inspect the skin carefully over the following pressure points: sacrum, trochanters, iliac crests, ischial tuberosities, knees, and heels. As the patient is turned, these areas should be cleansed very carefully with soap and water, dried gently, massaged lightly (except in areas that are portals for radiation therapy), and a bland oil or neutral ointment should be applied.

Decubitus-ulcer treatment requires adequate control of local pressure by placing the patient on a gel pad with a surrounding relief, foam mattress, or by surrounding the ulcer area or pressure points with polyurethane foam pads, or use of alternating pressure mattresses or beds, multiple bolsters, flotation beds, Stryker frames, or circle beds. Adequate debridement of slough and frequent changes of dry, soft, sterile dressings aid control or healing. Various dressings from sugar to dried plasma or red cells have been used with success. Topical hyperbaric oxygen may be beneficial to healing.

Pathologic Fractures

Primary or metastatic tumors involving bone destroy bony architecture, and pathologic fractures may threaten or occur. These lesions require appropriate orthopedic surgery, radiation therapy, and chemotherapy. All bones can be affected, but the fractures occur most commonly in the long bones, spine, pelvis, and ribs. Long-bone fractures are best treated by intramedullary nailing or by prosthetic insertions. Bone cement adds stability.

Hip replacement surgery allows postoperative weight-bearing activity earlier than pinning procedures for fractures. Austin-Moore prosthetic hips, without an artificial acetabular socket, will allow start of weight bearing by two to three weeks postsurgery. Acetabular replacement requires an additional two to three weeks of limited weight bearing. The degree of soft tissue healing and its support at the hip joint need consideration before starting the stress of weight bearing.

Any other diseases of the patient, such as obesity, hypertension, coronary insufficiency, chronic pulmonary insufficiency, need to be considered before ambulation is permitted. The amount of weight bearing permitted should be stipulated by the surgeon to conform to the limitations imposed by the type of surgical procedure performed or by the basic bone problem with consideration of the degree of postoperative soft tissue healing. An active exercise program for uninvolved extremities is important to maintain circulation and muscle strength and tone. Necessary restrictions of range of motion at the operated hip include limitation of flexion at the hip to no more than 80 to 90 degrees, and elimination of internal rotation and adduction beyond the midline.

The patient's age, tumor status and prognosis, possible presence of complications or other diseases, and other basic diagnoses need assessment in setting a time schedule for progression in activity.

Nutrition

Cancer itself and the effects of intensive radiation therapy and chemotherapy can induce systemic and local changes that deplete the nutritional status of the patients. These include serious weight loss, hypoproteinemia, vitamin and mineral deficiencies, and fluid and electrolyte imbalances, all of which often impose additional risks to the patient. Radiation therapy and chemotherapy can induce changes in the mouth and throughout the gastrointestinal tract with associated poor intake and malabsorbtion. For further information regarding nutrition and the patient with cancer see Chapter 45.

When nutritional therapy is indicated, patients need maximal tolerable programs of bed and bedside activity to prevent deterioration of strength, endurance, and range of joint motion. Instruction and assistance should be given in active programs of exercise, muscle setting without breath holding, and ambulatory activities within tolerance. Patients should be encouraged to repeat all activities, by themselves, several (four to five) times each day.

Special care must be given to any patient

with intravenous feeding or medication, naso-gastric intubation, gastrostomy, or jejunos-tomy to ensure that any physical or occupa-tional therapy program does not interfere with, or in any way disturb, the tubing, the timing of the set-up or the treatment, or any other aspect of such specific cancer care.

Communication and Counseling

Adequate counseling is an essential part of the concept of comprehensive medical care. This implies that concerned communication between physician and patient should start with the onset of treatment and then be main-tained. Communication and clinical care do not always receive equal application for the sick patient. Medical education has empha-sized the diagnosis and treatment of disease, overshadowing consideration of the particular complex of the interaction of the disease with each host.

Stimulation of patients' distrust and ill will is promoted by lack of defined concern by the physician and the failure to communicate well enough with the patient so that the latter feels both informed and party to the course of treat-ment. An attitude of superiority or withdrawal on the part of the physician is apt to be inter-preted by the patient in the light of personal anxiety and fears of the unknown.

Failure to receive adequate spoken commu-nication may be interpreted by the patient as rejection or abandonment. Misuse of speech develops distrust, suspicion, and depression. Good counseling embodies those qualities of personal understanding and empathy that re-veal to the patient that the physician is both aware of and interested in the problems. Counseling depends on the aggregate influ-ences upon the patient of the many variables that are part of the differences that make each of us an individual. These differences among people require that counseling as well as treat-ment be individualized. The hospitalized pa-tient surrenders freedom and individuality, and Von Doeltz (1971) reminds us that we are not dealing with diseases but with sick people. Unrealistic fear and mistrust are diminished directly by the degree of faith that patients place in what they are told. Mastrovito (1972) has noted the significant delusion commonly held by physicians that patients will believe what they are told in the face of contradictory nonverbal evidence.

The diagnosis or the fear of the diagnosis of cancer creates a crisis for the patient and, in turn, a crisis for the family. Advisory guidance, started early, will allay fears of the unknown and the related anxiety for the patient and fam-ily, and their confidence and cooperation will be improved. What patients believe they know about their diagnosis and treatment will influ-ence their course. Misinformation, or misin-terpretation of information, can alter compli-ance with and response to treatment.

Patients are not passive subjects under ma-nipulation by the physician. If they can be made informed and interested parties, they can be guided in a conscious and positive con-tribution to the success of their care, whether the goal of that care be prevention, restoration, support, or palliation.

Communication is a two-way process. Basic elements for the deliverer involve time, ability, and interest. The receiver may be open and eager or may be "shut down" by fear, denial, confusion, pain, or lack of understanding, or because of deficit in intellect or education and experience. Sutherland *et al.* (1952) under-score that the question of whether or not the physician should tell patients they have cancer cannot be (forthrightly) answered, because it presupposes a standard physician, a standard patient, and standard cancer, none of which exists. Verwoerdt (1966) declares instead that, "The real issue is not whether to tell or not to tell, but rather how to tell. Patient knowledge of the truth can grow gradually and should not be forced or denied."

Advice and communication must also in-clude the people upon whom the patient de-pends. Preventive aspects of counseling in-volve both correction and lessening of problems through proper informative under-standing and guidance of both the patient and the family. Patients recognize their role as con-sumers in the system of health care and may wish to participate in discussions and in some of the decisions concerning their care. To par-ticipate, they must have at least basic factual knowledge of their condition and prognosis. Uninformed fantasy can be worse than truth, and associated isolation makes the patient an outsider. The family becomes an accomplice to this "protective isolation."

Trachtenberg (unpublished presentations) feels that,

The patient as a consumer wants and deserves a greater share in his care and decisions. Frequently, when the professionals make the decision to protect the patient, the family, only too readily, will decide to do the same. Often it appears easier not to talk to the patient about the source of his symptomatology and the treatment planned, but rather to focus on semireassuring phrases that may indicate that we and the family are not listening to what he is saying. This evasion may make the patient an outsider to his family as well.

The physician is responsible for giving patients initial and ongoing information about their medical status. The rest of the hospital staff can then serve to make this knowledge tolerable to the patient by listening to the patient, by encouragement, and by guidance. It is imperative, therefore, that close intercommunication be maintained between physician and staff members to ensure uniformity of information and credibility for the patient. Truth is consistent, while fabrications wander and vary. Each member of the hospital team should be aware of his/her role in maintaining proper information and direction.

Counseling and communication are essentially synonyms. Communication requires understanding. If patients are to benefit, their understanding must be maintained, so that they can cope. As soon as the communication becomes vague, it becomes useless. Patients then resort to relatively frantic attempts at resolution of their confusion. When they understandably fail, they feel isolated, and anger, depression, and frustration increase progressively. False reassurances should be avoided, as the patient may well face marital problems, employment difficulties, or recurrence of disease. Anticipation for the future should be considered with understanding and with individual regard for personality, personal and sexual needs, age, and ability.

Counseling must be realistic and not escapist in intent. There must be sufficient reliable information to allow the patient to tolerate the course of the disease. This is especially true when cure cannot be expected. It is unfair to the patient to make any form of promise as to the end result of either effort or treatment. It is equally unfair to convey that without either treatment or effort much in the way of a satisfactory result can be expected. The patient needs encouragement couched in the language of positive direction. To counsel patients with cancer requires sufficient honesty incorporated in the communication with them to allow them to comprehend and to plan appropriately.

Cases of advanced disease or incurable cancer need careful consideration. Chance and probability can both be discussed, but removal of hope by the implication of abandonment, in the sense that "nothing more can be done," should never be allowed. Patients may well accept finality, but cannot accept being avoided by those upon whom they must depend.

The family needs to understand both the patient's feelings and their own. Crisis for the patient creates crisis for the family. Sharing of anxieties with the patient will increase understanding and reassurance. This is particularly true between husband and wife. Counseling must include guidance for patients in what to tell other important persons in their lives, particularly when these are children. The child needs constant reassurance that the patient is being cared for and that all treatment is organized to help, however severe the reaction may appear.

Counseling embraces all forms of communicative activities in the interactions among the physician, the staff, and the patient. The patient is an able interpreter of behavior and demeanor. Patients assess facial expression, hesitancy, evasiveness, or avoidance as confirmatory of their worst expectations. In contrast they will respond to warmth of personal attitude and to directness of approach with an interpretation of reassurance and support. To repeat, the physician's advice needs to be followed by adequate relay of information to the other members of the health care team to ensure consistency and reliability for the patient.

Counseling sessions for the patient should avoid being too long or too complex. Spontaneity is important, but structured presentations have value for all patients, and slides and charts add visual components to the discussion. Written or recorded directions and descriptions are, therefore, better than a single verbal explanation, however careful, to which the patient at that time may not be paying full attention, and for which there may be no other time for repetition. This latter problem must be expected in all counseling. Recordings or tapes can and should be prepared, covering the standard advice material such as hospital admission procedures. They will allow more attention to be given individual patients' specific problems by elimination of otherwise time-consuming, fundamental repetition.

It should be kept in mind that patients' interpretation of information received is limited by their own anxiety, any pain or discomfort, fatigue, or failure to follow the meaning or the continuum of what they hear. In addition, discussion without any adequate interval to digest its content with the patient's possible reluctance to question or disagree often is traumatic. The patient's interpretation is limited, from the physician's side, by the physician's technical language and lack of knowledge as to what or how much the patient understands, and a possible error of incompleteness, generated by the tedium of repetition.

Counseling the patient implies involvement, not avoidance. Personal contact itself is an important part of communication. The patient's hand should be firmly shaken and held for a moment of sincere contact. Look the patient squarely in the eyes. The approach should be serious, but with a smile, in the sense of warmth, concern, and friendship. The manner of approach should be positive and close.

Psychologic Problems

This subject was briefly addressed earlier in this chapter in the discussion of approaches to goals and phases of care. To further pursue the issue, Von Doeltz (1971) makes it clear that, "No one profession or person can meet the total needs of the patient and his family. There is need to work together in close cooperation." Some goals must be relinquished and other values postponed indefinitely. The staff must help both the patient and the family talk about anxieties and concerns, whenever the need arises. Such listening and discussion require tact.

The average patient will pass through phases of depression, anger, denial, and frustration, but will come to accept and comply when given appropriate interdisciplinary personal support. Staff intercommunication and mutual awareness of the patient's status are basic to such an effort.

A primary concern of the social phase of rehabilitation is the relationship of individuals to their environment. Success or failure in rehabilitation is usually determined by the individual's ability to adjust to the environment. The social worker's objective is to increase the patient's ability to deal effectively with the environment, economically, vocationally, and socially. Social work assistance answers two aims: first, to help the individual to adjust to the disease, the disability, the environment, and the rehabilitation process, and second, to make appropriate efforts to alter the physical and social environment to improve its suitability for the patient and to call in available sources of community assistance. For a more complete discussion, see Chapter 49.

Employment

A vocational outlet is important to patients who may otherwise fear that because of their illness or handicap their family will have to make serious sacrifices, or that they will cease to be economically independent.

A health history that lists cancer creates a complex issue for the returning worker. Public feelings of pessimism, defeat, or impending death are widely shared, and the reactions are both overt and covert. The American Cancer Society estimates that there is a serious discrimination problem for about 90% of patients trying to return to work. Employment and rehabilitation agencies have usually considered the patient with cancer to have no acceptable potential for a stipulated set of reasons. These reasons have been researched and are found to include the complexity of the disease, the associated disabilities related to both disease and treatment, the suspected mental, social, and occasional cosmetic problems, the actual problems of insurability, the expected problems of absenteeism, the occasional problems of communication, and the financial burdens presented. Employers' fears include prolonged sick leaves, increased costs of company health and life insurance and of other fringe benefits, and unacceptability of the employee to fellow workers.

Frequently, employer health services require a physical examination before returning to work. History of cancer or, particularly, residual evidence of treatment for cancer, often warps the judgment of the examiner. Taints of prejudice and misconception disallow a well-formulated prediction of the patient's productive capacity and future health status.

In the medical and personnel departments of most governmental and many large organizations and industries outdated policies exist that have either flatly rejected the job applicant with a history of cancer or demanded an impossible, disease-free waiting period of perhaps five years before consideration of eligibility. Employers and fellow employees basically fear the cancer patient, and all the more so if the patient has an obvious physical handicap or cosmetic deformity. Some are frightened by mistaken suspicion of contagion, others by expected loss of time or effort requiring assistance in coverage, or by suspected risk of performance safety. The human failing of intolerance of illness, physical handicap, or disfigurement turns fellow employees away from the patient, placing him or her in a position of isolation. Historically, the attitudes of the nondisabled have been overtly hostile toward the disabled. Ancient attitudes persist and interfere with acceptance of the patient with cancer.

Illness is believed to influence work, in the sense of its being utilized for secondary gains. Our culture permits release from responsibility and work as an accepted result of illness. The employer often fears this possibility in his consideration of an applicant for work or return to work.

Insurance benefits pose specific difficulties:

1. Group health insurance is automatically extended to the reemployed patients with cancer, but they may have a prolonged waiting period of perhaps 11 months before they can have this health coverage for any illness related to the cancer diagnosis. Also, an exclusion rider eliminating cancer-related problems may be attached to the policy. Personal health insurance is an even bigger problem and may be unavailable, or require a seven- to ten-year waiting period, or the policy may have a five-year rider excluding cancer.
2. An existing company fringe benefit of provision of group life insurance programs may actually be a barrier to employment of patients with cancer since employers may turn down a job applicant they fear is an expensive health risk.
3. This same attitude may affect the eligibility of the patient in the mind of the hiring agent when the latter thinks in terms of worker's compensation problems and premiums, since risks or implications of disease aggravation may be feared. Also, a history of cancer may cause the employer to wonder if the effects of the disease or its treatment have changed the patient's capabilities to perform the old or a new job, making the work hazardous.

Concerns arise about seniority, pension rights, or availability of the patient for transfer to another post. Promotion chances are reduced or disallowed when so shadowed. Misinformed judgment promotes the situation that any faults in performance, attendance, compliance, or whatever may be seized as reason to fire the patient or, at least, makes the work so distasteful as to encourage resignation.

Emotionally painful requirements for the patient who is partially disabled ramify even into such areas as qualification for benefits prescribed under the Social Security Disability Insurance Program. Here the applicant must demonstrate inability to perform "substantial gainful activity" because of "medically determinable" physical or mental impairment or impairments that can be expected to result in death or that have already lasted or can be expected to last a continuous period of 12 months. Criteria are often limited and unrealistic.

Problems arise when a patient with a history of cancer wishes to transfer within a company to another city or wishes to change jobs and join another firm. This may be unwise because of potential loss of insurance coverage and loss of job opportunity when the history of cancer is discovered.

In the family, as well as in the work setting, the patient's crisis can be precipitated by change itself. Change in performance ability and change in appearance resulting from the effects of illness, especially cancer, create such a crisis. Difficulty in finding employment is often demoralizing. Tension and strain in the family are increased by the effect of the patient's problems finding work.

Workers who have been off the job for any period of time are apt to be hard-pressed to meet basic living expenses. Their income from disability or unemployment does not meet their needs. This creates resistance to consideration of anything except an immediate job. The worker is apt to be unwilling to devote time and effort to vocational rehabilitation. A responsible worker must have exceptional faith in the ultimate success of any proffered rehabilitation program to undertake it. Additionally, the sympathetic understanding of the family is needed if success is to be achieved.

Patients' attitudes must be considered. As McKenna (1975) has stated,

Most patients are anxious to return to work, but there are exceptions. . . . Some who are close to retirement may elect to retire prematurely after cancer therapy. When cancer is diagnosed, some patients develop a feeling of hopelessness and despondency, and such a patient may give up and decide that he is no longer useful to himself, his family, and/or his community. This type of individual could be reluctant to return to work, even if his employer is anxious to have him do so.

McKenna has pointed out that,

. . . the cancer patient returnee to his community may find that the attitudes of his friends, relatives and family have changed. The patient's former role has changed to a different one, which he resents and does not understand. Public acceptance may range from pity to rejection to isolation.

This additional burden contributes to the difficulty in instituting vocational rehabilitation, if needed, and sometimes makes counseling frustrating or even impossible.

It has been determined that a large proportion of adults find it hard to accept a disability when it is their own. They tend to resist the undertaking of any special programs to prepare themselves for work. There is an opposing group, who, although they are willing to admit a disability, are all too apt to consider their productive capacity ended, and should they show any interest in work, they confine this to small, make-do jobs with few demands. Some patients resist the thoughts of testing, work trials, or training for fear of their own personal inadequacy being exposed. Proper counseling will correct many problems.

The Solutions. The potential to be able to work is present both for those cancer patients who can be expected to be cured and for those patients who must continue to live with and be treated for control of persistent disease. The inhospital treatment schedule should include full-team effort in bedside and rehabilitation department programs of physical therapy, occupational therapy, nutrition, pain control, psychologic assistance, social service, and vocational counseling. Help to ease difficulties of family strain and tension can be provided by both health and vocational agencies, especially when the patient can be referred to a treatment center which has a social service department. The medical social worker can provide the worker and the family with motivation and invaluable guidance and understanding of their predicament. Experience with industrial workers has revealed that prompt action was the factor of overriding importance in every case. Efforts should be made to prevent the involved worker and personnel from having to wait for time-consuming procedures with unclear relevance.

Social workers provide organized help and understanding when it is necessary to determine rights of reemployment, fringe benefits,

job duties, and working conditions. The social worker can also be of assistance in discussions between the physician and the representative of the patient's union, covering specific job details and recommendations based on accurate information. The social worker and the vocational and union counselors can aid in the solution of the problems of employer acceptance of a cancer diagnosis, possible limited ability for the patient in the practical matters of public transportation, a competitive labor market, and the occasional need for specialized job placement within the limitations of residual disability.

Both the physician and the employer must gain understanding of the patient's potential and the expertise to reconcile the patient's medical situation with job responsibilities. Even the patient with a limited time for work expectancy has hope for at least temporary employment or may need sheltered workshop placement. Common sense will dictate plans commensurate with the prognosis, rather than elimination of the patient as ineligible.

Most patients with cancer are able to return to their previous work situation and responsibilities. Some, however, are faced with specific restrictions or changes. Occasionally, neurologic deficits in function or sensation needed for a vocation may require retraining and rehabilitation before work is resumed.

Decisions to hire or not to hire patients with cancer must be made on an individual basis and not governed by an arbitrary, five-year-cure criterion. Consideration and preparation of the patient for employment demand realistic, goal-oriented, adequate provision of rehabilitation measures. Intelligent and early action can change the terms of the problem. If the patient must change his type of work because of persisting disability, or if by age level or other reasons he is to start working for the first time, the occupational therapist can give him prevocational guidance in choice of work. The social worker will aid immensely to help in motivation of the patient toward employment and in obtaining referral to vocational rehabilitation and community services. Vocational rehabilitation services can also guide the patient in the selection of a suitable work setting or type of work for which to train or retrain.

Additional guidance needs have been noted in adaptive vocational adjustment. Disabled workers must accept the fact of the disability and also the possibility of a vocational handicap. They must also believe that they need specialized combinations of services to overcome this vocational handicap. They must have faith in the success of the offered services, and they must also have the financial backing to meet the cost of their ongoing responsibilities while the services proceed. The families must share their belief and also be willing to accept the restrictions and financial problems during the course of the rehabilitation.

Community problems in aftercare following hospital discharge are often essential to patients in getting them back to their setting and to work. The reactions of the family to the patient and the diagnosis can be critical in terms of success or failure in rehabilitation and, therefore, to eligibility for employment. Family awareness and solidarity are needed in order for the patient to weather the storm.

REFERENCES

Abrams, R. D: The patient with cancer—His changing pattern of communication. *N. Engl. J. Med.,* **272:**317, 1966.

Adams, J.: Mutual help groups: Enhancing the coping ability of oncology clients. *Cancer Nurs.,* **2:**95, 1979.

American Cancer Society: *The Psychological Impact of Cancer.* Professional Educational Publication. American Cancer Society, New York, 1974.

American College of Surgeons, Commission on Cancer: *Guidelines for Cancer Care.* American College of Surgeons, Chicago, 1970.

American Thoracic Society, the Committee on Therapy: *Physical Adjuncts in the Treatment of Pulmonary Disease.* National Tuberculosis and Respiratory Diseases Association, New York, 1968.

Aronson, M.: How do patients accept life-sustaining devices? *Med. Surg. Rev.,* **6:**35, 1971.

Barckley, V.: What can I say to the cancer patients? *Nurs. Outlook,* **6:**316, 1958.

Boyarsky, S.; Labay, P. C.; Hanick, P.; Abramson, A. S.; and Boyarsky, R.: *Care of the Patient with Neurogenic Bladder.* Little, Brown & Company, Boston, 1980.

Brain, W. R., and Norris, F. H., Jr. (eds.): *The Remote Effects of Cancer on the Nervous System.* Contemporary Neurology Symposia, Vol 1. Grune & Stratton, Inc., New York, 1965.

Casswell, E. J.: In sickness and health. *Commentary,* **59:**6, 1970.

Christopherson, V. A.; Coulter, P. P.; and Wolanin, M. O.: *Rehabilitation Nursing. Perspectives and Applications.* McGraw-Hill, Inc., New York, 1974.

Cunnick, W. R.; Cromie, J. B.; Cortell, R. E.; *et al.:* Employing the cancer patient: A mutual responsibility. *J. Occup. Med.,* **16:**755–780, 1974.

Dietz, J. H., Jr.: Rehabilitation of the cancer patient: Its role in the scheme of comprehensive care. *Clin. Bull. Memorial Sloan-Kettering Cancer Center,* **4:**104, 1974.

Dietz, J. H., Jr.: How doctors can help solve cancer patients' employment problems. *Leg. Aspects Med. Pract.* **6:**25, 1978.

Dietz, J. H., Jr.: *Rehabilitation Oncology.* John Wiley & Sons, Inc., New York, 1981.

Dietz, J. H., Jr., and Rusk, H. A.: Rehabilitation. In Schwartz, S. I. (ed.): *Principles of Surgery,* 3rd ed. McGraw-Hill, Inc., New York, 1979.

Domanski, M.; Lipiec, K.; Rensel, S.; and Sherwin, K.: Comprehensive care of the chronically ill cancer patient: An inter-agency model. *Soc. Work Health Care,* **5:**59, 1979.

Dotson, T.: Only a ghost of a chance. *Texas Business,* pp. 18-23, August, 1977.

Dunphy, J. F.: Rising above suffering and death. *Bull. Am. Coll. Surg.,* **64:**10, 1979.

Egan, D. F.: *Fundamentals of Respiratory Therapy,* 2nd ed. The C. V. Mosby Company, St. Louis, 1975.

Entmacher, P. S.: Insurance for the cancer patient. *Cancer,* **36:**1, 1975.

Foley, K. M.: The management of pain of malignant origin. In Tyler, H. R., and Dawson, D. M. (ed.): *Current Neurology,* Vol. 2. Houghton Mifflin Company, Boston, 1979.

Frankel, H. L.: Bowel training. *Paraplegia,* **4:**254, 1967.

Freireich, E. J.: Supportive therapy in acute leukemia. In *Clinical Aspects of Acute Leukemia.* The American Cancer Society, New York, 1965.

Gaskell, D. V., and Webber, B. A.: *The Brompton Hospital Guide to Chest Physical Therapy,* 2nd ed. Blackwell, London, 1973.

Goldenberg, I. S.: Hospice: To humanize dying. *Bull. Am. Coll. Surg.,* **64:**6, 1979.

Healey, J. E. (ed.): *Ecology of the Cancer Patient.* The Interdisciplinary Communications Associates, Inc., Washington, D.C., 1970.

Hickey, R. G. (ed.): *Palliative Care of the Cancer Patient.* Little, Brown & Company, Boston, 1967.

Houde, R. W.: Medical treatment of oncological pain. In Bonica, J. J.; Procacci, P.; and Pagni, C. V. (eds.): *Recent Advances in Pain: Pathophysiology and Clinical Aspects.* Charles C Thomas, Publisher, Springfield, Illinois, 1974.

Klagsbrun, S. C.: Cancer, emotions and nurses. *Am. J. Psychiatry,* **126:**71, 1970.

Klein, R.: A crisis to grow on. *Cancer,* **6:**1660, 1971.

Krakoff, I. H.: The case for active treatment in patients with advanced cancer: Not everyone needs a hospice. *CA,* **29:**108, 1979.

Mastrovito, R. C.: Emotional considerations in cancer. *N.Y. State J. Med.,* **72:**2874. 1972.

McKenna, R. J.: Employment and insurability of the cancer patient, Part I, Treatment and rehabilitation. National Conference on Advances in Cancer Management. American Cancer Society and the National Cancer Institute, New York Proceedings, November 27, 1975.

McLeod, J. D.: Carcinomatous neuropathy. In Dyck, P. J.; Thomas, P. K.; and Lambert, E. H. (eds.): *Peripheral Neuropathy.* W. B. Saunders Company, Philadelphia, 1975.

Paul, T.; Katiyar, B. C.; Misra, S.; and Pant, G. C.: Carcinomatous neuromuscular syndromes: A clinical and quantitative electrophysiological study. *Brain,* **101:**53, 1978.

Petty, T. L.: *Intensive and Rehabilitative Respiratory Care,* 2nd ed. Lea & Febiger, Philadelphia, 1974.

Rizzo, R. F.: Hospice: Comprehensive terminal care. *N.Y. State J. Med.,* **78:**1902, 1978.

Rosenthal, S., and Kaufman, S.: Vincristine neurotoxicity. *Ann. Intern. Med.,* **80:**733, 1974.

Rubin, P. (ed.): *Clinical Oncology for Medical Students and Physicians,* 3rd ed. American Cancer Society, New York, 1971.

Saunders, C.: St. Christopher's Hospice. In Schneidman, E. S. (ed.): *Death: Current Perspectives.* Mayfield Publishing Company, Palo Alto, California, 1976.

Schottenfeld, D. (ed.): *Cancer Epidemiology Prevention.* Charles C Thomas, Publisher, Springfield, Illinois, 1975.

Stone, R. W.: Employing the recovered cancer patient. *Cancer,* **36:**1, 1975.

Stryker, R. P.: *Rehabilitation Aspects of Acute and Chronic Nursing Care.* W. B. Saunders Company, Philadelphia, 1972.

Sutherland, A.; Orbach, C. E.; and Dyk, R.: Psychological impact of cancer surgery. *Public Health Rep.,* **67:**1139, 1952.

Vanderpool, H. Y.: The ethics of terminal cancer. *J.A.M.A.,* **239:**850, 1978.

Verwoerdt, A.: *Communications with the Fatally Ill.* Charles C Thomas, Publisher, Springfield, Illinois, 1966.

Von Doeltz, D.: Helping the cancer patient: The minister and the social worker. *Pastoral Psychology,* Jan., pp. 35-40, 1971.

Wheatley, G. M., Cunnick, W. R.; Wright, B. P.; and van Keuren, D.: Proceedings: The employment of persons with a history of treatment for cancer. *Cancer,* **33:**441–445, 1974.

Index

Information provided in tables is indicated by the letter *t* following page numbers; illustrations are indicated by the letter *f* following page numbers.